Mark frequently used sections in your code book with these color-coded flags.

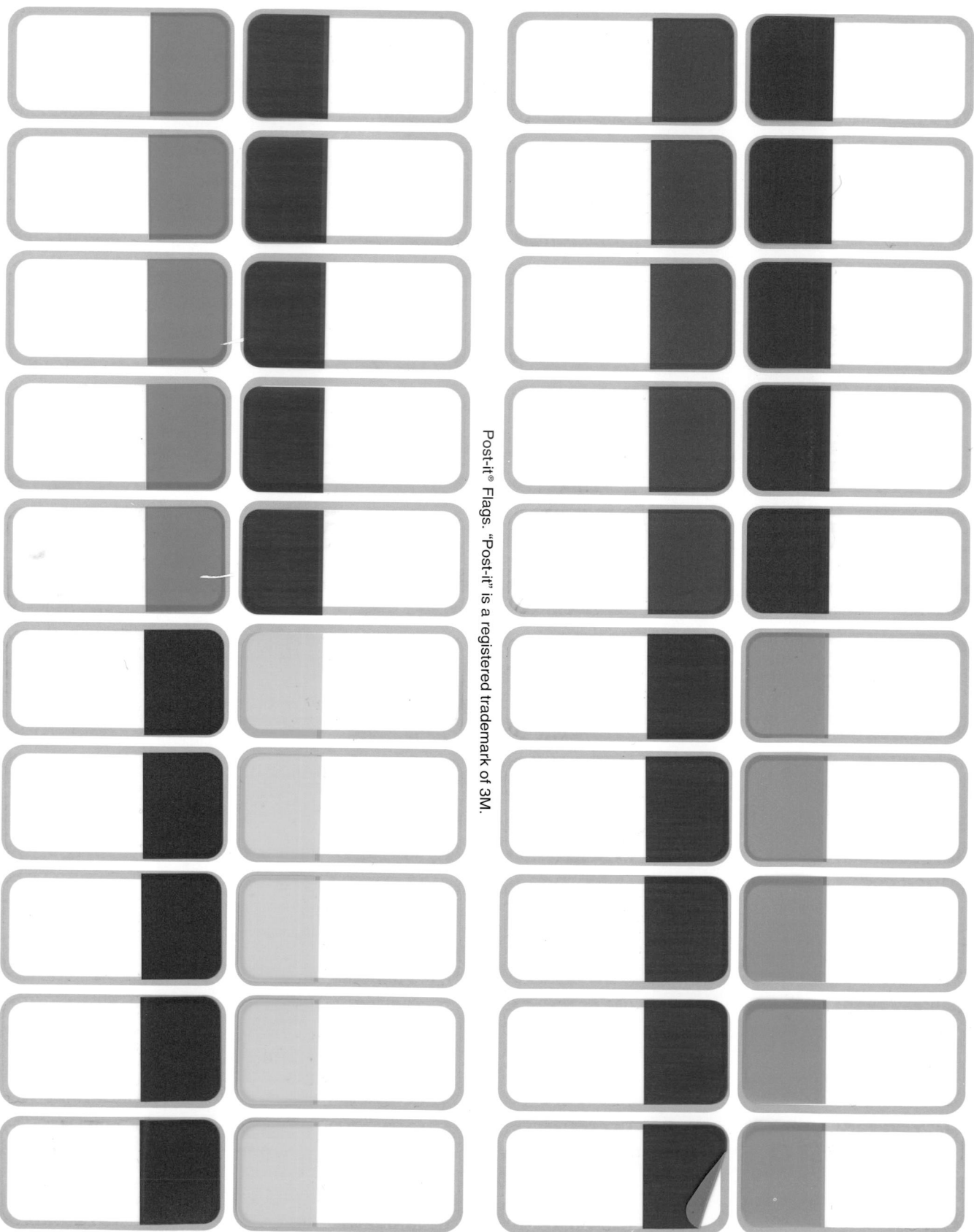

ICD-10-PCS
Code Book

2016

Anne B. Casto, RHIA, CCS
Consulting Editor

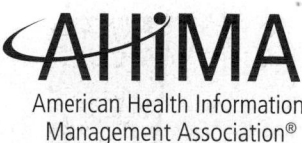

AHIMA
American Health Information
Management Association®

ISBN: 978-1-58426-524-5
AHIMA Product No.: AC222015

AHIMA Staff:
Megan Grennan, Senior Production Development Editor
Jason O. Malley, Vice President, Business and Innovation
Caitlin Wilson, Assistant Editor
Pamela Woolf, Director of Publications

The Centers for Medicare and Medicaid Services (CMS) and the National Center for Health Statistics (NCHS), two departments within the US Federal Government's Department of Health and Human Services (HHS) provide the *International Classification of Diseases, Tenth Revision, Clinical Modification* (ICD-10-CM) for coding and reporting. ICD-10-CM is the US modification to the World Health Organization's (WHO) International Classification of Diseases, Tenth Revision (ICD-10).

Coding Clinic for ICD-10-CM and ICD-10-PCS is a publication of the American Hospital Association (AHA).

Art pieces were created by Jason Isley and Cognition Studio, Inc, and are all copyright of the American Health Information Management Association.

The websites listed in this book were current and valid as of the date of publication. However, webpage addresses and the information on them may change at any time. The user is encouraged to perform his or her own general web searches to locate any site addresses listed here that are no longer valid.

For more information about AHIMA Press publications, including updates, visit http://www.ahima.org/publications/ updates.aspx.

American Health Information Management Association
233 North Michigan Avenue, 21st Floor
Chicago, Illinois 60601-5809
ahima.org

Contents

About the Consulting Editor

Anne B. Casto, RHIA, CCS, is the president of Casto Consulting, LLC. Casto Consulting, LLC is a consulting firm that provides services to hospitals and other healthcare stakeholders primarily in the areas of reimbursement and coding. Casto Consulting, LLC specializes in linking coding and billing practices to positive revenue cycle outcomes. Additionally, the firm provides guidance to consulting firms, healthcare organizations and healthcare insurers regarding reimbursement methodologies and Medicare regulations.

Prior to founding the firm, Ms. Casto was the program manager of the HIMS Division at The Ohio State University School of Allied Medical Professions. Ms. Casto taught healthcare reimbursement, ICD-9-CM coding, and CPT coding courses for several years. Additionally, Ms. Casto was responsible for curriculum revisions in the areas of chargemaster management, clinical data management, and healthcare reimbursement.

Additionally, Ms. Casto was the vice president of clinical information for Cleverley & Associates where she worked very closely with APC regulations and guidelines, preparing hospitals for the implementation of the Medicare OPPS. Ms. Casto was also the clinical information product manager for CHIPS/Ingenix. She joined CHIPS/Ingenix in 1998 and spent the majority of her time developing coding compliance products for the inpatient and outpatient settings.

Ms. Casto has been responsible for inpatient and outpatient coding activities in several large hospitals including Mt. Sinai Medical Center (NYC), Beth Israel Medical Center (NYC), and The Ohio State University. She worked extensively with CMI, quality measures, physician documentation, and coding accuracy efforts at these facilities.

Ms. Casto received her degree in Health Information Management at The Ohio State University in 1995. She received her Certified Coding Specialist credential in 1998 from the American Health Information Management Association. In 2009 Ms. Casto received her ICD-10-CM/PCS Trainer certificate from AHIMA. Ms. Casto is the co-author of an AHIMA-published text book entitled *Principles of Healthcare Reimbursement*. Additionally, Ms. Casto was a contributing author to the published AHIMA books: *Severity DRGs and Reimbursement; A MS-DRG Primer* and *Effective Management of Coding Services*. Most recently, Ms. Casto authored the AHIMA-published text entitled *The CDM Handbook*.

Ms. Casto received the AHIMA Legacy Award, part of the FORE Triumph Awards, in 2007 which honors a significant contribution to the knowledge base of the HIM field through an insightful publication. Additionally, Ms. Casto was honored with the Ohio Health Information Management Association's Distinguished Member Award in 2008 and the Ohio Health Information Management Association's Professional Achievement Award in 2011.

Acknowledgments

Many thanks to my family for their support during this project. Thanks to Dr. Susan White, The Ohio State University; your data manipulation skills are second to none. Thanks to Drew Beverick for providing valuable insight from the student perspective. I thank the reviewers for their thoughtful comments and suggestions. Many thanks to Linda Hyde and Jennifer Lame for their very thorough technical review of the book.

ICD-10-PCS Overview

The International Classification of Diseases, Tenth Revision, Procedure Coding System (ICD-10-PCS) was created to accompany the World Health Organization's (WHO) ICD-10 diagnosis classification. This coding system was developed to replace ICD-9-CM procedure codes for reporting inpatient procedures. Unlike the ICD-9-CM classification, ICD-10-PCS was designed to enable each code to have a standard structure and be very descriptive, and yet flexible enough to accommodate future needs.

History of ICD-10-PCS

The WHO has maintained the International Classification of Diseases (ICD) for recording cause of death since 1893. It has updated the ICD periodically to reflect new discoveries in epidemiology and changes in medical understanding of disease. The International Classification of Diseases Tenth Revision (ICD-10), published in 1992, is the latest revision of the ICD. The WHO authorized the National Center for Health Statistics (NCHS) to develop a clinical modification of ICD-10 for use in the United States. This version of ICD-10 is called ICD-10-CM, and is intended to replace the previous US clinical modification, ICD-9-CM, that has been in use since 1979. ICD-9-CM contains a procedure classification; ICD-10-CM does not.

The Centers for Medicare and Medicaid Services (CMS), the agency responsible for maintaining the inpatient procedure code set in the United States, contracted with 3M Health Information Systems in 1993 to design and then develop a procedure classification system to replace Volume 3 of ICD-9-CM. ICD-10-PCS is the result. ICD-10-PCS was initially released in 1998. It has been updated annually since that time.

ICD-10-PCS Design

ICD-10-PCS is fundamentally different from ICD-9-CM in its structure, organization, and capabilities. It was designed and developed to adhere to recommendations made by the National Committee on Vital and Health Statistics (NCVHS). It also incorporates input from a wide range of organizations, individual physicians, healthcare professionals, and researchers. Several structural attributes were recommended for a new procedure coding system. These attributes include a multiaxial structure, completeness, and expandability.

Multiaxial Structure

The key attribute that provides the framework for all other structural attributes is multiaxial code structure. *Multiaxial code structure* makes it possible for the ICD-10-PCS to be complete, expandable, and provide a high degree of flexibility and functionality.

ICD-10-PCS codes are composed of seven characters. Each character represents a category of information that can be specified about the procedure performed. A character defines both the category of information and its physical position in the code. A character's position can be understood as a semi-independent axis of classification that allows different specific values to be inserted into that space, and whose physical position remains stable. Within a defined code range, a character retains the general meaning that it confers on any value in that position.

Completeness

Completeness is considered a key structural attribute for a new procedure coding system. The specific recommendation for completeness included that a unique code be available for each significant procedure, that each code retain its unique definition, and that codes that have been deleted are not reused.

In Volume 3 of ICD-9-CM, procedures performed on many different body parts using different approaches or devices may be assigned to the same procedure code. In ICD-10-PCS, a unique code is constructed for every significantly different procedure.

Within each section, a character defines a consistent component of a code, and contains all applicable values for that character. The values define individual expressions (Open, Percutaneous) of the character's general meaning (approach) that are then used to construct unique procedure codes. Because all approaches by which a procedure is performed are assigned a separate approach value, every procedure which uses a different approach will have its own unique code. This is true of the other characters as well. The same procedure performed on a different body part has its own unique code; the same procedure performed using a different device has its own unique code, and so on.

Because ICD-10-PCS codes are constructed of individual values rather than lists of fixed codes and text descriptions, the unique, stable definition of a code in the system is retained. New values may be added to the system to represent a specific new approach or device or qualifier, but whole codes by design cannot be given new meanings and reused.

Expandability

Expandability was also recommended as a key structural attribute. The specific recommendation for expandability included that the system be capable of accommodating new procedures and technology and that these new codes could be added to the system without disrupting the existing structure.

ICD-10-PCS is designed to be easily updated as new codes are required for new procedures and new techniques. Changes to ICD-10-PCS can all be made within the existing structure because whole codes are not added. Instead, a new value for a character can be added to the system as needed. Likewise, an existing value for a character can be added to a table(s) in the system.

ICD-10-PCS Additional Characteristics

ICD-10-PCS possesses several additional characteristics in response to government and industry recommendations. These characteristics are

- Standardized terminology within the coding system
- Standardized level of specificity
- No diagnostic information
- No explicit "not otherwise specified" (NOS) code options
- Limited use of "not elsewhere classified" (NEC) code options

Standardized Terminology

Words commonly used in clinical vocabularies may have multiple meanings. This can cause confusion and result in inaccurate data. ICD-10-PCS is standardized and self-contained. Characters and values used in the system are defined in the system. For example, the word *excision* is used to describe a wide variety of surgical procedures. In ICD-10-PCS, the word *excision* describes a single, precise surgical objective, defined as "cutting out or off, without replacement, a portion of a body part."

No Eponyms or Common Procedure Names

The terminology used in ICD-10-PCS is standardized to provide precise and stable definitions of all procedures performed. This standardized terminology is used in all ICD-10-PCS code descriptions. As a result, ICD-10-PCS code descriptions do not include eponyms or common procedure names. Two examples from ICD-9-CM are

22.61, Excision of lesion of maxillary sinus with Caldwell-Luc approach

51.10, Endoscopic retrograde cholangiopancreatography [ERCP]

In ICD-10-PCS, physicians' names are not included in a code description, nor are procedures identified by common terms or acronyms such as appendectomy or CABG. Instead, such procedures are coded to the root operation that accurately identifies the objective of the procedure.

The procedures described in the preceding paragraph by ICD-9-CM codes are coded in ICD-10-PCS according to the root operation that matches the objective of the procedure. Here, the ICD-10-PCS equivalents would be Excision and Inspection, respectively. By relying on the universal objectives defined in root operations rather than eponyms or specific procedure titles that change or become obsolete, ICD-10-PCS preserves the capacity to define past, present, and future procedures accurately using stable terminology in the form of characters and values.

No Combination Codes

With rare exceptions, ICD-10-PCS does not define multiple procedures with one code. This is to preserve standardized terminology and consistency across the system. Procedures that are typically performed together but are distinct procedures may be defined by a single *combination code* in ICD-9-CM. An example of a combination code in ICD-9-CM is 28.3, Tonsillectomy with adenoidectomy.

A procedure that meets the reporting criteria for a separate procedure is coded separately in ICD-10-PCS. This allows the system to respond to changes in technology and medical practice with the maximum degree of stability and flexibility.

Standardized Level of Specificity

In ICD-9-CM, one code with its description and includes notes may encompass a vast number of procedure variations while another code defines a single specific procedure. ICD-10-PCS provides a standardized level of specificity for each code, so each code represents a single procedure variation.

The ICD-9-CM code 39.31, Suture of artery, does not specify the artery, whereas the code range 38.40–38.49, Resection of artery with replacement, provides a fourth-digit subclassification for specifying the artery by anatomical region (Thoracic, Abdominal, etc.). In ICD-10-PCS, the codes identifying all artery suture and artery replacement procedures possess the same degree of specificity. The ICD-9-CM examples above coded to their ICD-10-PCS equivalents would use the same artery body part values in all codes identifying the respective procedures.

In general, ICD-10-PCS code descriptions are much more specific than their ICD-9-CM counterparts, but sometimes an ICD-10-PCS code description is actually less specific. In most cases this is because the ICD-9-CM code contains diagnosis information. The standardized level of code specificity in ICD-10-PCS cannot always take account of these fluctuations in ICD-9-CM level of specificity. Instead, ICD-10-PCS provides a standardized level of specificity that can be predicted across the system.

Diagnosis Information Excluded

Another key feature of ICD-10-PCS is that information pertaining to a diagnosis is excluded from the code descriptions. ICD-9-CM often contains information about the diagnosis in its procedure codes. Adding diagnosis information limits the flexibility and functionality of a procedure coding system. It has the effect of placing a code "off limits" because the diagnosis in the medical record does not match the diagnosis in the procedure code description. The code cannot be used even though the procedural part of the code description precisely matches the procedure performed. Diagnosis information is not contained in any ICD-10-PCS code. The diagnosis codes, not the procedure codes, will specify the reason the procedure is performed.

NOS Code Options Restricted

ICD-9-CM often designates codes as "unspecified" or "not otherwise specified" (NOS) codes. By contrast, the standardized level of specificity designed into ICD-10-PCS restricts the use of broadly applicable NOS or unspecified code options in the system. A minimal level of specificity is required to construct a valid code.

Limited NEC Code Options

ICD-9-CM often designates codes as "not elsewhere classified" (NEC) or "other specified" versions of a procedure throughout the code set. NEC options are also provided in ICD-10-PCS, but only for specific, limited use.

In the Medical and Surgical section, two significant NEC options are the root operation value Q, Repair, and the device value Y, Other Device. The root operation Repair is a true NEC value. It is used only when the procedure performed is not one of the other root operations in the Medical and Surgical section. Other Device, on the other hand, is intended to be used to temporarily define new devices that do not have a specific value assigned, until one can be added to the system. No categories of medical or surgical devices are permanently classified to Other Device.

ICD-10-PCS Code Structure

Undergirding ICD-10-PCS is a logical, consistent structure that informs the system as a whole, down to the level of a single code. This means the process of constructing codes in ICD-10-PCS is also logical and consistent: the spaces of the code, called *characters* are filled with individual letters and numbers, called *values*.

Characters

All codes in ICD-10-PCS are seven characters long. Each character in the seven-character code represents an aspect of the procedure. The following are two examples of the code structure: one from the Medical and Surgical section and one from the Ancillary section.

Medical and Surgical Code Structure

Character 1	Character 2	Character 3	Character 4	Character 5	Character 6	Character 7
Section	Body System	Operation	Body Part	Approach	Device	Qualifier

Imaging Section Code Structure

Character 1	Character 2	Character 3	Character 4	Character 5	Character 6	Character 7
Section	Body System	Type	Body Part	Contrast	Qualifier	Qualifier

An ICD-10-PCS code is best understood as the result of a process rather than as an isolated, fixed quantity. The process consists of assigning values from among the valid choices for that part of the system, according to the rules governing the construction of codes.

Values

One of 34 possible values can be assigned to each character in a code: the numbers 0 through 9 and the alphabet (except the letters I and O, because they are easily confused with the numbers 1 and 0). A finished code looks like this: 02103D4.

This code is derived by choosing a specific value for each of the seven characters. Based on details about the procedure performed, values for each character specifying the section, body system, root operation, body part, approach, device, and qualifier are assigned. Because the definition of each character is a function of its physical position in the code, the same value placed in a different position in the code means something different. The value 0 in the first character means something different than 0 in the second character, or 0 in the third character, and so on.

Code Structure Example

The following example defines each character using the code 0LB50ZZ, Excision of right lower arm and wrist tendon, Open approach. This example comes from the Medical and Surgical section of ICD-10-PCS.

Character 1: Section

The first character in the code determines the broad procedure category, or section, where the code is found. In this example, the section is Medical and Surgical. 0 is the value that represents Medical and Surgical in the first character.

Character 1	Character 2	Character 3	Character 4	Character 5	Character 6	Character 7
Section	Body System	Root Operation	Body Part	Approach	Device	Qualifier
0						

Character 2: Body System

The second character defines the body system—the general physiological system or anatomical region involved. Examples of body systems include Lower Arteries, Central Nervous System, and Respiratory System. In this example, the body system is Tendons, represented by the value L.

Character 1	Character 2	Character 3	Character 4	Character 5	Character 6	Character 7
Section	Body System	Root Operation	Body Part	Approach	Device	Qualifier
0	**L**					

Character 3: Root Operation

The third character defines the root operation, or the objective of the procedure. Some examples of root operations are Bypass, Drainage, and Reattachment. In this example code, the root operation is Excision. When used in the third character of the code, the value B represents Excision.

Character 1	Character 2	Character 3	Character 4	Character 5	Character 6	Character 7
Section	Body System	Root Operation	Body Part	Approach	Device	Qualifier
0	**L**	**B**				

Character 4: Body Part

The fourth character defines the body part or specific anatomical site where the procedure was performed. The body system (second character) provides only a general indication of the procedure site. The body part and body system values together provide a precise description of the procedure site. Examples of body parts are Kidney, Tonsils, and

Thymus. In this example, the body part value is 5, Lower Arm and Wrist, Right. When the second character is L, the value 5 when used in the fourth character of the code represents the right lower arm and wrist tendon.

Character 1	Character 2	Character 3	Character 4	Character 5	Character 6	Character 7
Section	Body System	Root Operation	Body Part	Approach	Device	Qualifier
0	L	B	5			

Character 5: Approach

The fifth character defines the approach, or the technique used to reach the procedure site. Seven different approach values are used in the Medical and Surgical section to define the approach. Examples of approaches include Open and Percutaneous Endoscopic. In this example code, the approach is Open and is represented by the value 0.

Character 1	Character 2	Character 3	Character 4	Character 5	Character 6	Character 7
Section	Body System	Root Operation	Body Part	Approach	Device	Qualifier
0	L	B	5	0		

Character 6: Device

Depending on the procedure performed, there may be a device left in place at the end of the procedure. The sixth character defines the device. Device values fall into four basic categories:

- Grafts and Prostheses
- Implants
- Simple or Mechanical Appliances
- Electronic Appliances

In this example, there is no device used in the procedure. The value Z is used to represent No Device, as shown here:

Character 1	Character 2	Character 3	Character 4	Character 5	Character 6	Character 7
Section	Body System	Operation	Body Part	Approach	Device	Qualifier
0	L	B	5	0	Z	

Character 7: Qualifier

The seventh character defines a qualifier for the code. A qualifier specifies an additional attribute of the procedure, if applicable. Examples of qualifiers include Diagnostic and Stereotactic. Qualifier choices vary depending on the previous values selected. In this example, there is no specific qualifier applicable to this procedure, so the value is No Qualifier, represented by the letter Z.

Character 1	Character 2	Character 3	Character 4	Character 5	Character 6	Character 7
Section	Body System	Operation	Body Part	Approach	Device	Qualifier
0	L	B	5	0	Z	Z

0LB50ZZ is the complete specification of the procedure "Excision of right lower arm and wrist tendon, Open approach."

ICD-10-PCS Organization and Official Conventions

The *ICD-10-PCS Code Book, 2016 Edition* is based on the official International Classification of Diseases, Tenth Revision, Procedure Classification System, issued by the US Department of Health and Human Services (HHS) and CMS. This book is consistent with the content of the government's version of ICD-10-PCS and follows the official conventions.

Index

The Alphabetic Index is provided to assist the user with locating the appropriate table to construct procedure codes. Each table contains all the information required to construct valid procedure codes. Coders should not code from the PCS Index alone; the PCS code tables should always be consulted before assigning a PCS procedure code.

Main Terms

Main terms in the Alphabetic Index reflect the root operations, third character, of procedures. The Index includes not only root operation terms, but also other common procedural terms, anatomical sites, and device terms. The main terms are listed alphabetically. After the coder has located the correct main term and subterm in the Alphabetic Index, he or she is provided with the first three to four digits of the procedure code. The coder should then move to the Tables section of the code book and locate the appropriate table to complete the code construction. Even if the entire seven-digit code is provided in the Index, the coder should still reference the Tables to ensure the correct PCS code has been constructed.

See Reference

Common procedure terms are often listed with the *see* reference. The coder is instructed to follow the reference provided in order to locate the appropriate table to construct the code. For example, the *see* reference is present for the main term Colectomy. The Index excerpt is as follows:

Colectomy

see Excision, Gastrointestinal System 0DB

see Resection, Gastrointestinal System 0DT

In this example, the coder should review the definition of the root operations Excision and Resection to determine which is consistent with the medical record documentation. The coder should then proceed to the corresponding table as suggested by the *see* reference.

Use Reference

Anatomical site terms and device terms are often listed with the *use* reference. The coder is instructed to follow the reference provided in order to locate the appropriate main term for the procedure in question. For example, the *use* reference is present for the main term Inferior rectus muscle. The Index excerpt is as follows:

Inferior rectus muscle

use Muscle, Extraocular, Left

use Muscle, Extraocular, Right

In this example, the coder should identify the root operation for the procedure, and then look for the subterm that identifies the body part indicated in the *use* reference. For example, the procedure is excision of the inferior rectus muscle. The coder would locate the main term Excision. The Index excerpt is as follows:

Excision

Muscle

Extraocular

Left 08BM

Right 08BL

In this example, the coder knows that the Code Table 08B is the correct table because the previous review of the *use* reference identified that the inferior rectus muscle is and extraocular muscle. The coder can now proceed to the 08B Table to finish constructing the PCS code.

In addition to the *use* reference, the coder may also consult appendix D for Body Part Table or appendix E for the Device Table.

Code Tables

ICD-10-PCS contains 16 sections of Code Tables, represented by the numbers 0 through 9 and the letters B through D and F through H. The Tables are organized by general type of procedure. The three main sections of tables include:

1. **Medical and Surgical section**
   - Medical and Surgical (first character 0)

2. **Medical and Surgical Related sections**
   - Obstetrics (first character 1)

- Placement (first character 2)
- Administration (first character 3)
- Measurement and Monitoring (first character 4)
- Extracorporeal Assistance and Performance (first character 5)
- Extracorporeal Therapies (first character 6)
- Osteopathic (first character 7)
- Other Procedures (first character 8)
- Chiropractic (first character 9)

3. **Ancillary sections**
   - Imaging (first character B)
   - Nuclear Medicine (first character C)
   - Radiation Therapy (first character D)
   - Physical Rehabilitation and Diagnostic Audiology (first character F)
   - Mental Health (first character G)
   - Substance Abuse (first character H)
   - New Technology (first character X)

Each code table is defined by the first three characters of the PCS code. Each of these characters is displayed above the table. The table consists of all the options for characters 4 through 7. The root operation or root type, character 3, is present along with its official definition. Table 097 is provided here as an example of the table structure.

0 Medical and Surgical

9 Ear, Nose, Sinus

7 Dilation, Expanding an orifice or the lumen of a tubular body part

Body Part Character 4	Approach Character 5	Device Character 6	Qualifier Character 7
F Eustachian Tube, Right **G** Eustachian Tube, Left	**0** Open **7** Via Natural or Artificial Opening **8** Via Natural or Artificial Opening Endoscopic	**D** Intraluminal Device **Z** No Device	**Z** No Qualifier
F Eustachian Tube, Right **G** Eustachian Tube, Left	**3** Percutaneous **4** Percutaneous Endoscopic	**Z** No Device	**Z** No Qualifier

There can be multiple rows within the table for the first three characters, so the coder must carefully review all the applicable rows. Additionally, a table may cover multiple pages. Therefore, the coder must continue to review the code table options until the end of the table is reached to ensure the correct PCS code has been constructed.

Code Listing

Code Listings for the Medical and Surgical and Obstetrics sections are included in this manual to assist coders with ensuring that the intended code has been selected for reporting. The Code Listings are presented in alphanumeric order. Within the Code Listing, several additional conventions are included to assist coders with navigating the Medicare Code Editor (MCE) edits, official coding guidelines, and other reporting requirements such as the Inpatient Prospective Payment System (IPPS) Hospital-Acquired Conditions (HACs) related codes. The Code Listings are combined with the Tables section of the code book. In the Medical and Surgical section, the Code Listing appears after each body system. For the Obstetrics section, the Code Listing appears at the end of the section.

ICD-10-PCS Additional Conventions

The use of symbols has been added to this code book to alert the user to Medicare reimbursement logic and edits that are impacted by procedure coding. Some codes may be included in multiple reimbursement issues and, therefore, may have more than one symbol. For a quick reference review, the legend at the bottom of each page of the Code Listing (Medical/Surgical section and Obstetrics section) as well as the inside cover of the code book. The symbols are described in detail here.

Medicare Code Edits

Hospital inpatient Medicare claims paid under the IPPS are processed through the Medicare Code Editor (MCE) prior to payment by the Medicare administrative contractor (MAC). The code edits are intended to ensure that all claims processed by the MAC are accurate and complete. The information in this manual is based on the MCE v33.

Several of the MCE edits pertain to procedures. We have included identification of the codes included in these edits in this manual to assist users with preparing accurate and complete claims. The MCE edits included in this manual:

- Sex conflict
- Medicare non-covered procedures
- Medicare limited coverage procedures

Note: It is important to remember these edits are Medicare edits and may not apply to other third-party payers claim processing.

Sex Conflict Edit

The sex conflict edit is activated when the sex of the patient and the type of procedure performed does not match. The following symbols are used to identify female-only and male-only procedures.

> ♀ **Female-only** procedure: This symbol appears to the left of the applicable code in the code listing.

> ♂ **Male-only** procedure: This symbol appears to the left of the applicable code in the code listing.

Medicare Non-covered Procedure

Medicare does not reimburse for all ICD-10-PCS procedures. There are some procedures that are never reimbursed, and there are some procedures that are only reimbursed when certain specified diagnosis codes are also included on the claim. Non-covered procedures are designated by a red triangle symbol ▲ located next to the code description for the applicable code. If there is conditional logic for the non-coverage, it is provided to the right of the red triangle.

Medicare Limited Coverage Procedures

For certain procedures whose medical complexity and serious nature incur extraordinary associated costs, Medicare limits coverage to a portion of the cost. The limited coverage edit indicates this type of limited coverage. Limited coverage procedures are designated by a lime green triangle symbol ▲ located next to the code description for the applicable code. If there is conditional logic for the limited coverage, it is provided to the right of the lime green triangle.

MS-DRG Procedure Designations

The MS-DRG system is utilized within the IPPS to determine the unadjusted reimbursement amount for Medicare hospital inpatient claims. The MS-DRG Definitions Manual includes the logic for MS-DRG refinement and selection as well as logic based on the IPPS final rules released each August. The information in this manual is based on the MS-DRG v33. *Note:* It is important to remember that these edits are Medicare edits and may not apply to other third-party payers claim processing.

Non-Operating Room Procedures

Within the MS-DRG logic, CMS designates which procedures are operating room (OR) procedures and which procedures are non-OR procedures. Non-OR procedures do not impact the MS-DRG assignment; in the basic sense they do not covert medical MS-DRGs to surgical MS-DRGs. Once an encounter is determined as "surgical" specified OR procedures are utilized to refine the final MS-DRG assignment. Throughout the Medical and Surgical and Obstetrics sections, non-OR procedures are indicated with a purple dot ●. The purple dot symbol is located to the left of the applicable code in the code listing.

Hospital-Acquired Conditions Related Procedures

As part of the Medicare Value-Based Purchasing program, CMS has implemented a Paying for Value program entitled Hospital-Acquired Conditions (HACs) Reduction Program. This program is designed to reduce reimbursements to facilities where the value of the medical or surgical services have been comprised due to preventable conditions. Reimbursement for facilities with HAC scores in the lowest performance quartile will be reduced. In this manual, the HAC-associated

procedures are identified with an orange rectangle ▨ with HAC. The orange rectangle is located below the code description in the code listing. If there is conditional logic for the procedure code, it is included to the right of the orange rectangle.

Combination Codes Required

Within the MS-DRG logic CMS has designated codes that must be reported with specified other codes in order to fully report a complete procedure. For such procedures, such as simultaneous pancreas and kidney transplants, if the correct combination of codes is not reported, the desired MS-DRG will not be calculated for the encounter. Combination codes are identified with a green box with a plus sign in the middle ⊞. The green box with a code-specific note is located below the code description for applicable code in the code listing.

AHA *Coding Clinic for ICD-10-CM and ICD-10-PCS*

The American Hospital Association began publishing coding guidance for ICD-10-CM and ICD-10-PCS in the fourth quarter of 2012. In this code book we identify procedure codes that are discussed in the *Coding Clinic* guidance fourth quarter 2012 through first quarter 2015. Within the Code Listing the following sky blue note alerts the coder to review the AHA *Coding Clinic* prior to assignment of the code to ensure appropriate and accurate reporting. The quarter of publication, year and page number(s) are provided in the note.

AHA CC: 4Q; 2012; pg#-pg#

ICD-10-PCS Coding Guidelines

The ICD-10-PCS Coding Guidelines are presented here in the introduction and throughout this manual. Within the manual, the Medical and Surgical Section Guidelines are presented after the Introduction of the Medical and Surgical section. The Obstetric Section Guidelines are presented after the Introduction of the Obstetrics section.

Throughout the Code Listings, applicable guidelines are identified via an instruction note in order to remind users to reference the coding guidelines prior to code reporting. The instruction note *Review Coding Guideline...* followed by the guideline reference number is included after the section header for applicable sections or after the code description for applicable codes. It is imperative to review the ICD-10-PCS coding guidelines to ensure the procedure code being reported is accurate and complete.

ICD-10-PCS Official Guidelines for Coding and Reporting, 2016

The Centers for Medicare and Medicaid Services (CMS) and the National Center for Health Statistics (NCHS), two departments within the US federal government's Department of Health and Human Services (HHS) provide the following guidelines for coding and reporting using the International Classification of Diseases, 10th Revision, Procedure Coding System (ICD-10-PCS). These guidelines should be used as a companion document to the official version of the ICD-10-PCS as published on the CMS website. The ICD-10-PCS is a procedure classification published by the United States for classifying procedures performed in hospital inpatient health care settings.

These guidelines have been approved by the four organizations that make up the Cooperating Parties for the ICD-10-PCS: the American Hospital Association (AHA), the American Health Information Management Association (AHIMA), CMS, and NCHS.

These guidelines are a set of rules that have been developed to accompany and complement the official conventions and instructions provided within the ICD-10-PCS itself. The instructions and conventions of the classification take precedence over guidelines. These guidelines are based on the coding and sequencing instructions in the Tables, Index, and Definitions of ICD-10-PCS, but provide additional instruction. Adherence to these guidelines when assigning ICD-10-PCS procedure codes is required under the Health Insurance Portability and Accountability Act (HIPAA). The procedure codes have been adopted under HIPAA for hospital inpatient healthcare settings. A joint effort between the healthcare provider and the coder is essential to achieve complete and accurate documentation, code assignment, and reporting of diagnoses and procedures. These guidelines have been developed to assist both the healthcare provider and the coder in identifying those procedures that are to be reported. The importance of consistent, complete documentation in the medical record cannot be overemphasized. Without such documentation, accurate coding cannot be achieved.

Conventions

A1. ICD-10-PCS codes are composed of seven characters. Each character is an axis of classification that specifies information about the procedure performed. Within a defined code range, a character specifies the same type of information in that axis of classification.

Example: The fifth axis of classification specifies the approach in sections 0 through 4 and 7 through 9 of the system.

A2. One of 34 possible values can be assigned to each axis of classification in the seven-character code: they are the numbers 0 through 9 and the alphabet (except the letters I and O because they are easily confused with the numbers 1 and 0). The number of unique values used in an axis of classification differs as needed.

Example: Where the fifth axis of classification specifies the approach, seven different approach values are currently used to specify the approach.

A3. The valid values for an axis of classification can be added to as needed.

Example: If a significantly distinct type of device is used in a new procedure, a new device value can be added to the system.

A4. As with words in their context, the meaning of any single value is a combination of its axis of classification and any preceding values on which it may be dependent.

Example: The meaning of a body part value in the Medical and Surgical section is always dependent on the body system value. The body part value 0 in the Central Nervous body system specifies Brain and the body part value 0 in the Peripheral Nervous body system specifies Cervical Plexus.

A5. As the system is expanded to become increasingly detailed, more values will depend on preceding values for their meaning.

Example: In the Lower Joints body system, the device value 3 in the root operation Insertion specifies Infusion Device and the device value 3 in the root operation Replacement specifies Ceramic Synthetic Substitute.

A6. The purpose of the Alphabetic Index is to locate the appropriate table that contains all information necessary to construct a procedure code. The PCS Tables should always be consulted to find the most appropriate valid code.

A7. It is not required to consult the Index first before proceeding to the tables to complete the code. A valid code may be chosen directly from the Tables.

A8. All seven characters must be specified to be a valid code. If the documentation is incomplete for coding purposes, the physician should be queried for the necessary information.

A9. Within a PCS Table, valid codes include all combinations of choices in characters 4 through 7 contained in the same row of the table. In the example below, 0JHT3VZ is a valid code, and 0JHW3VZ is *not* a valid code.

Section:	0	Medical and Surgical
Body System:	J	Subcutaneous Tissue and Fascia
Operation:	H	Insertion: Putting in a nonbiological appliance that monitors, assists, performs, or prevents a physiological function but does not physically take the place of a body part

Body Part (4ᵗʰ)	Approach (5ᵗʰ)	Device (6ᵗʰ)	Qualifier (7ᵗʰ)
S Subcutaneous Tissue and Fascia, Head and Neck **V** Subcutaneous Tissue and Fascia, Upper Extremity **W** Subcutaneous Tissue and Fascia, Lower Extremity	**0** Open **3** Percutaneous	**1** Radioactive Element **3** Infusion Device	**Z** No Qualifier
T Subcutaneous Tissue and Fascia, Trunk	**0** Open **3** Percutaneous	**1** Radioactive Element **3** Infusion Device **V** Infusion Pump	**Z** No Qualifier

A10. "And," when used in a code description, means "and/or."

Example: Lower Arm and Wrist Muscle means lower arm and/or wrist muscle.

A11. Many of the terms used to construct PCS codes are defined within the system. It is the coder's responsibility to determine what the documentation in the medical record equates to in the PCS definitions. The physician is not expected to use the terms used in PCS code descriptions, nor is the coder required to query the physician when the correlation between the documentation and the defined PCS terms is clear.

Example: When the physician documents "partial resection" the coder can independently correlate "partial resection" to the root operation Excision without querying the physician for clarification.

Medical and Surgical Section Guidelines (section 0)

B2. Body System
General guidelines
B2.1a

The procedure codes in the general anatomical regions body systems should only be used when the procedure is performed on an anatomical region rather than a specific body part (e.g., root operations Control and Detachment, Drainage of a body cavity) or on the rare occasion when no information is available to support assignment of a code to a specific body part.

Example: Control of postoperative hemorrhage is coded to the root operation Control found in the general anatomical regions body systems.

B2.1b

Where the general body part values "upper" and "lower" are provided as an option in the Upper Arteries, Lower Arteries, Upper Veins, Lower Veins, Muscles and Tendons body systems, "upper" or "lower "specifies body parts located above or below the diaphragm respectively.

Example: Vein body parts above the diaphragm are found in the Upper Veins body system; vein body parts below the diaphragm are found in the Lower Veins body system.

B3. Root Operation
General guidelines
B3.1a

In order to determine the appropriate root operation, the full definition of the root operation as contained in the PCS Tables must be applied.

B3.1b

Components of a procedure specified in the root operation definition and explanation are not coded separately. Procedural steps necessary to reach the operative site and close the operative site, including anastomosis of a tubular body part, are also not coded separately.

Example: Resection of a joint as part of a joint replacement procedure is included in the root operation definition of Replacement and is not coded separately. Laparotomy performed to reach the site of an open liver biopsy is not coded separately. In a resection of sigmoid colon with anastomosis of descending colon to rectum, the anastomosis is not coded separately.

Multiple procedures
B3.2

During the same operative episode, multiple procedures are coded if:

    a. The same root operation is performed on different body parts as defined by distinct values of the body part character.

        Example: Diagnostic excision of liver and pancreas are coded separately.

    b. The same root operation is repeated at different body sites that are included in the same body part value.

        Example: Excision of the sartorius muscle and excision of the gracilis muscle are both included in the upper leg muscle body part value, and multiple procedures are coded.

    c. Multiple root operations with distinct objectives are performed on the same body part.

        Example: Destruction of sigmoid lesion and bypass of sigmoid colon are coded separately.

    d. The intended root operation is attempted using one approach, but is converted to a different approach.

        Example: Laparoscopic cholecystectomy converted to an open cholecystectomy is coded as percutaneous endoscopic Inspection and open Resection.

Discontinued procedures
B3.3

If the intended procedure is discontinued, code the procedure to the root operation performed. If a procedure is discontinued before any other root operation is performed, code the root operation Inspection of the body part or anatomical region inspected.

Example: A planned aortic valve replacement procedure is discontinued after the initial thoracotomy and before any incision is made in the heart muscle, when the patient becomes hemodynamically unstable. This procedure is coded as an open Inspection of the mediastinum.

Biopsy procedures

B3.4a

Biopsy procedures are coded using the root operations Excision, Extraction, or Drainage and the qualifier Diagnostic. The qualifier Diagnostic is used only for biopsies.

Examples: Fine needle aspiration biopsy of lung is coded to the root operation Drainage with the qualifier Diagnostic. Biopsy of bone marrow is coded to the root operation Extraction with the qualifier Diagnostic. Lymph node sampling for biopsy is coded to the root operation Excision with the qualifier Diagnostic.

Biopsy followed by more definitive treatment

B3.4b

If a diagnostic Excision, Extraction, or Drainage procedure (biopsy) is followed by a more definitive procedure, such as Destruction, Excision or Resection at the same procedure site, both the biopsy and the more definitive treatment are coded.

Example: Biopsy of breast followed by partial mastectomy at the same procedure site, both the biopsy and the partial mastectomy procedure are coded.

Overlapping body layers

B3.5

If the root operations Excision, Repair or Inspection are performed on overlapping layers of the musculoskeletal system, the body part specifying the deepest layer is coded.

Example: Excisional debridement that includes skin and subcutaneous tissue and muscle is coded to the muscle body part.

Bypass procedures

B3.6a

Bypass procedures are coded by identifying the body part bypassed "from" and the body part bypassed "to." The fourth character body part specifies the body part bypassed from, and the qualifier specifies the body part bypassed to.

Example: Bypass from stomach to jejunum, stomach is the body part and jejunum is the qualifier.

B3.6b

Coronary arteries are classified by number of distinct sites treated, rather than number of coronary arteries or anatomic name of a coronary artery (e.g., left anterior descending). Coronary artery bypass procedures are coded differently than other bypass procedures as described in the previous guideline. Rather than identifying the body part bypassed from, the body part identifies the number of coronary artery sites bypassed to, and the qualifier specifies the vessel bypassed from.

Example: Aortocoronary artery bypass of one site on the left anterior descending coronary artery and one site on the obtuse marginal coronary artery is classified in the body part axis of classification as two coronary artery sites and the qualifier specifies the aorta as the body part bypassed from.

B3.6c

If multiple coronary artery sites are bypassed, a separate procedure is coded for each coronary artery site that uses a different device and/or qualifier.

Example: Aortocoronary artery bypass and internal mammary coronary artery bypass are coded separately.

Control vs. more definitive root operations

B3.7

The root operation Control is defined as, "Stopping, or attempting to stop, postprocedural bleeding." If an attempt to stop postprocedural bleeding is initially unsuccessful, and to stop the bleeding requires performing any of the definitive root operations Bypass, Detachment, Excision, Extraction, Reposition, Replacement, or Resection, then that root operation is coded instead of Control.

Example: Resection of spleen to stop postprocedural bleeding is coded to Resection instead of Control.

Excision vs. Resection
B3.8

PCS contains specific body parts for anatomical subdivisions of a body part, such as lobes of the lungs or liver and regions of the intestine. Resection of the specific body part is coded whenever all of the body part is cut out or off, rather than coding Excision of a less specific body part.

Example: Left upper lung lobectomy is coded to Resection of Upper Lung Lobe, Left rather than Excision of Lung, Left.

Excision for graft
B3.9

If an autograft is obtained from a different body part in order to complete the objective of the procedure, a separate procedure is coded.

Example: Coronary bypass with excision of saphenous vein graft, excision of saphenous vein is coded separately.

Fusion procedures of the spine
B3.10a

The body part coded for a spinal vertebral joint(s) rendered immobile by a spinal fusion procedure is classified by the level of the spine (e.g. thoracic). There are distinct body part values for a single vertebral joint and for multiple vertebral joints at each spinal level.

Example: Body part values specify Lumbar Vertebral Joint, Lumbar Vertebral Joints, 2 or More and Lumbosacral Vertebral Joint.

B3.10b

If multiple vertebral joints are fused, a separate procedure is coded for each vertebral joint that uses a different device and/or qualifier.

Example: Fusion of lumbar vertebral joint, posterior approach, anterior column and fusion of lumbar vertebral joint, posterior approach, posterior column are coded separately.

B3.10c

Combinations of devices and materials are often used on a vertebral joint to render the joint immobile. When combinations of devices are used on the same vertebral joint, the device value coded for the procedure is as follows:

- If an interbody fusion device is used to render the joint immobile (alone or containing other material like bone graft), the procedure is coded with the device value Interbody Fusion Device
- If bone graft is the *only* device used to render the joint immobile, the procedure is coded with the device value Nonautologous Tissue Substitute or Autologous Tissue Substitute
- If a mixture of autologous and nonautologous bone graft (with or without biological or synthetic extenders or binders) is used to render the joint immobile, code the procedure with the device value Autologous Tissue Substitute

Examples: Fusion of a vertebral joint using a cage style interbody fusion device containing morsellized bone graft is coded to the device Interbody Fusion Device. Fusion of a vertebral joint using a bone dowel interbody fusion device made of cadaver bone and packed with a mixture of local morsellized bone and demineralized bone matrix is coded to the device Interbody Fusion Device.

Fusion of a vertebral joint using both autologous bone graft and bone bank bone graft is coded to the device Autologous Tissue Substitute.

Inspection procedures
B3.11a

Inspection of a body part(s) performed in order to achieve the objective of a procedure is not coded separately.

Example: Fiberoptic bronchoscopy performed for irrigation of bronchus, only the irrigation procedure is coded.

B3.11b

If multiple tubular body parts are inspected, the most distal body part inspected is coded. If multiple non-tubular body parts in a region are inspected, the body part that specifies the entire area inspected is coded.

Examples: Cystoureteroscopy with inspection of bladder and ureters is coded to the ureter body part value.

Exploratory laparotomy with general inspection of abdominal contents is coded to the peritoneal cavity body part value.

B3.11c

When both an Inspection procedure and another procedure are performed on the same body part during the same episode, if the Inspection procedure is performed using a different approach than the other procedure, the Inspection procedure is coded separately.

Example: Endoscopic Inspection of the duodenum is coded separately when open Excision of the duodenum is performed during the same procedural episode.

Occlusion vs. Restriction for vessel embolization procedures
B3.12

If the objective of an embolization procedure is to completely close a vessel, the root operation Occlusion is coded. If the objective of an embolization procedure is to narrow the lumen of a vessel, the root operation Restriction is coded.

Examples: Tumor embolization is coded to the root operation Occlusion, because the objective of the procedure is to cut off the blood supply to the vessel.

Embolization of a cerebral aneurysm is coded to the root operation Restriction, because the objective of the procedure is not to close off the vessel entirely, but to narrow the lumen of the vessel at the site of the aneurysm where it is abnormally wide.

Release procedures
B3.13

In the root operation Release, the body part value coded is the body part being freed and not the tissue being manipulated or cut to free the body part.

Example: Lysis of intestinal adhesions is coded to the specific intestine body part value.

Release vs. Division
B3.14

If the sole objective of the procedure is freeing a body part without cutting the body part, the root operation is Release. If the sole objective of the procedure is separating or transecting a body part, the root operation is Division.

Examples: Freeing a nerve root from surrounding scar tissue to relieve pain is coded to the root operation Release. Severing a nerve root to relieve pain is coded to the root operation Division.

Reposition for fracture treatment
B3.15

Reduction of a displaced fracture is coded to the root operation Reposition and the application of a cast or splint in conjunction with the Reposition procedure is not coded separately. Treatment of a nondisplaced fracture is coded to the procedure performed.

Examples: Casting of a nondisplaced fracture is coded to the root operation Immobilization in the Placement section.

Putting a pin in a nondisplaced fracture is coded to the root operation Insertion.

Transplantation vs. Administration
B3.16

Putting in a mature and functioning living body part taken from another individual or animal is coded to the root operation Transplantation. Putting in autologous or nonautologous cells is coded to the Administration section.

Example: Putting in autologous or nonautologous bone marrow, pancreatic islet cells or stem cells is coded to the Administration section.

B4. Body Part
General guidelines
B4.1a

If a procedure is performed on a portion of a body part that does not have a separate body part value, code the body part value corresponding to the whole body part.

Example: A procedure performed on the alveolar process of the mandible is coded to the mandible body part.

B4.1b

If the prefix "peri" is combined with a body part to identify the site of the procedure, and the site of the procedure is not further specified, then the procedure is coded to the body part named. This guideline applies only when a more specific body part value is not available.

Examples: A procedure site identified as perirenal is coded to the kidney body part when the site of the procedure is not further specified.

A procedure site described in the documentation as peri-urethral, and the documentation also indicates that it is the vulvar issue and not the urethral tissue that is the site of the procedure, then the procedure is coded to the vulva body part.

Branches of body parts
B4.2

Where a specific branch of a body part does not have its own body part value in PCS, the body part is coded to the closest proximal branch that has a specific body part value.

Example: A procedure performed on the mandibular branch of the trigeminal nerve is coded to the trigeminal nerve body part value.

Bilateral body part values
B4.3

Bilateral body part values are available for a limited number of body parts. If the identical procedure is performed on contralateral body parts, and a bilateral body part value exists for that body part, a single procedure is coded using the bilateral body part value. If no bilateral body part value exists, each procedure is coded separately using the appropriate body part value.

Example: The identical procedure performed on both fallopian tubes is coded once using the body part value Fallopian Tube, Bilateral. The identical procedure performed on both knee joints is coded twice using the body part values Knee Joint, Right and Knee Joint, Left.

Coronary arteries
B4.4

The coronary arteries are classified as a single body part that is further specified by number of sites treated and not by name or number of arteries. Separate body part values are used to specify the number of sites treated when the same procedure is performed on multiple sites in the coronary arteries.

Examples: Angioplasty of two distinct sites in the left anterior descending coronary artery with placement of two stents is coded as Dilation of Coronary Arteries, Two Sites, with Intraluminal Device.

Angioplasty of two distinct sites in the left anterior descending coronary artery, one with stent placed and one without, is coded separately as Dilation of Coronary Artery, One Site with Intraluminal Device, and Dilation of Coronary Artery, One Site with no device.

Tendons, ligaments, bursae and fascia near a joint
B4.5

Procedures performed on tendons, ligaments, bursae and fascia supporting a joint are coded to the body part in the respective body system that is the focus of the procedure. Procedures performed on joint structures themselves are coded to the body part in the joint body systems.

Example: Repair of the anterior cruciate ligament of the knee is coded to the knee bursaand ligament body part in the bursae and ligaments body system. Knee arthroscopy with shaving of articular cartilage is coded to the knee joint body part in the Lower Joints body system.

Skin, subcutaneous tissue and fascia overlying a joint
B4.6

If a procedure is performed on the skin, subcutaneous tissue or fascia overlying a joint, the procedure is coded to the following body part:

- Shoulder is coded to Upper Arm
- Elbow is coded to Lower Arm

- Wrist is coded to Lower Arm
- Hip is coded to Upper Leg
- Knee is coded to Lower Leg
- Ankle is coded to Foot

Fingers and toes
B4.7

If a body system does not contain a separate body part value for fingers, procedures performed on the fingers are coded to the body part value for the hand. If a body system does not contain a separate body part value for toes, procedures performed on the toes are coded to the body part value for the foot.

Example: Excision of finger muscle is coded to one of the hand muscle body part values in the Muscles body system.

Upper and lower intestinal tract
B4.8

In the Gastrointestinal body system, the general body part values Upper Intestinal Tract and Lower Intestinal Tract are provided as an option for the root operations Change, Inspection, Removal and Revision. Upper Intestinal Tract includes the portion of the gastrointestinal tract from the esophagus down to and including the duodenum, and Lower Intestinal Tract includes the portion of the gastrointestinal tract from the jejunum down to and including the rectum and anus.

Example: In the root operation Change table, change of a device in the jejunum is coded using the body part Lower Intestinal Tract.

B5. Approach
Open approach with percutaneous endoscopic assistance
B5.2

Procedures performed using the open approach with percutaneous endoscopic assistance are coded to the approach Open.

Example: Laparoscopic-assisted sigmoidectomy is coded to the approach Open.

External approach
B5.3a

Procedures performed within an orifice on structures that are visible without the aid of any instrumentation are coded to the approach External.

Example: Resection of tonsils is coded to the approach External.

B5.3b

Procedures performed indirectly by the application of external force through the intervening body layers are coded to the approach External.

Example: Closed reduction of fracture is coded to the approach External.

Percutaneous procedure via device
B5.4

Procedures performed percutaneously via a device placed for the procedure are coded to the approach Percutaneous.

Example: Fragmentation of kidney stone performed via percutaneous nephrostomy is coded to the approach Percutaneous.

B6. Device
General guidelines
B6.1a

A device is coded only if a device remains after the procedure is completed. If no device remains, the device value No Device is coded.

B6.1b

Materials such as sutures, ligatures, radiological markers and temporary post-operative wound drains are considered integral to the performance of a procedure and are not coded as devices.

B6.1c

Procedures performed on a device only and not on a body part are specified in the root operations Change, Irrigation, Removal and Revision, and are coded to the procedure performed.

Example: Irrigation of percutaneous nephrostomy tube is coded to the root operation
Irrigation of indwelling device in the Administration section.

Drainage device
B6.2

A separate procedure to put in a drainage device is coded to the root operation Drainage with the device value Drainage Device.

Obstetric Section Guidelines (section 1)
C. Obstetrics Section
Products of conception
C1

Procedures performed on the products of conception are coded to the Obstetrics section. Procedures performed on the pregnant female other than the products of conception are coded to the appropriate root operation in the Medical and Surgical section.

Example: Amniocentesis is coded to the products of conception body part in the Obstetrics section. Repair of obstetric urethral laceration is coded to the urethra body part in the Medical and Surgical section.

Procedures following delivery or abortion
C2

Procedures performed following a delivery or abortion for curettage of the endometrium or evacuation of retained products of conception are all coded in the Obstetrics section, to the root operation Extraction and the body part Products of Conception, Retained. Diagnostic or therapeutic dilation and curettage performed during times other than the postpartum or post-abortion period are all coded in the Medical and Surgical section, to the root operation Extraction and the body part Endometrium.

D. New Technology Section
General guidelines
D1

Section X codes are standalone codes. They are not supplemental codes. Section X codes fully represent the specific procedure described in the code title, and do not require any additional codes from other sections of ICD-10-PCS. When section X contains a code title which describes a specific new technology procedure, only that X code is reported for the procedure. There is no need to report a broader, non-specific code in another section of ICD-10-PCS.

Example: XW04321 Introduction of Ceftazidime-Avibactam Anti-infective into Central Vein, Percutaneous Approach, New Technology Group 1, can be coded to indicate that Ceftazidime-Avibactam Anti-infective was administered via a central vein. A separate code from table 3E0 in the Administration section of ICD-10-PCS is not coded in addition to this code.

Selection of Principal Procedure

The following instructions should be applied in the selection of principal procedure and clarification on the importance of the relation to the principal diagnosis when more than one procedure is performed:

1. Procedure performed for definitive treatment of both principal diagnosis and secondary diagnosis

    a. Sequence procedure performed for definitive treatment most related to principal diagnosis as principal procedure.

2. Procedure performed for definitive treatment and diagnostic procedures performed for both principal diagnosis and secondary diagnosis

    a. Sequence procedure performed for definitive treatment most related to principal diagnosis as principal procedure

3. A diagnostic procedure was performed for the principal diagnosis and a procedure is performed for definitive treatment of a secondary diagnosis.

    a. Sequence diagnostic procedure as principal procedure, since the procedure most related to the principal diagnosis takes precedence.

4. No procedures performed that are related to principal diagnosis; procedures performed for definitive treatment and diagnostic procedures were performed for secondary diagnosis

    a. Sequence procedure performed for definitive treatment of secondary diagnosis as principal procedure, since there are no procedures (definitive or nondefinitive treatment) related to principal diagnosis.

3

3f (Aortic) Bioprosthesis valve
  use Zooplastic Tissue in Heart and Great Vessels

A

Abdominal aortic plexus
  use Nerve, Abdominal Sympathetic
Abdominal esophagus
  use Esophagus, Lower
Abdominohysterectomy
  see Resection, Cervix 0UTC
  see Resection, Uterus 0UT9
Abdominoplasty
  see Alteration, Abdominal Wall 0W0F
  see Repair, Abdominal Wall 0WQF
  see Supplement, Abdominal Wall 0WUF
Abductor hallucis muscle
  use Muscle, Foot, Left
  use Muscle, Foot, Right
AbioCor® Total Replacement Heart
  use Synthetic Substitute
Ablation
  see Destruction
Abortion
  Abortifacient 10A07ZX
  Laminaria 10A07ZW
  Products of Conception 10A0
  Vacuum 10A07Z6
Abrasion
  see Extraction
Absolute Pro Vascular (OTW) Self-Expanding Stent System
  use Intraluminal Device
Accessory cephalic vein
  use Vein, Cephalic, Left
  use Vein, Cephalic, Right
Accessory obturator nerve
  use Nerve, Lumbar Plexus
Accessory phrenic nerve
  use Nerve, Phrenic
Accessory spleen
  use Spleen
Acculink (RX) Carotid Stent System
  use Intraluminal Device
Acellular Hydrated Dermis
  use Nonautologous Tissue Substitute
Acetabular cup
  use Liner in Lower Joints
Acetabulectomy
  see Excision, Lower Bones 0QB
  see Resection, Lower Bones 0QT
Acetabulofemoral joint
  use Joint, Hip, Left
  use Joint, Hip, Right
Acetabuloplasty
  see Repair, Lower Bones 0QQ
  see Replacement, Lower Bones 0QR
  see Supplement, Lower Bones 0QU
Achilles tendon
  use Tendon, Lower Leg, Left
  use Tendon, Lower Leg, Right
Achillorrhaphy
  see Repair, Tendons 0LQ
Achillotenotomy, achillotomy
  see Division, Tendons 0L8
  see Drainage, Tendons 0L9
Acromioclavicular ligament
  use Bursa and Ligament, Shoulder, Left
  use Bursa and Ligament, Shoulder, Right
Acromion (process)
  use Scapula, Left
  use Scapula, Right

Acromionectomy
  see Excision, Upper Joints 0RB
  see Resection, Upper Joints 0RT
Acromioplasty
  see Repair, Upper Joints 0RQ
  see Replacement, Upper Joints 0RR
  see Supplement, Upper Joints 0RU
Activa PC neurostimulator
  use Stimulator Generator, Multiple Array in 0JH
Activa RC neurostimulator
  use Stimulator Generator, Multiple Array Rechargeable in 0JH
Activa SC neurostimulator
  use Stimulator Generator, Single Array in 0JH
Activities of Daily Living Assessment
  F02
Activities of Daily Living Treatment
  F08
ACUITY™ Steerable Lead
  use Cardiac Lead, Defibrillator in 02H
  use Cardiac Lead, Pacemaker in 02H
Acupuncture
  Breast
    Anesthesia 8E0H300
    No Qualifier 8E0H30Z
  Integumentary System
    Anesthesia 8E0H300
    No Qualifier 8E0H30Z
Adductor brevis muscle
  use Muscle, Upper Leg, Left
  use Muscle, Upper Leg, Right
Adductor hallucis muscle
  use Muscle, Foot, Left
  use Muscle, Foot, Right
Adductor longus muscle
  use Muscle, Upper Leg, Left
  use Muscle, Upper Leg, Right
Adductor magnus muscle
  use Muscle, Upper Leg, Left
  use Muscle, Upper Leg, Right
Adenohypophysis
  use Gland, Pituitary
Adenoidectomy
  see Excision, Adenoids 0CBQ
  see Resection, Adenoids 0CTQ
Adenoidotomy
  see Drainage, Adenoids 0C9Q
Adhesiolysis
  see Release
Administration
  Blood products
    see Transfusion
  Other substance
    see Introduction of substance in or on
Adrenalectomy
  see Excision, Endocrine System 0GB
  see Resection, Endocrine System 0GT
Adrenalorrhaphy
  see Repair, Endocrine System 0GQ
Adrenalotomy
  see Drainage, Endocrine System 0G9
Advancement
  see Reposition
  see Transfer
Advisa (MRI)
  use Pacemaker, Dual Chamber in 0JH
AIGISRx Antibacterial Envelope
  use Anti-Infective Envelope

Alar ligament of axis
  use Bursa and Ligament, Head and Neck
Alimentation
  see Introduction of substance in or on
Alteration
  Abdominal Wall 0W0F
  Ankle Region
    Left 0Y0L
    Right 0Y0K
  Arm
    Lower
      Left 0X0F
      Right 0X0D
    Upper
      Left 0X09
      Right 0X08
  Axilla
    Left 0X05
    Right 0X04
  Back
    Lower 0W0L
    Upper 0W0K
  Breast
    Bilateral 0H0V
    Left 0H0U
    Right 0H0T
  Buttock
    Left 0Y01
    Right 0Y00
  Chest Wall 0W08
  Ear
    Bilateral 0902
    Left 0901
    Right 0900
  Elbow Region
    Left 0X0C
    Right 0X0B
  Extremity
    Lower
      Left 0Y0B
      Right 0Y09
    Upper
      Left 0X07
      Right 0X06
  Eyelid
    Lower
      Left 080R
      Right 080Q
    Upper
      Left 080P
      Right 080N
  Face 0W02
  Head 0W00
  Jaw
    Lower 0W05
    Upper 0W04
  Knee Region
    Left 0Y0G
    Right 0Y0F
  Leg
    Lower
      Left 0Y0J
      Right 0Y0H
    Upper
      Left 0Y0D
      Right 0Y0C
  Lip
    Lower 0C01X
    Upper 0C00X
  Neck 0W06
  Nose 090K
  Perineum
    Female 0W0N
    Male 0W0M

Alteration *(continued)*
  Shoulder Region
    Left 0X03
    Right 0X02
  Subcutaneous Tissue and Fascia
    Abdomen 0J08
    Back 0J07
    Buttock 0J09
    Chest 0J06
    Face 0J01
    Lower Arm
      Left 0J0H
      Right 0J0G
    Lower Leg
      Left 0J0P
      Right 0J0N
    Neck
      Anterior 0J04
      Posterior 0J05
    Upper Arm
      Left 0J0F
      Right 0J0D
    Upper Leg
      Left 0J0M
      Right 0J0L
  Wrist Region
    Left 0X0H
    Right 0X0G
Alveolar process of mandible
  use Mandible, Left
  use Mandible, Right
Alveolar process of maxilla
  use Maxilla, Left
  use Maxilla, Right
Alveolectomy
  see Excision, Head and Facial Bones 0NB
  see Resection, Head and Facial Bones 0NT
Alveoloplasty
  see Repair, Head and Facial Bones 0NQ
  see Replacement, Head and Facial Bones 0NR
  see Supplement, Head and Facial Bones 0NU
Alveolotomy
  see Division, Head and Facial Bones 0N8
  see Drainage, Head and Facial Bones 0N9
Ambulatory cardiac monitoring
  4A12X45
Amniocentesis
  see Drainage, Products of Conception 1090
Amnioinfusion
  see Introduction of substance in or on, Products of Conception 3E0E
Amnioscopy 10J08ZZ
Amniotomy
  see Drainage, Products of Conception 1090
AMPLATZER® Muscular VSD Occluder
  use Synthetic Substitute
Amputation
  see Detachment
AMS 800® Urinary Control System
  use Artificial Sphincter in Urinary System
Anal orifice
  use Anus
Analog radiography
  see Plain Radiography

Anastomosis
  see Bypass
Anatomical snuffbox
  use Muscle, Lower Arm and Wrist, Left
  use Muscle, Lower Arm and Wrist, Right
AneuRx® AAA Advantage®
  use Intraluminal Device
Angiectomy
  see Excision, Heart and Great Vessels 02B
  see Excision, Upper Arteries 03B
  see Excision, Lower Arteries 04B
  see Excision, Upper Veins 05B
  see Excision, Lower Veins 06B
Angiocardiography
  Combined right and left heart
    see Fluoroscopy, Heart, Right and Left B216
  Left Heart
    see Fluoroscopy, Heart, Left B215
  Right Heart
    see Fluoroscopy, Heart, Right B214
  SPY
    see Fluoroscopy, Heart B21
Angiography
  see Plain Radiography, Heart B20
  see Fluoroscopy, Heart B21
Angioplasty
  see Dilation, Heart and Great Vessels 027
  see Repair, Heart and Great Vessels 02Q
  see Replacement, Heart and Great Vessels 02R
  see Dilation, Upper Arteries 037
  see Repair, Upper Arteries 03Q
  see Replacement, Upper Arteries 03R
  see Dilation, Lower Arteries 047
  see Repair, Lower Arteries 04Q
  see Replacement, Lower Arteries 04R
  see Supplement, Heart and Great Vessels 02U
  see Supplement, Upper Arteries 03U
  see Supplement, Lower Arteries 04U
Angiorrhaphy
  see Repair, Heart and Great Vessels 02Q
  see Repair, Upper Arteries 03Q
  see Repair, Lower Arteries 04Q
Angioscopy
  02JY4ZZ
  03JY4ZZ
  04JY4ZZ
Angiotripsy
  see Occlusion, Upper Arteries 03L
  see Occlusion, Lower Arteries 04L
Angular artery
  use Artery, Face
Angular vein
  use Vein, Face, Left
  use Vein, Face, Right
Annular ligament
  use Bursa and Ligament, Elbow, Left
  use Bursa and Ligament, Elbow, Right
Annuloplasty
  see Repair, Heart and Great Vessels 02Q
  see Supplement, Heart and Great Vessels 02U
Annuloplasty ring
  use Synthetic Substitute

Anoplasty
  see Repair, Anus 0DQQ
  see Supplement, Anus 0DUQ
Anorectal junction
  use Rectum
Anoscopy 0DJD8ZZ
Ansa cervicalis
  use Nerve, Cervical Plexus
Antabuse therapy HZ93ZZZ
Antebrachial fascia
  use Subcutaneous Tissue and Fascia, Lower Arm, Left
  use Subcutaneous Tissue and Fascia, Lower Arm, Right
Anterior (pectoral) lymph node
  use Lymphatic, Axillary, Left
  use Lymphatic, Axillary, Right
Anterior cerebral artery
  use Artery, Intracranial
Anterior cerebral vein
  use Vein, Intracranial
Anterior choroidal artery
  use Artery, Intracranial
Anterior circumflex humeral artery
  use Artery, Axillary, Left
  use Artery, Axillary, Right
Anterior communicating artery
  use Artery, Intracranial
Anterior cruciate ligament (ACL)
  use Bursa and Ligament, Knee, Left
  use Bursa and Ligament, Knee, Right
Anterior crural nerve
  use Nerve, Femoral
Anterior facial vein
  use Vein, Face, Left
  use Vein, Face, Right
Anterior intercostal artery
  use Artery, Internal Mammary, Left
  use Artery, Internal Mammary, Right
Anterior interosseous nerve
  use Nerve, Median
Anterior lateral malleolar artery
  use Artery, Anterior Tibial, Left
  use Artery, Anterior Tibial, Right
Anterior lingual gland
  use Gland, Minor Salivary
Anterior medial malleolar artery
  use Artery, Anterior Tibial, Left
  use Artery, Anterior Tibial, Right
Anterior spinal artery
  use Artery, Vertebral, Left
  use Artery, Vertebral, Right
Anterior tibial recurrent artery
  use Artery, Anterior Tibial, Left
  use Artery, Anterior Tibial, Right
Anterior ulnar recurrent artery
  use Artery, Ulnar, Left
  use Artery, Ulnar, Right
Anterior vagal trunk
  use Nerve, Vagus
Anterior vertebral muscle
  use Muscle, Neck, Left
  use Muscle, Neck, Right
Antihelix
  use Ear, External, Bilateral
  use Ear, External, Left
  use Ear, External, Right
Antimicrobial envelope
  use Anti-Infective Envelope
Antitragus
  use Ear, External, Bilateral
  use Ear, External, Left
  use Ear, External, Right
Antrostomy
  see Drainage, Ear, Nose, Sinus 099
Antrotomy
  see Drainage, Ear, Nose, Sinus 099
Antrum of Highmore
  use Sinus, Maxillary, Left
  use Sinus, Maxillary, Right

Aortic annulus
  use Valve, Aortic
Aortic arch
  use Aorta, Thoracic
Aortic intercostal artery
  use Aorta, Thoracic
Aortography
  see Plain Radiography, Upper Arteries B30
  see Fluoroscopy, Upper Arteries B31
  see Plain Radiography, Lower Arteries B40
  see Fluoroscopy, Lower Arteries B41
Aortoplasty
  see Repair, Aorta, Thoracic 02QW
  see Replacement, Aorta, Thoracic 02RW
  see Supplement, Aorta, Thoracic 02UW
  see Repair, Aorta, Abdominal 04Q0
  see Replacement, Aorta, Abdominal 04R0
  see Supplement, Aorta, Abdominal 04U0
Apical (subclavicular) lymph node
  use Lymphatic, Axillary, Left
  use Lymphatic, Axillary, Right
Apneustic center
  use Pons
Appendectomy
  see Excision, Appendix 0DBJ
  see Resection, Appendix 0DTJ
Appendicolysis
  see Release, Appendix 0DNJ
Appendicotomy
  see Drainage, Appendix 0D9J
Application
  see Introduction of substance in or on
Aquapheresis 6A550Z3
Aqueduct of Sylvius
  use Cerebral Ventricle
Aqueous humour
  use Anterior Chamber, Left
  use Anterior Chamber, Right
Arachnoid mater, intracranial
  use Cerebral Meninges
Arachnoid mater, spinal
  use Spinal Meninges
Arcuate artery
  use Artery, Foot, Left
  use Artery, Foot, Right
Areola
  use Nipple, Left
  use Nipple, Right
AROM (artificial rupture of membranes) 10907ZC
Arterial canal (duct)
  use Artery, Pulmonary, Left
Arterial pulse tracing
  see Measurement, Arterial 4A03
Arteriectomy
  see Excision, Heart and Great Vessels 02B
  see Excision, Upper Arteries 03B
  see Excision, Lower Arteries 04B
Arteriography
  see Plain Radiography, Heart B20
  see Fluoroscopy, Heart B21
  see Plain Radiography, Upper Arteries B30
  see Fluoroscopy, Upper Arteries B31
  see Plain Radiography, Lower Arteries B40
  see Fluoroscopy, Lower Arteries B41
Arterioplasty
  see Repair, Heart and Great Vessels 02Q
  see Replacement, Heart and Great Vessels 02R
  see Repair, Upper Arteries 03Q

Arterioplasty *(continued)*
  see Replacement, Upper Arteries 03R
  see Repair, Lower Arteries 04Q
  see Replacement, Lower Arteries 04R
  see Supplement, Upper Arteries 03U
  see Supplement, Lower Arteries 04U
  see Supplement, Heart and Great Vessels 02U
Arteriorrhaphy
  see Repair, Heart and Great Vessels 02Q
  see Repair, Upper Arteries 03Q
  see Repair, Lower Arteries 04Q
Arterioscopy
  02JY4ZZ
  03JY4ZZ
  04JY4ZZ
Arthrectomy
  see Excision, Upper Joints 0RB
  see Resection, Upper Joints 0RT
  see Excision, Lower Joints 0SB
  see Resection, Lower Joints 0ST
Arthrocentesis
  see Drainage, Upper Joints 0R9
  see Drainage, Lower Joints 0S9
Arthrodesis
  see Fusion, Upper Joints 0RG
  see Fusion, Lower Joints 0SG
Arthrography
  see Plain Radiography, Skull and Facial Bones BN0
  see Plain Radiography, Non-Axial Upper Bones BP0
  see Plain Radiography, Non-Axial Lower Bones BQ0
Arthrolysis
  see Release, Upper Joints 0RN
  see Release, Lower Joints 0SN
Arthropexy
  see Repair, Upper Joints 0RQ
  see Reposition, Upper Joints 0RS
  see Repair, Lower Joints 0SQ
  see Reposition, Lower Joints 0SS
Arthroplasty
  see Repair, Upper Joints 0RQ
  see Replacement, Upper Joints 0RR
  see Repair, Lower Joints 0SQ
  see Replacement, Lower Joints 0SR
  see Supplement, Lower Joints 0SU
  see Supplement, Upper Joints 0RU
Arthroscopy
  see Inspection, Upper Joints 0RJ
  see Inspection, Lower Joints 0SJ
Arthrotomy
  see Drainage, Upper Joints 0R9
  see Drainage, Lower Joints 0S9
Artificial anal sphincter (AAS)
  use Artificial Sphincter in Gastrointestinal System
Artificial bowel sphincter (neosphincter)
  use Artificial Sphincter in Gastrointestinal System
Artificial Sphincter
  Insertion of device in
    Anus 0DHQ
    Bladder 0THB
    Bladder Neck 0THC
    Urethra 0THD
  Removal of device from
    Anus 0DPQ
    Bladder 0TPB
    Urethra 0TPD
  Revision of device in
    Anus 0DWQ
    Bladder 0TWB
    Urethra 0TWD
Artificial urinary sphincter (AUS)
  use Artificial Sphincter in Urinary System

Aryepiglottic fold
 use Larynx
Arytenoid cartilage
 use Larynx
Arytenoid muscle
 use Muscle, Neck, Left
 use Muscle, Neck, Right
Arytenoidectomy
 see Excision, Larynx 0CBS
Arytenoidopexy
 see Repair, Larynx 0CQS
Ascenda Intrathecal Catheter
 use Infusion Device
Ascending aorta
 use Aorta, Thoracic
Ascending palatine artery
 use Artery, Face
Ascending pharyngeal artery
 use Artery, External Carotid, Left
 use Artery, External Carotid, Right
Aspiration, fine needle
 Fluid or gas
  see Drainage
 Tissue
  see Excision
Assessment
 Activities of daily living
  see Activities of Daily Living
   Assessment, Rehabilitation F02
 Hearing
  see Hearing Assessment,
   Diagnostic Audiology F13
 Hearing aid
  see Hearing Aid Assessment,
   Diagnostic Audiology F14
 Motor function
  see Motor Function Assessment,
   Rehabilitation F01
 Nerve function
  see Motor Function Assessment,
   Rehabilitation F01
 Speech
  see Speech Assessment,
   Rehabilitation F00
 Vestibular
  see Vestibular Assessment,
   Diagnostic Audiology F15
 Vocational
  see Activities of Daily Living
   Treatment, Rehabilitation F08
Assistance
 Cardiac
  Continuous
   Balloon Pump 5A02210
   Impeller Pump 5A0221D
   Other Pump 5A02216
   Pulsatile Compression
    5A02215
  Intermittent
   Balloon Pump 5A02110
   Impeller Pump 5A0211D
   Other Pump 5A02116
   Pulsatile Compression
    5A02115
 Circulatory
  Continuous
   Hyperbaric 5A05221
   Supersaturated 5A0522C
  Intermittent
   Hyperbaric 5A05121
   Supersaturated 5A0512C
 Respiratory
  24-96 Consecutive Hours
   Continuous Negative Airway
    Pressure 5A09459
   Continuous Positive Airway
    Pressure 5A09457
   Intermittent Negative Airway
    Pressure 5A0945B
   Intermittent Positive Airway
    Pressure 5A09458
   No Qualifier 5A0945Z

Assistance *(continued)*
 Respiratory *(continued)*
  Greater than 96 Consecutive
   Hours
   Continuous Negative Airway
    Pressure 5A09559
   Continuous Positive Airway
    Pressure 5A09557
   Intermittent Negative Airway
    Pressure 5A0955B
   Intermittent Positive Airway
    Pressure 5A09558
   No Qualifier 5A0955Z
  Less than 24 Consecutive Hours
   Continuous Negative Airway
    Pressure 5A09359
   Continuous Positive Airway
    Pressure 5A09357
   Intermittent Negative Airway
    Pressure 5A0935B
   Intermittent Positive Airway
    Pressure 5A09358
   No Qualifier 5A0935Z
Assurant (Cobalt) stent
 use Intraluminal Device
Atherectomy
 see Extirpation, Heart and Great
  Vessels 02C
 see Extirpation, Upper Arteries 03C
 see Extirpation, Lower Arteries 04C
Atlantoaxial joint
 use Joint, Cervical Vertebral
Atmospheric Control 6A0Z
Atrioseptoplasty
 see Repair, Heart and Great Vessels
  02Q
 see Replacement, Heart and Great
  Vessels 02R
 see Supplement, Heart and Great
  Vessels 02U
Atrioventricular node
 use Conduction Mechanism
Atrium dextrum cordis
 use Atrium, Right
Atrium pulmonale
 use Atrium, Left
Attain Ability® lead
 use Cardiac Lead, Pacemaker in 02H
 use Cardiac Lead, Defibrillator in
  02H
Attain StarFix® (OTW) lead
 use Cardiac Lead, Defibrillator in
  02H
 use Cardiac Lead, Pacemaker in 02H
Audiology, diagnostic
 see Hearing Assessment, Diagnostic
  Audiology F13
 see Hearing Aid Assessment,
  Diagnostic Audiology F14
 see Vestibular Assessment,
  Diagnostic Audiology F15
Audiometry
 see Hearing Assessment, Diagnostic
  Audiology F13
Auditory tube
 use Eustachian Tube, Left
 use Eustachian Tube, Right
Auerbach's (myenteric) plexus
 use Nerve, Abdominal Sympathetic
Auricle
 use Ear, External, Bilateral
 use Ear, External, Left
 use Ear, External, Right
Auricularis muscle
 use Muscle, Head
Autograft
 use Autologous Tissue Substitute
Autologous artery graft
 use Autologous Arterial Tissue in
  Heart and Great Vessels
 use Autologous Arterial Tissue in
  Lower Arteries

Autologous artery graft *(continued)*
 use Autologous Arterial Tissue in
  Lower Veins
 use Autologous Arterial Tissue in
  Upper Arteries
 use Autologous Arterial Tissue in
  Upper Veins
Autologous vein graft
 use Autologous Venous Tissue in
  Heart and Great Vessels
 use Autologous Venous Tissue in
  Lower Arteries
 use Autologous Venous Tissue in
  Lower Veins
 use Autologous Venous Tissue in
  Upper Arteries
 use Autologous Venous Tissue in
  Upper Veins
Autotransfusion
 see Transfusion
Autotransplant
 Adrenal tissue
  see Reposition, Endocrine
   System 0GS
 Kidney
  see Reposition, Urinary System
   0TS
 Pancreatic tissue
  see Reposition, Pancreas 0FSG
 Parathyroid tissue
  see Reposition, Endocrine
   System 0GS
 Thyroid tissue
  see Reposition, Endocrine
   System 0GS
 Tooth
  see Reattachment, Mouth and
   Throat 0CM
Avulsion
 see Extraction
**Axial Lumbar Interbody Fusion
 System**
 use Interbody Fusion Device in
  Lower Joints
AxiaLIF® System
 use Interbody Fusion Device in
  Lower Joints
Axillary fascia
 use Subcutaneous Tissue and Fascia,
  Upper Arm, Left
 use Subcutaneous Tissue and Fascia,
  Upper Arm, Right
Axillary nerve
 use Nerve, Brachial Plexus

B

**BAK/C® Interbody Cervical Fusion
 System**
 use Interbody Fusion Device in
  Upper Joints
**BAL (bronchial alveolar lavage),
 diagnostic**
 see Drainage, Respiratory System
  0B9
Balanoplasty
 see Repair, Penis 0VQS
 see Supplement, Penis 0VUS
Balloon Pump
 Continuous, Output 5A02210
 Intermittent, Output 5A02110
Bandage, Elastic
 see Compression
Banding
 see Occlusion
 see Restriction
Bard® Composix® (E/X)(LP) mesh
 use Synthetic Substitute
Bard® Composix® Kugel® patch
 use Synthetic Substitute
Bard® Dulex™ mesh
 use Synthetic Substitute

Bard® Ventralex™ hernia patch
 use Synthetic Substitute
Barium swallow
 see Fluoroscopy, Gastrointestinal
  System BD1
**Baroreflex Activation Therapy®
 (BAT®)**
 Stimulator Generator in
  Subcutaneous Tissue and Fascia
 use Stimulator Lead in Upper
  Arteries
Bartholin's (greater vestibular) gland
 use Gland, Vestibular
Basal (internal) cerebral vein
 use Vein, Intracranial
Basal metabolic rate (BMR)
 see Measurement, Physiological
  Systems 4A0Z
Basal nuclei
 use Basal Ganglia
Basilar artery
 use Artery, Intracranial
Basis pontis
 use Pons
Beam Radiation
 Abdomen DW03
  Intraoperative DW033Z0
 Adrenal Gland DG02
  Intraoperative DG023Z0
 Bile Ducts DF02
  Intraoperative DF023Z0
 Bladder DT02
  Intraoperative DT023Z0
 Bone
  Intraoperative DP0C3Z0
  Other DP0C
 Bone Marrow D700
  Intraoperative D7003Z0
 Brain D000
  Intraoperative D0003Z0
 Brain Stem D001
  Intraoperative D0013Z0
 Breast
  Left DM00
   Intraoperative DM003Z0
  Right DM01
   Intraoperative DM013Z0
 Bronchus DB01
  Intraoperative DB013Z0
 Cervix DU01
  Intraoperative DU013Z0
 Chest DW02
  Intraoperative DW023Z0
 Chest Wall DB07
  Intraoperative DB073Z0
 Colon DD05
  Intraoperative DD053Z0
 Diaphragm DB08
  Intraoperative DB083Z0
 Duodenum DD02
  Intraoperative DD023Z0
 Ear D900
  Intraoperative D9003Z0
 Esophagus DD00
  Intraoperative DD003Z0
 Eye D800
  Intraoperative D8003Z0
 Femur DP09
  Intraoperative DP093Z0
 Fibula DP0B
  Intraoperative DP0B3Z0
 Gallbladder DF01
  Intraoperative DF013Z0
 Gland
  Adrenal DG02
   Intraoperative DG023Z0
  Parathyroid DG04
   Intraoperative DG043Z0
  Pituitary DG00
   Intraoperative DG003Z0
  Thyroid DG05
   Intraoperative DG053Z0

Beam Radiation (*continued*)
  Glands
    Intraoperative D9063Z0
    Salivary D906
  Head and Neck DW01
    Intraoperative DW013Z0
  Hemibody DW04
    Intraoperative DW043Z0
  Humerus DP06
    Intraoperative DP063Z0
  Hypopharynx D903
    Intraoperative D9033Z0
  Ileum DD04
    Intraoperative DD043Z0
  Jejunum DD03
    Intraoperative DD033Z0
  Kidney DT00
    Intraoperative DT003Z0
  Larynx D90B
    Intraoperative D90B3Z0
  Liver DF00
    Intraoperative DF003Z0
  Lung DB02
    Intraoperative DB023Z0
  Lymphatics
    Abdomen D706
      Intraoperative D7063Z0
    Axillary D704
      Intraoperative D7043Z0
    Inguinal D708
      Intraoperative D7083Z0
    Neck D703
      Intraoperative D7033Z0
    Pelvis D707
      Intraoperative D7073Z0
    Thorax D705
      Intraoperative D7053Z0
  Mandible DP03
    Intraoperative DP033Z0
  Maxilla DP02
    Intraoperative DP023Z0
  Mediastinum DB06
    Intraoperative DB063Z0
  Mouth D904
    Intraoperative D9043Z0
  Nasopharynx D90D
    Intraoperative D90D3Z0
  Neck and Head DW01
    Intraoperative DW013Z0
  Nerve
    Intraoperative D0073Z0
    Peripheral D007
  Nose D901
    Intraoperative D9013Z0
  Oropharynx D90F
    Intraoperative D90F3Z0
  Ovary DU00
    Intraoperative DU003Z0
  Palate
    Hard D908
      Intraoperative D9083Z0
    Soft D909
      Intraoperative D9093Z0
  Pancreas DF03
    Intraoperative DF033Z0
  Parathyroid Gland DG04
    Intraoperative DG043Z0
  Pelvic Bones DP08
    Intraoperative DP083Z0
  Pelvic Region DW06
    Intraoperative
      DW063Z0
  Pineal Body DG01
    Intraoperative DG013Z0
  Pituitary Gland DG00
    Intraoperative DG003Z0
  Pleura DB05
    Intraoperative DB053Z0
  Prostate DV00
    Intraoperative DV003Z0
  Radius DP07
    Intraoperative DP073Z0

Beam Radiation (*continued*)
  Rectum DD07
    Intraoperative DD073Z0
  Rib DP05
    Intraoperative DP053Z0
  Sinuses D907
    Intraoperative D9073Z0
  Skin
    Abdomen DH08
      Intraoperative DH083Z0
    Arm DH04
      Intraoperative DH043Z0
    Back DH07
      Intraoperative DH073Z0
    Buttock DH09
      Intraoperative DH093Z0
    Chest DH06
      Intraoperative DH063Z0
    Face DH02
      Intraoperative DH023Z0
    Leg DH0B
      Intraoperative DH0B3Z0
    Neck DH03
      Intraoperative DH033Z0
  Skull DP00
    Intraoperative DP003Z0
  Spinal Cord D006
    Intraoperative D0063Z0
  Spleen D702
    Intraoperative D7023Z0
  Sternum DP04
    Intraoperative DP043Z0
  Stomach DD01
    Intraoperative DD013Z0
  Testis DV01
    Intraoperative DV013Z0
  Thymus D701
    Intraoperative D7013Z0
  Thyroid Gland DG05
    Intraoperative DG053Z0
  Tibia DP0B
    Intraoperative DP0B3Z0
  Tongue D905
    Intraoperative D9053Z0
  Trachea DB00
    Intraoperative DB003Z0
  Ulna DP07
    Intraoperative DP073Z0
  Ureter DT01
    Intraoperative DT013Z0
  Urethra DT03
    Intraoperative DT033Z0
  Uterus DU02
    Intraoperative DU023Z0
  Whole Body DW05
    Intraoperative DW053Z0
Bedside swallow F00ZJWZ
Berlin Heart Ventricular Assist Device
  use Implantable Heart Assist System in Heart and Great Vessels
Biceps brachii muscle
  use Muscle, Upper Arm, Left
  use Muscle, Upper Arm, Right
Biceps femoris muscle
  use Muscle, Upper Leg, Left
  use Muscle, Upper Leg, Right
Bicipital aponeurosis
  use Subcutaneous Tissue and Fascia, Lower Arm, Left
  use Subcutaneous Tissue and Fascia, Lower Arm, Right
Bicuspid valve
  use Valve, Mitral
Bililite therapy
  see Ultraviolet Light Therapy, Skin 6A80
Bioactive embolization coil(s)
  use Intraluminal Device, Bioactive in Upper Arteries
Biofeedback GZC9ZZZ

Biopsy
  see Drainage with qualifier Diagnostic
  see Excision with qualifier Diagnostic
  Bone Marrow
    see Extraction with qualifier Diagnostic
BiPAP
  see Assistance, Respiratory v5A09
Bisection
  see Division
Biventricular external heart assist system
  use External Heart Assist System in Heart and Great Vessels
Blepharectomy
  see Excision, Eye 08B
  see Resection, Eye 08T
Blepharoplasty
  see Repair, Eye 08Q
  see Replacement, Eye 08R
  see Reposition, Eye 08S
  see Supplement, Eye 08U
Blepharorrhaphy
  see Repair, Eye 08Q
Blepharotomy
  see Drainage, Eye 089
Blinatumomab Antineoplastic Immunotherapy XW0
Block, Nerve, anesthetic injection 3E0T3CZ
Blood glucose monitoring system
  use Monitoring Device
Blood pressure
  see Measurement, Arterial 4A03
BMR (basal metabolic rate)
  see Measurement, Physiological Systems 4A0Z
Body of femur
  use Femoral Shaft, Left
  use Femoral Shaft, Right
Body of fibula
  use Fibula, Left
  use Fibula, Right
Bone anchored hearing device
  use Hearing Device, Bone Conduction in 09H
  use Hearing Device in Head and Facial Bones
Bone bank bone graft
  use Nonautologous Tissue Substitute
Bone Growth Stimulator
  Insertion of device in
  Bone
    Facial 0NHW
    Lower 0QHY
    Nasal 0NHB
    Upper 0PHY
    Skull 0NH0
  Removal of device from
  Bone
    Facial 0NPW
    Lower 0QPY
    Nasal 0NPB
    Upper 0PPY
    Skull 0NP0
  Revision of device in
  Bone
    Facial 0NWW
    Lower 0QWY
    Nasal 0NWB
    Upper 0PWY
    Skull 0NW0
Bone marrow transplant
  see Transfusion
Bone morphogenetic protein 2 (BMP 2)
  use Recombinant Bone Morphogenetic Protein
Bone screw (interlocking)(lag) (pedicle)(recessed)
  use Internal Fixation Device in Head and Facial Bones

Bone screw (*continued*)
  use Internal Fixation Device in Lower Bones
  use Internal Fixation Device in Upper Bones
Bony labyrinth
  use Ear, Inner, Left
  use Ear, Inner, Right
Bony orbit
  use Orbit, Left
  use Orbit, Right
Bony vestibule
  use Ear, Inner, Left
  use Ear, Inner, Right
Botallo's duct
  use Artery, Pulmonary, Left
Bovine pericardial valve
  use Zooplastic Tissue in Heart and Great Vessels
Bovine pericardium graft
  use Zooplastic Tissue in Heart and Great Vessels
BP (blood pressure)
  see Measurement, Arterial 4A03
Brachial (lateral) lymph node
  use Lymphatic, Axillary, Left
  use Lymphatic, Axillary, Right
Brachialis muscle
  use Muscle, Upper Arm, Left
  use Muscle, Upper Arm, Right
Brachiocephalic artery
  use Artery, Innominate
Brachiocephalic trunk
  use Artery, Innominate
Brachiocephalic vein
  use Vein, Innominate, Left
  use Vein, Innominate, Right
Brachioradialis muscle
  use Muscle, Lower Arm and Wrist, Left
  use Muscle, Lower Arm and Wrist, Right
Brachytherapy
  Abdomen DW13
  Adrenal Gland DG12
  Bile Ducts DF12
  Bladder DT12
  Bone Marrow D710
  Brain D010
  Brain Stem D011
  Breast
    Left DM10
    Right DM11
  Bronchus DB11
  Cervix DU11
  Chest DW12
  Chest Wall DB17
  Colon DD15
  Diaphragm DB18
  Duodenum DD12
  Ear D910
  Esophagus DD10
  Eye D810
  Gallbladder DF11
  Gland
    Adrenal DG12
    Parathyroid DG14
    Pituitary DG10
    Thyroid DG15
  Glands, Salivary D916
  Head and Neck DW11
  Hypopharynx D913
  Ileum DD14
  Jejunum DD13
  Kidney DT10
  Larynx D91B
  Liver DF10
  Lung DB12
  Lymphatics
    Abdomen D716
    Axillary D714
    Inguinal D718

Brachytherapy *(continued)*
　Lymphatics *(continued)*
　　Neck D713
　　Pelvis D717
　　Thorax D715
　Mediastinum DB16
　Mouth D914
　Nasopharynx D91D
　Neck and Head DW11
　Nerve, Peripheral D017
　Nose D911
　Oropharynx D91F
　Ovary DU10
　Palate
　　Hard D918
　　Soft D919
　Pancreas DF13
　Parathyroid Gland DG14
　Pelvic Region DW16
　Pineal Body DG11
　Pituitary Gland DG10
　Pleura DB15
　Prostate DV10
　Rectum DD17
　Sinuses D917
　Spinal Cord D016
　Spleen D712
　Stomach DD11
　Testis DV11
　Thymus D711
　Thyroid Gland DG15
　Tongue D915
　Trachea DB10
　Ureter DT11
　Urethra DT13
　Uterus DU12
Brachytherapy seeds
　use Radioactive Element
Broad ligament
　use Uterine Supporting Structure
Bronchial artery
　use Aorta, Thoracic
Bronchography
　see Fluoroscopy, Respiratory
　　System BB1
　see Plain Radiography, Respiratory
　　System BB0
Bronchoplasty
　see Repair, Respiratory System 0BQ
　see Supplement, Respiratory System
　　0BU
Bronchorrhaphy
　see Repair, Respiratory System 0BQ
Bronchoscopy 0BJ08ZZ
Bronchotomy
　see Drainage, Respiratory System
　　0B9
BRYAN® Cervical Disc System
　use Synthetic Substitute
Buccal gland
　use Buccal Mucosa
Buccinator lymph node
　use Lymphatic, Head
Buccinator muscle
　use Muscle, Facial
Buckling, scleral with implant
　see Supplement, Eye 08U
Bulbospongiosus muscle
　use Muscle, Perineum
Bulbourethral (Cowper's) gland
　use Urethra
Bundle of His
　use Conduction Mechanism
Bundle of Kent
　use Conduction Mechanism
Bunionectomy
　see Excision, Lower Bones 0QB
Bursectomy
　see Excision, Bursae and Ligaments
　　0MB
　see Resection, Bursae and
　　Ligaments 0MT

Bursocentesis
　see Drainage, Bursae and Ligaments
　　0M9
Bursography
　see Plain Radiography, Non-Axial
　　Upper Bones BP0
　see Plain Radiography, Non-Axial
　　Lower Bones BQ0
Bursotomy
　see Division, Bursae and Ligaments
　　0M8
　see Drainage, Bursae and Ligaments
　　0M9
BVS 5000 Ventricular Assist Device
　use External Heart Assist
　　System in Heart and Great
　　Vessels
Bypass
　Anterior Chamber
　　Left 08133
　　Right 08123
　Aorta
　　Abdominal 0410
　　Thoracic 021W
　Artery
　　Axillary
　　　Left 03160
　　　Right 03150
　　Brachial
　　　Left 03180
　　　Right 03170
　　Common Carotid
　　　Left 031J0
　　　Right 031H0
　　Common Iliac
　　　Left 041D
　　　Right 041C
　　Coronary
　　　Four or More Sites 0213
　　　One Site 0210
　　　Three Sites 0212
　　　Two Sites 0211
　　External Carotid
　　　Left 031N0
　　　Right 031M0
　　External Iliac
　　　Left 041J
　　　Right 041H
　　Femoral
　　　Left 041L
　　　Right 041K
　　Innominate 03120
　　Internal Carotid
　　　Left 031L0
　　　Right 031K0
　　Internal Iliac
　　　Left 041F
　　　Right 041E
　　Intracranial 031G0
　　Popliteal
　　　Left 041N
　　　Right 041M
　　Radial
　　　Left 031C0
　　　Right 031B0
　　Splenic 0414
　　Subclavian
　　　Left 03140
　　　Right 03130
　　Temporal
　　　Left 031T0
　　　Right 031S0
　　Ulnar
　　　Left 031A0
　　　Right 03190
　Atrium
　　Left 0217
　　Right 0216
　Bladder 0T1B
　Cavity, Cranial 0W110J
　Cecum 0D1H
　Cerebral Ventricle 0016

Bypass *(continued)*
　Colon
　　Ascending 0D1K
　　Descending 0D1M
　　Sigmoid 0D1N
　　Transverse 0D1L
　Duct
　　Common Bile 0F19
　　Cystic 0F18
　　Hepatic
　　　Left 0F16
　　　Right 0F15
　　Lacrimal
　　　Left 081Y
　　　Right 081X
　　Pancreatic 0F1D
　　　Accessory 0F1F
　Duodenum 0D19
　Ear
　　Left 091E0
　　Right 091D0
　Esophagus 0D15
　　Lower 0D13
　　Middle 0D12
　　Upper 0D11
　Fallopian Tube
　　Left 0U16
　　Right 0U15
　Gallbladder 0F14
　Ileum 0D1B
　Jejunum 0D1A
　Kidney Pelvis
　　Left 0T14
　　Right 0T13
　Pancreas 0F1G
　Pelvic Cavity 0W1J
　Peritoneal Cavity 0W1G
　Pleural Cavity
　　Left 0W1B
　　Right 0W19
　Spinal Canal 001U
　Stomach 0D16
　Trachea 0B11
　Ureter
　　Left 0T17
　　Right 0T16
　Ureters, Bilateral 0T18
　Vas Deferens
　　Bilateral 0V1Q
　　Left 0V1P
　　Right 0V1N
　Vein
　　Axillary
　　　Left 0518
　　　Right 0517
　　Azygos 0510
　　Basilic
　　　Left 051C
　　　Right 051B
　　Brachial
　　　Left 051A
　　　Right 0519
　　Cephalic
　　　Left 051F
　　　Right 051D
　　Colic 0617
　　Common Iliac
　　　Left 061D
　　　Right 061C
　　Esophageal 0613
　　External Iliac
　　　Left 061G
　　　Right 061F
　　External Jugular
　　　Left 051Q
　　　Right 051P
　　Face
　　　Left 051V
　　　Right 051T
　　Femoral
　　　Left 061N
　　　Right 061M

Bypass *(continued)*
　Vein *(continued)*
　　Foot
　　　Left 061V
　　　Right 061T
　　Gastric 0612
　　Greater Saphenous
　　　Left 061Q
　　　Right 061P
　　Hand
　　　Left 051H
　　　Right 051G
　　Hemiazygos 0511
　　Hepatic 0614
　　Hypogastric
　　　Left 061J
　　　Right 061H
　　Inferior Mesenteric 0616
　　Innominate
　　　Left 0514
　　　Right 0513
　　Internal Jugular
　　　Left 051N
　　　Right 051M
　　Intracranial 051L
　　Lesser Saphenous
　　　Left 061S
　　　Right 061R
　　Portal 0618
　　Renal
　　　Left 061B
　　　Right 0619
　　Splenic 0611
　　Subclavian
　　　Left 0516
　　　Right 0515
　　Superior Mesenteric 0615
　　Vertebral
　　　Left 051S
　　　Right 051R
　　Vena Cava
　　　Inferior 0610
　　　Superior 021V
　　Ventricle
　　　Left 021L
　　　Right 021K
Bypass, cardiopulmonary 5A1221Z

C

Caesarean section
　see Extraction, Products of Conception
　　10D0
Calcaneocuboid joint
　use Joint, Tarsal, Left
　use Joint, Tarsal, Right
Calcaneocuboid ligament
　use Bursa and Ligament, Foot, Left
　use Bursa and Ligament, Foot,
　　Right
Calcaneofibular ligament
　use Bursa and Ligament, Ankle,
　　Left
　use Bursa and Ligament, Ankle,
　　Right
Calcaneus
　use Tarsal, Left
　use Tarsal, Right
Cannulation
　see Bypass
　see Dilation
　see Drainage
　see Irrigation
Canthorrhaphy
　see Repair, Eye 08Q
Canthotomy
　see Release, Eye 08N
Capitate bone
　use Carpal, Left
　use Carpal, Right
Capsulectomy, lens
　see Excision, Eye 08B

Capsulorrhaphy, joint
  see Repair, Lower Joints 0SQ
  see Repair, Upper Joints 0RQ
Cardia
  use Esophagogastric Junction
Cardiac contractility modulation lead
  use Cardiac Lead in Heart and Great
    Vessels
Cardiac event recorder
  use Monitoring Device
Cardiac Lead
  Defibrillator
    Atrium
      Left 02H7
      Right 02H6
    Pericardium 02HN
    Vein, Coronary 02H4
    Ventricle
      Left 02HL
      Right 02HK
  Insertion of device in
    Atrium
      Left 02H7Z
      Right 02H6
    Pericardium 02HN
    Vein, Coronary 02H4
    Ventricle
      Left 02HL
      Right 02HK
  Pacemaker
    Atrium
      Left 02H7
      Right 02H6
    Pericardium 02HN
    Vein, Coronary 02H4
    Ventricle
      Left 02HL
      Right 02HK
  Removal of device from, Heart
    02PA
  Revision of device in, Heart 02WA
Cardiac plexus
  use Nerve, Thoracic Sympathetic
Cardiac Resynchronization
  Defibrillator Pulse Generator
  Abdomen 0JH8
  Chest 0JH6
Cardiac Resynchronization
  Pacemaker Pulse Generator
  Abdomen 0JH8
  Chest 0JH6
Cardiac resynchronization therapy
  (CRT) lead
  use Cardiac Lead, Defibrillator in
    02H
  use Cardiac Lead, Pacemaker in 02H
Cardiac Rhythm Related Device
  Insertion of device in
    Abdomen 0JH8
    Chest 0JH6
  Removal of device from,
    Subcutaneous Tissue and Fascia,
    Trunk 0JPT
  Revision of device in, Subcutaneous
    Tissue and Fascia, Trunk 0JWT
Cardiocentesis
  see Drainage, Pericardial Cavity
    0W9D
Cardioesophageal junction
  use Esophagogastric Junction
Cardiolysis
  see Release, Heart and Great Vessels
    02N
CardioMEMS® pressure sensor
  use Monitoring Device, Pressure
    Sensor in 02H
Cardiomyotomy
  see Division, Esophagogastric
    Junction 0D84
Cardioplegia
  see Introduction of substance in or
    on, Heart 3E08

Cardiorrhaphy
  see Repair, Heart and Great Vessels
    02Q
Cardioversion 5A2204Z
Caregiver Training F0FZ
Caroticotympanic artery
  use Artery, Internal Carotid, Left
  use Artery, Internal Carotid, Right
Carotid (artery) sinus (baroreceptor)
  lead
  use Stimulator Lead in Upper
    Arteries
Carotid glomus
  use Carotid Bodies, Bilateral
  use Carotid Body, Left
  use Carotid Body, Right
Carotid sinus
  use Artery, Internal Carotid, Left
  use Artery, Internal Carotid, Right
Carotid sinus nerve
  use Nerve, Glossopharyngeal
Carotid WALLSTENT® Monorail®
  Endoprosthesis
  use Intraluminal Device
Carpectomy
  see Excision, Upper Bones 0PB
  see Resection, Upper Bones 0PT
Carpometacarpal (CMC) joint
  use Joint, Metacarpocarpal, Left
  use Joint, Metacarpocarpal, Right
Carpometacarpal ligament
  use Bursa and Ligament, Hand, Left
  use Bursa and Ligament, Hand,
    Right
Casting
  see Immobilization
CAT scan
  see Computerized Tomography (CT
    Scan)
Catheterization
  see Dilation
  see Drainage
  Heart
    see Measurement, Cardiac 4A02
  see Irrigation
  see Insertion of device in
  Umbilical vein, for infusion
    06H033T
Cauda equina
  use Spinal Cord, Lumbar
Cauterization
  see Destruction
  see Repair
Cavernous plexus
  use Nerve, Head and Neck
    Sympathetic
Cecectomy
  see Excision, Cecum 0DBH
  see Resection, Cecum 0DTH
Cecocolostomy
  see Bypass, Gastrointestinal System
    0D1
  see Drainage, Gastrointestinal
    System 0D9
Cecopexy
  see Repair, Cecum 0DQH
  see Reposition, Cecum 0DSH
Cecoplication
  see Restriction, Cecum 0DVH
Cecorrhaphy
  see Repair, Cecum 0DQH
Cecostomy
  see Bypass, Cecum 0D1H
  see Drainage, Cecum 0D9H
Cecotomy
  see Drainage, Cecum 0D9H
Ceftazidime-Avibactam Anti-infective
  XW0
Celiac (solar) plexus
  use Nerve, Abdominal Sympathetic
Celiac ganglion
  use Nerve, Abdominal Sympathetic

Celiac lymph node
  use Lymphatic, Aortic
Celiac trunk
  use Artery, Celiac
Central axillary lymph node
  use Lymphatic, Axillary, Left
  use Lymphatic, Axillary, Right
Central venous pressure
  see Measurement, Venous 4A04
Centrimag® Blood Pump
  use External Heart Assist System in
    Heart and Great Vessels
Cephalogram BN00ZZZ
Cerclage
  see Restriction
Cerebral aqueduct (Sylvius)
  use Cerebral Ventricle
Cerebrum
  use Brain
Cervical esophagus
  use Esophagus, Upper
Cervical facet joint
  use Joint, Cervical Vertebral
  use Joint, Cervical Vertebral, 2 or
    more
Cervical ganglion
  use Nerve, Head and Neck
    Sympathetic
Cervical interspinous ligament
  use Bursa and Ligament, Head and
    Neck
Cervical intertransverse ligament
  use Bursa and Ligament, Head and
    Neck
Cervical ligamentum flavum
  use Bursa and Ligament, Head and
    Neck
Cervical lymph node
  use Lymphatic, Neck, Left
  use Lymphatic, Neck, Right
Cervicectomy
  see Excision, Cervix 0UBC
  see Resection, Cervix 0UTC
Cervicothoracic facet joint
  use Joint, Cervicothoracic
    Vertebral
Cesarean section
  see Extraction, Products of
    Conception 10D0
Change device in
  Abdominal Wall 0W2FX
  Back
    Lower 0W2LX
    Upper 0W2KX
  Bladder 0T2BX
  Bone
    Facial 0N2WX
    Lower 0Q2YX
    Nasal 0N2BX
    Upper 0P2YX
  Bone Marrow 072TX
  Brain 0020X
  Breast
    Left 0H2UX
    Right 0H2TX
  Bursa and Ligament
    Lower 0M2YX
    Upper 0M2XX
  Cavity, Cranial 0W21X
  Chest Wall 0W28X
  Cisterna Chyli 072LX
  Diaphragm 0B2TX
  Duct
    Hepatobiliary 0F2BX
    Pancreatic 0F2DX
  Ear
    Left 092JX
    Right 092HX
  Epididymis and Spermatic Cord
    0V2MX
  Extremity
    Lower

Change device in *(continued)*
  Extremity *(continued)*
    Lower *(continued)*
      Left 0Y2BX
      Right 0Y29X
    Upper
      Left 0X27X
      Right 0X26X
  Eye
    Left 0821X
    Right 0820X
  Face 0W22X
  Fallopian Tube 0U28X
  Gallbladder 0F24X
  Gland
    Adrenal 0G25X
    Endocrine 0G2SX
    Pituitary 0G20X
    Salivary 0C2AX
  Head 0W20X
  Intestinal Tract
    Lower 0D2DXUZ
    Upper 0D20XUZ
  Jaw
    Lower 0W25X
    Upper 0W24X
  Joint
    Lower 0S2YX
    Upper 0R2YX
  Kidney 0T25X
  Larynx 0C2SX
  Liver 0F20X
  Lung
    Left 0B2LX
    Right 0B2KX
  Lymphatic 072NX
    Thoracic Duct 072KX
  Mediastinum 0W2CX
  Mesentery 0D2VX
  Mouth and Throat 0C2YX
  Muscle
    Lower 0K2YX
    Upper 0K2XX
  Neck 0W26X
  Nerve
    Cranial 002EX
    Peripheral 012YX
  Nose 092KX
  Omentum 0D2UX
  Ovary 0U23X
  Pancreas 0F2GX
  Parathyroid Gland 0G2RX
  Pelvic Cavity 0W2JX
  Penis 0V2SX
  Pericardial Cavity 0W2DX
  Perineum
    Female 0W2NX
    Male 0W2MX
  Peritoneal Cavity 0W2GX
  Peritoneum 0D2WX
  Pineal Body 0G21X
  Pleura 0B2QX
  Pleural Cavity
    Left 0W2BX
    Right 0W29X
  Products of Conception 10207
  Prostate and Seminal Vesicles
    0V24X
  Retroperitoneum 0W2HX
  Scrotum and Tunica Vaginalis
    0V28X
  Sinus 092YX
  Skin 0H2PX
  Skull 0N20X
  Spinal Canal 002UX
  Spleen 072PX
  Subcutaneous Tissue and
    Fascia
    Head and Neck 0J2SX
    Lower Extremity 0J2WX
    Trunk 0J2TX
    Upper Extremity 0J2VX

Change device in (continued)
Tendon
Lower 0L2YX
Upper 0L2XX
Testis 0V2DX
Thymus 072MX
Thyroid Gland 0G2KX
Trachea 0B21
Tracheobronchial Tree 0B20X
Ureter 0T29X
Urethra 0T2DX
Uterus and Cervix 0U2DXHZ
Vagina and Cul-de-sac 0U2HXGZ
Vas Deferens 0V2RX
Vulva 0U2MX
Change device in or on
Abdominal Wall 2W03X
Anorectal 2Y03X5Z
Arm
Lower
Left 2W0DX
Right 2W0CX
Upper
Left 2W0BX
Right 2W0AX
Back 2W05X
Chest Wall 2W04X
Ear 2Y02X5Z
Extremity
Lower
Left 2W0MX
Right 2W0LX
Upper
Left 2W09X
Right 2W08X
Face 2W01X
Finger
Left 2W0KX
Right 2W0JX
Foot
Left 2W0TX
Right 2W0SX
Genital Tract, Female 2Y04X5Z
Hand
Left 2W0FX
Right 2W0EX
Head 2W00X
Inguinal Region
Left 2W07X
Right 2W06X
Leg
Lower
Left 2W0RX
Right 2W0QX
Upper
Left 2W0PX
Right 2W0NX
Mouth and Pharynx 2Y00X5Z
Nasal 2Y01X5Z
Neck 2W02X
Thumb
Left 2W0HX
Right 2W0GX
Toe
Left 2W0VX
Right 2W0UX
Urethra 2Y05X5Z
Chemoembolization
see Introduction of substance in
or on
Chemosurgery, Skin 3E00XTZ
Chemothalamectomy
see Destruction, Thalamus 0059
Chemotherapy, Infusion for cancer
see Introduction of substance in
or on
Chest x-ray
see Plain Radiography, Chest
BW03
Chiropractic Manipulation
Abdomen 9WB9X
Cervical 9WB1X

Chiropractic Manipulation (continued)
Extremities
Lower 9WB6X
Upper 9WB7X
Head 9WB0X
Lumbar 9WB3X
Pelvis 9WB5X
Rib Cage 9WB8X
Sacrum 9WB4X
Thoracic 9WB2X
Choana
use Nasopharynx
Cholangiogram
see Plain Radiography,
Hepatobiliary System and
Pancreas BF0
see Fluoroscopy, Hepatobiliary
System and Pancreas BF1
Cholecystectomy
see Excision, Gallbladder 0FB4
see Resection, Gallbladder 0FT4
Cholecystojejunostomy
see Bypass, Hepatobiliary System
and Pancreas 0F1
see Drainage, Hepatobiliary System
and Pancreas 0F9
Cholecystopexy
see Repair, Gallbladder 0FQ4
see Reposition, Gallbladder 0FS4
Cholecystoscopy 0FJ44ZZ
Cholecystostomy
see Drainage, Gallbladder 0F94
see Bypass, Gallbladder 0F14
Cholecystotomy
see Drainage, Gallbladder 0F94
Choledochectomy
see Excision, Hepatobiliary System
and Pancreas 0FB
see Resection, Hepatobiliary System
and Pancreas 0FT
Choledocholithotomy
see Extirpation, Duct, Common Bile
0FC9
Choledochoplasty
see Repair, Hepatobiliary System
and Pancreas 0FQ
see Replacement, Hepatobiliary
System and Pancreas 0FR
see Supplement, Hepatobiliary
System and Pancreas 0FU
Choledochoscopy 0FJB8ZZ
Choledochotomy
see Drainage, Hepatobiliary System
and Pancreas 0F9
Cholelithotomy
see Extirpation, Hepatobiliary
System and Pancreas 0FC
Chondrectomy
see Excision, Lower Joints 0SB
see Excision, Upper Joints 0RB
Knee
see Excision, Lower Joints 0SB
Semilunar cartilage
see Excision, Lower Joints 0SB
Chondroglossus muscle
use Muscle, Tongue, Palate, Pharynx
Chorda tympani
use Nerve, Facial
Chordotomy
see Division, Central Nervous
System 008
Choroid plexus
use Cerebral Ventricle
Choroidectomy
see Excision, Eye 08B
see Resection, Eye 08T
Ciliary body
use Eye, Left
use Eye, Right
Ciliary ganglion
use Nerve, Head and Neck
Sympathetic

Circle of Willis
use Artery, Intracranial
Circumcision 0VTTXZZ
Circumflex iliac artery
use Artery, Femoral, Left
use Artery, Femoral, Right
**Clamp and rod internal fixation
system (CRIF)**
use Internal Fixation Device in
Lower Bones
use Internal Fixation Device in Upper
Bones
Clamping
see Occlusion
Claustrum
use Basal Ganglia
Claviculectomy
see Excision, Upper Bones 0PB
see Resection, Upper Bones
0PT
Claviculotomy
see Division, Upper Bones 0P8
see Drainage, Upper Bones 0P9
Clipping, aneurysm
see Restriction using Extraluminal
Device
Clitorectomy, clitoridectomy
see Excision, Clitoris 0UBJ
see Resection, Clitoris 0UTJ
Clolar
use Clofarabine
Closure
see Occlusion
see Repair
Clysis
see Introduction of substance in
or on
Coagulation
see Destruction
CoAxia NeuroFlo catheter
use Intraluminal Device
**Cobalt/chromium head and
polyethylene socket**
use Synthetic Substitute, Metal on
Polyethylene in 0SR
Cobalt/chromium head and socket
use Synthetic Substitute, Metal in
0SR
Coccygeal body
use Coccygeal Glomus
Coccygeus muscle
use Muscle, Trunk, Left
use Muscle, Trunk, Right
Cochlea
use Ear, Inner, Left
use Ear, Inner, Right
**Cochlear implant (CI), multiple
channel (electrode)**
use Hearing Device, Multiple
Channel Cochlear Prosthesis
in 09H
**Cochlear implant (CI), single channel
(electrode)**
use Hearing Device, Single Channel
Cochlear Prosthesis in 09H
Cochlear Implant Treatment
F0BZ0
Cochlear nerve
use Nerve, Acoustic
COGNIS® CRT-D
use Cardiac Resynchronization
Defibrillator Pulse Generator
in 0JH
Colectomy
see Excision, Gastrointestinal System
0DB
see Resection, Gastrointestinal
System 0DT
Collapse
see Occlusion
Collection from
Breast, Breast Milk 8E0HX62

Collection from (continued)
Indwelling Device
Circulatory System
Blood 8C02X6K
Other Fluid 8C02X6L
Nervous System
Cerebrospinal Fluid
8C01X6J
Other Fluid 8C01X6L
Integumentary System, Breast Milk
8E0HX62
Reproductive System, Male, Sperm
8E0VX63
Colocentesis
see Drainage, Gastrointestinal
System 0D9
Colofixation
see Repair, Gastrointestinal System
0DQ
see Reposition, Gastrointestinal
System 0DS
Cololysis
see Release, Gastrointestinal System
0DN
Colonic Z-Stent®
use Intraluminal Device
Colonoscopy 0DJD8ZZ
Colopexy
see Repair, Gastrointestinal System
0DQ
see Reposition, Gastrointestinal
System 0DS
Coloplication
see Restriction, Gastrointestinal
System 0DV
Coloproctectomy
see Excision, Gastrointestinal
System 0DB
see Resection, Gastrointestinal
System 0DT
Coloproctostomy
see Bypass, Gastrointestinal System
0D1
see Drainage, Gastrointestinal
System 0D9
Colopuncture
see Drainage, Gastrointestinal
System 0D9
Colorrhaphy
see Repair, Gastrointestinal System
0DQ
Colostomy
see Bypass, Gastrointestinal System
0D1
see Drainage, Gastrointestinal
System 0D9
Colpectomy
see Excision, Vagina 0UBG
see Resection, Vagina 0UTG
Colpocentesis
see Drainage, Vagina 0U9G
Colpopexy
see Repair, Vagina 0UQG
see Reposition, Vagina 0USG
Colpoplasty
see Repair, Vagina 0UQG
see Supplement, Vagina 0UUG
Colporrhaphy
see Repair, Vagina 0UQG
Colposcopy 0UJH8ZZ
Columella
use Nose
Common digital vein
use Vein, Foot, Left
use Vein, Foot, Right
Common facial vein
use Vein, Face, Left
use Vein, Face, Right
Common fibular nerve
use Nerve, Peroneal
Common hepatic artery
use Artery, Hepatic

Common iliac (subaortic) lymph node
use Lymphatic, Pelvis
Common interosseous artery
use Artery, Ulnar, Left
use Artery, Ulnar, Right
Common peroneal nerve
use Nerve, Peroneal
Complete (SE) stent
use Intraluminal Device
Compression
see Restriction
Abdominal Wall 2W13X
Arm
 Lower
  Left 2W1DX
  Right 2W1CX
 Upper
  Left 2W1BX
  Right 2W1AX
Back 2W15X
Chest Wall 2W14X
Extremity
 Lower
  Left 2W1MX
  Right 2W1LX
 Upper
  Left 2W19X
  Right 2W18X
Face 2W11X
Finger
 Left 2W1KX
 Right 2W1JX
Foot
 Left 2W1TX
 Right 2W1SX
Hand
 Left 2W1FX
 Right 2W1EX
Head 2W10X
Inguinal Region
 Left 2W17X
 Right 2W16X
Leg
 Lower
  Left 2W1RX
  Right 2W1QX
 Upper
  Left 2W1PX
  Right 2W1NX
Neck 2W12X
Thumb
 Left 2W1HX
 Right 2W1GX
Toe
 Left 2W1VX
 Right 2W1UX
Computer Assisted Procedure
Extremity
 Lower
  No Qualifier 8E0YXBZ
  With Computerized
   Tomography 8E0YXBG
  With Fluoroscopy 8E0YXBF
  With Magnetic Resonance
   Imaging 8E0YXBH
 Upper
  No Qualifier 8E0XXBZ
  With Computerized
   Tomography 8E0XXBG
  With Fluoroscopy 8E0XXBF
  With Magnetic Resonance
   Imaging 8E0XXBH
Head and Neck Region
 No Qualifier 8E09XBZ
 With Computerized Tomography
  8E09XBG
 With Fluoroscopy 8E09XBF
 With Magnetic Resonance
  Imaging 8E09XBH
Trunk Region
 No Qualifier 8E0WXBZ

Computer Assisted Procedure *(continued)*
Trunk Region *(continued)*
 With Computerized Tomography
  8E0WXBG
 With Fluoroscopy 8E0WXBF
 With Magnetic Resonance
  Imaging 8E0WXBH
Computerized Tomography (CT Scan)
Abdomen BW20
 Chest and Pelvis BW25
Abdomen and Chest BW24
Abdomen and Pelvis BW21
Airway, Trachea BB2F
Ankle
 Left BQ2H
 Right BQ2G
Aorta
 Abdominal B420
  Intravascular Optical
   Coherence B420Z2Z
 Thoracic B320
  Intravascular Optical
   Coherence B320Z2Z
Arm
 Left BP2F
 Right BP2E
Artery
 Celiac B421
  Intravascular Optical
   Coherence B421Z2Z
 Common Carotid
  Bilateral B325
  Intravascular Optical
   Coherence B325Z2Z
 Coronary
  Bypass Graft
   Multiple B223
   Intravascular Optical
    Coherence B223Z2Z
  Multiple B221
   Intravascular Optical
    Coherence B221Z2Z
 Internal Carotid
  Bilateral B328
  Intravascular Optical
   Coherence B328Z2Z
 Intracranial B32R
  Intravascular Optical
   Coherence B32RZ2Z
 Lower Extremity
  Bilateral B42H
   Intravascular Optical
    Coherence B42HZ2Z
  Left B42G
   Intravascular Optical
    Coherence B42GZ2Z
  Right B42F
   Intravascular Optical
    Coherence B42FZ2Z
 Pelvic B42C
  Intravascular Optical
   Coherence B42CZ2Z
 Pulmonary
  Left B32T
   Intravascular Optical
    Coherence B32TZ2Z
  Right B32S
   Intravascular Optical
    Coherence B32SZ2Z
 Renal
  Bilateral B428
   Intravascular Optical
    Coherence B428Z2Z
  Transplant B42M
   Intravascular Optical
    Coherence
    B42MZ2Z
 Superior Mesenteric B424
  Intravascular Optical
   Coherence B424Z2Z

Computerized Tomography (CT Scan) *(continued)*
Artery *(continued)*
 Vertebral
  Bilateral B32G
  Intravascular Optical
   Coherence
   B32GZ2Z
Bladder BT20
Bone
 Facial BN25
 Temporal BN2F
Brain B020
Calcaneus
 Left BQ2K
 Right BQ2J
Cerebral Ventricle B028
Chest, Abdomen and Pelvis
 BW25
Chest and Abdomen BW24
Cisterna B027
Clavicle
 Left BP25
 Right BP24
Coccyx BR2F
Colon BD24
Ear B920
Elbow
 Left BP2H
 Right BP2G
Extremity
 Lower
  Left BQ2S
  Right BQ2R
 Upper
  Bilateral BP2V
  Left BP2U
  Right BP2T
Eye
 Bilateral B827
 Left B826
 Right B825
Femur
 Left BQ24
 Right BQ23
Fibula
 Left BQ2C
 Right BQ2B
Finger
 Left BP2S
 Right BP2R
Foot
 Left BQ2M
 Right BQ2L
Forearm
 Left BP2K
 Right BP2J
Gland
 Adrenal, Bilateral BG22
 Parathyroid BG23
 Parotid, Bilateral B926
 Salivary, Bilateral B92D
 Submandibular, Bilateral
  B929
 Thyroid BG24
Hand
 Left BP2P
 Right BP2N
Hands and Wrists, Bilateral BP2Q
Head BW28
Head and Neck BW29
Heart
 Intravascular Optical Coherence
  B226Z2Z
 Right and Left B226
Hepatobiliary System, All BF2C
Hip
 Left BQ21
 Right BQ20
Humerus
 Left BP2B
 Right BP2A

Computerized Tomography (CT Scan) *(continued)*
Intracranial Sinus B522
 Intravascular Optical Coherence
  B522Z2Z
Joint
 Acromioclavicular, Bilateral
  BP23
 Finger
  Left BP2DZZZ
  Right BP2CZZZ
 Foot
  Left BQ2Y
  Right BQ2X
 Hand
  Left BP2DZZZ
  Right BP2CZZZ
 Sacroiliac BR2D
 Sternoclavicular
  Bilateral BP22
  Left BP21
  Right BP20
 Temporomandibular, Bilateral
  BN29
 Toe
  Left BQ2Y
  Right BQ2X
Kidney
 Bilateral BT23
 Left BT22
 Right BT21
 Transplant BT29
Knee
 Left BQ28
 Right BQ27
Larynx B92J
Leg
 Left BQ2F
 Right BQ2D
Liver BF25
Liver and Spleen BF26
Lung, Bilateral BB24
Mandible BN26
Nasopharynx B92F
Neck BW2F
Neck and Head BW29
Orbit, Bilateral BN23
Oropharynx B92F
Pancreas BF27
Patella
 Left BQ2W
 Right BQ2V
Pelvic Region BW2G
Pelvis BR2C
 Chest and Abdomen BW25
Pelvis and Abdomen BW21
Pituitary Gland B029
Prostate BV23
Ribs
 Left BP2Y
 Right BP2X
Sacrum BR2F
Scapula
 Left BP27
 Right BP26
Sella Turcica B029
Shoulder
 Left BP29
 Right BP28
Sinus
 Intracranial B522
  Intravascular Optical
   Coherence B522Z2Z
 Paranasal B922
Skull BN20
Spinal Cord B02B
Spine
 Cervical BR20
 Lumbar BR29
 Thoracic BR27
Spleen and Liver BF26
Thorax BP2W

Computerized Tomography
(CT Scan) *(continued)*
Tibia
  Left BQ2C
  Right BQ2B
Toe
  Left BQ2Q
  Right BQ2P
Trachea BB2F
Tracheobronchial Tree
  Bilateral BB29
  Left BB28
  Right BB27
Vein
  Pelvic (Iliac)
    Left B52G
      Intravascular Optical
        Coherence B52GZ2Z
    Right B52F
      Intravascular Optical
        Coherence B52FZ2Z
  Pelvic (Iliac) Bilateral B52H
    Intravascular Optical
      Coherence B52HZ2Z
  Portal B52T
    Intravascular Optical
      Coherence B52TZ2Z
  Pulmonary
    Bilateral B52S
      Intravascular Optical
        Coherence B52SZ2Z
    Left B52R
      Intravascular Optical
        Coherence B52RZ2Z
    Right B52Q
      Intravascular Optical
        Coherence B52QZ2Z
  Renal
    Bilateral B52L
      Intravascular Optical
        Coherence B52LZ2Z
    Left B52K
      Intravascular Optical
        Coherence B52KZ2Z
    Right B52J
      Intravascular Optical
        Coherence B52JZ2Z
  Spanchnic B52T
    Intravascular Optical
      Coherence B52TZ2Z
Vena Cava
  Inferior B529
    Intravascular Optical
      Coherence B529Z2Z
  Superior B528
    Intravascular Optical
      Coherence B528Z2Z
Ventricle, Cerebral B028
Wrist
  Left BP2M
  Right BP2L
Concerto II CRT-D
use Cardiac Resynchronization
  Defibrillator Pulse Generator
  in 0JH
Condylectomy
see Excision, Head and Facial Bones
  0NB
see Excision, Lower Bones 0QB
see Excision, Upper Bones 0PB
Condyloid process
use Mandible, Left
use Mandible, Right
Condylotomy
see Division, Head and Facial Bones
  0N8
see Division, Lower Bones 0Q8
see Division, Upper Bones 0P8
see Drainage, Head and Facial
  Bones 0N9
see Drainage, Lower Bones 0Q9
see Drainage, Upper Bones 0P9

Condylysis
see Release, Head and Facial Bones
  0NN
see Release, Lower Bones 0QN
see Release, Upper Bones 0PN
Conization, cervix
see Excision, Uterus 0UB9
Conjunctivoplasty
see Repair, Eye 08Q
see Replacement, Eye 08R
CONSERVE® PLUS Total
Resurfacing Hip System
use Resurfacing Device in Lower
  Joints
Construction
Auricle, ear
  see Bypass, Urinary System 0T1
Ileal conduit
  see Replacement, Ear, Nose,
    Sinus 09R
Consulta CRT-D
use Cardiac Resynchronization
  Defibrillator Pulse Generator
  in 0JH
Consulta CRT-P
use Cardiac Resynchronization
  Pacemaker Pulse Generator in
  0JH
Contact Radiation
Abdomen DWY37ZZ
Adrenal Gland DGY27ZZ
Bile Ducts DFY27ZZ
Bladder DTY27ZZ
Bone, Other DPYC7ZZ
Brain D0Y07ZZ
Brain Stem D0Y17ZZ
Breast
  Left DMY07ZZ
  Right DMY17ZZ
Bronchus DBY17ZZ
Cervix DUY17ZZ
Chest DWY27ZZ
Chest Wall DBY77ZZ
Colon DDY57ZZ
Diaphragm DBY87ZZ
Duodenum DDY27ZZ
Ear D9Y07ZZ
Esophagus DDY07ZZ
Eye D8Y07ZZ
Femur DPY97ZZ
Fibula DPYB7ZZ
Gallbladder DFY17ZZ
Gland
  Adrenal DGY27ZZ
  Parathyroid DGY47ZZ
  Pituitary DGY07ZZ
  Thyroid DGY57ZZ
Glands, Salivary D9Y67ZZ
Head and Neck DWY17ZZ
Hemibody DWY47ZZ
Humerus DPY67ZZ
Hypopharynx D9Y37ZZ
Ileum DDY47ZZ
Jejunum DDY37ZZ
Kidney DTY07ZZ
Larynx D9YB7ZZ
Liver DFY07ZZ
Lung DBY27ZZ
Mandible DPY37ZZ
Maxilla DPY27ZZ
Mediastinum DBY67ZZ
Mouth D9Y47ZZ
Nasopharynx D9YD7ZZ
Neck and Head DWY17ZZ
Nerve, Peripheral D0Y77ZZ
Nose D9Y17ZZ
Oropharynx D9YF7ZZ
Ovary DUY07ZZ
Palate
  Hard D9Y87ZZ
  Soft D9Y97ZZ
Pancreas DFY37ZZ

Contact Radiation *(continued)*
Parathyroid Gland DGY47ZZ
Pelvic Bones DPY87ZZ
Pelvic Region DWY67ZZ
Pineal Body DGY17ZZ
Pituitary Gland DGY07ZZ
Pleura DBY57ZZ
Prostate DVY07ZZ
Radius DPY77ZZ
Rectum DDY77ZZ
Rib DPY57ZZ
Sinuses D9Y77ZZ
Skin
  Abdomen DHY87ZZ
  Arm DHY47ZZ
  Back DHY77ZZ
  Buttock DHY97ZZ
  Chest DHY67ZZ
  Face DHY27ZZ
  Leg DHYB7ZZ
  Neck DHY37ZZ
Skull DPY07ZZ
Spinal Cord D0Y67ZZ
Sternum DPY47ZZ
Stomach DDY17ZZ
Testis DVY17ZZ
Thyroid Gland DGY57ZZ
Tibia DPYB7ZZ
Tongue D9Y57ZZ
Trachea DBY07ZZ
Ulna DPY77ZZ
Ureter DTY17ZZ
Urethra DTY37ZZ
Uterus DUY27ZZ
Whole Body DWY57ZZ
CONTAK RENEWAL® 3 RF (HE)
CRT-D
use Cardiac Resynchronization
  Defibrillator Pulse Generator
  in 0JH
Contegra Pulmonary Valved Conduit
use Zooplastic Tissue in Heart and
  Great Vessels
Continuous Glucose Monitoring
(CGM) device
use Monitoring Device
Continuous Negative Airway
Pressure
24-96 Consecutive Hours,
  Ventilation 5A09459
Greater than 96 Consecutive Hours,
  Ventilation 5A09559
Less than 24 Consecutive Hours,
  Ventilation 5A09359
Continuous Positive Airway Pressure
24-96 Consecutive Hours,
  Ventilation 5A09457
Greater than 96 Consecutive Hours,
  Ventilation 5A09557
Less than 24 Consecutive Hours,
  Ventilation 5A09357
Contraceptive Device
Change device in, Uterus and Cervix
  0U2DXHZ
Insertion of device in
  Cervix 0UHC
  Subcutaneous Tissue and Fascia
    Abdomen 0JH8
    Chest 0JH6
    Lower Arm
      Left 0JHH
      Right 0JHG
    Lower Leg
      Left 0JHP
      Right 0JHN
    Upper Arm
      Left 0JHF
      Right 0JHD
    Upper Leg
      Left 0JHM
      Right 0JHL
  Uterus 0UH9

Contraceptive Device *(continued)*
Removal of device from
  Subcutaneous Tissue and Fascia
    Lower Extremity 0JPW
    Trunk 0JPT
    Upper Extremity 0JPV
  Uterus and Cervix 0UPD
Revision of device in
  Subcutaneous Tissue and Fascia
    Lower Extremity 0JWW
    Trunk 0JWT
    Upper Extremity 0JWV
  Uterus and Cervix 0UWD
Contractility Modulation Device
Abdomen 0JH8
Chest 0JH6
Control postprocedural bleeding in
Abdominal Wall 0W3F
Ankle Region
  Left 0Y3L
  Right 0Y3K
Arm
  Lower
    Left 0X3F
    Right 0X3D
  Upper
    Left 0X39
    Right 0X38
Axilla
  Left 0X35
  Right 0X34
Back
  Lower 0W3L
  Upper 0W3K
Buttock
  Left 0Y31
  Right 0Y30
Cavity, Cranial 0W31
Chest Wall 0W38
Elbow Region
  Left 0X3C
  Right 0X3B
Extremity
  Lower
    Left 0Y3B
    Right 0Y39
  Upper
    Left 0X37
    Right 0X36
Face 0W32
Femoral Region
  Left 0Y38
  Right 0Y37
Foot
  Left 0Y3N
  Right 0Y3M
Gastrointestinal Tract 0W3P
Genitourinary Tract 0W3R
Hand
  Left 0X3K
  Right 0X3J
Head 0W30
Inguinal Region
  Left 0Y36
  Right 0Y35
Jaw
  Lower 0W35
  Upper 0W34
Knee Region
  Left 0Y3G
  Right 0Y3F
Leg
  Lower
    Left 0Y3J
    Right 0Y3H
  Upper
    Left 0Y3D
    Right 0Y3C
Mediastinum 0W3C
Neck 0W36
Oral Cavity and Throat 0W33
Pelvic Cavity 0W3J

Control postprocedural bleeding in *(continued)*
  Pericardial Cavity 0W3D
  Perineum
    Female 0W3N
    Male 0W3M
  Peritoneal Cavity 0W3G
  Pleural Cavity
    Left 0W3B
    Right 0W39
  Respiratory Tract 0W3Q
  Retroperitoneum 0W3H
  Shoulder Region
    Left 0X33
    Right 0X32
  Wrist Region
    Left 0X3H
    Right 0X3G
Conus arteriosus
  use Ventricle, Right
Conus medullaris
  use Spinal Cord, Lumbar
Conversion
  Cardiac rhythm 5A2204Z
  Gastrostomy to jejunostomy feeding device
    see Insertion of device in, Jejunum 0DHA
Coracoacromial ligament
  use Bursa and Ligament, Shoulder, Left
  use Bursa and Ligament, Shoulder, Right
Coracobrachialis muscle
  use Muscle, Upper Arm, Left
  use Muscle, Upper Arm, Right
Coracoclavicular ligament
  use Bursa and Ligament, Shoulder, Left
  use Bursa and Ligament, Shoulder, Right
Coracohumeral ligament
  use Bursa and Ligament, Shoulder, Left
  use Bursa and Ligament, Shoulder, Right
Coracoid process
  use Scapula, Left
  use Scapula, Right
Cordotomy
  see Division, Central Nervous System 008
Core needle biopsy
  see Excision with qualifier Diagnostic
CoreValve transcatheter aortic valve
  use Zooplastic Tissue in Heart and Great Vessels
Cormet Hip Resurfacing System
  use Resurfacing Device in Lower Joints
Corniculate cartilage
  use Larynx
CoRoent® XL
  use Interbody Fusion Device in Lower Joints
Coronary arteriography
  see Fluoroscopy, Heart B21
  see Plain Radiography, Heart B20
Corox (OTW) Bipolar Lead
  use Cardiac Lead, Defibrillator in 02H
  use Cardiac Lead, Pacemaker in 02H
Corpus callosum
  use Brain
Corpus cavernosum
  use Penis
Corpus spongiosum
  use Penis
Corpus striatum
  use Basal Ganglia
Corrugator supercilii muscle
  use Muscle, Facial

Cortical strip neurostimulator lead
  use Neurostimulator Lead in Central Nervous System
Costatectomy
  see Excision, Upper Bones 0PB
  see Resection, Upper Bones 0PT
Costectomy
  see Excision, Upper Bones 0PB
  see Resection, Upper Bones 0PT
Costocervical trunk
  use Artery, Subclavian, Left
  use Artery, Subclavian, Right
Costochondrectomy
  see Excision, Upper Bones 0PB
  see Resection, Upper Bones 0PT
Costoclavicular ligament
  use Bursa and Ligament, Shoulder, Left
  use Bursa and Ligament, Shoulder, Right
Costosternoplasty
  see Repair, Upper Bones 0PQ
  see Replacement, Upper Bones 0PR
  see Supplement, Upper Bones 0PU
Costotomy
  see Division, Upper Bones 0P8
  see Drainage, Upper Bones 0P9
Costotransverse joint
  use Joint, Thoracic Vertebral
Costotransverse ligament
  use Bursa and Ligament, Thorax, Left
  use Bursa and Ligament, Thorax, Right
Costovertebral joint
  use Joint, Thoracic Vertebral
Costoxiphoid ligament
  use Bursa and Ligament, Thorax, Left
  use Bursa and Ligament, Thorax, Right
Counseling
  Family, for substance abuse, Other Family Counseling HZ63ZZZ
  Group
    12-Step HZ43ZZZ
    Behavioral HZ41ZZZ
    Cognitive HZ40ZZZ
    Cognitive-Behavioral HZ42ZZZ
    Confrontational HZ48ZZZ
    Continuing Care HZ49ZZZ
    Infectious Disease
      Post-Test HZ4CZZZ
      Pre-Test HZ4CZZZ
    Interpersonal HZ44ZZZ
    Motivational Enhancement HZ47ZZZ
    Psychoeducation HZ46ZZZ
    Spiritual HZ4BZZZ
    Vocational HZ45ZZZ
  Individual
    12-Step HZ33ZZZ
    Behavioral HZ31ZZZ
    Cognitive HZ30ZZZ
    Cognitive-Behavioral HZ32ZZZ
    Confrontational HZ38ZZZ
    Continuing Care HZ39ZZZ
    Infectious Disease
      Post-Test HZ3CZZZ
      Pre-Test HZ3CZZZ
    Interpersonal HZ34ZZZ
    Motivational Enhancement HZ37ZZZ
    Psychoeducation HZ36ZZZ
    Spiritual HZ3BZZZ
    Vocational HZ35ZZZ
  Mental Health Services
    Educational GZ60ZZZ
    Other Counseling GZ63ZZZ
    Vocational GZ61ZZZ

Countershock, cardiac 5A2204Z
Cowper's (bulbourethral) gland
  use Urethra
CPAP (continuous positive airway pressure)
  see Assistance, Respiratory 5A09
Craniectomy
  see Excision, Head and Facial Bones 0NB
  see Resection, Head and Facial Bones 0NT
Cranioplasty
  see Repair, Head and Facial Bones 0NQ
  see Replacement, Head and Facial Bones 0NR
  see Supplement, Head and Facial Bones 0NU
Craniotomy
  see Drainage, Central Nervous System 009
  see Division, Head and Facial Bones 0N8
  see Drainage, Head and Facial Bones 0N9
Creation
  Female 0W4N0
  Male 0W4M0
Cremaster muscle
  use Muscle, Perineum
Cribriform plate
  use Bone, Ethmoid, Left
  use Bone, Ethmoid, Right
Cricoid cartilage
  use Trachea
Cricoidectomy
  see Excision, Larynx 0CBS
Cricothyroid artery
  use Artery, Thyroid, Left
  use Artery, Thyroid, Right
Cricothyroid muscle
  use Muscle, Neck, Left
  use Muscle, Neck, Right
Crisis Intervention GZ2ZZZZ
Crural fascia
  use Subcutaneous Tissue and Fascia, Upper Leg, Left
  use Subcutaneous Tissue and Fascia, Upper Leg, Right
Crushing, nerve
  Cranial
    see Destruction, Central Nervous System 005
  Peripheral
    see Destruction, Peripheral Nervous System 015
Cryoablation
  see Destruction
Cryotherapy
  see Destruction
Cryptorchidectomy
  see Excision, Male Reproductive System 0VB
  see Resection, Male Reproductive System 0VT
Cryptorchiectomy
  see Excision, Male Reproductive System 0VB
  see Resection, Male Reproductive System 0VT
Cryptotomy
  see Division, Gastrointestinal System 0D8
  see Drainage, Gastrointestinal System 0D9
CT scan
  see Computerized Tomography (CT Scan)
CT sialogram
  see Computerized Tomography (CT Scan), Ear, Nose, Mouth and Throat B92

Cubital lymph node
  use Lymphatic, Upper Extremity, Left
  use Lymphatic, Upper Extremity, Right
Cubital nerve
  use Nerve, Ulnar
Cuboid bone
  use Tarsal, Left
  use Tarsal, Right
Cuboideonavicular joint
  use Joint, Tarsal, Left
  use Joint, Tarsal, Right
Culdocentesis
  see Drainage, Cul-de-sac 0U9F
Culdoplasty
  see Repair, Cul-de-sac 0UQF
  see Supplement, Cul-de-sac 0UUF
Culdoscopy 0UJH8ZZ
Culdotomy
  see Drainage, Cul-de-sac 0U9F
Culmen
  use Cerebellum
Cultured epidermal cell autograft
  use Autologous Tissue Substitute
Cuneiform cartilage
  use Larynx
Cuneonavicular joint
  use Joint, Tarsal, Left
  use Joint, Tarsal, Right
Cuneonavicular ligament
  use Bursa and Ligament, Foot, Left
  use Bursa and Ligament, Foot, Right
Curettage
  see Excision
  see Extraction
Cutaneous (transverse) cervical nerve
  use Nerve, Cervical Plexus
CVP (central venous pressure)
  see Measurement, Venous 4A04
Cyclodiathermy
  see Destruction, Eye 085
Cyclophotocoagulation
  see Destruction, Eye 085
CYPHER® Stent
  use Intraluminal Device, Drug-eluting in Heart and Great Vessels
Cystectomy
  see Excision, Bladder 0TBB
  see Resection, Bladder 0TTB
Cystocele repair
  see Repair, Subcutaneous Tissue and Fascia, Pelvic Region 0JQC
Cystography
  see Fluoroscopy, Urinary System BT1
  see Plain Radiography, Urinary System BT0
Cystolithotomy
  see Extirpation, Bladder 0TCB
Cystopexy
  see Repair, Bladder 0TQB
  see Reposition, Bladder 0TSB
Cystoplasty
  see Repair, Bladder 0TQB
  see Replacement, Bladder 0TRB
  see Supplement, Bladder 0TUB
Cystorrhaphy
  see Repair, Bladder 0TQB
Cystoscopy 0TJB8ZZ

Cystostomy
  see Bypass, Bladder 0T1B
Cystostomy tube
  use Drainage Device
Cystotomy
  see Drainage, Bladder 0T9B
Cystourethrography
  see Fluoroscopy, Urinary System BT1
  see Plain Radiography, Urinary System BT0
Cystourethroplasty
  see Repair, Urinary System 0TQ
  see Replacement, Urinary System 0TR
  see Supplement, Urinary System 0TU

D

DBS lead
  use Neurostimulator Lead in Central Nervous System
DeBakey Left Ventricular Assist Device
  use Implantable Heart Assist System in Heart and Great Vessels
Debridement
  Excisional
    see Excision
  Non-excisional
    see Extraction
Decompression, Circulatory 6A15
Decortication, lung
  see Extraction, Respiratory System 0BD
Deep brain neurostimulator lead
  use Neurostimulator Lead in Central Nervous System
Deep cervical fascia
  use Subcutaneous Tissue and Fascia, Neck, Anterior
Deep cervical vein
  use Vein, Vertebral, Left
  use Vein, Vertebral, Right
Deep circumflex iliac artery
  use Artery, External Iliac, Left
  use Artery, External Iliac, Right
Deep facial vein
  use Vein, Face, Left
  use Vein, Face, Right
Deep femoral (profunda femoris) vein
  use Vein, Femoral, Left
  use Vein, Femoral, Right
Deep femoral artery
  use Artery, Femoral, Left
  use Artery, Femoral, Right
Deep Inferior Epigastric Artery Perforator Flap
  Bilateral 0HRV077
  Left 0HRU077
  Right 0HRT077
Deep palmar arch
  use Artery, Hand, Left
  use Artery, Hand, Right
Deep transverse perineal muscle
  use Muscle, Perineum
Deferential artery
  use Artery, Internal Iliac, Left
  use Artery, Internal Iliac, Right
Defibrillator Generator
  Abdomen 0JH8
  Chest 0JH6
Delivery
  Cesarean
    see Extraction, Products of Conception 10D0
  Forceps
    see Extraction, Products of Conception 10D0
  Manually assisted 10E0XZZ

Delivery *(continued)*
  Products of Conception 10E0XZZ
  Vacuum assisted
    see Extraction, Products of Conception 10D0
Delta frame external fixator
  use External Fixation Device, Hybrid in 0PH
  use External Fixation Device, Hybrid in 0PS
  use External Fixation Device, Hybrid in 0QH
  use External Fixation Device, Hybrid in 0QS
Delta III Reverse shoulder prosthesis
  use Synthetic Substitute, Reverse Ball and Socket in 0RR
Deltoid fascia
  use Subcutaneous Tissue and Fascia, Upper Arm, Left
  use Subcutaneous Tissue and Fascia, Upper Arm, Right
Deltoid ligament
  use Bursa and Ligament, Ankle, Left
  use Bursa and Ligament, Ankle, Right
Deltoid muscle
  use Muscle, Shoulder, Left
  use Muscle, Shoulder, Right
Deltopectoral (infraclavicular) lymph node
  use Lymphatic, Upper Extremity, Left
  use Lymphatic, Upper Extremity, Right
Denervation
  Cranial nerve
    see Destruction, Central Nervous System 005
  Peripheral nerve
    see Destruction, Peripheral Nervous System 015
Densitometry
  Plain Radiography
    Femur
      Left BQ04ZZ1
      Right BQ03ZZ1
    Hip
      Left BQ01ZZ1
      Right BQ00ZZ1
    Spine
      Cervical BR00ZZ1
      Lumbar BR09ZZ1
      Thoracic BR07ZZ1
      Whole BR0GZZ1
  Ultrasonography
    Elbow
      Left BP4HZZ1
      Right BP4GZZ1
    Hand
      Left BP4PZZ1
      Right BP4NZZ1
    Shoulder
      Left BP49ZZ1
      Right BP48ZZ1
    Wrist
      Left BP4MZZ1
      Right BP4LZZ1
Denticulate (dentate) ligament
  use Spinal Meninges
Depressor anguli oris muscle
  use Muscle, Facial
Depressor labii inferioris muscle
  use Muscle, Facial
Depressor septi nasi muscle
  use Muscle, Facial
Depressor supercilii muscle
  use Muscle, Facial
Dermabrasion
  see Extraction, Skin and Breast 0HD

Dermis
  use Skin
Descending genicular artery
  use Artery, Femoral, Left
  use Artery, Femoral, Right
Destruction
  Acetabulum
    Left 0Q55
    Right 0Q54
  Adenoids 0C5Q
  Ampulla of Vater 0F5C
  Anal Sphincter 0D5R
  Anterior Chamber
    Left 08533ZZ
    Right 08523ZZ
  Anus 0D5Q
  Aorta
    Abdominal 0450
    Thoracic 025W
  Aortic Body 0G5D
  Appendix 0D5J
  Artery
    Anterior Tibial
      Left 045Q
      Right 045P
    Axillary
      Left 0356
      Right 0355
    Brachial
      Left 0358
      Right 0357
    Celiac 0451
    Colic
      Left 0457
      Middle 0458
      Right 0456
    Common Carotid
      Left 035J
      Right 035H
    Common Iliac
      Left 045D
      Right 045C
    External Carotid
      Left 035N
      Right 035M
    External Iliac
      Left 045J
      Right 045H
    Face 035R
    Femoral
      Left 045L
      Right 045K
    Foot
      Left 045W
      Right 045V
    Gastric 0452
    Hand
      Left 035F
      Right 035D
    Hepatic 0453
    Inferior Mesenteric 045B
    Innominate 0352
    Internal Carotid
      Left 035L
      Right 035K
    Internal Iliac
      Left 045F
      Right 045E
    Internal Mammary
      Left 0351
      Right 0350
    Intracranial 035G
    Lower 045Y
    Peroneal
      Left 045U
      Right 045T
    Popliteal
      Left 045N
      Right 045M
    Posterior Tibial
      Left 045S
      Right 045R

Destruction *(continued)*
  Artery *(continued)*
    Pulmonary
      Left 025R
      Right 025Q
    Pulmonary Trunk 025P
    Radial
      Left 035C
      Right 035B
    Renal
      Left 045A
      Right 0459
    Splenic 0454
    Subclavian
      Left 0354
      Right 0353
    Superior Mesenteric 0455
    Temporal
      Left 035T
      Right 035S
    Thyroid
      Left 035V
      Right 035U
    Ulnar
      Left 035A
      Right 0359
    Upper 035Y
    Vertebral
      Left 035Q
      Right 035P
  Atrium
    Left 0257
    Right 0256
  Auditory Ossicle
    Left 095A0ZZ
    Right 09590ZZ
  Basal Ganglia 0058
  Bladder 0T5B
  Bladder Neck 0T5C
  Bone
    Ethmoid
      Left 0N5G
      Right 0N5F
    Frontal
      Left 0N52
      Right 0N51
    Hyoid 0N5X
    Lacrimal
      Left 0N5J
      Right 0N5H
    Nasal 0N5B
    Occipital
      Left 0N58
      Right 0N57
    Palatine
      Left 0N5L
      Right 0N5K
    Parietal
      Left 0N54
      Right 0N53
    Pelvic
      Left 0Q53
      Right 0Q52
    Sphenoid
      Left 0N5D
      Right 0N5C
    Temporal
      Left 0N56
      Right 0N55
    Zygomatic
      Left 0N5N
      Right 0N5M
  Brain 0050
  Breast
    Bilateral 0H5V
    Left 0H5U
    Right 0H5T
  Bronchus
    Lingula 0B59
    Lower Lobe
      Left 0B5B
      Right 0B56

Destruction *(continued)*
Bronchus *(continued)*
  Main
    Left 0B57
    Right 0B53
  Middle Lobe, Right 0B55
  Upper Lobe
    Left 0B58
    Right 0B54
Buccal Mucosa 0C54
Bursa and Ligament
  Abdomen
    Left 0M5J
    Right 0M5H
  Ankle
    Left 0M5R
    Right 0M5Q
  Elbow
    Left 0M54
    Right 0M53
  Foot
    Left 0M5T
    Right 0M5S
  Hand
    Left 0M58
    Right 0M57
  Head and Neck 0M50
  Hip
    Left 0M5M
    Right 0M5L
  Knee
    Left 0M5P
    Right 0M5N
  Lower Extremity
    Left 0M5W
    Right 0M5V
  Perineum 0M5K
  Shoulder
    Left 0M52
    Right 0M51
  Thorax
    Left 0M5G
    Right 0M5F
  Trunk
    Left 0M5D
    Right 0M5C
  Upper Extremity
    Left 0M5B
    Right 0M59
  Wrist
    Left 0M56
    Right 0M55
Carina 0B52
Carotid Bodies, Bilateral 0G58
Carotid Body
  Left 0G56
  Right 0G57
Carpal
  Left 0P5N
  Right 0P5M
Cecum 0D5H
Cerebellum 005C
Cerebral Hemisphere 0057
Cerebral Meninges 0051
Cerebral Ventricle 0056
Cervix 0U5C
Chordae Tendineae 0259
Choroid
  Left 085B
  Right 085A
Cisterna Chyli 075L
Clavicle
  Left 0P5B
  Right 0P59
Clitoris 0U5J
Coccygeal Glomus 0G5B
Coccyx 0Q5S
Colon
  Ascending 0D5K
  Descending 0D5M
  Sigmoid 0D5N
  Transverse 0D5L

Destruction *(continued)*
Conduction Mechanism 0258
Conjunctiva
  Left 085TXZZ
  Right 085SXZZ
Cord
  Bilateral 0V5H
  Left 0V5G
  Right 0V5F
Cornea
  Left 0859XZZ
  Right 0858XZZ
Cul-de-sac 0U5F
Diaphragm
  Left 0B5S
  Right 0B5R
Disc
  Cervical Vertebral 0R53
  Cervicothoracic Vertebral 0R55
  Lumbar Vertebral 0S52
  Lumbosacral 0S54
  Thoracic Vertebral 0R59
  Thoracolumbar Vertebral
    0R5B
Duct
  Common Bile 0F59
  Cystic 0F58
  Hepatic
    Left 0F56
    Right 0F55
  Lacrimal
    Left 085Y
    Right 085X
  Pancreatic 0F5D
    Accessory 0F5F
  Parotid
    Left 0C5C
    Right 0C5B
Duodenum 0D59
Dura Mater 0052
Ear
  External
    Left 0951
    Right 0950
  External Auditory Canal
    Left 0954
    Right 0953
  Inner
    Left 095E0ZZ
    Right 095D0ZZ
  Middle
    Left 09560ZZ
    Right 09550ZZ
Endometrium 0U5B
Epididymis
  Bilateral 0V5L
  Left 0V5K
  Right 0V5J
Epiglottis 0C5R
Esophagogastric Junction 0D54
Esophagus 0D55
  Lower 0D53
  Middle 0D52
  Upper 0D51
Eustachian Tube
  Left 095G
  Right 095F
Eye
  Left 0851XZZ
  Right 0850XZZ
Eyelid
  Lower
    Left 085R
    Right 085Q
  Upper
    Left 085P
    Right 085N
Fallopian Tube
  Left 0U56
  Right 0U55
Fallopian Tubes, Bilateral
  0U57

Destruction *(continued)*
Femoral Shaft
  Left 0Q59
  Right 0Q58
Femur
  Lower
    Left 0Q5C
    Right 0Q5B
  Upper
    Left 0Q57
    Right 0Q56
Fibula
  Left 0Q5K
  Right 0Q5J
Finger Nail 0H5QXZZ
Gallbladder 0F54
Gingiva
  Lower 0C56
  Upper 0C55
Gland
  Adrenal
    Bilateral 0G54
    Left 0G52
    Right 0G53
  Lacrimal
    Left 085W
    Right 085V
  Minor Salivary 0C5J
  Parotid
    Left 0C59
    Right 0C58
  Pituitary 0G50
  Sublingual
    Left 0C5F
    Right 0C5D
  Submaxillary
    Left 0C5H
    Right 0C5G
  Vestibular 0U5L
Glenoid Cavity
  Left 0P58
  Right 0P57
Glomus Jugulare
  0G5C
Humeral Head
  Left 0P5D
  Right 0P5C
Humeral Shaft
  Left 0P5G
  Right 0P5F
Hymen 0U5K
Hypothalamus 005A
Ileocecal Valve 0D5C
Ileum 0D5B
Intestine
  Large 0D5E
    Left 0D5G
    Right 0D5F
  Small 0D58
Iris
  Left 085D3ZZ
  Right 085C3ZZ
Jejunum 0D5A
Joint
  Acromioclavicular
    Left 0R5H
    Right 0R5G
  Ankle
    Left 0S5G
    Right 0S5F
  Carpal
    Left 0R5R
    Right 0R5Q
  Cervical Vertebral 0R51
  Cervicothoracic Vertebral 0R54
  Coccygeal 0S56
  Elbow
    Left 0R5M
    Right 0R5L
  Finger Phalangeal
    Left 0R5X
    Right 0R5W

Destruction *(continued)*
Joint *(continued)*
  Hip
    Left 0S5B
    Right 0S59
  Knee
    Left 0S5D
    Right 0S5C
  Lumbar Vertebral 0S50
  Lumbosacral 0S53
  Metacarpocarpal
    Left 0R5T
    Right 0R5S
  Metacarpophalangeal
    Left 0R5V
    Right 0R5U
  Metatarsal-Phalangeal
    Left 0S5N
    Right 0S5M
  Metatarsal-Tarsal
    Left 0S5L
    Right 0S5K
  Occipital-cervical 0R50
  Sacrococcygeal 0S55
  Sacroiliac
    Left 0S58
    Right 0S57
  Shoulder
    Left 0R5K
    Right 0R5J
  Sternoclavicular
    Left 0R5F
    Right 0R5E
  Tarsal
    Left 0S5J
    Right 0S5H
  Temporomandibular
    Left 0R5D
    Right 0R5C
  Thoracic Vertebral 0R56
  Thoracolumbar Vertebral 0R5A
  Toe Phalangeal
    Left 0S5Q
    Right 0S5P
  Wrist
    Left 0R5P
    Right 0R5N
Kidney
  Left 0T51
  Right 0T50
Kidney Pelvis
  Left 0T54
  Right 0T53
Larynx 0C5S
Lens
  Left 085K3ZZ
  Right 085J3ZZ
Lip
  Lower 0C51
  Upper 0C50
Liver 0F50
  Left Lobe 0F52
  Right Lobe 0F51
Lung
  Bilateral 0B5M
  Left 0B5L
  Lower Lobe
    Left 0B5J
    Right 0B5F
  Middle Lobe, Right
    0B5D
  Right 0B5K
  Upper Lobe
    Left 0B5G
    Right 0B5C
Lung Lingula 0B5H
Lymphatic
  Aortic 075D
  Axillary
    Left 0756
    Right 0755
  Head 0750

Destruction *(continued)*
  Tendon *(continued)*
    Upper Arm *(continued)*
      Right 0L53
    Upper Leg
      Left 0L5M
      Right 0L5L
  Testis
    Bilateral 0V5C
    Left 0V5B
    Right 0V59
  Thalamus 0059
  Thymus 075M
  Thyroid Gland 0G5K
    Left Lobe 0G5G
    Right Lobe 0G5H
  Tibia
    Left 0Q5H
    Right 0Q5G
  Toe Nail 0H5RXZZ
  Tongue 0C57
  Tonsils 0C5P
  Tooth
    Lower 0C5X
    Upper 0C5W
  Trachea 0B51
  Tunica Vaginalis
    Left 0V57
    Right 0V56
  Turbinate, Nasal 095L
  Tympanic Membrane
    Left 0958
    Right 0957
  Ulna
    Left 0P5L
    Right 0P5K
  Ureter
    Left 0T57
    Right 0T56
  Urethra 0T5D
  Uterine Supporting Structure 0U54
  Uterus 0U59
  Uvula 0C5N
  Vagina 0U5G
  Valve
    Aortic 025F
    Mitral 025G
    Pulmonary 025H
    Tricuspid 025J
  Vas Deferens
    Bilateral 0V5Q
    Left 0V5P
    Right 0V5N
  Vein
    Axillary
      Left 0558
      Right 0557
    Azygos 0550
    Basilic
      Left 055C
      Right 055B
    Brachial
      Left 055A
      Right 0559
    Cephalic
      Left 055F
      Right 055D
    Colic 0657
    Common Iliac
      Left 065D
      Right 065C
    Coronary 0254
    Esophageal 0653
    External Iliac
      Left 065D
      Right 065F
    External Jugular
      Left 055Q
      Right 055P
    Face
      Left 055V
      Right 055T

Destruction *(continued)*
  Vein *(continued)*
    Femoral
      Left 065N
      Right 065M
    Foot
      Left 065V
      Right 065T
    Gastric 0652
    Greater Saphenous
      Left 065Q
      Right 065P
    Hand
      Left 055H
      Right 055G
    Hemiazygos 0551
    Hepatic 0654
    Hypogastric
      Left 065J
      Right 065H
    Inferior Mesenteric 0656
    Innominate
      Left 0554
      Right 0553
    Internal Jugular
      Left 055N
      Right 055M
    Intracranial 055L
    Lesser Saphenous
      Left 065S
      Right 065R
    Lower 065Y
    Portal 0658
    Pulmonary
      Left 025T
      Right 025S
    Renal
      Left 065B
      Right 0659
    Splenic 0651
    Subclavian
      Left 0556
      Right 0555
    Superior Mesenteric 0655
    Upper 055Y
    Vertebral
      Left 055S
      Right 055R
  Vena Cava
    Inferior 0650
    Superior 025V
  Ventricle
    Left 025L
    Right 025K
  Vertebra
    Cervical 0P53
    Lumbar 0Q50
    Thoracic 0P54
  Vesicle
    Bilateral 0V53
    Left 0V52
    Right 0V51
  Vitreous
    Left 08553ZZ
    Right 08543ZZ
  Vocal Cord
    Left 0C5V
    Right 0C5T
  Vulva 0U5M
Detachment
  Arm
    Lower
      Left 0X6F0Z
      Right 0X6D0Z
    Upper
      Left 0X690Z
      Right 0X680Z
  Elbow Region
    Left 0X6C0ZZ
    Right 0X6B0ZZ

Detachment *(continued)*
  Femoral Region
    Left 0Y680ZZ
    Right 0Y670ZZ
  Finger
    Index
      Left 0X6P0Z
      Right 0X6N0Z
    Little
      Left 0X6W0Z
      Right 0X6V0Z
    Middle
      Left 0X6R0Z
      Right 0X6Q0Z
    Ring
      Left 0X6T0Z
      Right 0X6S0Z
  Foot
    Left 0Y6N0Z
    Right 0Y6M0Z
  Forequarter
    Left 0X610ZZ
    Right 0X600ZZ
  Hand
    Left 0X6K0Z
    Right 0X6J0Z
  Hindquarter
    Bilateral 0Y640ZZ
    Left 0Y630ZZ
    Right 0Y620ZZ
  Knee Region
    Left 0Y6G0ZZ
    Right 0Y6F0ZZ
  Leg
    Lower
      Left 0Y6J0Z
      Right 0Y6H0Z
    Upper
      Left 0Y6D0Z
      Right 0Y6C0Z
  Shoulder Region
    Left 0X630ZZ
    Right 0X620ZZ
  Thumb
    Left 0X6M0Z
    Right 0X6L0Z
  Toe
    1st
      Left 0Y6Q0Z
      Right 0Y6P0Z
    2nd
      Left 0Y6S0Z
      Right 0Y6R0Z
    3rd
      Left 0Y6U0Z
      Right 0Y6T0Z
    4th
      Left 0Y6W0Z
      Right 0Y6V0Z
    5th
      Left 0Y6Y0Z
      Right 0Y6X0Z
Determination, Mental status
  GZ14ZZZ
Detorsion
  see Release
  see Reposition
Detoxification Services, for substance abuse HZ2ZZZZ
Device Fitting F0DZ
Diagnostic Audiology
  see Audiology, Diagnostic
Diagnostic imaging
  see Imaging, Diagnostic
Diagnostic radiology
  see Imaging, Diagnostic
Dialysis
  Hemodialysis 5A1D00Z
  Peritoneal 3E1M39Z
Diaphragma sellae
  use Dura Mater

Diaphragmatic pacemaker generator
  use Stimulator Generator in Subcutaneous Tissue and Fascia
Diaphragmatic Pacemaker Lead
  Insertion of device in
    Left 0BHS
    Right 0BHR
  Removal of device from, Diaphragm 0BPT
  Revision of device in, Diaphragm 0BWT
Digital radiography, plain
  see Plain Radiography
Dilation
  Ampulla of Vater 0F7C
  Anus 0D7Q
  Aorta
    Abdominal 0470
    Thoracic 027W
  Artery
    Anterior Tibial
      Left 047Q
      Right 047P
    Axillary
      Left 0376
      Right 0375
    Brachial
      Left 0378
      Right 0377
    Celiac 0471
    Colic
      Left 0477
      Middle 0478
      Right 0476
    Common Carotid
      Left 037J
      Right 037H
    Common Iliac
      Left 047D
      Right 047C
    Coronary
      Four or More Sites 0273
      One Site 0270
      Three Sites 0272
      Two Sites 0271
    External Carotid
      Left 037N
      Right 037M
    External Iliac
      Left 047J
      Right 047H
    Face 037R
    Femoral
      Left 047L
      Right 047K
    Foot
      Left 047W
      Right 047V
    Gastric 0472
    Hand
      Left 037F
      Right 037D
    Hepatic 0473
    Inferior Mesenteric 047B
    Innominate 0372
    Internal Carotid
      Left 037L
      Right 037K
    Internal Iliac
      Left 047F
      Right 047E
    Internal Mammary
      Left 0371
      Right 0370
    Intracranial 037G
    Lower 047Y
    Peroneal
      Left 047U
      Right 047T
    Popliteal
      Left 047N
      Right 047M

Dilation *(continued)*
  Artery *(continued)*
    Posterior Tibial
      Left 047S
      Right 047R
    Pulmonary
      Left 027R
      Right 027Q
    Pulmonary Trunk 027P
    Radial
      Left 037C
      Right 037B
    Renal
      Left 047A
      Right 0479
    Splenic 0474
    Subclavian
      Left 0374
      Right 0373
    Superior Mesenteric 0475
    Temporal
      Left 037T
      Right 037S
    Thyroid
      Left 037V
      Right 037U
    Ulnar
      Left 037A
      Right 0379
    Upper 037Y
    Vertebral
      Left 037Q
      Right 037P
  Bladder 0T7B
  Bladder Neck 0T7C
  Bronchus
    Lingula 0B79
    Lower Lobe
      Left 0B7B
      Right 0B76
    Main
      Left 0B77
      Right 0B73
    Middle Lobe, Right 0B75
    Upper Lobe
      Left 0B78
      Right 0B74
  Carina 0B72
  Cecum 0D7H
  Cervix 0U7C
  Colon
    Ascending 0D7K
    Descending 0D7M
    Sigmoid 0D7N
    Transverse 0D7L
  Duct
    Common Bile 0F79
    Cystic 0F78
    Hepatic
      Left 0F76
      Right 0F75
    Lacrimal
      Left 087Y
      Right 087X
    Pancreatic 0F7D
      Accessory 0F7F
    Parotid
      Left 0C7C
      Right 0C7B
  Duodenum 0D79
  Esophagogastric Junction 0D74
  Esophagus 0D75
    Lower 0D73
    Middle 0D72
    Upper 0D71
  Eustachian Tube
    Left 097G
    Right 097F
  Fallopian Tube
    Left 0U76
    Right 0U75
  Fallopian Tubes, Bilateral 0U77

Dilation *(continued)*
  Hymen 0U7K
  Ileocecal Valve 0D7C
  Ileum 0D7B
  Intestine
    Large 0D7E
      Left 0D7G
      Right 0D7F
    Small 0D78
  Jejunum 0D7A
  Kidney Pelvis
    Left 0T74
    Right 0T73
  Larynx 0C7S
  Pharynx 0C7M
  Rectum 0D7P
  Stomach 0D76
    Pylorus 0D77
  Trachea 0B71
  Ureter
    Left 0T77
    Right 0T76
  Ureters, Bilateral 0T78
  Urethra 0T7D
  Uterus 0U79
  Vagina 0U7G
  Valve
    Aortic 027F
    Mitral 027G
    Pulmonary 027H
    Tricuspid 027J
  Vas Deferens
    Bilateral 0V7Q
    Left 0V7P
    Right 0V7N
  Vein
    Axillary
      Left 0578
      Right 0577
    Azygos 0570
    Basilic
      Left 057C
      Right 057B
    Brachial
      Left 057A
      Right 0579
    Cephalic
      Left 057F
      Right 057D
    Colic 0677
    Common Iliac
      Left 067D
      Right 067C
    Esophageal 0673
    External Iliac
      Left 067G
      Right 067F
    External Jugular
      Left 057Q
      Right 057P
    Face
      Left 057V
      Right 057T
    Femoral
      Left 067N
      Right 067M
    Foot
      Left 067V
      Right 067T
    Gastric 0672
    Greater Saphenous
      Left 067Q
      Right 067P
    Hand
      Left 057H
      Right 057G
    Hemiazygos 0571
    Hepatic 0674
    Hypogastric
      Left 067J
      Right 067H
    Inferior Mesenteric 0676

Dilation *(continued)*
  Vein *(continued)*
    Innominate
      Left 0574
      Right 0573
    Internal Jugular
      Left 057N
      Right 057M
    Intracranial 057L
    Lesser Saphenous
      Left 067S
      Right 067R
    Lower 067Y
    Portal 0678
    Pulmonary
      Left 027T
      Right 027S
    Renal
      Left 067B
      Right 0679
    Splenic 0671
    Subclavian
      Left 0576
      Right 0575
    Superior Mesenteric 0675
    Upper 057Y
    Vertebral
      Left 057S
      Right 057R
  Vena Cava
    Inferior 0670
    Superior 027V
  Ventricle, Right 027K
Direct Lateral Interbody Fusion (DLIF) device
  use Interbody Fusion Device in Lower Joints
Disarticulation
  see Detachment
Discectomy, diskectomy
  see Excision, Lower Joints 0SB
  see Excision, Upper Joints 0RB
  see Resection, Lower Joints 0ST
  see Resection, Upper Joints 0RT
Discography
  see Fluoroscopy, Axial Skeleton, Except Skull and Facial Bones BR1
  see Plain Radiography, Axial Skeleton, Except Skull and Facial Bones BR0
Distal humerus
  use Humeral Shaft, Left
  use Humeral Shaft, Right
Distal humerus, involving joint
  use Joint, Elbow, Left
  use Joint, Elbow, Right
Distal radioulnar joint
  use Joint, Wrist, Left
  use Joint, Wrist, Right
Diversion
  see Bypass
Diverticulectomy
  see Excision, Gastrointestinal System 0DB
Division
  Acetabulum
    Left 0Q85
    Right 0Q84
  Anal Sphincter 0D8R
  Basal Ganglia 0088
  Bladder Neck 0T8C
  Bone
    Ethmoid
      Left 0N8G
      Right 0N8F
    Frontal
      Left 0N82
      Right 0N81
    Hyoid 0N8X

Division *(continued)*
  Bone *(continued)*
    Lacrimal
      Left 0N8J
      Right 0N8H
    Nasal 0N8B
    Occipital
      Left 0N88
      Right 0N87
    Palatine
      Left 0N8L
      Right 0N8K
    Parietal
      Left 0N84
      Right 0N83
    Pelvic
      Left 0Q83
      Right 0Q82
    Sphenoid
      Left 0N8D
      Right 0N8C
    Temporal
      Left 0N86
      Right 0N85
    Zygomatic
      Left 0N8N
      Right 0N8M
  Brain 0080
  Bursa and Ligament
    Abdomen
      Left 0M8J
      Right 0M8H
    Ankle
      Left 0M8R
      Right 0M8Q
    Elbow
      Left 0M84
      Right 0M83
    Foot
      Left 0M8T
      Right 0M8S
    Hand
      Left 0M88
      Right 0M87
    Head and Neck 0M80
    Hip
      Left 0M8M
      Right 0M8L
    Knee
      Left 0M8P
      Right 0M8N
    Lower Extremity
      Left 0M8W
      Right 0M8V
    Perineum 0M8K
    Shoulder
      Left 0M82
      Right 0M81
    Thorax
      Left 0M8G
      Right 0M8F
    Trunk
      Left 0M8D
      Right 0M8C
    Upper Extremity
      Left 0M8B
      Right 0M89
    Wrist
      Left 0M86
      Right 0M85
  Carpal
    Left 0P8N
    Right 0P8M
  Cerebral Hemisphere 0087
  Chordae Tendineae 0289
  Clavicle
    Left 0P8B
    Right 0P89
  Coccyx 0Q8S
  Conduction Mechanism 0288
  Esophagogastric Junction 0D84

Division *(continued)*
Femoral Shaft
    Left 0Q89
    Right 0Q88
Femur
    Lower
        Left 0Q8C
        Right 0Q8B
    Upper
        Left 0Q87
        Right 0Q86
Fibula
    Left 0Q8K
    Right 0Q8J
Gland, Pituitary 0G80
Glenoid Cavity
    Left 0P88
    Right 0P87
Humeral Head
    Left 0P8D
    Right 0P8C
Humeral Shaft
    Left 0P8G
    Right 0P8F
Hymen 0U8K
Kidneys, Bilateral 0T82
Mandible
    Left 0N8V
    Right 0N8T
Maxilla
    Left 0N8S
    Right 0N8R
Metacarpal
    Left 0P8Q
    Right 0P8P
Metatarsal
    Left 0Q8P
    Right 0Q8N
Muscle
    Abdomen
        Left 0K8L
        Right 0K8K
    Facial 0K81
    Foot
        Left 0K8W
        Right 0K8V
    Hand
        Left 0K8D
        Right 0K8C
    Head 0K80
    Hip
        Left 0K8P
        Right 0K8N
    Lower Arm and Wrist
        Left 0K8B
        Right 0K89
    Lower Leg
        Left 0K8T
        Right 0K8S
    Neck
        Left 0K83
        Right 0K82
    Papillary 028D
    Perineum 0K8M
    Shoulder
        Left 0K86
        Right 0K85
    Thorax
        Left 0K8J
        Right 0K8H
    Tongue, Palate, Pharynx 0K84
    Trunk
        Left 0K8G
        Right 0K8F
    Upper Arm
        Left 0K88
        Right 0K87
    Upper Leg
        Left 0K8R
        Right 0K8Q
Nerve
    Abdominal Sympathetic 018M

Division *(continued)*
Nerve *(continued)*
    Abducens 008L
    Accessory 008R
    Acoustic 008N
    Brachial Plexus 0183
    Cervical 0181
    Cervical Plexus 0180
    Facial 008M
    Femoral 018D
    Glossopharyngeal 008P
    Head and Neck Sympathetic
        018K
    Hypoglossal 008S
    Lumbar 018B
    Lumbar Plexus 0189
    Lumbar Sympathetic 018N
    Lumbosacral Plexus 018A
    Median 0185
    Oculomotor 008H
    Olfactory 008F
    Optic 008G
    Peroneal 018H
    Phrenic 0182
    Pudendal 018C
    Radial 0186
    Sacral 018R
    Sacral Plexus 018Q
    Sacral Sympathetic 018P
    Sciatic 018F
    Thoracic 0188
    Thoracic Sympathetic 018L
    Tibial 018G
    Trigeminal 008K
    Trochlear 008J
    Ulnar 0184
    Vagus 008Q
Orbit
    Left 0N8Q
    Right 0N8P
Ovary
    Bilateral 0U82
    Left 0U81
    Right 0U80
Pancreas 0F8G
Patella
    Left 0Q8F
    Right 0Q8D
Perineum, Female 0W8NXZZ
Phalanx
    Finger
        Left 0P8V
        Right 0P8T
    Thumb
        Left 0P8S
        Right 0P8R
    Toe
        Left 0Q8R
        Right 0Q8Q
Radius
    Left 0P8J
    Right 0P8H
Rib
    Left 0P82
    Right 0P81
Sacrum 0Q81
Scapula
    Left 0P86
    Right 0P85
Skin
    Abdomen 0H87XZZ
    Back 0H86XZZ
    Buttock 0H88XZZ
    Chest 0H85XZZ
    Ear
        Left 0H83XZZ
        Right 0H82XZZ
    Face 0H81XZZ
    Foot
        Left 0H8NXZZ
        Right 0H8MXZZ
    Genitalia 0H8AXZZ

Division *(continued)*
Skin *(continued)*
    Hand
        Left 0H8GXZZ
        Right 0H8FXZZ
    Lower Arm
        Left 0H8EXZZ
        Right 0H8DXZZ
    Lower Leg
        Left 0H8LXZZ
        Right 0H8KXZZ
    Neck 0H84XZZ
    Perineum 0H89XZZ
    Scalp 0H80XZZ
    Upper Arm
        Left 0H8CXZZ
        Right 0H8BXZZ
    Upper Leg
        Left 0H8JXZZ
        Right 0H8HXZZ
Skull 0N80
Spinal Cord
    Cervical 008W
    Lumbar 008Y
    Thoracic 008X
Sternum 0P80
Stomach, Pylorus 0D87
Subcutaneous Tissue and
    Fascia
    Abdomen 0J88
    Back 0J87
    Buttock 0J89
    Chest 0J86
    Face 0J81
    Foot
        Left 0J8R
        Right 0J8Q
    Hand
        Left 0J8K
        Right 0J8J
    Head and Neck 0J8S
    Lower Arm
        Left 0J8H
        Right 0J8G
    Lower Extremity 0J8W
    Lower Leg
        Left 0J8P
        Right 0J8N
    Neck
        Anterior 0J84
        Posterior 0J85
    Pelvic Region 0J8C
    Perineum 0J8B
    Scalp 0J80
    Trunk 0J8T
    Upper Arm
        Left 0J8F
        Right 0J8D
    Upper Extremity 0J8V
    Upper Leg
        Left 0J8M
        Right 0J8L
Tarsal
    Left 0Q8M
    Right 0Q8L
Tendon
    Abdomen
        Left 0L8G
        Right 0L8F
    Ankle
        Left 0L8T
        Right 0L8S
    Foot
        Left 0L8W
        Right 0L8V
    Hand
        Left 0L88
        Right 0L87
    Head and Neck 0L80
    Hip
        Left 0L8K
        Right 0L8J

Division *(continued)*
Tendon *(continued)*
    Knee
        Left 0L8R
        Right 0L8Q
    Lower Arm and Wrist
        Left 0L86
        Right 0L85
    Lower Leg
        Left 0L8P
        Right 0L8N
    Perineum 0L8H
    Shoulder
        Left 0L82
        Right 0L81
    Thorax
        Left 0L8D
        Right 0L8C
    Trunk
        Left 0L8B
        Right 0L89
    Upper Arm
        Left 0L84
        Right 0L83
    Upper Leg
        Left 0L8M
        Right 0L8L
Thyroid Gland Isthmus 0G8J
Tibia
    Left 0Q8H
    Right 0Q8G
Turbinate, Nasal 098L
Ulna
    Left 0P8L
    Right 0P8K
Uterine Supporting Structure
    0U84
Vertebra
    Cervical 0P83
    Lumbar 0Q80
    Thoracic 0P84
Doppler study
    see Ultrasonography
Dorsal digital nerve
    use Nerve, Radial
Dorsal metacarpal vein
    use Vein, Hand, Left
    use Vein, Hand, Right
Dorsal metatarsal artery
    use Artery, Foot, Left
    use Artery, Foot, Right
Dorsal metatarsal vein
    use Vein, Foot, Left
    use Vein, Foot, Right
Dorsal scapular artery
    use Artery, Subclavian, Left
    use Artery, Subclavian, Right
Dorsal scapular nerve
    use Nerve, Brachial Plexus
Dorsal venous arch
    use Vein, Foot, Left
    use Vein, Foot, Right
Dorsalis pedis artery
    use Artery, Anterior Tibial,
        Left
    use Artery, Anterior Tibial,
        Right
Drainage
    Abdominal Wall 0W9F
    Acetabulum
        Left 0Q95
        Right 0Q94
    Adenoids 0C9Q
    Ampulla of Vater 0F9C
    Anal Sphincter 0D9R
    Ankle Region
        Left 0Y9L
        Right 0Y9K
    Anterior Chamber
        Left 0893
        Right 0892
    Anus 0D9Q

Drainage *(continued)*

Palate
    Hard 0C92
    Soft 0C93
Pancreas 0F9G
Para-aortic Body 0G99
Paraganglion Extremity 0G9F
Parathyroid Gland 0G9R
    Inferior
        Left 0G9P
        Right 0G9N
    Multiple 0G9Q
    Superior
        Left 0G9M
        Right 0G9L
Patella
    Left 0Q9F
    Right 0Q9D
Pelvic Cavity 0W9J
Penis 0V9S
Pericardial Cavity 0W9D
Perineum
    Female 0W9N
    Male 0W9M
Peritoneal Cavity 0W9G
Peritoneum 0D9W
Phalanx
    Finger
        Left 0P9V
        Right 0P9T
    Thumb
        Left 0P9S
        Right 0P9R
    Toe
        Left 0Q9R
        Right 0Q9Q
Pharynx 0C9M
Pineal Body 0G91
Pleura
    Left 0B9P
    Right 0B9N
Pleural Cavity
    Left 0W9B
    Right 0W99
Pons 009B
Prepuce 0V9T
Products of Conception
    Amniotic Fluid
        Diagnostic 1090
        Therapeutic 1090
    Fetal Blood 1090
    Fetal Cerebrospinal Fluid
        1090
    Fetal Fluid, Other 1090
    Fluid, Other 1090
Prostate 0V90
Radius
    Left 0P9J
    Right 0P9H
Rectum 0D9P
Retina
    Left 089F
    Right 089E
Retinal Vessel
    Left 089H
    Right 089G
Retroperitoneum 0W9H
Rib
    Left 0P92
    Right 0P91
Sacrum 0Q91
Scapula
    Left 0P96
    Right 0P95
Sclera
    Left 0897
    Right 0896
Scrotum 0V95
Septum, Nasal 099M
Shoulder Region
    Left 0X93
    Right 0X92

Drainage *(continued)*

Sinus
    Accessory 099P
    Ethmoid
        Left 099V
        Right 099U
    Frontal
        Left 099T
        Right 099S
    Mastoid
        Left 099C
        Right 099B
    Maxillary
        Left 099R
        Right 099Q
    Sphenoid
        Left 099X
        Right 099W
Skin
    Abdomen 0H97
    Back 0H96
    Buttock 0H98
    Chest 0H95
    Ear
        Left 0H93
        Right 0H92
    Face 0H91
    Foot
        Left 0H9N
        Right 0H9M
    Genitalia 0H9A
    Hand
        Left 0H9G
        Right 0H9F
    Lower Arm
        Left 0H9E
        Right 0H9D
    Lower Leg
        Left 0H9L
        Right 0H9K
    Neck 0H94
    Perineum 0H99
    Scalp 0H90
    Upper Arm
        Left 0H9C
        Right 0H9B
    Upper Leg
        Left 0H9J
        Right 0H9H
Skull 0N90
Spinal Canal 009U
Spinal Cord
    Cervical 009W
    Lumbar 009Y
    Thoracic 009X
Spinal Meninges 009T
Spleen 079P
Sternum 0P90
Stomach 0D96
    Pylorus 0D97
Subarachnoid Space 0095
Subcutaneous Tissue and Fascia
    Abdomen 0J98
    Back 0J97
    Buttock 0J99
    Chest 0J96
    Face 0J91
    Foot
        Left 0J9R
        Right 0J9Q
    Hand
        Left 0J9K
        Right 0J9J
    Lower Arm
        Left 0J9H
        Right 0J9G
    Lower Leg
        Left 0J9P
        Right 0J9N
    Neck
        Anterior 0J94
        Posterior 0J95

Drainage *(continued)*

Subcutaneous Tissue and
    Fascia *(continued)*
    Pelvic Region 0J9C
    Perineum 0J9B
    Scalp 0J90
    Upper Arm
        Left 0J9F
        Right 0J9D
    Upper Leg
        Left 0J9M
        Right 0J9L
Subdural Space 0094
Tarsal
    Left 0Q9M
    Right 0Q9L
Tendon
    Abdomen
        Left 0L9G
        Right 0L9F
    Ankle
        Left 0L9T
        Right 0L9S
    Foot
        Left 0L9W
        Right 0L9V
    Hand
        Left 0L98
        Right 0L97
    Head and Neck 0L90
    Hip
        Left 0L9K
        Right 0L9J
    Knee
        Left 0L9R
        Right 0L9Q
    Lower Arm and Wrist
        Left 0L96
        Right 0L95
    Lower Leg
        Left 0L9P
        Right 0L9N
    Perineum 0L9H
    Shoulder
        Left 0L92
        Right 0L91
    Thorax
        Left 0L9D
        Right 0L9C
    Electrocautery
        Right 0L99
    Upper Arm
        Left 0L94
        Right 0L93
    Upper Leg
        Left 0L9M
        Right 0L9L
Testis
    Bilateral 0V9C
    Left 0V9B
    Right 0V99
Thalamus 0099
Thymus 079M
Thyroid Gland 0G9K
    Left Lobe 0G9G
    Right Lobe 0G9H
Tibia
    Left 0Q9H
    Right 0Q9G
Toe Nail 0H9R
Tongue 0C97
Tonsils 0C9P
Tooth
    Lower 0C9X
    Upper 0C9W
Trachea 0B91
Tunica Vaginalis
    Left 0V97
    Right 0V96
Turbinate, Nasal 099L
Tympanic Membrane
    Left 0998

Drainage *(continued)*

Tympanic Membrane *(continued)*
    Right 0997
Ulna
    Left 0P9L
    Right 0P9K
Ureter
    Left 0T97
    Right 0T96
Ureters, Bilateral 0T98
Urethra 0T9D
Uterine Supporting Structure 0U94
Uterus 0U99
Uvula 0C9N
Vagina 0U9G
Vas Deferens
    Bilateral 0V9Q
    Left 0V9P
    Right 0V9N
Vein
    Axillary
        Left 0598
        Right 0597
    Azygos 0590
    Basilic
        Left 059C
        Right 059B
    Brachial
        Left 059A
        Right 0599
    Cephalic
        Left 059F
        Right 059D
    Colic 0697
    Common Iliac
        Left 069D
        Right 069C
    Esophageal 0693
    External Iliac
        Left 069G
        Right 069F
    External Jugular
        Left 059Q
        Right 059P
    Face
        Left 059V
        Right 059T
    Femoral
        Left 069N
        Right 069M
    Foot
        Left 069V
        Right 069T
    Gastric 0692
    Greater Saphenous
        Left 069Q
        Right 069P
    Hand
        Left 059H
        Right 059G
    Hemiazygos 0591
    Hepatic 0694
    Hypogastric
        Left 069J
        Right 069H
    Inferior Mesenteric 0696
    Innominate
        Left 0594
        Right 0593
    Internal Jugular
        Left 059N
        Right 059M
    Intracranial 059L
    Lesser Saphenous
        Left 069S
        Right 069R
    Lower 069Y
    Portal 0698
    Renal
        Left 069B
        Right 0699
    Splenic 0691

Drainage *(continued)*
  Vein *(continued)*
    Subclavian
      Left 0596
      Right 0595
    Superior Mesenteric 0695
    Upper 059Y
    Vertebral
      Left 059S
      Right 059R
    Vena Cava, Inferior 0690
    Vertebra
      Cervical 0P93
      Lumbar 0Q90
      Thoracic 0P94
    Vesicle
      Bilateral 0V93
      Left 0V92
      Right 0V91
    Vitreous
      Left 0895
      Right 0894
    Vocal Cord
      Left 0C9V
      Right 0C9T
    Vulva 0U9M
    Wrist Region
      Left 0X9H
      Right 0X9G
Dressing
  Abdominal Wall 2W23X4Z
  Arm
    Lower
      Left 2W2DX4Z
      Right 2W2CX4Z
    Upper
      Left 2W2BX4Z
      Right 2W2AX4Z
  Back 2W25X4Z
  Chest Wall 2W24X4Z
  Extremity
    Lower
      Left 2W2MX4Z
      Right 2W2LX4Z
    Upper
      Left 2W29X4Z
      Right 2W28X4Z
  Face 2W21X4Z
  Finger
    Left 2W2KX4Z
    Right 2W2JX4Z
  Foot
    Left 2W2TX4Z
    Right 2W2SX4Z
  Hand
    Left 2W2FX4Z
    Right 2W2EX4Z
  Head 2W20X4Z
  Inguinal Region
    Left 2W27X4Z
    Right 2W26X4Z
  Leg
    Lower
      Left 2W2RX4Z
      Right 2W2QX4Z
    Upper
      Left 2W2PX4Z
      Right 2W2NX4Z
  Neck 2W22X4Z
  Thumb
    Left 2W2HX4Z
    Right 2W2GX4Z
  Toe
    Left 2W2VX4Z
    Right 2W2UX4Z
Driver stent (RX) (OTW)
  use Intraluminal Device
Drotrecogin alfa
  see Introduction of Recombinant
    Human-activated Protein C
Duct of Santorini
  use Duct, Pancreatic, Accessory

Duct of Wirsung
  use Duct, Pancreatic
Ductogram, mammary
  see Plain Radiography, Skin,
    Subcutaneous Tissue and
    Breast BH0
Ductography, mammary
  see Plain Radiography, Skin,
    Subcutaneous Tissue and Breast
    BH0
Ductus deferens
  use Vas Deferens
  use Vas Deferens, Bilateral
  use Vas Deferens, Left
  use Vas Deferens, Right
Duodenal ampulla
  use Ampulla of Vater
Duodenectomy
  see Excision, Duodenum 0DB9
  see Resection, Duodenum 0DT9
Duodenocholedochotomy
  see Drainage, Gallbladder 0F94
Duodenocystostomy
  see Bypass, Gallbladder 0F14
  see Drainage, Gallbladder 0F94
Duodenoenterostomy
  see Bypass, Gastrointestinal System
    0D1
  see Drainage, Gastrointestinal
    System 0D9
Duodenojejunal flexure
  use Jejunum
Duodenolysis
  see Release, Duodenum 0DN9
Duodenorrhaphy
  see Repair, Duodenum 0DQ9
Duodenostomy
  see Bypass, Duodenum 0D19
  see Drainage, Duodenum 0D99
Duodenotomy
  see Drainage, Duodenum 0D99
DuraHeart Left Ventricular Assist
    System
  use Implantable Heart Assist System
    in Heart and Great Vessels
Dural venous sinus
  use Vein, Intracranial
Dura mater, intracranial
  use Dura Mater
Dura mater, spinal
  use Spinal Meninges
Durata® Defibrillation Lead
  use Cardiac Lead, Defibrillator in 02H
Dynesys® Dynamic Stabilization
    System
  use Spinal Stabilization Device,
    Pedicle-Based in 0RH
  use Spinal Stabilization Device,
    Pedicle-Based in 0SH

E

E-Luminexx™ (Biliary)(Vascular)
    Stent
  use Intraluminal Device
Earlobe
  use Ear, External, Bilateral
  use Ear, External, Left
  use Ear, External, Right
Echocardiogram
  see Ultrasonography, Heart B24
Echography
  see Ultrasonography
ECMO
  see Performance, Circulatory 5A15
EEG (electroencephalogram)
  see Measurement, Central Nervous
    4A00
EGD (esophagog astroduodenscopy)
    0DJ08ZZ
Eighth cranial nerve
  use Nerve, Acoustic

Ejaculatory duct
  use Vas Deferens
  use Vas Deferens, Bilateral
  use Vas Deferens, Left
  use Vas Deferens, Right
EKG (electrocardiogram)
  see Measurement, Cardiac 4A02
Electrical bone growth stimulator
    (EBGS)
  use Bone Growth Stimulator in
    Head and Facial Bones
  use Bone Growth Stimulator in
    Lower Bones
  use Bone Growth Stimulator in
    Upper Bones
Electrical muscle stimulation (EMS)
    lead
  use Stimulator Lead in Muscles
Electrocautery
  Destruction
    see Destruction
  Repair
    see Repair
Electroconvulsive Therapy
  Bilateral-Multiple Seizure
    GZB3ZZZ
  Bilateral-Single Seizure GZB2ZZZ
  Electroconvulsive Therapy, Other
    GZB4ZZZ
  Unilateral-Multiple Seizure
    GZB1ZZZ
  Unilateral-Single Seizure GZB0ZZZ
Electroencephalogram (EEG)
  see Measurement, Central Nervous
    4A00
Electromagnetic Therapy
  Central Nervous 6A22
  Urinary 6A21
Electronic muscle stimulator lead
  use Stimulator Lead in Muscles
Electrophysiologic stimulation (EPS)
  see Measurement, Cardiac 4A02
Electroshock therapy
  see Electroconvulsive Therapy
Elevation, bone fragments, skull
  see Reposition, Head and Facial
    Bones 0NS
Eleventh cranial nerve
  use Nerve, Accessory
Embolectomy
  see Extirpation
Embolization
  see Occlusion
  see Restriction
Embolization coil(s)
  use Intraluminal Device
EMG (electromyogram)
  see Measurement, Musculoskeletal
    4A0F
Encephalon
  use Brain
Endarterectomy
  see Extirpation, Lower Arteries 04C
  see Extirpation, Upper Arteries 03C
Endeavor® (III)(IV) (Sprint)
    Zotarolimus-eluting Coronary
    Stent System
  use Intraluminal Device, Drug-
    eluting in Heart and Great
    Vessels
EndoSure® sensor
  use Monitoring Device, Pressure
    Sensor in 02H
ENDOTAK RELIANCE® (G)
    Defibrillation Lead
  use Cardiac Lead, Defibrillator in
    02H
Endotracheal tube (cuffed)(double-
    lumen)
  use Intraluminal Device,
    Endotracheal Airway in
    Respiratory System

Endurant® Endovascular Stent Graft
  use Intraluminal Device
Enlargement
  see Dilation
  see Repair
EnRhythm
  use Pacemaker, Dual Chamber in 0JH
Enterorrhaphy
  see Repair, Gastrointestinal System
    0DQ
Enterra gastric neurostimulator
  use Stimulator Generator, Multiple
    Array in 0JH
Enucleation
  Eyeball
    see Resection, Eye 08T
  Eyeball with prosthetic implant
    see Replacement, Eye 08R
Ependyma
  use Cerebral Ventricle
Epicel® cultured epidermal autograft
  use Autologous Tissue Substitute
Epic™ Stented Tissue Valve (aortic)
  use Zooplastic Tissue in Heart and
    Great Vessels
Epidermis
  use Skin
Epididymectomy
  see Excision, Male Reproductive
    System 0VB
  see Resection, Male Reproductive
    System 0VT
Epididymoplasty
  see Repair, Male Reproductive
    System 0VQ
  see Supplement, Male Reproductive
    System 0VU
Epididymorrhaphy
  see Repair, Male Reproductive
    System 0VQ
Epididymotomy
  see Drainage, Male Reproductive
    System 0V9
Epidural space, intracranial
  use Epidural Space
Epidural space, spinal
  use Spinal Canal
Epiphysiodesis
  see Fusion, Lower Joints 0SG
  see Fusion, Upper Joints 0RG
Epiploic foramen
  use Peritoneum
Epiretinal Visual Prosthesis
  Left 08H105Z
  Right 08H005Z
Episiorrhaphy
  see Repair, Perineum, Female
    0WQN
Episiotomy
  see Division, Perineum, Female
    0W8N
Epithalamus
  use Thalamus
Epitrochlear lymph node
  use Lymphatic, Upper Extremity,
    Left
  use Lymphatic, Upper Extremity,
    Right
EPS (electrophysiologic stimulation)
  see Measurement, Cardiac 4A02
Eptifibatide, infusion
  see Introduction of Platelet
    Inhibitor
ERCP (endoscopic retrograde
    cholangiopancreatography)
  see Fluoroscopy, Hepatobiliary
    System and Pancreas BF1
Erector spinae muscle
  use Muscle, Trunk, Left
  use Muscle, Trunk, Right
Esophageal artery
  use Aorta, Thoracic

Esophageal obturator airway (EOA)
  use Intraluminal Device, Airway in
    Gastrointestinal System
Esophageal plexus
  use Nerve, Thoracic Sympathetic
Esophagectomy
  see Excision, Gastrointestinal
    System 0DB
  see Resection, Gastrointestinal
    System 0DT
Esophagocoloplasty
  see Repair, Gastrointestinal System
    0DQ
  see Supplement, Gastrointestinal
    System 0DU
Esophagoenterostomy
  see Bypass, Gastrointestinal System
    0D1
  see Drainage, Gastrointestinal
    System 0D9
Esophagoesophagostomy
  see Bypass, Gastrointestinal System
    0D1
  see Drainage, Gastrointestinal
    System 0D9
Esophagogastrectomy
  see Excision, Gastrointestinal
    System 0DB
  see Resection, Gastrointestinal
    System 0DT
Esophagogastroduodenoscopy (EGD)
    0DJ08ZZ
Esophagogastroplasty
  see Repair, Gastrointestinal System
    0DQ
  see Supplement, Gastrointestinal
    System 0DU
Esophagogastroscopy 0DJ68ZZ
Esophagogastrostomy
  see Bypass, Gastrointestinal System
    0D1
  see Drainage, Gastrointestinal
    System 0D9
Esophagojejunoplasty
  see Supplement, Gastrointestinal
    System 0DU
Esophagojejunostomy
  see Bypass, Gastrointestinal System
    0D1
  see Drainage, Gastrointestinal
    System 0D9
Esophagomyotomy
  see Division, Esophagogastric
    Junction 0D84
Esophagoplasty
  see Repair, Gastrointestinal System
    0DQ
  see Replacement, Esophagus 0DR5
  see Supplement, Gastrointestinal
    System 0DU
Esophagoplication
  see Restriction, Gastrointestinal
    System 0DV
Esophagorrhaphy
  see Repair, Gastrointestinal System
    0DQ
Esophagoscopy 0DJ08ZZ
Esophagotomy
  see Drainage, Gastrointestinal
    System 0D9
Esteem® implantable hearing system
  use Hearing Device in Ear, Nose, Sinus
**ESWL (extracorporeal shock wave
    lithotripsy)**
  see Fragmentation
Ethmoidal air cell
  use Sinus, Ethmoid, Left
  use Sinus, Ethmoid, Right
Ethmoidectomy
  see Excision, Ear, Nose, Sinus 09B
  see Excision, Head and Facial Bones
    0NB

Ethmoidectomy *(continued)*
  see Resection, Ear, Nose,
    Sinus 09T
  see Resection, Head and Facial
    Bones 0NT
Ethmoidotomy
  see Drainage, Ear, Nose, Sinus 099
Evacuation
  Hematoma
    see Extirpation
  Other Fluid
    see Drainage
Evera (XT)(S)(DR/VR)
  use Defibrillator Generator in 0JH
Everolimus-eluting coronary stent
  use Intraluminal Device, Drug-
    eluting in Heart and Great
    Vessels
Evisceration
  Eyeball
    see Resection, Eye 08T
  Eyeball with prosthetic implant
    see Replacement, Eye 08R
**Ex-PRESS™ mini glaucoma
    shunt**
  use Synthetic Substitute
Examination
  see Inspection
Exchange
  see Change device in
Excision
  Abdominal Wall 0WBF
  Acetabulum
    Left 0QB5
    Right 0QB4
  Adenoids 0CBQ
  Ampulla of Vater 0FBC
  Anal Sphincter 0DBR
  Ankle Region
    Left 0YBL
    Right 0YBK
  Anus 0DBQ
  Aorta
    Abdominal 04B0
    Thoracic 02BW
  Aortic Body 0GBD
  Appendix 0DBJ
  Arm
    Lower
      Left 0XBF
      Right 0XBD
    Upper
      Left 0XB9
      Right 0XB8
  Artery
    Anterior Tibial
      Left 04BQ
      Right 04BP
    Axillary
      Left 03B6
      Right 03B5
    Brachial
      Left 03B8
      Right 03B7
    Celiac 04B1
    Colic
      Left 04B7
      Middle 04B8
      Right 04B6
    Common Carotid
      Left 03BJ
      Right 03BH
    Common Iliac
      Left 04BD
      Right 04BC
    External Carotid
      Left 03BN
      Right 03BM
    External Iliac
      Left 04BJ
      Right 04BH
    Face 03BR

Excision *(continued)*
  Artery *(continued)*
    Femoral
      Left 04BL
      Right 04BK
    Foot
      Left 04BW
      Right 04BV
    Gastric 04B2
    Hand
      Left 03BF
      Right 03BD
    Hepatic 04B3
    Inferior Mesenteric 04BB
    Innominate 03B2
    Internal Carotid
      Left 03BL
      Right 03BK
    Internal Iliac
      Left 04BF
      Right 04BE
    Internal Mammary
      Left 03B1
      Right 03B0
    Intracranial 03BG
    Lower 04BY
    Peroneal
      Left 04BU
      Right 04BT
    Popliteal
      Left 04BN
      Right 04BM
    Posterior Tibial
      Left 04BS
      Right 04BR
    Pulmonary
      Left 02BR
      Right 02BQ
    Pulmonary Trunk 02BP
    Radial
      Left 03BC
      Right 03BB
    Renal
      Left 04BA
      Right 04B9
    Splenic 04B4
    Subclavian
      Left 03B4
      Right 03B3
    Superior Mesenteric 04B5
    Temporal
      Left 03BT
      Right 03BS
    Thyroid
      Left 03BV
      Right 03BU
    Ulnar
      Left 03BA
      Right 03B9
    Upper 03BY
    Vertebral
      Left 03BQ
      Right 03BP
  Atrium
    Left 02B7
    Right 02B6
  Auditory Ossicle
    Left 09BA0Z
    Right 09B90Z
  Axilla
    Left 0XB5
    Right 0XB4
  Back
    Lower 0WBL
    Upper 0WBK
  Basal Ganglia 00B8
  Bladder 0TBB
  Bladder Neck 0TBC
  Bone
    Ethmoid
      Left 0NBG
      Right 0NBF

Excision *(continued)*
  Bone *(continued)*
    Frontal
      Left 0NB2
      Right 0NB1
    Hyoid 0NBX
    Lacrimal
      Left 0NBJ
      Right 0NBH
    Nasal 0NBB
    Occipital
      Left 0NB8
      Right 0NB7
    Palatine
      Left 0NBL
      Right 0NBK
    Parietal
      Left 0NB4
      Right 0NB3
    Pelvic
      Left 0QB3
      Right 0QB2
    Sphenoid
      Left 0NBD
      Right 0NBC
    Temporal
      Left 0NB6
      Right 0NB5
    Zygomatic
      Left 0NBN
      Right 0NBM
  Brain 00B0
  Breast
    Bilateral 0HBV
    Left 0HBU
    Right 0HBT
    Supernumerary 0HBY
  Bronchus
    Lingula 0BB9
    Lower Lobe
      Left 0BBB
      Right 0BB6
    Main
      Left 0BB7
      Right 0BB3
    Middle Lobe, Right
      0BB5
    Upper Lobe
      Left 0BB8
      Right 0BB4
  Buccal Mucosa 0CB4
  Bursa and Ligament
    Abdomen
      Left 0MBJ
      Right 0MBH
    Ankle
      Left 0MBR
      Right 0MBQ
    Elbow
      Left 0MB4
      Right 0MB3
    Foot
      Left 0MBT
      Right 0MBS
    Hand
      Left 0MB8
      Right 0MB7
    Head and Neck
      0MB0
    Hip
      Left 0MBM
      Right 0MBL
    Knee
      Left 0MBP
      Right 0MBN
    Lower Extremity
      Left 0MBW
      Right 0MBV
    Perineum 0MBK
    Shoulder
      Left 0MB2
      Right 0MB1

Bursa and Ligament
(continued)
Thorax
Left 0MBG
Right 0MBF
Trunk
Left 0MBD
Right 0MBC
Upper Extremity
Left 0MBB
Right 0MB9
Wrist
Left 0MB6
Right 0MB5
Buttock
Left 0YB1
Right 0YB0
Carina 0BB2
Carotid Bodies, Bilateral 0GB8
Carotid Body
Left 0GB6
Right 0GB7
Carpal
Left 0PBN
Right 0PBM
Cecum 0DBH
Cerebellum 00BC
Cerebral Hemisphere 00B7
Cerebral Meninges 00B1
Cerebral Ventricle 00B6
Cervix 0UBC
Chest Wall 0WB8
Chordae Tendineae 02B9
Choroid
Left 08BB
Right 08BA
Cisterna Chyli 07BL
Clavicle
Left 0PBB
Right 0PB9
Clitoris 0UBJ
Coccygeal Glomus 0GBB
Coccyx 0QBS
Colon
Ascending 0DBK
Descending 0DBM
Sigmoid 0DBN
Transverse 0DBL
Conduction Mechanism 02B8
Conjunctiva
Left 08BTXZ
Right 08BSXZ
Cord
Bilateral 0VBH
Left 0VBG
Right 0VBF
Cornea
Left 08B9XZ
Right 08B8XZ
Cul-de-sac 0UBF
Diaphragm
Left 0BBS
Right 0BBR
Disc
Cervical Vertebral 0RB3
Cervicothoracic Vertebral
0RB5
Lumbar Vertebral 0SB2
Lumbosacral 0SB4
Thoracic Vertebral 0RB9
Thoracolumbar Vertebral
0RBB
Duct
Common Bile 0FB9
Cystic 0FB8
Hepatic
Left 0FB6
Right 0FB5
Lacrimal
Left 08BY
Right 08BX

Duct *(continued)*
Pancreatic 0FBD
Accessory 0FBF
Parotid
Left 0CBC
Right 0CBB
Duodenum 0DB9
Dura Mater 00B2
Ear
External
Left 09B1
Right 09B0
External Auditory Canal
Left 09B4
Right 09B3
Inner
Left 09BE0Z
Right 09BD0Z
Middle
Left 09B60Z
Right 09B50Z
Elbow Region
Left 0XBC
Right 0XBB
Epididymis
Bilateral 0VBL
Left 0VBK
Right 0VBJ
Epiglottis 0CBR
Esophagogastric Junction
0DB4
Esophagus 0DB5
Lower 0DB3
Middle 0DB2
Upper 0DB1
Eustachian Tube
Left 09BG
Right 09BF
Extremity
Lower
Left 0YBB
Right 0YB9
Upper
Left 0XB7
Right 0XB6
Eye
Left 08B1
Right 08B0
Eyelid
Lower
Left 08BR
Right 08BQ
Upper
Left 08BP
Right 08BN
Face 0WB2
Fallopian Tube
Left 0UB6
Right 0UB5
Fallopian Tubes, Bilateral 0UB7
Femoral Region
Left 0YB8
Right 0YB7
Femoral Shaft
Left 0QB9
Right 0QB8
Femur
Lower
Left 0QBC
Right 0QBB
Upper
Left 0QB7
Right 0QB6
Fibula
Left 0QBK
Right 0QBJ
Finger Nail 0HBQXZ
Foot
Left 0YBN
Right 0YBM
Gallbladder 0FB4

Gingiva
Lower 0CB6
Upper 0CB5
Gland
Adrenal
Bilateral 0GB4
Left 0GB2
Right 0GB3
Lacrimal
Left 08BW
Right 08BV
Minor Salivary 0CBJ
Parotid
Left 0CB9
Right 0CB8
Pituitary 0GB0
Sublingual
Left 0CBF
Right 0CBD
Submaxillary
Left 0CBH
Right 0CBG
Vestibular 0UBL
Glenoid Cavity
Left 0PB8
Right 0PB7
Glomus Jugulare 0GBC
Hand
Left 0XBK
Right 0XBJ
Head 0WB0
Humeral Head
Left 0PBD
Right 0PBC
Humeral Shaft
Left 0PBG
Right 0PBF
Hymen 0UBK
Hypothalamus 00BA
Ileocecal Valve 0DBC
Ileum 0DBB
Inguinal Region
Left 0YB6
Right 0YB5
Intestine
Large 0DBE
Left 0DBG
Right 0DBF
Small 0DB8
Iris
Left 08BD3Z
Right 08BC3Z
Jaw
Lower 0WB5
Upper 0WB4
Jejunum 0DBA
Joint
Acromioclavicular
Left 0RBH
Right 0RBG
Ankle
Left 0SBG
Right 0SBF
Carpal
Left 0RBR
Right 0RBQ
Cervical Vertebral 0RB1
Cervicothoracic Vertebral 0RB4
Coccygeal 0SB6
Elbow
Left 0RBM
Right 0RBL
Finger Phalangeal
Left 0RBX
Right 0RBW
Hip
Left 0SBB
Right 0SB9
Knee
Left 0SBD
Right 0SBC

Joint *(continued)*
Lumbar Vertebral 0SB0
Lumbosacral 0SB3
Metacarpocarpal
Left 0RBT
Right 0RBS
Metacarpophalangeal
Left 0RBV
Right 0RBU
Metatarsal-Phalangeal
Left 0SBN
Right 0SBM
Metatarsal-Tarsal
Left 0SBL
Right 0SBK
Occipital-cervical 0RB0
Sacrococcygeal 0SB5
Sacroiliac
Left 0SB8
Right 0SB7
Shoulder
Left 0RBK
Right 0RBJ
Sternoclavicular
Left 0RBF
Right 0RBE
Tarsal
Left 0SBJ
Right 0SBH
Temporomandibular
Left 0RBD
Right 0RBC
Thoracic Vertebral 0RB6
Thoracolumbar Vertebral
0RBA
Toe Phalangeal
Left 0SBQ
Right 0SBP
Wrist
Left 0RBP
Right 0RBN
Kidney
Left 0TB1
Right 0TB0
Kidney Pelvis
Left 0TB4
Right 0TB3
Knee Region
Left 0YBG
Right 0YBF
Larynx 0CBS
Leg
Lower
Left 0YBJ
Right 0YBH
Upper
Left 0YBD
Right 0YBC
Lens
Left 08BK3Z
Right 08BJ3Z
Lip
Lower 0CB1
Upper 0CB0
Liver 0FB0
Left Lobe 0FB2
Right Lobe 0FB1
Lung
Bilateral 0BBM
Left 0BBL
Lower Lobe
Left 0BBJ
Right 0BBF
Middle Lobe, Right 0BBD
Right 0BBK
Upper Lobe
Left 0BBG
Right 0BBC
Lung Lingula 0BBH
Lymphatic
Aortic 07BD

Excision (continued)

Lymphatic (continued)
Axillary
Left 07B6
Right 07B5
Head 07B0
Inguinal
Left 07BJ
Right 07BH
Internal Mammary
Left 07B9
Right 07B8
Lower Extremity
Left 07BG
Right 07BF
Mesenteric 07BB
Neck
Left 07B2
Right 07B1
Pelvis 07BC
Thoracic Duct 07BK
Thorax 07B7
Upper Extremity
Left 07B4
Right 07B3
Mandible
Left 0NBV
Right 0NBT
Maxilla
Left 0NBS
Right 0NBR
Mediastinum 0WBC
Medulla Oblongata 00BD
Mesentery 0DBV
Metacarpal
Left 0PBQ
Right 0PBP
Metatarsal
Left 0QBP
Right 0QBN
Muscle
Abdomen
Left 0KBL
Right 0KBK
Extraocular
Left 08BM
Right 08BL
Facial 0KB1
Foot
Left 0KBW
Right 0KBV
Hand
Left 0KBD
Right 0KBC
Head 0KB0
Hip
Left 0KBP
Right 0KBN
Lower Arm and Wrist
Left 0KBB
Right 0KB9
Lower Leg
Left 0KBT
Right 0KBS
Neck
Left 0KB3
Right 0KB2
Papillary 02BD
Perineum 0KBM
Shoulder
Left 0KB6
Right 0KB5
Thorax
Left 0KBJ
Right 0KBH
Tongue, Palate, Pharynx 0KB4
Trunk
Left 0KBG
Right 0KBF
Upper Arm
Left 0KB8
Right 0KB7

Excision (continued)

Muscle (continued)
Upper Leg
Left 0KBR
Right 0KBQ
Nasopharynx 09BN
Neck 0WB6
Nerve
Abdominal Sympathetic 01BM
Abducens 00BL
Accessory 00BR
Acoustic 00BN
Brachial Plexus 01B3
Cervical 01B1
Cervical Plexus 01B0
Facial 00BM
Femoral 01BD
Glossopharyngeal 00BP
Head and Neck Sympathetic 01BK
Hypoglossal 00BS
Lumbar 01BB
Lumbar Plexus 01B9
Lumbar Sympathetic 01BN
Lumbosacral Plexus 01BA
Median 01B5
Oculomotor 00BH
Olfactory 00BF
Optic 00BG
Peroneal 01BH
Phrenic 01B2
Pudendal 01BC
Radial 01B6
Sacral 01BR
Sacral Plexus 01BQ
Sacral Sympathetic 01BP
Sciatic 01BF
Thoracic 01B8
Thoracic Sympathetic 01BL
Tibial 01BG
Trigeminal 00BK
Trochlear 00BJ
Ulnar 01B4
Vagus 00BQ
Nipple
Left 0HBX
Right 0HBW
Nose 09BK
Omentum
Greater 0DBS
Lesser 0DBT
Orbit
Left 0NBQ
Right 0NBP
Ovary
Bilateral 0UB2
Left 0UB1
Right 0UB0
Palate
Hard 0CB2
Soft 0CB3
Pancreas 0FBG
Para-aortic Body 0GB9
Paraganglion Extremity 0GBF
Parathyroid Gland 0GBR
Inferior
Left 0GBP
Right 0GBN
Multiple 0GBQ
Superior
Left 0GBM
Right 0GBL
Patella
Left 0QBF
Right 0QBD
Penis 0VBS
Pericardium 02BN
Perineum
Female 0WBN
Male 0WBM
Peritoneum 0DBW

Excision (continued)

Phalanx
Finger
Left 0PBV
Right 0PBT
Thumb
Left 0PBS
Right 0PBR
Toe
Left 0QBR
Right 0QBQ
Pharynx 0CBM
Pineal Body 0GB1
Pleura
Left 0BBP
Right 0BBN
Pons 00BB
Prepuce 0VBT
Prostate 0VB0
Radius
Left 0PBJ
Right 0PBH
Rectum 0DBP
Retina
Left 08BF3Z
Right 08BE3Z
Retroperitoneum 0WBH
Rib
Left 0PB2
Right 0PB1
Sacrum 0QB1
Scapula
Left 0PB6
Right 0PB5
Sclera
Left 08B7XZ
Right 08B6XZ
Scrotum 0VB5
Septum
Atrial 02B5
Nasal 09BM
Ventricular 02BM
Shoulder Region
Left 0XB3
Right 0XB2
Sinus
Accessory 09BP
Ethmoid
Left 09BV
Right 09BU
Frontal
Left 09BT
Right 09BS
Mastoid
Left 09BC
Right 09BB
Maxillary
Left 09BR
Right 09BQ
Sphenoid
Left 09BX
Right 09BW
Skin
Abdomen 0HB7XZ
Back 0HB6XZ
Buttock 0HB8XZ
Chest 0HB5XZ
Ear
Left 0HB3XZ
Right 0HB2XZ
Face 0HB1XZ
Foot
Left 0HBNXZ
Right 0HBMXZ
Genitalia 0HBAXZ
Hand
Left 0HBGXZ
Right 0HBFXZ
Lower Arm
Left 0HBEXZ
Right 0HBDXZ

Excision (continued)

Skin (continued)
Lower Leg
Left 0HBLXZ
Right 0HBKXZ
Neck 0HB4XZ
Perineum 0HB9XZ
Scalp 0HB0XZ
Upper Arm
Left 0HBCXZ
Right 0HBBXZ
Upper Leg
Left 0HBJXZ
Right 0HBHXZ
Skull 0NB0
Spinal Cord
Cervical 00BW
Lumbar 00BY
Thoracic 00BX
Spinal Meninges 00BT
Spleen 07BP
Sternum 0PB0
Stomach 0DB6
Pylorus 0DB7
Subcutaneous Tissue and Fascia
Abdomen 0JB8
Back 0JB7
Buttock 0JB9
Chest 0JB6
Face 0JB1
Foot
Left 0JBR
Right 0JBQ
Hand
Left 0JBK
Right 0JBJ
Lower Arm
Left 0JBH
Right 0JBG
Lower Leg
Left 0JBP
Right 0JBN
Neck
Anterior 0JB4
Posterior 0JB5
Pelvic Region 0JBC
Perineum 0JBB
Scalp 0JB0
Upper Arm
Left 0JBF
Right 0JBD
Upper Leg
Left 0JBM
Right 0JBL
Tarsal
Left 0QBM
Right 0QBL
Tendon
Abdomen
Left 0LBG
Right 0LBF
Ankle
Left 0LBT
Right 0LBS
Foot
Left 0LBW
Right 0LBV
Hand
Left 0LB8
Right 0LB7
Head and Neck 0LB0
Hip
Left 0LBK
Right 0LBJ
Knee
Left 0LBR
Right 0LBQ
Lower Arm and Wrist
Left 0LB6
Right 0LB5

Excision *(continued)*
  Tendon *(continued)*
    Lower Leg
      Left 0LBP
      Right 0LBN
    Perineum 0LBH
    Shoulder
      Left 0LB2
      Right 0LB1
    Thorax
      Left 0LBD
      Right 0LBC
    Trunk
      Left 0LBB
      Right 0LB9
    Upper Arm
      Left 0LB4
      Right 0LB3
    Upper Leg
      Left 0LBM
      Right 0LBL
  Testis
    Bilateral 0VBC
    Left 0VBB
    Right 0VB9
  Thalamus 00B9
  Thymus 07BM
  Thyroid Gland
    Left Lobe 0GBG
    Right Lobe 0GBH
  Tibia
    Left 0QBH
    Right 0QBG
  Toe Nail 0HBRXZ
  Tongue 0CB7
  Tonsils 0CBP
  Tooth
    Lower 0CBX
    Upper 0CBW
  Trachea 0BB1
  Tunica Vaginalis
    Left 0VB7
    Right 0VB6
  Turbinate, Nasal 09BL
  Tympanic Membrane
    Left 09B8
    Right 09B7
  Ulna
    Left 0PBL
    Right 0PBK
  Ureter
    Left 0TB7
    Right 0TB6
  Urethra 0TBD
  Uterine Supporting Structure 0UB4
  Uterus 0UB9
  Uvula 0CBN
  Vagina 0UBG
  Valve
    Aortic 02BF
    Mitral 02BG
    Pulmonary 02BH
    Tricuspid 02BJ
  Vas Deferens
    Bilateral 0VBQ
    Left 0VBP
    Right 0VBN
  Vein
    Axillary
      Left 05B8
      Right 05B7
    Azygos 05B0
    Basilic
      Left 05BC
      Right 05BB
    Brachial
      Left 05BA
      Right 05B9
    Cephalic
      Left 05BF
      Right 05BD
    Colic 06B7

Excision *(continued)*
  Vein *(continued)*
    Common Iliac
      Left 06BD
      Right 06BC
    Coronary 02B4
    Esophageal 06B3
    External Iliac
      Left 06BG
      Right 06BF
    External Jugular
      Left 05BQ
      Right 05BP
    Face
      Left 05BV
      Right 05BT
    Femoral
      Left 06BN
      Right 06BM
    Foot
      Left 06BV
      Right 06BT
    Gastric 06B2
    Greater Saphenous
      Left 06BQ
      Right 06BP
    Hand
      Left 05BH
      Right 05BG
    Hemiazygos 05B1
    Hepatic 06B4
    Hypogastric
      Left 06BJ
      Right 06BH
    Inferior Mesenteric 06B6
    Innominate
      Left 05B4
      Right 05B3
    Internal Jugular
      Left 05BN
      Right 05BM
    Intracranial 05BL
    Lesser Saphenous
      Left 06BS
      Right 06BR
    Lower 06BY
    Portal 06B8
    Pulmonary
      Left 02BT
      Right 02BS
    Renal
      Left 06BB
      Right 06B9
    Splenic 06B1
    Subclavian
      Left 05B6
      Right 05B5
    Superior Mesenteric 06B5
    Upper 05BY
    Vertebral
      Left 05BS
      Right 05BR
  Vena Cava
    Inferior 06B0
    Superior 02BV
  Ventricle
    Left 02BL
    Right 02BK
  Vertebra
    Cervical 0PB3
    Lumbar 0QB0
    Thoracic 0PB4
  Vesicle
    Bilateral 0VB3
    Left 0VB2
    Right 0VB1
  Vitreous
    Left 08B53Z
    Right 08B43Z
  Vocal Cord
    Left 0CBV
    Right 0CBT

Excision *(continued)*
  Vulva 0UBM
  Wrist Region
    Left 0XBH
    Right 0XBG
Exclusion, Left atrial appendage (LAA)
  see Occlusion, Atrium, Left 02L7
Exercise, rehabilitation
  see Motor Treatment, Rehabilitation F07
Exploration
  see Inspection
Express® (LD) Premounted Stent System
  use Intraluminal Device
Express® Biliary SD Monorail® Premounted Stent System
  use Intraluminal Device
Express® SD Renal Monorail® Premounted Stent System
  use Intraluminal Device
Extensor carpi radialis muscle
  use Muscle, Lower Arm and Wrist, Left
  use Muscle, Lower Arm and Wrist, Right
Extensor carpi ulnaris muscle
  use Muscle, Lower Arm and Wrist, Left
  use Muscle, Lower Arm and Wrist, Right
Extensor digitorum brevis muscle
  use Muscle, Foot, Left
  use Muscle, Foot, Right
Extensor digitorum longus muscle
  use Muscle, Lower Leg, Left
  use Muscle, Lower Leg, Right
Extensor hallucis brevis muscle
  use Muscle, Foot, Left
  use Muscle, Foot, Right
Extensor hallucis longus muscle
  use Muscle, Lower Leg, Left
  use Muscle, Lower Leg, Right
External anal sphincter
  use Anal Sphincter
External auditory meatus
  use Ear, External Auditory Canal, Left
  use Ear, External Auditory Canal, Right
External fixator
  use External Fixation Device in Head and Facial Bones
  use External Fixation Device in Lower Bones
  use External Fixation Device in Lower Joints
  use External Fixation Device in Upper Bones
  use External Fixation Device in Upper Joints
External maxillary artery
  use Artery, Face
External naris
  use Nose
External oblique aponeurosis
  use Subcutaneous Tissue and Fascia, Trunk
External oblique muscle
  use Muscle, Abdomen, Left
  use Muscle, Abdomen, Right
External popliteal nerve
  use Nerve, Peroneal
External pudendal artery
  use Artery, Femoral, Left
  use Artery, Femoral, Right
External pudendal vein
  use Vein, Greater Saphenous, Left
  use Vein, Greater Saphenous, Right

External urethral sphincter
  use Urethra
Extirpation
  Acetabulum
    Left 0QC5
    Right 0QC4
  Adenoids 0CCQ
  Ampulla of Vater 0FCC
  Anal Sphincter 0DCR
  Anterior Chamber
    Left 08C3
    Right 08C2
  Anus 0DCQ
  Aorta
    Abdominal 04C0
    Thoracic 02CW
  Aortic Body 0GCD
  Appendix 0DCJ
  Artery
    Anterior Tibial
      Left 04CQ
      Right 04CP
    Axillary
      Left 03C6
      Right 03C5
    Brachial
      Left 03C8
      Right 03C7
    Celiac 04C1
    Colic
      Left 04C7
      Middle 04C8
      Right 04C6
    Common Carotid
      Left 03CJ
      Right 03CH
    Common Iliac
      Left 04CD
      Right 04CC
    Coronary
      Four or More Sites 02C3
      One Site 02C0
      Three Sites 02C2
      Two Sites 02C1
    External Carotid
      Left 03CN
      Right 03CM
    External Iliac
      Left 04CJ
      Right 04CH
    Face 03CR
    Femoral
      Left 04CL
      Right 04CK
    Foot
      Left 04CW
      Right 04CV
    Gastric 04C2
    Hand
      Left 03CF
      Right 03CD
    Hepatic 04C3
    Inferior Mesenteric 04CB
    Innominate 03C2
    Internal Carotid
      Left 03CL
      Right 03CK
    Internal Iliac
      Left 04CF
      Right 04CE
    Internal Mammary
      Left 03C1
      Right 03C0
    Intracranial 03CG
    Lower 04CY
    Peroneal
      Left 04CU
      Right 04CT
    Popliteal
      Left 04CN
      Right 04CM

Extirpation *(continued)*
- Artery *(continued)*
  - Posterior Tibial
    - Left 04CS
    - Right 04CR
  - Pulmonary
    - Left 02CR
    - Right 02CQ
  - Pulmonary Trunk 02CP
  - Radial
    - Left 03CC
    - Right 03CB
  - Renal
    - Left 04CA
    - Right 04C9
  - Splenic 04C4
  - Subclavian
    - Left 03C4
    - Right 03C3
  - Superior Mesenteric 04C5
  - Temporal
    - Left 03CT
    - Right 03CS
  - Thyroid
    - Left 03CV
    - Right 03CU
  - Ulnar
    - Left 03CA
    - Right 03C9
  - Upper 03CY
  - Vertebral
    - Left 03CQ
    - Right 03CP
- Atrium
  - Left 02C7
  - Right 02C6
- Auditory Ossicle
  - Left 09CA0ZZ
  - Right 09C90ZZ
- Basal Ganglia 00C8
- Bladder 0TCB
- Bladder Neck 0TCC
- Bone
  - Ethmoid
    - Left 0NCG
    - Right 0NCF
  - Frontal
    - Left 0NC2
    - Right 0NC1
  - Hyoid 0NCX
  - Lacrimal
    - Left 0NCJ
    - Right 0NCH
  - Nasal 0NCB
  - Occipital
    - Left 0NC8
    - Right 0NC7
  - Palatine
    - Left 0NCL
    - Right 0NCK
  - Parietal
    - Left 0NC4
    - Right 0NC3
  - Pelvic
    - Left 0QC3
    - Right 0QC2
  - Sphenoid
    - Left 0NCD
    - Right 0NCC
  - Temporal
    - Left 0NC6
    - Right 0NC5
  - Zygomatic
    - Left 0NCN
    - Right 0NCM
- Brain 00C0
- Breast
  - Bilateral 0HCV
  - Left 0HCU
  - Right 0HCT
- Bronchus
  - Lingula 0BC9

- Bronchus *(continued)*
  - Lower Lobe
    - Left 0BCB
    - Right 0BC6
  - Main
    - Left 0BC7
    - Right 0BC3
  - Middle Lobe, Right 0BC5
  - Upper Lobe
    - Left 0BC8
    - Right 0BC4
- Buccal Mucosa 0CC4
- Bursa and Ligament
  - Abdomen
    - Left 0MCJ
    - Right 0MCH
  - Ankle
    - Left 0MCR
    - Right 0MCQ
  - Elbow
    - Left 0MC4
    - Right 0MC3
  - Foot
    - Left 0MCT
    - Right 0MCS
  - Hand
    - Left 0MC8
    - Right 0MC7
  - Head and Neck 0MC0
  - Hip
    - Left 0MCM
    - Right 0MCL
  - Knee
    - Left 0MCP
    - Right 0MCN
  - Lower Extremity
    - Left 0MCW
    - Right 0MCV
  - Perineum 0MCK
  - Shoulder
    - Left 0MC2
    - Right 0MC1
  - Thorax
    - Left 0MCG
    - Right 0MCF
  - Trunk
    - Left 0MCD
    - Right 0MCC
  - Upper Extremity
    - Left 0MCB
    - Right 0MC9
  - Wrist
    - Left 0MC6
    - Right 0MC5
- Carina 0BC2
- Carotid Bodies, Bilateral 0GC8
- Carotid Body
  - Left 0GC6
  - Right 0GC7
- Carpal
  - Left 0PCN
  - Right 0PCM
- Cavity, Cranial 0WC1
- Cecum 0DCH
- Cerebellum 00CC
- Cerebral Hemisphere 00C7
- Cerebral Meninges 00C1
- Cerebral Ventricle 00C6
- Cervix 0UCC
- Chordae Tendineae 02C9
- Choroid
  - Left 08CB
  - Right 08CA
- Cisterna Chyli 07CL
- Clavicle
  - Left 0PCB
  - Right 0PC9
- Clitoris 0UCJ
- Coccygeal Glomus 0GCB
- Coccyx 0QCS

- Colon
  - Ascending 0DCK
  - Descending 0DCM
  - Sigmoid 0DCN
  - Transverse 0DCL
- Conduction Mechanism 02C8
- Conjunctiva
  - Left 08CTXZZ
  - Right 08CSXZZ
- Cord
  - Bilateral 0VCH
  - Left 0VCG
  - Right 0VCF
- Cornea
  - Left 08C9XZZ
  - Right 08C8XZZ
- Cul-de-sac 0UCF
- Diaphragm
  - Left 0BCS
  - Right 0BCR
- Disc
  - Cervical Vertebral 0RC3
  - Cervicothoracic Vertebral 0RC5
  - Lumbar Vertebral 0SC2
  - Lumbosacral 0SC4
  - Thoracic Vertebral 0RC9
  - Thoracolumbar Vertebral 0RCB
- Duct
  - Common Bile 0FC9
  - Cystic 0FC8
  - Hepatic
    - Left 0FC6
    - Right 0FC5
  - Lacrimal
    - Left 08CY
    - Right 08CX
  - Pancreatic 0FCD
    - Accessory 0FCF
  - Parotid
    - Left 0CCC
    - Right 0CCB
- Duodenum 0DC9
- Dura Mater 00C2
- Ear
  - External
    - Left 09C1
    - Right 09C0
  - External Auditory Canal
    - Left 09C4
    - Right 09C3
  - Inner
    - Left 09CE0ZZ
    - Right 09CD0ZZ
  - Middle
    - Left 09C60ZZ
    - Right 09C50ZZ
- Endometrium 0UCB
- Epididymis
  - Bilateral 0VCL
  - Left 0VCK
  - Right 0VCJ
- Epidural Space 00C3
- Epiglottis 0CCR
- Esophagogastric Junction 0DC4
- Esophagus 0DC5
  - Lower 0DC3
  - Middle 0DC2
  - Upper 0DC1
- Eustachian Tube
  - Left 09CG
  - Right 09CF
- Eye
  - Left 08C1XZZ
  - Right 08C0XZZ
- Eyelid
  - Lower
    - Left 08CR
    - Right 08CQ
  - Upper
    - Left 08CP
    - Right 08CN

- Fallopian Tube
  - Left 0UC6
  - Right 0UC5
- Fallopian Tubes, Bilateral 0UC7
- Femoral Shaft
  - Left 0QC9
  - Right 0QC8
- Femur
  - Lower
    - Left 0QCC
    - Right 0QCB
  - Upper
    - Left 0QC7
    - Right 0QC6
- Fibula
  - Left 0QCK
  - Right 0QCJ
- Finger Nail 0HCQXZZ
- Gallbladder 0FC4
- Gastrointestinal Tract 0WCP
- Genitourinary Tract 0WCR
- Gingiva
  - Lower 0CC6
  - Upper 0CC5
- Gland
  - Adrenal
    - Bilateral 0GC4
    - Left 0GC2
    - Right 0GC3
  - Lacrimal
    - Left 08CW
    - Right 08CV
  - Minor Salivary 0CCJ
  - Parotid
    - Left 0CC9
    - Right 0CC8
  - Pituitary 0GC0
  - Sublingual
    - Left 0CCF
    - Right 0CCD
  - Submaxillary
    - Left 0CCH
    - Right 0CCG
  - Vestibular 0UCL
- Glenoid Cavity
  - Left 0PC8
  - Right 0PC7
- Glomus Jugulare 0GCC
- Humeral Head
  - Left 0PCD
  - Right 0PCC
- Humeral Shaft
  - Left 0PCG
  - Right 0PCF
- Hymen 0UCK
- Hypothalamus 00CA
- Ileocecal Valve 0DCC
- Ileum 0DCB
- Intestine
  - Large 0DCE
    - Left 0DCG
    - Right 0DCF
  - Small 0DC8
- Iris
  - Left 08CD
  - Right 08CC
- Jejunum 0DCA
- Joint
  - Acromioclavicular
    - Left 0RCH
    - Right 0RCG
  - Ankle
    - Left 0SCG
    - Right 0SCF
  - Carpal
    - Left 0RCR
    - Right 0RCQ
  - Cervical Vertebral 0RC1
  - Cervicothoracic Vertebral 0RC4
  - Coccygeal 0SC6

Joint (continued)
  Elbow
    Left 0RCM
    Right 0RCL
  Finger Phalangeal
    Left 0RCX
    Right 0RCW
  Hip
    Left 0SCB
    Right 0SC9
  Knee
    Left 0SCD
    Right 0SCC
  Lumbar Vertebral 0SC0
  Lumbosacral 0SC3
  Metacarpocarpal
    Left 0RCT
    Right 0RCS
  Metacarpophalangeal
    Left 0RCV
    Right 0RCU
  Metatarsal-Phalangeal
    Left 0SCN
    Right 0SCM
  Metatarsal-Tarsal
    Left 0SCL
    Right 0SCK
  Occipital-cervical 0RC0
  Sacrococcygeal 0SC5
  Sacroiliac
    Left 0SC8
    Right 0SC7
  Shoulder
    Left 0RCK
    Right 0RCJ
  Sternoclavicular
    Left 0RCF
    Right 0RCE
  Tarsal
    Left 0SCJ
    Right 0SCH
  Temporomandibular
    Left 0RCD
    Right 0RCC
  Thoracic Vertebral 0RC6
  Thoracolumbar Vertebral
    0RCA
  Toe Phalangeal
    Left 0SCQ
    Right 0SCP
  Wrist
    Left 0RCP
    Right 0RCN
Kidney
  Left 0TC1
  Right 0TC0
Kidney Pelvis
  Left 0TC4
  Right 0TC3
Larynx 0CCS
Lens
  Left 08CK
  Right 08CJ
Lip
  Lower 0CC1
  Upper 0CC0
Liver 0FC0
  Left Lobe 0FC2
  Right Lobe 0FC1
Lung
  Bilateral 0BCM
  Left 0BCL
  Lower Lobe
    Left 0BCJ
    Right 0BCF
  Middle Lobe, Right
    0BCD
  Right 0BCK
  Upper Lobe
    Left 0BCG
    Right 0BCC

Lung Lingula 0BCH
Lymphatic
  Aortic 07CD
  Axillary
    Left 07C6
    Right 07C5
  Head 07C0
  Inguinal
    Left 07CJ
    Right 07CH
  Internal Mammary
    Left 07C9
    Right 07C8
  Lower Extremity
    Left 07CG
    Right 07CF
  Mesenteric 07CB
  Neck
    Left 07C2
    Right 07C1
  Pelvis 07CC
  Thoracic Duct 07CK
  Thorax 07C7
  Upper Extremity
    Left 07C4
    Right 07C3
Mandible
  Left 0NCV
  Right 0NCT
Maxilla
  Left 0NCS
  Right 0NCR
Mediastinum 0WCC
Medulla Oblongata 00CD
Mesentery 0DCV
Metacarpal
  Left 0PCQ
  Right 0PCP
Metatarsal
  Left 0QCP
  Right 0QCN
Muscle
  Abdomen
    Left 0KCL
    Right 0KCK
  Extraocular
    Left 08CM
    Right 08CL
  Facial 0KC1
  Foot
    Left 0KCW
    Right 0KCV
  Hand
    Left 0KCD
    Right 0KCC
  Head 0KC0
  Hip
    Left 0KCP
    Right 0KCN
  Lower Arm and Wrist
    Left 0KCB
    Right 0KC9
  Lower Leg
    Left 0KCT
    Right 0KCS
  Neck
    Left 0KC3
    Right 0KC2
  Papillary 02CD
  Perineum 0KCM
  Shoulder
    Left 0KC6
    Right 0KC5
  Thorax
    Left 0KCJ
    Right 0KCH
  Tongue, Palate, Pharynx
    0KC4
  Trunk
    Left 0KCG
    Right 0KCF

Muscle (continued)
  Upper Arm
    Left 0KC8
    Right 0KC7
  Upper Leg
    Left 0KCR
    Right 0KCQ
Nasopharynx 09CN
Nerve
  Abdominal Sympathetic 01CM
  Abducens 00CL
  Accessory 00CR
  Acoustic 00CN
  Brachial Plexus 01C3
  Cervical 01C1
  Cervical Plexus 01C0
  Facial 00CM
  Femoral 01CD
  Glossopharyngeal 00CP
  Head and Neck Sympathetic 01CK
  Hypoglossal 00CS
  Lumbar 01CB
  Lumbar Plexus 01C9
  Lumbar Sympathetic 01CN
  Lumbosacral Plexus 01CA
  Median 01C5
  Oculomotor 00CH
  Olfactory 00CF
  Optic 00CG
  Peroneal 01CH
  Phrenic 01C2
  Pudendal 01CC
  Radial 01C6
  Sacral 01CR
  Sacral Plexus 01CQ
  Sacral Sympathetic 01CP
  Sciatic 01CF
  Thoracic 01C8
  Thoracic Sympathetic 01CL
  Tibial 01CG
  Trigeminal 00CK
  Trochlear 00CJ
  Ulnar 01C4
  Vagus 00CQ
Nipple
  Left 0HCX
  Right 0HCW
Nose 09CK
Omentum
  Greater 0DCS
  Lesser 0DCT
Oral Cavity and Throat 0WC3
Orbit
  Left 0NCQ
  Right 0NCP
Orbital Atherectomy Technology X2C
Ovary
  Bilateral 0UC2
  Left 0UC1
  Right 0UC0
Palate
  Hard 0CC2
  Soft 0CC3
Pancreas 0FCG
Para-aortic Body 0GC9
Paraganglion Extremity 0GCF
Parathyroid Gland 0GCR
  Inferior
    Left 0GCP
    Right 0GCN
  Multiple 0GCQ
  Superior
    Left 0GCM
    Right 0GCL
Patella
  Left 0QCF
  Right 0QCD
Pelvic Cavity 0WCJ
Penis 0VCS
Pericardial Cavity 0WCD
Pericardium 02CN

Peritoneal Cavity
  0WCG
Peritoneum 0DCW
Phalanx
  Finger
    Left 0PCV
    Right 0PCT
  Thumb
    Left 0PCS
    Right 0PCR
  Toe
    Left 0QCR
    Right 0QCQ
Pharynx 0CCM
Pineal Body 0GC1
Pleura
  Left 0BCP
  Right 0BCN
Pleural Cavity
  Left 0WCB
  Right 0WC9
Pons 00CB
Prepuce 0VCT
Prostate 0VC0
Radius
  Left 0PCJ
  Right 0PCH
Rectum 0DCP
Respiratory Tract
  0WCQ
Retina
  Left 08CF
  Right 08CE
Retinal Vessel
  Left 08CH
  Right 08CG
Rib
  Left 0PC2
  Right 0PC1
Sacrum 0QC1
Scapula
  Left 0PC6
  Right 0PC5
Sclera
  Left 08C7XZZ
  Right 08C6XZZ
Scrotum 0VC5
Septum
  Atrial 02C5
  Nasal 09CM
  Ventricular 02CM
Sinus
  Accessory 09CP
  Ethmoid
    Left 09CV
    Right 09CU
  Frontal
    Left 09CT
    Right 09CS
  Mastoid
    Left 09CC
    Right 09CB
  Maxillary
    Left 09CR
    Right 09CQ
  Sphenoid
    Left 09CX
    Right 09CW
Skin
  Abdomen 0HC7XZZ
  Back 0HC6XZZ
  Buttock 0HC8XZZ
  Chest 0HC5XZZ
  Ear
    Left 0HC3XZZ
    Right 0HC2XZZ
  Face 0HC1XZZ
  Foot
    Left 0HCNXZZ
    Right 0HCMXZZ
  Genitalia 0HCAXZZ

Extirpation *(continued)*
  Skin *(continued)*
    Hand
      Left 0HCGXZZ
      Right 0HCFXZZ
    Lower Arm
      Left 0HCEXZZ
      Right 0HCDXZZ
    Lower Leg
      Left 0HCLXZZ
      Right 0HCKXZZ
    Neck 0HC4XZZ
    Perineum 0HC9XZZ
    Scalp 0HC0XZZ
    Upper Arm
      Left 0HCCXZZ
      Right 0HCBXZZ
    Upper Leg
      Left 0HCJXZZ
      Right 0HCHXZZ
  Spinal Cord
    Cervical 00CW
    Lumbar 00CY
    Thoracic 00CX
  Spinal Meninges 00CT
  Spleen 07CP
  Sternum 0PC0
  Stomach 0DC6
    Pylorus 0DC7
  Subarachnoid Space 00C5
  Subcutaneous Tissue and Fascia
    Abdomen 0JC8
    Back 0JC7
    Buttock 0JC9
    Chest 0JC6
    Face 0JC1
    Foot
      Left 0JCR
      Right 0JCQ
    Hand
      Left 0JCK
      Right 0JCJ
    Lower Arm
      Left 0JCH
      Right 0JCG
    Lower Leg
      Left 0JCP
      Right 0JCN
    Neck
      Anterior 0JC4
      Posterior 0JC5
    Pelvic Region
      0JCC
    Perineum 0JCB
    Scalp 0JC0
    Upper Arm
      Left 0JCF
      Right 0JCD
    Upper Leg
      Left 0JCM
      Right 0JCL
  Subdural Space 00C4
  Tarsal
    Left 0QCM
    Right 0QCL
  Tendon
    Abdomen
      Left 0LCG
      Right 0LCF
    Ankle
      Left 0LCT
      Right 0LCS
    Foot
      Left 0LCW
      Right 0LCV
    Hand
      Left 0LC8
      Right 0LC7
    Head and Neck 0LC0
    Hip
      Left 0LCK
      Right 0LCJ

Extirpation *(continued)*
  Tendon *(continued)*
    Knee
      Left 0LCR
      Right 0LCQ
    Lower Arm and Wrist
      Left 0LC6
      Right 0LC5
    Lower Leg
      Left 0LCP
      Right 0LCN
    Perineum 0LCH
    Shoulder
      Left 0LC2
      Right 0LC1
    Thorax
      Left 0LCD
      Right 0LCC
    Trunk
      Left 0LCB
      Right 0LC9
    Upper Arm
      Left 0LC4
      Right 0LC3
    Upper Leg
      Left 0LCM
      Right 0LCL
  Testis
    Bilateral 0VCC
    Left 0VCB
    Right 0VC9
  Thalamus 00C9
  Thymus 07CM
  Thyroid Gland 0GCK
    Left Lobe 0GCG
    Right Lobe 0GCH
  Tibia
    Left 0QCH
    Right 0QCG
  Toe Nail 0HCRXZZ
  Tongue 0CC7
  Tonsils 0CCP
  Tooth
    Lower 0CCX
    Upper 0CCW
  Trachea 0BC1
  Tunica Vaginalis
    Left 0VC7
    Right 0VC6
  Turbinate, Nasal 09CL
  Tympanic Membrane
    Left 09C8
    Right 09C7
  Ulna
    Left 0PCL
    Right 0PCK
  Ureter
    Left 0TC7
    Right 0TC6
  Urethra 0TCD
  Uterine Supporting Structure
    0UC4
  Uterus 0UC9
  Uvula 0CCN
  Vagina 0UCG
  Valve
    Aortic 02CF
    Mitral 02CG
    Pulmonary 02CH
    Tricuspid 02CJ
  Vas Deferens
    Bilateral 0VCQ
    Left 0VCP
    Right 0VCN
  Vein
    Axillary
      Left 05C8
      Right 05C7
    Azygos 05C0
    Basilic
      Left 05CC
      Right 05CB

Extirpation *(continued)*
  Vein *(continued)*
    Brachial
      Left 05CA
      Right 05C9
    Cephalic
      Left 05CF
      Right 05CD
    Colic 06C7
    Common Iliac
      Left 06CD
      Right 06CC
    Coronary 02C4
    Esophageal 06C3
    External Iliac
      Left 06CG
      Right 06CF
    External Jugular
      Left 05CQ
      Right 05CP
    Face
      Left 05CV
      Right 05CT
    Femoral
      Left 06CN
      Right 06CM
    Foot
      Left 06CV
      Right 06CT
    Gastric 06C2
    Greater Saphenous
      Left 06CQ
      Right 06CP
    Hand
      Left 05CH
      Right 05CG
    Hemiazygos 05C1
    Hepatic 06C4
    Hypogastric
      Left 06CJ
      Right 06CH
    Inferior Mesenteric
      06C6
    Innominate
      Left 05C4
      Right 05C3
    Internal Jugular
      Left 05CN
      Right 05CM
    Intracranial 05CL
    Lesser Saphenous
      Left 06CS
      Right 06CR
    Lower 06CY
    Portal 06C8
    Pulmonary
      Left 02CT
      Right 02CS
    Renal
      Left 06CB
      Right 06C9
    Splenic 06C1
    Subclavian
      Left 05C6
      Right 05C5
    Superior Mesenteric 06C5
    Upper 05CY
    Vertebral
      Left 05CS
      Right 05CR
  Vena Cava
    Inferior 06C0
    Superior 02CV
  Ventricle
    Left 02CL
    Right 02CK
  Vertebra
    Cervical 0PC3
    Lumbar 0QC0
    Thoracic 0PC4
  Vesicle
    Bilateral 0VC3

Extirpation *(continued)*
  Vesicle *(continued)*
    Left 0VC2
    Right 0VC1
  Vitreous
    Left 08C5
    Right 08C4
  Vocal Cord
    Left 0CCV
    Right 0CCT
  Vulva 0UCM
Extracorporeal shock wave
  lithotripsy
  see Fragmentation
Extracranial-intracranial bypass
  (EC-IC)
  see Bypass, Upper Arteries
  031
Extraction
  Auditory Ossicle
    Left 09DA0ZZ
    Right 09D90ZZ
  Bone Marrow
    Iliac 07DR
    Sternum 07DQ
    Vertebral 07DS
  Bursa and Ligament
    Abdomen
      Left 0MDJ
      Right 0MDH
    Ankle
      Left 0MDR
      Right 0MDQ
    Elbow
      Left 0MD4
      Right 0MD3
    Foot
      Left 0MDT
      Right 0MDS
    Hand
      Left 0MD8
      Right 0MD7
    Head and Neck 0MD0
    Hip
      Left 0MDM
      Right 0MDL
    Knee
      Left 0MDP
      Right 0MDN
    Lower Extremity
      Left 0MDW
      Right 0MDV
    Perineum 0MDK
    Shoulder
      Left 0MD2
      Right 0MD1
    Thorax
      Left 0MDG
      Right 0MDF
    Trunk
      Left 0MDD
      Right 0MDC
    Upper Extremity
      Left 0MDB
      Right 0MD9
    Wrist
      Left 0MD6
      Right 0MD5
  Cerebral Meninges 00D1
  Cornea
    Left 08D9XZ
    Right 08D8XZ
  Dura Mater 00D2
  Endometrium 0UDB
  Finger Nail 0HDQXZZ
  Hair 0HDSXZZ
  Kidney
    Left 0TD1
    Right 0TD0
  Lens
    Left 08DK3ZZ
    Right 08DJ3ZZ

Extraction *(continued)*
- Nerve
  - Abdominal Sympathetic 01DM
  - Abducens 00DL
  - Accessory 00DR
  - Acoustic 00DN
  - Brachial Plexus 01D3
  - Cervical 01D1
  - Cervical Plexus 01D0
  - Facial 00DM
  - Femoral 01DD
  - Glossopharyngeal 00DP
  - Head and Neck Sympathetic 01DK
  - Hypoglossal 00DS
  - Lumbar 01DB
  - Lumbar Plexus 01D9
  - Lumbar Sympathetic 01DN
  - Lumbosacral Plexus 01DA
  - Median 01D5
  - Oculomotor 00DH
  - Olfactory 00DF
  - Optic 00DG
  - Peroneal 01DH
  - Phrenic 01D2
  - Pudendal 01DC
  - Radial 01D6
  - Sacral 01DR
  - Sacral Plexus 01DQ
  - Sacral Sympathetic 01DP
  - Sciatic 01DF
  - Thoracic 01D8
  - Thoracic Sympathetic 01DL
  - Tibial 01DG
  - Trigeminal 00DK
  - Trochlear 00DJ
  - Ulnar 01D4
  - Vagus 00DQ
- Ova 0UDN
- Pleura
  - Left 0BDP
  - Right 0BDN
- Products of Conception
  - Classical 10D00Z0
  - Ectopic 10D2
  - Extraperitoneal 10D00Z2
  - High Forceps 10D07Z5
  - Internal Version 10D07Z7
  - Low Cervical 10D00Z1
  - Low Forceps 10D07Z3
  - Mid Forceps 10D07Z4
  - Other 10D07Z8
  - Retained 10D1
  - Vacuum 10D07Z6
- Septum, Nasal 09DM
- Sinus
  - Accessory 09DP
  - Ethmoid
    - Left 09DV
    - Right 09DU
  - Frontal
    - Left 09DT
    - Right 09DS
  - Mastoid
    - Left 09DC
    - Right 09DB
  - Maxillary
    - Left 09DR
    - Right 09DQ
  - Sphenoid
    - Left 09DX
    - Right 09DW
- Skin
  - Abdomen 0HD7XZZ
  - Back 0HD6XZZ
  - Buttock 0HD8XZZ
- Skin
  - Chest 0HD5XZZ
  - Ear
    - Left 0HD3XZZ
    - Right 0HD2XZZ
  - Face 0HD1XZZ

Extraction *(continued)*
- Skin *(continued)*
  - Foot
    - Left 0HDNXZZ
    - Right 0HDMXZZ
  - Genitalia 0HDAXZZ
  - Hand
    - Left 0HDGXZZ
    - Right 0HDFXZZ
  - Lower Arm
    - Left 0HDEXZZ
    - Right 0HDDXZZ
  - Lower Leg
    - Left 0HDLXZZ
    - Right 0HDKXZZ
  - Neck 0HD4XZZ
  - Perineum 0HD9XZZ
  - Scalp 0HD0XZZ
  - Upper Arm
    - Left 0HDCXZZ
    - Right 0HDBXZZ
  - Upper Leg
    - Left 0HDJXZZ
    - Right 0HDHXZZ
- Spinal Meninges 00DT
- Subcutaneous Tissue and Fascia
  - Abdomen 0JD8
  - Back 0JD7
  - Buttock 0JD9
  - Chest 0JD6
  - Face 0JD1
  - Foot
    - Left 0JDR
    - Right 0JDQ
  - Hand
    - Left 0JDK
    - Right 0JDJ
  - Lower Arm
    - Left 0JDH
    - Right 0JDG
  - Lower Leg
    - Left 0JDP
    - Right 0JDN
  - Neck
    - Anterior 0JD4
    - Posterior 0JD5
  - Pelvic Region 0JDC
  - Perineum 0JDB
  - Scalp 0JD0
  - Upper Arm
    - Left 0JDF
    - Right 0JDD
  - Upper Leg
    - Left 0JDM
    - Right 0JDL
- Toe Nail 0HDRXZZ
- Tooth
  - Lower 0CDXXZ
  - Upper 0CDWXZ
- Turbinate, Nasal 09DL
- Tympanic Membrane
  - Left 09D8
  - Right 09D7
- Vein
  - Basilic
    - Left 05DC
    - Right 05DB
  - Brachial
    - Left 05DA
    - Right 05D9
  - Cephalic
    - Left 05DF
    - Right 05DD
  - Femoral
    - Left 06DN
    - Right 06DM
  - Foot
    - Left 06DV
    - Right 06DT
  - Greater Saphenous
    - Left 06DQ
    - Right 06DP

Extraction *(continued)*
- Vein *(continued)*
  - Hand
    - Left 05DH
    - Right 05DG
  - Lesser Saphenous
    - Left 06DS
    - Right 06DR
  - Lower 06DY
  - Upper 05DY
- Vocal Cord
  - Left 0CDV
  - Right 0CDT

Extradural space, intracranial
use Epidural Space
Extradural space, spinal
use Spinal Canal
EXtreme Lateral Interbody Fusion (XLIF) device
use Interbody Fusion Device in Lower Joints

F

Face lift
see Alteration, Face 0W02
Facet replacement spinal stabilization device
use Spinal Stabilization Device, Facet Replacement in 0RH
use Spinal Stabilization Device, Facet Replacement in 0SH
Facial artery
use Artery, Face
False vocal cord
use Larynx
Falx cerebri
use Dura Mater
Fascia lata
use Subcutaneous Tissue and Fascia, Upper Leg, Left
use Subcutaneous Tissue and Fascia, Upper Leg, Right
Fasciaplasty, fascioplasty
see Repair, Subcutaneous Tissue and Fascia 0JQ
see Replacement, Subcutaneous Tissue and Fascia 0JR
Fasciectomy
see Excision, Subcutaneous Tissue and Fascia 0JB
Fasciorrhaphy
see Repair, Subcutaneous Tissue and Fascia 0JQ
Fasciotomy
see Division, Subcutaneous Tissue and Fascia 0J8
see Drainage, Subcutaneous Tissue and Fascia 0J9
Feeding Device
- Change device in
  - Lower 0D2DXUZ
  - Upper 0D20XUZ
- Insertion of device in
  - Duodenum 0DH9
  - Esophagus 0DH5
  - Ileum 0DHB
  - Intestine, Small 0DH8
  - Jejunum 0DHA
  - Stomach 0DH6
- Removal of device from
  - Esophagus 0DP5
  - Intestinal Tract
    - Lower 0DPD
    - Upper 0DP0
  - Stomach 0DP6
- Revision of device in
  - Intestinal Tract
    - Lower 0DWD
    - Upper 0DW0
  - Stomach 0DW6

Femoral head
use Femur, Upper, Left
use Femur, Upper, Right
Femoral lymph node
use Lymphatic, Lower Extremity, Left
use Lymphatic, Lower Extremity, Right
Femoropatellar joint
use Joint, Knee, Left
use Joint, Knee, Left, Femoral Surface
use Joint, Knee, Right
use Joint, Knee, Right, Femoral Surface
Femorotibial joint
use Joint, Knee, Left
use Joint, Knee, Left, Tibial Surface
use Joint, Knee, Right
use Joint, Knee, Right, Tibial Surface
Fibular artery
use Artery, Peroneal, Left
use Artery, Peroneal, Right
Fibularis brevis muscle
use Muscle, Lower Leg, Left
use Muscle, Lower Leg, Right
Fibularis longus muscle
use Muscle, Lower Leg, Left
use Muscle, Lower Leg, Right
Fifth cranial nerve
use Nerve, Trigeminal
Fimbriectomy
see Excision, Female Reproductive System 0UB
see Resection, Female Reproductive System 0UT
Fine needle aspiration
- Fluid or gas
  - *see* Drainage
- Tissue
  - *see* Excision
First cranial nerve
use Nerve, Olfactory
First intercostal nerve
use Nerve, Brachial Plexus
Fistulization
see Bypass
see Drainage
see Repair
Fitting
- Arch bars, for fracture reduction
  - *see* Reposition, Mouth and Throat 0CS
- Arch bars, for immobilization
  - *see* Immobilization, Face 2W31
- Artificial limb
  - *see* Device Fitting, Rehabilitation F0D
- Hearing aid
  - *see* Device Fitting, Rehabilitation F0D
- Ocular prosthesis F0DZ8UZ
- Prosthesis, limb
  - *see* Device Fitting, Rehabilitation F0D
- Prosthesis, ocular F0DZ8UZ
Fixation, bone
- External, with fracture reduction
  - *see* Reposition
- External, without fracture reduction
  - *see* Insertion
- Internal, with fracture reduction
  - *see* Reposition
- Internal, without fracture reduction
  - *see* Insertion
FLAIR® Endovascular Stent Graft
use Intraluminal Device
Flexible Composite Mesh
use Synthetic Substitute
Flexor carpi radialis muscle
use Muscle, Lower Arm and Wrist, Left
use Muscle, Lower Arm and Wrist, Right

Flexor carpi ulnaris muscle
  use Muscle, Lower Arm and Wrist, Left
  use Muscle, Lower Arm and Wrist, Right
Flexor digitorum brevis muscle
  use Muscle, Foot, Left
  use Muscle, Foot, Right
Flexor digitorum longus muscle
  use Muscle, Lower Leg, Left
  use Muscle, Lower Leg, Right
Flexor hallucis brevis muscle
  use Muscle, Foot, Left
  use Muscle, Foot, Right
Flexor hallucis longus muscle
  use Muscle, Lower Leg, Left
  use Muscle, Lower Leg, Right
Flexor pollicis longus muscle
  use Muscle, Lower Arm and Wrist, Left
  use Muscle, Lower Arm and Wrist, Right
Fluoroscopy
  Abdomen and Pelvis BW11
  Airway, Upper BB1DZZZ
  Ankle
    Left BQ1
    Right BQ1G
  Aorta
    Abdominal B410
      Laser, Intraoperative B410
    Thoracic B310
      Laser, Intraoperative B310
    Thoraco-Abdominal B31P
      Laser, Intraoperative B31P
  Aorta and Bilateral Lower Extremity Arteries B41D
    Laser, Intraoperative B41D
  Arm
    Left BP1FZZZ
    Right BP1EZZZ
  Artery
    Brachiocephalic-Subclavian
      Right B311
        Laser, Intraoperative B311
    Bronchial B31L
      Laser, Intraoperative B31L
    Bypass Graft, Other B21F
    Cervico-Cerebral Arch B31Q
      Laser, Intraoperative B31Q
    Common Carotid
      Bilateral B315
        Laser, Intraoperative B315
      Left B314
        Laser, Intraoperative B314
      Right B313
        Laser, Intraoperative B313
    Coronary
      Bypass Graft
        Multiple B213
          Laser, Intraoperative B213
        Single B212
          Laser, Intraoperative B212
      Multiple B211
        Laser, Intraoperative B211
      Single B210
        Laser, Intraoperative B210
    External Carotid
      Bilateral B31C
        Laser, Intraoperative B31C
      Left B31B
        Laser, Intraoperative B31B
      Right B319
        Laser, Intraoperative B319
    Hepatic B412
      Laser, Intraoperative B412
    Inferior Mesenteric B415
      Laser, Intraoperative B415

Fluoroscopy *(continued)*
  Artery *(continued)*
    Intercostal B31L
      Laser, Intraoperative B31L
    Internal Carotid
      Bilateral B318
        Laser, Intraoperative B318
      Left B317
        Laser, Intraoperative B317
      Right B316
        Laser, Intraoperative B316
    Internal Mammary Bypass Graft
      Left B218
      Right B217
    Intra-Abdominal
      Laser, Intraoperative B41B
      Other B41B
    Intracranial B31R
      Laser, Intraoperative B31R
    Lower
      Laser, Intraoperative B41J
      Other B41J
    Lower Extremity
      Bilateral and Aorta B41D
        Laser, Intraoperative B41D
      Left B41G
        Laser, Intraoperative B41G
      Right B41F
        Laser, Intraoperative B41F
    Lumbar B419
      Laser, Intraoperative B419
    Pelvic B41C
      Laser, Intraoperative B41C
    Pulmonary
      Left B31T
        Laser, Intraoperative B31T
      Right B31S
        Laser, Intraoperative B31S
    Renal
      Bilateral B418
        Laser, Intraoperative B418
      Left B417
        Laser, Intraoperative B417
      Right B416
        Laser, Intraoperative B416
    Spinal B31M
      Laser, Intraoperative B31M
    Splenic B413
      Laser, Intraoperative B413
    Subclavian
      Laser, Intraoperative B312
      Left B312
    Superior Mesenteric B414
      Laser, Intraoperative B414
    Upper
      Laser, Intraoperative B31N
      Other B31N
    Upper Extremity
      Bilateral B31K
        Laser, Intraoperative B31K
      Left B31J
        Laser, Intraoperative B31J
      Right B31H
        Laser, Intraoperative B31H

Fluoroscopy *(continued)*
  Artery *(continued)*
    Vertebral
      Bilateral B31G
        Laser, Intraoperative B31G
      Left B31F
        Laser, Intraoperative B31F
      Right B31D
        Laser, Intraoperative B31D
  Bile Duct BF10
    Pancreatic Duct and Gallbladder BF14
  Bile Duct and Gallbladder BF13
  Biliary Duct BF11
  Bladder BT10
    Kidney and Ureter BT14
    Left BT1F
    Right BT1D
  Bladder and Urethra BT1B
  Bowel, Small BD1
  Calcaneus
    Left BQ1KZZZ
    Right BQ1JZZZ
  Clavicle
    Left BP15ZZZ
    Right BP14ZZZ
  Coccyx BR1F
  Colon BD14
  Corpora Cavernosa BV10
  Dialysis Fistula B51W
  Dialysis Shunt B51W
  Diaphragm BB16ZZZ
  Disc
    Cervical BR11
    Lumbar BR13
    Thoracic BR12
  Duodenum BD19
  Elbow
    Left BP1H
    Right BP1G
  Epiglottis B91G
  Esophagus BD11
  Extremity
    Lower BW1C
    Upper BW1J
  Facet Joint
    Cervical BR14
    Lumbar BR16
    Thoracic BR15
  Fallopian Tube
    Bilateral BU12
    Left BU11
    Right BU10
  Fallopian Tube and Uterus BU18
  Femur
    Left BQ14ZZZ
    Right BQ13ZZZ
  Finger
    Left BP1SZZZ
    Right BP1RZZZ
  Foot
    Left BQ1MZZZ
    Right BQ1LZZZ
  Forearm
    Left BP1KZZZ
    Right BP1JZZZ
  Gallbladder BF12
    Bile Duct and Pancreatic Duct BF14
  Gallbladder and Bile Duct BF13
  Gastrointestinal, Upper BD1
  Hand
    Left BP1PZZZ
    Right BP1NZZZ
  Head and Neck BW19
  Heart
    Left B215
    Right B214
    Right and Left B216

Fluoroscopy *(continued)*
  Hip
    Left BQ11
    Right BQ10
  Humerus
    Left BP1BZZZ
    Right BP1AZZZ
  Ileal Diversion Loop BT1C
  Ileal Loop, Ureters and Kidney BT1G
  Intracranial Sinus B512
  Joint
    Acromioclavicular, Bilateral BP13ZZZ
    Finger
      Left BP1D
      Right BP1C
    Foot
      Left BQ1Y
      Right BQ1X
    Hand
      Left BP1D
      Right BP1C
    Lumbosacral BR1B
    Sacroiliac BR1D
    Sternoclavicular
      Bilateral BP12ZZZ
      Left BP11ZZZ
      Right BP10ZZZ
    Temporomandibular
      Bilateral BN19
      Left BN18
      Right BN17
    Thoracolumbar BR18
    Toe
      Left BQ1Y
      Right BQ1X
  Kidney
    Bilateral BT13
    Ileal Loop and Ureter BT1G
    Left BT12
    Right BT11
    Ureter and Bladder BT14
      Left BT1F
      Right BT1D
  Knee
    Left BQ18
    Right BQ17
  Larynx B91J
  Leg
    Left BQ1FZZZ
    Right BQ1DZZZ
  Lung
    Bilateral BB14ZZZ
    Left BB13ZZZ
    Right BB12ZZZ
  Mediastinum BB1CZZZ
  Mouth BD1B
  Neck and Head BW19
  Oropharynx BD1B
  Pancreatic Duct BF1
    Gallbladder and Bile Buct BF14
  Patella
    Left BQ1WZZZ
    Right BQ1VZZZ
  Pelvis BR1C
  Pelvis and Abdomen BW11
  Pharynix B91G
  Ribs
    Left BP1YZZZ
    Right BP1XZZZ
  Sacrum BR1F
  Scapula
    Left BP17ZZZ
    Right BP16ZZZ
  Shoulder
    Left BP19
    Right BP18
  Sinus, Intracranial B512
  Spinal Cord B01B

Fluoroscopy *(continued)*
Spine
   Cervical BR10
   Lumbar BR19
   Thoracic BR17
   Whole BR1G
  Sternum BR1H
  Stomach BD12
  Toe
   Left BQ1QZZZ
   Right BQ1PZZZ
  Tracheobronchial Tree
   Bilateral BB19YZZ
   Left BB18YZZ
   Right BB17YZZ
  Ureter
   Ileal Loop and Kidney BT1G
   Kidney and Bladder BT14
    Left BT1F
    Right BT1D
   Left BT17
   Right BT16
  Urethra BT15
  Urethra and Bladder BT1B
  Uterus BU16
  Uterus and Fallopian Tube BU18
  Vagina BU19
  Vasa Vasorum BV18
  Vein
   Cerebellar B511
   Cerebral B511
   Epidural B510
   Jugular
    Bilateral B515
    Left B514
    Right B513
   Lower Extremity
    Bilateral B51D
    Left B51C
    Right B51B
   Other B51V
   Pelvic (Iliac)
    Left B51G
    Right B51F
   Pelvic (Iliac) Bilateral B51H
   Portal B51T
   Pulmonary
    Bilateral B51S
    Left B51R
    Right B51Q
   Renal
    Bilateral B51L
    Left B51K
    Right B51J
   Spanchnic B51T
   Subclavian
    Left B517
    Right B516
   Upper Extremity
    Bilateral B51P
    Left B51N
    Right B51M
  Vena Cava
   Inferior B519
   Superior B518
  Wrist
   Left BP1M
   Right BP1L

Fluoroscopy, laser intraoperative
  Fluoroscopy, Heart B21
  Fluoroscopy, Lower Arteries B41
  Fluoroscopy, Upper Arteries B31

Flushing
  see Irrigation

Foley catheter
  use Drainage Device

Foramen magnum
  use Bone, Occipital, Left
  use Bone, Occipital, Right

Foramen of Monro (intraventricular)
  use Cerebral Ventricle

Foreskin
  use Prepuce

Formula™ Balloon-Expandable Renal Stent System
  use Intraluminal Device

Fossa of Rosenmuller
  use Nasopharynx

Fourth cranial nerve
  use Nerve, Trochlear

Fourth ventricle
  use Cerebral Ventricle

Fovea
  use Retina, Left
  use Retina, Right

Fragmentation
  Ampulla of Vater 0FFC
  Anus 0DFQ
  Appendix 0DFJ
  Bladder 0TFB
  Bladder Neck 0TFC
  Bronchus
   Lingula 0BF9
   Lower Lobe
    Left 0BFB
    Right 0BF6
   Main
    Left 0BF7
    Right 0BF3
   Middle Lobe, Right 0BF5
   Upper Lobe
    Left 0BF8
    Right 0BF4
  Carina 0BF2
  Cavity, Cranial 0WF1
  Cecum 0DFH
  Cerebral Ventricle 00F6
  Colon
   Ascending 0DFK
   Descending 0DFM
   Sigmoid 0DFN
   Transverse 0DFL
  Duct
   Common Bile 0FF9
   Cystic 0FF8
   Hepatic
    Left 0FF6
    Right 0FF5
   Pancreatic 0FFD
    Accessory 0FFF
   Parotid
    Left 0CFC
    Right 0CFB
  Duodenum 0DF9
  Epidural Space 00F3
  Esophagus 0DF5
  Fallopian Tube
   Left 0UF6
   Right 0UF5
  Fallopian Tubes, Bilateral 0UF7
  Gallbladder 0FF4
  Gastrointestinal Tract 0WFP
  Genitourinary Tract 0WFR
  Ileum 0DFB
  Intestine
   Large 0DFE
    Left 0DFG
    Right 0DFF
   Small 0DF8
  Jejunum 0DFA
  Kidney Pelvis
   Left 0TF4
   Right 0TF3
  Mediastinum 0WFC
  Oral Cavity and Throat 0WF3
  Pelvic Cavity 0WFJ
  Pericardial Cavity 0WFD
  Pericardium 02FN
  Peritoneal Cavity 0WFG
  Pleural Cavity
   Left 0WFB
   Right 0WF9

Fragmentation *(continued)*
  Rectum 0DFP
  Respiratory Tract 0WFQ
  Spinal Canal 00FU
  Stomach 0DF6
  Subarachnoid Space 00F5
  Subdural Space 00F4
  Trachea 0BF1
  Ureter
   Left 0TF7
   Right 0TF6
  Urethra 0TFD
  Uterus 0UF9
  Vitreous
   Left 08F5
   Right 08F4

Freestyle (Stentless) Aortic Root Bioprosthesis
  use Zooplastic Tissue in Heart and Great Vessels

Frenectomy
  see Excision, Mouth and Throat 0CB
  see Resection, Mouth and Throat 0CT

Frenoplasty, frenuloplasty
  see Repair, Mouth and Throat 0CQ
  see Replacement, Mouth and Throat 0CR
  see Supplement, Mouth and Throat 0CU

Frenotomy
  see Drainage, Mouth and Throat 0C9
  see Release, Mouth and Throat 0CN

Frenulotomy
  see Drainage, Mouth and Throat 0C9
  see Release, Mouth and Throat 0CN

Frenulum labii inferioris
  use Lip, Lower

Frenulum labii superioris
  use Lip, Upper

Frenulum linguae
  use Tongue

Frenulumectomy
  see Excision, Mouth and Throat 0CB
  see Resection, Mouth and Throat 0CT

Frontal lobe
  use Cerebral Hemisphere

Frontal vein
  use Vein, Face, Left
  use Vein, Face, Right

Fulguration
  see Destruction

Fundoplication, gastroesophageal
  see Restriction, Esophagogastric Junction 0DV4

Fundus uteri
  use Uterus

Fusion
  Acromioclavicular
   Left 0RGH
   Right 0RGG
  Ankle
   Left 0SGG
   Right 0SGF
  Carpal
   Left 0RGR
   Right 0RGQ
  Cervical Vertebral 0RG1
   2 or more 0RG2
  Cervicothoracic Vertebral 0RG4
  Coccygeal 0SG6
  Elbow
   Left 0RGM
   Right 0RGL
  Finger Phalangeal
   Left 0RGX
   Right 0RGW
  Hip
   Left 0SGB
   Right 0SG9
  Knee
   Left 0SGD
   Right 0SGC

Fusion *(continued)*
  Lumbar Vertebral 0SG0
   2 or more 0SG1
  Lumbosacral 0SG3
  Metacarpocarpal
   Left 0RGT
   Right 0RGS
  Metacarpophalangeal
   Left 0RGV
   Right 0RGU
  Metatarsal-Phalangeal
   Left 0SGN
   Right 0SGM
  Metatarsal-Tarsal
   Left 0SGL
   Right 0SGK
  Occipital-cervical 0RG0
  Sacrococcygeal 0SG5
  Sacroiliac
   Left 0SG8
   Right 0SG7
  Shoulder
   Left 0RGK
   Right 0RGJ
  Sternoclavicular
   Left 0RGF
   Right 0RGE
  Tarsal
   Left 0SGJ
   Right 0SGH
  Temporomandibular
   Left 0RGD
   Right 0RGC
  Thoracic Vertebral 0RG6
   2 to 7 0RG7
   8 or more 0RG8
  Thoracolumbar Vertebral 0RGA
  Toe Phalangeal
   Left 0SGQ
   Right 0SGP
  Wrist
   Left 0RGP
   Right 0RGN

Fusion screw (compression)(lag) (locking)
  use Internal Fixation Device in Lower Joints
  use Internal Fixation Device in Upper Joints

G

Gait training
  see Motor Treatment, Rehabilitation F07

Galea aponeurotica
  use Subcutaneous Tissue and Fascia, Scalp

Ganglion impar (ganglion of Walther)
  use Nerve, Sacral Sympathetic

Ganglionectomy
  Destruction of lesion
   see Destruction
  Excision of lesion
   see Excision

Gasserian ganglion
  use Nerve, Trigeminal

Gastrectomy
  Partial
   see Excision, Stomach 0DB6
  Total
   see Resection, Stomach 0DT6
  Vertical (sleeve)
   see Excision, Stomach 0DB6

Gastric electrical stimulation (GES) lead
  use Stimulator Lead in Gastrointestinal System

Gastric lymph node
  use Lymphatic, Aortic

Gastric pacemaker lead
use Stimulator Lead in
Gastrointestinal System
Gastric plexus
use Nerve, Abdominal Sympathetic
Gastrocnemius muscle
use Muscle, Lower Leg, Left
use Muscle, Lower Leg, Right
Gastrocolic ligament
use Omentum, Greater
Gastrocolic omentum
use Omentum, Greater
Gastrocolostomy
see Bypass, Gastrointestinal
System 0D1
see Drainage, Gastrointestinal
System 0D9
Gastroduodenal artery
use Artery, Hepatic
Gastroduodenectomy
see Excision, Gastrointestinal
System 0DB
see Resection, Gastrointestinal
System 0DT
Gastroduodenoscopy 0DJ08ZZ
Gastroenteroplasty
see Repair, Gastrointestinal System
0DQ
see Supplement, Gastrointestinal
System 0DU
Gastroenterostomy
see Bypass, Gastrointestinal System
0D1
see Drainage, Gastrointestinal
System 0D9
Gastroesophageal (GE) junction
use Esophagogastric Junction
Gastrogastrostomy
see Bypass, Stomach 0D16
see Drainage, Stomach 0D96
Gastrohepatic omentum
use Omentum, Lesser
Gastrojejunostomy
see Bypass, Stomach 0D16
see Drainage, Stomach 0D96
Gastrolysis
see Release, Stomach 0DN6
Gastropexy
see Repair, Stomach 0DQ6
see Reposition, Stomach 0DS6
Gastrophrenic ligament
use Omentum, Greater
Gastroplasty
see Repair, Stomach 0DQ6
see Supplement, Stomach 0DU6
Gastroplication
see Restriction, Stomach 0DV6
Gastropylorectomy
see Excision, Gastrointestinal
System 0DB
Gastrorrhaphy
see Repair, Stomach 0DQ6
Gastroscopy 0DJ68ZZ
Gastrosplenic ligament
use Omentum, Greater
Gastrostomy
see Bypass, Stomach 0D16
see Drainage, Stomach 0D96
Gastrotomy
see Drainage, Stomach 0D96
Gemellus muscle
use Muscle, Hip, Left
use Muscle, Hip, Right
Geniculate ganglion
use Nerve, Facial
Geniculate nucleus
use Thalamus
Genioglossus muscle
use Muscle, Tongue, Palate,
Pharynx
Genioplasty
see Alteration, Jaw, Lower 0W05

Genitofemoral nerve
use Nerve, Lumbar Plexus
Gingivectomy
see Excision, Mouth and Throat
0CB
Gingivoplasty
see Repair, Mouth and Throat
0CQ
see Replacement, Mouth and Throat
0CR
see Supplement, Mouth and Throat
0CU
Glans penis
use Prepuce
Glenohumeral joint
use Joint, Shoulder, Left
use Joint, Shoulder, Right
Glenohumeral ligament
use Bursa and Ligament, Shoulder,
Left
use Bursa and Ligament, Shoulder,
Right
Glenoid fossa (of scapula)
use Glenoid Cavity, Left
use Glenoid Cavity, Right
Glenoid ligament (labrum)
use Shoulder Joint, Left
use Shoulder Joint, Right
Globus pallidus
use Basal Ganglia
Glomectomy
see Excision, Endocrine System
0GB
see Resection, Endocrine System
0GT
Glossectomy
see Excision, Tongue 0CB7
see Resection, Tongue 0CT7
Glossoepiglottic fold
use Epiglottis
Glossopexy
see Repair, Tongue 0CQ7
see Reposition, Tongue 0CS7
Glossoplasty
see Repair, Tongue 0CQ7
see Replacement, Tongue
0CR7
see Supplement, Tongue 0CU7
Glossorrhaphy
see Repair, Tongue 0CQ7
Glossotomy
see Drainage, Tongue 0C97
Glottis
use Larynx
Gluteal Artery Perforator Flap
Bilateral 0HRV079
Left 0HRU079
Right 0HRT079
Gluteal lymph node
use Lymphatic, Pelvis
Gluteal vein
use Vein, Hypogastric, Left
use Vein, Hypogastric, Right
Gluteus maximus muscle
use Muscle, Hip, Left
use Muscle, Hip, Right
Gluteus medius muscle
use Muscle, Hip, Left
use Muscle, Hip, Right
Gluteus minimus muscle
use Muscle, Hip, Left
use Muscle, Hip, Right
GORE® DUALMESH®
use Synthetic Substitute
Gracilis muscle
use Muscle, Upper Leg, Left
use Muscle, Upper Leg, Right
Graft
see Replacement
see Supplement
Great auricular nerve
use Nerve, Cervical Plexus

Great cerebral vein
use Vein, Intracranial
Great saphenous vein
use Vein, Greater Saphenous, Left
use Vein, Greater Saphenous, Right
Greater alar cartilage
use Nose
Greater occipital nerve
use Nerve, Cervical
Greater splanchnic nerve
use Nerve, Thoracic Sympathetic
Greater superficial petrosal nerve
use Nerve, Facial
Greater trochanter
use Femur, Upper, Left
use Femur, Upper, Right
Greater tuberosity
use Humeral Head, Left
use Humeral Head, Right
Greater vestibular (Bartholin's) gland
use Gland, Vestibular
Greater wing
use Bone, Sphenoid, Left
use Bone, Sphenoid, Right
Guedel airway
use Intraluminal Device, Airway in
Mouth and Throat
Guidance, catheter placement
EKG
see Measurement, Physiological
Systems 4A0
Fluoroscopy
see Fluoroscopy, Veins B51
Ultrasound
see Ultrasonography, Veins B54

H

Hallux
use Toe, 1st, Left
use Toe, 1st, Right
Hamate bone
use Carpal, Left
use Carpal, Right
**Hancock Bioprosthesis (aortic)
(mitral) valve**
use Zooplastic Tissue in Heart and
Great Vessels
**Hancock Bioprosthetic Valved
Conduit**
use Zooplastic Tissue in Heart and
Great Vessels
Harvesting, stem cells
see Pheresis, Circulatory 6A55
Head of fibula
use Fibula, Left
use Fibula, Right
Hearing Aid Assessment F14Z
Hearing Assessment F13Z
Hearing Device
Bone Conduction
Left 09HE
Right 09HD
Insertion of device in
Left 0NH6
Right 0NH5
Multiple Channel Cochlear
Prosthesis
Left 09HE
Right 09HD
Removal of device from, Skull 0NP0
Revision of device in, Skull 0NW0
Single Channel Cochlear Prosthesis
Left 09HE
Right 09HD
Hearing Treatment F09Z
Heart Assist System
External
Insertion of device in, Heart
02HA
Removal of device from, Heart
02PA

Heart Assist System *(continued)*
External *(continued)*
Revision of device in, Heart
02WA
Implantable
Insertion of device in, Heart
02HA
Removal of device from, Heart
02PA
Revision of device in, Heart
02WA
**HeartMate II® Left Ventricular Assist
Device (LVAD)**
use Implantable Heart Assist System
in Heart and Great Vessels
**HeartMate XVE® Left Ventricular
Assist Device (LVAD)**
use Implantable Heart Assist
System in Heart and Great
Vessels
**HeartMate® implantable heart assist
system**
see Insertion of device in, Heart
02HA
Helix
use Ear, External, Bilateral
use Ear, External, Left
use Ear, External, Right
Hemicolectomy
see Resection, Gastrointestinal
System 0DT
Hemicystectomy
see Excision, Urinary System 0TB
Hemigastrectomy
see Excision, Gastrointestinal
System 0DB
Hemiglossectomy
see Excision, Mouth and Throat
0CB
Hemilaminectomy
see Excision, Lower Bones 0QB
see Excision, Upper Bones 0PB
Hemilaminotomy
see Drainage, Lower Bones 0Q9
see Drainage, Upper Bones 0P9
see Excision, Lower Bones 0QB
see Excision, Upper Bones 0PB
see Release, Central Nervous
System 00N
see Release, Lower Bones 0QN
see Release, Peripheral Nervous
System 01N
see Release, Upper Bones 0PN
Hemilaryngectomy
see Excision, Larynx 0CBS
Hemimandibulectomy
see Excision, Head and Facial Bones
0NB
Hemimaxillectomy
see Excision, Head and Facial Bones
0NB
Hemipylorectomy
see Excision, Gastrointestinal
System 0DB
Hemispherectomy
see Excision, Central Nervous
System 00B
see Resection, Central Nervous
System 00T
Hemithyroidectomy
see Resection, Endocrine System
0GT
see Excision, Endocrine System
0GB
Hemodialysis 5A1D00Z
Hepatectomy
see Excision, Hepatobiliary System
and Pancreas 0FB
see Resection, Hepatobiliary System
and Pancreas 0FT
Hepatic artery proper
use Artery, Hepatic

Hepatic flexure
　use Colon, Ascending
Hepatic lymph node
　use Lymphatic, Aortic
Hepatic plexus
　use Nerve, Abdominal Sympathetic
Hepatic portal vein
　use Vein, Portal
Hepaticoduodenostomy
　see Bypass, Hepatobiliary System
　　and Pancreas 0F1
　see Drainage, Hepatobiliary System
　　and Pancreas 0F9
Hepaticotomy
　see Drainage, Hepatobiliary System
　　and Pancreas 0F9
Hepatocholedochostomy
　see Drainage, Duct, Common Bile
　　0F99
Hepatogastric ligament
　use Omentum, Lesser
Hepatopancreatic ampulla
　use Ampulla of Vater
Hepatopexy
　see Repair, Hepatobiliary System
　　and Pancreas 0FQ
　see Reposition, Hepatobiliary
　　System and Pancreas 0FS
Hepatorrhaphy
　see Repair, Hepatobiliary System
　　and Pancreas 0FQ
Hepatotomy
　see Drainage, Hepatobiliary System
　　and Pancreas 0F9
**Herculink (RX) Elite Renal Stent
　System**
　use Intraluminal Device
Herniorrhaphy
　see Repair, Anatomical Regions,
　　General 0WQ
　see Repair, Anatomical Regions,
　　Lower Extremities 0YQ
　with synthetic substitute
　see Supplement, Anatomical
　　Regions, General 0WU
　see Supplement, Anatomical
　　Regions, Lower Extremities
　　0YU
Hiip (joint) liner
　use Liner in Lower Joints
Holter monitoring 4A12X45
Holter valve ventricular shunt
　use Synthetic Substitute
Humeroradial joint
　use Joint, Elbow, Left
　use Joint, Elbow, Right
Humeroulnar joint
　use Joint, Elbow, Left
　use Joint, Elbow, Right
Humerus, distal
　use Humeral Shaft, Left
　use Humeral Shaft, Right
Hydrocelectomy
　see Excision, Male Reproductive
　　System 0VB
Hydrotherapy
　Assisted exercise in pool
　see Motor Treatment,
　　Rehabilitation F07
　Whirlpool
　see Activities of Daily Living
　　Treatment, Rehabilitation
　　F08
Hymenectomy
　see Excision, Hymen 0UBK
　see Resection, Hymen 0UTK
Hymenoplasty
　see Repair, Hymen 0UQK
　see Supplement, Hymen
　　0UUK
Hymenorrhaphy
　see Repair, Hymen 0UQK

Hymenotomy
　see Division, Hymen 0U8K
　see Drainage, Hymen 0U9K
Hyoglossus muscle
　use Muscle, Tongue, Palate, Pharynx
Hyoid artery
　use Artery, Thyroid, Left
　use Artery, Thyroid, Right
Hyperalimentation
　see Introduction of substance in
　　or on
Hyperbaric oxygenation
　Decompression sickness treatment
　see Decompression, Circulatory
　　6A15
　Wound treatment
　see Assistance, Circulatory
　　5A05
Hyperthermia
　Radiation Therapy
　　Abdomen DWY38ZZ
　　Adrenal Gland DGY28ZZ
　　Bile Ducts DFY28ZZ
　　Bladder DTY28ZZ
　　Bone, Other DPYC8ZZ
　　Bone Marrow D7Y08ZZ
　　Brain D0Y08ZZ
　　Brain Stem D0Y18ZZ
　　Breast
　　　Left DMY08ZZ
　　　Right DMY18ZZ
　　Bronchus DBY18ZZ
　　Cervix DUY18ZZ
　　Chest DWY28ZZ
　　Chest Wall DBY78ZZ
　　Colon DDY58ZZ
　　Diaphragm DBY88ZZ
　　Duodenum DDY28ZZ
　　Ear D9Y08ZZ
　　Esophagus DDY08ZZ
　　Eye D8Y08ZZ
　　Femur DPY98ZZ
　　Fibula DPYB8ZZ
　　Gallbladder DFY18ZZ
　　Gland
　　　Adrenal DGY28ZZ
　　　Parathyroid DGY48ZZ
　　　Pituitary DGY08ZZ
　　　Thyroid DGY58ZZ
　　Glands, Salivary D9Y68ZZ
　　Head and Neck DWY18ZZ
　　Hemibody DWY48ZZ
　　Humerus DPY68ZZ
　　Hypopharynx D9Y38ZZ
　　Ileum DDY48ZZ
　　Jejunum DDY38ZZ
　　Kidney DTY08ZZ
　　Larynx D9YB8ZZ
　　Liver DFY08ZZ
　　Lung DBY28ZZ
　　Lymphatics
　　　Abdomen D7Y68ZZ
　　　Axillary D7Y48ZZ
　　　Inguinal D7Y88ZZ
　　　Neck D7Y38ZZ
　　　Pelvis D7Y78ZZ
　　　Thorax D7Y58ZZ
　　Mandible DPY38ZZ
　　Maxilla DPY28ZZ
　　Mediastinum DBY68ZZ
　　Mouth D9Y48ZZ
　　Nasopharynx D9YD8ZZ
　　Neck and Head DWY18ZZ
　　Nerve, Peripheral D0Y78ZZ
　　Nose D9Y18ZZ
　　Oropharynx D9YF8ZZ
　　Ovary DUY08ZZ
　　Palate
　　　Hard D9Y88ZZ
　　　Soft D9Y98ZZ
　　Pancreas DFY38ZZ
　　Parathyroid Gland DGY48ZZ

Hyperthermia *(continued)*
　Radiation Therapy *(continued)*
　　Pelvic Bones DPY88ZZ
　　Pelvic Region DWY68ZZ
　　Pineal Body DGY18ZZ
　　Pituitary Gland DGY08ZZ
　　Pleura DBY58ZZ
　　Prostate DVY08ZZ
　　Radius DPY78ZZ
　　Rectum DDY78ZZ
　　Rib DPY58ZZ
　　Sinuses D9Y78ZZ
　　Skin
　　　Abdomen DHY88ZZ
　　　Arm DHY48ZZ
　　　Back DHY78ZZ
　　　Buttock DHY98ZZ
　　　Chest DHY68ZZ
　　　Face DHY28ZZ
　　　Leg DHYB8ZZ
　　　Neck DHY38ZZ
　　Skull DPY08ZZ
　　Spinal Cord D0Y68ZZ
　　Spleen D7Y28ZZ
　　Sternum DPY48ZZ
　　Stomach DDY18ZZ
　　Testis DVY18ZZ
　　Thymus D7Y18ZZ
　　Thyroid Gland DGY58ZZ
　　Tibia DPYB8ZZ
　　Tongue D9Y58ZZ
　　Trachea DBY08ZZ
　　Ulna DPY78ZZ
　　Ureter DTY18ZZ
　　Urethra DTY38ZZ
　　Uterus DUY28ZZ
　　Whole Body DWY58ZZ
　Whole Body 6A3Z
Hypnosis GZFZZZZZ
Hypogastric artery
　use Artery, Internal Iliac, Left
　use Artery, Internal Iliac, Right
Hypopharynx
　use Pharynx
Hypophysectomy
　see Excision, Gland, Pituitary
　　0GB0
　see Resection, Gland, Pituitary
　　0GT0
Hypophysis
　use Gland, Pituitary
Hypothalamotomy
　see Destruction, Thalamus 0059
Hypothenar muscle
　use Muscle, Hand, Left
　use Muscle, Hand, Right
Hypothermia, Whole Body 6A4Z
Hysterectomy
　supracervical
　see Resection, Uterus 0UT9
　total
　see Resection, Cervix 0UTC
　see Resection, Uterus 0UT9
Hysterolysis
　see Release, Uterus 0UN9
Hysteropexy
　see Repair, Uterus 0UQ9
　see Reposition, Uterus 0US9
Hysteroplasty
　see Repair, Uterus 0UQ9
Hysterorrhaphy
　see Repair, Uterus 0UQ9
Hysteroscopy 0UJD8ZZ
Hysterotomy
　see Drainage, Uterus 0U99
Hysterotrachelectomy
　see Resection, Cervix 0UTC
　see Resection, Uterus 0UT9
Hysterotracheloplasty
　see Repair, Uterus 0UQ9
Hysterotrachelorrhaphy
　see Repair, Uterus 0UQ9

I

IABP (Intra-aortic balloon pump)
　see Assistance, Cardiac 5A02
**IAEMT (Intraoperative anesthetic
　effect monitoring and
　titration)**
　see Monitoring, Central Nervous
　　4A10
**Idarucizumab, Dabigatran Reversal
　Agent** XW0
Ileal artery
　use Artery, Superior Mesenteric
Ileectomy
　see Excision, Ileum 0DBB
　see Resection, Ileum 0DTB
Ileocolic artery
　use Artery, Superior Mesenteric
Ileocolic vein
　use Vein, Colic
Ileopexy
　see Repair, Ileum 0DQB
　see Reposition, Ileum 0DSB
Ileorrhaphy
　see Repair, Ileum 0DQB
Ileoscopy 0DJD8ZZ
Ileostomy
　see Bypass, Ileum 0D1B
　see Drainage, Ileum 0D9B
Ileotomy
　see Drainage, Ileum 0D9B
Ileoureterostomy
　see Bypass, Urinary System 0T1
Iliac crest
　use Bone, Pelvic, Left
　use Bone, Pelvic, Right
Iliac fascia
　use Subcutaneous Tissue and Fascia,
　　Upper Leg, Left
　use Subcutaneous Tissue and Fascia,
　　Upper Leg, Right
Iliac lymph node
　use Lymphatic, Pelvis
Iliacus muscle
　use Muscle, Hip, Left
　use Muscle, Hip, Right
Iliofemoral ligament
　use Bursa and Ligament, Hip, Left
　use Bursa and Ligament, Hip, Right
Iliohypogastric nerve
　use Nerve, Lumbar Plexus
Ilioinguinal nerve
　use Nerve, Lumbar Plexus
Iliolumbar artery
　use Artery, Internal Iliac, Left
　use Artery, Internal Iliac, Right
Iliolumbar ligament
　use Bursa and Ligament, Trunk, Left
　use Bursa and Ligament, Trunk,
　　Right
Iliotibial tract (band)
　use Subcutaneous Tissue and Fascia,
　　Upper Leg, Left
　use Subcutaneous Tissue and Fascia,
　　Upper Leg, Right
Ilium
　use Bone, Pelvic, Left
　use Bone, Pelvic, Right
Ilizarov external fixator
　use External Fixation Device, Ring
　　in 0PH
　use External Fixation Device, Ring
　　in 0PS
　use External Fixation Device, Ring
　　in 0QH
　use External Fixation Device, Ring
　　in 0QS
Ilizarov-Vecklich device
　use External Fixation Device, Limb
　　Lengthening in 0QH
　use External Fixation Device, Limb
　　Lengthening in 0PH

Imaging, diagnostic
  see Computerized Tomography (CT Scan)
  see Fluoroscopy
  see Magnetic Resonance Imaging (MRI)
  see Plain Radiography
  see Ultrasonography
Immobilization
  Abdominal Wall 2W33X
  Arm
    Lower
      Left 2W3DX
      Right 2W3CX
    Upper
      Left 2W3BX
      Right 2W3AX
  Back 2W35X
  Chest Wall 2W34X
  Extremity
    Lower
      Left 2W3MX
      Right 2W3LX
    Upper
      Left 2W39X
      Right 2W38X
  Face 2W31X
  Finger
    Left 2W3KX
    Right 2W3JX
  Foot
    Left 2W3TX
    Right 2W3SX
  Hand
    Left 2W3FX
    Right 2W3EX
  Head 2W30X
  Inguinal Region
    Left 2W37X
    Right 2W36X
  Leg
    Lower
      Left 2W3RX
      Right 2W3QX
    Upper
      Left 2W3PX
      Right 2W3NX
  Neck 2W32X
  Thumb
    Left 2W3H
    Right 2W3GX
  Toe
    Left 2W3VX
    Right 2W3UX
Immunization
  see Introduction of Serum, Toxoid, and Vaccine
Immunotherapy
  see Introduction of Immunotherapeutic Substance
Immunotherapy, antineoplastic
  Interferon
    see Introduction of Low-dose Interleukin-2
  Interleukin-2, high-dose
    see Introduction of High-dose Interleukin-2
  Interleukin-2, low-dose
    see Introduction of Low-dose Interleukin-2
  Monoclonal antibody
    see Introduction of Monoclonal Antibody
  Proleukin, high-dose
    see Introduction of High-dose Interleukin-2
  Proleukin, low-dose
    see Introduction of Low-dose Interleukin-2
Impeller Pump
  Continuous, Output 5A0221D
  Intermittent, Output 5A0211D

Implantable cardioverter-defibrillator (ICD)
  use Defibrillator Generator in 0JH
Implantable drug infusion pump (anti-spasmodic) (chemotherapy)(pain)
  use Infusion Device, Pump in Subcutaneous Tissue and Fascia
Implantable glucose monitoring device
  use Monitoring Device
Implantable hemodynamic monitor (IHM)
  use Monitoring Device, Hemodynamic in 0JH
Implantable hemodynamic monitoring system (IHMS)
  use Monitoring Device, Hemodynamic in 0JH
Implantable Miniature Telescope™ (IMT)
  use Synthetic Substitute, Intraocular Telescope in 08R
Implantation
  see Insertion
  see Replacement
Implanted (venous)(access) port
  use Vascular Access Device, Reservoir in Subcutaneous Tissue and Fascia
IMV (intermittent mandatory ventilation)
  see Assistance, Respiratory 5A09
In Vitro Fertilization 8E0ZXY1
Incision, abscess
  see Drainage
Incudectomy
  see Excision, Ear, Nose, Sinus 09B
  see Resection, Ear, Nose, Sinus 09T
Incudopexy
  see Reposition, Ear, Nose, Sinus 09S
  see Repair, Ear, Nose, Sinus 09Q
Incus
  use Auditory Ossicle, Left
  use Auditory Ossicle, Right
Induction of labor
  Artificial rupture of membranes
    see Drainage, Pregnancy 109
  Oxytocin
    see Introduction of Hormone
InDura, intrathecal catheter (1P) (spinal)
  use Infusion Device
Inferior cardiac nerve
  use Nerve, Thoracic Sympathetic
Inferior cerebellar vein
  use Vein, Intracranial
Inferior cerebral vein
  use Vein, Intracranial
Inferior epigastric artery
  use Artery, External Iliac, Left
  use Artery, External Iliac, Right
Inferior epigastric lymph node
  use Lymphatic, Pelvis
Inferior genicular artery
  use Artery, Popliteal, Left
  use Artery, Popliteal, Right
Inferior gluteal artery
  use Artery, Internal Iliac, Left
  use Artery, Internal Iliac, Right
Inferior gluteal nerve
  use Nerve, Sacral Plexus
Inferior hypogastric plexus
  use Nerve, Abdominal Sympathetic
Inferior labial artery
  use Artery, Face
Inferior longitudinal muscle
  use Muscle, Tongue, Palate, Pharynx
Inferior mesenteric ganglion
  use Nerve, Abdominal Sympathetic

Inferior mesenteric lymph node
  use Lymphatic, Mesenteric
Inferior mesenteric plexus
  use Nerve, Abdominal Sympathetic
Inferior oblique muscle
  use Muscle, Extraocular, Left
  use Muscle, Extraocular, Right
Inferior pancreaticoduodenal artery
  use Artery, Superior Mesenteric
Inferior phrenic artery
  use Aorta, Abdominal
Inferior rectus muscle
  use Muscle, Extraocular, Left
  use Muscle, Extraocular, Right
Inferior suprarenal artery
  use Artery, Renal, Left
  use Artery, Renal, Right
Inferior tarsal plate
  use Eyelid, Lower, Left
  use Eyelid, Lower, Right
Inferior thyroid vein
  use Vein, Innominate, Left
  use Vein, Innominate, Right
Inferior tibiofibular joint
  use Joint, Ankle, Left
  use Joint, Ankle, Right
Inferior turbinate
  use Turbinate, Nasal
Inferior ulnar collateral artery
  use Artery, Brachial, Left
  use Artery, Brachial, Right
Inferior vesical artery
  use Artery, Internal Iliac, Left
  use Artery, Internal Iliac, Right
Infraauricular lymph node
  use Lymphatic, Head
Infraclavicular (deltopectoral) lymph node
  use Lymphatic, Upper Extremity, Left
  use Lymphatic, Upper Extremity, Right
Infrahyoid muscle
  use Muscle, Neck, Left
  use Muscle, Neck, Right
Infraparotid lymph node
  use Lymphatic, Head
Infraspinatus fascia
  use Subcutaneous Tissue and Fascia, Upper Arm, Left
  use Subcutaneous Tissue and Fascia, Upper Arm, Right
Infraspinatus muscle
  use Muscle, Shoulder, Left
  use Muscle, Shoulder, Right
Infundibulopelvic ligament
  use Uterine Supporting Structure
Infusion
  see Introduction of substance in or on
Infusion Device, Pump
  Insertion of device in
    Abdomen 0JH8
    Back 0JH7
    Chest 0JH6
    Lower Arm
      Left 0JHH
      Right 0JHG
    Lower Leg
      Left 0JHP
      Right 0JHN
    Trunk 0JHT
    Upper Arm
      Left 0JHF
      Right 0JHD
    Upper Leg
      Left 0JHM
      Right 0JHL
  Removal of device from
    Lower Extremity 0JPW
    Trunk 0JPT
    Upper Extremity 0JPV

Infusion Device, Pump *(continued)*
  Revision of device in
    Lower Extremity 0JWW
    Trunk 0JWT
    Upper Extremity 0JWV
Infusion, glucarpidase
  Central vein 3E043GQ
  Peripheral vein 3E033GQ
Inguinal canal
  use Inguinal Region, Bilateral
  use Inguinal Region, Left
  use Inguinal Region, Right
Inguinal triangle
  use Inguinal Region, Bilateral
  use Inguinal Region, Left
  use Inguinal Region, Right
Injection
  see Introduction of substance in or on
Injection reservoir, port
  use Vascular Access Device, Reservoir in Subcutaneous Tissue and Fascia
Injection reservoir, pump
  use Infusion Device, Pump in Subcutaneous Tissue and Fascia
Insemination, artificial 3E0P7LZ
Insertion
  Antimicrobial envelope
    see Introduction of Anti-infective
  Aqueous drainage shunt
    see Bypass, Eye 081
    see Drainage, Eye 089
  Products of Conception 10H0
  Spinal Stabilization Device
    see Insertion of device in, Upper Joints 0RH
    see Insertion of device in, Lower Joints 0SH
Insertion of device in
  Abdominal Wall 0WHF
  Acetabulum
    Left 0QH5
    Right 0QH4
  Anal Sphincter 0DHR
  Ankle Region
    Left 0YHL
    Right 0YHK
  Anus 0DHQ
  Aorta
    Abdominal 04H0
    Thoracic 02HW
  Arm
    Lower
      Left 0XHF
      Right 0XHD
    Upper
      Left 0XH9
      Right 0XH8
  Artery
    Anterior Tibial
      Left 04HQ
      Right 04HP
    Axillary
      Left 03H6
      Right 03H5
    Brachial
      Left 03H8
      Right 03H7
    Celiac 04H1
    Colic
      Left 04H7
      Middle 04H8
      Right 04H6
    Common Carotid
      Left 03HJ
      Right 03HH
    Common Iliac
      Left 04HD
      Right 04HC

Inspection (*continued*)

Inguinal Region
  Bilateral 0YJA
  Left 0YJ6
  Right 0YJ5
Intestinal Tract
  Lower 0DJD
  Upper 0DJ0
Jaw
  Lower 0WJ5
  Upper 0WJ4
Joint
  Acromioclavicular
    Left 0RJH
    Right 0RJG
  Ankle
    Left 0SJG
    Right 0SJF
  Carpal
    Left 0RJR
    Right 0RJQ
  Cervical Vertebral 0RJ1
  Cervicothoracic Vertebral
    0RJ4
  Coccygeal 0SJ6
  Elbow
    Left 0RJM
    Right 0RJL
  Finger Phalangeal
    Left 0RJX
    Right 0RJW
  Hip
    Left 0SJB
    Right 0SJ9
  Knee
    Left 0SJD
    Right 0SJC
  Lumbar Vertebral 0SJ0
  Lumbosacral 0SJ3
  Metacarpocarpal
    Left 0RJT
    Right 0RJS
  Metacarpophalangeal
    Left 0RJV
    Right 0RJU
  Metatarsal-Phalangeal
    Left 0SJN
    Right 0SJM
  Metatarsal-Tarsal
    Left 0SJL
    Right 0SJK
  Occipital-cervical 0RJ0
  Sacrococcygeal 0SJ5
  Sacroiliac
    Left 0SJ8
    Right 0SJ7
  Shoulder
    Left 0RJK
    Right 0RJJ
  Sternoclavicular
    Left 0RJF
    Right 0RJE
  Tarsal
    Left 0SJJ
    Right 0SJH
  Temporomandibular
    Left 0RJD
    Right 0RJC
  Thoracic Vertebral 0RJ6
  Thoracolumbar Vertebral
    0RJA
  Toe Phalangeal
    Left 0SJQ
    Right 0SJP
  Wrist
    Left 0RJP
    Right 0RJN
Kidney 0TJ5
Knee Region
  Left 0YJG
  Right 0YJF
Larynx 0CJS

Inspection (*continued*)

Leg
  Lower
    Left 0YJJ
    Right 0YJH
  Upper
    Left 0YJD
    Right 0YJC
Lens
  Left 08JKXZZ
  Right 08JJXZZ
Liver 0FJ0
Lung
  Left 0BJL
  Right 0BJK
Lymphatic 07JN
  Thoracic Duct 07JK
Mediastinum 0WJC
Mesentery 0DJV
Mouth and Throat 0CJY
Muscle
  Extraocular
    Left 08JM
    Right 08JL
  Lower 0KJY
  Upper 0KJX
Neck 0WJ6
Nerve
  Cranial 00JE
  Peripheral 01JY
Nose 09JK
Omentum 0DJU
Oral Cavity and Throat 0WJ3
Ovary 0UJ3
Pancreas 0FJG
Parathyroid Gland 0GJR
Pelvic Cavity 0WJJ
Penis 0VJS
Pericardial Cavity 0WJD
Perineum
  Female 0WJN
  Male 0WJM
Peritoneal Cavity 0WJG
Peritoneum 0DJW
Pineal Body 0GJ1
Pleura 0BJQ
Pleural Cavity
  Left 0WJB
  Right 0WJ9
Products of Conception 10J0
  Ectopic 10J2
  Retained 10J1
Prostate and Seminal Vesicles
  0VJ4
Respiratory Tract 0WJQ
Retroperitoneum 0WJH
Scrotum and Tunica Vaginalis
  0VJ8
Shoulder Region
  Left 0XJ3
  Right 0XJ2
Sinus 09JY
Skin 0HJPXZZ
Skull 0NJ0
Spinal Canal 00JU
Spinal Cord 00JV
Spleen 07JP
Stomach 0DJ6
Subcutaneous Tissue and Fascia
  Head and Neck 0JJS
  Lower Extremity 0JJW
  Trunk 0JJT
  Upper Extremity 0JJV
Tendon
  Lower 0LJY
  Upper 0LJX
Testis 0VJD
Thymus 07JM
Thyroid Gland 0GJK
Toe Nail 0HJRXZZ
Trachea 0BJ1
Tracheobronchial Tree 0BJ0

Inspection (*continued*)

Tympanic Membrane
  Left 09J8
  Right 09J7
Ureter 0TJ9
Urethra 0TJD
Uterus and Cervix 0UJD
Vagina and Cul-de-sac 0UJH
Vas Deferens 0VJR
Vein
  Lower 06JY
  Upper 05JY
Vulva 0UJM
Wrist Region
  Left 0XJH
  Right 0XJG
Instillation
  see Introduction of substance in
    or on
Insufflation
  see Introduction of substance in
    or on
Interatrial septum
  use Septum, Atrial
Interbody fusion (spine) cage
  use Interbody Fusion Device in
    Lower Joints
  use Interbody Fusion Device in
    Upper Joints
Intercarpal joint
  use Joint, Carpal, Left
  use Joint, Carpal, Right
Intercarpal ligament
  use Bursa and Ligament, Hand, Left
  use Bursa and Ligament, Hand,
    Right
Interclavicular ligament
  use Bursa and Ligament, Shoulder,
    Left
  use Bursa and Ligament, Shoulder,
    Right
Intercostal lymph node
  use Lymphatic, Thorax
Intercostal muscle
  use Muscle, Thorax, Left
  use Muscle, Thorax, Right
Intercostal nerve
  use Nerve, Thoracic
Intercostobrachial nerve
  use Nerve, Thoracic
Intercuneiform joint
  use Joint, Tarsal, Left
  use Joint, Tarsal, Right
Intercuneiform ligament
  use Bursa and Ligament, Foot, Left
  use Bursa and Ligament, Foot, Right
Intermediate cuneiform bone
  use Tarsal, Left
  use Tarsal, Right
**Intermittent mandatory
  ventilation**
  see Assistance, Respiratory 5A09
**Intermittent Negative Airway
  Pressure**
  24-96 Consecutive Hours,
    Ventilation 5A0945B
  Greater than 96 Consecutive Hours,
    Ventilation 5A0955B
  Less than 24 Consecutive Hours,
    Ventilation 5A0935B
Intermittent Positive Airway Pressure
  24-96 Consecutive Hours,
    Ventilation 5A09458
  Greater than 96 Consecutive Hours,
    Ventilation 5A09558
  Less than 24 Consecutive Hours,
    Ventilation 5A09358
**Intermittent positive pressure
  breathing**
  see Assistance, Respiratory 5A09
Internal anal sphincter
  use Anal Sphincter

Internal (basal) cerebral vein
  use Vein, Intracranial
Internal carotid plexus
  use Nerve, Head and Neck
    Sympathetic
Internal iliac vein
  use Vein, Hypogastric, Left
  use Vein, Hypogastric, Right
Internal maxillary artery
  use Artery, External Carotid, Left
  use Artery, External Carotid, Right
Internal naris
  use Nose
Internal oblique muscle
  use Muscle, Abdomen, Left
  use Muscle, Abdomen, Right
Internal pudendal artery
  use Artery, Internal Iliac, Left
  use Artery, Internal Iliac, Right
Internal pudendal vein
  use Vein, Hypogastric, Left
  use Vein, Hypogastric, Right
Internal thoracic artery
  use Artery, Internal Mammary, Left
  use Artery, Internal Mammary, Right
  use Artery, Subclavian, Left
  use Artery, Subclavian, Right
Internal urethral sphincter
  use Urethra
Interphalangeal (IP) joint
  use Joint, Finger Phalangeal, Left
  use Joint, Finger Phalangeal, Right
  use Joint, Toe Phalangeal, Left
  use Joint, Toe Phalangeal, Right
Interphalangeal ligament
  use Bursa and Ligament, Foot, Left
  use Bursa and Ligament, Foot, Right
  use Bursa and Ligament, Hand, Left
  use Bursa and Ligament, Hand, Right
**Interrogation, cardiac rhythm related
  device**
  Interrogation only
    see Measurement, Cardiac 4B02
  With cardiac function testing
    see Measurement, Cardiac 4A02
Interruption
  see Occlusion
Interspinalis muscle
  use Muscle, Trunk, Left
  use Muscle, Trunk, Right
Interspinous ligament
  use Bursa and Ligament, Head and
    Neck
  use Bursa and Ligament, Trunk,
    Left
  use Bursa and Ligament, Trunk,
    Right
**Interspinous process spinal
  stabilization device**
  use Spinal Stabilization Device,
    Interspinous Process in 0RH
  use Spinal Stabilization Device,
    Interspinous Process in 0SH
InterStim® Therapy lead
  use Neurostimulator Lead in
    Peripheral Nervous System
InterStim® Therapy neurostimulator
  use Stimulator Generator, Single
    Array in 0JH
Intertransversarius muscle
  use Muscle, Trunk, Left
  use Muscle, Trunk, Right
Intertransverse ligament
  use Bursa and Ligament, Trunk, Left
  use Bursa and Ligament, Trunk,
    Right
Interventricular foramen (Monro)
  use Cerebral Ventricle
Interventricular septum
  use Septum, Ventricular
Intestinal lymphatic trunk
  use Cisterna Chyli

Intraluminal Device
 Airway
  Esophagus 0DH5
  Mouth and Throat 0CHY
  Nasopharynx 09HN
 Bioactive
  Occlusion
   Common Carotid
    Left 03LJ
    Right 03LH
   External Carotid
    Left 03LN
    Right 03LM
   Internal Carotid
    Left 03LL
    Right 03LK
   Intracranial 03LG
   Vertebral
    Left 03LQ
    Right 03LP
  Restriction
   Common Carotid
    Left 03VJ
    Right 03VH
   External Carotid
    Left 03VN
    Right 03VM
   Internal Carotid
    Left 03VL
    Right 03VK
   Intracranial 03VG
   Vertebral
    Left 03VQ
    Right 03VP
 Endobronchial Valve
  Lingula 0BH9
  Lower Lobe
   Left 0BHB
   Right 0BH6
  Main
   Left 0BH7
   Right 0BH3
  Middle Lobe, Right 0BH5
  Upper Lobe
   Left 0BH8
   Right 0BH4
 Endotracheal Airway
  Change device in, Trachea
   0B21XEZ
  Insertion of device in, Trachea
   0BH1
 Pessary
  Change device in, Vagina and
   Cul-de-sac 0U2HXGZ
  Insertion of device in
   Cul-de-sac 0UHF
   Vagina 0UHG
Intramedullary (IM) rod (nail)
 use Internal Fixation Device,
  Intramedullary in Lower Bones
 use Internal Fixation Device,
  Intramedullary in Upper Bones
**Intramedullary skeletal kinetic
 distractor (ISKD)**
 use Internal Fixation Device,
  Intramedullary in Lower Bones
 use Internal Fixation Device,
  Intramedullary in Upper Bones
Intraocular Telescope
 Left 08RK30Z
 Right 08RJ30Z
**Intraoperative Knee Replacement
 Sensor** XR2
Intraoperative Radiation Therapy (IORT)
 Anus DDY8CZZ
 Bile Ducts DFY2CZZ
 Bladder DTY2CZZ
 Cervix DUY1CZZ
 Colon DDY5CZZ
 Duodenum DDY2CZZ
 Gallbladder DFY1CZZ
 Ileum DDY4CZZ

**Intraoperative Radiation Therapy
 (IORT)** *(continued)*
 Jejunum DDY3CZZ
 Kidney DTY0CZZ
 Larynx D9YBCZZ
 Liver DFY0CZZ
 Mouth D9Y4CZZ
 Nasopharynx D9YDCZZ
 Ovary DUY0CZZ
 Pancreas DFY3CZZ
 Pharynx D9YCCZZ
 Prostate DVY0CZZ
 Rectum DDY7CZZ
 Stomach DDY1CZZ
 Ureter DTY1CZZ
 Urethra DTY3CZZ
 Uterus DUY2CZZ
Intrauterine device (IUD)
 use Contraceptive Device in Female
  Reproductive System
Introduction of substance in or on
 Artery
  Central 3E06
   Analgesics 3E06
   Anesthetic, Intracirculatory
    3E06
   Anti-infective 3E06
   Anti-inflammatory 3E06
   Antiarrhythmic 3E06
   Antineoplastic 3E06
   Destructive Agent 3E06
   Diagnostic Substance, Other
    3E06
   Electrolytic Substance 3E06
   Hormone 3E06
   Hypnotics 3E06
   Immunotherapeutic 3E06
   Nutritional Substance 3E06
   Platelet Inhibitor 3E06
   Radioactive Substance 3E06
   Sedatives 3E06
   Serum 3E06
   Thrombolytic 3E06
   Toxoid 3E06
   Vaccine 3E06
   Vasopressor 3E06
   Water Balance Substance
    3E06
  Coronary 3E07
   Diagnostic Substance, Other
    3E07
   Platelet Inhibitor 3E07
   Thrombolytic 3E07
  Peripheral 3E05
   Analgesics 3E05
   Anesthetic, Intracirculatory
    3E05
   Anti-infective 3E052
   Anti-inflammatory 3E05
   Antiarrhythmic 3E05
   Antineoplastic 3E05
   Destructive Agent 3E05
   Diagnostic Substance, Other
    3E05
   Electrolytic Substance 3E05
   Hormone 3E05
   Hypnotics 3E05
   Immunotherapeutic 3E05
   Nutritional Substance 3E05
   Platelet Inhibitor 3E05
   Radioactive Substance 3E05
   Sedatives 3E05
   Serum 3E05
   Thrombolytic 3E05
   Toxoid 3E05
   Vaccine 3E05
   Vasopressor 3E05
   Water Balance Substance 3E05
 Biliary Tract 3E0J
  Analgesics 3E0J
  Anesthetic, Local 3E0J
  Anti-infective 3E0J

**Introduction of substance in or
 on** *(continued)*
 Biliary Tract 3E0J *(continued)*
  Anti-inflammatory 3E0J
  Antineoplastic 3E0J
  Destructive Agent 3E0J
  Diagnostic Substance, Other
   3E0J
  Electrolytic Substance 3E0J
  Gas 3E0J
  Hypnotics 3E0J
  Islet Cells, Pancreatic 3E0J
  Nutritional Substance 3E0J
  Radioactive Substance 3E0J
  Sedatives 3E0J
  Water Balance Substance 3E0J
 Bone 3E0V
  Analgesics 3E0V3NZ
  Anesthetic, Local 3E0V3BZ
  Anti-infective 3E0V32
  Anti-inflammatory 3E0V33Z
  Antineoplastic 3E0V30
  Destructive Agent 3E0V3TZ
  Diagnostic Substance, Other
   3E0V3KZ
  Electrolytic Substance 3E0V37Z
  Hypnotics 3E0V3NZ
  Nutritional Substance 3E0V36Z
  Radioactive Substance
   3E0V3HZ
  Sedatives 3E0V3NZ
  Water Balance Substance
   3E0V37Z
 Bone Marrow 3E0A3GC
  Antineoplastic 3E0A30
 Brain 3E0Q3GC
  Analgesics 3E0Q3NZ
  Anesthetic, Local 3E0Q3BZ
  Anti-infective 3E0Q32
  Anti-inflammatory 3E0Q33Z
  Antineoplastic 3E0Q
  Destructive Agent 3E0Q3TZ
  Diagnostic Substance, Other
   3E0Q3KZ
  Electrolytic Substance 3E0Q37Z
  Gas 3E0Q
  Hypnotics 3E0Q3NZ
  Nutritional Substance 3E0Q36Z
  Radioactive Substance
   3E0Q3HZ
  Sedatives 3E0Q3NZ
  Stem Cells
   Embryonic 3E0Q
   Somatic 3E0Q
  Water Balance Substance
   3E0Q37Z
 Cranial Cavity 3E0Q3GC
  Analgesics 3E0Q3NZ
  Anesthetic, Local 3E0Q3BZ
  Anti-infective 3E0Q32
  Anti-inflammatory 3E0Q33Z
  Antineoplastic 3E0Q
  Destructive Agent 3E0Q3TZ
  Diagnostic Substance, Other
   3E0Q3KZ
  Electrolytic Substance 3E0Q37Z
 Gas 3E0Q
  Hypnotics 3E0Q3NZ
  Nutritional Substance 3E0Q36Z
  Radioactive Substance
   3E0Q3HZ
  Sedatives 3E0Q3NZ
  Stem Cells
   Embryonic 3E0Q
   Somatic 3E0Q
  Water Balance Substance
   3E0Q37Z
 Ear 3E0B
  Analgesics 3E0B
  Anesthetic, Local 3E0B
  Anti-infective 3E0B
  Anti-inflammatory 3E0B

**Introduction of substance in or
 on** *(continued)*
 Ear 3E0B *(continued)*
  Antineoplastic 3E0B
  Destructive Agent 3E0B
  Diagnostic Substance, Other
   3E0B
  Hypnotics 3E0B
  Radioactive Substance 3E0B
  Sedatives 3E0B
 Epidural Space 3E0S3GC
  Analgesics 3E0S3NZ
  Anesthetic
   Local 3E0S3BZ
   Regional 3E0S3CZ
  Anti-infective 3E0S32
  Anti-inflammatory 3E0S33Z
  Antineoplastic 3E0S30
  Destructive Agent 3E0S3TZ
  Diagnostic Substance, Other
   3E0S3KZ
  Electrolytic Substance 3E0S37Z
  Gas 3E0S
  Hypnotics 3E0S3NZ
  Nutritional Substance 3E0S36Z
  Radioactive Substance 3E0S3HZ
  Sedatives 3E0S3NZ
  Water Balance Substance
   3E0S37Z
 Eye 3E0C
  Analgesics 3E0C
  Anesthetic, Local 3E0C
  Anti-infective 3E0C
  Anti-inflammatory 3E0C
  Antineoplastic 3E0C
  Destructive Agent 3E0C
  Diagnostic Substance, Other
   3E0C
  Gas 3E0C
  Hypnotics 3E0C
  Pigment 3E0C
  Radioactive Substance 3E0C
  Sedatives 3E0C
 Gastrointestinal Tract
  Lower 3E0H
   Analgesics 3E0H
   Anesthetic, Local 3E0H
   Anti-infective 3E0H
   Anti-inflammatory 3E0H
   Antineoplastic 3E0H
   Destructive Agent 3E0H
   Diagnostic Substance, Other
    3E0H
   Electrolytic Substance 3E0H
   Gas 3E0H
   Hypnotics 3E0H
   Nutritional Substance 3E0H
   Radioactive Substance 3E0H
   Sedatives 3E0H
   Water Balance Substance
    3E0H
  Upper 3E0G
   Analgesics 3E0G
   Anesthetic, Local 3E0G
   Anti-infective 3E0G
   Anti-inflammatory 3E0G
   Antineoplastic 3E0G
   Destructive Agent 3E0G
   Diagnostic Substance, Other
    3E0G
   Electrolytic Substance 3E0G
   Gas 3E0G
   Hypnotics 3E0G
   Nutritional Substance 3E0G
   Radioactive Substance 3E0G
   Sedatives 3E0G
   Water Balance Substance
    3E0G
 Genitourinary Tract 3E0K
  Analgesics 3E0K
  Anesthetic, Local 3E0K
  Anti-infective 3E0K

Laryngopexy
see Repair, Larynx 0CQS
Laryngopharynx
use Pharynx
Laryngoplasty
see Repair, Larynx 0CQS
see Replacement, Larynx 0CRS
see Supplement, Larynx 0CUS
Laryngorrhaphy
see Repair, Larynx 0CQS
Laryngoscopy 0CJS8ZZ
Laryngotomy
see Drainage, Larynx 0C9S
Laser Interstitial Thermal Therapy
Adrenal Gland DGY2KZZ
Anus DDY8KZZ
Bile Ducts DFY2KZZ
Brain D0Y0KZZ
Brain Stem D0Y1KZZ
Breast
    Left DMY0KZZ
    Right DMY1KZZ
Bronchus DBY1KZZ
Chest Wall DBY7KZZ
Colon DDY5KZZ
Diaphragm DBY8KZZ
Duodenum DDY2KZZ
Esophagus DDY0KZZ
Gallbladder DFY1KZZ
Gland
    Adrenal DGY2KZZ
    Parathyroid DGY4KZZ
    Pituitary DGY0KZZ
    Thyroid DGY5KZZ
Ileum DDY4KZZ
Jejunum DDY3KZZ
Liver DFY0KZZ
Lung DBY2KZZ
Mediastinum DBY6KZZ
Nerve, Peripheral D0Y7KZZ
Pancreas DFY3KZZ
Parathyroid Gland DGY4KZZ
Pineal Body DGY1KZZ
Pituitary Gland DGY0KZZ
Pleura DBY5KZZ
Prostate DVY0KZZ
Rectum DDY7KZZ
Spinal Cord D0Y6KZZ
Stomach DDY1KZZ
Thyroid Gland DGY5KZZ
Trachea DBY0KZZ
Lateral (brachial) lymph node
use Lymphatic, Axillary, Left
use Lymphatic, Axillary, Right
Lateral canthus
use Eyelid, Upper, Left
use Eyelid, Upper, Right
Lateral collateral ligament (LCL)
use Bursa and Ligament, Knee, Left
use Bursa and Ligament, Knee, Right
Lateral condyle of femur
use Femur, Lower, Left
use Femur, Lower, Right
Lateral condyle of tibia
use Tibia, Left
use Tibia, Right
Lateral cuneiform bone
use Tarsal, Left
use Tarsal, Right
Lateral epicondyle of femur
use Femur, Lower, Left
use Femur, Lower, Right
Lateral epicondyle of humerus
use Humeral Shaft, Left
use Humeral Shaft, Right
Lateral femoral cutaneous nerve
use Nerve, Lumbar Plexus
Lateral malleolus
use Fibula, Left
use Fibula, Right

Lateral meniscus
use Joint, Knee, Left
use Joint, Knee, Right
Lateral nasal cartilage
use Nose
Lateral plantar artery
use Artery, Foot, Left
use Artery, Foot, Right
Lateral plantar nerve
use Nerve, Tibial
Lateral rectus muscle
use Muscle, Extraocular, Left
use Muscle, Extraocular, Right
Lateral sacral artery
use Artery, Internal Iliac, Left
use Artery, Internal Iliac, Right
Lateral sacral vein
use Vein, Hypogastric, Left
use Vein, Hypogastric, Right
Lateral sural cutaneous nerve
use Nerve, Peroneal
Lateral tarsal artery
use Artery, Foot, Left
use Artery, Foot, Right
Lateral temporomandibular ligament
use Bursa and Ligament, Head and Neck
Lateral thoracic artery
use Artery, Axillary, Left
use Artery, Axillary, Right
Latissimus dorsi muscle
use Muscle, Trunk, Left
use Muscle, Trunk, Right
Latissimus Dorsi Myocutaneous Flap
Bilateral 0HRV075
Left 0HRU075
Right 0HRT075
Lavage
see Irrigation
bronchial alveolar, diagnostic
    see Drainage, Respiratory System 0B9
Least splanchnic nerve
use Nerve, Thoracic Sympathetic
Left ascending lumbar vein
use Vein, Hemiazygos
Left atrioventricular valve
use Valve, Mitral
Left auricular appendix
use Atrium, Left
Left colic vein
use Vein, Colic
Left coronary sulcus
use Heart, Left
Left gastric artery
use Artery, Gastric
Left gastroepiploic artery
use Artery, Splenic
Left gastroepiploic vein
use Vein, Splenic
Left inferior phrenic vein
use Vein, Renal, Left
Left inferior pulmonary vein
use Vein, Pulmonary, Left
Left jugular trunk
use Lymphatic, Thoracic Duct
Left lateral ventricle
use Cerebral Ventricle
Left ovarian vein
use Vein, Renal, Left
Left second lumbar vein
use Vein, Renal, Left
Left subclavian trunk
use Lymphatic, Thoracic Duct
Left subcostal vein
use Vein, Hemiazygos
Left superior pulmonary vein
use Vein, Pulmonary, Left
Left suprarenal vein
use Vein, Renal, Left
Left testicular vein
use Vein, Renal, Left

Lengthening
Bone, with device
    see Insertion of Limb Lengthening Device
Muscle, by incision
    see Division, Muscles 0K8
Tendon, by incision
    see Division, Tendons 0L8
Leptomeninges, intracranial
use Cerebral Meninges
Leptomeninges, spinal
use Spinal Meninges
Lesser alar cartilage
use Nose
Lesser occipital nerve
use Nerve, Cervical Plexus
Lesser splanchnic nerve
use Nerve, Thoracic Sympathetic
Lesser trochanter
use Femur, Upper, Left
use Femur, Upper, Right
Lesser tuberosity
use Humeral Head, Left
use Humeral Head, Right
Lesser wing
use Bone, Sphenoid, Left
use Bone, Sphenoid, Right
Leukopheresis, therapeutic
see Pheresis, Circulatory 6A55
Levator anguli oris muscle
use Muscle, Facial
Levator ani muscle
use Muscle, Trunk, Left
use Muscle, Trunk, Right
Levator labii superioris alaeque nasi muscle
use Muscle, Facial
Levator labii superioris muscle
use Muscle, Facial
Levator palpebrae superioris muscle
use Eyelid, Upper, Left
use Eyelid, Upper, Right
Levator scapulae muscle
use Muscle, Neck, Left
use Muscle, Neck, Right
Levator veli palatini muscle
use Muscle, Tongue, Palate, Pharynx
Levatores costarum muscle
use Muscle, Thorax, Left
use Muscle, Thorax, Right
LifeStent® (Flexstar)(XL) Vascular Stent System
use Intraluminal Device
Ligament of head of fibula
use Bursa and Ligament, Knee, Left
use Bursa and Ligament, Knee, Right
Ligament of the lateral malleolus
use Bursa and Ligament, Ankle, Left
use Bursa and Ligament, Ankle, Right
Ligamentum flavum
use Bursa and Ligament, Trunk, Left
use Bursa and Ligament, Trunk, Right
Ligation
see Occlusion
Ligation, hemorrhoid
see Occlusion, Lower Veins, Hemorrhoidal Plexus
Light Therapy GZJZZZZ
Liner
Removal of device from
Hip
    Left 0SPB09Z
    Right 0SP909Z
Knee
    Left 0SPD09Z
    Right 0SPC09Z

Liner (continued)
Revision of device in
Hip
    Left 0SWB09Z
    Right 0SW909Z
Knee
    Left 0SWD09Z
    Right 0SWC09Z
Supplement
Hip
    Left 0SUB09Z
        Acetabular Surface 0SUE09Z
        Femoral Surface 0SUS09Z
    Right 0SU909Z
        Acetabular Surface 0SUA09Z
        Femoral Surface 0SUR09Z
Knee
    Left 0SUD09
        Femoral Surface 0SUU09Z
        Tibial Surface 0SUW09Z
    Right 0SUC09
        Femoral Surface 0SUT09Z
        Tibial Surface 0SUV09Z
Lingual artery
use Artery, External Carotid, Left
use Artery, External Carotid, Right
Lingual tonsil
use Tongue
Lingulectomy, lung
see Excision, Lung Lingula 0BBH
see Resection, Lung Lingula 0BTH
Lithotripsy
see Fragmentation
with removal of fragments
    see Extirpation
LITT (laser interstitial thermal therapy)
see Laser Interstitial Thermal Therapy
LIVIAN™ CRT-D
use Cardiac Resynchronization Defibrillator Pulse Generator in 0JH
Lobectomy
see Excision, Central Nervous System 00B
see Excision, Endocrine System 0GB
see Excision, Hepatobiliary System and Pancreas 0FB
see Excision, Respiratory System 0BB
see Resection, Endocrine System 0GT
see Resection, Hepatobiliary System and Pancreas 0FT
see Resection, Respiratory System 0BT
Lobotomy
see Division, Brain 0080
Localization
see Map
see Imaging
Locus ceruleus
use Pons
Long thoracic nerve
use Nerve, Brachial Plexus
Loop ileostomy
see Bypass, Ileum 0D1B
Loop recorder, implantable
use Monitoring Device
Lower GI series
see Fluoroscopy, Colon BD14
Lumbar artery
use Aorta, Abdominal
Lumbar facet joint
use Joint, Lumbar Vertebral
Lumbar ganglion
use Nerve, Lumbar Sympathetic

Lumbar lymph node
  use Lymphatic, Aortic
Lumbar lymphatic trunk
  use Cisterna Chyli
Lumbar splanchnic nerve
  use Nerve, Lumbar Sympathetic
Lumbosacral facet joint
  use Joint, Lumbosacral
Lumbosacral trunk
  use Nerve, Lumbar
Lumpectomy
  see Excision
Lunate bone
  use Carpal, Left
  use Carpal, Right
Lunotriquetral ligament
  use Bursa and Ligament, Hand, Left
  use Bursa and Ligament, Hand,
    Right
Lymphadenectomy
  see Excision, Lymphatic and Hemic
    Systems 07B
  see Resection, Lymphatic and
    Hemic Systems 07T
Lymphadenotomy
  see Drainage, Lymphatic and Hemic
    Systems 079
Lymphangiectomy
  see Excision, Lymphatic and Hemic
    Systems 07B
  see Resection, Lymphatic and
    Hemic Systems 07T
Lymphangiogram
  see Plain Radiography, Lymphatic
    System B70
Lymphangioplasty
  see Repair, Lymphatic and Hemic
    Systems 07Q
  see Supplement, Lymphatic and
    Hemic Systems 07U
Lymphangiorrhaphy
  see Repair, Lymphatic and Hemic
    Systems 07Q
Lymphangiotomy
  see Drainage, Lymphatic and Hemic
    Systems 079
Lysis
  see Release

M

Macula
  use Retina, Left
  use Retina, Right
Magnet extraction, ocular foreign
    body
  see Extirpation, Eye 08C
Magnetic Resonance Imaging (MRI)
  Abdomen BW30
  Ankle
    Left BQ3H
    Right BQ3G
  Aorta
    Abdominal B430
    Thoracic B330
  Arm
    Left BP3F
    Right BP3E
  Artery
    Celiac B431
    Cervico-Cerebral Arch B33Q
    Common Carotid, Bilateral
      B335
    Coronary
      Bypass Graft, Multiple B233
      Multiple B231
    Internal Carotid, Bilateral B338
    Intracranial B33R
    Lower Extremity
      Bilateral B43H
      Left B43G
      Right B43F

Magnetic Resonance Imaging
    (MRI) *(continued)*
  Artery *(continued)*
    Pelvic B43C
    Renal, Bilateral B438
    Spinal B33M
    Superior Mesenteric B434
    Upper Extremity
      Bilateral B33K
      Left B33J
      Right B33H
    Vertebral, Bilateral B33G
  Bladder BT30
  Brachial Plexus BW3P
  Brain B030
  Breast
    Bilateral BH32
    Left BH31
    Right BH30
  Calcaneus
    Left BQ3K
    Right BQ3J
  Chest BW33Y
  Coccyx BR3F
  Connective Tissue
    Lower Extremity BL31
    Upper Extremity BL30
  Corpora Cavernosa BV30
  Disc
    Cervical BR31
    Lumbar BR33
    Thoracic BR32
  Ear B930
  Elbow
    Left BP3H
    Right BP3G
  Eye
    Bilateral B837
    Left B836
    Right B835
  Femur
    Left BQ34
    Right BQ33
  Fetal Abdomen BY33
  Fetal Extremity BY35
  Fetal Head BY30
  Fetal Heart BY31
  Fetal Spine BY34
  Fetal Thorax BY32
  Fetus, Whole BY36
  Foot
    Left BQ3M
    Right BQ3L
  Forearm
    Left BP3K
    Right BP3J
  Gland
    Adrenal, Bilateral BG32
    Parathyroid BG33
    Parotid, Bilateral B936
    Salivary, Bilateral B93D
    Submandibular, Bilateral
      B939
    Thyroid BG34
  Head BW38
  Heart, Right and Left B236
  Hip
    Left BQ31
    Right BQ30
  Intracranial Sinus B532
  Joint
    Finger
      Left BP3D
      Right BP3C
    Hand
      Left BP3D
      Right BP3C
    Temporomandibular, Bilateral
      BN39
  Kidney
    Bilateral BT33
    Left BT32

Magnetic Resonance Imaging
    (MRI) *(continued)*
  Kidney *(continued)*
    Right BT31
    Transplant BT39
  Knee
    Left BQ38
    Right BQ37
  Larynx B93J
  Leg
    Left BQ3F
    Right BQ3D
  Liver BF35
  Liver and Spleen BF36
  Lung Apices BB3G
  Nasopharynx B93F
  Neck BW3F
  Nerve
    Acoustic B03C
    Brachial Plexus BW3P
  Oropharynx B93F
  Ovary
    Bilateral BU35
    Left BU34
    Right BU33
  Ovary and Uterus BU3C
  Pancreas BF37
  Patella
    Left BQ3W
    Right BQ3V
  Pelvic Region BW3G
  Pelvis BR3C
  Pituitary Gland B039
  Plexus, Brachial BW3P
  Prostate BV33
  Retroperitoneum BW3H
  Sacrum BR3F
  Scrotum BV34
  Sella Turcica B039
  Shoulder
    Left BP39
    Right BP38
  Sinus
    Intracranial B532
    Paranasal B932
  Spinal Cord B03B
  Spine
    Cervical BR30
    Lumbar BR39
    Thoracic BR37
  Spleen and Liver BF36
  Subcutaneous Tissue
    Abdomen BH3H
    Extremity
      Lower BH3J
      Upper BH3F
    Head BH3D
    Neck BH3D
    Pelvis BH3H
    Thorax BH3G
  Tendon
    Lower Extremity BL33
    Upper Extremity BL32
  Testicle
    Bilateral BV37
    Left BV36
    Right BV35
  Toe
    Left BQ3Q
    Right BQ3P
  Uterus BU36
    Pregnant BU3B
  Uterus and Ovary BU3C
  Vagina BU39
  Vein
    Cerebellar B531
    Cerebral B531
    Jugular, Bilateral B535
    Lower Extremity
      Bilateral B53D
      Left B53C
      Right B53B

Magnetic Resonance Imaging
    (MRI) *(continued)*
  Vein *(continued)*
    Other B53V
    Pelvic (Iliac) Bilateral B53H
    Portal B53T
    Pulmonary, Bilateral B53S
    Renal, Bilateral B53L
    Spanchnic B53T
    Upper Extremity
      Bilateral B53P
      Left B53N
      Right B53M
  Vena Cava
    Inferior B539
    Superior B538
  Wrist
    Left BP3M
    Right BP3L
Malleotomy
  see Drainage, Ear, Nose, Sinus 099
Malleus
  use Auditory Ossicle, Left
  use Auditory Ossicle, Right
Mammaplasty, mammoplasty
  see Alteration, Skin and Breast 0H0
  see Repair, Skin and Breast 0HQ
  see Replacement, Skin and Breast
    0HR
  see Supplement, Skin and Breast
    0HU
Mammary duct
  use Breast, Bilateral
  use Breast, Left
  use Breast, Right
Mammary gland
  use Breast, Bilateral
  use Breast, Left
  use Breast, Right
Mammectomy
  see Excision, Skin and Breast 0HB
  see Resection, Skin and Breast 0HT
Mammillary body
  use Hypothalamus
Mammography
  see Plain Radiography, Skin,
    Subcutaneous Tissue and Breast
    BH0
Mammotomy
  see Drainage, Skin and Breast 0H9
Mandibular nerve
  use Nerve, Trigeminal
Mandibular notch
  use Mandible, Left
  use Mandible, Right
Mandibulectomy
  see Excision, Head and Facial Bones
    0NB
  see Resection, Head and Facial
    Bones 0NT
Manipulation
  Adhesions
    see Release
  Chiropractic
    see Chiropractic Manipulation
Manubrium
  use Sternum
Map
  Basal Ganglia 00K8
  Brain 00K0
  Cerebellum 00KC
  Cerebral Hemisphere 00K7
  Conduction Mechanism 02K8
  Hypothalamus 00KA
  Medulla Oblongata 00KD
  Pons 00KB
  Thalamus 00K9
Mapping
  Doppler ultrasound
    see Ultrasonography
  Electrocardiogram only
    see Measurement, Cardiac 4A02

Mark IV Breathing Pacemaker System
use Stimulator Generator in Subcutaneous Tissue and Fascia

Marsupialization
see Drainage
see Excision

Massage, cardiac
External 5A12012
Open 02QA0ZZ

Masseter muscle
use Muscle, Head

Masseteric fascia
use Subcutaneous Tissue and Fascia, Face

Mastectomy
see Excision, Skin and Breast 0HB
see Resection, Skin and Breast 0HT

Mastoid (postauricular) lymph node
use Lymphatic, Neck, Left
use Lymphatic, Neck, Right

Mastoid air cells
use Sinus, Mastoid, Left
use Sinus, Mastoid, Right

Mastoid process
use Bone, Temporal, Left
use Bone, Temporal, Right

Mastoidectomy
see Excision, Ear, Nose, Sinus 09B
see Resection, Ear, Nose, Sinus 09T

Mastoidotomy
see Drainage, Ear, Nose, Sinus 099

Mastopexy
see Repair, Skin and Breast 0HQ
see Reposition, Skin and Breast 0HS

Mastorrhaphy
see Repair, Skin and Breast 0HQ

Mastotomy
see Drainage, Skin and Breast 0H9

Maxillary artery
use Artery, External Carotid, Left
use Artery, External Carotid, Right

Maxillary nerve
use Nerve, Trigeminal

Maximo II DR (VR)
use Defibrillator Generator in 0JH

Maximo II DR CRT-D
use Cardiac Resynchronization Defibrillator Pulse Generator in 0JH

Measurement
Arterial
  Flow
    Coronary 4A03
    Peripheral 4A03
    Pulmonary 4A03
  Pressure
    Coronary 4A03
    Peripheral 4A03
    Pulmonary 4A03
    Thoracic, Other 4A03
  Pulse
    Coronary 4A03
    Peripheral 4A03
    Pulmonary 4A03
  Saturation, Peripheral 4A03
  Sound, Peripheral 4A03
Biliary
  Flow 4A0C
  Pressure 4A0C
Cardiac
  Action Currents 4A02
  Defibrillator 4B02XTZ
  Electrical Activity 4A02
    Guidance 4A02X4A
    No Qualifier 4A02X4Z
  Output 4A02
  Pacemaker 4B02XSZ
  Rate 4A02
  Rhythm 4A02

Measurement *(continued)*
Cardiac *(continued)*
  Sampling and Pressure
    Bilateral 4A02
    Left Heart 4A02
    Right Heart 4A02
  Sound 4A02
  Total Activity, Stress 4A02XM4
Central Nervous
  Conductivity 4A00
  Electrical Activity 4A00
  Pressure 4A000BZ
    Intracranial 4A00
  Saturation, Intracranial 4A00
  Stimulator 4B00XVZ
  Temperature, Intracranial 4A00
Circulatory, Volume 4A05XLZ
Gastrointestinal
  Motility 4A0B
  Pressure 4A0B
  Secretion 4A0B
Lymphatic
  Flow 4A06
  Pressure 4A06
Metabolism 4A0Z
Musculoskeletal
  Contractility 4A0F
  Stimulator 4B0FXVZ
Olfactory, Acuity 4A08X0Z
Peripheral Nervous
  Conductivity
    Motor 4A01
    Sensory 4A01
  Electrical Activity 4A01
  Stimulator 4B01XVZ
Products of Conception
  Cardiac
    Electrical Activity 4A0H
    Rate 4A0H
    Rhythm 4A0H
    Sound 4A0HH
  Nervous
    Conductivity 4A0J
    Electrical Activity 4A0J
    Pressure 4A0J
Respiratory
  Capacity 4A09
  Flow 4A09
  Pacemaker 4B09X
  Rate 4A09
  Resistance 4A09
  Total Activity 4A09
  Volume 4A09
Sleep 4A0ZXQZ
Temperature 4A0Z
Urinary
  Contractility 4A0D73Z
  Flow 4A0D75Z
  Pressure 4A0D7BZ
  Resistance 4A0D7DZ
  Volume 4A0D7LZ
Venous
  Flow
    Central 4A04
    Peripheral 4A04
    Portal 4A04
    Pulmonary 4A04
  Pressure
    Central 4A04
    Peripheral 4A04
    Portal 4A04
    Pulmonary 4A04
  Pulse
    Central 4A04
    Peripheral 4A04
    Portal 4A04
    Pulmonary 4A04
  Saturation, Peripheral 4A04
Visual
  Acuity 4A07X0Z
  Mobility 4A07X7Z
  Pressure 4A07XBZ

Meatoplasty, urethra
see Repair, Urethra 0TQD

Meatotomy
see Drainage, Urinary System 0T9

Mechanical ventilation
see Performance, Respiratory 5A19

Medial canthus
use Eyelid, Lower, Left
use Eyelid, Lower, Right

Medial collateral ligament (MCL)
use Bursa and Ligament, Knee, Left
use Bursa and Ligament, Knee, Right

Medial condyle of femur
use Femur, Lower, Left
use Femur, Lower, Right

Medial condyle of tibia
use Tibia, Left
use Tibia, Right

Medial cuneiform bone
use Tarsal, Left
use Tarsal, Right

Medial epicondyle of femur
use Femur, Lower, Left
use Femur, Lower, Right

Medial epicondyle of humerus
use Humeral Shaft, Left
use Humeral Shaft, Right

Medial malleolus
use Tibia, Left
use Tibia, Right

Medial meniscus
use Joint, Knee, Left
use Joint, Knee, Right

Medial plantar artery
use Artery, Foot, Left
use Artery, Foot, Right

Medial plantar nerve
use Nerve, Tibial

Medial popliteal nerve
use Nerve, Tibial

Medial rectus muscle
use Muscle, Extraocular, Left
use Muscle, Extraocular, Right

Medial sural cutaneous nerve
use Nerve, Tibial

Median antebrachial vein
use Vein, Basilic, Left
use Vein, Basilic, Right

Median cubital vein
use Vein, Basilic, Left
use Vein, Basilic, Right

Median sacral artery
use Aorta, Abdominal

Mediastinal lymph node
use Lymphatic, Thorax

Mediastinoscopy 0WJC4ZZ

Medication Management GZ3ZZZZ
for substance abuse
  Antabuse HZ83ZZZ
  Bupropion HZ87ZZZ
  Clonidine HZ86ZZZ
  Levo-alpha-acetyl-methadol (LAAM) HZ82ZZZ
  Methadone Maintenance HZ81ZZZ
  Naloxone HZ85ZZZ
  Naltrexone HZ84ZZZ
  Nicotine Replacement HZ80ZZZ
  Other Replacement Medication HZ89ZZZ
  Psychiatric Medication HZ88ZZZ

Meditation 8E0ZXY5

Meissner's (submucous) plexus
use Nerve, Abdominal Sympathetic

Melody® transcatheter pulmonary valve
use Zooplastic Tissue in Heart and Great Vessels

Membranous urethra
use Urethra

Meningeorrhaphy
see Repair, Cerebral Meninges 00Q1
see Repair, Spinal Meninges 00QT

Meniscectomy, knee
see Excision, Lower Joints 0SB

Mental foramen
use Mandible, Left
use Mandible, Right

Mentalis muscle
use Muscle, Facial

Mentoplasty
see Alteration, Jaw, Lower 0W05

Mesenterectomy
see Excision, Mesentery 0DBV

Mesenteriorrhaphy, mesenterorrhaphy
see Repair, Mesentery 0DQV

Mesenteriplication
see Repair, Mesentery 0DQV

Mesoappendix
use Mesentery

Mesocolon
use Mesentery

Metacarpal ligament
use Bursa and Ligament, Hand, Left
use Bursa and Ligament, Hand, Right

Metacarpophalangeal ligament
use Bursa and Ligament, Hand, Left
use Bursa and Ligament, Hand, Right

Metatarsal ligament
use Bursa and Ligament, Foot, Left
use Bursa and Ligament, Foot, Right

Metatarsectomy
see Excision, Lower Bones 0QB
see Resection, Lower Bones 0QT

Metatarsophalangeal (MTP) joint
use Joint, Metatarsal-Phalangeal, Left
use Joint, Metatarsal-Phalangeal, Right

Metatarsophalangeal ligament
use Bursa and Ligament, Foot, Left
use Bursa and Ligament, Foot, Right

Metathalamus
use Thalamus

Micro-Driver stent (RX) (OTW)
use Intraluminal Device

MicroMed HeartAssist
use Implantable Heart Assist System in Heart and Great Vessels

Micrus CERECYTE microcoil
use Intraluminal Device, Bioactive in Upper Arteries

Midcarpal joint
use Joint, Carpal, Left
use Joint, Carpal, Right

Middle cardiac nerve
use Nerve, Thoracic Sympathetic

Middle cerebral artery
use Artery, Intracranial

Middle cerebral vein
use Vein, Intracranial

Middle colic vein
use Vein, Colic

Middle genicular artery
use Artery, Popliteal, Left
use Artery, Popliteal, Right

Middle hemorrhoidal vein
use Vein, Hypogastric, Left
use Vein, Hypogastric, Right

Middle rectal artery
use Artery, Internal Iliac, Left
use Artery, Internal Iliac, Right

Middle suprarenal artery
use Aorta, Abdominal

Middle temporal artery
  use Artery, Temporal, Left
  use Artery, Temporal, Right
Middle turbinate
  use Turbinate, Nasal
MitraClip valve repair system
  use Synthetic Substitute
Mitral annulus
  use Valve, Mitral
Mitroflow® Aortic Pericardial Heart Valve
  use Zooplastic Tissue in Heart and Great Vessels
Mobilization, adhesions
  see Release
Molar gland
  use Buccal Mucosa
Monitoring
  Arterial
    Flow
      Coronary 4A13
      Peripheral 4A13
      Pulmonary 4A13
    Pressure
      Coronary 4A13
      Peripheral 4A13
      Pulmonary 4A13
    Pulse
      Coronary 4A13
      Peripheral 4A13
      Pulmonary 4A13
    Saturation, Peripheral 4A13
    Sound, Peripheral 4A13
  Cardiac
    Electrical Activity 4A12
      Ambulatory 4A12X45
      No Qualifier 4A12X4Z
    Output 4A12
    Rate 4A12
    Rhythm 4A12
    Sound 4A12
    Total Activity, Stress 4A12XM4
  Central Nervous
    Conductivity 4A10
    Electrical Activity
      Intraoperative 4A10
      No Qualifier 4A10
    Pressure 4A100BZ
      Intracranial 4A10
    Saturation, Intracranial 4A10
    Temperature, Intracranial 4A10
  Gastrointestinal
    Motility 4A1B
    Pressure 4A1B
    Secretion 4A1B
  Intraopertive Knee Replacement
    Sensor XR2
  Lymphatic
    Flow 4A16
    Pressure 4A16
  Peripheral Nervous
    Conductivity
      Motor 4A11
      Sensory 4A11
    Electrical Activity
      Intraoperative 4A11
      No Qualifier 4A11
  Products of Conception
    Cardiac
      Electrical Activity 4A1H
      Rate 4A1H
      Rhythm 4A1H
      Sound 4A1H
    Nervous
      Conductivity 4A1J
      Electrical Activity 4A1J
      Pressure 4A1J
  Respiratory
    Capacity 4A19
    Flow 4A19
    Rate 4A19
    Resistance 4A19

Monitoring *(continued)*
  Respiratory *(continued)*
    Volume 4A19
    Sleep 4A1ZXQZ
    Temperature 4A1Z
  Urinary
    Contractility 4A1D73Z
    Flow 4A1D75Z
    Pressure 4A1D7BZ
    Resistance 4A1D7DZ
    Volume 4A1D7LZ
  Venous
    Flow
      Central 4A14
      Peripheral 4A14
      Portal 4A14
      Pulmonary 4A14
    Pressure
      Central 4A14
      Peripheral 4A14
      Portal 4A14
      Pulmonary 4A14
    Pulse
      Central 4A14
      Peripheral 4A14
      Portal 4A14
      Pulmonary 4A14
    Saturation
      Central 4A14
      Portal 4A14
      Pulmonary 4A14
Monitoring Device, Hemodynamic
  Abdomen 0JH8
  Chest 0JH6
Mosaic Bioprosthesis (aortic) (mitral) valve
  use Zooplastic Tissue in Heart and Great Vessels
Motor Function Assessment F01
Motor Treatment F07
MR Angiography
  see Magnetic Resonance Imaging (MRI), Heart B23
  see Magnetic Resonance Imaging (MRI), Lower Arteries B43
  see Magnetic Resonance Imaging (MRI), Upper Arteries B33
MULTI-LINK (VISION)(MINI-VISION)(ULTRA) Coronary Stent System
  use Intraluminal Device
Multiple sleep latency test 4A0ZXQZ
Musculocutaneous nerve
  use Nerve, Brachial Plexus
Musculopexy
  see Repair, Muscles 0KQ
  see Reposition, Muscles 0KS
Musculophrenic artery
  use Artery, Internal Mammary, Left
  use Artery, Internal Mammary, Right
Musculoplasty
  see Repair, Muscles 0KQ
  see Supplement, Muscles 0KU
Musculorrhaphy
  see Repair, Muscles 0KQ
Musculospiral nerve
  use Nerve, Radial
Myectomy
  see Excision, Muscles 0KB
  see Resection, Muscles 0KT
Myelencephalon
  use Medulla Oblongata
Myelogram
  CT
    see Computerized Tomography (CT Scan), Central Nervous System B02
  MRI
    see Magnetic Resonance Imaging (MRI), Central Nervous System B03

Myenteric (Auerbach's) plexus
  use Nerve, Abdominal Sympathetic
Myomectomy
  see Excision, Female Reproductive System 0UB
Myometrium
  use Uterus
Myopexy
  see Repair, Muscles 0KQ
  see Reposition, Muscles 0KS
Myoplasty
  see Repair, Muscles 0KQ
  see Supplement, Muscles 0KU
Myorrhaphy
  see Repair, Muscles 0KQ
Myoscopy
  see Inspection, Muscles 0KJ
Myotomy
  see Division, Muscles 0K8
  see Drainage, Muscles 0K9
Myringectomy
  see Excision, Ear, Nose, Sinus 09B
  see Resection, Ear, Nose, Sinus 09T
Myringoplasty
  see Repair, Ear, Nose, Sinus 09Q
  see Replacement, Ear, Nose, Sinus 09R
  see Supplement, Ear, Nose, Sinus 09U
Myringostomy
  see Drainage, Ear, Nose, Sinus 099
Myringotomy
  see Drainage, Ear, Nose, Sinus 099

N

Nail bed
  use Finger Nail
  use Toe Nail
Nail plate
  use Finger Nail
  use Toe Nail
Narcosynthesis GZGZZZZ
Nasal cavity
  use Nose
Nasal concha
  use Turbinate, Nasal
Nasalis muscle
  use Muscle, Facial
Nasolacrimal duct
  use Duct, Lacrimal, Left
  use Duct, Lacrimal, Right
Nasopharyngeal airway (NPA)
  use Intraluminal Device, Airway in Ear, Nose, Sinus
Navicular bone
  use Tarsal, Left
  use Tarsal, Right
Near Infrared Spectroscopy, Circulatory System 8E023DZ
Neck of femur
  use Femur, Upper, Left
  use Femur, Upper, Right
Neck of humerus (anatomical) (surgical)
  use Humeral Head, Left
  use Humeral Head, Right
Nephrectomy
  see Excision, Urinary System 0TB
  see Resection, Urinary System 0TT
Nephrolithotomy
  see Extirpation, Urinary System 0TC
Nephrolysis
  see Release, Urinary System 0TN
Nephropexy
  see Repair, Urinary System 0TQ
  see Reposition, Urinary System 0TS
Nephroplasty
  see Repair, Urinary System 0TQ
  see Supplement, Urinary System 0TU

Nephropyeloureterostomy
  see Bypass, Urinary System 0T1
  see Drainage, Urinary System 0T9
Nephrorrhaphy
  see Repair, Urinary System 0TQ
Nephroscopy, transurethral 0TJ58ZZ
Nephrostomy
  see Bypass, Urinary System 0T1
  see Drainage, Urinary System 0T9
Nephrotomography
  see Fluoroscopy, Urinary System BT1
  see Plain Radiography, Urinary System BT0
Nephrotomy
  see Division, Urinary System 0T8
  see Drainage, Urinary System 0T9
Nerve conduction study
  see Measurement, Central Nervous 4A00
  see Measurement, Peripheral Nervous 4A01
Nerve Function Assessment F01
Nerve to the stapedius
  use Nerve, Facial
Nesiritide
  use Human B-type Natriuretic Peptide
Neurectomy
  see Excision, Central Nervous System 00B
  see Excision, Peripheral Nervous System 01B
Neurexeresis
  see Extraction, Central Nervous System 00D
  see Extraction, Peripheral Nervous System 01D
Neurohypophysis
  use Gland, Pituitary
Neurolysis
  see Release, Central Nervous System 00N
  see Release, Peripheral Nervous System 01N
Neuromuscular electrical stimulation (NEMS) lead
  use Stimulator Lead in Muscles
Neurophysiologic monitoring
  see Monitoring, Central Nervous 4A10
Neuroplasty
  see Repair, Central Nervous System 00Q
  see Repair, Peripheral Nervous System 01Q
  see Supplement, Central Nervous System 00U
  see Supplement, Peripheral Nervous System 01U
Neurorrhaphy
  see Repair, Central Nervous System 00Q
  see Repair, Peripheral Nervous System 01Q
Neurostimulator Generator
  Insertion of device in, Skull 0NH00NZ
  Removal of device from, Skull 0NP00NZ
  Revision of device in, Skull 0NW00NZ
Neurostimulator generator, multiple channel
  use Stimulator Generator, Multiple Array in 0JH
Neurostimulator generator, multiple channel rechargeable
  use Stimulator Generator, Multiple Array Rechargeable in 0JH

Neurostimulator generator, single channel
  use Stimulator Generator, Single Array in 0JH
Neurostimulator generator, single channel rechargeable
  use Stimulator Generator, Single Array Rechargeable in 0JH
Neurostimulator Lead
  Insertion of device in
    Brain 00H0
    Cerebral Ventricle 00H6
    Nerve
      Cranial 00HE
      Peripheral 01HY
    Spinal Canal 00HU
    Spinal Cord 00HV
  Removal of device from
    Brain 00P0
    Cerebral Ventricle 00P6
    Nerve
      Cranial 00PE
      Peripheral 01PY
    Spinal Canal 00PU
    Spinal Cord 00PV
  Revision of device in
    Brain 00W0
    Cerebral Ventricle 00W6
    Nerve
      Cranial 00WE
      Peripheral 01WY
    Spinal Canal 00WU
    Spinal Cord 00WV
Neurotomy
  see Division, Central Nervous System 008
  see Division, Peripheral Nervous System 018
Neurotripsy
  see Destruction, Central Nervous System 005
  see Destruction, Peripheral Nervous System 015
Neutralization plate
  use Internal Fixation Device in Head and Facial Bones
  use Internal Fixation Device in Lower Bones
  use Internal Fixation Device in Upper Bones
New Technology
  Blinatumomab Antineoplastic Immunotherapy XW0
  Ceftazidime-Avibactam Anti0infective XW0
  Idarucizumab, Dabigatran Reversal Agent XW0
  Intraoperative Knee Replacement Sensor XR2
  Isavuconazole Anti-infective XW0
  Orbital Atherectomy Technology X2C
Ninth cranial nerve
  use Nerve, Glossopharyngeal
Nitinol framed polymer mesh
  use Synthetic Substitute
Non-tunneled central venous catheter
  use Infusion Device
Nonimaging Nuclear Medicine Assay
  Bladder, Kidneys and Ureters CT63
  Blood C763
  Kidneys, Ureters and Bladder CT63
  Lymphatics and Hematologic System C76YYZZ
  Ureters, Kidneys and Bladder CT63
  Urinary System CT6YYZZ
Nonimaging Nuclear Medicine Probe
  Abdomen CW50
  Abdomen and Chest CW54
  Abdomen and Pelvis CW51
  Brain C050
  Central Nervous System C05YYZZ
  Chest CW53ZZ

Nonimaging Nuclear Medicine Probe *(continued)*
  Chest and Abdomen CW54
  Chest and Neck CW56
  Extremity
    Lower CP5PZZZ
    Upper CP5NZZZ
  Head and Neck CW5B
  Heart C25YYZZ
    Right and Left C256
  Lymphatics
    Head C75J
    Head and Neck C755
    Lower Extremity C75P
    Neck C75K
    Pelvic C75D
    Trunk C75M
    Upper Chest C75L
    Upper Extremity C75N
  Lymphatics and Hematologic System C75YYZZ
  Musculoskeletal System, Other CP5YYZZ
  Neck and Chest CW56
  Neck and Head CW5B
  Pelvic Region CW5J
  Pelvis and Abdomen CW51
  Spine CP55ZZZ
Nonimaging Nuclear Medicine Uptake
  Endocrine System CG4YYZZ
  Gland, Thyroid CG42
Nostril
  use Nose
Novacor Left Ventricular Assist Device
  use Implantable Heart Assist System in Heart and Great Vessels
Novation® Ceramic AHS® (Articulation Hip System)
  use Synthetic Substitute, Ceramic in 0SR
Nuclear medicine
  see Nonimaging Nuclear Medicine Assay
  see Nonimaging Nuclear Medicine Probe
  see Nonimaging Nuclear Medicine Uptake
  see Planar Nuclear Medicine Imaging
  see Positron Emission Tomographic (PET) Imaging
  see Systemic Nuclear Medicine Therapy
  see Tomographic (Tomo) Nuclear Medicine Imaging
Nuclear scintigraphy
  see Nuclear Medicine
Nutrition, concentrated substances
  Enteral infusion 3E0G36Z
  Parenteral (peripheral) infusion
    see Introduction of Nutritional Substance

O

Obliteration
  see Destruction
Obturator artery
  use Artery, Internal Iliac, Left
  use Artery, Internal Iliac, Right
Obturator lymph node
  use Lymphatic, Pelvis
Obturator muscle
  use Muscle, Hip, Left
  use Muscle, Hip, Right
Obturator nerve
  use Nerve, Lumbar Plexus
Obturator vein
  use Vein, Hypogastric, Left
  use Vein, Hypogastric, Right
Obtuse margin
  use Heart, Left
Occipital artery
  use Artery, External Carotid, Left
  use Artery, External Carotid, Right

Occipital lobe
  use Cerebral Hemisphere
Occipital lymph node
  use Lymphatic, Neck, Left
  use Lymphatic, Neck, Right
Occipitofrontalis muscle
  use Muscle, Facial
Occlusion
  Ampulla of Vater 0FLC
  Anus 0DLQ
  Aorta, Abdominal 04L0
  Artery
    Anterior Tibial
      Left 04LQ
      Right 04LP
    Axillary
      Left 03L6
      Right 03L5
    Brachial
      Left 03L8
      Right 03L7
    Celiac 04L1
    Colic
      Left 04L7
      Middle 04L8
      Right 04L6
    Common Carotid
      Left 03LJ
      Right 03LH
    Common Iliac
      Left 04LD
      Right 04LC
    External Carotid
      Left 03LN
      Right 03LM
    External Iliac
      Left 04LJ
      Right 04LH
    Face 03LR
    Femoral
      Left 04LL
      Right 04LK
    Foot
      Left 04LW
      Right 04LV
    Gastric 04L2
    Hand
      Left 03LF
      Right 03LD
    Hepatic 04L3
    Inferior Mesenteric 04LB
    Innominate 03L2
    Internal Carotid
      Left 03LL
      Right 03LK
    Internal Iliac
      Left 04LF
      Right 04LE
    Internal Mammary
      Left 03L1
      Right 03L0
    Intracranial 03LG
    Lower 04LY
    Peroneal
      Left 04LU
      Right 04LT
    Popliteal
      Left 04LN
      Right 04LM
    Posterior Tibial
      Left 04LS
      Right 04LR
    Pulmonary, Left 02LR
    Radial
      Left 03LC
      Right 03LB
    Renal
      Left 04LA
      Right 04L9
    Splenic 04L4
    Subclavian
      Left 03L4

Occlusion *(continued)*
    Subclavian *(continued)*
      Right 03L3
    Superior Mesenteric 04L5
    Temporal
      Left 03LT
      Right 03LS
    Thyroid
      Left 03LV
      Right 03LU
    Ulnar
      Left 03LA
      Right 03L9
    Upper 03LY
    Vertebral
      Left 03LQ
      Right 03LP
  Atrium, Left 02L7
  Bladder 0TLB
  Bladder Neck 0TLC
  Bronchus
    Lingula 0BL9
    Lower Lobe
      Left 0BLB
      Right 0BL6
    Main
      Left 0BL7
      Right 0BL3
    Middle Lobe, Right 0BL5
    Upper Lobe
      Left 0BL8
      Right 0BL4
  Carina 0BL2
  Cecum 0DLH
  Cisterna Chyli 07LL
  Colon
    Ascending 0DLK
    Descending 0DLM
    Sigmoid 0DLN
    Transverse 0DLL
  Cord
    Bilateral 0VLH
    Left 0VLG
    Right 0VLF
  Cul-dc-sac 0ULF
  Duct
    Common Bile 0FL9
    Cystic 0FL8
    Hepatic
      Left 0FL6
      Right 0FL5
    Lacrimal
      Left 08LY
      Right 08LX
    Pancreatic 0FLD
      Accessory 0FLF
    Parotid
      Left 0CLC
      Right 0CLB
  Duodenum 0DL9
  Esophagogastric Junction 0DL4
  Esophagus 0DL5
    Lower 0DL3
    Middle 0DL2
    Upper 0DL1
  Fallopian Tube
    Left 0UL6
    Right 0UL5
  Fallopian Tubes, Bilateral 0UL7
  Ileocecal Valve 0DLC
  Ileum 0DLB
  Intestine
    Large 0DLE
      Left 0DLG
      Right 0DLF
    Small 0DL8
  Jejunum 0DLA
  Kidney Pelvis
    Left 0TL4
    Right 0TL3
  Left atrial appendage (LAA)
    see Occlusion, Atrium, Left 02L7

Occlusion *(continued)*
  Lymphatic
    Aortic 07LD
    Axillary
      Left 07L6
      Right 07L5
    Head 07L0
    Inguinal
      Left 07LJ
      Right 07LH
    Internal Mammary
      Left 07L9
      Right 07L8
    Lower Extremity
      Left 07LG
      Right 07LF
    Mesenteric 07LB
    Neck
      Left 07L2
      Right 07L1
    Pelvis 07LC
    Thoracic Duct 07LK
    Thorax 07L7
    Upper Extremity
      Left 07L4
      Right 07L3
  Rectum 0DLP
  Stomach 0DL6
    Pylorus 0DL7
  Trachea 0BL1
  Ureter
    Left 0TL7
    Right 0TL6
  Urethra 0TLD
  Vagina 0ULG
  Vas Deferens
    Bilateral 0VLQ
    Left 0VLP
    Right 0VLN
  Vein
    Axillary
      Left 05L8
      Right 05L7
    Azygos 05L0
    Basilic
      Left 05LC
      Right 05LB
    Brachial
      Left 05LA
      Right 05L9
    Cephalic
      Left 05LF
      Right 05LD
    Colic 06L7
    Common Iliac
      Left 06LD
      Right 06LC
    Esophageal 06L3
    External Iliac
      Left 06LG
      Right 06LF
    External Jugular
      Left 05LQ
      Right 05LP
    Face
      Left 05LV
      Right 05LT
    Femoral
      Left 06LN
      Right 06LM
    Foot
      Left 06LV
      Right 06LT
    Gastric 06L2
    Greater Saphenous
      Left 06LQ
      Right 06LP
    Hand
      Left 05LH
      Right 05LG
    Hemiazygos 05L1
    Hepatic 06L4

Occlusion *(continued)*
  Vein *(continued)*
    Hypogastric
      Left 06LJ
      Right 06LH
    Inferior Mesenteric 06L6
    Innominate
      Left 05L4
      Right 05L3
    Internal Jugular
      Left 05LN
      Right 05LM
    Intracranial 05LL
    Lesser Saphenous
      Left 06LS
      Right 06LR
    Lower 06LY
    Portal 06L8
    Pulmonary
      Left 02LT
      Right 02LS
    Renal
      Left 06LB
      Right 06L9
    Splenic 06L1
    Subclavian
      Left 05L6
      Right 05L5
    Superior Mesenteric 06L5
    Upper 05LY
    Vertebral
      Left 05LS
      Right 05LR
  Vena Cava
    Inferior 06L0
    Superior 02LV
Occupational therapy
  see Activities of Daily Living
    Treatment, Rehabilitation
    F08
Odentectomy
  see Excision, Mouth and Throat
    0CB
  see Resection, Mouth and Throat
    0CT
Olecranon bursa
  use Bursa and Ligament, Elbow,
    Left
  use Bursa and Ligament, Elbow,
    Right
Olecranon process
  use Ulna, Left
  use Ulna, Right
Olfactory bulb
  use Nerve, Olfactory
Omentectomy, omentumectomy
  see Excision, Gastrointestinal
    System 0DB
  see Resection, Gastrointestinal
    System 0DT
Omentofixation
  see Repair, Gastrointestinal System
    0DQ
Omentoplasty
  see Repair, Gastrointestinal System
    0DQ
  see Replacement, Gastrointestinal
    System 0DR
  see Supplement, Gastrointestinal
    System 0DU
Omentorrhaphy
  see Repair, Gastrointestinal System
    0DQ
Omentotomy
  see Drainage, Gastrointestinal
    System 0D9
**Omnilink Elite Vascular Balloon
  Expandable Stent System**
  use Intraluminal Device
Onychectomy
  see Excision, Skin and Breast 0HB
  see Resection, Skin and Breast 0HT

Onychoplasty
  see Repair, Skin and Breast 0HQ
  see Replacement, Skin and Breast 0HR
Onychotomy
  see Drainage, Skin and Breast 0H9
Oophorectomy
  see Excision, Female Reproductive
    System 0UB
  see Resection, Female Reproductive
    System 0UT
Oophoropexy
  see Repair, Female Reproductive
    System 0UQ
  see Reposition, Female
    Reproductive System 0US
Oophoroplasty
  see Repair, Female Reproductive
    System 0UQ
  see Supplement, Female
    Reproductive System 0UU
Oophororrhaphy
  see Repair, Female Reproductive
    System 0UQ
Oophorostomy
  see Drainage, Female Reproductive
    System 0U9
Oophorotomy
  see Drainage, Female Reproductive
    System 0U9
  see Division, Female Reproductive
    System 0U8
Oophorrhaphy
  see Repair, Female Reproductive
    System 0UQ
Open Pivot (mechanical) valve
  use Synthetic Substitute
**Open Pivot Aortic Valve Graft
  (AVG)**
  use Synthetic Substitute
Ophthalmic artery
  use Artery, Internal Carotid, Left
  use Artery, Internal Carotid, Right
Ophthalmic nerve
  use Nerve, Trigeminal
Ophthalmic vein
  use Vein, Intracranial
Opponensplasty
  Tendon replacement
    see Replacement, Tendons 0LR
  Tendon transfer
    see Transfer, Tendons 0LX
Optic chiasma
  use Nerve, Optic
Optic disc
  use Retina, Left
  use Retina, Right
Optic foramen
  use Bone, Sphenoid, Left
  use Bone, Sphenoid, Right
**Optical coherence tomography,
  intravascular**
  see Computerized Tomography
    (CT Scan)
**Optimizer™ III implantable pulse
  generator**
  use Contractility Modulation Device
    in 0JH
Orbicularis oculi muscle
  use Eyelid, Upper, Left
  use Eyelid, Upper, Right
Orbicularis oris muscle
  use Muscle, Facial
Orbital Atherectomy Technology X2C
Orbital fascia
  use Subcutaneous Tissue and Fascia,
    Face
Orbital portion of ethmoid bone
  use Orbit, Left
  use Orbit, Right
Orbital portion of frontal bone
  use Orbit, Left
  use Orbit, Right

Orbital portion of lacrimal bone
  use Orbit, Left
  use Orbit, Right
Orbital portion of maxilla
  use Orbit, Left
  use Orbit, Right
Orbital portion of palatine bone
  use Orbit, Left
  use Orbit, Right
Orbital portion of sphenoid bone
  use Orbit, Left
  use Orbit, Right
Orbital portion of zygomatic bone
  use Orbit, Left
  use Orbit, Right
**Orchectomy, orchidectomy,
  orchiectomy**
  see Excision, Male Reproductive
    System 0VB
  see Resection, Male Reproductive
    System 0VT
Orchidoplasty, orchioplasty
  see Repair, Male Reproductive
    System 0VQ
  see Replacement, Male
    Reproductive System 0VR
  see Supplement, Male Reproductive
    System 0VU
Orchidorrhaphy, orchiorrhaphy
  see Repair, Male Reproductive
    System 0VQ
Orchidotomy, orchiotomy, orchotomy
  see Drainage, Male Reproductive
    System 0V9
Orchiopexy
  see Repair, Male Reproductive
    System 0VQ
  see Reposition, Male Reproductive
    System 0VS
Oropharyngeal airway (OPA)
  use Intraluminal Device, Airway in
    Mouth and Throat
Oropharynx
  use Pharynx
Ossicular chain
  use Auditory Ossicle, Left
  use Auditory Ossicle, Right
Ossiculectomy
  see Excision, Ear, Nose, Sinus 09B
  see Resection, Ear, Nose, Sinus
    09T
Ossiculotomy
  see Drainage, Ear, Nose, Sinus 099
Ostectomy
  see Excision, Head and Facial Bones
    0NB
  see Excision, Lower Bones 0QB
  see Excision, Upper Bones 0PB
  see Resection, Head and Facial
    Bones 0NT
  see Resection, Lower Bones 0QT
  see Resection, Upper Bones 0PT
Osteoclasis
  see Division, Head and Facial Bones
    0N8
  see Division, Lower Bones 0Q8
  see Division, Upper Bones 0P8
Osteolysis
  see Release, Head and Facial Bones
    0NN
  see Release, Lower Bones 0QN
  see Release, Upper Bones 0PN
Osteopathic Treatment
  Abdomen 7W09X
  Cervical 7W01X
  Extremity
    Lower 7W06X
    Upper 7W07X
  Head 7W00X
  Lumbar 7W03X
  Pelvis 7W05X
  Rib Cage 7W08X

Osteopathic Treatment *(continued)*
  Sacrum 7W04X
  Thoracic 7W02X
Osteopexy
  see Repair, Head and Facial Bones
    0NQ
  see Repair, Lower Bones 0QQ
  see Repair, Upper Bones 0PQ
  see Reposition, Head and Facial
    Bones 0NS
  see Reposition, Lower Bones 0QS
  see Reposition, Upper Bones 0PS
Osteoplasty
  see Repair, Head and Facial Bones
    0NQ
  see Repair, Lower Bones 0QQ
  see Repair, Upper Bones 0PQ
  see Replacement, Head and Facial
    Bones 0NR
  see Replacement, Lower Bones
    0QR
  see Replacement, Upper Bones 0PR
  see Supplement, Head and Facial
    Bones 0NU
  see Supplement, Lower Bones 0QU
  see Supplement, Upper Bones 0PU
Osteorrhaphy
  see Repair, Head and Facial Bones
    0NQ
  see Repair, Lower Bones 0QQ
  see Repair, Upper Bones 0PQ
Osteotomy, ostotomy
  see Division, Head and Facial Bones
    0N8
  see Division, Lower Bones 0Q8
  see Division, Upper Bones 0P8
  see Drainage, Head and Facial
    Bones 0N9
  see Drainage, Lower Bones 0Q9
  see Drainage, Upper Bones 0P9
Otic ganglion
  use Nerve, Head and Neck
    Sympathetic
Otoplasty
  see Repair, Ear, Nose, Sinus 09Q
  see Replacement, Ear, Nose, Sinus
    09R
  see Supplement, Ear, Nose, Sinus
    09U
Otoscopy
  see Inspection, Ear, Nose, Sinus
    09J
Oval window
  use Ear, Middle, Left
  use Ear, Middle, Right
Ovarian artery
  use Aorta, Abdominal
Ovarian ligament
  use Uterine Supporting
    Structure
Ovariectomy
  see Excision, Female Reproductive
    System 0UB
  see Resection, Female Reproductive
    System 0UT
Ovariocentesis
  see Drainage, Female Reproductive
    System 0U9
Ovariopexy
  see Repair, Female Reproductive
    System 0UQ
  see Reposition, Female
    Reproductive System 0US
Ovariotomy
  see Division, Female Reproductive
    System 0U8
  see Drainage, Female Reproductive
    System 0U9
Ovatio™ CRT-D
  use Cardiac Resynchronization
    Defibrillator Pulse Generator
    in 0JH

Oversewing
  Gastrointestinal ulcer
    see Repair, Gastrointestinal
      System 0DQ
  Pleural bleb
    see Repair, Respiratory System
      0BQ
Oviduct
  use Fallopian Tube, Left
  use Fallopian Tube, Right
Oxidized zirconium ceramic hip
  bearing surface
  use Synthetic Substitute, Ceramic on
    Polyethylene in 0SR
Oximetry, Fetal pulse 10H073Z
Oxygenation
  Extracorporeal membrane (ECMO)
    see Performance, Circulatory 5A15
  Hyperbaric
    see Assistance, Circulatory 5A05
  Supersaturated
    see Assistance, Circulatory 5A05

P

Pacemaker
  Dual Chamber
    Abdomen 0JH8
    Chest 0JH6
  Single Chamber
    Abdomen 0JH8
    Chest 0JH6
  Single Chamber Rate Responsive
    Abdomen 0JH8
    Chest 0JH6
Packing
  Abdominal Wall 2W43X5Z
  Anorectal 2Y43X5Z
  Arm
    Lower
      Left 2W4DX5Z
      Right 2W4CX5Z
    Upper
      Left 2W4BX5Z
      Right 2W4AX5Z
  Back 2W45X5Z
  Chest Wall 2W44X5Z
  Ear 2Y42X5Z
  Extremity
    Lower
      Left 2W4MX5Z
      Right 2W4LX5Z
    Upper
      Left 2W49X5Z
      Right 2W48X5Z
  Face 2W41X5Z
  Finger
    Left 2W4KX5Z
    Right 2W4JX5Z
  Foot
    Left 2W4TX5Z
    Right 2W4SX5Z
  Genital Tract, Female 2Y44X5Z
  Hand
    Left 2W4FX5Z
    Right 2W4EX5Z
  Head 2W40X5Z
  Inguinal Region
    Left 2W47X5Z
    Right 2W46X5Z
  Leg
    Lower
      Left 2W4RX5Z
      Right 2W4QX5Z
    Upper
      Left 2W4PX5Z
      Right 2W4NX5Z
  Mouth and Pharynx 2Y40X5Z
  Nasal 2Y41X5Z
  Neck 2W42X5Z
  Thumb
    Left 2W4HX5Z
    Right 2W4GX5Z

Packing *(continued)*
  Toe
    Left 2W4VX5Z
    Right 2W4UX5Z
  Urethra 2Y45X5Z
Paclitaxel-eluting coronary stent
  use Intraluminal Device, Drug-
    eluting in Heart and Great
    Vessels
Paclitaxel-eluting peripheral stent
  use Intraluminal Device, Drug-
    eluting in Lower Arteries
  use Intraluminal Device, Drug-
    eluting in Upper Arteries
Palatine gland
  use Buccal Mucosa
Palatine tonsil
  use Tonsils
Palatine uvula
  use Uvula
Palatoglossal muscle
  use Muscle, Tongue, Palate,
    Pharynx
Palatopharyngeal muscle
  use Muscle, Tongue, Palate,
    Pharynx
Palatoplasty
  see Repair, Mouth and Throat 0CQ
  see Replacement, Mouth and Throat
    0CR
  see Supplement, Mouth and Throat
    0CU
Palatorrhaphy
  see Repair, Mouth and Throat 0CQ
Palmar (volar) digital vein
  use Vein, Hand, Left
  use Vein, Hand, Right
Palmar (volar) metacarpal vein
  use Vein, Hand, Left
  use Vein, Hand, Right
Palmar cutaneous nerve
  use Nerve, Median
  use Nerve, Radial
Palmar fascia (aponeurosis)
  use Subcutaneous Tissue and Fascia,
    Hand, Left
  use Subcutaneous Tissue and Fascia,
    Hand, Right
Palmar interosseous muscle
  use Muscle, Hand, Left
  use Muscle, Hand, Right
Palmar ulnocarpal ligament
  use Bursa and Ligament, Wrist, Left
  use Bursa and Ligament, Wrist, Right
Palmaris longus muscle
  use Muscle, Lower Arm and Wrist,
    Left
  use Muscle, Lower Arm and Wrist,
    Right
Pancreatectomy
  see Excision, Pancreas 0FBG
  see Resection, Pancreas 0FTG
Pancreatic artery
  use Artery, Splenic
Pancreatic plexus
  use Nerve, Abdominal Sympathetic
Pancreatic vein
  use Vein, Splenic
Pancreaticoduodenostomy
  see Bypass, Hepatobiliary System
    and Pancreas 0F1
Pancreaticosplenic lymph node
  use Lymphatic, Aortic
Pancreatogram, endoscopic
  retrograde
  see Fluoroscopy, Pancreatic Duct
    BF18
Pancreatolithotomy
  see Extirpation, Pancreas 0FCG
Pancreatotomy
  see Division, Pancreas 0F8G
  see Drainage, Pancreas 0F9G

Panniculectomy
  see Excision, Abdominal Wall
    0WBF
  see Excision, Skin, Abdomen 0HB7
Paraaortic lymph node
  use Lymphatic, Aortic
Paracentesis
  Eye
    see Drainage, Eye 089
  Peritoneal Cavity
    see Drainage, Peritoneal Cavity
      0W9G
  Tympanum
    see Drainage, Ear, Nose, Sinus
      099
Pararectal lymph node
  use Lymphatic, Mesenteric
Parasternal lymph node
  use Lymphatic, Thorax
Parathyroidectomy
  see Excision, Endocrine System
    0GB
  see Resection, Endocrine System
    0GT
Paratracheal lymph node
  use Lymphatic, Thorax
Paraurethral (Skene's) gland
  use Gland, Vestibular
Parenteral nutrition, total
  see Introduction of Nutritional
    Substance
Parietal lobe
  use Cerebral Hemisphere
Parotid lymph node
  use Lymphatic, Head
Parotid plexus
  use Nerve, Facial
Parotidectomy
  see Excision, Mouth and Throat 0CB
  see Resection, Mouth and Throat
    0CT
Pars flaccida
  use Tympanic Membrane, Left
  use Tympanic Membrane, Right
Partial joint replacement
  Hip
    see Replacement, Lower Joints
      0SR
  Knee
    see Replacement, Lower Joints
      0SR
  Shoulder
    see Replacement, Upper Joints
      0RR
Partially absorbable mesh
  use Synthetic Substitute
Patch, blood, spinal 3E0S3GC
Patellapexy
  see Repair, Lower Bones 0QQ
  see Reposition, Lower Bones 0QS
Patellaplasty
  see Repair, Lower Bones 0QQ
  see Replacement, Lower Bones
    0QR
  see Supplement, Lower Bones 0QU
Patellar ligament
  use Bursa and Ligament, Knee, Left
  use Bursa and Ligament, Knee,
    Right
Patellar tendon
  use Tendon, Knee, Left
  use Tendon, Knee, Right
Patellectomy
  see Excision, Lower Bones 0QB
  see Resection, Lower Bones 0QT
Patellofemoral joint
  use Joint, Knee, Left
  use Joint, Knee, Left, Femoral
    Surface
  use Joint, Knee, Right
  use Joint, Knee, Right, Femoral
    Surface

Pectineus muscle
 use Muscle, Upper Leg, Left
 use Muscle, Upper Leg, Right
Pectoral (anterior) lymph node
 use Lymphatic, Axillary, Left
 use Lymphatic, Axillary, Right
Pectoral fascia
 use Subcutaneous Tissue and Fascia, Chest
Pectoralis major muscle
 use Muscle, Thorax, Left
 use Muscle, Thorax, Right
Pectoralis minor muscle
 use Muscle, Thorax, Left
 use Muscle, Thorax, Right
Pedicle-based dynamic stabilization device
 use Spinal Stabilization Device, Pedicle-Based in 0RH
 use Spinal Stabilization Device, Pedicle-Based in 0SH
PEEP (positive end expiratory pressure)
 see Assistance, Respiratory 5A09
PEG (percutaneous endoscopic gastrostomy) 0DH63UZ
PEJ (percutaneous endoscopic jejunostomy) 0DHA3UZ
Pelvic splanchnic nerve
 use Nerve, Abdominal Sympathetic
 use Nerve, Sacral Sympathetic
Penectomy
 see Excision, Male Reproductive System 0VB
 see Resection, Male Reproductive System 0VT
Penile urethra
 use Urethra
Percutaneous endoscopic gastrojejunostomy (PEG/J) tube
 use Feeding Device in Gastrointestinal System
Percutaneous endoscopic gastrostomy (PEG) tube
 use Feeding Device in Gastrointestinal System
Percutaneous nephrostomy catheter
 use Drainage Device
Percutaneous transluminal coronary angioplasty (PTCA)
 see Dilation, Heart and Great Vessels 027
Performance
 Biliary
  Multiple, Filtration 5A1C60Z
  Single, Filtration 5A1C00Z
 Cardiac
  Continuous
   Output 5A1221Z
   Pacing 5A1223Z
  Intermittent, Pacing 5A1213Z
  Single, Output, Manual 5A12012
 Circulatory, Continuous, Oxygenation, Membrane 5A15223
 Respiratory
  24-96 Consecutive Hours, Ventilation 5A1945Z
  Greater than 96 Consecutive Hours, Ventilation 5A1955Z
  Less than 24 Consecutive Hours, Ventilation 5A1935Z
  Single, Ventilation, Nonmechanical 5A19054
 Urinary
  Multiple, Filtration 5A1D60Z
  Single, Filtration 5A1D00Z

Perfusion
 see Introduction of substance in or on
Pericardiectomy
 see Excision, Pericardium 02BN
 see Resection, Pericardium 02TN
Pericardiocentesis
 see Drainage, Pericardial Cavity 0W9D
Pericardiolysis
 see Release, Pericardium 02NN
Pericardiophrenic artery
 use Artery, Internal Mammary, Left
 use Artery, Internal Mammary, Right
Pericardioplasty
 see Repair, Pericardium 02QN
 see Replacement, Pericardium 02RN
 see Supplement, Pericardium 02UN
Pericardiorrhaphy
 see Repair, Pericardium 02QN
Pericardiostomy
 see Drainage, Pericardial Cavity 0W9D
Pericardiotomy
 see Drainage, Pericardial Cavity 0W9D
Perimetrium
 use Uterus
Peripheral parenteral nutrition
 see Introduction of Nutritional Substance
Peripherally inserted central catheter (PICC)
 use Infusion Device
Peritoneal dialysis 3E1M39Z
Peritoneocentesis
 see Drainage, Peritoneal Cavity 0W9G
 see Drainage, Peritoneum 0D9W
Peritoneoplasty
 see Repair, Peritoneum 0DQW
 see Replacement, Peritoneum 0DRW
 see Supplement, Peritoneum 0DUW
Peritoneoscopy 0DJW4ZZ
Peritoneotomy
 see Drainage, Peritoneum 0D9W
Peritoneumectomy
 see Excision, Peritoneum 0DBW
Peroneus brevis muscle
 use Muscle, Lower Leg, Left
 use Muscle, Lower Leg, Right
Peroneus longus muscle
 use Muscle, Lower Leg, Left
 use Muscle, Lower Leg, Right
Pessary ring
 use Intraluminal Device, Pessary in Female Reproductive System
PET scan
 see Positron Emission Tomographic (PET) Imaging
Petrous part of temoporal bone
 use Bone, Temporal, Left
 use Bone, Temporal, Right
Phacoemulsification, lens
 With IOL implant
  see Replacement, Eye 08R
 Without IOL implant
  see Extraction, Eye 08D
Phalangectomy
 see Excision, Lower Bones 0QB
 see Excision, Upper Bones 0PB
 see Resection, Lower Bones 0QT
 see Resection, Upper Bones 0PT
Phallectomy
 see Excision, Penis 0VBS
 see Resection, Penis 0VTS
Phalloplasty
 see Repair, Penis 0VQS
 see Supplement, Penis 0VUS
Phallotomy
 see Drainage, Penis 0V9S

Pharmacotherapy, for substance abuse
 Antabuse HZ93ZZZ
 Bupropion HZ97ZZZ
 Clonidine HZ96ZZZ
 Levo-alpha-acetyl-methadol (LAAM) HZ92ZZZ
 Methadone Maintenance HZ91ZZZ
 Naloxone HZ95ZZZ
 Naltrexone HZ94ZZZ
 Nicotine Replacement HZ90ZZZ
 Psychiatric Medication HZ98ZZZ
 Replacement Medication, Other HZ99ZZZ
Pharyngeal constrictor muscle
 use Muscle, Tongue, Palate, Pharynx
Pharyngeal plexus
 use Nerve, Vagus
Pharyngeal recess
 use Nasopharynx
Pharyngeal tonsil
 use Adenoids
Pharyngogram
 see Fluoroscopy, Pharynix B91G
Pharyngoplasty
 see Repair, Mouth and Throat 0CQ
 see Replacement, Mouth and Throat 0CR
 see Supplement, Mouth and Throat 0CU
Pharyngorrhaphy
 see Repair, Mouth and Throat 0CQ
Pharyngotomy
 see Drainage, Mouth and Throat 0C9
Pharyngotympanic tube
 use Eustachian Tube, Left
 use Eustachian Tube, Right
Pheresis
 Erythrocytes 6A55
 Leukocytes 6A55
 Plasma 6A55
 Platelets 6A55
 Stem Cells
  Cord Blood 6A55
  Hematopoietic 6A55
Phlebectomy
 see Excision, Lower Veins 06B
 see Excision, Upper Veins 05B
 see Extraction, Lower Veins 06D
 see Extraction, Upper Veins 05D
Phlebography
 see Plain Radiography, Veins B50
 Impedance 4A04X51
Phleborrhaphy
 see Repair, Lower Veins 06Q
 see Repair, Upper Veins 05Q
Phlebotomy
 see Drainage, Lower Veins 069
 see Drainage, Upper Veins 059
Photocoagulation
 for Destruction
  see Destruction
 for Repair
  see Repair
Photopheresis, therapeutic
 see Phototherapy, Circulatory 6A65
Phototherapy
 Circulatory 6A65
 Skin 6A60
Phrenectomy, phrenoneurectomy
 see Excision, Nerve, Phrenic 01B2
Phrenemphraxis
 see Destruction, Nerve, Phrenic 0152

Phrenic nerve stimulator generator
 use Stimulator Generator in Subcutaneous Tissue and Fascia
Phrenic nerve stimulator lead
 use Diaphragmatic Pacemaker Lead in Respiratory System

Phreniclasis
 see Destruction, Nerve, Phrenic 0152
Phrenicoexeresis
 see Extraction, Nerve, Phrenic 01D2
Phrenicotomy
 see Division, Nerve, Phrenic 0182
Phrenicotripsy
 see Destruction, Nerve, Phrenic 0152
Phrenoplasty
 see Repair, Respiratory System 0BQ
 see Supplement, Respiratory System 0BU
Phrenotomy
 see Drainage, Respiratory System 0B9
Physiatry
 see Motor Treatment, Rehabilitation F07
Physical medicine
 see Motor Treatment, Rehabilitation F07
Physical therapy
 see Motor Treatment, Rehabilitation F07
PHYSIOMESH™ Flexible Composite Mesh
 use Synthetic Substitute
Pia mater, intracranial
 use Cerebral Meninges
Pia mater, spinal
 use Spinal Meninges
Pinealectomy
 see Excision, Pineal Body 0GB1
 see Resection, Pineal Body 0GT1
Pinealoscopy 0GJ14ZZ
Pinealotomy
 see Drainage, Pineal Body 0G91
Pinna
 use Ear, External, Bilateral
 use Ear, External, Left
 use Ear, External, Right
Pipeline™ Embolization device (PED)
 use Intraluminal Device
Piriform recess (sinus)
 use Pharynx
Piriformis muscle
 use Muscle, Hip, Right
 use Muscle, Hip, Left
Pisiform bone
 use Carpal, Left
 use Carpal, Right
Pisohamate ligament
 use Bursa and Ligament, Hand, Left
 use Bursa and Ligament, Hand, Right
Pisometacarpal ligament
 use Bursa and Ligament, Hand, Left
 use Bursa and Ligament, Hand, Right
Pituitectomy
 see Excision, Gland, Pituitary 0GB0
 see Resection, Gland, Pituitary 0GT0
Plain film radiology
 see Plain Radiography
Plain Radiography
 Abdomen BW00ZZZ
 Abdomen and Pelvis BW01ZZZ
 Abdominal Lymphatic
  Bilateral B701
  Unilateral B700
 Airway, Upper BB0DZZZ
 Ankle
  Left BQ0H
  Right BQ0G
 Aorta
  Abdominal B400
  Thoracic B300
  Thoraco-Abdominal B30P

Plain Radiography (*continued*)
  Vein (*continued*)
    Subclavian
      Left B507
      Right B506
    Upper Extremity
      Bilateral B50P
      Left B50N
      Right B50M
    Vena Cava
      Inferior B509
      Superior B508
    Whole Body BW0KZZZ
      Infant BW0MZZZ
    Whole Skeleton BW0LZZZ
    Wrist
      Left BP0M
      Right BP0L
Planar Nuclear Medicine Imaging
  Abdomen CW10
  Abdomen and Chest CW14
  Abdomen and Pelvis CW11
  Anatomical Regions, Multiple
    CW1YYZZ
  Anatomical Region, Other CW1ZZZZ
  Bladder, Kidneys and Ureters CT13
  Bladder and Ureters CT1H
  Blood C713
  Bone Marrow C710
  Brain C010
  Breast CH1YYZZ
    Bilateral CH12
    Left CH11
    Right CH10
  Bronchi and Lungs CB12
  Central Nervous System C01YYZZ
  Cerebrospinal Fluid C015
  Chest CW13
  Chest and Abdomen CW14
  Chest and Neck CW16
  Digestive System CD1YYZZ
  Ducts, Lacrimal, Bilateral C819
  Ear, Nose, Mouth and Throat
    C91YYZZ
  Endocrine System CG1YYZZ
  Extremity
    Lower CW1D
      Bilateral CP1F
      Left CP1D
      Right CP1C
    Upper CW1M
      Bilateral CP1B
      Left CP19
      Right CP18
  Eye C81YYZZ
  Gallbladder CF14
  Gastrointestinal Tract CD17
    Upper CD15
  Gland
    Adrenal, Bilateral CG14
    Parathyroid CG11
    Thyroid CG12
  Glands, Salivary, Bilateral C91B
  Head and Neck CW1B
  Heart C21YYZZ
    Right and Left C216
  Hepatobiliary System, All CF1C
  Hepatobiliary System and Pancreas
    CF1YYZZ
  Kidneys, Ureters and Bladder CT13
  Liver CF15
  Liver and Spleen CF16
  Lungs and Bronchi CB12
  Lymphatics
    Head C71J
    Head and Neck C715
    Lower Extremity C71P
    Neck C71K
    Pelvic C71D
    Trunk C71M
    Upper Chest C71L
    Upper Extremity C71N

Planar Nuclear Medicine Imaging
  CP1 (*continued*)
  Lymphatics and Hematologic
    System C71YYZZ
  Musculoskeletal System
    All CP1Z
    Other CP1YYZZ
  Myocardium C21G
  Neck and Chest CW16
  Neck and Head CW1B
  Pancreas and Hepatobiliary System
    CF1YYZZ
  Pelvic Region CW1J
  Pelvis CP16
  Pelvis and Abdomen CW11
  Pelvis and Spine CP17
  Reproductive System, Male
    CV1YYZZ
  Respiratory System CB1YYZZ
  Skin CH1YYZZ
  Skull CP11
  Spine CP15
  Spine and Pelvis CP17
  Spleen C712
  Spleen and Liver CF16
  Subcutaneous Tissue CH1YYZZ
  Testicles, Bilateral CV19
  Thorax CP14
  Ureters, Kidneys and Bladder CT13
  Ureters and Bladder CT1H
  Urinary System CT1YYZZ
  Veins C51YYZZ
    Central C51R
    Lower Extremity
      Bilateral C51D
      Left C51C
      Right C51B
    Upper Extremity
      Bilateral C51Q
      Left C51P
      Right C51N
  Whole Body CW1N
Plantar digital vein
  use Vein, Foot, Left
  use Vein, Foot, Right
Plantar fascia (aponeurosis)
  use Subcutaneous Tissue and Fascia,
    Foot, Left
  use Subcutaneous Tissue and Fascia,
    Foot, Right
Plantar metatarsal vein
  use Vein, Foot, Left
  use Vein, Foot, Right
Plantar venous arch
  use Vein, Foot, Left
  use Vein, Foot, Right
Plaque Radiation
  Abdomen DWY3FZZ
  Adrenal Gland DGY2FZZ
  Anus DDY8FZZ
  Bile Ducts DFY2FZZ
  Bladder DTY2FZZ
  Bone, Other DPYCFZZ
  Bone Marrow D7Y0FZZ
  Brain D0Y0FZZ
  Brain Stem D0Y1FZZ
  Breast
    Left DMY0FZZ
    Right DMY1FZZ
  Bronchus DBY1FZZ
  Cervix DUY1FZZ
  Chest DWY2FZZ
  Chest Wall DBY7FZZ
  Colon DDY5FZZ
  Diaphragm DBY8FZZ
  Duodenum DDY2FZZ
  Ear D9Y0FZZ
  Esophagus DDY0FZZ
  Eye D8Y0FZZ
  Femur DPY9FZZ
  Fibula DPYBFZZ
  Gallbladder DFY1FZZ

Plaque Radiation (*continued*)
  Gland
    Adrenal DGY2FZZ
    Parathyroid DGY4FZZ
    Pituitary DGY0FZZ
    Thyroid DGY5FZZ
  Glands, Salivary D9Y6FZZ
  Head and Neck DWY1FZZ
  Hemibody DWY4FZZ
  Humerus DPY6FZZ
  Ileum DDY4FZZ
  Jejunum DDY3FZZ
  Kidney DTY0FZZ
  Larynx D9YBFZZ
  Liver DFY0FZZ
  Lung DBY2FZZ
  Lymphatics
    Abdomen D7Y6FZZ
    Axillary D7Y4FZZ
    Inguinal D7Y8FZZ
    Neck D7Y3FZZ
    Pelvis D7Y7FZZ
    Thorax D7Y5FZZ
  Mandible DPY3FZZ
  Maxilla DPY2FZZ
  Mediastinum DBY6FZZ
  Mouth D9Y4FZZ
  Nasopharynx D9YDFZZ
  Neck and Head DWY1FZZ
  Nerve, Peripheral D0Y7FZZ
  Nose D9Y1FZZ
  Ovary DUY0FZZ
  Palate
    Hard D9Y8FZZ
    Soft D9Y9FZZ
  Pancreas DFY3FZZ
  Parathyroid Gland DGY4FZZ
  Pelvic Bones DPY8FZZ
  Pelvic Region DWY6FZZ
  Pharynx D9YCFZZ
  Pineal Body DGY1FZZ
  Pituitary Gland DGY0FZZ
  Pleura DBY5FZZ
  Prostate DVY0FZZ
  Radius DPY7FZZ
  Rectum DDY7FZZ
  Rib DPY5FZZ
  Sinuses D9Y7FZZ
  Skin
    Abdomen DHY8FZZ
    Arm DHY4FZZ
    Back DHY7FZZ
    Buttock DHY9FZZ
    Chest DHY6FZZ
    Face DHY2FZZ
    Foot DHYCFZZ
    Hand DHY5FZZ
    Leg DHYBFZZ
    Neck DHY3FZZ
  Skull DPY0FZZ
  Spinal Cord D0Y6FZZ
  Spleen D7Y2FZZ
  Sternum DPY4FZZ
  Stomach DDY1FZZ
  Testis DVY1FZZ
  Thymus D7Y1FZZ
  Thyroid Gland DGY5FZZ
  Tibia DPYBFZZ
  Tongue D9Y5FZZ
  Trachea DBY0FZZ
  Ulna DPY7FZZ
  Ureter DTY1FZZ
  Urethra DTY3FZZ
  Uterus DUY2FZZ
  Whole Body DWY5FZZ
Plasmapheresis, therapeutic
  6A550Z3
Plateletpheresis, therapeutic
  6A550Z2
Platysma muscle
  use Muscle, Neck, Left
  use Muscle, Neck, Right

Pleurectomy
  see Excision, Respiratory System
    0BB
  see Resection, Respiratory System
    0BT
Pleurocentesis
  see Drainage, Anatomical Regions,
    General 0W9
Pleurodesis, pleurosclerosis
  Chemical injection
    see Introduction of substance
      in or on, Pleural Cavity
      3E0L
  Surgical
    see Destruction, Respiratory
      System 0B5
Pleurolysis
  see Release, Respiratory System
    0BN
Pleuroscopy 0BJQ4ZZ
Pleurotomy
  see Drainage, Respiratory System
    0B9
Plica semilunaris
  use Conjunctiva, Left
  use Conjunctiva, Right
Plication
  see Restriction
Pneumectomy
  see Excision, Respiratory System
    0BB
  see Resection, Respiratory System
    0BT
Pneumocentesis
  see Drainage, Respiratory System
    0B9
Pneumogastric nerve
  use Nerve, Vagus
Pneumolysis
  see Release, Respiratory System
    0BN
Pneumonectomy
  see Resection, Respiratory System
    0BT
Pneumonolysis
  see Release, Respiratory System
    0BN
Pneumonopexy
  see Repair, Respiratory System 0BQ
  see Reposition, Respiratory System
    0BS
Pneumonorrhaphy
  see Repair, Respiratory System 0BQ
Pneumonotomy
  see Drainage, Respiratory System
    0B9
Pneumotaxic center
  use Pons
Pneumotomy
  see Drainage, Respiratory System
    0B9
Pollicization
  see Transfer, Anatomical Regions,
    Upper Extremities 0XX
Polyethylene socket
  use Synthetic Substitute,
    Polyethylene in 0SR
Polymethylmethacrylate (PMMA)
  use Synthetic Substitute
Polypectomy, gastrointestinal
  see Excision, Gastrointestinal
    System 0DB
Polypropylene mesh
  use Synthetic Substitute
Polysomnogram 4A1ZXQZ
Pontine tegmentum
  use Pons
Popliteal ligament
  use Bursa and Ligament, Knee,
    Left
  use Bursa and Ligament, Knee,
    Right

Popliteal lymph node
use Lymphatic, Lower Extremity, Left
use Lymphatic, Lower Extremity, Right
Popliteal vein
use Vein, Femoral, Left
use Vein, Femoral, Right
Popliteus muscle
use Muscle, Lower Leg, Left
use Muscle, Lower Leg, Right
Porcine (bioprosthetic) valve
use Zooplastic Tissue in Heart and Great Vessels
Positive end expiratory pressure
see Performance, Respiratory 5A19
Positron Emission Tomographic (PET) Imaging
Brain C030
Bronchi and Lungs CB32
Central Nervous System C03YYZZ
Heart C23YYZZ
Lungs and Bronchi CB32
Myocardium C23G
Respiratory System CB3YYZZ
Whole Body CW3NYZZ
Positron emission tomography
see Positron Emission Tomographic (PET) Imaging
Postauricular (mastoid) lymph node
use Lymphatic, Neck, Left
use Lymphatic, Neck, Right
Postcava
use Vena Cava, Inferior
Posterior (subscapular) lymph node
use Lymphatic, Axillary, Left
use Lymphatic, Axillary, Right
Posterior auricular artery
use Artery, External Carotid, Left
use Artery, External Carotid, Right
Posterior auricular nerve
use Nerve, Facial
Posterior auricular vein
use Vein, External Jugular, Left
use Vein, External Jugular, Right
Posterior cerebral artery
use Artery, Intracranial
Posterior chamber
use Eye, Left
use Eye, Right
Posterior circumflex humeral artery
use Artery, Axillary, Left
use Artery, Axillary, Right
Posterior communicating artery
use Artery, Intracranial
Posterior cruciate ligament (PCL)
use Bursa and Ligament, Knee, Left
use Bursa and Ligament, Knee, Right
Posterior facial (retromandibular) vein
use Vein, Face, Left
use Vein, Face, Right
Posterior femoral cutaneous nerve
use Nerve, Sacral Plexus
Posterior inferior cerebellar artery (PICA)
use Artery, Intracranial
Posterior interosseous nerve
use Nerve, Radial
Posterior labial nerve
use Nerve, Pudendal
Posterior scrotal nerve
use Nerve, Pudendal
Posterior spinal artery
use Artery, Vertebral, Left
use Artery, Vertebral, Right
Posterior tibial recurrent artery
use Artery, Anterior Tibial, Left
use Artery, Anterior Tibial, Right

Posterior ulnar recurrent artery
use Artery, Ulnar, Left
use Artery, Ulnar, Right
Posterior vagal trunk
use Nerve, Vagus
PPN (peripheral parenteral nutrition)
see Introduction of Nutritional Substance
Preauricular lymph node
use Lymphatic, Head
Precava
use Vena Cava, Superior
Prepatellar bursa
use Bursa and Ligament, Knee, Left
use Bursa and Ligament, Knee, Right
Preputiotomy
see Drainage, Male Reproductive System 0V9
Pressure support ventilation
see Performance, Respiratory 5A19
PRESTIGE® Cervical Disc
use Synthetic Substitute
Pretracheal fascia
use Subcutaneous Tissue and Fascia, Neck, Anterior
Prevertebral fascia
use Subcutaneous Tissue and Fascia, Neck, Posterior
PrimeAdvanced neurostimulator (SureScan)(MRI Safe)
use Stimulator Generator, Multiple Array in 0JH
Princeps pollicis artery
use Artery, Hand, Left
use Artery, Hand, Right
Probing, duct
Diagnostic
see Inspection
Dilation
see Dilation
PROCEED™ Ventral Patch
use Synthetic Substitute
Procerus muscle
use Muscle, Facial
Proctectomy
see Excision, Rectum 0DBP
see Resection, Rectum 0DTP
Proctoclysis
see Introduction of substance in or on, Gastrointestinal Tract, Lower 3E0H
Proctocolectomy
see Excision, Gastrointestinal System 0DB
see Resection, Gastrointestinal System 0DT
Proctocolpoplasty
see Repair, Gastrointestinal System 0DQ
see Supplement, Gastrointestinal System 0DU
Proctoperineoplasty
see Repair, Gastrointestinal System 0DQ
see Supplement, Gastrointestinal System 0DU
Proctoperineorrhaphy
see Repair, Gastrointestinal System 0DQ
Proctopexy
see Repair, Rectum 0DQP
see Reposition, Rectum 0DSP
Proctoplasty
see Repair, Rectum 0DQP
see Supplement, Rectum 0DUP
Proctorrhaphy
see Repair, Rectum 0DQP
Proctoscopy 0DJD8ZZ

Proctosigmoidectomy
see Excision, Gastrointestinal System 0DB
see Resection, Gastrointestinal System 0DT
Proctosigmoidoscopy 0DJD8ZZ
Proctostomy
see Drainage, Rectum 0D9P
Proctotomy
see Drainage, Rectum 0D9P
Prodisc-C
use Synthetic Substitute
Prodisc-L
use Synthetic Substitute
Production, atrial septal defect
see Excision, Septum, Atrial 02B5
Profunda brachii
use Artery, Brachial, Left
use Artery, Brachial, Right
Profunda femoris (deep femoral) vein
use Vein, Femoral, Left
use Vein, Femoral, Right
PROLENE Polypropylene Hernia System (PHS)
use Synthetic Substitute
Pronator quadratus muscle
use Muscle, Lower Arm and Wrist, Left
use Muscle, Lower Arm and Wrist, Right
Pronator teres muscle
use Muscle, Lower Arm and Wrist, Left
use Muscle, Lower Arm and Wrist, Right
Prostatectomy
see Excision, Prostate 0VB0
see Resection, Prostate 0VT0
Prostatic urethra
use Urethra
Prostatomy, prostatotomy
see Drainage, Prostate 0V90
Protecta XT CRT-D
use Cardiac Resynchronization Defibrillator Pulse Generator in 0JH
Protecta XT DR (XT VR)
use Defibrillator Generator in 0JH
Protégé® RX Carotid Stent System
use Intraluminal Device
Proximal radioulnar joint
use Joint, Elbow, Left
use Joint, Elbow, Right
Psoas muscle
use Muscle, Hip, Left
use Muscle, Hip, Right
PSV (pressure support ventilation)
see Performance, Respiratory 5A19
Psychoanalysis GZ54ZZZ
Psychological Tests
Cognitive Status GZ14ZZZ
Developmental GZ10ZZZ
Intellectual and Psychoeducational GZ12ZZZ
Neurobehavioral Status GZ14ZZZ
Neuropsychological GZ13ZZZ
Personality and Behavioral GZ11ZZZ
Psychotherapy
Family, Mental Health Services GZ72ZZZ
Group
GZHZZZZ
Mental Health Services GZHZZZZ
Individual
see Psychotherapy, Individual, Mental Health Services for substance abuse
12-Step HZ53ZZZ

Psychotherapy *(continued)*
see Psychotherapy, Individual, Mental Health Services for substance ab*use (continued)*
Behavioral HZ51ZZZ
Cognitive HZ50ZZZ
Cognitive-Behavioral HZ52ZZZ
Confrontational HZ58ZZZ
Interactive HZ55ZZZ
Interpersonal HZ54ZZZ
Motivational Enhancement HZ57ZZZ
Psychoanalysis HZ5BZZZ
Psychodynamic HZ5CZZZ
Psychoeducation HZ56ZZZ
Psychophysiological HZ5DZZZ
Supportive HZ59ZZZ
Mental Health Services
Behavioral GZ51ZZZ
Cognitive GZ52ZZZ
Cognitive-Behavioral GZ58ZZZ
Interactive GZ50ZZZ
Interpersonal GZ53ZZZ
Psychoanalysis GZ54ZZZ
Psychodynamic GZ55ZZZ
Psychophysiological GZ59ZZZ
Supportive GZ56ZZZ
PTCA (percutaneous transluminal coronary angioplasty)
see Dilation, Heart and Great Vessels 027
Pterygoid muscle
use Muscle, Head
Pterygoid process
use Bone, Sphenoid, Left
use Bone, Sphenoid, Right
Pterygopalatine (sphenopalatine) ganglion
use Nerve, Head and Neck Sympathetic
Pubic ligament
use Bursa and Ligament, Trunk, Left
use Bursa and Ligament, Trunk, Right
Pubis
use Bone, Pelvic, Left
use Bone, Pelvic, Right
Pubofemoral ligament
use Bursa and Ligament, Hip, Left
use Bursa and Ligament, Hip, Right
Pudendal nerve
use Nerve, Sacral Plexus
Pull-through, rectal
see Resection, Rectum 0DTP
Pulmoaortic canal
use Artery, Pulmonary, Left
Pulmonary annulus
use Valve, Pulmonary
Pulmonary artery wedge monitoring
see Monitoring, Arterial 4A13
Pulmonary plexus
use Nerve, Thoracic Sympathetic
use Nerve, Vagus
Pulmonic valve
use Valve, Pulmonary
Pulpectomy
see Excision, Mouth and Throat 0CB
Pulverization
see Fragmentation
Pulvinar
use Thalamus
Pump reservoir
use Infusion Device, Pump in Subcutaneous Tissue and Fascia
Punch biopsy
see Excision with qualifier Diagnostic

Reattachment (continued)

Leg (continued)
  Upper
    Left 0YMD0ZZ
    Right 0YMC0ZZ
Lip
  Lower 0CM10ZZ
  Upper 0CM00ZZ
Liver 0FM0
  Left Lobe 0FM2
  Right Lobe 0FM1
Lung
  Left 0BML0ZZ
  Lower Lobe
    Left 0BMJ0ZZ
    Right 0BMF0ZZ
  Middle Lobe, Right 0BMD0ZZ
  Right 0BMK0ZZ
  Upper Lobe
    Left 0BMG0ZZ
    Right 0BMC0ZZ
Lung Lingula 0BMH0ZZ
Muscle
  Abdomen
    Left 0KML
    Right 0KMK
  Facial 0KM1
  Foot
    Left 0KMW
    Right 0KMV
  Hand
    Left 0KMD
    Right 0KMC
  Head 0KM0
  Hip
    Left 0KMP
    Right 0KMN
  Lower Arm and Wrist
    Left 0KMB
    Right 0KM9
  Lower Leg
    Left 0KMT
    Right 0KMS
  Neck
    Left 0KM3
    Right 0KM2
  Perineum 0KMM
  Shoulder
    Left 0KM6
    Right 0KM5
  Thorax
    Left 0KMJ
    Right 0KMH
  Tongue, Palate, Pharynx 0KM4
  Trunk
    Left 0KMG
    Right 0KMF
  Upper Arm
    Left 0KM8
    Right 0KM7
  Upper Leg
    Left 0KMR
    Right 0KMQ
Neck 0WM60ZZ
Nipple
  Left 0HMXXZZ
  Right 0HMWXZZ
Nose 09MKXZZ
Ovary
  Bilateral 0UM2
  Left 0UM1
  Right 0UM0
Palate, Soft 0CM30ZZ
Pancreas 0FMG
Parathyroid Gland 0GMR
  Inferior
    Left 0GMP
    Right 0GMN
  Multiple 0GMQ
  Superior
    Left 0GMM
    Right 0GML

Reattachment (continued)

Penis 0VMSXZZ
Perineum
  Female 0WMN0ZZ
  Male 0WMM0ZZ
Rectum 0DMP
Scrotum 0VM5XZZ
Shoulder Region
  Left 0XM30ZZ
  Right 0XM20ZZ
Skin
  Abdomen 0HM7XZZ
  Back 0HM6XZZ
  Buttock 0HM8XZZ
  Chest 0HM5XZZ
  Ear
    Left 0HM3XZZ
    Right 0HM2XZZ
  Face 0HM1XZZ
  Foot
    Left 0HMNXZZ
    Right 0HMMXZZ
  Genitalia 0HMAXZZ
  Hand
    Left 0HMGXZZ
    Right 0HMFXZZ
  Lower Arm
    Left 0HMEXZZ
    Right 0HMDXZZ
  Lower Leg
    Left 0HMLXZZ
    Right 0HMKXZZ
  Neck 0HM4XZZ
  Perineum 0HM9XZZ
  Scalp 0HM0XZZ
  Upper Arm
    Left 0HMCXZZ
    Right 0HMBXZZ
  Upper Leg
    Left 0HMJXZZ
    Right 0HMHXZZ
Stomach 0DM6
Tendon
  Abdomen
    Left 0LMG
    Right 0LMF
  Ankle
    Left 0LMT
    Right 0LMS
  Foot
    Left 0LMW
    Right 0LMV
  Hand
    Left 0LM8
    Right 0LM7
  Head and Neck
    0LM0
  Hip
    Left 0LMK
    Right 0LMJ
  Knee
    Left 0LMR
    Right 0LMQ
  Lower Arm and Wrist
    Left 0LM6
    Right 0LM5
  Lower Leg
    Left 0LMP
    Right 0LMN
  Perineum 0LMH
  Shoulder
    Left 0LM2
    Right 0LM1
  Thorax
    Left 0LMD
    Right 0LMC
  Trunk
    Left 0LMB
    Right 0LM9
  Upper Arm
    Left 0LM4
    Right 0LM3

Reattachment (continued)

Tendon (continued)
  Upper Leg
    Left 0LMM
    Right 0LML
Testis
  Bilateral 0VMC
  Left 0VMB
  Right 0VM9
Thumb
  Left 0XMM0ZZ
  Right 0XML0ZZ
Thyroid Gland
  Left Lobe 0GMG
  Right Lobe 0GMH
Toe
  1st
    Left 0YMQ0ZZ
    Right 0YMP0ZZ
  2nd
    Left 0YMS0ZZ
    Right 0YMR0ZZ
  3rd
    Left 0YMU0ZZ
    Right 0YMT0ZZ
  4th
    Left 0YMW0ZZ
    Right 0YMV0ZZ
  5th
    Left 0YMY0ZZ
    Right 0YMX0ZZ
Tongue 0CM70ZZ
Tooth
  Lower 0CMX
  Upper 0CMW
Trachea 0BM10ZZ
Tunica Vaginalis
  Left 0VM7
  Right 0VM6
Ureter
  Left 0TM7
  Right 0TM6
Ureters, Bilateral 0TM8
Urethra 0TMD
Uterine Supporting Structure 0UM4
Uterus 0UM9
Uvula 0CMN0ZZ
Vagina 0UMG
Vulva 0UMMXZZ
Wrist Region
  Left 0XMH0ZZ
  Right 0XMG0ZZ
Rebound HRD® (Hernia Repair Device)
  use Synthetic Substitute
Recession
  see Repair
  see Reposition
Reclosure, disrupted abdominal wall
  0WQFXZZ
Reconstruction
  see Repair
  see Replacement
  see Supplement
Rectectomy
  see Excision, Rectum 0DBP
  see Resection, Rectum 0DTP
Rectocele repair
  see Repair, Subcutaneous Tissue and
    Fascia, Pelvic Region 0JQC
Rectopexy
  see Repair, Gastrointestinal System
    0DQ
  see Reposition, Gastrointestinal
    System 0DS
Rectoplasty
  see Repair, Gastrointestinal System
    0DQ
  see Supplement, Gastrointestinal
    System 0DU
Rectorrhaphy
  see Repair, Gastrointestinal System
    0DQ

Rectoscopy 0DJD8ZZ
Rectosigmoid junction
  use Colon, Sigmoid
Rectosigmoidectomy
  see Excision, Gastrointestinal
    System 0DB
  see Resection, Gastrointestinal
    System 0DT
Rectostomy
  see Drainage, Rectum 0D9P
Rectotomy
  see Drainage, Rectum 0D9P
Rectus abdominis muscle
  use Muscle, Abdomen, Left
  use Muscle, Abdomen, Right
Rectus femoris muscle
  use Muscle, Upper Leg, Left
  use Muscle, Upper Leg, Right
Recurrent laryngeal nerve
  use Nerve, Vagus
Reduction
  Dislocation
    see Reposition
  Fracture
    see Reposition
  Intussusception, intestinal
    see Reposition, Gastrointestinal
      System 0DS
  Mammoplasty
    see Excision, Skin and Breast 0HB
  Prolapse
    see Reposition
  Torsion
    see Reposition
  Volvulus, gastrointestinal
    see Reposition, Gastrointestinal
      System 0DS
Refusion
  see Fusion
Rehabilitation
  see Activities of Daily Living
    Assessment, Rehabilitation F02
  see Activities of Daily Living
    Treatment, Rehabilitation F08
  see Caregiver Training,
    Rehabilitation F0F
  see Cochlear Implant Treatment,
    Rehabilitation F0B
  see Device Fitting, Rehabilitation
    F0D
  see Hearing Treatment,
    Rehabilitation F09
  see Motor Function Assessment,
    Rehabilitation F01
  see Motor Treatment, Rehabilitation
    F07
  see Speech Assessment,
    Rehabilitation F00
  see Speech Treatment,
    Rehabilitation F06
  see Vestibular Treatment,
    Rehabilitation F0C
Reimplantation
  see Reattachment
  see Reposition
  see Transfer
Reinforcement
  see Repair
  see Supplement
Relaxation, scar tissue
  see Release
Release
  Acetabulum
    Left 0QN5
    Right 0QN4
  Adenoids 0CNQ
  Ampulla of Vater 0FNC
  Anal Sphincter 0DNR
  Anterior Chamber
    Left 08N33ZZ
    Right 08N23ZZ
  Anus 0DNQ

Removal of device from *(continued)*
  Vein
    Lower 06PY
    Upper 05PY
  Vertebra
    Cervical 0PP3
    Lumbar 0QP0
    Thoracic 0PP4
  Vulva 0UPM
Renal calyx
  use Kidney
  use Kidneys, Bilateral
  use Kidney, Left
  use Kidney, Right
Renal capsule
  use Kidney
  use Kidneys, Bilateral
  use Kidney, Left
  use Kidney, Right
Renal cortex
  use Kidney
  use Kidneys, Bilateral
  use Kidney, Left
  use Kidney, Right
Renal dialysis
  see Performance, Urinary 5A1D
Renal plexus
  use Nerve, Abdominal Sympathetic
Renal segment
  use Kidney
  use Kidneys, Bilateral
  use Kidney, Left
  use Kidney, Right
Renal segmental artery
  use Artery, Renal, Left
  use Artery, Renal, Right
Reopening, operative site
  Control of bleeding
    see Control postprocedural
      bleeding in
  Inspection only
    see Inspection
Repair
  Abdominal Wall 0WQF
  Acetabulum
    Left 0QQ5
    Right 0QQ4
  Adenoids 0CQQ
  Ampulla of Vater 0FQC
  Anal Sphincter 0DQR
  Ankle Region
    Left 0YQL
    Right 0YQK
  Anterior Chamber
    Left 08Q33
    Right 08Q23
  Anus 0DQQ
  Aorta
    Abdominal 04Q0
    Thoracic 02QW
  Aortic Body 0GQD
  Appendix 0DQJ
  Arm
    Lower
      Left 0XQF
      Right 0XQD
    Upper
      Left 0XQ9
      Right 0XQ8
  Artery
    Anterior Tibial
      Left 04QQ
      Right 04QP
    Axillary
      Left 03Q6
      Right 03Q5
    Brachial
      Left 03Q8
      Right 03Q7
    Celiac 04Q1
    Colic
      Left 04Q7

Repair *(continued)*
  Artery *(continued)*
    Colic *(continued)*
      Middle 04Q8
      Right 04Q6
    Common Carotid
      Left 03QJ
      Right 03QH
    Common Iliac
      Left 04QD
      Right 04QC
    Coronary
      Four or More Sites 02Q3
      One Site 02Q0
      Three Sites 02Q2
      Two Sites 02Q1
    External Carotid
      Left 03QN
      Right 03QM
    External Iliac
      Left 04QJ
      Right 04QH
    Face 03QR
    Femoral
      Left 04QL
      Right 04QK
    Foot
      Left 04QW
      Right 04QV
    Gastric 04Q2
    Hand
      Left 03QF
      Right 03QD
    Hepatic 04Q3
    Inferior Mesenteric 04QB
    Innominate 03Q2
    Internal Carotid
      Left 03QL
      Right 03QK
    Internal Iliac
      Left 04QF
      Right 04QE
    Internal Mammary
      Left 03Q1
      Right 03Q0
    Intracranial 03QG
    Lower 04QY
    Peroneal
      Left 04QU
      Right 04QT
    Popliteal
      Left 04QN
      Right 04QM
    Posterior Tibial
      Left 04QS
      Right 04QR
    Pulmonary
      Left 02QR
      Right 02QQ
    Pulmonary Trunk 02QP
    Radial
      Left 03QC
      Right 03QB
    Renal
      Left 04QA
      Right 04Q9
    Splenic 04Q4
    Subclavian
      Left 03Q4
      Right 03Q3
    Superior Mesenteric 04Q5
    Temporal
      Left 03QT
      Right 03QS
    Thyroid
      Left 03QV
      Right 03QU
    Ulnar
      Left 03QA
      Right 03Q9
    Upper 03QY
    Vertebral

Repair *(continued)*
  Artery *(continued)*
    Vertebral *(continued)*
      Left 03QQ
      Right 03QP
  Atrium
    Left 02Q7
    Right 02Q6
  Auditory Ossicle
    Left 09QA0
    Right 09Q90
  Axilla
    Left 0XQ5
    Right 0XQ4
  Back
    Lower 0WQL
    Upper 0WQK
  Basal Ganglia 00Q8
  Bladder 0TQB
  Bladder Neck 0TQC
  Bone
    Ethmoid
      Left 0NQG
      Right 0NQF
    Frontal
      Left 0NQ2
      Right 0NQ1
    Hyoid 0NQX
    Lacrimal
      Left 0NQJ
      Right 0NQH
    Nasal 0NQB
    Occipital
      Left 0NQ8
      Right 0NQ7
    Palatine
      Left 0NQL
      Right 0NQK
    Parietal
      Left 0NQ4
      Right 0NQ3
    Pelvic
      Left 0QQ3
      Right 0QQ2
    Sphenoid
      Left 0NQD
      Right 0NQC
    Temporal
      Left 0NQ6
      Right 0NQ
    Zygomatic
      Left 0NQN
      Right 0NQM
  Brain 00Q0
  Breast
    Bilateral 0HQV
    Left 0HQU
    Right 0HQT
    Supernumerary 0HQY
  Bronchus
    Lingula 0BQ9
    Lower Lobe
      Left 0BQB
      Right 0BQ6
    Main
      Left 0BQ7
      Right 0BQ3
    Middle Lobe, Right 0BQ5
    Upper Lobe
      Left 0BQ8
      Right 0BQ4
  Buccal Mucosa 0CQ4
  Bursa and Ligament
    Abdomen
      Left 0MQJ
      Right 0MQH
    Ankle
      Left 0MQR
      Right 0MQQ
    Elbow
      Left 0MQ4
      Right 0MQ3

Repair *(continued)*
  Bursa and Ligament *(continued)*
    Foot
      Left 0MQT
      Right 0MQS
    Hand
      Left 0MQ8
      Right 0MQ7
    Head and Neck 0MQ0
    Hip
      Left 0MQM
      Right 0MQL
    Knee
      Left 0MQP
      Right 0MQN
    Lower Extremity
      Left 0MQW
      Right 0MQV
    Perineum 0MQK
    Shoulder
      Left 0MQ2
      Right 0MQ1
    Thorax
      Left 0MQG
      Right 0MQF
    Trunk
      Left 0MQD
      Right 0MQC
    Upper Extremity
      Left 0MQB
      Right 0MQ9
    Wrist
      Left 0MQ6
      Right 0MQ5
  Buttock
    Left 0YQ1
    Right 0YQ0
  Carina 0BQ2
  Carotid Bodies, Bilateral 0GQ8
  Carotid Body
    Left 0GQ6
    Right 0GQ7
  Carpal
    Left 0PQN
    Right 0PQM
  Cecum 0DQH
  Cerebellum 00QC
  Cerebral Hemisphere 00Q7
  Cerebral Meninges 00Q1
  Cerebral Ventricle 00Q6
  Cervix 0UQC
  Chest Wall 0WQ8
  Chordae Tendineae 02Q9
  Choroid
    Left 08QB
    Right 08QA
  Cisterna Chyli 07QL
  Clavicle
    Left 0PQB
    Right 0PQ9
  Clitoris 0UQJ
  Coccygeal Glomus 0GQB
  Coccyx 0QQS
  Colon
    Ascending 0DQK
    Descending 0DQM
    Sigmoid 0DQN
    Transverse 0DQL
  Conduction Mechanism 02Q8
  Conjunctiva
    Left 08QTXZZ
    Right 08QSXZZ
  Cord
    Bilateral 0VQH
    Left 0VQG
    Right 0VQF
  Cornea
    Left 08Q9XZZ
    Right 08Q8XZZ
  Cul-de-sac 0UQF
  Diaphragm
    Left 0BQS

Repair *(continued)*

Diaphragm *(continued)*
    Right 0BQR
Disc
    Cervical Vertebral 0RQ3
    Cervicothoracic Vertebral 0RQ5
    Lumbar Vertebral 0SQ2
    Lumbosacral 0SQ4
    Thoracic Vertebral 0RQ9
    Thoracolumbar Vertebral 0RQB
Duct
    Common Bile 0FQ9
    Cystic 0FQ8
    Hepatic
        Left 0FQ6
        Right 0FQ5
    Lacrimal
        Left 08QY
        Right 08QX
    Pancreatic 0FQD
        Accessory 0FQF
    Parotid
        Left 0CQC
        Right 0CQB
Duodenum 0DQ9
Dura Mater 00Q2
Ear
    External
        Bilateral 09Q2
        Left 09Q1
        Right 09Q0
    External Auditory Canal
        Left 09Q4
        Right 09Q3
    Inner
        Left 09QE0ZZ
        Right 09QD0ZZ
    Middle
        Left 09Q60ZZ
        Right 09Q50ZZ
Elbow Region
    Left 0XQC
    Right 0XQB
Epididymis
    Bilateral 0VQL
    Left 0VQK
    Right 0VQJ
Epiglottis 0CQR
Esophagogastric Junction 0DQ4
Esophagus 0DQ5
    Lower 0DQ3
    Middle 0DQ2
    Upper 0DQ1
Eustachian Tube
    Left 09QG
    Right 09QF
Extremity
    Lower
        Left 0YQB
        Right 0YQ9
    Upper
        Left 0XQ7
        Right 0XQ6
Eye
    Left 08Q1XZZ
    Right 08Q0XZZ
Eyelid
    Lower
        Left 08QR
        Right 08QQ
    Upper
        Left 08QP
        Right 08QN
Face 0WQ2
Fallopian Tube
    Left 0UQ6
    Right 0UQ5
Fallopian Tubes, Bilateral 0UQ7
Femoral Region
    Bilateral 0YQE
    Left 0YQ8
    Right 0YQ7

Repair *(continued)*

Femoral Shaft
    Left 0QQ9
    Right 0QQ8
Femur
    Lower
        Left 0QQC
        Right 0QQB
    Upper
        Left 0QQ7
        Right 0QQ6
Fibula
    Left 0QQK
    Right 0QQJ
Finger
    Index
        Left 0XQP
        Right 0XQN
    Little
        Left 0XQW
        Right 0XQV
    Middle
        Left 0XQR
        Right 0XQQ
    Ring
        Left 0XQT
        Right 0XQS
Finger Nail 0HQQXZZ
Foot
    Left 0YQN
    Right 0YQM
Gallbladder 0FQ4
Gingiva
    Lower 0CQ6
    Upper 0CQ5
Gland
    Adrenal
        Bilateral 0GQ4
        Left 0GQ2
        Right 0GQ3
    Lacrimal
        Left 08QW
        Right 08QV
    Minor Salivary 0CQJ
    Parotid
        Left 0CQ9
        Right 0CQ8
    Pituitary 0GQ0
    Sublingual
        Left 0CQF
        Right 0CQD
    Submaxillary
        Left 0CQH
        Right 0CQG
    Vestibular 0UQL
Glenoid Cavity
    Left 0PQ8
    Right 0PQ7
Glomus Jugulare 0GQC
Hand
    Left 0XQK
    Right 0XQJ
Head 0WQ0
Heart 02QA
    Left 02QC
    Right 02QB
Humeral Head
    Left 0PQD
    Right 0PQC
Humeral Shaft
    Left 0PQG
    Right 0PQF
Hymen 0UQK
Hypothalamus 00QA
Ileocecal Valve 0DQC
Ileum 0DQB
Inguinal Region
    Bilateral 0YQA
    Left 0YQ6
    Right 0YQ5
Intestine
    Large 0DQE

Repair *(continued)*

Intestine *(continued)*
    Large 0DQE *(continued)*
        Left 0DQG
        Right 0DQF
    Small 0DQ8
Iris
    Left 08QD3ZZ
    Right 08QC3ZZ
Jaw
    Lower 0WQ5
    Upper 0WQ4
Jejunum 0DQA
Joint
    Acromioclavicular
        Left 0RQH
        Right 0RQG
    Ankle
        Left 0SQG
        Right 0SQF
    Carpal
        Left 0RQR
        Right 0RQQ
    Cervical Vertebral 0RQ1
    Cervicothoracic Vertebral 0RQ4
    Coccygeal 0SQ6
    Elbow
        Left 0RQM
        Right 0RQL
    Finger Phalangeal
        Left 0RQX
        Right 0RQW
    Hip
        Left 0SQB
        Right 0SQ9
    Knee
        Left 0SQD
        Right 0SQC
    Lumbar Vertebral 0SQ0
    Lumbosacral 0SQ3
    Metacarpocarpal
        Left 0RQT
        Right 0RQS
    Metacarpophalangeal
        Left 0RQV
        Right 0RQU
    Metatarsal-Phalangeal
        Left 0SQN
        Right 0SQM
    Metatarsal-Tarsal
        Left 0SQL
        Right 0SQK
    Occipital-cervical 0RQ0
    Sacrococcygeal 0SQ5
    Sacroiliac
        Left 0SQ8
        Right 0SQ7
    Shoulder
        Left 0RQK
        Right 0RQJ
    Sternoclavicular
        Left 0RQF
        Right 0RQE
    Tarsal
        Left 0SQJ
        Right 0SQH
    Temporomandibular
        Left 0RQD
        Right 0RQC
    Thoracic Vertebral 0RQ6
    Thoracolumbar Vertebral 0RQA
    Toe Phalangeal
        Left 0SQQ
        Right 0SQP
    Wrist
        Left 0RQP
        Right 0RQN
Kidney
    Left 0TQ1
    Right 0TQ0
Kidney Pelvis
    Left 0TQ4

Repair *(continued)*

Kidney Pelvis *(continued)*
    Right 0TQ3
Knee Region
    Left 0YQG
    Right 0YQF
Larynx 0CQS
Leg
    Lower
        Left 0YQJ
        Right 0YQH
    Upper
        Left 0YQD
        Right 0YQC
Lens
    Left 08QK3ZZ
    Right 08QJ3ZZ
Lip
    Lower 0CQ1
    Upper 0CQ0
Liver 0FQ0
    Left Lobe 0FQ2
    Right Lobe 0FQ1
Lung
    Bilateral 0BQM
    Left 0BQL
    Lower Lobe
        Left 0BQJ
        Right 0BQF
    Middle Lobe, Right 0BQD
    Right 0BQK
    Upper Lobe
        Left 0BQG
        Right 0BQC
Lung Lingula 0BQH
Lymphatic
    Aortic 07QD
    Axillary
        Left 07Q6
        Right 07Q5
    Head 07Q0
    Inguinal
        Left 07QJ
        Right 07QH
    Internal Mammary
        Left 07Q9
        Right 07Q8
    Lower Extremity
        Left 07QG
        Right 07QF
    Mesenteric 07QB
    Neck
        Left 07Q2
        Right 07Q1
    Pelvis 07QC
    Thoracic Duct 07QK
    Thorax 07Q7
    Upper Extremity
        Left 07Q4
        Right 07Q3
Mandible
    Left 0NQV
    Right 0NQT
Maxilla
    Left 0NQS
    Right 0NQR
Mediastinum 0WQC
Medulla Oblongata 00QD
Mesentery 0DQV
Metacarpal
    Left 0PQQ
    Right 0PQP
Metatarsal
    Left 0QQP
    Right 0QQN
Muscle
    Abdomen
        Left 0KQL
        Right 0KQK
    Extraocular
        Left 08QM
        Right 08QL

Repair *(continued)*

Muscle *(continued)*
Facial 0KQ1
Foot
Left 0KQW
Right 0KQV
Hand
Left 0KQD
Right 0KQC
Head 0KQ0
Hip
Left 0KQP
Right 0KQN
Lower Arm and Wrist
Left 0KQB
Right 0KQ9
Lower Leg
Left 0KQT
Right 0KQS
Neck
Left 0KQ3
Right 0KQ2
Papillary 02QD
Perineum 0KQM
Shoulder
Left 0KQ6
Right 0KQ5
Thorax
Left 0KQJ
Right 0KQH
Tongue, Palate, Pharynx 0KQ4
Trunk
Left 0KQG
Right 0KQF
Upper Arm
Left 0KQ8
Right 0KQ7
Upper Leg
Left 0KQR
Right 0KQQ
Nasopharynx 09QN
Neck 0WQ6
Nerve
Abdominal Sympathetic 01QM
Abducens 00QL
Accessory 00QR
Acoustic 00QN
Brachial Plexus 01Q3
Cervical 01Q1
Cervical Plexus 01Q0
Facial 00QM
Femoral 01QD
Glossopharyngeal 00QP
Head and Neck Sympathetic 01QK
Hypoglossal 00QS
Lumbar 01QB
Lumbar Plexus 01Q9
Lumbar Sympathetic 01QN
Lumbosacral Plexus 01QA
Median 01Q5
Oculomotor 00QH
Olfactory 00QF
Optic 00QG
Peroneal 01QH
Phrenic 01Q2
Pudendal 01QC
Radial 01Q6
Sacral 01QR
Sacral Plexus 01QQ
Sacral Sympathetic 01QP
Sciatic 01QF
Thoracic 01Q8
Thoracic Sympathetic 01QL
Tibial 01QG
Trigeminal 00QK
Trochlear 00QJ
Ulnar 01Q4
Vagus 00QQ
Nipple
Left 0HQX
Right 0HQW
Nose 09QK

Repair *(continued)*

Omentum
Greater 0DQS
Lesser 0DQT
Orbit
Left 0NQQ
Right 0NQP
Ovary
Bilateral 0UQ2
Left 0UQ1
Right 0UQ0
Palate
Hard 0CQ2
Soft 0CQ3
Pancreas 0FQG
Para-aortic Body 0GQ9
Paraganglion Extremity 0GQF
Parathyroid Gland 0GQR
Inferior
Left 0GQP
Right 0GQN
Multiple 0GQQ
Superior
Left 0GQM
Right 0GQL
Patella
Left 0QQF
Right 0QQD
Penis 0VQS
Pericardium 02QN
Perineum
Female 0WQN
Male 0WQM
Peritoneum 0DQW
Phalanx
Finger
Left 0PQV
Right 0PQT
Thumb
Left 0PQS
Right 0PQR
Toe
Left 0QQR
Right 0QQQ
Pharynx 0CQM
Pineal Body 0GQ1
Pleura
Left 0BQP
Right 0BQN
Pons 00QB
Prepuce 0VQT
Products of Conception 10Q0
Prostate 0VQ0
Radius
Left 0PQJ
Right 0PQH
Rectum 0DQP
Retina
Left 08QF3ZZ
Right 08QE3ZZ
Retinal Vessel
Left 08QH3ZZ
Right 08QG3ZZ
Rib
Left 0PQ2
Right 0PQ1
Sacrum 0QQ1
Scapula
Left 0PQ6
Right 0PQ5
Sclera
Left 08Q7XZZ
Right 08Q6XZZ
Scrotum 0VQ5
Septum
Atrial 02Q5
Nasal 09QM
Ventricular 02QM
Shoulder Region
Left 0XQ3
Right 0XQ2
Sinus

Repair *(continued)*

Sinus *(continued)*
Accessory 09QP
Ethmoid
Left 09QV
Right 09QU
Frontal
Left 09QT
Right 09QS
Mastoid
Left 09QC
Right 09QB
Maxillary
Left 09QR
Right 09QQ
Sphenoid
Left 09QX
Right 09QW
Skin
Abdomen 0HQ7XZZ
Back 0HQ6XZZ
Buttock 0HQ8XZZ
Chest 0HQ5XZZ
Ear
Left 0HQ3XZZ
Right 0HQ2XZZ
Face 0HQ1XZZ
Foot
Left 0HQNXZZ
Right 0HQMXZZ
Genitalia 0HQAXZZ
Hand
Left 0HQGXZZ
Right 0HQFXZZ
Lower Arm
Left 0HQEXZZ
Right 0HQDXZZ
Lower Leg
Left 0HQLXZZ
Right 0HQKXZZ
Neck 0HQ4XZZ
Perineum 0HQ9XZZ
Scalp 0HQ0XZZ
Upper Arm
Left 0HQCXZZ
Right 0HQBXZZ
Upper Leg
Left 0HQJXZZ
Right 0HQHXZZ
Skull 0NQ0
Spinal Cord
Cervical 00QW
Lumbar 00QY
Thoracic 00QX
Spinal Meninges 00QT
Spleen 07QP
Sternum 0PQ0
Stomach 0DQ6
Pylorus 0DQ7
Subcutaneous Tissue and Fascia
Abdomen 0JQ8
Back 0JQ7
Buttock 0JQ9
Chest 0JQ6
Face 0JQ1
Foot
Left 0JQR
Right 0JQQ
Hand
Left 0JQK
Right 0JQJ
Lower Arm
Left 0JQH
Right 0JQG
Lower Leg
Left 0JQP
Right 0JQN
Neck
Anterior 0JQ4
Posterior 0JQ5
Pelvic Region 0JQC
Perineum 0JQB

Repair *(continued)*

Subcutaneous Tissue and Fascia *(continued)*
Scalp 0JQ0
Upper Arm
Left 0JQF
Right 0JQD
Upper Leg
Left 0JQM
Right 0JQL
Tarsal
Left 0QQM
Right 0QQL
Tendon
Abdomen
Left 0LQG
Right 0LQF
Ankle
Left 0LQT
Right 0LQS
Foot
Left 0LQW
Right 0LQV
Hand
Left 0LQ8
Right 0LQ7
Head and Neck 0LQ0
Hip
Left 0LQK
Right 0LQJ
Knee
Left 0LQR
Right 0LQQ
Lower Arm and Wrist
Left 0LQ6
Right 0LQ5
Lower Leg
Left 0LQP
Right 0LQN
Perineum 0LQH
Shoulder
Left 0LQ2
Right 0LQ1
Thorax
Left 0LQD
Right 0LQC
Trunk
Left 0LQB
Right 0LQ9
Upper Arm
Left 0LQ4
Right 0LQ3
Upper Leg
Left 0LQM
Right 0LQL
Testis
Bilateral 0VQC
Left 0VQB
Right 0VQ9
Thalamus 00Q9
Thumb
Left 0XQM
Right 0XQL
Thymus 07QM
Thyroid Gland 0GQK
Left Lobe 0GQG
Right Lobe 0GQH
Thyroid Gland Isthmus 0GQJ
Tibia
Left 0QQH
Right 0QQG
Toe
1st
Left 0YQQ
Right 0YQP
2nd
Left 0YQS
Right 0YQR
3rd
Left 0YQU
Right 0YQT
4th

Repair *(continued)*
Toe *(continued)*
  4th *(continued)*
    Left 0YQW
    Right 0YQV
  5th
    Left 0YQY
    Right 0YQX
Toe Nail 0HQRXZZ
Tongue 0CQ7
Tonsils 0CQP
Tooth
  Lower 0CQX
  Upper 0CQW
Trachea 0BQ1
Tunica Vaginalis
  Left 0VQ7
  Right 0VQ6
  Turbinate, Nasal 09QL
Tympanic Membrane
  Left 09Q8
  Right 09Q7
Ulna
  Left 0PQL
  Right 0PQK
Ureter
  Left 0TQ7
  Right 0TQ6
Urethra 0TQD
Uterine Supporting Structure
  0UQ4
Uterus 0UQ9
Uvula 0CQN
Vagina 0UQG
Valve
  Aortic 02QF
  Mitral 02QG
  Pulmonary 02QH
  Tricuspid 02QJ
Vas Deferens
  Bilateral 0VQQ
  Left 0VQP
  Right 0VQN
Vein
  Axillary
    Left 05Q8
    Right 05Q7
  Azygos 05Q0
  Basilic
    Left 05QC
    Right 05QB
  Brachial
    Left 05QA
    Right 05Q9
  Cephalic
    Left 05QF
    Right 05QD
  Colic 06Q7
  Common Iliac
    Left 06QD
    Right 06QC
  Coronary 02Q4
  Esophageal 06Q3
  External Iliac
    Left 06QG
    Right 06QF
  External Jugular
    Left 05QQ
    Right 05QP
  Face
    Left 05QV
    Right 05QT
  Femoral
    Left 06QN
    Right 06QM
  Foot
    Left 06QV
    Right 06QT
  Gastric 06Q2
  Greater Saphenous
    Left 06QQ
    Right 06QP

Repair *(continued)*
Vein *(continued)*
  Hand
    Left 05QH
    Right 05QG
  Hemiazygos 05Q1
  Hepatic 06Q4
  Hypogastric
    Left 06QJ
    Right 06QH
  Inferior Mesenteric 06Q6
  Innominate
    Left 05Q4
    Right 05Q3
  Internal Jugular
    Left 05QN
    Right 05QM
  Intracranial 05QL
  Lesser Saphenous
    Left 06QS
    Right 06QR
  Lower 06QY
  Portal 06Q8
  Pulmonary
    Left 02QT
    Right 02QS
  Renal
    Left 06QB
    Right 06Q9
  Splenic 06Q1
  Subclavian
    Left 05Q6
    Right 05Q5
  Superior Mesenteric 06Q5
  Upper 05QY
  Vertebral
    Left 05QS
    Right 05QR
Vena Cava
  Inferior 06Q0
  Superior 02QV
Ventricle
  Left 02QL
  Right 02QK
Vertebra
  Cervical 0PQ3
  Lumbar 0QQ0
  Thoracic 0PQ4
Vesicle
  Bilateral 0VQ3
  Left 0VQ2
  Right 0VQ1
Vitreous
  Left 08Q53ZZ
  Right 08Q43ZZ
Vocal Cord
  Left 0CQV
  Right 0CQT
Vulva 0UQM
Wrist Region
  Left 0XQH
  Right 0XQG
Repair, obstetric laceration,
  periurethral 0UQMXZZ
Replacement
Acetabulum
  Left 0QR5
  Right 0QR4
Ampulla of Vater 0FRC
Anal Sphincter 0DRR
Aorta
  Abdominal 04R0
  Thoracic 02RW
Artery
  Anterior Tibial
    Left 04RQ
    Right 04RP
  Axillary
    Left 03R6
    Right 03R5
  Brachial
    Left 03R8

Replacement *(continued)*
Artery *(continued)*
  Brachial *(continued)*
    Right 03R7
  Celiac 04R1
  Colic
    Left 04R7
    Middle 04R8
    Right 04R6
  Common Carotid
    Left 03RJ
    Right 03RH
  Common Iliac
    Left 04RD
    Right 04RC
  External Carotid
    Left 03RN
    Right 03RM
  External Iliac
    Left 04RJ
    Right 04RH
  Face 03RR
  Femoral
    Left 04RL
    Right 04RK
  Foot
    Left 04RW
    Right 04RV
  Gastric 04R2
  Hand
    Left 03RF
    Right 03RD
  Hepatic 04R3
  Inferior Mesenteric 04RB
  Innominate 03R2
  Internal Carotid
    Left 03RL
    Right 03RK
  Internal Iliac
    Left 04RF
    Right 04RE
  Internal Mammary
    Left 03R1
    Right 03R0
  Intracranial 03RG
  Lower 04RY
  Peroneal
    Left 04RU
    Right 04RT
  Popliteal
    Left 04RN
    Right 04RM
  Posterior Tibial
    Left 04RS
    Right 04RR
  Pulmonary
    Left 02RR
    Right 02RQ
  Pulmonary Trunk 02RP
  Radial
    Left 03RC
    Right 03RB
  Renal
    Left 04RA
    Right 04R9
  Splenic 04R4
  Subclavian
    Left 03R4
    Right 03R3
  Superior Mesenteric 04R5
  Temporal
    Left 03RT
    Right 03RS
  Thyroid
    Left 03RV
    Right 03RU
  Ulnar
    Left 03RA
    Right 03R9
  Upper 03RY
  Vertebral
    Left 03RQ

Replacement *(continued)*
Artery *(continued)*
  Vertebral *(continued)*
    Right 03RP
Atrium
  Left 02R
  Right 02R6
Auditory Ossicle
  Left 09RA0
  Right 09R90
Bladder 0TRB
Bladder Neck 0TRC
Bone
  Ethmoid
    Left 0NRG
    Right 0NRF
  Frontal
    Left 0NR2
    Right 0NR1
  Hyoid 0NRX
  Lacrimal
    Left 0NRJ
    Right 0NRH
  Nasal 0NRB
  Occipital
    Left 0NR8
    Right 0NR7
  Palatine
    Left 0NRL
    Right 0NRK
  Parietal
    Left 0NR4
    Right 0NR3
  Pelvic
    Left 0QR3
    Right 0QR2
  Sphenoid
    Left 0NRD
    Right 0NRC
  Temporal
    Left 0NR6
    Right 0NR5
  Zygomatic
    Left 0NRN
    Right 0NRM
Breast
  Bilateral 0HRV
  Left 0HRU
  Right 0HRT
Buccal Mucosa 0CR4
Carpal
  Left 0PRN
  Right 0PRM
Chordae Tendineae 02R9
Choroid
  Left 08RB
  Right 08RA
Clavicle
  Left 0PRB
  Right 0PR9
Coccyx 0QRS
Conjunctiva
  Left 08RTX
  Right 08RSX
Cornea
  Left 08R9
  Right 08R8
Disc
  Cervical Vertebral 0RR30
  Cervicothoracic Vertebral 0RR50
  Lumbar Vertebral 0SR20
  Lumbosacral 0SR40
  Thoracic Vertebral 0RR90
  Thoracolumbar Vertebral 0RRB0
Duct
  Common Bile 0FR9
  Cystic 0FR8
  Hepatic
    Left 0FR6
    Right 0FR5
  Lacrimal
    Left 08RY

Replacement *(continued)*
- Duct *(continued)*
  - Lacrimal *(continued)*
    - Right 08RX
  - Pancreatic 0FRD
    - Accessory 0FRF
  - Parotid
    - Left 0CRC
    - Right 0CRB
- Ear
  - External
    - Bilateral 09R2
    - Left 09R1
    - Right 09R0
  - Inner
    - Left 09RE0
    - Right 09RD0
  - Middle
    - Left 09R60
    - Right 09R50
- Epiglottis 0CRR
- Esophagus 0DR5
- Eye
  - Left 08R1
  - Right 08R0
- Eyelid
  - Lower
    - Left 08RR
    - Right 08RQ
  - Upper
    - Left 08RP
    - Right 08RN
- Femoral Shaft
  - Left 0QR9
  - Right 0QR8
- Femur
  - Lower
    - Left 0QRC
    - Right 0QRB
  - Upper
    - Left 0QR7
    - Right 0QR6
- Fibula
  - Left 0QRK
  - Right 0QRJ
- Finger Nail 0HRQX
- Gingiva
  - Lower 0CR6
  - Upper 0CR5
- Glenoid Cavity
  - Left 0PR8
  - Right 0PR7
- Hair 0HRSX
- Humeral Head
  - Left 0PRD
  - Right 0PRC
- Humeral Shaft
  - Left 0PRG
  - Right 0PRF
- Iris
  - Left 08RD3
  - Right 08RC3
- Joint
  - Acromioclavicular
    - Left 0RRH0
    - Right 0RRG0
  - Ankle
    - Left 0SRG
    - Right 0SRF
  - Carpal
    - Left 0RRR0
    - Right 0RRQ0
  - Cervical Vertebral 0RR10
  - Cervicothoracic Vertebral 0RR40
  - Coccygeal 0SR60
  - Elbow
    - Left 0RRM0
    - Right 0RRL0
  - Finger Phalangeal
    - Left 0RRX0
    - Right 0RRW0

Replacement *(continued)*
- Joint *(continued)*
  - Hip
    - Left 0SRB
      - Acetabular Surface 0SRE
      - Femoral Surface 0SRS
    - Right 0SR9
      - Acetabular Surface 0SRA
      - Femoral Surface 0SRR
  - Knee
    - Left 0SRD
      - Femoral Surface 0SRU
      - Tibial Surface 0SRW
    - Right 0SRC
      - Femoral Surface 0SRT
      - Tibial Surface 0SRV
  - Lumbar Vertebral 0SR00
  - Lumbosacral 0SR30
  - Metacarpocarpal
    - Left 0RRT0
    - Right 0RRS0
  - Metacarpophalangeal
    - Left 0RRV0
    - Right 0RRU0
  - Metatarsal-Phalangeal
    - Left 0SRN0
    - Right 0SRM0
  - Metatarsal-Tarsal
    - Left 0SRL0
    - Right 0SRK0
  - Occipital-cervical 0RR00
  - Sacrococcygeal 0SR50
  - Sacroiliac
    - Left 0SR80
    - Right 0SR70
  - Shoulder
    - Left 0RRK
    - Right 0RRJ
  - Sternoclavicular
    - Left 0RRF0
    - Right 0RRE0
  - Tarsal
    - Left 0SRJ0
    - Right 0SRH0
  - Temporomandibular
    - Left 0RRD0
    - Right 0RRC0
  - Thoracic Vertebral 0RR60
  - Thoracolumbar Vertebral 0RRA0
  - Toe Phalangeal
    - Left 0SRQ0
    - Right 0SRP0
  - Wrist
    - Left 0RRP0
    - Right 0RRN0
- Kidney Pelvis
  - Left 0TR4
  - Right 0TR3
- Larynx 0CRS
- Lens
  - Left 08RK30Z
  - Right 08RJ30Z
- Lip
  - Lower 0CR1
  - Upper 0CR0
- Mandible
  - Left 0NRV
  - Right 0NRT
- Maxilla
  - Left 0NRS
  - Right 0NRR
- Mesentery 0DRV
- Metacarpal
  - Left 0PRQ
  - Right 0PRP
- Metatarsal
  - Left 0QRP
  - Right 0QR
- Muscle, Papillary 02RD
- Nasopharynx 09RN
- Nipple
  - Left 0HRX

Replacement *(continued)*
- Nipple *(continued)*
  - Right 0HRW
- Nose 09RK
- Omentum
  - Greater 0DRS
  - Lesser 0DRT
- Orbit
  - Left 0NRQ
  - Right 0NRP
- Palate
  - Hard 0CR2
  - Soft 0CR3
- Patella
  - Left 0QRF
  - Right 0QRD
- Pericardium 02RN
- Peritoneum 0DRW
- Phalanx
  - Finger
    - Left 0PRV
    - Right 0PRT
  - Thumb
    - Left 0PRS
    - Right 0PRR
  - Toe
    - Left 0QRR
    - Right 0QRQ
- Pharynx 0CRM
- Radius
  - Left 0PRJ
  - Right 0PRH
- Retinal Vessel
  - Left 08RH3
  - Right 08RG3
- Rib
  - Left 0PR2
  - Right 0PR1
- Sacrum 0QR1
- Scapula
  - Left 0PR6
  - Right 0PR5
- Sclera
  - Left 08R7X
  - Right 08R6X
- Septum
  - Atrial 02R5
  - Nasal 09RM
  - Ventricular 02RM
- Skin
  - Abdomen 0HR7
  - Back 0HR6
  - Buttock 0HR8
  - Chest 0HR5
  - Ear
    - Left 0HR3
    - Right 0HR2
  - Face 0HR1
  - Foot
    - Left 0HRN
    - Right 0HRM
  - Genitalia 0HRA
  - Hand
    - Left 0HRG
    - Right 0HRF
  - Lower Arm
    - Left 0HRE
    - Right 0HRD
  - Lower Leg
    - Left 0HRL
    - Right 0HRK
  - Neck 0HR4
  - Perineum 0HR9
  - Scalp 0HR0
  - Upper Arm
    - Left 0HRC
    - Right 0HRB
  - Upper Leg
    - Left 0HRJ
    - Right 0HRH
- Skull 0NR0
- Sternum 0PR0

Replacement *(continued)*
- Subcutaneous Tissue and Fascia
  - Abdomen 0JR8
  - Back 0JR7
  - Buttock 0JR9
  - Chest 0JR6
  - Face 0JR1
  - Foot
    - Left 0JRR
    - Right 0JRQ
  - Hand
    - Left 0JRK
    - Right 0JRJ
  - Lower Arm
    - Left 0JRH
    - Right 0JRG
  - Lower Leg
    - Left 0JRP
    - Right 0JRN
  - Neck
    - Anterior 0JR4
    - Posterior 0JR5
  - Pelvic Region 0JRC
  - Perineum 0JRB
  - Scalp 0JR0
  - Upper Arm
    - Left 0JRF
    - Right 0JRD
  - Upper Leg
    - Left 0JRM
    - Right 0JRL
- Tarsal
  - Left 0QRM
  - Right 0QRL
- Tendon
  - Abdomen
    - Left 0LRG
    - Right 0LRF
  - Ankle
    - Left 0LRT
    - Right 0LRS
  - Foot
    - Left 0LRW
    - Right 0LRV
  - Hand
    - Left 0LR8
    - Right 0LR7
  - Head and Neck 0LR0
  - Hip
    - Left 0LRK
    - Right 0LRJ
  - Knee
    - Left 0LRR
    - Right 0LRQ
  - Lower Arm and Wrist
    - Left 0LR6
    - Right 0LR5
  - Lower Leg
    - Left 0LRP
    - Right 0LRN
  - Perineum 0LRH
  - Shoulder
    - Left 0LR2
    - Right 0LR1
  - Thorax
    - Left 0LRD
    - Right 0LRC
  - Trunk
    - Left 0LRB
    - Right 0LR9
  - Upper Arm
    - Left 0LR4
    - Right 0LR3
  - Upper Leg
    - Left 0LRM
    - Right 0LRL
- Testis
  - Bilateral 0VRC0J
  - Left 0VRB0J
  - Right 0VR90J
- Thumb
  - Left 0XRM

Replacement *(continued)*
Thumb *(continued)*
    Right 0XRL
Tibia
    Left 0QRH
    Right 0QRG
Toe Nail 0HRRX
Tongue 0CR7
Tooth
    Lower 0CRX
    Upper 0CRW
Turbinate, Nasal 09RL
Tympanic Membrane
    Left 09R8
    Right 09R7
Ulna
    Left 0PRL
    Right 0PRK
Ureter
    Left 0TR7
    Right 0TR6
Urethra 0TRD
Uvula 0CRN
Valve
    Aortic 02RF
    Mitral 02RG
    Pulmonary 02RH
    Tricuspid 02RJ
Vein
    Axillary
        Left 05R8
        Right 05R7
    Azygos 05R0
    Basilic
        Left 05RC
        Right 05RB
    Brachial
        Left 05RA
        Right 05R9
    Cephalic
        Left 05RF
        Right 05RD
    Colic 06R7
    Common Iliac
        Left 06RD
        Right 06RC
    Esophageal 06R3
    External Iliac
        Left 06RG
        Right 06RF
    External Jugular
        Left 05RQ
        Right 05RP
    Face
        Left 05RV
        Right 05RT
    Femoral
        Left 06RN
        Right 06RM
    Foot
        Left 06RV
        Right 06RT
    Gastric 06R2
    Greater Saphenous
        Left 06RQ
        Right 06RP
    Hand
        Left 05RH
        Right 05RG
    Hemiazygos 05R1
    Hepatic 06R4
    Hypogastric
        Left 06RJ
        Right 06RH
    Inferior Mesenteric 06R6
    Innominate
        Left 05R4
        Right 05R3
    Internal Jugular
        Left 05RN
        Right 05RM
    Intracranial 05RL

Replacement *(continued)*
Vein *(continued)*
    Lesser Saphenous
        Left 06RS
        Right 06RR
    Lower 06RY
    Portal 06R8
    Pulmonary
        Left 02RT
        Right 02RS
    Renal
        Left 06RB
        Right 06R9
    Splenic 06R1
    Subclavian
        Left 05R6
        Right 05R5
    Superior Mesenteric 06R5
    Upper 05RY
    Vertebral
        Left 05RS
        Right 05RR
Vena Cava
    Inferior 06R0
    Superior 02RV
Ventricle
    Left 02RL
    Right 02RK
Vertebra
    Cervical 0PR3
    Lumbar 0QR0
    Thoracic 0PR4
Vitreous
    Left 08R53
    Right 08R43
Vocal Cord
    Left 0CRV
    Right 0CRT
Replacement, hip
Partial or total
    see Replacement, Lower Joints 0SR
Resurfacing only
    see Supplement, Lower Joints 0SU
Replantation
    see Reposition
Replantation, scalp
    see Reattachment, Skin, Scalp 0HM0
Reposition
Acetabulum
    Left 0QS5
    Right 0QS4
Ampulla of Vater 0FSC
Anus 0DSQ
Aorta
    Abdominal 04S0
    Thoracic 02SW0ZZ
Artery
    Anterior Tibial
        Left 04SQ
        Right 04SP
    Axillary
        Left 03S6
        Right 03S5
    Brachial
        Left 03S8
        Right 03S7
    Celiac 04S1
    Colic
        Left 04S7
        Middle 04S8
        Right 04S6
    Common Carotid
        Left 03SJ
        Right 03SH
    Common Iliac
        Left 04SD
        Right 04SC
    External Carotid
        Left 03SN
        Right 03SM
    External Iliac
        Left 04SJ

Reposition *(continued)*
Artery *(continued)*
    External Iliac *(continued)*
        Right 04SH
    Face 03SR
    Femoral
        Left 04SL
        Right 04SK
    Foot
        Left 04SW
        Right 04SV
    Gastric 04S2
    Hand
        Left 03SF
        Right 03SD
    Hepatic 04S3
    Inferior Mesenteric 04SB
    Innominate 03S2
    Internal Carotid
        Left 03SL
        Right 03SK
    Internal Iliac
        Left 04SF
        Right 04SE
    Internal Mammary
        Left 03S1
        Right 03S0
    Intracranial 03SG
    Lower 04SY
    Peroneal
        Left 04SU
        Right 04ST
    Popliteal
        Left 04SN
        Right 04SM
    Posterior Tibial
        Left 04SS
        Right 04SR
    Pulmonary
        Left 02SR0ZZ
        Right 02SQ0ZZ
    Pulmonary Trunk 02SP0ZZ
    Radial
        Left 03SC
        Right 03SB
    Renal
        Left 04SA
        Right 04S9
    Splenic 04S4
    Subclavian
        Left 03S4
        Right 03S3
    Superior Mesenteric 04S5
    Temporal
        Left 03ST
        Right 03SS
    Thyroid
        Left 03SV
        Right 03SU
    Ulnar
        Left 03SA
        Right 03S9
    Upper 03SY
    Vertebral
        Left 03SQ
        Right 03SP
Auditory Ossicle
    Left 09SA
    Right 09S9
Bladder 0TSB
Bladder Neck 0TSC
Bone
    Ethmoid
        Left 0NSG
        Right 0NSF
    Frontal
        Left 0NS2
        Right 0NS1
    Hyoid 0NSX
    Lacrimal
        Left 0NSJ
        Right 0NSH

Reposition *(continued)*
Bone *(continued)*
    Nasal 0NSB
    Occipital
        Left 0NS8
        Right 0NS7
    Palatine
        Left 0NSL
        Right 0NSK
    Parietal
        Left 0NS4
        Right 0NS3
    Pelvic
        Left 0QS3
        Right 0QS2
    Sphenoid
        Left 0NSD
        Right 0NSC
    Temporal
        Left 0NS6
        Right 0NS5
    Zygomatic
        Left 0NSN
        Right 0NSM
Breast
    Bilateral 0HSV0ZZ
    Left 0HSU0ZZ
    Right 0HST0ZZ
Bronchus
    Lingula 0BS90ZZ
    Lower Lobe
        Left 0BSB0ZZ
        Right 0BS60ZZ
    Main
        Left 0BS70ZZ
        Right 0BS30ZZ
    Middle Lobe, Right 0BS50ZZ
    Upper Lobe
        Left 0BS80ZZ
        Right 0BS40ZZ
Bursa and Ligament
    Abdomen
        Left 0MSJ
        Right 0MSH
    Ankle
        Left 0MSR
        Right 0MSQ
    Elbow
        Left 0MS4
        Right 0MS3
    Foot
        Left 0MST
        Right 0MSS
    Hand
        Left 0MS8
        Right 0MS7
    Head and Neck 0MS0
    Hip
        Left 0MSM
        Right 0MSL
    Knee
        Left 0MSP
        Right 0MSN
    Lower Extremity
        Left 0MSW
        Right 0MSV
    Perineum 0MSK
    Shoulder
        Left 0MS2
        Right 0MS1
    Thorax
        Left 0MSG
        Right 0MSF
    Trunk
        Left 0MSD
        Right 0MSC
    Upper Extremity
        Left 0MSB
        Right 0MS9
    Wrist
        Left 0MS6
        Right 0MS5

Reposition (continued)
Carina 0BS20ZZ
Carpal
  Left 0PSN
  Right 0PSM
Cecum 0DSH
Cervix 0USC
Clavicle
  Left 0PSB
  Right 0PS9
Coccyx 0QSS
Colon
  Ascending 0DSK
  Descending 0DSM
  Sigmoid 0DSN
  Transverse 0DSL
Cord
  Bilateral 0VSH
  Left 0VSG
  Right 0VSF
Cul-de-sac 0USF
Diaphragm
  Left 0BSS0ZZ
  Right 0BSR0ZZ
Duct
  Common Bile 0FS9
  Cystic 0FS8
  Hepatic
    Left 0FS6
    Right 0FS5
  Lacrimal
    Left 08SY
    Right 08SX
  Pancreatic 0FSD
    Accessory 0FSF
  Parotid
    Left 0CSC
    Right 0CSB
Duodenum 0DS9ZZ
Ear
  Bilateral 09S2ZZ
  Left 09S1ZZ
  Right 09S0ZZ
Epiglottis 0CSR
Esophagus 0DS5ZZ
Eustachian Tube
  Left 09SG
  Right 09SF
Eyelid
  Lower
    Left 08SR
    Right 08SQ
  Upper
    Left 08SP
    Right 08SN
Fallopian Tube
  Left 0US6
  Right 0US5
Fallopian Tubes, Bilateral 0US7
Femoral Shaft
  Left 0QS9
  Right 0QS8
Femur
  Lower
    Left 0QSC
    Right 0QSB
  Upper
    Left 0QS7
    Right 0QS6
Fibula
  Left 0QSK
  Right 0QSJ
Gallbladder 0FS4
Gland
  Adrenal
    Left 0GS2
    Right 0GS3
  Lacrimal
    Left 08SW
    Right 08SV
Glenoid Cavity
  Left 0PS8

Reposition (continued)
Glenoid Cavity (continued)
  Right 0PS7
Hair 0HSSXZZ
Humeral Head
  Left 0PSD
  Right 0PSC
Humeral Shaft
  Left 0PSG
  Right 0PSF
Ileum 0DSB
Iris
  Left 08SD3ZZ
  Right 08SC3ZZ
Jejunum 0DSAZZ
Joint
  Acromioclavicular
    Left 0RSHZ
    Right 0RSGZ
  Ankle
    Left 0SSG
    Right 0SSF
  Carpal
    Left 0RSR
    Right 0RSQ
  Cervical Vertebral 0RS1
  Cervicothoracic Vertebral 0RS4
  Coccygeal 0SS6
  Elbow
    Left 0RSM
    Right 0RSL
  Finger Phalangeal
    Left 0RSX
    Right 0RSW
  Hip
    Left 0SSB
    Right 0SS9
  Knee
    Left 0SSD
    Right 0SSC
  Lumbar Vertebral 0SS0
  Lumbosacral 0SS3
  Metacarpocarpal
    Left 0RST
    Right 0RSS
  Metacarpophalangeal
    Left 0RSV
    Right 0RSU
  Metatarsal-Phalangeal
    Left 0SSN
    Right 0SSM
  Metatarsal-Tarsal
    Left 0SSL
    Right 0SSK
  Occipital-cervical 0RS0
  Sacrococcygeal 0SS5
  Sacroiliac
    Left 0SS8
    Right 0SS7
  Shoulder
    Left 0RSK
    Right 0RSJ
  Sternoclavicular
    Left 0RSF
    Right 0RSE
  Tarsal
    Left 0SSJ
    Right 0SSH
  Temporomandibular
    Left 0RSD
    Right 0RSC
  Thoracic Vertebral 0RS6
  Thoracolumbar Vertebral 0RSA
  Toe Phalangeal
    Left 0SSQ
    Right 0SSP
  Wrist
    Left 0RSP
    Right 0RSN
Kidney
  Left 0TS1
  Right 0TS0

Reposition (continued)
Kidney Pelvis
  Left 0TS4
  Right 0TS3
Kidneys, Bilateral 0TS2
Lens
  Left 08SK3ZZ
  Right 08SJ3ZZ
Lip
  Lower 0CS1
  Upper 0CS0
Liver 0FS0
Lung
  Left 0BSL0ZZ
  Lower Lobe
    Left 0BSJ0ZZ
    Right 0BSF0ZZ
  Middle Lobe, Right 0BSD0ZZ
  Right 0BSK0ZZ
  Upper Lobe
    Left 0BSG0ZZ
    Right 0BSC0ZZ
Lung Lingula 0BSH0ZZ
Mandible
  Left 0NSV
  Right 0NST
Maxilla
  Left 0NSS
  Right 0NSR
Metacarpal
  Left 0PSQ
  Right 0PSP
Metatarsal
  Left 0QSP
  Right 0QSN
Muscle
  Abdomen
    Left 0KSL
    Right 0KSK
  Extraocular
    Left 08SM
    Right 08SL
  Facial 0KS1
  Foot
    Left 0KSW
    Right 0KSV
  Hand
    Left 0KSD
    Right 0KSC
  Head 0KS0
  Hip
    Left 0KSP
    Right 0KSN
  Lower Arm and Wrist
    Left 0KSB
    Right 0KS9
  Lower Leg
    Left 0KST
    Right 0KSS
  Neck
    Left 0KS3
    Right 0KS2
  Perineum 0KSM
  Shoulder
    Left 0KS6
    Right 0KS5
  Thorax
    Left 0KSJ
    Right 0KSH
  Tongue, Palate, Pharynx 0KS4
  Trunk
    Left 0KSG
    Right 0KSF
  Upper Arm
    Left 0KS8
    Right 0KS7
  Upper Leg
    Left 0KSR
    Right 0KSQ
Nerve
  Abducens 00SL
  Accessory 00SR

Reposition (continued)
Nerve (continued)
  Acoustic 00SN
  Brachial Plexus 01S3
  Cervical 01S1
  Cervical Plexus 01S0
  Facial 00SM
  Femoral 01SD
  Glossopharyngeal 00SP
  Hypoglossal 00SS
  Lumbar 01SB
  Lumbar Plexus 01S9
  Lumbosacral Plexus 01SA
  Median 01S5
  Oculomotor 00SH
  Olfactory 00SF
  Optic 00SG
  Peroneal 01SH
  Phrenic 01S2
  Pudendal 01SC
  Radial 01S6
  Sacral 01SR
  Sacral Plexus 01SQ
  Sciatic 01SF
  Thoracic 01S8
  Tibial 01SG
  Trigeminal 00SK
  Trochlear 00SJ
  Ulnar 01S4
  Vagus 00SQ
Nipple
  Left 0HSXXZZ
  Right 0HSWXZZ
Nose 09SK
Orbit
  Left 0NSQ
  Right 0NSP
Ovary
  Bilateral 0US2
  Left 0US1
  Right 0US0
Palate
  Hard 0CS2
  Soft 0CS3
Pancreas 0FSG
Parathyroid Gland 0GSR
  Inferior
    Left 0GSP
    Right 0GSN
  Multiple 0GSQ
  Superior
    Left 0GSM
    Right 0GSL
Patella
  Left 0QSF
  Right 0QSD
Phalanx
  Finger
    Left 0PSV
    Right 0PST
  Thumb
    Left 0PSS
    Right 0PSR
  Toe
    Left 0QSR
    Right 0QSQ
Products of Conception 10S0
  Ectopic 10S2
Radius
  Left 0PSJ
  Right 0PSH
Rectum 0DSP
Retinal Vessel
  Left 08SH3ZZ
  Right 08SG3ZZ
Rib
  Left 0PS2
  Right 0PS1
Sacrum 0QS1
Scapula
  Left 0PS6
  Right 0PS5

Reposition *(continued)*

Septum, Nasal 09SM
Skull 0NS0
Spinal Cord
    Cervical 00SW
    Lumbar 00SY
    Thoracic 00SX
Spleen 07SP0ZZ
Sternum 0PS0
Stomach 0DS6
Tarsal
    Left 0QSM
    Right 0QSL
Tendon
    Abdomen
        Left 0LSG
        Right 0LSF
    Ankle
        Left 0LST
        Right 0LSS
    Foot
        Left 0LSW
        Right 0LSV
    Hand
        Left 0LS8
        Right 0LS7
    Head and Neck 0LS0
    Hip
        Left 0LSK
        Right 0LSJ
    Knee
        Left 0LSR
        Right 0LSQ
    Lower Arm and Wrist
        Left 0LS6
        Right 0LS5
    Lower Leg
        Left 0LSP
        Right 0LSN
    Perineum 0LSH
    Shoulder
        Left 0LS2
        Right 0LS1
    Thorax
        Left 0LSD
        Right 0LSC
    Trunk
        Left 0LSB
        Right 0LS9
    Upper Arm
        Left 0LS4
        Right 0LS3
    Upper Leg
        Left 0LSM
        Right 0LSL
Testis
    Bilateral 0VSC
    Left 0VSB
    Right 0VS9
Thymus 07SM0ZZ
Thyroid Gland
    Left Lobe 0GSG
    Right Lobe 0GSH
Tibia
    Left 0QSH
    Right 0QSG
Tongue 0CS7
Tooth
    Lower 0CSX
    Upper 0CSW
Trachea 0BS10ZZ
Turbinate, Nasal 09SL
Tympanic Membrane
    Left 09S8
    Right 09S7
Ulna
    Left 0PSL
    Right 0PSK
Ureter
    Left 0TS7
    Right 0TS6
Ureters, Bilateral 0TS8

Reposition *(continued)*

Urethra 0TSD
Uterine Supporting Structure 0US4
Uterus 0US9
Uvula 0CSN
Vagina 0USG
Vein
    Axillary
        Left 05S8
        Right 05S7
    Azygos 05S0
    Basilic
        Left 05SC
        Right 05SB
    Brachial
        Left 05SA
        Right 05S9
    Cephalic
        Left 05SF
        Right 05SD
    Colic 06S7
    Common Iliac
        Left 06SD
        Right 06SC
    Esophageal 06S3
    External Iliac
        Left 06SG
        Right 06SF
    External Jugular
        Left 05SQ
        Right 05SP
    Face
        Left 05SV
        Right 05ST
    Femoral
        Left 06SN
        Right 06SM
    Foot
        Left 06SV
        Right 06ST
    Gastric 06S2
    Greater Saphenous
        Left 06SQ
        Right 06SP
    Hand
        Left 05SH
        Right 05SG
    Hemiazygos 05S1
    Hepatic 06S4
    Hypogastric
        Left 06SJ
        Right 06SH
    Inferior Mesenteric 06S6
    Innominate
        Left 05S4
        Right 05S3
    Internal Jugular
        Left 05SN
        Right 05SM
    Intracranial 05SL
    Lesser Saphenous
        Left 06SS
        Right 06SR
    Lower 06SY
    Portal 06S8
    Pulmonary
        Left 02ST0ZZ
        Right 02SS0ZZ
    Renal
        Left 06SB
        Right 06S9
    Splenic 06S1
    Subclavian
        Left 05S6
        Right 05S5
    Superior Mesenteric 06S5
    Upper 05SY
    Vertebral
        Left 05SS
        Right 05SR
Vena Cava
    Inferior 06S0

Reposition *(continued)*

Vena Cava *(continued)*
    Superior 02SV0ZZ
Vertebra
    Cervical 0PS3
    Lumbar 0QS0
    Thoracic 0PS4
Vocal Cord
    Left 0CSV
    Right 0CST

Resection

Acetabulum
    Left 0QT50ZZ
    Right 0QT40ZZ
Adenoids 0CTQ
Ampulla of Vater 0FTC
Anal Sphincter 0DTR
Anus 0DTQ
Aortic Body 0GTD
Appendix 0DTJ
Auditory Ossicle
    Left 09TA0ZZ
    Right 09T90ZZ
Bladder 0TTB
Bladder Neck 0TTC
Bone
    Ethmoid
        Left 0NTG0ZZ
        Right 0NTF0ZZ
    Frontal
        Left 0NT20ZZ
        Right 0NT10ZZ
    Hyoid 0NTX0ZZ
    Lacrimal
        Left 0NTJ0ZZ
        Right 0NTH0ZZ
    Nasal 0NTB0ZZ
    Occipital
        Left 0NT80ZZ
        Right 0NT70ZZ
    Palatine
        Left 0NTL0ZZ
        Right 0NTK0ZZ
    Parietal
        Left 0NT40ZZ
        Right 0NT30ZZ
    Pelvic
        Left 0QT30ZZ
        Right 0QT20ZZ
    Sphenoid
        Left 0NTD0ZZ
        Right 0NTC0ZZ
    Temporal
        Left 0NT60ZZ
        Right 0NT50ZZ
    Zygomatic
        Left 0NTN0ZZ
        Right 0NTM0ZZ
Breast
    Bilateral 0HTV0ZZ
    Left 0HTU0ZZ
    Right 0HTT0ZZ
    Supernumerary 0HTY0ZZ
Bronchus
    Lingula 0BT9
    Lower Lobe
        Left 0BTB
        Right 0BT6
    Main
        Left 0BT7
        Right 0BT3
    Middle Lobe, Right 0BT5
    Upper Lobe
        Left 0BT8
        Right 0BT4
Bursa and Ligament
    Abdomen
        Left 0MTJ
        Right 0MTH
    Ankle
        Left 0MTR
        Right 0MTQ

Resection *(continued)*

Bursa and Ligament *(continued)*
    Elbow
        Left 0MT4
        Right 0MT3
    Foot
        Left 0MTT
        Right 0MTS
    Hand
        Left 0MT8
        Right 0MT7
    Head and Neck 0MT0
    Hip
        Left 0MTM
        Right 0MTL
    Knee
        Left 0MTP
        Right 0MTN
    Lower Extremity
        Left 0MTW
        Right 0MTV
    Perineum 0MTK
    Shoulder
        Left 0MT2
        Right 0MT1
    Thorax
        Left 0MTG
        Right 0MTF
    Trunk
        Left 0MTD
        Right 0MTC
    Upper Extremity
        Left 0MTB
        Right 0MT9
    Wrist
        Left 0MT6
        Right 0MT5
Carina 0BT2
Carotid Bodies, Bilateral 0GT8
Carotid Body
    Left 0GT6
    Right 0GT7
Carpal
    Left 0PTN0ZZ
    Right 0PTM0ZZ
Cecum 0DTH
Cerebral Hemisphere 00T7
Cervix 0UTC
Chordae Tendineae 02T9
Cisterna Chyli 07TL
Clavicle
    Left 0PTB0ZZ
    Right 0PT90ZZ
Clitoris 0UTJ
Coccygeal Glomus 0GTB
Coccyx 0QTS0ZZ
Colon
    Ascending 0DTK
    Descending 0DTM
    Sigmoid 0DTN
    Transverse 0DTL
Conduction Mechanism 02T8
Cord
    Bilateral 0VTH
    Left 0VTG
    Right 0VTF
Cornea
    Left 08T9XZZ
    Right 08T8XZZ
Cul-de-sac 0UTF
Diaphragm
    Left 0BTS
    Right 0BTR
Disc
    Cervical Vertebral 0RT30ZZ
    Cervicothoracic Vertebral
        0RT50ZZ
    Lumbar Vertebral 0ST20ZZ
    Lumbosacral 0ST40ZZ
    Thoracic Vertebral 0RT90ZZ
    Thoracolumbar Vertebral
        0RTB0ZZ

Resection *(continued)*

Duct
Common Bile 0FT9
Cystic 0FT8
Hepatic
Left 0FT6
Right 0FT5
Lacrimal
Left 08TY
Right 08TX
Pancreatic 0FTD
Accessory 0FTF
Parotid
Left 0CTC0ZZ
Right 0CTB0ZZ
Duodenum 0DT9
Ear
External
Left 09T1
Right 09T0
Inner
Left 09TE0
Right 09TD0
Middle
Left 09T60
Right 09T50
Epididymis
Bilateral 0VTL
Left 0VTK
Right 0VTJ
Epiglottis 0CTR
Esophagogastric Junction 0DT4
Esophagus 0DT5
Lower 0DT3
Middle 0DT2
Upper 0DT1
Eustachian Tube
Left 09TG
Right 09TF
Eye
Left 08T1XZZ
Right 08T0XZZ
Eyelid
Lower
Left 08TR
Right 08TQ
Upper
Left 08TP
Right 08TN
Fallopian Tube
Left 0UT6
Right 0UT5
Fallopian Tubes, Bilateral 0UT7
Femoral Shaft
Left 0QT90ZZ
Right 0QT80ZZ
Femur
Lower
Left 0QTC0ZZ
Right 0QTB0ZZ
Upper
Left 0QT70ZZ
Right 0QT60ZZ
Fibula
Left 0QTK0ZZ
Right 0QTJ0ZZ
Finger Nail 0HTQXZZ
Gallbladder 0FT4
Gland
Adrenal
Bilateral 0GT4
Left 0GT2
Right 0GT3
Lacrimal
Left 08TW
Right 08TV
Minor Salivary 0CTJ0ZZ
Parotid
Left 0CT90ZZ
Right 0CT80ZZ
Pituitary 0GT0
Sublingual

Resection *(continued)*

Gland *(continued)*
Sublingual *(continued)*
Left 0CTF0ZZ
Right 0CTD0ZZ
Submaxillary
Left 0CTH0ZZ
Right 0CTG0ZZ
Vestibular 0UTL
Glenoid Cavity
Left 0PT80ZZ
Right 0PT70ZZ
Glomus Jugulare 0GTC
Humeral Head
Left 0PTD0ZZ
Right 0PTC0ZZ
Humeral Shaft
Left 0PTG0ZZ
Right 0PTF0ZZ
Hymen 0UTK
Ileocecal Valve 0DTC
Ileum 0DTB
Intestine
Large 0DTE
Left 0DTG
Right 0DTF
Small 0DT8
Iris
Left 08TD3ZZ
Right 08TC3ZZ
Jejunum 0DTA
Joint
Acromioclavicular
Left 0RTH0ZZ
Right 0RTG0ZZ
Ankle
Left 0STG0ZZ
Right 0STF0ZZ
Carpal
Left 0RTR0ZZ
Right 0RTQ0ZZ
Cervicothoracic Vertebral
0RT40ZZ
Coccygeal 0ST60ZZ
Elbow
Left 0RTM0ZZ
Right 0RTL0ZZ
Finger Phalangeal
Left 0RTX0ZZ
Right 0RTW0ZZ
Hip
Left 0STB0ZZ
Right 0ST90ZZ
Knee
Left 0STD0ZZ
Right 0STC0ZZ
Metacarpocarpal
Left 0RTT0ZZ
Right 0RTS0ZZ
Metacarpophalangeal
Left 0RTV0ZZ
Right 0RTU0ZZ
Metatarsal-Phalangeal
Left 0STN0ZZ
Right 0STM0ZZ
Metatarsal-Tarsal
Left 0STL0ZZ
Right 0STK0ZZ
Sacrococcygeal 0ST50ZZ
Sacroiliac
Left 0ST80ZZ
Right 0ST70ZZ
Shoulder
Left 0RTK0ZZ
Right 0RTJ0ZZ
Sternoclavicular
Left 0RTF0ZZ
Right 0RTE0ZZ
Tarsal
Left 0STJ0ZZ
Right 0STH0ZZ
Temporomandibular

Resection *(continued)*

Joint *(continued)*
Temporomandibular *(continued)*
Left 0RTD0ZZ
Right 0RTC0ZZ
Toe Phalangeal
Left 0STQ0ZZ
Right 0STP0ZZ
Wrist
Left 0RTP0ZZ
Right 0RTN0ZZ
Kidney
Left 0TT1
Right 0TT0
Kidney Pelvis
Left 0TT4
Right 0TT3
Kidneys, Bilateral 0TT2
Larynx 0CTS
Lens
Left 08TK3ZZ
Right 08TJ3ZZ
Lip
Lower 0CT1
Upper 0CT0
Liver 0FT0
Left Lobe 0FT2
Right Lobe 0FT1
Lung
Bilateral 0BTM
Left 0BTL
Lower Lobe
Left 0BTJ
Right 0BTF
Middle Lobe, Right 0BTD
Right 0BTK
Upper Lobe
Left 0BTG
Right 0BTC
Lung Lingula 0BTH
Lymphatic
Aortic 07TD
Axillary
Left 07T6
Right 07T5
Head 07T0
Inguinal
Left 07TJ
Right 07TH
Internal Mammary
Left 07T9
Right 07T8
Lower Extremity
Left 07TG
Right 07TF
Mesenteric 07TB
Neck
Left 07T2
Right 07T1
Pelvis 07TC
Thoracic Duct 07TK
Thorax 07T7
Upper Extremity
Left 07T4
Right 07T3
Mandible
Left 0NTV0ZZ
Right 0NTT0ZZ
Maxilla
Left 0NTS0ZZ
Right 0NTR0ZZ
Metacarpal
Left 0PTQ0ZZ
Right 0PTP0ZZ
Metatarsal
Left 0QTP0ZZ
Right 0QTN0ZZ
Muscle
Abdomen
Left 0KTL
Right 0KTK
Extraocular

Resection *(continued)*

Muscle *(continued)*
Extraocular *(continued)*
Left 08TM
Right 08TL
Facial 0KT1
Foot
Left 0KTW
Right 0KTV
Hand
Left 0KTD
Right 0KTC
Head 0KT0
Hip
Left 0KTP
Right 0KTN
Lower Arm and Wrist
Left 0KTB
Right 0KT9
Lower Leg
Left 0KTT
Right 0KTS
Neck
Left 0KT3
Right 0KT2
Papillary 02TD
Pcrincum 0KTM
Shoulder
Left 0KT6
Right 0KT5
Thorax
Left 0KTJ
Right 0KTH
Tongue, Palate, Pharynx 0KT4
Trunk
Left 0KTG
Right 0KTF
Upper Arm
Left 0KT8
Right 0KT7
Upper Leg
Left 0KTR
Right 0KTQ
Nasopharynx 09TN
Nipple
Left 0HTXXZZ
Right 0HTWXZZ
Nose 09TK
Omentum
Greater 0DTS
Lesser 0DTT
Orbit
Left 0NTQ0ZZ
Right 0NTP0ZZ
Ovary
Bilateral 0UT2
Left 0UT1
Right 0UT0
Palate
Hard 0CT2
Soft 0CT3
Pancreas 0FTG
Para-aortic Body 0GT9
Paraganglion Extremity
0GTF
Parathyroid Gland 0GTR
Inferior
Left 0GTP
Right 0GTN
Multiple 0GTQ
Superior
Left 0GTM
Right 0GTL
Patella
Left 0QTF0ZZ
Right 0QTD0ZZ
Penis 0VTS
Pericardium 02TN
Phalanx
Finger
Left 0PTV0ZZ
Right 0PTT0ZZ

Revision of device in (continued)

Joint (continued)
  Sacroiliac
    Left 0SW8
    Right 0SW7
  Shoulder
    Left 0RWK
    Right 0RWJ
  Sternoclavicular
    Left 0RWF
    Right 0RWE
  Tarsal
    Left 0SWJ
    Right 0SWH
  Temporomandibular
    Left 0RWD
    Right 0RWC
  Thoracic Vertebral 0RW6
  Thoracolumbar Vertebral 0RWA
  Toe Phalangeal
    Left 0SWQ
    Right 0SWP
  Wrist
    Left 0RWP
    Right 0RWN
Kidney 0TW5
Larynx 0CWS
Lens
  Left 08WKJ
  Right 08WJ
Liver 0FW0
Lung
  Left 0BWL
  Right 0BWK
Lymphatic 07WN
  Thoracic Duct 07WK
Mediastinum 0WWC
Mesentery 0DWV
Metacarpal
  Left 0PWQ
  Right 0PWP
Metatarsal
  Left 0QWP
  Right 0QWN
Mouth and Throat 0CWY
Muscle
  Extraocular
    Left 08WM
    Right 08WL
  Lower 0KWY
  Upper 0KWX
Neck 0WW6
Nerve
  Cranial 00WE
  Peripheral 01WY
Nose 09WK
Omentum 0DWU
Ovary 0UW3
Pancreas 0FWG
Parathyroid Gland 0GWR
Patella
  Left 0QWF
  Right 0QWD
Pelvic Cavity 0WWJ
Penis 0VWS
Pericardial Cavity 0WWD
Perineum
  Female 0WWN
  Male 0WWM
Peritoneal Cavity 0WWG
Peritoneum 0DWW
Phalanx
  Finger
    Left 0PWV
    Right 0PWT
  Thumb
    Left 0PWS
    Right 0PWR
  Toe
    Left 0QWR
    Right 0QWQ
Pineal Body 0GW10

Revision of device in (continued)

Pleura 0BWQ
Pleural Cavity
  Left 0WWB
  Right 0WW9
Prostate and Seminal Vesicles 0VW4
Radius
  Left 0PWJ
  Right 0PWH
Respiratory Tract 0WWQ
Retroperitoneum 0WWH
Rib
  Left 0PW2
  Right 0PW1
Sacrum 0QW1
Scapula
  Left 0PW6
  Right 0PW5
Scrotum and Tunica Vaginalis 0VW8
Septum
  Atrial 02W5
  Ventricular 02WM
Sinus 09WY0
Skin 0HWPX
Skull 0NW0
Spinal Canal 00WU
Spinal Cord 00WV
Spleen 07WP
Sternum 0PW0
Stomach 0DW6
Subcutaneous Tissue and Fascia
  Head and Neck 0JWS
  Lower Extremity 0JWW
  Trunk 0JWT
  Upper Extremity 0JWV
Tarsal
  Left 0QWM
  Right 0QWL
Tendon
  Lower 0LWY
  Upper 0LWX
Testis 0VWD
Thymus 07WM
Thyroid Gland 0GWK0
Tibia
  Left 0QWH
  Right 0QWG
Toe Nail 0HWRX
Trachea 0BW1F
Tracheobronchial Tree 0BW0
Tympanic Membrane
  Left 09W8
  Right 09W7
Ulna
  Left 0PWL
  Right 0PWK
Ureter 0TW9M
Urethra 0TWD
Uterus and Cervix 0UWD
Vagina and Cul-de-sac 0UWH
Valve
  Aortic 02WF
  Mitral 02WG
  Pulmonary 02WH
  Tricuspid 02WJ
Vas Deferens 0VWR
Vein
  Lower 06WY
  Upper 05WY
Vertebra
  Cervical 0PW3
  Lumbar 0QW0
  Thoracic 0PW4
Vulva 0UWM
Revo MRI™ SureScan® pacemaker
  use Pacemaker, Dual Chamber in 0JH
rhBMP-2
  use Recombinant Bone Morphogenetic Protein
Rheos® System device
  use Stimulator Generator in Subcutaneous Tissue and Fascia

Rheos® System lead
  use Stimulator Lead in Upper Arteries
Rhinopharynx
  use Nasopharynx
Rhinoplasty
  see Alteration, Nose 090K
  see Repair, Nose 09QK
  see Replacement, Nose 09RK
  see Supplement, Nose 09UK
Rhinorrhaphy
  see Repair, Nose 09QK
Rhinoscopy 09JKXZZ
Rhizotomy
  see Division, Central Nervous System 008
  see Division, Peripheral Nervous System 018
Rhomboid major muscle
  use Muscle, Trunk, Left
  use Muscle, Trunk, Right
Rhomboid minor muscle
  use Muscle, Trunk, Left
  use Muscle, Trunk, Right
Rhythm electrocardiogram
  see Measurement, Cardiac 4A02
Rhytidectomy
  see Face lift
Right ascending lumbar vein
  use Vein, Azygos
Right atrioventricular valve
  use Valve, Tricuspid
Right auricular appendix
  use Atrium, Right
Right colic vein
  use Vein, Colic
Right coronary sulcus
  use Heart, Right
Right gastric artery
  use Artery, Gastric
Right gastroepiploic vein
  use Vein, Superior Mesenteric
Right inferior phrenic vein
  use Vena Cava, Inferior
Right inferior pulmonary vein
  use Vein, Pulmonary, Right
Right jugular trunk
  use Lymphatic, Neck, Right
Right lateral ventricle
  use Cerebral Ventricle
Right lymphatic duct
  use Lymphatic, Neck, Right
Right ovarian vein
  use Vena Cava, Inferior
Right second lumbar vein
  use Vena Cava, Inferior
Right subclavian trunk
  use Lymphatic, Neck, Right
Right subcostal vein
  use Vein, Azygos
Right superior pulmonary vein
  use Vein, Pulmonary, Right
Right suprarenal vein
  use Vena Cava, Inferior
Right testicular vein
  use Vena Cava, Inferior
Rima glottidis
  use Larynx
Risorius muscle
  use Muscle, Facial
RNS System lead
  use Neurostimulator Lead in Central Nervous System
RNS system neurostimulator generator
  use Neurostimulator Generator in Head and Facial Bones
Robotic Assisted Procedure
  Extremity
    Lower 8E0Y
    Upper 8E0X
  Head and Neck Region 8E09
  Trunk Region 8E0W

Rotation of fetal head
  Forceps 10S07ZZ
  Manual 10S0XZZ
Round ligament of uterus
  use Uterine Supporting Structure
Round window
  use Ear, Inner, Left
  use Ear, Inner, Right
Roux-en-Y operation
  see Bypass, Gastrointestinal System 0D1
  see Bypass, Hepatobiliary System and Pancreas 0F1
Rupture
  Adhesions
    see Release
  Fluid collection
    see Drainage

S

Sacral ganglion
  use Nerve, Sacral Sympathetic
Sacral lymph node
  use Lymphatic, Pelvis
Sacral nerve modulation (SNM) lead
  use Stimulator Lead in Urinary System
Sacral neuromodulation lead
  use Stimulator Lead in Urinary System
Sacral splanchnic nerve
  use Nerve, Sacral Sympathetic
Sacrectomy
  see Excision, Lower Bones 0QB
Sacrococcygeal ligament
  use Bursa and Ligament, Trunk, Left
  use Bursa and Ligament, Trunk, Right
Sacrococcygeal symphysis
  use Joint, Sacrococcygeal
Sacroiliac ligament
  use Bursa and Ligament, Trunk, Left
  use Bursa and Ligament, Trunk, Right
Sacrospinous ligament
  use Bursa and Ligament, Trunk, Left
  use Bursa and Ligament, Trunk, Right
Sacrotuberous ligament
  use Bursa and Ligament, Trunk, Left
  use Bursa and Ligament, Trunk, Right
Salpingectomy
  see Excision, Female Reproductive System 0UB
  see Resection, Female Reproductive System 0UT
Salpingolysis
  see Release, Female Reproductive System 0UN
Salpingopexy
  see Repair, Female Reproductive System 0UQ
  see Reposition, Female Reproductive System 0US
Salpingopharyngeus muscle
  use Muscle, Tongue, Palate, Pharynx
Salpingoplasty
  see Repair, Female Reproductive System 0UQ
  see Supplement, Female Reproductive System 0UU
Salpingorrhaphy
  see Repair, Female Reproductive System 0UQ
Salpingoscopy 0UJ88ZZ
Salpingostomy
  see Drainage, Female Reproductive System 0U9

Salpingotomy
   see Drainage, Female Reproductive
     System 0U9
Salpinx
   use Fallopian Tube, Left
   use Fallopian Tube, Right
Saphenous nerve
   use Nerve, Femoral
SAPIEN transcatheter aortic valve
   use Zooplastic Tissue in Heart and
     Great Vessels
Sartorius muscle
   use Muscle, Upper Leg, Left
   use Muscle, Upper Leg, Right
Scalene muscle
   use Muscle, Neck, Left
   use Muscle, Neck, Right
Scan
   Computerized Tomography (CT)
     see Computerized Tomography
       (CT Scan)
   Radioisotope
     see Planar Nuclear Medicine
       Imaging
Scaphoid bone
   use Carpal, Left
   use Carpal, Right
Scapholunate ligament
   use Bursa and Ligament, Hand, Left
   use Bursa and Ligament, Hand,
     Right
Scaphotrapezium ligament
   use Bursa and Ligament, Hand, Left
   use Bursa and Ligament, Hand,
     Right
Scapulectomy
   see Excision, Upper Bones 0PB
   see Resection, Upper Bones 0PT
Scapulopexy
   see Repair, Upper Bones 0PQ
   see Reposition, Upper Bones 0PS
Scarpa's (vestibular) ganglion
   use Nerve, Acoustic
Sclerectomy
   see Excision, Eye 08B
Sclerotherapy, mechanical
   see Destruction
Sclerotomy
   see Drainage, Eye 089
Scrotectomy
   see Excision, Male Reproductive
     System 0VB
   see Resection, Male Reproductive
     System 0VT
Scrotoplasty
   see Repair, Male Reproductive
     System 0VQ
   see Supplement, Male Reproductive
     System 0VU
Scrotorrhaphy
   see Repair, Male Reproductive
     System 0VQ
Scrototomy
   see Drainage, Male Reproductive
     System 0V9
Sebaceous gland
   use Skin
Second cranial nerve
   use Nerve, Optic
Section, cesarean
   see Extraction, Pregnancy 10D
Secura (DR) (VR)
   use Defibrillator Generator in 0JH
Sella Turcica
   use Bone, Sphenoid, Left
   use Bone, Sphenoid, Right
Semicircular canal
   use Ear, Inner, Left
   use Ear, Inner, Right
Semimembranosus muscle
   use Muscle, Upper Leg, Left
   use Muscle, Upper Leg, Right

Semitendinosus muscle
   use Muscle, Upper Leg, Left
   use Muscle, Upper Leg, Right
Seprafilm
   use Adhesion Barrier
Septal cartilage
   use Septum, Nasal
Septectomy
   see Excision, Ear, Nose, Sinus 09B
   see Excision, Heart and Great
     Vessels 02B
   see Resection, Ear, Nose, Sinus 09T
   see Resection, Heart and Great
     Vessels 02T
Septoplasty
   see Repair, Ear, Nose, Sinus 09Q
   see Repair, Heart and Great Vessels
     02Q
   see Replacement, Ear, Nose, Sinus
     09R
   see Replacement, Heart and Great
     Vessels 02R
   see Reposition, Ear, Nose, Sinus 09S
   see Supplement, Ear, Nose, Sinus
     09U
   see Supplement, Heart and Great
     Vessels 02U
Septotomy
   see Drainage, Ear, Nose,
     Sinus 099
Sequestrectomy, bone
   see Extirpation
Serratus anterior muscle
   use Muscle, Thorax, Left
   use Muscle, Thorax, Right
Serratus posterior muscle
   use Muscle, Trunk, Left
   use Muscle, Trunk, Right
Seventh cranial nerve
   use Nerve, Facial
Sheffield hybrid external fixator
   use External Fixation Device,
     Hybrid in 0PH
   use External Fixation Device,
     Hybrid in 0PS
   use External Fixation Device,
     Hybrid in 0QH
   use External Fixation Device,
     Hybrid in 0QS
Sheffield ring external fixator
   use External Fixation Device, Ring
     in 0PH
   use External Fixation Device, Ring
     in 0PS
   use External Fixation Device, Ring
     in 0QH
   use External Fixation Device, Ring
     in 0QS
Shirodkar cervical cerclage 0UVC7ZZ
Shock Wave Therapy,
   Musculoskeletal 6A93
Short gastric artery
   use Artery, Splenic
Shortening
   see Excision
   see Repair
   see Reposition
Shunt creation
   see Bypass
Sialoadenectomy
   Complete
     see Resection, Mouth and Throat
       0CT
   Partial
     see Excision, Mouth and Throat
       0CB
Sialodochoplasty
   see Repair, Mouth and Throat 0CQ
   see Replacement, Mouth and Throat
     0CR
   see Supplement, Mouth and Throat
     0CU

Sialoectomy
   see Excision, Mouth and Throat 0CB
   see Resection, Mouth and Throat
     0CT
Sialography
   see Plain Radiography, Ear, Nose,
     Mouth and Throat B90
Sialolithotomy
   see Extirpation, Mouth and Throat
     0CC
Sigmoid artery
   use Artery, Inferior Mesenteric
Sigmoid flexure
   use Colon, Sigmoid
Sigmoid vein
   use Vein, Inferior Mesenteric
Sigmoidectomy
   see Excision, Gastrointestinal
     System 0DB
   see Resection, Gastrointestinal
     System 0DT
Sigmoidorrhaphy
   see Repair, Gastrointestinal System
     0DQ
Sigmoidoscopy 0DJD8ZZ
Sigmoidotomy
   see Drainage, Gastrointestinal
     System 0D9
Single lead pacemaker (atrium)
   (ventricle)
   use Pacemaker, Single Chamber
     in 0JH
Single lead rate responsive pacemaker
   (atrium)(ventricle)
   use Pacemaker, Single Chamber
     Rate Responsive in 0JH
Sinoatrial node
   use Conduction Mechanism
Sinogram
   Abdominal Wall
     see Fluoroscopy, Abdomen and
       Pelvis BW11
   Chest Wall
     see Plain Radiography, Chest
       BW03
   Retroperitoneum
     see Fluoroscopy, Abdomen and
       Pelvis BW11
Sinusectomy
   see Excision, Ear, Nose, Sinus 09B
   see Resection, Ear, Nose, Sinus 09T
Sinusoscopy 09JY4ZZ
Sinusotomy
   see Drainage, Ear, Nose, Sinus 099
Sinus venosus
   use Atrium, Right
Sirolimus-eluting coronary stent
   use Intraluminal Device, Drug-
     eluting in Heart and Great Vessels
Sixth cranial nerve
   use Nerve, Abducens
Size reduction, breast
   see Excision, Skin and Breast 0HB
SJM Biocor® Stented Valve System
   use Zooplastic Tissue in Heart and
     Great Vessels
Skene's (paraurethral) gland
   use Gland, Vestibular
Sling
   Fascial, orbicularis muscle (mouth)
     see Supplement, Muscle, Facial
       0KU1
   Levator muscle, for urethral
     suspension
     see Reposition, Bladder Neck
       0TSC
   Pubococcygeal, for urethral
     suspension
     see Reposition, Bladder Neck
       0TSC
   Rectum
     see Reposition, Rectum 0DSP

Small bowel series
   see Fluoroscopy, Bowel, Small
     BD13
Small saphenous vein
   use Vein, Lesser Saphenous, Left
   use Vein, Lesser Saphenous, Right
Snaring, polyp, colon
   see Excision, Gastrointestinal
     System 0DB
Solar (celiac) plexus
   use Nerve, Abdominal Sympathetic
Soleus muscle
   use Muscle, Lower Leg, Left
   use Muscle, Lower Leg, Right
Spacer
   Insertion of device in
     Disc
       Lumbar Vertebral 0SH2
       Lumbosacral 0SH4
     Joint
       Acromioclavicular
         Left 0RHH
         Right 0RHG
       Ankle
         Left 0SHG
         Right 0SHF
       Carpal
         Left 0RHR
         Right 0RHQ
       Cervical Vertebral 0RH1
       Cervicothoracic Vertebral
         0RH4
       Coccygeal 0SH6
       Elbow
         Left 0RHM
         Right 0RHL
       Finger Phalangeal
         Left 0RHX
         Right 0RHW
       Hip
         Left 0SHB
         Right 0SH9
       Knee
         Left 0SHD
         Right 0SHC
       Lumbar Vertebral 0SH0
       Lumbosacral 0SH3
       Metacarpocarpal
         Left 0RHT
         Right 0RHS
       Metacarpophalangeal
         Left 0RHV
         Right 0RHU
       Metatarsal-Phalangeal
         Left 0SHN
         Right 0SHM
       Metatarsal-Tarsal
         Left 0SHL
         Right 0SHK
       Occipital-cervical 0RH0
       Sacrococcygeal 0SH5
       Sacroiliac
         Left 0SH8
         Right 0SH7
       Shoulder
         Left 0RHK
         Right 0RHJ
       Sternoclavicular
         Left 0RHF
         Right 0RHE
       Tarsal
         Left 0SHJ
         Right 0SHH
       Temporomandibular
         Left 0RHD
         Right 0RHC
       Thoracic Vertebral 0RH6
       Thoracolumbar Vertebral
         0RHA
       Toe Phalangeal
         Left 0SHQ
         Right 0SHP

Spacer (continued)
Insertion of device in (continued)
Joint (continued)
Wrist
Left 0RHP
Right 0RHN
Removal of device from
Acromioclavicular
Left 0RPH
Right 0RPG
Ankle
Left 0SPG
Right 0SPF
Carpal
Left 0RPR
Right 0RPQ
Cervical Vertebral 0RP1
Cervicothoracic Vertebral 0RP4
Coccygeal 0SP6
Elbow
Left 0RPM
Right 0RPL
Finger Phalangeal
Left 0RPX
Right 0RPW
Hip
Left 0SPB
Right 0SP9
Knee
Left 0SPD
Right 0SPC
Lumbar Vertebral 0SP0
Lumbosacral 0SP3
Metacarpocarpal
Left 0RPT
Right 0RPS
Metacarpophalangeal
Left 0RPV
Right 0RPU
Metatarsal-Phalangeal
Left 0SPN
Right 0SPM
Metatarsal-Tarsal
Left 0SPL
Right 0SPK
Occipital-cervical 0RP0
Sacrococcygeal 0SP5
Sacroiliac
Left 0SP8
Right 0SP7
Shoulder
Left 0RPK
Right 0RPJ
Sternoclavicular
Left 0RPF
Right 0RPE
Tarsal
Left 0SPJ
Right 0SPH
Temporomandibular
Left 0RPD
Right 0RPC
Thoracic Vertebral 0RP6
Thoracolumbar Vertebral 0RPA
Toe Phalangeal
Left 0SPQ
Right 0SPP
Wrist
Left 0RPP
Right 0RPN
Revision of device in
Acromioclavicular
Left 0RWH
Right 0RWG
Ankle
Left 0SWG
Right 0SWF
Carpal
Left 0RWR
Right 0RWQ
Cervical Vertebral 0RW1

Spacer (continued)
Revision of device in (continued)
Cervicothoracic Vertebral 0RW4
Coccygeal 0SW6
Elbow
Left 0RWM
Right 0RWL
Finger Phalangeal
Left 0RWX
Right 0RWW
Hip
Left 0SWB
Right 0SW9
Knee
Left 0SWD
Right 0SWC
Lumbar Vertebral 0SW0
Lumbosacral 0SW3
Metacarpocarpal
Left 0RWT
Right 0RWS
Metacarpophalangeal
Left 0RWV
Right 0RWU
Metatarsal-Phalangeal
Left 0SWN
Right 0SWM
Metatarsal-Tarsal
Left 0SWL
Right 0SWK
Occipital-cervical 0RW0
Sacrococcygeal 0SW5
Sacroiliac
Left 0SW8
Right 0SW7
Shoulder
Left 0RWK
Right 0RWJ
Sternoclavicular
Left 0RWF
Right 0RWE
Tarsal
Left 0SWJ
Right 0SWH
Temporomandibular
Left 0RWD
Right 0RWC
Thoracic Vertebral 0RW6
Thoracolumbar Vertebral 0RWA
Toe Phalangeal
Left 0SWQ
Right 0SWP
Wrist
Left 0RWP
Right 0RWN
Spectroscopy
Intravascular 8E023DZ
Near infrared 8E023DZ
Speech Assessment F00
Speech therapy
see Speech Treatment,
Rehabilitation F06
Speech Treatment F06
Sphenoidectomy
see Excision, Ear, Nose, Sinus 09B
see Excision, Head and Facial Bones 0NB
see Resection, Ear, Nose, Sinus 09T
see Resection, Head and Facial Bones 0NT
Sphenoidotomy
see Drainage, Ear, Nose, Sinus 099
Sphenomandibular ligament
use Bursa and Ligament, Head and Neck
Sphenopalatine (pterygopalatine) ganglion
use Nerve, Head and Neck Sympathetic
Sphincterorrhaphy, anal
see Repair, Anal Sphincter 0DQR

Sphincterotomy, anal
see Division, Anal Sphincter 0D8R
see Drainage, Anal Sphincter 0D9R
Spinal cord neurostimulator lead
use Neurostimulator Lead in Central Nervous System
Spinal nerve, cervical
use Nerve, Cervical
Spinal nerve, lumbar
use Nerve, Lumbar
Spinal nerve, sacral
use Nerve, Sacral
Spinal nerve, thoracic
use Nerve, Thoracic
Spinal Stabilization Device
Facet Replacement
Cervical Vertebral 0RH1
Cervicothoracic Vertebral 0RH4
Lumbar Vertebral 0SH0
Lumbosacral 0SH3
Occipital-cervical 0RH0
Thoracic Vertebral 0RH6
Thoracolumbar Vertebral 0RHA
Interspinous Process
Cervical Vertebral 0RH1
Cervicothoracic Vertebral 0RH4
Lumbar Vertebral 0SH0
Lumbosacral 0SH3
Occipital-cervical 0RH0
Thoracic Vertebral 0RH6
Thoracolumbar Vertebral 0RHA
Pedicle-Based
Cervical Vertebral 0RH1
Cervicothoracic Vertebral 0RH4
Lumbar Vertebral 0SH0
Lumbosacral 0SH3
Occipital-cervical 0RH0
Thoracic Vertebral 0RH6
Thoracolumbar Vertebral 0RHA
Spinous process
use Vertebra, Cervical
use Vertebra, Lumbar
use Vertebra, Thoracic
Spiral ganglion
use Nerve, Acoustic
Spiration IBV™ Valve System
use Intraluminal Device, Endobronchial Valve in Respiratory System
Splenectomy
see Excision, Lymphatic and Hemic Systems 07B
see Resection, Lymphatic and Hemic Systems 07T
Splenic flexure
use Colon, Transverse
Splenic plexus
use Nerve, Abdominal Sympathetic
Splenius capitis muscle
use Muscle, Head
Splenius cervicis muscle
use Muscle, Neck, Left
use Muscle, Neck, Right
Splenolysis
see Release, Lymphatic and Hemic Systems 07N
Splenopexy
see Repair, Lymphatic and Hemic Systems 07Q
see Reposition, Lymphatic and Hemic Systems 07S
Splenoplasty
see Repair, Lymphatic and Hemic Systems 07Q
Splenorrhaphy
see Repair, Lymphatic and Hemic Systems 07Q
Splenotomy
see Drainage, Lymphatic and Hemic Systems 079
Splinting, musculoskeletal
see Immobilization, Anatomical Regions 2W3

Stapedectomy
see Excision, Ear, Nose, Sinus 09B
see Resection, Ear, Nose, Sinus 09T
Stapediolysis
see Release, Ear, Nose, Sinus 09N
Stapedioplasty
see Repair, Ear, Nose, Sinus 09Q
see Replacement, Ear, Nose, Sinus 09R
see Supplement, Ear, Nose, Sinus 09U
Stapedotomy
see Drainage, Ear, Nose, Sinus 099
Stapes
use Auditory Ossicle, Left
use Auditory Ossicle, Right
Stellate ganglion
use Nerve, Head and Neck Sympathetic
Stensen's duct
use Duct, Parotid, Left
use Duct, Parotid, Right
Stent, intraluminal (cardiovascular) (gastrointestinal) (hepatobiliary)(urinary)
use Intraluminal Device
Stented tissue valve
use Zooplastic Tissue in Heart and Great Vessels
Stereotactic Radiosurgery
Abdomen DW23
Adrenal Gland DG22
Bile Ducts DF22
Bladder DT22
Bone Marrow D720
Brain D020
Brain Stem D021
Breast
Left DM20
Right DM21
Bronchus DB21
Cervix DU21
Chest DW22
Chest Wall DB27
Colon DD25
Diaphragm DB28
Duodenum DD22
Ear D920
Esophagus DD20
Eye D820
Gallbladder DF21
Gamma Beam
Abdomen DW23JZZ
Adrenal Gland DG22JZZ
Bile Ducts DF22JZZ
Bladder DT22JZZ
Bone Marrow D720JZZ
Brain D020JZZ
Brain Stem D021JZZ
Breast
Left DM20JZZ
Right DM21JZZ
Bronchus DB21JZZ
Cervix DU21JZZ
Chest DW22JZZ
Chest Wall DB27JZZ
Colon DD25JZZ
Diaphragm DB28JZZ
Duodenum DD22JZZ
Ear D920JZZ
Esophagus DD20JZZ
Eye D820JZZ
Gallbladder DF21JZZ
Gland
Adrenal DG22JZZ
Parathyroid DG24JZZ
Pituitary DG20JZZ
Thyroid DG25JZZ
Glands, Salivary D926JZZ
Head and Neck DW21JZZ
Ileum DD24JZZ
Jejunum DD23JZZ

Stereotactic Radiosurgery *(continued)*
  Gamma Beam *(continued)*
    Kidney DT20JZZ
    Larynx D92BJZZ
    Liver DF20JZZ
    Lung DB22JZZ
    Lymphatics
      Abdomen D726JZZ
      Axillary D724JZZ
      Inguinal D728JZZ
      Neck D723JZZ
      Pelvis D727JZZ
      Thorax D725JZZ
    Mediastinum DB26JZZ
    Mouth D924JZZ
    Nasopharynx D92DJZZ
    Neck and Head DW21JZZ
    Nerve, Peripheral D027JZZ
    Nose D921JZZ
    Ovary DU20JZZ
    Palate
      Hard D928JZZ
      Soft D929JZZ
    Pancreas DF23JZZ
    Parathyroid Gland DG24JZZ
    Pelvic Region DW26JZZ
    Pharynx D92CJZZ
    Pineal Body DG21JZZ
    Pituitary Gland DG20JZZ
    Pleura DB25JZZ
    Prostate DV20JZZ
    Rectum DD27JZZ
    Sinuses D927JZZ
    Spinal Cord D026JZZ
    Spleen D722JZZ
    Stomach DD21JZZ
    Testis DV21JZZ
    Thymus D721JZZ
    Thyroid Gland DG25JZZ
    Tongue D925JZZ
    Trachea DB20JZZ
    Ureter DT21JZZ
    Urethra DT23JZZ
    Uterus DU22JZZ
  Gland
    Adrenal DG22
    Parathyroid DG24
    Pituitary DG20
    Thyroid DG25
  Glands, Salivary D926
  Head and Neck DW21
  Ileum DD24
  Jejunum DD23
  Kidney DT20
  Larynx D92B
  Liver DF20
  Lung DB22
  Lymphatics
    Abdomen D726
    Axillary D724
    Inguinal D728
    Neck D723
    Pelvis D727
    Thorax D725
  Mediastinum DB26
  Mouth D924
  Nasopharynx D92D
  Neck and Head DW21
  Nerve, Peripheral D027
  Nose D921
  Other Photon
    Abdomen DW23DZZ
    Adrenal Gland DG22DZZ
    Bile Ducts DF22DZZ
    Bladder DT22DZZ
    Bone Marrow D720DZZ
    Brain D020DZZ
    Brain Stem D021DZZ
    Breast
      Left DM20DZZ
      Right DM21DZZ
    Bronchus DB21DZZ

Stereotactic Radiosurgery *(continued)*
  Other Photon *(continued)*
    Cervix DU21DZZ
    Chest DW22DZZ
    Chest Wall DB27DZZ
    Colon DD25DZZ
    Diaphragm DB28DZZ
    Duodenum DD22DZZ
    Ear D920DZZ
    Esophagus DD20DZZ
    Eye D820DZZ
    Gallbladder DF21DZZ
    Gland
      Adrenal DG22DZZ
      Parathyroid DG24DZZ
      Pituitary DG20DZZ
      Thyroid DG25DZZ
    Glands, Salivary D926DZZ
    Head and Neck DW21DZZ
    Ileum DD24DZZ
    Jejunum DD23DZZ
    Kidney DT20DZZ
    Larynx D92BDZZ
    Liver DF20DZZ
    Lung DB22DZZ
    Lymphatics
      Abdomen D726DZZ
      Axillary D724DZZ
      Inguinal D728DZZ
      Neck D723DZZ
      Pelvis D727DZZ
      Thorax D725DZZ
    Mediastinum DB26DZZ
    Mouth D924DZZ
    Nasopharynx D92DDZZ
    Neck and Head DW21DZZ
    Nerve, Peripheral D027DZZ
    Nose D921DZZ
    Ovary DU20DZZ
    Palate
      Hard D928DZZ
      Soft D929DZZ
    Pancreas DF23DZZ
    Parathyroid Gland
      DG24DZZ
    Pelvic Region DW26DZZ
    Pharynx D92CDZZ
    Pineal Body DG21DZZ
    Pituitary Gland DG20DZZ
    Pleura DB25DZZ
    Prostate DV20DZZ
    Rectum DD27DZZ
    Sinuses D927DZZ
    Spinal Cord D026DZZ
    Spleen D722DZZ
    Stomach DD21DZZ
    Testis DV21DZZ
    Thymus D721DZZ
    Thyroid Gland DG25DZZ
    Tongue D925DZZ
    Trachea DB20DZZ
    Ureter DT21DZZ
    Urethra DT23DZZ
    Uterus DU22DZZ
  Ovary DU20
  Palate
    Hard D928
    Soft D929
  Pancreas DF23
  Parathyroid Gland DG24
  Particulate
    Abdomen DW23HZZ
    Adrenal Gland DG22HZZ
    Bile Ducts DF22HZZ
    Bladder DT22HZZ
    Bone Marrow D720HZZ
    Brain D020HZZ
    Brain Stem D021HZZ
    Breast
      Left DM20HZZ
      Right DM21HZZ
    Bronchus DB21HZZ

Stereotactic Radiosurgery *(continued)*
  Particulate *(continued)*
    Cervix DU21HZZ
    Chest DW22HZZ
    Chest Wall DB27HZZ
    Colon DD25HZZ
    Diaphragm DB28HZZ
    Duodenum DD22HZZ
    Ear D920HZZ
    Esophagus DD20HZZ
    Eye D820HZZ
    Gallbladder DF21HZZ
    Gland
      Adrenal DG22HZZ
      Parathyroid DG24HZZ
      Pituitary DG20HZZ
      Thyroid DG25HZZ
    Glands, Salivary D926HZZ
    Head and Neck DW21HZZ
    Ileum DD24HZZ
    Jejunum DD23HZZ
    Kidney DT20HZZ
    Larynx D92BHZZ
    Liver DF20HZZ
    Lung DB22HZZ
    Lymphatics
      Abdomen D726HZZ
      Axillary D724HZZ
      Inguinal D728HZZ
      Neck D723HZZ
      Pelvis D727HZZ
      Thorax D725HZZ
    Mediastinum DB26HZZ
    Mouth D924HZZ
    Nasopharynx D92DHZZ
    Neck and Head DW21HZZ
    Nerve, Peripheral D027HZZ
    Nose D921HZZ
    Ovary DU20HZZ
    Palate
      Hard D928HZZ
      Soft D929HZZ
    Pancreas DF23HZZ
    Parathyroid Gland DG24HZZ
    Pelvic Region DW26HZZ
    Pharynx D92CHZZ
    Pineal Body DG21HZZ
    Pituitary Gland DG20HZZ
    Pleura DB25HZZ
    Prostate DV20HZZ
    Rectum DD27HZZ
    Sinuses D927HZZ
    Spinal Cord D026HZZ
    Spleen D722HZZ
    Stomach DD21HZZ
    Testis DV21HZZ
    Thymus D721HZZ
    Thyroid Gland DG25HZZ
    Tongue D925HZZ
    Trachea DB20HZZ
    Ureter DT21HZZ
    Urethra DT23HZZ
    Uterus DU22HZZ
  Pelvic Region DW26
  Pharynx D92C
  Pineal Body DG21
  Pituitary Gland DG20
  Pleura DB25
  Prostate DV20
  Rectum DD27
  Sinuses D927
  Spinal Cord D026
  Spleen D722
  Stomach DD21
  Testis DV21
  Thymus D721
  Thyroid Gland DG25
  Tongue D925
  Trachea SB20
  Ureter DT21
  Urethra DT23
  Uterus DU22

Sternoclavicular ligament
  use Bursa and Ligament, Shoulder, Left
  use Bursa and Ligament, Shoulder, Right
Sternocleidomastoid artery
  use Artery, Thyroid, Left
  use Artery, Thyroid, Right
Sternocleidomastoid muscle
  use Muscle, Neck, Left
  use Muscle, Neck, Right
Sternocostal ligament
  use Bursa and Ligament, Thorax, Left
  use Bursa and Ligament, Thorax, Right
Sternotomy
  see Division, Sternum 0P80
  see Drainage, Sternum 0P90
Stimulation, cardiac
  Cardioversion 5A2204Z
  Electrophysiologic testing
    see Measurement, Cardiac 4A02
Stimulator Generator
  Insertion of device in
    Abdomen 0JH8
    Back 0JH7
    Chest 0JH6
  Multiple Array
    Abdomen 0JH8
    Back 0JH7
    Chest 0JH6
  Multiple Array Rechargeable
    Abdomen 0JH8
    Back 0JH7
    Chest 0JH6
  Removal of device from,
    Subcutaneous Tissue and Fascia, Trunk 0JPT
  Revision of device in, Subcutaneous Tissue and Fascia, Trunk 0JWT
  Single Array
    Abdomen 0JH8
    Back 0JH7
    Chest 0JH6
  Single Array Rechargeable
    Abdomen 0JH8
    Back 0JH7
    Chest 0JH6
Stimulator Lead
  Insertion of device in
    Anal Sphincter 0DHR
    Artery
      Left 03HL
      Right 03HK
    Bladder 0THB
    Muscle
      Lower 0KHY
      Upper 0KHX
    Stomach 0DH6
    Ureter 0TH9
  Removal of device from
    Anal Sphincter 0DPR
    Artery, Upper 03PY
    Bladder 0TPB
    Muscle
      Lower 0KPY
      Upper 0KPX
    Stomach 0DP6
    Ureter 0TP9
  Revision of device in
    Anal Sphincter 0DWR
    Artery, Upper 03WY
    Bladder 0TWB
    Muscle
      Lower 0KWY
      Upper 0KWX
    Stomach 0DW6
    Ureter 0TW9
Stoma
  Excision

Stoma *(continued)*
  Excision *(continued)*
    Abdominal Wall 0WBFXZ2
    Neck 0WB6XZ2
  Repair
    Abdominal Wall 0WQFXZ2
    Neck 0WQ6XZ2
Stomatoplasty
  see Repair, Mouth and Throat 0CQ
  see Replacement, Mouth and Throat
    0CR
  see Supplement, Mouth and Throat
    0CU
Stomatorrhaphy
  see Repair, Mouth and Throat 0CQ
Stratos LV
  use Cardiac Resynchronization
    Pacemaker Pulse Generator in 0JH
Stress test
  4A02XM4
  4A12XM4
Stripping
  see Extraction
Study
  Electrophysiologic stimulation, cardiac
    see Measurement, Cardiac 4A02
  Ocular motility 4A07X7Z
  Pulmonary airway flow measurement
    see Measurement, Respiratory 4A09
  Visual acuity 4A07X0Z
Styloglossus muscle
  use Muscle, Tongue, Palate, Pharynx
Stylomandibular ligament
  use Bursa and Ligament, Head and
    Neck
Stylopharyngeus muscle
  use Muscle, Tongue, Palate, Pharynx
Subacromial bursa
  use Bursa and Ligament, Shoulder, Left
  use Bursa and Ligament, Shoulder,
    Right
Subaortic (common iliac) lymph node
  use Lymphatic, Pelvis
Subarachnoid space, intracranial
  use Subarachnoid Space
Subarachnoid space, spinal
  use Spinal Canal
Subclavicular (apical) lymph node
  use Lymphatic, Axillary, Left
  use Lymphatic, Axillary, Right
Subclavius muscle
  use Muscle, Thorax, Left
  use Muscle, Thorax, Right
Subclavius nerve
  use Nerve, Brachial Plexus
Subcostal artery
  use Aorta, Thoracic
Subcostal muscle
  use Muscle, Thorax, Left
  use Muscle, Thorax, Right
Subcostal nerve
  use Nerve, Thoracic
Subcutaneous injection reservoir, port
  use Vascular Access Device,
    Reservoir in Subcutaneous
    Tissue and Fascia
Subcutaneous injection reservoir, pump
  use Infusion Device, Pump in
    Subcutaneous Tissue and Fascia
Subdermal progesterone implant
  use Contraceptive Device in
    Subcutaneous Tissue and Fascia
Subdural space, intracranial
  use Subdural Space
Subdural space, spinal
  use Spinal Canal
Submandibular ganglion
  use Nerve, Facial
  use Nerve, Head and Neck Sympathetic
Submandibular gland
  use Gland, Submaxillary, Left
  use Gland, Submaxillary, Right

Submandibular lymph node
  use Lymphatic, Head
Submaxillary ganglion
  use Nerve, Head and Neck
    Sympathetic
Submaxillary lymph node
  use Lymphatic, Head
Submental artery
  use Artery, Face
Submental lymph node
  use Lymphatic, Head
Submucous (Meissner's) plexus
  use Nerve, Abdominal Sympathetic
Suboccipital nerve
  use Nerve, Cervical
Suboccipital venous plexus
  use Vein, Vertebral, Left
  use Vein, Vertebral, Right
Subparotid lymph node
  use Lymphatic, Head
Subscapular (posterior) lymph node
  use Lymphatic, Axillary, Left
  use Lymphatic, Axillary, Right
Subscapular aponeurosis
  use Subcutaneous Tissue and Fascia,
    Upper Arm, Left
  use Subcutaneous Tissue and Fascia,
    Upper Arm, Right
Subscapular artery
  use Artery, Axillary, Left
  use Artery, Axillary, Right
Subscapularis muscle
  use Muscle, Shoulder, Left
  use Muscle, Shoulder, Right
Substance Abuse Treatment
  Counseling
    Family, for substance abuse, Other
      Family Counseling HZ63ZZZ
    Group
      12-Step HZ43ZZZ
      Behavioral HZ41ZZZ
      Cognitive HZ40ZZZ
      Cognitive-Behavioral
        HZ42ZZZ
      Confrontational HZ48ZZZ
      Continuing Care HZ49ZZZ
      Infectious Disease
        Post-Test HZ4CZZZ
        Pre-Test HZ4CZZZ
      Interpersonal HZ44ZZZ
      Motivational Enhancement
        HZ47ZZZ
      Psychoeducation HZ46ZZZ
      Spiritual HZ4BZZZ
      Vocational HZ45ZZZ
    Individual
      12-Step HZ33ZZZ
      Behavioral HZ31ZZZ
      Cognitive HZ30ZZZ
      Cognitive-Behavioral
        HZ32ZZZ
      Confrontational HZ38ZZZ
      Continuing Care HZ39ZZZ
      Infectious Disease
        Post-Test HZ3CZZZ
        Pre-Test HZ3CZZZ
      Interpersonal HZ34ZZZ
      Motivational Enhancement
        HZ37ZZZ
      Psychoeducation HZ36ZZZ
      Spiritual HZ3BZZZ
      Vocational HZ35ZZZ
    Detoxification Services, for
      substance abuse HZ2ZZZZ
    Medication Management
      Antabuse HZ83ZZZ
      Bupropion HZ87ZZZ
      Clonidine HZ86ZZZ
      Levo-alpha-acetyl-methadol
        (LAAM) HZ82ZZZ
      Methadone Maintenance
        HZ81ZZZ

Substance Abuse Treatment *(continued)*
  Medication Management *(continued)*
    Naloxone HZ85ZZZ
    Naltrexone HZ84ZZZ
    Nicotine Replacement HZ80ZZZ
    Other Replacement Medication
      HZ89ZZZ
    Psychiatric Medication HZ88ZZZ
  Pharmacotherapy
    Antabuse HZ93ZZZ
    Bupropion HZ97ZZZ
    Clonidine HZ96ZZZ
    Levo-alpha-acetyl-methadol
      (LAAM) HZ92ZZZ
    Methadone Maintenance HZ91ZZZ
    Naloxone HZ95ZZZ
    Naltrexone HZ94ZZZ
    Nicotine Replacement HZ90ZZZ
    Psychiatric Medication HZ98ZZZ
    Replacement Medication, Other
      HZ99ZZZ
  Psychotherapy
    12-Step HZ53ZZZ
    Behavioral HZ51ZZZ
    Cognitive HZ50ZZZ
    Cognitive-Behavioral HZ52ZZZ
    Confrontational HZ58ZZZ
    Interactive HZ55ZZZ
    Interpersonal HZ54ZZZ
    Motivational Enhancement
      HZ57ZZZ
    Psychoanalysis HZ5BZZZ
    Psychodynamic HZ5CZZZ
    Psychoeducation HZ56ZZZ
    Psychophysiological HZ5DZZZ
    Supportive HZ59ZZZ
Substantia nigra
  use Basal Ganglia
Subtalar (talocalcaneal) joint
  use Joint, Tarsal, Left
  use Joint, Tarsal, Right
Subtalar ligament
  use Bursa and Ligament, Foot, Left
  use Bursa and Ligament, Foot, Right
Subthalamic nucleus
  use Basal Ganglia
Suction curettage (D&C), nonobstetric
  see Extraction, Endometrium 0UDB
Suction curettage, obstetric post-delivery
  see Extraction, Products of
    Conception, Retained 10D1
Superficial circumflex iliac vein
  use Vein, Greater Saphenous, Left
  use Vein, Greater Saphenous, Right
Superficial epigastric artery
  use Artery, Femoral, Left
  use Artery, Femoral, Right
Superficial epigastric vein
  use Vein, Greater Saphenous, Left
  use Vein, Greater Saphenous, Right
Superficial Inferior Epigastric Artery
  Flap
  Bilateral 0HRV078
  Left 0HRU078
  Right 0HRT078
Superficial palmar arch
  use Artery, Hand, Left
  use Artery, Hand, Right
Superficial palmar venous arch
  use Vein, Hand, Left
  use Vein, Hand, Right
Superficial temporal artery
  use Artery, Temporal, Left
  use Artery, Temporal, Right
Superficial transverse perineal muscle
  use Muscle, Perineum
Superior cardiac nerve
  use Nerve, Thoracic Sympathetic
Superior cerebellar vein
  use Vein, Intracranial
Superior cerebral vein
  use Vein, Intracranial

Superior clunic (cluneal) nerve
  use Nerve, Lumbar
Superior epigastric artery
  use Artery, Internal Mammary, Left
  use Artery, Internal Mammary, Right
Superior genicular artery
  use Artery, Popliteal, Left
  use Artery, Popliteal, Right
Superior gluteal artery
  use Artery, Internal Iliac, Left
  use Artery, Internal Iliac, Right
Superior gluteal nerve
  use Nerve, Lumbar Plexus
Superior hypogastric plexus
  use Nerve, Abdominal Sympathetic
Superior labial artery
  use Artery, Face
Superior laryngeal artery
  use Artery, Thyroid, Left
  use Artery, Thyroid, Right
Superior laryngeal nerve
  use Nerve, Vagus
Superior longitudinal muscle
  use Muscle, Tongue, Palate, Pharynx
Superior mesenteric ganglion
  use Nerve, Abdominal Sympathetic
Superior mesenteric lymph node
  use Lymphatic, Mesenteric
Superior mesenteric plexus
  use Nerve, Abdominal Sympathetic
Superior oblique muscle
  use Muscle, Extraocular, Left
  use Muscle, Extraocular, Right
Superior olivary nucleus
  use Pons
Superior rectal artery
  use Artery, Inferior Mesenteric
Superior rectal vein
  use Vein, Inferior Mesenteric
Superior rectus muscle
  use Muscle, Extraocular, Left
  use Muscle, Extraocular, Right
Superior tarsal plate
  use Eyelid, Upper, Left
  use Eyelid, Upper, Right
Superior thoracic artery
  use Artery, Axillary, Left
  use Artery, Axillary, Right
Superior thyroid artery
  use External Carotid Artery, Left
  use External Carotid Artery, Right
  use Thyroid, Left
  use Thyroid, Right
Superior turbinate
  use Turbinate, Nasal
Superior ulnar collateral artery
  use Artery, Brachial, Left
  use Artery, Brachial, Right
Supplement
  Abdominal Wall 0WUF
  Acetabulum
    Left 0QU5
    Right 0QU4
  Ampulla of Vater 0FUC
  Anal Sphincter 0DUR
  Ankle Region
    Left 0YUL
    Right 0YUK
  Anus 0DUQ
  Aorta
    Abdominal 04U0
    Thoracic 02UW
  Arm
    Lower
      Left 0XUF
      Right 0XUD
    Upper
      Left 0XU9
      Right 0XU8
  Artery
    Anterior Tibial
      Left 04UQ

Finger (continued)
  Ring
    Left 0XUT
    Right 0XUS
Foot
  Left 0YUN
  Right 0YUM
Gingiva
  Lower 0CU6
  Upper 0CU5
Glenoid Cavity
  Left 0PU8
  Right 0PU7
Hand
  Left 0XUK
  Right 0XUJ
Head 0WU0
Heart 02UA
Humeral Head
  Left 0PUD
  Right 0PUC
Humeral Shaft
  Left 0PUG
  Right 0PUF
Hymen 0UUK
Ileocecal Valve 0DUC
Ileum 0DUB
Inguinal Region
  Bilateral 0YUA
  Left 0YU6
  Right 0YU5
Intestine
  Large 0DUE
    Left 0DUG
    Right 0DUF
  Small 0DU8
Iris
  Left 08UD
  Right 08UC
Jaw
  Lower 0WU5
  Upper 0WU4
Jejunum 0DUA
Joint
  Acromioclavicular
    Left 0RUH
    Right 0RUG
  Ankle
    Left 0SUG
    Right 0SUF
  Carpal
    Left 0RUR
    Right 0RUQ
  Cervical Vertebral 0RU1
  Cervicothoracic Vertebral 0RU4
  Coccygeal 0SU6
  Elbow
    Left 0RUM
    Right 0RUL
  Finger Phalangeal
    Left 0RUX
    Right 0RUW
  Hip
    Left 0SUB
      Acetabular Surface 0SUE
      Femoral Surface 0SUS
    Right 0SU9
      Acetabular Surface 0SUA
      Femoral Surface 0SUR
  Knee
    Left 0SUD
      Femoral Surface 0SUU09Z
      Tibial Surface 0SUW09Z
    Right 0SUC
      Femoral Surface 0SUT09Z
      Tibial Surface 0SUV09Z
  Lumbar Vertebral 0SU0
  Lumbosacral 0SU3
  Metacarpocarpal
    Left 0RUT
    Right 0RUS

Joint (continued)
  Metacarpophalangeal
    Left 0RUV
    Right 0RUU
  Metatarsal-Phalangeal
    Left 0SUN
    Right 0SUM
  Metatarsal-Tarsal
    Left 0SUL
    Right 0SUK
  Occipital-cervical 0RU0
  Sacrococcygeal 0SU5
  Sacroiliac
    Left 0SU8
    Right 0SU7
  Shoulder
    Left 0RUK
    Right 0RUJ
  Sternoclavicular
    Left 0RUF
    Right 0RUE
  Tarsal
    Left 0SUJ
    Right 0SUH
  Temporomandibular
    Left 0RUD
    Right 0RUC
  Thoracic Vertebral 0RU6
  Thoracolumbar Vertebral 0RUA
  Toe Phalangeal
    Left 0SUQ
    Right 0SUP
  Wrist
    Left 0RUP
    Right 0RUN
Kidney Pelvis
  Left 0TU4
  Right 0TU3
Knee Region
  Left 0YUG
  Right 0YUF
Larynx 0CUS
Leg
  Lower
    Left 0YUJ
    Right 0YUH
  Upper
    Left 0YUD
    Right 0YUC
Lip
  Lower 0CU1
  Upper 0CU0
Lymphatic
  Aortic 07UD
  Axillary
    Left 07U6
    Right 07U5
  Head 07U0
  Inguinal
    Left 07UJ
    Right 07UH
  Internal Mammary
    Left 07U9
    Right 07U8
  Lower Extremity
    Left 07UG
    Right 07UF
  Mesenteric 07UB
  Neck
    Left 07U2
    Right 07U1
  Pelvis 07UC
  Thoracic Duct
    07UK
  Thorax 07U7
  Upper Extremity
    Left 07U4
    Right 07U3
Mandible
  Left 0NUV
  Right 0NUT

Maxilla
  Left 0NUS
  Right 0NUR
Mediastinum 0WUC
Mesentery 0DUV
Metacarpal
  Left 0PUQ
  Right 0PUP
Metatarsal
  Left 0QUP
  Right 0QUN
Muscle
  Abdomen
    Left 0KUL
    Right 0KUK
  Extraocular
    Left 08UM
    Right 08UL
  Facial 0KU1
  Foot
    Left 0KUW
    Right 0KUV
  Hand
    Left 0KUD
    Right 0KUC
  Head 0KU0
  Hip
    Left 0KUP
    Right 0KUN
  Lower Arm and Wrist
    Left 0KUB
    Right 0KU9
  Lower Leg
    Left 0KUT
    Right 0KUS
  Neck
    Left 0KU3
    Right 0KU2
  Papillary 02UD
  Perineum 0KUM
  Shoulder
    Left 0KU6
    Right 0KU5
  Thorax
    Left 0KUJ
    Right 0KUH
  Tongue, Palate, Pharynx 0KU4
  Trunk
    Left 0KUG
    Right 0KUF
  Upper Arm
    Left 0KU8
    Right 0KU7
  Upper Leg
    Left 0KUR
    Right 0KUQ
Nasopharynx 09UN
Neck 0WU6
Nerve
  Abducens 00UL
  Accessory 00UR
  Acoustic 00UN
  Cervical 01U1
  Facial 00UM
  Femoral 01UD
  Glossopharyngeal 00UP
  Hypoglossal 00US
  Lumbar 01UB
  Median 01U5
  Oculomotor 00UH
  Olfactory 00UF
  Optic 00UG
  Peroneal 01UH
  Phrenic 01U2
  Pudendal 01UC
  Radial 01U6
  Sacral 01UR
  Sciatic 01UF
  Thoracic 01U8
  Tibial 01UG
  Trigeminal 00UK

Nerve (continued)
  Trochlear 00UJ
  Ulnar 01U4
  Vagus 00UQ
Nipple
  Left 0HUX
  Right 0HUW
Nose 09UK
Omentum
  Greater 0DUS
  Lesser 0DUT
Orbit
  Left 0NUQ
  Right 0NUP
Palate
  Hard 0CU2
  Soft 0CU3
Patella
  Left 0QUF
  Right 0QUD
Penis 0VUS
Pericardium 02UN
Perineum
  Female 0WUN
  Male 0WUM
Peritoneum 0DUW
Phalanx
  Finger
    Left 0PUV
    Right 0PUT
  Thumb
    Left 0PUS
    Right 0PUR
  Toe
    Left 0QUR
    Right 0QUQ
Pharynx 0CUM
Prepuce 0VUT
Radius
  Left 0PUJ
  Right 0PUH
Rectum 0DUP
Retina
  Left 08UF
  Right 08UE
Retinal Vessel
  Left 08UH
  Right 08UG
Rib
  Left 0PU2
  Right 0PU1
Sacrum 0QU1
Scapula
  Left 0PU6
  Right 0PU5
Scrotum 0VU5
Septum
  Atrial 02U5
  Nasal 09UM
  Ventricular 02UM
Shoulder Region
  Left 0XU3
  Right 0XU2
Skull 0NU0
Spinal Meninges 00UT
Sternum 0PU0
Stomach 0DU6
  Pylorus 0DU7
Subcutaneous Tissue and
  Fascia
    Abdomen 0JU8
    Back 0JU7
    Buttock 0JU9
    Chest 0JU6
    Face 0JU1
    Foot
      Left 0JUR
      Right 0JUQ
    Hand
      Left 0JUK
      Right 0JUJ

Takedown *(continued)*
  Stoma
    see Repair
Talent® Converter
  use Intraluminal Device
Talent® Occluder
  use Intraluminal Device
Talent® Stent Graft (abdominal) (thoracic)
  use Intraluminal Device
Talocalcaneal (subtalar) joint
  use Joint, Tarsal, Left
  use Joint, Tarsal, Right
Talocalcaneal ligament
  use Bursa and Ligament, Foot, Left
  use Bursa and Ligament, Foot, Right
Talocalcaneonavicular joint
  use Joint, Tarsal, Left
  use Joint, Tarsal, Right
Talocalcaneonavicular ligament
  use Bursa and Ligament, Foot, Left
  use Bursa and Ligament, Foot, Right
Talocrural joint
  use Joint, Ankle, Left
  use Joint, Ankle, Right
Talofibular ligament
  use Bursa and Ligament, Ankle, Left
  use Bursa and Ligament, Ankle, Right
Talus bone
  use Tarsal, Left
  use Tarsal, Right
TandemHeart® System
  use External Heart Assist System in Heart and Great Vessels
Tarsectomy
  see Excision, Lower Bones 0QB
  see Resection, Lower Bones 0QT
Tarsometatarsal joint
  use Joint, Metatarsal-Tarsal, Left
  use Joint, Metatarsal-Tarsal, Right
Tarsometatarsal ligament
  use Bursa and Ligament, Foot, Left
  use Bursa and Ligament, Foot, Right
Tarsorrhaphy
  see Repair, Eye 08Q
Tattooing
  Cornea 3E0CXMZ
  Skin
    see Introduction of substance in or on, Skin 3E00
TAXUS® Liberté® Paclitaxel-eluting Coronary Stent System
  use Intraluminal Device, Drug-eluting in Heart and Great Vessels
TBNA (transbronchial needle aspiration)
  see Drainage, Respiratory System 0B9
Telemetry 4A12X4Z
  Ambulatory 4A12X45
Temperature gradient study 4A0ZXKZ
Temporal lobe
  use Cerebral Hemisphere
Temporalis muscle
  use Muscle, Head
Temporoparietalis muscle
  use Muscle, Head
Tendolysis
  see Release, Tendons 0LN
Tendonectomy
  see Excision, Tendons 0LB
  see Resection, Tendons 0LT
Tendonoplasty, tenoplasty
  see Repair, Tendons 0LQ
  see Replacement, Tendons 0LR
  see Supplement, Tendons 0LU
Tendorrhaphy
  see Repair, Tendons 0LQ
Tendototomy
  see Division, Tendons 0L8
  see Drainage, Tendons 0L9

Tenectomy, tenonectomy
  see Excision, Tendons 0LB
  see Resection, Tendons 0LT
Tenolysis
  see Release, Tendons 0LN
Tenontorrhaphy
  see Repair, Tendons 0LQ
Tenontotomy
  see Division, Tendons 0L8
  see Drainage, Tendons 0L9
Tenorrhaphy
  see Repair, Tendons 0LQ
Tenosynovectomy
  see Excision, Tendons 0LB
  see Resection, Tendons 0LT
Tenotomy
  see Division, Tendons 0L8
  see Drainage, Tendons 0L9
Tensor fasciae latae muscle
  use Muscle, Hip, Left
  use Muscle, Hip, Right
Tensor veli palatini muscle
  use Muscle, Tongue, Palate, Pharynx
Tenth cranial nerve
  use Nerve, Vagus
Tentorium cerebelli
  use Dura Mater
Teres major muscle
  use Muscle, Shoulder, Left
  use Muscle, Shoulder, Right
Teres minor muscle
  use Muscle, Shoulder, Left
  use Muscle, Shoulder, Right
Termination of pregnancy
  Aspiration curettage 10A07ZZ
  Dilation and curettage 10A07ZZ
  Hysterotomy 10A00ZZ
  Intra-amniotic injection 10A03ZZ
  Laminaria 10A07ZW
  Vacuum 10A07Z6
Testectomy
  see Excision, Male Reproductive System 0VB
  see Resection, Male Reproductive System 0VT
Testicular artery
  use Aorta, Abdominal
Testing
  Glaucoma 4A07XBZ
  Hearing
    see Hearing Assessment, Diagnostic Audiology F13
  Mental health
    see Psychological Tests
  Muscle function, electromyography (EMG)
    see Measurement, Musculoskeletal 4A0F
  Muscle function, manual
    see Motor Function Assessment, Rehabilitation F01
  Neurophysiologic monitoring, intra-operative
    see Monitoring, Physiological Systems 4A1
  Range of motion
    see Motor Function Assessment, Rehabilitation F01
  Vestibular function
    see Vestibular Assessment, Diagnostic Audiology F15
Thalamectomy
  see Excision, Thalamus 00B9
Thalamotomy
  see Drainage, Thalamus 0099
Thenar muscle
  use Muscle, Hand, Left
  use Muscle, Hand, Right
Therapeutic Massage
  Musculoskeletal System 8E0KX1Z
  Reproductive System
    Prostate 8E0VX1C

Therapeutic Massage *(continued)*
  Reproductive System *(continued)*
    Rectum 8E0VX1D
Therapeutic occlusion coil(s)
  use Intraluminal Device
Thermography 4A0ZXKZ
Thermotherapy, prostate
  see Destruction, Prostate 0V50
Third cranial nerve
  use Nerve, Oculomotor
Third occipital nerve
  use Nerve, Cervical
Third ventricle
  use Cerebral Ventricle
Thoracectomy
  see Excision, Anatomical Regions, General 0WB
Thoracentesis
  see Drainage, Anatomical Regions, General 0W9
Thoracic aortic plexus
  use Nerve, Thoracic Sympathetic
Thoracic esophagus
  use Esophagus, Middle
Thoracic facet joint
  use Joint, Thoracic Vertebral
Thoracic ganglion
  use Nerve, Thoracic Sympathetic
Thoracoacromial artery
  use Artery, Axillary, Left
  use Artery, Axillary, Right
Thoracocentesis
  see Drainage, Anatomical Regions, General 0W9
Thoracolumbar facet joint
  use Joint, Thoracolumbar Vertebral
Thoracoplasty
  see Repair, Anatomical Regions, General 0WQ
  see Supplement, Anatomical Regions, General 0WU
Thoracostomy tube
  use Drainage Device
Thoracostomy, for lung collapse
  see Drainage, Respiratory System 0B9
Thoracotomy
  see Drainage, Anatomical Regions, General 0W9
Thoratec IVAD (Implantable Ventricular Assist Device)
  use Implantable Heart Assist System in Heart and Great Vessels
Thoratec Paracorporeal Ventricular Assist Device
  use External Heart Assist System in Heart and Great Vessels
Thrombectomy
  see Extirpation
Thymectomy
  see Excision, Lymphatic and Hemic Systems 07B
  see Resection, Lymphatic and Hemic Systems 07T
Thymopexy
  see Repair, Lymphatic and Hemic Systems 07Q
  see Reposition, Lymphatic and Hemic Systems 07S
Thymus gland
  use Thymus
Thyroarytenoid muscle
  use Muscle, Neck, Left
  use Muscle, Neck, Right
Thyrocervical trunk
  use Artery, Thyroid, Left
  use Artery, Thyroid, Right
Thyroid cartilage
  use Larynx
Thyroidectomy
  see Excision, Endocrine System 0GB
  see Resection, Endocrine System 0GT

Thyroidorrhaphy
  see Repair, Endocrine System 0GQ
Thyroidoscopy 0GJK4ZZ
Thyroidotomy
  see Drainage, Endocrine System 0G9
Tibial insert
  use Liner in Lower Joints
Tibialis anterior muscle
  use Muscle, Lower Leg, Left
  use Muscle, Lower Leg, Right
Tibialis posterior muscle
  use Muscle, Lower Leg, Left
  use Muscle, Lower Leg, Right
Tibiofemoral joint
  use Joint, Knee, Left
  use Joint, Knee, Left, Tibial Surface
  use Joint, Knee, Right
  use Joint, Knee, Right, Tibial Surface
TigerPaw® system for closure of left atrial appendage
  use Extraluminal Device
Tissue bank graft
  use Nonautologous Tissue Substitute
Tissue Expander
  Insertion of device in
    Breast
      Bilateral 0HHV
      Left 0HHU
      Right 0HHT
    Nipple
      Left 0HHX
      Right 0HHW
    Subcutaneous Tissue and Fascia
      Abdomen 0JH8
      Back 0JH7
      Buttock 0JH9
      Chest 0JH6
      Face 0JH1
      Foot
        Left 0JHR
        Right 0JHQ
      Hand
        Left 0JHK
        Right 0JHJ
      Lower Arm
        Left 0JHH
        Right 0JHG
      Lower Leg
        Left 0JHP
        Right 0JHN
      Neck
        Anterior 0JH4
        Posterior 0JH5
      Pelvic Region 0JHC
      Perineum 0JHB
      Scalp 0JH0
      Upper Arm
        Left 0JHF
        Right 0JHD
      Upper Leg
        Left 0JHM
        Right 0JHL
  Removal of device from
    Breast
      Left 0HPU
      Right 0HPT
    Subcutaneous Tissue and Fascia
      Head and Neck 0JPS
      Lower Extremity 0JPW
      Trunk 0JPT
      Upper Extremity 0JPV
  Revision of device in
    Breast
      Left 0HWU
      Right 0HWT
    Subcutaneous Tissue and Fascia
      Head and Neck 0JWS
      Lower Extremity 0JWW
      Trunk 0JWT
      Upper Extremity 0JWV
Tissue expander (inflatable)(injectable)
  use Tissue Expander in Skin and Breast

Tissue expander (inflatable)
(injectable) *(continued)*
  use Tissue Expander in Skin and
    Breast *(continued)*
  use Tissue Expander in
    Subcutaneous Tissue and Fascia
Tissue Plasminogen Activator (tPA)
(r-tPA)
  use Thrombolytic Other
Titanium Sternal Fixation System
(TSFS)
  use Internal Fixation Device, Rigid
    Plate in 0PS
  use Internal Fixation Device, Rigid
    Plate in 0PH
Tomographic (Tomo) Nuclear
Medicine Imaging
Abdomen CW20
Abdomen and Chest CW24
Abdomen and Pelvis CW21
Anatomical Regions, Multiple
  CW2YYZZ
Bladder, Kidneys and Ureters CT23
Brain C020
Breast CH2YYZZ
  Bilateral CH22
  Left CH21
  Right CH20
Bronchi and Lungs CB22
Central Nervous System C02YYZZ
Cerebrospinal Fluid C025
Chest CW23
Chest and Abdomen CW24
Chest and Neck CW26
Digestive System CD2YYZZ
Endocrine System CG2YYZZ
Extremity
  Lower CW2D
    Bilateral CP2F
    Left CP2D
    Right CP2C
  Upper CW2M
    Bilateral CP2B
    Left CP29
    Right CP28
Gallbladder CF24
Gastrointestinal Tract CD27
Gland, Parathyroid CG21
Head and Neck CW2B
Heart C22YYZZ
  Right and Left C226
Hepatobiliary System and Pancreas
  CF2YYZZ
Kidneys, Ureters and Bladder CT23
Liver CF25
Liver and Spleen CF26
Lungs and Bronchi CB22
Lymphatics and Hematologic
  System C72YYZZ
Musculoskeletal System, Other
  CP2YYZZ
Myocardium C22G
Neck and Chest CW26
Neck and Head CW2B
Pancreas and Hepatobiliary System
  CF2YYZZ
Pelvic Region CW2J
Pelvis CP26
Pelvis and Abdomen CW21
Pelvis and Spine CP27
Respiratory System CB2YYZZ
Skin CH2YYZZ
Skull CP21
Skull and Cervical Spine CP23
Spine
  Cervical CP22
  Cervical and Skull CP23
  Lumbar CP2H
  Thoracic CP2G
  Thoracolumbar CP2J
Spine and Pelvis CP27
Spleen C722

Tomographic (Tomo) Nuclear
Medicine Imaging *(continued)*
Spleen and Liver CF26
Subcutaneous Tissue CH2YYZZ
Thorax CP24
Ureters, Kidneys and Bladder CT23
Urinary System CT2YYZZ
Tomography, computerized
  see Computerized Tomography
    (CT Scan)
Tonometry 4A07XBZ
Tonsillectomy
  see Excision, Mouth and Throat 0CB
  see Resection, Mouth and Throat 0CT
Tonsillotomy
  see Drainage, Mouth and Throat 0C9
Total artificial (replacement) heart
  use Synthetic Substitute
Total parenteral nutrition (TPN)
  see Introduction of Nutritional
    Substance
Trachectomy
  see Excision, Trachea 0BB1
  see Resection, Trachea 0BT1
Trachelectomy
  see Excision, Cervix 0UBC
  see Resection, Cervix 0UTC
Trachelopexy
  see Repair, Cervix 0UQC
  see Reposition, Cervix 0USC
Tracheloplasty
  see Repair, Cervix 0UQC
Trachelorrhaphy
  see Repair, Cervix 0UQC
Trachelotomy
  see Drainage, Cervix 0U9C
Tracheobronchial lymph node
  use Lymphatic, Thorax
Tracheoesophageal fistulization
  0B110D6
Tracheolysis
  see Release, Respiratory System 0BN
Tracheoplasty
  see Repair, Respiratory System 0BQ
  see Supplement, Respiratory System
    0BU
Tracheorrhaphy
  see Repair, Respiratory System 0BQ
Tracheoscopy 0BJ18ZZ
Tracheostomy
  see Bypass, Respiratory System 0B1
Tracheostomy Device
  Bypass, Trachea 0B11
  Change device in, Trachea
    0B21XFZ
  Removal of device from, Trachea
    0BP1
  Revision of device in, Trachea 0BW1
Tracheostomy tube
  use Tracheostomy Device in
    Respiratory System
Tracheotomy
  see Drainage, Respiratory System 0B9
Traction
Abdominal Wall 2W63X
Arm
  Lower
    Left 2W6DX
    Right 2W6CX
  Upper
    Left 2W6BX
    Right 2W6AX
Back 2W65X
Chest Wall 2W64X
Extremity
  Lower
    Left 2W6MX
    Right 2W6LX
  Upper
    Left 2W69X
    Right 2W68X
Face 2W61X

Traction *(continued)*
Finger
  Left 2W6KX
  Right 2W6JX
Foot
  Left 2W6TX
  Right 2W6SX
Hand
  Left 2W6FXZ
  Right 2W6EXZ
Head 2W60X
Inguinal Region
  Left 2W67X
  Right 2W66X
Leg
  Lower
    Left 2W6RX
    Right 2W6QX
  Upper
    Left 2W6PX
    Right 2W6NX
Neck 2W62X
Thumb
  Left 2W6HX
  Right 2W6GX
Toe
  Left 2W6VX
  Right 2W6UX
Tractotomy
  see Division, Central Nervous
    System 008
Tragus
  use Ear, External, Bilateral
  use Ear, External, Left
  use Ear, External, Right
Training, caregiver
  see Caregiver Training
TRAM (transverse rectus abdominis
myocutaneous) flap
reconstruction
Free
  see Replacement, Skin and
    Breast 0HR
Pedicled
  see Transfer, Muscles 0KX
Transection
  see Division
Transfer
Buccal Mucosa 0CX4
Bursa and Ligament
  Abdomen
    Left 0MXJ
    Right 0MXH
  Ankle
    Left 0MXR
    Right 0MXQ
  Elbow
    Left 0MX4
    Right 0MX3
  Foot
    Left 0MXT
    Right 0MXS
  Hand
    Left 0MX8
    Right 0MX7
  Head and Neck 0MX0
  Hip
    Left 0MXM
    Right 0MXL
  Knee
    Left 0MXP
    Right 0MXN
  Lower Extremity
    Left 0MXW
    Right 0MXV
  Perineum 0MXK
  Shoulder
    Left 0MX2
    Right 0MX1
  Thorax
    Left 0MXG
    Right 0MXF

Transfer *(continued)*
Bursa and Ligament *(continued)*
  Trunk
    Left 0MXD
    Right 0MXC
  Upper Extremity
    Left 0MXB
    Right 0MX9
  Wrist
    Left 0MX6
    Right 0MX5
Finger
  Left 0XXP0ZM
  Right 0XXN0ZL
Gingiva
  Lower 0CX6
  Upper 0CX5
Intestine
  Large 0DXE
  Small 0DX8
Lip
  Lower 0CX1
  Upper 0CX0
Muscle
  Abdomen
    Left 0KXL
    Right 0KXK
  Extraocular
    Left 08XM
    Right 08XL
  Facial 0KX1
  Foot
    Left 0KXW
    Right 0KXV
  Hand
    Left 0KXD
    Right 0KXC
  Head 0KX0
  Hip
    Left 0KXP
    Right 0KXN
  Lower Arm and Wrist
    Left 0KXB
    Right 0KX9
  Lower Leg
    Left 0KXT
    Right 0KXS
  Neck
    Left 0KX3
    Right 0KX2
  Perineum 0KXM
  Shoulder
    Left 0KX6
    Right 0KX5
  Thorax
    Left 0KXJ
    Right 0KXH
  Tongue, Palate, Pharynx 0KX4
  Trunk
    Left 0KXG
    Right 0KXF
  Upper Arm
    Left 0KX8
    Right 0KX7
  Upper Leg
    Left 0KXR
    Right 0KXQ
Nerve
  Abducens 00XL
  Accessory 00XR
  Acoustic 00XN
  Cervical 01X1
  Facial 00XM
  Femoral 01XD
  Glossopharyngeal 00XP
  Hypoglossal 00XS
  Lumbar 01XB
  Median 01X5
  Oculomotor 00XH
  Olfactory 00XF
  Optic 00XG
  Peroneal 01XH

Transfer *(continued)*
Nerve *(continued)*
    Phrenic 01X2
    Pudendal 01XC
    Radial 01X6
    Sciatic 01XF
    Thoracic 01X8
    Tibial 01XG
    Trigeminal 00XK
    Trochlear 00XJ
    Ulnar 01X4
    Vagus 00XQ
Palate, Soft 0CX3
Skin
    Abdomen 0HX7XZZ
    Back 0HX6XZZ
    Buttock 0HX8XZZ
    Chest 0HX5XZZ
    Ear
        Left 0HX3XZZ
        Right 0HX2XZZ
    Face 0HX1XZZ
    Foot
        Left 0HXNXZZ
        Right 0HXMXZZ
    Genitalia 0HXAXZZ
    Hand
        Left 0HXGXZZ
        Right 0HXFXZZ
    Lower Arm
        Left 0HXEXZZ
        Right 0HXDXZZ
    Lower Leg
        Left 0HXLXZZ
        Right 0HXKXZZ
    Neck 0HX4XZZ
    Perineum 0HX9XZZ
    Scalp 0HX0XZZ
    Upper Arm
        Left 0HXCXZZ
        Right 0HXBXZZ
    Upper Leg
        Left 0HXJXZZ
        Right 0HXHXZZ
Stomach 0DX6
Subcutaneous Tissue and Fascia
    Abdomen 0JX8
    Back 0JX7
    Buttock 0JX9
    Chest 0JX6
    Face 0JX1
    Foot
        Left 0JXR
        Right 0JXQ
    Hand
        Left 0JXK
        Right 0JXJ
    Lower Arm
        Left 0JXH
        Right 0JXG
    Lower Leg
        Left 0JXP
        Right 0JXN
    Neck
        Anterior 0JX4
        Posterior 0JX5
    Pelvic Region 0JXC
    Perineum 0JXB
    Scalp 0JX0
    Upper Arm
        Left 0JXF
        Right 0JXD
    Upper Leg
        Left 0JXM
        Right 0JXL
Tendon
    Abdomen
        Left 0LXG
        Right 0LXF
    Ankle
        Left 0LXT
        Right 0LXS

Transfer *(continued)*
Tendon *(continued)*
    Foot
        Left 0LXW
        Right 0LXV
    Hand
        Left 0LX8
        Right 0LX7
    Head and Neck 0LX0
    Hip
        Left 0LXK
        Right 0LXJ
    Knee
        Left 0LXR
        Right 0LXQ
    Lower Arm and Wrist
        Left 0LX6
        Right 0LX5
    Lower Leg
        Left 0LXP
        Right 0LXN
    Perineum 0LXH
    Shoulder
        Left 0LX2
        Right 0LX1
    Thorax
        Left 0LXD
        Right 0LXC
    Trunk
        Left 0LXB
        Right 0LX9
    Upper Arm
        Left 0LX4
        Right 0LX3
    Upper Leg
        Left 0LXM
        Right 0LXL
Tongue 0CX7
Transfusion
Artery
    Central
        Antihemophilic Factors 3026
        Blood
            Platelets 3026
            Red Cells 3026
                Frozen 3026
            White Cells 3026
            Whole 3026
        Bone Marrow 3026
        Factor IX 3026
        Fibrinogen 3026
        Globulin 3026
        Plasma
            Fresh 3026
            Frozen 3026
        Plasma Cryoprecipitate 3026
        Serum Albumin 3026
        Stem Cells
            Cord Blood 3026
            Hematopoietic 3026
    Peripheral
        Antihemophilic Factors 3025
        Blood
            Platelets 3025
            Red Cells 3025
                Frozen 3025
            White Cells 3025
            Whole 3025
        Bone Marrow 3025
        Factor IX 3025
        Fibrinogen 3025
        Globulin 3025
        Plasma
            Fresh 3025
            Frozen 3025
        Plasma Cryoprecipitate 3025
        Serum Albumin 3025
        Stem Cells
            Cord Blood 3025
            Hematopoietic 3025
Products of Conception
    Antihemophilic Factors 3027

Transfusion *(continued)*
Products of Conception *(continued)*
    Blood
        Platelets 3027
        Red Cells 3027
            Frozen 3027
        White Cells 3027
        Whole 3027
    Factor IX 3027
    Fibrinogen 3027
    Globulin 3027
    Plasma
        Fresh 3027
        Frozen 3027
    Plasma Cryoprecipitate 3027
    Serum Albumin 3027
Vein
    4-Factor Prothrombin Complex
        Concentrate 3028
    Central
        Antihemophilic Factors 3024
        Blood
            Platelets 3024
            Red Cells 3024
                Frozen 3024
            White Cells 3024
            Whole 3024
        Bone Marrow 3024
        Factor IX 3024
        Fibrinogen 3024
        Globulin 3024
        Plasma
            Fresh 3024
            Frozen 3024
        Plasma Cryoprecipitate 3024
        Serum Albumin 3024
        Stem Cells
            Cord Blood 3024
            Embryonic 3024
            Hematopoietic 3024
    Peripheral
        Antihemophilic Factors 3023
        Blood
            Platelets 3023
            Red Cells 3023
                Frozen 3023
            White Cells 3023
            Whole 3023
        Bone Marrow 3023
        Factor IX 3023
        Fibrinogen 3023
        Globulin 3023
        Plasma
            Fresh 3023
            Frozen 3023
        Plasma Cryoprecipitate 3023
        Serum Albumin 3023
        Stem Cells
            Cord Blood 3023X
            Embryonic 3023
            Hematopoietic 3023
Transplantation
Esophagus 0DY50Z
Heart 02YA0Z
Intestine
    Large 0DYE0Z
    Small 0DY80Z
Kidney
    Left 0TY10Z
    Right 0TY00Z
Liver 0FY00Z
Lung
    Bilateral 0BYM0Z
    Left 0BYL0Z
    Lower Lobe
        Left 0BYJ0Z
        Right 0BYF0Z
    Middle Lobe, Right 0BYD0Z
    Right 0BYK0Z
    Upper Lobe
        Left 0BYG0Z
        Right 0BYC0Z

Transplantation *(continued)*
    Lung Lingula 0BYH0Z
Ovary
    Left 0UY10Z
    Right 0UY00Z
Pancreas 0FYG0Z
Products of Conception 10Y0
Spleen 07YP0Z
Stomach 0DY60Z
Thymus 07YM0Z
Transposition
see Reposition
see Transfer
Transversalis fascia
    use Subcutaneous Tissue and Fascia,
        Trunk
Transverse acetabular ligament
    use Bursa and Ligament, Hip, Left
    use Bursa and Ligament, Hip, Right
Transverse (cutaneous) cervical nerve
    use Nerve, Cervical Plexus
Transverse facial artery
    use Artery, Temporal, Left
    use Artery, Temporal, Right
Transverse humeral ligament
    use Bursa and Ligament, Shoulder,
        Left
    use Bursa and Ligament, Shoulder,
        Right
Transverse ligament of atlas
    use Bursa and Ligament, Head and
        Neck
Transverse Rectus Abdominis
    Myocutaneous Flap
    Replacement
        Bilateral 0HRV076
        Left 0HRU076
        Right 0HRT076
    Transfer
        Left 0KXL
        Right 0KXK
Transverse scapular ligament
    use Bursa and Ligament, Shoulder,
        Left
    use Bursa and Ligament, Shoulder,
        Right
Transverse thoracis muscle
    use Muscle, Thorax, Left
    use Muscle, Thorax, Right
Transversospinalis muscle
    use Muscle, Trunk, Left
    use Muscle, Trunk, Right
Transversus abdominis muscle
    use Muscle, Abdomen, Left
    use Muscle, Abdomen,
        Right
Trapezium bone
    use Carpal, Left
    use Carpal, Right
Trapezius muscle
    use Muscle, Trunk, Left
    use Muscle, Trunk, Right
Trapezoid bone
    use Carpal, Left
    use Carpal, Right
Triceps brachii muscle
    use Muscle, Upper Arm, Left
    use Muscle, Upper Arm, Right
Tricuspid annulus
    use Valve, Tricuspid
Trifacial nerve
    use Nerve, Trigeminal
Trifecta™ Valve (aortic)
    use Zooplastic Tissue in Heart and
        Great Vessels
Trigone of bladder
    use Bladder
Trimming, excisional
    see Excision
Triquetral bone
    use Carpal, Left
    use Carpal, Right

Trochanteric bursa
  use Bursa and Ligament, Hip, Left
  use Bursa and Ligament, Hip, Right
TUMT (Transurethral microwave thermotherapy of prostate) 0V507ZZ
TUNA (transurethral needle ablation of prostate) 0V507ZZ
Tunneled central venous catheter
  use Vascular Access Device in Subcutaneous Tissue and Fascia
Tunneled spinal (intrathecal) catheter
  use Infusion Device
Turbinectomy
  see Excision, Ear, Nose, Sinus 09B
  see Resection, Ear, Nose, Sinus 09T
Turbinoplasty
  see Repair, Ear, Nose, Sinus 09Q
  see Replacement, Ear, Nose, Sinus 09R
  see Supplement, Ear, Nose, Sinus 09U
Turbinotomy
  see Division, Ear, Nose, Sinus 098
  see Drainage, Ear, Nose, Sinus 099
TURP (transurethral resection of prostate)
  see Excision, Prostate 0VB0
  see Resection, Prostate 0VT0
Twelfth cranial nerve
  use Nerve, Hypoglossal
Two lead pacemaker
  use Pacemaker, Dual Chamber in 0JH
Tympanic cavity
  use Ear, Middle, Left
  use Ear, Middle, Right
Tympanic nerve
  use Nerve, Glossopharyngeal
Tympanic part of temporal bone
  use Bone, Temporal, Left
  use Bone, Temporal, Right
Tympanogram
  see Hearing Assessment, Diagnostic Audiology F13
Tympanoplasty
  see Repair, Ear, Nose, Sinus 09Q
  see Replacement, Ear, Nose, Sinus 09R
  see Supplement, Ear, Nose, Sinus 09U
Tympanosympathectomy
  see Excision, Nerve, Head and Neck Sympathetic 01BK
Tympanotomy
  see Drainage, Ear, Nose, Sinus 099

U

Ulnar collateral carpal ligament
  use Bursa and Ligament, Wrist, Left
  use Bursa and Ligament, Wrist, Right
Ulnar collateral ligament
  use Bursa and Ligament, Elbow, Left
  use Bursa and Ligament, Elbow, Right
Ulnar notch
  use Radius, Left
  use Radius, Right
Ulnar vein
  use Vein, Brachial, Left
  use Vein, Brachial, Right
Ultrafiltration
  Hemodialysis
    see Performance, Urinary 5A1D
  Therapeutic plasmapheresis
    see Pheresis, Circulatory 6A55
Ultraflex™ Precision Colonic Stent System
  use Intraluminal Device
ULTRAPRO Hernia System (UHS)
  use Synthetic Substitute
ULTRAPRO Partially Absorbable Lightweight Mesh
  use Synthetic Substitute

ULTRAPRO Plug
  use Synthetic Substitute
Ultrasonic osteogenic stimulator
  use Bone Growth Stimulator in Head and Facial Bones
  use Bone Growth Stimulator in Lower Bones
  use Bone Growth Stimulator in Upper Bones
Ultrasonography
  Abdomen BW40ZZZ
  Abdomen and Pelvis BW41ZZZ
  Abdominal Wall BH49ZZZ
  Aorta
    Abdominal, Intravascular B440ZZ3
    Thoracic, Intravascular B340ZZ3
  Appendix BD48ZZZ
  Artery
    Brachiocephalic-Subclavian, Right, Intravascular B341ZZ3
    Celiac and Mesenteric, Intravascular B44KZZ3
    Common Carotid
      Bilateral, Intravascular B345ZZ3
      Left, Intravascular B344ZZ3
      Right, Intravascular B343ZZ3
    Coronary
      Multiple B241YZZ
        Intravascular B241ZZ3
        Transesophageal B241ZZ4
      Single B240YZZ
        Intravascular B240ZZ3
        Transesophageal B240ZZ4
    Femoral, Intravascular B44LZZ3
    Inferior Mesenteric, Intravascular B445ZZ3
    Internal Carotid
      Bilateral, Intravascular B348ZZ3
      Left, Intravascular B347ZZ3
      Right, Intravascular B346ZZ3
    Intra-Abdominal, Other, Intravascular B44BZZ3
    Intracranial, Intravascular B34RZZ3
    Lower Extremity
      Bilateral, Intravascular B44HZZ3
      Left, Intravascular B44GZZ3
      Right, Intravascular B44FZZ3
    Mesenteric and Celiac, Intravascular B44KZZ3
    Ophthalmic, Intravascular B34VZZ3
    Penile, Intravascular B44NZZ3
    Pulmonary
      Left, Intravascular B34TZZ3
      Right, Intravascular B34SZZ3
    Renal
      Bilateral, Intravascular B448ZZ3
      Left, Intravascular B447ZZ3
      Right, Intravascular B446ZZ3
    Subclavian, Left, Intravascular B342ZZ3
    Superior Mesenteric, Intravascular B444ZZ3
    Upper Extremity
      Bilateral, Intravascular B34KZZ3
      Left, Intravascular B34JZZ3
      Right, Intravascular B34HZZ3
  Bile Duct BF40ZZZ

Ultrasonography *(continued)*
  Bile Duct and Gallbladder BF43ZZZ
  Bladder BT40ZZZ
    and Kidney BT4JZZZ
  Brain B040ZZZ
  Breast
    Bilateral BH42ZZZ
    Left BH41ZZZ
    Right BH40ZZZ
  Chest Wall BH4BZZZ
  Coccyx BR4FZZZ
  Connective Tissue
    Lower Extremity BL41ZZZ
    Upper Extremity BL40ZZZ
  Duodenum BD49ZZZ
  Elbow
    Left, Densitometry BP4HZZ1
    Right, Densitometry BP4GZZ1
  Esophagus BD41ZZZ
  Extremity
    Lower BH48ZZZ
    Upper BH47ZZZ
  Eye
    Bilateral B847ZZZ
    Left B846ZZZ
    Right B845ZZZ
  Fallopian Tube
    Bilateral BU42
    Left BU41
    Right BU40
  Fetal Umbilical Cord BY47ZZZ
  Fetus
    First Trimester, Multiple Gestation BY4BZZZ
    Second Trimester, Multiple Gestation BY4DZZZ
    Single
      First Trimester BY49ZZZ
      Second Trimester BY4CZZZ
      Third Trimester BY4FZZZ
    Third Trimester, Multiple Gestation BY4GZZZ
  Gallbladder BF42ZZZ
  Gallbladder and Bile Duct BF43ZZZ
  Gastrointestinal Tract BD47ZZZ
  Gland
    Adrenal
      Bilateral BG42ZZZ
      Left BG41ZZZ
      Right BG40ZZZ
    Parathyroid BG43ZZZ
    Thyroid BG44ZZZ
  Hand
    Left, Densitometry BP4PZZ1
    Right, Densitometry BP4NZZ1
  Head and Neck BH4CZZZ
  Heart
    Left B245YZZ
      Intravascular B245ZZ3
      Transesophageal B245ZZ4
    Pediatric B24DYZZ
      Intravascular B24DZZ3
      Transesophageal B24DZZ4
    Right B244YZZ
      Intravascular B244ZZ3
      Transesophageal B244ZZ4
    Right and Left B246YZZ
      Intravascular B246ZZ3
      Transesophageal B246ZZ4
  Heart with Aorta B24BYZZ
    Intravascular B24BZZ3
    Transesophageal B24BZZ4
  Hepatobiliary System, All BF4CZZZ
  Hip
    Bilateral BQ42ZZZ
    Left BQ41ZZZ
    Right BQ40ZZZ
  Kidney
    and Bladder BT4JZZZ
    Bilateral BT43ZZZ
    Left BT42ZZZ

Ultrasonography *(continued)*
  Kidney *(continued)*
    Right BT41ZZZ
    Transplant BT49ZZZ
  Knee
    Bilateral BQ49ZZZ
    Left BQ48ZZZ
    Right BQ47ZZZ
  Liver BF45ZZZ
  Liver and Spleen BF46ZZZ
  Mediastinum BB4CZZZ
  Neck BW4FZZZ
  Ovary
    Bilateral BU45
    Left BU44
    Right BU43
  Ovary and Uterus BU4C
  Pancreas BF47ZZZ
  Pelvic Region BW4GZZZ
  Pelvis and Abdomen BW41ZZZ
  Penis BV4BZZZ
  Pericardium B24CYZZ
    Intravascular B24CZZ3
    Transesophageal B24CZZ4
  Placenta BY48ZZZ
  Pleura BB4BZZZ
  Prostate and Seminal Vesicle BV49ZZZ
  Rectum BD4CZZZ
  Sacrum BR4FZZZ
  Scrotum BV44ZZZ
  Seminal Vesicle and Prostate BV49ZZZ
  Shoulder
    Left, Densitometry BP49ZZ1
    Right, Densitometry BP48ZZ1
  Spinal Cord B04BZZZ
  Spine
    Cervical BR40ZZZ
    Lumbar BR49ZZZ
    Thoracic BR47ZZZ
  Spleen and Liver BF46ZZZ
  Stomach BD42ZZZ
  Tendon
    Lower Extremity BL43ZZZ
    Upper Extremity BL42ZZZ
  Ureter
    Bilateral BT48ZZZ
    Left BT47ZZZ
    Right BT46ZZZ
  Urethra BT45ZZZ
  Uterus BU46
  Uterus and Ovary BU4C
  Vein
    Jugular
      Left, Intravascular B544ZZ3
      Right, Intravascular B543ZZ3
    Lower Extremity
      Bilateral, Intravascular B54DZZ3
      Left, Intravascular B54CZZ3
      Right, Intravascular B54BZZ3
    Portal, Intravascular B54TZZ3
    Renal
      Bilateral, Intravascular B54LZZ3
      Left, Intravascular B54KZZ3
      Right, Intravascular B54JZZ3
    Spanchnic, Intravascular B54TZZ3
    Subclavian
      Left, Intravascular B547ZZ3
      Right, Intravascular B546ZZ3

Ultrasonography (*continued*)
  Vein (*continued*)
    Upper Extremity
      Bilateral, Intravascular
        B54PZZ3
      Left, Intravascular B54NZZ3
      Right, Intravascular
        B54MZZ3
    Vena Cava
      Inferior, Intravascular B549ZZ3
      Superior, Intravascular B548ZZ3
    Wrist
      Left, Densitometry BP4MZZ1
      Right, Densitometry BP4LZZ1
Ultrasound bone healing system
  use Bone Growth Stimulator in
    Head and Facial Bones
  use Bone Growth Stimulator in
    Lower Bones
  use Bone Growth Stimulator in
    Upper Bones
Ultrasound Therapy
  Heart 6A75
  No Qualifier 6A75
  Vessels
    Head and Neck 6A75
    Other 6A75
    Peripheral 6A75
Ultraviolet Light Therapy, Skin
  6A80
Umbilical artery
  use Artery, Internal Iliac, Left
  use Artery, Internal Iliac, Right
Uniplanar external fixator
  use External Fixation Device,
    Monoplanar in 0PH
  use External Fixation Device,
    Monoplanar in 0PS
  use External Fixation Device,
    Monoplanar in 0QH
  use External Fixation Device,
    Monoplanar in 0QS
Upper GI series
  see Fluoroscopy, Gastrointestinal,
    Upper BD15
Ureteral orifice
  use Ureter
  use Ureter, Left
  use Ureter, Right
  use Ureters, Bilateral
Ureterectomy
  see Excision, Urinary System 0TB
  see Resection, Urinary System 0TT
Ureterocolostomy
  see Bypass, Urinary System 0T1
Ureterocystostomy
  see Bypass, Urinary System 0T1
Ureteroenterostomy
  see Bypass, Urinary System 0T1
Ureteroileostomy
  see Bypass, Urinary System 0T1
Ureterolithotomy
  see Extirpation, Urinary System
    0TC
Ureterolysis
  see Release, Urinary System 0TN
Ureteroneocystostomy
  see Bypass, Urinary System 0T1
  see Reposition, Urinary System
    0TS
Ureteropelvic junction (UPJ)
  use Kidney Pelvis, Left
  use Kidney Pelvis, Right
Ureteropexy
  see Repair, Urinary System 0TQ
  see Reposition, Urinary System 0TS
Ureteroplasty
  see Repair, Urinary System 0TQ
  see Replacement, Urinary System
    0TR
  see Supplement, Urinary System
    0TU

Ureteroplication
  see Restriction, Urinary System
    0TV
Ureteropyelography
  see Fluoroscopy, Urinary System
    BT1
Ureterorrhaphy
  see Repair, Urinary System 0TQ
Ureteroscopy 0TJ98ZZ
Ureterostomy
  see Bypass, Urinary System 0T1
  see Drainage, Urinary System 0T9
Ureterotomy
  see Drainage, Urinary System 0T9
Ureteroureterostomy
  see Bypass, Urinary System 0T1
Ureterovesical orifice
  use Ureter
  use Ureters, Bilateral
  use Ureter, Left
  use Ureter, Right
Urethral catheterization, indwelling
  0T9B70Z
Urethrectomy
  see Excision, Urethra 0TBD
  see Resection, Urethra 0TTD
Urethrolithotomy
  see Extirpation, Urethra 0TCD
Urethrolysis
  see Release, Urethra 0TND
Urethropexy
  see Repair, Urethra 0TQD
  see Reposition, Urethra 0TSD
Urethroplasty
  see Repair, Urethra 0TQD
  see Replacement, Urethra
    0TRD
  see Supplement, Urethra 0TUD
Urethrorrhaphy
  see Repair, Urethra 0TQD
Urethroscopy 0TJD8ZZ
Urethrotomy
  see Drainage, Urethra 0T9D
Urinary incontinence stimulator lead
  use Stimulator Lead in Urinary
    System
Urography
  see Fluoroscopy, Urinary System
    BT1
Uterine Artery
  use Artery, Internal Iliac, Left
  use Artery, Internal Iliac, Right
Uterine artery embolization (UAE)
  see Occlusion, Lower Arteries
    04L
Uterine cornu
  use Uterus
Uterine tube
  use Fallopian Tube, Left
  use Fallopian Tube, Right
Uterine vein
  use Vein, Hypogastric, Left
  use Vein, Hypogastric, Right
Uvulectomy
  see Excision, Uvula 0CBN
  see Resection, Uvula 0CTN
Uvulorrhaphy
  see Repair, Uvula 0CQN
Uvulotomy
  see Drainage, Uvula 0C9N

V

Vaccination
  see Introduction of Serum, Toxoid,
    and Vaccine
Vacuum extraction, obstetric
  10D07Z6
Vaginal artery
  use Artery, Internal Iliac, Left
  use Artery, Internal Iliac, Right

Vaginal pessary
  use Intraluminal Device, Pessary
    in Female Reproductive
    System
Vaginal vein
  use Vein, Hypogastric, Left
  use Vein, Hypogastric, Right
Vaginectomy
  see Excision, Vagina
    0UBG
  see Resection, Vagina
    0UTG
Vaginofixation
  see Repair, Vagina 0UQG
  see Reposition, Vagina 0USG
Vaginoplasty
  see Repair, Vagina 0UQG
  see Supplement, Vagina 0UUG
Vaginorrhaphy
  see Repair, Vagina 0UQG
Vaginoscopy 0UJH8ZZ
Vaginotomy
  see Drainage, Female
    Reproductive System
    0U9
Vagotomy
  see Division, Nerve, Vagus
    008Q
Valiant Thoracic Stent Graft
  use Intraluminal Device
Valvotomy, valvulotomy
  see Division, Heart and Great
    Vessels 028
  see Release, Heart and Great Vessels
    02N
Valvuloplasty
  see Repair, Heart and Great Vessels
    02Q
  see Replacement, Heart and Great
    Vessels 02R
  see Supplement, Heart and Great
    Vessels 02U
Vascular Access Device
  Insertion of device in
    Abdomen 0JH8
    Chest 0JH6
    Lower Arm
      Left 0JHH
      Right 0JHG
    Lower Leg
      Left 0JHP
      Right 0JHN
    Upper Arm
      Left 0JHF
      Right 0JHD
    Upper Leg
      Left 0JHM
      Right 0JHL
  Removal of device from
    Lower Extremity 0JPW
    Trunk 0JPT
    Upper Extremity 0JPV
  Reservoir
    Insertion of device in
      Abdomen 0JH8
      Chest 0JH6
      Lower Arm
        Left 0JHH
        Right 0JHG
      Lower Leg
        Left 0JHP
        Right 0JHN
      Upper Arm
        Left 0JHF
        Right 0JHD
      Upper Leg
        Left 0JHM
        Right 0JHL
    Removal of device from
      Lower Extremity 0JPW
      Trunk 0JPT
      Upper Extremity 0JPV

Vascular Access Device (*continued*)
  Reservoir (*continued*)
    Revision of device in
      Lower Extremity 0JWW
      Trunk 0JWT
      Upper Extremity 0JWV
  Revision of device in
    Lower Extremity 0JWW
    Trunk 0JWT
    Upper Extremity 0JWV
Vasectomy
  see Excision, Male Reproductive
    System 0VB
Vasography
  see Fluoroscopy, Male Reproductive
    System BV1
  see Plain Radiography, Male
    Reproductive System BV0
Vasoligation
  see Occlusion, Male Reproductive
    System 0VL
Vasorrhaphy
  see Repair, Male Reproductive
    System 0VQ
Vasostomy
  see Bypass, Male Reproductive
    System 0V1
Vasotomy
  Drainage
    see Drainage, Male
      Reproductive System 0V9
    see Occlusion, Male
      Reproductive System 0VL
  With ligation
Vasovasostomy
  see Repair, Male Reproductive
    System 0VQ
Vastus intermedius muscle
  use Muscle, Upper Leg, Left
  use Muscle, Upper Leg, Right
Vastus lateralis muscle
  use Muscle, Upper Leg, Left
  use Muscle, Upper Leg, Right
Vastus medialis muscle
  use Muscle, Upper Leg, Left
  use Muscle, Upper Leg, Right
VCG (vectorcardiogram)
  see Measurement, Cardiac 4A02
Vectra® Vascular Access Graft
  use Vascular Access Device in
    Subcutaneous Tissue and
    Fascia
Venectomy
  see Excision, Lower Veins 06B
  see Excision, Upper Veins 05B
Venography
  see Fluoroscopy, Veins B51
  see Plain Radiography, Veins B50
Venorrhaphy
  see Repair, Lower Veins 06Q
  see Repair, Upper Veins 05Q
Venotripsy
  see Occlusion, Lower Veins 06L
  see Occlusion, Upper Veins 05L
Ventricular fold
  use Larynx
Ventriculoatriostomy
  see Bypass, Central Nervous System
    001
Ventriculocisternostomy
  see Bypass, Central Nervous System
    001
Ventriculogram, cardiac
  Combined left and right heart
    see Fluoroscopy, Heart, Right
      and Left B216
  Left ventricle
    see Fluoroscopy, Heart, Left
      B215
  Right ventricle
    see Fluoroscopy, Heart, Right
      B214

Ventriculopuncture, through previously implanted catheter 8C01X6J
Ventriculoscopy 00J04ZZ
Ventriculostomy
  External drainage
    see Drainage, Cerebral Ventricle 0096
  Internal shunt
    see Bypass, Cerebral Ventricle 0016
Ventriculovenostomy
  see Bypass, Cerebral Ventricle 0016
Ventrio™ Hernia Patch
  use Synthetic Substitute
VEP (visual evoked potential) 4A07X0Z
Vermiform appendix
  use Appendix
Vermilion border
  use Lip, Lower
  use Lip, Upper
Versa
  use Pacemaker, Dual Chamber in 0JH
Version, obstetric
  External 10S0XZZ
  Internal 10S07ZZ
Vertebral arch
  use Vertebra, Cervical
  use Vertebra, Lumbar
  use Vertebra, Thoracic
Vertebral canal
  use Spinal Canal
Vertebral foramen
  use Vertebra, Cervical
  use Vertebra, Lumbar
  use Vertebra, Thoracic
Vertebral lamina
  use Vertebra, Cervical
  use Vertebra, Lumbar
  use Vertebra, Thoracic
Vertebral pedicle
  use Vertebra, Cervical
  use Vertebra, Lumbar
  use Vertebra, Thoracic
Vesical vein
  use Vein, Hypogastric, Left
  use Vein, Hypogastric, Right
Vesicotomy
  see Drainage, Urinary System 0T9

Vesiculectomy
  see Excision, Male Reproductive System 0VB
  see Resection, Male Reproductive System 0VT
Vesiculogram, seminal
  see Plain Radiography, Male Reproductive System BV0
Vesiculotomy
  see Drainage, Male Reproductive System 0V9
Vestibular (Scarpa's) ganglion
  use Nerve, Acoustic
Vestibular Assessment F15Z
Vestibular nerve
  use Nerve, Acoustic
Vestibular Treatment F0C
Vestibulocochlear nerve
  use Nerve, Acoustic
VH-IVUS (virtual histology intravascular ultrasound)
  see Ultrasonography, Heart B24
Virchow's (supraclavicular) lymph node
  use Lymphatic, Neck, Left
  use Lymphatic, Neck, Right
Virtuoso (II) (DR) (VR)
  use Defibrillator Generator in 0JH
Vitrectomy
  see Excision, Eye 08B
  see Resection, Eye 08T
Vitreous body
  use Vitreous, Left
  use Vitreous, Right
Viva (XT)(S)
  use Cardiac Resynchronization Defibrillator Pulse Generator in 0JH
Vocal fold
  use Vocal Cord, Left
  use Vocal Cord, Right
Vocational
  Assessment
  Retraining
    see Activities of Daily Living Assessment, Rehabilitation F02
    see Activities of Daily Living Treatment, Rehabilitation F08
Volar (palmar) digital vein
  use Vein, Hand, Left

Volar (palmar) digital vein *(continued)*
  use Vein, Hand, Right
Volar (palmar) metacarpal vein
  use Vein, Hand, Left
  use Vein, Hand, Right
Vomer bone
  use Septum, Nasal
Vomer of nasal septum
  use Bone, Nasal
Voraxaze
  use Glucarpidase
Vulvectomy
  see Excision, Female Reproductive System 0UB
  see Resection, Female Reproductive System 0UT

W

WALLSTENT® Endoprosthesis
  use Intraluminal Device
Washing
  see Irrigation
Wedge resection, pulmonary
  see Excision, Respiratory System 0BB
Window
  see Drainage
Wiring, dental 2W31X9Z

X

X-ray
  see Plain Radiography
X-STOP® Spacer
  use Spinal Stabilization Device, Interspinous Process in 0RH
  use Spinal Stabilization Device, Interspinous Process in 0SH
Xact Carotid Stent System
  use Intraluminal Device
Xenograft
  use Zooplastic Tissue in Heart and Great Vessels
XIENCE Everolimus Eluting Coronary Stent System
  use Intraluminal Device, Drug-eluting in Heart and Great Vessels

Xiphoid process
  use Sternum
XLIF® System
  use Interbody Fusion Device in Lower Joints

Y

Yoga Therapy 8E0ZXY4

Z

Z-plasty, skin for scar contracture
  see Release, Skin and Breast 0HN
Zenith Flex® AAA Endovascular Graft
  use Intraluminal Device
Zenith TX2® TAA Endovascular Graft
  use Intraluminal Device
Zenith® Renu™ AAA Ancillary Graft
  use Intraluminal Device
Zilver® PTX® (paclitaxel) Drug-Eluting Peripheral Stent
  use Intraluminal Device, Drug-eluting in Lower Arteries
  use Intraluminal Device, Drug-eluting in Upper Arteries
Zimmer® NexGen® LPS Mobile Bearing Knee
  use Synthetic Substitute
Zimmer® NexGen® LPS-Flex Mobile Knee
  use Synthetic Substitute
Zonule of Zinn
  use Lens, Left
  use Lens, Right
Zotarolimus-eluting coronary stent
  use Intraluminal Device, Drug-eluting in Heart and Great Vessels
Zygomatic process of frontal bone
  use Bone, Frontal, Left
  use Bone, Frontal, Right
Zygomatic process of temporal bone
  use Bone, Temporal, Left
  use Bone, Temporal, Right
Zygomaticus muscle
  use Muscle, Facial
Zyvox
  use Oxazolidinones

Within each section of ICD-10-PCS the characters have different meanings. The seven character meanings for the Medical and Surgical section are illustrated here through the procedure example of *Percutaneous needle core biopsy of the right kidney.*

Section	Body System	Root Operation	Body Part	Approach	Device	Qualifier
Med/Surg	Urinary	Excision	Kidney, Right	Percutaneous	None	Diagnostic
0	T	B	0	3	Z	X

Section (Character 1)

All Medical and Surgical procedure codes have a first character value of 0.

Body System (Character 2)

The alphanumeric character for the body system is placed in the second position. The following are the body systems applicable to the Medical and Surgical section.

Character Value	Character Value Description
0	Central Nervous System
1	Peripheral Nervous System
2	Heart and Great Vessels
3	Upper Arteries
4	Lower Arteries
5	Upper Veins
6	Lower Veins
7	Lymphatic and Hemic Systems
8	Eye
9	Ear, Nose, Sinus
B	Respiratory System
C	Mouth and Throat
D	Gastrointestinal System
F	Hepatobiliary System and Pancreas
G	Endocrine System
H	Skin and Breast
J	Subcutaneous Tissue and Fascia
K	Muscles
L	Tendons
M	Bursae and Ligaments
N	Head and Facial Bones
P	Upper Bones
Q	Lower Bones
R	Upper Joints
S	Lower Joints
T	Urinary System
U	Female Reproductive System
V	Male Reproductive System
W	Anatomical Regions, General
X	Anatomical Regions, Upper Extremities
Y	Anatomical Regions, Lower Extremities

Root Operations (Character 3)

The alphanumeric character value for root operations is placed in the third position. Listed below are the root operations applicable to the Medical and Surgical section with their associated meaning.

Character Value	Root Operation	Root Operation Definition
0	Alteration	Modifying the anatomic structure of a body part without affecting the function of the body part
1	Bypass	Altering the route of passage of the contents of a tubular body part
2	Change	Taking out or off a device from a body part and putting back an identical or similar device in or on the same body part without cutting or puncturing the skin or a mucous membrane
3	Control	Stopping, or attempting to stop, postprocedural bleeding
4	Creation	Making a new genital structure that does not take over the function of a body part
5	Destruction	Physical eradication of all or a portion of a body part by the direct use of energy, force, or a destructive agent
6	Detachment	Cutting off all or a portion of the upper or lower extremities
7	Dilation	Expanding an orifice or the lumen of a tubular body part
8	Division	Cutting into a body part, without draining fluids and/or gases from the body part, in order to separate or transect a body part
9	Drainage	Taking or letting out fluids and/or gases from a body part
B	Excision	Cutting out or off, without replacement, a portion of a body part
C	Extirpation	Taking or cutting out solid matter from a body part
D	Extraction	Pulling or stripping out or off all or a portion of a body part by the use of force
F	Fragmentation	Breaking solid matter in a body part into pieces
G	Fusion	Joining together portions of an articular body part rendering the articular body part immobile
H	Insertion	Putting in a nonbiological appliance that monitors, assists, performs, or prevents a physiological function but does not physically take the place of a body part
J	Inspection	Visually and/or manually exploring a body part
K	Map	Locating the route of passage of electrical impulses and/or locating functional areas in a body part
L	Occlusion	Completely closing an orifice or the lumen of a tubular body part
M	Reattachment	Putting back in or on all or a portion of a separated body part to its normal location or other suitable location
N	Release	Freeing a body part from an abnormal physical constraint by cutting or by the use of force
P	Removal	Taking out or off a device from a body part
Q	Repair	Restoring, to the extent possible, a body part to its normal anatomic structure and function
R	Replacement	Putting in or on biological or synthetic material that physically takes the place and/or function of all or a portion of a body part
S	Reposition	Moving to its normal location, or other suitable location, all or a portion of a body part
T	Resection	Cutting out or off, without replacement, all of a body part
V	Restriction	Partially closing an orifice or the lumen of a tubular body part
W	Revision	Correcting, to the extent possible, a portion of a malfunctioning device or the position of a displaced device
U	Supplement	Putting in or on biological or synthetic material that physically reinforces and/or augments the function of a portion of a body part
X	Transfer	Moving, without taking out, all or a portion of a body part to another location to take over the function of all or a portion of a body part
Y	Transplantation	Putting in or on all or a portion of a living body part taken from another individual or animal to physically take the place and/or function of all or a portion of a similar body part

Body Part (Character 4)

For each body system the applicable body part character values will be available for procedure code construction. An example of a body part for this section is the Large Intestines.

Approach (Character 5)

The approach is the technique used to reach the procedure site. The following are the approach character values for the Medical and Surgical section with the associated definitions.

Character Value	Approach	Approach Definition
0	Open	Cutting through the skin or mucous membrane and any other body layers necessary to expose the site of the procedure
3	Percutaneous	Entry, by puncture or minor incision, of instrumentation through the skin or mucous membrane and any other body layers necessary to reach the site of the procedure
4	Percutaneous Endoscopic	Entry, by puncture or minor incision, of instrumentation through the skin or mucous membrane and any other body layers necessary to reach and visualize the site of the procedure
7	Via Natural or Artificial Opening	Entry of instrumentation through a natural or artificial external opening to reach the site of the procedure
8	Via Natural or Artificial Opening Endoscopic	Entry of instrumentation through a natural or artificial external opening to reach and visualize the site of the procedure
F	Via Natural or Artificial Opening Percutaneous Endoscopic	Entry of instrumentation through a natural or artificial external opening to reach and visualize the site of the procedure, and entry, by puncture or minor incision, of instrumentation through the skin or mucous membrane and any other body layers necessary to aid in the performance of the procedure
X	External	Procedures performed directly on the skin or mucous membrane and procedures performed indirectly by the application of external force through the skin or mucous membrane

Device (Character 6)

Depending on the procedure performed there may or may not be a device used. There are several types of devices included in the Medical and Surgical section that fall into one of the four following categories.

- Electronic Appliances
- Grafts and Prostheses
- Implants
- Simple or Mechanical Appliances

When a device is not utilized during the procedure, the character value of Z should be reported.

If a coder is unsure of which option to select for the device utilized during the procedure, Appendix E can be used to guide the selection. For example, if the coder is in Table 02R (replacement of heart and great vessels) the coder can locate the device categories in Appendix E (Autologous Tissue Substitute, Zooplastic Tissue, Synthetic Substitute, and Nonautologous Tissue Substitue). For each of these categories brand name devices and other devices are listed. The coder should select the category in which the device utilized during the procedure is listed.

Qualifier (Character 7)

The qualifier represents an additional attribute for the procedure when applicable. In the preceding example of *Percutaneous needle core biopsy of the right kidney*, the qualifier of X was used to report that the biopsy procedure was diagnostic in nature. If there is no qualifier for a procedure, the Z character value should be reported.

Important Definitions for the Medical and Surgical Section

Medical Surgical Root Operation	Qualifier	Definition
Detachment of Upper and Lower Extremities (0X6 and 0Y6) Arms and Legs	1 – High	Amputation at the proximal portion of the shaft of the humerus or femur
	2 – Mid	Amputation at the middle portion of the shaft of the humerus or femur
	3 – Low	Amputation at the distal portion of the shaft of the humerus or femur
Detachment of Upper and Lower Extremities (0X6 and 0Y6) Fingers, Thumbs, and Toes	0 – Complete	Amputation at the metacarpophalangeal/metatarsal-phalangeal joint
	1 – High	Amputation anywhere along the proximal phalanx
	2 – Mid	Amputation through the proximal interphalangeal joint or anywhere along the middle phalanx
	3 – Low	Amputation through the distal interphalangeal joint or anywhere along the distal phalanx
Transplantation	0 – Allogeneic	Being genetically different although belonging to or obtained from the same species*
	1 – Syngeneic	Genetically identical or closely related, so as to allow tissue transplant; immunologically compatible*
	2 – Zooplastic	Surgical transfer of tissue from an animal to a human*

*Taken from The Free Dictionary by Farlex at www.thefreedictionary.com

Medical and Surgical Section Guidelines (section 0)

B2. Body System

General guidelines

B2.1a The procedure codes in the general anatomical regions body systems should only be used when the procedure is performed on an anatomical region rather than a specific body part (e.g., root operations Control and Detachment, Drainage of a body cavity) or on the rare occasion when no information is available to support assignment of a code to a specific body part.

Example: Control of postoperative hemorrhage is coded to the root operation Control found in the general anatomical regions body systems.

B2.1b Where the general body part values "upper" and "lower" are provided as an option in the Upper Arteries, Lower Arteries, Upper Veins, Lower Veins, Muscles and Tendons body systems, "upper" or "lower" specifies body parts located above or below the diaphragm respectively.

Example: Vein body parts above the diaphragm are found in the Upper Veins body system; vein body parts below the diaphragm are found in the Lower Veins body system.

B3. Root Operation

General guidelines

B3.1a In order to determine the appropriate root operation, the full definition of the root operation as contained in the PCS Tables must be applied.

B3.1b Components of a procedure specified in the root operation definition and explanation are not coded separately. Procedural steps necessary to reach the operative site and close the operative site, including anastomosis of a tubular body part, are also not coded separately.

Example: Resection of a joint as part of a joint replacement procedure is included in the root operation definition of Replacement and is not coded separately. Laparotomy performed to reach the site of an open liver biopsy is not coded separately. In a resection of sigmoid colon with anastomosis of descending colon to rectum, the anastomosis is not coded separately.

Multiple procedures

B3.2 During the same operative episode, multiple procedures are coded if:

a. The same root operation is performed on different body parts as defined by distinct values of the body part character.

Example: Diagnostic excision of liver and pancreas are coded separately.

b. The same root operation is repeated at different body sites that are included in the same body part value.

Example: Excision of the sartorius muscle and excision of the gracilis muscle are both included in the upper leg muscle body part value, and multiple procedures are coded.

c. Multiple root operations with distinct objectives are performed on the same body part.

Example: Destruction of sigmoid lesion and bypass of sigmoid colon are coded separately.

d. The intended root operation is attempted using one approach, but is converted to a different approach.

Example: Laparoscopic cholecystectomy converted to an open cholecystectomy is coded as percutaneous endoscopic Inspection and open Resection.

Discontinued procedures

B3.3 If the intended procedure is discontinued, code the procedure to the root operation performed. If a procedure is discontinued before any other root operation is performed, code the root operation Inspection of the body part or anatomical region inspected.

Example: A planned aortic valve replacement procedure is discontinued after the initial thoracotomy and before any incision is made in the heart muscle, when the patient becomes hemodynamically unstable. This procedure is coded as an open Inspection of the mediastinum.

Biopsy procedures

B3.4a Biopsy procedures are coded using the root operations Excision, Extraction, or Drainage and the qualifier Diagnostic. The qualifier Diagnostic is used only for biopsies.

Example: Fine needle aspiration biopsy of lung is coded to the root operation Drainage with the qualifier Diagnostic. Biopsy of bone marrow is coded to the root operation Extraction with the qualifier Diagnostic. Lymph node sampling for biopsy is coded to the root operation Excision with the qualifier Diagnostic.

Biopsy followed by more definitive treatment

B3.4b If a diagnostic Excision, Extraction, or Drainage procedure (biopsy) is followed by a more definitive procedure, such as Destruction, Excision or Resection at the same procedure site, both the biopsy and the more definitive treatment are coded.

Example: Biopsy of breast followed by partial mastectomy at the same procedure site, both the biopsy and the partial mastectomy procedure are coded.

Overlapping body layers

B3.5 If the root operations Excision, Repair or Inspection are performed on overlapping layers of the musculoskeletal system, the body part specifying the deepest layer is coded.

Example: Excisional debridement that includes skin and subcutaneous tissue and muscle is coded to the muscle body part.

Bypass procedures

B3.6a Bypass procedures are coded by identifying the body part bypassed "from" and the body part bypassed "to." The fourth character body part specifies the body part bypassed from, and the qualifier specifies the body part bypassed to.

Example: Bypass from stomach to jejunum, stomach is the body part and jejunum is the qualifier.

B3.6b Coronary arteries are classified by number of distinct sites treated, rather than number of coronary arteries or anatomic name of a coronary artery (e.g., left anterior descending). Coronary artery bypass procedures are coded differently than other bypass procedures as described in the previous guideline. Rather than identifying the body part bypassed from, the body part identifies the number of coronary artery sites bypassed to, and the qualifier specifies the vessel bypassed from.

Example: Aortocoronary artery bypass of one site on the left anterior descending coronary artery and one site on the obtuse marginal coronary artery is classified in the body part axis of classification as two coronary artery sites and the qualifier specifies the aorta as the body part bypassed from.

B3.6c If multiple coronary artery sites are bypassed, a separate procedure is coded for each coronary artery site that uses a different device and/or qualifier.

Example: Aortocoronary artery bypass and internal mammary coronary artery bypass are coded separately.

Control vs. more definitive root operations

B3.7 The root operation Control is defined as, "Stopping, or attempting to stop, postprocedural bleeding." If an attempt to stop postprocedural bleeding is initially unsuccessful, and to stop the bleeding requires performing any of the definitive root operations Bypass, Detachment, Excision, Extraction, Reposition, Replacement, or Resection, then that root operation is coded instead of Control.

Example: Resection of spleen to stop postprocedural bleeding is coded to Resection instead of Control.

Excision vs. Resection

B3.8 PCS contains specific body parts for anatomical subdivisions of a body part, such as lobes of the lungs or liver and regions of the intestine. Resection of the specific body part is coded whenever all of the body part is cut out or off, rather than coding Excision of a less specific body part.

Example: Left upper lung lobectomy is coded to Resection of Upper Lung Lobe, Left rather than Excision of Lung, Left.

Excision for graft

B3.9 If an autograft is obtained from a different body part in order to complete the objective of the procedure, a separate procedure is coded.

Example: Coronary bypass with excision of saphenous vein graft, excision of saphenous vein is coded separately.

Fusion procedures of the spine

B3.10a The body part coded for a spinal vertebral joint(s) rendered immobile by a spinal fusion procedure is classified by the level of the spine (e.g. thoracic). There are distinct body part values for a single vertebral joint and for multiple vertebral joints at each spinal level.

Example: Body part values specify Lumbar Vertebral Joint, Lumbar Vertebral Joints, 2 or More and Lumbosacral Vertebral Joint.

B3.10b If multiple vertebral joints are fused, a separate procedure is coded for each vertebral joint that uses a different device and/or qualifier.

Example: Fusion of lumbar vertebral joint, posterior approach, anterior column and fusion of lumbar vertebral joint, posterior approach, posterior column are coded separately.

B3.10c Combinations of devices and materials are often used on a vertebral joint to render the joint immobile. When combinations of devices are used on the same vertebral joint, the device value coded for the procedure is as follows:

- If an interbody fusion device is used to render the joint immobile (alone or containing other material like bone graft), the procedure is coded with the device value Interbody Fusion Device

- If bone graft is the only device used to render the joint immobile, the procedure is coded with the device value Nonautologous Tissue Substitute or Autologous Tissue Substitute
- If a mixture of autologous and nonautologous bone graft (with or without biological or synthetic extenders or binders) is used to render the joint immobile, code the procedure with the device value Autologous Tissue Substitute

Examples: Fusion of a vertebral joint using a cage style interbody fusion device containing morsellized bone graft is coded to the device Interbody Fusion Device.

Fusion of a vertebral joint using a bone dowel interbody fusion device made of cadaver bone and packed with a mixture of local morsellized bone and demineralized bone matrix is coded to the device Interbody Fusion Device.

Fusion of a vertebral joint using both autologous bone graft and bone bank bone graft is coded to the device Autologous Tissue Substitute.

Inspection procedures

B3.11a Inspection of a body part(s) performed in order to achieve the objective of a procedure is not coded separately.

Example: Fiberoptic bronchoscopy performed for irrigation of bronchus, only the irrigation procedure is coded.

B3.11b If multiple tubular body parts are inspected, the most distal body part inspected is coded. If multiple non-tubular body parts in a region are inspected, the body part that specifies the entire area inspected is coded.

Example: Cystoureteroscopy with inspection of bladder and ureters is coded to the ureter body part value.

Exploratory laparotomy with general inspection of abdominal contents is coded to the peritoneal cavity body part value.

B3.11c When both an Inspection procedure and another procedure are performed on the same body part during the same episode, if the Inspection procedure is performed using a different approach than the other procedure, the Inspection procedure is coded separately.

Example: Endoscopic Inspection of the duodenum is coded separately when open Excision of the duodenum is performed during the same procedural episode.

Occlusion vs. Restriction for vessel embolization procedures

B3.12 If the objective of an embolization procedure is to completely close a vessel, the root operation Occlusion is coded. If the objective of an embolization procedure is to narrow the lumen of a vessel, the root operation Restriction is coded.

Examples: Tumor embolization is coded to the root operation Occlusion, because the objective of the procedure is to cut off the blood supply to the vessel.

Embolization of a cerebral aneurysm is coded to the root operation Restriction, because the objective of the procedure is not to close off the vessel entirely, but to narrow the lumen of the vessel at the site of the aneurysm where it is abnormally wide.

Release procedures

B3.13 In the root operation Release, the body part value coded is the body part being freed and not the tissue being manipulated or cut to free the body part.

Example: Lysis of intestinal adhesions is coded to the specific intestine body part value.

Release vs. Division

B3.14 If the sole objective of the procedure is freeing a body part without cutting the body part, the root operation is Release. If the sole objective of the procedure is separating or transecting a body part, the root operation is Division.

Example: Freeing a nerve root from surrounding scar tissue to relieve pain is coded to the root operation Release. Severing a nerve root to relieve pain is coded to the root operation Division.

Reposition for fracture treatment

B3.15 Reduction of a displaced fracture is coded to the root operation Reposition and the application of a cast or splint in conjunction with the Reposition procedure is not coded separately. Treatment of a nondisplaced fracture is coded to the procedure performed.

Example: Putting a pin in a nondisplaced fracture is coded to the root operation Insertion.

Casting of a nondisplaced fracture is coded to the root operation Immobilization in the Placement section.

Transplantation vs. Administration

B3.16 Putting in a mature and functioning living body part taken from another individual or animal is coded to the root operation Transplantation. Putting in autologous or nonautologous cells is coded to the Administration section.

Example: Putting in autologous or nonautologous bone marrow, pancreatic islet cells or stem cells is coded to the Administration section.

B4. Body Part

General guidelines

B4.1a If a procedure is performed on a portion of a body part that does not have a separate body part value, code the body part value corresponding to the whole body part.

Example: A procedure performed on the alveolar process of the mandible is coded to the mandible body part.

B4.1b If the prefix "peri" is combined with a body part to identify the site of the procedure, and the site of the procedure is not further specified, then the procedure is coded to the body part named. This guideline applies only when a more specific body part value is not available.

Examples: A procedure site identified as perirenal is coded to the kidney body part when the site of the procedure is not further specified.

A procedure site described in the documentation as peri-urethral tissue, and the documentation also indicates that it is the vulvar tissue and not the urethral tissue that is the site of the procedure, then the procedure is coded to the vulva body part.

Branches of body parts

B4.2 Where a specific branch of a body part does not have its own body part value in PCS, the body part is coded to the closest proximal branch that has a specific body part value.

Example: A procedure performed on the mandibular branch of the trigeminal nerve is coded to the trigeminal nerve body part value.

Bilateral body part values

B4.3 Bilateral body part values are available for a limited number of body parts. If the identical procedure is performed on contralateral body parts, and a bilateral body part value exists for that body part, a single procedure is coded using the bilateral body part value. If no bilateral body part value exists, each procedure is coded separately using the appropriate body part value.

Example: The identical procedure performed on both fallopian tubes is coded once using the body part value Fallopian Tube, Bilateral. The identical procedure performed on both knee joints is coded twice using the body part values Knee Joint, Right and Knee Joint, Left.

Coronary arteries

B4.4 The coronary arteries are classified as a single body part that is further specified by number of sites treated and not by name or number of arteries. Separate body part values are used to specify the number of sites treated when the same procedure is performed on multiple sites in the coronary arteries.

Examples: Angioplasty of two distinct sites in the left anterior descending coronary artery with placement of two stents is coded as Dilation of Coronary Arteries, Two Sites, with Intraluminal Device.

Angioplasty of two distinct sites in the left anterior descending coronary artery, one with stent placed and one without, is coded separately as Dilation of Coronary Artery, One Site with Intraluminal Device, and Dilation of Coronary Artery, One Site with no device.

Tendons, ligaments, bursae and fascia near a joint

B4.5 Procedures performed on tendons, ligaments, bursae and fascia supporting a joint are coded to the body part in the respective body system that is the focus of the procedure. Procedures performed on joint structures themselves are coded to the body part in the joint body systems.

Example: Repair of the anterior cruciate ligament of the knee is coded to the knee bursae and ligament body part in the bursae and ligaments body system. Knee arthroscopy with shaving of articular cartilage is coded to the knee joint body part in the Lower Joints body system.

Skin, subcutaneous tissue and fascia overlying a joint

B4.6 If a procedure is performed on the skin, subcutaneous tissue or fascia overlying a joint, the procedure is coded to the following body part:

- Shoulder is coded to Upper Arm
- Elbow is coded to Lower Arm
- Wrist is coded to Lower Arm
- Hip is coded to Upper Leg
- Knee is coded to Lower Leg
- Ankle is coded to Foot

Fingers and toes

B4.7 If a body system does not contain a separate body part value for fingers, procedures performed on the fingers are coded to the body part value for the hand. If a body system does not contain a separate body part value for toes, procedures performed on the toes are coded to the body part value for the foot.

Example: Excision of finger muscle is coded to one of the hand muscle body part values in the Muscles body system.

Upper and lower intestinal tract

B4.8 In the Gastrointestinal body system, the general body part values Upper Intestinal Tract and Lower Intestinal Tract are provided as a option for the root operations Change, Inspection, Removal and Revision. Upper Intestinal Tract includes the portion of the gastrointestina tract from the esophagus down to and including the duodenum, and Lower Intestinal Tract includes the portion of the gastrointestinal trac from the jejunum down to and including the rectum and anus.

Example: In the root operation Change table, change of a device in the jejunum is coded using the body part Lower Intestinal Tract.

B5. Approach

Open approach with percutaneous endoscopic assistance

B5.2 Procedures performed using the open approach with percutaneous endoscopic assistance are coded to the approach Open.

Example: Laparoscopic-assisted sigmoidectomy is coded to the approach Open.

External approach

B5.3a Procedures performed within an orifice on structures that are visible without the aid of any instrumentation are coded to the approac External.

Example: Resection of tonsils is coded to the approach External.

B5.3b Procedures performed indirectly by the application of external force through the intervening body layers are coded to the approac External.

Example: Closed reduction of fracture is coded to the approach External.

Percutaneous procedure via device

B5.4 Procedures performed percutaneously via a device placed for the procedure are coded to the approach Percutaneous.

Example: Fragmentation of kidney stone performed via percutaneous nephrostomy is coded to the approach Percutaneous.

B6. Device
General guidelines

B6.1a A device is coded only if a device remains after the procedure is completed. If no device remains, the device value No Device is coded

B6.1b Materials such as sutures, ligatures, radiological markers and temporary post-operative wound drains are considered integral to th performance of a procedure and are not coded as devices.

B6.1c Procedures performed on a device only and not on a body part are specified in the root operations Change, Irrigation, Removal an Revision, and are coded to the procedure performed.

Example: Irrigation of percutaneous nephrostomy tube is coded to the root operation Irrigation of indwelling device in the Administratio section.

Drainage device

B6.2 A separate procedure to put in a drainage device is coded to the root operation Drainage with the device value Drainage Device.

Brain

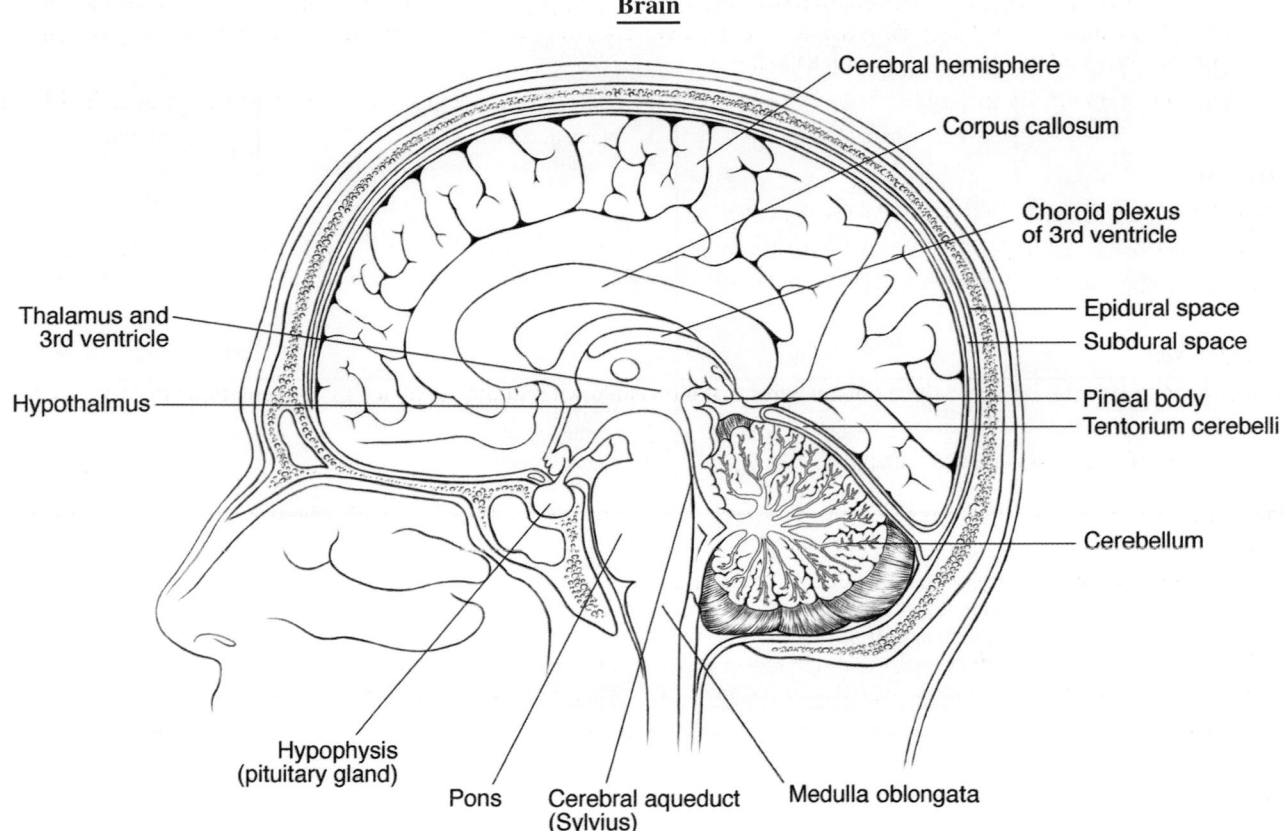

Cerebral hemisphere

Corpus callosum

Choroid plexus
of 3rd ventricle

Epidural space
Subdural space

Thalamus and
3rd ventricle

Hypothalmus

Pineal body
Tentorium cerebelli

Cerebellum

Hypophysis
(pituitary gland)

Pons

Cerebral aqueduct
(Sylvius)

Medulla oblongata

©AHIMA

Cranial Nerves

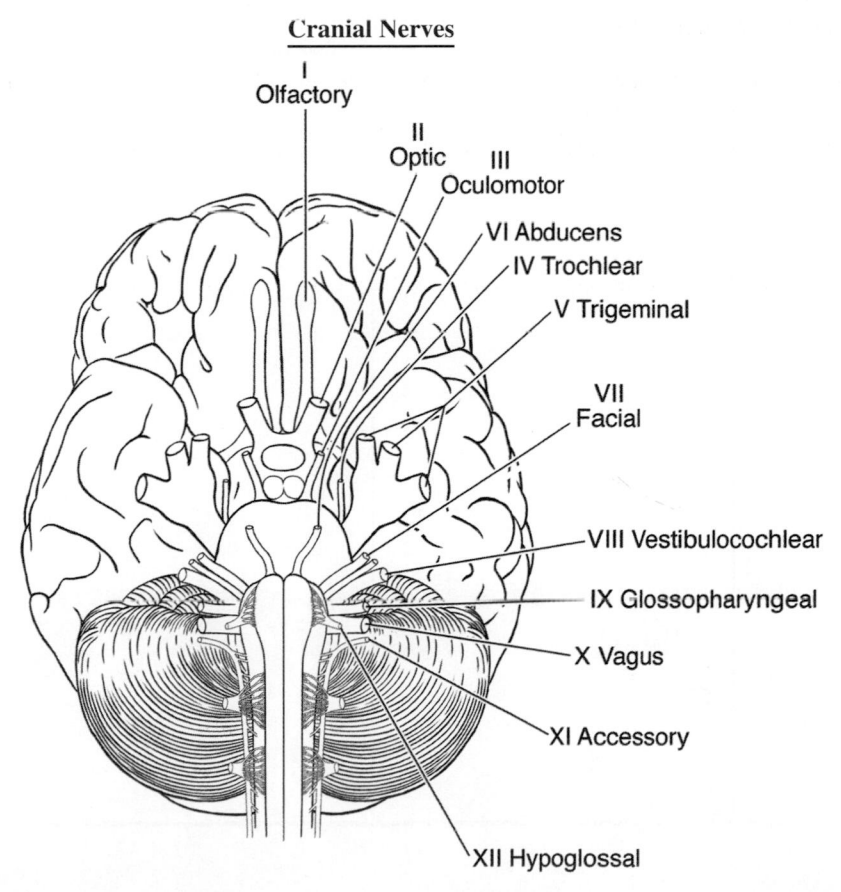

I
Olfactory

II
Optic

III
Oculomotor

VI Abducens

IV Trochlear

V Trigeminal

VII
Facial

VIII Vestibulocochlear

IX Glossopharyngeal

X Vagus

XI Accessory

XII Hypoglossal

©AHIMA

Central Nervous System Tables 001–00X

Section 0 **Medical and Surgical**
Body System 0 **Central Nervous System**
Operation 1 **Bypass:** Altering the route of passage of the contents of a tubular body part

Body Part (4ᵗʰ)	Approach (5ᵗʰ)	Device (6ᵗʰ)	Qualifier (7ᵗʰ)
6 Cerebral Ventricle	0 Open 3 Percutaneous	7 Autologous Tissue Substitute J Synthetic Substitute K Nonautologous Tissue Substitute	0 Nasopharynx 1 Mastoid Sinus 2 Atrium 3 Blood Vessel 4 Pleural Cavity 5 Intestine 6 Peritoneal Cavity 7 Urinary Tract 8 Bone Marrow B Cerebral Cisterns
U Spinal Canal	0 Open 3 Percutaneous	7 Autologous Tissue Substitute J Synthetic Substitute K Nonautologous Tissue Substitute	4 Pleural Cavity 6 Peritoneal Cavity 7 Urinary Tract 9 Fallopian Tube

Section 0 **Medical and Surgical**
Body System 0 **Central Nervous System**
Operation 2 **Change:** Taking out or off a device from a body part and putting back an identical or similar device in or on the same body part without cutting or puncturing the skin or a mucous membrane

Body Part (4ᵗʰ)	Approach (5ᵗʰ)	Device (6ᵗʰ)	Qualifier (7ᵗʰ)
0 Brain E Cranial Nerve U Spinal Canal	X External	0 Drainage Device Y Other Device	Z No Qualifier

Section 0 **Medical and Surgical**
Body System 0 **Central Nervous System**
Operation 5 **Destruction:** Physical eradication of all or a portion of a body part by the direct use of energy, force, or a destructive agent

Body Part (4ᵗʰ)	Approach (5ᵗʰ)	Device (6ᵗʰ)	Qualifier (7ᵗʰ)
0 Brain 1 Cerebral Meninges 2 Dura Mater 6 Cerebral Ventricle 7 Cerebral Hemisphere 8 Basal Ganglia 9 Thalamus A Hypothalamus B Pons C Cerebellum D Medulla Oblongata F Olfactory Nerve G Optic Nerve H Oculomotor Nerve J Trochlear Nerve K Trigeminal Nerve L Abducens Nerve M Facial Nerve N Acoustic Nerve P Glossopharyngeal Nerve Q Vagus Nerve R Accessory Nerve S Hypoglossal Nerve T Spinal Meninges W Cervical Spinal Cord X Thoracic Spinal Cord Y Lumbar Spinal Cord	0 Open 3 Percutaneous 4 Percutaneous Endoscopic	Z No Device	Z No Qualifier

Section	0	Medical and Surgical
Body System	0	Central Nervous System
Operation	8	**Division:** Cutting into a body part, without draining fluids and/or gases from the body part, in order to separate or transect a body part

Body Part (4th)	Approach (5th)	Device (6th)	Qualifier (7th)
0 Brain	0 Open	Z No Device	Z No Qualifier
7 Cerebral Hemisphere	3 Percutaneous		
8 Basal Ganglia	4 Percutaneous Endoscopic		
F Olfactory Nerve			
G Optic Nerve			
H Oculomotor Nerve			
J Trochlear Nerve			
K Trigeminal Nerve			
L Abducens Nerve			
M Facial Nerve			
N Acoustic Nerve			
P Glossopharyngeal Nerve			
Q Vagus Nerve			
R Accessory Nerve			
S Hypoglossal Nerve			
W Cervical Spinal Cord			
X Thoracic Spinal Cord			
Y Lumbar Spinal Cord			

Section	0	Medical and Surgical
Body System	0	Central Nervous System
Operation	9	**Drainage:** Taking or letting out fluids and/or gases from a body part

Body Part (4th)	Approach (5th)	Device (6th)	Qualifier (7th)
0 Brain	0 Open	0 Drainage Device	Z No Qualifier
1 Cerebral Meninges	3 Percutaneous		
2 Dura Mater	4 Percutaneous Endoscopic		
3 Epidural Space			
4 Subdural Space			
5 Subarachnoid Space			
6 Cerebral Ventricle			
7 Cerebral Hemisphere			
8 Basal Ganglia			
9 Thalamus			
A Hypothalamus			
B Pons			
C Cerebellum			
D Medulla Oblongata			
F Olfactory Nerve			
G Optic Nerve			
H Oculomotor Nerve			
J Trochlear Nerve			
K Trigeminal Nerve			
L Abducens Nerve			
M Facial Nerve			
N Acoustic Nerve			
P Glossopharyngeal Nerve			
Q Vagus Nerve			
R Accessory Nerve			
S Hypoglossal Nerve			
T Spinal Meninges			
U Spinal Canal			
W Cervical Spinal Cord			
X Thoracic Spinal Cord			
Y Lumbar Spinal Cord			

Continued →

Section	0	Medical and Surgical
Body System	0	Central Nervous System
Operation	9	**Drainage:** Taking or letting out fluids and/or gases from a body part

Body Part (4ᵗʰ)	Approach (5ᵗʰ)	Device (6ᵗʰ)	Qualifier (7ᵗʰ)
0 Brain	0 Open	Z No Device	X Diagnostic
1 Cerebral Meninges	3 Percutaneous		Z No Qualifier
2 Dura Mater	4 Percutaneous Endoscopic		
3 Epidural Space			
4 Subdural Space			
5 Subarachnoid Space			
6 Cerebral Ventricle			
7 Cerebral Hemisphere			
8 Basal Ganglia			
9 Thalamus			
A Hypothalamus			
B Pons			
C Cerebellum			
D Medulla Oblongata			
F Olfactory Nerve			
G Optic Nerve			
H Oculomotor Nerve			
J Trochlear Nerve			
K Trigeminal Nerve			
L Abducens Nerve			
M Facial Nerve			
N Acoustic Nerve			
P Glossopharyngeal Nerve			
Q Vagus Nerve			
R Accessory Nerve			
S Hypoglossal Nerve			
T Spinal Meninges			
U Spinal Canal			
W Cervical Spinal Cord			
X Thoracic Spinal Cord			
Y Lumbar Spinal Cord			

Section	0	Medical and Surgical
Body System	0	Central Nervous System
Operation	B	**Excision:** Cutting out or off, without replacement, a portion of a body part

Body Part (4ᵗʰ)	Approach (5ᵗʰ)	Device (6ᵗʰ)	Qualifier (7ᵗʰ)
0 Brain	0 Open	Z No Device	X Diagnostic
1 Cerebral Meninges	3 Percutaneous		Z No Qualifier
2 Dura Mater	4 Percutaneous Endoscopic		
6 Cerebral Ventricle			
7 Cerebral Hemisphere			
8 Basal Ganglia			
9 Thalamus			
A Hypothalamus			
B Pons			
C Cerebellum			
D Medulla Oblongata			
F Olfactory Nerve			
G Optic Nerve			
H Oculomotor Nerve			
J Trochlear Nerve			
K Trigeminal Nerve			
L Abducens Nerve			
M Facial Nerve			
N Acoustic Nerve			
P Glossopharyngeal Nerve			
Q Vagus Nerve			
R Accessory Nerve			
S Hypoglossal Nerve			
T Spinal Meninges			
W Cervical Spinal Cord			
X Thoracic Spinal Cord			
Y Lumbar Spinal Cord			

Section 0 **Medical and Surgical**
Body System 0 **Central Nervous System**
Operation C **Extirpation:** Taking or cutting out solid matter from a body part

Body Part (4th)	Approach (5th)	Device (6th)	Qualifier (7th)
0 Brain	0 Open	Z No Device	Z No Qualifier
1 Cerebral Meninges	3 Percutaneous		
2 Dura Mater	4 Percutaneous Endoscopic		
3 Epidural Space			
4 Subdural Space			
5 Subarachnoid Space			
6 Cerebral Ventricle			
7 Cerebral Hemisphere			
8 Basal Ganglia			
9 Thalamus			
A Hypothalamus			
B Pons			
C Cerebellum			
D Medulla Oblongata			
F Olfactory Nerve			
G Optic Nerve			
H Oculomotor Nerve			
J Trochlear Nerve			
K Trigeminal Nerve			
L Abducens Nerve			
M Facial Nerve			
N Acoustic Nerve			
P Glossopharyngeal Nerve			
Q Vagus Nerve			
R Accessory Nerve			
S Hypoglossal Nerve			
T Spinal Meninges			
W Cervical Spinal Cord			
X Thoracic Spinal Cord			
Y Lumbar Spinal Cord			

Section 0 **Medical and Surgical**
Body System 0 **Central Nervous System**
Operation D **Extraction:** Pulling or stripping out or off all or a portion of a body part by the use of force

Body Part (4th)	Approach (5th)	Device (6th)	Qualifier (7th)
1 Cerebral Meninges	0 Open	Z No Device	Z No Qualifier
2 Dura Mater	3 Percutaneous		
F Olfactory Nerve	4 Percutaneous Endoscopic		
G Optic Nerve			
H Oculomotor Nerve			
J Trochlear Nerve			
K Trigeminal Nerve			
L Abducens Nerve			
M Facial Nerve			
N Acoustic Nerve			
P Glossopharyngeal Nerve			
Q Vagus Nerve			
R Accessory Nerve			
S Hypoglossal Nerve			
T Spinal Meninges			

Section	0	Medical and Surgical
Body System	0	Central Nervous System
Operation	F	Fragmentation: Breaking solid matter in a body part into pieces

Body Part (4th)	Approach (5th)	Device (6th)	Qualifier (7th)
3 Epidural Space 4 Subdural Space 5 Subarachnoid Space 6 Cerebral Ventricle U Spinal Canal	0 Open 3 Percutaneous 4 Percutaneous Endoscopic X External	Z No Device	Z No Qualifier

Section	0	Medical and Surgical
Body System	0	Central Nervous System
Operation	H	Insertion: Putting in a nonbiological appliance that monitors, assists, performs, or prevents a physiological function but does not physically take the place of a body part

Body Part (4th)	Approach (5th)	Device (6th)	Qualifier (7th)
0 Brain 6 Cerebral Ventricle E Cranial Nerve U Spinal Canal V Spinal Cord	0 Open 3 Percutaneous 4 Percutaneous Endoscopic	2 Monitoring Device 3 Infusion Device M Neurostimulator Lead	Z No Qualifier

Section	0	Medical and Surgical
Body System	0	Central Nervous System
Operation	J	Inspection: Visually and/or manually exploring a body part

Body Part (4th)	Approach (5th)	Device (6th)	Qualifier (7th)
0 Brain E Cranial Nerve U Spinal Canal V Spinal Cord	0 Open 3 Percutaneous 4 Percutaneous Endoscopic	Z No Device	Z No Qualifier

Section	0	Medical and Surgical
Body System	0	Central Nervous System
Operation	K	Map: Locating the route of passage of electrical impulses and/or locating functional areas in a body part

Body Part (4th)	Approach (5th)	Device (6th)	Qualifier (7th)
0 Brain 7 Cerebral Hemisphere 8 Basal Ganglia 9 Thalamus A Hypothalamus B Pons C Cerebellum D Medulla Oblongata	0 Open 3 Percutaneous 4 Percutaneous Endoscopic	Z No Device	Z No Qualifier

Section | 0 | **Medical and Surgical**
Body System | 0 | **Central Nervous System**
Operation | N | **Release:** Freeing a body part from an abnormal physical constraint by cutting or by the use of force

Body Part (4th)	Approach (5th)	Device (6th)	Qualifier (7th)
0 Brain 1 Cerebral Meninges 2 Dura Mater 6 Cerebral Ventricle 7 Cerebral Hemisphere 8 Basal Ganglia 9 Thalamus A Hypothalamus B Pons C Cerebellum D Medulla Oblongata F Olfactory Nerve G Optic Nerve H Oculomotor Nerve J Trochlear Nerve K Trigeminal Nerve L Abducens Nerve M Facial Nerve N Acoustic Nerve P Glossopharyngeal Nerve Q Vagus Nerve R Accessory Nerve S Hypoglossal Nerve T Spinal Meninges W Cervical Spinal Cord X Thoracic Spinal Cord Y Lumbar Spinal Cord	0 Open 3 Percutaneous 4 Percutaneous Endoscopic	Z No Device	Z No Qualifier

Section | 0 | **Medical and Surgical**
Body System | 0 | **Central Nervous System**
Operation | P | **Removal:** Taking out or off a device from a body part

Body Part (4th)	Approach (5th)	Device (6th)	Qualifier (7th)
0 Brain V Spinal Cord	0 Open 3 Percutaneous 4 Percutaneous Endoscopic	0 Drainage Device 2 Monitoring Device 3 Infusion Device 7 Autologous Tissue Substitute J Synthetic Substitute K Nonautologous Tissue Substitute M Neurostimulator Lead	Z No Qualifier
0 Brain V Spinal Cord	X External	0 Drainage Device 2 Monitoring Device 3 Infusion Device M Neurostimulator Lead	Z No Qualifier
6 Cerebral Ventricle U Spinal Canal	0 Open 3 Percutaneous 4 Percutaneous Endoscopic	0 Drainage Device 2 Monitoring Device 3 Infusion Device J Synthetic Substitute M Neurostimulator Lead	Z No Qualifier
6 Cerebral Ventricle U Spinal Canal	X External	0 Drainage Device 2 Monitoring Device 3 Infusion Device M Neurostimulator Lead	Z No Qualifier
E Cranial Nerve	0 Open 3 Percutaneous 4 Percutaneous Endoscopic	0 Drainage Device 2 Monitoring Device 3 Infusion Device 7 Autologous Tissue Substitute M Neurostimulator Lead	Z No Qualifier

Continued →

Section	0	Medical and Surgical
Body System	0	Central Nervous System
Operation	P	Removal: Taking out or off a device from a body part

Body Part (4th)	Approach (5th)	Device (6th)	Qualifier (7th)
E Cranial Nerve	X External	0 Drainage Device 2 Monitoring Device 3 Infusion Device M Neurostimulator Lead	Z No Qualifier

Section	0	Medical and Surgical
Body System	0	Central Nervous System
Operation	Q	Repair: Restoring, to the extent possible, a body part to its normal anatomic structure and function

Body Part (4th)	Approach (5th)	Device (6th)	Qualifier (7th)
0 Brain 1 Cerebral Meninges 2 Dura Mater 6 Cerebral Ventricle 7 Cerebral Hemisphere 8 Basal Ganglia 9 Thalamus A Hypothalamus B Pons C Cerebellum D Medulla Oblongata F Olfactory Nerve G Optic Nerve H Oculomotor Nerve J Trochlear Nerve K Trigeminal Nerve L Abducens Nerve M Facial Nerve N Acoustic Nerve P Glossopharyngeal Nerve Q Vagus Nerve R Accessory Nerve S Hypoglossal Nerve T Spinal Meninges W Cervical Spinal Cord X Thoracic Spinal Cord Y Lumbar Spinal Cord	0 Open 3 Percutaneous 4 Percutaneous Endoscopic	Z No Device	Z No Qualifier

Section	0	Medical and Surgical
Body System	0	Central Nervous System
Operation	S	Reposition: Moving to its normal location, or other suitable location, all or a portion of a body part

Body Part (4th)	Approach (5th)	Device (6th)	Qualifier (7th)
F Olfactory Nerve G Optic Nerve H Oculomotor Nerve J Trochlear Nerve K Trigeminal Nerve L Abducens Nerve M Facial Nerve N Acoustic Nerve P Glossopharyngeal Nerve Q Vagus Nerve R Accessory Nerve S Hypoglossal Nerve W Cervical Spinal Cord X Thoracic Spinal Cord Y Lumbar Spinal Cord	0 Open 3 Percutaneous 4 Percutaneous Endoscopic	Z No Device	Z No Qualifier

Section	0	Medical and Surgical
Body System	0	Central Nervous System
Operation	T	**Resection:** Cutting out or off, without replacement, all of a body part

Body Part (4th)	Approach (5th)	Device (6th)	Qualifier (7th)
7 Cerebral Hemisphere	0 Open 3 Percutaneous 4 Percutaneous Endoscopic	Z No Device	Z No Qualifier

Section	0	Medical and Surgical
Body System	0	Central Nervous System
Operation	U	**Supplement:** Putting in or on biological or synthetic material that physically reinforces and/or augments the function of a portion of a body part

Body Part (4th)	Approach (5th)	Device (6th)	Qualifier (7th)
1 Cerebral Meninges 2 Dura Mater T Spinal Meninges	0 Open 3 Percutaneous 4 Percutaneous Endoscopic	7 Autologous Tissue Substitute J Synthetic Substitute K Nonautologous Tissue Substitute	Z No Qualifier
F Olfactory Nerve G Optic Nerve H Oculomotor Nerve J Trochlear Nerve K Trigeminal Nerve L Abducens Nerve M Facial Nerve N Acoustic Nerve P Glossopharyngeal Nerve Q Vagus Nerve R Accessory Nerve S Hypoglossal Nerve	0 Open 3 Percutaneous 4 Percutaneous Endoscopic	7 Autologous Tissue Substitute	Z No Qualifier

Section	0	Medical and Surgical
Body System	0	Central Nervous System
Operation	W	**Revision:** Correcting, to the extent possible, a portion of a malfunctioning device or the position of a displaced device

Body Part (4th)	Approach (5th)	Device (6th)	Qualifier (7th)
0 Brain V Spinal Cord	0 Open 3 Percutaneous 4 Percutaneous Endoscopic X External	0 Drainage Device 2 Monitoring Device 3 Infusion Device 7 Autologous Tissue Substitute J Synthetic Substitute K Nonautologous Tissue Substitute M Neurostimulator Lead	Z No Qualifier
6 Cerebral Ventricle U Spinal Canal	0 Open 3 Percutaneous 4 Percutaneous Endoscopic X External	0 Drainage Device 2 Monitoring Device 3 Infusion Device J Synthetic Substitute M Neurostimulator Lead	Z No Qualifier
E Cranial Nerve	0 Open 3 Percutaneous 4 Percutaneous Endoscopic X External	0 Drainage Device 2 Monitoring Device 3 Infusion Device 7 Autologous Tissue Substitute M Neurostimulator Lead	Z No Qualifier

Section	0	Medical and Surgical
Body System	0	Central Nervous System
Operation	X	**Transfer:** Moving, without taking out, all or a portion of a body part to another location to take over the function of all or a portion of a body part

Body Part (4th)	Approach (5th)	Device (6th)	Qualifier (7th)
F Olfactory Nerve G Optic Nerve H Oculomotor Nerve J Trochlear Nerve K Trigeminal Nerve L Abducens Nerve M Facial Nerve N Acoustic Nerve P Glossopharyngeal Nerve Q Vagus Nerve R Accessory Nerve S Hypoglossal Nerve	0 Open 4 Percutaneous Endoscopic	Z No Device	F Olfactory Nerve G Optic Nerve H Oculomotor Nerve J Trochlear Nerve K Trigeminal Nerve L Abducens Nerve M Facial Nerve N Acoustic Nerve P Glossopharyngeal Nerve Q Vagus Nerve R Accessory Nerve S Hypoglossal Nerve

Central Nervous System Code Listing 001–00X

001 – Central Nervous System, Bypass

Review Coding Guideline B3.6a

0016070 Bypass Cerebral Ventricle to Nasopharynx with Autologous Tissue Substitute, Open Approach

0016071 Bypass Cerebral Ventricle to Mastoid Sinus with Autologous Tissue Substitute, Open Approach

0016072 Bypass Cerebral Ventricle to Atrium with Autologous Tissue Substitute, Open Approach

0016073 Bypass Cerebral Ventricle to Blood Vessel with Autologous Tissue Substitute, Open Approach

0016074 Bypass Cerebral Ventricle to Pleural Cavity with Autologous Tissue Substitute, Open Approach

0016075 Bypass Cerebral Ventricle to Intestine with Autologous Tissue Substitute, Open Approach

0016076 Bypass Cerebral Ventricle to Peritoneal Cavity with Autologous Tissue Substitute, Open Approach

0016077 Bypass Cerebral Ventricle to Urinary Tract with Autologous Tissue Substitute, Open Approach

0016078 Bypass Cerebral Ventricle to Bone Marrow with Autologous Tissue Substitute, Open Approach

001607B Bypass Cerebral Ventricle to Cerebral Cisterns with Autologous Tissue Substitute, Open Approach

00160J0 Bypass Cerebral Ventricle to Nasopharynx with Synthetic Substitute, Open Approach

00160J1 Bypass Cerebral Ventricle to Mastoid Sinus with Synthetic Substitute, Open Approach

00160J2 Bypass Cerebral Ventricle to Atrium with Synthetic Substitute, Open Approach

00160J3 Bypass Cerebral Ventricle to Blood Vessel with Synthetic Substitute, Open Approach

00160J4 Bypass Cerebral Ventricle to Pleural Cavity with Synthetic Substitute, Open Approach

00160J5 Bypass Cerebral Ventricle to Intestine with Synthetic Substitute, Open Approach

00160J6 Bypass Cerebral Ventricle to Peritoneal Cavity with Synthetic Substitute, Open Approach

00160J7 Bypass Cerebral Ventricle to Urinary Tract with Synthetic Substitute, Open Approach

00160J8 Bypass Cerebral Ventricle to Bone Marrow with Synthetic Substitute, Open Approach

00160JB Bypass Cerebral Ventricle to Cerebral Cisterns with Synthetic Substitute, Open Approach

00160K0 Bypass Cerebral Ventricle to Nasopharynx with Nonautologous Tissue Substitute, Open Approach

00160K1 Bypass Cerebral Ventricle to Mastoid Sinus with Nonautologous Tissue Substitute, Open Approach

00160K2 Bypass Cerebral Ventricle to Atrium with Nonautologous Tissue Substitute, Open Approach

00160K3 Bypass Cerebral Ventricle to Blood Vessel with Nonautologous Tissue Substitute, Open Approach

00160K4 Bypass Cerebral Ventricle to Pleural Cavity with Nonautologous Tissue Substitute, Open Approach

00160K5 Bypass Cerebral Ventricle to Intestine with Nonautologous Tissue Substitute, Open Approach

00160K6 Bypass Cerebral Ventricle to Peritoneal Cavity with Nonautologous Tissue Substitute, Open Approach

00160K7 Bypass Cerebral Ventricle to Urinary Tract with Nonautologous Tissue Substitute, Open Approach

00160K8 Bypass Cerebral Ventricle to Bone Marrow with Nonautologous Tissue Substitute, Open Approach

00160KB Bypass Cerebral Ventricle to Cerebral Cisterns with Nonautologous Tissue Substitute, Open Approach

0016370 Bypass Cerebral Ventricle to Nasopharynx with Autologous Tissue Substitute, Percutaneous Approach

0016371 Bypass Cerebral Ventricle to Mastoid Sinus with Autologous Tissue Substitute, Percutaneous Approach

0016372 Bypass Cerebral Ventricle to Atrium with Autologous Tissue Substitute, Percutaneous Approach

0016373 Bypass Cerebral Ventricle to Blood Vessel with Autologous Tissue Substitute, Percutaneous Approach

0016374 Bypass Cerebral Ventricle to Pleural Cavity with Autologous Tissue Substitute, Percutaneous Approach

0016375 Bypass Cerebral Ventricle to Intestine with Autologous Tissue Substitute, Percutaneous Approach

0016376 Bypass Cerebral Ventricle to Peritoneal Cavity with Autologous Tissue Substitute, Percutaneous Approach

0016377 Bypass Cerebral Ventricle to Urinary Tract with Autologous Tissue Substitute, Percutaneous Approach

0016378 Bypass Cerebral Ventricle to Bone Marrow with Autologous Tissue Substitute, Percutaneous Approach

001637B Bypass Cerebral Ventricle to Cerebral Cisterns with Autologous Tissue Substitute, Percutaneous Approach

00163J0 Bypass Cerebral Ventricle to Nasopharynx with Synthetic Substitute, Percutaneous Approach

00163J1 Bypass Cerebral Ventricle to Mastoid Sinus with Synthetic Substitute, Percutaneous Approach

00163J2 Bypass Cerebral Ventricle to Atrium with Synthetic Substitute, Percutaneous Approach

00163J3 Bypass Cerebral Ventricle to Blood Vessel with Synthetic Substitute, Percutaneous Approach

00163J4 Bypass Cerebral Ventricle to Pleural Cavity with Synthetic Substitute, Percutaneous Approach

00163J5 Bypass Cerebral Ventricle to Intestine with Synthetic Substitute, Percutaneous Approach

00163J6 Bypass Cerebral Ventricle to Peritoneal Cavity with Synthetic Substitute, Percutaneous Approach
AHA CC: 2Q, 2013, 36-37

00163J7 Bypass Cerebral Ventricle to Urinary Tract with Synthetic Substitute, Percutaneous Approach

00163J8 Bypass Cerebral Ventricle to Bone Marrow with Synthetic Substitute, Percutaneous Approach

00163JB Bypass Cerebral Ventricle to Cerebral Cisterns with Synthetic Substitute, Percutaneous Approach

00163K0 Bypass Cerebral Ventricle to Nasopharynx with Nonautologous Tissue Substitute, Percutaneous Approach

0163K1   Bypass Cerebral Ventricle to Mastoid Sinus with Nonautologous Tissue Substitute, Percutaneous Approach

0163K2   Bypass Cerebral Ventricle to Atrium with Nonautologous Tissue Substitute, Percutaneous Approach

0163K3   Bypass Cerebral Ventricle to Blood Vessel with Nonautologous Tissue Substitute, Percutaneous Approach

0163K4   Bypass Cerebral Ventricle to Pleural Cavity with Nonautologous Tissue Substitute, Percutaneous Approach

0163K5   Bypass Cerebral Ventricle to Intestine with Nonautologous Tissue Substitute, Percutaneous Approach

0163K6   Bypass Cerebral Ventricle to Peritoneal Cavity with Nonautologous Tissue Substitute, Percutaneous Approach

0163K7   Bypass Cerebral Ventricle to Urinary Tract with Nonautologous Tissue Substitute, Percutaneous Approach

0163K8   Bypass Cerebral Ventricle to Bone Marrow with Nonautologous Tissue Substitute, Percutaneous Approach

0163KB   Bypass Cerebral Ventricle to Cerebral Cisterns with Nonautologous Tissue Substitute, Percutaneous Approach

01U074   Bypass Spinal Canal to Pleural Cavity with Autologous Tissue Substitute, Open Approach

01U076   Bypass Spinal Canal to Peritoneal Cavity with Autologous Tissue Substitute, Open Approach

001U077   Bypass Spinal Canal to Urinary Tract with Autologous Tissue Substitute, Open Approach

001U079   Bypass Spinal Canal to Fallopian Tube with Autologous Tissue Substitute, Open Approach

001U0J4   Bypass Spinal Canal to Pleural Cavity with Synthetic Substitute, Open Approach

001U0J6   Bypass Spinal Canal to Peritoneal Cavity with Synthetic Substitute, Open Approach

001U0J7   Bypass Spinal Canal to Urinary Tract with Synthetic Substitute, Open Approach

001U0J9   Bypass Spinal Canal to Fallopian Tube with Synthetic Substitute, Open Approach

001U0K4   Bypass Spinal Canal to Pleural Cavity with Nonautologous Tissue Substitute, Open Approach

001U0K6   Bypass Spinal Canal to Peritoneal Cavity with Nonautologous Tissue Substitute, Open Approach

001U0K7   Bypass Spinal Canal to Urinary Tract with Nonautologous Tissue Substitute, Open Approach

001U0K9   Bypass Spinal Canal to Fallopian Tube with Nonautologous Tissue Substitute, Open Approach

001U374   Bypass Spinal Canal to Pleural Cavity with Autologous Tissue Substitute, Percutaneous Approach

001U376   Bypass Spinal Canal to Peritoneal Cavity with Autologous Tissue Substitute, Percutaneous Approach

001U377   Bypass Spinal Canal to Urinary Tract with Autologous Tissue Substitute, Percutaneous Approach

001U379   Bypass Spinal Canal to Fallopian Tube with Autologous Tissue Substitute, Percutaneous Approach

001U3J4   Bypass Spinal Canal to Pleural Cavity with Synthetic Substitute, Percutaneous Approach

001U3J6   Bypass Spinal Canal to Peritoneal Cavity with Synthetic Substitute, Percutaneous Approach

001U3J7   Bypass Spinal Canal to Urinary Tract with Synthetic Substitute, Percutaneous Approach

001U3J9   Bypass Spinal Canal to Fallopian Tube with Synthetic Substitute, Percutaneous Approach

001U3K4   Bypass Spinal Canal to Pleural Cavity with Nonautologous Tissue Substitute, Percutaneous Approach

001U3K6   Bypass Spinal Canal to Peritoneal Cavity with Nonautologous Tissue Substitute, Percutaneous Approach

001U3K7   Bypass Spinal Canal to Urinary Tract with Nonautologous Tissue Substitute, Percutaneous Approach

001U3K9   Bypass Spinal Canal to Fallopian Tube with Nonautologous Tissue Substitute, Percutaneous Approach

002 – Central Nervous System, Change

Review Coding Guideline B6.1c

020X0Z   Change Drainage Device in Brain, External Approach

020XYZ   Change Other Device in Brain, External Approach

002EX0Z   Change Drainage Device in Cranial Nerve, External Approach

002EXYZ   Change Other Device in Cranial Nerve, External Approach

002UX0Z   Change Drainage Device in Spinal Canal, External Approach

002UXYZ   Change Other Device in Spinal Canal, External Approach

005 – Central Nervous System, Destruction

0500ZZ   Destruction of Brain, Open Approach

0503ZZ   Destruction of Brain, Percutaneous Approach

0504ZZ   Destruction of Brain, Percutaneous Endoscopic Approach

0510ZZ   Destruction of Cerebral Meninges, Open Approach

0513ZZ   Destruction of Cerebral Meninges, Percutaneous Approach

0514ZZ   Destruction of Cerebral Meninges, Percutaneous Endoscopic Approach

0520ZZ   Destruction of Dura Mater, Open Approach

0523ZZ   Destruction of Dura Mater, Percutaneous Approach

0524ZZ   Destruction of Dura Mater, Percutaneous Endoscopic Approach

0560ZZ   Destruction of Cerebral Ventricle, Open Approach

0563ZZ   Destruction of Cerebral Ventricle, Percutaneous Approach

0564ZZ   Destruction of Cerebral Ventricle, Percutaneous Endoscopic Approach

0570ZZ   Destruction of Cerebral Hemisphere, Open Approach

0573ZZ   Destruction of Cerebral Hemisphere, Percutaneous Approach

0574ZZ   Destruction of Cerebral Hemisphere, Percutaneous Endoscopic Approach

0580ZZ   Destruction of Basal Ganglia, Open Approach

0583ZZ   Destruction of Basal Ganglia, Percutaneous Approach

00584ZZ   Destruction of Basal Ganglia, Percutaneous Endoscopic Approach

00590ZZ   Destruction of Thalamus, Open Approach

00593ZZ   Destruction of Thalamus, Percutaneous Approach

00594ZZ   Destruction of Thalamus, Percutaneous Endoscopic Approach

005A0ZZ   Destruction of Hypothalamus, Open Approach

005A3ZZ   Destruction of Hypothalamus, Percutaneous Approach

005A4ZZ   Destruction of Hypothalamus, Percutaneous Endoscopic Approach

005B0ZZ   Destruction of Pons, Open Approach

005B3ZZ   Destruction of Pons, Percutaneous Approach

005B4ZZ   Destruction of Pons, Percutaneous Endoscopic Approach

005C0ZZ   Destruction of Cerebellum, Open Approach

005C3ZZ   Destruction of Cerebellum, Percutaneous Approach

005C4ZZ   Destruction of Cerebellum, Percutaneous Endoscopic Approach

005D0ZZ   Destruction of Medulla Oblongata, Open Approach

005D3ZZ   Destruction of Medulla Oblongata, Percutaneous Approach

005D4ZZ   Destruction of Medulla Oblongata, Percutaneous Endoscopic Approach

005F0ZZ   Destruction of Olfactory Nerve, Open Approach

005F3ZZ   Destruction of Olfactory Nerve, Percutaneous Approach

005F4ZZ   Destruction of Olfactory Nerve, Percutaneous Endoscopic Approach

005G0ZZ   Destruction of Optic Nerve, Open Approach

005G3ZZ   Destruction of Optic Nerve, Percutaneous Approach

005G4ZZ   Destruction of Optic Nerve, Percutaneous Endoscopic Approach

005H0ZZ   Destruction of Oculomotor Nerve, Open Approach

005H3ZZ   Destruction of Oculomotor Nerve, Percutaneous Approach

005H4ZZ   Destruction of Oculomotor Nerve, Percutaneous Endoscopic Approach

005J0ZZ   Destruction of Trochlear Nerve, Open Approach

005J3ZZ   Destruction of Trochlear Nerve, Percutaneous Approach

005J4ZZ   Destruction of Trochlear Nerve, Percutaneous Endoscopic Approach

005K0ZZ   Destruction of Trigeminal Nerve, Open Approach

005K3ZZ   Destruction of Trigeminal Nerve, Percutaneous Approach

005K4ZZ   Destruction of Trigeminal Nerve, Percutaneous Endoscopic Approach

005L0ZZ   Destruction of Abducens Nerve, Open Approach

005L3ZZ   Destruction of Abducens Nerve, Percutaneous Approach

Female-only   ♂ Male-only   ▲ Limited Coverage   ● Non-OR   ■ HAC-associated procedure   ▲ Non-covered procedures   ✚ Combination

005L4ZZ	Destruction of Abducens Nerve, Percutaneous Endoscopic Approach	005Q3ZZ	Destruction of Vagus Nerve, Percutaneous Approach	005W0ZZ	Destruction of Cervical Spinal Cord, Open Approach
005M0ZZ	Destruction of Facial Nerve, Open Approach	005Q4ZZ	Destruction of Vagus Nerve, Percutaneous Endoscopic Approach	005W3ZZ	Destruction of Cervical Spinal Cord, Percutaneous Approach
005M3ZZ	Destruction of Facial Nerve, Percutaneous Approach	005R0ZZ	Destruction of Accessory Nerve, Open Approach	005W4ZZ	Destruction of Cervical Spinal Cord, Percutaneous Endoscopic Approach
005M4ZZ	Destruction of Facial Nerve, Percutaneous Endoscopic Approach	005R3ZZ	Destruction of Accessory Nerve, Percutaneous Approach	005X0ZZ	Destruction of Thoracic Spinal Cord, Open Approach
005N0ZZ	Destruction of Acoustic Nerve, Open Approach	005R4ZZ	Destruction of Accessory Nerve, Percutaneous Endoscopic Approach	005X3ZZ	Destruction of Thoracic Spinal Cord, Percutaneous Approach
005N3ZZ	Destruction of Acoustic Nerve, Percutaneous Approach	005S0ZZ	Destruction of Hypoglossal Nerve, Open Approach	005X4ZZ	Destruction of Thoracic Spinal Cord, Percutaneous Endoscopic Approach
005N4ZZ	Destruction of Acoustic Nerve, Percutaneous Endoscopic Approach	005S3ZZ	Destruction of Hypoglossal Nerve, Percutaneous Approach	005Y0ZZ	Destruction of Lumbar Spinal Cord, Open Approach
005P0ZZ	Destruction of Glossopharyngeal Nerve, Open Approach	005S4ZZ	Destruction of Hypoglossal Nerve, Percutaneous Endoscopic Approach	005Y3ZZ	Destruction of Lumbar Spinal Cord, Percutaneous Approach
005P3ZZ	Destruction of Glossopharyngeal Nerve, Percutaneous Approach	005T0ZZ	Destruction of Spinal Meninges, Open Approach	005Y4ZZ	Destruction of Lumbar Spinal Cord, Percutaneous Endoscopic Approach
005P4ZZ	Destruction of Glossopharyngeal Nerve, Percutaneous Endoscopic Approach	005T3ZZ	Destruction of Spinal Meninges, Percutaneous Approach		
005Q0ZZ	Destruction of Vagus Nerve, Open Approach	005T4ZZ	Destruction of Spinal Meninges, Percutaneous Endoscopic Approach		

008 – Central Nervous System, Division

Review Coding Guideline B3.14

00800ZZ	Division of Brain, Open Approach	008J3ZZ	Division of Trochlear Nerve, Percutaneous Approach	008Q3ZZ	Division of Vagus Nerve, Percutaneous Approach
00803ZZ	Division of Brain, Percutaneous Approach	008J4ZZ	Division of Trochlear Nerve, Percutaneous Endoscopic Approach	008Q4ZZ	Division of Vagus Nerve, Percutaneous Endoscopic Approach
00804ZZ	Division of Brain, Percutaneous Endoscopic Approach	008K0ZZ	Division of Trigeminal Nerve, Open Approach	008R0ZZ	Division of Accessory Nerve, Open Approach
00870ZZ	Division of Cerebral Hemisphere, Open Approach	008K3ZZ	Division of Trigeminal Nerve, Percutaneous Approach	008R3ZZ	Division of Accessory Nerve, Percutaneous Approach
00873ZZ	Division of Cerebral Hemisphere, Percutaneous Approach	008K4ZZ	Division of Trigeminal Nerve, Percutaneous Endoscopic Approach	008R4ZZ	Division of Accessory Nerve, Percutaneous Endoscopic Approach
00874ZZ	Division of Cerebral Hemisphere, Percutaneous Endoscopic Approach	008L0ZZ	Division of Abducens Nerve, Open Approach	008S0ZZ	Division of Hypoglossal Nerve, Open Approach
00880ZZ	Division of Basal Ganglia, Open Approach	008L3ZZ	Division of Abducens Nerve, Percutaneous Approach	008S3ZZ	Division of Hypoglossal Nerve, Percutaneous Approach
00883ZZ	Division of Basal Ganglia, Percutaneous Approach	008L4ZZ	Division of Abducens Nerve, Percutaneous Endoscopic Approach	008S4ZZ	Division of Hypoglossal Nerve, Percutaneous Endoscopic Approach
00884ZZ	Division of Basal Ganglia, Percutaneous Endoscopic Approach	008M0ZZ	Division of Facial Nerve, Open Approach	008W0ZZ	Division of Cervical Spinal Cord, Open Approach
008F0ZZ	Division of Olfactory Nerve, Open Approach	008M3ZZ	Division of Facial Nerve, Percutaneous Approach	008W3ZZ	Division of Cervical Spinal Cord, Percutaneous Approach
008F3ZZ	Division of Olfactory Nerve, Percutaneous Approach	008M4ZZ	Division of Facial Nerve, Percutaneous Endoscopic Approach	008W4ZZ	Division of Cervical Spinal Cord, Percutaneous Endoscopic Approach
008F4ZZ	Division of Olfactory Nerve, Percutaneous Endoscopic Approach	008N0ZZ	Division of Acoustic Nerve, Open Approach	008X0ZZ	Division of Thoracic Spinal Cord, Open Approach
008G0ZZ	Division of Optic Nerve, Open Approach	008N3ZZ	Division of Acoustic Nerve, Percutaneous Approach	008X3ZZ	Division of Thoracic Spinal Cord, Percutaneous Approach
008G3ZZ	Division of Optic Nerve, Percutaneous Approach	008N4ZZ	Division of Acoustic Nerve, Percutaneous Endoscopic Approach	008X4ZZ	Division of Thoracic Spinal Cord, Percutaneous Endoscopic Approach
008G4ZZ	Division of Optic Nerve, Percutaneous Endoscopic Approach	008P0ZZ	Division of Glossopharyngeal Nerve, Open Approach	008Y0ZZ	Division of Lumbar Spinal Cord, Open Approach
008H0ZZ	Division of Oculomotor Nerve, Open Approach	008P3ZZ	Division of Glossopharyngeal Nerve, Percutaneous Approach	008Y3ZZ	Division of Lumbar Spinal Cord, Percutaneous Approach
008H3ZZ	Division of Oculomotor Nerve, Percutaneous Approach	008P4ZZ	Division of Glossopharyngeal Nerve, Percutaneous Endoscopic Approach	008Y4ZZ	Division of Lumbar Spinal Cord, Percutaneous Endoscopic Approach
008H4ZZ	Division of Oculomotor Nerve, Percutaneous Endoscopic Approach	008Q0ZZ	Division of Vagus Nerve, Open Approach		
008J0ZZ	Division of Trochlear Nerve, Open Approach				

009 – Central Nervous System, Drainage

Review Coding Guidelines B3.4a and B3.4b

Review Coding Guideline B6.2

009000Z	Drainage of Brain with Drainage Device, Open Approach	009040Z	Drainage of Brain with Drainage Device, Percutaneous Endoscopic Approach	00910ZX	Drainage of Cerebral Meninges, Open Approach, Diagnostic
00900ZX	Drainage of Brain, Open Approach, Diagnostic			00910ZZ	Drainage of Cerebral Meninges, Open Approach
00900ZZ	Drainage of Brain, Open Approach	00904ZX	Drainage of Brain, Percutaneous Endoscopic Approach, Diagnostic	009130Z	Drainage of Cerebral Meninges with Drainage Device, Percutaneous Approach
009030Z	Drainage of Brain with Drainage Device, Percutaneous Approach	00904ZZ	Drainage of Brain, Percutaneous Endoscopic Approach	00913ZX	Drainage of Cerebral Meninges, Percutaneous Approach, Diagnostic
00903ZX	Drainage of Brain, Percutaneous Approach, Diagnostic	009100Z	Drainage of Cerebral Meninges with Drainage Device, Open Approach	00913ZZ	Drainage of Cerebral Meninges, Percutaneous Approach
00903ZZ	Drainage of Brain, Percutaneous Approach				

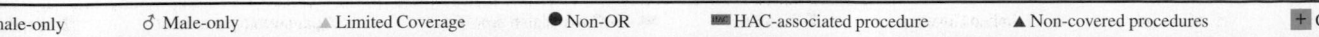

♀ Female-only   ♂ Male-only   ▲ Limited Coverage   ● Non-OR   ▨ HAC-associated procedure   ▲ Non-covered procedures   ✚ Combinatio

009140Z Drainage of Cerebral Meninges with Drainage Device, Percutaneous Endoscopic Approach

00914ZX Drainage of Cerebral Meninges, Percutaneous Endoscopic Approach, Diagnostic

00914ZZ Drainage of Cerebral Meninges, Percutaneous Endoscopic Approach

009200Z Drainage of Dura Mater with Drainage Device, Open Approach

00920ZX Drainage of Dura Mater, Open Approach, Diagnostic

00920ZZ Drainage of Dura Mater, Open Approach

009230Z Drainage of Dura Mater with Drainage Device, Percutaneous Approach

00923ZX Drainage of Dura Mater, Percutaneous Approach, Diagnostic

00923ZZ Drainage of Dura Mater, Percutaneous Approach

009240Z Drainage of Dura Mater with Drainage Device, Percutaneous Endoscopic Approach

00924ZX Drainage of Dura Mater, Percutaneous Endoscopic Approach, Diagnostic

00924ZZ Drainage of Dura Mater, Percutaneous Endoscopic Approach

009300Z Drainage of Epidural Space with Drainage Device, Open Approach

00930ZX Drainage of Epidural Space, Open Approach, Diagnostic

00930ZZ Drainage of Epidural Space, Open Approach

009330Z Drainage of Epidural Space with Drainage Device, Percutaneous Approach

00933ZX Drainage of Epidural Space, Percutaneous Approach, Diagnostic

00933ZZ Drainage of Epidural Space, Percutaneous Approach

009340Z Drainage of Epidural Space with Drainage Device, Percutaneous Endoscopic Approach

00934ZX Drainage of Epidural Space, Percutaneous Endoscopic Approach, Diagnostic

00934ZZ Drainage of Epidural Space, Percutaneous Endoscopic Approach

009400Z Drainage of Subdural Space with Drainage Device, Open Approach

00940ZX Drainage of Subdural Space, Open Approach, Diagnostic

00940ZZ Drainage of Subdural Space, Open Approach

009430Z Drainage of Subdural Space with Drainage Device, Percutaneous Approach

00943ZX Drainage of Subdural Space, Percutaneous Approach, Diagnostic

00943ZZ Drainage of Subdural Space, Percutaneous Approach

009440Z Drainage of Subdural Space with Drainage Device, Percutaneous Endoscopic Approach

00944ZX Drainage of Subdural Space, Percutaneous Endoscopic Approach, Diagnostic

00944ZZ Drainage of Subdural Space, Percutaneous Endoscopic Approach

009500Z Drainage of Subarachnoid Space with Drainage Device, Open Approach

00950ZX Drainage of Subarachnoid Space, Open Approach, Diagnostic

00950ZZ Drainage of Subarachnoid Space, Open Approach

009530Z Drainage of Subarachnoid Space with Drainage Device, Percutaneous Approach

00953ZX Drainage of Subarachnoid Space, Percutaneous Approach, Diagnostic

00953ZZ Drainage of Subarachnoid Space, Percutaneous Approach

009540Z Drainage of Subarachnoid Space with Drainage Device, Percutaneous Endoscopic Approach

00954ZX Drainage of Subarachnoid Space, Percutaneous Endoscopic Approach, Diagnostic

00954ZZ Drainage of Subarachnoid Space, Percutaneous Endoscopic Approach

009600Z Drainage of Cerebral Ventricle with Drainage Device, Open Approach

00960ZX Drainage of Cerebral Ventricle, Open Approach, Diagnostic

00960ZZ Drainage of Cerebral Ventricle, Open Approach

009630Z Drainage of Cerebral Ventricle with Drainage Device, Percutaneous Approach

00963ZX Drainage of Cerebral Ventricle, Percutaneous Approach, Diagnostic

00963ZZ Drainage of Cerebral Ventricle, Percutaneous Approach

009640Z Drainage of Cerebral Ventricle with Drainage Device, Percutaneous Endoscopic Approach

00964ZX Drainage of Cerebral Ventricle, Percutaneous Endoscopic Approach, Diagnostic

00964ZZ Drainage of Cerebral Ventricle, Percutaneous Endoscopic Approach

009700Z Drainage of Cerebral Hemisphere with Drainage Device, Open Approach

00970ZX Drainage of Cerebral Hemisphere, Open Approach, Diagnostic

00970ZZ Drainage of Cerebral Hemisphere, Open Approach

009730Z Drainage of Cerebral Hemisphere with Drainage Device, Percutaneous Approach

00973ZX Drainage of Cerebral Hemisphere, Percutaneous Approach, Diagnostic

00973ZZ Drainage of Cerebral Hemisphere, Percutaneous Approach

009740Z Drainage of Cerebral Hemisphere with Drainage Device, Percutaneous Endoscopic Approach

00974ZX Drainage of Cerebral Hemisphere, Percutaneous Endoscopic Approach, Diagnostic

00974ZZ Drainage of Cerebral Hemisphere, Percutaneous Endoscopic Approach

009800Z Drainage of Basal Ganglia with Drainage Device, Open Approach

00980ZX Drainage of Basal Ganglia, Open Approach, Diagnostic

00980ZZ Drainage of Basal Ganglia, Open Approach

009830Z Drainage of Basal Ganglia with Drainage Device, Percutaneous Approach

00983ZX Drainage of Basal Ganglia, Percutaneous Approach, Diagnostic

00983ZZ Drainage of Basal Ganglia, Percutaneous Approach

009840Z Drainage of Basal Ganglia with Drainage Device, Percutaneous Endoscopic Approach

00984ZX Drainage of Basal Ganglia, Percutaneous Endoscopic Approach, Diagnostic

00984ZZ Drainage of Basal Ganglia, Percutaneous Endoscopic Approach

009900Z Drainage of Thalamus with Drainage Device, Open Approach

00990ZX Drainage of Thalamus, Open Approach, Diagnostic

00990ZZ Drainage of Thalamus, Open Approach

009930Z Drainage of Thalamus with Drainage Device, Percutaneous Approach

00993ZX Drainage of Thalamus, Percutaneous Approach, Diagnostic

00993ZZ Drainage of Thalamus, Percutaneous Approach

009940Z Drainage of Thalamus with Drainage Device, Percutaneous Endoscopic Approach

00994ZX Drainage of Thalamus, Percutaneous Endoscopic Approach, Diagnostic

00994ZZ Drainage of Thalamus, Percutaneous Endoscopic Approach

009A00Z Drainage of Hypothalamus with Drainage Device, Open Approach

009A0ZX Drainage of Hypothalamus, Open Approach, Diagnostic

009A0ZZ Drainage of Hypothalamus, Open Approach

009A30Z Drainage of Hypothalamus with Drainage Device, Percutaneous Approach

009A3ZX Drainage of Hypothalamus, Percutaneous Approach, Diagnostic

009A3ZZ Drainage of Hypothalamus, Percutaneous Approach

009A40Z Drainage of Hypothalamus with Drainage Device, Percutaneous Endoscopic Approach

009A4ZX Drainage of Hypothalamus, Percutaneous Endoscopic Approach, Diagnostic

009A4ZZ Drainage of Hypothalamus, Percutaneous Endoscopic Approach

009B00Z Drainage of Pons with Drainage Device, Open Approach

009B0ZX Drainage of Pons, Open Approach, Diagnostic

009B0ZZ Drainage of Pons, Open Approach

009B30Z Drainage of Pons with Drainage Device, Percutaneous Approach

009B3ZX Drainage of Pons, Percutaneous Approach, Diagnostic

009B3ZZ Drainage of Pons, Percutaneous Approach

009B40Z Drainage of Pons with Drainage Device, Percutaneous Endoscopic Approach

009B4ZX Drainage of Pons, Percutaneous Endoscopic Approach, Diagnostic

009B4ZZ Drainage of Pons, Percutaneous Endoscopic Approach

009C00Z Drainage of Cerebellum with Drainage Device, Open Approach

009C0ZX Drainage of Cerebellum, Open Approach, Diagnostic

009C0ZZ Drainage of Cerebellum, Open Approach

009C30Z Drainage of Cerebellum with Drainage Device, Percutaneous Approach

009C3ZX Drainage of Cerebellum, Percutaneous Approach, Diagnostic

009C3ZZ Drainage of Cerebellum, Percutaneous Approach

009C40Z Drainage of Cerebellum with Drainage Device, Percutaneous Endoscopic Approach

009C4ZX Drainage of Cerebellum, Percutaneous Endoscopic Approach, Diagnostic

009C4ZZ Drainage of Cerebellum, Percutaneous Endoscopic Approach

009D00Z Drainage of Medulla Oblongata with Drainage Device, Open Approach

009D0ZX Drainage of Medulla Oblongata, Open Approach, Diagnostic

009D0ZZ Drainage of Medulla Oblongata, Open Approach

009D30Z Drainage of Medulla Oblongata with Drainage Device, Percutaneous Approach

009D3ZX Drainage of Medulla Oblongata, Percutaneous Approach, Diagnostic

009D3ZZ Drainage of Medulla Oblongata, Percutaneous Approach

009D40Z Drainage of Medulla Oblongata with Drainage Device, Percutaneous Endoscopic Approach

009D4ZX Drainage of Medulla Oblongata, Percutaneous Endoscopic Approach, Diagnostic

Female-only   ♂ Male-only   ▲ Limited Coverage   ● Non-OR   ■ HAC-associated procedure   ▲ Non-covered procedures   + Combination

009D4ZZ Drainage of Medulla Oblongata, Percutaneous Endoscopic Approach

009F00Z Drainage of Olfactory Nerve with Drainage Device, Open Approach

009F0ZX Drainage of Olfactory Nerve, Open Approach, Diagnostic

009F0ZZ Drainage of Olfactory Nerve, Open Approach

009F30Z Drainage of Olfactory Nerve with Drainage Device, Percutaneous Approach

009F3ZX Drainage of Olfactory Nerve, Percutaneous Approach, Diagnostic

009F3ZZ Drainage of Olfactory Nerve, Percutaneous Approach

009F40Z Drainage of Olfactory Nerve with Drainage Device, Percutaneous Endoscopic Approach

009F4ZX Drainage of Olfactory Nerve, Percutaneous Endoscopic Approach, Diagnostic

009F4ZZ Drainage of Olfactory Nerve, Percutaneous Endoscopic Approach

009G00Z Drainage of Optic Nerve with Drainage Device, Open Approach

009G0ZX Drainage of Optic Nerve, Open Approach, Diagnostic

009G0ZZ Drainage of Optic Nerve, Open Approach

009G30Z Drainage of Optic Nerve with Drainage Device, Percutaneous Approach

009G3ZX Drainage of Optic Nerve, Percutaneous Approach, Diagnostic

009G3ZZ Drainage of Optic Nerve, Percutaneous Approach

009G40Z Drainage of Optic Nerve with Drainage Device, Percutaneous Endoscopic Approach

009G4ZX Drainage of Optic Nerve, Percutaneous Endoscopic Approach, Diagnostic

009G4ZZ Drainage of Optic Nerve, Percutaneous Endoscopic Approach

009H00Z Drainage of Oculomotor Nerve with Drainage Device, Open Approach

009H0ZX Drainage of Oculomotor Nerve, Open Approach, Diagnostic

009H0ZZ Drainage of Oculomotor Nerve, Open Approach

009H30Z Drainage of Oculomotor Nerve with Drainage Device, Percutaneous Approach

009H3ZX Drainage of Oculomotor Nerve, Percutaneous Approach, Diagnostic

009H3ZZ Drainage of Oculomotor Nerve, Percutaneous Approach

009H40Z Drainage of Oculomotor Nerve with Drainage Device, Percutaneous Endoscopic Approach

009H4ZX Drainage of Oculomotor Nerve, Percutaneous Endoscopic Approach, Diagnostic

009H4ZZ Drainage of Oculomotor Nerve, Percutaneous Endoscopic Approach

009J00Z Drainage of Trochlear Nerve with Drainage Device, Open Approach

009J0ZX Drainage of Trochlear Nerve, Open Approach, Diagnostic

009J0ZZ Drainage of Trochlear Nerve, Open Approach

009J30Z Drainage of Trochlear Nerve with Drainage Device, Percutaneous Approach

009J3ZX Drainage of Trochlear Nerve, Percutaneous Approach, Diagnostic

009J3ZZ Drainage of Trochlear Nerve, Percutaneous Approach

009J40Z Drainage of Trochlear Nerve with Drainage Device, Percutaneous Endoscopic Approach

009J4ZX Drainage of Trochlear Nerve, Percutaneous Endoscopic Approach, Diagnostic

009J4ZZ Drainage of Trochlear Nerve, Percutaneous Endoscopic Approach

009K00Z Drainage of Trigeminal Nerve with Drainage Device, Open Approach

009K0ZX Drainage of Trigeminal Nerve, Open Approach, Diagnostic

009K0ZZ Drainage of Trigeminal Nerve, Open Approach

009K30Z Drainage of Trigeminal Nerve with Drainage Device, Percutaneous Approach

009K3ZX Drainage of Trigeminal Nerve, Percutaneous Approach, Diagnostic

009K3ZZ Drainage of Trigeminal Nerve, Percutaneous Approach

009K40Z Drainage of Trigeminal Nerve with Drainage Device, Percutaneous Endoscopic Approach

009K4ZX Drainage of Trigeminal Nerve, Percutaneous Endoscopic Approach, Diagnostic

009K4ZZ Drainage of Trigeminal Nerve, Percutaneous Endoscopic Approach

009L00Z Drainage of Abducens Nerve with Drainage Device, Open Approach

009L0ZX Drainage of Abducens Nerve, Open Approach, Diagnostic

009L0ZZ Drainage of Abducens Nerve, Open Approach

009L30Z Drainage of Abducens Nerve with Drainage Device, Percutaneous Approach

009L3ZX Drainage of Abducens Nerve, Percutaneous Approach, Diagnostic

009L3ZZ Drainage of Abducens Nerve, Percutaneous Approach

009L40Z Drainage of Abducens Nerve with Drainage Device, Percutaneous Endoscopic Approach

009L4ZX Drainage of Abducens Nerve, Percutaneous Endoscopic Approach, Diagnostic

009L4ZZ Drainage of Abducens Nerve, Percutaneous Endoscopic Approach

009M00Z Drainage of Facial Nerve with Drainage Device, Open Approach

009M0ZX Drainage of Facial Nerve, Open Approach, Diagnostic

009M0ZZ Drainage of Facial Nerve, Open Approach

009M30Z Drainage of Facial Nerve with Drainage Device, Percutaneous Approach

009M3ZX Drainage of Facial Nerve, Percutaneous Approach, Diagnostic

009M3ZZ Drainage of Facial Nerve, Percutaneous Approach

009M40Z Drainage of Facial Nerve with Drainage Device, Percutaneous Endoscopic Approach

009M4ZX Drainage of Facial Nerve, Percutaneous Endoscopic Approach, Diagnostic

009M4ZZ Drainage of Facial Nerve, Percutaneous Endoscopic Approach

009N00Z Drainage of Acoustic Nerve with Drainage Device, Open Approach

009N0ZX Drainage of Acoustic Nerve, Open Approach, Diagnostic

009N0ZZ Drainage of Acoustic Nerve, Open Approach

009N30Z Drainage of Acoustic Nerve with Drainage Device, Percutaneous Approach

009N3ZX Drainage of Acoustic Nerve, Percutaneous Approach, Diagnostic

009N3ZZ Drainage of Acoustic Nerve, Percutaneous Approach

009N40Z Drainage of Acoustic Nerve with Drainage Device, Percutaneous Endoscopic Approach

009N4ZX Drainage of Acoustic Nerve, Percutaneous Endoscopic Approach, Diagnostic

009N4ZZ Drainage of Acoustic Nerve, Percutaneous Endoscopic Approach

009P00Z Drainage of Glossopharyngeal Nerve with Drainage Device, Open Approach

009P0ZX Drainage of Glossopharyngeal Nerve, Open Approach, Diagnostic

009P0ZZ Drainage of Glossopharyngeal Nerve, Open Approach

009P30Z Drainage of Glossopharyngeal Nerve with Drainage Device, Percutaneous Approach

009P3ZX Drainage of Glossopharyngeal Nerve, Percutaneous Approach, Diagnostic

009P3ZZ Drainage of Glossopharyngeal Nerve, Percutaneous Approach

009P40Z Drainage of Glossopharyngeal Nerve with Drainage Device, Percutaneous Endoscopic Approach

009P4ZX Drainage of Glossopharyngeal Nerve, Percutaneous Endoscopic Approach, Diagnostic

009P4ZZ Drainage of Glossopharyngeal Nerve, Percutaneous Endoscopic Approach

009Q00Z Drainage of Vagus Nerve with Drainage Device, Open Approach

009Q0ZX Drainage of Vagus Nerve, Open Approach, Diagnostic

009Q0ZZ Drainage of Vagus Nerve, Open Approach

009Q30Z Drainage of Vagus Nerve with Drainage Device, Percutaneous Approach

009Q3ZX Drainage of Vagus Nerve, Percutaneous Approach, Diagnostic

009Q3ZZ Drainage of Vagus Nerve, Percutaneous Approach

009Q40Z Drainage of Vagus Nerve with Drainage Device, Percutaneous Endoscopic Approach

009Q4ZX Drainage of Vagus Nerve, Percutaneous Endoscopic Approach, Diagnostic

009Q4ZZ Drainage of Vagus Nerve, Percutaneous Endoscopic Approach

009R00Z Drainage of Accessory Nerve with Drainage Device, Open Approach

009R0ZX Drainage of Accessory Nerve, Open Approach, Diagnostic

009R0ZZ Drainage of Accessory Nerve, Open Approach

009R30Z Drainage of Accessory Nerve with Drainage Device, Percutaneous Approach

009R3ZX Drainage of Accessory Nerve, Percutaneous Approach, Diagnostic

009R3ZZ Drainage of Accessory Nerve, Percutaneous Approach

009R40Z Drainage of Accessory Nerve with Drainage Device, Percutaneous Endoscopic Approach

009R4ZX Drainage of Accessory Nerve, Percutaneous Endoscopic Approach, Diagnostic

009R4ZZ Drainage of Accessory Nerve, Percutaneous Endoscopic Approach

009S00Z Drainage of Hypoglossal Nerve with Drainage Device, Open Approach

009S0ZX Drainage of Hypoglossal Nerve, Open Approach, Diagnostic

009S0ZZ Drainage of Hypoglossal Nerve, Open Approach

009S30Z Drainage of Hypoglossal Nerve with Drainage Device, Percutaneous Approach

009S3ZX Drainage of Hypoglossal Nerve, Percutaneous Approach, Diagnostic

009S3ZZ Drainage of Hypoglossal Nerve, Percutaneous Approach

009S40Z Drainage of Hypoglossal Nerve with Drainage Device, Percutaneous Endoscopic Approach

009S4ZX Drainage of Hypoglossal Nerve, Percutaneous Endoscopic Approach, Diagnostic

009S4ZZ Drainage of Hypoglossal Nerve, Percutaneous Endoscopic Approach

009T00Z Drainage of Spinal Meninges with Drainage Device, Open Approach

09T0ZX Drainage of Spinal Meninges, Open Approach, Diagnostic

09T0ZZ Drainage of Spinal Meninges, Open Approach

09T30Z Drainage of Spinal Meninges with Drainage Device, Percutaneous Approach

09T3ZX Drainage of Spinal Meninges, Percutaneous Approach, Diagnostic

09T3ZZ Drainage of Spinal Meninges, Percutaneous Approach

09T40Z Drainage of Spinal Meninges with Drainage Device, Percutaneous Endoscopic Approach

09T4ZX Drainage of Spinal Meninges, Percutaneous Endoscopic Approach, Diagnostic

09T4ZZ Drainage of Spinal Meninges, Percutaneous Endoscopic Approach

09U00Z Drainage of Spinal Canal with Drainage Device, Open Approach

09U0ZX Drainage of Spinal Canal, Open Approach, Diagnostic

09U0ZZ Drainage of Spinal Canal, Open Approach

09U30Z Drainage of Spinal Canal with Drainage Device, Percutaneous Approach

009U3ZX Drainage of Spinal Canal, Percutaneous Approach, Diagnostic
AHA CC: 1Q, 2014, 8

09U3ZZ Drainage of Spinal Canal, Percutaneous Approach

09U40Z Drainage of Spinal Canal with Drainage Device, Percutaneous Endoscopic Approach

● 009U4ZX Drainage of Spinal Canal, Percutaneous Endoscopic Approach, Diagnostic

009U4ZZ Drainage of Spinal Canal, Percutaneous Endoscopic Approach

009W00Z Drainage of Cervical Spinal Cord with Drainage Device, Open Approach

009W0ZX Drainage of Cervical Spinal Cord, Open Approach, Diagnostic

009W0ZZ Drainage of Cervical Spinal Cord, Open Approach

009W30Z Drainage of Cervical Spinal Cord with Drainage Device, Percutaneous Approach

009W3ZX Drainage of Cervical Spinal Cord, Percutaneous Approach, Diagnostic

009W3ZZ Drainage of Cervical Spinal Cord, Percutaneous Approach

009W40Z Drainage of Cervical Spinal Cord with Drainage Device, Percutaneous Endoscopic Approach

009W4ZX Drainage of Cervical Spinal Cord, Percutaneous Endoscopic Approach, Diagnostic

009W4ZZ Drainage of Cervical Spinal Cord, Percutaneous Endoscopic Approach

009X00Z Drainage of Thoracic Spinal Cord with Drainage Device, Open Approach

009X0ZX Drainage of Thoracic Spinal Cord, Open Approach, Diagnostic

009X0ZZ Drainage of Thoracic Spinal Cord, Open Approach

009X30Z Drainage of Thoracic Spinal Cord with Drainage Device, Percutaneous Approach

009X3ZX Drainage of Thoracic Spinal Cord, Percutaneous Approach, Diagnostic

009X3ZZ Drainage of Thoracic Spinal Cord, Percutaneous Approach

009X40Z Drainage of Thoracic Spinal Cord with Drainage Device, Percutaneous Endoscopic Approach

009X4ZX Drainage of Thoracic Spinal Cord, Percutaneous Endoscopic Approach, Diagnostic

009X4ZZ Drainage of Thoracic Spinal Cord, Percutaneous Endoscopic Approach

009Y00Z Drainage of Lumbar Spinal Cord with Drainage Device, Open Approach

009Y0ZX Drainage of Lumbar Spinal Cord, Open Approach, Diagnostic

009Y0ZZ Drainage of Lumbar Spinal Cord, Open Approach

009Y30Z Drainage of Lumbar Spinal Cord with Drainage Device, Percutaneous Approach

009Y3ZX Drainage of Lumbar Spinal Cord, Percutaneous Approach, Diagnostic

009Y3ZZ Drainage of Lumbar Spinal Cord, Percutaneous Approach

009Y40Z Drainage of Lumbar Spinal Cord with Drainage Device, Percutaneous Endoscopic Approach

009Y4ZX Drainage of Lumbar Spinal Cord, Percutaneous Endoscopic Approach, Diagnostic

009Y4ZZ Drainage of Lumbar Spinal Cord, Percutaneous Endoscopic Approach

00B – Central Nervous System, Excision

Review Coding Guidelines B3.4a and B3.4b

Review Coding Guideline B3.8

00B00ZX Excision of Brain, Open Approach, Diagnostic
AHA CC: 1Q, 2015, 12-13

00B00ZZ Excision of Brain, Open Approach

00B03ZX Excision of Brain, Percutaneous Approach, Diagnostic

00B03ZZ Excision of Brain, Percutaneous Approach

00B04ZX Excision of Brain, Percutaneous Endoscopic Approach, Diagnostic

00B04ZZ Excision of Brain, Percutaneous Endoscopic Approach

00B10ZX Excision of Cerebral Meninges, Open Approach, Diagnostic

00B10ZZ Excision of Cerebral Meninges, Open Approach

00B13ZX Excision of Cerebral Meninges, Percutaneous Approach, Diagnostic

00B13ZZ Excision of Cerebral Meninges, Percutaneous Approach

00B14ZX Excision of Cerebral Meninges, Percutaneous Endoscopic Approach, Diagnostic

00B14ZZ Excision of Cerebral Meninges, Percutaneous Endoscopic Approach

00B20ZX Excision of Dura Mater, Open Approach, Diagnostic

00B20ZZ Excision of Dura Mater, Open Approach

00B23ZX Excision of Dura Mater, Percutaneous Approach, Diagnostic

00B23ZZ Excision of Dura Mater, Percutaneous Approach

00B24ZX Excision of Dura Mater, Percutaneous Endoscopic Approach, Diagnostic

00B24ZZ Excision of Dura Mater, Percutaneous Endoscopic Approach

00B60ZX Excision of Cerebral Ventricle, Open Approach, Diagnostic

00B60ZZ Excision of Cerebral Ventricle, Open Approach

00B63ZX Excision of Cerebral Ventricle, Percutaneous Approach, Diagnostic

00B63ZZ Excision of Cerebral Ventricle, Percutaneous Approach

00B64ZX Excision of Cerebral Ventricle, Percutaneous Endoscopic Approach, Diagnostic

00B64ZZ Excision of Cerebral Ventricle, Percutaneous Endoscopic Approach

00B70ZX Excision of Cerebral Hemisphere, Open Approach, Diagnostic

00B70ZZ Excision of Cerebral Hemisphere, Open Approach
AHA CC: 4Q, 2014, 34-35

00B73ZX Excision of Cerebral Hemisphere, Percutaneous Approach, Diagnostic

00B73ZZ Excision of Cerebral Hemisphere, Percutaneous Approach

00B74ZX Excision of Cerebral Hemisphere, Percutaneous Endoscopic Approach, Diagnostic

00B74ZZ Excision of Cerebral Hemisphere, Percutaneous Endoscopic Approach

00B80ZX Excision of Basal Ganglia, Open Approach, Diagnostic

00B80ZZ Excision of Basal Ganglia, Open Approach

00B83ZX Excision of Basal Ganglia, Percutaneous Approach, Diagnostic

00B83ZZ Excision of Basal Ganglia, Percutaneous Approach

00B84ZX Excision of Basal Ganglia, Percutaneous Endoscopic Approach, Diagnostic

00B84ZZ Excision of Basal Ganglia, Percutaneous Endoscopic Approach

00B90ZX Excision of Thalamus, Open Approach, Diagnostic

00B90ZZ Excision of Thalamus, Open Approach

00B93ZX Excision of Thalamus, Percutaneous Approach, Diagnostic

00B93ZZ Excision of Thalamus, Percutaneous Approach

00B94ZX Excision of Thalamus, Percutaneous Endoscopic Approach, Diagnostic

00B94ZZ Excision of Thalamus, Percutaneous Endoscopic Approach

00BA0ZX Excision of Hypothalamus, Open Approach, Diagnostic

00BA0ZZ Excision of Hypothalamus, Open Approach

00BA3ZX Excision of Hypothalamus, Percutaneous Approach, Diagnostic

00BA3ZZ Excision of Hypothalamus, Percutaneous Approach

00BA4ZX Excision of Hypothalamus, Percutaneous Endoscopic Approach, Diagnostic

00BA4ZZ Excision of Hypothalamus, Percutaneous Endoscopic Approach

00BB0ZX Excision of Pons, Open Approach, Diagnostic

00BB0ZZ Excision of Pons, Open Approach

00BB3ZX Excision of Pons, Percutaneous Approach, Diagnostic

00BB3ZZ Excision of Pons, Percutaneous Approach

00BB4ZX Excision of Pons, Percutaneous Endoscopic Approach, Diagnostic

00BB4ZZ Excision of Pons, Percutaneous Endoscopic Approach

00BC0ZX Excision of Cerebellum, Open Approach, Diagnostic

00BC0ZZ Excision of Cerebellum, Open Approach

00BC3ZX Excision of Cerebellum, Percutaneous Approach, Diagnostic

00BC3ZZ Excision of Cerebellum, Percutaneous Approach

00BC4ZX Excision of Cerebellum, Percutaneous Endoscopic Approach, Diagnostic

Female-only   ♂ Male-only   ▲ Limited Coverage   ● Non-OR   🅷🅰🅲 HAC-associated procedure   ▲ Non-covered procedures   ➕ Combination

00BC4ZZ	Excision of Cerebellum, Percutaneous Endoscopic Approach	**00BK4ZX**	Excision of Trigeminal Nerve, Percutaneous Endoscopic Approach, Diagnostic	**00BR4ZX**	Excision of Accessory Nerve, Percutaneous Endoscopic Approach, Diagnostic
00BD0ZX	Excision of Medulla Oblongata, Open Approach, Diagnostic	**00BK4ZZ**	Excision of Trigeminal Nerve, Percutaneous Endoscopic Approach	**00BR4ZZ**	Excision of Accessory Nerve, Percutaneous Endoscopic Approach
00BD0ZZ	Excision of Medulla Oblongata, Open Approach	**00BL0ZX**	Excision of Abducens Nerve, Open Approach, Diagnostic	**00BS0ZX**	Excision of Hypoglossal Nerve, Open Approach, Diagnostic
00BD3ZX	Excision of Medulla Oblongata, Percutaneous Approach, Diagnostic	**00BL0ZZ**	Excision of Abducens Nerve, Open Approach	**00BS0ZZ**	Excision of Hypoglossal Nerve, Open Approach
00BD3ZZ	Excision of Medulla Oblongata, Percutaneous Approach	**00BL3ZX**	Excision of Abducens Nerve, Percutaneous Approach, Diagnostic	**00BS3ZX**	Excision of Hypoglossal Nerve, Percutaneous Approach, Diagnostic
00BD4ZX	Excision of Medulla Oblongata, Percutaneous Endoscopic Approach, Diagnostic	**00BL3ZZ**	Excision of Abducens Nerve, Percutaneous Approach	**00BS3ZZ**	Excision of Hypoglossal Nerve, Percutaneous Approach
00BD4ZZ	Excision of Medulla Oblongata, Percutaneous Endoscopic Approach	**00BL4ZX**	Excision of Abducens Nerve, Percutaneous Endoscopic Approach, Diagnostic	**00BS4ZX**	Excision of Hypoglossal Nerve, Percutaneous Endoscopic Approach, Diagnostic
00BF0ZX	Excision of Olfactory Nerve, Open Approach, Diagnostic	**00BL4ZZ**	Excision of Abducens Nerve, Percutaneous Endoscopic Approach	**00BS4ZZ**	Excision of Hypoglossal Nerve, Percutaneous Endoscopic Approach
00BF0ZZ	Excision of Olfactory Nerve, Open Approach	**00BM0ZX**	Excision of Facial Nerve, Open Approach, Diagnostic	**00BT0ZX**	Excision of Spinal Meninges, Open Approach, Diagnostic
00BF3ZX	Excision of Olfactory Nerve, Percutaneous Approach, Diagnostic	**00BM0ZZ**	Excision of Facial Nerve, Open Approach	**00BT0ZZ**	Excision of Spinal Meninges, Open Approach
00BF3ZZ	Excision of Olfactory Nerve, Percutaneous Approach	**00BM3ZX**	Excision of Facial Nerve, Percutaneous Approach, Diagnostic	**00BT3ZX**	Excision of Spinal Meninges, Percutaneous Approach, Diagnostic
00BF4ZX	Excision of Olfactory Nerve, Percutaneous Endoscopic Approach, Diagnostic	**00BM3ZZ**	Excision of Facial Nerve, Percutaneous Approach	**00BT3ZZ**	Excision of Spinal Meninges, Percutaneous Approach
00BF4ZZ	Excision of Olfactory Nerve, Percutaneous Endoscopic Approach	**00BM4ZX**	Excision of Facial Nerve, Percutaneous Endoscopic Approach, Diagnostic	**00BT4ZX**	Excision of Spinal Meninges, Percutaneous Endoscopic Approach, Diagnostic
00BG0ZX	Excision of Optic Nerve, Open Approach, Diagnostic	**00BM4ZZ**	Excision of Facial Nerve, Percutaneous Endoscopic Approach	**00BT4ZZ**	Excision of Spinal Meninges, Percutaneous Endoscopic Approach
00BG0ZZ	Excision of Optic Nerve, Open Approach	**00BN0ZX**	Excision of Acoustic Nerve, Open Approach, Diagnostic	**00BW0ZX**	Excision of Cervical Spinal Cord, Open Approach, Diagnostic
00BG3ZX	Excision of Optic Nerve, Percutaneous Approach, Diagnostic	**00BN0ZZ**	Excision of Acoustic Nerve, Open Approach	**00BW0ZZ**	Excision of Cervical Spinal Cord, Open Approach
00BG3ZZ	Excision of Optic Nerve, Percutaneous Approach	**00BN3ZX**	Excision of Acoustic Nerve, Percutaneous Approach, Diagnostic	**00BW3ZX**	Excision of Cervical Spinal Cord, Percutaneous Approach, Diagnostic
00BG4ZX	Excision of Optic Nerve, Percutaneous Endoscopic Approach, Diagnostic	**00BN3ZZ**	Excision of Acoustic Nerve, Percutaneous Approach	**00BW3ZZ**	Excision of Cervical Spinal Cord, Percutaneous Approach
00BG4ZZ	Excision of Optic Nerve, Percutaneous Endoscopic Approach	**00BN4ZX**	Excision of Acoustic Nerve, Percutaneous Endoscopic Approach, Diagnostic	**00BW4ZX**	Excision of Cervical Spinal Cord, Percutaneous Endoscopic Approach, Diagnostic
00BH0ZX	Excision of Oculomotor Nerve, Open Approach, Diagnostic	**00BN4ZZ**	Excision of Acoustic Nerve, Percutaneous Endoscopic Approach	**00BW4ZZ**	Excision of Cervical Spinal Cord, Percutaneous Endoscopic Approach
00BH0ZZ	Excision of Oculomotor Nerve, Open Approach	**00BP0ZX**	Excision of Glossopharyngeal Nerve, Open Approach, Diagnostic	**00BX0ZX**	Excision of Thoracic Spinal Cord, Open Approach, Diagnostic
00BH3ZX	Excision of Oculomotor Nerve, Percutaneous Approach, Diagnostic	**00BP0ZZ**	Excision of Glossopharyngeal Nerve, Open Approach	**00BX0ZZ**	Excision of Thoracic Spinal Cord, Open Approach
00BH3ZZ	Excision of Oculomotor Nerve, Percutaneous Approach	**00BP3ZX**	Excision of Glossopharyngeal Nerve, Percutaneous Approach, Diagnostic	**00BX3ZX**	Excision of Thoracic Spinal Cord, Percutaneous Approach, Diagnostic
00BH4ZX	Excision of Oculomotor Nerve, Percutaneous Endoscopic Approach, Diagnostic	**00BP3ZZ**	Excision of Glossopharyngeal Nerve, Percutaneous Approach	**00BX3ZZ**	Excision of Thoracic Spinal Cord, Percutaneous Approach
00BH4ZZ	Excision of Oculomotor Nerve, Percutaneous Endoscopic Approach	**00BP4ZX**	Excision of Glossopharyngeal Nerve, Percutaneous Endoscopic Approach, Diagnostic	**00BX4ZX**	Excision of Thoracic Spinal Cord, Percutaneous Endoscopic Approach, Diagnostic
00BJ0ZX	Excision of Trochlear Nerve, Open Approach, Diagnostic	**00BP4ZZ**	Excision of Glossopharyngeal Nerve, Percutaneous Endoscopic Approach	**00BX4ZZ**	Excision of Thoracic Spinal Cord, Percutaneous Endoscopic Approach
00BJ0ZZ	Excision of Trochlear Nerve, Open Approach	**00BQ0ZX**	Excision of Vagus Nerve, Open Approach, Diagnostic	**00BY0ZX**	Excision of Lumbar Spinal Cord, Open Approach, Diagnostic
00BJ3ZX	Excision of Trochlear Nerve, Percutaneous Approach, Diagnostic	**00BQ0ZZ**	Excision of Vagus Nerve, Open Approach	**00BY0ZZ**	Excision of Lumbar Spinal Cord, Open Approach
00BJ3ZZ	Excision of Trochlear Nerve, Percutaneous Approach	**00BQ3ZX**	Excision of Vagus Nerve, Percutaneous Approach, Diagnostic		*AHA CC: 3Q, 2014, 24*
00BJ4ZX	Excision of Trochlear Nerve, Percutaneous Endoscopic Approach, Diagnostic	**00BQ3ZZ**	Excision of Vagus Nerve, Percutaneous Approach	**00BY3ZX**	Excision of Lumbar Spinal Cord, Percutaneous Approach, Diagnostic
00BJ4ZZ	Excision of Trochlear Nerve, Percutaneous Endoscopic Approach	**00BQ4ZX**	Excision of Vagus Nerve, Percutaneous Endoscopic Approach, Diagnostic	**00BY3ZZ**	Excision of Lumbar Spinal Cord, Percutaneous Approach
00BK0ZX	Excision of Trigeminal Nerve, Open Approach, Diagnostic	**00BQ4ZZ**	Excision of Vagus Nerve, Percutaneous Endoscopic Approach	**00BY4ZX**	Excision of Lumbar Spinal Cord, Percutaneous Endoscopic Approach, Diagnostic
00BK0ZZ	Excision of Trigeminal Nerve, Open Approach	**00BR0ZX**	Excision of Accessory Nerve, Open Approach, Diagnostic	**00BY4ZZ**	Excision of Lumbar Spinal Cord, Percutaneous Endoscopic Approach
00BK3ZX	Excision of Trigeminal Nerve, Percutaneous Approach, Diagnostic	**00BR0ZZ**	Excision of Accessory Nerve, Open Approach		
00BK3ZZ	Excision of Trigeminal Nerve, Percutaneous Approach	**00BR3ZX**	Excision of Accessory Nerve, Percutaneous Approach, Diagnostic		
		00BR3ZZ	Excision of Accessory Nerve, Percutaneous Approach		

00C – Central Nervous System, Extirpation

00C00ZZ	Extirpation of Matter from Brain, Open Approach	**00C03ZZ**	Extirpation of Matter from Brain, Percutaneous Approach	**00C04ZZ**	Extirpation of Matter from Brain, Percutaneous Endoscopic Approach
	AHA CC: 1Q, 2015, 12-13				

♀ Female-only　　♂ Male-only　　▲ Limited Coverage　　● Non-OR　　▨ HAC-associated procedure　　▲ Non-covered procedures　　✚ Combinatio

0C10ZZ	Extirpation of Matter from Cerebral Meninges, Open Approach
0C13ZZ	Extirpation of Matter from Cerebral Meninges, Percutaneous Approach
0C14ZZ	Extirpation of Matter from Cerebral Meninges, Percutaneous Endoscopic Approach
0C20ZZ	Extirpation of Matter from Dura Mater, Open Approach
0C23ZZ	Extirpation of Matter from Dura Mater, Percutaneous Approach
0C24ZZ	Extirpation of Matter from Dura Mater, Percutaneous Endoscopic Approach
0C30ZZ	Extirpation of Matter from Epidural Space, Open Approach
0C33ZZ	Extirpation of Matter from Epidural Space, Percutaneous Approach
0C34ZZ	Extirpation of Matter from Epidural Space, Percutaneous Endoscopic Approach
0C40ZZ	Extirpation of Matter from Subdural Space, Open Approach
0C43ZZ	Extirpation of Matter from Subdural Space, Percutaneous Approach
0C44ZZ	Extirpation of Matter from Subdural Space, Percutaneous Endoscopic Approach
0C50ZZ	Extirpation of Matter from Subarachnoid Space, Open Approach
0C53ZZ	Extirpation of Matter from Subarachnoid Space, Percutaneous Approach
0C54ZZ	Extirpation of Matter from Subarachnoid Space, Percutaneous Endoscopic Approach
0C60ZZ	Extirpation of Matter from Cerebral Ventricle, Open Approach
0C63ZZ	Extirpation of Matter from Cerebral Ventricle, Percutaneous Approach
0C64ZZ	Extirpation of Matter from Cerebral Ventricle, Percutaneous Endoscopic Approach
0C70ZZ	Extirpation of Matter from Cerebral Hemisphere, Open Approach
0C73ZZ	Extirpation of Matter from Cerebral Hemisphere, Percutaneous Approach
0C74ZZ	Extirpation of Matter from Cerebral Hemisphere, Percutaneous Endoscopic Approach
0C80ZZ	Extirpation of Matter from Basal Ganglia, Open Approach
0C83ZZ	Extirpation of Matter from Basal Ganglia, Percutaneous Approach
0C84ZZ	Extirpation of Matter from Basal Ganglia, Percutaneous Endoscopic Approach
0C90ZZ	Extirpation of Matter from Thalamus, Open Approach
0C93ZZ	Extirpation of Matter from Thalamus, Percutaneous Approach
0C94ZZ	Extirpation of Matter from Thalamus, Percutaneous Endoscopic Approach
0CA0ZZ	Extirpation of Matter from Hypothalamus, Open Approach
0CA3ZZ	Extirpation of Matter from Hypothalamus, Percutaneous Approach

00CA4ZZ	Extirpation of Matter from Hypothalamus, Percutaneous Endoscopic Approach
00CB0ZZ	Extirpation of Matter from Pons, Open Approach
00CB3ZZ	Extirpation of Matter from Pons, Percutaneous Approach
00CB4ZZ	Extirpation of Matter from Pons, Percutaneous Endoscopic Approach
00CC0ZZ	Extirpation of Matter from Cerebellum, Open Approach
00CC3ZZ	Extirpation of Matter from Cerebellum, Percutaneous Approach
00CC4ZZ	Extirpation of Matter from Cerebellum, Percutaneous Endoscopic Approach
00CD0ZZ	Extirpation of Matter from Medulla Oblongata, Open Approach
00CD3ZZ	Extirpation of Matter from Medulla Oblongata, Percutaneous Approach
00CD4ZZ	Extirpation of Matter from Medulla Oblongata, Percutaneous Endoscopic Approach
00CF0ZZ	Extirpation of Matter from Olfactory Nerve, Open Approach
00CF3ZZ	Extirpation of Matter from Olfactory Nerve, Percutaneous Approach
00CF4ZZ	Extirpation of Matter from Olfactory Nerve, Percutaneous Endoscopic Approach
00CG0ZZ	Extirpation of Matter from Optic Nerve, Open Approach
00CG3ZZ	Extirpation of Matter from Optic Nerve, Percutaneous Approach
00CG4ZZ	Extirpation of Matter from Optic Nerve, Percutaneous Endoscopic Approach
00CH0ZZ	Extirpation of Matter from Oculomotor Nerve, Open Approach
00CH3ZZ	Extirpation of Matter from Oculomotor Nerve, Percutaneous Approach
00CH4ZZ	Extirpation of Matter from Oculomotor Nerve, Percutaneous Endoscopic Approach
00CJ0ZZ	Extirpation of Matter from Trochlear Nerve, Open Approach
00CJ3ZZ	Extirpation of Matter from Trochlear Nerve, Percutaneous Approach
00CJ4ZZ	Extirpation of Matter from Trochlear Nerve, Percutaneous Endoscopic Approach
00CK0ZZ	Extirpation of Matter from Trigeminal Nerve, Open Approach
00CK3ZZ	Extirpation of Matter from Trigeminal Nerve, Percutaneous Approach
00CK4ZZ	Extirpation of Matter from Trigeminal Nerve, Percutaneous Endoscopic Approach
00CL0ZZ	Extirpation of Matter from Abducens Nerve, Open Approach
00CL3ZZ	Extirpation of Matter from Abducens Nerve, Percutaneous Approach
00CL4ZZ	Extirpation of Matter from Abducens Nerve, Percutaneous Endoscopic Approach
00CM0ZZ	Extirpation of Matter from Facial Nerve, Open Approach

00CM3ZZ	Extirpation of Matter from Facial Nerve, Percutaneous Approach
00CM4ZZ	Extirpation of Matter from Facial Nerve, Percutaneous Endoscopic Approach
00CN0ZZ	Extirpation of Matter from Acoustic Nerve, Open Approach
00CN3ZZ	Extirpation of Matter from Acoustic Nerve, Percutaneous Approach
00CN4ZZ	Extirpation of Matter from Acoustic Nerve, Percutaneous Endoscopic Approach
00CP0ZZ	Extirpation of Matter from Glossopharyngeal Nerve, Open Approach
00CP3ZZ	Extirpation of Matter from Glossopharyngeal Nerve, Percutaneous Approach
00CP4ZZ	Extirpation of Matter from Glossopharyngeal Nerve, Percutaneous Endoscopic Approach
00CQ0ZZ	Extirpation of Matter from Vagus Nerve, Open Approach
00CQ3ZZ	Extirpation of Matter from Vagus Nerve, Percutaneous Approach
00CQ4ZZ	Extirpation of Matter from Vagus Nerve, Percutaneous Endoscopic Approach
00CR0ZZ	Extirpation of Matter from Accessory Nerve, Open Approach
00CR3ZZ	Extirpation of Matter from Accessory Nerve, Percutaneous Approach
00CR4ZZ	Extirpation of Matter from Accessory Nerve, Percutaneous Endoscopic Approach
00CS0ZZ	Extirpation of Matter from Hypoglossal Nerve, Open Approach
00CS3ZZ	Extirpation of Matter from Hypoglossal Nerve, Percutaneous Approach
00CS4ZZ	Extirpation of Matter from Hypoglossal Nerve, Percutaneous Endoscopic Approach
00CT0ZZ	Extirpation of Matter from Spinal Meninges, Open Approach
00CT3ZZ	Extirpation of Matter from Spinal Meninges, Percutaneous Approach
00CT4ZZ	Extirpation of Matter from Spinal Meninges, Percutaneous Endoscopic Approach
00CW0ZZ	Extirpation of Matter from Cervical Spinal Cord, Open Approach
00CW3ZZ	Extirpation of Matter from Cervical Spinal Cord, Percutaneous Approach
00CW4ZZ	Extirpation of Matter from Cervical Spinal Cord, Percutaneous Endoscopic Approach
00CX0ZZ	Extirpation of Matter from Thoracic Spinal Cord, Open Approach
00CX3ZZ	Extirpation of Matter from Thoracic Spinal Cord, Percutaneous Approach
00CX4ZZ	Extirpation of Matter from Thoracic Spinal Cord, Percutaneous Endoscopic Approach
00CY0ZZ	Extirpation of Matter from Lumbar Spinal Cord, Open Approach
00CY3ZZ	Extirpation of Matter from Lumbar Spinal Cord, Percutaneous Approach
00CY4ZZ	Extirpation of Matter from Lumbar Spinal Cord, Percutaneous Endoscopic Approach

00D – Central Nervous System, Extraction

00D10ZZ	Extraction of Cerebral Meninges, Open Approach
00D13ZZ	Extraction of Cerebral Meninges, Percutaneous Approach
00D14ZZ	Extraction of Cerebral Meninges, Percutaneous Endoscopic Approach
00D20ZZ	Extraction of Dura Mater, Open Approach
00D23ZZ	Extraction of Dura Mater, Percutaneous Approach
00D24ZZ	Extraction of Dura Mater, Percutaneous Endoscopic Approach

00DF0ZZ	Extraction of Olfactory Nerve, Open Approach
00DF3ZZ	Extraction of Olfactory Nerve, Percutaneous Approach
00DF4ZZ	Extraction of Olfactory Nerve, Percutaneous Endoscopic Approach
00DG0ZZ	Extraction of Optic Nerve, Open Approach
00DG3ZZ	Extraction of Optic Nerve, Percutaneous Approach
00DG4ZZ	Extraction of Optic Nerve, Percutaneous Endoscopic Approach

00DH0ZZ	Extraction of Oculomotor Nerve, Open Approach
00DH3ZZ	Extraction of Oculomotor Nerve, Percutaneous Approach
00DH4ZZ	Extraction of Oculomotor Nerve, Percutaneous Endoscopic Approach
00DJ0ZZ	Extraction of Trochlear Nerve, Open Approach
00DJ3ZZ	Extraction of Trochlear Nerve, Percutaneous Approach

Female-only	♂ Male-only	▲ Limited Coverage	● Non-OR	▨ HAC-associated procedure	▲ Non-covered procedures	➕ Combination

00DJ4ZZ	Extraction of Trochlear Nerve, Percutaneous Endoscopic Approach
00DK0ZZ	Extraction of Trigeminal Nerve, Open Approach
00DK3ZZ	Extraction of Trigeminal Nerve, Percutaneous Approach
00DK4ZZ	Extraction of Trigeminal Nerve, Percutaneous Endoscopic Approach
00DL0ZZ	Extraction of Abducens Nerve, Open Approach
00DL3ZZ	Extraction of Abducens Nerve, Percutaneous Approach
00DL4ZZ	Extraction of Abducens Nerve, Percutaneous Endoscopic Approach
00DM0ZZ	Extraction of Facial Nerve, Open Approach
00DM3ZZ	Extraction of Facial Nerve, Percutaneous Approach
00DM4ZZ	Extraction of Facial Nerve, Percutaneous Endoscopic Approach
00DN0ZZ	Extraction of Acoustic Nerve, Open Approach
00DN3ZZ	Extraction of Acoustic Nerve, Percutaneous Approach
00DN4ZZ	Extraction of Acoustic Nerve, Percutaneous Endoscopic Approach
00DP0ZZ	Extraction of Glossopharyngeal Nerve, Open Approach
00DP3ZZ	Extraction of Glossopharyngeal Nerve, Percutaneous Approach
00DP4ZZ	Extraction of Glossopharyngeal Nerve, Percutaneous Endoscopic Approach
00DQ0ZZ	Extraction of Vagus Nerve, Open Approach
00DQ3ZZ	Extraction of Vagus Nerve, Percutaneous Approach
00DQ4ZZ	Extraction of Vagus Nerve, Percutaneous Endoscopic Approach
00DR0ZZ	Extraction of Accessory Nerve, Open Approach
00DR3ZZ	Extraction of Accessory Nerve, Percutaneous Approach
00DR4ZZ	Extraction of Accessory Nerve, Percutaneous Endoscopic Approach
00DS0ZZ	Extraction of Hypoglossal Nerve, Open Approach
00DS3ZZ	Extraction of Hypoglossal Nerve, Percutaneous Approach
00DS4ZZ	Extraction of Hypoglossal Nerve, Percutaneous Endoscopic Approach
00DT0ZZ	Extraction of Spinal Meninges, Open Approach
00DT3ZZ	Extraction of Spinal Meninges, Percutaneous Approach
00DT4ZZ	Extraction of Spinal Meninges, Percutaneous Endoscopic Approach

00F – Central Nervous System, Fragmentation

00F30ZZ	Fragmentation in Epidural Space, Open Approach
00F33ZZ	Fragmentation in Epidural Space, Percutaneous Approach
00F34ZZ	Fragmentation in Epidural Space, Percutaneous Endoscopic Approach
▲ 00F3XZZ	Fragmentation in Epidural Space, External Approach
00F40ZZ	Fragmentation in Subdural Space, Open Approach
00F43ZZ	Fragmentation in Subdural Space, Percutaneous Approach
00F44ZZ	Fragmentation in Subdural Space, Percutaneous Endoscopic Approach
▲ 00F4XZZ	Fragmentation in Subdural Space, External Approach
00F50ZZ	Fragmentation in Subarachnoid Space, Open Approach
00F53ZZ	Fragmentation in Subarachnoid Space, Percutaneous Approach
00F54ZZ	Fragmentation in Subarachnoid Space, Percutaneous Endoscopic Approach
▲ 00F5XZZ	Fragmentation in Subarachnoid Space, External Approach
00F60ZZ	Fragmentation in Cerebral Ventricle, Open Approach
00F63ZZ	Fragmentation in Cerebral Ventricle, Percutaneous Approach
00F64ZZ	Fragmentation in Cerebral Ventricle, Percutaneous Endoscopic Approach
▲ 00F6XZZ	Fragmentation in Cerebral Ventricle, External Approach
00FU0ZZ	Fragmentation in Spinal Canal, Open Approach
00FU3ZZ	Fragmentation in Spinal Canal, Percutaneous Approach
00FU4ZZ	Fragmentation in Spinal Canal, Percutaneous Endoscopic Approach
00FUXZZ	Fragmentation in Spinal Canal, External Approach

00H – Central Nervous System, Insertion

Review Coding Guideline B4.6

00H002Z	Insertion of Monitoring Device into Brain, Open Approach
00H003Z	Insertion of Infusion Device into Brain, Open Approach
00H00MZ	Insertion of Neurostimulator Lead into Brain, Open Approach
00H032Z	Insertion of Monitoring Device into Brain, Percutaneous Approach
00H033Z	Insertion of Infusion Device into Brain, Percutaneous Approach
00H03MZ	Insertion of Neurostimulator Lead into Brain, Percutaneous Approach
00H042Z	Insertion of Monitoring Device into Brain, Percutaneous Endoscopic Approach
00H043Z	Insertion of Infusion Device into Brain, Percutaneous Endoscopic Approach
00H04MZ	Insertion of Neurostimulator Lead into Brain, Percutaneous Endoscopic Approach
00H602Z	Insertion of Monitoring Device into Cerebral Ventricle, Open Approach
00H603Z	Insertion of Infusion Device into Cerebral Ventricle, Open Approach
00H60MZ	Insertion of Neurostimulator Lead into Cerebral Ventricle, Open Approach
00H632Z	Insertion of Monitoring Device into Cerebral Ventricle, Percutaneous Approach
00H633Z	Insertion of Infusion Device into Cerebral Ventricle, Percutaneous Approach
00H63MZ	Insertion of Neurostimulator Lead into Cerebral Ventricle, Percutaneous Approach
00H642Z	Insertion of Monitoring Device into Cerebral Ventricle, Percutaneous Endoscopic Approach
00H643Z	Insertion of Infusion Device into Cerebral Ventricle, Percutaneous Endoscopic Approach
00H64MZ	Insertion of Neurostimulator Lead into Cerebral Ventricle, Percutaneous Endoscopic Approach
00HE02Z	Insertion of Monitoring Device into Cranial Nerve, Open Approach
00HE03Z	Insertion of Infusion Device into Cranial Nerve, Open Approach
00HE0MZ	Insertion of Neurostimulator Lead into Cranial Nerve, Open Approach
00HE32Z	Insertion of Monitoring Device into Cranial Nerve, Percutaneous Approach
00HE33Z	Insertion of Infusion Device into Cranial Nerve, Percutaneous Approach
00HE3MZ	Insertion of Neurostimulator Lead into Cranial Nerve, Percutaneous Approach
00HE42Z	Insertion of Monitoring Device into Cranial Nerve, Percutaneous Endoscopic Approach
00HE43Z	Insertion of Infusion Device into Cranial Nerve, Percutaneous Endoscopic Approach
00HE4MZ	Insertion of Neurostimulator Lead into Cranial Nerve, Percutaneous Endoscopic Approach
00HU02Z	Insertion of Monitoring Device into Spinal Canal, Open Approach
00HU03Z	Insertion of Infusion Device into Spinal Canal, Open Approach
00HU0MZ	Insertion of Neurostimulator Lead into Spinal Canal, Open Approach
00HU32Z	Insertion of Monitoring Device into Spinal Canal, Percutaneous Approach
00HU33Z	Insertion of Infusion Device into Spinal Canal, Percutaneous Approach

AHA CC: 3Q, 2014, 19-20

00HU3MZ	Insertion of Neurostimulator Lead into Spinal Canal, Percutaneous Approach
00HU42Z	Insertion of Monitoring Device into Spinal Canal, Percutaneous Endoscopic Approach
00HU43Z	Insertion of Infusion Device into Spinal Canal, Percutaneous Endoscopic Approach
00HU4MZ	Insertion of Neurostimulator Lead into Spinal Canal, Percutaneous Endoscopic Approach
00HV02Z	Insertion of Monitoring Device into Spinal Cord, Open Approach
00HV03Z	Insertion of Infusion Device into Spinal Cord, Open Approach
00HV0MZ	Insertion of Neurostimulator Lead into Spinal Cord, Open Approach
00HV32Z	Insertion of Monitoring Device into Spinal Cord, Percutaneous Approach
00HV33Z	Insertion of Infusion Device into Spinal Cord, Percutaneous Approach
00HV3MZ	Insertion of Neurostimulator Lead into Spinal Cord, Percutaneous Approach
00HV42Z	Insertion of Monitoring Device into Spinal Cord, Percutaneous Endoscopic Approach
00HV43Z	Insertion of Infusion Device into Spinal Cord, Percutaneous Endoscopic Approach
00HV4MZ	Insertion of Neurostimulator Lead into Spinal Cord, Percutaneous Endoscopic Approach

00J – Central Nervous System, Inspection

Review Coding Guidelines B3.11a, B3.11b and B3.11c

00J00ZZ	Inspection of Brain, Open Approach	
00J03ZZ	Inspection of Brain, Percutaneous Approach	
00J04ZZ	Inspection of Brain, Percutaneous Endoscopic Approach	
00JE0ZZ	Inspection of Cranial Nerve, Open Approach	

00JE3ZZ	Inspection of Cranial Nerve, Percutaneous Approach
00JE4ZZ	Inspection of Cranial Nerve, Percutaneous Endoscopic Approach
00JU0ZZ	Inspection of Spinal Canal, Open Approach
00JU3ZZ	Inspection of Spinal Canal, Percutaneous Approach

00JU4ZZ	Inspection of Spinal Canal, Percutaneous Endoscopic Approach
00JV0ZZ	Inspection of Spinal Cord, Open Approach
00JV3ZZ	Inspection of Spinal Cord, Percutaneous Approach
00JV4ZZ	Inspection of Spinal Cord, Percutaneous Endoscopic Approach

00K – Central Nervous System, Map

00K00ZZ	Map Brain, Open Approach
00K03ZZ	Map Brain, Percutaneous Approach
00K04ZZ	Map Brain, Percutaneous Endoscopic Approach
00K70ZZ	Map Cerebral Hemisphere, Open Approach
00K73ZZ	Map Cerebral Hemisphere, Percutaneous Approach
00K74ZZ	Map Cerebral Hemisphere, Percutaneous Endoscopic Approach
00K80ZZ	Map Basal Ganglia, Open Approach
00K83ZZ	Map Basal Ganglia, Percutaneous Approach

00K84ZZ	Map Basal Ganglia, Percutaneous Endoscopic Approach
00K90ZZ	Map Thalamus, Open Approach
00K93ZZ	Map Thalamus, Percutaneous Approach
00K94ZZ	Map Thalamus, Percutaneous Endoscopic Approach
00KA0ZZ	Map Hypothalamus, Open Approach
00KA3ZZ	Map Hypothalamus, Percutaneous Approach
00KA4ZZ	Map Hypothalamus, Percutaneous Endoscopic Approach
00KB0ZZ	Map Pons, Open Approach
00KB3ZZ	Map Pons, Percutaneous Approach

00KB4ZZ	Map Pons, Percutaneous Endoscopic Approach
00KC0ZZ	Map Cerebellum, Open Approach
00KC3ZZ	Map Cerebellum, Percutaneous Approach
00KC4ZZ	Map Cerebellum, Percutaneous Endoscopic Approach
00KD0ZZ	Map Medulla Oblongata, Open Approach
00KD3ZZ	Map Medulla Oblongata, Percutaneous Approach
00KD4ZZ	Map Medulla Oblongata, Percutaneous Endoscopic Approach

00N – Central Nervous System, Release

Review Coding Guideline B3.13

Review Coding Guideline B3.14

00N00ZZ	Release Brain, Open Approach
00N03ZZ	Release Brain, Percutaneous Approach
00N04ZZ	Release Brain, Percutaneous Endoscopic Approach
00N10ZZ	Release Cerebral Meninges, Open Approach
00N13ZZ	Release Cerebral Meninges, Percutaneous Approach
00N14ZZ	Release Cerebral Meninges, Percutaneous Endoscopic Approach
00N20ZZ	Release Dura Mater, Open Approach
00N23ZZ	Release Dura Mater, Percutaneous Approach
00N24ZZ	Release Dura Mater, Percutaneous Endoscopic Approach
00N60ZZ	Release Cerebral Ventricle, Open Approach
00N63ZZ	Release Cerebral Ventricle, Percutaneous Approach
00N64ZZ	Release Cerebral Ventricle, Percutaneous Endoscopic Approach
00N70ZZ	Release Cerebral Hemisphere, Open Approach
00N73ZZ	Release Cerebral Hemisphere, Percutaneous Approach
00N74ZZ	Release Cerebral Hemisphere, Percutaneous Endoscopic Approach
00N80ZZ	Release Basal Ganglia, Open Approach
00N83ZZ	Release Basal Ganglia, Percutaneous Approach
00N84ZZ	Release Basal Ganglia, Percutaneous Endoscopic Approach
00N90ZZ	Release Thalamus, Open Approach
00N93ZZ	Release Thalamus, Percutaneous Approach
00N94ZZ	Release Thalamus, Percutaneous Endoscopic Approach
00NA0ZZ	Release Hypothalamus, Open Approach
00NA3ZZ	Release Hypothalamus, Percutaneous Approach
00NA4ZZ	Release Hypothalamus, Percutaneous Endoscopic Approach
00NB0ZZ	Release Pons, Open Approach

00NB3ZZ	Release Pons, Percutaneous Approach
00NB4ZZ	Release Pons, Percutaneous Endoscopic Approach
00NC0ZZ	Release Cerebellum, Open Approach
00NC3ZZ	Release Cerebellum, Percutaneous Approach
00NC4ZZ	Release Cerebellum, Percutaneous Endoscopic Approach
00ND0ZZ	Release Medulla Oblongata, Open Approach
00ND3ZZ	Release Medulla Oblongata, Percutaneous Approach
00ND4ZZ	Release Medulla Oblongata, Percutaneous Endoscopic Approach
00NF0ZZ	Release Olfactory Nerve, Open Approach
00NF3ZZ	Release Olfactory Nerve, Percutaneous Approach
00NF4ZZ	Release Olfactory Nerve, Percutaneous Endoscopic Approach
00NG0ZZ	Release Optic Nerve, Open Approach
00NG3ZZ	Release Optic Nerve, Percutaneous Approach
00NG4ZZ	Release Optic Nerve, Percutaneous Endoscopic Approach
00NH0ZZ	Release Oculomotor Nerve, Open Approach
00NH3ZZ	Release Oculomotor Nerve, Percutaneous Approach
00NH4ZZ	Release Oculomotor Nerve, Percutaneous Endoscopic Approach
00NJ0ZZ	Release Trochlear Nerve, Open Approach
00NJ3ZZ	Release Trochlear Nerve, Percutaneous Approach
00NJ4ZZ	Release Trochlear Nerve, Percutaneous Endoscopic Approach
00NK0ZZ	Release Trigeminal Nerve, Open Approach
00NK3ZZ	Release Trigeminal Nerve, Percutaneous Approach
00NK4ZZ	Release Trigeminal Nerve, Percutaneous Endoscopic Approach
00NL0ZZ	Release Abducens Nerve, Open Approach

00NL3ZZ	Release Abducens Nerve, Percutaneous Approach
00NL4ZZ	Release Abducens Nerve, Percutaneous Endoscopic Approach
00NM0ZZ	Release Facial Nerve, Open Approach
00NM3ZZ	Release Facial Nerve, Percutaneous Approach
00NM4ZZ	Release Facial Nerve, Percutaneous Endoscopic Approach
00NN0ZZ	Release Acoustic Nerve, Open Approach
00NN3ZZ	Release Acoustic Nerve, Percutaneous Approach
00NN4ZZ	Release Acoustic Nerve, Percutaneous Endoscopic Approach
00NP0ZZ	Release Glossopharyngeal Nerve, Open Approach
00NP3ZZ	Release Glossopharyngeal Nerve, Percutaneous Approach
00NP4ZZ	Release Glossopharyngeal Nerve, Percutaneous Endoscopic Approach
00NQ0ZZ	Release Vagus Nerve, Open Approach
00NQ3ZZ	Release Vagus Nerve, Percutaneous Approach
00NQ4ZZ	Release Vagus Nerve, Percutaneous Endoscopic Approach
00NR0ZZ	Release Accessory Nerve, Open Approach
00NR3ZZ	Release Accessory Nerve, Percutaneous Approach
00NR4ZZ	Release Accessory Nerve, Percutaneous Endoscopic Approach
00NS0ZZ	Release Hypoglossal Nerve, Open Approach
00NS3ZZ	Release Hypoglossal Nerve, Percutaneous Approach
00NS4ZZ	Release Hypoglossal Nerve, Percutaneous Endoscopic Approach
00NT0ZZ	Release Spinal Meninges, Open Approach
00NT3ZZ	Release Spinal Meninges, Percutaneous Approach
00NT4ZZ	Release Spinal Meninges, Percutaneous Endoscopic Approach
00NW0ZZ	Release Cervical Spinal Cord, Open Approach

Female-only   ♂ Male-only   ▲ Limited Coverage   ● Non-OR   ▨ HAC-associated procedure   ▲ Non-covered procedures   ✚ Combination

00NW3ZZ	Release Cervical Spinal Cord, Percutaneous Approach	
00NW4ZZ	Release Cervical Spinal Cord, Percutaneous Endoscopic Approach	
00NX0ZZ	Release Thoracic Spinal Cord, Open Approach	

00NX3ZZ	Release Thoracic Spinal Cord, Percutaneous Approach
00NX4ZZ	Release Thoracic Spinal Cord, Percutaneous Endoscopic Approach
00NY0ZZ	Release Lumbar Spinal Cord, Open Approach

AHA CC: 3Q, 2014, 24

00NY3ZZ	Release Lumbar Spinal Cord, Percutaneous Approach
00NY4ZZ	Release Lumbar Spinal Cord, Percutaneous Endoscopic Approach

00P – Central Nervous System, Removal

Review Coding Guideline B6.1c

00P000Z	Removal of Drainage Device from Brain, Open Approach
00P002Z	Removal of Monitoring Device from Brain, Open Approach
00P003Z	Removal of Infusion Device from Brain, Open Approach
00P007Z	Removal of Autologous Tissue Substitute from Brain, Open Approach
00P00JZ	Removal of Synthetic Substitute from Brain, Open Approach
00P00KZ	Removal of Nonautologous Tissue Substitute from Brain, Open Approach
00P00MZ	Removal of Neurostimulator Lead from Brain, Open Approach
00P030Z	Removal of Drainage Device from Brain, Percutaneous Approach
00P032Z	Removal of Monitoring Device from Brain, Percutaneous Approach
00P033Z	Removal of Infusion Device from Brain, Percutaneous Approach
00P037Z	Removal of Autologous Tissue Substitute from Brain, Percutaneous Approach
00P03JZ	Removal of Synthetic Substitute from Brain, Percutaneous Approach
00P03KZ	Removal of Nonautologous Tissue Substitute from Brain, Percutaneous Approach
00P03MZ	Removal of Neurostimulator Lead from Brain, Percutaneous Approach
00P040Z	Removal of Drainage Device from Brain, Percutaneous Endoscopic Approach
00P042Z	Removal of Monitoring Device from Brain, Percutaneous Endoscopic Approach
00P043Z	Removal of Infusion Device from Brain, Percutaneous Endoscopic Approach
00P047Z	Removal of Autologous Tissue Substitute from Brain, Percutaneous Endoscopic Approach
00P04JZ	Removal of Synthetic Substitute from Brain, Percutaneous Endoscopic Approach
00P04KZ	Removal of Nonautologous Tissue Substitute from Brain, Percutaneous Endoscopic Approach
00P04MZ	Removal of Neurostimulator Lead from Brain, Percutaneous Endoscopic Approach
00P0X0Z	Removal of Drainage Device from Brain, External Approach
00P0X2Z	Removal of Monitoring Device from Brain, External Approach
00P0X3Z	Removal of Infusion Device from Brain, External Approach
00P0XMZ	Removal of Neurostimulator Lead from Brain, External Approach
00P600Z	Removal of Drainage Device from Cerebral Ventricle, Open Approach
00P602Z	Removal of Monitoring Device from Cerebral Ventricle, Open Approach
00P603Z	Removal of Infusion Device from Cerebral Ventricle, Open Approach
00P60JZ	Removal of Synthetic Substitute from Cerebral Ventricle, Open Approach
00P60MZ	Removal of Neurostimulator Lead from Cerebral Ventricle, Open Approach
00P630Z	Removal of Drainage Device from Cerebral Ventricle, Percutaneous Approach
00P632Z	Removal of Monitoring Device from Cerebral Ventricle, Percutaneous Approach

00P633Z	Removal of Infusion Device from Cerebral Ventricle, Percutaneous Approach
00P63JZ	Removal of Synthetic Substitute from Cerebral Ventricle, Percutaneous Approach
00P63MZ	Removal of Neurostimulator Lead from Cerebral Ventricle, Percutaneous Approach
00P640Z	Removal of Drainage Device from Cerebral Ventricle, Percutaneous Endoscopic Approach
00P642Z	Removal of Monitoring Device from Cerebral Ventricle, Percutaneous Endoscopic Approach
00P643Z	Removal of Infusion Device from Cerebral Ventricle, Percutaneous Endoscopic Approach
00P64JZ	Removal of Synthetic Substitute from Cerebral Ventricle, Percutaneous Endoscopic Approach
00P64MZ	Removal of Neurostimulator Lead from Cerebral Ventricle, Percutaneous Endoscopic Approach
00P6X0Z	Removal of Drainage Device from Cerebral Ventricle, External Approach
00P6X2Z	Removal of Monitoring Device from Cerebral Ventricle, External Approach
00P6X3Z	Removal of Infusion Device from Cerebral Ventricle, External Approach
00P6XMZ	Removal of Neurostimulator Lead from Cerebral Ventricle, External Approach
00PE00Z	Removal of Drainage Device from Cranial Nerve, Open Approach
00PE02Z	Removal of Monitoring Device from Cranial Nerve, Open Approach
00PE03Z	Removal of Infusion Device from Cranial Nerve, Open Approach
00PE07Z	Removal of Autologous Tissue Substitute from Cranial Nerve, Open Approach
00PE0MZ	Removal of Neurostimulator Lead from Cranial Nerve, Open Approach
00PE30Z	Removal of Drainage Device from Cranial Nerve, Percutaneous Approach
00PE32Z	Removal of Monitoring Device from Cranial Nerve, Percutaneous Approach
00PE33Z	Removal of Infusion Device from Cranial Nerve, Percutaneous Approach
00PE37Z	Removal of Autologous Tissue Substitute from Cranial Nerve, Percutaneous Approach
00PE3MZ	Removal of Neurostimulator Lead from Cranial Nerve, Percutaneous Approach
00PE40Z	Removal of Drainage Device from Cranial Nerve, Percutaneous Endoscopic Approach
00PE42Z	Removal of Monitoring Device from Cranial Nerve, Percutaneous Endoscopic Approach
00PE43Z	Removal of Infusion Device from Cranial Nerve, Percutaneous Endoscopic Approach
00PE47Z	Removal of Autologous Tissue Substitute from Cranial Nerve, Percutaneous Endoscopic Approach
00PE4MZ	Removal of Neurostimulator Lead from Cranial Nerve, Percutaneous Endoscopic Approach
00PEX0Z	Removal of Drainage Device from Cranial Nerve, External Approach

00PEX2Z	Removal of Monitoring Device from Cranial Nerve, External Approach
00PEX3Z	Removal of Infusion Device from Cranial Nerve, External Approach
00PEXMZ	Removal of Neurostimulator Lead from Cranial Nerve, External Approach
00PU00Z	Removal of Drainage Device from Spinal Canal, Open Approach
00PU02Z	Removal of Monitoring Device from Spinal Canal, Open Approach
00PU03Z	Removal of Infusion Device from Spinal Canal, Open Approach

AHA CC: 3Q, 2014, 19-20

00PU0JZ	Removal of Synthetic Substitute from Spinal Canal, Open Approach
00PU0MZ	Removal of Neurostimulator Lead from Spinal Canal, Open Approach
00PU30Z	Removal of Drainage Device from Spinal Canal, Percutaneous Approach
00PU32Z	Removal of Monitoring Device from Spinal Canal, Percutaneous Approach
00PU33Z	Removal of Infusion Device from Spinal Canal, Percutaneous Approach
00PU3JZ	Removal of Synthetic Substitute from Spinal Canal, Percutaneous Approach
00PU3MZ	Removal of Neurostimulator Lead from Spinal Canal, Percutaneous Approach
00PU40Z	Removal of Drainage Device from Spinal Canal, Percutaneous Endoscopic Approach
00PU42Z	Removal of Monitoring Device from Spinal Canal, Percutaneous Endoscopic Approach
00PU43Z	Removal of Infusion Device from Spinal Canal, Percutaneous Endoscopic Approach
00PU4JZ	Removal of Synthetic Substitute from Spinal Canal, Percutaneous Endoscopic Approach
00PU4MZ	Removal of Neurostimulator Lead from Spinal Canal, Percutaneous Endoscopic Approach
00PUX0Z	Removal of Drainage Device from Spinal Canal, External Approach
00PUX2Z	Removal of Monitoring Device from Spinal Canal, External Approach
00PUX3Z	Removal of Infusion Device from Spinal Canal, External Approach
00PUXMZ	Removal of Neurostimulator Lead from Spinal Canal, External Approach
00PV00Z	Removal of Drainage Device from Spinal Cord, Open Approach
00PV02Z	Removal of Monitoring Device from Spinal Cord, Open Approach
00PV03Z	Removal of Infusion Device from Spinal Cord, Open Approach
00PV07Z	Removal of Autologous Tissue Substitute from Spinal Cord, Open Approach
00PV0JZ	Removal of Synthetic Substitute from Spinal Cord, Open Approach
00PV0KZ	Removal of Nonautologous Tissue Substitute from Spinal Cord, Open Approach
00PV0MZ	Removal of Neurostimulator Lead from Spinal Cord, Open Approach
00PV30Z	Removal of Drainage Device from Spinal Cord, Percutaneous Approach

♀ Female-only	♂ Male-only

▲ Limited Coverage   ● Non-OR   ▬ HAC-associated procedure   ▲ Non-covered procedures   ✚ Combination

00PV32Z Removal of Monitoring Device from Spinal Cord, Percutaneous Approach
00PV33Z Removal of Infusion Device from Spinal Cord, Percutaneous Approach
00PV37Z Removal of Autologous Tissue Substitute from Spinal Cord, Percutaneous Approach
00PV3JZ Removal of Synthetic Substitute from Spinal Cord, Percutaneous Approach
00PV3KZ Removal of Nonautologous Tissue Substitute from Spinal Cord, Percutaneous Approach
00PV3MZ Removal of Neurostimulator Lead from Spinal Cord, Percutaneous Approach

00PV40Z Removal of Drainage Device from Spinal Cord, Percutaneous Endoscopic Approach
00PV42Z Removal of Monitoring Device from Spinal Cord, Percutaneous Endoscopic Approach
00PV43Z Removal of Infusion Device from Spinal Cord, Percutaneous Endoscopic Approach
00PV47Z Removal of Autologous Tissue Substitute from Spinal Cord, Percutaneous Endoscopic Approach
00PV4JZ Removal of Synthetic Substitute from Spinal Cord, Percutaneous Endoscopic Approach

00PV4KZ Removal of Nonautologous Tissue Substitute from Spinal Cord, Percutaneous Endoscopic Approach
00PV4MZ Removal of Neurostimulator Lead from Spinal Cord, Percutaneous Endoscopic Approach
00PVX0Z Removal of Drainage Device from Spinal Cord, External Approach
00PVX2Z Removal of Monitoring Device from Spinal Cord, External Approach
00PVX3Z Removal of Infusion Device from Spinal Cord, External Approach
00PVXMZ Removal of Neurostimulator Lead from Spinal Cord, External Approach

00Q – Central Nervous System, Repair

00Q00ZZ Repair Brain, Open Approach
00Q03ZZ Repair Brain, Percutaneous Approach
00Q04ZZ Repair Brain, Percutaneous Endoscopic Approach
00Q10ZZ Repair Cerebral Meninges, Open Approach
00Q13ZZ Repair Cerebral Meninges, Percutaneous Approach
00Q14ZZ Repair Cerebral Meninges, Percutaneous Endoscopic Approach
00Q20ZZ Repair Dura Mater, Open Approach
AHA CC: 3Q, 2013, 25; 3Q, 2014, 7-8
00Q23ZZ Repair Dura Mater, Percutaneous Approach
00Q24ZZ Repair Dura Mater, Percutaneous Endoscopic Approach
00Q60ZZ Repair Cerebral Ventricle, Open Approach
00Q63ZZ Repair Cerebral Ventricle, Percutaneous Approach
00Q64ZZ Repair Cerebral Ventricle, Percutaneous Endoscopic Approach
00Q70ZZ Repair Cerebral Hemisphere, Open Approach
00Q73ZZ Repair Cerebral Hemisphere, Percutaneous Approach
00Q74ZZ Repair Cerebral Hemisphere, Percutaneous Endoscopic Approach
00Q80ZZ Repair Basal Ganglia, Open Approach
00Q83ZZ Repair Basal Ganglia, Percutaneous Approach
00Q84ZZ Repair Basal Ganglia, Percutaneous Endoscopic Approach
00Q90ZZ Repair Thalamus, Open Approach
00Q93ZZ Repair Thalamus, Percutaneous Approach
00Q94ZZ Repair Thalamus, Percutaneous Endoscopic Approach
00QA0ZZ Repair Hypothalamus, Open Approach
00QA3ZZ Repair Hypothalamus, Percutaneous Approach
00QA4ZZ Repair Hypothalamus, Percutaneous Endoscopic Approach
00QB0ZZ Repair Pons, Open Approach
00QB3ZZ Repair Pons, Percutaneous Approach
00QB4ZZ Repair Pons, Percutaneous Endoscopic Approach
00QC0ZZ Repair Cerebellum, Open Approach
00QC3ZZ Repair Cerebellum, Percutaneous Approach

00QC4ZZ Repair Cerebellum, Percutaneous Endoscopic Approach
00QD0ZZ Repair Medulla Oblongata, Open Approach
00QD3ZZ Repair Medulla Oblongata, Percutaneous Approach
00QD4ZZ Repair Medulla Oblongata, Percutaneous Endoscopic Approach
00QF0ZZ Repair Olfactory Nerve, Open Approach
00QF3ZZ Repair Olfactory Nerve, Percutaneous Approach
00QF4ZZ Repair Olfactory Nerve, Percutaneous Endoscopic Approach
00QG0ZZ Repair Optic Nerve, Open Approach
00QG3ZZ Repair Optic Nerve, Percutaneous Approach
00QG4ZZ Repair Optic Nerve, Percutaneous Endoscopic Approach
00QH0ZZ Repair Oculomotor Nerve, Open Approach
00QH3ZZ Repair Oculomotor Nerve, Percutaneous Approach
00QH4ZZ Repair Oculomotor Nerve, Percutaneous Endoscopic Approach
00QJ0ZZ Repair Trochlear Nerve, Open Approach
00QJ3ZZ Repair Trochlear Nerve, Percutaneous Approach
00QJ4ZZ Repair Trochlear Nerve, Percutaneous Endoscopic Approach
00QK0ZZ Repair Trigeminal Nerve, Open Approach
00QK3ZZ Repair Trigeminal Nerve, Percutaneous Approach
00QK4ZZ Repair Trigeminal Nerve, Percutaneous Endoscopic Approach
00QL0ZZ Repair Abducens Nerve, Open Approach
00QL3ZZ Repair Abducens Nerve, Percutaneous Approach
00QL4ZZ Repair Abducens Nerve, Percutaneous Endoscopic Approach
00QM0ZZ Repair Facial Nerve, Open Approach
00QM3ZZ Repair Facial Nerve, Percutaneous Approach
00QM4ZZ Repair Facial Nerve, Percutaneous Endoscopic Approach
00QN0ZZ Repair Acoustic Nerve, Open Approach
00QN3ZZ Repair Acoustic Nerve, Percutaneous Approach

00QN4ZZ Repair Acoustic Nerve, Percutaneous Endoscopic Approach
00QP0ZZ Repair Glossopharyngeal Nerve, Open Approach
00QP3ZZ Repair Glossopharyngeal Nerve, Percutaneous Approach
00QP4ZZ Repair Glossopharyngeal Nerve, Percutaneous Endoscopic Approach
00QQ0ZZ Repair Vagus Nerve, Open Approach
00QQ3ZZ Repair Vagus Nerve, Percutaneous Approach
00QQ4ZZ Repair Vagus Nerve, Percutaneous Endoscopic Approach
00QR0ZZ Repair Accessory Nerve, Open Approach
00QR3ZZ Repair Accessory Nerve, Percutaneous Approach
00QR4ZZ Repair Accessory Nerve, Percutaneous Endoscopic Approach
00QS0ZZ Repair Hypoglossal Nerve, Open Approach
00QS3ZZ Repair Hypoglossal Nerve, Percutaneous Approach
00QS4ZZ Repair Hypoglossal Nerve, Percutaneous Endoscopic Approach
00QT0ZZ Repair Spinal Meninges, Open Approach
00QT3ZZ Repair Spinal Meninges, Percutaneous Approach
00QT4ZZ Repair Spinal Meninges, Percutaneous Endoscopic Approach
00QW0ZZ Repair Cervical Spinal Cord, Open Approach
00QW3ZZ Repair Cervical Spinal Cord, Percutaneous Approach
00QW4ZZ Repair Cervical Spinal Cord, Percutaneous Endoscopic Approach
00QX0ZZ Repair Thoracic Spinal Cord, Open Approach
00QX3ZZ Repair Thoracic Spinal Cord, Percutaneous Approach
00QX4ZZ Repair Thoracic Spinal Cord, Percutaneous Endoscopic Approach
00QY0ZZ Repair Lumbar Spinal Cord, Open Approach
00QY3ZZ Repair Lumbar Spinal Cord, Percutaneous Approach
00QY4ZZ Repair Lumbar Spinal Cord, Percutaneous Endoscopic Approach

00S – Central Nervous System, Reposition

00SF0ZZ Reposition Olfactory Nerve, Open Approach
00SF3ZZ Reposition Olfactory Nerve, Percutaneous Approach
00SF4ZZ Reposition Olfactory Nerve, Percutaneous Endoscopic Approach
00SG0ZZ Reposition Optic Nerve, Open Approach
00SG3ZZ Reposition Optic Nerve, Percutaneous Approach
00SG4ZZ Reposition Optic Nerve, Percutaneous Endoscopic Approach

00SH0ZZ Reposition Oculomotor Nerve, Open Approach
00SH3ZZ Reposition Oculomotor Nerve, Percutaneous Approach
00SH4ZZ Reposition Oculomotor Nerve, Percutaneous Endoscopic Approach
00SJ0ZZ Reposition Trochlear Nerve, Open Approach
00SJ3ZZ Reposition Trochlear Nerve, Percutaneous Approach
00SJ4ZZ Reposition Trochlear Nerve, Percutaneous Endoscopic Approach

00SK0ZZ Reposition Trigeminal Nerve, Open Approach
00SK3ZZ Reposition Trigeminal Nerve, Percutaneous Approach
00SK4ZZ Reposition Trigeminal Nerve, Percutaneous Endoscopic Approach
00SL0ZZ Reposition Abducens Nerve, Open Approach
00SL3ZZ Reposition Abducens Nerve, Percutaneous Approach

Female-only   ♂ Male-only   ▲ Limited Coverage   ● Non-OR   ▥ HAC-associated procedure   ▲ Non-covered procedures   ✚ Combination

00SL4ZZ	Reposition Abducens Nerve, Percutaneous Endoscopic Approach	
00SM0ZZ	Reposition Facial Nerve, Open Approach	
	AHA CC: 4Q, 2014, 35	
00SM3ZZ	Reposition Facial Nerve, Percutaneous Approach	
00SM4ZZ	Reposition Facial Nerve, Percutaneous Endoscopic Approach	
00SN0ZZ	Reposition Acoustic Nerve, Open Approach	
00SN3ZZ	Reposition Acoustic Nerve, Percutaneous Approach	
00SN4ZZ	Reposition Acoustic Nerve, Percutaneous Endoscopic Approach	
00SP0ZZ	Reposition Glossopharyngeal Nerve, Open Approach	
00SP3ZZ	Reposition Glossopharyngeal Nerve, Percutaneous Approach	
00SP4ZZ	Reposition Glossopharyngeal Nerve, Percutaneous Endoscopic Approach	
00SQ0ZZ	Reposition Vagus Nerve, Open Approach	
00SQ3ZZ	Reposition Vagus Nerve, Percutaneous Approach	
00SQ4ZZ	Reposition Vagus Nerve, Percutaneous Endoscopic Approach	
00SR0ZZ	Reposition Accessory Nerve, Open Approach	
00SR3ZZ	Reposition Accessory Nerve, Percutaneous Approach	
00SR4ZZ	Reposition Accessory Nerve, Percutaneous Endoscopic Approach	
00SS0ZZ	Reposition Hypoglossal Nerve, Open Approach	
00SS3ZZ	Reposition Hypoglossal Nerve, Percutaneous Approach	
00SS4ZZ	Reposition Hypoglossal Nerve, Percutaneous Endoscopic Approach	
00SW0ZZ	Reposition Cervical Spinal Cord, Open Approach	
00SW3ZZ	Reposition Cervical Spinal Cord, Percutaneous Approach	
00SW4ZZ	Reposition Cervical Spinal Cord, Percutaneous Endoscopic Approach	
00SX0ZZ	Reposition Thoracic Spinal Cord, Open Approach	
00SX3ZZ	Reposition Thoracic Spinal Cord, Percutaneous Approach	
00SX4ZZ	Reposition Thoracic Spinal Cord, Percutaneous Endoscopic Approach	
00SY0ZZ	Reposition Lumbar Spinal Cord, Open Approach	
00SY3ZZ	Reposition Lumbar Spinal Cord, Percutaneous Approach	
00SY4ZZ	Reposition Lumbar Spinal Cord, Percutaneous Endoscopic Approach	

00T – Central Nervous System, Resection

Review Coding Guideline B3.8

00T70ZZ	Resection of Cerebral Hemisphere, Open Approach	
00T73ZZ	Resection of Cerebral Hemisphere, Percutaneous Approach	
00T74ZZ	Resection of Cerebral Hemisphere, Percutaneous Endoscopic Approach	

00U – Central Nervous System, Supplement

00U107Z	Supplement Cerebral Meninges with Autologous Tissue Substitute, Open Approach
00U10JZ	Supplement Cerebral Meninges with Synthetic Substitute, Open Approach
00U10KZ	Supplement Cerebral Meninges with Nonautologous Tissue Substitute, Open Approach
00U137Z	Supplement Cerebral Meninges with Autologous Tissue Substitute, Percutaneous Approach
00U13JZ	Supplement Cerebral Meninges with Synthetic Substitute, Percutaneous Approach
00U13KZ	Supplement Cerebral Meninges with Nonautologous Tissue Substitute, Percutaneous Approach
00U147Z	Supplement Cerebral Meninges with Autologous Tissue Substitute, Percutaneous Endoscopic Approach
00U14JZ	Supplement Cerebral Meninges with Synthetic Substitute, Percutaneous Endoscopic Approach
00U14KZ	Supplement Cerebral Meninges with Nonautologous Tissue Substitute, Percutaneous Endoscopic Approach
00U207Z	Supplement Dura Mater with Autologous Tissue Substitute, Open Approach
00U20JZ	Supplement Dura Mater with Synthetic Substitute, Open Approach
00U20KZ	Supplement Dura Mater with Nonautologous Tissue Substitute, Open Approach
00U237Z	Supplement Dura Mater with Autologous Tissue Substitute, Percutaneous Approach
00U23JZ	Supplement Dura Mater with Synthetic Substitute, Percutaneous Approach
00U23KZ	Supplement Dura Mater with Nonautologous Tissue Substitute, Percutaneous Approach
00U247Z	Supplement Dura Mater with Autologous Tissue Substitute, Percutaneous Endoscopic Approach
00U24JZ	Supplement Dura Mater with Synthetic Substitute, Percutaneous Endoscopic Approach
00U24KZ	Supplement Dura Mater with Nonautologous Tissue Substitute, Percutaneous Endoscopic Approach
00UF07Z	Supplement Olfactory Nerve with Autologous Tissue Substitute, Open Approach
00UF37Z	Supplement Olfactory Nerve with Autologous Tissue Substitute, Percutaneous Approach
00UF47Z	Supplement Olfactory Nerve with Autologous Tissue Substitute, Percutaneous Endoscopic Approach
00UG07Z	Supplement Optic Nerve with Autologous Tissue Substitute, Open Approach
00UG37Z	Supplement Optic Nerve with Autologous Tissue Substitute, Percutaneous Approach
00UG47Z	Supplement Optic Nerve with Autologous Tissue Substitute, Percutaneous Endoscopic Approach
00UH07Z	Supplement Oculomotor Nerve with Autologous Tissue Substitute, Open Approach
00UH37Z	Supplement Oculomotor Nerve with Autologous Tissue Substitute, Percutaneous Approach
00UH47Z	Supplement Oculomotor Nerve with Autologous Tissue Substitute, Percutaneous Endoscopic Approach
00UJ07Z	Supplement Trochlear Nerve with Autologous Tissue Substitute, Open Approach
00UJ37Z	Supplement Trochlear Nerve with Autologous Tissue Substitute, Percutaneous Approach
00UJ47Z	Supplement Trochlear Nerve with Autologous Tissue Substitute, Percutaneous Endoscopic Approach
00UK07Z	Supplement Trigeminal Nerve with Autologous Tissue Substitute, Open Approach
00UK37Z	Supplement Trigeminal Nerve with Autologous Tissue Substitute, Percutaneous Approach
00UK47Z	Supplement Trigeminal Nerve with Autologous Tissue Substitute, Percutaneous Endoscopic Approach
00UL07Z	Supplement Abducens Nerve with Autologous Tissue Substitute, Open Approach
00UL37Z	Supplement Abducens Nerve with Autologous Tissue Substitute, Percutaneous Approach
00UL47Z	Supplement Abducens Nerve with Autologous Tissue Substitute, Percutaneous Endoscopic Approach
00UM07Z	Supplement Facial Nerve with Autologous Tissue Substitute, Open Approach
00UM37Z	Supplement Facial Nerve with Autologous Tissue Substitute, Percutaneous Approach
00UM47Z	Supplement Facial Nerve with Autologous Tissue Substitute, Percutaneous Endoscopic Approach
00UN07Z	Supplement Acoustic Nerve with Autologous Tissue Substitute, Open Approach
00UN37Z	Supplement Acoustic Nerve with Autologous Tissue Substitute, Percutaneous Approach
00UN47Z	Supplement Acoustic Nerve with Autologous Tissue Substitute, Percutaneous Endoscopic Approach
00UP07Z	Supplement Glossopharyngeal Nerve with Autologous Tissue Substitute, Open Approach
00UP37Z	Supplement Glossopharyngeal Nerve with Autologous Tissue Substitute, Percutaneous Approach
00UP47Z	Supplement Glossopharyngeal Nerve with Autologous Tissue Substitute, Percutaneous Endoscopic Approach
00UQ07Z	Supplement Vagus Nerve with Autologous Tissue Substitute, Open Approach
00UQ37Z	Supplement Vagus Nerve with Autologous Tissue Substitute, Percutaneous Approach
00UQ47Z	Supplement Vagus Nerve with Autologous Tissue Substitute, Percutaneous Endoscopic Approach
00UR07Z	Supplement Accessory Nerve with Autologous Tissue Substitute, Open Approach
00UR37Z	Supplement Accessory Nerve with Autologous Tissue Substitute, Percutaneous Approach
00UR47Z	Supplement Accessory Nerve with Autologous Tissue Substitute, Percutaneous Endoscopic Approach
00US07Z	Supplement Hypoglossal Nerve with Autologous Tissue Substitute, Open Approach
00US37Z	Supplement Hypoglossal Nerve with Autologous Tissue Substitute, Percutaneous Approach

♀ Female-only   ♂ Male-only   ▲ Limited Coverage   ● Non-OR   ▨ HAC-associated procedure   ▲ Non-covered procedures   ✚ Combination

00US47Z Supplement Hypoglossal Nerve with Autologous Tissue Substitute, Percutaneous Endoscopic Approach

00UT07Z Supplement Spinal Meninges with Autologous Tissue Substitute, Open Approach

00UT0JZ Supplement Spinal Meninges with Synthetic Substitute, Open Approach

00UT0KZ Supplement Spinal Meninges with Nonautologous Tissue Substitute, Open Approach
AHA CC: 3Q, 2014, 24

00UT37Z Supplement Spinal Meninges with Autologous Tissue Substitute, Percutaneous Approach

00UT3JZ Supplement Spinal Meninges with Synthetic Substitute, Percutaneous Approach

00UT3KZ Supplement Spinal Meninges with Nonautologous Tissue Substitute, Percutaneous Approach

00UT47Z Supplement Spinal Meninges with Autologous Tissue Substitute, Percutaneous Endoscopic Approach

00UT4JZ Supplement Spinal Meninges with Synthetic Substitute, Percutaneous Endoscopic Approach

00UT4KZ Supplement Spinal Meninges with Nonautologous Tissue Substitute, Percutaneous Endoscopic Approach

0W – Central Nervous System, Revision

Review Coding Guideline B6.1c

00W000Z Revision of Drainage Device in Brain, Open Approach

00W002Z Revision of Monitoring Device in Brain, Open Approach

00W003Z Revision of Infusion Device in Brain, Open Approach

00W007Z Revision of Autologous Tissue Substitute in Brain, Open Approach

00W00JZ Revision of Synthetic Substitute in Brain, Open Approach

00W00KZ Revision of Nonautologous Tissue Substitute in Brain, Open Approach

00W00MZ Revision of Neurostimulator Lead in Brain, Open Approach

00W030Z Revision of Drainage Device in Brain, Percutaneous Approach

00W032Z Revision of Monitoring Device in Brain, Percutaneous Approach

00W033Z Revision of Infusion Device in Brain, Percutaneous Approach

00W037Z Revision of Autologous Tissue Substitute in Brain, Percutaneous Approach

00W03JZ Revision of Synthetic Substitute in Brain, Percutaneous Approach

00W03KZ Revision of Nonautologous Tissue Substitute in Brain, Percutaneous Approach

00W03MZ Revision of Neurostimulator Lead in Brain, Percutaneous Approach

00W040Z Revision of Drainage Device in Brain, Percutaneous Endoscopic Approach

00W042Z Revision of Monitoring Device in Brain, Percutaneous Endoscopic Approach

00W043Z Revision of Infusion Device in Brain, Percutaneous Endoscopic Approach

00W047Z Revision of Autologous Tissue Substitute in Brain, Percutaneous Endoscopic Approach

00W04JZ Revision of Synthetic Substitute in Brain, Percutaneous Endoscopic Approach

00W04KZ Revision of Nonautologous Tissue Substitute in Brain, Percutaneous Endoscopic Approach

00W04MZ Revision of Neurostimulator Lead in Brain, Percutaneous Endoscopic Approach

00W0X0Z Revision of Drainage Device in Brain, External Approach

00W0X2Z Revision of Monitoring Device in Brain, External Approach

00W0X3Z Revision of Infusion Device in Brain, External Approach

00W0X7Z Revision of Autologous Tissue Substitute in Brain, External Approach

00W0XJZ Revision of Synthetic Substitute in Brain, External Approach

00W0XKZ Revision of Nonautologous Tissue Substitute in Brain, External Approach

00W0XMZ Revision of Neurostimulator Lead in Brain, External Approach

00W600Z Revision of Drainage Device in Cerebral Ventricle, Open Approach

00W602Z Revision of Monitoring Device in Cerebral Ventricle, Open Approach

00W603Z Revision of Infusion Device in Cerebral Ventricle, Open Approach

00W60JZ Revision of Synthetic Substitute in Cerebral Ventricle, Open Approach

00W60MZ Revision of Neurostimulator Lead in Cerebral Ventricle, Open Approach

00W630Z Revision of Drainage Device in Cerebral Ventricle, Percutaneous Approach

00W632Z Revision of Monitoring Device in Cerebral Ventricle, Percutaneous Approach

00W633Z Revision of Infusion Device in Cerebral Ventricle, Percutaneous Approach

00W63JZ Revision of Synthetic Substitute in Cerebral Ventricle, Percutaneous Approach

00W63MZ Revision of Neurostimulator Lead in Cerebral Ventricle, Percutaneous Approach

00W640Z Revision of Drainage Device in Cerebral Ventricle, Percutaneous Endoscopic Approach

00W642Z Revision of Monitoring Device in Cerebral Ventricle, Percutaneous Endoscopic Approach

00W643Z Revision of Infusion Device in Cerebral Ventricle, Percutaneous Endoscopic Approach

00W64JZ Revision of Synthetic Substitute in Cerebral Ventricle, Percutaneous Endoscopic Approach

00W64MZ Revision of Neurostimulator Lead in Cerebral Ventricle, Percutaneous Endoscopic Approach

00W6X0Z Revision of Drainage Device in Cerebral Ventricle, External Approach

00W6X2Z Revision of Monitoring Device in Cerebral Ventricle, External Approach

00W6X3Z Revision of Infusion Device in Cerebral Ventricle, External Approach

00W6XJZ Revision of Synthetic Substitute in Cerebral Ventricle, External Approach

00W6XMZ Revision of Neurostimulator Lead in Cerebral Ventricle, External Approach

00WE00Z Revision of Drainage Device in Cranial Nerve, Open Approach

00WE02Z Revision of Monitoring Device in Cranial Nerve, Open Approach

00WE03Z Revision of Infusion Device in Cranial Nerve, Open Approach

00WE07Z Revision of Autologous Tissue Substitute in Cranial Nerve, Open Approach

00WE0MZ Revision of Neurostimulator Lead in Cranial Nerve, Open Approach

00WE30Z Revision of Drainage Device in Cranial Nerve, Percutaneous Approach

00WE32Z Revision of Monitoring Device in Cranial Nerve, Percutaneous Approach

00WE33Z Revision of Infusion Device in Cranial Nerve, Percutaneous Approach

00WE37Z Revision of Autologous Tissue Substitute in Cranial Nerve, Percutaneous Approach

00WE3MZ Revision of Neurostimulator Lead in Cranial Nerve, Percutaneous Approach

00WE40Z Revision of Drainage Device in Cranial Nerve, Percutaneous Endoscopic Approach

00WE42Z Revision of Monitoring Device in Cranial Nerve, Percutaneous Endoscopic Approach

00WE43Z Revision of Infusion Device in Cranial Nerve, Percutaneous Endoscopic Approach

00WE47Z Revision of Autologous Tissue Substitute in Cranial Nerve, Percutaneous Endoscopic Approach

00WE4MZ Revision of Neurostimulator Lead in Cranial Nerve, Percutaneous Endoscopic Approach

00WEX0Z Revision of Drainage Device in Cranial Nerve, External Approach

00WEX2Z Revision of Monitoring Device in Cranial Nerve, External Approach

00WEX3Z Revision of Infusion Device in Cranial Nerve, External Approach

00WEX7Z Revision of Autologous Tissue Substitute in Cranial Nerve, External Approach

00WEXMZ Revision of Neurostimulator Lead in Cranial Nerve, External Approach

00WU00Z Revision of Drainage Device in Spinal Canal, Open Approach

00WU02Z Revision of Monitoring Device in Spinal Canal, Open Approach

00WU03Z Revision of Infusion Device in Spinal Canal, Open Approach

00WU0JZ Revision of Synthetic Substitute in Spinal Canal, Open Approach

00WU0MZ Revision of Neurostimulator Lead in Spinal Canal, Open Approach

00WU30Z Revision of Drainage Device in Spinal Canal, Percutaneous Approach

00WU32Z Revision of Monitoring Device in Spinal Canal, Percutaneous Approach

00WU33Z Revision of Infusion Device in Spinal Canal, Percutaneous Approach

00WU3JZ Revision of Synthetic Substitute in Spinal Canal, Percutaneous Approach

00WU3MZ Revision of Neurostimulator Lead in Spinal Canal, Percutaneous Approach

00WU40Z Revision of Drainage Device in Spinal Canal, Percutaneous Endoscopic Approach

00WU42Z Revision of Monitoring Device in Spinal Canal, Percutaneous Endoscopic Approach

00WU43Z Revision of Infusion Device in Spinal Canal, Percutaneous Endoscopic Approach

00WU4JZ Revision of Synthetic Substitute in Spinal Canal, Percutaneous Endoscopic Approach

Female-only ♂ Male-only ▲ Limited Coverage ● Non-OR ▦ HAC-associated procedure ▲ Non-covered procedures ＋ Combination

00WU4MZ	Revision of Neurostimulator Lead in Spinal Canal, Percutaneous Endoscopic Approach
00WUX0Z	Revision of Drainage Device in Spinal Canal, External Approach
00WUX2Z	Revision of Monitoring Device in Spinal Canal, External Approach
00WUX3Z	Revision of Infusion Device in Spinal Canal, External Approach
00WUXJZ	Revision of Synthetic Substitute in Spinal Canal, External Approach
00WUXMZ	Revision of Neurostimulator Lead in Spinal Canal, External Approach
00WV00Z	Revision of Drainage Device in Spinal Cord, Open Approach
00WV02Z	Revision of Monitoring Device in Spinal Cord, Open Approach
00WV03Z	Revision of Infusion Device in Spinal Cord, Open Approach
00WV07Z	Revision of Autologous Tissue Substitute in Spinal Cord, Open Approach
00WV0JZ	Revision of Synthetic Substitute in Spinal Cord, Open Approach
00WV0KZ	Revision of Nonautologous Tissue Substitute in Spinal Cord, Open Approach
00WV0MZ	Revision of Neurostimulator Lead in Spinal Cord, Open Approach

00WV30Z	Revision of Drainage Device in Spinal Cord, Percutaneous Approach
00WV32Z	Revision of Monitoring Device in Spinal Cord, Percutaneous Approach
00WV33Z	Revision of Infusion Device in Spinal Cord, Percutaneous Approach
00WV37Z	Revision of Autologous Tissue Substitute in Spinal Cord, Percutaneous Approach
00WV3JZ	Revision of Synthetic Substitute in Spinal Cord, Percutaneous Approach
00WV3KZ	Revision of Nonautologous Tissue Substitute in Spinal Cord, Percutaneous Approach
00WV3MZ	Revision of Neurostimulator Lead in Spinal Cord, Percutaneous Approach
00WV40Z	Revision of Drainage Device in Spinal Cord, Percutaneous Endoscopic Approach
00WV42Z	Revision of Monitoring Device in Spinal Cord, Percutaneous Endoscopic Approach
00WV43Z	Revision of Infusion Device in Spinal Cord, Percutaneous Endoscopic Approach
00WV47Z	Revision of Autologous Tissue Substitute in Spinal Cord, Percutaneous Endoscopic Approach

00WV4JZ	Revision of Synthetic Substitute in Spinal Cord, Percutaneous Endoscopic Approach
00WV4KZ	Revision of Nonautologous Tissue Substitute in Spinal Cord, Percutaneous Endoscopic Approach
00WV4MZ	Revision of Neurostimulator Lead in Spinal Cord, Percutaneous Endoscopic Approach
00WVX0Z	Revision of Drainage Device in Spinal Cord, External Approach
00WVX2Z	Revision of Monitoring Device in Spinal Cord, External Approach
00WVX3Z	Revision of Infusion Device in Spinal Cord, External Approach
00WVX7Z	Revision of Autologous Tissue Substitute in Spinal Cord, External Approach
00WVXJZ	Revision of Synthetic Substitute in Spinal Cord, External Approach
00WVXKZ	Revision of Nonautologous Tissue Substitute in Spinal Cord, External Approach
00WVXMZ	Revision of Neurostimulator Lead in Spinal Cord, External Approach

00X – Central Nervous System, Transfer

00XF0ZF	Transfer Olfactory Nerve to Olfactory Nerve, Open Approach
00XF0ZG	Transfer Olfactory Nerve to Optic Nerve, Open Approach
00XF0ZH	Transfer Olfactory Nerve to Oculomotor Nerve, Open Approach
00XF0ZJ	Transfer Olfactory Nerve to Trochlear Nerve, Open Approach
00XF0ZK	Transfer Olfactory Nerve to Trigeminal Nerve, Open Approach
00XF0ZL	Transfer Olfactory Nerve to Abducens Nerve, Open Approach
00XF0ZM	Transfer Olfactory Nerve to Facial Nerve, Open Approach
00XF0ZN	Transfer Olfactory Nerve to Acoustic Nerve, Open Approach
00XF0ZP	Transfer Olfactory Nerve to Glossopharyngeal Nerve, Open Approach
00XF0ZQ	Transfer Olfactory Nerve to Vagus Nerve, Open Approach
00XF0ZR	Transfer Olfactory Nerve to Accessory Nerve, Open Approach
00XF0ZS	Transfer Olfactory Nerve to Hypoglossal Nerve, Open Approach
00XF4ZF	Transfer Olfactory Nerve to Olfactory Nerve, Percutaneous Endoscopic Approach
00XF4ZG	Transfer Olfactory Nerve to Optic Nerve, Percutaneous Endoscopic Approach
00XF4ZH	Transfer Olfactory Nerve to Oculomotor Nerve, Percutaneous Endoscopic Approach
00XF4ZJ	Transfer Olfactory Nerve to Trochlear Nerve, Percutaneous Endoscopic Approach
00XF4ZK	Transfer Olfactory Nerve to Trigeminal Nerve, Percutaneous Endoscopic Approach
00XF4ZL	Transfer Olfactory Nerve to Abducens Nerve, Percutaneous Endoscopic Approach
00XF4ZM	Transfer Olfactory Nerve to Facial Nerve, Percutaneous Endoscopic Approach
00XF4ZN	Transfer Olfactory Nerve to Acoustic Nerve, Percutaneous Endoscopic Approach

00XF4ZP	Transfer Olfactory Nerve to Glossopharyngeal Nerve, Percutaneous Endoscopic Approach
00XF4ZQ	Transfer Olfactory Nerve to Vagus Nerve, Percutaneous Endoscopic Approach
00XF4ZR	Transfer Olfactory Nerve to Accessory Nerve, Percutaneous Endoscopic Approach
00XF4ZS	Transfer Olfactory Nerve to Hypoglossal Nerve, Percutaneous Endoscopic Approach
00XG0ZF	Transfer Optic Nerve to Olfactory Nerve, Open Approach
00XG0ZG	Transfer Optic Nerve to Optic Nerve, Open Approach
00XG0ZH	Transfer Optic Nerve to Oculomotor Nerve, Open Approach
00XG0ZJ	Transfer Optic Nerve to Trochlear Nerve, Open Approach
00XG0ZK	Transfer Optic Nerve to Trigeminal Nerve, Open Approach
00XG0ZL	Transfer Optic Nerve to Abducens Nerve, Open Approach
00XG0ZM	Transfer Optic Nerve to Facial Nerve, Open Approach
00XG0ZN	Transfer Optic Nerve to Acoustic Nerve, Open Approach
00XG0ZP	Transfer Optic Nerve to Glossopharyngeal Nerve, Open Approach
00XG0ZQ	Transfer Optic Nerve to Vagus Nerve, Open Approach
00XG0ZR	Transfer Optic Nerve to Accessory Nerve, Open Approach
00XG0ZS	Transfer Optic Nerve to Hypoglossal Nerve, Open Approach
00XG4ZF	Transfer Optic Nerve to Olfactory Nerve, Percutaneous Endoscopic Approach
00XG4ZG	Transfer Optic Nerve to Optic Nerve, Percutaneous Endoscopic Approach
00XG4ZH	Transfer Optic Nerve to Oculomotor Nerve, Percutaneous Endoscopic Approach
00XG4ZJ	Transfer Optic Nerve to Trochlear Nerve, Percutaneous Endoscopic Approach

00XG4ZK	Transfer Optic Nerve to Trigeminal Nerve, Percutaneous Endoscopic Approach
00XG4ZL	Transfer Optic Nerve to Abducens Nerve, Percutaneous Endoscopic Approach
00XG4ZM	Transfer Optic Nerve to Facial Nerve, Percutaneous Endoscopic Approach
00XG4ZN	Transfer Optic Nerve to Acoustic Nerve, Percutaneous Endoscopic Approach
00XG4ZP	Transfer Optic Nerve to Glossopharyngeal Nerve, Percutaneous Endoscopic Approach
00XG4ZQ	Transfer Optic Nerve to Vagus Nerve, Percutaneous Endoscopic Approach
00XG4ZR	Transfer Optic Nerve to Accessory Nerve, Percutaneous Endoscopic Approach
00XG4ZS	Transfer Optic Nerve to Hypoglossal Nerve, Percutaneous Endoscopic Approach
00XH0ZF	Transfer Oculomotor Nerve to Olfactory Nerve, Open Approach
00XH0ZG	Transfer Oculomotor Nerve to Optic Nerve, Open Approach
00XH0ZH	Transfer Oculomotor Nerve to Oculomotor Nerve, Open Approach
00XH0ZJ	Transfer Oculomotor Nerve to Trochlear Nerve, Open Approach
00XH0ZK	Transfer Oculomotor Nerve to Trigeminal Nerve, Open Approach
00XH0ZL	Transfer Oculomotor Nerve to Abducens Nerve, Open Approach
00XH0ZM	Transfer Oculomotor Nerve to Facial Nerve, Open Approach
00XH0ZN	Transfer Oculomotor Nerve to Acoustic Nerve, Open Approach
00XH0ZP	Transfer Oculomotor Nerve to Glossopharyngeal Nerve, Open Approach
00XH0ZQ	Transfer Oculomotor Nerve to Vagus Nerve, Open Approach
00XH0ZR	Transfer Oculomotor Nerve to Accessory Nerve, Open Approach
00XH0ZS	Transfer Oculomotor Nerve to Hypoglossal Nerve, Open Approach
00XH4ZF	Transfer Oculomotor Nerve to Olfactory Nerve, Percutaneous Endoscopic Approach

0XH4ZG Transfer Oculomotor Nerve to Optic Nerve, Percutaneous Endoscopic Approach

0XH4ZH Transfer Oculomotor Nerve to Oculomotor Nerve, Percutaneous Endoscopic Approach

0XH4ZJ Transfer Oculomotor Nerve to Trochlear Nerve, Percutaneous Endoscopic Approach

0XH4ZK Transfer Oculomotor Nerve to Trigeminal Nerve, Percutaneous Endoscopic Approach

0XH4ZL Transfer Oculomotor Nerve to Abducens Nerve, Percutaneous Endoscopic Approach

0XH4ZM Transfer Oculomotor Nerve to Facial Nerve, Percutaneous Endoscopic Approach

0XH4ZN Transfer Oculomotor Nerve to Acoustic Nerve, Percutaneous Endoscopic Approach

0XH4ZP Transfer Oculomotor Nerve to Glossopharyngeal Nerve, Percutaneous Endoscopic Approach

0XH4ZQ Transfer Oculomotor Nerve to Vagus Nerve, Percutaneous Endoscopic Approach

0XH4ZR Transfer Oculomotor Nerve to Accessory Nerve, Percutaneous Endoscopic Approach

0XH4ZS Transfer Oculomotor Nerve to Hypoglossal Nerve, Percutaneous Endoscopic Approach

0XJ0ZF Transfer Trochlear Nerve to Olfactory Nerve, Open Approach

0XJ0ZG Transfer Trochlear Nerve to Optic Nerve, Open Approach

0XJ0ZH Transfer Trochlear Nerve to Oculomotor Nerve, Open Approach

0XJ0ZJ Transfer Trochlear Nerve to Trochlear Nerve, Open Approach

0XJ0ZK Transfer Trochlear Nerve to Trigeminal Nerve, Open Approach

0XJ0ZL Transfer Trochlear Nerve to Abducens Nerve, Open Approach

0XJ0ZM Transfer Trochlear Nerve to Facial Nerve, Open Approach

0XJ0ZN Transfer Trochlear Nerve to Acoustic Nerve, Open Approach

0XJ0ZP Transfer Trochlear Nerve to Glossopharyngeal Nerve, Open Approach

0XJ0ZQ Transfer Trochlear Nerve to Vagus Nerve, Open Approach

0XJ0ZR Transfer Trochlear Nerve to Accessory Nerve, Open Approach

0XJ0ZS Transfer Trochlear Nerve to Hypoglossal Nerve, Open Approach

0XJ4ZF Transfer Trochlear Nerve to Olfactory Nerve, Percutaneous Endoscopic Approach

0XJ4ZG Transfer Trochlear Nerve to Optic Nerve, Percutaneous Endoscopic Approach

0XJ4ZH Transfer Trochlear Nerve to Oculomotor Nerve, Percutaneous Endoscopic Approach

0XJ4ZJ Transfer Trochlear Nerve to Trochlear Nerve, Percutaneous Endoscopic Approach

0XJ4ZK Transfer Trochlear Nerve to Trigeminal Nerve, Percutaneous Endoscopic Approach

0XJ4ZL Transfer Trochlear Nerve to Abducens Nerve, Percutaneous Endoscopic Approach

0XJ4ZM Transfer Trochlear Nerve to Facial Nerve, Percutaneous Endoscopic Approach

00XJ4ZN Transfer Trochlear Nerve to Acoustic Nerve, Percutaneous Endoscopic Approach

00XJ4ZP Transfer Trochlear Nerve to Glossopharyngeal Nerve, Percutaneous Endoscopic Approach

00XJ4ZQ Transfer Trochlear Nerve to Vagus Nerve, Percutaneous Endoscopic Approach

00XJ4ZR Transfer Trochlear Nerve to Accessory Nerve, Percutaneous Endoscopic Approach

00XJ4ZS Transfer Trochlear Nerve to Hypoglossal Nerve, Percutaneous Endoscopic Approach

00XK0ZF Transfer Trigeminal Nerve to Olfactory Nerve, Open Approach

00XK0ZG Transfer Trigeminal Nerve to Optic Nerve, Open Approach

00XK0ZH Transfer Trigeminal Nerve to Oculomotor Nerve, Open Approach

00XK0ZJ Transfer Trigeminal Nerve to Trochlear Nerve, Open Approach

00XK0ZK Transfer Trigeminal Nerve to Trigeminal Nerve, Open Approach

00XK0ZL Transfer Trigeminal Nerve to Abducens Nerve, Open Approach

00XK0ZM Transfer Trigeminal Nerve to Facial Nerve, Open Approach

00XK0ZN Transfer Trigeminal Nerve to Acoustic Nerve, Open Approach

00XK0ZP Transfer Trigeminal Nerve to Glossopharyngeal Nerve, Open Approach

00XK0ZQ Transfer Trigeminal Nerve to Vagus Nerve, Open Approach

00XK0ZR Transfer Trigeminal Nerve to Accessory Nerve, Open Approach

00XK0ZS Transfer Trigeminal Nerve to Hypoglossal Nerve, Open Approach

00XK4ZF Transfer Trigeminal Nerve to Olfactory Nerve, Percutaneous Endoscopic Approach

00XK4ZG Transfer Trigeminal Nerve to Optic Nerve, Percutaneous Endoscopic Approach

00XK4ZH Transfer Trigeminal Nerve to Oculomotor Nerve, Percutaneous Endoscopic Approach

00XK4ZJ Transfer Trigeminal Nerve to Trochlear Nerve, Percutaneous Endoscopic Approach

00XK4ZK Transfer Trigeminal Nerve to Trigeminal Nerve, Percutaneous Endoscopic Approach

00XK4ZL Transfer Trigeminal Nerve to Abducens Nerve, Percutaneous Endoscopic Approach

00XK4ZM Transfer Trigeminal Nerve to Facial Nerve, Percutaneous Endoscopic Approach

00XK4ZN Transfer Trigeminal Nerve to Acoustic Nerve, Percutaneous Endoscopic Approach

00XK4ZP Transfer Trigeminal Nerve to Glossopharyngeal Nerve, Percutaneous Endoscopic Approach

00XK4ZQ Transfer Trigeminal Nerve to Vagus Nerve, Percutaneous Endoscopic Approach

00XK4ZR Transfer Trigeminal Nerve to Accessory Nerve, Percutaneous Endoscopic Approach

00XK4ZS Transfer Trigeminal Nerve to Hypoglossal Nerve, Percutaneous Endoscopic Approach

00XL0ZF Transfer Abducens Nerve to Olfactory Nerve, Open Approach

00XL0ZG Transfer Abducens Nerve to Optic Nerve, Open Approach

00XL0ZH Transfer Abducens Nerve to Oculomotor Nerve, Open Approach

00XL0ZJ Transfer Abducens Nerve to Trochlear Nerve, Open Approach

00XL0ZK Transfer Abducens Nerve to Trigeminal Nerve, Open Approach

00XL0ZL Transfer Abducens Nerve to Abducens Nerve, Open Approach

00XL0ZM Transfer Abducens Nerve to Facial Nerve, Open Approach

00XL0ZN Transfer Abducens Nerve to Acoustic Nerve, Open Approach

00XL0ZP Transfer Abducens Nerve to Glossopharyngeal Nerve, Open Approach

00XL0ZQ Transfer Abducens Nerve to Vagus Nerve, Open Approach

00XL0ZR Transfer Abducens Nerve to Accessory Nerve, Open Approach

00XL0ZS Transfer Abducens Nerve to Hypoglossal Nerve, Open Approach

00XL4ZF Transfer Abducens Nerve to Olfactory Nerve, Percutaneous Endoscopic Approach

00XL4ZG Transfer Abducens Nerve to Optic Nerve, Percutaneous Endoscopic Approach

00XL4ZH Transfer Abducens Nerve to Oculomotor Nerve, Percutaneous Endoscopic Approach

00XL4ZJ Transfer Abducens Nerve to Trochlear Nerve, Percutaneous Endoscopic Approach

00XL4ZK Transfer Abducens Nerve to Trigeminal Nerve, Percutaneous Endoscopic Approach

00XL4ZL Transfer Abducens Nerve to Abducens Nerve, Percutaneous Endoscopic Approach

00XL4ZM Transfer Abducens Nerve to Facial Nerve, Percutaneous Endoscopic Approach

00XL4ZN Transfer Abducens Nerve to Acoustic Nerve, Percutaneous Endoscopic Approach

00XL4ZP Transfer Abducens Nerve to Glossopharyngeal Nerve, Percutaneous Endoscopic Approach

00XL4ZQ Transfer Abducens Nerve to Vagus Nerve, Percutaneous Endoscopic Approach

00XL4ZR Transfer Abducens Nerve to Accessory Nerve, Percutaneous Endoscopic Approach

00XL4ZS Transfer Abducens Nerve to Hypoglossal Nerve, Percutaneous Endoscopic Approach

00XM0ZF Transfer Facial Nerve to Olfactory Nerve, Open Approach

00XM0ZG Transfer Facial Nerve to Optic Nerve, Open Approach

00XM0ZH Transfer Facial Nerve to Oculomotor Nerve, Open Approach

00XM0ZJ Transfer Facial Nerve to Trochlear Nerve, Open Approach

00XM0ZK Transfer Facial Nerve to Trigeminal Nerve, Open Approach

00XM0ZL Transfer Facial Nerve to Abducens Nerve, Open Approach

00XM0ZM Transfer Facial Nerve to Facial Nerve, Open Approach

00XM0ZN Transfer Facial Nerve to Acoustic Nerve, Open Approach

00XM0ZP Transfer Facial Nerve to Glossopharyngeal Nerve, Open Approach

00XM0ZQ Transfer Facial Nerve to Vagus Nerve, Open Approach

00XM0ZR Transfer Facial Nerve to Accessory Nerve, Open Approach

Female-only   ♂ Male-only   ▲ Limited Coverage   ● Non-OR   ▆▆ HAC-associated procedure   ▲ Non-covered procedures   ✚ Combination

00XM0ZS	Transfer Facial Nerve to Hypoglossal Nerve, Open Approach
00XM4ZF	Transfer Facial Nerve to Olfactory Nerve, Percutaneous Endoscopic Approach
00XM4ZG	Transfer Facial Nerve to Optic Nerve, Percutaneous Endoscopic Approach
00XM4ZH	Transfer Facial Nerve to Oculomotor Nerve, Percutaneous Endoscopic Approach
00XM4ZJ	Transfer Facial Nerve to Trochlear Nerve, Percutaneous Endoscopic Approach
00XM4ZK	Transfer Facial Nerve to Trigeminal Nerve, Percutaneous Endoscopic Approach
00XM4ZL	Transfer Facial Nerve to Abducens Nerve, Percutaneous Endoscopic Approach
00XM4ZM	Transfer Facial Nerve to Facial Nerve, Percutaneous Endoscopic Approach
00XM4ZN	Transfer Facial Nerve to Acoustic Nerve, Percutaneous Endoscopic Approach
00XM4ZP	Transfer Facial Nerve to Glossopharyngeal Nerve, Percutaneous Endoscopic Approach
00XM4ZQ	Transfer Facial Nerve to Vagus Nerve, Percutaneous Endoscopic Approach
00XM4ZR	Transfer Facial Nerve to Accessory Nerve, Percutaneous Endoscopic Approach
00XM4ZS	Transfer Facial Nerve to Hypoglossal Nerve, Percutaneous Endoscopic Approach
00XN0ZF	Transfer Acoustic Nerve to Olfactory Nerve, Open Approach
00XN0ZG	Transfer Acoustic Nerve to Optic Nerve, Open Approach
00XN0ZH	Transfer Acoustic Nerve to Oculomotor Nerve, Open Approach
00XN0ZJ	Transfer Acoustic Nerve to Trochlear Nerve, Open Approach
00XN0ZK	Transfer Acoustic Nerve to Trigeminal Nerve, Open Approach
00XN0ZL	Transfer Acoustic Nerve to Abducens Nerve, Open Approach
00XN0ZM	Transfer Acoustic Nerve to Facial Nerve, Open Approach
00XN0ZN	Transfer Acoustic Nerve to Acoustic Nerve, Open Approach
00XN0ZP	Transfer Acoustic Nerve to Glossopharyngeal Nerve, Open Approach
00XN0ZQ	Transfer Acoustic Nerve to Vagus Nerve, Open Approach
00XN0ZR	Transfer Acoustic Nerve to Accessory Nerve, Open Approach
00XN0ZS	Transfer Acoustic Nerve to Hypoglossal Nerve, Open Approach
00XN4ZF	Transfer Acoustic Nerve to Olfactory Nerve, Percutaneous Endoscopic Approach
00XN4ZG	Transfer Acoustic Nerve to Optic Nerve, Percutaneous Endoscopic Approach
00XN4ZH	Transfer Acoustic Nerve to Oculomotor Nerve, Percutaneous Endoscopic Approach
00XN4ZJ	Transfer Acoustic Nerve to Trochlear Nerve, Percutaneous Endoscopic Approach
00XN4ZK	Transfer Acoustic Nerve to Trigeminal Nerve, Percutaneous Endoscopic Approach
00XN4ZL	Transfer Acoustic Nerve to Abducens Nerve, Percutaneous Endoscopic Approach
00XN4ZM	Transfer Acoustic Nerve to Facial Nerve, Percutaneous Endoscopic Approach
00XN4ZN	Transfer Acoustic Nerve to Acoustic Nerve, Percutaneous Endoscopic Approach

00XN4ZP	Transfer Acoustic Nerve to Glossopharyngeal Nerve, Percutaneous Endoscopic Approach
00XN4ZQ	Transfer Acoustic Nerve to Vagus Nerve, Percutaneous Endoscopic Approach
00XN4ZR	Transfer Acoustic Nerve to Accessory Nerve, Percutaneous Endoscopic Approach
00XN4ZS	Transfer Acoustic Nerve to Hypoglossal Nerve, Percutaneous Endoscopic Approach
00XP0ZF	Transfer Glossopharyngeal Nerve to Olfactory Nerve, Open Approach
00XP0ZG	Transfer Glossopharyngeal Nerve to Optic Nerve, Open Approach
00XP0ZH	Transfer Glossopharyngeal Nerve to Oculomotor Nerve, Open Approach
00XP0ZJ	Transfer Glossopharyngeal Nerve to Trochlear Nerve, Open Approach
00XP0ZK	Transfer Glossopharyngeal Nerve to Trigeminal Nerve, Open Approach
00XP0ZL	Transfer Glossopharyngeal Nerve to Abducens Nerve, Open Approach
00XP0ZM	Transfer Glossopharyngeal Nerve to Facial Nerve, Open Approach
00XP0ZN	Transfer Glossopharyngeal Nerve to Acoustic Nerve, Open Approach
00XP0ZP	Transfer Glossopharyngeal Nerve to Glossopharyngeal Nerve, Open Approach
00XP0ZQ	Transfer Glossopharyngeal Nerve to Vagus Nerve, Open Approach
00XP0ZR	Transfer Glossopharyngeal Nerve to Accessory Nerve, Open Approach
00XP0ZS	Transfer Glossopharyngeal Nerve to Hypoglossal Nerve, Open Approach
00XP4ZF	Transfer Glossopharyngeal Nerve to Olfactory Nerve, Percutaneous Endoscopic Approach
00XP4ZG	Transfer Glossopharyngeal Nerve to Optic Nerve, Percutaneous Endoscopic Approach
00XP4ZH	Transfer Glossopharyngeal Nerve to Oculomotor Nerve, Percutaneous Endoscopic Approach
00XP4ZJ	Transfer Glossopharyngeal Nerve to Trochlear Nerve, Percutaneous Endoscopic Approach
00XP4ZK	Transfer Glossopharyngeal Nerve to Trigeminal Nerve, Percutaneous Endoscopic Approach
00XP4ZL	Transfer Glossopharyngeal Nerve to Abducens Nerve, Percutaneous Endoscopic Approach
00XP4ZM	Transfer Glossopharyngeal Nerve to Facial Nerve, Percutaneous Endoscopic Approach
00XP4ZN	Transfer Glossopharyngeal Nerve to Acoustic Nerve, Percutaneous Endoscopic Approach
00XP4ZP	Transfer Glossopharyngeal Nerve to Glossopharyngeal Nerve, Percutaneous Endoscopic Approach
00XP4ZQ	Transfer Glossopharyngeal Nerve to Vagus Nerve, Percutaneous Endoscopic Approach
00XP4ZR	Transfer Glossopharyngeal Nerve to Accessory Nerve, Percutaneous Endoscopic Approach
00XP4ZS	Transfer Glossopharyngeal Nerve to Hypoglossal Nerve, Percutaneous Endoscopic Approach
00XQ0ZF	Transfer Vagus Nerve to Olfactory Nerve, Open Approach
00XQ0ZG	Transfer Vagus Nerve to Optic Nerve, Open Approach
00XQ0ZH	Transfer Vagus Nerve to Oculomotor Nerve, Open Approach

00XQ0ZJ	Transfer Vagus Nerve to Trochlear Nerve, Open Approach
00XQ0ZK	Transfer Vagus Nerve to Trigeminal Nerve, Open Approach
00XQ0ZL	Transfer Vagus Nerve to Abducens Nerve, Open Approach
00XQ0ZM	Transfer Vagus Nerve to Facial Nerve, Open Approach
00XQ0ZN	Transfer Vagus Nerve to Acoustic Nerve, Open Approach
00XQ0ZP	Transfer Vagus Nerve to Glossopharyngeal Nerve, Open Approach
00XQ0ZQ	Transfer Vagus Nerve to Vagus Nerve, Open Approach
00XQ0ZR	Transfer Vagus Nerve to Accessory Nerve, Open Approach
00XQ0ZS	Transfer Vagus Nerve to Hypoglossal Nerve, Open Approach
00XQ4ZF	Transfer Vagus Nerve to Olfactory Nerve, Percutaneous Endoscopic Approach
00XQ4ZG	Transfer Vagus Nerve to Optic Nerve, Percutaneous Endoscopic Approach
00XQ4ZH	Transfer Vagus Nerve to Oculomotor Nerve, Percutaneous Endoscopic Approach
00XQ4ZJ	Transfer Vagus Nerve to Trochlear Nerve, Percutaneous Endoscopic Approach
00XQ4ZK	Transfer Vagus Nerve to Trigeminal Nerve, Percutaneous Endoscopic Approach
00XQ4ZL	Transfer Vagus Nerve to Abducens Nerve, Percutaneous Endoscopic Approach
00XQ4ZM	Transfer Vagus Nerve to Facial Nerve, Percutaneous Endoscopic Approach
00XQ4ZN	Transfer Vagus Nerve to Acoustic Nerve, Percutaneous Endoscopic Approach
00XQ4ZP	Transfer Vagus Nerve to Glossopharyngeal Nerve, Percutaneous Endoscopic Approach
00XQ4ZQ	Transfer Vagus Nerve to Vagus Nerve, Percutaneous Endoscopic Approach
00XQ4ZR	Transfer Vagus Nerve to Accessory Nerve, Percutaneous Endoscopic Approach
00XQ4ZS	Transfer Vagus Nerve to Hypoglossal Nerve, Percutaneous Endoscopic Approach
00XR0ZF	Transfer Accessory Nerve to Olfactory Nerve, Open Approach
00XR0ZG	Transfer Accessory Nerve to Optic Nerve, Open Approach
00XR0ZH	Transfer Accessory Nerve to Oculomotor Nerve, Open Approach
00XR0ZJ	Transfer Accessory Nerve to Trochlear Nerve, Open Approach
00XR0ZK	Transfer Accessory Nerve to Trigeminal Nerve, Open Approach
00XR0ZL	Transfer Accessory Nerve to Abducens Nerve, Open Approach
00XR0ZM	Transfer Accessory Nerve to Facial Nerve, Open Approach
00XR0ZN	Transfer Accessory Nerve to Acoustic Nerve, Open Approach
00XR0ZP	Transfer Accessory Nerve to Glossopharyngeal Nerve, Open Approach
00XR0ZQ	Transfer Accessory Nerve to Vagus Nerve, Open Approach
00XR0ZR	Transfer Accessory Nerve to Accessory Nerve, Open Approach
00XR0ZS	Transfer Accessory Nerve to Hypoglossal Nerve, Open Approach
00XR4ZF	Transfer Accessory Nerve to Olfactory Nerve, Percutaneous Endoscopic Approach
00XR4ZG	Transfer Accessory Nerve to Optic Nerve, Percutaneous Endoscopic Approach
00XR4ZH	Transfer Accessory Nerve to Oculomotor Nerve, Percutaneous Endoscopic Approach

00XR4ZJ	Transfer Accessory Nerve to Trochlear Nerve, Percutaneous Endoscopic Approach	**00XS0ZF**	Transfer Hypoglossal Nerve to Olfactory Nerve, Open Approach	**00XS4ZG**	Transfer Hypoglossal Nerve to Optic Nerve, Percutaneous Endoscopic Approach
00XR4ZK	Transfer Accessory Nerve to Trigeminal Nerve, Percutaneous Endoscopic Approach	**00XS0ZG**	Transfer Hypoglossal Nerve to Optic Nerve, Open Approach	**00XS4ZH**	Transfer Hypoglossal Nerve to Oculomotor Nerve, Percutaneous Endoscopic Approach
00XR4ZL	Transfer Accessory Nerve to Abducens Nerve, Percutaneous Endoscopic Approach	**00XS0ZH**	Transfer Hypoglossal Nerve to Oculomotor Nerve, Open Approach	**00XS4ZJ**	Transfer Hypoglossal Nerve to Trochlear Nerve, Percutaneous Endoscopic Approach
00XR4ZM	Transfer Accessory Nerve to Facial Nerve, Percutaneous Endoscopic Approach	**00XS0ZJ**	Transfer Hypoglossal Nerve to Trochlear Nerve, Open Approach	**00XS4ZK**	Transfer Hypoglossal Nerve to Trigeminal Nerve, Percutaneous Endoscopic Approach
00XR4ZN	Transfer Accessory Nerve to Acoustic Nerve, Percutaneous Endoscopic Approach	**00XS0ZK**	Transfer Hypoglossal Nerve to Trigeminal Nerve, Open Approach	**00XS4ZL**	Transfer Hypoglossal Nerve to Abducens Nerve, Percutaneous Endoscopic Approach
00XR4ZP	Transfer Accessory Nerve to Glossopharyngeal Nerve, Percutaneous Endoscopic Approach	**00XS0ZL**	Transfer Hypoglossal Nerve to Abducens Nerve, Open Approach	**00XS4ZM**	Transfer Hypoglossal Nerve to Facial Nerve, Percutaneous Endoscopic Approach
00XR4ZQ	Transfer Accessory Nerve to Vagus Nerve, Percutaneous Endoscopic Approach	**00XS0ZM**	Transfer Hypoglossal Nerve to Facial Nerve, Open Approach	**00XS4ZN**	Transfer Hypoglossal Nerve to Acoustic Nerve, Percutaneous Endoscopic Approach
00XR4ZR	Transfer Accessory Nerve to Accessory Nerve, Percutaneous Endoscopic Approach	**00XS0ZN**	Transfer Hypoglossal Nerve to Acoustic Nerve, Open Approach	**00XS4ZP**	Transfer Hypoglossal Nerve to Glossopharyngeal Nerve, Percutaneous Endoscopic Approach
00XR4ZS	Transfer Accessory Nerve to Hypoglossal Nerve, Percutaneous Endoscopic Approach	**00XS0ZP**	Transfer Hypoglossal Nerve to Glossopharyngeal Nerve, Open Approach	**00XS4ZQ**	Transfer Hypoglossal Nerve to Vagus Nerve, Percutaneous Endoscopic Approach
		00XS0ZQ	Transfer Hypoglossal Nerve to Vagus Nerve, Open Approach		
		00XS0ZR	Transfer Hypoglossal Nerve to Accessory Nerve, Open Approach		
		00XS0ZS	Transfer Hypoglossal Nerve to Hypoglossal Nerve, Open Approach		
		00XS4ZF	Transfer Hypoglossal Nerve to Olfactory Nerve, Percutaneous Endoscopic Approach		

♀ Female-only   ♂ Male-only   ▲ Limited Coverage   ● Non-OR   ▦ HAC-associated procedure   ▲ Non-covered procedures   ✚ Combination

Peripheral Nervous System

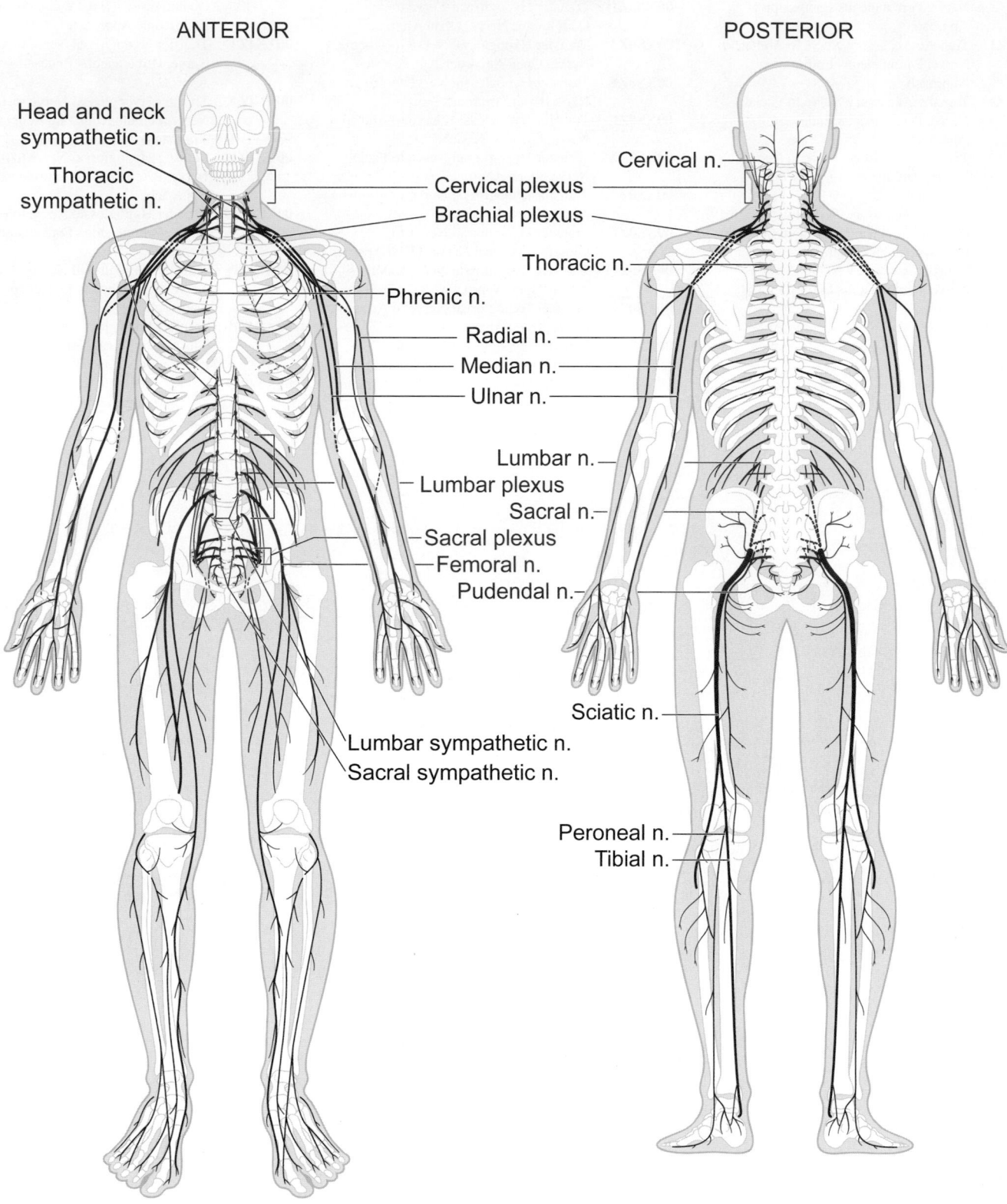

ANTERIOR   POSTERIOR

Head and neck sympathetic n.

Thoracic sympathetic n.

Cervical n.

Cervical plexus

Brachial plexus

Thoracic n.

Phrenic n.

Radial n.

Median n.

Ulnar n.

Lumbar n.

Lumbar plexus

Sacral n.

Sacral plexus

Femoral n.

Pudendal n.

Lumbar sympathetic n.

Sacral sympathetic n.

Sciatic n.

Peroneal n.

Tibial n.

©AHIMA

Spinal Column

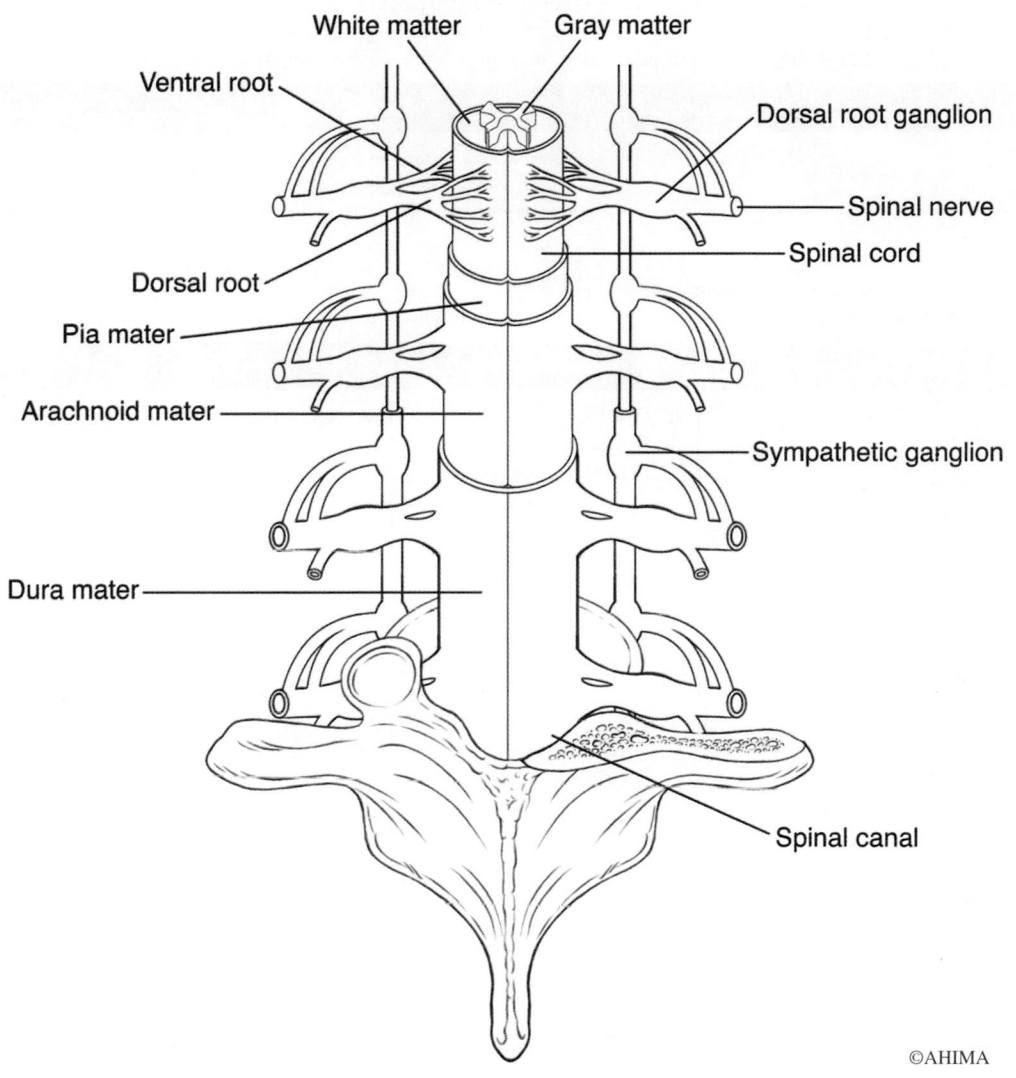

White matter

Gray matter

Ventral root

Dorsal root ganglion

Spinal nerve

Spinal cord

Dorsal root

Pia mater

Arachnoid mater

Sympathetic ganglion

Dura mater

Spinal canal

©AHIMA

Peripheral Nervous System Tables 012–01X

Section	0	Medical and Surgical
Body System	1	Peripheral Nervous System
Operation	2	**Change:** Taking out or off a device from a body part and putting back an identical or similar device in or on the same body part without cutting or puncturing the skin or a mucous membrane

Body Part (4th)	Approach (5th)	Device (6th)	Qualifier (7th)
Y Peripheral Nerve	X External	0 Drainage Device Y Other Device	Z No Qualifier

Section	0	Medical and Surgical
Body System	1	Peripheral Nervous System
Operation	5	**Destruction:** Physical eradication of all or a portion of a body part by the direct use of energy, force, or a destructive agent

Body Part (4th)	Approach (5th)	Device (6th)	Qualifier (7th)
0 Cervical Plexus 1 Cervical Nerve 2 Phrenic Nerve 3 Brachial Plexus 4 Ulnar Nerve 5 Median Nerve 6 Radial Nerve 8 Thoracic Nerve 9 Lumbar Plexus A Lumbosacral Plexus B Lumbar Nerve C Pudendal Nerve D Femoral Nerve F Sciatic Nerve G Tibial Nerve H Peroneal Nerve K Head and Neck Sympathetic Nerve L Thoracic Sympathetic Nerve M Abdominal Sympathetic Nerve N Lumbar Sympathetic Nerve P Sacral Sympathetic Nerve Q Sacral Plexus R Sacral Nerve	0 Open 3 Percutaneous 4 Percutaneous Endoscopic	Z No Device	Z No Qualifier

Section 0 **Medical and Surgical**
Body System 1 **Peripheral Nervous System**
Operation 8 **Division:** Cutting into a body part, without draining fluids and/or gases from the body part, in order to separate or transect a body part

Body Part (4ᵗʰ)	Approach (5ᵗʰ)	Device (6ᵗʰ)	Qualifier (7ᵗʰ)
0 Cervical Plexus	0 Open	Z No Device	Z No Qualifier
1 Cervical Nerve	3 Percutaneous		
2 Phrenic Nerve	4 Percutaneous Endoscopic		
3 Brachial Plexus			
4 Ulnar Nerve			
5 Median Nerve			
6 Radial Nerve			
8 Thoracic Nerve			
9 Lumbar Plexus			
A Lumbosacral Plexus			
B Lumbar Nerve			
C Pudendal Nerve			
D Femoral Nerve			
F Sciatic Nerve			
G Tibial Nerve			
H Peroneal Nerve			
K Head and Neck Sympathetic Nerve			
L Thoracic Sympathetic Nerve			
M Abdominal Sympathetic Nerve			
N Lumbar Sympathetic Nerve			
P Sacral Sympathetic Nerve			
Q Sacral Plexus			
R Sacral Nerve			

Section 0 **Medical and Surgical**
Body System 1 **Peripheral Nervous System**
Operation 9 **Drainage:** Taking or letting out fluids and/or gases from a body part

Body Part (4ᵗʰ)	Approach (5ᵗʰ)	Device (6ᵗʰ)	Qualifier (7ᵗʰ)
0 Cervical Plexus	0 Open	0 Drainage Device	Z No Qualifier
1 Cervical Nerve	3 Percutaneous		
2 Phrenic Nerve	4 Percutaneous Endoscopic		
3 Brachial Plexus			
4 Ulnar Nerve			
5 Median Nerve			
6 Radial Nerve			
8 Thoracic Nerve			
9 Lumbar Plexus			
A Lumbosacral Plexus			
B Lumbar Nerve			
C Pudendal Nerve			
D Femoral Nerve			
F Sciatic Nerve			
G Tibial Nerve			
H Peroneal Nerve			
K Head and Neck Sympathetic Nerve			
L Thoracic Sympathetic Nerve			
M Abdominal Sympathetic Nerve			
N Lumbar Sympathetic Nerve			
P Sacral Sympathetic Nerve			
Q Sacral Plexus			
R Sacral Nerve			

Continued →

Section	0	Medical and Surgical
Body System	1	Peripheral Nervous System
Operation	9	Drainage: Taking or letting out fluids and/or gases from a body part

Body Part (4th)	Approach (5th)	Device (6th)	Qualifier (7th)
0 Cervical Plexus 1 Cervical Nerve 2 Phrenic Nerve 3 Brachial Plexus 4 Ulnar Nerve 5 Median Nerve 6 Radial Nerve 8 Thoracic Nerve 9 Lumbar Plexus A Lumbosacral Plexus B Lumbar Nerve C Pudendal Nerve D Femoral Nerve F Sciatic Nerve G Tibial Nerve H Peroneal Nerve K Head and Neck Sympathetic Nerve L Thoracic Sympathetic Nerve M Abdominal Sympathetic Nerve N Lumbar Sympathetic Nerve P Sacral Sympathetic Nerve Q Sacral Plexus R Sacral Nerve	0 Open 3 Percutaneous 4 Percutaneous Endoscopic	Z No Device	X Diagnostic Z No Qualifier

Section	0	Medical and Surgical
Body System	1	Peripheral Nervous System
Operation	B	Excision: Cutting out or off, without replacement, a portion of a body part

Body Part (4th)	Approach (5th)	Device (6th)	Qualifier (7th)
0 Cervical Plexus 1 Cervical Nerve 2 Phrenic Nerve 3 Brachial Plexus 4 Ulnar Nerve 5 Median Nerve 6 Radial Nerve 8 Thoracic Nerve 9 Lumbar Plexus A Lumbosacral Plexus B Lumbar Nerve C Pudendal Nerve D Femoral Nerve F Sciatic Nerve G Tibial Nerve H Peroneal Nerve K Head and Neck Sympathetic Nerve L Thoracic Sympathetic Nerve M Abdominal Sympathetic Nerve N Lumbar Sympathetic Nerve P Sacral Sympathetic Nerve Q Sacral Plexus R Sacral Nerve	0 Open 3 Percutaneous 4 Percutaneous Endoscopic	Z No Device	X Diagnostic Z No Qualifier

Section 0 **Medical and Surgical**
Body System 1 **Peripheral Nervous System**
Operation C **Extirpation:** Taking or cutting out solid matter from a body part

Body Part (4th)	Approach (5th)	Device (6th)	Qualifier (7th)
0 Cervical Plexus 1 Cervical Nerve 2 Phrenic Nerve 3 Brachial Plexus 4 Ulnar Nerve 5 Median Nerve 6 Radial Nerve 8 Thoracic Nerve 9 Lumbar Plexus A Lumbosacral Plexus B Lumbar Nerve C Pudendal Nerve D Femoral Nerve F Sciatic Nerve G Tibial Nerve H Peroneal Nerve K Head and Neck Sympathetic Nerve L Thoracic Sympathetic Nerve M Abdominal Sympathetic Nerve N Lumbar Sympathetic Nerve P Sacral Sympathetic Nerve Q Sacral Plexus R Sacral Nerve	0 Open 3 Percutaneous 4 Percutaneous Endoscopic	Z No Device	Z No Qualifier

Section 0 **Medical and Surgical**
Body System 1 **Peripheral Nervous System**
Operation D **Extraction:** Pulling or stripping out or off all or a portion of a body part by the use of force

Body Part (4th)	Approach (5th)	Device (6th)	Qualifier (7th)
0 Cervical Plexus 1 Cervical Nerve 2 Phrenic Nerve 3 Brachial Plexus 4 Ulnar Nerve 5 Median Nerve 6 Radial Nerve 8 Thoracic Nerve 9 Lumbar Plexus A Lumbosacral Plexus B Lumbar Nerve C Pudendal Nerve D Femoral Nerve F Sciatic Nerve G Tibial Nerve H Peroneal Nerve K Head and Neck Sympathetic Nerve L Thoracic Sympathetic Nerve M Abdominal Sympathetic Nerve N Lumbar Sympathetic Nerve P Sacral Sympathetic Nerve Q Sacral Plexus R Sacral Nerve	0 Open 3 Percutaneous 4 Percutaneous Endoscopic	Z No Device	Z No Qualifier

Section	0	Medical and Surgical
Body System	1	Peripheral Nervous System
Operation	H	Insertion: Putting in a nonbiological appliance that monitors, assists, performs, or prevents a physiological function but does not physically take the place of a body part

Body Part (4th)	Approach (5th)	Device (6th)	Qualifier (7th)
Y Peripheral Nerve	0 Open 3 Percutaneous 4 Percutaneous Endoscopic	2 Monitoring Device M Neurostimulator Lead	Z No Qualifier

Section	0	Medical and Surgical
Body System	1	Peripheral Nervous System
Operation	J	Inspection: Visually and/or manually exploring a body part

Body Part (4th)	Approach (5th)	Device (6th)	Qualifier (7th)
Y Peripheral Nerve	0 Open 3 Percutaneous 4 Percutaneous Endoscopic	Z No Device	Z No Qualifier

Section	0	Medical and Surgical
Body System	1	Peripheral Nervous System
Operation	N	Release: Freeing a body part from an abnormal physical constraint by cutting or by the use of force

Body Part (4th)	Approach (5th)	Device (6th)	Qualifier (7th)
0 Cervical Plexus 1 Cervical Nerve 2 Phrenic Nerve 3 Brachial Plexus 4 Ulnar Nerve 5 Median Nerve 6 Radial Nerve 8 Thoracic Nerve 9 Lumbar Plexus A Lumbosacral Plexus B Lumbar Nerve C Pudendal Nerve D Femoral Nerve F Sciatic Nerve G Tibial Nerve H Peroneal Nerve K Head and Neck Sympathetic Nerve L Thoracic Sympathetic Nerve M Abdominal Sympathetic Nerve N Lumbar Sympathetic Nerve P Sacral Sympathetic Nerve Q Sacral Plexus R Sacral Nerve	0 Open 3 Percutaneous 4 Percutaneous Endoscopic	Z No Device	Z No Qualifier

Section	0	Medical and Surgical
Body System	1	Peripheral Nervous System
Operation	P	Removal: Taking out or off a device from a body part

Body Part (4th)	Approach (5th)	Device (6th)	Qualifier (7th)
Y Peripheral Nerve	0 Open 3 Percutaneous 4 Percutaneous Endoscopic	0 Drainage Device 2 Monitoring Device 7 Autologous Tissue Substitute M Neurostimulator Lead	Z No Qualifier
Y Peripheral Nerve	X External	0 Drainage Device 2 Monitoring Device M Neurostimulator Lead	Z No Qualifier

Section 0 **Medical and Surgical**
Body System 1 **Peripheral Nervous System**
Operation Q **Repair:** Restoring, to the extent possible, a body part to its normal anatomic structure and function

Body Part (4ᵗʰ)	Approach (5ᵗʰ)	Device (6ᵗʰ)	Qualifier (7ᵗʰ)
0 Cervical Plexus 1 Cervical Nerve 2 Phrenic Nerve 3 Brachial Plexus 4 Ulnar Nerve 5 Median Nerve 6 Radial Nerve 8 Thoracic Nerve 9 Lumbar Plexus A Lumbosacral Plexus B Lumbar Nerve C Pudendal Nerve D Femoral Nerve F Sciatic Nerve G Tibial Nerve H Peroneal Nerve K Head and Neck Sympathetic Nerve L Thoracic Sympathetic Nerve M Abdominal Sympathetic Nerve N Lumbar Sympathetic Nerve P Sacral Sympathetic Nerve Q Sacral Plexus R Sacral Nerve	0 Open 3 Percutaneous 4 Percutaneous Endoscopic	Z No Device	Z No Qualifier

Section 0 **Medical and Surgical**
Body System 1 **Peripheral Nervous System**
Operation S **Reposition:** Moving to its normal location, or other suitable location, all or a portion of a body part

Body Part (4ᵗʰ)	Approach (5ᵗʰ)	Device (6ᵗʰ)	Qualifier (7ᵗʰ)
0 Cervical Plexus 1 Cervical Nerve 2 Phrenic Nerve 3 Brachial Plexus 4 Ulnar Nerve 5 Median Nerve 6 Radial Nerve 8 Thoracic Nerve 9 Lumbar Plexus A Lumbosacral Plexus B Lumbar Nerve C Pudendal Nerve D Femoral Nerve F Sciatic Nerve G Tibial Nerve H Peroneal Nerve Q Sacral Plexus R Sacral Nerve	0 Open 3 Percutaneous 4 Percutaneous Endoscopic	Z No Device	Z No Qualifier

Section	0	Medical and Surgical
Body System	1	Peripheral Nervous System
Operation	U	**Supplement:** Putting in or on biological or synthetic material that physically reinforces and/or augments the function of a portion of a body part

Body Part (4th)	Approach (5th)	Device (6th)	Qualifier (7th)
1 Cervical Nerve 2 Phrenic Nerve 4 Ulnar Nerve 5 Median Nerve 6 Radial Nerve 8 Thoracic Nerve B Lumbar Nerve C Pudendal Nerve D Femoral Nerve F Sciatic Nerve G Tibial Nerve H Peroneal Nerve R Sacral Nerve	0 Open 3 Percutaneous 4 Percutaneous Endoscopic	7 Autologous Tissue Substitute	Z No Qualifier

Section	0	Medical and Surgical
Body System	1	Peripheral Nervous System
Operation	W	**Revision:** Correcting, to the extent possible, a portion of a malfunctioning device or the position of a displaced device

Body Part (4th)	Approach (5th)	Device (6th)	Qualifier (7th)
Y Peripheral Nerve	0 Open 3 Percutaneous 4 Percutaneous Endoscopic X External	0 Drainage Device 2 Monitoring Device 7 Autologous Tissue Substitute M Neurostimulator Lead	Z No Qualifier

Section	0	Medical and Surgical
Body System	1	Peripheral Nervous System
Operation	X	**Transfer:** Moving, without taking out, all or a portion of a body part to another location to take over the function of all or a portion of a body part

Body Part (4th)	Approach (5th)	Device (6th)	Qualifier (7th)
1 Cervical Nerve 2 Phrenic Nerve	0 Open 4 Percutaneous Endoscopic	Z No Device	1 Cervical Nerve 2 Phrenic Nerve
4 Ulnar Nerve 5 Median Nerve 6 Radial Nerve	0 Open 4 Percutaneous Endoscopic	Z No Device	4 Ulnar Nerve 5 Median Nerve 6 Radial Nerve
8 Thoracic Nerve	0 Open 4 Percutaneous Endoscopic	Z No Device	8 Thoracic Nerve
B Lumbar Nerve C Pudendal Nerve	0 Open 4 Percutaneous Endoscopic	Z No Device	B Lumbar Nerve C Perineal Nerve
D Femoral Nerve F Sciatic Nerve G Tibial Nerve H Peroneal Nerve	0 Open 4 Percutaneous Endoscopic	Z No Device	D Femoral Nerve F Sciatic Nerve G Tibial Nerve H Peroneal Nerve

Peripheral Nervous System Code Listing 012–01X

012 – Peripheral Nervous System, Change

Review Coding Guideline B6.1c

012YX0Z Change Drainage Device in Peripheral Nerve, External Approach

012YXYZ Change Other Device in Peripheral Nerve, External Approach

015 – Peripheral Nervous System, Destruction

01500ZZ Destruction of Cervical Plexus, Open Approach

01503ZZ Destruction of Cervical Plexus, Percutaneous Approach

01504ZZ Destruction of Cervical Plexus, Percutaneous Endoscopic Approach

♀ Female-only   ♂ Male-only   ▲ Limited Coverage   ● Non-OR   ▒ HAC-associated procedure   ▲ Non-covered procedures   + Combination

01510ZZ	Destruction of Cervical Nerve, Open Approach	
01513ZZ	Destruction of Cervical Nerve, Percutaneous Approach	
01514ZZ	Destruction of Cervical Nerve, Percutaneous Endoscopic Approach	
01520ZZ	Destruction of Phrenic Nerve, Open Approach	
01523ZZ	Destruction of Phrenic Nerve, Percutaneous Approach	
01524ZZ	Destruction of Phrenic Nerve, Percutaneous Endoscopic Approach	
01530ZZ	Destruction of Brachial Plexus, Open Approach	
01533ZZ	Destruction of Brachial Plexus, Percutaneous Approach	
01534ZZ	Destruction of Brachial Plexus, Percutaneous Endoscopic Approach	
01540ZZ	Destruction of Ulnar Nerve, Open Approach	
01543ZZ	Destruction of Ulnar Nerve, Percutaneous Approach	
01544ZZ	Destruction of Ulnar Nerve, Percutaneous Endoscopic Approach	
01550ZZ	Destruction of Median Nerve, Open Approach	
01553ZZ	Destruction of Median Nerve, Percutaneous Approach	
01554ZZ	Destruction of Median Nerve, Percutaneous Endoscopic Approach	
01560ZZ	Destruction of Radial Nerve, Open Approach	
01563ZZ	Destruction of Radial Nerve, Percutaneous Approach	
01564ZZ	Destruction of Radial Nerve, Percutaneous Endoscopic Approach	
01580ZZ	Destruction of Thoracic Nerve, Open Approach	
01583ZZ	Destruction of Thoracic Nerve, Percutaneous Approach	
01584ZZ	Destruction of Thoracic Nerve, Percutaneous Endoscopic Approach	
01590ZZ	Destruction of Lumbar Plexus, Open Approach	
01593ZZ	Destruction of Lumbar Plexus, Percutaneous Approach	

01594ZZ	Destruction of Lumbar Plexus, Percutaneous Endoscopic Approach
015A0ZZ	Destruction of Lumbosacral Plexus, Open Approach
015A3ZZ	Destruction of Lumbosacral Plexus, Percutaneous Approach
015A4ZZ	Destruction of Lumbosacral Plexus, Percutaneous Endoscopic Approach
015B0ZZ	Destruction of Lumbar Nerve, Open Approach
015B3ZZ	Destruction of Lumbar Nerve, Percutaneous Approach
015B4ZZ	Destruction of Lumbar Nerve, Percutaneous Endoscopic Approach
015C0ZZ	Destruction of Pudendal Nerve, Open Approach
015C3ZZ	Destruction of Pudendal Nerve, Percutaneous Approach
015C4ZZ	Destruction of Pudendal Nerve, Percutaneous Endoscopic Approach
015D0ZZ	Destruction of Femoral Nerve, Open Approach
015D3ZZ	Destruction of Femoral Nerve, Percutaneous Approach
015D4ZZ	Destruction of Femoral Nerve, Percutaneous Endoscopic Approach
015F0ZZ	Destruction of Sciatic Nerve, Open Approach
015F3ZZ	Destruction of Sciatic Nerve, Percutaneous Approach
015F4ZZ	Destruction of Sciatic Nerve, Percutaneous Endoscopic Approach
015G0ZZ	Destruction of Tibial Nerve, Open Approach
015G3ZZ	Destruction of Tibial Nerve, Percutaneous Approach
015G4ZZ	Destruction of Tibial Nerve, Percutaneous Endoscopic Approach
015H0ZZ	Destruction of Peroneal Nerve, Open Approach
015H3ZZ	Destruction of Peroneal Nerve, Percutaneous Approach
015H4ZZ	Destruction of Peroneal Nerve, Percutaneous Endoscopic Approach
015K0ZZ	Destruction of Head and Neck Sympathetic Nerve, Open Approach

015K3ZZ	Destruction of Head and Neck Sympathetic Nerve, Percutaneous Approach
015K4ZZ	Destruction of Head and Neck Sympathetic Nerve, Percutaneous Endoscopic Approach
015L0ZZ	Destruction of Thoracic Sympathetic Nerve, Open Approach
015L3ZZ	Destruction of Thoracic Sympathetic Nerve, Percutaneous Approach
015L4ZZ	Destruction of Thoracic Sympathetic Nerve, Percutaneous Endoscopic Approach
015M0ZZ	Destruction of Abdominal Sympathetic Nerve, Open Approach
015M3ZZ	Destruction of Abdominal Sympathetic Nerve, Percutaneous Approach
015M4ZZ	Destruction of Abdominal Sympathetic Nerve, Percutaneous Endoscopic Approach
015N0ZZ	Destruction of Lumbar Sympathetic Nerve, Open Approach
015N3ZZ	Destruction of Lumbar Sympathetic Nerve, Percutaneous Approach
015N4ZZ	Destruction of Lumbar Sympathetic Nerve, Percutaneous Endoscopic Approach
015P0ZZ	Destruction of Sacral Sympathetic Nerve, Open Approach
015P3ZZ	Destruction of Sacral Sympathetic Nerve, Percutaneous Approach
015P4ZZ	Destruction of Sacral Sympathetic Nerve, Percutaneous Endoscopic Approach
015Q0ZZ	Destruction of Sacral Plexus, Open Approach
015Q3ZZ	Destruction of Sacral Plexus, Percutaneous Approach
015Q4ZZ	Destruction of Sacral Plexus, Percutaneous Endoscopic Approach
015R0ZZ	Destruction of Sacral Nerve, Open Approach
015R3ZZ	Destruction of Sacral Nerve, Percutaneous Approach
015R4ZZ	Destruction of Sacral Nerve, Percutaneous Endoscopic Approach

018 – Peripheral Nervous System, Division

Review Coding Guideline B3.14

01800ZZ	Division of Cervical Plexus, Open Approach	
01803ZZ	Division of Cervical Plexus, Percutaneous Approach	
01804ZZ	Division of Cervical Plexus, Percutaneous Endoscopic Approach	
01810ZZ	Division of Cervical Nerve, Open Approach	
01813ZZ	Division of Cervical Nerve, Percutaneous Approach	
01814ZZ	Division of Cervical Nerve, Percutaneous Endoscopic Approach	
01820ZZ	Division of Phrenic Nerve, Open Approach	
01823ZZ	Division of Phrenic Nerve, Percutaneous Approach	
01824ZZ	Division of Phrenic Nerve, Percutaneous Endoscopic Approach	
01830ZZ	Division of Brachial Plexus, Open Approach	
01833ZZ	Division of Brachial Plexus, Percutaneous Approach	
01834ZZ	Division of Brachial Plexus, Percutaneous Endoscopic Approach	
01840ZZ	Division of Ulnar Nerve, Open Approach	

01843ZZ	Division of Ulnar Nerve, Percutaneous Approach
01844ZZ	Division of Ulnar Nerve, Percutaneous Endoscopic Approach
01850ZZ	Division of Median Nerve, Open Approach
01853ZZ	Division of Median Nerve, Percutaneous Approach
01854ZZ	Division of Median Nerve, Percutaneous Endoscopic Approach
01860ZZ	Division of Radial Nerve, Open Approach
01863ZZ	Division of Radial Nerve, Percutaneous Approach
01864ZZ	Division of Radial Nerve, Percutaneous Endoscopic Approach
01880ZZ	Division of Thoracic Nerve, Open Approach
01883ZZ	Division of Thoracic Nerve, Percutaneous Approach
01884ZZ	Division of Thoracic Nerve, Percutaneous Endoscopic Approach
01890ZZ	Division of Lumbar Plexus, Open Approach
01893ZZ	Division of Lumbar Plexus, Percutaneous Approach

01894ZZ	Division of Lumbar Plexus, Percutaneous Endoscopic Approach
018A0ZZ	Division of Lumbosacral Plexus, Open Approach
018A3ZZ	Division of Lumbosacral Plexus, Percutaneous Approach
018A4ZZ	Division of Lumbosacral Plexus, Percutaneous Endoscopic Approach
018B0ZZ	Division of Lumbar Nerve, Open Approach
018B3ZZ	Division of Lumbar Nerve, Percutaneous Approach
018B4ZZ	Division of Lumbar Nerve, Percutaneous Endoscopic Approach
018C0ZZ	Division of Pudendal Nerve, Open Approach
018C3ZZ	Division of Pudendal Nerve, Percutaneous Approach
018C4ZZ	Division of Pudendal Nerve, Percutaneous Endoscopic Approach
018D0ZZ	Division of Femoral Nerve, Open Approach
018D3ZZ	Division of Femoral Nerve, Percutaneous Approach
018D4ZZ	Division of Femoral Nerve, Percutaneous Endoscopic Approach

018F0ZZ	Division of Sciatic Nerve, Open Approach
018F3ZZ	Division of Sciatic Nerve, Percutaneous Approach
018F4ZZ	Division of Sciatic Nerve, Percutaneous Endoscopic Approach
018G0ZZ	Division of Tibial Nerve, Open Approach
018G3ZZ	Division of Tibial Nerve, Percutaneous Approach
018G4ZZ	Division of Tibial Nerve, Percutaneous Endoscopic Approach
018H0ZZ	Division of Peroneal Nerve, Open Approach
018H3ZZ	Division of Peroneal Nerve, Percutaneous Approach
018H4ZZ	Division of Peroneal Nerve, Percutaneous Endoscopic Approach
018K0ZZ	Division of Head and Neck Sympathetic Nerve, Open Approach
018K3ZZ	Division of Head and Neck Sympathetic Nerve, Percutaneous Approach

018K4ZZ	Division of Head and Neck Sympathetic Nerve, Percutaneous Endoscopic Approach
018L0ZZ	Division of Thoracic Sympathetic Nerve, Open Approach
018L3ZZ	Division of Thoracic Sympathetic Nerve, Percutaneous Approach
018L4ZZ	Division of Thoracic Sympathetic Nerve, Percutaneous Endoscopic Approach
018M0ZZ	Division of Abdominal Sympathetic Nerve, Open Approach
018M3ZZ	Division of Abdominal Sympathetic Nerve, Percutaneous Approach
018M4ZZ	Division of Abdominal Sympathetic Nerve, Percutaneous Endoscopic Approach
018N0ZZ	Division of Lumbar Sympathetic Nerve, Open Approach
018N3ZZ	Division of Lumbar Sympathetic Nerve, Percutaneous Approach

018N4ZZ	Division of Lumbar Sympathetic Nerve, Percutaneous Endoscopic Approach
018P0ZZ	Division of Sacral Sympathetic Nerve, Open Approach
018P3ZZ	Division of Sacral Sympathetic Nerve, Percutaneous Approach
018P4ZZ	Division of Sacral Sympathetic Nerve, Percutaneous Endoscopic Approach
018Q0ZZ	Division of Sacral Plexus, Open Approach
018Q3ZZ	Division of Sacral Plexus, Percutaneous Approach
018Q4ZZ	Division of Sacral Plexus, Percutaneous Endoscopic Approach
018R0ZZ	Division of Sacral Nerve, Open Approach
018R3ZZ	Division of Sacral Nerve, Percutaneous Approach
018R4ZZ	Division of Sacral Nerve, Percutaneous Endoscopic Approach

019 – Peripheral Nervous System, Drainage

Review Coding Guidelines B3.4a and B3.4b

Review Coding Guideline B6.2

019000Z	Drainage of Cervical Plexus with Drainage Device, Open Approach
01900ZX	Drainage of Cervical Plexus, Open Approach, Diagnostic
01900ZZ	Drainage of Cervical Plexus, Open Approach
019030Z	Drainage of Cervical Plexus with Drainage Device, Percutaneous Approach
01903ZX	Drainage of Cervical Plexus, Percutaneous Approach, Diagnostic
01903ZZ	Drainage of Cervical Plexus, Percutaneous Approach
019040Z	Drainage of Cervical Plexus with Drainage Device, Percutaneous Endoscopic Approach
01904ZX	Drainage of Cervical Plexus, Percutaneous Endoscopic Approach, Diagnostic
01904ZZ	Drainage of Cervical Plexus, Percutaneous Endoscopic Approach
019100Z	Drainage of Cervical Nerve with Drainage Device, Open Approach
01910ZX	Drainage of Cervical Nerve, Open Approach, Diagnostic
01910ZZ	Drainage of Cervical Nerve, Open Approach
019130Z	Drainage of Cervical Nerve with Drainage Device, Percutaneous Approach
01913ZX	Drainage of Cervical Nerve, Percutaneous Approach, Diagnostic
01913ZZ	Drainage of Cervical Nerve, Percutaneous Approach
019140Z	Drainage of Cervical Nerve with Drainage Device, Percutaneous Endoscopic Approach
01914ZX	Drainage of Cervical Nerve, Percutaneous Endoscopic Approach, Diagnostic
01914ZZ	Drainage of Cervical Nerve, Percutaneous Endoscopic Approach
019200Z	Drainage of Phrenic Nerve with Drainage Device, Open Approach
01920ZX	Drainage of Phrenic Nerve, Open Approach, Diagnostic
01920ZZ	Drainage of Phrenic Nerve, Open Approach
019230Z	Drainage of Phrenic Nerve with Drainage Device, Percutaneous Approach
01923ZX	Drainage of Phrenic Nerve, Percutaneous Approach, Diagnostic
01923ZZ	Drainage of Phrenic Nerve, Percutaneous Approach

019240Z	Drainage of Phrenic Nerve with Drainage Device, Percutaneous Endoscopic Approach
01924ZX	Drainage of Phrenic Nerve, Percutaneous Endoscopic Approach, Diagnostic
01924ZZ	Drainage of Phrenic Nerve, Percutaneous Endoscopic Approach
019300Z	Drainage of Brachial Plexus with Drainage Device, Open Approach
01930ZX	Drainage of Brachial Plexus, Open Approach, Diagnostic
01930ZZ	Drainage of Brachial Plexus, Open Approach
019330Z	Drainage of Brachial Plexus with Drainage Device, Percutaneous Approach
01933ZX	Drainage of Brachial Plexus, Percutaneous Approach, Diagnostic
01933ZZ	Drainage of Brachial Plexus, Percutaneous Approach
019340Z	Drainage of Brachial Plexus with Drainage Device, Percutaneous Endoscopic Approach
01934ZX	Drainage of Brachial Plexus, Percutaneous Endoscopic Approach, Diagnostic
01934ZZ	Drainage of Brachial Plexus, Percutaneous Endoscopic Approach
019400Z	Drainage of Ulnar Nerve with Drainage Device, Open Approach
01940ZX	Drainage of Ulnar Nerve, Open Approach, Diagnostic
01940ZZ	Drainage of Ulnar Nerve, Open Approach
019430Z	Drainage of Ulnar Nerve with Drainage Device, Percutaneous Approach
01943ZX	Drainage of Ulnar Nerve, Percutaneous Approach, Diagnostic
01943ZZ	Drainage of Ulnar Nerve, Percutaneous Approach
019440Z	Drainage of Ulnar Nerve with Drainage Device, Percutaneous Endoscopic Approach
01944ZX	Drainage of Ulnar Nerve, Percutaneous Endoscopic Approach, Diagnostic
01944ZZ	Drainage of Ulnar Nerve, Percutaneous Endoscopic Approach
019500Z	Drainage of Median Nerve with Drainage Device, Open Approach
01950ZX	Drainage of Median Nerve, Open Approach, Diagnostic
01950ZZ	Drainage of Median Nerve, Open Approach

019530Z	Drainage of Median Nerve with Drainage Device, Percutaneous Approach
01953ZX	Drainage of Median Nerve, Percutaneous Approach, Diagnostic
01953ZZ	Drainage of Median Nerve, Percutaneous Approach
019540Z	Drainage of Median Nerve with Drainage Device, Percutaneous Endoscopic Approach
01954ZX	Drainage of Median Nerve, Percutaneous Endoscopic Approach, Diagnostic
01954ZZ	Drainage of Median Nerve, Percutaneous Endoscopic Approach
019600Z	Drainage of Radial Nerve with Drainage Device, Open Approach
01960ZX	Drainage of Radial Nerve, Open Approach, Diagnostic
01960ZZ	Drainage of Radial Nerve, Open Approach
019630Z	Drainage of Radial Nerve with Drainage Device, Percutaneous Approach
01963ZX	Drainage of Radial Nerve, Percutaneous Approach, Diagnostic
01963ZZ	Drainage of Radial Nerve, Percutaneous Approach
019640Z	Drainage of Radial Nerve with Drainage Device, Percutaneous Endoscopic Approach
01964ZX	Drainage of Radial Nerve, Percutaneous Endoscopic Approach, Diagnostic
01964ZZ	Drainage of Radial Nerve, Percutaneous Endoscopic Approach
019800Z	Drainage of Thoracic Nerve with Drainage Device, Open Approach
01980ZX	Drainage of Thoracic Nerve, Open Approach, Diagnostic
01980ZZ	Drainage of Thoracic Nerve, Open Approach
019830Z	Drainage of Thoracic Nerve with Drainage Device, Percutaneous Approach
01983ZX	Drainage of Thoracic Nerve, Percutaneous Approach, Diagnostic
01983ZZ	Drainage of Thoracic Nerve, Percutaneous Approach
019840Z	Drainage of Thoracic Nerve with Drainage Device, Percutaneous Endoscopic Approach
01984ZX	Drainage of Thoracic Nerve, Percutaneous Endoscopic Approach, Diagnostic
01984ZZ	Drainage of Thoracic Nerve, Percutaneous Endoscopic Approach

019900Z	Drainage of Lumbar Plexus with Drainage Device, Open Approach	019D00Z	Drainage of Femoral Nerve with Drainage Device, Open Approach	019K0ZX	Drainage of Head and Neck Sympathetic Nerve, Open Approach, Diagnostic
01990ZX	Drainage of Lumbar Plexus, Open Approach, Diagnostic	019D0ZX	Drainage of Femoral Nerve, Open Approach, Diagnostic	019K0ZZ	Drainage of Head and Neck Sympathetic Nerve, Open Approach
01990ZZ	Drainage of Lumbar Plexus, Open Approach	019D0ZZ	Drainage of Femoral Nerve, Open Approach	019K30Z	Drainage of Head and Neck Sympathetic Nerve with Drainage Device, Percutaneous Approach
019930Z	Drainage of Lumbar Plexus with Drainage Device, Percutaneous Approach	019D30Z	Drainage of Femoral Nerve with Drainage Device, Percutaneous Approach		
01993ZX	Drainage of Lumbar Plexus, Percutaneous Approach, Diagnostic	019D3ZX	Drainage of Femoral Nerve, Percutaneous Approach, Diagnostic	019K3ZX	Drainage of Head and Neck Sympathetic Nerve, Percutaneous Approach, Diagnostic
01993ZZ	Drainage of Lumbar Plexus, Percutaneous Approach	019D3ZZ	Drainage of Femoral Nerve, Percutaneous Approach	019K3ZZ	Drainage of Head and Neck Sympathetic Nerve, Percutaneous Approach
019940Z	Drainage of Lumbar Plexus with Drainage Device, Percutaneous Endoscopic Approach	019D40Z	Drainage of Femoral Nerve with Drainage Device, Percutaneous Endoscopic Approach	019K40Z	Drainage of Head and Neck Sympathetic Nerve with Drainage Device, Percutaneous Endoscopic Approach
01994ZX	Drainage of Lumbar Plexus, Percutaneous Endoscopic Approach, Diagnostic	019D4ZX	Drainage of Femoral Nerve, Percutaneous Endoscopic Approach, Diagnostic	019K4ZX	Drainage of Head and Neck Sympathetic Nerve, Percutaneous Endoscopic Approach, Diagnostic
01994ZZ	Drainage of Lumbar Plexus, Percutaneous Endoscopic Approach	019D4ZZ	Drainage of Femoral Nerve, Percutaneous Endoscopic Approach	019K4ZZ	Drainage of Head and Neck Sympathetic Nerve, Percutaneous Endoscopic Approach
019A00Z	Drainage of Lumbosacral Plexus with Drainage Device, Open Approach	019F00Z	Drainage of Sciatic Nerve with Drainage Device, Open Approach	019L00Z	Drainage of Thoracic Sympathetic Nerve with Drainage Device, Open Approach
019A0ZX	Drainage of Lumbosacral Plexus, Open Approach, Diagnostic	019F0ZX	Drainage of Sciatic Nerve, Open Approach, Diagnostic	019L0ZX	Drainage of Thoracic Sympathetic Nerve, Open Approach, Diagnostic
019A0ZZ	Drainage of Lumbosacral Plexus, Open Approach	019F0ZZ	Drainage of Sciatic Nerve, Open Approach	019L0ZZ	Drainage of Thoracic Sympathetic Nerve, Open Approach
019A30Z	Drainage of Lumbosacral Plexus with Drainage Device, Percutaneous Approach	019F30Z	Drainage of Sciatic Nerve with Drainage Device, Percutaneous Approach	019L30Z	Drainage of Thoracic Sympathetic Nerve with Drainage Device, Percutaneous Approach
019A3ZX	Drainage of Lumbosacral Plexus, Percutaneous Approach, Diagnostic	019F3ZX	Drainage of Sciatic Nerve, Percutaneous Approach, Diagnostic	019L3ZX	Drainage of Thoracic Sympathetic Nerve, Percutaneous Approach, Diagnostic
019A3ZZ	Drainage of Lumbosacral Plexus, Percutaneous Approach	019F3ZZ	Drainage of Sciatic Nerve, Percutaneous Approach	019L3ZZ	Drainage of Thoracic Sympathetic Nerve, Percutaneous Approach
019A40Z	Drainage of Lumbosacral Plexus with Drainage Device, Percutaneous Endoscopic Approach	019F40Z	Drainage of Sciatic Nerve with Drainage Device, Percutaneous Endoscopic Approach	019L40Z	Drainage of Thoracic Sympathetic Nerve with Drainage Device, Percutaneous Endoscopic Approach
019A4ZX	Drainage of Lumbosacral Plexus, Percutaneous Endoscopic Approach, Diagnostic	019F4ZX	Drainage of Sciatic Nerve, Percutaneous Endoscopic Approach, Diagnostic	019L4ZX	Drainage of Thoracic Sympathetic Nerve, Percutaneous Endoscopic Approach, Diagnostic
019A4ZZ	Drainage of Lumbosacral Plexus, Percutaneous Endoscopic Approach	019F4ZZ	Drainage of Sciatic Nerve, Percutaneous Endoscopic Approach	019L4ZZ	Drainage of Thoracic Sympathetic Nerve, Percutaneous Endoscopic Approach
019B00Z	Drainage of Lumbar Nerve with Drainage Device, Open Approach	019G00Z	Drainage of Tibial Nerve with Drainage Device, Open Approach	019M00Z	Drainage of Abdominal Sympathetic Nerve with Drainage Device, Open Approach
019B0ZX	Drainage of Lumbar Nerve, Open Approach, Diagnostic	019G0ZX	Drainage of Tibial Nerve, Open Approach, Diagnostic	019M0ZX	Drainage of Abdominal Sympathetic Nerve, Open Approach, Diagnostic
019B0ZZ	Drainage of Lumbar Nerve, Open Approach	019G0ZZ	Drainage of Tibial Nerve, Open Approach	019M0ZZ	Drainage of Abdominal Sympathetic Nerve, Open Approach
019B30Z	Drainage of Lumbar Nerve with Drainage Device, Percutaneous Approach	019G30Z	Drainage of Tibial Nerve with Drainage Device, Percutaneous Approach	019M30Z	Drainage of Abdominal Sympathetic Nerve with Drainage Device, Percutaneous Approach
019B3ZX	Drainage of Lumbar Nerve, Percutaneous Approach, Diagnostic	019G3ZX	Drainage of Tibial Nerve, Percutaneous Approach, Diagnostic	019M3ZX	Drainage of Abdominal Sympathetic Nerve, Percutaneous Approach, Diagnostic
019B3ZZ	Drainage of Lumbar Nerve, Percutaneous Approach	019G3ZZ	Drainage of Tibial Nerve, Percutaneous Approach	019M3ZZ	Drainage of Abdominal Sympathetic Nerve, Percutaneous Approach
019B40Z	Drainage of Lumbar Nerve with Drainage Device, Percutaneous Endoscopic Approach	019G40Z	Drainage of Tibial Nerve with Drainage Device, Percutaneous Endoscopic Approach	019M40Z	Drainage of Abdominal Sympathetic Nerve with Drainage Device, Percutaneous Endoscopic Approach
019B4ZX	Drainage of Lumbar Nerve, Percutaneous Endoscopic Approach, Diagnostic	019G4ZX	Drainage of Tibial Nerve, Percutaneous Endoscopic Approach, Diagnostic	019M4ZX	Drainage of Abdominal Sympathetic Nerve, Percutaneous Endoscopic Approach, Diagnostic
019B4ZZ	Drainage of Lumbar Nerve, Percutaneous Endoscopic Approach	019G4ZZ	Drainage of Tibial Nerve, Percutaneous Endoscopic Approach	019M4ZZ	Drainage of Abdominal Sympathetic Nerve, Percutaneous Endoscopic Approach
019C00Z	Drainage of Pudendal Nerve with Drainage Device, Open Approach	019H00Z	Drainage of Peroneal Nerve with Drainage Device, Open Approach	019N00Z	Drainage of Lumbar Sympathetic Nerve with Drainage Device, Open Approach
019C0ZX	Drainage of Pudendal Nerve, Open Approach, Diagnostic	019H0ZX	Drainage of Peroneal Nerve, Open Approach, Diagnostic	019N0ZX	Drainage of Lumbar Sympathetic Nerve, Open Approach, Diagnostic
019C0ZZ	Drainage of Pudendal Nerve, Open Approach	019H0ZZ	Drainage of Peroneal Nerve, Open Approach	019N0ZZ	Drainage of Lumbar Sympathetic Nerve, Open Approach
019C30Z	Drainage of Pudendal Nerve with Drainage Device, Percutaneous Approach	019H30Z	Drainage of Peroneal Nerve with Drainage Device, Percutaneous Approach	019N30Z	Drainage of Lumbar Sympathetic Nerve with Drainage Device, Percutaneous Approach
019C3ZX	Drainage of Pudendal Nerve, Percutaneous Approach, Diagnostic	019H3ZX	Drainage of Peroneal Nerve, Percutaneous Approach, Diagnostic		
019C3ZZ	Drainage of Pudendal Nerve, Percutaneous Approach	019H3ZZ	Drainage of Peroneal Nerve, Percutaneous Approach	019N3ZX	Drainage of Lumbar Sympathetic Nerve, Percutaneous Approach, Diagnostic
019C40Z	Drainage of Pudendal Nerve with Drainage Device, Percutaneous Endoscopic Approach	019H40Z	Drainage of Peroneal Nerve with Drainage Device, Percutaneous Endoscopic Approach	019N3ZZ	Drainage of Lumbar Sympathetic Nerve, Percutaneous Approach
019C4ZX	Drainage of Pudendal Nerve, Percutaneous Endoscopic Approach, Diagnostic	019H4ZX	Drainage of Peroneal Nerve, Percutaneous Endoscopic Approach, Diagnostic		
019C4ZZ	Drainage of Pudendal Nerve, Percutaneous Endoscopic Approach	019H4ZZ	Drainage of Peroneal Nerve, Percutaneous Endoscopic Approach		
		019K00Z	Drainage of Head and Neck Sympathetic Nerve with Drainage Device, Open Approach		

145

♀ Female-only	♂ Male-only	▲ Limited Coverage	● Non-OR	▦ HAC-associated procedure	▲ Non-covered procedures	✚ Combination

019N40Z Drainage of Lumbar Sympathetic Nerve with Drainage Device, Percutaneous Endoscopic Approach

019N4ZX Drainage of Lumbar Sympathetic Nerve, Percutaneous Endoscopic Approach, Diagnostic

019N4ZZ Drainage of Lumbar Sympathetic Nerve, Percutaneous Endoscopic Approach

019P00Z Drainage of Sacral Sympathetic Nerve with Drainage Device, Open Approach

019P0ZX Drainage of Sacral Sympathetic Nerve, Open Approach, Diagnostic

019P0ZZ Drainage of Sacral Sympathetic Nerve, Open Approach

019P30Z Drainage of Sacral Sympathetic Nerve with Drainage Device, Percutaneous Approach

019P3ZX Drainage of Sacral Sympathetic Nerve, Percutaneous Approach, Diagnostic

019P3ZZ Drainage of Sacral Sympathetic Nerve, Percutaneous Approach

019P40Z Drainage of Sacral Sympathetic Nerve with Drainage Device, Percutaneous Endoscopic Approach

019P4ZX Drainage of Sacral Sympathetic Nerve, Percutaneous Endoscopic Approach, Diagnostic

019P4ZZ Drainage of Sacral Sympathetic Nerve, Percutaneous Endoscopic Approach

019Q00Z Drainage of Sacral Plexus with Drainage Device, Open Approach

019Q0ZX Drainage of Sacral Plexus, Open Approach, Diagnostic

019Q0ZZ Drainage of Sacral Plexus, Open Approach

019Q30Z Drainage of Sacral Plexus with Drainage Device, Percutaneous Approach

019Q3ZX Drainage of Sacral Plexus, Percutaneous Approach, Diagnostic

019Q3ZZ Drainage of Sacral Plexus, Percutaneous Approach

019Q40Z Drainage of Sacral Plexus with Drainage Device, Percutaneous Endoscopic Approach

019Q4ZX Drainage of Sacral Plexus, Percutaneous Endoscopic Approach, Diagnostic

019Q4ZZ Drainage of Sacral Plexus, Percutaneous Endoscopic Approach

019R00Z Drainage of Sacral Nerve with Drainage Device, Open Approach

019R0ZX Drainage of Sacral Nerve, Open Approach, Diagnostic

019R0ZZ Drainage of Sacral Nerve, Open Approach

019R30Z Drainage of Sacral Nerve with Drainage Device, Percutaneous Approach

019R3ZX Drainage of Sacral Nerve, Percutaneous Approach, Diagnostic

019R3ZZ Drainage of Sacral Nerve, Percutaneous Approach

019R40Z Drainage of Sacral Nerve with Drainage Device, Percutaneous Endoscopic Approach

019R4ZX Drainage of Sacral Nerve, Percutaneous Endoscopic Approach, Diagnostic

019R4ZZ Drainage of Sacral Nerve, Percutaneous Endoscopic Approach

01B – Peripheral Nervous System, Excision

Review Coding Guidelines B3.4a and B3.4b

Review Coding Guideline B3.8

01B00ZX Excision of Cervical Plexus, Open Approach, Diagnostic

01B00ZZ Excision of Cervical Plexus, Open Approach

01B03ZX Excision of Cervical Plexus, Percutaneous Approach, Diagnostic

01B03ZZ Excision of Cervical Plexus, Percutaneous Approach

01B04ZX Excision of Cervical Plexus, Percutaneous Endoscopic Approach, Diagnostic

01B04ZZ Excision of Cervical Plexus, Percutaneous Endoscopic Approach

01B10ZX Excision of Cervical Nerve, Open Approach, Diagnostic

01B10ZZ Excision of Cervical Nerve, Open Approach

01B13ZX Excision of Cervical Nerve, Percutaneous Approach, Diagnostic

01B13ZZ Excision of Cervical Nerve, Percutaneous Approach

01B14ZX Excision of Cervical Nerve, Percutaneous Endoscopic Approach, Diagnostic

01B14ZZ Excision of Cervical Nerve, Percutaneous Endoscopic Approach

01B20ZX Excision of Phrenic Nerve, Open Approach, Diagnostic

01B20ZZ Excision of Phrenic Nerve, Open Approach

01B23ZX Excision of Phrenic Nerve, Percutaneous Approach, Diagnostic

01B23ZZ Excision of Phrenic Nerve, Percutaneous Approach

01B24ZX Excision of Phrenic Nerve, Percutaneous Endoscopic Approach, Diagnostic

01B24ZZ Excision of Phrenic Nerve, Percutaneous Endoscopic Approach

01B30ZX Excision of Brachial Plexus, Open Approach, Diagnostic

01B30ZZ Excision of Brachial Plexus, Open Approach

01B33ZX Excision of Brachial Plexus, Percutaneous Approach, Diagnostic

01B33ZZ Excision of Brachial Plexus, Percutaneous Approach

01B34ZX Excision of Brachial Plexus, Percutaneous Endoscopic Approach, Diagnostic

01B34ZZ Excision of Brachial Plexus, Percutaneous Endoscopic Approach

01B40ZX Excision of Ulnar Nerve, Open Approach, Diagnostic

01B40ZZ Excision of Ulnar Nerve, Open Approach

01B43ZX Excision of Ulnar Nerve, Percutaneous Approach, Diagnostic

01B43ZZ Excision of Ulnar Nerve, Percutaneous Approach

01B44ZX Excision of Ulnar Nerve, Percutaneous Endoscopic Approach, Diagnostic

01B44ZZ Excision of Ulnar Nerve, Percutaneous Endoscopic Approach

01B50ZX Excision of Median Nerve, Open Approach, Diagnostic

01B50ZZ Excision of Median Nerve, Open Approach

01B53ZX Excision of Median Nerve, Percutaneous Approach, Diagnostic

01B53ZZ Excision of Median Nerve, Percutaneous Approach

01B54ZX Excision of Median Nerve, Percutaneous Endoscopic Approach, Diagnostic

01B54ZZ Excision of Median Nerve, Percutaneous Endoscopic Approach

01B60ZX Excision of Radial Nerve, Open Approach, Diagnostic

01B60ZZ Excision of Radial Nerve, Open Approach

01B63ZX Excision of Radial Nerve, Percutaneous Approach, Diagnostic

01B63ZZ Excision of Radial Nerve, Percutaneous Approach

01B64ZX Excision of Radial Nerve, Percutaneous Endoscopic Approach, Diagnostic

01B64ZZ Excision of Radial Nerve, Percutaneous Endoscopic Approach

01B80ZX Excision of Thoracic Nerve, Open Approach, Diagnostic

01B80ZZ Excision of Thoracic Nerve, Open Approach

01B83ZX Excision of Thoracic Nerve, Percutaneous Approach, Diagnostic

01B83ZZ Excision of Thoracic Nerve, Percutaneous Approach

01B84ZX Excision of Thoracic Nerve, Percutaneous Endoscopic Approach, Diagnostic

01B84ZZ Excision of Thoracic Nerve, Percutaneous Endoscopic Approach

01B90ZX Excision of Lumbar Plexus, Open Approach, Diagnostic

01B90ZZ Excision of Lumbar Plexus, Open Approach

01B93ZX Excision of Lumbar Plexus, Percutaneous Approach, Diagnostic

01B93ZZ Excision of Lumbar Plexus, Percutaneous Approach

01B94ZX Excision of Lumbar Plexus, Percutaneous Endoscopic Approach, Diagnostic

01B94ZZ Excision of Lumbar Plexus, Percutaneous Endoscopic Approach

01BA0ZX Excision of Lumbosacral Plexus, Open Approach, Diagnostic

01BA0ZZ Excision of Lumbosacral Plexus, Open Approach

01BA3ZX Excision of Lumbosacral Plexus, Percutaneous Approach, Diagnostic

01BA3ZZ Excision of Lumbosacral Plexus, Percutaneous Approach

01BA4ZX Excision of Lumbosacral Plexus, Percutaneous Endoscopic Approach, Diagnostic

01BA4ZZ Excision of Lumbosacral Plexus, Percutaneous Endoscopic Approach

01BB0ZX Excision of Lumbar Nerve, Open Approach, Diagnostic

01BB0ZZ Excision of Lumbar Nerve, Open Approach

01BB3ZX Excision of Lumbar Nerve, Percutaneous Approach, Diagnostic

01BB3ZZ Excision of Lumbar Nerve, Percutaneous Approach

01BB4ZX Excision of Lumbar Nerve, Percutaneous Endoscopic Approach, Diagnostic

01BB4ZZ Excision of Lumbar Nerve, Percutaneous Endoscopic Approach

01BC0ZX Excision of Pudendal Nerve, Open Approach, Diagnostic

01BC0ZZ Excision of Pudendal Nerve, Open Approach

01BC3ZX Excision of Pudendal Nerve, Percutaneous Approach, Diagnostic

01BC3ZZ Excision of Pudendal Nerve, Percutaneous Approach

01BC4ZX Excision of Pudendal Nerve, Percutaneous Endoscopic Approach, Diagnostic

01BC4ZZ Excision of Pudendal Nerve, Percutaneous Endoscopic Approach

♀ Female-only   ♂ Male-only   ▲ Limited Coverage   ● Non-OR   ■ HAC-associated procedure   ▲ Non-covered procedures   ✚ Combination

01BD0ZX	Excision of Femoral Nerve, Open Approach, Diagnostic
01BD0ZZ	Excision of Femoral Nerve, Open Approach
01BD3ZX	Excision of Femoral Nerve, Percutaneous Approach, Diagnostic
01BD3ZZ	Excision of Femoral Nerve, Percutaneous Approach
01BD4ZX	Excision of Femoral Nerve, Percutaneous Endoscopic Approach, Diagnostic
01BD4ZZ	Excision of Femoral Nerve, Percutaneous Endoscopic Approach
01BF0ZX	Excision of Sciatic Nerve, Open Approach, Diagnostic
01BF0ZZ	Excision of Sciatic Nerve, Open Approach
01BF3ZX	Excision of Sciatic Nerve, Percutaneous Approach, Diagnostic
01BF3ZZ	Excision of Sciatic Nerve, Percutaneous Approach
01BF4ZX	Excision of Sciatic Nerve, Percutaneous Endoscopic Approach, Diagnostic
01BF4ZZ	Excision of Sciatic Nerve, Percutaneous Endoscopic Approach
01BG0ZX	Excision of Tibial Nerve, Open Approach, Diagnostic
01BG0ZZ	Excision of Tibial Nerve, Open Approach
01BG3ZX	Excision of Tibial Nerve, Percutaneous Approach, Diagnostic
01BG3ZZ	Excision of Tibial Nerve, Percutaneous Approach
01BG4ZX	Excision of Tibial Nerve, Percutaneous Endoscopic Approach, Diagnostic
01BG4ZZ	Excision of Tibial Nerve, Percutaneous Endoscopic Approach
01BH0ZX	Excision of Peroneal Nerve, Open Approach, Diagnostic
01BH0ZZ	Excision of Peroneal Nerve, Open Approach
01BH3ZX	Excision of Peroneal Nerve, Percutaneous Approach, Diagnostic
01BH3ZZ	Excision of Peroneal Nerve, Percutaneous Approach
01BH4ZX	Excision of Peroneal Nerve, Percutaneous Endoscopic Approach, Diagnostic
01BH4ZZ	Excision of Peroneal Nerve, Percutaneous Endoscopic Approach
01BK0ZX	Excision of Head and Neck Sympathetic Nerve, Open Approach, Diagnostic
01BK0ZZ	Excision of Head and Neck Sympathetic Nerve, Open Approach
01BK3ZX	Excision of Head and Neck Sympathetic Nerve, Percutaneous Approach, Diagnostic
01BK3ZZ	Excision of Head and Neck Sympathetic Nerve, Percutaneous Approach
01BK4ZX	Excision of Head and Neck Sympathetic Nerve, Percutaneous Endoscopic Approach, Diagnostic
01BK4ZZ	Excision of Head and Neck Sympathetic Nerve, Percutaneous Endoscopic Approach
01BL0ZX	Excision of Thoracic Sympathetic Nerve, Open Approach, Diagnostic
01BL0ZZ	Excision of Thoracic Sympathetic Nerve, Open Approach
01BL3ZX	Excision of Thoracic Sympathetic Nerve, Percutaneous Approach, Diagnostic
01BL3ZZ	Excision of Thoracic Sympathetic Nerve, Percutaneous Approach
01BL4ZX	Excision of Thoracic Sympathetic Nerve, Percutaneous Endoscopic Approach, Diagnostic
01BL4ZZ	Excision of Thoracic Sympathetic Nerve, Percutaneous Endoscopic Approach
01BM0ZX	Excision of Abdominal Sympathetic Nerve, Open Approach, Diagnostic
01BM0ZZ	Excision of Abdominal Sympathetic Nerve, Open Approach
01BM3ZX	Excision of Abdominal Sympathetic Nerve, Percutaneous Approach, Diagnostic
01BM3ZZ	Excision of Abdominal Sympathetic Nerve, Percutaneous Approach
01BM4ZX	Excision of Abdominal Sympathetic Nerve, Percutaneous Endoscopic Approach, Diagnostic
01BM4ZZ	Excision of Abdominal Sympathetic Nerve, Percutaneous Endoscopic Approach
01BN0ZX	Excision of Lumbar Sympathetic Nerve, Open Approach, Diagnostic
01BN0ZZ	Excision of Lumbar Sympathetic Nerve, Open Approach
01BN3ZX	Excision of Lumbar Sympathetic Nerve, Percutaneous Approach, Diagnostic
01BN3ZZ	Excision of Lumbar Sympathetic Nerve, Percutaneous Approach
01BN4ZX	Excision of Lumbar Sympathetic Nerve, Percutaneous Endoscopic Approach, Diagnostic
01BN4ZZ	Excision of Lumbar Sympathetic Nerve, Percutaneous Endoscopic Approach
01BP0ZX	Excision of Sacral Sympathetic Nerve, Open Approach, Diagnostic
01BP0ZZ	Excision of Sacral Sympathetic Nerve, Open Approach
01BP3ZX	Excision of Sacral Sympathetic Nerve, Percutaneous Approach, Diagnostic
01BP3ZZ	Excision of Sacral Sympathetic Nerve, Percutaneous Approach
01BP4ZX	Excision of Sacral Sympathetic Nerve, Percutaneous Endoscopic Approach, Diagnostic
01BP4ZZ	Excision of Sacral Sympathetic Nerve, Percutaneous Endoscopic Approach
01BQ0ZX	Excision of Sacral Plexus, Open Approach, Diagnostic
01BQ0ZZ	Excision of Sacral Plexus, Open Approach
01BQ3ZX	Excision of Sacral Plexus, Percutaneous Approach, Diagnostic
01BQ3ZZ	Excision of Sacral Plexus, Percutaneous Approach
01BQ4ZX	Excision of Sacral Plexus, Percutaneous Endoscopic Approach, Diagnostic
01BQ4ZZ	Excision of Sacral Plexus, Percutaneous Endoscopic Approach
01BR0ZX	Excision of Sacral Nerve, Open Approach, Diagnostic
01BR0ZZ	Excision of Sacral Nerve, Open Approach
01BR3ZX	Excision of Sacral Nerve, Percutaneous Approach, Diagnostic
01BR3ZZ	Excision of Sacral Nerve, Percutaneous Approach
01BR4ZX	Excision of Sacral Nerve, Percutaneous Endoscopic Approach, Diagnostic
01BR4ZZ	Excision of Sacral Nerve, Percutaneous Endoscopic Approach

01C – Peripheral Nervous System, Extirpation

01C00ZZ	Extirpation of Matter from Cervical Plexus, Open Approach
01C03ZZ	Extirpation of Matter from Cervical Plexus, Percutaneous Approach
01C04ZZ	Extirpation of Matter from Cervical Plexus, Percutaneous Endoscopic Approach
01C10ZZ	Extirpation of Matter from Cervical Nerve, Open Approach
01C13ZZ	Extirpation of Matter from Cervical Nerve, Percutaneous Approach
01C14ZZ	Extirpation of Matter from Cervical Nerve, Percutaneous Endoscopic Approach
01C20ZZ	Extirpation of Matter from Phrenic Nerve, Open Approach
01C23ZZ	Extirpation of Matter from Phrenic Nerve, Percutaneous Approach
01C24ZZ	Extirpation of Matter from Phrenic Nerve, Percutaneous Endoscopic Approach
01C30ZZ	Extirpation of Matter from Brachial Plexus, Open Approach
01C33ZZ	Extirpation of Matter from Brachial Plexus, Percutaneous Approach
01C34ZZ	Extirpation of Matter from Brachial Plexus, Percutaneous Endoscopic Approach
01C40ZZ	Extirpation of Matter from Ulnar Nerve, Open Approach
01C43ZZ	Extirpation of Matter from Ulnar Nerve, Percutaneous Approach
01C44ZZ	Extirpation of Matter from Ulnar Nerve, Percutaneous Endoscopic Approach
01C50ZZ	Extirpation of Matter from Median Nerve, Open Approach
01C53ZZ	Extirpation of Matter from Median Nerve, Percutaneous Approach
01C54ZZ	Extirpation of Matter from Median Nerve, Percutaneous Endoscopic Approach
01C60ZZ	Extirpation of Matter from Radial Nerve, Open Approach
01C63ZZ	Extirpation of Matter from Radial Nerve, Percutaneous Approach
01C64ZZ	Extirpation of Matter from Radial Nerve, Percutaneous Endoscopic Approach
01C80ZZ	Extirpation of Matter from Thoracic Nerve, Open Approach
01C83ZZ	Extirpation of Matter from Thoracic Nerve, Percutaneous Approach
01C84ZZ	Extirpation of Matter from Thoracic Nerve, Percutaneous Endoscopic Approach
01C90ZZ	Extirpation of Matter from Lumbar Plexus, Open Approach
01C93ZZ	Extirpation of Matter from Lumbar Plexus, Percutaneous Approach
01C94ZZ	Extirpation of Matter from Lumbar Plexus, Percutaneous Endoscopic Approach
01CA0ZZ	Extirpation of Matter from Lumbosacral Plexus, Open Approach
01CA3ZZ	Extirpation of Matter from Lumbosacral Plexus, Percutaneous Approach
01CA4ZZ	Extirpation of Matter from Lumbosacral Plexus, Percutaneous Endoscopic Approach
01CB0ZZ	Extirpation of Matter from Lumbar Nerve, Open Approach
01CB3ZZ	Extirpation of Matter from Lumbar Nerve, Percutaneous Approach
01CB4ZZ	Extirpation of Matter from Lumbar Nerve, Percutaneous Endoscopic Approach
01CC0ZZ	Extirpation of Matter from Pudendal Nerve, Open Approach
01CC3ZZ	Extirpation of Matter from Pudendal Nerve, Percutaneous Approach
01CC4ZZ	Extirpation of Matter from Pudendal Nerve, Percutaneous Endoscopic Approach
01CD0ZZ	Extirpation of Matter from Femoral Nerve, Open Approach
01CD3ZZ	Extirpation of Matter from Femoral Nerve, Percutaneous Approach
01CD4ZZ	Extirpation of Matter from Femoral Nerve, Percutaneous Endoscopic Approach

♀ Female-only   ♂ Male-only   ▲ Limited Coverage   ● Non-OR   ▩ HAC-associated procedure   ▲ Non-covered procedures   ✚ Combination

01CF0ZZ Extirpation of Matter from Sciatic Nerve, Open Approach

01CF3ZZ Extirpation of Matter from Sciatic Nerve, Percutaneous Approach

01CF4ZZ Extirpation of Matter from Sciatic Nerve, Percutaneous Endoscopic Approach

01CG0ZZ Extirpation of Matter from Tibial Nerve, Open Approach

01CG3ZZ Extirpation of Matter from Tibial Nerve, Percutaneous Approach

01CG4ZZ Extirpation of Matter from Tibial Nerve, Percutaneous Endoscopic Approach

01CH0ZZ Extirpation of Matter from Peroneal Nerve, Open Approach

01CH3ZZ Extirpation of Matter from Peroneal Nerve, Percutaneous Approach

01CH4ZZ Extirpation of Matter from Peroneal Nerve, Percutaneous Endoscopic Approach

01CK0ZZ Extirpation of Matter from Head and Neck Sympathetic Nerve, Open Approach

01CK3ZZ Extirpation of Matter from Head and Neck Sympathetic Nerve, Percutaneous Approach

01CK4ZZ Extirpation of Matter from Head and Neck Sympathetic Nerve, Percutaneous Endoscopic Approach

01CL0ZZ Extirpation of Matter from Thoracic Sympathetic Nerve, Open Approach

01CL3ZZ Extirpation of Matter from Thoracic Sympathetic Nerve, Percutaneous Approach

01CL4ZZ Extirpation of Matter from Thoracic Sympathetic Nerve, Percutaneous Endoscopic Approach

01CM0ZZ Extirpation of Matter from Abdominal Sympathetic Nerve, Open Approach

01CM3ZZ Extirpation of Matter from Abdominal Sympathetic Nerve, Percutaneous Approach

01CM4ZZ Extirpation of Matter from Abdominal Sympathetic Nerve, Percutaneous Endoscopic Approach

01CN0ZZ Extirpation of Matter from Lumbar Sympathetic Nerve, Open Approach

01CN3ZZ Extirpation of Matter from Lumbar Sympathetic Nerve, Percutaneous Approach

01CN4ZZ Extirpation of Matter from Lumbar Sympathetic Nerve, Percutaneous Endoscopic Approach

01CP0ZZ Extirpation of Matter from Sacral Sympathetic Nerve, Open Approach

01CP3ZZ Extirpation of Matter from Sacral Sympathetic Nerve, Percutaneous Approach

01CP4ZZ Extirpation of Matter from Sacral Sympathetic Nerve, Percutaneous Endoscopic Approach

01CQ0ZZ Extirpation of Matter from Sacral Plexus, Open Approach

01CQ3ZZ Extirpation of Matter from Sacral Plexus, Percutaneous Approach

01CQ4ZZ Extirpation of Matter from Sacral Plexus, Percutaneous Endoscopic Approach

01CR0ZZ Extirpation of Matter from Sacral Nerve, Open Approach

01CR3ZZ Extirpation of Matter from Sacral Nerve, Percutaneous Approach

01CR4ZZ Extirpation of Matter from Sacral Nerve, Percutaneous Endoscopic Approach

01D – Peripheral Nervous System, Extraction

01D00ZZ Extraction of Cervical Plexus, Open Approach

01D03ZZ Extraction of Cervical Plexus, Percutaneous Approach

01D04ZZ Extraction of Cervical Plexus, Percutaneous Endoscopic Approach

01D10ZZ Extraction of Cervical Nerve, Open Approach

01D13ZZ Extraction of Cervical Nerve, Percutaneous Approach

01D14ZZ Extraction of Cervical Nerve, Percutaneous Endoscopic Approach

01D20ZZ Extraction of Phrenic Nerve, Open Approach

01D23ZZ Extraction of Phrenic Nerve, Percutaneous Approach

01D24ZZ Extraction of Phrenic Nerve, Percutaneous Endoscopic Approach

01D30ZZ Extraction of Brachial Plexus, Open Approach

01D33ZZ Extraction of Brachial Plexus, Percutaneous Approach

01D34ZZ Extraction of Brachial Plexus, Percutaneous Endoscopic Approach

01D40ZZ Extraction of Ulnar Nerve, Open Approach

01D43ZZ Extraction of Ulnar Nerve, Percutaneous Approach

01D44ZZ Extraction of Ulnar Nerve, Percutaneous Endoscopic Approach

01D50ZZ Extraction of Median Nerve, Open Approach

01D53ZZ Extraction of Median Nerve, Percutaneous Approach

01D54ZZ Extraction of Median Nerve, Percutaneous Endoscopic Approach

01D60ZZ Extraction of Radial Nerve, Open Approach

01D63ZZ Extraction of Radial Nerve, Percutaneous Approach

01D64ZZ Extraction of Radial Nerve, Percutaneous Endoscopic Approach

01D80ZZ Extraction of Thoracic Nerve, Open Approach

01D83ZZ Extraction of Thoracic Nerve, Percutaneous Approach

01D84ZZ Extraction of Thoracic Nerve, Percutaneous Endoscopic Approach

01D90ZZ Extraction of Lumbar Plexus, Open Approach

01D93ZZ Extraction of Lumbar Plexus, Percutaneous Approach

01D94ZZ Extraction of Lumbar Plexus, Percutaneous Endoscopic Approach

01DA0ZZ Extraction of Lumbosacral Plexus, Open Approach

01DA3ZZ Extraction of Lumbosacral Plexus, Percutaneous Approach

01DA4ZZ Extraction of Lumbosacral Plexus, Percutaneous Endoscopic Approach

01DB0ZZ Extraction of Lumbar Nerve, Open Approach

01DB3ZZ Extraction of Lumbar Nerve, Percutaneous Approach

01DB4ZZ Extraction of Lumbar Nerve, Percutaneous Endoscopic Approach

01DC0ZZ Extraction of Pudendal Nerve, Open Approach

01DC3ZZ Extraction of Pudendal Nerve, Percutaneous Approach

01DC4ZZ Extraction of Pudendal Nerve, Percutaneous Endoscopic Approach

01DD0ZZ Extraction of Femoral Nerve, Open Approach

01DD3ZZ Extraction of Femoral Nerve, Percutaneous Approach

01DD4ZZ Extraction of Femoral Nerve, Percutaneous Endoscopic Approach

01DF0ZZ Extraction of Sciatic Nerve, Open Approach

01DF3ZZ Extraction of Sciatic Nerve, Percutaneous Approach

01DF4ZZ Extraction of Sciatic Nerve, Percutaneous Endoscopic Approach

01DG0ZZ Extraction of Tibial Nerve, Open Approach

01DG3ZZ Extraction of Tibial Nerve, Percutaneous Approach

01DG4ZZ Extraction of Tibial Nerve, Percutaneous Endoscopic Approach

01DH0ZZ Extraction of Peroneal Nerve, Open Approach

01DH3ZZ Extraction of Peroneal Nerve, Percutaneous Approach

01DH4ZZ Extraction of Peroneal Nerve, Percutaneous Endoscopic Approach

01DK0ZZ Extraction of Head and Neck Sympathetic Nerve, Open Approach

01DK3ZZ Extraction of Head and Neck Sympathetic Nerve, Percutaneous Approach

01DK4ZZ Extraction of Head and Neck Sympathetic Nerve, Percutaneous Endoscopic Approach

01DL0ZZ Extraction of Thoracic Sympathetic Nerve, Open Approach

01DL3ZZ Extraction of Thoracic Sympathetic Nerve, Percutaneous Approach

01DL4ZZ Extraction of Thoracic Sympathetic Nerve, Percutaneous Endoscopic Approach

01DM0ZZ Extraction of Abdominal Sympathetic Nerve, Open Approach

01DM3ZZ Extraction of Abdominal Sympathetic Nerve, Percutaneous Approach

01DM4ZZ Extraction of Abdominal Sympathetic Nerve, Percutaneous Endoscopic Approach

01DN0ZZ Extraction of Lumbar Sympathetic Nerve, Open Approach

01DN3ZZ Extraction of Lumbar Sympathetic Nerve, Percutaneous Approach

01DN4ZZ Extraction of Lumbar Sympathetic Nerve, Percutaneous Endoscopic Approach

01DP0ZZ Extraction of Sacral Sympathetic Nerve, Open Approach

01DP3ZZ Extraction of Sacral Sympathetic Nerve, Percutaneous Approach

01DP4ZZ Extraction of Sacral Sympathetic Nerve, Percutaneous Endoscopic Approach

01DQ0ZZ Extraction of Sacral Plexus, Open Approach

01DQ3ZZ Extraction of Sacral Plexus, Percutaneous Approach

01DQ4ZZ Extraction of Sacral Plexus, Percutaneous Endoscopic Approach

01DR0ZZ Extraction of Sacral Nerve, Open Approach

01DR3ZZ Extraction of Sacral Nerve, Percutaneous Approach

01DR4ZZ Extraction of Sacral Nerve, Percutaneous Endoscopic Approach

1H – Peripheral Nervous System, Insertion

01HY02Z Insertion of Monitoring Device into Peripheral Nerve, Open Approach

01HY0MZ Insertion of Neurostimulator Lead into Peripheral Nerve, Open Approach

01HY32Z Insertion of Monitoring Device into Peripheral Nerve, Percutaneous Approach

01HY3MZ Insertion of Neurostimulator Lead into Peripheral Nerve, Percutaneous Approach

01HY42Z Insertion of Monitoring Device into Peripheral Nerve, Percutaneous Endoscopic Approach

01HY4MZ Insertion of Neurostimulator Lead into Peripheral Nerve, Percutaneous Endoscopic Approach

1J – Peripheral Nervous System, Inspection

Review Coding Guidelines B3.11a, B3.11b and B3.11c

01JY0ZZ Inspection of Peripheral Nerve, Open Approach

01JY3ZZ Inspection of Peripheral Nerve, Percutaneous Approach

01JY4ZZ Inspection of Peripheral Nerve, Percutaneous Endoscopic Approach

1N – Peripheral Nervous System, Release

Review Coding Guideline B3.13

Review Coding Guideline B3.14

01N00ZZ Release Cervical Plexus, Open Approach

01N03ZZ Release Cervical Plexus, Percutaneous Approach

01N04ZZ Release Cervical Plexus, Percutaneous Endoscopic Approach

01N10ZZ Release Cervical Nerve, Open Approach

01N13ZZ Release Cervical Nerve, Percutaneous Approach

01N14ZZ Release Cervical Nerve, Percutaneous Endoscopic Approach

01N20ZZ Release Phrenic Nerve, Open Approach

01N23ZZ Release Phrenic Nerve, Percutaneous Approach

01N24ZZ Release Phrenic Nerve, Percutaneous Endoscopic Approach

01N30ZZ Release Brachial Plexus, Open Approach

01N33ZZ Release Brachial Plexus, Percutaneous Approach

01N34ZZ Release Brachial Plexus, Percutaneous Endoscopic Approach

01N40ZZ Release Ulnar Nerve, Open Approach

01N43ZZ Release Ulnar Nerve, Percutaneous Approach

01N44ZZ Release Ulnar Nerve, Percutaneous Endoscopic Approach

01N50ZZ Release Median Nerve, Open Approach
AHA CC: 3Q, 2014, 33-34

01N53ZZ Release Median Nerve, Percutaneous Approach

01N54ZZ Release Median Nerve, Percutaneous Endoscopic Approach

01N60ZZ Release Radial Nerve, Open Approach

01N63ZZ Release Radial Nerve, Percutaneous Approach

01N64ZZ Release Radial Nerve, Percutaneous Endoscopic Approach

01N80ZZ Release Thoracic Nerve, Open Approach

01N83ZZ Release Thoracic Nerve, Percutaneous Approach

01N84ZZ Release Thoracic Nerve, Percutaneous Endoscopic Approach

01N90ZZ Release Lumbar Plexus, Open Approach

01N93ZZ Release Lumbar Plexus, Percutaneous Approach

01N94ZZ Release Lumbar Plexus, Percutaneous Endoscopic Approach

01NA0ZZ Release Lumbosacral Plexus, Open Approach

01NA3ZZ Release Lumbosacral Plexus, Percutaneous Approach

01NA4ZZ Release Lumbosacral Plexus, Percutaneous Endoscopic Approach

01NB0ZZ Release Lumbar Nerve, Open Approach

01NB3ZZ Release Lumbar Nerve, Percutaneous Approach

01NB4ZZ Release Lumbar Nerve, Percutaneous Endoscopic Approach

01NC0ZZ Release Pudendal Nerve, Open Approach

01NC3ZZ Release Pudendal Nerve, Percutaneous Approach

01NC4ZZ Release Pudendal Nerve, Percutaneous Endoscopic Approach

01ND0ZZ Release Femoral Nerve, Open Approach

01ND3ZZ Release Femoral Nerve, Percutaneous Approach

01ND4ZZ Release Femoral Nerve, Percutaneous Endoscopic Approach

01NF0ZZ Release Sciatic Nerve, Open Approach

01NF3ZZ Release Sciatic Nerve, Percutaneous Approach

01NF4ZZ Release Sciatic Nerve, Percutaneous Endoscopic Approach

01NG0ZZ Release Tibial Nerve, Open Approach

01NG3ZZ Release Tibial Nerve, Percutaneous Approach

01NG4ZZ Release Tibial Nerve, Percutaneous Endoscopic Approach

01NH0ZZ Release Peroneal Nerve, Open Approach

01NH3ZZ Release Peroneal Nerve, Percutaneous Approach

01NH4ZZ Release Peroneal Nerve, Percutaneous Endoscopic Approach

01NK0ZZ Release Head and Neck Sympathetic Nerve, Open Approach

01NK3ZZ Release Head and Neck Sympathetic Nerve, Percutaneous Approach

01NK4ZZ Release Head and Neck Sympathetic Nerve, Percutaneous Endoscopic Approach

01NL0ZZ Release Thoracic Sympathetic Nerve, Open Approach

01NL3ZZ Release Thoracic Sympathetic Nerve, Percutaneous Approach

01NL4ZZ Release Thoracic Sympathetic Nerve, Percutaneous Endoscopic Approach

01NM0ZZ Release Abdominal Sympathetic Nerve, Open Approach

01NM3ZZ Release Abdominal Sympathetic Nerve, Percutaneous Approach

01NM4ZZ Release Abdominal Sympathetic Nerve, Percutaneous Endoscopic Approach

01NN0ZZ Release Lumbar Sympathetic Nerve, Open Approach

01NN3ZZ Release Lumbar Sympathetic Nerve, Percutaneous Approach

01NN4ZZ Release Lumbar Sympathetic Nerve, Percutaneous Endoscopic Approach

01NP0ZZ Release Sacral Sympathetic Nerve, Open Approach

01NP3ZZ Release Sacral Sympathetic Nerve, Percutaneous Approach

01NP4ZZ Release Sacral Sympathetic Nerve, Percutaneous Endoscopic Approach

01NQ0ZZ Release Sacral Plexus, Open Approach

01NQ3ZZ Release Sacral Plexus, Percutaneous Approach

01NQ4ZZ Release Sacral Plexus, Percutaneous Endoscopic Approach

01NR0ZZ Release Sacral Nerve, Open Approach

01NR3ZZ Release Sacral Nerve, Percutaneous Approach

01NR4ZZ Release Sacral Nerve, Percutaneous Endoscopic Approach

01P – Peripheral Nervous System, Removal

Review Coding Guideline B6.1c

01PY00Z Removal of Drainage Device from Peripheral Nerve, Open Approach

01PY02Z Removal of Monitoring Device from Peripheral Nerve, Open Approach

01PY07Z Removal of Autologous Tissue Substitute from Peripheral Nerve, Open Approach

01PY0MZ Removal of Neurostimulator Lead from Peripheral Nerve, Open Approach

01PY30Z Removal of Drainage Device from Peripheral Nerve, Percutaneous Approach

01PY32Z Removal of Monitoring Device from Peripheral Nerve, Percutaneous Approach

01PY37Z Removal of Autologous Tissue Substitute from Peripheral Nerve, Percutaneous Approach

01PY3MZ Removal of Neurostimulator Lead from Peripheral Nerve, Percutaneous Approach

01PY40Z Removal of Drainage Device from Peripheral Nerve, Percutaneous Endoscopic Approach

01PY42Z Removal of Monitoring Device from Peripheral Nerve, Percutaneous Endoscopic Approach

01PY47Z Removal of Autologous Tissue Substitute from Peripheral Nerve, Percutaneous Endoscopic Approach

01PY4MZ Removal of Neurostimulator Lead from Peripheral Nerve, Percutaneous Endoscopic Approach

♀ Female-only   ♂ Male-only   ▲ Limited Coverage   ● Non-OR   ▨ HAC-associated procedure   ▲ Non-covered procedures   ✚ Combination

01PYX0Z Removal of Drainage Device from Peripheral Nerve, External Approach	**01PYX2Z** Removal of Monitoring Device from Peripheral Nerve, External Approach	**01PYXMZ** Removal of Neurostimulator Lead from Peripheral Nerve, External Approach

01Q – Peripheral Nervous System, Repair

01Q00ZZ Repair Cervical Plexus, Open Approach	**01Q93ZZ** Repair Lumbar Plexus, Percutaneous Approach	**01QK0ZZ** Repair Head and Neck Sympathetic Nerve, Open Approach
01Q03ZZ Repair Cervical Plexus, Percutaneous Approach	**01Q94ZZ** Repair Lumbar Plexus, Percutaneous Endoscopic Approach	**01QK3ZZ** Repair Head and Neck Sympathetic Nerve, Percutaneous Approach
01Q04ZZ Repair Cervical Plexus, Percutaneous Endoscopic Approach	**01QA0ZZ** Repair Lumbosacral Plexus, Open Approach	**01QK4ZZ** Repair Head and Neck Sympathetic Nerve, Percutaneous Endoscopic Approach
01Q10ZZ Repair Cervical Nerve, Open Approach	**01QA3ZZ** Repair Lumbosacral Plexus, Percutaneous Approach	**01QL0ZZ** Repair Thoracic Sympathetic Nerve, Open Approach
01Q13ZZ Repair Cervical Nerve, Percutaneous Approach	**01QA4ZZ** Repair Lumbosacral Plexus, Percutaneous Endoscopic Approach	**01QL3ZZ** Repair Thoracic Sympathetic Nerve, Percutaneous Approach
01Q14ZZ Repair Cervical Nerve, Percutaneous Endoscopic Approach	**01QB0ZZ** Repair Lumbar Nerve, Open Approach	**01QL4ZZ** Repair Thoracic Sympathetic Nerve, Percutaneous Endoscopic Approach
01Q20ZZ Repair Phrenic Nerve, Open Approach	**01QB3ZZ** Repair Lumbar Nerve, Percutaneous Approach	**01QM0ZZ** Repair Abdominal Sympathetic Nerve, Open Approach
01Q23ZZ Repair Phrenic Nerve, Percutaneous Approach	**01QB4ZZ** Repair Lumbar Nerve, Percutaneous Endoscopic Approach	**01QM3ZZ** Repair Abdominal Sympathetic Nerve, Percutaneous Approach
01Q24ZZ Repair Phrenic Nerve, Percutaneous Endoscopic Approach	**01QC0ZZ** Repair Pudendal Nerve, Open Approach	**01QM4ZZ** Repair Abdominal Sympathetic Nerve, Percutaneous Endoscopic Approach
01Q30ZZ Repair Brachial Plexus, Open Approach	**01QC3ZZ** Repair Pudendal Nerve, Percutaneous Approach	**01QN0ZZ** Repair Lumbar Sympathetic Nerve, Open Approach
01Q33ZZ Repair Brachial Plexus, Percutaneous Approach	**01QC4ZZ** Repair Pudendal Nerve, Percutaneous Endoscopic Approach	**01QN3ZZ** Repair Lumbar Sympathetic Nerve, Percutaneous Approach
01Q34ZZ Repair Brachial Plexus, Percutaneous Endoscopic Approach	**01QD0ZZ** Repair Femoral Nerve, Open Approach	**01QN4ZZ** Repair Lumbar Sympathetic Nerve, Percutaneous Endoscopic Approach
01Q40ZZ Repair Ulnar Nerve, Open Approach	**01QD3ZZ** Repair Femoral Nerve, Percutaneous Approach	**01QP0ZZ** Repair Sacral Sympathetic Nerve, Open Approach
01Q43ZZ Repair Ulnar Nerve, Percutaneous Approach	**01QD4ZZ** Repair Femoral Nerve, Percutaneous Endoscopic Approach	**01QP3ZZ** Repair Sacral Sympathetic Nerve, Percutaneous Approach
01Q44ZZ Repair Ulnar Nerve, Percutaneous Endoscopic Approach	**01QF0ZZ** Repair Sciatic Nerve, Open Approach	**01QP4ZZ** Repair Sacral Sympathetic Nerve, Percutaneous Endoscopic Approach
01Q50ZZ Repair Median Nerve, Open Approach	**01QF3ZZ** Repair Sciatic Nerve, Percutaneous Approach	**01QQ0ZZ** Repair Sacral Plexus, Open Approach
01Q53ZZ Repair Median Nerve, Percutaneous Approach	**01QF4ZZ** Repair Sciatic Nerve, Percutaneous Endoscopic Approach	**01QQ3ZZ** Repair Sacral Plexus, Percutaneous Approach
01Q54ZZ Repair Median Nerve, Percutaneous Endoscopic Approach	**01QG0ZZ** Repair Tibial Nerve, Open Approach	**01QQ4ZZ** Repair Sacral Plexus, Percutaneous Endoscopic Approach
01Q60ZZ Repair Radial Nerve, Open Approach	**01QG3ZZ** Repair Tibial Nerve, Percutaneous Approach	**01QR0ZZ** Repair Sacral Nerve, Open Approach
01Q63ZZ Repair Radial Nerve, Percutaneous Approach	**01QG4ZZ** Repair Tibial Nerve, Percutaneous Endoscopic Approach	**01QR3ZZ** Repair Sacral Nerve, Percutaneous Approach
01Q64ZZ Repair Radial Nerve, Percutaneous Endoscopic Approach	**01QH0ZZ** Repair Peroneal Nerve, Open Approach	**01QR4ZZ** Repair Sacral Nerve, Percutaneous Endoscopic Approach
01Q80ZZ Repair Thoracic Nerve, Open Approach	**01QH3ZZ** Repair Peroneal Nerve, Percutaneous Approach	
01Q83ZZ Repair Thoracic Nerve, Percutaneous Approach	**01QH4ZZ** Repair Peroneal Nerve, Percutaneous Endoscopic Approach	
01Q84ZZ Repair Thoracic Nerve, Percutaneous Endoscopic Approach		
01Q90ZZ Repair Lumbar Plexus, Open Approach		

01S – Peripheral Nervous System, Reposition

01S00ZZ Reposition Cervical Plexus, Open Approach	**01S50ZZ** Reposition Median Nerve, Open Approach	**01SB0ZZ** Reposition Lumbar Nerve, Open Approach
01S03ZZ Reposition Cervical Plexus, Percutaneous Approach	**01S53ZZ** Reposition Median Nerve, Percutaneous Approach	**01SB3ZZ** Reposition Lumbar Nerve, Percutaneous Approach
01S04ZZ Reposition Cervical Plexus, Percutaneous Endoscopic Approach	**01S54ZZ** Reposition Median Nerve, Percutaneous Endoscopic Approach	**01SB4ZZ** Reposition Lumbar Nerve, Percutaneous Endoscopic Approach
01S10ZZ Reposition Cervical Nerve, Open Approach	**01S60ZZ** Reposition Radial Nerve, Open Approach	**01SC0ZZ** Reposition Pudendal Nerve, Open Approach
01S13ZZ Reposition Cervical Nerve, Percutaneous Approach	**01S63ZZ** Reposition Radial Nerve, Percutaneous Approach	**01SC3ZZ** Reposition Pudendal Nerve, Percutaneous Approach
01S14ZZ Reposition Cervical Nerve, Percutaneous Endoscopic Approach	**01S64ZZ** Reposition Radial Nerve, Percutaneous Endoscopic Approach	**01SC4ZZ** Reposition Pudendal Nerve, Percutaneous Endoscopic Approach
01S20ZZ Reposition Phrenic Nerve, Open Approach	**01S80ZZ** Reposition Thoracic Nerve, Open Approach	**01SD0ZZ** Reposition Femoral Nerve, Open Approach
01S23ZZ Reposition Phrenic Nerve, Percutaneous Approach	**01S83ZZ** Reposition Thoracic Nerve, Percutaneous Approach	**01SD3ZZ** Reposition Femoral Nerve, Percutaneous Approach
01S24ZZ Reposition Phrenic Nerve, Percutaneous Endoscopic Approach	**01S84ZZ** Reposition Thoracic Nerve, Percutaneous Endoscopic Approach	**01SD4ZZ** Reposition Femoral Nerve, Percutaneous Endoscopic Approach
01S30ZZ Reposition Brachial Plexus, Open Approach	**01S90ZZ** Reposition Lumbar Plexus, Open Approach	**01SF0ZZ** Reposition Sciatic Nerve, Open Approach
01S33ZZ Reposition Brachial Plexus, Percutaneous Approach	**01S93ZZ** Reposition Lumbar Plexus, Percutaneous Approach	**01SF3ZZ** Reposition Sciatic Nerve, Percutaneous Approach
01S34ZZ Reposition Brachial Plexus, Percutaneous Endoscopic Approach	**01S94ZZ** Reposition Lumbar Plexus, Percutaneous Endoscopic Approach	**01SF4ZZ** Reposition Sciatic Nerve, Percutaneous Endoscopic Approach
01S40ZZ Reposition Ulnar Nerve, Open Approach	**01SA0ZZ** Reposition Lumbosacral Plexus, Open Approach	**01SG0ZZ** Reposition Tibial Nerve, Open Approach
01S43ZZ Reposition Ulnar Nerve, Percutaneous Approach	**01SA3ZZ** Reposition Lumbosacral Plexus, Percutaneous Approach	**01SG3ZZ** Reposition Tibial Nerve, Percutaneous Approach
01S44ZZ Reposition Ulnar Nerve, Percutaneous Endoscopic Approach	**01SA4ZZ** Reposition Lumbosacral Plexus, Percutaneous Endoscopic Approach	**01SG4ZZ** Reposition Tibial Nerve, Percutaneous Endoscopic Approach

♀ Female-only　　♂ Male-only　　▲ Limited Coverage　　● Non-OR　　▬ HAC-associated procedure　　▲ Non-covered procedures　　✚ Combination

01SH0ZZ Reposition Peroneal Nerve, Open Approach
01SH3ZZ Reposition Peroneal Nerve, Percutaneous Approach
01SH4ZZ Reposition Peroneal Nerve, Percutaneous Endoscopic Approach

01SQ0ZZ Reposition Sacral Plexus, Open Approach
01SQ3ZZ Reposition Sacral Plexus, Percutaneous Approach
01SQ4ZZ Reposition Sacral Plexus, Percutaneous Endoscopic Approach
01SR0ZZ Reposition Sacral Nerve, Open Approach

01SR3ZZ Reposition Sacral Nerve, Percutaneous Approach
01SR4ZZ Reposition Sacral Nerve, Percutaneous Endoscopic Approach

01U – Peripheral Nervous System, Supplement

01U107Z Supplement Cervical Nerve with Autologous Tissue Substitute, Open Approach
01U137Z Supplement Cervical Nerve with Autologous Tissue Substitute, Percutaneous Approach
01U147Z Supplement Cervical Nerve with Autologous Tissue Substitute, Percutaneous Endoscopic Approach
01U207Z Supplement Phrenic Nerve with Autologous Tissue Substitute, Open Approach
01U237Z Supplement Phrenic Nerve with Autologous Tissue Substitute, Percutaneous Approach
01U247Z Supplement Phrenic Nerve with Autologous Tissue Substitute, Percutaneous Endoscopic Approach
01U407Z Supplement Ulnar Nerve with Autologous Tissue Substitute, Open Approach
01U437Z Supplement Ulnar Nerve with Autologous Tissue Substitute, Percutaneous Approach
01U447Z Supplement Ulnar Nerve with Autologous Tissue Substitute, Percutaneous Endoscopic Approach
01U507Z Supplement Median Nerve with Autologous Tissue Substitute, Open Approach
01U537Z Supplement Median Nerve with Autologous Tissue Substitute, Percutaneous Approach
01U547Z Supplement Median Nerve with Autologous Tissue Substitute, Percutaneous Endoscopic Approach
01U607Z Supplement Radial Nerve with Autologous Tissue Substitute, Open Approach
01U637Z Supplement Radial Nerve with Autologous Tissue Substitute, Percutaneous Approach

01U647Z Supplement Radial Nerve with Autologous Tissue Substitute, Percutaneous Endoscopic Approach
01U807Z Supplement Thoracic Nerve with Autologous Tissue Substitute, Open Approach
01U837Z Supplement Thoracic Nerve with Autologous Tissue Substitute, Percutaneous Approach
01U847Z Supplement Thoracic Nerve with Autologous Tissue Substitute, Percutaneous Endoscopic Approach
01UB07Z Supplement Lumbar Nerve with Autologous Tissue Substitute, Open Approach
01UB37Z Supplement Lumbar Nerve with Autologous Tissue Substitute, Percutaneous Approach
01UB47Z Supplement Lumbar Nerve with Autologous Tissue Substitute, Percutaneous Endoscopic Approach
01UC07Z Supplement Pudendal Nerve with Autologous Tissue Substitute, Open Approach
01UC37Z Supplement Pudendal Nerve with Autologous Tissue Substitute, Percutaneous Approach
01UC47Z Supplement Pudendal Nerve with Autologous Tissue Substitute, Percutaneous Endoscopic Approach
01UD07Z Supplement Femoral Nerve with Autologous Tissue Substitute, Open Approach
01UD37Z Supplement Femoral Nerve with Autologous Tissue Substitute, Percutaneous Approach

01UD47Z Supplement Femoral Nerve with Autologous Tissue Substitute, Percutaneous Endoscopic Approach
01UF07Z Supplement Sciatic Nerve with Autologous Tissue Substitute, Open Approach
01UF37Z Supplement Sciatic Nerve with Autologous Tissue Substitute, Percutaneous Approach
01UF47Z Supplement Sciatic Nerve with Autologous Tissue Substitute, Percutaneous Endoscopic Approach
01UG07Z Supplement Tibial Nerve with Autologous Tissue Substitute, Open Approach
01UG37Z Supplement Tibial Nerve with Autologous Tissue Substitute, Percutaneous Approach
01UG47Z Supplement Tibial Nerve with Autologous Tissue Substitute, Percutaneous Endoscopic Approach
01UH07Z Supplement Peroneal Nerve with Autologous Tissue Substitute, Open Approach
01UH37Z Supplement Peroneal Nerve with Autologous Tissue Substitute, Percutaneous Approach
01UH47Z Supplement Peroneal Nerve with Autologous Tissue Substitute, Percutaneous Endoscopic Approach
01UR07Z Supplement Sacral Nerve with Autologous Tissue Substitute, Open Approach
01UR37Z Supplement Sacral Nerve with Autologous Tissue Substitute, Percutaneous Approach
01UR47Z Supplement Sacral Nerve with Autologous Tissue Substitute, Percutaneous Endoscopic Approach

01W – Peripheral Nervous System, Revision

Review Coding Guideline B6.1c

01WY00Z Revision of Drainage Device in Peripheral Nerve, Open Approach
01WY02Z Revision of Monitoring Device in Peripheral Nerve, Open Approach
01WY07Z Revision of Autologous Tissue Substitute in Peripheral Nerve, Open Approach
01WY0MZ Revision of Neurostimulator Lead in Peripheral Nerve, Open Approach
01WY30Z Revision of Drainage Device in Peripheral Nerve, Percutaneous Approach
01WY32Z Revision of Monitoring Device in Peripheral Nerve, Percutaneous Approach

01WY37Z Revision of Autologous Tissue Substitute in Peripheral Nerve, Percutaneous Approach
01WY3MZ Revision of Neurostimulator Lead in Peripheral Nerve, Percutaneous Approach
01WY40Z Revision of Drainage Device in Peripheral Nerve, Percutaneous Endoscopic Approach
01WY42Z Revision of Monitoring Device in Peripheral Nerve, Percutaneous Endoscopic Approach
01WY47Z Revision of Autologous Tissue Substitute in Peripheral Nerve, Percutaneous Endoscopic Approach

01WY4MZ Revision of Neurostimulator Lead in Peripheral Nerve, Percutaneous Endoscopic Approach
01WYX0Z Revision of Drainage Device in Peripheral Nerve, External Approach
01WYX2Z Revision of Monitoring Device in Peripheral Nerve, External Approach
01WYX7Z Revision of Autologous Tissue Substitute in Peripheral Nerve, External Approach
01WYXMZ Revision of Neurostimulator Lead in Peripheral Nerve, External Approach

01X – Peripheral Nervous System, Transfer

01X10Z1 Transfer Cervical Nerve to Cervical Nerve, Open Approach
01X10Z2 Transfer Cervical Nerve to Phrenic Nerve, Open Approach
01X14Z1 Transfer Cervical Nerve to Cervical Nerve, Percutaneous Endoscopic Approach

01X14Z2 Transfer Cervical Nerve to Phrenic Nerve, Percutaneous Endoscopic Approach
01X20Z1 Transfer Phrenic Nerve to Cervical Nerve, Open Approach
01X20Z2 Transfer Phrenic Nerve to Phrenic Nerve, Open Approach

01X24Z1 Transfer Phrenic Nerve to Cervical Nerve, Percutaneous Endoscopic Approach
01X24Z2 Transfer Phrenic Nerve to Phrenic Nerve, Percutaneous Endoscopic Approach
01X40Z4 Transfer Ulnar Nerve to Ulnar Nerve, Open Approach

♀ Female-only   ♂ Male-only   ▲ Limited Coverage   ● Non-OR   ▦ HAC-associated procedure   ▲ Non-covered procedures   ✚ Combination

01X40Z5	Transfer Ulnar Nerve to Median Nerve, Open Approach
01X40Z6	Transfer Ulnar Nerve to Radial Nerve, Open Approach
01X44Z4	Transfer Ulnar Nerve to Ulnar Nerve, Percutaneous Endoscopic Approach
01X44Z5	Transfer Ulnar Nerve to Median Nerve, Percutaneous Endoscopic Approach
01X44Z6	Transfer Ulnar Nerve to Radial Nerve, Percutaneous Endoscopic Approach
01X50Z4	Transfer Median Nerve to Ulnar Nerve, Open Approach
01X50Z5	Transfer Median Nerve to Median Nerve, Open Approach
01X50Z6	Transfer Median Nerve to Radial Nerve, Open Approach
01X54Z4	Transfer Median Nerve to Ulnar Nerve, Percutaneous Endoscopic Approach
01X54Z5	Transfer Median Nerve to Median Nerve, Percutaneous Endoscopic Approach
01X54Z6	Transfer Median Nerve to Radial Nerve, Percutaneous Endoscopic Approach
01X60Z4	Transfer Radial Nerve to Ulnar Nerve, Open Approach
01X60Z5	Transfer Radial Nerve to Median Nerve, Open Approach
01X60Z6	Transfer Radial Nerve to Radial Nerve, Open Approach
01X64Z4	Transfer Radial Nerve to Ulnar Nerve, Percutaneous Endoscopic Approach
01X64Z5	Transfer Radial Nerve to Median Nerve, Percutaneous Endoscopic Approach
01X64Z6	Transfer Radial Nerve to Radial Nerve, Percutaneous Endoscopic Approach
01X80Z8	Transfer Thoracic Nerve to Thoracic Nerve, Open Approach
01X84Z8	Transfer Thoracic Nerve to Thoracic Nerve, Percutaneous Endoscopic Approach
01XB0ZB	Transfer Lumbar Nerve to Lumbar Nerve, Open Approach
01XB0ZC	Transfer Lumbar Nerve to Perineal Nerve, Open Approach
01XB4ZB	Transfer Lumbar Nerve to Lumbar Nerve, Percutaneous Endoscopic Approach
01XB4ZC	Transfer Lumbar Nerve to Perineal Nerve, Percutaneous Endoscopic Approach
01XC0ZB	Transfer Pudendal Nerve to Lumbar Nerve, Open Approach
01XC0ZC	Transfer Pudendal Nerve to Perineal Nerve, Open Approach
01XC4ZB	Transfer Pudendal Nerve to Lumbar Nerve, Percutaneous Endoscopic Approach
01XC4ZC	Transfer Pudendal Nerve to Perineal Nerve, Percutaneous Endoscopic Approach
01XD0ZD	Transfer Femoral Nerve to Femoral Nerve, Open Approach
01XD0ZF	Transfer Femoral Nerve to Sciatic Nerve, Open Approach
01XD0ZG	Transfer Femoral Nerve to Tibial Nerve, Open Approach
01XD0ZH	Transfer Femoral Nerve to Peroneal Nerve, Open Approach
01XD4ZD	Transfer Femoral Nerve to Femoral Nerve, Percutaneous Endoscopic Approach
01XD4ZF	Transfer Femoral Nerve to Sciatic Nerve, Percutaneous Endoscopic Approach
01XD4ZG	Transfer Femoral Nerve to Tibial Nerve, Percutaneous Endoscopic Approach
01XD4ZH	Transfer Femoral Nerve to Peroneal Nerve, Percutaneous Endoscopic Approach
01XF0ZD	Transfer Sciatic Nerve to Femoral Nerve, Open Approach
01XF0ZF	Transfer Sciatic Nerve to Sciatic Nerve, Open Approach
01XF0ZG	Transfer Sciatic Nerve to Tibial Nerve, Open Approach
01XF0ZH	Transfer Sciatic Nerve to Peroneal Nerve, Open Approach
01XF4ZD	Transfer Sciatic Nerve to Femoral Nerve, Percutaneous Endoscopic Approach
01XF4ZF	Transfer Sciatic Nerve to Sciatic Nerve, Percutaneous Endoscopic Approach
01XF4ZG	Transfer Sciatic Nerve to Tibial Nerve, Percutaneous Endoscopic Approach
01XF4ZH	Transfer Sciatic Nerve to Peroneal Nerve, Percutaneous Endoscopic Approach
01XG0ZD	Transfer Tibial Nerve to Femoral Nerve, Open Approach
01XG0ZF	Transfer Tibial Nerve to Sciatic Nerve, Open Approach
01XG0ZG	Transfer Tibial Nerve to Tibial Nerve, Open Approach
01XG0ZH	Transfer Tibial Nerve to Peroneal Nerve, Open Approach
01XG4ZD	Transfer Tibial Nerve to Femoral Nerve, Percutaneous Endoscopic Approach
01XG4ZF	Transfer Tibial Nerve to Sciatic Nerve, Percutaneous Endoscopic Approach
01XG4ZG	Transfer Tibial Nerve to Tibial Nerve, Percutaneous Endoscopic Approach
01XG4ZH	Transfer Tibial Nerve to Peroneal Nerve, Percutaneous Endoscopic Approach
01XH0ZD	Transfer Peroneal Nerve to Femoral Nerve, Open Approach
01XH0ZF	Transfer Peroneal Nerve to Sciatic Nerve, Open Approach
01XH0ZG	Transfer Peroneal Nerve to Tibial Nerve, Open Approach
01XH0ZH	Transfer Peroneal Nerve to Peroneal Nerve, Open Approach
01XH4ZD	Transfer Peroneal Nerve to Femoral Nerve, Percutaneous Endoscopic Approach
01XH4ZF	Transfer Peroneal Nerve to Sciatic Nerve, Percutaneous Endoscopic Approach
01XH4ZG	Transfer Peroneal Nerve to Tibial Nerve, Percutaneous Endoscopic Approach
01XH4ZH	Transfer Peroneal Nerve to Peroneal Nerve, Percutaneous Endoscopic Approach

♀ Female-only   ♂ Male-only   ▲ Limited Coverage   ● Non-OR   ▨ HAC-associated procedure   ▲ Non-covered procedures   ✛ Combination

Heart

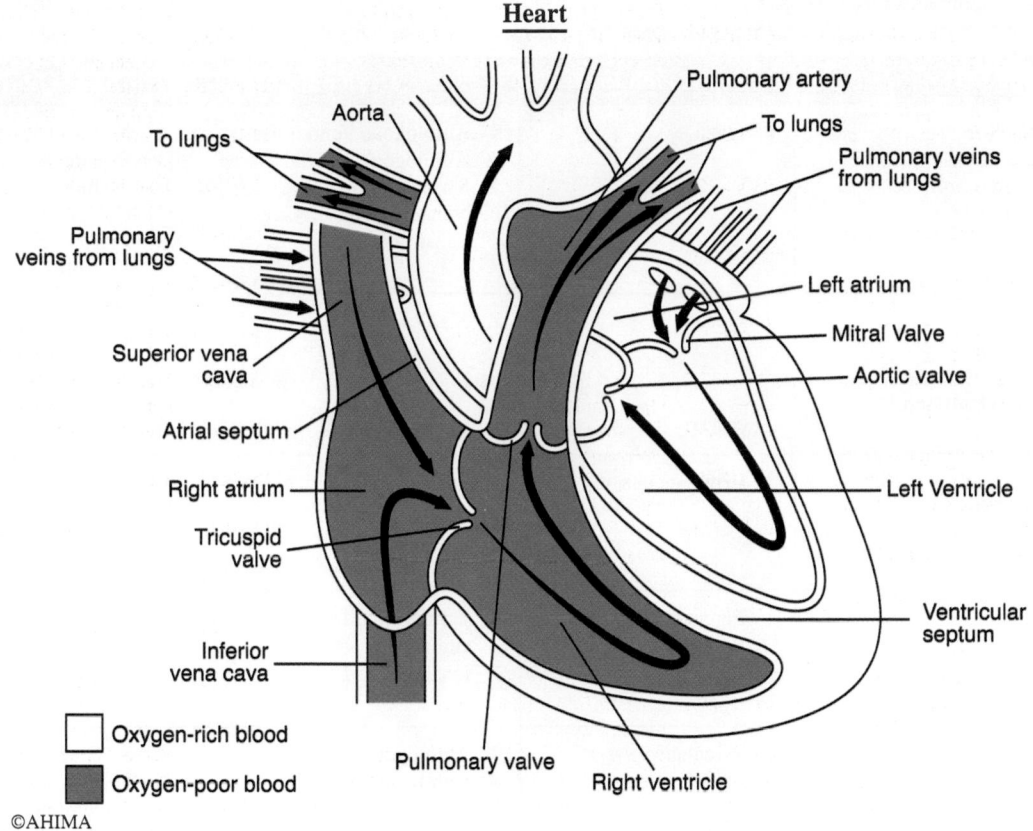

To lungs
Aorta
Pulmonary artery
To lungs
Pulmonary veins from lungs
Pulmonary veins from lungs
Left atrium
Mitral Valve
Superior vena cava
Aortic valve
Atrial septum
Right atrium
Left Ventricle
Tricuspid valve
Inferior vena cava
Ventricular septum
Oxygen-rich blood
Oxygen-poor blood
Pulmonary valve
Right ventricle
©AHIMA

Great Vessels of Heart

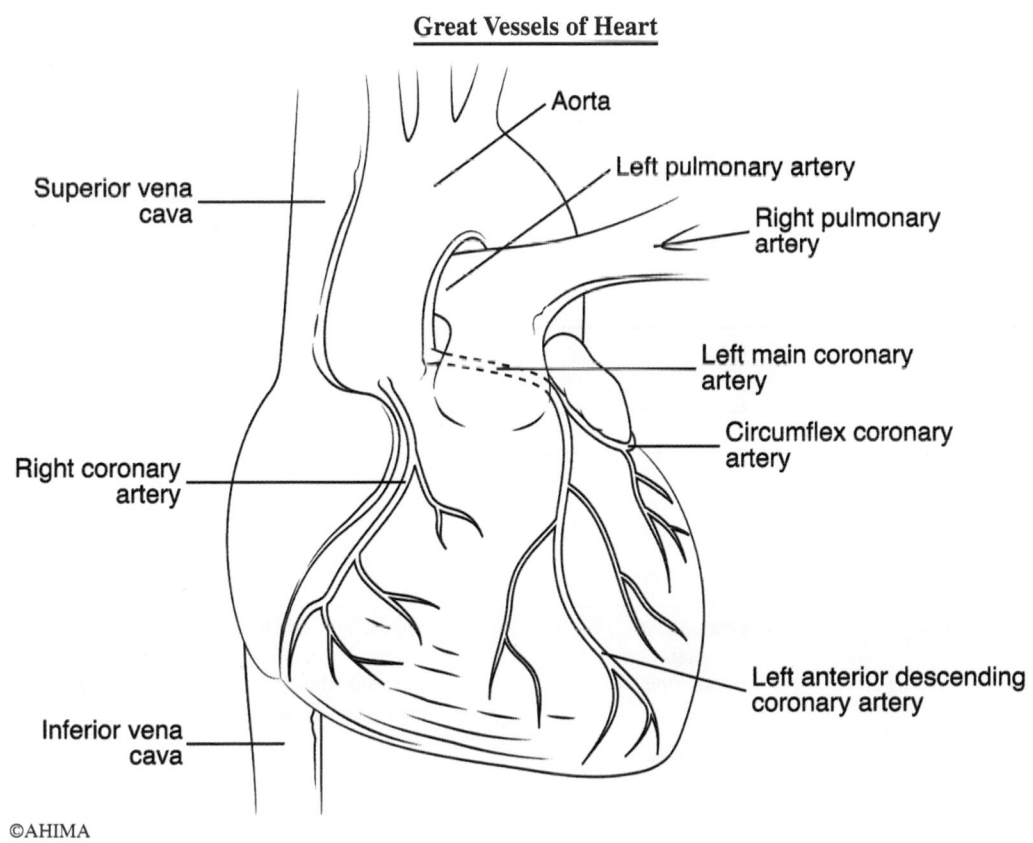

Aorta
Superior vena cava
Left pulmonary artery
Right pulmonary artery
Left main coronary artery
Right coronary artery
Circumflex coronary artery
Left anterior descending coronary artery
Inferior vena cava
©AHIMA

Heart and Great Vessels Tables 021–02Y

Section	0	Medical and Surgical
Body System	2	Heart and Great Vessels
Operation	1	**Bypass:** Altering the route of passage of the contents of a tubular body part

Body Part (4th)	Approach (5th)	Device (6th)	Qualifier (7th)
0 Coronary Artery, One Site 1 Coronary Artery, Two Sites 2 Coronary Artery, Three Sites 3 Coronary Artery, Four or More Sites	0 Open	9 Autologous Venous Tissue A Autologous Arterial Tissue J Synthetic Substitute K Nonautologous Tissue Substitute	3 Coronary Artery 8 Internal Mammary, Right 9 Internal Mammary, Left C Thoracic Artery F Abdominal Artery W Aorta
0 Coronary Artery, One Site 1 Coronary Artery, Two Sites 2 Coronary Artery, Three Sites 3 Coronary Artery, Four or More Sites	0 Open	Z No Device	3 Coronary Artery 8 Internal Mammary, Right 9 Internal Mammary, Left C Thoracic Artery F Abdominal Artery
0 Coronary Artery, One Site 1 Coronary Artery, Two Sites 2 Coronary Artery, Three Sites 3 Coronary Artery, Four or More Sites	3 Percutaneous	4 Intraluminal Device, Drug-eluting D Intraluminal Device	4 Coronary Vein
0 Coronary Artery, One Site 1 Coronary Artery, Two Sites 2 Coronary Artery, Three Sites 3 Coronary Artery, Four or More Sites	4 Percutaneous Endoscopic	4 Intraluminal Device, Drug-eluting D Intraluminal Device	4 Coronary Vein
0 Coronary Artery, One Site 1 Coronary Artery, Two Sites 2 Coronary Artery, Three Sites 3 Coronary Artery, Four or More Sites	4 Percutaneous Endoscopic	9 Autologous Venous Tissue A Autologous Arterial Tissue J Synthetic Substitute K Nonautologous Tissue Substitute	3 Coronary Artery 8 Internal Mammary, Right 9 Internal Mammary, Left C Thoracic Artery F Abdominal Artery W Aorta
0 Coronary Artery, One Site 1 Coronary Artery, Two Sites 2 Coronary Artery, Three Sites 3 Coronary Artery, Four or More Sites	4 Percutaneous Endoscopic	Z No Device	3 Coronary Artery 8 Internal Mammary, Right 9 Internal Mammary, Left C Thoracic Artery F Abdominal Artery
6 Atrium, Right	0 Open 4 Percutaneous Endoscopic	9 Autologous Venous Tissue A Autologous Arterial Tissue J Synthetic Substitute K Nonautologous Tissue Substitute	P Pulmonary Trunk Q Pulmonary Artery, Right R Pulmonary Artery, Left
6 Atrium, Right	0 Open 4 Percutaneous Endoscopic	Z No Device	7 Atrium, Left P Pulmonary Trunk Q Pulmonary Artery, Right R Pulmonary Artery, Left
7 Atrium, Left V Superior Vena Cava	0 Open 4 Percutaneous Endoscopic	9 Autologous Venous Tissue A Autologous Arterial Tissue J Synthetic Substitute K Nonautologous Tissue Substitute Z No Device	P Pulmonary Trunk Q Pulmonary Artery, Right R Pulmonary Artery, Left
K Ventricle, Right L Ventricle, Left	0 Open 4 Percutaneous Endoscopic	9 Autologous Venous Tissue A Autologous Arterial Tissue J Synthetic Substitute K Nonautologous Tissue Substitute	P Pulmonary Trunk Q Pulmonary Artery, Right R Pulmonary Artery, Left

Continued →

Section 0 Medical and Surgical
Body System 2 Heart and Great Vessels
Operation 1 **Bypass:** Altering the route of passage of the contents of a tubular body part

Body Part (4th)	Approach (5th)	Device (6th)	Qualifier (7th)
K Ventricle, Right L Ventricle, Left	0 Open 4 Percutaneous Endoscopic	Z No Device	5 Coronary Circulation 8 Internal Mammary, Right 9 Internal Mammary, Left C Thoracic Artery F Abdominal Artery P Pulmonary Trunk Q Pulmonary Artery, Right R Pulmonary Artery, Left W Aorta
W Thoracic Aorta	0 Open 4 Percutaneous Endoscopic	9 Autologous Venous Tissue A Autologous Arterial Tissue J Synthetic Substitute K Nonautologous Tissue Substitute Z No Device	B Subclavian D Carotid P Pulmonary Trunk Q Pulmonary Artery, Right R Pulmonary Artery, Left

Section 0 Medical and Surgical
Body System 2 Heart and Great Vessels
Operation 5 **Destruction:** Physical eradication of all or a portion of a body part by the direct use of energy, force, or a destructive agent

Body Part (4th)	Approach (5th)	Device (6th)	Qualifier (7th)
4 Coronary Vein 5 Atrial Septum 6 Atrium, Right 8 Conduction Mechanism 9 Chordae Tendineae D Papillary Muscle F Aortic Valve G Mitral Valve H Pulmonary Valve J Tricuspid Valve K Ventricle, Right L Ventricle, Left M Ventricular Septum N Pericardium P Pulmonary Trunk Q Pulmonary Artery, Right R Pulmonary Artery, Left S Pulmonary Vein, Right T Pulmonary Vein, Left V Superior Vena Cava W Thoracic Aorta	0 Open 3 Percutaneous 4 Percutaneous Endoscopic	Z No Device	Z No Qualifier
7 Atrium, Left	0 Open 3 Percutaneous 4 Percutaneous Endoscopic	Z No Device	K Left Atrial Appendage Z No Qualifier

Section 0 Medical and Surgical
Body System 2 Heart and Great Vessels
Operation 7 **Dilation:** Expanding an orifice or the lumen of a tubular body part

Body Part (4th)	Approach (5th)	Device (6th)	Qualifier (7th)
0 Coronary Artery, One Site 1 Coronary Artery, Two Sites 2 Coronary Artery, Three Sites 3 Coronary Artery, Four or More Sites	0 Open 3 Percutaneous 4 Percutaneous Endoscopic	4 Intraluminal Device, Drug-eluting D Intraluminal Device T Intraluminal Device, Radioactive Z No Device	6 Bifurcation Z No Qualifier

Continued →

Section   0   **Medical and Surgical**
Body System   2   **Heart and Great Vessels**
Operation   7   **Dilation:** Expanding an orifice or the lumen of a tubular body part

Body Part (4th)	Approach (5th)	Device (6th)	Qualifier (7th)
F Aortic Valve G Mitral Valve H Pulmonary Valve J Tricuspid Valve K Ventricle, Right P Pulmonary Trunk Q Pulmonary Artery, Right S Pulmonary Vein, Right T Pulmonary Vein, Left V Superior Vena Cava W Thoracic Aorta	0 Open 3 Percutaneous 4 Percutaneous Endoscopic	4 Intraluminal Device, Drug-eluting D Intraluminal Device Z No Device	Z No Qualifier
R Pulmonary Artery, Left	0 Open 3 Percutaneous 4 Percutaneous Endoscopic	4 Intraluminal Device, Drug-eluting D Intraluminal Device Z No Device	T Ductus Arteriosus Z No Qualifier

Section   0   **Medical and Surgical**
Body System   2   **Heart and Great Vessels**
Operation   8   **Division:** Cutting into a body part, without draining fluids and/or gases from the body part, in order to separate or transect a body part

Body Part (4th)	Approach (5th)	Device (6th)	Qualifier (7th)
8 Conduction Mechanism 9 Chordae Tendineae D Papillary Muscle	0 Open 3 Percutaneous 4 Percutaneous Endoscopic	Z No Device	Z No Qualifier

Section   0   **Medical and Surgical**
Body System   2   **Heart and Great Vessels**
Operation   B   **Excision:** Cutting out or off, without replacement, a portion of a body part

Body Part (4th)	Approach (5th)	Device (6th)	Qualifier (7th)
4 Coronary Vein 5 Atrial Septum 6 Atrium, Right 8 Conduction Mechanism 9 Chordae Tendineae D Papillary Muscle F Aortic Valve G Mitral Valve H Pulmonary Valve J Tricuspid Valve K Ventricle, Right L Ventricle, Left M Ventricular Septum N Pericardium P Pulmonary Trunk Q Pulmonary Artery, Right R Pulmonary Artery, Left S Pulmonary Vein, Right T Pulmonary Vein, Left V Superior Vena Cava W Thoracic Aorta	0 Open 3 Percutaneous 4 Percutaneous Endoscopic	Z No Device	X Diagnostic Z No Qualifier
7 Atrium, Left	0 Open 3 Percutaneous 4 Percutaneous Endoscopic	Z No Device	K Left Atrial Appendage X Diagnostic Z No Qualifier

Section	0	Medical and Surgical
Body System	2	Heart and Great Vessels
Operation	C	Extirpation: Taking or cutting out solid matter from a body part

Body Part (4th)	Approach (5th)	Device (6th)	Qualifier (7th)
0 Coronary Artery, One Site 1 Coronary Artery, Two Sites 2 Coronary Artery, Three Sites 3 Coronary Artery, Four or More Sites 4 Coronary Vein 5 Atrial Septum 6 Atrium, Right 7 Atrium, Left 8 Conduction Mechanism 9 Chordae Tendineae D Papillary Muscle F Aortic Valve G Mitral Valve H Pulmonary Valve J Tricuspid Valve K Ventricle, Right L Ventricle, Left M Ventricular Septum N Pericardium P Pulmonary Trunk Q Pulmonary Artery, Right R Pulmonary Artery, Left S Pulmonary Vein, Right T Pulmonary Vein, Left V Superior Vena Cava W Thoracic Aorta	0 Open 3 Percutaneous 4 Percutaneous Endoscopic	Z No Device	Z No Qualifier

Section	0	Medical and Surgical
Body System	2	Heart and Great Vessels
Operation	F	Fragmentation: Breaking solid matter in a body part into pieces

Body Part (4th)	Approach (5th)	Device (6th)	Qualifier (7th)
N Pericardium	0 Open 3 Percutaneous 4 Percutaneous Endoscopic X External	Z No Device	Z No Qualifier

Section	0	Medical and Surgical
Body System	2	Heart and Great Vessels
Operation	H	Insertion: Putting in a nonbiological appliance that monitors, assists, performs, or prevents a physiological function but does not physically take the place of a body part

Body Part (4th)	Approach (5th)	Device (6th)	Qualifier (7th)
4 Coronary Vein 6 Atrium, Right 7 Atrium, Left K Ventricle, Right L Ventricle, Left	0 Open 3 Percutaneous 4 Percutaneous Endoscopic	0 Monitoring Device, Pressure Sensor 2 Monitoring Device 3 Infusion Device D Intraluminal Device J Cardiac Lead, Pacemaker K Cardiac Lead, Defibrillator M Cardiac Lead	Z No Qualifier
A Heart	0 Open 3 Percutaneous 4 Percutaneous Endoscopic	Q Implantable Heart Assist System	Z No Qualifier

Continued →

Section	0	Medical and Surgical
Body System	2	Heart and Great Vessels
Operation	H	Insertion: Putting in a nonbiological appliance that monitors, assists, performs, or prevents a physiological function but does not physically take the place of a body part

Body Part (4th)	Approach (5th)	Device (6th)	Qualifier (7th)
A Heart	0 Open 3 Percutaneous 4 Percutaneous Endoscopic	R External Heart Assist System	S Biventricular Z No Qualifier
N Pericardium	0 Open 3 Percutaneous 4 Percutaneous Endoscopic	0 Monitoring Device, Pressure Sensor 2 Monitoring Device J Cardiac Lead, Pacemaker K Cardiac Lead, Defibrillator M Cardiac Lead	Z No Qualifier
P Pulmonary Trunk Q Pulmonary Artery, Right R Pulmonary Artery, Left S Pulmonary Vein, Right T Pulmonary Vein, Left V Superior Vena Cava W Thoracic Aorta	0 Open 3 Percutaneous 4 Percutaneous Endoscopic	0 Monitoring Device, Pressure Sensor 2 Monitoring Device 3 Infusion Device D Intraluminal Device	Z No Qualifier

Section	0	Medical and Surgical
Body System	2	Heart and Great Vessels
Operation	J	Inspection: Visually and/or manually exploring a body part

Body Part (4th)	Approach (5th)	Device (6th)	Qualifier (7th)
A Heart Y Great Vessel	0 Open 3 Percutaneous 4 Percutaneous Endoscopic	Z No Device	Z No Qualifier

Section	0	Medical and Surgical
Body System	2	Heart and Great Vessels
Operation	K	Map: Locating the route of passage of electrical impulses and/or locating functional areas in a body part

Body Part (4th)	Approach (5th)	Device (6th)	Qualifier (7th)
8 Conduction Mechanism	0 Open 3 Percutaneous 4 Percutaneous Endoscopic	Z No Device	Z No Qualifier

Section	0	Medical and Surgical
Body System	2	Heart and Great Vessels
Operation	L	Occlusion: Completely closing an orifice or the lumen of a tubular body part

Body Part (4th)	Approach (5th)	Device (6th)	Qualifier (7th)
7 Atrium, Left	0 Open 3 Percutaneous 4 Percutaneous Endoscopic	C Extraluminal Device D Intraluminal Device Z No Device	K Left Atrial Appendage
R Pulmonary Artery, Left	0 Open 3 Percutaneous 4 Percutaneous Endoscopic	C Extraluminal Device D Intraluminal Device Z No Device	T Ductus Arteriosus
S Pulmonary Vein, Right T Pulmonary Vein, Left V Superior Vena Cava	0 Open 3 Percutaneous 4 Percutaneous Endoscopic	C Extraluminal Device D Intraluminal Device Z No Device	Z No Qualifier

Section	0	Medical and Surgical
Body System	2	Heart and Great Vessels
Operation	N	Release: Freeing a body part from an abnormal physical constraint by cutting or by the use of force

Body Part (4th)	Approach (5th)	Device (6th)	Qualifier (7th)
4 Coronary Vein 5 Atrial Septum 6 Atrium, Right 7 Atrium, Left 8 Conduction Mechanism 9 Chordae Tendineae D Papillary Muscle F Aortic Valve G Mitral Valve H Pulmonary Valve J Tricuspid Valve K Ventricle, Right L Ventricle, Left M Ventricular Septum N Pericardium P Pulmonary Trunk Q Pulmonary Artery, Right R Pulmonary Artery, Left S Pulmonary Vein, Right T Pulmonary Vein, Left V Superior Vena Cava W Thoracic Aorta	0 Open 3 Percutaneous 4 Percutaneous Endoscopic	Z No Device	Z No Qualifier

Section	0	Medical and Surgical
Body System	2	Heart and Great Vessels
Operation	P	Removal: Taking out or off a device from a body part

Body Part (4th)	Approach (5th)	Device (6th)	Qualifier (7th)
A Heart	0 Open 3 Percutaneous 4 Percutaneous Endoscopic	2 Monitoring Device 3 Infusion Device 7 Autologous Tissue Substitute 8 Zooplastic Tissue C Extraluminal Device D Intraluminal Device J Synthetic Substitute K Nonautologous Tissue Substitute M Cardiac Lead Q Implantable Heart Assist System R External Heart Assist System	Z No Qualifier
A Heart	X External	2 Monitoring Device 3 Infusion Device D Intraluminal Device M Cardiac Lead	Z No Qualifier
Y Great Vessel	0 Open 3 Percutaneous 4 Percutaneous Endoscopic	2 Monitoring Device 3 Infusion Device 7 Autologous Tissue Substitute 8 Zooplastic Tissue C Extraluminal Device D Intraluminal Device J Synthetic Substitute K Nonautologous Tissue Substitute	Z No Qualifier
Y Great Vessel	X External	2 Monitoring Device 3 Infusion Device D Intraluminal Device	Z No Qualifier

Section	0	Medical and Surgical
Body System	2	Heart and Great Vessels
Operation	Q	**Repair:** Restoring, to the extent possible, a body part to its normal anatomic structure and function

Body Part (4th)	Approach (5th)	Device (6th)	Qualifier (7th)
0 Coronary Artery, One Site 1 Coronary Artery, Two Sites 2 Coronary Artery, Three Sites 3 Coronary Artery, Four or More Sites 4 Coronary Vein 5 Atrial Septum 6 Atrium, Right 7 Atrium, Left 8 Conduction Mechanism 9 Chordae Tendineae A Heart B Heart, Right C Heart, Left D Papillary Muscle F Aortic Valve G Mitral Valve H Pulmonary Valve J Tricuspid Valve K Ventricle, Right L Ventricle, Left M Ventricular Septum N Pericardium P Pulmonary Trunk Q Pulmonary Artery, Right R Pulmonary Artery, Left S Pulmonary Vein, Right T Pulmonary Vein, Left V Superior Vena Cava W Thoracic Aorta	0 Open 3 Percutaneous 4 Percutaneous Endoscopic	Z No Device	Z No Qualifier

Section	0	Medical and Surgical
Body System	2	Heart and Great Vessels
Operation	R	**Replacement:** Putting in or on biological or synthetic material that physically takes the place and/or function of all or a portion of a body part

Body Part (4th)	Approach (5th)	Device (6th)	Qualifier (7th)
5 Atrial Septum 6 Atrium, Right 7 Atrium, Left 9 Chordae Tendineae D Papillary Muscle J Tricuspid Valve K Ventricle, Right L Ventricle, Left M Ventricular Septum N Pericardium P Pulmonary Trunk Q Pulmonary Artery, Right R Pulmonary Artery, Left S Pulmonary Vein, Right T Pulmonary Vein, Left V Superior Vena Cava W Thoracic Aorta	0 Open 4 Percutaneous Endoscopic	7 Autologous Tissue Substitute 8 Zooplastic Tissue J Synthetic Substitute K Nonautologous Tissue Substitute	Z No Qualifier
F Aortic Valve G Mitral Valve H Pulmonary Valve	0 Open 4 Percutaneous Endoscopic	7 Autologous Tissue Substitute 8 Zooplastic Tissue J Synthetic Substitute K Nonautologous Tissue Substitute	Z No Qualifier

Continued →

Section	0	Medical and Surgical
Body System	2	Heart and Great Vessels
Operation	R	Replacement: Putting in or on biological or synthetic material that physically takes the place and/or function of all or a portion of a body part

Body Part (4th)	Approach (5th)	Device (6th)	Qualifier (7th)
F Aortic Valve G Mitral Valve H Pulmonary Valve	3 Percutaneous	7 Autologous Tissue Substitute 8 Zooplastic Tissue J Synthetic Substitute K Nonautologous Tissue Substitute	H Transapical Z No Qualifier

Section	0	Medical and Surgical
Body System	2	Heart and Great Vessels
Operation	S	Reposition: Moving to its normal location, or other suitable location, all or a portion of a body part

Body Part (4th)	Approach (5th)	Device (6th)	Qualifier (7th)
P Pulmonary Trunk Q Pulmonary Artery, Right R Pulmonary Artery, Left S Pulmonary Vein, Right T Pulmonary Vein, Left V Superior Vena Cava W Thoracic Aorta	0 Open	Z No Device	Z No Qualifier

Section	0	Medical and Surgical
Body System	2	Heart and Great Vessels
Operation	T	Resection: Cutting out or off, without replacement, all of a body part

Body Part (4th)	Approach (5th)	Device (6th)	Qualifier (7th)
5 Atrial Septum 8 Conduction Mechanism 9 Chordae Tendineae D Papillary Muscle H Pulmonary Valve M Ventricular Septum N Pericardium	0 Open 3 Percutaneous 4 Percutaneous Endoscopic	Z No Device	Z No Qualifier

Section	0	Medical and Surgical
Body System	2	Heart and Great Vessels
Operation	U	Supplement: Putting in or on biological or synthetic material that physically reinforces and/or augments the function of a portion of a body part

Body Part (4th)	Approach (5th)	Device (6th)	Qualifier (7th)
5 Atrial Septum 6 Atrium, Right 7 Atrium, Left 9 Chordae Tendineae A Heart D Papillary Muscle F Aortic Valve G Mitral Valve H Pulmonary Valve J Tricuspid Valve K Ventricle, Right L Ventricle, Left M Ventricular Septum N Pericardium P Pulmonary Trunk Q Pulmonary Artery, Right R Pulmonary Artery, Left S Pulmonary Vein, Right T Pulmonary Vein, Left V Superior Vena Cava W Thoracic Aorta	0 Open 3 Percutaneous 4 Percutaneous Endoscopic	7 Autologous Tissue Substitute 8 Zooplastic Tissue J Synthetic Substitute K Nonautologous Tissue Substitute	Z No Qualifier

Section	0	Medical and Surgical
Body System	2	Heart and Great Vessels
Operation	V	**Restriction:** Partially closing an orifice or the lumen of a tubular body part

Body Part (4th)	Approach (5th)	Device (6th)	Qualifier (7th)
A Heart	0 Open 3 Percutaneous 4 Percutaneous Endoscopic	C Extraluminal Device Z No Device	Z No Qualifier
P Pulmonary Trunk Q Pulmonary Artery, Right S Pulmonary Vein, Right T Pulmonary Vein, Left V Superior Vena Cava W Thoracic Aorta	0 Open 3 Percutaneous 4 Percutaneous Endoscopic	C Extraluminal Device D Intraluminal Device Z No Device	Z No Qualifier
R Pulmonary Artery, Left	0 Open 3 Percutaneous 4 Percutaneous Endoscopic	C Extraluminal Device D Intraluminal Device Z No Device	T Ductus Arteriosus Z No Qualifier

Section	0	Medical and Surgical
Body System	2	Heart and Great Vessels
Operation	W	**Revision:** Correcting, to the extent possible, a portion of a malfunctioning device or the position of a displaced device

Body Part (4th)	Approach (5th)	Device (6th)	Qualifier (7th)
5 Atrial Septum M Ventricular Septum	0 Open 4 Percutaneous Endoscopic	J Synthetic Substitute	Z No Qualifier
A Heart	0 Open 3 Percutaneous 4 Percutaneous Endoscopic X External	2 Monitoring Device 3 Infusion Device 7 Autologous Tissue Substitute 8 Zooplastic Tissue C Extraluminal Device D Intraluminal Device J Synthetic Substitute K Nonautologous Tissue Substitute M Cardiac Lead Q Implantable Heart Assist System R External Heart Assist System	Z No Qualifier
F Aortic Valve G Mitral Valve H Pulmonary Valve J Tricuspid Valve	0 Open 4 Percutaneous Endoscopic	7 Autologous Tissue Substitute 8 Zooplastic Tissue J Synthetic Substitute K Nonautologous Tissue Substitute	Z No Qualifier
Y Great Vessel	0 Open 3 Percutaneous 4 Percutaneous Endoscopic X External	2 Monitoring Device 3 Infusion Device 7 Autologous Tissue Substitute 8 Zooplastic Tissue C Extraluminal Device D Intraluminal Device J Synthetic Substitute K Nonautologous Tissue Substitute	Z No Qualifier

Section	0	Medical and Surgical
Body System	2	Heart and Great Vessels
Operation	Y	**Transplantation:** Putting in or on all or a portion of a living body part taken from another individual or animal to physically take the place and/or function of all or a portion of a similar body part

Body Part (4th)	Approach (5th)	Device (6th)	Qualifier (7th)
A Heart	0 Open	Z No Device	0 Allogeneic 1 Syngeneic 2 Zooplastic

021 – Heart and Great Vessels, Bypass

Review Coding Guideline B3.6a

For Bypass procedures involving the coronary arteries, review Coding Guidelines B3.6b and B3.6c

For Bypass procedures involving the coronary arteries, review Coding Guideline B4.4

0210093 Bypass Coronary Artery, One Site from Coronary Artery with Autologous Venous Tissue, Open Approach
- When reported with secondary diagnosis code J98.5

0210098 Bypass Coronary Artery, One Site from Right Internal Mammary with Autologous Venous Tissue, Open Approach
- When reported with secondary diagnosis code J98.5

0210099 Bypass Coronary Artery, One Site from Left Internal Mammary with Autologous Venous Tissue, Open Approach
- When reported with secondary diagnosis code J98.5

021009C Bypass Coronary Artery, One Site from Thoracic Artery with Autologous Venous Tissue, Open Approach
- When reported with secondary diagnosis code J98.5

021009F Bypass Coronary Artery, One Site from Abdominal Artery with Autologous Venous Tissue, Open Approach
- When reported with secondary diagnosis code J98.5

021009W Bypass Coronary Artery, One Site from Aorta with Autologous Venous Tissue, Open Approach
- When reported with secondary diagnosis code J98.5
  AHA CC: 1Q, 2014, 10-11

02100A3 Bypass Coronary Artery, One Site from Coronary Artery with Autologous Arterial Tissue, Open Approach
- When reported with secondary diagnosis code J98.5

02100A8 Bypass Coronary Artery, One Site from Right Internal Mammary with Autologous Arterial Tissue, Open Approach
- When reported with secondary diagnosis code J98.5

02100A9 Bypass Coronary Artery, One Site from Left Internal Mammary with Autologous Arterial Tissue, Open Approach
- When reported with secondary diagnosis code J98.5

02100AC Bypass Coronary Artery, One Site from Thoracic Artery with Autologous Arterial Tissue, Open Approach
- When reported with secondary diagnosis code J98.5

02100AF Bypass Coronary Artery, One Site from Abdominal Artery with Autologous Arterial Tissue, Open Approach
- When reported with secondary diagnosis code J98.5

02100AW Bypass Coronary Artery, One Site from Aorta with Autologous Arterial Tissue, Open Approach
- When reported with secondary diagnosis code J98.5

02100J3 Bypass Coronary Artery, One Site from Coronary Artery with Synthetic Substitute, Open Approach
- When reported with secondary diagnosis code J98.5

02100J8 Bypass Coronary Artery, One Site from Right Internal Mammary with Synthetic Substitute, Open Approach
- When reported with secondary diagnosis code J98.5

02100J9 Bypass Coronary Artery, One Site from Left Internal Mammary with Synthetic Substitute, Open Approach
- When reported with secondary diagnosis code J98.5

02100JC Bypass Coronary Artery, One Site from Thoracic Artery with Synthetic Substitute, Open Approach
- When reported with secondary diagnosis code J98.5

02100JF Bypass Coronary Artery, One Site from Abdominal Artery with Synthetic Substitute, Open Approach
- When reported with secondary diagnosis code J98.5

02100JW Bypass Coronary Artery, One Site from Aorta with Synthetic Substitute, Open Approach
- When reported with secondary diagnosis code J98.5

02100K3 Bypass Coronary Artery, One Site from Coronary Artery with Nonautologous Tissue Substitute, Open Approach
- When reported with secondary diagnosis code J98.5

02100K8 Bypass Coronary Artery, One Site from Right Internal Mammary with Nonautologous Tissue Substitute, Open Approach
- When reported with secondary diagnosis code J98.5

02100K9 Bypass Coronary Artery, One Site from Left Internal Mammary with Nonautologous Tissue Substitute, Open Approach
- When reported with secondary diagnosis code J98.5

02100KC Bypass Coronary Artery, One Site from Thoracic Artery with Nonautologous Tissue Substitute, Open Approach
- When reported with secondary diagnosis code J98.5

02100KF Bypass Coronary Artery, One Site from Abdominal Artery with Nonautologous Tissue Substitute, Open Approach
- When reported with secondary diagnosis code J98.5

02100KW Bypass Coronary Artery, One Site from Aorta with Nonautologous Tissue Substitute, Open Approach
- When reported with secondary diagnosis code J98.5

02100Z3 Bypass Coronary Artery, One Site from Coronary Artery, Open Approach
- When reported with secondary diagnosis code J98.5

02100Z8 Bypass Coronary Artery, One Site from Right Internal Mammary, Open Approach
- When reported with secondary diagnosis code J98.5

02100Z9 Bypass Coronary Artery, One Site from Left Internal Mammary, Open Approach
- When reported with secondary diagnosis code J98.5
  AHA CC: 3Q, 2014, 8, 20-21

02100ZC Bypass Coronary Artery, One Site from Thoracic Artery, Open Approach
- When reported with secondary diagnosis code J98.5

02100ZF Bypass Coronary Artery, One Site from Abdominal Artery, Open Approach
- When reported with secondary diagnosis code J98.5

0210344 Bypass Coronary Artery, One Site from Coronary Vein with Drug-eluting Intraluminal Device, Percutaneous Approach

02103D4 Bypass Coronary Artery, One Site from Coronary Vein with Intraluminal Device, Percutaneous Approach

0210444 Bypass Coronary Artery, One Site from Coronary Vein with Drug-eluting Intraluminal Device, Percutaneous Endoscopic Approach

0210493 Bypass Coronary Artery, One Site from Coronary Artery with Autologous Venous Tissue, Percutaneous Endoscopic Approach
- When reported with secondary diagnosis code J98.5

0210498 Bypass Coronary Artery, One Site from Right Internal Mammary with Autologous Venous Tissue, Percutaneous Endoscopic Approach
- When reported with secondary diagnosis code J98.5

0210499 Bypass Coronary Artery, One Site from Left Internal Mammary with Autologous Venous Tissue, Percutaneous Endoscopic Approach
- When reported with secondary diagnosis code J98.5

021049C Bypass Coronary Artery, One Site from Thoracic Artery with Autologous Venous Tissue, Percutaneous Endoscopic Approach
- When reported with secondary diagnosis code J98.5

021049F Bypass Coronary Artery, One Site from Abdominal Artery with Autologous Venous Tissue, Percutaneous Endoscopic Approach
- When reported with secondary diagnosis code J98.5

021049W Bypass Coronary Artery, One Site from Aorta with Autologous Venous Tissue, Percutaneous Endoscopic Approach
- When reported with secondary diagnosis code J98.5

02104A3 Bypass Coronary Artery, One Site from Coronary Artery with Autologous Arterial Tissue, Percutaneous Endoscopic Approach
- When reported with secondary diagnosis code J98.5

02104A8 Bypass Coronary Artery, One Site from Right Internal Mammary with Autologous Arterial Tissue, Percutaneous Endoscopic Approach
- When reported with secondary diagnosis code J98.5

02104A9 Bypass Coronary Artery, One Site from Left Internal Mammary with Autologous Arterial Tissue, Percutaneous Endoscopic Approach
- ᴴᴬᶜ When reported with secondary diagnosis code J98.5

02104AC Bypass Coronary Artery, One Site from Thoracic Artery with Autologous Arterial Tissue, Percutaneous Endoscopic Approach
- ᴴᴬᶜ When reported with secondary diagnosis code J98.5

02104AF Bypass Coronary Artery, One Site from Abdominal Artery with Autologous Arterial Tissue, Percutaneous Endoscopic Approach
- ᴴᴬᶜ When reported with secondary diagnosis code J98.5

02104AW Bypass Coronary Artery, One Site from Aorta with Autologous Arterial Tissue, Percutaneous Endoscopic Approach
- ᴴᴬᶜ When reported with secondary diagnosis code J98.5

02104D4 Bypass Coronary Artery, One Site from Coronary Vein with Intraluminal Device, Percutaneous Endoscopic Approach
- ᴴᴬᶜ When reported with secondary diagnosis code J98.5

02104J3 Bypass Coronary Artery, One Site from Coronary Artery with Synthetic Substitute, Percutaneous Endoscopic Approach
- ᴴᴬᶜ When reported with secondary diagnosis code J98.5

02104J8 Bypass Coronary Artery, One Site from Right Internal Mammary with Synthetic Substitute, Percutaneous Endoscopic Approach
- ᴴᴬᶜ When reported with secondary diagnosis code J98.5

02104J9 Bypass Coronary Artery, One Site from Left Internal Mammary with Synthetic Substitute, Percutaneous Endoscopic Approach
- ᴴᴬᶜ When reported with secondary diagnosis code J98.5

02104JC Bypass Coronary Artery, One Site from Thoracic Artery with Synthetic Substitute, Percutaneous Endoscopic Approach
- ᴴᴬᶜ When reported with secondary diagnosis code J98.5

02104JF Bypass Coronary Artery, One Site from Abdominal Artery with Synthetic Substitute, Percutaneous Endoscopic Approach
- ᴴᴬᶜ When reported with secondary diagnosis code J98.5

02104JW Bypass Coronary Artery, One Site from Aorta with Synthetic Substitute, Percutaneous Endoscopic Approach
- ᴴᴬᶜ When reported with secondary diagnosis code J98.5

02104K3 Bypass Coronary Artery, One Site from Coronary Artery with Nonautologous Tissue Substitute, Percutaneous Endoscopic Approach
- ᴴᴬᶜ When reported with secondary diagnosis code J98.5

02104K8 Bypass Coronary Artery, One Site from Right Internal Mammary with Nonautologous Tissue Substitute, Percutaneous Endoscopic Approach
- ᴴᴬᶜ When reported with secondary diagnosis code J98.5

02104K9 Bypass Coronary Artery, One Site from Left Internal Mammary with Nonautologous Tissue Substitute, Percutaneous Endoscopic Approach
- ᴴᴬᶜ When reported with secondary diagnosis code J98.5

02104KC Bypass Coronary Artery, One Site from Thoracic Artery with Nonautologous Tissue Substitute, Percutaneous Endoscopic Approach
- ᴴᴬᶜ When reported with secondary diagnosis code J98.5

02104KF Bypass Coronary Artery, One Site from Abdominal Artery with Nonautologous Tissue Substitute, Percutaneous Endoscopic Approach
- ᴴᴬᶜ When reported with secondary diagnosis code J98.5

02104KW Bypass Coronary Artery, One Site from Aorta with Nonautologous Tissue Substitute, Percutaneous Endoscopic Approach
- ᴴᴬᶜ When reported with secondary diagnosis code J98.5

02104Z3 Bypass Coronary Artery, One Site from Coronary Artery, Percutaneous Endoscopic Approach
- ᴴᴬᶜ When reported with secondary diagnosis code J98.5

02104Z8 Bypass Coronary Artery, One Site from Right Internal Mammary, Percutaneous Endoscopic Approach
- ᴴᴬᶜ When reported with secondary diagnosis code J98.5

02104Z9 Bypass Coronary Artery, One Site from Left Internal Mammary, Percutaneous Endoscopic Approach
- ᴴᴬᶜ When reported with secondary diagnosis code J98.5

02104ZC Bypass Coronary Artery, One Site from Thoracic Artery, Percutaneous Endoscopic Approach
- ᴴᴬᶜ When reported with secondary diagnosis code J98.5

02104ZF Bypass Coronary Artery, One Site from Abdominal Artery, Percutaneous Endoscopic Approach
- ᴴᴬᶜ When reported with secondary diagnosis code J98.5

0211093 Bypass Coronary Artery, Two Sites from Coronary Artery with Autologous Venous Tissue, Open Approach
- ᴴᴬᶜ When reported with secondary diagnosis code J98.5

0211098 Bypass Coronary Artery, Two Sites from Right Internal Mammary with Autologous Venous Tissue, Open Approach
- ᴴᴬᶜ When reported with secondary diagnosis code J98.5

0211099 Bypass Coronary Artery, Two Sites from Left Internal Mammary with Autologous Venous Tissue, Open Approach
- ᴴᴬᶜ When reported with secondary diagnosis code J98.5

021109C Bypass Coronary Artery, Two Sites from Thoracic Artery with Autologous Venous Tissue, Open Approach
- ᴴᴬᶜ When reported with secondary diagnosis code J98.5

021109F Bypass Coronary Artery, Two Sites from Abdominal Artery with Autologous Venous Tissue, Open Approach
- ᴴᴬᶜ When reported with secondary diagnosis code J98.5

021109W Bypass Coronary Artery, Two Sites from Aorta with Autologous Venous Tissue, Open Approach
- ᴴᴬᶜ When reported with secondary diagnosis code J98.5

AHA CC: 3Q, 2014, 20-21

02110A3 Bypass Coronary Artery, Two Sites from Coronary Artery with Autologous Arterial Tissue, Open Approach
- ᴴᴬᶜ When reported with secondary diagnosis code J98.5

02110A8 Bypass Coronary Artery, Two Sites from Right Internal Mammary with Autologous Arterial Tissue, Open Approach
- ᴴᴬᶜ When reported with secondary diagnosis code J98.5

02110A9 Bypass Coronary Artery, Two Sites from Left Internal Mammary with Autologous Arterial Tissue, Open Approach
- ᴴᴬᶜ When reported with secondary diagnosis code J98.5

02110AC Bypass Coronary Artery, Two Sites from Thoracic Artery with Autologous Arterial Tissue, Open Approach
- ᴴᴬᶜ When reported with secondary diagnosis code J98.5

02110AF Bypass Coronary Artery, Two Sites from Abdominal Artery with Autologous Arterial Tissue, Open Approach
- ᴴᴬᶜ When reported with secondary diagnosis code J98.5

02110AW Bypass Coronary Artery, Two Sites from Aorta with Autologous Arterial Tissue, Open Approach
- ᴴᴬᶜ When reported with secondary diagnosis code J98.5

02110J3 Bypass Coronary Artery, Two Sites from Coronary Artery with Synthetic Substitute, Open Approach
- ᴴᴬᶜ When reported with secondary diagnosis code J98.5

02110J8 Bypass Coronary Artery, Two Sites from Right Internal Mammary with Synthetic Substitute, Open Approach
- ᴴᴬᶜ When reported with secondary diagnosis code J98.5

02110J9 Bypass Coronary Artery, Two Sites from Left Internal Mammary with Synthetic Substitute, Open Approach
- ᴴᴬᶜ When reported with secondary diagnosis code J98.5

02110JC Bypass Coronary Artery, Two Sites from Thoracic Artery with Synthetic Substitute, Open Approach
- ᴴᴬᶜ When reported with secondary diagnosis code J98.5

02110JF Bypass Coronary Artery, Two Sites from Abdominal Artery with Synthetic Substitute, Open Approach
- ᴴᴬᶜ When reported with secondary diagnosis code J98.5

02110JW Bypass Coronary Artery, Two Sites from Aorta with Synthetic Substitute, Open Approach
- ᴴᴬᶜ When reported with secondary diagnosis code J98.5

02110K3 Bypass Coronary Artery, Two Sites from Coronary Artery with Nonautologous Tissue Substitute, Open Approach
- ᴴᴬᶜ When reported with secondary diagnosis code J98.5

02110K8 Bypass Coronary Artery, Two Sites from Right Internal Mammary with Nonautologous Tissue Substitute, Open Approach
- ᴴᴬᶜ When reported with secondary diagnosis code J98.5

02110K9 Bypass Coronary Artery, Two Sites from Left Internal Mammary with Nonautologous Tissue Substitute, Open Approach
- ᴴᴬᶜ When reported with secondary diagnosis code J98.5

02110KC Bypass Coronary Artery, Two Sites from Thoracic Artery with Nonautologous Tissue Substitute, Open Approach
- ᴴᴬᶜ When reported with secondary diagnosis code J98.5

♀ Female-only   ♂ Male-only   ▲ Limited Coverage   ● Non-OR   ᴴᴬᶜ HAC-associated procedure   ▲ Non-covered procedures   ➕ Combination

02110KF Bypass Coronary Artery, Two Sites from Abdominal Artery with Nonautologous Tissue Substitute, Open Approach
- When reported with secondary diagnosis code J98.5

02110KW Bypass Coronary Artery, Two Sites from Aorta with Nonautologous Tissue Substitute, Open Approach
- When reported with secondary diagnosis code J98.5

02110Z3 Bypass Coronary Artery, Two Sites from Coronary Artery, Open Approach
- When reported with secondary diagnosis code J98.5

02110Z8 Bypass Coronary Artery, Two Sites from Right Internal Mammary, Open Approach
- When reported with secondary diagnosis code J98.5

02110Z9 Bypass Coronary Artery, Two Sites from Left Internal Mammary, Open Approach
- When reported with secondary diagnosis code J98.5

02110ZC Bypass Coronary Artery, Two Sites from Thoracic Artery, Open Approach
- When reported with secondary diagnosis code J98.5

02110ZF Bypass Coronary Artery, Two Sites from Abdominal Artery, Open Approach
- When reported with secondary diagnosis code J98.5

0211344 Bypass Coronary Artery, Two Sites from Coronary Vein with Drug-eluting Intraluminal Device, Percutaneous Approach

02113D4 Bypass Coronary Artery, Two Sites from Coronary Vein with Intraluminal Device, Percutaneous Approach

0211444 Bypass Coronary Artery, Two Sites from Coronary Vein with Drug-eluting Intraluminal Device, Percutaneous Endoscopic Approach
- When reported with secondary diagnosis code J98.5

0211493 Bypass Coronary Artery, Two Sites from Coronary Artery with Autologous Venous Tissue, Percutaneous Endoscopic Approach
- When reported with secondary diagnosis code J98.5

0211498 Bypass Coronary Artery, Two Sites from Right Internal Mammary with Autologous Venous Tissue, Percutaneous Endoscopic Approach
- When reported with secondary diagnosis code J98.5

0211499 Bypass Coronary Artery, Two Sites from Left Internal Mammary with Autologous Venous Tissue, Percutaneous Endoscopic Approach
- When reported with secondary diagnosis code J98.5

021149C Bypass Coronary Artery, Two Sites from Thoracic Artery with Autologous Venous Tissue, Percutaneous Endoscopic Approach
- When reported with secondary diagnosis code J98.5

021149F Bypass Coronary Artery, Two Sites from Abdominal Artery with Autologous Venous Tissue, Percutaneous Endoscopic Approach
- When reported with secondary diagnosis code J98.5

021149W Bypass Coronary Artery, Two Sites from Aorta with Autologous Venous Tissue, Percutaneous Endoscopic Approach
- When reported with secondary diagnosis code J98.5

02114A3 Bypass Coronary Artery, Two Sites from Coronary Artery with Autologous Arterial Tissue, Percutaneous Endoscopic Approach
- When reported with secondary diagnosis code J98.5

02114A8 Bypass Coronary Artery, Two Sites from Right Internal Mammary with Autologous Arterial Tissue, Percutaneous Endoscopic Approach
- When reported with secondary diagnosis code J98.5

02114A9 Bypass Coronary Artery, Two Sites from Left Internal Mammary with Autologous Arterial Tissue, Percutaneous Endoscopic Approach
- When reported with secondary diagnosis code J98.5

02114AC Bypass Coronary Artery, Two Sites from Thoracic Artery with Autologous Arterial Tissue, Percutaneous Endoscopic Approach
- When reported with secondary diagnosis code J98.5

02114AF Bypass Coronary Artery, Two Sites from Abdominal Artery with Autologous Arterial Tissue, Percutaneous Endoscopic Approach
- When reported with secondary diagnosis code J98.5

02114AW Bypass Coronary Artery, Two Sites from Aorta with Autologous Arterial Tissue, Percutaneous Endoscopic Approach
- When reported with secondary diagnosis code J98.5

02114D4 Bypass Coronary Artery, Two Sites from Coronary Vein with Intraluminal Device, Percutaneous Endoscopic Approach

02114J3 Bypass Coronary Artery, Two Sites from Coronary Artery with Synthetic Substitute, Percutaneous Endoscopic Approach
- When reported with secondary diagnosis code J98.5

02114J8 Bypass Coronary Artery, Two Sites from Right Internal Mammary with Synthetic Substitute, Percutaneous Endoscopic Approach
- When reported with secondary diagnosis code J98.5

02114J9 Bypass Coronary Artery, Two Sites from Left Internal Mammary with Synthetic Substitute, Percutaneous Endoscopic Approach
- When reported with secondary diagnosis code J98.5

02114JC Bypass Coronary Artery, Two Sites from Thoracic Artery with Synthetic Substitute, Percutaneous Endoscopic Approach
- When reported with secondary diagnosis code J98.5

02114JF Bypass Coronary Artery, Two Sites from Abdominal Artery with Synthetic Substitute, Percutaneous Endoscopic Approach
- When reported with secondary diagnosis code J98.5

02114JW Bypass Coronary Artery, Two Sites from Aorta with Synthetic Substitute, Percutaneous Endoscopic Approach
- When reported with secondary diagnosis code J98.5

02114K3 Bypass Coronary Artery, Two Sites from Coronary Artery with Nonautologous Tissue Substitute, Percutaneous Endoscopic Approach
- When reported with secondary diagnosis code J98.5

02114K8 Bypass Coronary Artery, Two Sites from Right Internal Mammary with Nonautologous Tissue Substitute, Percutaneous Endoscopic Approach
- When reported with secondary diagnosis code J98.5

02114K9 Bypass Coronary Artery, Two Sites from Left Internal Mammary with Nonautologous Tissue Substitute, Percutaneous Endoscopic Approach
- When reported with secondary diagnosis code J98.5

02114KC Bypass Coronary Artery, Two Sites from Thoracic Artery with Nonautologous Tissue Substitute, Percutaneous Endoscopic Approach
- When reported with secondary diagnosis code J98.5

02114KF Bypass Coronary Artery, Two Sites from Abdominal Artery with Nonautologous Tissue Substitute, Percutaneous Endoscopic Approach
- When reported with secondary diagnosis code J98.5

02114KW Bypass Coronary Artery, Two Sites from Aorta with Nonautologous Tissue Substitute, Percutaneous Endoscopic Approach
- When reported with secondary diagnosis code J98.5

02114Z3 Bypass Coronary Artery, Two Sites from Coronary Artery, Percutaneous Endoscopic Approach
- When reported with secondary diagnosis code J98.5

02114Z8 Bypass Coronary Artery, Two Sites from Right Internal Mammary, Percutaneous Endoscopic Approach
- When reported with secondary diagnosis code J98.5

02114Z9 Bypass Coronary Artery, Two Sites from Left Internal Mammary, Percutaneous Endoscopic Approach
- When reported with secondary diagnosis code J98.5

02114ZC Bypass Coronary Artery, Two Sites from Thoracic Artery, Percutaneous Endoscopic Approach
- When reported with secondary diagnosis code J98.5

02114ZF Bypass Coronary Artery, Two Sites from Abdominal Artery, Percutaneous Endoscopic Approach
- When reported with secondary diagnosis code J98.5

0212093 Bypass Coronary Artery, Three Sites from Coronary Artery with Autologous Venous Tissue, Open Approach
- When reported with secondary diagnosis code J98.5

0212098 Bypass Coronary Artery, Three Sites from Right Internal Mammary with Autologous Venous Tissue, Open Approach
- When reported with secondary diagnosis code J98.5

0212099 Bypass Coronary Artery, Three Sites from Left Internal Mammary with Autologous Venous Tissue, Open Approach
- When reported with secondary diagnosis code J98.5

021209C Bypass Coronary Artery, Three Sites from Thoracic Artery with Autologous Venous Tissue, Open Approach
- When reported with secondary diagnosis code J98.5

021209F Bypass Coronary Artery, Three Sites from Abdominal Artery with Autologous Venous Tissue, Open Approach
HAC When reported with secondary diagnosis code J98.5

021209W Bypass Coronary Artery, Three Sites from Aorta with Autologous Venous Tissue, Open Approach
HAC When reported with secondary diagnosis code J98.5

02120A3 Bypass Coronary Artery, Three Sites from Coronary Artery with Autologous Arterial Tissue, Open Approach
HAC When reported with secondary diagnosis code J98.5

02120A8 Bypass Coronary Artery, Three Sites from Right Internal Mammary with Autologous Arterial Tissue, Open Approach
HAC When reported with secondary diagnosis code J98.5

02120A9 Bypass Coronary Artery, Three Sites from Left Internal Mammary with Autologous Arterial Tissue, Open Approach
HAC When reported with secondary diagnosis code J98.5

02120AC Bypass Coronary Artery, Three Sites from Thoracic Artery with Autologous Arterial Tissue, Open Approach
HAC When reported with secondary diagnosis code J98.5

02120AF Bypass Coronary Artery, Three Sites from Abdominal Artery with Autologous Arterial Tissue, Open Approach
HAC When reported with secondary diagnosis code J98.5

02120AW Bypass Coronary Artery, Three Sites from Aorta with Autologous Arterial Tissue, Open Approach
HAC When reported with secondary diagnosis code J98.5

02120J3 Bypass Coronary Artery, Three Sites from Coronary Artery with Synthetic Substitute, Open Approach
HAC When reported with secondary diagnosis code J98.5

02120J8 Bypass Coronary Artery, Three Sites from Right Internal Mammary with Synthetic Substitute, Open Approach
HAC When reported with secondary diagnosis code J98.5

02120J9 Bypass Coronary Artery, Three Sites from Left Internal Mammary with Synthetic Substitute, Open Approach
HAC When reported with secondary diagnosis code J98.5

02120JC Bypass Coronary Artery, Three Sites from Thoracic Artery with Synthetic Substitute, Open Approach
HAC When reported with secondary diagnosis code J98.5

02120JF Bypass Coronary Artery, Three Sites from Abdominal Artery with Synthetic Substitute, Open Approach
HAC When reported with secondary diagnosis code J98.5

02120JW Bypass Coronary Artery, Three Sites from Aorta with Synthetic Substitute, Open Approach
HAC When reported with secondary diagnosis code J98.5

02120K3 Bypass Coronary Artery, Three Sites from Coronary Artery with Nonautologous Tissue Substitute, Open Approach
HAC When reported with secondary diagnosis code J98.5

02120K8 Bypass Coronary Artery, Three Sites from Right Internal Mammary with Nonautologous Tissue Substitute, Open Approach
HAC When reported with secondary diagnosis code J98.5

02120K9 Bypass Coronary Artery, Three Sites from Left Internal Mammary with Nonautologous Tissue Substitute, Open Approach
HAC When reported with secondary diagnosis code J98.5

02120KC Bypass Coronary Artery, Three Sites from Thoracic Artery with Nonautologous Tissue Substitute, Open Approach
HAC When reported with secondary diagnosis code J98.5

02120KF Bypass Coronary Artery, Three Sites from Abdominal Artery with Nonautologous Tissue Substitute, Open Approach
HAC When reported with secondary diagnosis code J98.5

02120KW Bypass Coronary Artery, Three Sites from Aorta with Nonautologous Tissue Substitute, Open Approach
HAC When reported with secondary diagnosis code J98.5

02120Z3 Bypass Coronary Artery, Three Sites from Coronary Artery, Open Approach
HAC When reported with secondary diagnosis code J98.5

02120Z8 Bypass Coronary Artery, Three Sites from Right Internal Mammary, Open Approach
HAC When reported with secondary diagnosis code J98.5

02120Z9 Bypass Coronary Artery, Three Sites from Left Internal Mammary, Open Approach
HAC When reported with secondary diagnosis code J98.5

02120ZC Bypass Coronary Artery, Three Sites from Thoracic Artery, Open Approach
HAC When reported with secondary diagnosis code J98.5

02120ZF Bypass Coronary Artery, Three Sites from Abdominal Artery, Open Approach
HAC When reported with secondary diagnosis code J98.5

0212344 Bypass Coronary Artery, Three Sites from Coronary Vein with Drug-eluting Intraluminal Device, Percutaneous Approach

02123D4 Bypass Coronary Artery, Three Sites from Coronary Vein with Intraluminal Device, Percutaneous Approach

0212444 Bypass Coronary Artery, Three Sites from Coronary Vein with Drug-eluting Intraluminal Device, Percutaneous Endoscopic Approach

0212493 Bypass Coronary Artery, Three Sites from Coronary Artery with Autologous Venous Tissue, Percutaneous Endoscopic Approach
HAC When reported with secondary diagnosis code J98.5

0212498 Bypass Coronary Artery, Three Sites from Right Internal Mammary with Autologous Venous Tissue, Percutaneous Endoscopic Approach
HAC When reported with secondary diagnosis code J98.5

0212499 Bypass Coronary Artery, Three Sites from Left Internal Mammary with Autologous Venous Tissue, Percutaneous Endoscopic Approach
HAC When reported with secondary diagnosis code J98.5

021249C Bypass Coronary Artery, Three Sites from Thoracic Artery with Autologous Venous Tissue, Percutaneous Endoscopic Approach
HAC When reported with secondary diagnosis code J98.5

021249F Bypass Coronary Artery, Three Sites from Abdominal Artery with Autologous Venous Tissue, Percutaneous Endoscopic Approach
HAC When reported with secondary diagnosis code J98.5

021249W Bypass Coronary Artery, Three Sites from Aorta with Autologous Venous Tissue, Percutaneous Endoscopic Approach
HAC When reported with secondary diagnosis code J98.5

02124A3 Bypass Coronary Artery, Three Sites from Coronary Artery with Autologous Arterial Tissue, Percutaneous Endoscopic Approach
HAC When reported with secondary diagnosis code J98.5

02124A8 Bypass Coronary Artery, Three Sites from Right Internal Mammary with Autologous Arterial Tissue, Percutaneous Endoscopic Approach
HAC When reported with secondary diagnosis code J98.5

02124A9 Bypass Coronary Artery, Three Sites from Left Internal Mammary with Autologous Arterial Tissue, Percutaneous Endoscopic Approach
HAC When reported with secondary diagnosis code J98.5

02124AC Bypass Coronary Artery, Three Sites from Thoracic Artery with Autologous Arterial Tissue, Percutaneous Endoscopic Approach
HAC When reported with secondary diagnosis code J98.5

02124AF Bypass Coronary Artery, Three Sites from Abdominal Artery with Autologous Arterial Tissue, Percutaneous Endoscopic Approach
HAC When reported with secondary diagnosis code J98.5

02124AW Bypass Coronary Artery, Three Sites from Aorta with Autologous Arterial Tissue, Percutaneous Endoscopic Approach
HAC When reported with secondary diagnosis code J98.5

02124D4 Bypass Coronary Artery, Three Sites from Coronary Vein with Intraluminal Device, Percutaneous Endoscopic Approach
HAC When reported with secondary diagnosis code J98.5

02124J3 Bypass Coronary Artery, Three Sites from Coronary Artery with Synthetic Substitute, Percutaneous Endoscopic Approach
HAC When reported with secondary diagnosis code J98.5

02124J8 Bypass Coronary Artery, Three Sites from Right Internal Mammary with Synthetic Substitute, Percutaneous Endoscopic Approach
HAC When reported with secondary diagnosis code J98.5

02124J9 Bypass Coronary Artery, Three Sites from Left Internal Mammary with Synthetic Substitute, Percutaneous Endoscopic Approach
HAC When reported with secondary diagnosis code J98.5

♀ Female-only   ♂ Male-only   ▲ Limited Coverage   ● Non-OR   HAC HAC-associated procedure   ▲ Non-covered procedures   ✚ Combinatio

2124JC Bypass Coronary Artery, Three Sites from Thoracic Artery with Synthetic Substitute, Percutaneous Endoscopic Approach
- *When reported with secondary diagnosis code J98.5*

2124JF Bypass Coronary Artery, Three Sites from Abdominal Artery with Synthetic Substitute, Percutaneous Endoscopic Approach
- *When reported with secondary diagnosis code J98.5*

2124JW Bypass Coronary Artery, Three Sites from Aorta with Synthetic Substitute, Percutaneous Endoscopic Approach
- *When reported with secondary diagnosis code J98.5*

2124K3 Bypass Coronary Artery, Three Sites from Coronary Artery with Nonautologous Tissue Substitute, Percutaneous Endoscopic Approach
- *When reported with secondary diagnosis code J98.5*

2124K8 Bypass Coronary Artery, Three Sites from Right Internal Mammary with Nonautologous Tissue Substitute, Percutaneous Endoscopic Approach
- *When reported with secondary diagnosis code J98.5*

2124K9 Bypass Coronary Artery, Three Sites from Left Internal Mammary with Nonautologous Tissue Substitute, Percutaneous Endoscopic Approach
- *When reported with secondary diagnosis code J98.5*

2124KC Bypass Coronary Artery, Three Sites from Thoracic Artery with Nonautologous Tissue Substitute, Percutaneous Endoscopic Approach
- *When reported with secondary diagnosis code J98.5*

2124KF Bypass Coronary Artery, Three Sites from Abdominal Artery with Nonautologous Tissue Substitute, Percutaneous Endoscopic Approach
- *When reported with secondary diagnosis code J98.5*

2124KW Bypass Coronary Artery, Three Sites from Aorta with Nonautologous Tissue Substitute, Percutaneous Endoscopic Approach
- *When reported with secondary diagnosis code J98.5*

2124Z3 Bypass Coronary Artery, Three Sites from Coronary Artery, Percutaneous Endoscopic Approach
- *When reported with secondary diagnosis code J98.5*

2124Z8 Bypass Coronary Artery, Three Sites from Right Internal Mammary, Percutaneous Endoscopic Approach
- *When reported with secondary diagnosis code J98.5*

2124Z9 Bypass Coronary Artery, Three Sites from Left Internal Mammary, Percutaneous Endoscopic Approach
- *When reported with secondary diagnosis code J98.5*

2124ZC Bypass Coronary Artery, Three Sites from Thoracic Artery, Percutaneous Endoscopic Approach
- *When reported with secondary diagnosis code J98.5*

2124ZF Bypass Coronary Artery, Three Sites from Abdominal Artery, Percutaneous Endoscopic Approach
- *When reported with secondary diagnosis code J98.5*

0213093 Bypass Coronary Artery, Four or More Sites from Coronary Artery with Autologous Venous Tissue, Open Approach
- *When reported with secondary diagnosis code J98.5*

0213098 Bypass Coronary Artery, Four or More Sites from Right Internal Mammary with Autologous Venous Tissue, Open Approach
- *When reported with secondary diagnosis code J98.5*

0213099 Bypass Coronary Artery, Four or More Sites from Left Internal Mammary with Autologous Venous Tissue, Open Approach
- *When reported with secondary diagnosis code J98.5*

021309C Bypass Coronary Artery, Four or More Sites from Thoracic Artery with Autologous Venous Tissue, Open Approach
- *When reported with secondary diagnosis code J98.5*

021309F Bypass Coronary Artery, Four or More Sites from Abdominal Artery with Autologous Venous Tissue, Open Approach
- *When reported with secondary diagnosis code J98.5*

021309W Bypass Coronary Artery, Four or More Sites from Aorta with Autologous Venous Tissue, Open Approach
- *When reported with secondary diagnosis code J98.5*

02130A3 Bypass Coronary Artery, Four or More Sites from Coronary Artery with Autologous Arterial Tissue, Open Approach
- *When reported with secondary diagnosis code J98.5*

02130A8 Bypass Coronary Artery, Four or More Sites from Right Internal Mammary with Autologous Arterial Tissue, Open Approach
- *When reported with secondary diagnosis code J98.5*

02130A9 Bypass Coronary Artery, Four or More Sites from Left Internal Mammary with Autologous Arterial Tissue, Open Approach
- *When reported with secondary diagnosis code J98.5*

02130AC Bypass Coronary Artery, Four or More Sites from Thoracic Artery with Autologous Arterial Tissue, Open Approach
- *When reported with secondary diagnosis code J98.5*

02130AF Bypass Coronary Artery, Four or More Sites from Abdominal Artery with Autologous Arterial Tissue, Open Approach
- *When reported with secondary diagnosis code J98.5*

02130AW Bypass Coronary Artery, Four or More Sites from Aorta with Autologous Arterial Tissue, Open Approach
- *When reported with secondary diagnosis code J98.5*

02130J3 Bypass Coronary Artery, Four or More Sites from Coronary Artery with Synthetic Substitute, Open Approach
- *When reported with secondary diagnosis code J98.5*

02130J8 Bypass Coronary Artery, Four or More Sites from Right Internal Mammary with Synthetic Substitute, Open Approach
- *When reported with secondary diagnosis code J98.5*

02130J9 Bypass Coronary Artery, Four or More Sites from Left Internal Mammary with Synthetic Substitute, Open Approach
- *When reported with secondary diagnosis code J98.5*

02130JC Bypass Coronary Artery, Four or More Sites from Thoracic Artery with Synthetic Substitute, Open Approach
- *When reported with secondary diagnosis code J98.5*

02130JF Bypass Coronary Artery, Four or More Sites from Abdominal Artery with Synthetic Substitute, Open Approach
- *When reported with secondary diagnosis code J98.5*

02130JW Bypass Coronary Artery, Four or More Sites from Aorta with Synthetic Substitute, Open Approach
- *When reported with secondary diagnosis code J98.5*

02130K3 Bypass Coronary Artery, Four or More Sites from Coronary Artery with Nonautologous Tissue Substitute, Open Approach
- *When reported with secondary diagnosis code J98.5*

02130K8 Bypass Coronary Artery, Four or More Sites from Right Internal Mammary with Nonautologous Tissue Substitute, Open Approach
- *When reported with secondary diagnosis code J98.5*

02130K9 Bypass Coronary Artery, Four or More Sites from Left Internal Mammary with Nonautologous Tissue Substitute, Open Approach
- *When reported with secondary diagnosis code J98.5*

02130KC Bypass Coronary Artery, Four or More Sites from Thoracic Artery with Nonautologous Tissue Substitute, Open Approach
- *When reported with secondary diagnosis code J98.5*

02130KF Bypass Coronary Artery, Four or More Sites from Abdominal Artery with Nonautologous Tissue Substitute, Open Approach
- *When reported with secondary diagnosis code J98.5*

02130KW Bypass Coronary Artery, Four or More Sites from Aorta with Nonautologous Tissue Substitute, Open Approach
- *When reported with secondary diagnosis code J98.5*

02130Z3 Bypass Coronary Artery, Four or More Sites from Coronary Artery, Open Approach
- *When reported with secondary diagnosis code J98.5*

02130Z8 Bypass Coronary Artery, Four or More Sites from Right Internal Mammary, Open Approach
- *When reported with secondary diagnosis code J98.5*

02130Z9 Bypass Coronary Artery, Four or More Sites from Left Internal Mammary, Open Approach
- *When reported with secondary diagnosis code J98.5*

Female-only   ♂ Male-only   ▲ Limited Coverage   ● Non-OR   ▦ HAC-associated procedure   ▲ Non-covered procedures   ✚ Combination

02130ZC Bypass Coronary Artery, Four or More Sites from Thoracic Artery, Open Approach
- When reported with secondary diagnosis code J98.5

02130ZF Bypass Coronary Artery, Four or More Sites from Abdominal Artery, Open Approach
- When reported with secondary diagnosis code J98.5

0213344 Bypass Coronary Artery, Four or More Sites from Coronary Vein with Drug-eluting Intraluminal Device, Percutaneous Approach
- When reported with secondary diagnosis code J98.5

02133D4 Bypass Coronary Artery, Four or More Sites from Coronary Vein with Intraluminal Device, Percutaneous Approach
- When reported with secondary diagnosis code J98.5

0213444 Bypass Coronary Artery, Four or More Sites from Coronary Vein with Drug-eluting Intraluminal Device, Percutaneous Endoscopic Approach
- When reported with secondary diagnosis code J98.5

0213493 Bypass Coronary Artery, Four or More Sites from Coronary Artery with Autologous Venous Tissue, Percutaneous Endoscopic Approach
- When reported with secondary diagnosis code J98.5

0213498 Bypass Coronary Artery, Four or More Sites from Right Internal Mammary with Autologous Venous Tissue, Percutaneous Endoscopic Approach
- When reported with secondary diagnosis code J98.5

0213499 Bypass Coronary Artery, Four or More Sites from Left Internal Mammary with Autologous Venous Tissue, Percutaneous Endoscopic Approach
- When reported with secondary diagnosis code J98.5

021349C Bypass Coronary Artery, Four or More Sites from Thoracic Artery with Autologous Venous Tissue, Percutaneous Endoscopic Approach
- When reported with secondary diagnosis code J98.5

021349F Bypass Coronary Artery, Four or More Sites from Abdominal Artery with Autologous Venous Tissue, Percutaneous Endoscopic Approach
- When reported with secondary diagnosis code J98.5

021349W Bypass Coronary Artery, Four or More Sites from Aorta with Autologous Venous Tissue, Percutaneous Endoscopic Approach
- When reported with secondary diagnosis code J98.5

02134A3 Bypass Coronary Artery, Four or More Sites from Coronary Artery with Autologous Arterial Tissue, Percutaneous Endoscopic Approach
- When reported with secondary diagnosis code J98.5

02134A8 Bypass Coronary Artery, Four or More Sites from Right Internal Mammary with Autologous Arterial Tissue, Percutaneous Endoscopic Approach
- When reported with secondary diagnosis code J98.5

02134A9 Bypass Coronary Artery, Four or More Sites from Left Internal Mammary with Autologous Arterial Tissue, Percutaneous Endoscopic Approach
- When reported with secondary diagnosis code J98.5

02134AC Bypass Coronary Artery, Four or More Sites from Thoracic Artery with Autologous Arterial Tissue, Percutaneous Endoscopic Approach
- When reported with secondary diagnosis code J98.5

02134AF Bypass Coronary Artery, Four or More Sites from Abdominal Artery with Autologous Arterial Tissue, Percutaneous Endoscopic Approach
- When reported with secondary diagnosis code J98.5

02134AW Bypass Coronary Artery, Four or More Sites from Aorta with Autologous Arterial Tissue, Percutaneous Endoscopic Approach
- When reported with secondary diagnosis code J98.5

02134D4 Bypass Coronary Artery, Four or More Sites from Coronary Vein with Intraluminal Device, Percutaneous Endoscopic Approach
- When reported with secondary diagnosis code J98.5

02134J3 Bypass Coronary Artery, Four or More Sites from Coronary Artery with Synthetic Substitute, Percutaneous Endoscopic Approach
- When reported with secondary diagnosis code J98.5

02134J8 Bypass Coronary Artery, Four or More Sites from Right Internal Mammary with Synthetic Substitute, Percutaneous Endoscopic Approach
- When reported with secondary diagnosis code J98.5

02134J9 Bypass Coronary Artery, Four or More Sites from Left Internal Mammary with Synthetic Substitute, Percutaneous Endoscopic Approach
- When reported with secondary diagnosis code J98.5

02134JC Bypass Coronary Artery, Four or More Sites from Thoracic Artery with Synthetic Substitute, Percutaneous Endoscopic Approach
- When reported with secondary diagnosis code J98.5

02134JF Bypass Coronary Artery, Four or More Sites from Abdominal Artery with Synthetic Substitute, Percutaneous Endoscopic Approach
- When reported with secondary diagnosis code J98.5

02134JW Bypass Coronary Artery, Four or More Sites from Aorta with Synthetic Substitute, Percutaneous Endoscopic Approach
- When reported with secondary diagnosis code J98.5

02134K3 Bypass Coronary Artery, Four or More Sites from Coronary Artery with Nonautologous Tissue Substitute, Percutaneous Endoscopic Approach
- When reported with secondary diagnosis code J98.5

02134K8 Bypass Coronary Artery, Four or More Sites from Right Internal Mammary with Nonautologous Tissue Substitute, Percutaneous Endoscopic Approach
- When reported with secondary diagnosis code J98.5

02134K9 Bypass Coronary Artery, Four or More Sites from Left Internal Mammary with Nonautologous Tissue Substitute, Percutaneous Endoscopic Approach
- When reported with secondary diagnosis code J98.5

02134KC Bypass Coronary Artery, Four or More Sites from Thoracic Artery with Nonautologous Tissue Substitute, Percutaneous Endoscopic Approach
- When reported with secondary diagnosis code J98.5

02134KF Bypass Coronary Artery, Four or More Sites from Abdominal Artery with Nonautologous Tissue Substitute, Percutaneous Endoscopic Approach
- When reported with secondary diagnosis code J98.5

02134KW Bypass Coronary Artery, Four or More Sites from Aorta with Nonautologous Tissue Substitute, Percutaneous Endoscopic Approach
- When reported with secondary diagnosis code J98.5

02134Z3 Bypass Coronary Artery, Four or More Sites from Coronary Artery, Percutaneous Endoscopic Approach
- When reported with secondary diagnosis code J98.5

02134Z8 Bypass Coronary Artery, Four or More Sites from Right Internal Mammary, Percutaneous Endoscopic Approach
- When reported with secondary diagnosis code J98.5

02134Z9 Bypass Coronary Artery, Four or More Sites from Left Internal Mammary, Percutaneous Endoscopic Approach
- When reported with secondary diagnosis code J98.5

02134ZC Bypass Coronary Artery, Four or More Sites from Thoracic Artery, Percutaneous Endoscopic Approach
- When reported with secondary diagnosis code J98.5

02134ZF Bypass Coronary Artery, Four or More Sites from Abdominal Artery, Percutaneous Endoscopic Approach
- When reported with secondary diagnosis code J98.5

021609P Bypass Right Atrium to Pulmonary Trunk with Autologous Venous Tissue, Open Approach

021609Q Bypass Right Atrium to Right Pulmonary Artery with Autologous Venous Tissue, Open Approach

021609R Bypass Right Atrium to Left Pulmonary Artery with Autologous Venous Tissue, Open Approach

02160AP Bypass Right Atrium to Pulmonary Trunk with Autologous Arterial Tissue, Open Approach

02160AQ Bypass Right Atrium to Right Pulmonary Artery with Autologous Arterial Tissue, Open Approach

02160AR Bypass Right Atrium to Left Pulmonary Artery with Autologous Arterial Tissue, Open Approach

02160JP Bypass Right Atrium to Pulmonary Trunk with Synthetic Substitute, Open Approach

02160JQ Bypass Right Atrium to Right Pulmonary Artery with Synthetic Substitute, Open Approach
AHA CC: 3Q, 2014, 29

02160JR Bypass Right Atrium to Left Pulmonary Artery with Synthetic Substitute, Open Approach

♀ Female-only   ♂ Male-only   ▲ Limited Coverage   ● Non-OR   ▨ HAC-associated procedure   ▲ Non-covered procedures   ✛ Combination

2160KP Bypass Right Atrium to Pulmonary Trunk with Nonautologous Tissue Substitute, Open Approach

2160KQ Bypass Right Atrium to Right Pulmonary Artery with Nonautologous Tissue Substitute, Open Approach

2160KR Bypass Right Atrium to Left Pulmonary Artery with Nonautologous Tissue Substitute, Open Approach

2160Z7 Bypass Right Atrium to Left Atrium, Open Approach

2160ZP Bypass Right Atrium to Pulmonary Trunk, Open Approach

2160ZQ Bypass Right Atrium to Right Pulmonary Artery, Open Approach

2160ZR Bypass Right Atrium to Left Pulmonary Artery, Open Approach

21649P Bypass Right Atrium to Pulmonary Trunk with Autologous Venous Tissue, Percutaneous Endoscopic Approach

21649Q Bypass Right Atrium to Right Pulmonary Artery with Autologous Venous Tissue, Percutaneous Endoscopic Approach

21649R Bypass Right Atrium to Left Pulmonary Artery with Autologous Venous Tissue, Percutaneous Endoscopic Approach

2164AP Bypass Right Atrium to Pulmonary Trunk with Autologous Arterial Tissue, Percutaneous Endoscopic Approach

2164AQ Bypass Right Atrium to Right Pulmonary Artery with Autologous Arterial Tissue, Percutaneous Endoscopic Approach

2164AR Bypass Right Atrium to Left Pulmonary Artery with Autologous Arterial Tissue, Percutaneous Endoscopic Approach

2164JP Bypass Right Atrium to Pulmonary Trunk with Synthetic Substitute, Percutaneous Endoscopic Approach

2164JQ Bypass Right Atrium to Right Pulmonary Artery with Synthetic Substitute, Percutaneous Endoscopic Approach

2164JR Bypass Right Atrium to Left Pulmonary Artery with Synthetic Substitute, Percutaneous Endoscopic Approach

2164KP Bypass Right Atrium to Pulmonary Trunk with Nonautologous Tissue Substitute, Percutaneous Endoscopic Approach

2164KQ Bypass Right Atrium to Right Pulmonary Artery with Nonautologous Tissue Substitute, Percutaneous Endoscopic Approach

2164KR Bypass Right Atrium to Left Pulmonary Artery with Nonautologous Tissue Substitute, Percutaneous Endoscopic Approach

2164Z7 Bypass Right Atrium to Left Atrium, Percutaneous Endoscopic Approach

2164ZP Bypass Right Atrium to Pulmonary Trunk, Percutaneous Endoscopic Approach

2164ZQ Bypass Right Atrium to Right Pulmonary Artery, Percutaneous Endoscopic Approach

2164ZR Bypass Right Atrium to Left Pulmonary Artery, Percutaneous Endoscopic Approach

21709P Bypass Left Atrium to Pulmonary Trunk with Autologous Venous Tissue, Open Approach

21709Q Bypass Left Atrium to Right Pulmonary Artery with Autologous Venous Tissue, Open Approach

21709R Bypass Left Atrium to Left Pulmonary Artery with Autologous Venous Tissue, Open Approach

2170AP Bypass Left Atrium to Pulmonary Trunk with Autologous Arterial Tissue, Open Approach

02170AQ Bypass Left Atrium to Right Pulmonary Artery with Autologous Arterial Tissue, Open Approach

02170AR Bypass Left Atrium to Left Pulmonary Artery with Autologous Arterial Tissue, Open Approach

02170JP Bypass Left Atrium to Pulmonary Trunk with Synthetic Substitute, Open Approach

02170JQ Bypass Left Atrium to Right Pulmonary Artery with Synthetic Substitute, Open Approach

02170JR Bypass Left Atrium to Left Pulmonary Artery with Synthetic Substitute, Open Approach

02170KP Bypass Left Atrium to Pulmonary Trunk with Nonautologous Tissue Substitute, Open Approach

02170KQ Bypass Left Atrium to Right Pulmonary Artery with Nonautologous Tissue Substitute, Open Approach

02170KR Bypass Left Atrium to Left Pulmonary Artery with Nonautologous Tissue Substitute, Open Approach

02170ZP Bypass Left Atrium to Pulmonary Trunk, Open Approach

02170ZQ Bypass Left Atrium to Right Pulmonary Artery, Open Approach

02170ZR Bypass Left Atrium to Left Pulmonary Artery, Open Approach

021749P Bypass Left Atrium to Pulmonary Trunk with Autologous Venous Tissue, Percutaneous Endoscopic Approach

021749Q Bypass Left Atrium to Right Pulmonary Artery with Autologous Venous Tissue, Percutaneous Endoscopic Approach

021749R Bypass Left Atrium to Left Pulmonary Artery with Autologous Venous Tissue, Percutaneous Endoscopic Approach

02174AP Bypass Left Atrium to Pulmonary Trunk with Autologous Arterial Tissue, Percutaneous Endoscopic Approach

02174AQ Bypass Left Atrium to Right Pulmonary Artery with Autologous Arterial Tissue, Percutaneous Endoscopic Approach

02174AR Bypass Left Atrium to Left Pulmonary Artery with Autologous Arterial Tissue, Percutaneous Endoscopic Approach

02174JP Bypass Left Atrium to Pulmonary Trunk with Synthetic Substitute, Percutaneous Endoscopic Approach

02174JQ Bypass Left Atrium to Right Pulmonary Artery with Synthetic Substitute, Percutaneous Endoscopic Approach

02174JR Bypass Left Atrium to Left Pulmonary Artery with Synthetic Substitute, Percutaneous Endoscopic Approach

02174KP Bypass Left Atrium to Pulmonary Trunk with Nonautologous Tissue Substitute, Percutaneous Endoscopic Approach

02174KQ Bypass Left Atrium to Right Pulmonary Artery with Nonautologous Tissue Substitute, Percutaneous Endoscopic Approach

02174KR Bypass Left Atrium to Left Pulmonary Artery with Nonautologous Tissue Substitute, Percutaneous Endoscopic Approach

02174ZP Bypass Left Atrium to Pulmonary Trunk, Percutaneous Endoscopic Approach

02174ZQ Bypass Left Atrium to Right Pulmonary Artery, Percutaneous Endoscopic Approach

02174ZR Bypass Left Atrium to Left Pulmonary Artery, Percutaneous Endoscopic Approach

021K09P Bypass Right Ventricle to Pulmonary Trunk with Autologous Venous Tissue, Open Approach

021K09Q Bypass Right Ventricle to Right Pulmonary Artery with Autologous Venous Tissue, Open Approach

021K09R Bypass Right Ventricle to Left Pulmonary Artery with Autologous Venous Tissue, Open Approach

021K0AP Bypass Right Ventricle to Pulmonary Trunk with Autologous Arterial Tissue, Open Approach

021K0AQ Bypass Right Ventricle to Right Pulmonary Artery with Autologous Arterial Tissue, Open Approach

021K0AR Bypass Right Ventricle to Left Pulmonary Artery with Autologous Arterial Tissue, Open Approach

021K0JP Bypass Right Ventricle to Pulmonary Trunk with Synthetic Substitute, Open Approach

021K0JQ Bypass Right Ventricle to Right Pulmonary Artery with Synthetic Substitute, Open Approach

AHA CC: 3Q, 2014, 30

021K0JR Bypass Right Ventricle to Left Pulmonary Artery with Synthetic Substitute, Open Approach

021K0KP Bypass Right Ventricle to Pulmonary Trunk with Nonautologous Tissue Substitute, Open Approach

021K0KQ Bypass Right Ventricle to Right Pulmonary Artery with Nonautologous Tissue Substitute, Open Approach

021K0KR Bypass Right Ventricle to Left Pulmonary Artery with Nonautologous Tissue Substitute, Open Approach

021K0Z5 Bypass Right Ventricle to Coronary Circulation, Open Approach

021K0Z8 Bypass Right Ventricle to Right Internal Mammary, Open Approach

021K0Z9 Bypass Right Ventricle to Left Internal Mammary, Open Approach

021K0ZC Bypass Right Ventricle to Thoracic Artery, Open Approach

021K0ZF Bypass Right Ventricle to Abdominal Artery, Open Approach

021K0ZP Bypass Right Ventricle to Pulmonary Trunk, Open Approach

021K0ZQ Bypass Right Ventricle to Right Pulmonary Artery, Open Approach

021K0ZR Bypass Right Ventricle to Left Pulmonary Artery, Open Approach

021K0ZW Bypass Right Ventricle to Aorta, Open Approach

021K49P Bypass Right Ventricle to Pulmonary Trunk with Autologous Venous Tissue, Percutaneous Endoscopic Approach

021K49Q Bypass Right Ventricle to Right Pulmonary Artery with Autologous Venous Tissue, Percutaneous Endoscopic Approach

021K49R Bypass Right Ventricle to Left Pulmonary Artery with Autologous Venous Tissue, Percutaneous Endoscopic Approach

021K4AP Bypass Right Ventricle to Pulmonary Trunk with Autologous Arterial Tissue, Percutaneous Endoscopic Approach

021K4AQ Bypass Right Ventricle to Right Pulmonary Artery with Autologous Arterial Tissue, Percutaneous Endoscopic Approach

021K4AR Bypass Right Ventricle to Left Pulmonary Artery with Autologous Arterial Tissue, Percutaneous Endoscopic Approach

021K4JP Bypass Right Ventricle to Pulmonary Trunk with Synthetic Substitute, Percutaneous Endoscopic Approach

021K4JQ Bypass Right Ventricle to Right Pulmonary Artery with Synthetic Substitute, Percutaneous Endoscopic Approach

---

Female-only   ♂ Male-only   ▲ Limited Coverage   ● Non-OR   ▣ HAC-associated procedure   ▲ Non-covered procedures   ✚ Combination

021K4JR Bypass Right Ventricle to Left Pulmonary Artery with Synthetic Substitute, Percutaneous Endoscopic Approach

021K4KP Bypass Right Ventricle to Pulmonary Trunk with Nonautologous Tissue Substitute, Percutaneous Endoscopic Approach

021K4KQ Bypass Right Ventricle to Right Pulmonary Artery with Nonautologous Tissue Substitute, Percutaneous Endoscopic Approach

021K4KR Bypass Right Ventricle to Left Pulmonary Artery with Nonautologous Tissue Substitute, Percutaneous Endoscopic Approach

021K4Z5 Bypass Right Ventricle to Coronary Circulation, Percutaneous Endoscopic Approach

021K4Z8 Bypass Right Ventricle to Right Internal Mammary, Percutaneous Endoscopic Approach

021K4Z9 Bypass Right Ventricle to Left Internal Mammary, Percutaneous Endoscopic Approach

021K4ZC Bypass Right Ventricle to Thoracic Artery, Percutaneous Endoscopic Approach

021K4ZF Bypass Right Ventricle to Abdominal Artery, Percutaneous Endoscopic Approach

021K4ZP Bypass Right Ventricle to Pulmonary Trunk, Percutaneous Endoscopic Approach

021K4ZQ Bypass Right Ventricle to Right Pulmonary Artery, Percutaneous Endoscopic Approach

021K4ZR Bypass Right Ventricle to Left Pulmonary Artery, Percutaneous Endoscopic Approach

021K4ZW Bypass Right Ventricle to Aorta, Percutaneous Endoscopic Approach

021L09P Bypass Left Ventricle to Pulmonary Trunk with Autologous Venous Tissue, Open Approach

021L09Q Bypass Left Ventricle to Right Pulmonary Artery with Autologous Venous Tissue, Open Approach

021L09R Bypass Left Ventricle to Left Pulmonary Artery with Autologous Venous Tissue, Open Approach

021L0AP Bypass Left Ventricle to Pulmonary Trunk with Autologous Arterial Tissue, Open Approach

021L0AQ Bypass Left Ventricle to Right Pulmonary Artery with Autologous Arterial Tissue, Open Approach

021L0AR Bypass Left Ventricle to Left Pulmonary Artery with Autologous Arterial Tissue, Open Approach

021L0JP Bypass Left Ventricle to Pulmonary Trunk with Synthetic Substitute, Open Approach

021L0JQ Bypass Left Ventricle to Right Pulmonary Artery with Synthetic Substitute, Open Approach

021L0JR Bypass Left Ventricle to Left Pulmonary Artery with Synthetic Substitute, Open Approach

021L0KP Bypass Left Ventricle to Pulmonary Trunk with Nonautologous Tissue Substitute, Open Approach

021L0KQ Bypass Left Ventricle to Right Pulmonary Artery with Nonautologous Tissue Substitute, Open Approach

021L0KR Bypass Left Ventricle to Left Pulmonary Artery with Nonautologous Tissue Substitute, Open Approach

021L0Z5 Bypass Left Ventricle to Coronary Circulation, Open Approach

021L0Z8 Bypass Left Ventricle to Right Internal Mammary, Open Approach

021L0Z9 Bypass Left Ventricle to Left Internal Mammary, Open Approach

021L0ZC Bypass Left Ventricle to Thoracic Artery, Open Approach

021L0ZF Bypass Left Ventricle to Abdominal Artery, Open Approach

021L0ZP Bypass Left Ventricle to Pulmonary Trunk, Open Approach

021L0ZQ Bypass Left Ventricle to Right Pulmonary Artery, Open Approach

021L0ZR Bypass Left Ventricle to Left Pulmonary Artery, Open Approach

021L0ZW Bypass Left Ventricle to Aorta, Open Approach

021L49P Bypass Left Ventricle to Pulmonary Trunk with Autologous Venous Tissue, Percutaneous Endoscopic Approach

021L49Q Bypass Left Ventricle to Right Pulmonary Artery with Autologous Venous Tissue, Percutaneous Endoscopic Approach

021L49R Bypass Left Ventricle to Left Pulmonary Artery with Autologous Venous Tissue, Percutaneous Endoscopic Approach

021L4AP Bypass Left Ventricle to Pulmonary Trunk with Autologous Arterial Tissue, Percutaneous Endoscopic Approach

021L4AQ Bypass Left Ventricle to Right Pulmonary Artery with Autologous Arterial Tissue, Percutaneous Endoscopic Approach

021L4AR Bypass Left Ventricle to Left Pulmonary Artery with Autologous Arterial Tissue, Percutaneous Endoscopic Approach

021L4JP Bypass Left Ventricle to Pulmonary Trunk with Synthetic Substitute, Percutaneous Endoscopic Approach

021L4JQ Bypass Left Ventricle to Right Pulmonary Artery with Synthetic Substitute, Percutaneous Endoscopic Approach

021L4JR Bypass Left Ventricle to Left Pulmonary Artery with Synthetic Substitute, Percutaneous Endoscopic Approach

021L4KP Bypass Left Ventricle to Pulmonary Trunk with Nonautologous Tissue Substitute, Percutaneous Endoscopic Approach

021L4KQ Bypass Left Ventricle to Right Pulmonary Artery with Nonautologous Tissue Substitute, Percutaneous Endoscopic Approach

021L4KR Bypass Left Ventricle to Left Pulmonary Artery with Nonautologous Tissue Substitute, Percutaneous Endoscopic Approach

021L4Z5 Bypass Left Ventricle to Coronary Circulation, Percutaneous Endoscopic Approach

021L4Z8 Bypass Left Ventricle to Right Internal Mammary, Percutaneous Endoscopic Approach

021L4Z9 Bypass Left Ventricle to Left Internal Mammary, Percutaneous Endoscopic Approach

021L4ZC Bypass Left Ventricle to Thoracic Artery, Percutaneous Endoscopic Approach

021L4ZF Bypass Left Ventricle to Abdominal Artery, Percutaneous Endoscopic Approach

021L4ZP Bypass Left Ventricle to Pulmonary Trunk, Percutaneous Endoscopic Approach

021L4ZQ Bypass Left Ventricle to Right Pulmonary Artery, Percutaneous Endoscopic Approach

021L4ZR Bypass Left Ventricle to Left Pulmonary Artery, Percutaneous Endoscopic Approach

021L4ZW Bypass Left Ventricle to Aorta, Percutaneous Endoscopic Approach

021V09P Bypass Superior Vena Cava to Pulmonary Trunk with Autologous Venous Tissue, Open Approach

021V09Q Bypass Superior Vena Cava to Right Pulmonary Artery with Autologous Venous Tissue, Open Approach

021V09R Bypass Superior Vena Cava to Left Pulmonary Artery with Autologous Venous Tissue, Open Approach

021V0AP Bypass Superior Vena Cava to Pulmonary Trunk with Autologous Arterial Tissue, Open Approach

021V0AQ Bypass Superior Vena Cava to Right Pulmonary Artery with Autologous Arterial Tissue, Open Approach

021V0AR Bypass Superior Vena Cava to Left Pulmonary Artery with Autologous Arterial Tissue, Open Approach

021V0JP Bypass Superior Vena Cava to Pulmonary Trunk with Synthetic Substitute, Open Approach

021V0JQ Bypass Superior Vena Cava to Right Pulmonary Artery with Synthetic Substitute, Open Approach

021V0JR Bypass Superior Vena Cava to Left Pulmonary Artery with Synthetic Substitute, Open Approach

021V0KP Bypass Superior Vena Cava to Pulmonary Trunk with Nonautologous Tissue Substitute, Open Approach

021V0KQ Bypass Superior Vena Cava to Right Pulmonary Artery with Nonautologous Tissue Substitute, Open Approach

021V0KR Bypass Superior Vena Cava to Left Pulmonary Artery with Nonautologous Tissue Substitute, Open Approach

021V0ZP Bypass Superior Vena Cava to Pulmonary Trunk, Open Approach

021V0ZQ Bypass Superior Vena Cava to Right Pulmonary Artery, Open Approach

021V0ZR Bypass Superior Vena Cava to Left Pulmonary Artery, Open Approach

021V49P Bypass Superior Vena Cava to Pulmonary Trunk with Autologous Venous Tissue, Percutaneous Endoscopic Approach

021V49Q Bypass Superior Vena Cava to Right Pulmonary Artery with Autologous Venous Tissue, Percutaneous Endoscopic Approach

021V49R Bypass Superior Vena Cava to Left Pulmonary Artery with Autologous Venous Tissue, Percutaneous Endoscopic Approach

021V4AP Bypass Superior Vena Cava to Pulmonary Trunk with Autologous Arterial Tissue, Percutaneous Endoscopic Approach

021V4AQ Bypass Superior Vena Cava to Right Pulmonary Artery with Autologous Arterial Tissue, Percutaneous Endoscopic Approach

021V4AR Bypass Superior Vena Cava to Left Pulmonary Artery with Autologous Arterial Tissue, Percutaneous Endoscopic Approach

021V4JP Bypass Superior Vena Cava to Pulmonary Trunk with Synthetic Substitute, Percutaneous Endoscopic Approach

021V4JQ Bypass Superior Vena Cava to Right Pulmonary Artery with Synthetic Substitute, Percutaneous Endoscopic Approach

021V4JR Bypass Superior Vena Cava to Left Pulmonary Artery with Synthetic Substitute, Percutaneous Endoscopic Approach

021V4KP Bypass Superior Vena Cava to Pulmonary Trunk with Nonautologous Tissue Substitute, Percutaneous Endoscopic Approach

021V4KQ Bypass Superior Vena Cava to Right Pulmonary Artery with Nonautologous Tissue Substitute, Percutaneous Endoscopic Approach

1V4KR Bypass Superior Vena Cava to Left Pulmonary Artery with Nonautologous Tissue Substitute, Percutaneous Endoscopic Approach

1V4ZP Bypass Superior Vena Cava to Pulmonary Trunk, Percutaneous Endoscopic Approach

1V4ZQ Bypass Superior Vena Cava to Right Pulmonary Artery, Percutaneous Endoscopic Approach

1V4ZR Bypass Superior Vena Cava to Left Pulmonary Artery, Percutaneous Endoscopic Approach

1W09B Bypass Thoracic Aorta to Subclavian with Autologous Venous Tissue, Open Approach

1W09D Bypass Thoracic Aorta to Carotid with Autologous Venous Tissue, Open Approach

1W09P Bypass Thoracic Aorta to Pulmonary Trunk with Autologous Venous Tissue, Open Approach

1W09Q Bypass Thoracic Aorta to Right Pulmonary Artery with Autologous Venous Tissue, Open Approach

1W09R Bypass Thoracic Aorta to Left Pulmonary Artery with Autologous Venous Tissue, Open Approach

1W0AB Bypass Thoracic Aorta to Subclavian with Autologous Arterial Tissue, Open Approach

1W0AD Bypass Thoracic Aorta to Carotid with Autologous Arterial Tissue, Open Approach

1W0AP Bypass Thoracic Aorta to Pulmonary Trunk with Autologous Arterial Tissue, Open Approach

1W0AQ Bypass Thoracic Aorta to Right Pulmonary Artery with Autologous Arterial Tissue, Open Approach

1W0AR Bypass Thoracic Aorta to Left Pulmonary Artery with Autologous Arterial Tissue, Open Approach

1W0JB Bypass Thoracic Aorta to Subclavian with Synthetic Substitute, Open Approach

1W0JD Bypass Thoracic Aorta to Carotid with Synthetic Substitute, Open Approach

1W0JP Bypass Thoracic Aorta to Pulmonary Trunk with Synthetic Substitute, Open Approach

1W0JQ Bypass Thoracic Aorta to Right Pulmonary Artery with Synthetic Substitute, Open Approach

AHA CC: 3Q, 2014, 3

021W0JR Bypass Thoracic Aorta to Left Pulmonary Artery with Synthetic Substitute, Open Approach

021W0KB Bypass Thoracic Aorta to Subclavian with Nonautologous Tissue Substitute, Open Approach

021W0KD Bypass Thoracic Aorta to Carotid with Nonautologous Tissue Substitute, Open Approach

021W0KP Bypass Thoracic Aorta to Pulmonary Trunk with Nonautologous Tissue Substitute, Open Approach

021W0KQ Bypass Thoracic Aorta to Right Pulmonary Artery with Nonautologous Tissue Substitute, Open Approach

021W0KR Bypass Thoracic Aorta to Left Pulmonary Artery with Nonautologous Tissue Substitute, Open Approach

021W0ZB Bypass Thoracic Aorta to Subclavian, Open Approach

021W0ZD Bypass Thoracic Aorta to Carotid, Open Approach

021W0ZP Bypass Thoracic Aorta to Pulmonary Trunk, Open Approach

021W0ZQ Bypass Thoracic Aorta to Right Pulmonary Artery, Open Approach

021W0ZR Bypass Thoracic Aorta to Left Pulmonary Artery, Open Approach

021W49B Bypass Thoracic Aorta to Subclavian with Autologous Venous Tissue, Percutaneous Endoscopic Approach

021W49D Bypass Thoracic Aorta to Carotid with Autologous Venous Tissue, Percutaneous Endoscopic Approach

021W49P Bypass Thoracic Aorta to Pulmonary Trunk with Autologous Venous Tissue, Percutaneous Endoscopic Approach

021W49Q Bypass Thoracic Aorta to Right Pulmonary Artery with Autologous Venous Tissue, Percutaneous Endoscopic Approach

021W49R Bypass Thoracic Aorta to Left Pulmonary Artery with Autologous Venous Tissue, Percutaneous Endoscopic Approach

021W4AB Bypass Thoracic Aorta to Subclavian with Autologous Arterial Tissue, Percutaneous Endoscopic Approach

021W4AD Bypass Thoracic Aorta to Carotid with Autologous Arterial Tissue, Percutaneous Endoscopic Approach

021W4AP Bypass Thoracic Aorta to Pulmonary Trunk with Autologous Arterial Tissue, Percutaneous Endoscopic Approach

021W4AQ Bypass Thoracic Aorta to Right Pulmonary Artery with Autologous Arterial Tissue, Percutaneous Endoscopic Approach

021W4AR Bypass Thoracic Aorta to Left Pulmonary Artery with Autologous Arterial Tissue, Percutaneous Endoscopic Approach

021W4JB Bypass Thoracic Aorta to Subclavian with Synthetic Substitute, Percutaneous Endoscopic Approach

021W4JD Bypass Thoracic Aorta to Carotid with Synthetic Substitute, Percutaneous Endoscopic Approach

021W4JP Bypass Thoracic Aorta to Pulmonary Trunk with Synthetic Substitute, Percutaneous Endoscopic Approach

021W4JQ Bypass Thoracic Aorta to Right Pulmonary Artery with Synthetic Substitute, Percutaneous Endoscopic Approach

021W4JR Bypass Thoracic Aorta to Left Pulmonary Artery with Synthetic Substitute, Percutaneous Endoscopic Approach

021W4KB Bypass Thoracic Aorta to Subclavian with Nonautologous Tissue Substitute, Percutaneous Endoscopic Approach

021W4KD Bypass Thoracic Aorta to Carotid with Nonautologous Tissue Substitute, Percutaneous Endoscopic Approach

021W4KP Bypass Thoracic Aorta to Pulmonary Trunk with Nonautologous Tissue Substitute, Percutaneous Endoscopic Approach

021W4KQ Bypass Thoracic Aorta to Right Pulmonary Artery with Nonautologous Tissue Substitute, Percutaneous Endoscopic Approach

021W4KR Bypass Thoracic Aorta to Left Pulmonary Artery with Nonautologous Tissue Substitute, Percutaneous Endoscopic Approach

021W4ZB Bypass Thoracic Aorta to Subclavian, Percutaneous Endoscopic Approach

021W4ZD Bypass Thoracic Aorta to Carotid, Percutaneous Endoscopic Approach

021W4ZP Bypass Thoracic Aorta to Pulmonary Trunk, Percutaneous Endoscopic Approach

021W4ZQ Bypass Thoracic Aorta to Right Pulmonary Artery, Percutaneous Endoscopic Approach

021W4ZR Bypass Thoracic Aorta to Left Pulmonary Artery, Percutaneous Endoscopic Approach

25 – Heart and Great Vessels, Destruction

540ZZ Destruction of Coronary Vein, Open Approach

543ZZ Destruction of Coronary Vein, Percutaneous Approach

544ZZ Destruction of Coronary Vein, Percutaneous Endoscopic Approach

550ZZ Destruction of Atrial Septum, Open Approach

553ZZ Destruction of Atrial Septum, Percutaneous Approach

554ZZ Destruction of Atrial Septum, Percutaneous Endoscopic Approach

560ZZ Destruction of Right Atrium, Open Approach

563ZZ Destruction of Right Atrium, Percutaneous Approach

564ZZ Destruction of Right Atrium, Percutaneous Endoscopic Approach

02570ZK Destruction of Left Atrial Appendage, Open Approach

AHA CC: 3Q, 2014, 20-21

2570ZZ Destruction of Left Atrium, Open Approach

● **02573ZK** Destruction of Left Atrial Appendage, Percutaneous Approach

02573ZZ Destruction of Left Atrium, Percutaneous Approach

● **02574ZK** Destruction of Left Atrial Appendage, Percutaneous Endoscopic Approach

02574ZZ Destruction of Left Atrium, Percutaneous Endoscopic Approach

02580ZZ Destruction of Conduction Mechanism, Open Approach

02583ZZ Destruction of Conduction Mechanism, Percutaneous Approach

AHA CC: 3Q, 2014, 19; 4Q, 2014, 47-48

02584ZZ Destruction of Conduction Mechanism, Percutaneous Endoscopic Approach

02590ZZ Destruction of Chordae Tendineae, Open Approach

02593ZZ Destruction of Chordae Tendineae, Percutaneous Approach

02594ZZ Destruction of Chordae Tendineae, Percutaneous Endoscopic Approach

025D0ZZ Destruction of Papillary Muscle, Open Approach

025D3ZZ Destruction of Papillary Muscle, Percutaneous Approach

025D4ZZ Destruction of Papillary Muscle, Percutaneous Endoscopic Approach

025F0ZZ Destruction of Aortic Valve, Open Approach

025F3ZZ Destruction of Aortic Valve, Percutaneous Approach

025F4ZZ Destruction of Aortic Valve, Percutaneous Endoscopic Approach

025G0ZZ Destruction of Mitral Valve, Open Approach

025G3ZZ Destruction of Mitral Valve, Percutaneous Approach

025G4ZZ Destruction of Mitral Valve, Percutaneous Endoscopic Approach

025H0ZZ Destruction of Pulmonary Valve, Open Approach

025H3ZZ Destruction of Pulmonary Valve, Percutaneous Approach

Female-only   ♂ Male-only   ▲ Limited Coverage   ● Non-OR   ▦ HAC-associated procedure   ▲ Non-covered procedures   ✚ Combination

025H4ZZ	Destruction of Pulmonary Valve, Percutaneous Endoscopic Approach	
025J0ZZ	Destruction of Tricuspid Valve, Open Approach	
025J3ZZ	Destruction of Tricuspid Valve, Percutaneous Approach	
025J4ZZ	Destruction of Tricuspid Valve, Percutaneous Endoscopic Approach	
025K0ZZ	Destruction of Right Ventricle, Open Approach	
025K3ZZ	Destruction of Right Ventricle, Percutaneous Approach	
025K4ZZ	Destruction of Right Ventricle, Percutaneous Endoscopic Approach	
025L0ZZ	Destruction of Left Ventricle, Open Approach	
025L3ZZ	Destruction of Left Ventricle, Percutaneous Approach	
025L4ZZ	Destruction of Left Ventricle, Percutaneous Endoscopic Approach	
025M0ZZ	Destruction of Ventricular Septum, Open Approach	
025M3ZZ	Destruction of Ventricular Septum, Percutaneous Approach	
025M4ZZ	Destruction of Ventricular Septum, Percutaneous Endoscopic Approach	

025N0ZZ	Destruction of Pericardium, Open Approach
025N3ZZ	Destruction of Pericardium, Percutaneous Approach
025N4ZZ	Destruction of Pericardium, Percutaneous Endoscopic Approach
025P0ZZ	Destruction of Pulmonary Trunk, Open Approach
025P3ZZ	Destruction of Pulmonary Trunk, Percutaneous Approach
025P4ZZ	Destruction of Pulmonary Trunk, Percutaneous Endoscopic Approach
025Q0ZZ	Destruction of Right Pulmonary Artery, Open Approach
025Q3ZZ	Destruction of Right Pulmonary Artery, Percutaneous Approach
025Q4ZZ	Destruction of Right Pulmonary Artery, Percutaneous Endoscopic Approach
025R0ZZ	Destruction of Left Pulmonary Artery, Open Approach
025R3ZZ	Destruction of Left Pulmonary Artery, Percutaneous Approach
025R4ZZ	Destruction of Left Pulmonary Artery, Percutaneous Endoscopic Approach
025S0ZZ	Destruction of Right Pulmonary Vein, Open Approach

025S3ZZ	Destruction of Right Pulmonary Vein, Percutaneous Approach
025S4ZZ	Destruction of Right Pulmonary Vein, Percutaneous Endoscopic Approach
025T0ZZ	Destruction of Left Pulmonary Vein, Op Approach
025T3ZZ	Destruction of Left Pulmonary Vein, Percutaneous Approach
025T4ZZ	Destruction of Left Pulmonary Vein, Percutaneous Endoscopic Approach
025V0ZZ	Destruction of Superior Vena Cava, Ope Approach
025V3ZZ	Destruction of Superior Vena Cava, Percutaneous Approach
025V4ZZ	Destruction of Superior Vena Cava, Percutaneous Endoscopic Approach
025W0ZZ	Destruction of Thoracic Aorta, Open Approach
025W3ZZ	Destruction of Thoracic Aorta, Percutaneous Approach
025W4ZZ	Destruction of Thoracic Aorta, Percutaneous Endoscopic Approach

027 – Heart and Great Vessels, Dilation

For Dilation procedures involving the coronary arteries, Review Coding Guideline B4.4

0270046	Dilation of Coronary Artery, One Site, Bifurcation, with Drug-eluting Intraluminal Device, Open Approach
027004Z	Dilation of Coronary Artery, One Site with Drug-eluting Intraluminal Device, Open Approach
02700D6	Dilation of Coronary Artery, One Site, Bifurcation, with Intraluminal Device, Open Approach
02700DZ	Dilation of Coronary Artery, One Site with Intraluminal Device, Open Approach
02700T6	Dilation of Coronary Artery, One Site, Bifurcation, with Radioactive Intraluminal Device, Open Approach
02700TZ	Dilation of Coronary Artery, One Site with Radioactive Intraluminal Device, Open Approach
02700Z6	Dilation of Coronary Artery, One Site, Bifurcation, Open Approach
02700ZZ	Dilation of Coronary Artery, One Site, Open Approach
0270346	Dilation of Coronary Artery, One Site, Bifurcation, with Drug-eluting Intraluminal Device, Percutaneous Approach
027034Z	Dilation of Coronary Artery, One Site with Drug-eluting Intraluminal Device, Percutaneous Approach
	AHA CC: 2Q, 2014, 4
02703D6	Dilation of Coronary Artery, One Site, Bifurcation, with Intraluminal Device, Percutaneous Approach
02703DZ	Dilation of Coronary Artery, One Site with Intraluminal Device, Percutaneous Approach
02703T6	Dilation of Coronary Artery, One Site, Bifurcation, with Radioactive Intraluminal Device, Percutaneous Approach
02703TZ	Dilation of Coronary Artery, One Site with Radioactive Intraluminal Device, Percutaneous Approach
02703Z6	Dilation of Coronary Artery, One Site, Bifurcation, Percutaneous Approach
02703ZZ	Dilation of Coronary Artery, One Site, Percutaneous Approach
0270446	Dilation of Coronary Artery, One Site, Bifurcation, with Drug-eluting Intraluminal Device, Percutaneous Endoscopic Approach

027044Z	Dilation of Coronary Artery, One Site with Drug-eluting Intraluminal Device, Percutaneous Endoscopic Approach
02704D6	Dilation of Coronary Artery, One Site, Bifurcation, with Intraluminal Device, Percutaneous Endoscopic Approach
02704DZ	Dilation of Coronary Artery, One Site with Intraluminal Device, Percutaneous Endoscopic Approach
02704T6	Dilation of Coronary Artery, One Site, Bifurcation, with Radioactive Intraluminal Device, Percutaneous Endoscopic Approach
02704TZ	Dilation of Coronary Artery, One Site with Radioactive Intraluminal Device, Percutaneous Endoscopic Approach
02704Z6	Dilation of Coronary Artery, One Site, Bifurcation, Percutaneous Endoscopic Approach
02704ZZ	Dilation of Coronary Artery, One Site, Percutaneous Endoscopic Approach
0271046	Dilation of Coronary Artery, Two Sites, Bifurcation, with Drug-eluting Intraluminal Device, Open Approach
027104Z	Dilation of Coronary Artery, Two Sites with Drug-eluting Intraluminal Device, Open Approach
02710D6	Dilation of Coronary Artery, Two Sites, Bifurcation, with Intraluminal Device, Open Approach
02710DZ	Dilation of Coronary Artery, Two Sites with Intraluminal Device, Open Approach
02710T6	Dilation of Coronary Artery, Two Sites, Bifurcation, with Radioactive Intraluminal Device, Open Approach
02710TZ	Dilation of Coronary Artery, Two Sites with Radioactive Intraluminal Device, Open Approach
02710Z6	Dilation of Coronary Artery, Two Sites, Bifurcation, Open Approach
02710ZZ	Dilation of Coronary Artery, Two Sites, Open Approach
0271346	Dilation of Coronary Artery, Two Sites, Bifurcation, with Drug-eluting Intraluminal Device, Percutaneous Approach

027134Z	Dilation of Coronary Artery, Two Sites with Drug-eluting Intraluminal Device, Percutaneous Approach
02713D6	Dilation of Coronary Artery, Two Sites, Bifurcation, with Intraluminal Device, Percutaneous Approach
02713DZ	Dilation of Coronary Artery, Two Sites with Intraluminal Device, Percutaneous Approach
02713T6	Dilation of Coronary Artery, Two Sites, Bifurcation, with Radioactive Intralumir Device, Percutaneous Approach
02713TZ	Dilation of Coronary Artery, Two Sites with Radioactive Intraluminal Device, Percutaneous Approach
02713Z6	Dilation of Coronary Artery, Two Sites, Bifurcation, Percutaneous Approach
02713ZZ	Dilation of Coronary Artery, Two Sites, Percutaneous Approach
0271446	Dilation of Coronary Artery, Two Sites, Bifurcation, with Drug-eluting Intraluminal Device, Percutaneous Endoscopic Approach
027144Z	Dilation of Coronary Artery, Two Sites with Drug-eluting Intraluminal Device, Percutaneous Endoscopic Approach
02714D6	Dilation of Coronary Artery, Two Sites, Bifurcation, with Intraluminal Device, Percutaneous Endoscopic Approach
02714DZ	Dilation of Coronary Artery, Two Sites with Intraluminal Device, Percutaneous Endoscopic Approach
02714T6	Dilation of Coronary Artery, Two Sites, Bifurcation, with Radioactive Intralumir Device, Percutaneous Endoscopic Approach
02714TZ	Dilation of Coronary Artery, Two Sites with Radioactive Intraluminal Device, Percutaneous Endoscopic Approach
02714Z6	Dilation of Coronary Artery, Two Sites, Bifurcation, Percutaneous Endoscopic Approach
02714ZZ	Dilation of Coronary Artery, Two Sites, Percutaneous Endoscopic Approach
0272046	Dilation of Coronary Artery, Three Sites, Bifurcation, with Drug-eluting Intraluminal Device, Open Approach

♀ Female-only	♂ Male-only	▲ Limited Coverage	● Non-OR	▨ HAC-associated procedure	▲ Non-covered procedures	✚ Combinati

7204Z Dilation of Coronary Artery, Three Sites with Drug-eluting Intraluminal Device, Open Approach

720D6 Dilation of Coronary Artery, Three Sites, Bifurcation, with Intraluminal Device, Open Approach

720DZ Dilation of Coronary Artery, Three Sites with Intraluminal Device, Open Approach

720T6 Dilation of Coronary Artery, Three Sites, Bifurcation, with Radioactive Intraluminal Device, Open Approach

720TZ Dilation of Coronary Artery, Three Sites with Radioactive Intraluminal Device, Open Approach

720Z6 Dilation of Coronary Artery, Three Sites, Bifurcation, Open Approach

720ZZ Dilation of Coronary Artery, Three Sites, Open Approach

72346 Dilation of Coronary Artery, Three Sites, Bifurcation, with Drug-eluting Intraluminal Device, Percutaneous Approach

7234Z Dilation of Coronary Artery, Three Sites with Drug-eluting Intraluminal Device, Percutaneous Approach

723D6 Dilation of Coronary Artery, Three Sites, Bifurcation, with Intraluminal Device, Percutaneous Approach

723DZ Dilation of Coronary Artery, Three Sites with Intraluminal Device, Percutaneous Approach

723T6 Dilation of Coronary Artery, Three Sites, Bifurcation, with Radioactive Intraluminal Device, Percutaneous Approach

723TZ Dilation of Coronary Artery, Three Sites with Radioactive Intraluminal Device, Percutaneous Approach

723Z6 Dilation of Coronary Artery, Three Sites, Bifurcation, Percutaneous Approach

723ZZ Dilation of Coronary Artery, Three Sites, Percutaneous Approach

72446 Dilation of Coronary Artery, Three Sites, Bifurcation, with Drug-eluting Intraluminal Device, Percutaneous Endoscopic Approach

7244Z Dilation of Coronary Artery, Three Sites with Drug-eluting Intraluminal Device, Percutaneous Endoscopic Approach

724D6 Dilation of Coronary Artery, Three Sites, Bifurcation, with Intraluminal Device, Percutaneous Endoscopic Approach

724DZ Dilation of Coronary Artery, Three Sites with Intraluminal Device, Percutaneous Endoscopic Approach

724T6 Dilation of Coronary Artery, Three Sites, Bifurcation, with Radioactive Intraluminal Device, Percutaneous Endoscopic Approach

724TZ Dilation of Coronary Artery, Three Sites with Radioactive Intraluminal Device, Percutaneous Endoscopic Approach

724Z6 Dilation of Coronary Artery, Three Sites, Bifurcation, Percutaneous Endoscopic Approach

724ZZ Dilation of Coronary Artery, Three Sites, Percutaneous Endoscopic Approach

273046 Dilation of Coronary Artery, Four or More Sites, Bifurcation, with Drug-eluting Intraluminal Device, Open Approach

27304Z Dilation of Coronary Artery, Four or More Sites with Drug-eluting Intraluminal Device, Open Approach

2730D6 Dilation of Coronary Artery, Four or More Sites, Bifurcation, with Intraluminal Device, Open Approach

2730DZ Dilation of Coronary Artery, Four or More Sites with Intraluminal Device, Open Approach

02730T6 Dilation of Coronary Artery, Four or More Sites, Bifurcation, with Radioactive Intraluminal Device, Open Approach

02730TZ Dilation of Coronary Artery, Four or More Sites with Radioactive Intraluminal Device, Open Approach

02730Z6 Dilation of Coronary Artery, Four or More Sites, Bifurcation, Open Approach

02730ZZ Dilation of Coronary Artery, Four or More Sites, Open Approach

0273346 Dilation of Coronary Artery, Four or More Sites, Bifurcation, with Drug-eluting Intraluminal Device, Percutaneous Approach

027334Z Dilation of Coronary Artery, Four or More Sites with Drug-eluting Intraluminal Device, Percutaneous Approach

02733D6 Dilation of Coronary Artery, Four or More Sites, Bifurcation, with Intraluminal Device, Percutaneous Approach

02733DZ Dilation of Coronary Artery, Four or More Sites with Intraluminal Device, Percutaneous Approach

02733T6 Dilation of Coronary Artery, Four or More Sites, Bifurcation, with Radioactive Intraluminal Device, Percutaneous Approach

02733TZ Dilation of Coronary Artery, Four or More Sites with Radioactive Intraluminal Device, Percutaneous Approach

02733Z6 Dilation of Coronary Artery, Four or More Sites, Bifurcation, Percutaneous Approach

02733ZZ Dilation of Coronary Artery, Four or More Sites, Percutaneous Approach

0273446 Dilation of Coronary Artery, Four or More Sites, Bifurcation, with Drug-eluting Intraluminal Device, Percutaneous Endoscopic Approach

027344Z Dilation of Coronary Artery, Four or More Sites with Drug-eluting Intraluminal Device, Percutaneous Endoscopic Approach

02734D6 Dilation of Coronary Artery, Four or More Sites, Bifurcation, with Intraluminal Device, Percutaneous Endoscopic Approach

02734DZ Dilation of Coronary Artery, Four or More Sites with Intraluminal Device, Percutaneous Endoscopic Approach

02734T6 Dilation of Coronary Artery, Four or More Sites, Bifurcation, with Radioactive Intraluminal Device, Percutaneous Endoscopic Approach

02734TZ Dilation of Coronary Artery, Four or More Sites with Radioactive Intraluminal Device, Percutaneous Endoscopic Approach

02734Z6 Dilation of Coronary Artery, Four or More Sites, Bifurcation, Percutaneous Endoscopic Approach

02734ZZ Dilation of Coronary Artery, Four or More Sites, Percutaneous Endoscopic Approach

027F04Z Dilation of Aortic Valve with Drug-eluting Intraluminal Device, Open Approach

027F0DZ Dilation of Aortic Valve with Intraluminal Device, Open Approach

027F0ZZ Dilation of Aortic Valve, Open Approach

027F34Z Dilation of Aortic Valve with Drug-eluting Intraluminal Device, Percutaneous Approach

027F3DZ Dilation of Aortic Valve with Intraluminal Device, Percutaneous Approach

027F3ZZ Dilation of Aortic Valve, Percutaneous Approach

027F44Z Dilation of Aortic Valve with Drug-eluting Intraluminal Device, Percutaneous Endoscopic Approach

027F4DZ Dilation of Aortic Valve with Intraluminal Device, Percutaneous Endoscopic Approach

027F4ZZ Dilation of Aortic Valve, Percutaneous Endoscopic Approach

027G04Z Dilation of Mitral Valve with Drug-eluting Intraluminal Device, Open Approach

027G0DZ Dilation of Mitral Valve with Intraluminal Device, Open Approach

027G0ZZ Dilation of Mitral Valve, Open Approach

027G34Z Dilation of Mitral Valve with Drug-eluting Intraluminal Device, Percutaneous Approach

027G3DZ Dilation of Mitral Valve with Intraluminal Device, Percutaneous Approach

027G3ZZ Dilation of Mitral Valve, Percutaneous Approach

027G44Z Dilation of Mitral Valve with Drug-eluting Intraluminal Device, Percutaneous Endoscopic Approach

027G4DZ Dilation of Mitral Valve with Intraluminal Device, Percutaneous Endoscopic Approach

027G4ZZ Dilation of Mitral Valve, Percutaneous Endoscopic Approach

027H04Z Dilation of Pulmonary Valve with Drug-eluting Intraluminal Device, Open Approach

027H0DZ Dilation of Pulmonary Valve with Intraluminal Device, Open Approach

027H0ZZ Dilation of Pulmonary Valve, Open Approach

027H34Z Dilation of Pulmonary Valve with Drug-eluting Intraluminal Device, Percutaneous Approach

027H3DZ Dilation of Pulmonary Valve with Intraluminal Device, Percutaneous Approach

027H3ZZ Dilation of Pulmonary Valve, Percutaneous Approach

027H44Z Dilation of Pulmonary Valve with Drug-eluting Intraluminal Device, Percutaneous Endoscopic Approach

027H4DZ Dilation of Pulmonary Valve with Intraluminal Device, Percutaneous Endoscopic Approach

027H4ZZ Dilation of Pulmonary Valve, Percutaneous Endoscopic Approach

027J04Z Dilation of Tricuspid Valve with Drug-eluting Intraluminal Device, Open Approach

027J0DZ Dilation of Tricuspid Valve with Intraluminal Device, Open Approach

027J0ZZ Dilation of Tricuspid Valve, Open Approach

027J34Z Dilation of Tricuspid Valve with Drug-eluting Intraluminal Device, Percutaneous Approach

027J3DZ Dilation of Tricuspid Valve with Intraluminal Device, Percutaneous Approach

027J3ZZ Dilation of Tricuspid Valve, Percutaneous Approach

027J44Z Dilation of Tricuspid Valve with Drug-eluting Intraluminal Device, Percutaneous Endoscopic Approach

027J4DZ Dilation of Tricuspid Valve with Intraluminal Device, Percutaneous Endoscopic Approach

027J4ZZ Dilation of Tricuspid Valve, Percutaneous Endoscopic Approach

027K04Z Dilation of Right Ventricle with Drug-eluting Intraluminal Device, Open Approach

027K0DZ Dilation of Right Ventricle with Intraluminal Device, Open Approach

027K0ZZ Dilation of Right Ventricle, Open Approach

027K34Z	Dilation of Right Ventricle with Drug-eluting Intraluminal Device, Percutaneous Approach
027K3DZ	Dilation of Right Ventricle with Intraluminal Device, Percutaneous Approach
027K3ZZ	Dilation of Right Ventricle, Percutaneous Approach
027K44Z	Dilation of Right Ventricle with Drug-eluting Intraluminal Device, Percutaneous Endoscopic Approach
027K4DZ	Dilation of Right Ventricle with Intraluminal Device, Percutaneous Endoscopic Approach
027K4ZZ	Dilation of Right Ventricle, Percutaneous Endoscopic Approach
027P04Z	Dilation of Pulmonary Trunk with Drug-eluting Intraluminal Device, Open Approach
027P0DZ	Dilation of Pulmonary Trunk with Intraluminal Device, Open Approach
027P0ZZ	Dilation of Pulmonary Trunk, Open Approach
027P34Z	Dilation of Pulmonary Trunk with Drug-eluting Intraluminal Device, Percutaneous Approach
027P3DZ	Dilation of Pulmonary Trunk with Intraluminal Device, Percutaneous Approach
027P3ZZ	Dilation of Pulmonary Trunk, Percutaneous Approach
027P44Z	Dilation of Pulmonary Trunk with Drug-eluting Intraluminal Device, Percutaneous Endoscopic Approach
027P4DZ	Dilation of Pulmonary Trunk with Intraluminal Device, Percutaneous Endoscopic Approach
027P4ZZ	Dilation of Pulmonary Trunk, Percutaneous Endoscopic Approach
027Q04Z	Dilation of Right Pulmonary Artery with Drug-eluting Intraluminal Device, Open Approach
027Q0DZ	Dilation of Right Pulmonary Artery with Intraluminal Device, Open Approach
027Q0ZZ	Dilation of Right Pulmonary Artery, Open Approach
027Q34Z	Dilation of Right Pulmonary Artery with Drug-eluting Intraluminal Device, Percutaneous Approach
027Q3DZ	Dilation of Right Pulmonary Artery with Intraluminal Device, Percutaneous Approach
027Q3ZZ	Dilation of Right Pulmonary Artery, Percutaneous Approach
027Q44Z	Dilation of Right Pulmonary Artery with Drug-eluting Intraluminal Device, Percutaneous Endoscopic Approach
027Q4DZ	Dilation of Right Pulmonary Artery with Intraluminal Device, Percutaneous Endoscopic Approach
027Q4ZZ	Dilation of Right Pulmonary Artery, Percutaneous Endoscopic Approach
027R04T	Dilation of Ductus Arteriosus with Drug-eluting Intraluminal Device, Open Approach
027R04Z	Dilation of Left Pulmonary Artery with Drug-eluting Intraluminal Device, Open Approach

027R0DT	Dilation of Ductus Arteriosus with Intraluminal Device, Open Approach
027R0DZ	Dilation of Left Pulmonary Artery with Intraluminal Device, Open Approach
027R0ZT	Dilation of Ductus Arteriosus, Open Approach
027R0ZZ	Dilation of Left Pulmonary Artery, Open Approach
027R34T	Dilation of Ductus Arteriosus with Drug-eluting Intraluminal Device, Percutaneous Approach
027R34Z	Dilation of Left Pulmonary Artery with Drug-eluting Intraluminal Device, Percutaneous Approach
027R3DT	Dilation of Ductus Arteriosus with Intraluminal Device, Percutaneous Approach
027R3DZ	Dilation of Left Pulmonary Artery with Intraluminal Device, Percutaneous Approach
027R3ZT	Dilation of Ductus Arteriosus, Percutaneous Approach
027R3ZZ	Dilation of Left Pulmonary Artery, Percutaneous Approach
027R44T	Dilation of Ductus Arteriosus with Drug-eluting Intraluminal Device, Percutaneous Endoscopic Approach
027R44Z	Dilation of Left Pulmonary Artery with Drug-eluting Intraluminal Device, Percutaneous Endoscopic Approach
027R4DT	Dilation of Ductus Arteriosus with Intraluminal Device, Percutaneous Endoscopic Approach
027R4DZ	Dilation of Left Pulmonary Artery with Intraluminal Device, Percutaneous Endoscopic Approach
027R4ZT	Dilation of Ductus Arteriosus, Percutaneous Endoscopic Approach
027R4ZZ	Dilation of Left Pulmonary Artery, Percutaneous Endoscopic Approach
027S04Z	Dilation of Right Pulmonary Vein with Drug-eluting Intraluminal Device, Open Approach
027S0DZ	Dilation of Right Pulmonary Vein with Intraluminal Device, Open Approach
027S0ZZ	Dilation of Right Pulmonary Vein, Open Approach
027S34Z	Dilation of Right Pulmonary Vein with Drug-eluting Intraluminal Device, Percutaneous Approach
027S3DZ	Dilation of Right Pulmonary Vein with Intraluminal Device, Percutaneous Approach
027S3ZZ	Dilation of Right Pulmonary Vein, Percutaneous Approach
027S44Z	Dilation of Right Pulmonary Vein with Drug-eluting Intraluminal Device, Percutaneous Endoscopic Approach
027S4DZ	Dilation of Right Pulmonary Vein with Intraluminal Device, Percutaneous Endoscopic Approach
027S4ZZ	Dilation of Right Pulmonary Vein, Percutaneous Endoscopic Approach
027T04Z	Dilation of Left Pulmonary Vein with Drug-eluting Intraluminal Device, Open Approach

027T0DZ	Dilation of Left Pulmonary Vein with Intraluminal Device, Open Approach
027T0ZZ	Dilation of Left Pulmonary Vein, Open Approach
027T34Z	Dilation of Left Pulmonary Vein with Drug-eluting Intraluminal Device, Percutaneous Approach
027T3DZ	Dilation of Left Pulmonary Vein with Intraluminal Device, Percutaneous Approach
027T3ZZ	Dilation of Left Pulmonary Vein, Percutaneous Approach
027T44Z	Dilation of Left Pulmonary Vein with Drug-eluting Intraluminal Device, Percutaneous Endoscopic Approach
027T4DZ	Dilation of Left Pulmonary Vein with Intraluminal Device, Percutaneous Endoscopic Approach
027T4ZZ	Dilation of Left Pulmonary Vein, Percutaneous Endoscopic Approach
027V04Z	Dilation of Superior Vena Cava with Drug-eluting Intraluminal Device, Open Approach
027V0DZ	Dilation of Superior Vena Cava with Intraluminal Device, Open Approach
027V0ZZ	Dilation of Superior Vena Cava, Open Approach
027V34Z	Dilation of Superior Vena Cava with Drug-eluting Intraluminal Device, Percutaneous Approach
027V3DZ	Dilation of Superior Vena Cava with Intraluminal Device, Percutaneous Approach
027V3ZZ	Dilation of Superior Vena Cava, Percutaneous Approach
027V44Z	Dilation of Superior Vena Cava with Drug-eluting Intraluminal Device, Percutaneous Endoscopic Approach
027V4DZ	Dilation of Superior Vena Cava with Intraluminal Device, Percutaneous Endoscopic Approach
027V4ZZ	Dilation of Superior Vena Cava, Percutaneous Endoscopic Approach
027W04Z	Dilation of Thoracic Aorta with Drug-eluting Intraluminal Device, Open Approach
027W0DZ	Dilation of Thoracic Aorta with Intraluminal Device, Open Approach
027W0ZZ	Dilation of Thoracic Aorta, Open Approach
027W34Z	Dilation of Thoracic Aorta with Drug-eluting Intraluminal Device, Percutaneous Approach
027W3DZ	Dilation of Thoracic Aorta with Intraluminal Device, Percutaneous Approach
027W3ZZ	Dilation of Thoracic Aorta, Percutaneous Approach
027W44Z	Dilation of Thoracic Aorta with Drug-eluting Intraluminal Device, Percutaneous Endoscopic Approach
027W4DZ	Dilation of Thoracic Aorta with Intraluminal Device, Percutaneous Endoscopic Approach
027W4ZZ	Dilation of Thoracic Aorta, Percutaneous Endoscopic Approach

028 – Heart and Great Vessels, Division

Review Coding Guideline B3.14

02880ZZ	Division of Conduction Mechanism, Open Approach
02883ZZ	Division of Conduction Mechanism, Percutaneous Approach
02884ZZ	Division of Conduction Mechanism, Percutaneous Endoscopic Approach

02890ZZ	Division of Chordae Tendineae, Open Approach
02893ZZ	Division of Chordae Tendineae, Percutaneous Approach
02894ZZ	Division of Chordae Tendineae, Percutaneous Endoscopic Approach

028D0ZZ	Division of Papillary Muscle, Open Approach
028D3ZZ	Division of Papillary Muscle, Percutaneous Approach
028D4ZZ	Division of Papillary Muscle, Percutaneous Endoscopic Approach

B – Heart and Great Vessels, Excision

view Coding Guidelines B3.4a and B3.4b

view Coding Guideline B3.8

340ZX Excision of Coronary Vein, Open Approach, Diagnostic
340ZZ Excision of Coronary Vein, Open Approach
343ZX Excision of Coronary Vein, Percutaneous Approach, Diagnostic
343ZZ Excision of Coronary Vein, Percutaneous Approach
344ZX Excision of Coronary Vein, Percutaneous Endoscopic Approach, Diagnostic
344ZZ Excision of Coronary Vein, Percutaneous Endoscopic Approach
350ZX Excision of Atrial Septum, Open Approach, Diagnostic
350ZZ Excision of Atrial Septum, Open Approach
353ZX Excision of Atrial Septum, Percutaneous Approach, Diagnostic
353ZZ Excision of Atrial Septum, Percutaneous Approach
354ZX Excision of Atrial Septum, Percutaneous Endoscopic Approach, Diagnostic
354ZZ Excision of Atrial Septum, Percutaneous Endoscopic Approach
360ZX Excision of Right Atrium, Open Approach, Diagnostic
360ZZ Excision of Right Atrium, Open Approach
363ZX Excision of Right Atrium, Percutaneous Approach, Diagnostic
363ZZ Excision of Right Atrium, Percutaneous Approach
364ZX Excision of Right Atrium, Percutaneous Endoscopic Approach, Diagnostic
364ZZ Excision of Right Atrium, Percutaneous Endoscopic Approach
2B70ZK Excision of Left Atrial Appendage, Open Approach
B70ZX Excision of Left Atrium, Open Approach, Diagnostic
B70ZZ Excision of Left Atrium, Open Approach
2B73ZK Excision of Left Atrial Appendage, Percutaneous Approach
B73ZX Excision of Left Atrium, Percutaneous Approach, Diagnostic
B73ZZ Excision of Left Atrium, Percutaneous Approach
2B74ZK Excision of Left Atrial Appendage, Percutaneous Endoscopic Approach
B74ZX Excision of Left Atrium, Percutaneous Endoscopic Approach, Diagnostic
B74ZZ Excision of Left Atrium, Percutaneous Endoscopic Approach
B80ZX Excision of Conduction Mechanism, Open Approach, Diagnostic
B80ZZ Excision of Conduction Mechanism, Open Approach
2B83ZX Excision of Conduction Mechanism, Percutaneous Approach, Diagnostic
2B83ZZ Excision of Conduction Mechanism, Percutaneous Approach
2B84ZX Excision of Conduction Mechanism, Percutaneous Endoscopic Approach, Diagnostic
2B84ZZ Excision of Conduction Mechanism, Percutaneous Endoscopic Approach
2B90ZX Excision of Chordae Tendineae, Open Approach, Diagnostic
2B90ZZ Excision of Chordae Tendineae, Open Approach
2B93ZX Excision of Chordae Tendineae, Percutaneous Approach, Diagnostic
2B93ZZ Excision of Chordae Tendineae, Percutaneous Approach

02B94ZX Excision of Chordae Tendineae, Percutaneous Endoscopic Approach, Diagnostic
02B94ZZ Excision of Chordae Tendineae, Percutaneous Endoscopic Approach
02BD0ZX Excision of Papillary Muscle, Open Approach, Diagnostic
02BD0ZZ Excision of Papillary Muscle, Open Approach
02BD3ZX Excision of Papillary Muscle, Percutaneous Approach, Diagnostic
02BD3ZZ Excision of Papillary Muscle, Percutaneous Approach
02BD4ZX Excision of Papillary Muscle, Percutaneous Endoscopic Approach, Diagnostic
02BD4ZZ Excision of Papillary Muscle, Percutaneous Endoscopic Approach
02BF0ZX Excision of Aortic Valve, Open Approach, Diagnostic
02BF0ZZ Excision of Aortic Valve, Open Approach
02BF3ZX Excision of Aortic Valve, Percutaneous Approach, Diagnostic
02BF3ZZ Excision of Aortic Valve, Percutaneous Approach
02BF4ZX Excision of Aortic Valve, Percutaneous Endoscopic Approach, Diagnostic
02BF4ZZ Excision of Aortic Valve, Percutaneous Endoscopic Approach
02BG0ZX Excision of Mitral Valve, Open Approach, Diagnostic
02BG0ZZ Excision of Mitral Valve, Open Approach
02BG3ZX Excision of Mitral Valve, Percutaneous Approach, Diagnostic
02BG3ZZ Excision of Mitral Valve, Percutaneous Approach
02BG4ZX Excision of Mitral Valve, Percutaneous Endoscopic Approach, Diagnostic
02BG4ZZ Excision of Mitral Valve, Percutaneous Endoscopic Approach
02BH0ZX Excision of Pulmonary Valve, Open Approach, Diagnostic
02BH0ZZ Excision of Pulmonary Valve, Open Approach
02BH3ZX Excision of Pulmonary Valve, Percutaneous Approach, Diagnostic
02BH3ZZ Excision of Pulmonary Valve, Percutaneous Approach
02BH4ZX Excision of Pulmonary Valve, Percutaneous Endoscopic Approach, Diagnostic
02BH4ZZ Excision of Pulmonary Valve, Percutaneous Endoscopic Approach
02BJ0ZX Excision of Tricuspid Valve, Open Approach, Diagnostic
02BJ0ZZ Excision of Tricuspid Valve, Open Approach
02BJ3ZX Excision of Tricuspid Valve, Percutaneous Approach, Diagnostic
02BJ3ZZ Excision of Tricuspid Valve, Percutaneous Approach
02BJ4ZX Excision of Tricuspid Valve, Percutaneous Endoscopic Approach, Diagnostic
02BJ4ZZ Excision of Tricuspid Valve, Percutaneous Endoscopic Approach
02BK0ZX Excision of Right Ventricle, Open Approach, Diagnostic
▲ 02BK0ZZ Excision of Right Ventricle, Open Approach
02BK3ZX Excision of Right Ventricle, Percutaneous Approach, Diagnostic

▲ 02BK3ZZ Excision of Right Ventricle, Percutaneous Approach
02BK4ZX Excision of Right Ventricle, Percutaneous Endoscopic Approach, Diagnostic
▲ 02BK4ZZ Excision of Right Ventricle, Percutaneous Endoscopic Approach
02BL0ZX Excision of Left Ventricle, Open Approach, Diagnostic
▲ 02BL0ZZ Excision of Left Ventricle, Open Approach
02BL3ZX Excision of Left Ventricle, Percutaneous Approach, Diagnostic
▲ 02BL3ZZ Excision of Left Ventricle, Percutaneous Approach
02BL4ZX Excision of Left Ventricle, Percutaneous Endoscopic Approach, Diagnostic
▲ 02BL4ZZ Excision of Left Ventricle, Percutaneous Endoscopic Approach
02BM0ZX Excision of Ventricular Septum, Open Approach, Diagnostic
02BM0ZZ Excision of Ventricular Septum, Open Approach
02BM3ZX Excision of Ventricular Septum, Percutaneous Approach, Diagnostic
02BM3ZZ Excision of Ventricular Septum, Percutaneous Approach
02BM4ZX Excision of Ventricular Septum, Percutaneous Endoscopic Approach, Diagnostic
02BM4ZZ Excision of Ventricular Septum, Percutaneous Endoscopic Approach
02BN0ZX Excision of Pericardium, Open Approach, Diagnostic
02BN0ZZ Excision of Pericardium, Open Approach
02BN3ZX Excision of Pericardium, Percutaneous Approach, Diagnostic
02BN3ZZ Excision of Pericardium, Percutaneous Approach
02BN4ZX Excision of Pericardium, Percutaneous Endoscopic Approach, Diagnostic
02BN4ZZ Excision of Pericardium, Percutaneous Endoscopic Approach
02BP0ZX Excision of Pulmonary Trunk, Open Approach, Diagnostic
02BP0ZZ Excision of Pulmonary Trunk, Open Approach
02BP3ZX Excision of Pulmonary Trunk, Percutaneous Approach, Diagnostic
02BP3ZZ Excision of Pulmonary Trunk, Percutaneous Approach
02BP4ZX Excision of Pulmonary Trunk, Percutaneous Endoscopic Approach, Diagnostic
02BP4ZZ Excision of Pulmonary Trunk, Percutaneous Endoscopic Approach
02BQ0ZX Excision of Right Pulmonary Artery, Open Approach, Diagnostic
02BQ0ZZ Excision of Right Pulmonary Artery, Open Approach
02BQ3ZX Excision of Right Pulmonary Artery, Percutaneous Approach, Diagnostic
02BQ3ZZ Excision of Right Pulmonary Artery, Percutaneous Approach
02BQ4ZX Excision of Right Pulmonary Artery, Percutaneous Endoscopic Approach, Diagnostic
02BQ4ZZ Excision of Right Pulmonary Artery, Percutaneous Endoscopic Approach
02BR0ZX Excision of Left Pulmonary Artery, Open Approach, Diagnostic
02BR0ZZ Excision of Left Pulmonary Artery, Open Approach

Female-only   ♂ Male-only   ▲ Limited Coverage   ● Non-OR   HAC-associated procedure   ▲ Non-covered procedures   + Combination

02BR3ZX Excision of Left Pulmonary Artery, Percutaneous Approach, Diagnostic

02BR3ZZ Excision of Left Pulmonary Artery, Percutaneous Approach

02BR4ZX Excision of Left Pulmonary Artery, Percutaneous Endoscopic Approach, Diagnostic

02BR4ZZ Excision of Left Pulmonary Artery, Percutaneous Endoscopic Approach

02BS0ZX Excision of Right Pulmonary Vein, Open Approach, Diagnostic

02BS0ZZ Excision of Right Pulmonary Vein, Open Approach

02BS3ZX Excision of Right Pulmonary Vein, Percutaneous Approach, Diagnostic

02BS3ZZ Excision of Right Pulmonary Vein, Percutaneous Approach

02BS4ZX Excision of Right Pulmonary Vein, Percutaneous Endoscopic Approach, Diagnostic

02BS4ZZ Excision of Right Pulmonary Vein, Percutaneous Endoscopic Approach

02BT0ZX Excision of Left Pulmonary Vein, Open Approach, Diagnostic

02BT0ZZ Excision of Left Pulmonary Vein, Open Approach

02BT3ZX Excision of Left Pulmonary Vein, Percutaneous Approach, Diagnostic

02BT3ZZ Excision of Left Pulmonary Vein, Percutaneous Approach

02BT4ZX Excision of Left Pulmonary Vein, Percutaneous Endoscopic Approach, Diagnostic

02BT4ZZ Excision of Left Pulmonary Vein, Percutaneous Endoscopic Approach

02BV0ZX Excision of Superior Vena Cava, Open Approach, Diagnostic

02BV0ZZ Excision of Superior Vena Cava, Open Approach

02BV3ZX Excision of Superior Vena Cava, Percutaneous Approach, Diagnostic

02BV3ZZ Excision of Superior Vena Cava, Percutaneous Approach

02BV4ZX Excision of Superior Vena Cava, Percutaneous Endoscopic Approach, Diagnostic

02BV4ZZ Excision of Superior Vena Cava, Percutaneous Endoscopic Approach

02BW0ZX Excision of Thoracic Aorta, Open Approach, Diagnostic

02BW0ZZ Excision of Thoracic Aorta, Open Appro

02BW3ZX Excision of Thoracic Aorta, Percutaneo Approach, Diagnostic

02BW3ZZ Excision of Thoracic Aorta, Percutaneo Approach

02BW4ZX Excision of Thoracic Aorta, Percutaneo Endoscopic Approach, Diagnostic

02BW4ZZ Excision of Thoracic Aorta, Percutaneo Endoscopic Approach

02C – Heart and Great Vessels, Extirpation

For Extirpation procedures involving coronary arteries, Review Coding Guideline B4.4

02C00ZZ Extirpation of Matter from Coronary Artery, One Site, Open Approach

02C03ZZ Extirpation of Matter from Coronary Artery, One Site, Percutaneous Approach

02C04ZZ Extirpation of Matter from Coronary Artery, One Site, Percutaneous Endoscopic Approach

02C10ZZ Extirpation of Matter from Coronary Artery, Two Sites, Open Approach

02C13ZZ Extirpation of Matter from Coronary Artery, Two Sites, Percutaneous Approach

02C14ZZ Extirpation of Matter from Coronary Artery, Two Sites, Percutaneous Endoscopic Approach

02C20ZZ Extirpation of Matter from Coronary Artery, Three Sites, Open Approach

02C23ZZ Extirpation of Matter from Coronary Artery, Three Sites, Percutaneous Approach

02C24ZZ Extirpation of Matter from Coronary Artery, Three Sites, Percutaneous Endoscopic Approach

02C30ZZ Extirpation of Matter from Coronary Artery, Four or More Sites, Open Approach

02C33ZZ Extirpation of Matter from Coronary Artery, Four or More Sites, Percutaneous Approach

02C34ZZ Extirpation of Matter from Coronary Artery, Four or More Sites, Percutaneous Endoscopic Approach

02C40ZZ Extirpation of Matter from Coronary Vein, Open Approach

02C43ZZ Extirpation of Matter from Coronary Vein, Percutaneous Approach

02C44ZZ Extirpation of Matter from Coronary Vein, Percutaneous Endoscopic Approach

02C50ZZ Extirpation of Matter from Atrial Septum, Open Approach

02C53ZZ Extirpation of Matter from Atrial Septum, Percutaneous Approach

02C54ZZ Extirpation of Matter from Atrial Septum, Percutaneous Endoscopic Approach

02C60ZZ Extirpation of Matter from Right Atrium, Open Approach

02C63ZZ Extirpation of Matter from Right Atrium, Percutaneous Approach

02C64ZZ Extirpation of Matter from Right Atrium, Percutaneous Endoscopic Approach

02C70ZZ Extirpation of Matter from Left Atrium, Open Approach

02C73ZZ Extirpation of Matter from Left Atrium, Percutaneous Approach

02C74ZZ Extirpation of Matter from Left Atrium, Percutaneous Endoscopic Approach

02C80ZZ Extirpation of Matter from Conduction Mechanism, Open Approach

02C83ZZ Extirpation of Matter from Conduction Mechanism, Percutaneous Approach

02C84ZZ Extirpation of Matter from Conduction Mechanism, Percutaneous Endoscopic Approach

02C90ZZ Extirpation of Matter from Chordae Tendineae, Open Approach

02C93ZZ Extirpation of Matter from Chordae Tendineae, Percutaneous Approach

02C94ZZ Extirpation of Matter from Chordae Tendineae, Percutaneous Endoscopic Approach

02CD0ZZ Extirpation of Matter from Papillary Muscle, Open Approach

02CD3ZZ Extirpation of Matter from Papillary Muscle, Percutaneous Approach

02CD4ZZ Extirpation of Matter from Papillary Muscle, Percutaneous Endoscopic Approach

02CF0ZZ Extirpation of Matter from Aortic Valve, Open Approach

02CF3ZZ Extirpation of Matter from Aortic Valve, Percutaneous Approach

02CF4ZZ Extirpation of Matter from Aortic Valve, Percutaneous Endoscopic Approach

02CG0ZZ Extirpation of Matter from Mitral Valve, Open Approach

02CG3ZZ Extirpation of Matter from Mitral Valve, Percutaneous Approach

02CG4ZZ Extirpation of Matter from Mitral Valve, Percutaneous Endoscopic Approach

02CH0ZZ Extirpation of Matter from Pulmonary Valve, Open Approach

02CH3ZZ Extirpation of Matter from Pulmonary Valve, Percutaneous Approach

02CH4ZZ Extirpation of Matter from Pulmonary Valve, Percutaneous Endoscopic Approach

02CJ0ZZ Extirpation of Matter from Tricuspid Valve, Open Approach

02CJ3ZZ Extirpation of Matter from Tricuspid Valve, Percutaneous Approach

02CJ4ZZ Extirpation of Matter from Tricuspid Valve, Percutaneous Endoscopic Approach

02CK0ZZ Extirpation of Matter from Right Ventricle, Open Approach

02CK3ZZ Extirpation of Matter from Right Ventricle, Percutaneous Approach

02CK4ZZ Extirpation of Matter from Right Ventricle, Percutaneous Endoscopic Approach

02CL0ZZ Extirpation of Matter from Left Ventricl Open Approach

02CL3ZZ Extirpation of Matter from Left Ventricl Percutaneous Approach

02CL4ZZ Extirpation of Matter from Left Ventricl Percutaneous Endoscopic Approach

02CM0ZZ Extirpation of Matter from Ventricular Septum, Open Approach

02CM3ZZ Extirpation of Matter from Ventricular Septum, Percutaneous Approach

02CM4ZZ Extirpation of Matter from Ventricular Septum, Percutaneous Endoscopic Approach

02CN0ZZ Extirpation of Matter from Pericardium, Open Approach

02CN3ZZ Extirpation of Matter from Pericardium, Percutaneous Approach

02CN4ZZ Extirpation of Matter from Pericardium, Percutaneous Endoscopic Approach

02CP0ZZ Extirpation of Matter from Pulmonary Trunk, Open Approach

02CP3ZZ Extirpation of Matter from Pulmonary Trunk, Percutaneous Approach

02CP4ZZ Extirpation of Matter from Pulmonary Trunk, Percutaneous Endoscopic Approach

02CQ0ZZ Extirpation of Matter from Right Pulmonary Artery, Open Approach

02CQ3ZZ Extirpation of Matter from Right Pulmonary Artery, Percutaneous Approa

02CQ4ZZ Extirpation of Matter from Right Pulmonary Artery, Percutaneous Endoscopic Approach

02CR0ZZ Extirpation of Matter from Left Pulmona Artery, Open Approach

02CR3ZZ Extirpation of Matter from Left Pulmona Artery, Percutaneous Approach

02CR4ZZ Extirpation of Matter from Left Pulmona Artery, Percutaneous Endoscopic Approach

02CS0ZZ Extirpation of Matter from Right Pulmonary Vein, Open Approach

02CS3ZZ Extirpation of Matter from Right Pulmonary Vein, Percutaneous Approach

02CS4ZZ Extirpation of Matter from Right Pulmonary Vein, Percutaneous Endoscop Approach

02CT0ZZ Extirpation of Matter from Left Pulmona Vein, Open Approach

02CT3ZZ Extirpation of Matter from Left Pulmona Vein, Percutaneous Approach

02CT4ZZ Extirpation of Matter from Left Pulmona Vein, Percutaneous Endoscopic Approac

♀ Female-only   ♂ Male-only   ▲ Limited Coverage   ● Non-OR   ▥ HAC-associated procedure   ▲ Non-covered procedures   ✚ Combinati

CV0ZZ Extirpation of Matter from Superior Vena Cava, Open Approach

CV3ZZ Extirpation of Matter from Superior Vena Cava, Percutaneous Approach

02CV4ZZ Extirpation of Matter from Superior Vena Cava, Percutaneous Endoscopic Approach

02CW0ZZ Extirpation of Matter from Thoracic Aorta, Open Approach

02CW3ZZ Extirpation of Matter from Thoracic Aorta, Percutaneous Approach

02CW4ZZ Extirpation of Matter from Thoracic Aorta, Percutaneous Endoscopic Approach

'F – Heart and Great Vessels, Fragmentation

FN0ZZ Fragmentation in Pericardium, Open Approach

FN3ZZ Fragmentation in Pericardium, Percutaneous Approach

02FN4ZZ Fragmentation in Pericardium, Percutaneous Endoscopic Approach

▲ 02FNXZZ Fragmentation in Pericardium, External Approach

'H – Heart and Great Vessels, Insertion

H400Z Insertion of Pressure Sensor Monitoring Device into Coronary Vein, Open Approach

H402Z Insertion of Monitoring Device into Coronary Vein, Open Approach

H403Z Insertion of Infusion Device into Coronary Vein, Open Approach

H40DZ Insertion of Intraluminal Device into Coronary Vein, Open Approach

2H40JZ Insertion of Pacemaker Lead into Coronary Vein, Open Approach

+ Lead device when reported with an Insertion of a pacemaker device or cardiac rhythm related device (6th character 4, 5, 6 or P) into the chest or abdomen subcutaneous tissue and fascia. *See table 0JH to construct the Insertion code.* When a device is replaced, also report the Removal of a cardiac rhythm related device (6th character P) from the trunk subcutaneous tissue and fascia. *See table 0JP to construct the Removal code.*

H40KZ Insertion of Defibrillator Lead into Coronary Vein, Open Approach

2H40MZ Insertion of Cardiac Lead into Coronary Vein, Open Approach

+ Lead device when reported with an Insertion of a pacemaker device or cardiac rhythm related device (6th character 4, 5, 6 or P) into the chest or abdomen subcutaneous tissue and fascia. *See table 0JH to construct the Insertion code.* When a device is replaced, also report the Removal of a cardiac rhythm related device (6th character P) from the trunk subcutaneous tissue and fascia. *See table 0JP to construct the Removal code.*

2H430Z Insertion of Pressure Sensor Monitoring Device into Coronary Vein, Percutaneous Approach

2H432Z Insertion of Monitoring Device into Coronary Vein, Percutaneous Approach

2H433Z Insertion of Infusion Device into Coronary Vein, Percutaneous Approach

2H43DZ Insertion of Intraluminal Device into Coronary Vein, Percutaneous Approach

2H43JZ Insertion of Pacemaker Lead into Coronary Vein, Percutaneous Approach

▪ With a secondary diagnosis code of K68.11, T81.4XXA, T82.6XXA, T82.7XXA

2H43KZ Insertion of Defibrillator Lead into Coronary Vein, Percutaneous Approach

▪ With a secondary diagnosis code of K68.11, T81.4XXA, T82.6XXA, T82.7XXA

2H43MZ Insertion of Cardiac Lead into Coronary Vein, Percutaneous Approach

▪ With a secondary diagnosis code of K68.11, T81.4XXA, T82.6XXA, T82.7XXA

2H440Z Insertion of Pressure Sensor Monitoring Device into Coronary Vein, Percutaneous Endoscopic Approach

2H442Z Insertion of Monitoring Device into Coronary Vein, Percutaneous Endoscopic Approach

02H443Z Insertion of Infusion Device into Coronary Vein, Percutaneous Endoscopic Approach

02H44DZ Insertion of Intraluminal Device into Coronary Vein, Percutaneous Endoscopic Approach

● 02H44JZ Insertion of Pacemaker Lead into Coronary Vein, Percutaneous Endoscopic Approach

+ Lead device when reported with an Insertion of a pacemaker device or cardiac rhythm related device (6th character 4, 5, 6 or P) into the chest or abdomen subcutaneous tissue and fascia. *See table 0JH to construct the Insertion code.* When a device is replaced, also report the Removal of a cardiac rhythm related device (6th character P) from the trunk subcutaneous tissue and fascia. *See table 0JP to construct the Removal code.*

02H44KZ Insertion of Defibrillator Lead into Coronary Vein, Percutaneous Endoscopic Approach

● 02H44MZ Insertion of Cardiac Lead into Coronary Vein, Percutaneous Endoscopic Approach

+ Lead device when reported with an Insertion of a pacemaker device or cardiac rhythm related device (6th character 4, 5, 6 or P) into the chest or abdomen subcutaneous tissue and fascia. *See table 0JH to construct the Insertion code.* When a device is replaced, also report the Removal of a cardiac rhythm related device (6th character P) from the trunk subcutaneous tissue and fascia. *See table 0JP to construct the Removal code.*

02H600Z Insertion of Pressure Sensor Monitoring Device into Right Atrium, Open Approach

02H602Z Insertion of Monitoring Device into Right Atrium, Open Approach

02H603Z Insertion of Infusion Device into Right Atrium, Open Approach

02H60DZ Insertion of Intraluminal Device into Right Atrium, Open Approach

● 02H60JZ Insertion of Pacemaker Lead into Right Atrium, Open Approach

+ Lead device when reported with an Insertion of a pacemaker device or cardiac rhythm related device (6th character 4, 5, 6 or P) into the chest or abdomen subcutaneous tissue and fascia. *See table 0JH to construct the Insertion code.* When a device is replaced, also report the Removal of a cardiac rhythm related device (6th character P) from the trunk subcutaneous tissue and fascia. *See table 0JP to construct the Removal code.*

02H60KZ Insertion of Defibrillator Lead into Right Atrium, Open Approach

+ Lead device when reported with an Insertion of a defibrillator generator (6th character 8) into the chest or abdomen subcutaneous tissue and fascia. *See table 0JH to construct the Insertion code.*

● 02H60MZ Insertion of Cardiac Lead into Right Atrium, Open Approach

+ Lead device when reported with an Insertion of a pacemaker device or cardiac rhythm related device (6th character 4, 5, 6 or P) into the chest or abdomen subcutaneous tissue and fascia. *See table 0JH to construct the Insertion code.* When a device is replaced, also report the Removal of a cardiac rhythm related device (6th character P) from the trunk subcutaneous tissue and fascia. *See table 0JP to construct the Removal code.*

02H630Z Insertion of Pressure Sensor Monitoring Device into Right Atrium, Percutaneous Approach

02H632Z Insertion of Monitoring Device into Right Atrium, Percutaneous Approach

● 02H633Z Insertion of Infusion Device into Right Atrium, Percutaneous Approach

02H63DZ Insertion of Intraluminal Device into Right Atrium, Percutaneous Approach

● 02H63JZ Insertion of Pacemaker Lead into Right Atrium, Percutaneous Approach

▪ With a secondary diagnosis code of K68.11, T81.4XXA, T82.6XXA, T82.7XXA

+ Lead device when reported with an Insertion of a pacemaker device or cardiac rhythm related device (6th character 4, 5, 6 or P) into the chest or abdomen subcutaneous tissue and fascia. *See table 0JH to construct the Insertion code.* When a device is replaced, also report the removal of a cardiac rhythm related device (6th character P) from the trunk subcutaneous tissue and fascia. *See table 0JP to construct the Removal code.* When a cardiac lead is replaced, also report the removal of cardiac lead (6th character M) from the heart. *See table 02P to construct the Removal code.*

02H63KZ Insertion of Defibrillator Lead into Right Atrium, Percutaneous Approach

+ Lead device when reported with an Insertion of a defibrillator generator (6th character 8) into the chest or abdomen subcutaneous tissue and fascia. *See table 0JH to construct the Insertion code.*

02H63MZ Insertion of Cardiac Lead into Right Atrium, Percutaneous Approach

+ Lead device when reported with an Insertion of a pacemaker device or cardiac rhythm related device (6th character 4, 5, 6 or P) into the chest or abdomen subcutaneous tissue and fascia. *See table 0JH to construct the Insertion code.* When a device is replaced, also report the Removal of a cardiac rhythm related device (6th character P) from the trunk subcutaneous tissue and fascia. *See table 0JP to construct the Removal code.*

▪ With a secondary diagnosis code of K68.11, T81.4XXA, T82.6XXA, T82.7XXA

Female-only   ♂ Male-only   ▲ Limited Coverage   ● Non-OR   ▪ HAC-associated procedure   ▲ Non-covered procedures   + Combination

02H640Z Insertion of Pressure Sensor Monitoring Device into Right Atrium, Percutaneous Endoscopic Approach

02H642Z Insertion of Monitoring Device into Right Atrium, Percutaneous Endoscopic Approach

02H643Z Insertion of Infusion Device into Right Atrium, Percutaneous Endoscopic Approach

02H64DZ Insertion of Intraluminal Device into Right Atrium, Percutaneous Endoscopic Approach

● **02H64JZ** Insertion of Pacemaker Lead into Right Atrium, Percutaneous Endoscopic Approach

➕ Lead device when reported with an Insertion of a pacemaker device or cardiac rhythm related device (6th character 4, 5, 6 or P) into the chest or abdomen subcutaneous tissue and fascia. *See table 0JH to construct the Insertion code. When a device is replaced, also report the Removal of a cardiac rhythm related device (6th character P) from the trunk subcutaneous tissue and fascia. See table 0JP to construct the Removal code.*

02H64KZ Insertion of Defibrillator Lead into Right Atrium, Percutaneous Endoscopic Approach

➕ Lead device when reported with an Insertion of a defibrillator generator (6th character 8) into the chest or abdomen subcutaneous tissue and fascia. *See table 0JH to construct the Insertion code.*

● **02H64MZ** Insertion of Cardiac Lead into Right Atrium, Percutaneous Endoscopic Approach

➕ Lead device when reported with an Insertion of a pacemaker device or cardiac rhythm related device (6th character 4, 5, 6 or P) into the chest or abdomen subcutaneous tissue and fascia. *See table 0JH to construct the Insertion code. When a device is replaced, also report the Removal of a cardiac rhythm related device (6th character P) from the trunk subcutaneous tissue and fascia. See table 0JP to construct the Removal code.*

02H700Z Insertion of Pressure Sensor Monitoring Device into Left Atrium, Open Approach

02H702Z Insertion of Monitoring Device into Left Atrium, Open Approach

02H703Z Insertion of Infusion Device into Left Atrium, Open Approach

02H70DZ Insertion of Intraluminal Device into Left Atrium, Open Approach

● **02H70JZ** Insertion of Pacemaker Lead into Left Atrium, Open Approach

➕ Lead device when reported with an Insertion of a pacemaker device or cardiac rhythm related device (6th character 4, 5, 6 or P) into the chest or abdomen subcutaneous tissue and fascia. *See table 0JH to construct the Insertion code. When a device is replaced, also report the Removal of a cardiac rhythm related device (6th character P) from the trunk subcutaneous tissue and fascia. See table 0JP to construct the Removal code.*

02H70KZ Insertion of Defibrillator Lead into Left Atrium, Open Approach

➕ Lead device when reported with an Insertion of a defibrillator generator (6th character 8) into the chest or abdomen subcutaneous tissue and fascia. *See table 0JH to construct the Insertion code.*

● **02H70MZ** Insertion of Cardiac Lead into Left Atrium, Open Approach

➕ Lead device when reported with an Insertion of a pacemaker device or cardiac rhythm related device (6th character 4, 5, 6 or P) into the chest or abdomen subcutaneous tissue and fascia. *See table 0JH to construct the Insertion code. When a device is replaced, also report the Removal of a cardiac rhythm related device (6th character P) from the trunk subcutaneous tissue and fascia. See table 0JP to construct the Removal code.*

02H730Z Insertion of Pressure Sensor Monitoring Device into Left Atrium, Percutaneous Approach

02H732Z Insertion of Monitoring Device into Left Atrium, Percutaneous Approach

02H733Z Insertion of Infusion Device into Left Atrium, Percutaneous Approach

02H73DZ Insertion of Intraluminal Device into Left Atrium, Percutaneous Approach

● **02H73JZ** Insertion of Pacemaker Lead into Left Atrium, Percutaneous Approach

▨ With a secondary diagnosis code of K68.11, T81.4XXA, T82.6XXA, T82.7XXA

➕ Lead device when reported with an Insertion of a pacemaker device or cardiac rhythm related device (6th character 4, 5, 6 or P) into the chest or abdomen subcutaneous tissue and fascia. *See table 0JH to construct the Insertion code. When a device is replaced, also report the removal of a cardiac rhythm related device (6th character P) from the trunk subcutaneous tissue and fascia. See table 0JP to construct the Removal code. When a cardiac lead is replaced, also report the removal of cardiac lead (6th character M) from the heart. See table 02P to construct the Removal code.*

02H73KZ Insertion of Defibrillator Lead into Left Atrium, Percutaneous Approach

➕ Lead device when reported with an Insertion of a defibrillator generator (6th character 8) into the chest or abdomen subcutaneous tissue and fascia. *See table 0JH to construct the Insertion code.*

02H73MZ Insertion of Cardiac Lead into Left Atrium, Percutaneous Approach

▨ With a secondary diagnosis code of K68.11, T81.4XXA, T82.6XXA, T82.7XXA

➕ Lead device when reported with an Insertion of a pacemaker device or cardiac rhythm related device (6th character 4, 5, 6 or P) into the chest or abdomen subcutaneous tissue and fascia. *See table 0JH to construct the Insertion code. When a device is replaced, also report the Removal of a cardiac rhythm related device (6th character P) from the trunk subcutaneous tissue and fascia. See table 0JP to construct the Removal code.*

02H740Z Insertion of Pressure Sensor Monitoring Device into Left Atrium, Percutaneous Endoscopic Approach

02H742Z Insertion of Monitoring Device into Left Atrium, Percutaneous Endoscopic Approach

02H743Z Insertion of Infusion Device into Left Atrium, Percutaneous Endoscopic Approach

02H74DZ Insertion of Intraluminal Device into Left Atrium, Percutaneous Endoscopic Approach

● **02H74JZ** Insertion of Pacemaker Lead into Left Atrium, Percutaneous Endoscopic Approach

➕ Lead device when reported with an Insertion of a pacemaker device or cardiac rhythm related device (6th character 4, 5, 6 or P) into the chest or abdomen subcutaneous tissue and fascia. *See table 0JH to construct the Insertion code. When a device is replaced, also report the Removal of a cardiac rhythm related device (6th character P) from the trunk subcutaneous tissue and fascia. See table 0JP to construct the Removal code.*

02H74KZ Insertion of Defibrillator Lead into Left Atrium, Percutaneous Endoscopic Approach

➕ Lead device when reported with an Insertion of a defibrillator generator (6th character 8) into the chest or abdomen subcutaneous tissue and fascia. *See table 0JH to construct the Insertion code.*

● **02H74MZ** Insertion of Cardiac Lead into Left Atrium, Percutaneous Endoscopic Approach

➕ Lead device when reported with an Insertion of a pacemaker device or cardiac rhythm related device (6th character 4, 5, 6 or P) into the chest or abdomen subcutaneous tissue and fascia. *See table 0JH to construct the Insertion code. When a device is replaced, also report the Removal of a cardiac rhythm related device (6th character P) from the trunk subcutaneous tissue and fascia. See table 0JP to construct the Removal code.*

▲ **02HA0QZ** Insertion of Implantable Heart Assist System into Heart, Open Approach

02HA0RS Insertion of Biventricular External Heart Assist System into Heart, Open Approach

➕ Heart assist system replacement when reported with a removal of an external heart assist system (6th character R) from the heart. *See table 02P to construct the Removal code.*

02HA0RZ Insertion of External Heart Assist System into Heart, Open Approach

➕ Heart assist system replacement when reported with a removal of an external heart assist system (6th character R) from the heart. *See table 02P to construct the Removal code.*

▲ **02HA3QZ** Insertion of Implantable Heart Assist System into Heart, Percutaneous Approach

02HA3RS Insertion of Biventricular External Heart Assist System into Heart, Percutaneous Approach

➕ Heart assist system replacement when reported with a removal of an external heart assist system (6th character R) from the heart. *See table 02P to construct the Removal code.*

02HA3RZ Insertion of External Heart Assist System into Heart, Percutaneous Approach

➕ Heart assist system replacement when reported with a removal of an external heart assist system (6th character R) from the heart. *See table 02P to construct the Removal code.*

▲ **02HA4QZ** Insertion of Implantable Heart Assist System into Heart, Percutaneous Endoscopic Approach

02HA4RS Insertion of Biventricular External Heart Assist System into Heart, Percutaneous Endoscopic Approach

➕ Heart assist system replacement when reported with a removal of an external heart assist system (6th character R) from the heart. *See table 02P to construct the Removal code.*

A4RZ Insertion of External Heart Assist System into Heart, Percutaneous Endoscopic Approach

+ Heart assist system replacement when reported with a removal of an external heart assist system (6th character R) from the heart. *See table 02P to construct the Removal code.*

1K00Z Insertion of Pressure Sensor Monitoring Device into Right Ventricle, Open Approach

+ Intracardiac lead device when reported with an Insertion of a hemodynamic monitoring device (6th character 0) into the chest or abdomen sucutaneous tissue and fascia. *See table 0JH to construct the Insertion code.*

IK02Z Insertion of Monitoring Device into Right Ventricle, Open Approach

+ Intracardiac lead device when reported with an Insertion of a hemodynamic monitoring device (6th character 0) into the chest or abdomen sucutaneous tissue and fascia. *See table 0JH to construct the Insertion code.*

IK03Z Insertion of Infusion Device into Right Ventricle, Open Approach

HK0DZ Insertion of Intraluminal Device into Right Ventricle, Open Approach

2HK0JZ Insertion of Pacemaker Lead into Right Ventricle, Open Approach

+ Lead device when reported with an Insertion of a pacemaker device or cardiac rhythm related device (6th character 4, 5, 6 or P) into the chest or abdomen subcutaneous tissue and fascia. *See table 0JH to construct the Insertion code.* When a device is replaced, also report the Removal of a cardiac rhythm related device (6th character P) from the trunk subcutaneous tissue and fascia. *See table 0JP to construct the Removal code.*

HK0KZ Insertion of Defibrillator Lead into Right Ventricle, Open Approach

+ Lead device when reported with an Insertion of a defibrillator generator (6th character 8 or 9) into the chest or abdomen subcutaneous tissue and fascia. *See table 0JH to construct the Insertion code.*

2HK0MZ Insertion of Cardiac Lead into Right Ventricle, Open Approach

+ Lead device when reported with an Insertion of a pacemaker device or cardiac rhythm related device (6th character 4, 5, 6 or P) into the chest or abdomen subcutaneous tissue and fascia. *See table 0JH to construct the Insertion code.* When a device is replaced, also report the Removal of a cardiac rhythm related device (6th character P) from the trunk subcutaneous tissue and fascia. *See table 0JP to construct the Removal code.*

HK30Z Insertion of Pressure Sensor Monitoring Device into Right Ventricle, Percutaneous Approach

+ Intracardiac lead device when reported with an Insertion of a hemodynamic monitoring device (6th character 0) into the chest or abdomen sucutaneous tissue and fascia. *See table 0JH to construct the Insertion code.*

2HK32Z Insertion of Monitoring Device into Right Ventricle, Percutaneous Approach

+ Intracardiac lead device when reported with an Insertion of a hemodynamic monitoring device (6th character 0) into the chest or abdomen sucutaneous tissue

and fascia. *See table 0JH to construct the Insertion code.*

● **02HK33Z** Insertion of Infusion Device into Right Ventricle, Percutaneous Approach

02HK3DZ Insertion of Intraluminal Device into Right Ventricle, Percutaneous Approach

● **02HK3JZ** Insertion of Pacemaker Lead into Right Ventricle, Percutaneous Approach

HAC With a secondary diagnosis code of K68.11, T81.4XXA, T82.6XXA, T82.7XXA

+ Lead device when reported with an Insertion of a pacemaker device or cardiac rhythm related device (6th character 4, 5, 6 or P) into the chest or abdomen subcutaneous tissue and fascia. See table 0JH to construct the Insertion code. When a device is replaced, also report the removal of a cardiac rhythm related device (6th character P) from the trunk subcutaneous tissue and fascia. See table 0JP to construct the Removal code. When a cardiac lead is replaced, also report the removal of cardiac lead (6th character M) from the heart. *See table 02P to construct the Removal code.*

02HK3KZ Insertion of Defibrillator Lead into Right Ventricle, Percutaneous Approach

+ Lead device when reported with an Insertion of a defibrillator generator (6th character 8 or 9) into the chest or abdomen subcutaneous tissue and fascia. *See table 0JH to construct the Insertion code.*

● **02HK3MZ** Insertion of Cardiac Lead into Right Ventricle, Percutaneous Approach

+ Lead device when reported with an Insertion of a pacemaker device or cardiac rhythm related device (6th character 4, 5, 6 or P) into the chest or abdomen subcutaneous tissue and fascia. *See table 0JH to construct the Insertion code.* When a device is replaced, also report the Removal of a cardiac rhythm related device (6th character P) from the trunk subcutaneous tissue and fascia. *See table 0JP to construct the Removal code.*

02HK40Z Insertion of Pressure Sensor Monitoring Device into Right Ventricle, Percutaneous Endoscopic Approach

+ Intracardiac lead device when reported with an Insertion of a hemodynamic monitoring device (6th character 0) into the chest or abdomen sucutaneous tissue and fascia. *See table 0JH to construct the Insertion code.*

02HK42Z Insertion of Monitoring Device into Right Ventricle, Percutaneous Endoscopic Approach

+ Intracardiac lead device when reported with an Insertion of a hemodynamic monitoring device (6th character 0) into the chest or abdomen sucutaneous tissue and fascia. *See table 0JH to construct the Insertion code.*

02HK43Z Insertion of Infusion Device into Right Ventricle, Percutaneous Endoscopic Approach

02HK4DZ Insertion of Intraluminal Device into Right Ventricle, Percutaneous Endoscopic Approach

● **02HK4JZ** Insertion of Pacemaker Lead into Right Ventricle, Percutaneous Endoscopic Approach

+ Lead device when reported with an Insertion of a pacemaker device or cardiac rhythm related device (6th character 4, 5, 6 or P) into the chest or abdomen subcutaneous tissue and fascia. *See table*

0JH to construct the Insertion code. When a device is replaced, also report the Removal of a cardiac rhythm related device (6th character P) from the trunk subcutaneous tissue and fascia. *See table 0JP to construct the Removal code.*

02HK4KZ Insertion of Defibrillator Lead into Right Ventricle, Percutaneous Endoscopic Approach

+ Lead device when reported with an Insertion of a defibrillator generator (6th character 8 or 9) into the chest or abdomen subcutaneous tissue and fascia. *See table 0JH to construct the Insertion code.*

● **02HK4MZ** Insertion of Cardiac Lead into Right Ventricle, Percutaneous Endoscopic Approach

+ Lead device when reported with an Insertion of a pacemaker device or cardiac rhythm related device (6th character 4, 5, 6 or P) into the chest or abdomen subcutaneous tissue and fascia. *See table 0JH to construct the Insertion code.* When a device is replaced, also report the Removal of a cardiac rhythm related device (6th character P) from the trunk subcutaneous tissue and fascia. *See table 0JP to construct the Removal code.*

02HL00Z Insertion of Pressure Sensor Monitoring Device into Left Ventricle, Open Approach

02HL02Z Insertion of Monitoring Device into Left Ventricle, Open Approach

02HL03Z Insertion of Infusion Device into Left Ventricle, Open Approach

02HL0DZ Insertion of Intraluminal Device into Left Ventricle, Open Approach

● **02HL0JZ** Insertion of Pacemaker Lead into Left Ventricle, Open Approach

+ Lead device when reported with an Insertion of a pacemaker device or cardiac rhythm related device (6th character 4, 5, 6 or P) into the chest or abdomen subcutaneous tissue and fascia. *See table 0JH to construct the Insertion code.* When a device is replaced, also report the Removal of a cardiac rhythm related device (6th character P) from the trunk subcutaneous tissue and fascia. *See table 0JP to construct the Removal code.*

02HL0KZ Insertion of Defibrillator Lead into Left Ventricle, Open Approach

+ Lead device when reported with an Insertion of a defibrillator generator (6th character 8 or 9) into the chest or abdomen subcutaneous tissue and fascia. *See table 0JH to construct the Insertion code.*

● **02HL0MZ** Insertion of Cardiac Lead into Left Ventricle, Open Approach

+ Lead device when reported with an Insertion of a pacemaker device, cardiac rhythm related device or contractility modulation device (6th character 4, 5, 6, M or P) into the chest or abdomen subcutaneous tissue and fascia. *See table 0JH to construct the Insertion code.* When a device is replaced, also report the Removal of a cardiac rhythm related device (6th character P) from the trunk subcutaneous tissue and fascia. *See table 0JP to construct the Removal code.*

02HL30Z Insertion of Pressure Sensor Monitoring Device into Left Ventricle, Percutaneous Approach

02HL32Z Insertion of Monitoring Device into Left Ventricle, Percutaneous Approach

Female-only   ♂ Male-only   ▲ Limited Coverage   ● Non-OR   HAC HAC-associated procedure   ▲ Non-covered procedures   + Combination

02HL33Z Insertion of Infusion Device into Left Ventricle, Percutaneous Approach

02HL3DZ Insertion of Intraluminal Device into Left Ventricle, Percutaneous Approach

● **02HL3JZ** Insertion of Pacemaker Lead into Left Ventricle, Percutaneous Approach

    ■ With a secondary diagnosis code of K68.11, T81.4XXA, T82.6XXA, T82.7XXA

    + Lead device when reported with an Insertion of a pacemaker device or cardiac rhythm related device (6th character 4, 5, 6 or P) into the chest or abdomen subcutaneous tissue and fascia. *See table 0JH to construct the Insertion code. When a device is replaced, also report the removal of a cardiac rhythm related device (6th character P) from the trunk subcutaneous tissue and fascia. See table 0JP to construct the Removal code. When a cardiac lead is replaced, also report the removal of cardiac lead (6th character M) from the heart. See table 02P to construct the Removal code.*

02HL3KZ Insertion of Defibrillator Lead into Left Ventricle, Percutaneous Approach

    + Lead device when reported with an Insertion of a defibrillator generator (6th character 8 or 9) into the chest or abdomen subcutaneous tissue and fascia. *See table 0JH to construct the Insertion code.*

● **02HL3MZ** Insertion of Cardiac Lead into Left Ventricle, Percutaneous Approach

    + Lead device when reported with an Insertion of a pacemaker device, cardiac rhythm related device or contractility modulation device (6th character 4, 5, 6, M or P) into the chest or abdomen subcutaneous tissue and fascia. *See table 0JH to construct the Insertion code. When a device is replaced, also report the Removal of a cardiac rhythm related device (6th character P) from the trunk subcutaneous tissue and fascia. See table 0JP to construct the Removal code.*

02HL40Z Insertion of Pressure Sensor Monitoring Device into Left Ventricle, Percutaneous Endoscopic Approach

02HL42Z Insertion of Monitoring Device into Left Ventricle, Percutaneous Endoscopic Approach

02HL43Z Insertion of Infusion Device into Left Ventricle, Percutaneous Endoscopic Approach

02HL4DZ Insertion of Intraluminal Device into Left Ventricle, Percutaneous Endoscopic Approach

● **02HL4JZ** Insertion of Pacemaker Lead into Left Ventricle, Percutaneous Endoscopic Approach

    + Lead device when reported with an Insertion of a pacemaker device or cardiac rhythm related device (6th character 4, 5, 6 or P) into the chest or abdomen subcutaneous tissue and fascia. *See table 0JH to construct the Insertion code. When a device is replaced, also report the Removal of a cardiac rhythm related device (6th character P) from the trunk subcutaneous tissue and fascia. See table 0JP to construct the Removal code.*

02HL4KZ Insertion of Defibrillator Lead into Left Ventricle, Percutaneous Endoscopic Approach

● **02HL4MZ** Insertion of Cardiac Lead into Left Ventricle, Percutaneous Endoscopic Approach

    + Lead device when reported with an Insertion of a pacemaker device or cardiac rhythm related device (6th character 4, 5, 6 or P) into the chest or abdomen subcutaneous tissue and fascia. *See table 0JH to construct the Insertion code. When a device is replaced, also report the Removal of a cardiac rhythm related device (6th character P) from the trunk subcutaneous tissue and fascia. See table 0JP to construct the Removal code.*

02HN00Z Insertion of Pressure Sensor Monitoring Device into Pericardium, Open Approach

02HN02Z Insertion of Monitoring Device into Pericardium, Open Approach

02HN0JZ Insertion of Pacemaker Lead into Pericardium, Open Approach

    ■ With a secondary diagnosis code of K68.11, T81.4XXA, T82.6XXA, T82.7XXA

    + Lead device when reported with an Insertion of a pacemaker device or cardiac rhythm related device (6th character 4, 5, 6 or P) into the chest or abdomen subcutaneous tissue and fascia. *See table 0JH to construct the Insertion code. When a device is replaced, also report the Removal of a cardiac rhythm related device (6th character P) from the trunk subcutaneous tissue and fascia. See table 0JP to construct the Removal code.*

02HN0KZ Insertion of Defibrillator Lead into Pericardium, Open Approach

02HN0MZ Insertion of Cardiac Lead into Pericardium, Open Approach

    ■ With a secondary diagnosis code of K68.11, T81.4XXA, T82.6XXA, T82.7XXA

    + Lead device when reported with an Insertion of a pacemaker device, cardiac rhythm related device or contractility modulation device (6th character 4, 5, 6, M or P) into the chest or abdomen subcutaneous tissue and fascia. *See table 0JH to construct the Insertion code. When a device is replaced, also report the Removal of a cardiac rhythm related device (6th character P) from the trunk subcutaneous tissue and fascia. See table 0JP to construct the Removal code.*

02HN30Z Insertion of Pressure Sensor Monitoring Device into Pericardium, Percutaneous Approach

02HN32Z Insertion of Monitoring Device into Pericardium, Percutaneous Approach

02HN3JZ Insertion of Pacemaker Lead into Pericardium, Percutaneous Approach

    ■ With a secondary diagnosis code of K68.11, T81.4XXA, T82.6XXA, T82.7XXA

    + Lead device when reported with an Insertion of a pacemaker device or cardiac rhythm related device (6th character 4, 5, 6 or P) into the chest or abdomen subcutaneous tissue and fascia. *See table 0JH to construct the Insertion code. When a device is replaced, also report the Removal of a cardiac rhythm related device (6th character P) from the trunk subcutaneous tissue and fascia. See table 0JP to construct the Removal code.*

02HN3KZ Insertion of Defibrillator Lead into Pericardium, Percutaneous Approach

02HN3MZ Insertion of Cardiac Lead into Pericardium, Percutaneous Approach

    ■ With a secondary diagnosis code of K68.11, T81.4XXA, T82.6XXA, T82.7XXA

02HN40Z Insertion of Pressure Sensor Monitoring Device into Pericardium, Percutaneous Endoscopic Approach

02HN42Z Insertion of Monitoring Device into Pericardium, Percutaneous Endoscopic Approach

02HN4JZ Insertion of Pacemaker Lead into Pericardium, Percutaneous Endoscopic Approach

    ■ With a secondary diagnosis code of K68.11, T81.4XXA, T82.6XXA, T82.7XXA

    + Lead device when reported with an Insertion of a pacemaker device or cardiac rhythm related device (6th character 4, 5, 6 or P) into the chest or abdomen subcutaneous tissue and fascia. *See table 0JH to construct the Insertion code. When a device is replaced, also report the Removal of a cardiac rhythm related device (6th character P) from the trunk subcutaneous tissue and fascia. See table 0JP to construct the Removal code.*

02HN4KZ Insertion of Defibrillator Lead into Pericardium, Percutaneous Endoscopic Approach

02HN4MZ Insertion of Cardiac Lead into Pericardium, Percutaneous Endoscopic Approach

    ■ With a secondary diagnosis code of K68.11, T81.4XXA, T82.6XXA, T82.7XXA

    + Lead device when reported with an Insertion of a pacemaker device or cardiac rhythm related device (6th character 4, 5, 6 or P) into the chest or abdomen subcutaneous tissue and fascia. *See table 0JH to construct the Insertion code. When a device is replaced, also report the Removal of a cardiac rhythm related device (6th character P) from the trunk subcutaneous tissue and fascia. See table 0JP to construct the Removal code.*

02HP00Z Insertion of Pressure Sensor Monitoring Device into Pulmonary Trunk, Open Approach

02HP02Z Insertion of Monitoring Device into Pulmonary Trunk, Open Approach

02HP03Z Insertion of Infusion Device into Pulmonary Trunk, Open Approach

02HP0DZ Insertion of Intraluminal Device into Pulmonary Trunk, Open Approach

02HP30Z Insertion of Pressure Sensor Monitoring Device into Pulmonary Trunk, Percutaneous Approach

02HP32Z Insertion of Monitoring Device into Pulmonary Trunk, Percutaneous Approach

02HP33Z Insertion of Infusion Device into Pulmonary Trunk, Percutaneous Approach

02HP3DZ Insertion of Intraluminal Device into Pulmonary Trunk, Percutaneous Approach

02HP40Z Insertion of Pressure Sensor Monitoring Device into Pulmonary Trunk, Percutaneous Endoscopic Approach

02HP42Z Insertion of Monitoring Device into Pulmonary Trunk, Percutaneous Endoscopic Approach

P43Z	Insertion of Infusion Device into Pulmonary Trunk, Percutaneous Endoscopic Approach
P4DZ	Insertion of Intraluminal Device into Pulmonary Trunk, Percutaneous Endoscopic Approach
Q00Z	Insertion of Pressure Sensor Monitoring Device into Right Pulmonary Artery, Open Approach
Q02Z	Insertion of Monitoring Device into Right Pulmonary Artery, Open Approach
Q03Z	Insertion of Infusion Device into Right Pulmonary Artery, Open Approach
Q0DZ	Insertion of Intraluminal Device into Right Pulmonary Artery, Open Approach
Q30Z	Insertion of Pressure Sensor Monitoring Device into Right Pulmonary Artery, Percutaneous Approach
Q32Z	Insertion of Monitoring Device into Right Pulmonary Artery, Percutaneous Approach
Q33Z	Insertion of Infusion Device into Right Pulmonary Artery, Percutaneous Approach
Q3DZ	Insertion of Intraluminal Device into Right Pulmonary Artery, Percutaneous Approach
Q40Z	Insertion of Pressure Sensor Monitoring Device into Right Pulmonary Artery, Percutaneous Endoscopic Approach
Q42Z	Insertion of Monitoring Device into Right Pulmonary Artery, Percutaneous Endoscopic Approach
Q43Z	Insertion of Infusion Device into Right Pulmonary Artery, Percutaneous Endoscopic Approach
Q4DZ	Insertion of Intraluminal Device into Right Pulmonary Artery, Percutaneous Endoscopic Approach
R00Z	Insertion of Pressure Sensor Monitoring Device into Left Pulmonary Artery, Open Approach
R02Z	Insertion of Monitoring Device into Left Pulmonary Artery, Open Approach
R03Z	Insertion of Infusion Device into Left Pulmonary Artery, Open Approach
R0DZ	Insertion of Intraluminal Device into Left Pulmonary Artery, Open Approach
R30Z	Insertion of Pressure Sensor Monitoring Device into Left Pulmonary Artery, Percutaneous Approach
R32Z	Insertion of Monitoring Device into Left Pulmonary Artery, Percutaneous Approach
R33Z	Insertion of Infusion Device into Left Pulmonary Artery, Percutaneous Approach
R3DZ	Insertion of Intraluminal Device into Left Pulmonary Artery, Percutaneous Approach
R40Z	Insertion of Pressure Sensor Monitoring Device into Left Pulmonary Artery, Percutaneous Endoscopic Approach

02HR42Z	Insertion of Monitoring Device into Left Pulmonary Artery, Percutaneous Endoscopic Approach
02HR43Z	Insertion of Infusion Device into Left Pulmonary Artery, Percutaneous Endoscopic Approach
02HR4DZ	Insertion of Intraluminal Device into Left Pulmonary Artery, Percutaneous Endoscopic Approach
02HS00Z	Insertion of Pressure Sensor Monitoring Device into Right Pulmonary Vein, Open Approach
02HS02Z	Insertion of Monitoring Device into Right Pulmonary Vein, Open Approach
02HS03Z	Insertion of Infusion Device into Right Pulmonary Vein, Open Approach
02HS0DZ	Insertion of Intraluminal Device into Right Pulmonary Vein, Open Approach
02HS30Z	Insertion of Pressure Sensor Monitoring Device into Right Pulmonary Vein, Percutaneous Approach
02HS32Z	Insertion of Monitoring Device into Right Pulmonary Vein, Percutaneous Approach
02HS33Z	Insertion of Infusion Device into Right Pulmonary Vein, Percutaneous Approach
02HS3DZ	Insertion of Intraluminal Device into Right Pulmonary Vein, Percutaneous Approach
02HS40Z	Insertion of Pressure Sensor Monitoring Device into Right Pulmonary Vein, Percutaneous Endoscopic Approach
02HS42Z	Insertion of Monitoring Device into Right Pulmonary Vein, Percutaneous Endoscopic Approach
02HS43Z	Insertion of Infusion Device into Right Pulmonary Vein, Percutaneous Endoscopic Approach
02HS4DZ	Insertion of Intraluminal Device into Right Pulmonary Vein, Percutaneous Endoscopic Approach
02HT00Z	Insertion of Pressure Sensor Monitoring Device into Left Pulmonary Vein, Open Approach
02HT02Z	Insertion of Monitoring Device into Left Pulmonary Vein, Open Approach
02HT03Z	Insertion of Infusion Device into Left Pulmonary Vein, Open Approach
02HT0DZ	Insertion of Intraluminal Device into Left Pulmonary Vein, Open Approach
02HT30Z	Insertion of Pressure Sensor Monitoring Device into Left Pulmonary Vein, Percutaneous Approach
02HT32Z	Insertion of Monitoring Device into Left Pulmonary Vein, Percutaneous Approach
02HT33Z	Insertion of Infusion Device into Left Pulmonary Vein, Percutaneous Approach
02HT3DZ	Insertion of Intraluminal Device into Left Pulmonary Vein, Percutaneous Approach
02HT40Z	Insertion of Pressure Sensor Monitoring Device into Left Pulmonary Vein, Percutaneous Endoscopic Approach

02HT42Z	Insertion of Monitoring Device into Left Pulmonary Vein, Percutaneous Endoscopic Approach
02HT43Z	Insertion of Infusion Device into Left Pulmonary Vein, Percutaneous Endoscopic Approach
02HT4DZ	Insertion of Intraluminal Device into Left Pulmonary Vein, Percutaneous Endoscopic Approach
02HV00Z	Insertion of Pressure Sensor Monitoring Device into Superior Vena Cava, Open Approach
02HV02Z	Insertion of Monitoring Device into Superior Vena Cava, Open Approach
02HV03Z	Insertion of Infusion Device into Superior Vena Cava, Open Approach
02HV0DZ	Insertion of Intraluminal Device into Superior Vena Cava, Open Approach
02HV30Z	Insertion of Pressure Sensor Monitoring Device into Superior Vena Cava, Percutaneous Approach
02HV32Z	Insertion of Monitoring Device into Superior Vena Cava, Percutaneous Approach
02HV33Z	Insertion of Infusion Device into Superior Vena Cava, Percutaneous Approach
	AHA CC: 3Q, 2013, 18
02HV3DZ	Insertion of Intraluminal Device into Superior Vena Cava, Percutaneous Approach
02HV40Z	Insertion of Pressure Sensor Monitoring Device into Superior Vena Cava, Percutaneous Endoscopic Approach
02HV42Z	Insertion of Monitoring Device into Superior Vena Cava, Percutaneous Endoscopic Approach
02HV43Z	Insertion of Infusion Device into Superior Vena Cava, Percutaneous Endoscopic Approach
02HV4DZ	Insertion of Intraluminal Device into Superior Vena Cava, Percutaneous Endoscopic Approach
02HW00Z	Insertion of Pressure Sensor Monitoring Device into Thoracic Aorta, Open Approach
02HW02Z	Insertion of Monitoring Device into Thoracic Aorta, Open Approach
02HW03Z	Insertion of Infusion Device into Thoracic Aorta, Open Approach
02HW0DZ	Insertion of Intraluminal Device into Thoracic Aorta, Open Approach
02HW30Z	Insertion of Pressure Sensor Monitoring Device into Thoracic Aorta, Percutaneous Approach
02HW32Z	Insertion of Monitoring Device into Thoracic Aorta, Percutaneous Approach
02HW33Z	Insertion of Infusion Device into Thoracic Aorta, Percutaneous Approach
02HW3DZ	Insertion of Intraluminal Device into Thoracic Aorta, Percutaneous Approach

J – Heart and Great Vessels, Inspection

Review Coding Guidelines B3.11a, B3.11b and B3.11c

JA0ZZ	Inspection of Heart, Open Approach
JA3ZZ	Inspection of Heart, Percutaneous Approach

02JA4ZZ	Inspection of Heart, Percutaneous Endoscopic Approach
02JY0ZZ	Inspection of Great Vessel, Open Approach

02JY3ZZ	Inspection of Great Vessel, Percutaneous Approach
02JY4ZZ	Inspection of Great Vessel, Percutaneous Endoscopic Approach

K – Heart and Great Vessels, Map

2K80ZZ	Map Conduction Mechanism, Open Approach

●	02K83ZZ	Map Conduction Mechanism, Percutaneous Approach

●	02K84ZZ	Map Conduction Mechanism, Percutaneous Endoscopic Approach

♀ Female-only   ♂ Male-only   ▲ Limited Coverage   ● Non-OR   ▬ HAC-associated procedure   ▲ Non-covered procedures   ✚ Combination

02L – Heart and Great Vessels, Occlusion

● **02L70CK** Occlusion of Left Atrial Appendage with Extraluminal Device, Open Approach
AHA CC: 3Q, 2014, 20-21

● **02L70DK** Occlusion of Left Atrial Appendage with Intraluminal Device, Open Approach

● **02L70ZK** Occlusion of Left Atrial Appendage, Open Approach

● **02L73CK** Occlusion of Left Atrial Appendage with Extraluminal Device, Percutaneous Approach

● **02L73DK** Occlusion of Left Atrial Appendage with Intraluminal Device, Percutaneous Approach

● **02L73ZK** Occlusion of Left Atrial Appendage, Percutaneous Approach

● **02L74CK** Occlusion of Left Atrial Appendage with Extraluminal Device, Percutaneous Endoscopic Approach

● **02L74DK** Occlusion of Left Atrial Appendage with Intraluminal Device, Percutaneous Endoscopic Approach

● **02L74ZK** Occlusion of Left Atrial Appendage, Percutaneous Endoscopic Approach

02LR0CT Occlusion of Ductus Arteriosus with Extraluminal Device, Open Approach

02LR0DT Occlusion of Ductus Arteriosus with Intraluminal Device, Open Approach

02LR0ZT Occlusion of Ductus Arteriosus, Open Approach

02LR3CT Occlusion of Ductus Arteriosus with Extraluminal Device, Percutaneous Approach

02LR3DT Occlusion of Ductus Arteriosus with Intraluminal Device, Percutaneous Approach

02LR3ZT Occlusion of Ductus Arteriosus, Percutaneous Approach

02LR4CT Occlusion of Ductus Arteriosus with Extraluminal Device, Percutaneous Endoscopic Approach

02LR4DT Occlusion of Ductus Arteriosus with Intraluminal Device, Percutaneous Endoscopic Approach

02LR4ZT Occlusion of Ductus Arteriosus, Percutaneous Endoscopic Approach

02LS0CZ Occlusion of Right Pulmonary Vein with Extraluminal Device, Open Approach

02LS0DZ Occlusion of Right Pulmonary Vein with Intraluminal Device, Open Approach

02LS0ZZ Occlusion of Right Pulmonary Vein, Open Approach

02LS3CZ Occlusion of Right Pulmonary Vein with Extraluminal Device, Percutaneous Approach

02LS3DZ Occlusion of Right Pulmonary Vein with Intraluminal Device, Percutaneous Approach

02LS3ZZ Occlusion of Right Pulmonary Vein, Percutaneous Approach

02LS4CZ Occlusion of Right Pulmonary Vein with Extraluminal Device, Percutaneous Endoscopic Approach

02LS4DZ Occlusion of Right Pulmonary Vein with Intraluminal Device, Percutaneous Endoscopic Approach

02LS4ZZ Occlusion of Right Pulmonary Vein, Percutaneous Endoscopic Approach

02LT0CZ Occlusion of Left Pulmonary Vein with Extraluminal Device, Open Approach

02LT0DZ Occlusion of Left Pulmonary Vein with Intraluminal Device, Open Approach

02LT0ZZ Occlusion of Left Pulmonary Vein, Open Approach

02LT3CZ Occlusion of Left Pulmonary Vein with Extraluminal Device, Percutaneous Approach

02LT3DZ Occlusion of Left Pulmonary Vein with Intraluminal Device, Percutaneous Approach

02LT3ZZ Occlusion of Left Pulmonary Vein, Percutaneous Approach

02LT4CZ Occlusion of Left Pulmonary Vein with Extraluminal Device, Percutaneous Endoscopic Approach

02LT4DZ Occlusion of Left Pulmonary Vein with Intraluminal Device, Percutaneous Endoscopic Approach

02LT4ZZ Occlusion of Left Pulmonary Vein, Percutaneous Endoscopic Approach

02LV0CZ Occlusion of Superior Vena Cava with Extraluminal Device, Open Approach

02LV0DZ Occlusion of Superior Vena Cava with Intraluminal Device, Open Approach

02LV0ZZ Occlusion of Superior Vena Cava, Open Approach

02LV3CZ Occlusion of Superior Vena Cava with Extraluminal Device, Percutaneous Approach

02LV3DZ Occlusion of Superior Vena Cava with Intraluminal Device, Percutaneous Approach

02LV3ZZ Occlusion of Superior Vena Cava, Percutaneous Approach

02LV4CZ Occlusion of Superior Vena Cava with Extraluminal Device, Percutaneous Endoscopic Approach

02LV4DZ Occlusion of Superior Vena Cava with Intraluminal Device, Percutaneous Endoscopic Approach

02LV4ZZ Occlusion of Superior Vena Cava, Percutaneous Endoscopic Approach

02N – Heart and Great Vessels, Release

Review Coding Guideline B3.13

Review Coding Guideline B3.14

02N40ZZ Release Coronary Vein, Open Approach

02N43ZZ Release Coronary Vein, Percutaneous Approach

02N44ZZ Release Coronary Vein, Percutaneous Endoscopic Approach

02N50ZZ Release Atrial Septum, Open Approach

02N53ZZ Release Atrial Septum, Percutaneous Approach

02N54ZZ Release Atrial Septum, Percutaneous Endoscopic Approach

02N60ZZ Release Right Atrium, Open Approach

02N63ZZ Release Right Atrium, Percutaneous Approach

02N64ZZ Release Right Atrium, Percutaneous Endoscopic Approach

02N70ZZ Release Left Atrium, Open Approach

02N73ZZ Release Left Atrium, Percutaneous Approach

02N74ZZ Release Left Atrium, Percutaneous Endoscopic Approach

02N80ZZ Release Conduction Mechanism, Open Approach

02N83ZZ Release Conduction Mechanism, Percutaneous Approach

02N84ZZ Release Conduction Mechanism, Percutaneous Endoscopic Approach

02N90ZZ Release Chordae Tendineae, Open Approach

02N93ZZ Release Chordae Tendineae, Percutaneous Approach

02N94ZZ Release Chordae Tendineae, Percutaneous Endoscopic Approach

02ND0ZZ Release Papillary Muscle, Open Approach

02ND3ZZ Release Papillary Muscle, Percutaneous Approach

02ND4ZZ Release Papillary Muscle, Percutaneous Endoscopic Approach

02NF0ZZ Release Aortic Valve, Open Approach

02NF3ZZ Release Aortic Valve, Percutaneous Approach

02NF4ZZ Release Aortic Valve, Percutaneous Endoscopic Approach

02NG0ZZ Release Mitral Valve, Open Approach

02NG3ZZ Release Mitral Valve, Percutaneous Approach

02NG4ZZ Release Mitral Valve, Percutaneous Endoscopic Approach

02NH0ZZ Release Pulmonary Valve, Open Approach

02NH3ZZ Release Pulmonary Valve, Percutaneous Approach

02NH4ZZ Release Pulmonary Valve, Percutaneous Endoscopic Approach

02NJ0ZZ Release Tricuspid Valve, Open Approach

02NJ3ZZ Release Tricuspid Valve, Percutaneous Approach

02NJ4ZZ Release Tricuspid Valve, Percutaneous Endoscopic Approach

02NK0ZZ Release Right Ventricle, Open Approach
AHA CC: 3Q, 2014, 16-17

02NK3ZZ Release Right Ventricle, Percutaneous Approach

02NK4ZZ Release Right Ventricle, Percutaneous Endoscopic Approach

02NL0ZZ Release Left Ventricle, Open Approach

02NL3ZZ Release Left Ventricle, Percutaneous Approach

02NL4ZZ Release Left Ventricle, Percutaneous Endoscopic Approach

02NM0ZZ Release Ventricular Septum, Open Approach

02NM3ZZ Release Ventricular Septum, Percutaneous Approach

02NM4ZZ Release Ventricular Septum, Percutaneous Endoscopic Approach

02NN0ZZ Release Pericardium, Open Approach

02NN3ZZ Release Pericardium, Percutaneous Approach

02NN4ZZ Release Pericardium, Percutaneous Endoscopic Approach

02NP0ZZ Release Pulmonary Trunk, Open Approach

02NP3ZZ Release Pulmonary Trunk, Percutaneous Approach

02NP4ZZ Release Pulmonary Trunk, Percutaneous Endoscopic Approach

02NQ0ZZ Release Right Pulmonary Artery, Open Approach

02NQ3ZZ Release Right Pulmonary Artery, Percutaneous Approach

02NQ4ZZ Release Right Pulmonary Artery, Percutaneous Endoscopic Approach

♀ Female-only　　♂ Male-only　　▲ Limited Coverage　　● Non-OR　　HAC-associated procedure　　▲ Non-covered procedures　　+ Combination

NR0ZZ Release Left Pulmonary Artery, Open Approach

NR3ZZ Release Left Pulmonary Artery, Percutaneous Approach

NR4ZZ Release Left Pulmonary Artery, Percutaneous Endoscopic Approach

NS0ZZ Release Right Pulmonary Vein, Open Approach

NS3ZZ Release Right Pulmonary Vein, Percutaneous Approach

02NS4ZZ Release Right Pulmonary Vein, Percutaneous Endoscopic Approach

02NT0ZZ Release Left Pulmonary Vein, Open Approach

02NT3ZZ Release Left Pulmonary Vein, Percutaneous Approach

02NT4ZZ Release Left Pulmonary Vein, Percutaneous Endoscopic Approach

02NV0ZZ Release Superior Vena Cava, Open Approach

02NV3ZZ Release Superior Vena Cava, Percutaneous Approach

02NV4ZZ Release Superior Vena Cava, Percutaneous Endoscopic Approach

02NW0ZZ Release Thoracic Aorta, Open Approach

02NW3ZZ Release Thoracic Aorta, Percutaneous Approach

02NW4ZZ Release Thoracic Aorta, Percutaneous Endoscopic Approach

P – Heart and Great Vessels, Removal

view Coding Guideline B6.1c

PA02Z Removal of Monitoring Device from Heart, Open Approach

PA03Z Removal of Infusion Device from Heart, Open Approach

PA07Z Removal of Autologous Tissue Substitute from Heart, Open Approach

PA08Z Removal of Zooplastic Tissue from Heart, Open Approach

PA0CZ Removal of Extraluminal Device from Heart, Open Approach

PA0DZ Removal of Intraluminal Device from Heart, Open Approach

PA0JZ Removal of Synthetic Substitute from Heart, Open Approach

PA0KZ Removal of Nonautologous Tissue Substitute from Heart, Open Approach

PA0MZ Removal of Cardiac Lead from Heart, Open Approach

HAC With a secondary diagnosis code of K68.11, T81.4XXA, T82.6XXA, T82.7XXA

PA0QZ Removal of Implantable Heart Assist System from Heart, Open Approach

PA0RZ Removal of External Heart Assist System from Heart, Open Approach

PA32Z Removal of Monitoring Device from Heart, Percutaneous Approach

PA33Z Removal of Infusion Device from Heart, Percutaneous Approach

PA37Z Removal of Autologous Tissue Substitute from Heart, Percutaneous Approach

PA38Z Removal of Zooplastic Tissue from Heart, Percutaneous Approach

PA3CZ Removal of Extraluminal Device from Heart, Percutaneous Approach

PA3DZ Removal of Intraluminal Device from Heart, Percutaneous Approach

PA3JZ Removal of Synthetic Substitute from Heart, Percutaneous Approach

PA3KZ Removal of Nonautologous Tissue Substitute from Heart, Percutaneous Approach

PA3MZ Removal of Cardiac Lead from Heart, Percutaneous Approach

HAC With a secondary diagnosis code of K68.11, T81.4XXA, T82.6XXA, T82.7XXA

PA3QZ Removal of Implantable Heart Assist System from Heart, Percutaneous Approach

PA3RZ Removal of External Heart Assist System from Heart, Percutaneous Approach

02PA42Z Removal of Monitoring Device from Heart, Percutaneous Endoscopic Approach

02PA43Z Removal of Infusion Device from Heart, Percutaneous Endoscopic Approach

02PA47Z Removal of Autologous Tissue Substitute from Heart, Percutaneous Endoscopic Approach

02PA48Z Removal of Zooplastic Tissue from Heart, Percutaneous Endoscopic Approach

02PA4CZ Removal of Extraluminal Device from Heart, Percutaneous Endoscopic Approach

02PA4DZ Removal of Intraluminal Device from Heart, Percutaneous Endoscopic Approach

02PA4JZ Removal of Synthetic Substitute from Heart, Percutaneous Endoscopic Approach

02PA4KZ Removal of Nonautologous Tissue Substitute from Heart, Percutaneous Endoscopic Approach

02PA4MZ Removal of Cardiac Lead from Heart, Percutaneous Endoscopic Approach

HAC With a secondary diagnosis code of K68.11, T81.4XXA, T82.6XXA, T82.7XXA

02PA4QZ Removal of Implantable Heart Assist System from Heart, Percutaneous Endoscopic Approach

02PA4RZ Removal of External Heart Assist System from Heart, Percutaneous Endoscopic Approach

02PAX2Z Removal of Monitoring Device from Heart, External Approach

02PAX3Z Removal of Infusion Device from Heart, External Approach

02PAXDZ Removal of Intraluminal Device from Heart, External Approach

02PAXMZ Removal of Cardiac Lead from Heart, External Approach

HAC With a secondary diagnosis code of K68.11, T81.4XXA, T82.6XXA, T82.7XXA

02PY02Z Removal of Monitoring Device from Great Vessel, Open Approach

02PY03Z Removal of Infusion Device from Great Vessel, Open Approach

02PY07Z Removal of Autologous Tissue Substitute from Great Vessel, Open Approach

02PY08Z Removal of Zooplastic Tissue from Great Vessel, Open Approach

02PY0CZ Removal of Extraluminal Device from Great Vessel, Open Approach

02PY0DZ Removal of Intraluminal Device from Great Vessel, Open Approach

02PY0JZ Removal of Synthetic Substitute from Great Vessel, Open Approach

02PY0KZ Removal of Nonautologous Tissue Substitute from Great Vessel, Open Approach

02PY32Z Removal of Monitoring Device from Great Vessel, Percutaneous Approach

02PY33Z Removal of Infusion Device from Great Vessel, Percutaneous Approach

02PY37Z Removal of Autologous Tissue Substitute from Great Vessel, Percutaneous Approach

02PY38Z Removal of Zooplastic Tissue from Great Vessel, Percutaneous Approach

02PY3CZ Removal of Extraluminal Device from Great Vessel, Percutaneous Approach

02PY3DZ Removal of Intraluminal Device from Great Vessel, Percutaneous Approach

02PY3JZ Removal of Synthetic Substitute from Great Vessel, Percutaneous Approach

02PY3KZ Removal of Nonautologous Tissue Substitute from Great Vessel, Percutaneous Approach

02PY42Z Removal of Monitoring Device from Great Vessel, Percutaneous Endoscopic Approach

02PY43Z Removal of Infusion Device from Great Vessel, Percutaneous Endoscopic Approach

02PY47Z Removal of Autologous Tissue Substitute from Great Vessel, Percutaneous Endoscopic Approach

02PY48Z Removal of Zooplastic Tissue from Great Vessel, Percutaneous Endoscopic Approach

02PY4CZ Removal of Extraluminal Device from Great Vessel, Percutaneous Endoscopic Approach

02PY4DZ Removal of Intraluminal Device from Great Vessel, Percutaneous Endoscopic Approach

02PY4JZ Removal of Synthetic Substitute from Great Vessel, Percutaneous Endoscopic Approach

02PY4KZ Removal of Nonautologous Tissue Substitute from Great Vessel, Percutaneous Endoscopic Approach

02PYX2Z Removal of Monitoring Device from Great Vessel, External Approach

02PYX3Z Removal of Infusion Device from Great Vessel, External Approach

02PYXDZ Removal of Intraluminal Device from Great Vessel, External Approach

2Q – Heart and Great Vessels, Repair

or Repair of coronary arteries, Review Coding Guideline B4.4

Q00ZZ Repair Coronary Artery, One Site, Open Approach

Q03ZZ Repair Coronary Artery, One Site, Percutaneous Approach

02Q04ZZ Repair Coronary Artery, One Site, Percutaneous Endoscopic Approach

02Q10ZZ Repair Coronary Artery, Two Sites, Open Approach

02Q13ZZ Repair Coronary Artery, Two Sites, Percutaneous Approach

02Q14ZZ Repair Coronary Artery, Two Sites, Percutaneous Endoscopic Approach

♀ Female-only   ♂ Male-only   ▲ Limited Coverage   ● Non-OR   HAC HAC-associated procedure   ▲ Non-covered procedures   ✚ Combination

02Q20ZZ	Repair Coronary Artery, Three Sites, Open Approach
02Q23ZZ	Repair Coronary Artery, Three Sites, Percutaneous Approach
02Q24ZZ	Repair Coronary Artery, Three Sites, Percutaneous Endoscopic Approach
02Q30ZZ	Repair Coronary Artery, Four or More Sites, Open Approach
02Q33ZZ	Repair Coronary Artery, Four or More Sites, Percutaneous Approach
02Q34ZZ	Repair Coronary Artery, Four or More Sites, Percutaneous Endoscopic Approach
02Q40ZZ	Repair Coronary Vein, Open Approach
02Q43ZZ	Repair Coronary Vein, Percutaneous Approach
02Q44ZZ	Repair Coronary Vein, Percutaneous Endoscopic Approach
02Q50ZZ	Repair Atrial Septum, Open Approach
02Q53ZZ	Repair Atrial Septum, Percutaneous Approach
02Q54ZZ	Repair Atrial Septum, Percutaneous Endoscopic Approach
02Q60ZZ	Repair Right Atrium, Open Approach
02Q63ZZ	Repair Right Atrium, Percutaneous Approach
02Q64ZZ	Repair Right Atrium, Percutaneous Endoscopic Approach
02Q70ZZ	Repair Left Atrium, Open Approach
02Q73ZZ	Repair Left Atrium, Percutaneous Approach
02Q74ZZ	Repair Left Atrium, Percutaneous Endoscopic Approach
02Q80ZZ	Repair Conduction Mechanism, Open Approach
02Q83ZZ	Repair Conduction Mechanism, Percutaneous Approach
02Q84ZZ	Repair Conduction Mechanism, Percutaneous Endoscopic Approach
02Q90ZZ	Repair Chordae Tendineae, Open Approach
02Q93ZZ	Repair Chordae Tendineae, Percutaneous Approach
02Q94ZZ	Repair Chordae Tendineae, Percutaneous Endoscopic Approach
02QA0ZZ	Repair Heart, Open Approach
02QA3ZZ	Repair Heart, Percutaneous Approach
02QA4ZZ	Repair Heart, Percutaneous Endoscopic Approach
02QB0ZZ	Repair Right Heart, Open Approach
02QB3ZZ	Repair Right Heart, Percutaneous Approach
02QB4ZZ	Repair Right Heart, Percutaneous Endoscopic Approach
02QC0ZZ	Repair Left Heart, Open Approach
02QC3ZZ	Repair Left Heart, Percutaneous Approach
02QC4ZZ	Repair Left Heart, Percutaneous Endoscopic Approach
02QD0ZZ	Repair Papillary Muscle, Open Approach
02QD3ZZ	Repair Papillary Muscle, Percutaneous Approach
02QD4ZZ	Repair Papillary Muscle, Percutaneous Endoscopic Approach
02QF0ZZ	Repair Aortic Valve, Open Approach
02QF3ZZ	Repair Aortic Valve, Percutaneous Approach
02QF4ZZ	Repair Aortic Valve, Percutaneous Endoscopic Approach
02QG0ZZ	Repair Mitral Valve, Open Approach
02QG3ZZ	Repair Mitral Valve, Percutaneous Approach
02QG4ZZ	Repair Mitral Valve, Percutaneous Endoscopic Approach
02QH0ZZ	Repair Pulmonary Valve, Open Approach
02QH3ZZ	Repair Pulmonary Valve, Percutaneous Approach
02QH4ZZ	Repair Pulmonary Valve, Percutaneous Endoscopic Approach
02QJ0ZZ	Repair Tricuspid Valve, Open Approach
02QJ3ZZ	Repair Tricuspid Valve, Percutaneous Approach
02QJ4ZZ	Repair Tricuspid Valve, Percutaneous Endoscopic Approach
02QK0ZZ	Repair Right Ventricle, Open Approach
02QK3ZZ	Repair Right Ventricle, Percutaneous Approach
02QK4ZZ	Repair Right Ventricle, Percutaneous Endoscopic Approach
02QL0ZZ	Repair Left Ventricle, Open Approach
02QL3ZZ	Repair Left Ventricle, Percutaneous Approach
02QL4ZZ	Repair Left Ventricle, Percutaneous Endoscopic Approach
02QM0ZZ	Repair Ventricular Septum, Open Approach
02QM3ZZ	Repair Ventricular Septum, Percutaneous Approach
02QM4ZZ	Repair Ventricular Septum, Percutaneous Endoscopic Approach
02QN0ZZ	Repair Pericardium, Open Approach
02QN3ZZ	Repair Pericardium, Percutaneous Approach
02QN4ZZ	Repair Pericardium, Percutaneous Endoscopic Approach
02QP0ZZ	Repair Pulmonary Trunk, Open Approach
02QP3ZZ	Repair Pulmonary Trunk, Percutaneous Approach
02QP4ZZ	Repair Pulmonary Trunk, Percutaneous Endoscopic Approach
02QQ0ZZ	Repair Right Pulmonary Artery, Open Approach
02QQ3ZZ	Repair Right Pulmonary Artery, Percutaneous Approach
02QQ4ZZ	Repair Right Pulmonary Artery, Percutaneous Endoscopic Approach
02QR0ZZ	Repair Left Pulmonary Artery, Open Approach
02QR3ZZ	Repair Left Pulmonary Artery, Percutaneous Approach
02QR4ZZ	Repair Left Pulmonary Artery, Percutaneous Endoscopic Approach
02QS0ZZ	Repair Right Pulmonary Vein, Open Approach
02QS3ZZ	Repair Right Pulmonary Vein, Percutaneous Approach
02QS4ZZ	Repair Right Pulmonary Vein, Percutaneous Endoscopic Approach
02QT0ZZ	Repair Left Pulmonary Vein, Open Approach
02QT3ZZ	Repair Left Pulmonary Vein, Percutaneous Approach
02QT4ZZ	Repair Left Pulmonary Vein, Percutaneous Endoscopic Approach
02QV0ZZ	Repair Superior Vena Cava, Open Approach
02QV3ZZ	Repair Superior Vena Cava, Percutaneous Approach
02QV4ZZ	Repair Superior Vena Cava, Percutaneous Endoscopic Approach
02QW0ZZ	Repair Thoracic Aorta, Open Approach
02QW3ZZ	Repair Thoracic Aorta, Percutaneous Approach
02QW4ZZ	Repair Thoracic Aorta, Percutaneous Endoscopic Approach

02R – Heart and Great Vessels, Replacement

02R507Z	Replacement of Atrial Septum with Autologous Tissue Substitute, Open Approach
02R508Z	Replacement of Atrial Septum with Zooplastic Tissue, Open Approach
02R50JZ	Replacement of Atrial Septum with Synthetic Substitute, Open Approach
02R50KZ	Replacement of Atrial Septum with Nonautologous Tissue Substitute, Open Approach
02R547Z	Replacement of Atrial Septum with Autologous Tissue Substitute, Percutaneous Endoscopic Approach
02R548Z	Replacement of Atrial Septum with Zooplastic Tissue, Percutaneous Endoscopic Approach
02R54JZ	Replacement of Atrial Septum with Synthetic Substitute, Percutaneous Endoscopic Approach
02R54KZ	Replacement of Atrial Septum with Nonautologous Tissue Substitute, Percutaneous Endoscopic Approach
02R607Z	Replacement of Right Atrium with Autologous Tissue Substitute, Open Approach
02R608Z	Replacement of Right Atrium with Zooplastic Tissue, Open Approach
02R60JZ	Replacement of Right Atrium with Synthetic Substitute, Open Approach
02R60KZ	Replacement of Right Atrium with Nonautologous Tissue Substitute, Open Approach
02R647Z	Replacement of Right Atrium with Autologous Tissue Substitute, Percutaneous Endoscopic Approach
02R648Z	Replacement of Right Atrium with Zooplastic Tissue, Percutaneous Endoscopic Approach
02R64JZ	Replacement of Right Atrium with Synthetic Substitute, Percutaneous Endoscopic Approach
02R64KZ	Replacement of Right Atrium with Nonautologous Tissue Substitute, Percutaneous Endoscopic Approach
02R707Z	Replacement of Left Atrium with Autologous Tissue Substitute, Open Approach
02R708Z	Replacement of Left Atrium with Zooplastic Tissue, Open Approach
02R70JZ	Replacement of Left Atrium with Synthetic Substitute, Open Approach
02R70KZ	Replacement of Left Atrium with Nonautologous Tissue Substitute, Open Approach
02R747Z	Replacement of Left Atrium with Autologous Tissue Substitute, Percutaneous Endoscopic Approach
02R748Z	Replacement of Left Atrium with Zooplastic Tissue, Percutaneous Endoscopic Approach
02R74JZ	Replacement of Left Atrium with Synthetic Substitute, Percutaneous Endoscopic Approach
02R74KZ	Replacement of Left Atrium with Nonautologous Tissue Substitute, Percutaneous Endoscopic Approach
02R907Z	Replacement of Chordae Tendineae with Autologous Tissue Substitute, Open Approach
02R908Z	Replacement of Chordae Tendineae with Zooplastic Tissue, Open Approach
02R90JZ	Replacement of Chordae Tendineae with Synthetic Substitute, Open Approach
02R90KZ	Replacement of Chordae Tendineae with Nonautologous Tissue Substitute, Open Approach
02R947Z	Replacement of Chordae Tendineae with Autologous Tissue Substitute, Percutaneous Endoscopic Approach

♀ Female-only   ♂ Male-only   ▲ Limited Coverage   ● Non-OR   ▰ HAC-associated procedure   ▲ Non-covered procedures   ✚ Combination

948Z Replacement of Chordae Tendineae with Zooplastic Tissue, Percutaneous Endoscopic Approach

94JZ Replacement of Chordae Tendineae with Synthetic Substitute, Percutaneous Endoscopic Approach

94KZ Replacement of Chordae Tendineae with Nonautologous Tissue Substitute, Percutaneous Endoscopic Approach

D07Z Replacement of Papillary Muscle with Autologous Tissue Substitute, Open Approach

D08Z Replacement of Papillary Muscle with Zooplastic Tissue, Open Approach

D0JZ Replacement of Papillary Muscle with Synthetic Substitute, Open Approach

D0KZ Replacement of Papillary Muscle with Nonautologous Tissue Substitute, Open Approach

D47Z Replacement of Papillary Muscle with Autologous Tissue Substitute, Percutaneous Endoscopic Approach

D48Z Replacement of Papillary Muscle with Zooplastic Tissue, Percutaneous Endoscopic Approach

D4JZ Replacement of Papillary Muscle with Synthetic Substitute, Percutaneous Endoscopic Approach

D4KZ Replacement of Papillary Muscle with Nonautologous Tissue Substitute, Percutaneous Endoscopic Approach

F07Z Replacement of Aortic Valve with Autologous Tissue Substitute, Open Approach

F08Z Replacement of Aortic Valve with Zooplastic Tissue, Open Approach

F0JZ Replacement of Aortic Valve with Synthetic Substitute, Open Approach

F0KZ Replacement of Aortic Valve with Nonautologous Tissue Substitute, Open Approach

F37H Replacement of Aortic Valve with Autologous Tissue Substitute, Transapical, Percutaneous Approach

F37Z Replacement of Aortic Valve with Autologous Tissue Substitute, Percutaneous Approach

F38H Replacement of Aortic Valve with Zooplastic Tissue, Transapical, Percutaneous Approach

F38Z Replacement of Aortic Valve with Zooplastic Tissue, Percutaneous Approach

F3JH Replacement of Aortic Valve with Synthetic Substitute, Transapical, Percutaneous Approach

F3JZ Replacement of Aortic Valve with Synthetic Substitute, Percutaneous Approach

F3KH Replacement of Aortic Valve with Nonautologous Tissue Substitute, Transapical, Percutaneous Approach

F3KZ Replacement of Aortic Valve with Nonautologous Tissue Substitute, Percutaneous Approach

F47Z Replacement of Aortic Valve with Autologous Tissue Substitute, Percutaneous Endoscopic Approach

F48Z Replacement of Aortic Valve with Zooplastic Tissue, Percutaneous Endoscopic Approach

F4JZ Replacement of Aortic Valve with Synthetic Substitute, Percutaneous Endoscopic Approach

F4KZ Replacement of Aortic Valve with Nonautologous Tissue Substitute, Percutaneous Endoscopic Approach

02RG07Z Replacement of Mitral Valve with Autologous Tissue Substitute, Open Approach

02RG08Z Replacement of Mitral Valve with Zooplastic Tissue, Open Approach

02RG0JZ Replacement of Mitral Valve with Synthetic Substitute, Open Approach

02RG0KZ Replacement of Mitral Valve with Nonautologous Tissue Substitute, Open Approach

02RG37H Replacement of Mitral Valve with Autologous Tissue Substitute, Transapical, Percutaneous Approach

02RG37Z Replacement of Mitral Valve with Autologous Tissue Substitute, Percutaneous Approach

02RG38H Replacement of Mitral Valve with Zooplastic Tissue, Transapical, Percutaneous Approach

02RG38Z Replacement of Mitral Valve with Zooplastic Tissue, Percutaneous Approach

02RG3JH Replacement of Mitral Valve with Synthetic Substitute, Transapical, Percutaneous Approach

02RG3JZ Replacement of Mitral Valve with Synthetic Substitute, Percutaneous Approach

02RG3KH Replacement of Mitral Valve with Nonautologous Tissue Substitute, Transapical, Percutaneous Approach

02RG3KZ Replacement of Mitral Valve with Nonautologous Tissue Substitute, Percutaneous Approach

02RG47Z Replacement of Mitral Valve with Autologous Tissue Substitute, Percutaneous Endoscopic Approach

02RG48Z Replacement of Mitral Valve with Zooplastic Tissue, Percutaneous Endoscopic Approach

02RG4JZ Replacement of Mitral Valve with Synthetic Substitute, Percutaneous Endoscopic Approach

02RG4KZ Replacement of Mitral Valve with Nonautologous Tissue Substitute, Percutaneous Endoscopic Approach

02RH07Z Replacement of Pulmonary Valve with Autologous Tissue Substitute, Open Approach

02RH08Z Replacement of Pulmonary Valve with Zooplastic Tissue, Open Approach

02RH0JZ Replacement of Pulmonary Valve with Synthetic Substitute, Open Approach

02RH0KZ Replacement of Pulmonary Valve with Nonautologous Tissue Substitute, Open Approach

02RH37H Replacement of Pulmonary Valve with Autologous Tissue Substitute, Transapical, Percutaneous Approach

02RH37Z Replacement of Pulmonary Valve with Autologous Tissue Substitute, Percutaneous Approach

02RH38H Replacement of Pulmonary Valve with Zooplastic Tissue, Transapical, Percutaneous Approach

02RH38Z Replacement of Pulmonary Valve with Zooplastic Tissue, Percutaneous Approach

02RH3JH Replacement of Pulmonary Valve with Synthetic Substitute, Transapical, Percutaneous Approach

02RH3JZ Replacement of Pulmonary Valve with Synthetic Substitute, Percutaneous Approach

02RH3KH Replacement of Pulmonary Valve with Nonautologous Tissue Substitute, Transapical, Percutaneous Approach

02RH3KZ Replacement of Pulmonary Valve with Nonautologous Tissue Substitute, Percutaneous Approach

02RH47Z Replacement of Pulmonary Valve with Autologous Tissue Substitute, Percutaneous Endoscopic Approach

02RH48Z Replacement of Pulmonary Valve with Zooplastic Tissue, Percutaneous Endoscopic Approach

02RH4JZ Replacement of Pulmonary Valve with Synthetic Substitute, Percutaneous Endoscopic Approach

02RH4KZ Replacement of Pulmonary Valve with Nonautologous Tissue Substitute, Percutaneous Endoscopic Approach

02RJ07Z Replacement of Tricuspid Valve with Autologous Tissue Substitute, Open Approach

02RJ08Z Replacement of Tricuspid Valve with Zooplastic Tissue, Open Approach

02RJ0JZ Replacement of Tricuspid Valve with Synthetic Substitute, Open Approach

02RJ0KZ Replacement of Tricuspid Valve with Nonautologous Tissue Substitute, Open Approach

02RJ47Z Replacement of Tricuspid Valve with Autologous Tissue Substitute, Percutaneous Endoscopic Approach

02RJ48Z Replacement of Tricuspid Valve with Zooplastic Tissue, Percutaneous Endoscopic Approach

02RJ4JZ Replacement of Tricuspid Valve with Synthetic Substitute, Percutaneous Endoscopic Approach

02RJ4KZ Replacement of Tricuspid Valve with Nonautologous Tissue Substitute, Percutaneous Endoscopic Approach

02RK07Z Replacement of Right Ventricle with Autologous Tissue Substitute, Open Approach

02RK08Z Replacement of Right Ventricle with Zooplastic Tissue, Open Approach

02RK0JZ Replacement of Right Ventricle with Synthetic Substitute, Open Approach
▲ *When reported with 02RL0JZ and diagnosis code Z00.6*

02RK0KZ Replacement of Right Ventricle with Nonautologous Tissue Substitute, Open Approach

02RK47Z Replacement of Right Ventricle with Autologous Tissue Substitute, Percutaneous Endoscopic Approach

02RK48Z Replacement of Right Ventricle with Zooplastic Tissue, Percutaneous Endoscopic Approach

02RK4JZ Replacement of Right Ventricle with Synthetic Substitute, Percutaneous Endoscopic Approach

02RK4KZ Replacement of Right Ventricle with Nonautologous Tissue Substitute, Percutaneous Endoscopic Approach

02RL07Z Replacement of Left Ventricle with Autologous Tissue Substitute, Open Approach

02RL08Z Replacement of Left Ventricle with Zooplastic Tissue, Open Approach

02RL0JZ Replacement of Left Ventricle with Synthetic Substitute, Open Approach
▲ *When reported with 02RK0JZ and diagnosis code Z00.6*

02RL0KZ Replacement of Left Ventricle with Nonautologous Tissue Substitute, Open Approach

02RL47Z Replacement of Left Ventricle with Autologous Tissue Substitute, Percutaneous Endoscopic Approach

02RL48Z Replacement of Left Ventricle with Zooplastic Tissue, Percutaneous Endoscopic Approach

02RL4JZ Replacement of Left Ventricle with Synthetic Substitute, Percutaneous Endoscopic Approach

02RL4KZ Replacement of Left Ventricle with Nonautologous Tissue Substitute, Percutaneous Endoscopic Approach

02RM07Z Replacement of Ventricular Septum with Autologous Tissue Substitute, Open Approach

02RM08Z Replacement of Ventricular Septum with Zooplastic Tissue, Open Approach

02RM0JZ Replacement of Ventricular Septum with Synthetic Substitute, Open Approach

02RM0KZ Replacement of Ventricular Septum with Nonautologous Tissue Substitute, Open Approach

02RM47Z Replacement of Ventricular Septum with Autologous Tissue Substitute, Percutaneous Endoscopic Approach

02RM48Z Replacement of Ventricular Septum with Zooplastic Tissue, Percutaneous Endoscopic Approach

02RM4JZ Replacement of Ventricular Septum with Synthetic Substitute, Percutaneous Endoscopic Approach

02RM4KZ Replacement of Ventricular Septum with Nonautologous Tissue Substitute, Percutaneous Endoscopic Approach

02RN07Z Replacement of Pericardium with Autologous Tissue Substitute, Open Approach

02RN08Z Replacement of Pericardium with Zooplastic Tissue, Open Approach

02RN0JZ Replacement of Pericardium with Synthetic Substitute, Open Approach

02RN0KZ Replacement of Pericardium with Nonautologous Tissue Substitute, Open Approach

02RN47Z Replacement of Pericardium with Autologous Tissue Substitute, Percutaneous Endoscopic Approach

02RN48Z Replacement of Pericardium with Zooplastic Tissue, Percutaneous Endoscopic Approach

02RN4JZ Replacement of Pericardium with Synthetic Substitute, Percutaneous Endoscopic Approach

02RN4KZ Replacement of Pericardium with Nonautologous Tissue Substitute, Percutaneous Endoscopic Approach

02RP07Z Replacement of Pulmonary Trunk with Autologous Tissue Substitute, Open Approach

02RP08Z Replacement of Pulmonary Trunk with Zooplastic Tissue, Open Approach

02RP0JZ Replacement of Pulmonary Trunk with Synthetic Substitute, Open Approach

02RP0KZ Replacement of Pulmonary Trunk with Nonautologous Tissue Substitute, Open Approach

02RP47Z Replacement of Pulmonary Trunk with Autologous Tissue Substitute, Percutaneous Endoscopic Approach

02RP48Z Replacement of Pulmonary Trunk with Zooplastic Tissue, Percutaneous Endoscopic Approach

02RP4JZ Replacement of Pulmonary Trunk with Synthetic Substitute, Percutaneous Endoscopic Approach

02RP4KZ Replacement of Pulmonary Trunk with Nonautologous Tissue Substitute, Percutaneous Endoscopic Approach

02RQ07Z Replacement of Right Pulmonary Artery with Autologous Tissue Substitute, Open Approach

02RQ08Z Replacement of Right Pulmonary Artery with Zooplastic Tissue, Open Approach

02RQ0JZ Replacement of Right Pulmonary Artery with Synthetic Substitute, Open Approach

02RQ0KZ Replacement of Right Pulmonary Artery with Nonautologous Tissue Substitute, Open Approach

02RQ47Z Replacement of Right Pulmonary Artery with Autologous Tissue Substitute, Percutaneous Endoscopic Approach

02RQ48Z Replacement of Right Pulmonary Artery with Zooplastic Tissue, Percutaneous Endoscopic Approach

02RQ4JZ Replacement of Right Pulmonary Artery with Synthetic Substitute, Percutaneous Endoscopic Approach

02RQ4KZ Replacement of Right Pulmonary Artery with Nonautologous Tissue Substitute, Percutaneous Endoscopic Approach

02RR07Z Replacement of Left Pulmonary Artery with Autologous Tissue Substitute, Open Approach

02RR08Z Replacement of Left Pulmonary Artery with Zooplastic Tissue, Open Approach

02RR0JZ Replacement of Left Pulmonary Artery with Synthetic Substitute, Open Approach

02RR0KZ Replacement of Left Pulmonary Artery with Nonautologous Tissue Substitute, Open Approach

02RR47Z Replacement of Left Pulmonary Artery with Autologous Tissue Substitute, Percutaneous Endoscopic Approach

02RR48Z Replacement of Left Pulmonary Artery with Zooplastic Tissue, Percutaneous Endoscopic Approach

02RR4JZ Replacement of Left Pulmonary Artery with Synthetic Substitute, Percutaneous Endoscopic Approach

02RR4KZ Replacement of Left Pulmonary Artery with Nonautologous Tissue Substitute, Percutaneous Endoscopic Approach

02RS07Z Replacement of Right Pulmonary Vein with Autologous Tissue Substitute, Open Approach

02RS08Z Replacement of Right Pulmonary Vein with Zooplastic Tissue, Open Approach

02RS0JZ Replacement of Right Pulmonary Vein with Synthetic Substitute, Open Approach

02RS0KZ Replacement of Right Pulmonary Vein with Nonautologous Tissue Substitute, Open Approach

02RS47Z Replacement of Right Pulmonary Vein with Autologous Tissue Substitute, Percutaneous Endoscopic Approach

02RS48Z Replacement of Right Pulmonary Vein with Zooplastic Tissue, Percutaneous Endoscopic Approach

02RS4JZ Replacement of Right Pulmonary Vein with Synthetic Substitute, Percutaneous Endoscopic Approach

02RS4KZ Replacement of Right Pulmonary Vein with Nonautologous Tissue Substitute, Percutaneous Endoscopic Approach

02RT07Z Replacement of Left Pulmonary Vein with Autologous Tissue Substitute, Open Approach

02RT08Z Replacement of Left Pulmonary Vein with Zooplastic Tissue, Open Approach

02RT0JZ Replacement of Left Pulmonary Vein with Synthetic Substitute, Open Approach

02RT0KZ Replacement of Left Pulmonary Vein with Nonautologous Tissue Substitute, Open Approach

02RT47Z Replacement of Left Pulmonary Vein with Autologous Tissue Substitute, Percutaneous Endoscopic Approach

02RT48Z Replacement of Left Pulmonary Vein with Zooplastic Tissue, Percutaneous Endoscopic Approach

02RT4JZ Replacement of Left Pulmonary Vein with Synthetic Substitute, Percutaneous Endoscopic Approach

02RT4KZ Replacement of Left Pulmonary Vein with Nonautologous Tissue Substitute, Percutaneous Endoscopic Approach

02RV07Z Replacement of Superior Vena Cava with Autologous Tissue Substitute, Open Approach

02RV08Z Replacement of Superior Vena Cava with Zooplastic Tissue, Open Approach

02RV0JZ Replacement of Superior Vena Cava with Synthetic Substitute, Open Approach

02RV0KZ Replacement of Superior Vena Cava with Nonautologous Tissue Substitute, Open Approach

02RV47Z Replacement of Superior Vena Cava with Autologous Tissue Substitute, Percutaneous Endoscopic Approach

02RV48Z Replacement of Superior Vena Cava with Zooplastic Tissue, Percutaneous Endoscopic Approach

02RV4JZ Replacement of Superior Vena Cava with Synthetic Substitute, Percutaneous Endoscopic Approach

02RV4KZ Replacement of Superior Vena Cava with Nonautologous Tissue Substitute, Percutaneous Endoscopic Approach

02RW07Z Replacement of Thoracic Aorta with Autologous Tissue Substitute, Open Approach

02RW08Z Replacement of Thoracic Aorta with Zooplastic Tissue, Open Approach

02RW0JZ Replacement of Thoracic Aorta with Synthetic Substitute, Open Approach

02RW0KZ Replacement of Thoracic Aorta with Nonautologous Tissue Substitute, Open Approach

AHA CC: 1Q, 2014, 10-11

02RW47Z Replacement of Thoracic Aorta with Autologous Tissue Substitute, Percutaneous Endoscopic Approach

02RW48Z Replacement of Thoracic Aorta with Zooplastic Tissue, Percutaneous Endoscopic Approach

02RW4JZ Replacement of Thoracic Aorta with Synthetic Substitute, Percutaneous Endoscopic Approach

02RW4KZ Replacement of Thoracic Aorta with Nonautologous Tissue Substitute, Percutaneous Endoscopic Approach

02S – Heart and Great Vessels, Reposition

02SP0ZZ Reposition Pulmonary Trunk, Open Approach

02SQ0ZZ Reposition Right Pulmonary Artery, Open Approach

02SR0ZZ Reposition Left Pulmonary Artery, Open Approach

02SS0ZZ Reposition Right Pulmonary Vein, Open Approach

02ST0ZZ Reposition Left Pulmonary Vein, Open Approach

02SV0ZZ Reposition Superior Vena Cava, Open Approach

02SW0ZZ Reposition Thoracic Aorta, Open Approach

♀ Female-only   ♂ Male-only   ▲ Limited Coverage   ● Non-OR   ▨ HAC-associated procedure   ▲ Non-covered procedures   ➕ Combinati

T – Heart and Great Vessels, Resection

iew Coding Guideline B3.8

50ZZ Resection of Atrial Septum, Open Approach

53ZZ Resection of Atrial Septum, Percutaneous Approach

54ZZ Resection of Atrial Septum, Percutaneous Endoscopic Approach

80ZZ Resection of Conduction Mechanism, Open Approach

83ZZ Resection of Conduction Mechanism, Percutaneous Approach

84ZZ Resection of Conduction Mechanism, Percutaneous Endoscopic Approach

90ZZ Resection of Chordae Tendineae, Open Approach

02T93ZZ Resection of Chordae Tendineae, Percutaneous Approach

02T94ZZ Resection of Chordae Tendineae, Percutaneous Endoscopic Approach

02TD0ZZ Resection of Papillary Muscle, Open Approach

02TD3ZZ Resection of Papillary Muscle, Percutaneous Approach

02TD4ZZ Resection of Papillary Muscle, Percutaneous Endoscopic Approach

02TH0ZZ Resection of Pulmonary Valve, Open Approach

02TH3ZZ Resection of Pulmonary Valve, Percutaneous Approach

02TH4ZZ Resection of Pulmonary Valve, Percutaneous Endoscopic Approach

02TM0ZZ Resection of Ventricular Septum, Open Approach

02TM3ZZ Resection of Ventricular Septum, Percutaneous Approach

02TM4ZZ Resection of Ventricular Septum, Percutaneous Endoscopic Approach

02TN0ZZ Resection of Pericardium, Open Approach

02TN3ZZ Resection of Pericardium, Percutaneous Approach

02TN4ZZ Resection of Pericardium, Percutaneous Endoscopic Approach

U – Heart and Great Vessels, Supplement

507Z Supplement Atrial Septum with Autologous Tissue Substitute, Open Approach

508Z Supplement Atrial Septum with Zooplastic Tissue, Open Approach

50JZ Supplement Atrial Septum with Synthetic Substitute, Open Approach

50KZ Supplement Atrial Septum with Nonautologous Tissue Substitute, Open Approach

537Z Supplement Atrial Septum with Autologous Tissue Substitute, Percutaneous Approach

538Z Supplement Atrial Septum with Zooplastic Tissue, Percutaneous Approach

53JZ Supplement Atrial Septum with Synthetic Substitute, Percutaneous Approach

53KZ Supplement Atrial Septum with Nonautologous Tissue Substitute, Percutaneous Approach

547Z Supplement Atrial Septum with Autologous Tissue Substitute, Percutaneous Endoscopic Approach

548Z Supplement Atrial Septum with Zooplastic Tissue, Percutaneous Endoscopic Approach

54JZ Supplement Atrial Septum with Synthetic Substitute, Percutaneous Endoscopic Approach

54KZ Supplement Atrial Septum with Nonautologous Tissue Substitute, Percutaneous Endoscopic Approach

607Z Supplement Right Atrium with Autologous Tissue Substitute, Open Approach

U608Z Supplement Right Atrium with Zooplastic Tissue, Open Approach

U60JZ Supplement Right Atrium with Synthetic Substitute, Open Approach

U60KZ Supplement Right Atrium with Nonautologous Tissue Substitute, Open Approach

U637Z Supplement Right Atrium with Autologous Tissue Substitute, Percutaneous Approach

U638Z Supplement Right Atrium with Zooplastic Tissue, Percutaneous Approach

U63JZ Supplement Right Atrium with Synthetic Substitute, Percutaneous Approach

U63KZ Supplement Right Atrium with Nonautologous Tissue Substitute, Percutaneous Approach

U647Z Supplement Right Atrium with Autologous Tissue Substitute, Percutaneous Endoscopic Approach

U648Z Supplement Right Atrium with Zooplastic Tissue, Percutaneous Endoscopic Approach

02U64JZ Supplement Right Atrium with Synthetic Substitute, Percutaneous Endoscopic Approach

02U64KZ Supplement Right Atrium with Nonautologous Tissue Substitute, Percutaneous Endoscopic Approach

02U707Z Supplement Left Atrium with Autologous Tissue Substitute, Open Approach

02U708Z Supplement Left Atrium with Zooplastic Tissue, Open Approach

02U70JZ Supplement Left Atrium with Synthetic Substitute, Open Approach

02U70KZ Supplement Left Atrium with Nonautologous Tissue Substitute, Open Approach

02U737Z Supplement Left Atrium with Autologous Tissue Substitute, Percutaneous Approach

02U738Z Supplement Left Atrium with Zooplastic Tissue, Percutaneous Approach

● **02U73JZ** Supplement Left Atrium with Synthetic Substitute, Percutaneous Approach

02U73KZ Supplement Left Atrium with Nonautologous Tissue Substitute, Percutaneous Approach

02U747Z Supplement Left Atrium with Autologous Tissue Substitute, Percutaneous Endoscopic Approach

02U748Z Supplement Left Atrium with Zooplastic Tissue, Percutaneous Endoscopic Approach

● **02U74JZ** Supplement Left Atrium with Synthetic Substitute, Percutaneous Endoscopic Approach

02U74KZ Supplement Left Atrium with Nonautologous Tissue Substitute, Percutaneous Endoscopic Approach

02U907Z Supplement Chordae Tendineae with Autologous Tissue Substitute, Open Approach

02U908Z Supplement Chordae Tendineae with Zooplastic Tissue, Open Approach

02U90JZ Supplement Chordae Tendineae with Synthetic Substitute, Open Approach

02U90KZ Supplement Chordae Tendineae with Nonautologous Tissue Substitute, Open Approach

02U937Z Supplement Chordae Tendineae with Autologous Tissue Substitute, Percutaneous Approach

02U938Z Supplement Chordae Tendineae with Zooplastic Tissue, Percutaneous Approach

02U93JZ Supplement Chordae Tendineae with Synthetic Substitute, Percutaneous Approach

02U93KZ Supplement Chordae Tendineae with Nonautologous Tissue Substitute, Percutaneous Approach

02U947Z Supplement Chordae Tendineae with Autologous Tissue Substitute, Percutaneous Endoscopic Approach

02U948Z Supplement Chordae Tendineae with Zooplastic Tissue, Percutaneous Endoscopic Approach

02U94JZ Supplement Chordae Tendineae with Synthetic Substitute, Percutaneous Endoscopic Approach

02U94KZ Supplement Chordae Tendineae with Nonautologous Tissue Substitute, Percutaneous Endoscopic Approach

02UA07Z Supplement Heart with Autologous Tissue Substitute, Open Approach

02UA08Z Supplement Heart with Zooplastic Tissue, Open Approach

02UA0JZ Supplement Heart with Synthetic Substitute, Open Approach

02UA0KZ Supplement Heart with Nonautologous Tissue Substitute, Open Approach

02UA37Z Supplement Heart with Autologous Tissue Substitute, Percutaneous Approach

02UA38Z Supplement Heart with Zooplastic Tissue, Percutaneous Approach

02UA3JZ Supplement Heart with Synthetic Substitute, Percutaneous Approach

02UA3KZ Supplement Heart with Nonautologous Tissue Substitute, Percutaneous Approach

02UA47Z Supplement Heart with Autologous Tissue Substitute, Percutaneous Endoscopic Approach

02UA48Z Supplement Heart with Zooplastic Tissue, Percutaneous Endoscopic Approach

02UA4JZ Supplement Heart with Synthetic Substitute, Percutaneous Endoscopic Approach

02UA4KZ Supplement Heart with Nonautologous Tissue Substitute, Percutaneous Endoscopic Approach

02UD07Z Supplement Papillary Muscle with Autologous Tissue Substitute, Open Approach

02UD08Z Supplement Papillary Muscle with Zooplastic Tissue, Open Approach

02UD0JZ Supplement Papillary Muscle with Synthetic Substitute, Open Approach

02UD0KZ Supplement Papillary Muscle with Nonautologous Tissue Substitute, Open Approach

02UD37Z Supplement Papillary Muscle with Autologous Tissue Substitute, Percutaneous Approach

02UD38Z Supplement Papillary Muscle with Zooplastic Tissue, Percutaneous Approach

02UD3JZ Supplement Papillary Muscle with Synthetic Substitute, Percutaneous Approach

♀ Female-only ♂ Male-only ▲ Limited Coverage ● Non-OR ▬ HAC-associated procedure ▲ Non-covered procedures ✛ Combination

02UD3KZ	Supplement Papillary Muscle with Nonautologous Tissue Substitute, Percutaneous Approach	02UH08Z	Supplement Pulmonary Valve with Zooplastic Tissue, Open Approach	02UK38Z	Supplement Right Ventricle with Zooplastic Tissue, Percutaneous Approach
02UD47Z	Supplement Papillary Muscle with Autologous Tissue Substitute, Percutaneous Endoscopic Approach	02UH0JZ	Supplement Pulmonary Valve with Synthetic Substitute, Open Approach	02UK3JZ	Supplement Right Ventricle with Synthetic Substitute, Percutaneous Approach
02UD48Z	Supplement Papillary Muscle with Zooplastic Tissue, Percutaneous Endoscopic Approach	02UH0KZ	Supplement Pulmonary Valve with Nonautologous Tissue Substitute, Open Approach	02UK3KZ	Supplement Right Ventricle with Nonautologous Tissue Substitute, Percutaneous Approach
02UD4JZ	Supplement Papillary Muscle with Synthetic Substitute, Percutaneous Endoscopic Approach	02UH37Z	Supplement Pulmonary Valve with Autologous Tissue Substitute, Percutaneous Approach	02UK47Z	Supplement Right Ventricle with Autologous Tissue Substitute, Percutaneous Endoscopic Approach
02UD4KZ	Supplement Papillary Muscle with Nonautologous Tissue Substitute, Percutaneous Endoscopic Approach	02UH38Z	Supplement Pulmonary Valve with Zooplastic Tissue, Percutaneous Approach	02UK48Z	Supplement Right Ventricle with Zooplastic Tissue, Percutaneous Endoscopic Approach
02UF07Z	Supplement Aortic Valve with Autologous Tissue Substitute, Open Approach	02UH3JZ	Supplement Pulmonary Valve with Synthetic Substitute, Percutaneous Approach	02UK4JZ	Supplement Right Ventricle with Synthetic Substitute, Percutaneous Endoscopic Approach
02UF08Z	Supplement Aortic Valve with Zooplastic Tissue, Open Approach	02UH3KZ	Supplement Pulmonary Valve with Nonautologous Tissue Substitute, Percutaneous Approach	02UK4KZ	Supplement Right Ventricle with Nonautologous Tissue Substitute, Percutaneous Endoscopic Approach
02UF0JZ	Supplement Aortic Valve with Synthetic Substitute, Open Approach	02UH47Z	Supplement Pulmonary Valve with Autologous Tissue Substitute, Percutaneous Endoscopic Approach	02UL07Z	Supplement Left Ventricle with Autologous Tissue Substitute, Open Approach
02UF0KZ	Supplement Aortic Valve with Nonautologous Tissue Substitute, Open Approach	02UH48Z	Supplement Pulmonary Valve with Zooplastic Tissue, Percutaneous Endoscopic Approach	02UL08Z	Supplement Left Ventricle with Zooplas Tissue, Open Approach
02UF37Z	Supplement Aortic Valve with Autologous Tissue Substitute, Percutaneous Approach	02UH4JZ	Supplement Pulmonary Valve with Synthetic Substitute, Percutaneous Endoscopic Approach	02UL0JZ	Supplement Left Ventricle with Synthe Substitute, Open Approach
02UF38Z	Supplement Aortic Valve with Zooplastic Tissue, Percutaneous Approach	02UH4KZ	Supplement Pulmonary Valve with Nonautologous Tissue Substitute, Percutaneous Endoscopic Approach	02UL0KZ	Supplement Left Ventricle with Nonautologous Tissue Substitute, Open Approach
02UF3JZ	Supplement Aortic Valve with Synthetic Substitute, Percutaneous Approach	02UJ07Z	Supplement Tricuspid Valve with Autologous Tissue Substitute, Open Approach	02UL37Z	Supplement Left Ventricle with Autologous Tissue Substitute, Percutaneous Approach
02UF3KZ	Supplement Aortic Valve with Nonautologous Tissue Substitute, Percutaneous Approach	02UJ08Z	Supplement Tricuspid Valve with Zooplastic Tissue, Open Approach	02UL38Z	Supplement Left Ventricle with Zooplas Tissue, Percutaneous Approach
02UF47Z	Supplement Aortic Valve with Autologous Tissue Substitute, Percutaneous Endoscopic Approach	02UJ0JZ	Supplement Tricuspid Valve with Synthetic Substitute, Open Approach	02UL3JZ	Supplement Left Ventricle with Synthe Substitute, Percutaneous Approach
02UF48Z	Supplement Aortic Valve with Zooplastic Tissue, Percutaneous Endoscopic Approach	02UJ0KZ	Supplement Tricuspid Valve with Nonautologous Tissue Substitute, Open Approach	02UL3KZ	Supplement Left Ventricle with Nonautologous Tissue Substitute, Percutaneous Approach
02UF4JZ	Supplement Aortic Valve with Synthetic Substitute, Percutaneous Endoscopic Approach	02UJ37Z	Supplement Tricuspid Valve with Autologous Tissue Substitute, Percutaneous Approach	02UL47Z	Supplement Left Ventricle with Autologous Tissue Substitute, Percutaneous Endoscopic Approach
02UF4KZ	Supplement Aortic Valve with Nonautologous Tissue Substitute, Percutaneous Endoscopic Approach	02UJ38Z	Supplement Tricuspid Valve with Zooplastic Tissue, Percutaneous Approach	02UL48Z	Supplement Left Ventricle with Zooplas Tissue, Percutaneous Endoscopic Approach
02UG07Z	Supplement Mitral Valve with Autologous Tissue Substitute, Open Approach	02UJ3JZ	Supplement Tricuspid Valve with Synthetic Substitute, Percutaneous Approach	02UL4JZ	Supplement Left Ventricle with Synthet Substitute, Percutaneous Endoscopic Approach
02UG08Z	Supplement Mitral Valve with Zooplastic Tissue, Open Approach	02UJ3KZ	Supplement Tricuspid Valve with Nonautologous Tissue Substitute, Percutaneous Approach	02UL4KZ	Supplement Left Ventricle with Nonautologous Tissue Substitute, Percutaneous Endoscopic Approach
02UG0JZ	Supplement Mitral Valve with Synthetic Substitute, Open Approach	02UJ47Z	Supplement Tricuspid Valve with Autologous Tissue Substitute, Percutaneous Endoscopic Approach	02UM07Z	Supplement Ventricular Septum with Autologous Tissue Substitute, Open Approach
02UG0KZ	Supplement Mitral Valve with Nonautologous Tissue Substitute, Open Approach	02UJ48Z	Supplement Tricuspid Valve with Zooplastic Tissue, Percutaneous Endoscopic Approach	02UM08Z	Supplement Ventricular Septum with Zooplastic Tissue, Open Approach
02UG37Z	Supplement Mitral Valve with Autologous Tissue Substitute, Percutaneous Approach	02UJ4JZ	Supplement Tricuspid Valve with Synthetic Substitute, Percutaneous Endoscopic Approach	02UM0JZ	Supplement Ventricular Septum with Synthetic Substitute, Open Approach
02UG38Z	Supplement Mitral Valve with Zooplastic Tissue, Percutaneous Approach			*AHA CC: 3Q, 2014, 16-17*	
02UG3JZ	Supplement Mitral Valve with Synthetic Substitute, Percutaneous Approach	02UJ4KZ	Supplement Tricuspid Valve with Nonautologous Tissue Substitute, Percutaneous Endoscopic Approach	02UM0KZ	Supplement Ventricular Septum with Nonautologous Tissue Substitute, Open Approach
02UG3KZ	Supplement Mitral Valve with Nonautologous Tissue Substitute, Percutaneous Approach	02UK07Z	Supplement Right Ventricle with Autologous Tissue Substitute, Open Approach	02UM37Z	Supplement Ventricular Septum with Autologous Tissue Substitute, Percutaneous Approach
02UG47Z	Supplement Mitral Valve with Autologous Tissue Substitute, Percutaneous Endoscopic Approach	02UK08Z	Supplement Right Ventricle with Zooplastic Tissue, Open Approach	02UM38Z	Supplement Ventricular Septum with Zooplastic Tissue, Percutaneous Approac
02UG48Z	Supplement Mitral Valve with Zooplastic Tissue, Percutaneous Endoscopic Approach	02UK0JZ	Supplement Right Ventricle with Synthetic Substitute, Open Approach	02UM3JZ	Supplement Ventricular Septum with Synthetic Substitute, Percutaneous Approach
02UG4JZ	Supplement Mitral Valve with Synthetic Substitute, Percutaneous Endoscopic Approach	02UK0KZ	Supplement Right Ventricle with Nonautologous Tissue Substitute, Open Approach	02UM3KZ	Supplement Ventricular Septum with Nonautologous Tissue Substitute, Percutaneous Approach
02UG4KZ	Supplement Mitral Valve with Nonautologous Tissue Substitute, Percutaneous Endoscopic Approach	02UK37Z	Supplement Right Ventricle with Autologous Tissue Substitute, Percutaneous Approach	02UM47Z	Supplement Ventricular Septum with Autologous Tissue Substitute, Percutaneous Endoscopic Approach
02UH07Z	Supplement Pulmonary Valve with Autologous Tissue Substitute, Open Approach				

♀ Female-only   ♂ Male-only   ▲ Limited Coverage   ● Non-OR   ▨ HAC-associated procedure   ▲ Non-covered procedures   ✚ Combinati

UM48Z Supplement Ventricular Septum with Zooplastic Tissue, Percutaneous Endoscopic Approach

UM4JZ Supplement Ventricular Septum with Synthetic Substitute, Percutaneous Endoscopic Approach

UM4KZ Supplement Ventricular Septum with Nonautologous Tissue Substitute, Percutaneous Endoscopic Approach

UN07Z Supplement Pericardium with Autologous Tissue Substitute, Open Approach

UN08Z Supplement Pericardium with Zooplastic Tissue, Open Approach

UN0JZ Supplement Pericardium with Synthetic Substitute, Open Approach

UN0KZ Supplement Pericardium with Nonautologous Tissue Substitute, Open Approach

UN37Z Supplement Pericardium with Autologous Tissue Substitute, Percutaneous Approach

UN38Z Supplement Pericardium with Zooplastic Tissue, Percutaneous Approach

UN3JZ Supplement Pericardium with Synthetic Substitute, Percutaneous Approach

UN3KZ Supplement Pericardium with Nonautologous Tissue Substitute, Percutaneous Approach

UN47Z Supplement Pericardium with Autologous Tissue Substitute, Percutaneous Endoscopic Approach

UN48Z Supplement Pericardium with Zooplastic Tissue, Percutaneous Endoscopic Approach

UN4JZ Supplement Pericardium with Synthetic Substitute, Percutaneous Endoscopic Approach

UN4KZ Supplement Pericardium with Nonautologous Tissue Substitute, Percutaneous Endoscopic Approach

UP07Z Supplement Pulmonary Trunk with Autologous Tissue Substitute, Open Approach

UP08Z Supplement Pulmonary Trunk with Zooplastic Tissue, Open Approach

UP0JZ Supplement Pulmonary Trunk with Synthetic Substitute, Open Approach

UP0KZ Supplement Pulmonary Trunk with Nonautologous Tissue Substitute, Open Approach

UP37Z Supplement Pulmonary Trunk with Autologous Tissue Substitute, Percutaneous Approach

UP38Z Supplement Pulmonary Trunk with Zooplastic Tissue, Percutaneous Approach

UP3JZ Supplement Pulmonary Trunk with Synthetic Substitute, Percutaneous Approach

UP3KZ Supplement Pulmonary Trunk with Nonautologous Tissue Substitute, Percutaneous Approach

UP47Z Supplement Pulmonary Trunk with Autologous Tissue Substitute, Percutaneous Endoscopic Approach

UP48Z Supplement Pulmonary Trunk with Zooplastic Tissue, Percutaneous Endoscopic Approach

UP4JZ Supplement Pulmonary Trunk with Synthetic Substitute, Percutaneous Endoscopic Approach

UP4KZ Supplement Pulmonary Trunk with Nonautologous Tissue Substitute, Percutaneous Endoscopic Approach

UQ07Z Supplement Right Pulmonary Artery with Autologous Tissue Substitute, Open Approach

UQ08Z Supplement Right Pulmonary Artery with Zooplastic Tissue, Open Approach

02UQ0JZ Supplement Right Pulmonary Artery with Synthetic Substitute, Open Approach

02UQ0KZ Supplement Right Pulmonary Artery with Nonautologous Tissue Substitute, Open Approach

02UQ37Z Supplement Right Pulmonary Artery with Autologous Tissue Substitute, Percutaneous Approach

02UQ38Z Supplement Right Pulmonary Artery with Zooplastic Tissue, Percutaneous Approach

02UQ3JZ Supplement Right Pulmonary Artery with Synthetic Substitute, Percutaneous Approach

02UQ3KZ Supplement Right Pulmonary Artery with Nonautologous Tissue Substitute, Percutaneous Approach

02UQ47Z Supplement Right Pulmonary Artery with Autologous Tissue Substitute, Percutaneous Endoscopic Approach

02UQ48Z Supplement Right Pulmonary Artery with Zooplastic Tissue, Percutaneous Endoscopic Approach

02UQ4JZ Supplement Right Pulmonary Artery with Synthetic Substitute, Percutaneous Endoscopic Approach

02UQ4KZ Supplement Right Pulmonary Artery with Nonautologous Tissue Substitute, Percutaneous Endoscopic Approach

02UR07Z Supplement Left Pulmonary Artery with Autologous Tissue Substitute, Open Approach

02UR08Z Supplement Left Pulmonary Artery with Zooplastic Tissue, Open Approach

02UR0JZ Supplement Left Pulmonary Artery with Synthetic Substitute, Open Approach

02UR0KZ Supplement Left Pulmonary Artery with Nonautologous Tissue Substitute, Open Approach

02UR37Z Supplement Left Pulmonary Artery with Autologous Tissue Substitute, Percutaneous Approach

02UR38Z Supplement Left Pulmonary Artery with Zooplastic Tissue, Percutaneous Approach

02UR3JZ Supplement Left Pulmonary Artery with Synthetic Substitute, Percutaneous Approach

02UR3KZ Supplement Left Pulmonary Artery with Nonautologous Tissue Substitute, Percutaneous Approach

02UR47Z Supplement Left Pulmonary Artery with Autologous Tissue Substitute, Percutaneous Endoscopic Approach

02UR48Z Supplement Left Pulmonary Artery with Zooplastic Tissue, Percutaneous Endoscopic Approach

02UR4JZ Supplement Left Pulmonary Artery with Synthetic Substitute, Percutaneous Endoscopic Approach

02UR4KZ Supplement Left Pulmonary Artery with Nonautologous Tissue Substitute, Percutaneous Endoscopic Approach

02US07Z Supplement Right Pulmonary Vein with Autologous Tissue Substitute, Open Approach

02US08Z Supplement Right Pulmonary Vein with Zooplastic Tissue, Open Approach

02US0JZ Supplement Right Pulmonary Vein with Synthetic Substitute, Open Approach

02US0KZ Supplement Right Pulmonary Vein with Nonautologous Tissue Substitute, Open Approach

02US37Z Supplement Right Pulmonary Vein with Autologous Tissue Substitute, Percutaneous Approach

02US38Z Supplement Right Pulmonary Vein with Zooplastic Tissue, Percutaneous Approach

02US3JZ Supplement Right Pulmonary Vein with Synthetic Substitute, Percutaneous Approach

02US3KZ Supplement Right Pulmonary Vein with Nonautologous Tissue Substitute, Percutaneous Approach

02US47Z Supplement Right Pulmonary Vein with Autologous Tissue Substitute, Percutaneous Endoscopic Approach

02US48Z Supplement Right Pulmonary Vein with Zooplastic Tissue, Percutaneous Endoscopic Approach

02US4JZ Supplement Right Pulmonary Vein with Synthetic Substitute, Percutaneous Endoscopic Approach

02US4KZ Supplement Right Pulmonary Vein with Nonautologous Tissue Substitute, Percutaneous Endoscopic Approach

02UT07Z Supplement Left Pulmonary Vein with Autologous Tissue Substitute, Open Approach

02UT08Z Supplement Left Pulmonary Vein with Zooplastic Tissue, Open Approach

02UT0JZ Supplement Left Pulmonary Vein with Synthetic Substitute, Open Approach

02UT0KZ Supplement Left Pulmonary Vein with Nonautologous Tissue Substitute, Open Approach

02UT37Z Supplement Left Pulmonary Vein with Autologous Tissue Substitute, Percutaneous Approach

02UT38Z Supplement Left Pulmonary Vein with Zooplastic Tissue, Percutaneous Approach

02UT3JZ Supplement Left Pulmonary Vein with Synthetic Substitute, Percutaneous Approach

02UT3KZ Supplement Left Pulmonary Vein with Nonautologous Tissue Substitute, Percutaneous Approach

02UT47Z Supplement Left Pulmonary Vein with Autologous Tissue Substitute, Percutaneous Endoscopic Approach

02UT48Z Supplement Left Pulmonary Vein with Zooplastic Tissue, Percutaneous Endoscopic Approach

02UT4JZ Supplement Left Pulmonary Vein with Synthetic Substitute, Percutaneous Endoscopic Approach

02UT4KZ Supplement Left Pulmonary Vein with Nonautologous Tissue Substitute, Percutaneous Endoscopic Approach

02UV07Z Supplement Superior Vena Cava with Autologous Tissue Substitute, Open Approach

02UV08Z Supplement Superior Vena Cava with Zooplastic Tissue, Open Approach

02UV0JZ Supplement Superior Vena Cava with Synthetic Substitute, Open Approach

02UV0KZ Supplement Superior Vena Cava with Nonautologous Tissue Substitute, Open Approach

02UV37Z Supplement Superior Vena Cava with Autologous Tissue Substitute, Percutaneous Approach

02UV38Z Supplement Superior Vena Cava with Zooplastic Tissue, Percutaneous Approach

02UV3JZ Supplement Superior Vena Cava with Synthetic Substitute, Percutaneous Approach

02UV3KZ Supplement Superior Vena Cava with Nonautologous Tissue Substitute, Percutaneous Approach

02UV47Z Supplement Superior Vena Cava with Autologous Tissue Substitute, Percutaneous Endoscopic Approach

02UV48Z Supplement Superior Vena Cava with Zooplastic Tissue, Percutaneous Endoscopic Approach

02UV4JZ Supplement Superior Vena Cava with Synthetic Substitute, Percutaneous Endoscopic Approach

Female-only   ♂ Male-only   ▲ Limited Coverage   ● Non-OR   ▥ HAC-associated procedure   ▲ Non-covered procedures   ✛ Combination

02UV4KZ	Supplement Superior Vena Cava with Nonautologous Tissue Substitute, Percutaneous Endoscopic Approach
02UW07Z	Supplement Thoracic Aorta with Autologous Tissue Substitute, Open Approach
02UW08Z	Supplement Thoracic Aorta with Zooplastic Tissue, Open Approach
02UW0JZ	Supplement Thoracic Aorta with Synthetic Substitute, Open Approach
02UW0KZ	Supplement Thoracic Aorta with Nonautologous Tissue Substitute, Open Approach
02UW37Z	Supplement Thoracic Aorta with Autologous Tissue Substitute, Percutaneous Approach
02UW38Z	Supplement Thoracic Aorta with Zooplastic Tissue, Percutaneous Approach
02UW3JZ	Supplement Thoracic Aorta with Synthetic Substitute, Percutaneous Approach
02UW3KZ	Supplement Thoracic Aorta with Nonautologous Tissue Substitute, Percutaneous Approach
02UW47Z	Supplement Thoracic Aorta with Autologous Tissue Substitute, Percutaneous Endoscopic Approach
02UW48Z	Supplement Thoracic Aorta with Zooplastic Tissue, Percutaneous Endoscopic Approach
02UW4JZ	Supplement Thoracic Aorta with Synthetic Substitute, Percutaneous Endoscopic Approach
02UW4KZ	Supplement Thoracic Aorta with Nonautologous Tissue Substitute, Percutaneous Endoscopic Approach

02V – Heart and Great Vessels, Restriction

02VA0CZ	Restriction of Heart with Extraluminal Device, Open Approach
02VA0ZZ	Restriction of Heart, Open Approach
02VA3CZ	Restriction of Heart with Extraluminal Device, Percutaneous Approach
02VA3ZZ	Restriction of Heart, Percutaneous Approach
02VA4CZ	Restriction of Heart with Extraluminal Device, Percutaneous Endoscopic Approach
02VA4ZZ	Restriction of Heart, Percutaneous Endoscopic Approach
02VP0CZ	Restriction of Pulmonary Trunk with Extraluminal Device, Open Approach
02VP0DZ	Restriction of Pulmonary Trunk with Intraluminal Device, Open Approach
02VP0ZZ	Restriction of Pulmonary Trunk, Open Approach
02VP3CZ	Restriction of Pulmonary Trunk with Extraluminal Device, Percutaneous Approach
02VP3DZ	Restriction of Pulmonary Trunk with Intraluminal Device, Percutaneous Approach
02VP3ZZ	Restriction of Pulmonary Trunk, Percutaneous Approach
02VP4CZ	Restriction of Pulmonary Trunk with Extraluminal Device, Percutaneous Endoscopic Approach
02VP4DZ	Restriction of Pulmonary Trunk with Intraluminal Device, Percutaneous Endoscopic Approach
02VP4ZZ	Restriction of Pulmonary Trunk, Percutaneous Endoscopic Approach
02VQ0CZ	Restriction of Right Pulmonary Artery with Extraluminal Device, Open Approach
02VQ0DZ	Restriction of Right Pulmonary Artery with Intraluminal Device, Open Approach
02VQ0ZZ	Restriction of Right Pulmonary Artery, Open Approach
02VQ3CZ	Restriction of Right Pulmonary Artery with Extraluminal Device, Percutaneous Approach
02VQ3DZ	Restriction of Right Pulmonary Artery with Intraluminal Device, Percutaneous Approach
02VQ3ZZ	Restriction of Right Pulmonary Artery, Percutaneous Approach
02VQ4CZ	Restriction of Right Pulmonary Artery with Extraluminal Device, Percutaneous Endoscopic Approach
02VQ4DZ	Restriction of Right Pulmonary Artery with Intraluminal Device, Percutaneous Endoscopic Approach
02VQ4ZZ	Restriction of Right Pulmonary Artery, Percutaneous Endoscopic Approach
02VR0CT	Restriction of Ductus Arteriosus with Extraluminal Device, Open Approach
02VR0CZ	Restriction of Left Pulmonary Artery with Extraluminal Device, Open Approach
02VR0DT	Restriction of Ductus Arteriosus with Intraluminal Device, Open Approach
02VR0DZ	Restriction of Left Pulmonary Artery with Intraluminal Device, Open Approach
02VR0ZT	Restriction of Ductus Arteriosus, Open Approach
02VR0ZZ	Restriction of Left Pulmonary Artery, Open Approach
02VR3CT	Restriction of Ductus Arteriosus with Extraluminal Device, Percutaneous Approach
02VR3CZ	Restriction of Left Pulmonary Artery with Extraluminal Device, Percutaneous Approach
02VR3DT	Restriction of Ductus Arteriosus with Intraluminal Device, Percutaneous Approach
02VR3DZ	Restriction of Left Pulmonary Artery with Intraluminal Device, Percutaneous Approach
02VR3ZT	Restriction of Ductus Arteriosus, Percutaneous Approach
02VR3ZZ	Restriction of Left Pulmonary Artery, Percutaneous Approach
02VR4CT	Restriction of Ductus Arteriosus with Extraluminal Device, Percutaneous Endoscopic Approach
02VR4CZ	Restriction of Left Pulmonary Artery with Extraluminal Device, Percutaneous Endoscopic Approach
02VR4DT	Restriction of Ductus Arteriosus with Intraluminal Device, Percutaneous Endoscopic Approach
02VR4DZ	Restriction of Left Pulmonary Artery with Intraluminal Device, Percutaneous Endoscopic Approach
02VR4ZT	Restriction of Ductus Arteriosus, Percutaneous Endoscopic Approach
02VR4ZZ	Restriction of Left Pulmonary Artery, Percutaneous Endoscopic Approach
02VS0CZ	Restriction of Right Pulmonary Vein with Extraluminal Device, Open Approach
02VS0DZ	Restriction of Right Pulmonary Vein with Intraluminal Device, Open Approach
02VS0ZZ	Restriction of Right Pulmonary Vein, Open Approach
02VS3CZ	Restriction of Right Pulmonary Vein with Extraluminal Device, Percutaneous Approach
02VS3DZ	Restriction of Right Pulmonary Vein with Intraluminal Device, Percutaneous Approach
02VS3ZZ	Restriction of Right Pulmonary Vein, Percutaneous Approach
02VS4CZ	Restriction of Right Pulmonary Vein with Extraluminal Device, Percutaneous Endoscopic Approach
02VS4DZ	Restriction of Right Pulmonary Vein with Intraluminal Device, Percutaneous Endoscopic Approach
02VS4ZZ	Restriction of Right Pulmonary Vein, Percutaneous Endoscopic Approach
02VT0CZ	Restriction of Left Pulmonary Vein with Extraluminal Device, Open Approach
02VT0DZ	Restriction of Left Pulmonary Vein with Intraluminal Device, Open Approach
02VT0ZZ	Restriction of Left Pulmonary Vein, Open Approach
02VT3CZ	Restriction of Left Pulmonary Vein with Extraluminal Device, Percutaneous Approach
02VT3DZ	Restriction of Left Pulmonary Vein with Intraluminal Device, Percutaneous Approach
02VT3ZZ	Restriction of Left Pulmonary Vein, Percutaneous Approach
02VT4CZ	Restriction of Left Pulmonary Vein with Extraluminal Device, Percutaneous Endoscopic Approach
02VT4DZ	Restriction of Left Pulmonary Vein with Intraluminal Device, Percutaneous Endoscopic Approach
02VT4ZZ	Restriction of Left Pulmonary Vein, Percutaneous Endoscopic Approach
02VV0CZ	Restriction of Superior Vena Cava with Extraluminal Device, Open Approach
02VV0DZ	Restriction of Superior Vena Cava with Intraluminal Device, Open Approach
02VV0ZZ	Restriction of Superior Vena Cava, Open Approach
02VV3CZ	Restriction of Superior Vena Cava with Extraluminal Device, Percutaneous Approach
02VV3DZ	Restriction of Superior Vena Cava with Intraluminal Device, Percutaneous Approach
02VV3ZZ	Restriction of Superior Vena Cava, Percutaneous Approach
02VV4CZ	Restriction of Superior Vena Cava with Extraluminal Device, Percutaneous Endoscopic Approach
02VV4DZ	Restriction of Superior Vena Cava with Intraluminal Device, Percutaneous Endoscopic Approach
02VV4ZZ	Restriction of Superior Vena Cava, Percutaneous Endoscopic Approach
02VW0CZ	Restriction of Thoracic Aorta with Extraluminal Device, Open Approach
02VW0DZ	Restriction of Thoracic Aorta with Intraluminal Device, Open Approach
02VW0ZZ	Restriction of Thoracic Aorta, Open Approach
02VW3CZ	Restriction of Thoracic Aorta with Extraluminal Device, Percutaneous Approach
02VW3DZ	Restriction of Thoracic Aorta with Intraluminal Device, Percutaneous Approach
02VW3ZZ	Restriction of Thoracic Aorta, Percutaneous Approach
02VW4CZ	Restriction of Thoracic Aorta with Extraluminal Device, Percutaneous Endoscopic Approach
02VW4DZ	Restriction of Thoracic Aorta with Intraluminal Device, Percutaneous Endoscopic Approach
02VW4ZZ	Restriction of Thoracic Aorta, Percutaneous Endoscopic Approach

♀ Female-only   ♂ Male-only   ▲ Limited Coverage   ● Non-OR   ▦ HAC-associated procedure   ▲ Non-covered procedures   ✚ Combinati

W – Heart and Great Vessels, Revision

view Coding Guideline B6.1c

W50JZ Revision of Synthetic Substitute in Atrial Septum, Open Approach

W54JZ Revision of Synthetic Substitute in Atrial Septum, Percutaneous Endoscopic Approach

WA02Z Revision of Monitoring Device in Heart, Open Approach

WA03Z Revision of Infusion Device in Heart, Open Approach

WA07Z Revision of Autologous Tissue Substitute in Heart, Open Approach

WA08Z Revision of Zooplastic Tissue in Heart, Open Approach

WA0CZ Revision of Extraluminal Device in Heart, Open Approach

WA0DZ Revision of Intraluminal Device in Heart, Open Approach

2WA0JZ Revision of Synthetic Substitute in Heart, Open Approach

WA0KZ Revision of Nonautologous Tissue Substitute in Heart, Open Approach

WA0MZ Revision of Cardiac Lead in Heart, Open Approach
- With a secondary diagnosis code of K68.11, T81.4XXA, T82.6XXA, T82.7XXA

2WA0QZ Revision of Implantable Heart Assist System in Heart, Open Approach
- + Heart assist system replacement when reported with a removal of an external heart assist system (6th character R) from the heart. *See table 02P to construct the Removal code.*

WA0RZ Revision of External Heart Assist System in Heart, Open Approach
- + Heart assist system replacement when reported with a removal of an external heart assist system (6th character R) from the heart. *See table 02P to construct the Removal code.*

WA32Z Revision of Monitoring Device in Heart, Percutaneous Approach

WA33Z Revision of Infusion Device in Heart, Percutaneous Approach

WA37Z Revision of Autologous Tissue Substitute in Heart, Percutaneous Approach

WA38Z Revision of Zooplastic Tissue in Heart, Percutaneous Approach

WA3CZ Revision of Extraluminal Device in Heart, Percutaneous Approach

WA3DZ Revision of Intraluminal Device in Heart, Percutaneous Approach

WA3JZ Revision of Synthetic Substitute in Heart, Percutaneous Approach
- *AHA CC: 3Q, 2014, 31-32*

WA3KZ Revision of Nonautologous Tissue Substitute in Heart, Percutaneous Approach

WA3MZ Revision of Cardiac Lead in Heart, Percutaneous Approach
- With a secondary diagnosis code of K68.11, T81.4XXA, T82.6XXA, T82.7XXA

2WA3QZ Revision of Implantable Heart Assist System in Heart, Percutaneous Approach
- + Heart assist system replacement when reported with a removal of an external heart assist system (6th character R) from the heart. *See table 02P to construct the Removal code.*

WA3RZ Revision of External Heart Assist System in Heart, Percutaneous Approach
- + Heart assist system replacement when reported with a removal of an external heart assist system (6th character R) from the heart. *See table 02P to construct the Removal code.*

02WA42Z Revision of Monitoring Device in Heart, Percutaneous Endoscopic Approach

02WA43Z Revision of Infusion Device in Heart, Percutaneous Endoscopic Approach

02WA47Z Revision of Autologous Tissue Substitute in Heart, Percutaneous Endoscopic Approach

02WA48Z Revision of Zooplastic Tissue in Heart, Percutaneous Endoscopic Approach

02WA4CZ Revision of Extraluminal Device in Heart, Percutaneous Endoscopic Approach

02WA4DZ Revision of Intraluminal Device in Heart, Percutaneous Endoscopic Approach

02WA4JZ Revision of Synthetic Substitute in Heart, Percutaneous Endoscopic Approach

02WA4KZ Revision of Nonautologous Tissue Substitute in Heart, Percutaneous Endoscopic Approach

02WA4MZ Revision of Cardiac Lead in Heart, Percutaneous Endoscopic Approach
- With a secondary diagnosis code of K68.11, T81.4XXA, T82.6XXA, T82.7XXA

▲ 02WA4QZ Revision of Implantable Heart Assist System in Heart, Percutaneous Endoscopic Approach
- + Heart assist system replacement when reported with a removal of an external heart assist system (6th character R) from the heart. *See table 02P to construct the Removal code.*

02WA4RZ Revision of External Heart Assist System in Heart, Percutaneous Endoscopic Approach
- + Heart assist system replacement when reported with a removal of an external heart assist system (6th character R) from the heart. *See table 02P to construct the Removal code.*

02WAX2Z Revision of Monitoring Device in Heart, External Approach

02WAX3Z Revision of Infusion Device in Heart, External Approach

02WAX7Z Revision of Autologous Tissue Substitute in Heart, External Approach

02WAX8Z Revision of Zooplastic Tissue in Heart, External Approach

02WAXCZ Revision of Extraluminal Device in Heart, External Approach

02WAXDZ Revision of Intraluminal Device in Heart, External Approach

02WAXJZ Revision of Synthetic Substitute in Heart, External Approach

02WAXKZ Revision of Nonautologous Tissue Substitute in Heart, External Approach

02WAXMZ Revision of Cardiac Lead in Heart, External Approach

02WAXQZ Revision of Implantable Heart Assist System in Heart, External Approach

02WAXRZ Revision of External Heart Assist System in Heart, External Approach

02WF07Z Revision of Autologous Tissue Substitute in Aortic Valve, Open Approach

02WF08Z Revision of Zooplastic Tissue in Aortic Valve, Open Approach

02WF0JZ Revision of Synthetic Substitute in Aortic Valve, Open Approach

02WF0KZ Revision of Nonautologous Tissue Substitute in Aortic Valve, Open Approach

02WF47Z Revision of Autologous Tissue Substitute in Aortic Valve, Percutaneous Endoscopic Approach

02WF48Z Revision of Zooplastic Tissue in Aortic Valve, Percutaneous Endoscopic Approach

02WF4JZ Revision of Synthetic Substitute in Aortic Valve, Percutaneous Endoscopic Approach

02WF4KZ Revision of Nonautologous Tissue Substitute in Aortic Valve, Percutaneous Endoscopic Approach

02WG07Z Revision of Autologous Tissue Substitute in Mitral Valve, Open Approach

02WG08Z Revision of Zooplastic Tissue in Mitral Valve, Open Approach

02WG0JZ Revision of Synthetic Substitute in Mitral Valve, Open Approach

02WG0KZ Revision of Nonautologous Tissue Substitute in Mitral Valve, Open Approach

02WG47Z Revision of Autologous Tissue Substitute in Mitral Valve, Percutaneous Endoscopic Approach

02WG48Z Revision of Zooplastic Tissue in Mitral Valve, Percutaneous Endoscopic Approach

02WG4JZ Revision of Synthetic Substitute in Mitral Valve, Percutaneous Endoscopic Approach

02WG4KZ Revision of Nonautologous Tissue Substitute in Mitral Valve, Percutaneous Endoscopic Approach

02WH07Z Revision of Autologous Tissue Substitute in Pulmonary Valve, Open Approach

02WH08Z Revision of Zooplastic Tissue in Pulmonary Valve, Open Approach

02WH0JZ Revision of Synthetic Substitute in Pulmonary Valve, Open Approach

02WH0KZ Revision of Nonautologous Tissue Substitute in Pulmonary Valve, Open Approach

02WH47Z Revision of Autologous Tissue Substitute in Pulmonary Valve, Percutaneous Endoscopic Approach

02WH48Z Revision of Zooplastic Tissue in Pulmonary Valve, Percutaneous Endoscopic Approach

02WH4JZ Revision of Synthetic Substitute in Pulmonary Valve, Percutaneous Endoscopic Approach

02WH4KZ Revision of Nonautologous Tissue Substitute in Pulmonary Valve, Percutaneous Endoscopic Approach

02WJ07Z Revision of Autologous Tissue Substitute in Tricuspid Valve, Open Approach

02WJ08Z Revision of Zooplastic Tissue in Tricuspid Valve, Open Approach

02WJ0JZ Revision of Synthetic Substitute in Tricuspid Valve, Open Approach

02WJ0KZ Revision of Nonautologous Tissue Substitute in Tricuspid Valve, Open Approach

02WJ47Z Revision of Autologous Tissue Substitute in Tricuspid Valve, Percutaneous Endoscopic Approach

02WJ48Z Revision of Zooplastic Tissue in Tricuspid Valve, Percutaneous Endoscopic Approach

02WJ4JZ Revision of Synthetic Substitute in Tricuspid Valve, Percutaneous Endoscopic Approach

02WJ4KZ Revision of Nonautologous Tissue Substitute in Tricuspid Valve, Percutaneous Endoscopic Approach

02WM0JZ Revision of Synthetic Substitute in Ventricular Septum, Open Approach

♀ Female-only ♂ Male-only ▲ Limited Coverage ● Non-OR ▨ HAC-associated procedure ▲ Non-covered procedures + Combination

02WM4JZ	Revision of Synthetic Substitute in Ventricular Septum, Percutaneous Endoscopic Approach
02WY02Z	Revision of Monitoring Device in Great Vessel, Open Approach
02WY03Z	Revision of Infusion Device in Great Vessel, Open Approach
02WY07Z	Revision of Autologous Tissue Substitute in Great Vessel, Open Approach
02WY08Z	Revision of Zooplastic Tissue in Great Vessel, Open Approach
02WY0CZ	Revision of Extraluminal Device in Great Vessel, Open Approach
02WY0DZ	Revision of Intraluminal Device in Great Vessel, Open Approach
02WY0JZ	Revision of Synthetic Substitute in Great Vessel, Open Approach
02WY0KZ	Revision of Nonautologous Tissue Substitute in Great Vessel, Open Approach
02WY32Z	Revision of Monitoring Device in Great Vessel, Percutaneous Approach
02WY33Z	Revision of Infusion Device in Great Vessel, Percutaneous Approach
02WY37Z	Revision of Autologous Tissue Substitute in Great Vessel, Percutaneous Approach

02WY38Z	Revision of Zooplastic Tissue in Great Vessel, Percutaneous Approach
02WY3CZ	Revision of Extraluminal Device in Great Vessel, Percutaneous Approach
02WY3DZ	Revision of Intraluminal Device in Great Vessel, Percutaneous Approach
02WY3JZ	Revision of Synthetic Substitute in Great Vessel, Percutaneous Approach
02WY3KZ	Revision of Nonautologous Tissue Substitute in Great Vessel, Percutaneous Approach
02WY42Z	Revision of Monitoring Device in Great Vessel, Percutaneous Endoscopic Approach
02WY43Z	Revision of Infusion Device in Great Vessel, Percutaneous Endoscopic Approach
02WY47Z	Revision of Autologous Tissue Substitute in Great Vessel, Percutaneous Endoscopic Approach
02WY48Z	Revision of Zooplastic Tissue in Great Vessel, Percutaneous Endoscopic Approach
02WY4CZ	Revision of Extraluminal Device in Great Vessel, Percutaneous Endoscopic Approach

02WY4DZ	Revision of Intraluminal Device in Great Vessel, Percutaneous Endoscopic Approach
02WY4JZ	Revision of Synthetic Substitute in Great Vessel, Percutaneous Endoscopic Approach
02WY4KZ	Revision of Nonautologous Tissue Substitute in Great Vessel, Percutaneous Endoscopic Approach
02WYX2Z	Revision of Monitoring Device in Great Vessel, External Approach
02WYX3Z	Revision of Infusion Device in Great Vessel, External Approach
02WYX7Z	Revision of Autologous Tissue Substitute in Great Vessel, External Approach
02WYX8Z	Revision of Zooplastic Tissue in Great Vessel, External Approach
02WYXCZ	Revision of Extraluminal Device in Great Vessel, External Approach
02WYXDZ	Revision of Intraluminal Device in Great Vessel, External Approach
02WYXJZ	Revision of Synthetic Substitute in Great Vessel, External Approach
02WYXKZ	Revision of Nonautologous Tissue Substitute in Great Vessel, External Approach

02Y – Heart and Great Vessels, Transplantation

Review Coding Guideline B3.16

| ▲ 02YA0Z0 | Transplantation of Heart, Allogeneic, Open Approach |
| | AHA CC: 3Q, 2013, 18-19 |

| ▲ 02YA0Z1 | Transplantation of Heart, Syngeneic, Open Approach |

| ▲ 02YA0Z2 | Transplantation of Heart, Zooplastic, Open Approach |

♀ Female-only   ♂ Male-only   ▲ Limited Coverage   ● Non-OR   HAC HAC-associated procedure   ▲ Non-covered procedures   + Combinat

Arteries

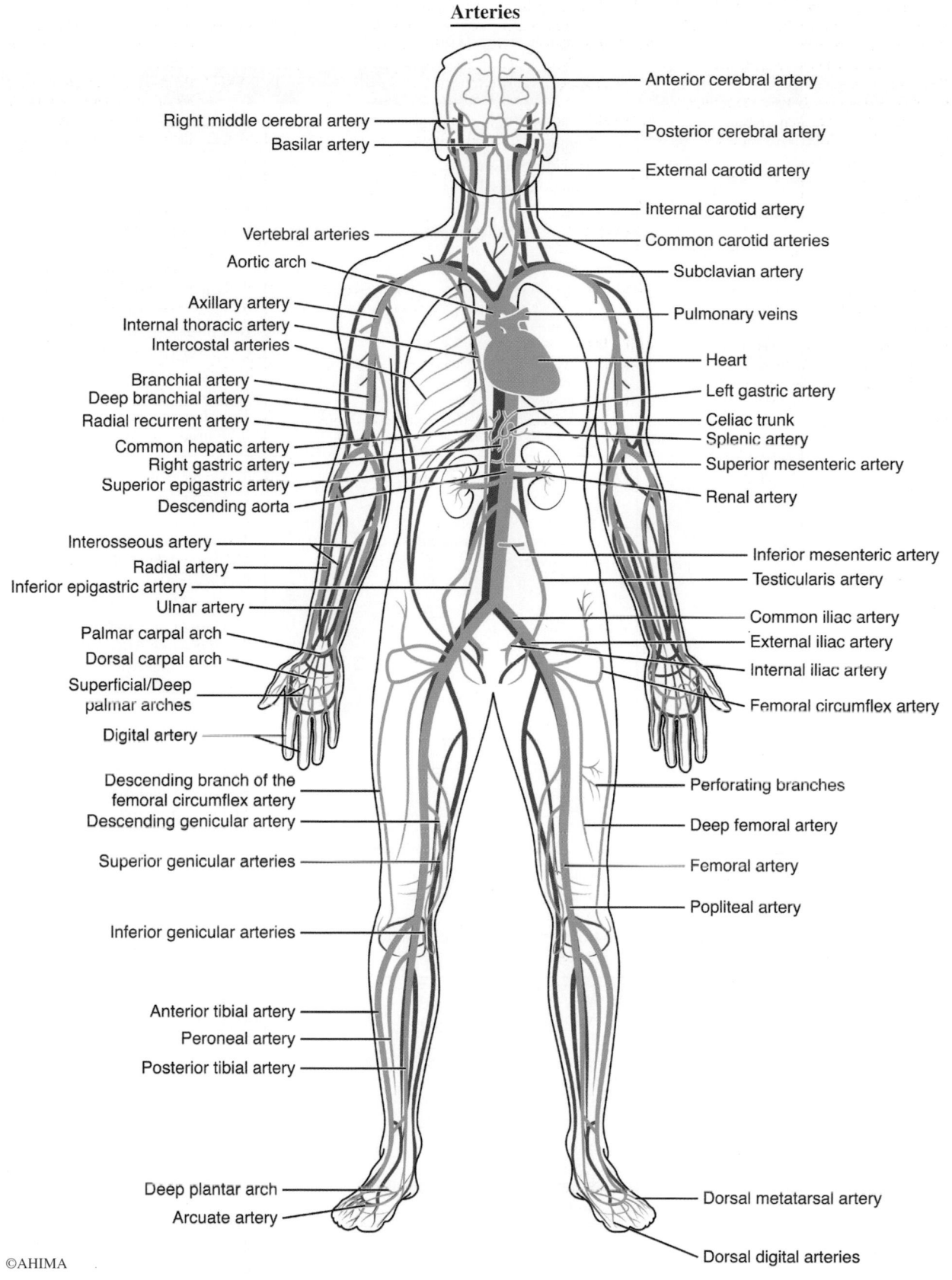

Anterior cerebral artery

Right middle cerebral artery

Posterior cerebral artery

Basilar artery

External carotid artery

Internal carotid artery

Vertebral arteries

Common carotid arteries

Aortic arch

Subclavian artery

Axillary artery

Pulmonary veins

Internal thoracic artery

Intercostal arteries

Heart

Branchial artery

Left gastric artery

Deep branchial artery

Celiac trunk

Radial recurrent artery

Splenic artery

Common hepatic artery

Superior mesenteric artery

Right gastric artery

Superior epigastric artery

Renal artery

Descending aorta

Interosseous artery

Inferior mesenteric artery

Radial artery

Testicularis artery

Inferior epigastric artery

Ulnar artery

Common iliac artery

Palmar carpal arch

External iliac artery

Dorsal carpal arch

Internal iliac artery

Superficial/Deep
palmar arches

Femoral circumflex artery

Digital artery

Descending branch of the
femoral circumflex artery

Perforating branches

Descending genicular artery

Deep femoral artery

Superior genicular arteries

Femoral artery

Popliteal artery

Inferior genicular arteries

Anterior tibial artery

Peroneal artery

Posterior tibial artery

Deep plantar arch

Dorsal metatarsal artery

Arcuate artery

Dorsal digital arteries

©AHIMA

Section	0	Medical and Surgical
Body System	3	Upper Arteries
Operation	1	Bypass: Altering the route of passage of the contents of a tubular body part

Body Part (4ᵗʰ)	Approach (5ᵗʰ)	Device (6ᵗʰ)	Qualifier (7ᵗʰ)
2 Innominate Artery 5 Axillary Artery, Right 6 Axillary Artery, Left	0 Open	9 Autologous Venous Tissue A Autologous Arterial Tissue J Synthetic Substitute K Nonautologous Tissue Substitute Z No Device	0 Upper Arm Artery, Right 1 Upper Arm Artery, Left 2 Upper Arm Artery, Bilateral 3 Lower Arm Artery, Right 4 Lower Arm Artery, Left 5 Lower Arm Artery, Bilateral 6 Upper Leg Artery, Right 7 Upper Leg Artery, Left 8 Upper Leg Artery, Bilateral 9 Lower Leg Artery, Right B Lower Leg Artery, Left C Lower Leg Artery, Bilateral D Upper Arm Vein F Lower Arm Vein J Extracranial Artery, Right K Extracranial Artery, Left
3 Subclavian Artery, Right 4 Subclavian Artery, Left	0 Open	9 Autologous Venous Tissue A Autologous Arterial Tissue J Synthetic Substitute K Nonautologous Tissue Substitute Z No Device	0 Upper Arm Artery, Right 1 Upper Arm Artery, Left 2 Upper Arm Artery, Bilateral 3 Lower Arm Artery, Right 4 Lower Arm Artery, Left 5 Lower Arm Artery, Bilateral 6 Upper Leg Artery, Right 7 Upper Leg Artery, Left 8 Upper Leg Artery, Bilateral 9 Lower Leg Artery, Right B Lower Leg Artery, Left C Lower Leg Artery, Bilateral D Upper Arm Vein F Lower Arm Vein J Extracranial Artery, Right K Extracranial Artery, Left M Pulmonary Artery, Right N Pulmonary Artery, Left
7 Brachial Artery, Right	0 Open	9 Autologous Venous Tissue A Autologous Arterial Tissue J Synthetic Substitute K Nonautologous Tissue Substitute Z No Device	0 Upper Arm Artery, Right 3 Lower Arm Artery, Right D Upper Arm Vein F Lower Arm Vein
8 Brachial Artery, Left	0 Open	9 Autologous Venous Tissue A Autologous Arterial Tissue J Synthetic Substitute K Nonautologous Tissue Substitute Z No Device	1 Upper Arm Artery, Left 4 Lower Arm Artery, Left D Upper Arm Vein F Lower Arm Vein
9 Ulnar Artery, Right B Radial Artery, Right	0 Open	9 Autologous Venous Tissue A Autologous Arterial Tissue J Synthetic Substitute K Nonautologous Tissue Substitute Z No Device	3 Lower Arm Artery, Right F Lower Arm Vein
A Ulnar Artery, Left C Radial Artery, Left	0 Open	9 Autologous Venous Tissue A Autologous Arterial Tissue J Synthetic Substitute K Nonautologous Tissue Substitute Z No Device	4 Lower Arm Artery, Left F Lower Arm Vein

Continued →

Section 0 Medical and Surgical
Body System 3 Upper Arteries
Operation 1 Bypass: Altering the route of passage of the contents of a tubular body part

Body Part (4th)	Approach (5th)	Device (6th)	Qualifier (7th)
G Intracranial Artery S Temporal Artery, Right T Temporal Artery, Left	0 Open	9 Autologous Venous Tissue A Autologous Arterial Tissue J Synthetic Substitute K Nonautologous Tissue Substitute Z No Device	G Intracranial Artery
H Common Carotid Artery, Right	0 Open	9 Autologous Venous Tissue A Autologous Arterial Tissue J Synthetic Substitute K Nonautologous Tissue Substitute Z No Device	G Intracranial Artery J Extracranial Artery, Right
J Common Carotid Artery, Left	0 Open	9 Autologous Venous Tissue A Autologous Arterial Tissue J Synthetic Substitute K Nonautologous Tissue Substitute Z No Device	G Intracranial Artery K Extracranial Artery, Left
K Internal Carotid Artery, Right M External Carotid Artery, Right	0 Open	9 Autologous Venous Tissue A Autologous Arterial Tissue J Synthetic Substitute K Nonautologous Tissue Substitute Z No Device	J Extracranial Artery, Right
L Internal Carotid Artery, Left N External Carotid Artery, Left	0 Open	9 Autologous Venous Tissue A Autologous Arterial Tissue J Synthetic Substitute K Nonautologous Tissue Substitute Z No Device	K Extracranial Artery, Left

Section 0 Medical and Surgical
Body System 3 Upper Arteries
Operation 5 Destruction: Physical eradication of all or a portion of a body part by the direct use of energy, force, or a destructive agent

Body Part (4th)	Approach (5th)	Device (6th)	Qualifier (7th)
0 Internal Mammary Artery, Right 1 Internal Mammary Artery, Left 2 Innominate Artery 3 Subclavian Artery, Right 4 Subclavian Artery, Left 5 Axillary Artery, Right 6 Axillary Artery, Left 7 Brachial Artery, Right 8 Brachial Artery, Left 9 Ulnar Artery, Right A Ulnar Artery, Left B Radial Artery, Right C Radial Artery, Left D Hand Artery, Right F Hand Artery, Left G Intracranial Artery H Common Carotid Artery, Right J Common Carotid Artery, Left K Internal Carotid Artery, Right L Internal Carotid Artery, Left M External Carotid Artery, Right N External Carotid Artery, Left P Vertebral Artery, Right	0 Open 3 Percutaneous 4 Percutaneous Endoscopic	Z No Device	Z No Qualifier

Continued →

195

Section	**0**	**Medical and Surgical**	
Body System	**3**	**Upper Arteries**	
Operation	**5**	**Destruction:** Physical eradication of all or a portion of a body part by the direct use of energy, force, or a destructive agent	

Body Part (4th)	Approach (5th)	Device (6th)	Qualifier (7th)
Q Vertebral Artery, Left **R** Face Artery **S** Temporal Artery, Right **T** Temporal Artery, Left **U** Thyroid Artery, Right **V** Thyroid Artery, Left **Y** Upper Artery			

Section	**0**	**Medical and Surgical**	
Body System	**3**	**Upper Arteries**	
Operation	**7**	**Dilation:** Expanding an orifice or the lumen of a tubular body part	

Body Part (4th)	Approach (5th)	Device (6th)	Qualifier (7th)
0 Internal Mammary Artery, Right **1** Internal Mammary Artery, Left **2** Innominate Artery **3** Subclavian Artery, Right **4** Subclavian Artery, Left **5** Axillary Artery, Right **6** Axillary Artery, Left **7** Brachial Artery, Right **8** Brachial Artery, Left **9** Ulnar Artery, Right **A** Ulnar Artery, Left **B** Radial Artery, Right **C** Radial Artery, Left **D** Hand Artery, Right **F** Hand Artery, Left **G** Intracranial Artery **H** Common Carotid Artery, Right **J** Common Carotid Artery, Left **K** Internal Carotid Artery, Right **L** Internal Carotid Artery, Left **M** External Carotid Artery, Right **N** External Carotid Artery, Left **P** Vertebral Artery, Right **Q** Vertebral Artery, Left **R** Face Artery **S** Temporal Artery, Right **T** Temporal Artery, Left **U** Thyroid Artery, Right **V** Thyroid Artery, Left **Y** Upper Artery	**0** Open **3** Percutaneous **4** Percutaneous Endoscopic	**4** Intraluminal Device, Drug-eluting **D** Intraluminal Device **Z** No Device	**Z** No Qualifier

Section	0	Medical and Surgical
Body System	3	Upper Arteries
Operation	9	Drainage: Taking or letting out fluids and/or gases from a body part

Body Part (4th)	Approach (5th)	Device (6th)	Qualifier (7th)
0 Internal Mammary Artery, Right	0 Open	0 Drainage Device	Z No Qualifier
1 Internal Mammary Artery, Left	3 Percutaneous		
2 Innominate Artery	4 Percutaneous Endoscopic		
3 Subclavian Artery, Right			
4 Subclavian Artery, Left			
5 Axillary Artery, Right			
6 Axillary Artery, Left			
7 Brachial Artery, Right			
8 Brachial Artery, Left			
9 Ulnar Artery, Right			
A Ulnar Artery, Left			
B Radial Artery, Right			
C Radial Artery, Left			
D Hand Artery, Right			
F Hand Artery, Left			
G Intracranial Artery			
H Common Carotid Artery, Right			
J Common Carotid Artery, Left			
K Internal Carotid Artery, Right			
L Internal Carotid Artery, Left			
M External Carotid Artery, Right			
N External Carotid Artery, Left			
P Vertebral Artery, Right			
Q Vertebral Artery, Left			
R Face Artery			
S Temporal Artery, Right			
T Temporal Artery, Left			
U Thyroid Artery, Right			
V Thyroid Artery, Left			
Y Upper Artery			
0 Internal Mammary Artery, Right	0 Open	Z No Device	X Diagnostic
1 Internal Mammary Artery, Left	3 Percutaneous		Z No Qualifier
2 Innominate Artery	4 Percutaneous Endoscopic		
3 Subclavian Artery, Right			
4 Subclavian Artery, Left			
5 Axillary Artery, Right			
6 Axillary Artery, Left			
7 Brachial Artery, Right			
8 Brachial Artery, Left			
9 Ulnar Artery, Right			
A Ulnar Artery, Left			
B Radial Artery, Right			
C Radial Artery, Left			
D Hand Artery, Right			
F Hand Artery, Left			
G Intracranial Artery			
H Common Carotid Artery, Right			
J Common Carotid Artery, Left			
K Internal Carotid Artery, Right			
L Internal Carotid Artery, Left			
M External Carotid Artery, Right			
N External Carotid Artery, Left			
P Vertebral Artery, Right			
Q Vertebral Artery, Left			
R Face Artery			
S Temporal Artery, Right			
T Temporal Artery, Left			
U Thyroid Artery, Right			
V Thyroid Artery, Left			
Y Upper Artery			

Section	0	Medical and Surgical
Body System	3	Upper Arteries
Operation	B	**Excision:** Cutting out or off, without replacement, a portion of a body part

Body Part (4th)	Approach (5th)	Device (6th)	Qualifier (7th)
0 Internal Mammary Artery, Right	0 Open	Z No Device	X Diagnostic
1 Internal Mammary Artery, Left	3 Percutaneous		Z No Qualifier
2 Innominate Artery	4 Percutaneous Endoscopic		
3 Subclavian Artery, Right			
4 Subclavian Artery, Left			
5 Axillary Artery, Right			
6 Axillary Artery, Left			
7 Brachial Artery, Right			
8 Brachial Artery, Left			
9 Ulnar Artery, Right			
A Ulnar Artery, Left			
B Radial Artery, Right			
C Radial Artery, Left			
D Hand Artery, Right			
F Hand Artery, Left			
G Intracranial Artery			
H Common Carotid Artery, Right			
J Common Carotid Artery, Left			
K Internal Carotid Artery, Right			
L Internal Carotid Artery, Left			
M External Carotid Artery, Right			
N External Carotid Artery, Left			
P Vertebral Artery, Right			
Q Vertebral Artery, Left			
R Face Artery			
S Temporal Artery, Right			
T Temporal Artery, Left			
U Thyroid Artery, Right			
V Thyroid Artery, Left			
Y Upper Artery			

Section	0	Medical and Surgical
Body System	3	Upper Arteries
Operation	C	**Extirpation:** Taking or cutting out solid matter from a body part

Body Part (4th)	Approach (5th)	Device (6th)	Qualifier (7th)
0 Internal Mammary Artery, Right	0 Open	Z No Device	Z No Qualifier
1 Internal Mammary Artery, Left	3 Percutaneous		
2 Innominate Artery	4 Percutaneous Endoscopic		
3 Subclavian Artery, Right			
4 Subclavian Artery, Left			
5 Axillary Artery, Right			
6 Axillary Artery, Left			
7 Brachial Artery, Right			
8 Brachial Artery, Left			
9 Ulnar Artery, Right			
A Ulnar Artery, Left			
B Radial Artery, Right			
C Radial Artery, Left			
D Hand Artery, Right			
F Hand Artery, Left			
G Intracranial Artery			
H Common Carotid Artery, Right			
J Common Carotid Artery, Left			
K Internal Carotid Artery, Right			
L Internal Carotid Artery, Left			
M External Carotid Artery, Right			
N External Carotid Artery, Left			
P Vertebral Artery, Right			
Q Vertebral Artery, Left			
R Face Artery			
S Temporal Artery, Right			
T Temporal Artery, Left			
U Thyroid Artery, Right			
V Thyroid Artery, Left			
Y Upper Artery			

Section | 0 | Medical and Surgical
Body System | 3 | Upper Arteries
Operation | H | Insertion: Putting in a nonbiological appliance that monitors, assists, performs, or prevents a physiological function but does not physically take the place of a body part

Body Part (4th)	Approach (5th)	Device (6th)	Qualifier (7th)
0 Internal Mammary Artery, Right 1 Internal Mammary Artery, Left 2 Innominate Artery 3 Subclavian Artery, Right 4 Subclavian Artery, Left 5 Axillary Artery, Right 6 Axillary Artery, Left 7 Brachial Artery, Right 8 Brachial Artery, Left 9 Ulnar Artery, Right A Ulnar Artery, Left B Radial Artery, Right C Radial Artery, Left D Hand Artery, Right F Hand Artery, Left G Intracranial Artery H Common Carotid Artery, Right J Common Carotid Artery, Left M External Carotid Artery, Right N External Carotid Artery, Left P Vertebral Artery, Right Q Vertebral Artery, Left R Face Artery S Temporal Artery, Right T Temporal Artery, Left U Thyroid Artery, Right V Thyroid Artery, Left	0 Open 3 Percutaneous 4 Percutaneous Endoscopic	3 Infusion Device D Intraluminal Device	Z No Qualifier
K Internal Carotid Artery, Right L Internal Carotid Artery, Left	0 Open 3 Percutaneous 4 Percutaneous Endoscopic	3 Infusion Device D Intraluminal Device M Stimulator Lead	Z No Qualifier
Y Upper Artery	0 Open 3 Percutaneous 4 Percutaneous Endoscopic	2 Monitoring Device 3 Infusion Device D Intraluminal Device	Z No Qualifier

Section | 0 | Medical and Surgical
Body System | 3 | Upper Arteries
Operation | J | Inspection: Visually and/or manually exploring a body part

Body Part (4th)	Approach (5th)	Device (6th)	Qualifier (7th)
Y Upper Artery	0 Open 3 Percutaneous 4 Percutaneous Endoscopic X External	Z No Device	Z No Qualifier

Section   0   **Medical and Surgical**
Body System   3   **Upper Arteries**
Operation   L   **Occlusion:** Completely closing an orifice or the lumen of a tubular body part

Body Part (4th)	Approach (5th)	Device (6th)	Qualifier (7th)
0 Internal Mammary Artery, Right 1 Internal Mammary Artery, Left 2 Innominate Artery 3 Subclavian Artery, Right 4 Subclavian Artery, Left 5 Axillary Artery, Right 6 Axillary Artery, Left 7 Brachial Artery, Right 8 Brachial Artery, Left 9 Ulnar Artery, Right A Ulnar Artery, Left B Radial Artery, Right C Radial Artery, Left D Hand Artery, Right F Hand Artery, Left R Face Artery S Temporal Artery, Right T Temporal Artery, Left U Thyroid Artery, Right V Thyroid Artery, Left Y Upper Artery	0 Open 3 Percutaneous 4 Percutaneous Endoscopic	C Extraluminal Device D Intraluminal Device Z No Device	Z No Qualifier
G Intracranial Artery H Common Carotid Artery, Right J Common Carotid Artery, Left K Internal Carotid Artery, Right L Internal Carotid Artery, Left M External Carotid Artery, Right N External Carotid Artery, Left P Vertebral Artery, Right Q Vertebral Artery, Left	0 Open 3 Percutaneous 4 Percutaneous Endoscopic	B Intraluminal Device, Bioactive C Extraluminal Device D Intraluminal Device Z No Device	Z No Qualifier

Section   0   **Medical and Surgical**
Body System   3   **Upper Arteries**
Operation   N   **Release:** Freeing a body part from an abnormal physical constraint by cutting or by the use of force

Body Part (4th)	Approach (5th)	Device (6th)	Qualifier (7th)
0 Internal Mammary Artery, Right 1 Internal Mammary Artery, Left 2 Innominate Artery 3 Subclavian Artery, Right 4 Subclavian Artery, Left 5 Axillary Artery, Right 6 Axillary Artery, Left 7 Brachial Artery, Right 8 Brachial Artery, Left 9 Ulnar Artery, Right A Ulnar Artery, Left B Radial Artery, Right C Radial Artery, Left D Hand Artery, Right F Hand Artery, Left G Intracranial Artery H Common Carotid Artery, Right J Common Carotid Artery, Left K Internal Carotid Artery, Right L Internal Carotid Artery, Left M External Carotid Artery, Right N External Carotid Artery, Left P Vertebral Artery, Right Q Vertebral Artery, Left R Face Artery S Temporal Artery, Right T Temporal Artery, Left U Thyroid Artery, Right V Thyroid Artery, Left Y Upper Artery	0 Open 3 Percutaneous 4 Percutaneous Endoscopic	Z No Device	Z No Qualifier

ction	0	Medical and Surgical	
dy System	3	Upper Arteries	
eration	P	**Removal:** Taking out or off a device from a body part	

Body Part (4th)	Approach (5th)	Device (6th)	Qualifier (7th)
Y Upper Artery	0 Open 3 Percutaneous 4 Percutaneous Endoscopic	0 Drainage Device 2 Monitoring Device 3 Infusion Device 7 Autologous Tissue Substitute C Extraluminal Device D Intraluminal Device J Synthetic Substitute K Nonautologous Tissue Substitute M Stimulator Lead	Z No Qualifier
Y Upper Artery	X External	0 Drainage Device 2 Monitoring Device 3 Infusion Device D Intraluminal Device M Stimulator Lead	Z No Qualifier

ction	0	Medical and Surgical	
dy System	3	Upper Arteries	
eration	Q	**Repair:** Restoring, to the extent possible, a body part to its normal anatomic structure and function	

Body Part (4th)	Approach (5th)	Device (6th)	Qualifier (7th)
0 Internal Mammary Artery, Right 1 Internal Mammary Artery, Left 2 Innominate Artery 3 Subclavian Artery, Right 4 Subclavian Artery, Left 5 Axillary Artery, Right 6 Axillary Artery, Left 7 Brachial Artery, Right 8 Brachial Artery, Left 9 Ulnar Artery, Right A Ulnar Artery, Left B Radial Artery, Right C Radial Artery, Left D Hand Artery, Right F Hand Artery, Left G Intracranial Artery H Common Carotid Artery, Right J Common Carotid Artery, Left K Internal Carotid Artery, Right L Internal Carotid Artery, Left M External Carotid Artery, Right N External Carotid Artery, Left P Vertebral Artery, Right Q Vertebral Artery, Left R Face Artery S Temporal Artery, Right T Temporal Artery, Left U Thyroid Artery, Right V Thyroid Artery, Left Y Upper Artery	0 Open 3 Percutaneous 4 Percutaneous Endoscopic	Z No Device	Z No Qualifier

Section	0	Medical and Surgical
Body System	3	Upper Arteries
Operation	R	Replacement: Putting in or on biological or synthetic material that physically takes the place and/or function of all or a portion of a body part

Body Part (4th)	Approach (5th)	Device (6th)	Qualifier (7th)
0 Internal Mammary Artery, Right	0 Open	7 Autologous Tissue Substitute	Z No Qualifier
1 Internal Mammary Artery, Left	4 Percutaneous Endoscopic	J Synthetic Substitute	
2 Innominate Artery		K Nonautologous Tissue Substitute	
3 Subclavian Artery, Right			
4 Subclavian Artery, Left			
5 Axillary Artery, Right			
6 Axillary Artery, Left			
7 Brachial Artery, Right			
8 Brachial Artery, Left			
9 Ulnar Artery, Right			
A Ulnar Artery, Left			
B Radial Artery, Right			
C Radial Artery, Left			
D Hand Artery, Right			
F Hand Artery, Left			
G Intracranial Artery			
H Common Carotid Artery, Right			
J Common Carotid Artery, Left			
K Internal Carotid Artery, Right			
L Internal Carotid Artery, Left			
M External Carotid Artery, Right			
N External Carotid Artery, Left			
P Vertebral Artery, Right			
Q Vertebral Artery, Left			
R Face Artery			
S Temporal Artery, Right			
T Temporal Artery, Left			
U Thyroid Artery, Right			
V Thyroid Artery, Left			
Y Upper Artery			

Section	0	Medical and Surgical
Body System	3	Upper Arteries
Operation	S	Reposition: Moving to its normal location, or other suitable location, all or a portion of a body part

Body Part (4th)	Approach (5th)	Device (6th)	Qualifier (7th)
0 Internal Mammary Artery, Right	0 Open	Z No Device	Z No Qualifier
1 Internal Mammary Artery, Left	3 Percutaneous		
2 Innominate Artery	4 Percutaneous Endoscopic		
3 Subclavian Artery, Right			
4 Subclavian Artery, Left			
5 Axillary Artery, Right			
6 Axillary Artery, Left			
7 Brachial Artery, Right			
8 Brachial Artery, Left			
9 Ulnar Artery, Right			
A Ulnar Artery, Left			
B Radial Artery, Right			
C Radial Artery, Left			
D Hand Artery, Right			
F Hand Artery, Left			
G Intracranial Artery			
H Common Carotid Artery, Right			
J Common Carotid Artery, Left			
K Internal Carotid Artery, Right			
L Internal Carotid Artery, Left			
M External Carotid Artery, Right			
N External Carotid Artery, Left			
P Vertebral Artery, Right			
Q Vertebral Artery, Left			
R Face Artery			
S Temporal Artery, Right			
T Temporal Artery, Left			
U Thyroid Artery, Right			
V Thyroid Artery, Left			
Y Upper Artery			

Section	0 Medical and Surgical
Body System	3 Upper Arteries
Operation	U Supplement: Putting in or on biological or synthetic material that physically reinforces and/or augments the function of a portion of a body part

Body Part (4th)	Approach (5th)	Device (6th)	Qualifier (7th)
0 Internal Mammary Artery, Right	0 Open	7 Autologous Tissue Substitute	Z No Qualifier
1 Internal Mammary Artery, Left	3 Percutaneous	J Synthetic Substitute	
2 Innominate Artery	4 Percutaneous Endoscopic	K Nonautologous Tissue Substitute	
3 Subclavian Artery, Right			
4 Subclavian Artery, Left			
5 Axillary Artery, Right			
6 Axillary Artery, Left			
7 Brachial Artery, Right			
8 Brachial Artery, Left			
9 Ulnar Artery, Right			
A Ulnar Artery, Left			
B Radial Artery, Right			
C Radial Artery, Left			
D Hand Artery, Right			
F Hand Artery, Left			
G Intracranial Artery			
H Common Carotid Artery, Right			
J Common Carotid Artery, Left			
K Internal Carotid Artery, Right			
L Internal Carotid Artery, Left			
M External Carotid Artery, Right			
N External Carotid Artery, Left			
P Vertebral Artery, Right			
Q Vertebral Artery, Left			
R Face Artery			
S Temporal Artery, Right			
T Temporal Artery, Left			
U Thyroid Artery, Right			
V Thyroid Artery, Left			
Y Upper Artery			

Section	0	Medical and Surgical
Body System	3	Upper Arteries
Operation	V	**Restriction:** Partially closing an orifice or the lumen of a tubular body part

Body Part (4ᵗʰ)	Approach (5ᵗʰ)	Device (6ᵗʰ)	Qualifier (7ᵗʰ)
0 Internal Mammary Artery, Right 1 Internal Mammary Artery, Left 2 Innominate Artery 3 Subclavian Artery, Right 4 Subclavian Artery, Left 5 Axillary Artery, Right 6 Axillary Artery, Left 7 Brachial Artery, Right 8 Brachial Artery, Left 9 Ulnar Artery, Right A Ulnar Artery, Left B Radial Artery, Right C Radial Artery, Left D Hand Artery, Right F Hand Artery, Left R Face Artery S Temporal Artery, Right T Temporal Artery, Left U Thyroid Artery, Right V Thyroid Artery, Left Y Upper Artery	0 Open 3 Percutaneous 4 Percutaneous Endoscopic	C Extraluminal Device D Intraluminal Device Z No Device	Z No Qualifier
G Intracranial Artery H Common Carotid Artery, Right J Common Carotid Artery, Left K Internal Carotid Artery, Right L Internal Carotid Artery, Left M External Carotid Artery, Right N External Carotid Artery, Left P Vertebral Artery, Right Q Vertebral Artery, Left	0 Open 3 Percutaneous 4 Percutaneous Endoscopic	B Intraluminal Device, Bioactive C Extraluminal Device D Intraluminal Device Z No Device	Z No Qualifier

Section	0	Medical and Surgical
Body System	3	Upper Arteries
Operation	W	**Revision:** Correcting, to the extent possible, a portion of a malfunctioning device or the position of a displaced device

Body Part (4ᵗʰ)	Approach (5ᵗʰ)	Device (6ᵗʰ)	Qualifier (7ᵗʰ)
Y Upper Artery	0 Open 3 Percutaneous 4 Percutaneous Endoscopic X External	0 Drainage Device 2 Monitoring Device 3 Infusion Device 7 Autologous Tissue Substitute C Extraluminal Device D Intraluminal Device J Synthetic Substitute K Nonautologous Tissue Substitute M Stimulator Lead	Z No Qualifier

Upper Arteries Code Listing 031–03W

031 – Upper Arteries, Bypass

Review Coding Guideline B3.6a

0312090	Bypass Innominate Artery to Right Upper Arm Artery with Autologous Venous Tissue, Open Approach	**0312093**	Bypass Innominate Artery to Right Lower Arm Artery with Autologous Venous Tissue, Open Approach	**0312096**	Bypass Innominate Artery to Right Uppe Leg Artery with Autologous Venous Tissue, Open Approach
0312091	Bypass Innominate Artery to Left Upper Arm Artery with Autologous Venous Tissue, Open Approach	**0312094**	Bypass Innominate Artery to Left Lower Arm Artery with Autologous Venous Tissue, Open Approach	**0312097**	Bypass Innominate Artery to Left Upper Leg Artery with Autologous Venous Tissue, Open Approach
0312092	Bypass Innominate Artery to Bilateral Upper Arm Artery with Autologous Venous Tissue, Open Approach	**0312095**	Bypass Innominate Artery to Bilateral Lower Arm Artery with Autologous Venous Tissue, Open Approach	**0312098**	Bypass Innominate Artery to Bilateral Upper Leg Artery with Autologous Venou Tissue, Open Approach

312099 Bypass Innominate Artery to Right Lower Leg Artery with Autologous Venous Tissue, Open Approach

31209B Bypass Innominate Artery to Left Lower Leg Artery with Autologous Venous Tissue, Open Approach

31209C Bypass Innominate Artery to Bilateral Lower Leg Artery with Autologous Venous Tissue, Open Approach

31209D Bypass Innominate Artery to Upper Arm Vein with Autologous Venous Tissue, Open Approach

31209F Bypass Innominate Artery to Lower Arm Vein with Autologous Venous Tissue, Open Approach

31209J Bypass Innominate Artery to Right Extracranial Artery with Autologous Venous Tissue, Open Approach

31209K Bypass Innominate Artery to Left Extracranial Artery with Autologous Venous Tissue, Open Approach

3120A0 Bypass Innominate Artery to Right Upper Arm Artery with Autologous Arterial Tissue, Open Approach

3120A1 Bypass Innominate Artery to Left Upper Arm Artery with Autologous Arterial Tissue, Open Approach

3120A2 Bypass Innominate Artery to Bilateral Upper Arm Artery with Autologous Arterial Tissue, Open Approach

3120A3 Bypass Innominate Artery to Right Lower Arm Artery with Autologous Arterial Tissue, Open Approach

3120A4 Bypass Innominate Artery to Left Lower Arm Artery with Autologous Arterial Tissue, Open Approach

3120A5 Bypass Innominate Artery to Bilateral Lower Arm Artery with Autologous Arterial Tissue, Open Approach

3120A6 Bypass Innominate Artery to Right Upper Leg Artery with Autologous Arterial Tissue, Open Approach

3120A7 Bypass Innominate Artery to Left Upper Leg Artery with Autologous Arterial Tissue, Open Approach

3120A8 Bypass Innominate Artery to Bilateral Upper Leg Artery with Autologous Arterial Tissue, Open Approach

3120A9 Bypass Innominate Artery to Right Lower Leg Artery with Autologous Arterial Tissue, Open Approach

3120AB Bypass Innominate Artery to Left Lower Leg Artery with Autologous Arterial Tissue, Open Approach

3120AC Bypass Innominate Artery to Bilateral Lower Leg Artery with Autologous Arterial Tissue, Open Approach

3120AD Bypass Innominate Artery to Upper Arm Vein with Autologous Arterial Tissue, Open Approach

3120AF Bypass Innominate Artery to Lower Arm Vein with Autologous Arterial Tissue, Open Approach

3120AJ Bypass Innominate Artery to Right Extracranial Artery with Autologous Arterial Tissue, Open Approach

3120AK Bypass Innominate Artery to Left Extracranial Artery with Autologous Arterial Tissue, Open Approach

3120J0 Bypass Innominate Artery to Right Upper Arm Artery with Synthetic Substitute, Open Approach

3120J1 Bypass Innominate Artery to Left Upper Arm Artery with Synthetic Substitute, Open Approach

03120J2 Bypass Innominate Artery to Bilateral Upper Arm Artery with Synthetic Substitute, Open Approach

03120J3 Bypass Innominate Artery to Right Lower Arm Artery with Synthetic Substitute, Open Approach

03120J4 Bypass Innominate Artery to Left Lower Arm Artery with Synthetic Substitute, Open Approach

03120J5 Bypass Innominate Artery to Bilateral Lower Arm Artery with Synthetic Substitute, Open Approach

03120J6 Bypass Innominate Artery to Right Upper Leg Artery with Synthetic Substitute, Open Approach

03120J7 Bypass Innominate Artery to Left Upper Leg Artery with Synthetic Substitute, Open Approach

03120J8 Bypass Innominate Artery to Bilateral Upper Leg Artery with Synthetic Substitute, Open Approach

03120J9 Bypass Innominate Artery to Right Lower Leg Artery with Synthetic Substitute, Open Approach

03120JB Bypass Innominate Artery to Left Lower Leg Artery with Synthetic Substitute, Open Approach

03120JC Bypass Innominate Artery to Bilateral Lower Leg Artery with Synthetic Substitute, Open Approach

03120JD Bypass Innominate Artery to Upper Arm Vein with Synthetic Substitute, Open Approach

03120JF Bypass Innominate Artery to Lower Arm Vein with Synthetic Substitute, Open Approach

03120JJ Bypass Innominate Artery to Right Extracranial Artery with Synthetic Substitute, Open Approach

03120JK Bypass Innominate Artery to Left Extracranial Artery with Synthetic Substitute, Open Approach

03120K0 Bypass Innominate Artery to Right Upper Arm Artery with Nonautologous Tissue Substitute, Open Approach

03120K1 Bypass Innominate Artery to Left Upper Arm Artery with Nonautologous Tissue Substitute, Open Approach

03120K2 Bypass Innominate Artery to Bilateral Upper Arm Artery with Nonautologous Tissue Substitute, Open Approach

03120K3 Bypass Innominate Artery to Right Lower Arm Artery with Nonautologous Tissue Substitute, Open Approach

03120K4 Bypass Innominate Artery to Left Lower Arm Artery with Nonautologous Tissue Substitute, Open Approach

03120K5 Bypass Innominate Artery to Bilateral Lower Arm Artery with Nonautologous Tissue Substitute, Open Approach

03120K6 Bypass Innominate Artery to Right Upper Leg Artery with Nonautologous Tissue Substitute, Open Approach

03120K7 Bypass Innominate Artery to Left Upper Leg Artery with Nonautologous Tissue Substitute, Open Approach

03120K8 Bypass Innominate Artery to Bilateral Upper Leg Artery with Nonautologous Tissue Substitute, Open Approach

03120K9 Bypass Innominate Artery to Right Lower Leg Artery with Nonautologous Tissue Substitute, Open Approach

03120KB Bypass Innominate Artery to Left Lower Leg Artery with Nonautologous Tissue Substitute, Open Approach

03120KC Bypass Innominate Artery to Bilateral Lower Leg Artery with Nonautologous Tissue Substitute, Open Approach

03120KD Bypass Innominate Artery to Upper Arm Vein with Nonautologous Tissue Substitute, Open Approach

03120KF Bypass Innominate Artery to Lower Arm Vein with Nonautologous Tissue Substitute, Open Approach

03120KJ Bypass Innominate Artery to Right Extracranial Artery with Nonautologous Tissue Substitute, Open Approach

03120KK Bypass Innominate Artery to Left Extracranial Artery with Nonautologous Tissue Substitute, Open Approach

03120Z0 Bypass Innominate Artery to Right Upper Arm Artery, Open Approach

03120Z1 Bypass Innominate Artery to Left Upper Arm Artery, Open Approach

03120Z2 Bypass Innominate Artery to Bilateral Upper Arm Artery, Open Approach

03120Z3 Bypass Innominate Artery to Right Lower Arm Artery, Open Approach

03120Z4 Bypass Innominate Artery to Left Lower Arm Artery, Open Approach

03120Z5 Bypass Innominate Artery to Bilateral Lower Arm Artery, Open Approach

03120Z6 Bypass Innominate Artery to Right Upper Leg Artery, Open Approach

03120Z7 Bypass Innominate Artery to Left Upper Leg Artery, Open Approach

03120Z8 Bypass Innominate Artery to Bilateral Upper Leg Artery, Open Approach

03120Z9 Bypass Innominate Artery to Right Lower Leg Artery, Open Approach

03120ZB Bypass Innominate Artery to Left Lower Leg Artery, Open Approach

03120ZC Bypass Innominate Artery to Bilateral Lower Leg Artery, Open Approach

03120ZD Bypass Innominate Artery to Upper Arm Vein, Open Approach

03120ZF Bypass Innominate Artery to Lower Arm Vein, Open Approach

03120ZJ Bypass Innominate Artery to Right Extracranial Artery, Open Approach

03120ZK Bypass Innominate Artery to Left Extracranial Artery, Open Approach

0313090 Bypass Right Subclavian Artery to Right Upper Arm Artery with Autologous Venous Tissue, Open Approach

0313091 Bypass Right Subclavian Artery to Left Upper Arm Artery with Autologous Venous Tissue, Open Approach

0313092 Bypass Right Subclavian Artery to Bilateral Upper Arm Artery with Autologous Venous Tissue, Open Approach

0313093 Bypass Right Subclavian Artery to Right Lower Arm Artery with Autologous Venous Tissue, Open Approach

0313094 Bypass Right Subclavian Artery to Left Lower Arm Artery with Autologous Venous Tissue, Open Approach

0313095 Bypass Right Subclavian Artery to Bilateral Lower Arm Artery with Autologous Venous Tissue, Open Approach

0313096 Bypass Right Subclavian Artery to Right Upper Leg Artery with Autologous Venous Tissue, Open Approach

0313097 Bypass Right Subclavian Artery to Left Upper Leg Artery with Autologous Venous Tissue, Open Approach

0313098 Bypass Right Subclavian Artery to Bilateral Upper Leg Artery with Autologous Venous Tissue, Open Approach

0313099 Bypass Right Subclavian Artery to Right Lower Leg Artery with Autologous Venous Tissue, Open Approach

031309B Bypass Right Subclavian Artery to Left Lower Leg Artery with Autologous Venous Tissue, Open Approach

031309C Bypass Right Subclavian Artery to Bilateral Lower Leg Artery with Autologous Venous Tissue, Open Approach

031309D Bypass Right Subclavian Artery to Upper Arm Vein with Autologous Venous Tissue, Open Approach

031309F Bypass Right Subclavian Artery to Lower Arm Vein with Autologous Venous Tissue, Open Approach

031309J Bypass Right Subclavian Artery to Right Extracranial Artery with Autologous Venous Tissue, Open Approach

031309K Bypass Right Subclavian Artery to Left Extracranial Artery with Autologous Venous Tissue, Open Approach

031309M Bypass Right Subclavian Artery to Right Pulmonary Artery with Autologous Venous Tissue, Open Approach

031309N Bypass Right Subclavian Artery to Left Pulmonary Artery with Autologous Venous Tissue, Open Approach

03130A0 Bypass Right Subclavian Artery to Right Upper Arm Artery with Autologous Arterial Tissue, Open Approach

03130A1 Bypass Right Subclavian Artery to Left Upper Arm Artery with Autologous Arterial Tissue, Open Approach

03130A2 Bypass Right Subclavian Artery to Bilateral Upper Arm Artery with Autologous Arterial Tissue, Open Approach

03130A3 Bypass Right Subclavian Artery to Right Lower Arm Artery with Autologous Arterial Tissue, Open Approach

03130A4 Bypass Right Subclavian Artery to Left Lower Arm Artery with Autologous Arterial Tissue, Open Approach

03130A5 Bypass Right Subclavian Artery to Bilateral Lower Arm Artery with Autologous Arterial Tissue, Open Approach

03130A6 Bypass Right Subclavian Artery to Right Upper Leg Artery with Autologous Arterial Tissue, Open Approach

03130A7 Bypass Right Subclavian Artery to Left Upper Leg Artery with Autologous Arterial Tissue, Open Approach

03130A8 Bypass Right Subclavian Artery to Bilateral Upper Leg Artery with Autologous Arterial Tissue, Open Approach

03130A9 Bypass Right Subclavian Artery to Right Lower Leg Artery with Autologous Arterial Tissue, Open Approach

03130AB Bypass Right Subclavian Artery to Left Lower Leg Artery with Autologous Arterial Tissue, Open Approach

03130AC Bypass Right Subclavian Artery to Bilateral Lower Leg Artery with Autologous Arterial Tissue, Open Approach

03130AD Bypass Right Subclavian Artery to Upper Arm Vein with Autologous Arterial Tissue, Open Approach

03130AF Bypass Right Subclavian Artery to Lower Arm Vein with Autologous Arterial Tissue, Open Approach

03130AJ Bypass Right Subclavian Artery to Right Extracranial Artery with Autologous Arterial Tissue, Open Approach

03130AK Bypass Right Subclavian Artery to Left Extracranial Artery with Autologous Arterial Tissue, Open Approach

03130AM Bypass Right Subclavian Artery to Right Pulmonary Artery with Autologous Arterial Tissue, Open Approach

03130AN Bypass Right Subclavian Artery to Left Pulmonary Artery with Autologous Arterial Tissue, Open Approach

03130J0 Bypass Right Subclavian Artery to Right Upper Arm Artery with Synthetic Substitute, Open Approach

03130J1 Bypass Right Subclavian Artery to Left Upper Arm Artery with Synthetic Substitute, Open Approach

03130J2 Bypass Right Subclavian Artery to Bilateral Upper Arm Artery with Synthetic Substitute, Open Approach

03130J3 Bypass Right Subclavian Artery to Right Lower Arm Artery with Synthetic Substitute, Open Approach

03130J4 Bypass Right Subclavian Artery to Left Lower Arm Artery with Synthetic Substitute, Open Approach

03130J5 Bypass Right Subclavian Artery to Bilateral Lower Arm Artery with Synthetic Substitute, Open Approach

03130J6 Bypass Right Subclavian Artery to Right Upper Leg Artery with Synthetic Substitute, Open Approach

03130J7 Bypass Right Subclavian Artery to Left Upper Leg Artery with Synthetic Substitute, Open Approach

03130J8 Bypass Right Subclavian Artery to Bilateral Upper Leg Artery with Synthetic Substitute, Open Approach

03130J9 Bypass Right Subclavian Artery to Right Lower Leg Artery with Synthetic Substitute, Open Approach

03130JB Bypass Right Subclavian Artery to Left Lower Leg Artery with Synthetic Substitute, Open Approach

03130JC Bypass Right Subclavian Artery to Bilateral Lower Leg Artery with Synthetic Substitute, Open Approach

03130JD Bypass Right Subclavian Artery to Upper Arm Vein with Synthetic Substitute, Open Approach

03130JF Bypass Right Subclavian Artery to Lower Arm Vein with Synthetic Substitute, Open Approach

03130JJ Bypass Right Subclavian Artery to Right Extracranial Artery with Synthetic Substitute, Open Approach

03130JK Bypass Right Subclavian Artery to Left Extracranial Artery with Synthetic Substitute, Open Approach

03130JM Bypass Right Subclavian Artery to Right Pulmonary Artery with Synthetic Substitute, Open Approach

03130JN Bypass Right Subclavian Artery to Left Pulmonary Artery with Synthetic Substitute, Open Approach

03130K0 Bypass Right Subclavian Artery to Right Upper Arm Artery with Nonautologous Tissue Substitute, Open Approach

03130K1 Bypass Right Subclavian Artery to Left Upper Arm Artery with Nonautologous Tissue Substitute, Open Approach

03130K2 Bypass Right Subclavian Artery to Bilateral Upper Arm Artery with Nonautologous Tissue Substitute, Open Approach

03130K3 Bypass Right Subclavian Artery to Right Lower Arm Artery with Nonautologous Tissue Substitute, Open Approach

03130K4 Bypass Right Subclavian Artery to Left Lower Arm Artery with Nonautologous Tissue Substitute, Open Approach

03130K5 Bypass Right Subclavian Artery to Bilateral Lower Arm Artery with Nonautologous Tissue Substitute, Open Approach

03130K6 Bypass Right Subclavian Artery to Right Upper Leg Artery with Nonautologous Tissue Substitute, Open Approach

03130K7 Bypass Right Subclavian Artery to Left Upper Leg Artery with Nonautologous Tissue Substitute, Open Approach

03130K8 Bypass Right Subclavian Artery to Bilateral Upper Leg Artery with Nonautologous Tissue Substitute, Open Approach

03130K9 Bypass Right Subclavian Artery to Right Lower Leg Artery with Nonautologous Tissue Substitute, Open Approach

03130KB Bypass Right Subclavian Artery to Left Lower Leg Artery with Nonautologous Tissue Substitute, Open Approach

03130KC Bypass Right Subclavian Artery to Bilateral Lower Leg Artery with Nonautologous Tissue Substitute, Open Approach

03130KD Bypass Right Subclavian Artery to Upper Arm Vein with Nonautologous Tissue Substitute, Open Approach

03130KF Bypass Right Subclavian Artery to Lower Arm Vein with Nonautologous Tissue Substitute, Open Approach

03130KJ Bypass Right Subclavian Artery to Right Extracranial Artery with Nonautologous Tissue Substitute, Open Approach

03130KK Bypass Right Subclavian Artery to Left Extracranial Artery with Nonautologous Tissue Substitute, Open Approach

03130KM Bypass Right Subclavian Artery to Right Pulmonary Artery with Nonautologous Tissue Substitute, Open Approach

03130KN Bypass Right Subclavian Artery to Left Pulmonary Artery with Nonautologous Tissue Substitute, Open Approach

03130Z0 Bypass Right Subclavian Artery to Right Upper Arm Artery, Open Approach

03130Z1 Bypass Right Subclavian Artery to Left Upper Arm Artery, Open Approach

03130Z2 Bypass Right Subclavian Artery to Bilateral Upper Arm Artery, Open Approach

03130Z3 Bypass Right Subclavian Artery to Right Lower Arm Artery, Open Approach

03130Z4 Bypass Right Subclavian Artery to Left Lower Arm Artery, Open Approach

03130Z5 Bypass Right Subclavian Artery to Bilateral Lower Arm Artery, Open Approach

03130Z6 Bypass Right Subclavian Artery to Right Upper Leg Artery, Open Approach

03130Z7 Bypass Right Subclavian Artery to Left Upper Leg Artery, Open Approach

03130Z8 Bypass Right Subclavian Artery to Bilateral Upper Leg Artery, Open Approach

03130Z9 Bypass Right Subclavian Artery to Right Lower Leg Artery, Open Approach

03130ZB Bypass Right Subclavian Artery to Left Lower Leg Artery, Open Approach

03130ZC Bypass Right Subclavian Artery to Bilateral Lower Leg Artery, Open Approach

03130ZD Bypass Right Subclavian Artery to Upper Arm Vein, Open Approach

03130ZF Bypass Right Subclavian Artery to Lower Arm Vein, Open Approach

03130ZJ Bypass Right Subclavian Artery to Right Extracranial Artery, Open Approach

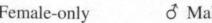

♀ Female-only   ♂ Male-only   ▲ Limited Coverage   ● Non-OR   ▥ HAC-associated procedure   ▲ Non-covered procedures   ✚ Combination

03130ZK	Bypass Right Subclavian Artery to Left Extracranial Artery, Open Approach
03130ZM	Bypass Right Subclavian Artery to Right Pulmonary Artery, Open Approach
03130ZN	Bypass Right Subclavian Artery to Left Pulmonary Artery, Open Approach
0314090	Bypass Left Subclavian Artery to Right Upper Arm Artery with Autologous Venous Tissue, Open Approach
0314091	Bypass Left Subclavian Artery to Left Upper Arm Artery with Autologous Venous Tissue, Open Approach
0314092	Bypass Left Subclavian Artery to Bilateral Upper Arm Artery with Autologous Venous Tissue, Open Approach
0314093	Bypass Left Subclavian Artery to Right Lower Arm Artery with Autologous Venous Tissue, Open Approach
0314094	Bypass Left Subclavian Artery to Left Lower Arm Artery with Autologous Venous Tissue, Open Approach
0314095	Bypass Left Subclavian Artery to Bilateral Lower Arm Artery with Autologous Venous Tissue, Open Approach
0314096	Bypass Left Subclavian Artery to Right Upper Leg Artery with Autologous Venous Tissue, Open Approach
0314097	Bypass Left Subclavian Artery to Left Upper Leg Artery with Autologous Venous Tissue, Open Approach
0314098	Bypass Left Subclavian Artery to Bilateral Upper Leg Artery with Autologous Venous Tissue, Open Approach
0314099	Bypass Left Subclavian Artery to Right Lower Leg Artery with Autologous Venous Tissue, Open Approach
031409B	Bypass Left Subclavian Artery to Left Lower Leg Artery with Autologous Venous Tissue, Open Approach
031409C	Bypass Left Subclavian Artery to Bilateral Lower Leg Artery with Autologous Venous Tissue, Open Approach
031409D	Bypass Left Subclavian Artery to Upper Arm Vein with Autologous Venous Tissue, Open Approach
031409F	Bypass Left Subclavian Artery to Lower Arm Vein with Autologous Venous Tissue, Open Approach
031409J	Bypass Left Subclavian Artery to Right Extracranial Artery with Autologous Venous Tissue, Open Approach
031409K	Bypass Left Subclavian Artery to Left Extracranial Artery with Autologous Venous Tissue, Open Approach
031409M	Bypass Left Subclavian Artery to Right Pulmonary Artery with Autologous Venous Tissue, Open Approach
031409N	Bypass Left Subclavian Artery to Left Pulmonary Artery with Autologous Venous Tissue, Open Approach
03140A0	Bypass Left Subclavian Artery to Right Upper Arm Artery with Autologous Arterial Tissue, Open Approach
03140A1	Bypass Left Subclavian Artery to Left Upper Arm Artery with Autologous Arterial Tissue, Open Approach
03140A2	Bypass Left Subclavian Artery to Bilateral Upper Arm Artery with Autologous Arterial Tissue, Open Approach
03140A3	Bypass Left Subclavian Artery to Right Lower Arm Artery with Autologous Arterial Tissue, Open Approach
03140A4	Bypass Left Subclavian Artery to Left Lower Arm Artery with Autologous Arterial Tissue, Open Approach
03140A5	Bypass Left Subclavian Artery to Bilateral Lower Arm Artery with Autologous Arterial Tissue, Open Approach

03140A6	Bypass Left Subclavian Artery to Right Upper Leg Artery with Autologous Arterial Tissue, Open Approach
03140A7	Bypass Left Subclavian Artery to Left Upper Leg Artery with Autologous Arterial Tissue, Open Approach
03140A8	Bypass Left Subclavian Artery to Bilateral Upper Leg Artery with Autologous Arterial Tissue, Open Approach
03140A9	Bypass Left Subclavian Artery to Right Lower Leg Artery with Autologous Arterial Tissue, Open Approach
03140AB	Bypass Left Subclavian Artery to Left Lower Leg Artery with Autologous Arterial Tissue, Open Approach
03140AC	Bypass Left Subclavian Artery to Bilateral Lower Leg Artery with Autologous Arterial Tissue, Open Approach
03140AD	Bypass Left Subclavian Artery to Upper Arm Vein with Autologous Arterial Tissue, Open Approach
03140AF	Bypass Left Subclavian Artery to Lower Arm Vein with Autologous Arterial Tissue, Open Approach
03140AJ	Bypass Left Subclavian Artery to Right Extracranial Artery with Autologous Arterial Tissue, Open Approach
03140AK	Bypass Left Subclavian Artery to Left Extracranial Artery with Autologous Arterial Tissue, Open Approach
03140AM	Bypass Left Subclavian Artery to Right Pulmonary Artery with Autologous Arterial Tissue, Open Approach
03140AN	Bypass Left Subclavian Artery to Left Pulmonary Artery with Autologous Arterial Tissue, Open Approach
03140J0	Bypass Left Subclavian Artery to Right Upper Arm Artery with Synthetic Substitute, Open Approach
03140J1	Bypass Left Subclavian Artery to Left Upper Arm Artery with Synthetic Substitute, Open Approach
03140J2	Bypass Left Subclavian Artery to Bilateral Upper Arm Artery with Synthetic Substitute, Open Approach
03140J3	Bypass Left Subclavian Artery to Right Lower Arm Artery with Synthetic Substitute, Open Approach
03140J4	Bypass Left Subclavian Artery to Left Lower Arm Artery with Synthetic Substitute, Open Approach
03140J5	Bypass Left Subclavian Artery to Bilateral Lower Arm Artery with Synthetic Substitute, Open Approach
03140J6	Bypass Left Subclavian Artery to Right Upper Leg Artery with Synthetic Substitute, Open Approach
03140J7	Bypass Left Subclavian Artery to Left Upper Leg Artery with Synthetic Substitute, Open Approach
03140J8	Bypass Left Subclavian Artery to Bilateral Upper Leg Artery with Synthetic Substitute, Open Approach
03140J9	Bypass Left Subclavian Artery to Right Lower Leg Artery with Synthetic Substitute, Open Approach
03140JB	Bypass Left Subclavian Artery to Left Lower Leg Artery with Synthetic Substitute, Open Approach
03140JC	Bypass Left Subclavian Artery to Bilateral Lower Leg Artery with Synthetic Substitute, Open Approach
03140JD	Bypass Left Subclavian Artery to Upper Arm Vein with Synthetic Substitute, Open Approach
03140JF	Bypass Left Subclavian Artery to Lower Arm Vein with Synthetic Substitute, Open Approach

03140JJ	Bypass Left Subclavian Artery to Right Extracranial Artery with Synthetic Substitute, Open Approach
03140JK	Bypass Left Subclavian Artery to Left Extracranial Artery with Synthetic Substitute, Open Approach
03140JM	Bypass Left Subclavian Artery to Right Pulmonary Artery with Synthetic Substitute, Open Approach
03140JN	Bypass Left Subclavian Artery to Left Pulmonary Artery with Synthetic Substitute, Open Approach
03140K0	Bypass Left Subclavian Artery to Right Upper Arm Artery with Nonautologous Tissue Substitute, Open Approach
03140K1	Bypass Left Subclavian Artery to Left Upper Arm Artery with Nonautologous Tissue Substitute, Open Approach
03140K2	Bypass Left Subclavian Artery to Bilateral Upper Arm Artery with Nonautologous Tissue Substitute, Open Approach
03140K3	Bypass Left Subclavian Artery to Right Lower Arm Artery with Nonautologous Tissue Substitute, Open Approach
03140K4	Bypass Left Subclavian Artery to Left Lower Arm Artery with Nonautologous Tissue Substitute, Open Approach
03140K5	Bypass Left Subclavian Artery to Bilateral Lower Arm Artery with Nonautologous Tissue Substitute, Open Approach
03140K6	Bypass Left Subclavian Artery to Right Upper Leg Artery with Nonautologous Tissue Substitute, Open Approach
03140K7	Bypass Left Subclavian Artery to Left Upper Leg Artery with Nonautologous Tissue Substitute, Open Approach
03140K8	Bypass Left Subclavian Artery to Bilateral Upper Leg Artery with Nonautologous Tissue Substitute, Open Approach
03140K9	Bypass Left Subclavian Artery to Right Lower Leg Artery with Nonautologous Tissue Substitute, Open Approach
03140KB	Bypass Left Subclavian Artery to Left Lower Leg Artery with Nonautologous Tissue Substitute, Open Approach
03140KC	Bypass Left Subclavian Artery to Bilateral Lower Leg Artery with Nonautologous Tissue Substitute, Open Approach
03140KD	Bypass Left Subclavian Artery to Upper Arm Vein with Nonautologous Tissue Substitute, Open Approach
03140KF	Bypass Left Subclavian Artery to Lower Arm Vein with Nonautologous Tissue Substitute, Open Approach
03140KJ	Bypass Left Subclavian Artery to Right Extracranial Artery with Nonautologous Tissue Substitute, Open Approach
03140KK	Bypass Left Subclavian Artery to Left Extracranial Artery with Nonautologous Tissue Substitute, Open Approach
03140KM	Bypass Left Subclavian Artery to Right Pulmonary Artery with Nonautologous Tissue Substitute, Open Approach
03140KN	Bypass Left Subclavian Artery to Left Pulmonary Artery with Nonautologous Tissue Substitute, Open Approach
03140Z0	Bypass Left Subclavian Artery to Right Upper Arm Artery, Open Approach
03140Z1	Bypass Left Subclavian Artery to Left Upper Arm Artery, Open Approach
03140Z2	Bypass Left Subclavian Artery to Bilateral Upper Arm Artery, Open Approach
03140Z3	Bypass Left Subclavian Artery to Right Lower Arm Artery, Open Approach
03140Z4	Bypass Left Subclavian Artery to Left Lower Arm Artery, Open Approach
03140Z5	Bypass Left Subclavian Artery to Bilateral Lower Arm Artery, Open Approach

03140Z6	Bypass Left Subclavian Artery to Right Upper Leg Artery, Open Approach
03140Z7	Bypass Left Subclavian Artery to Left Upper Leg Artery, Open Approach
03140Z8	Bypass Left Subclavian Artery to Bilateral Upper Leg Artery, Open Approach
03140Z9	Bypass Left Subclavian Artery to Right Lower Leg Artery, Open Approach
03140ZB	Bypass Left Subclavian Artery to Left Lower Leg Artery, Open Approach
03140ZC	Bypass Left Subclavian Artery to Bilateral Lower Leg Artery, Open Approach
03140ZD	Bypass Left Subclavian Artery to Upper Arm Vein, Open Approach
03140ZF	Bypass Left Subclavian Artery to Lower Arm Vein, Open Approach
03140ZJ	Bypass Left Subclavian Artery to Right Extracranial Artery, Open Approach
03140ZK	Bypass Left Subclavian Artery to Left Extracranial Artery, Open Approach
03140ZM	Bypass Left Subclavian Artery to Right Pulmonary Artery, Open Approach
03140ZN	Bypass Left Subclavian Artery to Left Pulmonary Artery, Open Approach
0315090	Bypass Right Axillary Artery to Right Upper Arm Artery with Autologous Venous Tissue, Open Approach
0315091	Bypass Right Axillary Artery to Left Upper Arm Artery with Autologous Venous Tissue, Open Approach
0315092	Bypass Right Axillary Artery to Bilateral Upper Arm Artery with Autologous Venous Tissue, Open Approach
0315093	Bypass Right Axillary Artery to Right Lower Arm Artery with Autologous Venous Tissue, Open Approach
0315094	Bypass Right Axillary Artery to Left Lower Arm Artery with Autologous Venous Tissue, Open Approach
0315095	Bypass Right Axillary Artery to Bilateral Lower Arm Artery with Autologous Venous Tissue, Open Approach
0315096	Bypass Right Axillary Artery to Right Upper Leg Artery with Autologous Venous Tissue, Open Approach
0315097	Bypass Right Axillary Artery to Left Upper Leg Artery with Autologous Venous Tissue, Open Approach
0315098	Bypass Right Axillary Artery to Bilateral Upper Leg Artery with Autologous Venous Tissue, Open Approach
0315099	Bypass Right Axillary Artery to Right Lower Leg Artery with Autologous Venous Tissue, Open Approach
031509B	Bypass Right Axillary Artery to Left Lower Leg Artery with Autologous Venous Tissue, Open Approach
031509C	Bypass Right Axillary Artery to Bilateral Lower Leg Artery with Autologous Venous Tissue, Open Approach
031509D	Bypass Right Axillary Artery to Upper Arm Vein with Autologous Venous Tissue, Open Approach
031509F	Bypass Right Axillary Artery to Lower Arm Vein with Autologous Venous Tissue, Open Approach
031509J	Bypass Right Axillary Artery to Right Extracranial Artery with Autologous Venous Tissue, Open Approach
031509K	Bypass Right Axillary Artery to Left Extracranial Artery with Autologous Venous Tissue, Open Approach
03150A0	Bypass Right Axillary Artery to Right Upper Arm Artery with Autologous Arterial Tissue, Open Approach
03150A1	Bypass Right Axillary Artery to Left Upper Arm Artery with Autologous Arterial Tissue, Open Approach
03150A2	Bypass Right Axillary Artery to Bilateral Upper Arm Artery with Autologous Arterial Tissue, Open Approach
03150A3	Bypass Right Axillary Artery to Right Lower Arm Artery with Autologous Arterial Tissue, Open Approach
03150A4	Bypass Right Axillary Artery to Left Lower Arm Artery with Autologous Arterial Tissue, Open Approach
03150A5	Bypass Right Axillary Artery to Bilateral Lower Arm Artery with Autologous Arterial Tissue, Open Approach
03150A6	Bypass Right Axillary Artery to Right Upper Leg Artery with Autologous Arterial Tissue, Open Approach
03150A7	Bypass Right Axillary Artery to Left Upper Leg Artery with Autologous Arterial Tissue, Open Approach
03150A8	Bypass Right Axillary Artery to Bilateral Upper Leg Artery with Autologous Arterial Tissue, Open Approach
03150A9	Bypass Right Axillary Artery to Right Lower Leg Artery with Autologous Arterial Tissue, Open Approach
03150AB	Bypass Right Axillary Artery to Left Lower Leg Artery with Autologous Arterial Tissue, Open Approach
03150AC	Bypass Right Axillary Artery to Bilateral Lower Leg Artery with Autologous Arterial Tissue, Open Approach
03150AD	Bypass Right Axillary Artery to Upper Arm Vein with Autologous Arterial Tissue, Open Approach
03150AF	Bypass Right Axillary Artery to Lower Arm Vein with Autologous Arterial Tissue, Open Approach
03150AJ	Bypass Right Axillary Artery to Right Extracranial Artery with Autologous Arterial Tissue, Open Approach
03150AK	Bypass Right Axillary Artery to Left Extracranial Artery with Autologous Arterial Tissue, Open Approach
03150J0	Bypass Right Axillary Artery to Right Upper Arm Artery with Synthetic Substitute, Open Approach
03150J1	Bypass Right Axillary Artery to Left Upper Arm Artery with Synthetic Substitute, Open Approach
03150J2	Bypass Right Axillary Artery to Bilateral Upper Arm Artery with Synthetic Substitute, Open Approach
03150J3	Bypass Right Axillary Artery to Right Lower Arm Artery with Synthetic Substitute, Open Approach
03150J4	Bypass Right Axillary Artery to Left Lower Arm Artery with Synthetic Substitute, Open Approach
03150J5	Bypass Right Axillary Artery to Bilateral Lower Arm Artery with Synthetic Substitute, Open Approach
03150J6	Bypass Right Axillary Artery to Right Upper Leg Artery with Synthetic Substitute, Open Approach
03150J7	Bypass Right Axillary Artery to Left Upper Leg Artery with Synthetic Substitute, Open Approach
03150J8	Bypass Right Axillary Artery to Bilateral Upper Leg Artery with Synthetic Substitute, Open Approach
03150J9	Bypass Right Axillary Artery to Right Lower Leg Artery with Synthetic Substitute, Open Approach
03150JB	Bypass Right Axillary Artery to Left Lower Leg Artery with Synthetic Substitute, Open Approach
03150JC	Bypass Right Axillary Artery to Bilateral Lower Leg Artery with Synthetic Substitute, Open Approach
03150JD	Bypass Right Axillary Artery to Upper Arm Vein with Synthetic Substitute, Open Approach
03150JF	Bypass Right Axillary Artery to Lower Arm Vein with Synthetic Substitute, Open Approach
03150JJ	Bypass Right Axillary Artery to Right Extracranial Artery with Synthetic Substitute, Open Approach
03150JK	Bypass Right Axillary Artery to Left Extracranial Artery with Synthetic Substitute, Open Approach
03150K0	Bypass Right Axillary Artery to Right Upper Arm Artery with Nonautologous Tissue Substitute, Open Approach
03150K1	Bypass Right Axillary Artery to Left Upper Arm Artery with Nonautologous Tissue Substitute, Open Approach
03150K2	Bypass Right Axillary Artery to Bilateral Upper Arm Artery with Nonautologous Tissue Substitute, Open Approach
03150K3	Bypass Right Axillary Artery to Right Lower Arm Artery with Nonautologous Tissue Substitute, Open Approach
03150K4	Bypass Right Axillary Artery to Left Lower Arm Artery with Nonautologous Tissue Substitute, Open Approach
03150K5	Bypass Right Axillary Artery to Bilateral Lower Arm Artery with Nonautologous Tissue Substitute, Open Approach
03150K6	Bypass Right Axillary Artery to Right Upper Leg Artery with Nonautologous Tissue Substitute, Open Approach
03150K7	Bypass Right Axillary Artery to Left Upper Leg Artery with Nonautologous Tissue Substitute, Open Approach
03150K8	Bypass Right Axillary Artery to Bilateral Upper Leg Artery with Nonautologous Tissue Substitute, Open Approach
03150K9	Bypass Right Axillary Artery to Right Lower Leg Artery with Nonautologous Tissue Substitute, Open Approach
03150KB	Bypass Right Axillary Artery to Left Lower Leg Artery with Nonautologous Tissue Substitute, Open Approach
03150KC	Bypass Right Axillary Artery to Bilateral Lower Leg Artery with Nonautologous Tissue Substitute, Open Approach
03150KD	Bypass Right Axillary Artery to Upper Arm Vein with Nonautologous Tissue Substitute, Open Approach
03150KF	Bypass Right Axillary Artery to Lower Arm Vein with Nonautologous Tissue Substitute, Open Approach
03150KJ	Bypass Right Axillary Artery to Right Extracranial Artery with Nonautologous Tissue Substitute, Open Approach
03150KK	Bypass Right Axillary Artery to Left Extracranial Artery with Nonautologous Tissue Substitute, Open Approach
03150Z0	Bypass Right Axillary Artery to Right Upper Arm Artery, Open Approach
03150Z1	Bypass Right Axillary Artery to Left Upper Arm Artery, Open Approach
03150Z2	Bypass Right Axillary Artery to Bilateral Upper Arm Artery, Open Approach
03150Z3	Bypass Right Axillary Artery to Right Lower Arm Artery, Open Approach
03150Z4	Bypass Right Axillary Artery to Left Lower Arm Artery, Open Approach
03150Z5	Bypass Right Axillary Artery to Bilateral Lower Arm Artery, Open Approach
03150Z6	Bypass Right Axillary Artery to Right Upper Leg Artery, Open Approach
03150Z7	Bypass Right Axillary Artery to Left Upper Leg Artery, Open Approach

♀ Female-only   ♂ Male-only   ▲ Limited Coverage   ● Non-OR   ▪ HAC-associated procedure   ▲ Non-covered procedures   ✚ Combination

3150Z8	Bypass Right Axillary Artery to Bilateral Upper Leg Artery, Open Approach
3150Z9	Bypass Right Axillary Artery to Right Lower Leg Artery, Open Approach
3150ZB	Bypass Right Axillary Artery to Left Lower Leg Artery, Open Approach
3150ZC	Bypass Right Axillary Artery to Bilateral Lower Leg Artery, Open Approach
3150ZD	Bypass Right Axillary Artery to Upper Arm Vein, Open Approach
3150ZF	Bypass Right Axillary Artery to Lower Arm Vein, Open Approach
3150ZJ	Bypass Right Axillary Artery to Right Extracranial Artery, Open Approach
3150ZK	Bypass Right Axillary Artery to Left Extracranial Artery, Open Approach
316090	Bypass Left Axillary Artery to Right Upper Arm Artery with Autologous Venous Tissue, Open Approach
316091	Bypass Left Axillary Artery to Left Upper Arm Artery with Autologous Venous Tissue, Open Approach
316092	Bypass Left Axillary Artery to Bilateral Upper Arm Artery with Autologous Venous Tissue, Open Approach
316093	Bypass Left Axillary Artery to Right Lower Arm Artery with Autologous Venous Tissue, Open Approach
316094	Bypass Left Axillary Artery to Left Lower Arm Artery with Autologous Venous Tissue, Open Approach
316095	Bypass Left Axillary Artery to Bilateral Lower Arm Artery with Autologous Venous Tissue, Open Approach
316096	Bypass Left Axillary Artery to Right Upper Leg Artery with Autologous Venous Tissue, Open Approach
316097	Bypass Left Axillary Artery to Left Upper Leg Artery with Autologous Venous Tissue, Open Approach
316098	Bypass Left Axillary Artery to Bilateral Upper Leg Artery with Autologous Venous Tissue, Open Approach
316099	Bypass Left Axillary Artery to Right Lower Leg Artery with Autologous Venous Tissue, Open Approach
31609B	Bypass Left Axillary Artery to Left Lower Leg Artery with Autologous Venous Tissue, Open Approach
31609C	Bypass Left Axillary Artery to Bilateral Lower Leg Artery with Autologous Venous Tissue, Open Approach
31609D	Bypass Left Axillary Artery to Upper Arm Vein with Autologous Venous Tissue, Open Approach
31609F	Bypass Left Axillary Artery to Lower Arm Vein with Autologous Venous Tissue, Open Approach
31609J	Bypass Left Axillary Artery to Right Extracranial Artery with Autologous Venous Tissue, Open Approach
31609K	Bypass Left Axillary Artery to Left Extracranial Artery with Autologous Venous Tissue, Open Approach
3160A0	Bypass Left Axillary Artery to Right Upper Arm Artery with Autologous Arterial Tissue, Open Approach
3160A1	Bypass Left Axillary Artery to Left Upper Arm Artery with Autologous Arterial Tissue, Open Approach
3160A2	Bypass Left Axillary Artery to Bilateral Upper Arm Artery with Autologous Arterial Tissue, Open Approach
3160A3	Bypass Left Axillary Artery to Right Lower Arm Artery with Autologous Arterial Tissue, Open Approach
03160A4	Bypass Left Axillary Artery to Left Lower Arm Artery with Autologous Arterial Tissue, Open Approach
03160A5	Bypass Left Axillary Artery to Bilateral Lower Arm Artery with Autologous Arterial Tissue, Open Approach
03160A6	Bypass Left Axillary Artery to Right Upper Leg Artery with Autologous Arterial Tissue, Open Approach
03160A7	Bypass Left Axillary Artery to Left Upper Leg Artery with Autologous Arterial Tissue, Open Approach
03160A8	Bypass Left Axillary Artery to Bilateral Upper Leg Artery with Autologous Arterial Tissue, Open Approach
03160A9	Bypass Left Axillary Artery to Right Lower Leg Artery with Autologous Arterial Tissue, Open Approach
03160AB	Bypass Left Axillary Artery to Left Lower Leg Artery with Autologous Arterial Tissue, Open Approach
03160AC	Bypass Left Axillary Artery to Bilateral Lower Leg Artery with Autologous Arterial Tissue, Open Approach
03160AD	Bypass Left Axillary Artery to Upper Arm Vein with Autologous Arterial Tissue, Open Approach
03160AF	Bypass Left Axillary Artery to Lower Arm Vein with Autologous Arterial Tissue, Open Approach
03160AJ	Bypass Left Axillary Artery to Right Extracranial Artery with Autologous Arterial Tissue, Open Approach
03160AK	Bypass Left Axillary Artery to Left Extracranial Artery with Autologous Arterial Tissue, Open Approach
03160J0	Bypass Left Axillary Artery to Right Upper Arm Artery with Synthetic Substitute, Open Approach
03160J1	Bypass Left Axillary Artery to Left Upper Arm Artery with Synthetic Substitute, Open Approach
03160J2	Bypass Left Axillary Artery to Bilateral Upper Arm Artery with Synthetic Substitute, Open Approach
03160J3	Bypass Left Axillary Artery to Right Lower Arm Artery with Synthetic Substitute, Open Approach
03160J4	Bypass Left Axillary Artery to Left Lower Arm Artery with Synthetic Substitute, Open Approach
03160J5	Bypass Left Axillary Artery to Bilateral Lower Arm Artery with Synthetic Substitute, Open Approach
03160J6	Bypass Left Axillary Artery to Right Upper Leg Artery with Synthetic Substitute, Open Approach
03160J7	Bypass Left Axillary Artery to Left Upper Leg Artery with Synthetic Substitute, Open Approach
03160J8	Bypass Left Axillary Artery to Bilateral Upper Leg Artery with Synthetic Substitute, Open Approach
03160J9	Bypass Left Axillary Artery to Right Lower Leg Artery with Synthetic Substitute, Open Approach
03160JB	Bypass Left Axillary Artery to Left Lower Leg Artery with Synthetic Substitute, Open Approach
03160JC	Bypass Left Axillary Artery to Bilateral Lower Leg Artery with Synthetic Substitute, Open Approach
03160JD	Bypass Left Axillary Artery to Upper Arm Vein with Synthetic Substitute, Open Approach
03160JF	Bypass Left Axillary Artery to Lower Arm Vein with Synthetic Substitute, Open Approach
03160JJ	Bypass Left Axillary Artery to Right Extracranial Artery with Synthetic Substitute, Open Approach
03160JK	Bypass Left Axillary Artery to Left Extracranial Artery with Synthetic Substitute, Open Approach
03160K0	Bypass Left Axillary Artery to Right Upper Arm Artery with Nonautologous Tissue Substitute, Open Approach
03160K1	Bypass Left Axillary Artery to Left Upper Arm Artery with Nonautologous Tissue Substitute, Open Approach
03160K2	Bypass Left Axillary Artery to Bilateral Upper Arm Artery with Nonautologous Tissue Substitute, Open Approach
03160K3	Bypass Left Axillary Artery to Right Lower Arm Artery with Nonautologous Tissue Substitute, Open Approach
03160K4	Bypass Left Axillary Artery to Left Lower Arm Artery with Nonautologous Tissue Substitute, Open Approach
03160K5	Bypass Left Axillary Artery to Bilateral Lower Arm Artery with Nonautologous Tissue Substitute, Open Approach
03160K6	Bypass Left Axillary Artery to Right Upper Leg Artery with Nonautologous Tissue Substitute, Open Approach
03160K7	Bypass Left Axillary Artery to Left Upper Leg Artery with Nonautologous Tissue Substitute, Open Approach
03160K8	Bypass Left Axillary Artery to Bilateral Upper Leg Artery with Nonautologous Tissue Substitute, Open Approach
03160K9	Bypass Left Axillary Artery to Right Lower Leg Artery with Nonautologous Tissue Substitute, Open Approach
03160KB	Bypass Left Axillary Artery to Left Lower Leg Artery with Nonautologous Tissue Substitute, Open Approach
03160KC	Bypass Left Axillary Artery to Bilateral Lower Leg Artery with Nonautologous Tissue Substitute, Open Approach
03160KD	Bypass Left Axillary Artery to Upper Arm Vein with Nonautologous Tissue Substitute, Open Approach
03160KF	Bypass Left Axillary Artery to Lower Arm Vein with Nonautologous Tissue Substitute, Open Approach
03160KJ	Bypass Left Axillary Artery to Right Extracranial Artery with Nonautologous Tissue Substitute, Open Approach
03160KK	Bypass Left Axillary Artery to Left Extracranial Artery with Nonautologous Tissue Substitute, Open Approach
03160Z0	Bypass Left Axillary Artery to Right Upper Arm Artery, Open Approach
03160Z1	Bypass Left Axillary Artery to Left Upper Arm Artery, Open Approach
03160Z2	Bypass Left Axillary Artery to Bilateral Upper Arm Artery, Open Approach
03160Z3	Bypass Left Axillary Artery to Right Lower Arm Artery, Open Approach
03160Z4	Bypass Left Axillary Artery to Left Lower Arm Artery, Open Approach
03160Z5	Bypass Left Axillary Artery to Bilateral Lower Arm Artery, Open Approach
03160Z6	Bypass Left Axillary Artery to Right Upper Leg Artery, Open Approach
03160Z7	Bypass Left Axillary Artery to Left Upper Leg Artery, Open Approach
03160Z8	Bypass Left Axillary Artery to Bilateral Upper Leg Artery, Open Approach
03160Z9	Bypass Left Axillary Artery to Right Lower Leg Artery, Open Approach
03160ZB	Bypass Left Axillary Artery to Left Lower Leg Artery, Open Approach

209

Female-only	♂ Male-only	▲ Limited Coverage	● Non-OR	▦ HAC-associated procedure	▲ Non-covered procedures	✛ Combination

03160ZC Bypass Left Axillary Artery to Bilateral Lower Leg Artery, Open Approach

03160ZD Bypass Left Axillary Artery to Upper Arm Vein, Open Approach

03160ZF Bypass Left Axillary Artery to Lower Arm Vein, Open Approach

03160ZJ Bypass Left Axillary Artery to Right Extracranial Artery, Open Approach

03160ZK Bypass Left Axillary Artery to Left Extracranial Artery, Open Approach

0317090 Bypass Right Brachial Artery to Right Upper Arm Artery with Autologous Venous Tissue, Open Approach

0317093 Bypass Right Brachial Artery to Right Lower Arm Artery with Autologous Venous Tissue, Open Approach

031709D Bypass Right Brachial Artery to Upper Arm Vein with Autologous Venous Tissue, Open Approach

031709F Bypass Right Brachial Artery to Lower Arm Vein with Autologous Venous Tissue, Open Approach

03170A0 Bypass Right Brachial Artery to Right Upper Arm Artery with Autologous Arterial Tissue, Open Approach

03170A3 Bypass Right Brachial Artery to Right Lower Arm Artery with Autologous Arterial Tissue, Open Approach

03170AD Bypass Right Brachial Artery to Upper Arm Vein with Autologous Arterial Tissue, Open Approach

03170AF Bypass Right Brachial Artery to Lower Arm Vein with Autologous Arterial Tissue, Open Approach

03170J0 Bypass Right Brachial Artery to Right Upper Arm Artery with Synthetic Substitute, Open Approach

03170J3 Bypass Right Brachial Artery to Right Lower Arm Artery with Synthetic Substitute, Open Approach

03170JD Bypass Right Brachial Artery to Upper Arm Vein with Synthetic Substitute, Open Approach

03170JF Bypass Right Brachial Artery to Lower Arm Vein with Synthetic Substitute, Open Approach

03170K0 Bypass Right Brachial Artery to Right Upper Arm Artery with Nonautologous Tissue Substitute, Open Approach

03170K3 Bypass Right Brachial Artery to Right Lower Arm Artery with Nonautologous Tissue Substitute, Open Approach

03170KD Bypass Right Brachial Artery to Upper Arm Vein with Nonautologous Tissue Substitute, Open Approach

03170KF Bypass Right Brachial Artery to Lower Arm Vein with Nonautologous Tissue Substitute, Open Approach

03170Z0 Bypass Right Brachial Artery to Right Upper Arm Artery, Open Approach

03170Z3 Bypass Right Brachial Artery to Right Lower Arm Artery, Open Approach

03170ZD Bypass Right Brachial Artery to Upper Arm Vein, Open Approach
AHA CC: 4Q, 2013, 125-126

03170ZF Bypass Right Brachial Artery to Lower Arm Vein, Open Approach

0318091 Bypass Left Brachial Artery to Left Upper Arm Artery with Autologous Venous Tissue, Open Approach

0318094 Bypass Left Brachial Artery to Left Lower Arm Artery with Autologous Venous Tissue, Open Approach

031809D Bypass Left Brachial Artery to Upper Arm Vein with Autologous Venous Tissue, Open Approach

031809F Bypass Left Brachial Artery to Lower Arm Vein with Autologous Venous Tissue, Open Approach

03180A1 Bypass Left Brachial Artery to Left Upper Arm Artery with Autologous Arterial Tissue, Open Approach

03180A4 Bypass Left Brachial Artery to Left Lower Arm Artery with Autologous Arterial Tissue, Open Approach

03180AD Bypass Left Brachial Artery to Upper Arm Vein with Autologous Arterial Tissue, Open Approach

03180AF Bypass Left Brachial Artery to Lower Arm Vein with Autologous Arterial Tissue, Open Approach

03180J1 Bypass Left Brachial Artery to Left Upper Arm Artery with Synthetic Substitute, Open Approach

03180J4 Bypass Left Brachial Artery to Left Lower Arm Artery with Synthetic Substitute, Open Approach

03180JD Bypass Left Brachial Artery to Upper Arm Vein with Synthetic Substitute, Open Approach

03180JF Bypass Left Brachial Artery to Lower Arm Vein with Synthetic Substitute, Open Approach

03180K1 Bypass Left Brachial Artery to Left Upper Arm Artery with Nonautologous Tissue Substitute, Open Approach

03180K4 Bypass Left Brachial Artery to Left Lower Arm Artery with Nonautologous Tissue Substitute, Open Approach

03180KD Bypass Left Brachial Artery to Upper Arm Vein with Nonautologous Tissue Substitute, Open Approach

03180KF Bypass Left Brachial Artery to Lower Arm Vein with Nonautologous Tissue Substitute, Open Approach

03180Z1 Bypass Left Brachial Artery to Left Upper Arm Artery, Open Approach

03180Z4 Bypass Left Brachial Artery to Left Lower Arm Artery, Open Approach

03180ZD Bypass Left Brachial Artery to Upper Arm Vein, Open Approach

03180ZF Bypass Left Brachial Artery to Lower Arm Vein, Open Approach

0319093 Bypass Right Ulnar Artery to Right Lower Arm Artery with Autologous Venous Tissue, Open Approach

031909F Bypass Right Ulnar Artery to Lower Arm Vein with Autologous Venous Tissue, Open Approach

03190A3 Bypass Right Ulnar Artery to Right Lower Arm Artery with Autologous Arterial Tissue, Open Approach

03190AF Bypass Right Ulnar Artery to Lower Arm Vein with Autologous Arterial Tissue, Open Approach

03190J3 Bypass Right Ulnar Artery to Right Lower Arm Artery with Synthetic Substitute, Open Approach

03190JF Bypass Right Ulnar Artery to Lower Arm Vein with Synthetic Substitute, Open Approach

03190K3 Bypass Right Ulnar Artery to Right Lower Arm Artery with Nonautologous Tissue Substitute, Open Approach

03190KF Bypass Right Ulnar Artery to Lower Arm Vein with Nonautologous Tissue Substitute, Open Approach

03190Z3 Bypass Right Ulnar Artery to Right Lower Arm Artery, Open Approach

03190ZF Bypass Right Ulnar Artery to Lower Arm Vein, Open Approach

031A094 Bypass Left Ulnar Artery to Left Lower Arm Artery with Autologous Venous Tissue, Open Approach

031A09F Bypass Left Ulnar Artery to Lower Arm Vein with Autologous Venous Tissue, Open Approach

031A0A4 Bypass Left Ulnar Artery to Left Lower Arm Artery with Autologous Arterial Tissue, Open Approach

031A0AF Bypass Left Ulnar Artery to Lower Arm Vein with Autologous Arterial Tissue, Open Approach

031A0J4 Bypass Left Ulnar Artery to Left Lower Arm Artery with Synthetic Substitute, Open Approach

031A0JF Bypass Left Ulnar Artery to Lower Arm Vein with Synthetic Substitute, Open Approach

031A0K4 Bypass Left Ulnar Artery to Left Lower Arm Artery with Nonautologous Tissue Substitute, Open Approach

031A0KF Bypass Left Ulnar Artery to Lower Arm Vein with Nonautologous Tissue Substitute, Open Approach

031A0Z4 Bypass Left Ulnar Artery to Left Lower Arm Artery, Open Approach

031A0ZF Bypass Left Ulnar Artery to Lower Arm Vein, Open Approach

031B093 Bypass Right Radial Artery to Right Lower Arm Artery with Autologous Venous Tissue, Open Approach

031B09F Bypass Right Radial Artery to Lower Arm Vein with Autologous Venous Tissue, Open Approach

031B0A3 Bypass Right Radial Artery to Right Lower Arm Artery with Autologous Arterial Tissue, Open Approach

031B0AF Bypass Right Radial Artery to Lower Arm Vein with Autologous Arterial Tissue, Open Approach

031B0J3 Bypass Right Radial Artery to Right Lower Arm Artery with Synthetic Substitute, Open Approach

031B0JF Bypass Right Radial Artery to Lower Arm Vein with Synthetic Substitute, Open Approach

031B0K3 Bypass Right Radial Artery to Right Lower Arm Artery with Nonautologous Tissue Substitute, Open Approach

031B0KF Bypass Right Radial Artery to Lower Arm Vein with Nonautologous Tissue Substitute, Open Approach

031B0Z3 Bypass Right Radial Artery to Right Lower Arm Artery, Open Approach

031B0ZF Bypass Right Radial Artery to Lower Arm Vein, Open Approach

031C094 Bypass Left Radial Artery to Left Lower Arm Artery with Autologous Venous Tissue, Open Approach

031C09F Bypass Left Radial Artery to Lower Arm Vein with Autologous Venous Tissue, Open Approach

031C0A4 Bypass Left Radial Artery to Left Lower Arm Artery with Autologous Arterial Tissue, Open Approach

031C0AF Bypass Left Radial Artery to Lower Arm Vein with Autologous Arterial Tissue, Open Approach

031C0J4 Bypass Left Radial Artery to Left Lower Arm Artery with Synthetic Substitute, Open Approach

031C0JF Bypass Left Radial Artery to Lower Arm Vein with Synthetic Substitute, Open Approach

031C0K4 Bypass Left Radial Artery to Left Lower Arm Artery with Nonautologous Tissue Substitute, Open Approach

031C0KF Bypass Left Radial Artery to Lower Arm Vein with Nonautologous Tissue Substitute, Open Approach

031C0Z4 Bypass Left Radial Artery to Left Lower Arm Artery, Open Approach

031C0ZF Bypass Left Radial Artery to Lower Arm Vein, Open Approach
AHA CC: 1Q, 2013, 27-28

031G09G Bypass Intracranial Artery to Intracranial Artery with Autologous Venous Tissue, Open Approach

031G0AG Bypass Intracranial Artery to Intracranial Artery with Autologous Arterial Tissue, Open Approach

031G0JG Bypass Intracranial Artery to Intracranial Artery with Synthetic Substitute, Open Approach

031G0KG Bypass Intracranial Artery to Intracranial Artery with Nonautologous Tissue Substitute, Open Approach

031G0ZG Bypass Intracranial Artery to Intracranial Artery, Open Approach

031H09G Bypass Right Common Carotid Artery to Intracranial Artery with Autologous Venous Tissue, Open Approach

031H09J Bypass Right Common Carotid Artery to Right Extracranial Artery with Autologous Venous Tissue, Open Approach

031H0AG Bypass Right Common Carotid Artery to Intracranial Artery with Autologous Arterial Tissue, Open Approach

031H0AJ Bypass Right Common Carotid Artery to Right Extracranial Artery with Autologous Arterial Tissue, Open Approach

031H0JG Bypass Right Common Carotid Artery to Intracranial Artery with Synthetic Substitute, Open Approach

031H0JJ Bypass Right Common Carotid Artery to Right Extracranial Artery with Synthetic Substitute, Open Approach

031H0KG Bypass Right Common Carotid Artery to Intracranial Artery with Nonautologous Tissue Substitute, Open Approach

031H0KJ Bypass Right Common Carotid Artery to Right Extracranial Artery with Nonautologous Tissue Substitute, Open Approach

031H0ZG Bypass Right Common Carotid Artery to Intracranial Artery, Open Approach

031H0ZJ Bypass Right Common Carotid Artery to Right Extracranial Artery, Open Approach

031J09G Bypass Left Common Carotid Artery to Intracranial Artery with Autologous Venous Tissue, Open Approach

031J09K Bypass Left Common Carotid Artery to Left Extracranial Artery with Autologous Venous Tissue, Open Approach

▲ 031J0AG Bypass Left Common Carotid Artery to Intracranial Artery with Autologous Arterial Tissue, Open Approach

031J0AK Bypass Left Common Carotid Artery to Left Extracranial Artery with Autologous Arterial Tissue, Open Approach

▲ 031J0JG Bypass Left Common Carotid Artery to Intracranial Artery with Synthetic Substitute, Open Approach

031J0JK Bypass Left Common Carotid Artery to Left Extracranial Artery with Synthetic Substitute, Open Approach

▲ 031J0KG Bypass Left Common Carotid Artery to Intracranial Artery with Nonautologous Tissue Substitute, Open Approach

031J0KK Bypass Left Common Carotid Artery to Left Extracranial Artery with Nonautologous Tissue Substitute, Open Approach

▲ 031J0ZG Bypass Left Common Carotid Artery to Intracranial Artery, Open Approach

031J0ZK Bypass Left Common Carotid Artery to Left Extracranial Artery, Open Approach

031K09J Bypass Right Internal Carotid Artery to Right Extracranial Artery with Autologous Venous Tissue, Open Approach

031K0AJ Bypass Right Internal Carotid Artery to Right Extracranial Artery with Autologous Arterial Tissue, Open Approach

031K0JJ Bypass Right Internal Carotid Artery to Right Extracranial Artery with Synthetic Substitute, Open Approach

031K0KJ Bypass Right Internal Carotid Artery to Right Extracranial Artery with Nonautologous Tissue Substitute, Open Approach

031K0ZJ Bypass Right Internal Carotid Artery to Right Extracranial Artery, Open Approach

031L09K Bypass Left Internal Carotid Artery to Left Extracranial Artery with Autologous Venous Tissue, Open Approach

031L0AK Bypass Left Internal Carotid Artery to Left Extracranial Artery with Autologous Arterial Tissue, Open Approach

031L0JK Bypass Left Internal Carotid Artery to Left Extracranial Artery with Synthetic Substitute, Open Approach

031L0KK Bypass Left Internal Carotid Artery to Left Extracranial Artery with Nonautologous Tissue Substitute, Open Approach

031L0ZK Bypass Left Internal Carotid Artery to Left Extracranial Artery, Open Approach

031M09J Bypass Right External Carotid Artery to Right Extracranial Artery with Autologous Venous Tissue, Open Approach

031M0AJ Bypass Right External Carotid Artery to Right Extracranial Artery with Autologous Arterial Tissue, Open Approach

031M0JJ Bypass Right External Carotid Artery to Right Extracranial Artery with Synthetic Substitute, Open Approach

031M0KJ Bypass Right External Carotid Artery to Right Extracranial Artery with Nonautologous Tissue Substitute, Open Approach

031M0ZJ Bypass Right External Carotid Artery to Right Extracranial Artery, Open Approach

031N09K Bypass Left External Carotid Artery to Left Extracranial Artery with Autologous Venous Tissue, Open Approach

031N0AK Bypass Left External Carotid Artery to Left Extracranial Artery with Autologous Arterial Tissue, Open Approach

031N0JK Bypass Left External Carotid Artery to Left Extracranial Artery with Synthetic Substitute, Open Approach

031N0KK Bypass Left External Carotid Artery to Left Extracranial Artery with Nonautologous Tissue Substitute, Open Approach

031N0ZK Bypass Left External Carotid Artery to Left Extracranial Artery, Open Approach

▲ 031S09G Bypass Right Temporal Artery to Intracranial Artery with Autologous Venous Tissue, Open Approach

▲ 031S0AG Bypass Right Temporal Artery to Intracranial Artery with Autologous Arterial Tissue, Open Approach

▲ 031S0JG Bypass Right Temporal Artery to Intracranial Artery with Synthetic Substitute, Open Approach

▲ 031S0KG Bypass Right Temporal Artery to Intracranial Artery with Nonautologous Tissue Substitute, Open Approach

▲ 031S0ZG Bypass Right Temporal Artery to Intracranial Artery, Open Approach

▲ 031T09G Bypass Left Temporal Artery to Intracranial Artery with Autologous Venous Tissue, Open Approach

▲ 031T0AG Bypass Left Temporal Artery to Intracranial Artery with Autologous Arterial Tissue, Open Approach

▲ 031T0JG Bypass Left Temporal Artery to Intracranial Artery with Synthetic Substitute, Open Approach

▲ 031T0KG Bypass Left Temporal Artery to Intracranial Artery with Nonautologous Tissue Substitute, Open Approach

▲ 031T0ZG Bypass Left Temporal Artery to Intracranial Artery, Open Approach

035 – Upper Arteries, Destruction

0350ZZ Destruction of Right Internal Mammary Artery, Open Approach

03503ZZ Destruction of Right Internal Mammary Artery, Percutaneous Approach

03504ZZ Destruction of Right Internal Mammary Artery, Percutaneous Endoscopic Approach

03510ZZ Destruction of Left Internal Mammary Artery, Open Approach

03513ZZ Destruction of Left Internal Mammary Artery, Percutaneous Approach

03514ZZ Destruction of Left Internal Mammary Artery, Percutaneous Endoscopic Approach

03520ZZ Destruction of Innominate Artery, Open Approach

03523ZZ Destruction of Innominate Artery, Percutaneous Approach

03524ZZ Destruction of Innominate Artery, Percutaneous Endoscopic Approach

03530ZZ Destruction of Right Subclavian Artery, Open Approach

03533ZZ Destruction of Right Subclavian Artery, Percutaneous Approach

03534ZZ Destruction of Right Subclavian Artery, Percutaneous Endoscopic Approach

03540ZZ Destruction of Left Subclavian Artery, Open Approach

03543ZZ Destruction of Left Subclavian Artery, Percutaneous Approach

03544ZZ Destruction of Left Subclavian Artery, Percutaneous Endoscopic Approach

♀ Female-only   ♂ Male-only   ▲ Limited Coverage   ● Non-OR   ■ HAC-associated procedure   ▲ Non-covered procedures   ✚ Combination

03550ZZ Destruction of Right Axillary Artery, Open Approach
03553ZZ Destruction of Right Axillary Artery, Percutaneous Approach
03554ZZ Destruction of Right Axillary Artery, Percutaneous Endoscopic Approach
03560ZZ Destruction of Left Axillary Artery, Open Approach
03563ZZ Destruction of Left Axillary Artery, Percutaneous Approach
03564ZZ Destruction of Left Axillary Artery, Percutaneous Endoscopic Approach
03570ZZ Destruction of Right Brachial Artery, Open Approach
03573ZZ Destruction of Right Brachial Artery, Percutaneous Approach
03574ZZ Destruction of Right Brachial Artery, Percutaneous Endoscopic Approach
03580ZZ Destruction of Left Brachial Artery, Open Approach
03583ZZ Destruction of Left Brachial Artery, Percutaneous Approach
03584ZZ Destruction of Left Brachial Artery, Percutaneous Endoscopic Approach
03590ZZ Destruction of Right Ulnar Artery, Open Approach
03593ZZ Destruction of Right Ulnar Artery, Percutaneous Approach
03594ZZ Destruction of Right Ulnar Artery, Percutaneous Endoscopic Approach
035A0ZZ Destruction of Left Ulnar Artery, Open Approach
035A3ZZ Destruction of Left Ulnar Artery, Percutaneous Approach
035A4ZZ Destruction of Left Ulnar Artery, Percutaneous Endoscopic Approach
035B0ZZ Destruction of Right Radial Artery, Open Approach
035B3ZZ Destruction of Right Radial Artery, Percutaneous Approach
035B4ZZ Destruction of Right Radial Artery, Percutaneous Endoscopic Approach
035C0ZZ Destruction of Left Radial Artery, Open Approach
035C3ZZ Destruction of Left Radial Artery, Percutaneous Approach
035C4ZZ Destruction of Left Radial Artery, Percutaneous Endoscopic Approach
035D0ZZ Destruction of Right Hand Artery, Open Approach

035D3ZZ Destruction of Right Hand Artery, Percutaneous Approach
035D4ZZ Destruction of Right Hand Artery, Percutaneous Endoscopic Approach
035F0ZZ Destruction of Left Hand Artery, Open Approach
035F3ZZ Destruction of Left Hand Artery, Percutaneous Approach
035F4ZZ Destruction of Left Hand Artery, Percutaneous Endoscopic Approach
035G0ZZ Destruction of Intracranial Artery, Open Approach
035G3ZZ Destruction of Intracranial Artery, Percutaneous Approach
035G4ZZ Destruction of Intracranial Artery, Percutaneous Endoscopic Approach
035H0ZZ Destruction of Right Common Carotid Artery, Open Approach
035H3ZZ Destruction of Right Common Carotid Artery, Percutaneous Approach
035H4ZZ Destruction of Right Common Carotid Artery, Percutaneous Endoscopic Approach
035J0ZZ Destruction of Left Common Carotid Artery, Open Approach
035J3ZZ Destruction of Left Common Carotid Artery, Percutaneous Approach
035J4ZZ Destruction of Left Common Carotid Artery, Percutaneous Endoscopic Approach
035K0ZZ Destruction of Right Internal Carotid Artery, Open Approach
035K3ZZ Destruction of Right Internal Carotid Artery, Percutaneous Approach
035K4ZZ Destruction of Right Internal Carotid Artery, Percutaneous Endoscopic Approach
035L0ZZ Destruction of Left Internal Carotid Artery, Open Approach
035L3ZZ Destruction of Left Internal Carotid Artery, Percutaneous Approach
035L4ZZ Destruction of Left Internal Carotid Artery, Percutaneous Endoscopic Approach
035M0ZZ Destruction of Right External Carotid Artery, Open Approach
035M3ZZ Destruction of Right External Carotid Artery, Percutaneous Approach
035M4ZZ Destruction of Right External Carotid Artery, Percutaneous Endoscopic Approach
035N0ZZ Destruction of Left External Carotid Artery, Open Approach
035N3ZZ Destruction of Left External Carotid Artery, Percutaneous Approach

035N4ZZ Destruction of Left External Carotid Artery, Percutaneous Endoscopic Approach
035P0ZZ Destruction of Right Vertebral Artery, Open Approach
035P3ZZ Destruction of Right Vertebral Artery, Percutaneous Approach
035P4ZZ Destruction of Right Vertebral Artery, Percutaneous Endoscopic Approach
035Q0ZZ Destruction of Left Vertebral Artery, Open Approach
035Q3ZZ Destruction of Left Vertebral Artery, Percutaneous Approach
035Q4ZZ Destruction of Left Vertebral Artery, Percutaneous Endoscopic Approach
035R0ZZ Destruction of Face Artery, Open Approach
035R3ZZ Destruction of Face Artery, Percutaneous Approach
035R4ZZ Destruction of Face Artery, Percutaneous Endoscopic Approach
035S0ZZ Destruction of Right Temporal Artery, Open Approach
035S3ZZ Destruction of Right Temporal Artery, Percutaneous Approach
035S4ZZ Destruction of Right Temporal Artery, Percutaneous Endoscopic Approach
035T0ZZ Destruction of Left Temporal Artery, Open Approach
035T3ZZ Destruction of Left Temporal Artery, Percutaneous Approach
035T4ZZ Destruction of Left Temporal Artery, Percutaneous Endoscopic Approach
035U0ZZ Destruction of Right Thyroid Artery, Open Approach
035U3ZZ Destruction of Right Thyroid Artery, Percutaneous Approach
035U4ZZ Destruction of Right Thyroid Artery, Percutaneous Endoscopic Approach
035V0ZZ Destruction of Left Thyroid Artery, Open Approach
035V3ZZ Destruction of Left Thyroid Artery, Percutaneous Approach
035V4ZZ Destruction of Left Thyroid Artery, Percutaneous Endoscopic Approach
035Y0ZZ Destruction of Upper Artery, Open Approach
035Y3ZZ Destruction of Upper Artery, Percutaneous Approach
035Y4ZZ Destruction of Upper Artery, Percutaneous Endoscopic Approach

037 – Upper Arteries, Dilation

037004Z Dilation of Right Internal Mammary Artery with Drug-eluting Intraluminal Device, Open Approach
03700DZ Dilation of Right Internal Mammary Artery with Intraluminal Device, Open Approach
03700ZZ Dilation of Right Internal Mammary Artery, Open Approach
037034Z Dilation of Right Internal Mammary Artery with Drug-eluting Intraluminal Device, Percutaneous Approach
03703DZ Dilation of Right Internal Mammary Artery with Intraluminal Device, Percutaneous Approach
03703ZZ Dilation of Right Internal Mammary Artery, Percutaneous Approach
037044Z Dilation of Right Internal Mammary Artery with Drug-eluting Intraluminal Device, Percutaneous Endoscopic Approach

03704DZ Dilation of Right Internal Mammary Artery with Intraluminal Device, Percutaneous Endoscopic Approach
03704ZZ Dilation of Right Internal Mammary Artery, Percutaneous Endoscopic Approach
037104Z Dilation of Left Internal Mammary Artery with Drug-eluting Intraluminal Device, Open Approach
03710DZ Dilation of Left Internal Mammary Artery with Intraluminal Device, Open Approach
03710ZZ Dilation of Left Internal Mammary Artery, Open Approach
037134Z Dilation of Left Internal Mammary Artery with Drug-eluting Intraluminal Device, Percutaneous Approach
03713DZ Dilation of Left Internal Mammary Artery with Intraluminal Device, Percutaneous Approach

03713ZZ Dilation of Left Internal Mammary Artery, Percutaneous Approach
037144Z Dilation of Left Internal Mammary Artery with Drug-eluting Intraluminal Device, Percutaneous Endoscopic Approach
03714DZ Dilation of Left Internal Mammary Artery with Intraluminal Device, Percutaneous Endoscopic Approach
03714ZZ Dilation of Left Internal Mammary Artery, Percutaneous Endoscopic Approach
037204Z Dilation of Innominate Artery with Drug-eluting Intraluminal Device, Open Approach
03720DZ Dilation of Innominate Artery with Intraluminal Device, Open Approach
03720ZZ Dilation of Innominate Artery, Open Approach
037234Z Dilation of Innominate Artery with Drug-eluting Intraluminal Device, Percutaneous Approach

3723DZ Dilation of Innominate Artery with Intraluminal Device, Percutaneous Approach

3723ZZ Dilation of Innominate Artery, Percutaneous Approach

37244Z Dilation of Innominate Artery with Drug-eluting Intraluminal Device, Percutaneous Endoscopic Approach

3724DZ Dilation of Innominate Artery with Intraluminal Device, Percutaneous Endoscopic Approach

3724ZZ Dilation of Innominate Artery, Percutaneous Endoscopic Approach

37304Z Dilation of Right Subclavian Artery with Drug-eluting Intraluminal Device, Open Approach

3730DZ Dilation of Right Subclavian Artery with Intraluminal Device, Open Approach

3730ZZ Dilation of Right Subclavian Artery, Open Approach

37334Z Dilation of Right Subclavian Artery with Drug-eluting Intraluminal Device, Percutaneous Approach

3733DZ Dilation of Right Subclavian Artery with Intraluminal Device, Percutaneous Approach

3733ZZ Dilation of Right Subclavian Artery, Percutaneous Approach

37344Z Dilation of Right Subclavian Artery with Drug-eluting Intraluminal Device, Percutaneous Endoscopic Approach

3734DZ Dilation of Right Subclavian Artery with Intraluminal Device, Percutaneous Endoscopic Approach

3734ZZ Dilation of Right Subclavian Artery, Percutaneous Endoscopic Approach

37404Z Dilation of Left Subclavian Artery with Drug-eluting Intraluminal Device, Open Approach

3740DZ Dilation of Left Subclavian Artery with Intraluminal Device, Open Approach

3740ZZ Dilation of Left Subclavian Artery, Open Approach

37434Z Dilation of Left Subclavian Artery with Drug-eluting Intraluminal Device, Percutaneous Approach

3743DZ Dilation of Left Subclavian Artery with Intraluminal Device, Percutaneous Approach

3743ZZ Dilation of Left Subclavian Artery, Percutaneous Approach

37444Z Dilation of Left Subclavian Artery with Drug-eluting Intraluminal Device, Percutaneous Endoscopic Approach

3744DZ Dilation of Left Subclavian Artery with Intraluminal Device, Percutaneous Endoscopic Approach

3744ZZ Dilation of Left Subclavian Artery, Percutaneous Endoscopic Approach

37504Z Dilation of Right Axillary Artery with Drug-eluting Intraluminal Device, Open Approach

3750DZ Dilation of Right Axillary Artery with Intraluminal Device, Open Approach

3750ZZ Dilation of Right Axillary Artery, Open Approach

37534Z Dilation of Right Axillary Artery with Drug-eluting Intraluminal Device, Percutaneous Approach

3753DZ Dilation of Right Axillary Artery with Intraluminal Device, Percutaneous Approach

3753ZZ Dilation of Right Axillary Artery, Percutaneous Approach

37544Z Dilation of Right Axillary Artery with Drug-eluting Intraluminal Device, Percutaneous Endoscopic Approach

03754DZ Dilation of Right Axillary Artery with Intraluminal Device, Percutaneous Endoscopic Approach

03754ZZ Dilation of Right Axillary Artery, Percutaneous Endoscopic Approach

037604Z Dilation of Left Axillary Artery with Drug-eluting Intraluminal Device, Open Approach

03760DZ Dilation of Left Axillary Artery with Intraluminal Device, Open Approach

03760ZZ Dilation of Left Axillary Artery, Open Approach

037634Z Dilation of Left Axillary Artery with Drug-eluting Intraluminal Device, Percutaneous Approach

03763DZ Dilation of Left Axillary Artery with Intraluminal Device, Percutaneous Approach

03763ZZ Dilation of Left Axillary Artery, Percutaneous Approach

037644Z Dilation of Left Axillary Artery with Drug-eluting Intraluminal Device, Percutaneous Endoscopic Approach

03764DZ Dilation of Left Axillary Artery with Intraluminal Device, Percutaneous Endoscopic Approach

03764ZZ Dilation of Left Axillary Artery, Percutaneous Endoscopic Approach

037704Z Dilation of Right Brachial Artery with Drug-eluting Intraluminal Device, Open Approach

03770DZ Dilation of Right Brachial Artery with Intraluminal Device, Open Approach

03770ZZ Dilation of Right Brachial Artery, Open Approach

037734Z Dilation of Right Brachial Artery with Drug-eluting Intraluminal Device, Percutaneous Approach

03773DZ Dilation of Right Brachial Artery with Intraluminal Device, Percutaneous Approach

03773ZZ Dilation of Right Brachial Artery, Percutaneous Approach

037744Z Dilation of Right Brachial Artery with Drug-eluting Intraluminal Device, Percutaneous Endoscopic Approach

03774DZ Dilation of Right Brachial Artery with Intraluminal Device, Percutaneous Endoscopic Approach

03774ZZ Dilation of Right Brachial Artery, Percutaneous Endoscopic Approach

037804Z Dilation of Left Brachial Artery with Drug-eluting Intraluminal Device, Open Approach

03780DZ Dilation of Left Brachial Artery with Intraluminal Device, Open Approach

03780ZZ Dilation of Left Brachial Artery, Open Approach

037834Z Dilation of Left Brachial Artery with Drug-eluting Intraluminal Device, Percutaneous Approach

03783DZ Dilation of Left Brachial Artery with Intraluminal Device, Percutaneous Approach

03783ZZ Dilation of Left Brachial Artery, Percutaneous Approach

037844Z Dilation of Left Brachial Artery with Drug-eluting Intraluminal Device, Percutaneous Endoscopic Approach

03784DZ Dilation of Left Brachial Artery with Intraluminal Device, Percutaneous Endoscopic Approach

03784ZZ Dilation of Left Brachial Artery, Percutaneous Endoscopic Approach

037904Z Dilation of Right Ulnar Artery with Drug-eluting Intraluminal Device, Open Approach

03790DZ Dilation of Right Ulnar Artery with Intraluminal Device, Open Approach

03790ZZ Dilation of Right Ulnar Artery, Open Approach

037934Z Dilation of Right Ulnar Artery with Drug-eluting Intraluminal Device, Percutaneous Approach

03793DZ Dilation of Right Ulnar Artery with Intraluminal Device, Percutaneous Approach

03793ZZ Dilation of Right Ulnar Artery, Percutaneous Approach

037944Z Dilation of Right Ulnar Artery with Drug-eluting Intraluminal Device, Percutaneous Endoscopic Approach

03794DZ Dilation of Right Ulnar Artery with Intraluminal Device, Percutaneous Endoscopic Approach

03794ZZ Dilation of Right Ulnar Artery, Percutaneous Endoscopic Approach

037A04Z Dilation of Left Ulnar Artery with Drug-eluting Intraluminal Device, Open Approach

037A0DZ Dilation of Left Ulnar Artery with Intraluminal Device, Open Approach

037A0ZZ Dilation of Left Ulnar Artery, Open Approach

037A34Z Dilation of Left Ulnar Artery with Drug-eluting Intraluminal Device, Percutaneous Approach

037A3DZ Dilation of Left Ulnar Artery with Intraluminal Device, Percutaneous Approach

037A3ZZ Dilation of Left Ulnar Artery, Percutaneous Approach

037A44Z Dilation of Left Ulnar Artery with Drug-eluting Intraluminal Device, Percutaneous Endoscopic Approach

037A4DZ Dilation of Left Ulnar Artery with Intraluminal Device, Percutaneous Endoscopic Approach

037A4ZZ Dilation of Left Ulnar Artery, Percutaneous Endoscopic Approach

037B04Z Dilation of Right Radial Artery with Drug-eluting Intraluminal Device, Open Approach

037B0DZ Dilation of Right Radial Artery with Intraluminal Device, Open Approach

037B0ZZ Dilation of Right Radial Artery, Open Approach

037B34Z Dilation of Right Radial Artery with Drug-eluting Intraluminal Device, Percutaneous Approach

037B3DZ Dilation of Right Radial Artery with Intraluminal Device, Percutaneous Approach

037B3ZZ Dilation of Right Radial Artery, Percutaneous Approach

037B44Z Dilation of Right Radial Artery with Drug-eluting Intraluminal Device, Percutaneous Endoscopic Approach

037B4DZ Dilation of Right Radial Artery with Intraluminal Device, Percutaneous Endoscopic Approach

037B4ZZ Dilation of Right Radial Artery, Percutaneous Endoscopic Approach

037C04Z Dilation of Left Radial Artery with Drug-eluting Intraluminal Device, Open Approach

037C0DZ Dilation of Left Radial Artery with Intraluminal Device, Open Approach

037C0ZZ Dilation of Left Radial Artery, Open Approach

037C34Z Dilation of Left Radial Artery with Drug-eluting Intraluminal Device, Percutaneous Approach

♀ Female-only   ♂ Male-only   ▲ Limited Coverage   ● Non-OR   ▬ HAC-associated procedure   ▲ Non-covered procedures   ✚ Combination

037C3DZ Dilation of Left Radial Artery with Intraluminal Device, Percutaneous Approach

037C3ZZ Dilation of Left Radial Artery, Percutaneous Approach

037C44Z Dilation of Left Radial Artery with Drug-eluting Intraluminal Device, Percutaneous Endoscopic Approach

037C4DZ Dilation of Left Radial Artery with Intraluminal Device, Percutaneous Endoscopic Approach

037C4ZZ Dilation of Left Radial Artery, Percutaneous Endoscopic Approach

037D04Z Dilation of Right Hand Artery with Drug-eluting Intraluminal Device, Open Approach

037D0DZ Dilation of Right Hand Artery with Intraluminal Device, Open Approach

037D0ZZ Dilation of Right Hand Artery, Open Approach

037D34Z Dilation of Right Hand Artery with Drug-eluting Intraluminal Device, Percutaneous Approach

037D3DZ Dilation of Right Hand Artery with Intraluminal Device, Percutaneous Approach

037D3ZZ Dilation of Right Hand Artery, Percutaneous Approach

037D44Z Dilation of Right Hand Artery with Drug-eluting Intraluminal Device, Percutaneous Endoscopic Approach

037D4DZ Dilation of Right Hand Artery with Intraluminal Device, Percutaneous Endoscopic Approach

037D4ZZ Dilation of Right Hand Artery, Percutaneous Endoscopic Approach

037F04Z Dilation of Left Hand Artery with Drug-eluting Intraluminal Device, Open Approach

037F0DZ Dilation of Left Hand Artery with Intraluminal Device, Open Approach

037F0ZZ Dilation of Left Hand Artery, Open Approach

037F34Z Dilation of Left Hand Artery with Drug-eluting Intraluminal Device, Percutaneous Approach

037F3DZ Dilation of Left Hand Artery with Intraluminal Device, Percutaneous Approach

037F3ZZ Dilation of Left Hand Artery, Percutaneous Approach

037F44Z Dilation of Left Hand Artery with Drug-eluting Intraluminal Device, Percutaneous Endoscopic Approach

037F4DZ Dilation of Left Hand Artery with Intraluminal Device, Percutaneous Endoscopic Approach

037F4ZZ Dilation of Left Hand Artery, Percutaneous Endoscopic Approach

037G04Z Dilation of Intracranial Artery with Drug-eluting Intraluminal Device, Open Approach

037G0DZ Dilation of Intracranial Artery with Intraluminal Device, Open Approach

037G0ZZ Dilation of Intracranial Artery, Open Approach

037G34Z Dilation of Intracranial Artery with Drug-eluting Intraluminal Device, Percutaneous Approach

037G3DZ Dilation of Intracranial Artery with Intraluminal Device, Percutaneous Approach

▲ **037G3ZZ** Dilation of Intracranial Artery, Percutaneous Approach

037G44Z Dilation of Intracranial Artery with Drug-eluting Intraluminal Device, Percutaneous Endoscopic Approach

037G4DZ Dilation of Intracranial Artery with Intraluminal Device, Percutaneous Endoscopic Approach

▲ **037G4ZZ** Dilation of Intracranial Artery, Percutaneous Endoscopic Approach

037H04Z Dilation of Right Common Carotid Artery with Drug-eluting Intraluminal Device, Open Approach

037H0DZ Dilation of Right Common Carotid Artery with Intraluminal Device, Open Approach

037H0ZZ Dilation of Right Common Carotid Artery, Open Approach

037H34Z Dilation of Right Common Carotid Artery with Drug-eluting Intraluminal Device, Percutaneous Approach

037H3DZ Dilation of Right Common Carotid Artery with Intraluminal Device, Percutaneous Approach

037H3ZZ Dilation of Right Common Carotid Artery, Percutaneous Approach

037H44Z Dilation of Right Common Carotid Artery with Drug-eluting Intraluminal Device, Percutaneous Endoscopic Approach

037H4DZ Dilation of Right Common Carotid Artery with Intraluminal Device, Percutaneous Endoscopic Approach

037H4ZZ Dilation of Right Common Carotid Artery, Percutaneous Endoscopic Approach

037J04Z Dilation of Left Common Carotid Artery with Drug-eluting Intraluminal Device, Open Approach

037J0DZ Dilation of Left Common Carotid Artery with Intraluminal Device, Open Approach

037J0ZZ Dilation of Left Common Carotid Artery, Open Approach

037J34Z Dilation of Left Common Carotid Artery with Drug-eluting Intraluminal Device, Percutaneous Approach

037J3DZ Dilation of Left Common Carotid Artery with Intraluminal Device, Percutaneous Approach

037J3ZZ Dilation of Left Common Carotid Artery, Percutaneous Approach

037J44Z Dilation of Left Common Carotid Artery with Drug-eluting Intraluminal Device, Percutaneous Endoscopic Approach

037J4DZ Dilation of Left Common Carotid Artery with Intraluminal Device, Percutaneous Endoscopic Approach

037J4ZZ Dilation of Left Common Carotid Artery, Percutaneous Endoscopic Approach

037K04Z Dilation of Right Internal Carotid Artery with Drug-eluting Intraluminal Device, Open Approach

037K0DZ Dilation of Right Internal Carotid Artery with Intraluminal Device, Open Approach

037K0ZZ Dilation of Right Internal Carotid Artery, Open Approach

037K34Z Dilation of Right Internal Carotid Artery with Drug-eluting Intraluminal Device, Percutaneous Approach

037K3DZ Dilation of Right Internal Carotid Artery with Intraluminal Device, Percutaneous Approach

037K3ZZ Dilation of Right Internal Carotid Artery, Percutaneous Approach

037K44Z Dilation of Right Internal Carotid Artery with Drug-eluting Intraluminal Device, Percutaneous Endoscopic Approach

037K4DZ Dilation of Right Internal Carotid Artery with Intraluminal Device, Percutaneous Endoscopic Approach

037K4ZZ Dilation of Right Internal Carotid Artery, Percutaneous Endoscopic Approach

037L04Z Dilation of Left Internal Carotid Artery with Drug-eluting Intraluminal Device, Open Approach

037L0DZ Dilation of Left Internal Carotid Artery with Intraluminal Device, Open Approach

037L0ZZ Dilation of Left Internal Carotid Artery, Open Approach

037L34Z Dilation of Left Internal Carotid Artery with Drug-eluting Intraluminal Device, Percutaneous Approach

037L3DZ Dilation of Left Internal Carotid Artery with Intraluminal Device, Percutaneous Approach

037L3ZZ Dilation of Left Internal Carotid Artery, Percutaneous Approach

037L44Z Dilation of Left Internal Carotid Artery with Drug-eluting Intraluminal Device, Percutaneous Endoscopic Approach

037L4DZ Dilation of Left Internal Carotid Artery with Intraluminal Device, Percutaneous Endoscopic Approach

037L4ZZ Dilation of Left Internal Carotid Artery, Percutaneous Endoscopic Approach

037M04Z Dilation of Right External Carotid Artery with Drug-eluting Intraluminal Device, Open Approach

037M0DZ Dilation of Right External Carotid Artery with Intraluminal Device, Open Approach

037M0ZZ Dilation of Right External Carotid Artery, Open Approach

037M34Z Dilation of Right External Carotid Artery with Drug-eluting Intraluminal Device, Percutaneous Approach

037M3DZ Dilation of Right External Carotid Artery with Intraluminal Device, Percutaneous Approach

037M3ZZ Dilation of Right External Carotid Artery, Percutaneous Approach

037M44Z Dilation of Right External Carotid Artery with Drug-eluting Intraluminal Device, Percutaneous Endoscopic Approach

037M4DZ Dilation of Right External Carotid Artery with Intraluminal Device, Percutaneous Endoscopic Approach

037M4ZZ Dilation of Right External Carotid Artery, Percutaneous Endoscopic Approach

037N04Z Dilation of Left External Carotid Artery with Drug-eluting Intraluminal Device, Open Approach

037N0DZ Dilation of Left External Carotid Artery with Intraluminal Device, Open Approach

037N0ZZ Dilation of Left External Carotid Artery, Open Approach

037N34Z Dilation of Left External Carotid Artery with Drug-eluting Intraluminal Device, Percutaneous Approach

037N3DZ Dilation of Left External Carotid Artery with Intraluminal Device, Percutaneous Approach

037N3ZZ Dilation of Left External Carotid Artery, Percutaneous Approach

037N44Z Dilation of Left External Carotid Artery with Drug-eluting Intraluminal Device, Percutaneous Endoscopic Approach

037N4DZ Dilation of Left External Carotid Artery with Intraluminal Device, Percutaneous Endoscopic Approach

037N4ZZ Dilation of Left External Carotid Artery, Percutaneous Endoscopic Approach

037P04Z Dilation of Right Vertebral Artery with Drug-eluting Intraluminal Device, Open Approach

037P0DZ Dilation of Right Vertebral Artery with Intraluminal Device, Open Approach

037P0ZZ Dilation of Right Vertebral Artery, Open Approach

037P34Z Dilation of Right Vertebral Artery with Drug-eluting Intraluminal Device, Percutaneous Approach

7P3DZ	Dilation of Right Vertebral Artery with Intraluminal Device, Percutaneous Approach
7P3ZZ	Dilation of Right Vertebral Artery, Percutaneous Approach
7P44Z	Dilation of Right Vertebral Artery with Drug-eluting Intraluminal Device, Percutaneous Endoscopic Approach
7P4DZ	Dilation of Right Vertebral Artery with Intraluminal Device, Percutaneous Endoscopic Approach
7P4ZZ	Dilation of Right Vertebral Artery, Percutaneous Endoscopic Approach
7Q04Z	Dilation of Left Vertebral Artery with Drug-eluting Intraluminal Device, Open Approach
7Q0DZ	Dilation of Left Vertebral Artery with Intraluminal Device, Open Approach
7Q0ZZ	Dilation of Left Vertebral Artery, Open Approach
7Q34Z	Dilation of Left Vertebral Artery with Drug-eluting Intraluminal Device, Percutaneous Approach
7Q3DZ	Dilation of Left Vertebral Artery with Intraluminal Device, Percutaneous Approach
7Q3ZZ	Dilation of Left Vertebral Artery, Percutaneous Approach
7Q44Z	Dilation of Left Vertebral Artery with Drug-eluting Intraluminal Device, Percutaneous Endoscopic Approach
7Q4DZ	Dilation of Left Vertebral Artery with Intraluminal Device, Percutaneous Endoscopic Approach
7Q4ZZ	Dilation of Left Vertebral Artery, Percutaneous Endoscopic Approach
37R04Z	Dilation of Face Artery with Drug-eluting Intraluminal Device, Open Approach
37R0DZ	Dilation of Face Artery with Intraluminal Device, Open Approach
37R0ZZ	Dilation of Face Artery, Open Approach
37R34Z	Dilation of Face Artery with Drug-eluting Intraluminal Device, Percutaneous Approach
37R3DZ	Dilation of Face Artery with Intraluminal Device, Percutaneous Approach
37R3ZZ	Dilation of Face Artery, Percutaneous Approach
37R44Z	Dilation of Face Artery with Drug-eluting Intraluminal Device, Percutaneous Endoscopic Approach
37R4DZ	Dilation of Face Artery with Intraluminal Device, Percutaneous Endoscopic Approach
37R4ZZ	Dilation of Face Artery, Percutaneous Endoscopic Approach

037S04Z	Dilation of Right Temporal Artery with Drug-eluting Intraluminal Device, Open Approach
037S0DZ	Dilation of Right Temporal Artery with Intraluminal Device, Open Approach
037S0ZZ	Dilation of Right Temporal Artery, Open Approach
037S34Z	Dilation of Right Temporal Artery with Drug-eluting Intraluminal Device, Percutaneous Approach
037S3DZ	Dilation of Right Temporal Artery with Intraluminal Device, Percutaneous Approach
037S3ZZ	Dilation of Right Temporal Artery, Percutaneous Approach
037S44Z	Dilation of Right Temporal Artery with Drug-eluting Intraluminal Device, Percutaneous Endoscopic Approach
037S4DZ	Dilation of Right Temporal Artery with Intraluminal Device, Percutaneous Endoscopic Approach
037S4ZZ	Dilation of Right Temporal Artery, Percutaneous Endoscopic Approach
037T04Z	Dilation of Left Temporal Artery with Drug-eluting Intraluminal Device, Open Approach
037T0DZ	Dilation of Left Temporal Artery with Intraluminal Device, Open Approach
037T0ZZ	Dilation of Left Temporal Artery, Open Approach
037T34Z	Dilation of Left Temporal Artery with Drug-eluting Intraluminal Device, Percutaneous Approach
037T3DZ	Dilation of Left Temporal Artery with Intraluminal Device, Percutaneous Approach
037T3ZZ	Dilation of Left Temporal Artery, Percutaneous Approach
037T44Z	Dilation of Left Temporal Artery with Drug-eluting Intraluminal Device, Percutaneous Endoscopic Approach
037T4DZ	Dilation of Left Temporal Artery with Intraluminal Device, Percutaneous Endoscopic Approach
037T4ZZ	Dilation of Left Temporal Artery, Percutaneous Endoscopic Approach
037U04Z	Dilation of Right Thyroid Artery with Drug-eluting Intraluminal Device, Open Approach
037U0DZ	Dilation of Right Thyroid Artery with Intraluminal Device, Open Approach
037U0ZZ	Dilation of Right Thyroid Artery, Open Approach
037U34Z	Dilation of Right Thyroid Artery with Drug-eluting Intraluminal Device, Percutaneous Approach

037U3DZ	Dilation of Right Thyroid Artery with Intraluminal Device, Percutaneous Approach
037U3ZZ	Dilation of Right Thyroid Artery, Percutaneous Approach
037U44Z	Dilation of Right Thyroid Artery with Drug-eluting Intraluminal Device, Percutaneous Endoscopic Approach
037U4DZ	Dilation of Right Thyroid Artery with Intraluminal Device, Percutaneous Endoscopic Approach
037U4ZZ	Dilation of Right Thyroid Artery, Percutaneous Endoscopic Approach
037V04Z	Dilation of Left Thyroid Artery with Drug-eluting Intraluminal Device, Open Approach
037V0DZ	Dilation of Left Thyroid Artery with Intraluminal Device, Open Approach
037V0ZZ	Dilation of Left Thyroid Artery, Open Approach
037V34Z	Dilation of Left Thyroid Artery with Drug-eluting Intraluminal Device, Percutaneous Approach
037V3DZ	Dilation of Left Thyroid Artery with Intraluminal Device, Percutaneous Approach
037V3ZZ	Dilation of Left Thyroid Artery, Percutaneous Approach
037V44Z	Dilation of Left Thyroid Artery with Drug-eluting Intraluminal Device, Percutaneous Endoscopic Approach
037V4DZ	Dilation of Left Thyroid Artery with Intraluminal Device, Percutaneous Endoscopic Approach
037V4ZZ	Dilation of Left Thyroid Artery, Percutaneous Endoscopic Approach
037Y04Z	Dilation of Upper Artery with Drug-eluting Intraluminal Device, Open Approach
037Y0DZ	Dilation of Upper Artery with Intraluminal Device, Open Approach
037Y0ZZ	Dilation of Upper Artery, Open Approach
037Y34Z	Dilation of Upper Artery with Drug-eluting Intraluminal Device, Percutaneous Approach
037Y3DZ	Dilation of Upper Artery with Intraluminal Device, Percutaneous Approach
037Y3ZZ	Dilation of Upper Artery, Percutaneous Approach
037Y44Z	Dilation of Upper Artery with Drug-eluting Intraluminal Device, Percutaneous Endoscopic Approach
037Y4DZ	Dilation of Upper Artery with Intraluminal Device, Percutaneous Endoscopic Approach
037Y4ZZ	Dilation of Upper Artery, Percutaneous Endoscopic Approach

39 – Upper Arteries, Drainage

Review Coding Guidelines B3.4a and B3.4b

Review Coding Guideline B6.2

39000Z	Drainage of Right Internal Mammary Artery with Drainage Device, Open Approach
3900ZX	Drainage of Right Internal Mammary Artery, Open Approach, Diagnostic
3900ZZ	Drainage of Right Internal Mammary Artery, Open Approach
39030Z	Drainage of Right Internal Mammary Artery with Drainage Device, Percutaneous Approach
3903ZX	Drainage of Right Internal Mammary Artery, Percutaneous Approach, Diagnostic

03903ZZ	Drainage of Right Internal Mammary Artery, Percutaneous Approach
039040Z	Drainage of Right Internal Mammary Artery with Drainage Device, Percutaneous Endoscopic Approach
03904ZX	Drainage of Right Internal Mammary Artery, Percutaneous Endoscopic Approach, Diagnostic
03904ZZ	Drainage of Right Internal Mammary Artery, Percutaneous Endoscopic Approach
039100Z	Drainage of Left Internal Mammary Artery with Drainage Device, Open Approach

03910ZX	Drainage of Left Internal Mammary Artery, Open Approach, Diagnostic
03910ZZ	Drainage of Left Internal Mammary Artery, Open Approach
039130Z	Drainage of Left Internal Mammary Artery with Drainage Device, Percutaneous Approach
03913ZX	Drainage of Left Internal Mammary Artery, Percutaneous Approach, Diagnostic
03913ZZ	Drainage of Left Internal Mammary Artery, Percutaneous Approach

Female-only	♂ Male-only	▲ Limited Coverage	● Non-OR	▬ HAC-associated procedure	▲ Non-covered procedures	✛ Combination

039140Z Drainage of Left Internal Mammary Artery with Drainage Device, Percutaneous Endoscopic Approach

03914ZX Drainage of Left Internal Mammary Artery, Percutaneous Endoscopic Approach, Diagnostic

03914ZZ Drainage of Left Internal Mammary Artery, Percutaneous Endoscopic Approach

039200Z Drainage of Innominate Artery with Drainage Device, Open Approach

03920ZX Drainage of Innominate Artery, Open Approach, Diagnostic

03920ZZ Drainage of Innominate Artery, Open Approach

039230Z Drainage of Innominate Artery with Drainage Device, Percutaneous Approach

03923ZX Drainage of Innominate Artery, Percutaneous Approach, Diagnostic

03923ZZ Drainage of Innominate Artery, Percutaneous Approach

039240Z Drainage of Innominate Artery with Drainage Device, Percutaneous Endoscopic Approach

03924ZX Drainage of Innominate Artery, Percutaneous Endoscopic Approach, Diagnostic

03924ZZ Drainage of Innominate Artery, Percutaneous Endoscopic Approach

039300Z Drainage of Right Subclavian Artery with Drainage Device, Open Approach

03930ZX Drainage of Right Subclavian Artery, Open Approach, Diagnostic

03930ZZ Drainage of Right Subclavian Artery, Open Approach

039330Z Drainage of Right Subclavian Artery with Drainage Device, Percutaneous Approach

03933ZX Drainage of Right Subclavian Artery, Percutaneous Approach, Diagnostic

03933ZZ Drainage of Right Subclavian Artery, Percutaneous Approach

039340Z Drainage of Right Subclavian Artery with Drainage Device, Percutaneous Endoscopic Approach

03934ZX Drainage of Right Subclavian Artery, Percutaneous Endoscopic Approach, Diagnostic

03934ZZ Drainage of Right Subclavian Artery, Percutaneous Endoscopic Approach

039400Z Drainage of Left Subclavian Artery with Drainage Device, Open Approach

03940ZX Drainage of Left Subclavian Artery, Open Approach, Diagnostic

03940ZZ Drainage of Left Subclavian Artery, Open Approach

039430Z Drainage of Left Subclavian Artery with Drainage Device, Percutaneous Approach

03943ZX Drainage of Left Subclavian Artery, Percutaneous Approach, Diagnostic

03943ZZ Drainage of Left Subclavian Artery, Percutaneous Approach

039440Z Drainage of Left Subclavian Artery with Drainage Device, Percutaneous Endoscopic Approach

03944ZX Drainage of Left Subclavian Artery, Percutaneous Endoscopic Approach, Diagnostic

03944ZZ Drainage of Left Subclavian Artery, Percutaneous Endoscopic Approach

039500Z Drainage of Right Axillary Artery with Drainage Device, Open Approach

03950ZX Drainage of Right Axillary Artery, Open Approach, Diagnostic

03950ZZ Drainage of Right Axillary Artery, Open Approach

039530Z Drainage of Right Axillary Artery with Drainage Device, Percutaneous Approach

03953ZX Drainage of Right Axillary Artery, Percutaneous Approach, Diagnostic

03953ZZ Drainage of Right Axillary Artery, Percutaneous Approach

039540Z Drainage of Right Axillary Artery with Drainage Device, Percutaneous Endoscopic Approach

03954ZX Drainage of Right Axillary Artery, Percutaneous Endoscopic Approach, Diagnostic

03954ZZ Drainage of Right Axillary Artery, Percutaneous Endoscopic Approach

039600Z Drainage of Left Axillary Artery with Drainage Device, Open Approach

03960ZX Drainage of Left Axillary Artery, Open Approach, Diagnostic

03960ZZ Drainage of Left Axillary Artery, Open Approach

039630Z Drainage of Left Axillary Artery with Drainage Device, Percutaneous Approach

03963ZX Drainage of Left Axillary Artery, Percutaneous Approach, Diagnostic

03963ZZ Drainage of Left Axillary Artery, Percutaneous Approach

039640Z Drainage of Left Axillary Artery with Drainage Device, Percutaneous Endoscopic Approach

03964ZX Drainage of Left Axillary Artery, Percutaneous Endoscopic Approach, Diagnostic

03964ZZ Drainage of Left Axillary Artery, Percutaneous Endoscopic Approach

039700Z Drainage of Right Brachial Artery with Drainage Device, Open Approach

03970ZX Drainage of Right Brachial Artery, Open Approach, Diagnostic

03970ZZ Drainage of Right Brachial Artery, Open Approach

039730Z Drainage of Right Brachial Artery with Drainage Device, Percutaneous Approach

03973ZX Drainage of Right Brachial Artery, Percutaneous Approach, Diagnostic

03973ZZ Drainage of Right Brachial Artery, Percutaneous Approach

039740Z Drainage of Right Brachial Artery with Drainage Device, Percutaneous Endoscopic Approach

03974ZX Drainage of Right Brachial Artery, Percutaneous Endoscopic Approach, Diagnostic

03974ZZ Drainage of Right Brachial Artery, Percutaneous Endoscopic Approach

039800Z Drainage of Left Brachial Artery with Drainage Device, Open Approach

03980ZX Drainage of Left Brachial Artery, Open Approach, Diagnostic

03980ZZ Drainage of Left Brachial Artery, Open Approach

039830Z Drainage of Left Brachial Artery with Drainage Device, Percutaneous Approach

03983ZX Drainage of Left Brachial Artery, Percutaneous Approach, Diagnostic

03983ZZ Drainage of Left Brachial Artery, Percutaneous Approach

039840Z Drainage of Left Brachial Artery with Drainage Device, Percutaneous Endoscopic Approach

03984ZX Drainage of Left Brachial Artery, Percutaneous Endoscopic Approach, Diagnostic

03984ZZ Drainage of Left Brachial Artery, Percutaneous Endoscopic Approach

039900Z Drainage of Right Ulnar Artery with Drainage Device, Open Approach

03990ZX Drainage of Right Ulnar Artery, Open Approach, Diagnostic

03990ZZ Drainage of Right Ulnar Artery, Open Approach

039930Z Drainage of Right Ulnar Artery with Drainage Device, Percutaneous Approach

03993ZX Drainage of Right Ulnar Artery, Percutaneous Approach, Diagnostic

03993ZZ Drainage of Right Ulnar Artery, Percutaneous Approach

039940Z Drainage of Right Ulnar Artery with Drainage Device, Percutaneous Endoscopic Approach

03994ZX Drainage of Right Ulnar Artery, Percutaneous Endoscopic Approach, Diagnostic

03994ZZ Drainage of Right Ulnar Artery, Percutaneous Endoscopic Approach

039A00Z Drainage of Left Ulnar Artery with Drainage Device, Open Approach

039A0ZX Drainage of Left Ulnar Artery, Open Approach, Diagnostic

039A0ZZ Drainage of Left Ulnar Artery, Open Approach

039A30Z Drainage of Left Ulnar Artery with Drainage Device, Percutaneous Approach

039A3ZX Drainage of Left Ulnar Artery, Percutaneous Approach, Diagnostic

039A3ZZ Drainage of Left Ulnar Artery, Percutaneous Approach

039A40Z Drainage of Left Ulnar Artery with Drainage Device, Percutaneous Endoscopic Approach

039A4ZX Drainage of Left Ulnar Artery, Percutaneous Endoscopic Approach, Diagnostic

039A4ZZ Drainage of Left Ulnar Artery, Percutaneous Endoscopic Approach

039B00Z Drainage of Right Radial Artery with Drainage Device, Open Approach

039B0ZX Drainage of Right Radial Artery, Open Approach, Diagnostic

039B0ZZ Drainage of Right Radial Artery, Open Approach

039B30Z Drainage of Right Radial Artery with Drainage Device, Percutaneous Approach

039B3ZX Drainage of Right Radial Artery, Percutaneous Approach, Diagnostic

039B3ZZ Drainage of Right Radial Artery, Percutaneous Approach

039B40Z Drainage of Right Radial Artery with Drainage Device, Percutaneous Endoscopic Approach

039B4ZX Drainage of Right Radial Artery, Percutaneous Endoscopic Approach, Diagnostic

039B4ZZ Drainage of Right Radial Artery, Percutaneous Endoscopic Approach

039C00Z Drainage of Left Radial Artery with Drainage Device, Open Approach

039C0ZX Drainage of Left Radial Artery, Open Approach, Diagnostic

039C0ZZ Drainage of Left Radial Artery, Open Approach

039C30Z Drainage of Left Radial Artery with Drainage Device, Percutaneous Approach

039C3ZX Drainage of Left Radial Artery, Percutaneous Approach, Diagnostic

039C3ZZ Drainage of Left Radial Artery, Percutaneous Approach

039C40Z Drainage of Left Radial Artery with Drainage Device, Percutaneous Endoscopic Approach

039C4ZX Drainage of Left Radial Artery, Percutaneous Endoscopic Approach, Diagnostic

039C4ZZ Drainage of Left Radial Artery, Percutaneous Endoscopic Approach

039D00Z Drainage of Right Hand Artery with Drainage Device, Open Approach

039D0ZX Drainage of Right Hand Artery, Open Approach, Diagnostic

♀ Female-only   ♂ Male-only   ▲ Limited Coverage   ● Non-OR   ▨ HAC-associated procedure   ▲ Non-covered procedures   ✚ Combination

39D0ZZ Drainage of Right Hand Artery, Open Approach

39D30Z Drainage of Right Hand Artery with Drainage Device, Percutaneous Approach

39D3ZX Drainage of Right Hand Artery, Percutaneous Approach, Diagnostic

39D3ZZ Drainage of Right Hand Artery, Percutaneous Approach

39D40Z Drainage of Right Hand Artery with Drainage Device, Percutaneous Endoscopic Approach

39D4ZX Drainage of Right Hand Artery, Percutaneous Endoscopic Approach, Diagnostic

39D4ZZ Drainage of Right Hand Artery, Percutaneous Endoscopic Approach

39F00Z Drainage of Left Hand Artery with Drainage Device, Open Approach

39F0ZX Drainage of Left Hand Artery, Open Approach, Diagnostic

39F0ZZ Drainage of Left Hand Artery, Open Approach

39F30Z Drainage of Left Hand Artery with Drainage Device, Percutaneous Approach

39F3ZX Drainage of Left Hand Artery, Percutaneous Approach, Diagnostic

39F3ZZ Drainage of Left Hand Artery, Percutaneous Approach

39F40Z Drainage of Left Hand Artery with Drainage Device, Percutaneous Endoscopic Approach

39F4ZX Drainage of Left Hand Artery, Percutaneous Endoscopic Approach, Diagnostic

39F4ZZ Drainage of Left Hand Artery, Percutaneous Endoscopic Approach

39G00Z Drainage of Intracranial Artery with Drainage Device, Open Approach

39G0ZX Drainage of Intracranial Artery, Open Approach, Diagnostic

39G0ZZ Drainage of Intracranial Artery, Open Approach

39G30Z Drainage of Intracranial Artery with Drainage Device, Percutaneous Approach

39G3ZX Drainage of Intracranial Artery, Percutaneous Approach, Diagnostic

39G3ZZ Drainage of Intracranial Artery, Percutaneous Approach

39G40Z Drainage of Intracranial Artery with Drainage Device, Percutaneous Endoscopic Approach

39G4ZX Drainage of Intracranial Artery, Percutaneous Endoscopic Approach, Diagnostic

39G4ZZ Drainage of Intracranial Artery, Percutaneous Endoscopic Approach

39H00Z Drainage of Right Common Carotid Artery with Drainage Device, Open Approach

39H0ZX Drainage of Right Common Carotid Artery, Open Approach, Diagnostic

39H0ZZ Drainage of Right Common Carotid Artery, Open Approach

39H30Z Drainage of Right Common Carotid Artery with Drainage Device, Percutaneous Approach

39H3ZX Drainage of Right Common Carotid Artery, Percutaneous Approach, Diagnostic

39H3ZZ Drainage of Right Common Carotid Artery, Percutaneous Approach

39H40Z Drainage of Right Common Carotid Artery with Drainage Device, Percutaneous Endoscopic Approach

39H4ZX Drainage of Right Common Carotid Artery, Percutaneous Endoscopic Approach, Diagnostic

39H4ZZ Drainage of Right Common Carotid Artery, Percutaneous Endoscopic Approach

039J00Z Drainage of Left Common Carotid Artery with Drainage Device, Open Approach

039J0ZX Drainage of Left Common Carotid Artery, Open Approach, Diagnostic

039J0ZZ Drainage of Left Common Carotid Artery, Open Approach

039J30Z Drainage of Left Common Carotid Artery with Drainage Device, Percutaneous Approach

039J3ZX Drainage of Left Common Carotid Artery, Percutaneous Approach, Diagnostic

039J3ZZ Drainage of Left Common Carotid Artery, Percutaneous Approach

039J40Z Drainage of Left Common Carotid Artery with Drainage Device, Percutaneous Endoscopic Approach

039J4ZX Drainage of Left Common Carotid Artery, Percutaneous Endoscopic Approach, Diagnostic

039J4ZZ Drainage of Left Common Carotid Artery, Percutaneous Endoscopic Approach

039K00Z Drainage of Right Internal Carotid Artery with Drainage Device, Open Approach

039K0ZX Drainage of Right Internal Carotid Artery, Open Approach, Diagnostic

039K0ZZ Drainage of Right Internal Carotid Artery, Open Approach

039K30Z Drainage of Right Internal Carotid Artery with Drainage Device, Percutaneous Approach

039K3ZX Drainage of Right Internal Carotid Artery, Percutaneous Approach, Diagnostic

039K3ZZ Drainage of Right Internal Carotid Artery, Percutaneous Approach

039K40Z Drainage of Right Internal Carotid Artery with Drainage Device, Percutaneous Endoscopic Approach

039K4ZX Drainage of Right Internal Carotid Artery, Percutaneous Endoscopic Approach, Diagnostic

039K4ZZ Drainage of Right Internal Carotid Artery, Percutaneous Endoscopic Approach

039L00Z Drainage of Left Internal Carotid Artery with Drainage Device, Open Approach

039L0ZX Drainage of Left Internal Carotid Artery, Open Approach, Diagnostic

039L0ZZ Drainage of Left Internal Carotid Artery, Open Approach

039L30Z Drainage of Left Internal Carotid Artery with Drainage Device, Percutaneous Approach

039L3ZX Drainage of Left Internal Carotid Artery, Percutaneous Approach, Diagnostic

039L3ZZ Drainage of Left Internal Carotid Artery, Percutaneous Approach

039L40Z Drainage of Left Internal Carotid Artery with Drainage Device, Percutaneous Endoscopic Approach

039L4ZX Drainage of Left Internal Carotid Artery, Percutaneous Endoscopic Approach, Diagnostic

039L4ZZ Drainage of Left Internal Carotid Artery, Percutaneous Endoscopic Approach

039M00Z Drainage of Right External Carotid Artery with Drainage Device, Open Approach

039M0ZX Drainage of Right External Carotid Artery, Open Approach, Diagnostic

039M0ZZ Drainage of Right External Carotid Artery, Open Approach

039M30Z Drainage of Right External Carotid Artery with Drainage Device, Percutaneous Approach

039M3ZX Drainage of Right External Carotid Artery, Percutaneous Approach, Diagnostic

039M3ZZ Drainage of Right External Carotid Artery, Percutaneous Approach

039M40Z Drainage of Right External Carotid Artery with Drainage Device, Percutaneous Endoscopic Approach

039M4ZX Drainage of Right External Carotid Artery, Percutaneous Endoscopic Approach, Diagnostic

039M4ZZ Drainage of Right External Carotid Artery, Percutaneous Endoscopic Approach

039N00Z Drainage of Left External Carotid Artery with Drainage Device, Open Approach

039N0ZX Drainage of Left External Carotid Artery, Open Approach, Diagnostic

039N0ZZ Drainage of Left External Carotid Artery, Open Approach

039N30Z Drainage of Left External Carotid Artery with Drainage Device, Percutaneous Approach

039N3ZX Drainage of Left External Carotid Artery, Percutaneous Approach, Diagnostic

039N3ZZ Drainage of Left External Carotid Artery, Percutaneous Approach

039N40Z Drainage of Left External Carotid Artery with Drainage Device, Percutaneous Endoscopic Approach

039N4ZX Drainage of Left External Carotid Artery, Percutaneous Endoscopic Approach, Diagnostic

039N4ZZ Drainage of Left External Carotid Artery, Percutaneous Endoscopic Approach

039P00Z Drainage of Right Vertebral Artery with Drainage Device, Open Approach

039P0ZX Drainage of Right Vertebral Artery, Open Approach, Diagnostic

039P0ZZ Drainage of Right Vertebral Artery, Open Approach

039P30Z Drainage of Right Vertebral Artery with Drainage Device, Percutaneous Approach

039P3ZX Drainage of Right Vertebral Artery, Percutaneous Approach, Diagnostic

039P3ZZ Drainage of Right Vertebral Artery, Percutaneous Approach

039P40Z Drainage of Right Vertebral Artery with Drainage Device, Percutaneous Endoscopic Approach

039P4ZX Drainage of Right Vertebral Artery, Percutaneous Endoscopic Approach, Diagnostic

039P4ZZ Drainage of Right Vertebral Artery, Percutaneous Endoscopic Approach

039Q00Z Drainage of Left Vertebral Artery with Drainage Device, Open Approach

039Q0ZX Drainage of Left Vertebral Artery, Open Approach, Diagnostic

039Q0ZZ Drainage of Left Vertebral Artery, Open Approach

039Q30Z Drainage of Left Vertebral Artery with Drainage Device, Percutaneous Approach

039Q3ZX Drainage of Left Vertebral Artery, Percutaneous Approach, Diagnostic

039Q3ZZ Drainage of Left Vertebral Artery, Percutaneous Approach

039Q40Z Drainage of Left Vertebral Artery with Drainage Device, Percutaneous Endoscopic Approach

039Q4ZX Drainage of Left Vertebral Artery, Percutaneous Endoscopic Approach, Diagnostic

039Q4ZZ Drainage of Left Vertebral Artery, Percutaneous Endoscopic Approach

039R00Z Drainage of Face Artery with Drainage Device, Open Approach

039R0ZX Drainage of Face Artery, Open Approach, Diagnostic

039R0ZZ Drainage of Face Artery, Open Approach

039R30Z Drainage of Face Artery with Drainage Device, Percutaneous Approach

039R3ZX Drainage of Face Artery, Percutaneous Approach, Diagnostic

♀ Female-only   ♂ Male-only   ▲ Limited Coverage   ● Non-OR   HAC-associated procedure   ▲ Non-covered procedures   ✚ Combination

039R3ZZ Drainage of Face Artery, Percutaneous Approach

039R40Z Drainage of Face Artery with Drainage Device, Percutaneous Endoscopic Approach

039R4ZX Drainage of Face Artery, Percutaneous Endoscopic Approach, Diagnostic

039R4ZZ Drainage of Face Artery, Percutaneous Endoscopic Approach

039S00Z Drainage of Right Temporal Artery with Drainage Device, Open Approach

039S0ZX Drainage of Right Temporal Artery, Open Approach, Diagnostic

039S0ZZ Drainage of Right Temporal Artery, Open Approach

039S30Z Drainage of Right Temporal Artery with Drainage Device, Percutaneous Approach

039S3ZX Drainage of Right Temporal Artery, Percutaneous Approach, Diagnostic

039S3ZZ Drainage of Right Temporal Artery, Percutaneous Approach

039S40Z Drainage of Right Temporal Artery with Drainage Device, Percutaneous Endoscopic Approach

039S4ZX Drainage of Right Temporal Artery, Percutaneous Endoscopic Approach, Diagnostic

039S4ZZ Drainage of Right Temporal Artery, Percutaneous Endoscopic Approach

039T00Z Drainage of Left Temporal Artery with Drainage Device, Open Approach

039T0ZX Drainage of Left Temporal Artery, Open Approach, Diagnostic

039T0ZZ Drainage of Left Temporal Artery, Open Approach

039T30Z Drainage of Left Temporal Artery with Drainage Device, Percutaneous Approach

039T3ZX Drainage of Left Temporal Artery, Percutaneous Approach, Diagnostic

039T3ZZ Drainage of Left Temporal Artery, Percutaneous Approach

039T40Z Drainage of Left Temporal Artery with Drainage Device, Percutaneous Endoscopic Approach

039T4ZX Drainage of Left Temporal Artery, Percutaneous Endoscopic Approach, Diagnostic

039T4ZZ Drainage of Left Temporal Artery, Percutaneous Endoscopic Approach

039U00Z Drainage of Right Thyroid Artery with Drainage Device, Open Approach

039U0ZX Drainage of Right Thyroid Artery, Open Approach, Diagnostic

039U0ZZ Drainage of Right Thyroid Artery, Open Approach

039U30Z Drainage of Right Thyroid Artery with Drainage Device, Percutaneous Approach

039U3ZX Drainage of Right Thyroid Artery, Percutaneous Approach, Diagnostic

039U3ZZ Drainage of Right Thyroid Artery, Percutaneous Approach

039U40Z Drainage of Right Thyroid Artery with Drainage Device, Percutaneous Endoscopic Approach

039U4ZX Drainage of Right Thyroid Artery, Percutaneous Endoscopic Approach, Diagnostic

039U4ZZ Drainage of Right Thyroid Artery, Percutaneous Endoscopic Approach

039V00Z Drainage of Left Thyroid Artery with Drainage Device, Open Approach

039V0ZX Drainage of Left Thyroid Artery, Open Approach, Diagnostic

039V0ZZ Drainage of Left Thyroid Artery, Open Approach

039V30Z Drainage of Left Thyroid Artery with Drainage Device, Percutaneous Approach

039V3ZX Drainage of Left Thyroid Artery, Percutaneous Approach, Diagnostic

039V3ZZ Drainage of Left Thyroid Artery, Percutaneous Approach

039V40Z Drainage of Left Thyroid Artery with Drainage Device, Percutaneous Endoscopic Approach

039V4ZX Drainage of Left Thyroid Artery, Percutaneous Endoscopic Approach, Diagnostic

039V4ZZ Drainage of Left Thyroid Artery, Percutaneous Endoscopic Approach

039Y00Z Drainage of Upper Artery with Drainage Device, Open Approach

039Y0ZX Drainage of Upper Artery, Open Approach, Diagnostic

039Y0ZZ Drainage of Upper Artery, Open Approach

039Y30Z Drainage of Upper Artery with Drainage Device, Percutaneous Approach

039Y3ZX Drainage of Upper Artery, Percutaneous Approach, Diagnostic

039Y3ZZ Drainage of Upper Artery, Percutaneous Approach

039Y40Z Drainage of Upper Artery with Drainage Device, Percutaneous Endoscopic Approach

039Y4ZX Drainage of Upper Artery, Percutaneous Endoscopic Approach, Diagnostic

039Y4ZZ Drainage of Upper Artery, Percutaneous Endoscopic Approach

03B – Upper Arteries, Excision

Review Coding Guidelines B3.4a and B3.4b

Review Coding Guideline B3.8

03B00ZX Excision of Right Internal Mammary Artery, Open Approach, Diagnostic

03B00ZZ Excision of Right Internal Mammary Artery, Open Approach

03B03ZX Excision of Right Internal Mammary Artery, Percutaneous Approach, Diagnostic

03B03ZZ Excision of Right Internal Mammary Artery, Percutaneous Approach

03B04ZX Excision of Right Internal Mammary Artery, Percutaneous Endoscopic Approach, Diagnostic

03B04ZZ Excision of Right Internal Mammary Artery, Percutaneous Endoscopic Approach

03B10ZX Excision of Left Internal Mammary Artery, Open Approach, Diagnostic

03B10ZZ Excision of Left Internal Mammary Artery, Open Approach

03B13ZX Excision of Left Internal Mammary Artery, Percutaneous Approach, Diagnostic

03B13ZZ Excision of Left Internal Mammary Artery, Percutaneous Approach

03B14ZX Excision of Left Internal Mammary Artery, Percutaneous Endoscopic Approach, Diagnostic

03B14ZZ Excision of Left Internal Mammary Artery, Percutaneous Endoscopic Approach

03B20ZX Excision of Innominate Artery, Open Approach, Diagnostic

03B20ZZ Excision of Innominate Artery, Open Approach

03B23ZX Excision of Innominate Artery, Percutaneous Approach, Diagnostic

03B23ZZ Excision of Innominate Artery, Percutaneous Approach

03B24ZX Excision of Innominate Artery, Percutaneous Endoscopic Approach, Diagnostic

03B24ZZ Excision of Innominate Artery, Percutaneous Endoscopic Approach

03B30ZX Excision of Right Subclavian Artery, Open Approach, Diagnostic

03B30ZZ Excision of Right Subclavian Artery, Open Approach

03B33ZX Excision of Right Subclavian Artery, Percutaneous Approach, Diagnostic

03B33ZZ Excision of Right Subclavian Artery, Percutaneous Approach

03B34ZX Excision of Right Subclavian Artery, Percutaneous Endoscopic Approach, Diagnostic

03B34ZZ Excision of Right Subclavian Artery, Percutaneous Endoscopic Approach

03B40ZX Excision of Left Subclavian Artery, Open Approach, Diagnostic

03B40ZZ Excision of Left Subclavian Artery, Open Approach

03B43ZX Excision of Left Subclavian Artery, Percutaneous Approach, Diagnostic

03B43ZZ Excision of Left Subclavian Artery, Percutaneous Approach

03B44ZX Excision of Left Subclavian Artery, Percutaneous Endoscopic Approach, Diagnostic

03B44ZZ Excision of Left Subclavian Artery, Percutaneous Endoscopic Approach

03B50ZX Excision of Right Axillary Artery, Open Approach, Diagnostic

03B50ZZ Excision of Right Axillary Artery, Open Approach

03B53ZX Excision of Right Axillary Artery, Percutaneous Approach, Diagnostic

03B53ZZ Excision of Right Axillary Artery, Percutaneous Approach

03B54ZX Excision of Right Axillary Artery, Percutaneous Endoscopic Approach, Diagnostic

03B54ZZ Excision of Right Axillary Artery, Percutaneous Endoscopic Approach

03B60ZX Excision of Left Axillary Artery, Open Approach, Diagnostic

03B60ZZ Excision of Left Axillary Artery, Open Approach

03B63ZX Excision of Left Axillary Artery, Percutaneous Approach, Diagnostic

03B63ZZ Excision of Left Axillary Artery, Percutaneous Approach

03B64ZX Excision of Left Axillary Artery, Percutaneous Endoscopic Approach, Diagnostic

03B64ZZ Excision of Left Axillary Artery, Percutaneous Endoscopic Approach

03B70ZX Excision of Right Brachial Artery, Open Approach, Diagnostic

03B70ZZ Excision of Right Brachial Artery, Open Approach

03B73ZX Excision of Right Brachial Artery, Percutaneous Approach, Diagnostic

03B73ZZ Excision of Right Brachial Artery, Percutaneous Approach

03B74ZX Excision of Right Brachial Artery, Percutaneous Endoscopic Approach, Diagnostic

03B74ZZ Excision of Right Brachial Artery, Percutaneous Endoscopic Approach

03B80ZX Excision of Left Brachial Artery, Open Approach, Diagnostic

03B80ZZ Excision of Left Brachial Artery, Open Approach

03B83ZX Excision of Left Brachial Artery, Percutaneous Approach, Diagnostic

03B83ZZ Excision of Left Brachial Artery, Percutaneous Approach

03B84ZX Excision of Left Brachial Artery, Percutaneous Endoscopic Approach, Diagnostic

03B84ZZ Excision of Left Brachial Artery, Percutaneous Endoscopic Approach

03B90ZX Excision of Right Ulnar Artery, Open Approach, Diagnostic

03B90ZZ Excision of Right Ulnar Artery, Open Approach

03B93ZX Excision of Right Ulnar Artery, Percutaneous Approach, Diagnostic

03B93ZZ Excision of Right Ulnar Artery, Percutaneous Approach

03B94ZX Excision of Right Ulnar Artery, Percutaneous Endoscopic Approach, Diagnostic

03B94ZZ Excision of Right Ulnar Artery, Percutaneous Endoscopic Approach

03BA0ZX Excision of Left Ulnar Artery, Open Approach, Diagnostic

03BA0ZZ Excision of Left Ulnar Artery, Open Approach

03BA3ZX Excision of Left Ulnar Artery, Percutaneous Approach, Diagnostic

03BA3ZZ Excision of Left Ulnar Artery, Percutaneous Approach

03BA4ZX Excision of Left Ulnar Artery, Percutaneous Endoscopic Approach, Diagnostic

03BA4ZZ Excision of Left Ulnar Artery, Percutaneous Endoscopic Approach

03BB0ZX Excision of Right Radial Artery, Open Approach, Diagnostic

03BB0ZZ Excision of Right Radial Artery, Open Approach

03BB3ZX Excision of Right Radial Artery, Percutaneous Approach, Diagnostic

03BB3ZZ Excision of Right Radial Artery, Percutaneous Approach

03BB4ZX Excision of Right Radial Artery, Percutaneous Endoscopic Approach, Diagnostic

03BB4ZZ Excision of Right Radial Artery, Percutaneous Endoscopic Approach

03BC0ZX Excision of Left Radial Artery, Open Approach, Diagnostic

03BC0ZZ Excision of Left Radial Artery, Open Approach

03BC3ZX Excision of Left Radial Artery, Percutaneous Approach, Diagnostic

03BC3ZZ Excision of Left Radial Artery, Percutaneous Approach

03BC4ZX Excision of Left Radial Artery, Percutaneous Endoscopic Approach, Diagnostic

03BC4ZZ Excision of Left Radial Artery, Percutaneous Endoscopic Approach

03BD0ZX Excision of Right Hand Artery, Open Approach, Diagnostic

03BD0ZZ Excision of Right Hand Artery, Open Approach

03BD3ZX Excision of Right Hand Artery, Percutaneous Approach, Diagnostic

03BD3ZZ Excision of Right Hand Artery, Percutaneous Approach

03BD4ZX Excision of Right Hand Artery, Percutaneous Endoscopic Approach, Diagnostic

03BD4ZZ Excision of Right Hand Artery, Percutaneous Endoscopic Approach

03BF0ZX Excision of Left Hand Artery, Open Approach, Diagnostic

03BF0ZZ Excision of Left Hand Artery, Open Approach

03BF3ZX Excision of Left Hand Artery, Percutaneous Approach, Diagnostic

03BF3ZZ Excision of Left Hand Artery, Percutaneous Approach

03BF4ZX Excision of Left Hand Artery, Percutaneous Endoscopic Approach, Diagnostic

03BF4ZZ Excision of Left Hand Artery, Percutaneous Endoscopic Approach

03BG0ZX Excision of Intracranial Artery, Open Approach, Diagnostic

03BG0ZZ Excision of Intracranial Artery, Open Approach

03BG3ZX Excision of Intracranial Artery, Percutaneous Approach, Diagnostic

03BG3ZZ Excision of Intracranial Artery, Percutaneous Approach

03BG4ZX Excision of Intracranial Artery, Percutaneous Endoscopic Approach, Diagnostic

03BG4ZZ Excision of Intracranial Artery, Percutaneous Endoscopic Approach

03BH0ZX Excision of Right Common Carotid Artery, Open Approach, Diagnostic

03BH0ZZ Excision of Right Common Carotid Artery, Open Approach

03BH3ZX Excision of Right Common Carotid Artery, Percutaneous Approach, Diagnostic

03BH3ZZ Excision of Right Common Carotid Artery, Percutaneous Approach

03BH4ZX Excision of Right Common Carotid Artery, Percutaneous Endoscopic Approach, Diagnostic

03BH4ZZ Excision of Right Common Carotid Artery, Percutaneous Endoscopic Approach

03BJ0ZX Excision of Left Common Carotid Artery, Open Approach, Diagnostic

03BJ0ZZ Excision of Left Common Carotid Artery, Open Approach

03BJ3ZX Excision of Left Common Carotid Artery, Percutaneous Approach, Diagnostic

03BJ3ZZ Excision of Left Common Carotid Artery, Percutaneous Approach

03BJ4ZX Excision of Left Common Carotid Artery, Percutaneous Endoscopic Approach, Diagnostic

03BJ4ZZ Excision of Left Common Carotid Artery, Percutaneous Endoscopic Approach

03BK0ZX Excision of Right Internal Carotid Artery, Open Approach, Diagnostic

03BK0ZZ Excision of Right Internal Carotid Artery, Open Approach

03BK3ZX Excision of Right Internal Carotid Artery, Percutaneous Approach, Diagnostic

03BK3ZZ Excision of Right Internal Carotid Artery, Percutaneous Approach

03BK4ZX Excision of Right Internal Carotid Artery, Percutaneous Endoscopic Approach, Diagnostic

03BK4ZZ Excision of Right Internal Carotid Artery, Percutaneous Endoscopic Approach

03BL0ZX Excision of Left Internal Carotid Artery, Open Approach, Diagnostic

03BL0ZZ Excision of Left Internal Carotid Artery, Open Approach

03BL3ZX Excision of Left Internal Carotid Artery, Percutaneous Approach, Diagnostic

03BL3ZZ Excision of Left Internal Carotid Artery, Percutaneous Approach

03BL4ZX Excision of Left Internal Carotid Artery, Percutaneous Endoscopic Approach, Diagnostic

03BL4ZZ Excision of Left Internal Carotid Artery, Percutaneous Endoscopic Approach

03BM0ZX Excision of Right External Carotid Artery, Open Approach, Diagnostic

03BM0ZZ Excision of Right External Carotid Artery, Open Approach

03BM3ZX Excision of Right External Carotid Artery, Percutaneous Approach, Diagnostic

03BM3ZZ Excision of Right External Carotid Artery, Percutaneous Approach

03BM4ZX Excision of Right External Carotid Artery, Percutaneous Endoscopic Approach, Diagnostic

03BM4ZZ Excision of Right External Carotid Artery, Percutaneous Endoscopic Approach

03BN0ZX Excision of Left External Carotid Artery, Open Approach, Diagnostic

03BN0ZZ Excision of Left External Carotid Artery, Open Approach

03BN3ZX Excision of Left External Carotid Artery, Percutaneous Approach, Diagnostic

03BN3ZZ Excision of Left External Carotid Artery, Percutaneous Approach

03BN4ZX Excision of Left External Carotid Artery, Percutaneous Endoscopic Approach, Diagnostic

03BN4ZZ Excision of Left External Carotid Artery, Percutaneous Endoscopic Approach

03BP0ZX Excision of Right Vertebral Artery, Open Approach, Diagnostic

03BP0ZZ Excision of Right Vertebral Artery, Open Approach

03BP3ZX Excision of Right Vertebral Artery, Percutaneous Approach, Diagnostic

03BP3ZZ Excision of Right Vertebral Artery, Percutaneous Approach

03BP4ZX Excision of Right Vertebral Artery, Percutaneous Endoscopic Approach, Diagnostic

03BP4ZZ Excision of Right Vertebral Artery, Percutaneous Endoscopic Approach

03BQ0ZX Excision of Left Vertebral Artery, Open Approach, Diagnostic

03BQ0ZZ Excision of Left Vertebral Artery, Open Approach

03BQ3ZX Excision of Left Vertebral Artery, Percutaneous Approach, Diagnostic

03BQ3ZZ Excision of Left Vertebral Artery, Percutaneous Approach

03BQ4ZX Excision of Left Vertebral Artery, Percutaneous Endoscopic Approach, Diagnostic

03BQ4ZZ Excision of Left Vertebral Artery, Percutaneous Endoscopic Approach

03BR0ZX Excision of Face Artery, Open Approach, Diagnostic

03BR0ZZ Excision of Face Artery, Open Approach

03BR3ZX Excision of Face Artery, Percutaneous Approach, Diagnostic

03BR3ZZ Excision of Face Artery, Percutaneous Approach

03BR4ZX Excision of Face Artery, Percutaneous Endoscopic Approach, Diagnostic

03BR4ZZ Excision of Face Artery, Percutaneous Endoscopic Approach

03BS0ZX Excision of Right Temporal Artery, Open Approach, Diagnostic

03BS0ZZ Excision of Right Temporal Artery, Open Approach

03BS3ZX Excision of Right Temporal Artery, Percutaneous Approach, Diagnostic

219

♀ Female-only   ♂ Male-only   ▲ Limited Coverage   ● Non-OR   ▧ HAC-associated procedure   ▲ Non-covered procedures   ✚ Combination

03BS3ZZ Excision of Right Temporal Artery, Percutaneous Approach
03BS4ZX Excision of Right Temporal Artery, Percutaneous Endoscopic Approach, Diagnostic
03BS4ZZ Excision of Right Temporal Artery, Percutaneous Endoscopic Approach
03BT0ZX Excision of Left Temporal Artery, Open Approach, Diagnostic
03BT0ZZ Excision of Left Temporal Artery, Open Approach
03BT3ZX Excision of Left Temporal Artery, Percutaneous Approach, Diagnostic
03BT3ZZ Excision of Left Temporal Artery, Percutaneous Approach
03BT4ZX Excision of Left Temporal Artery, Percutaneous Endoscopic Approach, Diagnostic
03BT4ZZ Excision of Left Temporal Artery, Percutaneous Endoscopic Approach

03BU0ZX Excision of Right Thyroid Artery, Open Approach, Diagnostic
03BU0ZZ Excision of Right Thyroid Artery, Open Approach
03BU3ZX Excision of Right Thyroid Artery, Percutaneous Approach, Diagnostic
03BU3ZZ Excision of Right Thyroid Artery, Percutaneous Approach
03BU4ZX Excision of Right Thyroid Artery, Percutaneous Endoscopic Approach, Diagnostic
03BU4ZZ Excision of Right Thyroid Artery, Percutaneous Endoscopic Approach
03BV0ZX Excision of Left Thyroid Artery, Open Approach, Diagnostic
03BV0ZZ Excision of Left Thyroid Artery, Open Approach
03BV3ZX Excision of Left Thyroid Artery, Percutaneous Approach, Diagnostic

03BV3ZZ Excision of Left Thyroid Artery, Percutaneous Approach
03BV4ZX Excision of Left Thyroid Artery, Percutaneous Endoscopic Approach, Diagnostic
03BV4ZZ Excision of Left Thyroid Artery, Percutaneous Endoscopic Approach
03BY0ZX Excision of Upper Artery, Open Approach, Diagnostic
03BY0ZZ Excision of Upper Artery, Open Approach
03BY3ZX Excision of Upper Artery, Percutaneous Approach, Diagnostic
03BY3ZZ Excision of Upper Artery, Percutaneous Approach
03BY4ZX Excision of Upper Artery, Percutaneous Endoscopic Approach, Diagnostic
03BY4ZZ Excision of Upper Artery, Percutaneous Endoscopic Approach

03C – Upper Arteries, Extirpation

03C00ZZ Extirpation of Matter from Right Internal Mammary Artery, Open Approach
03C03ZZ Extirpation of Matter from Right Internal Mammary Artery, Percutaneous Approach
03C04ZZ Extirpation of Matter from Right Internal Mammary Artery, Percutaneous Endoscopic Approach
03C10ZZ Extirpation of Matter from Left Internal Mammary Artery, Open Approach
03C13ZZ Extirpation of Matter from Left Internal Mammary Artery, Percutaneous Approach
03C14ZZ Extirpation of Matter from Left Internal Mammary Artery, Percutaneous Endoscopic Approach
03C20ZZ Extirpation of Matter from Innominate Artery, Open Approach
03C23ZZ Extirpation of Matter from Innominate Artery, Percutaneous Approach
03C24ZZ Extirpation of Matter from Innominate Artery, Percutaneous Endoscopic Approach
03C30ZZ Extirpation of Matter from Right Subclavian Artery, Open Approach
03C33ZZ Extirpation of Matter from Right Subclavian Artery, Percutaneous Approach
03C34ZZ Extirpation of Matter from Right Subclavian Artery, Percutaneous Endoscopic Approach
03C40ZZ Extirpation of Matter from Left Subclavian Artery, Open Approach
03C43ZZ Extirpation of Matter from Left Subclavian Artery, Percutaneous Approach
03C44ZZ Extirpation of Matter from Left Subclavian Artery, Percutaneous Endoscopic Approach
03C50ZZ Extirpation of Matter from Right Axillary Artery, Open Approach
03C53ZZ Extirpation of Matter from Right Axillary Artery, Percutaneous Approach
03C54ZZ Extirpation of Matter from Right Axillary Artery, Percutaneous Endoscopic Approach
03C60ZZ Extirpation of Matter from Left Axillary Artery, Open Approach
03C63ZZ Extirpation of Matter from Left Axillary Artery, Percutaneous Approach
03C64ZZ Extirpation of Matter from Left Axillary Artery, Percutaneous Endoscopic Approach
03C70ZZ Extirpation of Matter from Right Brachial Artery, Open Approach
03C73ZZ Extirpation of Matter from Right Brachial Artery, Percutaneous Approach

03C74ZZ Extirpation of Matter from Right Brachial Artery, Percutaneous Endoscopic Approach
03C80ZZ Extirpation of Matter from Left Brachial Artery, Open Approach
03C83ZZ Extirpation of Matter from Left Brachial Artery, Percutaneous Approach
03C84ZZ Extirpation of Matter from Left Brachial Artery, Percutaneous Endoscopic Approach
03C90ZZ Extirpation of Matter from Right Ulnar Artery, Open Approach
03C93ZZ Extirpation of Matter from Right Ulnar Artery, Percutaneous Approach
03C94ZZ Extirpation of Matter from Right Ulnar Artery, Percutaneous Endoscopic Approach
03CA0ZZ Extirpation of Matter from Left Ulnar Artery, Open Approach
03CA3ZZ Extirpation of Matter from Left Ulnar Artery, Percutaneous Approach
03CA4ZZ Extirpation of Matter from Left Ulnar Artery, Percutaneous Endoscopic Approach
03CB0ZZ Extirpation of Matter from Right Radial Artery, Open Approach
03CB3ZZ Extirpation of Matter from Right Radial Artery, Percutaneous Approach
03CB4ZZ Extirpation of Matter from Right Radial Artery, Percutaneous Endoscopic Approach
03CC0ZZ Extirpation of Matter from Left Radial Artery, Open Approach
03CC3ZZ Extirpation of Matter from Left Radial Artery, Percutaneous Approach
03CC4ZZ Extirpation of Matter from Left Radial Artery, Percutaneous Endoscopic Approach
03CD0ZZ Extirpation of Matter from Right Hand Artery, Open Approach
03CD3ZZ Extirpation of Matter from Right Hand Artery, Percutaneous Approach
03CD4ZZ Extirpation of Matter from Right Hand Artery, Percutaneous Endoscopic Approach
03CF0ZZ Extirpation of Matter from Left Hand Artery, Open Approach
03CF3ZZ Extirpation of Matter from Left Hand Artery, Percutaneous Approach
03CF4ZZ Extirpation of Matter from Left Hand Artery, Percutaneous Endoscopic Approach
03CG0ZZ Extirpation of Matter from Intracranial Artery, Open Approach

▲ 03CG3ZZ Extirpation of Matter from Intracranial Artery, Percutaneous Approach
▲ 03CG4ZZ Extirpation of Matter from Intracranial Artery, Percutaneous Endoscopic Approach
03CH0ZZ Extirpation of Matter from Right Common Carotid Artery, Open Approach
03CH3ZZ Extirpation of Matter from Right Common Carotid Artery, Percutaneous Approach
03CH4ZZ Extirpation of Matter from Right Common Carotid Artery, Percutaneous Endoscopic Approach
03CJ0ZZ Extirpation of Matter from Left Common Carotid Artery, Open Approach
03CJ3ZZ Extirpation of Matter from Left Common Carotid Artery, Percutaneous Approach
03CJ4ZZ Extirpation of Matter from Left Common Carotid Artery, Percutaneous Endoscopic Approach
03CK0ZZ Extirpation of Matter from Right Internal Carotid Artery, Open Approach
03CK3ZZ Extirpation of Matter from Right Internal Carotid Artery, Percutaneous Approach
03CK4ZZ Extirpation of Matter from Right Internal Carotid Artery, Percutaneous Endoscopic Approach
03CL0ZZ Extirpation of Matter from Left Internal Carotid Artery, Open Approach
03CL3ZZ Extirpation of Matter from Left Internal Carotid Artery, Percutaneous Approach
03CL4ZZ Extirpation of Matter from Left Internal Carotid Artery, Percutaneous Endoscopic Approach
03CM0ZZ Extirpation of Matter from Right External Carotid Artery, Open Approach
03CM3ZZ Extirpation of Matter from Right External Carotid Artery, Percutaneous Approach
03CM4ZZ Extirpation of Matter from Right External Carotid Artery, Percutaneous Endoscopic Approach
03CN0ZZ Extirpation of Matter from Left External Carotid Artery, Open Approach
03CN3ZZ Extirpation of Matter from Left External Carotid Artery, Percutaneous Approach
03CN4ZZ Extirpation of Matter from Left External Carotid Artery, Percutaneous Endoscopic Approach
03CP0ZZ Extirpation of Matter from Right Vertebral Artery, Open Approach
03CP3ZZ Extirpation of Matter from Right Vertebral Artery, Percutaneous Approach
03CP4ZZ Extirpation of Matter from Right Vertebral Artery, Percutaneous Endoscopic Approach

CQ0ZZ Extirpation of Matter from Left Vertebral Artery, Open Approach

CQ3ZZ Extirpation of Matter from Left Vertebral Artery, Percutaneous Approach

CQ4ZZ Extirpation of Matter from Left Vertebral Artery, Percutaneous Endoscopic Approach

CR0ZZ Extirpation of Matter from Face Artery, Open Approach

CR3ZZ Extirpation of Matter from Face Artery, Percutaneous Approach

CR4ZZ Extirpation of Matter from Face Artery, Percutaneous Endoscopic Approach

CS0ZZ Extirpation of Matter from Right Temporal Artery, Open Approach

03CS3ZZ Extirpation of Matter from Right Temporal Artery, Percutaneous Approach

03CS4ZZ Extirpation of Matter from Right Temporal Artery, Percutaneous Endoscopic Approach

03CT0ZZ Extirpation of Matter from Left Temporal Artery, Open Approach

03CT3ZZ Extirpation of Matter from Left Temporal Artery, Percutaneous Approach

03CT4ZZ Extirpation of Matter from Left Temporal Artery, Percutaneous Endoscopic Approach

03CU0ZZ Extirpation of Matter from Right Thyroid Artery, Open Approach

03CU3ZZ Extirpation of Matter from Right Thyroid Artery, Percutaneous Approach

03CU4ZZ Extirpation of Matter from Right Thyroid Artery, Percutaneous Endoscopic Approach

03CV0ZZ Extirpation of Matter from Left Thyroid Artery, Open Approach

03CV3ZZ Extirpation of Matter from Left Thyroid Artery, Percutaneous Approach

03CV4ZZ Extirpation of Matter from Left Thyroid Artery, Percutaneous Endoscopic Approach

03CY0ZZ Extirpation of Matter from Upper Artery, Open Approach

03CY3ZZ Extirpation of Matter from Upper Artery, Percutaneous Approach

03CY4ZZ Extirpation of Matter from Upper Artery, Percutaneous Endoscopic Approach

3H – Upper Arteries, Insertion

H003Z Insertion of Infusion Device into Right Internal Mammary Artery, Open Approach

H00DZ Insertion of Intraluminal Device into Right Internal Mammary Artery, Open Approach

H033Z Insertion of Infusion Device into Right Internal Mammary Artery, Percutaneous Approach

H03DZ Insertion of Intraluminal Device into Right Internal Mammary Artery, Percutaneous Approach

H043Z Insertion of Infusion Device into Right Internal Mammary Artery, Percutaneous Endoscopic Approach

H04DZ Insertion of Intraluminal Device into Right Internal Mammary Artery, Percutaneous Endoscopic Approach

H103Z Insertion of Infusion Device into Left Internal Mammary Artery, Open Approach

H10DZ Insertion of Intraluminal Device into Left Internal Mammary Artery, Open Approach

H133Z Insertion of Infusion Device into Left Internal Mammary Artery, Percutaneous Approach

H13DZ Insertion of Intraluminal Device into Left Internal Mammary Artery, Percutaneous Approach

H143Z Insertion of Infusion Device into Left Internal Mammary Artery, Percutaneous Endoscopic Approach

H14DZ Insertion of Intraluminal Device into Left Internal Mammary Artery, Percutaneous Endoscopic Approach

3H203Z Insertion of Infusion Device into Innominate Artery, Open Approach

3H20DZ Insertion of Intraluminal Device into Innominate Artery, Open Approach

3H233Z Insertion of Infusion Device into Innominate Artery, Percutaneous Approach

3H23DZ Insertion of Intraluminal Device into Innominate Artery, Percutaneous Approach

3H243Z Insertion of Infusion Device into Innominate Artery, Percutaneous Endoscopic Approach

3H24DZ Insertion of Intraluminal Device into Innominate Artery, Percutaneous Endoscopic Approach

3H303Z Insertion of Infusion Device into Right Subclavian Artery, Open Approach

3H30DZ Insertion of Intraluminal Device into Right Subclavian Artery, Open Approach

3H333Z Insertion of Infusion Device into Right Subclavian Artery, Percutaneous Approach

3H33DZ Insertion of Intraluminal Device into Right Subclavian Artery, Percutaneous Approach

3H343Z Insertion of Infusion Device into Right Subclavian Artery, Percutaneous Endoscopic Approach

03H34DZ Insertion of Intraluminal Device into Right Subclavian Artery, Percutaneous Endoscopic Approach

03H403Z Insertion of Infusion Device into Left Subclavian Artery, Open Approach

03H40DZ Insertion of Intraluminal Device into Left Subclavian Artery, Open Approach

03H433Z Insertion of Infusion Device into Left Subclavian Artery, Percutaneous Approach

03H43DZ Insertion of Intraluminal Device into Left Subclavian Artery, Percutaneous Approach

03H443Z Insertion of Infusion Device into Left Subclavian Artery, Percutaneous Endoscopic Approach

03H44DZ Insertion of Intraluminal Device into Left Subclavian Artery, Percutaneous Endoscopic Approach

03H503Z Insertion of Infusion Device into Right Axillary Artery, Open Approach

03H50DZ Insertion of Intraluminal Device into Right Axillary Artery, Open Approach

03H533Z Insertion of Infusion Device into Right Axillary Artery, Percutaneous Approach

03H53DZ Insertion of Intraluminal Device into Right Axillary Artery, Percutaneous Approach

03H543Z Insertion of Infusion Device into Right Axillary Artery, Percutaneous Endoscopic Approach

03H54DZ Insertion of Intraluminal Device into Right Axillary Artery, Percutaneous Endoscopic Approach

03H603Z Insertion of Infusion Device into Left Axillary Artery, Open Approach

03H60DZ Insertion of Intraluminal Device into Left Axillary Artery, Open Approach

03H633Z Insertion of Infusion Device into Left Axillary Artery, Percutaneous Approach

03H63DZ Insertion of Intraluminal Device into Left Axillary Artery, Percutaneous Approach

03H643Z Insertion of Infusion Device into Left Axillary Artery, Percutaneous Endoscopic Approach

03H64DZ Insertion of Intraluminal Device into Left Axillary Artery, Percutaneous Endoscopic Approach

03H703Z Insertion of Infusion Device into Right Brachial Artery, Open Approach

03H70DZ Insertion of Intraluminal Device into Right Brachial Artery, Open Approach

03H733Z Insertion of Infusion Device into Right Brachial Artery, Percutaneous Approach

03H73DZ Insertion of Intraluminal Device into Right Brachial Artery, Percutaneous Approach

03H743Z Insertion of Infusion Device into Right Brachial Artery, Percutaneous Endoscopic Approach

03H74DZ Insertion of Intraluminal Device into Right Brachial Artery, Percutaneous Endoscopic Approach

03H803Z Insertion of Infusion Device into Left Brachial Artery, Open Approach

03H80DZ Insertion of Intraluminal Device into Left Brachial Artery, Open Approach

03H833Z Insertion of Infusion Device into Left Brachial Artery, Percutaneous Approach

03H83DZ Insertion of Intraluminal Device into Left Brachial Artery, Percutaneous Approach

03H843Z Insertion of Infusion Device into Left Brachial Artery, Percutaneous Endoscopic Approach

03H84DZ Insertion of Intraluminal Device into Left Brachial Artery, Percutaneous Endoscopic Approach

03H903Z Insertion of Infusion Device into Right Ulnar Artery, Open Approach

03H90DZ Insertion of Intraluminal Device into Right Ulnar Artery, Open Approach

03H933Z Insertion of Infusion Device into Right Ulnar Artery, Percutaneous Approach

03H93DZ Insertion of Intraluminal Device into Right Ulnar Artery, Percutaneous Approach

03H943Z Insertion of Infusion Device into Right Ulnar Artery, Percutaneous Endoscopic Approach

03H94DZ Insertion of Intraluminal Device into Right Ulnar Artery, Percutaneous Endoscopic Approach

03HA03Z Insertion of Infusion Device into Left Ulnar Artery, Open Approach

03HA0DZ Insertion of Intraluminal Device into Left Ulnar Artery, Open Approach

03HA33Z Insertion of Infusion Device into Left Ulnar Artery, Percutaneous Approach

03HA3DZ Insertion of Intraluminal Device into Left Ulnar Artery, Percutaneous Approach

03HA43Z Insertion of Infusion Device into Left Ulnar Artery, Percutaneous Endoscopic Approach

03HA4DZ Insertion of Intraluminal Device into Left Ulnar Artery, Percutaneous Endoscopic Approach

03HB03Z Insertion of Infusion Device into Right Radial Artery, Open Approach

03HB0DZ Insertion of Intraluminal Device into Right Radial Artery, Open Approach

03HB33Z Insertion of Infusion Device into Right Radial Artery, Percutaneous Approach

03HB3DZ Insertion of Intraluminal Device into Right Radial Artery, Percutaneous Approach

03HB43Z Insertion of Infusion Device into Right Radial Artery, Percutaneous Endoscopic Approach

03HB4DZ Insertion of Intraluminal Device into Right Radial Artery, Percutaneous Endoscopic Approach

03HC03Z Insertion of Infusion Device into Left Radial Artery, Open Approach

♀ Female-only ♂ Male-only ▲ Limited Coverage ● Non-OR ■ HAC-associated procedure ▲ Non-covered procedures ✚ Combination

03HC0DZ Insertion of Intraluminal Device into Left Radial Artery, Open Approach

03HC33Z Insertion of Infusion Device into Left Radial Artery, Percutaneous Approach

03HC3DZ Insertion of Intraluminal Device into Left Radial Artery, Percutaneous Approach

03HC43Z Insertion of Infusion Device into Left Radial Artery, Percutaneous Endoscopic Approach

03HC4DZ Insertion of Intraluminal Device into Left Radial Artery, Percutaneous Endoscopic Approach

03HD03Z Insertion of Infusion Device into Right Hand Artery, Open Approach

03HD0DZ Insertion of Intraluminal Device into Right Hand Artery, Open Approach

03HD33Z Insertion of Infusion Device into Right Hand Artery, Percutaneous Approach

03HD3DZ Insertion of Intraluminal Device into Right Hand Artery, Percutaneous Approach

03HD43Z Insertion of Infusion Device into Right Hand Artery, Percutaneous Endoscopic Approach

03HD4DZ Insertion of Intraluminal Device into Right Hand Artery, Percutaneous Endoscopic Approach

03HF03Z Insertion of Infusion Device into Left Hand Artery, Open Approach

03HF0DZ Insertion of Intraluminal Device into Left Hand Artery, Open Approach

03HF33Z Insertion of Infusion Device into Left Hand Artery, Percutaneous Approach

03HF3DZ Insertion of Intraluminal Device into Left Hand Artery, Percutaneous Approach

03HF43Z Insertion of Infusion Device into Left Hand Artery, Percutaneous Endoscopic Approach

03HF4DZ Insertion of Intraluminal Device into Left Hand Artery, Percutaneous Endoscopic Approach

03HG03Z Insertion of Infusion Device into Intracranial Artery, Open Approach

03HG0DZ Insertion of Intraluminal Device into Intracranial Artery, Open Approach

03HG33Z Insertion of Infusion Device into Intracranial Artery, Percutaneous Approach

03HG3DZ Insertion of Intraluminal Device into Intracranial Artery, Percutaneous Approach

03HG43Z Insertion of Infusion Device into Intracranial Artery, Percutaneous Endoscopic Approach

03HG4DZ Insertion of Intraluminal Device into Intracranial Artery, Percutaneous Endoscopic Approach

03HH03Z Insertion of Infusion Device into Right Common Carotid Artery, Open Approach

03HH0DZ Insertion of Intraluminal Device into Right Common Carotid Artery, Open Approach

03HH33Z Insertion of Infusion Device into Right Common Carotid Artery, Percutaneous Approach

03HH3DZ Insertion of Intraluminal Device into Right Common Carotid Artery, Percutaneous Approach

03HH43Z Insertion of Infusion Device into Right Common Carotid Artery, Percutaneous Endoscopic Approach

03HH4DZ Insertion of Intraluminal Device into Right Common Carotid Artery, Percutaneous Endoscopic Approach

03HJ03Z Insertion of Infusion Device into Left Common Carotid Artery, Open Approach

03HJ0DZ Insertion of Intraluminal Device into Left Common Carotid Artery, Open Approach

03HJ33Z Insertion of Infusion Device into Left Common Carotid Artery, Percutaneous Approach

03HJ3DZ Insertion of Intraluminal Device into Left Common Carotid Artery, Percutaneous Approach

03HJ43Z Insertion of Infusion Device into Left Common Carotid Artery, Percutaneous Endoscopic Approach

03HJ4DZ Insertion of Intraluminal Device into Left Common Carotid Artery, Percutaneous Endoscopic Approach

03HK03Z Insertion of Infusion Device into Right Internal Carotid Artery, Open Approach

03HK0DZ Insertion of Intraluminal Device into Right Internal Carotid Artery, Open Approach

03HK0MZ Insertion of Stimulator Lead into Right Internal Carotid Artery, Open Approach

03HK33Z Insertion of Infusion Device into Right Internal Carotid Artery, Percutaneous Approach

03HK3DZ Insertion of Intraluminal Device into Right Internal Carotid Artery, Percutaneous Approach

03HK3MZ Insertion of Stimulator Lead into Right Internal Carotid Artery, Percutaneous Approach

03HK43Z Insertion of Infusion Device into Right Internal Carotid Artery, Percutaneous Endoscopic Approach

03HK4DZ Insertion of Intraluminal Device into Right Internal Carotid Artery, Percutaneous Endoscopic Approach

03HK4MZ Insertion of Stimulator Lead into Right Internal Carotid Artery, Percutaneous Endoscopic Approach

03HL03Z Insertion of Infusion Device into Left Internal Carotid Artery, Open Approach

03HL0DZ Insertion of Intraluminal Device into Left Internal Carotid Artery, Open Approach

03HL0MZ Insertion of Stimulator Lead into Left Internal Carotid Artery, Open Approach

03HL33Z Insertion of Infusion Device into Left Internal Carotid Artery, Percutaneous Approach

03HL3DZ Insertion of Intraluminal Device into Left Internal Carotid Artery, Percutaneous Approach

03HL3MZ Insertion of Stimulator Lead into Left Internal Carotid Artery, Percutaneous Approach

03HL43Z Insertion of Infusion Device into Left Internal Carotid Artery, Percutaneous Endoscopic Approach

03HL4DZ Insertion of Intraluminal Device into Left Internal Carotid Artery, Percutaneous Endoscopic Approach

03HL4MZ Insertion of Stimulator Lead into Left Internal Carotid Artery, Percutaneous Endoscopic Approach

03HM03Z Insertion of Infusion Device into Right External Carotid Artery, Open Approach

03HM0DZ Insertion of Intraluminal Device into Right External Carotid Artery, Open Approach

03HM33Z Insertion of Infusion Device into Right External Carotid Artery, Percutaneous Approach

03HM3DZ Insertion of Intraluminal Device into Right External Carotid Artery, Percutaneous Approach

03HM43Z Insertion of Infusion Device into Right External Carotid Artery, Percutaneous Endoscopic Approach

03HM4DZ Insertion of Intraluminal Device into Right External Carotid Artery, Percutaneous Endoscopic Approach

03HN03Z Insertion of Infusion Device into Left External Carotid Artery, Open Approach

03HN0DZ Insertion of Intraluminal Device into Left External Carotid Artery, Open Approach

03HN33Z Insertion of Infusion Device into Left External Carotid Artery, Percutaneous Approach

03HN3DZ Insertion of Intraluminal Device into Left External Carotid Artery, Percutaneous Approach

03HN43Z Insertion of Infusion Device into Left External Carotid Artery, Percutaneous Endoscopic Approach

03HN4DZ Insertion of Intraluminal Device into Left External Carotid Artery, Percutaneous Endoscopic Approach

03HP03Z Insertion of Infusion Device into Right Vertebral Artery, Open Approach

03HP0DZ Insertion of Intraluminal Device into Right Vertebral Artery, Open Approach

03HP33Z Insertion of Infusion Device into Right Vertebral Artery, Percutaneous Approach

03HP3DZ Insertion of Intraluminal Device into Right Vertebral Artery, Percutaneous Approach

03HP43Z Insertion of Infusion Device into Right Vertebral Artery, Percutaneous Endoscopic Approach

03HP4DZ Insertion of Intraluminal Device into Right Vertebral Artery, Percutaneous Endoscopic Approach

03HQ03Z Insertion of Infusion Device into Left Vertebral Artery, Open Approach

03HQ0DZ Insertion of Intraluminal Device into Left Vertebral Artery, Open Approach

03HQ33Z Insertion of Infusion Device into Left Vertebral Artery, Percutaneous Approach

03HQ3DZ Insertion of Intraluminal Device into Left Vertebral Artery, Percutaneous Approach

03HQ43Z Insertion of Infusion Device into Left Vertebral Artery, Percutaneous Endoscopic Approach

03HQ4DZ Insertion of Intraluminal Device into Left Vertebral Artery, Percutaneous Endoscopic Approach

03HR03Z Insertion of Infusion Device into Face Artery, Open Approach

03HR0DZ Insertion of Intraluminal Device into Face Artery, Open Approach

03HR33Z Insertion of Infusion Device into Face Artery, Percutaneous Approach

03HR3DZ Insertion of Intraluminal Device into Face Artery, Percutaneous Approach

03HR43Z Insertion of Infusion Device into Face Artery, Percutaneous Endoscopic Approach

03HR4DZ Insertion of Intraluminal Device into Face Artery, Percutaneous Endoscopic Approach

03HS03Z Insertion of Infusion Device into Right Temporal Artery, Open Approach

03HS0DZ Insertion of Intraluminal Device into Right Temporal Artery, Open Approach

03HS33Z Insertion of Infusion Device into Right Temporal Artery, Percutaneous Approach

03HS3DZ Insertion of Intraluminal Device into Right Temporal Artery, Percutaneous Approach

03HS43Z Insertion of Infusion Device into Right Temporal Artery, Percutaneous Endoscopic Approach

03HS4DZ Insertion of Intraluminal Device into Right Temporal Artery, Percutaneous Endoscopic Approach

03HT03Z Insertion of Infusion Device into Left Temporal Artery, Open Approach

03HT0DZ Insertion of Intraluminal Device into Left Temporal Artery, Open Approach

03HT33Z Insertion of Infusion Device into Left Temporal Artery, Percutaneous Approach

03HT3DZ Insertion of Intraluminal Device into Left Temporal Artery, Percutaneous Approach

03HT43Z Insertion of Infusion Device into Left Temporal Artery, Percutaneous Endoscopic Approach

03HT4DZ Insertion of Intraluminal Device into Left Temporal Artery, Percutaneous Endoscopic Approach

03HU03Z Insertion of Infusion Device into Right Thyroid Artery, Open Approach

03HU0DZ Insertion of Intraluminal Device into Right Thyroid Artery, Open Approach

03HU33Z Insertion of Infusion Device into Right Thyroid Artery, Percutaneous Approach

03HU3DZ Insertion of Intraluminal Device into Right Thyroid Artery, Percutaneous Approach

03HU43Z Insertion of Infusion Device into Right Thyroid Artery, Percutaneous Endoscopic Approach

03HU4DZ Insertion of Intraluminal Device into Right Thyroid Artery, Percutaneous Endoscopic Approach

03HV03Z Insertion of Infusion Device into Left Thyroid Artery, Open Approach

03HV0DZ Insertion of Intraluminal Device into Left Thyroid Artery, Open Approach

03HV33Z Insertion of Infusion Device into Left Thyroid Artery, Percutaneous Approach

03HV3DZ Insertion of Intraluminal Device into Left Thyroid Artery, Percutaneous Approach

03HV43Z Insertion of Infusion Device into Left Thyroid Artery, Percutaneous Endoscopic Approach

03HV4DZ Insertion of Intraluminal Device into Left Thyroid Artery, Percutaneous Endoscopic Approach

03HY02Z Insertion of Monitoring Device into Upper Artery, Open Approach

03HY03Z Insertion of Infusion Device into Upper Artery, Open Approach

03HY0DZ Insertion of Intraluminal Device into Upper Artery, Open Approach

03HY32Z Insertion of Monitoring Device into Upper Artery, Percutaneous Approach

03HY33Z Insertion of Infusion Device into Upper Artery, Percutaneous Approach

03HY3DZ Insertion of Intraluminal Device into Upper Artery, Percutaneous Approach

03HY42Z Insertion of Monitoring Device into Upper Artery, Percutaneous Endoscopic Approach

03HY43Z Insertion of Infusion Device into Upper Artery, Percutaneous Endoscopic Approach

03HY4DZ Insertion of Intraluminal Device into Upper Artery, Percutaneous Endoscopic Approach

3J – Upper Arteries, Inspection

Review Coding Guidelines B3.11a, B3.11b and B3.11c

03JY0ZZ Inspection of Upper Artery, Open Approach
AHA CC: 1Q, 2015, 29

03JY3ZZ Inspection of Upper Artery, Percutaneous Approach

03JY4ZZ Inspection of Upper Artery, Percutaneous Endoscopic Approach

03JYXZZ Inspection of Upper Artery, External Approach

3L – Upper Arteries, Occlusion

Review Coding Guideline B3.12

03L00CZ Occlusion of Right Internal Mammary Artery with Extraluminal Device, Open Approach

03L00DZ Occlusion of Right Internal Mammary Artery with Intraluminal Device, Open Approach

03L00ZZ Occlusion of Right Internal Mammary Artery, Open Approach

03L03CZ Occlusion of Right Internal Mammary Artery with Extraluminal Device, Percutaneous Approach

03L03DZ Occlusion of Right Internal Mammary Artery with Intraluminal Device, Percutaneous Approach

03L03ZZ Occlusion of Right Internal Mammary Artery, Percutaneous Approach

03L04CZ Occlusion of Right Internal Mammary Artery with Extraluminal Device, Percutaneous Endoscopic Approach

03L04DZ Occlusion of Right Internal Mammary Artery with Intraluminal Device, Percutaneous Endoscopic Approach

03L04ZZ Occlusion of Right Internal Mammary Artery, Percutaneous Endoscopic Approach

03L10CZ Occlusion of Left Internal Mammary Artery with Extraluminal Device, Open Approach

03L10DZ Occlusion of Left Internal Mammary Artery with Intraluminal Device, Open Approach

03L10ZZ Occlusion of Left Internal Mammary Artery, Open Approach

03L13CZ Occlusion of Left Internal Mammary Artery with Extraluminal Device, Percutaneous Approach

03L13DZ Occlusion of Left Internal Mammary Artery with Intraluminal Device, Percutaneous Approach

03L13ZZ Occlusion of Left Internal Mammary Artery, Percutaneous Approach

03L14CZ Occlusion of Left Internal Mammary Artery with Extraluminal Device, Percutaneous Endoscopic Approach

03L14DZ Occlusion of Left Internal Mammary Artery with Intraluminal Device, Percutaneous Endoscopic Approach

03L14ZZ Occlusion of Left Internal Mammary Artery, Percutaneous Endoscopic Approach

03L20CZ Occlusion of Innominate Artery with Extraluminal Device, Open Approach

03L20DZ Occlusion of Innominate Artery with Intraluminal Device, Open Approach

03L20ZZ Occlusion of Innominate Artery, Open Approach

03L23CZ Occlusion of Innominate Artery with Extraluminal Device, Percutaneous Approach

03L23DZ Occlusion of Innominate Artery with Intraluminal Device, Percutaneous Approach

03L23ZZ Occlusion of Innominate Artery, Percutaneous Approach

03L24CZ Occlusion of Innominate Artery with Extraluminal Device, Percutaneous Endoscopic Approach

03L24DZ Occlusion of Innominate Artery with Intraluminal Device, Percutaneous Endoscopic Approach

03L24ZZ Occlusion of Innominate Artery, Percutaneous Endoscopic Approach

03L30CZ Occlusion of Right Subclavian Artery with Extraluminal Device, Open Approach

03L30DZ Occlusion of Right Subclavian Artery with Intraluminal Device, Open Approach

03L30ZZ Occlusion of Right Subclavian Artery, Open Approach

03L33CZ Occlusion of Right Subclavian Artery with Extraluminal Device, Percutaneous Approach

03L33DZ Occlusion of Right Subclavian Artery with Intraluminal Device, Percutaneous Approach

03L33ZZ Occlusion of Right Subclavian Artery, Percutaneous Approach

03L34CZ Occlusion of Right Subclavian Artery with Extraluminal Device, Percutaneous Endoscopic Approach

03L34DZ Occlusion of Right Subclavian Artery with Intraluminal Device, Percutaneous Endoscopic Approach

03L34ZZ Occlusion of Right Subclavian Artery, Percutaneous Endoscopic Approach

03L40CZ Occlusion of Left Subclavian Artery with Extraluminal Device, Open Approach

03L40DZ Occlusion of Left Subclavian Artery with Intraluminal Device, Open Approach

03L40ZZ Occlusion of Left Subclavian Artery, Open Approach

03L43CZ Occlusion of Left Subclavian Artery with Extraluminal Device, Percutaneous Approach

03L43DZ Occlusion of Left Subclavian Artery with Intraluminal Device, Percutaneous Approach

03L43ZZ Occlusion of Left Subclavian Artery, Percutaneous Approach

03L44CZ Occlusion of Left Subclavian Artery with Extraluminal Device, Percutaneous Endoscopic Approach

03L44DZ Occlusion of Left Subclavian Artery with Intraluminal Device, Percutaneous Endoscopic Approach

03L44ZZ Occlusion of Left Subclavian Artery, Percutaneous Endoscopic Approach

03L50CZ Occlusion of Right Axillary Artery with Extraluminal Device, Open Approach

03L50DZ Occlusion of Right Axillary Artery with Intraluminal Device, Open Approach

03L50ZZ Occlusion of Right Axillary Artery, Open Approach

03L53CZ Occlusion of Right Axillary Artery with Extraluminal Device, Percutaneous Approach

03L53DZ Occlusion of Right Axillary Artery with Intraluminal Device, Percutaneous Approach

03L53ZZ Occlusion of Right Axillary Artery, Percutaneous Approach

03L54CZ Occlusion of Right Axillary Artery with Extraluminal Device, Percutaneous Endoscopic Approach

223

03L54DZ Occlusion of Right Axillary Artery with Intraluminal Device, Percutaneous Endoscopic Approach
03L54ZZ Occlusion of Right Axillary Artery, Percutaneous Endoscopic Approach
03L60CZ Occlusion of Left Axillary Artery with Extraluminal Device, Open Approach
03L60DZ Occlusion of Left Axillary Artery with Intraluminal Device, Open Approach
03L60ZZ Occlusion of Left Axillary Artery, Open Approach
03L63CZ Occlusion of Left Axillary Artery with Extraluminal Device, Percutaneous Approach
03L63DZ Occlusion of Left Axillary Artery with Intraluminal Device, Percutaneous Approach
03L63ZZ Occlusion of Left Axillary Artery, Percutaneous Approach
03L64CZ Occlusion of Left Axillary Artery with Extraluminal Device, Percutaneous Endoscopic Approach
03L64DZ Occlusion of Left Axillary Artery with Intraluminal Device, Percutaneous Endoscopic Approach
03L64ZZ Occlusion of Left Axillary Artery, Percutaneous Endoscopic Approach
03L70CZ Occlusion of Right Brachial Artery with Extraluminal Device, Open Approach
03L70DZ Occlusion of Right Brachial Artery with Intraluminal Device, Open Approach
03L70ZZ Occlusion of Right Brachial Artery, Open Approach
03L73CZ Occlusion of Right Brachial Artery with Extraluminal Device, Percutaneous Approach
03L73DZ Occlusion of Right Brachial Artery with Intraluminal Device, Percutaneous Approach
03L73ZZ Occlusion of Right Brachial Artery, Percutaneous Approach
03L74CZ Occlusion of Right Brachial Artery with Extraluminal Device, Percutaneous Endoscopic Approach
03L74DZ Occlusion of Right Brachial Artery with Intraluminal Device, Percutaneous Endoscopic Approach
03L74ZZ Occlusion of Right Brachial Artery, Percutaneous Endoscopic Approach
03L80CZ Occlusion of Left Brachial Artery with Extraluminal Device, Open Approach
03L80DZ Occlusion of Left Brachial Artery with Intraluminal Device, Open Approach
03L80ZZ Occlusion of Left Brachial Artery, Open Approach
03L83CZ Occlusion of Left Brachial Artery with Extraluminal Device, Percutaneous Approach
03L83DZ Occlusion of Left Brachial Artery with Intraluminal Device, Percutaneous Approach
03L83ZZ Occlusion of Left Brachial Artery, Percutaneous Approach
03L84CZ Occlusion of Left Brachial Artery with Extraluminal Device, Percutaneous Endoscopic Approach
03L84DZ Occlusion of Left Brachial Artery with Intraluminal Device, Percutaneous Endoscopic Approach
03L84ZZ Occlusion of Left Brachial Artery, Percutaneous Endoscopic Approach
03L90CZ Occlusion of Right Ulnar Artery with Extraluminal Device, Open Approach
03L90DZ Occlusion of Right Ulnar Artery with Intraluminal Device, Open Approach
03L90ZZ Occlusion of Right Ulnar Artery, Open Approach

03L93CZ Occlusion of Right Ulnar Artery with Extraluminal Device, Percutaneous Approach
03L93DZ Occlusion of Right Ulnar Artery with Intraluminal Device, Percutaneous Approach
03L93ZZ Occlusion of Right Ulnar Artery, Percutaneous Approach
03L94CZ Occlusion of Right Ulnar Artery with Extraluminal Device, Percutaneous Endoscopic Approach
03L94DZ Occlusion of Right Ulnar Artery with Intraluminal Device, Percutaneous Endoscopic Approach
03L94ZZ Occlusion of Right Ulnar Artery, Percutaneous Endoscopic Approach
03LA0CZ Occlusion of Left Ulnar Artery with Extraluminal Device, Open Approach
03LA0DZ Occlusion of Left Ulnar Artery with Intraluminal Device, Open Approach
03LA0ZZ Occlusion of Left Ulnar Artery, Open Approach
03LA3CZ Occlusion of Left Ulnar Artery with Extraluminal Device, Percutaneous Approach
03LA3DZ Occlusion of Left Ulnar Artery with Intraluminal Device, Percutaneous Approach
03LA3ZZ Occlusion of Left Ulnar Artery, Percutaneous Approach
03LA4CZ Occlusion of Left Ulnar Artery with Extraluminal Device, Percutaneous Endoscopic Approach
03LA4DZ Occlusion of Left Ulnar Artery with Intraluminal Device, Percutaneous Endoscopic Approach
03LA4ZZ Occlusion of Left Ulnar Artery, Percutaneous Endoscopic Approach
03LB0CZ Occlusion of Right Radial Artery with Extraluminal Device, Open Approach
03LB0DZ Occlusion of Right Radial Artery with Intraluminal Device, Open Approach
03LB0ZZ Occlusion of Right Radial Artery, Open Approach
03LB3CZ Occlusion of Right Radial Artery with Extraluminal Device, Percutaneous Approach
03LB3DZ Occlusion of Right Radial Artery with Intraluminal Device, Percutaneous Approach
03LB3ZZ Occlusion of Right Radial Artery, Percutaneous Approach
03LB4CZ Occlusion of Right Radial Artery with Extraluminal Device, Percutaneous Endoscopic Approach
03LB4DZ Occlusion of Right Radial Artery with Intraluminal Device, Percutaneous Endoscopic Approach
03LB4ZZ Occlusion of Right Radial Artery, Percutaneous Endoscopic Approach
03LC0CZ Occlusion of Left Radial Artery with Extraluminal Device, Open Approach
03LC0DZ Occlusion of Left Radial Artery with Intraluminal Device, Open Approach
03LC0ZZ Occlusion of Left Radial Artery, Open Approach
03LC3CZ Occlusion of Left Radial Artery with Extraluminal Device, Percutaneous Approach
03LC3DZ Occlusion of Left Radial Artery with Intraluminal Device, Percutaneous Approach
03LC3ZZ Occlusion of Left Radial Artery, Percutaneous Approach
03LC4CZ Occlusion of Left Radial Artery with Extraluminal Device, Percutaneous Endoscopic Approach

03LC4DZ Occlusion of Left Radial Artery with Intraluminal Device, Percutaneous Endoscopic Approach
03LC4ZZ Occlusion of Left Radial Artery, Percutaneous Endoscopic Approach
03LD0CZ Occlusion of Right Hand Artery with Extraluminal Device, Open Approach
03LD0DZ Occlusion of Right Hand Artery with Intraluminal Device, Open Approach
03LD0ZZ Occlusion of Right Hand Artery, Open Approach
03LD3CZ Occlusion of Right Hand Artery with Extraluminal Device, Percutaneous Approach
03LD3DZ Occlusion of Right Hand Artery with Intraluminal Device, Percutaneous Approach
03LD3ZZ Occlusion of Right Hand Artery, Percutaneous Approach
03LD4CZ Occlusion of Right Hand Artery with Extraluminal Device, Percutaneous Endoscopic Approach
03LD4DZ Occlusion of Right Hand Artery with Intraluminal Device, Percutaneous Endoscopic Approach
03LD4ZZ Occlusion of Right Hand Artery, Percutaneous Endoscopic Approach
03LF0CZ Occlusion of Left Hand Artery with Extraluminal Device, Open Approach
03LF0DZ Occlusion of Left Hand Artery with Intraluminal Device, Open Approach
03LF0ZZ Occlusion of Left Hand Artery, Open Approach
03LF3CZ Occlusion of Left Hand Artery with Extraluminal Device, Percutaneous Approach
03LF3DZ Occlusion of Left Hand Artery with Intraluminal Device, Percutaneous Approach
03LF3ZZ Occlusion of Left Hand Artery, Percutaneous Approach
03LF4CZ Occlusion of Left Hand Artery with Extraluminal Device, Percutaneous Endoscopic Approach
03LF4DZ Occlusion of Left Hand Artery with Intraluminal Device, Percutaneous Endoscopic Approach
03LF4ZZ Occlusion of Left Hand Artery, Percutaneous Endoscopic Approach
03LG0BZ Occlusion of Intracranial Artery with Bioactive Intraluminal Device, Open Approach
03LG0CZ Occlusion of Intracranial Artery with Extraluminal Device, Open Approach
03LG0DZ Occlusion of Intracranial Artery with Intraluminal Device, Open Approach
03LG0ZZ Occlusion of Intracranial Artery, Open Approach
03LG3BZ Occlusion of Intracranial Artery with Bioactive Intraluminal Device, Percutaneous Approach
03LG3CZ Occlusion of Intracranial Artery with Extraluminal Device, Percutaneous Approach
03LG3DZ Occlusion of Intracranial Artery with Intraluminal Device, Percutaneous Approach
AHA CC: 4Q, 2014, 37
03LG3ZZ Occlusion of Intracranial Artery, Percutaneous Approach
03LG4BZ Occlusion of Intracranial Artery with Bioactive Intraluminal Device, Percutaneous Endoscopic Approach
03LG4CZ Occlusion of Intracranial Artery with Extraluminal Device, Percutaneous Endoscopic Approach
03LG4DZ Occlusion of Intracranial Artery with Intraluminal Device, Percutaneous Endoscopic Approach

03LG4ZZ	Occlusion of Intracranial Artery, Percutaneous Endoscopic Approach
03LH0BZ	Occlusion of Right Common Carotid Artery with Bioactive Intraluminal Device, Open Approach
03LH0CZ	Occlusion of Right Common Carotid Artery with Extraluminal Device, Open Approach
03LH0DZ	Occlusion of Right Common Carotid Artery with Intraluminal Device, Open Approach
03LH0ZZ	Occlusion of Right Common Carotid Artery, Open Approach
03LH3BZ	Occlusion of Right Common Carotid Artery with Bioactive Intraluminal Device, Percutaneous Approach
03LH3CZ	Occlusion of Right Common Carotid Artery with Extraluminal Device, Percutaneous Approach
03LH3DZ	Occlusion of Right Common Carotid Artery with Intraluminal Device, Percutaneous Approach
03LH3ZZ	Occlusion of Right Common Carotid Artery, Percutaneous Approach
03LH4BZ	Occlusion of Right Common Carotid Artery with Bioactive Intraluminal Device, Percutaneous Endoscopic Approach
03LH4CZ	Occlusion of Right Common Carotid Artery with Extraluminal Device, Percutaneous Endoscopic Approach
03LH4DZ	Occlusion of Right Common Carotid Artery with Intraluminal Device, Percutaneous Endoscopic Approach
03LH4ZZ	Occlusion of Right Common Carotid Artery, Percutaneous Endoscopic Approach
03LJ0BZ	Occlusion of Left Common Carotid Artery with Bioactive Intraluminal Device, Open Approach
03LJ0CZ	Occlusion of Left Common Carotid Artery with Extraluminal Device, Open Approach
03LJ0DZ	Occlusion of Left Common Carotid Artery with Intraluminal Device, Open Approach
03LJ0ZZ	Occlusion of Left Common Carotid Artery, Open Approach
03LJ3BZ	Occlusion of Left Common Carotid Artery with Bioactive Intraluminal Device, Percutaneous Approach
03LJ3CZ	Occlusion of Left Common Carotid Artery with Extraluminal Device, Percutaneous Approach
03LJ3DZ	Occlusion of Left Common Carotid Artery with Intraluminal Device, Percutaneous Approach
03LJ3ZZ	Occlusion of Left Common Carotid Artery, Percutaneous Approach
03LJ4BZ	Occlusion of Left Common Carotid Artery with Bioactive Intraluminal Device, Percutaneous Endoscopic Approach
03LJ4CZ	Occlusion of Left Common Carotid Artery with Extraluminal Device, Percutaneous Endoscopic Approach
03LJ4DZ	Occlusion of Left Common Carotid Artery with Intraluminal Device, Percutaneous Endoscopic Approach
03LJ4ZZ	Occlusion of Left Common Carotid Artery, Percutaneous Endoscopic Approach
03LK0BZ	Occlusion of Right Internal Carotid Artery with Bioactive Intraluminal Device, Open Approach
03LK0CZ	Occlusion of Right Internal Carotid Artery with Extraluminal Device, Open Approach
03LK0DZ	Occlusion of Right Internal Carotid Artery with Intraluminal Device, Open Approach
03LK0ZZ	Occlusion of Right Internal Carotid Artery, Open Approach
03LK3BZ	Occlusion of Right Internal Carotid Artery with Bioactive Intraluminal Device, Percutaneous Approach
03LK3CZ	Occlusion of Right Internal Carotid Artery with Extraluminal Device, Percutaneous Approach
03LK3DZ	Occlusion of Right Internal Carotid Artery with Intraluminal Device, Percutaneous Approach
03LK3ZZ	Occlusion of Right Internal Carotid Artery, Percutaneous Approach
03LK4BZ	Occlusion of Right Internal Carotid Artery with Bioactive Intraluminal Device, Percutaneous Endoscopic Approach
03LK4CZ	Occlusion of Right Internal Carotid Artery with Extraluminal Device, Percutaneous Endoscopic Approach
03LK4DZ	Occlusion of Right Internal Carotid Artery with Intraluminal Device, Percutaneous Endoscopic Approach
03LK4ZZ	Occlusion of Right Internal Carotid Artery, Percutaneous Endoscopic Approach
03LL0BZ	Occlusion of Left Internal Carotid Artery with Bioactive Intraluminal Device, Open Approach
03LL0CZ	Occlusion of Left Internal Carotid Artery with Extraluminal Device, Open Approach
03LL0DZ	Occlusion of Left Internal Carotid Artery with Intraluminal Device, Open Approach
03LL0ZZ	Occlusion of Left Internal Carotid Artery, Open Approach
03LL3BZ	Occlusion of Left Internal Carotid Artery with Bioactive Intraluminal Device, Percutaneous Approach
03LL3CZ	Occlusion of Left Internal Carotid Artery with Extraluminal Device, Percutaneous Approach
03LL3DZ	Occlusion of Left Internal Carotid Artery with Intraluminal Device, Percutaneous Approach
03LL3ZZ	Occlusion of Left Internal Carotid Artery, Percutaneous Approach
03LL4BZ	Occlusion of Left Internal Carotid Artery with Bioactive Intraluminal Device, Percutaneous Endoscopic Approach
03LL4CZ	Occlusion of Left Internal Carotid Artery with Extraluminal Device, Percutaneous Endoscopic Approach
03LL4DZ	Occlusion of Left Internal Carotid Artery with Intraluminal Device, Percutaneous Endoscopic Approach
03LL4ZZ	Occlusion of Left Internal Carotid Artery, Percutaneous Endoscopic Approach
03LM0BZ	Occlusion of Right External Carotid Artery with Bioactive Intraluminal Device, Open Approach
03LM0CZ	Occlusion of Right External Carotid Artery with Extraluminal Device, Open Approach
03LM0DZ	Occlusion of Right External Carotid Artery with Intraluminal Device, Open Approach
03LM0ZZ	Occlusion of Right External Carotid Artery, Open Approach
03LM3BZ	Occlusion of Right External Carotid Artery with Bioactive Intraluminal Device, Percutaneous Approach
03LM3CZ	Occlusion of Right External Carotid Artery with Extraluminal Device, Percutaneous Approach
03LM3DZ	Occlusion of Right External Carotid Artery with Intraluminal Device, Percutaneous Approach
03LM3ZZ	Occlusion of Right External Carotid Artery, Percutaneous Approach
03LM4BZ	Occlusion of Right External Carotid Artery with Bioactive Intraluminal Device, Percutaneous Endoscopic Approach
03LM4CZ	Occlusion of Right External Carotid Artery with Extraluminal Device, Percutaneous Endoscopic Approach
03LM4DZ	Occlusion of Right External Carotid Artery with Intraluminal Device, Percutaneous Endoscopic Approach
03LM4ZZ	Occlusion of Right External Carotid Artery, Percutaneous Endoscopic Approach
03LN0BZ	Occlusion of Left External Carotid Artery with Bioactive Intraluminal Device, Open Approach
03LN0CZ	Occlusion of Left External Carotid Artery with Extraluminal Device, Open Approach
03LN0DZ	Occlusion of Left External Carotid Artery with Intraluminal Device, Open Approach
03LN0ZZ	Occlusion of Left External Carotid Artery, Open Approach
03LN3BZ	Occlusion of Left External Carotid Artery with Bioactive Intraluminal Device, Percutaneous Approach
03LN3CZ	Occlusion of Left External Carotid Artery with Extraluminal Device, Percutaneous Approach
03LN3DZ	Occlusion of Left External Carotid Artery with Intraluminal Device, Percutaneous Approach
03LN3ZZ	Occlusion of Left External Carotid Artery, Percutaneous Approach
03LN4BZ	Occlusion of Left External Carotid Artery with Bioactive Intraluminal Device, Percutaneous Endoscopic Approach
03LN4CZ	Occlusion of Left External Carotid Artery with Extraluminal Device, Percutaneous Endoscopic Approach
03LN4DZ	Occlusion of Left External Carotid Artery with Intraluminal Device, Percutaneous Endoscopic Approach
03LN4ZZ	Occlusion of Left External Carotid Artery, Percutaneous Endoscopic Approach
03LP0BZ	Occlusion of Right Vertebral Artery with Bioactive Intraluminal Device, Open Approach
03LP0CZ	Occlusion of Right Vertebral Artery with Extraluminal Device, Open Approach
03LP0DZ	Occlusion of Right Vertebral Artery with Intraluminal Device, Open Approach
03LP0ZZ	Occlusion of Right Vertebral Artery, Open Approach
03LP3BZ	Occlusion of Right Vertebral Artery with Bioactive Intraluminal Device, Percutaneous Approach
03LP3CZ	Occlusion of Right Vertebral Artery with Extraluminal Device, Percutaneous Approach
03LP3DZ	Occlusion of Right Vertebral Artery with Intraluminal Device, Percutaneous Approach
03LP3ZZ	Occlusion of Right Vertebral Artery, Percutaneous Approach
03LP4BZ	Occlusion of Right Vertebral Artery with Bioactive Intraluminal Device, Percutaneous Endoscopic Approach
03LP4CZ	Occlusion of Right Vertebral Artery with Extraluminal Device, Percutaneous Endoscopic Approach
03LP4DZ	Occlusion of Right Vertebral Artery with Intraluminal Device, Percutaneous Endoscopic Approach
03LP4ZZ	Occlusion of Right Vertebral Artery, Percutaneous Endoscopic Approach
03LQ0BZ	Occlusion of Left Vertebral Artery with Bioactive Intraluminal Device, Open Approach
03LQ0CZ	Occlusion of Left Vertebral Artery with Extraluminal Device, Open Approach
03LQ0DZ	Occlusion of Left Vertebral Artery with Intraluminal Device, Open Approach

Female-only   ♂ Male-only   ▲ Limited Coverage   ● Non-OR   ▧ HAC-associated procedure   ▲ Non-covered procedures   ✚ Combination

03LQ0ZZ	Occlusion of Left Vertebral Artery, Open Approach	03LS3CZ	Occlusion of Right Temporal Artery with Extraluminal Device, Percutaneous Approach	03LU4CZ	Occlusion of Right Thyroid Artery with Extraluminal Device, Percutaneous Endoscopic Approach
03LQ3BZ	Occlusion of Left Vertebral Artery with Bioactive Intraluminal Device, Percutaneous Approach	03LS3DZ	Occlusion of Right Temporal Artery with Intraluminal Device, Percutaneous Approach	03LU4DZ	Occlusion of Right Thyroid Artery with Intraluminal Device, Percutaneous Endoscopic Approach
03LQ3CZ	Occlusion of Left Vertebral Artery with Extraluminal Device, Percutaneous Approach	03LS3ZZ	Occlusion of Right Temporal Artery, Percutaneous Approach	03LU4ZZ	Occlusion of Right Thyroid Artery, Percutaneous Endoscopic Approach
03LQ3DZ	Occlusion of Left Vertebral Artery with Intraluminal Device, Percutaneous Approach	03LS4CZ	Occlusion of Right Temporal Artery with Extraluminal Device, Percutaneous Endoscopic Approach	03LV0CZ	Occlusion of Left Thyroid Artery with Extraluminal Device, Open Approach
03LQ3ZZ	Occlusion of Left Vertebral Artery, Percutaneous Approach	03LS4DZ	Occlusion of Right Temporal Artery with Intraluminal Device, Percutaneous Endoscopic Approach	03LV0DZ	Occlusion of Left Thyroid Artery with Intraluminal Device, Open Approach
03LQ4BZ	Occlusion of Left Vertebral Artery with Bioactive Intraluminal Device, Percutaneous Endoscopic Approach	03LS4ZZ	Occlusion of Right Temporal Artery, Percutaneous Endoscopic Approach	03LV0ZZ	Occlusion of Left Thyroid Artery, Open Approach
03LQ4CZ	Occlusion of Left Vertebral Artery with Extraluminal Device, Percutaneous Endoscopic Approach	03LT0CZ	Occlusion of Left Temporal Artery with Extraluminal Device, Open Approach	03LV3CZ	Occlusion of Left Thyroid Artery with Extraluminal Device, Percutaneous Approach
03LQ4DZ	Occlusion of Left Vertebral Artery with Intraluminal Device, Percutaneous Endoscopic Approach	03LT0DZ	Occlusion of Left Temporal Artery with Intraluminal Device, Open Approach	03LV3DZ	Occlusion of Left Thyroid Artery with Intraluminal Device, Percutaneous Approach
03LQ4ZZ	Occlusion of Left Vertebral Artery, Percutaneous Endoscopic Approach	03LT0ZZ	Occlusion of Left Temporal Artery, Open Approach	03LV3ZZ	Occlusion of Left Thyroid Artery, Percutaneous Approach
03LR0CZ	Occlusion of Face Artery with Extraluminal Device, Open Approach	03LT3CZ	Occlusion of Left Temporal Artery with Extraluminal Device, Percutaneous Approach	03LV4CZ	Occlusion of Left Thyroid Artery with Extraluminal Device, Percutaneous Endoscopic Approach
03LR0DZ	Occlusion of Face Artery with Intraluminal Device, Open Approach	03LT3DZ	Occlusion of Left Temporal Artery with Intraluminal Device, Percutaneous Approach	03LV4DZ	Occlusion of Left Thyroid Artery with Intraluminal Device, Percutaneous Endoscopic Approach
03LR0ZZ	Occlusion of Face Artery, Open Approach	03LT3ZZ	Occlusion of Left Temporal Artery, Percutaneous Approach	03LV4ZZ	Occlusion of Left Thyroid Artery, Percutaneous Endoscopic Approach
03LR3CZ	Occlusion of Face Artery with Extraluminal Device, Percutaneous Approach	03LT4CZ	Occlusion of Left Temporal Artery with Extraluminal Device, Percutaneous Endoscopic Approach	03LY0CZ	Occlusion of Upper Artery with Extraluminal Device, Open Approach
03LR3DZ	Occlusion of Face Artery with Intraluminal Device, Percutaneous Approach	03LT4DZ	Occlusion of Left Temporal Artery with Intraluminal Device, Percutaneous Endoscopic Approach	03LY0DZ	Occlusion of Upper Artery with Intraluminal Device, Open Approach
03LR3ZZ	Occlusion of Face Artery, Percutaneous Approach	03LT4ZZ	Occlusion of Left Temporal Artery, Percutaneous Endoscopic Approach	03LY0ZZ	Occlusion of Upper Artery, Open Approach
03LR4CZ	Occlusion of Face Artery with Extraluminal Device, Percutaneous Endoscopic Approach	03LU0CZ	Occlusion of Right Thyroid Artery with Extraluminal Device, Open Approach	03LY3CZ	Occlusion of Upper Artery with Extraluminal Device, Percutaneous Approach
03LR4DZ	Occlusion of Face Artery with Intraluminal Device, Percutaneous Endoscopic Approach	03LU0DZ	Occlusion of Right Thyroid Artery with Intraluminal Device, Open Approach	03LY3DZ	Occlusion of Upper Artery with Intraluminal Device, Percutaneous Approach
03LR4ZZ	Occlusion of Face Artery, Percutaneous Endoscopic Approach	03LU0ZZ	Occlusion of Right Thyroid Artery, Open Approach	03LY3ZZ	Occlusion of Upper Artery, Percutaneous Approach
03LS0CZ	Occlusion of Right Temporal Artery with Extraluminal Device, Open Approach	03LU3CZ	Occlusion of Right Thyroid Artery with Extraluminal Device, Percutaneous Approach	03LY4CZ	Occlusion of Upper Artery with Extraluminal Device, Percutaneous Endoscopic Approach
03LS0DZ	Occlusion of Right Temporal Artery with Intraluminal Device, Open Approach	03LU3DZ	Occlusion of Right Thyroid Artery with Intraluminal Device, Percutaneous Approach	03LY4DZ	Occlusion of Upper Artery with Intraluminal Device, Percutaneous Endoscopic Approach
03LS0ZZ	Occlusion of Right Temporal Artery, Open Approach	03LU3ZZ	Occlusion of Right Thyroid Artery, Percutaneous Approach	03LY4ZZ	Occlusion of Upper Artery, Percutaneous Endoscopic Approach

03N – Upper Arteries, Release

Review Coding Guidelines B3.13 and B3.14

03N00ZZ	Release Right Internal Mammary Artery, Open Approach	03N33ZZ	Release Right Subclavian Artery, Percutaneous Approach	03N64ZZ	Release Left Axillary Artery, Percutaneous Endoscopic Approach
03N03ZZ	Release Right Internal Mammary Artery, Percutaneous Approach	03N34ZZ	Release Right Subclavian Artery, Percutaneous Endoscopic Approach	03N70ZZ	Release Right Brachial Artery, Open Approach
03N04ZZ	Release Right Internal Mammary Artery, Percutaneous Endoscopic Approach	03N40ZZ	Release Left Subclavian Artery, Open Approach	03N73ZZ	Release Right Brachial Artery, Percutaneous Approach
03N10ZZ	Release Left Internal Mammary Artery, Open Approach	03N43ZZ	Release Left Subclavian Artery, Percutaneous Approach	03N74ZZ	Release Right Brachial Artery, Percutaneous Endoscopic Approach
03N13ZZ	Release Left Internal Mammary Artery, Percutaneous Approach	03N44ZZ	Release Left Subclavian Artery, Percutaneous Endoscopic Approach	03N80ZZ	Release Left Brachial Artery, Open Approach
03N14ZZ	Release Left Internal Mammary Artery, Percutaneous Endoscopic Approach	03N50ZZ	Release Right Axillary Artery, Open Approach	03N83ZZ	Release Left Brachial Artery, Percutaneous Approach
03N20ZZ	Release Innominate Artery, Open Approach	03N53ZZ	Release Right Axillary Artery, Percutaneous Approach	03N84ZZ	Release Left Brachial Artery, Percutaneous Endoscopic Approach
03N23ZZ	Release Innominate Artery, Percutaneous Approach	03N54ZZ	Release Right Axillary Artery, Percutaneous Endoscopic Approach	03N90ZZ	Release Right Ulnar Artery, Open Approach
03N24ZZ	Release Innominate Artery, Percutaneous Endoscopic Approach	03N60ZZ	Release Left Axillary Artery, Open Approach	03N93ZZ	Release Right Ulnar Artery, Percutaneous Approach
03N30ZZ	Release Right Subclavian Artery, Open Approach	03N63ZZ	Release Left Axillary Artery, Percutaneous Approach	03N94ZZ	Release Right Ulnar Artery, Percutaneous Endoscopic Approach

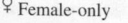

♀ Female-only   ♂ Male-only   ▲ Limited Coverage   ● Non-OR   ▨ HAC-associated procedure   ▲ Non-covered procedures   ✚ Combination

NA0ZZ	Release Left Ulnar Artery, Open Approach	03NH4ZZ	Release Right Common Carotid Artery, Percutaneous Endoscopic Approach	03NQ3ZZ	Release Left Vertebral Artery, Percutaneous Approach
NA3ZZ	Release Left Ulnar Artery, Percutaneous Approach	03NJ0ZZ	Release Left Common Carotid Artery, Open Approach	03NQ4ZZ	Release Left Vertebral Artery, Percutaneous Endoscopic Approach
NA4ZZ	Release Left Ulnar Artery, Percutaneous Endoscopic Approach	03NJ3ZZ	Release Left Common Carotid Artery, Percutaneous Approach	03NR0ZZ	Release Face Artery, Open Approach
NB0ZZ	Release Right Radial Artery, Open Approach	03NJ4ZZ	Release Left Common Carotid Artery, Percutaneous Endoscopic Approach	03NR3ZZ	Release Face Artery, Percutaneous Approach
NB3ZZ	Release Right Radial Artery, Percutaneous Approach	03NK0ZZ	Release Right Internal Carotid Artery, Open Approach	03NR4ZZ	Release Face Artery, Percutaneous Endoscopic Approach
NB4ZZ	Release Right Radial Artery, Percutaneous Endoscopic Approach	03NK3ZZ	Release Right Internal Carotid Artery, Percutaneous Approach	03NS0ZZ	Release Right Temporal Artery, Open Approach
NC0ZZ	Release Left Radial Artery, Open Approach	03NK4ZZ	Release Right Internal Carotid Artery, Percutaneous Endoscopic Approach	03NS3ZZ	Release Right Temporal Artery, Percutaneous Approach
NC3ZZ	Release Left Radial Artery, Percutaneous Approach	03NL0ZZ	Release Left Internal Carotid Artery, Open Approach	03NS4ZZ	Release Right Temporal Artery, Percutaneous Endoscopic Approach
NC4ZZ	Release Left Radial Artery, Percutaneous Endoscopic Approach	03NL3ZZ	Release Left Internal Carotid Artery, Percutaneous Approach	03NT0ZZ	Release Left Temporal Artery, Open Approach
ND0ZZ	Release Right Hand Artery, Open Approach	03NL4ZZ	Release Left Internal Carotid Artery, Percutaneous Endoscopic Approach	03NT3ZZ	Release Left Temporal Artery, Percutaneous Approach
ND3ZZ	Release Right Hand Artery, Percutaneous Approach	03NM0ZZ	Release Right External Carotid Artery, Open Approach	03NT4ZZ	Release Left Temporal Artery, Percutaneous Endoscopic Approach
ND4ZZ	Release Right Hand Artery, Percutaneous Endoscopic Approach	03NM3ZZ	Release Right External Carotid Artery, Percutaneous Approach	03NU0ZZ	Release Right Thyroid Artery, Open Approach
NF0ZZ	Release Left Hand Artery, Open Approach	03NM4ZZ	Release Right External Carotid Artery, Percutaneous Endoscopic Approach	03NU3ZZ	Release Right Thyroid Artery, Percutaneous Approach
NF3ZZ	Release Left Hand Artery, Percutaneous Approach	03NN0ZZ	Release Left External Carotid Artery, Open Approach	03NU4ZZ	Release Right Thyroid Artery, Percutaneous Endoscopic Approach
NF4ZZ	Release Left Hand Artery, Percutaneous Endoscopic Approach	03NN3ZZ	Release Left External Carotid Artery, Percutaneous Approach	03NV0ZZ	Release Left Thyroid Artery, Open Approach
NG0ZZ	Release Intracranial Artery, Open Approach	03NN4ZZ	Release Left External Carotid Artery, Percutaneous Endoscopic Approach	03NV3ZZ	Release Left Thyroid Artery, Percutaneous Approach
NG3ZZ	Release Intracranial Artery, Percutaneous Approach	03NP0ZZ	Release Right Vertebral Artery, Open Approach	03NV4ZZ	Release Left Thyroid Artery, Percutaneous Endoscopic Approach
NG4ZZ	Release Intracranial Artery, Percutaneous Endoscopic Approach	03NP3ZZ	Release Right Vertebral Artery, Percutaneous Approach	03NY0ZZ	Release Upper Artery, Open Approach
NH0ZZ	Release Right Common Carotid Artery, Open Approach	03NP4ZZ	Release Right Vertebral Artery, Percutaneous Endoscopic Approach	03NY3ZZ	Release Upper Artery, Percutaneous Approach
NH3ZZ	Release Right Common Carotid Artery, Percutaneous Approach	03NQ0ZZ	Release Left Vertebral Artery, Open Approach	03NY4ZZ	Release Upper Artery, Percutaneous Endoscopic Approach

3P – Upper Arteries, Removal

eview Coding Guideline B6.1c

3PY00Z	Removal of Drainage Device from Upper Artery, Open Approach	03PY37Z	Removal of Autologous Tissue Substitute from Upper Artery, Percutaneous Approach	03PY4CZ	Removal of Extraluminal Device from Upper Artery, Percutaneous Endoscopic Approach
3PY02Z	Removal of Monitoring Device from Upper Artery, Open Approach	03PY3CZ	Removal of Extraluminal Device from Upper Artery, Percutaneous Approach	03PY4DZ	Removal of Intraluminal Device from Upper Artery, Percutaneous Endoscopic Approach
3PY03Z	Removal of Infusion Device from Upper Artery, Open Approach	03PY3DZ	Removal of Intraluminal Device from Upper Artery, Percutaneous Approach	03PY4JZ	Removal of Synthetic Substitute from Upper Artery, Percutaneous Endoscopic Approach
3PY07Z	Removal of Autologous Tissue Substitute from Upper Artery, Open Approach	03PY3JZ	Removal of Synthetic Substitute from Upper Artery, Percutaneous Approach	03PY4KZ	Removal of Nonautologous Tissue Substitute from Upper Artery, Percutaneous Endoscopic Approach
3PY0CZ	Removal of Extraluminal Device from Upper Artery, Open Approach	03PY3KZ	Removal of Nonautologous Tissue Substitute from Upper Artery, Percutaneous Approach		
3PY0DZ	Removal of Intraluminal Device from Upper Artery, Open Approach	03PY3MZ	Removal of Stimulator Lead from Upper Artery, Percutaneous Approach	03PY4MZ	Removal of Stimulator Lead from Upper Artery, Percutaneous Endoscopic Approach
3PY0JZ	Removal of Synthetic Substitute from Upper Artery, Open Approach	03PY40Z	Removal of Drainage Device from Upper Artery, Percutaneous Endoscopic Approach	03PYX0Z	Removal of Drainage Device from Upper Artery, External Approach
3PY0KZ	Removal of Nonautologous Tissue Substitute from Upper Artery, Open Approach	03PY42Z	Removal of Monitoring Device from Upper Artery, Percutaneous Endoscopic Approach	03PYX2Z	Removal of Monitoring Device from Upper Artery, External Approach
3PY0MZ	Removal of Stimulator Lead from Upper Artery, Open Approach	03PY43Z	Removal of Infusion Device from Upper Artery, Percutaneous Endoscopic Approach	03PYX3Z	Removal of Infusion Device from Upper Artery, External Approach
3PY30Z	Removal of Drainage Device from Upper Artery, Percutaneous Approach			03PYXDZ	Removal of Intraluminal Device from Upper Artery, External Approach
3PY32Z	Removal of Monitoring Device from Upper Artery, Percutaneous Approach	03PY47Z	Removal of Autologous Tissue Substitute from Upper Artery, Percutaneous Endoscopic Approach	03PYXMZ	Removal of Stimulator Lead from Upper Artery, External Approach
3PY33Z	Removal of Infusion Device from Upper Artery, Percutaneous Approach				

3Q – Upper Arteries, Repair

3Q00ZZ	Repair Right Internal Mammary Artery, Open Approach	03Q04ZZ	Repair Right Internal Mammary Artery, Percutaneous Endoscopic Approach	03Q13ZZ	Repair Left Internal Mammary Artery, Percutaneous Approach
3Q03ZZ	Repair Right Internal Mammary Artery, Percutaneous Approach	03Q10ZZ	Repair Left Internal Mammary Artery, Open Approach	03Q14ZZ	Repair Left Internal Mammary Artery, Percutaneous Endoscopic Approach

Female-only	♂ Male-only	▲ Limited Coverage	● Non-OR	▦ HAC-associated procedure	▲ Non-covered procedures	✚ Combination

03Q20ZZ	Repair Innominate Artery, Open Approach
03Q23ZZ	Repair Innominate Artery, Percutaneous Approach
03Q24ZZ	Repair Innominate Artery, Percutaneous Endoscopic Approach
03Q30ZZ	Repair Right Subclavian Artery, Open Approach
03Q33ZZ	Repair Right Subclavian Artery, Percutaneous Approach
03Q34ZZ	Repair Right Subclavian Artery, Percutaneous Endoscopic Approach
03Q40ZZ	Repair Left Subclavian Artery, Open Approach
03Q43ZZ	Repair Left Subclavian Artery, Percutaneous Approach
03Q44ZZ	Repair Left Subclavian Artery, Percutaneous Endoscopic Approach
03Q50ZZ	Repair Right Axillary Artery, Open Approach
03Q53ZZ	Repair Right Axillary Artery, Percutaneous Approach
03Q54ZZ	Repair Right Axillary Artery, Percutaneous Endoscopic Approach
03Q60ZZ	Repair Left Axillary Artery, Open Approach
03Q63ZZ	Repair Left Axillary Artery, Percutaneous Approach
03Q64ZZ	Repair Left Axillary Artery, Percutaneous Endoscopic Approach
03Q70ZZ	Repair Right Brachial Artery, Open Approach
03Q73ZZ	Repair Right Brachial Artery, Percutaneous Approach
03Q74ZZ	Repair Right Brachial Artery, Percutaneous Endoscopic Approach
03Q80ZZ	Repair Left Brachial Artery, Open Approach
03Q83ZZ	Repair Left Brachial Artery, Percutaneous Approach
03Q84ZZ	Repair Left Brachial Artery, Percutaneous Endoscopic Approach
03Q90ZZ	Repair Right Ulnar Artery, Open Approach
03Q93ZZ	Repair Right Ulnar Artery, Percutaneous Approach
03Q94ZZ	Repair Right Ulnar Artery, Percutaneous Endoscopic Approach
03QA0ZZ	Repair Left Ulnar Artery, Open Approach
03QA3ZZ	Repair Left Ulnar Artery, Percutaneous Approach
03QA4ZZ	Repair Left Ulnar Artery, Percutaneous Endoscopic Approach
03QB0ZZ	Repair Right Radial Artery, Open Approach
03QB3ZZ	Repair Right Radial Artery, Percutaneous Approach

03QB4ZZ	Repair Right Radial Artery, Percutaneous Endoscopic Approach
03QC0ZZ	Repair Left Radial Artery, Open Approach
03QC3ZZ	Repair Left Radial Artery, Percutaneous Approach
03QC4ZZ	Repair Left Radial Artery, Percutaneous Endoscopic Approach
03QD0ZZ	Repair Right Hand Artery, Open Approach
03QD3ZZ	Repair Right Hand Artery, Percutaneous Approach
03QD4ZZ	Repair Right Hand Artery, Percutaneous Endoscopic Approach
03QF0ZZ	Repair Left Hand Artery, Open Approach
03QF3ZZ	Repair Left Hand Artery, Percutaneous Approach
03QF4ZZ	Repair Left Hand Artery, Percutaneous Endoscopic Approach
03QG0ZZ	Repair Intracranial Artery, Open Approach
03QG3ZZ	Repair Intracranial Artery, Percutaneous Approach
03QG4ZZ	Repair Intracranial Artery, Percutaneous Endoscopic Approach
03QH0ZZ	Repair Right Common Carotid Artery, Open Approach
03QH3ZZ	Repair Right Common Carotid Artery, Percutaneous Approach
03QH4ZZ	Repair Right Common Carotid Artery, Percutaneous Endoscopic Approach
03QJ0ZZ	Repair Left Common Carotid Artery, Open Approach
03QJ3ZZ	Repair Left Common Carotid Artery, Percutaneous Approach
03QJ4ZZ	Repair Left Common Carotid Artery, Percutaneous Endoscopic Approach
03QK0ZZ	Repair Right Internal Carotid Artery, Open Approach
03QK3ZZ	Repair Right Internal Carotid Artery, Percutaneous Approach
03QK4ZZ	Repair Right Internal Carotid Artery, Percutaneous Endoscopic Approach
03QL0ZZ	Repair Left Internal Carotid Artery, Open Approach
03QL3ZZ	Repair Left Internal Carotid Artery, Percutaneous Approach
03QL4ZZ	Repair Left Internal Carotid Artery, Percutaneous Endoscopic Approach
03QM0ZZ	Repair Right External Carotid Artery, Open Approach
03QM3ZZ	Repair Right External Carotid Artery, Percutaneous Approach
03QM4ZZ	Repair Right External Carotid Artery, Percutaneous Endoscopic Approach

03QN0ZZ	Repair Left External Carotid Artery, Open Approach
03QN3ZZ	Repair Left External Carotid Artery, Percutaneous Approach
03QN4ZZ	Repair Left External Carotid Artery, Percutaneous Endoscopic Approach
03QP0ZZ	Repair Right Vertebral Artery, Open Approach
03QP3ZZ	Repair Right Vertebral Artery, Percutaneous Approach
03QP4ZZ	Repair Right Vertebral Artery, Percutaneous Endoscopic Approach
03QQ0ZZ	Repair Left Vertebral Artery, Open Approach
03QQ3ZZ	Repair Left Vertebral Artery, Percutaneous Approach
03QQ4ZZ	Repair Left Vertebral Artery, Percutaneous Endoscopic Approach
03QR0ZZ	Repair Face Artery, Open Approach
03QR3ZZ	Repair Face Artery, Percutaneous Approach
03QR4ZZ	Repair Face Artery, Percutaneous Endoscopic Approach
03QS0ZZ	Repair Right Temporal Artery, Open Approach
03QS3ZZ	Repair Right Temporal Artery, Percutaneous Approach
03QS4ZZ	Repair Right Temporal Artery, Percutaneous Endoscopic Approach
03QT0ZZ	Repair Left Temporal Artery, Open Approach
03QT3ZZ	Repair Left Temporal Artery, Percutaneous Approach
03QT4ZZ	Repair Left Temporal Artery, Percutaneous Endoscopic Approach
03QU0ZZ	Repair Right Thyroid Artery, Open Approach
03QU3ZZ	Repair Right Thyroid Artery, Percutaneous Approach
03QU4ZZ	Repair Right Thyroid Artery, Percutaneous Endoscopic Approach
03QV0ZZ	Repair Left Thyroid Artery, Open Approach
03QV3ZZ	Repair Left Thyroid Artery, Percutaneous Approach
03QV4ZZ	Repair Left Thyroid Artery, Percutaneous Endoscopic Approach
03QY0ZZ	Repair Upper Artery, Open Approach
03QY3ZZ	Repair Upper Artery, Percutaneous Approach
03QY4ZZ	Repair Upper Artery, Percutaneous Endoscopic Approach

03R – Upper Arteries, Replacement

03R007Z	Replacement of Right Internal Mammary Artery with Autologous Tissue Substitute, Open Approach
03R00JZ	Replacement of Right Internal Mammary Artery with Synthetic Substitute, Open Approach
03R00KZ	Replacement of Right Internal Mammary Artery with Nonautologous Tissue Substitute, Open Approach
03R047Z	Replacement of Right Internal Mammary Artery with Autologous Tissue Substitute, Percutaneous Endoscopic Approach
03R04JZ	Replacement of Right Internal Mammary Artery with Synthetic Substitute, Percutaneous Endoscopic Approach
03R04KZ	Replacement of Right Internal Mammary Artery with Nonautologous Tissue Substitute, Percutaneous Endoscopic Approach
03R107Z	Replacement of Left Internal Mammary Artery with Autologous Tissue Substitute, Open Approach

03R10JZ	Replacement of Left Internal Mammary Artery with Synthetic Substitute, Open Approach
03R10KZ	Replacement of Left Internal Mammary Artery with Nonautologous Tissue Substitute, Open Approach
03R147Z	Replacement of Left Internal Mammary Artery with Autologous Tissue Substitute, Percutaneous Endoscopic Approach
03R14JZ	Replacement of Left Internal Mammary Artery with Synthetic Substitute, Percutaneous Endoscopic Approach
03R14KZ	Replacement of Left Internal Mammary Artery with Nonautologous Tissue Substitute, Percutaneous Endoscopic Approach
03R207Z	Replacement of Innominate Artery with Autologous Tissue Substitute, Open Approach
03R20JZ	Replacement of Innominate Artery with Synthetic Substitute, Open Approach

03R20KZ	Replacement of Innominate Artery with Nonautologous Tissue Substitute, Open Approach
03R247Z	Replacement of Innominate Artery with Autologous Tissue Substitute, Percutaneous Endoscopic Approach
03R24JZ	Replacement of Innominate Artery with Synthetic Substitute, Percutaneous Endoscopic Approach
03R24KZ	Replacement of Innominate Artery with Nonautologous Tissue Substitute, Percutaneous Endoscopic Approach
03R307Z	Replacement of Right Subclavian Artery with Autologous Tissue Substitute, Open Approach
03R30JZ	Replacement of Right Subclavian Artery with Synthetic Substitute, Open Approach
03R30KZ	Replacement of Right Subclavian Artery with Nonautologous Tissue Substitute, Open Approach

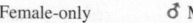

♀ Female-only   ♂ Male-only   ▲ Limited Coverage   ● Non-OR   ▬ HAC-associated procedure   ▲ Non-covered procedures   ✛ Combination

03R347Z Replacement of Right Subclavian Artery with Autologous Tissue Substitute, Percutaneous Endoscopic Approach

03R34JZ Replacement of Right Subclavian Artery with Synthetic Substitute, Percutaneous Endoscopic Approach

03R34KZ Replacement of Right Subclavian Artery with Nonautologous Tissue Substitute, Percutaneous Endoscopic Approach

03R407Z Replacement of Left Subclavian Artery with Autologous Tissue Substitute, Open Approach

03R40JZ Replacement of Left Subclavian Artery with Synthetic Substitute, Open Approach

03R40KZ Replacement of Left Subclavian Artery with Nonautologous Tissue Substitute, Open Approach

03R447Z Replacement of Left Subclavian Artery with Autologous Tissue Substitute, Percutaneous Endoscopic Approach

03R44JZ Replacement of Left Subclavian Artery with Synthetic Substitute, Percutaneous Endoscopic Approach

03R44KZ Replacement of Left Subclavian Artery with Nonautologous Tissue Substitute, Percutaneous Endoscopic Approach

03R507Z Replacement of Right Axillary Artery with Autologous Tissue Substitute, Open Approach

03R50JZ Replacement of Right Axillary Artery with Synthetic Substitute, Open Approach

03R50KZ Replacement of Right Axillary Artery with Nonautologous Tissue Substitute, Open Approach

03R547Z Replacement of Right Axillary Artery with Autologous Tissue Substitute, Percutaneous Endoscopic Approach

03R54JZ Replacement of Right Axillary Artery with Synthetic Substitute, Percutaneous Endoscopic Approach

03R54KZ Replacement of Right Axillary Artery with Nonautologous Tissue Substitute, Percutaneous Endoscopic Approach

03R607Z Replacement of Left Axillary Artery with Autologous Tissue Substitute, Open Approach

03R60JZ Replacement of Left Axillary Artery with Synthetic Substitute, Open Approach

03R60KZ Replacement of Left Axillary Artery with Nonautologous Tissue Substitute, Open Approach

03R647Z Replacement of Left Axillary Artery with Autologous Tissue Substitute, Percutaneous Endoscopic Approach

03R64JZ Replacement of Left Axillary Artery with Synthetic Substitute, Percutaneous Endoscopic Approach

03R64KZ Replacement of Left Axillary Artery with Nonautologous Tissue Substitute, Percutaneous Endoscopic Approach

03R707Z Replacement of Right Brachial Artery with Autologous Tissue Substitute, Open Approach

03R70JZ Replacement of Right Brachial Artery with Synthetic Substitute, Open Approach

03R70KZ Replacement of Right Brachial Artery with Nonautologous Tissue Substitute, Open Approach

03R747Z Replacement of Right Brachial Artery with Autologous Tissue Substitute, Percutaneous Endoscopic Approach

03R74JZ Replacement of Right Brachial Artery with Synthetic Substitute, Percutaneous Endoscopic Approach

03R74KZ Replacement of Right Brachial Artery with Nonautologous Tissue Substitute, Percutaneous Endoscopic Approach

03R807Z Replacement of Left Brachial Artery with Autologous Tissue Substitute, Open Approach

03R80JZ Replacement of Left Brachial Artery with Synthetic Substitute, Open Approach

03R80KZ Replacement of Left Brachial Artery with Nonautologous Tissue Substitute, Open Approach

03R847Z Replacement of Left Brachial Artery with Autologous Tissue Substitute, Percutaneous Endoscopic Approach

03R84JZ Replacement of Left Brachial Artery with Synthetic Substitute, Percutaneous Endoscopic Approach

03R84KZ Replacement of Left Brachial Artery with Nonautologous Tissue Substitute, Percutaneous Endoscopic Approach

03R907Z Replacement of Right Ulnar Artery with Autologous Tissue Substitute, Open Approach

03R90JZ Replacement of Right Ulnar Artery with Synthetic Substitute, Open Approach

03R90KZ Replacement of Right Ulnar Artery with Nonautologous Tissue Substitute, Open Approach

03R947Z Replacement of Right Ulnar Artery with Autologous Tissue Substitute, Percutaneous Endoscopic Approach

03R94JZ Replacement of Right Ulnar Artery with Synthetic Substitute, Percutaneous Endoscopic Approach

03R94KZ Replacement of Right Ulnar Artery with Nonautologous Tissue Substitute, Percutaneous Endoscopic Approach

03RA07Z Replacement of Left Ulnar Artery with Autologous Tissue Substitute, Open Approach

03RA0JZ Replacement of Left Ulnar Artery with Synthetic Substitute, Open Approach

03RA0KZ Replacement of Left Ulnar Artery with Nonautologous Tissue Substitute, Open Approach

03RA47Z Replacement of Left Ulnar Artery with Autologous Tissue Substitute, Percutaneous Endoscopic Approach

03RA4JZ Replacement of Left Ulnar Artery with Synthetic Substitute, Percutaneous Endoscopic Approach

03RA4KZ Replacement of Left Ulnar Artery with Nonautologous Tissue Substitute, Percutaneous Endoscopic Approach

03RB07Z Replacement of Right Radial Artery with Autologous Tissue Substitute, Open Approach

03RB0JZ Replacement of Right Radial Artery with Synthetic Substitute, Open Approach

03RB0KZ Replacement of Right Radial Artery with Nonautologous Tissue Substitute, Open Approach

03RB47Z Replacement of Right Radial Artery with Autologous Tissue Substitute, Percutaneous Endoscopic Approach

03RB4JZ Replacement of Right Radial Artery with Synthetic Substitute, Percutaneous Endoscopic Approach

03RB4KZ Replacement of Right Radial Artery with Nonautologous Tissue Substitute, Percutaneous Endoscopic Approach

03RC07Z Replacement of Left Radial Artery with Autologous Tissue Substitute, Open Approach

03RC0JZ Replacement of Left Radial Artery with Synthetic Substitute, Open Approach

03RC0KZ Replacement of Left Radial Artery with Nonautologous Tissue Substitute, Open Approach

03RC47Z Replacement of Left Radial Artery with Autologous Tissue Substitute, Percutaneous Endoscopic Approach

03RC4JZ Replacement of Left Radial Artery with Synthetic Substitute, Percutaneous Endoscopic Approach

03RC4KZ Replacement of Left Radial Artery with Nonautologous Tissue Substitute, Percutaneous Endoscopic Approach

03RD07Z Replacement of Right Hand Artery with Autologous Tissue Substitute, Open Approach

03RD0JZ Replacement of Right Hand Artery with Synthetic Substitute, Open Approach

03RD0KZ Replacement of Right Hand Artery with Nonautologous Tissue Substitute, Open Approach

03RD47Z Replacement of Right Hand Artery with Autologous Tissue Substitute, Percutaneous Endoscopic Approach

03RD4JZ Replacement of Right Hand Artery with Synthetic Substitute, Percutaneous Endoscopic Approach

03RD4KZ Replacement of Right Hand Artery with Nonautologous Tissue Substitute, Percutaneous Endoscopic Approach

03RF07Z Replacement of Left Hand Artery with Autologous Tissue Substitute, Open Approach

03RF0JZ Replacement of Left Hand Artery with Synthetic Substitute, Open Approach

03RF0KZ Replacement of Left Hand Artery with Nonautologous Tissue Substitute, Open Approach

03RF47Z Replacement of Left Hand Artery with Autologous Tissue Substitute, Percutaneous Endoscopic Approach

03RF4JZ Replacement of Left Hand Artery with Synthetic Substitute, Percutaneous Endoscopic Approach

03RF4KZ Replacement of Left Hand Artery with Nonautologous Tissue Substitute, Percutaneous Endoscopic Approach

03RG07Z Replacement of Intracranial Artery with Autologous Tissue Substitute, Open Approach

03RG0JZ Replacement of Intracranial Artery with Synthetic Substitute, Open Approach

03RG0KZ Replacement of Intracranial Artery with Nonautologous Tissue Substitute, Open Approach

03RG47Z Replacement of Intracranial Artery with Autologous Tissue Substitute, Percutaneous Endoscopic Approach

03RG4JZ Replacement of Intracranial Artery with Synthetic Substitute, Percutaneous Endoscopic Approach

03RG4KZ Replacement of Intracranial Artery with Nonautologous Tissue Substitute, Percutaneous Endoscopic Approach

03RH07Z Replacement of Right Common Carotid Artery with Autologous Tissue Substitute, Open Approach

03RH0JZ Replacement of Right Common Carotid Artery with Synthetic Substitute, Open Approach

03RH0KZ Replacement of Right Common Carotid Artery with Nonautologous Tissue Substitute, Open Approach

03RH47Z Replacement of Right Common Carotid Artery with Autologous Tissue Substitute, Percutaneous Endoscopic Approach

03RH4JZ Replacement of Right Common Carotid Artery with Synthetic Substitute, Percutaneous Endoscopic Approach

03RH4KZ Replacement of Right Common Carotid Artery with Nonautologous Tissue Substitute, Percutaneous Endoscopic Approach

03RJ07Z Replacement of Left Common Carotid Artery with Autologous Tissue Substitute, Open Approach

03RJ0JZ Replacement of Left Common Carotid Artery with Synthetic Substitute, Open Approach

03RJ0KZ Replacement of Left Common Carotid Artery with Nonautologous Tissue Substitute, Open Approach

03RJ47Z Replacement of Left Common Carotid Artery with Autologous Tissue Substitute, Percutaneous Endoscopic Approach

03RJ4JZ Replacement of Left Common Carotid Artery with Synthetic Substitute, Percutaneous Endoscopic Approach

03RJ4KZ Replacement of Left Common Carotid Artery with Nonautologous Tissue Substitute, Percutaneous Endoscopic Approach

03RK07Z Replacement of Right Internal Carotid Artery with Autologous Tissue Substitute, Open Approach

03RK0JZ Replacement of Right Internal Carotid Artery with Synthetic Substitute, Open Approach

03RK0KZ Replacement of Right Internal Carotid Artery with Nonautologous Tissue Substitute, Open Approach

03RK47Z Replacement of Right Internal Carotid Artery with Autologous Tissue Substitute, Percutaneous Endoscopic Approach

03RK4JZ Replacement of Right Internal Carotid Artery with Synthetic Substitute, Percutaneous Endoscopic Approach

03RK4KZ Replacement of Right Internal Carotid Artery with Nonautologous Tissue Substitute, Percutaneous Endoscopic Approach

03RL07Z Replacement of Left Internal Carotid Artery with Autologous Tissue Substitute, Open Approach

03RL0JZ Replacement of Left Internal Carotid Artery with Synthetic Substitute, Open Approach

03RL0KZ Replacement of Left Internal Carotid Artery with Nonautologous Tissue Substitute, Open Approach

03RL47Z Replacement of Left Internal Carotid Artery with Autologous Tissue Substitute, Percutaneous Endoscopic Approach

03RL4JZ Replacement of Left Internal Carotid Artery with Synthetic Substitute, Percutaneous Endoscopic Approach

03RL4KZ Replacement of Left Internal Carotid Artery with Nonautologous Tissue Substitute, Percutaneous Endoscopic Approach

03RM07Z Replacement of Right External Carotid Artery with Autologous Tissue Substitute, Open Approach

03RM0JZ Replacement of Right External Carotid Artery with Synthetic Substitute, Open Approach

03RM0KZ Replacement of Right External Carotid Artery with Nonautologous Tissue Substitute, Open Approach

03RM47Z Replacement of Right External Carotid Artery with Autologous Tissue Substitute, Percutaneous Endoscopic Approach

03RM4JZ Replacement of Right External Carotid Artery with Synthetic Substitute, Percutaneous Endoscopic Approach

03RM4KZ Replacement of Right External Carotid Artery with Nonautologous Tissue Substitute, Percutaneous Endoscopic Approach

03RN07Z Replacement of Left External Carotid Artery with Autologous Tissue Substitute, Open Approach

03RN0JZ Replacement of Left External Carotid Artery with Synthetic Substitute, Open Approach

03RN0KZ Replacement of Left External Carotid Artery with Nonautologous Tissue Substitute, Open Approach

03RN47Z Replacement of Left External Carotid Artery with Autologous Tissue Substitute, Percutaneous Endoscopic Approach

03RN4JZ Replacement of Left External Carotid Artery with Synthetic Substitute, Percutaneous Endoscopic Approach

03RN4KZ Replacement of Left External Carotid Artery with Nonautologous Tissue Substitute, Percutaneous Endoscopic Approach

03RP07Z Replacement of Right Vertebral Artery with Autologous Tissue Substitute, Open Approach

03RP0JZ Replacement of Right Vertebral Artery with Synthetic Substitute, Open Approach

03RP0KZ Replacement of Right Vertebral Artery with Nonautologous Tissue Substitute, Open Approach

03RP47Z Replacement of Right Vertebral Artery with Autologous Tissue Substitute, Percutaneous Endoscopic Approach

03RP4JZ Replacement of Right Vertebral Artery with Synthetic Substitute, Percutaneous Endoscopic Approach

03RP4KZ Replacement of Right Vertebral Artery with Nonautologous Tissue Substitute, Percutaneous Endoscopic Approach

03RQ07Z Replacement of Left Vertebral Artery with Autologous Tissue Substitute, Open Approach

03RQ0JZ Replacement of Left Vertebral Artery with Synthetic Substitute, Open Approach

03RQ0KZ Replacement of Left Vertebral Artery with Nonautologous Tissue Substitute, Open Approach

03RQ47Z Replacement of Left Vertebral Artery with Autologous Tissue Substitute, Percutaneous Endoscopic Approach

03RQ4JZ Replacement of Left Vertebral Artery with Synthetic Substitute, Percutaneous Endoscopic Approach

03RQ4KZ Replacement of Left Vertebral Artery with Nonautologous Tissue Substitute, Percutaneous Endoscopic Approach

03RR07Z Replacement of Face Artery with Autologous Tissue Substitute, Open Approach

03RR0JZ Replacement of Face Artery with Synthetic Substitute, Open Approach

03RR0KZ Replacement of Face Artery with Nonautologous Tissue Substitute, Open Approach

03RR47Z Replacement of Face Artery with Autologous Tissue Substitute, Percutaneous Endoscopic Approach

03RR4JZ Replacement of Face Artery with Synthetic Substitute, Percutaneous Endoscopic Approach

03RR4KZ Replacement of Face Artery with Nonautologous Tissue Substitute, Percutaneous Endoscopic Approach

03RS07Z Replacement of Right Temporal Artery with Autologous Tissue Substitute, Open Approach

03RS0JZ Replacement of Right Temporal Artery with Synthetic Substitute, Open Approach

03RS0KZ Replacement of Right Temporal Artery with Nonautologous Tissue Substitute, Open Approach

03RS47Z Replacement of Right Temporal Artery with Autologous Tissue Substitute, Percutaneous Endoscopic Approach

03RS4JZ Replacement of Right Temporal Artery with Synthetic Substitute, Percutaneous Endoscopic Approach

03RS4KZ Replacement of Right Temporal Artery with Nonautologous Tissue Substitute, Percutaneous Endoscopic Approach

03RT07Z Replacement of Left Temporal Artery with Autologous Tissue Substitute, Open Approach

03RT0JZ Replacement of Left Temporal Artery with Synthetic Substitute, Open Approach

03RT0KZ Replacement of Left Temporal Artery with Nonautologous Tissue Substitute, Open Approach

03RT47Z Replacement of Left Temporal Artery with Autologous Tissue Substitute, Percutaneous Endoscopic Approach

03RT4JZ Replacement of Left Temporal Artery with Synthetic Substitute, Percutaneous Endoscopic Approach

03RT4KZ Replacement of Left Temporal Artery with Nonautologous Tissue Substitute, Percutaneous Endoscopic Approach

03RU07Z Replacement of Right Thyroid Artery with Autologous Tissue Substitute, Open Approach

03RU0JZ Replacement of Right Thyroid Artery with Synthetic Substitute, Open Approach

03RU0KZ Replacement of Right Thyroid Artery with Nonautologous Tissue Substitute, Open Approach

03RU47Z Replacement of Right Thyroid Artery with Autologous Tissue Substitute, Percutaneous Endoscopic Approach

03RU4JZ Replacement of Right Thyroid Artery with Synthetic Substitute, Percutaneous Endoscopic Approach

03RU4KZ Replacement of Right Thyroid Artery with Nonautologous Tissue Substitute, Percutaneous Endoscopic Approach

03RV07Z Replacement of Left Thyroid Artery with Autologous Tissue Substitute, Open Approach

03RV0JZ Replacement of Left Thyroid Artery with Synthetic Substitute, Open Approach

03RV0KZ Replacement of Left Thyroid Artery with Nonautologous Tissue Substitute, Open Approach

03RV47Z Replacement of Left Thyroid Artery with Autologous Tissue Substitute, Percutaneous Endoscopic Approach

03RV4JZ Replacement of Left Thyroid Artery with Synthetic Substitute, Percutaneous Endoscopic Approach

03RV4KZ Replacement of Left Thyroid Artery with Nonautologous Tissue Substitute, Percutaneous Endoscopic Approach

03RY07Z Replacement of Upper Artery with Autologous Tissue Substitute, Open Approach

03RY0JZ Replacement of Upper Artery with Synthetic Substitute, Open Approach

03RY0KZ Replacement of Upper Artery with Nonautologous Tissue Substitute, Open Approach

♀ Female-only   ♂ Male-only   ▲ Limited Coverage   ● Non-OR   ▨ HAC-associated procedure   ▲ Non-covered procedures   ✚ Combinatic

03RY47Z	Replacement of Upper Artery with Autologous Tissue Substitute, Percutaneous Endoscopic Approach
03RY4JZ	Replacement of Upper Artery with Synthetic Substitute, Percutaneous Endoscopic Approach
03RY4KZ	Replacement of Upper Artery with Nonautologous Tissue Substitute, Percutaneous Endoscopic Approach

3S – Upper Arteries, Reposition

03S00ZZ	Reposition Right Internal Mammary Artery, Open Approach
03S03ZZ	Reposition Right Internal Mammary Artery, Percutaneous Approach
03S04ZZ	Reposition Right Internal Mammary Artery, Percutaneous Endoscopic Approach
03S10ZZ	Reposition Left Internal Mammary Artery, Open Approach
03S13ZZ	Reposition Left Internal Mammary Artery, Percutaneous Approach
03S14ZZ	Reposition Left Internal Mammary Artery, Percutaneous Endoscopic Approach
03S20ZZ	Reposition Innominate Artery, Open Approach
03S23ZZ	Reposition Innominate Artery, Percutaneous Approach
03S24ZZ	Reposition Innominate Artery, Percutaneous Endoscopic Approach
03S30ZZ	Reposition Right Subclavian Artery, Open Approach
03S33ZZ	Reposition Right Subclavian Artery, Percutaneous Approach
03S34ZZ	Reposition Right Subclavian Artery, Percutaneous Endoscopic Approach
03S40ZZ	Reposition Left Subclavian Artery, Open Approach
03S43ZZ	Reposition Left Subclavian Artery, Percutaneous Approach
03S44ZZ	Reposition Left Subclavian Artery, Percutaneous Endoscopic Approach
03S50ZZ	Reposition Right Axillary Artery, Open Approach
03S53ZZ	Reposition Right Axillary Artery, Percutaneous Approach
03S54ZZ	Reposition Right Axillary Artery, Percutaneous Endoscopic Approach
03S60ZZ	Reposition Left Axillary Artery, Open Approach
03S63ZZ	Reposition Left Axillary Artery, Percutaneous Approach
03S64ZZ	Reposition Left Axillary Artery, Percutaneous Endoscopic Approach
03S70ZZ	Reposition Right Brachial Artery, Open Approach
03S73ZZ	Reposition Right Brachial Artery, Percutaneous Approach
03S74ZZ	Reposition Right Brachial Artery, Percutaneous Endoscopic Approach
03S80ZZ	Reposition Left Brachial Artery, Open Approach
03S83ZZ	Reposition Left Brachial Artery, Percutaneous Approach
03S84ZZ	Reposition Left Brachial Artery, Percutaneous Endoscopic Approach
03S90ZZ	Reposition Right Ulnar Artery, Open Approach
03S93ZZ	Reposition Right Ulnar Artery, Percutaneous Approach
03S94ZZ	Reposition Right Ulnar Artery, Percutaneous Endoscopic Approach
03SA0ZZ	Reposition Left Ulnar Artery, Open Approach
03SA3ZZ	Reposition Left Ulnar Artery, Percutaneous Approach
03SA4ZZ	Reposition Left Ulnar Artery, Percutaneous Endoscopic Approach
03SB0ZZ	Reposition Right Radial Artery, Open Approach
03SB3ZZ	Reposition Right Radial Artery, Percutaneous Approach
03SB4ZZ	Reposition Right Radial Artery, Percutaneous Endoscopic Approach
03SC0ZZ	Reposition Left Radial Artery, Open Approach
03SC3ZZ	Reposition Left Radial Artery, Percutaneous Approach
03SC4ZZ	Reposition Left Radial Artery, Percutaneous Endoscopic Approach
03SD0ZZ	Reposition Right Hand Artery, Open Approach
03SD3ZZ	Reposition Right Hand Artery, Percutaneous Approach
03SD4ZZ	Reposition Right Hand Artery, Percutaneous Endoscopic Approach
03SF0ZZ	Reposition Left Hand Artery, Open Approach
03SF3ZZ	Reposition Left Hand Artery, Percutaneous Approach
03SF4ZZ	Reposition Left Hand Artery, Percutaneous Endoscopic Approach
03SG0ZZ	Reposition Intracranial Artery, Open Approach
03SG3ZZ	Reposition Intracranial Artery, Percutaneous Approach
03SG4ZZ	Reposition Intracranial Artery, Percutaneous Endoscopic Approach
03SH0ZZ	Reposition Right Common Carotid Artery, Open Approach
03SH3ZZ	Reposition Right Common Carotid Artery, Percutaneous Approach
03SH4ZZ	Reposition Right Common Carotid Artery, Percutaneous Endoscopic Approach
03SJ0ZZ	Reposition Left Common Carotid Artery, Open Approach
03SJ3ZZ	Reposition Left Common Carotid Artery, Percutaneous Approach
03SJ4ZZ	Reposition Left Common Carotid Artery, Percutaneous Endoscopic Approach
03SK0ZZ	Reposition Right Internal Carotid Artery, Open Approach
03SK3ZZ	Reposition Right Internal Carotid Artery, Percutaneous Approach
03SK4ZZ	Reposition Right Internal Carotid Artery, Percutaneous Endoscopic Approach
03SL0ZZ	Reposition Left Internal Carotid Artery, Open Approach
03SL3ZZ	Reposition Left Internal Carotid Artery, Percutaneous Approach
03SL4ZZ	Reposition Left Internal Carotid Artery, Percutaneous Endoscopic Approach
03SM0ZZ	Reposition Right External Carotid Artery, Open Approach
03SM3ZZ	Reposition Right External Carotid Artery, Percutaneous Approach
03SM4ZZ	Reposition Right External Carotid Artery, Percutaneous Endoscopic Approach
03SN0ZZ	Reposition Left External Carotid Artery, Open Approach
03SN3ZZ	Reposition Left External Carotid Artery, Percutaneous Approach
03SN4ZZ	Reposition Left External Carotid Artery, Percutaneous Endoscopic Approach
03SP0ZZ	Reposition Right Vertebral Artery, Open Approach
03SP3ZZ	Reposition Right Vertebral Artery, Percutaneous Approach
03SP4ZZ	Reposition Right Vertebral Artery, Percutaneous Endoscopic Approach
03SQ0ZZ	Reposition Left Vertebral Artery, Open Approach
03SQ3ZZ	Reposition Left Vertebral Artery, Percutaneous Approach
03SQ4ZZ	Reposition Left Vertebral Artery, Percutaneous Endoscopic Approach
03SR0ZZ	Reposition Face Artery, Open Approach
03SR3ZZ	Reposition Face Artery, Percutaneous Approach
03SR4ZZ	Reposition Face Artery, Percutaneous Endoscopic Approach
03SS0ZZ	Reposition Right Temporal Artery, Open Approach
03SS3ZZ	Reposition Right Temporal Artery, Percutaneous Approach
03SS4ZZ	Reposition Right Temporal Artery, Percutaneous Endoscopic Approach
03ST0ZZ	Reposition Left Temporal Artery, Open Approach
03ST3ZZ	Reposition Left Temporal Artery, Percutaneous Approach
03ST4ZZ	Reposition Left Temporal Artery, Percutaneous Endoscopic Approach
03SU0ZZ	Reposition Right Thyroid Artery, Open Approach
03SU3ZZ	Reposition Right Thyroid Artery, Percutaneous Approach
03SU4ZZ	Reposition Right Thyroid Artery, Percutaneous Endoscopic Approach
03SV0ZZ	Reposition Left Thyroid Artery, Open Approach
03SV3ZZ	Reposition Left Thyroid Artery, Percutaneous Approach
03SV4ZZ	Reposition Left Thyroid Artery, Percutaneous Endoscopic Approach
03SY0ZZ	Reposition Upper Artery, Open Approach
03SY3ZZ	Reposition Upper Artery, Percutaneous Approach
03SY4ZZ	Reposition Upper Artery, Percutaneous Endoscopic Approach

3U – Upper Arteries, Supplement

03U007Z	Supplement Right Internal Mammary Artery with Autologous Tissue Substitute, Open Approach
03U00JZ	Supplement Right Internal Mammary Artery with Synthetic Substitute, Open Approach
03U00KZ	Supplement Right Internal Mammary Artery with Nonautologous Tissue Substitute, Open Approach
03U037Z	Supplement Right Internal Mammary Artery with Autologous Tissue Substitute, Percutaneous Approach
03U03JZ	Supplement Right Internal Mammary Artery with Synthetic Substitute, Percutaneous Approach
03U03KZ	Supplement Right Internal Mammary Artery with Nonautologous Tissue Substitute, Percutaneous Approach
03U047Z	Supplement Right Internal Mammary Artery with Autologous Tissue Substitute, Percutaneous Endoscopic Approach
03U04JZ	Supplement Right Internal Mammary Artery with Synthetic Substitute, Percutaneous Endoscopic Approach

Female-only　♂ Male-only　▲ Limited Coverage　● Non-OR　HAC-associated procedure　▲ Non-covered procedures　✚ Combination

03U04KZ Supplement Right Internal Mammary Artery with Nonautologous Tissue Substitute, Percutaneous Endoscopic Approach

03U107Z Supplement Left Internal Mammary Artery with Autologous Tissue Substitute, Open Approach

03U10JZ Supplement Left Internal Mammary Artery with Synthetic Substitute, Open Approach

03U10KZ Supplement Left Internal Mammary Artery with Nonautologous Tissue Substitute, Open Approach

03U137Z Supplement Left Internal Mammary Artery with Autologous Tissue Substitute, Percutaneous Approach

03U13JZ Supplement Left Internal Mammary Artery with Synthetic Substitute, Percutaneous Approach

03U13KZ Supplement Left Internal Mammary Artery with Nonautologous Tissue Substitute, Percutaneous Approach

03U147Z Supplement Left Internal Mammary Artery with Autologous Tissue Substitute, Percutaneous Endoscopic Approach

03U14JZ Supplement Left Internal Mammary Artery with Synthetic Substitute, Percutaneous Endoscopic Approach

03U14KZ Supplement Left Internal Mammary Artery with Nonautologous Tissue Substitute, Percutaneous Endoscopic Approach

03U207Z Supplement Innominate Artery with Autologous Tissue Substitute, Open Approach

03U20JZ Supplement Innominate Artery with Synthetic Substitute, Open Approach

03U20KZ Supplement Innominate Artery with Nonautologous Tissue Substitute, Open Approach

03U237Z Supplement Innominate Artery with Autologous Tissue Substitute, Percutaneous Approach

03U23JZ Supplement Innominate Artery with Synthetic Substitute, Percutaneous Approach

03U23KZ Supplement Innominate Artery with Nonautologous Tissue Substitute, Percutaneous Approach

03U247Z Supplement Innominate Artery with Autologous Tissue Substitute, Percutaneous Endoscopic Approach

03U24JZ Supplement Innominate Artery with Synthetic Substitute, Percutaneous Endoscopic Approach

03U24KZ Supplement Innominate Artery with Nonautologous Tissue Substitute, Percutaneous Endoscopic Approach

03U307Z Supplement Right Subclavian Artery with Autologous Tissue Substitute, Open Approach

03U30JZ Supplement Right Subclavian Artery with Synthetic Substitute, Open Approach

03U30KZ Supplement Right Subclavian Artery with Nonautologous Tissue Substitute, Open Approach

03U337Z Supplement Right Subclavian Artery with Autologous Tissue Substitute, Percutaneous Approach

03U33JZ Supplement Right Subclavian Artery with Synthetic Substitute, Percutaneous Approach

03U33KZ Supplement Right Subclavian Artery with Nonautologous Tissue Substitute, Percutaneous Approach

03U347Z Supplement Right Subclavian Artery with Autologous Tissue Substitute, Percutaneous Endoscopic Approach

03U34JZ Supplement Right Subclavian Artery with Synthetic Substitute, Percutaneous Endoscopic Approach

03U34KZ Supplement Right Subclavian Artery with Nonautologous Tissue Substitute, Percutaneous Endoscopic Approach

03U407Z Supplement Left Subclavian Artery with Autologous Tissue Substitute, Open Approach

03U40JZ Supplement Left Subclavian Artery with Synthetic Substitute, Open Approach

03U40KZ Supplement Left Subclavian Artery with Nonautologous Tissue Substitute, Open Approach

03U437Z Supplement Left Subclavian Artery with Autologous Tissue Substitute, Percutaneous Approach

03U43JZ Supplement Left Subclavian Artery with Synthetic Substitute, Percutaneous Approach

03U43KZ Supplement Left Subclavian Artery with Nonautologous Tissue Substitute, Percutaneous Approach

03U447Z Supplement Left Subclavian Artery with Autologous Tissue Substitute, Percutaneous Endoscopic Approach

03U44JZ Supplement Left Subclavian Artery with Synthetic Substitute, Percutaneous Endoscopic Approach

03U44KZ Supplement Left Subclavian Artery with Nonautologous Tissue Substitute, Percutaneous Endoscopic Approach

03U507Z Supplement Right Axillary Artery with Autologous Tissue Substitute, Open Approach

03U50JZ Supplement Right Axillary Artery with Synthetic Substitute, Open Approach

03U50KZ Supplement Right Axillary Artery with Nonautologous Tissue Substitute, Open Approach

03U537Z Supplement Right Axillary Artery with Autologous Tissue Substitute, Percutaneous Approach

03U53JZ Supplement Right Axillary Artery with Synthetic Substitute, Percutaneous Approach

03U53KZ Supplement Right Axillary Artery with Nonautologous Tissue Substitute, Percutaneous Approach

03U547Z Supplement Right Axillary Artery with Autologous Tissue Substitute, Percutaneous Endoscopic Approach

03U54JZ Supplement Right Axillary Artery with Synthetic Substitute, Percutaneous Endoscopic Approach

03U54KZ Supplement Right Axillary Artery with Nonautologous Tissue Substitute, Percutaneous Endoscopic Approach

03U607Z Supplement Left Axillary Artery with Autologous Tissue Substitute, Open Approach

03U60JZ Supplement Left Axillary Artery with Synthetic Substitute, Open Approach

03U60KZ Supplement Left Axillary Artery with Nonautologous Tissue Substitute, Open Approach

03U637Z Supplement Left Axillary Artery with Autologous Tissue Substitute, Percutaneous Approach

03U63JZ Supplement Left Axillary Artery with Synthetic Substitute, Percutaneous Approach

03U63KZ Supplement Left Axillary Artery with Nonautologous Tissue Substitute, Percutaneous Approach

03U647Z Supplement Left Axillary Artery with Autologous Tissue Substitute, Percutaneous Endoscopic Approach

03U64JZ Supplement Left Axillary Artery with Synthetic Substitute, Percutaneous Endoscopic Approach

03U64KZ Supplement Left Axillary Artery with Nonautologous Tissue Substitute, Percutaneous Endoscopic Approach

03U707Z Supplement Right Brachial Artery with Autologous Tissue Substitute, Open Approach

03U70JZ Supplement Right Brachial Artery with Synthetic Substitute, Open Approach

03U70KZ Supplement Right Brachial Artery with Nonautologous Tissue Substitute, Open Approach

03U737Z Supplement Right Brachial Artery with Autologous Tissue Substitute, Percutaneous Approach

03U73JZ Supplement Right Brachial Artery with Synthetic Substitute, Percutaneous Approach

03U73KZ Supplement Right Brachial Artery with Nonautologous Tissue Substitute, Percutaneous Approach

03U747Z Supplement Right Brachial Artery with Autologous Tissue Substitute, Percutaneous Endoscopic Approach

03U74JZ Supplement Right Brachial Artery with Synthetic Substitute, Percutaneous Endoscopic Approach

03U74KZ Supplement Right Brachial Artery with Nonautologous Tissue Substitute, Percutaneous Endoscopic Approach

03U807Z Supplement Left Brachial Artery with Autologous Tissue Substitute, Open Approach

03U80JZ Supplement Left Brachial Artery with Synthetic Substitute, Open Approach

03U80KZ Supplement Left Brachial Artery with Nonautologous Tissue Substitute, Open Approach

03U837Z Supplement Left Brachial Artery with Autologous Tissue Substitute, Percutaneous Approach

03U83JZ Supplement Left Brachial Artery with Synthetic Substitute, Percutaneous Approach

03U83KZ Supplement Left Brachial Artery with Nonautologous Tissue Substitute, Percutaneous Approach

03U847Z Supplement Left Brachial Artery with Autologous Tissue Substitute, Percutaneous Endoscopic Approach

03U84JZ Supplement Left Brachial Artery with Synthetic Substitute, Percutaneous Endoscopic Approach

03U84KZ Supplement Left Brachial Artery with Nonautologous Tissue Substitute, Percutaneous Endoscopic Approach

03U907Z Supplement Right Ulnar Artery with Autologous Tissue Substitute, Open Approach

03U90JZ Supplement Right Ulnar Artery with Synthetic Substitute, Open Approach

03U90KZ Supplement Right Ulnar Artery with Nonautologous Tissue Substitute, Open Approach

03U937Z Supplement Right Ulnar Artery with Autologous Tissue Substitute, Percutaneous Approach

03U93JZ Supplement Right Ulnar Artery with Synthetic Substitute, Percutaneous Approach

03U93KZ Supplement Right Ulnar Artery with Nonautologous Tissue Substitute, Percutaneous Approach

03U947Z Supplement Right Ulnar Artery with Autologous Tissue Substitute, Percutaneous Endoscopic Approach

03U94JZ Supplement Right Ulnar Artery with Synthetic Substitute, Percutaneous Endoscopic Approach

03U94KZ Supplement Right Ulnar Artery with Nonautologous Tissue Substitute, Percutaneous Endoscopic Approach

03UA07Z Supplement Left Ulnar Artery with Autologous Tissue Substitute, Open Approach

03UA0JZ Supplement Left Ulnar Artery with Synthetic Substitute, Open Approach

03UA0KZ Supplement Left Ulnar Artery with Nonautologous Tissue Substitute, Open Approach

03UA37Z Supplement Left Ulnar Artery with Autologous Tissue Substitute, Percutaneous Approach

03UA3JZ Supplement Left Ulnar Artery with Synthetic Substitute, Percutaneous Approach

03UA3KZ Supplement Left Ulnar Artery with Nonautologous Tissue Substitute, Percutaneous Approach

03UA47Z Supplement Left Ulnar Artery with Autologous Tissue Substitute, Percutaneous Endoscopic Approach

03UA4JZ Supplement Left Ulnar Artery with Synthetic Substitute, Percutaneous Endoscopic Approach

03UA4KZ Supplement Left Ulnar Artery with Nonautologous Tissue Substitute, Percutaneous Endoscopic Approach

03UB07Z Supplement Right Radial Artery with Autologous Tissue Substitute, Open Approach

03UB0JZ Supplement Right Radial Artery with Synthetic Substitute, Open Approach

03UB0KZ Supplement Right Radial Artery with Nonautologous Tissue Substitute, Open Approach

03UB37Z Supplement Right Radial Artery with Autologous Tissue Substitute, Percutaneous Approach

03UB3JZ Supplement Right Radial Artery with Synthetic Substitute, Percutaneous Approach

03UB3KZ Supplement Right Radial Artery with Nonautologous Tissue Substitute, Percutaneous Approach

03UB47Z Supplement Right Radial Artery with Autologous Tissue Substitute, Percutaneous Endoscopic Approach

03UB4JZ Supplement Right Radial Artery with Synthetic Substitute, Percutaneous Endoscopic Approach

03UB4KZ Supplement Right Radial Artery with Nonautologous Tissue Substitute, Percutaneous Endoscopic Approach

03UC07Z Supplement Left Radial Artery with Autologous Tissue Substitute, Open Approach

03UC0JZ Supplement Left Radial Artery with Synthetic Substitute, Open Approach

03UC0KZ Supplement Left Radial Artery with Nonautologous Tissue Substitute, Open Approach

03UC37Z Supplement Left Radial Artery with Autologous Tissue Substitute, Percutaneous Approach

03UC3JZ Supplement Left Radial Artery with Synthetic Substitute, Percutaneous Approach

03UC3KZ Supplement Left Radial Artery with Nonautologous Tissue Substitute, Percutaneous Approach

03UC47Z Supplement Left Radial Artery with Autologous Tissue Substitute, Percutaneous Endoscopic Approach

03UC4JZ Supplement Left Radial Artery with Synthetic Substitute, Percutaneous Endoscopic Approach

03UC4KZ Supplement Left Radial Artery with Nonautologous Tissue Substitute, Percutaneous Endoscopic Approach

03UD07Z Supplement Right Hand Artery with Autologous Tissue Substitute, Open Approach

03UD0JZ Supplement Right Hand Artery with Synthetic Substitute, Open Approach

03UD0KZ Supplement Right Hand Artery with Nonautologous Tissue Substitute, Open Approach

03UD37Z Supplement Right Hand Artery with Autologous Tissue Substitute, Percutaneous Approach

03UD3JZ Supplement Right Hand Artery with Synthetic Substitute, Percutaneous Approach

03UD3KZ Supplement Right Hand Artery with Nonautologous Tissue Substitute, Percutaneous Approach

03UD47Z Supplement Right Hand Artery with Autologous Tissue Substitute, Percutaneous Endoscopic Approach

03UD4JZ Supplement Right Hand Artery with Synthetic Substitute, Percutaneous Endoscopic Approach

03UD4KZ Supplement Right Hand Artery with Nonautologous Tissue Substitute, Percutaneous Endoscopic Approach

03UF07Z Supplement Left Hand Artery with Autologous Tissue Substitute, Open Approach

03UF0JZ Supplement Left Hand Artery with Synthetic Substitute, Open Approach

03UF0KZ Supplement Left Hand Artery with Nonautologous Tissue Substitute, Open Approach

03UF37Z Supplement Left Hand Artery with Autologous Tissue Substitute, Percutaneous Approach

03UF3JZ Supplement Left Hand Artery with Synthetic Substitute, Percutaneous Approach

03UF3KZ Supplement Left Hand Artery with Nonautologous Tissue Substitute, Percutaneous Approach

03UF47Z Supplement Left Hand Artery with Autologous Tissue Substitute, Percutaneous Endoscopic Approach

03UF4JZ Supplement Left Hand Artery with Synthetic Substitute, Percutaneous Endoscopic Approach

03UF4KZ Supplement Left Hand Artery with Nonautologous Tissue Substitute, Percutaneous Endoscopic Approach

03UG07Z Supplement Intracranial Artery with Autologous Tissue Substitute, Open Approach

03UG0JZ Supplement Intracranial Artery with Synthetic Substitute, Open Approach

03UG0KZ Supplement Intracranial Artery with Nonautologous Tissue Substitute, Open Approach

03UG37Z Supplement Intracranial Artery with Autologous Tissue Substitute, Percutaneous Approach

03UG3JZ Supplement Intracranial Artery with Synthetic Substitute, Percutaneous Approach

03UG3KZ Supplement Intracranial Artery with Nonautologous Tissue Substitute, Percutaneous Approach

03UG47Z Supplement Intracranial Artery with Autologous Tissue Substitute, Percutaneous Endoscopic Approach

03UG4JZ Supplement Intracranial Artery with Synthetic Substitute, Percutaneous Endoscopic Approach

03UG4KZ Supplement Intracranial Artery with Nonautologous Tissue Substitute, Percutaneous Endoscopic Approach

03UH07Z Supplement Right Common Carotid Artery with Autologous Tissue Substitute, Open Approach

03UH0JZ Supplement Right Common Carotid Artery with Synthetic Substitute, Open Approach

03UH0KZ Supplement Right Common Carotid Artery with Nonautologous Tissue Substitute, Open Approach

03UH37Z Supplement Right Common Carotid Artery with Autologous Tissue Substitute, Percutaneous Approach

03UH3JZ Supplement Right Common Carotid Artery with Synthetic Substitute, Percutaneous Approach

03UH3KZ Supplement Right Common Carotid Artery with Nonautologous Tissue Substitute, Percutaneous Approach

03UH47Z Supplement Right Common Carotid Artery with Autologous Tissue Substitute, Percutaneous Endoscopic Approach

03UH4JZ Supplement Right Common Carotid Artery with Synthetic Substitute, Percutaneous Endoscopic Approach

03UH4KZ Supplement Right Common Carotid Artery with Nonautologous Tissue Substitute, Percutaneous Endoscopic Approach

03UJ07Z Supplement Left Common Carotid Artery with Autologous Tissue Substitute, Open Approach

03UJ0JZ Supplement Left Common Carotid Artery with Synthetic Substitute, Open Approach

03UJ0KZ Supplement Left Common Carotid Artery with Nonautologous Tissue Substitute, Open Approach

03UJ37Z Supplement Left Common Carotid Artery with Autologous Tissue Substitute, Percutaneous Approach

03UJ3JZ Supplement Left Common Carotid Artery with Synthetic Substitute, Percutaneous Approach

03UJ3KZ Supplement Left Common Carotid Artery with Nonautologous Tissue Substitute, Percutaneous Approach

03UJ47Z Supplement Left Common Carotid Artery with Autologous Tissue Substitute, Percutaneous Endoscopic Approach

03UJ4JZ Supplement Left Common Carotid Artery with Synthetic Substitute, Percutaneous Endoscopic Approach

03UJ4KZ Supplement Left Common Carotid Artery with Nonautologous Tissue Substitute, Percutaneous Endoscopic Approach

03UK07Z Supplement Right Internal Carotid Artery with Autologous Tissue Substitute, Open Approach

03UK0JZ Supplement Right Internal Carotid Artery with Synthetic Substitute, Open Approach

03UK0KZ Supplement Right Internal Carotid Artery with Nonautologous Tissue Substitute, Open Approach

03UK37Z Supplement Right Internal Carotid Artery with Autologous Tissue Substitute, Percutaneous Approach

03UK3JZ Supplement Right Internal Carotid Artery with Synthetic Substitute, Percutaneous Approach

03UK3KZ Supplement Right Internal Carotid Artery with Nonautologous Tissue Substitute, Percutaneous Approach

Female-only   ♂ Male-only   ▲ Limited Coverage   ● Non-OR   ▨ HAC-associated procedure   ▲ Non-covered procedures   ✚ Combination

03UK47Z Supplement Right Internal Carotid Artery with Autologous Tissue Substitute, Percutaneous Endoscopic Approach

03UK4JZ Supplement Right Internal Carotid Artery with Synthetic Substitute, Percutaneous Endoscopic Approach

03UK4KZ Supplement Right Internal Carotid Artery with Nonautologous Tissue Substitute, Percutaneous Endoscopic Approach

03UL07Z Supplement Left Internal Carotid Artery with Autologous Tissue Substitute, Open Approach

03UL0JZ Supplement Left Internal Carotid Artery with Synthetic Substitute, Open Approach

03UL0KZ Supplement Left Internal Carotid Artery with Nonautologous Tissue Substitute, Open Approach

03UL37Z Supplement Left Internal Carotid Artery with Autologous Tissue Substitute, Percutaneous Approach

03UL3JZ Supplement Left Internal Carotid Artery with Synthetic Substitute, Percutaneous Approach

03UL3KZ Supplement Left Internal Carotid Artery with Nonautologous Tissue Substitute, Percutaneous Approach

03UL47Z Supplement Left Internal Carotid Artery with Autologous Tissue Substitute, Percutaneous Endoscopic Approach

03UL4JZ Supplement Left Internal Carotid Artery with Synthetic Substitute, Percutaneous Endoscopic Approach

03UL4KZ Supplement Left Internal Carotid Artery with Nonautologous Tissue Substitute, Percutaneous Endoscopic Approach

03UM07Z Supplement Right External Carotid Artery with Autologous Tissue Substitute, Open Approach

03UM0JZ Supplement Right External Carotid Artery with Synthetic Substitute, Open Approach

03UM0KZ Supplement Right External Carotid Artery with Nonautologous Tissue Substitute, Open Approach

03UM37Z Supplement Right External Carotid Artery with Autologous Tissue Substitute, Percutaneous Approach

03UM3JZ Supplement Right External Carotid Artery with Synthetic Substitute, Percutaneous Approach

03UM3KZ Supplement Right External Carotid Artery with Nonautologous Tissue Substitute, Percutaneous Approach

03UM47Z Supplement Right External Carotid Artery with Autologous Tissue Substitute, Percutaneous Endoscopic Approach

03UM4JZ Supplement Right External Carotid Artery with Synthetic Substitute, Percutaneous Endoscopic Approach

03UM4KZ Supplement Right External Carotid Artery with Nonautologous Tissue Substitute, Percutaneous Endoscopic Approach

03UN07Z Supplement Left External Carotid Artery with Autologous Tissue Substitute, Open Approach

03UN0JZ Supplement Left External Carotid Artery with Synthetic Substitute, Open Approach

03UN0KZ Supplement Left External Carotid Artery with Nonautologous Tissue Substitute, Open Approach

03UN37Z Supplement Left External Carotid Artery with Autologous Tissue Substitute, Percutaneous Approach

03UN3JZ Supplement Left External Carotid Artery with Synthetic Substitute, Percutaneous Approach

03UN3KZ Supplement Left External Carotid Artery with Nonautologous Tissue Substitute, Percutaneous Approach

03UN47Z Supplement Left External Carotid Artery with Autologous Tissue Substitute, Percutaneous Endoscopic Approach

03UN4JZ Supplement Left External Carotid Artery with Synthetic Substitute, Percutaneous Endoscopic Approach

03UN4KZ Supplement Left External Carotid Artery with Nonautologous Tissue Substitute, Percutaneous Endoscopic Approach

03UP07Z Supplement Right Vertebral Artery with Autologous Tissue Substitute, Open Approach

03UP0JZ Supplement Right Vertebral Artery with Synthetic Substitute, Open Approach

03UP0KZ Supplement Right Vertebral Artery with Nonautologous Tissue Substitute, Open Approach

03UP37Z Supplement Right Vertebral Artery with Autologous Tissue Substitute, Percutaneous Approach

03UP3JZ Supplement Right Vertebral Artery with Synthetic Substitute, Percutaneous Approach

03UP3KZ Supplement Right Vertebral Artery with Nonautologous Tissue Substitute, Percutaneous Approach

03UP47Z Supplement Right Vertebral Artery with Autologous Tissue Substitute, Percutaneous Endoscopic Approach

03UP4JZ Supplement Right Vertebral Artery with Synthetic Substitute, Percutaneous Endoscopic Approach

03UP4KZ Supplement Right Vertebral Artery with Nonautologous Tissue Substitute, Percutaneous Endoscopic Approach

03UQ07Z Supplement Left Vertebral Artery with Autologous Tissue Substitute, Open Approach

03UQ0JZ Supplement Left Vertebral Artery with Synthetic Substitute, Open Approach

03UQ0KZ Supplement Left Vertebral Artery with Nonautologous Tissue Substitute, Open Approach

03UQ37Z Supplement Left Vertebral Artery with Autologous Tissue Substitute, Percutaneous Approach

03UQ3JZ Supplement Left Vertebral Artery with Synthetic Substitute, Percutaneous Approach

03UQ3KZ Supplement Left Vertebral Artery with Nonautologous Tissue Substitute, Percutaneous Approach

03UQ47Z Supplement Left Vertebral Artery with Autologous Tissue Substitute, Percutaneous Endoscopic Approach

03UQ4JZ Supplement Left Vertebral Artery with Synthetic Substitute, Percutaneous Endoscopic Approach

03UQ4KZ Supplement Left Vertebral Artery with Nonautologous Tissue Substitute, Percutaneous Endoscopic Approach

03UR07Z Supplement Face Artery with Autologous Tissue Substitute, Open Approach

03UR0JZ Supplement Face Artery with Synthetic Substitute, Open Approach

03UR0KZ Supplement Face Artery with Nonautologous Tissue Substitute, Open Approach

03UR37Z Supplement Face Artery with Autologous Tissue Substitute, Percutaneous Approach

03UR3JZ Supplement Face Artery with Synthetic Substitute, Percutaneous Approach

03UR3KZ Supplement Face Artery with Nonautologous Tissue Substitute, Percutaneous Approach

03UR47Z Supplement Face Artery with Autologous Tissue Substitute, Percutaneous Endoscopic Approach

03UR4JZ Supplement Face Artery with Synthetic Substitute, Percutaneous Endoscopic Approach

03UR4KZ Supplement Face Artery with Nonautologous Tissue Substitute, Percutaneous Endoscopic Approach

03US07Z Supplement Right Temporal Artery with Autologous Tissue Substitute, Open Approach

03US0JZ Supplement Right Temporal Artery with Synthetic Substitute, Open Approach

03US0KZ Supplement Right Temporal Artery with Nonautologous Tissue Substitute, Open Approach

03US37Z Supplement Right Temporal Artery with Autologous Tissue Substitute, Percutaneous Approach

03US3JZ Supplement Right Temporal Artery with Synthetic Substitute, Percutaneous Approach

03US3KZ Supplement Right Temporal Artery with Nonautologous Tissue Substitute, Percutaneous Approach

03US47Z Supplement Right Temporal Artery with Autologous Tissue Substitute, Percutaneous Endoscopic Approach

03US4JZ Supplement Right Temporal Artery with Synthetic Substitute, Percutaneous Endoscopic Approach

03US4KZ Supplement Right Temporal Artery with Nonautologous Tissue Substitute, Percutaneous Endoscopic Approach

03UT07Z Supplement Left Temporal Artery with Autologous Tissue Substitute, Open Approach

03UT0JZ Supplement Left Temporal Artery with Synthetic Substitute, Open Approach

03UT0KZ Supplement Left Temporal Artery with Nonautologous Tissue Substitute, Open Approach

03UT37Z Supplement Left Temporal Artery with Autologous Tissue Substitute, Percutaneous Approach

03UT3JZ Supplement Left Temporal Artery with Synthetic Substitute, Percutaneous Approach

03UT3KZ Supplement Left Temporal Artery with Nonautologous Tissue Substitute, Percutaneous Approach

03UT47Z Supplement Left Temporal Artery with Autologous Tissue Substitute, Percutaneous Endoscopic Approach

03UT4JZ Supplement Left Temporal Artery with Synthetic Substitute, Percutaneous Endoscopic Approach

03UT4KZ Supplement Left Temporal Artery with Nonautologous Tissue Substitute, Percutaneous Endoscopic Approach

03UU07Z Supplement Right Thyroid Artery with Autologous Tissue Substitute, Open Approach

03UU0JZ Supplement Right Thyroid Artery with Synthetic Substitute, Open Approach

03UU0KZ Supplement Right Thyroid Artery with Nonautologous Tissue Substitute, Open Approach

03UU37Z Supplement Right Thyroid Artery with Autologous Tissue Substitute, Percutaneous Approach

03UU3JZ Supplement Right Thyroid Artery with Synthetic Substitute, Percutaneous Approach

03UU3KZ Supplement Right Thyroid Artery with Nonautologous Tissue Substitute, Percutaneous Approach

03UU47Z Supplement Right Thyroid Artery with Autologous Tissue Substitute, Percutaneous Endoscopic Approach

♀ Female-only   ♂ Male-only   ▲ Limited Coverage   ● Non-OR   ▦ HAC-associated procedure   ▲ Non-covered procedures   ✚ Combinati

JU4JZ Supplement Right Thyroid Artery with Synthetic Substitute, Percutaneous Endoscopic Approach
JU4KZ Supplement Right Thyroid Artery with Nonautologous Tissue Substitute, Percutaneous Endoscopic Approach
JV07Z Supplement Left Thyroid Artery with Autologous Tissue Substitute, Open Approach
JV0JZ Supplement Left Thyroid Artery with Synthetic Substitute, Open Approach
JV0KZ Supplement Left Thyroid Artery with Nonautologous Tissue Substitute, Open Approach
JV37Z Supplement Left Thyroid Artery with Autologous Tissue Substitute, Percutaneous Approach

03UV3JZ Supplement Left Thyroid Artery with Synthetic Substitute, Percutaneous Approach
03UV3KZ Supplement Left Thyroid Artery with Nonautologous Tissue Substitute, Percutaneous Approach
03UV47Z Supplement Left Thyroid Artery with Autologous Tissue Substitute, Percutaneous Endoscopic Approach
03UV4JZ Supplement Left Thyroid Artery with Synthetic Substitute, Percutaneous Endoscopic Approach
03UV4KZ Supplement Left Thyroid Artery with Nonautologous Tissue Substitute, Percutaneous Endoscopic Approach
03UY07Z Supplement Upper Artery with Autologous Tissue Substitute, Open Approach
03UY0JZ Supplement Upper Artery with Synthetic Substitute, Open Approach

03UY0KZ Supplement Upper Artery with Nonautologous Tissue Substitute, Open Approach
03UY37Z Supplement Upper Artery with Autologous Tissue Substitute, Percutaneous Approach
03UY3JZ Supplement Upper Artery with Synthetic Substitute, Percutaneous Approach
03UY3KZ Supplement Upper Artery with Nonautologous Tissue Substitute, Percutaneous Approach
03UY47Z Supplement Upper Artery with Autologous Tissue Substitute, Percutaneous Endoscopic Approach
03UY4JZ Supplement Upper Artery with Synthetic Substitute, Percutaneous Endoscopic Approach
03UY4KZ Supplement Upper Artery with Nonautologous Tissue Substitute, Percutaneous Endoscopic Approach

V – Upper Arteries, Restriction

view Coding Guideline B3.12

V00CZ Restriction of Right Internal Mammary Artery with Extraluminal Device, Open Approach
V00DZ Restriction of Right Internal Mammary Artery with Intraluminal Device, Open Approach
V00ZZ Restriction of Right Internal Mammary Artery, Open Approach
V03CZ Restriction of Right Internal Mammary Artery with Extraluminal Device, Percutaneous Approach
V03DZ Restriction of Right Internal Mammary Artery with Intraluminal Device, Percutaneous Approach
V03ZZ Restriction of Right Internal Mammary Artery, Percutaneous Approach
V04CZ Restriction of Right Internal Mammary Artery with Extraluminal Device, Percutaneous Endoscopic Approach
V04DZ Restriction of Right Internal Mammary Artery with Intraluminal Device, Percutaneous Endoscopic Approach
V04ZZ Restriction of Right Internal Mammary Artery, Percutaneous Endoscopic Approach
V10CZ Restriction of Left Internal Mammary Artery with Extraluminal Device, Open Approach
V10DZ Restriction of Left Internal Mammary Artery with Intraluminal Device, Open Approach
V10ZZ Restriction of Left Internal Mammary Artery, Open Approach
V13CZ Restriction of Left Internal Mammary Artery with Extraluminal Device, Percutaneous Approach
V13DZ Restriction of Left Internal Mammary Artery with Intraluminal Device, Percutaneous Approach
V13ZZ Restriction of Left Internal Mammary Artery, Percutaneous Approach
V14CZ Restriction of Left Internal Mammary Artery with Extraluminal Device, Percutaneous Endoscopic Approach
V14DZ Restriction of Left Internal Mammary Artery with Intraluminal Device, Percutaneous Endoscopic Approach
V14ZZ Restriction of Left Internal Mammary Artery, Percutaneous Endoscopic Approach
V20CZ Restriction of Innominate Artery with Extraluminal Device, Open Approach
V20DZ Restriction of Innominate Artery with Intraluminal Device, Open Approach

03V20ZZ Restriction of Innominate Artery, Open Approach
03V23CZ Restriction of Innominate Artery with Extraluminal Device, Percutaneous Approach
03V23DZ Restriction of Innominate Artery with Intraluminal Device, Percutaneous Approach
03V23ZZ Restriction of Innominate Artery, Percutaneous Approach
03V24CZ Restriction of Innominate Artery with Extraluminal Device, Percutaneous Endoscopic Approach
03V24DZ Restriction of Innominate Artery with Intraluminal Device, Percutaneous Endoscopic Approach
03V24ZZ Restriction of Innominate Artery, Percutaneous Endoscopic Approach
03V30CZ Restriction of Right Subclavian Artery with Extraluminal Device, Open Approach
03V30DZ Restriction of Right Subclavian Artery with Intraluminal Device, Open Approach
03V30ZZ Restriction of Right Subclavian Artery, Open Approach
03V33CZ Restriction of Right Subclavian Artery with Extraluminal Device, Percutaneous Approach
03V33DZ Restriction of Right Subclavian Artery with Intraluminal Device, Percutaneous Approach
03V33ZZ Restriction of Right Subclavian Artery, Percutaneous Approach
03V34CZ Restriction of Right Subclavian Artery with Extraluminal Device, Percutaneous Endoscopic Approach
03V34DZ Restriction of Right Subclavian Artery with Intraluminal Device, Percutaneous Endoscopic Approach
03V34ZZ Restriction of Right Subclavian Artery, Percutaneous Endoscopic Approach
03V40CZ Restriction of Left Subclavian Artery with Extraluminal Device, Open Approach
03V40DZ Restriction of Left Subclavian Artery with Intraluminal Device, Open Approach
03V40ZZ Restriction of Left Subclavian Artery, Open Approach
03V43CZ Restriction of Left Subclavian Artery with Extraluminal Device, Percutaneous Approach
03V43DZ Restriction of Left Subclavian Artery with Intraluminal Device, Percutaneous Approach
03V43ZZ Restriction of Left Subclavian Artery, Percutaneous Approach

03V44CZ Restriction of Left Subclavian Artery with Extraluminal Device, Percutaneous Endoscopic Approach
03V44DZ Restriction of Left Subclavian Artery with Intraluminal Device, Percutaneous Endoscopic Approach
03V44ZZ Restriction of Left Subclavian Artery, Percutaneous Endoscopic Approach
03V50CZ Restriction of Right Axillary Artery with Extraluminal Device, Open Approach
03V50DZ Restriction of Right Axillary Artery with Intraluminal Device, Open Approach
03V50ZZ Restriction of Right Axillary Artery, Open Approach
03V53CZ Restriction of Right Axillary Artery with Extraluminal Device, Percutaneous Approach
03V53DZ Restriction of Right Axillary Artery with Intraluminal Device, Percutaneous Approach
03V53ZZ Restriction of Right Axillary Artery, Percutaneous Approach
03V54CZ Restriction of Right Axillary Artery with Extraluminal Device, Percutaneous Endoscopic Approach
03V54DZ Restriction of Right Axillary Artery with Intraluminal Device, Percutaneous Endoscopic Approach
03V54ZZ Restriction of Right Axillary Artery, Percutaneous Endoscopic Approach
03V60CZ Restriction of Left Axillary Artery with Extraluminal Device, Open Approach
03V60DZ Restriction of Left Axillary Artery with Intraluminal Device, Open Approach
03V60ZZ Restriction of Left Axillary Artery, Open Approach
03V63CZ Restriction of Left Axillary Artery with Extraluminal Device, Percutaneous Approach
03V63DZ Restriction of Left Axillary Artery with Intraluminal Device, Percutaneous Approach
03V63ZZ Restriction of Left Axillary Artery, Percutaneous Approach
03V64CZ Restriction of Left Axillary Artery with Extraluminal Device, Percutaneous Endoscopic Approach
03V64DZ Restriction of Left Axillary Artery with Intraluminal Device, Percutaneous Endoscopic Approach
03V64ZZ Restriction of Left Axillary Artery, Percutaneous Endoscopic Approach
03V70CZ Restriction of Right Brachial Artery with Extraluminal Device, Open Approach

♀ Female-only ♂ Male-only ▲ Limited Coverage ● Non-OR ▨ HAC-associated procedure ▲ Non-covered procedures ➕ Combination

03V70DZ Restriction of Right Brachial Artery with Intraluminal Device, Open Approach

03V70ZZ Restriction of Right Brachial Artery, Open Approach

03V73CZ Restriction of Right Brachial Artery with Extraluminal Device, Percutaneous Approach

03V73DZ Restriction of Right Brachial Artery with Intraluminal Device, Percutaneous Approach

03V73ZZ Restriction of Right Brachial Artery, Percutaneous Approach

03V74CZ Restriction of Right Brachial Artery with Extraluminal Device, Percutaneous Endoscopic Approach

03V74DZ Restriction of Right Brachial Artery with Intraluminal Device, Percutaneous Endoscopic Approach

03V74ZZ Restriction of Right Brachial Artery, Percutaneous Endoscopic Approach

03V80CZ Restriction of Left Brachial Artery with Extraluminal Device, Open Approach

03V80DZ Restriction of Left Brachial Artery with Intraluminal Device, Open Approach

03V80ZZ Restriction of Left Brachial Artery, Open Approach

03V83CZ Restriction of Left Brachial Artery with Extraluminal Device, Percutaneous Approach

03V83DZ Restriction of Left Brachial Artery with Intraluminal Device, Percutaneous Approach

03V83ZZ Restriction of Left Brachial Artery, Percutaneous Approach

03V84CZ Restriction of Left Brachial Artery with Extraluminal Device, Percutaneous Endoscopic Approach

03V84DZ Restriction of Left Brachial Artery with Intraluminal Device, Percutaneous Endoscopic Approach

03V84ZZ Restriction of Left Brachial Artery, Percutaneous Endoscopic Approach

03V90CZ Restriction of Right Ulnar Artery with Extraluminal Device, Open Approach

03V90DZ Restriction of Right Ulnar Artery with Intraluminal Device, Open Approach

03V90ZZ Restriction of Right Ulnar Artery, Open Approach

03V93CZ Restriction of Right Ulnar Artery with Extraluminal Device, Percutaneous Approach

03V93DZ Restriction of Right Ulnar Artery with Intraluminal Device, Percutaneous Approach

03V93ZZ Restriction of Right Ulnar Artery, Percutaneous Approach

03V94CZ Restriction of Right Ulnar Artery with Extraluminal Device, Percutaneous Endoscopic Approach

03V94DZ Restriction of Right Ulnar Artery with Intraluminal Device, Percutaneous Endoscopic Approach

03V94ZZ Restriction of Right Ulnar Artery, Percutaneous Endoscopic Approach

03VA0CZ Restriction of Left Ulnar Artery with Extraluminal Device, Open Approach

03VA0DZ Restriction of Left Ulnar Artery with Intraluminal Device, Open Approach

03VA0ZZ Restriction of Left Ulnar Artery, Open Approach

03VA3CZ Restriction of Left Ulnar Artery with Extraluminal Device, Percutaneous Approach

03VA3DZ Restriction of Left Ulnar Artery with Intraluminal Device, Percutaneous Approach

03VA3ZZ Restriction of Left Ulnar Artery, Percutaneous Approach

03VA4CZ Restriction of Left Ulnar Artery with Extraluminal Device, Percutaneous Endoscopic Approach

03VA4DZ Restriction of Left Ulnar Artery with Intraluminal Device, Percutaneous Endoscopic Approach

03VA4ZZ Restriction of Left Ulnar Artery, Percutaneous Endoscopic Approach

03VB0CZ Restriction of Right Radial Artery with Extraluminal Device, Open Approach

03VB0DZ Restriction of Right Radial Artery with Intraluminal Device, Open Approach

03VB0ZZ Restriction of Right Radial Artery, Open Approach

03VB3CZ Restriction of Right Radial Artery with Extraluminal Device, Percutaneous Approach

03VB3DZ Restriction of Right Radial Artery with Intraluminal Device, Percutaneous Approach

03VB3ZZ Restriction of Right Radial Artery, Percutaneous Approach

03VB4CZ Restriction of Right Radial Artery with Extraluminal Device, Percutaneous Endoscopic Approach

03VB4DZ Restriction of Right Radial Artery with Intraluminal Device, Percutaneous Endoscopic Approach

03VB4ZZ Restriction of Right Radial Artery, Percutaneous Endoscopic Approach

03VC0CZ Restriction of Left Radial Artery with Extraluminal Device, Open Approach

03VC0DZ Restriction of Left Radial Artery with Intraluminal Device, Open Approach

03VC0ZZ Restriction of Left Radial Artery, Open Approach

03VC3CZ Restriction of Left Radial Artery with Extraluminal Device, Percutaneous Approach

03VC3DZ Restriction of Left Radial Artery with Intraluminal Device, Percutaneous Approach

03VC3ZZ Restriction of Left Radial Artery, Percutaneous Approach

03VC4CZ Restriction of Left Radial Artery with Extraluminal Device, Percutaneous Endoscopic Approach

03VC4DZ Restriction of Left Radial Artery with Intraluminal Device, Percutaneous Endoscopic Approach

03VC4ZZ Restriction of Left Radial Artery, Percutaneous Endoscopic Approach

03VD0CZ Restriction of Right Hand Artery with Extraluminal Device, Open Approach

03VD0DZ Restriction of Right Hand Artery with Intraluminal Device, Open Approach

03VD0ZZ Restriction of Right Hand Artery, Open Approach

03VD3CZ Restriction of Right Hand Artery with Extraluminal Device, Percutaneous Approach

03VD3DZ Restriction of Right Hand Artery with Intraluminal Device, Percutaneous Approach

03VD3ZZ Restriction of Right Hand Artery, Percutaneous Approach

03VD4CZ Restriction of Right Hand Artery with Extraluminal Device, Percutaneous Endoscopic Approach

03VD4DZ Restriction of Right Hand Artery with Intraluminal Device, Percutaneous Endoscopic Approach

03VD4ZZ Restriction of Right Hand Artery, Percutaneous Endoscopic Approach

03VF0CZ Restriction of Left Hand Artery with Extraluminal Device, Open Approach

03VF0DZ Restriction of Left Hand Artery with Intraluminal Device, Open Approach

03VF0ZZ Restriction of Left Hand Artery, Open Approach

03VF3CZ Restriction of Left Hand Artery with Extraluminal Device, Percutaneous Approach

03VF3DZ Restriction of Left Hand Artery with Intraluminal Device, Percutaneous Approach

03VF3ZZ Restriction of Left Hand Artery, Percutaneous Approach

03VF4CZ Restriction of Left Hand Artery with Extraluminal Device, Percutaneous Endoscopic Approach

03VF4DZ Restriction of Left Hand Artery with Intraluminal Device, Percutaneous Endoscopic Approach

03VF4ZZ Restriction of Left Hand Artery, Percutaneous Endoscopic Approach

03VG0BZ Restriction of Intracranial Artery with Bioactive Intraluminal Device, Open Approach

03VG0CZ Restriction of Intracranial Artery with Extraluminal Device, Open Approach

03VG0DZ Restriction of Intracranial Artery with Intraluminal Device, Open Approach

03VG0ZZ Restriction of Intracranial Artery, Open Approach

03VG3BZ Restriction of Intracranial Artery with Bioactive Intraluminal Device, Percutaneous Approach

03VG3CZ Restriction of Intracranial Artery with Extraluminal Device, Percutaneous Approach

03VG3DZ Restriction of Intracranial Artery with Intraluminal Device, Percutaneous Approach

03VG3ZZ Restriction of Intracranial Artery, Percutaneous Approach

03VG4BZ Restriction of Intracranial Artery with Bioactive Intraluminal Device, Percutaneous Endoscopic Approach

03VG4CZ Restriction of Intracranial Artery with Extraluminal Device, Percutaneous Endoscopic Approach

03VG4DZ Restriction of Intracranial Artery with Intraluminal Device, Percutaneous Endoscopic Approach

03VG4ZZ Restriction of Intracranial Artery, Percutaneous Endoscopic Approach

03VH0BZ Restriction of Right Common Carotid Artery with Bioactive Intraluminal Device, Open Approach

03VH0CZ Restriction of Right Common Carotid Artery with Extraluminal Device, Open Approach

03VH0DZ Restriction of Right Common Carotid Artery with Intraluminal Device, Open Approach

03VH0ZZ Restriction of Right Common Carotid Artery, Open Approach

03VH3BZ Restriction of Right Common Carotid Artery with Bioactive Intraluminal Device, Percutaneous Approach

03VH3CZ Restriction of Right Common Carotid Artery with Extraluminal Device, Percutaneous Approach

03VH3DZ Restriction of Right Common Carotid Artery with Intraluminal Device, Percutaneous Approach

03VH3ZZ Restriction of Right Common Carotid Artery, Percutaneous Approach

03VH4BZ Restriction of Right Common Carotid Artery with Bioactive Intraluminal Device, Percutaneous Endoscopic Approach

03VH4CZ Restriction of Right Common Carotid Artery with Extraluminal Device, Percutaneous Endoscopic Approach

H4DZ Restriction of Right Common Carotid Artery with Intraluminal Device, Percutaneous Endoscopic Approach

H4ZZ Restriction of Right Common Carotid Artery, Percutaneous Endoscopic Approach

J0BZ Restriction of Left Common Carotid Artery with Bioactive Intraluminal Device, Open Approach

J0CZ Restriction of Left Common Carotid Artery with Extraluminal Device, Open Approach

J0DZ Restriction of Left Common Carotid Artery with Intraluminal Device, Open Approach

J0ZZ Restriction of Left Common Carotid Artery, Open Approach

J3BZ Restriction of Left Common Carotid Artery with Bioactive Intraluminal Device, Percutaneous Approach

J3CZ Restriction of Left Common Carotid Artery with Extraluminal Device, Percutaneous Approach

J3DZ Restriction of Left Common Carotid Artery with Intraluminal Device, Percutaneous Approach

J3ZZ Restriction of Left Common Carotid Artery, Percutaneous Approach

J4BZ Restriction of Left Common Carotid Artery with Bioactive Intraluminal Device, Percutaneous Endoscopic Approach

J4CZ Restriction of Left Common Carotid Artery with Extraluminal Device, Percutaneous Endoscopic Approach

J4DZ Restriction of Left Common Carotid Artery with Intraluminal Device, Percutaneous Endoscopic Approach

J4ZZ Restriction of Left Common Carotid Artery, Percutaneous Endoscopic Approach

VK0BZ Restriction of Right Internal Carotid Artery with Bioactive Intraluminal Device, Open Approach

VK0CZ Restriction of Right Internal Carotid Artery with Extraluminal Device, Open Approach

VK0DZ Restriction of Right Internal Carotid Artery with Intraluminal Device, Open Approach

VK0ZZ Restriction of Right Internal Carotid Artery, Open Approach

VK3BZ Restriction of Right Internal Carotid Artery with Bioactive Intraluminal Device, Percutaneous Approach

VK3CZ Restriction of Right Internal Carotid Artery with Extraluminal Device, Percutaneous Approach

VK3DZ Restriction of Right Internal Carotid Artery with Intraluminal Device, Percutaneous Approach

VK3ZZ Restriction of Right Internal Carotid Artery, Percutaneous Approach

VK4BZ Restriction of Right Internal Carotid Artery with Bioactive Intraluminal Device, Percutaneous Endoscopic Approach

VK4CZ Restriction of Right Internal Carotid Artery with Extraluminal Device, Percutaneous Endoscopic Approach

VK4DZ Restriction of Right Internal Carotid Artery with Intraluminal Device, Percutaneous Endoscopic Approach

VK4ZZ Restriction of Right Internal Carotid Artery, Percutaneous Endoscopic Approach

3VL0BZ Restriction of Left Internal Carotid Artery with Bioactive Intraluminal Device, Open Approach

03VL0CZ Restriction of Left Internal Carotid Artery with Extraluminal Device, Open Approach

03VL0DZ Restriction of Left Internal Carotid Artery with Intraluminal Device, Open Approach

03VL0ZZ Restriction of Left Internal Carotid Artery, Open Approach

03VL3BZ Restriction of Left Internal Carotid Artery with Bioactive Intraluminal Device, Percutaneous Approach

03VL3CZ Restriction of Left Internal Carotid Artery with Extraluminal Device, Percutaneous Approach

03VL3DZ Restriction of Left Internal Carotid Artery with Intraluminal Device, Percutaneous Approach

03VL3ZZ Restriction of Left Internal Carotid Artery, Percutaneous Approach

03VL4BZ Restriction of Left Internal Carotid Artery with Bioactive Intraluminal Device, Percutaneous Endoscopic Approach

03VL4CZ Restriction of Left Internal Carotid Artery with Extraluminal Device, Percutaneous Endoscopic Approach

03VL4DZ Restriction of Left Internal Carotid Artery with Intraluminal Device, Percutaneous Endoscopic Approach

03VL4ZZ Restriction of Left Internal Carotid Artery, Percutaneous Endoscopic Approach

03VM0BZ Restriction of Right External Carotid Artery with Bioactive Intraluminal Device, Open Approach

03VM0CZ Restriction of Right External Carotid Artery with Extraluminal Device, Open Approach

03VM0DZ Restriction of Right External Carotid Artery with Intraluminal Device, Open Approach

03VM0ZZ Restriction of Right External Carotid Artery, Open Approach

03VM3BZ Restriction of Right External Carotid Artery with Bioactive Intraluminal Device, Percutaneous Approach

03VM3CZ Restriction of Right External Carotid Artery with Extraluminal Device, Percutaneous Approach

03VM3DZ Restriction of Right External Carotid Artery with Intraluminal Device, Percutaneous Approach

03VM3ZZ Restriction of Right External Carotid Artery, Percutaneous Approach

03VM4BZ Restriction of Right External Carotid Artery with Bioactive Intraluminal Device, Percutaneous Endoscopic Approach

03VM4CZ Restriction of Right External Carotid Artery with Extraluminal Device, Percutaneous Endoscopic Approach

03VM4DZ Restriction of Right External Carotid Artery with Intraluminal Device, Percutaneous Endoscopic Approach

03VM4ZZ Restriction of Right External Carotid Artery, Percutaneous Endoscopic Approach

03VN0BZ Restriction of Left External Carotid Artery with Bioactive Intraluminal Device, Open Approach

03VN0CZ Restriction of Left External Carotid Artery with Extraluminal Device, Open Approach

03VN0DZ Restriction of Left External Carotid Artery with Intraluminal Device, Open Approach

03VN0ZZ Restriction of Left External Carotid Artery, Open Approach

03VN3BZ Restriction of Left External Carotid Artery with Bioactive Intraluminal Device, Percutaneous Approach

03VN3CZ Restriction of Left External Carotid Artery with Extraluminal Device, Percutaneous Approach

03VN3DZ Restriction of Left External Carotid Artery with Intraluminal Device, Percutaneous Approach

03VN3ZZ Restriction of Left External Carotid Artery, Percutaneous Approach

03VN4BZ Restriction of Left External Carotid Artery with Bioactive Intraluminal Device, Percutaneous Endoscopic Approach

03VN4CZ Restriction of Left External Carotid Artery with Extraluminal Device, Percutaneous Endoscopic Approach

03VN4DZ Restriction of Left External Carotid Artery with Intraluminal Device, Percutaneous Endoscopic Approach

03VN4ZZ Restriction of Left External Carotid Artery, Percutaneous Endoscopic Approach

03VP0BZ Restriction of Right Vertebral Artery with Bioactive Intraluminal Device, Open Approach

03VP0CZ Restriction of Right Vertebral Artery with Extraluminal Device, Open Approach

03VP0DZ Restriction of Right Vertebral Artery with Intraluminal Device, Open Approach

03VP0ZZ Restriction of Right Vertebral Artery, Open Approach

03VP3BZ Restriction of Right Vertebral Artery with Bioactive Intraluminal Device, Percutaneous Approach

03VP3CZ Restriction of Right Vertebral Artery with Extraluminal Device, Percutaneous Approach

03VP3DZ Restriction of Right Vertebral Artery with Intraluminal Device, Percutaneous Approach

03VP3ZZ Restriction of Right Vertebral Artery, Percutaneous Approach

03VP4BZ Restriction of Right Vertebral Artery with Bioactive Intraluminal Device, Percutaneous Endoscopic Approach

03VP4CZ Restriction of Right Vertebral Artery with Extraluminal Device, Percutaneous Endoscopic Approach

03VP4DZ Restriction of Right Vertebral Artery with Intraluminal Device, Percutaneous Endoscopic Approach

03VP4ZZ Restriction of Right Vertebral Artery, Percutaneous Endoscopic Approach

03VQ0BZ Restriction of Left Vertebral Artery with Bioactive Intraluminal Device, Open Approach

03VQ0CZ Restriction of Left Vertebral Artery with Extraluminal Device, Open Approach

03VQ0DZ Restriction of Left Vertebral Artery with Intraluminal Device, Open Approach

03VQ0ZZ Restriction of Left Vertebral Artery, Open Approach

03VQ3BZ Restriction of Left Vertebral Artery with Bioactive Intraluminal Device, Percutaneous Approach

03VQ3CZ Restriction of Left Vertebral Artery with Extraluminal Device, Percutaneous Approach

03VQ3DZ Restriction of Left Vertebral Artery with Intraluminal Device, Percutaneous Approach

03VQ3ZZ Restriction of Left Vertebral Artery, Percutaneous Approach

03VQ4BZ Restriction of Left Vertebral Artery with Bioactive Intraluminal Device, Percutaneous Endoscopic Approach

03VQ4CZ Restriction of Left Vertebral Artery with Extraluminal Device, Percutaneous Endoscopic Approach

03VQ4DZ Restriction of Left Vertebral Artery with Intraluminal Device, Percutaneous Endoscopic Approach

♀ Female-only   ♂ Male-only   ▲ Limited Coverage   ● Non-OR   ▨ HAC-associated procedure   ▲ Non-covered procedures   ✛ Combination

03VQ4ZZ	Restriction of Left Vertebral Artery, Percutaneous Endoscopic Approach
03VR0CZ	Restriction of Face Artery with Extraluminal Device, Open Approach
03VR0DZ	Restriction of Face Artery with Intraluminal Device, Open Approach
03VR0ZZ	Restriction of Face Artery, Open Approach
03VR3CZ	Restriction of Face Artery with Extraluminal Device, Percutaneous Approach
03VR3DZ	Restriction of Face Artery with Intraluminal Device, Percutaneous Approach
03VR3ZZ	Restriction of Face Artery, Percutaneous Approach
03VR4CZ	Restriction of Face Artery with Extraluminal Device, Percutaneous Endoscopic Approach
03VR4DZ	Restriction of Face Artery with Intraluminal Device, Percutaneous Endoscopic Approach
03VR4ZZ	Restriction of Face Artery, Percutaneous Endoscopic Approach
03VS0CZ	Restriction of Right Temporal Artery with Extraluminal Device, Open Approach
03VS0DZ	Restriction of Right Temporal Artery with Intraluminal Device, Open Approach
03VS0ZZ	Restriction of Right Temporal Artery, Open Approach
03VS3CZ	Restriction of Right Temporal Artery with Extraluminal Device, Percutaneous Approach
03VS3DZ	Restriction of Right Temporal Artery with Intraluminal Device, Percutaneous Approach
03VS3ZZ	Restriction of Right Temporal Artery, Percutaneous Approach
03VS4CZ	Restriction of Right Temporal Artery with Extraluminal Device, Percutaneous Endoscopic Approach
03VS4DZ	Restriction of Right Temporal Artery with Intraluminal Device, Percutaneous Endoscopic Approach
03VS4ZZ	Restriction of Right Temporal Artery, Percutaneous Endoscopic Approach
03VT0CZ	Restriction of Left Temporal Artery with Extraluminal Device, Open Approach
03VT0DZ	Restriction of Left Temporal Artery with Intraluminal Device, Open Approach
03VT0ZZ	Restriction of Left Temporal Artery, Open Approach
03VT3CZ	Restriction of Left Temporal Artery with Extraluminal Device, Percutaneous Approach
03VT3DZ	Restriction of Left Temporal Artery with Intraluminal Device, Percutaneous Approach
03VT3ZZ	Restriction of Left Temporal Artery, Percutaneous Approach
03VT4CZ	Restriction of Left Temporal Artery with Extraluminal Device, Percutaneous Endoscopic Approach
03VT4DZ	Restriction of Left Temporal Artery with Intraluminal Device, Percutaneous Endoscopic Approach
03VT4ZZ	Restriction of Left Temporal Artery, Percutaneous Endoscopic Approach
03VU0CZ	Restriction of Right Thyroid Artery with Extraluminal Device, Open Approach
03VU0DZ	Restriction of Right Thyroid Artery with Intraluminal Device, Open Approach
03VU0ZZ	Restriction of Right Thyroid Artery, Open Approach
03VU3CZ	Restriction of Right Thyroid Artery with Extraluminal Device, Percutaneous Approach
03VU3DZ	Restriction of Right Thyroid Artery with Intraluminal Device, Percutaneous Approach
03VU3ZZ	Restriction of Right Thyroid Artery, Percutaneous Approach
03VU4CZ	Restriction of Right Thyroid Artery with Extraluminal Device, Percutaneous Endoscopic Approach
03VU4DZ	Restriction of Right Thyroid Artery with Intraluminal Device, Percutaneous Endoscopic Approach
03VU4ZZ	Restriction of Right Thyroid Artery, Percutaneous Endoscopic Approach
03VV0CZ	Restriction of Left Thyroid Artery with Extraluminal Device, Open Approach
03VV0DZ	Restriction of Left Thyroid Artery with Intraluminal Device, Open Approach
03VV0ZZ	Restriction of Left Thyroid Artery, Open Approach
03VV3CZ	Restriction of Left Thyroid Artery with Extraluminal Device, Percutaneous Approach
03VV3DZ	Restriction of Left Thyroid Artery with Intraluminal Device, Percutaneous Approach
03VV3ZZ	Restriction of Left Thyroid Artery, Percutaneous Approach
03VV4CZ	Restriction of Left Thyroid Artery with Extraluminal Device, Percutaneous Endoscopic Approach
03VV4DZ	Restriction of Left Thyroid Artery with Intraluminal Device, Percutaneous Endoscopic Approach
03VV4ZZ	Restriction of Left Thyroid Artery, Percutaneous Endoscopic Approach
03VY0CZ	Restriction of Upper Artery with Extraluminal Device, Open Approach
03VY0DZ	Restriction of Upper Artery with Intraluminal Device, Open Approach
03VY0ZZ	Restriction of Upper Artery, Open Approach
03VY3CZ	Restriction of Upper Artery with Extraluminal Device, Percutaneous Approach
03VY3DZ	Restriction of Upper Artery with Intraluminal Device, Percutaneous Approach
03VY3ZZ	Restriction of Upper Artery, Percutaneous Approach
03VY4CZ	Restriction of Upper Artery with Extraluminal Device, Percutaneous Endoscopic Approach
03VY4DZ	Restriction of Upper Artery with Intraluminal Device, Percutaneous Endoscopic Approach
03VY4ZZ	Restriction of Upper Artery, Percutaneous Endoscopic Approach

03W – Upper Arteries, Revision

Review Coding Guideline B6.1c

03WY00Z	Revision of Drainage Device in Upper Artery, Open Approach
03WY02Z	Revision of Monitoring Device in Upper Artery, Open Approach
03WY03Z	Revision of Infusion Device in Upper Artery, Open Approach
03WY07Z	Revision of Autologous Tissue Substitute in Upper Artery, Open Approach
03WY0CZ	Revision of Extraluminal Device in Upper Artery, Open Approach
03WY0DZ	Revision of Intraluminal Device in Upper Artery, Open Approach
03WY0JZ	Revision of Synthetic Substitute in Upper Artery, Open Approach
03WY0KZ	Revision of Nonautologous Tissue Substitute in Upper Artery, Open Approach
03WY0MZ	Revision of Stimulator Lead in Upper Artery, Open Approach
03WY30Z	Revision of Drainage Device in Upper Artery, Percutaneous Approach
03WY32Z	Revision of Monitoring Device in Upper Artery, Percutaneous Approach
03WY33Z	Revision of Infusion Device in Upper Artery, Percutaneous Approach
03WY37Z	Revision of Autologous Tissue Substitute in Upper Artery, Percutaneous Approach
03WY3CZ	Revision of Extraluminal Device in Upper Artery, Percutaneous Approach
03WY3DZ	Revision of Intraluminal Device in Upper Artery, Percutaneous Approach *AHA CC: 1Q, 2015, 32-33*
03WY3JZ	Revision of Synthetic Substitute in Upper Artery, Percutaneous Approach
03WY3KZ	Revision of Nonautologous Tissue Substitute in Upper Artery, Percutaneous Approach
03WY3MZ	Revision of Stimulator Lead in Upper Artery, Percutaneous Approach
03WY40Z	Revision of Drainage Device in Upper Artery, Percutaneous Endoscopic Approach
03WY42Z	Revision of Monitoring Device in Upper Artery, Percutaneous Endoscopic Approach
03WY43Z	Revision of Infusion Device in Upper Artery, Percutaneous Endoscopic Approach
03WY47Z	Revision of Autologous Tissue Substitute in Upper Artery, Percutaneous Endoscopic Approach
03WY4CZ	Revision of Extraluminal Device in Upper Artery, Percutaneous Endoscopic Approach
03WY4DZ	Revision of Intraluminal Device in Upper Artery, Percutaneous Endoscopic Approach
03WY4JZ	Revision of Synthetic Substitute in Upper Artery, Percutaneous Endoscopic Approach
03WY4KZ	Revision of Nonautologous Tissue Substitute in Upper Artery, Percutaneous Endoscopic Approach
03WY4MZ	Revision of Stimulator Lead in Upper Artery, Percutaneous Endoscopic Approach
03WYX0Z	Revision of Drainage Device in Upper Artery, External Approach
03WYX2Z	Revision of Monitoring Device in Upper Artery, External Approach
03WYX3Z	Revision of Infusion Device in Upper Artery, External Approach
03WYX7Z	Revision of Autologous Tissue Substitute in Upper Artery, External Approach
03WYXCZ	Revision of Extraluminal Device in Upper Artery, External Approach
03WYXDZ	Revision of Intraluminal Device in Upper Artery, External Approach
03WYXJZ	Revision of Synthetic Substitute in Upper Artery, External Approach
03WYXKZ	Revision of Nonautologous Tissue Substitute in Upper Artery, External Approach
03WYXMZ	Revision of Stimulator Lead in Upper Artery, External Approach

Arteries

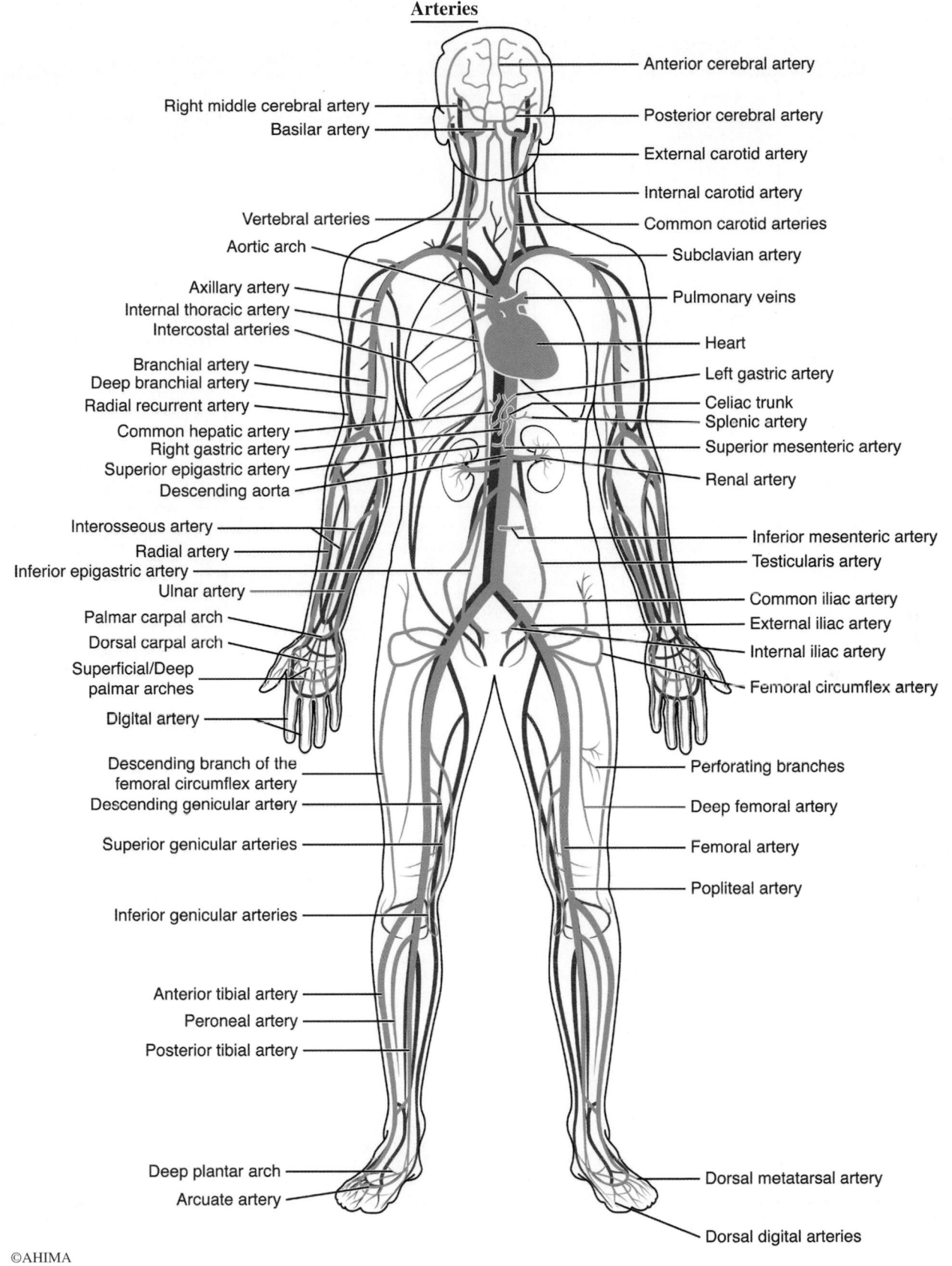

Anterior cerebral artery

Right middle cerebral artery

Basilar artery

Posterior cerebral artery

External carotid artery

Internal carotid artery

Vertebral arteries

Common carotid arteries

Aortic arch

Subclavian artery

Axillary artery

Pulmonary veins

Internal thoracic artery

Intercostal arteries

Heart

Branchial artery

Left gastric artery

Deep branchial artery

Celiac trunk

Radial recurrent artery

Splenic artery

Common hepatic artery

Superior mesenteric artery

Right gastric artery

Superior epigastric artery

Renal artery

Descending aorta

Interosseous artery

Inferior mesenteric artery

Radial artery

Testicularis artery

Inferior epigastric artery

Ulnar artery

Common iliac artery

External iliac artery

Palmar carpal arch

Internal iliac artery

Dorsal carpal arch

Femoral circumflex artery

Superficial/Deep
palmar arches

Digital artery

Descending branch of the
femoral circumflex artery

Perforating branches

Descending genicular artery

Deep femoral artery

Superior genicular arteries

Femoral artery

Popliteal artery

Inferior genicular arteries

Anterior tibial artery

Peroneal artery

Posterior tibial artery

Deep plantar arch

Dorsal metatarsal artery

Arcuate artery

Dorsal digital arteries

©AHIMA

Section	0	Medical and Surgical
Body System	4	Lower Arteries
Operation	1	**Bypass:** Altering the route of passage of the contents of a tubular body part

Body Part (4th)	Approach (5th)	Device (6th)	Qualifier (7th)
0 Abdominal Aorta C Common Iliac Artery, Right D Common Iliac Artery, Left	0 Open 4 Percutaneous Endoscopic	9 Autologous Venous Tissue A Autologous Arterial Tissue J Synthetic Substitute K Nonautologous Tissue Substitute Z No Device	0 Abdominal Aorta 1 Celiac Artery 2 Mesenteric Artery 3 Renal Artery, Right 4 Renal Artery, Left 5 Renal Artery, Bilateral 6 Common Iliac Artery, Right 7 Common Iliac Artery, Left 8 Common Iliac Arteries, Bilateral 9 Internal Iliac Artery, Right B Internal Iliac Artery, Left C Internal Iliac Arteries, Bilateral D External Iliac Artery, Right F External Iliac Artery, Left G External Iliac Arteries, Bilateral H Femoral Artery, Right J Femoral Artery, Left K Femoral Arteries, Bilateral Q Lower Extremity Artery R Lower Artery
4 Splenic Artery	0 Open 4 Percutaneous Endoscopic	9 Autologous Venous Tissue A Autologous Arterial Tissue J Synthetic Substitute K Nonautologous Tissue Substitute Z No Device	3 Renal Artery, Right 4 Renal Artery, Left 5 Renal Artery, Bilateral
E Internal Iliac Artery, Right F Internal Iliac Artery, Left H External Iliac Artery, Right J External Iliac Artery, Left	0 Open 4 Percutaneous Endoscopic	9 Autologous Venous Tissue A Autologous Arterial Tissue J Synthetic Substitute K Nonautologous Tissue Substitute Z No Device	9 Internal Iliac Artery, Right B Internal Iliac Artery, Left C Internal Iliac Arteries, Bilateral D External Iliac Artery, Right F External Iliac Artery, Left G External Iliac Arteries, Bilateral H Femoral Artery, Right J Femoral Artery, Left K Femoral Arteries, Bilateral P Foot Artery Q Lower Extremity Artery
K Femoral Artery, Right L Femoral Artery, Left	0 Open 4 Percutaneous Endoscopic	9 Autologous Venous Tissue A Autologous Arterial Tissue J Synthetic Substitute K Nonautologous Tissue Substitute Z No Device	H Femoral Artery, Right J Femoral Artery, Left K Femoral Arteries, Bilateral L Popliteal Artery M Peroneal Artery N Posterior Tibial Artery P Foot Artery Q Lower Extremity Artery S Lower Extremity Vein
M Popliteal Artery, Right N Popliteal Artery, Left	0 Open 4 Percutaneous Endoscopic	9 Autologous Venous Tissue A Autologous Arterial Tissue J Synthetic Substitute K Nonautologous Tissue Substitute Z No Device	L Popliteal Artery M Peroneal Artery P Foot Artery Q Lower Extremity Artery S Lower Extremity Vein

tion	0	**Medical and Surgical**	
~~y~~ System	4	**Lower Arteries**	
eration	5	**Destruction:** Physical eradication of all or a portion of a body part by the direct use of energy, force, or a destructive agent	

Body Part (4ᵗʰ)	Approach (5ᵗʰ)	Device (6ᵗʰ)	Qualifier (7ᵗʰ)
Abdominal Aorta Celiac Artery Gastric Artery Hepatic Artery Splenic Artery Superior Mesenteric Artery Colic Artery, Right Colic Artery, Left Colic Artery, Middle Renal Artery, Right Renal Artery, Left Inferior Mesenteric Artery Common Iliac Artery, Right Common Iliac Artery, Left Internal Iliac Artery, Right Internal Iliac Artery, Left External Iliac Artery, Right External Iliac Artery, Left Femoral Artery, Right Femoral Artery, Left Popliteal Artery, Right Popliteal Artery, Left Anterior Tibial Artery, Right Anterior Tibial Artery, Left Posterior Tibial Artery, Right Posterior Tibial Artery, Left Peroneal Artery, Right Peroneal Artery, Left Foot Artery, Right Foot Artery, Left Lower Artery	0 Open 3 Percutaneous 4 Percutaneous Endoscopic	**Z** No Device	**Z** No Qualifier

Section	**0** **Medical and Surgical**
Body System	**4** **Lower Arteries**
Operation	**7** **Dilation:** Expanding an orifice or the lumen of a tubular body part

Body Part (4th)	Approach (5th)	Device (6th)	Qualifier (7th)
0 Abdominal Aorta **1** Celiac Artery **2** Gastric Artery **3** Hepatic Artery **4** Splenic Artery **5** Superior Mesenteric Artery **6** Colic Artery, Right **7** Colic Artery, Left **8** Colic Artery, Middle **9** Renal Artery, Right **A** Renal Artery, Left **B** Inferior Mesenteric Artery **C** Common Iliac Artery, Right **D** Common Iliac Artery, Left **E** Internal Iliac Artery, Right **F** Internal Iliac Artery, Left **H** External Iliac Artery, Right **J** External Iliac Artery, Left **P** Anterior Tibial Artery, Right **Q** Anterior Tibial Artery, Left **R** Posterior Tibial Artery, Right **S** Posterior Tibial Artery, Left **T** Peroneal Artery, Right **U** Peroneal Artery, Left **V** Foot Artery, Right **W** Foot Artery, Left **Y** Lower Artery	**0** Open **3** Percutaneous **4** Percutaneous Endoscopic	**4** Intraluminal Device, Drug-eluting **D** Intraluminal Device **Z** No Device	**Z** No Qualifier
K Femoral Artery, Right **L** Femoral Artery, Left **M** Popliteal Artery, Right **N** Popliteal Artery, Left	**0** Open **3** Percutaneous **4** Percutaneous Endoscopic	**4** Intraluminal Device, Drug-eluting **D** Intraluminal Device **Z** No Device	**1** Drug-Coated Balloon **Z** No Qualifier

tion	**0**	**Medical and Surgical**	
ly System	**4**	**Lower Arteries**	
eration	**9**	**Drainage:** Taking or letting out fluids and/or gases from a body part	

Body Part (4th)	Approach (5th)	Device (6th)	Qualifier (7th)
Abdominal Aorta Celiac Artery Gastric Artery Hepatic Artery Splenic Artery Superior Mesenteric Artery Colic Artery, Right Colic Artery, Left Colic Artery, Middle Renal Artery, Right Renal Artery, Left Inferior Mesenteric Artery Common Iliac Artery, Right Common Iliac Artery, Left Internal Iliac Artery, Right Internal Iliac Artery, Left External Iliac Artery, Right External Iliac Artery, Left Femoral Artery, Right Femoral Artery, Left Popliteal Artery, Right Popliteal Artery, Left Anterior Tibial Artery, Right Anterior Tibial Artery, Left Posterior Tibial Artery, Right Posterior Tibial Artery, Left Peroneal Artery, Right Peroneal Artery, Left Foot Artery, Right Foot Artery, Left Lower Artery	**0** Open **3** Percutaneous **4** Percutaneous Endoscopic	**0** Drainage Device	**Z** No Qualifier
1 Abdominal Aorta Celiac Artery **2** Gastric Artery **3** Hepatic Artery **4** Splenic Artery **5** Superior Mesenteric Artery **6** Colic Artery, Right **7** Colic Artery, Left **8** Colic Artery, Middle **9** Renal Artery, Right **A** Renal Artery, Left **B** Inferior Mesenteric Artery **C** Common Iliac Artery, Right **D** Common Iliac Artery, Left **E** Internal Iliac Artery, Right **F** Internal Iliac Artery, Left **H** External Iliac Artery, Right **J** External Iliac Artery, Left **K** Femoral Artery, Right **L** Femoral Artery, Left **M** Popliteal Artery, Right **N** Popliteal Artery, Left **P** Anterior Tibial Artery, Right **Q** Anterior Tibial Artery, Left **R** Posterior Tibial Artery, Right **S** Posterior Tibial Artery, Left **T** Peroneal Artery, Right **U** Peroneal Artery, Left **V** Foot Artery, Right **W** Foot Artery, Left **Y** Lower Artery	**0** Open **3** Percutaneous **4** Percutaneous Endoscopic	**Z** No Device	**X** Diagnostic **Z** No Qualifier

Section	0	**Medical and Surgical**
Body System	4	**Lower Arteries**
Operation	B	**Excision:** Cutting out or off, without replacement, a portion of a body part

Body Part (4th)	Approach (5th)	Device (6th)	Qualifier (7th)
0 Abdominal Aorta	0 Open	Z No Device	X Diagnostic
1 Celiac Artery	3 Percutaneous		Z No Qualifier
2 Gastric Artery	4 Percutaneous Endoscopic		
3 Hepatic Artery			
4 Splenic Artery			
5 Superior Mesenteric Artery			
6 Colic Artery, Right			
7 Colic Artery, Left			
8 Colic Artery, Middle			
9 Renal Artery, Right			
A Renal Artery, Left			
B Inferior Mesenteric Artery			
C Common Iliac Artery, Right			
D Common Iliac Artery, Left			
E Internal Iliac Artery, Right			
F Internal Iliac Artery, Left			
H External Iliac Artery, Right			
J External Iliac Artery, Left			
K Femoral Artery, Right			
L Femoral Artery, Left			
M Popliteal Artery, Right			
N Popliteal Artery, Left			
P Anterior Tibial Artery, Right			
Q Anterior Tibial Artery, Left			
R Posterior Tibial Artery, Right			
S Posterior Tibial Artery, Left			
T Peroneal Artery, Right			
U Peroneal Artery, Left			
V Foot Artery, Right			
W Foot Artery, Left			
Y Lower Artery			

tion	**0**	**Medical and Surgical**	
dy System	**4**	**Lower Arteries**	
eration	**C**	**Extirpation:** Taking or cutting out solid matter from a body part	

Body Part (4ᵗʰ)	Approach (5ᵗʰ)	Device (6ᵗʰ)	Qualifier (7ᵗʰ)
Abdominal Aorta Celiac Artery Gastric Artery Hepatic Artery Splenic Artery Superior Mesenteric Artery Colic Artery, Right Colic Artery, Left Colic Artery, Middle Renal Artery, Right Renal Artery, Left Inferior Mesenteric Artery Common Iliac Artery, Right Common Iliac Artery, Left Internal Iliac Artery, Right Internal Iliac Artery, Left External Iliac Artery, Right External Iliac Artery, Left Femoral Artery, Right Femoral Artery, Left Popliteal Artery, Right Popliteal Artery, Left Anterior Tibial Artery, Right Anterior Tibial Artery, Left Posterior Tibial Artery, Right Posterior Tibial Artery, Left Peroneal Artery, Right Peroneal Artery, Left Foot Artery, Right Foot Artery, Left Lower Artery	**0** Open **3** Percutaneous **4** Percutaneous Endoscopic	**Z** No Device	**Z** No Qualifier

tion	**0**	**Medical and Surgical**	
dy System	**4**	**Lower Arteries**	
eration	**H**	**Insertion:** Putting in a nonbiological appliance that monitors, assists, performs, or prevents a physiological function but does not physically take the place of a body part	

Body Part (4ᵗʰ)	Approach (5ᵗʰ)	Device (6ᵗʰ)	Qualifier (7ᵗʰ)
Abdominal Aorta Lower Artery	**0** Open **3** Percutaneous **4** Percutaneous Endoscopic	**2** Monitoring Device **3** Infusion Device **D** Intraluminal Device	**Z** No Qualifier

Continued →

Section   **0**   **Medical and Surgical**
Body System   **4**   **Lower Arteries**
Operation   **H**   **Insertion:** Putting in a nonbiological appliance that monitors, assists, performs, or prevents a physiological function but do∙ not physically take the place of a body part

Body Part (4ᵗʰ)	Approach (5ᵗʰ)	Device (6ᵗʰ)	Qualifier (7ᵗʰ)
1 Celiac Artery	0 Open	3 Infusion Device	Z No Qualifier
2 Gastric Artery	3 Percutaneous	D Intraluminal Device	
3 Hepatic Artery	4 Percutaneous Endoscopic		
4 Splenic Artery			
5 Superior Mesenteric Artery			
6 Colic Artery, Right			
7 Colic Artery, Left			
8 Colic Artery, Middle			
9 Renal Artery, Right			
A Renal Artery, Left			
B Inferior Mesenteric Artery			
C Common Iliac Artery, Right			
D Common Iliac Artery, Left			
E Internal Iliac Artery, Right			
F Internal Iliac Artery, Left			
H External Iliac Artery, Right			
J External Iliac Artery, Left			
K Femoral Artery, Right			
L Femoral Artery, Left			
M Popliteal Artery, Right			
N Popliteal Artery, Left			
P Anterior Tibial Artery, Right			
Q Anterior Tibial Artery, Left			
R Posterior Tibial Artery, Right			
S Posterior Tibial Artery, Left			
T Peroneal Artery, Right			
U Peroneal Artery, Left			
V Foot Artery, Right			
W Foot Artery, Left			

Section   **0**   **Medical and Surgical**
Body System   **4**   **Lower Arteries**
Operation   **J**   **Inspection:** Visually and/or manually exploring a body part

Body Part (4ᵗʰ)	Approach (5ᵗʰ)	Device (6ᵗʰ)	Qualifier (7ᵗʰ)
Y Lower Artery	0 Open	Z No Device	Z No Qualifier
	3 Percutaneous		
	4 Percutaneous Endoscopic		
	X External		

tion	0	Medical and Surgical
ly System	4	Lower Arteries
eration	L	Occlusion: Completely closing an orifice or the lumen of a tubular body part

Body Part (4th)	Approach (5th)	Device (6th)	Qualifier (7th)
Abdominal Aorta Celiac Artery Gastric Artery Hepatic Artery Splenic Artery Superior Mesenteric Artery Colic Artery, Right Colic Artery, Left Colic Artery, Middle Renal Artery, Right Renal Artery, Left Inferior Mesenteric Artery Common Iliac Artery, Right Common Iliac Artery, Left External Iliac Artery, Right External Iliac Artery, Left Femoral Artery, Right Femoral Artery, Left Popliteal Artery, Right Popliteal Artery, Left Anterior Tibial Artery, Right Anterior Tibial Artery, Left Posterior Tibial Artery, Right Posterior Tibial Artery, Left Peroneal Artery, Right Peroneal Artery, Left Foot Artery, Right Foot Artery, Left Lower Artery	0 Open 3 Percutaneous 4 Percutaneous Endoscopic	C Extraluminal Device D Intraluminal Device Z No Device	Z No Qualifier
Internal Iliac Artery, Right	0 Open 3 Percutaneous 4 Percutaneous Endoscopic	C Extraluminal Device D Intraluminal Device Z No Device	T Uterine Artery, Right Z No Qualifier
Internal Iliac Artery, Left	0 Open 3 Percutaneous 4 Percutaneous Endoscopic	C Extraluminal Device D Intraluminal Device Z No Device	U Uterine Artery, Left Z No Qualifier

Section	0	Medical and Surgical
Body System	4	Lower Arteries
Operation	N	Release: Freeing a body part from an abnormal physical constraint by cutting or by the use of force

Body Part (4th)	Approach (5th)	Device (6th)	Qualifier (7th)
0 Abdominal Aorta 1 Celiac Artery 2 Gastric Artery 3 Hepatic Artery 4 Splenic Artery 5 Superior Mesenteric Artery 6 Colic Artery, Right 7 Colic Artery, Left 8 Colic Artery, Middle 9 Renal Artery, Right A Renal Artery, Left B Inferior Mesenteric Artery C Common Iliac Artery, Right D Common Iliac Artery, Left E Internal Iliac Artery, Right F Internal Iliac Artery, Left H External Iliac Artery, Right J External Iliac Artery, Left K Femoral Artery, Right L Femoral Artery, Left M Popliteal Artery, Right N Popliteal Artery, Left P Anterior Tibial Artery, Right Q Anterior Tibial Artery, Left R Posterior Tibial Artery, Right S Posterior Tibial Artery, Left T Peroneal Artery, Right U Peroneal Artery, Left V Foot Artery, Right W Foot Artery, Left Y Lower Artery	0 Open 3 Percutaneous 4 Percutaneous Endoscopic	Z No Device	Z No Qualifier

Section	0	Medical and Surgical
Body System	4	Lower Arteries
Operation	P	Removal: Taking out or off a device from a body part

Body Part (4th)	Approach (5th)	Device (6th)	Qualifier (7th)
Y Lower Artery	0 Open 3 Percutaneous 4 Percutaneous Endoscopic	0 Drainage Device 2 Monitoring Device 3 Infusion Device 7 Autologous Tissue Substitute C Extraluminal Device D Intraluminal Device J Synthetic Substitute K Nonautologous Tissue Substitute	Z No Qualifier
Y Lower Artery	X External	0 Drainage Device 1 Radioactive Element 2 Monitoring Device 3 Infusion Device D Intraluminal Device	Z No Qualifier

Section   0   **Medical and Surgical**
Body System   4   **Lower Arteries**
Operation   Q   **Repair:** Restoring, to the extent possible, a body part to its normal anatomic structure and function

Body Part (4th)	Approach (5th)	Device (6th)	Qualifier (7th)
0 Abdominal Aorta 1 Celiac Artery 2 Gastric Artery 3 Hepatic Artery 4 Splenic Artery 5 Superior Mesenteric Artery 6 Colic Artery, Right 7 Colic Artery, Left 8 Colic Artery, Middle 9 Renal Artery, Right A Renal Artery, Left B Inferior Mesenteric Artery C Common Iliac Artery, Right D Common Iliac Artery, Left E Internal Iliac Artery, Right F Internal Iliac Artery, Left H External Iliac Artery, Right J External Iliac Artery, Left K Femoral Artery, Right L Femoral Artery, Left M Popliteal Artery, Right N Popliteal Artery, Left P Anterior Tibial Artery, Right Q Anterior Tibial Artery, Left R Posterior Tibial Artery, Right S Posterior Tibial Artery, Left T Peroneal Artery, Right U Peroneal Artery, Left V Foot Artery, Right W Foot Artery, Left Y Lower Artery	0 Open 3 Percutaneous 4 Percutaneous Endoscopic	Z No Device	Z No Qualifier

Section   0   **Medical and Surgical**
Body System   4   **Lower Arteries**
Operation   R   **Replacement:** Putting in or on biological or synthetic material that physically takes the place and/or function of all or a portion of a body part

Body Part (4ᵗʰ)	Approach (5ᵗʰ)	Device (6ᵗʰ)	Qualifier (7ᵗʰ)
0 Abdominal Aorta 1 Celiac Artery 2 Gastric Artery 3 Hepatic Artery 4 Splenic Artery 5 Superior Mesenteric Artery 6 Colic Artery, Right 7 Colic Artery, Left 8 Colic Artery, Middle 9 Renal Artery, Right A Renal Artery, Left B Inferior Mesenteric Artery C Common Iliac Artery, Right D Common Iliac Artery, Left E Internal Iliac Artery, Right F Internal Iliac Artery, Left H External Iliac Artery, Right J External Iliac Artery, Left K Femoral Artery, Right L Femoral Artery, Left M Popliteal Artery, Right N Popliteal Artery, Left P Anterior Tibial Artery, Right Q Anterior Tibial Artery, Left R Posterior Tibial Artery, Right S Posterior Tibial Artery, Left T Peroneal Artery, Right U Peroneal Artery, Left V Foot Artery, Right W Foot Artery, Left Y Lower Artery	0 Open 4 Percutaneous Endoscopic	7 Autologous Tissue Substitute J Synthetic Substitute K Nonautologous Tissue Substitute	Z No Qualifier

tion	0	Medical and Surgical
ly System	4	Lower Arteries
eration	S	**Reposition:** Moving to its normal location, or other suitable location, all or a portion of a body part

Body Part (4th)	Approach (5th)	Device (6th)	Qualifier (7th)
Abdominal Aorta Celiac Artery Gastric Artery Hepatic Artery Splenic Artery Superior Mesenteric Artery Colic Artery, Right Colic Artery, Left Colic Artery, Middle Renal Artery, Right Renal Artery, Left Inferior Mesenteric Artery Common Iliac Artery, Right Common Iliac Artery, Left Internal Iliac Artery, Right Internal Iliac Artery, Left External Iliac Artery, Right External Iliac Artery, Left Femoral Artery, Right Femoral Artery, Left Popliteal Artery, Right Popliteal Artery, Left Anterior Tibial Artery, Right Anterior Tibial Artery, Left Posterior Tibial Artery, Right Posterior Tibial Artery, Left Peroneal Artery, Right Peroneal Artery, Left Foot Artery, Right Foot Artery, Left Lower Artery	0 Open 3 Percutaneous 4 Percutaneous Endoscopic	Z No Device	Z No Qualifier

Section 0 **Medical and Surgical**
Body System 4 **Lower Arteries**
Operation U **Supplement:** Putting in or on biological or synthetic material that physically reinforces and/or augments the function of a portion of a body part

Body Part (4th)	Approach (5th)	Device (6th)	Qualifier (7th)
0 Abdominal Aorta 1 Celiac Artery 2 Gastric Artery 3 Hepatic Artery 4 Splenic Artery 5 Superior Mesenteric Artery 6 Colic Artery, Right 7 Colic Artery, Left 8 Colic Artery, Middle 9 Renal Artery, Right A Renal Artery, Left B Inferior Mesenteric Artery C Common Iliac Artery, Right D Common Iliac Artery, Left E Internal Iliac Artery, Right F Internal Iliac Artery, Left H External Iliac Artery, Right J External Iliac Artery, Left K Femoral Artery, Right L Femoral Artery, Left M Popliteal Artery, Right N Popliteal Artery, Left P Anterior Tibial Artery, Right Q Anterior Tibial Artery, Left R Posterior Tibial Artery, Right S Posterior Tibial Artery, Left T Peroneal Artery, Right U Peroneal Artery, Left V Foot Artery, Right W Foot Artery, Left Y Lower Artery	0 Open 3 Percutaneous 4 Percutaneous Endoscopic	7 Autologous Tissue Substitute J Synthetic Substitute K Nonautologous Tissue Substitute	Z No Qualifier

Section 0 **Medical and Surgical**
Body System 4 **Lower Arteries**
Operation V **Restriction:** Partially closing an orifice or the lumen of a tubular body part

Body Part (4th)	Approach (5th)	Device (6th)	Qualifier (7th)
0 Abdominal Aorta	0 Open 3 Percutaneous 4 Percutaneous Endoscopic	C Extraluminal Device Z No Device	Z No Qualifier
0 Abdominal Aorta	0 Open 3 Percutaneous 4 Percutaneous Endoscopic	D Intraluminal Device	J Temporary Z No Qualifier

Continued →

ction	0	**Medical and Surgical**
dy System	4	**Lower Arteries**
eration	V	**Restriction:** Partially closing an orifice or the lumen of a tubular body part

Body Part (4ᵗʰ)	Approach (5ᵗʰ)	Device (6ᵗʰ)	Qualifier (7ᵗʰ)
1 Celiac Artery 2 Gastric Artery 3 Hepatic Artery 4 Splenic Artery 5 Superior Mesenteric Artery 6 Colic Artery, Right 7 Colic Artery, Left 8 Colic Artery, Middle 9 Renal Artery, Right A Renal Artery, Left B Inferior Mesenteric Artery C Common Iliac Artery, Right D Common Iliac Artery, Left E Internal Iliac Artery, Right F Internal Iliac Artery, Left H External Iliac Artery, Right J External Iliac Artery, Left K Femoral Artery, Right L Femoral Artery, Left M Popliteal Artery, Right N Popliteal Artery, Left P Anterior Tibial Artery, Right Q Anterior Tibial Artery, Left R Posterior Tibial Artery, Right S Posterior Tibial Artery, Left T Peroneal Artery, Right U Peroneal Artery, Left V Foot Artery, Right W Foot Artery, Left Y Lower Artery	0 Open 3 Percutaneous 4 Percutaneous Endoscopic	C Extraluminal Device D Intraluminal Device Z No Device	Z No Qualifier

ction	0	**Medical and Surgical**
dy System	4	**Lower Arteries**
eration	W	**Revision:** Correcting, to the extent possible, a portion of a malfunctioning device or the position of a displaced device

Body Part (4ᵗʰ)	Approach (5ᵗʰ)	Device (6ᵗʰ)	Qualifier (7ᵗʰ)
Y Lower Artery	0 Open 3 Percutaneous 4 Percutaneous Endoscopic X External	0 Drainage Device 2 Monitoring Device 3 Infusion Device 7 Autologous Tissue Substitute C Extraluminal Device D Intraluminal Device J Synthetic Substitute K Nonautologous Tissue Substitute	Z No Qualifier

Lower Arteries Code Listing 041–04W

041 – Lower Arteries, Bypass

Review Coding Guideline B3.6a

410090	Bypass Abdominal Aorta to Abdominal Aorta with Autologous Venous Tissue, Open Approach	
410091	Bypass Abdominal Aorta to Celiac Artery with Autologous Venous Tissue, Open Approach	
410092	Bypass Abdominal Aorta to Mesenteric Artery with Autologous Venous Tissue, Open Approach	
410093	Bypass Abdominal Aorta to Right Renal Artery with Autologous Venous Tissue, Open Approach	
0410094	Bypass Abdominal Aorta to Left Renal Artery with Autologous Venous Tissue, Open Approach	
0410095	Bypass Abdominal Aorta to Bilateral Renal Artery with Autologous Venous Tissue, Open Approach	
0410096	Bypass Abdominal Aorta to Right Common Iliac Artery with Autologous Venous Tissue, Open Approach	
0410097	Bypass Abdominal Aorta to Left Common Iliac Artery with Autologous Venous Tissue, Open Approach	
0410098	Bypass Abdominal Aorta to Bilateral Common Iliac Arteries with Autologous Venous Tissue, Open Approach	
0410099	Bypass Abdominal Aorta to Right Internal Iliac Artery with Autologous Venous Tissue, Open Approach	
041009B	Bypass Abdominal Aorta to Left Internal Iliac Artery with Autologous Venous Tissue, Open Approach	
041009C	Bypass Abdominal Aorta to Bilateral Internal Iliac Arteries with Autologous Venous Tissue, Open Approach	

253

041009D	Bypass Abdominal Aorta to Right External Iliac Artery with Autologous Venous Tissue, Open Approach
041009F	Bypass Abdominal Aorta to Left External Iliac Artery with Autologous Venous Tissue, Open Approach
041009G	Bypass Abdominal Aorta to Bilateral External Iliac Arteries with Autologous Venous Tissue, Open Approach
041009H	Bypass Abdominal Aorta to Right Femoral Artery with Autologous Venous Tissue, Open Approach
041009J	Bypass Abdominal Aorta to Left Femoral Artery with Autologous Venous Tissue, Open Approach
041009K	Bypass Abdominal Aorta to Bilateral Femoral Arteries with Autologous Venous Tissue, Open Approach
041009Q	Bypass Abdominal Aorta to Lower Extremity Artery with Autologous Venous Tissue, Open Approach
041009R	Bypass Abdominal Aorta to Lower Artery with Autologous Venous Tissue, Open Approach
04100A0	Bypass Abdominal Aorta to Abdominal Aorta with Autologous Arterial Tissue, Open Approach
04100A1	Bypass Abdominal Aorta to Celiac Artery with Autologous Arterial Tissue, Open Approach
04100A2	Bypass Abdominal Aorta to Mesenteric Artery with Autologous Arterial Tissue, Open Approach
04100A3	Bypass Abdominal Aorta to Right Renal Artery with Autologous Arterial Tissue, Open Approach
04100A4	Bypass Abdominal Aorta to Left Renal Artery with Autologous Arterial Tissue, Open Approach
04100A5	Bypass Abdominal Aorta to Bilateral Renal Artery with Autologous Arterial Tissue, Open Approach
04100A6	Bypass Abdominal Aorta to Right Common Iliac Artery with Autologous Arterial Tissue, Open Approach
04100A7	Bypass Abdominal Aorta to Left Common Iliac Artery with Autologous Arterial Tissue, Open Approach
04100A8	Bypass Abdominal Aorta to Bilateral Common Iliac Arteries with Autologous Arterial Tissue, Open Approach
04100A9	Bypass Abdominal Aorta to Right Internal Iliac Artery with Autologous Arterial Tissue, Open Approach
04100AB	Bypass Abdominal Aorta to Left Internal Iliac Artery with Autologous Arterial Tissue, Open Approach
04100AC	Bypass Abdominal Aorta to Bilateral Internal Iliac Arteries with Autologous Arterial Tissue, Open Approach
04100AD	Bypass Abdominal Aorta to Right External Iliac Artery with Autologous Arterial Tissue, Open Approach
04100AF	Bypass Abdominal Aorta to Left External Iliac Artery with Autologous Arterial Tissue, Open Approach
04100AG	Bypass Abdominal Aorta to Bilateral External Iliac Arteries with Autologous Arterial Tissue, Open Approach
04100AH	Bypass Abdominal Aorta to Right Femoral Artery with Autologous Arterial Tissue, Open Approach
04100AJ	Bypass Abdominal Aorta to Left Femoral Artery with Autologous Arterial Tissue, Open Approach
04100AK	Bypass Abdominal Aorta to Bilateral Femoral Arteries with Autologous Arterial Tissue, Open Approach
04100AQ	Bypass Abdominal Aorta to Lower Extremity Artery with Autologous Arterial Tissue, Open Approach
04100AR	Bypass Abdominal Aorta to Lower Artery with Autologous Arterial Tissue, Open Approach
04100J0	Bypass Abdominal Aorta to Abdominal Aorta with Synthetic Substitute, Open Approach
04100J1	Bypass Abdominal Aorta to Celiac Artery with Synthetic Substitute, Open Approach
04100J2	Bypass Abdominal Aorta to Mesenteric Artery with Synthetic Substitute, Open Approach
04100J3	Bypass Abdominal Aorta to Right Renal Artery with Synthetic Substitute, Open Approach
04100J4	Bypass Abdominal Aorta to Left Renal Artery with Synthetic Substitute, Open Approach
04100J5	Bypass Abdominal Aorta to Bilateral Renal Artery with Synthetic Substitute, Open Approach
04100J6	Bypass Abdominal Aorta to Right Common Iliac Artery with Synthetic Substitute, Open Approach
04100J7	Bypass Abdominal Aorta to Left Common Iliac Artery with Synthetic Substitute, Open Approach
04100J8	Bypass Abdominal Aorta to Bilateral Common Iliac Arteries with Synthetic Substitute, Open Approach
04100J9	Bypass Abdominal Aorta to Right Internal Iliac Artery with Synthetic Substitute, Open Approach
04100JB	Bypass Abdominal Aorta to Left Internal Iliac Artery with Synthetic Substitute, Open Approach
04100JC	Bypass Abdominal Aorta to Bilateral Internal Iliac Arteries with Synthetic Substitute, Open Approach
04100JD	Bypass Abdominal Aorta to Right External Iliac Artery with Synthetic Substitute, Open Approach
04100JF	Bypass Abdominal Aorta to Left External Iliac Artery with Synthetic Substitute, Open Approach
04100JG	Bypass Abdominal Aorta to Bilateral External Iliac Arteries with Synthetic Substitute, Open Approach
04100JH	Bypass Abdominal Aorta to Right Femoral Artery with Synthetic Substitute, Open Approach
04100JJ	Bypass Abdominal Aorta to Left Femoral Artery with Synthetic Substitute, Open Approach
04100JK	Bypass Abdominal Aorta to Bilateral Femoral Arteries with Synthetic Substitute, Open Approach
04100JQ	Bypass Abdominal Aorta to Lower Extremity Artery with Synthetic Substitute, Open Approach
04100JR	Bypass Abdominal Aorta to Lower Artery with Synthetic Substitute, Open Approach
04100K0	Bypass Abdominal Aorta to Abdominal Aorta with Nonautologous Tissue Substitute, Open Approach
04100K1	Bypass Abdominal Aorta to Celiac Artery with Nonautologous Tissue Substitute, Open Approach
04100K2	Bypass Abdominal Aorta to Mesenteric Artery with Nonautologous Tissue Substitute, Open Approach
04100K3	Bypass Abdominal Aorta to Right Renal Artery with Nonautologous Tissue Substitute, Open Approach
04100K4	Bypass Abdominal Aorta to Left Renal Artery with Nonautologous Tissue Substitute, Open Approach
04100K5	Bypass Abdominal Aorta to Bilateral Renal Artery with Nonautologous Tissue Substitute, Open Approach
04100K6	Bypass Abdominal Aorta to Right Common Iliac Artery with Nonautologous Tissue Substitute, Open Approach
04100K7	Bypass Abdominal Aorta to Left Common Iliac Artery with Nonautologous Tissue Substitute, Open Approach
04100K8	Bypass Abdominal Aorta to Bilateral Common Iliac Arteries with Nonautologous Tissue Substitute, Open Approach
04100K9	Bypass Abdominal Aorta to Right Internal Iliac Artery with Nonautologous Tissue Substitute, Open Approach
04100KB	Bypass Abdominal Aorta to Left Internal Iliac Artery with Nonautologous Tissue Substitute, Open Approach
04100KC	Bypass Abdominal Aorta to Bilateral Internal Iliac Arteries with Nonautologous Tissue Substitute, Open Approach
04100KD	Bypass Abdominal Aorta to Right External Iliac Artery with Nonautologous Tissue Substitute, Open Approach
04100KF	Bypass Abdominal Aorta to Left External Iliac Artery with Nonautologous Tissue Substitute, Open Approach
04100KG	Bypass Abdominal Aorta to Bilateral External Iliac Arteries with Nonautologous Tissue Substitute, Open Approach
04100KH	Bypass Abdominal Aorta to Right Femoral Artery with Nonautologous Tissue Substitute, Open Approach
04100KJ	Bypass Abdominal Aorta to Left Femoral Artery with Nonautologous Tissue Substitute, Open Approach
04100KK	Bypass Abdominal Aorta to Bilateral Femoral Arteries with Nonautologous Tissue Substitute, Open Approach
04100KQ	Bypass Abdominal Aorta to Lower Extremity Artery with Nonautologous Tissue Substitute, Open Approach
04100KR	Bypass Abdominal Aorta to Lower Artery with Nonautologous Tissue Substitute, Open Approach
04100Z0	Bypass Abdominal Aorta to Abdominal Aorta, Open Approach
04100Z1	Bypass Abdominal Aorta to Celiac Artery, Open Approach
04100Z2	Bypass Abdominal Aorta to Mesenteric Artery, Open Approach
04100Z3	Bypass Abdominal Aorta to Right Renal Artery, Open Approach
04100Z4	Bypass Abdominal Aorta to Left Renal Artery, Open Approach
04100Z5	Bypass Abdominal Aorta to Bilateral Renal Artery, Open Approach
04100Z6	Bypass Abdominal Aorta to Right Common Iliac Artery, Open Approach
04100Z7	Bypass Abdominal Aorta to Left Common Iliac Artery, Open Approach
04100Z8	Bypass Abdominal Aorta to Bilateral Common Iliac Arteries, Open Approach
04100Z9	Bypass Abdominal Aorta to Right Internal Iliac Artery, Open Approach
04100ZB	Bypass Abdominal Aorta to Left Internal Iliac Artery, Open Approach
04100ZC	Bypass Abdominal Aorta to Bilateral Internal Iliac Arteries, Open Approach

♀ Female-only　　♂ Male-only　　▲ Limited Coverage　　● Non-OR　　HAC HAC-associated procedure　　▲ Non-covered procedures　　+ Combination

00ZD Bypass Abdominal Aorta to Right External Iliac Artery, Open Approach

00ZF Bypass Abdominal Aorta to Left External Iliac Artery, Open Approach

00ZG Bypass Abdominal Aorta to Bilateral External Iliac Arteries, Open Approach

00ZH Bypass Abdominal Aorta to Right Femoral Artery, Open Approach

00ZJ Bypass Abdominal Aorta to Left Femoral Artery, Open Approach

00ZK Bypass Abdominal Aorta to Bilateral Femoral Arteries, Open Approach

00ZQ Bypass Abdominal Aorta to Lower Extremity Artery, Open Approach

00ZR Bypass Abdominal Aorta to Lower Artery, Open Approach

0490 Bypass Abdominal Aorta to Abdominal Aorta with Autologous Venous Tissue, Percutaneous Endoscopic Approach

0491 Bypass Abdominal Aorta to Celiac Artery with Autologous Venous Tissue, Percutaneous Endoscopic Approach

0492 Bypass Abdominal Aorta to Mesenteric Artery with Autologous Venous Tissue, Percutaneous Endoscopic Approach

0493 Bypass Abdominal Aorta to Right Renal Artery with Autologous Venous Tissue, Percutaneous Endoscopic Approach

0494 Bypass Abdominal Aorta to Left Renal Artery with Autologous Venous Tissue, Percutaneous Endoscopic Approach

0495 Bypass Abdominal Aorta to Bilateral Renal Artery with Autologous Venous Tissue, Percutaneous Endoscopic Approach

0496 Bypass Abdominal Aorta to Right Common Iliac Artery with Autologous Venous Tissue, Percutaneous Endoscopic Approach

0497 Bypass Abdominal Aorta to Left Common Iliac Artery with Autologous Venous Tissue, Percutaneous Endoscopic Approach

0498 Bypass Abdominal Aorta to Bilateral Common Iliac Arteries with Autologous Venous Tissue, Percutaneous Endoscopic Approach

0499 Bypass Abdominal Aorta to Right Internal Iliac Artery with Autologous Venous Tissue, Percutaneous Endoscopic Approach

1049B Bypass Abdominal Aorta to Left Internal Iliac Artery with Autologous Venous Tissue, Percutaneous Endoscopic Approach

1049C Bypass Abdominal Aorta to Bilateral Internal Iliac Arteries with Autologous Venous Tissue, Percutaneous Endoscopic Approach

1049D Bypass Abdominal Aorta to Right External Iliac Artery with Autologous Venous Tissue, Percutaneous Endoscopic Approach

1049F Bypass Abdominal Aorta to Left External Iliac Artery with Autologous Venous Tissue, Percutaneous Endoscopic Approach

1049G Bypass Abdominal Aorta to Bilateral External Iliac Arteries with Autologous Venous Tissue, Percutaneous Endoscopic Approach

1049H Bypass Abdominal Aorta to Right Femoral Artery with Autologous Venous Tissue, Percutaneous Endoscopic Approach

1049J Bypass Abdominal Aorta to Left Femoral Artery with Autologous Venous Tissue, Percutaneous Endoscopic Approach

041049K Bypass Abdominal Aorta to Bilateral Femoral Arteries with Autologous Venous Tissue, Percutaneous Endoscopic Approach

041049Q Bypass Abdominal Aorta to Lower Extremity Artery with Autologous Venous Tissue, Percutaneous Endoscopic Approach

041049R Bypass Abdominal Aorta to Lower Artery with Autologous Venous Tissue, Percutaneous Endoscopic Approach

04104A0 Bypass Abdominal Aorta to Abdominal Aorta with Autologous Arterial Tissue, Percutaneous Endoscopic Approach

04104A1 Bypass Abdominal Aorta to Celiac Artery with Autologous Arterial Tissue, Percutaneous Endoscopic Approach

04104A2 Bypass Abdominal Aorta to Mesenteric Artery with Autologous Arterial Tissue, Percutaneous Endoscopic Approach

04104A3 Bypass Abdominal Aorta to Right Renal Artery with Autologous Arterial Tissue, Percutaneous Endoscopic Approach

04104A4 Bypass Abdominal Aorta to Left Renal Artery with Autologous Arterial Tissue, Percutaneous Endoscopic Approach

04104A5 Bypass Abdominal Aorta to Bilateral Renal Artery with Autologous Arterial Tissue, Percutaneous Endoscopic Approach

04104A6 Bypass Abdominal Aorta to Right Common Iliac Artery with Autologous Arterial Tissue, Percutaneous Endoscopic Approach

04104A7 Bypass Abdominal Aorta to Left Common Iliac Artery with Autologous Arterial Tissue, Percutaneous Endoscopic Approach

04104A8 Bypass Abdominal Aorta to Bilateral Common Iliac Arteries with Autologous Arterial Tissue, Percutaneous Endoscopic Approach

04104A9 Bypass Abdominal Aorta to Right Internal Iliac Artery with Autologous Arterial Tissue, Percutaneous Endoscopic Approach

04104AB Bypass Abdominal Aorta to Left Internal Iliac Artery with Autologous Arterial Tissue, Percutaneous Endoscopic Approach

04104AC Bypass Abdominal Aorta to Bilateral Internal Iliac Arteries with Autologous Arterial Tissue, Percutaneous Endoscopic Approach

04104AD Bypass Abdominal Aorta to Right External Iliac Artery with Autologous Arterial Tissue, Percutaneous Endoscopic Approach

04104AF Bypass Abdominal Aorta to Left External Iliac Artery with Autologous Arterial Tissue, Percutaneous Endoscopic Approach

04104AG Bypass Abdominal Aorta to Bilateral External Iliac Arteries with Autologous Arterial Tissue, Percutaneous Endoscopic Approach

04104AH Bypass Abdominal Aorta to Right Femoral Artery with Autologous Arterial Tissue, Percutaneous Endoscopic Approach

04104AJ Bypass Abdominal Aorta to Left Femoral Artery with Autologous Arterial Tissue, Percutaneous Endoscopic Approach

04104AK Bypass Abdominal Aorta to Bilateral Femoral Arteries with Autologous Arterial Tissue, Percutaneous Endoscopic Approach

04104AQ Bypass Abdominal Aorta to Lower Extremity Artery with Autologous Arterial Tissue, Percutaneous Endoscopic Approach

04104AR Bypass Abdominal Aorta to Lower Artery with Autologous Arterial Tissue, Percutaneous Endoscopic Approach

04104J0 Bypass Abdominal Aorta to Abdominal Aorta with Synthetic Substitute, Percutaneous Endoscopic Approach

04104J1 Bypass Abdominal Aorta to Celiac Artery with Synthetic Substitute, Percutaneous Endoscopic Approach

04104J2 Bypass Abdominal Aorta to Mesenteric Artery with Synthetic Substitute, Percutaneous Endoscopic Approach

04104J3 Bypass Abdominal Aorta to Right Renal Artery with Synthetic Substitute, Percutaneous Endoscopic Approach

04104J4 Bypass Abdominal Aorta to Left Renal Artery with Synthetic Substitute, Percutaneous Endoscopic Approach

04104J5 Bypass Abdominal Aorta to Bilateral Renal Artery with Synthetic Substitute, Percutaneous Endoscopic Approach

04104J6 Bypass Abdominal Aorta to Right Common Iliac Artery with Synthetic Substitute, Percutaneous Endoscopic Approach

04104J7 Bypass Abdominal Aorta to Left Common Iliac Artery with Synthetic Substitute, Percutaneous Endoscopic Approach

04104J8 Bypass Abdominal Aorta to Bilateral Common Iliac Arteries with Synthetic Substitute, Percutaneous Endoscopic Approach

04104J9 Bypass Abdominal Aorta to Right Internal Iliac Artery with Synthetic Substitute, Percutaneous Endoscopic Approach

04104JB Bypass Abdominal Aorta to Left Internal Iliac Artery with Synthetic Substitute, Percutaneous Endoscopic Approach

04104JC Bypass Abdominal Aorta to Bilateral Internal Iliac Arteries with Synthetic Substitute, Percutaneous Endoscopic Approach

04104JD Bypass Abdominal Aorta to Right External Iliac Artery with Synthetic Substitute, Percutaneous Endoscopic Approach

04104JF Bypass Abdominal Aorta to Left External Iliac Artery with Synthetic Substitute, Percutaneous Endoscopic Approach

04104JG Bypass Abdominal Aorta to Bilateral External Iliac Arteries with Synthetic Substitute, Percutaneous Endoscopic Approach

04104JH Bypass Abdominal Aorta to Right Femoral Artery with Synthetic Substitute, Percutaneous Endoscopic Approach

04104JJ Bypass Abdominal Aorta to Left Femoral Artery with Synthetic Substitute, Percutaneous Endoscopic Approach

04104JK Bypass Abdominal Aorta to Bilateral Femoral Arteries with Synthetic Substitute, Percutaneous Endoscopic Approach

04104JQ Bypass Abdominal Aorta to Lower Extremity Artery with Synthetic Substitute, Percutaneous Endoscopic Approach

04104JR Bypass Abdominal Aorta to Lower Artery with Synthetic Substitute, Percutaneous Endoscopic Approach

04104K0 Bypass Abdominal Aorta to Abdominal Aorta with Nonautologous Tissue Substitute, Percutaneous Endoscopic Approach

04104K1 Bypass Abdominal Aorta to Celiac Artery with Nonautologous Tissue Substitute, Percutaneous Endoscopic Approach

04104K2 Bypass Abdominal Aorta to Mesenteric Artery with Nonautologous Tissue Substitute, Percutaneous Endoscopic Approach

04104K3 Bypass Abdominal Aorta to Right Renal Artery with Nonautologous Tissue Substitute, Percutaneous Endoscopic Approach

04104K4 Bypass Abdominal Aorta to Left Renal Artery with Nonautologous Tissue Substitute, Percutaneous Endoscopic Approach

04104K5 Bypass Abdominal Aorta to Bilateral Renal Artery with Nonautologous Tissue Substitute, Percutaneous Endoscopic Approach

04104K6 Bypass Abdominal Aorta to Right Common Iliac Artery with Nonautologous Tissue Substitute, Percutaneous Endoscopic Approach

04104K7 Bypass Abdominal Aorta to Left Common Iliac Artery with Nonautologous Tissue Substitute, Percutaneous Endoscopic Approach

04104K8 Bypass Abdominal Aorta to Bilateral Common Iliac Arteries with Nonautologous Tissue Substitute, Percutaneous Endoscopic Approach

04104K9 Bypass Abdominal Aorta to Right Internal Iliac Artery with Nonautologous Tissue Substitute, Percutaneous Endoscopic Approach

04104KB Bypass Abdominal Aorta to Left Internal Iliac Artery with Nonautologous Tissue Substitute, Percutaneous Endoscopic Approach

04104KC Bypass Abdominal Aorta to Bilateral Internal Iliac Arteries with Nonautologous Tissue Substitute, Percutaneous Endoscopic Approach

04104KD Bypass Abdominal Aorta to Right External Iliac Artery with Nonautologous Tissue Substitute, Percutaneous Endoscopic Approach

04104KF Bypass Abdominal Aorta to Left External Iliac Artery with Nonautologous Tissue Substitute, Percutaneous Endoscopic Approach

04104KG Bypass Abdominal Aorta to Bilateral External Iliac Arteries with Nonautologous Tissue Substitute, Percutaneous Endoscopic Approach

04104KH Bypass Abdominal Aorta to Right Femoral Artery with Nonautologous Tissue Substitute, Percutaneous Endoscopic Approach

04104KJ Bypass Abdominal Aorta to Left Femoral Artery with Nonautologous Tissue Substitute, Percutaneous Endoscopic Approach

04104KK Bypass Abdominal Aorta to Bilateral Femoral Arteries with Nonautologous Tissue Substitute, Percutaneous Endoscopic Approach

04104KQ Bypass Abdominal Aorta to Lower Extremity Artery with Nonautologous Tissue Substitute, Percutaneous Endoscopic Approach

04104KR Bypass Abdominal Aorta to Lower Artery with Nonautologous Tissue Substitute, Percutaneous Endoscopic Approach

04104Z0 Bypass Abdominal Aorta to Abdominal Aorta, Percutaneous Endoscopic Approach

04104Z1 Bypass Abdominal Aorta to Celiac Artery, Percutaneous Endoscopic Approach

04104Z2 Bypass Abdominal Aorta to Mesenteric Artery, Percutaneous Endoscopic Approach

04104Z3 Bypass Abdominal Aorta to Right Renal Artery, Percutaneous Endoscopic Approach

04104Z4 Bypass Abdominal Aorta to Left Renal Artery, Percutaneous Endoscopic Approach

04104Z5 Bypass Abdominal Aorta to Bilateral Renal Artery, Percutaneous Endoscopic Approach

04104Z6 Bypass Abdominal Aorta to Right Common Iliac Artery, Percutaneous Endoscopic Approach

04104Z7 Bypass Abdominal Aorta to Left Common Iliac Artery, Percutaneous Endoscopic Approach

04104Z8 Bypass Abdominal Aorta to Bilateral Common Iliac Arteries, Percutaneous Endoscopic Approach

04104Z9 Bypass Abdominal Aorta to Right Internal Iliac Artery, Percutaneous Endoscopic Approach

04104ZB Bypass Abdominal Aorta to Left Internal Iliac Artery, Percutaneous Endoscopic Approach

04104ZC Bypass Abdominal Aorta to Bilateral Internal Iliac Arteries, Percutaneous Endoscopic Approach

04104ZD Bypass Abdominal Aorta to Right External Iliac Artery, Percutaneous Endoscopic Approach

04104ZF Bypass Abdominal Aorta to Left External Iliac Artery, Percutaneous Endoscopic Approach

04104ZG Bypass Abdominal Aorta to Bilateral External Iliac Arteries, Percutaneous Endoscopic Approach

04104ZH Bypass Abdominal Aorta to Right Femoral Artery, Percutaneous Endoscopic Approach

04104ZJ Bypass Abdominal Aorta to Left Femoral Artery, Percutaneous Endoscopic Approach

04104ZK Bypass Abdominal Aorta to Bilateral Femoral Arteries, Percutaneous Endoscopic Approach

04104ZQ Bypass Abdominal Aorta to Lower Extremity Artery, Percutaneous Endoscopic Approach

04104ZR Bypass Abdominal Aorta to Lower Artery, Percutaneous Endoscopic Approach

0414093 Bypass Splenic Artery to Right Renal Artery with Autologous Venous Tissue, Open Approach

0414094 Bypass Splenic Artery to Left Renal Artery with Autologous Venous Tissue, Open Approach

0414095 Bypass Splenic Artery to Bilateral Renal Artery with Autologous Venous Tissue, Open Approach

04140A3 Bypass Splenic Artery to Right Renal Artery with Autologous Arterial Tissue, Open Approach

04140A4 Bypass Splenic Artery to Left Renal Artery with Autologous Arterial Tissue, Open Approach

04140A5 Bypass Splenic Artery to Bilateral Renal Artery with Autologous Arterial Tissue, Open Approach

04140J3 Bypass Splenic Artery to Right Renal Artery with Synthetic Substitute, Open Approach

04140J4 Bypass Splenic Artery to Left Renal Artery with Synthetic Substitute, Open Approach

04140J5 Bypass Splenic Artery to Bilateral Renal Artery with Synthetic Substitute, Open Approach

04140K3 Bypass Splenic Artery to Right Renal Artery with Nonautologous Tissue Substitute, Open Approach

04140K4 Bypass Splenic Artery to Left Renal Artery with Nonautologous Tissue Substitute, Open Approach

04140K5 Bypass Splenic Artery to Bilateral Renal Artery with Nonautologous Tissue Substitute, Open Approach

04140Z3 Bypass Splenic Artery to Right Renal Artery, Open Approach

04140Z4 Bypass Splenic Artery to Left Renal Artery, Open Approach

04140Z5 Bypass Splenic Artery to Bilateral Renal Artery, Open Approach

414493 Bypass Splenic Artery to Right Renal Artery with Autologous Venous Tissue, Percutaneous Endoscopic Approach

0414494 Bypass Splenic Artery to Left Renal Artery with Autologous Venous Tissue, Percutaneous Endoscopic Approach

0414495 Bypass Splenic Artery to Bilateral Renal Artery with Autologous Venous Tissue, Percutaneous Endoscopic Approach

04144A3 Bypass Splenic Artery to Right Renal Artery with Autologous Arterial Tissue, Percutaneous Endoscopic Approach

04144A4 Bypass Splenic Artery to Left Renal Artery with Autologous Arterial Tissue, Percutaneous Endoscopic Approach

04144A5 Bypass Splenic Artery to Bilateral Renal Artery with Autologous Arterial Tissue, Percutaneous Endoscopic Approach

04144J3 Bypass Splenic Artery to Right Renal Artery with Synthetic Substitute, Percutaneous Endoscopic Approach

04144J4 Bypass Splenic Artery to Left Renal Artery with Synthetic Substitute, Percutaneous Endoscopic Approach

04144J5 Bypass Splenic Artery to Bilateral Renal Artery with Synthetic Substitute, Percutaneous Endoscopic Approach

04144K3 Bypass Splenic Artery to Right Renal Artery with Nonautologous Tissue Substitute, Percutaneous Endoscopic Approach

04144K4 Bypass Splenic Artery to Left Renal Artery with Nonautologous Tissue Substitute, Percutaneous Endoscopic Approach

04144K5 Bypass Splenic Artery to Bilateral Renal Artery with Nonautologous Tissue Substitute, Percutaneous Endoscopic Approach

04144Z3 Bypass Splenic Artery to Right Renal Artery, Percutaneous Endoscopic Approach

04144Z4 Bypass Splenic Artery to Left Renal Artery, Percutaneous Endoscopic Approach

04144Z5 Bypass Splenic Artery to Bilateral Renal Artery, Percutaneous Endoscopic Approach

041C090 Bypass Right Common Iliac Artery to Abdominal Aorta with Autologous Venous Tissue, Open Approach

041C091 Bypass Right Common Iliac Artery to Celiac Artery with Autologous Venous Tissue, Open Approach

041C092 Bypass Right Common Iliac Artery to Mesenteric Artery with Autologous Venous Tissue, Open Approach

041C093 Bypass Right Common Iliac Artery to Right Renal Artery with Autologous Venous Tissue, Open Approach

041C094 Bypass Right Common Iliac Artery to Left Renal Artery with Autologous Venous Tissue, Open Approach

♀ Female-only   ♂ Male-only   ▲ Limited Coverage   ● Non-OR   ▥ HAC-associated procedure   ▲ Non-covered procedures   ✛ Combinati

C095 Bypass Right Common Iliac Artery to Bilateral Renal Artery with Autologous Venous Tissue, Open Approach

C096 Bypass Right Common Iliac Artery to Right Common Iliac Artery with Autologous Venous Tissue, Open Approach

C097 Bypass Right Common Iliac Artery to Left Common Iliac Artery with Autologous Venous Tissue, Open Approach

C098 Bypass Right Common Iliac Artery to Bilateral Common Iliac Arteries with Autologous Venous Tissue, Open Approach

C099 Bypass Right Common Iliac Artery to Right Internal Iliac Artery with Autologous Venous Tissue, Open Approach

C09B Bypass Right Common Iliac Artery to Left Internal Iliac Artery with Autologous Venous Tissue, Open Approach

C09C Bypass Right Common Iliac Artery to Bilateral Internal Iliac Arteries with Autologous Venous Tissue, Open Approach

C09D Bypass Right Common Iliac Artery to Right External Iliac Artery with Autologous Venous Tissue, Open Approach

C09F Bypass Right Common Iliac Artery to Left External Iliac Artery with Autologous Venous Tissue, Open Approach

C09G Bypass Right Common Iliac Artery to Bilateral External Iliac Arteries with Autologous Venous Tissue, Open Approach

C09H Bypass Right Common Iliac Artery to Right Femoral Artery with Autologous Venous Tissue, Open Approach

C09J Bypass Right Common Iliac Artery to Left Femoral Artery with Autologous Venous Tissue, Open Approach

C09K Bypass Right Common Iliac Artery to Bilateral Femoral Arteries with Autologous Venous Tissue, Open Approach

C09Q Bypass Right Common Iliac Artery to Lower Extremity Artery with Autologous Venous Tissue, Open Approach

C09R Bypass Right Common Iliac Artery to Lower Artery with Autologous Venous Tissue, Open Approach

C0A0 Bypass Right Common Iliac Artery to Abdominal Aorta with Autologous Arterial Tissue, Open Approach

C0A1 Bypass Right Common Iliac Artery to Celiac Artery with Autologous Arterial Tissue, Open Approach

C0A2 Bypass Right Common Iliac Artery to Mesenteric Artery with Autologous Arterial Tissue, Open Approach

C0A3 Bypass Right Common Iliac Artery to Right Renal Artery with Autologous Arterial Tissue, Open Approach

1C0A4 Bypass Right Common Iliac Artery to Left Renal Artery with Autologous Arterial Tissue, Open Approach

1C0A5 Bypass Right Common Iliac Artery to Bilateral Renal Artery with Autologous Arterial Tissue, Open Approach

1C0A6 Bypass Right Common Iliac Artery to Right Common Iliac Artery with Autologous Arterial Tissue, Open Approach

1C0A7 Bypass Right Common Iliac Artery to Left Common Iliac Artery with Autologous Arterial Tissue, Open Approach

1C0A8 Bypass Right Common Iliac Artery to Bilateral Common Iliac Arteries with Autologous Arterial Tissue, Open Approach

041C0A9 Bypass Right Common Iliac Artery to Right Internal Iliac Artery with Autologous Arterial Tissue, Open Approach

041C0AB Bypass Right Common Iliac Artery to Left Internal Iliac Artery with Autologous Arterial Tissue, Open Approach

041C0AC Bypass Right Common Iliac Artery to Bilateral Internal Iliac Arteries with Autologous Arterial Tissue, Open Approach

041C0AD Bypass Right Common Iliac Artery to Right External Iliac Artery with Autologous Arterial Tissue, Open Approach

041C0AF Bypass Right Common Iliac Artery to Left External Iliac Artery with Autologous Arterial Tissue, Open Approach

041C0AG Bypass Right Common Iliac Artery to Bilateral External Iliac Arteries with Autologous Arterial Tissue, Open Approach

041C0AH Bypass Right Common Iliac Artery to Right Femoral Artery with Autologous Arterial Tissue, Open Approach

041C0AJ Bypass Right Common Iliac Artery to Left Femoral Artery with Autologous Arterial Tissue, Open Approach

041C0AK Bypass Right Common Iliac Artery to Bilateral Femoral Arteries with Autologous Arterial Tissue, Open Approach

041C0AQ Bypass Right Common Iliac Artery to Lower Extremity Artery with Autologous Arterial Tissue, Open Approach

041C0AR Bypass Right Common Iliac Artery to Lower Artery with Autologous Arterial Tissue, Open Approach

041C0J0 Bypass Right Common Iliac Artery to Abdominal Aorta with Synthetic Substitute, Open Approach

041C0J1 Bypass Right Common Iliac Artery to Celiac Artery with Synthetic Substitute, Open Approach

041C0J2 Bypass Right Common Iliac Artery to Mesenteric Artery with Synthetic Substitute, Open Approach

041C0J3 Bypass Right Common Iliac Artery to Right Renal Artery with Synthetic Substitute, Open Approach

041C0J4 Bypass Right Common Iliac Artery to Left Renal Artery with Synthetic Substitute, Open Approach

041C0J5 Bypass Right Common Iliac Artery to Bilateral Renal Artery with Synthetic Substitute, Open Approach

041C0J6 Bypass Right Common Iliac Artery to Right Common Iliac Artery with Synthetic Substitute, Open Approach

041C0J7 Bypass Right Common Iliac Artery to Left Common Iliac Artery with Synthetic Substitute, Open Approach

041C0J8 Bypass Right Common Iliac Artery to Bilateral Common Iliac Arteries with Synthetic Substitute, Open Approach

041C0J9 Bypass Right Common Iliac Artery to Right Internal Iliac Artery with Synthetic Substitute, Open Approach

041C0JB Bypass Right Common Iliac Artery to Left Internal Iliac Artery with Synthetic Substitute, Open Approach

041C0JC Bypass Right Common Iliac Artery to Bilateral Internal Iliac Arteries with Synthetic Substitute, Open Approach

041C0JD Bypass Right Common Iliac Artery to Right External Iliac Artery with Synthetic Substitute, Open Approach

041C0JF Bypass Right Common Iliac Artery to Left External Iliac Artery with Synthetic Substitute, Open Approach

041C0JG Bypass Right Common Iliac Artery to Bilateral External Iliac Arteries with Synthetic Substitute, Open Approach

041C0JH Bypass Right Common Iliac Artery to Right Femoral Artery with Synthetic Substitute, Open Approach

041C0JJ Bypass Right Common Iliac Artery to Left Femoral Artery with Synthetic Substitute, Open Approach

041C0JK Bypass Right Common Iliac Artery to Bilateral Femoral Arteries with Synthetic Substitute, Open Approach

041C0JQ Bypass Right Common Iliac Artery to Lower Extremity Artery with Synthetic Substitute, Open Approach

041C0JR Bypass Right Common Iliac Artery to Lower Artery with Synthetic Substitute, Open Approach

041C0K0 Bypass Right Common Iliac Artery to Abdominal Aorta with Nonautologous Tissue Substitute, Open Approach

041C0K1 Bypass Right Common Iliac Artery to Celiac Artery with Nonautologous Tissue Substitute, Open Approach

041C0K2 Bypass Right Common Iliac Artery to Mesenteric Artery with Nonautologous Tissue Substitute, Open Approach

041C0K3 Bypass Right Common Iliac Artery to Right Renal Artery with Nonautologous Tissue Substitute, Open Approach

041C0K4 Bypass Right Common Iliac Artery to Left Renal Artery with Nonautologous Tissue Substitute, Open Approach

041C0K5 Bypass Right Common Iliac Artery to Bilateral Renal Artery with Nonautologous Tissue Substitute, Open Approach

041C0K6 Bypass Right Common Iliac Artery to Right Common Iliac Artery with Nonautologous Tissue Substitute, Open Approach

041C0K7 Bypass Right Common Iliac Artery to Left Common Iliac Artery with Nonautologous Tissue Substitute, Open Approach

041C0K8 Bypass Right Common Iliac Artery to Bilateral Common Iliac Arteries with Nonautologous Tissue Substitute, Open Approach

041C0K9 Bypass Right Common Iliac Artery to Right Internal Iliac Artery with Nonautologous Tissue Substitute, Open Approach

041C0KB Bypass Right Common Iliac Artery to Left Internal Iliac Artery with Nonautologous Tissue Substitute, Open Approach

041C0KC Bypass Right Common Iliac Artery to Bilateral Internal Iliac Arteries with Nonautologous Tissue Substitute, Open Approach

041C0KD Bypass Right Common Iliac Artery to Right External Iliac Artery with Nonautologous Tissue Substitute, Open Approach

041C0KF Bypass Right Common Iliac Artery to Left External Iliac Artery with Nonautologous Tissue Substitute, Open Approach

041C0KG Bypass Right Common Iliac Artery to Bilateral External Iliac Arteries with Nonautologous Tissue Substitute, Open Approach

Female-only   ♂ Male-only   ▲ Limited Coverage   ● Non-OR   ▩ HAC-associated procedure   ▲ Non-covered procedures   ➕ Combination

041C0KH   Bypass Right Common Iliac Artery to Right Femoral Artery with Nonautologous Tissue Substitute, Open Approach

041C0KJ   Bypass Right Common Iliac Artery to Left Femoral Artery with Nonautologous Tissue Substitute, Open Approach

041C0KK   Bypass Right Common Iliac Artery to Bilateral Femoral Arteries with Nonautologous Tissue Substitute, Open Approach

041C0KQ   Bypass Right Common Iliac Artery to Lower Extremity Artery with Nonautologous Tissue Substitute, Open Approach

041C0KR   Bypass Right Common Iliac Artery to Lower Artery with Nonautologous Tissue Substitute, Open Approach

041C0Z0   Bypass Right Common Iliac Artery to Abdominal Aorta, Open Approach

041C0Z1   Bypass Right Common Iliac Artery to Celiac Artery, Open Approach

041C0Z2   Bypass Right Common Iliac Artery to Mesenteric Artery, Open Approach

041C0Z3   Bypass Right Common Iliac Artery to Right Renal Artery, Open Approach

041C0Z4   Bypass Right Common Iliac Artery to Left Renal Artery, Open Approach

041C0Z5   Bypass Right Common Iliac Artery to Bilateral Renal Artery, Open Approach

041C0Z6   Bypass Right Common Iliac Artery to Right Common Iliac Artery, Open Approach

041C0Z7   Bypass Right Common Iliac Artery to Left Common Iliac Artery, Open Approach

041C0Z8   Bypass Right Common Iliac Artery to Bilateral Common Iliac Arteries, Open Approach

041C0Z9   Bypass Right Common Iliac Artery to Right Internal Iliac Artery, Open Approach

041C0ZB   Bypass Right Common Iliac Artery to Left Internal Iliac Artery, Open Approach

041C0ZC   Bypass Right Common Iliac Artery to Bilateral Internal Iliac Arteries, Open Approach

041C0ZD   Bypass Right Common Iliac Artery to Right External Iliac Artery, Open Approach

041C0ZF   Bypass Right Common Iliac Artery to Left External Iliac Artery, Open Approach

041C0ZG   Bypass Right Common Iliac Artery to Bilateral External Iliac Arteries, Open Approach

041C0ZH   Bypass Right Common Iliac Artery to Right Femoral Artery, Open Approach

041C0ZJ   Bypass Right Common Iliac Artery to Left Femoral Artery, Open Approach

041C0ZK   Bypass Right Common Iliac Artery to Bilateral Femoral Arteries, Open Approach

041C0ZQ   Bypass Right Common Iliac Artery to Lower Extremity Artery, Open Approach

041C0ZR   Bypass Right Common Iliac Artery to Lower Artery, Open Approach

041C490   Bypass Right Common Iliac Artery to Abdominal Aorta with Autologous Venous Tissue, Percutaneous Endoscopic Approach

041C491   Bypass Right Common Iliac Artery to Celiac Artery with Autologous Venous Tissue, Percutaneous Endoscopic Approach

041C492   Bypass Right Common Iliac Artery to Mesenteric Artery with Autologous Venous Tissue, Percutaneous Endoscopic Approach

041C493   Bypass Right Common Iliac Artery to Right Renal Artery with Autologous Venous Tissue, Percutaneous Endoscopic Approach

041C494   Bypass Right Common Iliac Artery to Left Renal Artery with Autologous Venous Tissue, Percutaneous Endoscopic Approach

041C495   Bypass Right Common Iliac Artery to Bilateral Renal Artery with Autologous Venous Tissue, Percutaneous Endoscopic Approach

041C496   Bypass Right Common Iliac Artery to Right Common Iliac Artery with Autologous Venous Tissue, Percutaneous Endoscopic Approach

041C497   Bypass Right Common Iliac Artery to Left Common Iliac Artery with Autologous Venous Tissue, Percutaneous Endoscopic Approach

041C498   Bypass Right Common Iliac Artery to Bilateral Common Iliac Arteries with Autologous Venous Tissue, Percutaneous Endoscopic Approach

041C499   Bypass Right Common Iliac Artery to Right Internal Iliac Artery with Autologous Venous Tissue, Percutaneous Endoscopic Approach

041C49B   Bypass Right Common Iliac Artery to Left Internal Iliac Artery with Autologous Venous Tissue, Percutaneous Endoscopic Approach

041C49C   Bypass Right Common Iliac Artery to Bilateral Internal Iliac Arteries with Autologous Venous Tissue, Percutaneous Endoscopic Approach

041C49D   Bypass Right Common Iliac Artery to Right External Iliac Artery with Autologous Venous Tissue, Percutaneous Endoscopic Approach

041C49F   Bypass Right Common Iliac Artery to Left External Iliac Artery with Autologous Venous Tissue, Percutaneous Endoscopic Approach

041C49G   Bypass Right Common Iliac Artery to Bilateral External Iliac Arteries with Autologous Venous Tissue, Percutaneous Endoscopic Approach

041C49H   Bypass Right Common Iliac Artery to Right Femoral Artery with Autologous Venous Tissue, Percutaneous Endoscopic Approach

041C49J   Bypass Right Common Iliac Artery to Left Femoral Artery with Autologous Venous Tissue, Percutaneous Endoscopic Approach

041C49K   Bypass Right Common Iliac Artery to Bilateral Femoral Arteries with Autologous Venous Tissue, Percutaneous Endoscopic Approach

041C49Q   Bypass Right Common Iliac Artery to Lower Extremity Artery with Autologous Venous Tissue, Percutaneous Endoscopic Approach

041C49R   Bypass Right Common Iliac Artery to Lower Artery with Autologous Venous Tissue, Percutaneous Endoscopic Approach

041C4A0   Bypass Right Common Iliac Artery to Abdominal Aorta with Autologous Arterial Tissue, Percutaneous Endoscopic Approach

041C4A1   Bypass Right Common Iliac Artery to Celiac Artery with Autologous Arterial Tissue, Percutaneous Endoscopic Approach

041C4A2   Bypass Right Common Iliac Artery to Mesenteric Artery with Autologous Arterial Tissue, Percutaneous Endoscopic Approach

041C4A3   Bypass Right Common Iliac Artery to Right Renal Artery with Autologous Arterial Tissue, Percutaneous Endoscopic Approach

041C4A4   Bypass Right Common Iliac Artery to Left Renal Artery with Autologous Arterial Tissue, Percutaneous Endoscopic Approach

041C4A5   Bypass Right Common Iliac Artery to Bilateral Renal Artery with Autologous Arterial Tissue, Percutaneous Endoscopic Approach

041C4A6   Bypass Right Common Iliac Artery to Right Common Iliac Artery with Autologous Arterial Tissue, Percutaneous Endoscopic Approach

041C4A7   Bypass Right Common Iliac Artery to Left Common Iliac Artery with Autologous Arterial Tissue, Percutaneous Endoscopic Approach

041C4A8   Bypass Right Common Iliac Artery to Bilateral Common Iliac Arteries with Autologous Arterial Tissue, Percutaneous Endoscopic Approach

041C4A9   Bypass Right Common Iliac Artery to Right Internal Iliac Artery with Autologous Arterial Tissue, Percutaneous Endoscopic Approach

041C4AB   Bypass Right Common Iliac Artery to Left Internal Iliac Artery with Autologous Arterial Tissue, Percutaneous Endoscopic Approach

041C4AC   Bypass Right Common Iliac Artery to Bilateral Internal Iliac Arteries with Autologous Arterial Tissue, Percutaneous Endoscopic Approach

041C4AD   Bypass Right Common Iliac Artery to Right External Iliac Artery with Autologous Arterial Tissue, Percutaneous Endoscopic Approach

041C4AF   Bypass Right Common Iliac Artery to Left External Iliac Artery with Autologous Arterial Tissue, Percutaneous Endoscopic Approach

041C4AG   Bypass Right Common Iliac Artery to Bilateral External Iliac Arteries with Autologous Arterial Tissue, Percutaneous Endoscopic Approach

041C4AH   Bypass Right Common Iliac Artery to Right Femoral Artery with Autologous Arterial Tissue, Percutaneous Endoscopic Approach

041C4AJ   Bypass Right Common Iliac Artery to Left Femoral Artery with Autologous Arterial Tissue, Percutaneous Endoscopic Approach

041C4AK   Bypass Right Common Iliac Artery to Bilateral Femoral Arteries with Autologous Arterial Tissue, Percutaneous Endoscopic Approach

041C4AQ   Bypass Right Common Iliac Artery to Lower Extremity Artery with Autologous Arterial Tissue, Percutaneous Endoscopic Approach

041C4AR   Bypass Right Common Iliac Artery to Lower Artery with Autologous Arterial Tissue, Percutaneous Endoscopic Approach

041C4J0   Bypass Right Common Iliac Artery to Abdominal Aorta with Synthetic Substitute, Percutaneous Endoscopic Approach

041C4J1   Bypass Right Common Iliac Artery to Celiac Artery with Synthetic Substitute, Percutaneous Endoscopic Approach

041C4J2 Bypass Right Common Iliac Artery to Mesenteric Artery with Synthetic Substitute, Percutaneous Endoscopic Approach

041C4J3 Bypass Right Common Iliac Artery to Right Renal Artery with Synthetic Substitute, Percutaneous Endoscopic Approach

041C4J4 Bypass Right Common Iliac Artery to Left Renal Artery with Synthetic Substitute, Percutaneous Endoscopic Approach

041C4J5 Bypass Right Common Iliac Artery to Bilateral Renal Artery with Synthetic Substitute, Percutaneous Endoscopic Approach

041C4J6 Bypass Right Common Iliac Artery to Right Common Iliac Artery with Synthetic Substitute, Percutaneous Endoscopic Approach

041C4J7 Bypass Right Common Iliac Artery to Left Common Iliac Artery with Synthetic Substitute, Percutaneous Endoscopic Approach

041C4J8 Bypass Right Common Iliac Artery to Bilateral Common Iliac Arteries with Synthetic Substitute, Percutaneous Endoscopic Approach

041C4J9 Bypass Right Common Iliac Artery to Right Internal Iliac Artery with Synthetic Substitute, Percutaneous Endoscopic Approach

041C4JB Bypass Right Common Iliac Artery to Left Internal Iliac Artery with Synthetic Substitute, Percutaneous Endoscopic Approach

041C4JC Bypass Right Common Iliac Artery to Bilateral Internal Iliac Arteries with Synthetic Substitute, Percutaneous Endoscopic Approach

041C4JD Bypass Right Common Iliac Artery to Right External Iliac Artery with Synthetic Substitute, Percutaneous Endoscopic Approach

041C4JF Bypass Right Common Iliac Artery to Left External Iliac Artery with Synthetic Substitute, Percutaneous Endoscopic Approach

041C4JG Bypass Right Common Iliac Artery to Bilateral External Iliac Arteries with Synthetic Substitute, Percutaneous Endoscopic Approach

041C4JH Bypass Right Common Iliac Artery to Right Femoral Artery with Synthetic Substitute, Percutaneous Endoscopic Approach

041C4JJ Bypass Right Common Iliac Artery to Left Femoral Artery with Synthetic Substitute, Percutaneous Endoscopic Approach

041C4JK Bypass Right Common Iliac Artery to Bilateral Femoral Arteries with Synthetic Substitute, Percutaneous Endoscopic Approach

041C4JQ Bypass Right Common Iliac Artery to Lower Extremity Artery with Synthetic Substitute, Percutaneous Endoscopic Approach

041C4JR Bypass Right Common Iliac Artery to Lower Artery with Synthetic Substitute, Percutaneous Endoscopic Approach

041C4K0 Bypass Right Common Iliac Artery to Abdominal Aorta with Nonautologous Tissue Substitute, Percutaneous Endoscopic Approach

041C4K1 Bypass Right Common Iliac Artery to Celiac Artery with Nonautologous Tissue Substitute, Percutaneous Endoscopic Approach

041C4K2 Bypass Right Common Iliac Artery to Mesenteric Artery with Nonautologous Tissue Substitute, Percutaneous Endoscopic Approach

041C4K3 Bypass Right Common Iliac Artery to Right Renal Artery with Nonautologous Tissue Substitute, Percutaneous Endoscopic Approach

041C4K4 Bypass Right Common Iliac Artery to Left Renal Artery with Nonautologous Tissue Substitute, Percutaneous Endoscopic Approach

041C4K5 Bypass Right Common Iliac Artery to Bilateral Renal Artery with Nonautologous Tissue Substitute, Percutaneous Endoscopic Approach

041C4K6 Bypass Right Common Iliac Artery to Right Common Iliac Artery with Nonautologous Tissue Substitute, Percutaneous Endoscopic Approach

041C4K7 Bypass Right Common Iliac Artery to Left Common Iliac Artery with Nonautologous Tissue Substitute, Percutaneous Endoscopic Approach

041C4K8 Bypass Right Common Iliac Artery to Bilateral Common Iliac Arteries with Nonautologous Tissue Substitute, Percutaneous Endoscopic Approach

041C4K9 Bypass Right Common Iliac Artery to Right Internal Iliac Artery with Nonautologous Tissue Substitute, Percutaneous Endoscopic Approach

041C4KB Bypass Right Common Iliac Artery to Left Internal Iliac Artery with Nonautologous Tissue Substitute, Percutaneous Endoscopic Approach

041C4KC Bypass Right Common Iliac Artery to Bilateral Internal Iliac Arteries with Nonautologous Tissue Substitute, Percutaneous Endoscopic Approach

041C4KD Bypass Right Common Iliac Artery to Right External Iliac Artery with Nonautologous Tissue Substitute, Percutaneous Endoscopic Approach

041C4KF Bypass Right Common Iliac Artery to Left External Iliac Artery with Nonautologous Tissue Substitute, Percutaneous Endoscopic Approach

041C4KG Bypass Right Common Iliac Artery to Bilateral External Iliac Arteries with Nonautologous Tissue Substitute, Percutaneous Endoscopic Approach

041C4KH Bypass Right Common Iliac Artery to Right Femoral Artery with Nonautologous Tissue Substitute, Percutaneous Endoscopic Approach

041C4KJ Bypass Right Common Iliac Artery to Left Femoral Artery with Nonautologous Tissue Substitute, Percutaneous Endoscopic Approach

041C4KK Bypass Right Common Iliac Artery to Bilateral Femoral Arteries with Nonautologous Tissue Substitute, Percutaneous Endoscopic Approach

041C4KQ Bypass Right Common Iliac Artery to Lower Extremity Artery with Nonautologous Tissue Substitute, Percutaneous Endoscopic Approach

041C4KR Bypass Right Common Iliac Artery to Lower Artery with Nonautologous Tissue Substitute, Percutaneous Endoscopic Approach

041C4Z0 Bypass Right Common Iliac Artery to Abdominal Aorta, Percutaneous Endoscopic Approach

041C4Z1 Bypass Right Common Iliac Artery to Celiac Artery, Percutaneous Endoscopic Approach

041C4Z2 Bypass Right Common Iliac Artery to Mesenteric Artery, Percutaneous Endoscopic Approach

041C4Z3 Bypass Right Common Iliac Artery to Right Renal Artery, Percutaneous Endoscopic Approach

041C4Z4 Bypass Right Common Iliac Artery to Left Renal Artery, Percutaneous Endoscopic Approach

041C4Z5 Bypass Right Common Iliac Artery to Bilateral Renal Artery, Percutaneous Endoscopic Approach

041C4Z6 Bypass Right Common Iliac Artery to Right Common Iliac Artery, Percutaneous Endoscopic Approach

041C4Z7 Bypass Right Common Iliac Artery to Left Common Iliac Artery, Percutaneous Endoscopic Approach

041C4Z8 Bypass Right Common Iliac Artery to Bilateral Common Iliac Arteries, Percutaneous Endoscopic Approach

041C4Z9 Bypass Right Common Iliac Artery to Right Internal Iliac Artery, Percutaneous Endoscopic Approach

041C4ZB Bypass Right Common Iliac Artery to Left Internal Iliac Artery, Percutaneous Endoscopic Approach

041C4ZC Bypass Right Common Iliac Artery to Bilateral Internal Iliac Arteries, Percutaneous Endoscopic Approach

041C4ZD Bypass Right Common Iliac Artery to Right External Iliac Artery, Percutaneous Endoscopic Approach

041C4ZF Bypass Right Common Iliac Artery to Left External Iliac Artery, Percutaneous Endoscopic Approach

041C4ZG Bypass Right Common Iliac Artery to Bilateral External Iliac Arteries, Percutaneous Endoscopic Approach

041C4ZH Bypass Right Common Iliac Artery to Right Femoral Artery, Percutaneous Endoscopic Approach

041C4ZJ Bypass Right Common Iliac Artery to Left Femoral Artery, Percutaneous Endoscopic Approach

041C4ZK Bypass Right Common Iliac Artery to Bilateral Femoral Arteries, Percutaneous Endoscopic Approach

041C4ZQ Bypass Right Common Iliac Artery to Lower Extremity Artery, Percutaneous Endoscopic Approach

041C4ZR Bypass Right Common Iliac Artery to Lower Artery, Percutaneous Endoscopic Approach

041D090 Bypass Left Common Iliac Artery to Abdominal Aorta with Autologous Venous Tissue, Open Approach

041D091 Bypass Left Common Iliac Artery to Celiac Artery with Autologous Venous Tissue, Open Approach

041D092 Bypass Left Common Iliac Artery to Mesenteric Artery with Autologous Venous Tissue, Open Approach

041D093 Bypass Left Common Iliac Artery to Right Renal Artery with Autologous Venous Tissue, Open Approach

041D094 Bypass Left Common Iliac Artery to Left Renal Artery with Autologous Venous Tissue, Open Approach

041D095 Bypass Left Common Iliac Artery to Bilateral Renal Artery with Autologous Venous Tissue, Open Approach

041D096 Bypass Left Common Iliac Artery to Right Common Iliac Artery with Autologous Venous Tissue, Open Approach

041D097 Bypass Left Common Iliac Artery to Left Common Iliac Artery with Autologous Venous Tissue, Open Approach

♀ Female-only   ♂ Male-only   ▲ Limited Coverage   ● Non-OR   █ HAC-associated procedure   ▲ Non-covered procedures   ✚ Combination

041D098 Bypass Left Common Iliac Artery to Bilateral Common Iliac Arteries with Autologous Venous Tissue, Open Approach

041D099 Bypass Left Common Iliac Artery to Right Internal Iliac Artery with Autologous Venous Tissue, Open Approach

041D09B Bypass Left Common Iliac Artery to Left Internal Iliac Artery with Autologous Venous Tissue, Open Approach

041D09C Bypass Left Common Iliac Artery to Bilateral Internal Iliac Arteries with Autologous Venous Tissue, Open Approach

041D09D Bypass Left Common Iliac Artery to Right External Iliac Artery with Autologous Venous Tissue, Open Approach

041D09F Bypass Left Common Iliac Artery to Left External Iliac Artery with Autologous Venous Tissue, Open Approach

041D09G Bypass Left Common Iliac Artery to Bilateral External Iliac Arteries with Autologous Venous Tissue, Open Approach

041D09H Bypass Left Common Iliac Artery to Right Femoral Artery with Autologous Venous Tissue, Open Approach

041D09J Bypass Left Common Iliac Artery to Left Femoral Artery with Autologous Venous Tissue, Open Approach

041D09K Bypass Left Common Iliac Artery to Bilateral Femoral Arteries with Autologous Venous Tissue, Open Approach

041D09Q Bypass Left Common Iliac Artery to Lower Extremity Artery with Autologous Venous Tissue, Open Approach

041D09R Bypass Left Common Iliac Artery to Lower Artery with Autologous Venous Tissue, Open Approach

041D0A0 Bypass Left Common Iliac Artery to Abdominal Aorta with Autologous Arterial Tissue, Open Approach

041D0A1 Bypass Left Common Iliac Artery to Celiac Artery with Autologous Arterial Tissue, Open Approach

041D0A2 Bypass Left Common Iliac Artery to Mesenteric Artery with Autologous Arterial Tissue, Open Approach

041D0A3 Bypass Left Common Iliac Artery to Right Renal Artery with Autologous Arterial Tissue, Open Approach

041D0A4 Bypass Left Common Iliac Artery to Left Renal Artery with Autologous Arterial Tissue, Open Approach

041D0A5 Bypass Left Common Iliac Artery to Bilateral Renal Artery with Autologous Arterial Tissue, Open Approach

041D0A6 Bypass Left Common Iliac Artery to Right Common Iliac Artery with Autologous Arterial Tissue, Open Approach

041D0A7 Bypass Left Common Iliac Artery to Left Common Iliac Artery with Autologous Arterial Tissue, Open Approach

041D0A8 Bypass Left Common Iliac Artery to Bilateral Common Iliac Arteries with Autologous Arterial Tissue, Open Approach

041D0A9 Bypass Left Common Iliac Artery to Right Internal Iliac Artery with Autologous Arterial Tissue, Open Approach

041D0AB Bypass Left Common Iliac Artery to Left Internal Iliac Artery with Autologous Arterial Tissue, Open Approach

041D0AC Bypass Left Common Iliac Artery to Bilateral Internal Iliac Arteries with Autologous Arterial Tissue, Open Approach

041D0AD Bypass Left Common Iliac Artery to Right External Iliac Artery with Autologous Arterial Tissue, Open Approach

041D0AF Bypass Left Common Iliac Artery to Left External Iliac Artery with Autologous Arterial Tissue, Open Approach

041D0AG Bypass Left Common Iliac Artery to Bilateral External Iliac Arteries with Autologous Arterial Tissue, Open Approach

041D0AH Bypass Left Common Iliac Artery to Right Femoral Artery with Autologous Arterial Tissue, Open Approach

041D0AJ Bypass Left Common Iliac Artery to Left Femoral Artery with Autologous Arterial Tissue, Open Approach

041D0AK Bypass Left Common Iliac Artery to Bilateral Femoral Arteries with Autologous Arterial Tissue, Open Approach

041D0AQ Bypass Left Common Iliac Artery to Lower Extremity Artery with Autologous Arterial Tissue, Open Approach

041D0AR Bypass Left Common Iliac Artery to Lower Artery with Autologous Arterial Tissue, Open Approach

041D0J0 Bypass Left Common Iliac Artery to Abdominal Aorta with Synthetic Substitute, Open Approach

041D0J1 Bypass Left Common Iliac Artery to Celiac Artery with Synthetic Substitute, Open Approach

041D0J2 Bypass Left Common Iliac Artery to Mesenteric Artery with Synthetic Substitute, Open Approach

041D0J3 Bypass Left Common Iliac Artery to Right Renal Artery with Synthetic Substitute, Open Approach

041D0J4 Bypass Left Common Iliac Artery to Left Renal Artery with Synthetic Substitute, Open Approach

041D0J5 Bypass Left Common Iliac Artery to Bilateral Renal Artery with Synthetic Substitute, Open Approach

041D0J6 Bypass Left Common Iliac Artery to Right Common Iliac Artery with Synthetic Substitute, Open Approach

041D0J7 Bypass Left Common Iliac Artery to Left Common Iliac Artery with Synthetic Substitute, Open Approach

041D0J8 Bypass Left Common Iliac Artery to Bilateral Common Iliac Arteries with Synthetic Substitute, Open Approach

041D0J9 Bypass Left Common Iliac Artery to Right Internal Iliac Artery with Synthetic Substitute, Open Approach

041D0JB Bypass Left Common Iliac Artery to Left Internal Iliac Artery with Synthetic Substitute, Open Approach

041D0JC Bypass Left Common Iliac Artery to Bilateral Internal Iliac Arteries with Synthetic Substitute, Open Approach

041D0JD Bypass Left Common Iliac Artery to Right External Iliac Artery with Synthetic Substitute, Open Approach

041D0JF Bypass Left Common Iliac Artery to Left External Iliac Artery with Synthetic Substitute, Open Approach

041D0JG Bypass Left Common Iliac Artery to Bilateral External Iliac Arteries with Synthetic Substitute, Open Approach

041D0JH Bypass Left Common Iliac Artery to Right Femoral Artery with Synthetic Substitute, Open Approach

041D0JJ Bypass Left Common Iliac Artery to Left Femoral Artery with Synthetic Substitute, Open Approach

041D0JK Bypass Left Common Iliac Artery to Bilateral Femoral Arteries with Synthetic Substitute, Open Approach

041D0JQ Bypass Left Common Iliac Artery to Lower Extremity Artery with Synthetic Substitute, Open Approach

041D0JR Bypass Left Common Iliac Artery to Lower Artery with Synthetic Substitute, Open Approach

041D0K0 Bypass Left Common Iliac Artery to Abdominal Aorta with Nonautologous Tissue Substitute, Open Approach

041D0K1 Bypass Left Common Iliac Artery to Celiac Artery with Nonautologous Tissue Substitute, Open Approach

041D0K2 Bypass Left Common Iliac Artery to Mesenteric Artery with Nonautologous Tissue Substitute, Open Approach

041D0K3 Bypass Left Common Iliac Artery to Right Renal Artery with Nonautologous Tissue Substitute, Open Approach

041D0K4 Bypass Left Common Iliac Artery to Left Renal Artery with Nonautologous Tissue Substitute, Open Approach

041D0K5 Bypass Left Common Iliac Artery to Bilateral Renal Artery with Nonautologous Tissue Substitute, Open Approach

041D0K6 Bypass Left Common Iliac Artery to Right Common Iliac Artery with Nonautologous Tissue Substitute, Open Approach

041D0K7 Bypass Left Common Iliac Artery to Left Common Iliac Artery with Nonautologous Tissue Substitute, Open Approach

041D0K8 Bypass Left Common Iliac Artery to Bilateral Common Iliac Arteries with Nonautologous Tissue Substitute, Open Approach

041D0K9 Bypass Left Common Iliac Artery to Right Internal Iliac Artery with Nonautologous Tissue Substitute, Open Approach

041D0KB Bypass Left Common Iliac Artery to Left Internal Iliac Artery with Nonautologous Tissue Substitute, Open Approach

041D0KC Bypass Left Common Iliac Artery to Bilateral Internal Iliac Arteries with Nonautologous Tissue Substitute, Open Approach

041D0KD Bypass Left Common Iliac Artery to Right External Iliac Artery with Nonautologous Tissue Substitute, Open Approach

041D0KF Bypass Left Common Iliac Artery to Left External Iliac Artery with Nonautologous Tissue Substitute, Open Approach

041D0KG Bypass Left Common Iliac Artery to Bilateral External Iliac Arteries with Nonautologous Tissue Substitute, Open Approach

041D0KH Bypass Left Common Iliac Artery to Right Femoral Artery with Nonautologous Tissue Substitute, Open Approach

041D0KJ Bypass Left Common Iliac Artery to Left Femoral Artery with Nonautologous Tissue Substitute, Open Approach

041D0KK Bypass Left Common Iliac Artery to Bilateral Femoral Arteries with Nonautologous Tissue Substitute, Open Approach

041D0KQ Bypass Left Common Iliac Artery to Lower Extremity Artery with Nonautologous Tissue Substitute, Open Approach

041D0KR Bypass Left Common Iliac Artery to Lower Artery with Nonautologous Tissue Substitute, Open Approach

041D0Z0 Bypass Left Common Iliac Artery to Abdominal Aorta, Open Approach

041D0Z1 Bypass Left Common Iliac Artery to Celiac Artery, Open Approach

D0Z2 Bypass Left Common Iliac Artery to Mesenteric Artery, Open Approach

D0Z3 Bypass Left Common Iliac Artery to Right Renal Artery, Open Approach

D0Z4 Bypass Left Common Iliac Artery to Left Renal Artery, Open Approach

D0Z5 Bypass Left Common Iliac Artery to Bilateral Renal Artery, Open Approach

D0Z6 Bypass Left Common Iliac Artery to Right Common Iliac Artery, Open Approach

D0Z7 Bypass Left Common Iliac Artery to Left Common Iliac Artery, Open Approach

D0Z8 Bypass Left Common Iliac Artery to Bilateral Common Iliac Arteries, Open Approach

D0Z9 Bypass Left Common Iliac Artery to Right Internal Iliac Artery, Open Approach

D0ZB Bypass Left Common Iliac Artery to Left Internal Iliac Artery, Open Approach

D0ZC Bypass Left Common Iliac Artery to Bilateral Internal Iliac Arteries, Open Approach

D0ZD Bypass Left Common Iliac Artery to Right External Iliac Artery, Open Approach

D0ZF Bypass Left Common Iliac Artery to Left External Iliac Artery, Open Approach

D0ZG Bypass Left Common Iliac Artery to Bilateral External Iliac Arteries, Open Approach

D0ZH Bypass Left Common Iliac Artery to Right Femoral Artery, Open Approach

D0ZJ Bypass Left Common Iliac Artery to Left Femoral Artery, Open Approach

D0ZK Bypass Left Common Iliac Artery to Bilateral Femoral Arteries, Open Approach

D0ZQ Bypass Left Common Iliac Artery to Lower Extremity Artery, Open Approach

D0ZR Bypass Left Common Iliac Artery to Lower Artery, Open Approach

D490 Bypass Left Common Iliac Artery to Abdominal Aorta with Autologous Venous Tissue, Percutaneous Endoscopic Approach

D491 Bypass Left Common Iliac Artery to Celiac Artery with Autologous Venous Tissue, Percutaneous Endoscopic Approach

D492 Bypass Left Common Iliac Artery to Mesenteric Artery with Autologous Venous Tissue, Percutaneous Endoscopic Approach

D493 Bypass Left Common Iliac Artery to Right Renal Artery with Autologous Venous Tissue, Percutaneous Endoscopic Approach

D494 Bypass Left Common Iliac Artery to Left Renal Artery with Autologous Venous Tissue, Percutaneous Endoscopic Approach

D495 Bypass Left Common Iliac Artery to Bilateral Renal Artery with Autologous Venous Tissue, Percutaneous Endoscopic Approach

D496 Bypass Left Common Iliac Artery to Right Common Iliac Artery with Autologous Venous Tissue, Percutaneous Endoscopic Approach

D497 Bypass Left Common Iliac Artery to Left Common Iliac Artery with Autologous Venous Tissue, Percutaneous Endoscopic Approach

D498 Bypass Left Common Iliac Artery to Bilateral Common Iliac Arteries with Autologous Venous Tissue, Percutaneous Endoscopic Approach

D499 Bypass Left Common Iliac Artery to Right Internal Iliac Artery with Autologous Venous Tissue, Percutaneous Endoscopic Approach

041D49B Bypass Left Common Iliac Artery to Left Internal Iliac Artery with Autologous Venous Tissue, Percutaneous Endoscopic Approach

041D49C Bypass Left Common Iliac Artery to Bilateral Internal Iliac Arteries with Autologous Venous Tissue, Percutaneous Endoscopic Approach

041D49D Bypass Left Common Iliac Artery to Right External Iliac Artery with Autologous Venous Tissue, Percutaneous Endoscopic Approach

041D49F Bypass Left Common Iliac Artery to Left External Iliac Artery with Autologous Venous Tissue, Percutaneous Endoscopic Approach

041D49G Bypass Left Common Iliac Artery to Bilateral External Iliac Arteries with Autologous Venous Tissue, Percutaneous Endoscopic Approach

041D49H Bypass Left Common Iliac Artery to Right Femoral Artery with Autologous Venous Tissue, Percutaneous Endoscopic Approach

041D49J Bypass Left Common Iliac Artery to Left Femoral Artery with Autologous Venous Tissue, Percutaneous Endoscopic Approach

041D49K Bypass Left Common Iliac Artery to Bilateral Femoral Arteries with Autologous Venous Tissue, Percutaneous Endoscopic Approach

041D49Q Bypass Left Common Iliac Artery to Lower Extremity Artery with Autologous Venous Tissue, Percutaneous Endoscopic Approach

041D49R Bypass Left Common Iliac Artery to Lower Artery with Autologous Venous Tissue, Percutaneous Endoscopic Approach

041D4A0 Bypass Left Common Iliac Artery to Abdominal Aorta with Autologous Arterial Tissue, Percutaneous Endoscopic Approach

041D4A1 Bypass Left Common Iliac Artery to Celiac Artery with Autologous Arterial Tissue, Percutaneous Endoscopic Approach

041D4A2 Bypass Left Common Iliac Artery to Mesenteric Artery with Autologous Arterial Tissue, Percutaneous Endoscopic Approach

041D4A3 Bypass Left Common Iliac Artery to Right Renal Artery with Autologous Arterial Tissue, Percutaneous Endoscopic Approach

041D4A4 Bypass Left Common Iliac Artery to Left Renal Artery with Autologous Arterial Tissue, Percutaneous Endoscopic Approach

041D4A5 Bypass Left Common Iliac Artery to Bilateral Renal Artery with Autologous Arterial Tissue, Percutaneous Endoscopic Approach

041D4A6 Bypass Left Common Iliac Artery to Right Common Iliac Artery with Autologous Arterial Tissue, Percutaneous Endoscopic Approach

041D4A7 Bypass Left Common Iliac Artery to Left Common Iliac Artery with Autologous Arterial Tissue, Percutaneous Endoscopic Approach

041D4A8 Bypass Left Common Iliac Artery to Bilateral Common Iliac Arteries with Autologous Arterial Tissue, Percutaneous Endoscopic Approach

041D4A9 Bypass Left Common Iliac Artery to Right Internal Iliac Artery with Autologous Arterial Tissue, Percutaneous Endoscopic Approach

041D4AB Bypass Left Common Iliac Artery to Left Internal Iliac Artery with Autologous Arterial Tissue, Percutaneous Endoscopic Approach

041D4AC Bypass Left Common Iliac Artery to Bilateral Internal Iliac Arteries with Autologous Arterial Tissue, Percutaneous Endoscopic Approach

041D4AD Bypass Left Common Iliac Artery to Right External Iliac Artery with Autologous Arterial Tissue, Percutaneous Endoscopic Approach

041D4AF Bypass Left Common Iliac Artery to Left External Iliac Artery with Autologous Arterial Tissue, Percutaneous Endoscopic Approach

041D4AG Bypass Left Common Iliac Artery to Bilateral External Iliac Arteries with Autologous Arterial Tissue, Percutaneous Endoscopic Approach

041D4AH Bypass Left Common Iliac Artery to Right Femoral Artery with Autologous Arterial Tissue, Percutaneous Endoscopic Approach

041D4AJ Bypass Left Common Iliac Artery to Left Femoral Artery with Autologous Arterial Tissue, Percutaneous Endoscopic Approach

041D4AK Bypass Left Common Iliac Artery to Bilateral Femoral Arteries with Autologous Arterial Tissue, Percutaneous Endoscopic Approach

041D4AQ Bypass Left Common Iliac Artery to Lower Extremity Artery with Autologous Arterial Tissue, Percutaneous Endoscopic Approach

041D4AR Bypass Left Common Iliac Artery to Lower Artery with Autologous Arterial Tissue, Percutaneous Endoscopic Approach

041D4J0 Bypass Left Common Iliac Artery to Abdominal Aorta with Synthetic Substitute, Percutaneous Endoscopic Approach

041D4J1 Bypass Left Common Iliac Artery to Celiac Artery with Synthetic Substitute, Percutaneous Endoscopic Approach

041D4J2 Bypass Left Common Iliac Artery to Mesenteric Artery with Synthetic Substitute, Percutaneous Endoscopic Approach

041D4J3 Bypass Left Common Iliac Artery to Right Renal Artery with Synthetic Substitute, Percutaneous Endoscopic Approach

041D4J4 Bypass Left Common Iliac Artery to Left Renal Artery with Synthetic Substitute, Percutaneous Endoscopic Approach

041D4J5 Bypass Left Common Iliac Artery to Bilateral Renal Artery with Synthetic Substitute, Percutaneous Endoscopic Approach

041D4J6 Bypass Left Common Iliac Artery to Right Common Iliac Artery with Synthetic Substitute, Percutaneous Endoscopic Approach

041D4J7 Bypass Left Common Iliac Artery to Left Common Iliac Artery with Synthetic Substitute, Percutaneous Endoscopic Approach

041D4J8 Bypass Left Common Iliac Artery to Bilateral Common Iliac Arteries with Synthetic Substitute, Percutaneous Endoscopic Approach

Female-only   ♂ Male-only   ▲ Limited Coverage   ● Non-OR   ▬ HAC-associated procedure   ▲ Non-covered procedures   ✚ Combination

041D4J9 Bypass Left Common Iliac Artery to Right Internal Iliac Artery with Synthetic Substitute, Percutaneous Endoscopic Approach

041D4JB Bypass Left Common Iliac Artery to Left Internal Iliac Artery with Synthetic Substitute, Percutaneous Endoscopic Approach

041D4JC Bypass Left Common Iliac Artery to Bilateral Internal Iliac Arteries with Synthetic Substitute, Percutaneous Endoscopic Approach

041D4JD Bypass Left Common Iliac Artery to Right External Iliac Artery with Synthetic Substitute, Percutaneous Endoscopic Approach

041D4JF Bypass Left Common Iliac Artery to Left External Iliac Artery with Synthetic Substitute, Percutaneous Endoscopic Approach

041D4JG Bypass Left Common Iliac Artery to Bilateral External Iliac Arteries with Synthetic Substitute, Percutaneous Endoscopic Approach

041D4JH Bypass Left Common Iliac Artery to Right Femoral Artery with Synthetic Substitute, Percutaneous Endoscopic Approach

041D4JJ Bypass Left Common Iliac Artery to Left Femoral Artery with Synthetic Substitute, Percutaneous Endoscopic Approach

041D4JK Bypass Left Common Iliac Artery to Bilateral Femoral Arteries with Synthetic Substitute, Percutaneous Endoscopic Approach

041D4JQ Bypass Left Common Iliac Artery to Lower Extremity Artery with Synthetic Substitute, Percutaneous Endoscopic Approach

041D4JR Bypass Left Common Iliac Artery to Lower Artery with Synthetic Substitute, Percutaneous Endoscopic Approach

041D4K0 Bypass Left Common Iliac Artery to Abdominal Aorta with Nonautologous Tissue Substitute, Percutaneous Endoscopic Approach

041D4K1 Bypass Left Common Iliac Artery to Celiac Artery with Nonautologous Tissue Substitute, Percutaneous Endoscopic Approach

041D4K2 Bypass Left Common Iliac Artery to Mesenteric Artery with Nonautologous Tissue Substitute, Percutaneous Endoscopic Approach

041D4K3 Bypass Left Common Iliac Artery to Right Renal Artery with Nonautologous Tissue Substitute, Percutaneous Endoscopic Approach

041D4K4 Bypass Left Common Iliac Artery to Left Renal Artery with Nonautologous Tissue Substitute, Percutaneous Endoscopic Approach

041D4K5 Bypass Left Common Iliac Artery to Bilateral Renal Artery with Nonautologous Tissue Substitute, Percutaneous Endoscopic Approach

041D4K6 Bypass Left Common Iliac Artery to Right Common Iliac Artery with Nonautologous Tissue Substitute, Percutaneous Endoscopic Approach

041D4K7 Bypass Left Common Iliac Artery to Left Common Iliac Artery with Nonautologous Tissue Substitute, Percutaneous Endoscopic Approach

041D4K8 Bypass Left Common Iliac Artery to Bilateral Common Iliac Arteries with Nonautologous Tissue Substitute, Percutaneous Endoscopic Approach

041D4K9 Bypass Left Common Iliac Artery to Right Internal Iliac Artery with Nonautologous Tissue Substitute, Percutaneous Endoscopic Approach

041D4KB Bypass Left Common Iliac Artery to Left Internal Iliac Artery with Nonautologous Tissue Substitute, Percutaneous Endoscopic Approach

041D4KC Bypass Left Common Iliac Artery to Bilateral Internal Iliac Arteries with Nonautologous Tissue Substitute, Percutaneous Endoscopic Approach

041D4KD Bypass Left Common Iliac Artery to Right External Iliac Artery with Nonautologous Tissue Substitute, Percutaneous Endoscopic Approach

041D4KF Bypass Left Common Iliac Artery to Left External Iliac Artery with Nonautologous Tissue Substitute, Percutaneous Endoscopic Approach

041D4KG Bypass Left Common Iliac Artery to Bilateral External Iliac Arteries with Nonautologous Tissue Substitute, Percutaneous Endoscopic Approach

041D4KH Bypass Left Common Iliac Artery to Right Femoral Artery with Nonautologous Tissue Substitute, Percutaneous Endoscopic Approach

041D4KJ Bypass Left Common Iliac Artery to Left Femoral Artery with Nonautologous Tissue Substitute, Percutaneous Endoscopic Approach

041D4KK Bypass Left Common Iliac Artery to Bilateral Femoral Arteries with Nonautologous Tissue Substitute, Percutaneous Endoscopic Approach

041D4KQ Bypass Left Common Iliac Artery to Lower Extremity Artery with Nonautologous Tissue Substitute, Percutaneous Endoscopic Approach

041D4KR Bypass Left Common Iliac Artery to Lower Artery with Nonautologous Tissue Substitute, Percutaneous Endoscopic Approach

041D4Z0 Bypass Left Common Iliac Artery to Abdominal Aorta, Percutaneous Endoscopic Approach

041D4Z1 Bypass Left Common Iliac Artery to Celiac Artery, Percutaneous Endoscopic Approach

041D4Z2 Bypass Left Common Iliac Artery to Mesenteric Artery, Percutaneous Endoscopic Approach

041D4Z3 Bypass Left Common Iliac Artery to Right Renal Artery, Percutaneous Endoscopic Approach

041D4Z4 Bypass Left Common Iliac Artery to Left Renal Artery, Percutaneous Endoscopic Approach

041D4Z5 Bypass Left Common Iliac Artery to Bilateral Renal Artery, Percutaneous Endoscopic Approach

041D4Z6 Bypass Left Common Iliac Artery to Right Common Iliac Artery, Percutaneous Endoscopic Approach

041D4Z7 Bypass Left Common Iliac Artery to Left Common Iliac Artery, Percutaneous Endoscopic Approach

041D4Z8 Bypass Left Common Iliac Artery to Bilateral Common Iliac Arteries, Percutaneous Endoscopic Approach

041D4Z9 Bypass Left Common Iliac Artery to Right Internal Iliac Artery, Percutaneous Endoscopic Approach

041D4ZB Bypass Left Common Iliac Artery to Left Internal Iliac Artery, Percutaneous Endoscopic Approach

041D4ZC Bypass Left Common Iliac Artery to Bilateral Internal Iliac Arteries, Percutaneous Endoscopic Approach

041D4ZD Bypass Left Common Iliac Artery to Right External Iliac Artery, Percutaneous Endoscopic Approach

041D4ZF Bypass Left Common Iliac Artery to Left External Iliac Artery, Percutaneous Endoscopic Approach

041D4ZG Bypass Left Common Iliac Artery to Bilateral External Iliac Arteries, Percutaneous Endoscopic Approach

041D4ZH Bypass Left Common Iliac Artery to Right Femoral Artery, Percutaneous Endoscopic Approach

041D4ZJ Bypass Left Common Iliac Artery to Left Femoral Artery, Percutaneous Endoscopic Approach

041D4ZK Bypass Left Common Iliac Artery to Bilateral Femoral Arteries, Percutaneous Endoscopic Approach

041D4ZQ Bypass Left Common Iliac Artery to Lower Extremity Artery, Percutaneous Endoscopic Approach

041D4ZR Bypass Left Common Iliac Artery to Lower Artery, Percutaneous Endoscopic Approach

041E099 Bypass Right Internal Iliac Artery to Right Internal Iliac Artery with Autologous Venous Tissue, Open Approach

041E09B Bypass Right Internal Iliac Artery to Left Internal Iliac Artery with Autologous Venous Tissue, Open Approach

041E09C Bypass Right Internal Iliac Artery to Bilateral Internal Iliac Arteries with Autologous Venous Tissue, Open Approach

041E09D Bypass Right Internal Iliac Artery to Right External Iliac Artery with Autologous Venous Tissue, Open Approach

041E09F Bypass Right Internal Iliac Artery to Left External Iliac Artery with Autologous Venous Tissue, Open Approach

041E09G Bypass Right Internal Iliac Artery to Bilateral External Iliac Arteries with Autologous Venous Tissue, Open Approach

041E09H Bypass Right Internal Iliac Artery to Right Femoral Artery with Autologous Venous Tissue, Open Approach

041E09J Bypass Right Internal Iliac Artery to Left Femoral Artery with Autologous Venous Tissue, Open Approach

041E09K Bypass Right Internal Iliac Artery to Bilateral Femoral Arteries with Autologous Venous Tissue, Open Approach

041E09P Bypass Right Internal Iliac Artery to Foot Artery with Autologous Venous Tissue, Open Approach

041E09Q Bypass Right Internal Iliac Artery to Lower Extremity Artery with Autologous Venous Tissue, Open Approach

041E0A9 Bypass Right Internal Iliac Artery to Right Internal Iliac Artery with Autologous Arterial Tissue, Open Approach

041E0AB Bypass Right Internal Iliac Artery to Left Internal Iliac Artery with Autologous Arterial Tissue, Open Approach

041E0AC Bypass Right Internal Iliac Artery to Bilateral Internal Iliac Arteries with Autologous Arterial Tissue, Open Approach

041E0AD Bypass Right Internal Iliac Artery to Right External Iliac Artery with Autologous Arterial Tissue, Open Approach

E0AF Bypass Right Internal Iliac Artery to Left External Iliac Artery with Autologous Arterial Tissue, Open Approach	**041E0KH** Bypass Right Internal Iliac Artery to Right Femoral Artery with Nonautologous Tissue Substitute, Open Approach	**041E49P** Bypass Right Internal Iliac Artery to Foot Artery with Autologous Venous Tissue, Percutaneous Endoscopic Approach
E0AG Bypass Right Internal Iliac Artery to Bilateral External Iliac Arteries with Autologous Arterial Tissue, Open Approach	**041E0KJ** Bypass Right Internal Iliac Artery to Left Femoral Artery with Nonautologous Tissue Substitute, Open Approach	**041E49Q** Bypass Right Internal Iliac Artery to Lower Extremity Artery with Autologous Venous Tissue, Percutaneous Endoscopic Approach
E0AH Bypass Right Internal Iliac Artery to Right Femoral Artery with Autologous Arterial Tissue, Open Approach	**041E0KK** Bypass Right Internal Iliac Artery to Bilateral Femoral Arteries with Nonautologous Tissue Substitute, Open Approach	**041E4A9** Bypass Right Internal Iliac Artery to Right Internal Iliac Artery with Autologous Arterial Tissue, Percutaneous Endoscopic Approach
E0AJ Bypass Right Internal Iliac Artery to Left Femoral Artery with Autologous Arterial Tissue, Open Approach	**041E0KP** Bypass Right Internal Iliac Artery to Foot Artery with Nonautologous Tissue Substitute, Open Approach	**041E4AB** Bypass Right Internal Iliac Artery to Left Internal Iliac Artery with Autologous Arterial Tissue, Percutaneous Endoscopic Approach
E0AK Bypass Right Internal Iliac Artery to Bilateral Femoral Arteries with Autologous Arterial Tissue, Open Approach	**041E0KQ** Bypass Right Internal Iliac Artery to Lower Extremity Artery with Nonautologous Tissue Substitute, Open Approach	**041E4AC** Bypass Right Internal Iliac Artery to Bilateral Internal Iliac Arteries with Autologous Arterial Tissue, Percutaneous Endoscopic Approach
E0AP Bypass Right Internal Iliac Artery to Foot Artery with Autologous Arterial Tissue, Open Approach	**041E0Z9** Bypass Right Internal Iliac Artery to Right Internal Iliac Artery, Open Approach	**041E4AD** Bypass Right Internal Iliac Artery to Right External Iliac Artery with Autologous Arterial Tissue, Percutaneous Endoscopic Approach
E0AQ Bypass Right Internal Iliac Artery to Lower Extremity Artery with Autologous Arterial Tissue, Open Approach	**041E0ZB** Bypass Right Internal Iliac Artery to Left Internal Iliac Artery, Open Approach	**041E4AF** Bypass Right Internal Iliac Artery to Left External Iliac Artery with Autologous Arterial Tissue, Percutaneous Endoscopic Approach
E0J9 Bypass Right Internal Iliac Artery to Right Internal Iliac Artery with Synthetic Substitute, Open Approach	**041E0ZC** Bypass Right Internal Iliac Artery to Bilateral Internal Iliac Arteries, Open Approach	**041E4AG** Bypass Right Internal Iliac Artery to Bilateral External Iliac Arteries with Autologous Arterial Tissue, Percutaneous Endoscopic Approach
E0JB Bypass Right Internal Iliac Artery to Left Internal Iliac Artery with Synthetic Substitute, Open Approach	**041E0ZD** Bypass Right Internal Iliac Artery to Right External Iliac Artery, Open Approach	**041E4AH** Bypass Right Internal Iliac Artery to Right Femoral Artery with Autologous Arterial Tissue, Percutaneous Endoscopic Approach
E0JC Bypass Right Internal Iliac Artery to Bilateral Internal Iliac Arteries with Synthetic Substitute, Open Approach	**041E0ZF** Bypass Right Internal Iliac Artery to Left External Iliac Artery, Open Approach	**041E4AJ** Bypass Right Internal Iliac Artery to Left Femoral Artery with Autologous Arterial Tissue, Percutaneous Endoscopic Approach
E0JD Bypass Right Internal Iliac Artery to Right External Iliac Artery with Synthetic Substitute, Open Approach	**041E0ZG** Bypass Right Internal Iliac Artery to Bilateral External Iliac Arteries, Open Approach	**041E4AK** Bypass Right Internal Iliac Artery to Bilateral Femoral Arteries with Autologous Arterial Tissue, Percutaneous Endoscopic Approach
E0JF Bypass Right Internal Iliac Artery to Left External Iliac Artery with Synthetic Substitute, Open Approach	**041E0ZH** Bypass Right Internal Iliac Artery to Right Femoral Artery, Open Approach	**041E4AP** Bypass Right Internal Iliac Artery to Foot Artery with Autologous Arterial Tissue, Percutaneous Endoscopic Approach
E0JG Bypass Right Internal Iliac Artery to Bilateral External Iliac Arteries with Synthetic Substitute, Open Approach	**041E0ZJ** Bypass Right Internal Iliac Artery to Left Femoral Artery, Open Approach	**041E4AQ** Bypass Right Internal Iliac Artery to Lower Extremity Artery with Autologous Arterial Tissue, Percutaneous Endoscopic Approach
E0JH Bypass Right Internal Iliac Artery to Right Femoral Artery with Synthetic Substitute, Open Approach	**041E0ZK** Bypass Right Internal Iliac Artery to Bilateral Femoral Arteries, Open Approach	**041E4J9** Bypass Right Internal Iliac Artery to Right Internal Iliac Artery with Synthetic Substitute, Percutaneous Endoscopic Approach
E0JJ Bypass Right Internal Iliac Artery to Left Femoral Artery with Synthetic Substitute, Open Approach	**041E0ZP** Bypass Right Internal Iliac Artery to Foot Artery, Open Approach	**041E4JB** Bypass Right Internal Iliac Artery to Left Internal Iliac Artery with Synthetic Substitute, Percutaneous Endoscopic Approach
E0JK Bypass Right Internal Iliac Artery to Bilateral Femoral Arteries with Synthetic Substitute, Open Approach	**041E0ZQ** Bypass Right Internal Iliac Artery to Lower Extremity Artery, Open Approach	**041E4JC** Bypass Right Internal Iliac Artery to Bilateral Internal Iliac Arteries with Synthetic Substitute, Percutaneous Endoscopic Approach
E0JP Bypass Right Internal Iliac Artery to Foot Artery with Synthetic Substitute, Open Approach	**041E499** Bypass Right Internal Iliac Artery to Right Internal Iliac Artery with Autologous Venous Tissue, Percutaneous Endoscopic Approach	**041E4JD** Bypass Right Internal Iliac Artery to Right External Iliac Artery with Synthetic Substitute, Percutaneous Endoscopic Approach
E0JQ Bypass Right Internal Iliac Artery to Lower Extremity Artery with Synthetic Substitute, Open Approach	**041E49B** Bypass Right Internal Iliac Artery to Left Internal Iliac Artery with Autologous Venous Tissue, Percutaneous Endoscopic Approach	**041E4JF** Bypass Right Internal Iliac Artery to Left External Iliac Artery with Synthetic Substitute, Percutaneous Endoscopic Approach
E0K9 Bypass Right Internal Iliac Artery to Right Internal Iliac Artery with Nonautologous Tissue Substitute, Open Approach	**041E49C** Bypass Right Internal Iliac Artery to Bilateral Internal Iliac Arteries with Autologous Venous Tissue, Percutaneous Endoscopic Approach	**041E4JG** Bypass Right Internal Iliac Artery to Bilateral External Iliac Arteries with Synthetic Substitute, Percutaneous Endoscopic Approach
E0KB Bypass Right Internal Iliac Artery to Left Internal Iliac Artery with Nonautologous Tissue Substitute, Open Approach	**041E49D** Bypass Right Internal Iliac Artery to Right External Iliac Artery with Autologous Venous Tissue, Percutaneous Endoscopic Approach	**041E4JH** Bypass Right Internal Iliac Artery to Right Femoral Artery with Synthetic Substitute, Percutaneous Endoscopic Approach
E0KC Bypass Right Internal Iliac Artery to Bilateral Internal Iliac Arteries with Nonautologous Tissue Substitute, Open Approach	**041E49F** Bypass Right Internal Iliac Artery to Left External Iliac Artery with Autologous Venous Tissue, Percutaneous Endoscopic Approach	
E0KD Bypass Right Internal Iliac Artery to Right External Iliac Artery with Nonautologous Tissue Substitute, Open Approach	**041E49G** Bypass Right Internal Iliac Artery to Bilateral External Iliac Arteries with Autologous Venous Tissue, Percutaneous Endoscopic Approach	
E0KF Bypass Right Internal Iliac Artery to Left External Iliac Artery with Nonautologous Tissue Substitute, Open Approach	**041E49H** Bypass Right Internal Iliac Artery to Right Femoral Artery with Autologous Venous Tissue, Percutaneous Endoscopic Approach	
E0KG Bypass Right Internal Iliac Artery to Bilateral External Iliac Arteries with Nonautologous Tissue Substitute, Open Approach	**041E49J** Bypass Right Internal Iliac Artery to Left Femoral Artery with Autologous Venous Tissue, Percutaneous Endoscopic Approach	
	041E49K Bypass Right Internal Iliac Artery to Bilateral Femoral Arteries with Autologous Venous Tissue, Percutaneous Endoscopic Approach	

♀ Female-only   ♂ Male-only   ▲ Limited Coverage   ● Non-OR   HAC HAC-associated procedure   ▲ Non-covered procedures   + Combination

041E4JJ Bypass Right Internal Iliac Artery to Left Femoral Artery with Synthetic Substitute, Percutaneous Endoscopic Approach

041E4JK Bypass Right Internal Iliac Artery to Bilateral Femoral Arteries with Synthetic Substitute, Percutaneous Endoscopic Approach

041E4JP Bypass Right Internal Iliac Artery to Foot Artery with Synthetic Substitute, Percutaneous Endoscopic Approach

041E4JQ Bypass Right Internal Iliac Artery to Lower Extremity Artery with Synthetic Substitute, Percutaneous Endoscopic Approach

041E4K9 Bypass Right Internal Iliac Artery to Right Internal Iliac Artery with Nonautologous Tissue Substitute, Percutaneous Endoscopic Approach

041E4KB Bypass Right Internal Iliac Artery to Left Internal Iliac Artery with Nonautologous Tissue Substitute, Percutaneous Endoscopic Approach

041E4KC Bypass Right Internal Iliac Artery to Bilateral Internal Iliac Arteries with Nonautologous Tissue Substitute, Percutaneous Endoscopic Approach

041E4KD Bypass Right Internal Iliac Artery to Right External Iliac Artery with Nonautologous Tissue Substitute, Percutaneous Endoscopic Approach

041E4KF Bypass Right Internal Iliac Artery to Left External Iliac Artery with Nonautologous Tissue Substitute, Percutaneous Endoscopic Approach

041E4KG Bypass Right Internal Iliac Artery to Bilateral External Iliac Arteries with Nonautologous Tissue Substitute, Percutaneous Endoscopic Approach

041E4KH Bypass Right Internal Iliac Artery to Right Femoral Artery with Nonautologous Tissue Substitute, Percutaneous Endoscopic Approach

041E4KJ Bypass Right Internal Iliac Artery to Left Femoral Artery with Nonautologous Tissue Substitute, Percutaneous Endoscopic Approach

041E4KK Bypass Right Internal Iliac Artery to Bilateral Femoral Arteries with Nonautologous Tissue Substitute, Percutaneous Endoscopic Approach

041E4KP Bypass Right Internal Iliac Artery to Foot Artery with Nonautologous Tissue Substitute, Percutaneous Endoscopic Approach

041E4KQ Bypass Right Internal Iliac Artery to Lower Extremity Artery with Nonautologous Tissue Substitute, Percutaneous Endoscopic Approach

041E4Z9 Bypass Right Internal Iliac Artery to Right Internal Iliac Artery, Percutaneous Endoscopic Approach

041E4ZB Bypass Right Internal Iliac Artery to Left Internal Iliac Artery, Percutaneous Endoscopic Approach

041E4ZC Bypass Right Internal Iliac Artery to Bilateral Internal Iliac Arteries, Percutaneous Endoscopic Approach

041E4ZD Bypass Right Internal Iliac Artery to Right External Iliac Artery, Percutaneous Endoscopic Approach

041E4ZF Bypass Right Internal Iliac Artery to Left External Iliac Artery, Percutaneous Endoscopic Approach

041E4ZG Bypass Right Internal Iliac Artery to Bilateral External Iliac Arteries, Percutaneous Endoscopic Approach

041E4ZH Bypass Right Internal Iliac Artery to Right Femoral Artery, Percutaneous Endoscopic Approach

041E4ZJ Bypass Right Internal Iliac Artery to Left Femoral Artery, Percutaneous Endoscopic Approach

041E4ZK Bypass Right Internal Iliac Artery to Bilateral Femoral Arteries, Percutaneous Endoscopic Approach

041E4ZP Bypass Right Internal Iliac Artery to Foot Artery, Percutaneous Endoscopic Approach

041E4ZQ Bypass Right Internal Iliac Artery to Lower Extremity Artery, Percutaneous Endoscopic Approach

041F099 Bypass Left Internal Iliac Artery to Right Internal Iliac Artery with Autologous Venous Tissue, Open Approach

041F09B Bypass Left Internal Iliac Artery to Left Internal Iliac Artery with Autologous Venous Tissue, Open Approach

041F09C Bypass Left Internal Iliac Artery to Bilateral Internal Iliac Arteries with Autologous Venous Tissue, Open Approach

041F09D Bypass Left Internal Iliac Artery to Right External Iliac Artery with Autologous Venous Tissue, Open Approach

041F09F Bypass Left Internal Iliac Artery to Left External Iliac Artery with Autologous Venous Tissue, Open Approach

041F09G Bypass Left Internal Iliac Artery to Bilateral External Iliac Arteries with Autologous Venous Tissue, Open Approach

041F09H Bypass Left Internal Iliac Artery to Right Femoral Artery with Autologous Venous Tissue, Open Approach

041F09J Bypass Left Internal Iliac Artery to Left Femoral Artery with Autologous Venous Tissue, Open Approach

041F09K Bypass Left Internal Iliac Artery to Bilateral Femoral Arteries with Autologous Venous Tissue, Open Approach

041F09P Bypass Left Internal Iliac Artery to Foot Artery with Autologous Venous Tissue, Open Approach

041F09Q Bypass Left Internal Iliac Artery to Lower Extremity Artery with Autologous Venous Tissue, Open Approach

041F0A9 Bypass Left Internal Iliac Artery to Right Internal Iliac Artery with Autologous Arterial Tissue, Open Approach

041F0AB Bypass Left Internal Iliac Artery to Left Internal Iliac Artery with Autologous Arterial Tissue, Open Approach

041F0AC Bypass Left Internal Iliac Artery to Bilateral Internal Iliac Arteries with Autologous Arterial Tissue, Open Approach

041F0AD Bypass Left Internal Iliac Artery to Right External Iliac Artery with Autologous Arterial Tissue, Open Approach

041F0AF Bypass Left Internal Iliac Artery to Left External Iliac Artery with Autologous Arterial Tissue, Open Approach

041F0AG Bypass Left Internal Iliac Artery to Bilateral External Iliac Arteries with Autologous Arterial Tissue, Open Approach

041F0AH Bypass Left Internal Iliac Artery to Right Femoral Artery with Autologous Arterial Tissue, Open Approach

041F0AJ Bypass Left Internal Iliac Artery to Left Femoral Artery with Autologous Arterial Tissue, Open Approach

041F0AK Bypass Left Internal Iliac Artery to Bilateral Femoral Arteries with Autologous Arterial Tissue, Open Approach

041F0AP Bypass Left Internal Iliac Artery to Foot Artery with Autologous Arterial Tissue, Open Approach

041F0AQ Bypass Left Internal Iliac Artery to Lower Extremity Artery with Autologous Arterial Tissue, Open Approach

041F0J9 Bypass Left Internal Iliac Artery to Right Internal Iliac Artery with Synthetic Substitute, Open Approach

041F0JB Bypass Left Internal Iliac Artery to Left Internal Iliac Artery with Synthetic Substitute, Open Approach

041F0JC Bypass Left Internal Iliac Artery to Bilateral Internal Iliac Arteries with Synthetic Substitute, Open Approach

041F0JD Bypass Left Internal Iliac Artery to Right External Iliac Artery with Synthetic Substitute, Open Approach

041F0JF Bypass Left Internal Iliac Artery to Left External Iliac Artery with Synthetic Substitute, Open Approach

041F0JG Bypass Left Internal Iliac Artery to Bilateral External Iliac Arteries with Synthetic Substitute, Open Approach

041F0JH Bypass Left Internal Iliac Artery to Right Femoral Artery with Synthetic Substitute, Open Approach

041F0JJ Bypass Left Internal Iliac Artery to Left Femoral Artery with Synthetic Substitute, Open Approach

041F0JK Bypass Left Internal Iliac Artery to Bilateral Femoral Arteries with Synthetic Substitute, Open Approach

041F0JP Bypass Left Internal Iliac Artery to Foot Artery with Synthetic Substitute, Open Approach

041F0JQ Bypass Left Internal Iliac Artery to Lower Extremity Artery with Synthetic Substitute, Open Approach

041F0K9 Bypass Left Internal Iliac Artery to Right Internal Iliac Artery with Nonautologous Tissue Substitute, Open Approach

041F0KB Bypass Left Internal Iliac Artery to Left Internal Iliac Artery with Nonautologous Tissue Substitute, Open Approach

041F0KC Bypass Left Internal Iliac Artery to Bilateral Internal Iliac Arteries with Nonautologous Tissue Substitute, Open Approach

041F0KD Bypass Left Internal Iliac Artery to Right External Iliac Artery with Nonautologous Tissue Substitute, Open Approach

041F0KF Bypass Left Internal Iliac Artery to Left External Iliac Artery with Nonautologous Tissue Substitute, Open Approach

041F0KG Bypass Left Internal Iliac Artery to Bilateral External Iliac Arteries with Nonautologous Tissue Substitute, Open Approach

041F0KH Bypass Left Internal Iliac Artery to Right Femoral Artery with Nonautologous Tissue Substitute, Open Approach

041F0KJ Bypass Left Internal Iliac Artery to Left Femoral Artery with Nonautologous Tissue Substitute, Open Approach

041F0KK Bypass Left Internal Iliac Artery to Bilateral Femoral Arteries with Nonautologous Tissue Substitute, Open Approach

041F0KP Bypass Left Internal Iliac Artery to Foot Artery with Nonautologous Tissue Substitute, Open Approach

041F0KQ	Bypass Left Internal Iliac Artery to Lower Extremity Artery with Nonautologous Tissue Substitute, Open Approach
041F0Z9	Bypass Left Internal Iliac Artery to Right Internal Iliac Artery, Open Approach
041F0ZB	Bypass Left Internal Iliac Artery to Left Internal Iliac Artery, Open Approach
041F0ZC	Bypass Left Internal Iliac Artery to Bilateral Internal Iliac Arteries, Open Approach
041F0ZD	Bypass Left Internal Iliac Artery to Right External Iliac Artery, Open Approach
041F0ZF	Bypass Left Internal Iliac Artery to Left External Iliac Artery, Open Approach
041F0ZG	Bypass Left Internal Iliac Artery to Bilateral External Iliac Arteries, Open Approach
041F0ZH	Bypass Left Internal Iliac Artery to Right Femoral Artery, Open Approach
041F0ZJ	Bypass Left Internal Iliac Artery to Left Femoral Artery, Open Approach
041F0ZK	Bypass Left Internal Iliac Artery to Bilateral Femoral Arteries, Open Approach
041F0ZP	Bypass Left Internal Iliac Artery to Foot Artery, Open Approach
041F0ZQ	Bypass Left Internal Iliac Artery to Lower Extremity Artery, Open Approach
041F499	Bypass Left Internal Iliac Artery to Right Internal Iliac Artery with Autologous Venous Tissue, Percutaneous Endoscopic Approach
041F49B	Bypass Left Internal Iliac Artery to Left Internal Iliac Artery with Autologous Venous Tissue, Percutaneous Endoscopic Approach
041F49C	Bypass Left Internal Iliac Artery to Bilateral Internal Iliac Arteries with Autologous Venous Tissue, Percutaneous Endoscopic Approach
041F49D	Bypass Left Internal Iliac Artery to Right External Iliac Artery with Autologous Venous Tissue, Percutaneous Endoscopic Approach
041F49F	Bypass Left Internal Iliac Artery to Left External Iliac Artery with Autologous Venous Tissue, Percutaneous Endoscopic Approach
041F49G	Bypass Left Internal Iliac Artery to Bilateral External Iliac Arteries with Autologous Venous Tissue, Percutaneous Endoscopic Approach
041F49H	Bypass Left Internal Iliac Artery to Right Femoral Artery with Autologous Venous Tissue, Percutaneous Endoscopic Approach
041F49J	Bypass Left Internal Iliac Artery to Left Femoral Artery with Autologous Venous Tissue, Percutaneous Endoscopic Approach
041F49K	Bypass Left Internal Iliac Artery to Bilateral Femoral Arteries with Autologous Venous Tissue, Percutaneous Endoscopic Approach
041F49P	Bypass Left Internal Iliac Artery to Foot Artery with Autologous Venous Tissue, Percutaneous Endoscopic Approach
041F49Q	Bypass Left Internal Iliac Artery to Lower Extremity Artery with Autologous Venous Tissue, Percutaneous Endoscopic Approach
041F4A9	Bypass Left Internal Iliac Artery to Right Internal Iliac Artery with Autologous Arterial Tissue, Percutaneous Endoscopic Approach
041F4AB	Bypass Left Internal Iliac Artery to Left Internal Iliac Artery with Autologous Arterial Tissue, Percutaneous Endoscopic Approach
041F4AC	Bypass Left Internal Iliac Artery to Bilateral Internal Iliac Arteries with Autologous Arterial Tissue, Percutaneous Endoscopic Approach
041F4AD	Bypass Left Internal Iliac Artery to Right External Iliac Artery with Autologous Arterial Tissue, Percutaneous Endoscopic Approach
041F4AF	Bypass Left Internal Iliac Artery to Left External Iliac Artery with Autologous Arterial Tissue, Percutaneous Endoscopic Approach
041F4AG	Bypass Left Internal Iliac Artery to Bilateral External Iliac Arteries with Autologous Arterial Tissue, Percutaneous Endoscopic Approach
041F4AH	Bypass Left Internal Iliac Artery to Right Femoral Artery with Autologous Arterial Tissue, Percutaneous Endoscopic Approach
041F4AJ	Bypass Left Internal Iliac Artery to Left Femoral Artery with Autologous Arterial Tissue, Percutaneous Endoscopic Approach
041F4AK	Bypass Left Internal Iliac Artery to Bilateral Femoral Arteries with Autologous Arterial Tissue, Percutaneous Endoscopic Approach
041F4AP	Bypass Left Internal Iliac Artery to Foot Artery with Autologous Arterial Tissue, Percutaneous Endoscopic Approach
041F4AQ	Bypass Left Internal Iliac Artery to Lower Extremity Artery with Autologous Arterial Tissue, Percutaneous Endoscopic Approach
041F4J9	Bypass Left Internal Iliac Artery to Right Internal Iliac Artery with Synthetic Substitute, Percutaneous Endoscopic Approach
041F4JB	Bypass Left Internal Iliac Artery to Left Internal Iliac Artery with Synthetic Substitute, Percutaneous Endoscopic Approach
041F4JC	Bypass Left Internal Iliac Artery to Bilateral Internal Iliac Arteries with Synthetic Substitute, Percutaneous Endoscopic Approach
041F4JD	Bypass Left Internal Iliac Artery to Right External Iliac Artery with Synthetic Substitute, Percutaneous Endoscopic Approach
041F4JF	Bypass Left Internal Iliac Artery to Left External Iliac Artery with Synthetic Substitute, Percutaneous Endoscopic Approach
041F4JG	Bypass Left Internal Iliac Artery to Bilateral External Iliac Arteries with Synthetic Substitute, Percutaneous Endoscopic Approach
041F4JH	Bypass Left Internal Iliac Artery to Right Femoral Artery with Synthetic Substitute, Percutaneous Endoscopic Approach
041F4JJ	Bypass Left Internal Iliac Artery to Left Femoral Artery with Synthetic Substitute, Percutaneous Endoscopic Approach
041F4JK	Bypass Left Internal Iliac Artery to Bilateral Femoral Arteries with Synthetic Substitute, Percutaneous Endoscopic Approach
041F4JP	Bypass Left Internal Iliac Artery to Foot Artery with Synthetic Substitute, Percutaneous Endoscopic Approach
041F4JQ	Bypass Left Internal Iliac Artery to Lower Extremity Artery with Synthetic Substitute, Percutaneous Endoscopic Approach
041F4K9	Bypass Left Internal Iliac Artery to Right Internal Iliac Artery with Nonautologous Tissue Substitute, Percutaneous Endoscopic Approach
041F4KB	Bypass Left Internal Iliac Artery to Left Internal Iliac Artery with Nonautologous Tissue Substitute, Percutaneous Endoscopic Approach
041F4KC	Bypass Left Internal Iliac Artery to Bilateral Internal Iliac Arteries with Nonautologous Tissue Substitute, Percutaneous Endoscopic Approach
041F4KD	Bypass Left Internal Iliac Artery to Right External Iliac Artery with Nonautologous Tissue Substitute, Percutaneous Endoscopic Approach
041F4KF	Bypass Left Internal Iliac Artery to Left External Iliac Artery with Nonautologous Tissue Substitute, Percutaneous Endoscopic Approach
041F4KG	Bypass Left Internal Iliac Artery to Bilateral External Iliac Arteries with Nonautologous Tissue Substitute, Percutaneous Endoscopic Approach
041F4KH	Bypass Left Internal Iliac Artery to Right Femoral Artery with Nonautologous Tissue Substitute, Percutaneous Endoscopic Approach
041F4KJ	Bypass Left Internal Iliac Artery to Left Femoral Artery with Nonautologous Tissue Substitute, Percutaneous Endoscopic Approach
041F4KK	Bypass Left Internal Iliac Artery to Bilateral Femoral Arteries with Nonautologous Tissue Substitute, Percutaneous Endoscopic Approach
041F4KP	Bypass Left Internal Iliac Artery to Foot Artery with Nonautologous Tissue Substitute, Percutaneous Endoscopic Approach
041F4KQ	Bypass Left Internal Iliac Artery to Lower Extremity Artery with Nonautologous Tissue Substitute, Percutaneous Endoscopic Approach
041F4Z9	Bypass Left Internal Iliac Artery to Right Internal Iliac Artery, Percutaneous Endoscopic Approach
041F4ZB	Bypass Left Internal Iliac Artery to Left Internal Iliac Artery, Percutaneous Endoscopic Approach
041F4ZC	Bypass Left Internal Iliac Artery to Bilateral Internal Iliac Arteries, Percutaneous Endoscopic Approach
041F4ZD	Bypass Left Internal Iliac Artery to Right External Iliac Artery, Percutaneous Endoscopic Approach
041F4ZF	Bypass Left Internal Iliac Artery to Left External Iliac Artery, Percutaneous Endoscopic Approach
041F4ZG	Bypass Left Internal Iliac Artery to Bilateral External Iliac Arteries, Percutaneous Endoscopic Approach
041F4ZH	Bypass Left Internal Iliac Artery to Right Femoral Artery, Percutaneous Endoscopic Approach
041F4ZJ	Bypass Left Internal Iliac Artery to Left Femoral Artery, Percutaneous Endoscopic Approach
041F4ZK	Bypass Left Internal Iliac Artery to Bilateral Femoral Arteries, Percutaneous Endoscopic Approach
041F4ZP	Bypass Left Internal Iliac Artery to Foot Artery, Percutaneous Endoscopic Approach
041F4ZQ	Bypass Left Internal Iliac Artery to Lower Extremity Artery, Percutaneous Endoscopic Approach

Female-only ♂ Male-only ▲ Limited Coverage ● Non-OR ▬ HAC-associated procedure ▲ Non-covered procedures ✛ Combination

041H099 Bypass Right External Iliac Artery to Right Internal Iliac Artery with Autologous Venous Tissue, Open Approach

041H09B Bypass Right External Iliac Artery to Left Internal Iliac Artery with Autologous Venous Tissue, Open Approach

041H09C Bypass Right External Iliac Artery to Bilateral Internal Iliac Arteries with Autologous Venous Tissue, Open Approach

041H09D Bypass Right External Iliac Artery to Right External Iliac Artery with Autologous Venous Tissue, Open Approach

041H09F Bypass Right External Iliac Artery to Left External Iliac Artery with Autologous Venous Tissue, Open Approach

041H09G Bypass Right External Iliac Artery to Bilateral External Iliac Arteries with Autologous Venous Tissue, Open Approach

041H09H Bypass Right External Iliac Artery to Right Femoral Artery with Autologous Venous Tissue, Open Approach

041H09J Bypass Right External Iliac Artery to Left Femoral Artery with Autologous Venous Tissue, Open Approach

041H09K Bypass Right External Iliac Artery to Bilateral Femoral Arteries with Autologous Venous Tissue, Open Approach

041H09P Bypass Right External Iliac Artery to Foot Artery with Autologous Venous Tissue, Open Approach

041H09Q Bypass Right External Iliac Artery to Lower Extremity Artery with Autologous Venous Tissue, Open Approach

041H0A9 Bypass Right External Iliac Artery to Right Internal Iliac Artery with Autologous Arterial Tissue, Open Approach

041H0AB Bypass Right External Iliac Artery to Left Internal Iliac Artery with Autologous Arterial Tissue, Open Approach

041H0AC Bypass Right External Iliac Artery to Bilateral Internal Iliac Arteries with Autologous Arterial Tissue, Open Approach

041H0AD Bypass Right External Iliac Artery to Right External Iliac Artery with Autologous Arterial Tissue, Open Approach

041H0AF Bypass Right External Iliac Artery to Left External Iliac Artery with Autologous Arterial Tissue, Open Approach

041H0AG Bypass Right External Iliac Artery to Bilateral External Iliac Arteries with Autologous Arterial Tissue, Open Approach

041H0AH Bypass Right External Iliac Artery to Right Femoral Artery with Autologous Arterial Tissue, Open Approach

041H0AJ Bypass Right External Iliac Artery to Left Femoral Artery with Autologous Arterial Tissue, Open Approach

041H0AK Bypass Right External Iliac Artery to Bilateral Femoral Arteries with Autologous Arterial Tissue, Open Approach

041H0AP Bypass Right External Iliac Artery to Foot Artery with Autologous Arterial Tissue, Open Approach

041H0AQ Bypass Right External Iliac Artery to Lower Extremity Artery with Autologous Arterial Tissue, Open Approach

041H0J9 Bypass Right External Iliac Artery to Right Internal Iliac Artery with Synthetic Substitute, Open Approach

041H0JB Bypass Right External Iliac Artery to Left Internal Iliac Artery with Synthetic Substitute, Open Approach

041H0JC Bypass Right External Iliac Artery to Bilateral Internal Iliac Arteries with Synthetic Substitute, Open Approach

041H0JD Bypass Right External Iliac Artery to Right External Iliac Artery with Synthetic Substitute, Open Approach

041H0JF Bypass Right External Iliac Artery to Left External Iliac Artery with Synthetic Substitute, Open Approach

041H0JG Bypass Right External Iliac Artery to Bilateral External Iliac Arteries with Synthetic Substitute, Open Approach

041H0JH Bypass Right External Iliac Artery to Right Femoral Artery with Synthetic Substitute, Open Approach

041H0JJ Bypass Right External Iliac Artery to Left Femoral Artery with Synthetic Substitute, Open Approach

041H0JK Bypass Right External Iliac Artery to Bilateral Femoral Arteries with Synthetic Substitute, Open Approach

041H0JP Bypass Right External Iliac Artery to Foot Artery with Synthetic Substitute, Open Approach

041H0JQ Bypass Right External Iliac Artery to Lower Extremity Artery with Synthetic Substitute, Open Approach

041H0K9 Bypass Right External Iliac Artery to Right Internal Iliac Artery with Nonautologous Tissue Substitute, Open Approach

041H0KB Bypass Right External Iliac Artery to Left Internal Iliac Artery with Nonautologous Tissue Substitute, Open Approach

041H0KC Bypass Right External Iliac Artery to Bilateral Internal Iliac Arteries with Nonautologous Tissue Substitute, Open Approach

041H0KD Bypass Right External Iliac Artery to Right External Iliac Artery with Nonautologous Tissue Substitute, Open Approach

041H0KF Bypass Right External Iliac Artery to Left External Iliac Artery with Nonautologous Tissue Substitute, Open Approach

041H0KG Bypass Right External Iliac Artery to Bilateral External Iliac Arteries with Nonautologous Tissue Substitute, Open Approach

041H0KH Bypass Right External Iliac Artery to Right Femoral Artery with Nonautologous Tissue Substitute, Open Approach

041H0KJ Bypass Right External Iliac Artery to Left Femoral Artery with Nonautologous Tissue Substitute, Open Approach

041H0KK Bypass Right External Iliac Artery to Bilateral Femoral Arteries with Nonautologous Tissue Substitute, Open Approach

041H0KP Bypass Right External Iliac Artery to Foot Artery with Nonautologous Tissue Substitute, Open Approach

041H0KQ Bypass Right External Iliac Artery to Lower Extremity Artery with Nonautologous Tissue Substitute, Open Approach

041H0Z9 Bypass Right External Iliac Artery to Right Internal Iliac Artery, Open Approach

041H0ZB Bypass Right External Iliac Artery to Left Internal Iliac Artery, Open Approach

041H0ZC Bypass Right External Iliac Artery to Bilateral Internal Iliac Arteries, Open Approach

041H0ZD Bypass Right External Iliac Artery to Right External Iliac Artery, Open Approach

041H0ZF Bypass Right External Iliac Artery to Left External Iliac Artery, Open Approach

041H0ZG Bypass Right External Iliac Artery to Bilateral External Iliac Arteries, Open Approach

041H0ZH Bypass Right External Iliac Artery to Right Femoral Artery, Open Approach

041H0ZJ Bypass Right External Iliac Artery to Left Femoral Artery, Open Approach

041H0ZK Bypass Right External Iliac Artery to Bilateral Femoral Arteries, Open Approach

041H0ZP Bypass Right External Iliac Artery to Foot Artery, Open Approach

041H0ZQ Bypass Right External Iliac Artery to Lower Extremity Artery, Open Approach

041H499 Bypass Right External Iliac Artery to Right Internal Iliac Artery with Autologous Venous Tissue, Percutaneous Endoscopic Approach

041H49B Bypass Right External Iliac Artery to Left Internal Iliac Artery with Autologous Venous Tissue, Percutaneous Endoscopic Approach

041H49C Bypass Right External Iliac Artery to Bilateral Internal Iliac Arteries with Autologous Venous Tissue, Percutaneous Endoscopic Approach

041H49D Bypass Right External Iliac Artery to Right External Iliac Artery with Autologous Venous Tissue, Percutaneous Endoscopic Approach

041H49F Bypass Right External Iliac Artery to Left External Iliac Artery with Autologous Venous Tissue, Percutaneous Endoscopic Approach

041H49G Bypass Right External Iliac Artery to Bilateral External Iliac Arteries with Autologous Venous Tissue, Percutaneous Endoscopic Approach

041H49H Bypass Right External Iliac Artery to Right Femoral Artery with Autologous Venous Tissue, Percutaneous Endoscopic Approach

041H49J Bypass Right External Iliac Artery to Left Femoral Artery with Autologous Venous Tissue, Percutaneous Endoscopic Approach

041H49K Bypass Right External Iliac Artery to Bilateral Femoral Arteries with Autologous Venous Tissue, Percutaneous Endoscopic Approach

041H49P Bypass Right External Iliac Artery to Foot Artery with Autologous Venous Tissue, Percutaneous Endoscopic Approach

041H49Q Bypass Right External Iliac Artery to Lower Extremity Artery with Autologous Venous Tissue, Percutaneous Endoscopic Approach

041H4A9 Bypass Right External Iliac Artery to Right Internal Iliac Artery with Autologous Arterial Tissue, Percutaneous Endoscopic Approach

041H4AB Bypass Right External Iliac Artery to Left Internal Iliac Artery with Autologous Arterial Tissue, Percutaneous Endoscopic Approach

041H4AC Bypass Right External Iliac Artery to Bilateral Internal Iliac Arteries with Autologous Arterial Tissue, Percutaneous Endoscopic Approach

♀ Female-only　　♂ Male-only　　▲ Limited Coverage　　● Non-OR　　▓ HAC-associated procedure　　▲ Non-covered procedures　　✚ Combinatio

1H4AD Bypass Right External Iliac Artery to Right External Iliac Artery with Autologous Arterial Tissue, Percutaneous Endoscopic Approach

1H4AF Bypass Right External Iliac Artery to Left External Iliac Artery with Autologous Arterial Tissue, Percutaneous Endoscopic Approach

1H4AG Bypass Right External Iliac Artery to Bilateral External Iliac Arteries with Autologous Arterial Tissue, Percutaneous Endoscopic Approach

1H4AH Bypass Right External Iliac Artery to Right Femoral Artery with Autologous Arterial Tissue, Percutaneous Endoscopic Approach

1H4AJ Bypass Right External Iliac Artery to Left Femoral Artery with Autologous Arterial Tissue, Percutaneous Endoscopic Approach

1H4AK Bypass Right External Iliac Artery to Bilateral Femoral Arteries with Autologous Arterial Tissue, Percutaneous Endoscopic Approach

1H4AP Bypass Right External Iliac Artery to Foot Artery with Autologous Arterial Tissue, Percutaneous Endoscopic Approach

1H4AQ Bypass Right External Iliac Artery to Lower Extremity Artery with Autologous Arterial Tissue, Percutaneous Endoscopic Approach

1H4J9 Bypass Right External Iliac Artery to Right Internal Iliac Artery with Synthetic Substitute, Percutaneous Endoscopic Approach

1H4JB Bypass Right External Iliac Artery to Left Internal Iliac Artery with Synthetic Substitute, Percutaneous Endoscopic Approach

1H4JC Bypass Right External Iliac Artery to Bilateral Internal Iliac Arteries with Synthetic Substitute, Percutaneous Endoscopic Approach

1H4JD Bypass Right External Iliac Artery to Right External Iliac Artery with Synthetic Substitute, Percutaneous Endoscopic Approach

1H4JF Bypass Right External Iliac Artery to Left External Iliac Artery with Synthetic Substitute, Percutaneous Endoscopic Approach

1H4JG Bypass Right External Iliac Artery to Bilateral External Iliac Arteries with Synthetic Substitute, Percutaneous Endoscopic Approach

1H4JH Bypass Right External Iliac Artery to Right Femoral Artery with Synthetic Substitute, Percutaneous Endoscopic Approach

1H4JJ Bypass Right External Iliac Artery to Left Femoral Artery with Synthetic Substitute, Percutaneous Endoscopic Approach

1H4JK Bypass Right External Iliac Artery to Bilateral Femoral Arteries with Synthetic Substitute, Percutaneous Endoscopic Approach

1H4JP Bypass Right External Iliac Artery to Foot Artery with Synthetic Substitute, Percutaneous Endoscopic Approach

1H4JQ Bypass Right External Iliac Artery to Lower Extremity Artery with Synthetic Substitute, Percutaneous Endoscopic Approach

1H4K9 Bypass Right External Iliac Artery to Right Internal Iliac Artery with

Nonautologous Tissue Substitute, Percutaneous Endoscopic Approach

041H4KB Bypass Right External Iliac Artery to Left Internal Iliac Artery with Nonautologous Tissue Substitute, Percutaneous Endoscopic Approach

041H4KC Bypass Right External Iliac Artery to Bilateral Internal Iliac Arteries with Nonautologous Tissue Substitute, Percutaneous Endoscopic Approach

041H4KD Bypass Right External Iliac Artery to Right External Iliac Artery with Nonautologous Tissue Substitute, Percutaneous Endoscopic Approach

041H4KF Bypass Right External Iliac Artery to Left External Iliac Artery with Nonautologous Tissue Substitute, Percutaneous Endoscopic Approach

041H4KG Bypass Right External Iliac Artery to Bilateral External Iliac Arteries with Nonautologous Tissue Substitute, Percutaneous Endoscopic Approach

041H4KH Bypass Right External Iliac Artery to Right Femoral Artery with Nonautologous Tissue Substitute, Percutaneous Endoscopic Approach

041H4KJ Bypass Right External Iliac Artery to Left Femoral Artery with Nonautologous Tissue Substitute, Percutaneous Endoscopic Approach

041H4KK Bypass Right External Iliac Artery to Bilateral Femoral Arteries with Nonautologous Tissue Substitute, Percutaneous Endoscopic Approach

041H4KP Bypass Right External Iliac Artery to Foot Artery with Nonautologous Tissue Substitute, Percutaneous Endoscopic Approach

041H4KQ Bypass Right External Iliac Artery to Lower Extremity Artery with Nonautologous Tissue Substitute, Percutaneous Endoscopic Approach

041H4Z9 Bypass Right External Iliac Artery to Right Internal Iliac Artery, Percutaneous Endoscopic Approach

041H4ZB Bypass Right External Iliac Artery to Left Internal Iliac Artery, Percutaneous Endoscopic Approach

041H4ZC Bypass Right External Iliac Artery to Bilateral Internal Iliac Arteries, Percutaneous Endoscopic Approach

041H4ZD Bypass Right External Iliac Artery to Right External Iliac Artery, Percutaneous Endoscopic Approach

041H4ZF Bypass Right External Iliac Artery to Left External Iliac Artery, Percutaneous Endoscopic Approach

041H4ZG Bypass Right External Iliac Artery to Bilateral External Iliac Arteries, Percutaneous Endoscopic Approach

041H4ZH Bypass Right External Iliac Artery to Right Femoral Artery, Percutaneous Endoscopic Approach

041H4ZJ Bypass Right External Iliac Artery to Left Femoral Artery, Percutaneous Endoscopic Approach

041H4ZK Bypass Right External Iliac Artery to Bilateral Femoral Arteries, Percutaneous Endoscopic Approach

041H4ZP Bypass Right External Iliac Artery to Foot Artery, Percutaneous Endoscopic Approach

041H4ZQ Bypass Right External Iliac Artery to Lower Extremity Artery, Percutaneous Endoscopic Approach

041J099 Bypass Left External Iliac Artery to Right Internal Iliac Artery with

Autologous Venous Tissue, Open Approach

041J09B Bypass Left External Iliac Artery to Left Internal Iliac Artery with Autologous Venous Tissue, Open Approach

041J09C Bypass Left External Iliac Artery to Bilateral Internal Iliac Arteries with Autologous Venous Tissue, Open Approach

041J09D Bypass Left External Iliac Artery to Right External Iliac Artery with Autologous Venous Tissue, Open Approach

041J09F Bypass Left External Iliac Artery to Left External Iliac Artery with Autologous Venous Tissue, Open Approach

041J09G Bypass Left External Iliac Artery to Bilateral External Iliac Arteries with Autologous Venous Tissue, Open Approach

041J09H Bypass Left External Iliac Artery to Right Femoral Artery with Autologous Venous Tissue, Open Approach

041J09J Bypass Left External Iliac Artery to Left Femoral Artery with Autologous Venous Tissue, Open Approach

041J09K Bypass Left External Iliac Artery to Bilateral Femoral Arteries with Autologous Venous Tissue, Open Approach

041J09P Bypass Left External Iliac Artery to Foot Artery with Autologous Venous Tissue, Open Approach

041J09Q Bypass Left External Iliac Artery to Lower Extremity Artery with Autologous Venous Tissue, Open Approach

041J0A9 Bypass Left External Iliac Artery to Right Internal Iliac Artery with Autologous Arterial Tissue, Open Approach

041J0AB Bypass Left External Iliac Artery to Left Internal Iliac Artery with Autologous Arterial Tissue, Open Approach

041J0AC Bypass Left External Iliac Artery to Bilateral Internal Iliac Arteries with Autologous Arterial Tissue, Open Approach

041J0AD Bypass Left External Iliac Artery to Right External Iliac Artery with Autologous Arterial Tissue, Open Approach

041J0AF Bypass Left External Iliac Artery to Left External Iliac Artery with Autologous Arterial Tissue, Open Approach

041J0AG Bypass Left External Iliac Artery to Bilateral External Iliac Arteries with Autologous Arterial Tissue, Open Approach

041J0AH Bypass Left External Iliac Artery to Right Femoral Artery with Autologous Arterial Tissue, Open Approach

041J0AJ Bypass Left External Iliac Artery to Left Femoral Artery with Autologous Arterial Tissue, Open Approach

041J0AK Bypass Left External Iliac Artery to Bilateral Femoral Arteries with Autologous Arterial Tissue, Open Approach

041J0AP Bypass Left External Iliac Artery to Foot Artery with Autologous Arterial Tissue, Open Approach

041J0AQ Bypass Left External Iliac Artery to Lower Extremity Artery with Autologous Arterial Tissue, Open Approach

041J0J9 Bypass Left External Iliac Artery to Right Internal Iliac Artery with Synthetic Substitute, Open Approach

041J0JB Bypass Left External Iliac Artery to Left Internal Iliac Artery with Synthetic Substitute, Open Approach

Female-only   ♂ Male-only   ▲ Limited Coverage   ● Non-OR   ▬ HAC-associated procedure   ▲ Non-covered procedures   ✚ Combination

041J0JC Bypass Left External Iliac Artery to Bilateral Internal Iliac Arteries with Synthetic Substitute, Open Approach

041J0JD Bypass Left External Iliac Artery to Right External Iliac Artery with Synthetic Substitute, Open Approach

041J0JF Bypass Left External Iliac Artery to Left External Iliac Artery with Synthetic Substitute, Open Approach

041J0JG Bypass Left External Iliac Artery to Bilateral External Iliac Arteries with Synthetic Substitute, Open Approach

041J0JH Bypass Left External Iliac Artery to Right Femoral Artery with Synthetic Substitute, Open Approach

041J0JJ Bypass Left External Iliac Artery to Left Femoral Artery with Synthetic Substitute, Open Approach

041J0JK Bypass Left External Iliac Artery to Bilateral Femoral Arteries with Synthetic Substitute, Open Approach

041J0JP Bypass Left External Iliac Artery to Foot Artery with Synthetic Substitute, Open Approach

041J0JQ Bypass Left External Iliac Artery to Lower Extremity Artery with Synthetic Substitute, Open Approach

041J0K9 Bypass Left External Iliac Artery to Right Internal Iliac Artery with Nonautologous Tissue Substitute, Open Approach

041J0KB Bypass Left External Iliac Artery to Left Internal Iliac Artery with Nonautologous Tissue Substitute, Open Approach

041J0KC Bypass Left External Iliac Artery to Bilateral Internal Iliac Arteries with Nonautologous Tissue Substitute, Open Approach

041J0KD Bypass Left External Iliac Artery to Right External Iliac Artery with Nonautologous Tissue Substitute, Open Approach

041J0KF Bypass Left External Iliac Artery to Left External Iliac Artery with Nonautologous Tissue Substitute, Open Approach

041J0KG Bypass Left External Iliac Artery to Bilateral External Iliac Arteries with Nonautologous Tissue Substitute, Open Approach

041J0KH Bypass Left External Iliac Artery to Right Femoral Artery with Nonautologous Tissue Substitute, Open Approach

041J0KJ Bypass Left External Iliac Artery to Left Femoral Artery with Nonautologous Tissue Substitute, Open Approach

041J0KK Bypass Left External Iliac Artery to Bilateral Femoral Arteries with Nonautologous Tissue Substitute, Open Approach

041J0KP Bypass Left External Iliac Artery to Foot Artery with Nonautologous Tissue Substitute, Open Approach

041J0KQ Bypass Left External Iliac Artery to Lower Extremity Artery with Nonautologous Tissue Substitute, Open Approach

041J0Z9 Bypass Left External Iliac Artery to Right Internal Iliac Artery, Open Approach

041J0ZB Bypass Left External Iliac Artery to Left Internal Iliac Artery, Open Approach

041J0ZC Bypass Left External Iliac Artery to Bilateral Internal Iliac Arteries, Open Approach

041J0ZD Bypass Left External Iliac Artery to Right External Iliac Artery, Open Approach

041J0ZF Bypass Left External Iliac Artery to Left External Iliac Artery, Open Approach

041J0ZG Bypass Left External Iliac Artery to Bilateral External Iliac Arteries, Open Approach

041J0ZH Bypass Left External Iliac Artery to Right Femoral Artery, Open Approach

041J0ZJ Bypass Left External Iliac Artery to Left Femoral Artery, Open Approach

041J0ZK Bypass Left External Iliac Artery to Bilateral Femoral Arteries, Open Approach

041J0ZP Bypass Left External Iliac Artery to Foot Artery, Open Approach

041J0ZQ Bypass Left External Iliac Artery to Lower Extremity Artery, Open Approach

041J499 Bypass Left External Iliac Artery to Right Internal Iliac Artery with Autologous Venous Tissue, Percutaneous Endoscopic Approach

041J49B Bypass Left External Iliac Artery to Left Internal Iliac Artery with Autologous Venous Tissue, Percutaneous Endoscopic Approach

041J49C Bypass Left External Iliac Artery to Bilateral Internal Iliac Arteries with Autologous Venous Tissue, Percutaneous Endoscopic Approach

041J49D Bypass Left External Iliac Artery to Right External Iliac Artery with Autologous Venous Tissue, Percutaneous Endoscopic Approach

041J49F Bypass Left External Iliac Artery to Left External Iliac Artery with Autologous Venous Tissue, Percutaneous Endoscopic Approach

041J49G Bypass Left External Iliac Artery to Bilateral External Iliac Arteries with Autologous Venous Tissue, Percutaneous Endoscopic Approach

041J49H Bypass Left External Iliac Artery to Right Femoral Artery with Autologous Venous Tissue, Percutaneous Endoscopic Approach

041J49J Bypass Left External Iliac Artery to Left Femoral Artery with Autologous Venous Tissue, Percutaneous Endoscopic Approach

041J49K Bypass Left External Iliac Artery to Bilateral Femoral Arteries with Autologous Venous Tissue, Percutaneous Endoscopic Approach

041J49P Bypass Left External Iliac Artery to Foot Artery with Autologous Venous Tissue, Percutaneous Endoscopic Approach

041J49Q Bypass Left External Iliac Artery to Lower Extremity Artery with Autologous Venous Tissue, Percutaneous Endoscopic Approach

041J4A9 Bypass Left External Iliac Artery to Right Internal Iliac Artery with Autologous Arterial Tissue, Percutaneous Endoscopic Approach

041J4AB Bypass Left External Iliac Artery to Left Internal Iliac Artery with Autologous Arterial Tissue, Percutaneous Endoscopic Approach

041J4AC Bypass Left External Iliac Artery to Bilateral Internal Iliac Arteries with Autologous Arterial Tissue, Percutaneous Endoscopic Approach

041J4AD Bypass Left External Iliac Artery to Right External Iliac Artery with Autologous Arterial Tissue, Percutaneous Endoscopic Approach

041J4AF Bypass Left External Iliac Artery to Left External Iliac Artery with Autologous Arterial Tissue, Percutaneous Endoscopic Approach

041J4AG Bypass Left External Iliac Artery to Bilateral External Iliac Arteries with Autologous Arterial Tissue, Percutaneous Endoscopic Approach

041J4AH Bypass Left External Iliac Artery to Right Femoral Artery with Autologous Arterial Tissue, Percutaneous Endoscopic Approach

041J4AJ Bypass Left External Iliac Artery to Left Femoral Artery with Autologous Arterial Tissue, Percutaneous Endoscopic Approach

041J4AK Bypass Left External Iliac Artery to Bilateral Femoral Arteries with Autologous Arterial Tissue, Percutaneous Endoscopic Approach

041J4AP Bypass Left External Iliac Artery to Foot Artery with Autologous Arterial Tissue, Percutaneous Endoscopic Approach

041J4AQ Bypass Left External Iliac Artery to Lower Extremity Artery with Autologous Arterial Tissue, Percutaneous Endoscopic Approach

041J4J9 Bypass Left External Iliac Artery to Right Internal Iliac Artery with Synthetic Substitute, Percutaneous Endoscopic Approach

041J4JB Bypass Left External Iliac Artery to Left Internal Iliac Artery with Synthetic Substitute, Percutaneous Endoscopic Approach

041J4JC Bypass Left External Iliac Artery to Bilateral Internal Iliac Arteries with Synthetic Substitute, Percutaneous Endoscopic Approach

041J4JD Bypass Left External Iliac Artery to Right External Iliac Artery with Synthetic Substitute, Percutaneous Endoscopic Approach

041J4JF Bypass Left External Iliac Artery to Left External Iliac Artery with Synthetic Substitute, Percutaneous Endoscopic Approach

041J4JG Bypass Left External Iliac Artery to Bilateral External Iliac Arteries with Synthetic Substitute, Percutaneous Endoscopic Approach

041J4JH Bypass Left External Iliac Artery to Right Femoral Artery with Synthetic Substitute, Percutaneous Endoscopic Approach

041J4JJ Bypass Left External Iliac Artery to Left Femoral Artery with Synthetic Substitute, Percutaneous Endoscopic Approach

041J4JK Bypass Left External Iliac Artery to Bilateral Femoral Arteries with Synthetic Substitute, Percutaneous Endoscopic Approach

041J4JP Bypass Left External Iliac Artery to Foot Artery with Synthetic Substitute, Percutaneous Endoscopic Approach

041J4JQ Bypass Left External Iliac Artery to Lower Extremity Artery with Synthetic Substitute, Percutaneous Endoscopic Approach

041J4K9 Bypass Left External Iliac Artery to Right Internal Iliac Artery with Nonautologous Tissue Substitute, Percutaneous Endoscopic Approach

041J4KB Bypass Left External Iliac Artery to Left Internal Iliac Artery with Nonautologous Tissue Substitute, Percutaneous Endoscopic Approach

041J4KC Bypass Left External Iliac Artery to Bilateral Internal Iliac Arteries with Nonautologous Tissue Substitute, Percutaneous Endoscopic Approach

041J4KD Bypass Left External Iliac Artery to Right External Iliac Artery with Nonautologous Tissue Substitute, Percutaneous Endoscopic Approach

041J4KF Bypass Left External Iliac Artery to Left External Iliac Artery with Nonautologous Tissue Substitute, Percutaneous Endoscopic Approach

041J4KG Bypass Left External Iliac Artery to Bilateral External Iliac Arteries with Nonautologous Tissue Substitute, Percutaneous Endoscopic Approach

041J4KH Bypass Left External Iliac Artery to Right Femoral Artery with Nonautologous Tissue Substitute, Percutaneous Endoscopic Approach

041J4KJ Bypass Left External Iliac Artery to Left Femoral Artery with Nonautologous Tissue Substitute, Percutaneous Endoscopic Approach

041J4KK Bypass Left External Iliac Artery to Bilateral Femoral Arteries with Nonautologous Tissue Substitute, Percutaneous Endoscopic Approach

041J4KP Bypass Left External Iliac Artery to Foot Artery with Nonautologous Tissue Substitute, Percutaneous Endoscopic Approach

041J4KQ Bypass Left External Iliac Artery to Lower Extremity Artery with Nonautologous Tissue Substitute, Percutaneous Endoscopic Approach

041J4Z9 Bypass Left External Iliac Artery to Right Internal Iliac Artery, Percutaneous Endoscopic Approach

041J4ZB Bypass Left External Iliac Artery to Left Internal Iliac Artery, Percutaneous Endoscopic Approach

041J4ZC Bypass Left External Iliac Artery to Bilateral Internal Iliac Arteries, Percutaneous Endoscopic Approach

041J4ZD Bypass Left External Iliac Artery to Right External Iliac Artery, Percutaneous Endoscopic Approach

041J4ZF Bypass Left External Iliac Artery to Left External Iliac Artery, Percutaneous Endoscopic Approach

041J4ZG Bypass Left External Iliac Artery to Bilateral External Iliac Arteries, Percutaneous Endoscopic Approach

041J4ZH Bypass Left External Iliac Artery to Right Femoral Artery, Percutaneous Endoscopic Approach

041J4ZJ Bypass Left External Iliac Artery to Left Femoral Artery, Percutaneous Endoscopic Approach

041J4ZK Bypass Left External Iliac Artery to Bilateral Femoral Arteries, Percutaneous Endoscopic Approach

041J4ZP Bypass Left External Iliac Artery to Foot Artery, Percutaneous Endoscopic Approach

041J4ZQ Bypass Left External Iliac Artery to Lower Extremity Artery, Percutaneous Endoscopic Approach

041K09H Bypass Right Femoral Artery to Right Femoral Artery with Autologous Venous Tissue, Open Approach

041K09J Bypass Right Femoral Artery to Left Femoral Artery with Autologous Venous Tissue, Open Approach

041K09K Bypass Right Femoral Artery to Bilateral Femoral Arteries with Autologous Venous Tissue, Open Approach

041K09L Bypass Right Femoral Artery to Popliteal Artery with Autologous Venous Tissue, Open Approach

041K09M Bypass Right Femoral Artery to Peroneal Artery with Autologous Venous Tissue, Open Approach

041K09N Bypass Right Femoral Artery to Posterior Tibial Artery with Autologous Venous Tissue, Open Approach

041K09P Bypass Right Femoral Artery to Foot Artery with Autologous Venous Tissue, Open Approach

041K09Q Bypass Right Femoral Artery to Lower Extremity Artery with Autologous Venous Tissue, Open Approach

041K09S Bypass Right Femoral Artery to Lower Extremity Vein with Autologous Venous Tissue, Open Approach

041K0AH Bypass Right Femoral Artery to Right Femoral Artery with Autologous Arterial Tissue, Open Approach

041K0AJ Bypass Right Femoral Artery to Left Femoral Artery with Autologous Arterial Tissue, Open Approach

041K0AK Bypass Right Femoral Artery to Bilateral Femoral Arteries with Autologous Arterial Tissue, Open Approach

041K0AL Bypass Right Femoral Artery to Popliteal Artery with Autologous Arterial Tissue, Open Approach

041K0AM Bypass Right Femoral Artery to Peroneal Artery with Autologous Arterial Tissue, Open Approach

041K0AN Bypass Right Femoral Artery to Posterior Tibial Artery with Autologous Arterial Tissue, Open Approach

041K0AP Bypass Right Femoral Artery to Foot Artery with Autologous Arterial Tissue, Open Approach

041K0AQ Bypass Right Femoral Artery to Lower Extremity Artery with Autologous Arterial Tissue, Open Approach

041K0AS Bypass Right Femoral Artery to Lower Extremity Vein with Autologous Arterial Tissue, Open Approach

041K0JH Bypass Right Femoral Artery to Right Femoral Artery with Synthetic Substitute, Open Approach

041K0JJ Bypass Right Femoral Artery to Left Femoral Artery with Synthetic Substitute, Open Approach

041K0JK Bypass Right Femoral Artery to Bilateral Femoral Arteries with Synthetic Substitute, Open Approach

041K0JL Bypass Right Femoral Artery to Popliteal Artery with Synthetic Substitute, Open Approach

041K0JM Bypass Right Femoral Artery to Peroneal Artery with Synthetic Substitute, Open Approach

041K0JN Bypass Right Femoral Artery to Posterior Tibial Artery with Synthetic Substitute, Open Approach

041K0JP Bypass Right Femoral Artery to Foot Artery with Synthetic Substitute, Open Approach

041K0JQ Bypass Right Femoral Artery to Lower Extremity Artery with Synthetic Substitute, Open Approach

041K0JS Bypass Right Femoral Artery to Lower Extremity Vein with Synthetic Substitute, Open Approach

041K0KH Bypass Right Femoral Artery to Right Femoral Artery with Nonautologous Tissue Substitute, Open Approach

041K0KJ Bypass Right Femoral Artery to Left Femoral Artery with Nonautologous Tissue Substitute, Open Approach

041K0KK Bypass Right Femoral Artery to Bilateral Femoral Arteries with Nonautologous Tissue Substitute, Open Approach

041K0KL Bypass Right Femoral Artery to Popliteal Artery with Nonautologous Tissue Substitute, Open Approach

041K0KM Bypass Right Femoral Artery to Peroneal Artery with Nonautologous Tissue Substitute, Open Approach

041K0KN Bypass Right Femoral Artery to Posterior Tibial Artery with Nonautologous Tissue Substitute, Open Approach

041K0KP Bypass Right Femoral Artery to Foot Artery with Nonautologous Tissue Substitute, Open Approach

041K0KQ Bypass Right Femoral Artery to Lower Extremity Artery with Nonautologous Tissue Substitute, Open Approach

041K0KS Bypass Right Femoral Artery to Lower Extremity Vein with Nonautologous Tissue Substitute, Open Approach

041K0ZH Bypass Right Femoral Artery to Right Femoral Artery, Open Approach

041K0ZJ Bypass Right Femoral Artery to Left Femoral Artery, Open Approach

041K0ZK Bypass Right Femoral Artery to Bilateral Femoral Arteries, Open Approach

041K0ZL Bypass Right Femoral Artery to Popliteal Artery, Open Approach

041K0ZM Bypass Right Femoral Artery to Peroneal Artery, Open Approach

041K0ZN Bypass Right Femoral Artery to Posterior Tibial Artery, Open Approach

041K0ZP Bypass Right Femoral Artery to Foot Artery, Open Approach

041K0ZQ Bypass Right Femoral Artery to Lower Extremity Artery, Open Approach

041K0ZS Bypass Right Femoral Artery to Lower Extremity Vein, Open Approach

041K49H Bypass Right Femoral Artery to Right Femoral Artery with Autologous Venous Tissue, Percutaneous Endoscopic Approach

041K49J Bypass Right Femoral Artery to Left Femoral Artery with Autologous Venous Tissue, Percutaneous Endoscopic Approach

041K49K Bypass Right Femoral Artery to Bilateral Femoral Arteries with Autologous Venous Tissue, Percutaneous Endoscopic Approach

041K49L Bypass Right Femoral Artery to Popliteal Artery with Autologous Venous Tissue, Percutaneous Endoscopic Approach

041K49M Bypass Right Femoral Artery to Peroneal Artery with Autologous Venous Tissue, Percutaneous Endoscopic Approach

041K49N Bypass Right Femoral Artery to Posterior Tibial Artery with Autologous Venous Tissue, Percutaneous Endoscopic Approach

041K49P Bypass Right Femoral Artery to Foot Artery with Autologous Venous Tissue, Percutaneous Endoscopic Approach

041K49Q Bypass Right Femoral Artery to Lower Extremity Artery with Autologous Venous Tissue, Percutaneous Endoscopic Approach

041K49S Bypass Right Femoral Artery to Lower Extremity Vein with Autologous Venous Tissue, Percutaneous Endoscopic Approach

041K4AH Bypass Right Femoral Artery to Right Femoral Artery with Autologous Arterial Tissue, Percutaneous Endoscopic Approach

041K4AJ Bypass Right Femoral Artery to Left Femoral Artery with Autologous Arterial Tissue, Percutaneous Endoscopic Approach

041K4AK Bypass Right Femoral Artery to Bilateral Femoral Arteries with Autologous Arterial Tissue, Percutaneous Endoscopic Approach

Female-only   ♂ Male-only   ▲ Limited Coverage   ● Non-OR   ■ HAC-associated procedure   ▲ Non-covered procedures   ✚ Combination

041K4AL Bypass Right Femoral Artery to Popliteal Artery with Autologous Arterial Tissue, Percutaneous Endoscopic Approach

041K4AM Bypass Right Femoral Artery to Peroneal Artery with Autologous Arterial Tissue, Percutaneous Endoscopic Approach

041K4AN Bypass Right Femoral Artery to Posterior Tibial Artery with Autologous Arterial Tissue, Percutaneous Endoscopic Approach

041K4AP Bypass Right Femoral Artery to Foot Artery with Autologous Arterial Tissue, Percutaneous Endoscopic Approach

041K4AQ Bypass Right Femoral Artery to Lower Extremity Artery with Autologous Arterial Tissue, Percutaneous Endoscopic Approach

041K4AS Bypass Right Femoral Artery to Lower Extremity Vein with Autologous Arterial Tissue, Percutaneous Endoscopic Approach

041K4JH Bypass Right Femoral Artery to Right Femoral Artery with Synthetic Substitute, Percutaneous Endoscopic Approach

041K4JJ Bypass Right Femoral Artery to Left Femoral Artery with Synthetic Substitute, Percutaneous Endoscopic Approach

041K4JK Bypass Right Femoral Artery to Bilateral Femoral Arteries with Synthetic Substitute, Percutaneous Endoscopic Approach

041K4JL Bypass Right Femoral Artery to Popliteal Artery with Synthetic Substitute, Percutaneous Endoscopic Approach

041K4JM Bypass Right Femoral Artery to Peroneal Artery with Synthetic Substitute, Percutaneous Endoscopic Approach

041K4JN Bypass Right Femoral Artery to Posterior Tibial Artery with Synthetic Substitute, Percutaneous Endoscopic Approach

041K4JP Bypass Right Femoral Artery to Foot Artery with Synthetic Substitute, Percutaneous Endoscopic Approach

041K4JQ Bypass Right Femoral Artery to Lower Extremity Artery with Synthetic Substitute, Percutaneous Endoscopic Approach

041K4JS Bypass Right Femoral Artery to Lower Extremity Vein with Synthetic Substitute, Percutaneous Endoscopic Approach

041K4KH Bypass Right Femoral Artery to Right Femoral Artery with Nonautologous Tissue Substitute, Percutaneous Endoscopic Approach

041K4KJ Bypass Right Femoral Artery to Left Femoral Artery with Nonautologous Tissue Substitute, Percutaneous Endoscopic Approach

041K4KK Bypass Right Femoral Artery to Bilateral Femoral Arteries with Nonautologous Tissue Substitute, Percutaneous Endoscopic Approach

041K4KL Bypass Right Femoral Artery to Popliteal Artery with Nonautologous Tissue Substitute, Percutaneous Endoscopic Approach

041K4KM Bypass Right Femoral Artery to Peroneal Artery with Nonautologous Tissue Substitute, Percutaneous Endoscopic Approach

041K4KN Bypass Right Femoral Artery to Posterior Tibial Artery with Nonautologous Tissue Substitute, Percutaneous Endoscopic Approach

041K4KP Bypass Right Femoral Artery to Foot Artery with Nonautologous Tissue Substitute, Percutaneous Endoscopic Approach

041K4KQ Bypass Right Femoral Artery to Lower Extremity Artery with Nonautologous Tissue Substitute, Percutaneous Endoscopic Approach

041K4KS Bypass Right Femoral Artery to Lower Extremity Vein with Nonautologous Tissue Substitute, Percutaneous Endoscopic Approach

041K4ZH Bypass Right Femoral Artery to Right Femoral Artery, Percutaneous Endoscopic Approach

041K4ZJ Bypass Right Femoral Artery to Left Femoral Artery, Percutaneous Endoscopic Approach

041K4ZK Bypass Right Femoral Artery to Bilateral Femoral Arteries, Percutaneous Endoscopic Approach

041K4ZL Bypass Right Femoral Artery to Popliteal Artery, Percutaneous Endoscopic Approach

041K4ZM Bypass Right Femoral Artery to Peroneal Artery, Percutaneous Endoscopic Approach

041K4ZN Bypass Right Femoral Artery to Posterior Tibial Artery, Percutaneous Endoscopic Approach

041K4ZP Bypass Right Femoral Artery to Foot Artery, Percutaneous Endoscopic Approach

041K4ZQ Bypass Right Femoral Artery to Lower Extremity Artery, Percutaneous Endoscopic Approach

041K4ZS Bypass Right Femoral Artery to Lower Extremity Vein, Percutaneous Endoscopic Approach

041L09H Bypass Left Femoral Artery to Right Femoral Artery with Autologous Venous Tissue, Open Approach

041L09J Bypass Left Femoral Artery to Left Femoral Artery with Autologous Venous Tissue, Open Approach

041L09K Bypass Left Femoral Artery to Bilateral Femoral Arteries with Autologous Venous Tissue, Open Approach

041L09L Bypass Left Femoral Artery to Popliteal Artery with Autologous Venous Tissue, Open Approach

041L09M Bypass Left Femoral Artery to Peroneal Artery with Autologous Venous Tissue, Open Approach

041L09N Bypass Left Femoral Artery to Posterior Tibial Artery with Autologous Venous Tissue, Open Approach

041L09P Bypass Left Femoral Artery to Foot Artery with Autologous Venous Tissue, Open Approach

041L09Q Bypass Left Femoral Artery to Lower Extremity Artery with Autologous Venous Tissue, Open Approach

041L09S Bypass Left Femoral Artery to Lower Extremity Vein with Autologous Venous Tissue, Open Approach

041L0AH Bypass Left Femoral Artery to Right Femoral Artery with Autologous Arterial Tissue, Open Approach

041L0AJ Bypass Left Femoral Artery to Left Femoral Artery with Autologous Arterial Tissue, Open Approach

041L0AK Bypass Left Femoral Artery to Bilateral Femoral Arteries with Autologous Arterial Tissue, Open Approach

041L0AL Bypass Left Femoral Artery to Popliteal Artery with Autologous Arterial Tissue, Open Approach

041L0AM Bypass Left Femoral Artery to Peroneal Artery with Autologous Arterial Tissue, Open Approach

041L0AN Bypass Left Femoral Artery to Posterior Tibial Artery with Autologous Arterial Tissue, Open Approach

041L0AP Bypass Left Femoral Artery to Foot Artery with Autologous Arterial Tissue, Open Approach

041L0AQ Bypass Left Femoral Artery to Lower Extremity Artery with Autologous Arterial Tissue, Open Approach

041L0AS Bypass Left Femoral Artery to Lower Extremity Vein with Autologous Arterial Tissue, Open Approach

041L0JH Bypass Left Femoral Artery to Right Femoral Artery with Synthetic Substitute, Open Approach

041L0JJ Bypass Left Femoral Artery to Left Femoral Artery with Synthetic Substitute, Open Approach

041L0JK Bypass Left Femoral Artery to Bilateral Femoral Arteries with Synthetic Substitute, Open Approach

041L0JL Bypass Left Femoral Artery to Popliteal Artery with Synthetic Substitute, Open Approach

041L0JM Bypass Left Femoral Artery to Peroneal Artery with Synthetic Substitute, Open Approach

041L0JN Bypass Left Femoral Artery to Posterior Tibial Artery with Synthetic Substitute, Open Approach

041L0JP Bypass Left Femoral Artery to Foot Artery with Synthetic Substitute, Open Approach

041L0JQ Bypass Left Femoral Artery to Lower Extremity Artery with Synthetic Substitute, Open Approach

041L0JS Bypass Left Femoral Artery to Lower Extremity Vein with Synthetic Substitute, Open Approach

041L0KH Bypass Left Femoral Artery to Right Femoral Artery with Nonautologous Tissue Substitute, Open Approach

041L0KJ Bypass Left Femoral Artery to Left Femoral Artery with Nonautologous Tissue Substitute, Open Approach

041L0KK Bypass Left Femoral Artery to Bilateral Femoral Arteries with Nonautologous Tissue Substitute, Open Approach

041L0KL Bypass Left Femoral Artery to Popliteal Artery with Nonautologous Tissue Substitute, Open Approach

041L0KM Bypass Left Femoral Artery to Peroneal Artery with Nonautologous Tissue Substitute, Open Approach

041L0KN Bypass Left Femoral Artery to Posterior Tibial Artery with Nonautologous Tissue Substitute, Open Approach

041L0KP Bypass Left Femoral Artery to Foot Artery with Nonautologous Tissue Substitute, Open Approach

041L0KQ Bypass Left Femoral Artery to Lower Extremity Artery with Nonautologous Tissue Substitute, Open Approach

041L0KS Bypass Left Femoral Artery to Lower Extremity Vein with Nonautologous Tissue Substitute, Open Approach

041L0ZH Bypass Left Femoral Artery to Right Femoral Artery, Open Approach

041L0ZJ Bypass Left Femoral Artery to Left Femoral Artery, Open Approach

041L0ZK Bypass Left Femoral Artery to Bilateral Femoral Arteries, Open Approach

041L0ZL Bypass Left Femoral Artery to Popliteal Artery, Open Approach

041L0ZM Bypass Left Femoral Artery to Peroneal Artery, Open Approach

041L0ZN Bypass Left Femoral Artery to Posterior Tibial Artery, Open Approach

041L0ZP Bypass Left Femoral Artery to Foot Artery, Open Approach

041L0ZQ Bypass Left Femoral Artery to Lower Extremity Artery, Open Approach

041L0ZS Bypass Left Femoral Artery to Lower Extremity Vein, Open Approach

041L49H Bypass Left Femoral Artery to Right Femoral Artery with Autologous Venous Tissue, Percutaneous Endoscopic Approach

041L49J Bypass Left Femoral Artery to Left Femoral Artery with Autologous Venous Tissue, Percutaneous Endoscopic Approach

041L49K Bypass Left Femoral Artery to Bilateral Femoral Arteries with Autologous Venous Tissue, Percutaneous Endoscopic Approach

041L49L Bypass Left Femoral Artery to Popliteal Artery with Autologous Venous Tissue, Percutaneous Endoscopic Approach

041L49M Bypass Left Femoral Artery to Peroneal Artery with Autologous Venous Tissue, Percutaneous Endoscopic Approach

041L49N Bypass Left Femoral Artery to Posterior Tibial Artery with Autologous Venous Tissue, Percutaneous Endoscopic Approach

041L49P Bypass Left Femoral Artery to Foot Artery with Autologous Venous Tissue, Percutaneous Endoscopic Approach

041L49Q Bypass Left Femoral Artery to Lower Extremity Artery with Autologous Venous Tissue, Percutaneous Endoscopic Approach

041L49S Bypass Left Femoral Artery to Lower Extremity Vein with Autologous Venous Tissue, Percutaneous Endoscopic Approach

041L4AH Bypass Left Femoral Artery to Right Femoral Artery with Autologous Arterial Tissue, Percutaneous Endoscopic Approach

041L4AJ Bypass Left Femoral Artery to Left Femoral Artery with Autologous Arterial Tissue, Percutaneous Endoscopic Approach

041L4AK Bypass Left Femoral Artery to Bilateral Femoral Arteries with Autologous Arterial Tissue, Percutaneous Endoscopic Approach

041L4AL Bypass Left Femoral Artery to Popliteal Artery with Autologous Arterial Tissue, Percutaneous Endoscopic Approach

041L4AM Bypass Left Femoral Artery to Peroneal Artery with Autologous Arterial Tissue, Percutaneous Endoscopic Approach

041L4AN Bypass Left Femoral Artery to Posterior Tibial Artery with Autologous Arterial Tissue, Percutaneous Endoscopic Approach

041L4AP Bypass Left Femoral Artery to Foot Artery with Autologous Arterial Tissue, Percutaneous Endoscopic Approach

041L4AQ Bypass Left Femoral Artery to Lower Extremity Artery with Autologous Arterial Tissue, Percutaneous Endoscopic Approach

041L4AS Bypass Left Femoral Artery to Lower Extremity Vein with Autologous Arterial Tissue, Percutaneous Endoscopic Approach

041L4JH Bypass Left Femoral Artery to Right Femoral Artery with Synthetic Substitute, Percutaneous Endoscopic Approach

041L4JJ Bypass Left Femoral Artery to Left Femoral Artery with Synthetic Substitute, Percutaneous Endoscopic Approach

041L4JK Bypass Left Femoral Artery to Bilateral Femoral Arteries with Synthetic Substitute, Percutaneous Endoscopic Approach

041L4JL Bypass Left Femoral Artery to Popliteal Artery with Synthetic Substitute, Percutaneous Endoscopic Approach

041L4JM Bypass Left Femoral Artery to Peroneal Artery with Synthetic Substitute, Percutaneous Endoscopic Approach

041L4JN Bypass Left Femoral Artery to Posterior Tibial Artery with Synthetic Substitute, Percutaneous Endoscopic Approach

041L4JP Bypass Left Femoral Artery to Foot Artery with Synthetic Substitute, Percutaneous Endoscopic Approach

041L4JQ Bypass Left Femoral Artery to Lower Extremity Artery with Synthetic Substitute, Percutaneous Endoscopic Approach

041L4JS Bypass Left Femoral Artery to Lower Extremity Vein with Synthetic Substitute, Percutaneous Endoscopic Approach

041L4KH Bypass Left Femoral Artery to Right Femoral Artery with Nonautologous Tissue Substitute, Percutaneous Endoscopic Approach

041L4KJ Bypass Left Femoral Artery to Left Femoral Artery with Nonautologous Tissue Substitute, Percutaneous Endoscopic Approach

041L4KK Bypass Left Femoral Artery to Bilateral Femoral Arteries with Nonautologous Tissue Substitute, Percutaneous Endoscopic Approach

041L4KL Bypass Left Femoral Artery to Popliteal Artery with Nonautologous Tissue Substitute, Percutaneous Endoscopic Approach

041L4KM Bypass Left Femoral Artery to Peroneal Artery with Nonautologous Tissue Substitute, Percutaneous Endoscopic Approach

041L4KN Bypass Left Femoral Artery to Posterior Tibial Artery with Nonautologous Tissue Substitute, Percutaneous Endoscopic Approach

041L4KP Bypass Left Femoral Artery to Foot Artery with Nonautologous Tissue Substitute, Percutaneous Endoscopic Approach

041L4KQ Bypass Left Femoral Artery to Lower Extremity Artery with Nonautologous Tissue Substitute, Percutaneous Endoscopic Approach

041L4KS Bypass Left Femoral Artery to Lower Extremity Vein with Nonautologous Tissue Substitute, Percutaneous Endoscopic Approach

041L4ZH Bypass Left Femoral Artery to Right Femoral Artery, Percutaneous Endoscopic Approach

041L4ZJ Bypass Left Femoral Artery to Left Femoral Artery, Percutaneous Endoscopic Approach

041L4ZK Bypass Left Femoral Artery to Bilateral Femoral Arteries, Percutaneous Endoscopic Approach

041L4ZL Bypass Left Femoral Artery to Popliteal Artery, Percutaneous Endoscopic Approach

041L4ZM Bypass Left Femoral Artery to Peroneal Artery, Percutaneous Endoscopic Approach

041L4ZN Bypass Left Femoral Artery to Posterior Tibial Artery, Percutaneous Endoscopic Approach

041L4ZP Bypass Left Femoral Artery to Foot Artery, Percutaneous Endoscopic Approach

041L4ZQ Bypass Left Femoral Artery to Lower Extremity Artery, Percutaneous Endoscopic Approach

041L4ZS Bypass Left Femoral Artery to Lower Extremity Vein, Percutaneous Endoscopic Approach

041M09L Bypass Right Popliteal Artery to Popliteal Artery with Autologous Venous Tissue, Open Approach

041M09M Bypass Right Popliteal Artery to Peroneal Artery with Autologous Venous Tissue, Open Approach

041M09P Bypass Right Popliteal Artery to Foot Artery with Autologous Venous Tissue, Open Approach

041M09Q Bypass Right Popliteal Artery to Lower Extremity Artery with Autologous Venous Tissue, Open Approach

041M09S Bypass Right Popliteal Artery to Lower Extremity Vein with Autologous Venous Tissue, Open Approach

041M0AL Bypass Right Popliteal Artery to Popliteal Artery with Autologous Arterial Tissue, Open Approach

041M0AM Bypass Right Popliteal Artery to Peroneal Artery with Autologous Arterial Tissue, Open Approach

041M0AP Bypass Right Popliteal Artery to Foot Artery with Autologous Arterial Tissue, Open Approach

041M0AQ Bypass Right Popliteal Artery to Lower Extremity Artery with Autologous Arterial Tissue, Open Approach

041M0AS Bypass Right Popliteal Artery to Lower Extremity Vein with Autologous Arterial Tissue, Open Approach

041M0JL Bypass Right Popliteal Artery to Popliteal Artery with Synthetic Substitute, Open Approach

041M0JM Bypass Right Popliteal Artery to Peroneal Artery with Synthetic Substitute, Open Approach

041M0JP Bypass Right Popliteal Artery to Foot Artery with Synthetic Substitute, Open Approach

041M0JQ Bypass Right Popliteal Artery to Lower Extremity Artery with Synthetic Substitute, Open Approach

041M0JS Bypass Right Popliteal Artery to Lower Extremity Vein with Synthetic Substitute, Open Approach

041M0KL Bypass Right Popliteal Artery to Popliteal Artery with Nonautologous Tissue Substitute, Open Approach

041M0KM Bypass Right Popliteal Artery to Peroneal Artery with Nonautologous Tissue Substitute, Open Approach

041M0KP Bypass Right Popliteal Artery to Foot Artery with Nonautologous Tissue Substitute, Open Approach

♀ Female-only   ♂ Male-only   ▲ Limited Coverage   ● Non-OR   ▦ HAC-associated procedure   ▲ Non-covered procedures   ➕ Combination

041M0KQ	Bypass Right Popliteal Artery to Lower Extremity Artery with Nonautologous Tissue Substitute, Open Approach
041M0KS	Bypass Right Popliteal Artery to Lower Extremity Vein with Nonautologous Tissue Substitute, Open Approach
041M0ZL	Bypass Right Popliteal Artery to Popliteal Artery, Open Approach
041M0ZM	Bypass Right Popliteal Artery to Peroneal Artery, Open Approach
041M0ZP	Bypass Right Popliteal Artery to Foot Artery, Open Approach
041M0ZQ	Bypass Right Popliteal Artery to Lower Extremity Artery, Open Approach
041M0ZS	Bypass Right Popliteal Artery to Lower Extremity Vein, Open Approach
041M49L	Bypass Right Popliteal Artery to Popliteal Artery with Autologous Venous Tissue, Percutaneous Endoscopic Approach
041M49M	Bypass Right Popliteal Artery to Peroneal Artery with Autologous Venous Tissue, Percutaneous Endoscopic Approach
041M49P	Bypass Right Popliteal Artery to Foot Artery with Autologous Venous Tissue, Percutaneous Endoscopic Approach
041M49Q	Bypass Right Popliteal Artery to Lower Extremity Artery with Autologous Venous Tissue, Percutaneous Endoscopic Approach
041M49S	Bypass Right Popliteal Artery to Lower Extremity Vein with Autologous Venous Tissue, Percutaneous Endoscopic Approach
041M4AL	Bypass Right Popliteal Artery to Popliteal Artery with Autologous Arterial Tissue, Percutaneous Endoscopic Approach
041M4AM	Bypass Right Popliteal Artery to Peroneal Artery with Autologous Arterial Tissue, Percutaneous Endoscopic Approach
041M4AP	Bypass Right Popliteal Artery to Foot Artery with Autologous Arterial Tissue, Percutaneous Endoscopic Approach
041M4AQ	Bypass Right Popliteal Artery to Lower Extremity Artery with Autologous Arterial Tissue, Percutaneous Endoscopic Approach
041M4AS	Bypass Right Popliteal Artery to Lower Extremity Vein with Autologous Arterial Tissue, Percutaneous Endoscopic Approach
041M4JL	Bypass Right Popliteal Artery to Popliteal Artery with Synthetic Substitute, Percutaneous Endoscopic Approach
041M4JM	Bypass Right Popliteal Artery to Peroneal Artery with Synthetic Substitute, Percutaneous Endoscopic Approach
041M4JP	Bypass Right Popliteal Artery to Foot Artery with Synthetic Substitute, Percutaneous Endoscopic Approach
041M4JQ	Bypass Right Popliteal Artery to Lower Extremity Artery with Synthetic Substitute, Percutaneous Endoscopic Approach
041M4JS	Bypass Right Popliteal Artery to Lower Extremity Vein with Synthetic Substitute, Percutaneous Endoscopic Approach
041M4KL	Bypass Right Popliteal Artery to Popliteal Artery with Nonautologous Tissue Substitute, Percutaneous Endoscopic Approach
041M4KM	Bypass Right Popliteal Artery to Peroneal Artery with Nonautologous Tissue Substitute, Percutaneous Endoscopic Approach
041M4KP	Bypass Right Popliteal Artery to Foot Artery with Nonautologous Tissue Substitute, Percutaneous Endoscopic Approach
041M4KQ	Bypass Right Popliteal Artery to Lower Extremity Artery with Nonautologous Tissue Substitute, Percutaneous Endoscopic Approach
041M4KS	Bypass Right Popliteal Artery to Lower Extremity Vein with Nonautologous Tissue Substitute, Percutaneous Endoscopic Approach
041M4ZL	Bypass Right Popliteal Artery to Popliteal Artery, Percutaneous Endoscopic Approach
041M4ZM	Bypass Right Popliteal Artery to Peroneal Artery, Percutaneous Endoscopic Approach
041M4ZP	Bypass Right Popliteal Artery to Foot Artery, Percutaneous Endoscopic Approach
041M4ZQ	Bypass Right Popliteal Artery to Lower Extremity Artery, Percutaneous Endoscopic Approach
041M4ZS	Bypass Right Popliteal Artery to Lower Extremity Vein, Percutaneous Endoscopic Approach
041N09L	Bypass Left Popliteal Artery to Popliteal Artery with Autologous Venous Tissue, Open Approach
041N09M	Bypass Left Popliteal Artery to Peroneal Artery with Autologous Venous Tissue, Open Approach
041N09P	Bypass Left Popliteal Artery to Foot Artery with Autologous Venous Tissue, Open Approach
041N09Q	Bypass Left Popliteal Artery to Lower Extremity Artery with Autologous Venous Tissue, Open Approach
041N09S	Bypass Left Popliteal Artery to Lower Extremity Vein with Autologous Venous Tissue, Open Approach
041N0AL	Bypass Left Popliteal Artery to Popliteal Artery with Autologous Arterial Tissue, Open Approach
041N0AM	Bypass Left Popliteal Artery to Peroneal Artery with Autologous Arterial Tissue, Open Approach
041N0AP	Bypass Left Popliteal Artery to Foot Artery with Autologous Arterial Tissue, Open Approach
041N0AQ	Bypass Left Popliteal Artery to Lower Extremity Artery with Autologous Arterial Tissue, Open Approach
041N0AS	Bypass Left Popliteal Artery to Lower Extremity Vein with Autologous Arterial Tissue, Open Approach
041N0JL	Bypass Left Popliteal Artery to Popliteal Artery with Synthetic Substitute, Open Approach
041N0JM	Bypass Left Popliteal Artery to Peroneal Artery with Synthetic Substitute, Open Approach
041N0JP	Bypass Left Popliteal Artery to Foot Artery with Synthetic Substitute, Open Approach
041N0JQ	Bypass Left Popliteal Artery to Lower Extremity Artery with Synthetic Substitute, Open Approach
041N0JS	Bypass Left Popliteal Artery to Lower Extremity Vein with Synthetic Substitute, Open Approach
041N0KL	Bypass Left Popliteal Artery to Popliteal Artery with Nonautologous Tissue Substitute, Open Approach
041N0KM	Bypass Left Popliteal Artery to Peroneal Artery with Nonautologous Tissue Substitute, Open Approach
041N0KP	Bypass Left Popliteal Artery to Foot Artery with Nonautologous Tissue Substitute, Open Approach
041N0KQ	Bypass Left Popliteal Artery to Lower Extremity Artery with Nonautologous Tissue Substitute, Open Approach
041N0KS	Bypass Left Popliteal Artery to Lower Extremity Vein with Nonautologous Tissue Substitute, Open Approach
041N0ZL	Bypass Left Popliteal Artery to Popliteal Artery, Open Approach
041N0ZM	Bypass Left Popliteal Artery to Peroneal Artery, Open Approach
041N0ZP	Bypass Left Popliteal Artery to Foot Artery, Open Approach
041N0ZQ	Bypass Left Popliteal Artery to Lower Extremity Artery, Open Approach
041N0ZS	Bypass Left Popliteal Artery to Lower Extremity Vein, Open Approach
041N49L	Bypass Left Popliteal Artery to Popliteal Artery with Autologous Venous Tissue, Percutaneous Endoscopic Approach
041N49M	Bypass Left Popliteal Artery to Peroneal Artery with Autologous Venous Tissue, Percutaneous Endoscopic Approach
041N49P	Bypass Left Popliteal Artery to Foot Artery with Autologous Venous Tissue, Percutaneous Endoscopic Approach
041N49Q	Bypass Left Popliteal Artery to Lower Extremity Artery with Autologous Venous Tissue, Percutaneous Endoscopic Approach
041N49S	Bypass Left Popliteal Artery to Lower Extremity Vein with Autologous Venous Tissue, Percutaneous Endoscopic Approach
041N4AL	Bypass Left Popliteal Artery to Popliteal Artery with Autologous Arterial Tissue, Percutaneous Endoscopic Approach
041N4AM	Bypass Left Popliteal Artery to Peroneal Artery with Autologous Arterial Tissue, Percutaneous Endoscopic Approach
041N4AP	Bypass Left Popliteal Artery to Foot Artery with Autologous Arterial Tissue, Percutaneous Endoscopic Approach
041N4AQ	Bypass Left Popliteal Artery to Lower Extremity Artery with Autologous Arterial Tissue, Percutaneous Endoscopic Approach
041N4AS	Bypass Left Popliteal Artery to Lower Extremity Vein with Autologous Arterial Tissue, Percutaneous Endoscopic Approach
041N4JL	Bypass Left Popliteal Artery to Popliteal Artery with Synthetic Substitute, Percutaneous Endoscopic Approach
041N4JM	Bypass Left Popliteal Artery to Peroneal Artery with Synthetic Substitute, Percutaneous Endoscopic Approach
041N4JP	Bypass Left Popliteal Artery to Foot Artery with Synthetic Substitute, Percutaneous Endoscopic Approach
041N4JQ	Bypass Left Popliteal Artery to Lower Extremity Artery with Synthetic Substitute, Percutaneous Endoscopic Approach
041N4JS	Bypass Left Popliteal Artery to Lower Extremity Vein with Synthetic Substitute, Percutaneous Endoscopic Approach
041N4KL	Bypass Left Popliteal Artery to Popliteal Artery with Nonautologous Tissue Substitute, Percutaneous Endoscopic Approach
041N4KM	Bypass Left Popliteal Artery to Peroneal Artery with Nonautologous Tissue Substitute, Percutaneous Endoscopic Approach

Code	Description	Code	Description	Code	Description
N4KP	Bypass Left Popliteal Artery to Foot Artery with Nonautologous Tissue Substitute, Percutaneous Endoscopic Approach		Nonautologous Tissue Substitute, Percutaneous Endoscopic Approach	041N4ZP	Bypass Left Popliteal Artery to Foot Artery, Percutaneous Endoscopic Approach
N4KQ	Bypass Left Popliteal Artery to Lower Extremity Artery with Nonautologous Tissue Substitute, Percutaneous Endoscopic Approach	041N4ZL	Bypass Left Popliteal Artery to Popliteal Artery, Percutaneous Endoscopic Approach	041N4ZQ	Bypass Left Popliteal Artery to Lower Extremity Artery, Percutaneous Endoscopic Approach
N4KS	Bypass Left Popliteal Artery to Lower Extremity Vein with	041N4ZM	Bypass Left Popliteal Artery to Peroneal Artery, Percutaneous Endoscopic Approach	041N4ZS	Bypass Left Popliteal Artery to Lower Extremity Vein, Percutaneous Endoscopic Approach

5 – Lower Arteries, Destruction

Code	Description	Code	Description	Code	Description
600ZZ	Destruction of Abdominal Aorta, Open Approach	045A3ZZ	Destruction of Left Renal Artery, Percutaneous Approach	045M4ZZ	Destruction of Right Popliteal Artery, Percutaneous Endoscopic Approach
603ZZ	Destruction of Abdominal Aorta, Percutaneous Approach	045A4ZZ	Destruction of Left Renal Artery, Percutaneous Endoscopic Approach	045N0ZZ	Destruction of Left Popliteal Artery, Open Approach
604ZZ	Destruction of Abdominal Aorta, Percutaneous Endoscopic Approach	045B0ZZ	Destruction of Inferior Mesenteric Artery, Open Approach	045N3ZZ	Destruction of Left Popliteal Artery, Percutaneous Approach
610ZZ	Destruction of Celiac Artery, Open Approach	045B3ZZ	Destruction of Inferior Mesenteric Artery, Percutaneous Approach	045N4ZZ	Destruction of Left Popliteal Artery, Percutaneous Endoscopic Approach
613ZZ	Destruction of Celiac Artery, Percutaneous Approach	045B4ZZ	Destruction of Inferior Mesenteric Artery, Percutaneous Endoscopic Approach	045P0ZZ	Destruction of Right Anterior Tibial Artery, Open Approach
614ZZ	Destruction of Celiac Artery, Percutaneous Endoscopic Approach	045C0ZZ	Destruction of Right Common Iliac Artery, Open Approach	045P3ZZ	Destruction of Right Anterior Tibial Artery, Percutaneous Approach
620ZZ	Destruction of Gastric Artery, Open Approach	045C3ZZ	Destruction of Right Common Iliac Artery, Percutaneous Approach	045P4ZZ	Destruction of Right Anterior Tibial Artery, Percutaneous Endoscopic Approach
623ZZ	Destruction of Gastric Artery, Percutaneous Approach	045C4ZZ	Destruction of Right Common Iliac Artery, Percutaneous Endoscopic Approach	045Q0ZZ	Destruction of Left Anterior Tibial Artery, Open Approach
624ZZ	Destruction of Gastric Artery, Percutaneous Endoscopic Approach	045D0ZZ	Destruction of Left Common Iliac Artery, Open Approach	045Q3ZZ	Destruction of Left Anterior Tibial Artery, Percutaneous Approach
630ZZ	Destruction of Hepatic Artery, Open Approach	045D3ZZ	Destruction of Left Common Iliac Artery, Percutaneous Approach	045Q4ZZ	Destruction of Left Anterior Tibial Artery, Percutaneous Endoscopic Approach
633ZZ	Destruction of Hepatic Artery, Percutaneous Approach	045D4ZZ	Destruction of Left Common Iliac Artery, Percutaneous Endoscopic Approach	045R0ZZ	Destruction of Right Posterior Tibial Artery, Open Approach
634ZZ	Destruction of Hepatic Artery, Percutaneous Endoscopic Approach	045E0ZZ	Destruction of Right Internal Iliac Artery, Open Approach	045R3ZZ	Destruction of Right Posterior Tibial Artery, Percutaneous Approach
640ZZ	Destruction of Splenic Artery, Open Approach	045E3ZZ	Destruction of Right Internal Iliac Artery, Percutaneous Approach	045R4ZZ	Destruction of Right Posterior Tibial Artery, Percutaneous Endoscopic Approach
643ZZ	Destruction of Splenic Artery, Percutaneous Approach	045E4ZZ	Destruction of Right Internal Iliac Artery, Percutaneous Endoscopic Approach	045S0ZZ	Destruction of Left Posterior Tibial Artery, Open Approach
644ZZ	Destruction of Splenic Artery, Percutaneous Endoscopic Approach	045F0ZZ	Destruction of Left Internal Iliac Artery, Open Approach	045S3ZZ	Destruction of Left Posterior Tibial Artery, Percutaneous Approach
650ZZ	Destruction of Superior Mesenteric Artery, Open Approach	045F3ZZ	Destruction of Left Internal Iliac Artery, Percutaneous Approach	045S4ZZ	Destruction of Left Posterior Tibial Artery, Percutaneous Endoscopic Approach
653ZZ	Destruction of Superior Mesenteric Artery, Percutaneous Approach	045F4ZZ	Destruction of Left Internal Iliac Artery, Percutaneous Endoscopic Approach	045T0ZZ	Destruction of Right Peroneal Artery, Open Approach
654ZZ	Destruction of Superior Mesenteric Artery, Percutaneous Endoscopic Approach	045H0ZZ	Destruction of Right External Iliac Artery, Open Approach	045T3ZZ	Destruction of Right Peroneal Artery, Percutaneous Approach
660ZZ	Destruction of Right Colic Artery, Open Approach	045H3ZZ	Destruction of Right External Iliac Artery, Percutaneous Approach	045T4ZZ	Destruction of Right Peroneal Artery, Percutaneous Endoscopic Approach
663ZZ	Destruction of Right Colic Artery, Percutaneous Approach	045H4ZZ	Destruction of Right External Iliac Artery, Percutaneous Endoscopic Approach	045U0ZZ	Destruction of Left Peroneal Artery, Open Approach
664ZZ	Destruction of Right Colic Artery, Percutaneous Endoscopic Approach	045J0ZZ	Destruction of Left External Iliac Artery, Open Approach	045U3ZZ	Destruction of Left Peroneal Artery, Percutaneous Approach
670ZZ	Destruction of Left Colic Artery, Open Approach	045J3ZZ	Destruction of Left External Iliac Artery, Percutaneous Approach	045U4ZZ	Destruction of Left Peroneal Artery, Percutaneous Endoscopic Approach
673ZZ	Destruction of Left Colic Artery, Percutaneous Approach	045J4ZZ	Destruction of Left External Iliac Artery, Percutaneous Endoscopic Approach	045V0ZZ	Destruction of Right Foot Artery, Open Approach
674ZZ	Destruction of Left Colic Artery, Percutaneous Endoscopic Approach	045K0ZZ	Destruction of Right Femoral Artery, Open Approach	045V3ZZ	Destruction of Right Foot Artery, Percutaneous Approach
680ZZ	Destruction of Middle Colic Artery, Open Approach	045K3ZZ	Destruction of Right Femoral Artery, Percutaneous Approach	045V4ZZ	Destruction of Right Foot Artery, Percutaneous Endoscopic Approach
683ZZ	Destruction of Middle Colic Artery, Percutaneous Approach	045K4ZZ	Destruction of Right Femoral Artery, Percutaneous Endoscopic Approach	045W0ZZ	Destruction of Left Foot Artery, Open Approach
684ZZ	Destruction of Middle Colic Artery, Percutaneous Endoscopic Approach	045L0ZZ	Destruction of Left Femoral Artery, Open Approach	045W3ZZ	Destruction of Left Foot Artery, Percutaneous Approach
690ZZ	Destruction of Right Renal Artery, Open Approach	045L3ZZ	Destruction of Left Femoral Artery, Percutaneous Approach	045W4ZZ	Destruction of Left Foot Artery, Percutaneous Endoscopic Approach
693ZZ	Destruction of Right Renal Artery, Percutaneous Approach	045L4ZZ	Destruction of Left Femoral Artery, Percutaneous Endoscopic Approach	045Y0ZZ	Destruction of Lower Artery, Open Approach
694ZZ	Destruction of Right Renal Artery, Percutaneous Endoscopic Approach	045M0ZZ	Destruction of Right Popliteal Artery, Open Approach	045Y3ZZ	Destruction of Lower Artery, Percutaneous Approach
5A0ZZ	Destruction of Left Renal Artery, Open Approach	045M3ZZ	Destruction of Right Popliteal Artery, Percutaneous Approach	045Y4ZZ	Destruction of Lower Artery, Percutaneous Endoscopic Approach

Female-only   ♂ Male-only   ▲ Limited Coverage   ● Non-OR   ■ HAC-associated procedure   ▲ Non-covered procedures   + Combination

047 – Lower Arteries, Dilation

047004Z   Dilation of Abdominal Aorta with Drug-eluting Intraluminal Device, Open Approach

04700DZ   Dilation of Abdominal Aorta with Intraluminal Device, Open Approach

04700ZZ   Dilation of Abdominal Aorta, Open Approach

047034Z   Dilation of Abdominal Aorta with Drug-eluting Intraluminal Device, Percutaneous Approach

04703DZ   Dilation of Abdominal Aorta with Intraluminal Device, Percutaneous Approach

04703ZZ   Dilation of Abdominal Aorta, Percutaneous Approach

047044Z   Dilation of Abdominal Aorta with Drug-eluting Intraluminal Device, Percutaneous Endoscopic Approach

04704DZ   Dilation of Abdominal Aorta with Intraluminal Device, Percutaneous Endoscopic Approach

04704ZZ   Dilation of Abdominal Aorta, Percutaneous Endoscopic Approach

047104Z   Dilation of Celiac Artery with Drug-eluting Intraluminal Device, Open Approach

04710DZ   Dilation of Celiac Artery with Intraluminal Device, Open Approach

04710ZZ   Dilation of Celiac Artery, Open Approach

047134Z   Dilation of Celiac Artery with Drug-eluting Intraluminal Device, Percutaneous Approach

04713DZ   Dilation of Celiac Artery with Intraluminal Device, Percutaneous Approach

04713ZZ   Dilation of Celiac Artery, Percutaneous Approach

047144Z   Dilation of Celiac Artery with Drug-eluting Intraluminal Device, Percutaneous Endoscopic Approach

04714DZ   Dilation of Celiac Artery with Intraluminal Device, Percutaneous Endoscopic Approach

04714ZZ   Dilation of Celiac Artery, Percutaneous Endoscopic Approach

047204Z   Dilation of Gastric Artery with Drug-eluting Intraluminal Device, Open Approach

04720DZ   Dilation of Gastric Artery with Intraluminal Device, Open Approach

04720ZZ   Dilation of Gastric Artery, Open Approach

047234Z   Dilation of Gastric Artery with Drug-eluting Intraluminal Device, Percutaneous Approach

04723DZ   Dilation of Gastric Artery with Intraluminal Device, Percutaneous Approach

04723ZZ   Dilation of Gastric Artery, Percutaneous Approach

047244Z   Dilation of Gastric Artery with Drug-eluting Intraluminal Device, Percutaneous Endoscopic Approach

04724DZ   Dilation of Gastric Artery with Intraluminal Device, Percutaneous Endoscopic Approach

04724ZZ   Dilation of Gastric Artery, Percutaneous Endoscopic Approach

047304Z   Dilation of Hepatic Artery with Drug-eluting Intraluminal Device, Open Approach

04730DZ   Dilation of Hepatic Artery with Intraluminal Device, Open Approach

04730ZZ   Dilation of Hepatic Artery, Open Approach

047334Z   Dilation of Hepatic Artery with Drug-eluting Intraluminal Device, Percutaneous Approach

04733DZ   Dilation of Hepatic Artery with Intraluminal Device, Percutaneous Approach

04733ZZ   Dilation of Hepatic Artery, Percutaneous Approach

047344Z   Dilation of Hepatic Artery with Drug-eluting Intraluminal Device, Percutaneous Endoscopic Approach

04734DZ   Dilation of Hepatic Artery with Intraluminal Device, Percutaneous Endoscopic Approach

04734ZZ   Dilation of Hepatic Artery, Percutaneous Endoscopic Approach

047404Z   Dilation of Splenic Artery with Drug-eluting Intraluminal Device, Open Approach

04740DZ   Dilation of Splenic Artery with Intraluminal Device, Open Approach

04740ZZ   Dilation of Splenic Artery, Open Approach

047434Z   Dilation of Splenic Artery with Drug-eluting Intraluminal Device, Percutaneous Approach

04743DZ   Dilation of Splenic Artery with Intraluminal Device, Percutaneous Approach

04743ZZ   Dilation of Splenic Artery, Percutaneous Approach

047444Z   Dilation of Splenic Artery with Drug-eluting Intraluminal Device, Percutaneous Endoscopic Approach

04744DZ   Dilation of Splenic Artery with Intraluminal Device, Percutaneous Endoscopic Approach

04744ZZ   Dilation of Splenic Artery, Percutaneous Endoscopic Approach

047504Z   Dilation of Superior Mesenteric Artery with Drug-eluting Intraluminal Device, Open Approach

04750DZ   Dilation of Superior Mesenteric Artery with Intraluminal Device, Open Approach

04750ZZ   Dilation of Superior Mesenteric Artery, Open Approach

047534Z   Dilation of Superior Mesenteric Artery with Drug-eluting Intraluminal Device, Percutaneous Approach

04753DZ   Dilation of Superior Mesenteric Artery with Intraluminal Device, Percutaneous Approach

04753ZZ   Dilation of Superior Mesenteric Artery, Percutaneous Approach

047544Z   Dilation of Superior Mesenteric Artery with Drug-eluting Intraluminal Device, Percutaneous Endoscopic Approach

04754DZ   Dilation of Superior Mesenteric Artery with Intraluminal Device, Percutaneous Endoscopic Approach

04754ZZ   Dilation of Superior Mesenteric Artery, Percutaneous Endoscopic Approach

047604Z   Dilation of Right Colic Artery with Drug-eluting Intraluminal Device, Open Approach

04760DZ   Dilation of Right Colic Artery with Intraluminal Device, Open Approach

04760ZZ   Dilation of Right Colic Artery, Open Approach

047634Z   Dilation of Right Colic Artery with Drug-eluting Intraluminal Device, Percutaneous Approach

04763DZ   Dilation of Right Colic Artery with Intraluminal Device, Percutaneous Approach

04763ZZ   Dilation of Right Colic Artery, Percutaneous Approach

047644Z   Dilation of Right Colic Artery with Drug-eluting Intraluminal Device, Percutaneous Endoscopic Approach

04764DZ   Dilation of Right Colic Artery with Intraluminal Device, Percutaneous Endoscopic Approach

04764ZZ   Dilation of Right Colic Artery, Percutaneous Endoscopic Approach

047704Z   Dilation of Left Colic Artery with Drug-eluting Intraluminal Device, Open Approach

04770DZ   Dilation of Left Colic Artery with Intraluminal Device, Open Approach

04770ZZ   Dilation of Left Colic Artery, Open Approach

047734Z   Dilation of Left Colic Artery with Drug-eluting Intraluminal Device, Percutaneous Approach

04773DZ   Dilation of Left Colic Artery with Intraluminal Device, Percutaneous Approach

04773ZZ   Dilation of Left Colic Artery, Percutaneous Approach

047744Z   Dilation of Left Colic Artery with Drug-eluting Intraluminal Device, Percutaneous Endoscopic Approach

04774DZ   Dilation of Left Colic Artery with Intraluminal Device, Percutaneous Endoscopic Approach

04774ZZ   Dilation of Left Colic Artery, Percutaneous Endoscopic Approach

047804Z   Dilation of Middle Colic Artery with Drug-eluting Intraluminal Device, Open Approach

04780DZ   Dilation of Middle Colic Artery with Intraluminal Device, Open Approach

04780ZZ   Dilation of Middle Colic Artery, Open Approach

047834Z   Dilation of Middle Colic Artery with Drug-eluting Intraluminal Device, Percutaneous Approach

04783DZ   Dilation of Middle Colic Artery with Intraluminal Device, Percutaneous Approach

04783ZZ   Dilation of Middle Colic Artery, Percutaneous Approach

047844Z   Dilation of Middle Colic Artery with Drug-eluting Intraluminal Device, Percutaneous Endoscopic Approach

04784DZ   Dilation of Middle Colic Artery with Intraluminal Device, Percutaneous Endoscopic Approach

04784ZZ   Dilation of Middle Colic Artery, Percutaneous Endoscopic Approach

047904Z   Dilation of Right Renal Artery with Drug-eluting Intraluminal Device, Open Approach

04790DZ   Dilation of Right Renal Artery with Intraluminal Device, Open Approach

04790ZZ   Dilation of Right Renal Artery, Open Approach

047934Z   Dilation of Right Renal Artery with Drug-eluting Intraluminal Device, Percutaneous Approach

04793DZ   Dilation of Right Renal Artery with Intraluminal Device, Percutaneous Approach

04793ZZ   Dilation of Right Renal Artery, Percutaneous Approach

047944Z   Dilation of Right Renal Artery with Drug-eluting Intraluminal Device, Percutaneous Endoscopic Approach

794DZ Dilation of Right Renal Artery with Intraluminal Device, Percutaneous Endoscopic Approach

794ZZ Dilation of Right Renal Artery, Percutaneous Endoscopic Approach

7A04Z Dilation of Left Renal Artery with Drug-eluting Intraluminal Device, Open Approach

7A0DZ Dilation of Left Renal Artery with Intraluminal Device, Open Approach

7A0ZZ Dilation of Left Renal Artery, Open Approach

7A34Z Dilation of Left Renal Artery with Drug-eluting Intraluminal Device, Percutaneous Approach

7A3DZ Dilation of Left Renal Artery with Intraluminal Device, Percutaneous Approach

7A3ZZ Dilation of Left Renal Artery, Percutaneous Approach

7A44Z Dilation of Left Renal Artery with Drug-eluting Intraluminal Device, Percutaneous Endoscopic Approach

7A4DZ Dilation of Left Renal Artery with Intraluminal Device, Percutaneous Endoscopic Approach

7A4ZZ Dilation of Left Renal Artery, Percutaneous Endoscopic Approach

7B04Z Dilation of Inferior Mesenteric Artery with Drug-eluting Intraluminal Device, Open Approach

7B0DZ Dilation of Inferior Mesenteric Artery with Intraluminal Device, Open Approach

7B0ZZ Dilation of Inferior Mesenteric Artery, Open Approach

7B34Z Dilation of Inferior Mesenteric Artery with Drug-eluting Intraluminal Device, Percutaneous Approach

7B3DZ Dilation of Inferior Mesenteric Artery with Intraluminal Device, Percutaneous Approach

7B3ZZ Dilation of Inferior Mesenteric Artery, Percutaneous Approach

7B44Z Dilation of Inferior Mesenteric Artery with Drug-eluting Intraluminal Device, Percutaneous Endoscopic Approach

7B4DZ Dilation of Inferior Mesenteric Artery with Intraluminal Device, Percutaneous Endoscopic Approach

7B4ZZ Dilation of Inferior Mesenteric Artery, Percutaneous Endoscopic Approach

47C04Z Dilation of Right Common Iliac Artery with Drug-eluting Intraluminal Device, Open Approach

47C0DZ Dilation of Right Common Iliac Artery with Intraluminal Device, Open Approach

47C0ZZ Dilation of Right Common Iliac Artery, Open Approach

47C34Z Dilation of Right Common Iliac Artery with Drug-eluting Intraluminal Device, Percutaneous Approach

47C3DZ Dilation of Right Common Iliac Artery with Intraluminal Device, Percutaneous Approach

47C3ZZ Dilation of Right Common Iliac Artery, Percutaneous Approach

47C44Z Dilation of Right Common Iliac Artery with Drug-eluting Intraluminal Device, Percutaneous Endoscopic Approach

47C4DZ Dilation of Right Common Iliac Artery with Intraluminal Device, Percutaneous Endoscopic Approach

47C4ZZ Dilation of Right Common Iliac Artery, Percutaneous Endoscopic Approach

047D04Z Dilation of Left Common Iliac Artery with Drug-eluting Intraluminal Device, Open Approach

047D0DZ Dilation of Left Common Iliac Artery with Intraluminal Device, Open Approach

047D0ZZ Dilation of Left Common Iliac Artery, Open Approach

047D34Z Dilation of Left Common Iliac Artery with Drug-eluting Intraluminal Device, Percutaneous Approach

047D3DZ Dilation of Left Common Iliac Artery with Intraluminal Device, Percutaneous Approach

047D3ZZ Dilation of Left Common Iliac Artery, Percutaneous Approach

047D44Z Dilation of Left Common Iliac Artery with Drug-eluting Intraluminal Device, Percutaneous Endoscopic Approach

047D4DZ Dilation of Left Common Iliac Artery with Intraluminal Device, Percutaneous Endoscopic Approach

047D4ZZ Dilation of Left Common Iliac Artery, Percutaneous Endoscopic Approach

047E04Z Dilation of Right Internal Iliac Artery with Drug-eluting Intraluminal Device, Open Approach

047E0DZ Dilation of Right Internal Iliac Artery with Intraluminal Device, Open Approach

047E0ZZ Dilation of Right Internal Iliac Artery, Open Approach

047E34Z Dilation of Right Internal Iliac Artery with Drug-eluting Intraluminal Device, Percutaneous Approach

047E3DZ Dilation of Right Internal Iliac Artery with Intraluminal Device, Percutaneous Approach

047E3ZZ Dilation of Right Internal Iliac Artery, Percutaneous Approach

047E44Z Dilation of Right Internal Iliac Artery with Drug-eluting Intraluminal Device, Percutaneous Endoscopic Approach

047E4DZ Dilation of Right Internal Iliac Artery with Intraluminal Device, Percutaneous Endoscopic Approach

047E4ZZ Dilation of Right Internal Iliac Artery, Percutaneous Endoscopic Approach

047F04Z Dilation of Left Internal Iliac Artery with Drug-eluting Intraluminal Device, Open Approach

047F0DZ Dilation of Left Internal Iliac Artery with Intraluminal Device, Open Approach

047F0ZZ Dilation of Left Internal Iliac Artery, Open Approach

047F34Z Dilation of Left Internal Iliac Artery with Drug-eluting Intraluminal Device, Percutaneous Approach

047F3DZ Dilation of Left Internal Iliac Artery with Intraluminal Device, Percutaneous Approach

047F3ZZ Dilation of Left Internal Iliac Artery, Percutaneous Approach

047F44Z Dilation of Left Internal Iliac Artery with Drug-eluting Intraluminal Device, Percutaneous Endoscopic Approach

047F4DZ Dilation of Left Internal Iliac Artery with Intraluminal Device, Percutaneous Endoscopic Approach

047F4ZZ Dilation of Left Internal Iliac Artery, Percutaneous Endoscopic Approach

047H04Z Dilation of Right External Iliac Artery with Drug-eluting Intraluminal Device, Open Approach

047H0DZ Dilation of Right External Iliac Artery with Intraluminal Device, Open Approach

047H0ZZ Dilation of Right External Iliac Artery, Open Approach

047H34Z Dilation of Right External Iliac Artery with Drug-eluting Intraluminal Device, Percutaneous Approach

047H3DZ Dilation of Right External Iliac Artery with Intraluminal Device, Percutaneous Approach

047H3ZZ Dilation of Right External Iliac Artery, Percutaneous Approach

047H44Z Dilation of Right External Iliac Artery with Drug-eluting Intraluminal Device, Percutaneous Endoscopic Approach

047H4DZ Dilation of Right External Iliac Artery with Intraluminal Device, Percutaneous Endoscopic Approach

047H4ZZ Dilation of Right External Iliac Artery, Percutaneous Endoscopic Approach

047J04Z Dilation of Left External Iliac Artery with Drug-eluting Intraluminal Device, Open Approach

047J0DZ Dilation of Left External Iliac Artery with Intraluminal Device, Open Approach

047J0ZZ Dilation of Left External Iliac Artery, Open Approach

047J34Z Dilation of Left External Iliac Artery with Drug-eluting Intraluminal Device, Percutaneous Approach

047J3DZ Dilation of Left External Iliac Artery with Intraluminal Device, Percutaneous Approach

047J3ZZ Dilation of Left External Iliac Artery, Percutaneous Approach

047J44Z Dilation of Left External Iliac Artery with Drug-eluting Intraluminal Device, Percutaneous Endoscopic Approach

047J4DZ Dilation of Left External Iliac Artery with Intraluminal Device, Percutaneous Endoscopic Approach

047J4ZZ Dilation of Left External Iliac Artery, Percutaneous Endoscopic Approach

047K041 Dilation of Right Femoral Artery with Drug-eluting Intraluminal Device, using Drug-Coated Balloon, Open Approach

047K04Z Dilation of Right Femoral Artery with Drug-eluting Intraluminal Device, Open Approach

047K0D1 Dilation of Right Femoral Artery with Intraluminal Device, using Drug-Coated Balloon, Open Approach

047K0DZ Dilation of Right Femoral Artery with Intraluminal Device, Open Approach

047K0Z1 Dilation of Right Femoral Artery using Drug-Coated Balloon, Open Approach

047K0ZZ Dilation of Right Femoral Artery, Open Approach

047K341 Dilation of Right Femoral Artery with Drug-eluting Intraluminal Device, using Drug-Coated Balloon, Percutaneous Approach

047K34Z Dilation of Right Femoral Artery with Drug-eluting Intraluminal Device, Percutaneous Approach

047K3D1 Dilation of Right Femoral Artery with Intraluminal Device, using Drug-Coated Balloon, Percutaneous Approach

047K3DZ Dilation of Right Femoral Artery with Intraluminal Device, Percutaneous Approach

047K3Z1 Dilation of Right Femoral Artery using Drug-Coated Balloon, Percutaneous Approach

047K3ZZ Dilation of Right Femoral Artery, Percutaneous Approach

047K441 Dilation of Right Femoral Artery with Drug-eluting Intraluminal Device, using Drug-Coated Balloon, Percutaneous Endoscopic Approach

Female-only   ♂ Male-only   ▲ Limited Coverage   ● Non-OR   ■ HAC-associated procedure   ▲ Non-covered procedures   ✚ Combination

047K44Z Dilation of Right Femoral Artery with Drug-eluting Intraluminal Device, Percutaneous Endoscopic Approach

047K4D1 Dilation of Right Femoral Artery with Intraluminal Device, using Drug-Coated Balloon, Percutaneous Endoscopic Approach

047K4DZ Dilation of Right Femoral Artery with Intraluminal Device, Percutaneous Endoscopic Approach

047K4Z1 Dilation of Right Femoral Artery using Drug-Coated Balloon, Percutaneous Endoscopic Approach

047K4ZZ Dilation of Right Femoral Artery, Percutaneous Endoscopic Approach

047L041 Dilation of Left Femoral Artery with Drug-eluting Intraluminal Device, using Drug-Coated Balloon, Open Approach

047L04Z Dilation of Left Femoral Artery with Drug-eluting Intraluminal Device, Open Approach

047L0D1 Dilation of Left Femoral Artery with Intraluminal Device, using Drug-Coated Balloon, Open Approach

047L0DZ Dilation of Left Femoral Artery with Intraluminal Device, Open Approach

047L0Z1 Dilation of Left Femoral Artery using Drug-Coated Balloon, Open Approach

047L0ZZ Dilation of Left Femoral Artery, Open Approach

047L341 Dilation of Left Femoral Artery with Drug-eluting Intraluminal Device, using Drug-Coated Balloon, Percutaneous Approach

047L34Z Dilation of Left Femoral Artery with Drug-eluting Intraluminal Device, Percutaneous Approach

047L3D1 Dilation of Left Femoral Artery with Intraluminal Device, using Drug-Coated Balloon, Percutaneous Approach

047L3DZ Dilation of Left Femoral Artery with Intraluminal Device, Percutaneous Approach

047L3Z1 Dilation of Left Femoral Artery using Drug-Coated Balloon, Percutaneous Approach

047L3ZZ Dilation of Left Femoral Artery, Percutaneous Approach

047L441 Dilation of Left Femoral Artery with Drug-eluting Intraluminal Device, using Drug-Coated Balloon, Percutaneous Endoscopic Approach

047L44Z Dilation of Left Femoral Artery with Drug-eluting Intraluminal Device, Percutaneous Endoscopic Approach

047L4D1 Dilation of Left Femoral Artery with Intraluminal Device, using Drug-Coated Balloon, Percutaneous Endoscopic Approach

047L4DZ Dilation of Left Femoral Artery with Intraluminal Device, Percutaneous Endoscopic Approach

047L4Z1 Dilation of Left Femoral Artery using Drug-Coated Balloon, Percutaneous Endoscopic Approach

047L4ZZ Dilation of Left Femoral Artery, Percutaneous Endoscopic Approach

047M041 Dilation of Right Popliteal Artery with Drug-eluting Intraluminal Device, using Drug-Coated Balloon, Open Approach

047M04Z Dilation of Right Popliteal Artery with Drug-eluting Intraluminal Device, Open Approach

047M0D1 Dilation of Right Popliteal Artery with Intraluminal Device, using Drug-Coated Balloon, Open Approach

047M0DZ Dilation of Right Popliteal Artery with Intraluminal Device, Open Approach

047M0Z1 Dilation of Right Popliteal Artery using Drug-Coated Balloon, Open Approach

047M0ZZ Dilation of Right Popliteal Artery, Open Approach

047M341 Dilation of Right Popliteal Artery with Drug-eluting Intraluminal Device, using Drug-Coated Balloon, Percutaneous Approach

047M34Z Dilation of Right Popliteal Artery with Drug-eluting Intraluminal Device, Percutaneous Approach

047M3D1 Dilation of Right Popliteal Artery with Intraluminal Device, using Drug-Coated Balloon, Percutaneous Approach

047M3DZ Dilation of Right Popliteal Artery with Intraluminal Device, Percutaneous Approach

047M3Z1 Dilation of Right Popliteal Artery using Drug-Coated Balloon, Percutaneous Approach

047M3ZZ Dilation of Right Popliteal Artery, Percutaneous Approach

047M441 Dilation of Right Popliteal Artery with Drug-eluting Intraluminal Device, using Drug-Coated Balloon, Percutaneous Endoscopic Approach

047M44Z Dilation of Right Popliteal Artery with Drug-eluting Intraluminal Device, Percutaneous Endoscopic Approach

047M4D1 Dilation of Right Popliteal Artery with Intraluminal Device, using Drug-Coated Balloon, Percutaneous Endoscopic Approach

047M4DZ Dilation of Right Popliteal Artery with Intraluminal Device, Percutaneous Endoscopic Approach

047M4Z1 Dilation of Right Popliteal Artery using Drug-Coated Balloon, Percutaneous Endoscopic Approach

047M4ZZ Dilation of Right Popliteal Artery, Percutaneous Endoscopic Approach

047N041 Dilation of Left Popliteal Artery with Drug-eluting Intraluminal Device, using Drug-Coated Balloon, Open Approach

047N04Z Dilation of Left Popliteal Artery with Drug-eluting Intraluminal Device, Open Approach

047N0D1 Dilation of Left Popliteal Artery with Intraluminal Device, using Drug-Coated Balloon, Open Approach

047N0DZ Dilation of Left Popliteal Artery with Intraluminal Device, Open Approach

047N0Z1 Dilation of Left Popliteal Artery using Drug-Coated Balloon, Open Approach

047N0ZZ Dilation of Left Popliteal Artery, Open Approach

047N341 Dilation of Left Popliteal Artery with Drug-eluting Intraluminal Device, using Drug-Coated Balloon, Percutaneous Approach

047N34Z Dilation of Left Popliteal Artery with Drug-eluting Intraluminal Device, Percutaneous Approach

047N3D1 Dilation of Left Popliteal Artery with Intraluminal Device, using Drug-Coated Balloon, Percutaneous Approach

047N3DZ Dilation of Left Popliteal Artery with Intraluminal Device, Percutaneous Approach

047N3Z1 Dilation of Left Popliteal Artery using Drug-Coated Balloon, Percutaneous Approach

047N3ZZ Dilation of Left Popliteal Artery, Percutaneous Approach

047N441 Dilation of Left Popliteal Artery with Drug-eluting Intraluminal Device, using Drug-Coated Balloon, Percutaneous Endoscopic Approach

047N44Z Dilation of Left Popliteal Artery with Drug-eluting Intraluminal Device, Percutaneous Endoscopic Approach

047N4D1 Dilation of Left Popliteal Artery with Intraluminal Device, using Drug-Coated Balloon, Percutaneous Endoscopic Approach

047N4DZ Dilation of Left Popliteal Artery with Intraluminal Device, Percutaneous Endoscopic Approach

047N4Z1 Dilation of Left Popliteal Artery using Drug-Coated Balloon, Percutaneous Endoscopic Approach

047N4ZZ Dilation of Left Popliteal Artery, Percutaneous Endoscopic Approach

047P04Z Dilation of Right Anterior Tibial Artery with Drug-eluting Intraluminal Device, Open Approach

047P0DZ Dilation of Right Anterior Tibial Artery with Intraluminal Device, Open Approach

047P0ZZ Dilation of Right Anterior Tibial Artery, Open Approach

047P34Z Dilation of Right Anterior Tibial Artery with Drug-eluting Intraluminal Device, Percutaneous Approach

047P3DZ Dilation of Right Anterior Tibial Artery with Intraluminal Device, Percutaneous Approach

047P3ZZ Dilation of Right Anterior Tibial Artery, Percutaneous Approach

047P44Z Dilation of Right Anterior Tibial Artery with Drug-eluting Intraluminal Device, Percutaneous Endoscopic Approach

047P4DZ Dilation of Right Anterior Tibial Artery with Intraluminal Device, Percutaneous Endoscopic Approach

047P4ZZ Dilation of Right Anterior Tibial Artery, Percutaneous Endoscopic Approach

047Q04Z Dilation of Left Anterior Tibial Artery with Drug-eluting Intraluminal Device, Open Approach

047Q0DZ Dilation of Left Anterior Tibial Artery with Intraluminal Device, Open Approach

047Q0ZZ Dilation of Left Anterior Tibial Artery, Open Approach

047Q34Z Dilation of Left Anterior Tibial Artery with Drug-eluting Intraluminal Device, Percutaneous Approach

047Q3DZ Dilation of Left Anterior Tibial Artery with Intraluminal Device, Percutaneous Approach

047Q3ZZ Dilation of Left Anterior Tibial Artery, Percutaneous Approach

047Q44Z Dilation of Left Anterior Tibial Artery with Drug-eluting Intraluminal Device, Percutaneous Endoscopic Approach

047Q4DZ Dilation of Left Anterior Tibial Artery with Intraluminal Device, Percutaneous Endoscopic Approach

047Q4ZZ Dilation of Left Anterior Tibial Artery, Percutaneous Endoscopic Approach

047R04Z Dilation of Right Posterior Tibial Artery with Drug-eluting Intraluminal Device, Open Approach

047R0DZ Dilation of Right Posterior Tibial Artery with Intraluminal Device, Open Approach

7R0ZZ	Dilation of Right Posterior Tibial Artery, Open Approach	047T3DZ	Dilation of Right Peroneal Artery with Intraluminal Device, Percutaneous Approach	047V44Z	Dilation of Right Foot Artery with Drug-eluting Intraluminal Device, Percutaneous Endoscopic Approach
7R34Z	Dilation of Right Posterior Tibial Artery with Drug-eluting Intraluminal Device, Percutaneous Approach	047T3ZZ	Dilation of Right Peroneal Artery, Percutaneous Approach	047V4DZ	Dilation of Right Foot Artery with Intraluminal Device, Percutaneous Endoscopic Approach
7R3DZ	Dilation of Right Posterior Tibial Artery with Intraluminal Device, Percutaneous Approach	047T44Z	Dilation of Right Peroneal Artery with Drug-eluting Intraluminal Device, Percutaneous Endoscopic Approach	047V4ZZ	Dilation of Right Foot Artery, Percutaneous Endoscopic Approach
7R3ZZ	Dilation of Right Posterior Tibial Artery, Percutaneous Approach	047T4DZ	Dilation of Right Peroneal Artery with Intraluminal Device, Percutaneous Endoscopic Approach	047W04Z	Dilation of Left Foot Artery with Drug-eluting Intraluminal Device, Open Approach
7R44Z	Dilation of Right Posterior Tibial Artery with Drug-eluting Intraluminal Device, Percutaneous Endoscopic Approach	047T4ZZ	Dilation of Right Peroneal Artery, Percutaneous Endoscopic Approach	047W0DZ	Dilation of Left Foot Artery with Intraluminal Device, Open Approach
7R4DZ	Dilation of Right Posterior Tibial Artery with Intraluminal Device, Percutaneous Endoscopic Approach	047U04Z	Dilation of Left Peroneal Artery with Drug-eluting Intraluminal Device, Open Approach	047W0ZZ	Dilation of Left Foot Artery, Open Approach
7R4ZZ	Dilation of Right Posterior Tibial Artery, Percutaneous Endoscopic Approach	047U0DZ	Dilation of Left Peroneal Artery with Intraluminal Device, Open Approach	047W34Z	Dilation of Left Foot Artery with Drug-eluting Intraluminal Device, Percutaneous Approach
7S04Z	Dilation of Left Posterior Tibial Artery with Drug-eluting Intraluminal Device, Open Approach	047U0ZZ	Dilation of Left Peroneal Artery, Open Approach	047W3DZ	Dilation of Left Foot Artery with Intraluminal Device, Percutaneous Approach
7S0DZ	Dilation of Left Posterior Tibial Artery with Intraluminal Device, Open Approach	047U34Z	Dilation of Left Peroneal Artery with Drug-eluting Intraluminal Device, Percutaneous Approach	047W3ZZ	Dilation of Left Foot Artery, Percutaneous Approach
7S0ZZ	Dilation of Left Posterior Tibial Artery, Open Approach	047U3DZ	Dilation of Left Peroneal Artery with Intraluminal Device, Percutaneous Approach	047W44Z	Dilation of Left Foot Artery with Drug-eluting Intraluminal Device, Percutaneous Endoscopic Approach
7S34Z	Dilation of Left Posterior Tibial Artery with Drug-eluting Intraluminal Device, Percutaneous Approach	047U3ZZ	Dilation of Left Peroneal Artery, Percutaneous Approach	047W4DZ	Dilation of Left Foot Artery with Intraluminal Device, Percutaneous Endoscopic Approach
7S3DZ	Dilation of Left Posterior Tibial Artery with Intraluminal Device, Percutaneous Approach	047U44Z	Dilation of Left Peroneal Artery with Drug-eluting Intraluminal Device, Percutaneous Endoscopic Approach	047W4ZZ	Dilation of Left Foot Artery, Percutaneous Endoscopic Approach
7S3ZZ	Dilation of Left Posterior Tibial Artery, Percutaneous Approach	047U4DZ	Dilation of Left Peroneal Artery with Intraluminal Device, Percutaneous Endoscopic Approach	047Y04Z	Dilation of Lower Artery with Drug-eluting Intraluminal Device, Open Approach
7S44Z	Dilation of Left Posterior Tibial Artery with Drug-eluting Intraluminal Device, Percutaneous Endoscopic Approach	047U4ZZ	Dilation of Left Peroneal Artery, Percutaneous Endoscopic Approach	047Y0DZ	Dilation of Lower Artery with Intraluminal Device, Open Approach
7S4DZ	Dilation of Left Posterior Tibial Artery with Intraluminal Device, Percutaneous Endoscopic Approach	047V04Z	Dilation of Right Foot Artery with Drug-eluting Intraluminal Device, Open Approach	047Y0ZZ	Dilation of Lower Artery, Open Approach
7S4ZZ	Dilation of Left Posterior Tibial Artery, Percutaneous Endoscopic Approach	047V0DZ	Dilation of Right Foot Artery with Intraluminal Device, Open Approach	047Y34Z	Dilation of Lower Artery with Drug-eluting Intraluminal Device, Percutaneous Approach
7T04Z	Dilation of Right Peroneal Artery with Drug-eluting Intraluminal Device, Open Approach	047V0ZZ	Dilation of Right Foot Artery, Open Approach	047Y3DZ	Dilation of Lower Artery with Intraluminal Device, Percutaneous Approach
7T0DZ	Dilation of Right Peroneal Artery with Intraluminal Device, Open Approach	047V34Z	Dilation of Right Foot Artery with Drug-eluting Intraluminal Device, Percutaneous Approach	047Y3ZZ	Dilation of Lower Artery, Percutaneous Approach
7T0ZZ	Dilation of Right Peroneal Artery, Open Approach	047V3DZ	Dilation of Right Foot Artery with Intraluminal Device, Percutaneous Approach	047Y44Z	Dilation of Lower Artery with Drug-eluting Intraluminal Device, Percutaneous Endoscopic Approach
7T34Z	Dilation of Right Peroneal Artery with Drug-eluting Intraluminal Device, Percutaneous Approach	047V3ZZ	Dilation of Right Foot Artery, Percutaneous Approach	047Y4DZ	Dilation of Lower Artery with Intraluminal Device, Percutaneous Endoscopic Approach
				047Y4ZZ	Dilation of Lower Artery, Percutaneous Endoscopic Approach

49 – Lower Arteries, Drainage

Review Coding Guidelines B3.4a and B3.4b

Review Coding Guideline B6.2

49000Z	Drainage of Abdominal Aorta with Drainage Device, Open Approach	04904ZX	Drainage of Abdominal Aorta, Percutaneous Endoscopic Approach, Diagnostic	04913ZZ	Drainage of Celiac Artery, Percutaneous Approach
4900ZX	Drainage of Abdominal Aorta, Open Approach, Diagnostic	04904ZZ	Drainage of Abdominal Aorta, Percutaneous Endoscopic Approach	049140Z	Drainage of Celiac Artery with Drainage Device, Percutaneous Endoscopic Approach
4900ZZ	Drainage of Abdominal Aorta, Open Approach	049100Z	Drainage of Celiac Artery with Drainage Device, Open Approach	04914ZX	Drainage of Celiac Artery, Percutaneous Endoscopic Approach, Diagnostic
49030Z	Drainage of Abdominal Aorta with Drainage Device, Percutaneous Approach	04910ZX	Drainage of Celiac Artery, Open Approach, Diagnostic	04914ZZ	Drainage of Celiac Artery, Percutaneous Endoscopic Approach
4903ZX	Drainage of Abdominal Aorta, Percutaneous Approach, Diagnostic	04910ZZ	Drainage of Celiac Artery, Open Approach	049200Z	Drainage of Gastric Artery with Drainage Device, Open Approach
4903ZZ	Drainage of Abdominal Aorta, Percutaneous Approach	049130Z	Drainage of Celiac Artery with Drainage Device, Percutaneous Approach	04920ZX	Drainage of Gastric Artery, Open Approach, Diagnostic
49040Z	Drainage of Abdominal Aorta with Drainage Device, Percutaneous Endoscopic Approach	04913ZX	Drainage of Celiac Artery, Percutaneous Approach, Diagnostic	04920ZZ	Drainage of Gastric Artery, Open Approach

Female-only	♂ Male-only	▲ Limited Coverage	● Non-OR	▬ HAC-associated procedure	▲ Non-covered procedures	✚ Combination

049230Z	Drainage of Gastric Artery with Drainage Device, Percutaneous Approach
04923ZX	Drainage of Gastric Artery, Percutaneous Approach, Diagnostic
04923ZZ	Drainage of Gastric Artery, Percutaneous Approach
049240Z	Drainage of Gastric Artery with Drainage Device, Percutaneous Endoscopic Approach
04924ZX	Drainage of Gastric Artery, Percutaneous Endoscopic Approach, Diagnostic
04924ZZ	Drainage of Gastric Artery, Percutaneous Endoscopic Approach
049300Z	Drainage of Hepatic Artery with Drainage Device, Open Approach
04930ZX	Drainage of Hepatic Artery, Open Approach, Diagnostic
04930ZZ	Drainage of Hepatic Artery, Open Approach
049330Z	Drainage of Hepatic Artery with Drainage Device, Percutaneous Approach
04933ZX	Drainage of Hepatic Artery, Percutaneous Approach, Diagnostic
04933ZZ	Drainage of Hepatic Artery, Percutaneous Approach
049340Z	Drainage of Hepatic Artery with Drainage Device, Percutaneous Endoscopic Approach
04934ZX	Drainage of Hepatic Artery, Percutaneous Endoscopic Approach, Diagnostic
04934ZZ	Drainage of Hepatic Artery, Percutaneous Endoscopic Approach
049400Z	Drainage of Splenic Artery with Drainage Device, Open Approach
04940ZX	Drainage of Splenic Artery, Open Approach, Diagnostic
04940ZZ	Drainage of Splenic Artery, Open Approach
049430Z	Drainage of Splenic Artery with Drainage Device, Percutaneous Approach
04943ZX	Drainage of Splenic Artery, Percutaneous Approach, Diagnostic
04943ZZ	Drainage of Splenic Artery, Percutaneous Approach
049440Z	Drainage of Splenic Artery with Drainage Device, Percutaneous Endoscopic Approach
04944ZX	Drainage of Splenic Artery, Percutaneous Endoscopic Approach, Diagnostic
04944ZZ	Drainage of Splenic Artery, Percutaneous Endoscopic Approach
049500Z	Drainage of Superior Mesenteric Artery with Drainage Device, Open Approach
04950ZX	Drainage of Superior Mesenteric Artery, Open Approach, Diagnostic
04950ZZ	Drainage of Superior Mesenteric Artery, Open Approach
049530Z	Drainage of Superior Mesenteric Artery with Drainage Device, Percutaneous Approach
04953ZX	Drainage of Superior Mesenteric Artery, Percutaneous Approach, Diagnostic
04953ZZ	Drainage of Superior Mesenteric Artery, Percutaneous Approach
049540Z	Drainage of Superior Mesenteric Artery with Drainage Device, Percutaneous Endoscopic Approach
04954ZX	Drainage of Superior Mesenteric Artery, Percutaneous Endoscopic Approach, Diagnostic
04954ZZ	Drainage of Superior Mesenteric Artery, Percutaneous Endoscopic Approach
049600Z	Drainage of Right Colic Artery with Drainage Device, Open Approach
04960ZX	Drainage of Right Colic Artery, Open Approach, Diagnostic
04960ZZ	Drainage of Right Colic Artery, Open Approach
049630Z	Drainage of Right Colic Artery with Drainage Device, Percutaneous Approach
04963ZX	Drainage of Right Colic Artery, Percutaneous Approach, Diagnostic
04963ZZ	Drainage of Right Colic Artery, Percutaneous Approach
049640Z	Drainage of Right Colic Artery with Drainage Device, Percutaneous Endoscopic Approach
04964ZX	Drainage of Right Colic Artery, Percutaneous Endoscopic Approach, Diagnostic
04964ZZ	Drainage of Right Colic Artery, Percutaneous Endoscopic Approach
049700Z	Drainage of Left Colic Artery with Drainage Device, Open Approach
04970ZX	Drainage of Left Colic Artery, Open Approach, Diagnostic
04970ZZ	Drainage of Left Colic Artery, Open Approach
049730Z	Drainage of Left Colic Artery with Drainage Device, Percutaneous Approach
04973ZX	Drainage of Left Colic Artery, Percutaneous Approach, Diagnostic
04973ZZ	Drainage of Left Colic Artery, Percutaneous Approach
049740Z	Drainage of Left Colic Artery with Drainage Device, Percutaneous Endoscopic Approach
04974ZX	Drainage of Left Colic Artery, Percutaneous Endoscopic Approach, Diagnostic
04974ZZ	Drainage of Left Colic Artery, Percutaneous Endoscopic Approach
049800Z	Drainage of Middle Colic Artery with Drainage Device, Open Approach
04980ZX	Drainage of Middle Colic Artery, Open Approach, Diagnostic
04980ZZ	Drainage of Middle Colic Artery, Open Approach
049830Z	Drainage of Middle Colic Artery with Drainage Device, Percutaneous Approach
04983ZX	Drainage of Middle Colic Artery, Percutaneous Approach, Diagnostic
04983ZZ	Drainage of Middle Colic Artery, Percutaneous Approach
049840Z	Drainage of Middle Colic Artery with Drainage Device, Percutaneous Endoscopic Approach
04984ZX	Drainage of Middle Colic Artery, Percutaneous Endoscopic Approach, Diagnostic
04984ZZ	Drainage of Middle Colic Artery, Percutaneous Endoscopic Approach
049900Z	Drainage of Right Renal Artery with Drainage Device, Open Approach
04990ZX	Drainage of Right Renal Artery, Open Approach, Diagnostic
04990ZZ	Drainage of Right Renal Artery, Open Approach
049930Z	Drainage of Right Renal Artery with Drainage Device, Percutaneous Approach
04993ZX	Drainage of Right Renal Artery, Percutaneous Approach, Diagnostic
04993ZZ	Drainage of Right Renal Artery, Percutaneous Approach
049940Z	Drainage of Right Renal Artery with Drainage Device, Percutaneous Endoscopic Approach
04994ZX	Drainage of Right Renal Artery, Percutaneous Endoscopic Approach, Diagnostic
04994ZZ	Drainage of Right Renal Artery, Percutaneous Endoscopic Approach
049A00Z	Drainage of Left Renal Artery with Drainage Device, Open Approach
049A0ZX	Drainage of Left Renal Artery, Open Approach, Diagnostic
049A0ZZ	Drainage of Left Renal Artery, Open Approach
049A30Z	Drainage of Left Renal Artery with Drainage Device, Percutaneous Approach
049A3ZX	Drainage of Left Renal Artery, Percutaneous Approach, Diagnostic
049A3ZZ	Drainage of Left Renal Artery, Percutaneous Approach
049A40Z	Drainage of Left Renal Artery with Drainage Device, Percutaneous Endoscopic Approach
049A4ZX	Drainage of Left Renal Artery, Percutaneous Endoscopic Approach, Diagnostic
049A4ZZ	Drainage of Left Renal Artery, Percutaneous Endoscopic Approach
049B00Z	Drainage of Inferior Mesenteric Artery with Drainage Device, Open Approach
049B0ZX	Drainage of Inferior Mesenteric Artery, Open Approach, Diagnostic
049B0ZZ	Drainage of Inferior Mesenteric Artery, Open Approach
049B30Z	Drainage of Inferior Mesenteric Artery with Drainage Device, Percutaneous Approach
049B3ZX	Drainage of Inferior Mesenteric Artery, Percutaneous Approach, Diagnostic
049B3ZZ	Drainage of Inferior Mesenteric Artery, Percutaneous Approach
049B40Z	Drainage of Inferior Mesenteric Artery with Drainage Device, Percutaneous Endoscopic Approach
049B4ZX	Drainage of Inferior Mesenteric Artery, Percutaneous Endoscopic Approach, Diagnostic
049B4ZZ	Drainage of Inferior Mesenteric Artery, Percutaneous Endoscopic Approach
049C00Z	Drainage of Right Common Iliac Artery with Drainage Device, Open Approach
049C0ZX	Drainage of Right Common Iliac Artery, Open Approach, Diagnostic
049C0ZZ	Drainage of Right Common Iliac Artery, Open Approach
049C30Z	Drainage of Right Common Iliac Artery with Drainage Device, Percutaneous Approach
049C3ZX	Drainage of Right Common Iliac Artery, Percutaneous Approach, Diagnostic
049C3ZZ	Drainage of Right Common Iliac Artery, Percutaneous Approach
049C40Z	Drainage of Right Common Iliac Artery with Drainage Device, Percutaneous Endoscopic Approach
049C4ZX	Drainage of Right Common Iliac Artery, Percutaneous Endoscopic Approach, Diagnostic
049C4ZZ	Drainage of Right Common Iliac Artery, Percutaneous Endoscopic Approach
049D00Z	Drainage of Left Common Iliac Artery with Drainage Device, Open Approach
049D0ZX	Drainage of Left Common Iliac Artery, Open Approach, Diagnostic
049D0ZZ	Drainage of Left Common Iliac Artery, Open Approach
049D30Z	Drainage of Left Common Iliac Artery with Drainage Device, Percutaneous Approach
049D3ZX	Drainage of Left Common Iliac Artery, Percutaneous Approach, Diagnostic
049D3ZZ	Drainage of Left Common Iliac Artery, Percutaneous Approach
049D40Z	Drainage of Left Common Iliac Artery with Drainage Device, Percutaneous Endoscopic Approach

♀ Female-only   ♂ Male-only   ▲ Limited Coverage   ● Non-OR   ▥ HAC-associated procedure   ▲ Non-covered procedures   ✚ Combination

D4ZX Drainage of Left Common Iliac Artery, Percutaneous Endoscopic Approach, Diagnostic

D4ZZ Drainage of Left Common Iliac Artery, Percutaneous Endoscopic Approach

E00Z Drainage of Right Internal Iliac Artery with Drainage Device, Open Approach

E0ZX Drainage of Right Internal Iliac Artery, Open Approach, Diagnostic

E0ZZ Drainage of Right Internal Iliac Artery, Open Approach

E30Z Drainage of Right Internal Iliac Artery with Drainage Device, Percutaneous Approach

E3ZX Drainage of Right Internal Iliac Artery, Percutaneous Approach, Diagnostic

E3ZZ Drainage of Right Internal Iliac Artery, Percutaneous Approach

E40Z Drainage of Right Internal Iliac Artery with Drainage Device, Percutaneous Endoscopic Approach

E4ZX Drainage of Right Internal Iliac Artery, Percutaneous Endoscopic Approach, Diagnostic

E4ZZ Drainage of Right Internal Iliac Artery, Percutaneous Endoscopic Approach

F00Z Drainage of Left Internal Iliac Artery with Drainage Device, Open Approach

F0ZX Drainage of Left Internal Iliac Artery, Open Approach, Diagnostic

F0ZZ Drainage of Left Internal Iliac Artery, Open Approach

F30Z Drainage of Left Internal Iliac Artery with Drainage Device, Percutaneous Approach

F3ZX Drainage of Left Internal Iliac Artery, Percutaneous Approach, Diagnostic

F3ZZ Drainage of Left Internal Iliac Artery, Percutaneous Approach

F40Z Drainage of Left Internal Iliac Artery with Drainage Device, Percutaneous Endoscopic Approach

F4ZX Drainage of Left Internal Iliac Artery, Percutaneous Endoscopic Approach, Diagnostic

F4ZZ Drainage of Left Internal Iliac Artery, Percutaneous Endoscopic Approach

H00Z Drainage of Right External Iliac Artery with Drainage Device, Open Approach

H0ZX Drainage of Right External Iliac Artery, Open Approach, Diagnostic

H0ZZ Drainage of Right External Iliac Artery, Open Approach

H30Z Drainage of Right External Iliac Artery with Drainage Device, Percutaneous Approach

9H3ZX Drainage of Right External Iliac Artery, Percutaneous Approach, Diagnostic

9H3ZZ Drainage of Right External Iliac Artery, Percutaneous Approach

9H40Z Drainage of Right External Iliac Artery with Drainage Device, Percutaneous Endoscopic Approach

9H4ZX Drainage of Right External Iliac Artery, Percutaneous Endoscopic Approach, Diagnostic

9H4ZZ Drainage of Right External Iliac Artery, Percutaneous Endoscopic Approach

49J00Z Drainage of Left External Iliac Artery with Drainage Device, Open Approach

49J0ZX Drainage of Left External Iliac Artery, Open Approach, Diagnostic

49J0ZZ Drainage of Left External Iliac Artery, Open Approach

49J30Z Drainage of Left External Iliac Artery with Drainage Device, Percutaneous Approach

49J3ZX Drainage of Left External Iliac Artery, Percutaneous Approach, Diagnostic

049J3ZZ Drainage of Left External Iliac Artery, Percutaneous Approach

049J40Z Drainage of Left External Iliac Artery with Drainage Device, Percutaneous Endoscopic Approach

049J4ZX Drainage of Left External Iliac Artery, Percutaneous Endoscopic Approach, Diagnostic

049J4ZZ Drainage of Left External Iliac Artery, Percutaneous Endoscopic Approach

049K00Z Drainage of Right Femoral Artery with Drainage Device, Open Approach

049K0ZX Drainage of Right Femoral Artery, Open Approach, Diagnostic

049K0ZZ Drainage of Right Femoral Artery, Open Approach

049K30Z Drainage of Right Femoral Artery with Drainage Device, Percutaneous Approach

049K3ZX Drainage of Right Femoral Artery, Percutaneous Approach, Diagnostic

049K3ZZ Drainage of Right Femoral Artery, Percutaneous Approach

049K40Z Drainage of Right Femoral Artery with Drainage Device, Percutaneous Endoscopic Approach

049K4ZX Drainage of Right Femoral Artery, Percutaneous Endoscopic Approach, Diagnostic

049K4ZZ Drainage of Right Femoral Artery, Percutaneous Endoscopic Approach

049L00Z Drainage of Left Femoral Artery with Drainage Device, Open Approach

049L0ZX Drainage of Left Femoral Artery, Open Approach, Diagnostic

049L0ZZ Drainage of Left Femoral Artery, Open Approach

049L30Z Drainage of Left Femoral Artery with Drainage Device, Percutaneous Approach

049L3ZX Drainage of Left Femoral Artery, Percutaneous Approach, Diagnostic

049L3ZZ Drainage of Left Femoral Artery, Percutaneous Approach

049L40Z Drainage of Left Femoral Artery with Drainage Device, Percutaneous Endoscopic Approach

049L4ZX Drainage of Left Femoral Artery, Percutaneous Endoscopic Approach, Diagnostic

049L4ZZ Drainage of Left Femoral Artery, Percutaneous Endoscopic Approach

049M00Z Drainage of Right Popliteal Artery with Drainage Device, Open Approach

049M0ZX Drainage of Right Popliteal Artery, Open Approach, Diagnostic

049M0ZZ Drainage of Right Popliteal Artery, Open Approach

049M30Z Drainage of Right Popliteal Artery with Drainage Device, Percutaneous Approach

049M3ZX Drainage of Right Popliteal Artery, Percutaneous Approach, Diagnostic

049M3ZZ Drainage of Right Popliteal Artery, Percutaneous Approach

049M40Z Drainage of Right Popliteal Artery with Drainage Device, Percutaneous Endoscopic Approach

049M4ZX Drainage of Right Popliteal Artery, Percutaneous Endoscopic Approach, Diagnostic

049M4ZZ Drainage of Right Popliteal Artery, Percutaneous Endoscopic Approach

049N00Z Drainage of Left Popliteal Artery with Drainage Device, Open Approach

049N0ZX Drainage of Left Popliteal Artery, Open Approach, Diagnostic

049N0ZZ Drainage of Left Popliteal Artery, Open Approach

049N30Z Drainage of Left Popliteal Artery with Drainage Device, Percutaneous Approach

049N3ZX Drainage of Left Popliteal Artery, Percutaneous Approach, Diagnostic

049N3ZZ Drainage of Left Popliteal Artery, Percutaneous Approach

049N40Z Drainage of Left Popliteal Artery with Drainage Device, Percutaneous Endoscopic Approach

049N4ZX Drainage of Left Popliteal Artery, Percutaneous Endoscopic Approach, Diagnostic

049N4ZZ Drainage of Left Popliteal Artery, Percutaneous Endoscopic Approach

049P00Z Drainage of Right Anterior Tibial Artery with Drainage Device, Open Approach

049P0ZX Drainage of Right Anterior Tibial Artery, Open Approach, Diagnostic

049P0ZZ Drainage of Right Anterior Tibial Artery, Open Approach

049P30Z Drainage of Right Anterior Tibial Artery with Drainage Device, Percutaneous Approach

049P3ZX Drainage of Right Anterior Tibial Artery, Percutaneous Approach, Diagnostic

049P3ZZ Drainage of Right Anterior Tibial Artery, Percutaneous Approach

049P40Z Drainage of Right Anterior Tibial Artery with Drainage Device, Percutaneous Endoscopic Approach

049P4ZX Drainage of Right Anterior Tibial Artery, Percutaneous Endoscopic Approach, Diagnostic

049P4ZZ Drainage of Right Anterior Tibial Artery, Percutaneous Endoscopic Approach

049Q00Z Drainage of Left Anterior Tibial Artery with Drainage Device, Open Approach

049Q0ZX Drainage of Left Anterior Tibial Artery, Open Approach, Diagnostic

049Q0ZZ Drainage of Left Anterior Tibial Artery, Open Approach

049Q30Z Drainage of Left Anterior Tibial Artery with Drainage Device, Percutaneous Approach

049Q3ZX Drainage of Left Anterior Tibial Artery, Percutaneous Approach, Diagnostic

049Q3ZZ Drainage of Left Anterior Tibial Artery, Percutaneous Approach

049Q40Z Drainage of Left Anterior Tibial Artery with Drainage Device, Percutaneous Endoscopic Approach

049Q4ZX Drainage of Left Anterior Tibial Artery, Percutaneous Endoscopic Approach, Diagnostic

049Q4ZZ Drainage of Left Anterior Tibial Artery, Percutaneous Endoscopic Approach

049R00Z Drainage of Right Posterior Tibial Artery with Drainage Device, Open Approach

049R0ZX Drainage of Right Posterior Tibial Artery, Open Approach, Diagnostic

049R0ZZ Drainage of Right Posterior Tibial Artery, Open Approach

049R30Z Drainage of Right Posterior Tibial Artery with Drainage Device, Percutaneous Approach

049R3ZX Drainage of Right Posterior Tibial Artery, Percutaneous Approach, Diagnostic

049R3ZZ Drainage of Right Posterior Tibial Artery, Percutaneous Approach

049R40Z Drainage of Right Posterior Tibial Artery with Drainage Device, Percutaneous Endoscopic Approach

049R4ZX Drainage of Right Posterior Tibial Artery, Percutaneous Endoscopic Approach, Diagnostic

049R4ZZ Drainage of Right Posterior Tibial Artery, Percutaneous Endoscopic Approach

Female-only   ♂ Male-only   ▲ Limited Coverage   ● Non-OR   ▦ HAC-associated procedure   ▲ Non-covered procedures   ✚ Combination

049S00Z Drainage of Left Posterior Tibial Artery with Drainage Device, Open Approach	**049T4ZZ** Drainage of Right Peroneal Artery, Percutaneous Endoscopic Approach	**049V4ZZ** Drainage of Right Foot Artery, Percutaneous Endoscopic Approach
049S0ZX Drainage of Left Posterior Tibial Artery, Open Approach, Diagnostic	**049U00Z** Drainage of Left Peroneal Artery with Drainage Device, Open Approach	**049W00Z** Drainage of Left Foot Artery with Drainage Device, Open Approach
049S0ZZ Drainage of Left Posterior Tibial Artery, Open Approach	**049U0ZX** Drainage of Left Peroneal Artery, Open Approach, Diagnostic	**049W0ZX** Drainage of Left Foot Artery, Open Approach, Diagnostic
049S30Z Drainage of Left Posterior Tibial Artery with Drainage Device, Percutaneous Approach	**049U0ZZ** Drainage of Left Peroneal Artery, Open Approach	**049W0ZZ** Drainage of Left Foot Artery, Open Approach
049S3ZX Drainage of Left Posterior Tibial Artery, Percutaneous Approach, Diagnostic	**049U30Z** Drainage of Left Peroneal Artery with Drainage Device, Percutaneous Approach	**049W30Z** Drainage of Left Foot Artery with Drainage Device, Percutaneous Approach
049S3ZZ Drainage of Left Posterior Tibial Artery, Percutaneous Approach	**049U3ZX** Drainage of Left Peroneal Artery, Percutaneous Approach, Diagnostic	**049W3ZX** Drainage of Left Foot Artery, Percutaneous Approach, Diagnostic
049S40Z Drainage of Left Posterior Tibial Artery with Drainage Device, Percutaneous Endoscopic Approach	**049U3ZZ** Drainage of Left Peroneal Artery, Percutaneous Approach	**049W3ZZ** Drainage of Left Foot Artery, Percutaneous Approach
049S4ZX Drainage of Left Posterior Tibial Artery, Percutaneous Endoscopic Approach, Diagnostic	**049U40Z** Drainage of Left Peroneal Artery with Drainage Device, Percutaneous Endoscopic Approach	**049W40Z** Drainage of Left Foot Artery with Drainage Device, Percutaneous Endoscopic Approach
049S4ZZ Drainage of Left Posterior Tibial Artery, Percutaneous Endoscopic Approach	**049U4ZX** Drainage of Left Peroneal Artery, Percutaneous Endoscopic Approach, Diagnostic	**049W4ZX** Drainage of Left Foot Artery, Percutaneous Endoscopic Approach, Diagnostic
049T00Z Drainage of Right Peroneal Artery with Drainage Device, Open Approach	**049U4ZZ** Drainage of Left Peroneal Artery, Percutaneous Endoscopic Approach	**049W4ZZ** Drainage of Left Foot Artery, Percutaneous Endoscopic Approach
049T0ZX Drainage of Right Peroneal Artery, Open Approach, Diagnostic	**049V00Z** Drainage of Right Foot Artery with Drainage Device, Open Approach	**049Y00Z** Drainage of Lower Artery with Drainage Device, Open Approach
049T0ZZ Drainage of Right Peroneal Artery, Open Approach	**049V0ZX** Drainage of Right Foot Artery, Open Approach, Diagnostic	**049Y0ZX** Drainage of Lower Artery, Open Approach, Diagnostic
049T30Z Drainage of Right Peroneal Artery with Drainage Device, Percutaneous Approach	**049V0ZZ** Drainage of Right Foot Artery, Open Approach	**049Y0ZZ** Drainage of Lower Artery, Open Approach
049T3ZX Drainage of Right Peroneal Artery, Percutaneous Approach, Diagnostic	**049V30Z** Drainage of Right Foot Artery with Drainage Device, Percutaneous Approach	**049Y30Z** Drainage of Lower Artery with Drainage Device, Percutaneous Approach
049T3ZZ Drainage of Right Peroneal Artery, Percutaneous Approach	**049V3ZX** Drainage of Right Foot Artery, Percutaneous Approach, Diagnostic	**049Y3ZX** Drainage of Lower Artery, Percutaneous Approach, Diagnostic
049T40Z Drainage of Right Peroneal Artery with Drainage Device, Percutaneous Endoscopic Approach	**049V3ZZ** Drainage of Right Foot Artery, Percutaneous Approach	**049Y3ZZ** Drainage of Lower Artery, Percutaneous Approach
049T4ZX Drainage of Right Peroneal Artery, Percutaneous Endoscopic Approach, Diagnostic	**049V40Z** Drainage of Right Foot Artery with Drainage Device, Percutaneous Endoscopic Approach	**049Y40Z** Drainage of Lower Artery with Drainage Device, Percutaneous Endoscopic Approach
	049V4ZX Drainage of Right Foot Artery, Percutaneous Endoscopic Approach, Diagnostic	**049Y4ZX** Drainage of Lower Artery, Percutaneous Endoscopic Approach, Diagnostic
		049Y4ZZ Drainage of Lower Artery, Percutaneous Endoscopic Approach

04B – Lower Arteries, Excision

Review Coding Guidelines B3.4a and B3.4b

Review Coding Guideline B3.8

04B00ZX Excision of Abdominal Aorta, Open Approach, Diagnostic	**04B23ZZ** Excision of Gastric Artery, Percutaneous Approach	**04B50ZX** Excision of Superior Mesenteric Artery, Open Approach, Diagnostic
04B00ZZ Excision of Abdominal Aorta, Open Approach	**04B24ZX** Excision of Gastric Artery, Percutaneous Endoscopic Approach, Diagnostic	**04B50ZZ** Excision of Superior Mesenteric Artery, Open Approach
04B03ZX Excision of Abdominal Aorta, Percutaneous Approach, Diagnostic	**04B24ZZ** Excision of Gastric Artery, Percutaneous Endoscopic Approach	**04B53ZX** Excision of Superior Mesenteric Artery, Percutaneous Approach, Diagnostic
04B03ZZ Excision of Abdominal Aorta, Percutaneous Approach	**04B30ZX** Excision of Hepatic Artery, Open Approach, Diagnostic	**04B53ZZ** Excision of Superior Mesenteric Artery, Percutaneous Approach
04B04ZX Excision of Abdominal Aorta, Percutaneous Endoscopic Approach, Diagnostic	**04B30ZZ** Excision of Hepatic Artcry, Open Approach	**04B54ZX** Excision of Superior Mesenteric Artery, Percutaneous Endoscopic Approach, Diagnostic
04B04ZZ Excision of Abdominal Aorta, Percutaneous Endoscopic Approach	**04B33ZX** Excision of Hepatic Artery, Percutaneous Approach, Diagnostic	**04B54ZZ** Excision of Superior Mesenteric Artery, Percutaneous Endoscopic Approach
04B10ZX Excision of Celiac Artery, Open Approach, Diagnostic	**04B33ZZ** Excision of Hepatic Artery, Percutaneous Approach	**04B60ZX** Excision of Right Colic Artery, Open Approach, Diagnostic
04B10ZZ Excision of Celiac Artery, Open Approach	**04B34ZX** Excision of Hepatic Artery, Percutaneous Endoscopic Approach, Diagnostic	**04B60ZZ** Excision of Right Colic Artery, Open Approach
04B13ZX Excision of Celiac Artery, Percutaneous Approach, Diagnostic	**04B34ZZ** Excision of Hepatic Artery, Percutaneous Endoscopic Approach	**04B63ZX** Excision of Right Colic Artery, Percutaneous Approach, Diagnostic
04B13ZZ Excision of Celiac Artery, Percutaneous Approach	**04B40ZX** Excision of Splenic Artery, Open Approach, Diagnostic	**04B63ZZ** Excision of Right Colic Artery, Percutaneous Approach
04B14ZX Excision of Celiac Artery, Percutaneous Endoscopic Approach, Diagnostic	**04B40ZZ** Excision of Splenic Artery, Open Approach	**04B64ZX** Excision of Right Colic Artery, Percutaneous Endoscopic Approach, Diagnostic
04B14ZZ Excision of Celiac Artery, Percutaneous Endoscopic Approach	**04B43ZX** Excision of Splenic Artery, Percutaneous Approach, Diagnostic	**04B64ZZ** Excision of Right Colic Artery, Percutaneous Endoscopic Approach
04B20ZX Excision of Gastric Artery, Open Approach, Diagnostic	**04B43ZZ** Excision of Splenic Artery, Percutaneous Approach	**04B70ZX** Excision of Left Colic Artery, Open Approach, Diagnostic
04B20ZZ Excision of Gastric Artery, Open Approach	**04B44ZX** Excision of Splenic Artery, Percutaneous Endoscopic Approach, Diagnostic	**04B70ZZ** Excision of Left Colic Artery, Open Approach
04B23ZX Excision of Gastric Artery, Percutaneous Approach, Diagnostic	**04B44ZZ** Excision of Splenic Artery, Percutaneous Endoscopic Approach	

♀ Female-only   ♂ Male-only   ▲ Limited Coverage   ● Non-OR   ▦ HAC-associated procedure   ▲ Non-covered procedures   ✚ Combinatio

4B73ZX	Excision of Left Colic Artery, Percutaneous Approach, Diagnostic	
4B73ZZ	Excision of Left Colic Artery, Percutaneous Approach	
4B74ZX	Excision of Left Colic Artery, Percutaneous Endoscopic Approach, Diagnostic	
4B74ZZ	Excision of Left Colic Artery, Percutaneous Endoscopic Approach	
4B80ZX	Excision of Middle Colic Artery, Open Approach, Diagnostic	
4B80ZZ	Excision of Middle Colic Artery, Open Approach	
4B83ZX	Excision of Middle Colic Artery, Percutaneous Approach, Diagnostic	
4B83ZZ	Excision of Middle Colic Artery, Percutaneous Approach	
4B84ZX	Excision of Middle Colic Artery, Percutaneous Endoscopic Approach, Diagnostic	
4B84ZZ	Excision of Middle Colic Artery, Percutaneous Endoscopic Approach	
4B90ZX	Excision of Right Renal Artery, Open Approach, Diagnostic	
4B90ZZ	Excision of Right Renal Artery, Open Approach	
4B93ZX	Excision of Right Renal Artery, Percutaneous Approach, Diagnostic	
4B93ZZ	Excision of Right Renal Artery, Percutaneous Approach	
4B94ZX	Excision of Right Renal Artery, Percutaneous Endoscopic Approach, Diagnostic	
4B94ZZ	Excision of Right Renal Artery, Percutaneous Endoscopic Approach	
4BA0ZX	Excision of Left Renal Artery, Open Approach, Diagnostic	
4BA0ZZ	Excision of Left Renal Artery, Open Approach	
4BA3ZX	Excision of Left Renal Artery, Percutaneous Approach, Diagnostic	
4BA3ZZ	Excision of Left Renal Artery, Percutaneous Approach	
4BA4ZX	Excision of Left Renal Artery, Percutaneous Endoscopic Approach, Diagnostic	
4BA4ZZ	Excision of Left Renal Artery, Percutaneous Endoscopic Approach	
4BB0ZX	Excision of Inferior Mesenteric Artery, Open Approach, Diagnostic	
4BB0ZZ	Excision of Inferior Mesenteric Artery, Open Approach	
4BB3ZX	Excision of Inferior Mesenteric Artery, Percutaneous Approach, Diagnostic	
4BB3ZZ	Excision of Inferior Mesenteric Artery, Percutaneous Approach	
4BB4ZX	Excision of Inferior Mesenteric Artery, Percutaneous Endoscopic Approach, Diagnostic	
4BB4ZZ	Excision of Inferior Mesenteric Artery, Percutaneous Endoscopic Approach	
04BC0ZX	Excision of Right Common Iliac Artery, Open Approach, Diagnostic	
04BC0ZZ	Excision of Right Common Iliac Artery, Open Approach	
04BC3ZX	Excision of Right Common Iliac Artery, Percutaneous Approach, Diagnostic	
04BC3ZZ	Excision of Right Common Iliac Artery, Percutaneous Approach	
04BC4ZX	Excision of Right Common Iliac Artery, Percutaneous Endoscopic Approach, Diagnostic	
04BC4ZZ	Excision of Right Common Iliac Artery, Percutaneous Endoscopic Approach	
04BD0ZX	Excision of Left Common Iliac Artery, Open Approach, Diagnostic	

04BD0ZZ	Excision of Left Common Iliac Artery, Open Approach
04BD3ZX	Excision of Left Common Iliac Artery, Percutaneous Approach, Diagnostic
04BD3ZZ	Excision of Left Common Iliac Artery, Percutaneous Approach
04BD4ZX	Excision of Left Common Iliac Artery, Percutaneous Endoscopic Approach, Diagnostic
04BD4ZZ	Excision of Left Common Iliac Artery, Percutaneous Endoscopic Approach
04BE0ZX	Excision of Right Internal Iliac Artery, Open Approach, Diagnostic
04BE0ZZ	Excision of Right Internal Iliac Artery, Open Approach
04BE3ZX	Excision of Right Internal Iliac Artery, Percutaneous Approach, Diagnostic
04BE3ZZ	Excision of Right Internal Iliac Artery, Percutaneous Approach
04BE4ZX	Excision of Right Internal Iliac Artery, Percutaneous Endoscopic Approach, Diagnostic
04BE4ZZ	Excision of Right Internal Iliac Artery, Percutaneous Endoscopic Approach
04BF0ZX	Excision of Left Internal Iliac Artery, Open Approach, Diagnostic
04BF0ZZ	Excision of Left Internal Iliac Artery, Open Approach
04BF3ZX	Excision of Left Internal Iliac Artery, Percutaneous Approach, Diagnostic
04BF3ZZ	Excision of Left Internal Iliac Artery, Percutaneous Approach
04BF4ZX	Excision of Left Internal Iliac Artery, Percutaneous Endoscopic Approach, Diagnostic
04BF4ZZ	Excision of Left Internal Iliac Artery, Percutaneous Endoscopic Approach
04BH0ZX	Excision of Right External Iliac Artery, Open Approach, Diagnostic
04BH0ZZ	Excision of Right External Iliac Artery, Open Approach
04BH3ZX	Excision of Right External Iliac Artery, Percutaneous Approach, Diagnostic
04BH3ZZ	Excision of Right External Iliac Artery, Percutaneous Approach
04BH4ZX	Excision of Right External Iliac Artery, Percutaneous Endoscopic Approach, Diagnostic
04BH4ZZ	Excision of Right External Iliac Artery, Percutaneous Endoscopic Approach
04BJ0ZX	Excision of Left External Iliac Artery, Open Approach, Diagnostic
04BJ0ZZ	Excision of Left External Iliac Artery, Open Approach
04BJ3ZX	Excision of Left External Iliac Artery, Percutaneous Approach, Diagnostic
04BJ3ZZ	Excision of Left External Iliac Artery, Percutaneous Approach
04BJ4ZX	Excision of Left External Iliac Artery, Percutaneous Endoscopic Approach, Diagnostic
04BJ4ZZ	Excision of Left External Iliac Artery, Percutaneous Endoscopic Approach
04BK0ZX	Excision of Right Femoral Artery, Open Approach, Diagnostic
04BL4ZZ	Excision of Left Femoral Artery, Percutaneous Endoscopic Approach
04BM0ZX	Excision of Right Popliteal Artery, Open Approach, Diagnostic
04BM0ZZ	Excision of Right Popliteal Artery, Open Approach
04BM3ZX	Excision of Right Popliteal Artery, Percutaneous Approach, Diagnostic
04BM3ZZ	Excision of Right Popliteal Artery, Percutaneous Approach

04BM4ZX	Excision of Right Popliteal Artery, Percutaneous Endoscopic Approach, Diagnostic
04BM4ZZ	Excision of Right Popliteal Artery, Percutaneous Endoscopic Approach
04BN0ZX	Excision of Left Popliteal Artery, Open Approach, Diagnostic
04BN0ZZ	Excision of Left Popliteal Artery, Open Approach
04BN3ZX	Excision of Left Popliteal Artery, Percutaneous Approach, Diagnostic
04BN3ZZ	Excision of Left Popliteal Artery, Percutaneous Approach
04BN4ZX	Excision of Left Popliteal Artery, Percutaneous Endoscopic Approach, Diagnostic
04BN4ZZ	Excision of Left Popliteal Artery, Percutaneous Endoscopic Approach
04BP0ZX	Excision of Right Anterior Tibial Artery, Open Approach, Diagnostic
04BP0ZZ	Excision of Right Anterior Tibial Artery, Open Approach
04BP3ZX	Excision of Right Anterior Tibial Artery, Percutaneous Approach, Diagnostic
04BP3ZZ	Excision of Right Anterior Tibial Artery, Percutaneous Approach
04BP4ZX	Excision of Right Anterior Tibial Artery, Percutaneous Endoscopic Approach, Diagnostic
04BP4ZZ	Excision of Right Anterior Tibial Artery, Percutaneous Endoscopic Approach
04BQ0ZX	Excision of Left Anterior Tibial Artery, Open Approach, Diagnostic
04BQ0ZZ	Excision of Left Anterior Tibial Artery, Open Approach
04BQ3ZX	Excision of Left Anterior Tibial Artery, Percutaneous Approach, Diagnostic
04BQ3ZZ	Excision of Left Anterior Tibial Artery, Percutaneous Approach
04BQ4ZX	Excision of Left Anterior Tibial Artery, Percutaneous Endoscopic Approach, Diagnostic
04BQ4ZZ	Excision of Left Anterior Tibial Artery, Percutaneous Endoscopic Approach
04BR0ZX	Excision of Right Posterior Tibial Artery, Open Approach, Diagnostic
04BR0ZZ	Excision of Right Posterior Tibial Artery, Open Approach
04BR3ZX	Excision of Right Posterior Tibial Artery, Percutaneous Approach, Diagnostic
04BR3ZZ	Excision of Right Posterior Tibial Artery, Percutaneous Approach
04BR4ZX	Excision of Right Posterior Tibial Artery, Percutaneous Endoscopic Approach, Diagnostic
04BR4ZZ	Excision of Right Posterior Tibial Artery, Percutaneous Endoscopic Approach
04BS0ZX	Excision of Left Posterior Tibial Artery, Open Approach, Diagnostic
04BS0ZZ	Excision of Left Posterior Tibial Artery, Open Approach
04BS3ZX	Excision of Left Posterior Tibial Artery, Percutaneous Approach, Diagnostic
04BS3ZZ	Excision of Left Posterior Tibial Artery, Percutaneous Approach
04BS4ZX	Excision of Left Posterior Tibial Artery, Percutaneous Endoscopic Approach, Diagnostic
04BS4ZZ	Excision of Left Posterior Tibial Artery, Percutaneous Endoscopic Approach
04BT0ZX	Excision of Right Peroneal Artery, Open Approach, Diagnostic
04BT0ZZ	Excision of Right Peroneal Artery, Open Approach

♀ Female-only   ♂ Male-only   ▲ Limited Coverage   ● Non-OR   🔲 HAC-associated procedure   ▲ Non-covered procedures   ➕ Combination

04BT3ZX Excision of Right Peroneal Artery, Percutaneous Approach, Diagnostic

04BT3ZZ Excision of Right Peroneal Artery, Percutaneous Approach

04BT4ZX Excision of Right Peroneal Artery, Percutaneous Endoscopic Approach, Diagnostic

04BT4ZZ Excision of Right Peroneal Artery, Percutaneous Endoscopic Approach

04BU0ZX Excision of Left Peroneal Artery, Open Approach, Diagnostic

04BU0ZZ Excision of Left Peroneal Artery, Open Approach

04BU3ZX Excision of Left Peroneal Artery, Percutaneous Approach, Diagnostic

04BU3ZZ Excision of Left Peroneal Artery, Percutaneous Approach

04BU4ZX Excision of Left Peroneal Artery, Percutaneous Endoscopic Approach, Diagnostic

04BU4ZZ Excision of Left Peroneal Artery, Percutaneous Endoscopic Approach

04BV0ZX Excision of Right Foot Artery, Open Approach, Diagnostic

04BV0ZZ Excision of Right Foot Artery, Open Approach

04BV3ZX Excision of Right Foot Artery, Percutaneous Approach, Diagnostic

04BV3ZZ Excision of Right Foot Artery, Percutaneous Approach

04BV4ZX Excision of Right Foot Artery, Percutaneous Endoscopic Approach, Diagnostic

04BV4ZZ Excision of Right Foot Artery, Percutaneous Endoscopic Approach

04BW0ZX Excision of Left Foot Artery, Open Approach, Diagnostic

04BW0ZZ Excision of Left Foot Artery, Open Approach

04BW3ZX Excision of Left Foot Artery, Percutaneous Approach, Diagnostic

04BW3ZZ Excision of Left Foot Artery, Percutaneous Approach

04BW4ZX Excision of Left Foot Artery, Percutaneous Endoscopic Approach, Diagnostic

04BW4ZZ Excision of Left Foot Artery, Percutaneous Endoscopic Approach

04BY0ZX Excision of Lower Artery, Open Approach, Diagnostic

04BY0ZZ Excision of Lower Artery, Open Approach

04BY3ZX Excision of Lower Artery, Percutaneous Approach, Diagnostic

04BY3ZZ Excision of Lower Artery, Percutaneous Approach

04BY4ZX Excision of Lower Artery, Percutaneous Endoscopic Approach, Diagnostic

04BY4ZZ Excision of Lower Artery, Percutaneous Endoscopic Approach

04C – Lower Arteries, Extirpation

04C00ZZ Extirpation of Matter from Abdominal Aorta, Open Approach

04C03ZZ Extirpation of Matter from Abdominal Aorta, Percutaneous Approach

04C04ZZ Extirpation of Matter from Abdominal Aorta, Percutaneous Endoscopic Approach

04C10ZZ Extirpation of Matter from Celiac Artery, Open Approach

04C13ZZ Extirpation of Matter from Celiac Artery, Percutaneous Approach

04C14ZZ Extirpation of Matter from Celiac Artery, Percutaneous Endoscopic Approach

04C20ZZ Extirpation of Matter from Gastric Artery, Open Approach

04C23ZZ Extirpation of Matter from Gastric Artery, Percutaneous Approach

04C24ZZ Extirpation of Matter from Gastric Artery, Percutaneous Endoscopic Approach

04C30ZZ Extirpation of Matter from Hepatic Artery, Open Approach

04C33ZZ Extirpation of Matter from Hepatic Artery, Percutaneous Approach

04C34ZZ Extirpation of Matter from Hepatic Artery, Percutaneous Endoscopic Approach

04C40ZZ Extirpation of Matter from Splenic Artery, Open Approach

04C43ZZ Extirpation of Matter from Splenic Artery, Percutaneous Approach

04C44ZZ Extirpation of Matter from Splenic Artery, Percutaneous Endoscopic Approach

04C50ZZ Extirpation of Matter from Superior Mesenteric Artery, Open Approach

04C53ZZ Extirpation of Matter from Superior Mesenteric Artery, Percutaneous Approach

04C54ZZ Extirpation of Matter from Superior Mesenteric Artery, Percutaneous Endoscopic Approach

04C60ZZ Extirpation of Matter from Right Colic Artery, Open Approach

04C63ZZ Extirpation of Matter from Right Colic Artery, Percutaneous Approach

04C64ZZ Extirpation of Matter from Right Colic Artery, Percutaneous Endoscopic Approach

04C70ZZ Extirpation of Matter from Left Colic Artery, Open Approach

04C73ZZ Extirpation of Matter from Left Colic Artery, Percutaneous Approach

04C74ZZ Extirpation of Matter from Left Colic Artery, Percutaneous Endoscopic Approach

04C80ZZ Extirpation of Matter from Middle Colic Artery, Open Approach

04C83ZZ Extirpation of Matter from Middle Colic Artery, Percutaneous Approach

04C84ZZ Extirpation of Matter from Middle Colic Artery, Percutaneous Endoscopic Approach

04C90ZZ Extirpation of Matter from Right Renal Artery, Open Approach

04C93ZZ Extirpation of Matter from Right Renal Artery, Percutaneous Approach

04C94ZZ Extirpation of Matter from Right Renal Artery, Percutaneous Endoscopic Approach

04CA0ZZ Extirpation of Matter from Left Renal Artery, Open Approach

04CA3ZZ Extirpation of Matter from Left Renal Artery, Percutaneous Approach

04CA4ZZ Extirpation of Matter from Left Renal Artery, Percutaneous Endoscopic Approach

04CB0ZZ Extirpation of Matter from Inferior Mesenteric Artery, Open Approach

04CB3ZZ Extirpation of Matter from Inferior Mesenteric Artery, Percutaneous Approach

04CB4ZZ Extirpation of Matter from Inferior Mesenteric Artery, Percutaneous Endoscopic Approach

04CC0ZZ Extirpation of Matter from Right Common Iliac Artery, Open Approach

04CC3ZZ Extirpation of Matter from Right Common Iliac Artery, Percutaneous Approach

04CC4ZZ Extirpation of Matter from Right Common Iliac Artery, Percutaneous Endoscopic Approach

04CD0ZZ Extirpation of Matter from Left Common Iliac Artery, Open Approach

04CD3ZZ Extirpation of Matter from Left Common Iliac Artery, Percutaneous Approach

04CD4ZZ Extirpation of Matter from Left Common Iliac Artery, Percutaneous Endoscopic Approach

04CE0ZZ Extirpation of Matter from Right Internal Iliac Artery, Open Approach

04CE3ZZ Extirpation of Matter from Right Internal Iliac Artery, Percutaneous Approach

04CE4ZZ Extirpation of Matter from Right Internal Iliac Artery, Percutaneous Endoscopic Approach

04CF0ZZ Extirpation of Matter from Left Internal Iliac Artery, Open Approach

04CF3ZZ Extirpation of Matter from Left Internal Iliac Artery, Percutaneous Approach

04CF4ZZ Extirpation of Matter from Left Internal Iliac Artery, Percutaneous Endoscopic Approach

04CH0ZZ Extirpation of Matter from Right External Iliac Artery, Open Approach

04CH3ZZ Extirpation of Matter from Right External Iliac Artery, Percutaneous Approach

04CH4ZZ Extirpation of Matter from Right External Iliac Artery, Percutaneous Endoscopic Approach

04CJ0ZZ Extirpation of Matter from Left External Iliac Artery, Open Approach

04CJ3ZZ Extirpation of Matter from Left External Iliac Artery, Percutaneous Approach

04CJ4ZZ Extirpation of Matter from Left External Iliac Artery, Percutaneous Endoscopic Approach

04CK0ZZ Extirpation of Matter from Right Femoral Artery, Open Approach

04CK3ZZ Extirpation of Matter from Right Femoral Artery, Percutaneous Approach

04CK4ZZ Extirpation of Matter from Right Femoral Artery, Percutaneous Endoscopic Approach

04CL0ZZ Extirpation of Matter from Left Femoral Artery, Open Approach

04CL3ZZ Extirpation of Matter from Left Femoral Artery, Percutaneous Approach

AHA CC: 1Q, 2015, 36

04CL4ZZ Extirpation of Matter from Left Femoral Artery, Percutaneous Endoscopic Approach

04CM0ZZ Extirpation of Matter from Right Popliteal Artery, Open Approach

04CM3ZZ Extirpation of Matter from Right Popliteal Artery, Percutaneous Approach

04CM4ZZ Extirpation of Matter from Right Popliteal Artery, Percutaneous Endoscopic Approach

04CN0ZZ Extirpation of Matter from Left Popliteal Artery, Open Approach

04CN3ZZ Extirpation of Matter from Left Popliteal Artery, Percutaneous Approach

04CN4ZZ Extirpation of Matter from Left Popliteal Artery, Percutaneous Endoscopic Approach

04CP0ZZ Extirpation of Matter from Right Anterior Tibial Artery, Open Approach

04CP3ZZ Extirpation of Matter from Right Anterior Tibial Artery, Percutaneous Approach

♀ Female-only   ♂ Male-only   ▲ Limited Coverage   ● Non-OR   ▬ HAC-associated procedure   ▲ Non-covered procedures   ✚ Combination

04CP4ZZ Extirpation of Matter from Right Anterior Tibial Artery, Percutaneous Endoscopic Approach

4CQ0ZZ Extirpation of Matter from Left Anterior Tibial Artery, Open Approach

4CQ3ZZ Extirpation of Matter from Left Anterior Tibial Artery, Percutaneous Approach

4CQ4ZZ Extirpation of Matter from Left Anterior Tibial Artery, Percutaneous Endoscopic Approach

4CR0ZZ Extirpation of Matter from Right Posterior Tibial Artery, Open Approach

4CR3ZZ Extirpation of Matter from Right Posterior Tibial Artery, Percutaneous Approach

4CR4ZZ Extirpation of Matter from Right Posterior Tibial Artery, Percutaneous Endoscopic Approach

4CS0ZZ Extirpation of Matter from Left Posterior Tibial Artery, Open Approach

04CS3ZZ Extirpation of Matter from Left Posterior Tibial Artery, Percutaneous Approach

04CS4ZZ Extirpation of Matter from Left Posterior Tibial Artery, Percutaneous Endoscopic Approach

04CT0ZZ Extirpation of Matter from Right Peroneal Artery, Open Approach

04CT3ZZ Extirpation of Matter from Right Peroneal Artery, Percutaneous Approach

04CT4ZZ Extirpation of Matter from Right Peroneal Artery, Percutaneous Endoscopic Approach

04CU0ZZ Extirpation of Matter from Left Peroneal Artery, Open Approach

04CU3ZZ Extirpation of Matter from Left Peroneal Artery, Percutaneous Approach

04CU4ZZ Extirpation of Matter from Left Peroneal Artery, Percutaneous Endoscopic Approach

04CV0ZZ Extirpation of Matter from Right Foot Artery, Open Approach

04CV3ZZ Extirpation of Matter from Right Foot Artery, Percutaneous Approach

04CV4ZZ Extirpation of Matter from Right Foot Artery, Percutaneous Endoscopic Approach

04CW0ZZ Extirpation of Matter from Left Foot Artery, Open Approach

04CW3ZZ Extirpation of Matter from Left Foot Artery, Percutaneous Approach

04CW4ZZ Extirpation of Matter from Left Foot Artery, Percutaneous Endoscopic Approach

04CY0ZZ Extirpation of Matter from Lower Artery, Open Approach

04CY3ZZ Extirpation of Matter from Lower Artery, Percutaneous Approach

04CY4ZZ Extirpation of Matter from Lower Artery, Percutaneous Endoscopic Approach

4H – Lower Arteries, Insertion

4H002Z Insertion of Monitoring Device into Abdominal Aorta, Open Approach

4H003Z Insertion of Infusion Device into Abdominal Aorta, Open Approach

4H00DZ Insertion of Intraluminal Device into Abdominal Aorta, Open Approach

4H032Z Insertion of Monitoring Device into Abdominal Aorta, Percutaneous Approach

4H033Z Insertion of Infusion Device into Abdominal Aorta, Percutaneous Approach

4H03DZ Insertion of Intraluminal Device into Abdominal Aorta, Percutaneous Approach

4H042Z Insertion of Monitoring Device into Abdominal Aorta, Percutaneous Endoscopic Approach

4H043Z Insertion of Infusion Device into Abdominal Aorta, Percutaneous Endoscopic Approach

4H04DZ Insertion of Intraluminal Device into Abdominal Aorta, Percutaneous Endoscopic Approach

4H103Z Insertion of Infusion Device into Celiac Artery, Open Approach

4H110DZ Insertion of Intraluminal Device into Celiac Artery, Open Approach

4H133Z Insertion of Infusion Device into Celiac Artery, Percutaneous Approach

4H13DZ Insertion of Intraluminal Device into Celiac Artery, Percutaneous Approach

4H143Z Insertion of Infusion Device into Celiac Artery, Percutaneous Endoscopic Approach

4H14DZ Insertion of Intraluminal Device into Celiac Artery, Percutaneous Endoscopic Approach

04H203Z Insertion of Infusion Device into Gastric Artery, Open Approach

4H20DZ Insertion of Intraluminal Device into Gastric Artery, Open Approach

4H233Z Insertion of Infusion Device into Gastric Artery, Percutaneous Approach

4H23DZ Insertion of Intraluminal Device into Gastric Artery, Percutaneous Approach

4H243Z Insertion of Infusion Device into Gastric Artery, Percutaneous Endoscopic Approach

4H24DZ Insertion of Intraluminal Device into Gastric Artery, Percutaneous Endoscopic Approach

4H303Z Insertion of Infusion Device into Hepatic Artery, Open Approach

04H30DZ Insertion of Intraluminal Device into Hepatic Artery, Open Approach

04H333Z Insertion of Infusion Device into Hepatic Artery, Percutaneous Approach

04H33DZ Insertion of Intraluminal Device into Hepatic Artery, Percutaneous Approach

04H343Z Insertion of Infusion Device into Hepatic Artery, Percutaneous Endoscopic Approach

04H34DZ Insertion of Intraluminal Device into Hepatic Artery, Percutaneous Endoscopic Approach

04H403Z Insertion of Infusion Device into Splenic Artery, Open Approach

04H40DZ Insertion of Intraluminal Device into Splenic Artery, Open Approach

04H433Z Insertion of Infusion Device into Splenic Artery, Percutaneous Approach

04H43DZ Insertion of Intraluminal Device into Splenic Artery, Percutaneous Approach

04H443Z Insertion of Infusion Device into Splenic Artery, Percutaneous Endoscopic Approach

04H44DZ Insertion of Intraluminal Device into Splenic Artery, Percutaneous Endoscopic Approach

04H503Z Insertion of Infusion Device into Superior Mesenteric Artery, Open Approach

04H50DZ Insertion of Intraluminal Device into Superior Mesenteric Artery, Open Approach

04H533Z Insertion of Infusion Device into Superior Mesenteric Artery, Percutaneous Approach

04H53DZ Insertion of Intraluminal Device into Superior Mesenteric Artery, Percutaneous Approach

04H543Z Insertion of Infusion Device into Superior Mesenteric Artery, Percutaneous Endoscopic Approach

04H54DZ Insertion of Intraluminal Device into Superior Mesenteric Artery, Percutaneous Endoscopic Approach

04H603Z Insertion of Infusion Device into Right Colic Artery, Open Approach

04H60DZ Insertion of Intraluminal Device into Right Colic Artery, Open Approach

04H633Z Insertion of Infusion Device into Right Colic Artery, Percutaneous Approach

04H63DZ Insertion of Intraluminal Device into Right Colic Artery, Percutaneous Approach

04H643Z Insertion of Infusion Device into Right Colic Artery, Percutaneous Endoscopic Approach

04H64DZ Insertion of Intraluminal Device into Right Colic Artery, Percutaneous Endoscopic Approach

04H703Z Insertion of Infusion Device into Left Colic Artery, Open Approach

04H70DZ Insertion of Intraluminal Device into Left Colic Artery, Open Approach

04H733Z Insertion of Infusion Device into Left Colic Artery, Percutaneous Approach

04H73DZ Insertion of Intraluminal Device into Left Colic Artery, Percutaneous Approach

04H743Z Insertion of Infusion Device into Left Colic Artery, Percutaneous Endoscopic Approach

04H74DZ Insertion of Intraluminal Device into Left Colic Artery, Percutaneous Endoscopic Approach

04H803Z Insertion of Infusion Device into Middle Colic Artery, Open Approach

04H80DZ Insertion of Intraluminal Device into Middle Colic Artery, Open Approach

04H833Z Insertion of Infusion Device into Middle Colic Artery, Percutaneous Approach

04H83DZ Insertion of Intraluminal Device into Middle Colic Artery, Percutaneous Approach

04H843Z Insertion of Infusion Device into Middle Colic Artery, Percutaneous Endoscopic Approach

04H84DZ Insertion of Intraluminal Device into Middle Colic Artery, Percutaneous Endoscopic Approach

04H903Z Insertion of Infusion Device into Right Renal Artery, Open Approach

04H90DZ Insertion of Intraluminal Device into Right Renal Artery, Open Approach

04H933Z Insertion of Infusion Device into Right Renal Artery, Percutaneous Approach

04H93DZ Insertion of Intraluminal Device into Right Renal Artery, Percutaneous Approach

04H943Z Insertion of Infusion Device into Right Renal Artery, Percutaneous Endoscopic Approach

04H94DZ Insertion of Intraluminal Device into Right Renal Artery, Percutaneous Endoscopic Approach

04HA03Z Insertion of Infusion Device into Left Renal Artery, Open Approach

♀ Female-only ♂ Male-only ▲ Limited Coverage ● Non-OR ▥ HAC-associated procedure ▲ Non-covered procedures ✚ Combination

04HA0DZ Insertion of Intraluminal Device into Left Renal Artery, Open Approach

04HA33Z Insertion of Infusion Device into Left Renal Artery, Percutaneous Approach

04HA3DZ Insertion of Intraluminal Device into Left Renal Artery, Percutaneous Approach

04HA43Z Insertion of Infusion Device into Left Renal Artery, Percutaneous Endoscopic Approach

04HA4DZ Insertion of Intraluminal Device into Left Renal Artery, Percutaneous Endoscopic Approach

04HB03Z Insertion of Infusion Device into Inferior Mesenteric Artery, Open Approach

04HB0DZ Insertion of Intraluminal Device into Inferior Mesenteric Artery, Open Approach

04HB33Z Insertion of Infusion Device into Inferior Mesenteric Artery, Percutaneous Approach

04HB3DZ Insertion of Intraluminal Device into Inferior Mesenteric Artery, Percutaneous Approach

04HB43Z Insertion of Infusion Device into Inferior Mesenteric Artery, Percutaneous Endoscopic Approach

04HB4DZ Insertion of Intraluminal Device into Inferior Mesenteric Artery, Percutaneous Endoscopic Approach

04HC03Z Insertion of Infusion Device into Right Common Iliac Artery, Open Approach

04HC0DZ Insertion of Intraluminal Device into Right Common Iliac Artery, Open Approach

04HC33Z Insertion of Infusion Device into Right Common Iliac Artery, Percutaneous Approach

04HC3DZ Insertion of Intraluminal Device into Right Common Iliac Artery, Percutaneous Approach

04HC43Z Insertion of Infusion Device into Right Common Iliac Artery, Percutaneous Endoscopic Approach

04HC4DZ Insertion of Intraluminal Device into Right Common Iliac Artery, Percutaneous Endoscopic Approach

04HD03Z Insertion of Infusion Device into Left Common Iliac Artery, Open Approach

04HD0DZ Insertion of Intraluminal Device into Left Common Iliac Artery, Open Approach

04HD33Z Insertion of Infusion Device into Left Common Iliac Artery, Percutaneous Approach

04HD3DZ Insertion of Intraluminal Device into Left Common Iliac Artery, Percutaneous Approach

04HD43Z Insertion of Infusion Device into Left Common Iliac Artery, Percutaneous Endoscopic Approach

04HD4DZ Insertion of Intraluminal Device into Left Common Iliac Artery, Percutaneous Endoscopic Approach

04HE03Z Insertion of Infusion Device into Right Internal Iliac Artery, Open Approach

04HE0DZ Insertion of Intraluminal Device into Right Internal Iliac Artery, Open Approach

04HE33Z Insertion of Infusion Device into Right Internal Iliac Artery, Percutaneous Approach

04HE3DZ Insertion of Intraluminal Device into Right Internal Iliac Artery, Percutaneous Approach

04HE43Z Insertion of Infusion Device into Right Internal Iliac Artery, Percutaneous Endoscopic Approach

04HE4DZ Insertion of Intraluminal Device into Right Internal Iliac Artery, Percutaneous Endoscopic Approach

04HF03Z Insertion of Infusion Device into Left Internal Iliac Artery, Open Approach

04HF0DZ Insertion of Intraluminal Device into Left Internal Iliac Artery, Open Approach

04HF33Z Insertion of Infusion Device into Left Internal Iliac Artery, Percutaneous Approach

04HF3DZ Insertion of Intraluminal Device into Left Internal Iliac Artery, Percutaneous Approach

04HF43Z Insertion of Infusion Device into Left Internal Iliac Artery, Percutaneous Endoscopic Approach

04HF4DZ Insertion of Intraluminal Device into Left Internal Iliac Artery, Percutaneous Endoscopic Approach

04HH03Z Insertion of Infusion Device into Right External Iliac Artery, Open Approach

04HH0DZ Insertion of Intraluminal Device into Right External Iliac Artery, Open Approach

04HH33Z Insertion of Infusion Device into Right External Iliac Artery, Percutaneous Approach

04HH3DZ Insertion of Intraluminal Device into Right External Iliac Artery, Percutaneous Approach

04HH43Z Insertion of Infusion Device into Right External Iliac Artery, Percutaneous Endoscopic Approach

04HH4DZ Insertion of Intraluminal Device into Right External Iliac Artery, Percutaneous Endoscopic Approach

04HJ03Z Insertion of Infusion Device into Left External Iliac Artery, Open Approach

04HJ0DZ Insertion of Intraluminal Device into Left External Iliac Artery, Open Approach

04HJ33Z Insertion of Infusion Device into Left External Iliac Artery, Percutaneous Approach

04HJ3DZ Insertion of Intraluminal Device into Left External Iliac Artery, Percutaneous Approach

04HJ43Z Insertion of Infusion Device into Left External Iliac Artery, Percutaneous Endoscopic Approach

04HJ4DZ Insertion of Intraluminal Device into Left External Iliac Artery, Percutaneous Endoscopic Approach

04HK03Z Insertion of Infusion Device into Right Femoral Artery, Open Approach

04HK0DZ Insertion of Intraluminal Device into Right Femoral Artery, Open Approach

04HK33Z Insertion of Infusion Device into Right Femoral Artery, Percutaneous Approach

04HK3DZ Insertion of Intraluminal Device into Right Femoral Artery, Percutaneous Approach

04HK43Z Insertion of Infusion Device into Right Femoral Artery, Percutaneous Endoscopic Approach

04HK4DZ Insertion of Intraluminal Device into Right Femoral Artery, Percutaneous Endoscopic Approach

04HL03Z Insertion of Infusion Device into Left Femoral Artery, Open Approach

04HL0DZ Insertion of Intraluminal Device into Left Femoral Artery, Open Approach

04HL33Z Insertion of Infusion Device into Left Femoral Artery, Percutaneous Approach

04HL3DZ Insertion of Intraluminal Device into Left Femoral Artery, Percutaneous Approach

04HL43Z Insertion of Infusion Device into Left Femoral Artery, Percutaneous Endoscopic Approach

04HL4DZ Insertion of Intraluminal Device into Left Femoral Artery, Percutaneous Endoscopic Approach

04HM03Z Insertion of Infusion Device into Right Popliteal Artery, Open Approach

04HM0DZ Insertion of Intraluminal Device into Right Popliteal Artery, Open Approach

04HM33Z Insertion of Infusion Device into Right Popliteal Artery, Percutaneous Approach

04HM3DZ Insertion of Intraluminal Device into Right Popliteal Artery, Percutaneous Approach

04HM43Z Insertion of Infusion Device into Right Popliteal Artery, Percutaneous Endoscopic Approach

04HM4DZ Insertion of Intraluminal Device into Right Popliteal Artery, Percutaneous Endoscopic Approach

04HN03Z Insertion of Infusion Device into Left Popliteal Artery, Open Approach

04HN0DZ Insertion of Intraluminal Device into Left Popliteal Artery, Open Approach

04HN33Z Insertion of Infusion Device into Left Popliteal Artery, Percutaneous Approach

04HN3DZ Insertion of Intraluminal Device into Left Popliteal Artery, Percutaneous Approach

04HN43Z Insertion of Infusion Device into Left Popliteal Artery, Percutaneous Endoscopic Approach

04HN4DZ Insertion of Intraluminal Device into Left Popliteal Artery, Percutaneous Endoscopic Approach

04HP03Z Insertion of Infusion Device into Right Anterior Tibial Artery, Open Approach

04HP0DZ Insertion of Intraluminal Device into Right Anterior Tibial Artery, Open Approach

04HP33Z Insertion of Infusion Device into Right Anterior Tibial Artery, Percutaneous Approach

04HP3DZ Insertion of Intraluminal Device into Right Anterior Tibial Artery, Percutaneous Approach

04HP43Z Insertion of Infusion Device into Right Anterior Tibial Artery, Percutaneous Endoscopic Approach

04HP4DZ Insertion of Intraluminal Device into Right Anterior Tibial Artery, Percutaneous Endoscopic Approach

04HQ03Z Insertion of Infusion Device into Left Anterior Tibial Artery, Open Approach

04HQ0DZ Insertion of Intraluminal Device into Left Anterior Tibial Artery, Open Approach

04HQ33Z Insertion of Infusion Device into Left Anterior Tibial Artery, Percutaneous Approach

04HQ3DZ Insertion of Intraluminal Device into Left Anterior Tibial Artery, Percutaneous Approach

04HQ43Z Insertion of Infusion Device into Left Anterior Tibial Artery, Percutaneous Endoscopic Approach

04HQ4DZ Insertion of Intraluminal Device into Left Anterior Tibial Artery, Percutaneous Endoscopic Approach

04HR03Z Insertion of Infusion Device into Right Posterior Tibial Artery, Open Approach

04HR0DZ Insertion of Intraluminal Device into Right Posterior Tibial Artery, Open Approach

04HR33Z Insertion of Infusion Device into Right Posterior Tibial Artery, Percutaneous Approach

04HR3DZ Insertion of Intraluminal Device into Right Posterior Tibial Artery, Percutaneous Approach

04HR43Z Insertion of Infusion Device into Right Posterior Tibial Artery, Percutaneous Endoscopic Approach

04HR4DZ Insertion of Intraluminal Device into Right Posterior Tibial Artery, Percutaneous Endoscopic Approach

04HS03Z Insertion of Infusion Device into Left Posterior Tibial Artery, Open Approach

♀ Female-only   ♂ Male-only   ▲ Limited Coverage   ● Non-OR   ▦ HAC-associated procedure   ▲ Non-covered procedures   ✚ Combination

0DZ Insertion of Intraluminal Device into Left Posterior Tibial Artery, Open Approach

S33Z Insertion of Infusion Device into Left Posterior Tibial Artery, Percutaneous Approach

S3DZ Insertion of Intraluminal Device into Left Posterior Tibial Artery, Percutaneous Approach

S43Z Insertion of Infusion Device into Left Posterior Tibial Artery, Percutaneous Endoscopic Approach

S4DZ Insertion of Intraluminal Device into Left Posterior Tibial Artery, Percutaneous Endoscopic Approach

T03Z Insertion of Infusion Device into Right Peroneal Artery, Open Approach

T0DZ Insertion of Intraluminal Device into Right Peroneal Artery, Open Approach

T33Z Insertion of Infusion Device into Right Peroneal Artery, Percutaneous Approach

T3DZ Insertion of Intraluminal Device into Right Peroneal Artery, Percutaneous Approach

T43Z Insertion of Infusion Device into Right Peroneal Artery, Percutaneous Endoscopic Approach

T4DZ Insertion of Intraluminal Device into Right Peroneal Artery, Percutaneous Endoscopic Approach

U03Z Insertion of Infusion Device into Left Peroneal Artery, Open Approach

04HU0DZ Insertion of Intraluminal Device into Left Peroneal Artery, Open Approach

04HU33Z Insertion of Infusion Device into Left Peroneal Artery, Percutaneous Approach

04HU3DZ Insertion of Intraluminal Device into Left Peroneal Artery, Percutaneous Approach

04HU43Z Insertion of Infusion Device into Left Peroneal Artery, Percutaneous Endoscopic Approach

04HU4DZ Insertion of Intraluminal Device into Left Peroneal Artery, Percutaneous Endoscopic Approach

04HV03Z Insertion of Infusion Device into Right Foot Artery, Open Approach

04HV0DZ Insertion of Intraluminal Device into Right Foot Artery, Open Approach

04HV33Z Insertion of Infusion Device into Right Foot Artery, Percutaneous Approach

04HV3DZ Insertion of Intraluminal Device into Right Foot Artery, Percutaneous Approach

04HV43Z Insertion of Infusion Device into Right Foot Artery, Percutaneous Endoscopic Approach

04HV4DZ Insertion of Intraluminal Device into Right Foot Artery, Percutaneous Endoscopic Approach

04HW03Z Insertion of Infusion Device into Left Foot Artery, Open Approach

04HW0DZ Insertion of Intraluminal Device into Left Foot Artery, Open Approach

04HW33Z Insertion of Infusion Device into Left Foot Artery, Percutaneous Approach

04HW3DZ Insertion of Intraluminal Device into Left Foot Artery, Percutaneous Approach

04HW43Z Insertion of Infusion Device into Left Foot Artery, Percutaneous Endoscopic Approach

04HW4DZ Insertion of Intraluminal Device into Left Foot Artery, Percutaneous Endoscopic Approach

04HY02Z Insertion of Monitoring Device into Lower Artery, Open Approach

04HY03Z Insertion of Infusion Device into Lower Artery, Open Approach

04HY0DZ Insertion of Intraluminal Device into Lower Artery, Open Approach

04HY32Z Insertion of Monitoring Device into Lower Artery, Percutaneous Approach

04HY33Z Insertion of Infusion Device into Lower Artery, Percutaneous Approach

04HY3DZ Insertion of Intraluminal Device into Lower Artery, Percutaneous Approach

04HY42Z Insertion of Monitoring Device into Lower Artery, Percutaneous Endoscopic Approach

04HY43Z Insertion of Infusion Device into Lower Artery, Percutaneous Endoscopic Approach

04HY4DZ Insertion of Intraluminal Device into Lower Artery, Percutaneous Endoscopic Approach

J – Lower Arteries, Inspection

view Coding Guidelines B3.11a, B3.11b and B3.11c

JY0ZZ Inspection of Lower Artery, Open Approach

JY3ZZ Inspection of Lower Artery, Percutaneous Approach

04JY4ZZ Inspection of Lower Artery, Percutaneous Endoscopic Approach

04JYXZZ Inspection of Lower Artery, External Approach

L – Lower Arteries, Occlusion

view Coding Guideline B3.12

L00CZ Occlusion of Abdominal Aorta with Extraluminal Device, Open Approach

L00DZ Occlusion of Abdominal Aorta with Intraluminal Device, Open Approach

L00ZZ Occlusion of Abdominal Aorta, Open Approach

L03CZ Occlusion of Abdominal Aorta with Extraluminal Device, Percutaneous Approach

L03DZ Occlusion of Abdominal Aorta with Intraluminal Device, Percutaneous Approach

L03ZZ Occlusion of Abdominal Aorta, Percutaneous Approach

L04CZ Occlusion of Abdominal Aorta with Extraluminal Device, Percutaneous Endoscopic Approach

L04DZ Occlusion of Abdominal Aorta with Intraluminal Device, Percutaneous Endoscopic Approach

L04ZZ Occlusion of Abdominal Aorta, Percutaneous Endoscopic Approach

L10CZ Occlusion of Celiac Artery with Extraluminal Device, Open Approach

L10DZ Occlusion of Celiac Artery with Intraluminal Device, Open Approach

L10ZZ Occlusion of Celiac Artery, Open Approach

L13CZ Occlusion of Celiac Artery with Extraluminal Device, Percutaneous Approach

04L13DZ Occlusion of Celiac Artery with Intraluminal Device, Percutaneous Approach

04L13ZZ Occlusion of Celiac Artery, Percutaneous Approach

04L14CZ Occlusion of Celiac Artery with Extraluminal Device, Percutaneous Endoscopic Approach

04L14DZ Occlusion of Celiac Artery with Intraluminal Device, Percutaneous Endoscopic Approach

04L14ZZ Occlusion of Celiac Artery, Percutaneous Endoscopic Approach

04L20CZ Occlusion of Gastric Artery with Extraluminal Device, Open Approach

04L20DZ Occlusion of Gastric Artery with Intraluminal Device, Open Approach

04L20ZZ Occlusion of Gastric Artery, Open Approach

04L23CZ Occlusion of Gastric Artery with Extraluminal Device, Percutaneous Approach

04L23DZ Occlusion of Gastric Artery with Intraluminal Device, Percutaneous Approach

04L23ZZ Occlusion of Gastric Artery, Percutaneous Approach

04L24CZ Occlusion of Gastric Artery with Extraluminal Device, Percutaneous Endoscopic Approach

04L24DZ Occlusion of Gastric Artery with Intraluminal Device, Percutaneous Endoscopic Approach

04L24ZZ Occlusion of Gastric Artery, Percutaneous Endoscopic Approach

04L30CZ Occlusion of Hepatic Artery with Extraluminal Device, Open Approach

04L30DZ Occlusion of Hepatic Artery with Intraluminal Device, Open Approach

04L30ZZ Occlusion of Hepatic Artery, Open Approach

04L33CZ Occlusion of Hepatic Artery with Extraluminal Device, Percutaneous Approach

04L33DZ Occlusion of Hepatic Artery with Intraluminal Device, Percutaneous Approach

AHA CC: 3Q, 2014, 26-27

04L33ZZ Occlusion of Hepatic Artery, Percutaneous Approach

04L34CZ Occlusion of Hepatic Artery with Extraluminal Device, Percutaneous Endoscopic Approach

04L34DZ Occlusion of Hepatic Artery with Intraluminal Device, Percutaneous Endoscopic Approach

04L34ZZ Occlusion of Hepatic Artery, Percutaneous Endoscopic Approach

04L40CZ Occlusion of Splenic Artery with Extraluminal Device, Open Approach

04L40DZ Occlusion of Splenic Artery with Intraluminal Device, Open Approach

04L40ZZ Occlusion of Splenic Artery, Open Approach

04L43CZ Occlusion of Splenic Artery with Extraluminal Device, Percutaneous Approach

04L43DZ Occlusion of Splenic Artery with Intraluminal Device, Percutaneous Approach

04L43ZZ Occlusion of Splenic Artery, Percutaneous Approach

04L44CZ Occlusion of Splenic Artery with Extraluminal Device, Percutaneous Endoscopic Approach

04L44DZ Occlusion of Splenic Artery with Intraluminal Device, Percutaneous Endoscopic Approach

04L44ZZ Occlusion of Splenic Artery, Percutaneous Endoscopic Approach

04L50CZ Occlusion of Superior Mesenteric Artery with Extraluminal Device, Open Approach

04L50DZ Occlusion of Superior Mesenteric Artery with Intraluminal Device, Open Approach

04L50ZZ Occlusion of Superior Mesenteric Artery, Open Approach

04L53CZ Occlusion of Superior Mesenteric Artery with Extraluminal Device, Percutaneous Approach

04L53DZ Occlusion of Superior Mesenteric Artery with Intraluminal Device, Percutaneous Approach

04L53ZZ Occlusion of Superior Mesenteric Artery, Percutaneous Approach

04L54CZ Occlusion of Superior Mesenteric Artery with Extraluminal Device, Percutaneous Endoscopic Approach

04L54DZ Occlusion of Superior Mesenteric Artery with Intraluminal Device, Percutaneous Endoscopic Approach

04L54ZZ Occlusion of Superior Mesenteric Artery, Percutaneous Endoscopic Approach

04L60CZ Occlusion of Right Colic Artery with Extraluminal Device, Open Approach

04L60DZ Occlusion of Right Colic Artery with Intraluminal Device, Open Approach

04L60ZZ Occlusion of Right Colic Artery, Open Approach

04L63CZ Occlusion of Right Colic Artery with Extraluminal Device, Percutaneous Approach

04L63DZ Occlusion of Right Colic Artery with Intraluminal Device, Percutaneous Approach

04L63ZZ Occlusion of Right Colic Artery, Percutaneous Approach

04L64CZ Occlusion of Right Colic Artcry with Extraluminal Device, Percutaneous Endoscopic Approach

04L64DZ Occlusion of Right Colic Artery with Intraluminal Device, Percutaneous Endoscopic Approach

04L64ZZ Occlusion of Right Colic Artery, Percutaneous Endoscopic Approach

04L70CZ Occlusion of Left Colic Artery with Extraluminal Device, Open Approach

04L70DZ Occlusion of Left Colic Artery with Intraluminal Device, Open Approach

04L70ZZ Occlusion of Left Colic Artery, Open Approach

04L73CZ Occlusion of Left Colic Artery with Extraluminal Device, Percutaneous Approach

04L73DZ Occlusion of Left Colic Artery with Intraluminal Device, Percutaneous Approach
AHA CC: 1Q, 2014, 24

04L73ZZ Occlusion of Left Colic Artery, Percutaneous Approach

04L74CZ Occlusion of Left Colic Artery with Extraluminal Device, Percutaneous Endoscopic Approach

04L74DZ Occlusion of Left Colic Artery with Intraluminal Device, Percutaneous Endoscopic Approach

04L74ZZ Occlusion of Left Colic Artery, Percutaneous Endoscopic Approach

04L80CZ Occlusion of Middle Colic Artery with Extraluminal Device, Open Approach

04L80DZ Occlusion of Middle Colic Artery with Intraluminal Device, Open Approach

04L80ZZ Occlusion of Middle Colic Artery, Open Approach

04L83CZ Occlusion of Middle Colic Artery with Extraluminal Device, Percutaneous Approach

04L83DZ Occlusion of Middle Colic Artery with Intraluminal Device, Percutaneous Approach

04L83ZZ Occlusion of Middle Colic Artery, Percutaneous Approach

04L84CZ Occlusion of Middle Colic Artery with Extraluminal Device, Percutaneous Endoscopic Approach

04L84DZ Occlusion of Middle Colic Artery with Intraluminal Device, Percutaneous Endoscopic Approach

04L84ZZ Occlusion of Middle Colic Artery, Percutaneous Endoscopic Approach

04L90CZ Occlusion of Right Renal Artery with Extraluminal Device, Open Approach

04L90DZ Occlusion of Right Renal Artery with Intraluminal Device, Open Approach

04L90ZZ Occlusion of Right Renal Artery, Open Approach

04L93CZ Occlusion of Right Renal Artery with Extraluminal Device, Percutaneous Approach

04L93DZ Occlusion of Right Renal Artery with Intraluminal Device, Percutaneous Approach

04L93ZZ Occlusion of Right Renal Artery, Percutaneous Approach

04L94CZ Occlusion of Right Renal Artery with Extraluminal Device, Percutaneous Endoscopic Approach

04L94DZ Occlusion of Right Renal Artery with Intraluminal Device, Percutaneous Endoscopic Approach

04L94ZZ Occlusion of Right Renal Artery, Percutaneous Endoscopic Approach

04LA0CZ Occlusion of Left Renal Artery with Extraluminal Device, Open Approach

04LA0DZ Occlusion of Left Renal Artery with Intraluminal Device, Open Approach

04LA0ZZ Occlusion of Left Renal Artery, Open Approach

04LA3CZ Occlusion of Left Renal Artery with Extraluminal Device, Percutaneous Approach

04LA3DZ Occlusion of Left Renal Artery with Intraluminal Device, Percutaneous Approach

04LA3ZZ Occlusion of Left Renal Artery, Percutaneous Approach

04LA4CZ Occlusion of Left Renal Artery with Extraluminal Device, Percutaneous Endoscopic Approach

04LA4DZ Occlusion of Left Renal Artery with Intraluminal Device, Percutaneous Endoscopic Approach

04LA4ZZ Occlusion of Left Renal Artery, Percutaneous Endoscopic Approach

04LB0CZ Occlusion of Inferior Mesenteric Artery with Extraluminal Device, Open Approach

04LB0DZ Occlusion of Inferior Mesenteric Artery with Intraluminal Device, Open Approach

04LB0ZZ Occlusion of Inferior Mesenteric Artery, Open Approach

04LB3CZ Occlusion of Inferior Mesenteric Artery with Extraluminal Device, Percutaneous Approach

04LB3DZ Occlusion of Inferior Mesenteric Artery with Intraluminal Device, Percutaneous Approach
AHA CC: 1Q, 2014, 24

04LB3ZZ Occlusion of Inferior Mesenteric Artery, Percutaneous Approach

04LB4CZ Occlusion of Inferior Mesenteric Artery with Extraluminal Device, Percutaneous Endoscopic Approach

04LB4DZ Occlusion of Inferior Mesenteric Artery with Intraluminal Device, Percutaneous Endoscopic Approach

04LB4ZZ Occlusion of Inferior Mesenteric Artery, Percutaneous Endoscopic Approach

04LC0CZ Occlusion of Right Common Iliac Artery with Extraluminal Device, Open Approach

04LC0DZ Occlusion of Right Common Iliac Artery with Intraluminal Device, Open Approach

04LC0ZZ Occlusion of Right Common Iliac Artery, Open Approach

04LC3CZ Occlusion of Right Common Iliac Artery with Extraluminal Device, Percutaneous Approach

04LC3DZ Occlusion of Right Common Iliac Artery with Intraluminal Device, Percutaneous Approach

04LC3ZZ Occlusion of Right Common Iliac Artery, Percutaneous Approach

04LC4CZ Occlusion of Right Common Iliac Artery with Extraluminal Device, Percutaneous Endoscopic Approach

04LC4DZ Occlusion of Right Common Iliac Artery with Intraluminal Device, Percutaneous Endoscopic Approach

04LC4ZZ Occlusion of Right Common Iliac Artery, Percutaneous Endoscopic Approach

04LD0CZ Occlusion of Left Common Iliac Artery with Extraluminal Device, Open Approach

04LD0DZ Occlusion of Left Common Iliac Artery with Intraluminal Device, Open Approach

04LD0ZZ Occlusion of Left Common Iliac Artery, Open Approach

04LD3CZ Occlusion of Left Common Iliac Artery with Extraluminal Device, Percutaneous Approach

04LD3DZ Occlusion of Left Common Iliac Artery with Intraluminal Device, Percutaneous Approach

04LD3ZZ Occlusion of Left Common Iliac Artery, Percutaneous Approach

04LD4CZ Occlusion of Left Common Iliac Artery with Extraluminal Device, Percutaneous Endoscopic Approach

04LD4DZ Occlusion of Left Common Iliac Artery with Intraluminal Device, Percutaneous Endoscopic Approach

04LD4ZZ Occlusion of Left Common Iliac Artery, Percutaneous Endoscopic Approach

♀ 04LE0CT Occlusion of Right Uterine Artery with Extraluminal Device, Open Approach

04LE0CZ Occlusion of Right Internal Iliac Artery with Extraluminal Device, Open Approach

♀ 04LE0DT Occlusion of Right Uterine Artery with Intraluminal Device, Open Approach

04LE0DZ Occlusion of Right Internal Iliac Artery with Intraluminal Device, Open Approach

♀ 04LE0ZT Occlusion of Right Uterine Artery, Open Approach

04LE0ZZ Occlusion of Right Internal Iliac Artery, Open Approach

♀ 04LE3CT Occlusion of Right Uterine Artery with Extraluminal Device, Percutaneous Approach

Medical and Surgical, Lower Arteries Code Listings

E3CZ Occlusion of Right Internal Iliac Artery with Extraluminal Device, Percutaneous Approach

LE3DT Occlusion of Right Uterine Artery with Intraluminal Device, Percutaneous Approach

E3DZ Occlusion of Right Internal Iliac Artery with Intraluminal Device, Percutaneous Approach

LE3ZT Occlusion of Right Uterine Artery, Percutaneous Approach

E3ZZ Occlusion of Right Internal Iliac Artery, Percutaneous Approach

LE4CT Occlusion of Right Uterine Artery with Extraluminal Device, Percutaneous Endoscopic Approach

E4CZ Occlusion of Right Internal Iliac Artery with Extraluminal Device, Percutaneous Endoscopic Approach

LE4DT Occlusion of Right Uterine Artery with Intraluminal Device, Percutaneous Endoscopic Approach

E4DZ Occlusion of Right Internal Iliac Artery with Intraluminal Device, Percutaneous Endoscopic Approach

LE4ZT Occlusion of Right Uterine Artery, Percutaneous Endoscopic Approach

E4ZZ Occlusion of Right Internal Iliac Artery, Percutaneous Endoscopic Approach

LF0CU Occlusion of Left Uterine Artery with Extraluminal Device, Open Approach

F0CZ Occlusion of Left Internal Iliac Artery with Extraluminal Device, Open Approach

LF0DU Occlusion of Left Uterine Artery with Intraluminal Device, Open Approach

F0DZ Occlusion of Left Internal Iliac Artery with Intraluminal Device, Open Approach

LF0ZU Occlusion of Left Uterine Artery, Open Approach

F0ZZ Occlusion of Left Internal Iliac Artery, Open Approach

LF3CU Occlusion of Left Uterine Artery with Extraluminal Device, Percutaneous Approach

LF3CZ Occlusion of Left Internal Iliac Artery with Extraluminal Device, Percutaneous Approach

LF3DU Occlusion of Left Uterine Artery with Intraluminal Device, Percutaneous Approach

LF3DZ Occlusion of Left Internal Iliac Artery with Intraluminal Device, Percutaneous Approach

LF3ZU Occlusion of Left Uterine Artery, Percutaneous Approach

LF3ZZ Occlusion of Left Internal Iliac Artery, Percutaneous Approach

LF4CU Occlusion of Left Uterine Artery with Extraluminal Device, Percutaneous Endoscopic Approach

LF4CZ Occlusion of Left Internal Iliac Artery with Extraluminal Device, Percutaneous Endoscopic Approach

LF4DU Occlusion of Left Uterine Artery with Intraluminal Device, Percutaneous Endoscopic Approach

LF4DZ Occlusion of Left Internal Iliac Artery with Intraluminal Device, Percutaneous Endoscopic Approach

LF4ZU Occlusion of Left Uterine Artery, Percutaneous Endoscopic Approach

LF4ZZ Occlusion of Left Internal Iliac Artery, Percutaneous Endoscopic Approach

LH0CZ Occlusion of Right External Iliac Artery with Extraluminal Device, Open Approach

04LH0DZ Occlusion of Right External Iliac Artery with Intraluminal Device, Open Approach

04LH0ZZ Occlusion of Right External Iliac Artery, Open Approach

04LH3CZ Occlusion of Right External Iliac Artery with Extraluminal Device, Percutaneous Approach

04LH3DZ Occlusion of Right External Iliac Artery with Intraluminal Device, Percutaneous Approach

04LH3ZZ Occlusion of Right External Iliac Artery, Percutaneous Approach

04LH4CZ Occlusion of Right External Iliac Artery with Extraluminal Device, Percutaneous Endoscopic Approach

04LH4DZ Occlusion of Right External Iliac Artery with Intraluminal Device, Percutaneous Endoscopic Approach

04LH4ZZ Occlusion of Right External Iliac Artery, Percutaneous Endoscopic Approach

04LJ0CZ Occlusion of Left External Iliac Artery with Extraluminal Device, Open Approach

04LJ0DZ Occlusion of Left External Iliac Artery with Intraluminal Device, Open Approach

04LJ0ZZ Occlusion of Left External Iliac Artery, Open Approach

04LJ3CZ Occlusion of Left External Iliac Artery with Extraluminal Device, Percutaneous Approach

04LJ3DZ Occlusion of Left External Iliac Artery with Intraluminal Device, Percutaneous Approach

04LJ3ZZ Occlusion of Left External Iliac Artery, Percutaneous Approach

04LJ4CZ Occlusion of Left External Iliac Artery with Extraluminal Device, Percutaneous Endoscopic Approach

04LJ4DZ Occlusion of Left External Iliac Artery with Intraluminal Device, Percutaneous Endoscopic Approach

04LJ4ZZ Occlusion of Left External Iliac Artery, Percutaneous Endoscopic Approach

04LK0CZ Occlusion of Right Femoral Artery with Extraluminal Device, Open Approach

04LK0DZ Occlusion of Right Femoral Artery with Intraluminal Device, Open Approach

04LK0ZZ Occlusion of Right Femoral Artery, Open Approach

04LK3CZ Occlusion of Right Femoral Artery with Extraluminal Device, Percutaneous Approach

04LK3DZ Occlusion of Right Femoral Artery with Intraluminal Device, Percutaneous Approach

04LK3ZZ Occlusion of Right Femoral Artery, Percutaneous Approach

04LK4CZ Occlusion of Right Femoral Artery with Extraluminal Device, Percutaneous Endoscopic Approach

04LK4DZ Occlusion of Right Femoral Artery with Intraluminal Device, Percutaneous Endoscopic Approach

04LK4ZZ Occlusion of Right Femoral Artery, Percutaneous Endoscopic Approach

04LL0CZ Occlusion of Left Femoral Artery with Extraluminal Device, Open Approach

04LL0DZ Occlusion of Left Femoral Artery with Intraluminal Device, Open Approach

04LL0ZZ Occlusion of Left Femoral Artery, Open Approach

04LL3CZ Occlusion of Left Femoral Artery with Extraluminal Device, Percutaneous Approach

04LL3DZ Occlusion of Left Femoral Artery with Intraluminal Device, Percutaneous Approach

04LL3ZZ Occlusion of Left Femoral Artery, Percutaneous Approach

04LL4CZ Occlusion of Left Femoral Artery with Extraluminal Device, Percutaneous Endoscopic Approach

04LL4DZ Occlusion of Left Femoral Artery with Intraluminal Device, Percutaneous Endoscopic Approach

04LL4ZZ Occlusion of Left Femoral Artery, Percutaneous Endoscopic Approach

04LM0CZ Occlusion of Right Popliteal Artery with Extraluminal Device, Open Approach

04LM0DZ Occlusion of Right Popliteal Artery with Intraluminal Device, Open Approach

04LM0ZZ Occlusion of Right Popliteal Artery, Open Approach

04LM3CZ Occlusion of Right Popliteal Artery with Extraluminal Device, Percutaneous Approach

04LM3DZ Occlusion of Right Popliteal Artery with Intraluminal Device, Percutaneous Approach

04LM3ZZ Occlusion of Right Popliteal Artery, Percutaneous Approach

04LM4CZ Occlusion of Right Popliteal Artery with Extraluminal Device, Percutaneous Endoscopic Approach

04LM4DZ Occlusion of Right Popliteal Artery with Intraluminal Device, Percutaneous Endoscopic Approach

04LM4ZZ Occlusion of Right Popliteal Artery, Percutaneous Endoscopic Approach

04LN0CZ Occlusion of Left Popliteal Artery with Extraluminal Device, Open Approach

04LN0DZ Occlusion of Left Popliteal Artery with Intraluminal Device, Open Approach

04LN0ZZ Occlusion of Left Popliteal Artery, Open Approach

04LN3CZ Occlusion of Left Popliteal Artery with Extraluminal Device, Percutaneous Approach

04LN3DZ Occlusion of Left Popliteal Artery with Intraluminal Device, Percutaneous Approach

04LN3ZZ Occlusion of Left Popliteal Artery, Percutaneous Approach

04LN4CZ Occlusion of Left Popliteal Artery with Extraluminal Device, Percutaneous Endoscopic Approach

04LN4DZ Occlusion of Left Popliteal Artery with Intraluminal Device, Percutaneous Endoscopic Approach

04LN4ZZ Occlusion of Left Popliteal Artery, Percutaneous Endoscopic Approach

04LP0CZ Occlusion of Right Anterior Tibial Artery with Extraluminal Device, Open Approach

04LP0DZ Occlusion of Right Anterior Tibial Artery with Intraluminal Device, Open Approach

04LP0ZZ Occlusion of Right Anterior Tibial Artery, Open Approach

04LP3CZ Occlusion of Right Anterior Tibial Artery with Extraluminal Device, Percutaneous Approach

04LP3DZ Occlusion of Right Anterior Tibial Artery with Intraluminal Device, Percutaneous Approach

04LP3ZZ Occlusion of Right Anterior Tibial Artery, Percutaneous Approach

04LP4CZ Occlusion of Right Anterior Tibial Artery with Extraluminal Device, Percutaneous Endoscopic Approach

04LP4DZ Occlusion of Right Anterior Tibial Artery with Intraluminal Device, Percutaneous Endoscopic Approach

04LP4ZZ Occlusion of Right Anterior Tibial Artery, Percutaneous Endoscopic Approach

04LQ0CZ Occlusion of Left Anterior Tibial Artery with Extraluminal Device, Open Approach

Female-only   ♂ Male-only   ▲ Limited Coverage   ● Non-OR   ▦ HAC-associated procedure   ▲ Non-covered procedures   + Combination

04LQ0DZ Occlusion of Left Anterior Tibial Artery with Intraluminal Device, Open Approach

04LQ0ZZ Occlusion of Left Anterior Tibial Artery, Open Approach

04LQ3CZ Occlusion of Left Anterior Tibial Artery with Extraluminal Device, Percutaneous Approach

04LQ3DZ Occlusion of Left Anterior Tibial Artery with Intraluminal Device, Percutaneous Approach

04LQ3ZZ Occlusion of Left Anterior Tibial Artery, Percutaneous Approach

04LQ4CZ Occlusion of Left Anterior Tibial Artery with Extraluminal Device, Percutaneous Endoscopic Approach

04LQ4DZ Occlusion of Left Anterior Tibial Artery with Intraluminal Device, Percutaneous Endoscopic Approach

04LQ4ZZ Occlusion of Left Anterior Tibial Artery, Percutaneous Endoscopic Approach

04LR0CZ Occlusion of Right Posterior Tibial Artery with Extraluminal Device, Open Approach

04LR0DZ Occlusion of Right Posterior Tibial Artery with Intraluminal Device, Open Approach

04LR0ZZ Occlusion of Right Posterior Tibial Artery, Open Approach

04LR3CZ Occlusion of Right Posterior Tibial Artery with Extraluminal Device, Percutaneous Approach

04LR3DZ Occlusion of Right Posterior Tibial Artery with Intraluminal Device, Percutaneous Approach

04LR3ZZ Occlusion of Right Posterior Tibial Artery, Percutaneous Approach

04LR4CZ Occlusion of Right Posterior Tibial Artery with Extraluminal Device, Percutaneous Endoscopic Approach

04LR4DZ Occlusion of Right Posterior Tibial Artery with Intraluminal Device, Percutaneous Endoscopic Approach

04LR4ZZ Occlusion of Right Posterior Tibial Artery, Percutaneous Endoscopic Approach

04LS0CZ Occlusion of Left Posterior Tibial Artery with Extraluminal Device, Open Approach

04LS0DZ Occlusion of Left Posterior Tibial Artery with Intraluminal Device, Open Approach

04LS0ZZ Occlusion of Left Posterior Tibial Artery, Open Approach

04LS3CZ Occlusion of Left Posterior Tibial Artery with Extraluminal Device, Percutaneous Approach

04LS3DZ Occlusion of Left Posterior Tibial Artery with Intraluminal Device, Percutaneous Approach

04LS3ZZ Occlusion of Left Posterior Tibial Artery, Percutaneous Approach

04LS4CZ Occlusion of Left Posterior Tibial Artery with Extraluminal Device, Percutaneous Endoscopic Approach

04LS4DZ Occlusion of Left Posterior Tibial Artery with Intraluminal Device, Percutaneous Endoscopic Approach

04LS4ZZ Occlusion of Left Posterior Tibial Artery, Percutaneous Endoscopic Approach

04LT0CZ Occlusion of Right Peroneal Artery with Extraluminal Device, Open Approach

04LT0DZ Occlusion of Right Peroneal Artery with Intraluminal Device, Open Approach

04LT0ZZ Occlusion of Right Peroneal Artery, Open Approach

04LT3CZ Occlusion of Right Peroneal Artery with Extraluminal Device, Percutaneous Approach

04LT3DZ Occlusion of Right Peroneal Artery with Intraluminal Device, Percutaneous Approach

04LT3ZZ Occlusion of Right Peroneal Artery, Percutaneous Approach

04LT4CZ Occlusion of Right Peroneal Artery with Extraluminal Device, Percutaneous Endoscopic Approach

04LT4DZ Occlusion of Right Peroneal Artery with Intraluminal Device, Percutaneous Endoscopic Approach

04LT4ZZ Occlusion of Right Peroneal Artery, Percutaneous Endoscopic Approach

04LU0CZ Occlusion of Left Peroneal Artery with Extraluminal Device, Open Approach

04LU0DZ Occlusion of Left Peroneal Artery with Intraluminal Device, Open Approach

04LU0ZZ Occlusion of Left Peroneal Artery, Open Approach

04LU3CZ Occlusion of Left Peroneal Artery with Extraluminal Device, Percutaneous Approach

04LU3DZ Occlusion of Left Peroneal Artery with Intraluminal Device, Percutaneous Approach

04LU3ZZ Occlusion of Left Peroneal Artery, Percutaneous Approach

04LU4CZ Occlusion of Left Peroneal Artery with Extraluminal Device, Percutaneous Endoscopic Approach

04LU4DZ Occlusion of Left Peroneal Artery with Intraluminal Device, Percutaneous Endoscopic Approach

04LU4ZZ Occlusion of Left Peroneal Artery, Percutaneous Endoscopic Approach

04LV0CZ Occlusion of Right Foot Artery with Extraluminal Device, Open Approach

04LV0DZ Occlusion of Right Foot Artery with Intraluminal Device, Open Approach

04LV0ZZ Occlusion of Right Foot Artery, Open Approach

04LV3CZ Occlusion of Right Foot Artery with Extraluminal Device, Percutaneous Approach

04LV3DZ Occlusion of Right Foot Artery with Intraluminal Device, Percutaneous Approach

04LV3ZZ Occlusion of Right Foot Artery, Percutaneous Approach

04LV4CZ Occlusion of Right Foot Artery with Extraluminal Device, Percutaneous Endoscopic Approach

04LV4DZ Occlusion of Right Foot Artery with Intraluminal Device, Percutaneous Endoscopic Approach

04LV4ZZ Occlusion of Right Foot Artery, Percutaneous Endoscopic Approach

04LW0CZ Occlusion of Left Foot Artery with Extraluminal Device, Open Approach

04LW0DZ Occlusion of Left Foot Artery with Intraluminal Device, Open Approach

04LW0ZZ Occlusion of Left Foot Artery, Open Approach

04LW3CZ Occlusion of Left Foot Artery with Extraluminal Device, Percutaneous Approach

04LW3DZ Occlusion of Left Foot Artery with Intraluminal Device, Percutaneous Approach

04LW3ZZ Occlusion of Left Foot Artery, Percutaneous Approach

04LW4CZ Occlusion of Left Foot Artery with Extraluminal Device, Percutaneous Endoscopic Approach

04LW4DZ Occlusion of Left Foot Artery with Intraluminal Device, Percutaneous Endoscopic Approach

04LW4ZZ Occlusion of Left Foot Artery, Percutaneous Endoscopic Approach

04LY0CZ Occlusion of Lower Artery with Extraluminal Device, Open Approach

04LY0DZ Occlusion of Lower Artery with Intraluminal Device, Open Approach

04LY0ZZ Occlusion of Lower Artery, Open Approach

04LY3CZ Occlusion of Lower Artery with Extraluminal Device, Percutaneous Approach

04LY3DZ Occlusion of Lower Artery with Intraluminal Device, Percutaneous Approach

04LY3ZZ Occlusion of Lower Artery, Percutaneous Approach

04LY4CZ Occlusion of Lower Artery with Extraluminal Device, Percutaneous Endoscopic Approach

04LY4DZ Occlusion of Lower Artery with Intraluminal Device, Percutaneous Endoscopic Approach

04LY4ZZ Occlusion of Lower Artery, Percutaneous Endoscopic Approach

04N – Lower Arteries, Release

Review Coding Guidelines B3.13 and B3.14

04N00ZZ Release Abdominal Aorta, Open Approach

04N03ZZ Release Abdominal Aorta, Percutaneous Approach

04N04ZZ Release Abdominal Aorta, Percutaneous Endoscopic Approach

04N10ZZ Release Celiac Artery, Open Approach

04N13ZZ Release Celiac Artery, Percutaneous Approach

04N14ZZ Release Celiac Artery, Percutaneous Endoscopic Approach

04N20ZZ Release Gastric Artery, Open Approach

04N23ZZ Release Gastric Artery, Percutaneous Approach

04N24ZZ Release Gastric Artery, Percutaneous Endoscopic Approach

04N30ZZ Release Hepatic Artery, Open Approach

04N33ZZ Release Hepatic Artery, Percutaneous Approach

04N34ZZ Release Hepatic Artery, Percutaneous Endoscopic Approach

04N40ZZ Release Splenic Artery, Open Approach

04N43ZZ Release Splenic Artery, Percutaneous Approach

04N44ZZ Release Splenic Artery, Percutaneous Endoscopic Approach

04N50ZZ Release Superior Mesenteric Artery, Open Approach

04N53ZZ Release Superior Mesenteric Artery, Percutaneous Approach

04N54ZZ Release Superior Mesenteric Artery, Percutaneous Endoscopic Approach

04N60ZZ Release Right Colic Artery, Open Approach

04N63ZZ Release Right Colic Artery, Percutaneous Approach

04N64ZZ Release Right Colic Artery, Percutaneous Endoscopic Approach

04N70ZZ Release Left Colic Artery, Open Approach

04N73ZZ Release Left Colic Artery, Percutaneous Approach

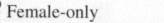

♀ Female-only ♂ Male-only ▲ Limited Coverage ● Non-OR ▥ HAC-associated procedure ▲ Non-covered procedures ✛ Combinati

N74ZZ	Release Left Colic Artery, Percutaneous Endoscopic Approach	04NF3ZZ	Release Left Internal Iliac Artery, Percutaneous Approach	04NQ0ZZ	Release Left Anterior Tibial Artery, Open Approach
N80ZZ	Release Middle Colic Artery, Open Approach	04NF4ZZ	Release Left Internal Iliac Artery, Percutaneous Endoscopic Approach	04NQ3ZZ	Release Left Anterior Tibial Artery, Percutaneous Approach
N83ZZ	Release Middle Colic Artery, Percutaneous Approach	04NH0ZZ	Release Right External Iliac Artery, Open Approach	04NQ4ZZ	Release Left Anterior Tibial Artery, Percutaneous Endoscopic Approach
N84ZZ	Release Middle Colic Artery, Percutaneous Endoscopic Approach	04NH3ZZ	Release Right External Iliac Artery, Percutaneous Approach	04NR0ZZ	Release Right Posterior Tibial Artery, Open Approach
N90ZZ	Release Right Renal Artery, Open Approach	04NH4ZZ	Release Right External Iliac Artery, Percutaneous Endoscopic Approach	04NR3ZZ	Release Right Posterior Tibial Artery, Percutaneous Approach
N93ZZ	Release Right Renal Artery, Percutaneous Approach	04NJ0ZZ	Release Left External Iliac Artery, Open Approach	04NR4ZZ	Release Right Posterior Tibial Artery, Percutaneous Endoscopic Approach
N94ZZ	Release Right Renal Artery, Percutaneous Endoscopic Approach	04NJ3ZZ	Release Left External Iliac Artery, Percutaneous Approach	04NS0ZZ	Release Left Posterior Tibial Artery, Open Approach
4NA0ZZ	Release Left Renal Artery, Open Approach	04NJ4ZZ	Release Left External Iliac Artery, Percutaneous Endoscopic Approach	04NS3ZZ	Release Left Posterior Tibial Artery, Percutaneous Approach
4NA3ZZ	Release Left Renal Artery, Percutaneous Approach	04NK0ZZ	Release Right Femoral Artery, Open Approach	04NS4ZZ	Release Left Posterior Tibial Artery, Percutaneous Endoscopic Approach
4NA4ZZ	Release Left Renal Artery, Percutaneous Endoscopic Approach	04NK3ZZ	Release Right Femoral Artery, Percutaneous Approach	04NT0ZZ	Release Right Peroneal Artery, Open Approach
4NB0ZZ	Release Inferior Mesenteric Artery, Open Approach	04NK4ZZ	Release Right Femoral Artery, Percutaneous Endoscopic Approach	04NT3ZZ	Release Right Peroneal Artery, Percutaneous Approach
4NB3ZZ	Release Inferior Mesenteric Artery, Percutaneous Approach	04NL0ZZ	Release Left Femoral Artery, Open Approach	04NT4ZZ	Release Right Peroneal Artery, Percutaneous Endoscopic Approach
4NB4ZZ	Release Inferior Mesenteric Artery, Percutaneous Endoscopic Approach	04NL3ZZ	Release Left Femoral Artery, Percutaneous Approach	04NU0ZZ	Release Left Peroneal Artery, Open Approach
4NC0ZZ	Release Right Common Iliac Artery, Open Approach	04NL4ZZ	Release Left Femoral Artery, Percutaneous Endoscopic Approach	04NU3ZZ	Release Left Peroneal Artery, Percutaneous Approach
4NC3ZZ	Release Right Common Iliac Artery, Percutaneous Approach	04NM0ZZ	Release Right Popliteal Artery, Open Approach	04NU4ZZ	Release Left Peroneal Artery, Percutaneous Endoscopic Approach
4NC4ZZ	Release Right Common Iliac Artery, Percutaneous Endoscopic Approach	04NM3ZZ	Release Right Popliteal Artery, Percutaneous Approach	04NV0ZZ	Release Right Foot Artery, Open Approach
4ND0ZZ	Release Left Common Iliac Artery, Open Approach	04NM4ZZ	Release Right Popliteal Artery, Percutaneous Endoscopic Approach	04NV3ZZ	Release Right Foot Artery, Percutaneous Approach
4ND3ZZ	Release Left Common Iliac Artery, Percutaneous Approach	04NN0ZZ	Release Left Popliteal Artery, Open Approach	04NV4ZZ	Release Right Foot Artery, Percutaneous Endoscopic Approach
4ND4ZZ	Release Left Common Iliac Artery, Percutaneous Endoscopic Approach	04NN3ZZ	Release Left Popliteal Artery, Percutaneous Approach	04NW0ZZ	Release Left Foot Artery, Open Approach
4NE0ZZ	Release Right Internal Iliac Artery, Open Approach	04NN4ZZ	Release Left Popliteal Artery, Percutaneous Endoscopic Approach	04NW3ZZ	Release Left Foot Artery, Percutaneous Approach
4NE3ZZ	Release Right Internal Iliac Artery, Percutaneous Approach	04NP0ZZ	Release Right Anterior Tibial Artery, Open Approach	04NW4ZZ	Release Left Foot Artery, Percutaneous Endoscopic Approach
4NE4ZZ	Release Right Internal Iliac Artery, Percutaneous Endoscopic Approach	04NP3ZZ	Release Right Anterior Tibial Artery, Percutaneous Approach	04NY0ZZ	Release Lower Artery, Open Approach
4NF0ZZ	Release Left Internal Iliac Artery, Open Approach	04NP4ZZ	Release Right Anterior Tibial Artery, Percutaneous Endoscopic Approach	04NY3ZZ	Release Lower Artery, Percutaneous Approach
				04NY4ZZ	Release Lower Artery, Percutaneous Endoscopic Approach

4P – Lower Arteries, Removal

Review Coding Guideline B6.1c

4PY00Z	Removal of Drainage Device from Lower Artery, Open Approach	04PY37Z	Removal of Autologous Tissue Substitute from Lower Artery, Percutaneous Approach	04PY4CZ	Removal of Extraluminal Device from Lower Artery, Percutaneous Endoscopic Approach
4PY02Z	Removal of Monitoring Device from Lower Artery, Open Approach	04PY3CZ	Removal of Extraluminal Device from Lower Artery, Percutaneous Approach	04PY4DZ	Removal of Intraluminal Device from Lower Artery, Percutaneous Endoscopic Approach
4PY03Z	Removal of Infusion Device from Lower Artery, Open Approach	04PY3DZ	Removal of Intraluminal Device from Lower Artery, Percutaneous Approach	04PY4JZ	Removal of Synthetic Substitute from Lower Artery, Percutaneous Endoscopic Approach
4PY07Z	Removal of Autologous Tissue Substitute from Lower Artery, Open Approach	04PY3JZ	Removal of Synthetic Substitute from Lower Artery, Percutaneous Approach	04PY4KZ	Removal of Nonautologous Tissue Substitute from Lower Artery, Percutaneous Endoscopic Approach
4PY0CZ	Removal of Extraluminal Device from Lower Artery, Open Approach	04PY3KZ	Removal of Nonautologous Tissue Substitute from Lower Artery, Percutaneous Approach	04PYX0Z	Removal of Drainage Device from Lower Artery, External Approach
4PY0DZ	Removal of Intraluminal Device from Lower Artery, Open Approach	04PY40Z	Removal of Drainage Device from Lower Artery, Percutaneous Endoscopic Approach	04PYX1Z	Removal of Radioactive Element from Lower Artery, External Approach
4PY0JZ	Removal of Synthetic Substitute from Lower Artery, Open Approach	04PY42Z	Removal of Monitoring Device from Lower Artery, Percutaneous Endoscopic Approach	04PYX2Z	Removal of Monitoring Device from Lower Artery, External Approach
4PY0KZ	Removal of Nonautologous Tissue Substitute from Lower Artery, Open Approach	04PY43Z	Removal of Infusion Device from Lower Artery, Percutaneous Endoscopic Approach	04PYX3Z	Removal of Infusion Device from Lower Artery, External Approach
4PY30Z	Removal of Drainage Device from Lower Artery, Percutaneous Approach	04PY47Z	Removal of Autologous Tissue Substitute from Lower Artery, Percutaneous Endoscopic Approach	04PYXDZ	Removal of Intraluminal Device from Lower Artery, External Approach
4PY32Z	Removal of Monitoring Device from Lower Artery, Percutaneous Approach				
4PY33Z	Removal of Infusion Device from Lower Artery, Percutaneous Approach				

♀ Female-only	♂ Male-only	▲ Limited Coverage	● Non-OR	▥ HAC-associated procedure	▲ Non-covered procedures	✚ Combination

04Q – Lower Arteries, Repair

04Q00ZZ Repair Abdominal Aorta, Open Approach

04Q03ZZ Repair Abdominal Aorta, Percutaneous Approach

04Q04ZZ Repair Abdominal Aorta, Percutaneous Endoscopic Approach

04Q10ZZ Repair Celiac Artery, Open Approach

04Q13ZZ Repair Celiac Artery, Percutaneous Approach

04Q14ZZ Repair Celiac Artery, Percutaneous Endoscopic Approach

04Q20ZZ Repair Gastric Artery, Open Approach

04Q23ZZ Repair Gastric Artery, Percutaneous Approach

04Q24ZZ Repair Gastric Artery, Percutaneous Endoscopic Approach

04Q30ZZ Repair Hepatic Artery, Open Approach

04Q33ZZ Repair Hepatic Artery, Percutaneous Approach

04Q34ZZ Repair Hepatic Artery, Percutaneous Endoscopic Approach

04Q40ZZ Repair Splenic Artery, Open Approach

04Q43ZZ Repair Splenic Artery, Percutaneous Approach

04Q44ZZ Repair Splenic Artery, Percutaneous Endoscopic Approach

04Q50ZZ Repair Superior Mesenteric Artery, Open Approach

04Q53ZZ Repair Superior Mesenteric Artery, Percutaneous Approach

04Q54ZZ Repair Superior Mesenteric Artery, Percutaneous Endoscopic Approach

04Q60ZZ Repair Right Colic Artery, Open Approach

04Q63ZZ Repair Right Colic Artery, Percutaneous Approach

04Q64ZZ Repair Right Colic Artery, Percutaneous Endoscopic Approach

04Q70ZZ Repair Left Colic Artery, Open Approach

04Q73ZZ Repair Left Colic Artery, Percutaneous Approach

04Q74ZZ Repair Left Colic Artery, Percutaneous Endoscopic Approach

04Q80ZZ Repair Middle Colic Artery, Open Approach

04Q83ZZ Repair Middle Colic Artery, Percutaneous Approach

04Q84ZZ Repair Middle Colic Artery, Percutaneous Endoscopic Approach

04Q90ZZ Repair Right Renal Artery, Open Approach

04Q93ZZ Repair Right Renal Artery, Percutaneous Approach

04Q94ZZ Repair Right Renal Artery, Percutaneous Endoscopic Approach

04QA0ZZ Repair Left Renal Artery, Open Approach

04QA3ZZ Repair Left Renal Artery, Percutaneous Approach

04QA4ZZ Repair Left Renal Artery, Percutaneous Endoscopic Approach

04QB0ZZ Repair Inferior Mesenteric Artery, Open Approach

04QB3ZZ Repair Inferior Mesenteric Artery, Percutaneous Approach

04QB4ZZ Repair Inferior Mesenteric Artery, Percutaneous Endoscopic Approach

04QC0ZZ Repair Right Common Iliac Artery, Open Approach

04QC3ZZ Repair Right Common Iliac Artery, Percutaneous Approach

04QC4ZZ Repair Right Common Iliac Artery, Percutaneous Endoscopic Approach

04QD0ZZ Repair Left Common Iliac Artery, Open Approach

04QD3ZZ Repair Left Common Iliac Artery, Percutaneous Approach

04QD4ZZ Repair Left Common Iliac Artery, Percutaneous Endoscopic Approach

04QE0ZZ Repair Right Internal Iliac Artery, Open Approach

04QE3ZZ Repair Right Internal Iliac Artery, Percutaneous Approach

04QE4ZZ Repair Right Internal Iliac Artery, Percutaneous Endoscopic Approach

04QF0ZZ Repair Left Internal Iliac Artery, Open Approach

04QF3ZZ Repair Left Internal Iliac Artery, Percutaneous Approach

04QF4ZZ Repair Left Internal Iliac Artery, Percutaneous Endoscopic Approach

04QH0ZZ Repair Right External Iliac Artery, Open Approach

04QH3ZZ Repair Right External Iliac Artery, Percutaneous Approach

04QH4ZZ Repair Right External Iliac Artery, Percutaneous Endoscopic Approach

04QJ0ZZ Repair Left External Iliac Artery, Open Approach

04QJ3ZZ Repair Left External Iliac Artery, Percutaneous Approach

04QJ4ZZ Repair Left External Iliac Artery, Percutaneous Endoscopic Approach

04QK0ZZ Repair Right Femoral Artery, Open Approach

AHA CC: 1Q, 2014, 21-22

04QK3ZZ Repair Right Femoral Artery, Percutaneous Approach

04QK4ZZ Repair Right Femoral Artery, Percutaneous Endoscopic Approach

04QL0ZZ Repair Left Femoral Artery, Open Approach

04QL3ZZ Repair Left Femoral Artery, Percutaneous Approach

04QL4ZZ Repair Left Femoral Artery, Percutancous Endoscopic Approach

04QM0ZZ Repair Right Popliteal Artery, Open Approach

04QM3ZZ Repair Right Popliteal Artery, Percutaneous Approach

04QM4ZZ Repair Right Popliteal Artery, Percutaneous Endoscopic Approach

04QN0ZZ Repair Left Popliteal Artery, Open Approach

04QN3ZZ Repair Left Popliteal Artery, Percutaneous Approach

04QN4ZZ Repair Left Popliteal Artery, Percutaneous Endoscopic Approach

04QP0ZZ Repair Right Anterior Tibial Artery, Open Approach

04QP3ZZ Repair Right Anterior Tibial Artery, Percutaneous Approach

04QP4ZZ Repair Right Anterior Tibial Artery, Percutaneous Endoscopic Approach

04QQ0ZZ Repair Left Anterior Tibial Artery, Open Approach

04QQ3ZZ Repair Left Anterior Tibial Artery, Percutaneous Approach

04QQ4ZZ Repair Left Anterior Tibial Artery, Percutaneous Endoscopic Approach

04QR0ZZ Repair Right Posterior Tibial Artery, Open Approach

04QR3ZZ Repair Right Posterior Tibial Artery, Percutaneous Approach

04QR4ZZ Repair Right Posterior Tibial Artery, Percutaneous Endoscopic Approach

04QS0ZZ Repair Left Posterior Tibial Artery, Open Approach

04QS3ZZ Repair Left Posterior Tibial Artery, Percutaneous Approach

04QS4ZZ Repair Left Posterior Tibial Artery, Percutaneous Endoscopic Approach

04QT0ZZ Repair Right Peroneal Artery, Open Approach

04QT3ZZ Repair Right Peroneal Artery, Percutaneous Approach

04QT4ZZ Repair Right Peroneal Artery, Percutaneous Endoscopic Approach

04QU0ZZ Repair Left Peroneal Artery, Open Approach

04QU3ZZ Repair Left Peroneal Artery, Percutaneous Approach

04QU4ZZ Repair Left Peroneal Artery, Percutaneous Endoscopic Approach

04QV0ZZ Repair Right Foot Artery, Open Approach

04QV3ZZ Repair Right Foot Artery, Percutaneous Approach

04QV4ZZ Repair Right Foot Artery, Percutaneous Endoscopic Approach

04QW0ZZ Repair Left Foot Artery, Open Approach

04QW3ZZ Repair Left Foot Artery, Percutaneous Approach

04QW4ZZ Repair Left Foot Artery, Percutaneous Endoscopic Approach

04QY0ZZ Repair Lower Artery, Open Approach

04QY3ZZ Repair Lower Artery, Percutaneous Approach

04QY4ZZ Repair Lower Artery, Percutaneous Endoscopic Approach

04R – Lower Arteries, Replacement

04R007Z Replacement of Abdominal Aorta with Autologous Tissue Substitute, Open Approach

04R00JZ Replacement of Abdominal Aorta with Synthetic Substitute, Open Approach

04R00KZ Replacement of Abdominal Aorta with Nonautologous Tissue Substitute, Open Approach

04R047Z Replacement of Abdominal Aorta with Autologous Tissue Substitute, Percutaneous Endoscopic Approach

04R04JZ Replacement of Abdominal Aorta with Synthetic Substitute, Percutaneous Endoscopic Approach

04R04KZ Replacement of Abdominal Aorta with Nonautologous Tissue Substitute, Percutaneous Endoscopic Approach

04R107Z Replacement of Celiac Artery with Autologous Tissue Substitute, Open Approach

04R10JZ Replacement of Celiac Artery with Synthetic Substitute, Open Approach

04R10KZ Replacement of Celiac Artery with Nonautologous Tissue Substitute, Open Approach

04R147Z Replacement of Celiac Artery with Autologous Tissue Substitute, Percutaneous Endoscopic Approach

04R14JZ Replacement of Celiac Artery with Synthetic Substitute, Percutaneous Endoscopic Approach

04R14KZ Replacement of Celiac Artery with Nonautologous Tissue Substitute, Percutaneous Endoscopic Approach

04R207Z Replacement of Gastric Artery with Autologous Tissue Substitute, Open Approach

04R20JZ Replacement of Gastric Artery with Synthetic Substitute, Open Approach

♀ Female-only   ♂ Male-only   ▲ Limited Coverage   ● Non-OR   ▦ HAC-associated procedure   ▲ Non-covered procedures   ✚ Combination

04R20KZ	Replacement of Gastric Artery with Nonautologous Tissue Substitute, Open Approach
04R247Z	Replacement of Gastric Artery with Autologous Tissue Substitute, Percutaneous Endoscopic Approach
04R24JZ	Replacement of Gastric Artery with Synthetic Substitute, Percutaneous Endoscopic Approach
04R24KZ	Replacement of Gastric Artery with Nonautologous Tissue Substitute, Percutaneous Endoscopic Approach
04R307Z	Replacement of Hepatic Artery with Autologous Tissue Substitute, Open Approach
04R30JZ	Replacement of Hepatic Artery with Synthetic Substitute, Open Approach
04R30KZ	Replacement of Hepatic Artery with Nonautologous Tissue Substitute, Open Approach
04R347Z	Replacement of Hepatic Artery with Autologous Tissue Substitute, Percutaneous Endoscopic Approach
04R34JZ	Replacement of Hepatic Artery with Synthetic Substitute, Percutaneous Endoscopic Approach
04R34KZ	Replacement of Hepatic Artery with Nonautologous Tissue Substitute, Percutaneous Endoscopic Approach
04R407Z	Replacement of Splenic Artery with Autologous Tissue Substitute, Open Approach
04R40JZ	Replacement of Splenic Artery with Synthetic Substitute, Open Approach
04R40KZ	Replacement of Splenic Artery with Nonautologous Tissue Substitute, Open Approach
04R447Z	Replacement of Splenic Artery with Autologous Tissue Substitute, Percutaneous Endoscopic Approach
04R44JZ	Replacement of Splenic Artery with Synthetic Substitute, Percutaneous Endoscopic Approach
04R44KZ	Replacement of Splenic Artery with Nonautologous Tissue Substitute, Percutaneous Endoscopic Approach
04R507Z	Replacement of Superior Mesenteric Artery with Autologous Tissue Substitute, Open Approach
04R50JZ	Replacement of Superior Mesenteric Artery with Synthetic Substitute, Open Approach
04R50KZ	Replacement of Superior Mesenteric Artery with Nonautologous Tissue Substitute, Open Approach
04R547Z	Replacement of Superior Mesenteric Artery with Autologous Tissue Substitute, Percutaneous Endoscopic Approach
04R54JZ	Replacement of Superior Mesenteric Artery with Synthetic Substitute, Percutaneous Endoscopic Approach
04R54KZ	Replacement of Superior Mesenteric Artery with Nonautologous Tissue Substitute, Percutaneous Endoscopic Approach
04R607Z	Replacement of Right Colic Artery with Autologous Tissue Substitute, Open Approach
04R60JZ	Replacement of Right Colic Artery with Synthetic Substitute, Open Approach
04R60KZ	Replacement of Right Colic Artery with Nonautologous Tissue Substitute, Open Approach
04R647Z	Replacement of Right Colic Artery with Autologous Tissue Substitute, Percutaneous Endoscopic Approach
04R64JZ	Replacement of Right Colic Artery with Synthetic Substitute, Percutaneous Endoscopic Approach
04R64KZ	Replacement of Right Colic Artery with Nonautologous Tissue Substitute, Percutaneous Endoscopic Approach
04R707Z	Replacement of Left Colic Artery with Autologous Tissue Substitute, Open Approach
04R70JZ	Replacement of Left Colic Artery with Synthetic Substitute, Open Approach
04R70KZ	Replacement of Left Colic Artery with Nonautologous Tissue Substitute, Open Approach
04R747Z	Replacement of Left Colic Artery with Autologous Tissue Substitute, Percutaneous Endoscopic Approach
04R74JZ	Replacement of Left Colic Artery with Synthetic Substitute, Percutaneous Endoscopic Approach
04R74KZ	Replacement of Left Colic Artery with Nonautologous Tissue Substitute, Percutaneous Endoscopic Approach
04R807Z	Replacement of Middle Colic Artery with Autologous Tissue Substitute, Open Approach
04R80JZ	Replacement of Middle Colic Artery with Synthetic Substitute, Open Approach
04R80KZ	Replacement of Middle Colic Artery with Nonautologous Tissue Substitute, Open Approach
04R847Z	Replacement of Middle Colic Artery with Autologous Tissue Substitute, Percutaneous Endoscopic Approach
04R84JZ	Replacement of Middle Colic Artery with Synthetic Substitute, Percutaneous Endoscopic Approach
04R84KZ	Replacement of Middle Colic Artery with Nonautologous Tissue Substitute, Percutaneous Endoscopic Approach
04R907Z	Replacement of Right Renal Artery with Autologous Tissue Substitute, Open Approach
04R90JZ	Replacement of Right Renal Artery with Synthetic Substitute, Open Approach
04R90KZ	Replacement of Right Renal Artery with Nonautologous Tissue Substitute, Open Approach
04R947Z	Replacement of Right Renal Artery with Autologous Tissue Substitute, Percutaneous Endoscopic Approach
04R94JZ	Replacement of Right Renal Artery with Synthetic Substitute, Percutaneous Endoscopic Approach
04R94KZ	Replacement of Right Renal Artery with Nonautologous Tissue Substitute, Percutaneous Endoscopic Approach
04RA07Z	Replacement of Left Renal Artery with Autologous Tissue Substitute, Open Approach
04RA0JZ	Replacement of Left Renal Artery with Synthetic Substitute, Open Approach
04RA0KZ	Replacement of Left Renal Artery with Nonautologous Tissue Substitute, Open Approach
04RA47Z	Replacement of Left Renal Artery with Autologous Tissue Substitute, Percutaneous Endoscopic Approach
04RA4JZ	Replacement of Left Renal Artery with Synthetic Substitute, Percutaneous Endoscopic Approach
04RA4KZ	Replacement of Left Renal Artery with Nonautologous Tissue Substitute, Percutaneous Endoscopic Approach
04RB07Z	Replacement of Inferior Mesenteric Artery with Autologous Tissue Substitute, Open Approach
04RB0JZ	Replacement of Inferior Mesenteric Artery with Synthetic Substitute, Open Approach
04RB0KZ	Replacement of Inferior Mesenteric Artery with Nonautologous Tissue Substitute, Open Approach
04RB47Z	Replacement of Inferior Mesenteric Artery with Autologous Tissue Substitute, Percutaneous Endoscopic Approach
04RB4JZ	Replacement of Inferior Mesenteric Artery with Synthetic Substitute, Percutaneous Endoscopic Approach
04RB4KZ	Replacement of Inferior Mesenteric Artery with Nonautologous Tissue Substitute, Percutaneous Endoscopic Approach
04RC07Z	Replacement of Right Common Iliac Artery with Autologous Tissue Substitute, Open Approach
04RC0JZ	Replacement of Right Common Iliac Artery with Synthetic Substitute, Open Approach
04RC0KZ	Replacement of Right Common Iliac Artery with Nonautologous Tissue Substitute, Open Approach
04RC47Z	Replacement of Right Common Iliac Artery with Autologous Tissue Substitute, Percutaneous Endoscopic Approach
04RC4JZ	Replacement of Right Common Iliac Artery with Synthetic Substitute, Percutaneous Endoscopic Approach
04RC4KZ	Replacement of Right Common Iliac Artery with Nonautologous Tissue Substitute, Percutaneous Endoscopic Approach
04RD07Z	Replacement of Left Common Iliac Artery with Autologous Tissue Substitute, Open Approach
04RD0JZ	Replacement of Left Common Iliac Artery with Synthetic Substitute, Open Approach
04RD0KZ	Replacement of Left Common Iliac Artery with Nonautologous Tissue Substitute, Open Approach
04RD47Z	Replacement of Left Common Iliac Artery with Autologous Tissue Substitute, Percutaneous Endoscopic Approach
04RD4JZ	Replacement of Left Common Iliac Artery with Synthetic Substitute, Percutaneous Endoscopic Approach
04RD4KZ	Replacement of Left Common Iliac Artery with Nonautologous Tissue Substitute, Percutaneous Endoscopic Approach
04RE07Z	Replacement of Right Internal Iliac Artery with Autologous Tissue Substitute, Open Approach
04RE0JZ	Replacement of Right Internal Iliac Artery with Synthetic Substitute, Open Approach
04RE0KZ	Replacement of Right Internal Iliac Artery with Nonautologous Tissue Substitute, Open Approach
04RE47Z	Replacement of Right Internal Iliac Artery with Autologous Tissue Substitute, Percutaneous Endoscopic Approach
04RE4JZ	Replacement of Right Internal Iliac Artery with Synthetic Substitute, Percutaneous Endoscopic Approach
04RE4KZ	Replacement of Right Internal Iliac Artery with Nonautologous Tissue Substitute, Percutaneous Endoscopic Approach
04RF07Z	Replacement of Left Internal Iliac Artery with Autologous Tissue Substitute, Open Approach
04RF0JZ	Replacement of Left Internal Iliac Artery with Synthetic Substitute, Open Approach
04RF0KZ	Replacement of Left Internal Iliac Artery with Nonautologous Tissue Substitute, Open Approach

291

04RF47Z Replacement of Left Internal Iliac Artery with Autologous Tissue Substitute, Percutaneous Endoscopic Approach

04RF4JZ Replacement of Left Internal Iliac Artery with Synthetic Substitute, Percutaneous Endoscopic Approach

04RF4KZ Replacement of Left Internal Iliac Artery with Nonautologous Tissue Substitute, Percutaneous Endoscopic Approach

04RH07Z Replacement of Right External Iliac Artery with Autologous Tissue Substitute, Open Approach

04RH0JZ Replacement of Right External Iliac Artery with Synthetic Substitute, Open Approach

04RH0KZ Replacement of Right External Iliac Artery with Nonautologous Tissue Substitute, Open Approach

04RH47Z Replacement of Right External Iliac Artery with Autologous Tissue Substitute, Percutaneous Endoscopic Approach

04RH4JZ Replacement of Right External Iliac Artery with Synthetic Substitute, Percutaneous Endoscopic Approach

04RH4KZ Replacement of Right External Iliac Artery with Nonautologous Tissue Substitute, Percutaneous Endoscopic Approach

04RJ07Z Replacement of Left External Iliac Artery with Autologous Tissue Substitute, Open Approach

04RJ0JZ Replacement of Left External Iliac Artery with Synthetic Substitute, Open Approach

04RJ0KZ Replacement of Left External Iliac Artery with Nonautologous Tissue Substitute, Open Approach

04RJ47Z Replacement of Left External Iliac Artery with Autologous Tissue Substitute, Percutaneous Endoscopic Approach

04RJ4JZ Replacement of Left External Iliac Artery with Synthetic Substitute, Percutaneous Endoscopic Approach

04RJ4KZ Replacement of Left External Iliac Artery with Nonautologous Tissue Substitute, Percutaneous Endoscopic Approach

04RK07Z Replacement of Right Femoral Artery with Autologous Tissue Substitute, Open Approach

04RK0JZ Replacement of Right Femoral Artery with Synthetic Substitute, Open Approach

04RK0KZ Replacement of Right Femoral Artery with Nonautologous Tissue Substitute, Open Approach

04RK47Z Replacement of Right Femoral Artery with Autologous Tissue Substitute, Percutaneous Endoscopic Approach

04RK4JZ Replacement of Right Femoral Artery with Synthetic Substitute, Percutaneous Endoscopic Approach

04RK4KZ Replacement of Right Femoral Artery with Nonautologous Tissue Substitute, Percutaneous Endoscopic Approach

04RL07Z Replacement of Left Femoral Artery with Autologous Tissue Substitute, Open Approach

04RL0JZ Replacement of Left Femoral Artery with Synthetic Substitute, Open Approach

04RL0KZ Replacement of Left Femoral Artery with Nonautologous Tissue Substitute, Open Approach

04RL47Z Replacement of Left Femoral Artery with Autologous Tissue Substitute, Percutaneous Endoscopic Approach

04RL4JZ Replacement of Left Femoral Artery with Synthetic Substitute, Percutaneous Endoscopic Approach

04RL4KZ Replacement of Left Femoral Artery with Nonautologous Tissue Substitute, Percutaneous Endoscopic Approach

04RM07Z Replacement of Right Popliteal Artery with Autologous Tissue Substitute, Open Approach

04RM0JZ Replacement of Right Popliteal Artery with Synthetic Substitute, Open Approach

04RM0KZ Replacement of Right Popliteal Artery with Nonautologous Tissue Substitute, Open Approach

04RM47Z Replacement of Right Popliteal Artery with Autologous Tissue Substitute, Percutaneous Endoscopic Approach

04RM4JZ Replacement of Right Popliteal Artery with Synthetic Substitute, Percutaneous Endoscopic Approach

04RM4KZ Replacement of Right Popliteal Artery with Nonautologous Tissue Substitute, Percutaneous Endoscopic Approach

04RN07Z Replacement of Left Popliteal Artery with Autologous Tissue Substitute, Open Approach

04RN0JZ Replacement of Left Popliteal Artery with Synthetic Substitute, Open Approach

04RN0KZ Replacement of Left Popliteal Artery with Nonautologous Tissue Substitute, Open Approach

04RN47Z Replacement of Left Popliteal Artery with Autologous Tissue Substitute, Percutaneous Endoscopic Approach

04RN4JZ Replacement of Left Popliteal Artery with Synthetic Substitute, Percutaneous Endoscopic Approach

04RN4KZ Replacement of Left Popliteal Artery with Nonautologous Tissue Substitute, Percutaneous Endoscopic Approach

04RP07Z Replacement of Right Anterior Tibial Artery with Autologous Tissue Substitute, Open Approach

04RP0JZ Replacement of Right Anterior Tibial Artery with Synthetic Substitute, Open Approach

04RP0KZ Replacement of Right Anterior Tibial Artery with Nonautologous Tissue Substitute, Open Approach

04RP47Z Replacement of Right Anterior Tibial Artery with Autologous Tissue Substitute, Percutaneous Endoscopic Approach

04RP4JZ Replacement of Right Anterior Tibial Artery with Synthetic Substitute, Percutaneous Endoscopic Approach

04RP4KZ Replacement of Right Anterior Tibial Artery with Nonautologous Tissue Substitute, Percutaneous Endoscopic Approach

04RQ07Z Replacement of Left Anterior Tibial Artery with Autologous Tissue Substitute, Open Approach

04RQ0JZ Replacement of Left Anterior Tibial Artery with Synthetic Substitute, Open Approach

04RQ0KZ Replacement of Left Anterior Tibial Artery with Nonautologous Tissue Substitute, Open Approach

04RQ47Z Replacement of Left Anterior Tibial Artery with Autologous Tissue Substitute, Percutaneous Endoscopic Approach

04RQ4JZ Replacement of Left Anterior Tibial Artery with Synthetic Substitute, Percutaneous Endoscopic Approach

04RQ4KZ Replacement of Left Anterior Tibial Artery with Nonautologous Tissue Substitute, Percutaneous Endoscopic Approach

04RR07Z Replacement of Right Posterior Tibial Artery with Autologous Tissue Substitute, Open Approach

04RR0JZ Replacement of Right Posterior Tibial Artery with Synthetic Substitute, Open Approach

04RR0KZ Replacement of Right Posterior Tibial Artery with Nonautologous Tissue Substitute, Open Approach

04RR47Z Replacement of Right Posterior Tibial Artery with Autologous Tissue Substitute, Percutaneous Endoscopic Approach

04RR4JZ Replacement of Right Posterior Tibial Artery with Synthetic Substitute, Percutaneous Endoscopic Approach

04RR4KZ Replacement of Right Posterior Tibial Artery with Nonautologous Tissue Substitute, Percutaneous Endoscopic Approach

04RS07Z Replacement of Left Posterior Tibial Artery with Autologous Tissue Substitute, Open Approach

04RS0JZ Replacement of Left Posterior Tibial Artery with Synthetic Substitute, Open Approach

04RS0KZ Replacement of Left Posterior Tibial Artery with Nonautologous Tissue Substitute, Open Approach

04RS47Z Replacement of Left Posterior Tibial Artery with Autologous Tissue Substitute, Percutaneous Endoscopic Approach

04RS4JZ Replacement of Left Posterior Tibial Artery with Synthetic Substitute, Percutaneous Endoscopic Approach

04RS4KZ Replacement of Left Posterior Tibial Artery with Nonautologous Tissue Substitute, Percutaneous Endoscopic Approach

04RT07Z Replacement of Right Peroneal Artery with Autologous Tissue Substitute, Open Approach

04RT0JZ Replacement of Right Peroneal Artery with Synthetic Substitute, Open Approach

04RT0KZ Replacement of Right Peroneal Artery with Nonautologous Tissue Substitute, Open Approach

04RT47Z Replacement of Right Peroneal Artery with Autologous Tissue Substitute, Percutaneous Endoscopic Approach

04RT4JZ Replacement of Right Peroneal Artery with Synthetic Substitute, Percutaneous Endoscopic Approach

04RT4KZ Replacement of Right Peroneal Artery with Nonautologous Tissue Substitute, Percutaneous Endoscopic Approach

04RU07Z Replacement of Left Peroneal Artery with Autologous Tissue Substitute, Open Approach

04RU0JZ Replacement of Left Peroneal Artery with Synthetic Substitute, Open Approach

04RU0KZ Replacement of Left Peroneal Artery with Nonautologous Tissue Substitute, Open Approach

04RU47Z Replacement of Left Peroneal Artery with Autologous Tissue Substitute, Percutaneous Endoscopic Approach

04RU4JZ Replacement of Left Peroneal Artery with Synthetic Substitute, Percutaneous Endoscopic Approach

04RU4KZ Replacement of Left Peroneal Artery with Nonautologous Tissue Substitute, Percutaneous Endoscopic Approach

04RV07Z Replacement of Right Foot Artery with Autologous Tissue Substitute, Open Approach

04RV0JZ Replacement of Right Foot Artery with Synthetic Substitute, Open Approach

04RV0KZ Replacement of Right Foot Artery with Nonautologous Tissue Substitute, Open Approach

04RV47Z Replacement of Right Foot Artery with Autologous Tissue Substitute, Percutaneous Endoscopic Approach

♀ Female-only   ♂ Male-only   ▲ Limited Coverage   ● Non-OR   ▨ HAC-associated procedure   ▲ Non-covered procedures   ✚ Combinatio

RV4JZ   Replacement of Right Foot Artery with Synthetic Substitute, Percutaneous Endoscopic Approach

RV4KZ   Replacement of Right Foot Artery with Nonautologous Tissue Substitute, Percutaneous Endoscopic Approach

RW07Z   Replacement of Left Foot Artery with Autologous Tissue Substitute, Open Approach

RW0JZ   Replacement of Left Foot Artery with Synthetic Substitute, Open Approach

RW0KZ   Replacement of Left Foot Artery with Nonautologous Tissue Substitute, Open Approach

04RW47Z   Replacement of Left Foot Artery with Autologous Tissue Substitute, Percutaneous Endoscopic Approach

04RW4JZ   Replacement of Left Foot Artery with Synthetic Substitute, Percutaneous Endoscopic Approach

04RW4KZ   Replacement of Left Foot Artery with Nonautologous Tissue Substitute, Percutaneous Endoscopic Approach

04RY07Z   Replacement of Lower Artery with Autologous Tissue Substitute, Open Approach

04RY0JZ   Replacement of Lower Artery with Synthetic Substitute, Open Approach

04RY0KZ   Replacement of Lower Artery with Nonautologous Tissue Substitute, Open Approach

04RY47Z   Replacement of Lower Artery with Autologous Tissue Substitute, Percutaneous Endoscopic Approach

04RY4JZ   Replacement of Lower Artery with Synthetic Substitute, Percutaneous Endoscopic Approach

04RY4KZ   Replacement of Lower Artery with Nonautologous Tissue Substitute, Percutaneous Endoscopic Approach

'S – Lower Arteries, Reposition

S00ZZ   Reposition Abdominal Aorta, Open Approach

S03ZZ   Reposition Abdominal Aorta, Percutaneous Approach

S04ZZ   Reposition Abdominal Aorta, Percutaneous Endoscopic Approach

S10ZZ   Reposition Celiac Artery, Open Approach

S13ZZ   Reposition Celiac Artery, Percutaneous Approach

S14ZZ   Reposition Celiac Artery, Percutaneous Endoscopic Approach

S20ZZ   Reposition Gastric Artery, Open Approach

S23ZZ   Reposition Gastric Artery, Percutaneous Approach

S24ZZ   Reposition Gastric Artery, Percutaneous Endoscopic Approach

S30ZZ   Reposition Hepatic Artery, Open Approach

S33ZZ   Reposition Hepatic Artery, Percutaneous Approach

S34ZZ   Reposition Hepatic Artery, Percutaneous Endoscopic Approach

S40ZZ   Reposition Splenic Artery, Open Approach

S43ZZ   Reposition Splenic Artery, Percutaneous Approach

S44ZZ   Reposition Splenic Artery, Percutaneous Endoscopic Approach

S50ZZ   Reposition Superior Mesenteric Artery, Open Approach

S53ZZ   Reposition Superior Mesenteric Artery, Percutaneous Approach

S54ZZ   Reposition Superior Mesenteric Artery, Percutaneous Endoscopic Approach

S60ZZ   Reposition Right Colic Artery, Open Approach

S63ZZ   Reposition Right Colic Artery, Percutaneous Approach

S64ZZ   Reposition Right Colic Artery, Percutaneous Endoscopic Approach

S70ZZ   Reposition Left Colic Artery, Open Approach

S73ZZ   Reposition Left Colic Artery, Percutaneous Approach

S74ZZ   Reposition Left Colic Artery, Percutaneous Endoscopic Approach

S80ZZ   Reposition Middle Colic Artery, Open Approach

S83ZZ   Reposition Middle Colic Artery, Percutaneous Approach

S84ZZ   Reposition Middle Colic Artery, Percutaneous Endoscopic Approach

S90ZZ   Reposition Right Renal Artery, Open Approach

S93ZZ   Reposition Right Renal Artery, Percutaneous Approach

S94ZZ   Reposition Right Renal Artery, Percutaneous Endoscopic Approach

SA0ZZ   Reposition Left Renal Artery, Open Approach

SA3ZZ   Reposition Left Renal Artery, Percutaneous Approach

04SA4ZZ   Reposition Left Renal Artery, Percutaneous Endoscopic Approach

04SB0ZZ   Reposition Inferior Mesenteric Artery, Open Approach

04SB3ZZ   Reposition Inferior Mesenteric Artery, Percutaneous Approach

04SB4ZZ   Reposition Inferior Mesenteric Artery, Percutaneous Endoscopic Approach

04SC0ZZ   Reposition Right Common Iliac Artery, Open Approach

04SC3ZZ   Reposition Right Common Iliac Artery, Percutaneous Approach

04SC4ZZ   Reposition Right Common Iliac Artery, Percutaneous Endoscopic Approach

04SD0ZZ   Reposition Left Common Iliac Artery, Open Approach

04SD3ZZ   Reposition Left Common Iliac Artery, Percutaneous Approach

04SD4ZZ   Reposition Left Common Iliac Artery, Percutaneous Endoscopic Approach

04SE0ZZ   Reposition Right Internal Iliac Artery, Open Approach

04SE3ZZ   Reposition Right Internal Iliac Artery, Percutaneous Approach

04SE4ZZ   Reposition Right Internal Iliac Artery, Percutaneous Endoscopic Approach

04SF0ZZ   Reposition Left Internal Iliac Artery, Open Approach

04SF3ZZ   Reposition Left Internal Iliac Artery, Percutaneous Approach

04SF4ZZ   Reposition Left Internal Iliac Artery, Percutaneous Endoscopic Approach

04SH0ZZ   Reposition Right External Iliac Artery, Open Approach

04SH3ZZ   Reposition Right External Iliac Artery, Percutaneous Approach

04SH4ZZ   Reposition Right External Iliac Artery, Percutaneous Endoscopic Approach

04SJ0ZZ   Reposition Left External Iliac Artery, Open Approach

04SJ3ZZ   Reposition Left External Iliac Artery, Percutaneous Approach

04SJ4ZZ   Reposition Left External Iliac Artery, Percutaneous Endoscopic Approach

04SK0ZZ   Reposition Right Femoral Artery, Open Approach

04SK3ZZ   Reposition Right Femoral Artery, Percutaneous Approach

04SK4ZZ   Reposition Right Femoral Artery, Percutaneous Endoscopic Approach

04SL0ZZ   Reposition Left Femoral Artery, Open Approach

04SL3ZZ   Reposition Left Femoral Artery, Percutaneous Approach

04SL4ZZ   Reposition Left Femoral Artery, Percutaneous Endoscopic Approach

04SM0ZZ   Reposition Right Popliteal Artery, Open Approach

04SM3ZZ   Reposition Right Popliteal Artery, Percutaneous Approach

04SM4ZZ   Reposition Right Popliteal Artery, Percutaneous Endoscopic Approach

04SN0ZZ   Reposition Left Popliteal Artery, Open Approach

04SN3ZZ   Reposition Left Popliteal Artery, Percutaneous Approach

04SN4ZZ   Reposition Left Popliteal Artery, Percutaneous Endoscopic Approach

04SP0ZZ   Reposition Right Anterior Tibial Artery, Open Approach

04SP3ZZ   Reposition Right Anterior Tibial Artery, Percutaneous Approach

04SP4ZZ   Reposition Right Anterior Tibial Artery, Percutaneous Endoscopic Approach

04SQ0ZZ   Reposition Left Anterior Tibial Artery, Open Approach

04SQ3ZZ   Reposition Left Anterior Tibial Artery, Percutaneous Approach

04SQ4ZZ   Reposition Left Anterior Tibial Artery, Percutaneous Endoscopic Approach

04SR0ZZ   Reposition Right Posterior Tibial Artery, Open Approach

04SR3ZZ   Reposition Right Posterior Tibial Artery, Percutaneous Approach

04SR4ZZ   Reposition Right Posterior Tibial Artery, Percutaneous Endoscopic Approach

04SS0ZZ   Reposition Left Posterior Tibial Artery, Open Approach

04SS3ZZ   Reposition Left Posterior Tibial Artery, Percutaneous Approach

04SS4ZZ   Reposition Left Posterior Tibial Artery, Percutaneous Endoscopic Approach

04ST0ZZ   Reposition Right Peroneal Artery, Open Approach

04ST3ZZ   Reposition Right Peroneal Artery, Percutaneous Approach

04ST4ZZ   Reposition Right Peroneal Artery, Percutaneous Endoscopic Approach

04SU0ZZ   Reposition Left Peroneal Artery, Open Approach

04SU3ZZ   Reposition Left Peroneal Artery, Percutaneous Approach

04SU4ZZ   Reposition Left Peroneal Artery, Percutaneous Endoscopic Approach

04SV0ZZ   Reposition Right Foot Artery, Open Approach

04SV3ZZ   Reposition Right Foot Artery, Percutaneous Approach

04SV4ZZ   Reposition Right Foot Artery, Percutaneous Endoscopic Approach

04SW0ZZ   Reposition Left Foot Artery, Open Approach

04SW3ZZ   Reposition Left Foot Artery, Percutaneous Approach

04SW4ZZ   Reposition Left Foot Artery, Percutaneous Endoscopic Approach

04SY0ZZ   Reposition Lower Artery, Open Approach

04SY3ZZ   Reposition Lower Artery, Percutaneous Approach

04SY4ZZ   Reposition Lower Artery, Percutaneous Endoscopic Approach

| Female-only | ♂ Male-only | ▲ Limited Coverage | ● Non-OR | ▥ HAC-associated procedure | ▲ Non-covered procedures | ▤ Combination |

04U007Z Supplement Abdominal Aorta with Autologous Tissue Substitute, Open Approach

04U00JZ Supplement Abdominal Aorta with Synthetic Substitute, Open Approach

04U00KZ Supplement Abdominal Aorta with Nonautologous Tissue Substitute, Open Approach

04U037Z Supplement Abdominal Aorta with Autologous Tissue Substitute, Percutaneous Approach

04U03JZ Supplement Abdominal Aorta with Synthetic Substitute, Percutaneous Approach

04U03KZ Supplement Abdominal Aorta with Nonautologous Tissue Substitute, Percutaneous Approach

04U047Z Supplement Abdominal Aorta with Autologous Tissue Substitute, Percutaneous Endoscopic Approach

04U04JZ Supplement Abdominal Aorta with Synthetic Substitute, Percutaneous Endoscopic Approach

04U04KZ Supplement Abdominal Aorta with Nonautologous Tissue Substitute, Percutaneous Endoscopic Approach

04U107Z Supplement Celiac Artery with Autologous Tissue Substitute, Open Approach

04U10JZ Supplement Celiac Artery with Synthetic Substitute, Open Approach

04U10KZ Supplement Celiac Artery with Nonautologous Tissue Substitute, Open Approach

04U137Z Supplement Celiac Artery with Autologous Tissue Substitute, Percutaneous Approach

04U13JZ Supplement Celiac Artery with Synthetic Substitute, Percutaneous Approach

04U13KZ Supplement Celiac Artery with Nonautologous Tissue Substitute, Percutaneous Approach

04U147Z Supplement Celiac Artery with Autologous Tissue Substitute, Percutaneous Endoscopic Approach

04U14JZ Supplement Celiac Artery with Synthetic Substitute, Percutaneous Endoscopic Approach

04U14KZ Supplement Celiac Artery with Nonautologous Tissue Substitute, Percutaneous Endoscopic Approach

04U207Z Supplement Gastric Artery with Autologous Tissue Substitute, Open Approach

04U20JZ Supplement Gastric Artery with Synthetic Substitute, Open Approach

04U20KZ Supplement Gastric Artery with Nonautologous Tissue Substitute, Open Approach

04U237Z Supplement Gastric Artery with Autologous Tissue Substitute, Percutaneous Approach

04U23JZ Supplement Gastric Artery with Synthetic Substitute, Percutaneous Approach

04U23KZ Supplement Gastric Artery with Nonautologous Tissue Substitute, Percutaneous Approach

04U247Z Supplement Gastric Artery with Autologous Tissue Substitute, Percutaneous Endoscopic Approach

04U24JZ Supplement Gastric Artery with Synthetic Substitute, Percutaneous Endoscopic Approach

04U24KZ Supplement Gastric Artery with Nonautologous Tissue Substitute, Percutaneous Endoscopic Approach

04U307Z Supplement Hepatic Artery with Autologous Tissue Substitute, Open Approach

04U30JZ Supplement Hepatic Artery with Synthetic Substitute, Open Approach

04U30KZ Supplement Hepatic Artery with Nonautologous Tissue Substitute, Open Approach

04U337Z Supplement Hepatic Artery with Autologous Tissue Substitute, Percutaneous Approach

04U33JZ Supplement Hepatic Artery with Synthetic Substitute, Percutaneous Approach

04U33KZ Supplement Hepatic Artery with Nonautologous Tissue Substitute, Percutaneous Approach

04U347Z Supplement Hepatic Artery with Autologous Tissue Substitute, Percutaneous Endoscopic Approach

04U34JZ Supplement Hepatic Artery with Synthetic Substitute, Percutaneous Endoscopic Approach

04U34KZ Supplement Hepatic Artery with Nonautologous Tissue Substitute, Percutaneous Endoscopic Approach

04U407Z Supplement Splenic Artery with Autologous Tissue Substitute, Open Approach

04U40JZ Supplement Splenic Artery with Synthetic Substitute, Open Approach

04U40KZ Supplement Splenic Artery with Nonautologous Tissue Substitute, Open Approach

04U437Z Supplement Splenic Artery with Autologous Tissue Substitute, Percutaneous Approach

04U43JZ Supplement Splenic Artery with Synthetic Substitute, Percutaneous Approach

04U43KZ Supplement Splenic Artery with Nonautologous Tissue Substitute, Percutaneous Approach

04U447Z Supplement Splenic Artery with Autologous Tissue Substitute, Percutaneous Endoscopic Approach

04U44JZ Supplement Splenic Artery with Synthetic Substitute, Percutaneous Endoscopic Approach

04U44KZ Supplement Splenic Artery with Nonautologous Tissue Substitute, Percutaneous Endoscopic Approach

04U507Z Supplement Superior Mesenteric Artery with Autologous Tissue Substitute, Open Approach

04U50JZ Supplement Superior Mesenteric Artery with Synthetic Substitute, Open Approach

04U50KZ Supplement Superior Mesenteric Artery with Nonautologous Tissue Substitute, Open Approach

04U537Z Supplement Superior Mesenteric Artery with Autologous Tissue Substitute, Percutaneous Approach

04U53JZ Supplement Superior Mesenteric Artery with Synthetic Substitute, Percutaneous Approach

04U53KZ Supplement Superior Mesenteric Artery with Nonautologous Tissue Substitute, Percutaneous Approach

04U547Z Supplement Superior Mesenteric Artery with Autologous Tissue Substitute, Percutaneous Endoscopic Approach

04U54JZ Supplement Superior Mesenteric Artery with Synthetic Substitute, Percutaneous Endoscopic Approach

04U54KZ Supplement Superior Mesenteric Artery with Nonautologous Tissue Substitute, Percutaneous Endoscopic Approach

04U607Z Supplement Right Colic Artery with Autologous Tissue Substitute, Open Approach

04U60JZ Supplement Right Colic Artery with Synthetic Substitute, Open Approach

04U60KZ Supplement Right Colic Artery with Nonautologous Tissue Substitute, Open Approach

04U637Z Supplement Right Colic Artery with Autologous Tissue Substitute, Percutaneous Approach

04U63JZ Supplement Right Colic Artery with Synthetic Substitute, Percutaneous Approach

04U63KZ Supplement Right Colic Artery with Nonautologous Tissue Substitute, Percutaneous Approach

04U647Z Supplement Right Colic Artery with Autologous Tissue Substitute, Percutaneous Endoscopic Approach

04U64JZ Supplement Right Colic Artery with Synthetic Substitute, Percutaneous Endoscopic Approach

04U64KZ Supplement Right Colic Artery with Nonautologous Tissue Substitute, Percutaneous Endoscopic Approach

04U707Z Supplement Left Colic Artery with Autologous Tissue Substitute, Open Approach

04U70JZ Supplement Left Colic Artery with Synthetic Substitute, Open Approach

04U70KZ Supplement Left Colic Artery with Nonautologous Tissue Substitute, Open Approach

04U737Z Supplement Left Colic Artery with Autologous Tissue Substitute, Percutaneous Approach

04U73JZ Supplement Left Colic Artery with Synthetic Substitute, Percutaneous Approach

04U73KZ Supplement Left Colic Artery with Nonautologous Tissue Substitute, Percutaneous Approach

04U747Z Supplement Left Colic Artery with Autologous Tissue Substitute, Percutaneous Endoscopic Approach

04U74JZ Supplement Left Colic Artery with Synthetic Substitute, Percutaneous Endoscopic Approach

04U74KZ Supplement Left Colic Artery with Nonautologous Tissue Substitute, Percutaneous Endoscopic Approach

04U807Z Supplement Middle Colic Artery with Autologous Tissue Substitute, Open Approach

04U80JZ Supplement Middle Colic Artery with Synthetic Substitute, Open Approach

04U80KZ Supplement Middle Colic Artery with Nonautologous Tissue Substitute, Open Approach

04U837Z Supplement Middle Colic Artery with Autologous Tissue Substitute, Percutaneous Approach

04U83JZ Supplement Middle Colic Artery with Synthetic Substitute, Percutaneous Approach

04U83KZ Supplement Middle Colic Artery with Nonautologous Tissue Substitute, Percutaneous Approach

04U847Z Supplement Middle Colic Artery with Autologous Tissue Substitute, Percutaneous Endoscopic Approach

04U84JZ Supplement Middle Colic Artery with Synthetic Substitute, Percutaneous Endoscopic Approach

04U84KZ Supplement Middle Colic Artery with Nonautologous Tissue Substitute, Percutaneous Endoscopic Approach

04U907Z Supplement Right Renal Artery with Autologous Tissue Substitute, Open Approach

04U90JZ Supplement Right Renal Artery with Synthetic Substitute, Open Approach

04U90KZ Supplement Right Renal Artery with Nonautologous Tissue Substitute, Open Approach

04U937Z Supplement Right Renal Artery with Autologous Tissue Substitute, Percutaneous Approach

04U93JZ Supplement Right Renal Artery with Synthetic Substitute, Percutaneous Approach

04U93KZ Supplement Right Renal Artery with Nonautologous Tissue Substitute, Percutaneous Approach

04U947Z Supplement Right Renal Artery with Autologous Tissue Substitute, Percutaneous Endoscopic Approach

04U94JZ Supplement Right Renal Artery with Synthetic Substitute, Percutaneous Endoscopic Approach

04U94KZ Supplement Right Renal Artery with Nonautologous Tissue Substitute, Percutaneous Endoscopic Approach

04UA07Z Supplement Left Renal Artery with Autologous Tissue Substitute, Open Approach

04UA0JZ Supplement Left Renal Artery with Synthetic Substitute, Open Approach

04UA0KZ Supplement Left Renal Artery with Nonautologous Tissue Substitute, Open Approach

04UA37Z Supplement Left Renal Artery with Autologous Tissue Substitute, Percutaneous Approach

04UA3JZ Supplement Left Renal Artery with Synthetic Substitute, Percutaneous Approach

04UA3KZ Supplement Left Renal Artery with Nonautologous Tissue Substitute, Percutaneous Approach

04UA47Z Supplement Left Renal Artery with Autologous Tissue Substitute, Percutaneous Endoscopic Approach

04UA4JZ Supplement Left Renal Artery with Synthetic Substitute, Percutaneous Endoscopic Approach

04UA4KZ Supplement Left Renal Artery with Nonautologous Tissue Substitute, Percutaneous Endoscopic Approach

04UB07Z Supplement Inferior Mesenteric Artery with Autologous Tissue Substitute, Open Approach

04UB0JZ Supplement Inferior Mesenteric Artery with Synthetic Substitute, Open Approach

04UB0KZ Supplement Inferior Mesenteric Artery with Nonautologous Tissue Substitute, Open Approach

04UB37Z Supplement Inferior Mesenteric Artery with Autologous Tissue Substitute, Percutaneous Approach

04UB3JZ Supplement Inferior Mesenteric Artery with Synthetic Substitute, Percutaneous Approach

04UB3KZ Supplement Inferior Mesenteric Artery with Nonautologous Tissue Substitute, Percutaneous Approach

04UB47Z Supplement Inferior Mesenteric Artery with Autologous Tissue Substitute, Percutaneous Endoscopic Approach

04UB4JZ Supplement Inferior Mesenteric Artery with Synthetic Substitute, Percutaneous Endoscopic Approach

04UB4KZ Supplement Inferior Mesenteric Artery with Nonautologous Tissue Substitute, Percutaneous Endoscopic Approach

04UC07Z Supplement Right Common Iliac Artery with Autologous Tissue Substitute, Open Approach

04UC0JZ Supplement Right Common Iliac Artery with Synthetic Substitute, Open Approach

04UC0KZ Supplement Right Common Iliac Artery with Nonautologous Tissue Substitute, Open Approach

04UC37Z Supplement Right Common Iliac Artery with Autologous Tissue Substitute, Percutaneous Approach

04UC3JZ Supplement Right Common Iliac Artery with Synthetic Substitute, Percutaneous Approach

04UC3KZ Supplement Right Common Iliac Artery with Nonautologous Tissue Substitute, Percutaneous Approach

04UC47Z Supplement Right Common Iliac Artery with Autologous Tissue Substitute, Percutaneous Endoscopic Approach

04UC4JZ Supplement Right Common Iliac Artery with Synthetic Substitute, Percutaneous Endoscopic Approach

04UC4KZ Supplement Right Common Iliac Artery with Nonautologous Tissue Substitute, Percutaneous Endoscopic Approach

04UD07Z Supplement Left Common Iliac Artery with Autologous Tissue Substitute, Open Approach

04UD0JZ Supplement Left Common Iliac Artery with Synthetic Substitute, Open Approach

04UD0KZ Supplement Left Common Iliac Artery with Nonautologous Tissue Substitute, Open Approach

04UD37Z Supplement Left Common Iliac Artery with Autologous Tissue Substitute, Percutaneous Approach

04UD3JZ Supplement Left Common Iliac Artery with Synthetic Substitute, Percutaneous Approach

04UD3KZ Supplement Left Common Iliac Artery with Nonautologous Tissue Substitute, Percutaneous Approach

04UD47Z Supplement Left Common Iliac Artery with Autologous Tissue Substitute, Percutaneous Endoscopic Approach

04UD4JZ Supplement Left Common Iliac Artery with Synthetic Substitute, Percutaneous Endoscopic Approach

04UD4KZ Supplement Left Common Iliac Artery with Nonautologous Tissue Substitute, Percutaneous Endoscopic Approach

04UE07Z Supplement Right Internal Iliac Artery with Autologous Tissue Substitute, Open Approach

04UE0JZ Supplement Right Internal Iliac Artery with Synthetic Substitute, Open Approach

04UE0KZ Supplement Right Internal Iliac Artery with Nonautologous Tissue Substitute, Open Approach

04UE37Z Supplement Right Internal Iliac Artery with Autologous Tissue Substitute, Percutaneous Approach

04UE3JZ Supplement Right Internal Iliac Artery with Synthetic Substitute, Percutaneous Approach

04UE3KZ Supplement Right Internal Iliac Artery with Nonautologous Tissue Substitute, Percutaneous Approach

04UE47Z Supplement Right Internal Iliac Artery with Autologous Tissue Substitute, Percutaneous Endoscopic Approach

04UE4JZ Supplement Right Internal Iliac Artery with Synthetic Substitute, Percutaneous Endoscopic Approach

04UE4KZ Supplement Right Internal Iliac Artery with Nonautologous Tissue Substitute, Percutaneous Endoscopic Approach

04UF07Z Supplement Left Internal Iliac Artery with Autologous Tissue Substitute, Open Approach

04UF0JZ Supplement Left Internal Iliac Artery with Synthetic Substitute, Open Approach

04UF0KZ Supplement Left Internal Iliac Artery with Nonautologous Tissue Substitute, Open Approach

04UF37Z Supplement Left Internal Iliac Artery with Autologous Tissue Substitute, Percutaneous Approach

04UF3JZ Supplement Left Internal Iliac Artery with Synthetic Substitute, Percutaneous Approach

04UF3KZ Supplement Left Internal Iliac Artery with Nonautologous Tissue Substitute, Percutaneous Approach

04UF47Z Supplement Left Internal Iliac Artery with Autologous Tissue Substitute, Percutaneous Endoscopic Approach

04UF4JZ Supplement Left Internal Iliac Artery with Synthetic Substitute, Percutaneous Endoscopic Approach

04UF4KZ Supplement Left Internal Iliac Artery with Nonautologous Tissue Substitute, Percutaneous Endoscopic Approach

04UH07Z Supplement Right External Iliac Artery with Autologous Tissue Substitute, Open Approach

04UH0JZ Supplement Right External Iliac Artery with Synthetic Substitute, Open Approach

04UH0KZ Supplement Right External Iliac Artery with Nonautologous Tissue Substitute, Open Approach

04UH37Z Supplement Right External Iliac Artery with Autologous Tissue Substitute, Percutaneous Approach

04UH3JZ Supplement Right External Iliac Artery with Synthetic Substitute, Percutaneous Approach

04UH3KZ Supplement Right External Iliac Artery with Nonautologous Tissue Substitute, Percutaneous Approach

04UH47Z Supplement Right External Iliac Artery with Autologous Tissue Substitute, Percutaneous Endoscopic Approach

04UH4JZ Supplement Right External Iliac Artery with Synthetic Substitute, Percutaneous Endoscopic Approach

04UH4KZ Supplement Right External Iliac Artery with Nonautologous Tissue Substitute, Percutaneous Endoscopic Approach

04UJ07Z Supplement Left External Iliac Artery with Autologous Tissue Substitute, Open Approach

04UJ0JZ Supplement Left External Iliac Artery with Synthetic Substitute, Open Approach

04UJ0KZ Supplement Left External Iliac Artery with Nonautologous Tissue Substitute, Open Approach

Female-only   ♂ Male-only   ▲ Limited Coverage   ● Non-OR   ■ HAC-associated procedure   ▲ Non-covered procedures   ✛ Combination

04UJ37Z Supplement Left External Iliac Artery with Autologous Tissue Substitute, Percutaneous Approach

04UJ3JZ Supplement Left External Iliac Artery with Synthetic Substitute, Percutaneous Approach

04UJ3KZ Supplement Left External Iliac Artery with Nonautologous Tissue Substitute, Percutaneous Approach

04UJ47Z Supplement Left External Iliac Artery with Autologous Tissue Substitute, Percutaneous Endoscopic Approach

04UJ4JZ Supplement Left External Iliac Artery with Synthetic Substitute, Percutaneous Endoscopic Approach

04UJ4KZ Supplement Left External Iliac Artery with Nonautologous Tissue Substitute, Percutaneous Endoscopic Approach

04UK07Z Supplement Right Femoral Artery with Autologous Tissue Substitute, Open Approach

04UK0JZ Supplement Right Femoral Artery with Synthetic Substitute, Open Approach

04UK0KZ Supplement Right Femoral Artery with Nonautologous Tissue Substitute, Open Approach
AHA CC: 4Q, 2014, 37-38

04UK37Z Supplement Right Femoral Artery with Autologous Tissue Substitute, Percutaneous Approach

04UK3JZ Supplement Right Femoral Artery with Synthetic Substitute, Percutaneous Approach
AHA CC: 1Q, 2014, 22-23

04UK3KZ Supplement Right Femoral Artery with Nonautologous Tissue Substitute, Percutaneous Approach

04UK47Z Supplement Right Femoral Artery with Autologous Tissue Substitute, Percutaneous Endoscopic Approach

04UK4JZ Supplement Right Femoral Artery with Synthetic Substitute, Percutaneous Endoscopic Approach

04UK4KZ Supplement Right Femoral Artery with Nonautologous Tissue Substitute, Percutaneous Endoscopic Approach

04UL07Z Supplement Left Femoral Artery with Autologous Tissue Substitute, Open Approach

04UL0JZ Supplement Left Femoral Artery with Synthetic Substitute, Open Approach

04UL0KZ Supplement Left Femoral Artery with Nonautologous Tissue Substitute, Open Approach

04UL37Z Supplement Left Femoral Artery with Autologous Tissue Substitute, Percutaneous Approach

04UL3JZ Supplement Left Femoral Artery with Synthetic Substitute, Percutaneous Approach

04UL3KZ Supplement Left Femoral Artery with Nonautologous Tissue Substitute, Percutaneous Approach

04UL47Z Supplement Left Femoral Artery with Autologous Tissue Substitute, Percutaneous Endoscopic Approach

04UL4JZ Supplement Left Femoral Artery with Synthetic Substitute, Percutaneous Endoscopic Approach

04UL4KZ Supplement Left Femoral Artery with Nonautologous Tissue Substitute, Percutaneous Endoscopic Approach

04UM07Z Supplement Right Popliteal Artery with Autologous Tissue Substitute, Open Approach

04UM0JZ Supplement Right Popliteal Artery with Synthetic Substitute, Open Approach

04UM0KZ Supplement Right Popliteal Artery with Nonautologous Tissue Substitute, Open Approach

04UM37Z Supplement Right Popliteal Artery with Autologous Tissue Substitute, Percutaneous Approach

04UM3JZ Supplement Right Popliteal Artery with Synthetic Substitute, Percutaneous Approach

04UM3KZ Supplement Right Popliteal Artery with Nonautologous Tissue Substitute, Percutaneous Approach

04UM47Z Supplement Right Popliteal Artery with Autologous Tissue Substitute, Percutaneous Endoscopic Approach

04UM4JZ Supplement Right Popliteal Artery with Synthetic Substitute, Percutaneous Endoscopic Approach

04UM4KZ Supplement Right Popliteal Artery with Nonautologous Tissue Substitute, Percutaneous Endoscopic Approach

04UN07Z Supplement Left Popliteal Artery with Autologous Tissue Substitute, Open Approach

04UN0JZ Supplement Left Popliteal Artery with Synthetic Substitute, Open Approach

04UN0KZ Supplement Left Popliteal Artery with Nonautologous Tissue Substitute, Open Approach

04UN37Z Supplement Left Popliteal Artery with Autologous Tissue Substitute, Percutaneous Approach

04UN3JZ Supplement Left Popliteal Artery with Synthetic Substitute, Percutaneous Approach

04UN3KZ Supplement Left Popliteal Artery with Nonautologous Tissue Substitute, Percutaneous Approach

04UN47Z Supplement Left Popliteal Artery with Autologous Tissue Substitute, Percutaneous Endoscopic Approach

04UN4JZ Supplement Left Popliteal Artery with Synthetic Substitute, Percutaneous Endoscopic Approach

04UN4KZ Supplement Left Popliteal Artery with Nonautologous Tissue Substitute, Percutaneous Endoscopic Approach

04UP07Z Supplement Right Anterior Tibial Artery with Autologous Tissue Substitute, Open Approach

04UP0JZ Supplement Right Anterior Tibial Artery with Synthetic Substitute, Open Approach

04UP0KZ Supplement Right Anterior Tibial Artery with Nonautologous Tissue Substitute, Open Approach

04UP37Z Supplement Right Anterior Tibial Artery with Autologous Tissue Substitute, Percutaneous Approach

04UP3JZ Supplement Right Anterior Tibial Artery with Synthetic Substitute, Percutaneous Approach

04UP3KZ Supplement Right Anterior Tibial Artery with Nonautologous Tissue Substitute, Percutaneous Approach

04UP47Z Supplement Right Anterior Tibial Artery with Autologous Tissue Substitute, Percutaneous Endoscopic Approach

04UP4JZ Supplement Right Anterior Tibial Artery with Synthetic Substitute, Percutaneous Endoscopic Approach

04UP4KZ Supplement Right Anterior Tibial Artery with Nonautologous Tissue Substitute, Percutaneous Endoscopic Approach

04UQ07Z Supplement Left Anterior Tibial Artery with Autologous Tissue Substitute, Open Approach

04UQ0JZ Supplement Left Anterior Tibial Artery with Synthetic Substitute, Open Approach

04UQ0KZ Supplement Left Anterior Tibial Artery with Nonautologous Tissue Substitute, Open Approach

04UQ37Z Supplement Left Anterior Tibial Artery with Autologous Tissue Substitute, Percutaneous Approach

04UQ3JZ Supplement Left Anterior Tibial Artery with Synthetic Substitute, Percutaneous Approach

04UQ3KZ Supplement Left Anterior Tibial Artery with Nonautologous Tissue Substitute, Percutaneous Approach

04UQ47Z Supplement Left Anterior Tibial Artery with Autologous Tissue Substitute, Percutaneous Endoscopic Approach

04UQ4JZ Supplement Left Anterior Tibial Artery with Synthetic Substitute, Percutaneous Endoscopic Approach

04UQ4KZ Supplement Left Anterior Tibial Artery with Nonautologous Tissue Substitute, Percutaneous Endoscopic Approach

04UR07Z Supplement Right Posterior Tibial Artery with Autologous Tissue Substitute, Open Approach

04UR0JZ Supplement Right Posterior Tibial Artery with Synthetic Substitute, Open Approach

04UR0KZ Supplement Right Posterior Tibial Artery with Nonautologous Tissue Substitute, Open Approach

04UR37Z Supplement Right Posterior Tibial Artery with Autologous Tissue Substitute, Percutaneous Approach

04UR3JZ Supplement Right Posterior Tibial Artery with Synthetic Substitute, Percutaneous Approach

04UR3KZ Supplement Right Posterior Tibial Artery with Nonautologous Tissue Substitute, Percutaneous Approach

04UR47Z Supplement Right Posterior Tibial Artery with Autologous Tissue Substitute, Percutaneous Endoscopic Approach

04UR4JZ Supplement Right Posterior Tibial Artery with Synthetic Substitute, Percutaneous Endoscopic Approach

04UR4KZ Supplement Right Posterior Tibial Artery with Nonautologous Tissue Substitute, Percutaneous Endoscopic Approach

04US07Z Supplement Left Posterior Tibial Artery with Autologous Tissue Substitute, Open Approach

04US0JZ Supplement Left Posterior Tibial Artery with Synthetic Substitute, Open Approach

04US0KZ Supplement Left Posterior Tibial Artery with Nonautologous Tissue Substitute, Open Approach

04US37Z Supplement Left Posterior Tibial Artery with Autologous Tissue Substitute, Percutaneous Approach

04US3JZ Supplement Left Posterior Tibial Artery with Synthetic Substitute, Percutaneous Approach

04US3KZ Supplement Left Posterior Tibial Artery with Nonautologous Tissue Substitute, Percutaneous Approach

04US47Z Supplement Left Posterior Tibial Artery with Autologous Tissue Substitute, Percutaneous Endoscopic Approach

04US4JZ Supplement Left Posterior Tibial Artery with Synthetic Substitute, Percutaneous Endoscopic Approach

S4KZ	Supplement Left Posterior Tibial Artery with Nonautologous Tissue Substitute, Percutaneous Endoscopic Approach
T07Z	Supplement Right Peroneal Artery with Autologous Tissue Substitute, Open Approach
T0JZ	Supplement Right Peroneal Artery with Synthetic Substitute, Open Approach
T0KZ	Supplement Right Peroneal Artery with Nonautologous Tissue Substitute, Open Approach
T37Z	Supplement Right Peroneal Artery with Autologous Tissue Substitute, Percutaneous Approach
T3JZ	Supplement Right Peroneal Artery with Synthetic Substitute, Percutaneous Approach
T3KZ	Supplement Right Peroneal Artery with Nonautologous Tissue Substitute, Percutaneous Approach
T47Z	Supplement Right Peroneal Artery with Autologous Tissue Substitute, Percutaneous Endoscopic Approach
T4JZ	Supplement Right Peroneal Artery with Synthetic Substitute, Percutaneous Endoscopic Approach
T4KZ	Supplement Right Peroneal Artery with Nonautologous Tissue Substitute, Percutaneous Endoscopic Approach
U07Z	Supplement Left Peroneal Artery with Autologous Tissue Substitute, Open Approach
U0JZ	Supplement Left Peroneal Artery with Synthetic Substitute, Open Approach
U0KZ	Supplement Left Peroneal Artery with Nonautologous Tissue Substitute, Open Approach
U37Z	Supplement Left Peroneal Artery with Autologous Tissue Substitute, Percutaneous Approach
U3JZ	Supplement Left Peroneal Artery with Synthetic Substitute, Percutaneous Approach
U3KZ	Supplement Left Peroneal Artery with Nonautologous Tissue Substitute, Percutaneous Approach

04UU47Z	Supplement Left Peroneal Artery with Autologous Tissue Substitute, Percutaneous Endoscopic Approach
04UU4JZ	Supplement Left Peroneal Artery with Synthetic Substitute, Percutaneous Endoscopic Approach
04UU4KZ	Supplement Left Peroneal Artery with Nonautologous Tissue Substitute, Percutaneous Endoscopic Approach
04UV07Z	Supplement Right Foot Artery with Autologous Tissue Substitute, Open Approach
04UV0JZ	Supplement Right Foot Artery with Synthetic Substitute, Open Approach
04UV0KZ	Supplement Right Foot Artery with Nonautologous Tissue Substitute, Open Approach
04UV37Z	Supplement Right Foot Artery with Autologous Tissue Substitute, Percutaneous Approach
04UV3JZ	Supplement Right Foot Artery with Synthetic Substitute, Percutaneous Approach
04UV3KZ	Supplement Right Foot Artery with Nonautologous Tissue Substitute, Percutaneous Approach
04UV47Z	Supplement Right Foot Artery with Autologous Tissue Substitute, Percutaneous Endoscopic Approach
04UV4JZ	Supplement Right Foot Artery with Synthetic Substitute, Percutaneous Endoscopic Approach
04UV4KZ	Supplement Right Foot Artery with Nonautologous Tissue Substitute, Percutaneous Endoscopic Approach
04UW07Z	Supplement Left Foot Artery with Autologous Tissue Substitute, Open Approach
04UW0JZ	Supplement Left Foot Artery with Synthetic Substitute, Open Approach
04UW0KZ	Supplement Left Foot Artery with Nonautologous Tissue Substitute, Open Approach
04UW37Z	Supplement Left Foot Artery with Autologous Tissue Substitute, Percutaneous Approach

04UW3JZ	Supplement Left Foot Artery with Synthetic Substitute, Percutaneous Approach
04UW3KZ	Supplement Left Foot Artery with Nonautologous Tissue Substitute, Percutaneous Approach
04UW47Z	Supplement Left Foot Artery with Autologous Tissue Substitute, Percutaneous Endoscopic Approach
04UW4JZ	Supplement Left Foot Artery with Synthetic Substitute, Percutaneous Endoscopic Approach
04UW4KZ	Supplement Left Foot Artery with Nonautologous Tissue Substitute, Percutaneous Endoscopic Approach
04UY07Z	Supplement Lower Artery with Autologous Tissue Substitute, Open Approach
04UY0JZ	Supplement Lower Artery with Synthetic Substitute, Open Approach
04UY0KZ	Supplement Lower Artery with Nonautologous Tissue Substitute, Open Approach
04UY37Z	Supplement Lower Artery with Autologous Tissue Substitute, Percutaneous Approach
04UY3JZ	Supplement Lower Artery with Synthetic Substitute, Percutaneous Approach
04UY3KZ	Supplement Lower Artery with Nonautologous Tissue Substitute, Percutaneous Approach
04UY47Z	Supplement Lower Artery with Autologous Tissue Substitute, Percutaneous Endoscopic Approach
04UY4JZ	Supplement Lower Artery with Synthetic Substitute, Percutaneous Endoscopic Approach
04UY4KZ	Supplement Lower Artery with Nonautologous Tissue Substitute, Percutaneous Endoscopic Approach

V – Lower Arteries, Restriction

view Coding Guideline B3.12

V00CZ	Restriction of Abdominal Aorta with Extraluminal Device, Open Approach
V00DJ	Restriction of Abdominal Aorta with Intraluminal Device, Temporary, Open Approach
V00DZ	Restriction of Abdominal Aorta with Intraluminal Device, Open Approach
V00ZZ	Restriction of Abdominal Aorta, Open Approach
V03CZ	Restriction of Abdominal Aorta with Extraluminal Device, Percutaneous Approach
V03DJ	Restriction of Abdominal Aorta with Intraluminal Device, Temporary, Percutaneous Approach
V03DZ	Restriction of Abdominal Aorta with Intraluminal Device, Percutaneous Approach
	AHA CC: 1Q, 2014, 9
V03ZZ	Restriction of Abdominal Aorta, Percutaneous Approach
V04CZ	Restriction of Abdominal Aorta with Extraluminal Device, Percutaneous Endoscopic Approach

04V04DJ	Restriction of Abdominal Aorta with Intraluminal Device, Temporary, Percutaneous Endoscopic Approach
04V04DZ	Restriction of Abdominal Aorta with Intraluminal Device, Percutaneous Endoscopic Approach
04V04ZZ	Restriction of Abdominal Aorta, Percutaneous Endoscopic Approach
04V10CZ	Restriction of Celiac Artery with Extraluminal Device, Open Approach
04V10DZ	Restriction of Celiac Artery with Intraluminal Device, Open Approach
04V10ZZ	Restriction of Celiac Artery, Open Approach
04V13CZ	Restriction of Celiac Artery with Extraluminal Device, Percutaneous Approach
04V13DZ	Restriction of Celiac Artery with Intraluminal Device, Percutaneous Approach
04V13ZZ	Restriction of Celiac Artery, Percutaneous Approach

04V14CZ	Restriction of Celiac Artery with Extraluminal Device, Percutaneous Endoscopic Approach
04V14DZ	Restriction of Celiac Artery with Intraluminal Device, Percutaneous Endoscopic Approach
04V14ZZ	Restriction of Celiac Artery, Percutaneous Endoscopic Approach
04V20CZ	Restriction of Gastric Artery with Extraluminal Device, Open Approach
04V20DZ	Restriction of Gastric Artery with Intraluminal Device, Open Approach
04V20ZZ	Restriction of Gastric Artery, Open Approach
04V23CZ	Restriction of Gastric Artery with Extraluminal Device, Percutaneous Approach
04V23DZ	Restriction of Gastric Artery with Intraluminal Device, Percutaneous Approach
04V23ZZ	Restriction of Gastric Artery, Percutaneous Approach
04V24CZ	Restriction of Gastric Artery with Extraluminal Device, Percutaneous Endoscopic Approach

04V24DZ Restriction of Gastric Artery with Intraluminal Device, Percutaneous Endoscopic Approach

04V24ZZ Restriction of Gastric Artery, Percutaneous Endoscopic Approach

04V30CZ Restriction of Hepatic Artery with Extraluminal Device, Open Approach

04V30DZ Restriction of Hepatic Artery with Intraluminal Device, Open Approach

04V30ZZ Restriction of Hepatic Artery, Open Approach

04V33CZ Restriction of Hepatic Artery with Extraluminal Device, Percutaneous Approach

04V33DZ Restriction of Hepatic Artery with Intraluminal Device, Percutaneous Approach

04V33ZZ Restriction of Hepatic Artery, Percutaneous Approach

04V34CZ Restriction of Hepatic Artery with Extraluminal Device, Percutaneous Endoscopic Approach

04V34DZ Restriction of Hepatic Artery with Intraluminal Device, Percutaneous Endoscopic Approach

04V34ZZ Restriction of Hepatic Artery, Percutaneous Endoscopic Approach

04V40CZ Restriction of Splenic Artery with Extraluminal Device, Open Approach

04V40DZ Restriction of Splenic Artery with Intraluminal Device, Open Approach

04V40ZZ Restriction of Splenic Artery, Open Approach

04V43CZ Restriction of Splenic Artery with Extraluminal Device, Percutaneous Approach

04V43DZ Restriction of Splenic Artery with Intraluminal Device, Percutaneous Approach

04V43ZZ Restriction of Splenic Artery, Percutaneous Approach

04V44CZ Restriction of Splenic Artery with Extraluminal Device, Percutaneous Endoscopic Approach

04V44DZ Restriction of Splenic Artery with Intraluminal Device, Percutaneous Endoscopic Approach

04V44ZZ Restriction of Splenic Artery, Percutaneous Endoscopic Approach

04V50CZ Restriction of Superior Mesenteric Artery with Extraluminal Device, Open Approach

04V50DZ Restriction of Superior Mesenteric Artery with Intraluminal Device, Open Approach

04V50ZZ Restriction of Superior Mesenteric Artery, Open Approach

04V53CZ Restriction of Superior Mesenteric Artery with Extraluminal Device, Percutaneous Approach

04V53DZ Restriction of Superior Mesenteric Artery with Intraluminal Device, Percutaneous Approach

04V53ZZ Restriction of Superior Mesenteric Artery, Percutaneous Approach

04V54CZ Restriction of Superior Mesenteric Artery with Extraluminal Device, Percutaneous Endoscopic Approach

04V54DZ Restriction of Superior Mesenteric Artery with Intraluminal Device, Percutaneous Endoscopic Approach

04V54ZZ Restriction of Superior Mesenteric Artery, Percutaneous Endoscopic Approach

04V60CZ Restriction of Right Colic Artery with Extraluminal Device, Open Approach

04V60DZ Restriction of Right Colic Artery with Intraluminal Device, Open Approach

04V60ZZ Restriction of Right Colic Artery, Open Approach

04V63CZ Restriction of Right Colic Artery with Extraluminal Device, Percutaneous Approach

04V63DZ Restriction of Right Colic Artery with Intraluminal Device, Percutaneous Approach

04V63ZZ Restriction of Right Colic Artery, Percutaneous Approach

04V64CZ Restriction of Right Colic Artery with Extraluminal Device, Percutaneous Endoscopic Approach

04V64DZ Restriction of Right Colic Artery with Intraluminal Device, Percutaneous Endoscopic Approach

04V64ZZ Restriction of Right Colic Artery, Percutaneous Endoscopic Approach

04V70CZ Restriction of Left Colic Artery with Extraluminal Device, Open Approach

04V70DZ Restriction of Left Colic Artery with Intraluminal Device, Open Approach

04V70ZZ Restriction of Left Colic Artery, Open Approach

04V73CZ Restriction of Left Colic Artery with Extraluminal Device, Percutaneous Approach

04V73DZ Restriction of Left Colic Artery with Intraluminal Device, Percutaneous Approach

04V73ZZ Restriction of Left Colic Artery, Percutaneous Approach

04V74CZ Restriction of Left Colic Artery with Extraluminal Device, Percutaneous Endoscopic Approach

04V74DZ Restriction of Left Colic Artery with Intraluminal Device, Percutaneous Endoscopic Approach

04V74ZZ Restriction of Left Colic Artery, Percutaneous Endoscopic Approach

04V80CZ Restriction of Middle Colic Artery with Extraluminal Device, Open Approach

04V80DZ Restriction of Middle Colic Artery with Intraluminal Device, Open Approach

04V80ZZ Restriction of Middle Colic Artery, Open Approach

04V83CZ Restriction of Middle Colic Artery with Extraluminal Device, Percutaneous Approach

04V83DZ Restriction of Middle Colic Artery with Intraluminal Device, Percutaneous Approach

04V83ZZ Restriction of Middle Colic Artery, Percutaneous Approach

04V84CZ Restriction of Middle Colic Artery with Extraluminal Device, Percutaneous Endoscopic Approach

04V84DZ Restriction of Middle Colic Artery with Intraluminal Device, Percutaneous Endoscopic Approach

04V84ZZ Restriction of Middle Colic Artery, Percutaneous Endoscopic Approach

04V90CZ Restriction of Right Renal Artery with Extraluminal Device, Open Approach

04V90DZ Restriction of Right Renal Artery with Intraluminal Device, Open Approach

04V90ZZ Restriction of Right Renal Artery, Open Approach

04V93CZ Restriction of Right Renal Artery with Extraluminal Device, Percutaneous Approach

04V93DZ Restriction of Right Renal Artery with Intraluminal Device, Percutaneous Approach

04V93ZZ Restriction of Right Renal Artery, Percutaneous Approach

04V94CZ Restriction of Right Renal Artery with Extraluminal Device, Percutaneous Endoscopic Approach

04V94DZ Restriction of Right Renal Artery with Intraluminal Device, Percutaneous Endoscopic Approach

04V94ZZ Restriction of Right Renal Artery, Percutaneous Endoscopic Approach

04VA0CZ Restriction of Left Renal Artery with Extraluminal Device, Open Approach

04VA0DZ Restriction of Left Renal Artery with Intraluminal Device, Open Approach

04VA0ZZ Restriction of Left Renal Artery, Open Approach

04VA3CZ Restriction of Left Renal Artery with Extraluminal Device, Percutaneous Approach

04VA3DZ Restriction of Left Renal Artery with Intraluminal Device, Percutaneous Approach

04VA3ZZ Restriction of Left Renal Artery, Percutaneous Approach

04VA4CZ Restriction of Left Renal Artery with Extraluminal Device, Percutaneous Endoscopic Approach

04VA4DZ Restriction of Left Renal Artery with Intraluminal Device, Percutaneous Endoscopic Approach

04VA4ZZ Restriction of Left Renal Artery, Percutaneous Endoscopic Approach

04VB0CZ Restriction of Inferior Mesenteric Artery with Extraluminal Device, Open Approach

04VB0DZ Restriction of Inferior Mesenteric Artery with Intraluminal Device, Open Approach

04VB0ZZ Restriction of Inferior Mesenteric Artery, Open Approach

04VB3CZ Restriction of Inferior Mesenteric Artery with Extraluminal Device, Percutaneous Approach

04VB3DZ Restriction of Inferior Mesenteric Artery with Intraluminal Device, Percutaneous Approach

04VB3ZZ Restriction of Inferior Mesenteric Artery, Percutaneous Approach

04VB4CZ Restriction of Inferior Mesenteric Artery with Extraluminal Device, Percutaneous Endoscopic Approach

04VB4DZ Restriction of Inferior Mesenteric Artery with Intraluminal Device, Percutaneous Endoscopic Approach

04VB4ZZ Restriction of Inferior Mesenteric Artery, Percutaneous Endoscopic Approach

04VC0CZ Restriction of Right Common Iliac Artery with Extraluminal Device, Open Approach

04VC0DZ Restriction of Right Common Iliac Artery with Intraluminal Device, Open Approach

04VC0ZZ Restriction of Right Common Iliac Artery, Open Approach

04VC3CZ Restriction of Right Common Iliac Artery with Extraluminal Device, Percutaneous Approach

04VC3DZ Restriction of Right Common Iliac Artery with Intraluminal Device, Percutaneous Approach

04VC3ZZ Restriction of Right Common Iliac Artery, Percutaneous Approach

04VC4CZ Restriction of Right Common Iliac Artery with Extraluminal Device, Percutaneous Endoscopic Approach

04VC4DZ Restriction of Right Common Iliac Artery with Intraluminal Device, Percutaneous Endoscopic Approach

04VC4ZZ Restriction of Right Common Iliac Artery, Percutaneous Endoscopic Approach

04VD0CZ Restriction of Left Common Iliac Artery with Extraluminal Device, Open Approach

04VD0DZ Restriction of Left Common Iliac Artery with Intraluminal Device, Open Approach

04VD0ZZ Restriction of Left Common Iliac Artery, Open Approach

04VD3CZ Restriction of Left Common Iliac Artery with Extraluminal Device, Percutaneous Approach

04VD3DZ Restriction of Left Common Iliac Artery with Intraluminal Device, Percutaneous Approach

04VD3ZZ Restriction of Left Common Iliac Artery, Percutaneous Approach

04VD4CZ Restriction of Left Common Iliac Artery with Extraluminal Device, Percutaneous Endoscopic Approach

04VD4DZ Restriction of Left Common Iliac Artery with Intraluminal Device, Percutaneous Endoscopic Approach

04VD4ZZ Restriction of Left Common Iliac Artery, Percutaneous Endoscopic Approach

04VE0CZ Restriction of Right Internal Iliac Artery with Extraluminal Device, Open Approach

04VE0DZ Restriction of Right Internal Iliac Artery with Intraluminal Device, Open Approach

04VE0ZZ Restriction of Right Internal Iliac Artery, Open Approach

04VE3CZ Restriction of Right Internal Iliac Artery with Extraluminal Device, Percutaneous Approach

04VE3DZ Restriction of Right Internal Iliac Artery with Intraluminal Device, Percutaneous Approach

04VE3ZZ Restriction of Right Internal Iliac Artery, Percutaneous Approach

04VE4CZ Restriction of Right Internal Iliac Artery with Extraluminal Device, Percutaneous Endoscopic Approach

04VE4DZ Restriction of Right Internal Iliac Artery with Intraluminal Device, Percutaneous Endoscopic Approach

04VE4ZZ Restriction of Right Internal Iliac Artery, Percutaneous Endoscopic Approach

04VF0CZ Restriction of Left Internal Iliac Artery with Extraluminal Device, Open Approach

04VF0DZ Restriction of Left Internal Iliac Artery with Intraluminal Device, Open Approach

04VF0ZZ Restriction of Left Internal Iliac Artery, Open Approach

04VF3CZ Restriction of Left Internal Iliac Artery with Extraluminal Device, Percutaneous Approach

04VF3DZ Restriction of Left Internal Iliac Artery with Intraluminal Device, Percutaneous Approach

04VF3ZZ Restriction of Left Internal Iliac Artery, Percutaneous Approach

04VF4CZ Restriction of Left Internal Iliac Artery with Extraluminal Device, Percutaneous Endoscopic Approach

04VF4DZ Restriction of Left Internal Iliac Artery with Intraluminal Device, Percutaneous Endoscopic Approach

04VF4ZZ Restriction of Left Internal Iliac Artery, Percutaneous Endoscopic Approach

04VH0CZ Restriction of Right External Iliac Artery with Extraluminal Device, Open Approach

04VH0DZ Restriction of Right External Iliac Artery with Intraluminal Device, Open Approach

04VH0ZZ Restriction of Right External Iliac Artery, Open Approach

04VH3CZ Restriction of Right Common Iliac Artery with Extraluminal Device, Percutaneous Approach

04VH3DZ Restriction of Right External Iliac Artery with Intraluminal Device, Percutaneous Approach

04VH3ZZ Restriction of Right External Iliac Artery, Percutaneous Approach

04VH4CZ Restriction of Right External Iliac Artery with Extraluminal Device, Percutaneous Endoscopic Approach

04VH4DZ Restriction of Right External Iliac Artery with Intraluminal Device, Percutaneous Endoscopic Approach

04VH4ZZ Restriction of Right External Iliac Artery, Percutaneous Endoscopic Approach

04VJ0CZ Restriction of Left External Iliac Artery with Extraluminal Device, Open Approach

04VJ0DZ Restriction of Left External Iliac Artery with Intraluminal Device, Open Approach

04VJ0ZZ Restriction of Left External Iliac Artery, Open Approach

04VJ3CZ Restriction of Left External Iliac Artery with Extraluminal Device, Percutaneous Approach

04VJ3DZ Restriction of Left External Iliac Artery with Intraluminal Device, Percutaneous Approach

04VJ3ZZ Restriction of Left External Iliac Artery, Percutaneous Approach

04VJ4CZ Restriction of Left External Iliac Artery with Extraluminal Device, Percutaneous Endoscopic Approach

04VJ4DZ Restriction of Left External Iliac Artery with Intraluminal Device, Percutaneous Endoscopic Approach

04VJ4ZZ Restriction of Left External Iliac Artery, Percutaneous Endoscopic Approach

04VK0CZ Restriction of Right Femoral Artery with Extraluminal Device, Open Approach

04VK0DZ Restriction of Right Femoral Artery with Intraluminal Device, Open Approach

04VK0ZZ Restriction of Right Femoral Artery, Open Approach

04VK3CZ Restriction of Right Femoral Artery with Extraluminal Device, Percutaneous Approach

04VK3DZ Restriction of Right Femoral Artery with Intraluminal Device, Percutaneous Approach

04VK3ZZ Restriction of Right Femoral Artery, Percutaneous Approach

04VK4CZ Restriction of Right Femoral Artery with Extraluminal Device, Percutaneous Endoscopic Approach

04VK4DZ Restriction of Right Femoral Artery with Intraluminal Device, Percutaneous Endoscopic Approach

04VK4ZZ Restriction of Right Femoral Artery, Percutaneous Endoscopic Approach

04VL0CZ Restriction of Left Femoral Artery with Extraluminal Device, Open Approach

04VL0DZ Restriction of Left Femoral Artery with Intraluminal Device, Open Approach

04VL0ZZ Restriction of Left Femoral Artery, Open Approach

04VL3CZ Restriction of Left Femoral Artery with Extraluminal Device, Percutaneous Approach

04VL3DZ Restriction of Left Femoral Artery with Intraluminal Device, Percutaneous Approach

04VL3ZZ Restriction of Left Femoral Artery, Percutaneous Approach

04VL4CZ Restriction of Left Femoral Artery with Extraluminal Device, Percutaneous Endoscopic Approach

04VL4DZ Restriction of Left Femoral Artery with Intraluminal Device, Percutaneous Endoscopic Approach

04VL4ZZ Restriction of Left Femoral Artery, Percutaneous Endoscopic Approach

04VM0CZ Restriction of Right Popliteal Artery with Extraluminal Device, Open Approach

04VM0DZ Restriction of Right Popliteal Artery with Intraluminal Device, Open Approach

04VM0ZZ Restriction of Right Popliteal Artery, Open Approach

04VM3CZ Restriction of Right Popliteal Artery with Extraluminal Device, Percutaneous Approach

04VM3DZ Restriction of Right Popliteal Artery with Intraluminal Device, Percutaneous Approach

04VM3ZZ Restriction of Right Popliteal Artery, Percutaneous Approach

04VM4CZ Restriction of Right Popliteal Artery with Extraluminal Device, Percutaneous Endoscopic Approach

04VM4DZ Restriction of Right Popliteal Artery with Intraluminal Device, Percutaneous Endoscopic Approach

04VM4ZZ Restriction of Right Popliteal Artery, Percutaneous Endoscopic Approach

04VN0CZ Restriction of Left Popliteal Artery with Extraluminal Device, Open Approach

04VN0DZ Restriction of Left Popliteal Artery with Intraluminal Device, Open Approach

04VN0ZZ Restriction of Left Popliteal Artery, Open Approach

04VN3CZ Restriction of Left Popliteal Artery with Extraluminal Device, Percutaneous Approach

04VN3DZ Restriction of Left Popliteal Artery with Intraluminal Device, Percutaneous Approach

04VN3ZZ Restriction of Left Popliteal Artery, Percutaneous Approach

04VN4CZ Restriction of Left Popliteal Artery with Extraluminal Device, Percutaneous Endoscopic Approach

04VN4DZ Restriction of Left Popliteal Artery with Intraluminal Device, Percutaneous Endoscopic Approach

04VN4ZZ Restriction of Left Popliteal Artery, Percutaneous Endoscopic Approach

04VP0CZ Restriction of Right Anterior Tibial Artery with Extraluminal Device, Open Approach

04VP0DZ Restriction of Right Anterior Tibial Artery with Intraluminal Device, Open Approach

04VP0ZZ Restriction of Right Anterior Tibial Artery, Open Approach

04VP3CZ Restriction of Right Anterior Tibial Artery with Extraluminal Device, Percutaneous Approach

04VP3DZ Restriction of Right Anterior Tibial Artery with Intraluminal Device, Percutaneous Approach

04VP3ZZ Restriction of Right Anterior Tibial Artery, Percutaneous Approach

04VP4CZ Restriction of Right Anterior Tibial Artery with Extraluminal Device, Percutaneous Endoscopic Approach

04VP4DZ Restriction of Right Anterior Tibial Artery with Intraluminal Device, Percutaneous Endoscopic Approach

04VP4ZZ Restriction of Right Anterior Tibial Artery, Percutaneous Endoscopic Approach

04VQ0CZ Restriction of Left Anterior Tibial Artery with Extraluminal Device, Open Approach

04VQ0DZ Restriction of Left Anterior Tibial Artery with Intraluminal Device, Open Approach

♀ Female-only   ♂ Male-only   ▲ Limited Coverage   ● Non-OR   ▥ HAC-associated procedure   ▲ Non-covered procedures   ✚ Combination

04VQ0ZZ Restriction of Left Anterior Tibial Artery, Open Approach

04VQ3CZ Restriction of Left Anterior Tibial Artery with Extraluminal Device, Percutaneous Approach

04VQ3DZ Restriction of Left Anterior Tibial Artery with Intraluminal Device, Percutaneous Approach

04VQ3ZZ Restriction of Left Anterior Tibial Artery, Percutaneous Approach

04VQ4CZ Restriction of Left Anterior Tibial Artery with Extraluminal Device, Percutaneous Endoscopic Approach

04VQ4DZ Restriction of Left Anterior Tibial Artery with Intraluminal Device, Percutaneous Endoscopic Approach

04VQ4ZZ Restriction of Left Anterior Tibial Artery, Percutaneous Endoscopic Approach

04VR0CZ Restriction of Right Posterior Tibial Artery with Extraluminal Device, Open Approach

04VR0DZ Restriction of Right Posterior Tibial Artery with Intraluminal Device, Open Approach

04VR0ZZ Restriction of Right Posterior Tibial Artery, Open Approach

04VR3CZ Restriction of Right Posterior Tibial Artery with Extraluminal Device, Percutaneous Approach

04VR3DZ Restriction of Right Posterior Tibial Artery with Intraluminal Device, Percutaneous Approach

04VR3ZZ Restriction of Right Posterior Tibial Artery, Percutaneous Approach

04VR4CZ Restriction of Right Posterior Tibial Artery with Extraluminal Device, Percutaneous Endoscopic Approach

04VR4DZ Restriction of Right Posterior Tibial Artery with Intraluminal Device, Percutaneous Endoscopic Approach

04VR4ZZ Restriction of Right Posterior Tibial Artery, Percutaneous Endoscopic Approach

04VS0CZ Restriction of Left Posterior Tibial Artery with Extraluminal Device, Open Approach

04VS0DZ Restriction of Left Posterior Tibial Artery with Intraluminal Device, Open Approach

04VS0ZZ Restriction of Left Posterior Tibial Artery, Open Approach

04VS3CZ Restriction of Left Posterior Tibial Artery with Extraluminal Device, Percutaneous Approach

04VS3DZ Restriction of Left Posterior Tibial Artery with Intraluminal Device, Percutaneous Approach

04VS3ZZ Restriction of Left Posterior Tibial Artery, Percutaneous Approach

04VS4CZ Restriction of Left Posterior Tibial Artery with Extraluminal Device, Percutaneous Endoscopic Approach

04VS4DZ Restriction of Left Posterior Tibial Artery with Intraluminal Device, Percutaneous Endoscopic Approach

04VS4ZZ Restriction of Left Posterior Tibial Artery, Percutaneous Endoscopic Approach

04VT0CZ Restriction of Right Peroneal Artery with Extraluminal Device, Open Approach

04VT0DZ Restriction of Right Peroneal Artery with Intraluminal Device, Open Approach

04VT0ZZ Restriction of Right Peroneal Artery, Open Approach

04VT3CZ Restriction of Right Peroneal Artery with Extraluminal Device, Percutaneous Approach

04VT3DZ Restriction of Right Peroneal Artery with Intraluminal Device, Percutaneous Approach

04VT3ZZ Restriction of Right Peroneal Artery, Percutaneous Approach

04VT4CZ Restriction of Right Peroneal Artery with Extraluminal Device, Percutaneous Endoscopic Approach

04VT4DZ Restriction of Right Peroneal Artery with Intraluminal Device, Percutaneous Endoscopic Approach

04VT4ZZ Restriction of Right Peroneal Artery, Percutaneous Endoscopic Approach

04VU0CZ Restriction of Left Peroneal Artery with Extraluminal Device, Open Approach

04VU0DZ Restriction of Left Peroneal Artery with Intraluminal Device, Open Approach

04VU0ZZ Restriction of Left Peroneal Artery, Open Approach

04VU3CZ Restriction of Left Peroneal Artery with Extraluminal Device, Percutaneous Approach

04VU3DZ Restriction of Left Peroneal Artery with Intraluminal Device, Percutaneous Approach

04VU3ZZ Restriction of Left Peroneal Artery, Percutaneous Approach

04VU4CZ Restriction of Left Peroneal Artery with Extraluminal Device, Percutaneous Endoscopic Approach

04VU4DZ Restriction of Left Peroneal Artery with Intraluminal Device, Percutaneous Endoscopic Approach

04VU4ZZ Restriction of Left Peroneal Artery, Percutaneous Endoscopic Approach

04VV0CZ Restriction of Right Foot Artery with Extraluminal Device, Open Approach

04VV0DZ Restriction of Right Foot Artery with Intraluminal Device, Open Approach

04VV0ZZ Restriction of Right Foot Artery, Open Approach

04VV3CZ Restriction of Right Foot Artery with Extraluminal Device, Percutaneous Approach

04VV3DZ Restriction of Right Foot Artery with Intraluminal Device, Percutaneous Approach

04VV3ZZ Restriction of Right Foot Artery, Percutaneous Approach

04VV4CZ Restriction of Right Foot Artery with Extraluminal Device, Percutaneous Endoscopic Approach

04VV4DZ Restriction of Right Foot Artery with Intraluminal Device, Percutaneous Endoscopic Approach

04VV4ZZ Restriction of Right Foot Artery, Percutaneous Endoscopic Approach

04VW0CZ Restriction of Left Foot Artery with Extraluminal Device, Open Approach

04VW0DZ Restriction of Left Foot Artery with Intraluminal Device, Open Approach

04VW0ZZ Restriction of Left Foot Artery, Open Approach

04VW3CZ Restriction of Left Foot Artery with Extraluminal Device, Percutaneous Approach

04VW3DZ Restriction of Left Foot Artery with Intraluminal Device, Percutaneous Approach

04VW3ZZ Restriction of Left Foot Artery, Percutaneous Approach

04VW4CZ Restriction of Left Foot Artery with Extraluminal Device, Percutaneous Endoscopic Approach

04VW4DZ Restriction of Left Foot Artery with Intraluminal Device, Percutaneous Endoscopic Approach

04VW4ZZ Restriction of Left Foot Artery, Percutaneous Endoscopic Approach

04VY0CZ Restriction of Lower Artery with Extraluminal Device, Open Approach

04VY0DZ Restriction of Lower Artery with Intraluminal Device, Open Approach

04VY0ZZ Restriction of Lower Artery, Open Approach

04VY3CZ Restriction of Lower Artery with Extraluminal Device, Percutaneous Approach

04VY3DZ Restriction of Lower Artery with Intraluminal Device, Percutaneous Approach

04VY3ZZ Restriction of Lower Artery, Percutaneous Approach

04VY4CZ Restriction of Lower Artery with Extraluminal Device, Percutaneous Endoscopic Approach

04VY4DZ Restriction of Lower Artery with Intraluminal Device, Percutaneous Endoscopic Approach

04VY4ZZ Restriction of Lower Artery, Percutaneous Endoscopic Approach

04W – Lower Arteries, Revision

Review Coding Guideline B6.1c

04WY00Z Revision of Drainage Device in Lower Artery, Open Approach

04WY02Z Revision of Monitoring Device in Lower Artery, Open Approach

04WY03Z Revision of Infusion Device in Lower Artery, Open Approach

04WY07Z Revision of Autologous Tissue Substitute in Lower Artery, Open Approach
AHA CC: 1Q, 2015, 36-37

04WY0CZ Revision of Extraluminal Device in Lower Artery, Open Approach

04WY0DZ Revision of Intraluminal Device in Lower Artery, Open Approach

04WY0JZ Revision of Synthetic Substitute in Lower Artery, Open Approach

04WY0KZ Revision of Nonautologous Tissue Substitute in Lower Artery, Open Approach

04WY30Z Revision of Drainage Device in Lower Artery, Percutaneous Approach

♀ Female-only   ♂ Male-only   ▲ Limited Coverage   ● Non-OR   ▥ HAC-associated procedure   ▲ Non-covered procedures   ✚ Combinat

Y32Z	Revision of Monitoring Device in Lower Artery, Percutaneous Approach	**04WY42Z**	Revision of Monitoring Device in Lower Artery, Percutaneous Endoscopic Approach	**04WYX0Z**	Revision of Drainage Device in Lower Artery, External Approach
Y33Z	Revision of Infusion Device in Lower Artery, Percutaneous Approach	**04WY43Z**	Revision of Infusion Device in Lower Artery, Percutaneous Endoscopic Approach	**04WYX2Z**	Revision of Monitoring Device in Lower Artery, External Approach
Y37Z	Revision of Autologous Tissue Substitute in Lower Artery, Percutaneous Approach	**04WY47Z**	Revision of Autologous Tissue Substitute in Lower Artery, Percutaneous Endoscopic Approach	**04WYX3Z**	Revision of Infusion Device in Lower Artery, External Approach
	AHA CC: 1Q, 2014, 26			**04WYX7Z**	Revision of Autologous Tissue Substitute in Lower Artery, External Approach
Y3CZ	Revision of Extraluminal Device in Lower Artery, Percutaneous Approach	**04WY4CZ**	Revision of Extraluminal Device in Lower Artery, Percutaneous Endoscopic Approach		
Y3DZ	Revision of Intraluminal Device in Lower Artery, Percutaneous Approach	**04WY4DZ**	Revision of Intraluminal Device in Lower Artery, Percutaneous Endoscopic Approach	**04WYXCZ**	Revision of Extraluminal Device in Lower Artery, External Approach
	AHA CC: 1Q, 2014, 9-10			**04WYXDZ**	Revision of Intraluminal Device in Lower Artery, External Approach
Y3JZ	Revision of Synthetic Substitute in Lower Artery, Percutaneous Approach	**04WY4JZ**	Revision of Synthetic Substitute in Lower Artery, Percutaneous Endoscopic Approach	**04WYXJZ**	Revision of Synthetic Substitute in Lower Artery, External Approach
Y3KZ	Revision of Nonautologous Tissue Substitute in Lower Artery, Percutaneous Approach	**04WY4KZ**	Revision of Nonautologous Tissue Substitute in Lower Artery, Percutaneous Endoscopic Approach	**04WYXKZ**	Revision of Nonautologous Tissue Substitute in Lower Artery, External Approach
Y40Z	Revision of Drainage Device in Lower Artery, Percutaneous Endoscopic Approach				

Veins

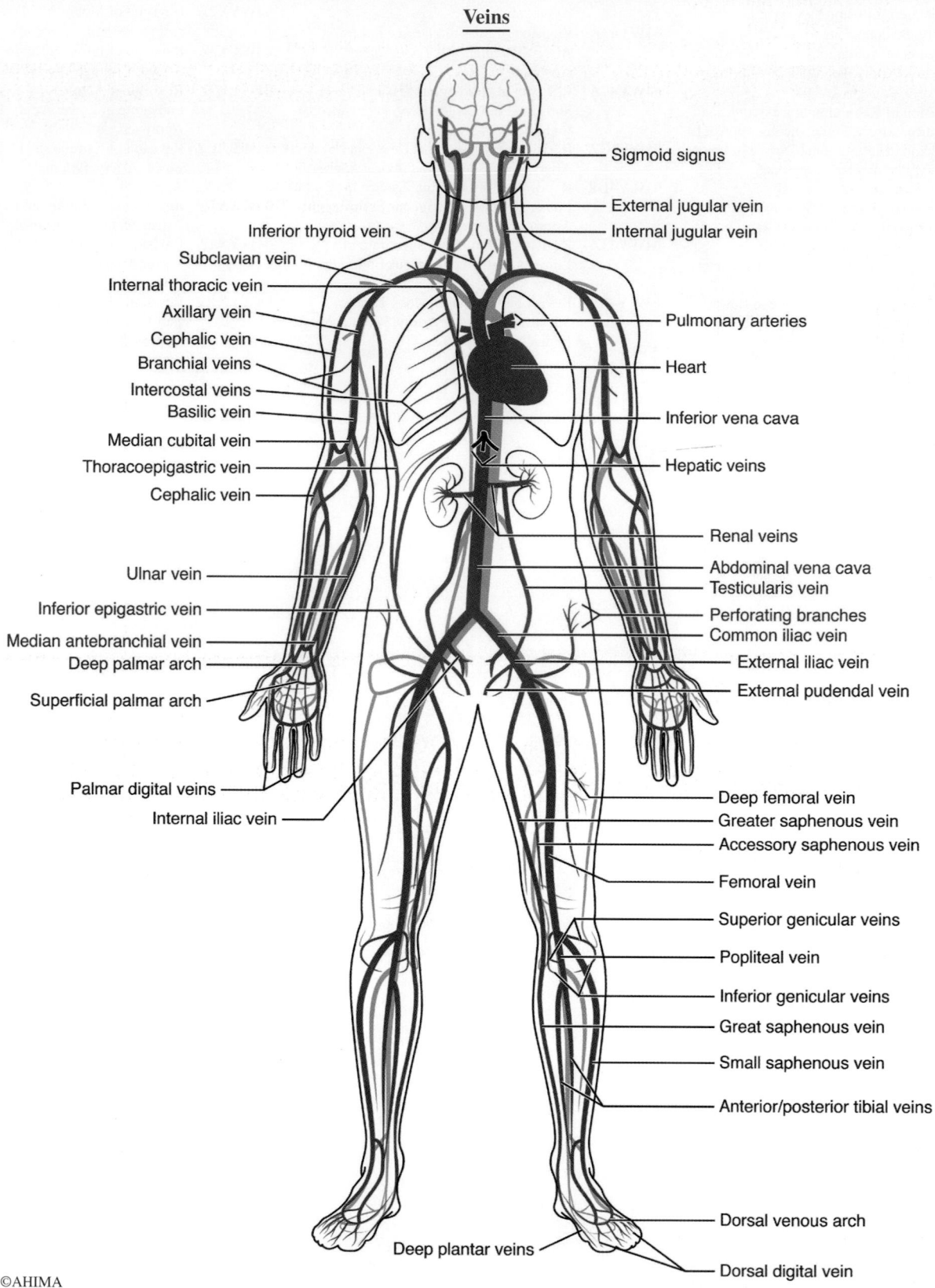

Sigmoid signus

External jugular vein

Internal jugular vein

Inferior thyroid vein

Subclavian vein

Internal thoracic vein

Axillary vein

Cephalic vein

Branchial veins

Intercostal veins

Basilic vein

Median cubital vein

Thoracoepigastric vein

Cephalic vein

Pulmonary arteries

Heart

Inferior vena cava

Hepatic veins

Renal veins

Abdominal vena cava

Testicularis vein

Perforating branches

Common iliac vein

External iliac vein

External pudendal vein

Ulnar vein

Inferior epigastric vein

Median antebranchial vein

Deep palmar arch

Superficial palmar arch

Palmar digital veins

Internal iliac vein

Deep femoral vein

Greater saphenous vein

Accessory saphenous vein

Femoral vein

Superior genicular veins

Popliteal vein

Inferior genicular veins

Great saphenous vein

Small saphenous vein

Anterior/posterior tibial veins

Dorsal venous arch

Deep plantar veins

Dorsal digital vein

©AHIMA

tion	0	Medical and Surgical
dy System	5	Upper Veins
eration	1	**Bypass:** Altering the route of passage of the contents of a tubular body part

Body Part (4th)	Approach (5th)	Device (6th)	Qualifier (7th)
Azygos Vein Hemiazygos Vein Innominate Vein, Right Innominate Vein, Left Subclavian Vein, Right Subclavian Vein, Left Axillary Vein, Right Axillary Vein, Left Brachial Vein, Right Brachial Vein, Left Basilic Vein, Right Basilic Vein, Left Cephalic Vein, Right Cephalic Vein, Left Hand Vein, Right Hand Vein, Left Intracranial Vein Internal Jugular Vein, Right Internal Jugular Vein, Left External Jugular Vein, Right External Jugular Vein, Left Vertebral Vein, Right Vertebral Vein, Left Face Vein, Right Face Vein, Left	0 Open 4 Percutaneous Endoscopic	7 Autologous Tissue Substitute 9 Autologous Venous Tissue A Autologous Arterial Tissue J Synthetic Substitute K Nonautologous Tissue Substitute Z No Device	Y Upper Vein

ction	0	Medical and Surgical
dy System	5	Upper Veins
eration	5	**Destruction:** Physical eradication of all or a portion of a body part by the direct use of energy, force, or a destructive agent

Body Part (4th)	Approach (5th)	Device (6th)	Qualifier (7th)
Azygos Vein Hemiazygos Vein Innominate Vein, Right Innominate Vein, Left Subclavian Vein, Right Subclavian Vein, Left Axillary Vein, Right Axillary Vein, Left Brachial Vein, Right Brachial Vein, Left Basilic Vein, Right Basilic Vein, Left Cephalic Vein, Right Cephalic Vein, Left Hand Vein, Right Hand Vein, Left Intracranial Vein Internal Jugular Vein, Right Internal Jugular Vein, Left External Jugular Vein, Right External Jugular Vein, Left Vertebral Vein, Right Vertebral Vein, Left Face Vein, Right Face Vein, Left Upper Vein	0 Open 3 Percutaneous 4 Percutaneous Endoscopic	Z No Device	Z No Qualifier

Section   **0**   **Medical and Surgical**
Body System   **5**   **Upper Veins**
Operation   **7**   **Dilation:** Expanding an orifice or the lumen of a tubular body part

Body Part (4th)	Approach (5th)	Device (6th)	Qualifier (7th)
0 Azygos Vein	0 Open	D Intraluminal Device	Z No Qualifier
1 Hemiazygos Vein	3 Percutaneous	Z No Device	
3 Innominate Vein, Right	4 Percutaneous Endoscopic		
4 Innominate Vein, Left			
5 Subclavian Vein, Right			
6 Subclavian Vein, Left			
7 Axillary Vein, Right			
8 Axillary Vein, Left			
9 Brachial Vein, Right			
A Brachial Vein, Left			
B Basilic Vein, Right			
C Basilic Vein, Left			
D Cephalic Vein, Right			
F Cephalic Vein, Left			
G Hand Vein, Right			
H Hand Vein, Left			
L Intracranial Vein			
M Internal Jugular Vein, Right			
N Internal Jugular Vein, Left			
P External Jugular Vein, Right			
Q External Jugular Vein, Left			
R Vertebral Vein, Right			
S Vertebral Vein, Left			
T Face Vein, Right			
V Face Vein, Left			
Y Upper Vein			

Section   **0**   **Medical and Surgical**
Body System   **5**   **Upper Veins**
Operation   **9**   **Drainage:** Taking or letting out fluids and/or gases from a body part

Body Part (4th)	Approach (5th)	Device (6th)	Qualifier (7th)
0 Azygos Vein	0 Open	0 Drainage Device	Z No Qualifier
1 Hemiazygos Vein	3 Percutaneous		
3 Innominate Vein, Right	4 Percutaneous Endoscopic		
4 Innominate Vein, Left			
5 Subclavian Vein, Right			
6 Subclavian Vein, Left			
7 Axillary Vein, Right			
8 Axillary Vein, Left			
9 Brachial Vein, Right			
A Brachial Vein, Left			
B Basilic Vein, Right			
C Basilic Vein, Left			
D Cephalic Vein, Right			
F Cephalic Vein, Left			
G Hand Vein, Right			
H Hand Vein, Left			
L Intracranial Vein			
M Internal Jugular Vein, Right			
N Internal Jugular Vein, Left			
P External Jugular Vein, Right			
Q External Jugular Vein, Left			
R Vertebral Vein, Right			
S Vertebral Vein, Left			
T Face Vein, Right			
V Face Vein, Left			
Y Upper Vein			

Continued →

ction	0	**Medical and Surgical**
dy System	5	**Upper Veins**
eration	9	**Drainage:** Taking or letting out fluids and/or gases from a body part

Body Part (4ᵗʰ)	Approach (5ᵗʰ)	Device (6ᵗʰ)	Qualifier (7ᵗʰ)
Azygos Vein Hemiazygos Vein Innominate Vein, Right Innominate Vein, Left Subclavian Vein, Right Subclavian Vein, Left Axillary Vein, Right Axillary Vein, Left Brachial Vein, Right Brachial Vein, Left Basilic Vein, Right Basilic Vein, Left Cephalic Vein, Right Cephalic Vein, Left Hand Vein, Right Hand Vein, Left Intracranial Vein Internal Jugular Vein, Right Internal Jugular Vein, Left External Jugular Vein, Right External Jugular Vein, Left Vertebral Vein, Right Vertebral Vein, Left Face Vein, Right Face Vein, Left Upper Vein	**0** Open **3** Percutaneous **4** Percutaneous Endoscopic	**Z** No Device	**X** Diagnostic **Z** No Qualifier

ction	0	**Medical and Surgical**
dy System	5	**Upper Veins**
eration	B	**Excision:** Cutting out or off, without replacement, a portion of a body part

Body Part (4ᵗʰ)	Approach (5ᵗʰ)	Device (6ᵗʰ)	Qualifier (7ᵗʰ)
0 Azygos Vein **1** Hemiazygos Vein **3** Innominate Vein, Right **4** Innominate Vein, Left **5** Subclavian Vein, Right **6** Subclavian Vein, Left **7** Axillary Vein, Right **8** Axillary Vein, Left **9** Brachial Vein, Right **A** Brachial Vein, Left **B** Basilic Vein, Right **C** Basilic Vein, Left **D** Cephalic Vein, Right **F** Cephalic Vein, Left **G** Hand Vein, Right **H** Hand Vein, Left **L** Intracranial Vein **M** Internal Jugular Vein, Right **N** Internal Jugular Vein, Left **P** External Jugular Vein, Right **Q** External Jugular Vein, Left **R** Vertebral Vein, Right **S** Vertebral Vein, Left **T** Face Vein, Right **V** Face Vein, Left **Y** Upper Vein	**0** Open **3** Percutaneous **4** Percutaneous Endoscopic	**Z** No Device	**X** Diagnostic **Z** No Qualifier

Section	0	Medical and Surgical
Body System	5	Upper Veins
Operation	C	Extirpation: Taking or cutting out solid matter from a body part

Body Part (4th)	Approach (5th)	Device (6th)	Qualifier (7th)
0 Azygos Vein	0 Open	Z No Device	Z No Qualifier
1 Hemiazygos Vein	3 Percutaneous		
3 Innominate Vein, Right	4 Percutaneous Endoscopic		
4 Innominate Vein, Left			
5 Subclavian Vein, Right			
6 Subclavian Vein, Left			
7 Axillary Vein, Right			
8 Axillary Vein, Left			
9 Brachial Vein, Right			
A Brachial Vein, Left			
B Basilic Vein, Right			
C Basilic Vein, Left			
D Cephalic Vein, Right			
F Cephalic Vein, Left			
G Hand Vein, Right			
H Hand Vein, Left			
L Intracranial Vein			
M Internal Jugular Vein, Right			
N Internal Jugular Vein, Left			
P External Jugular Vein, Right			
Q External Jugular Vein, Left			
R Vertebral Vein, Right			
S Vertebral Vein, Left			
T Face Vein, Right			
V Face Vein, Left			
Y Upper Vein			

Section	0	Medical and Surgical
Body System	5	Upper Veins
Operation	D	Extraction: Pulling or stripping out or off all or a portion of a body part by the use of force

Body Part (4th)	Approach (5th)	Device (6th)	Qualifier (7th)
9 Brachial Vein, Right	0 Open	Z No Device	Z No Qualifier
A Brachial Vein, Left	3 Percutaneous		
B Basilic Vein, Right			
C Basilic Vein, Left			
D Cephalic Vein, Right			
F Cephalic Vein, Left			
G Hand Vein, Right			
H Hand Vein, Left			
Y Upper Vein			

tion | 0 | **Medical and Surgical**
dy System | 5 | **Upper Veins**
eration | H | **Insertion:** Putting in a nonbiological appliance that monitors, assists, performs, or prevents a physiological function but does not physically take the place of a body part

Body Part (4th)	Approach (5th)	Device (6th)	Qualifier (7th)
Azygos Vein Hemiazygos Vein Innominate Vein, Right Innominate Vein, Left Subclavian Vein, Right Subclavian Vein, Left Axillary Vein, Right Axillary Vein, Left Brachial Vein, Right Brachial Vein, Left Basilic Vein, Right Basilic Vein, Left Cephalic Vein, Right Cephalic Vein, Left Hand Vein, Right Hand Vein, Left Intracranial Vein Internal Jugular Vein, Right Internal Jugular Vein, Left External Jugular Vein, Right External Jugular Vein, Left Vertebral Vein, Right Vertebral Vein, Left Face Vein, Right Face Vein, Left	0 Open 3 Percutaneous 4 Percutaneous Endoscopic	3 Infusion Device D Intraluminal Device	Z No Qualifier
Y Upper Vein	0 Open 3 Percutaneous 4 Percutaneous Endoscopic	2 Monitoring Device 3 Infusion Device D Intraluminal Device	Z No Qualifier

ction | 0 | **Medical and Surgical**
dy System | 5 | **Upper Veins**
eration | J | **Inspection:** Visually and/or manually exploring a body part

Body Part (4th)	Approach (5th)	Device (6th)	Qualifier (7th)
Y Upper Vein	0 Open 3 Percutaneous 4 Percutaneous Endoscopic X External	Z No Device	Z No Qualifier

Section	0	Medical and Surgical		
Body System	5	Upper Veins		
Operation	L	Occlusion: Completely closing an orifice or the lumen of a tubular body part		

Body Part (4th)	Approach (5th)	Device (6th)	Qualifier (7th)
0 Azygos Vein 1 Hemiazygos Vein 3 Innominate Vein, Right 4 Innominate Vein, Left 5 Subclavian Vein, Right 6 Subclavian Vein, Left 7 Axillary Vein, Right 8 Axillary Vein, Left 9 Brachial Vein, Right A Brachial Vein, Left B Basilic Vein, Right C Basilic Vein, Left D Cephalic Vein, Right F Cephalic Vein, Left G Hand Vein, Right H Hand Vein, Left L Intracranial Vein M Internal Jugular Vein, Right N Internal Jugular Vein, Left P External Jugular Vein, Right Q External Jugular Vein, Left R Vertebral Vein, Right S Vertebral Vein, Left T Face Vein, Right V Face Vein, Left Y Upper Vein	0 Open 3 Percutaneous 4 Percutaneous Endoscopic	C Extraluminal Device D Intraluminal Device Z No Device	Z No Qualifier

Section	0	Medical and Surgical		
Body System	5	Upper Veins		
Operation	N	Release: Freeing a body part from an abnormal physical constraint by cutting or by the use of force		

Body Part (4th)	Approach (5th)	Device (6th)	Qualifier (7th)
0 Azygos Vein 1 Hemiazygos Vein 3 Innominate Vein, Right 4 Innominate Vein, Left 5 Subclavian Vein, Right 6 Subclavian Vein, Left 7 Axillary Vein, Right 8 Axillary Vein, Left 9 Brachial Vein, Right A Brachial Vein, Left B Basilic Vein, Right C Basilic Vein, Left D Cephalic Vein, Right F Cephalic Vein, Left G Hand Vein, Right H Hand Vein, Left L Intracranial Vein M Internal Jugular Vein, Right N Internal Jugular Vein, Left P External Jugular Vein, Right Q External Jugular Vein, Left R Vertebral Vein, Right S Vertebral Vein, Left T Face Vein, Right V Face Vein, Left Y Upper Vein	0 Open 3 Percutaneous 4 Percutaneous Endoscopic	Z No Device	Z No Qualifier

tion	0	**Medical and Surgical**
dy System	5	**Upper Veins**
eration	P	**Removal:** Taking out or off a device from a body part

Body Part (4ᵗʰ)	Approach (5ᵗʰ)	Device (6ᵗʰ)	Qualifier (7ᵗʰ)
⸗ Upper Vein	0 Open 3 Percutaneous 4 Percutaneous Endoscopic	0 Drainage Device 2 Monitoring Device 3 Infusion Device 7 Autologous Tissue Substitute C Extraluminal Device D Intraluminal Device J Synthetic Substitute K Nonautologous Tissue Substitute	Z No Qualifier
⸗ Upper Vein	X External	0 Drainage Device 2 Monitoring Device 3 Infusion Device D Intraluminal Device	Z No Qualifier

tion	0	**Medical and Surgical**
dy System	5	**Upper Veins**
eration	Q	**Repair:** Restoring, to the extent possible, a body part to its normal anatomic structure and function

Body Part (4ᵗʰ)	Approach (5ᵗʰ)	Device (6ᵗʰ)	Qualifier (7ᵗʰ)
Azygos Vein Hemiazygos Vein Innominate Vein, Right Innominate Vein, Left Subclavian Vein, Right Subclavian Vein, Left Axillary Vein, Right Axillary Vein, Left Brachial Vein, Right Brachial Vein, Left Basilic Vein, Right Basilic Vein, Left Cephalic Vein, Right Cephalic Vein, Left Hand Vein, Right Hand Vein, Left Intracranial Vein Internal Jugular Vein, Right Internal Jugular Vein, Left External Jugular Vein, Right External Jugular Vein, Left Vertebral Vein, Right Vertebral Vein, Left Face Vein, Right Face Vein, Left Upper Vein	0 Open 3 Percutaneous 4 Percutaneous Endoscopic	Z No Device	Z No Qualifier

Section	0	Medical and Surgical
Body System	5	Upper Veins
Operation	R	**Replacement:** Putting in or on biological or synthetic material that physically takes the place and/or function of all or a portion of a body part

Body Part (4th)	Approach (5th)	Device (6th)	Qualifier (7th)
0 Azygos Vein	0 Open	7 Autologous Tissue Substitute	Z No Qualifier
1 Hemiazygos Vein	4 Percutaneous Endoscopic	J Synthetic Substitute	
3 Innominate Vein, Right		K Nonautologous Tissue Substitute	
4 Innominate Vein, Left			
5 Subclavian Vein, Right			
6 Subclavian Vein, Left			
7 Axillary Vein, Right			
8 Axillary Vein, Left			
9 Brachial Vein, Right			
A Brachial Vein, Left			
B Basilic Vein, Right			
C Basilic Vein, Left			
D Cephalic Vein, Right			
F Cephalic Vein, Left			
G Hand Vein, Right			
H Hand Vein, Left			
L Intracranial Vein			
M Internal Jugular Vein, Right			
N Internal Jugular Vein, Left			
P External Jugular Vein, Right			
Q External Jugular Vein, Left			
R Vertebral Vein, Right			
S Vertebral Vein, Left			
T Face Vein, Right			
V Face Vein, Left			
Y Upper Vein			

Section	0	Medical and Surgical
Body System	5	Upper Veins
Operation	S	**Reposition:** Moving to its normal location, or other suitable location, all or a portion of a body part

Body Part (4th)	Approach (5th)	Device (6th)	Qualifier (7th)
0 Azygos Vein	0 Open	Z No Device	Z No Qualifier
1 Hemiazygos Vein	3 Percutaneous		
3 Innominate Vein, Right	4 Percutaneous Endoscopic		
4 Innominate Vein, Left			
5 Subclavian Vein, Right			
6 Subclavian Vein, Left			
7 Axillary Vein, Right			
8 Axillary Vein, Left			
9 Brachial Vein, Right			
A Brachial Vein, Left			
B Basilic Vein, Right			
C Basilic Vein, Left			
D Cephalic Vein, Right			
F Cephalic Vein, Left			
G Hand Vein, Right			
H Hand Vein, Left			
L Intracranial Vein			
M Internal Jugular Vein, Right			
N Internal Jugular Vein, Left			
P External Jugular Vein, Right			
Q External Jugular Vein, Left			
R Vertebral Vein, Right			
S Vertebral Vein, Left			
T Face Vein, Right			
V Face Vein, Left			
Y Upper Vein			

Section 0 Medical and Surgical
Body System 5 Upper Veins
Operation U Supplement: Putting in or on biological or synthetic material that physically reinforces and/or augments the function of a portion of a body part

Body Part (4th)	Approach (5th)	Device (6th)	Qualifier (7th)
Azygos Vein	0 Open	7 Autologous Tissue Substitute	Z No Qualifier
Hemiazygos Vein	3 Percutaneous	J Synthetic Substitute	
Innominate Vein, Right	4 Percutaneous Endoscopic	K Nonautologous Tissue Substitute	
Innominate Vein, Left			
Subclavian Vein, Right			
Subclavian Vein, Left			
Axillary Vein, Right			
Axillary Vein, Left			
Brachial Vein, Right			
Brachial Vein, Left			
Basilic Vein, Right			
Basilic Vein, Left			
Cephalic Vein, Right			
Cephalic Vein, Left			
Hand Vein, Right			
Hand Vein, Left			
Intracranial Vein			
Internal Jugular Vein, Right			
Internal Jugular Vein, Left			
External Jugular Vein, Right			
External Jugular Vein, Left			
Vertebral Vein, Right			
Vertebral Vein, Left			
Face Vein, Right			
Face Vein, Left			
Upper Vein			

Section 0 Medical and Surgical
Body System 5 Upper Veins
Operation V Restriction: Partially closing an orifice or the lumen of a tubular body part

Body Part (4th)	Approach (5th)	Device (6th)	Qualifier (7th)
Azygos Vein	0 Open	C Extraluminal Device	Z No Qualifier
Hemiazygos Vein	3 Percutaneous	D Intraluminal Device	
Innominate Vein, Right	4 Percutaneous Endoscopic	Z No Device	
Innominate Vein, Left			
Subclavian Vein, Right			
Subclavian Vein, Left			
Axillary Vein, Right			
Axillary Vein, Left			
Brachial Vein, Right			
Brachial Vein, Left			
Basilic Vein, Right			
Basilic Vein, Left			
Cephalic Vein, Right			
Cephalic Vein, Left			
Hand Vein, Right			
Hand Vein, Left			
Intracranial Vein			
Internal Jugular Vein, Right			
Internal Jugular Vein, Left			
External Jugular Vein, Right			
External Jugular Vein, Left			
Vertebral Vein, Right			
Vertebral Vein, Left			
Face Vein, Right			
Face Vein, Left			
Upper Vein			

Section   0   Medical and Surgical
Body System   5   Upper Veins
Operation   W   Revision: Correcting, to the extent possible, a portion of a malfunctioning device or the position of a displaced device

Body Part (4ᵗʰ)	Approach (5ᵗʰ)	Device (6ᵗʰ)	Qualifier (7ᵗʰ)
Y Upper Vein	0 Open 3 Percutaneous 4 Percutaneous Endoscopic X External	0 Drainage Device 2 Monitoring Device 3 Infusion Device 7 Autologous Tissue Substitute C Extraluminal Device D Intraluminal Device J Synthetic Substitute K Nonautologous Tissue Substitute	Z No Qualifier

Upper Veins Code Listing 051–05W

051 – Upper Veins, Bypass

Review Coding Guideline B3.6a

051007Y Bypass Azygos Vein to Upper Vein with Autologous Tissue Substitute, Open Approach

051009Y Bypass Azygos Vein to Upper Vein with Autologous Venous Tissue, Open Approach

05100AY Bypass Azygos Vein to Upper Vein with Autologous Arterial Tissue, Open Approach

05100JY Bypass Azygos Vein to Upper Vein with Synthetic Substitute, Open Approach

05100KY Bypass Azygos Vein to Upper Vein with Nonautologous Tissue Substitute, Open Approach

05100ZY Bypass Azygos Vein to Upper Vein, Open Approach

051047Y Bypass Azygos Vein to Upper Vein with Autologous Tissue Substitute, Percutaneous Endoscopic Approach

051049Y Bypass Azygos Vein to Upper Vein with Autologous Venous Tissue, Percutaneous Endoscopic Approach

05104AY Bypass Azygos Vein to Upper Vein with Autologous Arterial Tissue, Percutaneous Endoscopic Approach

05104JY Bypass Azygos Vein to Upper Vein with Synthetic Substitute, Percutaneous Endoscopic Approach

05104KY Bypass Azygos Vein to Upper Vein with Nonautologous Tissue Substitute, Percutaneous Endoscopic Approach

05104ZY Bypass Azygos Vein to Upper Vein, Percutaneous Endoscopic Approach

051107Y Bypass Hemiazygos Vein to Upper Vein with Autologous Tissue Substitute, Open Approach

051109Y Bypass Hemiazygos Vein to Upper Vein with Autologous Venous Tissue, Open Approach

05110AY Bypass Hemiazygos Vein to Upper Vein with Autologous Arterial Tissue, Open Approach

05110JY Bypass Hemiazygos Vein to Upper Vein with Synthetic Substitute, Open Approach

05110KY Bypass Hemiazygos Vein to Upper Vein with Nonautologous Tissue Substitute, Open Approach

05110ZY Bypass Hemiazygos Vein to Upper Vein, Open Approach

051147Y Bypass Hemiazygos Vein to Upper Vein with Autologous Tissue Substitute, Percutaneous Endoscopic Approach

051149Y Bypass Hemiazygos Vein to Upper Vein with Autologous Venous Tissue, Percutaneous Endoscopic Approach

05114AY Bypass Hemiazygos Vein to Upper Vein with Autologous Arterial Tissue, Percutaneous Endoscopic Approach

05114JY Bypass Hemiazygos Vein to Upper Vein with Synthetic Substitute, Percutaneous Endoscopic Approach

05114KY Bypass Hemiazygos Vein to Upper Vein with Nonautologous Tissue Substitute, Percutaneous Endoscopic Approach

05114ZY Bypass Hemiazygos Vein to Upper Vein, Percutaneous Endoscopic Approach

051307Y Bypass Right Innominate Vein to Upper Vein with Autologous Tissue Substitute, Open Approach

051309Y Bypass Right Innominate Vein to Upper Vein with Autologous Venous Tissue, Open Approach

05130AY Bypass Right Innominate Vein to Upper Vein with Autologous Arterial Tissue, Open Approach

05130JY Bypass Right Innominate Vein to Upper Vein with Synthetic Substitute, Open Approach

05130KY Bypass Right Innominate Vein to Upper Vein with Nonautologous Tissue Substitute, Open Approach

05130ZY Bypass Right Innominate Vein to Upper Vein, Open Approach

051347Y Bypass Right Innominate Vein to Upper Vein with Autologous Tissue Substitute, Percutaneous Endoscopic Approach

051349Y Bypass Right Innominate Vein to Upper Vein with Autologous Venous Tissue, Percutaneous Endoscopic Approach

05134AY Bypass Right Innominate Vein to Upper Vein with Autologous Arterial Tissue, Percutaneous Endoscopic Approach

05134JY Bypass Right Innominate Vein to Upper Vein with Synthetic Substitute, Percutaneous Endoscopic Approach

05134KY Bypass Right Innominate Vein to Upper Vein with Nonautologous Tissue Substitute, Percutaneous Endoscopic Approach

05134ZY Bypass Right Innominate Vein to Upper Vein, Percutaneous Endoscopic Approach

051407Y Bypass Left Innominate Vein to Upper Vein with Autologous Tissue Substitute, Open Approach

051409Y Bypass Left Innominate Vein to Upper Vein with Autologous Venous Tissue, Open Approach

05140AY Bypass Left Innominate Vein to Upper Vein with Autologous Arterial Tissue, Open Approach

05140JY Bypass Left Innominate Vein to Upper Vein with Synthetic Substitute, Open Approach

05140KY Bypass Left Innominate Vein to Upper Vein with Nonautologous Tissue Substitute, Open Approach

05140ZY Bypass Left Innominate Vein to Upper Vein, Open Approach

051447Y Bypass Left Innominate Vein to Upper Vein with Autologous Tissue Substitute, Percutaneous Endoscopic Approach

051449Y Bypass Left Innominate Vein to Upper Vein with Autologous Venous Tissue, Percutaneous Endoscopic Approach

05144AY Bypass Left Innominate Vein to Upper Vein with Autologous Arterial Tissue, Percutaneous Endoscopic Approach

05144JY Bypass Left Innominate Vein to Upper Vein with Synthetic Substitute, Percutaneous Endoscopic Approach

05144KY Bypass Left Innominate Vein to Upper Vein with Nonautologous Tissue Substitute, Percutaneous Endoscopic Approach

05144ZY Bypass Left Innominate Vein to Upper Vein, Percutaneous Endoscopic Approach

051507Y Bypass Right Subclavian Vein to Upper Vein with Autologous Tissue Substitute, Open Approach

051509Y Bypass Right Subclavian Vein to Upper Vein with Autologous Venous Tissue, Open Approach

05150AY Bypass Right Subclavian Vein to Upper Vein with Autologous Arterial Tissue, Open Approach

05150JY Bypass Right Subclavian Vein to Upper Vein with Synthetic Substitute, Open Approach

05150KY Bypass Right Subclavian Vein to Upper Vein with Nonautologous Tissue Substitute, Open Approach

05150ZY Bypass Right Subclavian Vein to Upper Vein, Open Approach

051547Y Bypass Right Subclavian Vein to Upper Vein with Autologous Tissue Substitute, Percutaneous Endoscopic Approach

051549Y Bypass Right Subclavian Vein to Upper Vein with Autologous Venous Tissue, Percutaneous Endoscopic Approach

05154AY Bypass Right Subclavian Vein to Upper Vein with Autologous Arterial Tissue, Percutaneous Endoscopic Approach

05154JY Bypass Right Subclavian Vein to Upper Vein with Synthetic Substitute, Percutaneous Endoscopic Approach

♀ Female-only   ♂ Male-only   ▲ Limited Coverage   ● Non-OR   ▨ HAC-associated procedure   ▲ Non-covered procedures   ✛ Combinati

4KY Bypass Right Subclavian Vein to Upper Vein with Nonautologous Tissue Substitute, Percutaneous Endoscopic Approach

4ZY Bypass Right Subclavian Vein to Upper Vein, Percutaneous Endoscopic Approach

07Y Bypass Left Subclavian Vein to Upper Vein with Autologous Tissue Substitute, Open Approach

09Y Bypass Left Subclavian Vein to Upper Vein with Autologous Venous Tissue, Open Approach

0AY Bypass Left Subclavian Vein to Upper Vein with Autologous Arterial Tissue, Open Approach

0JY Bypass Left Subclavian Vein to Upper Vein with Synthetic Substitute, Open Approach

0KY Bypass Left Subclavian Vein to Upper Vein with Nonautologous Tissue Substitute, Open Approach

0ZY Bypass Left Subclavian Vein to Upper Vein, Open Approach

47Y Bypass Left Subclavian Vein to Upper Vein with Autologous Tissue Substitute, Percutaneous Endoscopic Approach

49Y Bypass Left Subclavian Vein to Upper Vein with Autologous Venous Tissue, Percutaneous Endoscopic Approach

4AY Bypass Left Subclavian Vein to Upper Vein with Autologous Arterial Tissue, Percutaneous Endoscopic Approach

4JY Bypass Left Subclavian Vein to Upper Vein with Synthetic Substitute, Percutaneous Endoscopic Approach

4KY Bypass Left Subclavian Vein to Upper Vein with Nonautologous Tissue Substitute, Percutaneous Endoscopic Approach

4ZY Bypass Left Subclavian Vein to Upper Vein, Percutaneous Endoscopic Approach

707Y Bypass Right Axillary Vein to Upper Vein with Autologous Tissue Substitute, Open Approach

709Y Bypass Right Axillary Vein to Upper Vein with Autologous Venous Tissue, Open Approach

70AY Bypass Right Axillary Vein to Upper Vein with Autologous Arterial Tissue, Open Approach

70JY Bypass Right Axillary Vein to Upper Vein with Synthetic Substitute, Open Approach

70KY Bypass Right Axillary Vein to Upper Vein with Nonautologous Tissue Substitute, Open Approach

70ZY Bypass Right Axillary Vein to Upper Vein, Open Approach

747Y Bypass Right Axillary Vein to Upper Vein with Autologous Tissue Substitute, Percutaneous Endoscopic Approach

749Y Bypass Right Axillary Vein to Upper Vein with Autologous Venous Tissue, Percutaneous Endoscopic Approach

74AY Bypass Right Axillary Vein to Upper Vein with Autologous Arterial Tissue, Percutaneous Endoscopic Approach

74JY Bypass Right Axillary Vein to Upper Vein with Synthetic Substitute, Percutaneous Endoscopic Approach

74KY Bypass Right Axillary Vein to Upper Vein with Nonautologous Tissue Substitute, Percutaneous Endoscopic Approach

74ZY Bypass Right Axillary Vein to Upper Vein, Percutaneous Endoscopic Approach

807Y Bypass Left Axillary Vein to Upper Vein with Autologous Tissue Substitute, Open Approach

809Y Bypass Left Axillary Vein to Upper Vein with Autologous Venous Tissue, Open Approach

05180AY Bypass Left Axillary Vein to Upper Vein with Autologous Arterial Tissue, Open Approach

05180JY Bypass Left Axillary Vein to Upper Vein with Synthetic Substitute, Open Approach

05180KY Bypass Left Axillary Vein to Upper Vein with Nonautologous Tissue Substitute, Open Approach

05180ZY Bypass Left Axillary Vein to Upper Vein, Open Approach

051847Y Bypass Left Axillary Vein to Upper Vein with Autologous Tissue Substitute, Percutaneous Endoscopic Approach

051849Y Bypass Left Axillary Vein to Upper Vein with Autologous Venous Tissue, Percutaneous Endoscopic Approach

05184AY Bypass Left Axillary Vein to Upper Vein with Autologous Arterial Tissue, Percutaneous Endoscopic Approach

05184JY Bypass Left Axillary Vein to Upper Vein with Synthetic Substitute, Percutaneous Endoscopic Approach

05184KY Bypass Left Axillary Vein to Upper Vein with Nonautologous Tissue Substitute, Percutaneous Endoscopic Approach

05184ZY Bypass Left Axillary Vein to Upper Vein, Percutaneous Endoscopic Approach

051907Y Bypass Right Brachial Vein to Upper Vein with Autologous Tissue Substitute, Open Approach

051909Y Bypass Right Brachial Vein to Upper Vein with Autologous Venous Tissue, Open Approach

05190AY Bypass Right Brachial Vein to Upper Vein with Autologous Arterial Tissue, Open Approach

05190JY Bypass Right Brachial Vein to Upper Vein with Synthetic Substitute, Open Approach

05190KY Bypass Right Brachial Vein to Upper Vein with Nonautologous Tissue Substitute, Open Approach

05190ZY Bypass Right Brachial Vein to Upper Vein, Open Approach

051947Y Bypass Right Brachial Vein to Upper Vein with Autologous Tissue Substitute, Percutaneous Endoscopic Approach

051949Y Bypass Right Brachial Vein to Upper Vein with Autologous Venous Tissue, Percutaneous Endoscopic Approach

05194AY Bypass Right Brachial Vein to Upper Vein with Autologous Arterial Tissue, Percutaneous Endoscopic Approach

05194JY Bypass Right Brachial Vein to Upper Vein with Synthetic Substitute, Percutaneous Endoscopic Approach

05194KY Bypass Right Brachial Vein to Upper Vein with Nonautologous Tissue Substitute, Percutaneous Endoscopic Approach

05194ZY Bypass Right Brachial Vein to Upper Vein, Percutaneous Endoscopic Approach

051A07Y Bypass Left Brachial Vein to Upper Vein with Autologous Tissue Substitute, Open Approach

051A09Y Bypass Left Brachial Vein to Upper Vein with Autologous Venous Tissue, Open Approach

051A0AY Bypass Left Brachial Vein to Upper Vein with Autologous Arterial Tissue, Open Approach

051A0JY Bypass Left Brachial Vein to Upper Vein with Synthetic Substitute, Open Approach

051A0KY Bypass Left Brachial Vein to Upper Vein with Nonautologous Tissue Substitute, Open Approach

051A0ZY Bypass Left Brachial Vein to Upper Vein, Open Approach

051A47Y Bypass Left Brachial Vein to Upper Vein with Autologous Tissue Substitute, Percutaneous Endoscopic Approach

051A49Y Bypass Left Brachial Vein to Upper Vein with Autologous Venous Tissue, Percutaneous Endoscopic Approach

051A4AY Bypass Left Brachial Vein to Upper Vein with Autologous Arterial Tissue, Percutaneous Endoscopic Approach

051A4JY Bypass Left Brachial Vein to Upper Vein with Synthetic Substitute, Percutaneous Endoscopic Approach

051A4KY Bypass Left Brachial Vein to Upper Vein with Nonautologous Tissue Substitute, Percutaneous Endoscopic Approach

051A4ZY Bypass Left Brachial Vein to Upper Vein, Percutaneous Endoscopic Approach

051B07Y Bypass Right Basilic Vein to Upper Vein with Autologous Tissue Substitute, Open Approach

051B09Y Bypass Right Basilic Vein to Upper Vein with Autologous Venous Tissue, Open Approach

051B0AY Bypass Right Basilic Vein to Upper Vein with Autologous Arterial Tissue, Open Approach

051B0JY Bypass Right Basilic Vein to Upper Vein with Synthetic Substitute, Open Approach

051B0KY Bypass Right Basilic Vein to Upper Vein with Nonautologous Tissue Substitute, Open Approach

051B0ZY Bypass Right Basilic Vein to Upper Vein, Open Approach

051B47Y Bypass Right Basilic Vein to Upper Vein with Autologous Tissue Substitute, Percutaneous Endoscopic Approach

051B49Y Bypass Right Basilic Vein to Upper Vein with Autologous Venous Tissue, Percutaneous Endoscopic Approach

051B4AY Bypass Right Basilic Vein to Upper Vein with Autologous Arterial Tissue, Percutaneous Endoscopic Approach

051B4JY Bypass Right Basilic Vein to Upper Vein with Synthetic Substitute, Percutaneous Endoscopic Approach

051B4KY Bypass Right Basilic Vein to Upper Vein with Nonautologous Tissue Substitute, Percutaneous Endoscopic Approach

051B4ZY Bypass Right Basilic Vein to Upper Vein, Percutaneous Endoscopic Approach

051C07Y Bypass Left Basilic Vein to Upper Vein with Autologous Tissue Substitute, Open Approach

051C09Y Bypass Left Basilic Vein to Upper Vein with Autologous Venous Tissue, Open Approach

051C0AY Bypass Left Basilic Vein to Upper Vein with Autologous Arterial Tissue, Open Approach

051C0JY Bypass Left Basilic Vein to Upper Vein with Synthetic Substitute, Open Approach

051C0KY Bypass Left Basilic Vein to Upper Vein with Nonautologous Tissue Substitute, Open Approach

051C0ZY Bypass Left Basilic Vein to Upper Vein, Open Approach

051C47Y Bypass Left Basilic Vein to Upper Vein with Autologous Tissue Substitute, Percutaneous Endoscopic Approach

051C49Y Bypass Left Basilic Vein to Upper Vein with Autologous Venous Tissue, Percutaneous Endoscopic Approach

051C4AY Bypass Left Basilic Vein to Upper Vein with Autologous Arterial Tissue, Percutaneous Endoscopic Approach

051C4JY Bypass Left Basilic Vein to Upper Vein with Synthetic Substitute, Percutaneous Endoscopic Approach

051C4KY Bypass Left Basilic Vein to Upper Vein with Nonautologous Tissue Substitute, Percutaneous Endoscopic Approach

051C4ZY Bypass Left Basilic Vein to Upper Vein, Percutaneous Endoscopic Approach

051D07Y Bypass Right Cephalic Vein to Upper Vein with Autologous Tissue Substitute, Open Approach

051D09Y Bypass Right Cephalic Vein to Upper Vein with Autologous Venous Tissue, Open Approach

051D0AY Bypass Right Cephalic Vein to Upper Vein with Autologous Arterial Tissue, Open Approach

051D0JY Bypass Right Cephalic Vein to Upper Vein with Synthetic Substitute, Open Approach

051D0KY Bypass Right Cephalic Vein to Upper Vein with Nonautologous Tissue Substitute, Open Approach

051D0ZY Bypass Right Cephalic Vein to Upper Vein, Open Approach

051D47Y Bypass Right Cephalic Vein to Upper Vein with Autologous Tissue Substitute, Percutaneous Endoscopic Approach

051D49Y Bypass Right Cephalic Vein to Upper Vein with Autologous Venous Tissue, Percutaneous Endoscopic Approach

051D4AY Bypass Right Cephalic Vein to Upper Vein with Autologous Arterial Tissue, Percutaneous Endoscopic Approach

051D4JY Bypass Right Cephalic Vein to Upper Vein with Synthetic Substitute, Percutaneous Endoscopic Approach

051D4KY Bypass Right Cephalic Vein to Upper Vein with Nonautologous Tissue Substitute, Percutaneous Endoscopic Approach

051D4ZY Bypass Right Cephalic Vein to Upper Vein, Percutaneous Endoscopic Approach

051F07Y Bypass Left Cephalic Vein to Upper Vein with Autologous Tissue Substitute, Open Approach

051F09Y Bypass Left Cephalic Vein to Upper Vein with Autologous Venous Tissue, Open Approach

051F0AY Bypass Left Cephalic Vein to Upper Vein with Autologous Arterial Tissue, Open Approach

051F0JY Bypass Left Cephalic Vein to Upper Vein with Synthetic Substitute, Open Approach

051F0KY Bypass Left Cephalic Vein to Upper Vein with Nonautologous Tissue Substitute, Open Approach

051F0ZY Bypass Left Cephalic Vein to Upper Vein, Open Approach

051F47Y Bypass Left Cephalic Vein to Upper Vein with Autologous Tissue Substitute, Percutaneous Endoscopic Approach

051F49Y Bypass Left Cephalic Vein to Upper Vein with Autologous Venous Tissue, Percutaneous Endoscopic Approach

051F4AY Bypass Left Cephalic Vein to Upper Vein with Autologous Arterial Tissue, Percutaneous Endoscopic Approach

051F4JY Bypass Left Cephalic Vein to Upper Vein with Synthetic Substitute, Percutaneous Endoscopic Approach

051F4KY Bypass Left Cephalic Vein to Upper Vein with Nonautologous Tissue Substitute, Percutaneous Endoscopic Approach

051F4ZY Bypass Left Cephalic Vein to Upper Vein, Percutaneous Endoscopic Approach

051G07Y Bypass Right Hand Vein to Upper Vein with Autologous Tissue Substitute, Open Approach

051G09Y Bypass Right Hand Vein to Upper Vein with Autologous Venous Tissue, Open Approach

051G0AY Bypass Right Hand Vein to Upper Vein with Autologous Arterial Tissue, Open Approach

051G0JY Bypass Right Hand Vein to Upper Vein with Synthetic Substitute, Open Approach

051G0KY Bypass Right Hand Vein to Upper Vein with Nonautologous Tissue Substitute, Open Approach

051G0ZY Bypass Right Hand Vein to Upper Vein, Open Approach

051G47Y Bypass Right Hand Vein to Upper Vein with Autologous Tissue Substitute, Percutaneous Endoscopic Approach

051G49Y Bypass Right Hand Vein to Upper Vein with Autologous Venous Tissue, Percutaneous Endoscopic Approach

051G4AY Bypass Right Hand Vein to Upper Vein with Autologous Arterial Tissue, Percutaneous Endoscopic Approach

051G4JY Bypass Right Hand Vein to Upper Vein with Synthetic Substitute, Percutaneous Endoscopic Approach

051G4KY Bypass Right Hand Vein to Upper Vein with Nonautologous Tissue Substitute, Percutaneous Endoscopic Approach

051G4ZY Bypass Right Hand Vein to Upper Vein, Percutaneous Endoscopic Approach

051H07Y Bypass Left Hand Vein to Upper Vein with Autologous Tissue Substitute, Open Approach

051H09Y Bypass Left Hand Vein to Upper Vein with Autologous Venous Tissue, Open Approach

051H0AY Bypass Left Hand Vein to Upper Vein with Autologous Arterial Tissue, Open Approach

051H0JY Bypass Left Hand Vein to Upper Vein with Synthetic Substitute, Open Approach

051H0KY Bypass Left Hand Vein to Upper Vein with Nonautologous Tissue Substitute, Open Approach

051H0ZY Bypass Left Hand Vein to Upper Vein, Open Approach

051H47Y Bypass Left Hand Vein to Upper Vein with Autologous Tissue Substitute, Percutaneous Endoscopic Approach

051H49Y Bypass Left Hand Vein to Upper Vein with Autologous Venous Tissue, Percutaneous Endoscopic Approach

051H4AY Bypass Left Hand Vein to Upper Vein with Autologous Arterial Tissue, Percutaneous Endoscopic Approach

051H4JY Bypass Left Hand Vein to Upper Vein with Synthetic Substitute, Percutaneous Endoscopic Approach

051H4KY Bypass Left Hand Vein to Upper Vein with Nonautologous Tissue Substitute, Percutaneous Endoscopic Approach

051H4ZY Bypass Left Hand Vein to Upper Vein, Percutaneous Endoscopic Approach

051L07Y Bypass Intracranial Vein to Upper Vein with Autologous Tissue Substitute, Open Approach

051L09Y Bypass Intracranial Vein to Upper Vein with Autologous Venous Tissue, Open Approach

051L0AY Bypass Intracranial Vein to Upper Vein with Autologous Arterial Tissue, Open Approach

051L0JY Bypass Intracranial Vein to Upper Vein with Synthetic Substitute, Open Approach

051L0KY Bypass Intracranial Vein to Upper Vein with Nonautologous Tissue Substitute, Open Approach

051L0ZY Bypass Intracranial Vein to Upper Vein, Open Approach

051L47Y Bypass Intracranial Vein to Upper Vein with Autologous Tissue Substitute, Percutaneous Endoscopic Approach

051L49Y Bypass Intracranial Vein to Upper Vein with Autologous Venous Tissue, Percutaneous Endoscopic Approach

051L4AY Bypass Intracranial Vein to Upper Vein with Autologous Arterial Tissue, Percutaneous Endoscopic Approach

051L4JY Bypass Intracranial Vein to Upper Vein with Synthetic Substitute, Percutaneous Endoscopic Approach

051L4KY Bypass Intracranial Vein to Upper Vein with Nonautologous Tissue Substitute, Percutaneous Endoscopic Approach

051L4ZY Bypass Intracranial Vein to Upper Vein, Percutaneous Endoscopic Approach

051M07Y Bypass Right Internal Jugular Vein to Upper Vein with Autologous Tissue Substitute, Open Approach

051M09Y Bypass Right Internal Jugular Vein to Upper Vein with Autologous Venous Tissue, Open Approach

051M0AY Bypass Right Internal Jugular Vein to Upper Vein with Autologous Arterial Tissue, Open Approach

051M0JY Bypass Right Internal Jugular Vein to Upper Vein with Synthetic Substitute, Open Approach

051M0KY Bypass Right Internal Jugular Vein to Upper Vein with Nonautologous Tissue Substitute, Open Approach

051M0ZY Bypass Right Internal Jugular Vein to Upper Vein, Open Approach

051M47Y Bypass Right Internal Jugular Vein to Upper Vein with Autologous Tissue Substitute, Percutaneous Endoscopic Approach

051M49Y Bypass Right Internal Jugular Vein to Upper Vein with Autologous Venous Tissue, Percutaneous Endoscopic Approach

051M4AY Bypass Right Internal Jugular Vein to Upper Vein with Autologous Arterial Tissue, Percutaneous Endoscopic Approach

051M4JY Bypass Right Internal Jugular Vein to Upper Vein with Synthetic Substitute, Percutaneous Endoscopic Approach

051M4KY Bypass Right Internal Jugular Vein to Upper Vein with Nonautologous Tissue Substitute, Percutaneous Endoscopic Approach

051M4ZY Bypass Right Internal Jugular Vein to Upper Vein, Percutaneous Endoscopic Approach

051N07Y Bypass Left Internal Jugular Vein to Upper Vein with Autologous Tissue Substitute, Open Approach

051N09Y Bypass Left Internal Jugular Vein to Upper Vein with Autologous Venous Tissue, Open Approach

051N0AY Bypass Left Internal Jugular Vein to Upper Vein with Autologous Arterial Tissue, Open Approach

051N0JY Bypass Left Internal Jugular Vein to Upper Vein with Synthetic Substitute, Open Approach

051N0KY Bypass Left Internal Jugular Vein to Upper Vein with Nonautologous Tissue Substitute, Open Approach

051N0ZY Bypass Left Internal Jugular Vein to Upper Vein, Open Approach

051N47Y Bypass Left Internal Jugular Vein to Upper Vein with Autologous Tissue Substitute, Percutaneous Endoscopic Approach

♀ Female-only   ♂ Male-only   ▲ Limited Coverage   ● Non-OR   ▦ HAC-associated procedure   ▲ Non-covered procedures   ✚ Combination

49Y Bypass Left Internal Jugular Vein to Upper Vein with Autologous Venous Tissue, Percutaneous Endoscopic Approach	**051Q49Y** Bypass Left External Jugular Vein to Upper Vein with Autologous Venous Tissue, Percutaneous Endoscopic Approach	**051S4JY** Bypass Left Vertebral Vein to Upper Vein with Synthetic Substitute, Percutaneous Endoscopic Approach
4AY Bypass Left Internal Jugular Vein to Upper Vein with Autologous Arterial Tissue, Percutaneous Endoscopic Approach	**051Q4AY** Bypass Left External Jugular Vein to Upper Vein with Autologous Arterial Tissue, Percutaneous Endoscopic Approach	**051S4KY** Bypass Left Vertebral Vein to Upper Vein with Nonautologous Tissue Substitute, Percutaneous Endoscopic Approach
4JY Bypass Left Internal Jugular Vein to Upper Vein with Synthetic Substitute, Percutaneous Endoscopic Approach	**051Q4JY** Bypass Left External Jugular Vein to Upper Vein with Synthetic Substitute, Percutaneous Endoscopic Approach	**051S4ZY** Bypass Left Vertebral Vein to Upper Vein, Percutaneous Endoscopic Approach
4KY Bypass Left Internal Jugular Vein to Upper Vein with Nonautologous Tissue Substitute, Percutaneous Endoscopic Approach	**051Q4KY** Bypass Left External Jugular Vein to Upper Vein with Nonautologous Tissue Substitute, Percutaneous Endoscopic Approach	**051T07Y** Bypass Right Face Vein to Upper Vein with Autologous Tissue Substitute, Open Approach
4ZY Bypass Left Internal Jugular Vein to Upper Vein, Percutaneous Endoscopic Approach	**051Q4ZY** Bypass Left External Jugular Vein to Upper Vein, Percutaneous Endoscopic Approach	**051T09Y** Bypass Right Face Vein to Upper Vein with Autologous Venous Tissue, Open Approach
07Y Bypass Right External Jugular Vein to Upper Vein with Autologous Tissue Substitute, Open Approach	**051R07Y** Bypass Right Vertebral Vein to Upper Vein with Autologous Tissue Substitute, Open Approach	**051T0AY** Bypass Right Face Vein to Upper Vein with Autologous Arterial Tissue, Open Approach
09Y Bypass Right External Jugular Vein to Upper Vein with Autologous Venous Tissue, Open Approach	**051R09Y** Bypass Right Vertebral Vein to Upper Vein with Autologous Venous Tissue, Open Approach	**051T0JY** Bypass Right Face Vein to Upper Vein with Synthetic Substitute, Open Approach
0AY Bypass Right External Jugular Vein to Upper Vein with Autologous Arterial Tissue, Open Approach	**051R0AY** Bypass Right Vertebral Vein to Upper Vein with Autologous Arterial Tissue, Open Approach	**051T0KY** Bypass Right Face Vein to Upper Vein with Nonautologous Tissue Substitute, Open Approach
0JY Bypass Right External Jugular Vein to Upper Vein with Synthetic Substitute, Open Approach	**051R0JY** Bypass Right Vertebral Vein to Upper Vein with Synthetic Substitute, Open Approach	**051T0ZY** Bypass Right Face Vein to Upper Vein, Open Approach
0KY Bypass Right External Jugular Vein to Upper Vein with Nonautologous Tissue Substitute, Open Approach	**051R0KY** Bypass Right Vertebral Vein to Upper Vein with Nonautologous Tissue Substitute, Open Approach	**051T47Y** Bypass Right Face Vein to Upper Vein with Autologous Tissue Substitute, Percutaneous Endoscopic Approach
0ZY Bypass Right External Jugular Vein to Upper Vein, Open Approach	**051R0ZY** Bypass Right Vertebral Vein to Upper Vein, Open Approach	**051T49Y** Bypass Right Face Vein to Upper Vein with Autologous Venous Tissue, Percutaneous Endoscopic Approach
47Y Bypass Right External Jugular Vein to Upper Vein with Autologous Tissue Substitute, Percutaneous Endoscopic Approach	**051R47Y** Bypass Right Vertebral Vein to Upper Vein with Autologous Tissue Substitute, Percutaneous Endoscopic Approach	**051T4AY** Bypass Right Face Vein to Upper Vein with Autologous Arterial Tissue, Percutaneous Endoscopic Approach
49Y Bypass Right External Jugular Vein to Upper Vein with Autologous Venous Tissue, Percutaneous Endoscopic Approach	**051R49Y** Bypass Right Vertebral Vein to Upper Vein with Autologous Venous Tissue, Percutaneous Endoscopic Approach	**051T4JY** Bypass Right Face Vein to Upper Vein with Synthetic Substitute, Percutaneous Endoscopic Approach
4AY Bypass Right External Jugular Vein to Upper Vein with Autologous Arterial Tissue, Percutaneous Endoscopic Approach	**051R4AY** Bypass Right Vertebral Vein to Upper Vein with Autologous Arterial Tissue, Percutaneous Endoscopic Approach	**051T4KY** Bypass Right Face Vein to Upper Vein with Nonautologous Tissue Substitute, Percutaneous Endoscopic Approach
4JY Bypass Right External Jugular Vein to Upper Vein with Synthetic Substitute, Percutaneous Endoscopic Approach	**051R4JY** Bypass Right Vertebral Vein to Upper Vein with Synthetic Substitute, Percutaneous Endoscopic Approach	**051T4ZY** Bypass Right Face Vein to Upper Vein, Percutaneous Endoscopic Approach
4KY Bypass Right External Jugular Vein to Upper Vein with Nonautologous Tissue Substitute, Percutaneous Endoscopic Approach	**051R4KY** Bypass Right Vertebral Vein to Upper Vein with Nonautologous Tissue Substitute, Percutaneous Endoscopic Approach	**051V07Y** Bypass Left Face Vein to Upper Vein with Autologous Tissue Substitute, Open Approach
4ZY Bypass Right External Jugular Vein to Upper Vein, Percutaneous Endoscopic Approach	**051R4ZY** Bypass Right Vertebral Vein to Upper Vein, Percutaneous Endoscopic Approach	**051V09Y** Bypass Left Face Vein to Upper Vein with Autologous Venous Tissue, Open Approach
Q07Y Bypass Left External Jugular Vein to Upper Vein with Autologous Tissue Substitute, Open Approach	**051S07Y** Bypass Left Vertebral Vein to Upper Vein with Autologous Tissue Substitute, Open Approach	**051V0AY** Bypass Left Face Vein to Upper Vein with Autologous Arterial Tissue, Open Approach
Q09Y Bypass Left External Jugular Vein to Upper Vein with Autologous Venous Tissue, Open Approach	**051S09Y** Bypass Left Vertebral Vein to Upper Vein with Autologous Venous Tissue, Open Approach	**051V0JY** Bypass Left Face Vein to Upper Vein with Synthetic Substitute, Open Approach
Q0AY Bypass Left External Jugular Vein to Upper Vein with Autologous Arterial Tissue, Open Approach	**051S0AY** Bypass Left Vertebral Vein to Upper Vein with Autologous Arterial Tissue, Open Approach	**051V0KY** Bypass Left Face Vein to Upper Vein with Nonautologous Tissue Substitute, Open Approach
Q0JY Bypass Left External Jugular Vein to Upper Vein with Synthetic Substitute, Open Approach	**051S0JY** Bypass Left Vertebral Vein to Upper Vein with Synthetic Substitute, Open Approach	**051V0ZY** Bypass Left Face Vein to Upper Vein, Open Approach
Q0KY Bypass Left External Jugular Vein to Upper Vein with Nonautologous Tissue Substitute, Open Approach	**051S0KY** Bypass Left Vertebral Vein to Upper Vein with Nonautologous Tissue Substitute, Open Approach	**051V47Y** Bypass Left Face Vein to Upper Vein with Autologous Tissue Substitute, Percutaneous Endoscopic Approach
Q0ZY Bypass Left External Jugular Vein to Upper Vein, Open Approach	**051S0ZY** Bypass Left Vertebral Vein to Upper Vein, Open Approach	**051V49Y** Bypass Left Face Vein to Upper Vein with Autologous Venous Tissue, Percutaneous Endoscopic Approach
Q47Y Bypass Left External Jugular Vein to Upper Vein with Autologous Tissue Substitute, Percutaneous Endoscopic Approach	**051S47Y** Bypass Left Vertebral Vein to Upper Vein with Autologous Tissue Substitute, Percutaneous Endoscopic Approach	**051V4AY** Bypass Left Face Vein to Upper Vein with Autologous Arterial Tissue, Percutaneous Endoscopic Approach
	051S49Y Bypass Left Vertebral Vein to Upper Vein with Autologous Venous Tissue, Percutaneous Endoscopic Approach	**051V4JY** Bypass Left Face Vein to Upper Vein with Synthetic Substitute, Percutaneous Endoscopic Approach
	051S4AY Bypass Left Vertebral Vein to Upper Vein with Autologous Arterial Tissue, Percutaneous Endoscopic Approach	**051V4KY** Bypass Left Face Vein to Upper Vein with Nonautologous Tissue Substitute, Percutaneous Endoscopic Approach
		051V4ZY Bypass Left Face Vein to Upper Vein, Percutaneous Endoscopic Approach

315

055 – Upper Veins, Destruction

05500ZZ Destruction of Azygos Vein, Open Approach

05503ZZ Destruction of Azygos Vein, Percutaneous Approach

05504ZZ Destruction of Azygos Vein, Percutaneous Endoscopic Approach

05510ZZ Destruction of Hemiazygos Vein, Open Approach

05513ZZ Destruction of Hemiazygos Vein, Percutaneous Approach

05514ZZ Destruction of Hemiazygos Vein, Percutaneous Endoscopic Approach

05530ZZ Destruction of Right Innominate Vein, Open Approach

05533ZZ Destruction of Right Innominate Vein, Percutaneous Approach

05534ZZ Destruction of Right Innominate Vein, Percutaneous Endoscopic Approach

05540ZZ Destruction of Left Innominate Vein, Open Approach

05543ZZ Destruction of Left Innominate Vein, Percutaneous Approach

05544ZZ Destruction of Left Innominate Vein, Percutaneous Endoscopic Approach

05550ZZ Destruction of Right Subclavian Vein, Open Approach

05553ZZ Destruction of Right Subclavian Vein, Percutaneous Approach

05554ZZ Destruction of Right Subclavian Vein, Percutaneous Endoscopic Approach

05560ZZ Destruction of Left Subclavian Vein, Open Approach

05563ZZ Destruction of Left Subclavian Vein, Percutaneous Approach

05564ZZ Destruction of Left Subclavian Vein, Percutaneous Endoscopic Approach

05570ZZ Destruction of Right Axillary Vein, Open Approach

05573ZZ Destruction of Right Axillary Vein, Percutaneous Approach

05574ZZ Destruction of Right Axillary Vein, Percutaneous Endoscopic Approach

05580ZZ Destruction of Left Axillary Vein, Open Approach

05583ZZ Destruction of Left Axillary Vein, Percutaneous Approach

05584ZZ Destruction of Left Axillary Vein, Percutaneous Endoscopic Approach

05590ZZ Destruction of Right Brachial Vein, Open Approach

05593ZZ Destruction of Right Brachial Vein, Percutaneous Approach

05594ZZ Destruction of Right Brachial Vein, Percutaneous Endoscopic Approach

055A0ZZ Destruction of Left Brachial Vein, Open Approach

055A3ZZ Destruction of Left Brachial Vein, Percutaneous Approach

055A4ZZ Destruction of Left Brachial Vein, Percutaneous Endoscopic Approach

055B0ZZ Destruction of Right Basilic Vein, Open Approach

055B3ZZ Destruction of Right Basilic Vein, Percutaneous Approach

055B4ZZ Destruction of Right Basilic Vein, Percutaneous Endoscopic Approach

055C0ZZ Destruction of Left Basilic Vein, Open Approach

055C3ZZ Destruction of Left Basilic Vein, Percutaneous Approach

055C4ZZ Destruction of Left Basilic Vein, Percutaneous Endoscopic Approach

055D0ZZ Destruction of Right Cephalic Vein, Open Approach

055D3ZZ Destruction of Right Cephalic Vein, Percutaneous Approach

055D4ZZ Destruction of Right Cephalic Vein, Percutaneous Endoscopic Approach

055F0ZZ Destruction of Left Cephalic Vein, Open Approach

055F3ZZ Destruction of Left Cephalic Vein, Percutaneous Approach

055F4ZZ Destruction of Left Cephalic Vein, Percutaneous Endoscopic Approach

055G0ZZ Destruction of Right Hand Vein, Open Approach

055G3ZZ Destruction of Right Hand Vein, Percutaneous Approach

055G4ZZ Destruction of Right Hand Vein, Percutaneous Endoscopic Approach

055H0ZZ Destruction of Left Hand Vein, Open Approach

055H3ZZ Destruction of Left Hand Vein, Percutaneous Approach

055H4ZZ Destruction of Left Hand Vein, Percutaneous Endoscopic Approach

055L0ZZ Destruction of Intracranial Vein, Open Approach

055L3ZZ Destruction of Intracranial Vein, Percutaneous Approach

055L4ZZ Destruction of Intracranial Vein, Percutaneous Endoscopic Approach

055M0ZZ Destruction of Right Internal Jugular Vein, Open Approach

055M3ZZ Destruction of Right Internal Jugular Vein, Percutaneous Approach

055M4ZZ Destruction of Right Internal Jugular Vein, Percutaneous Endoscopic Approach

055N0ZZ Destruction of Left Internal Jugular Vein, Open Approach

055N3ZZ Destruction of Left Internal Jugular Vein, Percutaneous Approach

055N4ZZ Destruction of Left Internal Jugular Vein, Percutaneous Endoscopic Approach

055P0ZZ Destruction of Right External Jugular Vein, Open Approach

055P3ZZ Destruction of Right External Jugular Vein, Percutaneous Approach

055P4ZZ Destruction of Right External Jugular Vein, Percutaneous Endoscopic Approach

055Q0ZZ Destruction of Left External Jugular Vein, Open Approach

055Q3ZZ Destruction of Left External Jugular Vein, Percutaneous Approach

055Q4ZZ Destruction of Left External Jugular Vein, Percutaneous Endoscopic Approach

055R0ZZ Destruction of Right Vertebral Vein, Open Approach

055R3ZZ Destruction of Right Vertebral Vein, Percutaneous Approach

055R4ZZ Destruction of Right Vertebral Vein, Percutaneous Endoscopic Approach

055S0ZZ Destruction of Left Vertebral Vein, Open Approach

055S3ZZ Destruction of Left Vertebral Vein, Percutaneous Approach

055S4ZZ Destruction of Left Vertebral Vein, Percutaneous Endoscopic Approach

055T0ZZ Destruction of Right Face Vein, Open Approach

055T3ZZ Destruction of Right Face Vein, Percutaneous Approach

055T4ZZ Destruction of Right Face Vein, Percutaneous Endoscopic Approach

055V0ZZ Destruction of Left Face Vein, Open Approach

055V3ZZ Destruction of Left Face Vein, Percutaneous Approach

055V4ZZ Destruction of Left Face Vein, Percutaneous Endoscopic Approach

055Y0ZZ Destruction of Upper Vein, Open Approach

055Y3ZZ Destruction of Upper Vein, Percutaneous Approach

055Y4ZZ Destruction of Upper Vein, Percutaneous Endoscopic Approach

057 – Upper Veins, Dilation

05700DZ Dilation of Azygos Vein with Intraluminal Device, Open Approach

05700ZZ Dilation of Azygos Vein, Open Approach

05703DZ Dilation of Azygos Vein with Intraluminal Device, Percutaneous Approach

05703ZZ Dilation of Azygos Vein, Percutaneous Approach

05704DZ Dilation of Azygos Vein with Intraluminal Device, Percutaneous Endoscopic Approach

05704ZZ Dilation of Azygos Vein, Percutaneous Endoscopic Approach

05710DZ Dilation of Hemiazygos Vein with Intraluminal Device, Open Approach

05710ZZ Dilation of Hemiazygos Vein, Open Approach

05713DZ Dilation of Hemiazygos Vein with Intraluminal Device, Percutaneous Approach

05713ZZ Dilation of Hemiazygos Vein, Percutaneous Approach

05714DZ Dilation of Hemiazygos Vein with Intraluminal Device, Percutaneous Endoscopic Approach

05714ZZ Dilation of Hemiazygos Vein, Percutaneous Endoscopic Approach

05730DZ Dilation of Right Innominate Vein with Intraluminal Device, Open Approach

05730ZZ Dilation of Right Innominate Vein, Open Approach

05733DZ Dilation of Right Innominate Vein with Intraluminal Device, Percutaneous Approach

05733ZZ Dilation of Right Innominate Vein, Percutaneous Approach

05734DZ Dilation of Right Innominate Vein with Intraluminal Device, Percutaneous Endoscopic Approach

05734ZZ Dilation of Right Innominate Vein, Percutaneous Endoscopic Approach

05740DZ Dilation of Left Innominate Vein with Intraluminal Device, Open Approach

05740ZZ Dilation of Left Innominate Vein, Open Approach

05743DZ Dilation of Left Innominate Vein with Intraluminal Device, Percutaneous Approach

05743ZZ Dilation of Left Innominate Vein, Percutaneous Approach

05744DZ Dilation of Left Innominate Vein with Intraluminal Device, Percutaneous Endoscopic Approach

05744ZZ Dilation of Left Innominate Vein, Percutaneous Endoscopic Approach

05750DZ Dilation of Right Subclavian Vein with Intraluminal Device, Open Approach

♀ Female-only   ♂ Male-only   ▲ Limited Coverage   ● Non-OR   ▦ HAC-associated procedure   ▲ Non-covered procedures   ✚ Combina

050ZZ	Dilation of Right Subclavian Vein, Open Approach	
053DZ	Dilation of Right Subclavian Vein with Intraluminal Device, Percutaneous Approach	
053ZZ	Dilation of Right Subclavian Vein, Percutaneous Approach	
054DZ	Dilation of Right Subclavian Vein with Intraluminal Device, Percutaneous Endoscopic Approach	
054ZZ	Dilation of Right Subclavian Vein, Percutaneous Endoscopic Approach	
060DZ	Dilation of Left Subclavian Vein with Intraluminal Device, Open Approach	
060ZZ	Dilation of Left Subclavian Vein, Open Approach	
063DZ	Dilation of Left Subclavian Vein with Intraluminal Device, Percutaneous Approach	
063ZZ	Dilation of Left Subclavian Vein, Percutaneous Approach	
064DZ	Dilation of Left Subclavian Vein with Intraluminal Device, Percutaneous Endoscopic Approach	
064ZZ	Dilation of Left Subclavian Vein, Percutaneous Endoscopic Approach	
070DZ	Dilation of Right Axillary Vein with Intraluminal Device, Open Approach	
070ZZ	Dilation of Right Axillary Vein, Open Approach	
073DZ	Dilation of Right Axillary Vein with Intraluminal Device, Percutaneous Approach	
073ZZ	Dilation of Right Axillary Vein, Percutaneous Approach	
074DZ	Dilation of Right Axillary Vein with Intraluminal Device, Percutaneous Endoscopic Approach	
074ZZ	Dilation of Right Axillary Vein, Percutaneous Endoscopic Approach	
080DZ	Dilation of Left Axillary Vein with Intraluminal Device, Open Approach	
080ZZ	Dilation of Left Axillary Vein, Open Approach	
083DZ	Dilation of Left Axillary Vein with Intraluminal Device, Percutaneous Approach	
083ZZ	Dilation of Left Axillary Vein, Percutaneous Approach	
084DZ	Dilation of Left Axillary Vein with Intraluminal Device, Percutaneous Endoscopic Approach	
084ZZ	Dilation of Left Axillary Vein, Percutaneous Endoscopic Approach	
090DZ	Dilation of Right Brachial Vein with Intraluminal Device, Open Approach	
090ZZ	Dilation of Right Brachial Vein, Open Approach	
093DZ	Dilation of Right Brachial Vein with Intraluminal Device, Percutaneous Approach	
093ZZ	Dilation of Right Brachial Vein, Percutaneous Approach	
094DZ	Dilation of Right Brachial Vein with Intraluminal Device, Percutaneous Endoscopic Approach	
094ZZ	Dilation of Right Brachial Vein, Percutaneous Endoscopic Approach	
07A0DZ	Dilation of Left Brachial Vein with Intraluminal Device, Open Approach	
07A0ZZ	Dilation of Left Brachial Vein, Open Approach	
07A3DZ	Dilation of Left Brachial Vein with Intraluminal Device, Percutaneous Approach	
07A3ZZ	Dilation of Left Brachial Vein, Percutaneous Approach	

057A4DZ	Dilation of Left Brachial Vein with Intraluminal Device, Percutaneous Endoscopic Approach
057A4ZZ	Dilation of Left Brachial Vein, Percutaneous Endoscopic Approach
057B0DZ	Dilation of Right Basilic Vein with Intraluminal Device, Open Approach
057B0ZZ	Dilation of Right Basilic Vein, Open Approach
057B3DZ	Dilation of Right Basilic Vein with Intraluminal Device, Percutaneous Approach
057B3ZZ	Dilation of Right Basilic Vein, Percutaneous Approach
057B4DZ	Dilation of Right Basilic Vein with Intraluminal Device, Percutaneous Endoscopic Approach
057B4ZZ	Dilation of Right Basilic Vein, Percutaneous Endoscopic Approach
057C0DZ	Dilation of Left Basilic Vein with Intraluminal Device, Open Approach
057C0ZZ	Dilation of Left Basilic Vein, Open Approach
057C3DZ	Dilation of Left Basilic Vein with Intraluminal Device, Percutaneous Approach
057C3ZZ	Dilation of Left Basilic Vein, Percutaneous Approach
057C4DZ	Dilation of Left Basilic Vein with Intraluminal Device, Percutaneous Endoscopic Approach
057C4ZZ	Dilation of Left Basilic Vein, Percutaneous Endoscopic Approach
057D0DZ	Dilation of Right Cephalic Vein with Intraluminal Device, Open Approach
057D0ZZ	Dilation of Right Cephalic Vein, Open Approach
057D3DZ	Dilation of Right Cephalic Vein with Intraluminal Device, Percutaneous Approach
057D3ZZ	Dilation of Right Cephalic Vein, Percutaneous Approach
057D4DZ	Dilation of Right Cephalic Vein with Intraluminal Device, Percutaneous Endoscopic Approach
057D4ZZ	Dilation of Right Cephalic Vein, Percutaneous Endoscopic Approach
057F0DZ	Dilation of Left Cephalic Vein with Intraluminal Device, Open Approach
057F0ZZ	Dilation of Left Cephalic Vein, Open Approach
057F3DZ	Dilation of Left Cephalic Vein with Intraluminal Device, Percutaneous Approach
057F3ZZ	Dilation of Left Cephalic Vein, Percutaneous Approach
057F4DZ	Dilation of Left Cephalic Vein with Intraluminal Device, Percutaneous Endoscopic Approach
057F4ZZ	Dilation of Left Cephalic Vein, Percutaneous Endoscopic Approach
057G0DZ	Dilation of Right Hand Vein with Intraluminal Device, Open Approach
057G0ZZ	Dilation of Right Hand Vein, Open Approach
057G3DZ	Dilation of Right Hand Vein with Intraluminal Device, Percutaneous Approach
057G3ZZ	Dilation of Right Hand Vein, Percutaneous Approach
057G4DZ	Dilation of Right Hand Vein with Intraluminal Device, Percutaneous Endoscopic Approach
057G4ZZ	Dilation of Right Hand Vein, Percutaneous Endoscopic Approach
057H0DZ	Dilation of Left Hand Vein with Intraluminal Device, Open Approach

057H0ZZ	Dilation of Left Hand Vein, Open Approach
057H3DZ	Dilation of Left Hand Vein with Intraluminal Device, Percutaneous Approach
057H3ZZ	Dilation of Left Hand Vein, Percutaneous Approach
057H4DZ	Dilation of Left Hand Vein with Intraluminal Device, Percutaneous Endoscopic Approach
057H4ZZ	Dilation of Left Hand Vein, Percutaneous Endoscopic Approach
057L0DZ	Dilation of Intracranial Vein with Intraluminal Device, Open Approach
057L0ZZ	Dilation of Intracranial Vein, Open Approach
057L3DZ	Dilation of Intracranial Vein with Intraluminal Device, Percutaneous Approach
▲ **057L3ZZ**	Dilation of Intracranial Vein, Percutaneous Approach
057L4DZ	Dilation of Intracranial Vein with Intraluminal Device, Percutaneous Endoscopic Approach
▲ **057L4ZZ**	Dilation of Intracranial Vein, Percutaneous Endoscopic Approach
057M0DZ	Dilation of Right Internal Jugular Vein with Intraluminal Device, Open Approach
057M0ZZ	Dilation of Right Internal Jugular Vein, Open Approach
057M3DZ	Dilation of Right Internal Jugular Vein with Intraluminal Device, Percutaneous Approach
057M3ZZ	Dilation of Right Internal Jugular Vein, Percutaneous Approach
057M4DZ	Dilation of Right Internal Jugular Vein with Intraluminal Device, Percutaneous Endoscopic Approach
057M4ZZ	Dilation of Right Internal Jugular Vein, Percutaneous Endoscopic Approach
057N0DZ	Dilation of Left Internal Jugular Vein with Intraluminal Device, Open Approach
057N0ZZ	Dilation of Left Internal Jugular Vein, Open Approach
057N3DZ	Dilation of Left Internal Jugular Vein with Intraluminal Device, Percutaneous Approach
057N3ZZ	Dilation of Left Internal Jugular Vein, Percutaneous Approach
057N4DZ	Dilation of Left Internal Jugular Vein with Intraluminal Device, Percutaneous Endoscopic Approach
057N4ZZ	Dilation of Left Internal Jugular Vein, Percutaneous Endoscopic Approach
057P0DZ	Dilation of Right External Jugular Vein with Intraluminal Device, Open Approach
057P0ZZ	Dilation of Right External Jugular Vein, Open Approach
057P3DZ	Dilation of Right External Jugular Vein with Intraluminal Device, Percutaneous Approach
057P3ZZ	Dilation of Right External Jugular Vein, Percutaneous Approach
057P4DZ	Dilation of Right External Jugular Vein with Intraluminal Device, Percutaneous Endoscopic Approach
057P4ZZ	Dilation of Right External Jugular Vein, Percutaneous Endoscopic Approach
057Q0DZ	Dilation of Left External Jugular Vein with Intraluminal Device, Open Approach
057Q0ZZ	Dilation of Left External Jugular Vein, Open Approach
057Q3DZ	Dilation of Left External Jugular Vein with Intraluminal Device, Percutaneous Approach
057Q3ZZ	Dilation of Left External Jugular Vein, Percutaneous Approach

♀ Female-only	♂ Male-only	▲ Limited Coverage	● Non-OR	▨ HAC-associated procedure	▲ Non-covered procedures	✚ Combination

057Q4DZ	Dilation of Left External Jugular Vein with Intraluminal Device, Percutaneous Endoscopic Approach	**057S3DZ**	Dilation of Left Vertebral Vein with Intraluminal Device, Percutaneous Approach	**057V0DZ**	Dilation of Left Face Vein with Intraluminal Device, Open Approach
057Q4ZZ	Dilation of Left External Jugular Vein, Percutaneous Endoscopic Approach	**057S3ZZ**	Dilation of Left Vertebral Vein, Percutaneous Approach	**057V0ZZ**	Dilation of Left Face Vein, Open Appro
057R0DZ	Dilation of Right Vertebral Vein with Intraluminal Device, Open Approach	**057S4DZ**	Dilation of Left Vertebral Vein with Intraluminal Device, Percutaneous Endoscopic Approach	**057V3DZ**	Dilation of Left Face Vein with Intraluminal Device, Percutaneous Approach
057R0ZZ	Dilation of Right Vertebral Vein, Open Approach	**057S4ZZ**	Dilation of Left Vertebral Vein, Percutaneous Endoscopic Approach	**057V3ZZ**	Dilation of Left Face Vein, Percutaneou Approach
057R3DZ	Dilation of Right Vertebral Vein with Intraluminal Device, Percutaneous Approach	**057T0DZ**	Dilation of Right Face Vein with Intraluminal Device, Open Approach	**057V4DZ**	Dilation of Left Face Vein with Intraluminal Device, Percutaneous Endoscopic Approach
057R3ZZ	Dilation of Right Vertebral Vein, Percutaneous Approach	**057T0ZZ**	Dilation of Right Face Vein, Open Approach	**057V4ZZ**	Dilation of Left Face Vein, Percutaneou Endoscopic Approach
057R4DZ	Dilation of Right Vertebral Vein with Intraluminal Device, Percutaneous Endoscopic Approach	**057T3DZ**	Dilation of Right Face Vein with Intraluminal Device, Percutaneous Approach	**057Y0DZ**	Dilation of Upper Vein with Intralumina Device, Open Approach
057R4ZZ	Dilation of Right Vertebral Vein, Percutaneous Endoscopic Approach	**057T3ZZ**	Dilation of Right Face Vein, Percutaneous Approach	**057Y0ZZ**	Dilation of Upper Vein, Open Approach
057S0DZ	Dilation of Left Vertebral Vein with Intraluminal Device, Open Approach	**057T4DZ**	Dilation of Right Face Vein with Intraluminal Device, Percutaneous Endoscopic Approach	**057Y3DZ**	Dilation of Upper Vein with Intralumina Device, Percutaneous Approach
057S0ZZ	Dilation of Left Vertebral Vein, Open Approach	**057T4ZZ**	Dilation of Right Face Vein, Percutaneous Endoscopic Approach	**057Y3ZZ**	Dilation of Upper Vein, Percutaneous Approach
				057Y4DZ	Dilation of Upper Vein with Intralumina Device, Percutaneous Endoscopic Approach
				057Y4ZZ	Dilation of Upper Vein, Percutaneous Endoscopic Approach

059 – Upper Veins, Drainage

Review Coding Guidelines B3.4a and B3.4b

Review Coding Guideline B6.2

059000Z	Drainage of Azygos Vein with Drainage Device, Open Approach	**05933ZX**	Drainage of Right Innominate Vein, Percutaneous Approach, Diagnostic	**059540Z**	Drainage of Right Subclavian Vein with Drainage Device, Percutaneous Endoscopic Approach
05900ZX	Drainage of Azygos Vein, Open Approach, Diagnostic	**05933ZZ**	Drainage of Right Innominate Vein, Percutaneous Approach	**05954ZX**	Drainage of Right Subclavian Vein, Percutaneous Endoscopic Approach, Diagnostic
05900ZZ	Drainage of Azygos Vein, Open Approach	**059340Z**	Drainage of Right Innominate Vein with Drainage Device, Percutaneous Endoscopic Approach	**05954ZZ**	Drainage of Right Subclavian Vein, Percutaneous Endoscopic Approach
059030Z	Drainage of Azygos Vein with Drainage Device, Percutaneous Approach	**05934ZX**	Drainage of Right Innominate Vein, Percutaneous Endoscopic Approach, Diagnostic	**059600Z**	Drainage of Left Subclavian Vein with Drainage Device, Open Approach
05903ZX	Drainage of Azygos Vein, Percutaneous Approach, Diagnostic	**05934ZZ**	Drainage of Right Innominate Vein, Percutaneous Endoscopic Approach	**05960ZX**	Drainage of Left Subclavian Vein, Open Approach, Diagnostic
05903ZZ	Drainage of Azygos Vein, Percutaneous Approach	**059400Z**	Drainage of Left Innominate Vein with Drainage Device, Open Approach	**05960ZZ**	Drainage of Left Subclavian Vein, Open Approach
059040Z	Drainage of Azygos Vein with Drainage Device, Percutaneous Endoscopic Approach	**05940ZX**	Drainage of Left Innominate Vein, Open Approach, Diagnostic	**059630Z**	Drainage of Left Subclavian Vein with Drainage Device, Percutaneous Approac
05904ZX	Drainage of Azygos Vein, Percutaneous Endoscopic Approach, Diagnostic	**05940ZZ**	Drainage of Left Innominate Vein, Open Approach	**05963ZX**	Drainage of Left Subclavian Vein, Percutaneous Approach, Diagnostic
05904ZZ	Drainage of Azygos Vein, Percutaneous Endoscopic Approach	**059430Z**	Drainage of Left Innominate Vein with Drainage Device, Percutaneous Approach	**05963ZZ**	Drainage of Left Subclavian Vein, Percutaneous Approach
059100Z	Drainage of Hemiazygos Vein with Drainage Device, Open Approach	**05943ZX**	Drainage of Left Innominate Vein, Percutaneous Approach, Diagnostic	**059640Z**	Drainage of Left Subclavian Vein with Drainage Device, Percutaneous Endoscopic Approach
05910ZX	Drainage of Hemiazygos Vein, Open Approach, Diagnostic	**05943ZZ**	Drainage of Left Innominate Vein, Percutaneous Approach	**05964ZX**	Drainage of Left Subclavian Vein, Percutaneous Endoscopic Approach, Diagnostic
05910ZZ	Drainage of Hemiazygos Vein, Open Approach	**059440Z**	Drainage of Left Innominate Vein with Drainage Device, Percutaneous Endoscopic Approach	**05964ZZ**	Drainage of Left Subclavian Vein, Percutaneous Endoscopic Approach
059130Z	Drainage of Hemiazygos Vein with Drainage Device, Percutaneous Approach	**05944ZX**	Drainage of Left Innominate Vein, Percutaneous Endoscopic Approach, Diagnostic	**059700Z**	Drainage of Right Axillary Vein with Drainage Device, Open Approach
05913ZX	Drainage of Hemiazygos Vein, Percutaneous Approach, Diagnostic	**05944ZZ**	Drainage of Left Innominate Vein, Percutaneous Endoscopic Approach	**05970ZX**	Drainage of Right Axillary Vein, Open Approach, Diagnostic
05913ZZ	Drainage of Hemiazygos Vein, Percutaneous Approach	**059500Z**	Drainage of Right Subclavian Vein with Drainage Device, Open Approach	**05970ZZ**	Drainage of Right Axillary Vein, Open Approach
059140Z	Drainage of Hemiazygos Vein with Drainage Device, Percutaneous Endoscopic Approach	**05950ZX**	Drainage of Right Subclavian Vein, Open Approach, Diagnostic	**059730Z**	Drainage of Right Axillary Vein with Drainage Device, Percutaneous Approac
05914ZX	Drainage of Hemiazygos Vein, Percutaneous Endoscopic Approach, Diagnostic	**05950ZZ**	Drainage of Right Subclavian Vein, Open Approach	**05973ZX**	Drainage of Right Axillary Vein, Percutaneous Approach, Diagnostic
05914ZZ	Drainage of Hemiazygos Vein, Percutaneous Endoscopic Approach	**059530Z**	Drainage of Right Subclavian Vein with Drainage Device, Percutaneous Approach	**05973ZZ**	Drainage of Right Axillary Vein, Percutaneous Approach
059300Z	Drainage of Right Innominate Vein with Drainage Device, Open Approach	**05953ZX**	Drainage of Right Subclavian Vein, Percutaneous Approach, Diagnostic	**059740Z**	Drainage of Right Axillary Vein with Drainage Device, Percutaneous Endoscopic Approach
05930ZX	Drainage of Right Innominate Vein, Open Approach, Diagnostic	**05953ZZ**	Drainage of Right Subclavian Vein, Percutaneous Approach	**05974ZX**	Drainage of Right Axillary Vein, Percutaneous Endoscopic Approach, Diagnostic
05930ZZ	Drainage of Right Innominate Vein, Open Approach				
059330Z	Drainage of Right Innominate Vein with Drainage Device, Percutaneous Approach				

74ZZ	Drainage of Right Axillary Vein, Percutaneous Endoscopic Approach
800Z	Drainage of Left Axillary Vein with Drainage Device, Open Approach
80ZX	Drainage of Left Axillary Vein, Open Approach, Diagnostic
80ZZ	Drainage of Left Axillary Vein, Open Approach
830Z	Drainage of Left Axillary Vein with Drainage Device, Percutaneous Approach
83ZX	Drainage of Left Axillary Vein, Percutaneous Approach, Diagnostic
83ZZ	Drainage of Left Axillary Vein, Percutaneous Approach
840Z	Drainage of Left Axillary Vein with Drainage Device, Percutaneous Endoscopic Approach
84ZX	Drainage of Left Axillary Vein, Percutaneous Endoscopic Approach, Diagnostic
84ZZ	Drainage of Left Axillary Vein, Percutaneous Endoscopic Approach
900Z	Drainage of Right Brachial Vein with Drainage Device, Open Approach
90ZX	Drainage of Right Brachial Vein, Open Approach, Diagnostic
90ZZ	Drainage of Right Brachial Vein, Open Approach
930Z	Drainage of Right Brachial Vein with Drainage Device, Percutaneous Approach
93ZX	Drainage of Right Brachial Vein, Percutaneous Approach, Diagnostic
93ZZ	Drainage of Right Brachial Vein, Percutaneous Approach
940Z	Drainage of Right Brachial Vein with Drainage Device, Percutaneous Endoscopic Approach
94ZX	Drainage of Right Brachial Vein, Percutaneous Endoscopic Approach, Diagnostic
94ZZ	Drainage of Right Brachial Vein, Percutaneous Endoscopic Approach
A00Z	Drainage of Left Brachial Vein with Drainage Device, Open Approach
A0ZX	Drainage of Left Brachial Vein, Open Approach, Diagnostic
A0ZZ	Drainage of Left Brachial Vein, Open Approach
A30Z	Drainage of Left Brachial Vein with Drainage Device, Percutaneous Approach
A3ZX	Drainage of Left Brachial Vein, Percutaneous Approach, Diagnostic
A3ZZ	Drainage of Left Brachial Vein, Percutaneous Approach
A40Z	Drainage of Left Brachial Vein with Drainage Device, Percutaneous Endoscopic Approach
A4ZX	Drainage of Left Brachial Vein, Percutaneous Endoscopic Approach, Diagnostic
A4ZZ	Drainage of Left Brachial Vein, Percutaneous Endoscopic Approach
B00Z	Drainage of Right Basilic Vein with Drainage Device, Open Approach
B0ZX	Drainage of Right Basilic Vein, Open Approach, Diagnostic
B0ZZ	Drainage of Right Basilic Vein, Open Approach
B30Z	Drainage of Right Basilic Vein with Drainage Device, Percutaneous Approach
B3ZX	Drainage of Right Basilic Vein, Percutaneous Approach, Diagnostic
B3ZZ	Drainage of Right Basilic Vein, Percutaneous Approach
B40Z	Drainage of Right Basilic Vein with Drainage Device, Percutaneous Endoscopic Approach

059B4ZX	Drainage of Right Basilic Vein, Percutaneous Endoscopic Approach, Diagnostic
059B4ZZ	Drainage of Right Basilic Vein, Percutaneous Endoscopic Approach
059C00Z	Drainage of Left Basilic Vein with Drainage Device, Open Approach
059C0ZX	Drainage of Left Basilic Vein, Open Approach, Diagnostic
059C0ZZ	Drainage of Left Basilic Vein, Open Approach
059C30Z	Drainage of Left Basilic Vein with Drainage Device, Percutaneous Approach
059C3ZX	Drainage of Left Basilic Vein, Percutaneous Approach, Diagnostic
059C3ZZ	Drainage of Left Basilic Vein, Percutaneous Approach
059C40Z	Drainage of Left Basilic Vein with Drainage Device, Percutaneous Endoscopic Approach
059C4ZX	Drainage of Left Basilic Vein, Percutaneous Endoscopic Approach, Diagnostic
059C4ZZ	Drainage of Left Basilic Vein, Percutaneous Endoscopic Approach
059D00Z	Drainage of Right Cephalic Vein with Drainage Device, Open Approach
059D0ZX	Drainage of Right Cephalic Vein, Open Approach, Diagnostic
059D0ZZ	Drainage of Right Cephalic Vein, Open Approach
059D30Z	Drainage of Right Cephalic Vein with Drainage Device, Percutaneous Approach
059D3ZX	Drainage of Right Cephalic Vein, Percutaneous Approach, Diagnostic
059D3ZZ	Drainage of Right Cephalic Vein, Percutaneous Approach
059D40Z	Drainage of Right Cephalic Vein with Drainage Device, Percutaneous Endoscopic Approach
059D4ZX	Drainage of Right Cephalic Vein, Percutaneous Endoscopic Approach, Diagnostic
059D4ZZ	Drainage of Right Cephalic Vein, Percutaneous Endoscopic Approach
059F00Z	Drainage of Left Cephalic Vein with Drainage Device, Open Approach
059F0ZX	Drainage of Left Cephalic Vein, Open Approach, Diagnostic
059F0ZZ	Drainage of Left Cephalic Vein, Open Approach
059F30Z	Drainage of Left Cephalic Vein with Drainage Device, Percutaneous Approach
059F3ZX	Drainage of Left Cephalic Vein, Percutaneous Approach, Diagnostic
059F3ZZ	Drainage of Left Cephalic Vein, Percutaneous Approach
059F40Z	Drainage of Left Cephalic Vein with Drainage Device, Percutaneous Endoscopic Approach
059F4ZX	Drainage of Left Cephalic Vein, Percutaneous Endoscopic Approach, Diagnostic
059F4ZZ	Drainage of Left Cephalic Vein, Percutaneous Endoscopic Approach
059G00Z	Drainage of Right Hand Vein with Drainage Device, Open Approach
059G0ZX	Drainage of Right Hand Vein, Open Approach, Diagnostic
059G0ZZ	Drainage of Right Hand Vein, Open Approach
059G30Z	Drainage of Right Hand Vein with Drainage Device, Percutaneous Approach
059G3ZX	Drainage of Right Hand Vein, Percutaneous Approach, Diagnostic
059G3ZZ	Drainage of Right Hand Vein, Percutaneous Approach

059G40Z	Drainage of Right Hand Vein with Drainage Device, Percutaneous Endoscopic Approach
059G4ZX	Drainage of Right Hand Vein, Percutaneous Endoscopic Approach, Diagnostic
059G4ZZ	Drainage of Right Hand Vein, Percutaneous Endoscopic Approach
059H00Z	Drainage of Left Hand Vein with Drainage Device, Open Approach
059H0ZX	Drainage of Left Hand Vein, Open Approach, Diagnostic
059H0ZZ	Drainage of Left Hand Vein, Open Approach
059H30Z	Drainage of Left Hand Vein with Drainage Device, Percutaneous Approach
059H3ZX	Drainage of Left Hand Vein, Percutaneous Approach, Diagnostic
059H3ZZ	Drainage of Left Hand Vein, Percutaneous Approach
059H40Z	Drainage of Left Hand Vein with Drainage Device, Percutaneous Endoscopic Approach
059H4ZX	Drainage of Left Hand Vein, Percutaneous Endoscopic Approach, Diagnostic
059H4ZZ	Drainage of Left Hand Vein, Percutaneous Endoscopic Approach
059L00Z	Drainage of Intracranial Vein with Drainage Device, Open Approach
059L0ZX	Drainage of Intracranial Vein, Open Approach, Diagnostic
059L0ZZ	Drainage of Intracranial Vein, Open Approach
059L30Z	Drainage of Intracranial Vein with Drainage Device, Percutaneous Approach
059L3ZX	Drainage of Intracranial Vein, Percutaneous Approach, Diagnostic
059L3ZZ	Drainage of Intracranial Vein, Percutaneous Approach
059L40Z	Drainage of Intracranial Vein with Drainage Device, Percutaneous Endoscopic Approach
059L4ZX	Drainage of Intracranial Vein, Percutaneous Endoscopic Approach, Diagnostic
059L4ZZ	Drainage of Intracranial Vein, Percutaneous Endoscopic Approach
059M00Z	Drainage of Right Internal Jugular Vein with Drainage Device, Open Approach
059M0ZX	Drainage of Right Internal Jugular Vein, Open Approach, Diagnostic
059M0ZZ	Drainage of Right Internal Jugular Vein, Open Approach
059M30Z	Drainage of Right Internal Jugular Vein with Drainage Device, Percutaneous Approach
059M3ZX	Drainage of Right Internal Jugular Vein, Percutaneous Approach, Diagnostic
059M3ZZ	Drainage of Right Internal Jugular Vein, Percutaneous Approach
059M40Z	Drainage of Right Internal Jugular Vein with Drainage Device, Percutaneous Endoscopic Approach
059M4ZX	Drainage of Right Internal Jugular Vein, Percutaneous Endoscopic Approach, Diagnostic
059M4ZZ	Drainage of Right Internal Jugular Vein, Percutaneous Endoscopic Approach
059N00Z	Drainage of Left Internal Jugular Vein with Drainage Device, Open Approach
059N0ZX	Drainage of Left Internal Jugular Vein, Open Approach, Diagnostic
059N0ZZ	Drainage of Left Internal Jugular Vein, Open Approach
059N30Z	Drainage of Left Internal Jugular Vein with Drainage Device, Percutaneous Approach
059N3ZX	Drainage of Left Internal Jugular Vein, Percutaneous Approach, Diagnostic

319

059N3ZZ Drainage of Left Internal Jugular Vein, Percutaneous Approach

059N40Z Drainage of Left Internal Jugular Vein with Drainage Device, Percutaneous Endoscopic Approach

059N4ZX Drainage of Left Internal Jugular Vein, Percutaneous Endoscopic Approach, Diagnostic

059N4ZZ Drainage of Left Internal Jugular Vein, Percutaneous Endoscopic Approach

059P00Z Drainage of Right External Jugular Vein with Drainage Device, Open Approach

059P0ZX Drainage of Right External Jugular Vein, Open Approach, Diagnostic

059P0ZZ Drainage of Right External Jugular Vein, Open Approach

059P30Z Drainage of Right External Jugular Vein with Drainage Device, Percutaneous Approach

059P3ZX Drainage of Right External Jugular Vein, Percutaneous Approach, Diagnostic

059P3ZZ Drainage of Right External Jugular Vein, Percutaneous Approach

059P40Z Drainage of Right External Jugular Vein with Drainage Device, Percutaneous Endoscopic Approach

059P4ZX Drainage of Right External Jugular Vein, Percutaneous Endoscopic Approach, Diagnostic

059P4ZZ Drainage of Right External Jugular Vein, Percutaneous Endoscopic Approach

059Q00Z Drainage of Left External Jugular Vein with Drainage Device, Open Approach

059Q0ZX Drainage of Left External Jugular Vein, Open Approach, Diagnostic

059Q0ZZ Drainage of Left External Jugular Vein, Open Approach

059Q30Z Drainage of Left External Jugular Vein with Drainage Device, Percutaneous Approach

059Q3ZX Drainage of Left External Jugular Vein, Percutaneous Approach, Diagnostic

059Q3ZZ Drainage of Left External Jugular Vein, Percutaneous Approach

059Q40Z Drainage of Left External Jugular Vein with Drainage Device, Percutaneous Endoscopic Approach

059Q4ZX Drainage of Left External Jugular Vein, Percutaneous Endoscopic Approach, Diagnostic

059Q4ZZ Drainage of Left External Jugular Vein, Percutaneous Endoscopic Approach

059R00Z Drainage of Right Vertebral Vein with Drainage Device, Open Approach

059R0ZX Drainage of Right Vertebral Vein, Open Approach, Diagnostic

059R0ZZ Drainage of Right Vertebral Vein, Open Approach

059R30Z Drainage of Right Vertebral Vein with Drainage Device, Percutaneous Approach

059R3ZX Drainage of Right Vertebral Vein, Percutaneous Approach, Diagnostic

059R3ZZ Drainage of Right Vertebral Vein, Percutaneous Approach

059R40Z Drainage of Right Vertebral Vein with Drainage Device, Percutaneous Endoscopic Approach

059R4ZX Drainage of Right Vertebral Vein, Percutaneous Endoscopic Approach, Diagnostic

059R4ZZ Drainage of Right Vertebral Vein, Percutaneous Endoscopic Approach

059S00Z Drainage of Left Vertebral Vein with Drainage Device, Open Approach

059S0ZX Drainage of Left Vertebral Vein, Open Approach, Diagnostic

059S0ZZ Drainage of Left Vertebral Vein, Open Approach

059S30Z Drainage of Left Vertebral Vein with Drainage Device, Percutaneous Approach

059S3ZX Drainage of Left Vertebral Vein, Percutaneous Approach, Diagnostic

059S3ZZ Drainage of Left Vertebral Vein, Percutaneous Approach

059S40Z Drainage of Left Vertebral Vein with Drainage Device, Percutaneous Endoscopic Approach

059S4ZX Drainage of Left Vertebral Vein, Percutaneous Endoscopic Approach, Diagnostic

059S4ZZ Drainage of Left Vertebral Vein, Percutaneous Endoscopic Approach

059T00Z Drainage of Right Face Vein with Drainage Device, Open Approach

059T0ZX Drainage of Right Face Vein, Open Approach, Diagnostic

059T0ZZ Drainage of Right Face Vein, Open Approach

059T30Z Drainage of Right Face Vein with Drainage Device, Percutaneous Approach

059T3ZX Drainage of Right Face Vein, Percutaneous Approach, Diagnostic

059T3ZZ Drainage of Right Face Vein, Percutaneous Approach

059T40Z Drainage of Right Face Vein with Drainage Device, Percutaneous Endoscopic Approach

059T4ZX Drainage of Right Face Vein, Percutaneous Endoscopic Approach, Diagnostic

059T4ZZ Drainage of Right Face Vein, Percutaneous Endoscopic Approach

059V00Z Drainage of Left Face Vein with Drainage Device, Open Approach

059V0ZX Drainage of Left Face Vein, Open Approach, Diagnostic

059V0ZZ Drainage of Left Face Vein, Open Approach

059V30Z Drainage of Left Face Vein with Drainage Device, Percutaneous Approach

059V3ZX Drainage of Left Face Vein, Percutaneous Approach, Diagnostic

059V3ZZ Drainage of Left Face Vein, Percutaneous Approach

059V40Z Drainage of Left Face Vein with Drainage Device, Percutaneous Endoscopic Approach

059V4ZX Drainage of Left Face Vein, Percutaneous Endoscopic Approach, Diagnostic

059V4ZZ Drainage of Left Face Vein, Percutaneous Endoscopic Approach

059Y00Z Drainage of Upper Vein with Drainage Device, Open Approach

059Y0ZX Drainage of Upper Vein, Open Approach, Diagnostic

059Y0ZZ Drainage of Upper Vein, Open Approach

059Y30Z Drainage of Upper Vein with Drainage Device, Percutaneous Approach

059Y3ZX Drainage of Upper Vein, Percutaneous Approach, Diagnostic

059Y3ZZ Drainage of Upper Vein, Percutaneous Approach

059Y40Z Drainage of Upper Vein with Drainage Device, Percutaneous Endoscopic Approach

059Y4ZX Drainage of Upper Vein, Percutaneous Endoscopic Approach, Diagnostic

059Y4ZZ Drainage of Upper Vein, Percutaneous Endoscopic Approach

05B – Upper Veins, Excision

Review Coding Guidelines B3.4a and B3.4b

Review Coding Guideline B3.8

05B00ZX Excision of Azygos Vein, Open Approach, Diagnostic

05B00ZZ Excision of Azygos Vein, Open Approach

05B03ZX Excision of Azygos Vein, Percutaneous Approach, Diagnostic

05B03ZZ Excision of Azygos Vein, Percutaneous Approach

05B04ZX Excision of Azygos Vein, Percutaneous Endoscopic Approach, Diagnostic

05B04ZZ Excision of Azygos Vein, Percutaneous Endoscopic Approach

05B10ZX Excision of Hemiazygos Vein, Open Approach, Diagnostic

05B10ZZ Excision of Hemiazygos Vein, Open Approach

05B13ZX Excision of Hemiazygos Vein, Percutaneous Approach, Diagnostic

05B13ZZ Excision of Hemiazygos Vein, Percutaneous Approach

05B14ZX Excision of Hemiazygos Vein, Percutaneous Endoscopic Approach, Diagnostic

05B14ZZ Excision of Hemiazygos Vein, Percutaneous Endoscopic Approach

05B30ZX Excision of Right Innominate Vein, Open Approach, Diagnostic

05B30ZZ Excision of Right Innominate Vein, Open Approach

05B33ZX Excision of Right Innominate Vein, Percutaneous Approach, Diagnostic

05B33ZZ Excision of Right Innominate Vein, Percutaneous Approach

05B34ZX Excision of Right Innominate Vein, Percutaneous Endoscopic Approach, Diagnostic

05B34ZZ Excision of Right Innominate Vein, Percutaneous Endoscopic Approach

05B40ZX Excision of Left Innominate Vein, Open Approach, Diagnostic

05B40ZZ Excision of Left Innominate Vein, Open Approach

05B43ZX Excision of Left Innominate Vein, Percutaneous Approach, Diagnostic

05B43ZZ Excision of Left Innominate Vein, Percutaneous Approach

05B44ZX Excision of Left Innominate Vein, Percutaneous Endoscopic Approach, Diagnostic

05B44ZZ Excision of Left Innominate Vein, Percutaneous Endoscopic Approach

05B50ZX Excision of Right Subclavian Vein, Open Approach, Diagnostic

05B50ZZ Excision of Right Subclavian Vein, Open Approach

05B53ZX Excision of Right Subclavian Vein, Percutaneous Approach, Diagnostic

05B53ZZ Excision of Right Subclavian Vein, Percutaneous Approach

54ZX Excision of Right Subclavian Vein, Percutaneous Endoscopic Approach, Diagnostic

54ZZ Excision of Right Subclavian Vein, Percutaneous Endoscopic Approach

60ZX Excision of Left Subclavian Vein, Open Approach, Diagnostic

60ZZ Excision of Left Subclavian Vein, Open Approach

63ZX Excision of Left Subclavian Vein, Percutaneous Approach, Diagnostic

63ZZ Excision of Left Subclavian Vein, Percutaneous Approach

64ZX Excision of Left Subclavian Vein, Percutaneous Endoscopic Approach, Diagnostic

64ZZ Excision of Left Subclavian Vein, Percutaneous Endoscopic Approach

70ZX Excision of Right Axillary Vein, Open Approach, Diagnostic

70ZZ Excision of Right Axillary Vein, Open Approach

73ZX Excision of Right Axillary Vein, Percutaneous Approach, Diagnostic

73ZZ Excision of Right Axillary Vein, Percutaneous Approach

74ZX Excision of Right Axillary Vein, Percutaneous Endoscopic Approach, Diagnostic

74ZZ Excision of Right Axillary Vein, Percutaneous Endoscopic Approach

80ZX Excision of Left Axillary Vein, Open Approach, Diagnostic

80ZZ Excision of Left Axillary Vein, Open Approach

83ZX Excision of Left Axillary Vein, Percutaneous Approach, Diagnostic

83ZZ Excision of Left Axillary Vein, Percutaneous Approach

84ZX Excision of Left Axillary Vein, Percutaneous Endoscopic Approach, Diagnostic

84ZZ Excision of Left Axillary Vein, Percutaneous Endoscopic Approach

90ZX Excision of Right Brachial Vein, Open Approach, Diagnostic

90ZZ Excision of Right Brachial Vein, Open Approach

93ZX Excision of Right Brachial Vein, Percutaneous Approach, Diagnostic

93ZZ Excision of Right Brachial Vein, Percutaneous Approach

94ZX Excision of Right Brachial Vein, Percutaneous Endoscopic Approach, Diagnostic

94ZZ Excision of Right Brachial Vein, Percutaneous Endoscopic Approach

A0ZX Excision of Left Brachial Vein, Open Approach, Diagnostic

A0ZZ Excision of Left Brachial Vein, Open Approach

A3ZX Excision of Left Brachial Vein, Percutaneous Approach, Diagnostic

A3ZZ Excision of Left Brachial Vein, Percutaneous Approach

A4ZX Excision of Left Brachial Vein, Percutaneous Endoscopic Approach, Diagnostic

A4ZZ Excision of Left Brachial Vein, Percutaneous Endoscopic Approach

B0ZX Excision of Right Basilic Vein, Open Approach, Diagnostic

B0ZZ Excision of Right Basilic Vein, Open Approach

B3ZX Excision of Right Basilic Vein, Percutaneous Approach, Diagnostic

B3ZZ Excision of Right Basilic Vein, Percutaneous Approach

05BB4ZX Excision of Right Basilic Vein, Percutaneous Endoscopic Approach, Diagnostic

05BB4ZZ Excision of Right Basilic Vein, Percutaneous Endoscopic Approach

05BC0ZX Excision of Left Basilic Vein, Open Approach, Diagnostic

05BC0ZZ Excision of Left Basilic Vein, Open Approach

05BC3ZX Excision of Left Basilic Vein, Percutaneous Approach, Diagnostic

05BC3ZZ Excision of Left Basilic Vein, Percutaneous Approach

05BC4ZX Excision of Left Basilic Vein, Percutaneous Endoscopic Approach, Diagnostic

05BC4ZZ Excision of Left Basilic Vein, Percutaneous Endoscopic Approach

05BD0ZX Excision of Right Cephalic Vein, Open Approach, Diagnostic

05BD0ZZ Excision of Right Cephalic Vein, Open Approach

05BD3ZX Excision of Right Cephalic Vein, Percutaneous Approach, Diagnostic

05BD3ZZ Excision of Right Cephalic Vein, Percutaneous Approach

05BD4ZX Excision of Right Cephalic Vein, Percutaneous Endoscopic Approach, Diagnostic

05BD4ZZ Excision of Right Cephalic Vein, Percutaneous Endoscopic Approach

05BF0ZX Excision of Left Cephalic Vein, Open Approach, Diagnostic

05BF0ZZ Excision of Left Cephalic Vein, Open Approach

05BF3ZX Excision of Left Cephalic Vein, Percutaneous Approach, Diagnostic

05BF3ZZ Excision of Left Cephalic Vein, Percutaneous Approach

05BF4ZX Excision of Left Cephalic Vein, Percutaneous Endoscopic Approach, Diagnostic

05BF4ZZ Excision of Left Cephalic Vein, Percutaneous Endoscopic Approach

05BG0ZX Excision of Right Hand Vein, Open Approach, Diagnostic

05BG0ZZ Excision of Right Hand Vein, Open Approach

05BG3ZX Excision of Right Hand Vein, Percutaneous Approach, Diagnostic

05BG3ZZ Excision of Right Hand Vein, Percutaneous Approach

05BG4ZX Excision of Right Hand Vein, Percutaneous Endoscopic Approach, Diagnostic

05BG4ZZ Excision of Right Hand Vein, Percutaneous Endoscopic Approach

05BH0ZX Excision of Left Hand Vein, Open Approach, Diagnostic

05BH0ZZ Excision of Left Hand Vein, Open Approach

05BH3ZX Excision of Left Hand Vein, Percutaneous Approach, Diagnostic

05BH3ZZ Excision of Left Hand Vein, Percutaneous Approach

05BH4ZX Excision of Left Hand Vein, Percutaneous Endoscopic Approach, Diagnostic

05BH4ZZ Excision of Left Hand Vein, Percutaneous Endoscopic Approach

05BL0ZX Excision of Intracranial Vein, Open Approach, Diagnostic

05BL0ZZ Excision of Intracranial Vein, Open Approach

05BL3ZX Excision of Intracranial Vein, Percutaneous Approach, Diagnostic

05BL3ZZ Excision of Intracranial Vein, Percutaneous Approach

05BL4ZX Excision of Intracranial Vein, Percutaneous Endoscopic Approach, Diagnostic

05BL4ZZ Excision of Intracranial Vein, Percutaneous Endoscopic Approach

05BM0ZX Excision of Right Internal Jugular Vein, Open Approach, Diagnostic

05BM0ZZ Excision of Right Internal Jugular Vein, Open Approach

05BM3ZX Excision of Right Internal Jugular Vein, Percutaneous Approach, Diagnostic

05BM3ZZ Excision of Right Internal Jugular Vein, Percutaneous Approach

05BM4ZX Excision of Right Internal Jugular Vein, Percutaneous Endoscopic Approach, Diagnostic

05BM4ZZ Excision of Right Internal Jugular Vein, Percutaneous Endoscopic Approach

05BN0ZX Excision of Left Internal Jugular Vein, Open Approach, Diagnostic

05BN0ZZ Excision of Left Internal Jugular Vein, Open Approach

05BN3ZX Excision of Left Internal Jugular Vein, Percutaneous Approach, Diagnostic

05BN3ZZ Excision of Left Internal Jugular Vein, Percutaneous Approach

05BN4ZX Excision of Left Internal Jugular Vein, Percutaneous Endoscopic Approach, Diagnostic

05BN4ZZ Excision of Left Internal Jugular Vein, Percutaneous Endoscopic Approach

05BP0ZX Excision of Right External Jugular Vein, Open Approach, Diagnostic

05BP0ZZ Excision of Right External Jugular Vein, Open Approach

05BP3ZX Excision of Right External Jugular Vein, Percutaneous Approach, Diagnostic

05BP3ZZ Excision of Right External Jugular Vein, Percutaneous Approach

05BP4ZX Excision of Right External Jugular Vein, Percutaneous Endoscopic Approach, Diagnostic

05BP4ZZ Excision of Right External Jugular Vein, Percutaneous Endoscopic Approach

05BQ0ZX Excision of Left External Jugular Vein, Open Approach, Diagnostic

05BQ0ZZ Excision of Left External Jugular Vein, Open Approach

05BQ3ZX Excision of Left External Jugular Vein, Percutaneous Approach, Diagnostic

05BQ3ZZ Excision of Left External Jugular Vein, Percutaneous Approach

05BQ4ZX Excision of Left External Jugular Vein, Percutaneous Endoscopic Approach, Diagnostic

05BQ4ZZ Excision of Left External Jugular Vein, Percutaneous Endoscopic Approach

05BR0ZX Excision of Right Vertebral Vein, Open Approach, Diagnostic

05BR0ZZ Excision of Right Vertebral Vein, Open Approach

05BR3ZX Excision of Right Vertebral Vein, Percutaneous Approach, Diagnostic

05BR3ZZ Excision of Right Vertebral Vein, Percutaneous Approach

05BR4ZX Excision of Right Vertebral Vein, Percutaneous Endoscopic Approach, Diagnostic

05BR4ZZ Excision of Right Vertebral Vein, Percutaneous Endoscopic Approach

05BS0ZX Excision of Left Vertebral Vein, Open Approach, Diagnostic

05BS0ZZ Excision of Left Vertebral Vein, Open Approach

05BS3ZX Excision of Left Vertebral Vein, Percutaneous Approach, Diagnostic

05BS3ZZ Excision of Left Vertebral Vein, Percutaneous Approach

05BS4ZX	Excision of Left Vertebral Vein, Percutaneous Endoscopic Approach, Diagnostic	05BT4ZX	Excision of Right Face Vein, Percutaneous Endoscopic Approach, Diagnostic
05BS4ZZ	Excision of Left Vertebral Vein, Percutaneous Endoscopic Approach	05BT4ZZ	Excision of Right Face Vein, Percutaneous Endoscopic Approach
05BT0ZX	Excision of Right Face Vein, Open Approach, Diagnostic	05BV0ZX	Excision of Left Face Vein, Open Approach, Diagnostic
05BT0ZZ	Excision of Right Face Vein, Open Approach	05BV0ZZ	Excision of Left Face Vein, Open Approach
05BT3ZX	Excision of Right Face Vein, Percutaneous Approach, Diagnostic	05BV3ZX	Excision of Left Face Vein, Percutaneous Approach, Diagnostic
05BT3ZZ	Excision of Right Face Vein, Percutaneous Approach	05BV3ZZ	Excision of Left Face Vein, Percutaneous Approach
		05BV4ZX	Excision of Left Face Vein, Percutaneous Endoscopic Approach, Diagnostic

05BV4ZZ Excision of Left Face Vein, Percutaneous Endoscopic Approach
05BY0ZX Excision of Upper Vein, Open Approach, Diagnostic
05BY0ZZ Excision of Upper Vein, Open Approach
05BY3ZX Excision of Upper Vein, Percutaneous Approach, Diagnostic
05BY3ZZ Excision of Upper Vein, Percutaneous Approach
05BY4ZX Excision of Upper Vein, Percutaneous Endoscopic Approach, Diagnostic
05BY4ZZ Excision of Upper Vein, Percutaneous Endoscopic Approach

05C – Upper Veins, Extirpation

05C00ZZ Extirpation of Matter from Azygos Vein, Open Approach
05C03ZZ Extirpation of Matter from Azygos Vein, Percutaneous Approach
05C04ZZ Extirpation of Matter from Azygos Vein, Percutaneous Endoscopic Approach
05C10ZZ Extirpation of Matter from Hemiazygos Vein, Open Approach
05C13ZZ Extirpation of Matter from Hemiazygos Vein, Percutaneous Approach
05C14ZZ Extirpation of Matter from Hemiazygos Vein, Percutaneous Endoscopic Approach
05C30ZZ Extirpation of Matter from Right Innominate Vein, Open Approach
05C33ZZ Extirpation of Matter from Right Innominate Vein, Percutaneous Approach
05C34ZZ Extirpation of Matter from Right Innominate Vein, Percutaneous Endoscopic Approach
05C40ZZ Extirpation of Matter from Left Innominate Vein, Open Approach
05C43ZZ Extirpation of Matter from Left Innominate Vein, Percutaneous Approach
05C44ZZ Extirpation of Matter from Left Innominate Vein, Percutaneous Endoscopic Approach
05C50ZZ Extirpation of Matter from Right Subclavian Vein, Open Approach
05C53ZZ Extirpation of Matter from Right Subclavian Vein, Percutaneous Approach
05C54ZZ Extirpation of Matter from Right Subclavian Vein, Percutaneous Endoscopic Approach
05C60ZZ Extirpation of Matter from Left Subclavian Vein, Open Approach
05C63ZZ Extirpation of Matter from Left Subclavian Vein, Percutaneous Approach
05C64ZZ Extirpation of Matter from Left Subclavian Vein, Percutaneous Endoscopic Approach
05C70ZZ Extirpation of Matter from Right Axillary Vein, Open Approach
05C73ZZ Extirpation of Matter from Right Axillary Vein, Percutaneous Approach
05C74ZZ Extirpation of Matter from Right Axillary Vein, Percutaneous Endoscopic Approach
05C80ZZ Extirpation of Matter from Left Axillary Vein, Open Approach
05C83ZZ Extirpation of Matter from Left Axillary Vein, Percutaneous Approach
05C84ZZ Extirpation of Matter from Left Axillary Vein, Percutaneous Endoscopic Approach
05C90ZZ Extirpation of Matter from Right Brachial Vein, Open Approach
05C93ZZ Extirpation of Matter from Right Brachial Vein, Percutaneous Approach

05C94ZZ Extirpation of Matter from Right Brachial Vein, Percutaneous Endoscopic Approach
05CA0ZZ Extirpation of Matter from Left Brachial Vein, Open Approach
05CA3ZZ Extirpation of Matter from Left Brachial Vein, Percutaneous Approach
05CA4ZZ Extirpation of Matter from Left Brachial Vein, Percutaneous Endoscopic Approach
05CB0ZZ Extirpation of Matter from Right Basilic Vein, Open Approach
05CB3ZZ Extirpation of Matter from Right Basilic Vein, Percutaneous Approach
05CB4ZZ Extirpation of Matter from Right Basilic Vein, Percutaneous Endoscopic Approach
05CC0ZZ Extirpation of Matter from Left Basilic Vein, Open Approach
05CC3ZZ Extirpation of Matter from Left Basilic Vein, Percutaneous Approach
05CC4ZZ Extirpation of Matter from Left Basilic Vein, Percutaneous Endoscopic Approach
05CD0ZZ Extirpation of Matter from Right Cephalic Vein, Open Approach
05CD3ZZ Extirpation of Matter from Right Cephalic Vein, Percutaneous Approach
05CD4ZZ Extirpation of Matter from Right Cephalic Vein, Percutaneous Endoscopic Approach
05CF0ZZ Extirpation of Matter from Left Cephalic Vein, Open Approach
05CF3ZZ Extirpation of Matter from Left Cephalic Vein, Percutaneous Approach
05CF4ZZ Extirpation of Matter from Left Cephalic Vein, Percutaneous Endoscopic Approach
05CG0ZZ Extirpation of Matter from Right Hand Vein, Open Approach
05CG3ZZ Extirpation of Matter from Right Hand Vein, Percutaneous Approach
05CG4ZZ Extirpation of Matter from Right Hand Vein, Percutaneous Endoscopic Approach
05CH0ZZ Extirpation of Matter from Left Hand Vein, Open Approach
05CH3ZZ Extirpation of Matter from Left Hand Vein, Percutaneous Approach
05CH4ZZ Extirpation of Matter from Left Hand Vein, Percutaneous Endoscopic Approach
05CL0ZZ Extirpation of Matter from Intracranial Vein, Open Approach
▲ 05CL3ZZ Extirpation of Matter from Intracranial Vein, Percutaneous Approach
▲ 05CL4ZZ Extirpation of Matter from Intracranial Vein, Percutaneous Endoscopic Approach
05CM0ZZ Extirpation of Matter from Right Internal Jugular Vein, Open Approach
05CM3ZZ Extirpation of Matter from Right Internal Jugular Vein, Percutaneous Approach

05CM4ZZ Extirpation of Matter from Right Internal Jugular Vein, Percutaneous Endoscopic Approach
05CN0ZZ Extirpation of Matter from Left Internal Jugular Vein, Open Approach
05CN3ZZ Extirpation of Matter from Left Internal Jugular Vein, Percutaneous Approach
05CN4ZZ Extirpation of Matter from Left Internal Jugular Vein, Percutaneous Endoscopic Approach
05CP0ZZ Extirpation of Matter from Right External Jugular Vein, Open Approach
05CP3ZZ Extirpation of Matter from Right External Jugular Vein, Percutaneous Approach
05CP4ZZ Extirpation of Matter from Right External Jugular Vein, Percutaneous Endoscopic Approach
05CQ0ZZ Extirpation of Matter from Left External Jugular Vein, Open Approach
05CQ3ZZ Extirpation of Matter from Left External Jugular Vein, Percutaneous Approach
05CQ4ZZ Extirpation of Matter from Left External Jugular Vein, Percutaneous Endoscopic Approach
05CR0ZZ Extirpation of Matter from Right Vertebral Vein, Open Approach
05CR3ZZ Extirpation of Matter from Right Vertebral Vein, Percutaneous Approach
05CR4ZZ Extirpation of Matter from Right Vertebral Vein, Percutaneous Endoscopic Approach
05CS0ZZ Extirpation of Matter from Left Vertebral Vein, Open Approach
05CS3ZZ Extirpation of Matter from Left Vertebral Vein, Percutaneous Approach
05CS4ZZ Extirpation of Matter from Left Vertebral Vein, Percutaneous Endoscopic Approach
05CT0ZZ Extirpation of Matter from Right Face Vein, Open Approach
05CT3ZZ Extirpation of Matter from Right Face Vein, Percutaneous Approach
05CT4ZZ Extirpation of Matter from Right Face Vein, Percutaneous Endoscopic Approach
05CV0ZZ Extirpation of Matter from Left Face Vein, Open Approach
05CV3ZZ Extirpation of Matter from Left Face Vein, Percutaneous Approach
05CV4ZZ Extirpation of Matter from Left Face Vein, Percutaneous Endoscopic Approach
05CY0ZZ Extirpation of Matter from Upper Vein, Open Approach
05CY3ZZ Extirpation of Matter from Upper Vein, Percutaneous Approach
05CY4ZZ Extirpation of Matter from Upper Vein, Percutaneous Endoscopic Approach

05D – Upper Veins, Extraction

05D90ZZ	Extraction of Right Brachial Vein, Open Approach	05D93ZZ	Extraction of Right Brachial Vein, Percutaneous Approach	05DA0ZZ	Extraction of Left Brachial Vein, Open Approach

A3ZZ	Extraction of Left Brachial Vein, Percutaneous Approach
B0ZZ	Extraction of Right Basilic Vein, Open Approach
B3ZZ	Extraction of Right Basilic Vein, Percutaneous Approach
C0ZZ	Extraction of Left Basilic Vein, Open Approach
C3ZZ	Extraction of Left Basilic Vein, Percutaneous Approach

05DD0ZZ Extraction of Right Cephalic Vein, Open Approach
05DD3ZZ Extraction of Right Cephalic Vein, Percutaneous Approach
05DF0ZZ Extraction of Left Cephalic Vein, Open Approach
05DF3ZZ Extraction of Left Cephalic Vein, Percutaneous Approach
05DG0ZZ Extraction of Right Hand Vein, Open Approach

05DG3ZZ Extraction of Right Hand Vein, Percutaneous Approach
05DH0ZZ Extraction of Left Hand Vein, Open Approach
05DH3ZZ Extraction of Left Hand Vein, Percutaneous Approach
05DY0ZZ Extraction of Upper Vein, Open Approach
05DY3ZZ Extraction of Upper Vein, Percutaneous Approach

H – Upper Veins, Insertion

003Z Insertion of Infusion Device into Azygos Vein, Open Approach
00DZ Insertion of Intraluminal Device into Azygos Vein, Open Approach
033Z Insertion of Infusion Device into Azygos Vein, Percutaneous Approach
03DZ Insertion of Intraluminal Device into Azygos Vein, Percutaneous Approach
043Z Insertion of Infusion Device into Azygos Vein, Percutaneous Endoscopic Approach
04DZ Insertion of Intraluminal Device into Azygos Vein, Percutaneous Endoscopic Approach
103Z Insertion of Infusion Device into Hemiazygos Vein, Open Approach
10DZ Insertion of Intraluminal Device into Hemiazygos Vein, Open Approach
133Z Insertion of Infusion Device into Hemiazygos Vein, Percutaneous Approach
13DZ Insertion of Intraluminal Device into Hemiazygos Vein, Percutaneous Approach
143Z Insertion of Infusion Device into Hemiazygos Vein, Percutaneous Endoscopic Approach
14DZ Insertion of Intraluminal Device into Hemiazygos Vein, Percutaneous Endoscopic Approach
1303Z Insertion of Infusion Device into Right Innominate Vein, Open Approach
130DZ Insertion of Intraluminal Device into Right Innominate Vein, Open Approach
1333Z Insertion of Infusion Device into Right Innominate Vein, Percutaneous Approach
133DZ Insertion of Intraluminal Device into Right Innominate Vein, Percutaneous Approach
1343Z Insertion of Infusion Device into Right Innominate Vein, Percutaneous Endoscopic Approach
134DZ Insertion of Intraluminal Device into Right Innominate Vein, Percutaneous Endoscopic Approach
1403Z Insertion of Infusion Device into Left Innominate Vein, Open Approach
140DZ Insertion of Intraluminal Device into Left Innominate Vein, Open Approach
1433Z Insertion of Infusion Device into Left Innominate Vein, Percutaneous Approach
143DZ Insertion of Intraluminal Device into Left Innominate Vein, Percutaneous Approach
1443Z Insertion of Infusion Device into Left Innominate Vein, Percutaneous Endoscopic Approach
144DZ Insertion of Intraluminal Device into Left Innominate Vein, Percutaneous Endoscopic Approach
H503Z Insertion of Infusion Device into Right Subclavian Vein, Open Approach
H50DZ Insertion of Intraluminal Device into Right Subclavian Vein, Open Approach

● 05H533Z Insertion of Infusion Device into Right Subclavian Vein, Percutaneous Approach
05H53DZ Insertion of Intraluminal Device into Right Subclavian Vein, Percutaneous Approach
05H543Z Insertion of Infusion Device into Right Subclavian Vein, Percutaneous Endoscopic Approach
05H54DZ Insertion of Intraluminal Device into Right Subclavian Vein, Percutaneous Endoscopic Approach
05H603Z Insertion of Infusion Device into Left Subclavian Vein, Open Approach
05H60DZ Insertion of Intraluminal Device into Left Subclavian Vein, Open Approach
● 05H633Z Insertion of Infusion Device into Left Subclavian Vein, Percutaneous Approach
05H63DZ Insertion of Intraluminal Device into Left Subclavian Vein, Percutaneous Approach
05H643Z Insertion of Infusion Device into Left Subclavian Vein, Percutaneous Endoscopic Approach
05H64DZ Insertion of Intraluminal Device into Left Subclavian Vein, Percutaneous Endoscopic Approach
05H703Z Insertion of Infusion Device into Right Axillary Vein, Open Approach
05H70DZ Insertion of Intraluminal Device into Right Axillary Vein, Open Approach
05H733Z Insertion of Infusion Device into Right Axillary Vein, Percutaneous Approach
05H73DZ Insertion of Intraluminal Device into Right Axillary Vein, Percutaneous Approach
05H743Z Insertion of Infusion Device into Right Axillary Vein, Percutaneous Endoscopic Approach
05H74DZ Insertion of Intraluminal Device into Right Axillary Vein, Percutaneous Endoscopic Approach
05H803Z Insertion of Infusion Device into Left Axillary Vein, Open Approach
05H80DZ Insertion of Intraluminal Device into Left Axillary Vein, Open Approach
05H833Z Insertion of Infusion Device into Left Axillary Vein, Percutaneous Approach
05H83DZ Insertion of Intraluminal Device into Left Axillary Vein, Percutaneous Approach
05H843Z Insertion of Infusion Device into Left Axillary Vein, Percutaneous Endoscopic Approach
05H84DZ Insertion of Intraluminal Device into Left Axillary Vein, Percutaneous Endoscopic Approach
05H903Z Insertion of Infusion Device into Right Brachial Vein, Open Approach
05H90DZ Insertion of Intraluminal Device into Right Brachial Vein, Open Approach
05H933Z Insertion of Infusion Device into Right Brachial Vein, Percutaneous Approach
05H93DZ Insertion of Intraluminal Device into Right Brachial Vein, Percutaneous Approach

05H943Z Insertion of Infusion Device into Right Brachial Vein, Percutaneous Endoscopic Approach
05H94DZ Insertion of Intraluminal Device into Right Brachial Vein, Percutaneous Endoscopic Approach
05HA03Z Insertion of Infusion Device into Left Brachial Vein, Open Approach
05HA0DZ Insertion of Intraluminal Device into Left Brachial Vein, Open Approach
05HA33Z Insertion of Infusion Device into Left Brachial Vein, Percutaneous Approach
05HA3DZ Insertion of Intraluminal Device into Left Brachial Vein, Percutaneous Approach
05HA43Z Insertion of Infusion Device into Left Brachial Vein, Percutaneous Endoscopic Approach
05HA4DZ Insertion of Intraluminal Device into Left Brachial Vein, Percutaneous Endoscopic Approach
05HB03Z Insertion of Infusion Device into Right Basilic Vein, Open Approach
05HB0DZ Insertion of Intraluminal Device into Right Basilic Vein, Open Approach
05HB33Z Insertion of Infusion Device into Right Basilic Vein, Percutaneous Approach
05HB3DZ Insertion of Intraluminal Device into Right Basilic Vein, Percutaneous Approach
05HB43Z Insertion of Infusion Device into Right Basilic Vein, Percutaneous Endoscopic Approach
05HB4DZ Insertion of Intraluminal Device into Right Basilic Vein, Percutaneous Endoscopic Approach
05HC03Z Insertion of Infusion Device into Left Basilic Vein, Open Approach
05HC0DZ Insertion of Intraluminal Device into Left Basilic Vein, Open Approach
05HC33Z Insertion of Infusion Device into Left Basilic Vein, Percutaneous Approach
05HC3DZ Insertion of Intraluminal Device into Left Basilic Vein, Percutaneous Approach
05HC43Z Insertion of Infusion Device into Left Basilic Vein, Percutaneous Endoscopic Approach
05HC4DZ Insertion of Intraluminal Device into Left Basilic Vein, Percutaneous Endoscopic Approach
05HD03Z Insertion of Infusion Device into Right Cephalic Vein, Open Approach
05HD0DZ Insertion of Intraluminal Device into Right Cephalic Vein, Open Approach
05HD33Z Insertion of Infusion Device into Right Cephalic Vein, Percutaneous Approach
05HD3DZ Insertion of Intraluminal Device into Right Cephalic Vein, Percutaneous Approach
05HD43Z Insertion of Infusion Device into Right Cephalic Vein, Percutaneous Endoscopic Approach

♀ Female-only	♂ Male-only	▲ Limited Coverage	● Non-OR	HAC HAC-associated procedure	▲ Non-covered procedures	✚ Combination

05HD4DZ Insertion of Intraluminal Device into Right Cephalic Vein, Percutaneous Endoscopic Approach

05HF03Z Insertion of Infusion Device into Left Cephalic Vein, Open Approach

05HF0DZ Insertion of Intraluminal Device into Left Cephalic Vein, Open Approach

05HF33Z Insertion of Infusion Device into Left Cephalic Vein, Percutaneous Approach

05HF3DZ Insertion of Intraluminal Device into Left Cephalic Vein, Percutaneous Approach

05HF43Z Insertion of Infusion Device into Left Cephalic Vein, Percutaneous Endoscopic Approach

05HF4DZ Insertion of Intraluminal Device into Left Cephalic Vein, Percutaneous Endoscopic Approach

05HG03Z Insertion of Infusion Device into Right Hand Vein, Open Approach

05HG0DZ Insertion of Intraluminal Device into Right Hand Vein, Open Approach

05HG33Z Insertion of Infusion Device into Right Hand Vein, Percutaneous Approach

05HG3DZ Insertion of Intraluminal Device into Right Hand Vein, Percutaneous Approach

05HG43Z Insertion of Infusion Device into Right Hand Vein, Percutaneous Endoscopic Approach

05HG4DZ Insertion of Intraluminal Device into Right Hand Vein, Percutaneous Endoscopic Approach

05HH03Z Insertion of Infusion Device into Left Hand Vein, Open Approach

05HH0DZ Insertion of Intraluminal Device into Left Hand Vein, Open Approach

05HH33Z Insertion of Infusion Device into Left Hand Vein, Percutaneous Approach

05HH3DZ Insertion of Intraluminal Device into Left Hand Vein, Percutaneous Approach

05HH43Z Insertion of Infusion Device into Left Hand Vein, Percutaneous Endoscopic Approach

05HH4DZ Insertion of Intraluminal Device into Left Hand Vein, Percutaneous Endoscopic Approach

05HL03Z Insertion of Infusion Device into Intracranial Vein, Open Approach

05HL0DZ Insertion of Intraluminal Device into Intracranial Vein, Open Approach

05HL33Z Insertion of Infusion Device into Intracranial Vein, Percutaneous Approach

05HL3DZ Insertion of Intraluminal Device into Intracranial Vein, Percutaneous Approach

05HL43Z Insertion of Infusion Device into Intracranial Vein, Percutaneous Endoscopic Approach

05HL4DZ Insertion of Intraluminal Device into Intracranial Vein, Percutaneous Endoscopic Approach

05HM03Z Insertion of Infusion Device into Right Internal Jugular Vein, Open Approach

05HM0DZ Insertion of Intraluminal Device into Right Internal Jugular Vein, Open Approach

● 05HM33Z Insertion of Infusion Device into Right Internal Jugular Vein, Percutaneous Approach

    ▨ With secondary diagnosis code J95.811

05HM3DZ Insertion of Intraluminal Device into Right Internal Jugular Vein, Percutaneous Approach

05HM43Z Insertion of Infusion Device into Right Internal Jugular Vein, Percutaneous Endoscopic Approach

05HM4DZ Insertion of Intraluminal Device into Right Internal Jugular Vein, Percutaneous Endoscopic Approach

05HN03Z Insertion of Infusion Device into Left Internal Jugular Vein, Open Approach

05HN0DZ Insertion of Intraluminal Device into Left Internal Jugular Vein, Open Approach

● 05HN33Z Insertion of Infusion Device into Left Internal Jugular Vein, Percutaneous Approach

    ▨ With secondary diagnosis code J95.811

05HN3DZ Insertion of Intraluminal Device into Left Internal Jugular Vein, Percutaneous Approach

05HN43Z Insertion of Infusion Device into Left Internal Jugular Vein, Percutaneous Endoscopic Approach

05HN4DZ Insertion of Intraluminal Device into Left Internal Jugular Vein, Percutaneous Endoscopic Approach

05HP03Z Insertion of Infusion Device into Right External Jugular Vein, Open Approach

05HP0DZ Insertion of Intraluminal Device into Right External Jugular Vein, Open Approach

● 05HP33Z Insertion of Infusion Device into Right External Jugular Vein, Percutaneous Approach

    ▨ With secondary diagnosis code J95.811

05HP3DZ Insertion of Intraluminal Device into Right External Jugular Vein, Percutaneous Approach

05HP43Z Insertion of Infusion Device into Right External Jugular Vein, Percutaneous Endoscopic Approach

05HP4DZ Insertion of Intraluminal Device into Right External Jugular Vein, Percutaneous Endoscopic Approach

05HQ03Z Insertion of Infusion Device into Left External Jugular Vein, Open Approach

05HQ0DZ Insertion of Intraluminal Device into Left External Jugular Vein, Open Approach

● 05HQ33Z Insertion of Infusion Device into Left External Jugular Vein, Percutaneous Approach

    ▨ With secondary diagnosis code J95.811

05HQ3DZ Insertion of Intraluminal Device into Left External Jugular Vein, Percutaneous Approach

05HQ43Z Insertion of Infusion Device into Left External Jugular Vein, Percutaneous Endoscopic Approach

05HQ4DZ Insertion of Intraluminal Device into Left External Jugular Vein, Percutaneous Endoscopic Approach

05HR03Z Insertion of Infusion Device into Right Vertebral Vein, Open Approach

05HR0DZ Insertion of Intraluminal Device into Right Vertebral Vein, Open Approach

05HR33Z Insertion of Infusion Device into Right Vertebral Vein, Percutaneous Approach

05HR3DZ Insertion of Intraluminal Device into Right Vertebral Vein, Percutaneous Approach

05HR43Z Insertion of Infusion Device into Right Vertebral Vein, Percutaneous Endoscopic Approach

05HR4DZ Insertion of Intraluminal Device into Right Vertebral Vein, Percutaneous Endoscopic Approach

05HS03Z Insertion of Infusion Device into Left Vertebral Vein, Open Approach

05HS0DZ Insertion of Intraluminal Device into Left Vertebral Vein, Open Approach

05HS33Z Insertion of Infusion Device into Left Vertebral Vein, Percutaneous Approach

05HS3DZ Insertion of Intraluminal Device into Left Vertebral Vein, Percutaneous Approach

05HS43Z Insertion of Infusion Device into Left Vertebral Vein, Percutaneous Endoscopic Approach

05HS4DZ Insertion of Intraluminal Device into Left Vertebral Vein, Percutaneous Endoscopic Approach

05HT03Z Insertion of Infusion Device into Right Face Vein, Open Approach

05HT0DZ Insertion of Intraluminal Device into Right Face Vein, Open Approach

05HT33Z Insertion of Infusion Device into Right Face Vein, Percutaneous Approach

05HT3DZ Insertion of Intraluminal Device into Right Face Vein, Percutaneous Approach

05HT43Z Insertion of Infusion Device into Right Face Vein, Percutaneous Endoscopic Approach

05HT4DZ Insertion of Intraluminal Device into Right Face Vein, Percutaneous Endoscopic Approach

05HV03Z Insertion of Infusion Device into Left Face Vein, Open Approach

05HV0DZ Insertion of Intraluminal Device into Left Face Vein, Open Approach

05HV33Z Insertion of Infusion Device into Left Face Vein, Percutaneous Approach

05HV3DZ Insertion of Intraluminal Device into Left Face Vein, Percutaneous Approach

05HV43Z Insertion of Infusion Device into Left Face Vein, Percutaneous Endoscopic Approach

05HV4DZ Insertion of Intraluminal Device into Left Face Vein, Percutaneous Endoscopic Approach

05HY02Z Insertion of Monitoring Device into Upper Vein, Open Approach

05HY03Z Insertion of Infusion Device into Upper Vein, Open Approach

05HY0DZ Insertion of Intraluminal Device into Upper Vein, Open Approach

05HY32Z Insertion of Monitoring Device into Upper Vein, Percutaneous Approach

05HY33Z Insertion of Infusion Device into Upper Vein, Percutaneous Approach

05HY3DZ Insertion of Intraluminal Device into Upper Vein, Percutaneous Approach

05HY42Z Insertion of Monitoring Device into Upper Vein, Percutaneous Endoscopic Approach

05HY43Z Insertion of Infusion Device into Upper Vein, Percutaneous Endoscopic Approach

05HY4DZ Insertion of Intraluminal Device into Upper Vein, Percutaneous Endoscopic Approach

05J – Upper Veins, Inspection

Review Coding Guidelines B3.11a, B3.11b and B3.11c

05JY0ZZ Inspection of Upper Vein, Open Approach

05JY3ZZ Inspection of Upper Vein, Percutaneous Approach

05JY4ZZ Inspection of Upper Vein, Percutaneous Endoscopic Approach

05JYXZZ Inspection of Upper Vein, External Approach

♀ Female-only   ♂ Male-only   ▲ Limited Coverage   ● Non-OR   ▨ HAC-associated procedure   ▲ Non-covered procedures   ✚ Combina

– Upper Veins, Occlusion

iew Coding Guideline B3.12

00CZ	Occlusion of Azygos Vein with Extraluminal Device, Open Approach
00DZ	Occlusion of Azygos Vein with Intraluminal Device, Open Approach
00ZZ	Occlusion of Azygos Vein, Open Approach
03CZ	Occlusion of Azygos Vein with Extraluminal Device, Percutaneous Approach
03DZ	Occlusion of Azygos Vein with Intraluminal Device, Percutaneous Approach
03ZZ	Occlusion of Azygos Vein, Percutaneous Approach
04CZ	Occlusion of Azygos Vein with Extraluminal Device, Percutaneous Endoscopic Approach
04DZ	Occlusion of Azygos Vein with Intraluminal Device, Percutaneous Endoscopic Approach
04ZZ	Occlusion of Azygos Vein, Percutaneous Endoscopic Approach
10CZ	Occlusion of Hemiazygos Vein with Extraluminal Device, Open Approach
10DZ	Occlusion of Hemiazygos Vein with Intraluminal Device, Open Approach
10ZZ	Occlusion of Hemiazygos Vein, Open Approach
13CZ	Occlusion of Hemiazygos Vein with Extraluminal Device, Percutaneous Approach
13DZ	Occlusion of Hemiazygos Vein with Intraluminal Device, Percutaneous Approach
13ZZ	Occlusion of Hemiazygos Vein, Percutaneous Approach
14CZ	Occlusion of Hemiazygos Vein with Extraluminal Device, Percutaneous Endoscopic Approach
14DZ	Occlusion of Hemiazygos Vein with Intraluminal Device, Percutaneous Endoscopic Approach
14ZZ	Occlusion of Hemiazygos Vein, Percutaneous Endoscopic Approach
30CZ	Occlusion of Right Innominate Vein with Extraluminal Device, Open Approach
30DZ	Occlusion of Right Innominate Vein with Intraluminal Device, Open Approach
30ZZ	Occlusion of Right Innominate Vein, Open Approach
33CZ	Occlusion of Right Innominate Vein with Extraluminal Device, Percutaneous Approach
33DZ	Occlusion of Right Innominate Vein with Intraluminal Device, Percutaneous Approach
33ZZ	Occlusion of Right Innominate Vein, Percutaneous Approach
34CZ	Occlusion of Right Innominate Vein with Extraluminal Device, Percutaneous Endoscopic Approach
34DZ	Occlusion of Right Innominate Vein with Intraluminal Device, Percutaneous Endoscopic Approach
34ZZ	Occlusion of Right Innominate Vein, Percutaneous Endoscopic Approach
40CZ	Occlusion of Left Innominate Vein with Extraluminal Device, Open Approach
40DZ	Occlusion of Left Innominate Vein with Intraluminal Device, Open Approach
40ZZ	Occlusion of Left Innominate Vein, Open Approach
05L43CZ	Occlusion of Left Innominate Vein with Extraluminal Device, Percutaneous Approach
05L43DZ	Occlusion of Left Innominate Vein with Intraluminal Device, Percutaneous Approach
05L43ZZ	Occlusion of Left Innominate Vein, Percutaneous Approach
05L44CZ	Occlusion of Left Innominate Vein with Extraluminal Device, Percutaneous Endoscopic Approach
05L44DZ	Occlusion of Left Innominate Vein with Intraluminal Device, Percutaneous Endoscopic Approach
05L44ZZ	Occlusion of Left Innominate Vein, Percutaneous Endoscopic Approach
05L50CZ	Occlusion of Right Subclavian Vein with Extraluminal Device, Open Approach
05L50DZ	Occlusion of Right Subclavian Vein with Intraluminal Device, Open Approach
05L50ZZ	Occlusion of Right Subclavian Vein, Open Approach
05L53CZ	Occlusion of Right Subclavian Vein with Extraluminal Device, Percutaneous Approach
05L53DZ	Occlusion of Right Subclavian Vein with Intraluminal Device, Percutaneous Approach
05L53ZZ	Occlusion of Right Subclavian Vein, Percutaneous Approach
05L54CZ	Occlusion of Right Subclavian Vein with Extraluminal Device, Percutaneous Endoscopic Approach
05L54DZ	Occlusion of Right Subclavian Vein with Intraluminal Device, Percutaneous Endoscopic Approach
05L54ZZ	Occlusion of Right Subclavian Vein, Percutaneous Endoscopic Approach
05L60CZ	Occlusion of Left Subclavian Vein with Extraluminal Device, Open Approach
05L60DZ	Occlusion of Left Subclavian Vein with Intraluminal Device, Open Approach
05L60ZZ	Occlusion of Left Subclavian Vein, Open Approach
05L63CZ	Occlusion of Left Subclavian Vein with Extraluminal Device, Percutaneous Approach
05L63DZ	Occlusion of Left Subclavian Vein with Intraluminal Device, Percutaneous Approach
05L63ZZ	Occlusion of Left Subclavian Vein, Percutaneous Approach
05L64CZ	Occlusion of Left Subclavian Vein with Extraluminal Device, Percutaneous Endoscopic Approach
05L64DZ	Occlusion of Left Subclavian Vein with Intraluminal Device, Percutaneous Endoscopic Approach
05L64ZZ	Occlusion of Left Subclavian Vein, Percutaneous Endoscopic Approach
05L70CZ	Occlusion of Right Axillary Vein with Extraluminal Device, Open Approach
05L70DZ	Occlusion of Right Axillary Vein with Intraluminal Device, Open Approach
05L70ZZ	Occlusion of Right Axillary Vein, Open Approach
05L73CZ	Occlusion of Right Axillary Vein with Extraluminal Device, Percutaneous Approach
05L73DZ	Occlusion of Right Axillary Vein with Intraluminal Device, Percutaneous Approach
05L73ZZ	Occlusion of Right Axillary Vein, Percutaneous Approach
05L74CZ	Occlusion of Right Axillary Vein with Extraluminal Device, Percutaneous Endoscopic Approach
05L74DZ	Occlusion of Right Axillary Vein with Intraluminal Device, Percutaneous Endoscopic Approach
05L74ZZ	Occlusion of Right Axillary Vein, Percutaneous Endoscopic Approach
05L80CZ	Occlusion of Left Axillary Vein with Extraluminal Device, Open Approach
05L80DZ	Occlusion of Left Axillary Vein with Intraluminal Device, Open Approach
05L80ZZ	Occlusion of Left Axillary Vein, Open Approach
05L83CZ	Occlusion of Left Axillary Vein with Extraluminal Device, Percutaneous Approach
05L83DZ	Occlusion of Left Axillary Vein with Intraluminal Device, Percutaneous Approach
05L83ZZ	Occlusion of Left Axillary Vein, Percutaneous Approach
05L84CZ	Occlusion of Left Axillary Vein with Extraluminal Device, Percutaneous Endoscopic Approach
05L84DZ	Occlusion of Left Axillary Vein with Intraluminal Device, Percutaneous Endoscopic Approach
05L84ZZ	Occlusion of Left Axillary Vein, Percutaneous Endoscopic Approach
05L90CZ	Occlusion of Right Brachial Vein with Extraluminal Device, Open Approach
05L90DZ	Occlusion of Right Brachial Vein with Intraluminal Device, Open Approach
05L90ZZ	Occlusion of Right Brachial Vein, Open Approach
05L93CZ	Occlusion of Right Brachial Vein with Extraluminal Device, Percutaneous Approach
05L93DZ	Occlusion of Right Brachial Vein with Intraluminal Device, Percutaneous Approach
05L93ZZ	Occlusion of Right Brachial Vein, Percutaneous Approach
05L94CZ	Occlusion of Right Brachial Vein with Extraluminal Device, Percutaneous Endoscopic Approach
05L94DZ	Occlusion of Right Brachial Vein with Intraluminal Device, Percutaneous Endoscopic Approach
05L94ZZ	Occlusion of Right Brachial Vein, Percutaneous Endoscopic Approach
05LA0CZ	Occlusion of Left Brachial Vein with Extraluminal Device, Open Approach
05LA0DZ	Occlusion of Left Brachial Vein with Intraluminal Device, Open Approach
05LA0ZZ	Occlusion of Left Brachial Vein, Open Approach
05LA3CZ	Occlusion of Left Brachial Vein with Extraluminal Device, Percutaneous Approach
05LA3DZ	Occlusion of Left Brachial Vein with Intraluminal Device, Percutaneous Approach
05LA3ZZ	Occlusion of Left Brachial Vein, Percutaneous Approach
05LA4CZ	Occlusion of Left Brachial Vein with Extraluminal Device, Percutaneous Endoscopic Approach

emale-only   ♂ Male-only   ▲ Limited Coverage   ● Non-OR   ▨ HAC-associated procedure   ▲ Non-covered procedures   ✛ Combination

05LA4DZ Occlusion of Left Brachial Vein with Intraluminal Device, Percutaneous Endoscopic Approach

05LA4ZZ Occlusion of Left Brachial Vein, Percutaneous Endoscopic Approach

05LB0CZ Occlusion of Right Basilic Vein with Extraluminal Device, Open Approach

05LB0DZ Occlusion of Right Basilic Vein with Intraluminal Device, Open Approach

05LB0ZZ Occlusion of Right Basilic Vein, Open Approach

05LB3CZ Occlusion of Right Basilic Vein with Extraluminal Device, Percutaneous Approach

05LB3DZ Occlusion of Right Basilic Vein with Intraluminal Device, Percutaneous Approach

05LB3ZZ Occlusion of Right Basilic Vein, Percutaneous Approach

05LB4CZ Occlusion of Right Basilic Vein with Extraluminal Device, Percutaneous Endoscopic Approach

05LB4DZ Occlusion of Right Basilic Vein with Intraluminal Device, Percutaneous Endoscopic Approach

05LB4ZZ Occlusion of Right Basilic Vein, Percutaneous Endoscopic Approach

05LC0CZ Occlusion of Left Basilic Vein with Extraluminal Device, Open Approach

05LC0DZ Occlusion of Left Basilic Vein with Intraluminal Device, Open Approach

05LC0ZZ Occlusion of Left Basilic Vein, Open Approach

05LC3CZ Occlusion of Left Basilic Vein with Extraluminal Device, Percutaneous Approach

05LC3DZ Occlusion of Left Basilic Vein with Intraluminal Device, Percutaneous Approach

05LC3ZZ Occlusion of Left Basilic Vein, Percutaneous Approach

05LC4CZ Occlusion of Left Basilic Vein with Extraluminal Device, Percutaneous Endoscopic Approach

05LC4DZ Occlusion of Left Basilic Vein with Intraluminal Device, Percutaneous Endoscopic Approach

05LC4ZZ Occlusion of Left Basilic Vein, Percutaneous Endoscopic Approach

05LD0CZ Occlusion of Right Cephalic Vein with Extraluminal Device, Open Approach

05LD0DZ Occlusion of Right Cephalic Vein with Intraluminal Device, Open Approach

05LD0ZZ Occlusion of Right Cephalic Vein, Open Approach

05LD3CZ Occlusion of Right Cephalic Vein with Extraluminal Device, Percutaneous Approach

05LD3DZ Occlusion of Right Cephalic Vein with Intraluminal Device, Percutaneous Approach

05LD3ZZ Occlusion of Right Cephalic Vein, Percutaneous Approach

05LD4CZ Occlusion of Right Cephalic Vein with Extraluminal Device, Percutaneous Endoscopic Approach

05LD4DZ Occlusion of Right Cephalic Vein with Intraluminal Device, Percutaneous Endoscopic Approach

05LD4ZZ Occlusion of Right Cephalic Vein, Percutaneous Endoscopic Approach

05LF0CZ Occlusion of Left Cephalic Vein with Extraluminal Device, Open Approach

05LF0DZ Occlusion of Left Cephalic Vein with Intraluminal Device, Open Approach

05LF0ZZ Occlusion of Left Cephalic Vein, Open Approach

05LF3CZ Occlusion of Left Cephalic Vein with Extraluminal Device, Percutaneous Approach

05LF3DZ Occlusion of Left Cephalic Vein with Intraluminal Device, Percutaneous Approach

05LF3ZZ Occlusion of Left Cephalic Vein, Percutaneous Approach

05LF4CZ Occlusion of Left Cephalic Vein with Extraluminal Device, Percutaneous Endoscopic Approach

05LF4DZ Occlusion of Left Cephalic Vein with Intraluminal Device, Percutaneous Endoscopic Approach

05LF4ZZ Occlusion of Left Cephalic Vein, Percutaneous Endoscopic Approach

05LG0CZ Occlusion of Right Hand Vein with Extraluminal Device, Open Approach

05LG0DZ Occlusion of Right Hand Vein with Intraluminal Device, Open Approach

05LG0ZZ Occlusion of Right Hand Vein, Open Approach

05LG3CZ Occlusion of Right Hand Vein with Extraluminal Device, Percutaneous Approach

05LG3DZ Occlusion of Right Hand Vein with Intraluminal Device, Percutaneous Approach

05LG3ZZ Occlusion of Right Hand Vein, Percutaneous Approach

05LG4CZ Occlusion of Right Hand Vein with Extraluminal Device, Percutaneous Endoscopic Approach

05LG4DZ Occlusion of Right Hand Vein with Intraluminal Device, Percutaneous Endoscopic Approach

05LG4ZZ Occlusion of Right Hand Vein, Percutaneous Endoscopic Approach

05LH0CZ Occlusion of Left Hand Vein with Extraluminal Device, Open Approach

05LH0DZ Occlusion of Left Hand Vein with Intraluminal Device, Open Approach

05LH0ZZ Occlusion of Left Hand Vein, Open Approach

05LH3CZ Occlusion of Left Hand Vein with Extraluminal Device, Percutaneous Approach

05LH3DZ Occlusion of Left Hand Vein with Intraluminal Device, Percutaneous Approach

05LH3ZZ Occlusion of Left Hand Vein, Percutaneous Approach

05LH4CZ Occlusion of Left Hand Vein with Extraluminal Device, Percutaneous Endoscopic Approach

05LH4DZ Occlusion of Left Hand Vein with Intraluminal Device, Percutaneous Endoscopic Approach

05LH4ZZ Occlusion of Left Hand Vein, Percutaneous Endoscopic Approach

05LL0CZ Occlusion of Intracranial Vein with Extraluminal Device, Open Approach

05LL0DZ Occlusion of Intracranial Vein with Intraluminal Device, Open Approach

05LL0ZZ Occlusion of Intracranial Vein, Open Approach

05LL3CZ Occlusion of Intracranial Vein with Extraluminal Device, Percutaneous Approach

05LL3DZ Occlusion of Intracranial Vein with Intraluminal Device, Percutaneous Approach

05LL3ZZ Occlusion of Intracranial Vein, Percutaneous Approach

05LL4CZ Occlusion of Intracranial Vein with Extraluminal Device, Percutaneous Endoscopic Approach

05LL4DZ Occlusion of Intracranial Vein with Intraluminal Device, Percutaneous Endoscopic Approach

05LL4ZZ Occlusion of Intracranial Vein, Percutaneous Endoscopic Approach

05LM0CZ Occlusion of Right Internal Jugular Vein with Extraluminal Device, Open Approach

05LM0DZ Occlusion of Right Internal Jugular Vein with Intraluminal Device, Open Approach

05LM0ZZ Occlusion of Right Internal Jugular Vein, Open Approach

05LM3CZ Occlusion of Right Internal Jugular Vein with Extraluminal Device, Percutaneous Approach

05LM3DZ Occlusion of Right Internal Jugular Vein with Intraluminal Device, Percutaneous Approach

05LM3ZZ Occlusion of Right Internal Jugular Vein, Percutaneous Approach

05LM4CZ Occlusion of Right Internal Jugular Vein with Extraluminal Device, Percutaneous Endoscopic Approach

05LM4DZ Occlusion of Right Internal Jugular Vein with Intraluminal Device, Percutaneous Endoscopic Approach

05LM4ZZ Occlusion of Right Internal Jugular Vein, Percutaneous Endoscopic Approach

05LN0CZ Occlusion of Left Internal Jugular Vein with Extraluminal Device, Open Approach

05LN0DZ Occlusion of Left Internal Jugular Vein with Intraluminal Device, Open Approach

05LN0ZZ Occlusion of Left Internal Jugular Vein, Open Approach

05LN3CZ Occlusion of Left Internal Jugular Vein with Extraluminal Device, Percutaneous Approach

05LN3DZ Occlusion of Left Internal Jugular Vein with Intraluminal Device, Percutaneous Approach

05LN3ZZ Occlusion of Left Internal Jugular Vein, Percutaneous Approach

05LN4CZ Occlusion of Left Internal Jugular Vein with Extraluminal Device, Percutaneous Endoscopic Approach

05LN4DZ Occlusion of Left Internal Jugular Vein with Intraluminal Device, Percutaneous Endoscopic Approach

05LN4ZZ Occlusion of Left Internal Jugular Vein, Percutaneous Endoscopic Approach

05LP0CZ Occlusion of Right External Jugular Vein with Extraluminal Device, Open Approach

05LP0DZ Occlusion of Right External Jugular Vein with Intraluminal Device, Open Approach

05LP0ZZ Occlusion of Right External Jugular Vein, Open Approach

05LP3CZ Occlusion of Right External Jugular Vein with Extraluminal Device, Percutaneous Approach

05LP3DZ Occlusion of Right External Jugular Vein with Intraluminal Device, Percutaneous Approach

05LP3ZZ Occlusion of Right External Jugular Vein, Percutaneous Approach

05LP4CZ Occlusion of Right External Jugular Vein with Extraluminal Device, Percutaneous Endoscopic Approach

05LP4DZ Occlusion of Right External Jugular Vein with Intraluminal Device, Percutaneous Endoscopic Approach

05LP4ZZ Occlusion of Right External Jugular Vein, Percutaneous Endoscopic Approach

Q0CZ Occlusion of Left External Jugular Vein with Extraluminal Device, Open Approach

Q0DZ Occlusion of Left External Jugular Vein with Intraluminal Device, Open Approach

Q0ZZ Occlusion of Left External Jugular Vein, Open Approach

Q3CZ Occlusion of Left External Jugular Vein with Extraluminal Device, Percutaneous Approach

Q3DZ Occlusion of Left External Jugular Vein with Intraluminal Device, Percutaneous Approach

Q3ZZ Occlusion of Left External Jugular Vein, Percutaneous Approach

Q4CZ Occlusion of Left External Jugular Vein with Extraluminal Device, Percutaneous Endoscopic Approach

Q4DZ Occlusion of Left External Jugular Vein with Intraluminal Device, Percutaneous Endoscopic Approach

Q4ZZ Occlusion of Left External Jugular Vein, Percutaneous Endoscopic Approach

R0CZ Occlusion of Right Vertebral Vein with Extraluminal Device, Open Approach

R0DZ Occlusion of Right Vertebral Vein with Intraluminal Device, Open Approach

R0ZZ Occlusion of Right Vertebral Vein, Open Approach

R3CZ Occlusion of Right Vertebral Vein with Extraluminal Device, Percutaneous Approach

R3DZ Occlusion of Right Vertebral Vein with Intraluminal Device, Percutaneous Approach

R3ZZ Occlusion of Right Vertebral Vein, Percutaneous Approach

R4CZ Occlusion of Right Vertebral Vein with Extraluminal Device, Percutaneous Endoscopic Approach

R4DZ Occlusion of Right Vertebral Vein with Intraluminal Device, Percutaneous Endoscopic Approach

05LR4ZZ Occlusion of Right Vertebral Vein, Percutaneous Endoscopic Approach

05LS0CZ Occlusion of Left Vertebral Vein with Extraluminal Device, Open Approach

05LS0DZ Occlusion of Left Vertebral Vein with Intraluminal Device, Open Approach

05LS0ZZ Occlusion of Left Vertebral Vein, Open Approach

05LS3CZ Occlusion of Left Vertebral Vein with Extraluminal Device, Percutaneous Approach

05LS3DZ Occlusion of Left Vertebral Vein with Intraluminal Device, Percutaneous Approach

05LS3ZZ Occlusion of Left Vertebral Vein, Percutaneous Approach

05LS4CZ Occlusion of Left Vertebral Vein with Extraluminal Device, Percutaneous Endoscopic Approach

05LS4DZ Occlusion of Left Vertebral Vein with Intraluminal Device, Percutaneous Endoscopic Approach

05LS4ZZ Occlusion of Left Vertebral Vein, Percutaneous Endoscopic Approach

05LT0CZ Occlusion of Right Face Vein with Extraluminal Device, Open Approach

05LT0DZ Occlusion of Right Face Vein with Intraluminal Device, Open Approach

05LT0ZZ Occlusion of Right Face Vein, Open Approach

05LT3CZ Occlusion of Right Face Vein with Extraluminal Device, Percutaneous Approach

05LT3DZ Occlusion of Right Face Vein with Intraluminal Device, Percutaneous Approach

05LT3ZZ Occlusion of Right Face Vein, Percutaneous Approach

05LT4CZ Occlusion of Right Face Vein with Extraluminal Device, Percutaneous Endoscopic Approach

05LT4DZ Occlusion of Right Face Vein with Intraluminal Device, Percutaneous Endoscopic Approach

05LT4ZZ Occlusion of Right Face Vein, Percutaneous Endoscopic Approach

05LV0CZ Occlusion of Left Face Vein with Extraluminal Device, Open Approach

05LV0DZ Occlusion of Left Face Vein with Intraluminal Device, Open Approach

05LV0ZZ Occlusion of Left Face Vein, Open Approach

05LV3CZ Occlusion of Left Face Vein with Extraluminal Device, Percutaneous Approach

05LV3DZ Occlusion of Left Face Vein with Intraluminal Device, Percutaneous Approach

05LV3ZZ Occlusion of Left Face Vein, Percutaneous Approach

05LV4CZ Occlusion of Left Face Vein with Extraluminal Device, Percutaneous Endoscopic Approach

05LV4DZ Occlusion of Left Face Vein with Intraluminal Device, Percutaneous Endoscopic Approach

05LV4ZZ Occlusion of Left Face Vein, Percutaneous Endoscopic Approach

05LY0CZ Occlusion of Upper Vein with Extraluminal Device, Open Approach

05LY0DZ Occlusion of Upper Vein with Intraluminal Device, Open Approach

05LY0ZZ Occlusion of Upper Vein, Open Approach

05LY3CZ Occlusion of Upper Vein with Extraluminal Device, Percutaneous Approach

05LY3DZ Occlusion of Upper Vein with Intraluminal Device, Percutaneous Approach

05LY3ZZ Occlusion of Upper Vein, Percutaneous Approach

05LY4CZ Occlusion of Upper Vein with Extraluminal Device, Percutaneous Endoscopic Approach

05LY4DZ Occlusion of Upper Vein with Intraluminal Device, Percutaneous Endoscopic Approach

05LY4ZZ Occlusion of Upper Vein, Percutaneous Endoscopic Approach

N – Upper Veins, Release

Review Coding Guidelines B3.13 and B3.14

N00ZZ Release Azygos Vein, Open Approach

N03ZZ Release Azygos Vein, Percutaneous Approach

N04ZZ Release Azygos Vein, Percutaneous Endoscopic Approach

N10ZZ Release Hemiazygos Vein, Open Approach

N13ZZ Release Hemiazygos Vein, Percutaneous Approach

N14ZZ Release Hemiazygos Vein, Percutaneous Endoscopic Approach

N30ZZ Release Right Innominate Vein, Open Approach

N33ZZ Release Right Innominate Vein, Percutaneous Approach

N34ZZ Release Right Innominate Vein, Percutaneous Endoscopic Approach

N40ZZ Release Left Innominate Vein, Open Approach

N43ZZ Release Left Innominate Vein, Percutaneous Approach

N44ZZ Release Left Innominate Vein, Percutaneous Endoscopic Approach

N50ZZ Release Right Subclavian Vein, Open Approach

N53ZZ Release Right Subclavian Vein, Percutaneous Approach

05N54ZZ Release Right Subclavian Vein, Percutaneous Endoscopic Approach

05N60ZZ Release Left Subclavian Vein, Open Approach

05N63ZZ Release Left Subclavian Vein, Percutaneous Approach

05N64ZZ Release Left Subclavian Vein, Percutaneous Endoscopic Approach

05N70ZZ Release Right Axillary Vein, Open Approach

05N73ZZ Release Right Axillary Vein, Percutaneous Approach

05N74ZZ Release Right Axillary Vein, Percutaneous Endoscopic Approach

05N80ZZ Release Left Axillary Vein, Open Approach

05N83ZZ Release Left Axillary Vein, Percutaneous Approach

05N84ZZ Release Left Axillary Vein, Percutaneous Endoscopic Approach

05N90ZZ Release Right Brachial Vein, Open Approach

05N93ZZ Release Right Brachial Vein, Percutaneous Approach

05N94ZZ Release Right Brachial Vein, Percutaneous Endoscopic Approach

05NA0ZZ Release Left Brachial Vein, Open Approach

05NA3ZZ Release Left Brachial Vein, Percutaneous Approach

05NA4ZZ Release Left Brachial Vein, Percutaneous Endoscopic Approach

05NB0ZZ Release Right Basilic Vein, Open Approach

05NB3ZZ Release Right Basilic Vein, Percutaneous Approach

05NB4ZZ Release Right Basilic Vein, Percutaneous Endoscopic Approach

05NC0ZZ Release Left Basilic Vein, Open Approach

05NC3ZZ Release Left Basilic Vein, Percutaneous Approach

05NC4ZZ Release Left Basilic Vein, Percutaneous Endoscopic Approach

05ND0ZZ Release Right Cephalic Vein, Open Approach

05ND3ZZ Release Right Cephalic Vein, Percutaneous Approach

05ND4ZZ Release Right Cephalic Vein, Percutaneous Endoscopic Approach

05NF0ZZ Release Left Cephalic Vein, Open Approach

05NF3ZZ Release Left Cephalic Vein, Percutaneous Approach

emale-only ♂ Male-only ▲ Limited Coverage ● Non-OR ▨ HAC-associated procedure ▲ Non-covered procedures ✚ Combination

05NF4ZZ	Release Left Cephalic Vein, Percutaneous Endoscopic Approach	
05NG0ZZ	Release Right Hand Vein, Open Approach	
05NG3ZZ	Release Right Hand Vein, Percutaneous Approach	
05NG4ZZ	Release Right Hand Vein, Percutaneous Endoscopic Approach	
05NH0ZZ	Release Left Hand Vein, Open Approach	
05NH3ZZ	Release Left Hand Vein, Percutaneous Approach	
05NH4ZZ	Release Left Hand Vein, Percutaneous Endoscopic Approach	
05NL0ZZ	Release Intracranial Vein, Open Approach	
05NL3ZZ	Release Intracranial Vein, Percutaneous Approach	
05NL4ZZ	Release Intracranial Vein, Percutaneous Endoscopic Approach	
05NM0ZZ	Release Right Internal Jugular Vein, Open Approach	
05NM3ZZ	Release Right Internal Jugular Vein, Percutaneous Approach	
05NM4ZZ	Release Right Internal Jugular Vein, Percutaneous Endoscopic Approach	

05NN0ZZ	Release Left Internal Jugular Vein, Open Approach
05NN3ZZ	Release Left Internal Jugular Vein, Percutaneous Approach
05NN4ZZ	Release Left Internal Jugular Vein, Percutaneous Endoscopic Approach
05NP0ZZ	Release Right External Jugular Vein, Open Approach
05NP3ZZ	Release Right External Jugular Vein, Percutaneous Approach
05NP4ZZ	Release Right External Jugular Vein, Percutaneous Endoscopic Approach
05NQ0ZZ	Release Left External Jugular Vein, Open Approach
05NQ3ZZ	Release Left External Jugular Vein, Percutaneous Approach
05NQ4ZZ	Release Left External Jugular Vein, Percutaneous Endoscopic Approach
05NR0ZZ	Release Right Vertebral Vein, Open Approach
05NR3ZZ	Release Right Vertebral Vein, Percutaneous Approach

05NR4ZZ	Release Right Vertebral Vein, Percutaneous Endoscopic Approach
05NS0ZZ	Release Left Vertebral Vein, Open Approach
05NS3ZZ	Release Left Vertebral Vein, Percutaneous Approach
05NS4ZZ	Release Left Vertebral Vein, Percutaneous Endoscopic Approach
05NT0ZZ	Release Right Face Vein, Open Approach
05NT3ZZ	Release Right Face Vein, Percutaneous Approach
05NT4ZZ	Release Right Face Vein, Percutaneous Endoscopic Approach
05NV0ZZ	Release Left Face Vein, Open Approach
05NV3ZZ	Release Left Face Vein, Percutaneous Approach
05NV4ZZ	Release Left Face Vein, Percutaneous Endoscopic Approach
05NY0ZZ	Release Upper Vein, Open Approach
05NY3ZZ	Release Upper Vein, Percutaneous Approach
05NY4ZZ	Release Upper Vein, Percutaneous Endoscopic Approach

05P – Upper Veins, Removal

Review Coding Guideline B6.1c

05PY00Z	Removal of Drainage Device from Upper Vein, Open Approach
05PY02Z	Removal of Monitoring Device from Upper Vein, Open Approach
05PY03Z	Removal of Infusion Device from Upper Vein, Open Approach
05PY07Z	Removal of Autologous Tissue Substitute from Upper Vein, Open Approach
05PY0CZ	Removal of Extraluminal Device from Upper Vein, Open Approach
05PY0DZ	Removal of Intraluminal Device from Upper Vein, Open Approach
05PY0JZ	Removal of Synthetic Substitute from Upper Vein, Open Approach
05PY0KZ	Removal of Nonautologous Tissue Substitute from Upper Vein, Open Approach
05PY30Z	Removal of Drainage Device from Upper Vein, Percutaneous Approach
05PY32Z	Removal of Monitoring Device from Upper Vein, Percutaneous Approach
05PY33Z	Removal of Infusion Device from Upper Vein, Percutaneous Approach

05PY37Z	Removal of Autologous Tissue Substitute from Upper Vein, Percutaneous Approach
05PY3CZ	Removal of Extraluminal Device from Upper Vein, Percutaneous Approach
05PY3DZ	Removal of Intraluminal Device from Upper Vein, Percutaneous Approach
05PY3JZ	Removal of Synthetic Substitute from Upper Vein, Percutaneous Approach
05PY3KZ	Removal of Nonautologous Tissue Substitute from Upper Vein, Percutaneous Approach
05PY40Z	Removal of Drainage Device from Upper Vein, Percutaneous Endoscopic Approach
05PY42Z	Removal of Monitoring Device from Upper Vein, Percutaneous Endoscopic Approach
05PY43Z	Removal of Infusion Device from Upper Vein, Percutaneous Endoscopic Approach

05PY47Z	Removal of Autologous Tissue Substitute from Upper Vein, Percutaneous Endoscopic Approach
05PY4CZ	Removal of Extraluminal Device from Upper Vein, Percutaneous Endoscopic Approach
05PY4DZ	Removal of Intraluminal Device from Upper Vein, Percutaneous Endoscopic Approach
05PY4JZ	Removal of Synthetic Substitute from Upper Vein, Percutaneous Endoscopic Approach
05PY4KZ	Removal of Nonautologous Tissue Substitute from Upper Vein, Percutaneous Endoscopic Approach
05PYX0Z	Removal of Drainage Device from Upper Vein, External Approach
05PYX2Z	Removal of Monitoring Device from Upper Vein, External Approach
05PYX3Z	Removal of Infusion Device from Upper Vein, External Approach
05PYXDZ	Removal of Intraluminal Device from Upper Vein, External Approach

05Q – Upper Veins, Repair

05Q00ZZ	Repair Azygos Vein, Open Approach
05Q03ZZ	Repair Azygos Vein, Percutaneous Approach
05Q04ZZ	Repair Azygos Vein, Percutaneous Endoscopic Approach
05Q10ZZ	Repair Hemiazygos Vein, Open Approach
05Q13ZZ	Repair Hemiazygos Vein, Percutaneous Approach
05Q14ZZ	Repair Hemiazygos Vein, Percutaneous Endoscopic Approach
05Q30ZZ	Repair Right Innominate Vein, Open Approach
05Q33ZZ	Repair Right Innominate Vein, Percutaneous Approach
05Q34ZZ	Repair Right Innominate Vein, Percutaneous Endoscopic Approach
05Q40ZZ	Repair Left Innominate Vein, Open Approach
05Q43ZZ	Repair Left Innominate Vein, Percutaneous Approach
05Q44ZZ	Repair Left Innominate Vein, Percutaneous Endoscopic Approach
05Q50ZZ	Repair Right Subclavian Vein, Open Approach

05Q53ZZ	Repair Right Subclavian Vein, Percutaneous Approach
05Q54ZZ	Repair Right Subclavian Vein, Percutaneous Endoscopic Approach
05Q60ZZ	Repair Left Subclavian Vein, Open Approach
05Q63ZZ	Repair Left Subclavian Vein, Percutaneous Approach
05Q64ZZ	Repair Left Subclavian Vein, Percutaneous Endoscopic Approach
05Q70ZZ	Repair Right Axillary Vein, Open Approach
05Q73ZZ	Repair Right Axillary Vein, Percutaneous Approach
05Q74ZZ	Repair Right Axillary Vein, Percutaneous Endoscopic Approach
05Q80ZZ	Repair Left Axillary Vein, Open Approach
05Q83ZZ	Repair Left Axillary Vein, Percutaneous Approach
05Q84ZZ	Repair Left Axillary Vein, Percutaneous Endoscopic Approach
05Q90ZZ	Repair Right Brachial Vein, Open Approach
05Q93ZZ	Repair Right Brachial Vein, Percutaneous Approach

05Q94ZZ	Repair Right Brachial Vein, Percutaneous Endoscopic Approach
05QA0ZZ	Repair Left Brachial Vein, Open Approach
05QA3ZZ	Repair Left Brachial Vein, Percutaneous Approach
05QA4ZZ	Repair Left Brachial Vein, Percutaneous Endoscopic Approach
05QB0ZZ	Repair Right Basilic Vein, Open Approach
05QB3ZZ	Repair Right Basilic Vein, Percutaneous Approach
05QB4ZZ	Repair Right Basilic Vein, Percutaneous Endoscopic Approach
05QC0ZZ	Repair Left Basilic Vein, Open Approach
05QC3ZZ	Repair Left Basilic Vein, Percutaneous Approach
05QC4ZZ	Repair Left Basilic Vein, Percutaneous Endoscopic Approach
05QD0ZZ	Repair Right Cephalic Vein, Open Approach
05QD3ZZ	Repair Right Cephalic Vein, Percutaneous Approach
05QD4ZZ	Repair Right Cephalic Vein, Percutaneous Endoscopic Approach
05QF0ZZ	Repair Left Cephalic Vein, Open Approach

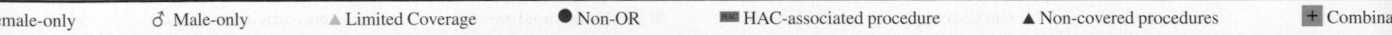

♀ Female-only   ♂ Male-only   ▲ Limited Coverage   ● Non-OR   ▦ HAC-associated procedure   ▲ Non-covered procedures   ✚ Combination

QF3ZZ Repair Left Cephalic Vein, Percutaneous Approach
QF4ZZ Repair Left Cephalic Vein, Percutaneous Endoscopic Approach
QG0ZZ Repair Right Hand Vein, Open Approach
QG3ZZ Repair Right Hand Vein, Percutaneous Approach
QG4ZZ Repair Right Hand Vein, Percutaneous Endoscopic Approach
QH0ZZ Repair Left Hand Vein, Open Approach
QH3ZZ Repair Left Hand Vein, Percutaneous Approach
QH4ZZ Repair Left Hand Vein, Percutaneous Endoscopic Approach
QL0ZZ Repair Intracranial Vein, Open Approach
QL3ZZ Repair Intracranial Vein, Percutaneous Approach
QL4ZZ Repair Intracranial Vein, Percutaneous Endoscopic Approach
QM0ZZ Repair Right Internal Jugular Vein, Open Approach
QM3ZZ Repair Right Internal Jugular Vein, Percutaneous Approach

05QM4ZZ Repair Right Internal Jugular Vein, Percutaneous Endoscopic Approach
05QN0ZZ Repair Left Internal Jugular Vein, Open Approach
05QN3ZZ Repair Left Internal Jugular Vein, Percutaneous Approach
05QN4ZZ Repair Left Internal Jugular Vein, Percutaneous Endoscopic Approach
05QP0ZZ Repair Right External Jugular Vein, Open Approach
05QP3ZZ Repair Right External Jugular Vein, Percutaneous Approach
05QP4ZZ Repair Right External Jugular Vein, Percutaneous Endoscopic Approach
05QQ0ZZ Repair Left External Jugular Vein, Open Approach
05QQ3ZZ Repair Left External Jugular Vein, Percutaneous Approach
05QQ4ZZ Repair Left External Jugular Vein, Percutaneous Endoscopic Approach
05QR0ZZ Repair Right Vertebral Vein, Open Approach
05QR3ZZ Repair Right Vertebral Vein, Percutaneous Approach

05QR4ZZ Repair Right Vertebral Vein, Percutaneous Endoscopic Approach
05QS0ZZ Repair Left Vertebral Vein, Open Approach
05QS3ZZ Repair Left Vertebral Vein, Percutaneous Approach
05QS4ZZ Repair Left Vertebral Vein, Percutaneous Endoscopic Approach
05QT0ZZ Repair Right Face Vein, Open Approach
05QT3ZZ Repair Right Face Vein, Percutaneous Approach
05QT4ZZ Repair Right Face Vein, Percutaneous Endoscopic Approach
05QV0ZZ Repair Left Face Vein, Open Approach
05QV3ZZ Repair Left Face Vein, Percutaneous Approach
05QV4ZZ Repair Left Face Vein, Percutaneous Endoscopic Approach
05QY0ZZ Repair Upper Vein, Open Approach
05QY3ZZ Repair Upper Vein, Percutaneous Approach
05QY4ZZ Repair Upper Vein, Percutaneous Endoscopic Approach

R – Upper Veins, Replacement

R007Z Replacement of Azygos Vein with Autologous Tissue Substitute, Open Approach
R00JZ Replacement of Azygos Vein with Synthetic Substitute, Open Approach
R00KZ Replacement of Azygos Vein with Nonautologous Tissue Substitute, Open Approach
R047Z Replacement of Azygos Vein with Autologous Tissue Substitute, Percutaneous Endoscopic Approach
R04JZ Replacement of Azygos Vein with Synthetic Substitute, Percutaneous Endoscopic Approach
R04KZ Replacement of Azygos Vein with Nonautologous Tissue Substitute, Percutaneous Endoscopic Approach
R107Z Replacement of Hemiazygos Vein with Autologous Tissue Substitute, Open Approach
R10JZ Replacement of Hemiazygos Vein with Synthetic Substitute, Open Approach
R10KZ Replacement of Hemiazygos Vein with Nonautologous Tissue Substitute, Open Approach
R147Z Replacement of Hemiazygos Vein with Autologous Tissue Substitute, Percutaneous Endoscopic Approach
R14JZ Replacement of Hemiazygos Vein with Synthetic Substitute, Percutaneous Endoscopic Approach
R14KZ Replacement of Hemiazygos Vein with Nonautologous Tissue Substitute, Percutaneous Endoscopic Approach
R307Z Replacement of Right Innominate Vein with Autologous Tissue Substitute, Open Approach
R30JZ Replacement of Right Innominate Vein with Synthetic Substitute, Open Approach
R30KZ Replacement of Right Innominate Vein with Nonautologous Tissue Substitute, Open Approach
R347Z Replacement of Right Innominate Vein with Autologous Tissue Substitute, Percutaneous Endoscopic Approach
R34JZ Replacement of Right Innominate Vein with Synthetic Substitute, Percutaneous Endoscopic Approach
R34KZ Replacement of Right Innominate Vein with Nonautologous Tissue Substitute, Percutaneous Endoscopic Approach

05R407Z Replacement of Left Innominate Vein with Autologous Tissue Substitute, Open Approach
05R40JZ Replacement of Left Innominate Vein with Synthetic Substitute, Open Approach
05R40KZ Replacement of Left Innominate Vein with Nonautologous Tissue Substitute, Open Approach
05R447Z Replacement of Left Innominate Vein with Autologous Tissue Substitute, Percutaneous Endoscopic Approach
05R44JZ Replacement of Left Innominate Vein with Synthetic Substitute, Percutaneous Endoscopic Approach
05R44KZ Replacement of Left Innominate Vein with Nonautologous Tissue Substitute, Percutaneous Endoscopic Approach
05R507Z Replacement of Right Subclavian Vein with Autologous Tissue Substitute, Open Approach
05R50JZ Replacement of Right Subclavian Vein with Synthetic Substitute, Open Approach
05R50KZ Replacement of Right Subclavian Vein with Nonautologous Tissue Substitute, Open Approach
05R547Z Replacement of Right Subclavian Vein with Autologous Tissue Substitute, Percutaneous Endoscopic Approach
05R54JZ Replacement of Right Subclavian Vein with Synthetic Substitute, Percutaneous Endoscopic Approach
05R54KZ Replacement of Right Subclavian Vein with Nonautologous Tissue Substitute, Percutaneous Endoscopic Approach
05R607Z Replacement of Left Subclavian Vein with Autologous Tissue Substitute, Open Approach
05R60JZ Replacement of Left Subclavian Vein with Synthetic Substitute, Open Approach
05R60KZ Replacement of Left Subclavian Vein with Nonautologous Tissue Substitute, Open Approach
05R647Z Replacement of Left Subclavian Vein with Autologous Tissue Substitute, Percutaneous Endoscopic Approach
05R64JZ Replacement of Left Subclavian Vein with Synthetic Substitute, Percutaneous Endoscopic Approach
05R64KZ Replacement of Left Subclavian Vein with Nonautologous Tissue Substitute, Percutaneous Endoscopic Approach

05R707Z Replacement of Right Axillary Vein with Autologous Tissue Substitute, Open Approach
05R70JZ Replacement of Right Axillary Vein with Synthetic Substitute, Open Approach
05R70KZ Replacement of Right Axillary Vein with Nonautologous Tissue Substitute, Open Approach
05R747Z Replacement of Right Axillary Vein with Autologous Tissue Substitute, Percutaneous Endoscopic Approach
05R74JZ Replacement of Right Axillary Vein with Synthetic Substitute, Percutaneous Endoscopic Approach
05R74KZ Replacement of Right Axillary Vein with Nonautologous Tissue Substitute, Percutaneous Endoscopic Approach
05R807Z Replacement of Left Axillary Vein with Autologous Tissue Substitute, Open Approach
05R80JZ Replacement of Left Axillary Vein with Synthetic Substitute, Open Approach
05R80KZ Replacement of Left Axillary Vein with Nonautologous Tissue Substitute, Open Approach
05R847Z Replacement of Left Axillary Vein with Autologous Tissue Substitute, Percutaneous Endoscopic Approach
05R84JZ Replacement of Left Axillary Vein with Synthetic Substitute, Percutaneous Endoscopic Approach
05R84KZ Replacement of Left Axillary Vein with Nonautologous Tissue Substitute, Percutaneous Endoscopic Approach
05R907Z Replacement of Right Brachial Vein with Autologous Tissue Substitute, Open Approach
05R90JZ Replacement of Right Brachial Vein with Synthetic Substitute, Open Approach
05R90KZ Replacement of Right Brachial Vein with Nonautologous Tissue Substitute, Open Approach
05R947Z Replacement of Right Brachial Vein with Autologous Tissue Substitute, Percutaneous Endoscopic Approach
05R94JZ Replacement of Right Brachial Vein with Synthetic Substitute, Percutaneous Endoscopic Approach
05R94KZ Replacement of Right Brachial Vein with Nonautologous Tissue Substitute, Percutaneous Endoscopic Approach

Female-only   ♂ Male-only   ▲ Limited Coverage   ● Non-OR   ▥ HAC-associated procedure   ▲ Non-covered procedures   ✚ Combination

05RA07Z Replacement of Left Brachial Vein with Autologous Tissue Substitute, Open Approach

05RA0JZ Replacement of Left Brachial Vein with Synthetic Substitute, Open Approach

05RA0KZ Replacement of Left Brachial Vein with Nonautologous Tissue Substitute, Open Approach

05RA47Z Replacement of Left Brachial Vein with Autologous Tissue Substitute, Percutaneous Endoscopic Approach

05RA4JZ Replacement of Left Brachial Vein with Synthetic Substitute, Percutaneous Endoscopic Approach

05RA4KZ Replacement of Left Brachial Vein with Nonautologous Tissue Substitute, Percutaneous Endoscopic Approach

05RB07Z Replacement of Right Basilic Vein with Autologous Tissue Substitute, Open Approach

05RB0JZ Replacement of Right Basilic Vein with Synthetic Substitute, Open Approach

05RB0KZ Replacement of Right Basilic Vein with Nonautologous Tissue Substitute, Open Approach

05RB47Z Replacement of Right Basilic Vein with Autologous Tissue Substitute, Percutaneous Endoscopic Approach

05RB4JZ Replacement of Right Basilic Vein with Synthetic Substitute, Percutaneous Endoscopic Approach

05RB4KZ Replacement of Right Basilic Vein with Nonautologous Tissue Substitute, Percutaneous Endoscopic Approach

05RC07Z Replacement of Left Basilic Vein with Autologous Tissue Substitute, Open Approach

05RC0JZ Replacement of Left Basilic Vein with Synthetic Substitute, Open Approach

05RC0KZ Replacement of Left Basilic Vein with Nonautologous Tissue Substitute, Open Approach

05RC47Z Replacement of Left Basilic Vein with Autologous Tissue Substitute, Percutaneous Endoscopic Approach

05RC4JZ Replacement of Left Basilic Vein with Synthetic Substitute, Percutaneous Endoscopic Approach

05RC4KZ Replacement of Left Basilic Vein with Nonautologous Tissue Substitute, Percutaneous Endoscopic Approach

05RD07Z Replacement of Right Cephalic Vein with Autologous Tissue Substitute, Open Approach

05RD0JZ Replacement of Right Cephalic Vein with Synthetic Substitute, Open Approach

05RD0KZ Replacement of Right Cephalic Vein with Nonautologous Tissue Substitute, Open Approach

05RD47Z Replacement of Right Cephalic Vein with Autologous Tissue Substitute, Percutaneous Endoscopic Approach

05RD4JZ Replacement of Right Cephalic Vein with Synthetic Substitute, Percutaneous Endoscopic Approach

05RD4KZ Replacement of Right Cephalic Vein with Nonautologous Tissue Substitute, Percutaneous Endoscopic Approach

05RF07Z Replacement of Left Cephalic Vein with Autologous Tissue Substitute, Open Approach

05RF0JZ Replacement of Left Cephalic Vein with Synthetic Substitute, Open Approach

05RF0KZ Replacement of Left Cephalic Vein with Nonautologous Tissue Substitute, Open Approach

05RF47Z Replacement of Left Cephalic Vein with Autologous Tissue Substitute, Percutaneous Endoscopic Approach

05RF4JZ Replacement of Left Cephalic Vein with Synthetic Substitute, Percutaneous Endoscopic Approach

05RF4KZ Replacement of Left Cephalic Vein with Nonautologous Tissue Substitute, Percutaneous Endoscopic Approach

05RG07Z Replacement of Right Hand Vein with Autologous Tissue Substitute, Open Approach

05RG0JZ Replacement of Right Hand Vein with Synthetic Substitute, Open Approach

05RG0KZ Replacement of Right Hand Vein with Nonautologous Tissue Substitute, Open Approach

05RG47Z Replacement of Right Hand Vein with Autologous Tissue Substitute, Percutaneous Endoscopic Approach

05RG4JZ Replacement of Right Hand Vein with Synthetic Substitute, Percutaneous Endoscopic Approach

05RG4KZ Replacement of Right Hand Vein with Nonautologous Tissue Substitute, Percutaneous Endoscopic Approach

05RH07Z Replacement of Left Hand Vein with Autologous Tissue Substitute, Open Approach

05RH0JZ Replacement of Left Hand Vein with Synthetic Substitute, Open Approach

05RH0KZ Replacement of Left Hand Vein with Nonautologous Tissue Substitute, Open Approach

05RH47Z Replacement of Left Hand Vein with Autologous Tissue Substitute, Percutaneous Endoscopic Approach

05RH4JZ Replacement of Left Hand Vein with Synthetic Substitute, Percutaneous Endoscopic Approach

05RH4KZ Replacement of Left Hand Vein with Nonautologous Tissue Substitute, Percutaneous Endoscopic Approach

05RL07Z Replacement of Intracranial Vein with Autologous Tissue Substitute, Open Approach

05RL0JZ Replacement of Intracranial Vein with Synthetic Substitute, Open Approach

05RL0KZ Replacement of Intracranial Vein with Nonautologous Tissue Substitute, Open Approach

05RL47Z Replacement of Intracranial Vein with Autologous Tissue Substitute, Percutaneous Endoscopic Approach

05RL4JZ Replacement of Intracranial Vein with Synthetic Substitute, Percutancous Endoscopic Approach

05RL4KZ Replacement of Intracranial Vein with Nonautologous Tissue Substitute, Percutaneous Endoscopic Approach

05RM07Z Replacement of Right Internal Jugular Vein with Autologous Tissue Substitute, Open Approach

05RM0JZ Replacement of Right Internal Jugular Vein with Synthetic Substitute, Open Approach

05RM0KZ Replacement of Right Internal Jugular Vein with Nonautologous Tissue Substitute, Open Approach

05RM47Z Replacement of Right Internal Jugular Vein with Autologous Tissue Substitute, Percutaneous Endoscopic Approach

05RM4JZ Replacement of Right Internal Jugular Vein with Synthetic Substitute, Percutaneous Endoscopic Approach

05RM4KZ Replacement of Right Internal Jugular Vein with Nonautologous Tissue

Substitute, Percutaneous Endoscopic Approach

05RN07Z Replacement of Left Internal Jugular Ve with Autologous Tissue Substitute, Ope Approach

05RN0JZ Replacement of Left Internal Jugular Ve with Synthetic Substitute, Open Approa

05RN0KZ Replacement of Left Internal Jugular Ve with Nonautologous Tissue Substitute, Open Approach

05RN47Z Replacement of Left Internal Jugular Vein with Autologous Tissue Substitute, Percutaneous Endoscopic Approach

05RN4JZ Replacement of Left Internal Jugular Ve with Synthetic Substitute, Percutaneous Endoscopic Approach

05RN4KZ Replacement of Left Internal Jugular Ve with Nonautologous Tissue Substitute, Percutaneous Endoscopic Approach

05RP07Z Replacement of Right External Jugular Vein with Autologous Tissue Substitute, Open Approach

05RP0JZ Replacement of Right External Jugular Vein with Synthetic Substitute, Open Approach

05RP0KZ Replacement of Right External Jugular Vein with Nonautologous Tissue Substitute, Open Approach

05RP47Z Replacement of Right External Jugular Vein with Autologous Tissue Substitute, Percutaneous Endoscopic Approach

05RP4JZ Replacement of Right External Jugular Vein with Synthetic Substitute, Percutaneous Endoscopic Approach

05RP4KZ Replacement of Right External Jugular Vein with Nonautologous Tissue Substitute, Percutaneous Endoscopic Approach

05RQ07Z Replacement of Left External Jugular Ve with Autologous Tissue Substitute, Oper Approach

05RQ0JZ Replacement of Left External Jugular Ve with Synthetic Substitute, Open Approac

05RQ0KZ Replacement of Left External Jugular Ve with Nonautologous Tissue Substitute, Open Approach

05RQ47Z Replacement of Left External Jugular Vein with Autologous Tissue Substitute, Percutaneous Endoscopic Approach

05RQ4JZ Replacement of Left External Jugular Ve with Synthetic Substitute, Percutaneous Endoscopic Approach

05RQ4KZ Replacement of Left External Jugular Ve with Nonautologous Tissue Substitute, Percutaneous Endoscopic Approach

05RR07Z Replacement of Right Vertebral Vein with Autologous Tissue Substitute, Open Approach

05RR0JZ Replacement of Right Vertebral Vein with Synthetic Substitute, Open Approach

05RR0KZ Replacement of Right Vertebral Vein with Nonautologous Tissue Substitute, Open Approach

05RR47Z Replacement of Right Vertebral Vein with Autologous Tissue Substitute, Percutaneous Endoscopic Approach

05RR4JZ Replacement of Right Vertebral Vein with Synthetic Substitute, Percutaneous Endoscopic Approach

05RR4KZ Replacement of Right Vertebral Vein with Nonautologous Tissue Substitute, Percutaneous Endoscopic Approach

05RS07Z Replacement of Left Vertebral Vein with Autologous Tissue Substitute, Open Approach

05RS0JZ Replacement of Left Vertebral Vein with Synthetic Substitute, Open Approach

RS0KZ	Replacement of Left Vertebral Vein with Nonautologous Tissue Substitute, Open Approach
RS47Z	Replacement of Left Vertebral Vein with Autologous Tissue Substitute, Percutaneous Endoscopic Approach
RS4JZ	Replacement of Left Vertebral Vein with Synthetic Substitute, Percutaneous Endoscopic Approach
RS4KZ	Replacement of Left Vertebral Vein with Nonautologous Tissue Substitute, Percutaneous Endoscopic Approach
RT07Z	Replacement of Right Face Vein with Autologous Tissue Substitute, Open Approach
RT0JZ	Replacement of Right Face Vein with Synthetic Substitute, Open Approach
RT0KZ	Replacement of Right Face Vein with Nonautologous Tissue Substitute, Open Approach
RT47Z	Replacement of Right Face Vein with Autologous Tissue Substitute, Percutaneous Endoscopic Approach

05RT4JZ	Replacement of Right Face Vein with Synthetic Substitute, Percutaneous Endoscopic Approach
05RT4KZ	Replacement of Right Face Vein with Nonautologous Tissue Substitute, Percutaneous Endoscopic Approach
05RV07Z	Replacement of Left Face Vein with Autologous Tissue Substitute, Open Approach
05RV0JZ	Replacement of Left Face Vein with Synthetic Substitute, Open Approach
05RV0KZ	Replacement of Left Face Vein with Nonautologous Tissue Substitute, Open Approach
05RV47Z	Replacement of Left Face Vein with Autologous Tissue Substitute, Percutaneous Endoscopic Approach
05RV4JZ	Replacement of Left Face Vein with Synthetic Substitute, Percutaneous Endoscopic Approach
05RV4KZ	Replacement of Left Face Vein with Nonautologous Tissue Substitute, Percutaneous Endoscopic Approach

05RY07Z	Replacement of Upper Vein with Autologous Tissue Substitute, Open Approach
05RY0JZ	Replacement of Upper Vein with Synthetic Substitute, Open Approach
05RY0KZ	Replacement of Upper Vein with Nonautologous Tissue Substitute, Open Approach
05RY47Z	Replacement of Upper Vein with Autologous Tissue Substitute, Percutaneous Endoscopic Approach
05RY4JZ	Replacement of Upper Vein with Synthetic Substitute, Percutaneous Endoscopic Approach
05RY4KZ	Replacement of Upper Vein with Nonautologous Tissue Substitute, Percutaneous Endoscopic Approach

5S – Upper Veins, Reposition

S00ZZ	Reposition Azygos Vein, Open Approach
S03ZZ	Reposition Azygos Vein, Percutaneous Approach
S04ZZ	Reposition Azygos Vein, Percutaneous Endoscopic Approach
S10ZZ	Reposition Hemiazygos Vein, Open Approach
S13ZZ	Reposition Hemiazygos Vein, Percutaneous Approach
S14ZZ	Reposition Hemiazygos Vein, Percutaneous Endoscopic Approach
S30ZZ	Reposition Right Innominate Vein, Open Approach
S33ZZ	Reposition Right Innominate Vein, Percutaneous Approach
S34ZZ	Reposition Right Innominate Vein, Percutaneous Endoscopic Approach
S40ZZ	Reposition Left Innominate Vein, Open Approach
S43ZZ	Reposition Left Innominate Vein, Percutaneous Approach
S44ZZ	Reposition Left Innominate Vein, Percutaneous Endoscopic Approach
S50ZZ	Reposition Right Subclavian Vein, Open Approach
S53ZZ	Reposition Right Subclavian Vein, Percutaneous Approach
S54ZZ	Reposition Right Subclavian Vein, Percutaneous Endoscopic Approach
S60ZZ	Reposition Left Subclavian Vein, Open Approach
S63ZZ	Reposition Left Subclavian Vein, Percutaneous Approach
S64ZZ	Reposition Left Subclavian Vein, Percutaneous Endoscopic Approach
S70ZZ	Reposition Right Axillary Vein, Open Approach
S73ZZ	Reposition Right Axillary Vein, Percutaneous Approach
S74ZZ	Reposition Right Axillary Vein, Percutaneous Endoscopic Approach
S80ZZ	Reposition Left Axillary Vein, Open Approach
S83ZZ	Reposition Left Axillary Vein, Percutaneous Approach
S84ZZ	Reposition Left Axillary Vein, Percutaneous Endoscopic Approach
S90ZZ	Reposition Right Brachial Vein, Open Approach
S93ZZ	Reposition Right Brachial Vein, Percutaneous Approach

05S94ZZ	Reposition Right Brachial Vein, Percutaneous Endoscopic Approach
05SA0ZZ	Reposition Left Brachial Vein, Open Approach
05SA3ZZ	Reposition Left Brachial Vein, Percutaneous Approach
05SA4ZZ	Reposition Left Brachial Vein, Percutaneous Endoscopic Approach
05SB0ZZ	Reposition Right Basilic Vein, Open Approach
05SB3ZZ	Reposition Right Basilic Vein, Percutaneous Approach
05SB4ZZ	Reposition Right Basilic Vein, Percutaneous Endoscopic Approach
05SC0ZZ	Reposition Left Basilic Vein, Open Approach
05SC3ZZ	Reposition Left Basilic Vein, Percutaneous Approach
05SC4ZZ	Reposition Left Basilic Vein, Percutaneous Endoscopic Approach
05SD0ZZ	Reposition Right Cephalic Vein, Open Approach

AHA CC: 4Q, 2013, 125-126

05SD3ZZ	Reposition Right Cephalic Vein, Percutaneous Approach
05SD4ZZ	Reposition Right Cephalic Vein, Percutaneous Endoscopic Approach
05SF0ZZ	Reposition Left Cephalic Vein, Open Approach
05SF3ZZ	Reposition Left Cephalic Vein, Percutaneous Approach
05SF4ZZ	Reposition Left Cephalic Vein, Percutaneous Endoscopic Approach
05SG0ZZ	Reposition Right Hand Vein, Open Approach
05SG3ZZ	Reposition Right Hand Vein, Percutaneous Approach
05SG4ZZ	Reposition Right Hand Vein, Percutaneous Endoscopic Approach
05SH0ZZ	Reposition Left Hand Vein, Open Approach
05SH3ZZ	Reposition Left Hand Vein, Percutaneous Approach
05SH4ZZ	Reposition Left Hand Vein, Percutaneous Endoscopic Approach
05SL0ZZ	Reposition Intracranial Vein, Open Approach
05SL3ZZ	Reposition Intracranial Vein, Percutaneous Approach
05SL4ZZ	Reposition Intracranial Vein, Percutaneous Endoscopic Approach
05SM0ZZ	Reposition Right Internal Jugular Vein, Open Approach

05SM3ZZ	Reposition Right Internal Jugular Vein, Percutaneous Approach
05SM4ZZ	Reposition Right Internal Jugular Vein, Percutaneous Endoscopic Approach
05SN0ZZ	Reposition Left Internal Jugular Vein, Open Approach
05SN3ZZ	Reposition Left Internal Jugular Vein, Percutaneous Approach
05SN4ZZ	Reposition Left Internal Jugular Vein, Percutaneous Endoscopic Approach
05SP0ZZ	Reposition Right External Jugular Vein, Open Approach
05SP3ZZ	Reposition Right External Jugular Vein, Percutaneous Approach
05SP4ZZ	Reposition Right External Jugular Vein, Percutaneous Endoscopic Approach
05SQ0ZZ	Reposition Left External Jugular Vein, Open Approach
05SQ3ZZ	Reposition Left External Jugular Vein, Percutaneous Approach
05SQ4ZZ	Reposition Left External Jugular Vein, Percutaneous Endoscopic Approach
05SR0ZZ	Reposition Right Vertebral Vein, Open Approach
05SR3ZZ	Reposition Right Vertebral Vein, Percutaneous Approach
05SR4ZZ	Reposition Right Vertebral Vein, Percutaneous Endoscopic Approach
05SS0ZZ	Reposition Left Vertebral Vein, Open Approach
05SS3ZZ	Reposition Left Vertebral Vein, Percutaneous Approach
05SS4ZZ	Reposition Left Vertebral Vein, Percutaneous Endoscopic Approach
05ST0ZZ	Reposition Right Face Vein, Open Approach
05ST3ZZ	Reposition Right Face Vein, Percutaneous Approach
05ST4ZZ	Reposition Right Face Vein, Percutaneous Endoscopic Approach
05SV0ZZ	Reposition Left Face Vein, Open Approach
05SV3ZZ	Reposition Left Face Vein, Percutaneous Approach
05SV4ZZ	Reposition Left Face Vein, Percutaneous Endoscopic Approach
05SY0ZZ	Reposition Upper Vein, Open Approach
05SY3ZZ	Reposition Upper Vein, Percutaneous Approach
05SY4ZZ	Reposition Upper Vein, Percutaneous Endoscopic Approach

♀ Female-only	♂ Male-only	▲ Limited Coverage	● Non-OR	▨ HAC-associated procedure	▲ Non-covered procedures	✛ Combination

05U – Upper Veins, Supplement

05U007Z Supplement Azygos Vein with Autologous Tissue Substitute, Open Approach
05U00JZ Supplement Azygos Vein with Synthetic Substitute, Open Approach
05U00KZ Supplement Azygos Vein with Nonautologous Tissue Substitute, Open Approach
05U037Z Supplement Azygos Vein with Autologous Tissue Substitute, Percutaneous Approach
05U03JZ Supplement Azygos Vein with Synthetic Substitute, Percutaneous Approach
05U03KZ Supplement Azygos Vein with Nonautologous Tissue Substitute, Percutaneous Approach
05U047Z Supplement Azygos Vein with Autologous Tissue Substitute, Percutaneous Endoscopic Approach
05U04JZ Supplement Azygos Vein with Synthetic Substitute, Percutaneous Endoscopic Approach
05U04KZ Supplement Azygos Vein with Nonautologous Tissue Substitute, Percutaneous Endoscopic Approach
05U107Z Supplement Hemiazygos Vein with Autologous Tissue Substitute, Open Approach
05U10JZ Supplement Hemiazygos Vein with Synthetic Substitute, Open Approach
05U10KZ Supplement Hemiazygos Vein with Nonautologous Tissue Substitute, Open Approach
05U137Z Supplement Hemiazygos Vein with Autologous Tissue Substitute, Percutaneous Approach
05U13JZ Supplement Hemiazygos Vein with Synthetic Substitute, Percutaneous Approach
05U13KZ Supplement Hemiazygos Vein with Nonautologous Tissue Substitute, Percutaneous Approach
05U147Z Supplement Hemiazygos Vein with Autologous Tissue Substitute, Percutaneous Endoscopic Approach
05U14JZ Supplement Hemiazygos Vein with Synthetic Substitute, Percutaneous Endoscopic Approach
05U14KZ Supplement Hemiazygos Vein with Nonautologous Tissue Substitute, Percutaneous Endoscopic Approach
05U307Z Supplement Right Innominate Vein with Autologous Tissue Substitute, Open Approach
05U30JZ Supplement Right Innominate Vein with Synthetic Substitute, Open Approach
05U30KZ Supplement Right Innominate Vein with Nonautologous Tissue Substitute, Open Approach
05U337Z Supplement Right Innominate Vein with Autologous Tissue Substitute, Percutaneous Approach
05U33JZ Supplement Right Innominate Vein with Synthetic Substitute, Percutaneous Approach
05U33KZ Supplement Right Innominate Vein with Nonautologous Tissue Substitute, Percutaneous Approach
05U347Z Supplement Right Innominate Vein with Autologous Tissue Substitute, Percutaneous Endoscopic Approach
05U34JZ Supplement Right Innominate Vein with Synthetic Substitute, Percutaneous Endoscopic Approach
05U34KZ Supplement Right Innominate Vein with Nonautologous Tissue Substitute, Percutaneous Endoscopic Approach

05U407Z Supplement Left Innominate Vein with Autologous Tissue Substitute, Open Approach
05U40JZ Supplement Left Innominate Vein with Synthetic Substitute, Open Approach
05U40KZ Supplement Left Innominate Vein with Nonautologous Tissue Substitute, Open Approach
05U437Z Supplement Left Innominate Vein with Autologous Tissue Substitute, Percutaneous Approach
05U43JZ Supplement Left Innominate Vein with Synthetic Substitute, Percutaneous Approach
05U43KZ Supplement Left Innominate Vein with Nonautologous Tissue Substitute, Percutaneous Approach
05U447Z Supplement Left Innominate Vein with Autologous Tissue Substitute, Percutaneous Endoscopic Approach
05U44JZ Supplement Left Innominate Vein with Synthetic Substitute, Percutaneous Endoscopic Approach
05U44KZ Supplement Left Innominate Vein with Nonautologous Tissue Substitute, Percutaneous Endoscopic Approach
05U507Z Supplement Right Subclavian Vein with Autologous Tissue Substitute, Open Approach
05U50JZ Supplement Right Subclavian Vein with Synthetic Substitute, Open Approach
05U50KZ Supplement Right Subclavian Vein with Nonautologous Tissue Substitute, Open Approach
05U537Z Supplement Right Subclavian Vein with Autologous Tissue Substitute, Percutaneous Approach
05U53JZ Supplement Right Subclavian Vein with Synthetic Substitute, Percutaneous Approach
05U53KZ Supplement Right Subclavian Vein with Nonautologous Tissue Substitute, Percutaneous Approach
05U547Z Supplement Right Subclavian Vein with Autologous Tissue Substitute, Percutaneous Endoscopic Approach
05U54JZ Supplement Right Subclavian Vein with Synthetic Substitute, Percutaneous Endoscopic Approach
05U54KZ Supplement Right Subclavian Vein with Nonautologous Tissue Substitute, Percutaneous Endoscopic Approach
05U607Z Supplement Left Subclavian Vein with Autologous Tissue Substitute, Open Approach
05U60JZ Supplement Left Subclavian Vein with Synthetic Substitute, Open Approach
05U60KZ Supplement Left Subclavian Vein with Nonautologous Tissue Substitute, Open Approach
05U637Z Supplement Left Subclavian Vein with Autologous Tissue Substitute, Percutaneous Approach
05U63JZ Supplement Left Subclavian Vein with Synthetic Substitute, Percutaneous Approach
05U63KZ Supplement Left Subclavian Vein with Nonautologous Tissue Substitute, Percutaneous Approach
05U647Z Supplement Left Subclavian Vein with Autologous Tissue Substitute, Percutaneous Endoscopic Approach
05U64JZ Supplement Left Subclavian Vein with Synthetic Substitute, Percutaneous Endoscopic Approach
05U64KZ Supplement Left Subclavian Vein with Nonautologous Tissue Substitute, Percutaneous Endoscopic Approach

05U707Z Supplement Right Axillary Vein with Autologous Tissue Substitute, Open Approach
05U70JZ Supplement Right Axillary Vein with Synthetic Substitute, Open Approach
05U70KZ Supplement Right Axillary Vein with Nonautologous Tissue Substitute, Open Approach
05U737Z Supplement Right Axillary Vein with Autologous Tissue Substitute, Percutaneous Approach
05U73JZ Supplement Right Axillary Vein with Synthetic Substitute, Percutaneous Approach
05U73KZ Supplement Right Axillary Vein with Nonautologous Tissue Substitute, Percutaneous Approach
05U747Z Supplement Right Axillary Vein with Autologous Tissue Substitute, Percutaneous Endoscopic Approach
05U74JZ Supplement Right Axillary Vein with Synthetic Substitute, Percutaneous Endoscopic Approach
05U74KZ Supplement Right Axillary Vein with Nonautologous Tissue Substitute, Percutaneous Endoscopic Approach
05U807Z Supplement Left Axillary Vein with Autologous Tissue Substitute, Open Approach
05U80JZ Supplement Left Axillary Vein with Synthetic Substitute, Open Approach
05U80KZ Supplement Left Axillary Vein with Nonautologous Tissue Substitute, Open Approach
05U837Z Supplement Left Axillary Vein with Autologous Tissue Substitute, Percutaneous Approach
05U83JZ Supplement Left Axillary Vein with Synthetic Substitute, Percutaneous Approach
05U83KZ Supplement Left Axillary Vein with Nonautologous Tissue Substitute, Percutaneous Approach
05U847Z Supplement Left Axillary Vein with Autologous Tissue Substitute, Percutaneous Endoscopic Approach
05U84JZ Supplement Left Axillary Vein with Synthetic Substitute, Percutaneous Endoscopic Approach
05U84KZ Supplement Left Axillary Vein with Nonautologous Tissue Substitute, Percutaneous Endoscopic Approach
05U907Z Supplement Right Brachial Vein with Autologous Tissue Substitute, Open Approach
05U90JZ Supplement Right Brachial Vein with Synthetic Substitute, Open Approach
05U90KZ Supplement Right Brachial Vein with Nonautologous Tissue Substitute, Open Approach
05U937Z Supplement Right Brachial Vein with Autologous Tissue Substitute, Percutaneous Approach
05U93JZ Supplement Right Brachial Vein with Synthetic Substitute, Percutaneous Approach
05U93KZ Supplement Right Brachial Vein with Nonautologous Tissue Substitute, Percutaneous Approach
05U947Z Supplement Right Brachial Vein with Autologous Tissue Substitute, Percutaneous Endoscopic Approach
05U94JZ Supplement Right Brachial Vein with Synthetic Substitute, Percutaneous Endoscopic Approach

♀ Female-only   ♂ Male-only   ▲ Limited Coverage   ● Non-OR   ▆ HAC-associated procedure   ▲ Non-covered procedures   ✛ Combination

J94KZ Supplement Right Brachial Vein with Nonautologous Tissue Substitute, Percutaneous Endoscopic Approach

JA07Z Supplement Left Brachial Vein with Autologous Tissue Substitute, Open Approach

JA0JZ Supplement Left Brachial Vein with Synthetic Substitute, Open Approach

JA0KZ Supplement Left Brachial Vein with Nonautologous Tissue Substitute, Open Approach

JA37Z Supplement Left Brachial Vein with Autologous Tissue Substitute, Percutaneous Approach

JA3JZ Supplement Left Brachial Vein with Synthetic Substitute, Percutaneous Approach

JA3KZ Supplement Left Brachial Vein with Nonautologous Tissue Substitute, Percutaneous Approach

JA47Z Supplement Left Brachial Vein with Autologous Tissue Substitute, Percutaneous Endoscopic Approach

JA4JZ Supplement Left Brachial Vein with Synthetic Substitute, Percutaneous Endoscopic Approach

JA4KZ Supplement Left Brachial Vein with Nonautologous Tissue Substitute, Percutaneous Endoscopic Approach

UB07Z Supplement Right Basilic Vein with Autologous Tissue Substitute, Open Approach

UB0JZ Supplement Right Basilic Vein with Synthetic Substitute, Open Approach

UB0KZ Supplement Right Basilic Vein with Nonautologous Tissue Substitute, Open Approach

UB37Z Supplement Right Basilic Vein with Autologous Tissue Substitute, Percutaneous Approach

UB3JZ Supplement Right Basilic Vein with Synthetic Substitute, Percutaneous Approach

UB3KZ Supplement Right Basilic Vein with Nonautologous Tissue Substitute, Percutaneous Approach

UB47Z Supplement Right Basilic Vein with Autologous Tissue Substitute, Percutaneous Endoscopic Approach

UB4JZ Supplement Right Basilic Vein with Synthetic Substitute, Percutaneous Endoscopic Approach

UB4KZ Supplement Right Basilic Vein with Nonautologous Tissue Substitute, Percutaneous Endoscopic Approach

UC07Z Supplement Left Basilic Vein with Autologous Tissue Substitute, Open Approach

UC0JZ Supplement Left Basilic Vein with Synthetic Substitute, Open Approach

UC0KZ Supplement Left Basilic Vein with Nonautologous Tissue Substitute, Open Approach

UC37Z Supplement Left Basilic Vein with Autologous Tissue Substitute, Percutaneous Approach

UC3JZ Supplement Left Basilic Vein with Synthetic Substitute, Percutaneous Approach

UC3KZ Supplement Left Basilic Vein with Nonautologous Tissue Substitute, Percutaneous Approach

UC47Z Supplement Left Basilic Vein with Autologous Tissue Substitute, Percutaneous Endoscopic Approach

UC4JZ Supplement Left Basilic Vein with Synthetic Substitute, Percutaneous Endoscopic Approach

05UC4KZ Supplement Left Basilic Vein with Nonautologous Tissue Substitute, Percutaneous Endoscopic Approach

05UD07Z Supplement Right Cephalic Vein with Autologous Tissue Substitute, Open Approach

05UD0JZ Supplement Right Cephalic Vein with Synthetic Substitute, Open Approach

05UD0KZ Supplement Right Cephalic Vein with Nonautologous Tissue Substitute, Open Approach

05UD37Z Supplement Right Cephalic Vein with Autologous Tissue Substitute, Percutaneous Approach

05UD3JZ Supplement Right Cephalic Vein with Synthetic Substitute, Percutaneous Approach

05UD3KZ Supplement Right Cephalic Vein with Nonautologous Tissue Substitute, Percutaneous Approach

05UD47Z Supplement Right Cephalic Vein with Autologous Tissue Substitute, Percutaneous Endoscopic Approach

05UD4JZ Supplement Right Cephalic Vein with Synthetic Substitute, Percutaneous Endoscopic Approach

05UD4KZ Supplement Right Cephalic Vein with Nonautologous Tissue Substitute, Percutaneous Endoscopic Approach

05UF07Z Supplement Left Cephalic Vein with Autologous Tissue Substitute, Open Approach

05UF0JZ Supplement Left Cephalic Vein with Synthetic Substitute, Open Approach

05UF0KZ Supplement Left Cephalic Vein with Nonautologous Tissue Substitute, Open Approach

05UF37Z Supplement Left Cephalic Vein with Autologous Tissue Substitute, Percutaneous Approach

05UF3JZ Supplement Left Cephalic Vein with Synthetic Substitute, Percutaneous Approach

05UF3KZ Supplement Left Cephalic Vein with Nonautologous Tissue Substitute, Percutaneous Approach

05UF47Z Supplement Left Cephalic Vein with Autologous Tissue Substitute, Percutaneous Endoscopic Approach

05UF4JZ Supplement Left Cephalic Vein with Synthetic Substitute, Percutaneous Endoscopic Approach

05UF4KZ Supplement Left Cephalic Vein with Nonautologous Tissue Substitute, Percutaneous Endoscopic Approach

05UG07Z Supplement Right Hand Vein with Autologous Tissue Substitute, Open Approach

05UG0JZ Supplement Right Hand Vein with Synthetic Substitute, Open Approach

05UG0KZ Supplement Right Hand Vein with Nonautologous Tissue Substitute, Open Approach

05UG37Z Supplement Right Hand Vein with Autologous Tissue Substitute, Percutaneous Approach

05UG3JZ Supplement Right Hand Vein with Synthetic Substitute, Percutaneous Approach

05UG3KZ Supplement Right Hand Vein with Nonautologous Tissue Substitute, Percutaneous Approach

05UG47Z Supplement Right Hand Vein with Autologous Tissue Substitute, Percutaneous Endoscopic Approach

05UG4JZ Supplement Right Hand Vein with Synthetic Substitute, Percutaneous Endoscopic Approach

05UG4KZ Supplement Right Hand Vein with Nonautologous Tissue Substitute, Percutaneous Endoscopic Approach

05UH07Z Supplement Left Hand Vein with Autologous Tissue Substitute, Open Approach

05UH0JZ Supplement Left Hand Vein with Synthetic Substitute, Open Approach

05UH0KZ Supplement Left Hand Vein with Nonautologous Tissue Substitute, Open Approach

05UH37Z Supplement Left Hand Vein with Autologous Tissue Substitute, Percutaneous Approach

05UH3JZ Supplement Left Hand Vein with Synthetic Substitute, Percutaneous Approach

05UH3KZ Supplement Left Hand Vein with Nonautologous Tissue Substitute, Percutaneous Approach

05UH47Z Supplement Left Hand Vein with Autologous Tissue Substitute, Percutaneous Endoscopic Approach

05UH4JZ Supplement Left Hand Vein with Synthetic Substitute, Percutaneous Endoscopic Approach

05UH4KZ Supplement Left Hand Vein with Nonautologous Tissue Substitute, Percutaneous Endoscopic Approach

05UL07Z Supplement Intracranial Vein with Autologous Tissue Substitute, Open Approach

05UL0JZ Supplement Intracranial Vein with Synthetic Substitute, Open Approach

05UL0KZ Supplement Intracranial Vein with Nonautologous Tissue Substitute, Open Approach

05UL37Z Supplement Intracranial Vein with Autologous Tissue Substitute, Percutaneous Approach

05UL3JZ Supplement Intracranial Vein with Synthetic Substitute, Percutaneous Approach

05UL3KZ Supplement Intracranial Vein with Nonautologous Tissue Substitute, Percutaneous Approach

05UL47Z Supplement Intracranial Vein with Autologous Tissue Substitute, Percutaneous Endoscopic Approach

05UL4JZ Supplement Intracranial Vein with Synthetic Substitute, Percutaneous Endoscopic Approach

05UL4KZ Supplement Intracranial Vein with Nonautologous Tissue Substitute, Percutaneous Endoscopic Approach

05UM07Z Supplement Right Internal Jugular Vein with Autologous Tissue Substitute, Open Approach

05UM0JZ Supplement Right Internal Jugular Vein with Synthetic Substitute, Open Approach

05UM0KZ Supplement Right Internal Jugular Vein with Nonautologous Tissue Substitute, Open Approach

05UM37Z Supplement Right Internal Jugular Vein with Autologous Tissue Substitute, Percutaneous Approach

05UM3JZ Supplement Right Internal Jugular Vein with Synthetic Substitute, Percutaneous Approach

05UM3KZ Supplement Right Internal Jugular Vein with Nonautologous Tissue Substitute, Percutaneous Approach

05UM47Z Supplement Right Internal Jugular Vein with Autologous Tissue Substitute, Percutaneous Endoscopic Approach

05UM4JZ Supplement Right Internal Jugular Vein with Synthetic Substitute, Percutaneous Endoscopic Approach

Female-only   ♂ Male-only   ▲ Limited Coverage   ● Non-OR   ▨ HAC-associated procedure   ▲ Non-covered procedures   ✚ Combination

05UM4KZ Supplement Right Internal Jugular Vein with Nonautologous Tissue Substitute, Percutaneous Endoscopic Approach

05UN07Z Supplement Left Internal Jugular Vein with Autologous Tissue Substitute, Open Approach

05UN0JZ Supplement Left Internal Jugular Vein with Synthetic Substitute, Open Approach

05UN0KZ Supplement Left Internal Jugular Vein with Nonautologous Tissue Substitute, Open Approach

05UN37Z Supplement Left Internal Jugular Vein with Autologous Tissue Substitute, Percutaneous Approach

05UN3JZ Supplement Left Internal Jugular Vein with Synthetic Substitute, Percutaneous Approach

05UN3KZ Supplement Left Internal Jugular Vein with Nonautologous Tissue Substitute, Percutaneous Approach

05UN47Z Supplement Left Internal Jugular Vein with Autologous Tissue Substitute, Percutaneous Endoscopic Approach

05UN4JZ Supplement Left Internal Jugular Vein with Synthetic Substitute, Percutaneous Endoscopic Approach

05UN4KZ Supplement Left Internal Jugular Vein with Nonautologous Tissue Substitute, Percutaneous Endoscopic Approach

05UP07Z Supplement Right External Jugular Vein with Autologous Tissue Substitute, Open Approach

05UP0JZ Supplement Right External Jugular Vein with Synthetic Substitute, Open Approach

05UP0KZ Supplement Right External Jugular Vein with Nonautologous Tissue Substitute, Open Approach

05UP37Z Supplement Right External Jugular Vein with Autologous Tissue Substitute, Percutaneous Approach

05UP3JZ Supplement Right External Jugular Vein with Synthetic Substitute, Percutaneous Approach

05UP3KZ Supplement Right External Jugular Vein with Nonautologous Tissue Substitute, Percutaneous Approach

05UP47Z Supplement Right External Jugular Vein with Autologous Tissue Substitute, Percutaneous Endoscopic Approach

05UP4JZ Supplement Right External Jugular Vein with Synthetic Substitute, Percutaneous Endoscopic Approach

05UP4KZ Supplement Right External Jugular Vein with Nonautologous Tissue Substitute, Percutaneous Endoscopic Approach

05UQ07Z Supplement Left External Jugular Vein with Autologous Tissue Substitute, Open Approach

05UQ0JZ Supplement Left External Jugular Vein with Synthetic Substitute, Open Approach

05UQ0KZ Supplement Left External Jugular Vein with Nonautologous Tissue Substitute, Open Approach

05UQ37Z Supplement Left External Jugular Vein with Autologous Tissue Substitute, Percutaneous Approach

05UQ3JZ Supplement Left External Jugular Vein with Synthetic Substitute, Percutaneous Approach

05UQ3KZ Supplement Left External Jugular Vein with Nonautologous Tissue Substitute, Percutaneous Approach

05UQ47Z Supplement Left External Jugular Vein with Autologous Tissue Substitute, Percutaneous Endoscopic Approach

05UQ4JZ Supplement Left External Jugular Vein with Synthetic Substitute, Percutaneous Endoscopic Approach

05UQ4KZ Supplement Left External Jugular Vein with Nonautologous Tissue Substitute, Percutaneous Endoscopic Approach

05UR07Z Supplement Right Vertebral Vein with Autologous Tissue Substitute, Open Approach

05UR0JZ Supplement Right Vertebral Vein with Synthetic Substitute, Open Approach

05UR0KZ Supplement Right Vertebral Vein with Nonautologous Tissue Substitute, Open Approach

05UR37Z Supplement Right Vertebral Vein with Autologous Tissue Substitute, Percutaneous Approach

05UR3JZ Supplement Right Vertebral Vein with Synthetic Substitute, Percutaneous Approach

05UR3KZ Supplement Right Vertebral Vein with Nonautologous Tissue Substitute, Percutaneous Approach

05UR47Z Supplement Right Vertebral Vein with Autologous Tissue Substitute, Percutaneous Endoscopic Approach

05UR4JZ Supplement Right Vertebral Vein with Synthetic Substitute, Percutaneous Endoscopic Approach

05UR4KZ Supplement Right Vertebral Vein with Nonautologous Tissue Substitute, Percutaneous Endoscopic Approach

05US07Z Supplement Left Vertebral Vein with Autologous Tissue Substitute, Open Approach

05US0JZ Supplement Left Vertebral Vein with Synthetic Substitute, Open Approach

05US0KZ Supplement Left Vertebral Vein with Nonautologous Tissue Substitute, Open Approach

05US37Z Supplement Left Vertebral Vein with Autologous Tissue Substitute, Percutaneous Approach

05US3JZ Supplement Left Vertebral Vein with Synthetic Substitute, Percutaneous Approach

05US3KZ Supplement Left Vertebral Vein with Nonautologous Tissue Substitute, Percutaneous Approach

05US47Z Supplement Left Vertebral Vein with Autologous Tissue Substitute, Percutaneous Endoscopic Approach

05US4JZ Supplement Left Vertebral Vein with Synthetic Substitute, Percutaneous Endoscopic Approach

05US4KZ Supplement Left Vertebral Vein with Nonautologous Tissue Substitute, Percutaneous Endoscopic Approach

05UT07Z Supplement Right Face Vein with Autologous Tissue Substitute, Open Approach

05UT0JZ Supplement Right Face Vein with Synthetic Substitute, Open Approach

05UT0KZ Supplement Right Face Vein with Nonautologous Tissue Substitute, Open Approach

05UT37Z Supplement Right Face Vein with Autologous Tissue Substitute, Percutaneous Approach

05UT3JZ Supplement Right Face Vein with Synthetic Substitute, Percutaneous Approach

05UT3KZ Supplement Right Face Vein with Nonautologous Tissue Substitute, Percutaneous Approach

05UT47Z Supplement Right Face Vein with Autologous Tissue Substitute, Percutaneous Endoscopic Approach

05UT4JZ Supplement Right Face Vein with Synthetic Substitute, Percutaneous Endoscopic Approach

05UT4KZ Supplement Right Face Vein with Nonautologous Tissue Substitute, Percutaneous Endoscopic Approach

05UV07Z Supplement Left Face Vein with Autologous Tissue Substitute, Open Approach

05UV0JZ Supplement Left Face Vein with Synthetic Substitute, Open Approach

05UV0KZ Supplement Left Face Vein with Nonautologous Tissue Substitute, Open Approach

05UV37Z Supplement Left Face Vein with Autologous Tissue Substitute, Percutaneous Approach

05UV3JZ Supplement Left Face Vein with Synthetic Substitute, Percutaneous Approach

05UV3KZ Supplement Left Face Vein with Nonautologous Tissue Substitute, Percutaneous Approach

05UV47Z Supplement Left Face Vein with Autologous Tissue Substitute, Percutaneous Endoscopic Approach

05UV4JZ Supplement Left Face Vein with Synthetic Substitute, Percutaneous Endoscopic Approach

05UV4KZ Supplement Left Face Vein with Nonautologous Tissue Substitute, Percutaneous Endoscopic Approach

05UY07Z Supplement Upper Vein with Autologous Tissue Substitute, Open Approach

05UY0JZ Supplement Upper Vein with Synthetic Substitute, Open Approach

05UY0KZ Supplement Upper Vein with Nonautologous Tissue Substitute, Open Approach

05UY37Z Supplement Upper Vein with Autologous Tissue Substitute, Percutaneous Approach

05UY3JZ Supplement Upper Vein with Synthetic Substitute, Percutaneous Approach

05UY3KZ Supplement Upper Vein with Nonautologous Tissue Substitute, Percutaneous Approach

05UY47Z Supplement Upper Vein with Autologous Tissue Substitute, Percutaneous Endoscopic Approach

05UY4JZ Supplement Upper Vein with Synthetic Substitute, Percutaneous Endoscopic Approach

05UY4KZ Supplement Upper Vein with Nonautologous Tissue Substitute, Percutaneous Endoscopic Approach

05V – Upper Veins, Restriction

Review Coding Guideline B3.12

05V00CZ Restriction of Azygos Vein with Extraluminal Device, Open Approach

05V00DZ Restriction of Azygos Vein with Intraluminal Device, Open Approach

05V00ZZ Restriction of Azygos Vein, Open Approach

05V03CZ Restriction of Azygos Vein with Extraluminal Device, Percutaneous Approach

05V03DZ Restriction of Azygos Vein with Intraluminal Device, Percutaneous Approach

♀ Female-only   ♂ Male-only   ▲ Limited Coverage   ● Non-OR   ▨ HAC-associated procedure   ▲ Non-covered procedures   ✚ Combination

V03ZZ Restriction of Azygos Vein, Percutaneous Approach

V04CZ Restriction of Azygos Vein with Extraluminal Device, Percutaneous Endoscopic Approach

V04DZ Restriction of Azygos Vein with Intraluminal Device, Percutaneous Endoscopic Approach

V04ZZ Restriction of Azygos Vein, Percutaneous Endoscopic Approach

V10CZ Restriction of Hemiazygos Vein with Extraluminal Device, Open Approach

V10DZ Restriction of Hemiazygos Vein with Intraluminal Device, Open Approach

V10ZZ Restriction of Hemiazygos Vein, Open Approach

V13CZ Restriction of Hemiazygos Vein with Extraluminal Device, Percutaneous Approach

V13DZ Restriction of Hemiazygos Vein with Intraluminal Device, Percutaneous Approach

V13ZZ Restriction of Hemiazygos Vein, Percutaneous Approach

V14CZ Restriction of Hemiazygos Vein with Extraluminal Device, Percutaneous Endoscopic Approach

V14DZ Restriction of Hemiazygos Vein with Intraluminal Device, Percutaneous Endoscopic Approach

V14ZZ Restriction of Hemiazygos Vein, Percutaneous Endoscopic Approach

5V30CZ Restriction of Right Innominate Vein with Extraluminal Device, Open Approach

5V30DZ Restriction of Right Innominate Vein with Intraluminal Device, Open Approach

5V30ZZ Restriction of Right Innominate Vein, Open Approach

5V33CZ Restriction of Right Innominate Vein with Extraluminal Device, Percutaneous Approach

5V33DZ Restriction of Right Innominate Vein with Intraluminal Device, Percutaneous Approach

5V33ZZ Restriction of Right Innominate Vein, Percutaneous Approach

5V34CZ Restriction of Right Innominate Vein with Extraluminal Device, Percutaneous Endoscopic Approach

5V34DZ Restriction of Right Innominate Vein with Intraluminal Device, Percutaneous Endoscopic Approach

5V34ZZ Restriction of Right Innominate Vein, Percutaneous Endoscopic Approach

5V40CZ Restriction of Left Innominate Vein with Extraluminal Device, Open Approach

5V40DZ Restriction of Left Innominate Vein with Intraluminal Device, Open Approach

5V40ZZ Restriction of Left Innominate Vein, Open Approach

5V43CZ Restriction of Left Innominate Vein with Extraluminal Device, Percutaneous Approach

05V43DZ Restriction of Left Innominate Vein with Intraluminal Device, Percutaneous Approach

05V43ZZ Restriction of Left Innominate Vein, Percutaneous Approach

05V44CZ Restriction of Left Innominate Vein with Extraluminal Device, Percutaneous Endoscopic Approach

05V44DZ Restriction of Left Innominate Vein with Intraluminal Device, Percutaneous Endoscopic Approach

05V44ZZ Restriction of Left Innominate Vein, Percutaneous Endoscopic Approach

05V50CZ Restriction of Right Subclavian Vein with Extraluminal Device, Open Approach

05V50DZ Restriction of Right Subclavian Vein with Intraluminal Device, Open Approach

05V50ZZ Restriction of Right Subclavian Vein, Open Approach

05V53CZ Restriction of Right Subclavian Vein with Extraluminal Device, Percutaneous Approach

05V53DZ Restriction of Right Subclavian Vein with Intraluminal Device, Percutaneous Approach

05V53ZZ Restriction of Right Subclavian Vein, Percutaneous Approach

05V54CZ Restriction of Right Subclavian Vein with Extraluminal Device, Percutaneous Endoscopic Approach

05V54DZ Restriction of Right Subclavian Vein with Intraluminal Device, Percutaneous Endoscopic Approach

05V54ZZ Restriction of Right Subclavian Vein, Percutaneous Endoscopic Approach

05V60CZ Restriction of Left Subclavian Vein with Extraluminal Device, Open Approach

05V60DZ Restriction of Left Subclavian Vein with Intraluminal Device, Open Approach

05V60ZZ Restriction of Left Subclavian Vein, Open Approach

05V63CZ Restriction of Left Subclavian Vein with Extraluminal Device, Percutaneous Approach

05V63DZ Restriction of Left Subclavian Vein with Intraluminal Device, Percutaneous Approach

05V63ZZ Restriction of Left Subclavian Vein, Percutaneous Approach

05V64CZ Restriction of Left Subclavian Vein with Extraluminal Device, Percutaneous Endoscopic Approach

05V64DZ Restriction of Left Subclavian Vein with Intraluminal Device, Percutaneous Endoscopic Approach

05V64ZZ Restriction of Left Subclavian Vein, Percutaneous Endoscopic Approach

05V70CZ Restriction of Right Axillary Vein with Extraluminal Device, Open Approach

05V70DZ Restriction of Right Axillary Vein with Intraluminal Device, Open Approach

05V70ZZ Restriction of Right Axillary Vein, Open Approach

05V73CZ Restriction of Right Axillary Vein with Extraluminal Device, Percutaneous Approach

05V73DZ Restriction of Right Axillary Vein with Intraluminal Device, Percutaneous Approach

05V73ZZ Restriction of Right Axillary Vein, Percutaneous Approach

05V74CZ Restriction of Right Axillary Vein with Extraluminal Device, Percutaneous Endoscopic Approach

05V74DZ Restriction of Right Axillary Vein with Intraluminal Device, Percutaneous Endoscopic Approach

05V74ZZ Restriction of Right Axillary Vein, Percutaneous Endoscopic Approach

05V80CZ Restriction of Left Axillary Vein with Extraluminal Device, Open Approach

05V80DZ Restriction of Left Axillary Vein with Intraluminal Device, Open Approach

05V80ZZ Restriction of Left Axillary Vein, Open Approach

05V83CZ Restriction of Left Axillary Vein with Extraluminal Device, Percutaneous Approach

05V83DZ Restriction of Left Axillary Vein with Intraluminal Device, Percutaneous Approach

05V83ZZ Restriction of Left Axillary Vein, Percutaneous Approach

05V84CZ Restriction of Left Axillary Vein with Extraluminal Device, Percutaneous Endoscopic Approach

05V84DZ Restriction of Left Axillary Vein with Intraluminal Device, Percutaneous Endoscopic Approach

05V84ZZ Restriction of Left Axillary Vein, Percutaneous Endoscopic Approach

05V90CZ Restriction of Right Brachial Vein with Extraluminal Device, Open Approach

05V90DZ Restriction of Right Brachial Vein with Intraluminal Device, Open Approach

05V90ZZ Restriction of Right Brachial Vein, Open Approach

05V93CZ Restriction of Right Brachial Vein with Extraluminal Device, Percutaneous Approach

05V93DZ Restriction of Right Brachial Vein with Intraluminal Device, Percutaneous Approach

05V93ZZ Restriction of Right Brachial Vein, Percutaneous Approach

05V94CZ Restriction of Right Brachial Vein with Extraluminal Device, Percutaneous Endoscopic Approach

05V94DZ Restriction of Right Brachial Vein with Intraluminal Device, Percutaneous Endoscopic Approach

05V94ZZ Restriction of Right Brachial Vein, Percutaneous Endoscopic Approach

05VA0CZ Restriction of Left Brachial Vein with Extraluminal Device, Open Approach

05VA0DZ Restriction of Left Brachial Vein with Intraluminal Device, Open Approach

05VA0ZZ Restriction of Left Brachial Vein, Open Approach

05VA3CZ Restriction of Left Brachial Vein with Extraluminal Device, Percutaneous Approach

05VA3DZ Restriction of Left Brachial Vein with Intraluminal Device, Percutaneous Approach

05VA3ZZ Restriction of Left Brachial Vein, Percutaneous Approach

05VA4CZ Restriction of Left Brachial Vein with Extraluminal Device, Percutaneous Endoscopic Approach

05VA4DZ Restriction of Left Brachial Vein with Intraluminal Device, Percutaneous Endoscopic Approach

05VA4ZZ Restriction of Left Brachial Vein, Percutaneous Endoscopic Approach

05VB0CZ Restriction of Right Basilic Vein with Extraluminal Device, Open Approach

05VB0DZ Restriction of Right Basilic Vein with Intraluminal Device, Open Approach

05VB0ZZ Restriction of Right Basilic Vein, Open Approach

05VB3CZ Restriction of Right Basilic Vein with Extraluminal Device, Percutaneous Approach

05VB3DZ Restriction of Right Basilic Vein with Intraluminal Device, Percutaneous Approach

05VB3ZZ Restriction of Right Basilic Vein, Percutaneous Approach

05VB4CZ Restriction of Right Basilic Vein with Extraluminal Device, Percutaneous Endoscopic Approach

05VB4DZ Restriction of Right Basilic Vein with Intraluminal Device, Percutaneous Endoscopic Approach

05VB4ZZ Restriction of Right Basilic Vein, Percutaneous Endoscopic Approach

05VC0CZ Restriction of Left Basilic Vein with Extraluminal Device, Open Approach

♀ Female-only   ♂ Male-only   ▲ Limited Coverage   ● Non-OR   ▥ HAC-associated procedure   ▲ Non-covered procedures   ➕ Combination

05VC0DZ Restriction of Left Basilic Vein with Intraluminal Device, Open Approach

05VC0ZZ Restriction of Left Basilic Vein, Open Approach

05VC3CZ Restriction of Left Basilic Vein with Extraluminal Device, Percutaneous Approach

05VC3DZ Restriction of Left Basilic Vein with Intraluminal Device, Percutaneous Approach

05VC3ZZ Restriction of Left Basilic Vein, Percutaneous Approach

05VC4CZ Restriction of Left Basilic Vein with Extraluminal Device, Percutaneous Endoscopic Approach

05VC4DZ Restriction of Left Basilic Vein with Intraluminal Device, Percutaneous Endoscopic Approach

05VC4ZZ Restriction of Left Basilic Vein, Percutaneous Endoscopic Approach

05VD0CZ Restriction of Right Cephalic Vein with Extraluminal Device, Open Approach

05VD0DZ Restriction of Right Cephalic Vein with Intraluminal Device, Open Approach

05VD0ZZ Restriction of Right Cephalic Vein, Open Approach

05VD3CZ Restriction of Right Cephalic Vein with Extraluminal Device, Percutaneous Approach

05VD3DZ Restriction of Right Cephalic Vein with Intraluminal Device, Percutaneous Approach

05VD3ZZ Restriction of Right Cephalic Vein, Percutaneous Approach

05VD4CZ Restriction of Right Cephalic Vein with Extraluminal Device, Percutaneous Endoscopic Approach

05VD4DZ Restriction of Right Cephalic Vein with Intraluminal Device, Percutaneous Endoscopic Approach

05VD4ZZ Restriction of Right Cephalic Vein, Percutaneous Endoscopic Approach

05VF0CZ Restriction of Left Cephalic Vein with Extraluminal Device, Open Approach

05VF0DZ Restriction of Left Cephalic Vein with Intraluminal Device, Open Approach

05VF0ZZ Restriction of Left Cephalic Vein, Open Approach

05VF3CZ Restriction of Left Cephalic Vein with Extraluminal Device, Percutaneous Approach

05VF3DZ Restriction of Left Cephalic Vein with Intraluminal Device, Percutaneous Approach

05VF3ZZ Restriction of Left Cephalic Vein, Percutaneous Approach

05VF4CZ Restriction of Left Cephalic Vein with Extraluminal Device, Percutaneous Endoscopic Approach

05VF4DZ Restriction of Left Cephalic Vein with Intraluminal Device, Percutaneous Endoscopic Approach

05VF4ZZ Restriction of Left Cephalic Vein, Percutaneous Endoscopic Approach

05VG0CZ Restriction of Right Hand Vein with Extraluminal Device, Open Approach

05VG0DZ Restriction of Right Hand Vein with Intraluminal Device, Open Approach

05VG0ZZ Restriction of Right Hand Vein, Open Approach

05VG3CZ Restriction of Right Hand Vein with Extraluminal Device, Percutaneous Approach

05VG3DZ Restriction of Right Hand Vein with Intraluminal Device, Percutaneous Approach

05VG3ZZ Restriction of Right Hand Vein, Percutaneous Approach

05VG4CZ Restriction of Right Hand Vein with Extraluminal Device, Percutaneous Endoscopic Approach

05VG4DZ Restriction of Right Hand Vein with Intraluminal Device, Percutaneous Endoscopic Approach

05VG4ZZ Restriction of Right Hand Vein, Percutaneous Endoscopic Approach

05VH0CZ Restriction of Left Hand Vein with Extraluminal Device, Open Approach

05VH0DZ Restriction of Left Hand Vein with Intraluminal Device, Open Approach

05VH0ZZ Restriction of Left Hand Vein, Open Approach

05VH3CZ Restriction of Left Hand Vein with Extraluminal Device, Percutaneous Approach

05VH3DZ Restriction of Left Hand Vein with Intraluminal Device, Percutaneous Approach

05VH3ZZ Restriction of Left Hand Vein, Percutaneous Approach

05VH4CZ Restriction of Left Hand Vein with Extraluminal Device, Percutaneous Endoscopic Approach

05VH4DZ Restriction of Left Hand Vein with Intraluminal Device, Percutaneous Endoscopic Approach

05VH4ZZ Restriction of Left Hand Vein, Percutaneous Endoscopic Approach

05VL0CZ Restriction of Intracranial Vein with Extraluminal Device, Open Approach

05VL0DZ Restriction of Intracranial Vein with Intraluminal Device, Open Approach

05VL0ZZ Restriction of Intracranial Vein, Open Approach

05VL3CZ Restriction of Intracranial Vein with Extraluminal Device, Percutaneous Approach

05VL3DZ Restriction of Intracranial Vein with Intraluminal Device, Percutaneous Approach

05VL3ZZ Restriction of Intracranial Vein, Percutaneous Approach

05VL4CZ Restriction of Intracranial Vein with Extraluminal Device, Percutaneous Endoscopic Approach

05VL4DZ Restriction of Intracranial Vein with Intraluminal Device, Percutaneous Endoscopic Approach

05VL4ZZ Restriction of Intracranial Vein, Percutaneous Endoscopic Approach

05VM0CZ Restriction of Right Internal Jugular Vein with Extraluminal Device, Open Approach

05VM0DZ Restriction of Right Internal Jugular Vein with Intraluminal Device, Open Approach

05VM0ZZ Restriction of Right Internal Jugular Vein, Open Approach

05VM3CZ Restriction of Right Internal Jugular Vein with Extraluminal Device, Percutaneous Approach

05VM3DZ Restriction of Right Internal Jugular Vein with Intraluminal Device, Percutaneous Approach

05VM3ZZ Restriction of Right Internal Jugular Vein, Percutaneous Approach

05VM4CZ Restriction of Right Internal Jugular Vein with Extraluminal Device, Percutaneous Endoscopic Approach

05VM4DZ Restriction of Right Internal Jugular Vein with Intraluminal Device, Percutaneous Endoscopic Approach

05VM4ZZ Restriction of Right Internal Jugular Vein, Percutaneous Endoscopic Approach

05VN0CZ Restriction of Left Internal Jugular Vein with Extraluminal Device, Open Approach

05VN0DZ Restriction of Left Internal Jugular Vein with Intraluminal Device, Open Approach

05VN0ZZ Restriction of Left Internal Jugular Vein, Open Approach

05VN3CZ Restriction of Left Internal Jugular Vein with Extraluminal Device, Percutaneous Approach

05VN3DZ Restriction of Left Internal Jugular Vein with Intraluminal Device, Percutaneous Approach

05VN3ZZ Restriction of Left Internal Jugular Vein, Percutaneous Approach

05VN4CZ Restriction of Left Internal Jugular Vein with Extraluminal Device, Percutaneous Endoscopic Approach

05VN4DZ Restriction of Left Internal Jugular Vein with Intraluminal Device, Percutaneous Endoscopic Approach

05VN4ZZ Restriction of Left Internal Jugular Vein, Percutaneous Endoscopic Approach

05VP0CZ Restriction of Right External Jugular Vein with Extraluminal Device, Open Approach

05VP0DZ Restriction of Right External Jugular Vein with Intraluminal Device, Open Approach

05VP0ZZ Restriction of Right External Jugular Vein, Open Approach

05VP3CZ Restriction of Right External Jugular Vein with Extraluminal Device, Percutaneous Approach

05VP3DZ Restriction of Right External Jugular Vein with Intraluminal Device, Percutaneous Approach

05VP3ZZ Restriction of Right External Jugular Vein, Percutaneous Approach

05VP4CZ Restriction of Right External Jugular Vein with Extraluminal Device, Percutaneous Endoscopic Approach

05VP4DZ Restriction of Right External Jugular Vein with Intraluminal Device, Percutaneous Endoscopic Approach

05VP4ZZ Restriction of Right External Jugular Vein Percutaneous Endoscopic Approach

05VQ0CZ Restriction of Left External Jugular Vein with Extraluminal Device, Open Approach

05VQ0DZ Restriction of Left External Jugular Vein with Intraluminal Device, Open Approach

05VQ0ZZ Restriction of Left External Jugular Vein, Open Approach

05VQ3CZ Restriction of Left External Jugular Vein with Extraluminal Device, Percutaneous Approach

05VQ3DZ Restriction of Left External Jugular Vein with Intraluminal Device, Percutaneous Approach

05VQ3ZZ Restriction of Left External Jugular Vein, Percutaneous Approach

05VQ4CZ Restriction of Left External Jugular Vein with Extraluminal Device, Percutaneous Endoscopic Approach

05VQ4DZ Restriction of Left External Jugular Vein with Intraluminal Device, Percutaneous Endoscopic Approach

05VQ4ZZ Restriction of Left External Jugular Vein, Percutaneous Endoscopic Approach

05VR0CZ Restriction of Right Vertebral Vein with Extraluminal Device, Open Approach

05VR0DZ Restriction of Right Vertebral Vein with Intraluminal Device, Open Approach

05VR0ZZ Restriction of Right Vertebral Vein, Open Approach

05VR3CZ Restriction of Right Vertebral Vein with Extraluminal Device, Percutaneous Approach

05VR3DZ Restriction of Right Vertebral Vein with Intraluminal Device, Percutaneous Approach

05VR3ZZ Restriction of Right Vertebral Vein, Percutaneous Approach

♀ Female-only ♂ Male-only ▲ Limited Coverage ● Non-OR ▥ HAC-associated procedure ▲ Non-covered procedures ✚ Combination

R4CZ	Restriction of Right Vertebral Vein with Extraluminal Device, Percutaneous Endoscopic Approach
R4DZ	Restriction of Right Vertebral Vein with Intraluminal Device, Percutaneous Endoscopic Approach
R4ZZ	Restriction of Right Vertebral Vein, Percutaneous Endoscopic Approach
S0CZ	Restriction of Left Vertebral Vein with Extraluminal Device, Open Approach
S0DZ	Restriction of Left Vertebral Vein with Intraluminal Device, Open Approach
S0ZZ	Restriction of Left Vertebral Vein, Open Approach
S3CZ	Restriction of Left Vertebral Vein with Extraluminal Device, Percutaneous Approach
S3DZ	Restriction of Left Vertebral Vein with Intraluminal Device, Percutaneous Approach
S3ZZ	Restriction of Left Vertebral Vein, Percutaneous Approach
S4CZ	Restriction of Left Vertebral Vein with Extraluminal Device, Percutaneous Endoscopic Approach
S4DZ	Restriction of Left Vertebral Vein with Intraluminal Device, Percutaneous Endoscopic Approach
S4ZZ	Restriction of Left Vertebral Vein, Percutaneous Endoscopic Approach
VT0CZ	Restriction of Right Face Vein with Extraluminal Device, Open Approach

05VT0DZ	Restriction of Right Face Vein with Intraluminal Device, Open Approach
05VT0ZZ	Restriction of Right Face Vein, Open Approach
05VT3CZ	Restriction of Right Face Vein with Extraluminal Device, Percutaneous Approach
05VT3DZ	Restriction of Right Face Vein with Intraluminal Device, Percutaneous Approach
05VT3ZZ	Restriction of Right Face Vein, Percutaneous Approach
05VT4CZ	Restriction of Right Face Vein with Extraluminal Device, Percutaneous Endoscopic Approach
05VT4DZ	Restriction of Right Face Vein with Intraluminal Device, Percutaneous Endoscopic Approach
05VT4ZZ	Restriction of Right Face Vein, Percutaneous Endoscopic Approach
05VV0CZ	Restriction of Left Face Vein with Extraluminal Device, Open Approach
05VV0DZ	Restriction of Left Face Vein with Intraluminal Device, Open Approach
05VV0ZZ	Restriction of Left Face Vein, Open Approach
05VV3CZ	Restriction of Left Face Vein with Extraluminal Device, Percutaneous Approach
05VV3DZ	Restriction of Left Face Vein with Intraluminal Device, Percutaneous Approach

05VV3ZZ	Restriction of Left Face Vein, Percutaneous Approach
05VV4CZ	Restriction of Left Face Vein with Extraluminal Device, Percutaneous Endoscopic Approach
05VV4DZ	Restriction of Left Face Vein with Intraluminal Device, Percutaneous Endoscopic Approach
05VV4ZZ	Restriction of Left Face Vein, Percutaneous Endoscopic Approach
05VY0CZ	Restriction of Upper Vein with Extraluminal Device, Open Approach
05VY0DZ	Restriction of Upper Vein with Intraluminal Device, Open Approach
05VY0ZZ	Restriction of Upper Vein, Open Approach
05VY3CZ	Restriction of Upper Vein with Extraluminal Device, Percutaneous Approach
05VY3DZ	Restriction of Upper Vein with Intraluminal Device, Percutaneous Approach
05VY3ZZ	Restriction of Upper Vein, Percutaneous Approach
05VY4CZ	Restriction of Upper Vein with Extraluminal Device, Percutaneous Endoscopic Approach
05VY4DZ	Restriction of Upper Vein with Intraluminal Device, Percutaneous Endoscopic Approach
05VY4ZZ	Restriction of Upper Vein, Percutaneous Endoscopic Approach

5W – Upper Veins, Revision

Review Coding Guideline B6.1c

WY00Z	Revision of Drainage Device in Upper Vein, Open Approach
WY02Z	Revision of Monitoring Device in Upper Vein, Open Approach
WY03Z	Revision of Infusion Device in Upper Vein, Open Approach
WY07Z	Revision of Autologous Tissue Substitute in Upper Vein, Open Approach
WY0CZ	Revision of Extraluminal Device in Upper Vein, Open Approach
WY0DZ	Revision of Intraluminal Device in Upper Vein, Open Approach
WY0JZ	Revision of Synthetic Substitute in Upper Vein, Open Approach
WY0KZ	Revision of Nonautologous Tissue Substitute in Upper Vein, Open Approach
WY30Z	Revision of Drainage Device in Upper Vein, Percutaneous Approach
WY32Z	Revision of Monitoring Device in Upper Vein, Percutaneous Approach
WY33Z	Revision of Infusion Device in Upper Vein, Percutaneous Approach
WY37Z	Revision of Autologous Tissue Substitute in Upper Vein, Percutaneous Approach

05WY3CZ	Revision of Extraluminal Device in Upper Vein, Percutaneous Approach
05WY3DZ	Revision of Intraluminal Device in Upper Vein, Percutaneous Approach
05WY3JZ	Revision of Synthetic Substitute in Upper Vein, Percutaneous Approach
05WY3KZ	Revision of Nonautologous Tissue Substitute in Upper Vein, Percutaneous Approach
05WY40Z	Revision of Drainage Device in Upper Vein, Percutaneous Endoscopic Approach
05WY42Z	Revision of Monitoring Device in Upper Vein, Percutaneous Endoscopic Approach
05WY43Z	Revision of Infusion Device in Upper Vein, Percutaneous Endoscopic Approach
05WY47Z	Revision of Autologous Tissue Substitute in Upper Vein, Percutaneous Endoscopic Approach
05WY4CZ	Revision of Extraluminal Device in Upper Vein, Percutaneous Endoscopic Approach
05WY4DZ	Revision of Intraluminal Device in Upper Vein, Percutaneous Endoscopic Approach

05WY4JZ	Revision of Synthetic Substitute in Upper Vein, Percutaneous Endoscopic Approach
05WY4KZ	Revision of Nonautologous Tissue Substitute in Upper Vein, Percutaneous Endoscopic Approach
05WYX0Z	Revision of Drainage Device in Upper Vein, External Approach
05WYX2Z	Revision of Monitoring Device in Upper Vein, External Approach
05WYX3Z	Revision of Infusion Device in Upper Vein, External Approach
05WYX7Z	Revision of Autologous Tissue Substitute in Upper Vein, External Approach
05WYXCZ	Revision of Extraluminal Device in Upper Vein, External Approach
05WYXDZ	Revision of Intraluminal Device in Upper Vein, External Approach
05WYXJZ	Revision of Synthetic Substitute in Upper Vein, External Approach
05WYXKZ	Revision of Nonautologous Tissue Substitute in Upper Vein, External Approach

♀ Female-only   ♂ Male-only   ▲ Limited Coverage   ● Non-OR   ▨ HAC-associated procedure   ▲ Non-covered procedures   ✚ Combination

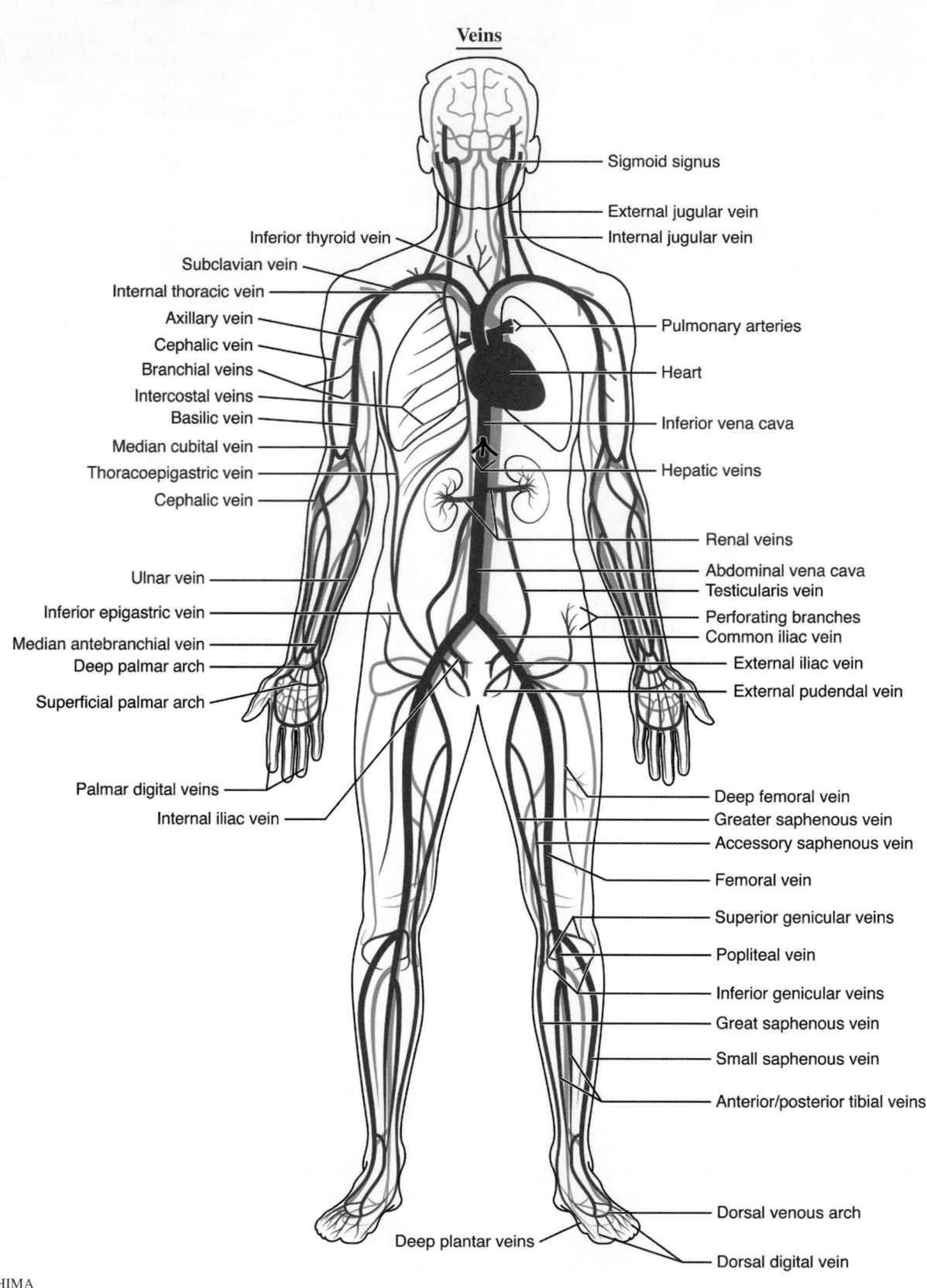

Veins

Sigmoid signus

External jugular vein

Internal jugular vein

Inferior thyroid vein

Subclavian vein

Internal thoracic vein

Axillary vein

Cephalic vein

Branchial veins

Intercostal veins

Basilic vein

Median cubital vein

Thoracoepigastric vein

Cephalic vein

Pulmonary arteries

Heart

Inferior vena cava

Hepatic veins

Renal veins

Ulnar vein

Inferior epigastric vein

Median antebranchial vein

Deep palmar arch

Superficial palmar arch

Abdominal vena cava

Testicularis vein

Perforating branches

Common iliac vein

External iliac vein

External pudendal vein

Palmar digital veins

Internal iliac vein

Deep femoral vein

Greater saphenous vein

Accessory saphenous vein

Femoral vein

Superior genicular veins

Popliteal vein

Inferior genicular veins

Great saphenous vein

Small saphenous vein

Anterior/posterior tibial veins

Dorsal venous arch

Deep plantar veins

Dorsal digital vein

©AHIMA

ower Veins Tables 061–06W

ection	0	**Medical and Surgical**	
ody System	6	**Lower Veins**	
peration	1	**Bypass:** Altering the route of passage of the contents of a tubular body part	

Body Part (4th)	Approach (5th)	Device (6th)	Qualifier (7th)
0 Inferior Vena Cava	0 Open 4 Percutaneous Endoscopic	7 Autologous Tissue Substitute 9 Autologous Venous Tissue A Autologous Arterial Tissue J Synthetic Substitute K Nonautologous Tissue Substitute Z No Device	5 Superior Mesenteric Vein 6 Inferior Mesenteric Vein Y Lower Vein
1 Splenic Vein	0 Open 4 Percutaneous Endoscopic	7 Autologous Tissue Substitute 9 Autologous Venous Tissue A Autologous Arterial Tissue J Synthetic Substitute K Nonautologous Tissue Substitute Z No Device	9 Renal Vein, Right B Renal Vein, Left Y Lower Vein
2 Gastric Vein 3 Esophageal Vein 4 Hepatic Vein 5 Superior Mesenteric Vein 6 Inferior Mesenteric Vein 7 Colic Vein 9 Renal Vein, Right B Renal Vein, Left C Common Iliac Vein, Right D Common Iliac Vein, Left F External Iliac Vein, Right G External Iliac Vein, Left H Hypogastric Vein, Right J Hypogastric Vein, Left M Femoral Vein, Right N Femoral Vein, Left P Greater Saphenous Vein, Right Q Greater Saphenous Vein, Left R Lesser Saphenous Vein, Right S Lesser Saphenous Vein, Left T Foot Vein, Right V Foot Vein, Left	0 Open 4 Percutaneous Endoscopic	7 Autologous Tissue Substitute 9 Autologous Venous Tissue A Autologous Arterial Tissue J Synthetic Substitute K Nonautologous Tissue Substitute Z No Device	Y Lower Vein
8 Portal Vein	0 Open	7 Autologous Tissue Substitute 9 Autologous Venous Tissue A Autologous Arterial Tissue J Synthetic Substitute K Nonautologous Tissue Substitute Z No Device	9 Renal Vein, Right B Renal Vein, Left Y Lower Vein
8 Portal Vein	3 Percutaneous	D Intraluminal Device	Y Lower Vein
8 Portal Vein	4 Percutaneous Endoscopic	7 Autologous Tissue Substitute 9 Autologous Venous Tissue A Autologous Arterial Tissue J Synthetic Substitute K Nonautologous Tissue Substitute Z No Device	9 Renal Vein, Right B Renal Vein, Left Y Lower Vein
8 Portal Vein	4 Percutaneous Endoscopic	D Intraluminal Device	Y Lower Vein

Section	0	Medical and Surgical
Body System	6	Lower Veins
Operation	5	Destruction: Physical eradication of all or a portion of a body part by the direct use of energy, force, or a destructive agent

Body Part (4th)	Approach (5th)	Device (6th)	Qualifier (7th)
0 Inferior Vena Cava 1 Splenic Vein 2 Gastric Vein 3 Esophageal Vein 4 Hepatic Vein 5 Superior Mesenteric Vein 6 Inferior Mesenteric Vein 7 Colic Vein 8 Portal Vein 9 Renal Vein, Right B Renal Vein, Left C Common Iliac Vein, Right D Common Iliac Vein, Left F External Iliac Vein, Right G External Iliac Vein, Left H Hypogastric Vein, Right J Hypogastric Vein, Left M Femoral Vein, Right N Femoral Vein, Left P Greater Saphenous Vein, Right Q Greater Saphenous Vein, Left R Lesser Saphenous Vein, Right S Lesser Saphenous Vein, Left T Foot Vein, Right V Foot Vein, Left	0 Open 3 Percutaneous 4 Percutaneous Endoscopic	Z No Device	Z No Qualifier
Y Lower Vein	0 Open 3 Percutaneous 4 Percutaneous Endoscopic	Z No Device	C Hemorrhoidal Plexus Z No Qualifier

Section	0	Medical and Surgical
Body System	6	Lower Veins
Operation	7	Dilation: Expanding an orifice or the lumen of a tubular body part

Body Part (4th)	Approach (5th)	Device (6th)	Qualifier (7th)
0 Inferior Vena Cava 1 Splenic Vein 2 Gastric Vein 3 Esophageal Vein 4 Hepatic Vein 5 Superior Mesenteric Vein 6 Inferior Mesenteric Vein 7 Colic Vein 8 Portal Vein 9 Renal Vein, Right B Renal Vein, Left C Common Iliac Vein, Right D Common Iliac Vein, Left F External Iliac Vein, Right G External Iliac Vein, Left H Hypogastric Vein, Right J Hypogastric Vein, Left M Femoral Vein, Right N Femoral Vein, Left P Greater Saphenous Vein, Right Q Greater Saphenous Vein, Left R Lesser Saphenous Vein, Right S Lesser Saphenous Vein, Left T Foot Vein, Right V Foot Vein, Left Y Lower Vein	0 Open 3 Percutaneous 4 Percutaneous Endoscopic	D Intraluminal Device Z No Device	Z No Qualifier

Section   **0**   **Medical and Surgical**
Body System   **6**   **Lower Veins**
Operation   **9**   **Drainage:** Taking or letting out fluids and/or gases from a body part

Body Part (4th)	Approach (5th)	Device (6th)	Qualifier (7th)
0 Inferior Vena Cava	**0** Open	**0** Drainage Device	**Z** No Qualifier
1 Splenic Vein	**3** Percutaneous		
2 Gastric Vein	**4** Percutaneous Endoscopic		
3 Esophageal Vein			
4 Hepatic Vein			
5 Superior Mesenteric Vein			
6 Inferior Mesenteric Vein			
7 Colic Vein			
8 Portal Vein			
9 Renal Vein, Right			
B Renal Vein, Left			
C Common Iliac Vein, Right			
D Common Iliac Vein, Left			
F External Iliac Vein, Right			
G External Iliac Vein, Left			
H Hypogastric Vein, Right			
J Hypogastric Vein, Left			
M Femoral Vein, Right			
N Femoral Vein, Left			
P Greater Saphenous Vein, Right			
Q Greater Saphenous Vein, Left			
R Lesser Saphenous Vein, Right			
S Lesser Saphenous Vein, Left			
T Foot Vein, Right			
V Foot Vein, Left			
Y Lower Vein			
0 Inferior Vena Cava	**0** Open	**Z** No Device	**X** Diagnostic
1 Splenic Vein	**3** Percutaneous		**Z** No Qualifier
2 Gastric Vein	**4** Percutaneous Endoscopic		
3 Esophageal Vein			
4 Hepatic Vein			
5 Superior Mesenteric Vein			
6 Inferior Mesenteric Vein			
7 Colic Vein			
8 Portal Vein			
9 Renal Vein, Right			
B Renal Vein, Left			
C Common Iliac Vein, Right			
D Common Iliac Vein, Left			
F External Iliac Vein, Right			
G External Iliac Vein, Left			
H Hypogastric Vein, Right			
J Hypogastric Vein, Left			
M Femoral Vein, Right			
N Femoral Vein, Left			
P Greater Saphenous Vein, Right			
Q Greater Saphenous Vein, Left			
R Lesser Saphenous Vein, Right			
S Lesser Saphenous Vein, Left			
T Foot Vein, Right			
V Foot Vein, Left			
Y Lower Vein			

Section	0	Medical and Surgical
Body System	6	Lower Veins
Operation	B	**Excision:** Cutting out or off, without replacement, a portion of a body part

Body Part (4th)	Approach (5th)	Device (6th)	Qualifier (7th)
0 Inferior Vena Cava 1 Splenic Vein 2 Gastric Vein 3 Esophageal Vein 4 Hepatic Vein 5 Superior Mesenteric Vein 6 Inferior Mesenteric Vein 7 Colic Vein 8 Portal Vein 9 Renal Vein, Right B Renal Vein, Left C Common Iliac Vein, Right D Common Iliac Vein, Left F External Iliac Vein, Right G External Iliac Vein, Left H Hypogastric Vein, Right J Hypogastric Vein, Left M Femoral Vein, Right N Femoral Vein, Left P Greater Saphenous Vein, Right Q Greater Saphenous Vein, Left R Lesser Saphenous Vein, Right S Lesser Saphenous Vein, Left T Foot Vein, Right V Foot Vein, Left	0 Open 3 Percutaneous 4 Percutaneous Endoscopic	Z No Device	X Diagnostic Z No Qualifier
Y Lower Vein	0 Open 3 Percutaneous 4 Percutaneous Endoscopic	Z No Device	C Hemorrhoidal Plexus X Diagnostic Z No Qualifier

Section	0	Medical and Surgical
Body System	6	Lower Veins
Operation	C	**Extirpation:** Taking or cutting out solid matter from a body part

Body Part (4th)	Approach (5th)	Device (6th)	Qualifier (7th)
0 Inferior Vena Cava 1 Splenic Vein 2 Gastric Vein 3 Esophageal Vein 4 Hepatic Vein 5 Superior Mesenteric Vein 6 Inferior Mesenteric Vein 7 Colic Vein 8 Portal Vein 9 Renal Vein, Right B Renal Vein, Left C Common Iliac Vein, Right D Common Iliac Vein, Left F External Iliac Vein, Right G External Iliac Vein, Left H Hypogastric Vein, Right J Hypogastric Vein, Left M Femoral Vein, Right N Femoral Vein, Left P Greater Saphenous Vein, Right Q Greater Saphenous Vein, Left R Lesser Saphenous Vein, Right S Lesser Saphenous Vein, Left T Foot Vein, Right V Foot Vein, Left Y Lower Vein	0 Open 3 Percutaneous 4 Percutaneous Endoscopic	Z No Device	Z No Qualifier

tion   0   **Medical and Surgical**
dy System   6   **Lower Veins**
eration   D   **Extraction:** Pulling or stripping out or off all or a portion of a body part by the use of force

Body Part (4th)	Approach (5th)	Device (6th)	Qualifier (7th)
1 Femoral Vein, Right N Femoral Vein, Left P Greater Saphenous Vein, Right Q Greater Saphenous Vein, Left R Lesser Saphenous Vein, Right Lesser Saphenous Vein, Left T Foot Vein, Right V Foot Vein, Left Y Lower Vein	0 Open 3 Percutaneous 4 Percutaneous Endoscopic	Z No Device	Z No Qualifier

ction   0   **Medical and Surgical**
dy System   6   **Lower Veins**
eration   H   **Insertion:** Putting in a nonbiological appliance that monitors, assists, performs, or prevents a physiological function but does not physically take the place of a body part

Body Part (4th)	Approach (5th)	Device (6th)	Qualifier (7th)
0 Inferior Vena Cava	0 Open 3 Percutaneous	3 Infusion Device	T Via Umbilical Vein Z No Qualifier
0 Inferior Vena Cava	0 Open 3 Percutaneous	D Intraluminal Device	Z No Qualifier
0 Inferior Vena Cava	4 Percutaneous Endoscopic	3 Infusion Device D Intraluminal Device	Z No Qualifier
1 Splenic Vein 2 Gastric Vein 3 Esophageal Vein 4 Hepatic Vein 5 Superior Mesenteric Vein 6 Inferior Mesenteric Vein 7 Colic Vein 8 Portal Vein 9 Renal Vein, Right B Renal Vein, Left C Common Iliac Vein, Right D Common Iliac Vein, Left F External Iliac Vein, Right G External Iliac Vein, Left H Hypogastric Vein, Right J Hypogastric Vein, Left M Femoral Vein, Right N Femoral Vein, Left P Greater Saphenous Vein, Right Q Greater Saphenous Vein, Left R Lesser Saphenous Vein, Right S Lesser Saphenous Vein, Left T Foot Vein, Right V Foot Vein, Left	0 Open 3 Percutaneous 4 Percutaneous Endoscopic	3 Infusion Device D Intraluminal Device	Z No Qualifier
Y Lower Vein	0 Open 3 Percutaneous 4 Percutaneous Endoscopic	2 Monitoring Device 3 Infusion Device D Intraluminal Device	Z No Qualifier

Section	0	Medical and Surgical
Body System	6	Lower Veins
Operation	J	**Inspection:** Visually and/or manually exploring a body part

Body Part (4th)	Approach (5th)	Device (6th)	Qualifier (7th)
Y Lower Vein	0 Open 3 Percutaneous 4 Percutaneous Endoscopic X External	Z No Device	Z No Qualifier

Section	0	Medical and Surgical
Body System	6	Lower Veins
Operation	L	**Occlusion:** Completely closing an orifice or the lumen of a tubular body part

Body Part (4th)	Approach (5th)	Device (6th)	Qualifier (7th)
0 Inferior Vena Cava 1 Splenic Vein 2 Gastric Vein 3 Esophageal Vein 4 Hepatic Vein 5 Superior Mesenteric Vein 6 Inferior Mesenteric Vein 7 Colic Vein 8 Portal Vein 9 Renal Vein, Right B Renal Vein, Left C Common Iliac Vein, Right D Common Iliac Vein, Left F External Iliac Vein, Right G External Iliac Vein, Left H Hypogastric Vein, Right J Hypogastric Vein, Left M Femoral Vein, Right N Femoral Vein, Left P Greater Saphenous Vein, Right Q Greater Saphenous Vein, Left R Lesser Saphenous Vein, Right S Lesser Saphenous Vein, Left T Foot Vein, Right V Foot Vein, Left	0 Open 3 Percutaneous 4 Percutaneous Endoscopic	C Extraluminal Device D Intraluminal Device Z No Device	Z No Qualifier
Y Lower Vein	0 Open 3 Percutaneous 4 Percutaneous Endoscopic	C Extraluminal Device D Intraluminal Device Z No Device	C Hemorrhoidal Plexus Z No Qualifier

Section	0	Medical and Surgical
Body System	6	Lower Veins
Operation	N	Release: Freeing a body part from an abnormal physical constraint by cutting or by the use of force

Body Part (4th)	Approach (5th)	Device (6th)	Qualifier (7th)
0 Inferior Vena Cava 1 Splenic Vein 2 Gastric Vein 3 Esophageal Vein 4 Hepatic Vein 5 Superior Mesenteric Vein 6 Inferior Mesenteric Vein 7 Colic Vein 8 Portal Vein 9 Renal Vein, Right B Renal Vein, Left C Common Iliac Vein, Right D Common Iliac Vein, Left F External Iliac Vein, Right G External Iliac Vein, Left H Hypogastric Vein, Right J Hypogastric Vein, Left M Femoral Vein, Right N Femoral Vein, Left P Greater Saphenous Vein, Right Q Greater Saphenous Vein, Left R Lesser Saphenous Vein, Right S Lesser Saphenous Vein, Left T Foot Vein, Right V Foot Vein, Left Y Lower Vein	0 Open 3 Percutaneous 4 Percutaneous Endoscopic	Z No Device	Z No Qualifier

Section	0	Medical and Surgical
Body System	6	Lower Veins
Operation	P	Removal: Taking out or off a device from a body part

Body Part (4th)	Approach (5th)	Device (6th)	Qualifier (7th)
Y Lower Vein	0 Open 3 Percutaneous 4 Percutaneous Endoscopic	0 Drainage Device 2 Monitoring Device 3 Infusion Device 7 Autologous Tissue Substitute C Extraluminal Device D Intraluminal Device J Synthetic Substitute K Nonautologous Tissue Substitute	Z No Qualifier
Y Lower Vein	X External	0 Drainage Device 2 Monitoring Device 3 Infusion Device D Intraluminal Device	Z No Qualifier

Section	0	Medical and Surgical
Body System	6	Lower Veins
Operation	Q	Repair: Restoring, to the extent possible, a body part to its normal anatomic structure and function

Body Part (4th)	Approach (5th)	Device (6th)	Qualifier (7th)
0 Inferior Vena Cava	0 Open	Z No Device	Z No Qualifier
1 Splenic Vein	3 Percutaneous		
2 Gastric Vein	4 Percutaneous Endoscopic		
3 Esophageal Vein			
4 Hepatic Vein			
5 Superior Mesenteric Vein			
6 Inferior Mesenteric Vein			
7 Colic Vein			
8 Portal Vein			
9 Renal Vein, Right			
B Renal Vein, Left			
C Common Iliac Vein, Right			
D Common Iliac Vein, Left			
F External Iliac Vein, Right			
G External Iliac Vein, Left			
H Hypogastric Vein, Right			
J Hypogastric Vein, Left			
M Femoral Vein, Right			
N Femoral Vein, Left			
P Greater Saphenous Vein, Right			
Q Greater Saphenous Vein, Left			
R Lesser Saphenous Vein, Right			
S Lesser Saphenous Vein, Left			
T Foot Vein, Right			
V Foot Vein, Left			
Y Lower Vein			

Section	0	Medical and Surgical
Body System	6	Lower Veins
Operation	R	Replacement: Putting in or on biological or synthetic material that physically takes the place and/or function of all or a portion of a body part

Body Part (4th)	Approach (5th)	Device (6th)	Qualifier (7th)
0 Inferior Vena Cava	0 Open	7 Autologous Tissue Substitute	Z No Qualifier
1 Splenic Vein	4 Percutaneous Endoscopic	J Synthetic Substitute	
2 Gastric Vein		K Nonautologous Tissue Substitute	
3 Esophageal Vein			
4 Hepatic Vein			
5 Superior Mesenteric Vein			
6 Inferior Mesenteric Vein			
7 Colic Vein			
8 Portal Vein			
9 Renal Vein, Right			
B Renal Vein, Left			
C Common Iliac Vein, Right			
D Common Iliac Vein, Left			
F External Iliac Vein, Right			
G External Iliac Vein, Left			
H Hypogastric Vein, Right			
J Hypogastric Vein, Left			
M Femoral Vein, Right			
N Femoral Vein, Left			
P Greater Saphenous Vein, Right			
Q Greater Saphenous Vein, Left			
R Lesser Saphenous Vein, Right			
S Lesser Saphenous Vein, Left			
T Foot Vein, Right			
V Foot Vein, Left			
Y Lower Vein			

Section   0   **Medical and Surgical**
Body System   6   **Lower Veins**
Operation   S   **Reposition:** Moving to its normal location, or other suitable location, all or a portion of a body part

Body Part (4ᵗʰ)	Approach (5ᵗʰ)	Device (6ᵗʰ)	Qualifier (7ᵗʰ)
0 Inferior Vena Cava	0 Open	Z No Device	Z No Qualifier
1 Splenic Vein	3 Percutaneous		
2 Gastric Vein	4 Percutaneous Endoscopic		
3 Esophageal Vein			
4 Hepatic Vein			
5 Superior Mesenteric Vein			
6 Inferior Mesenteric Vein			
7 Colic Vein			
8 Portal Vein			
9 Renal Vein, Right			
B Renal Vein, Left			
C Common Iliac Vein, Right			
D Common Iliac Vein, Left			
F External Iliac Vein, Right			
G External Iliac Vein, Left			
H Hypogastric Vein, Right			
J Hypogastric Vein, Left			
M Femoral Vein, Right			
N Femoral Vein, Left			
P Greater Saphenous Vein, Right			
Q Greater Saphenous Vein, Left			
R Lesser Saphenous Vein, Right			
S Lesser Saphenous Vein, Left			
T Foot Vein, Right			
V Foot Vein, Left			
Y Lower Vein			

Section   0   **Medical and Surgical**
Body System   6   **Lower Veins**
Operation   U   **Supplement:** Putting in or on biological or synthetic material that physically reinforces and/or augments the function of a portion of a body part

Body Part (4ᵗʰ)	Approach (5ᵗʰ)	Device (6ᵗʰ)	Qualifier (7ᵗʰ)
0 Inferior Vena Cava	0 Open	7 Autologous Tissue Substitute	Z No Qualifier
1 Splenic Vein	3 Percutaneous	J Synthetic Substitute	
2 Gastric Vein	4 Percutaneous Endoscopic	K Nonautologous Tissue Substitute	
3 Esophageal Vein			
4 Hepatic Vein			
5 Superior Mesenteric Vein			
6 Inferior Mesenteric Vein			
7 Colic Vein			
8 Portal Vein			
9 Renal Vein, Right			
B Renal Vein, Left			
C Common Iliac Vein, Right			
D Common Iliac Vein, Left			
F External Iliac Vein, Right			
G External Iliac Vein, Left			
H Hypogastric Vein, Right			
J Hypogastric Vein, Left			
M Femoral Vein, Right			
N Femoral Vein, Left			
P Greater Saphenous Vein, Right			
Q Greater Saphenous Vein, Left			
R Lesser Saphenous Vein, Right			
S Lesser Saphenous Vein, Left			
T Foot Vein, Right			
V Foot Vein, Left			
Y Lower Vein			

Section	0	Medical and Surgical
Body System	6	Lower Veins
Operation	V	**Restriction:** Partially closing an orifice or the lumen of a tubular body part

Body Part (4ᵗʰ)	Approach (5ᵗʰ)	Device (6ᵗʰ)	Qualifier (7ᵗʰ)
0 Inferior Vena Cava 1 Splenic Vein 2 Gastric Vein 3 Esophageal Vein 4 Hepatic Vein 5 Superior Mesenteric Vein 6 Inferior Mesenteric Vein 7 Colic Vein 8 Portal Vein 9 Renal Vein, Right B Renal Vein, Left C Common Iliac Vein, Right D Common Iliac Vein, Left F External Iliac Vein, Right G External Iliac Vein, Left H Hypogastric Vein, Right J Hypogastric Vein, Left M Femoral Vein, Right N Femoral Vein, Left P Greater Saphenous Vein, Right Q Greater Saphenous Vein, Left R Lesser Saphenous Vein, Right S Lesser Saphenous Vein, Left T Foot Vein, Right V Foot Vein, Left Y Lower Vein	0 Open 3 Percutaneous 4 Percutaneous Endoscopic	C Extraluminal Device D Intraluminal Device Z No Device	Z No Qualifier

Section	0	Medical and Surgical
Body System	6	Lower Veins
Operation	W	**Revision:** Correcting, to the extent possible, a portion of a malfunctioning device or the position of a displaced device

Body Part (4ᵗʰ)	Approach (5ᵗʰ)	Device (6ᵗʰ)	Qualifier (7ᵗʰ)
Y Lower Vein	0 Open 3 Percutaneous 4 Percutaneous Endoscopic X External	0 Drainage Device 2 Monitoring Device 3 Infusion Device 7 Autologous Tissue Substitute C Extraluminal Device D Intraluminal Device J Synthetic Substitute K Nonautologous Tissue Substitute	Z No Qualifier

Lower Veins Code Listing 061–06W

061 – Lower Veins, Bypass

Review Coding Guideline B3.6a

0610075	Bypass Inferior Vena Cava to Superior Mesenteric Vein with Autologous Tissue Substitute, Open Approach	**06100A5**	Bypass Inferior Vena Cava to Superior Mesenteric Vein with Autologous Arterial Tissue, Open Approach
0610076	Bypass Inferior Vena Cava to Inferior Mesenteric Vein with Autologous Tissue Substitute, Open Approach	**06100A6**	Bypass Inferior Vena Cava to Inferior Mesenteric Vein with Autologous Arterial Tissue, Open Approach
061007Y	Bypass Inferior Vena Cava to Lower Vein with Autologous Tissue Substitute, Open Approach	**06100AY**	Bypass Inferior Vena Cava to Lower Vein with Autologous Arterial Tissue, Open Approach
0610095	Bypass Inferior Vena Cava to Superior Mesenteric Vein with Autologous Venous Tissue, Open Approach	**06100J5**	Bypass Inferior Vena Cava to Superior Mesenteric Vein with Synthetic Substitute, Open Approach
0610096	Bypass Inferior Vena Cava to Inferior Mesenteric Vein with Autologous Venous Tissue, Open Approach	**06100J6**	Bypass Inferior Vena Cava to Inferior Mesenteric Vein with Synthetic Substitute, Open Approach
061009Y	Bypass Inferior Vena Cava to Lower Vein with Autologous Venous Tissue, Open Approach	**06100JY**	Bypass Inferior Vena Cava to Lower Vein with Synthetic Substitute, Open Approach

06100K5	Bypass Inferior Vena Cava to Superior Mesenteric Vein with Nonautologous Tissue Substitute, Open Approach
06100K6	Bypass Inferior Vena Cava to Inferior Mesenteric Vein with Nonautologous Tissue Substitute, Open Approach
06100KY	Bypass Inferior Vena Cava to Lower Vein with Nonautologous Tissue Substitute, Open Approach
06100Z5	Bypass Inferior Vena Cava to Superior Mesenteric Vein, Open Approach
06100Z6	Bypass Inferior Vena Cava to Inferior Mesenteric Vein, Open Approach
06100ZY	Bypass Inferior Vena Cava to Lower Vein, Open Approach
0610475	Bypass Inferior Vena Cava to Superior Mesenteric Vein with Autologous Tissue

Substitute, Percutaneous Endoscopic
Approach

.0476 Bypass Inferior Vena Cava to Inferior
Mesenteric Vein with Autologous Tissue
Substitute, Percutaneous Endoscopic
Approach

.047Y Bypass Inferior Vena Cava to Lower
Vein with Autologous Tissue Substitute,
Percutaneous Endoscopic Approach

.0495 Bypass Inferior Vena Cava to Superior
Mesenteric Vein with Autologous
Venous Tissue, Percutaneous Endoscopic
Approach

.0496 Bypass Inferior Vena Cava to Inferior
Mesenteric Vein with Autologous
Venous Tissue, Percutaneous Endoscopic
Approach

.049Y Bypass Inferior Vena Cava to Lower
Vein with Autologous Venous Tissue,
Percutaneous Endoscopic Approach

.104A5 Bypass Inferior Vena Cava to Superior
Mesenteric Vein with Autologous
Arterial Tissue, Percutaneous Endoscopic
Approach

.104A6 Bypass Inferior Vena Cava to Inferior
Mesenteric Vein with Autologous
Arterial Tissue, Percutaneous Endoscopic
Approach

104AY Bypass Inferior Vena Cava to Lower
Vein with Autologous Arterial Tissue,
Percutaneous Endoscopic Approach

104J5 Bypass Inferior Vena Cava to Superior
Mesenteric Vein with Synthetic Substitute,
Percutaneous Endoscopic Approach

104J6 Bypass Inferior Vena Cava to Inferior
Mesenteric Vein with Synthetic Substitute,
Percutaneous Endoscopic Approach

104JY Bypass Inferior Vena Cava to Lower Vein
with Synthetic Substitute, Percutaneous
Endoscopic Approach

.104K5 Bypass Inferior Vena Cava to Superior
Mesenteric Vein with Nonautologous
Tissue Substitute, Percutaneous
Endoscopic Approach

.104K6 Bypass Inferior Vena Cava to Inferior
Mesenteric Vein with Nonautologous
Tissue Substitute, Percutaneous
Endoscopic Approach

.104KY Bypass Inferior Vena Cava to Lower Vein
with Nonautologous Tissue Substitute,
Percutaneous Endoscopic Approach

.104Z5 Bypass Inferior Vena Cava to Superior
Mesenteric Vein, Percutaneous Endoscopic
Approach

.104Z6 Bypass Inferior Vena Cava to Inferior
Mesenteric Vein, Percutaneous Endoscopic
Approach

.104ZY Bypass Inferior Vena Cava to Lower Vein,
Percutaneous Endoscopic Approach

.611079 Bypass Splenic Vein to Right Renal Vein
with Autologous Tissue Substitute, Open
Approach

.61107B Bypass Splenic Vein to Left Renal Vein
with Autologous Tissue Substitute, Open
Approach

.61107Y Bypass Splenic Vein to Lower Vein with
Autologous Tissue Substitute, Open
Approach

.611099 Bypass Splenic Vein to Right Renal Vein
with Autologous Venous Tissue, Open
Approach

.61109B Bypass Splenic Vein to Left Renal Vein
with Autologous Venous Tissue, Open
Approach

.61109Y Bypass Splenic Vein to Lower Vein
with Autologous Venous Tissue, Open
Approach

06110A9 Bypass Splenic Vein to Right Renal Vein
with Autologous Arterial Tissue, Open
Approach

06110AB Bypass Splenic Vein to Left Renal Vein
with Autologous Arterial Tissue, Open
Approach

06110AY Bypass Splenic Vein to Lower Vein
with Autologous Arterial Tissue, Open
Approach

06110J9 Bypass Splenic Vein to Right Renal
Vein with Synthetic Substitute, Open
Approach

06110JB Bypass Splenic Vein to Left Renal Vein
with Synthetic Substitute, Open Approach

06110JY Bypass Splenic Vein to Lower Vein with
Synthetic Substitute, Open Approach

06110K9 Bypass Splenic Vein to Right Renal Vein
with Nonautologous Tissue Substitute,
Open Approach

06110KB Bypass Splenic Vein to Left Renal Vein
with Nonautologous Tissue Substitute,
Open Approach

06110KY Bypass Splenic Vein to Lower Vein with
Nonautologous Tissue Substitute, Open
Approach

06110Z9 Bypass Splenic Vein to Right Renal Vein,
Open Approach

06110ZB Bypass Splenic Vein to Left Renal Vein,
Open Approach

06110ZY Bypass Splenic Vein to Lower Vein, Open
Approach

0611479 Bypass Splenic Vein to Right Renal
Vein with Autologous Tissue Substitute,
Percutaneous Endoscopic Approach

061147B Bypass Splenic Vein to Left Renal Vein
with Autologous Tissue Substitute,
Percutaneous Endoscopic Approach

061147Y Bypass Splenic Vein to Lower Vein
with Autologous Tissue Substitute,
Percutaneous Endoscopic Approach

0611499 Bypass Splenic Vein to Right Renal Vein
with Autologous Venous
Tissue, Percutaneous Endoscopic
Approach

061149B Bypass Splenic Vein to Left Renal
Vein with Autologous Venous Tissue,
Percutaneous Endoscopic Approach

061149Y Bypass Splenic Vein to Lower Vein with
Autologous Venous Tissue, Percutaneous
Endoscopic Approach

06114A9 Bypass Splenic Vein to Right Renal
Vein with Autologous Arterial Tissue,
Percutaneous Endoscopic Approach

06114AB Bypass Splenic Vein to Left Renal
Vein with Autologous Arterial Tissue,
Percutaneous Endoscopic Approach

06114AY Bypass Splenic Vein to Lower Vein with
Autologous Arterial Tissue, Percutaneous
Endoscopic Approach

06114J9 Bypass Splenic Vein to Right Renal Vein
with Synthetic Substitute, Percutaneous
Endoscopic Approach

06114JB Bypass Splenic Vein to Left Renal Vein
with Synthetic Substitute, Percutaneous
Endoscopic Approach

06114JY Bypass Splenic Vein to Lower Vein
with Synthetic Substitute, Percutaneous
Endoscopic Approach

06114K9 Bypass Splenic Vein to Right Renal Vein
with Nonautologous Tissue Substitute,
Percutaneous Endoscopic Approach

06114KB Bypass Splenic Vein to Left Renal Vein
with Nonautologous Tissue Substitute,
Percutaneous Endoscopic Approach

06114KY Bypass Splenic Vein to Lower Vein
with Nonautologous Tissue Substitute,
Percutaneous Endoscopic Approach

06114Z9 Bypass Splenic Vein to Right Renal Vein,
Percutaneous Endoscopic Approach

06114ZB Bypass Splenic Vein to Left Renal Vein,
Percutaneous Endoscopic Approach

06114ZY Bypass Splenic Vein to Lower Vein,
Percutaneous Endoscopic Approach

061207Y Bypass Gastric Vein to Lower Vein with
Autologous Tissue Substitute, Open
Approach

061209Y Bypass Gastric Vein to Lower Vein
with Autologous Venous Tissue, Open
Approach

06120AY Bypass Gastric Vein to Lower Vein
with Autologous Arterial Tissue, Open
Approach

06120JY Bypass Gastric Vein to Lower Vein with
Synthetic Substitute, Open Approach

06120KY Bypass Gastric Vein to Lower Vein with
Nonautologous Tissue Substitute, Open
Approach

06120ZY Bypass Gastric Vein to Lower Vein, Open
Approach

061247Y Bypass Gastric Vein to Lower Vein
with Autologous Tissue Substitute,
Percutaneous Endoscopic Approach

061249Y Bypass Gastric Vein to Lower Vein with
Autologous Venous Tissue, Percutaneous
Endoscopic Approach

06124AY Bypass Gastric Vein to Lower Vein with
Autologous Arterial Tissue, Percutaneous
Endoscopic Approach

06124JY Bypass Gastric Vein to Lower Vein
with Synthetic Substitute, Percutaneous
Endoscopic Approach

06124KY Bypass Gastric Vein to Lower
Vein with Nonautologous Tissue
Substitute, Percutaneous Endoscopic
Approach

06124ZY Bypass Gastric Vein to Lower Vein,
Percutaneous Endoscopic Approach

061307Y Bypass Esophageal Vein to Lower Vein
with Autologous Tissue Substitute, Open
Approach

061309Y Bypass Esophageal Vein to Lower Vein
with Autologous Venous Tissue, Open
Approach

06130AY Bypass Esophageal Vein to Lower Vein
with Autologous Arterial Tissue, Open
Approach

06130JY Bypass Esophageal Vein to Lower
Vein with Synthetic Substitute, Open
Approach

06130KY Bypass Esophageal Vein to Lower Vein
with Nonautologous Tissue Substitute,
Open Approach

06130ZY Bypass Esophageal Vein to Lower Vein,
Open Approach

061347Y Bypass Esophageal Vein to Lower Vein
with Autologous Tissue Substitute,
Percutaneous Endoscopic Approach

061349Y Bypass Esophageal Vein to Lower
Vein with Autologous Venous Tissue,
Percutaneous Endoscopic Approach

06134AY Bypass Esophageal Vein to Lower
Vein with Autologous Arterial Tissue,
Percutaneous Endoscopic Approach

06134JY Bypass Esophageal Vein to Lower Vein
with Synthetic Substitute, Percutaneous
Endoscopic Approach

06134KY Bypass Esophageal Vein to Lower Vein
with Nonautologous Tissue Substitute,
Percutaneous Endoscopic Approach

06134ZY Bypass Esophageal Vein to Lower Vein,
Percutaneous Endoscopic Approach

061407Y Bypass Hepatic Vein to Lower Vein with
Autologous Tissue Substitute, Open
Approach

Female-only   ♂ Male-only   ▲ Limited Coverage   ● Non-OR   ■ HAC-associated procedure   ▲ Non-covered procedures   ✚ Combination

061409Y Bypass Hepatic Vein to Lower Vein with Autologous Venous Tissue, Open Approach

06140AY Bypass Hepatic Vein to Lower Vein with Autologous Arterial Tissue, Open Approach

06140JY Bypass Hepatic Vein to Lower Vein with Synthetic Substitute, Open Approach

06140KY Bypass Hepatic Vein to Lower Vein with Nonautologous Tissue Substitute, Open Approach

06140ZY Bypass Hepatic Vein to Lower Vein, Open Approach

061447Y Bypass Hepatic Vein to Lower Vein with Autologous Tissue Substitute, Percutaneous Endoscopic Approach

061449Y Bypass Hepatic Vein to Lower Vein with Autologous Venous Tissue, Percutaneous Endoscopic Approach

06144AY Bypass Hepatic Vein to Lower Vein with Autologous Arterial Tissue, Percutaneous Endoscopic Approach

06144JY Bypass Hepatic Vein to Lower Vein with Synthetic Substitute, Percutaneous Endoscopic Approach

06144KY Bypass Hepatic Vein to Lower Vein with Nonautologous Tissue Substitute, Percutaneous Endoscopic Approach

06144ZY Bypass Hepatic Vein to Lower Vein, Percutaneous Endoscopic Approach

061507Y Bypass Superior Mesenteric Vein to Lower Vein with Autologous Tissue Substitute, Open Approach

061509Y Bypass Superior Mesenteric Vein to Lower Vein with Autologous Venous Tissue, Open Approach

06150AY Bypass Superior Mesenteric Vein to Lower Vein with Autologous Arterial Tissue, Open Approach

06150JY Bypass Superior Mesenteric Vein to Lower Vein with Synthetic Substitute, Open Approach

06150KY Bypass Superior Mesenteric Vein to Lower Vein with Nonautologous Tissue Substitute, Open Approach

06150ZY Bypass Superior Mesenteric Vein to Lower Vein, Open Approach

061547Y Bypass Superior Mesenteric Vein to Lower Vein with Autologous Tissue Substitute, Percutaneous Endoscopic Approach

061549Y Bypass Superior Mesenteric Vein to Lower Vein with Autologous Venous Tissue, Percutaneous Endoscopic Approach

06154AY Bypass Superior Mesenteric Vein to Lower Vein with Autologous Arterial Tissue, Percutaneous Endoscopic Approach

06154JY Bypass Superior Mesenteric Vein to Lower Vein with Synthetic Substitute, Percutaneous Endoscopic Approach

06154KY Bypass Superior Mesenteric Vein to Lower Vein with Nonautologous Tissue Substitute, Percutaneous Endoscopic Approach

06154ZY Bypass Superior Mesenteric Vein to Lower Vein, Percutaneous Endoscopic Approach

061607Y Bypass Inferior Mesenteric Vein to Lower Vein with Autologous Tissue Substitute, Open Approach

061609Y Bypass Inferior Mesenteric Vein to Lower Vein with Autologous Venous Tissue, Open Approach

06160AY Bypass Inferior Mesenteric Vein to Lower Vein with Autologous Arterial Tissue, Open Approach

06160JY Bypass Inferior Mesenteric Vein to Lower Vein with Synthetic Substitute, Open Approach

06160KY Bypass Inferior Mesenteric Vein to Lower Vein with Nonautologous Tissue Substitute, Open Approach

06160ZY Bypass Inferior Mesenteric Vein to Lower Vein, Open Approach

061647Y Bypass Inferior Mesenteric Vein to Lower Vein with Autologous Tissue Substitute, Percutaneous Endoscopic Approach

061649Y Bypass Inferior Mesenteric Vein to Lower Vein with Autologous Venous Tissue, Percutaneous Endoscopic Approach

06164AY Bypass Inferior Mesenteric Vein to Lower Vein with Autologous Arterial Tissue, Percutaneous Endoscopic Approach

06164JY Bypass Inferior Mesenteric Vein to Lower Vein with Synthetic Substitute, Percutaneous Endoscopic Approach

06164KY Bypass Inferior Mesenteric Vein to Lower Vein with Nonautologous Tissue Substitute, Percutaneous Endoscopic Approach

06164ZY Bypass Inferior Mesenteric Vein to Lower Vein, Percutaneous Endoscopic Approach

061707Y Bypass Colic Vein to Lower Vein with Autologous Tissue Substitute, Open Approach

061709Y Bypass Colic Vein to Lower Vein with Autologous Venous Tissue, Open Approach

06170AY Bypass Colic Vein to Lower Vein with Autologous Arterial Tissue, Open Approach

06170JY Bypass Colic Vein to Lower Vein with Synthetic Substitute, Open Approach

06170KY Bypass Colic Vein to Lower Vein with Nonautologous Tissue Substitute, Open Approach

06170ZY Bypass Colic Vein to Lower Vein, Open Approach

061747Y Bypass Colic Vein to Lower Vein with Autologous Tissue Substitute, Percutaneous Endoscopic Approach

061749Y Bypass Colic Vein to Lower Vein with Autologous Venous Tissue, Percutaneous Endoscopic Approach

06174AY Bypass Colic Vein to Lower Vein with Autologous Arterial Tissue, Percutaneous Endoscopic Approach

06174JY Bypass Colic Vein to Lower Vein with Synthetic Substitute, Percutaneous Endoscopic Approach

06174KY Bypass Colic Vein to Lower Vein with Nonautologous Tissue Substitute, Percutaneous Endoscopic Approach

06174ZY Bypass Colic Vein to Lower Vein, Percutaneous Endoscopic Approach

0618079 Bypass Portal Vein to Right Renal Vein with Autologous Tissue Substitute, Open Approach

061807B Bypass Portal Vein to Left Renal Vein with Autologous Tissue Substitute, Open Approach

061807Y Bypass Portal Vein to Lower Vein with Autologous Tissue Substitute, Open Approach

0618099 Bypass Portal Vein to Right Renal Vein with Autologous Venous Tissue, Open Approach

061809B Bypass Portal Vein to Left Renal Vein with Autologous Venous Tissue, Open Approach

061809Y Bypass Portal Vein to Lower Vein with Autologous Venous Tissue, Open Approach

06180A9 Bypass Portal Vein to Right Renal Vein with Autologous Arterial Tissue, Open Approach

06180AB Bypass Portal Vein to Left Renal Vein with Autologous Arterial Tissue, Open Approach

06180AY Bypass Portal Vein to Lower Vein with Autologous Arterial Tissue, Open Approach

06180J9 Bypass Portal Vein to Right Renal Vein with Synthetic Substitute, Open Approach

06180JB Bypass Portal Vein to Left Renal Vein with Synthetic Substitute, Open Approach

06180JY Bypass Portal Vein to Lower Vein with Synthetic Substitute, Open Approach

06180K9 Bypass Portal Vein to Right Renal Vein with Nonautologous Tissue Substitute, Open Approach

06180KB Bypass Portal Vein to Left Renal Vein with Nonautologous Tissue Substitute, Open Approach

06180KY Bypass Portal Vein to Lower Vein with Nonautologous Tissue Substitute, Open Approach

06180Z9 Bypass Portal Vein to Right Renal Vein, Open Approach

06180ZB Bypass Portal Vein to Left Renal Vein, Open Approach

06180ZY Bypass Portal Vein to Lower Vein, Open Approach

06183DY Bypass Portal Vein to Lower Vein with Intraluminal Device, Percutaneous Approach

0618479 Bypass Portal Vein to Right Renal Vein with Autologous Tissue Substitute, Percutaneous Endoscopic Approach

061847B Bypass Portal Vein to Left Renal Vein with Autologous Tissue Substitute, Percutaneous Endoscopic Approach

061847Y Bypass Portal Vein to Lower Vein with Autologous Tissue Substitute, Percutaneous Endoscopic Approach

0618499 Bypass Portal Vein to Right Renal Vein with Autologous Venous Tissue, Percutaneous Endoscopic Approach

061849B Bypass Portal Vein to Left Renal Vein with Autologous Venous Tissue, Percutaneous Endoscopic Approach

061849Y Bypass Portal Vein to Lower Vein with Autologous Venous Tissue, Percutaneous Endoscopic Approach

06184A9 Bypass Portal Vein to Right Renal Vein with Autologous Arterial Tissue, Percutaneous Endoscopic Approach

06184AB Bypass Portal Vein to Left Renal Vein with Autologous Arterial Tissue, Percutaneous Endoscopic Approach

06184AY Bypass Portal Vein to Lower Vein with Autologous Arterial Tissue, Percutaneous Endoscopic Approach

06184DY Bypass Portal Vein to Lower Vein with Intraluminal Device, Percutaneous Endoscopic Approach

06184J9 Bypass Portal Vein to Right Renal Vein with Synthetic Substitute, Percutaneous Endoscopic Approach

06184JB Bypass Portal Vein to Left Renal Vein with Synthetic Substitute, Percutaneous Endoscopic Approach

06184JY Bypass Portal Vein to Lower Vein with Synthetic Substitute, Percutaneous Endoscopic Approach

06184K9 Bypass Portal Vein to Right Renal Vein with Nonautologous Tissue Substitute, Percutaneous Endoscopic Approach

06184KB Bypass Portal Vein to Left Renal Vein with Nonautologous Tissue Substitute, Percutaneous Endoscopic Approach

4KY Bypass Portal Vein to Lower Vein with Nonautologous Tissue Substitute, Percutaneous Endoscopic Approach

4Z9 Bypass Portal Vein to Right Renal Vein, Percutaneous Endoscopic Approach

4ZB Bypass Portal Vein to Left Renal Vein, Percutaneous Endoscopic Approach

4ZY Bypass Portal Vein to Lower Vein, Percutaneous Endoscopic Approach

907Y Bypass Right Renal Vein to Lower Vein with Autologous Tissue Substitute, Open Approach

909Y Bypass Right Renal Vein to Lower Vein with Autologous Venous Tissue, Open Approach

90AY Bypass Right Renal Vein to Lower Vein with Autologous Arterial Tissue, Open Approach

90JY Bypass Right Renal Vein to Lower Vein with Synthetic Substitute, Open Approach

90KY Bypass Right Renal Vein to Lower Vein with Nonautologous Tissue Substitute, Open Approach

90ZY Bypass Right Renal Vein to Lower Vein, Open Approach

947Y Bypass Right Renal Vein to Lower Vein with Autologous Tissue Substitute, Percutaneous Endoscopic Approach

949Y Bypass Right Renal Vein to Lower Vein with Autologous Venous Tissue, Percutaneous Endoscopic Approach

94AY Bypass Right Renal Vein to Lower Vein with Autologous Arterial Tissue, Percutaneous Endoscopic Approach

94JY Bypass Right Renal Vein to Lower Vein with Synthetic Substitute, Percutaneous Endoscopic Approach

94KY Bypass Right Renal Vein to Lower Vein with Nonautologous Tissue Substitute, Percutaneous Endoscopic Approach

94ZY Bypass Right Renal Vein to Lower Vein, Percutaneous Endoscopic Approach

B07Y Bypass Left Renal Vein to Lower Vein with Autologous Tissue Substitute, Open Approach

B09Y Bypass Left Renal Vein to Lower Vein with Autologous Venous Tissue, Open Approach

B0AY Bypass Left Renal Vein to Lower Vein with Autologous Arterial Tissue, Open Approach

B0JY Bypass Left Renal Vein to Lower Vein with Synthetic Substitute, Open Approach

B0KY Bypass Left Renal Vein to Lower Vein with Nonautologous Tissue Substitute, Open Approach

B0ZY Bypass Left Renal Vein to Lower Vein, Open Approach

1B47Y Bypass Left Renal Vein to Lower Vein with Autologous Tissue Substitute, Percutaneous Endoscopic Approach

1B49Y Bypass Left Renal Vein to Lower Vein with Autologous Venous Tissue, Percutaneous Endoscopic Approach

1B4AY Bypass Left Renal Vein to Lower Vein with Autologous Arterial Tissue, Percutaneous Endoscopic Approach

1B4JY Bypass Left Renal Vein to Lower Vein with Synthetic Substitute, Percutaneous Endoscopic Approach

1B4KY Bypass Left Renal Vein to Lower Vein with Nonautologous Tissue Substitute, Percutaneous Endoscopic Approach

1B4ZY Bypass Left Renal Vein to Lower Vein, Percutaneous Endoscopic Approach

061C07Y Bypass Right Common Iliac Vein to Lower Vein with Autologous Tissue Substitute, Open Approach

061C09Y Bypass Right Common Iliac Vein to Lower Vein with Autologous Venous Tissue, Open Approach

061C0AY Bypass Right Common Iliac Vein to Lower Vein with Autologous Arterial Tissue, Open Approach

061C0JY Bypass Right Common Iliac Vein to Lower Vein with Synthetic Substitute, Open Approach

061C0KY Bypass Right Common Iliac Vein to Lower Vein with Nonautologous Tissue Substitute, Open Approach

061C0ZY Bypass Right Common Iliac Vein to Lower Vein, Open Approach

061C47Y Bypass Right Common Iliac Vein to Lower Vein with Autologous Tissue Substitute, Percutaneous Endoscopic Approach

061C49Y Bypass Right Common Iliac Vein to Lower Vein with Autologous Venous Tissue, Percutaneous Endoscopic Approach

061C4AY Bypass Right Common Iliac Vein to Lower Vein with Autologous Arterial Tissue, Percutaneous Endoscopic Approach

061C4JY Bypass Right Common Iliac Vein to Lower Vein with Synthetic Substitute, Percutaneous Endoscopic Approach

061C4KY Bypass Right Common Iliac Vein to Lower Vein with Nonautologous Tissue Substitute, Percutaneous Endoscopic Approach

061C4ZY Bypass Right Common Iliac Vein to Lower Vein, Percutaneous Endoscopic Approach

061D07Y Bypass Left Common Iliac Vein to Lower Vein with Autologous Tissue Substitute, Open Approach

061D09Y Bypass Left Common Iliac Vein to Lower Vein with Autologous Venous Tissue, Open Approach

061D0AY Bypass Left Common Iliac Vein to Lower Vein with Autologous Arterial Tissue, Open Approach

061D0JY Bypass Left Common Iliac Vein to Lower Vein with Synthetic Substitute, Open Approach

061D0KY Bypass Left Common Iliac Vein to Lower Vein with Nonautologous Tissue Substitute, Open Approach

061D0ZY Bypass Left Common Iliac Vein to Lower Vein, Open Approach

061D47Y Bypass Left Common Iliac Vein to Lower Vein with Autologous Tissue Substitute, Percutaneous Endoscopic Approach

061D49Y Bypass Left Common Iliac Vein to Lower Vein with Autologous Venous Tissue, Percutaneous Endoscopic Approach

061D4AY Bypass Left Common Iliac Vein to Lower Vein with Autologous Arterial Tissue, Percutaneous Endoscopic Approach

061D4JY Bypass Left Common Iliac Vein to Lower Vein with Synthetic Substitute, Percutaneous Endoscopic Approach

061D4KY Bypass Left Common Iliac Vein to Lower Vein with Nonautologous Tissue Substitute, Percutaneous Endoscopic Approach

061D4ZY Bypass Left Common Iliac Vein to Lower Vein, Percutaneous Endoscopic Approach

061F07Y Bypass Right External Iliac Vein to Lower Vein with Autologous Tissue Substitute, Open Approach

061F09Y Bypass Right External Iliac Vein to Lower Vein with Autologous Venous Tissue, Open Approach

061F0AY Bypass Right External Iliac Vein to Lower Vein with Autologous Arterial Tissue, Open Approach

061F0JY Bypass Right External Iliac Vein to Lower Vein with Synthetic Substitute, Open Approach

061F0KY Bypass Right External Iliac Vein to Lower Vein with Nonautologous Tissue Substitute, Open Approach

061F0ZY Bypass Right External Iliac Vein to Lower Vein, Open Approach

061F47Y Bypass Right External Iliac Vein to Lower Vein with Autologous Tissue Substitute, Percutaneous Endoscopic Approach

061F49Y Bypass Right External Iliac Vein to Lower Vein with Autologous Venous Tissue, Percutaneous Endoscopic Approach

061F4AY Bypass Right External Iliac Vein to Lower Vein with Autologous Arterial Tissue, Percutaneous Endoscopic Approach

061F4JY Bypass Right External Iliac Vein to Lower Vein with Synthetic Substitute, Percutaneous Endoscopic Approach

061F4KY Bypass Right External Iliac Vein to Lower Vein with Nonautologous Tissue Substitute, Percutaneous Endoscopic Approach

061F4ZY Bypass Right External Iliac Vein to Lower Vein, Percutaneous Endoscopic Approach

061G07Y Bypass Left External Iliac Vein to Lower Vein with Autologous Tissue Substitute, Open Approach

061G09Y Bypass Left External Iliac Vein to Lower Vein with Autologous Venous Tissue, Open Approach

061G0AY Bypass Left External Iliac Vein to Lower Vein with Autologous Arterial Tissue, Open Approach

061G0JY Bypass Left External Iliac Vein to Lower Vein with Synthetic Substitute, Open Approach

061G0KY Bypass Left External Iliac Vein to Lower Vein with Nonautologous Tissue Substitute, Open Approach

061G0ZY Bypass Left External Iliac Vein to Lower Vein, Open Approach

061G47Y Bypass Left External Iliac Vein to Lower Vein with Autologous Tissue Substitute, Percutaneous Endoscopic Approach

061G49Y Bypass Left External Iliac Vein to Lower Vein with Autologous Venous Tissue, Percutaneous Endoscopic Approach

061G4AY Bypass Left External Iliac Vein to Lower Vein with Autologous Arterial Tissue, Percutaneous Endoscopic Approach

061G4JY Bypass Left External Iliac Vein to Lower Vein with Synthetic Substitute, Percutaneous Endoscopic Approach

061G4KY Bypass Left External Iliac Vein to Lower Vein with Nonautologous Tissue Substitute, Percutaneous Endoscopic Approach

061G4ZY Bypass Left External Iliac Vein to Lower Vein, Percutaneous Endoscopic Approach

061H07Y Bypass Right Hypogastric Vein to Lower Vein with Autologous Tissue Substitute, Open Approach

061H09Y Bypass Right Hypogastric Vein to Lower Vein with Autologous Venous Tissue, Open Approach

061H0AY Bypass Right Hypogastric Vein to Lower Vein with Autologous Arterial Tissue, Open Approach

061H0JY Bypass Right Hypogastric Vein to Lower Vein with Synthetic Substitute, Open Approach

♀ Female-only   ♂ Male-only   ▲ Limited Coverage   ● Non-OR   ▦ HAC-associated procedure   ▲ Non-covered procedures   ✛ Combination

061H0KY Bypass Right Hypogastric Vein to Lower Vein with Nonautologous Tissue Substitute, Open Approach

061H0ZY Bypass Right Hypogastric Vein to Lower Vein, Open Approach

061H47Y Bypass Right Hypogastric Vein to Lower Vein with Autologous Tissue Substitute, Percutaneous Endoscopic Approach

061H49Y Bypass Right Hypogastric Vein to Lower Vein with Autologous Venous Tissue, Percutaneous Endoscopic Approach

061H4AY Bypass Right Hypogastric Vein to Lower Vein with Autologous Arterial Tissue, Percutaneous Endoscopic Approach

061H4JY Bypass Right Hypogastric Vein to Lower Vein with Synthetic Substitute, Percutaneous Endoscopic Approach

061H4KY Bypass Right Hypogastric Vein to Lower Vein with Nonautologous Tissue Substitute, Percutaneous Endoscopic Approach

061H4ZY Bypass Right Hypogastric Vein to Lower Vein, Percutaneous Endoscopic Approach

061J07Y Bypass Left Hypogastric Vein to Lower Vein with Autologous Tissue Substitute, Open Approach

061J09Y Bypass Left Hypogastric Vein to Lower Vein with Autologous Venous Tissue, Open Approach

061J0AY Bypass Left Hypogastric Vein to Lower Vein with Autologous Arterial Tissue, Open Approach

061J0JY Bypass Left Hypogastric Vein to Lower Vein with Synthetic Substitute, Open Approach

061J0KY Bypass Left Hypogastric Vein to Lower Vein with Nonautologous Tissue Substitute, Open Approach

061J0ZY Bypass Left Hypogastric Vein to Lower Vein, Open Approach

061J47Y Bypass Left Hypogastric Vein to Lower Vein with Autologous Tissue Substitute, Percutaneous Endoscopic Approach

061J49Y Bypass Left Hypogastric Vein to Lower Vein with Autologous Venous Tissue, Percutaneous Endoscopic Approach

061J4AY Bypass Left Hypogastric Vein to Lower Vein with Autologous Arterial Tissue, Percutaneous Endoscopic Approach

061J4JY Bypass Left Hypogastric Vein to Lower Vein with Synthetic Substitute, Percutaneous Endoscopic Approach

061J4KY Bypass Left Hypogastric Vein to Lower Vein with Nonautologous Tissue Substitute, Percutaneous Endoscopic Approach

061J4ZY Bypass Left Hypogastric Vein to Lower Vein, Percutaneous Endoscopic Approach

061M07Y Bypass Right Femoral Vein to Lower Vein with Autologous Tissue Substitute, Open Approach

061M09Y Bypass Right Femoral Vein to Lower Vein with Autologous Venous Tissue, Open Approach

061M0AY Bypass Right Femoral Vein to Lower Vein with Autologous Arterial Tissue, Open Approach

061M0JY Bypass Right Femoral Vein to Lower Vein with Synthetic Substitute, Open Approach

061M0KY Bypass Right Femoral Vein to Lower Vein with Nonautologous Tissue Substitute, Open Approach

061M0ZY Bypass Right Femoral Vein to Lower Vein, Open Approach

061M47Y Bypass Right Femoral Vein to Lower Vein with Autologous Tissue Substitute, Percutaneous Endoscopic Approach

061M49Y Bypass Right Femoral Vein to Lower Vein with Autologous Venous Tissue, Percutaneous Endoscopic Approach

061M4AY Bypass Right Femoral Vein to Lower Vein with Autologous Arterial Tissue, Percutaneous Endoscopic Approach

061M4JY Bypass Right Femoral Vein to Lower Vein with Synthetic Substitute, Percutaneous Endoscopic Approach

061M4KY Bypass Right Femoral Vein to Lower Vein with Nonautologous Tissue Substitute, Percutaneous Endoscopic Approach

061M4ZY Bypass Right Femoral Vein to Lower Vein, Percutaneous Endoscopic Approach

061N07Y Bypass Left Femoral Vein to Lower Vein with Autologous Tissue Substitute, Open Approach

061N09Y Bypass Left Femoral Vein to Lower Vein with Autologous Venous Tissue, Open Approach

061N0AY Bypass Left Femoral Vein to Lower Vein with Autologous Arterial Tissue, Open Approach

061N0JY Bypass Left Femoral Vein to Lower Vein with Synthetic Substitute, Open Approach

061N0KY Bypass Left Femoral Vein to Lower Vein with Nonautologous Tissue Substitute, Open Approach

061N0ZY Bypass Left Femoral Vein to Lower Vein, Open Approach

061N47Y Bypass Left Femoral Vein to Lower Vein with Autologous Tissue Substitute, Percutaneous Endoscopic Approach

061N49Y Bypass Left Femoral Vein to Lower Vein with Autologous Venous Tissue, Percutaneous Endoscopic Approach

061N4AY Bypass Left Femoral Vein to Lower Vein with Autologous Arterial Tissue, Percutaneous Endoscopic Approach

061N4JY Bypass Left Femoral Vein to Lower Vein with Synthetic Substitute, Percutaneous Endoscopic Approach

061N4KY Bypass Left Femoral Vein to Lower Vein with Nonautologous Tissue Substitute, Percutaneous Endoscopic Approach

061N4ZY Bypass Left Femoral Vein to Lower Vein, Percutaneous Endoscopic Approach

061P07Y Bypass Right Greater Saphenous Vein to Lower Vein with Autologous Tissue Substitute, Open Approach

061P09Y Bypass Right Greater Saphenous Vein to Lower Vein with Autologous Venous Tissue, Open Approach

061P0AY Bypass Right Greater Saphenous Vein to Lower Vein with Autologous Arterial Tissue, Open Approach

061P0JY Bypass Right Greater Saphenous Vein to Lower Vein with Synthetic Substitute, Open Approach

061P0KY Bypass Right Greater Saphenous Vein to Lower Vein with Nonautologous Tissue Substitute, Open Approach

061P0ZY Bypass Right Greater Saphenous Vein to Lower Vein, Open Approach

061P47Y Bypass Right Greater Saphenous Vein to Lower Vein with Autologous Tissue Substitute, Percutaneous Endoscopic Approach

061P49Y Bypass Right Greater Saphenous Vein to Lower Vein with Autologous Venous Tissue, Percutaneous Endoscopic Approach

061P4AY Bypass Right Greater Saphenous Vein to Lower Vein with Autologous Arterial Tissue, Percutaneous Endoscopic Approach

061P4JY Bypass Right Greater Saphenous Vein to Lower Vein with Synthetic Substitute, Percutaneous Endoscopic Approach

061P4KY Bypass Right Greater Saphenous Vein to Lower Vein with Nonautologous Tissue Substitute, Percutaneous Endoscopic Approach

061P4ZY Bypass Right Greater Saphenous Vein to Lower Vein, Percutaneous Endoscopic Approach

061Q07Y Bypass Left Greater Saphenous Vein to Lower Vein with Autologous Tissue Substitute, Open Approach

061Q09Y Bypass Left Greater Saphenous Vein to Lower Vein with Autologous Venous Tissue, Open Approach

061Q0AY Bypass Left Greater Saphenous Vein to Lower Vein with Autologous Arterial Tissue, Open Approach

061Q0JY Bypass Left Greater Saphenous Vein to Lower Vein with Synthetic Substitute, Open Approach

061Q0KY Bypass Left Greater Saphenous Vein to Lower Vein with Nonautologous Tissue Substitute, Open Approach

061Q0ZY Bypass Left Greater Saphenous Vein to Lower Vein, Open Approach

061Q47Y Bypass Left Greater Saphenous Vein to Lower Vein with Autologous Tissue Substitute, Percutaneous Endoscopic Approach

061Q49Y Bypass Left Greater Saphenous Vein to Lower Vein with Autologous Venous Tissue, Percutaneous Endoscopic Approach

061Q4AY Bypass Left Greater Saphenous Vein to Lower Vein with Autologous Arterial Tissue, Percutaneous Endoscopic Approach

061Q4JY Bypass Left Greater Saphenous Vein to Lower Vein with Synthetic Substitute, Percutaneous Endoscopic Approach

061Q4KY Bypass Left Greater Saphenous Vein to Lower Vein with Nonautologous Tissue Substitute, Percutaneous Endoscopic Approach

061Q4ZY Bypass Left Greater Saphenous Vein to Lower Vein, Percutaneous Endoscopic Approach

061R07Y Bypass Right Lesser Saphenous Vein to Lower Vein with Autologous Tissue Substitute, Open Approach

061R09Y Bypass Right Lesser Saphenous Vein to Lower Vein with Autologous Venous Tissue, Open Approach

061R0AY Bypass Right Lesser Saphenous Vein to Lower Vein with Autologous Arterial Tissue, Open Approach

061R0JY Bypass Right Lesser Saphenous Vein to Lower Vein with Synthetic Substitute, Open Approach

061R0KY Bypass Right Lesser Saphenous Vein to Lower Vein with Nonautologous Tissue Substitute, Open Approach

061R0ZY Bypass Right Lesser Saphenous Vein to Lower Vein, Open Approach

061R47Y Bypass Right Lesser Saphenous Vein to Lower Vein with Autologous Tissue Substitute, Percutaneous Endoscopic Approach

061R49Y Bypass Right Lesser Saphenous Vein to Lower Vein with Autologous Venous Tissue, Percutaneous Endoscopic Approach

061R4AY Bypass Right Lesser Saphenous Vein to Lower Vein with Autologous Arterial Tissue, Percutaneous Endoscopic Approach

061R4JY Bypass Right Lesser Saphenous Vein to Lower Vein with Synthetic Substitute, Percutaneous Endoscopic Approach

♀ Female-only   ♂ Male-only   ▲ Limited Coverage   ● Non-OR   ▬ HAC-associated procedure   ▲ Non-covered procedures   + Combinati

R4KY	Bypass Right Lesser Saphenous Vein to Lower Vein with Nonautologous Tissue Substitute, Percutaneous Endoscopic Approach
R4ZY	Bypass Right Lesser Saphenous Vein to Lower Vein, Percutaneous Endoscopic Approach
S07Y	Bypass Left Lesser Saphenous Vein to Lower Vein with Autologous Tissue Substitute, Open Approach
S09Y	Bypass Left Lesser Saphenous Vein to Lower Vein with Autologous Venous Tissue, Open Approach
S0AY	Bypass Left Lesser Saphenous Vein to Lower Vein with Autologous Arterial Tissue, Open Approach
S0JY	Bypass Left Lesser Saphenous Vein to Lower Vein with Synthetic Substitute, Open Approach
S0KY	Bypass Left Lesser Saphenous Vein to Lower Vein with Nonautologous Tissue Substitute, Open Approach
S0ZY	Bypass Left Lesser Saphenous Vein to Lower Vein, Open Approach
S47Y	Bypass Left Lesser Saphenous Vein to Lower Vein with Autologous Tissue Substitute, Percutaneous Endoscopic Approach
S49Y	Bypass Left Lesser Saphenous Vein to Lower Vein with Autologous Venous Tissue, Percutaneous Endoscopic Approach
S4AY	Bypass Left Lesser Saphenous Vein to Lower Vein with Autologous Arterial Tissue, Percutaneous Endoscopic Approach
S4JY	Bypass Left Lesser Saphenous Vein to Lower Vein with Synthetic Substitute, Percutaneous Endoscopic Approach

061S4KY	Bypass Left Lesser Saphenous Vein to Lower Vein with Nonautologous Tissue Substitute, Percutaneous Endoscopic Approach
061S4ZY	Bypass Left Lesser Saphenous Vein to Lower Vein, Percutaneous Endoscopic Approach
061T07Y	Bypass Right Foot Vein to Lower Vein with Autologous Tissue Substitute, Open Approach
061T09Y	Bypass Right Foot Vein to Lower Vein with Autologous Venous Tissue, Open Approach
061T0AY	Bypass Right Foot Vein to Lower Vein with Autologous Arterial Tissue, Open Approach
061T0JY	Bypass Right Foot Vein to Lower Vein with Synthetic Substitute, Open Approach
061T0KY	Bypass Right Foot Vein to Lower Vein with Nonautologous Tissue Substitute, Open Approach
061T0ZY	Bypass Right Foot Vein to Lower Vein, Open Approach
061T47Y	Bypass Right Foot Vein to Lower Vein with Autologous Tissue Substitute, Percutaneous Endoscopic Approach
061T49Y	Bypass Right Foot Vein to Lower Vein with Autologous Venous Tissue, Percutaneous Endoscopic Approach
061T4AY	Bypass Right Foot Vein to Lower Vein with Autologous Arterial Tissue, Percutaneous Endoscopic Approach
061T4JY	Bypass Right Foot Vein to Lower Vein with Synthetic Substitute, Percutaneous Endoscopic Approach
061T4KY	Bypass Right Foot Vein to Lower Vein with Nonautologous Tissue Substitute, Percutaneous Endoscopic Approach

061T4ZY	Bypass Right Foot Vein to Lower Vein, Percutaneous Endoscopic Approach
061V07Y	Bypass Left Foot Vein to Lower Vein with Autologous Tissue Substitute, Open Approach
061V09Y	Bypass Left Foot Vein to Lower Vein with Autologous Venous Tissue, Open Approach
061V0AY	Bypass Left Foot Vein to Lower Vein with Autologous Arterial Tissue, Open Approach
061V0JY	Bypass Left Foot Vein to Lower Vein with Synthetic Substitute, Open Approach
061V0KY	Bypass Left Foot Vein to Lower Vein with Nonautologous Tissue Substitute, Open Approach
061V0ZY	Bypass Left Foot Vein to Lower Vein, Open Approach
061V47Y	Bypass Left Foot Vein to Lower Vein with Autologous Tissue Substitute, Percutaneous Endoscopic Approach
061V49Y	Bypass Left Foot Vein to Lower Vein with Autologous Venous Tissue, Percutaneous Endoscopic Approach
061V4AY	Bypass Left Foot Vein to Lower Vein with Autologous Arterial Tissue, Percutaneous Endoscopic Approach
061V4JY	Bypass Left Foot Vein to Lower Vein with Synthetic Substitute, Percutaneous Endoscopic Approach
061V4KY	Bypass Left Foot Vein to Lower Vein with Nonautologous Tissue Substitute, Percutaneous Endoscopic Approach
061V4ZY	Bypass Left Foot Vein to Lower Vein, Percutaneous Endoscopic Approach

65 – Lower Veins, Destruction

500ZZ	Destruction of Inferior Vena Cava, Open Approach
503ZZ	Destruction of Inferior Vena Cava, Percutaneous Approach
504ZZ	Destruction of Inferior Vena Cava, Percutaneous Endoscopic Approach
510ZZ	Destruction of Splenic Vein, Open Approach
513ZZ	Destruction of Splenic Vein, Percutaneous Approach
514ZZ	Destruction of Splenic Vein, Percutaneous Endoscopic Approach
520ZZ	Destruction of Gastric Vein, Open Approach
523ZZ	Destruction of Gastric Vein, Percutaneous Approach
524ZZ	Destruction of Gastric Vein, Percutaneous Endoscopic Approach
530ZZ	Destruction of Esophageal Vein, Open Approach
533ZZ	Destruction of Esophageal Vein, Percutaneous Approach
534ZZ	Destruction of Esophageal Vein, Percutaneous Endoscopic Approach
540ZZ	Destruction of Hepatic Vein, Open Approach
543ZZ	Destruction of Hepatic Vein, Percutaneous Approach
544ZZ	Destruction of Hepatic Vein, Percutaneous Endoscopic Approach
550ZZ	Destruction of Superior Mesenteric Vein, Open Approach
553ZZ	Destruction of Superior Mesenteric Vein, Percutaneous Approach
554ZZ	Destruction of Superior Mesenteric Vein, Percutaneous Endoscopic Approach

06560ZZ	Destruction of Inferior Mesenteric Vein, Open Approach
06563ZZ	Destruction of Inferior Mesenteric Vein, Percutaneous Approach
06564ZZ	Destruction of Inferior Mesenteric Vein, Percutaneous Endoscopic Approach
06570ZZ	Destruction of Colic Vein, Open Approach
06573ZZ	Destruction of Colic Vein, Percutaneous Approach
06574ZZ	Destruction of Colic Vein, Percutaneous Endoscopic Approach
06580ZZ	Destruction of Portal Vein, Open Approach
06583ZZ	Destruction of Portal Vein, Percutaneous Approach
06584ZZ	Destruction of Portal Vein, Percutaneous Endoscopic Approach
06590ZZ	Destruction of Right Renal Vein, Open Approach
06593ZZ	Destruction of Right Renal Vein, Percutaneous Approach
06594ZZ	Destruction of Right Renal Vein, Percutaneous Endoscopic Approach
065B0ZZ	Destruction of Left Renal Vein, Open Approach
065B3ZZ	Destruction of Left Renal Vein, Percutaneous Approach
065B4ZZ	Destruction of Left Renal Vein, Percutaneous Endoscopic Approach
065C0ZZ	Destruction of Right Common Iliac Vein, Open Approach
065C3ZZ	Destruction of Right Common Iliac Vein, Percutaneous Approach
065C4ZZ	Destruction of Right Common Iliac Vein, Percutaneous Endoscopic Approach
065D0ZZ	Destruction of Left Common Iliac Vein, Open Approach

065D3ZZ	Destruction of Left Common Iliac Vein, Percutaneous Approach
065D4ZZ	Destruction of Left Common Iliac Vein, Percutaneous Endoscopic Approach
065F0ZZ	Destruction of Right External Iliac Vein, Open Approach
065F3ZZ	Destruction of Right External Iliac Vein, Percutaneous Approach
065F4ZZ	Destruction of Right External Iliac Vein, Percutaneous Endoscopic Approach
065G0ZZ	Destruction of Left External Iliac Vein, Open Approach
065G3ZZ	Destruction of Left External Iliac Vein, Percutaneous Approach
065G4ZZ	Destruction of Left External Iliac Vein, Percutaneous Endoscopic Approach
065H0ZZ	Destruction of Right Hypogastric Vein, Open Approach
065H3ZZ	Destruction of Right Hypogastric Vein, Percutaneous Approach
065H4ZZ	Destruction of Right Hypogastric Vein, Percutaneous Endoscopic Approach
065J0ZZ	Destruction of Left Hypogastric Vein, Open Approach
065J3ZZ	Destruction of Left Hypogastric Vein, Percutaneous Approach
065J4ZZ	Destruction of Left Hypogastric Vein, Percutaneous Endoscopic Approach
065M0ZZ	Destruction of Right Femoral Vein, Open Approach
065M3ZZ	Destruction of Right Femoral Vein, Percutaneous Approach
065M4ZZ	Destruction of Right Femoral Vein, Percutaneous Endoscopic Approach
065N0ZZ	Destruction of Left Femoral Vein, Open Approach

Female-only	♂ Male-only	▲ Limited Coverage	● Non-OR	▨ HAC-associated procedure	▲ Non-covered procedures	✚ Combination

065N3ZZ	Destruction of Left Femoral Vein, Percutaneous Approach	065R3ZZ	Destruction of Right Lesser Saphenous Vein, Percutaneous Approach	065V3ZZ	Destruction of Left Foot Vein, Percutaneous Approach
065N4ZZ	Destruction of Left Femoral Vein, Percutaneous Endoscopic Approach	065R4ZZ	Destruction of Right Lesser Saphenous Vein, Percutaneous Endoscopic Approach	065V4ZZ	Destruction of Left Foot Vein, Percutaneous Endoscopic Approach
065P0ZZ	Destruction of Right Greater Saphenous Vein, Open Approach	065S0ZZ	Destruction of Left Lesser Saphenous Vein, Open Approach	065Y0ZC	Destruction of Hemorrhoidal Plexus, Open Approach
065P3ZZ	Destruction of Right Greater Saphenous Vein, Percutaneous Approach	065S3ZZ	Destruction of Left Lesser Saphenous Vein, Percutaneous Approach	065Y0ZZ	Destruction of Lower Vein, Open Approach
065P4ZZ	Destruction of Right Greater Saphenous Vein, Percutaneous Endoscopic Approach	065S4ZZ	Destruction of Left Lesser Saphenous Vein, Percutaneous Endoscopic Approach	065Y3ZC	Destruction of Hemorrhoidal Plexus, Percutaneous Approach
065Q0ZZ	Destruction of Left Greater Saphenous Vein, Open Approach	065T0ZZ	Destruction of Right Foot Vein, Open Approach	065Y3ZZ	Destruction of Lower Vein, Percutaneous Approach
065Q3ZZ	Destruction of Left Greater Saphenous Vein, Percutaneous Approach	065T3ZZ	Destruction of Right Foot Vein, Percutaneous Approach	065Y4ZC	Destruction of Hemorrhoidal Plexus, Percutaneous Endoscopic Approach
065Q4ZZ	Destruction of Left Greater Saphenous Vein, Percutaneous Endoscopic Approach	065T4ZZ	Destruction of Right Foot Vein, Percutaneous Endoscopic Approach	065Y4ZZ	Destruction of Lower Vein, Percutaneous Endoscopic Approach
065R0ZZ	Destruction of Right Lesser Saphenous Vein, Open Approach	065V0ZZ	Destruction of Left Foot Vein, Open Approach		

067 – Lower Veins, Dilation

06700DZ	Dilation of Inferior Vena Cava with Intraluminal Device, Open Approach	06743DZ	Dilation of Hepatic Vein with Intraluminal Device, Percutaneous Approach	06784DZ	Dilation of Portal Vein with Intraluminal Device, Percutaneous Endoscopic Approach
06700ZZ	Dilation of Inferior Vena Cava, Open Approach	06743ZZ	Dilation of Hepatic Vein, Percutaneous Approach	06784ZZ	Dilation of Portal Vein, Percutaneous Endoscopic Approach
06703DZ	Dilation of Inferior Vena Cava with Intraluminal Device, Percutaneous Approach	06744DZ	Dilation of Hepatic Vein with Intraluminal Device, Percutaneous Endoscopic Approach	06790DZ	Dilation of Right Renal Vein with Intraluminal Device, Open Approach
06703ZZ	Dilation of Inferior Vena Cava, Percutaneous Approach	06744ZZ	Dilation of Hepatic Vein, Percutaneous Endoscopic Approach	06790ZZ	Dilation of Right Renal Vein, Open Approach
06704DZ	Dilation of Inferior Vena Cava with Intraluminal Device, Percutaneous Endoscopic Approach	06750DZ	Dilation of Superior Mesenteric Vein with Intraluminal Device, Open Approach	06793DZ	Dilation of Right Renal Vein with Intraluminal Device, Percutaneous Approach
06704ZZ	Dilation of Inferior Vena Cava, Percutaneous Endoscopic Approach	06750ZZ	Dilation of Superior Mesenteric Vein, Open Approach	06793ZZ	Dilation of Right Renal Vein, Percutaneous Approach
06710DZ	Dilation of Splenic Vein with Intraluminal Device, Open Approach	06753DZ	Dilation of Superior Mesenteric Vein with Intraluminal Device, Percutaneous Approach	06794DZ	Dilation of Right Renal Vein with Intraluminal Device, Percutaneous Endoscopic Approach
06710ZZ	Dilation of Splenic Vein, Open Approach	06753ZZ	Dilation of Superior Mesenteric Vein, Percutaneous Approach	06794ZZ	Dilation of Right Renal Vein, Percutaneous Endoscopic Approach
06713DZ	Dilation of Splenic Vein with Intraluminal Device, Percutaneous Approach	06754DZ	Dilation of Superior Mesenteric Vein with Intraluminal Device, Percutaneous Endoscopic Approach	067B0DZ	Dilation of Left Renal Vein with Intraluminal Device, Open Approach
06713ZZ	Dilation of Splenic Vein, Percutaneous Approach	06754ZZ	Dilation of Superior Mesenteric Vein, Percutaneous Endoscopic Approach	067B0ZZ	Dilation of Left Renal Vein, Open Approach
06714DZ	Dilation of Splenic Vein with Intraluminal Device, Percutaneous Endoscopic Approach	06760DZ	Dilation of Inferior Mesenteric Vein with Intraluminal Device, Open Approach	067B3DZ	Dilation of Left Renal Vein with Intraluminal Device, Percutaneous Approach
06714ZZ	Dilation of Splenic Vein, Percutaneous Endoscopic Approach	06760ZZ	Dilation of Inferior Mesenteric Vein, Open Approach	067B3ZZ	Dilation of Left Renal Vein, Percutaneous Approach
06720DZ	Dilation of Gastric Vein with Intraluminal Device, Open Approach	06763DZ	Dilation of Inferior Mesenteric Vein with Intraluminal Device, Percutaneous Approach	067B4DZ	Dilation of Left Renal Vein with Intraluminal Device, Percutaneous Endoscopic Approach
06720ZZ	Dilation of Gastric Vein, Open Approach	06763ZZ	Dilation of Inferior Mesenteric Vein, Percutaneous Approach	067B4ZZ	Dilation of Left Renal Vein, Percutaneous Endoscopic Approach
06723DZ	Dilation of Gastric Vein with Intraluminal Device, Percutaneous Approach	06764DZ	Dilation of Inferior Mesenteric Vein with Intraluminal Device, Percutaneous Endoscopic Approach	067C0DZ	Dilation of Right Common Iliac Vein with Intraluminal Device, Open Approach
06723ZZ	Dilation of Gastric Vein, Percutaneous Approach	06764ZZ	Dilation of Inferior Mesenteric Vein, Percutaneous Endoscopic Approach	067C0ZZ	Dilation of Right Common Iliac Vein, Open Approach
06724DZ	Dilation of Gastric Vein with Intraluminal Device, Percutaneous Endoscopic Approach	06770DZ	Dilation of Colic Vein with Intraluminal Device, Open Approach	067C3DZ	Dilation of Right Common Iliac Vein with Intraluminal Device, Percutaneous Approach
06724ZZ	Dilation of Gastric Vein, Percutaneous Endoscopic Approach	06770ZZ	Dilation of Colic Vein, Open Approach	067C3ZZ	Dilation of Right Common Iliac Vein, Percutaneous Approach
06730DZ	Dilation of Esophageal Vein with Intraluminal Device, Open Approach	06773DZ	Dilation of Colic Vein with Intraluminal Device, Percutaneous Approach	067C4DZ	Dilation of Right Common Iliac Vein with Intraluminal Device, Percutaneous Endoscopic Approach
06730ZZ	Dilation of Esophageal Vein, Open Approach	06773ZZ	Dilation of Colic Vein, Percutaneous Approach	067C4ZZ	Dilation of Right Common Iliac Vein, Percutaneous Endoscopic Approach
06733DZ	Dilation of Esophageal Vein with Intraluminal Device, Percutaneous Approach	06774DZ	Dilation of Colic Vein with Intraluminal Device, Percutaneous Endoscopic Approach	067D0DZ	Dilation of Left Common Iliac Vein with Intraluminal Device, Open Approach
06733ZZ	Dilation of Esophageal Vein, Percutaneous Approach	06774ZZ	Dilation of Colic Vein, Percutaneous Endoscopic Approach	067D0ZZ	Dilation of Left Common Iliac Vein, Open Approach
06734DZ	Dilation of Esophageal Vein with Intraluminal Device, Percutaneous Endoscopic Approach	06780DZ	Dilation of Portal Vein with Intraluminal Device, Open Approach	067D3DZ	Dilation of Left Common Iliac Vein with Intraluminal Device, Percutaneous Approach
06734ZZ	Dilation of Esophageal Vein, Percutaneous Endoscopic Approach	06780ZZ	Dilation of Portal Vein, Open Approach	067D3ZZ	Dilation of Left Common Iliac Vein, Percutaneous Approach
06740DZ	Dilation of Hepatic Vein with Intraluminal Device, Open Approach	06783DZ	Dilation of Portal Vein with Intraluminal Device, Percutaneous Approach		
06740ZZ	Dilation of Hepatic Vein, Open Approach	06783ZZ	Dilation of Portal Vein, Percutaneous Approach		

♀ Female-only   ♂ Male-only   ▲ Limited Coverage   ● Non-OR   ▇ HAC-associated procedure   ▲ Non-covered procedures   ✚ Combination

▸4DZ	Dilation of Left Common Iliac Vein with Intraluminal Device, Percutaneous Endoscopic Approach
▸4ZZ	Dilation of Left Common Iliac Vein, Percutaneous Endoscopic Approach
▸0DZ	Dilation of Right External Iliac Vein with Intraluminal Device, Open Approach
▸0ZZ	Dilation of Right External Iliac Vein, Open Approach
▸3DZ	Dilation of Right External Iliac Vein with Intraluminal Device, Percutaneous Approach
▸3ZZ	Dilation of Right External Iliac Vein, Percutaneous Approach
▸4DZ	Dilation of Right External Iliac Vein with Intraluminal Device, Percutaneous Endoscopic Approach
▸4ZZ	Dilation of Right External Iliac Vein, Percutaneous Endoscopic Approach
▸0DZ	Dilation of Left External Iliac Vein with Intraluminal Device, Open Approach
▸0ZZ	Dilation of Left External Iliac Vein, Open Approach
▸3DZ	Dilation of Left External Iliac Vein with Intraluminal Device, Percutaneous Approach
▸3ZZ	Dilation of Left External Iliac Vein, Percutaneous Approach
▸4DZ	Dilation of Left External Iliac Vein with Intraluminal Device, Percutaneous Endoscopic Approach
▸4ZZ	Dilation of Left External Iliac Vein, Percutaneous Endoscopic Approach
▸0DZ	Dilation of Right Hypogastric Vein with Intraluminal Device, Open Approach
▸0ZZ	Dilation of Right Hypogastric Vein, Open Approach
▸3DZ	Dilation of Right Hypogastric Vein with Intraluminal Device, Percutaneous Approach
▸3ZZ	Dilation of Right Hypogastric Vein, Percutaneous Approach
▸4DZ	Dilation of Right Hypogastric Vein with Intraluminal Device, Percutaneous Endoscopic Approach
▸4ZZ	Dilation of Right Hypogastric Vein, Percutaneous Endoscopic Approach
▸0DZ	Dilation of Left Hypogastric Vein with Intraluminal Device, Open Approach
▸0ZZ	Dilation of Left Hypogastric Vein, Open Approach
▸3DZ	Dilation of Left Hypogastric Vein with Intraluminal Device, Percutaneous Approach
▸3ZZ	Dilation of Left Hypogastric Vein, Percutaneous Approach
▸4DZ	Dilation of Left Hypogastric Vein with Intraluminal Device, Percutaneous Endoscopic Approach
▸4ZZ	Dilation of Left Hypogastric Vein, Percutaneous Endoscopic Approach
▸M0DZ	Dilation of Right Femoral Vein with Intraluminal Device, Open Approach

067M0ZZ	Dilation of Right Femoral Vein, Open Approach
067M3DZ	Dilation of Right Femoral Vein with Intraluminal Device, Percutaneous Approach
067M3ZZ	Dilation of Right Femoral Vein, Percutaneous Approach
067M4DZ	Dilation of Right Femoral Vein with Intraluminal Device, Percutaneous Endoscopic Approach
067M4ZZ	Dilation of Right Femoral Vein, Percutaneous Endoscopic Approach
067N0DZ	Dilation of Left Femoral Vein with Intraluminal Device, Open Approach
067N0ZZ	Dilation of Left Femoral Vein, Open Approach
067N3DZ	Dilation of Left Femoral Vein with Intraluminal Device, Percutaneous Approach
067N3ZZ	Dilation of Left Femoral Vein, Percutaneous Approach
067N4DZ	Dilation of Left Femoral Vein with Intraluminal Device, Percutaneous Endoscopic Approach
067N4ZZ	Dilation of Left Femoral Vein, Percutaneous Endoscopic Approach
067P0DZ	Dilation of Right Greater Saphenous Vein with Intraluminal Device, Open Approach
067P0ZZ	Dilation of Right Greater Saphenous Vein, Open Approach
067P3DZ	Dilation of Right Greater Saphenous Vein with Intraluminal Device, Percutaneous Approach
067P3ZZ	Dilation of Right Greater Saphenous Vein, Percutaneous Approach
067P4DZ	Dilation of Right Greater Saphenous Vein with Intraluminal Device, Percutaneous Endoscopic Approach
067P4ZZ	Dilation of Right Greater Saphenous Vein, Percutaneous Endoscopic Approach
067Q0DZ	Dilation of Left Greater Saphenous Vein with Intraluminal Device, Open Approach
067Q0ZZ	Dilation of Left Greater Saphenous Vein, Open Approach
067Q3DZ	Dilation of Left Greater Saphenous Vein with Intraluminal Device, Percutaneous Approach
067Q3ZZ	Dilation of Left Greater Saphenous Vein, Percutaneous Approach
067Q4DZ	Dilation of Left Greater Saphenous Vein with Intraluminal Device, Percutaneous Endoscopic Approach
067Q4ZZ	Dilation of Left Greater Saphenous Vein, Percutaneous Endoscopic Approach
067R0DZ	Dilation of Right Lesser Saphenous Vein with Intraluminal Device, Open Approach
067R0ZZ	Dilation of Right Lesser Saphenous Vein, Open Approach

067R3DZ	Dilation of Right Lesser Saphenous Vein with Intraluminal Device, Percutaneous Approach
067R3ZZ	Dilation of Right Lesser Saphenous Vein, Percutaneous Approach
067R4DZ	Dilation of Right Lesser Saphenous Vein with Intraluminal Device, Percutaneous Endoscopic Approach
067R4ZZ	Dilation of Right Lesser Saphenous Vein, Percutaneous Endoscopic Approach
067S0DZ	Dilation of Left Lesser Saphenous Vein with Intraluminal Device, Open Approach
067S0ZZ	Dilation of Left Lesser Saphenous Vein, Open Approach
067S3DZ	Dilation of Left Lesser Saphenous Vein with Intraluminal Device, Percutaneous Approach
067S3ZZ	Dilation of Left Lesser Saphenous Vein, Percutaneous Approach
067S4DZ	Dilation of Left Lesser Saphenous Vein with Intraluminal Device, Percutaneous Endoscopic Approach
067S4ZZ	Dilation of Left Lesser Saphenous Vein, Percutaneous Endoscopic Approach
067T0DZ	Dilation of Right Foot Vein with Intraluminal Device, Open Approach
067T0ZZ	Dilation of Right Foot Vein, Open Approach
067T3DZ	Dilation of Right Foot Vein with Intraluminal Device, Percutaneous Approach
067T3ZZ	Dilation of Right Foot Vein, Percutaneous Approach
067T4DZ	Dilation of Right Foot Vein with Intraluminal Device, Percutaneous Endoscopic Approach
067T4ZZ	Dilation of Right Foot Vein, Percutaneous Endoscopic Approach
067V0DZ	Dilation of Left Foot Vein with Intraluminal Device, Open Approach
067V0ZZ	Dilation of Left Foot Vein, Open Approach
067V3DZ	Dilation of Left Foot Vein with Intraluminal Device, Percutaneous Approach
067V3ZZ	Dilation of Left Foot Vein, Percutaneous Approach
067V4DZ	Dilation of Left Foot Vein with Intraluminal Device, Percutaneous Endoscopic Approach
067V4ZZ	Dilation of Left Foot Vein, Percutaneous Endoscopic Approach
067Y0DZ	Dilation of Lower Vein with Intraluminal Device, Open Approach
067Y0ZZ	Dilation of Lower Vein, Open Approach
067Y3DZ	Dilation of Lower Vein with Intraluminal Device, Percutaneous Approach
067Y3ZZ	Dilation of Lower Vein, Percutaneous Approach
067Y4DZ	Dilation of Lower Vein with Intraluminal Device, Percutaneous Endoscopic Approach
067Y4ZZ	Dilation of Lower Vein, Percutaneous Endoscopic Approach

9 – Lower Veins, Drainage

view Coding Guidelines B3.4a and B3.4b

view Coding Guideline B6.2

▸000Z	Drainage of Inferior Vena Cava with Drainage Device, Open Approach
▸00ZX	Drainage of Inferior Vena Cava, Open Approach, Diagnostic
▸00ZZ	Drainage of Inferior Vena Cava, Open Approach
▸030Z	Drainage of Inferior Vena Cava with Drainage Device, Percutaneous Approach

06903ZX	Drainage of Inferior Vena Cava, Percutaneous Approach, Diagnostic
06903ZZ	Drainage of Inferior Vena Cava, Percutaneous Approach
069040Z	Drainage of Inferior Vena Cava with Drainage Device, Percutaneous Endoscopic Approach

06904ZX	Drainage of Inferior Vena Cava, Percutaneous Endoscopic Approach, Diagnostic
06904ZZ	Drainage of Inferior Vena Cava, Percutaneous Endoscopic Approach
069100Z	Drainage of Splenic Vein with Drainage Device, Open Approach

♀ Female-only	♂ Male-only	▲ Limited Coverage	● Non-OR	▦ HAC-associated procedure	▲ Non-covered procedures	✚ Combination

Code	Description	Code	Description	Code	Description
06910ZX	Drainage of Splenic Vein, Open Approach, Diagnostic	069530Z	Drainage of Superior Mesenteric Vein with Drainage Device, Percutaneous Approach	06993ZX	Drainage of Right Renal Vein, Percutaneous Approach, Diagnostic
06910ZZ	Drainage of Splenic Vein, Open Approach	06953ZX	Drainage of Superior Mesenteric Vein, Percutaneous Approach, Diagnostic	06993ZZ	Drainage of Right Renal Vein, Percutaneous Approach
069130Z	Drainage of Splenic Vein with Drainage Device, Percutaneous Approach	06953ZZ	Drainage of Superior Mesenteric Vein, Percutaneous Approach	069940Z	Drainage of Right Renal Vein with Drainage Device, Percutaneous Endoscopic Approach
06913ZX	Drainage of Splenic Vein, Percutaneous Approach, Diagnostic	069540Z	Drainage of Superior Mesenteric Vein with Drainage Device, Percutaneous Endoscopic Approach	06994ZX	Drainage of Right Renal Vein, Percutaneous Endoscopic Approach, Diagnostic
06913ZZ	Drainage of Splenic Vein, Percutaneous Approach	06954ZX	Drainage of Superior Mesenteric Vein, Percutaneous Endoscopic Approach, Diagnostic	06994ZZ	Drainage of Right Renal Vein, Percutaneous Endoscopic Approach
069140Z	Drainage of Splenic Vein with Drainage Device, Percutaneous Endoscopic Approach	06954ZZ	Drainage of Superior Mesenteric Vein, Percutaneous Endoscopic Approach	069B00Z	Drainage of Left Renal Vein with Drainage Device, Open Approach
06914ZX	Drainage of Splenic Vein, Percutaneous Endoscopic Approach, Diagnostic	069600Z	Drainage of Inferior Mesenteric Vein with Drainage Device, Open Approach	069B0ZX	Drainage of Left Renal Vein, Open Approach, Diagnostic
06914ZZ	Drainage of Splenic Vein, Percutaneous Endoscopic Approach	06960ZX	Drainage of Inferior Mesenteric Vein, Open Approach, Diagnostic	069B0ZZ	Drainage of Left Renal Vein, Open Approach
069200Z	Drainage of Gastric Vein with Drainage Device, Open Approach	06960ZZ	Drainage of Inferior Mesenteric Vein, Open Approach	069B30Z	Drainage of Left Renal Vein with Drainage Device, Percutaneous Approach
06920ZX	Drainage of Gastric Vein, Open Approach, Diagnostic	069630Z	Drainage of Inferior Mesenteric Vein with Drainage Device, Percutaneous Approach	069B3ZX	Drainage of Left Renal Vein, Percutaneous Approach, Diagnostic
06920ZZ	Drainage of Gastric Vein, Open Approach	06963ZX	Drainage of Inferior Mesenteric Vein, Percutaneous Approach, Diagnostic	069B3ZZ	Drainage of Left Renal Vein, Percutaneous Approach
069230Z	Drainage of Gastric Vein with Drainage Device, Percutaneous Approach	06963ZZ	Drainage of Inferior Mesenteric Vein, Percutaneous Approach	069B40Z	Drainage of Left Renal Vein with Drainage Device, Percutaneous Endoscopic Approach
06923ZX	Drainage of Gastric Vein, Percutaneous Approach, Diagnostic	069640Z	Drainage of Inferior Mesenteric Vein with Drainage Device, Percutaneous Endoscopic Approach	069B4ZX	Drainage of Left Renal Vein, Percutaneous Endoscopic Approach, Diagnostic
06923ZZ	Drainage of Gastric Vein, Percutaneous Approach	06964ZX	Drainage of Inferior Mesenteric Vein, Percutaneous Endoscopic Approach, Diagnostic	069B4ZZ	Drainage of Left Renal Vein, Percutaneous Endoscopic Approach
069240Z	Drainage of Gastric Vein with Drainage Device, Percutaneous Endoscopic Approach	06964ZZ	Drainage of Inferior Mesenteric Vein, Percutaneous Endoscopic Approach	069C00Z	Drainage of Right Common Iliac Vein with Drainage Device, Open Approach
06924ZX	Drainage of Gastric Vein, Percutaneous Endoscopic Approach, Diagnostic	069700Z	Drainage of Colic Vein with Drainage Device, Open Approach	069C0ZX	Drainage of Right Common Iliac Vein, Open Approach, Diagnostic
06924ZZ	Drainage of Gastric Vein, Percutaneous Endoscopic Approach	06970ZX	Drainage of Colic Vein, Open Approach, Diagnostic	069C0ZZ	Drainage of Right Common Iliac Vein, Open Approach
069300Z	Drainage of Esophageal Vein with Drainage Device, Open Approach	06970ZZ	Drainage of Colic Vein, Open Approach	069C30Z	Drainage of Right Common Iliac Vein with Drainage Device, Percutaneous Approach
06930ZX	Drainage of Esophageal Vein, Open Approach, Diagnostic	069730Z	Drainage of Colic Vein with Drainage Device, Percutaneous Approach	069C3ZX	Drainage of Right Common Iliac Vein, Percutaneous Approach, Diagnostic
06930ZZ	Drainage of Esophageal Vein, Open Approach	06973ZX	Drainage of Colic Vein, Percutaneous Approach, Diagnostic	069C3ZZ	Drainage of Right Common Iliac Vein, Percutaneous Approach
069330Z	Drainage of Esophageal Vein with Drainage Device, Percutaneous Approach	06973ZZ	Drainage of Colic Vein, Percutaneous Approach	069C40Z	Drainage of Right Common Iliac Vein with Drainage Device, Percutaneous Endoscopic Approach
06933ZX	Drainage of Esophageal Vein, Percutaneous Approach, Diagnostic	069740Z	Drainage of Colic Vein with Drainage Device, Percutaneous Endoscopic Approach	069C4ZX	Drainage of Right Common Iliac Vein, Percutaneous Endoscopic Approach, Diagnostic
06933ZZ	Drainage of Esophageal Vein, Percutaneous Approach	06974ZX	Drainage of Colic Vein, Percutaneous Endoscopic Approach, Diagnostic	069C4ZZ	Drainage of Right Common Iliac Vein, Percutaneous Endoscopic Approach
069340Z	Drainage of Esophageal Vein with Drainage Device, Percutaneous Endoscopic Approach	06974ZZ	Drainage of Colic Vein, Percutaneous Endoscopic Approach	069D00Z	Drainage of Left Common Iliac Vein with Drainage Device, Open Approach
06934ZX	Drainage of Esophageal Vein, Percutaneous Endoscopic Approach, Diagnostic	069800Z	Drainage of Portal Vein with Drainage Device, Open Approach	069D0ZX	Drainage of Left Common Iliac Vein, Open Approach, Diagnostic
06934ZZ	Drainage of Esophageal Vein, Percutaneous Endoscopic Approach	06980ZX	Drainage of Portal Vein, Open Approach, Diagnostic	069D0ZZ	Drainage of Left Common Iliac Vein, Open Approach
069400Z	Drainage of Hepatic Vein with Drainage Device, Open Approach	06980ZZ	Drainage of Portal Vein, Open Approach	069D30Z	Drainage of Left Common Iliac Vein with Drainage Device, Percutaneous Approach
06940ZX	Drainage of Hepatic Vein, Open Approach, Diagnostic	069830Z	Drainage of Portal Vein with Drainage Device, Percutaneous Approach	069D3ZX	Drainage of Left Common Iliac Vein, Percutaneous Approach, Diagnostic
06940ZZ	Drainage of Hepatic Vein, Open Approach	06983ZX	Drainage of Portal Vein, Percutaneous Approach, Diagnostic	069D3ZZ	Drainage of Left Common Iliac Vein, Percutaneous Approach
069430Z	Drainage of Hepatic Vein with Drainage Device, Percutaneous Approach	06983ZZ	Drainage of Portal Vein, Percutaneous Approach	069D40Z	Drainage of Left Common Iliac Vein with Drainage Device, Percutaneous Endoscopic Approach
06943ZX	Drainage of Hepatic Vein, Percutaneous Approach, Diagnostic	069840Z	Drainage of Portal Vein with Drainage Device, Percutaneous Endoscopic Approach	069D4ZX	Drainage of Left Common Iliac Vein, Percutaneous Endoscopic Approach, Diagnostic
06943ZZ	Drainage of Hepatic Vein, Percutaneous Approach	06984ZX	Drainage of Portal Vein, Percutaneous Endoscopic Approach, Diagnostic	069D4ZZ	Drainage of Left Common Iliac Vein, Percutaneous Endoscopic Approach
069440Z	Drainage of Hepatic Vein with Drainage Device, Percutaneous Endoscopic Approach	06984ZZ	Drainage of Portal Vein, Percutaneous Endoscopic Approach	069F00Z	Drainage of Right External Iliac Vein with Drainage Device, Open Approach
06944ZX	Drainage of Hepatic Vein, Percutaneous Endoscopic Approach, Diagnostic	069900Z	Drainage of Right Renal Vein with Drainage Device, Open Approach	069F0ZX	Drainage of Right External Iliac Vein, Open Approach, Diagnostic
06944ZZ	Drainage of Hepatic Vein, Percutaneous Endoscopic Approach	06990ZX	Drainage of Right Renal Vein, Open Approach, Diagnostic	069F0ZZ	Drainage of Right External Iliac Vein, Open Approach
069500Z	Drainage of Superior Mesenteric Vein with Drainage Device, Open Approach	06990ZZ	Drainage of Right Renal Vein, Open Approach		
06950ZX	Drainage of Superior Mesenteric Vein, Open Approach, Diagnostic	069930Z	Drainage of Right Renal Vein with Drainage Device, Percutaneous Approach		
06950ZZ	Drainage of Superior Mesenteric Vein, Open Approach				

♀ Female-only   ♂ Male-only   ▲ Limited Coverage   ● Non-OR   ▬ HAC-associated procedure   ▲ Non-covered procedures   ✚ Combinat

`30Z`	Drainage of Right External Iliac Vein with Drainage Device, Percutaneous Approach
`3ZX`	Drainage of Right External Iliac Vein, Percutaneous Approach, Diagnostic
`3ZZ`	Drainage of Right External Iliac Vein, Percutaneous Approach
`40Z`	Drainage of Right External Iliac Vein with Drainage Device, Percutaneous Endoscopic Approach
`4ZX`	Drainage of Right External Iliac Vein, Percutaneous Endoscopic Approach, Diagnostic
`4ZZ`	Drainage of Right External Iliac Vein, Percutaneous Endoscopic Approach
`G00Z`	Drainage of Left External Iliac Vein with Drainage Device, Open Approach
`G0ZX`	Drainage of Left External Iliac Vein, Open Approach, Diagnostic
`G0ZZ`	Drainage of Left External Iliac Vein, Open Approach
`G30Z`	Drainage of Left External Iliac Vein with Drainage Device, Percutaneous Approach
`G3ZX`	Drainage of Left External Iliac Vein, Percutaneous Approach, Diagnostic
`G3ZZ`	Drainage of Left External Iliac Vein, Percutaneous Approach
`G40Z`	Drainage of Left External Iliac Vein with Drainage Device, Percutaneous Endoscopic Approach
`G4ZX`	Drainage of Left External Iliac Vein, Percutaneous Endoscopic Approach, Diagnostic
`G4ZZ`	Drainage of Left External Iliac Vein, Percutaneous Endoscopic Approach
`H00Z`	Drainage of Right Hypogastric Vein with Drainage Device, Open Approach
`H0ZX`	Drainage of Right Hypogastric Vein, Open Approach, Diagnostic
`H0ZZ`	Drainage of Right Hypogastric Vein, Open Approach
`H30Z`	Drainage of Right Hypogastric Vein with Drainage Device, Percutaneous Approach
`H3ZX`	Drainage of Right Hypogastric Vein, Percutaneous Approach, Diagnostic
`H3ZZ`	Drainage of Right Hypogastric Vein, Percutaneous Approach
`H40Z`	Drainage of Right Hypogastric Vein with Drainage Device, Percutaneous Endoscopic Approach
`H4ZX`	Drainage of Right Hypogastric Vein, Percutaneous Endoscopic Approach, Diagnostic
`H4ZZ`	Drainage of Right Hypogastric Vein, Percutaneous Endoscopic Approach
`J00Z`	Drainage of Left Hypogastric Vein with Drainage Device, Open Approach
`J0ZX`	Drainage of Left Hypogastric Vein, Open Approach, Diagnostic
`J0ZZ`	Drainage of Left Hypogastric Vein, Open Approach
`J30Z`	Drainage of Left Hypogastric Vein with Drainage Device, Percutaneous Approach
`J3ZX`	Drainage of Left Hypogastric Vein, Percutaneous Approach, Diagnostic
`J3ZZ`	Drainage of Left Hypogastric Vein, Percutaneous Approach
`J40Z`	Drainage of Left Hypogastric Vein with Drainage Device, Percutaneous Endoscopic Approach
`J4ZX`	Drainage of Left Hypogastric Vein, Percutaneous Endoscopic Approach, Diagnostic
`J4ZZ`	Drainage of Left Hypogastric Vein, Percutaneous Endoscopic Approach
`M00Z`	Drainage of Right Femoral Vein with Drainage Device, Open Approach
`M0ZX`	Drainage of Right Femoral Vein, Open Approach, Diagnostic
069M0ZZ	Drainage of Right Femoral Vein, Open Approach
069M30Z	Drainage of Right Femoral Vein with Drainage Device, Percutaneous Approach
069M3ZX	Drainage of Right Femoral Vein, Percutaneous Approach, Diagnostic
069M3ZZ	Drainage of Right Femoral Vein, Percutaneous Approach
069M40Z	Drainage of Right Femoral Vein with Drainage Device, Percutaneous Endoscopic Approach
069M4ZX	Drainage of Right Femoral Vein, Percutaneous Endoscopic Approach, Diagnostic
069M4ZZ	Drainage of Right Femoral Vein, Percutaneous Endoscopic Approach
069N00Z	Drainage of Left Femoral Vein with Drainage Device, Open Approach
069N0ZX	Drainage of Left Femoral Vein, Open Approach, Diagnostic
069N0ZZ	Drainage of Left Femoral Vein, Open Approach
069N30Z	Drainage of Left Femoral Vein with Drainage Device, Percutaneous Approach
069N3ZX	Drainage of Left Femoral Vein, Percutaneous Approach, Diagnostic
069N3ZZ	Drainage of Left Femoral Vein, Percutaneous Approach
069N40Z	Drainage of Left Femoral Vein with Drainage Device, Percutaneous Endoscopic Approach
069N4ZX	Drainage of Left Femoral Vein, Percutaneous Endoscopic Approach, Diagnostic
069N4ZZ	Drainage of Left Femoral Vein, Percutaneous Endoscopic Approach
069P00Z	Drainage of Right Greater Saphenous Vein with Drainage Device, Open Approach
069P0ZX	Drainage of Right Greater Saphenous Vein, Open Approach, Diagnostic
069P0ZZ	Drainage of Right Greater Saphenous Vein, Open Approach
069P30Z	Drainage of Right Greater Saphenous Vein with Drainage Device, Percutaneous Approach
069P3ZX	Drainage of Right Greater Saphenous Vein, Percutaneous Approach, Diagnostic
069P3ZZ	Drainage of Right Greater Saphenous Vein, Percutaneous Approach
069P40Z	Drainage of Right Greater Saphenous Vein with Drainage Device, Percutaneous Endoscopic Approach
069P4ZX	Drainage of Right Greater Saphenous Vein, Percutaneous Endoscopic Approach, Diagnostic
069P4ZZ	Drainage of Right Greater Saphenous Vein, Percutaneous Endoscopic Approach
069Q00Z	Drainage of Left Greater Saphenous Vein with Drainage Device, Open Approach
069Q0ZX	Drainage of Left Greater Saphenous Vein, Open Approach, Diagnostic
069Q0ZZ	Drainage of Left Greater Saphenous Vein, Open Approach
069Q30Z	Drainage of Left Greater Saphenous Vein with Drainage Device, Percutaneous Approach
069Q3ZX	Drainage of Left Greater Saphenous Vein, Percutaneous Approach, Diagnostic
069Q3ZZ	Drainage of Left Greater Saphenous Vein, Percutaneous Approach
069Q40Z	Drainage of Left Greater Saphenous Vein with Drainage Device, Percutaneous Endoscopic Approach
069Q4ZX	Drainage of Left Greater Saphenous Vein, Percutaneous Endoscopic Approach, Diagnostic
069Q4ZZ	Drainage of Left Greater Saphenous Vein, Percutaneous Endoscopic Approach
069R00Z	Drainage of Right Lesser Saphenous Vein with Drainage Device, Open Approach
069R0ZX	Drainage of Right Lesser Saphenous Vein, Open Approach, Diagnostic
069R0ZZ	Drainage of Right Lesser Saphenous Vein, Open Approach
069R30Z	Drainage of Right Lesser Saphenous Vein with Drainage Device, Percutaneous Approach
069R3ZX	Drainage of Right Lesser Saphenous Vein, Percutaneous Approach, Diagnostic
069R3ZZ	Drainage of Right Lesser Saphenous Vein, Percutaneous Approach
069R40Z	Drainage of Right Lesser Saphenous Vein with Drainage Device, Percutaneous Endoscopic Approach
069R4ZX	Drainage of Right Lesser Saphenous Vein, Percutaneous Endoscopic Approach, Diagnostic
069R4ZZ	Drainage of Right Lesser Saphenous Vein, Percutaneous Endoscopic Approach
069S00Z	Drainage of Left Lesser Saphenous Vein with Drainage Device, Open Approach
069S0ZX	Drainage of Left Lesser Saphenous Vein, Open Approach, Diagnostic
069S0ZZ	Drainage of Left Lesser Saphenous Vein, Open Approach
069S30Z	Drainage of Left Lesser Saphenous Vein with Drainage Device, Percutaneous Approach
069S3ZX	Drainage of Left Lesser Saphenous Vein, Percutaneous Approach, Diagnostic
069S3ZZ	Drainage of Left Lesser Saphenous Vein, Percutaneous Approach
069S40Z	Drainage of Left Lesser Saphenous Vein with Drainage Device, Percutaneous Endoscopic Approach
069S4ZX	Drainage of Left Lesser Saphenous Vein, Percutaneous Endoscopic Approach, Diagnostic
069S4ZZ	Drainage of Left Lesser Saphenous Vein, Percutaneous Endoscopic Approach
069T00Z	Drainage of Right Foot Vein with Drainage Device, Open Approach
069T0ZX	Drainage of Right Foot Vein, Open Approach, Diagnostic
069T0ZZ	Drainage of Right Foot Vein, Open Approach
069T30Z	Drainage of Right Foot Vein with Drainage Device, Percutaneous Approach
069T3ZX	Drainage of Right Foot Vein, Percutaneous Approach, Diagnostic
069T3ZZ	Drainage of Right Foot Vein, Percutaneous Approach
069T40Z	Drainage of Right Foot Vein with Drainage Device, Percutaneous Endoscopic Approach
069T4ZX	Drainage of Right Foot Vein, Percutaneous Endoscopic Approach, Diagnostic
069T4ZZ	Drainage of Right Foot Vein, Percutaneous Endoscopic Approach
069V00Z	Drainage of Left Foot Vein with Drainage Device, Open Approach
069V0ZX	Drainage of Left Foot Vein, Open Approach, Diagnostic
069V0ZZ	Drainage of Left Foot Vein, Open Approach
069V30Z	Drainage of Left Foot Vein with Drainage Device, Percutaneous Approach
069V3ZX	Drainage of Left Foot Vein, Percutaneous Approach, Diagnostic
069V3ZZ	Drainage of Left Foot Vein, Percutaneous Approach
069V40Z	Drainage of Left Foot Vein with Drainage Device, Percutaneous Endoscopic Approach
069V4ZX	Drainage of Left Foot Vein, Percutaneous Endoscopic Approach, Diagnostic

069V4ZZ	Drainage of Left Foot Vein, Percutaneous Endoscopic Approach	069Y30Z	Drainage of Lower Vein with Drainage Device, Percutaneous Approach	069Y40Z	Drainage of Lower Vein with Drainage Device, Percutaneous Endoscopic Approach
069Y00Z	Drainage of Lower Vein with Drainage Device, Open Approach	069Y3ZX	Drainage of Lower Vein, Percutaneous Approach, Diagnostic	069Y4ZX	Drainage of Lower Vein, Percutaneous Endoscopic Approach, Diagnostic
069Y0ZX	Drainage of Lower Vein, Open Approach, Diagnostic	069Y3ZZ	Drainage of Lower Vein, Percutaneous Approach	069Y4ZZ	Drainage of Lower Vein, Percutaneous Endoscopic Approach
069Y0ZZ	Drainage of Lower Vein, Open Approach				

06B – Lower Veins, Excision

Review Coding Guidelines B3.4a and B3.4b

Review Coding Guideline B3.8

06B00ZX	Excision of Inferior Vena Cava, Open Approach, Diagnostic	06B53ZX	Excision of Superior Mesenteric Vein, Percutaneous Approach, Diagnostic	06BB3ZZ	Excision of Left Renal Vein, Percutane... Approach
06B00ZZ	Excision of Inferior Vena Cava, Open Approach	06B53ZZ	Excision of Superior Mesenteric Vein, Percutaneous Approach	06BB4ZX	Excision of Left Renal Vein, Percutane... Endoscopic Approach, Diagnostic
06B03ZX	Excision of Inferior Vena Cava, Percutaneous Approach, Diagnostic	06B54ZX	Excision of Superior Mesenteric Vein, Percutaneous Endoscopic Approach, Diagnostic	06BB4ZZ	Excision of Left Renal Vein, Percutane... Endoscopic Approach
06B03ZZ	Excision of Inferior Vena Cava, Percutaneous Approach	06B54ZZ	Excision of Superior Mesenteric Vein, Percutaneous Endoscopic Approach	06BC0ZX	Excision of Right Common Iliac Vein, Open Approach, Diagnostic
06B04ZX	Excision of Inferior Vena Cava, Percutaneous Endoscopic Approach, Diagnostic	06B60ZX	Excision of Inferior Mesenteric Vein, Open Approach, Diagnostic	06BC0ZZ	Excision of Right Common Iliac Vein, Open Approach
06B04ZZ	Excision of Inferior Vena Cava, Percutaneous Endoscopic Approach	06B60ZZ	Excision of Inferior Mesenteric Vein, Open Approach	06BC3ZX	Excision of Right Common Iliac Vein, Percutaneous Approach, Diagnostic
06B10ZX	Excision of Splenic Vein, Open Approach, Diagnostic	06B63ZX	Excision of Inferior Mesenteric Vein, Percutaneous Approach, Diagnostic	06BC3ZZ	Excision of Right Common Iliac Vein, Percutaneous Approach
06B10ZZ	Excision of Splenic Vein, Open Approach	06B63ZZ	Excision of Inferior Mesenteric Vein, Percutaneous Approach	06BC4ZX	Excision of Right Common Iliac Vein, Percutaneous Endoscopic Approach, Diagnostic
06B13ZX	Excision of Splenic Vein, Percutaneous Approach, Diagnostic	06B64ZX	Excision of Inferior Mesenteric Vein, Percutaneous Endoscopic Approach, Diagnostic	06BC4ZZ	Excision of Right Common Iliac Vein, Percutaneous Endoscopic Approach
06B13ZZ	Excision of Splenic Vein, Percutaneous Approach	06B64ZZ	Excision of Inferior Mesenteric Vein, Percutaneous Endoscopic Approach	06BD0ZX	Excision of Left Common Iliac Vein, C... Approach, Diagnostic
06B14ZX	Excision of Splenic Vein, Percutaneous Endoscopic Approach, Diagnostic	06B70ZX	Excision of Colic Vein, Open Approach, Diagnostic	06BD0ZZ	Excision of Left Common Iliac Vein, C... Approach
06B14ZZ	Excision of Splenic Vein, Percutaneous Endoscopic Approach	06B70ZZ	Excision of Colic Vein, Open Approach	06BD3ZX	Excision of Left Common Iliac Vein, Percutaneous Approach, Diagnostic
06B20ZX	Excision of Gastric Vein, Open Approach, Diagnostic	06B73ZX	Excision of Colic Vein, Percutaneous Approach, Diagnostic	06BD3ZZ	Excision of Left Common Iliac Vein, Percutaneous Approach
06B20ZZ	Excision of Gastric Vein, Open Approach	06B73ZZ	Excision of Colic Vein, Percutaneous Approach	06BD4ZX	Excision of Left Common Iliac Vein, Percutaneous Endoscopic Approach, Diagnostic
06B23ZX	Excision of Gastric Vein, Percutaneous Approach, Diagnostic	06B74ZX	Excision of Colic Vein, Percutaneous Endoscopic Approach, Diagnostic	06BD4ZZ	Excision of Left Common Iliac Vein, Percutaneous Endoscopic Approach
06B23ZZ	Excision of Gastric Vein, Percutaneous Approach	06B74ZZ	Excision of Colic Vein, Percutaneous Endoscopic Approach	06BF0ZX	Excision of Right External Iliac Vein, Open Approach, Diagnostic
06B24ZX	Excision of Gastric Vein, Percutaneous Endoscopic Approach, Diagnostic	06B80ZX	Excision of Portal Vein, Open Approach, Diagnostic	06BF0ZZ	Excision of Right External Iliac Vein, Open Approach
06B24ZZ	Excision of Gastric Vein, Percutaneous Endoscopic Approach	06B80ZZ	Excision of Portal Vein, Open Approach	06BF3ZX	Excision of Right External Iliac Vein, Percutaneous Approach, Diagnostic
06B30ZX	Excision of Esophageal Vein, Open Approach, Diagnostic	06B83ZX	Excision of Portal Vein, Percutaneous Approach, Diagnostic	06BF3ZZ	Excision of Right External Iliac Vein, Percutaneous Approach
06B30ZZ	Excision of Esophageal Vein, Open Approach	06B83ZZ	Excision of Portal Vein, Percutaneous Approach	06BF4ZX	Excision of Right External Iliac Vein, Percutaneous Endoscopic Approach, Diagnostic
06B33ZX	Excision of Esophageal Vein, Percutaneous Approach, Diagnostic	06B84ZX	Excision of Portal Vein, Percutaneous Endoscopic Approach, Diagnostic	06BF4ZZ	Excision of Right External Iliac Vein, Percutaneous Endoscopic Approach
06B33ZZ	Excision of Esophageal Vein, Percutaneous Approach	06B84ZZ	Excision of Portal Vein, Percutaneous Endoscopic Approach	06BG0ZX	Excision of Left External Iliac Vein, Op... Approach, Diagnostic
06B34ZX	Excision of Esophageal Vein, Percutaneous Endoscopic Approach, Diagnostic	06B90ZX	Excision of Right Renal Vein, Open Approach, Diagnostic	06BG0ZZ	Excision of Left External Iliac Vein, Op... Approach
06B34ZZ	Excision of Esophageal Vein, Percutaneous Endoscopic Approach	06B90ZZ	Excision of Right Renal Vein, Open Approach	06BG3ZX	Excision of Left External Iliac Vein, Percutaneous Approach, Diagnostic
06B40ZX	Excision of Hepatic Vein, Open Approach, Diagnostic	06B93ZX	Excision of Right Renal Vein, Percutaneous Approach, Diagnostic	06BG3ZZ	Excision of Left External Iliac Vein, Percutaneous Approach
06B40ZZ	Excision of Hepatic Vein, Open Approach	06B93ZZ	Excision of Right Renal Vein, Percutaneous Approach	06BG4ZX	Excision of Left External Iliac Vein, Percutaneous Endoscopic Approach, Diagnostic
06B43ZX	Excision of Hepatic Vein, Percutaneous Approach, Diagnostic	06B94ZX	Excision of Right Renal Vein, Percutaneous Endoscopic Approach, Diagnostic	06BG4ZZ	Excision of Left External Iliac Vein, Percutaneous Endoscopic Approach
06B43ZZ	Excision of Hepatic Vein, Percutaneous Approach	06B94ZZ	Excision of Right Renal Vein, Percutaneous Endoscopic Approach	06BH0ZX	Excision of Right Hypogastric Vein, Op... Approach, Diagnostic
06B44ZX	Excision of Hepatic Vein, Percutaneous Endoscopic Approach, Diagnostic	06BB0ZX	Excision of Left Renal Vein, Open Approach, Diagnostic	06BH0ZZ	Excision of Right Hypogastric Vein, Op... Approach
06B44ZZ	Excision of Hepatic Vein, Percutaneous Endoscopic Approach	06BB0ZZ	Excision of Left Renal Vein, Open Approach		
06B50ZX	Excision of Superior Mesenteric Vein, Open Approach, Diagnostic	06BB3ZX	Excision of Left Renal Vein, Percutaneous Approach, Diagnostic		
06B50ZZ	Excision of Superior Mesenteric Vein, Open Approach				

BH3ZX	Excision of Right Hypogastric Vein, Percutaneous Approach, Diagnostic
BH3ZZ	Excision of Right Hypogastric Vein, Percutaneous Approach
BH4ZX	Excision of Right Hypogastric Vein, Percutaneous Endoscopic Approach, Diagnostic
BH4ZZ	Excision of Right Hypogastric Vein, Percutaneous Endoscopic Approach
3J0ZX	Excision of Left Hypogastric Vein, Open Approach, Diagnostic
3J0ZZ	Excision of Left Hypogastric Vein, Open Approach
BJ3ZX	Excision of Left Hypogastric Vein, Percutaneous Approach, Diagnostic
BJ3ZZ	Excision of Left Hypogastric Vein, Percutaneous Approach
BJ4ZX	Excision of Left Hypogastric Vein, Percutaneous Endoscopic Approach, Diagnostic
BJ4ZZ	Excision of Left Hypogastric Vein, Percutaneous Endoscopic Approach
BM0ZX	Excision of Right Femoral Vein, Open Approach, Diagnostic
BM0ZZ	Excision of Right Femoral Vein, Open Approach
BM3ZX	Excision of Right Femoral Vein, Percutaneous Approach, Diagnostic
BM3ZZ	Excision of Right Femoral Vein, Percutaneous Approach
BM4ZX	Excision of Right Femoral Vein, Percutaneous Endoscopic Approach, Diagnostic
BM4ZZ	Excision of Right Femoral Vein, Percutaneous Endoscopic Approach
BN0ZX	Excision of Left Femoral Vein, Open Approach, Diagnostic
BN0ZZ	Excision of Left Femoral Vein, Open Approach
BN3ZX	Excision of Left Femoral Vein, Percutaneous Approach, Diagnostic
BN3ZZ	Excision of Left Femoral Vein, Percutaneous Approach
BN4ZX	Excision of Left Femoral Vein, Percutaneous Endoscopic Approach, Diagnostic
BN4ZZ	Excision of Left Femoral Vein, Percutaneous Endoscopic Approach

06BP0ZX	Excision of Right Greater Saphenous Vein, Open Approach, Diagnostic
06BP0ZZ	Excision of Right Greater Saphenous Vein, Open Approach
	AHA CC: 1Q, 2014, 10-11
06BP3ZX	Excision of Right Greater Saphenous Vein, Percutaneous Approach, Diagnostic
06BP3ZZ	Excision of Right Greater Saphenous Vein, Percutaneous Approach
06BP4ZX	Excision of Right Greater Saphenous Vein, Percutaneous Endoscopic Approach, Diagnostic
06BP4ZZ	Excision of Right Greater Saphenous Vein, Percutaneous Endoscopic Approach
	AHA CC: 3Q, 2014, 20-21
06BQ0ZX	Excision of Left Greater Saphenous Vein, Open Approach, Diagnostic
06BQ0ZZ	Excision of Left Greater Saphenous Vein, Open Approach
06BQ3ZX	Excision of Left Greater Saphenous Vein, Percutaneous Approach, Diagnostic
06BQ3ZZ	Excision of Left Greater Saphenous Vein, Percutaneous Approach
06BQ4ZX	Excision of Left Greater Saphenous Vein, Percutaneous Endoscopic Approach, Diagnostic
06BQ4ZZ	Excision of Left Greater Saphenous Vein, Percutaneous Endoscopic Approach
	AHA CC: 3Q, 2014, 20-21
06BR0ZX	Excision of Right Lesser Saphenous Vein, Open Approach, Diagnostic
06BR0ZZ	Excision of Right Lesser Saphenous Vein, Open Approach
06BR3ZX	Excision of Right Lesser Saphenous Vein, Percutaneous Approach, Diagnostic
06BR3ZZ	Excision of Right Lesser Saphenous Vein, Percutaneous Approach
06BR4ZX	Excision of Right Lesser Saphenous Vein, Percutaneous Endoscopic Approach, Diagnostic
06BR4ZZ	Excision of Right Lesser Saphenous Vein, Percutaneous Endoscopic Approach
06BS0ZX	Excision of Left Lesser Saphenous Vein, Open Approach, Diagnostic
06BS0ZZ	Excision of Left Lesser Saphenous Vein, Open Approach
06BS3ZX	Excision of Left Lesser Saphenous Vein, Percutaneous Approach, Diagnostic

06BS3ZZ	Excision of Left Lesser Saphenous Vein, Percutaneous Approach
06BS4ZX	Excision of Left Lesser Saphenous Vein, Percutaneous Endoscopic Approach, Diagnostic
06BS4ZZ	Excision of Left Lesser Saphenous Vein, Percutaneous Endoscopic Approach
06BT0ZX	Excision of Right Foot Vein, Open Approach, Diagnostic
06BT0ZZ	Excision of Right Foot Vein, Open Approach
06BT3ZX	Excision of Right Foot Vein, Percutaneous Approach, Diagnostic
06BT3ZZ	Excision of Right Foot Vein, Percutaneous Approach
06BT4ZX	Excision of Right Foot Vein, Percutaneous Endoscopic Approach, Diagnostic
06BT4ZZ	Excision of Right Foot Vein, Percutaneous Endoscopic Approach
06BV0ZX	Excision of Left Foot Vein, Open Approach, Diagnostic
06BV0ZZ	Excision of Left Foot Vein, Open Approach
06BV3ZX	Excision of Left Foot Vein, Percutaneous Approach, Diagnostic
06BV3ZZ	Excision of Left Foot Vein, Percutaneous Approach
06BV4ZX	Excision of Left Foot Vein, Percutaneous Endoscopic Approach, Diagnostic
06BV4ZZ	Excision of Left Foot Vein, Percutaneous Endoscopic Approach
06BY0ZC	Excision of Hemorrhoidal Plexus, Open Approach
06BY0ZX	Excision of Lower Vein, Open Approach, Diagnostic
06BY0ZZ	Excision of Lower Vein, Open Approach
06BY3ZC	Excision of Hemorrhoidal Plexus, Percutaneous Approach
06BY3ZX	Excision of Lower Vein, Percutaneous Approach, Diagnostic
06BY3ZZ	Excision of Lower Vein, Percutaneous Approach
06BY4ZC	Excision of Hemorrhoidal Plexus, Percutaneous Endoscopic Approach
06BY4ZX	Excision of Lower Vein, Percutaneous Endoscopic Approach, Diagnostic
06BY4ZZ	Excision of Lower Vein, Percutaneous Endoscopic Approach

6C – Lower Veins, Extirpation

C00ZZ	Extirpation of Matter from Inferior Vena Cava, Open Approach
C03ZZ	Extirpation of Matter from Inferior Vena Cava, Percutaneous Approach
C04ZZ	Extirpation of Matter from Inferior Vena Cava, Percutaneous Endoscopic Approach
C10ZZ	Extirpation of Matter from Splenic Vein, Open Approach
C13ZZ	Extirpation of Matter from Splenic Vein, Percutaneous Approach
C14ZZ	Extirpation of Matter from Splenic Vein, Percutaneous Endoscopic Approach
C20ZZ	Extirpation of Matter from Gastric Vein, Open Approach
C23ZZ	Extirpation of Matter from Gastric Vein, Percutaneous Approach
C24ZZ	Extirpation of Matter from Gastric Vein, Percutaneous Endoscopic Approach
C30ZZ	Extirpation of Matter from Esophageal Vein, Open Approach
C33ZZ	Extirpation of Matter from Esophageal Vein, Percutaneous Approach
C34ZZ	Extirpation of Matter from Esophageal Vein, Percutaneous Endoscopic Approach

06C40ZZ	Extirpation of Matter from Hepatic Vein, Open Approach
06C43ZZ	Extirpation of Matter from Hepatic Vein, Percutaneous Approach
06C44ZZ	Extirpation of Matter from Hepatic Vein, Percutaneous Endoscopic Approach
06C50ZZ	Extirpation of Matter from Superior Mesenteric Vein, Open Approach
06C53ZZ	Extirpation of Matter from Superior Mesenteric Vein, Percutaneous Approach
06C54ZZ	Extirpation of Matter from Superior Mesenteric Vein, Percutaneous Endoscopic Approach
06C60ZZ	Extirpation of Matter from Inferior Mesenteric Vein, Open Approach
06C63ZZ	Extirpation of Matter from Inferior Mesenteric Vein, Percutaneous Approach
06C64ZZ	Extirpation of Matter from Inferior Mesenteric Vein, Percutaneous Endoscopic Approach
06C70ZZ	Extirpation of Matter from Colic Vein, Open Approach
06C73ZZ	Extirpation of Matter from Colic Vein, Percutaneous Approach
06C74ZZ	Extirpation of Matter from Colic Vein, Percutaneous Endoscopic Approach

06C80ZZ	Extirpation of Matter from Portal Vein, Open Approach
06C83ZZ	Extirpation of Matter from Portal Vein, Percutaneous Approach
06C84ZZ	Extirpation of Matter from Portal Vein, Percutaneous Endoscopic Approach
06C90ZZ	Extirpation of Matter from Right Renal Vein, Open Approach
06C93ZZ	Extirpation of Matter from Right Renal Vein, Percutaneous Approach
06C94ZZ	Extirpation of Matter from Right Renal Vein, Percutaneous Endoscopic Approach
06CB0ZZ	Extirpation of Matter from Left Renal Vein, Open Approach
06CB3ZZ	Extirpation of Matter from Left Renal Vein, Percutaneous Approach
06CB4ZZ	Extirpation of Matter from Left Renal Vein, Percutaneous Endoscopic Approach
06CC0ZZ	Extirpation of Matter from Right Common Iliac Vein, Open Approach
06CC3ZZ	Extirpation of Matter from Right Common Iliac Vein, Percutaneous Approach
06CC4ZZ	Extirpation of Matter from Right Common Iliac Vein, Percutaneous Endoscopic Approach

Female-only	♂ Male-only	▲ Limited Coverage	● Non-OR	▓ HAC-associated procedure	▲ Non-covered procedures	✛ Combination

06CD0ZZ	Extirpation of Matter from Left Common Iliac Vein, Open Approach	
06CD3ZZ	Extirpation of Matter from Left Common Iliac Vein, Percutaneous Approach	
06CD4ZZ	Extirpation of Matter from Left Common Iliac Vein, Percutaneous Endoscopic Approach	
06CF0ZZ	Extirpation of Matter from Right External Iliac Vein, Open Approach	
06CF3ZZ	Extirpation of Matter from Right External Iliac Vein, Percutaneous Approach	
06CF4ZZ	Extirpation of Matter from Right External Iliac Vein, Percutaneous Endoscopic Approach	
06CG0ZZ	Extirpation of Matter from Left External Iliac Vein, Open Approach	
06CG3ZZ	Extirpation of Matter from Left External Iliac Vein, Percutaneous Approach	
06CG4ZZ	Extirpation of Matter from Left External Iliac Vein, Percutaneous Endoscopic Approach	
06CH0ZZ	Extirpation of Matter from Right Hypogastric Vein, Open Approach	
06CH3ZZ	Extirpation of Matter from Right Hypogastric Vein, Percutaneous Approach	
06CH4ZZ	Extirpation of Matter from Right Hypogastric Vein, Percutaneous Endoscopic Approach	
06CJ0ZZ	Extirpation of Matter from Left Hypogastric Vein, Open Approach	

06CJ3ZZ Extirpation of Matter from Left Hypogastric Vein, Percutaneous Approach

06CJ4ZZ Extirpation of Matter from Left Hypogastric Vein, Percutaneous Endoscopic Approach

06CM0ZZ Extirpation of Matter from Right Femoral Vein, Open Approach

06CM3ZZ Extirpation of Matter from Right Femoral Vein, Percutaneous Approach

06CM4ZZ Extirpation of Matter from Right Femoral Vein, Percutaneous Endoscopic Approach

06CN0ZZ Extirpation of Matter from Left Femoral Vein, Open Approach

06CN3ZZ Extirpation of Matter from Left Femoral Vein, Percutaneous Approach

06CN4ZZ Extirpation of Matter from Left Femoral Vein, Percutaneous Endoscopic Approach

06CP0ZZ Extirpation of Matter from Right Greater Saphenous Vein, Open Approach

06CP3ZZ Extirpation of Matter from Right Greater Saphenous Vein, Percutaneous Approach

06CP4ZZ Extirpation of Matter from Right Greater Saphenous Vein, Percutaneous Endoscopic Approach

06CQ0ZZ Extirpation of Matter from Left Greater Saphenous Vein, Open Approach

06CQ3ZZ Extirpation of Matter from Left Greater Saphenous Vein, Percutaneous Approach

06CQ4ZZ Extirpation of Matter from Left Greater Saphenous Vein, Percutaneous Endoscopic Approach

06CR0ZZ Extirpation of Matter from Right Lesser Saphenous Vein, Open Approach

06CR3ZZ Extirpation of Matter from Right Lesser Saphenous Vein, Percutaneous Approac...

06CR4ZZ Extirpation of Matter from Right Lesser Saphenous Vein, Percutaneous Endosco... Approach

06CS0ZZ Extirpation of Matter from Left Lesser Saphenous Vein, Open Approach...

06CS3ZZ Extirpation of Matter from Left Lesser Saphenous Vein, Percutaneous Approac...

06CS4ZZ Extirpation of Matter from Left Lesser Saphenous Vein, Percutaneous Endosco... Approach

06CT0ZZ Extirpation of Matter from Right Foot Vein, Open Approach

06CT3ZZ Extirpation of Matter from Right Foot Vein, Percutaneous Approach

06CT4ZZ Extirpation of Matter from Right Foot Vein, Percutaneous Endoscopic Approac...

06CV0ZZ Extirpation of Matter from Left Foot Ve... Open Approach

06CV3ZZ Extirpation of Matter from Left Foot Ve... Percutaneous Approach

06CV4ZZ Extirpation of Matter from Left Foot Ve... Percutaneous Endoscopic Approach

06CY0ZZ Extirpation of Matter from Lower Vein, Open Approach

06CY3ZZ Extirpation of Matter from Lower Vein, Percutaneous Approach

06CY4ZZ Extirpation of Matter from Lower Vein, Percutaneous Endoscopic Approach

06D – Lower Veins, Extraction

06DM0ZZ Extraction of Right Femoral Vein, Open Approach

06DM3ZZ Extraction of Right Femoral Vein, Percutaneous Approach

06DM4ZZ Extraction of Right Femoral Vein, Percutaneous Endoscopic Approach

06DN0ZZ Extraction of Left Femoral Vein, Open Approach

06DN3ZZ Extraction of Left Femoral Vein, Percutaneous Approach

06DN4ZZ Extraction of Left Femoral Vein, Percutaneous Endoscopic Approach

06DP0ZZ Extraction of Right Greater Saphenous Vein, Open Approach

06DP3ZZ Extraction of Right Greater Saphenous Vein, Percutaneous Approach

06DP4ZZ Extraction of Right Greater Saphenous Vein, Percutaneous Endoscopic Approach

06DQ0ZZ Extraction of Left Greater Saphenous Vein, Open Approach

06DQ3ZZ Extraction of Left Greater Saphenous Vein, Percutaneous Approach

06DQ4ZZ Extraction of Left Greater Saphenous Vein, Percutaneous Endoscopic Approach

06DR0ZZ Extraction of Right Lesser Saphenous Vein, Open Approach

06DR3ZZ Extraction of Right Lesser Saphenous Vein, Percutaneous Approach

06DR4ZZ Extraction of Right Lesser Saphenous Vein, Percutaneous Endoscopic Approach

06DS0ZZ Extraction of Left Lesser Saphenous Vein, Open Approach

06DS3ZZ Extraction of Left Lesser Saphenous Vein, Percutaneous Approach

06DS4ZZ Extraction of Left Lesser Saphenous Vein, Percutaneous Endoscopic Approach

06DT0ZZ Extraction of Right Foot Vein, Open Approach

06DT3ZZ Extraction of Right Foot Vein, Percutaneous Approach

06DT4ZZ Extraction of Right Foot Vein, Percutaneous Endoscopic Approach

06DV0ZZ Extraction of Left Foot Vein, Open Approach

06DV3ZZ Extraction of Left Foot Vein, Percutaneo... Approach

06DV4ZZ Extraction of Left Foot Vein, Percutaneo... Endoscopic Approach

06DY0ZZ Extraction of Lower Vein, Open Approac...

06DY3ZZ Extraction of Lower Vein, Percutaneous Approach

06DY4ZZ Extraction of Lower Vein, Percutaneous Endoscopic Approach

06H – Lower Veins, Insertion

06H003T Insertion of Infusion Device, Via Umbilical Vein, into Inferior Vena Cava, Open Approach

06H003Z Insertion of Infusion Device into Inferior Vena Cava, Open Approach

06H00DZ Insertion of Intraluminal Device into Inferior Vena Cava, Open Approach

06H033T Insertion of Infusion Device, Via Umbilical Vein, into Inferior Vena Cava, Percutaneous Approach

06H033Z Insertion of Infusion Device into Inferior Vena Cava, Percutaneous Approach

AHA CC: 3Q, 2013, 18-19

06H03DZ Insertion of Intraluminal Device into Inferior Vena Cava, Percutaneous Approach

06H043Z Insertion of Infusion Device into Inferior Vena Cava, Percutaneous Endoscopic Approach

06H04DZ Insertion of Intraluminal Device into Inferior Vena Cava, Percutaneous Endoscopic Approach

06H103Z Insertion of Infusion Device into Splenic Vein, Open Approach

06H10DZ Insertion of Intraluminal Device into Splenic Vein, Open Approach

06H133Z Insertion of Infusion Device into Splenic Vein, Percutaneous Approach

06H13DZ Insertion of Intraluminal Device into Splenic Vein, Percutaneous Approach

06H143Z Insertion of Infusion Device into Splenic Vein, Percutaneous Endoscopic Approach

06H14DZ Insertion of Intraluminal Device into Splenic Vein, Percutaneous Endoscopic Approach

06H203Z Insertion of Infusion Device into Gastric Vein, Open Approach

06H20DZ Insertion of Intraluminal Device into Gastric Vein, Open Approach

06H233Z Insertion of Infusion Device into Gastric Vein, Percutaneous Approach

06H23DZ Insertion of Intraluminal Device into Gastric Vein, Percutaneous Approach

06H243Z Insertion of Infusion Device into Gastric Vein, Percutaneous Endoscopic Approach...

06H24DZ Insertion of Intraluminal Device into Gastric Vein, Percutaneous Endoscopic Approach

06H303Z Insertion of Infusion Device into Esophageal Vein, Open Approach

06H30DZ Insertion of Intraluminal Device into Esophageal Vein, Open Approach

06H333Z Insertion of Infusion Device into Esophageal Vein, Percutaneous Approach...

06H33DZ Insertion of Intraluminal Device into Esophageal Vein, Percutaneous Approach...

06H343Z Insertion of Infusion Device into Esophageal Vein, Percutaneous Endoscopic Approach

06H34DZ Insertion of Intraluminal Device into Esophageal Vein, Percutaneous Endoscopic Approach

06H403Z Insertion of Infusion Device into Hepatic Vein, Open Approach

40DZ Insertion of Intraluminal Device into Hepatic Vein, Open Approach

433Z Insertion of Infusion Device into Hepatic Vein, Percutaneous Approach

43DZ Insertion of Intraluminal Device into Hepatic Vein, Percutaneous Approach

443Z Insertion of Infusion Device into Hepatic Vein, Percutaneous Endoscopic Approach

44DZ Insertion of Intraluminal Device into Hepatic Vein, Percutaneous Endoscopic Approach

503Z Insertion of Infusion Device into Superior Mesenteric Vein, Open Approach

50DZ Insertion of Intraluminal Device into Superior Mesenteric Vein, Open Approach

533Z Insertion of Infusion Device into Superior Mesenteric Vein, Percutaneous Approach

53DZ Insertion of Intraluminal Device into Superior Mesenteric Vein, Percutaneous Approach

543Z Insertion of Infusion Device into Superior Mesenteric Vein, Percutaneous Endoscopic Approach

54DZ Insertion of Intraluminal Device into Superior Mesenteric Vein, Percutaneous Endoscopic Approach

603Z Insertion of Infusion Device into Inferior Mesenteric Vein, Open Approach

60DZ Insertion of Intraluminal Device into Inferior Mesenteric Vein, Open Approach

633Z Insertion of Infusion Device into Inferior Mesenteric Vein, Percutaneous Approach

63DZ Insertion of Intraluminal Device into Inferior Mesenteric Vein, Percutaneous Approach

643Z Insertion of Infusion Device into Inferior Mesenteric Vein, Percutaneous Endoscopic Approach

64DZ Insertion of Intraluminal Device into Inferior Mesenteric Vein, Percutaneous Endoscopic Approach

703Z Insertion of Infusion Device into Colic Vein, Open Approach

70DZ Insertion of Intraluminal Device into Colic Vein, Open Approach

733Z Insertion of Infusion Device into Colic Vein, Percutaneous Approach

73DZ Insertion of Intraluminal Device into Colic Vein, Percutaneous Approach

743Z Insertion of Infusion Device into Colic Vein, Percutaneous Endoscopic Approach

74DZ Insertion of Intraluminal Device into Colic Vein, Percutaneous Endoscopic Approach

803Z Insertion of Infusion Device into Portal Vein, Open Approach

80DZ Insertion of Intraluminal Device into Portal Vein, Open Approach

833Z Insertion of Infusion Device into Portal Vein, Percutaneous Approach

83DZ Insertion of Intraluminal Device into Portal Vein, Percutaneous Approach

843Z Insertion of Infusion Device into Portal Vein, Percutaneous Endoscopic Approach

84DZ Insertion of Intraluminal Device into Portal Vein, Percutaneous Endoscopic Approach

903Z Insertion of Infusion Device into Right Renal Vein, Open Approach

90DZ Insertion of Intraluminal Device into Right Renal Vein, Open Approach

933Z Insertion of Infusion Device into Right Renal Vein, Percutaneous Approach

93DZ Insertion of Intraluminal Device into Right Renal Vein, Percutaneous Approach

943Z Insertion of Infusion Device into Right Renal Vein, Percutaneous Endoscopic Approach

06H94DZ Insertion of Intraluminal Device into Right Renal Vein, Percutaneous Endoscopic Approach

06HB03Z Insertion of Infusion Device into Left Renal Vein, Open Approach

06HB0DZ Insertion of Intraluminal Device into Left Renal Vein, Open Approach

06HB33Z Insertion of Infusion Device into Left Renal Vein, Percutaneous Approach

06HB3DZ Insertion of Intraluminal Device into Left Renal Vein, Percutaneous Approach

06HB43Z Insertion of Infusion Device into Left Renal Vein, Percutaneous Endoscopic Approach

06HB4DZ Insertion of Intraluminal Device into Left Renal Vein, Percutaneous Endoscopic Approach

06HC03Z Insertion of Infusion Device into Right Common Iliac Vein, Open Approach

06HC0DZ Insertion of Intraluminal Device into Right Common Iliac Vein, Open Approach

06HC33Z Insertion of Infusion Device into Right Common Iliac Vein, Percutaneous Approach

06HC3DZ Insertion of Intraluminal Device into Right Common Iliac Vein, Percutaneous Approach

06HC43Z Insertion of Infusion Device into Right Common Iliac Vein, Percutaneous Endoscopic Approach

06HC4DZ Insertion of Intraluminal Device into Right Common Iliac Vein, Percutaneous Endoscopic Approach

06HD03Z Insertion of Infusion Device into Left Common Iliac Vein, Open Approach

● **06HD0DZ** Insertion of Intraluminal Device into Left Common Iliac Vein, Open Approach

06HD33Z Insertion of Infusion Device into Left Common Iliac Vein, Percutaneous Approach

06HD3DZ Insertion of Intraluminal Device into Left Common Iliac Vein, Percutaneous Approach

06HD43Z Insertion of Infusion Device into Left Common Iliac Vein, Percutaneous Endoscopic Approach

06HD4DZ Insertion of Intraluminal Device into Left Common Iliac Vein, Percutaneous Endoscopic Approach

06HF03Z Insertion of Infusion Device into Right External Iliac Vein, Open Approach

06HF0DZ Insertion of Intraluminal Device into Right External Iliac Vein, Open Approach

06HF33Z Insertion of Infusion Device into Right External Iliac Vein, Percutaneous Approach

06HF3DZ Insertion of Intraluminal Device into Right External Iliac Vein, Percutaneous Approach

06HF43Z Insertion of Infusion Device into Right External Iliac Vein, Percutaneous Endoscopic Approach

06HF4DZ Insertion of Intraluminal Device into Right External Iliac Vein, Percutaneous Endoscopic Approach

06HG03Z Insertion of Infusion Device into Left External Iliac Vein, Open Approach

06HG0DZ Insertion of Intraluminal Device into Left External Iliac Vein, Open Approach

06HG33Z Insertion of Infusion Device into Left External Iliac Vein, Percutaneous Approach

06HG3DZ Insertion of Intraluminal Device into Left External Iliac Vein, Percutaneous Approach

06HG43Z Insertion of Infusion Device into Left External Iliac Vein, Percutaneous Endoscopic Approach

06HG4DZ Insertion of Intraluminal Device into Left External Iliac Vein, Percutaneous Endoscopic Approach

06HH03Z Insertion of Infusion Device into Right Hypogastric Vein, Open Approach

06HH0DZ Insertion of Intraluminal Device into Right Hypogastric Vein, Open Approach

06HH33Z Insertion of Infusion Device into Right Hypogastric Vein, Percutaneous Approach

06HH3DZ Insertion of Intraluminal Device into Right Hypogastric Vein, Percutaneous Approach

06HH43Z Insertion of Infusion Device into Right Hypogastric Vein, Percutaneous Endoscopic Approach

06HH4DZ Insertion of Intraluminal Device into Right Hypogastric Vein, Percutaneous Endoscopic Approach

06HJ03Z Insertion of Infusion Device into Left Hypogastric Vein, Open Approach

06HJ0DZ Insertion of Intraluminal Device into Left Hypogastric Vein, Open Approach

06HJ33Z Insertion of Infusion Device into Left Hypogastric Vein, Percutaneous Approach

06HJ3DZ Insertion of Intraluminal Device into Left Hypogastric Vein, Percutaneous Approach

06HJ43Z Insertion of Infusion Device into Left Hypogastric Vein, Percutaneous Endoscopic Approach

06HJ4DZ Insertion of Intraluminal Device into Left Hypogastric Vein, Percutaneous Endoscopic Approach

06HM03Z Insertion of Infusion Device into Right Femoral Vein, Open Approach

06HM0DZ Insertion of Intraluminal Device into Right Femoral Vein, Open Approach

● **06HM33Z** Insertion of Infusion Device into Right Femoral Vein, Percutaneous Approach

06HM3DZ Insertion of Intraluminal Device into Right Femoral Vein, Percutaneous Approach

06HM43Z Insertion of Infusion Device into Right Femoral Vein, Percutaneous Endoscopic Approach

06HM4DZ Insertion of Intraluminal Device into Right Femoral Vein, Percutaneous Endoscopic Approach

06HN03Z Insertion of Infusion Device into Left Femoral Vein, Open Approach

06HN0DZ Insertion of Intraluminal Device into Left Femoral Vein, Open Approach

● **06HN33Z** Insertion of Infusion Device into Left Femoral Vein, Percutaneous Approach

06HN3DZ Insertion of Intraluminal Device into Left Femoral Vein, Percutaneous Approach

06HN43Z Insertion of Infusion Device into Left Femoral Vein, Percutaneous Endoscopic Approach

06HN4DZ Insertion of Intraluminal Device into Left Femoral Vein, Percutaneous Endoscopic Approach

06HP03Z Insertion of Infusion Device into Right Greater Saphenous Vein, Open Approach

06HP0DZ Insertion of Intraluminal Device into Right Greater Saphenous Vein, Open Approach

06HP33Z Insertion of Infusion Device into Right Greater Saphenous Vein, Percutaneous Approach

06HP3DZ Insertion of Intraluminal Device into Right Greater Saphenous Vein, Percutaneous Approach

06HP43Z Insertion of Infusion Device into Right Greater Saphenous Vein, Percutaneous Endoscopic Approach

06HP4DZ Insertion of Intraluminal Device into Right Greater Saphenous Vein, Percutaneous Endoscopic Approach

06HQ03Z Insertion of Infusion Device into Left Greater Saphenous Vein, Open Approach

emale-only   ♂ Male-only   ▲ Limited Coverage   ● Non-OR   ▦ HAC-associated procedure   ▲ Non-covered procedures   ✚ Combination

06HQ0DZ Insertion of Intraluminal Device into Left Greater Saphenous Vein, Open Approach

06HQ33Z Insertion of Infusion Device into Left Greater Saphenous Vein, Percutaneous Approach

06HQ3DZ Insertion of Intraluminal Device into Left Greater Saphenous Vein, Percutaneous Approach

06HQ43Z Insertion of Infusion Device into Left Greater Saphenous Vein, Percutaneous Endoscopic Approach

06HQ4DZ Insertion of Intraluminal Device into Left Greater Saphenous Vein, Percutaneous Endoscopic Approach

06HR03Z Insertion of Infusion Device into Right Lesser Saphenous Vein, Open Approach

06HR0DZ Insertion of Intraluminal Device into Right Lesser Saphenous Vein, Open Approach

06HR33Z Insertion of Infusion Device into Right Lesser Saphenous Vein, Percutaneous Approach

06HR3DZ Insertion of Intraluminal Device into Right Lesser Saphenous Vein, Percutaneous Approach

06HR43Z Insertion of Infusion Device into Right Lesser Saphenous Vein, Percutaneous Endoscopic Approach

06HR4DZ Insertion of Intraluminal Device into Right Lesser Saphenous Vein, Percutaneous Endoscopic Approach

06HS03Z Insertion of Infusion Device into Left Lesser Saphenous Vein, Open Approach

06HS0DZ Insertion of Intraluminal Device into Left Lesser Saphenous Vein, Open Approach

06HS33Z Insertion of Infusion Device into Left Lesser Saphenous Vein, Percutaneous Approach

06HS3DZ Insertion of Intraluminal Device into Left Lesser Saphenous Vein, Percutaneous Approach

06HS43Z Insertion of Infusion Device into Left Lesser Saphenous Vein, Percutaneous Endoscopic Approach

06HS4DZ Insertion of Intraluminal Device into Left Lesser Saphenous Vein, Percutaneous Endoscopic Approach

06HT03Z Insertion of Infusion Device into Right Foot Vein, Open Approach

06HT0DZ Insertion of Intraluminal Device into Right Foot Vein, Open Approach

06HT33Z Insertion of Infusion Device into Right Foot Vein, Percutaneous Approach

06HT3DZ Insertion of Intraluminal Device into Right Foot Vein, Percutaneous Approach

06HT43Z Insertion of Infusion Device into Right Foot Vein, Percutaneous Endoscopic Approach

06HT4DZ Insertion of Intraluminal Device into Right Foot Vein, Percutaneous Endoscopic Approach

06HV03Z Insertion of Infusion Device into Left Foot Vein, Open Approach

06HV0DZ Insertion of Intraluminal Device into Left Foot Vein, Open Approach

06HV33Z Insertion of Infusion Device into Left Vein, Percutaneous Approach

06HV3DZ Insertion of Intraluminal Device into I Foot Vein, Percutaneous Approach

06HV43Z Insertion of Infusion Device into Left Foot Vein, Percutaneous Endoscopic Approach

06HV4DZ Insertion of Intraluminal Device into Left Foot Vein, Percutaneous Endosco Approach

06HY02Z Insertion of Monitoring Device into L< Vein, Open Approach

06HY03Z Insertion of Infusion Device into Low< Vein, Open Approach

06HY0DZ Insertion of Intraluminal Device into Lower Vein, Open Approach

06HY32Z Insertion of Monitoring Device into L< Vein, Percutaneous Approach

06HY33Z Insertion of Infusion Device into Low< Vein, Percutaneous Approach

06HY3DZ Insertion of Intraluminal Device into Lower Vein, Percutaneous Approach

06HY42Z Insertion of Monitoring Device into Lower Vein, Percutaneous Endoscopic Approach

06HY43Z Insertion of Infusion Device into Lower Vein, Percutaneous Endoscopic Approach

06HY4DZ Insertion of Intraluminal Device into Lower Vein, Percutaneous Endoscopic Approach

06J – Lower Veins, Inspection

Review Coding Guidelines B3.11a, B3.11b and B3.11c

06JY0ZZ Inspection of Lower Vein, Open Approach

06JY3ZZ Inspection of Lower Vein, Percutaneous Approach

06JY4ZZ Inspection of Lower Vein, Percutaneous Endoscopic Approach

06JYXZZ Inspection of Lower Vein, External Approach

06L – Lower Veins, Occlusion

Review Coding Guideline B3.12

06L00CZ Occlusion of Inferior Vena Cava with Extraluminal Device, Open Approach

06L00DZ Occlusion of Inferior Vena Cava with Intraluminal Device, Open Approach

06L00ZZ Occlusion of Inferior Vena Cava, Open Approach

06L03CZ Occlusion of Inferior Vena Cava with Extraluminal Device, Percutaneous Approach

06L03DZ Occlusion of Inferior Vena Cava with Intraluminal Device, Percutaneous Approach

06L03ZZ Occlusion of Inferior Vena Cava, Percutaneous Approach

06L04CZ Occlusion of Inferior Vena Cava with Extraluminal Device, Percutaneous Endoscopic Approach

06L04DZ Occlusion of Inferior Vena Cava with Intraluminal Device, Percutaneous Endoscopic Approach

06L04ZZ Occlusion of Inferior Vena Cava, Percutaneous Endoscopic Approach

06L10CZ Occlusion of Splenic Vein with Extraluminal Device, Open Approach

06L10DZ Occlusion of Splenic Vein with Intraluminal Device, Open Approach

06L10ZZ Occlusion of Splenic Vein, Open Approach

06L13CZ Occlusion of Splenic Vein with Extraluminal Device, Percutaneous Approach

06L13DZ Occlusion of Splenic Vein with Intraluminal Device, Percutaneous Approach

06L13ZZ Occlusion of Splenic Vein, Percutaneous Approach

06L14CZ Occlusion of Splenic Vein with Extraluminal Device, Percutaneous Endoscopic Approach

06L14DZ Occlusion of Splenic Vein with Intraluminal Device, Percutaneous Endoscopic Approach

06L14ZZ Occlusion of Splenic Vein, Percutaneous Endoscopic Approach

06L20CZ Occlusion of Gastric Vein with Extraluminal Device, Open Approach

06L20DZ Occlusion of Gastric Vein with Intraluminal Device, Open Approach

06L20ZZ Occlusion of Gastric Vein, Open Approach

06L23CZ Occlusion of Gastric Vein with Extraluminal Device, Percutaneous Approach

06L23DZ Occlusion of Gastric Vein with Intraluminal Device, Percutaneous Approach

06L23ZZ Occlusion of Gastric Vein, Percutaneous Approach

06L24CZ Occlusion of Gastric Vein with Extraluminal Device, Percutaneous Endoscopic Approach

06L24DZ Occlusion of Gastric Vein with Intraluminal Device, Percutaneous Endoscopic Approach

06L24ZZ Occlusion of Gastric Vein, Percutaneous Endoscopic Approach

06L30CZ Occlusion of Esophageal Vein with Extraluminal Device, Open Approach

06L30DZ Occlusion of Esophageal Vein with Intraluminal Device, Open Approach

06L30ZZ Occlusion of Esophageal Vein, Open Approach

06L33CZ Occlusion of Esophageal Vein with Extraluminal Device, Percutaneous Approach

06L33DZ Occlusion of Esophageal Vein with Intraluminal Device, Percutaneous Approach

06L33ZZ Occlusion of Esophageal Vein, Percutaneous Approach

06L34CZ Occlusion of Esophageal Vein with Extraluminal Device, Percutaneous Endoscopic Approach

AHA CC: 4Q, 2013, 112-113

06L34DZ Occlusion of Esophageal Vein with Intraluminal Device, Percutaneous Endoscopic Approach

06L34ZZ Occlusion of Esophageal Vein, Percutaneous Endoscopic Approach

06L40CZ Occlusion of Hepatic Vein with Extraluminal Device, Open Approach

06L40DZ Occlusion of Hepatic Vein with Intraluminal Device, Open Approach

06L40ZZ Occlusion of Hepatic Vein, Open Approach

06L43CZ Occlusion of Hepatic Vein with Extraluminal Device, Percutaneous Approach

06L43DZ Occlusion of Hepatic Vein with Intraluminal Device, Percutaneous Approach

43ZZ Occlusion of Hepatic Vein, Percutaneous Approach

44CZ Occlusion of Hepatic Vein with Extraluminal Device, Percutaneous Endoscopic Approach

44DZ Occlusion of Hepatic Vein with Intraluminal Device, Percutaneous Endoscopic Approach

44ZZ Occlusion of Hepatic Vein, Percutaneous Endoscopic Approach

50CZ Occlusion of Superior Mesenteric Vein with Extraluminal Device, Open Approach

50DZ Occlusion of Superior Mesenteric Vein with Intraluminal Device, Open Approach

50ZZ Occlusion of Superior Mesenteric Vein, Open Approach

53CZ Occlusion of Superior Mesenteric Vein with Extraluminal Device, Percutaneous Approach

53DZ Occlusion of Superior Mesenteric Vein with Intraluminal Device, Percutaneous Approach

53ZZ Occlusion of Superior Mesenteric Vein, Percutaneous Approach

54CZ Occlusion of Superior Mesenteric Vein with Extraluminal Device, Percutaneous Endoscopic Approach

54DZ Occlusion of Superior Mesenteric Vein with Intraluminal Device, Percutaneous Endoscopic Approach

54ZZ Occlusion of Superior Mesenteric Vein, Percutaneous Endoscopic Approach

L60CZ Occlusion of Inferior Mesenteric Vein with Extraluminal Device, Open Approach

L60DZ Occlusion of Inferior Mesenteric Vein with Intraluminal Device, Open Approach

L60ZZ Occlusion of Inferior Mesenteric Vein, Open Approach

L63CZ Occlusion of Inferior Mesenteric Vein with Extraluminal Device, Percutaneous Approach

L63DZ Occlusion of Inferior Mesenteric Vein with Intraluminal Device, Percutaneous Approach

L63ZZ Occlusion of Inferior Mesenteric Vein, Percutaneous Approach

L64CZ Occlusion of Inferior Mesenteric Vein with Extraluminal Device, Percutaneous Endoscopic Approach

L64DZ Occlusion of Inferior Mesenteric Vein with Intraluminal Device, Percutaneous Endoscopic Approach

L64ZZ Occlusion of Inferior Mesenteric Vein, Percutaneous Endoscopic Approach

L70CZ Occlusion of Colic Vein with Extraluminal Device, Open Approach

L70DZ Occlusion of Colic Vein with Intraluminal Device, Open Approach

L70ZZ Occlusion of Colic Vein, Open Approach

L73CZ Occlusion of Colic Vein with Extraluminal Device, Percutaneous Approach

L73DZ Occlusion of Colic Vein with Intraluminal Device, Percutaneous Approach

L73ZZ Occlusion of Colic Vein, Percutaneous Approach

L74CZ Occlusion of Colic Vein with Extraluminal Device, Percutaneous Endoscopic Approach

L74DZ Occlusion of Colic Vein with Intraluminal Device, Percutaneous Endoscopic Approach

L74ZZ Occlusion of Colic Vein, Percutaneous Endoscopic Approach

L80CZ Occlusion of Portal Vein with Extraluminal Device, Open Approach

L80DZ Occlusion of Portal Vein with Intraluminal Device, Open Approach

L80ZZ Occlusion of Portal Vein, Open Approach

06L83CZ Occlusion of Portal Vein with Extraluminal Device, Percutaneous Approach

06L83DZ Occlusion of Portal Vein with Intraluminal Device, Percutaneous Approach

06L83ZZ Occlusion of Portal Vein, Percutaneous Approach

06L84CZ Occlusion of Portal Vein with Extraluminal Device, Percutaneous Endoscopic Approach

06L84DZ Occlusion of Portal Vein with Intraluminal Device, Percutaneous Endoscopic Approach

06L84ZZ Occlusion of Portal Vein, Percutaneous Endoscopic Approach

06L90CZ Occlusion of Right Renal Vein with Extraluminal Device, Open Approach

06L90DZ Occlusion of Right Renal Vein with Intraluminal Device, Open Approach

06L90ZZ Occlusion of Right Renal Vein, Open Approach

06L93CZ Occlusion of Right Renal Vein with Extraluminal Device, Percutaneous Approach

06L93DZ Occlusion of Right Renal Vein with Intraluminal Device, Percutaneous Approach

06L93ZZ Occlusion of Right Renal Vein, Percutaneous Approach

06L94CZ Occlusion of Right Renal Vein with Extraluminal Device, Percutaneous Endoscopic Approach

06L94DZ Occlusion of Right Renal Vein with Intraluminal Device, Percutaneous Endoscopic Approach

06L94ZZ Occlusion of Right Renal Vein, Percutaneous Endoscopic Approach

06LB0CZ Occlusion of Left Renal Vein with Extraluminal Device, Open Approach

06LB0DZ Occlusion of Left Renal Vein with Intraluminal Device, Open Approach

06LB0ZZ Occlusion of Left Renal Vein, Open Approach

06LB3CZ Occlusion of Left Renal Vein with Extraluminal Device, Percutaneous Approach

06LB3DZ Occlusion of Left Renal Vein with Intraluminal Device, Percutaneous Approach

06LB3ZZ Occlusion of Left Renal Vein, Percutaneous Approach

06LB4CZ Occlusion of Left Renal Vein with Extraluminal Device, Percutaneous Endoscopic Approach

06LB4DZ Occlusion of Left Renal Vein with Intraluminal Device, Percutaneous Endoscopic Approach

06LB4ZZ Occlusion of Left Renal Vein, Percutaneous Endoscopic Approach

06LC0CZ Occlusion of Right Common Iliac Vein with Extraluminal Device, Open Approach

06LC0DZ Occlusion of Right Common Iliac Vein with Intraluminal Device, Open Approach

06LC0ZZ Occlusion of Right Common Iliac Vein, Open Approach

06LC3CZ Occlusion of Right Common Iliac Vein with Extraluminal Device, Percutaneous Approach

06LC3DZ Occlusion of Right Common Iliac Vein with Intraluminal Device, Percutaneous Approach

06LC3ZZ Occlusion of Right Common Iliac Vein, Percutaneous Approach

06LC4CZ Occlusion of Right Common Iliac Vein with Extraluminal Device, Percutaneous Endoscopic Approach

06LC4DZ Occlusion of Right Common Iliac Vein with Intraluminal Device, Percutaneous Endoscopic Approach

06LC4ZZ Occlusion of Right Common Iliac Vein, Percutaneous Endoscopic Approach

06LD0CZ Occlusion of Left Common Iliac Vein with Extraluminal Device, Open Approach

06LD0DZ Occlusion of Left Common Iliac Vein with Intraluminal Device, Open Approach

06LD0ZZ Occlusion of Left Common Iliac Vein, Open Approach

06LD3CZ Occlusion of Left Common Iliac Vein with Extraluminal Device, Percutaneous Approach

06LD3DZ Occlusion of Left Common Iliac Vein with Intraluminal Device, Percutaneous Approach

06LD3ZZ Occlusion of Left Common Iliac Vein, Percutaneous Approach

06LD4CZ Occlusion of Left Common Iliac Vein with Extraluminal Device, Percutaneous Endoscopic Approach

06LD4DZ Occlusion of Left Common Iliac Vein with Intraluminal Device, Percutaneous Endoscopic Approach

06LD4ZZ Occlusion of Left Common Iliac Vein, Percutaneous Endoscopic Approach

06LF0CZ Occlusion of Right External Iliac Vein with Extraluminal Device, Open Approach

06LF0DZ Occlusion of Right External Iliac Vein with Intraluminal Device, Open Approach

06LF0ZZ Occlusion of Right External Iliac Vein, Open Approach

06LF3CZ Occlusion of Right External Iliac Vein with Extraluminal Device, Percutaneous Approach

06LF3DZ Occlusion of Right External Iliac Vein with Intraluminal Device, Percutaneous Approach

06LF3ZZ Occlusion of Right External Iliac Vein, Percutaneous Approach

06LF4CZ Occlusion of Right External Iliac Vein with Extraluminal Device, Percutaneous Endoscopic Approach

06LF4DZ Occlusion of Right External Iliac Vein with Intraluminal Device, Percutaneous Endoscopic Approach

06LF4ZZ Occlusion of Right External Iliac Vein, Percutaneous Endoscopic Approach

06LG0CZ Occlusion of Left External Iliac Vein with Extraluminal Device, Open Approach

06LG0DZ Occlusion of Left External Iliac Vein with Intraluminal Device, Open Approach

06LG0ZZ Occlusion of Left External Iliac Vein, Open Approach

06LG3CZ Occlusion of Left External Iliac Vein with Extraluminal Device, Percutaneous Approach

06LG3DZ Occlusion of Left External Iliac Vein with Intraluminal Device, Percutaneous Approach

06LG3ZZ Occlusion of Left External Iliac Vein, Percutaneous Approach

06LG4CZ Occlusion of Left External Iliac Vein with Extraluminal Device, Percutaneous Endoscopic Approach

06LG4DZ Occlusion of Left External Iliac Vein with Intraluminal Device, Percutaneous Endoscopic Approach

06LG4ZZ Occlusion of Left External Iliac Vein, Percutaneous Endoscopic Approach

06LH0CZ Occlusion of Right Hypogastric Vein with Extraluminal Device, Open Approach

06LH0DZ Occlusion of Right Hypogastric Vein with Intraluminal Device, Open Approach

06LH0ZZ Occlusion of Right Hypogastric Vein, Open Approach

Female-only   ♂ Male-only   ▲ Limited Coverage   ● Non-OR   ▬ HAC-associated procedure   ▲ Non-covered procedures   ✚ Combination

06LH3CZ Occlusion of Right Hypogastric Vein with Extraluminal Device, Percutaneous Approach

06LH3DZ Occlusion of Right Hypogastric Vein with Intraluminal Device, Percutaneous Approach

06LH3ZZ Occlusion of Right Hypogastric Vein, Percutaneous Approach

06LH4CZ Occlusion of Right Hypogastric Vein with Extraluminal Device, Percutaneous Endoscopic Approach

06LH4DZ Occlusion of Right Hypogastric Vein with Intraluminal Device, Percutaneous Endoscopic Approach

06LH4ZZ Occlusion of Right Hypogastric Vein, Percutaneous Endoscopic Approach

06LJ0CZ Occlusion of Left Hypogastric Vein with Extraluminal Device, Open Approach

06LJ0DZ Occlusion of Left Hypogastric Vein with Intraluminal Device, Open Approach

06LJ0ZZ Occlusion of Left Hypogastric Vein, Open Approach

06LJ3CZ Occlusion of Left Hypogastric Vein with Extraluminal Device, Percutaneous Approach

06LJ3DZ Occlusion of Left Hypogastric Vein with Intraluminal Device, Percutaneous Approach

06LJ3ZZ Occlusion of Left Hypogastric Vein, Percutaneous Approach

06LJ4CZ Occlusion of Left Hypogastric Vein with Extraluminal Device, Percutaneous Endoscopic Approach

06LJ4DZ Occlusion of Left Hypogastric Vein with Intraluminal Device, Percutaneous Endoscopic Approach

06LJ4ZZ Occlusion of Left Hypogastric Vein, Percutaneous Endoscopic Approach

06LM0CZ Occlusion of Right Femoral Vein with Extraluminal Device, Open Approach

06LM0DZ Occlusion of Right Femoral Vein with Intraluminal Device, Open Approach

06LM0ZZ Occlusion of Right Femoral Vein, Open Approach

06LM3CZ Occlusion of Right Femoral Vein with Extraluminal Device, Percutaneous Approach

06LM3DZ Occlusion of Right Femoral Vein with Intraluminal Device, Percutaneous Approach

06LM3ZZ Occlusion of Right Femoral Vein, Percutaneous Approach

06LM4CZ Occlusion of Right Femoral Vein with Extraluminal Device, Percutaneous Endoscopic Approach

06LM4DZ Occlusion of Right Femoral Vein with Intraluminal Device, Percutaneous Endoscopic Approach

06LM4ZZ Occlusion of Right Femoral Vein, Percutaneous Endoscopic Approach

06LN0CZ Occlusion of Left Femoral Vein with Extraluminal Device, Open Approach

06LN0DZ Occlusion of Left Femoral Vein with Intraluminal Device, Open Approach

06LN0ZZ Occlusion of Left Femoral Vein, Open Approach

06LN3CZ Occlusion of Left Femoral Vein with Extraluminal Device, Percutaneous Approach

06LN3DZ Occlusion of Left Femoral Vein with Intraluminal Device, Percutaneous Approach

06LN3ZZ Occlusion of Left Femoral Vein, Percutaneous Approach

06LN4CZ Occlusion of Left Femoral Vein with Extraluminal Device, Percutaneous Endoscopic Approach

06LN4DZ Occlusion of Left Femoral Vein with Intraluminal Device, Percutaneous Endoscopic Approach

06LN4ZZ Occlusion of Left Femoral Vein, Percutaneous Endoscopic Approach

06LP0CZ Occlusion of Right Greater Saphenous Vein with Extraluminal Device, Open Approach

06LP0DZ Occlusion of Right Greater Saphenous Vein with Intraluminal Device, Open Approach

06LP0ZZ Occlusion of Right Greater Saphenous Vein, Open Approach

06LP3CZ Occlusion of Right Greater Saphenous Vein with Extraluminal Device, Percutaneous Approach

06LP3DZ Occlusion of Right Greater Saphenous Vein with Intraluminal Device, Percutaneous Approach

06LP3ZZ Occlusion of Right Greater Saphenous Vein, Percutaneous Approach

06LP4CZ Occlusion of Right Greater Saphenous Vein with Extraluminal Device, Percutaneous Endoscopic Approach

06LP4DZ Occlusion of Right Greater Saphenous Vein with Intraluminal Device, Percutaneous Endoscopic Approach

06LP4ZZ Occlusion of Right Greater Saphenous Vein, Percutaneous Endoscopic Approach

06LQ0CZ Occlusion of Left Greater Saphenous Vein with Extraluminal Device, Open Approach

06LQ0DZ Occlusion of Left Greater Saphenous Vein with Intraluminal Device, Open Approach

06LQ0ZZ Occlusion of Left Greater Saphenous Vein, Open Approach

06LQ3CZ Occlusion of Left Greater Saphenous Vein with Extraluminal Device, Percutaneous Approach

06LQ3DZ Occlusion of Left Greater Saphenous Vein with Intraluminal Device, Percutaneous Approach

06LQ3ZZ Occlusion of Left Greater Saphenous Vein, Percutaneous Approach

06LQ4CZ Occlusion of Left Greater Saphenous Vein with Extraluminal Device, Percutaneous Endoscopic Approach

06LQ4DZ Occlusion of Left Greater Saphenous Vein with Intraluminal Device, Percutaneous Endoscopic Approach

06LQ4ZZ Occlusion of Left Greater Saphenous Vein, Percutaneous Endoscopic Approach

06LR0CZ Occlusion of Right Lesser Saphenous Vein with Extraluminal Device, Open Approach

06LR0DZ Occlusion of Right Lesser Saphenous Vein with Intraluminal Device, Open Approach

06LR0ZZ Occlusion of Right Lesser Saphenous Vein, Open Approach

06LR3CZ Occlusion of Right Lesser Saphenous Vein with Extraluminal Device, Percutaneous Approach

06LR3DZ Occlusion of Right Lesser Saphenous Vein with Intraluminal Device, Percutaneous Approach

06LR3ZZ Occlusion of Right Lesser Saphenous Vein, Percutaneous Approach

06LR4CZ Occlusion of Right Lesser Saphenous Vein with Extraluminal Device, Percutaneous Endoscopic Approach

06LR4DZ Occlusion of Right Lesser Saphenous Vein with Intraluminal Device, Percutaneous Endoscopic Approach

06LR4ZZ Occlusion of Right Lesser Saphenous Vein, Percutaneous Endoscopic Approach

06LS0CZ Occlusion of Left Lesser Saphenous Vein with Extraluminal Device, Open Approach

06LS0DZ Occlusion of Left Lesser Saphenous Ve with Intraluminal Device, Open Appro

06LS0ZZ Occlusion of Left Lesser Saphenous Ve Open Approach

06LS3CZ Occlusion of Left Lesser Saphenous Ve with Extraluminal Device, Percutaneou Approach

06LS3DZ Occlusion of Left Lesser Saphenous Ve with Intraluminal Device, Percutaneous Approach

06LS3ZZ Occlusion of Left Lesser Saphenous Ve Percutaneous Approach

06LS4CZ Occlusion of Left Lesser Saphenous Ve with Extraluminal Device, Percutaneou Endoscopic Approach

06LS4DZ Occlusion of Left Lesser Saphenous Ve with Intraluminal Device, Percutaneous Endoscopic Approach

06LS4ZZ Occlusion of Left Lesser Saphenous Ve Percutaneous Endoscopic Approach

06LT0CZ Occlusion of Right Foot Vein with Extraluminal Device, Open Approach

06LT0DZ Occlusion of Right Foot Vein with Intraluminal Device, Open Approach

06LT0ZZ Occlusion of Right Foot Vein, Open Approach

06LT3CZ Occlusion of Right Foot Vein with Extraluminal Device, Percutaneous Approach

06LT3DZ Occlusion of Right Foot Vein with Intraluminal Device, Percutaneous Approach

06LT3ZZ Occlusion of Right Foot Vein, Percutaneous Approach

06LT4CZ Occlusion of Right Foot Vein with Extraluminal Device, Percutaneous Endoscopic Approach

06LT4DZ Occlusion of Right Foot Vein with Intraluminal Device, Percutaneous Endoscopic Approach

06LT4ZZ Occlusion of Right Foot Vein, Percutaneous Endoscopic Approach

06LV0CZ Occlusion of Left Foot Vein with Extraluminal Device, Open Approach

06LV0DZ Occlusion of Left Foot Vein with Intraluminal Device, Open Approach

06LV0ZZ Occlusion of Left Foot Vein, Open Approach

06LV3CZ Occlusion of Left Foot Vein with Extraluminal Device, Percutaneous Approach

06LV3DZ Occlusion of Left Foot Vein with Intraluminal Device, Percutaneous Approach

06LV3ZZ Occlusion of Left Foot Vein, Percutaneo Approach

06LV4CZ Occlusion of Left Foot Vein with Extraluminal Device, Percutaneous Endoscopic Approach

06LV4DZ Occlusion of Left Foot Vein with Intraluminal Device, Percutaneous Endoscopic Approach

06LV4ZZ Occlusion of Left Foot Vein, Percutaneo Endoscopic Approach

06LY0CC Occlusion of Hemorrhoidal Plexus with Extraluminal Device, Open Approach

06LY0CZ Occlusion of Lower Vein with Extraluminal Device, Open Approach

06LY0DC Occlusion of Hemorrhoidal Plexus with Intraluminal Device, Open Approach

06LY0DZ Occlusion of Lower Vein with Intralumin Device, Open Approach

06LY0ZC Occlusion of Hemorrhoidal Plexus, Open Approach

06LY0ZZ Occlusion of Lower Vein, Open Approac

'3CC Occlusion of Hemorrhoidal Plexus with Extraluminal Device, Percutaneous Approach
'3CZ Occlusion of Lower Vein with Extraluminal Device, Percutaneous Approach
'3DC Occlusion of Hemorrhoidal Plexus with Intraluminal Device, Percutaneous Approach
'3DZ Occlusion of Lower Vein with Intraluminal Device, Percutaneous Approach

06LY3ZC Occlusion of Hemorrhoidal Plexus, Percutaneous Approach
06LY3ZZ Occlusion of Lower Vein, Percutaneous Approach
06LY4CC Occlusion of Hemorrhoidal Plexus with Extraluminal Device, Percutaneous Endoscopic Approach
06LY4CZ Occlusion of Lower Vein with Extraluminal Device, Percutaneous Endoscopic Approach

06LY4DC Occlusion of Hemorrhoidal Plexus with Intraluminal Device, Percutaneous Endoscopic Approach
06LY4DZ Occlusion of Lower Vein with Intraluminal Device, Percutaneous Endoscopic Approach
06LY4ZC Occlusion of Hemorrhoidal Plexus, Percutaneous Endoscopic Approach
06LY4ZZ Occlusion of Lower Vein, Percutaneous Endoscopic Approach

N – Lower Veins, Release

Review Coding Guidelines B3.13 and B3.14

00ZZ Release Inferior Vena Cava, Open Approach
03ZZ Release Inferior Vena Cava, Percutaneous Approach
04ZZ Release Inferior Vena Cava, Percutaneous Endoscopic Approach
10ZZ Release Splenic Vein, Open Approach
13ZZ Release Splenic Vein, Percutaneous Approach
14ZZ Release Splenic Vein, Percutaneous Endoscopic Approach
20ZZ Release Gastric Vein, Open Approach
23ZZ Release Gastric Vein, Percutaneous Approach
24ZZ Release Gastric Vein, Percutaneous Endoscopic Approach
30ZZ Release Esophageal Vein, Open Approach
33ZZ Release Esophageal Vein, Percutaneous Approach
34ZZ Release Esophageal Vein, Percutaneous Endoscopic Approach
40ZZ Release Hepatic Vein, Open Approach
43ZZ Release Hepatic Vein, Percutaneous Approach
44ZZ Release Hepatic Vein, Percutaneous Endoscopic Approach
50ZZ Release Superior Mesenteric Vein, Open Approach
53ZZ Release Superior Mesenteric Vein, Percutaneous Approach
54ZZ Release Superior Mesenteric Vein, Percutaneous Endoscopic Approach
60ZZ Release Inferior Mesenteric Vein, Open Approach
63ZZ Release Inferior Mesenteric Vein, Percutaneous Approach
64ZZ Release Inferior Mesenteric Vein, Percutaneous Endoscopic Approach
70ZZ Release Colic Vein, Open Approach
73ZZ Release Colic Vein, Percutaneous Approach
74ZZ Release Colic Vein, Percutaneous Endoscopic Approach
80ZZ Release Portal Vein, Open Approach
83ZZ Release Portal Vein, Percutaneous Approach
84ZZ Release Portal Vein, Percutaneous Endoscopic Approach

06N90ZZ Release Right Renal Vein, Open Approach
06N93ZZ Release Right Renal Vein, Percutaneous Approach
06N94ZZ Release Right Renal Vein, Percutaneous Endoscopic Approach
06NB0ZZ Release Left Renal Vein, Open Approach
06NB3ZZ Release Left Renal Vein, Percutaneous Approach
06NB4ZZ Release Left Renal Vein, Percutaneous Endoscopic Approach
06NC0ZZ Release Right Common Iliac Vein, Open Approach
06NC3ZZ Release Right Common Iliac Vein, Percutaneous Approach
06NC4ZZ Release Right Common Iliac Vein, Percutaneous Endoscopic Approach
06ND0ZZ Release Left Common Iliac Vein, Open Approach
06ND3ZZ Release Left Common Iliac Vein, Percutaneous Approach
06ND4ZZ Release Left Common Iliac Vein, Percutaneous Endoscopic Approach
06NF0ZZ Release Right External Iliac Vein, Open Approach
06NF3ZZ Release Right External Iliac Vein, Percutaneous Approach
06NF4ZZ Release Right External Iliac Vein, Percutaneous Endoscopic Approach
06NG0ZZ Release Left External Iliac Vein, Open Approach
06NG3ZZ Release Left External Iliac Vein, Percutaneous Approach
06NG4ZZ Release Left External Iliac Vein, Percutaneous Endoscopic Approach
06NH0ZZ Release Right Hypogastric Vein, Open Approach
06NH3ZZ Release Right Hypogastric Vein, Percutaneous Approach
06NH4ZZ Release Right Hypogastric Vein, Percutaneous Endoscopic Approach
06NJ0ZZ Release Left Hypogastric Vein, Open Approach
06NJ3ZZ Release Left Hypogastric Vein, Percutaneous Approach
06NJ4ZZ Release Left Hypogastric Vein, Percutaneous Endoscopic Approach
06NM0ZZ Release Right Femoral Vein, Open Approach

06NM3ZZ Release Right Femoral Vein, Percutaneous Approach
06NM4ZZ Release Right Femoral Vein, Percutaneous Endoscopic Approach
06NN0ZZ Release Left Femoral Vein, Open Approach
06NN3ZZ Release Left Femoral Vein, Percutaneous Approach
06NN4ZZ Release Left Femoral Vein, Percutaneous Endoscopic Approach
06NP0ZZ Release Right Greater Saphenous Vein, Open Approach
06NP3ZZ Release Right Greater Saphenous Vein, Percutaneous Approach
06NP4ZZ Release Right Greater Saphenous Vein, Percutaneous Endoscopic Approach
06NQ0ZZ Release Left Greater Saphenous Vein, Open Approach
06NQ3ZZ Release Left Greater Saphenous Vein, Percutaneous Approach
06NQ4ZZ Release Left Greater Saphenous Vein, Percutaneous Endoscopic Approach
06NR0ZZ Release Right Lesser Saphenous Vein, Open Approach
06NR3ZZ Release Right Lesser Saphenous Vein, Percutaneous Approach
06NR4ZZ Release Right Lesser Saphenous Vein, Percutaneous Endoscopic Approach
06NS0ZZ Release Left Lesser Saphenous Vein, Open Approach
06NS3ZZ Release Left Lesser Saphenous Vein, Percutaneous Approach
06NS4ZZ Release Left Lesser Saphenous Vein, Percutaneous Endoscopic Approach
06NT0ZZ Release Right Foot Vein, Open Approach
06NT3ZZ Release Right Foot Vein, Percutaneous Approach
06NT4ZZ Release Right Foot Vein, Percutaneous Endoscopic Approach
06NV0ZZ Release Left Foot Vein, Open Approach
06NV3ZZ Release Left Foot Vein, Percutaneous Approach
06NV4ZZ Release Left Foot Vein, Percutaneous Endoscopic Approach
06NY0ZZ Release Lower Vein, Open Approach
06NY3ZZ Release Lower Vein, Percutaneous Approach
06NY4ZZ Release Lower Vein, Percutaneous Endoscopic Approach

P – Lower Veins, Removal

Review Coding Guideline B6.1c

PY00Z Removal of Drainage Device from Lower Vein, Open Approach
PY02Z Removal of Monitoring Device from Lower Vein, Open Approach
PY03Z Removal of Infusion Device from Lower Vein, Open Approach
PY07Z Removal of Autologous Tissue Substitute from Lower Vein, Open Approach

06PY0CZ Removal of Extraluminal Device from Lower Vein, Open Approach
06PY0DZ Removal of Intraluminal Device from Lower Vein, Open Approach
06PY0JZ Removal of Synthetic Substitute from Lower Vein, Open Approach

06PY0KZ Removal of Nonautologous Tissue Substitute from Lower Vein, Open Approach
06PY30Z Removal of Drainage Device from Lower Vein, Percutaneous Approach
06PY32Z Removal of Monitoring Device from Lower Vein, Percutaneous Approach

♀ Female-only   ♂ Male-only   ▲ Limited Coverage   ● Non-OR   ▩ HAC-associated procedure   ▲ Non-covered procedures   ✚ Combination

06PY33Z Removal of Infusion Device from Lower Vein, Percutaneous Approach
06PY37Z Removal of Autologous Tissue Substitute from Lower Vein, Percutaneous Approach
06PY3CZ Removal of Extraluminal Device from Lower Vein, Percutaneous Approach
06PY3DZ Removal of Intraluminal Device from Lower Vein, Percutaneous Approach
06PY3JZ Removal of Synthetic Substitute from Lower Vein, Percutaneous Approach
06PY3KZ Removal of Nonautologous Tissue Substitute from Lower Vein, Percutaneous Approach
06PY40Z Removal of Drainage Device from Lower Vein, Percutaneous Endoscopic Approach

06PY42Z Removal of Monitoring Device from Lower Vein, Percutaneous Endoscopic Approach
06PY43Z Removal of Infusion Device from Lower Vein, Percutaneous Endoscopic Approach
06PY47Z Removal of Autologous Tissue Substitute from Lower Vein, Percutaneous Endoscopic Approach
06PY4CZ Removal of Extraluminal Device from Lower Vein, Percutaneous Endoscopic Approach
06PY4DZ Removal of Intraluminal Device from Lower Vein, Percutaneous Endoscopic Approach

06PY4JZ Removal of Synthetic Substitute from Lower Vein, Percutaneous Endoscopic Approach
06PY4KZ Removal of Nonautologous Tissue Substitute from Lower Vein, Percutaneous Endoscopic Approach
06PYX0Z Removal of Drainage Device from Lower Vein, External Approach
06PYX2Z Removal of Monitoring Device from Lower Vein, External Approach
06PYX3Z Removal of Infusion Device from Lower Vein, External Approach
06PYXDZ Removal of Intraluminal Device from Lower Vein, External Approach

06Q – Lower Veins, Repair

06Q00ZZ Repair Inferior Vena Cava, Open Approach
06Q03ZZ Repair Inferior Vena Cava, Percutaneous Approach
06Q04ZZ Repair Inferior Vena Cava, Percutaneous Endoscopic Approach
06Q10ZZ Repair Splenic Vein, Open Approach
06Q13ZZ Repair Splenic Vein, Percutaneous Approach
06Q14ZZ Repair Splenic Vein, Percutaneous Endoscopic Approach
06Q20ZZ Repair Gastric Vein, Open Approach
06Q23ZZ Repair Gastric Vein, Percutaneous Approach
06Q24ZZ Repair Gastric Vein, Percutaneous Endoscopic Approach
06Q30ZZ Repair Esophageal Vein, Open Approach
06Q33ZZ Repair Esophageal Vein, Percutaneous Approach
06Q34ZZ Repair Esophageal Vein, Percutaneous Endoscopic Approach
06Q40ZZ Repair Hepatic Vein, Open Approach
06Q43ZZ Repair Hepatic Vein, Percutaneous Approach
06Q44ZZ Repair Hepatic Vein, Percutaneous Endoscopic Approach
06Q50ZZ Repair Superior Mesenteric Vein, Open Approach
06Q53ZZ Repair Superior Mesenteric Vein, Percutaneous Approach
06Q54ZZ Repair Superior Mesenteric Vein, Percutaneous Endoscopic Approach
06Q60ZZ Repair Inferior Mesenteric Vein, Open Approach
06Q63ZZ Repair Inferior Mesenteric Vein, Percutaneous Approach
06Q64ZZ Repair Inferior Mesenteric Vein, Percutaneous Endoscopic Approach
06Q70ZZ Repair Colic Vein, Open Approach
06Q73ZZ Repair Colic Vein, Percutaneous Approach
06Q74ZZ Repair Colic Vein, Percutaneous Endoscopic Approach
06Q80ZZ Repair Portal Vein, Open Approach
06Q83ZZ Repair Portal Vein, Percutaneous Approach
06Q84ZZ Repair Portal Vein, Percutaneous Endoscopic Approach
06Q90ZZ Repair Right Renal Vein, Open Approach

06Q93ZZ Repair Right Renal Vein, Percutaneous Approach
06Q94ZZ Repair Right Renal Vein, Percutaneous Endoscopic Approach
06QB0ZZ Repair Left Renal Vein, Open Approach
06QB3ZZ Repair Left Renal Vein, Percutaneous Approach
06QB4ZZ Repair Left Renal Vein, Percutaneous Endoscopic Approach
06QC0ZZ Repair Right Common Iliac Vein, Open Approach
06QC3ZZ Repair Right Common Iliac Vein, Percutaneous Approach
06QC4ZZ Repair Right Common Iliac Vein, Percutaneous Endoscopic Approach
06QD0ZZ Repair Left Common Iliac Vein, Open Approach
06QD3ZZ Repair Left Common Iliac Vein, Percutaneous Approach
06QD4ZZ Repair Left Common Iliac Vein, Percutaneous Endoscopic Approach
06QF0ZZ Repair Right External Iliac Vein, Open Approach
06QF3ZZ Repair Right External Iliac Vein, Percutaneous Approach
06QF4ZZ Repair Right External Iliac Vein, Percutaneous Endoscopic Approach
06QG0ZZ Repair Left External Iliac Vein, Open Approach
06QG3ZZ Repair Left External Iliac Vein, Percutaneous Approach
06QG4ZZ Repair Left External Iliac Vein, Percutaneous Endoscopic Approach
06QH0ZZ Repair Right Hypogastric Vein, Open Approach
06QH3ZZ Repair Right Hypogastric Vein, Percutaneous Approach
06QH4ZZ Repair Right Hypogastric Vein, Percutaneous Endoscopic Approach
06QJ0ZZ Repair Left Hypogastric Vein, Open Approach
06QJ3ZZ Repair Left Hypogastric Vein, Percutaneous Approach
06QJ4ZZ Repair Left Hypogastric Vein, Percutaneous Endoscopic Approach
06QM0ZZ Repair Right Femoral Vein, Open Approach

06QM3ZZ Repair Right Femoral Vein, Percutaneous Approach
06QM4ZZ Repair Right Femoral Vein, Percutaneous Endoscopic Approach
06QN0ZZ Repair Left Femoral Vein, Open Approach
06QN3ZZ Repair Left Femoral Vein, Percutaneous Approach
06QN4ZZ Repair Left Femoral Vein, Percutaneous Endoscopic Approach
06QP0ZZ Repair Right Greater Saphenous Vein, Open Approach
06QP3ZZ Repair Right Greater Saphenous Vein, Percutaneous Approach
06QP4ZZ Repair Right Greater Saphenous Vein, Percutaneous Endoscopic Approach
06QQ0ZZ Repair Left Greater Saphenous Vein, Open Approach
06QQ3ZZ Repair Left Greater Saphenous Vein, Percutaneous Approach
06QQ4ZZ Repair Left Greater Saphenous Vein, Percutaneous Endoscopic Approach
06QR0ZZ Repair Right Lesser Saphenous Vein, Open Approach
06QR3ZZ Repair Right Lesser Saphenous Vein, Percutaneous Approach
06QR4ZZ Repair Right Lesser Saphenous Vein, Percutaneous Endoscopic Approach
06QS0ZZ Repair Left Lesser Saphenous Vein, Open Approach
06QS3ZZ Repair Left Lesser Saphenous Vein, Percutaneous Approach
06QS4ZZ Repair Left Lesser Saphenous Vein, Percutaneous Endoscopic Approach
06QT0ZZ Repair Right Foot Vein, Open Approach
06QT3ZZ Repair Right Foot Vein, Percutaneous Approach
06QT4ZZ Repair Right Foot Vein, Percutaneous Endoscopic Approach
06QV0ZZ Repair Left Foot Vein, Open Approach
06QV3ZZ Repair Left Foot Vein, Percutaneous Approach
06QV4ZZ Repair Left Foot Vein, Percutaneous Endoscopic Approach
06QY0ZZ Repair Lower Vein, Open Approach
06QY3ZZ Repair Lower Vein, Percutaneous Approach
06QY4ZZ Repair Lower Vein, Percutaneous Endoscopic Approach

06R – Lower Veins, Replacement

06R007Z Replacement of Inferior Vena Cava with Autologous Tissue Substitute, Open Approach
06R00JZ Replacement of Inferior Vena Cava with Synthetic Substitute, Open Approach
06R00KZ Replacement of Inferior Vena Cava with Nonautologous Tissue Substitute, Open Approach

06R047Z Replacement of Inferior Vena Cava with Autologous Tissue Substitute, Percutaneous Endoscopic Approach
06R04JZ Replacement of Inferior Vena Cava with Synthetic Substitute, Percutaneous Endoscopic Approach
06R04KZ Replacement of Inferior Vena Cava with Nonautologous Tissue Substitute, Percutaneous Endoscopic Approach

06R107Z Replacement of Splenic Vein with Autologous Tissue Substitute, Open Approach
06R10JZ Replacement of Splenic Vein with Synthetic Substitute, Open Approach
06R10KZ Replacement of Splenic Vein with Nonautologous Tissue Substitute, Open Approach

♀ Female-only   ♂ Male-only   ▲ Limited Coverage   ● Non-OR   ▨ HAC-associated procedure   ▲ Non-covered procedures   ✛ Combinati

47Z Replacement of Splenic Vein with Autologous Tissue Substitute, Percutaneous Endoscopic Approach

4JZ Replacement of Splenic Vein with Synthetic Substitute, Percutaneous Endoscopic Approach

4KZ Replacement of Splenic Vein with Nonautologous Tissue Substitute, Percutaneous Endoscopic Approach

207Z Replacement of Gastric Vein with Autologous Tissue Substitute, Open Approach

20JZ Replacement of Gastric Vein with Synthetic Substitute, Open Approach

20KZ Replacement of Gastric Vein with Nonautologous Tissue Substitute, Open Approach

247Z Replacement of Gastric Vein with Autologous Tissue Substitute, Percutaneous Endoscopic Approach

24JZ Replacement of Gastric Vein with Synthetic Substitute, Percutaneous Endoscopic Approach

24KZ Replacement of Gastric Vein with Nonautologous Tissue Substitute, Percutaneous Endoscopic Approach

307Z Replacement of Esophageal Vein with Autologous Tissue Substitute, Open Approach

30JZ Replacement of Esophageal Vein with Synthetic Substitute, Open Approach

30KZ Replacement of Esophageal Vein with Nonautologous Tissue Substitute, Open Approach

347Z Replacement of Esophageal Vein with Autologous Tissue Substitute, Percutaneous Endoscopic Approach

34JZ Replacement of Esophageal Vein with Synthetic Substitute, Percutaneous Endoscopic Approach

34KZ Replacement of Esophageal Vein with Nonautologous Tissue Substitute, Percutaneous Endoscopic Approach

407Z Replacement of Hepatic Vein with Autologous Tissue Substitute, Open Approach

40JZ Replacement of Hepatic Vein with Synthetic Substitute, Open Approach

40KZ Replacement of Hepatic Vein with Nonautologous Tissue Substitute, Open Approach

447Z Replacement of Hepatic Vein with Autologous Tissue Substitute, Percutaneous Endoscopic Approach

44JZ Replacement of Hepatic Vein with Synthetic Substitute, Percutaneous Endoscopic Approach

44KZ Replacement of Hepatic Vein with Nonautologous Tissue Substitute, Percutaneous Endoscopic Approach

R507Z Replacement of Superior Mesenteric Vein with Autologous Tissue Substitute, Open Approach

R50JZ Replacement of Superior Mesenteric Vein with Synthetic Substitute, Open Approach

R50KZ Replacement of Superior Mesenteric Vein with Nonautologous Tissue Substitute, Open Approach

R547Z Replacement of Superior Mesenteric Vein with Autologous Tissue Substitute, Percutaneous Endoscopic Approach

R54JZ Replacement of Superior Mesenteric Vein with Synthetic Substitute, Percutaneous Endoscopic Approach

R54KZ Replacement of Superior Mesenteric Vein with Nonautologous Tissue Substitute, Percutaneous Endoscopic Approach

06R607Z Replacement of Inferior Mesenteric Vein with Autologous Tissue Substitute, Open Approach

06R60JZ Replacement of Inferior Mesenteric Vein with Synthetic Substitute, Open Approach

06R60KZ Replacement of Inferior Mesenteric Vein with Nonautologous Tissue Substitute, Open Approach

06R647Z Replacement of Inferior Mesenteric Vein with Autologous Tissue Substitute, Percutaneous Endoscopic Approach

06R64JZ Replacement of Inferior Mesenteric Vein with Synthetic Substitute, Percutaneous Endoscopic Approach

06R64KZ Replacement of Inferior Mesenteric Vein with Nonautologous Tissue Substitute, Percutaneous Endoscopic Approach

06R707Z Replacement of Colic Vein with Autologous Tissue Substitute, Open Approach

06R70JZ Replacement of Colic Vein with Synthetic Substitute, Open Approach

06R70KZ Replacement of Colic Vein with Nonautologous Tissue Substitute, Open Approach

06R747Z Replacement of Colic Vein with Autologous Tissue Substitute, Percutaneous Endoscopic Approach

06R74JZ Replacement of Colic Vein with Synthetic Substitute, Percutaneous Endoscopic Approach

06R74KZ Replacement of Colic Vein with Nonautologous Tissue Substitute, Percutaneous Endoscopic Approach

06R807Z Replacement of Portal Vein with Autologous Tissue Substitute, Open Approach

06R80JZ Replacement of Portal Vein with Synthetic Substitute, Open Approach

06R80KZ Replacement of Portal Vein with Nonautologous Tissue Substitute, Open Approach

06R847Z Replacement of Portal Vein with Autologous Tissue Substitute, Percutaneous Endoscopic Approach

06R84JZ Replacement of Portal Vein with Synthetic Substitute, Percutaneous Endoscopic Approach

06R84KZ Replacement of Portal Vein with Nonautologous Tissue Substitute, Percutaneous Endoscopic Approach

06R907Z Replacement of Right Renal Vein with Autologous Tissue Substitute, Open Approach

06R90JZ Replacement of Right Renal Vein with Synthetic Substitute, Open Approach

06R90KZ Replacement of Right Renal Vein with Nonautologous Tissue Substitute, Open Approach

06R947Z Replacement of Right Renal Vein with Autologous Tissue Substitute, Percutaneous Endoscopic Approach

06R94JZ Replacement of Right Renal Vein with Synthetic Substitute, Percutaneous Endoscopic Approach

06R94KZ Replacement of Right Renal Vein with Nonautologous Tissue Substitute, Percutaneous Endoscopic Approach

06RB07Z Replacement of Left Renal Vein with Autologous Tissue Substitute, Open Approach

06RB0JZ Replacement of Left Renal Vein with Synthetic Substitute, Open Approach

06RB0KZ Replacement of Left Renal Vein with Nonautologous Tissue Substitute, Open Approach

06RB47Z Replacement of Left Renal Vein with Autologous Tissue Substitute, Percutaneous Endoscopic Approach

06RB4JZ Replacement of Left Renal Vein with Synthetic Substitute, Percutaneous Endoscopic Approach

06RB4KZ Replacement of Left Renal Vein with Nonautologous Tissue Substitute, Percutaneous Endoscopic Approach

06RC07Z Replacement of Right Common Iliac Vein with Autologous Tissue Substitute, Open Approach

06RC0JZ Replacement of Right Common Iliac Vein with Synthetic Substitute, Open Approach

06RC0KZ Replacement of Right Common Iliac Vein with Nonautologous Tissue Substitute, Open Approach

06RC47Z Replacement of Right Common Iliac Vein with Autologous Tissue Substitute, Percutaneous Endoscopic Approach

06RC4JZ Replacement of Right Common Iliac Vein with Synthetic Substitute, Percutaneous Endoscopic Approach

06RC4KZ Replacement of Right Common Iliac Vein with Nonautologous Tissue Substitute, Percutaneous Endoscopic Approach

06RD07Z Replacement of Left Common Iliac Vein with Autologous Tissue Substitute, Open Approach

06RD0JZ Replacement of Left Common Iliac Vein with Synthetic Substitute, Open Approach

06RD0KZ Replacement of Left Common Iliac Vein with Nonautologous Tissue Substitute, Open Approach

06RD47Z Replacement of Left Common Iliac Vein with Autologous Tissue Substitute, Percutaneous Endoscopic Approach

06RD4JZ Replacement of Left Common Iliac Vein with Synthetic Substitute, Percutaneous Endoscopic Approach

06RD4KZ Replacement of Left Common Iliac Vein with Nonautologous Tissue Substitute, Percutaneous Endoscopic Approach

06RF07Z Replacement of Right External Iliac Vein with Autologous Tissue Substitute, Open Approach

06RF0JZ Replacement of Right External Iliac Vein with Synthetic Substitute, Open Approach

06RF0KZ Replacement of Right External Iliac Vein with Nonautologous Tissue Substitute, Open Approach

06RF47Z Replacement of Right External Iliac Vein with Autologous Tissue Substitute, Percutaneous Endoscopic Approach

06RF4JZ Replacement of Right External Iliac Vein with Synthetic Substitute, Percutaneous Endoscopic Approach

06RF4KZ Replacement of Right External Iliac Vein with Nonautologous Tissue Substitute, Percutaneous Endoscopic Approach

06RG07Z Replacement of Left External Iliac Vein with Autologous Tissue Substitute, Open Approach

06RG0JZ Replacement of Left External Iliac Vein with Synthetic Substitute, Open Approach

06RG0KZ Replacement of Left External Iliac Vein with Nonautologous Tissue Substitute, Open Approach

06RG47Z Replacement of Left External Iliac Vein with Autologous Tissue Substitute, Percutaneous Endoscopic Approach

06RG4JZ Replacement of Left External Iliac Vein with Synthetic Substitute, Percutaneous Endoscopic Approach

♀ Female-only   ♂ Male-only   ▲ Limited Coverage   ● Non-OR   ▥ HAC-associated procedure   ▲ Non-covered procedures   + Combination

06RG4KZ Replacement of Left External Iliac Vein with Nonautologous Tissue Substitute, Percutaneous Endoscopic Approach

06RH07Z Replacement of Right Hypogastric Vein with Autologous Tissue Substitute, Open Approach

06RH0JZ Replacement of Right Hypogastric Vein with Synthetic Substitute, Open Approach

06RH0KZ Replacement of Right Hypogastric Vein with Nonautologous Tissue Substitute, Open Approach

06RH47Z Replacement of Right Hypogastric Vein with Autologous Tissue Substitute, Percutaneous Endoscopic Approach

06RH4JZ Replacement of Right Hypogastric Vein with Synthetic Substitute, Percutaneous Endoscopic Approach

06RH4KZ Replacement of Right Hypogastric Vein with Nonautologous Tissue Substitute, Percutaneous Endoscopic Approach

06RJ07Z Replacement of Left Hypogastric Vein with Autologous Tissue Substitute, Open Approach

06RJ0JZ Replacement of Left Hypogastric Vein with Synthetic Substitute, Open Approach

06RJ0KZ Replacement of Left Hypogastric Vein with Nonautologous Tissue Substitute, Open Approach

06RJ47Z Replacement of Left Hypogastric Vein with Autologous Tissue Substitute, Percutaneous Endoscopic Approach

06RJ4JZ Replacement of Left Hypogastric Vein with Synthetic Substitute, Percutaneous Endoscopic Approach

06RJ4KZ Replacement of Left Hypogastric Vein with Nonautologous Tissue Substitute, Percutaneous Endoscopic Approach

06RM07Z Replacement of Right Femoral Vein with Autologous Tissue Substitute, Open Approach

06RM0JZ Replacement of Right Femoral Vein with Synthetic Substitute, Open Approach

06RM0KZ Replacement of Right Femoral Vein with Nonautologous Tissue Substitute, Open Approach

06RM47Z Replacement of Right Femoral Vein with Autologous Tissue Substitute, Percutaneous Endoscopic Approach

06RM4JZ Replacement of Right Femoral Vein with Synthetic Substitute, Percutaneous Endoscopic Approach

06RM4KZ Replacement of Right Femoral Vein with Nonautologous Tissue Substitute, Percutaneous Endoscopic Approach

06RN07Z Replacement of Left Femoral Vein with Autologous Tissue Substitute, Open Approach

06RN0JZ Replacement of Left Femoral Vein with Synthetic Substitute, Open Approach

06RN0KZ Replacement of Left Femoral Vein with Nonautologous Tissue Substitute, Open Approach

06RN47Z Replacement of Left Femoral Vein with Autologous Tissue Substitute, Percutaneous Endoscopic Approach

06RN4JZ Replacement of Left Femoral Vein with Synthetic Substitute, Percutaneous Endoscopic Approach

06RN4KZ Replacement of Left Femoral Vein with Nonautologous Tissue Substitute, Percutaneous Endoscopic Approach

06RP07Z Replacement of Right Greater Saphenous Vein with Autologous Tissue Substitute, Open Approach

06RP0JZ Replacement of Right Greater Saphenous Vein with Synthetic Substitute, Open Approach

06RP0KZ Replacement of Right Greater Saphenous Vein with Nonautologous Tissue Substitute, Open Approach

06RP47Z Replacement of Right Greater Saphenous Vein with Autologous Tissue Substitute, Percutaneous Endoscopic Approach

06RP4JZ Replacement of Right Greater Saphenous Vein with Synthetic Substitute, Percutaneous Endoscopic Approach

06RP4KZ Replacement of Right Greater Saphenous Vein with Nonautologous Tissue Substitute, Percutaneous Endoscopic Approach

06RQ07Z Replacement of Left Greater Saphenous Vein with Autologous Tissue Substitute, Open Approach

06RQ0JZ Replacement of Left Greater Saphenous Vein with Synthetic Substitute, Open Approach

06RQ0KZ Replacement of Left Greater Saphenous Vein with Nonautologous Tissue Substitute, Open Approach

06RQ47Z Replacement of Left Greater Saphenous Vein with Autologous Tissue Substitute, Percutaneous Endoscopic Approach

06RQ4JZ Replacement of Left Greater Saphenous Vein with Synthetic Substitute, Percutaneous Endoscopic Approach

06RQ4KZ Replacement of Left Greater Saphenous Vein with Nonautologous Tissue Substitute, Percutaneous Endoscopic Approach

06RR07Z Replacement of Right Lesser Saphenous Vein with Autologous Tissue Substitute, Open Approach

06RR0JZ Replacement of Right Lesser Saphenous Vein with Synthetic Substitute, Open Approach

06RR0KZ Replacement of Right Lesser Saphenous Vein with Nonautologous Tissue Substitute, Open Approach

06RR47Z Replacement of Right Lesser Saphenous Vein with Autologous Tissue Substitute, Percutaneous Endoscopic Approach

06RR4JZ Replacement of Right Lesser Saphenous Vein with Synthetic Substitute, Percutaneous Endoscopic Approach

06RR4KZ Replacement of Right Lesser Saphenous Vein with Nonautologous Tissue Substitute, Percutaneous Endoscopic Approach

06RS07Z Replacement of Left Lesser Saphenous Vein with Autologous Tissue Substitute, Open Approach

06RS0JZ Replacement of Left Lesser Saphenous Vein with Synthetic Substitute, Open Approach

06RS0KZ Replacement of Left Lesser Saphenous Vein with Nonautologous Tissue Substitute, Open Approach

06RS47Z Replacement of Left Lesser Saphenous Vein with Autologous Tissue Substitute, Percutaneous Endoscopic Approach

06RS4JZ Replacement of Left Lesser Saphenous Vein with Synthetic Substitute, Percutaneous Endoscopic Approach

06RS4KZ Replacement of Left Lesser Saphenous Vein with Nonautologous Tissue Substitute, Percutaneous Endoscopic Approach

06RT07Z Replacement of Right Foot Vein with Autologous Tissue Substitute, Open Approach

06RT0JZ Replacement of Right Foot Vein with Synthetic Substitute, Open Approach

06RT0KZ Replacement of Right Foot Vein with Nonautologous Tissue Substitute, Open Approach

06RT47Z Replacement of Right Foot Vein with Autologous Tissue Substitute, Percutaneous Endoscopic Approach

06RT4JZ Replacement of Right Foot Vein with Synthetic Substitute, Percutaneous Endoscopic Approach

06RT4KZ Replacement of Right Foot Vein with Nonautologous Tissue Substitute, Percutaneous Endoscopic Approach

06RV07Z Replacement of Left Foot Vein with Autologous Tissue Substitute, Open Approach

06RV0JZ Replacement of Left Foot Vein with Synthetic Substitute, Open Approach

06RV0KZ Replacement of Left Foot Vein with Nonautologous Tissue Substitute, Open Approach

06RV47Z Replacement of Left Foot Vein with Autologous Tissue Substitute, Percutaneous Endoscopic Approach

06RV4JZ Replacement of Left Foot Vein with Synthetic Substitute, Percutaneous Endoscopic Approach

06RV4KZ Replacement of Left Foot Vein with Nonautologous Tissue Substitute, Percutaneous Endoscopic Approach

06RY07Z Replacement of Lower Vein with Autologous Tissue Substitute, Open Approach

06RY0JZ Replacement of Lower Vein with Synthetic Substitute, Open Approach

06RY0KZ Replacement of Lower Vein with Nonautologous Tissue Substitute, Open Approach

06RY47Z Replacement of Lower Vein with Autologous Tissue Substitute, Percutaneous Endoscopic Approach

06RY4JZ Replacement of Lower Vein with Synthetic Substitute, Percutaneous Endoscopic Approach

06RY4KZ Replacement of Lower Vein with Nonautologous Tissue Substitute, Percutaneous Endoscopic Approach

06S – Lower Veins, Reposition

06S00ZZ Reposition Inferior Vena Cava, Open Approach

06S03ZZ Reposition Inferior Vena Cava, Percutaneous Approach

06S04ZZ Reposition Inferior Vena Cava, Percutaneous Endoscopic Approach

06S10ZZ Reposition Splenic Vein, Open Approach

06S13ZZ Reposition Splenic Vein, Percutaneous Approach

06S14ZZ Reposition Splenic Vein, Percutaneous Endoscopic Approach

06S20ZZ Reposition Gastric Vein, Open Approach

06S23ZZ Reposition Gastric Vein, Percutaneous Approach

06S24ZZ Reposition Gastric Vein, Percutaneous Endoscopic Approach

06S30ZZ Reposition Esophageal Vein, Open Approach

06S33ZZ Reposition Esophageal Vein, Percutaneous Approach

06S34ZZ Reposition Esophageal Vein, Percutaneous Endoscopic Approach

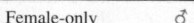

♀ Female-only　♂ Male-only　▲ Limited Coverage　● Non-OR　▨ HAC-associated procedure　▲ Non-covered procedures　✚ Combination

40ZZ	Reposition Hepatic Vein, Open Approach
43ZZ	Reposition Hepatic Vein, Percutaneous Approach
44ZZ	Reposition Hepatic Vein, Percutaneous Endoscopic Approach
50ZZ	Reposition Superior Mesenteric Vein, Open Approach
53ZZ	Reposition Superior Mesenteric Vein, Percutaneous Approach
54ZZ	Reposition Superior Mesenteric Vein, Percutaneous Endoscopic Approach
60ZZ	Reposition Inferior Mesenteric Vein, Open Approach
63ZZ	Reposition Inferior Mesenteric Vein, Percutaneous Approach
64ZZ	Reposition Inferior Mesenteric Vein, Percutaneous Endoscopic Approach
70ZZ	Reposition Colic Vein, Open Approach
73ZZ	Reposition Colic Vein, Percutaneous Approach
74ZZ	Reposition Colic Vein, Percutaneous Endoscopic Approach
80ZZ	Reposition Portal Vein, Open Approach
83ZZ	Reposition Portal Vein, Percutaneous Approach
84ZZ	Reposition Portal Vein, Percutaneous Endoscopic Approach
90ZZ	Reposition Right Renal Vein, Open Approach
93ZZ	Reposition Right Renal Vein, Percutaneous Approach
94ZZ	Reposition Right Renal Vein, Percutaneous Endoscopic Approach
SB0ZZ	Reposition Left Renal Vein, Open Approach
SB3ZZ	Reposition Left Renal Vein, Percutaneous Approach
SB4ZZ	Reposition Left Renal Vein, Percutaneous Endoscopic Approach
SC0ZZ	Reposition Right Common Iliac Vein, Open Approach
SC3ZZ	Reposition Right Common Iliac Vein, Percutaneous Approach

06SC4ZZ	Reposition Right Common Iliac Vein, Percutaneous Endoscopic Approach
06SD0ZZ	Reposition Left Common Iliac Vein, Open Approach
06SD3ZZ	Reposition Left Common Iliac Vein, Percutaneous Approach
06SD4ZZ	Reposition Left Common Iliac Vein, Percutaneous Endoscopic Approach
06SF0ZZ	Reposition Right External Iliac Vein, Open Approach
06SF3ZZ	Reposition Right External Iliac Vein, Percutaneous Approach
06SF4ZZ	Reposition Right External Iliac Vein, Percutaneous Endoscopic Approach
06SG0ZZ	Reposition Left External Iliac Vein, Open Approach
06SG3ZZ	Reposition Left External Iliac Vein, Percutaneous Approach
06SG4ZZ	Reposition Left External Iliac Vein, Percutaneous Endoscopic Approach
06SH0ZZ	Reposition Right Hypogastric Vein, Open Approach
06SH3ZZ	Reposition Right Hypogastric Vein, Percutaneous Approach
06SH4ZZ	Reposition Right Hypogastric Vein, Percutaneous Endoscopic Approach
06SJ0ZZ	Reposition Left Hypogastric Vein, Open Approach
06SJ3ZZ	Reposition Left Hypogastric Vein, Percutaneous Approach
06SJ4ZZ	Reposition Left Hypogastric Vein, Percutaneous Endoscopic Approach
06SM0ZZ	Reposition Right Femoral Vein, Open Approach
06SM3ZZ	Reposition Right Femoral Vein, Percutaneous Approach
06SM4ZZ	Reposition Right Femoral Vein, Percutaneous Endoscopic Approach
06SN0ZZ	Reposition Left Femoral Vein, Open Approach
06SN3ZZ	Reposition Left Femoral Vein, Percutaneous Approach

06SN4ZZ	Reposition Left Femoral Vein, Percutaneous Endoscopic Approach
06SP0ZZ	Reposition Right Greater Saphenous Vein, Open Approach
06SP3ZZ	Reposition Right Greater Saphenous Vein, Percutaneous Approach
06SP4ZZ	Reposition Right Greater Saphenous Vein, Percutaneous Endoscopic Approach
06SQ0ZZ	Reposition Left Greater Saphenous Vein, Open Approach
06SQ3ZZ	Reposition Left Greater Saphenous Vein, Percutaneous Approach
06SQ4ZZ	Reposition Left Greater Saphenous Vein, Percutaneous Endoscopic Approach
06SR0ZZ	Reposition Right Lesser Saphenous Vein, Open Approach
06SR3ZZ	Reposition Right Lesser Saphenous Vein, Percutaneous Approach
06SR4ZZ	Reposition Right Lesser Saphenous Vein, Percutaneous Endoscopic Approach
06SS0ZZ	Reposition Left Lesser Saphenous Vein, Open Approach
06SS3ZZ	Reposition Left Lesser Saphenous Vein, Percutaneous Approach
06SS4ZZ	Reposition Left Lesser Saphenous Vein, Percutaneous Endoscopic Approach
06ST0ZZ	Reposition Right Foot Vein, Open Approach
06ST3ZZ	Reposition Right Foot Vein, Percutaneous Approach
06ST4ZZ	Reposition Right Foot Vein, Percutaneous Endoscopic Approach
06SV0ZZ	Reposition Left Foot Vein, Open Approach
06SV3ZZ	Reposition Left Foot Vein, Percutaneous Approach
06SV4ZZ	Reposition Left Foot Vein, Percutaneous Endoscopic Approach
06SY0ZZ	Reposition Lower Vein, Open Approach
06SY3ZZ	Reposition Lower Vein, Percutaneous Approach
06SY4ZZ	Reposition Lower Vein, Percutaneous Endoscopic Approach

6U – Lower Veins, Supplement

U007Z	Supplement Inferior Vena Cava with Autologous Tissue Substitute, Open Approach
U00JZ	Supplement Inferior Vena Cava with Synthetic Substitute, Open Approach
U00KZ	Supplement Inferior Vena Cava with Nonautologous Tissue Substitute, Open Approach
U037Z	Supplement Inferior Vena Cava with Autologous Tissue Substitute, Percutaneous Approach
U03JZ	Supplement Inferior Vena Cava with Synthetic Substitute, Percutaneous Approach
U03KZ	Supplement Inferior Vena Cava with Nonautologous Tissue Substitute, Percutaneous Approach
U047Z	Supplement Inferior Vena Cava with Autologous Tissue Substitute, Percutaneous Endoscopic Approach
U04JZ	Supplement Inferior Vena Cava with Synthetic Substitute, Percutaneous Endoscopic Approach
U04KZ	Supplement Inferior Vena Cava with Nonautologous Tissue Substitute, Percutaneous Endoscopic Approach
6U107Z	Supplement Splenic Vein with Autologous Tissue Substitute, Open Approach
6U10JZ	Supplement Splenic Vein with Synthetic Substitute, Open Approach

06U10KZ	Supplement Splenic Vein with Nonautologous Tissue Substitute, Open Approach
06U137Z	Supplement Splenic Vein with Autologous Tissue Substitute, Percutaneous Approach
06U13JZ	Supplement Splenic Vein with Synthetic Substitute, Percutaneous Approach
06U13KZ	Supplement Splenic Vein with Nonautologous Tissue Substitute, Percutaneous Approach
06U147Z	Supplement Splenic Vein with Autologous Tissue Substitute, Percutaneous Endoscopic Approach
06U14JZ	Supplement Splenic Vein with Synthetic Substitute, Percutaneous Endoscopic Approach
06U14KZ	Supplement Splenic Vein with Nonautologous Tissue Substitute, Percutaneous Endoscopic Approach
06U207Z	Supplement Gastric Vein with Autologous Tissue Substitute, Open Approach
06U20JZ	Supplement Gastric Vein with Synthetic Substitute, Open Approach
06U20KZ	Supplement Gastric Vein with Nonautologous Tissue Substitute, Open Approach
06U237Z	Supplement Gastric Vein with Autologous Tissue Substitute, Percutaneous Approach
06U23JZ	Supplement Gastric Vein with Synthetic Substitute, Percutaneous Approach

06U23KZ	Supplement Gastric Vein with Nonautologous Tissue Substitute, Percutaneous Approach
06U247Z	Supplement Gastric Vein with Autologous Tissue Substitute, Percutaneous Endoscopic Approach
06U24JZ	Supplement Gastric Vein with Synthetic Substitute, Percutaneous Endoscopic Approach
06U24KZ	Supplement Gastric Vein with Nonautologous Tissue Substitute, Percutaneous Endoscopic Approach
06U307Z	Supplement Esophageal Vein with Autologous Tissue Substitute, Open Approach
06U30JZ	Supplement Esophageal Vein with Synthetic Substitute, Open Approach
06U30KZ	Supplement Esophageal Vein with Nonautologous Tissue Substitute, Open Approach
06U337Z	Supplement Esophageal Vein with Autologous Tissue Substitute, Percutaneous Approach
06U33JZ	Supplement Esophageal Vein with Synthetic Substitute, Percutaneous Approach
06U33KZ	Supplement Esophageal Vein with Nonautologous Tissue Substitute, Percutaneous Approach
06U347Z	Supplement Esophageal Vein with Autologous Tissue Substitute, Percutaneous Endoscopic Approach

Female-only   ♂ Male-only   ▲ Limited Coverage   ● Non-OR   ▧ HAC-associated procedure   ▲ Non-covered procedures   + Combination

06U34JZ	Supplement Esophageal Vein with Synthetic Substitute, Percutaneous Endoscopic Approach
06U34KZ	Supplement Esophageal Vein with Nonautologous Tissue Substitute, Percutaneous Endoscopic Approach
06U407Z	Supplement Hepatic Vein with Autologous Tissue Substitute, Open Approach
06U40JZ	Supplement Hepatic Vein with Synthetic Substitute, Open Approach
06U40KZ	Supplement Hepatic Vein with Nonautologous Tissue Substitute, Open Approach
06U437Z	Supplement Hepatic Vein with Autologous Tissue Substitute, Percutaneous Approach
06U43JZ	Supplement Hepatic Vein with Synthetic Substitute, Percutaneous Approach
06U43KZ	Supplement Hepatic Vein with Nonautologous Tissue Substitute, Percutaneous Approach
06U447Z	Supplement Hepatic Vein with Autologous Tissue Substitute, Percutaneous Endoscopic Approach
06U44JZ	Supplement Hepatic Vein with Synthetic Substitute, Percutaneous Endoscopic Approach
06U44KZ	Supplement Hepatic Vein with Nonautologous Tissue Substitute, Percutaneous Endoscopic Approach
06U507Z	Supplement Superior Mesenteric Vein with Autologous Tissue Substitute, Open Approach
06U50JZ	Supplement Superior Mesenteric Vein with Synthetic Substitute, Open Approach
06U50KZ	Supplement Superior Mesenteric Vein with Nonautologous Tissue Substitute, Open Approach
06U537Z	Supplement Superior Mesenteric Vein with Autologous Tissue Substitute, Percutaneous Approach
06U53JZ	Supplement Superior Mesenteric Vein with Synthetic Substitute, Percutaneous Approach
06U53KZ	Supplement Superior Mesenteric Vein with Nonautologous Tissue Substitute, Percutaneous Approach
06U547Z	Supplement Superior Mesenteric Vein with Autologous Tissue Substitute, Percutaneous Endoscopic Approach
06U54JZ	Supplement Superior Mesenteric Vein with Synthetic Substitute, Percutaneous Endoscopic Approach
06U54KZ	Supplement Superior Mesenteric Vein with Nonautologous Tissue Substitute, Percutaneous Endoscopic Approach
06U607Z	Supplement Inferior Mesenteric Vein with Autologous Tissue Substitute, Open Approach
06U60JZ	Supplement Inferior Mesenteric Vein with Synthetic Substitute, Open Approach
06U60KZ	Supplement Inferior Mesenteric Vein with Nonautologous Tissue Substitute, Open Approach
06U637Z	Supplement Inferior Mesenteric Vein with Autologous Tissue Substitute, Percutaneous Approach
06U63JZ	Supplement Inferior Mesenteric Vein with Synthetic Substitute, Percutaneous Approach
06U63KZ	Supplement Inferior Mesenteric Vein with Nonautologous Tissue Substitute, Percutaneous Approach
06U647Z	Supplement Inferior Mesenteric Vein with Autologous Tissue Substitute, Percutaneous Endoscopic Approach
06U64JZ	Supplement Inferior Mesenteric Vein with Synthetic Substitute, Percutaneous Endoscopic Approach
06U64KZ	Supplement Inferior Mesenteric Vein with Nonautologous Tissue Substitute, Percutaneous Endoscopic Approach
06U707Z	Supplement Colic Vein with Autologous Tissue Substitute, Open Approach
06U70JZ	Supplement Colic Vein with Synthetic Substitute, Open Approach
06U70KZ	Supplement Colic Vein with Nonautologous Tissue Substitute, Open Approach
06U737Z	Supplement Colic Vein with Autologous Tissue Substitute, Percutaneous Approach
06U73JZ	Supplement Colic Vein with Synthetic Substitute, Percutaneous Approach
06U73KZ	Supplement Colic Vein with Nonautologous Tissue Substitute, Percutaneous Approach
06U747Z	Supplement Colic Vein with Autologous Tissue Substitute, Percutaneous Endoscopic Approach
06U74JZ	Supplement Colic Vein with Synthetic Substitute, Percutaneous Endoscopic Approach
06U74KZ	Supplement Colic Vein with Nonautologous Tissue Substitute, Percutaneous Endoscopic Approach
06U807Z	Supplement Portal Vein with Autologous Tissue Substitute, Open Approach
06U80JZ	Supplement Portal Vein with Synthetic Substitute, Open Approach
06U80KZ	Supplement Portal Vein with Nonautologous Tissue Substitute, Open Approach
06U837Z	Supplement Portal Vein with Autologous Tissue Substitute, Percutaneous Approach
06U83JZ	Supplement Portal Vein with Synthetic Substitute, Percutaneous Approach
06U83KZ	Supplement Portal Vein with Nonautologous Tissue Substitute, Percutaneous Approach
06U847Z	Supplement Portal Vein with Autologous Tissue Substitute, Percutaneous Endoscopic Approach
06U84JZ	Supplement Portal Vein with Synthetic Substitute, Percutaneous Endoscopic Approach
06U84KZ	Supplement Portal Vein with Nonautologous Tissue Substitute, Percutaneous Endoscopic Approach
06U907Z	Supplement Right Renal Vein with Autologous Tissue Substitute, Open Approach
06U90JZ	Supplement Right Renal Vein with Synthetic Substitute, Open Approach
06U90KZ	Supplement Right Renal Vein with Nonautologous Tissue Substitute, Open Approach
06U937Z	Supplement Right Renal Vein with Autologous Tissue Substitute, Percutaneous Approach
06U93JZ	Supplement Right Renal Vein with Synthetic Substitute, Percutaneous Approach
06U93KZ	Supplement Right Renal Vein with Nonautologous Tissue Substitute, Percutaneous Approach
06U947Z	Supplement Right Renal Vein with Autologous Tissue Substitute, Percutaneous Endoscopic Approach
06U94JZ	Supplement Right Renal Vein with Synthetic Substitute, Percutaneous Endoscopic Approach
06U94KZ	Supplement Right Renal Vein with Nonautologous Tissue Substitute, Percutaneous Endoscopic Approach
06UB07Z	Supplement Left Renal Vein with Autologous Tissue Substitute, Open Approach
06UB0JZ	Supplement Left Renal Vein with Synthetic Substitute, Open Approach
06UB0KZ	Supplement Left Renal Vein with Nonautologous Tissue Substitute, Open Approach
06UB37Z	Supplement Left Renal Vein with Autologous Tissue Substitute, Percutaneous Approach
06UB3JZ	Supplement Left Renal Vein with Synthetic Substitute, Percutaneous Approach
06UB3KZ	Supplement Left Renal Vein with Nonautologous Tissue Substitute, Percutaneous Approach
06UB47Z	Supplement Left Renal Vein with Autologous Tissue Substitute, Percutaneous Endoscopic Approach
06UB4JZ	Supplement Left Renal Vein with Synthetic Substitute, Percutaneous Endoscopic Approach
06UB4KZ	Supplement Left Renal Vein with Nonautologous Tissue Substitute, Percutaneous Endoscopic Approach
06UC07Z	Supplement Right Common Iliac Vein with Autologous Tissue Substitute, Open Approach
06UC0JZ	Supplement Right Common Iliac Vein with Synthetic Substitute, Open Approach
06UC0KZ	Supplement Right Common Iliac Vein with Nonautologous Tissue Substitute, Open Approach
06UC37Z	Supplement Right Common Iliac Vein with Autologous Tissue Substitute, Percutaneous Approach
06UC3JZ	Supplement Right Common Iliac Vein with Synthetic Substitute, Percutaneous Approach
06UC3KZ	Supplement Right Common Iliac Vein with Nonautologous Tissue Substitute, Percutaneous Approach
06UC47Z	Supplement Right Common Iliac Vein with Autologous Tissue Substitute, Percutaneous Endoscopic Approach
06UC4JZ	Supplement Right Common Iliac Vein with Synthetic Substitute, Percutaneous Endoscopic Approach
06UC4KZ	Supplement Right Common Iliac Vein with Nonautologous Tissue Substitute, Percutaneous Endoscopic Approach
06UD07Z	Supplement Left Common Iliac Vein with Autologous Tissue Substitute, Open Approach
06UD0JZ	Supplement Left Common Iliac Vein with Synthetic Substitute, Open Approach
06UD0KZ	Supplement Left Common Iliac Vein with Nonautologous Tissue Substitute, Open Approach
06UD37Z	Supplement Left Common Iliac Vein with Autologous Tissue Substitute, Percutaneous Approach
06UD3JZ	Supplement Left Common Iliac Vein with Synthetic Substitute, Percutaneous Approach
06UD3KZ	Supplement Left Common Iliac Vein with Nonautologous Tissue Substitute, Percutaneous Approach
06UD47Z	Supplement Left Common Iliac Vein with Autologous Tissue Substitute, Percutaneous Endoscopic Approach
06UD4JZ	Supplement Left Common Iliac Vein with Synthetic Substitute, Percutaneous Endoscopic Approach
06UD4KZ	Supplement Left Common Iliac Vein with Nonautologous Tissue Substitute, Percutaneous Endoscopic Approach
06UF07Z	Supplement Right External Iliac Vein with Autologous Tissue Substitute, Open Approach

♀ Female-only   ♂ Male-only   ▲ Limited Coverage   ● Non-OR   ▨ HAC-associated procedure   ▲ Non-covered procedures   ✚ Combination

F0JZ	Supplement Right External Iliac Vein with Synthetic Substitute, Open Approach
F0KZ	Supplement Right External Iliac Vein with Nonautologous Tissue Substitute, Open Approach
F37Z	Supplement Right External Iliac Vein with Autologous Tissue Substitute, Percutaneous Approach
F3JZ	Supplement Right External Iliac Vein with Synthetic Substitute, Percutaneous Approach
F3KZ	Supplement Right External Iliac Vein with Nonautologous Tissue Substitute, Percutaneous Approach
F47Z	Supplement Right External Iliac Vein with Autologous Tissue Substitute, Percutaneous Endoscopic Approach
F4JZ	Supplement Right External Iliac Vein with Synthetic Substitute, Percutaneous Endoscopic Approach
F4KZ	Supplement Right External Iliac Vein with Nonautologous Tissue Substitute, Percutaneous Endoscopic Approach
JG07Z	Supplement Left External Iliac Vein with Autologous Tissue Substitute, Open Approach
JG0JZ	Supplement Left External Iliac Vein with Synthetic Substitute, Open Approach
JG0KZ	Supplement Left External Iliac Vein with Nonautologous Tissue Substitute, Open Approach
JG37Z	Supplement Left External Iliac Vein with Autologous Tissue Substitute, Percutaneous Approach
JG3JZ	Supplement Left External Iliac Vein with Synthetic Substitute, Percutaneous Approach
UG3KZ	Supplement Left External Iliac Vein with Nonautologous Tissue Substitute, Percutaneous Approach
UG47Z	Supplement Left External Iliac Vein with Autologous Tissue Substitute, Percutaneous Endoscopic Approach
UG4JZ	Supplement Left External Iliac Vein with Synthetic Substitute, Percutaneous Endoscopic Approach
UG4KZ	Supplement Left External Iliac Vein with Nonautologous Tissue Substitute, Percutaneous Endoscopic Approach
UH07Z	Supplement Right Hypogastric Vein with Autologous Tissue Substitute, Open Approach
UH0JZ	Supplement Right Hypogastric Vein with Synthetic Substitute, Open Approach
UH0KZ	Supplement Right Hypogastric Vein with Nonautologous Tissue Substitute, Open Approach
UH37Z	Supplement Right Hypogastric Vein with Autologous Tissue Substitute, Percutaneous Approach
UH3JZ	Supplement Right Hypogastric Vein with Synthetic Substitute, Percutaneous Approach
UH3KZ	Supplement Right Hypogastric Vein with Nonautologous Tissue Substitute, Percutaneous Approach
UH47Z	Supplement Right Hypogastric Vein with Autologous Tissue Substitute, Percutaneous Endoscopic Approach
UH4JZ	Supplement Right Hypogastric Vein with Synthetic Substitute, Percutaneous Endoscopic Approach
UH4KZ	Supplement Right Hypogastric Vein with Nonautologous Tissue Substitute, Percutaneous Endoscopic Approach
UJ07Z	Supplement Left Hypogastric Vein with Autologous Tissue Substitute, Open Approach

06UJ0JZ	Supplement Left Hypogastric Vein with Synthetic Substitute, Open Approach
06UJ0KZ	Supplement Left Hypogastric Vein with Nonautologous Tissue Substitute, Open Approach
06UJ37Z	Supplement Left Hypogastric Vein with Autologous Tissue Substitute, Percutaneous Approach
06UJ3JZ	Supplement Left Hypogastric Vein with Synthetic Substitute, Percutaneous Approach
06UJ3KZ	Supplement Left Hypogastric Vein with Nonautologous Tissue Substitute, Percutaneous Approach
06UJ47Z	Supplement Left Hypogastric Vein with Autologous Tissue Substitute, Percutaneous Endoscopic Approach
06UJ4JZ	Supplement Left Hypogastric Vein with Synthetic Substitute, Percutaneous Endoscopic Approach
06UJ4KZ	Supplement Left Hypogastric Vein with Nonautologous Tissue Substitute, Percutaneous Endoscopic Approach
06UM07Z	Supplement Right Femoral Vein with Autologous Tissue Substitute, Open Approach
06UM0JZ	Supplement Right Femoral Vein with Synthetic Substitute, Open Approach
06UM0KZ	Supplement Right Femoral Vein with Nonautologous Tissue Substitute, Open Approach
06UM37Z	Supplement Right Femoral Vein with Autologous Tissue Substitute, Percutaneous Approach
06UM3JZ	Supplement Right Femoral Vein with Synthetic Substitute, Percutaneous Approach
06UM3KZ	Supplement Right Femoral Vein with Nonautologous Tissue Substitute, Percutaneous Approach
06UM47Z	Supplement Right Femoral Vein with Autologous Tissue Substitute, Percutaneous Endoscopic Approach
06UM4JZ	Supplement Right Femoral Vein with Synthetic Substitute, Percutaneous Endoscopic Approach
06UM4KZ	Supplement Right Femoral Vein with Nonautologous Tissue Substitute, Percutaneous Endoscopic Approach
06UN07Z	Supplement Left Femoral Vein with Autologous Tissue Substitute, Open Approach
06UN0JZ	Supplement Left Femoral Vein with Synthetic Substitute, Open Approach
06UN0KZ	Supplement Left Femoral Vein with Nonautologous Tissue Substitute, Open Approach
06UN37Z	Supplement Left Femoral Vein with Autologous Tissue Substitute, Percutaneous Approach
06UN3JZ	Supplement Left Femoral Vein with Synthetic Substitute, Percutaneous Approach
06UN3KZ	Supplement Left Femoral Vein with Nonautologous Tissue Substitute, Percutaneous Approach
06UN47Z	Supplement Left Femoral Vein with Autologous Tissue Substitute, Percutaneous Endoscopic Approach
06UN4JZ	Supplement Left Femoral Vein with Synthetic Substitute, Percutaneous Endoscopic Approach
06UN4KZ	Supplement Left Femoral Vein with Nonautologous Tissue Substitute, Percutaneous Endoscopic Approach
06UP07Z	Supplement Right Greater Saphenous Vein with Autologous Tissue Substitute, Open Approach

06UP0JZ	Supplement Right Greater Saphenous Vein with Synthetic Substitute, Open Approach
06UP0KZ	Supplement Right Greater Saphenous Vein with Nonautologous Tissue Substitute, Open Approach
06UP37Z	Supplement Right Greater Saphenous Vein with Autologous Tissue Substitute, Percutaneous Approach
06UP3JZ	Supplement Right Greater Saphenous Vein with Synthetic Substitute, Percutaneous Approach
06UP3KZ	Supplement Right Greater Saphenous Vein with Nonautologous Tissue Substitute, Percutaneous Approach
06UP47Z	Supplement Right Greater Saphenous Vein with Autologous Tissue Substitute, Percutaneous Endoscopic Approach
06UP4JZ	Supplement Right Greater Saphenous Vein with Synthetic Substitute, Percutaneous Endoscopic Approach
06UP4KZ	Supplement Right Greater Saphenous Vein with Nonautologous Tissue Substitute, Percutaneous Endoscopic Approach
06UQ07Z	Supplement Left Greater Saphenous Vein with Autologous Tissue Substitute, Open Approach
06UQ0JZ	Supplement Left Greater Saphenous Vein with Synthetic Substitute, Open Approach
06UQ0KZ	Supplement Left Greater Saphenous Vein with Nonautologous Tissue Substitute, Open Approach
06UQ37Z	Supplement Left Greater Saphenous Vein with Autologous Tissue Substitute, Percutaneous Approach
06UQ3JZ	Supplement Left Greater Saphenous Vein with Synthetic Substitute, Percutaneous Approach
06UQ3KZ	Supplement Left Greater Saphenous Vein with Nonautologous Tissue Substitute, Percutaneous Approach
06UQ47Z	Supplement Left Greater Saphenous Vein with Autologous Tissue Substitute, Percutaneous Endoscopic Approach
06UQ4JZ	Supplement Left Greater Saphenous Vein with Synthetic Substitute, Percutaneous Endoscopic Approach
06UQ4KZ	Supplement Left Greater Saphenous Vein with Nonautologous Tissue Substitute, Percutaneous Endoscopic Approach
06UR07Z	Supplement Right Lesser Saphenous Vein with Autologous Tissue Substitute, Open Approach
06UR0JZ	Supplement Right Lesser Saphenous Vein with Synthetic Substitute, Open Approach
06UR0KZ	Supplement Right Lesser Saphenous Vein with Nonautologous Tissue Substitute, Open Approach
06UR37Z	Supplement Right Lesser Saphenous Vein with Autologous Tissue Substitute, Percutaneous Approach
06UR3JZ	Supplement Right Lesser Saphenous Vein with Synthetic Substitute, Percutaneous Approach
06UR3KZ	Supplement Right Lesser Saphenous Vein with Nonautologous Tissue Substitute, Percutaneous Approach
06UR47Z	Supplement Right Lesser Saphenous Vein with Autologous Tissue Substitute, Percutaneous Endoscopic Approach
06UR4JZ	Supplement Right Lesser Saphenous Vein with Synthetic Substitute, Percutaneous Endoscopic Approach
06UR4KZ	Supplement Right Lesser Saphenous Vein with Nonautologous Tissue Substitute, Percutaneous Endoscopic Approach

Female-only   ♂ Male-only   ▲ Limited Coverage   ● Non-OR   ▨ HAC-associated procedure   ▲ Non-covered procedures   ✚ Combination

06US07Z Supplement Left Lesser Saphenous Vein with Autologous Tissue Substitute, Open Approach

06US0JZ Supplement Left Lesser Saphenous Vein with Synthetic Substitute, Open Approach

06US0KZ Supplement Left Lesser Saphenous Vein with Nonautologous Tissue Substitute, Open Approach

06US37Z Supplement Left Lesser Saphenous Vein with Autologous Tissue Substitute, Percutaneous Approach

06US3JZ Supplement Left Lesser Saphenous Vein with Synthetic Substitute, Percutaneous Approach

06US3KZ Supplement Left Lesser Saphenous Vein with Nonautologous Tissue Substitute, Percutaneous Approach

06US47Z Supplement Left Lesser Saphenous Vein with Autologous Tissue Substitute, Percutaneous Endoscopic Approach

06US4JZ Supplement Left Lesser Saphenous Vein with Synthetic Substitute, Percutaneous Endoscopic Approach

06US4KZ Supplement Left Lesser Saphenous Vein with Nonautologous Tissue Substitute, Percutaneous Endoscopic Approach

06UT07Z Supplement Right Foot Vein with Autologous Tissue Substitute, Open Approach

06UT0JZ Supplement Right Foot Vein with Synthetic Substitute, Open Approach

06UT0KZ Supplement Right Foot Vein with Nonautologous Tissue Substitute, Open Approach

06UT37Z Supplement Right Foot Vein with Autologous Tissue Substitute, Percutaneous Approach

06UT3JZ Supplement Right Foot Vein with Synthetic Substitute, Percutaneous Approach

06UT3KZ Supplement Right Foot Vein with Nonautologous Tissue Substitute, Percutaneous Approach

06UT47Z Supplement Right Foot Vein with Autologous Tissue Substitute, Percutaneous Endoscopic Approach

06UT4JZ Supplement Right Foot Vein with Synthetic Substitute, Percutaneous Endoscopic Approach

06UT4KZ Supplement Right Foot Vein with Nonautologous Tissue Substitute, Percutaneous Endoscopic Approach

06UV07Z Supplement Left Foot Vein with Autologous Tissue Substitute, Open Approach

06UV0JZ Supplement Left Foot Vein with Synthetic Substitute, Open Approach

06UV0KZ Supplement Left Foot Vein with Nonautologous Tissue Substitute, Open Approach

06UV37Z Supplement Left Foot Vein with Autologous Tissue Substitute, Percutaneous Approach

06UV3JZ Supplement Left Foot Vein with Synthetic Substitute, Percutaneous Approach

06UV3KZ Supplement Left Foot Vein with Nonautologous Tissue Substitute, Percutaneous Approach

06UV47Z Supplement Left Foot Vein with Autologous Tissue Substitute, Percutaneous Endoscopic Approach

06UV4JZ Supplement Left Foot Vein with Synthetic Substitute, Percutaneous Endoscopic Approach

06UV4KZ Supplement Left Foot Vein with Nonautologous Tissue Substitute, Percutaneous Endoscopic Approach

06UY07Z Supplement Lower Vein with Autologous Tissue Substitute, Open Approach

06UY0JZ Supplement Lower Vein with Synthetic Substitute, Open Approach

06UY0KZ Supplement Lower Vein with Nonautologous Tissue Substitute, Open Approach

06UY37Z Supplement Lower Vein with Autologous Tissue Substitute, Percutaneous Approach

06UY3JZ Supplement Lower Vein with Synthetic Substitute, Percutaneous Approach

06UY3KZ Supplement Lower Vein with Nonautologous Tissue Substitute, Percutaneous Approach

06UY47Z Supplement Lower Vein with Autologous Tissue Substitute, Percutaneous Endoscopic Approach

06UY4JZ Supplement Lower Vein with Synthetic Substitute, Percutaneous Endoscopic Approach

06UY4KZ Supplement Lower Vein with Nonautologous Tissue Substitute, Percutaneous Endoscopic Approach

06V – Lower Veins, Restriction

Review Coding Guideline B3.12

06V00CZ Restriction of Inferior Vena Cava with Extraluminal Device, Open Approach

06V00DZ Restriction of Inferior Vena Cava with Intraluminal Device, Open Approach

06V00ZZ Restriction of Inferior Vena Cava, Open Approach

06V03CZ Restriction of Inferior Vena Cava with Extraluminal Device, Percutaneous Approach

06V03DZ Restriction of Inferior Vena Cava with Intraluminal Device, Percutaneous Approach

06V03ZZ Restriction of Inferior Vena Cava, Percutaneous Approach

06V04CZ Restriction of Inferior Vena Cava with Extraluminal Device, Percutaneous Endoscopic Approach

06V04DZ Restriction of Inferior Vena Cava with Intraluminal Device, Percutaneous Endoscopic Approach

06V04ZZ Restriction of Inferior Vena Cava, Percutaneous Endoscopic Approach

06V10CZ Restriction of Splenic Vein with Extraluminal Device, Open Approach

06V10DZ Restriction of Splenic Vein with Intraluminal Device, Open Approach

06V10ZZ Restriction of Splenic Vein, Open Approach

06V13CZ Restriction of Splenic Vein with Extraluminal Device, Percutaneous Approach

06V13DZ Restriction of Splenic Vein with Intraluminal Device, Percutaneous Approach

06V13ZZ Restriction of Splenic Vein, Percutaneous Approach

06V14CZ Restriction of Splenic Vein with Extraluminal Device, Percutaneous Endoscopic Approach

06V14DZ Restriction of Splenic Vein with Intraluminal Device, Percutaneous Endoscopic Approach

06V14ZZ Restriction of Splenic Vein, Percutaneous Endoscopic Approach

06V20CZ Restriction of Gastric Vein with Extraluminal Device, Open Approach

06V20DZ Restriction of Gastric Vein with Intraluminal Device, Open Approach

06V20ZZ Restriction of Gastric Vein, Open Approach

06V23CZ Restriction of Gastric Vein with Extraluminal Device, Percutaneous Approach

06V23DZ Restriction of Gastric Vein with Intraluminal Device, Percutaneous Approach

06V23ZZ Restriction of Gastric Vein, Percutaneous Approach

06V24CZ Restriction of Gastric Vein with Extraluminal Device, Percutaneous Endoscopic Approach

06V24DZ Restriction of Gastric Vein with Intraluminal Device, Percutaneous Endoscopic Approach

06V24ZZ Restriction of Gastric Vein, Percutaneous Endoscopic Approach

06V30CZ Restriction of Esophageal Vein with Extraluminal Device, Open Approach

06V30DZ Restriction of Esophageal Vein with Intraluminal Device, Open Approach

06V30ZZ Restriction of Esophageal Vein, Open Approach

06V33CZ Restriction of Esophageal Vein with Extraluminal Device, Percutaneous Approach

06V33DZ Restriction of Esophageal Vein with Intraluminal Device, Percutaneous Approach

06V33ZZ Restriction of Esophageal Vein, Percutaneous Approach

06V34CZ Restriction of Esophageal Vein with Extraluminal Device, Percutaneous Endoscopic Approach

06V34DZ Restriction of Esophageal Vein with Intraluminal Device, Percutaneous Endoscopic Approach

06V34ZZ Restriction of Esophageal Vein, Percutaneous Endoscopic Approach

06V40CZ Restriction of Hepatic Vein with Extraluminal Device, Open Approach

06V40DZ Restriction of Hepatic Vein with Intraluminal Device, Open Approach

06V40ZZ Restriction of Hepatic Vein, Open Approach

06V43CZ Restriction of Hepatic Vein with Extraluminal Device, Percutaneous Approach

06V43DZ Restriction of Hepatic Vein with Intraluminal Device, Percutaneous Approach

06V43ZZ Restriction of Hepatic Vein, Percutaneous Approach

06V44CZ Restriction of Hepatic Vein with Extraluminal Device, Percutaneous Endoscopic Approach

06V44DZ Restriction of Hepatic Vein with Intraluminal Device, Percutaneous Endoscopic Approach

♀ Female-only ♂ Male-only ▲ Limited Coverage ● Non-OR ▰▰ HAC-associated procedure ▲ Non-covered procedures ✚ Combinatio

44ZZ Restriction of Hepatic Vein, Percutaneous Endoscopic Approach

50CZ Restriction of Superior Mesenteric Vein with Extraluminal Device, Open Approach

50DZ Restriction of Superior Mesenteric Vein with Intraluminal Device, Open Approach

50ZZ Restriction of Superior Mesenteric Vein, Open Approach

53CZ Restriction of Superior Mesenteric Vein with Extraluminal Device, Percutaneous Approach

53DZ Restriction of Superior Mesenteric Vein with Intraluminal Device, Percutaneous Approach

53ZZ Restriction of Superior Mesenteric Vein, Percutaneous Approach

54CZ Restriction of Superior Mesenteric Vein with Extraluminal Device, Percutaneous Endoscopic Approach

54DZ Restriction of Superior Mesenteric Vein with Intraluminal Device, Percutaneous Endoscopic Approach

54ZZ Restriction of Superior Mesenteric Vein, Percutaneous Endoscopic Approach

60CZ Restriction of Inferior Mesenteric Vein with Extraluminal Device, Open Approach

60DZ Restriction of Inferior Mesenteric Vein with Intraluminal Device, Open Approach

60ZZ Restriction of Inferior Mesenteric Vein, Open Approach

63CZ Restriction of Inferior Mesenteric Vein with Extraluminal Device, Percutaneous Approach

63DZ Restriction of Inferior Mesenteric Vein with Intraluminal Device, Percutaneous Approach

63ZZ Restriction of Inferior Mesenteric Vein, Percutaneous Approach

64CZ Restriction of Inferior Mesenteric Vein with Extraluminal Device, Percutaneous Endoscopic Approach

64DZ Restriction of Inferior Mesenteric Vein with Intraluminal Device, Percutaneous Endoscopic Approach

64ZZ Restriction of Inferior Mesenteric Vein, Percutaneous Endoscopic Approach

V70CZ Restriction of Colic Vein with Extraluminal Device, Open Approach

V70DZ Restriction of Colic Vein with Intraluminal Device, Open Approach

V70ZZ Restriction of Colic Vein, Open Approach

V73CZ Restriction of Colic Vein with Extraluminal Device, Percutaneous Approach

V73DZ Restriction of Colic Vein with Intraluminal Device, Percutaneous Approach

V73ZZ Restriction of Colic Vein, Percutaneous Approach

V74CZ Restriction of Colic Vein with Extraluminal Device, Percutaneous Endoscopic Approach

V74DZ Restriction of Colic Vein with Intraluminal Device, Percutaneous Endoscopic Approach

V74ZZ Restriction of Colic Vein, Percutaneous Endoscopic Approach

V80CZ Restriction of Portal Vein with Extraluminal Device, Open Approach

V80DZ Restriction of Portal Vein with Intraluminal Device, Open Approach

V80ZZ Restriction of Portal Vein, Open Approach

V83CZ Restriction of Portal Vein with Extraluminal Device, Percutaneous Approach

V83DZ Restriction of Portal Vein with Intraluminal Device, Percutaneous Approach

06V83ZZ Restriction of Portal Vein, Percutaneous Approach

06V84CZ Restriction of Portal Vein with Extraluminal Device, Percutaneous Endoscopic Approach

06V84DZ Restriction of Portal Vein with Intraluminal Device, Percutaneous Endoscopic Approach

06V84ZZ Restriction of Portal Vein, Percutaneous Endoscopic Approach

06V90CZ Restriction of Right Renal Vein with Extraluminal Device, Open Approach

06V90DZ Restriction of Right Renal Vein with Intraluminal Device, Open Approach

06V90ZZ Restriction of Right Renal Vein, Open Approach

06V93CZ Restriction of Right Renal Vein with Extraluminal Device, Percutaneous Approach

06V93DZ Restriction of Right Renal Vein with Intraluminal Device, Percutaneous Approach

06V93ZZ Restriction of Right Renal Vein, Percutaneous Approach

06V94CZ Restriction of Right Renal Vein with Extraluminal Device, Percutaneous Endoscopic Approach

06V94DZ Restriction of Right Renal Vein with Intraluminal Device, Percutaneous Endoscopic Approach

06V94ZZ Restriction of Right Renal Vein, Percutaneous Endoscopic Approach

06VB0CZ Restriction of Left Renal Vein with Extraluminal Device, Open Approach

06VB0DZ Restriction of Left Renal Vein with Intraluminal Device, Open Approach

06VB0ZZ Restriction of Left Renal Vein, Open Approach

06VB3CZ Restriction of Left Renal Vein with Extraluminal Device, Percutaneous Approach

06VB3DZ Restriction of Left Renal Vein with Intraluminal Device, Percutaneous Approach

06VB3ZZ Restriction of Left Renal Vein, Percutaneous Approach

06VB4CZ Restriction of Left Renal Vein with Extraluminal Device, Percutaneous Endoscopic Approach

06VB4DZ Restriction of Left Renal Vein with Intraluminal Device, Percutaneous Endoscopic Approach

06VB4ZZ Restriction of Left Renal Vein, Percutaneous Endoscopic Approach

06VC0CZ Restriction of Right Common Iliac Vein with Extraluminal Device, Open Approach

06VC0DZ Restriction of Right Common Iliac Vein with Intraluminal Device, Open Approach

06VC0ZZ Restriction of Right Common Iliac Vein, Open Approach

06VC3CZ Restriction of Right Common Iliac Vein with Extraluminal Device, Percutaneous Approach

06VC3DZ Restriction of Right Common Iliac Vein with Intraluminal Device, Percutaneous Approach

06VC3ZZ Restriction of Right Common Iliac Vein, Percutaneous Approach

06VC4CZ Restriction of Right Common Iliac Vein with Extraluminal Device, Percutaneous Endoscopic Approach

06VC4DZ Restriction of Right Common Iliac Vein with Intraluminal Device, Percutaneous Endoscopic Approach

06VC4ZZ Restriction of Right Common Iliac Vein, Percutaneous Endoscopic Approach

06VD0CZ Restriction of Left Common Iliac Vein with Extraluminal Device, Open Approach

06VD0DZ Restriction of Left Common Iliac Vein with Intraluminal Device, Open Approach

06VD0ZZ Restriction of Left Common Iliac Vein, Open Approach

06VD3CZ Restriction of Left Common Iliac Vein with Extraluminal Device, Percutaneous Approach

06VD3DZ Restriction of Left Common Iliac Vein with Intraluminal Device, Percutaneous Approach

06VD3ZZ Restriction of Left Common Iliac Vein, Percutaneous Approach

06VD4CZ Restriction of Left Common Iliac Vein with Extraluminal Device, Percutaneous Endoscopic Approach

06VD4DZ Restriction of Left Common Iliac Vein with Intraluminal Device, Percutaneous Endoscopic Approach

06VD4ZZ Restriction of Left Common Iliac Vein, Percutaneous Endoscopic Approach

06VF0CZ Restriction of Right External Iliac Vein with Extraluminal Device, Open Approach

06VF0DZ Restriction of Right External Iliac Vein with Intraluminal Device, Open Approach

06VF0ZZ Restriction of Right External Iliac Vein, Open Approach

06VF3CZ Restriction of Right External Iliac Vein with Extraluminal Device, Percutaneous Approach

06VF3DZ Restriction of Right External Iliac Vein with Intraluminal Device, Percutaneous Approach

06VF3ZZ Restriction of Right External Iliac Vein, Percutaneous Approach

06VF4CZ Restriction of Right External Iliac Vein with Extraluminal Device, Percutaneous Endoscopic Approach

06VF4DZ Restriction of Right External Iliac Vein with Intraluminal Device, Percutaneous Endoscopic Approach

06VF4ZZ Restriction of Right External Iliac Vein, Percutaneous Endoscopic Approach

06VG0CZ Restriction of Left External Iliac Vein with Extraluminal Device, Open Approach

06VG0DZ Restriction of Left External Iliac Vein with Intraluminal Device, Open Approach

06VG0ZZ Restriction of Left External Iliac Vein, Open Approach

06VG3CZ Restriction of Left External Iliac Vein with Extraluminal Device, Percutaneous Approach

06VG3DZ Restriction of Left External Iliac Vein with Intraluminal Device, Percutaneous Approach

06VG3ZZ Restriction of Left External Iliac Vein, Percutaneous Approach

06VG4CZ Restriction of Left External Iliac Vein with Extraluminal Device, Percutaneous Endoscopic Approach

06VG4DZ Restriction of Left External Iliac Vein with Intraluminal Device, Percutaneous Endoscopic Approach

06VG4ZZ Restriction of Left External Iliac Vein, Percutaneous Endoscopic Approach

06VH0CZ Restriction of Right Hypogastric Vein with Extraluminal Device, Open Approach

06VH0DZ Restriction of Right Hypogastric Vein with Intraluminal Device, Open Approach

06VH0ZZ Restriction of Right Hypogastric Vein, Open Approach

06VH3CZ Restriction of Right Hypogastric Vein with Extraluminal Device, Percutaneous Approach

06VH3DZ Restriction of Right Hypogastric Vein with Intraluminal Device, Percutaneous Approach

06VH3ZZ Restriction of Right Hypogastric Vein, Percutaneous Approach

♀ Female-only   ♂ Male-only   ▲ Limited Coverage   ● Non-OR   ▥ HAC-associated procedure   ▲ Non-covered procedures   ✚ Combination

06VH4CZ Restriction of Right Hypogastric Vein with Extraluminal Device, Percutaneous Endoscopic Approach

06VH4DZ Restriction of Right Hypogastric Vein with Intraluminal Device, Percutaneous Endoscopic Approach

06VH4ZZ Restriction of Right Hypogastric Vein, Percutaneous Endoscopic Approach

06VJ0CZ Restriction of Left Hypogastric Vein with Extraluminal Device, Open Approach

06VJ0DZ Restriction of Left Hypogastric Vein with Intraluminal Device, Open Approach

06VJ0ZZ Restriction of Left Hypogastric Vein, Open Approach

06VJ3CZ Restriction of Left Hypogastric Vein with Extraluminal Device, Percutaneous Approach

06VJ3DZ Restriction of Left Hypogastric Vein with Intraluminal Device, Percutaneous Approach

06VJ3ZZ Restriction of Left Hypogastric Vein, Percutaneous Approach

06VJ4CZ Restriction of Left Hypogastric Vein with Extraluminal Device, Percutaneous Endoscopic Approach

06VJ4DZ Restriction of Left Hypogastric Vein with Intraluminal Device, Percutaneous Endoscopic Approach

06VJ4ZZ Restriction of Left Hypogastric Vein, Percutaneous Endoscopic Approach

06VM0CZ Restriction of Right Femoral Vein with Extraluminal Device, Open Approach

06VM0DZ Restriction of Right Femoral Vein with Intraluminal Device, Open Approach

06VM0ZZ Restriction of Right Femoral Vein, Open Approach

06VM3CZ Restriction of Right Femoral Vein with Extraluminal Device, Percutaneous Approach

06VM3DZ Restriction of Right Femoral Vein with Intraluminal Device, Percutaneous Approach

06VM3ZZ Restriction of Right Femoral Vein, Percutaneous Approach

06VM4CZ Restriction of Right Femoral Vein with Extraluminal Device, Percutaneous Endoscopic Approach

06VM4DZ Restriction of Right Femoral Vein with Intraluminal Device, Percutaneous Endoscopic Approach

06VM4ZZ Restriction of Right Femoral Vein, Percutaneous Endoscopic Approach

06VN0CZ Restriction of Left Femoral Vein with Extraluminal Device, Open Approach

06VN0DZ Restriction of Left Femoral Vein with Intraluminal Device, Open Approach

06VN0ZZ Restriction of Left Femoral Vein, Open Approach

06VN3CZ Restriction of Left Femoral Vein with Extraluminal Device, Percutaneous Approach

06VN3DZ Restriction of Left Femoral Vein with Intraluminal Device, Percutaneous Approach

06VN3ZZ Restriction of Left Femoral Vein, Percutaneous Approach

06VN4CZ Restriction of Left Femoral Vein with Extraluminal Device, Percutaneous Endoscopic Approach

06VN4DZ Restriction of Left Femoral Vein with Intraluminal Device, Percutaneous Endoscopic Approach

06VN4ZZ Restriction of Left Femoral Vein, Percutaneous Endoscopic Approach

06VP0CZ Restriction of Right Greater Saphenous Vein with Extraluminal Device, Open Approach

06VP0DZ Restriction of Right Greater Saphenous Vein with Intraluminal Device, Open Approach

06VP0ZZ Restriction of Right Greater Saphenous Vein, Open Approach

06VP3CZ Restriction of Right Greater Saphenous Vein with Extraluminal Device, Percutaneous Approach

06VP3DZ Restriction of Right Greater Saphenous Vein with Intraluminal Device, Percutaneous Approach

06VP3ZZ Restriction of Right Greater Saphenous Vein, Percutaneous Approach

06VP4CZ Restriction of Right Greater Saphenous Vein with Extraluminal Device, Percutaneous Endoscopic Approach

06VP4DZ Restriction of Right Greater Saphenous Vein with Intraluminal Device, Percutaneous Endoscopic Approach

06VP4ZZ Restriction of Right Greater Saphenous Vein, Percutaneous Endoscopic Approach

06VQ0CZ Restriction of Left Greater Saphenous Vein with Extraluminal Device, Open Approach

06VQ0DZ Restriction of Left Greater Saphenous Vein with Intraluminal Device, Open Approach

06VQ0ZZ Restriction of Left Greater Saphenous Vein, Open Approach

06VQ3CZ Restriction of Left Greater Saphenous Vein with Extraluminal Device, Percutaneous Approach

06VQ3DZ Restriction of Left Greater Saphenous Vein with Intraluminal Device, Percutaneous Approach

06VQ3ZZ Restriction of Left Greater Saphenous Vein, Percutaneous Approach

06VQ4CZ Restriction of Left Greater Saphenous Vein with Extraluminal Device, Percutaneous Endoscopic Approach

06VQ4DZ Restriction of Left Greater Saphenous Vein with Intraluminal Device, Percutaneous Endoscopic Approach

06VQ4ZZ Restriction of Left Greater Saphenous Vein, Percutaneous Endoscopic Approach

06VR0CZ Restriction of Right Lesser Saphenous Vein with Extraluminal Device, Open Approach

06VR0DZ Restriction of Right Lesser Saphenous Vein with Intraluminal Device, Open Approach

06VR0ZZ Restriction of Right Lesser Saphenous Vein, Open Approach

06VR3CZ Restriction of Right Lesser Saphenous Vein with Extraluminal Device, Percutaneous Approach

06VR3DZ Restriction of Right Lesser Saphenous Vein with Intraluminal Device, Percutaneous Approach

06VR3ZZ Restriction of Right Lesser Saphenous Vein, Percutaneous Approach

06VR4CZ Restriction of Right Lesser Saphenous Vein with Extraluminal Device, Percutaneous Endoscopic Approach

06VR4DZ Restriction of Right Lesser Saphenous Vein with Intraluminal Device, Percutaneous Endoscopic Approach

06VR4ZZ Restriction of Right Lesser Saphenous Vein, Percutaneous Endoscopic Approach

06VS0CZ Restriction of Left Lesser Saphenous Vein with Extraluminal Device, Open Approach

06VS0DZ Restriction of Left Lesser Saphenous Vein with Intraluminal Device, Open Approach

06VS0ZZ Restriction of Left Lesser Saphenous Vein, Open Approach

06VS3CZ Restriction of Left Lesser Saphenous Vein with Extraluminal Device, Percutaneous Approach

06VS3DZ Restriction of Left Lesser Saphenous Vein with Intraluminal Device, Percutaneous Approach

06VS3ZZ Restriction of Left Lesser Saphenous Vein, Percutaneous Approach

06VS4CZ Restriction of Left Lesser Saphenous Vein with Extraluminal Device, Percutaneous Endoscopic Approach

06VS4DZ Restriction of Left Lesser Saphenous Vein with Intraluminal Device, Percutaneous Endoscopic Approach

06VS4ZZ Restriction of Left Lesser Saphenous Vein, Percutaneous Endoscopic Approach

06VT0CZ Restriction of Right Foot Vein with Extraluminal Device, Open Approach

06VT0DZ Restriction of Right Foot Vein with Intraluminal Device, Open Approach

06VT0ZZ Restriction of Right Foot Vein, Open Approach

06VT3CZ Restriction of Right Foot Vein with Extraluminal Device, Percutaneous Approach

06VT3DZ Restriction of Right Foot Vein with Intraluminal Device, Percutaneous Approach

06VT3ZZ Restriction of Right Foot Vein, Percutaneous Approach

06VT4CZ Restriction of Right Foot Vein with Extraluminal Device, Percutaneous Endoscopic Approach

06VT4DZ Restriction of Right Foot Vein with Intraluminal Device, Percutaneous Endoscopic Approach

06VT4ZZ Restriction of Right Foot Vein, Percutaneous Endoscopic Approach

06VV0CZ Restriction of Left Foot Vein with Extraluminal Device, Open Approach

06VV0DZ Restriction of Left Foot Vein with Intraluminal Device, Open Approach

06VV0ZZ Restriction of Left Foot Vein, Open Approach

06VV3CZ Restriction of Left Foot Vein with Extraluminal Device, Percutaneous Approach

06VV3DZ Restriction of Left Foot Vein with Intraluminal Device, Percutaneous Approach

06VV3ZZ Restriction of Left Foot Vein, Percutaneous Approach

06VV4CZ Restriction of Left Foot Vein with Extraluminal Device, Percutaneous Endoscopic Approach

06VV4DZ Restriction of Left Foot Vein with Intraluminal Device, Percutaneous Endoscopic Approach

06VV4ZZ Restriction of Left Foot Vein, Percutaneous Endoscopic Approach

06VY0CZ Restriction of Lower Vein with Extraluminal Device, Open Approach

06VY0DZ Restriction of Lower Vein with Intraluminal Device, Open Approach

06VY0ZZ Restriction of Lower Vein, Open Approach

06VY3CZ Restriction of Lower Vein with Extraluminal Device, Percutaneous Approach

06VY3DZ Restriction of Lower Vein with Intraluminal Device, Percutaneous Approach

06VY3ZZ Restriction of Lower Vein, Percutaneous Approach

Y4CZ	Restriction of Lower Vein with Extraluminal Device, Percutaneous Endoscopic Approach
06VY4DZ	Restriction of Lower Vein with Intraluminal Device, Percutaneous Endoscopic Approach
06VY4ZZ	Restriction of Lower Vein, Percutaneous Endoscopic Approach

W – Lower Veins, Revision

iew Coding Guideline B6.1c

VY00Z	Revision of Drainage Device in Lower Vein, Open Approach
VY02Z	Revision of Monitoring Device in Lower Vein, Open Approach
VY03Z	Revision of Infusion Device in Lower Vein, Open Approach
VY07Z	Revision of Autologous Tissue Substitute in Lower Vein, Open Approach
VY0CZ	Revision of Extraluminal Device in Lower Vein, Open Approach
VY0DZ	Revision of Intraluminal Device in Lower Vein, Open Approach
VY0JZ	Revision of Synthetic Substitute in Lower Vein, Open Approach
VY0KZ	Revision of Nonautologous Tissue Substitute in Lower Vein, Open Approach
VY30Z	Revision of Drainage Device in Lower Vein, Percutaneous Approach
VY32Z	Revision of Monitoring Device in Lower Vein, Percutaneous Approach
VY33Z	Revision of Infusion Device in Lower Vein, Percutaneous Approach
VY37Z	Revision of Autologous Tissue Substitute in Lower Vein, Percutaneous Approach

06WY3CZ	Revision of Extraluminal Device in Lower Vein, Percutaneous Approach
06WY3DZ	Revision of Intraluminal Device in Lower Vein, Percutaneous Approach
	AHA CC: 3Q, 2014, 25-26
06WY3JZ	Revision of Synthetic Substitute in Lower Vein, Percutaneous Approach
06WY3KZ	Revision of Nonautologous Tissue Substitute in Lower Vein, Percutaneous Approach
06WY40Z	Revision of Drainage Device in Lower Vein, Percutaneous Endoscopic Approach
06WY42Z	Revision of Monitoring Device in Lower Vein, Percutaneous Endoscopic Approach
06WY43Z	Revision of Infusion Device in Lower Vein, Percutaneous Endoscopic Approach
06WY47Z	Revision of Autologous Tissue Substitute in Lower Vein, Percutaneous Endoscopic Approach
06WY4CZ	Revision of Extraluminal Device in Lower Vein, Percutaneous Endoscopic Approach
06WY4DZ	Revision of Intraluminal Device in Lower Vein, Percutaneous Endoscopic Approach

06WY4JZ	Revision of Synthetic Substitute in Lower Vein, Percutaneous Endoscopic Approach
06WY4KZ	Revision of Nonautologous Tissue Substitute in Lower Vein, Percutaneous Endoscopic Approach
06WYX0Z	Revision of Drainage Device in Lower Vein, External Approach
06WYX2Z	Revision of Monitoring Device in Lower Vein, External Approach
06WYX3Z	Revision of Infusion Device in Lower Vein, External Approach
06WYX7Z	Revision of Autologous Tissue Substitute in Lower Vein, External Approach
06WYXCZ	Revision of Extraluminal Device in Lower Vein, External Approach
06WYXDZ	Revision of Intraluminal Device in Lower Vein, External Approach
06WYXJZ	Revision of Synthetic Substitute in Lower Vein, External Approach
06WYXKZ	Revision of Nonautologous Tissue Substitute in Lower Vein, External Approach

♀ Female-only	♂ Male-only	▲ Limited Coverage	● Non-OR	⬛ HAC-associated procedure	▲ Non-covered procedures	➕ Combination

Lymphatic System

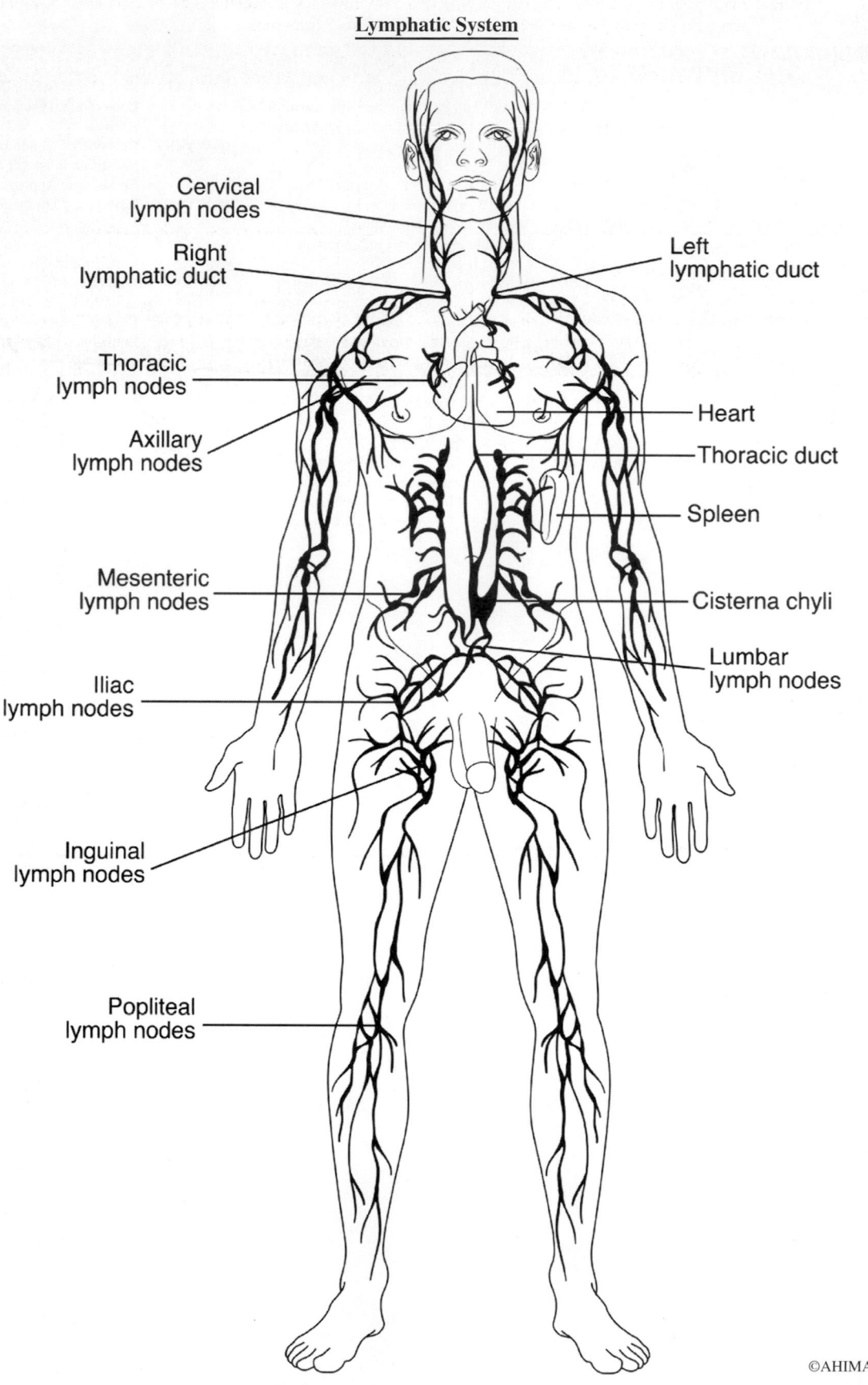

Cervical
lymph nodes

Right
lymphatic duct

Thoracic
lymph nodes

Axillary
lymph nodes

Mesenteric
lymph nodes

Iliac
lymph nodes

Inguinal
lymph nodes

Popliteal
lymph nodes

Left
lymphatic duct

Heart

Thoracic duct

Spleen

Cisterna chyli

Lumbar
lymph nodes

©AHIMA

ion	**0**	**Medical and Surgical**
y System	**7**	**Lymphatic and Hemic Systems**
ration	**2**	**Change:** Taking out or off a device from a body part and putting back an identical or similar device in or on the same body part without cutting or puncturing the skin or a mucous membrane

Body Part (4th)	Approach (5th)	Device (6th)	Qualifier (7th)
Thoracic Duct	**X** External	**0** Drainage Device	**Z** No Qualifier
Cisterna Chyli		**Y** Other Device	
Thymus			
Lymphatic			
Spleen			
Bone Marrow			

ion	**0**	**Medical and Surgical**
y System	**7**	**Lymphatic and Hemic Systems**
ration	**5**	**Destruction:** Physical eradication of all or a portion of a body part by the direct use of energy, force, or a destructive agent

Body Part (4th)	Approach (5th)	Device (6th)	Qualifier (7th)
Lymphatic, Head	**0** Open	**Z** No Device	**Z** No Qualifier
Lymphatic, Right Neck	**3** Percutaneous		
Lymphatic, Left Neck	**4** Percutaneous Endoscopic		
Lymphatic, Right Upper Extremity			
Lymphatic, Left Upper Extremity			
Lymphatic, Right Axillary			
Lymphatic, Left Axillary			
Lymphatic, Thorax			
Lymphatic, Internal Mammary, Right			
Lymphatic, Internal Mammary, Left			
Lymphatic, Mesenteric			
Lymphatic, Pelvis			
Lymphatic, Aortic			
Lymphatic, Right Lower Extremity			
Lymphatic, Left Lower Extremity			
Lymphatic, Right Inguinal			
Lymphatic, Left Inguinal			
Thoracic Duct			
Cisterna Chyli			
Thymus			
Spleen			

Section   **0**   **Medical and Surgical**
Body System   **7**   **Lymphatic and Hemic Systems**
Operation   **9**   **Drainage:** Taking or letting out fluids and/or gases from a body part

Body Part (4ᵗʰ)	Approach (5ᵗʰ)	Device (6ᵗʰ)	Qualifier (7ᵗʰ)
0 Lymphatic, Head 1 Lymphatic, Right Neck 2 Lymphatic, Left Neck 3 Lymphatic, Right Upper Extremity 4 Lymphatic, Left Upper Extremity 5 Lymphatic, Right Axillary 6 Lymphatic, Left Axillary 7 Lymphatic, Thorax 8 Lymphatic, Internal Mammary, Right 9 Lymphatic, Internal Mammary, Left B Lymphatic, Mesenteric C Lymphatic, Pelvis D Lymphatic, Aortic F Lymphatic, Right Lower Extremity G Lymphatic, Left Lower Extremity H Lymphatic, Right Inguinal J Lymphatic, Left Inguinal K Thoracic Duct L Cisterna Chyli M Thymus P Spleen T Bone Marrow	0 Open 3 Percutaneous 4 Percutaneous Endoscopic	0 Drainage Device	Z No Qualifier
0 Lymphatic, Head 1 Lymphatic, Right Neck 2 Lymphatic, Left Neck 3 Lymphatic, Right Upper Extremity 4 Lymphatic, Left Upper Extremity 5 Lymphatic, Right Axillary 6 Lymphatic, Left Axillary 7 Lymphatic, Thorax 8 Lymphatic, Internal Mammary, Right 9 Lymphatic, Internal Mammary, Left B Lymphatic, Mesenteric C Lymphatic, Pelvis D Lymphatic, Aortic F Lymphatic, Right Lower Extremity G Lymphatic, Left Lower Extremity H Lymphatic, Right Inguinal J Lymphatic, Left Inguinal K Thoracic Duct L Cisterna Chyli M Thymus P Spleen T Bone Marrow	0 Open 3 Percutaneous 4 Percutaneous Endoscopic	Z No Device	X Diagnostic Z No Qualifier

Section | 0 | **Medical and Surgical**
Body System | 7 | **Lymphatic and Hemic Systems**
Operation | B | **Excision:** Cutting out or off, without replacement, a portion of a body part

Body Part (4ᵗʰ)	Approach (5ᵗʰ)	Device (6ᵗʰ)	Qualifier (7ᵗʰ)
Lymphatic, Head Lymphatic, Right Neck Lymphatic, Left Neck Lymphatic, Right Upper Extremity Lymphatic, Left Upper Extremity Lymphatic, Right Axillary Lymphatic, Left Axillary Lymphatic, Thorax Lymphatic, Internal Mammary, Right Lymphatic, Internal Mammary, Left Lymphatic, Mesenteric Lymphatic, Pelvis Lymphatic, Aortic Lymphatic, Right Lower Extremity Lymphatic, Left Lower Extremity Lymphatic, Right Inguinal Lymphatic, Left Inguinal Thoracic Duct Cisterna Chyli Thymus Spleen	**0** Open **3** Percutaneous **4** Percutaneous Endoscopic	**Z** No Device	**X** Diagnostic **Z** No Qualifier

Section | 0 | **Medical and Surgical**
Body System | 7 | **Lymphatic and Hemic Systems**
Operation | C | **Extirpation:** Taking or cutting out solid matter from a body part

Body Part (4ᵗʰ)	Approach (5ᵗʰ)	Device (6ᵗʰ)	Qualifier (7ᵗʰ)
Lymphatic, Head Lymphatic, Right Neck Lymphatic, Left Neck Lymphatic, Right Upper Extremity Lymphatic, Left Upper Extremity Lymphatic, Right Axillary Lymphatic, Left Axillary Lymphatic, Thorax Lymphatic, Internal Mammary, Right Lymphatic, Internal Mammary, Left Lymphatic, Mesenteric Lymphatic, Pelvis Lymphatic, Aortic Lymphatic, Right Lower Extremity Lymphatic, Left Lower Extremity Lymphatic, Right Inguinal Lymphatic, Left Inguinal Thoracic Duct Cisterna Chyli Thymus Spleen	**0** Open **3** Percutaneous **4** Percutaneous Endoscopic	**Z** No Device	**Z** No Qualifier

Section | 0 | **Medical and Surgical**
Body System | 7 | **Lymphatic and Hemic Systems**
Operation | D | **Extraction:** Pulling or stripping out or off all or a portion of a body part by the use of force

Body Part (4ᵗʰ)	Approach (5ᵗʰ)	Device (6ᵗʰ)	Qualifier (7ᵗʰ)
Bone Marrow, Sternum Bone Marrow, Iliac Bone Marrow, Vertebral	**0** Open **3** Percutaneous	**Z** No Device	**X** Diagnostic **Z** No Qualifier

Section	0	Medical and Surgical
Body System	7	Lymphatic and Hemic Systems
Operation	H	**Insertion:** Putting in a nonbiological appliance that monitors, assists, performs, or prevents a physiological function but d... not physically take the place of a body part

Body Part (4th)	Approach (5th)	Device (6th)	Qualifier (7th)
K Thoracic Duct L Cisterna Chyli M Thymus N Lymphatic P Spleen	0 Open 3 Percutaneous 4 Percutaneous Endoscopic	3 Infusion Device	Z No Qualifier

Section	0	Medical and Surgical
Body System	7	Lymphatic and Hemic Systems
Operation	J	**Inspection:** Visually and/or manually exploring a body part

Body Part (4th)	Approach (5th)	Device (6th)	Qualifier (7th)
K Thoracic Duct L Cisterna Chyli M Thymus T Bone Marrow	0 Open 3 Percutaneous 4 Percutaneous Endoscopic	Z No Device	Z No Qualifier
N Lymphatic P Spleen	0 Open 3 Percutaneous 4 Percutaneous Endoscopic X External	Z No Device	Z No Qualifier

Section	0	Medical and Surgical
Body System	7	Lymphatic and Hemic Systems
Operation	L	**Occlusion:** Completely closing an orifice or the lumen of a tubular body part

Body Part (4th)	Approach (5th)	Device (6th)	Qualifier (7th)
0 Lymphatic, Head 1 Lymphatic, Right Neck 2 Lymphatic, Left Neck 3 Lymphatic, Right Upper Extremity 4 Lymphatic, Left Upper Extremity 5 Lymphatic, Right Axillary 6 Lymphatic, Left Axillary 7 Lymphatic, Thorax 8 Lymphatic, Internal Mammary, Right 9 Lymphatic, Internal Mammary, Left B Lymphatic, Mesenteric C Lymphatic, Pelvis D Lymphatic, Aortic F Lymphatic, Right Lower Extremity G Lymphatic, Left Lower Extremity H Lymphatic, Right Inguinal J Lymphatic, Left Inguinal K Thoracic Duct L Cisterna Chyli	0 Open 3 Percutaneous 4 Percutaneous Endoscopic	C Extraluminal Device D Intraluminal Device Z No Device	Z No Qualifier

tion	0	Medical and Surgical		
ly System	7	Lymphatic and Hemic Systems		
ration	N	Release: Freeing a body part from an abnormal physical constraint by cutting or by the use of force		

Body Part (4th)	Approach (5th)	Device (6th)	Qualifier (7th)
Lymphatic, Head Lymphatic, Right Neck Lymphatic, Left Neck Lymphatic, Right Upper Extremity Lymphatic, Left Upper Extremity Lymphatic, Right Axillary Lymphatic, Left Axillary Lymphatic, Thorax Lymphatic, Internal Mammary, Right Lymphatic, Internal Mammary, Left Lymphatic, Mesenteric Lymphatic, Pelvis Lymphatic, Aortic Lymphatic, Right Lower Extremity Lymphatic, Left Lower Extremity Lymphatic, Right Inguinal Lymphatic, Left Inguinal Thoracic Duct Cisterna Chyli Thymus Spleen	0 Open 3 Percutaneous 4 Percutaneous Endoscopic	Z No Device	Z No Qualifier

tion	0	Medical and Surgical		
ly System	7	Lymphatic and Hemic Systems		
ration	P	Removal: Taking out or off a device from a body part		

Body Part (4th)	Approach (5th)	Device (6th)	Qualifier (7th)
Thoracic Duct Cisterna Chyli Lymphatic	0 Open 3 Percutaneous 4 Percutaneous Endoscopic	0 Drainage Device 3 Infusion Device 7 Autologous Tissue Substitute C Extraluminal Device D Intraluminal Device J Synthetic Substitute K Nonautologous Tissue Substitute	Z No Qualifier
Thoracic Duct Cisterna Chyli Lymphatic	X External	0 Drainage Device 3 Infusion Device D Intraluminal Device	Z No Qualifier
Thymus Spleen	0 Open 3 Percutaneous 4 Percutaneous Endoscopic X External	0 Drainage Device 3 Infusion Device	Z No Qualifier
Bone Marrow	0 Open 3 Percutaneous 4 Percutaneous Endoscopic X External	0 Drainage Device	Z No Qualifier

Section	0	Medical and Surgical
Body System	7	Lymphatic and Hemic Systems
Operation	Q	Repair: Restoring, to the extent possible, a body part to its normal anatomic structure and function

Body Part (4ᵗʰ)	Approach (5ᵗʰ)	Device (6ᵗʰ)	Qualifier (7ᵗʰ)
0 Lymphatic, Head 1 Lymphatic, Right Neck 2 Lymphatic, Left Neck 3 Lymphatic, Right Upper Extremity 4 Lymphatic, Left Upper Extremity 5 Lymphatic, Right Axillary 6 Lymphatic, Left Axillary 7 Lymphatic, Thorax 8 Lymphatic, Internal Mammary, Right 9 Lymphatic, Internal Mammary, Left B Lymphatic, Mesenteric C Lymphatic, Pelvis D Lymphatic, Aortic F Lymphatic, Right Lower Extremity G Lymphatic, Left Lower Extremity H Lymphatic, Right Inguinal J Lymphatic, Left Inguinal K Thoracic Duct L Cisterna Chyli M Thymus P Spleen	0 Open 3 Percutaneous 4 Percutaneous Endoscopic	Z No Device	Z No Qualifier

Section	0	Medical and Surgical
Body System	7	Lymphatic and Hemic Systems
Operation	S	Reposition: Moving to its normal location, or other suitable location, all or a portion of a body part

Body Part (4ᵗʰ)	Approach (5ᵗʰ)	Device (6ᵗʰ)	Qualifier (7ᵗʰ)
M Thymus P Spleen	0 Open	Z No Device	Z No Qualifier

Section	0	Medical and Surgical
Body System	7	Lymphatic and Hemic Systems
Operation	T	Resection: Cutting out or off, without replacement, all of a body part

Body Part (4ᵗʰ)	Approach (5ᵗʰ)	Device (6ᵗʰ)	Qualifier (7ᵗʰ)
0 Lymphatic, Head 1 Lymphatic, Right Neck 2 Lymphatic, Left Neck 3 Lymphatic, Right Upper Extremity 4 Lymphatic, Left Upper Extremity 5 Lymphatic, Right Axillary 6 Lymphatic, Left Axillary 7 Lymphatic, Thorax 8 Lymphatic, Internal Mammary, Right 9 Lymphatic, Internal Mammary, Left B Lymphatic, Mesenteric C Lymphatic, Pelvis D Lymphatic, Aortic F Lymphatic, Right Lower Extremity G Lymphatic, Left Lower Extremity H Lymphatic, Right Inguinal J Lymphatic, Left Inguinal K Thoracic Duct L Cisterna Chyli M Thymus P Spleen	0 Open 4 Percutaneous Endoscopic	Z No Device	Z No Qualifier

	0	Medical and Surgical
ion	0	Medical and Surgical
y System	7	Lymphatic and Hemic Systems
ration	U	**Supplement:** Putting in or on biological or synthetic material that physically reinforces and/or augments the function of a portion of a body part

Body Part (4th)	Approach (5th)	Device (6th)	Qualifier (7th)
Lymphatic, Head Lymphatic, Right Neck Lymphatic, Left Neck Lymphatic, Right Upper Extremity Lymphatic, Left Upper Extremity Lymphatic, Right Axillary Lymphatic, Left Axillary Lymphatic, Thorax Lymphatic, Internal Mammary, Right Lymphatic, Internal Mammary, Left Lymphatic, Mesenteric Lymphatic, Pelvis Lymphatic, Aortic Lymphatic, Right Lower Extremity Lymphatic, Left Lower Extremity Lymphatic, Right Inguinal Lymphatic, Left Inguinal Thoracic Duct Cisterna Chyli	0 Open 4 Percutaneous Endoscopic	7 Autologous Tissue Substitute J Synthetic Substitute K Nonautologous Tissue Substitute	Z No Qualifier

tion	0	Medical and Surgical
ly System	7	Lymphatic and Hemic Systems
eration	V	**Restriction:** Partially closing an orifice or the lumen of a tubular body part

Body Part (4th)	Approach (5th)	Device (6th)	Qualifier (7th)
Lymphatic, Head Lymphatic, Right Neck Lymphatic, Left Neck Lymphatic, Right Upper Extremity Lymphatic, Left Upper Extremity Lymphatic, Right Axillary Lymphatic, Left Axillary Lymphatic, Thorax Lymphatic, Internal Mammary, Right Lymphatic, Internal Mammary, Left Lymphatic, Mesenteric Lymphatic, Pelvis Lymphatic, Aortic Lymphatic, Right Lower Extremity Lymphatic, Left Lower Extremity Lymphatic, Right Inguinal Lymphatic, Left Inguinal Thoracic Duct Cisterna Chyli	0 Open 3 Percutaneous 4 Percutaneous Endoscopic	C Extraluminal Device D Intraluminal Device Z No Device	Z No Qualifier

tion	0	Medical and Surgical
ly System	7	Lymphatic and Hemic Systems
eration	W	**Revision:** Correcting, to the extent possible, a portion of a malfunctioning device or the position of a displaced device

Body Part (4th)	Approach (5th)	Device (6th)	Qualifier (7th)
Thoracic Duct Cisterna Chyli Lymphatic	0 Open 3 Percutaneous 4 Percutaneous Endoscopic X External	0 Drainage Device 3 Infusion Device 7 Autologous Tissue Substitute C Extraluminal Device D Intraluminal Device J Synthetic Substitute K Nonautologous Tissue Substitute	Z No Qualifier

Continued →

		Section	0	Medical and Surgical
		Body System	7	Lymphatic and Hemic Systems
		Operation	W	Revision: Correcting, to the extent possible, a portion of a malfunctioning device or the position of a displaced device

Body Part (4th)	Approach (5th)	Device (6th)	Qualifier (7th)
M Thymus P Spleen	0 Open 3 Percutaneous 4 Percutaneous Endoscopic X External	0 Drainage Device 3 Infusion Device	Z No Qualifier
T Bone Marrow	0 Open 3 Percutaneous 4 Percutaneous Endoscopic X External	0 Drainage Device	Z No Qualifier

		Section	0	Medical and Surgical
		Body System	7	Lymphatic and Hemic Systems
		Operation	Y	Transplantation: Putting in or on all or a portion of a living body part taken from another individual or animal to physical[ ] take the place and/or function of all or a portion of a similar body part

Body Part (4th)	Approach (5th)	Device (6th)	Qualifier (7th)
M Thymus P Spleen	0 Open	Z No Device	0 Allogeneic 1 Syngeneic 2 Zooplastic

Lymphatic and Hemic Systems Code Listing 072–07Y

072 – Lymphatic and Hemic Systems, Change

Review Coding Guideline B6.1c

072KX0Z Change Drainage Device in Thoracic Duct, External Approach
072KXYZ Change Other Device in Thoracic Duct, External Approach
072LX0Z Change Drainage Device in Cisterna Chyli, External Approach
072LXYZ Change Other Device in Cisterna Chyli, External Approach

072MX0Z Change Drainage Device in Thymus, External Approach
072MXYZ Change Other Device in Thymus, External Approach
072NX0Z Change Drainage Device in Lymphatic, External Approach
072NXYZ Change Other Device in Lymphatic, External Approach

072PX0Z Change Drainage Device in Spleen, External Approach
072PXYZ Change Other Device in Spleen, Exter[ ] Approach
072TX0Z Change Drainage Device in Bone Mar[ ] External Approach
072TXYZ Change Other Device in Bone Marrow, External Approach

075 – Lymphatic and Hemic Systems, Destruction

07500ZZ Destruction of Head Lymphatic, Open Approach
07503ZZ Destruction of Head Lymphatic, Percutaneous Approach
07504ZZ Destruction of Head Lymphatic, Percutaneous Endoscopic Approach
07510ZZ Destruction of Right Neck Lymphatic, Open Approach
07513ZZ Destruction of Right Neck Lymphatic, Percutaneous Approach
07514ZZ Destruction of Right Neck Lymphatic, Percutaneous Endoscopic Approach
07520ZZ Destruction of Left Neck Lymphatic, Open Approach
07523ZZ Destruction of Left Neck Lymphatic, Percutaneous Approach
07524ZZ Destruction of Left Neck Lymphatic, Percutaneous Endoscopic Approach
07530ZZ Destruction of Right Upper Extremity Lymphatic, Open Approach
07533ZZ Destruction of Right Upper Extremity Lymphatic, Percutaneous Approach
07534ZZ Destruction of Right Upper Extremity Lymphatic, Percutaneous Endoscopic Approach

07540ZZ Destruction of Left Upper Extremity Lymphatic, Open Approach
07543ZZ Destruction of Left Upper Extremity Lymphatic, Percutaneous Approach
07544ZZ Destruction of Left Upper Extremity Lymphatic, Percutaneous Endoscopic Approach
07550ZZ Destruction of Right Axillary Lymphatic, Open Approach
07553ZZ Destruction of Right Axillary Lymphatic, Percutaneous Approach
07554ZZ Destruction of Right Axillary Lymphatic, Percutaneous Endoscopic Approach
07560ZZ Destruction of Left Axillary Lymphatic, Open Approach
07563ZZ Destruction of Left Axillary Lymphatic, Percutaneous Approach
07564ZZ Destruction of Left Axillary Lymphatic, Percutaneous Endoscopic Approach
07570ZZ Destruction of Thorax Lymphatic, Open Approach
07573ZZ Destruction of Thorax Lymphatic, Percutaneous Approach
07574ZZ Destruction of Thorax Lymphatic, Percutaneous Endoscopic Approach

07580ZZ Destruction of Right Internal Mammar[ ] Lymphatic, Open Approach
07583ZZ Destruction of Right Internal Mammary Lymphatic, Percutaneous Approach
07584ZZ Destruction of Right Internal Mammar[ ] Lymphatic, Percutaneous Endoscopic Approach
07590ZZ Destruction of Left Internal Mammary Lymphatic, Open Approach
07593ZZ Destruction of Left Internal Mammary Lymphatic, Percutaneous Approach
07594ZZ Destruction of Left Internal Mammary Lymphatic, Percutaneous Endoscopic Approach
075B0ZZ Destruction of Mesenteric Lymphatic, Open Approach
075B3ZZ Destruction of Mesenteric Lymphatic, Percutaneous Approach
075B4ZZ Destruction of Mesenteric Lymphatic, Percutaneous Endoscopic Approach
075C0ZZ Destruction of Pelvis Lymphatic, Open Approach
075C3ZZ Destruction of Pelvis Lymphatic, Percutaneous Approach

C4ZZ	Destruction of Pelvis Lymphatic, Percutaneous Endoscopic Approach
D0ZZ	Destruction of Aortic Lymphatic, Open Approach
D3ZZ	Destruction of Aortic Lymphatic, Percutaneous Approach
D4ZZ	Destruction of Aortic Lymphatic, Percutaneous Endoscopic Approach
F0ZZ	Destruction of Right Lower Extremity Lymphatic, Open Approach
F3ZZ	Destruction of Right Lower Extremity Lymphatic, Percutaneous Approach
F4ZZ	Destruction of Right Lower Extremity Lymphatic, Percutaneous Endoscopic Approach
G0ZZ	Destruction of Left Lower Extremity Lymphatic, Open Approach
G3ZZ	Destruction of Left Lower Extremity Lymphatic, Percutaneous Approach

075G4ZZ	Destruction of Left Lower Extremity Lymphatic, Percutaneous Endoscopic Approach
075H0ZZ	Destruction of Right Inguinal Lymphatic, Open Approach
075H3ZZ	Destruction of Right Inguinal Lymphatic, Percutaneous Approach
075H4ZZ	Destruction of Right Inguinal Lymphatic, Percutaneous Endoscopic Approach
075J0ZZ	Destruction of Left Inguinal Lymphatic, Open Approach
075J3ZZ	Destruction of Left Inguinal Lymphatic, Percutaneous Approach
075J4ZZ	Destruction of Left Inguinal Lymphatic, Percutaneous Endoscopic Approach
075K0ZZ	Destruction of Thoracic Duct, Open Approach
075K3ZZ	Destruction of Thoracic Duct, Percutaneous Approach

075K4ZZ	Destruction of Thoracic Duct, Percutaneous Endoscopic Approach
075L0ZZ	Destruction of Cisterna Chyli, Open Approach
075L3ZZ	Destruction of Cisterna Chyli, Percutaneous Approach
075L4ZZ	Destruction of Cisterna Chyli, Percutaneous Endoscopic Approach
075M0ZZ	Destruction of Thymus, Open Approach
075M3ZZ	Destruction of Thymus, Percutaneous Approach
075M4ZZ	Destruction of Thymus, Percutaneous Endoscopic Approach
075P0ZZ	Destruction of Spleen, Open Approach
075P3ZZ	Destruction of Spleen, Percutaneous Approach
075P4ZZ	Destruction of Spleen, Percutaneous Endoscopic Approach

9 – Lymphatic and Hemic Systems, Drainage

view Coding Guidelines B3.4a and B3.4b

view Coding Guideline B6.2

000Z	Drainage of Head Lymphatic with Drainage Device, Open Approach
00ZX	Drainage of Head Lymphatic, Open Approach, Diagnostic
00ZZ	Drainage of Head Lymphatic, Open Approach
030Z	Drainage of Head Lymphatic with Drainage Device, Percutaneous Approach
003ZX	Drainage of Head Lymphatic, Percutaneous Approach, Diagnostic
003ZZ	Drainage of Head Lymphatic, Percutaneous Approach
040Z	Drainage of Head Lymphatic with Drainage Device, Percutaneous Endoscopic Approach
004ZX	Drainage of Head Lymphatic, Percutaneous Endoscopic Approach, Diagnostic
004ZZ	Drainage of Head Lymphatic, Percutaneous Endoscopic Approach
0100Z	Drainage of Right Neck Lymphatic with Drainage Device, Open Approach
010ZX	Drainage of Right Neck Lymphatic, Open Approach, Diagnostic
010ZZ	Drainage of Right Neck Lymphatic, Open Approach
0130Z	Drainage of Right Neck Lymphatic with Drainage Device, Percutaneous Approach
013ZX	Drainage of Right Neck Lymphatic, Percutaneous Approach, Diagnostic
013ZZ	Drainage of Right Neck Lymphatic, Percutaneous Approach
0140Z	Drainage of Right Neck Lymphatic with Drainage Device, Percutaneous Endoscopic Approach
014ZX	Drainage of Right Neck Lymphatic, Percutaneous Endoscopic Approach, Diagnostic
014ZZ	Drainage of Right Neck Lymphatic, Percutaneous Endoscopic Approach
0200Z	Drainage of Left Neck Lymphatic with Drainage Device, Open Approach
020ZX	Drainage of Left Neck Lymphatic, Open Approach, Diagnostic
020ZZ	Drainage of Left Neck Lymphatic, Open Approach
0230Z	Drainage of Left Neck Lymphatic with Drainage Device, Percutaneous Approach
923ZX	Drainage of Left Neck Lymphatic, Percutaneous Approach, Diagnostic

07923ZZ	Drainage of Left Neck Lymphatic, Percutaneous Approach
079240Z	Drainage of Left Neck Lymphatic with Drainage Device, Percutaneous Endoscopic Approach
07924ZX	Drainage of Left Neck Lymphatic, Percutaneous Endoscopic Approach, Diagnostic
07924ZZ	Drainage of Left Neck Lymphatic, Percutaneous Endoscopic Approach
079300Z	Drainage of Right Upper Extremity Lymphatic with Drainage Device, Open Approach
07930ZX	Drainage of Right Upper Extremity Lymphatic, Open Approach, Diagnostic
07930ZZ	Drainage of Right Upper Extremity Lymphatic, Open Approach
079330Z	Drainage of Right Upper Extremity Lymphatic with Drainage Device, Percutaneous Approach
07933ZX	Drainage of Right Upper Extremity Lymphatic, Percutaneous Approach, Diagnostic
07933ZZ	Drainage of Right Upper Extremity Lymphatic, Percutaneous Approach
079340Z	Drainage of Right Upper Extremity Lymphatic with Drainage Device, Percutaneous Endoscopic Approach
07934ZX	Drainage of Right Upper Extremity Lymphatic, Percutaneous Endoscopic Approach, Diagnostic
07934ZZ	Drainage of Right Upper Extremity Lymphatic, Percutaneous Endoscopic Approach
079400Z	Drainage of Left Upper Extremity Lymphatic with Drainage Device, Open Approach
07940ZX	Drainage of Left Upper Extremity Lymphatic, Open Approach, Diagnostic
07940ZZ	Drainage of Left Upper Extremity Lymphatic, Open Approach
079430Z	Drainage of Left Upper Extremity Lymphatic with Drainage Device, Percutaneous Approach
07943ZX	Drainage of Left Upper Extremity Lymphatic, Percutaneous Approach, Diagnostic
07943ZZ	Drainage of Left Upper Extremity Lymphatic, Percutaneous Approach

079440Z	Drainage of Left Upper Extremity Lymphatic with Drainage Device, Percutaneous Endoscopic Approach
07944ZX	Drainage of Left Upper Extremity Lymphatic, Percutaneous Endoscopic Approach, Diagnostic
07944ZZ	Drainage of Left Upper Extremity Lymphatic, Percutaneous Endoscopic Approach
079500Z	Drainage of Right Axillary Lymphatic with Drainage Device, Open Approach
07950ZX	Drainage of Right Axillary Lymphatic, Open Approach, Diagnostic
07950ZZ	Drainage of Right Axillary Lymphatic, Open Approach
079530Z	Drainage of Right Axillary Lymphatic with Drainage Device, Percutaneous Approach
07953ZX	Drainage of Right Axillary Lymphatic, Percutaneous Approach, Diagnostic
07953ZZ	Drainage of Right Axillary Lymphatic, Percutaneous Approach
079540Z	Drainage of Right Axillary Lymphatic with Drainage Device, Percutaneous Endoscopic Approach
07954ZX	Drainage of Right Axillary Lymphatic, Percutaneous Endoscopic Approach, Diagnostic
07954ZZ	Drainage of Right Axillary Lymphatic, Percutaneous Endoscopic Approach
079600Z	Drainage of Left Axillary Lymphatic with Drainage Device, Open Approach
07960ZX	Drainage of Left Axillary Lymphatic, Open Approach, Diagnostic
07960ZZ	Drainage of Left Axillary Lymphatic, Open Approach
079630Z	Drainage of Left Axillary Lymphatic with Drainage Device, Percutaneous Approach
07963ZX	Drainage of Left Axillary Lymphatic, Percutaneous Approach, Diagnostic
07963ZZ	Drainage of Left Axillary Lymphatic, Percutaneous Approach
079640Z	Drainage of Left Axillary Lymphatic with Drainage Device, Percutaneous Endoscopic Approach
07964ZX	Drainage of Left Axillary Lymphatic, Percutaneous Endoscopic Approach, Diagnostic
07964ZZ	Drainage of Left Axillary Lymphatic, Percutaneous Endoscopic Approach

Female-only	♂ Male-only	▲ Limited Coverage	● Non-OR	▦ HAC-associated procedure	▲ Non-covered procedures	✛ Combination

079700Z Drainage of Thorax Lymphatic with Drainage Device, Open Approach
07970ZX Drainage of Thorax Lymphatic, Open Approach, Diagnostic
07970ZZ Drainage of Thorax Lymphatic, Open Approach
079730Z Drainage of Thorax Lymphatic with Drainage Device, Percutaneous Approach
07973ZX Drainage of Thorax Lymphatic, Percutaneous Approach, Diagnostic
07973ZZ Drainage of Thorax Lymphatic, Percutaneous Approach
079740Z Drainage of Thorax Lymphatic with Drainage Device, Percutaneous Endoscopic Approach
07974ZX Drainage of Thorax Lymphatic, Percutaneous Endoscopic Approach, Diagnostic
07974ZZ Drainage of Thorax Lymphatic, Percutaneous Endoscopic Approach
079800Z Drainage of Right Internal Mammary Lymphatic with Drainage Device, Open Approach
07980ZX Drainage of Right Internal Mammary Lymphatic, Open Approach, Diagnostic
07980ZZ Drainage of Right Internal Mammary Lymphatic, Open Approach
079830Z Drainage of Right Internal Mammary Lymphatic with Drainage Device, Percutaneous Approach
07983ZX Drainage of Right Internal Mammary Lymphatic, Percutaneous Approach, Diagnostic
07983ZZ Drainage of Right Internal Mammary Lymphatic, Percutaneous Approach
079840Z Drainage of Right Internal Mammary Lymphatic with Drainage Device, Percutaneous Endoscopic Approach
07984ZX Drainage of Right Internal Mammary Lymphatic, Percutaneous Endoscopic Approach, Diagnostic
07984ZZ Drainage of Right Internal Mammary Lymphatic, Percutaneous Endoscopic Approach
079900Z Drainage of Left Internal Mammary Lymphatic with Drainage Device, Open Approach
07990ZX Drainage of Left Internal Mammary Lymphatic, Open Approach, Diagnostic
07990ZZ Drainage of Left Internal Mammary Lymphatic, Open Approach
079930Z Drainage of Left Internal Mammary Lymphatic with Drainage Device, Percutaneous Approach
07993ZX Drainage of Left Internal Mammary Lymphatic, Percutaneous Approach, Diagnostic
07993ZZ Drainage of Left Internal Mammary Lymphatic, Percutaneous Approach
079940Z Drainage of Left Internal Mammary Lymphatic with Drainage Device, Percutaneous Endoscopic Approach
07994ZX Drainage of Left Internal Mammary Lymphatic, Percutaneous Endoscopic Approach, Diagnostic
07994ZZ Drainage of Left Internal Mammary Lymphatic, Percutaneous Endoscopic Approach
079B00Z Drainage of Mesenteric Lymphatic with Drainage Device, Open Approach
079B0ZX Drainage of Mesenteric Lymphatic, Open Approach, Diagnostic
079B0ZZ Drainage of Mesenteric Lymphatic, Open Approach

079B30Z Drainage of Mesenteric Lymphatic with Drainage Device, Percutaneous Approach
079B3ZX Drainage of Mesenteric Lymphatic, Percutaneous Approach, Diagnostic
079B3ZZ Drainage of Mesenteric Lymphatic, Percutaneous Approach
079B40Z Drainage of Mesenteric Lymphatic with Drainage Device, Percutaneous Endoscopic Approach
079B4ZX Drainage of Mesenteric Lymphatic, Percutaneous Endoscopic Approach, Diagnostic
079B4ZZ Drainage of Mesenteric Lymphatic, Percutaneous Endoscopic Approach
079C00Z Drainage of Pelvis Lymphatic with Drainage Device, Open Approach
079C0ZX Drainage of Pelvis Lymphatic, Open Approach, Diagnostic
079C0ZZ Drainage of Pelvis Lymphatic, Open Approach
079C30Z Drainage of Pelvis Lymphatic with Drainage Device, Percutaneous Approach
079C3ZX Drainage of Pelvis Lymphatic, Percutaneous Approach, Diagnostic
079C3ZZ Drainage of Pelvis Lymphatic, Percutaneous Approach
079C40Z Drainage of Pelvis Lymphatic with Drainage Device, Percutaneous Endoscopic Approach
079C4ZX Drainage of Pelvis Lymphatic, Percutaneous Endoscopic Approach, Diagnostic
079C4ZZ Drainage of Pelvis Lymphatic, Percutaneous Endoscopic Approach
079D00Z Drainage of Aortic Lymphatic with Drainage Device, Open Approach
079D0ZX Drainage of Aortic Lymphatic, Open Approach, Diagnostic
079D0ZZ Drainage of Aortic Lymphatic, Open Approach
079D30Z Drainage of Aortic Lymphatic with Drainage Device, Percutaneous Approach
079D3ZX Drainage of Aortic Lymphatic, Percutaneous Approach, Diagnostic
079D3ZZ Drainage of Aortic Lymphatic, Percutaneous Approach
079D40Z Drainage of Aortic Lymphatic with Drainage Device, Percutaneous Endoscopic Approach
079D4ZX Drainage of Aortic Lymphatic, Percutaneous Endoscopic Approach, Diagnostic
079D4ZZ Drainage of Aortic Lymphatic, Percutaneous Endoscopic Approach
079F00Z Drainage of Right Lower Extremity Lymphatic with Drainage Device, Open Approach
079F0ZX Drainage of Right Lower Extremity Lymphatic, Open Approach, Diagnostic
079F0ZZ Drainage of Right Lower Extremity Lymphatic, Open Approach
079F30Z Drainage of Right Lower Extremity Lymphatic with Drainage Device, Percutaneous Approach
079F3ZX Drainage of Right Lower Extremity Lymphatic, Percutaneous Approach, Diagnostic
079F3ZZ Drainage of Right Lower Extremity Lymphatic, Percutaneous Approach
079F40Z Drainage of Right Lower Extremity Lymphatic with Drainage Device, Percutaneous Endoscopic Approach
079F4ZX Drainage of Right Lower Extremity Lymphatic, Percutaneous Endoscopic Approach, Diagnostic

079F4ZZ Drainage of Right Lower Extremity Lymphatic, Percutaneous Endoscopic Approach
079G00Z Drainage of Left Lower Extremity Lymphatic with Drainage Device, Open Approach
079G0ZX Drainage of Left Lower Extremity Lymphatic, Open Approach, Diagnostic
079G0ZZ Drainage of Left Lower Extremity Lymphatic, Open Approach
079G30Z Drainage of Left Lower Extremity Lymphatic with Drainage Device, Percutaneous Approach
079G3ZX Drainage of Left Lower Extremity Lymphatic, Percutaneous Approach, Diagnostic
079G3ZZ Drainage of Left Lower Extremity Lymphatic, Percutaneous Approach
079G40Z Drainage of Left Lower Extremity Lymphatic with Drainage Device, Percutaneous Endoscopic Approach
079G4ZX Drainage of Left Lower Extremity Lymphatic, Percutaneous Endoscopic Approach, Diagnostic
079G4ZZ Drainage of Left Lower Extremity Lymphatic, Percutaneous Endoscopic Approach
079H00Z Drainage of Right Inguinal Lymphatic with Drainage Device, Open Approach
079H0ZX Drainage of Right Inguinal Lymphatic, Open Approach, Diagnostic
079H0ZZ Drainage of Right Inguinal Lymphatic, Open Approach
079H30Z Drainage of Right Inguinal Lymphatic with Drainage Device, Percutaneous Approach
079H3ZX Drainage of Right Inguinal Lymphatic, Percutaneous Approach, Diagnostic
079H3ZZ Drainage of Right Inguinal Lymphatic, Percutaneous Approach
079H40Z Drainage of Right Inguinal Lymphatic with Drainage Device, Percutaneous Endoscopic Approach
079H4ZX Drainage of Right Inguinal Lymphatic, Percutaneous Endoscopic Approach, Diagnostic
079H4ZZ Drainage of Right Inguinal Lymphatic, Percutaneous Endoscopic Approach
079J00Z Drainage of Left Inguinal Lymphatic with Drainage Device, Open Approach
079J0ZX Drainage of Left Inguinal Lymphatic, Open Approach, Diagnostic
079J0ZZ Drainage of Left Inguinal Lymphatic, Open Approach
079J30Z Drainage of Left Inguinal Lymphatic with Drainage Device, Percutaneous Approach
079J3ZX Drainage of Left Inguinal Lymphatic, Percutaneous Approach, Diagnostic
079J3ZZ Drainage of Left Inguinal Lymphatic, Percutaneous Approach
079J40Z Drainage of Left Inguinal Lymphatic with Drainage Device, Percutaneous Endoscopic Approach
079J4ZX Drainage of Left Inguinal Lymphatic, Percutaneous Endoscopic Approach, Diagnostic
079J4ZZ Drainage of Left Inguinal Lymphatic, Percutaneous Endoscopic Approach
079K00Z Drainage of Thoracic Duct with Drainage Device, Open Approach
079K0ZX Drainage of Thoracic Duct, Open Approach, Diagnostic
079K0ZZ Drainage of Thoracic Duct, Open Approach

K30Z Drainage of Thoracic Duct with Drainage Device, Percutaneous Approach
K3XZ Drainage of Thoracic Duct, Percutaneous Approach, Diagnostic
K3ZZ Drainage of Thoracic Duct, Percutaneous Approach
K40Z Drainage of Thoracic Duct with Drainage Device, Percutaneous Endoscopic Approach
K4XZ Drainage of Thoracic Duct, Percutaneous Endoscopic Approach, Diagnostic
K4ZZ Drainage of Thoracic Duct, Percutaneous Endoscopic Approach
L00Z Drainage of Cisterna Chyli with Drainage Device, Open Approach
L0XZ Drainage of Cisterna Chyli, Open Approach, Diagnostic
L0ZZ Drainage of Cisterna Chyli, Open Approach
L30Z Drainage of Cisterna Chyli with Drainage Device, Percutaneous Approach
L3XZ Drainage of Cisterna Chyli, Percutaneous Approach, Diagnostic
L3ZZ Drainage of Cisterna Chyli, Percutaneous Approach
L40Z Drainage of Cisterna Chyli with Drainage Device, Percutaneous Endoscopic Approach
L4XZ Drainage of Cisterna Chyli, Percutaneous Endoscopic Approach, Diagnostic

079L4ZZ Drainage of Cisterna Chyli, Percutaneous Endoscopic Approach
079M00Z Drainage of Thymus with Drainage Device, Open Approach
079M0XZ Drainage of Thymus, Open Approach, Diagnostic
079M0ZZ Drainage of Thymus, Open Approach
079M30Z Drainage of Thymus with Drainage Device, Percutaneous Approach
079M3XZ Drainage of Thymus, Percutaneous Approach, Diagnostic
079M3ZZ Drainage of Thymus, Percutaneous Approach
079M40Z Drainage of Thymus with Drainage Device, Percutaneous Endoscopic Approach
079M4XZ Drainage of Thymus, Percutaneous Endoscopic Approach, Diagnostic
079M4ZZ Drainage of Thymus, Percutaneous Endoscopic Approach
079P00Z Drainage of Spleen with Drainage Device, Open Approach
079P0XZ Drainage of Spleen, Open Approach, Diagnostic
079P0ZZ Drainage of Spleen, Open Approach
079P30Z Drainage of Spleen with Drainage Device, Percutaneous Approach
079P3XZ Drainage of Spleen, Percutaneous Approach, Diagnostic

079P3ZZ Drainage of Spleen, Percutaneous Approach
079P40Z Drainage of Spleen with Drainage Device, Percutaneous Endoscopic Approach
079P4XZ Drainage of Spleen, Percutaneous Endoscopic Approach, Diagnostic
079P4ZZ Drainage of Spleen, Percutaneous Endoscopic Approach
079T00Z Drainage of Bone Marrow with Drainage Device, Open Approach
079T0XZ Drainage of Bone Marrow, Open Approach, Diagnostic
079T0ZZ Drainage of Bone Marrow, Open Approach
079T30Z Drainage of Bone Marrow with Drainage Device, Percutaneous Approach
079T3XZ Drainage of Bone Marrow, Percutaneous Approach, Diagnostic
079T3ZZ Drainage of Bone Marrow, Percutaneous Approach
079T40Z Drainage of Bone Marrow with Drainage Device, Percutaneous Endoscopic Approach
079T4XZ Drainage of Bone Marrow, Percutaneous Endoscopic Approach, Diagnostic
079T4ZZ Drainage of Bone Marrow, Percutaneous Endoscopic Approach

'B – Lymphatic and Hemic Systems, Excision

Review Coding Guidelines B3.4a and B3.4b

Review Coding Guideline B3.8

B00ZX Excision of Head Lymphatic, Open Approach, Diagnostic
B00ZZ Excision of Head Lymphatic, Open Approach
B03ZX Excision of Head Lymphatic, Percutaneous Approach, Diagnostic
B03ZZ Excision of Head Lymphatic, Percutaneous Approach
B04ZX Excision of Head Lymphatic, Percutaneous Endoscopic Approach, Diagnostic
B04ZZ Excision of Head Lymphatic, Percutaneous Endoscopic Approach
B10ZX Excision of Right Neck Lymphatic, Open Approach, Diagnostic
B10ZZ Excision of Right Neck Lymphatic, Open Approach
B13ZX Excision of Right Neck Lymphatic, Percutaneous Approach, Diagnostic
B13ZZ Excision of Right Neck Lymphatic, Percutaneous Approach
B14ZX Excision of Right Neck Lymphatic, Percutaneous Endoscopic Approach, Diagnostic
B14ZZ Excision of Right Neck Lymphatic, Percutaneous Endoscopic Approach
B20ZX Excision of Left Neck Lymphatic, Open Approach, Diagnostic
B20ZZ Excision of Left Neck Lymphatic, Open Approach
B23ZX Excision of Left Neck Lymphatic, Percutaneous Approach, Diagnostic
B23ZZ Excision of Left Neck Lymphatic, Percutaneous Approach
B24ZX Excision of Left Neck Lymphatic, Percutaneous Endoscopic Approach, Diagnostic

07B24ZZ Excision of Left Neck Lymphatic, Percutaneous Endoscopic Approach
07B30ZX Excision of Right Upper Extremity Lymphatic, Open Approach, Diagnostic
07B30ZZ Excision of Right Upper Extremity Lymphatic, Open Approach
07B33ZX Excision of Right Upper Extremity Lymphatic, Percutaneous Approach, Diagnostic
07B33ZZ Excision of Right Upper Extremity Lymphatic, Percutaneous Approach
07B34ZX Excision of Right Upper Extremity Lymphatic, Percutaneous Endoscopic Approach, Diagnostic
07B34ZZ Excision of Right Upper Extremity Lymphatic, Percutaneous Endoscopic Approach
07B40ZX Excision of Left Upper Extremity Lymphatic, Open Approach, Diagnostic
07B40ZZ Excision of Left Upper Extremity Lymphatic, Open Approach
07B43ZX Excision of Left Upper Extremity Lymphatic, Percutaneous Approach, Diagnostic
07B43ZZ Excision of Left Upper Extremity Lymphatic, Percutaneous Approach
07B44ZX Excision of Left Upper Extremity Lymphatic, Percutaneous Endoscopic Approach, Diagnostic
07B44ZZ Excision of Left Upper Extremity Lymphatic, Percutaneous Endoscopic Approach
07B50ZX Excision of Right Axillary Lymphatic, Open Approach, Diagnostic
07B50ZZ Excision of Right Axillary Lymphatic, Open Approach
07B53ZX Excision of Right Axillary Lymphatic, Percutaneous Approach, Diagnostic

07B53ZZ Excision of Right Axillary Lymphatic, Percutaneous Approach
07B54ZX Excision of Right Axillary Lymphatic, Percutaneous Endoscopic Approach, Diagnostic
07B54ZZ Excision of Right Axillary Lymphatic, Percutaneous Endoscopic Approach
07B60ZX Excision of Left Axillary Lymphatic, Open Approach, Diagnostic
07B60ZZ Excision of Left Axillary Lymphatic, Open Approach
07B63ZX Excision of Left Axillary Lymphatic, Percutaneous Approach, Diagnostic
07B63ZZ Excision of Left Axillary Lymphatic, Percutaneous Approach
07B64ZX Excision of Left Axillary Lymphatic, Percutaneous Endoscopic Approach, Diagnostic
07B64ZZ Excision of Left Axillary Lymphatic, Percutaneous Endoscopic Approach
07B70ZX Excision of Thorax Lymphatic, Open Approach, Diagnostic
07B70ZZ Excision of Thorax Lymphatic, Open Approach
07B73ZX Excision of Thorax Lymphatic, Percutaneous Approach, Diagnostic
07B73ZZ Excision of Thorax Lymphatic, Percutaneous Approach
07B74ZX Excision of Thorax Lymphatic, Percutaneous Endoscopic Approach, Diagnostic
AHA CC: 1Q, 2014, 20-21, 26; 3Q, 2014, 10-11
07B74ZZ Excision of Thorax Lymphatic, Percutaneous Endoscopic Approach
07B80ZX Excision of Right Internal Mammary Lymphatic, Open Approach, Diagnostic
07B80ZZ Excision of Right Internal Mammary Lymphatic, Open Approach

Female-only   ♂ Male-only   ▲ Limited Coverage   ● Non-OR   ▦ HAC-associated procedure   ▲ Non-covered procedures   ✚ Combination

07B83ZX Excision of Right Internal Mammary Lymphatic, Percutaneous Approach, Diagnostic

07B83ZZ Excision of Right Internal Mammary Lymphatic, Percutaneous Approach

07B84ZX Excision of Right Internal Mammary Lymphatic, Percutaneous Endoscopic Approach, Diagnostic

07B84ZZ Excision of Right Internal Mammary Lymphatic, Percutaneous Endoscopic Approach

07B90ZX Excision of Left Internal Mammary Lymphatic, Open Approach, Diagnostic

07B90ZZ Excision of Left Internal Mammary Lymphatic, Open Approach

07B93ZX Excision of Left Internal Mammary Lymphatic, Percutaneous Approach, Diagnostic

07B93ZZ Excision of Left Internal Mammary Lymphatic, Percutaneous Approach

07B94ZX Excision of Left Internal Mammary Lymphatic, Percutaneous Endoscopic Approach, Diagnostic

07B94ZZ Excision of Left Internal Mammary Lymphatic, Percutaneous Endoscopic Approach

07BB0ZX Excision of Mesenteric Lymphatic, Open Approach, Diagnostic

07BB0ZZ Excision of Mesenteric Lymphatic, Open Approach

07BB3ZX Excision of Mesenteric Lymphatic, Percutaneous Approach, Diagnostic

07BB3ZZ Excision of Mesenteric Lymphatic, Percutaneous Approach

07BB4ZX Excision of Mesenteric Lymphatic, Percutaneous Endoscopic Approach, Diagnostic

07BB4ZZ Excision of Mesenteric Lymphatic, Percutaneous Endoscopic Approach

07BC0ZX Excision of Pelvis Lymphatic, Open Approach, Diagnostic

07BC0ZZ Excision of Pelvis Lymphatic, Open Approach

07BC3ZX Excision of Pelvis Lymphatic, Percutaneous Approach, Diagnostic

07BC3ZZ Excision of Pelvis Lymphatic, Percutaneous Approach

07BC4ZX Excision of Pelvis Lymphatic, Percutaneous Endoscopic Approach, Diagnostic

07BC4ZZ Excision of Pelvis Lymphatic, Percutaneous Endoscopic Approach

07BD0ZX Excision of Aortic Lymphatic, Open Approach, Diagnostic

07BD0ZZ Excision of Aortic Lymphatic, Open Approach

07BD3ZX Excision of Aortic Lymphatic, Percutaneous Approach, Diagnostic

07BD3ZZ Excision of Aortic Lymphatic, Percutaneous Approach

07BD4ZX Excision of Aortic Lymphatic, Percutaneous Endoscopic Approach, Diagnostic

07BD4ZZ Excision of Aortic Lymphatic, Percutaneous Endoscopic Approach

07BF0ZX Excision of Right Lower Extremity Lymphatic, Open Approach, Diagnostic

07BF0ZZ Excision of Right Lower Extremity Lymphatic, Open Approach

07BF3ZX Excision of Right Lower Extremity Lymphatic, Percutaneous Approach, Diagnostic

07BF3ZZ Excision of Right Lower Extremity Lymphatic, Percutaneous Approach

07BF4ZX Excision of Right Lower Extremity Lymphatic, Percutaneous Endoscopic Approach, Diagnostic

07BF4ZZ Excision of Right Lower Extremity Lymphatic, Percutaneous Endoscopic Approach

07BG0ZX Excision of Left Lower Extremity Lymphatic, Open Approach, Diagnostic

07BG0ZZ Excision of Left Lower Extremity Lymphatic, Open Approach

07BG3ZX Excision of Left Lower Extremity Lymphatic, Percutaneous Approach, Diagnostic

07BG3ZZ Excision of Left Lower Extremity Lymphatic, Percutaneous Approach

07BG4ZX Excision of Left Lower Extremity Lymphatic, Percutaneous Endoscopic Approach, Diagnostic

07BG4ZZ Excision of Left Lower Extremity Lymphatic, Percutaneous Endoscopic Approach

07BH0ZX Excision of Right Inguinal Lymphatic, Open Approach, Diagnostic

07BH0ZZ Excision of Right Inguinal Lymphatic, Open Approach

➕ Radical vulvectomy when reported with resection of vulva. *See table 0UT to construct the Resection code.*

07BH3ZX Excision of Right Inguinal Lymphatic, Percutaneous Approach, Diagnostic

07BH3ZZ Excision of Right Inguinal Lymphatic, Percutaneous Approach

07BH4ZX Excision of Right Inguinal Lymphatic, Percutaneous Endoscopic Approach, Diagnostic

07BH4ZZ Excision of Right Inguinal Lymphatic, Percutaneous Endoscopic Approach

➕ Radical vulvectomy when reported with resection of vulva. *See table 0UT to construct the Resection code.*

07BJ0ZX Excision of Left Inguinal Lymphatic, Open Approach, Diagnostic

07BJ0ZZ Excision of Left Inguinal Lymphatic, Open Approach

➕ Radical vulvectomy when reported with resection of vulva. *See table 0UT to construct the Resection code.*

07BJ3ZX Excision of Left Inguinal Lymphatic, Percutaneous Approach, Diagnostic

07BJ3ZZ Excision of Left Inguinal Lymphatic, Percutaneous Approach

07BJ4ZX Excision of Left Inguinal Lymphatic, Percutaneous Endoscopic Approach, Diagnostic

07BJ4ZZ Excision of Left Inguinal Lymphatic, Percutaneous Endoscopic Approach

➕ Radical vulvectomy when reported with resection of vulva. *See table 0UT to construct the Resection code.*

07BK0ZX Excision of Thoracic Duct, Open Approach, Diagnostic

07BK0ZZ Excision of Thoracic Duct, Open Approach

07BK3ZX Excision of Thoracic Duct, Percutaneous Approach, Diagnostic

07BK3ZZ Excision of Thoracic Duct, Percutaneous Approach

07BK4ZX Excision of Thoracic Duct, Percutaneous Endoscopic Approach, Diagnostic

07BK4ZZ Excision of Thoracic Duct, Percutaneous Endoscopic Approach

07BL0ZX Excision of Cisterna Chyli, Open Approach, Diagnostic

07BL0ZZ Excision of Cisterna Chyli, Open Approach

07BL3ZX Excision of Cisterna Chyli, Percutaneous Approach, Diagnostic

07BL3ZZ Excision of Cisterna Chyli, Percutaneous Approach

07BL4ZX Excision of Cisterna Chyli, Percutaneous Endoscopic Approach, Diagnostic

07BL4ZZ Excision of Cisterna Chyli, Percutaneous Endoscopic Approach

07BM0ZX Excision of Thymus, Open Approach, Diagnostic

07BM0ZZ Excision of Thymus, Open Approach

07BM3ZX Excision of Thymus, Percutaneous Approach, Diagnostic

07BM3ZZ Excision of Thymus, Percutaneous Approach

07BM4ZX Excision of Thymus, Percutaneous Endoscopic Approach, Diagnostic

07BM4ZZ Excision of Thymus, Percutaneous Endoscopic Approach

07BP0ZX Excision of Spleen, Open Approach, Diagnostic

07BP0ZZ Excision of Spleen, Open Approach

07BP3ZX Excision of Spleen, Percutaneous Approach, Diagnostic

07BP3ZZ Excision of Spleen, Percutaneous Approach

07BP4ZX Excision of Spleen, Percutaneous Endoscopic Approach, Diagnostic

07BP4ZZ Excision of Spleen, Percutaneous Endoscopic Approach

07C – Lymphatic and Hemic Systems, Extirpation

07C00ZZ Extirpation of Matter from Head Lymphatic, Open Approach

07C03ZZ Extirpation of Matter from Head Lymphatic, Percutaneous Approach

07C04ZZ Extirpation of Matter from Head Lymphatic, Percutaneous Endoscopic Approach

07C10ZZ Extirpation of Matter from Right Neck Lymphatic, Open Approach

07C13ZZ Extirpation of Matter from Right Neck Lymphatic, Percutaneous Approach

07C14ZZ Extirpation of Matter from Right Neck Lymphatic, Percutaneous Endoscopic Approach

07C20ZZ Extirpation of Matter from Left Neck Lymphatic, Open Approach

07C23ZZ Extirpation of Matter from Left Neck Lymphatic, Percutaneous Approach

07C24ZZ Extirpation of Matter from Left Neck Lymphatic, Percutaneous Endoscopic Approach

07C30ZZ Extirpation of Matter from Right Upper Extremity Lymphatic, Open Approach

07C33ZZ Extirpation of Matter from Right Upper Extremity Lymphatic, Percutaneous Approach

07C34ZZ Extirpation of Matter from Right Upper Extremity Lymphatic, Percutaneous Endoscopic Approach

07C40ZZ Extirpation of Matter from Left Upper Extremity Lymphatic, Open Approach

07C43ZZ Extirpation of Matter from Left Upper Extremity Lymphatic, Percutaneous Approach

07C44ZZ Extirpation of Matter from Left Upper Extremity Lymphatic, Percutaneous Endoscopic Approach

07C50ZZ Extirpation of Matter from Right Axillary Lymphatic, Open Approach

07C53ZZ Extirpation of Matter from Right Axillary Lymphatic, Percutaneous Approach

07C54ZZ Extirpation of Matter from Right Axillary Lymphatic, Percutaneous Endoscopic Approach

07C60ZZ Extirpation of Matter from Left Axillary Lymphatic, Open Approach

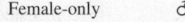

♀ Female-only   ♂ Male-only   ▲ Limited Coverage   ● Non-OR   ▬ HAC-associated procedure   ▲ Non-covered procedures   ➕ Combinati

C63ZZ Extirpation of Matter from Left Axillary Lymphatic, Percutaneous Approach

C64ZZ Extirpation of Matter from Left Axillary Lymphatic, Percutaneous Endoscopic Approach

C70ZZ Extirpation of Matter from Thorax Lymphatic, Open Approach

C73ZZ Extirpation of Matter from Thorax Lymphatic, Percutaneous Approach

C74ZZ Extirpation of Matter from Thorax Lymphatic, Percutaneous Endoscopic Approach

C80ZZ Extirpation of Matter from Right Internal Mammary Lymphatic, Open Approach

C83ZZ Extirpation of Matter from Right Internal Mammary Lymphatic, Percutaneous Approach

C84ZZ Extirpation of Matter from Right Internal Mammary Lymphatic, Percutaneous Endoscopic Approach

C90ZZ Extirpation of Matter from Left Internal Mammary Lymphatic, Open Approach

C93ZZ Extirpation of Matter from Left Internal Mammary Lymphatic, Percutaneous Approach

C94ZZ Extirpation of Matter from Left Internal Mammary Lymphatic, Percutaneous Endoscopic Approach

CB0ZZ Extirpation of Matter from Mesenteric Lymphatic, Open Approach

CB3ZZ Extirpation of Matter from Mesenteric Lymphatic, Percutaneous Approach

CB4ZZ Extirpation of Matter from Mesenteric Lymphatic, Percutaneous Endoscopic Approach

07CC0ZZ Extirpation of Matter from Pelvis Lymphatic, Open Approach

07CC3ZZ Extirpation of Matter from Pelvis Lymphatic, Percutaneous Approach

07CC4ZZ Extirpation of Matter from Pelvis Lymphatic, Percutaneous Endoscopic Approach

07CD0ZZ Extirpation of Matter from Aortic Lymphatic, Open Approach

07CD3ZZ Extirpation of Matter from Aortic Lymphatic, Percutaneous Approach

07CD4ZZ Extirpation of Matter from Aortic Lymphatic, Percutaneous Endoscopic Approach

07CF0ZZ Extirpation of Matter from Right Lower Extremity Lymphatic, Open Approach

07CF3ZZ Extirpation of Matter from Right Lower Extremity Lymphatic, Percutaneous Approach

07CF4ZZ Extirpation of Matter from Right Lower Extremity Lymphatic, Percutaneous Endoscopic Approach

07CG0ZZ Extirpation of Matter from Left Lower Extremity Lymphatic, Open Approach

07CG3ZZ Extirpation of Matter from Left Lower Extremity Lymphatic, Percutaneous Approach

07CG4ZZ Extirpation of Matter from Left Lower Extremity Lymphatic, Percutaneous Endoscopic Approach

07CH0ZZ Extirpation of Matter from Right Inguinal Lymphatic, Open Approach

07CH3ZZ Extirpation of Matter from Right Inguinal Lymphatic, Percutaneous Approach

07CH4ZZ Extirpation of Matter from Right Inguinal Lymphatic, Percutaneous Endoscopic Approach

07CJ0ZZ Extirpation of Matter from Left Inguinal Lymphatic, Open Approach

07CJ3ZZ Extirpation of Matter from Left Inguinal Lymphatic, Percutaneous Approach

07CJ4ZZ Extirpation of Matter from Left Inguinal Lymphatic, Percutaneous Endoscopic Approach

07CK0ZZ Extirpation of Matter from Thoracic Duct, Open Approach

07CK3ZZ Extirpation of Matter from Thoracic Duct, Percutaneous Approach

07CK4ZZ Extirpation of Matter from Thoracic Duct, Percutaneous Endoscopic Approach

07CL0ZZ Extirpation of Matter from Cisterna Chyli, Open Approach

07CL3ZZ Extirpation of Matter from Cisterna Chyli, Percutaneous Approach

07CL4ZZ Extirpation of Matter from Cisterna Chyli, Percutaneous Endoscopic Approach

07CM0ZZ Extirpation of Matter from Thymus, Open Approach

07CM3ZZ Extirpation of Matter from Thymus, Percutaneous Approach

07CM4ZZ Extirpation of Matter from Thymus, Percutaneous Endoscopic Approach

07CP0ZZ Extirpation of Matter from Spleen, Open Approach

07CP3ZZ Extirpation of Matter from Spleen, Percutaneous Approach

07CP4ZZ Extirpation of Matter from Spleen, Percutaneous Endoscopic Approach

7D – Lymphatic and Hemic Systems, Extraction

Review Coding Guidelines B3.4a and B3.4b

DQ0ZX Extraction of Sternum Bone Marrow, Open Approach, Diagnostic

DQ0ZZ Extraction of Sternum Bone Marrow, Open Approach

DQ3ZX Extraction of Sternum Bone Marrow, Percutaneous Approach, Diagnostic

DQ3ZZ Extraction of Sternum Bone Marrow, Percutaneous Approach

07DR0ZX Extraction of Iliac Bone Marrow, Open Approach, Diagnostic

07DR0ZZ Extraction of Iliac Bone Marrow, Open Approach

07DR3ZX Extraction of Iliac Bone Marrow, Percutaneous Approach, Diagnostic

07DR3ZZ Extraction of Iliac Bone Marrow, Percutaneous Approach

07DS0ZX Extraction of Vertebral Bone Marrow, Open Approach, Diagnostic

07DS0ZZ Extraction of Vertebral Bone Marrow, Open Approach

07DS3ZX Extraction of Vertebral Bone Marrow, Percutaneous Approach, Diagnostic

07DS3ZZ Extraction of Vertebral Bone Marrow, Percutaneous Approach

7H – Lymphatic and Hemic Systems, Insertion

HK03Z Insertion of Infusion Device into Thoracic Duct, Open Approach

HK33Z Insertion of Infusion Device into Thoracic Duct, Percutaneous Approach

HK43Z Insertion of Infusion Device into Thoracic Duct, Percutaneous Endoscopic Approach

HL03Z Insertion of Infusion Device into Cisterna Chyli, Open Approach

HL33Z Insertion of Infusion Device into Cisterna Chyli, Percutaneous Approach

07HL43Z Insertion of Infusion Device into Cisterna Chyli, Percutaneous Endoscopic Approach

07HM03Z Insertion of Infusion Device into Thymus, Open Approach

07HM33Z Insertion of Infusion Device into Thymus, Percutaneous Approach

07HM43Z Insertion of Infusion Device into Thymus, Percutaneous Endoscopic Approach

07HN03Z Insertion of Infusion Device into Lymphatic, Open Approach

07HN33Z Insertion of Infusion Device into Lymphatic, Percutaneous Approach

07HN43Z Insertion of Infusion Device into Lymphatic, Percutaneous Endoscopic Approach

07HP03Z Insertion of Infusion Device into Spleen, Open Approach

07HP33Z Insertion of Infusion Device into Spleen, Percutaneous Approach

07HP43Z Insertion of Infusion Device into Spleen, Percutaneous Endoscopic Approach

7J – Lymphatic and Hemic Systems, Inspection

Review Coding Guidelines B3.11a, B3.11b and B3.11c

JK0ZZ Inspection of Thoracic Duct, Open Approach

JK3ZZ Inspection of Thoracic Duct, Percutaneous Approach

JK4ZZ Inspection of Thoracic Duct, Percutaneous Endoscopic Approach

JL0ZZ Inspection of Cisterna Chyli, Open Approach

07JL3ZZ Inspection of Cisterna Chyli, Percutaneous Approach

07JL4ZZ Inspection of Cisterna Chyli, Percutaneous Endoscopic Approach

07JM0ZZ Inspection of Thymus, Open Approach

07JM3ZZ Inspection of Thymus, Percutaneous Approach

07JM4ZZ Inspection of Thymus, Percutaneous Endoscopic Approach

07JN0ZZ Inspection of Lymphatic, Open Approach

07JN3ZZ Inspection of Lymphatic, Percutaneous Approach

07JN4ZZ Inspection of Lymphatic, Percutaneous Endoscopic Approach

07JNXZZ Inspection of Lymphatic, External Approach

07JP0ZZ Inspection of Spleen, Open Approach

07JP3ZZ   Inspection of Spleen, Percutaneous Approach

07JP4ZZ   Inspection of Spleen, Percutaneous Endoscopic Approach

07JPXZZ   Inspection of Spleen, External Approach

07JT0ZZ   Inspection of Bone Marrow, Open Approach

07JT3ZZ   Inspection of Bone Marrow, Percutaneous Approach

07JT4ZZ   Inspection of Bone Marrow, Percutaneous Endoscopic Approach

07L – Lymphatic and Hemic Systems, Occlusion

07L00CZ   Occlusion of Head Lymphatic with Extraluminal Device, Open Approach

07L00DZ   Occlusion of Head Lymphatic with Intraluminal Device, Open Approach

07L00ZZ   Occlusion of Head Lymphatic, Open Approach

07L03CZ   Occlusion of Head Lymphatic with Extraluminal Device, Percutaneous Approach

07L03DZ   Occlusion of Head Lymphatic with Intraluminal Device, Percutaneous Approach

07L03ZZ   Occlusion of Head Lymphatic, Percutaneous Approach

07L04CZ   Occlusion of Head Lymphatic with Extraluminal Device, Percutaneous Endoscopic Approach

07L04DZ   Occlusion of Head Lymphatic with Intraluminal Device, Percutaneous Endoscopic Approach

07L04ZZ   Occlusion of Head Lymphatic, Percutaneous Endoscopic Approach

07L10CZ   Occlusion of Right Neck Lymphatic with Extraluminal Device, Open Approach

07L10DZ   Occlusion of Right Neck Lymphatic with Intraluminal Device, Open Approach

07L10ZZ   Occlusion of Right Neck Lymphatic, Open Approach

07L13CZ   Occlusion of Right Neck Lymphatic with Extraluminal Device, Percutaneous Approach

07L13DZ   Occlusion of Right Neck Lymphatic with Intraluminal Device, Percutaneous Approach

07L13ZZ   Occlusion of Right Neck Lymphatic, Percutaneous Approach

07L14CZ   Occlusion of Right Neck Lymphatic with Extraluminal Device, Percutaneous Endoscopic Approach

07L14DZ   Occlusion of Right Neck Lymphatic with Intraluminal Device, Percutaneous Endoscopic Approach

07L14ZZ   Occlusion of Right Neck Lymphatic, Percutaneous Endoscopic Approach

07L20CZ   Occlusion of Left Neck Lymphatic with Extraluminal Device, Open Approach

07L20DZ   Occlusion of Left Neck Lymphatic with Intraluminal Device, Open Approach

07L20ZZ   Occlusion of Left Neck Lymphatic, Open Approach

07L23CZ   Occlusion of Left Neck Lymphatic with Extraluminal Device, Percutaneous Approach

07L23DZ   Occlusion of Left Neck Lymphatic with Intraluminal Device, Percutaneous Approach

07L23ZZ   Occlusion of Left Neck Lymphatic, Percutaneous Approach

07L24CZ   Occlusion of Left Neck Lymphatic with Extraluminal Device, Percutaneous Endoscopic Approach

07L24DZ   Occlusion of Left Neck Lymphatic with Intraluminal Device, Percutaneous Endoscopic Approach

07L24ZZ   Occlusion of Left Neck Lymphatic, Percutaneous Endoscopic Approach

07L30CZ   Occlusion of Right Upper Extremity Lymphatic with Extraluminal Device, Open Approach

07L30DZ   Occlusion of Right Upper Extremity Lymphatic with Intraluminal Device, Open Approach

07L30ZZ   Occlusion of Right Upper Extremity Lymphatic, Open Approach

07L33CZ   Occlusion of Right Upper Extremity Lymphatic with Extraluminal Device, Percutaneous Approach

07L33DZ   Occlusion of Right Upper Extremity Lymphatic with Intraluminal Device, Percutaneous Approach

07L33ZZ   Occlusion of Right Upper Extremity Lymphatic, Percutaneous Approach

07L34CZ   Occlusion of Right Upper Extremity Lymphatic with Extraluminal Device, Percutaneous Endoscopic Approach

07L34DZ   Occlusion of Right Upper Extremity Lymphatic with Intraluminal Device, Percutaneous Endoscopic Approach

07L34ZZ   Occlusion of Right Upper Extremity Lymphatic, Percutaneous Endoscopic Approach

07L40CZ   Occlusion of Left Upper Extremity Lymphatic with Extraluminal Device, Open Approach

07L40DZ   Occlusion of Left Upper Extremity Lymphatic with Intraluminal Device, Open Approach

07L40ZZ   Occlusion of Left Upper Extremity Lymphatic, Open Approach

07L43CZ   Occlusion of Left Upper Extremity Lymphatic with Extraluminal Device, Percutaneous Approach

07L43DZ   Occlusion of Left Upper Extremity Lymphatic with Intraluminal Device, Percutaneous Approach

07L43ZZ   Occlusion of Left Upper Extremity Lymphatic, Percutaneous Approach

07L44CZ   Occlusion of Left Upper Extremity Lymphatic with Extraluminal Device, Percutaneous Endoscopic Approach

07L44DZ   Occlusion of Left Upper Extremity Lymphatic with Intraluminal Device, Percutaneous Endoscopic Approach

07L44ZZ   Occlusion of Left Upper Extremity Lymphatic, Percutaneous Endoscopic Approach

07L50CZ   Occlusion of Right Axillary Lymphatic with Extraluminal Device, Open Approach

07L50DZ   Occlusion of Right Axillary Lymphatic with Intraluminal Device, Open Approach

07L50ZZ   Occlusion of Right Axillary Lymphatic, Open Approach

07L53CZ   Occlusion of Right Axillary Lymphatic with Extraluminal Device, Percutaneous Approach

07L53DZ   Occlusion of Right Axillary Lymphatic with Intraluminal Device, Percutaneous Approach

07L53ZZ   Occlusion of Right Axillary Lymphatic, Percutaneous Approach

07L54CZ   Occlusion of Right Axillary Lymphatic with Extraluminal Device, Percutaneous Endoscopic Approach

07L54DZ   Occlusion of Right Axillary Lymphatic with Intraluminal Device, Percutaneous Endoscopic Approach

07L54ZZ   Occlusion of Right Axillary Lymphatic, Percutaneous Endoscopic Approach

07L60CZ   Occlusion of Left Axillary Lymphatic with Extraluminal Device, Open Approach

07L60DZ   Occlusion of Left Axillary Lymphatic with Intraluminal Device, Open Approach

07L60ZZ   Occlusion of Left Axillary Lymphatic, Open Approach

07L63CZ   Occlusion of Left Axillary Lymphatic with Extraluminal Device, Percutaneous Approach

07L63DZ   Occlusion of Left Axillary Lymphatic with Intraluminal Device, Percutaneous Approach

07L63ZZ   Occlusion of Left Axillary Lymphatic, Percutaneous Approach

07L64CZ   Occlusion of Left Axillary Lymphatic with Extraluminal Device, Percutaneous Endoscopic Approach

07L64DZ   Occlusion of Left Axillary Lymphatic with Intraluminal Device, Percutaneous Endoscopic Approach

07L64ZZ   Occlusion of Left Axillary Lymphatic, Percutaneous Endoscopic Approach

07L70CZ   Occlusion of Thorax Lymphatic with Extraluminal Device, Open Approach

07L70DZ   Occlusion of Thorax Lymphatic with Intraluminal Device, Open Approach

07L70ZZ   Occlusion of Thorax Lymphatic, Open Approach

07L73CZ   Occlusion of Thorax Lymphatic with Extraluminal Device, Percutaneous Approach

07L73DZ   Occlusion of Thorax Lymphatic with Intraluminal Device, Percutaneous Approach

07L73ZZ   Occlusion of Thorax Lymphatic, Percutaneous Approach

07L74CZ   Occlusion of Thorax Lymphatic with Extraluminal Device, Percutaneous Endoscopic Approach

07L74DZ   Occlusion of Thorax Lymphatic with Intraluminal Device, Percutaneous Endoscopic Approach

07L74ZZ   Occlusion of Thorax Lymphatic, Percutaneous Endoscopic Approach

07L80CZ   Occlusion of Right Internal Mammary Lymphatic with Extraluminal Device, Open Approach

07L80DZ   Occlusion of Right Internal Mammary Lymphatic with Intraluminal Device, Op Approach

07L80ZZ   Occlusion of Right Internal Mammary Lymphatic, Open Approach

07L83CZ   Occlusion of Right Internal Mammary Lymphatic with Extraluminal Device, Percutaneous Approach

07L83DZ   Occlusion of Right Internal Mammary Lymphatic with Intraluminal Device, Percutaneous Approach

07L83ZZ   Occlusion of Right Internal Mammary Lymphatic, Percutaneous Approach

07L84CZ   Occlusion of Right Internal Mammary Lymphatic with Extraluminal Device, Percutaneous Endoscopic Approach

07L84DZ   Occlusion of Right Internal Mammary Lymphatic with Intraluminal Device, Percutaneous Endoscopic Approach

07L84ZZ   Occlusion of Right Internal Mammary Lymphatic, Percutaneous Endoscopic Approach

♀ Female-only   ♂ Male-only   ▲ Limited Coverage   ● Non-OR   ▦ HAC-associated procedure   ▲ Non-covered procedures   ✚ Combinatio

07L90CZ	Occlusion of Left Internal Mammary Lymphatic with Extraluminal Device, Open Approach
07L90DZ	Occlusion of Left Internal Mammary Lymphatic with Intraluminal Device, Open Approach
07L90ZZ	Occlusion of Left Internal Mammary Lymphatic, Open Approach
07L93CZ	Occlusion of Left Internal Mammary Lymphatic with Extraluminal Device, Percutaneous Approach
07L93DZ	Occlusion of Left Internal Mammary Lymphatic with Intraluminal Device, Percutaneous Approach
07L93ZZ	Occlusion of Left Internal Mammary Lymphatic, Percutaneous Approach
07L94CZ	Occlusion of Left Internal Mammary Lymphatic with Extraluminal Device, Percutaneous Endoscopic Approach
07L94DZ	Occlusion of Left Internal Mammary Lymphatic with Intraluminal Device, Percutaneous Endoscopic Approach
07L94ZZ	Occlusion of Left Internal Mammary Lymphatic, Percutaneous Endoscopic Approach
07LB0CZ	Occlusion of Mesenteric Lymphatic with Extraluminal Device, Open Approach
07LB0DZ	Occlusion of Mesenteric Lymphatic with Intraluminal Device, Open Approach
07LB0ZZ	Occlusion of Mesenteric Lymphatic, Open Approach
07LB3CZ	Occlusion of Mesenteric Lymphatic with Extraluminal Device, Percutaneous Approach
07LB3DZ	Occlusion of Mesenteric Lymphatic with Intraluminal Device, Percutaneous Approach
07LB3ZZ	Occlusion of Mesenteric Lymphatic, Percutaneous Approach
07LB4CZ	Occlusion of Mesenteric Lymphatic with Extraluminal Device, Percutaneous Endoscopic Approach
07LB4DZ	Occlusion of Mesenteric Lymphatic with Intraluminal Device, Percutaneous Endoscopic Approach
07LB4ZZ	Occlusion of Mesenteric Lymphatic, Percutaneous Endoscopic Approach
07LC0CZ	Occlusion of Pelvis Lymphatic with Extraluminal Device, Open Approach
07LC0DZ	Occlusion of Pelvis Lymphatic with Intraluminal Device, Open Approach
07LC0ZZ	Occlusion of Pelvis Lymphatic, Open Approach
07LC3CZ	Occlusion of Pelvis Lymphatic with Extraluminal Device, Percutaneous Approach
07LC3DZ	Occlusion of Pelvis Lymphatic with Intraluminal Device, Percutaneous Approach
07LC3ZZ	Occlusion of Pelvis Lymphatic, Percutaneous Approach
07LC4CZ	Occlusion of Pelvis Lymphatic with Extraluminal Device, Percutaneous Endoscopic Approach
07LC4DZ	Occlusion of Pelvis Lymphatic with Intraluminal Device, Percutaneous Endoscopic Approach
07LC4ZZ	Occlusion of Pelvis Lymphatic, Percutaneous Endoscopic Approach
07LD0CZ	Occlusion of Aortic Lymphatic with Extraluminal Device, Open Approach
07LD0DZ	Occlusion of Aortic Lymphatic with Intraluminal Device, Open Approach
07LD0ZZ	Occlusion of Aortic Lymphatic, Open Approach
07LD3CZ	Occlusion of Aortic Lymphatic with Extraluminal Device, Percutaneous Approach
07LD3DZ	Occlusion of Aortic Lymphatic with Intraluminal Device, Percutaneous Approach
07LD3ZZ	Occlusion of Aortic Lymphatic, Percutaneous Approach
07LD4CZ	Occlusion of Aortic Lymphatic with Extraluminal Device, Percutaneous Endoscopic Approach
07LD4DZ	Occlusion of Aortic Lymphatic with Intraluminal Device, Percutaneous Endoscopic Approach
07LD4ZZ	Occlusion of Aortic Lymphatic, Percutaneous Endoscopic Approach
07LF0CZ	Occlusion of Right Lower Extremity Lymphatic with Extraluminal Device, Open Approach
07LF0DZ	Occlusion of Right Lower Extremity Lymphatic with Intraluminal Device, Open Approach
07LF0ZZ	Occlusion of Right Lower Extremity Lymphatic, Open Approach
07LF3CZ	Occlusion of Right Lower Extremity Lymphatic with Extraluminal Device, Percutaneous Approach
07LF3DZ	Occlusion of Right Lower Extremity Lymphatic with Intraluminal Device, Percutaneous Approach
07LF3ZZ	Occlusion of Right Lower Extremity Lymphatic, Percutaneous Approach
07LF4CZ	Occlusion of Right Lower Extremity Lymphatic with Extraluminal Device, Percutaneous Endoscopic Approach
07LF4DZ	Occlusion of Right Lower Extremity Lymphatic with Intraluminal Device, Percutaneous Endoscopic Approach
07LF4ZZ	Occlusion of Right Lower Extremity Lymphatic, Percutaneous Endoscopic Approach
07LG0CZ	Occlusion of Left Lower Extremity Lymphatic with Extraluminal Device, Open Approach
07LG0DZ	Occlusion of Left Lower Extremity Lymphatic with Intraluminal Device, Open Approach
07LG0ZZ	Occlusion of Left Lower Extremity Lymphatic, Open Approach
07LG3CZ	Occlusion of Left Lower Extremity Lymphatic with Extraluminal Device, Percutaneous Approach
07LG3DZ	Occlusion of Left Lower Extremity Lymphatic with Intraluminal Device, Percutaneous Approach
07LG3ZZ	Occlusion of Left Lower Extremity Lymphatic, Percutaneous Approach
07LG4CZ	Occlusion of Left Lower Extremity Lymphatic with Extraluminal Device, Percutaneous Endoscopic Approach
07LG4DZ	Occlusion of Left Lower Extremity Lymphatic with Intraluminal Device, Percutaneous Endoscopic Approach
07LG4ZZ	Occlusion of Left Lower Extremity Lymphatic, Percutaneous Endoscopic Approach
07LH0CZ	Occlusion of Right Inguinal Lymphatic with Extraluminal Device, Open Approach
07LH0DZ	Occlusion of Right Inguinal Lymphatic with Intraluminal Device, Open Approach
07LH0ZZ	Occlusion of Right Inguinal Lymphatic, Open Approach
07LH3CZ	Occlusion of Right Inguinal Lymphatic with Extraluminal Device, Percutaneous Approach
07LH3DZ	Occlusion of Right Inguinal Lymphatic with Intraluminal Device, Percutaneous Approach
07LH3ZZ	Occlusion of Right Inguinal Lymphatic, Percutaneous Approach
07LH4CZ	Occlusion of Right Inguinal Lymphatic with Extraluminal Device, Percutaneous Endoscopic Approach
07LH4DZ	Occlusion of Right Inguinal Lymphatic with Intraluminal Device, Percutaneous Endoscopic Approach
07LH4ZZ	Occlusion of Right Inguinal Lymphatic, Percutaneous Endoscopic Approach
07LJ0CZ	Occlusion of Left Inguinal Lymphatic with Extraluminal Device, Open Approach
07LJ0DZ	Occlusion of Left Inguinal Lymphatic with Intraluminal Device, Open Approach
07LJ0ZZ	Occlusion of Left Inguinal Lymphatic, Open Approach
07LJ3CZ	Occlusion of Left Inguinal Lymphatic with Extraluminal Device, Percutaneous Approach
07LJ3DZ	Occlusion of Left Inguinal Lymphatic with Intraluminal Device, Percutaneous Approach
07LJ3ZZ	Occlusion of Left Inguinal Lymphatic, Percutaneous Approach
07LJ4CZ	Occlusion of Left Inguinal Lymphatic with Extraluminal Device, Percutaneous Endoscopic Approach
07LJ4DZ	Occlusion of Left Inguinal Lymphatic with Intraluminal Device, Percutaneous Endoscopic Approach
07LJ4ZZ	Occlusion of Left Inguinal Lymphatic, Percutaneous Endoscopic Approach
07LK0CZ	Occlusion of Thoracic Duct with Extraluminal Device, Open Approach
07LK0DZ	Occlusion of Thoracic Duct with Intraluminal Device, Open Approach
07LK0ZZ	Occlusion of Thoracic Duct, Open Approach
07LK3CZ	Occlusion of Thoracic Duct with Extraluminal Device, Percutaneous Approach
07LK3DZ	Occlusion of Thoracic Duct with Intraluminal Device, Percutaneous Approach
07LK3ZZ	Occlusion of Thoracic Duct, Percutaneous Approach
07LK4CZ	Occlusion of Thoracic Duct with Extraluminal Device, Percutaneous Endoscopic Approach
07LK4DZ	Occlusion of Thoracic Duct with Intraluminal Device, Percutaneous Endoscopic Approach
07LK4ZZ	Occlusion of Thoracic Duct, Percutaneous Endoscopic Approach
07LL0CZ	Occlusion of Cisterna Chyli with Extraluminal Device, Open Approach
07LL0DZ	Occlusion of Cisterna Chyli with Intraluminal Device, Open Approach
07LL0ZZ	Occlusion of Cisterna Chyli, Open Approach
07LL3CZ	Occlusion of Cisterna Chyli with Extraluminal Device, Percutaneous Approach
07LL3DZ	Occlusion of Cisterna Chyli with Intraluminal Device, Percutaneous Approach
07LL3ZZ	Occlusion of Cisterna Chyli, Percutaneous Approach
07LL4CZ	Occlusion of Cisterna Chyli with Extraluminal Device, Percutaneous Endoscopic Approach
07LL4DZ	Occlusion of Cisterna Chyli with Intraluminal Device, Percutaneous Endoscopic Approach
07LL4ZZ	Occlusion of Cisterna Chyli, Percutaneous Endoscopic Approach

Female-only   ♂ Male-only   ▲ Limited Coverage   ● Non-OR   ▥ HAC-associated procedure   ▲ Non-covered procedures   ✚ Combination

07N – Lymphatic and Hemic Systems, Release

Review Coding Guidelines B3.13 and B3.14

07N00ZZ   Release Head Lymphatic, Open Approach
07N03ZZ   Release Head Lymphatic, Percutaneous Approach
07N04ZZ   Release Head Lymphatic, Percutaneous Endoscopic Approach
07N10ZZ   Release Right Neck Lymphatic, Open Approach
07N13ZZ   Release Right Neck Lymphatic, Percutaneous Approach
07N14ZZ   Release Right Neck Lymphatic, Percutaneous Endoscopic Approach
07N20ZZ   Release Left Neck Lymphatic, Open Approach
07N23ZZ   Release Left Neck Lymphatic, Percutaneous Approach
07N24ZZ   Release Left Neck Lymphatic, Percutaneous Endoscopic Approach
07N30ZZ   Release Right Upper Extremity Lymphatic, Open Approach
07N33ZZ   Release Right Upper Extremity Lymphatic, Percutaneous Approach
07N34ZZ   Release Right Upper Extremity Lymphatic, Percutaneous Endoscopic Approach
07N40ZZ   Release Left Upper Extremity Lymphatic, Open Approach
07N43ZZ   Release Left Upper Extremity Lymphatic, Percutaneous Approach
07N44ZZ   Release Left Upper Extremity Lymphatic, Percutaneous Endoscopic Approach
07N50ZZ   Release Right Axillary Lymphatic, Open Approach
07N53ZZ   Release Right Axillary Lymphatic, Percutaneous Approach
07N54ZZ   Release Right Axillary Lymphatic, Percutaneous Endoscopic Approach
07N60ZZ   Release Left Axillary Lymphatic, Open Approach
07N63ZZ   Release Left Axillary Lymphatic, Percutaneous Approach
07N64ZZ   Release Left Axillary Lymphatic, Percutaneous Endoscopic Approach

07N70ZZ   Release Thorax Lymphatic, Open Approach
07N73ZZ   Release Thorax Lymphatic, Percutaneous Approach
07N74ZZ   Release Thorax Lymphatic, Percutaneous Endoscopic Approach
07N80ZZ   Release Right Internal Mammary Lymphatic, Open Approach
07N83ZZ   Release Right Internal Mammary Lymphatic, Percutaneous Approach
07N84ZZ   Release Right Internal Mammary Lymphatic, Percutaneous Endoscopic Approach
07N90ZZ   Release Left Internal Mammary Lymphatic, Open Approach
07N93ZZ   Release Left Internal Mammary Lymphatic, Percutaneous Approach
07N94ZZ   Release Left Internal Mammary Lymphatic, Percutaneous Endoscopic Approach
07NB0ZZ   Release Mesenteric Lymphatic, Open Approach
07NB3ZZ   Release Mesenteric Lymphatic, Percutaneous Approach
07NB4ZZ   Release Mesenteric Lymphatic, Percutaneous Endoscopic Approach
07NC0ZZ   Release Pelvis Lymphatic, Open Approach
07NC3ZZ   Release Pelvis Lymphatic, Percutaneous Approach
07NC4ZZ   Release Pelvis Lymphatic, Percutaneous Endoscopic Approach
07ND0ZZ   Release Aortic Lymphatic, Open Approach
07ND3ZZ   Release Aortic Lymphatic, Percutaneous Approach
07ND4ZZ   Release Aortic Lymphatic, Percutaneous Endoscopic Approach
07NF0ZZ   Release Right Lower Extremity Lymphatic, Open Approach

07NF3ZZ   Release Right Lower Extremity Lymphatic, Percutaneous Approach
07NF4ZZ   Release Right Lower Extremity Lymphatic, Percutaneous Endoscopic Approach
07NG0ZZ   Release Left Lower Extremity Lymphat Open Approach
07NG3ZZ   Release Left Lower Extremity Lymphat Percutaneous Approach
07NG4ZZ   Release Left Lower Extremity Lymphat Percutaneous Endoscopic Approach
07NH0ZZ   Release Right Inguinal Lymphatic, Ope Approach
07NH3ZZ   Release Right Inguinal Lymphatic, Percutaneous Approach
07NH4ZZ   Release Right Inguinal Lymphatic, Percutaneous Endoscopic Approach
07NJ0ZZ   Release Left Inguinal Lymphatic, Open Approach
07NJ3ZZ   Release Left Inguinal Lymphatic, Percutaneous Approach
07NJ4ZZ   Release Left Inguinal Lymphatic, Percutaneous Endoscopic Approach
07NK0ZZ   Release Thoracic Duct, Open Approach
07NK3ZZ   Release Thoracic Duct, Percutaneous Approach
07NK4ZZ   Release Thoracic Duct, Percutaneous Endoscopic Approach
07NL0ZZ   Release Cisterna Chyli, Open Approach
07NL3ZZ   Release Cisterna Chyli, Percutaneous Approach
07NL4ZZ   Release Cisterna Chyli, Percutaneous Endoscopic Approach
07NM0ZZ   Release Thymus, Open Approach
07NM3ZZ   Release Thymus, Percutaneous Approach
07NM4ZZ   Release Thymus, Percutaneous Endoscopic Approach
07NP0ZZ   Release Spleen, Open Approach
07NP3ZZ   Release Spleen, Percutaneous Approach
07NP4ZZ   Release Spleen, Percutaneous Endoscopi Approach

07P – Lymphatic and Hemic Systems, Removal

Review Coding Guideline B6.1c

07PK00Z   Removal of Drainage Device from Thoracic Duct, Open Approach
07PK03Z   Removal of Infusion Device from Thoracic Duct, Open Approach
07PK07Z   Removal of Autologous Tissue Substitute from Thoracic Duct, Open Approach
07PK0CZ   Removal of Extraluminal Device from Thoracic Duct, Open Approach
07PK0DZ   Removal of Intraluminal Device from Thoracic Duct, Open Approach
07PK0JZ   Removal of Synthetic Substitute from Thoracic Duct, Open Approach
07PK0KZ   Removal of Nonautologous Tissue Substitute from Thoracic Duct, Open Approach
07PK30Z   Removal of Drainage Device from Thoracic Duct, Percutaneous Approach
07PK33Z   Removal of Infusion Device from Thoracic Duct, Percutaneous Approach
07PK37Z   Removal of Autologous Tissue Substitute from Thoracic Duct, Percutaneous Approach
07PK3CZ   Removal of Extraluminal Device from Thoracic Duct, Percutaneous Approach
07PK3DZ   Removal of Intraluminal Device from Thoracic Duct, Percutaneous Approach

07PK3JZ   Removal of Synthetic Substitute from Thoracic Duct, Percutaneous Approach
07PK3KZ   Removal of Nonautologous Tissue Substitute from Thoracic Duct, Percutaneous Approach
07PK40Z   Removal of Drainage Device from Thoracic Duct, Percutaneous Endoscopic Approach
07PK43Z   Removal of Infusion Device from Thoracic Duct, Percutaneous Endoscopic Approach
07PK47Z   Removal of Autologous Tissue Substitute from Thoracic Duct, Percutaneous Endoscopic Approach
07PK4CZ   Removal of Extraluminal Device from Thoracic Duct, Percutaneous Endoscopic Approach
07PK4DZ   Removal of Intraluminal Device from Thoracic Duct, Percutaneous Endoscopic Approach
07PK4JZ   Removal of Synthetic Substitute from Thoracic Duct, Percutaneous Endoscopic Approach
07PK4KZ   Removal of Nonautologous Tissue Substitute from Thoracic Duct, Percutaneous Endoscopic Approach

07PKX0Z   Removal of Drainage Device from Thoracic Duct, External Approach
07PKX3Z   Removal of Infusion Device from Thoracic Duct, External Approach
07PKXDZ   Removal of Intraluminal Device from Thoracic Duct, External Approach
07PL00Z   Removal of Drainage Device from Cisterna Chyli, Open Approach
07PL03Z   Removal of Infusion Device from Cistern Chyli, Open Approach
07PL07Z   Removal of Autologous Tissue Substitute from Cisterna Chyli, Open Approach
07PL0CZ   Removal of Extraluminal Device from Cisterna Chyli, Open Approach
07PL0DZ   Removal of Intraluminal Device from Cisterna Chyli, Open Approach
07PL0JZ   Removal of Synthetic Substitute from Cisterna Chyli, Open Approach
07PL0KZ   Removal of Nonautologous Tissue Substitute from Cisterna Chyli, Open Approach
07PL30Z   Removal of Drainage Device from Cisterna Chyli, Percutaneous Approach
07PL33Z   Removal of Infusion Device from Cistern Chyli, Percutaneous Approach

♀ Female-only   ♂ Male-only   ▲ Limited Coverage   ● Non-OR   ▥ HAC-associated procedure   ▲ Non-covered procedures   ✚ Combinatic

.37Z   Removal of Autologous Tissue Substitute from Cisterna Chyli, Percutaneous Approach

.3CZ   Removal of Extraluminal Device from Cisterna Chyli, Percutaneous Approach

.3DZ   Removal of Intraluminal Device from Cisterna Chyli, Percutaneous Approach

.3JZ   Removal of Synthetic Substitute from Cisterna Chyli, Percutaneous Approach

.3KZ   Removal of Nonautologous Tissue Substitute from Cisterna Chyli, Percutaneous Approach

.40Z   Removal of Drainage Device from Cisterna Chyli, Percutaneous Endoscopic Approach

.43Z   Removal of Infusion Device from Cisterna Chyli, Percutaneous Endoscopic Approach

.47Z   Removal of Autologous Tissue Substitute from Cisterna Chyli, Percutaneous Endoscopic Approach

.4CZ   Removal of Extraluminal Device from Cisterna Chyli, Percutaneous Endoscopic Approach

.4DZ   Removal of Intraluminal Device from Cisterna Chyli, Percutaneous Endoscopic Approach

.4JZ   Removal of Synthetic Substitute from Cisterna Chyli, Percutaneous Endoscopic Approach

.4KZ   Removal of Nonautologous Tissue Substitute from Cisterna Chyli, Percutaneous Endoscopic Approach

.X0Z   Removal of Drainage Device from Cisterna Chyli, External Approach

.X3Z   Removal of Infusion Device from Cisterna Chyli, External Approach

.XDZ   Removal of Intraluminal Device from Cisterna Chyli, External Approach

.M00Z   Removal of Drainage Device from Thymus, Open Approach

.M03Z   Removal of Infusion Device from Thymus, Open Approach

.M30Z   Removal of Drainage Device from Thymus, Percutaneous Approach

.M33Z   Removal of Infusion Device from Thymus, Percutaneous Approach

07PM40Z   Removal of Drainage Device from Thymus, Percutaneous Endoscopic Approach

07PM43Z   Removal of Infusion Device from Thymus, Percutaneous Endoscopic Approach

07PMX0Z   Removal of Drainage Device from Thymus, External Approach

07PMX3Z   Removal of Infusion Device from Thymus, External Approach

07PN00Z   Removal of Drainage Device from Lymphatic, Open Approach

07PN03Z   Removal of Infusion Device from Lymphatic, Open Approach

07PN07Z   Removal of Autologous Tissue Substitute from Lymphatic, Open Approach

07PN0CZ   Removal of Extraluminal Device from Lymphatic, Open Approach

07PN0DZ   Removal of Intraluminal Device from Lymphatic, Open Approach

07PN0JZ   Removal of Synthetic Substitute from Lymphatic, Open Approach

07PN0KZ   Removal of Nonautologous Tissue Substitute from Lymphatic, Open Approach

07PN30Z   Removal of Drainage Device from Lymphatic, Percutaneous Approach

07PN33Z   Removal of Infusion Device from Lymphatic, Percutaneous Approach

07PN37Z   Removal of Autologous Tissue Substitute from Lymphatic, Percutaneous Approach

07PN3CZ   Removal of Extraluminal Device from Lymphatic, Percutaneous Approach

07PN3DZ   Removal of Intraluminal Device from Lymphatic, Percutaneous Approach

07PN3JZ   Removal of Synthetic Substitute from Lymphatic, Percutaneous Approach

07PN3KZ   Removal of Nonautologous Tissue Substitute from Lymphatic, Percutaneous Approach

07PN40Z   Removal of Drainage Device from Lymphatic, Percutaneous Endoscopic Approach

07PN43Z   Removal of Infusion Device from Lymphatic, Percutaneous Endoscopic Approach

07PN47Z   Removal of Autologous Tissue Substitute from Lymphatic, Percutaneous Endoscopic Approach

07PN4CZ   Removal of Extraluminal Device from Lymphatic, Percutaneous Endoscopic Approach

07PN4DZ   Removal of Intraluminal Device from Lymphatic, Percutaneous Endoscopic Approach

07PN4JZ   Removal of Synthetic Substitute from Lymphatic, Percutaneous Endoscopic Approach

07PN4KZ   Removal of Nonautologous Tissue Substitute from Lymphatic, Percutaneous Endoscopic Approach

07PNX0Z   Removal of Drainage Device from Lymphatic, External Approach

07PNX3Z   Removal of Infusion Device from Lymphatic, External Approach

07PNXDZ   Removal of Intraluminal Device from Lymphatic, External Approach

07PP00Z   Removal of Drainage Device from Spleen, Open Approach

07PP03Z   Removal of Infusion Device from Spleen, Open Approach

07PP30Z   Removal of Drainage Device from Spleen, Percutaneous Approach

07PP33Z   Removal of Infusion Device from Spleen, Percutaneous Approach

07PP40Z   Removal of Drainage Device from Spleen, Percutaneous Endoscopic Approach

07PP43Z   Removal of Infusion Device from Spleen, Percutaneous Endoscopic Approach

07PPX0Z   Removal of Drainage Device from Spleen, External Approach

07PPX3Z   Removal of Infusion Device from Spleen, External Approach

07PT00Z   Removal of Drainage Device from Bone Marrow, Open Approach

07PT30Z   Removal of Drainage Device from Bone Marrow, Percutaneous Approach

07PT40Z   Removal of Drainage Device from Bone Marrow, Percutaneous Endoscopic Approach

07PTX0Z   Removal of Drainage Device from Bone Marrow, External Approach

Q – Lymphatic and Hemic Systems, Repair

.Q00ZZ   Repair Head Lymphatic, Open Approach

.Q03ZZ   Repair Head Lymphatic, Percutaneous Approach

.Q04ZZ   Repair Head Lymphatic, Percutaneous Endoscopic Approach

.Q10ZZ   Repair Right Neck Lymphatic, Open Approach

.Q13ZZ   Repair Right Neck Lymphatic, Percutaneous Approach

.Q14ZZ   Repair Right Neck Lymphatic, Percutaneous Endoscopic Approach

.Q20ZZ   Repair Left Neck Lymphatic, Open Approach

.Q23ZZ   Repair Left Neck Lymphatic, Percutaneous Approach

.Q24ZZ   Repair Left Neck Lymphatic, Percutaneous Endoscopic Approach

.Q30ZZ   Repair Right Upper Extremity Lymphatic, Open Approach

.Q33ZZ   Repair Right Upper Extremity Lymphatic, Percutaneous Approach

.Q34ZZ   Repair Right Upper Extremity Lymphatic, Percutaneous Endoscopic Approach

.Q40ZZ   Repair Left Upper Extremity Lymphatic, Open Approach

07Q43ZZ   Repair Left Upper Extremity Lymphatic, Percutaneous Approach

07Q44ZZ   Repair Left Upper Extremity Lymphatic, Percutaneous Endoscopic Approach

07Q50ZZ   Repair Right Axillary Lymphatic, Open Approach

07Q53ZZ   Repair Right Axillary Lymphatic, Percutaneous Approach

07Q54ZZ   Repair Right Axillary Lymphatic, Percutaneous Endoscopic Approach

07Q60ZZ   Repair Left Axillary Lymphatic, Open Approach

07Q63ZZ   Repair Left Axillary Lymphatic, Percutaneous Approach

07Q64ZZ   Repair Left Axillary Lymphatic, Percutaneous Endoscopic Approach

07Q70ZZ   Repair Thorax Lymphatic, Open Approach

07Q73ZZ   Repair Thorax Lymphatic, Percutaneous Approach

07Q74ZZ   Repair Thorax Lymphatic, Percutaneous Endoscopic Approach

07Q80ZZ   Repair Right Internal Mammary Lymphatic, Open Approach

07Q83ZZ   Repair Right Internal Mammary Lymphatic, Percutaneous Approach

07Q84ZZ   Repair Right Internal Mammary Lymphatic, Percutaneous Endoscopic Approach

07Q90ZZ   Repair Left Internal Mammary Lymphatic, Open Approach

07Q93ZZ   Repair Left Internal Mammary Lymphatic, Percutaneous Approach

07Q94ZZ   Repair Left Internal Mammary Lymphatic, Percutaneous Endoscopic Approach

07QB0ZZ   Repair Mesenteric Lymphatic, Open Approach

07QB3ZZ   Repair Mesenteric Lymphatic, Percutaneous Approach

07QB4ZZ   Repair Mesenteric Lymphatic, Percutaneous Endoscopic Approach

07QC0ZZ   Repair Pelvis Lymphatic, Open Approach

07QC3ZZ   Repair Pelvis Lymphatic, Percutaneous Approach

07QC4ZZ   Repair Pelvis Lymphatic, Percutaneous Endoscopic Approach

07QD0ZZ   Repair Aortic Lymphatic, Open Approach

07QD3ZZ   Repair Aortic Lymphatic, Percutaneous Approach

07QD4ZZ   Repair Aortic Lymphatic, Percutaneous Endoscopic Approach

♀ Female-only   ♂ Male-only   ▲ Limited Coverage   ● Non-OR   HAC HAC-associated procedure   ▲ Non-covered procedures   ✚ Combination

07QF0ZZ Repair Right Lower Extremity Lymphatic, Open Approach	**07QH3ZZ** Repair Right Inguinal Lymphatic, Percutaneous Approach	**07QL0ZZ** Repair Cisterna Chyli, Open Approach
07QF3ZZ Repair Right Lower Extremity Lymphatic, Percutaneous Approach	**07QH4ZZ** Repair Right Inguinal Lymphatic, Percutaneous Endoscopic Approach	**07QL3ZZ** Repair Cisterna Chyli, Percutaneous Approach
07QF4ZZ Repair Right Lower Extremity Lymphatic, Percutaneous Endoscopic Approach	**07QJ0ZZ** Repair Left Inguinal Lymphatic, Open Approach	**07QL4ZZ** Repair Cisterna Chyli, Percutaneous Endoscopic Approach
07QG0ZZ Repair Left Lower Extremity Lymphatic, Open Approach	**07QJ3ZZ** Repair Left Inguinal Lymphatic, Percutaneous Approach	**07QM0ZZ** Repair Thymus, Open Approach
07QG3ZZ Repair Left Lower Extremity Lymphatic, Percutaneous Approach	**07QJ4ZZ** Repair Left Inguinal Lymphatic, Percutaneous Endoscopic Approach	**07QM3ZZ** Repair Thymus, Percutaneous Approac
07QG4ZZ Repair Left Lower Extremity Lymphatic, Percutaneous Endoscopic Approach	**07QK0ZZ** Repair Thoracic Duct, Open Approach	**07QM4ZZ** Repair Thymus, Percutaneous Endosco Approach
07QH0ZZ Repair Right Inguinal Lymphatic, Open Approach	**07QK3ZZ** Repair Thoracic Duct, Percutaneous Approach	**07QP0ZZ** Repair Spleen, Open Approach
	07QK4ZZ Repair Thoracic Duct, Percutaneous Endoscopic Approach	**07QP3ZZ** Repair Spleen, Percutaneous Approach
		07QP4ZZ Repair Spleen, Percutaneous Endoscop Approach

07S – Lymphatic and Hemic Systems, Reposition

07SM0ZZ Reposition Thymus, Open Approach	**07SP0ZZ** Reposition Spleen, Open Approach

07T – Lymphatic and Hemic Systems, Resection

Review Coding Guideline B3.8

07T00ZZ Resection of Head Lymphatic, Open Approach	⊞ Mastectomy procedure when reported with resection of breast. *See table 0HT to construct the Resection of breast code. See table 0KT to construct the Resection of thorax muscle code if applicable. See table 07T to report additional lymph node resections.*	**07TF0ZZ** Resection of Right Lower Extremity Lymphatic, Open Approach
07T04ZZ Resection of Head Lymphatic, Percutaneous Endoscopic Approach		**07TF4ZZ** Resection of Right Lower Extremity Lymphatic, Percutaneous Endoscopic Approach
07T10ZZ Resection of Right Neck Lymphatic, Open Approach		**07TG0ZZ** Resection of Left Lower Extremity Lymphatic, Open Approach
AHA CC: 3Q, 2014, 9-10	**07T64ZZ** Resection of Left Axillary Lymphatic, Percutaneous Endoscopic Approach	**07TG4ZZ** Resection of Left Lower Extremity Lymphatic, Percutaneous Endoscopic Approach
07T14ZZ Resection of Right Neck Lymphatic, Percutaneous Endoscopic Approach	**07T70ZZ** Resection of Thorax Lymphatic, Open Approach	**07TH0ZZ** Resection of Right Inguinal Lymphatic Open Approach
07T20ZZ Resection of Left Neck Lymphatic, Open Approach	**07T74ZZ** Resection of Thorax Lymphatic, Percutaneous Endoscopic Approach	**07TH4ZZ** Resection of Right Inguinal Lymphatic Percutaneous Endoscopic Approach
AHA CC: 3Q, 2014, 9-10	**07T80ZZ** Resection of Right Internal Mammary Lymphatic, Open Approach	**07TJ0ZZ** Resection of Left Inguinal Lymphatic, Open Approach
07T24ZZ Resection of Left Neck Lymphatic, Percutaneous Endoscopic Approach	**07T84ZZ** Resection of Right Internal Mammary Lymphatic, Percutaneous Endoscopic Approach	**07TJ4ZZ** Resection of Left Inguinal Lymphatic, Percutaneous Endoscopic Approach
07T30ZZ Resection of Right Upper Extremity Lymphatic, Open Approach	**07T90ZZ** Resection of Left Internal Mammary Lymphatic, Open Approach	**07TK0ZZ** Resection of Thoracic Duct, Open Approach
07T34ZZ Resection of Right Upper Extremity Lymphatic, Percutaneous Endoscopic Approach	**07T94ZZ** Resection of Left Internal Mammary Lymphatic, Percutaneous Endoscopic Approach	**07TK4ZZ** Resection of Thoracic Duct, Percutaneo Endoscopic Approach
07T40ZZ Resection of Left Upper Extremity Lymphatic, Open Approach	**07TB0ZZ** Resection of Mesenteric Lymphatic, Open Approach	**07TL0ZZ** Resection of Cisterna Chyli, Open Approach
07T44ZZ Resection of Left Upper Extremity Lymphatic, Percutaneous Endoscopic Approach	**07TB4ZZ** Resection of Mesenteric Lymphatic, Percutaneous Endoscopic Approach	**07TL4ZZ** Resection of Cisterna Chyli, Percutane Endoscopic Approach
07T50ZZ Resection of Right Axillary Lymphatic, Open Approach	**07TC0ZZ** Resection of Pelvis Lymphatic, Open Approach	**07TM0ZZ** Resection of Thymus, Open Approach
⊞ Mastectomy procedure when reported with resection of breast. *See table 0HT to construct the Resection of breast code. See table 0KT to construct the Resection of thorax muscle code if applicable. See table 07T to report additional lymph node resections.*	**07TC4ZZ** Resection of Pelvis Lymphatic, Percutaneous Endoscopic Approach	*AHA CC: 3Q, 2014, 16-17*
		07TM4ZZ Resection of Thymus, Percutaneous Endoscopic Approach
	07TD0ZZ Resection of Aortic Lymphatic, Open Approach	**07TP0ZZ** Resection of Spleen, Open Approach
07T54ZZ Resection of Right Axillary Lymphatic, Percutaneous Endoscopic Approach	**07TD4ZZ** Resection of Aortic Lymphatic, Percutaneous Endoscopic Approach	**07TP4ZZ** Resection of Spleen, Percutaneous Endoscopic Approach
07T60ZZ Resection of Left Axillary Lymphatic, Open Approach		

07U – Lymphatic and Hemic Systems, Supplement

07U007Z Supplement Head Lymphatic with Autologous Tissue Substitute, Open Approach	**07U107Z** Supplement Right Neck Lymphatic with Autologous Tissue Substitute, Open Approach	**07U207Z** Supplement Left Neck Lymphatic with Autologous Tissue Substitute, Open Approach
07U00JZ Supplement Head Lymphatic with Synthetic Substitute, Open Approach	**07U10JZ** Supplement Right Neck Lymphatic with Synthetic Substitute, Open Approach	**07U20JZ** Supplement Left Neck Lymphatic with Synthetic Substitute, Open Approach
07U00KZ Supplement Head Lymphatic with Nonautologous Tissue Substitute, Open Approach	**07U10KZ** Supplement Right Neck Lymphatic with Nonautologous Tissue Substitute, Open Approach	**07U20KZ** Supplement Left Neck Lymphatic with Nonautologous Tissue Substitute, Open Approach
07U047Z Supplement Head Lymphatic with Autologous Tissue Substitute, Percutaneous Endoscopic Approach	**07U147Z** Supplement Right Neck Lymphatic with Autologous Tissue Substitute, Percutaneous Endoscopic Approach	**07U247Z** Supplement Left Neck Lymphatic with Autologous Tissue Substitute, Percutaneous Endoscopic Approach
07U04JZ Supplement Head Lymphatic with Synthetic Substitute, Percutaneous Endoscopic Approach	**07U14JZ** Supplement Right Neck Lymphatic with Synthetic Substitute, Percutaneous Endoscopic Approach	**07U24JZ** Supplement Left Neck Lymphatic with Synthetic Substitute, Percutaneous Endoscopic Approach
07U04KZ Supplement Head Lymphatic with Nonautologous Tissue Substitute, Percutaneous Endoscopic Approach	**07U14KZ** Supplement Right Neck Lymphatic with Nonautologous Tissue Substitute, Percutaneous Endoscopic Approach	**07U24KZ** Supplement Left Neck Lymphatic with Nonautologous Tissue Substitute, Percutaneous Endoscopic Approach

♀ Female-only   ♂ Male-only   ▲ Limited Coverage   ● Non-OR   ▬ HAC-associated procedure   ▲ Non-covered procedures   ⊞ Combinat

307Z Supplement Right Upper Extremity Lymphatic with Autologous Tissue Substitute, Open Approach

30JZ Supplement Right Upper Extremity Lymphatic with Synthetic Substitute, Open Approach

30KZ Supplement Right Upper Extremity Lymphatic with Nonautologous Tissue Substitute, Open Approach

347Z Supplement Right Upper Extremity Lymphatic with Autologous Tissue Substitute, Percutaneous Endoscopic Approach

34JZ Supplement Right Upper Extremity Lymphatic with Synthetic Substitute, Percutaneous Endoscopic Approach

34KZ Supplement Right Upper Extremity Lymphatic with Nonautologous Tissue Substitute, Percutaneous Endoscopic Approach

J407Z Supplement Left Upper Extremity Lymphatic with Autologous Tissue Substitute, Open Approach

J40JZ Supplement Left Upper Extremity Lymphatic with Synthetic Substitute, Open Approach

J40KZ Supplement Left Upper Extremity Lymphatic with Nonautologous Tissue Substitute, Open Approach

J447Z Supplement Left Upper Extremity Lymphatic with Autologous Tissue Substitute, Percutaneous Endoscopic Approach

J44JZ Supplement Left Upper Extremity Lymphatic with Synthetic Substitute, Percutaneous Endoscopic Approach

J44KZ Supplement Left Upper Extremity Lymphatic with Nonautologous Tissue Substitute, Percutaneous Endoscopic Approach

J507Z Supplement Right Axillary Lymphatic with Autologous Tissue Substitute, Open Approach

U50JZ Supplement Right Axillary Lymphatic with Synthetic Substitute, Open Approach

U50KZ Supplement Right Axillary Lymphatic with Nonautologous Tissue Substitute, Open Approach

U547Z Supplement Right Axillary Lymphatic with Autologous Tissue Substitute, Percutaneous Endoscopic Approach

U54JZ Supplement Right Axillary Lymphatic with Synthetic Substitute, Percutaneous Endoscopic Approach

U54KZ Supplement Right Axillary Lymphatic with Nonautologous Tissue Substitute, Percutaneous Endoscopic Approach

U607Z Supplement Left Axillary Lymphatic with Autologous Tissue Substitute, Open Approach

U60JZ Supplement Left Axillary Lymphatic with Synthetic Substitute, Open Approach

U60KZ Supplement Left Axillary Lymphatic with Nonautologous Tissue Substitute, Open Approach

U647Z Supplement Left Axillary Lymphatic with Autologous Tissue Substitute, Percutaneous Endoscopic Approach

U64JZ Supplement Left Axillary Lymphatic with Synthetic Substitute, Percutaneous Endoscopic Approach

U64KZ Supplement Left Axillary Lymphatic with Nonautologous Tissue Substitute, Percutaneous Endoscopic Approach

U707Z Supplement Thorax Lymphatic with Autologous Tissue Substitute, Open Approach

U70JZ Supplement Thorax Lymphatic with Synthetic Substitute, Open Approach

07U70KZ Supplement Thorax Lymphatic with Nonautologous Tissue Substitute, Open Approach

07U747Z Supplement Thorax Lymphatic with Autologous Tissue Substitute, Percutaneous Endoscopic Approach

07U74JZ Supplement Thorax Lymphatic with Synthetic Substitute, Percutaneous Endoscopic Approach

07U74KZ Supplement Thorax Lymphatic with Nonautologous Tissue Substitute, Percutaneous Endoscopic Approach

07U807Z Supplement Right Internal Mammary Lymphatic with Autologous Tissue Substitute, Open Approach

07U80JZ Supplement Right Internal Mammary Lymphatic with Synthetic Substitute, Open Approach

07U80KZ Supplement Right Internal Mammary Lymphatic with Nonautologous Tissue Substitute, Open Approach

07U847Z Supplement Right Internal Mammary Lymphatic with Autologous Tissue Substitute, Percutaneous Endoscopic Approach

07U84JZ Supplement Right Internal Mammary Lymphatic with Synthetic Substitute, Percutaneous Endoscopic Approach

07U84KZ Supplement Right Internal Mammary Lymphatic with Nonautologous Tissue Substitute, Percutaneous Endoscopic Approach

07U907Z Supplement Left Internal Mammary Lymphatic with Autologous Tissue Substitute, Open Approach

07U90JZ Supplement Left Internal Mammary Lymphatic with Synthetic Substitute, Open Approach

07U90KZ Supplement Left Internal Mammary Lymphatic with Nonautologous Tissue Substitute, Open Approach

07U947Z Supplement Left Internal Mammary Lymphatic with Autologous Tissue Substitute, Percutaneous Endoscopic Approach

07U94JZ Supplement Left Internal Mammary Lymphatic with Synthetic Substitute, Percutaneous Endoscopic Approach

07U94KZ Supplement Left Internal Mammary Lymphatic with Nonautologous Tissue Substitute, Percutaneous Endoscopic Approach

07UB07Z Supplement Mesenteric Lymphatic with Autologous Tissue Substitute, Open Approach

07UB0JZ Supplement Mesenteric Lymphatic with Synthetic Substitute, Open Approach

07UB0KZ Supplement Mesenteric Lymphatic with Nonautologous Tissue Substitute, Open Approach

07UB47Z Supplement Mesenteric Lymphatic with Autologous Tissue Substitute, Percutaneous Endoscopic Approach

07UB4JZ Supplement Mesenteric Lymphatic with Synthetic Substitute, Percutaneous Endoscopic Approach

07UB4KZ Supplement Mesenteric Lymphatic with Nonautologous Tissue Substitute, Percutaneous Endoscopic Approach

07UC07Z Supplement Pelvis Lymphatic with Autologous Tissue Substitute, Open Approach

07UC0JZ Supplement Pelvis Lymphatic with Synthetic Substitute, Open Approach

07UC0KZ Supplement Pelvis Lymphatic with Nonautologous Tissue Substitute, Open Approach

07UC47Z Supplement Pelvis Lymphatic with Autologous Tissue Substitute, Percutaneous Endoscopic Approach

07UC4JZ Supplement Pelvis Lymphatic with Synthetic Substitute, Percutaneous Endoscopic Approach

07UC4KZ Supplement Pelvis Lymphatic with Nonautologous Tissue Substitute, Percutaneous Endoscopic Approach

07UD07Z Supplement Aortic Lymphatic with Autologous Tissue Substitute, Open Approach

07UD0JZ Supplement Aortic Lymphatic with Synthetic Substitute, Open Approach

07UD0KZ Supplement Aortic Lymphatic with Nonautologous Tissue Substitute, Open Approach

07UD47Z Supplement Aortic Lymphatic with Autologous Tissue Substitute, Percutaneous Endoscopic Approach

07UD4JZ Supplement Aortic Lymphatic with Synthetic Substitute, Percutaneous Endoscopic Approach

07UD4KZ Supplement Aortic Lymphatic with Nonautologous Tissue Substitute, Percutaneous Endoscopic Approach

07UF07Z Supplement Right Lower Extremity Lymphatic with Autologous Tissue Substitute, Open Approach

07UF0JZ Supplement Right Lower Extremity Lymphatic with Synthetic Substitute, Open Approach

07UF0KZ Supplement Right Lower Extremity Lymphatic with Nonautologous Tissue Substitute, Open Approach

07UF47Z Supplement Right Lower Extremity Lymphatic with Autologous Tissue Substitute, Percutaneous Endoscopic Approach

07UF4JZ Supplement Right Lower Extremity Lymphatic with Synthetic Substitute, Percutaneous Endoscopic Approach

07UF4KZ Supplement Right Lower Extremity Lymphatic with Nonautologous Tissue Substitute, Percutaneous Endoscopic Approach

07UG07Z Supplement Left Lower Extremity Lymphatic with Autologous Tissue Substitute, Open Approach

07UG0JZ Supplement Left Lower Extremity Lymphatic with Synthetic Substitute, Open Approach

07UG0KZ Supplement Left Lower Extremity Lymphatic with Nonautologous Tissue Substitute, Open Approach

07UG47Z Supplement Left Lower Extremity Lymphatic with Autologous Tissue Substitute, Percutaneous Endoscopic Approach

07UG4JZ Supplement Left Lower Extremity Lymphatic with Synthetic Substitute, Percutaneous Endoscopic Approach

07UG4KZ Supplement Left Lower Extremity Lymphatic with Nonautologous Tissue Substitute, Percutaneous Endoscopic Approach

07UH07Z Supplement Right Inguinal Lymphatic with Autologous Tissue Substitute, Open Approach

07UH0JZ Supplement Right Inguinal Lymphatic with Synthetic Substitute, Open Approach

07UH0KZ Supplement Right Inguinal Lymphatic with Nonautologous Tissue Substitute, Open Approach

07UH47Z Supplement Right Inguinal Lymphatic with Autologous Tissue Substitute, Percutaneous Endoscopic Approach

07UH4JZ Supplement Right Inguinal Lymphatic with Synthetic Substitute, Percutaneous Endoscopic Approach

07UH4KZ Supplement Right Inguinal Lymphatic with Nonautologous Tissue Substitute, Percutaneous Endoscopic Approach

07UJ07Z Supplement Left Inguinal Lymphatic with Autologous Tissue Substitute, Open Approach

07UJ0JZ Supplement Left Inguinal Lymphatic with Synthetic Substitute, Open Approach

07UJ0KZ Supplement Left Inguinal Lymphatic with Nonautologous Tissue Substitute, Open Approach

07UJ47Z Supplement Left Inguinal Lymphatic with Autologous Tissue Substitute, Percutaneous Endoscopic Approach

07UJ4JZ Supplement Left Inguinal Lymphatic with Synthetic Substitute, Percutaneous Endoscopic Approach

07UJ4KZ Supplement Left Inguinal Lymphatic with Nonautologous Tissue Substitute, Percutaneous Endoscopic Approach

07UK07Z Supplement Thoracic Duct with Autologous Tissue Substitute, Open Approach

07UK0JZ Supplement Thoracic Duct with Synthetic Substitute, Open Approach

07UK0KZ Supplement Thoracic Duct with Nonautologous Tissue Substitute, Open Approach

07UK47Z Supplement Thoracic Duct with Autologous Tissue Substitute, Percutaneous Endoscopic Approach

07UK4JZ Supplement Thoracic Duct with Synthetic Substitute, Percutaneous Endoscopic Approach

07UK4KZ Supplement Thoracic Duct with Nonautologous Tissue Substitute, Percutaneous Endoscopic Approach

07UL07Z Supplement Cisterna Chyli with Autologous Tissue Substitute, Open Approach

07UL0JZ Supplement Cisterna Chyli with Synthetic Substitute, Open Approach

07UL0KZ Supplement Cisterna Chyli with Nonautologous Tissue Substitute, Open Approach

07UL47Z Supplement Cisterna Chyli with Autologous Tissue Substitute, Percutaneous Endoscopic Approach

07UL4JZ Supplement Cisterna Chyli with Synthetic Substitute, Percutaneous Endoscopic Approach

07UL4KZ Supplement Cisterna Chyli with Nonautologous Tissue Substitute, Percutaneous Endoscopic Approach

07V – Lymphatic and Hemic Systems, Restriction

07V00CZ Restriction of Head Lymphatic with Extraluminal Device, Open Approach

07V00DZ Restriction of Head Lymphatic with Intraluminal Device, Open Approach

07V00ZZ Restriction of Head Lymphatic, Open Approach

07V03CZ Restriction of Head Lymphatic with Extraluminal Device, Percutaneous Approach

07V03DZ Restriction of Head Lymphatic with Intraluminal Device, Percutaneous Approach

07V03ZZ Restriction of Head Lymphatic, Percutaneous Approach

07V04CZ Restriction of Head Lymphatic with Extraluminal Device, Percutaneous Endoscopic Approach

07V04DZ Restriction of Head Lymphatic with Intraluminal Device, Percutaneous Endoscopic Approach

07V04ZZ Restriction of Head Lymphatic, Percutaneous Endoscopic Approach

07V10CZ Restriction of Right Neck Lymphatic with Extraluminal Device, Open Approach

07V10DZ Restriction of Right Neck Lymphatic with Intraluminal Device, Open Approach

07V10ZZ Restriction of Right Neck Lymphatic, Open Approach

07V13CZ Restriction of Right Neck Lymphatic with Extraluminal Device, Percutaneous Approach

07V13DZ Restriction of Right Neck Lymphatic with Intraluminal Device, Percutaneous Approach

07V13ZZ Restriction of Right Neck Lymphatic, Percutaneous Approach

07V14CZ Restriction of Right Neck Lymphatic with Extraluminal Device, Percutaneous Endoscopic Approach

07V14DZ Restriction of Right Neck Lymphatic with Intraluminal Device, Percutaneous Endoscopic Approach

07V14ZZ Restriction of Right Neck Lymphatic, Percutaneous Endoscopic Approach

07V20CZ Restriction of Left Neck Lymphatic with Extraluminal Device, Open Approach

07V20DZ Restriction of Left Neck Lymphatic with Intraluminal Device, Open Approach

07V20ZZ Restriction of Left Neck Lymphatic, Open Approach

07V23CZ Restriction of Left Neck Lymphatic with Extraluminal Device, Percutaneous Approach

07V23DZ Restriction of Left Neck Lymphatic with Intraluminal Device, Percutaneous Approach

07V23ZZ Restriction of Left Neck Lymphatic, Percutaneous Approach

07V24CZ Restriction of Left Neck Lymphatic with Extraluminal Device, Percutaneous Endoscopic Approach

07V24DZ Restriction of Left Neck Lymphatic with Intraluminal Device, Percutaneous Endoscopic Approach

07V24ZZ Restriction of Left Neck Lymphatic, Percutaneous Endoscopic Approach

07V30CZ Restriction of Right Upper Extremity Lymphatic with Extraluminal Device, Open Approach

07V30DZ Restriction of Right Upper Extremity Lymphatic with Intraluminal Device, Open Approach

07V30ZZ Restriction of Right Upper Extremity Lymphatic, Open Approach

07V33CZ Restriction of Right Upper Extremity Lymphatic with Extraluminal Device, Percutaneous Approach

07V33DZ Restriction of Right Upper Extremity Lymphatic with Intraluminal Device, Percutaneous Approach

07V33ZZ Restriction of Right Upper Extremity Lymphatic, Percutaneous Approach

07V34CZ Restriction of Right Upper Extremity Lymphatic with Extraluminal Device, Percutaneous Endoscopic Approach

07V34DZ Restriction of Right Upper Extremity Lymphatic with Intraluminal Device, Percutaneous Endoscopic Approach

07V34ZZ Restriction of Right Upper Extremity Lymphatic, Percutaneous Endoscopic Approach

07V40CZ Restriction of Left Upper Extremity Lymphatic with Extraluminal Device, Open Approach

07V40DZ Restriction of Left Upper Extremity Lymphatic with Intraluminal Device, Open Approach

07V40ZZ Restriction of Left Upper Extremity Lymphatic, Open Approach

07V43CZ Restriction of Left Upper Extremity Lymphatic with Extraluminal Device, Percutaneous Approach

07V43DZ Restriction of Left Upper Extremity Lymphatic with Intraluminal Device, Percutaneous Approach

07V43ZZ Restriction of Left Upper Extremity Lymphatic, Percutaneous Approach

07V44CZ Restriction of Left Upper Extremity Lymphatic with Extraluminal Device, Percutaneous Endoscopic Approach

07V44DZ Restriction of Left Upper Extremity Lymphatic with Intraluminal Device, Percutaneous Endoscopic Approach

07V44ZZ Restriction of Left Upper Extremity Lymphatic, Percutaneous Endoscopic Approach

07V50CZ Restriction of Right Axillary Lymphatic with Extraluminal Device, Open Approach

07V50DZ Restriction of Right Axillary Lymphatic with Intraluminal Device, Open Approach

07V50ZZ Restriction of Right Axillary Lymphatic, Open Approach

07V53CZ Restriction of Right Axillary Lymphatic with Extraluminal Device, Percutaneous Approach

07V53DZ Restriction of Right Axillary Lymphatic with Intraluminal Device, Percutaneous Approach

07V53ZZ Restriction of Right Axillary Lymphatic, Percutaneous Approach

07V54CZ Restriction of Right Axillary Lymphatic with Extraluminal Device, Percutaneous Endoscopic Approach

07V54DZ Restriction of Right Axillary Lymphatic with Intraluminal Device, Percutaneous Endoscopic Approach

07V54ZZ Restriction of Right Axillary Lymphatic, Percutaneous Endoscopic Approach

07V60CZ Restriction of Left Axillary Lymphatic with Extraluminal Device, Open Approach

07V60DZ Restriction of Left Axillary Lymphatic with Intraluminal Device, Open Approach

07V60ZZ Restriction of Left Axillary Lymphatic, Open Approach

07V63CZ Restriction of Left Axillary Lymphatic with Extraluminal Device, Percutaneous Approach

07V63DZ Restriction of Left Axillary Lymphatic with Intraluminal Device, Percutaneous Approach

07V63ZZ Restriction of Left Axillary Lymphatic, Percutaneous Approach

64CZ	Restriction of Left Axillary Lymphatic with Extraluminal Device, Percutaneous Endoscopic Approach
64DZ	Restriction of Left Axillary Lymphatic with Intraluminal Device, Percutaneous Endoscopic Approach
64ZZ	Restriction of Left Axillary Lymphatic, Percutaneous Endoscopic Approach
70CZ	Restriction of Thorax Lymphatic with Extraluminal Device, Open Approach
70DZ	Restriction of Thorax Lymphatic with Intraluminal Device, Open Approach
70ZZ	Restriction of Thorax Lymphatic, Open Approach
73CZ	Restriction of Thorax Lymphatic with Extraluminal Device, Percutaneous Approach
73DZ	Restriction of Thorax Lymphatic with Intraluminal Device, Percutaneous Approach
73ZZ	Restriction of Thorax Lymphatic, Percutaneous Approach
74CZ	Restriction of Thorax Lymphatic with Extraluminal Device, Percutaneous Endoscopic Approach
74DZ	Restriction of Thorax Lymphatic with Intraluminal Device, Percutaneous Endoscopic Approach
74ZZ	Restriction of Thorax Lymphatic, Percutaneous Endoscopic Approach
80CZ	Restriction of Right Internal Mammary Lymphatic with Extraluminal Device, Open Approach
80DZ	Restriction of Right Internal Mammary Lymphatic with Intraluminal Device, Open Approach
80ZZ	Restriction of Right Internal Mammary Lymphatic, Open Approach
V83CZ	Restriction of Right Internal Mammary Lymphatic with Extraluminal Device, Percutaneous Approach
V83DZ	Restriction of Right Internal Mammary Lymphatic with Intraluminal Device, Percutaneous Approach
V83ZZ	Restriction of Right Internal Mammary Lymphatic, Percutaneous Approach
V84CZ	Restriction of Right Internal Mammary Lymphatic with Extraluminal Device, Percutaneous Endoscopic Approach
V84DZ	Restriction of Right Internal Mammary Lymphatic with Intraluminal Device, Percutaneous Endoscopic Approach
V84ZZ	Restriction of Right Internal Mammary Lymphatic, Percutaneous Endoscopic Approach
V90CZ	Restriction of Left Internal Mammary Lymphatic with Extraluminal Device, Open Approach
V90DZ	Restriction of Left Internal Mammary Lymphatic with Intraluminal Device, Open Approach
V90ZZ	Restriction of Left Internal Mammary Lymphatic, Open Approach
V93CZ	Restriction of Left Internal Mammary Lymphatic with Extraluminal Device, Percutaneous Approach
V93DZ	Restriction of Left Internal Mammary Lymphatic with Intraluminal Device, Percutaneous Approach
V93ZZ	Restriction of Left Internal Mammary Lymphatic, Percutaneous Approach
V94CZ	Restriction of Left Internal Mammary Lymphatic with Extraluminal Device, Percutaneous Endoscopic Approach
V94DZ	Restriction of Left Internal Mammary Lymphatic with Intraluminal Device, Percutaneous Endoscopic Approach
07V94ZZ	Restriction of Left Internal Mammary Lymphatic, Percutaneous Endoscopic Approach
07VB0CZ	Restriction of Mesenteric Lymphatic with Extraluminal Device, Open Approach
07VB0DZ	Restriction of Mesenteric Lymphatic with Intraluminal Device, Open Approach
07VB0ZZ	Restriction of Mesenteric Lymphatic, Open Approach
07VB3CZ	Restriction of Mesenteric Lymphatic with Extraluminal Device, Percutaneous Approach
07VB3DZ	Restriction of Mesenteric Lymphatic with Intraluminal Device, Percutaneous Approach
07VB3ZZ	Restriction of Mesenteric Lymphatic, Percutaneous Approach
07VB4CZ	Restriction of Mesenteric Lymphatic with Extraluminal Device, Percutaneous Endoscopic Approach
07VB4DZ	Restriction of Mesenteric Lymphatic with Intraluminal Device, Percutaneous Endoscopic Approach
07VB4ZZ	Restriction of Mesenteric Lymphatic, Percutaneous Endoscopic Approach
07VC0CZ	Restriction of Pelvis Lymphatic with Extraluminal Device, Open Approach
07VC0DZ	Restriction of Pelvis Lymphatic with Intraluminal Device, Open Approach
07VC0ZZ	Restriction of Pelvis Lymphatic, Open Approach
07VC3CZ	Restriction of Pelvis Lymphatic with Extraluminal Device, Percutaneous Approach
07VC3DZ	Restriction of Pelvis Lymphatic with Intraluminal Device, Percutaneous Approach
07VC3ZZ	Restriction of Pelvis Lymphatic, Percutaneous Approach
07VC4CZ	Restriction of Pelvis Lymphatic with Extraluminal Device, Percutaneous Endoscopic Approach
07VC4DZ	Restriction of Pelvis Lymphatic with Intraluminal Device, Percutaneous Endoscopic Approach
07VC4ZZ	Restriction of Pelvis Lymphatic, Percutaneous Endoscopic Approach
07VD0CZ	Restriction of Aortic Lymphatic with Extraluminal Device, Open Approach
07VD0DZ	Restriction of Aortic Lymphatic with Intraluminal Device, Open Approach
07VD0ZZ	Restriction of Aortic Lymphatic, Open Approach
07VD3CZ	Restriction of Aortic Lymphatic with Extraluminal Device, Percutaneous Approach
07VD3DZ	Restriction of Aortic Lymphatic with Intraluminal Device, Percutaneous Approach
07VD3ZZ	Restriction of Aortic Lymphatic, Percutaneous Approach
07VD4CZ	Restriction of Aortic Lymphatic with Extraluminal Device, Percutaneous Endoscopic Approach
07VD4DZ	Restriction of Aortic Lymphatic with Intraluminal Device, Percutaneous Endoscopic Approach
07VD4ZZ	Restriction of Aortic Lymphatic, Percutaneous Endoscopic Approach
07VF0CZ	Restriction of Right Lower Extremity Lymphatic with Extraluminal Device, Open Approach
07VF0DZ	Restriction of Right Lower Extremity Lymphatic with Intraluminal Device, Open Approach
07VF0ZZ	Restriction of Right Lower Extremity Lymphatic, Open Approach
07VF3CZ	Restriction of Right Lower Extremity Lymphatic with Extraluminal Device, Percutaneous Approach
07VF3DZ	Restriction of Right Lower Extremity Lymphatic with Intraluminal Device, Percutaneous Approach
07VF3ZZ	Restriction of Right Lower Extremity Lymphatic, Percutaneous Approach
07VF4CZ	Restriction of Right Lower Extremity Lymphatic with Extraluminal Device, Percutaneous Endoscopic Approach
07VF4DZ	Restriction of Right Lower Extremity Lymphatic with Intraluminal Device, Percutaneous Endoscopic Approach
07VF4ZZ	Restriction of Right Lower Extremity Lymphatic, Percutaneous Endoscopic Approach
07VG0CZ	Restriction of Left Lower Extremity Lymphatic with Extraluminal Device, Open Approach
07VG0DZ	Restriction of Left Lower Extremity Lymphatic with Intraluminal Device, Open Approach
07VG0ZZ	Restriction of Left Lower Extremity Lymphatic, Open Approach
07VG3CZ	Restriction of Left Lower Extremity Lymphatic with Extraluminal Device, Percutaneous Approach
07VG3DZ	Restriction of Left Lower Extremity Lymphatic with Intraluminal Device, Percutaneous Approach
07VG3ZZ	Restriction of Left Lower Extremity Lymphatic, Percutaneous Approach
07VG4CZ	Restriction of Left Lower Extremity Lymphatic with Extraluminal Device, Percutaneous Endoscopic Approach
07VG4DZ	Restriction of Left Lower Extremity Lymphatic with Intraluminal Device, Percutaneous Endoscopic Approach
07VG4ZZ	Restriction of Left Lower Extremity Lymphatic, Percutaneous Endoscopic Approach
07VH0CZ	Restriction of Right Inguinal Lymphatic with Extraluminal Device, Open Approach
07VH0DZ	Restriction of Right Inguinal Lymphatic with Intraluminal Device, Open Approach
07VH0ZZ	Restriction of Right Inguinal Lymphatic, Open Approach
07VH3CZ	Restriction of Right Inguinal Lymphatic with Extraluminal Device, Percutaneous Approach
07VH3DZ	Restriction of Right Inguinal Lymphatic with Intraluminal Device, Percutaneous Approach
07VH3ZZ	Restriction of Right Inguinal Lymphatic, Percutaneous Approach
07VH4CZ	Restriction of Right Inguinal Lymphatic with Extraluminal Device, Percutaneous Endoscopic Approach
07VH4DZ	Restriction of Right Inguinal Lymphatic with Intraluminal Device, Percutaneous Endoscopic Approach
07VH4ZZ	Restriction of Right Inguinal Lymphatic, Percutaneous Endoscopic Approach
07VJ0CZ	Restriction of Left Inguinal Lymphatic with Extraluminal Device, Open Approach
07VJ0DZ	Restriction of Left Inguinal Lymphatic with Intraluminal Device, Open Approach
07VJ0ZZ	Restriction of Left Inguinal Lymphatic, Open Approach
07VJ3CZ	Restriction of Left Inguinal Lymphatic with Extraluminal Device, Percutaneous Approach

397

Female-only   ♂ Male-only   ▲ Limited Coverage   ● Non-OR   ▥ HAC-associated procedure   ▲ Non-covered procedures   + Combination

07VJ3DZ   Restriction of Left Inguinal Lymphatic with Intraluminal Device, Percutaneous Approach

07VJ3ZZ   Restriction of Left Inguinal Lymphatic, Percutaneous Approach

07VJ4CZ   Restriction of Left Inguinal Lymphatic with Extraluminal Device, Percutaneous Endoscopic Approach

07VJ4DZ   Restriction of Left Inguinal Lymphatic with Intraluminal Device, Percutaneous Endoscopic Approach

07VJ4ZZ   Restriction of Left Inguinal Lymphatic, Percutaneous Endoscopic Approach

07VK0CZ   Restriction of Thoracic Duct with Extraluminal Device, Open Approach

07VK0DZ   Restriction of Thoracic Duct with Intraluminal Device, Open Approach

07VK0ZZ   Restriction of Thoracic Duct, Open Approach

07VK3CZ   Restriction of Thoracic Duct with Extraluminal Device, Percutaneous Approach

07VK3DZ   Restriction of Thoracic Duct with Intraluminal Device, Percutaneous Approach

07VK3ZZ   Restriction of Thoracic Duct, Percutaneous Approach

07VK4CZ   Restriction of Thoracic Duct with Extraluminal Device, Percutaneous Endoscopic Approach

07VK4DZ   Restriction of Thoracic Duct with Intraluminal Device, Percutaneous Endoscopic Approach

07VK4ZZ   Restriction of Thoracic Duct, Percutaneous Endoscopic Approach

07VL0CZ   Restriction of Cisterna Chyli with Extraluminal Device, Open Approach

07VL0DZ   Restriction of Cisterna Chyli with Intraluminal Device, Open Approach

07VL0ZZ   Restriction of Cisterna Chyli, Open Approach

07VL3CZ   Restriction of Cisterna Chyli with Extraluminal Device, Percutaneous Approach

07VL3DZ   Restriction of Cisterna Chyli with Intraluminal Device, Percutaneous Approach

07VL3ZZ   Restriction of Cisterna Chyli, Percutaneous Approach

07VL4CZ   Restriction of Cisterna Chyli with Extraluminal Device, Percutaneous Endoscopic Approach

07VL4DZ   Restriction of Cisterna Chyli with Intraluminal Device, Percutaneous Endoscopic Approach

07VL4ZZ   Restriction of Cisterna Chyli, Percutaneous Endoscopic Approach

07W – Lymphatic and Hemic Systems, Revision

Review Coding Guideline B6.1c

07WK00Z   Revision of Drainage Device in Thoracic Duct, Open Approach

07WK03Z   Revision of Infusion Device in Thoracic Duct, Open Approach

07WK07Z   Revision of Autologous Tissue Substitute in Thoracic Duct, Open Approach

07WK0CZ   Revision of Extraluminal Device in Thoracic Duct, Open Approach

07WK0DZ   Revision of Intraluminal Device in Thoracic Duct, Open Approach

07WK0JZ   Revision of Synthetic Substitute in Thoracic Duct, Open Approach

07WK0KZ   Revision of Nonautologous Tissue Substitute in Thoracic Duct, Open Approach

07WK30Z   Revision of Drainage Device in Thoracic Duct, Percutaneous Approach

07WK33Z   Revision of Infusion Device in Thoracic Duct, Percutaneous Approach

07WK37Z   Revision of Autologous Tissue Substitute in Thoracic Duct, Percutaneous Approach

07WK3CZ   Revision of Extraluminal Device in Thoracic Duct, Percutaneous Approach

07WK3DZ   Revision of Intraluminal Device in Thoracic Duct, Percutaneous Approach

07WK3JZ   Revision of Synthetic Substitute in Thoracic Duct, Percutaneous Approach

07WK3KZ   Revision of Nonautologous Tissue Substitute in Thoracic Duct, Percutaneous Approach

07WK40Z   Revision of Drainage Device in Thoracic Duct, Percutaneous Endoscopic Approach

07WK43Z   Revision of Infusion Device in Thoracic Duct, Percutaneous Endoscopic Approach

07WK47Z   Revision of Autologous Tissue Substitute in Thoracic Duct, Percutaneous Endoscopic Approach

07WK4CZ   Revision of Extraluminal Device in Thoracic Duct, Percutaneous Endoscopic Approach

07WK4DZ   Revision of Intraluminal Device in Thoracic Duct, Percutaneous Endoscopic Approach

07WK4JZ   Revision of Synthetic Substitute in Thoracic Duct, Percutaneous Endoscopic Approach

07WK4KZ   Revision of Nonautologous Tissue Substitute in Thoracic Duct, Percutaneous Endoscopic Approach

07WKX0Z   Revision of Drainage Device in Thoracic Duct, External Approach

07WKX3Z   Revision of Infusion Device in Thoracic Duct, External Approach

07WKX7Z   Revision of Autologous Tissue Substitute in Thoracic Duct, External Approach

07WKXCZ   Revision of Extraluminal Device in Thoracic Duct, External Approach

07WKXDZ   Revision of Intraluminal Device in Thoracic Duct, External Approach

07WKXJZ   Revision of Synthetic Substitute in Thoracic Duct, External Approach

07WKXKZ   Revision of Nonautologous Tissue Substitute in Thoracic Duct, External Approach

07WL00Z   Revision of Drainage Device in Cisterna Chyli, Open Approach

07WL03Z   Revision of Infusion Device in Cisterna Chyli, Open Approach

07WL07Z   Revision of Autologous Tissue Substitute in Cisterna Chyli, Open Approach

07WL0CZ   Revision of Extraluminal Device in Cisterna Chyli, Open Approach

07WL0DZ   Revision of Intraluminal Device in Cisterna Chyli, Open Approach

07WL0JZ   Revision of Synthetic Substitute in Cisterna Chyli, Open Approach

07WL0KZ   Revision of Nonautologous Tissue Substitute in Cisterna Chyli, Open Approach

07WL30Z   Revision of Drainage Device in Cisterna Chyli, Percutaneous Approach

07WL33Z   Revision of Infusion Device in Cisterna Chyli, Percutaneous Approach

07WL37Z   Revision of Autologous Tissue Substitute in Cisterna Chyli, Percutaneous Approach

07WL3CZ   Revision of Extraluminal Device in Cisterna Chyli, Percutaneous Approach

07WL3DZ   Revision of Intraluminal Device in Cisterna Chyli, Percutaneous Approach

07WL3JZ   Revision of Synthetic Substitute in Cisterna Chyli, Percutaneous Approach

07WL3KZ   Revision of Nonautologous Tissue Substitute in Cisterna Chyli, Percutaneous Approach

07WL40Z   Revision of Drainage Device in Cisterna Chyli, Percutaneous Endoscopic Approach

07WL43Z   Revision of Infusion Device in Cisterna Chyli, Percutaneous Endoscopic Approach

07WL47Z   Revision of Autologous Tissue Substit in Cisterna Chyli, Percutaneous Endoscopic Approach

07WL4CZ   Revision of Extraluminal Device in Cisterna Chyli, Percutaneous Endosco Approach

07WL4DZ   Revision of Intraluminal Device in Cisterna Chyli, Percutaneous Endosco Approach

07WL4JZ   Revision of Synthetic Substitute in Cisterna Chyli, Percutaneous Endosco Approach

07WL4KZ   Revision of Nonautologous Tissue Substitute in Cisterna Chyli, Percutaneous Endoscopic Approach

07WLX0Z   Revision of Drainage Device in Cistern Chyli, External Approach

07WLX3Z   Revision of Infusion Device in Cistern Chyli, External Approach

07WLX7Z   Revision of Autologous Tissue Substit in Cisterna Chyli, External Approach

07WLXCZ   Revision of Extraluminal Device in Cisterna Chyli, External Approach

07WLXDZ   Revision of Intraluminal Device in Cisterna Chyli, External Approach

07WLXJZ   Revision of Synthetic Substitute in Cisterna Chyli, External Approach

07WLXKZ   Revision of Nonautologous Tissue Substitute in Cisterna Chyli, External Approach

07WM00Z   Revision of Drainage Device in Thymu Open Approach

07WM03Z   Revision of Infusion Device in Thymus Open Approach

07WM30Z   Revision of Drainage Device in Thymu Percutaneous Approach

07WM33Z   Revision of Infusion Device in Thymus Percutaneous Approach

07WM40Z   Revision of Drainage Device in Thymu Percutaneous Endoscopic Approach

07WM43Z   Revision of Infusion Device in Thymus Percutaneous Endoscopic Approach

07WMX0Z   Revision of Drainage Device in Thymu External Approach

07WMX3Z   Revision of Infusion Device in Thymus External Approach

07WN00Z   Revision of Drainage Device in Lymphatic, Open Approach

07WN03Z   Revision of Infusion Device in Lymphatic, Open Approach

07WN07Z   Revision of Autologous Tissue Substitu in Lymphatic, Open Approach

♀ Female-only   ♂ Male-only   ▲ Limited Coverage   ● Non-OR   ▩ HAC-associated procedure   ▲ Non-covered procedures   ✛ Combinati

WN0CZ	Revision of Extraluminal Device in Lymphatic, Open Approach	07WN47Z	Revision of Autologous Tissue Substitute in Lymphatic, Percutaneous Endoscopic Approach	07WNXKZ	Revision of Nonautologous Tissue Substitute in Lymphatic, External Approach
WN0DZ	Revision of Intraluminal Device in Lymphatic, Open Approach	07WN4CZ	Revision of Extraluminal Device in Lymphatic, Percutaneous Endoscopic Approach	07WP00Z	Revision of Drainage Device in Spleen, Open Approach
WN0JZ	Revision of Synthetic Substitute in Lymphatic, Open Approach	07WN4DZ	Revision of Intraluminal Device in Lymphatic, Percutaneous Endoscopic Approach	07WP03Z	Revision of Infusion Device in Spleen, Open Approach
WN0KZ	Revision of Nonautologous Tissue Substitute in Lymphatic, Open Approach	07WN4JZ	Revision of Synthetic Substitute in Lymphatic, Percutaneous Endoscopic Approach	07WP30Z	Revision of Drainage Device in Spleen, Percutaneous Approach
WN30Z	Revision of Drainage Device in Lymphatic, Percutaneous Approach	07WN4KZ	Revision of Nonautologous Tissue Substitute in Lymphatic, Percutaneous Endoscopic Approach	07WP33Z	Revision of Infusion Device in Spleen, Percutaneous Approach
WN33Z	Revision of Infusion Device in Lymphatic, Percutaneous Approach	07WNX0Z	Revision of Drainage Device in Lymphatic, External Approach	07WP40Z	Revision of Drainage Device in Spleen, Percutaneous Endoscopic Approach
WN37Z	Revision of Autologous Tissue Substitute in Lymphatic, Percutaneous Approach	07WNX3Z	Revision of Infusion Device in Lymphatic, External Approach	07WP43Z	Revision of Infusion Device in Spleen, Percutaneous Endoscopic Approach
WN3CZ	Revision of Extraluminal Device in Lymphatic, Percutaneous Approach	07WNX7Z	Revision of Autologous Tissue Substitute in Lymphatic, External Approach	07WPX0Z	Revision of Drainage Device in Spleen, External Approach
WN3DZ	Revision of Intraluminal Device in Lymphatic, Percutaneous Approach	07WNXCZ	Revision of Extraluminal Device in Lymphatic, External Approach	07WPX3Z	Revision of Infusion Device in Spleen, External Approach
WN3JZ	Revision of Synthetic Substitute in Lymphatic, Percutaneous Approach	07WNXDZ	Revision of Intraluminal Device in Lymphatic, External Approach	07WT00Z	Revision of Drainage Device in Bone Marrow, Open Approach
WN3KZ	Revision of Nonautologous Tissue Substitute in Lymphatic, Percutaneous Approach	07WNXJZ	Revision of Synthetic Substitute in Lymphatic, External Approach	07WT30Z	Revision of Drainage Device in Bone Marrow, Percutaneous Approach
WN40Z	Revision of Drainage Device in Lymphatic, Percutaneous Endoscopic Approach			07WT40Z	Revision of Drainage Device in Bone Marrow, Percutaneous Endoscopic Approach
WN43Z	Revision of Infusion Device in Lymphatic, Percutaneous Endoscopic Approach			07WTX0Z	Revision of Drainage Device in Bone Marrow, External Approach

7Y – Lymphatic and Hemic Systems, Transplantation

eview Coding Guideline B3.16

YM0Z0	Transplantation of Thymus, Allogeneic, Open Approach	07YM0Z2	Transplantation of Thymus, Zooplastic, Open Approach	07YP0Z1	Transplantation of Spleen, Syngeneic, Open Approach
YM0Z1	Transplantation of Thymus, Syngeneic, Open Approach	07YP0Z0	Transplantation of Spleen, Allogeneic, Open Approach	07YP0Z2	Transplantation of Spleen, Zooplastic, Open Approach

Female-only	♂ Male-only	▲ Limited Coverage	● Non-OR	▥ HAC-associated procedure	▲ Non-covered procedures	➕ Combination

Eye

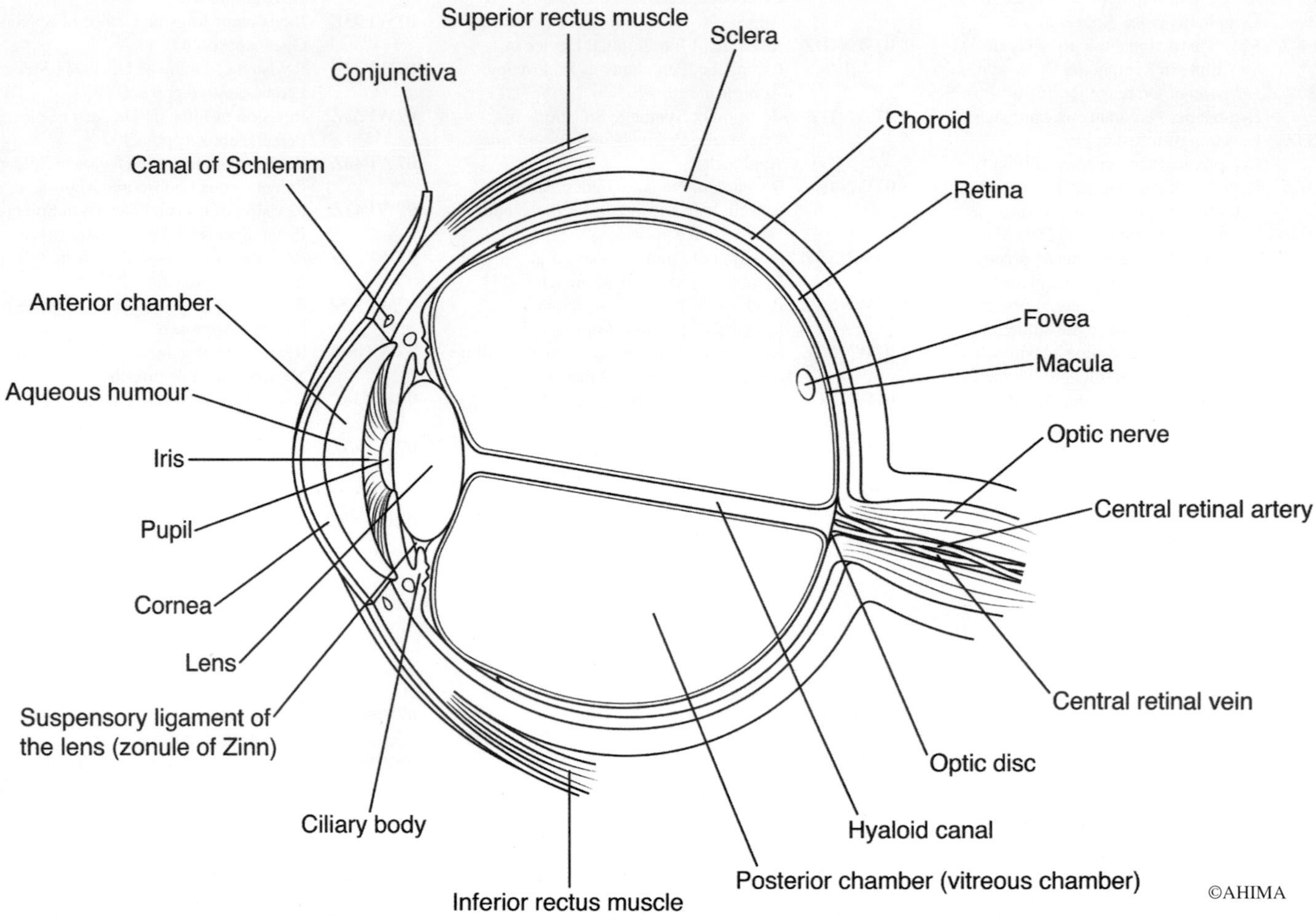

Superior rectus muscle

Conjunctiva

Sclera

Choroid

Retina

Canal of Schlemm

Anterior chamber

Fovea

Macula

Aqueous humour

Optic nerve

Iris

Central retinal artery

Pupil

Cornea

Lens

Central retinal vein

Suspensory ligament of
the lens (zonule of Zinn)

Optic disc

Ciliary body

Hyaloid canal

Inferior rectus muscle

Posterior chamber (vitreous chamber)

©AHIMA

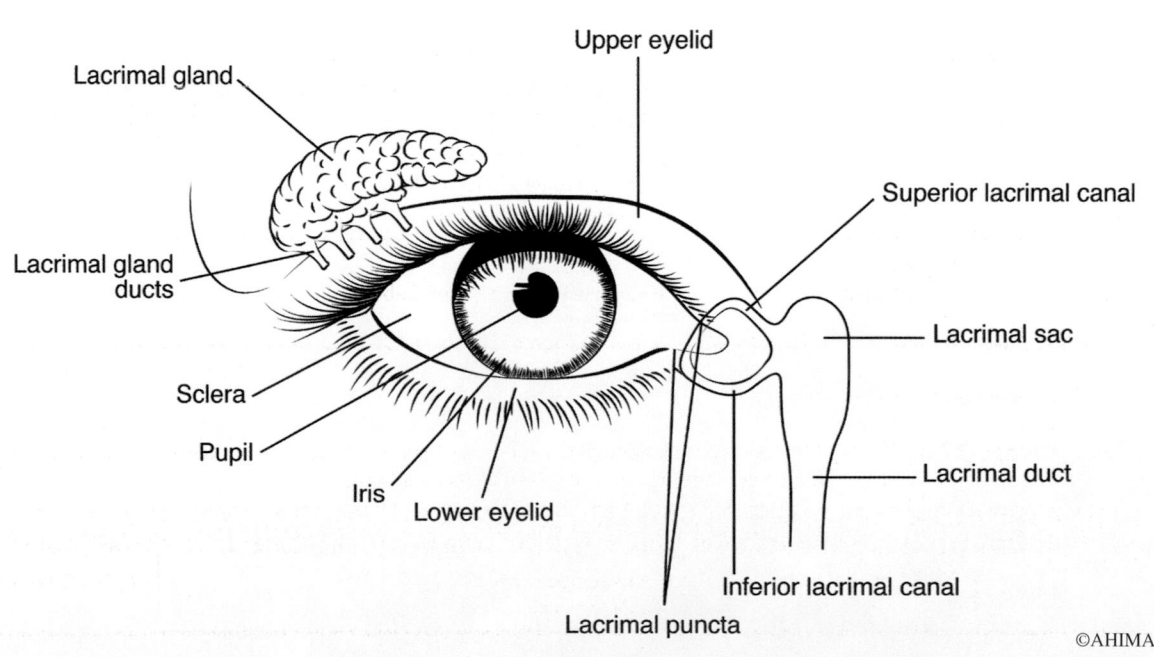

Lacrimal gland

Upper eyelid

Superior lacrimal canal

Lacrimal gland
ducts

Lacrimal sac

Sclera

Pupil

Iris Lower eyelid

Inferior lacrimal canal

Lacrimal puncta

Lacrimal duct

©AHIMA

Eye Muscles

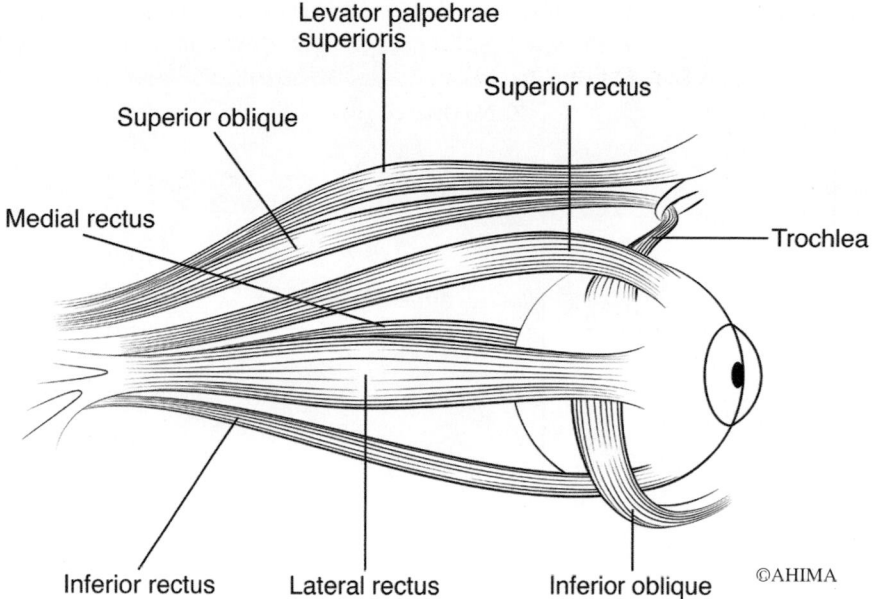

Levator palpebrae
superioris

Superior rectus

Superior oblique

Medial rectus

Trochlea

Inferior rectus

Lateral rectus

Inferior oblique

©AHIMA

Eye Tables 080–08X

Section	0	Medical and Surgical
Body System	8	Eye
Operation	0	**Alteration:** Modifying the anatomic structure of a body part without affecting the function of the body part

Body Part (4th)	Approach (5th)	Device (6th)	Qualifier (7th)
N Upper Eyelid, Right P Upper Eyelid, Left Q Lower Eyelid, Right R Lower Eyelid, Left	0 Open 3 Percutaneous X External	7 Autologous Tissue Substitute J Synthetic Substitute K Nonautologous Tissue Substitute Z No Device	Z No Qualifier

Section	0	Medical and Surgical
Body System	8	Eye
Operation	1	**Bypass:** Altering the route of passage of the contents of a tubular body part

Body Part (4th)	Approach (5th)	Device (6th)	Qualifier (7th)
2 Anterior Chamber, Right 3 Anterior Chamber, Left	3 Percutaneous	J Synthetic Substitute K Nonautologous Tissue Substitute Z No Device	4 Sclera
X Lacrimal Duct, Right Y Lacrimal Duct, Left	0 Open 3 Percutaneous	J Synthetic Substitute K Nonautologous Tissue Substitute Z No Device	3 Nasal Cavity

Section	0	Medical and Surgical
Body System	8	Eye
Operation	2	**Change:** Taking out or off a device from a body part and putting back an identical or similar device in or on the same body part without cutting or puncturing the skin or a mucous membrane

Body Part (4th)	Approach (5th)	Device (6th)	Qualifier (7th)
0 Eye, Right 1 Eye, Left	X External	0 Drainage Device Y Other Device	Z No Qualifier

Section 0 **Medical and Surgical**
Body System 8 **Eye**
Operation 5 **Destruction:** Physical eradication of all or a portion of a body part by the direct use of energy, force, or a destructive agent

Body Part (4th)	Approach (5th)	Device (6th)	Qualifier (7th)
0 Eye, Right 1 Eye, Left 6 Sclera, Right 7 Sclera, Left 8 Cornea, Right 9 Cornea, Left S Conjunctiva, Right T Conjunctiva, Left	X External	Z No Device	Z No Qualifier
2 Anterior Chamber, Right 3 Anterior Chamber, Left 4 Vitreous, Right 5 Vitreous, Left C Iris, Right D Iris, Left E Retina, Right F Retina, Left G Retinal Vessel, Right H Retinal Vessel, Left J Lens, Right K Lens, Left	3 Percutaneous	Z No Device	Z No Qualifier
A Choroid, Right B Choroid, Left L Extraocular Muscle, Right M Extraocular Muscle, Left V Lacrimal Gland, Right W Lacrimal Gland, Left	0 Open 3 Percutaneous	Z No Device	Z No Qualifier
N Upper Eyelid, Right P Upper Eyelid, Left Q Lower Eyelid, Right R Lower Eyelid, Left	0 Open 3 Percutaneous X External	Z No Device	Z No Qualifier
X Lacrimal Duct, Right Y Lacrimal Duct, Left	0 Open 3 Percutaneous 7 Via Natural or Artificial Opening 8 Via Natural or Artificial Opening Endoscopic	Z No Device	Z No Qualifier

Section 0 **Medical and Surgical**
Body System 8 **Eye**
Operation 7 **Dilation:** Expanding an orifice or the lumen of a tubular body part

Body Part (4th)	Approach (5th)	Device (6th)	Qualifier (7th)
X Lacrimal Duct, Right Y Lacrimal Duct, Left	0 Open 3 Percutaneous 7 Via Natural or Artificial Opening 8 Via Natural or Artificial Opening Endoscopic	D Intraluminal Device Z No Device	Z No Qualifier

ction	0	Medical and Surgical	
ody System	8	Eye	
peration	9	**Drainage:** Taking or letting out fluids and/or gases from a body part	

Body Part (4th)	Approach (5th)	Device (6th)	Qualifier (7th)
0 Eye, Right 1 Eye, Left 6 Sclera, Right 7 Sclera, Left 8 Cornea, Right 9 Cornea, Left S Conjunctiva, Right T Conjunctiva, Left	X External	0 Drainage Device	Z No Qualifier
0 Eye, Right 1 Eye, Left 6 Sclera, Right 7 Sclera, Left 8 Cornea, Right 9 Cornea, Left S Conjunctiva, Right T Conjunctiva, Left	X External	Z No Device	X Diagnostic Z No Qualifier
2 Anterior Chamber, Right 3 Anterior Chamber, Left 4 Vitreous, Right 5 Vitreous, Left C Iris, Right D Iris, Left E Retina, Right F Retina, Left G Retinal Vessel, Right H Retinal Vessel, Left J Lens, Right K Lens, Left	3 Percutaneous	0 Drainage Device	Z No Qualifier
2 Anterior Chamber, Right 3 Anterior Chamber, Left 4 Vitreous, Right 5 Vitreous, Left C Iris, Right D Iris, Left E Retina, Right F Retina, Left G Retinal Vessel, Right H Retinal Vessel, Left J Lens, Right K Lens, Left	3 Percutaneous	Z No Device	X Diagnostic Z No Qualifier
A Choroid, Right B Choroid, Left L Extraocular Muscle, Right M Extraocular Muscle, Left V Lacrimal Gland, Right W Lacrimal Gland, Left	0 Open 3 Percutaneous	0 Drainage Device	Z No Qualifier
A Choroid, Right B Choroid, Left L Extraocular Muscle, Right M Extraocular Muscle, Left V Lacrimal Gland, Right W Lacrimal Gland, Left	0 Open 3 Percutaneous	Z No Device	X Diagnostic Z No Qualifier
N Upper Eyelid, Right P Upper Eyelid, Left Q Lower Eyelid, Right R Lower Eyelid, Left	0 Open 3 Percutaneous X External	0 Drainage Device	Z No Qualifier

Continued →

Section	0	Medical and Surgical
Body System	8	Eye
Operation	9	**Drainage:** Taking or letting out fluids and/or gases from a body part

Body Part (4th)	Approach (5th)	Device (6th)	Qualifier (7th)
N Upper Eyelid, Right P Upper Eyelid, Left Q Lower Eyelid, Right R Lower Eyelid, Left	0 Open 3 Percutaneous X External	Z No Device	X Diagnostic Z No Qualifier
X Lacrimal Duct, Right Y Lacrimal Duct, Left	0 Open 3 Percutaneous 7 Via Natural or Artificial Opening 8 Via Natural or Artificial Opening Endoscopic	0 Drainage Device	Z No Qualifier
X Lacrimal Duct, Right Y Lacrimal Duct, Left	0 Open 3 Percutaneous 7 Via Natural or Artificial Opening 8 Via Natural or Artificial Opening Endoscopic	Z No Device	X Diagnostic Z No Qualifier

Section	0	Medical and Surgical
Body System	8	Eye
Operation	B	**Excision:** Cutting out or off, without replacement, a portion of a body part

Body Part (4th)	Approach (5th)	Device (6th)	Qualifier (7th)
0 Eye, Right 1 Eye, Left N Upper Eyelid, Right P Upper Eyelid, Left Q Lower Eyelid, Right R Lower Eyelid, Left	0 Open 3 Percutaneous X External	Z No Device	X Diagnostic Z No Qualifier
4 Vitreous, Right 5 Vitreous, Left C Iris, Right D Iris, Left E Retina, Right F Retina, Left J Lens, Right K Lens, Left	3 Percutaneous	Z No Device	X Diagnostic Z No Qualifier
6 Sclera, Right 7 Sclera, Left 8 Cornea, Right 9 Cornea, Left S Conjunctiva, Right T Conjunctiva, Left	X External	Z No Device	X Diagnostic Z No Qualifier
A Choroid, Right B Choroid, Left L Extraocular Muscle, Right M Extraocular Muscle, Left V Lacrimal Gland, Right W Lacrimal Gland, Left	0 Open 3 Percutaneous	Z No Device	X Diagnostic Z No Qualifier
X Lacrimal Duct, Right Y Lacrimal Duct, Left	0 Open 3 Percutaneous 7 Via Natural or Artificial Opening 8 Via Natural or Artificial Opening Endoscopic	Z No Device	X Diagnostic Z No Qualifier

Section 0 Medical and Surgical
Body System 8 Eye
Operation C **Extirpation:** Taking or cutting out solid matter from a body part

Body Part (4th)	Approach (5th)	Device (6th)	Qualifier (7th)
0 Eye, Right 1 Eye, Left 6 Sclera, Right 7 Sclera, Left 8 Cornea, Right 9 Cornea, Left S Conjunctiva, Right T Conjunctiva, Left	X External	Z No Device	Z No Qualifier
2 Anterior Chamber, Right 3 Anterior Chamber, Left 4 Vitreous, Right 5 Vitreous, Left C Iris, Right D Iris, Left E Retina, Right F Retina, Left G Retinal Vessel, Right	3 Percutaneous X External	Z No Device	Z No Qualifier
0 Eye, Right 1 Eye, Left 6 Sclera, Right 7 Sclera, Left 8 Cornea, Right 9 Cornea, Left S Conjunctiva, Right T Conjunctiva, Left	X External	Z No Device	Z No Qualifier
2 Anterior Chamber, Right 3 Anterior Chamber, Left 4 Vitreous, Right 5 Vitreous, Left C Iris, Right D Iris, Left E Retina, Right F Retina, Left G Retinal Vessel, Right H Retinal Vessel, Left J Lens, Right K Lens, Left	3 Percutaneous X External	Z No Device	Z No Qualifier
A Choroid, Right B Choroid, Left L Extraocular Muscle, Right M Extraocular Muscle, Left N Upper Eyelid, Right P Upper Eyelid, Left Q Lower Eyelid, Right R Lower Eyelid, Left V Lacrimal Gland, Right W Lacrimal Gland, Left	0 Open 3 Percutaneous X External	Z No Device	Z No Qualifier
X Lacrimal Duct, Right Y Lacrimal Duct, Left	0 Open 3 Percutaneous 7 Via Natural or Artificial Opening 8 Via Natural or Artificial Opening Endoscopic	Z No Device	Z No Qualifier

Section	0	Medical and Surgical
Body System	8	Eye
Operation	D	**Extraction:** Pulling or stripping out or off all or a portion of a body part by the use of force

Body Part (4ᵗʰ)	Approach (5ᵗʰ)	Device (6ᵗʰ)	Qualifier (7ᵗʰ)
8 Cornea, Right 9 Cornea, Left	X External	Z No Device	X Diagnostic Z No Qualifier
J Lens, Right K Lens, Left	3 Percutaneous	Z No Device	Z No Qualifier

Section	0	Medical and Surgical
Body System	8	Eye
Operation	F	**Fragmentation:** Breaking solid matter in a body part into pieces

Body Part (4ᵗʰ)	Approach (5ᵗʰ)	Device (6ᵗʰ)	Qualifier (7ᵗʰ)
4 Vitreous, Right 5 Vitreous, Left	3 Percutaneous X External	Z No Device	Z No Qualifier

Section	0	Medical and Surgical
Body System	8	Eye
Operation	H	**Insertion:** Putting in a nonbiological appliance that monitors, assists, performs, or prevents a physiological function but does not physically take the place of a body part

Body Part (4ᵗʰ)	Approach (5ᵗʰ)	Device (6ᵗʰ)	Qualifier (7ᵗʰ)
0 Eye, Right 1 Eye, Left	0 Open	5 Epiretinal Visual Prosthesis	Z No Qualifier
0 Eye, Right 1 Eye, Left	3 Percutaneous X External	1 Radioactive Element 3 Infusion Device	Z No Qualifier

Section	0	Medical and Surgical
Body System	8	Eye
Operation	J	**Inspection:** Visually and/or manually exploring a body part

Body Part (4ᵗʰ)	Approach (5ᵗʰ)	Device (6ᵗʰ)	Qualifier (7ᵗʰ)
0 Eye, Right 1 Eye, Left J Lens, Right K Lens, Left	X External	Z No Device	Z No Qualifier
L Extraocular Muscle, Right M Extraocular Muscle, Left	0 Open X External	Z No Device	Z No Qualifier

Section	0	Medical and Surgical
Body System	8	Eye
Operation	L	**Occlusion:** Completely closing an orifice or the lumen of a tubular body part

Body Part (4ᵗʰ)	Approach (5ᵗʰ)	Device (6ᵗʰ)	Qualifier (7ᵗʰ)
X Lacrimal Duct, Right Y Lacrimal Duct, Left	0 Open 3 Percutaneous	C Extraluminal Device D Intraluminal Device Z No Device	Z No Qualifier
X Lacrimal Duct, Right Y Lacrimal Duct, Left	7 Via Natural or Artificial Opening 8 Via Natural or Artificial Opening Endoscopic	D Intraluminal Device Z No Device	Z No Qualifier

Section	0	Medical and Surgical
Body System	8	Eye
Operation	M	Reattachment: Putting back in or on all or a portion of a separated body part to its normal location or other suitable location

Body Part (4th)	Approach (5th)	Device (6th)	Qualifier (7th)
N Upper Eyelid, Right P Upper Eyelid, Left Q Lower Eyelid, Right R Lower Eyelid, Left	X External	Z No Device	Z No Qualifier

Section	0	Medical and Surgical
Body System	8	Eye
Operation	N	Release: Freeing a body part from an abnormal physical constraint by cutting or by the use of force

Body Part (4th)	Approach (5th)	Device (6th)	Qualifier (7th)
0 Eye, Right 1 Eye, Left 6 Sclera, Right 7 Sclera, Left 8 Cornea, Right 9 Cornea, Left S Conjunctiva, Right T Conjunctiva, Left	X External	Z No Device	Z No Qualifier
2 Anterior Chamber, Right 3 Anterior Chamber, Left 4 Vitreous, Right 5 Vitreous, Left C Iris, Right D Iris, Left E Retina, Right F Retina, Left G Retinal Vessel, Right H Retinal Vessel, Left J Lens, Right K Lens, Left	3 Percutaneous	Z No Device	Z No Qualifier
A Choroid, Right B Choroid, Left L Extraocular Muscle, Right M Extraocular Muscle, Left V Lacrimal Gland, Right W Lacrimal Gland, Left	0 Open 3 Percutaneous	Z No Device	Z No Qualifier
N Upper Eyelid, Right P Upper Eyelid, Left Q Lower Eyelid, Right R Lower Eyelid, Left	0 Open 3 Percutaneous X External	Z No Device	Z No Qualifier
X Lacrimal Duct, Right Y Lacrimal Duct, Left	0 Open 3 Percutaneous 7 Via Natural or Artificial Opening 8 Via Natural or Artificial Opening Endoscopic	Z No Device	Z No Qualifier

Section   0   **Medical and Surgical**
Body System   8   **Eye**
Operation   P   **Removal:** Taking out or off a device from a body part

Body Part (4ᵗʰ)	Approach (5ᵗʰ)	Device (6ᵗʰ)	Qualifier (7ᵗʰ)
0 Eye, Right 1 Eye, Left	0 Open 3 Percutaneous 7 Via Natural or Artificial Opening 8 Via Natural or Artificial Opening Endoscopic X External	0 Drainage Device 1 Radioactive Element 3 Infusion Device 7 Autologous Tissue Substitute C Extraluminal Device D Intraluminal Device J Synthetic Substitute K Nonautologous Tissue Substitute	Z No Qualifier
J Lens, Right K Lens, Left	3 Percutaneous	J Synthetic Substitute	Z No Qualifier
L Extraocular Muscle, Right M Extraocular Muscle, Left	0 Open 3 Percutaneous	0 Drainage Device 7 Autologous Tissue Substitute J Synthetic Substitute K Nonautologous Tissue Substitute	Z No Qualifier

Section   0   **Medical and Surgical**
Body System   8   **Eye**
Operation   Q   **Repair:** Restoring, to the extent possible, a body part to its normal anatomic structure and function

Body Part (4ᵗʰ)	Approach (5ᵗʰ)	Device (6ᵗʰ)	Qualifier (7ᵗʰ)
0 Eye, Right 1 Eye, Left 6 Sclera, Right 7 Sclera, Left 8 Cornea, Right 9 Cornea, Left S Conjunctiva, Right T Conjunctiva, Left	X External	Z No Device	Z No Qualifier
2 Anterior Chamber, Right 3 Anterior Chamber, Left 4 Vitreous, Right 5 Vitreous, Left C Iris, Right D Iris, Left E Retina, Right F Retina, Left G Retinal Vessel, Right H Retinal Vessel, Left J Lens, Right K Lens, Left	3 Percutaneous	Z No Device	Z No Qualifier
A Choroid, Right B Choroid, Left L Extraocular Muscle, Right M Extraocular Muscle, Left V Lacrimal Gland, Right W Lacrimal Gland, Left	0 Open 3 Percutaneous	Z No Device	Z No Qualifier
N Upper Eyelid, Right P Upper Eyelid, Left Q Lower Eyelid, Right R Lower Eyelid, Left	0 Open 3 Percutaneous X External	Z No Device	Z No Qualifier
X Lacrimal Duct, Right Y Lacrimal Duct, Left	0 Open 3 Percutaneous 7 Via Natural or Artificial Opening 8 Via Natural or Artificial Opening Endoscopic	Z No Device	Z No Qualifier

Section | 0 | Medical and Surgical
Body System | 8 | Eye
Operation | R | Replacement: Putting in or on biological or synthetic material that physically takes the place and/or function of all or a portion of a body part

Body Part (4th)	Approach (5th)	Device (6th)	Qualifier (7th)
9 Eye, Right 1 Eye, Left A Choroid, Right B Choroid, Left	0 Open 3 Percutaneous	7 Autologous Tissue Substitute J Synthetic Substitute K Nonautologous Tissue Substitute	Z No Qualifier
4 Vitreous, Right 5 Vitreous, Left C Iris, Right D Iris, Left G Retinal Vessel, Right H Retinal Vessel, Left	3 Percutaneous	7 Autologous Tissue Substitute J Synthetic Substitute K Nonautologous Tissue Substitute	Z No Qualifier
0 Eye, Right 1 Eye, Left A Choroid, Right B Choroid, Left	0 Open 3 Percutaneous	7 Autologous Tissue Substitute J Synthetic Substitute K Nonautologous Tissue Substitute	Z No Qualifier
4 Vitreous, Right 5 Vitreous, Left C Iris, Right D Iris, Left G Retinal Vessel, Right H Retinal Vessel, Left	3 Percutaneous	7 Autologous Tissue Substitute J Synthetic Substitute K Nonautologous Tissue Substitute	Z No Qualifier
6 Sclera, Right 7 Sclera, Left S Conjunctiva, Right T Conjunctiva, Left	X External	7 Autologous Tissue Substitute J Synthetic Substitute K Nonautologous Tissue Substitute	Z No Qualifier
8 Cornea, Right 9 Cornea, Left	3 Percutaneous X External	7 Autologous Tissue Substitute J Synthetic Substitute K Nonautologous Tissue Substitute	Z No Qualifier
J Lens, Right K Lens, Left	3 Percutaneous	0 Synthetic Substitute, Intraocular Telescope 7 Autologous Tissue Substitute J Synthetic Substitute K Nonautologous Tissue Substitute	Z No Qualifier
N Upper Eyelid, Right P Upper Eyelid, Left Q Lower Eyelid, Right R Lower Eyelid, Left	0 Open 3 Percutaneous X External	7 Autologous Tissue Substitute J Synthetic Substitute K Nonautologous Tissue Substitute	Z No Qualifier
X Lacrimal Duct, Right Y Lacrimal Duct, Left	0 Open 3 Percutaneous 7 Via Natural or Artificial Opening 8 Via Natural or Artificial Opening Endoscopic	7 Autologous Tissue Substitute J Synthetic Substitute K Nonautologous Tissue Substitute	Z No Qualifier

Section	0	Medical and Surgical
Body System	8	Eye
Operation	S	**Reposition:** Moving to its normal location, or other suitable location, all or a portion of a body part

Body Part (4th)	Approach (5th)	Device (6th)	Qualifier (7th)
C Iris, Right D Iris, Left G Retinal Vessel, Right H Retinal Vessel, Left J Lens, Right K Lens, Left	3 Percutaneous	Z No Device	Z No Qualifier
L Extraocular Muscle, Right M Extraocular Muscle, Left V Lacrimal Gland, Right W Lacrimal Gland, Left	0 Open 3 Percutaneous	Z No Device	Z No Qualifier
N Upper Eyelid, Right P Upper Eyelid, Left Q Lower Eyelid, Right R Lower Eyelid, Left	0 Open 3 Percutaneous X External	Z No Device	Z No Qualifier
X Lacrimal Duct, Right Y Lacrimal Duct, Left	0 Open 3 Percutaneous 7 Via Natural or Artificial Opening 8 Via Natural or Artificial Opening Endoscopic	Z No Device	Z No Qualifier

Section	0	Medical and Surgical
Body System	8	Eye
Operation	T	**Resection:** Cutting out or off, without replacement, all of a body part

Body Part (4th)	Approach (5th)	Device (6th)	Qualifier (7th)
0 Eye, Right 1 Eye, Left 8 Cornea, Right 9 Cornea, Left	X External	Z No Device	Z No Qualifier
4 Vitreous, Right 5 Vitreous, Left C Iris, Right D Iris, Left J Lens, Right K Lens, Left	3 Percutaneous	Z No Device	Z No Qualifier
L Extraocular Muscle, Right M Extraocular Muscle, Left V Lacrimal Gland, Right W Lacrimal Gland, Left	0 Open 3 Percutaneous	Z No Device	Z No Qualifier
N Upper Eyelid, Right P Upper Eyelid, Left Q Lower Eyelid, Right R Lower Eyelid, Left	0 Open X External	Z No Device	Z No Qualifier
X Lacrimal Duct, Right Y Lacrimal Duct, Left	0 Open 3 Percutaneous 7 Via Natural or Artificial Opening 8 Via Natural or Artificial Opening Endoscopic	Z No Device	Z No Qualifier

Section	0	Medical and Surgical
Body System	8	Eye
Operation	U	Supplement: Putting in or on biological or synthetic material that physically reinforces and/or augments the function of a portion of a body part

Body Part (4th)	Approach (5th)	Device (6th)	Qualifier (7th)
Eye, Right Eye, Left Iris, Right Iris, Left Retina, Right Retina, Left Retinal Vessel, Right Retinal Vessel, Left Extraocular Muscle, Right M Extraocular Muscle, Left	0 Open 3 Percutaneous	7 Autologous Tissue Substitute J Synthetic Substitute K Nonautologous Tissue Substitute	Z No Qualifier
Cornea, Right Cornea, Left N Upper Eyelid, Right Upper Eyelid, Left Q Lower Eyelid, Right R Lower Eyelid, Left	0 Open 3 Percutaneous X External	7 Autologous Tissue Substitute J Synthetic Substitute K Nonautologous Tissue Substitute	Z No Qualifier
X Lacrimal Duct, Right Y Lacrimal Duct, Left	0 Open 3 Percutaneous 7 Via Natural or Artificial Opening 8 Via Natural or Artificial Opening Endoscopic	7 Autologous Tissue Substitute J Synthetic Substitute K Nonautologous Tissue Substitute	Z No Qualifier

Section	0	Medical and Surgical
Body System	8	Eye
Operation	V	Restriction: Partially closing an orifice or the lumen of a tubular body part

Body Part (4th)	Approach (5th)	Device (6th)	Qualifier (7th)
X Lacrimal Duct, Right Y Lacrimal Duct, Left	0 Open 3 Percutaneous	C Extraluminal Device D Intraluminal Device Z No Device	Z No Qualifier
X Lacrimal Duct, Right Y Lacrimal Duct, Left	7 Via Natural or Artificial Opening 8 Via Natural or Artificial Opening Endoscopic	D Intraluminal Device Z No Device	Z No Qualifier

Section	0	Medical and Surgical
Body System	8	Eye
Operation	W	Revision: Correcting, to the extent possible, a portion of a malfunctioning device or the position of a displaced device

Body Part (4th)	Approach (5th)	Device (6th)	Qualifier (7th)
0 Eye, Right 1 Eye, Left	0 Open 3 Percutaneous 7 Via Natural or Artificial Opening 8 Via Natural or Artificial Opening Endoscopic X External	0 Drainage Device 3 Infusion Device 7 Autologous Tissue Substitute C Extraluminal Device D Intraluminal Device J Synthetic Substitute K Nonautologous Tissue Substitute	Z No Qualifier
J Lens, Right K Lens, Left	3 Percutaneous X External	J Synthetic Substitute	Z No Qualifier
L Extraocular Muscle, Right M Extraocular Muscle, Left	0 Open 3 Percutaneous	0 Drainage Device 7 Autologous Tissue Substitute J Synthetic Substitute K Nonautologous Tissue Substitute	Z No Qualifier

Section	0	Medical and Surgical
Body System	8	Eye
Operation	X	**Transfer:** Moving, without taking out, all or a portion of a body part to another location to take over the function of all or a portion of a body part

Body Part (4th)	Approach (5th)	Device (6th)	Qualifier (7th)
L Extraocular Muscle, Right **M** Extraocular Muscle, Left	**0** Open **3** Percutaneous	**Z** No Device	**Z** No Qualifier

Eye Code Listing 080–08X

080 – Eye, Alteration

080N07Z Alteration of Right Upper Eyelid with Autologous Tissue Substitute, Open Approach

080N0JZ Alteration of Right Upper Eyelid with Synthetic Substitute, Open Approach

080N0KZ Alteration of Right Upper Eyelid with Nonautologous Tissue Substitute, Open Approach

080N0ZZ Alteration of Right Upper Eyelid, Open Approach

080N37Z Alteration of Right Upper Eyelid with Autologous Tissue Substitute, Percutaneous Approach

080N3JZ Alteration of Right Upper Eyelid with Synthetic Substitute, Percutaneous Approach

080N3KZ Alteration of Right Upper Eyelid with Nonautologous Tissue Substitute, Percutaneous Approach

080N3ZZ Alteration of Right Upper Eyelid, Percutaneous Approach

080NX7Z Alteration of Right Upper Eyelid with Autologous Tissue Substitute, External Approach

080NXJZ Alteration of Right Upper Eyelid with Synthetic Substitute, External Approach

080NXKZ Alteration of Right Upper Eyelid with Nonautologous Tissue Substitute, External Approach

080NXZZ Alteration of Right Upper Eyelid, External Approach

080P07Z Alteration of Left Upper Eyelid with Autologous Tissue Substitute, Open Approach

080P0JZ Alteration of Left Upper Eyelid with Synthetic Substitute, Open Approach

080P0KZ Alteration of Left Upper Eyelid with Nonautologous Tissue Substitute, Open Approach

080P0ZZ Alteration of Left Upper Eyelid, Open Approach

080P37Z Alteration of Left Upper Eyelid with Autologous Tissue Substitute, Percutaneous Approach

080P3JZ Alteration of Left Upper Eyelid with Synthetic Substitute, Percutaneous Approach

080P3KZ Alteration of Left Upper Eyelid with Nonautologous Tissue Substitute, Percutaneous Approach

080P3ZZ Alteration of Left Upper Eyelid, Percutaneous Approach

080PX7Z Alteration of Left Upper Eyelid with Autologous Tissue Substitute, External Approach

080PXJZ Alteration of Left Upper Eyelid with Synthetic Substitute, External Approach

080PXKZ Alteration of Left Upper Eyelid with Nonautologous Tissue Substitute, External Approach

080PXZZ Alteration of Left Upper Eyelid, External Approach

080Q07Z Alteration of Right Lower Eyelid with Autologous Tissue Substitute, Open Approach

080Q0JZ Alteration of Right Lower Eyelid with Synthetic Substitute, Open Approach

080Q0KZ Alteration of Right Lower Eyelid with Nonautologous Tissue Substitute, Open Approach

080Q0ZZ Alteration of Right Lower Eyelid, Open Approach

080Q37Z Alteration of Right Lower Eyelid with Autologous Tissue Substitute, Percutaneous Approach

080Q3JZ Alteration of Right Lower Eyelid with Synthetic Substitute, Percutaneous Approach

080Q3KZ Alteration of Right Lower Eyelid with Nonautologous Tissue Substitute, Percutaneous Approach

080Q3ZZ Alteration of Right Lower Eyelid, Percutaneous Approach

080QX7Z Alteration of Right Lower Eyelid with Autologous Tissue Substitute, External Approach

080QXJZ Alteration of Right Lower Eyelid with Synthetic Substitute, External Approach

080QXKZ Alteration of Right Lower Eyelid with Nonautologous Tissue Substitute, External Approach

080QXZZ Alteration of Right Lower Eyelid, External Approach

080R07Z Alteration of Left Lower Eyelid with Autologous Tissue Substitute, Open Approach

080R0JZ Alteration of Left Lower Eyelid with Synthetic Substitute, Open Approach

080R0KZ Alteration of Left Lower Eyelid with Nonautologous Tissue Substitute, Open Approach

080R0ZZ Alteration of Left Lower Eyelid, Open Approach

080R37Z Alteration of Left Lower Eyelid with Autologous Tissue Substitute, Percutaneous Approach

080R3JZ Alteration of Left Lower Eyelid with Synthetic Substitute, Percutaneous Approach

080R3KZ Alteration of Left Lower Eyelid with Nonautologous Tissue Substitute, Percutaneous Approach

080R3ZZ Alteration of Left Lower Eyelid, Percutaneous Approach

080RX7Z Alteration of Left Lower Eyelid with Autologous Tissue Substitute, External Approach

080RXJZ Alteration of Left Lower Eyelid with Synthetic Substitute, External Approach

080RXKZ Alteration of Left Lower Eyelid with Nonautologous Tissue Substitute, External Approach

080RXZZ Alteration of Left Lower Eyelid, External Approach

081 – Eye, Bypass

Review Coding Guideline B3.6a

08123J4 Bypass Right Anterior Chamber to Sclera with Synthetic Substitute, Percutaneous Approach

08123K4 Bypass Right Anterior Chamber to Sclera with Nonautologous Tissue Substitute, Percutaneous Approach

08123Z4 Bypass Right Anterior Chamber to Sclera, Percutaneous Approach

08133J4 Bypass Left Anterior Chamber to Sclera with Synthetic Substitute, Percutaneous Approach

08133K4 Bypass Left Anterior Chamber to Sclera with Nonautologous Tissue Substitute, Percutaneous Approach

08133Z4 Bypass Left Anterior Chamber to Sclera, Percutaneous Approach

081X0J3 Bypass Right Lacrimal Duct to Nasal Cavity with Synthetic Substitute, Open Approach

081X0K3 Bypass Right Lacrimal Duct to Nasal Cavity with Nonautologous Tissue Substitute, Open Approach

081X0Z3 Bypass Right Lacrimal Duct to Nasal Cavity, Open Approach

081X3J3 Bypass Right Lacrimal Duct to Nasal Cavity with Synthetic Substitute, Percutaneous Approach

081X3K3 Bypass Right Lacrimal Duct to Nasal Cavity with Nonautologous Tissue Substitute, Percutaneous Approach

081X3Z3 Bypass Right Lacrimal Duct to Nasal Cavity, Percutaneous Approach

081Y0J3 Bypass Left Lacrimal Duct to Nasal Cavity with Synthetic Substitute, Open Approach

081Y0K3 Bypass Left Lacrimal Duct to Nasal Cavity with Nonautologous Tissue Substitute, Open Approach

081Y0Z3 Bypass Left Lacrimal Duct to Nasal Cavity, Open Approach

081Y3J3 Bypass Left Lacrimal Duct to Nasal Cavity with Synthetic Substitute, Percutaneous Approach

081Y3K3 Bypass Left Lacrimal Duct to Nasal Cavity with Nonautologous Tissue Substitute, Percutaneous Approach

081Y3Z3 Bypass Left Lacrimal Duct to Nasal Cavity, Percutaneous Approach

♀ Female-only   ♂ Male-only   ▲ Limited Coverage   ● Non-OR   HAC-associated procedure   ▲ Non-covered procedures   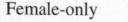 Combinatio

2 – Eye, Change

Review Coding Guideline B6.1c

0X0Z	Change Drainage Device in Right Eye, External Approach	**0821X0Z**	Change Drainage Device in Left Eye, External Approach
0XYZ	Change Other Device in Right Eye, External Approach	**0821XYZ**	Change Other Device in Left Eye, External Approach

5 – Eye, Destruction

0XZZ	Destruction of Right Eye, External Approach	**085G3ZZ**	Destruction of Right Retinal Vessel, Percutaneous Approach	**085R3ZZ**	Destruction of Left Lower Eyelid, Percutaneous Approach
1XZZ	Destruction of Left Eye, External Approach	**085H3ZZ**	Destruction of Left Retinal Vessel, Percutaneous Approach	**085RXZZ**	Destruction of Left Lower Eyelid, External Approach
23ZZ	Destruction of Right Anterior Chamber, Percutaneous Approach	**085J3ZZ**	Destruction of Right Lens, Percutaneous Approach	**085SXZZ**	Destruction of Right Conjunctiva, External Approach
33ZZ	Destruction of Left Anterior Chamber, Percutaneous Approach	**085K3ZZ**	Destruction of Left Lens, Percutaneous Approach	**085TXZZ**	Destruction of Left Conjunctiva, External Approach
43ZZ	Destruction of Right Vitreous, Percutaneous Approach	**085L0ZZ**	Destruction of Right Extraocular Muscle, Open Approach	**085V0ZZ**	Destruction of Right Lacrimal Gland, Open Approach
53ZZ	Destruction of Left Vitreous, Percutaneous Approach	**085L3ZZ**	Destruction of Right Extraocular Muscle, Percutaneous Approach	**085V3ZZ**	Destruction of Right Lacrimal Gland, Percutaneous Approach
56XZZ	Destruction of Right Sclera, External Approach	**085M0ZZ**	Destruction of Left Extraocular Muscle, Open Approach	**085W0ZZ**	Destruction of Left Lacrimal Gland, Open Approach
57XZZ	Destruction of Left Sclera, External Approach	**085M3ZZ**	Destruction of Left Extraocular Muscle, Percutaneous Approach	**085W3ZZ**	Destruction of Left Lacrimal Gland, Percutaneous Approach
58XZZ	Destruction of Right Cornea, External Approach	**085N0ZZ**	Destruction of Right Upper Eyelid, Open Approach	**085X0ZZ**	Destruction of Right Lacrimal Duct, Open Approach
59XZZ	Destruction of Left Cornea, External Approach	**085N3ZZ**	Destruction of Right Upper Eyelid, Percutaneous Approach	**085X3ZZ**	Destruction of Right Lacrimal Duct, Percutaneous Approach
5A0ZZ	Destruction of Right Choroid, Open Approach	**085NXZZ**	Destruction of Right Upper Eyelid, External Approach	**085X7ZZ**	Destruction of Right Lacrimal Duct, Via Natural or Artificial Opening
5A3ZZ	Destruction of Right Choroid, Percutaneous Approach	**085P0ZZ**	Destruction of Left Upper Eyelid, Open Approach	**085X8ZZ**	Destruction of Right Lacrimal Duct, Via Natural or Artificial Opening Endoscopic
5B0ZZ	Destruction of Left Choroid, Open Approach	**085P3ZZ**	Destruction of Left Upper Eyelid, Percutaneous Approach	**085Y0ZZ**	Destruction of Left Lacrimal Duct, Open Approach
5B3ZZ	Destruction of Left Choroid, Percutaneous Approach	**085PXZZ**	Destruction of Left Upper Eyelid, External Approach	**085Y3ZZ**	Destruction of Left Lacrimal Duct, Percutaneous Approach
5C3ZZ	Destruction of Right Iris, Percutaneous Approach	**085Q0ZZ**	Destruction of Right Lower Eyelid, Open Approach	**085Y7ZZ**	Destruction of Left Lacrimal Duct, Via Natural or Artificial Opening
5D3ZZ	Destruction of Left Iris, Percutaneous Approach	**085Q3ZZ**	Destruction of Right Lower Eyelid, Percutaneous Approach	**085Y8ZZ**	Destruction of Left Lacrimal Duct, Via Natural or Artificial Opening Endoscopic
5E3ZZ	Destruction of Right Retina, Percutaneous Approach	**085QXZZ**	Destruction of Right Lower Eyelid, External Approach		
5F3ZZ	Destruction of Left Retina, Percutaneous Approach	**085R0ZZ**	Destruction of Left Lower Eyelid, Open Approach		

87 – Eye, Dilation

7X0DZ	Dilation of Right Lacrimal Duct with Intraluminal Device, Open Approach	**087X8DZ**	Dilation of Right Lacrimal Duct with Intraluminal Device, Via Natural or Artificial Opening Endoscopic	**087Y7DZ**	Dilation of Left Lacrimal Duct with Intraluminal Device, Via Natural or Artificial Opening
7X0ZZ	Dilation of Right Lacrimal Duct, Open Approach	**087X8ZZ**	Dilation of Right Lacrimal Duct, Via Natural or Artificial Opening Endoscopic	**087Y7ZZ**	Dilation of Left Lacrimal Duct, Via Natural or Artificial Opening
7X3DZ	Dilation of Right Lacrimal Duct with Intraluminal Device, Percutaneous Approach	**087Y0DZ**	Dilation of Left Lacrimal Duct with Intraluminal Device, Open Approach	**087Y8DZ**	Dilation of Left Lacrimal Duct with Intraluminal Device, Via Natural or Artificial Opening Endoscopic
7X3ZZ	Dilation of Right Lacrimal Duct, Percutaneous Approach	**087Y0ZZ**	Dilation of Left Lacrimal Duct, Open Approach	**087Y8ZZ**	Dilation of Left Lacrimal Duct, Via Natural or Artificial Opening Endoscopic
7X7DZ	Dilation of Right Lacrimal Duct with Intraluminal Device, Via Natural or Artificial Opening	**087Y3DZ**	Dilation of Left Lacrimal Duct with Intraluminal Device, Percutaneous Approach		
7X7ZZ	Dilation of Right Lacrimal Duct, Via Natural or Artificial Opening	**087Y3ZZ**	Dilation of Left Lacrimal Duct, Percutaneous Approach		

89 – Eye, Drainage

Review Coding Guidelines B3.4a and B3.4b

Review Coding Guideline B6.2

890X0Z	Drainage of Right Eye with Drainage Device, External Approach	**0891XZX**	Drainage of Left Eye, External Approach, Diagnostic	**08923ZZ**	Drainage of Right Anterior Chamber, Percutaneous Approach
890XZX	Drainage of Right Eye, External Approach, Diagnostic	**0891XZZ**	Drainage of Left Eye, External Approach	**089330Z**	Drainage of Left Anterior Chamber with Drainage Device, Percutaneous Approach
890XZZ	Drainage of Right Eye, External Approach	**089230Z**	Drainage of Right Anterior Chamber with Drainage Device, Percutaneous Approach		
891X0Z	Drainage of Left Eye with Drainage Device, External Approach	**08923ZX**	Drainage of Right Anterior Chamber, Percutaneous Approach, Diagnostic	**08933ZX**	Drainage of Left Anterior Chamber, Percutaneous Approach, Diagnostic

Female-only	♂ Male-only	▲ Limited Coverage	● Non-OR	▥ HAC-associated procedure	▲ Non-covered procedures	✚ Combination

08933ZZ	Drainage of Left Anterior Chamber, Percutaneous Approach	**089E3ZZ**	Drainage of Right Retina, Percutaneous Approach	**089P0ZX**	Drainage of Left Upper Eyelid, Open Approach, Diagnostic
089430Z	Drainage of Right Vitreous with Drainage Device, Percutaneous Approach	**089F30Z**	Drainage of Left Retina with Drainage Device, Percutaneous Approach	**089P0ZZ**	Drainage of Left Upper Eyelid, Open Approach
08943ZX	Drainage of Right Vitreous, Percutaneous Approach, Diagnostic	**089F3ZX**	Drainage of Left Retina, Percutaneous Approach, Diagnostic	**089P30Z**	Drainage of Left Upper Eyelid with Drainage Device, Percutaneous Approach
08943ZZ	Drainage of Right Vitreous, Percutaneous Approach	**089F3ZZ**	Drainage of Left Retina, Percutaneous Approach	**089P3ZX**	Drainage of Left Upper Eyelid, Percutaneous Approach, Diagnostic
089530Z	Drainage of Left Vitreous with Drainage Device, Percutaneous Approach	**089G30Z**	Drainage of Right Retinal Vessel with Drainage Device, Percutaneous Approach	**089P3ZZ**	Drainage of Left Upper Eyelid, Percutaneous Approach
08953ZX	Drainage of Left Vitreous, Percutaneous Approach, Diagnostic	**089G3ZX**	Drainage of Right Retinal Vessel, Percutaneous Approach, Diagnostic	**089PX0Z**	Drainage of Left Upper Eyelid with Drainage Device, External Approach
08953ZZ	Drainage of Left Vitreous, Percutaneous Approach	**089G3ZZ**	Drainage of Right Retinal Vessel, Percutaneous Approach	**089PXZX**	Drainage of Left Upper Eyelid, External Approach, Diagnostic
0896X0Z	Drainage of Right Sclera with Drainage Device, External Approach	**089H30Z**	Drainage of Left Retinal Vessel with Drainage Device, Percutaneous Approach	**089PXZZ**	Drainage of Left Upper Eyelid, External Approach
0896XZX	Drainage of Right Sclera, External Approach, Diagnostic	**089H3ZX**	Drainage of Left Retinal Vessel, Percutaneous Approach, Diagnostic	**089Q00Z**	Drainage of Right Lower Eyelid with Drainage Device, Open Approach
0896XZZ	Drainage of Right Sclera, External Approach	**089H3ZZ**	Drainage of Left Retinal Vessel, Percutaneous Approach	**089Q0ZX**	Drainage of Right Lower Eyelid, Open Approach, Diagnostic
0897X0Z	Drainage of Left Sclera with Drainage Device, External Approach	**089J30Z**	Drainage of Right Lens with Drainage Device, Percutaneous Approach	**089Q0ZZ**	Drainage of Right Lower Eyelid, Open Approach
0897XZX	Drainage of Left Sclera, External Approach, Diagnostic	**089J3ZX**	Drainage of Right Lens, Percutaneous Approach, Diagnostic	**089Q30Z**	Drainage of Right Lower Eyelid with Drainage Device, Percutaneous Approach
0897XZZ	Drainage of Left Sclera, External Approach	**089J3ZZ**	Drainage of Right Lens, Percutaneous Approach	**089Q3ZX**	Drainage of Right Lower Eyelid, Percutaneous Approach, Diagnostic
0898X0Z	Drainage of Right Cornea with Drainage Device, External Approach	**089K30Z**	Drainage of Left Lens with Drainage Device, Percutaneous Approach	**089Q3ZZ**	Drainage of Right Lower Eyelid, Percutaneous Approach
0898XZX	Drainage of Right Cornea, External Approach, Diagnostic	**089K3ZX**	Drainage of Left Lens, Percutaneous Approach, Diagnostic	**089QX0Z**	Drainage of Right Lower Eyelid with Drainage Device, External Approach
0898XZZ	Drainage of Right Cornea, External Approach	**089K3ZZ**	Drainage of Left Lens, Percutaneous Approach	**089QXZX**	Drainage of Right Lower Eyelid, External Approach, Diagnostic
0899X0Z	Drainage of Left Cornea with Drainage Device, External Approach	**089L00Z**	Drainage of Right Extraocular Muscle with Drainage Device, Open Approach	**089QXZZ**	Drainage of Right Lower Eyelid, External Approach
0899XZX	Drainage of Left Cornea, External Approach, Diagnostic	**089L0ZX**	Drainage of Right Extraocular Muscle, Open Approach, Diagnostic	**089R00Z**	Drainage of Left Lower Eyelid with Drainage Device, Open Approach
0899XZZ	Drainage of Left Cornea, External Approach	**089L0ZZ**	Drainage of Right Extraocular Muscle, Open Approach	**089R0ZX**	Drainage of Left Lower Eyelid, Open Approach, Diagnostic
089A00Z	Drainage of Right Choroid with Drainage Device, Open Approach	**089L30Z**	Drainage of Right Extraocular Muscle with Drainage Device, Percutaneous Approach	**089R0ZZ**	Drainage of Left Lower Eyelid, Open Approach
089A0ZX	Drainage of Right Choroid, Open Approach, Diagnostic	**089L3ZX**	Drainage of Right Extraocular Muscle, Percutaneous Approach, Diagnostic	**089R30Z**	Drainage of Left Lower Eyelid with Drainage Device, Percutaneous Approach
089A0ZZ	Drainage of Right Choroid, Open Approach	**089L3ZZ**	Drainage of Right Extraocular Muscle, Percutaneous Approach	**089R3ZX**	Drainage of Left Lower Eyelid, Percutaneous Approach, Diagnostic
089A30Z	Drainage of Right Choroid with Drainage Device, Percutaneous Approach	**089M00Z**	Drainage of Left Extraocular Muscle with Drainage Device, Open Approach	**089R3ZZ**	Drainage of Left Lower Eyelid, Percutaneous Approach
089A3ZX	Drainage of Right Choroid, Percutaneous Approach, Diagnostic	**089M0ZX**	Drainage of Left Extraocular Muscle, Open Approach, Diagnostic	**089RX0Z**	Drainage of Left Lower Eyelid with Drainage Device, External Approach
089A3ZZ	Drainage of Right Choroid, Percutaneous Approach	**089M0ZZ**	Drainage of Left Extraocular Muscle, Open Approach	**089RXZX**	Drainage of Left Lower Eyelid, External Approach, Diagnostic
089B00Z	Drainage of Left Choroid with Drainage Device, Open Approach	**089M30Z**	Drainage of Left Extraocular Muscle with Drainage Device, Percutaneous Approach	**089RXZZ**	Drainage of Left Lower Eyelid, External Approach
089B0ZX	Drainage of Left Choroid, Open Approach, Diagnostic	**089M3ZX**	Drainage of Left Extraocular Muscle, Percutaneous Approach, Diagnostic	**089SX0Z**	Drainage of Right Conjunctiva with Drainage Device, External Approach
089B0ZZ	Drainage of Left Choroid, Open Approach	**089M3ZZ**	Drainage of Left Extraocular Muscle, Percutaneous Approach	**089SXZX**	Drainage of Right Conjunctiva, External Approach, Diagnostic
089B30Z	Drainage of Left Choroid with Drainage Device, Percutaneous Approach	**089N00Z**	Drainage of Right Upper Eyelid with Drainage Device, Open Approach	**089SXZZ**	Drainage of Right Conjunctiva, External Approach
089B3ZX	Drainage of Left Choroid, Percutaneous Approach, Diagnostic	**089N0ZX**	Drainage of Right Upper Eyelid, Open Approach, Diagnostic	**089TX0Z**	Drainage of Left Conjunctiva with Drainage Device, External Approach
089B3ZZ	Drainage of Left Choroid, Percutaneous Approach	**089N0ZZ**	Drainage of Right Upper Eyelid, Open Approach	**089TXZX**	Drainage of Left Conjunctiva, External Approach, Diagnostic
089C30Z	Drainage of Right Iris with Drainage Device, Percutaneous Approach	**089N30Z**	Drainage of Right Upper Eyelid with Drainage Device, Percutaneous Approach	**089TXZZ**	Drainage of Left Conjunctiva, External Approach
089C3ZX	Drainage of Right Iris, Percutaneous Approach, Diagnostic	**089N3ZX**	Drainage of Right Upper Eyelid, Percutaneous Approach, Diagnostic	**089V00Z**	Drainage of Right Lacrimal Gland with Drainage Device, Open Approach
089C3ZZ	Drainage of Right Iris, Percutaneous Approach	**089N3ZZ**	Drainage of Right Upper Eyelid, Percutaneous Approach	**089V0ZX**	Drainage of Right Lacrimal Gland, Open Approach, Diagnostic
089D30Z	Drainage of Left Iris with Drainage Device, Percutaneous Approach	**089NX0Z**	Drainage of Right Upper Eyelid with Drainage Device, External Approach	**089V0ZZ**	Drainage of Right Lacrimal Gland, Open Approach
089D3ZX	Drainage of Left Iris, Percutaneous Approach, Diagnostic	**089NXZX**	Drainage of Right Upper Eyelid, External Approach, Diagnostic	**089V30Z**	Drainage of Right Lacrimal Gland with Drainage Device, Percutaneous Approach
089D3ZZ	Drainage of Left Iris, Percutaneous Approach	**089NXZZ**	Drainage of Right Upper Eyelid, External Approach	**089V3ZX**	Drainage of Right Lacrimal Gland, Percutaneous Approach, Diagnostic
089E30Z	Drainage of Right Retina with Drainage Device, Percutaneous Approach	**089P00Z**	Drainage of Left Upper Eyelid with Drainage Device, Open Approach	**089V3ZZ**	Drainage of Right Lacrimal Gland, Percutaneous Approach
089E3ZX	Drainage of Right Retina, Percutaneous Approach, Diagnostic				

♀ Female-only　　♂ Male-only　　▲ Limited Coverage　　● Non-OR　　■ HAC-associated procedure　　▲ Non-covered procedures　　✚ Combination

W00Z Drainage of Left Lacrimal Gland with Drainage Device, Open Approach	**089X3ZZ** Drainage of Right Lacrimal Duct, Percutaneous Approach	**089Y30Z** Drainage of Left Lacrimal Duct with Drainage Device, Percutaneous Approach
W0ZX Drainage of Left Lacrimal Gland, Open Approach, Diagnostic	**089X70Z** Drainage of Right Lacrimal Duct with Drainage Device, Via Natural or Artificial Opening	**089Y3ZX** Drainage of Left Lacrimal Duct, Percutaneous Approach, Diagnostic
W0ZZ Drainage of Left Lacrimal Gland, Open Approach	**089X7ZX** Drainage of Right Lacrimal Duct, Via Natural or Artificial Opening, Diagnostic	**089Y3ZZ** Drainage of Left Lacrimal Duct, Percutaneous Approach
W30Z Drainage of Left Lacrimal Gland with Drainage Device, Percutaneous Approach	**089X7ZZ** Drainage of Right Lacrimal Duct, Via Natural or Artificial Opening	**089Y70Z** Drainage of Left Lacrimal Duct with Drainage Device, Via Natural or Artificial Opening
W3ZX Drainage of Left Lacrimal Gland, Percutaneous Approach, Diagnostic	**089X80Z** Drainage of Right Lacrimal Duct with Drainage Device, Via Natural or Artificial Opening Endoscopic	**089Y7ZX** Drainage of Left Lacrimal Duct, Via Natural or Artificial Opening, Diagnostic
W3ZZ Drainage of Left Lacrimal Gland, Percutaneous Approach	**089X8ZX** Drainage of Right Lacrimal Duct, Via Natural or Artificial Opening Endoscopic, Diagnostic	**089Y7ZZ** Drainage of Left Lacrimal Duct, Via Natural or Artificial Opening
X00Z Drainage of Right Lacrimal Duct with Drainage Device, Open Approach	**089X8ZZ** Drainage of Right Lacrimal Duct, Via Natural or Artificial Opening Endoscopic	**089Y80Z** Drainage of Left Lacrimal Duct with Drainage Device, Via Natural or Artificial Opening Endoscopic
X0ZX Drainage of Right Lacrimal Duct, Open Approach, Diagnostic	**089Y00Z** Drainage of Left Lacrimal Duct with Drainage Device, Open Approach	**089Y8ZX** Drainage of Left Lacrimal Duct, Via Natural or Artificial Opening Endoscopic, Diagnostic
X0ZZ Drainage of Right Lacrimal Duct, Open Approach	**089Y0ZX** Drainage of Left Lacrimal Duct, Open Approach, Diagnostic	**089Y8ZZ** Drainage of Left Lacrimal Duct, Via Natural or Artificial Opening Endoscopic
X30Z Drainage of Right Lacrimal Duct with Drainage Device, Percutaneous Approach	**089Y0ZZ** Drainage of Left Lacrimal Duct, Open Approach	
X3ZX Drainage of Right Lacrimal Duct, Percutaneous Approach, Diagnostic		

B – Eye, Excision

view Coding Guidelines B3.4a and B3.4b

view Coding Guideline B3.8

800ZX Excision of Right Eye, Open Approach, Diagnostic	**08BA0ZX** Excision of Right Choroid, Open Approach, Diagnostic	**08BM0ZX** Excision of Left Extraocular Muscle, Open Approach, Diagnostic
800ZZ Excision of Right Eye, Open Approach	**08BA0ZZ** Excision of Right Choroid, Open Approach	**08BM0ZZ** Excision of Left Extraocular Muscle, Open Approach
803ZX Excision of Right Eye, Percutaneous Approach, Diagnostic	**08BA3ZX** Excision of Right Choroid, Percutaneous Approach, Diagnostic	**08BM3ZX** Excision of Left Extraocular Muscle, Percutaneous Approach, Diagnostic
803ZZ Excision of Right Eye, Percutaneous Approach	**08BA3ZZ** Excision of Right Choroid, Percutaneous Approach	**08BM3ZZ** Excision of Left Extraocular Muscle, Percutaneous Approach
80XZX Excision of Right Eye, External Approach, Diagnostic	**08BB0ZX** Excision of Left Choroid, Open Approach, Diagnostic	**08BN0ZX** Excision of Right Upper Eyelid, Open Approach, Diagnostic
80XZZ Excision of Right Eye, External Approach	**08BB0ZZ** Excision of Left Choroid, Open Approach	**08BN0ZZ** Excision of Right Upper Eyelid, Open Approach
810ZX Excision of Left Eye, Open Approach, Diagnostic	**08BB3ZX** Excision of Left Choroid, Percutaneous Approach, Diagnostic	**08BN3ZX** Excision of Right Upper Eyelid, Percutaneous Approach, Diagnostic
810ZZ Excision of Left Eye, Open Approach	**08BB3ZZ** Excision of Left Choroid, Percutaneous Approach	**08BN3ZZ** Excision of Right Upper Eyelid, Percutaneous Approach
813ZX Excision of Left Eye, Percutaneous Approach, Diagnostic	**08BC3ZX** Excision of Right Iris, Percutaneous Approach, Diagnostic	**08BNXZX** Excision of Right Upper Eyelid, External Approach, Diagnostic
813ZZ Excision of Left Eye, Percutaneous Approach	**08BC3ZZ** Excision of Right Iris, Percutaneous Approach	**08BNXZZ** Excision of Right Upper Eyelid, External Approach
81XZX Excision of Left Eye, External Approach, Diagnostic	**08BD3ZX** Excision of Left Iris, Percutaneous Approach, Diagnostic	**08BP0ZX** Excision of Left Upper Eyelid, Open Approach, Diagnostic
81XZZ Excision of Left Eye, External Approach	**08BD3ZZ** Excision of Left Iris, Percutaneous Approach	**08BP0ZZ** Excision of Left Upper Eyelid, Open Approach
843ZX Excision of Right Vitreous, Percutaneous Approach, Diagnostic	**08BE3ZX** Excision of Right Retina, Percutaneous Approach, Diagnostic	**08BP3ZX** Excision of Left Upper Eyelid, Percutaneous Approach, Diagnostic
843ZZ Excision of Right Vitreous, Percutaneous Approach	**08BE3ZZ** Excision of Right Retina, Percutaneous Approach	**08BP3ZZ** Excision of Left Upper Eyelid, Percutaneous Approach
AHA CC: 4Q, 2014, 36-37	**08BF3ZX** Excision of Left Retina, Percutaneous Approach, Diagnostic	**08BPXZX** Excision of Left Upper Eyelid, External Approach, Diagnostic
853ZX Excision of Left Vitreous, Percutaneous Approach, Diagnostic	**08BF3ZZ** Excision of Left Retina, Percutaneous Approach	**08BPXZZ** Excision of Left Upper Eyelid, External Approach
853ZZ Excision of Left Vitreous, Percutaneous Approach	**08BJ3ZX** Excision of Right Lens, Percutaneous Approach, Diagnostic	**08BQ0ZX** Excision of Right Lower Eyelid, Open Approach, Diagnostic
AHA CC: 4Q, 2014, 35-36	**08BJ3ZZ** Excision of Right Lens, Percutaneous Approach	**08BQ0ZZ** Excision of Right Lower Eyelid, Open Approach
B6XZX Excision of Right Sclera, External Approach, Diagnostic	**08BK3ZX** Excision of Left Lens, Percutaneous Approach, Diagnostic	**08BQ3ZX** Excision of Right Lower Eyelid, Percutaneous Approach, Diagnostic
B6XZZ Excision of Right Sclera, External Approach	**08BK3ZZ** Excision of Left Lens, Percutaneous Approach	**08BQ3ZZ** Excision of Right Lower Eyelid, Percutaneous Approach
B7XZX Excision of Left Sclera, External Approach, Diagnostic	**08BL0ZX** Excision of Right Extraocular Muscle, Open Approach, Diagnostic	**08BQXZX** Excision of Right Lower Eyelid, External Approach, Diagnostic
B7XZZ Excision of Left Sclera, External Approach	**08BL0ZZ** Excision of Right Extraocular Muscle, Open Approach	**08BQXZZ** Excision of Right Lower Eyelid, External Approach
B8XZX Excision of Right Cornea, External Approach, Diagnostic	**08BL3ZX** Excision of Right Extraocular Muscle, Percutaneous Approach, Diagnostic	**08BR0ZX** Excision of Left Lower Eyelid, Open Approach, Diagnostic
B8XZZ Excision of Right Cornea, External Approach	**08BL3ZZ** Excision of Right Extraocular Muscle, Percutaneous Approach	
B9XZX Excision of Left Cornea, External Approach, Diagnostic		
B9XZZ Excision of Left Cornea, External Approach		

415

Female-only	♂ Male-only	▲ Limited Coverage	● Non-OR	▨ HAC-associated procedure	▲ Non-covered procedures	✚ Combination

08BR0ZZ Excision of Left Lower Eyelid, Open Approach

08BR3ZX Excision of Left Lower Eyelid, Percutaneous Approach, Diagnostic

08BR3ZZ Excision of Left Lower Eyelid, Percutaneous Approach

08BRXZX Excision of Left Lower Eyelid, External Approach, Diagnostic

08BRXZZ Excision of Left Lower Eyelid, External Approach

08BSXZX Excision of Right Conjunctiva, External Approach, Diagnostic

08BSXZZ Excision of Right Conjunctiva, External Approach

08BTXZX Excision of Left Conjunctiva, External Approach, Diagnostic

08BTXZZ Excision of Left Conjunctiva, External Approach

08BV0ZX Excision of Right Lacrimal Gland, Open Approach, Diagnostic

08BV0ZZ Excision of Right Lacrimal Gland, Open Approach

08BV3ZX Excision of Right Lacrimal Gland, Percutaneous Approach, Diagnostic

08BV3ZZ Excision of Right Lacrimal Gland, Percutaneous Approach

08BW0ZX Excision of Left Lacrimal Gland, Open Approach, Diagnostic

08BW0ZZ Excision of Left Lacrimal Gland, Open Approach

08BW3ZX Excision of Left Lacrimal Gland, Percutaneous Approach, Diagnostic

08BW3ZZ Excision of Left Lacrimal Gland, Percutaneous Approach

08BX0ZX Excision of Right Lacrimal Duct, Open Approach, Diagnostic

08BX0ZZ Excision of Right Lacrimal Duct, Open Approach

08BX3ZX Excision of Right Lacrimal Duct, Percutaneous Approach, Diagnostic

08BX3ZZ Excision of Right Lacrimal Duct, Percutaneous Approach

08BX7ZX Excision of Right Lacrimal Duct, Via Natural or Artificial Opening, Diagnostic

08BX7ZZ Excision of Right Lacrimal Duct, Via Natural or Artificial Opening

08BX8ZX Excision of Right Lacrimal Duct, Via Natural or Artificial Opening Endoscopic Diagnostic

08BX8ZZ Excision of Right Lacrimal Duct, Via Natural or Artificial Opening Endoscopic

08BY0ZX Excision of Left Lacrimal Duct, Open Approach, Diagnostic

08BY0ZZ Excision of Left Lacrimal Duct, Open Approach

08BY3ZX Excision of Left Lacrimal Duct, Percutaneous Approach, Diagnostic

08BY3ZZ Excision of Left Lacrimal Duct, Percutaneous Approach

08BY7ZX Excision of Left Lacrimal Duct, Via Natural or Artificial Opening, Diagnostic

08BY7ZZ Excision of Left Lacrimal Duct, Via Natural or Artificial Opening

08BY8ZX Excision of Left Lacrimal Duct, Via Natural or Artificial Opening Endoscopic Diagnostic

08BY8ZZ Excision of Left Lacrimal Duct, Via Natural or Artificial Opening Endoscopic

08C – Eye, Extirpation

08C0XZZ Extirpation of Matter from Right Eye, External Approach

08C1XZZ Extirpation of Matter from Left Eye, External Approach

08C23ZZ Extirpation of Matter from Right Anterior Chamber, Percutaneous Approach

08C2XZZ Extirpation of Matter from Right Anterior Chamber, External Approach

08C33ZZ Extirpation of Matter from Left Anterior Chamber, Percutaneous Approach

08C3XZZ Extirpation of Matter from Left Anterior Chamber, External Approach

08C43ZZ Extirpation of Matter from Right Vitreous, Percutaneous Approach

08C4XZZ Extirpation of Matter from Right Vitreous, External Approach

08C53ZZ Extirpation of Matter from Left Vitreous, Percutaneous Approach

08C5XZZ Extirpation of Matter from Left Vitreous, External Approach

08C6XZZ Extirpation of Matter from Right Sclera, External Approach

08C7XZZ Extirpation of Matter from Left Sclera, External Approach

08C8XZZ Extirpation of Matter from Right Cornea, External Approach

08C9XZZ Extirpation of Matter from Left Cornea, External Approach

08CA0ZZ Extirpation of Matter from Right Choroid, Open Approach

08CA3ZZ Extirpation of Matter from Right Choroid, Percutaneous Approach

08CAXZZ Extirpation of Matter from Right Choroid, External Approach

08CB0ZZ Extirpation of Matter from Left Choroid, Open Approach

08CB3ZZ Extirpation of Matter from Left Choroid, Percutaneous Approach

08CBXZZ Extirpation of Matter from Left Choroid, External Approach

08CC3ZZ Extirpation of Matter from Right Iris, Percutaneous Approach

08CCXZZ Extirpation of Matter from Right Iris, External Approach

08CD3ZZ Extirpation of Matter from Left Iris, Percutaneous Approach

08CDXZZ Extirpation of Matter from Left Iris, External Approach

08CE3ZZ Extirpation of Matter from Right Retina, Percutaneous Approach

08CEXZZ Extirpation of Matter from Right Retina, External Approach

08CF3ZZ Extirpation of Matter from Left Retina, Percutaneous Approach

08CFXZZ Extirpation of Matter from Left Retina, External Approach

08CG3ZZ Extirpation of Matter from Right Retinal Vessel, Percutaneous Approach

08CGXZZ Extirpation of Matter from Right Retinal Vessel, External Approach

08CH3ZZ Extirpation of Matter from Left Retinal Vessel, Percutaneous Approach

08CHXZZ Extirpation of Matter from Left Retinal Vessel, External Approach

08CJ3ZZ Extirpation of Matter from Right Lens, Percutaneous Approach

08CJXZZ Extirpation of Matter from Right Lens, External Approach

08CK3ZZ Extirpation of Matter from Left Lens, Percutaneous Approach

08CKXZZ Extirpation of Matter from Left Lens, External Approach

08CL0ZZ Extirpation of Matter from Right Extraocular Muscle, Open Approach

08CL3ZZ Extirpation of Matter from Right Extraocular Muscle, Percutaneous Approach

08CLXZZ Extirpation of Matter from Right Extraocular Muscle, External Approach

08CM0ZZ Extirpation of Matter from Left Extraocular Muscle, Open Approach

08CM3ZZ Extirpation of Matter from Left Extraocular Muscle, Percutaneous Approach

08CMXZZ Extirpation of Matter from Left Extraocular Muscle, External Approach

08CN0ZZ Extirpation of Matter from Right Upper Eyelid, Open Approach

08CN3ZZ Extirpation of Matter from Right Upper Eyelid, Percutaneous Approach

08CNXZZ Extirpation of Matter from Right Upper Eyelid, External Approach

08CP0ZZ Extirpation of Matter from Left Upper Eyelid, Open Approach

08CP3ZZ Extirpation of Matter from Left Upper Eyelid, Percutaneous Approach

08CPXZZ Extirpation of Matter from Left Upper Eyelid, External Approach

08CQ0ZZ Extirpation of Matter from Right Lower Eyelid, Open Approach

08CQ3ZZ Extirpation of Matter from Right Lower Eyelid, Percutaneous Approach

08CQXZZ Extirpation of Matter from Right Lower Eyelid, External Approach

08CR0ZZ Extirpation of Matter from Left Lower Eyelid, Open Approach

08CR3ZZ Extirpation of Matter from Left Lower Eyelid, Percutaneous Approach

08CRXZZ Extirpation of Matter from Left Lower Eyelid, External Approach

08CSXZZ Extirpation of Matter from Right Conjunctiva, External Approach

08CTXZZ Extirpation of Matter from Left Conjunctiva, External Approach

08CV0ZZ Extirpation of Matter from Right Lacrimal Gland, Open Approach

08CV3ZZ Extirpation of Matter from Right Lacrimal Gland, Percutaneous Approach

08CVXZZ Extirpation of Matter from Right Lacrimal Gland, External Approach

08CW0ZZ Extirpation of Matter from Left Lacrimal Gland, Open Approach

08CW3ZZ Extirpation of Matter from Left Lacrimal Gland, Percutaneous Approach

08CWXZZ Extirpation of Matter from Left Lacrimal Gland, External Approach

08CX0ZZ Extirpation of Matter from Right Lacrimal Duct, Open Approach

08CX3ZZ Extirpation of Matter from Right Lacrimal Duct, Percutaneous Approach

08CX7ZZ Extirpation of Matter from Right Lacrimal Duct, Via Natural or Artificial Opening

08CX8ZZ Extirpation of Matter from Right Lacrimal Duct, Via Natural or Artificial Opening Endoscopic

08CY0ZZ Extirpation of Matter from Left Lacrimal Duct, Open Approach

08CY3ZZ Extirpation of Matter from Left Lacrimal Duct, Percutaneous Approach

08CY7ZZ Extirpation of Matter from Left Lacrimal Duct, Via Natural or Artificial Opening

08CY8ZZ Extirpation of Matter from Left Lacrimal Duct, Via Natural or Artificial Opening Endoscopic

---

♀ Female-only   ♂ Male-only   ▲ Limited Coverage   ● Non-OR   ▦ HAC-associated procedure   ▲ Non-covered procedures   ✚ Combination

D – Eye, Extraction

view Coding Guidelines B3.4a and B3.4b

8XZX	Extraction of Right Cornea, External Approach, Diagnostic	08D9XZX	Extraction of Left Cornea, External Approach, Diagnostic	08DJ3ZZ	Extraction of Right Lens, Percutaneous Approach
8XZZ	Extraction of Right Cornea, External Approach	08D9XZZ	Extraction of Left Cornea, External Approach	08DK3ZZ	Extraction of Left Lens, Percutaneous Approach

F – Eye, Fragmentation

43ZZ	Fragmentation in Right Vitreous, Percutaneous Approach	08F53ZZ	Fragmentation in Left Vitreous, Percutaneous Approach
3F4XZZ	Fragmentation in Right Vitreous, External Approach	▲08F5XZZ	Fragmentation in Left Vitreous, External Approach

H – Eye, Insertion

4005Z	Insertion of Epiretinal Visual Prosthesis into Right Eye, Open Approach	08H0X3Z	Insertion of Infusion Device into Right Eye, External Approach	08H1X1Z	Insertion of Radioactive Element into Left Eye, External Approach
I031Z	Insertion of Radioactive Element into Right Eye, Percutaneous Approach	08H105Z	Insertion of Epiretinal Visual Prosthesis into Left Eye, Open Approach	08H1X3Z	Insertion of Infusion Device into Left Eye, External Approach
I033Z	Insertion of Infusion Device into Right Eye, Percutaneous Approach	08H131Z	Insertion of Radioactive Element into Left Eye, Percutaneous Approach		
I0X1Z	Insertion of Radioactive Element into Right Eye, External Approach	08H133Z	Insertion of Infusion Device into Left Eye, Percutaneous Approach		

J – Eye, Inspection

view Coding Guidelines B3.11a, B3.11b and B3.11c

40XZZ	Inspection of Right Eye, External Approach	08JKXZZ	Inspection of Left Lens, External Approach	08JM0ZZ	Inspection of Left Extraocular Muscle, Open Approach
	AHA CC: 1Q, 2015, 35-36	08JL0ZZ	Inspection of Right Extraocular Muscle, Open Approach	08JMXZZ	Inspection of Left Extraocular Muscle, External Approach
1XZZ	Inspection of Left Eye, External Approach	08JLXZZ	Inspection of Right Extraocular Muscle, External Approach		
JXZZ	Inspection of Right Lens, External Approach				

L – Eye, Occlusion

LX0CZ	Occlusion of Right Lacrimal Duct with Extraluminal Device, Open Approach	08LX7ZZ	Occlusion of Right Lacrimal Duct, Via Natural or Artificial Opening	08LY3DZ	Occlusion of Left Lacrimal Duct with Intraluminal Device, Percutaneous Approach
LX0DZ	Occlusion of Right Lacrimal Duct with Intraluminal Device, Open Approach	08LX8DZ	Occlusion of Right Lacrimal Duct with Intraluminal Device, Via Natural or Artificial Opening Endoscopic	08LY3ZZ	Occlusion of Left Lacrimal Duct, Percutaneous Approach
LX0ZZ	Occlusion of Right Lacrimal Duct, Open Approach	08LX8ZZ	Occlusion of Right Lacrimal Duct, Via Natural or Artificial Opening Endoscopic	08LY7DZ	Occlusion of Left Lacrimal Duct with Intraluminal Device, Via Natural or Artificial Opening
LX3CZ	Occlusion of Right Lacrimal Duct with Extraluminal Device, Percutaneous Approach	08LY0CZ	Occlusion of Left Lacrimal Duct with Extraluminal Device, Open Approach	08LY7ZZ	Occlusion of Left Lacrimal Duct, Via Natural or Artificial Opening
LX3DZ	Occlusion of Right Lacrimal Duct with Intraluminal Device, Percutaneous Approach	08LY0DZ	Occlusion of Left Lacrimal Duct with Intraluminal Device, Open Approach	08LY8DZ	Occlusion of Left Lacrimal Duct with Intraluminal Device, Via Natural or Artificial Opening Endoscopic
LX3ZZ	Occlusion of Right Lacrimal Duct, Percutaneous Approach	08LY0ZZ	Occlusion of Left Lacrimal Duct, Open Approach	08LY8ZZ	Occlusion of Left Lacrimal Duct, Via Natural or Artificial Opening Endoscopic
LX7DZ	Occlusion of Right Lacrimal Duct with Intraluminal Device, Via Natural or Artificial Opening	08LY3CZ	Occlusion of Left Lacrimal Duct with Extraluminal Device, Percutaneous Approach		

M – Eye, Reattachment

MNXZZ	Reattachment of Right Upper Eyelid, External Approach	08MQXZZ	Reattachment of Right Lower Eyelid, External Approach
MPXZZ	Reattachment of Left Upper Eyelid, External Approach	08MRXZZ	Reattachment of Left Lower Eyelid, External Approach

8N – Eye, Release

eview Coding Guidelines B3.13 and B3.14

3N0XZZ	Release Right Eye, External Approach	08N53ZZ	Release Left Vitreous, Percutaneous Approach	08NA3ZZ	Release Right Choroid, Percutaneous Approach
N1XZZ	Release Left Eye, External Approach	08N6XZZ	Release Right Sclera, External Approach	08NB0ZZ	Release Left Choroid, Open Approach
N23ZZ	Release Right Anterior Chamber, Percutaneous Approach	08N7XZZ	Release Left Sclera, External Approach	08NB3ZZ	Release Left Choroid, Percutaneous Approach
N33ZZ	Release Left Anterior Chamber, Percutaneous Approach	08N8XZZ	Release Right Cornea, External Approach	08NC3ZZ	Release Right Iris, Percutaneous Approach
N43ZZ	Release Right Vitreous, Percutaneous Approach	08N9XZZ	Release Left Cornea, External Approach	08ND3ZZ	Release Left Iris, Percutaneous Approach
		08NA0ZZ	Release Right Choroid, Open Approach		

Female-only   ♂ Male-only   ▲ Limited Coverage   ● Non-OR   HAC-associated procedure   ▲ Non-covered procedures   ✚ Combination

08NE3ZZ	Release Right Retina, Percutaneous Approach
08NF3ZZ	Release Left Retina, Percutaneous Approach
08NG3ZZ	Release Right Retinal Vessel, Percutaneous Approach
08NH3ZZ	Release Left Retinal Vessel, Percutaneous Approach
08NJ3ZZ	Release Right Lens, Percutaneous Approach
08NK3ZZ	Release Left Lens, Percutaneous Approach
08NL0ZZ	Release Right Extraocular Muscle, Open Approach
08NL3ZZ	Release Right Extraocular Muscle, Percutaneous Approach
08NM0ZZ	Release Left Extraocular Muscle, Open Approach
08NM3ZZ	Release Left Extraocular Muscle, Percutaneous Approach
08NN0ZZ	Release Right Upper Eyelid, Open Approach
08NN3ZZ	Release Right Upper Eyelid, Percutaneous Approach
08NNXZZ	Release Right Upper Eyelid, External Approach
08NP0ZZ	Release Left Upper Eyelid, Open Approach
08NP3ZZ	Release Left Upper Eyelid, Percutaneous Approach
08NPXZZ	Release Left Upper Eyelid, External Approach
08NQ0ZZ	Release Right Lower Eyelid, Open Approach
08NQ3ZZ	Release Right Lower Eyelid, Percutaneous Approach
08NQXZZ	Release Right Lower Eyelid, External Approach
08NR0ZZ	Release Left Lower Eyelid, Open Approach
08NR3ZZ	Release Left Lower Eyelid, Percutaneous Approach
08NRXZZ	Release Left Lower Eyelid, External Approach
08NSXZZ	Release Right Conjunctiva, External Approach
08NTXZZ	Release Left Conjunctiva, External Approach
08NV0ZZ	Release Right Lacrimal Gland, Open Approach
08NV3ZZ	Release Right Lacrimal Gland, Percutaneous Approach
08NW0ZZ	Release Left Lacrimal Gland, Open Approach
08NW3ZZ	Release Left Lacrimal Gland, Percutaneous Approach
08NX0ZZ	Release Right Lacrimal Duct, Open Approach
08NX3ZZ	Release Right Lacrimal Duct, Percutaneous Approach
08NX7ZZ	Release Right Lacrimal Duct, Via Natural or Artificial Opening
08NX8ZZ	Release Right Lacrimal Duct, Via Natural or Artificial Opening Endoscopic
08NY0ZZ	Release Left Lacrimal Duct, Open Approach
08NY3ZZ	Release Left Lacrimal Duct, Percutaneous Approach
08NY7ZZ	Release Left Lacrimal Duct, Via Natural or Artificial Opening
08NY8ZZ	Release Left Lacrimal Duct, Via Natural or Artificial Opening Endoscopic

08P – Eye, Removal

Review Coding Guideline B6.1c

08P000Z	Removal of Drainage Device from Right Eye, Open Approach
08P001Z	Removal of Radioactive Element from Right Eye, Open Approach
08P003Z	Removal of Infusion Device from Right Eye, Open Approach
08P007Z	Removal of Autologous Tissue Substitute from Right Eye, Open Approach
08P00CZ	Removal of Extraluminal Device from Right Eye, Open Approach
08P00DZ	Removal of Intraluminal Device from Right Eye, Open Approach
08P00JZ	Removal of Synthetic Substitute from Right Eye, Open Approach
08P00KZ	Removal of Nonautologous Tissue Substitute from Right Eye, Open Approach
08P030Z	Removal of Drainage Device from Right Eye, Percutaneous Approach
08P031Z	Removal of Radioactive Element from Right Eye, Percutaneous Approach
08P033Z	Removal of Infusion Device from Right Eye, Percutaneous Approach
08P037Z	Removal of Autologous Tissue Substitute from Right Eye, Percutaneous Approach
08P03CZ	Removal of Extraluminal Device from Right Eye, Percutaneous Approach
08P03DZ	Removal of Intraluminal Device from Right Eye, Percutaneous Approach
08P03JZ	Removal of Synthetic Substitute from Right Eye, Percutaneous Approach
08P03KZ	Removal of Nonautologous Tissue Substitute from Right Eye, Percutaneous Approach
08P070Z	Removal of Drainage Device from Right Eye, Via Natural or Artificial Opening
08P071Z	Removal of Radioactive Element from Right Eye, Via Natural or Artificial Opening
08P073Z	Removal of Infusion Device from Right Eye, Via Natural or Artificial Opening
08P077Z	Removal of Autologous Tissue Substitute from Right Eye, Via Natural or Artificial Opening
08P07CZ	Removal of Extraluminal Device from Right Eye, Via Natural or Artificial Opening
08P07DZ	Removal of Intraluminal Device from Right Eye, Via Natural or Artificial Opening
08P07JZ	Removal of Synthetic Substitute from Right Eye, Via Natural or Artificial Opening
08P07KZ	Removal of Nonautologous Tissue Substitute from Right Eye, Via Natural or Artificial Opening
08P080Z	Removal of Drainage Device from Right Eye, Via Natural or Artificial Opening Endoscopic
08P081Z	Removal of Radioactive Element from Right Eye, Via Natural or Artificial Opening Endoscopic
08P083Z	Removal of Infusion Device from Right Eye, Via Natural or Artificial Opening Endoscopic
08P087Z	Removal of Autologous Tissue Substitute from Right Eye, Via Natural or Artificial Opening Endoscopic
08P08CZ	Removal of Extraluminal Device from Right Eye, Via Natural or Artificial Opening Endoscopic
08P08DZ	Removal of Intraluminal Device from Right Eye, Via Natural or Artificial Opening Endoscopic
08P08JZ	Removal of Synthetic Substitute from Right Eye, Via Natural or Artificial Opening Endoscopic
08P08KZ	Removal of Nonautologous Tissue Substitute from Right Eye, Via Natural or Artificial Opening Endoscopic
08P0X0Z	Removal of Drainage Device from Right Eye, External Approach
08P0X1Z	Removal of Radioactive Element from Right Eye, External Approach
08P0X3Z	Removal of Infusion Device from Right Eye, External Approach
08P0X7Z	Removal of Autologous Tissue Substitute from Right Eye, External Approach
08P0XCZ	Removal of Extraluminal Device from Right Eye, External Approach
08P0XDZ	Removal of Intraluminal Device from Right Eye, External Approach
08P0XJZ	Removal of Synthetic Substitute from Right Eye, External Approach
08P0XKZ	Removal of Nonautologous Tissue Substitute from Right Eye, External Approach
08P100Z	Removal of Drainage Device from Left Eye, Open Approach
08P101Z	Removal of Radioactive Element from Left Eye, Open Approach
08P103Z	Removal of Infusion Device from Left Eye, Open Approach
08P107Z	Removal of Autologous Tissue Substitute from Left Eye, Open Approach
08P10CZ	Removal of Extraluminal Device from Left Eye, Open Approach
08P10DZ	Removal of Intraluminal Device from Left Eye, Open Approach
08P10JZ	Removal of Synthetic Substitute from Left Eye, Open Approach
08P10KZ	Removal of Nonautologous Tissue Substitute from Left Eye, Open Approach
08P130Z	Removal of Drainage Device from Left Eye, Percutaneous Approach
08P131Z	Removal of Radioactive Element from Left Eye, Percutaneous Approach
08P133Z	Removal of Infusion Device from Left Eye, Percutaneous Approach
08P137Z	Removal of Autologous Tissue Substitute from Left Eye, Percutaneous Approach
08P13CZ	Removal of Extraluminal Device from Left Eye, Percutaneous Approach
08P13DZ	Removal of Intraluminal Device from Left Eye, Percutaneous Approach
08P13JZ	Removal of Synthetic Substitute from Left Eye, Percutaneous Approach
08P13KZ	Removal of Nonautologous Tissue Substitute from Left Eye, Percutaneous Approach
08P170Z	Removal of Drainage Device from Left Eye, Via Natural or Artificial Opening
08P171Z	Removal of Radioactive Element from Left Eye, Via Natural or Artificial Opening
08P173Z	Removal of Infusion Device from Left Eye, Via Natural or Artificial Opening
08P177Z	Removal of Autologous Tissue Substitute from Left Eye, Via Natural or Artificial Opening
08P17CZ	Removal of Extraluminal Device from Left Eye, Via Natural or Artificial Opening

♀ Female-only   ♂ Male-only   ▲ Limited Coverage   ● Non-OR   ▨▨ HAC-associated procedure   ▲ Non-covered procedures   ✚ Combination

...7DZ	Removal of Intraluminal Device from Left Eye, Via Natural or Artificial Opening	08P1X1Z	Removal of Radioactive Element from Left Eye, External Approach	08PL37Z	Removal of Autologous Tissue Substitute from Right Extraocular Muscle, Percutaneous Approach

...7DZ Removal of Intraluminal Device from Left Eye, Via Natural or Artificial Opening

...7JZ Removal of Synthetic Substitute from Left Eye, Via Natural or Artificial Opening

...7KZ Removal of Nonautologous Tissue Substitute from Left Eye, Via Natural or Artificial Opening

...80Z Removal of Drainage Device from Left Eye, Via Natural or Artificial Opening Endoscopic

...81Z Removal of Radioactive Element from Left Eye, Via Natural or Artificial Opening

...83Z Removal of Infusion Device from Left Eye, Via Natural or Artificial Opening Endoscopic

...87Z Removal of Autologous Tissue Substitute from Left Eye, Via Natural or Artificial Opening Endoscopic

...8CZ Removal of Extraluminal Device from Left Eye, Via Natural or Artificial Opening Endoscopic

...8DZ Removal of Intraluminal Device from Left Eye, Via Natural or Artificial Opening Endoscopic

...8JZ Removal of Synthetic Substitute from Left Eye, Via Natural or Artificial Opening Endoscopic

...18KZ Removal of Nonautologous Tissue Substitute from Left Eye, Via Natural or Artificial Opening Endoscopic

...1X0Z Removal of Drainage Device from Left Eye, External Approach

08P1X3Z Removal of Infusion Device from Left Eye, External Approach

08P1X7Z Removal of Autologous Tissue Substitute from Left Eye, External Approach

08P1XCZ Removal of Extraluminal Device from Left Eye, External Approach

08P1XDZ Removal of Intraluminal Device from Left Eye, External Approach

08P1XJZ Removal of Synthetic Substitute from Left Eye, External Approach

08P1XKZ Removal of Nonautologous Tissue Substitute from Left Eye, External Approach

08PJ3JZ Removal of Synthetic Substitute from Right Lens, Percutaneous Approach

08PK3JZ Removal of Synthetic Substitute from Left Lens, Percutaneous Approach

08PL00Z Removal of Drainage Device from Right Extraocular Muscle, Open Approach

08PL07Z Removal of Autologous Tissue Substitute from Right Extraocular Muscle, Open Approach

08PL0JZ Removal of Synthetic Substitute from Right Extraocular Muscle, Open Approach

08PL0KZ Removal of Nonautologous Tissue Substitute from Right Extraocular Muscle, Open Approach

08PL30Z Removal of Drainage Device from Right Extraocular Muscle, Percutaneous Approach

08PL3JZ Removal of Synthetic Substitute from Right Extraocular Muscle, Percutaneous Approach

08PL3KZ Removal of Nonautologous Tissue Substitute from Right Extraocular Muscle, Percutaneous Approach

08PM00Z Removal of Drainage Device from Left Extraocular Muscle, Open Approach

08PM07Z Removal of Autologous Tissue Substitute from Left Extraocular Muscle, Open Approach

08PM0JZ Removal of Synthetic Substitute from Left Extraocular Muscle, Open Approach

08PM0KZ Removal of Nonautologous Tissue Substitute from Left Extraocular Muscle, Open Approach

08PM30Z Removal of Drainage Device from Left Extraocular Muscle, Percutaneous Approach

08PM37Z Removal of Autologous Tissue Substitute from Left Extraocular Muscle, Percutaneous Approach

08PM3JZ Removal of Synthetic Substitute from Left Extraocular Muscle, Percutaneous Approach

08PM3KZ Removal of Nonautologous Tissue Substitute from Left Extraocular Muscle, Percutaneous Approach

Q – Eye, Repair

...0XZZ Repair Right Eye, External Approach

...1XZZ Repair Left Eye, External Approach

...23ZZ Repair Right Anterior Chamber, Percutaneous Approach

...33ZZ Repair Left Anterior Chamber, Percutaneous Approach

...43ZZ Repair Right Vitreous, Percutaneous Approach

...53ZZ Repair Left Vitreous, Percutaneous Approach

...6XZZ Repair Right Sclera, External Approach

...7XZZ Repair Left Sclera, External Approach

08Q8XZZ Repair Right Cornea, External Approach

08Q9XZZ Repair Left Cornea, External Approach

...A0ZZ Repair Right Choroid, Open Approach

...A3ZZ Repair Right Choroid, Percutaneous Approach

...B0ZZ Repair Left Choroid, Open Approach

...B3ZZ Repair Left Choroid, Percutaneous Approach

...C3ZZ Repair Right Iris, Percutaneous Approach

...D3ZZ Repair Left Iris, Percutaneous Approach

...E3ZZ Repair Right Retina, Percutaneous Approach

...F3ZZ Repair Left Retina, Percutaneous Approach

...G3ZZ Repair Right Retinal Vessel, Percutaneous Approach

...H3ZZ Repair Left Retinal Vessel, Percutaneous Approach

08QJ3ZZ Repair Right Lens, Percutaneous Approach

08QK3ZZ Repair Left Lens, Percutaneous Approach

08QL0ZZ Repair Right Extraocular Muscle, Open Approach

08QL3ZZ Repair Right Extraocular Muscle, Percutaneous Approach

08QM0ZZ Repair Left Extraocular Muscle, Open Approach

08QM3ZZ Repair Left Extraocular Muscle, Percutaneous Approach

08QN0ZZ Repair Right Upper Eyelid, Open Approach

08QN3ZZ Repair Right Upper Eyelid, Percutaneous Approach

08QNXZZ Repair Right Upper Eyelid, External Approach

08QP0ZZ Repair Left Upper Eyelid, Open Approach

08QP3ZZ Repair Left Upper Eyelid, Percutaneous Approach

08QPXZZ Repair Left Upper Eyelid, External Approach

08QQ0ZZ Repair Right Lower Eyelid, Open Approach

08QQ3ZZ Repair Right Lower Eyelid, Percutaneous Approach

08QQXZZ Repair Right Lower Eyelid, External Approach

08QR0ZZ Repair Left Lower Eyelid, Open Approach

08QR3ZZ Repair Left Lower Eyelid, Percutaneous Approach

08QRXZZ Repair Left Lower Eyelid, External Approach

08QSXZZ Repair Right Conjunctiva, External Approach

08QTXZZ Repair Left Conjunctiva, External Approach

08QV0ZZ Repair Right Lacrimal Gland, Open Approach

08QV3ZZ Repair Right Lacrimal Gland, Percutaneous Approach

08QW0ZZ Repair Left Lacrimal Gland, Open Approach

08QW3ZZ Repair Left Lacrimal Gland, Percutaneous Approach

08QX0ZZ Repair Right Lacrimal Duct, Open Approach

08QX3ZZ Repair Right Lacrimal Duct, Percutaneous Approach

08QX7ZZ Repair Right Lacrimal Duct, Via Natural or Artificial Opening

08QX8ZZ Repair Right Lacrimal Duct, Via Natural or Artificial Opening Endoscopic

08QY0ZZ Repair Left Lacrimal Duct, Open Approach

08QY3ZZ Repair Left Lacrimal Duct, Percutaneous Approach

08QY7ZZ Repair Left Lacrimal Duct, Via Natural or Artificial Opening

08QY8ZZ Repair Left Lacrimal Duct, Via Natural or Artificial Opening Endoscopic

R – Eye, Replacement

...R007Z Replacement of Right Eye with Autologous Tissue Substitute, Open Approach

...R00JZ Replacement of Right Eye with Synthetic Substitute, Open Approach

08R00KZ Replacement of Right Eye with Nonautologous Tissue Substitute, Open Approach

08R037Z Replacement of Right Eye with Autologous Tissue Substitute, Percutaneous Approach

08R03JZ Replacement of Right Eye with Synthetic Substitute, Percutaneous Approach

08R03KZ Replacement of Right Eye with Nonautologous Tissue Substitute, Percutaneous Approach

Female-only ♂ Male-only ▲ Limited Coverage ● Non-OR ■ HAC-associated procedure ▲ Non-covered procedures ✚ Combination

08R107Z	Replacement of Left Eye with Autologous Tissue Substitute, Open Approach
08R10JZ	Replacement of Left Eye with Synthetic Substitute, Open Approach
08R10KZ	Replacement of Left Eye with Nonautologous Tissue Substitute, Open Approach
08R137Z	Replacement of Left Eye with Autologous Tissue Substitute, Percutaneous Approach
08R13JZ	Replacement of Left Eye with Synthetic Substitute, Percutaneous Approach
08R13KZ	Replacement of Left Eye with Nonautologous Tissue Substitute, Percutaneous Approach
08R437Z	Replacement of Right Vitreous with Autologous Tissue Substitute, Percutaneous Approach
08R43JZ	Replacement of Right Vitreous with Synthetic Substitute, Percutaneous Approach
08R43KZ	Replacement of Right Vitreous with Nonautologous Tissue Substitute, Percutaneous Approach
08R537Z	Replacement of Left Vitreous with Autologous Tissue Substitute, Percutaneous Approach
08R53JZ	Replacement of Left Vitreous with Synthetic Substitute, Percutaneous Approach
08R53KZ	Replacement of Left Vitreous with Nonautologous Tissue Substitute, Percutaneous Approach
08R6X7Z	Replacement of Right Sclera with Autologous Tissue Substitute, External Approach
08R6XJZ	Replacement of Right Sclera with Synthetic Substitute, External Approach
08R6XKZ	Replacement of Right Sclera with Nonautologous Tissue Substitute, External Approach
08R7X7Z	Replacement of Left Sclera with Autologous Tissue Substitute, External Approach
08R7XJZ	Replacement of Left Sclera with Synthetic Substitute, External Approach
08R7XKZ	Replacement of Left Sclera with Nonautologous Tissue Substitute, External Approach
08R837Z	Replacement of Right Cornea with Autologous Tissue Substitute, Percutaneous Approach
08R83JZ	Replacement of Right Cornea with Synthetic Substitute, Percutaneous Approach
08R83KZ	Replacement of Right Cornea with Nonautologous Tissue Substitute, Percutaneous Approach
08R8X7Z	Replacement of Right Cornea with Autologous Tissue Substitute, External Approach
08R8XJZ	Replacement of Right Cornea with Synthetic Substitute, External Approach
08R8XKZ	Replacement of Right Cornea with Nonautologous Tissue Substitute, External Approach
08R937Z	Replacement of Left Cornea with Autologous Tissue Substitute, Percutaneous Approach
08R93JZ	Replacement of Left Cornea with Synthetic Substitute, Percutaneous Approach
08R93KZ	Replacement of Left Cornea with Nonautologous Tissue Substitute, Percutaneous Approach
08R9X7Z	Replacement of Left Cornea with Autologous Tissue Substitute, External Approach

08R9XJZ	Replacement of Left Cornea with Synthetic Substitute, External Approach
08R9XKZ	Replacement of Left Cornea with Nonautologous Tissue Substitute, External Approach
08RA07Z	Replacement of Right Choroid with Autologous Tissue Substitute, Open Approach
08RA0JZ	Replacement of Right Choroid with Synthetic Substitute, Open Approach
08RA0KZ	Replacement of Right Choroid with Nonautologous Tissue Substitute, Open Approach
08RA37Z	Replacement of Right Choroid with Autologous Tissue Substitute, Percutaneous Approach
08RA3JZ	Replacement of Right Choroid with Synthetic Substitute, Percutaneous Approach
08RA3KZ	Replacement of Right Choroid with Nonautologous Tissue Substitute, Percutaneous Approach
08RB07Z	Replacement of Left Choroid with Autologous Tissue Substitute, Open Approach
08RB0JZ	Replacement of Left Choroid with Synthetic Substitute, Open Approach
08RB0KZ	Replacement of Left Choroid with Nonautologous Tissue Substitute, Open Approach
08RB37Z	Replacement of Left Choroid with Autologous Tissue Substitute, Percutaneous Approach
08RB3JZ	Replacement of Left Choroid with Synthetic Substitute, Percutaneous Approach
08RB3KZ	Replacement of Left Choroid with Nonautologous Tissue Substitute, Percutaneous Approach
08RC37Z	Replacement of Right Iris with Autologous Tissue Substitute, Percutaneous Approach
08RC3JZ	Replacement of Right Iris with Synthetic Substitute, Percutaneous Approach
08RC3KZ	Replacement of Right Iris with Nonautologous Tissue Substitute, Percutaneous Approach
08RD37Z	Replacement of Left Iris with Autologous Tissue Substitute, Percutaneous Approach
08RD3JZ	Replacement of Left Iris with Synthetic Substitute, Percutaneous Approach
08RD3KZ	Replacement of Left Iris with Nonautologous Tissue Substitute, Percutaneous Approach
08RG37Z	Replacement of Right Retinal Vessel with Autologous Tissue Substitute, Percutaneous Approach
08RG3JZ	Replacement of Right Retinal Vessel with Synthetic Substitute, Percutaneous Approach
08RG3KZ	Replacement of Right Retinal Vessel with Nonautologous Tissue Substitute, Percutaneous Approach
08RH37Z	Replacement of Left Retinal Vessel with Autologous Tissue Substitute, Percutaneous Approach
08RH3JZ	Replacement of Left Retinal Vessel with Synthetic Substitute, Percutaneous Approach
08RH3KZ	Replacement of Left Retinal Vessel with Nonautologous Tissue Substitute, Percutaneous Approach
08RJ30Z	Replacement of Right Lens with Intraocular Telescope, Percutaneous Approach
08RJ37Z	Replacement of Right Lens with Autologous Tissue Substitute, Percutaneous Approach

08RJ3JZ	Replacement of Right Lens with Synthetic Substitute, Percutaneous Approach
08RJ3KZ	Replacement of Right Lens with Nonautologous Tissue Substitute, Percutaneous Approach
08RK30Z	Replacement of Left Lens with Intraocular Telescope, Percutaneous Approach
08RK37Z	Replacement of Left Lens with Autologous Tissue Substitute, Percutaneous Approach
08RK3JZ	Replacement of Left Lens with Synthetic Substitute, Percutaneous Approach
08RK3KZ	Replacement of Left Lens with Nonautologous Tissue Substitute, Percutaneous Approach
08RN07Z	Replacement of Right Upper Eyelid with Autologous Tissue Substitute, Open Approach
08RN0JZ	Replacement of Right Upper Eyelid with Synthetic Substitute, Open Approach
08RN0KZ	Replacement of Right Upper Eyelid with Nonautologous Tissue Substitute, Open Approach
08RN37Z	Replacement of Right Upper Eyelid with Autologous Tissue Substitute, Percutaneous Approach
08RN3JZ	Replacement of Right Upper Eyelid with Synthetic Substitute, Percutaneous Approach
08RN3KZ	Replacement of Right Upper Eyelid with Nonautologous Tissue Substitute, Percutaneous Approach
08RNX7Z	Replacement of Right Upper Eyelid with Autologous Tissue Substitute, External Approach
08RNXJZ	Replacement of Right Upper Eyelid with Synthetic Substitute, External Approach
08RNXKZ	Replacement of Right Upper Eyelid with Nonautologous Tissue Substitute, External Approach
08RP07Z	Replacement of Left Upper Eyelid with Autologous Tissue Substitute, Open Approach
08RP0JZ	Replacement of Left Upper Eyelid with Synthetic Substitute, Open Approach
08RP0KZ	Replacement of Left Upper Eyelid with Nonautologous Tissue Substitute, Open Approach
08RP37Z	Replacement of Left Upper Eyelid with Autologous Tissue Substitute, Percutaneous Approach
08RP3JZ	Replacement of Left Upper Eyelid with Synthetic Substitute, Percutaneous Approach
08RP3KZ	Replacement of Left Upper Eyelid with Nonautologous Tissue Substitute, Percutaneous Approach
08RPX7Z	Replacement of Left Upper Eyelid with Autologous Tissue Substitute, External Approach
08RPXJZ	Replacement of Left Upper Eyelid with Synthetic Substitute, External Approach
08RPXKZ	Replacement of Left Upper Eyelid with Nonautologous Tissue Substitute, External Approach
08RQ07Z	Replacement of Right Lower Eyelid with Autologous Tissue Substitute, Open Approach
08RQ0JZ	Replacement of Right Lower Eyelid with Synthetic Substitute, Open Approach
08RQ0KZ	Replacement of Right Lower Eyelid with Nonautologous Tissue Substitute, Open Approach
08RQ37Z	Replacement of Right Lower Eyelid with Autologous Tissue Substitute, Percutaneous Approach

♀ Female-only   ♂ Male-only   ▲ Limited Coverage   ● Non-OR   ▰ HAC-associated procedure   ▲ Non-covered procedures   ✚ Combinat

Q3JZ	Replacement of Right Lower Eyelid with Synthetic Substitute, Percutaneous Approach
Q3KZ	Replacement of Right Lower Eyelid with Nonautologous Tissue Substitute, Percutaneous Approach
QX7Z	Replacement of Right Lower Eyelid with Autologous Tissue Substitute, External Approach
QXJZ	Replacement of Right Lower Eyelid with Synthetic Substitute, External Approach
QXKZ	Replacement of Right Lower Eyelid with Nonautologous Tissue Substitute, External Approach
R07Z	Replacement of Left Lower Eyelid with Autologous Tissue Substitute, Open Approach
R0JZ	Replacement of Left Lower Eyelid with Synthetic Substitute, Open Approach
R0KZ	Replacement of Left Lower Eyelid with Nonautologous Tissue Substitute, Open Approach
R37Z	Replacement of Left Lower Eyelid with Autologous Tissue Substitute, Percutaneous Approach
R3JZ	Replacement of Left Lower Eyelid with Synthetic Substitute, Percutaneous Approach
R3KZ	Replacement of Left Lower Eyelid with Nonautologous Tissue Substitute, Percutaneous Approach
RX7Z	Replacement of Left Lower Eyelid with Autologous Tissue Substitute, External Approach
RXJZ	Replacement of Left Lower Eyelid with Synthetic Substitute, External Approach
RXKZ	Replacement of Left Lower Eyelid with Nonautologous Tissue Substitute, External Approach
RSX7Z	Replacement of Right Conjunctiva with Autologous Tissue Substitute, External Approach

08RSXJZ	Replacement of Right Conjunctiva with Synthetic Substitute, External Approach
08RSXKZ	Replacement of Right Conjunctiva with Nonautologous Tissue Substitute, External Approach
08RTX7Z	Replacement of Left Conjunctiva with Autologous Tissue Substitute, External Approach
08RTXJZ	Replacement of Left Conjunctiva with Synthetic Substitute, External Approach
08RTXKZ	Replacement of Left Conjunctiva with Nonautologous Tissue Substitute, External Approach
08RX07Z	Replacement of Right Lacrimal Duct with Autologous Tissue Substitute, Open Approach
08RX0JZ	Replacement of Right Lacrimal Duct with Synthetic Substitute, Open Approach
08RX0KZ	Replacement of Right Lacrimal Duct with Nonautologous Tissue Substitute, Open Approach
08RX37Z	Replacement of Right Lacrimal Duct with Autologous Tissue Substitute, Percutaneous Approach
08RX3JZ	Replacement of Right Lacrimal Duct with Synthetic Substitute, Percutaneous Approach
08RX3KZ	Replacement of Right Lacrimal Duct with Nonautologous Tissue Substitute, Percutaneous Approach
08RX77Z	Replacement of Right Lacrimal Duct with Autologous Tissue Substitute, Via Natural or Artificial Opening
08RX7JZ	Replacement of Right Lacrimal Duct with Synthetic Substitute, Via Natural or Artificial Opening
08RX7KZ	Replacement of Right Lacrimal Duct with Nonautologous Tissue Substitute, Via Natural or Artificial Opening
08RX87Z	Replacement of Right Lacrimal Duct with Autologous Tissue Substitute, Via Natural or Artificial Opening Endoscopic

08RX8JZ	Replacement of Right Lacrimal Duct with Synthetic Substitute, Via Natural or Artificial Opening Endoscopic
08RX8KZ	Replacement of Right Lacrimal Duct with Nonautologous Tissue Substitute, Via Natural or Artificial Opening Endoscopic
08RY07Z	Replacement of Left Lacrimal Duct with Autologous Tissue Substitute, Open Approach
08RY0JZ	Replacement of Left Lacrimal Duct with Synthetic Substitute, Open Approach
08RY0KZ	Replacement of Left Lacrimal Duct with Nonautologous Tissue Substitute, Open Approach
08RY37Z	Replacement of Left Lacrimal Duct with Autologous Tissue Substitute, Percutaneous Approach
08RY3JZ	Replacement of Left Lacrimal Duct with Synthetic Substitute, Percutaneous Approach
08RY3KZ	Replacement of Left Lacrimal Duct with Nonautologous Tissue Substitute, Percutaneous Approach
08RY77Z	Replacement of Left Lacrimal Duct with Autologous Tissue Substitute, Via Natural or Artificial Opening
08RY7JZ	Replacement of Left Lacrimal Duct with Synthetic Substitute, Via Natural or Artificial Opening
08RY7KZ	Replacement of Left Lacrimal Duct with Nonautologous Tissue Substitute, Via Natural or Artificial Opening
08RY87Z	Replacement of Left Lacrimal Duct with Autologous Tissue Substitute, Via Natural or Artificial Opening Endoscopic
08RY8JZ	Replacement of Left Lacrimal Duct with Synthetic Substitute, Via Natural or Artificial Opening Endoscopic
08RY8KZ	Replacement of Left Lacrimal Duct with Nonautologous Tissue Substitute, Via Natural or Artificial Opening Endoscopic

S – Eye, Reposition

C3ZZ	Reposition Right Iris, Percutaneous Approach
D3ZZ	Reposition Left Iris, Percutaneous Approach
G3ZZ	Reposition Right Retinal Vessel, Percutaneous Approach
H3ZZ	Reposition Left Retinal Vessel, Percutaneous Approach
J3ZZ	Reposition Right Lens, Percutaneous Approach
K3ZZ	Reposition Left Lens, Percutaneous Approach
L0ZZ	Reposition Right Extraocular Muscle, Open Approach
L3ZZ	Reposition Right Extraocular Muscle, Percutaneous Approach
M0ZZ	Reposition Left Extraocular Muscle, Open Approach
M3ZZ	Reposition Left Extraocular Muscle, Percutaneous Approach
N0ZZ	Reposition Right Upper Eyelid, Open Approach
N3ZZ	Reposition Right Upper Eyelid, Percutaneous Approach

08SNXZZ	Reposition Right Upper Eyelid, External Approach
08SP0ZZ	Reposition Left Upper Eyelid, Open Approach
08SP3ZZ	Reposition Left Upper Eyelid, Percutaneous Approach
08SPXZZ	Reposition Left Upper Eyelid, External Approach
08SQ0ZZ	Reposition Right Lower Eyelid, Open Approach
08SQ3ZZ	Reposition Right Lower Eyelid, Percutaneous Approach
08SQXZZ	Reposition Right Lower Eyelid, External Approach
08SR0ZZ	Reposition Left Lower Eyelid, Open Approach
08SR3ZZ	Reposition Left Lower Eyelid, Percutaneous Approach
08SRXZZ	Reposition Left Lower Eyelid, External Approach
08SV0ZZ	Reposition Right Lacrimal Gland, Open Approach
08SV3ZZ	Reposition Right Lacrimal Gland, Percutaneous Approach

08SW0ZZ	Reposition Left Lacrimal Gland, Open Approach
08SW3ZZ	Reposition Left Lacrimal Gland, Percutaneous Approach
08SX0ZZ	Reposition Right Lacrimal Duct, Open Approach
08SX3ZZ	Reposition Right Lacrimal Duct, Percutaneous Approach
08SX7ZZ	Reposition Right Lacrimal Duct, Via Natural or Artificial Opening
08SX8ZZ	Reposition Right Lacrimal Duct, Via Natural or Artificial Opening Endoscopic
08SY0ZZ	Reposition Left Lacrimal Duct, Open Approach
08SY3ZZ	Reposition Left Lacrimal Duct, Percutaneous Approach
08SY7ZZ	Reposition Left Lacrimal Duct, Via Natural or Artificial Opening
08SY8ZZ	Reposition Left Lacrimal Duct, Via Natural or Artificial Opening Endoscopic

T – Eye, Resection

Review Coding Guideline B3.8

T0XZZ	Resection of Right Eye, External Approach
T1XZZ	Resection of Left Eye, External Approach

08T43ZZ	Resection of Right Vitreous, Percutaneous Approach

08T53ZZ	Resection of Left Vitreous, Percutaneous Approach

♀ Female-only   ♂ Male-only   ▲ Limited Coverage   ● Non-OR   ■ HAC-associated procedure   ▲ Non-covered procedures   ✚ Combination

08T8XZZ	Resection of Right Cornea, External Approach
08T9XZZ	Resection of Left Cornea, External Approach
08TC3ZZ	Resection of Right Iris, Percutaneous Approach
08TD3ZZ	Resection of Left Iris, Percutaneous Approach
08TJ3ZZ	Resection of Right Lens, Percutaneous Approach
08TK3ZZ	Resection of Left Lens, Percutaneous Approach
08TL0ZZ	Resection of Right Extraocular Muscle, Open Approach
08TL3ZZ	Resection of Right Extraocular Muscle, Percutaneous Approach
08TM0ZZ	Resection of Left Extraocular Muscle, Open Approach
08TM3ZZ	Resection of Left Extraocular Muscle, Percutaneous Approach

08TN0ZZ	Resection of Right Upper Eyelid, Open Approach
08TNXZZ	Resection of Right Upper Eyelid, External Approach
08TP0ZZ	Resection of Left Upper Eyelid, Open Approach
08TPXZZ	Resection of Left Upper Eyelid, External Approach
08TQ0ZZ	Resection of Right Lower Eyelid, Open Approach
08TQXZZ	Resection of Right Lower Eyelid, External Approach
08TR0ZZ	Resection of Left Lower Eyelid, Open Approach
08TRXZZ	Resection of Left Lower Eyelid, External Approach
08TV0ZZ	Resection of Right Lacrimal Gland, Open Approach
08TV3ZZ	Resection of Right Lacrimal Gland, Percutaneous Approach

08TW0ZZ	Resection of Left Lacrimal Gland, Open Approach
08TW3ZZ	Resection of Left Lacrimal Gland, Percutaneous Approach
08TX0ZZ	Resection of Right Lacrimal Duct, Open Approach
08TX3ZZ	Resection of Right Lacrimal Duct, Percutaneous Approach
08TX7ZZ	Resection of Right Lacrimal Duct, Via Natural or Artificial Opening
08TX8ZZ	Resection of Right Lacrimal Duct, Via Natural or Artificial Opening Endoscopic
08TY0ZZ	Resection of Left Lacrimal Duct, Open Approach
08TY3ZZ	Resection of Left Lacrimal Duct, Percutaneous Approach
08TY7ZZ	Resection of Left Lacrimal Duct, Via Natural or Artificial Opening
08TY8ZZ	Resection of Left Lacrimal Duct, Via Natural or Artificial Opening Endoscopic

08U – Eye, Supplement

08U007Z	Supplement of Right Eye with Autologous Tissue Substitute, Open Approach
08U00JZ	Supplement of Right Eye with Synthetic Substitute, Open Approach
08U00KZ	Supplement of Right Eye with Nonautologous Tissue Substitute, Open Approach
08U037Z	Supplement of Right Eye with Autologous Tissue Substitute, Percutaneous Approach
08U03JZ	Supplement of Right Eye with Synthetic Substitute, Percutaneous Approach
08U03KZ	Supplement of Right Eye with Nonautologous Tissue Substitute, Percutaneous Approach
08U107Z	Supplement of Left Eye with Autologous Tissue Substitute, Open Approach
08U10JZ	Supplement of Left Eye with Synthetic Substitute, Open Approach
08U10KZ	Supplement of Left Eye with Nonautologous Tissue Substitute, Open Approach
08U137Z	Supplement of Left Eye with Autologous Tissue Substitute, Percutaneous Approach
08U13JZ	Supplement of Left Eye with Synthetic Substitute, Percutaneous Approach
08U13KZ	Supplement of Left Eye with Nonautologous Tissue Substitute, Percutaneous Approach
08U807Z	Supplement Right Cornea with Autologous Tissue Substitute, Open Approach
08U80JZ	Supplement Right Cornea with Synthetic Substitute, Open Approach
▲ **08U80KZ**	Supplement Right Cornea with Nonautologous Tissue Substitute, Open Approach
08U837Z	Supplement Right Cornea with Autologous Tissue Substitute, Percutaneous Approach
08U83JZ	Supplement Right Cornea with Synthetic Substitute, Percutaneous Approach
▲ **08U83KZ**	Supplement Right Cornea with Nonautologous Tissue Substitute, Percutaneous Approach
08U8X7Z	Supplement Right Cornea with Autologous Tissue Substitute, External Approach
08U8XJZ	Supplement Right Cornea with Synthetic Substitute, External Approach
▲ **08U8XKZ**	Supplement Right Cornea with Nonautologous Tissue Substitute, External Approach
08U907Z	Supplement Left Cornea with Autologous Tissue Substitute, Open Approach

08U90JZ	Supplement Left Cornea with Synthetic Substitute, Open Approach
▲ **08U90KZ**	Supplement Left Cornea with Nonautologous Tissue Substitute, Open Approach
08U937Z	Supplement Left Cornea with Autologous Tissue Substitute, Percutaneous Approach
08U93JZ	Supplement Left Cornea with Synthetic Substitute, Percutaneous Approach
▲ **08U93KZ**	Supplement Left Cornea with Nonautologous Tissue Substitute, Percutaneous Approach
08U9X7Z	Supplement Left Cornea with Autologous Tissue Substitute, External Approach
08U9XJZ	Supplement Left Cornea with Synthetic Substitute, External Approach
▲ **08U9XKZ**	Supplement Left Cornea with Nonautologous Tissue Substitute, External Approach
	AHA CC: 3Q, 2014, 31
08UC07Z	Supplement Right Iris with Autologous Tissue Substitute, Open Approach
08UC0JZ	Supplement Right Iris with Synthetic Substitute, Open Approach
08UC0KZ	Supplement Right Iris with Nonautologous Tissue Substitute, Open Approach
08UC37Z	Supplement Right Iris with Autologous Tissue Substitute, Percutaneous Approach
08UC3JZ	Supplement Right Iris with Synthetic Substitute, Percutaneous Approach
08UC3KZ	Supplement Right Iris with Nonautologous Tissue Substitute, Percutaneous Approach
08UD07Z	Supplement Left Iris with Autologous Tissue Substitute, Open Approach
08UD0JZ	Supplement Left Iris with Synthetic Substitute, Open Approach
08UD0KZ	Supplement Left Iris with Nonautologous Tissue Substitute, Open Approach
08UD37Z	Supplement Left Iris with Autologous Tissue Substitute, Percutaneous Approach
08UD3JZ	Supplement Left Iris with Synthetic Substitute, Percutaneous Approach
08UD3KZ	Supplement Left Iris with Nonautologous Tissue Substitute, Percutaneous Approach
08UE07Z	Supplement Right Retina with Autologous Tissue Substitute, Open Approach
08UE0JZ	Supplement Right Retina with Synthetic Substitute, Open Approach
08UE0KZ	Supplement Right Retina with Nonautologous Tissue Substitute, Open Approach
08UE37Z	Supplement Right Retina with Autologous Tissue Substitute, Percutaneous Approach
08UE3JZ	Supplement Right Retina with Synthetic Substitute, Percutaneous Approach

08UE3KZ	Supplement Right Retina with Nonautologous Tissue Substitute, Percutaneous Approach
08UF07Z	Supplement Left Retina with Autologous Tissue Substitute, Open Approach
08UF0JZ	Supplement Left Retina with Synthetic Substitute, Open Approach
08UF0KZ	Supplement Left Retina with Nonautologous Tissue Substitute, Open Approach
08UF37Z	Supplement Left Retina with Autologous Tissue Substitute, Percutaneous Approach
08UF3JZ	Supplement Left Retina with Synthetic Substitute, Percutaneous Approach
08UF3KZ	Supplement Left Retina with Nonautologous Tissue Substitute, Percutaneous Approach
08UG07Z	Supplement Right Retinal Vessel with Autologous Tissue Substitute, Open Approach
08UG0JZ	Supplement Right Retinal Vessel with Synthetic Substitute, Open Approach
08UG0KZ	Supplement Right Retinal Vessel with Nonautologous Tissue Substitute, Open Approach
08UG37Z	Supplement Right Retinal Vessel with Autologous Tissue Substitute, Percutaneous Approach
08UG3JZ	Supplement Right Retinal Vessel with Synthetic Substitute, Percutaneous Approach
08UG3KZ	Supplement Right Retinal Vessel with Nonautologous Tissue Substitute, Percutaneous Approach
08UH07Z	Supplement Left Retinal Vessel with Autologous Tissue Substitute, Open Approach
08UH0JZ	Supplement Left Retinal Vessel with Synthetic Substitute, Open Approach
08UH0KZ	Supplement Left Retinal Vessel with Nonautologous Tissue Substitute, Open Approach
08UH37Z	Supplement Left Retinal Vessel with Autologous Tissue Substitute, Percutaneous Approach
08UH3JZ	Supplement Left Retinal Vessel with Synthetic Substitute, Percutaneous Approach
08UH3KZ	Supplement Left Retinal Vessel with Nonautologous Tissue Substitute, Percutaneous Approach
08UL07Z	Supplement Right Extraocular Muscle with Autologous Tissue Substitute, Open Approach

L0JZ	Supplement Right Extraocular Muscle with Synthetic Substitute, Open Approach	
L0KZ	Supplement Right Extraocular Muscle with Nonautologous Tissue Substitute, Open Approach	
L37Z	Supplement Right Extraocular Muscle with Autologous Tissue Substitute, Percutaneous Approach	
L3JZ	Supplement Right Extraocular Muscle with Synthetic Substitute, Percutaneous Approach	
L3KZ	Supplement Right Extraocular Muscle with Nonautologous Tissue Substitute, Percutaneous Approach	

08UP3JZ Supplement Left Upper Eyelid with Synthetic Substitute, Percutaneous Approach

08UP3KZ Supplement Left Upper Eyelid with Nonautologous Tissue Substitute, Percutaneous Approach

08UPX7Z Supplement Left Upper Eyelid with Autologous Tissue Substitute, External Approach

08UPXJZ Supplement Left Upper Eyelid with Synthetic Substitute, External Approach

08UPXKZ Supplement Left Upper Eyelid with Nonautologous Tissue Substitute, External Approach

08UQ07Z Supplement Right Lower Eyelid with Autologous Tissue Substitute, Open Approach

08UQ0JZ Supplement Right Lower Eyelid with Synthetic Substitute, Open Approach

08UQ0KZ Supplement Right Lower Eyelid with Nonautologous Tissue Substitute, Open Approach

08UQ37Z Supplement Right Lower Eyelid with Autologous Tissue Substitute, Percutaneous Approach

08UQ3JZ Supplement Right Lower Eyelid with Synthetic Substitute, Percutaneous Approach

08UQ3KZ Supplement Right Lower Eyelid with Nonautologous Tissue Substitute, Percutaneous Approach

08UQX7Z Supplement Right Lower Eyelid with Autologous Tissue Substitute, External Approach

08UQXJZ Supplement Right Lower Eyelid with Synthetic Substitute, External Approach

08UQXKZ Supplement Right Lower Eyelid with Nonautologous Tissue Substitute, External Approach

08UR07Z Supplement Left Lower Eyelid with Autologous Tissue Substitute, Open Approach

08UR0JZ Supplement Left Lower Eyelid with Synthetic Substitute, Open Approach

08UR0KZ Supplement Left Lower Eyelid with Nonautologous Tissue Substitute, Open Approach

08UR37Z Supplement Left Lower Eyelid with Autologous Tissue Substitute, Percutaneous Approach

08UR3JZ Supplement Left Lower Eyelid with Synthetic Substitute, Percutaneous Approach

08UR3KZ Supplement Left Lower Eyelid with Nonautologous Tissue Substitute, Percutaneous Approach

08URX7Z Supplement Left Lower Eyelid with Autologous Tissue Substitute, External Approach

08URXJZ Supplement Left Lower Eyelid with Synthetic Substitute, External Approach

08URXKZ Supplement Left Lower Eyelid with Nonautologous Tissue Substitute, External Approach

08UX07Z Supplement Right Lacrimal Duct with Autologous Tissue Substitute, Open Approach

08UX0JZ Supplement Right Lacrimal Duct with Synthetic Substitute, Open Approach

M07Z Supplement Left Extraocular Muscle with Autologous Tissue Substitute, Open Approach

M0JZ Supplement Left Extraocular Muscle with Synthetic Substitute, Open Approach

M0KZ Supplement Left Extraocular Muscle with Nonautologous Tissue Substitute, Open Approach

M37Z Supplement Left Extraocular Muscle with Autologous Tissue Substitute, Percutaneous Approach

M3JZ Supplement Left Extraocular Muscle with Synthetic Substitute, Percutaneous Approach

M3KZ Supplement Left Extraocular Muscle with Nonautologous Tissue Substitute, Percutaneous Approach

N07Z Supplement Right Upper Eyelid with Autologous Tissue Substitute, Open Approach

N0JZ Supplement Right Upper Eyelid with Synthetic Substitute, Open Approach

N0KZ Supplement Right Upper Eyelid with Nonautologous Tissue Substitute, Open Approach

N37Z Supplement Right Upper Eyelid with Autologous Tissue Substitute, Percutaneous Approach

N3JZ Supplement Right Upper Eyelid with Synthetic Substitute, Percutaneous Approach

N3KZ Supplement Right Upper Eyelid with Nonautologous Tissue Substitute, Percutaneous Approach

NX7Z Supplement Right Upper Eyelid with Autologous Tissue Substitute, External Approach

NXJZ Supplement Right Upper Eyelid with Synthetic Substitute, External Approach

NXKZ Supplement Right Upper Eyelid with Nonautologous Tissue Substitute, External Approach

UP07Z Supplement Left Upper Eyelid with Autologous Tissue Substitute, Open Approach

UP0JZ Supplement Left Upper Eyelid with Synthetic Substitute, Open Approach

UP0KZ Supplement Left Upper Eyelid with Nonautologous Tissue Substitute, Open Approach

UP37Z Supplement Left Upper Eyelid with Autologous Tissue Substitute, Percutaneous Approach

08UX0KZ Supplement Right Lacrimal Duct with Nonautologous Tissue Substitute, Open Approach

08UX37Z Supplement Right Lacrimal Duct with Autologous Tissue Substitute, Percutaneous Approach

08UX3JZ Supplement Right Lacrimal Duct with Synthetic Substitute, Percutaneous Approach

08UX3KZ Supplement Right Lacrimal Duct with Nonautologous Tissue Substitute, Percutaneous Approach

08UX77Z Supplement Right Lacrimal Duct with Autologous Tissue Substitute, Via Natural or Artificial Opening

08UX7JZ Supplement Right Lacrimal Duct with Synthetic Substitute, Via Natural or Artificial Opening

08UX7KZ Supplement Right Lacrimal Duct with Nonautologous Tissue Substitute, Via Natural or Artificial Opening

08UX87Z Supplement Right Lacrimal Duct with Autologous Tissue Substitute, Via Natural or Artificial Opening Endoscopic

08UX8JZ Supplement Right Lacrimal Duct with Synthetic Substitute, Via Natural or Artificial Opening Endoscopic

08UX8KZ Supplement Right Lacrimal Duct with Nonautologous Tissue Substitute, Via Natural or Artificial Opening Endoscopic

08UY07Z Supplement Left Lacrimal Duct with Autologous Tissue Substitute, Open Approach

08UY0JZ Supplement Left Lacrimal Duct with Synthetic Substitute, Open Approach

08UY0KZ Supplement Left Lacrimal Duct with Nonautologous Tissue Substitute, Open Approach

08UY37Z Supplement Left Lacrimal Duct with Autologous Tissue Substitute, Percutaneous Approach

08UY3JZ Supplement Left Lacrimal Duct with Synthetic Substitute, Percutaneous Approach

08UY3KZ Supplement Left Lacrimal Duct with Nonautologous Tissue Substitute, Percutaneous Approach

08UY77Z Supplement Left Lacrimal Duct with Autologous Tissue Substitute, Via Natural or Artificial Opening

08UY7JZ Supplement Left Lacrimal Duct with Synthetic Substitute, Via Natural or Artificial Opening

08UY7KZ Supplement Left Lacrimal Duct with Nonautologous Tissue Substitute, Via Natural or Artificial Opening

08UY87Z Supplement Left Lacrimal Duct with Autologous Tissue Substitute, Via Natural or Artificial Opening Endoscopic

08UY8JZ Supplement Left Lacrimal Duct with Synthetic Substitute, Via Natural or Artificial Opening Endoscopic

08UY8KZ Supplement Left Lacrimal Duct with Nonautologous Tissue Substitute, Via Natural or Artificial Opening Endoscopic

8V – Eye, Restriction

VX0CZ Restriction of Right Lacrimal Duct with Extraluminal Device, Open Approach

VX0DZ Restriction of Right Lacrimal Duct with Intraluminal Device, Open Approach

08VX0ZZ Restriction of Right Lacrimal Duct, Open Approach

08VX3CZ Restriction of Right Lacrimal Duct with Extraluminal Device, Percutaneous Approach

08VX3DZ Restriction of Right Lacrimal Duct with Intraluminal Device, Percutaneous Approach

08VX3ZZ Restriction of Right Lacrimal Duct, Percutaneous Approach

Female-only	♂ Male-only	▲ Limited Coverage	● Non-OR	▨ HAC-associated procedure	▲ Non-covered procedures	✚ Combination

08VX7DZ Restriction of Right Lacrimal Duct with Intraluminal Device, Via Natural or Artificial Opening

08VX7ZZ Restriction of Right Lacrimal Duct, Via Natural or Artificial Opening

08VX8DZ Restriction of Right Lacrimal Duct with Intraluminal Device, Via Natural or Artificial Opening Endoscopic

08VX8ZZ Restriction of Right Lacrimal Duct, Via Natural or Artificial Opening Endoscopic

08VY0CZ Restriction of Left Lacrimal Duct with Extraluminal Device, Open Approach

08VY0DZ Restriction of Left Lacrimal Duct with Intraluminal Device, Open Approach

08VY0ZZ Restriction of Left Lacrimal Duct, Open Approach

08VY3CZ Restriction of Left Lacrimal Duct with Extraluminal Device, Percutaneous Approach

08VY3DZ Restriction of Left Lacrimal Duct with Intraluminal Device, Percutaneous Approach

08VY3ZZ Restriction of Left Lacrimal Duct, Percutaneous Approach

08VY7DZ Restriction of Left Lacrimal Duct with Intraluminal Device, Via Natural or Artificial Opening

08VY7ZZ Restriction of Left Lacrimal Duct, Via Natural or Artificial Opening

08VY8DZ Restriction of Left Lacrimal Duct with Intraluminal Device, Via Natural or Artificial Opening Endoscopic

08VY8ZZ Restriction of Left Lacrimal Duct, Via Natural or Artificial Opening Endoscopic

08W – Eye, Revision

Review Coding Guideline B6.1c

08W000Z Revision of Drainage Device in Right Eye, Open Approach

08W003Z Revision of Infusion Device in Right Eye, Open Approach

08W007Z Revision of Autologous Tissue Substitute in Right Eye, Open Approach

08W00CZ Revision of Extraluminal Device in Right Eye, Open Approach

08W00DZ Revision of Intraluminal Device in Right Eye, Open Approach

08W00JZ Revision of Synthetic Substitute in Right Eye, Open Approach

08W00KZ Revision of Nonautologous Tissue Substitute in Right Eye, Open Approach

08W030Z Revision of Drainage Device in Right Eye, Percutaneous Approach

08W033Z Revision of Infusion Device in Right Eye, Percutaneous Approach

08W037Z Revision of Autologous Tissue Substitute in Right Eye, Percutaneous Approach

08W03CZ Revision of Extraluminal Device in Right Eye, Percutaneous Approach

08W03DZ Revision of Intraluminal Device in Right Eye, Percutaneous Approach

08W03JZ Revision of Synthetic Substitute in Right Eye, Percutaneous Approach

08W03KZ Revision of Nonautologous Tissue Substitute in Right Eye, Percutaneous Approach

08W070Z Revision of Drainage Device in Right Eye, Via Natural or Artificial Opening

08W073Z Revision of Infusion Device in Right Eye, Via Natural or Artificial Opening

08W077Z Revision of Autologous Tissue Substitute in Right Eye, Via Natural or Artificial Opening

08W07CZ Revision of Extraluminal Device in Right Eye, Via Natural or Artificial Opening

08W07DZ Revision of Intraluminal Device in Right Eye, Via Natural or Artificial Opening

08W07JZ Revision of Synthetic Substitute in Right Eye, Via Natural or Artificial Opening

08W07KZ Revision of Nonautologous Tissue Substitute in Right Eye, Via Natural or Artificial Opening

08W080Z Revision of Drainage Device in Right Eye, Via Natural or Artificial Opening Endoscopic

08W083Z Revision of Infusion Device in Right Eye, Via Natural or Artificial Opening Endoscopic

08W087Z Revision of Autologous Tissue Substitute in Right Eye, Via Natural or Artificial Opening Endoscopic

08W08CZ Revision of Extraluminal Device in Right Eye, Via Natural or Artificial Opening Endoscopic

08W08DZ Revision of Intraluminal Device in Right Eye, Via Natural or Artificial Opening Endoscopic

08W08JZ Revision of Synthetic Substitute in Right Eye, Via Natural or Artificial Opening Endoscopic

08W08KZ Revision of Nonautologous Tissue Substitute in Right Eye, Via Natural or Artificial Opening Endoscopic

08W0X0Z Revision of Drainage Device in Right Eye, External Approach

08W0X3Z Revision of Infusion Device in Right Eye, External Approach

08W0X7Z Revision of Autologous Tissue Substitute in Right Eye, External Approach

08W0XCZ Revision of Extraluminal Device in Right Eye, External Approach

08W0XDZ Revision of Intraluminal Device in Right Eye, External Approach

08W0XJZ Revision of Synthetic Substitute in Right Eye, External Approach

08W0XKZ Revision of Nonautologous Tissue Substitute in Right Eye, External Approach

08W100Z Revision of Drainage Device in Left Eye, Open Approach

08W103Z Revision of Infusion Device in Left Eye, Open Approach

08W107Z Revision of Autologous Tissue Substitute in Left Eye, Open Approach

08W10CZ Revision of Extraluminal Device in Left Eye, Open Approach

08W10DZ Revision of Intraluminal Device in Left Eye, Open Approach

08W10JZ Revision of Synthetic Substitute in Left Eye, Open Approach

08W10KZ Revision of Nonautologous Tissue Substitute in Left Eye, Open Approach

08W130Z Revision of Drainage Device in Left Eye, Percutaneous Approach

08W133Z Revision of Infusion Device in Left Eye, Percutaneous Approach

08W137Z Revision of Autologous Tissue Substitute in Left Eye, Percutaneous Approach

08W13CZ Revision of Extraluminal Device in Left Eye, Percutaneous Approach

08W13DZ Revision of Intraluminal Device in Left Eye, Percutaneous Approach

08W13JZ Revision of Synthetic Substitute in Left Eye, Percutaneous Approach

08W13KZ Revision of Nonautologous Tissue Substitute in Left Eye, Percutaneous Approach

08W170Z Revision of Drainage Device in Left Eye, Via Natural or Artificial Opening

08W173Z Revision of Infusion Device in Left Eye, Via Natural or Artificial Opening

08W177Z Revision of Autologous Tissue Substitute in Left Eye, Via Natural or Artificial Opening

08W17CZ Revision of Extraluminal Device in Left Eye, Via Natural or Artificial Opening

08W17DZ Revision of Intraluminal Device in Left Eye, Via Natural or Artificial Opening

08W17JZ Revision of Synthetic Substitute in Left Eye, Via Natural or Artificial Opening

08W17KZ Revision of Nonautologous Tissue Substitute in Left Eye, Via Natural or Artificial Opening

08W180Z Revision of Drainage Device in Left Eye, Via Natural or Artificial Opening Endoscopic

08W183Z Revision of Infusion Device in Left Eye, Via Natural or Artificial Opening Endoscopic

08W187Z Revision of Autologous Tissue Substitute in Left Eye, Via Natural or Artificial Opening Endoscopic

08W18CZ Revision of Extraluminal Device in Left Eye, Via Natural or Artificial Opening Endoscopic

08W18DZ Revision of Intraluminal Device in Left Eye, Via Natural or Artificial Opening Endoscopic

08W18JZ Revision of Synthetic Substitute in Left Eye, Via Natural or Artificial Opening Endoscopic

08W18KZ Revision of Nonautologous Tissue Substitute in Left Eye, Via Natural or Artificial Opening Endoscopic

08W1X0Z Revision of Drainage Device in Left Eye, External Approach

08W1X3Z Revision of Infusion Device in Left Eye, External Approach

08W1X7Z Revision of Autologous Tissue Substitute in Left Eye, External Approach

08W1XCZ Revision of Extraluminal Device in Left Eye, External Approach

08W1XDZ Revision of Intraluminal Device in Left Eye, External Approach

08W1XJZ Revision of Synthetic Substitute in Left Eye, External Approach

08W1XKZ Revision of Nonautologous Tissue Substitute in Left Eye, External Approach

08WJ3JZ Revision of Synthetic Substitute in Right Lens, Percutaneous Approach

08WJXJZ Revision of Synthetic Substitute in Right Lens, External Approach

08WK3JZ Revision of Synthetic Substitute in Left Lens, Percutaneous Approach

08WKXJZ Revision of Synthetic Substitute in Left Lens, External Approach

08WL00Z Revision of Drainage Device in Right Extraocular Muscle, Open Approach

08WL07Z Revision of Autologous Tissue Substitute in Right Extraocular Muscle, Open Approach

08WL0JZ Revision of Synthetic Substitute in Right Extraocular Muscle, Open Approach

08WL0KZ Revision of Nonautologous Tissue Substitute in Right Extraocular Muscle, Open Approach

L30Z	Revision of Drainage Device in Right Extraocular Muscle, Percutaneous Approach	08WM00Z	Revision of Drainage Device in Left Extraocular Muscle, Open Approach	08WM30Z	Revision of Drainage Device in Left Extraocular Muscle, Percutaneous Approach
L37Z	Revision of Autologous Tissue Substitute in Right Extraocular Muscle, Percutaneous Approach	08WM07Z	Revision of Autologous Tissue Substitute in Left Extraocular Muscle, Open Approach	08WM37Z	Revision of Autologous Tissue Substitute in Left Extraocular Muscle, Percutaneous Approach
L3JZ	Revision of Synthetic Substitute in Right Extraocular Muscle, Percutaneous Approach	08WM0JZ	Revision of Synthetic Substitute in Left Extraocular Muscle, Open Approach	08WM3JZ	Revision of Synthetic Substitute in Left Extraocular Muscle, Percutaneous Approach
L3KZ	Revision of Nonautologous Tissue Substitute in Right Extraocular Muscle, Percutaneous Approach	08WM0KZ	Revision of Nonautologous Tissue Substitute in Left Extraocular Muscle, Open Approach	08WM3KZ	Revision of Nonautologous Tissue Substitute in Left Extraocular Muscle, Percutaneous Approach

X – Eye, Transfer

L0ZZ	Transfer Right Extraocular Muscle, Open Approach	08XM0ZZ	Transfer Left Extraocular Muscle, Open Approach
L3ZZ	Transfer Right Extraocular Muscle, Percutaneous Approach	08XM3ZZ	Transfer Left Extraocular Muscle, Percutaneous Approach

Nose and Sinus

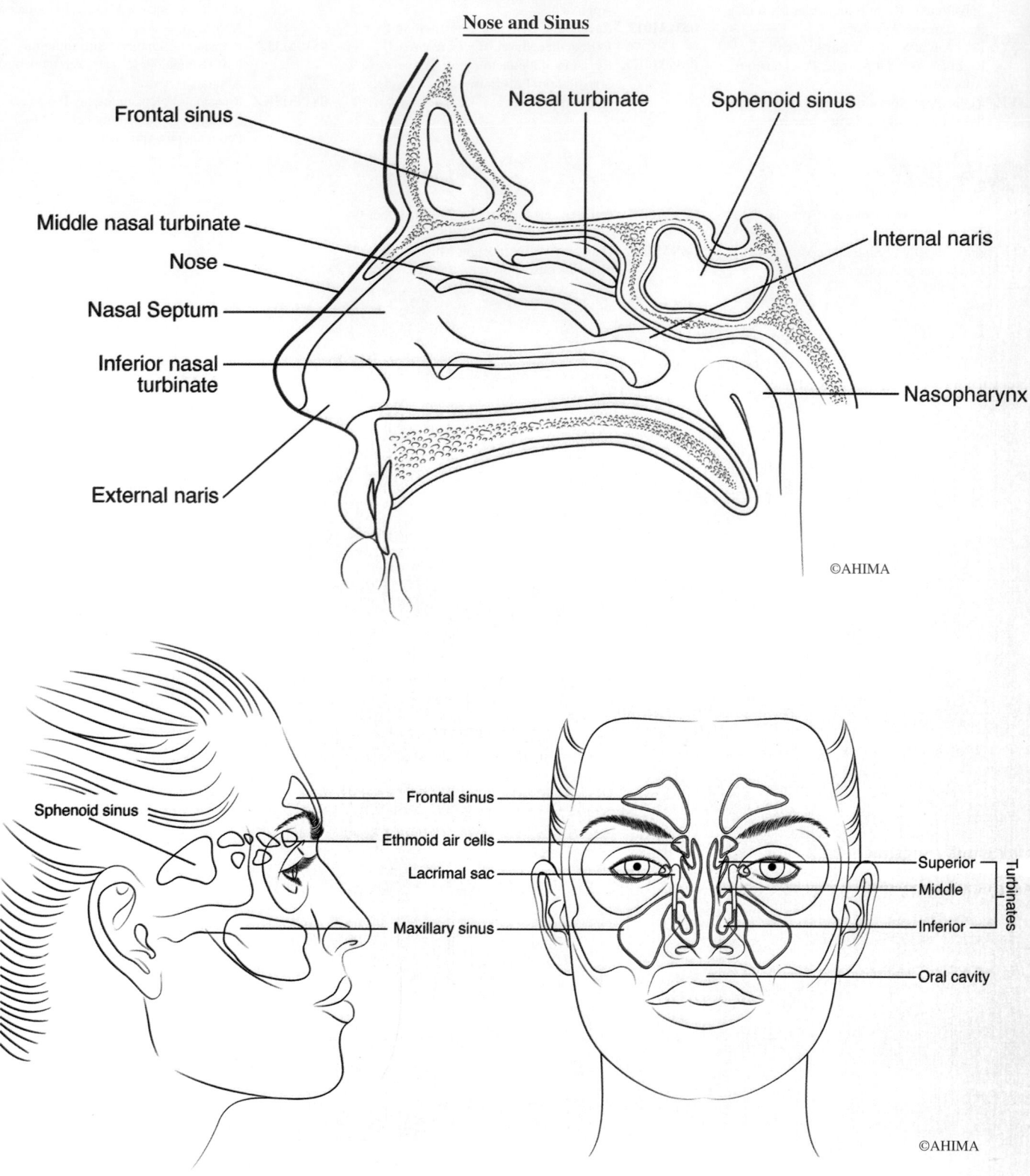

Frontal sinus

Nasal turbinate

Sphenoid sinus

Middle nasal turbinate

Nose

Nasal Septum

Inferior nasal turbinate

External naris

Internal naris

Nasopharynx

©AHIMA

Sphenoid sinus

Frontal sinus

Ethmoid air cells

Lacrimal sac

Maxillary sinus

Superior

Middle

Inferior

Turbinates

Oral cavity

©AHIMA

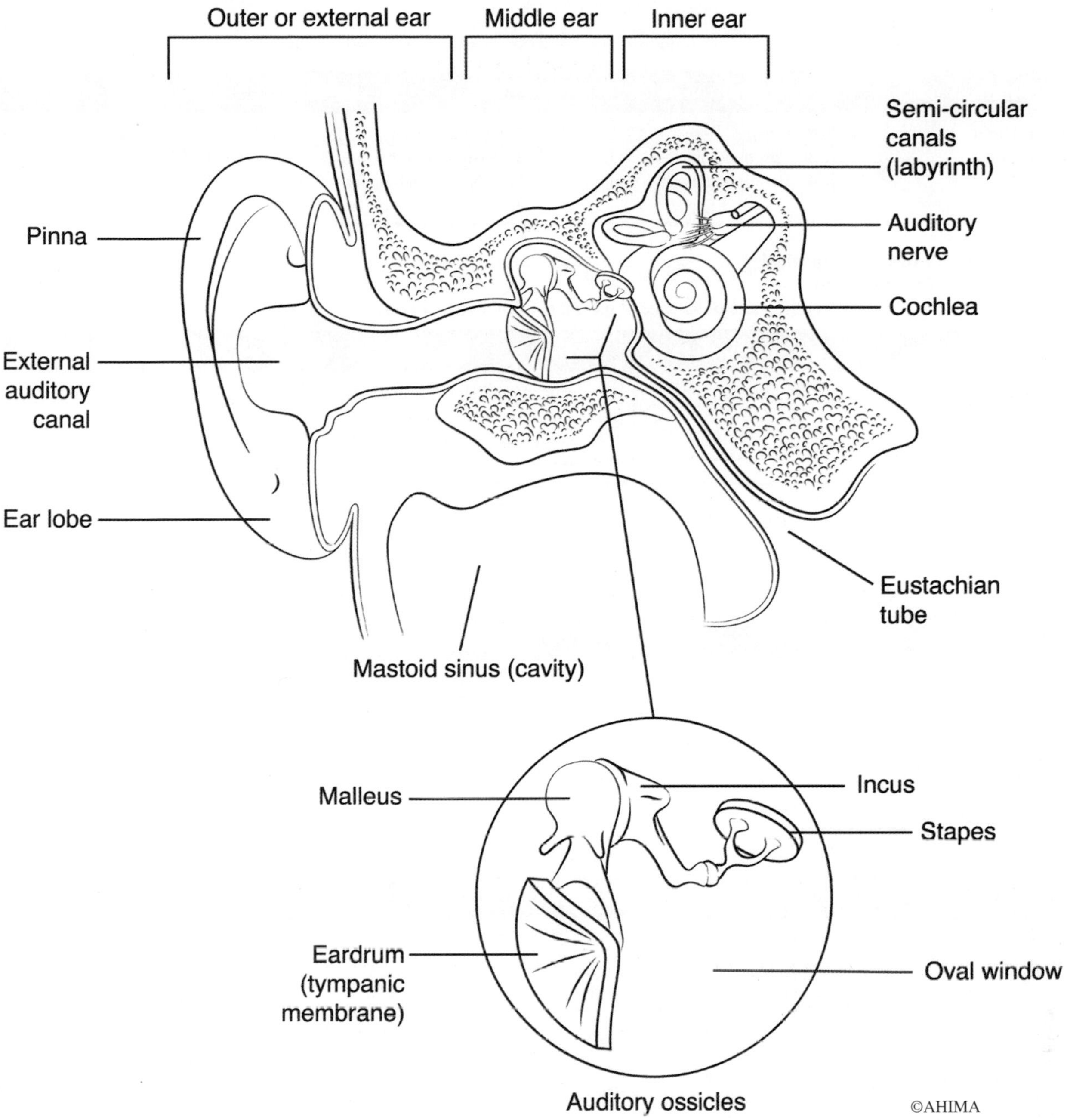

Ear

Outer or external ear | Middle ear | Inner ear

Pinna

External auditory canal

Ear lobe

Mastoid sinus (cavity)

Semi-circular canals (labyrinth)

Auditory nerve

Cochlea

Eustachian tube

Malleus

Eardrum (tympanic membrane)

Incus

Stapes

Oval window

Auditory ossicles

©AHIMA

Ear, Nose, Sinus Tables 090–09W

Section	0	Medical and Surgical
Body System	9	Ear, Nose, Sinus
Operation	0	Alteration: Modifying the anatomic structure of a body part without affecting the function of the body part

Body Part (4th)	Approach (5th)	Device (6th)	Qualifier (7th)
0 External Ear, Right 1 External Ear, Left 2 External Ear, Bilateral K Nose	0 Open 3 Percutaneous 4 Percutaneous Endoscopic X External	7 Autologous Tissue Substitute J Synthetic Substitute K Nonautologous Tissue Substitute Z No Device	Z No Qualifier

Section	0	Medical and Surgical
Body System	9	Ear, Nose, Sinus
Operation	1	Bypass: Altering the route of passage of the contents of a tubular body part

Body Part (4th)	Approach (5th)	Device (6th)	Qualifier (7th)
D Inner Ear, Right E Inner Ear, Left	0 Open	7 Autologous Tissue Substitute J Synthetic Substitute K Nonautologous Tissue Substitute Z No Device	0 Endolymphatic

Section	0	Medical and Surgical
Body System	9	Ear, Nose, Sinus
Operation	2	Change: Taking out or off a device from a body part and putting back an identical or similar device in or on the same body part without cutting or puncturing the skin or a mucous membrane

Body Part (4th)	Approach (5th)	Device (6th)	Qualifier (7th)
H Ear, Right J Ear, Left K Nose Y Sinus	X External	0 Drainage Device Y Other Device	Z No Qualifier

Section	0	Medical and Surgical
Body System	9	Ear, Nose, Sinus
Operation	5	Destruction: Physical eradication of all or a portion of a body part by the direct use of energy, force, or a destructive agent

Body Part (4th)	Approach (5th)	Device (6th)	Qualifier (7th)
0 External Ear, Right 1 External Ear, Left K Nose	0 Open 3 Percutaneous 4 Percutaneous Endoscopic X External	Z No Device	Z No Qualifier
3 External Auditory Canal, Right 4 External Auditory Canal, Left	0 Open 3 Percutaneous 4 Percutaneous Endoscopic 7 Via Natural or Artificial Opening 8 Via Natural or Artificial Opening Endoscopic X External	Z No Device	Z No Qualifier
5 Middle Ear, Right 6 Middle Ear, Left 9 Auditory Ossicle, Right A Auditory Ossicle, Left D Inner Ear, Right E Inner Ear, Left	0 Open	Z No Device	Z No Qualifier
7 Tympanic Membrane, Right 8 Tympanic Membrane, Left F Eustachian Tube, Right G Eustachian Tube, Left L Nasal Turbinate N Nasopharynx	0 Open 3 Percutaneous 4 Percutaneous Endoscopic 7 Via Natural or Artificial Opening 8 Via Natural or Artificial Opening Endoscopic	Z No Device	Z No Qualifier

Continued →

ion	0	Medical and Surgical
y System	9	Ear, Nose, Sinus
ration	5	**Destruction:** Physical eradication of all or a portion of a body part by the direct use of energy, force, or a destructive agent

Body Part (4th)	Approach (5th)	Device (6th)	Qualifier (7th)
Mastoid Sinus, Right Mastoid Sinus, Left Nasal Septum Accessory Sinus Maxillary Sinus, Right Maxillary Sinus, Left Frontal Sinus, Right Frontal Sinus, Left Ethmoid Sinus, Right Ethmoid Sinus, Left Sphenoid Sinus, Right Sphenoid Sinus, Left	**0** Open **3** Percutaneous **4** Percutaneous Endoscopic	**Z** No Device	**Z** No Qualifier

tion	0	Medical and Surgical
dy System	9	Ear, Nose, Sinus
eration	7	**Dilation:** Expanding an orifice or the lumen of a tubular body part

Body Part (4th)	Approach (5th)	Device (6th)	Qualifier (7th)
Eustachian Tube, Right Eustachian Tube, Left	**0** Open **7** Via Natural or Artificial Opening **8** Via Natural or Artificial Opening Endoscopic	**D** Intraluminal Device **Z** No Device	**Z** No Qualifier
Eustachian Tube, Right Eustachian Tube, Left	**3** Percutaneous **4** Percutaneous Endoscopic	**Z** No Device	**Z** No Qualifier

tion	0	Medical and Surgical
dy System	9	Ear, Nose, Sinus
eration	8	**Division:** Cutting into a body part, without draining fluids and/or gases from the body part, in order to separate or transect a body part

Body Part (4th)	Approach (5th)	Device (6th)	Qualifier (7th)
Nasal Turbinate	**0** Open **3** Percutaneous **4** Percutaneous Endoscopic **7** Via Natural or Artificial Opening **8** Via Natural or Artificial Opening Endoscopic	**Z** No Device	**Z** No Qualifier

ction	0	Medical and Surgical
dy System	9	Ear, Nose, Sinus
eration	9	**Drainage:** Taking or letting out fluids and/or gases from a body part

Body Part (4th)	Approach (5th)	Device (6th)	Qualifier (7th)
0 External Ear, Right 1 External Ear, Left K Nose	**0** Open **3** Percutaneous **4** Percutaneous Endoscopic **X** External	**0** Drainage Device	**Z** No Qualifier
0 External Ear, Right 1 External Ear, Left K Nose	**0** Open **3** Percutaneous **4** Percutaneous Endoscopic **X** External	**Z** No Device	**X** Diagnostic **Z** No Qualifier
3 External Auditory Canal, Right 4 External Auditory Canal, Left	**0** Open **3** Percutaneous **4** Percutaneous Endoscopic **7** Via Natural or Artificial Opening **8** Via Natural or Artificial Opening Endoscopic **X** External	**0** Drainage Device	**Z** No Qualifier

Continued →

Section 0 Medical and Surgical
Body System 9 Ear, Nose, Sinus
Operation 9 Drainage: Taking or letting out fluids and/or gases from a body part

Body Part (4th)	Approach (5th)	Device (6th)	Qualifier (7th)
3 External Auditory Canal, Right 4 External Auditory Canal, Left	0 Open 3 Percutaneous 4 Percutaneous Endoscopic 7 Via Natural or Artificial Opening 8 Via Natural or Artificial Opening Endoscopic X External	Z No Device	X Diagnostic Z No Qualifier
5 Middle Ear, Right 6 Middle Ear, Left 9 Auditory Ossicle, Right A Auditory Ossicle, Left D Inner Ear, Right E Inner Ear, Left	0 Open	0 Drainage Device	Z No Qualifier
5 Middle Ear, Right 6 Middle Ear, Left 9 Auditory Ossicle, Right A Auditory Ossicle, Left D Inner Ear, Right E Inner Ear, Left	0 Open	Z No Device	X Diagnostic Z No Qualifier
7 Tympanic Membrane, Right 8 Tympanic Membrane, Left F Eustachian Tube, Right G Eustachian Tube, Left L Nasal Turbinate N Nasopharynx	0 Open 3 Percutaneous 4 Percutaneous Endoscopic 7 Via Natural or Artificial Opening 8 Via Natural or Artificial Opening Endoscopic	0 Drainage Device	Z No Qualifier
7 Tympanic Membrane, Right 8 Tympanic Membrane, Left F Eustachian Tube, Right G Eustachian Tube, Left L Nasal Turbinate N Nasopharynx	0 Open 3 Percutaneous 4 Percutaneous Endoscopic 7 Via Natural or Artificial Opening 8 Via Natural or Artificial Opening Endoscopic	Z No Device	X Diagnostic Z No Qualifier
B Mastoid Sinus, Right C Mastoid Sinus, Left M Nasal Septum P Accessory Sinus Q Maxillary Sinus, Right R Maxillary Sinus, Left S Frontal Sinus, Right T Frontal Sinus, Left U Ethmoid Sinus, Right V Ethmoid Sinus, Left W Sphenoid Sinus, Right X Sphenoid Sinus, Left	0 Open 3 Percutaneous 4 Percutaneous Endoscopic	0 Drainage Device	Z No Qualifier
B Mastoid Sinus, Right C Mastoid Sinus, Left M Nasal Septum P Accessory Sinus Q Maxillary Sinus, Right R Maxillary Sinus, Left S Frontal Sinus, Right T Frontal Sinus, Left U Ethmoid Sinus, Right V Ethmoid Sinus, Left W Sphenoid Sinus, Right X Sphenoid Sinus, Left	0 Open 3 Percutaneous 4 Percutaneous Endoscopic	Z No Device	X Diagnostic Z No Qualifier

tion   0   **Medical and Surgical**
ly System   9   **Ear, Nose, Sinus**
eration   B   **Excision:** Cutting out or off, without replacement, a portion of a body part

Body Part (4th)	Approach (5th)	Device (6th)	Qualifier (7th)
External Ear, Right External Ear, Left Nose	0 Open 3 Percutaneous 4 Percutaneous Endoscopic X External	Z No Device	X Diagnostic Z No Qualifier
External Auditory Canal, Right External Auditory Canal, Left	0 Open 3 Percutaneous 4 Percutaneous Endoscopic 7 Via Natural or Artificial Opening 8 Via Natural or Artificial Opening Endoscopic X External	Z No Device	X Diagnostic Z No Qualifier
Middle Ear, Right Middle Ear, Left Auditory Ossicle, Right Auditory Ossicle, Left Inner Ear, Right Inner Ear, Left	0 Open	Z No Device	X Diagnostic Z No Qualifier
Tympanic Membrane, Right Tympanic Membrane, Left Eustachian Tube, Right Eustachian Tube, Left Nasal Turbinate Nasopharynx	0 Open 3 Percutaneous 4 Percutaneous Endoscopic 7 Via Natural or Artificial Opening 8 Via Natural or Artificial Opening Endoscopic	Z No Device	X Diagnostic Z No Qualifier
Mastoid Sinus, Right Mastoid Sinus, Left Nasal Septum Accessory Sinus Maxillary Sinus, Right Maxillary Sinus, Left Frontal Sinus, Right Frontal Sinus, Left Ethmoid Sinus, Right Ethmoid Sinus, Left Sphenoid Sinus, Right Sphenoid Sinus, Left	0 Open 3 Percutaneous 4 Percutaneous Endoscopic	Z No Device	X Diagnostic Z No Qualifier

ction   0   **Medical and Surgical**
dy System   9   **Ear, Nose, Sinus**
eration   C   **Extirpation:** Taking or cutting out solid matter from a body part

Body Part (4th)	Approach (5th)	Device (6th)	Qualifier (7th)
0 External Ear, Right 1 External Ear, Left K Nose	0 Open 3 Percutaneous 4 Percutaneous Endoscopic X External	Z No Device	Z No Qualifier
3 External Auditory Canal, Right 4 External Auditory Canal, Left	0 Open 3 Percutaneous 4 Percutaneous Endoscopic 7 Via Natural or Artificial Opening 8 Via Natural or Artificial Opening Endoscopic X External	Z No Device	Z No Qualifier

Continued →

Section	0	Medical and Surgical
Body System	9	Ear, Nose, Sinus
Operation	C	Extirpation: Taking or cutting out solid matter from a body part

Body Part (4th)	Approach (5th)	Device (6th)	Qualifier (7th)
5 Middle Ear, Right 6 Middle Ear, Left 9 Auditory Ossicle, Right A Auditory Ossicle, Left D Inner Ear, Right E Inner Ear, Left	0 Open	Z No Device	Z No Qualifier
7 Tympanic Membrane, Right 8 Tympanic Membrane, Left F Eustachian Tube, Right G Eustachian Tube, Left L Nasal Turbinate N Nasopharynx	0 Open 3 Percutaneous 4 Percutaneous Endoscopic 7 Via Natural or Artificial Opening 8 Via Natural or Artificial Opening Endoscopic	Z No Device	Z No Qualifier
B Mastoid Sinus, Right C Mastoid Sinus, Left M Nasal Septum P Accessory Sinus Q Maxillary Sinus, Right R Maxillary Sinus, Left S Frontal Sinus, Right T Frontal Sinus, Left U Ethmoid Sinus, Right V Ethmoid Sinus, Left W Sphenoid Sinus, Right X Sphenoid Sinus, Left	0 Open 3 Percutaneous 4 Percutaneous Endoscopic	Z No Device	Z No Qualifier

Section	0	Medical and Surgical
Body System	9	Ear, Nose, Sinus
Operation	D	Extraction: Pulling or stripping out or off all or a portion of a body part by the use of force

Body Part (4th)	Approach (5th)	Device (6th)	Qualifier (7th)
7 Tympanic Membrane, Right 8 Tympanic Membrane, Left L Nasal Turbinate	0 Open 3 Percutaneous 4 Percutaneous Endoscopic 7 Via Natural or Artificial Opening 8 Via Natural or Artificial Opening Endoscopic	Z No Device	Z No Qualifier
9 Auditory Ossicle, Right A Auditory Ossicle, Left	0 Open	Z No Device	Z No Qualifier
B Mastoid Sinus, Right C Mastoid Sinus, Left M Nasal Septum P Accessory Sinus Q Maxillary Sinus, Right R Maxillary Sinus, Left S Frontal Sinus, Right T Frontal Sinus, Left U Ethmoid Sinus, Right V Ethmoid Sinus, Left W Sphenoid Sinus, Right X Sphenoid Sinus, Left	0 Open 3 Percutaneous 4 Percutaneous Endoscopic	Z No Device	Z No Qualifier

on	0	Medical and Surgical
System	9	Ear, Nose, Sinus
ration	H	**Insertion:** Putting in a nonbiological appliance that monitors, assists, performs, or prevents a physiological function but does not physically take the place of a body part

Body Part (4th)	Approach (5th)	Device (6th)	Qualifier (7th)
Inner Ear, Right Inner Ear, Left	0 Open 3 Percutaneous 4 Percutaneous Endoscopic	4 Hearing Device, Bone Conduction 5 Hearing Device, Single Channel Cochlear Prosthesis 6 Hearing Device, Multiple Channel Cochlear Prosthesis S Hearing Device	Z No Qualifier
Nasopharynx	7 Via Natural or Artificial Opening 8 Via Natural or Artificial Opening Endoscopic	B Intraluminal Device, Airway	Z No Qualifier

ion	0	Medical and Surgical
y System	9	Ear, Nose, Sinus
ration	J	**Inspection:** Visually and/or manually exploring a body part

Body Part (4th)	Approach (5th)	Device (6th)	Qualifier (7th)
Tympanic Membrane, Right Tympanic Membrane, Left Ear, Right Ear, Left	0 Open 3 Percutaneous 4 Percutaneous Endoscopic 7 Via Natural or Artificial Opening 8 Via Natural or Artificial Opening Endoscopic X External	Z No Device	Z No Qualifier
Inner Ear, Right Inner Ear, Left Nose Sinus	0 Open 3 Percutaneous 4 Percutaneous Endoscopic X External	Z No Device	Z No Qualifier

tion	0	Medical and Surgical
ly System	9	Ear, Nose, Sinus
eration	M	**Reattachment:** Putting back in or on all or a portion of a separated body part to its normal location or other suitable location

Body Part (4th)	Approach (5th)	Device (6th)	Qualifier (7th)
External Ear, Right External Ear, Left Nose	X External	Z No Device	Z No Qualifier

tion	0	Medical and Surgical
ly System	9	Ear, Nose, Sinus
eration	N	**Release:** Freeing a body part from an abnormal physical constraint by cutting or by the use of force

Body Part (4th)	Approach (5th)	Device (6th)	Qualifier (7th)
External Ear, Right External Ear, Left Nose	0 Open 3 Percutaneous 4 Percutaneous Endoscopic X External	Z No Device	Z No Qualifier
External Auditory Canal, Right External Auditory Canal, Left	0 Open 3 Percutaneous 4 Percutaneous Endoscopic 7 Via Natural or Artificial Opening 8 Via Natural or Artificial Opening Endoscopic X External	Z No Device	Z No Qualifier

Continued →

Section	0	Medical and Surgical
Body System	9	Ear, Nose, Sinus
Operation	N	Release: Freeing a body part from an abnormal physical constraint by cutting or by the use of force

Body Part (4th)	Approach (5th)	Device (6th)	Qualifier (7th)
5 Middle Ear, Right 6 Middle Ear, Left 9 Auditory Ossicle, Right A Auditory Ossicle, Left D Inner Ear, Right E Inner Ear, Left	0 Open	Z No Device	Z No Qualifier
7 Tympanic Membrane, Right 8 Tympanic Membrane, Left F Eustachian Tube, Right G Eustachian Tube, Left L Nasal Turbinate N Nasopharynx	0 Open 3 Percutaneous 4 Percutaneous Endoscopic 7 Via Natural or Artificial Opening 8 Via Natural or Artificial Opening Endoscopic	Z No Device	Z No Qualifier
B Mastoid Sinus, Right C Mastoid Sinus, Left M Nasal Septum P Accessory Sinus Q Maxillary Sinus, Right R Maxillary Sinus, Left S Frontal Sinus, Right T Frontal Sinus, Left U Ethmoid Sinus, Right V Ethmoid Sinus, Left W Sphenoid Sinus, Right X Sphenoid Sinus, Left	0 Open 3 Percutaneous 4 Percutaneous Endoscopic	Z No Device	Z No Qualifier

Section	0	Medical and Surgical
Body System	9	Ear, Nose, Sinus
Operation	P	Removal: Taking out or off a device from a body part

Body Part (4th)	Approach (5th)	Device (6th)	Qualifier (7th)
7 Tympanic Membrane, Right 8 Tympanic Membrane, Left	0 Open 7 Via Natural or Artificial Opening 8 Via Natural or Artificial Opening Endoscopic X External	0 Drainage Device	Z No Qualifier
D Inner Ear, Right E Inner Ear, Left	0 Open 7 Via Natural or Artificial Opening 8 Via Natural or Artificial Opening Endoscopic	S Hearing Device	Z No Qualifier
H Ear, Right J Ear, Left K Nose	0 Open 3 Percutaneous 4 Percutaneous Endoscopic 7 Via Natural or Artificial Opening 8 Via Natural or Artificial Opening Endoscopic X External	0 Drainage Device 7 Autologous Tissue Substitute D Intraluminal Device J Synthetic Substitute K Nonautologous Tissue Substitute	Z No Qualifier
Y Sinus	0 Open 3 Percutaneous 4 Percutaneous Endoscopic X External	0 Drainage Device	Z No Qualifier

	0	Medical and Surgical
	9	Ear, Nose, Sinus
	Q	**Repair:** Restoring, to the extent possible, a body part to its normal anatomic structure and function

Body Part (4th)	Approach (5th)	Device (6th)	Qualifier (7th)
External Ear, Right External Ear, Left External Ear, Bilateral Nose	0 Open 3 Percutaneous 4 Percutaneous Endoscopic X External	Z No Device	Z No Qualifier
External Auditory Canal, Right External Auditory Canal, Left Eustachian Tube, Right Eustachian Tube, Left	0 Open 3 Percutaneous 4 Percutaneous Endoscopic 7 Via Natural or Artificial Opening 8 Via Natural or Artificial Opening Endoscopic X External	Z No Device	Z No Qualifier
Middle Ear, Right Middle Ear, Left Auditory Ossicle, Right Auditory Ossicle, Left Inner Ear, Right Inner Ear, Left	0 Open	Z No Device	Z No Qualifier
Tympanic Membrane, Right Tympanic Membrane, Left Nasal Turbinate Nasopharynx	0 Open 3 Percutaneous 4 Percutaneous Endoscopic 7 Via Natural or Artificial Opening 8 Via Natural or Artificial Opening Endoscopic	Z No Device	Z No Qualifier
Mastoid Sinus, Right Mastoid Sinus, Left Nasal Septum Accessory Sinus Maxillary Sinus, Right Maxillary Sinus, Left Frontal Sinus, Right Frontal Sinus, Left Ethmoid Sinus, Right Ethmoid Sinus, Left Sphenoid Sinus, Right Sphenoid Sinus, Left	0 Open 3 Percutaneous 4 Percutaneous Endoscopic	Z No Device	Z No Qualifier

	0	Medical and Surgical
	9	Ear, Nose, Sinus
	R	**Replacement:** Putting in or on biological or synthetic material that physically takes the place and/or function of all or a portion of a body part

Body Part (4th)	Approach (5th)	Device (6th)	Qualifier (7th)
External Ear, Right External Ear, Left External Ear, Bilateral Nose	0 Open X External	7 Autologous Tissue Substitute J Synthetic Substitute K Nonautologous Tissue Substitute	Z No Qualifier
Middle Ear, Right Middle Ear, Left Auditory Ossicle, Right Auditory Ossicle, Left Inner Ear, Right Inner Ear, Left	0 Open	7 Autologous Tissue Substitute J Synthetic Substitute K Nonautologous Tissue Substitute	Z No Qualifier
Tympanic Membrane, Right Tympanic Membrane, Left Nasopharynx	0 Open 7 Via Natural or Artificial Opening 8 Via Natural or Artificial Opening Endoscopic	7 Autologous Tissue Substitute J Synthetic Substitute K Nonautologous Tissue Substitute	Z No Qualifier

Continued →

Section	0	Medical and Surgical
Body System	9	Ear, Nose, Sinus
Operation	R	**Replacement:** Putting in or on biological or synthetic material that physically takes the place and/or function of all or a portion of a body part

Body Part (4th)	Approach (5th)	Device (6th)	Qualifier (7th)
L Nasal Turbinate	0 Open 3 Percutaneous 4 Percutaneous Endoscopic 7 Via Natural or Artificial Opening 8 Via Natural or Artificial Opening Endoscopic	7 Autologous Tissue Substitute J Synthetic Substitute K Nonautologous Tissue Substitute	Z No Qualifier
M Nasal Septum	0 Open 3 Percutaneous 4 Percutaneous Endoscopic	7 Autologous Tissue Substitute J Synthetic Substitute K Nonautologous Tissue Substitute	Z No Qualifier

Section	0	Medical and Surgical
Body System	9	Ear, Nose, Sinus
Operation	S	**Reposition:** Moving to its normal location, or other suitable location, all or a portion of a body part

Body Part (4th)	Approach (5th)	Device (6th)	Qualifier (7th)
0 External Ear, Right 1 External Ear, Left 2 External Ear, Bilateral K Nose	0 Open 4 Percutaneous Endoscopic X External	Z No Device	Z No Qualifier
7 Tympanic Membrane, Right 8 Tympanic Membrane, Left F Eustachian Tube, Right G Eustachian Tube, Left L Nasal Turbinate	0 Open 4 Percutaneous Endoscopic 7 Via Natural or Artificial Opening 8 Via Natural or Artificial Opening Endoscopic	Z No Device	Z No Qualifier
9 Auditory Ossicle, Right A Auditory Ossicle, Left M Nasal Septum	0 Open 4 Percutaneous Endoscopic	Z No Device	Z No Qualifier

Section	0	Medical and Surgical
Body System	9	Ear, Nose, Sinus
Operation	T	**Resection:** Cutting out or off, without replacement, all of a body part

Body Part (4th)	Approach (5th)	Device (6th)	Qualifier (7th)
0 External Ear, Right 1 External Ear, Left K Nose	0 Open 4 Percutaneous Endoscopic X External	Z No Device	Z No Qualifier
5 Middle Ear, Right 6 Middle Ear, Left 9 Auditory Ossicle, Right A Auditory Ossicle, Left D Inner Ear, Right E Inner Ear, Left	0 Open	Z No Device	Z No Qualifier
7 Tympanic Membrane, Right 8 Tympanic Membrane, Left F Eustachian Tube, Right G Eustachian Tube, Left L Nasal Turbinate N Nasopharynx	0 Open 4 Percutaneous Endoscopic 7 Via Natural or Artificial Opening 8 Via Natural or Artificial Opening Endoscopic	Z No Device	Z No Qualifier

Continued –

	0	Medical and Surgical
System	9	Ear, Nose, Sinus
ation	T	**Resection:** Cutting out or off, without replacement, all of a body part

Body Part (4th)	Approach (5th)	Device (6th)	Qualifier (7th)
Mastoid Sinus, Right Mastoid Sinus, Left Nasal Septum Accessory Sinus Maxillary Sinus, Right Maxillary Sinus, Left Frontal Sinus, Right Frontal Sinus, Left Ethmoid Sinus, Right Ethmoid Sinus, Left Sphenoid Sinus, Right Sphenoid Sinus, Left	**0** Open **4** Percutaneous Endoscopic	**Z** No Device	**Z** No Qualifier

	0	Medical and Surgical
y System	9	Ear, Nose, Sinus
ration	U	**Supplement:** Putting in or on biological or synthetic material that physically reinforces and/or augments the function of a portion of a body part

Body Part (4th)	Approach (5th)	Device (6th)	Qualifier (7th)
External Ear, Right External Ear, Left External Ear, Bilateral Nose	**0** Open **X** External	**7** Autologous Tissue Substitute **J** Synthetic Substitute **K** Nonautologous Tissue Substitute	**Z** No Qualifier
Middle Ear, Right Middle Ear, Left Auditory Ossicle, Right Auditory Ossicle, Left Inner Ear, Right Inner Ear, Left	**0** Open	**7** Autologous Tissue Substitute **J** Synthetic Substitute **K** Nonautologous Tissue Substitute	**Z** No Qualifier
Tympanic Membrane, Right Tympanic Membrane, Left Nasopharynx	**0** Open **7** Via Natural or Artificial Opening **8** Via Natural or Artificial Opening Endoscopic	**7** Autologous Tissue Substitute **J** Synthetic Substitute **K** Nonautologous Tissue Substitute	**Z** No Qualifier
Nasal Turbinate	**0** Open **3** Percutaneous **4** Percutaneous Endoscopic **7** Via Natural or Artificial Opening **8** Via Natural or Artificial Opening Endoscopic	**7** Autologous Tissue Substitute **J** Synthetic Substitute **K** Nonautologous Tissue Substitute	**Z** No Qualifier
Nasal Septum	**0** Open **3** Percutaneous **4** Percutaneous Endoscopic	**7** Autologous Tissue Substitute **J** Synthetic Substitute **K** Nonautologous Tissue Substitute	**Z** No Qualifier

	0	Medical and Surgical
dy System	9	Ear, Nose, Sinus
eration	W	**Revision:** Correcting, to the extent possible, a portion of a malfunctioning device or the position of a displaced device

Body Part (4th)	Approach (5th)	Device (6th)	Qualifier (7th)
Tympanic Membrane, Right Tympanic Membrane, Left Auditory Ossicle, Right Auditory Ossicle, Left	**0** Open **7** Via Natural or Artificial Opening **8** Via Natural or Artificial Opening Endoscopic	**7** Autologous Tissue Substitute **J** Synthetic Substitute **K** Nonautologous Tissue Substitute	**Z** No Qualifier
Inner Ear, Right Inner Ear, Left	**0** Open **7** Via Natural or Artificial Opening **8** Via Natural or Artificial Opening Endoscopic	**S** Hearing Device	**Z** No Qualifier

Continued →

	Section	0	Medical and Surgical
	Body System	9	Ear, Nose, Sinus
	Operation	W	Revision: Correcting, to the extent possible, a portion of a malfunctioning device or the position of a displaced device

Body Part (4th)	Approach (5th)	Device (6th)	Qualifier (7th)
H Ear, Right J Ear, Left K Nose	0 Open 3 Percutaneous 4 Percutaneous Endoscopic 7 Via Natural or Artificial Opening 8 Via Natural or Artificial Opening Endoscopic X External	0 Drainage Device 7 Autologous Tissue Substitute D Intraluminal Device J Synthetic Substitute K Nonautologous Tissue Substitute	Z No Qualifier
Y Sinus	0 Open 3 Percutaneous 4 Percutaneous Endoscopic X External	0 Drainage Device	Z No Qualifier

Ear, Nose, Sinus Code Listing 090–09W

090 – Ear, Nose, Sinus, Alteration

090007Z Alteration of Right External Ear with Autologous Tissue Substitute, Open Approach

09000JZ Alteration of Right External Ear with Synthetic Substitute, Open Approach

09000KZ Alteration of Right External Ear with Nonautologous Tissue Substitute, Open Approach

09000ZZ Alteration of Right External Ear, Open Approach

090037Z Alteration of Right External Ear with Autologous Tissue Substitute, Percutaneous Approach

09003JZ Alteration of Right External Ear with Synthetic Substitute, Percutaneous Approach

09003KZ Alteration of Right External Ear with Nonautologous Tissue Substitute, Percutaneous Approach

09003ZZ Alteration of Right External Ear, Percutaneous Approach

090047Z Alteration of Right External Ear with Autologous Tissue Substitute, Percutaneous Endoscopic Approach

09004JZ Alteration of Right External Ear with Synthetic Substitute, Percutaneous Endoscopic Approach

09004KZ Alteration of Right External Ear with Nonautologous Tissue Substitute, Percutaneous Endoscopic Approach

09004ZZ Alteration of Right External Ear, Percutaneous Endoscopic Approach

0900X7Z Alteration of Right External Ear with Autologous Tissue Substitute, External Approach

0900XJZ Alteration of Right External Ear with Synthetic Substitute, External Approach

0900XKZ Alteration of Right External Ear with Nonautologous Tissue Substitute, External Approach

0900XZZ Alteration of Right External Ear, External Approach

090107Z Alteration of Left External Ear with Autologous Tissue Substitute, Open Approach

09010JZ Alteration of Left External Ear with Synthetic Substitute, Open Approach

09010KZ Alteration of Left External Ear with Nonautologous Tissue Substitute, Open Approach

09010ZZ Alteration of Left External Ear, Open Approach

090137Z Alteration of Left External Ear with Autologous Tissue Substitute, Percutaneous Approach

09013JZ Alteration of Left External Ear with Synthetic Substitute, Percutaneous Approach

09013KZ Alteration of Left External Ear with Nonautologous Tissue Substitute, Percutaneous Approach

09013ZZ Alteration of Left External Ear, Percutaneous Approach

090147Z Alteration of Left External Ear with Autologous Tissue Substitute, Percutaneous Endoscopic Approach

09014JZ Alteration of Left External Ear with Synthetic Substitute, Percutaneous Endoscopic Approach

09014KZ Alteration of Left External Ear with Nonautologous Tissue Substitute, Percutaneous Endoscopic Approach

09014ZZ Alteration of Left External Ear, Percutaneous Endoscopic Approach

0901X7Z Alteration of Left External Ear with Autologous Tissue Substitute, External Approach

0901XJZ Alteration of Left External Ear with Synthetic Substitute, External Approach

0901XKZ Alteration of Left External Ear with Nonautologous Tissue Substitute, External Approach

0901XZZ Alteration of Left External Ear, External Approach

090207Z Alteration of Bilateral External Ear with Autologous Tissue Substitute, Open Approach

09020JZ Alteration of Bilateral External Ear with Synthetic Substitute, Open Approach

09020KZ Alteration of Bilateral External Ear with Nonautologous Tissue Substitute, Open Approach

09020ZZ Alteration of Bilateral External Ear, Open Approach

090237Z Alteration of Bilateral External Ear with Autologous Tissue Substitute, Percutaneous Approach

09023JZ Alteration of Bilateral External Ear with Synthetic Substitute, Percutaneous Approach

09023KZ Alteration of Bilateral External Ear with Nonautologous Tissue Substitute, Percutaneous Approach

09023ZZ Alteration of Bilateral External Ear, Percutaneous Approach

090247Z Alteration of Bilateral External Ear with Autologous Tissue Substitute, Percutaneous Endoscopic Approach

09024JZ Alteration of Bilateral External Ear with Synthetic Substitute, Percutaneou Endoscopic Approach

09024KZ Alteration of Bilateral External Ear with Nonautologous Tissue Substitute, Percutaneous Endoscopic Approach

09024ZZ Alteration of Bilateral External Ear, Percutaneous Endoscopic Approach

0902X7Z Alteration of Bilateral External Ear wi Autologous Tissue Substitute, Externa Approach

0902XJZ Alteration of Bilateral External Ear wi Synthetic Substitute, External Approac

0902XKZ Alteration of Bilateral External Ear wi Nonautologous Tissue Substitute, Exte Approach

0902XZZ Alteration of Bilateral External Ear, External Approach

090K07Z Alteration of Nose with Autologous Tis Substitute, Open Approach

090K0JZ Alteration of Nose with Synthetic Substitute, Open Approach

090K0KZ Alteration of Nose with Nonautologous Tissue Substitute, Open Approach

090K0ZZ Alteration of Nose, Open Approach

090K37Z Alteration of Nose with Autologous Tis Substitute, Percutaneous Approach

090K3JZ Alteration of Nose with Synthetic Substitute, Percutaneous Approach

090K3KZ Alteration of Nose with Nonautologous Tissue Substitute, Percutaneous Approa

090K3ZZ Alteration of Nose, Percutaneous Approach

090K47Z Alteration of Nose with Autologous Tis Substitute, Percutaneous Endoscopic Approach

090K4JZ Alteration of Nose with Synthetic Substit Percutaneous Endoscopic Approach

090K4KZ Alteration of Nose with Nonautologous Tissue Substitute, Percutaneous Endoscopic Approach

090K4ZZ Alteration of Nose, Percutaneous Endoscopic Approach

090KX7Z Alteration of Nose with Autologous Tiss Substitute, External Approach

090KXJZ Alteration of Nose with Synthetic Substitute, External Approach

090KXKZ Alteration of Nose with Nonautologous Tissue Substitute, External Approach

090KXZZ Alteration of Nose, External Approach

– Ear, Nose, Sinus, Bypass

ew Coding Guideline B3.6a

070 Bypass Right Inner Ear to Endolymphatic with Autologous Tissue Substitute, Open Approach	**091D0Z0** Bypass Right Inner Ear to Endolymphatic, Open Approach	**091E0K0** Bypass Left Inner Ear to Endolymphatic with Nonautologous Tissue Substitute, Open Approach
0J0 Bypass Right Inner Ear to Endolymphatic with Synthetic Substitute, Open Approach	**091E070** Bypass Left Inner Ear to Endolymphatic with Autologous Tissue Substitute, Open Approach	**091E0Z0** Bypass Left Inner Ear to Endolymphatic, Open Approach
0K0 Bypass Right Inner Ear to Endolymphatic with Nonautologous Tissue Substitute, Open Approach	**091E0J0** Bypass Left Inner Ear to Endolymphatic with Synthetic Substitute, Open Approach	

– Ear, Nose, Sinus, Change

iew Coding Guideline B6.1c

IX0Z Change Drainage Device in Right Ear, External Approach	**092JXYZ** Change Other Device in Left Ear, External Approach	**092YX0Z** Change Drainage Device in Sinus, External Approach
IXYZ Change Other Device in Right Ear, External Approach	**092KX0Z** Change Drainage Device in Nose, External Approach	**092YXYZ** Change Other Device in Sinus, External Approach
X0Z Change Drainage Device in Left Ear, External Approach	**092KXYZ** Change Other Device in Nose, External Approach	

– Ear, Nose, Sinus, Destruction

0ZZ Destruction of Right External Ear, Open Approach	**09574ZZ** Destruction of Right Tympanic Membrane, Percutaneous Endoscopic Approach	**095G3ZZ** Destruction of Left Eustachian Tube, Percutaneous Approach
3ZZ Destruction of Right External Ear, Percutaneous Approach	**09577ZZ** Destruction of Right Tympanic Membrane, Via Natural or Artificial Opening	**095G4ZZ** Destruction of Left Eustachian Tube, Percutaneous Endoscopic Approach
4ZZ Destruction of Right External Ear, Percutaneous Endoscopic Approach	**09578ZZ** Destruction of Right Tympanic Membrane, Via Natural or Artificial Opening Endoscopic	**095G7ZZ** Destruction of Left Eustachian Tube, Via Natural or Artificial Opening
XZZ Destruction of Right External Ear, External Approach	**09580ZZ** Destruction of Left Tympanic Membrane, Open Approach	**095G8ZZ** Destruction of Left Eustachian Tube, Via Natural or Artificial Opening Endoscopic
0ZZ Destruction of Left External Ear, Open Approach	**09583ZZ** Destruction of Left Tympanic Membrane, Percutaneous Approach	**095K0ZZ** Destruction of Nose, Open Approach
3ZZ Destruction of Left External Ear, Percutaneous Approach	**09584ZZ** Destruction of Left Tympanic Membrane, Percutaneous Endoscopic Approach	**095K3ZZ** Destruction of Nose, Percutaneous Approach
4ZZ Destruction of Left External Ear, Percutaneous Endoscopic Approach	**09587ZZ** Destruction of Left Tympanic Membrane, Via Natural or Artificial Opening	**095K4ZZ** Destruction of Nose, Percutaneous Endoscopic Approach
XZZ Destruction of Left External Ear, External Approach	**09588ZZ** Destruction of Left Tympanic Membrane, Via Natural or Artificial Opening Endoscopic	**095KXZZ** Destruction of Nose, External Approach
30ZZ Destruction of Right External Auditory Canal, Open Approach	**09590ZZ** Destruction of Right Auditory Ossicle, Open Approach	**095L0ZZ** Destruction of Nasal Turbinate, Open Approach
33ZZ Destruction of Right External Auditory Canal, Percutaneous Approach	**095A0ZZ** Destruction of Left Auditory Ossicle, Open Approach	**095L3ZZ** Destruction of Nasal Turbinate, Percutaneous Approach
34ZZ Destruction of Right External Auditory Canal, Percutaneous Endoscopic Approach	**095B0ZZ** Destruction of Right Mastoid Sinus, Open Approach	**095L4ZZ** Destruction of Nasal Turbinate, Percutaneous Endoscopic Approach
37ZZ Destruction of Right External Auditory Canal, Via Natural or Artificial Opening	**095B3ZZ** Destruction of Right Mastoid Sinus, Percutaneous Approach	**095L7ZZ** Destruction of Nasal Turbinate, Via Natural or Artificial Opening
38ZZ Destruction of Right External Auditory Canal, Via Natural or Artificial Opening Endoscopic	**095B4ZZ** Destruction of Right Mastoid Sinus, Percutaneous Endoscopic Approach	**095L8ZZ** Destruction of Nasal Turbinate, Via Natural or Artificial Opening Endoscopic
3XZZ Destruction of Right External Auditory Canal, External Approach	**095C0ZZ** Destruction of Left Mastoid Sinus, Open Approach	**095M0ZZ** Destruction of Nasal Septum, Open Approach
40ZZ Destruction of Left External Auditory Canal, Open Approach	**095C3ZZ** Destruction of Left Mastoid Sinus, Percutaneous Approach	**095M3ZZ** Destruction of Nasal Septum, Percutaneous Approach
43ZZ Destruction of Left External Auditory Canal, Percutaneous Approach	**095C4ZZ** Destruction of Left Mastoid Sinus, Percutaneous Endoscopic Approach	**095M4ZZ** Destruction of Nasal Septum, Percutaneous Endoscopic Approach
44ZZ Destruction of Left External Auditory Canal, Percutaneous Endoscopic Approach	**095D0ZZ** Destruction of Right Inner Ear, Open Approach	**095N0ZZ** Destruction of Nasopharynx, Open Approach
47ZZ Destruction of Left External Auditory Canal, Via Natural or Artificial Opening	**095E0ZZ** Destruction of Left Inner Ear, Open Approach	**095N3ZZ** Destruction of Nasopharynx, Percutaneous Approach
48ZZ Destruction of Left External Auditory Canal, Via Natural or Artificial Opening Endoscopic	**095F0ZZ** Destruction of Right Eustachian Tube, Open Approach	**095N4ZZ** Destruction of Nasopharynx, Percutaneous Endoscopic Approach
4XZZ Destruction of Left External Auditory Canal, External Approach	**095F3ZZ** Destruction of Right Eustachian Tube, Percutaneous Approach	**095N7ZZ** Destruction of Nasopharynx, Via Natural or Artificial Opening
550ZZ Destruction of Right Middle Ear, Open Approach	**095F4ZZ** Destruction of Right Eustachian Tube, Percutaneous Endoscopic Approach	**095N8ZZ** Destruction of Nasopharynx, Via Natural or Artificial Opening Endoscopic
560ZZ Destruction of Left Middle Ear, Open Approach	**095F7ZZ** Destruction of Right Eustachian Tube, Via Natural or Artificial Opening	**095P0ZZ** Destruction of Accessory Sinus, Open Approach
570ZZ Destruction of Right Tympanic Membrane, Open Approach	**095F8ZZ** Destruction of Right Eustachian Tube, Via Natural or Artificial Opening Endoscopic	**095P3ZZ** Destruction of Accessory Sinus, Percutaneous Approach
573ZZ Destruction of Right Tympanic Membrane, Percutaneous Approach	**095G0ZZ** Destruction of Left Eustachian Tube, Open Approach	**095P4ZZ** Destruction of Accessory Sinus, Percutaneous Endoscopic Approach
		095Q0ZZ Destruction of Right Maxillary Sinus, Open Approach
		095Q3ZZ Destruction of Right Maxillary Sinus, Percutaneous Approach

Female-only   ♂ Male-only   ▲ Limited Coverage   ● Non-OR   ▦ HAC-associated procedure   ▲ Non-covered procedures   ✚ Combination

095Q4ZZ Destruction of Right Maxillary Sinus, Percutaneous Endoscopic Approach	**095T3ZZ** Destruction of Left Frontal Sinus, Percutaneous Approach	**095W0ZZ** Destruction of Right Sphenoid Sinus, Open Approach
095R0ZZ Destruction of Left Maxillary Sinus, Open Approach	**095T4ZZ** Destruction of Left Frontal Sinus, Percutaneous Endoscopic Approach	**095W3ZZ** Destruction of Right Sphenoid Sinus, Percutaneous Approach
095R3ZZ Destruction of Left Maxillary Sinus, Percutaneous Approach	**095U0ZZ** Destruction of Right Ethmoid Sinus, Open Approach	**095W4ZZ** Destruction of Right Sphenoid Sinus, Percutaneous Endoscopic Approach
095R4ZZ Destruction of Left Maxillary Sinus, Percutaneous Endoscopic Approach	**095U3ZZ** Destruction of Right Ethmoid Sinus, Percutaneous Approach	**095X0ZZ** Destruction of Left Sphenoid Sinus, Open Approach
095S0ZZ Destruction of Right Frontal Sinus, Open Approach	**095U4ZZ** Destruction of Right Ethmoid Sinus, Percutaneous Endoscopic Approach	**095X3ZZ** Destruction of Left Sphenoid Sinus, Percutaneous Approach
095S3ZZ Destruction of Right Frontal Sinus, Percutaneous Approach	**095V0ZZ** Destruction of Left Ethmoid Sinus, Open Approach	**095X4ZZ** Destruction of Left Sphenoid Sinus, Percutaneous Endoscopic Approach
095S4ZZ Destruction of Right Frontal Sinus, Percutaneous Endoscopic Approach	**095V3ZZ** Destruction of Left Ethmoid Sinus, Percutaneous Approach	
095T0ZZ Destruction of Left Frontal Sinus, Open Approach	**095V4ZZ** Destruction of Left Ethmoid Sinus, Percutaneous Endoscopic Approach	

097 – Ear, Nose, Sinus, Dilation

097F0DZ Dilation of Right Eustachian Tube with Intraluminal Device, Open Approach	**097F8DZ** Dilation of Right Eustachian Tube with Intraluminal Device, Via Natural or Artificial Opening Endoscopic	**097G7DZ** Dilation of Left Eustachian Tube with Intraluminal Device, Via Natural or Artificial Opening
097F0ZZ Dilation of Right Eustachian Tube, Open Approach	**097F8ZZ** Dilation of Right Eustachian Tube, Via Natural or Artificial Opening Endoscopic	**097G7ZZ** Dilation of Left Eustachian Tube, Via Natural or Artificial Opening
097F3ZZ Dilation of Right Eustachian Tube, Percutaneous Approach	**097G0DZ** Dilation of Left Eustachian Tube with Intraluminal Device, Open Approach	**097G8DZ** Dilation of Left Eustachian Tube with Intraluminal Device, Via Natural or Artificial Opening Endoscopic
097F4ZZ Dilation of Right Eustachian Tube, Percutaneous Endoscopic Approach	**097G0ZZ** Dilation of Left Eustachian Tube, Open Approach	**097G8ZZ** Dilation of Left Eustachian Tube, Via Natural or Artificial Opening Endoscopic
097F7DZ Dilation of Right Eustachian Tube with Intraluminal Device, Via Natural or Artificial Opening	**097G3ZZ** Dilation of Left Eustachian Tube, Percutaneous Approach	
097F7ZZ Dilation of Right Eustachian Tube, Via Natural or Artificial Opening	**097G4ZZ** Dilation of Left Eustachian Tube, Percutaneous Endoscopic Approach	

098 – Ear, Nose, Sinus, Division

098L0ZZ Division of Nasal Turbinate, Open Approach	**098L4ZZ** Division of Nasal Turbinate, Percutaneous Endoscopic Approach	**098L8ZZ** Division of Nasal Turbinate, Via Natural or Artificial Opening Endoscopic
098L3ZZ Division of Nasal Turbinate, Percutaneous Approach	**098L7ZZ** Division of Nasal Turbinate, Via Natural or Artificial Opening	

099 – Ear, Nose, Sinus, Drainage

Review Coding Guidelines B3.4a and B3.4b

Review Coding Guideline B6.2

099000Z Drainage of Right External Ear with Drainage Device, Open Approach	**09910ZZ** Drainage of Left External Ear, Open Approach	**09933ZX** Drainage of Right External Auditory Canal, Percutaneous Approach, Diagnostic
09900ZX Drainage of Right External Ear, Open Approach, Diagnostic	**099130Z** Drainage of Left External Ear with Drainage Device, Percutaneous Approach	**09933ZZ** Drainage of Right External Auditory Canal, Percutaneous Approach
09900ZZ Drainage of Right External Ear, Open Approach	**09913ZX** Drainage of Left External Ear, Percutaneous Approach, Diagnostic	**099340Z** Drainage of Right External Auditory Canal with Drainage Device, Percutaneous Endoscopic Approach
099030Z Drainage of Right External Ear with Drainage Device, Percutaneous Approach	**09913ZZ** Drainage of Left External Ear, Percutaneous Approach	**09934ZX** Drainage of Right External Auditory Canal, Percutaneous Endoscopic Approach, Diagnostic
09903ZX Drainage of Right External Ear, Percutaneous Approach, Diagnostic	**099140Z** Drainage of Left External Ear with Drainage Device, Percutaneous Endoscopic Approach	**09934ZZ** Drainage of Right External Auditory Canal, Percutaneous Endoscopic Approach
09903ZZ Drainage of Right External Ear, Percutaneous Approach	**09914ZX** Drainage of Left External Ear, Percutaneous Endoscopic Approach, Diagnostic	**099370Z** Drainage of Right External Auditory Canal with Drainage Device, Via Natural or Artificial Opening
099040Z Drainage of Right External Ear with Drainage Device, Percutaneous Endoscopic Approach	**09914ZZ** Drainage of Left External Ear, Percutaneous Endoscopic Approach	**09937ZX** Drainage of Right External Auditory Canal, Via Natural or Artificial Opening, Diagnostic
09904ZX Drainage of Right External Ear, Percutaneous Endoscopic Approach, Diagnostic	**0991X0Z** Drainage of Left External Ear with Drainage Device, External Approach	**09937ZZ** Drainage of Right External Auditory Canal, Via Natural or Artificial Opening
09904ZZ Drainage of Right External Ear, Percutaneous Endoscopic Approach	**0991XZX** Drainage of Left External Ear, External Approach, Diagnostic	**099380Z** Drainage of Right External Auditory Canal with Drainage Device, Via Natural or Artificial Opening Endoscopic
0990X0Z Drainage of Right External Ear with Drainage Device, External Approach	**0991XZZ** Drainage of Left External Ear, External Approach	**09938ZX** Drainage of Right External Auditory Canal, Via Natural or Artificial Opening Endoscopic, Diagnostic
0990XZX Drainage of Right External Ear, External Approach, Diagnostic	**099300Z** Drainage of Right External Auditory Canal with Drainage Device, Open Approach	**09938ZZ** Drainage of Right External Auditory Canal, Via Natural or Artificial Opening Endoscopic
0990XZZ Drainage of Right External Ear, External Approach	**09930ZX** Drainage of Right External Auditory Canal, Open Approach, Diagnostic	
099100Z Drainage of Left External Ear with Drainage Device, Open Approach	**09930ZZ** Drainage of Right External Auditory Canal, Open Approach	
09910ZX Drainage of Left External Ear, Open Approach, Diagnostic	**099330Z** Drainage of Right External Auditory Canal with Drainage Device, Percutaneous Approach	

X0Z Drainage of Right External Auditory Canal with Drainage Device, External Approach	**099740Z** Drainage of Right Tympanic Membrane with Drainage Device, Percutaneous Endoscopic Approach	**099B0ZX** Drainage of Right Mastoid Sinus, Open Approach, Diagnostic
XZX Drainage of Right External Auditory Canal, External Approach, Diagnostic	**09974ZX** Drainage of Right Tympanic Membrane, Percutaneous Endoscopic Approach, Diagnostic	**099B0ZZ** Drainage of Right Mastoid Sinus, Open Approach
XZZ Drainage of Right External Auditory Canal, External Approach	**09974ZZ** Drainage of Right Tympanic Membrane, Percutaneous Endoscopic Approach	**099B30Z** Drainage of Right Mastoid Sinus with Drainage Device, Percutaneous Approach
400Z Drainage of Left External Auditory Canal with Drainage Device, Open Approach	**099770Z** Drainage of Right Tympanic Membrane with Drainage Device, Via Natural or Artificial Opening	**099B3ZX** Drainage of Right Mastoid Sinus, Percutaneous Approach, Diagnostic
40ZX Drainage of Left External Auditory Canal, Open Approach, Diagnostic	**09977ZX** Drainage of Right Tympanic Membrane, Via Natural or Artificial Opening, Diagnostic	**099B3ZZ** Drainage of Right Mastoid Sinus, Percutaneous Approach
40ZZ Drainage of Left External Auditory Canal, Open Approach	**09977ZZ** Drainage of Right Tympanic Membrane, Via Natural or Artificial Opening	**099B40Z** Drainage of Right Mastoid Sinus with Drainage Device, Percutaneous Endoscopic Approach
430Z Drainage of Left External Auditory Canal with Drainage Device, Percutaneous Approach	**099780Z** Drainage of Right Tympanic Membrane with Drainage Device, Via Natural or Artificial Opening Endoscopic	**099B4ZX** Drainage of Right Mastoid Sinus, Percutaneous Endoscopic Approach, Diagnostic
43ZX Drainage of Left External Auditory Canal, Percutaneous Approach, Diagnostic	**09978ZX** Drainage of Right Tympanic Membrane, Via Natural or Artificial Opening Endoscopic, Diagnostic	**099B4ZZ** Drainage of Right Mastoid Sinus, Percutaneous Endoscopic Approach
43ZZ Drainage of Left External Auditory Canal, Percutaneous Approach	**09978ZZ** Drainage of Right Tympanic Membrane, Via Natural or Artificial Opening Endoscopic	**099C00Z** Drainage of Left Mastoid Sinus with Drainage Device, Open Approach
440Z Drainage of Left External Auditory Canal with Drainage Device, Percutaneous Endoscopic Approach	**099800Z** Drainage of Left Tympanic Membrane with Drainage Device, Open Approach	**099C0ZX** Drainage of Left Mastoid Sinus, Open Approach, Diagnostic
44ZX Drainage of Left External Auditory Canal, Percutaneous Endoscopic Approach, Diagnostic	**09980ZX** Drainage of Left Tympanic Membrane, Open Approach, Diagnostic	**099C0ZZ** Drainage of Left Mastoid Sinus, Open Approach
44ZZ Drainage of Left External Auditory Canal, Percutaneous Endoscopic Approach	**09980ZZ** Drainage of Left Tympanic Membrane, Open Approach	**099C30Z** Drainage of Left Mastoid Sinus with Drainage Device, Percutaneous Approach
470Z Drainage of Left External Auditory Canal with Drainage Device, Via Natural or Artificial Opening	**099830Z** Drainage of Left Tympanic Membrane with Drainage Device, Percutaneous Approach	**099C3ZX** Drainage of Left Mastoid Sinus, Percutaneous Approach, Diagnostic
47ZX Drainage of Left External Auditory Canal, Via Natural or Artificial Opening, Diagnostic	**09983ZX** Drainage of Left Tympanic Membrane, Percutaneous Approach, Diagnostic	**099C3ZZ** Drainage of Left Mastoid Sinus, Percutaneous Approach
47ZZ Drainage of Left External Auditory Canal, Via Natural or Artificial Opening	**09983ZZ** Drainage of Left Tympanic Membrane, Percutaneous Approach	**099C40Z** Drainage of Left Mastoid Sinus with Drainage Device, Percutaneous Endoscopic Approach
480Z Drainage of Left External Auditory Canal with Drainage Device, Via Natural or Artificial Opening Endoscopic	**099840Z** Drainage of Left Tympanic Membrane with Drainage Device, Percutaneous Endoscopic Approach	**099C4ZX** Drainage of Left Mastoid Sinus, Percutaneous Endoscopic Approach, Diagnostic
48ZX Drainage of Left External Auditory Canal, Via Natural or Artificial Opening Endoscopic, Diagnostic	**09984ZX** Drainage of Left Tympanic Membrane, Percutaneous Endoscopic Approach, Diagnostic	**099C4ZZ** Drainage of Left Mastoid Sinus, Percutaneous Endoscopic Approach
48ZZ Drainage of Left External Auditory Canal, Via Natural or Artificial Opening Endoscopic	**09984ZZ** Drainage of Left Tympanic Membrane, Percutaneous Endoscopic Approach	**099D00Z** Drainage of Right Inner Ear with Drainage Device, Open Approach
4X0Z Drainage of Left External Auditory Canal with Drainage Device, External Approach	**099870Z** Drainage of Left Tympanic Membrane with Drainage Device, Via Natural or Artificial Opening	**099D0ZX** Drainage of Right Inner Ear, Open Approach, Diagnostic
4XZX Drainage of Left External Auditory Canal, External Approach, Diagnostic	**09987ZX** Drainage of Left Tympanic Membrane, Via Natural or Artificial Opening, Diagnostic	**099D0ZZ** Drainage of Right Inner Ear, Open Approach
4XZZ Drainage of Left External Auditory Canal, External Approach	**09987ZZ** Drainage of Left Tympanic Membrane, Via Natural or Artificial Opening	**099E00Z** Drainage of Left Inner Ear with Drainage Device, Open Approach
9500Z Drainage of Right Middle Ear with Drainage Device, Open Approach	**099880Z** Drainage of Left Tympanic Membrane with Drainage Device, Via Natural or Artificial Opening Endoscopic	**099E0ZX** Drainage of Left Inner Ear, Open Approach, Diagnostic
950ZX Drainage of Right Middle Ear, Open Approach, Diagnostic	**09988ZX** Drainage of Left Tympanic Membrane, Via Natural or Artificial Opening Endoscopic, Diagnostic	**099E0ZZ** Drainage of Left Inner Ear, Open Approach
950ZZ Drainage of Right Middle Ear, Open Approach	**09988ZZ** Drainage of Left Tympanic Membrane, Via Natural or Artificial Opening Endoscopic	**099F00Z** Drainage of Right Eustachian Tube with Drainage Device, Open Approach
9600Z Drainage of Left Middle Ear with Drainage Device, Open Approach	**099900Z** Drainage of Right Auditory Ossicle with Drainage Device, Open Approach	**099F0ZX** Drainage of Right Eustachian Tube, Open Approach, Diagnostic
960ZX Drainage of Left Middle Ear, Open Approach, Diagnostic	**09990ZX** Drainage of Right Auditory Ossicle, Open Approach, Diagnostic	**099F0ZZ** Drainage of Right Eustachian Tube, Open Approach
960ZZ Drainage of Left Middle Ear, Open Approach	**09990ZZ** Drainage of Right Auditory Ossicle, Open Approach	**099F30Z** Drainage of Right Eustachian Tube with Drainage Device, Percutaneous Approach
9700Z Drainage of Right Tympanic Membrane with Drainage Device, Open Approach	**099A00Z** Drainage of Left Auditory Ossicle with Drainage Device, Open Approach	**099F3ZX** Drainage of Right Eustachian Tube, Percutaneous Approach, Diagnostic
970ZX Drainage of Right Tympanic Membrane, Open Approach, Diagnostic	**099A0ZX** Drainage of Left Auditory Ossicle, Open Approach, Diagnostic	**099F3ZZ** Drainage of Right Eustachian Tube, Percutaneous Approach
970ZZ Drainage of Right Tympanic Membrane, Open Approach	**099A0ZZ** Drainage of Left Auditory Ossicle, Open Approach	**099F40Z** Drainage of Right Eustachian Tube with Drainage Device, Percutaneous Endoscopic Approach
9730Z Drainage of Right Tympanic Membrane with Drainage Device, Percutaneous Approach	**099B00Z** Drainage of Right Mastoid Sinus with Drainage Device, Open Approach	**099F4ZX** Drainage of Right Eustachian Tube, Percutaneous Endoscopic Approach, Diagnostic
973ZX Drainage of Right Tympanic Membrane, Percutaneous Approach, Diagnostic		**099F4ZZ** Drainage of Right Eustachian Tube, Percutaneous Endoscopic Approach
9973ZZ Drainage of Right Tympanic Membrane, Percutaneous Approach		**099F70Z** Drainage of Right Eustachian Tube with Drainage Device, Via Natural or Artificial Opening
		099F7ZX Drainage of Right Eustachian Tube, Via Natural or Artificial Opening, Diagnostic
		099F7ZZ Drainage of Right Eustachian Tube, Via Natural or Artificial Opening

441

099F80Z Drainage of Right Eustachian Tube with Drainage Device, Via Natural or Artificial Opening Endoscopic

099F8ZX Drainage of Right Eustachian Tube, Via Natural or Artificial Opening Endoscopic, Diagnostic

099F8ZZ Drainage of Right Eustachian Tube, Via Natural or Artificial Opening Endoscopic

099G00Z Drainage of Left Eustachian Tube with Drainage Device, Open Approach

099G0ZX Drainage of Left Eustachian Tube, Open Approach, Diagnostic

099G0ZZ Drainage of Left Eustachian Tube, Open Approach

099G30Z Drainage of Left Eustachian Tube with Drainage Device, Percutaneous Approach

099G3ZX Drainage of Left Eustachian Tube, Percutaneous Approach, Diagnostic

099G3ZZ Drainage of Left Eustachian Tube, Percutaneous Approach

099G40Z Drainage of Left Eustachian Tube with Drainage Device, Percutaneous Endoscopic Approach

099G4ZX Drainage of Left Eustachian Tube, Percutaneous Endoscopic Approach, Diagnostic

099G4ZZ Drainage of Left Eustachian Tube, Percutaneous Endoscopic Approach

099G70Z Drainage of Left Eustachian Tube with Drainage Device, Via Natural or Artificial Opening

099G7ZX Drainage of Left Eustachian Tube, Via Natural or Artificial Opening, Diagnostic

099G7ZZ Drainage of Left Eustachian Tube, Via Natural or Artificial Opening

099G80Z Drainage of Left Eustachian Tube with Drainage Device, Via Natural or Artificial Opening Endoscopic

099G8ZX Drainage of Left Eustachian Tube, Via Natural or Artificial Opening Endoscopic, Diagnostic

099G8ZZ Drainage of Left Eustachian Tube, Via Natural or Artificial Opening Endoscopic

099K00Z Drainage of Nose with Drainage Device, Open Approach

099K0ZX Drainage of Nose, Open Approach, Diagnostic

099K0ZZ Drainage of Nose, Open Approach

099K30Z Drainage of Nose with Drainage Device, Percutaneous Approach

099K3ZX Drainage of Nose, Percutaneous Approach, Diagnostic

099K3ZZ Drainage of Nose, Percutaneous Approach

099K40Z Drainage of Nose with Drainage Device, Percutaneous Endoscopic Approach

099K4ZX Drainage of Nose, Percutaneous Endoscopic Approach, Diagnostic

099K4ZZ Drainage of Nose, Percutaneous Endoscopic Approach

099KX0Z Drainage of Nose with Drainage Device, External Approach

099KXZX Drainage of Nose, External Approach, Diagnostic

099KXZZ Drainage of Nose, External Approach

099L00Z Drainage of Nasal Turbinate with Drainage Device, Open Approach

099L0ZX Drainage of Nasal Turbinate, Open Approach, Diagnostic

099L0ZZ Drainage of Nasal Turbinate, Open Approach

099L30Z Drainage of Nasal Turbinate with Drainage Device, Percutaneous Approach

099L3ZX Drainage of Nasal Turbinate, Percutaneous Approach, Diagnostic

099L3ZZ Drainage of Nasal Turbinate, Percutaneous Approach

099L40Z Drainage of Nasal Turbinate with Drainage Device, Percutaneous Endoscopic Approach

099L4ZX Drainage of Nasal Turbinate, Percutaneous Endoscopic Approach, Diagnostic

099L4ZZ Drainage of Nasal Turbinate, Percutaneous Endoscopic Approach

099L70Z Drainage of Nasal Turbinate with Drainage Device, Via Natural or Artificial Opening

099L7ZX Drainage of Nasal Turbinate, Via Natural or Artificial Opening, Diagnostic

099L7ZZ Drainage of Nasal Turbinate, Via Natural or Artificial Opening

099L80Z Drainage of Nasal Turbinate with Drainage Device, Via Natural or Artificial Opening Endoscopic

099L8ZX Drainage of Nasal Turbinate, Via Natural or Artificial Opening Endoscopic, Diagnostic

099L8ZZ Drainage of Nasal Turbinate, Via Natural or Artificial Opening Endoscopic

099M00Z Drainage of Nasal Septum with Drainage Device, Open Approach

099M0ZX Drainage of Nasal Septum, Open Approach, Diagnostic

099M0ZZ Drainage of Nasal Septum, Open Approach

099M30Z Drainage of Nasal Septum with Drainage Device, Percutaneous Approach

099M3ZX Drainage of Nasal Septum, Percutaneous Approach, Diagnostic

099M3ZZ Drainage of Nasal Septum, Percutaneous Approach

099M40Z Drainage of Nasal Septum with Drainage Device, Percutaneous Endoscopic Approach

099M4ZX Drainage of Nasal Septum, Percutaneous Endoscopic Approach, Diagnostic

099M4ZZ Drainage of Nasal Septum, Percutaneous Endoscopic Approach

099N00Z Drainage of Nasopharynx with Drainage Device, Open Approach

099N0ZX Drainage of Nasopharynx, Open Approach, Diagnostic

099N0ZZ Drainage of Nasopharynx, Open Approach

099N30Z Drainage of Nasopharynx with Drainage Device, Percutaneous Approach

099N3ZX Drainage of Nasopharynx, Percutaneous Approach, Diagnostic

099N3ZZ Drainage of Nasopharynx, Percutaneous Approach

099N40Z Drainage of Nasopharynx with Drainage Device, Percutaneous Endoscopic Approach

099N4ZX Drainage of Nasopharynx, Percutaneous Endoscopic Approach, Diagnostic

099N4ZZ Drainage of Nasopharynx, Percutaneous Endoscopic Approach

099N70Z Drainage of Nasopharynx with Drainage Device, Via Natural or Artificial Opening

099N7ZX Drainage of Nasopharynx, Via Natural or Artificial Opening, Diagnostic

099N7ZZ Drainage of Nasopharynx, Via Natural or Artificial Opening

099N80Z Drainage of Nasopharynx with Drainage Device, Via Natural or Artificial Opening Endoscopic

099N8ZX Drainage of Nasopharynx, Via Natural or Artificial Opening Endoscopic, Diagnostic

099N8ZZ Drainage of Nasopharynx, Via Natural or Artificial Opening Endoscopic

099P00Z Drainage of Accessory Sinus with Drainage Device, Open Approach

099P0ZX Drainage of Accessory Sinus, Open Approach, Diagnostic

099P0ZZ Drainage of Accessory Sinus, Open Approach

099P30Z Drainage of Accessory Sinus with Drainage Device, Percutaneous Appro

099P3ZX Drainage of Accessory Sinus, Percutaneous Approach, Diagnostic

099P3ZZ Drainage of Accessory Sinus, Percutaneous Approach

099P40Z Drainage of Accessory Sinus with Drainage Device, Percutaneous Endoscopic Approach

099P4ZX Drainage of Accessory Sinus, Percutaneous Endoscopic Approach, Diagnostic

099P4ZZ Drainage of Accessory Sinus, Percutaneous Endoscopic Approach

099Q00Z Drainage of Right Maxillary Sinus wit Drainage Device, Open Approach

099Q0ZX Drainage of Right Maxillary Sinus, Op Approach, Diagnostic

099Q0ZZ Drainage of Right Maxillary Sinus, Op Approach

099Q30Z Drainage of Right Maxillary Sinus with Drainage Device, Percutaneous Approach

099Q3ZX Drainage of Right Maxillary Sinus, Percutaneous Approach, Diagnostic

099Q3ZZ Drainage of Right Maxillary Sinus, Percutaneous Approach

099Q40Z Drainage of Right Maxillary Sinus with Drainage Device, Percutaneous Endoscopic Approach

099Q4ZX Drainage of Right Maxillary Sinus, Percutaneous Endoscopic Approach, Diagnostic

099Q4ZZ Drainage of Right Maxillary Sinus, Percutaneous Endoscopic Approach

099R00Z Drainage of Left Maxillary Sinus with Drainage Device, Open Approach

099R0ZX Drainage of Left Maxillary Sinus, Open Approach, Diagnostic

099R0ZZ Drainage of Left Maxillary Sinus, Open Approach

099R30Z Drainage of Left Maxillary Sinus with Drainage Device, Percutaneous Approac

099R3ZX Drainage of Left Maxillary Sinus, Percutaneous Approach, Diagnostic

099R3ZZ Drainage of Left Maxillary Sinus, Percutaneous Approach

099R40Z Drainage of Left Maxillary Sinus with Drainage Device, Percutaneous Endoscopic Approach

099R4ZX Drainage of Left Maxillary Sinus, Percutaneous Endoscopic Approach, Diagnostic

099R4ZZ Drainage of Left Maxillary Sinus, Percutaneous Endoscopic Approach

099S00Z Drainage of Right Frontal Sinus with Drainage Device, Open Approach

099S0ZX Drainage of Right Frontal Sinus, Open Approach, Diagnostic

099S0ZZ Drainage of Right Frontal Sinus, Open Approach

099S30Z Drainage of Right Frontal Sinus with Drainage Device, Percutaneous Approac

099S3ZX Drainage of Right Frontal Sinus, Percutaneous Approach, Diagnostic

099S3ZZ Drainage of Right Frontal Sinus, Percutaneous Approach

099S40Z Drainage of Right Frontal Sinus with Drainage Device, Percutaneous Endoscopic Approach

099S4ZX Drainage of Right Frontal Sinus, Percutaneous Endoscopic Approach, Diagnostic

099S4ZZ Drainage of Right Frontal Sinus, Percutaneous Endoscopic Approach

♀ Female-only   ♂ Male-only   ▲ Limited Coverage   ● Non-OR   ■ HAC-associated procedure   ▲ Non-covered procedures   ✛ Combinatic

00Z	Drainage of Left Frontal Sinus with Drainage Device, Open Approach
0ZX	Drainage of Left Frontal Sinus, Open Approach, Diagnostic
0ZZ	Drainage of Left Frontal Sinus, Open Approach
30Z	Drainage of Left Frontal Sinus with Drainage Device, Percutaneous Approach
3ZX	Drainage of Left Frontal Sinus, Percutaneous Approach, Diagnostic
3ZZ	Drainage of Left Frontal Sinus, Percutaneous Approach
40Z	Drainage of Left Frontal Sinus with Drainage Device, Percutaneous Endoscopic Approach
4ZX	Drainage of Left Frontal Sinus, Percutaneous Endoscopic Approach, Diagnostic
4ZZ	Drainage of Left Frontal Sinus, Percutaneous Endoscopic Approach
J00Z	Drainage of Right Ethmoid Sinus with Drainage Device, Open Approach
J0ZX	Drainage of Right Ethmoid Sinus, Open Approach, Diagnostic
J0ZZ	Drainage of Right Ethmoid Sinus, Open Approach
U30Z	Drainage of Right Ethmoid Sinus with Drainage Device, Percutaneous Approach
U3ZX	Drainage of Right Ethmoid Sinus, Percutaneous Approach, Diagnostic
U3ZZ	Drainage of Right Ethmoid Sinus, Percutaneous Approach

099U40Z	Drainage of Right Ethmoid Sinus with Drainage Device, Percutaneous Endoscopic Approach
099U4ZX	Drainage of Right Ethmoid Sinus, Percutaneous Endoscopic Approach, Diagnostic
099U4ZZ	Drainage of Right Ethmoid Sinus, Percutaneous Endoscopic Approach
099V00Z	Drainage of Left Ethmoid Sinus with Drainage Device, Open Approach
099V0ZX	Drainage of Left Ethmoid Sinus, Open Approach, Diagnostic
099V0ZZ	Drainage of Left Ethmoid Sinus, Open Approach
099V30Z	Drainage of Left Ethmoid Sinus with Drainage Device, Percutaneous Approach
099V3ZX	Drainage of Left Ethmoid Sinus, Percutaneous Approach, Diagnostic
099V3ZZ	Drainage of Left Ethmoid Sinus, Percutaneous Approach
099V40Z	Drainage of Left Ethmoid Sinus with Drainage Device, Percutaneous Endoscopic Approach
099V4ZX	Drainage of Left Ethmoid Sinus, Percutaneous Endoscopic Approach, Diagnostic
099V4ZZ	Drainage of Left Ethmoid Sinus, Percutaneous Endoscopic Approach
099W00Z	Drainage of Right Sphenoid Sinus with Drainage Device, Open Approach
099W0ZX	Drainage of Right Sphenoid Sinus, Open Approach, Diagnostic
099W0ZZ	Drainage of Right Sphenoid Sinus, Open Approach

099W30Z	Drainage of Right Sphenoid Sinus with Drainage Device, Percutaneous Approach
099W3ZX	Drainage of Right Sphenoid Sinus, Percutaneous Approach, Diagnostic
099W3ZZ	Drainage of Right Sphenoid Sinus, Percutaneous Approach
099W40Z	Drainage of Right Sphenoid Sinus with Drainage Device, Percutaneous Endoscopic Approach
099W4ZX	Drainage of Right Sphenoid Sinus, Percutaneous Endoscopic Approach, Diagnostic
099W4ZZ	Drainage of Right Sphenoid Sinus, Percutaneous Endoscopic Approach
099X00Z	Drainage of Left Sphenoid Sinus with Drainage Device, Open Approach
099X0ZX	Drainage of Left Sphenoid Sinus, Open Approach, Diagnostic
099X0ZZ	Drainage of Left Sphenoid Sinus, Open Approach
099X30Z	Drainage of Left Sphenoid Sinus with Drainage Device, Percutaneous Approach
099X3ZX	Drainage of Left Sphenoid Sinus, Percutaneous Approach, Diagnostic
099X3ZZ	Drainage of Left Sphenoid Sinus, Percutaneous Approach
099X40Z	Drainage of Left Sphenoid Sinus with Drainage Device, Percutaneous Endoscopic Approach
099X4ZX	Drainage of Left Sphenoid Sinus, Percutaneous Endoscopic Approach, Diagnostic
099X4ZZ	Drainage of Left Sphenoid Sinus, Percutaneous Endoscopic Approach

B – Ear, Nose, Sinus, Excision

Review Coding Guidelines B3.4a and B3.4b

Review Coding Guideline B3.8

00ZX	Excision of Right External Ear, Open Approach, Diagnostic
00ZZ	Excision of Right External Ear, Open Approach
03ZX	Excision of Right External Ear, Percutaneous Approach, Diagnostic
03ZZ	Excision of Right External Ear, Percutaneous Approach
04ZX	Excision of Right External Ear, Percutaneous Endoscopic Approach, Diagnostic
04ZZ	Excision of Right External Ear, Percutaneous Endoscopic Approach
0XZX	Excision of Right External Ear, External Approach, Diagnostic
0XZZ	Excision of Right External Ear, External Approach
B10ZX	Excision of Left External Ear, Open Approach, Diagnostic
B10ZZ	Excision of Left External Ear, Open Approach
B13ZX	Excision of Left External Ear, Percutaneous Approach, Diagnostic
B13ZZ	Excision of Left External Ear, Percutaneous Approach
B14ZX	Excision of Left External Ear, Percutaneous Endoscopic Approach, Diagnostic
B14ZZ	Excision of Left External Ear, Percutaneous Endoscopic Approach
B1XZX	Excision of Left External Ear, External Approach, Diagnostic
B1XZZ	Excision of Left External Ear, External Approach
B30ZX	Excision of Right External Auditory Canal, Open Approach, Diagnostic

09B30ZZ	Excision of Right External Auditory Canal, Open Approach
09B33ZX	Excision of Right External Auditory Canal, Percutaneous Approach, Diagnostic
09B33ZZ	Excision of Right External Auditory Canal, Percutaneous Approach
09B34ZX	Excision of Right External Auditory Canal, Percutaneous Endoscopic Approach, Diagnostic
09B34ZZ	Excision of Right External Auditory Canal, Percutaneous Endoscopic Approach
09B37ZX	Excision of Right External Auditory Canal, Via Natural or Artificial Opening, Diagnostic
09B37ZZ	Excision of Right External Auditory Canal, Via Natural or Artificial Opening
09B38ZX	Excision of Right External Auditory Canal, Via Natural or Artificial Opening Endoscopic, Diagnostic
09B38ZZ	Excision of Right External Auditory Canal, Via Natural or Artificial Opening Endoscopic
09B3XZX	Excision of Right External Auditory Canal, External Approach, Diagnostic
09B3XZZ	Excision of Right External Auditory Canal, External Approach
09B40ZX	Excision of Left External Auditory Canal, Open Approach, Diagnostic
09B40ZZ	Excision of Left External Auditory Canal, Open Approach
09B43ZX	Excision of Left External Auditory Canal, Percutaneous Approach, Diagnostic
09B43ZZ	Excision of Left External Auditory Canal, Percutaneous Approach

09B44ZX	Excision of Left External Auditory Canal, Percutaneous Endoscopic Approach, Diagnostic
09B44ZZ	Excision of Left External Auditory Canal, Percutaneous Endoscopic Approach
09B47ZX	Excision of Left External Auditory Canal, Via Natural or Artificial Opening, Diagnostic
09B47ZZ	Excision of Left External Auditory Canal, Via Natural or Artificial Opening
09B48ZX	Excision of Left External Auditory Canal, Via Natural or Artificial Opening Endoscopic, Diagnostic
09B48ZZ	Excision of Left External Auditory Canal, Via Natural or Artificial Opening Endoscopic
09B4XZX	Excision of Left External Auditory Canal, External Approach, Diagnostic
09B4XZZ	Excision of Left External Auditory Canal, External Approach
09B50ZX	Excision of Right Middle Ear, Open Approach, Diagnostic
09B50ZZ	Excision of Right Middle Ear, Open Approach
09B60ZX	Excision of Left Middle Ear, Open Approach, Diagnostic
09B60ZZ	Excision of Left Middle Ear, Open Approach
09B70ZX	Excision of Right Tympanic Membrane, Open Approach, Diagnostic
09B70ZZ	Excision of Right Tympanic Membrane, Open Approach
09B73ZX	Excision of Right Tympanic Membrane, Percutaneous Approach, Diagnostic
09B73ZZ	Excision of Right Tympanic Membrane, Percutaneous Approach

Female-only   ♂ Male-only   ▲ Limited Coverage   ● Non-OR   ▦ HAC-associated procedure   ▲ Non-covered procedures   ✛ Combination

09B74ZX	Excision of Right Tympanic Membrane, Percutaneous Endoscopic Approach, Diagnostic
09B74ZZ	Excision of Right Tympanic Membrane, Percutaneous Endoscopic Approach
09B77ZX	Excision of Right Tympanic Membrane, Via Natural or Artificial Opening, Diagnostic
09B77ZZ	Excision of Right Tympanic Membrane, Via Natural or Artificial Opening
09B78ZX	Excision of Right Tympanic Membrane, Via Natural or Artificial Opening Endoscopic, Diagnostic
09B78ZZ	Excision of Right Tympanic Membrane, Via Natural or Artificial Opening Endoscopic
09B80ZX	Excision of Left Tympanic Membrane, Open Approach, Diagnostic
09B80ZZ	Excision of Left Tympanic Membrane, Open Approach
09B83ZX	Excision of Left Tympanic Membrane, Percutaneous Approach, Diagnostic
09B83ZZ	Excision of Left Tympanic Membrane, Percutaneous Approach
09B84ZX	Excision of Left Tympanic Membrane, Percutaneous Endoscopic Approach, Diagnostic
09B84ZZ	Excision of Left Tympanic Membrane, Percutaneous Endoscopic Approach
09B87ZX	Excision of Left Tympanic Membrane, Via Natural or Artificial Opening, Diagnostic
09B87ZZ	Excision of Left Tympanic Membrane, Via Natural or Artificial Opening
09B88ZX	Excision of Left Tympanic Membrane, Via Natural or Artificial Opening Endoscopic, Diagnostic
09B88ZZ	Excision of Left Tympanic Membrane, Via Natural or Artificial Opening Endoscopic
09B90ZX	Excision of Right Auditory Ossicle, Open Approach, Diagnostic
09B90ZZ	Excision of Right Auditory Ossicle, Open Approach
09BA0ZX	Excision of Left Auditory Ossicle, Open Approach, Diagnostic
09BA0ZZ	Excision of Left Auditory Ossicle, Open Approach
09BB0ZX	Excision of Right Mastoid Sinus, Open Approach, Diagnostic
09BB0ZZ	Excision of Right Mastoid Sinus, Open Approach
09BB3ZX	Excision of Right Mastoid Sinus, Percutaneous Approach, Diagnostic
09BB3ZZ	Excision of Right Mastoid Sinus, Percutaneous Approach
09BB4ZX	Excision of Right Mastoid Sinus, Percutaneous Endoscopic Approach, Diagnostic
09BB4ZZ	Excision of Right Mastoid Sinus, Percutaneous Endoscopic Approach
09BC0ZX	Excision of Left Mastoid Sinus, Open Approach, Diagnostic
09BC0ZZ	Excision of Left Mastoid Sinus, Open Approach
09BC3ZX	Excision of Left Mastoid Sinus, Percutaneous Approach, Diagnostic
09BC3ZZ	Excision of Left Mastoid Sinus, Percutaneous Approach
09BC4ZX	Excision of Left Mastoid Sinus, Percutaneous Endoscopic Approach, Diagnostic
09BC4ZZ	Excision of Left Mastoid Sinus, Percutaneous Endoscopic Approach
09BD0ZX	Excision of Right Inner Ear, Open Approach, Diagnostic
09BD0ZZ	Excision of Right Inner Ear, Open Approach
09BE0ZX	Excision of Left Inner Ear, Open Approach, Diagnostic
09BE0ZZ	Excision of Left Inner Ear, Open Approach
09BF0ZX	Excision of Right Eustachian Tube, Open Approach, Diagnostic
09BF0ZZ	Excision of Right Eustachian Tube, Open Approach
09BF3ZX	Excision of Right Eustachian Tube, Percutaneous Approach, Diagnostic
09BF3ZZ	Excision of Right Eustachian Tube, Percutaneous Approach
09BF4ZX	Excision of Right Eustachian Tube, Percutaneous Endoscopic Approach, Diagnostic
09BF4ZZ	Excision of Right Eustachian Tube, Percutaneous Endoscopic Approach
09BF7ZX	Excision of Right Eustachian Tube, Via Natural or Artificial Opening, Diagnostic
09BF7ZZ	Excision of Right Eustachian Tube, Via Natural or Artificial Opening
09BF8ZX	Excision of Right Eustachian Tube, Via Natural or Artificial Opening Endoscopic, Diagnostic
09BF8ZZ	Excision of Right Eustachian Tube, Via Natural or Artificial Opening Endoscopic
09BG0ZX	Excision of Left Eustachian Tube, Open Approach, Diagnostic
09BG0ZZ	Excision of Left Eustachian Tube, Open Approach
09BG3ZX	Excision of Left Eustachian Tube, Percutaneous Approach, Diagnostic
09BG3ZZ	Excision of Left Eustachian Tube, Percutaneous Approach
09BG4ZX	Excision of Left Eustachian Tube, Percutaneous Endoscopic Approach, Diagnostic
09BG4ZZ	Excision of Left Eustachian Tube, Percutaneous Endoscopic Approach
09BG7ZX	Excision of Left Eustachian Tube, Via Natural or Artificial Opening, Diagnostic
09BG7ZZ	Excision of Left Eustachian Tube, Via Natural or Artificial Opening
09BG8ZX	Excision of Left Eustachian Tube, Via Natural or Artificial Opening Endoscopic, Diagnostic
09BG8ZZ	Excision of Left Eustachian Tube, Via Natural or Artificial Opening Endoscopic
09BK0ZX	Excision of Nose, Open Approach, Diagnostic
09BK0ZZ	Excision of Nose, Open Approach
09BK3ZX	Excision of Nose, Percutaneous Approach, Diagnostic
09BK3ZZ	Excision of Nose, Percutaneous Approach
09BK4ZX	Excision of Nose, Percutaneous Endoscopic Approach, Diagnostic
09BK4ZZ	Excision of Nose, Percutaneous Endoscopic Approach
09BKXZX	Excision of Nose, External Approach, Diagnostic
09BKXZZ	Excision of Nose, External Approach
09BL0ZX	Excision of Nasal Turbinate, Open Approach, Diagnostic
09BL0ZZ	Excision of Nasal Turbinate, Open Approach
09BL3ZX	Excision of Nasal Turbinate, Percutaneous Approach, Diagnostic
09BL3ZZ	Excision of Nasal Turbinate, Percutaneous Approach
09BL4ZX	Excision of Nasal Turbinate, Percutaneous Endoscopic Approach, Diagnostic
09BL4ZZ	Excision of Nasal Turbinate, Percutaneous Endoscopic Approach
09BL7ZX	Excision of Nasal Turbinate, Via Natural or Artificial Opening, Diagnostic
09BL7ZZ	Excision of Nasal Turbinate, Via Natural or Artificial Opening
09BL8ZX	Excision of Nasal Turbinate, Via Natu or Artificial Opening Endoscopic, Diagnostic
09BL8ZZ	Excision of Nasal Turbinate, Via Natu or Artificial Opening Endoscopic
09BM0ZX	Excision of Nasal Septum, Open Approach, Diagnostic
09BM0ZZ	Excision of Nasal Septum, Open App
09BM3ZX	Excision of Nasal Septum, Percutane Approach, Diagnostic
09BM3ZZ	Excision of Nasal Septum, Percutane Approach
09BM4ZX	Excision of Nasal Septum, Percutane Endoscopic Approach, Diagnostic
09BM4ZZ	Excision of Nasal Septum, Percutane Endoscopic Approach
09BN0ZX	Excision of Nasopharynx, Open App Diagnostic
09BN0ZZ	Excision of Nasopharynx, Open App
09BN3ZX	Excision of Nasopharynx, Percutane Approach, Diagnostic
09BN3ZZ	Excision of Nasopharynx, Percutane Approach
09BN4ZX	Excision of Nasopharynx, Percutane Endoscopic Approach, Diagnostic
09BN4ZZ	Excision of Nasopharynx, Percutane Endoscopic Approach
09BN7ZX	Excision of Nasopharynx, Via Natural Artificial Opening, Diagnostic
09BN7ZZ	Excision of Nasopharynx, Via Natural Artificial Opening
09BN8ZX	Excision of Nasopharynx, Via Natural Artificial Opening Endoscopic, Diagno
09BN8ZZ	Excision of Nasopharynx, Via Natural Artificial Opening Endoscopic
09BP0ZX	Excision of Accessory Sinus, Open Approach, Diagnostic
09BP0ZZ	Excision of Accessory Sinus, Open Approach
09BP3ZX	Excision of Accessory Sinus, Percutane Approach, Diagnostic
09BP3ZZ	Excision of Accessory Sinus, Percutane Approach
09BP4ZX	Excision of Accessory Sinus, Percutane Endoscopic Approach, Diagnostic
09BP4ZZ	Excision of Accessory Sinus, Percutane Endoscopic Approach
09BQ0ZX	Excision of Right Maxillary Sinus, Ope Approach, Diagnostic
09BQ0ZZ	Excision of Right Maxillary Sinus, Ope Approach
09BQ3ZX	Excision of Right Maxillary Sinus, Percutaneous Approach, Diagnostic
09BQ3ZZ	Excision of Right Maxillary Sinus, Percutaneous Approach
09BQ4ZX	Excision of Right Maxillary Sinus, Percutaneous Endoscopic Approach, Diagnostic
09BQ4ZZ	Excision of Right Maxillary Sinus, Percutaneous Endoscopic Approach
09BR0ZX	Excision of Left Maxillary Sinus, Open Approach, Diagnostic
09BR0ZZ	Excision of Left Maxillary Sinus, Open Approach
09BR3ZX	Excision of Left Maxillary Sinus, Percutaneous Approach, Diagnostic
09BR3ZZ	Excision of Left Maxillary Sinus, Percutaneous Approach
09BR4ZX	Excision of Left Maxillary Sinus, Percutaneous Endoscopic Approach, Diagnostic
09BR4ZZ	Excision of Left Maxillary Sinus, Percutaneous Endoscopic Approach
09BS0ZX	Excision of Right Frontal Sinus, Open Approach, Diagnostic
09BS0ZZ	Excision of Right Frontal Sinus, Open Approach

♀ Female-only	♂ Male-only	▲ Limited Coverage	● Non-OR	▦ HAC-associated procedure	▲ Non-covered procedures	+ Combinati

S3ZX	Excision of Right Frontal Sinus, Percutaneous Approach, Diagnostic	09BU3ZX	Excision of Right Ethmoid Sinus, Percutaneous Approach, Diagnostic	09BW3ZX	Excision of Right Sphenoid Sinus, Percutaneous Approach, Diagnostic
S3ZZ	Excision of Right Frontal Sinus, Percutaneous Approach	09BU3ZZ	Excision of Right Ethmoid Sinus, Percutaneous Approach	09BW3ZZ	Excision of Right Sphenoid Sinus, Percutaneous Approach
S4ZX	Excision of Right Frontal Sinus, Percutaneous Endoscopic Approach, Diagnostic	09BU4ZX	Excision of Right Ethmoid Sinus, Percutaneous Endoscopic Approach, Diagnostic	09BW4ZX	Excision of Right Sphenoid Sinus, Percutaneous Endoscopic Approach, Diagnostic
S4ZZ	Excision of Right Frontal Sinus, Percutaneous Endoscopic Approach	09BU4ZZ	Excision of Right Ethmoid Sinus, Percutaneous Endoscopic Approach	09BW4ZZ	Excision of Right Sphenoid Sinus, Percutaneous Endoscopic Approach
T0ZX	Excision of Left Frontal Sinus, Open Approach, Diagnostic	09BV0ZX	Excision of Left Ethmoid Sinus, Open Approach, Diagnostic	09BX0ZX	Excision of Left Sphenoid Sinus, Open Approach, Diagnostic
T0ZZ	Excision of Left Frontal Sinus, Open Approach	09BV0ZZ	Excision of Left Ethmoid Sinus, Open Approach	09BX0ZZ	Excision of Left Sphenoid Sinus, Open Approach
T3ZX	Excision of Left Frontal Sinus, Percutaneous Approach, Diagnostic	09BV3ZX	Excision of Left Ethmoid Sinus, Percutaneous Approach, Diagnostic	09BX3ZX	Excision of Left Sphenoid Sinus, Percutaneous Approach, Diagnostic
T3ZZ	Excision of Left Frontal Sinus, Percutaneous Approach	09BV3ZZ	Excision of Left Ethmoid Sinus, Percutaneous Approach	09BX3ZZ	Excision of Left Sphenoid Sinus, Percutaneous Approach
T4ZX	Excision of Left Frontal Sinus, Percutaneous Endoscopic Approach, Diagnostic	09BV4ZX	Excision of Left Ethmoid Sinus, Percutaneous Endoscopic Approach, Diagnostic	09BX4ZX	Excision of Left Sphenoid Sinus, Percutaneous Endoscopic Approach, Diagnostic
T4ZZ	Excision of Left Frontal Sinus, Percutaneous Endoscopic Approach	09BV4ZZ	Excision of Left Ethmoid Sinus, Percutaneous Endoscopic Approach	09BX4ZZ	Excision of Left Sphenoid Sinus, Percutaneous Endoscopic Approach
U0ZX	Excision of Right Ethmoid Sinus, Open Approach, Diagnostic	09BW0ZX	Excision of Right Sphenoid Sinus, Open Approach, Diagnostic		
U0ZZ	Excision of Right Ethmoid Sinus, Open Approach	09BW0ZZ	Excision of Right Sphenoid Sinus, Open Approach		

C – Ear, Nose, Sinus, Extirpation

00ZZ	Extirpation of Matter from Right External Ear, Open Approach	09C60ZZ	Extirpation of Matter from Left Middle Ear, Open Approach	09CE0ZZ	Extirpation of Matter from Left Inner Ear, Open Approach
03ZZ	Extirpation of Matter from Right External Ear, Percutaneous Approach	09C70ZZ	Extirpation of Matter from Right Tympanic Membrane, Open Approach	09CF0ZZ	Extirpation of Matter from Right Eustachian Tube, Open Approach
04ZZ	Extirpation of Matter from Right External Ear, Percutaneous Endoscopic Approach	09C73ZZ	Extirpation of Matter from Right Tympanic Membrane, Percutaneous Approach	09CF3ZZ	Extirpation of Matter from Right Eustachian Tube, Percutaneous Approach
0XZZ	Extirpation of Matter from Right External Ear, External Approach	09C74ZZ	Extirpation of Matter from Right Tympanic Membrane, Percutaneous Endoscopic Approach	09CF4ZZ	Extirpation of Matter from Right Eustachian Tube, Percutaneous Endoscopic Approach
10ZZ	Extirpation of Matter from Left External Ear, Open Approach	09C77ZZ	Extirpation of Matter from Right Tympanic Membrane, Via Natural or Artificial Opening	09CF7ZZ	Extirpation of Matter from Right Eustachian Tube, Via Natural or Artificial Opening
13ZZ	Extirpation of Matter from Left External Ear, Percutaneous Approach	09C78ZZ	Extirpation of Matter from Right Tympanic Membrane, Via Natural or Artificial Opening Endoscopic	09CF8ZZ	Extirpation of Matter from Right Eustachian Tube, Via Natural or Artificial Opening Endoscopic
14ZZ	Extirpation of Matter from Left External Ear, Percutaneous Endoscopic Approach	09C80ZZ	Extirpation of Matter from Left Tympanic Membrane, Open Approach	09CG0ZZ	Extirpation of Matter from Left Eustachian Tube, Open Approach
1XZZ	Extirpation of Matter from Left External Ear, External Approach	09C83ZZ	Extirpation of Matter from Left Tympanic Membrane, Percutaneous Approach	09CG3ZZ	Extirpation of Matter from Left Eustachian Tube, Percutaneous Approach
30ZZ	Extirpation of Matter from Right External Auditory Canal, Open Approach	09C84ZZ	Extirpation of Matter from Left Tympanic Membrane, Percutaneous Endoscopic Approach	09CG4ZZ	Extirpation of Matter from Left Eustachian Tube, Percutaneous Endoscopic Approach
33ZZ	Extirpation of Matter from Right External Auditory Canal, Percutaneous Approach	09C87ZZ	Extirpation of Matter from Left Tympanic Membrane, Via Natural or Artificial Opening	09CG7ZZ	Extirpation of Matter from Left Eustachian Tube, Via Natural or Artificial Opening
34ZZ	Extirpation of Matter from Right External Auditory Canal, Percutaneous Endoscopic Approach	09C88ZZ	Extirpation of Matter from Left Tympanic Membrane, Via Natural or Artificial Opening Endoscopic	09CG8ZZ	Extirpation of Matter from Left Eustachian Tube, Via Natural or Artificial Opening Endoscopic
37ZZ	Extirpation of Matter from Right External Auditory Canal, Via Natural or Artificial Opening	09C90ZZ	Extirpation of Matter from Right Auditory Ossicle, Open Approach	09CK0ZZ	Extirpation of Matter from Nose, Open Approach
38ZZ	Extirpation of Matter from Right External Auditory Canal, Via Natural or Artificial Opening Endoscopic	09CA0ZZ	Extirpation of Matter from Left Auditory Ossicle, Open Approach	09CK3ZZ	Extirpation of Matter from Nose, Percutaneous Approach
3XZZ	Extirpation of Matter from Right External Auditory Canal, External Approach	09CB0ZZ	Extirpation of Matter from Right Mastoid Sinus, Open Approach	09CK4ZZ	Extirpation of Matter from Nose, Percutaneous Endoscopic Approach
40ZZ	Extirpation of Matter from Left External Auditory Canal, Open Approach	09CB3ZZ	Extirpation of Matter from Right Mastoid Sinus, Percutaneous Approach	09CKXZZ	Extirpation of Matter from Nose, External Approach
43ZZ	Extirpation of Matter from Left External Auditory Canal, Percutaneous Approach	09CB4ZZ	Extirpation of Matter from Right Mastoid Sinus, Percutaneous Endoscopic Approach	09CL0ZZ	Extirpation of Matter from Nasal Turbinate, Open Approach
44ZZ	Extirpation of Matter from Left External Auditory Canal, Percutaneous Endoscopic Approach	09CC0ZZ	Extirpation of Matter from Left Mastoid Sinus, Open Approach	09CL3ZZ	Extirpation of Matter from Nasal Turbinate, Percutaneous Approach
47ZZ	Extirpation of Matter from Left External Auditory Canal, Via Natural or Artificial Opening	09CC3ZZ	Extirpation of Matter from Left Mastoid Sinus, Percutaneous Approach	09CL4ZZ	Extirpation of Matter from Nasal Turbinate, Percutaneous Endoscopic Approach
48ZZ	Extirpation of Matter from Left External Auditory Canal, Via Natural or Artificial Opening Endoscopic	09CC4ZZ	Extirpation of Matter from Left Mastoid Sinus, Percutaneous Endoscopic Approach	09CL7ZZ	Extirpation of Matter from Nasal Turbinate, Via Natural or Artificial Opening
4XZZ	Extirpation of Matter from Left External Auditory Canal, External Approach	09CD0ZZ	Extirpation of Matter from Right Inner Ear, Open Approach	09CL8ZZ	Extirpation of Matter from Nasal Turbinate, Via Natural or Artificial Opening Endoscopic
C50ZZ	Extirpation of Matter from Right Middle Ear, Open Approach				

Female-only   ♂ Male-only   ▲ Limited Coverage   ● Non-OR   ▦ HAC-associated procedure   ▲ Non-covered procedures   ✚ Combination

09CM0ZZ Extirpation of Matter from Nasal Septum, Open Approach

09CM3ZZ Extirpation of Matter from Nasal Septum, Percutaneous Approach

09CM4ZZ Extirpation of Matter from Nasal Septum, Percutaneous Endoscopic Approach

09CN0ZZ Extirpation of Matter from Nasopharynx, Open Approach

09CN3ZZ Extirpation of Matter from Nasopharynx, Percutaneous Approach

09CN4ZZ Extirpation of Matter from Nasopharynx, Percutaneous Endoscopic Approach

09CN7ZZ Extirpation of Matter from Nasopharynx, Via Natural or Artificial Opening

09CN8ZZ Extirpation of Matter from Nasopharynx, Via Natural or Artificial Opening Endoscopic

09CP0ZZ Extirpation of Matter from Accessory Sinus, Open Approach

09CP3ZZ Extirpation of Matter from Accessory Sinus, Percutaneous Approach

09CP4ZZ Extirpation of Matter from Accessory Sinus, Percutaneous Endoscopic Approach

09CQ0ZZ Extirpation of Matter from Right Maxillary Sinus, Open Approach

09CQ3ZZ Extirpation of Matter from Right Maxillary Sinus, Percutaneous Approach

09CQ4ZZ Extirpation of Matter from Right Maxillary Sinus, Percutaneous Endoscopic Approach

09CR0ZZ Extirpation of Matter from Left Maxillary Sinus, Open Approach

09CR3ZZ Extirpation of Matter from Left Maxillary Sinus, Percutaneous Approach

09CR4ZZ Extirpation of Matter from Left Maxillary Sinus, Percutaneous Endoscopic Approach

09CS0ZZ Extirpation of Matter from Right Frontal Sinus, Open Approach

09CS3ZZ Extirpation of Matter from Right Frontal Sinus, Percutaneous Approach

09CS4ZZ Extirpation of Matter from Right Frontal Sinus, Percutaneous Endoscopic Approach

09CT0ZZ Extirpation of Matter from Left Frontal Sinus, Open Approach

09CT3ZZ Extirpation of Matter from Left Frontal Sinus, Percutaneous Approach

09CT4ZZ Extirpation of Matter from Left Frontal Sinus, Percutaneous Endoscopic Approach

09CU0ZZ Extirpation of Matter from Right Ethmoid Sinus, Open Approach

09CU3ZZ Extirpation of Matter from Right Ethm┄ Sinus, Percutaneous Approach

09CU4ZZ Extirpation of Matter from Right Ethm┄ Sinus, Percutaneous Endoscopic Appr┄

09CV0ZZ Extirpation of Matter from Left Ethm┄ Sinus, Open Approach

09CV3ZZ Extirpation of Matter from Left Ethm┄ Sinus, Percutaneous Approach

09CV4ZZ Extirpation of Matter from Left Ethm┄ Sinus, Percutaneous Endoscopic Appr┄

09CW0ZZ Extirpation of Matter from Right Sphe┄ Sinus, Open Approach

09CW3ZZ Extirpation of Matter from Right Sphe┄ Sinus, Percutaneous Approach

09CW4ZZ Extirpation of Matter from Right Sphe┄ Sinus, Percutaneous Endoscopic Appr┄

09CX0ZZ Extirpation of Matter from Left Sphen┄ Sinus, Open Approach

09CX3ZZ Extirpation of Matter from Left Sphen┄ Sinus, Percutaneous Approach

09CX4ZZ Extirpation of Matter from Left Sphen┄ Sinus, Percutaneous Endoscopic Appr┄

09D – Ear, Nose, Sinus, Extraction

09D70ZZ Extraction of Right Tympanic Membrane, Open Approach

09D73ZZ Extraction of Right Tympanic Membrane, Percutaneous Approach

09D74ZZ Extraction of Right Tympanic Membrane, Percutaneous Endoscopic Approach

09D77ZZ Extraction of Right Tympanic Membrane, Via Natural or Artificial Opening

09D78ZZ Extraction of Right Tympanic Membrane, Via Natural or Artificial Opening Endoscopic

09D80ZZ Extraction of Left Tympanic Membrane, Open Approach

09D83ZZ Extraction of Left Tympanic Membrane, Percutaneous Approach

09D84ZZ Extraction of Left Tympanic Membrane, Percutaneous Endoscopic Approach

09D87ZZ Extraction of Left Tympanic Membrane, Via Natural or Artificial Opening

09D88ZZ Extraction of Left Tympanic Membrane, Via Natural or Artificial Opening Endoscopic

09D90ZZ Extraction of Right Auditory Ossicle, Open Approach

09DA0ZZ Extraction of Left Auditory Ossicle, Open Approach

09DB0ZZ Extraction of Right Mastoid Sinus, Open Approach

09DB3ZZ Extraction of Right Mastoid Sinus, Percutaneous Approach

09DB4ZZ Extraction of Right Mastoid Sinus, Percutaneous Endoscopic Approach

09DC0ZZ Extraction of Left Mastoid Sinus, Open Approach

09DC3ZZ Extraction of Left Mastoid Sinus, Percutaneous Approach

09DC4ZZ Extraction of Left Mastoid Sinus, Percutaneous Endoscopic Approach

09DL0ZZ Extraction of Nasal Turbinate, Open Approach

09DL3ZZ Extraction of Nasal Turbinate, Percutaneous Approach

09DL4ZZ Extraction of Nasal Turbinate, Percutaneous Endoscopic Approach

09DL7ZZ Extraction of Nasal Turbinate, Via Natural or Artificial Opening

09DL8ZZ Extraction of Nasal Turbinate, Via Natural or Artificial Opening Endoscopic

09DM0ZZ Extraction of Nasal Septum, Open Approach

09DM3ZZ Extraction of Nasal Septum, Percutaneous Approach

09DM4ZZ Extraction of Nasal Septum, Percutaneous Endoscopic Approach

09DP0ZZ Extraction of Accessory Sinus, Open Approach

09DP3ZZ Extraction of Accessory Sinus, Percutaneous Approach

09DP4ZZ Extraction of Accessory Sinus, Percutaneous Endoscopic Approach

09DQ0ZZ Extraction of Right Maxillary Sinus, Open Approach

09DQ3ZZ Extraction of Right Maxillary Sinus, Percutaneous Approach

09DQ4ZZ Extraction of Right Maxillary Sinus, Percutaneous Endoscopic Approach

09DR0ZZ Extraction of Left Maxillary Sinus, Open Approach

09DR3ZZ Extraction of Left Maxillary Sinus, Percutaneous Approach

09DR4ZZ Extraction of Left Maxillary Sinus, Percutaneous Endoscopic Approach

09DS0ZZ Extraction of Right Frontal Sinus, Ope┄ Approach

09DS3ZZ Extraction of Right Frontal Sinus, Percutaneous Approach

09DS4ZZ Extraction of Right Frontal Sinus, Percutaneous Endoscopic Approach

09DT0ZZ Extraction of Left Frontal Sinus, Open Approach

09DT3ZZ Extraction of Left Frontal Sinus, Percutaneous Approach

09DT4ZZ Extraction of Left Frontal Sinus, Percutaneous Endoscopic Approach

09DU0ZZ Extraction of Right Ethmoid Sinus, Op┄ Approach

09DU3ZZ Extraction of Right Ethmoid Sinus, Percutaneous Approach

09DU4ZZ Extraction of Right Ethmoid Sinus, Percutaneous Endoscopic Approach

09DV0ZZ Extraction of Left Ethmoid Sinus, Ope┄ Approach

09DV3ZZ Extraction of Left Ethmoid Sinus, Percutaneous Approach

09DV4ZZ Extraction of Left Ethmoid Sinus, Percutaneous Endoscopic Approach

09DW0ZZ Extraction of Right Sphenoid Sinus, Op┄ Approach

09DW3ZZ Extraction of Right Sphenoid Sinus, Percutaneous Approach

09DW4ZZ Extraction of Right Sphenoid Sinus, Percutaneous Endoscopic Approach

09DX0ZZ Extraction of Left Sphenoid Sinus, Ope┄ Approach

09DX3ZZ Extraction of Left Sphenoid Sinus, Percutaneous Approach

09DX4ZZ Extraction of Left Sphenoid Sinus, Percutaneous Endoscopic Approach

09H – Ear, Nose, Sinus, Insertion

09HD04Z Insertion of Bone Conduction Hearing Device into Right Inner Ear, Open Approach

09HD05Z Insertion of Single Channel Cochlear Prosthesis into Right Inner Ear, Open Approach

09HD06Z Insertion of Multiple Channel Cochlear Prosthesis into Right Inner Ear, Open Approach

09HD0SZ Insertion of Hearing Device into Right Inner Ear, Open Approach

09HD34Z Insertion of Bone Conduction Hearing Device into Right Inner Ear, Percutaneous Approach

09HD35Z Insertion of Single Channel Cochlear Prosthesis into Right Inner Ear, Percutaneous Approach

09HD36Z Insertion of Multiple Channel Cochlear Prosthesis into Right Inner Ear, Percutaneous Approach

09HD3SZ Insertion of Hearing Device into Right Inner Ear, Percutaneous Approach

09HD44Z Insertion of Bone Conduction Hearing Device into Right Inner Ear, Percutaneous Endoscopic Approach

09HD45Z Insertion of Single Channel Cochlear Prosthesis into Right Inner Ear, Percutaneous Endoscopic Approach

09HD46Z Insertion of Multiple Channel Cochlear Prosthesis into Right Inner Ear, Percutaneous Endoscopic Approach

♀ Female-only   ♂ Male-only   ▲ Limited Coverage   ● Non-OR   ▰ HAC-associated procedure   ▲ Non-covered procedures   ✛ Combina┄

D4SZ Insertion of Hearing Device into Right Inner Ear, Percutaneous Endoscopic Approach	**09HE34Z** Insertion of Bone Conduction Hearing Device into Left Inner Ear, Percutaneous Approach	**09HE45Z** Insertion of Single Channel Cochlear Prosthesis into Left Inner Ear, Percutaneous Endoscopic Approach
E04Z Insertion of Bone Conduction Hearing Device into Left Inner Ear, Open Approach	**09HE35Z** Insertion of Single Channel Cochlear Prosthesis into Left Inner Ear, Percutaneous Approach	**09HE46Z** Insertion of Multiple Channel Cochlear Prosthesis into Left Inner Ear, Percutaneous Endoscopic Approach
E05Z Insertion of Single Channel Cochlear Prosthesis into Left Inner Ear, Open Approach	**09HE36Z** Insertion of Multiple Channel Cochlear Prosthesis into Left Inner Ear, Percutaneous Approach	**09HE4SZ** Insertion of Hearing Device into Left Inner Ear, Percutaneous Endoscopic Approach
E06Z Insertion of Multiple Channel Cochlear Prosthesis into Left Inner Ear, Open Approach	**09HE3SZ** Insertion of Hearing Device into Left Inner Ear, Percutaneous Approach	**09HN7BZ** Insertion of Airway into Nasopharynx, Via Natural or Artificial Opening
E0SZ Insertion of Hearing Device into Left Inner Ear, Open Approach	**09HE44Z** Insertion of Bone Conduction Hearing Device into Left Inner Ear, Percutaneous Endoscopic Approach	**09HN8BZ** Insertion of Airway into Nasopharynx, Via Natural or Artificial Opening Endoscopic

J – Ear, Nose, Sinus, Inspection

view Coding Guidelines B3.11a, B3.11b and B3.11c

70ZZ Inspection of Right Tympanic Membrane, Open Approach	**09JD0ZZ** Inspection of Right Inner Ear, Open Approach	**09JHXZZ** Inspection of Right Ear, External Approach
73ZZ Inspection of Right Tympanic Membrane, Percutaneous Approach	**09JD3ZZ** Inspection of Right Inner Ear, Percutaneous Approach	**09JJ0ZZ** Inspection of Left Ear, Open Approach
74ZZ Inspection of Right Tympanic Membrane, Percutaneous Endoscopic Approach	**09JD4ZZ** Inspection of Right Inner Ear, Percutaneous Endoscopic Approach	**09JJ3ZZ** Inspection of Left Ear, Percutaneous Approach
77ZZ Inspection of Right Tympanic Membrane, Via Natural or Artificial Opening	**09JDXZZ** Inspection of Right Inner Ear, External Approach	**09JJ4ZZ** Inspection of Left Ear, Percutaneous Endoscopic Approach
78ZZ Inspection of Right Tympanic Membrane, Via Natural or Artificial Opening Endoscopic	**09JE0ZZ** Inspection of Left Inner Ear, Open Approach	**09JJ7ZZ** Inspection of Left Ear, Via Natural or Artificial Opening
7XZZ Inspection of Right Tympanic Membrane, External Approach	**09JE3ZZ** Inspection of Left Inner Ear, Percutaneous Approach	**09JJ8ZZ** Inspection of Left Ear, Via Natural or Artificial Opening Endoscopic
80ZZ Inspection of Left Tympanic Membrane, Open Approach	**09JE4ZZ** Inspection of Left Inner Ear, Percutaneous Endoscopic Approach	**09JJXZZ** Inspection of Left Ear, External Approach
83ZZ Inspection of Left Tympanic Membrane, Percutaneous Approach	**09JEXZZ** Inspection of Left Inner Ear, External Approach	**09JK0ZZ** Inspection of Nose, Open Approach
84ZZ Inspection of Left Tympanic Membrane, Percutaneous Endoscopic Approach	**09JH0ZZ** Inspection of Right Ear, Open Approach	**09JK3ZZ** Inspection of Nose, Percutaneous Approach
87ZZ Inspection of Left Tympanic Membrane, Via Natural or Artificial Opening	**09JH3ZZ** Inspection of Right Ear, Percutaneous Approach	**09JK4ZZ** Inspection of Nose, Percutaneous Endoscopic Approach
88ZZ Inspection of Left Tympanic Membrane, Via Natural or Artificial Opening Endoscopic	**09JH4ZZ** Inspection of Right Ear, Percutaneous Endoscopic Approach	**09JKXZZ** Inspection of Nose, External Approach
8XZZ Inspection of Left Tympanic Membrane, External Approach	**09JH7ZZ** Inspection of Right Ear, Via Natural or Artificial Opening	**09JY0ZZ** Inspection of Sinus, Open Approach
	09JH8ZZ Inspection of Right Ear, Via Natural or Artificial Opening Endoscopic	**09JY3ZZ** Inspection of Sinus, Percutaneous Approach
		09JY4ZZ Inspection of Sinus, Percutaneous Endoscopic Approach
		09JYXZZ Inspection of Sinus, External Approach

M – Ear, Nose, Sinus, Reattachment

M0XZZ Reattachment of Right External Ear, External Approach	**09M1XZZ** Reattachment of Left External Ear, External Approach	**09MKXZZ** Reattachment of Nose, External Approach

N – Ear, Nose, Sinus, Release

view Coding Guidelines B3.13 and B3.14

N00ZZ Release Right External Ear, Open Approach	**09N38ZZ** Release Right External Auditory Canal, Via Natural or Artificial Opening Endoscopic	**09N73ZZ** Release Right Tympanic Membrane, Percutaneous Approach
N03ZZ Release Right External Ear, Percutaneous Approach		**09N74ZZ** Release Right Tympanic Membrane, Percutaneous Endoscopic Approach
N04ZZ Release Right External Ear, Percutaneous Endoscopic Approach	**09N3XZZ** Release Right External Auditory Canal, External Approach	**09N77ZZ** Release Right Tympanic Membrane, Via Natural or Artificial Opening
N0XZZ Release Right External Ear, External Approach	**09N40ZZ** Release Left External Auditory Canal, Open Approach	**09N78ZZ** Release Right Tympanic Membrane, Via Natural or Artificial Opening Endoscopic
N10ZZ Release Left External Ear, Open Approach	**09N43ZZ** Release Left External Auditory Canal, Percutaneous Approach	**09N80ZZ** Release Left Tympanic Membrane, Open Approach
N13ZZ Release Left External Ear, Percutaneous Approach	**09N44ZZ** Release Left External Auditory Canal, Percutaneous Endoscopic Approach	**09N83ZZ** Release Left Tympanic Membrane, Percutaneous Approach
N14ZZ Release Left External Ear, Percutaneous Endoscopic Approach	**09N47ZZ** Release Left External Auditory Canal, Via Natural or Artificial Opening	**09N84ZZ** Release Left Tympanic Membrane, Percutaneous Endoscopic Approach
N1XZZ Release Left External Ear, External Approach	**09N48ZZ** Release Left External Auditory Canal, Via Natural or Artificial Opening Endoscopic	**09N87ZZ** Release Left Tympanic Membrane, Via Natural or Artificial Opening
N30ZZ Release Right External Auditory Canal, Open Approach	**09N4XZZ** Release Left External Auditory Canal, External Approach	**09N88ZZ** Release Left Tympanic Membrane, Via Natural or Artificial Opening Endoscopic
N33ZZ Release Right External Auditory Canal, Percutaneous Approach	**09N50ZZ** Release Right Middle Ear, Open Approach	**09N90ZZ** Release Right Auditory Ossicle, Open Approach
N34SZ Release Right External Auditory Canal, Percutaneous Endoscopic Approach	**09N60ZZ** Release Left Middle Ear, Open Approach	**09NA0ZZ** Release Left Auditory Ossicle, Open Approach
N37ZZ Release Right External Auditory Canal, Via Natural or Artificial Opening	**09N70ZZ** Release Right Tympanic Membrane, Open Approach	

♀ Female-only	♂ Male-only	▲ Limited Coverage	● Non-OR	▬ HAC-associated procedure	▲ Non-covered procedures	✚ Combination

09NB0ZZ	Release Right Mastoid Sinus, Open Approach	09NL0ZZ	Release Nasal Turbinate, Open Approach	09NR4ZZ	Release Left Maxillary Sinus, Percutaneous Endoscopic Approach
09NB3ZZ	Release Right Mastoid Sinus, Percutaneous Approach	09NL3ZZ	Release Nasal Turbinate, Percutaneous Approach	09NS0ZZ	Release Right Frontal Sinus, Open Approach
09NB4ZZ	Release Right Mastoid Sinus, Percutaneous Endoscopic Approach	09NL4ZZ	Release Nasal Turbinate, Percutaneous Endoscopic Approach	09NS3ZZ	Release Right Frontal Sinus, Percutane Approach
09NC0ZZ	Release Left Mastoid Sinus, Open Approach	09NL7ZZ	Release Nasal Turbinate, Via Natural or Artificial Opening	09NS4ZZ	Release Right Frontal Sinus, Percutane Endoscopic Approach
09NC3ZZ	Release Left Mastoid Sinus, Percutaneous Approach	09NL8ZZ	Release Nasal Turbinate, Via Natural or Artificial Opening Endoscopic	09NT0ZZ	Release Left Frontal Sinus, Open Approach
09NC4ZZ	Release Left Mastoid Sinus, Percutaneous Endoscopic Approach	09NM0ZZ	Release Nasal Septum, Open Approach	09NT3ZZ	Release Left Frontal Sinus, Percutaneo Approach
09ND0ZZ	Release Right Inner Ear, Open Approach	09NM3ZZ	Release Nasal Septum, Percutaneous Approach	09NT4ZZ	Release Left Frontal Sinus, Percutaneo Endoscopic Approach
09NE0ZZ	Release Left Inner Ear, Open Approach	09NM4ZZ	Release Nasal Septum, Percutaneous Endoscopic Approach	09NU0ZZ	Release Right Ethmoid Sinus, Open Approach
09NF0ZZ	Release Right Eustachian Tube, Open Approach	09NN0ZZ	Release Nasopharynx, Open Approach	09NU3ZZ	Release Right Ethmoid Sinus, Percutaneous Approach
09NF3ZZ	Release Right Eustachian Tube, Percutaneous Approach	09NN3ZZ	Release Nasopharynx, Percutaneous Approach	09NU4ZZ	Release Right Ethmoid Sinus, Percutaneous Endoscopic Approach
09NF4ZZ	Release Right Eustachian Tube, Percutaneous Endoscopic Approach	09NN4ZZ	Release Nasopharynx, Percutaneous Endoscopic Approach	09NV0ZZ	Release Left Ethmoid Sinus, Open Approach
09NF7ZZ	Release Right Eustachian Tube, Via Natural or Artificial Opening	09NN7ZZ	Release Nasopharynx, Via Natural or Artificial Opening	09NV3ZZ	Release Left Ethmoid Sinus, Percutane Approach
09NF8ZZ	Release Right Eustachian Tube, Via Natural or Artificial Opening Endoscopic	09NN8ZZ	Release Nasopharynx, Via Natural or Artificial Opening Endoscopic	09NV4ZZ	Release Left Ethmoid Sinus, Percutane Endoscopic Approach
09NG0ZZ	Release Left Eustachian Tube, Open Approach	09NP0ZZ	Release Accessory Sinus, Open Approach	09NW0ZZ	Release Right Sphenoid Sinus, Open Approach
09NG3ZZ	Release Left Eustachian Tube, Percutaneous Approach	09NP3ZZ	Release Accessory Sinus, Percutaneous Approach	09NW3ZZ	Release Right Sphenoid Sinus, Percutaneous Approach
09NG4ZZ	Release Left Eustachian Tube, Percutaneous Endoscopic Approach	09NP4ZZ	Release Accessory Sinus, Percutaneous Endoscopic Approach	09NW4ZZ	Release Right Sphenoid Sinus, Percutaneous Endoscopic Approach
09NG7ZZ	Release Left Eustachian Tube, Via Natural or Artificial Opening	09NQ0ZZ	Release Right Maxillary Sinus, Open Approach	09NX0ZZ	Release Left Sphenoid Sinus, Open Approach
09NG8ZZ	Release Left Eustachian Tube, Via Natural or Artificial Opening Endoscopic	09NQ3ZZ	Release Right Maxillary Sinus, Percutaneous Approach	09NX3ZZ	Release Left Sphenoid Sinus, Percutaneous Approach
09NK0ZZ	Release Nose, Open Approach	09NQ4ZZ	Release Right Maxillary Sinus, Percutaneous Endoscopic Approach	09NX4ZZ	Release Left Sphenoid Sinus, Percutaneous Endoscopic Approach
09NK3ZZ	Release Nose, Percutaneous Approach	09NR0ZZ	Release Left Maxillary Sinus, Open Approach		
09NK4ZZ	Release Nose, Percutaneous Endoscopic Approach	09NR3ZZ	Release Left Maxillary Sinus, Percutaneous Approach		
09NKXZZ	Release Nose, External Approach				

09P – Ear, Nose, Sinus, Removal

Review Coding Guideline B6.1c

09P700Z	Removal of Drainage Device from Right Tympanic Membrane, Open Approach	09PE7SZ	Removal of Hearing Device from Left Inner Ear, Via Natural or Artificial Opening	09PH4DZ	Removal of Intraluminal Device from Right Ear, Percutaneous Endoscopic Approach
09P770Z	Removal of Drainage Device from Right Tympanic Membrane, Via Natural or Artificial Opening	09PE8SZ	Removal of Hearing Device from Left Inner Ear, Via Natural or Artificial Opening Endoscopic	09PH4JZ	Removal of Synthetic Substitute from Right Ear, Percutaneous Endoscopic Approach
09P780Z	Removal of Drainage Device from Right Tympanic Membrane, Via Natural or Artificial Opening Endoscopic	09PH00Z	Removal of Drainage Device from Right Ear, Open Approach	09PH4KZ	Removal of Nonautologous Tissue Substitute from Right Ear, Percutaneous Endoscopic Approach
09P7X0Z	Removal of Drainage Device from Right Tympanic Membrane, External Approach	09PH07Z	Removal of Autologous Tissue Substitute from Right Ear, Open Approach	09PH70Z	Removal of Drainage Device from Right Ear, Via Natural or Artificial Opening
09P800Z	Removal of Drainage Device from Left Tympanic Membrane, Open Approach	09PH0DZ	Removal of Intraluminal Device from Right Ear, Open Approach	09PH77Z	Removal of Autologous Tissue Substitu from Right Ear, Via Natural or Artificial Opening
09P870Z	Removal of Drainage Device from Left Tympanic Membrane, Via Natural or Artificial Opening	09PH0JZ	Removal of Synthetic Substitute from Right Ear, Open Approach	09PH7DZ	Removal of Intraluminal Device from Right Ear, Via Natural or Artificial Opening
09P880Z	Removal of Drainage Device from Left Tympanic Membrane, Via Natural or Artificial Opening Endoscopic	09PH0KZ	Removal of Nonautologous Tissue Substitute from Right Ear, Open Approach	09PH7JZ	Removal of Synthetic Substitute from Right Ear, Via Natural or Artificial Opening
09P8X0Z	Removal of Drainage Device from Left Tympanic Membrane, External Approach	09PH30Z	Removal of Drainage Device from Right Ear, Percutaneous Approach	09PH7KZ	Removal of Nonautologous Tissue Substitute from Right Ear, Via Natural o Artificial Opening
09PD0SZ	Removal of Hearing Device from Right Inner Ear, Open Approach	09PH37Z	Removal of Autologous Tissue Substitute from Right Ear, Percutaneous Approach	09PH80Z	Removal of Drainage Device from Righ Ear, Via Natural or Artificial Opening Endoscopic
09PD7SZ	Removal of Hearing Device from Right Inner Ear, Via Natural or Artificial Opening	09PH3DZ	Removal of Intraluminal Device from Right Ear, Percutaneous Approach	09PH87Z	Removal of Autologous Tissue Substitut from Right Ear, Via Natural or Artificial Opening Endoscopic
09PD8SZ	Removal of Hearing Device from Right Inner Ear, Via Natural or Artificial Opening Endoscopic	09PH3JZ	Removal of Synthetic Substitute from Right Ear, Percutaneous Approach	09PH8DZ	Removal of Intraluminal Device from Right Ear, Via Natural or Artificial Opening Endoscopic
09PE0SZ	Removal of Hearing Device from Left Inner Ear, Open Approach	09PH3KZ	Removal of Nonautologous Tissue Substitute from Right Ear, Percutaneous Approach		
		09PH40Z	Removal of Drainage Device from Right Ear, Percutaneous Endoscopic Approach		
		09PH47Z	Removal of Autologous Tissue Substitute from Right Ear, Percutaneous Endoscopic Approach		

H8JZ Removal of Synthetic Substitute from Right Ear, Via Natural or Artificial Opening Endoscopic

H8KZ Removal of Nonautologous Tissue Substitute from Right Ear, Via Natural or Artificial Opening Endoscopic

HX0Z Removal of Drainage Device from Right Ear, External Approach

HX7Z Removal of Autologous Tissue Substitute from Right Ear, External Approach

HXDZ Removal of Intraluminal Device from Right Ear, External Approach

HXJZ Removal of Synthetic Substitute from Right Ear, External Approach

HXKZ Removal of Nonautologous Tissue Substitute from Right Ear, External Approach

J00Z Removal of Drainage Device from Left Ear, Open Approach

J07Z Removal of Autologous Tissue Substitute from Left Ear, Open Approach

J0DZ Removal of Intraluminal Device from Left Ear, Open Approach

J0JZ Removal of Synthetic Substitute from Left Ear, Open Approach

J0KZ Removal of Nonautologous Tissue Substitute from Left Ear, Open Approach

J30Z Removal of Drainage Device from Left Ear, Percutaneous Approach

J37Z Removal of Autologous Tissue Substitute from Left Ear, Percutaneous Approach

J3DZ Removal of Intraluminal Device from Left Ear, Percutaneous Approach

J3JZ Removal of Synthetic Substitute from Left Ear, Percutaneous Approach

J3KZ Removal of Nonautologous Tissue Substitute from Left Ear, Percutaneous Approach

J40Z Removal of Drainage Device from Left Ear, Percutaneous Endoscopic Approach

J47Z Removal of Autologous Tissue Substitute from Left Ear, Percutaneous Endoscopic Approach

J4DZ Removal of Intraluminal Device from Left Ear, Percutaneous Endoscopic Approach

J4JZ Removal of Synthetic Substitute from Left Ear, Percutaneous Endoscopic Approach

J4KZ Removal of Nonautologous Tissue Substitute from Left Ear, Percutaneous Endoscopic Approach

J70Z Removal of Drainage Device from Left Ear, Via Natural or Artificial Opening

J77Z Removal of Autologous Tissue Substitute from Left Ear, Via Natural or Artificial Opening

09PJ7DZ Removal of Intraluminal Device from Left Ear, Via Natural or Artificial Opening

09PJ7JZ Removal of Synthetic Substitute from Left Ear, Via Natural or Artificial Opening

09PJ7KZ Removal of Nonautologous Tissue Substitute from Left Ear, Via Natural or Artificial Opening

09PJ80Z Removal of Drainage Device from Left Ear, Via Natural or Artificial Opening Endoscopic

09PJ87Z Removal of Autologous Tissue Substitute from Left Ear, Via Natural or Artificial Opening Endoscopic

09PJ8DZ Removal of Intraluminal Device from Left Ear, Via Natural or Artificial Opening Endoscopic

09PJ8JZ Removal of Synthetic Substitute from Left Ear, Via Natural or Artificial Opening Endoscopic

09PJ8KZ Removal of Nonautologous Tissue Substitute from Left Ear, Via Natural or Artificial Opening Endoscopic

09PJX0Z Removal of Drainage Device from Left Ear, External Approach

09PJX7Z Removal of Autologous Tissue Substitute from Left Ear, External Approach

09PJXDZ Removal of Intraluminal Device from Left Ear, External Approach

09PJXJZ Removal of Synthetic Substitute from Left Ear, External Approach

09PJXKZ Removal of Nonautologous Tissue Substitute from Left Ear, External Approach

09PK00Z Removal of Drainage Device from Nose, Open Approach

09PK07Z Removal of Autologous Tissue Substitute from Nose, Open Approach

09PK0DZ Removal of Intraluminal Device from Nose, Open Approach

09PK0JZ Removal of Synthetic Substitute from Nose, Open Approach

09PK0KZ Removal of Nonautologous Tissue Substitute from Nose, Open Approach

09PK30Z Removal of Drainage Device from Nose, Percutaneous Approach

09PK37Z Removal of Autologous Tissue Substitute from Nose, Percutaneous Approach

09PK3DZ Removal of Intraluminal Device from Nose, Percutaneous Approach

09PK3JZ Removal of Synthetic Substitute from Nose, Percutaneous Approach

09PK3KZ Removal of Nonautologous Tissue Substitute from Nose, Percutaneous Approach

09PK40Z Removal of Drainage Device from Nose, Percutaneous Endoscopic Approach

09PK47Z Removal of Autologous Tissue Substitute from Nose, Percutaneous Endoscopic Approach

09PK4DZ Removal of Intraluminal Device from Nose, Percutaneous Endoscopic Approach

09PK4JZ Removal of Synthetic Substitute from Nose, Percutaneous Endoscopic Approach

09PK4KZ Removal of Nonautologous Tissue Substitute from Nose, Percutaneous Endoscopic Approach

09PK70Z Removal of Drainage Device from Nose, Via Natural or Artificial Opening

09PK77Z Removal of Autologous Tissue Substitute from Nose, Via Natural or Artificial Opening

09PK7DZ Removal of Intraluminal Device from Nose, Via Natural or Artificial Opening

09PK7JZ Removal of Synthetic Substitute from Nose, Via Natural or Artificial Opening

09PK7KZ Removal of Nonautologous Tissue Substitute from Nose, Via Natural or Artificial Opening

09PK80Z Removal of Drainage Device from Nose, Via Natural or Artificial Opening Endoscopic

09PK87Z Removal of Autologous Tissue Substitute from Nose, Via Natural or Artificial Opening Endoscopic

09PK8DZ Removal of Intraluminal Device from Nose, Via Natural or Artificial Opening Endoscopic

09PK8JZ Removal of Synthetic Substitute from Nose, Via Natural or Artificial Opening Endoscopic

09PK8KZ Removal of Nonautologous Tissue Substitute from Nose, Via Natural or Artificial Opening Endoscopic

09PKX0Z Removal of Drainage Device from Nose, External Approach

09PKX7Z Removal of Autologous Tissue Substitute from Nose, External Approach

09PKXDZ Removal of Intraluminal Device from Nose, External Approach

09PKXJZ Removal of Synthetic Substitute from Nose, External Approach

09PKXKZ Removal of Nonautologous Tissue Substitute from Nose, External Approach

09PY00Z Removal of Drainage Device from Sinus, Open Approach

09PY30Z Removal of Drainage Device from Sinus, Percutaneous Approach

09PY40Z Removal of Drainage Device from Sinus, Percutaneous Endoscopic Approach

09PYX0Z Removal of Drainage Device from Sinus, External Approach

Q – Ear, Nose, Sinus, Repair

Q00ZZ Repair Right External Ear, Open Approach

Q03ZZ Repair Right External Ear, Percutaneous Approach

Q04ZZ Repair Right External Ear, Percutaneous Endoscopic Approach

Q0XZZ Repair Right External Ear, External Approach

Q10ZZ Repair Left External Ear, Open Approach

Q13ZZ Repair Left External Ear, Percutaneous Approach

Q14ZZ Repair Left External Ear, Percutaneous Endoscopic Approach

Q1XZZ Repair Left External Ear, External Approach

Q20ZZ Repair Bilateral External Ear, Open Approach

Q23ZZ Repair Bilateral External Ear, Percutaneous Approach

09Q24ZZ Repair Bilateral External Ear, Percutaneous Endoscopic Approach

09Q2XZZ Repair Bilateral External Ear, External Approach

09Q30ZZ Repair Right External Auditory Canal, Open Approach

09Q33ZZ Repair Right External Auditory Canal, Percutaneous Approach

09Q34ZZ Repair Right External Auditory Canal, Percutaneous Endoscopic Approach

09Q37ZZ Repair Right External Auditory Canal, Via Natural or Artificial Opening

09Q38ZZ Repair Right External Auditory Canal, Via Natural or Artificial Opening Endoscopic

09Q3XZZ Repair Right External Auditory Canal, External Approach

09Q40ZZ Repair Left External Auditory Canal, Open Approach

09Q43ZZ Repair Left External Auditory Canal, Percutaneous Approach

09Q44ZZ Repair Left External Auditory Canal, Percutaneous Endoscopic Approach

09Q47ZZ Repair Left External Auditory Canal, Via Natural or Artificial Opening

09Q48ZZ Repair Left External Auditory Canal, Via Natural or Artificial Opening Endoscopic

09Q4XZZ Repair Left External Auditory Canal, External Approach

09Q50ZZ Repair Right Middle Ear, Open Approach

09Q60ZZ Repair Left Middle Ear, Open Approach

09Q70ZZ Repair Right Tympanic Membrane, Open Approach

09Q73ZZ Repair Right Tympanic Membrane, Percutaneous Approach

09Q74ZZ	Repair Right Tympanic Membrane, Percutaneous Endoscopic Approach	09QG3ZZ	Repair Left Eustachian Tube, Percutaneous Approach	09QQ3ZZ	Repair Right Maxillary Sinus, Percutaneous Approach
09Q77ZZ	Repair Right Tympanic Membrane, Via Natural or Artificial Opening	09QG4ZZ	Repair Left Eustachian Tube, Percutaneous Endoscopic Approach	09QQ4ZZ	Repair Right Maxillary Sinus, Percutaneous Endoscopic Approach
09Q78ZZ	Repair Right Tympanic Membrane, Via Natural or Artificial Opening Endoscopic	09QG7ZZ	Repair Left Eustachian Tube, Via Natural or Artificial Opening	09QR0ZZ	Repair Left Maxillary Sinus, Open Approach
09Q80ZZ	Repair Left Tympanic Membrane, Open Approach	09QG8ZZ	Repair Left Eustachian Tube, Via Natural or Artificial Opening Endoscopic	09QR3ZZ	Repair Left Maxillary Sinus, Percutane Approach
09Q83ZZ	Repair Left Tympanic Membrane, Percutaneous Approach	09QGXZZ	Repair Left Eustachian Tube, External Approach	09QR4ZZ	Repair Left Maxillary Sinus, Percutane Endoscopic Approach
09Q84ZZ	Repair Left Tympanic Membrane, Percutaneous Endoscopic Approach	09QK0ZZ	Repair Nose, Open Approach	09QS0ZZ	Repair Right Frontal Sinus, Open Approach
09Q87ZZ	Repair Left Tympanic Membrane, Via Natural or Artificial Opening	09QK3ZZ	Repair Nose, Percutaneous Approach	09QS3ZZ	Repair Right Frontal Sinus, Percutaned Approach
09Q88ZZ	Repair Left Tympanic Membrane, Via Natural or Artificial Opening Endoscopic	09QK4ZZ	Repair Nose, Percutaneous Endoscopic Approach	09QS4ZZ	Repair Right Frontal Sinus, Percutaned Endoscopic Approach
09Q90ZZ	Repair Right Auditory Ossicle, Open Approach		*AHA CC: 4Q, 2014, 20-21*	09QT0ZZ	Repair Left Frontal Sinus, Open Appro
09QA0ZZ	Repair Left Auditory Ossicle, Open Approach	09QL0ZZ	Repair Nasal Turbinate, Open Approach	09QT3ZZ	Repair Left Frontal Sinus, Percutaneou Approach
09QB0ZZ	Repair Right Mastoid Sinus, Open Approach	09QL3ZZ	Repair Nasal Turbinate, Percutaneous Approach	09QT4ZZ	Repair Left Frontal Sinus, Percutaneou Endoscopic Approach
09QB3ZZ	Repair Right Mastoid Sinus, Percutaneous Approach	09QL4ZZ	Repair Nasal Turbinate, Percutaneous Endoscopic Approach		*AHA CC: 4Q, 2013, 114*
09QB4ZZ	Repair Right Mastoid Sinus, Percutaneous Endoscopic Approach	09QL7ZZ	Repair Nasal Turbinate, Via Natural or Artificial Opening	09QU0ZZ	Repair Right Ethmoid Sinus, Open Approach
09QC0ZZ	Repair Left Mastoid Sinus, Open Approach	09QL8ZZ	Repair Nasal Turbinate, Via Natural or Artificial Opening Endoscopic	09QU3ZZ	Repair Right Ethmoid Sinus, Percutane Approach
09QC3ZZ	Repair Left Mastoid Sinus, Percutaneous Approach	09QM0ZZ	Repair Nasal Septum, Open Approach	09QU4ZZ	Repair Right Ethmoid Sinus, Percutane Endoscopic Approach
09QC4ZZ	Repair Left Mastoid Sinus, Percutaneous Endoscopic Approach	09QM3ZZ	Repair Nasal Septum, Percutaneous Approach	09QV0ZZ	Repair Left Ethmoid Sinus, Open Approach
09QD0ZZ	Repair Right Inner Ear, Open Approach	09QM4ZZ	Repair Nasal Septum, Percutaneous Endoscopic Approach	09QV3ZZ	Repair Left Ethmoid Sinus, Percutaneo Approach
09QE0ZZ	Repair Left Inner Ear, Open Approach	09QN0ZZ	Repair Nasopharynx, Open Approach	09QV4ZZ	Repair Left Ethmoid Sinus, Percutaneo Endoscopic Approach
09QF0ZZ	Repair Right Eustachian Tube, Open Approach	09QN3ZZ	Repair Nasopharynx, Percutaneous Approach	09QW0ZZ	Repair Right Sphenoid Sinus, Open Approach
09QF3ZZ	Repair Right Eustachian Tube, Percutaneous Approach	09QN4ZZ	Repair Nasopharynx, Percutaneous Endoscopic Approach		*AHA CC: 3Q, 2014, 22-23*
09QF4ZZ	Repair Right Eustachian Tube, Percutaneous Endoscopic Approach	09QN7ZZ	Repair Nasopharynx, Via Natural or Artificial Opening	09QW3ZZ	Repair Right Sphenoid Sinus, Percutaneous Approach
09QF7ZZ	Repair Right Eustachian Tube, Via Natural or Artificial Opening	09QN8ZZ	Repair Nasopharynx, Via Natural or Artificial Opening Endoscopic	09QW4ZZ	Repair Right Sphenoid Sinus, Percutaneous Endoscopic Approach
09QF8ZZ	Repair Right Eustachian Tube, Via Natural or Artificial Opening Endoscopic	09QP0ZZ	Repair Accessory Sinus, Open Approach	09QX0ZZ	Repair Left Sphenoid Sinus, Open Approach
09QFXZZ	Repair Right Eustachian Tube, External Approach	09QP3ZZ	Repair Accessory Sinus, Percutaneous Approach		*AHA CC: 3Q, 2014, 22-23*
09QG0ZZ	Repair Left Eustachian Tube, Open Approach	09QP4ZZ	Repair Accessory Sinus, Percutaneous Endoscopic Approach	09QX3ZZ	Repair Left Sphenoid Sinus, Percutaned Approach
		09QQ0ZZ	Repair Right Maxillary Sinus, Open Approach	09QX4ZZ	Repair Left Sphenoid Sinus, Percutaned Endoscopic Approach

09R – Ear, Nose, Sinus, Replacement

09R007Z	Replacement of Right External Ear with Autologous Tissue Substitute, Open Approach	09R1X7Z	Replacement of Left External Ear with Autologous Tissue Substitute, External Approach	09R507Z	Replacement of Right Middle Ear with Autologous Tissue Substitute, Open Approach
09R00JZ	Replacement of Right External Ear with Synthetic Substitute, Open Approach	09R1XJZ	Replacement of Left External Ear with Synthetic Substitute, External Approach	09R50JZ	Replacement of Right Middle Ear with Synthetic Substitute, Open Approach
09R00KZ	Replacement of Right External Ear with Nonautologous Tissue Substitute, Open Approach	09R1XKZ	Replacement of Left External Ear with Nonautologous Tissue Substitute, External Approach	09R50KZ	Replacement of Right Middle Ear with Nonautologous Tissue Substitute, Open Approach
09R0X7Z	Replacement of Right External Ear with Autologous Tissue Substitute, External Approach	09R207Z	Replacement of Bilateral External Ear with Autologous Tissue Substitute, Open Approach	09R607Z	Replacement of Left Middle Ear with Autologous Tissue Substitute, Open Approach
09R0XJZ	Replacement of Right External Ear with Synthetic Substitute, External Approach	09R20JZ	Replacement of Bilateral External Ear with Synthetic Substitute, Open Approach	09R60JZ	Replacement of Left Middle Ear with Synthetic Substitute, Open Approach
09R0XKZ	Replacement of Right External Ear with Nonautologous Tissue Substitute, External Approach	09R20KZ	Replacement of Bilateral External Ear with Nonautologous Tissue Substitute, Open Approach	09R60KZ	Replacement of Left Middle Ear with Nonautologous Tissue Substitute, Open Approach
09R107Z	Replacement of Left External Ear with Autologous Tissue Substitute, Open Approach	09R2X7Z	Replacement of Bilateral External Ear with Autologous Tissue Substitute, External Approach	09R707Z	Replacement of Right Tympanic Membrane with Autologous Tissue Substitute, Open Approach
09R10JZ	Replacement of Left External Ear with Synthetic Substitute, Open Approach	09R2XJZ	Replacement of Bilateral External Ear with Synthetic Substitute, External Approach	09R70JZ	Replacement of Right Tympanic Membrane with Synthetic Substitute, Open Approach
09R10KZ	Replacement of Left External Ear with Nonautologous Tissue Substitute, Open Approach	09R2XKZ	Replacement of Bilateral External Ear with Nonautologous Tissue Substitute, External Approach	09R70KZ	Replacement of Right Tympanic Membrane with Nonautologous Tissue Substitute, Open Approach

♀ Female-only	♂ Male-only	▲ Limited Coverage	● Non-OR	▰ HAC-associated procedure

▲ Non-covered procedures ✚ Combinat

777Z Replacement of Right Tympanic Membrane with Autologous Tissue Substitute, Via Natural or Artificial Opening

77JZ Replacement of Right Tympanic Membrane with Synthetic Substitute, Via Natural or Artificial Opening

77KZ Replacement of Right Tympanic Membrane with Nonautologous Tissue Substitute, Via Natural or Artificial Opening

787Z Replacement of Right Tympanic Membrane with Autologous Tissue Substitute, Via Natural or Artificial Opening Endoscopic

78JZ Replacement of Right Tympanic Membrane with Synthetic Substitute, Via Natural or Artificial Opening Endoscopic

78KZ Replacement of Right Tympanic Membrane with Nonautologous Tissue Substitute, Via Natural or Artificial Opening Endoscopic

807Z Replacement of Left Tympanic Membrane with Autologous Tissue Substitute, Open Approach

80JZ Replacement of Left Tympanic Membrane with Synthetic Substitute, Open Approach

80KZ Replacement of Left Tympanic Membrane with Nonautologous Tissue Substitute, Open Approach

877Z Replacement of Left Tympanic Membrane with Autologous Tissue Substitute, Via Natural or Artificial Opening

87JZ Replacement of Left Tympanic Membrane with Synthetic Substitute, Via Natural or Artificial Opening

87KZ Replacement of Left Tympanic Membrane with Nonautologous Tissue Substitute, Via Natural or Artificial Opening

887Z Replacement of Left Tympanic Membrane with Autologous Tissue Substitute, Via Natural or Artificial Opening Endoscopic

88JZ Replacement of Left Tympanic Membrane with Synthetic Substitute, Via Natural or Artificial Opening Endoscopic

88KZ Replacement of Left Tympanic Membrane with Nonautologous Tissue Substitute, Via Natural or Artificial Opening Endoscopic

R907Z Replacement of Right Auditory Ossicle with Autologous Tissue Substitute, Open Approach

R90JZ Replacement of Right Auditory Ossicle with Synthetic Substitute, Open Approach

R90KZ Replacement of Right Auditory Ossicle with Nonautologous Tissue Substitute, Open Approach

RA07Z Replacement of Left Auditory Ossicle with Autologous Tissue Substitute, Open Approach

RA0JZ Replacement of Left Auditory Ossicle with Synthetic Substitute, Open Approach

RA0KZ Replacement of Left Auditory Ossicle with Nonautologous Tissue Substitute, Open Approach

09RD07Z Replacement of Right Inner Ear with Autologous Tissue Substitute, Open Approach

09RD0JZ Replacement of Right Inner Ear with Synthetic Substitute, Open Approach

09RD0KZ Replacement of Right Inner Ear with Nonautologous Tissue Substitute, Open Approach

09RE07Z Replacement of Left Inner Ear with Autologous Tissue Substitute, Open Approach

09RE0JZ Replacement of Left Inner Ear with Synthetic Substitute, Open Approach

09RE0KZ Replacement of Left Inner Ear with Nonautologous Tissue Substitute, Open Approach

09RK07Z Replacement of Nose with Autologous Tissue Substitute, Open Approach

09RK0JZ Replacement of Nose with Synthetic Substitute, Open Approach

09RK0KZ Replacement of Nose with Nonautologous Tissue Substitute, Open Approach

09RKX7Z Replacement of Nose with Autologous Tissue Substitute, External Approach

09RKXJZ Replacement of Nose with Synthetic Substitute, External Approach

09RKXKZ Replacement of Nose with Nonautologous Tissue Substitute, External Approach

09RL07Z Replacement of Nasal Turbinate with Autologous Tissue Substitute, Open Approach

09RL0JZ Replacement of Nasal Turbinate with Synthetic Substitute, Open Approach

09RL0KZ Replacement of Nasal Turbinate with Nonautologous Tissue Substitute, Open Approach

09RL37Z Replacement of Nasal Turbinate with Autologous Tissue Substitute, Percutaneous Approach

09RL3JZ Replacement of Nasal Turbinate with Synthetic Substitute, Percutaneous Approach

09RL3KZ Replacement of Nasal Turbinate with Nonautologous Tissue Substitute, Percutaneous Approach

09RL47Z Replacement of Nasal Turbinate with Autologous Tissue Substitute, Percutaneous Endoscopic Approach

09RL4JZ Replacement of Nasal Turbinate with Synthetic Substitute, Percutaneous Endoscopic Approach

09RL4KZ Replacement of Nasal Turbinate with Nonautologous Tissue Substitute, Percutaneous Endoscopic Approach

09RL77Z Replacement of Nasal Turbinate with Autologous Tissue Substitute, Via Natural or Artificial Opening

09RL7JZ Replacement of Nasal Turbinate with Synthetic Substitute, Via Natural or Artificial Opening

09RL7KZ Replacement of Nasal Turbinate with Nonautologous Tissue Substitute, Via Natural or Artificial Opening

09RL87Z Replacement of Nasal Turbinate with Autologous Tissue Substitute, Via Natural or Artificial Opening Endoscopic

09RL8JZ Replacement of Nasal Turbinate with Synthetic Substitute, Via Natural or Artificial Opening Endoscopic

09RL8KZ Replacement of Nasal Turbinate with Nonautologous Tissue Substitute, Via Natural or Artificial Opening Endoscopic

09RM07Z Replacement of Nasal Septum with Autologous Tissue Substitute, Open Approach

09RM0JZ Replacement of Nasal Septum with Synthetic Substitute, Open Approach

09RM0KZ Replacement of Nasal Septum with Nonautologous Tissue Substitute, Open Approach

09RM37Z Replacement of Nasal Septum with Autologous Tissue Substitute, Percutaneous Approach

09RM3JZ Replacement of Nasal Septum with Synthetic Substitute, Percutaneous Approach

09RM3KZ Replacement of Nasal Septum with Nonautologous Tissue Substitute, Percutaneous Approach

09RM47Z Replacement of Nasal Septum with Autologous Tissue Substitute, Percutaneous Endoscopic Approach

09RM4JZ Replacement of Nasal Septum with Synthetic Substitute, Percutaneous Endoscopic Approach

09RM4KZ Replacement of Nasal Septum with Nonautologous Tissue Substitute, Percutaneous Endoscopic Approach

09RN07Z Replacement of Nasopharynx with Autologous Tissue Substitute, Open Approach

09RN0JZ Replacement of Nasopharynx with Synthetic Substitute, Open Approach

09RN0KZ Replacement of Nasopharynx with Nonautologous Tissue Substitute, Open Approach

09RN77Z Replacement of Nasopharynx with Autologous Tissue Substitute, Via Natural or Artificial Opening

09RN7JZ Replacement of Nasopharynx with Synthetic Substitute, Via Natural or Artificial Opening

09RN7KZ Replacement of Nasopharynx with Nonautologous Tissue Substitute, Via Natural or Artificial Opening

09RN87Z Replacement of Nasopharynx with Autologous Tissue Substitute, Via Natural or Artificial Opening Endoscopic

09RN8JZ Replacement of Nasopharynx with Synthetic Substitute, Via Natural or Artificial Opening Endoscopic

09RN8KZ Replacement of Nasopharynx with Nonautologous Tissue Substitute, Via Natural or Artificial Opening Endoscopic

0S – Ear, Nose, Sinus, Reposition

S00ZZ Reposition Right External Ear, Open Approach

S04ZZ Reposition Right External Ear, Percutaneous Endoscopic Approach

S0XZZ Reposition Right External Ear, External Approach

S10ZZ Reposition Left External Ear, Open Approach

S14ZZ Reposition Left External Ear, Percutaneous Endoscopic Approach

09S1XZZ Reposition Left External Ear, External Approach

09S20ZZ Reposition Bilateral External Ear, Open Approach

09S24ZZ Reposition Bilateral External Ear, Percutaneous Endoscopic Approach

09S2XZZ Reposition Bilateral External Ear, External Approach

09S70ZZ Reposition Right Tympanic Membrane, Open Approach

09S74ZZ Reposition Right Tympanic Membrane, Percutaneous Endoscopic Approach

09S77ZZ Reposition Right Tympanic Membrane, Via Natural or Artificial Opening

09S78ZZ Reposition Right Tympanic Membrane, Via Natural or Artificial Opening Endoscopic

09S80ZZ Reposition Left Tympanic Membrane, Open Approach

Female-only   ♂ Male-only   ▲ Limited Coverage   ● Non-OR   ▦ HAC-associated procedure   ▲ Non-covered procedures   + Combination

09S84ZZ Reposition Left Tympanic Membrane, Percutaneous Endoscopic Approach	**09SF4ZZ** Reposition Right Eustachian Tube, Percutaneous Endoscopic Approach	**09SK4ZZ** Reposition Nose, Percutaneous Endoscopic Approach
09S87ZZ Reposition Left Tympanic Membrane, Via Natural or Artificial Opening	**09SF7ZZ** Reposition Right Eustachian Tube, Via Natural or Artificial Opening	**09SKXZZ** Reposition Nose, External Approach
09S88ZZ Reposition Left Tympanic Membrane, Via Natural or Artificial Opening Endoscopic	**09SF8ZZ** Reposition Right Eustachian Tube, Via Natural or Artificial Opening Endoscopic	**09SL0ZZ** Reposition Nasal Turbinate, Open Approach
09S90ZZ Reposition Right Auditory Ossicle, Open Approach	**09SG0ZZ** Reposition Left Eustachian Tube, Open Approach	**09SL4ZZ** Reposition Nasal Turbinate, Percutaneous Endoscopic Approach
09S94ZZ Reposition Right Auditory Ossicle, Percutaneous Endoscopic Approach	**09SG4ZZ** Reposition Left Eustachian Tube, Percutaneous Endoscopic Approach	**09SL7ZZ** Reposition Nasal Turbinate, Via Natural Artificial Opening
09SA0ZZ Reposition Left Auditory Ossicle, Open Approach	**09SG7ZZ** Reposition Left Eustachian Tube, Via Natural or Artificial Opening	**09SL8ZZ** Reposition Nasal Turbinate, Via Natural Artificial Opening Endoscopic
09SA4ZZ Reposition Left Auditory Ossicle, Percutaneous Endoscopic Approach	**09SG8ZZ** Reposition Left Eustachian Tube, Via Natural or Artificial Opening Endoscopic	**09SM0ZZ** Reposition Nasal Septum, Open Appro
09SF0ZZ Reposition Right Eustachian Tube, Open Approach	**09SK0ZZ** Reposition Nose, Open Approach	**09SM4ZZ** Reposition Nasal Septum, Percutaneou Endoscopic Approach

09T – Ear, Nose, Sinus, Resection

Review Coding Guideline B3.8

09T00ZZ Resection of Right External Ear, Open Approach	**09TC0ZZ** Resection of Left Mastoid Sinus, Open Approach	**09TN4ZZ** Resection of Nasopharynx, Percutaneo Endoscopic Approach
09T04ZZ Resection of Right External Ear, Percutaneous Endoscopic Approach	**09TC4ZZ** Resection of Left Mastoid Sinus, Percutaneous Endoscopic Approach	**09TN7ZZ** Resection of Nasopharynx, Via Natural Artificial Opening
09T0XZZ Resection of Right External Ear, External Approach	**09TD0ZZ** Resection of Right Inner Ear, Open Approach	**09TN8ZZ** Resection of Nasopharynx, Via Natural Artificial Opening Endoscopic
09T10ZZ Resection of Left External Ear, Open Approach	**09TE0ZZ** Resection of Left Inner Ear, Open Approach	**09TP0ZZ** Resection of Accessory Sinus, Open Approach
09T14ZZ Resection of Left External Ear, Percutaneous Endoscopic Approach	**09TF0ZZ** Resection of Right Eustachian Tube, Open Approach	**09TP4ZZ** Resection of Accessory Sinus, Percutaneous Endoscopic Approach
09T1XZZ Resection of Left External Ear, External Approach	**09TF4ZZ** Resection of Right Eustachian Tube, Percutaneous Endoscopic Approach	**09TQ0ZZ** Resection of Right Maxillary Sinus, Op Approach
09T50ZZ Resection of Right Middle Ear, Open Approach	**09TF7ZZ** Resection of Right Eustachian Tube, Via Natural or Artificial Opening	**09TQ4ZZ** Resection of Right Maxillary Sinus, Percutaneous Endoscopic Approach
09T60ZZ Resection of Left Middle Ear, Open Approach	**09TF8ZZ** Resection of Right Eustachian Tube, Via Natural or Artificial Opening Endoscopic	**09TR0ZZ** Resection of Left Maxillary Sinus, Ope Approach
09T70ZZ Resection of Right Tympanic Membrane, Open Approach	**09TG0ZZ** Resection of Left Eustachian Tube, Open Approach	**09TR4ZZ** Resection of Left Maxillary Sinus, Percutaneous Endoscopic Approach
09T74ZZ Resection of Right Tympanic Membrane, Percutaneous Endoscopic Approach	**09TG4ZZ** Resection of Left Eustachian Tube, Percutaneous Endoscopic Approach	**09TS0ZZ** Resection of Right Frontal Sinus, Open Approach
09T77ZZ Resection of Right Tympanic Membrane, Via Natural or Artificial Opening	**09TG7ZZ** Resection of Left Eustachian Tube, Via Natural or Artificial Opening	**09TS4ZZ** Resection of Right Frontal Sinus, Percutaneous Endoscopic Approach
09T78ZZ Resection of Right Tympanic Membrane, Via Natural or Artificial Opening Endoscopic	**09TG8ZZ** Resection of Left Eustachian Tube, Via Natural or Artificial Opening Endoscopic	**09TT0ZZ** Resection of Left Frontal Sinus, Open Approach
09T80ZZ Resection of Left Tympanic Membrane, Open Approach	**09TK0ZZ** Resection of Nose, Open Approach	**09TT4ZZ** Resection of Left Frontal Sinus, Percutaneous Endoscopic Approach
09T84ZZ Resection of Left Tympanic Membrane, Percutaneous Endoscopic Approach	**09TK4ZZ** Resection of Nose, Percutaneous Endoscopic Approach	**09TU0ZZ** Resection of Right Ethmoid Sinus, Ope Approach
09T87ZZ Resection of Left Tympanic Membrane, Via Natural or Artificial Opening	**09TKXZZ** Resection of Nose, External Approach	**09TU4ZZ** Resection of Right Ethmoid Sinus, Percutaneous Endoscopic Approach
09T88ZZ Resection of Left Tympanic Membrane, Via Natural or Artificial Opening Endoscopic	**09TL0ZZ** Resection of Nasal Turbinate, Open Approach	**09TV0ZZ** Resection of Left Ethmoid Sinus, Open Approach
09T90ZZ Resection of Right Auditory Ossicle, Open Approach	**09TL4ZZ** Resection of Nasal Turbinate, Percutaneous Endoscopic Approach	**09TV4ZZ** Resection of Left Ethmoid Sinus, Percutaneous Endoscopic Approach
09TA0ZZ Resection of Left Auditory Ossicle, Open Approach	**09TL7ZZ** Resection of Nasal Turbinate, Via Natural or Artificial Opening	**09TW0ZZ** Resection of Right Sphenoid Sinus, Ope Approach
09TB0ZZ Resection of Right Mastoid Sinus, Open Approach	**09TL8ZZ** Resection of Nasal Turbinate, Via Natural or Artificial Opening Endoscopic	**09TW4ZZ** Resection of Right Sphenoid Sinus, Percutaneous Endoscopic Approach
09TB4ZZ Resection of Right Mastoid Sinus, Percutaneous Endoscopic Approach	**09TM0ZZ** Resection of Nasal Septum, Open Approach	**09TX0ZZ** Resection of Left Sphenoid Sinus, Open Approach
	09TM4ZZ Resection of Nasal Septum, Percutaneous Endoscopic Approach	**09TX4ZZ** Resection of Left Sphenoid Sinus, Percutaneous Endoscopic Approach
	09TN0ZZ Resection of Nasopharynx, Open Approach	

09U – Ear, Nose, Sinus, Supplement

09U007Z Supplement Right External Ear with Autologous Tissue Substitute, Open Approach	**09U0XJZ** Supplement Right External Ear with Synthetic Substitute, External Approach	**09U10KZ** Supplement Left External Ear with Nonautologous Tissue Substitute, Open Approach
09U00JZ Supplement Right External Ear with Synthetic Substitute, Open Approach	**09U0XKZ** Supplement Right External Ear with Nonautologous Tissue Substitute, External Approach	**09U1X7Z** Supplement Left External Ear with Autologous Tissue Substitute, External Approach
09U00KZ Supplement Right External Ear with Nonautologous Tissue Substitute, Open Approach	**09U107Z** Supplement Left External Ear with Autologous Tissue Substitute, Open Approach	**09U1XJZ** Supplement Left External Ear with Synthetic Substitute, External Approach
09U0X7Z Supplement Right External Ear with Autologous Tissue Substitute, External Approach	**09U10JZ** Supplement Left External Ear with Synthetic Substitute, Open Approach	**09U1XKZ** Supplement Left External Ear with Nonautologous Tissue Substitute, Extern Approach

♀ Female-only ♂ Male-only ▲ Limited Coverage ● Non-OR ᴴᴬᶜ HAC-associated procedure ▲ Non-covered procedures ✚ Combinati

207Z	Supplement Bilateral External Ear with Autologous Tissue Substitute, Open Approach
20JZ	Supplement Bilateral External Ear with Synthetic Substitute, Open Approach
20KZ	Supplement Bilateral External Ear with Nonautologous Tissue Substitute, Open Approach
2X7Z	Supplement Bilateral External Ear with Autologous Tissue Substitute, External Approach
2XJZ	Supplement Bilateral External Ear with Synthetic Substitute, External Approach
2XKZ	Supplement Bilateral External Ear with Nonautologous Tissue Substitute, External Approach
507Z	Supplement Right Middle Ear with Autologous Tissue Substitute, Open Approach
50JZ	Supplement Right Middle Ear with Synthetic Substitute, Open Approach
50KZ	Supplement Right Middle Ear with Nonautologous Tissue Substitute, Open Approach
J607Z	Supplement Left Middle Ear with Autologous Tissue Substitute, Open Approach
J60JZ	Supplement Left Middle Ear with Synthetic Substitute, Open Approach
J60KZ	Supplement Left Middle Ear with Nonautologous Tissue Substitute, Open Approach
J707Z	Supplement Right Tympanic Membrane with Autologous Tissue Substitute, Open Approach
J70JZ	Supplement Right Tympanic Membrane with Synthetic Substitute, Open Approach
J70KZ	Supplement Right Tympanic Membrane with Nonautologous Tissue Substitute, Open Approach
J777Z	Supplement Right Tympanic Membrane with Autologous Tissue Substitute, Via Natural or Artificial Opening
J77JZ	Supplement Right Tympanic Membrane with Synthetic Substitute, Via Natural or Artificial Opening
J77KZ	Supplement Right Tympanic Membrane with Nonautologous Tissue Substitute, Via Natural or Artificial Opening
U787Z	Supplement Right Tympanic Membrane with Autologous Tissue Substitute, Via Natural or Artificial Opening Endoscopic
U78JZ	Supplement Right Tympanic Membrane with Synthetic Substitute, Via Natural or Artificial Opening Endoscopic
U78KZ	Supplement Right Tympanic Membrane with Nonautologous Tissue Substitute, Via Natural or Artificial Opening Endoscopic
U807Z	Supplement Left Tympanic Membrane with Autologous Tissue Substitute, Open Approach
U80JZ	Supplement Left Tympanic Membrane with Synthetic Substitute, Open Approach
U80KZ	Supplement Left Tympanic Membrane with Nonautologous Tissue Substitute, Open Approach
U877Z	Supplement Left Tympanic Membrane with Autologous Tissue Substitute, Via Natural or Artificial Opening
U87JZ	Supplement Left Tympanic Membrane with Synthetic Substitute, Via Natural or Artificial Opening
U87KZ	Supplement Left Tympanic Membrane with Nonautologous Tissue Substitute, Via Natural or Artificial Opening
09U887Z	Supplement Left Tympanic Membrane with Autologous Tissue Substitute, Via Natural or Artificial Opening Endoscopic
09U88JZ	Supplement Left Tympanic Membrane with Synthetic Substitute, Via Natural or Artificial Opening Endoscopic
09U88KZ	Supplement Left Tympanic Membrane with Nonautologous Tissue Substitute, Via Natural or Artificial Opening Endoscopic
09U907Z	Supplement Right Auditory Ossicle with Autologous Tissue Substitute, Open Approach
09U90JZ	Supplement Right Auditory Ossicle with Synthetic Substitute, Open Approach
09U90KZ	Supplement Right Auditory Ossicle with Nonautologous Tissue Substitute, Open Approach
09UA07Z	Supplement Left Auditory Ossicle with Autologous Tissue Substitute, Open Approach
09UA0JZ	Supplement Left Auditory Ossicle with Synthetic Substitute, Open Approach
09UA0KZ	Supplement Left Auditory Ossicle with Nonautologous Tissue Substitute, Open Approach
09UD07Z	Supplement Right Inner Ear with Autologous Tissue Substitute, Open Approach
09UD0JZ	Supplement Right Inner Ear with Synthetic Substitute, Open Approach
09UD0KZ	Supplement Right Inner Ear with Nonautologous Tissue Substitute, Open Approach
09UE07Z	Supplement Left Inner Ear with Autologous Tissue Substitute, Open Approach
09UE0JZ	Supplement Left Inner Ear with Synthetic Substitute, Open Approach
09UE0KZ	Supplement Left Inner Ear with Nonautologous Tissue Substitute, Open Approach
09UK07Z	Supplement Nose with Autologous Tissue Substitute, Open Approach
09UK0JZ	Supplement Nose with Synthetic Substitute, Open Approach
09UK0KZ	Supplement Nose with Nonautologous Tissue Substitute, Open Approach
09UKX7Z	Supplement Nose with Autologous Tissue Substitute, External Approach
09UKXJZ	Supplement Nose with Synthetic Substitute, External Approach
09UKXKZ	Supplement Nose with Nonautologous Tissue Substitute, External Approach
09UL07Z	Supplement Nasal Turbinate with Autologous Tissue Substitute, Open Approach
09UL0JZ	Supplement Nasal Turbinate with Synthetic Substitute, Open Approach
09UL0KZ	Supplement Nasal Turbinate with Nonautologous Tissue Substitute, Open Approach
09UL37Z	Supplement Nasal Turbinate with Autologous Tissue Substitute, Percutaneous Approach
09UL3JZ	Supplement Nasal Turbinate with Synthetic Substitute, Percutaneous Approach
09UL3KZ	Supplement Nasal Turbinate with Nonautologous Tissue Substitute, Percutaneous Approach
09UL47Z	Supplement Nasal Turbinate with Autologous Tissue Substitute, Percutaneous Endoscopic Approach
09UL4JZ	Supplement Nasal Turbinate with Synthetic Substitute, Percutaneous Endoscopic Approach
09UL4KZ	Supplement Nasal Turbinate with Nonautologous Tissue Substitute, Percutaneous Endoscopic Approach
09UL77Z	Supplement Nasal Turbinate with Autologous Tissue Substitute, Via Natural or Artificial Opening
09UL7JZ	Supplement Nasal Turbinate with Synthetic Substitute, Via Natural or Artificial Opening
09UL7KZ	Supplement Nasal Turbinate with Nonautologous Tissue Substitute, Via Natural or Artificial Opening
09UL87Z	Supplement Nasal Turbinate with Autologous Tissue Substitute, Via Natural or Artificial Opening Endoscopic
09UL8JZ	Supplement Nasal Turbinate with Synthetic Substitute, Via Natural or Artificial Opening Endoscopic
09UL8KZ	Supplement Nasal Turbinate with Nonautologous Tissue Substitute, Via Natural or Artificial Opening Endoscopic
09UM07Z	Supplement Nasal Septum with Autologous Tissue Substitute, Open Approach
09UM0JZ	Supplement Nasal Septum with Synthetic Substitute, Open Approach
09UM0KZ	Supplement Nasal Septum with Nonautologous Tissue Substitute, Open Approach
09UM37Z	Supplement Nasal Septum with Autologous Tissue Substitute, Percutaneous Approach
09UM3JZ	Supplement Nasal Septum with Synthetic Substitute, Percutaneous Approach
09UM3KZ	Supplement Nasal Septum with Nonautologous Tissue Substitute, Percutaneous Approach
09UM47Z	Supplement Nasal Septum with Autologous Tissue Substitute, Percutaneous Endoscopic Approach
09UM4JZ	Supplement Nasal Septum with Synthetic Substitute, Percutaneous Endoscopic Approach
09UM4KZ	Supplement Nasal Septum with Nonautologous Tissue Substitute, Percutaneous Endoscopic Approach
09UN07Z	Supplement Nasopharynx with Autologous Tissue Substitute, Open Approach
09UN0JZ	Supplement Nasopharynx with Synthetic Substitute, Open Approach
09UN0KZ	Supplement Nasopharynx with Nonautologous Tissue Substitute, Open Approach
09UN77Z	Supplement Nasopharynx with Autologous Tissue Substitute, Via Natural or Artificial Opening
09UN7JZ	Supplement Nasopharynx with Synthetic Substitute, Via Natural or Artificial Opening
09UN7KZ	Supplement Nasopharynx with Nonautologous Tissue Substitute, Via Natural or Artificial Opening
09UN87Z	Supplement Nasopharynx with Autologous Tissue Substitute, Via Natural or Artificial Opening Endoscopic
09UN8JZ	Supplement Nasopharynx with Synthetic Substitute, Via Natural or Artificial Opening Endoscopic
09UN8KZ	Supplement Nasopharynx with Nonautologous Tissue Substitute, Via Natural or Artificial Opening Endoscopic

453

♀ Female-only ♂ Male-only ▲ Limited Coverage ● Non-OR ▧ HAC-associated procedure ▲ Non-covered procedures ✚ Combination

09W – Ear, Nose, Sinus, Revision

Review Coding Guideline B6.1c

09W707Z Revision of Autologous Tissue Substitute in Right Tympanic Membrane, Open Approach

09W70JZ Revision of Synthetic Substitute in Right Tympanic Membrane, Open Approach

09W70KZ Revision of Nonautologous Tissue Substitute in Right Tympanic Membrane, Open Approach

09W777Z Revision of Autologous Tissue Substitute in Right Tympanic Membrane, Via Natural or Artificial Opening

09W77JZ Revision of Synthetic Substitute in Right Tympanic Membrane, Via Natural or Artificial Opening

09W77KZ Revision of Nonautologous Tissue Substitute in Right Tympanic Membrane, Via Natural or Artificial Opening

09W787Z Revision of Autologous Tissue Substitute in Right Tympanic Membrane, Via Natural or Artificial Opening Endoscopic

09W78JZ Revision of Synthetic Substitute in Right Tympanic Membrane, Via Natural or Artificial Opening Endoscopic

09W78KZ Revision of Nonautologous Tissue Substitute in Right Tympanic Membrane, Via Natural or Artificial Opening Endoscopic

09W807Z Revision of Autologous Tissue Substitute in Left Tympanic Membrane, Open Approach

09W80JZ Revision of Synthetic Substitute in Left Tympanic Membrane, Open Approach

09W80KZ Revision of Nonautologous Tissue Substitute in Left Tympanic Membrane, Open Approach

09W877Z Revision of Autologous Tissue Substitute in Left Tympanic Membrane, Via Natural or Artificial Opening

09W87JZ Revision of Synthetic Substitute in Left Tympanic Membrane, Via Natural or Artificial Opening

09W87KZ Revision of Nonautologous Tissue Substitute in Left Tympanic Membrane, Via Natural or Artificial Opening

09W887Z Revision of Autologous Tissue Substitute in Left Tympanic Membrane, Via Natural or Artificial Opening Endoscopic

09W88JZ Revision of Synthetic Substitute in Left Tympanic Membrane, Via Natural or Artificial Opening Endoscopic

09W88KZ Revision of Nonautologous Tissue Substitute in Left Tympanic Membrane, Via Natural or Artificial Opening Endoscopic

09W907Z Revision of Autologous Tissue Substitute in Right Auditory Ossicle, Open Approach

09W90JZ Revision of Synthetic Substitute in Right Auditory Ossicle, Open Approach

09W90KZ Revision of Nonautologous Tissue Substitute in Right Auditory Ossicle, Open Approach

09W977Z Revision of Autologous Tissue Substitute in Right Auditory Ossicle, Via Natural or Artificial Opening

09W97JZ Revision of Synthetic Substitute in Right Auditory Ossicle, Via Natural or Artificial Opening

09W97KZ Revision of Nonautologous Tissue Substitute in Right Auditory Ossicle, Via Natural or Artificial Opening

09W987Z Revision of Autologous Tissue Substitute in Right Auditory Ossicle, Via Natural or Artificial Opening Endoscopic

09W98JZ Revision of Synthetic Substitute in Right Auditory Ossicle, Via Natural or Artificial Opening Endoscopic

09W98KZ Revision of Nonautologous Tissue Substitute in Right Auditory Ossicle, Via Natural or Artificial Opening Endoscopic

09WA07Z Revision of Autologous Tissue Substitute in Left Auditory Ossicle, Open Approach

09WA0JZ Revision of Synthetic Substitute in Left Auditory Ossicle, Open Approach

09WA0KZ Revision of Nonautologous Tissue Substitute in Left Auditory Ossicle, Open Approach

09WA77Z Revision of Autologous Tissue Substitute in Left Auditory Ossicle, Via Natural or Artificial Opening

09WA7JZ Revision of Synthetic Substitute in Left Auditory Ossicle, Via Natural or Artificial Opening

09WA7KZ Revision of Nonautologous Tissue Substitute in Left Auditory Ossicle, Via Natural or Artificial Opening

09WA87Z Revision of Autologous Tissue Substitute in Left Auditory Ossicle, Via Natural or Artificial Opening Endoscopic

09WA8JZ Revision of Synthetic Substitute in Left Auditory Ossicle, Via Natural or Artificial Opening Endoscopic

09WA8KZ Revision of Nonautologous Tissue Substitute in Left Auditory Ossicle, Via Natural or Artificial Opening Endoscopic

09WD0SZ Revision of Hearing Device in Right Inner Ear, Open Approach

09WD7SZ Revision of Hearing Device in Right Inner Ear, Via Natural or Artificial Opening

09WD8SZ Revision of Hearing Device in Right Inner Ear, Via Natural or Artificial Opening Endoscopic

09WE0SZ Revision of Hearing Device in Left Inner Ear, Open Approach

09WE7SZ Revision of Hearing Device in Left Inner Ear, Via Natural or Artificial Opening

09WE8SZ Revision of Hearing Device in Left Inner Ear, Via Natural or Artificial Opening Endoscopic

09WH00Z Revision of Drainage Device in Right Ear, Open Approach

09WH07Z Revision of Autologous Tissue Substitute in Right Ear, Open Approach

09WH0DZ Revision of Intraluminal Device in Right Ear, Open Approach

09WH0JZ Revision of Synthetic Substitute in Right Ear, Open Approach

09WH0KZ Revision of Nonautologous Tissue Substitute in Right Ear, Open Approach

09WH30Z Revision of Drainage Device in Right Ear, Percutaneous Approach

09WH37Z Revision of Autologous Tissue Substitute in Right Ear, Percutaneous Approach

09WH3DZ Revision of Intraluminal Device in Right Ear, Percutaneous Approach

09WH3JZ Revision of Synthetic Substitute in Right Ear, Percutaneous Approach

09WH3KZ Revision of Nonautologous Tissue Substitute in Right Ear, Percutaneous Approach

09WH40Z Revision of Drainage Device in Right Ear, Percutaneous Endoscopic Approach

09WH47Z Revision of Autologous Tissue Substitute in Right Ear, Percutaneous Endoscopic Approach

09WH4DZ Revision of Intraluminal Device in Right Ear, Percutaneous Endoscopic Approach

09WH4JZ Revision of Synthetic Substitute in Ri... Ear, Percutaneous Endoscopic Approa...

09WH4KZ Revision of Nonautologous Tissue Substitute in Right Ear, Percutaneous Endoscopic Approach

09WH70Z Revision of Drainage Device in Right Ear, Via Natural or Artificial Opening

09WH77Z Revision of Autologous Tissue Substi... in Right Ear, Via Natural or Artificial Opening

09WH7DZ Revision of Intraluminal Device in Rig... Ear, Via Natural or Artificial Opening

09WH7JZ Revision of Synthetic Substitute in Ri... Ear, Via Natural or Artificial Opening

09WH7KZ Revision of Nonautologous Tissue Substitute in Right Ear, Via Natural or Artificial Opening

09WH80Z Revision of Drainage Device in Right Ear, Via Natural or Artificial Opening Endoscopic

09WH87Z Revision of Autologous Tissue Substi... in Right Ear, Via Natural or Artificial Opening Endoscopic

09WH8DZ Revision of Intraluminal Device in Rig... Ear, Via Natural or Artificial Opening Endoscopic

09WH8JZ Revision of Synthetic Substitute in Ri... Ear, Via Natural or Artificial Opening Endoscopic

09WH8KZ Revision of Nonautologous Tissue Substitute in Right Ear, Via Natural or Artificial Opening Endoscopic

09WHX0Z Revision of Drainage Device in Right Ear, External Approach

09WHX7Z Revision of Autologous Tissue Substi... in Right Ear, External Approach

09WHXDZ Revision of Intraluminal Device in Rig... Ear, External Approach

09WHXJZ Revision of Synthetic Substitute in Rig... Ear, External Approach

09WHXKZ Revision of Nonautologous Tissue Substitute in Right Ear, External Approach

09WJ00Z Revision of Drainage Device in Left E... Open Approach

09WJ07Z Revision of Autologous Tissue Substitu... in Left Ear, Open Approach

09WJ0DZ Revision of Intraluminal Device in Lef... Ear, Open Approach

09WJ0JZ Revision of Synthetic Substitute in Lef... Ear, Open Approach

09WJ0KZ Revision of Nonautologous Tissue Substitute in Left Ear, Open Approach

09WJ30Z Revision of Drainage Device in Left E... Percutaneous Approach

09WJ37Z Revision of Autologous Tissue Substitu... in Left Ear, Percutaneous Approach

09WJ3DZ Revision of Intraluminal Device in Lef... Ear, Percutaneous Approach

09WJ3JZ Revision of Synthetic Substitute in Lef... Ear, Percutaneous Approach

09WJ3KZ Revision of Nonautologous Tissue Substitute in Left Ear, Percutaneous Approach

09WJ40Z Revision of Drainage Device in Left E... Percutaneous Endoscopic Approach

09WJ47Z Revision of Autologous Tissue Substitu... in Left Ear, Percutaneous Endoscopic Approach

09WJ4DZ Revision of Intraluminal Device in Left Ear, Percutaneous Endoscopic Approac...

09WJ4JZ Revision of Synthetic Substitute in Left Ear, Percutaneous Endoscopic Approac...

J4KZ	Revision of Nonautologous Tissue Substitute in Left Ear, Percutaneous Endoscopic Approach
J70Z	Revision of Drainage Device in Left Ear, Via Natural or Artificial Opening
J77Z	Revision of Autologous Tissue Substitute in Left Ear, Via Natural or Artificial Opening
J7DZ	Revision of Intraluminal Device in Left Ear, Via Natural or Artificial Opening
J7JZ	Revision of Synthetic Substitute in Left Ear, Via Natural or Artificial Opening
J7KZ	Revision of Nonautologous Tissue Substitute in Left Ear, Via Natural or Artificial Opening
J80Z	Revision of Drainage Device in Left Ear, Via Natural or Artificial Opening Endoscopic
J87Z	Revision of Autologous Tissue Substitute in Left Ear, Via Natural or Artificial Opening Endoscopic
J8DZ	Revision of Intraluminal Device in Left Ear, Via Natural or Artificial Opening Endoscopic
J8JZ	Revision of Synthetic Substitute in Left Ear, Via Natural or Artificial Opening Endoscopic
J8KZ	Revision of Nonautologous Tissue Substitute in Left Ear, Via Natural or Artificial Opening Endoscopic
JX0Z	Revision of Drainage Device in Left Ear, External Approach
JX7Z	Revision of Autologous Tissue Substitute in Left Ear, External Approach
JXDZ	Revision of Intraluminal Device in Left Ear, External Approach
JXJZ	Revision of Synthetic Substitute in Left Ear, External Approach

09WJXKZ	Revision of Nonautologous Tissue Substitute in Left Ear, External Approach
09WK00Z	Revision of Drainage Device in Nose, Open Approach
09WK07Z	Revision of Autologous Tissue Substitute in Nose, Open Approach
09WK0DZ	Revision of Intraluminal Device in Nose, Open Approach
09WK0JZ	Revision of Synthetic Substitute in Nose, Open Approach
09WK0KZ	Revision of Nonautologous Tissue Substitute in Nose, Open Approach
09WK30Z	Revision of Drainage Device in Nose, Percutaneous Approach
09WK37Z	Revision of Autologous Tissue Substitute in Nose, Percutaneous Approach
09WK3DZ	Revision of Intraluminal Device in Nose, Percutaneous Approach
09WK3JZ	Revision of Synthetic Substitute in Nose, Percutaneous Approach
09WK3KZ	Revision of Nonautologous Tissue Substitute in Nose, Percutaneous Approach
09WK40Z	Revision of Drainage Device in Nose, Percutaneous Endoscopic Approach
09WK47Z	Revision of Autologous Tissue Substitute in Nose, Percutaneous Endoscopic Approach
09WK4DZ	Revision of Intraluminal Device in Nose, Percutaneous Endoscopic Approach
09WK4JZ	Revision of Synthetic Substitute in Nose, Percutaneous Endoscopic Approach
09WK4KZ	Revision of Nonautologous Tissue Substitute in Nose, Percutaneous Endoscopic Approach
09WK70Z	Revision of Drainage Device in Nose, Via Natural or Artificial Opening
09WK77Z	Revision of Autologous Tissue Substitute in Nose, Via Natural or Artificial Opening

09WK7DZ	Revision of Intraluminal Device in Nose, Via Natural or Artificial Opening
09WK7JZ	Revision of Synthetic Substitute in Nose, Via Natural or Artificial Opening
09WK7KZ	Revision of Nonautologous Tissue Substitute in Nose, Via Natural or Artificial Opening
09WK80Z	Revision of Drainage Device in Nose, Via Natural or Artificial Opening Endoscopic
09WK87Z	Revision of Autologous Tissue Substitute in Nose, Via Natural or Artificial Opening Endoscopic
09WK8DZ	Revision of Intraluminal Device in Nose, Via Natural or Artificial Opening Endoscopic
09WK8JZ	Revision of Synthetic Substitute in Nose, Via Natural or Artificial Opening Endoscopic
09WK8KZ	Revision of Nonautologous Tissue Substitute in Nose, Via Natural or Artificial Opening Endoscopic
09WKX0Z	Revision of Drainage Device in Nose, External Approach
09WKX7Z	Revision of Autologous Tissue Substitute in Nose, External Approach
09WKXDZ	Revision of Intraluminal Device in Nose, External Approach
09WKXJZ	Revision of Synthetic Substitute in Nose, External Approach
09WKXKZ	Revision of Nonautologous Tissue Substitute in Nose, External Approach
09WY00Z	Revision of Drainage Device in Sinus, Open Approach
09WY30Z	Revision of Drainage Device in Sinus, Percutaneous Approach
09WY40Z	Revision of Drainage Device in Sinus, Percutaneous Endoscopic Approach
09WYX0Z	Revision of Drainage Device in Sinus, External Approach

Lungs

Right   Left

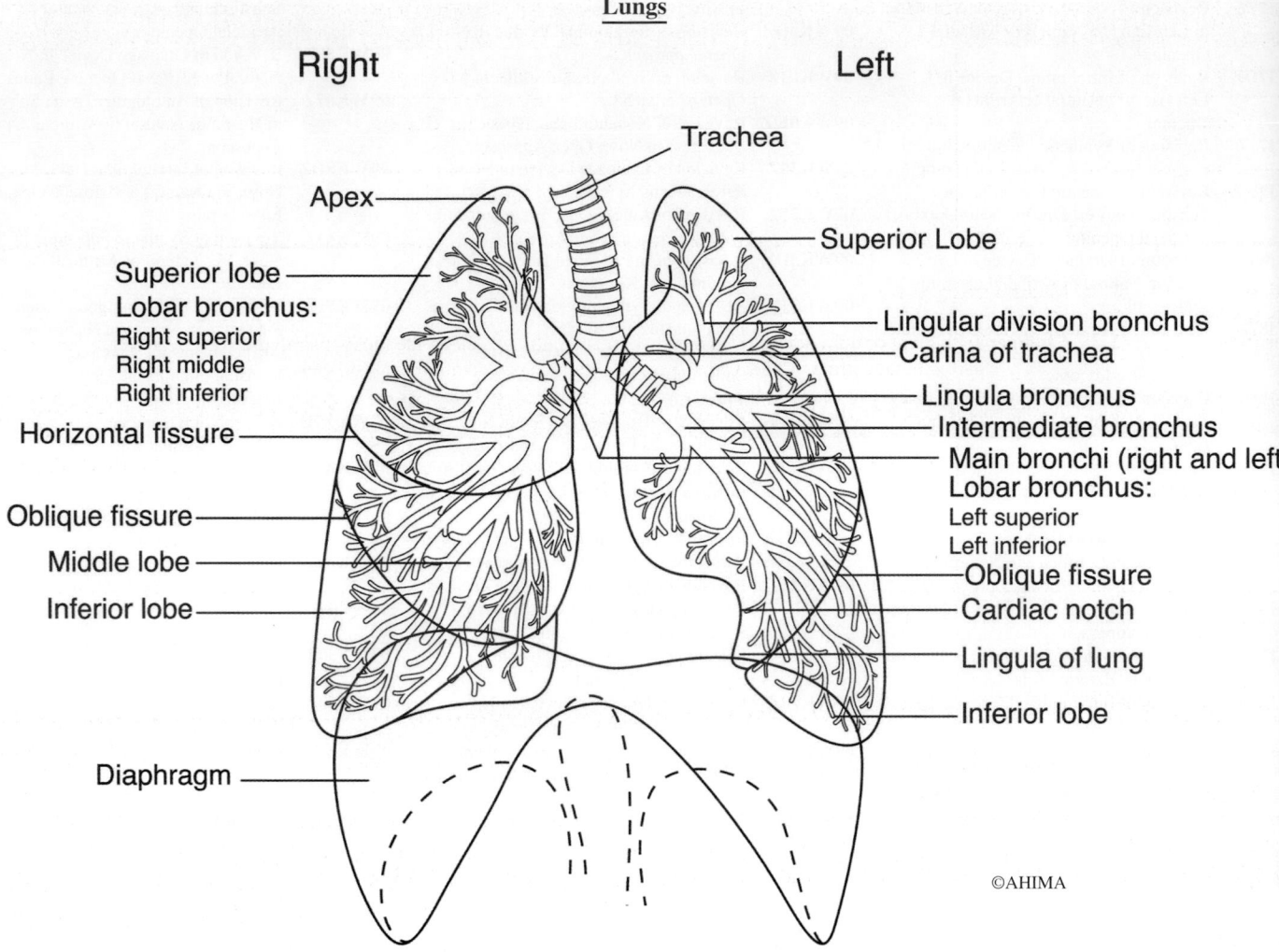

Trachea

Apex

Superior Lobe

Superior lobe
Lobar bronchus:
Right superior
Right middle
Right inferior

Lingular division bronchus
Carina of trachea

Horizontal fissure

Lingula bronchus
Intermediate bronchus
Main bronchi (right and left)
Lobar bronchus:
Left superior
Left inferior

Oblique fissure

Oblique fissure

Middle lobe

Cardiac notch

Inferior lobe

Lingula of lung

Inferior lobe

Diaphragm

©AHIMA

tion	0	Medical and Surgical
dy System	B	Respiratory System
eration	1	Bypass: Altering the route of passage of the contents of a tubular body part

Body Part (4th)	Approach (5th)	Device (6th)	Qualifier (7th)
Trachea	0 Open	D Intraluminal Device	6 Esophagus
Trachea	0 Open	F Tracheostomy Device Z No Device	4 Cutaneous
Trachea	3 Percutaneous 4 Percutaneous Endoscopic	F Tracheostomy Device Z No Device	4 Cutaneous

tion	0	Medical and Surgical
dy System	B	Respiratory System
eration	2	Change: Taking out or off a device from a body part and putting back an identical or similar device in or on the same body part without cutting or puncturing the skin or a mucous membrane

Body Part (4th)	Approach (5th)	Device (6th)	Qualifier (7th)
Tracheobronchial Tree Lung, Right Lung, Left Pleura Diaphragm	X External	0 Drainage Device Y Other Device	Z No Qualifier
Trachea	X External	0 Drainage Device E Intraluminal Device, Endotracheal Airway F Tracheostomy Device Y Other Device	Z No Qualifier

tion	0	Medical and Surgical
dy System	B	Respiratory System
eration	5	Destruction: Physical eradication of all or a portion of a body part by the direct use of energy, force, or a destructive agent

Body Part (4th)	Approach (5th)	Device (6th)	Qualifier (7th)
1 Trachea 2 Carina 3 Main Bronchus, Right 4 Upper Lobe Bronchus, Right 5 Middle Lobe Bronchus, Right 6 Lower Lobe Bronchus, Right 7 Main Bronchus, Left 8 Upper Lobe Bronchus, Left 9 Lingula Bronchus B Lower Lobe Bronchus, Left C Upper Lung Lobe, Right D Middle Lung Lobe, Right F Lower Lung Lobe, Right G Upper Lung Lobe, Left H Lung Lingula J Lower Lung Lobe, Left K Lung, Right L Lung, Left M Lungs, Bilateral	0 Open 3 Percutaneous 4 Percutaneous Endoscopic 7 Via Natural or Artificial Opening 8 Via Natural or Artificial Opening Endoscopic	Z No Device	Z No Qualifier
N Pleura, Right P Pleura, Left R Diaphragm, Right S Diaphragm, Left	0 Open 3 Percutaneous 4 Percutaneous Endoscopic	Z No Device	Z No Qualifier

Section	0	Medical and Surgical
Body System	B	Respiratory System
Operation	7	Dilation: Expanding an orifice or the lumen of a tubular body part

Body Part (4th)	Approach (5th)	Device (6th)	Qualifier (7th)
1 Trachea 2 Carina 3 Main Bronchus, Right 4 Upper Lobe Bronchus, Right 5 Middle Lobe Bronchus, Right 6 Lower Lobe Bronchus, Right 7 Main Bronchus, Left 8 Upper Lobe Bronchus, Left 9 Lingula Bronchus B Lower Lobe Bronchus, Left	0 Open 3 Percutaneous 4 Percutaneous Endoscopic 7 Via Natural or Artificial Opening 8 Via Natural or Artificial Opening Endoscopic	D Intraluminal Device Z No Device	Z No Qualifier

Section	0	Medical and Surgical
Body System	B	Respiratory System
Operation	9	Drainage: Taking or letting out fluids and/or gases from a body part

Body Part (4th)	Approach (5th)	Device (6th)	Qualifier (7th)
1 Trachea 2 Carina 3 Main Bronchus, Right 4 Upper Lobe Bronchus, Right 5 Middle Lobe Bronchus, Right 6 Lower Lobe Bronchus, Right 7 Main Bronchus, Left 8 Upper Lobe Bronchus, Left 9 Lingula Bronchus B Lower Lobe Bronchus, Left C Upper Lung Lobe, Right D Middle Lung Lobe, Right F Lower Lung Lobe, Right G Upper Lung Lobe, Left H Lung Lingula J Lower Lung Lobe, Left K Lung, Right L Lung, Left M Lungs, Bilateral	0 Open 3 Percutaneous 4 Percutaneous Endoscopic 7 Via Natural or Artificial Opening 8 Via Natural or Artificial Opening Endoscopic	0 Drainage Device	Z No Qualifier
1 Trachea 2 Carina 3 Main Bronchus, Right 4 Upper Lobe Bronchus, Right 5 Middle Lobe Bronchus, Right 6 Lower Lobe Bronchus, Right 7 Main Bronchus, Left 8 Upper Lobe Bronchus, Left 9 Lingula Bronchus B Lower Lobe Bronchus, Left C Upper Lung Lobe, Right D Middle Lung Lobe, Right F Lower Lung Lobe, Right G Upper Lung Lobe, Left H Lung Lingula J Lower Lung Lobe, Left K Lung, Right L Lung, Left M Lungs, Bilateral	0 Open 3 Percutaneous 4 Percutaneous Endoscopic 7 Via Natural or Artificial Opening 8 Via Natural or Artificial Opening Endoscopic	Z No Device	X Diagnostic Z No Qualifier
N Pleura, Right P Pleura, Left R Diaphragm, Right S Diaphragm, Left	0 Open 3 Percutaneous 4 Percutaneous Endoscopic	0 Drainage Device	Z No Qualifier

Continued →

Section 0 Medical and Surgical
Body System B Respiratory System
Operation 9 **Drainage:** Taking or letting out fluids and/or gases from a body part

Body Part (4ᵗʰ)	Approach (5ᵗʰ)	Device (6ᵗʰ)	Qualifier (7ᵗʰ)
Pleura, Right Pleura, Left Diaphragm, Right Diaphragm, Left	0 Open 3 Percutaneous 4 Percutaneous Endoscopic	Z No Device	X Diagnostic Z No Qualifier

Section 0 Medical and Surgical
Body System B Respiratory System
Operation B **Excision:** Cutting out or off, without replacement, a portion of a body part

Body Part (4ᵗʰ)	Approach (5ᵗʰ)	Device (6ᵗʰ)	Qualifier (7ᵗʰ)
Trachea Carina Main Bronchus, Right Upper Lobe Bronchus, Right Middle Lobe Bronchus, Right Lower Lobe Bronchus, Right Main Bronchus, Left Upper Lobe Bronchus, Left Lingula Bronchus Lower Lobe Bronchus, Left Upper Lung Lobe, Right Middle Lung Lobe, Right Lower Lung Lobe, Right Upper Lung Lobe, Left Lung Lingula Lower Lung Lobe, Left Lung, Right Lung, Left Lungs, Bilateral	0 Open 3 Percutaneous 4 Percutaneous Endoscopic 7 Via Natural or Artificial Opening 8 Via Natural or Artificial Opening Endoscopic	Z No Device	X Diagnostic Z No Qualifier
Pleura, Right Pleura, Left Diaphragm, Right Diaphragm, Left	0 Open 3 Percutaneous 4 Percutaneous Endoscopic	Z No Device	X Diagnostic Z No Qualifier

Section 0 Medical and Surgical
Body System B Respiratory System
Operation C **Extirpation:** Taking or cutting out solid matter from a body part

Body Part (4ᵗʰ)	Approach (5ᵗʰ)	Device (6ᵗʰ)	Qualifier (7ᵗʰ)
1 Trachea 2 Carina 3 Main Bronchus, Right 4 Upper Lobe Bronchus, Right 5 Middle Lobe Bronchus, Right 6 Lower Lobe Bronchus, Right 7 Main Bronchus, Left 8 Upper Lobe Bronchus, Left 9 Lingula Bronchus B Lower Lobe Bronchus, Left C Upper Lung Lobe, Right D Middle Lung Lobe, Right F Lower Lung Lobe, Right G Upper Lung Lobe, Left H Lung Lingula J Lower Lung Lobe, Left K Lung, Right L Lung, Left M Lungs, Bilateral	0 Open 3 Percutaneous 4 Percutaneous Endoscopic 7 Via Natural or Artificial Opening 8 Via Natural or Artificial Opening Endoscopic	Z No Device	Z No Qualifier

Continued →

Section	0	Medical and Surgical
Body System	B	Respiratory System
Operation	C	**Extirpation:** Taking or cutting out solid matter from a body part

Body Part (4th)	Approach (5th)	Device (6th)	Qualifier (7th)
N Pleura, Right P Pleura, Left R Diaphragm, Right S Diaphragm, Left	0 Open 3 Percutaneous 4 Percutaneous Endoscopic	Z No Device	Z No Qualifier

Section	0	Medical and Surgical
Body System	B	Respiratory System
Operation	D	**Extraction:** Pulling or stripping out or off all or a portion of a body part by the use of force

Body Part (4th)	Approach (5th)	Device (6th)	Qualifier (7th)
N Pleura, Right P Pleura, Left	0 Open 3 Percutaneous 4 Percutaneous Endoscopic	Z No Device	X Diagnostic Z No Qualifier

Section	0	Medical and Surgical
Body System	B	Respiratory System
Operation	F	**Fragmentation:** Breaking solid matter in a body part into pieces

Body Part (4th)	Approach (5th)	Device (6th)	Qualifier (7th)
1 Trachea 2 Carina 3 Main Bronchus, Right 4 Upper Lobe Bronchus, Right 5 Middle Lobe Bronchus, Right 6 Lower Lobe Bronchus, Right 7 Main Bronchus, Left 8 Upper Lobe Bronchus, Left 9 Lingula Bronchus B Lower Lobe Bronchus, Left	0 Open 3 Percutaneous 4 Percutaneous Endoscopic 7 Via Natural or Artificial Opening 8 Via Natural or Artificial Opening Endoscopic X External	Z No Device	Z No Qualifier

Section	0	Medical and Surgical
Body System	B	Respiratory System
Operation	H	**Insertion:** Putting in a nonbiological appliance that monitors, assists, performs, or prevents a physiological function but doe not physically take the place of a body part

Body Part (4th)	Approach (5th)	Device (6th)	Qualifier (7th)
0 Tracheobronchial Tree	0 Open 3 Percutaneous 4 Percutaneous Endoscopic 7 Via Natural or Artificial Opening 8 Via Natural or Artificial Opening Endoscopic	1 Radioactive Element 2 Monitoring Device 3 Infusion Device D Intraluminal Device	Z No Qualifier
1 Trachea	0 Open	2 Monitoring Device D Intraluminal Device	Z No Qualifier
1 Trachea	3 Percutaneous	D Intraluminal Device E Intraluminal Device, Endotracheal Airway	Z No Qualifier
1 Trachea	4 Percutaneous Endoscopic	D Intraluminal Device	Z No Qualifier
1 Trachea	7 Via Natural or Artificial Opening 8 Via Natural or Artificial Opening Endoscopic	2 Monitoring Device D Intraluminal Device E Intraluminal Device, Endotracheal Airway	Z No Qualifier

Continued →

Section 0 Medical and Surgical
Body System B Respiratory System
Operation H Insertion: Putting in a nonbiological appliance that monitors, assists, performs, or prevents a physiological function but does not physically take the place of a body part

Body Part (4th)	Approach (5th)	Device (6th)	Qualifier (7th)
Main Bronchus, Right Upper Lobe Bronchus, Right Middle Lobe Bronchus, Right Lower Lobe Bronchus, Right Main Bronchus, Left Upper Lobe Bronchus, Left Lingula Bronchus Lower Lobe Bronchus, Left	0 Open 3 Percutaneous 4 Percutaneous Endoscopic 7 Via Natural or Artificial Opening 8 Via Natural or Artificial Opening Endoscopic	G Intraluminal Device, Endobronchial Valve	Z No Qualifier
Lung, Right Lung, Left	0 Open 3 Percutaneous 4 Percutaneous Endoscopic 7 Via Natural or Artificial Opening 8 Via Natural or Artificial Opening Endoscopic	1 Radioactive Element 2 Monitoring Device 3 Infusion Device	Z No Qualifier
Diaphragm, Right Diaphragm, Left	0 Open 3 Percutaneous 4 Percutaneous Endoscopic	2 Monitoring Device M Diaphragmatic Pacemaker Lead	Z No Qualifier

Section 0 Medical and Surgical
Body System B Respiratory System
Operation J Inspection: Visually and/or manually exploring a body part

Body Part (4th)	Approach (5th)	Device (6th)	Qualifier (7th)
Tracheobronchial Tree Trachea Lung, Right Lung, Left Pleura Diaphragm	0 Open 3 Percutaneous 4 Percutaneous Endoscopic 7 Via Natural or Artificial Opening 8 Via Natural or Artificial Opening Endoscopic X External	Z No Device	Z No Qualifier

Section 0 Medical and Surgical
Body System B Respiratory System
Operation L Occlusion: Completely closing an orifice or the lumen of a tubular body part

Body Part (4th)	Approach (5th)	Device (6th)	Qualifier (7th)
1 Trachea 2 Carina 3 Main Bronchus, Right 4 Upper Lobe Bronchus, Right 5 Middle Lobe Bronchus, Right 6 Lower Lobe Bronchus, Right 7 Main Bronchus, Left 8 Upper Lobe Bronchus, Left 9 Lingula Bronchus B Lower Lobe Bronchus, Left	0 Open 3 Percutaneous 4 Percutaneous Endoscopic	C Extraluminal Device D Intraluminal Device Z No Device	Z No Qualifier
1 Trachea 2 Carina 3 Main Bronchus, Right 4 Upper Lobe Bronchus, Right 5 Middle Lobe Bronchus, Right 6 Lower Lobe Bronchus, Right 7 Main Bronchus, Left 8 Upper Lobe Bronchus, Left 9 Lingula Bronchus B Lower Lobe Bronchus, Left	7 Via Natural or Artificial Opening 8 Via Natural or Artificial Opening Endoscopic	D Intraluminal Device Z No Device	Z No Qualifier

Section	0	Medical and Surgical
Body System	B	Respiratory System
Operation	M	**Reattachment:** Putting back in or on all or a portion of a separated body part to its normal location or other suitable locatio

Body Part (4ᵗʰ)	Approach (5ᵗʰ)	Device (6ᵗʰ)	Qualifier (7ᵗʰ)
1 Trachea 2 Carina 3 Main Bronchus, Right 4 Upper Lobe Bronchus, Right 5 Middle Lobe Bronchus, Right 6 Lower Lobe Bronchus, Right 7 Main Bronchus, Left 8 Upper Lobe Bronchus, Left 9 Lingula Bronchus B Lower Lobe Bronchus, Left C Upper Lung Lobe, Right D Middle Lung Lobe, Right F Lower Lung Lobe, Right G Upper Lung Lobe, Left H Lung Lingula J Lower Lung Lobe, Left K Lung, Right L Lung, Left R Diaphragm, Right S Diaphragm, Left	0 Open	Z No Device	Z No Qualifier

Section	0	Medical and Surgical
Body System	B	Respiratory System
Operation	N	**Release:** Freeing a body part from an abnormal physical constraint by cutting or by the use of force

Body Part (4ᵗʰ)	Approach (5ᵗʰ)	Device (6ᵗʰ)	Qualifier (7ᵗʰ)
1 Trachea 2 Carina 3 Main Bronchus, Right 4 Upper Lobe Bronchus, Right 5 Middle Lobe Bronchus, Right 6 Lower Lobe Bronchus, Right 7 Main Bronchus, Left 8 Upper Lobe Bronchus, Left 9 Lingula Bronchus B Lower Lobe Bronchus, Left C Upper Lung Lobe, Right D Middle Lung Lobe, Right F Lower Lung Lobe, Right G Upper Lung Lobe, Left H Lung Lingula J Lower Lung Lobe, Left K Lung, Right L Lung, Left M Lungs, Bilateral	0 Open 3 Percutaneous 4 Percutaneous Endoscopic 7 Via Natural or Artificial Opening 8 Via Natural or Artificial Opening Endoscopic	Z No Device	Z No Qualifier
N Pleura, Right P Pleura, Left R Diaphragm, Right S Diaphragm, Left	0 Open 3 Percutaneous 4 Percutaneous Endoscopic	Z No Device	Z No Qualifier

	0	Medical and Surgical
...ion		
...y System	B	Respiratory System
...ration	P	**Removal:** Taking out or off a device from a body part

Body Part (4ᵗʰ)	Approach (5ᵗʰ)	Device (6ᵗʰ)	Qualifier (7ᵗʰ)
Tracheobronchial Tree	0 Open 3 Percutaneous 4 Percutaneous Endoscopic 7 Via Natural or Artificial Opening 8 Via Natural or Artificial Opening Endoscopic	0 Drainage Device 1 Radioactive Element 2 Monitoring Device 3 Infusion Device 7 Autologous Tissue Substitute C Extraluminal Device D Intraluminal Device J Synthetic Substitute K Nonautologous Tissue Substitute	Z No Qualifier
Tracheobronchial Tree	X External	0 Drainage Device 1 Radioactive Element 2 Monitoring Device 3 Infusion Device D Intraluminal Device	Z No Qualifier
Trachea	0 Open 3 Percutaneous 4 Percutaneous Endoscopic 7 Via Natural or Artificial Opening 8 Via Natural or Artificial Opening Endoscopic	0 Drainage Device 2 Monitoring Device 7 Autologous Tissue Substitute C Extraluminal Device D Intraluminal Device F Tracheostomy Device J Synthetic Substitute K Nonautologous Tissue Substitute	Z No Qualifier
Trachea	X External	0 Drainage Device 2 Monitoring Device D Intraluminal Device F Tracheostomy Device	Z No Qualifier
...K Lung, Right ...L Lung, Left	0 Open 3 Percutaneous 4 Percutaneous Endoscopic 7 Via Natural or Artificial Opening 8 Via Natural or Artificial Opening Endoscopic X External	0 Drainage Device 1 Radioactive Element 2 Monitoring Device 3 Infusion Device	Z No Qualifier
...Q Pleura	0 Open 3 Percutaneous 4 Percutaneous Endoscopic 7 Via Natural or Artificial Opening 8 Via Natural or Artificial Opening Endoscopic X External	0 Drainage Device 1 Radioactive Element 2 Monitoring Device	Z No Qualifier
...T Diaphragm	0 Open 3 Percutaneous 4 Percutaneous Endoscopic 7 Via Natural or Artificial Opening 8 Via Natural or Artificial Opening Endoscopic	0 Drainage Device 2 Monitoring Device 7 Autologous Tissue Substitute J Synthetic Substitute K Nonautologous Tissue Substitute M Diaphragmatic Pacemaker Lead	Z No Qualifier
...T Diaphragm	X External	0 Drainage Device 2 Monitoring Device M Diaphragmatic Pacemaker Lead	Z No Qualifier

Section   **0**   **Medical and Surgical**
Body System   **B**   **Respiratory System**
Operation   **Q**   **Repair:** Restoring, to the extent possible, a body part to its normal anatomic structure and function

Body Part (4th)	Approach (5th)	Device (6th)	Qualifier (7th)
1 Trachea 2 Carina 3 Main Bronchus, Right 4 Upper Lobe Bronchus, Right 5 Middle Lobe Bronchus, Right 6 Lower Lobe Bronchus, Right 7 Main Bronchus, Left 8 Upper Lobe Bronchus, Left 9 Lingula Bronchus B Lower Lobe Bronchus, Left C Upper Lung Lobe, Right D Middle Lung Lobe, Right F Lower Lung Lobe, Right G Upper Lung Lobe, Left H Lung Lingula J Lower Lung Lobe, Left K Lung, Right L Lung, Left M Lungs, Bilateral	0 Open 3 Percutaneous 4 Percutaneous Endoscopic 7 Via Natural or Artificial Opening 8 Via Natural or Artificial Opening Endoscopic	Z No Device	Z No Qualifier
N Pleura, Right P Pleura, Left R Diaphragm, Right S Diaphragm, Left	0 Open 3 Percutaneous 4 Percutaneous Endoscopic	Z No Device	Z No Qualifier

Section   **0**   **Medical and Surgical**
Body System   **B**   **Respiratory System**
Operation   **S**   **Reposition:** Moving to its normal location, or other suitable location, all or a portion of a body part

Body Part (4th)	Approach (5th)	Device (6th)	Qualifier (7th)
1 Trachea 2 Carina 3 Main Bronchus, Right 4 Upper Lobe Bronchus, Right 5 Middle Lobe Bronchus, Right 6 Lower Lobe Bronchus, Right 7 Main Bronchus, Left 8 Upper Lobe Bronchus, Left 9 Lingula Bronchus B Lower Lobe Bronchus, Left C Upper Lung Lobe, Right D Middle Lung Lobe, Right F Lower Lung Lobe, Right G Upper Lung Lobe, Left H Lung Lingula J Lower Lung Lobe, Left K Lung, Right L Lung, Left R Diaphragm, Right S Diaphragm, Left	0 Open	Z No Device	Z No Qualifier

Section 0 Medical and Surgical
Body System B Respiratory System
Operation T Resection: Cutting out or off, without replacement, all of a body part

Body Part (4th)	Approach (5th)	Device (6th)	Qualifier (7th)
1 Trachea	0 Open	Z No Device	Z No Qualifier
2 Carina	4 Percutaneous Endoscopic		
3 Main Bronchus, Right			
4 Upper Lobe Bronchus, Right			
5 Middle Lobe Bronchus, Right			
6 Lower Lobe Bronchus, Right			
7 Main Bronchus, Left			
8 Upper Lobe Bronchus, Left			
9 Lingula Bronchus			
B Lower Lobe Bronchus, Left			
C Upper Lung Lobe, Right			
D Middle Lung Lobe, Right			
F Lower Lung Lobe, Right			
G Upper Lung Lobe, Left			
H Lung Lingula			
J Lower Lung Lobe, Left			
K Lung, Right			
L Lung, Left			
M Lungs, Bilateral			
R Diaphragm, Right			
S Diaphragm, Left			

Section 0 Medical and Surgical
Body System B Respiratory System
Operation U Supplement: Putting in or on biological or synthetic material that physically reinforces and/or augments the function of a portion of a body part

Body Part (4th)	Approach (5th)	Device (6th)	Qualifier (7th)
1 Trachea	0 Open	7 Autologous Tissue Substitute	Z No Qualifier
2 Carina	4 Percutaneous Endoscopic	J Synthetic Substitute	
3 Main Bronchus, Right		K Nonautologous Tissue Substitute	
4 Upper Lobe Bronchus, Right			
5 Middle Lobe Bronchus, Right			
6 Lower Lobe Bronchus, Right			
7 Main Bronchus, Left			
8 Upper Lobe Bronchus, Left			
9 Lingula Bronchus			
B Lower Lobe Bronchus, Left			
R Diaphragm, Right			
S Diaphragm, Left			

Section 0 Medical and Surgical
Body System B Respiratory System
Operation V Restriction: Partially closing an orifice or the lumen of a tubular body part

Body Part (4th)	Approach (5th)	Device (6th)	Qualifier (7th)
1 Trachea	0 Open	C Extraluminal Device	Z No Qualifier
2 Carina	3 Percutaneous	D Intraluminal Device	
3 Main Bronchus, Right	4 Percutaneous Endoscopic	Z No Device	
4 Upper Lobe Bronchus, Right			
5 Middle Lobe Bronchus, Right			
6 Lower Lobe Bronchus, Right			
7 Main Bronchus, Left			
8 Upper Lobe Bronchus, Left			
9 Lingula Bronchus			
B Lower Lobe Bronchus, Left			

Continued →

Section	0	Medical and Surgical
Body System	B	Respiratory System
Operation	V	Restriction: Partially closing an orifice or the lumen of a tubular body part

Body Part (4th)	Approach (5th)	Device (6th)	Qualifier (7th)
1 Trachea 2 Carina 3 Main Bronchus, Right 4 Upper Lobe Bronchus, Right 5 Middle Lobe Bronchus, Right 6 Lower Lobe Bronchus, Right 7 Main Bronchus, Left 8 Upper Lobe Bronchus, Left 9 Lingula Bronchus B Lower Lobe Bronchus, Left	7 Via Natural or Artificial Opening 8 Via Natural or Artificial Opening Endoscopic	D Intraluminal Device Z No Device	Z No Qualifier

Section	0	Medical and Surgical
Body System	B	Respiratory System
Operation	W	Revision: Correcting, to the extent possible, a portion of a malfunctioning device or the position of a displaced device

Body Part (4th)	Approach (5th)	Device (6th)	Qualifier (7th)
0 Tracheobronchial Tree	0 Open 3 Percutaneous 4 Percutaneous Endoscopic 7 Via Natural or Artificial Opening 8 Via Natural or Artificial Opening Endoscopic X External	0 Drainage Device 2 Monitoring Device 3 Infusion Device 7 Autologous Tissue Substitute C Extraluminal Device D Intraluminal Device J Synthetic Substitute K Nonautologous Tissue Substitute	Z No Qualifier
1 Trachea	0 Open 3 Percutaneous 4 Percutaneous Endoscopic 7 Via Natural or Artificial Opening 8 Via Natural or Artificial Opening Endoscopic X External	0 Drainage Device 2 Monitoring Device 7 Autologous Tissue Substitute C Extraluminal Device D Intraluminal Device F Tracheostomy Device J Synthetic Substitute K Nonautologous Tissue Substitute	Z No Qualifier
K Lung, Right L Lung, Left	0 Open 3 Percutaneous 4 Percutaneous Endoscopic 7 Via Natural or Artificial Opening 8 Via Natural or Artificial Opening Endoscopic X External	0 Drainage Device 2 Monitoring Device 3 Infusion Device	Z No Qualifier
Q Pleura	0 Open 3 Percutaneous 4 Percutaneous Endoscopic 7 Via Natural or Artificial Opening 8 Via Natural or Artificial Opening Endoscopic X External	0 Drainage Device 2 Monitoring Device	Z No Qualifier
T Diaphragm	0 Open 3 Percutaneous 4 Percutaneous Endoscopic 7 Via Natural or Artificial Opening 8 Via Natural or Artificial Opening Endoscopic X External	0 Drainage Device 2 Monitoring Device 7 Autologous Tissue Substitute J Synthetic Substitute K Nonautologous Tissue Substitute M Diaphragmatic Pacemaker Lead	Z No Qualifier

		Medical and Surgical
·tion	**0**	**Medical and Surgical**
·dy System	**B**	**Respiratory System**
·eration	**Y**	**Transplantation:** Putting in or on all or a portion of a living body part taken from another individual or animal to physically take the place and/or function of all or a portion of a similar body part

Body Part (4th)	Approach (5th)	Device (6th)	Qualifier (7th)
C Upper Lung Lobe, Right D Middle Lung Lobe, Right F Lower Lung Lobe, Right G Upper Lung Lobe, Left H Lung Lingula J Lower Lung Lobe, Left K Lung, Right L Lung, Left M Lungs, Bilateral	**0** Open	**Z** No Device	**0** Allogeneic **1** Syngeneic **2** Zooplastic

·espiratory System Code Listing 0B1–0BY

·31 – Respiratory System, Bypass

·*eview Coding Guideline B3.6a*

·110D6	Bypass Trachea to Esophagus with Intraluminal Device, Open Approach	● **0B113F4**	Bypass Trachea to Cutaneous with Tracheostomy Device, Percutaneous Approach
·110F4	Bypass Trachea to Cutaneous with Tracheostomy Device, Open Approach	● **0B113Z4**	Bypass Trachea to Cutaneous, Percutaneous Approach
·110Z4	Bypass Trachea to Cutaneous, Open Approach		

0B114F4 Bypass Trachea to Cutaneous with Tracheostomy Device, Percutaneous Endoscopic Approach

0B114Z4 Bypass Trachea to Cutaneous, Percutaneous Endoscopic Approach

·B2 – Respiratory System, Change

·*eview Coding Guideline B6.1c*

·320X0Z	Change Drainage Device in Tracheobronchial Tree, External Approach	**0B21XYZ**	Change Other Device in Trachea, External Approach
·320XYZ	Change Other Device in Tracheobronchial Tree, External Approach	**0B2KX0Z**	Change Drainage Device in Right Lung, External Approach
·321X0Z	Change Drainage Device in Trachea, External Approach	**0B2KXYZ**	Change Other Device in Right Lung, External Approach
·321XEZ	Change Endotracheal Airway in Trachea, External Approach	**0B2LX0Z**	Change Drainage Device in Left Lung, External Approach
·321XFZ	Change Tracheostomy Device in Trachea, External Approach	**0B2LXYZ**	Change Other Device in Left Lung, External Approach

0B2QX0Z Change Drainage Device in Pleura, External Approach

0B2QXYZ Change Other Device in Pleura, External Approach

0B2TX0Z Change Drainage Device in Diaphragm, External Approach

0B2TXYZ Change Other Device in Diaphragm, External Approach

·B5 – Respiratory System, Destruction

·3510ZZ	Destruction of Trachea, Open Approach	**0B540ZZ**	Destruction of Right Upper Lobe Bronchus, Open Approach	**0B563ZZ**	Destruction of Right Lower Lobe Bronchus, Percutaneous Approach
·3513ZZ	Destruction of Trachea, Percutaneous Approach	**0B543ZZ**	Destruction of Right Upper Lobe Bronchus, Percutaneous Approach	**0B564ZZ**	Destruction of Right Lower Lobe Bronchus, Percutaneous Endoscopic Approach
·3514ZZ	Destruction of Trachea, Percutaneous Endoscopic Approach	**0B544ZZ**	Destruction of Right Upper Lobe Bronchus, Percutaneous Endoscopic Approach	**0B567ZZ**	Destruction of Right Lower Lobe Bronchus, Via Natural or Artificial Opening
·3517ZZ	Destruction of Trachea, Via Natural or Artificial Opening	**0B547ZZ**	Destruction of Right Upper Lobe Bronchus, Via Natural or Artificial Opening	**0B568ZZ**	Destruction of Right Lower Lobe Bronchus, Via Natural or Artificial Opening Endoscopic
·3518ZZ	Destruction of Trachea, Via Natural or Artificial Opening Endoscopic	**0B548ZZ**	Destruction of Right Upper Lobe Bronchus, Via Natural or Artificial Opening Endoscopic	**0B570ZZ**	Destruction of Left Main Bronchus, Open Approach
·3520ZZ	Destruction of Carina, Open Approach	**0B550ZZ**	Destruction of Right Middle Lobe Bronchus, Open Approach	**0B573ZZ**	Destruction of Left Main Bronchus, Percutaneous Approach
·3523ZZ	Destruction of Carina, Percutaneous Approach	**0B553ZZ**	Destruction of Right Middle Lobe Bronchus, Percutaneous Approach	**0B574ZZ**	Destruction of Left Main Bronchus, Percutaneous Endoscopic Approach
·3524ZZ	Destruction of Carina, Percutaneous Endoscopic Approach	**0B554ZZ**	Destruction of Right Middle Lobe Bronchus, Percutaneous Endoscopic Approach	**0B577ZZ**	Destruction of Left Main Bronchus, Via Natural or Artificial Opening
·3527ZZ	Destruction of Carina, Via Natural or Artificial Opening	**0B557ZZ**	Destruction of Right Middle Lobe Bronchus, Via Natural or Artificial Opening	**0B578ZZ**	Destruction of Left Main Bronchus, Via Natural or Artificial Opening Endoscopic
·3528ZZ	Destruction of Carina, Via Natural or Artificial Opening Endoscopic	**0B558ZZ**	Destruction of Right Middle Lobe Bronchus, Via Natural or Artificial Opening Endoscopic	**0B580ZZ**	Destruction of Left Upper Lobe Bronchus, Open Approach
·3530ZZ	Destruction of Right Main Bronchus, Open Approach	**0B560ZZ**	Destruction of Right Lower Lobe Bronchus, Open Approach	**0B583ZZ**	Destruction of Left Upper Lobe Bronchus, Percutaneous Approach
·3533ZZ	Destruction of Right Main Bronchus, Percutaneous Approach			**0B584ZZ**	Destruction of Left Upper Lobe Bronchus, Percutaneous Endoscopic Approach
·3534ZZ	Destruction of Right Main Bronchus, Percutaneous Endoscopic Approach				
·3537ZZ	Destruction of Right Main Bronchus, Via Natural or Artificial Opening				
·3538ZZ	Destruction of Right Main Bronchus, Via Natural or Artificial Opening Endoscopic				

♀ Female-only	♂ Male-only	▲ Limited Coverage	● Non-OR	▦ HAC-associated procedure	▲ Non-covered procedures	⊞ Combination

0B587ZZ Destruction of Left Upper Lobe Bronchus, Via Natural or Artificial Opening

0B588ZZ Destruction of Left Upper Lobe Bronchus, Via Natural or Artificial Opening Endoscopic

0B590ZZ Destruction of Lingula Bronchus, Open Approach

0B593ZZ Destruction of Lingula Bronchus, Percutaneous Approach

0B594ZZ Destruction of Lingula Bronchus, Percutaneous Endoscopic Approach

0B597ZZ Destruction of Lingula Bronchus, Via Natural or Artificial Opening

0B598ZZ Destruction of Lingula Bronchus, Via Natural or Artificial Opening Endoscopic

0B5B0ZZ Destruction of Left Lower Lobe Bronchus, Open Approach

0B5B3ZZ Destruction of Left Lower Lobe Bronchus, Percutaneous Approach

0B5B4ZZ Destruction of Left Lower Lobe Bronchus, Percutaneous Endoscopic Approach

0B5B7ZZ Destruction of Left Lower Lobe Bronchus, Via Natural or Artificial Opening

0B5B8ZZ Destruction of Left Lower Lobe Bronchus, Via Natural or Artificial Opening Endoscopic

0B5C0ZZ Destruction of Right Upper Lung Lobe, Open Approach

0B5C3ZZ Destruction of Right Upper Lung Lobe, Percutaneous Approach

0B5C4ZZ Destruction of Right Upper Lung Lobe, Percutaneous Endoscopic Approach

0B5C7ZZ Destruction of Right Upper Lung Lobe, Via Natural or Artificial Opening

0B5C8ZZ Destruction of Right Upper Lung Lobe, Via Natural or Artificial Opening Endoscopic

0B5D0ZZ Destruction of Right Middle Lung Lobe, Open Approach

0B5D3ZZ Destruction of Right Middle Lung Lobe, Percutaneous Approach

0B5D4ZZ Destruction of Right Middle Lung Lobe, Percutaneous Endoscopic Approach

0B5D7ZZ Destruction of Right Middle Lung Lobe, Via Natural or Artificial Opening

0B5D8ZZ Destruction of Right Middle Lung Lobe, Via Natural or Artificial Opening Endoscopic

0B5F0ZZ Destruction of Right Lower Lung Lobe, Open Approach

0B5F3ZZ Destruction of Right Lower Lung Lobe, Percutaneous Approach

0B5F4ZZ Destruction of Right Lower Lung Lobe, Percutaneous Endoscopic Approach

0B5F7ZZ Destruction of Right Lower Lung Lobe, Via Natural or Artificial Opening

0B5F8ZZ Destruction of Right Lower Lung Lobe, Via Natural or Artificial Opening Endoscopic

0B5G0ZZ Destruction of Left Upper Lung Lobe, Open Approach

0B5G3ZZ Destruction of Left Upper Lung Lobe, Percutaneous Approach

0B5G4ZZ Destruction of Left Upper Lung Lobe, Percutaneous Endoscopic Approach

0B5G7ZZ Destruction of Left Upper Lung Lobe, Via Natural or Artificial Opening

0B5G8ZZ Destruction of Left Upper Lung Lobe, Via Natural or Artificial Opening Endoscopic

0B5H0ZZ Destruction of Lung Lingula, Open Approach

0B5H3ZZ Destruction of Lung Lingula, Percutaneous Approach

0B5H4ZZ Destruction of Lung Lingula, Percutaneous Endoscopic Approach

0B5H7ZZ Destruction of Lung Lingula, Via Natural or Artificial Opening

0B5H8ZZ Destruction of Lung Lingula, Via Natural or Artificial Opening Endoscopic

0B5J0ZZ Destruction of Left Lower Lung Lobe, Open Approach

0B5J3ZZ Destruction of Left Lower Lung Lobe, Percutaneous Approach

0B5J4ZZ Destruction of Left Lower Lung Lobe, Percutaneous Endoscopic Approach

0B5J7ZZ Destruction of Left Lower Lung Lobe, Via Natural or Artificial Opening

0B5J8ZZ Destruction of Left Lower Lung Lobe, Via Natural or Artificial Opening Endoscopic

0B5K0ZZ Destruction of Right Lung, Open Approach

0B5K3ZZ Destruction of Right Lung, Percutaneous Approach

0B5K4ZZ Destruction of Right Lung, Percutaneous Endoscopic Approach

0B5K7ZZ Destruction of Right Lung, Via Natural Artificial Opening

0B5K8ZZ Destruction of Right Lung, Via Natural Artificial Opening Endoscopic

0B5L0ZZ Destruction of Left Lung, Open Approach

0B5L3ZZ Destruction of Left Lung, Percutaneous Approach

0B5L4ZZ Destruction of Left Lung, Percutaneous Endoscopic Approach

0B5L7ZZ Destruction of Left Lung, Via Natural o Artificial Opening

0B5L8ZZ Destruction of Left Lung, Via Natural o Artificial Opening Endoscopic

0B5M0ZZ Destruction of Bilateral Lungs, Open Approach

0B5M3ZZ Destruction of Bilateral Lungs, Percutaneous Approach

0B5M4ZZ Destruction of Bilateral Lungs, Percutaneous Endoscopic Approach

0B5M7ZZ Destruction of Bilateral Lungs, Via Natural or Artificial Opening

0B5M8ZZ Destruction of Bilateral Lungs, Via Natural or Artificial Opening Endoscopi

0B5N0ZZ Destruction of Right Pleura, Open Approach

0B5N3ZZ Destruction of Right Pleura, Percutaneo Approach

0B5N4ZZ Destruction of Right Pleura, Percutaneo Endoscopic Approach

0B5P0ZZ Destruction of Left Pleura, Open Approach

0B5P3ZZ Destruction of Left Pleura, Percutaneous Approach

0B5P4ZZ Destruction of Left Pleura, Percutaneous Endoscopic Approach

0B5R0ZZ Destruction of Right Diaphragm, Open Approach

0B5R3ZZ Destruction of Right Diaphragm, Percutaneous Approach

0B5R4ZZ Destruction of Right Diaphragm, Percutaneous Endoscopic Approach

0B5S0ZZ Destruction of Left Diaphragm, Open Approach

0B5S3ZZ Destruction of Left Diaphragm, Percutaneous Approach

0B5S4ZZ Destruction of Left Diaphragm, Percutaneous Endoscopic Approach

0B7 – Respiratory System, Dilation

0B710DZ Dilation of Trachea with Intraluminal Device, Open Approach

0B710ZZ Dilation of Trachea, Open Approach

0B713DZ Dilation of Trachea with Intraluminal Device, Percutaneous Approach

0B713ZZ Dilation of Trachea, Percutaneous Approach

0B714DZ Dilation of Trachea with Intraluminal Device, Percutaneous Endoscopic Approach

0B714ZZ Dilation of Trachea, Percutaneous Endoscopic Approach

0B717DZ Dilation of Trachea with Intraluminal Device, Via Natural or Artificial Opening

0B717ZZ Dilation of Trachea, Via Natural or Artificial Opening

0B718DZ Dilation of Trachea with Intraluminal Device, Via Natural or Artificial Opening Endoscopic

0B718ZZ Dilation of Trachea, Via Natural or Artificial Opening Endoscopic

0B720DZ Dilation of Carina with Intraluminal Device, Open Approach

0B720ZZ Dilation of Carina, Open Approach

0B723DZ Dilation of Carina with Intraluminal Device, Percutaneous Approach

0B723ZZ Dilation of Carina, Percutaneous Approach

0B724DZ Dilation of Carina with Intraluminal Device, Percutaneous Endoscopic Approach

0B724ZZ Dilation of Carina, Percutaneous Endoscopic Approach

0B727DZ Dilation of Carina with Intraluminal Device, Via Natural or Artificial Opening

0B727ZZ Dilation of Carina, Via Natural or Artificial Opening

0B728DZ Dilation of Carina with Intraluminal Device, Via Natural or Artificial Opening Endoscopic

0B728ZZ Dilation of Carina, Via Natural or Artificial Opening Endoscopic

0B730DZ Dilation of Right Main Bronchus with Intraluminal Device, Open Approach

0B730ZZ Dilation of Right Main Bronchus, Open Approach

0B733DZ Dilation of Right Main Bronchus with Intraluminal Device, Percutaneous Approach

0B733ZZ Dilation of Right Main Bronchus, Percutaneous Approach

0B734DZ Dilation of Right Main Bronchus with Intraluminal Device, Percutaneous Endoscopic Approach

0B734ZZ Dilation of Right Main Bronchus, Percutaneous Endoscopic Approach

0B737DZ Dilation of Right Main Bronchus with Intraluminal Device, Via Natural or Artificial Opening

0B737ZZ Dilation of Right Main Bronchus, Via Natural or Artificial Opening

0B738DZ Dilation of Right Main Bronchus with Intraluminal Device, Via Natural or Artificial Opening Endoscopic

0B738ZZ Dilation of Right Main Bronchus, Via Natural or Artificial Opening Endoscopic

0B740DZ Dilation of Right Upper Lobe Bronchus with Intraluminal Device, Open Approach

0B740ZZ Dilation of Right Upper Lobe Bronchus, Open Approach

0B743DZ Dilation of Right Upper Lobe Bronchus with Intraluminal Device, Percutaneous Approach

0B743ZZ Dilation of Right Upper Lobe Bronchus, Percutaneous Approach

0B744DZ Dilation of Right Upper Lobe Bronchus with Intraluminal Device, Percutaneous Endoscopic Approach

0B744ZZ Dilation of Right Upper Lobe Bronchus, Percutaneous Endoscopic Approach

♀ Female-only   ♂ Male-only   ▲ Limited Coverage   ● Non-OR   ▦ HAC-associated procedure   ▲ Non-covered procedures   ✚ Combination

'47DZ	Dilation of Right Upper Lobe Bronchus with Intraluminal Device, Via Natural or Artificial Opening
'47ZZ	Dilation of Right Upper Lobe Bronchus, Via Natural or Artificial Opening
'48DZ	Dilation of Right Upper Lobe Bronchus with Intraluminal Device, Via Natural or Artificial Opening Endoscopic
'48ZZ	Dilation of Right Upper Lobe Bronchus, Via Natural or Artificial Opening Endoscopic
'50DZ	Dilation of Right Middle Lobe Bronchus with Intraluminal Device, Open Approach
'50ZZ	Dilation of Right Middle Lobe Bronchus, Open Approach
'53DZ	Dilation of Right Middle Lobe Bronchus with Intraluminal Device, Percutaneous Approach
'53ZZ	Dilation of Right Middle Lobe Bronchus, Percutaneous Approach
'54DZ	Dilation of Right Middle Lobe Bronchus with Intraluminal Device, Percutaneous Endoscopic Approach
'54ZZ	Dilation of Right Middle Lobe Bronchus, Percutaneous Endoscopic Approach
'57DZ	Dilation of Right Middle Lobe Bronchus with Intraluminal Device, Via Natural or Artificial Opening
'57ZZ	Dilation of Right Middle Lobe Bronchus, Via Natural or Artificial Opening
'758DZ	Dilation of Right Middle Lobe Bronchus with Intraluminal Device, Via Natural or Artificial Opening Endoscopic
'758ZZ	Dilation of Right Middle Lobe Bronchus, Via Natural or Artificial Opening Endoscopic
'760DZ	Dilation of Right Lower Lobe Bronchus with Intraluminal Device, Open Approach
'760ZZ	Dilation of Right Lower Lobe Bronchus, Open Approach
'763DZ	Dilation of Right Lower Lobe Bronchus with Intraluminal Device, Percutaneous Approach
'763ZZ	Dilation of Right Lower Lobe Bronchus, Percutaneous Approach
'764DZ	Dilation of Right Lower Lobe Bronchus with Intraluminal Device, Percutaneous Endoscopic Approach
'764ZZ	Dilation of Right Lower Lobe Bronchus, Percutaneous Endoscopic Approach
'767DZ	Dilation of Right Lower Lobe Bronchus with Intraluminal Device, Via Natural or Artificial Opening
'767ZZ	Dilation of Right Lower Lobe Bronchus, Via Natural or Artificial Opening

0B768DZ	Dilation of Right Lower Lobe Bronchus with Intraluminal Device, Via Natural or Artificial Opening Endoscopic
0B768ZZ	Dilation of Right Lower Lobe Bronchus, Via Natural or Artificial Opening Endoscopic
0B770DZ	Dilation of Left Main Bronchus with Intraluminal Device, Open Approach
0B770ZZ	Dilation of Left Main Bronchus, Open Approach
0B773DZ	Dilation of Left Main Bronchus with Intraluminal Device, Percutaneous Approach
0B773ZZ	Dilation of Left Main Bronchus, Percutaneous Approach
0B774DZ	Dilation of Left Main Bronchus with Intraluminal Device, Percutaneous Endoscopic Approach
0B774ZZ	Dilation of Left Main Bronchus, Percutaneous Endoscopic Approach
0B777DZ	Dilation of Left Main Bronchus with Intraluminal Device, Via Natural or Artificial Opening
0B777ZZ	Dilation of Left Main Bronchus, Via Natural or Artificial Opening
0B778DZ	Dilation of Left Main Bronchus with Intraluminal Device, Via Natural or Artificial Opening Endoscopic
0B778ZZ	Dilation of Left Main Bronchus, Via Natural or Artificial Opening Endoscopic
0B780DZ	Dilation of Left Upper Lobe Bronchus with Intraluminal Device, Open Approach
0B780ZZ	Dilation of Left Upper Lobe Bronchus, Open Approach
0B783DZ	Dilation of Left Upper Lobe Bronchus with Intraluminal Device, Percutaneous Approach
0B783ZZ	Dilation of Left Upper Lobe Bronchus, Percutaneous Approach
0B784DZ	Dilation of Left Upper Lobe Bronchus with Intraluminal Device, Percutaneous Endoscopic Approach
0B784ZZ	Dilation of Left Upper Lobe Bronchus, Percutaneous Endoscopic Approach
0B787DZ	Dilation of Left Upper Lobe Bronchus with Intraluminal Device, Via Natural or Artificial Opening
0B787ZZ	Dilation of Left Upper Lobe Bronchus, Via Natural or Artificial Opening
0B788DZ	Dilation of Left Upper Lobe Bronchus with Intraluminal Device, Via Natural or Artificial Opening Endoscopic
0B788ZZ	Dilation of Left Upper Lobe Bronchus, Via Natural or Artificial Opening Endoscopic

0B790DZ	Dilation of Lingula Bronchus with Intraluminal Device, Open Approach
0B790ZZ	Dilation of Lingula Bronchus, Open Approach
0B793DZ	Dilation of Lingula Bronchus with Intraluminal Device, Percutaneous Approach
0B793ZZ	Dilation of Lingula Bronchus, Percutaneous Approach
0B794DZ	Dilation of Lingula Bronchus with Intraluminal Device, Percutaneous Endoscopic Approach
0B794ZZ	Dilation of Lingula Bronchus, Percutaneous Endoscopic Approach
0B797DZ	Dilation of Lingula Bronchus with Intraluminal Device, Via Natural or Artificial Opening
0B797ZZ	Dilation of Lingula Bronchus, Via Natural or Artificial Opening
0B798DZ	Dilation of Lingula Bronchus with Intraluminal Device, Via Natural or Artificial Opening Endoscopic
0B798ZZ	Dilation of Lingula Bronchus, Via Natural or Artificial Opening Endoscopic
0B7B0DZ	Dilation of Left Lower Lobe Bronchus with Intraluminal Device, Open Approach
0B7B0ZZ	Dilation of Left Lower Lobe Bronchus, Open Approach
0B7B3DZ	Dilation of Left Lower Lobe Bronchus with Intraluminal Device, Percutaneous Approach
0B7B3ZZ	Dilation of Left Lower Lobe Bronchus, Percutaneous Approach
0B7B4DZ	Dilation of Left Lower Lobe Bronchus with Intraluminal Device, Percutaneous Endoscopic Approach
0B7B4ZZ	Dilation of Left Lower Lobe Bronchus, Percutaneous Endoscopic Approach
0B7B7DZ	Dilation of Left Lower Lobe Bronchus with Intraluminal Device, Via Natural or Artificial Opening
0B7B7ZZ	Dilation of Left Lower Lobe Bronchus, Via Natural or Artificial Opening
0B7B8DZ	Dilation of Left Lower Lobe Bronchus with Intraluminal Device, Via Natural or Artificial Opening Endoscopic
0B7B8ZZ	Dilation of Left Lower Lobe Bronchus, Via Natural or Artificial Opening Endoscopic

0B9 – Respiratory System, Drainage

Review Coding Guidelines B3.4a and B3.4b

Review Coding Guideline B6.2

0B9100Z	Drainage of Trachea with Drainage Device, Open Approach
0B910ZX	Drainage of Trachea, Open Approach, Diagnostic
0B910ZZ	Drainage of Trachea, Open Approach
0B9130Z	Drainage of Trachea with Drainage Device, Percutaneous Approach
0B913ZX	Drainage of Trachea, Percutaneous Approach, Diagnostic
0B913ZZ	Drainage of Trachea, Percutaneous Approach
0B9140Z	Drainage of Trachea with Drainage Device, Percutaneous Endoscopic Approach

0B914ZX	Drainage of Trachea, Percutaneous Endoscopic Approach, Diagnostic
0B914ZZ	Drainage of Trachea, Percutaneous Endoscopic Approach
0B9170Z	Drainage of Trachea with Drainage Device, Via Natural or Artificial Opening
0B917ZX	Drainage of Trachea, Via Natural or Artificial Opening, Diagnostic
0B917ZZ	Drainage of Trachea, Via Natural or Artificial Opening
0B9180Z	Drainage of Trachea with Drainage Device, Via Natural or Artificial Opening Endoscopic

0B918ZX	Drainage of Trachea, Via Natural or Artificial Opening Endoscopic, Diagnostic
0B918ZZ	Drainage of Trachea, Via Natural or Artificial Opening Endoscopic
0B9200Z	Drainage of Carina with Drainage Device, Open Approach
0B920ZX	Drainage of Carina, Open Approach, Diagnostic
0B920ZZ	Drainage of Carina, Open Approach
0B9230Z	Drainage of Carina with Drainage Device, Percutaneous Approach
0B923ZX	Drainage of Carina, Percutaneous Approach, Diagnostic
0B923ZZ	Drainage of Carina, Percutaneous Approach

♀ Female-only　　♂ Male-only　　▲ Limited Coverage　　● Non-OR　　▥ HAC-associated procedure　　▲ Non-covered procedures　　✛ Combination

0B9240Z Drainage of Carina with Drainage Device, Percutaneous Endoscopic Approach

0B924ZX Drainage of Carina, Percutaneous Endoscopic Approach, Diagnostic

0B924ZZ Drainage of Carina, Percutaneous Endoscopic Approach

0B9270Z Drainage of Carina with Drainage Device, Via Natural or Artificial Opening

0B927ZX Drainage of Carina, Via Natural or Artificial Opening, Diagnostic

0B927ZZ Drainage of Carina, Via Natural or Artificial Opening

0B9280Z Drainage of Carina with Drainage Device, Via Natural or Artificial Opening Endoscopic

0B928ZX Drainage of Carina, Via Natural or Artificial Opening Endoscopic, Diagnostic

0B928ZZ Drainage of Carina, Via Natural or Artificial Opening Endoscopic

0B9300Z Drainage of Right Main Bronchus with Drainage Device, Open Approach

0B930ZX Drainage of Right Main Bronchus, Open Approach, Diagnostic

0B930ZZ Drainage of Right Main Bronchus, Open Approach

0B9330Z Drainage of Right Main Bronchus with Drainage Device, Percutaneous Approach

0B933ZX Drainage of Right Main Bronchus, Percutaneous Approach, Diagnostic

0B933ZZ Drainage of Right Main Bronchus, Percutaneous Approach

0B9340Z Drainage of Right Main Bronchus with Drainage Device, Percutaneous Endoscopic Approach

0B934ZX Drainage of Right Main Bronchus, Percutaneous Endoscopic Approach, Diagnostic

0B934ZZ Drainage of Right Main Bronchus, Percutaneous Endoscopic Approach

0B9370Z Drainage of Right Main Bronchus with Drainage Device, Via Natural or Artificial Opening

0B937ZX Drainage of Right Main Bronchus, Via Natural or Artificial Opening, Diagnostic

0B937ZZ Drainage of Right Main Bronchus, Via Natural or Artificial Opening

0B9380Z Drainage of Right Main Bronchus with Drainage Device, Via Natural or Artificial Opening Endoscopic

0B938ZX Drainage of Right Main Bronchus, Via Natural or Artificial Opening Endoscopic, Diagnostic

0B938ZZ Drainage of Right Main Bronchus, Via Natural or Artificial Opening Endoscopic

0B9400Z Drainage of Right Upper Lobe Bronchus with Drainage Device, Open Approach

0B940ZX Drainage of Right Upper Lobe Bronchus, Open Approach, Diagnostic

0B940ZZ Drainage of Right Upper Lobe Bronchus, Open Approach

0B9430Z Drainage of Right Upper Lobe Bronchus with Drainage Device, Percutaneous Approach

0B943ZX Drainage of Right Upper Lobe Bronchus, Percutaneous Approach, Diagnostic

0B943ZZ Drainage of Right Upper Lobe Bronchus, Percutaneous Approach

0B9440Z Drainage of Right Upper Lobe Bronchus with Drainage Device, Percutaneous Endoscopic Approach

0B944ZX Drainage of Right Upper Lobe Bronchus, Percutaneous Endoscopic Approach, Diagnostic

0B944ZZ Drainage of Right Upper Lobe Bronchus, Percutaneous Endoscopic Approach

0B9470Z Drainage of Right Upper Lobe Bronchus with Drainage Device, Via Natural or Artificial Opening

0B947ZX Drainage of Right Upper Lobe Bronchus, Via Natural or Artificial Opening, Diagnostic

0B947ZZ Drainage of Right Upper Lobe Bronchus, Via Natural or Artificial Opening

0B9480Z Drainage of Right Upper Lobe Bronchus with Drainage Device, Via Natural or Artificial Opening Endoscopic

0B948ZX Drainage of Right Upper Lobe Bronchus, Via Natural or Artificial Opening Endoscopic, Diagnostic

0B948ZZ Drainage of Right Upper Lobe Bronchus, Via Natural or Artificial Opening Endoscopic

0B9500Z Drainage of Right Middle Lobe Bronchus with Drainage Device, Open Approach

0B950ZX Drainage of Right Middle Lobe Bronchus, Open Approach, Diagnostic

0B950ZZ Drainage of Right Middle Lobe Bronchus, Open Approach

0B9530Z Drainage of Right Middle Lobe Bronchus with Drainage Device, Percutaneous Approach

0B953ZX Drainage of Right Middle Lobe Bronchus, Percutaneous Approach, Diagnostic

0B953ZZ Drainage of Right Middle Lobe Bronchus, Percutaneous Approach

0B9540Z Drainage of Right Middle Lobe Bronchus with Drainage Device, Percutaneous Endoscopic Approach

0B954ZX Drainage of Right Middle Lobe Bronchus, Percutaneous Endoscopic Approach, Diagnostic

0B954ZZ Drainage of Right Middle Lobe Bronchus, Percutaneous Endoscopic Approach

0B9570Z Drainage of Right Middle Lobe Bronchus with Drainage Device, Via Natural or Artificial Opening

0B957ZX Drainage of Right Middle Lobe Bronchus, Via Natural or Artificial Opening, Diagnostic

0B957ZZ Drainage of Right Middle Lobe Bronchus, Via Natural or Artificial Opening

0B9580Z Drainage of Right Middle Lobe Bronchus with Drainage Device, Via Natural or Artificial Opening Endoscopic

0B958ZX Drainage of Right Middle Lobe Bronchus, Via Natural or Artificial Opening Endoscopic, Diagnostic

0B958ZZ Drainage of Right Middle Lobe Bronchus, Via Natural or Artificial Opening Endoscopic

0B9600Z Drainage of Right Lower Lobe Bronchus with Drainage Device, Open Approach

0B960ZX Drainage of Right Lower Lobe Bronchus, Open Approach, Diagnostic

0B960ZZ Drainage of Right Lower Lobe Bronchus, Open Approach

0B9630Z Drainage of Right Lower Lobe Bronchus with Drainage Device, Percutaneous Approach

0B963ZX Drainage of Right Lower Lobe Bronchus, Percutaneous Approach, Diagnostic

0B963ZZ Drainage of Right Lower Lobe Bronchus, Percutaneous Approach

0B9640Z Drainage of Right Lower Lobe Bronchus with Drainage Device, Percutaneous Endoscopic Approach

0B964ZX Drainage of Right Lower Lobe Bronchus, Percutaneous Endoscopic Approach, Diagnostic

0B964ZZ Drainage of Right Lower Lobe Bronchus, Percutaneous Endoscopic Approach

0B9670Z Drainage of Right Lower Lobe Bronchus with Drainage Device, Via Natural or Artificial Opening

0B967ZX Drainage of Right Lower Lobe Bronchus, Via Natural or Artificial Opening, Diagnostic

0B967ZZ Drainage of Right Lower Lobe Bronchus, Via Natural or Artificial Opening

0B9680Z Drainage of Right Lower Lobe Bronchus with Drainage Device, Via Natural or Artificial Opening Endoscopic

0B968ZX Drainage of Right Lower Lobe Bronchus, Via Natural or Artificial Opening Endoscopic, Diagnostic

0B968ZZ Drainage of Right Lower Lobe Bronchus, Via Natural or Artificial Opening Endoscopic

0B9700Z Drainage of Left Main Bronchus with Drainage Device, Open Approach

0B970ZX Drainage of Left Main Bronchus, Open Approach, Diagnostic

0B970ZZ Drainage of Left Main Bronchus, Open Approach

0B9730Z Drainage of Left Main Bronchus with Drainage Device, Percutaneous Approach

0B973ZX Drainage of Left Main Bronchus, Percutaneous Approach, Diagnostic

0B973ZZ Drainage of Left Main Bronchus, Percutaneous Approach

0B9740Z Drainage of Left Main Bronchus with Drainage Device, Percutaneous Endoscopic Approach

0B974ZX Drainage of Left Main Bronchus, Percutaneous Endoscopic Approach, Diagnostic

0B974ZZ Drainage of Left Main Bronchus, Percutaneous Endoscopic Approach

0B9770Z Drainage of Left Main Bronchus with Drainage Device, Via Natural or Artificial Opening

0B977ZX Drainage of Left Main Bronchus, Via Natural or Artificial Opening, Diagnostic

0B977ZZ Drainage of Left Main Bronchus, Via Natural or Artificial Opening

0B9780Z Drainage of Left Main Bronchus with Drainage Device, Via Natural or Artificial Opening Endoscopic

0B978ZX Drainage of Left Main Bronchus, Via Natural or Artificial Opening Endoscopic Diagnostic

0B978ZZ Drainage of Left Main Bronchus, Via Natural or Artificial Opening Endoscopic

0B9800Z Drainage of Left Upper Lobe Bronchus with Drainage Device, Open Approach

0B980ZX Drainage of Left Upper Lobe Bronchus, Open Approach, Diagnostic

0B980ZZ Drainage of Left Upper Lobe Bronchus, Open Approach

0B9830Z Drainage of Left Upper Lobe Bronchus with Drainage Device, Percutaneous Approach

0B983ZX Drainage of Left Upper Lobe Bronchus, Percutaneous Approach, Diagnostic

0B983ZZ Drainage of Left Upper Lobe Bronchus, Percutaneous Approach

0B9840Z Drainage of Left Upper Lobe Bronchus with Drainage Device, Percutaneous Endoscopic Approach

0B984ZX Drainage of Left Upper Lobe Bronchus, Percutaneous Endoscopic Approach, Diagnostic

0B984ZZ Drainage of Left Upper Lobe Bronchus, Percutaneous Endoscopic Approach

0B9870Z Drainage of Left Upper Lobe Bronchus with Drainage Device, Via Natural or Artificial Opening

0B987ZX	Drainage of Left Upper Lobe Bronchus, Via Natural or Artificial Opening, Diagnostic
0B987ZZ	Drainage of Left Upper Lobe Bronchus, Via Natural or Artificial Opening
0B9880Z	Drainage of Left Upper Lobe Bronchus with Drainage Device, Via Natural or Artificial Opening Endoscopic
0B988ZX	Drainage of Left Upper Lobe Bronchus, Via Natural or Artificial Opening Endoscopic, Diagnostic
0B988ZZ	Drainage of Left Upper Lobe Bronchus, Via Natural or Artificial Opening Endoscopic
0B9900Z	Drainage of Lingula Bronchus with Drainage Device, Open Approach
0B990ZX	Drainage of Lingula Bronchus, Open Approach, Diagnostic
0B990ZZ	Drainage of Lingula Bronchus, Open Approach
0B9930Z	Drainage of Lingula Bronchus with Drainage Device, Percutaneous Approach
0B993ZX	Drainage of Lingula Bronchus, Percutaneous Approach, Diagnostic
0B993ZZ	Drainage of Lingula Bronchus, Percutaneous Approach
0B9940Z	Drainage of Lingula Bronchus with Drainage Device, Percutaneous Endoscopic Approach
0B994ZX	Drainage of Lingula Bronchus, Percutaneous Endoscopic Approach, Diagnostic
0B994ZZ	Drainage of Lingula Bronchus, Percutaneous Endoscopic Approach
0B9970Z	Drainage of Lingula Bronchus with Drainage Device, Via Natural or Artificial Opening
0B997ZX	Drainage of Lingula Bronchus, Via Natural or Artificial Opening, Diagnostic
0B997ZZ	Drainage of Lingula Bronchus, Via Natural or Artificial Opening
0B9980Z	Drainage of Lingula Bronchus with Drainage Device, Via Natural or Artificial Opening Endoscopic
0B998ZX	Drainage of Lingula Bronchus, Via Natural or Artificial Opening Endoscopic, Diagnostic
0B998ZZ	Drainage of Lingula Bronchus, Via Natural or Artificial Opening Endoscopic
0B9B00Z	Drainage of Left Lower Lobe Bronchus with Drainage Device, Open Approach
0B9B0ZX	Drainage of Left Lower Lobe Bronchus, Open Approach, Diagnostic
0B9B0ZZ	Drainage of Left Lower Lobe Bronchus, Open Approach
0B9B30Z	Drainage of Left Lower Lobe Bronchus with Drainage Device, Percutaneous Approach
0B9B3ZX	Drainage of Left Lower Lobe Bronchus, Percutaneous Approach, Diagnostic
0B9B3ZZ	Drainage of Left Lower Lobe Bronchus, Percutaneous Approach
0B9B40Z	Drainage of Left Lower Lobe Bronchus with Drainage Device, Percutaneous Endoscopic Approach
0B9B4ZX	Drainage of Left Lower Lobe Bronchus, Percutaneous Endoscopic Approach, Diagnostic
0B9B4ZZ	Drainage of Left Lower Lobe Bronchus, Percutaneous Endoscopic Approach
0B9B70Z	Drainage of Left Lower Lobe Bronchus with Drainage Device, Via Natural or Artificial Opening
0B9B7ZX	Drainage of Left Lower Lobe Bronchus, Via Natural or Artificial Opening, Diagnostic
0B9B7ZZ	Drainage of Left Lower Lobe Bronchus, Via Natural or Artificial Opening
0B9B80Z	Drainage of Left Lower Lobe Bronchus with Drainage Device, Via Natural or Artificial Opening Endoscopic
0B9B8ZX	Drainage of Left Lower Lobe Bronchus, Via Natural or Artificial Opening Endoscopic, Diagnostic
0B9B8ZZ	Drainage of Left Lower Lobe Bronchus, Via Natural or Artificial Opening Endoscopic
0B9C00Z	Drainage of Right Upper Lung Lobe with Drainage Device, Open Approach
0B9C0ZX	Drainage of Right Upper Lung Lobe, Open Approach, Diagnostic
0B9C0ZZ	Drainage of Right Upper Lung Lobe, Open Approach
0B9C30Z	Drainage of Right Upper Lung Lobe with Drainage Device, Percutaneous Approach
0B9C3ZX	Drainage of Right Upper Lung Lobe, Percutaneous Approach, Diagnostic
0B9C3ZZ	Drainage of Right Upper Lung Lobe, Percutaneous Approach
0B9C40Z	Drainage of Right Upper Lung Lobe with Drainage Device, Percutaneous Endoscopic Approach
0B9C4ZX	Drainage of Right Upper Lung Lobe, Percutaneous Endoscopic Approach, Diagnostic
0B9C4ZZ	Drainage of Right Upper Lung Lobe, Percutaneous Endoscopic Approach
0B9C70Z	Drainage of Right Upper Lung Lobe with Drainage Device, Via Natural or Artificial Opening
0B9C7ZX	Drainage of Right Upper Lung Lobe, Via Natural or Artificial Opening, Diagnostic
0B9C7ZZ	Drainage of Right Upper Lung Lobe, Via Natural or Artificial Opening
0B9C80Z	Drainage of Right Upper Lung Lobe with Drainage Device, Via Natural or Artificial Opening Endoscopic
0B9C8ZX	Drainage of Right Upper Lung Lobe, Via Natural or Artificial Opening Endoscopic, Diagnostic
0B9C8ZZ	Drainage of Right Upper Lung Lobe, Via Natural or Artificial Opening Endoscopic
0B9D00Z	Drainage of Right Middle Lung Lobe with Drainage Device, Open Approach
0B9D0ZX	Drainage of Right Middle Lung Lobe, Open Approach, Diagnostic
0B9D0ZZ	Drainage of Right Middle Lung Lobe, Open Approach
0B9D30Z	Drainage of Right Middle Lung Lobe with Drainage Device, Percutaneous Approach
0B9D3ZX	Drainage of Right Middle Lung Lobe, Percutaneous Approach, Diagnostic
0B9D3ZZ	Drainage of Right Middle Lung Lobe, Percutaneous Approach
0B9D40Z	Drainage of Right Middle Lung Lobe with Drainage Device, Percutaneous Endoscopic Approach
0B9D4ZX	Drainage of Right Middle Lung Lobe, Percutaneous Endoscopic Approach, Diagnostic
0B9D4ZZ	Drainage of Right Middle Lung Lobe, Percutaneous Endoscopic Approach
0B9D70Z	Drainage of Right Middle Lung Lobe with Drainage Device, Via Natural or Artificial Opening
0B9D7ZX	Drainage of Right Middle Lung Lobe, Via Natural or Artificial Opening, Diagnostic
0B9D7ZZ	Drainage of Right Middle Lung Lobe, Via Natural or Artificial Opening
0B9D80Z	Drainage of Right Middle Lung Lobe with Drainage Device, Via Natural or Artificial Opening Endoscopic
0B9D8ZX	Drainage of Right Middle Lung Lobe, Via Natural or Artificial Opening Endoscopic, Diagnostic
0B9D8ZZ	Drainage of Right Middle Lung Lobe, Via Natural or Artificial Opening Endoscopic
0B9F00Z	Drainage of Right Lower Lung Lobe with Drainage Device, Open Approach
0B9F0ZX	Drainage of Right Lower Lung Lobe, Open Approach, Diagnostic
0B9F0ZZ	Drainage of Right Lower Lung Lobe, Open Approach
0B9F30Z	Drainage of Right Lower Lung Lobe with Drainage Device, Percutaneous Approach
0B9F3ZX	Drainage of Right Lower Lung Lobe, Percutaneous Approach, Diagnostic
0B9F3ZZ	Drainage of Right Lower Lung Lobe, Percutaneous Approach
0B9F40Z	Drainage of Right Lower Lung Lobe with Drainage Device, Percutaneous Endoscopic Approach
0B9F4ZX	Drainage of Right Lower Lung Lobe, Percutaneous Endoscopic Approach, Diagnostic
0B9F4ZZ	Drainage of Right Lower Lung Lobe, Percutaneous Endoscopic Approach
0B9F70Z	Drainage of Right Lower Lung Lobe with Drainage Device, Via Natural or Artificial Opening
0B9F7ZX	Drainage of Right Lower Lung Lobe, Via Natural or Artificial Opening, Diagnostic
0B9F7ZZ	Drainage of Right Lower Lung Lobe, Via Natural or Artificial Opening
0B9F80Z	Drainage of Right Lower Lung Lobe with Drainage Device, Via Natural or Artificial Opening Endoscopic
0B9F8ZX	Drainage of Right Lower Lung Lobe, Via Natural or Artificial Opening Endoscopic, Diagnostic
0B9F8ZZ	Drainage of Right Lower Lung Lobe, Via Natural or Artificial Opening Endoscopic
0B9G00Z	Drainage of Left Upper Lung Lobe with Drainage Device, Open Approach
0B9G0ZX	Drainage of Left Upper Lung Lobe, Open Approach, Diagnostic
0B9G0ZZ	Drainage of Left Upper Lung Lobe, Open Approach
0B9G30Z	Drainage of Left Upper Lung Lobe with Drainage Device, Percutaneous Approach
0B9G3ZX	Drainage of Left Upper Lung Lobe, Percutaneous Approach, Diagnostic
0B9G3ZZ	Drainage of Left Upper Lung Lobe, Percutaneous Approach
0B9G40Z	Drainage of Left Upper Lung Lobe with Drainage Device, Percutaneous Endoscopic Approach
0B9G4ZX	Drainage of Left Upper Lung Lobe, Percutaneous Endoscopic Approach, Diagnostic
0B9G4ZZ	Drainage of Left Upper Lung Lobe, Percutaneous Endoscopic Approach
0B9G70Z	Drainage of Left Upper Lung Lobe with Drainage Device, Via Natural or Artificial Opening
0B9G7ZX	Drainage of Left Upper Lung Lobe, Via Natural or Artificial Opening, Diagnostic
0B9G7ZZ	Drainage of Left Upper Lung Lobe, Via Natural or Artificial Opening
0B9G80Z	Drainage of Left Upper Lung Lobe with Drainage Device, Via Natural or Artificial Opening Endoscopic
0B9G8ZX	Drainage of Left Upper Lung Lobe, Via Natural or Artificial Opening Endoscopic, Diagnostic
0B9G8ZZ	Drainage of Left Upper Lung Lobe, Via Natural or Artificial Opening Endoscopic
0B9H00Z	Drainage of Lung Lingula with Drainage Device, Open Approach

0B9H0ZX Drainage of Lung Lingula, Open Approach, Diagnostic

0B9H0ZZ Drainage of Lung Lingula, Open Approach

0B9H30Z Drainage of Lung Lingula with Drainage Device, Percutaneous Approach

0B9H3ZX Drainage of Lung Lingula, Percutaneous Approach, Diagnostic

0B9H3ZZ Drainage of Lung Lingula, Percutaneous Approach

0B9H40Z Drainage of Lung Lingula with Drainage Device, Percutaneous Endoscopic Approach

0B9H4ZX Drainage of Lung Lingula, Percutaneous Endoscopic Approach, Diagnostic

0B9H4ZZ Drainage of Lung Lingula, Percutaneous Endoscopic Approach

0B9H70Z Drainage of Lung Lingula with Drainage Device, Via Natural or Artificial Opening

0B9H7ZX Drainage of Lung Lingula, Via Natural or Artificial Opening, Diagnostic

0B9H7ZZ Drainage of Lung Lingula, Via Natural or Artificial Opening

0B9H80Z Drainage of Lung Lingula with Drainage Device, Via Natural or Artificial Opening Endoscopic

0B9H8ZX Drainage of Lung Lingula, Via Natural or Artificial Opening Endoscopic, Diagnostic

0B9H8ZZ Drainage of Lung Lingula, Via Natural or Artificial Opening Endoscopic

0B9J00Z Drainage of Left Lower Lung Lobe with Drainage Device, Open Approach

0B9J0ZX Drainage of Left Lower Lung Lobe, Open Approach, Diagnostic

0B9J0ZZ Drainage of Left Lower Lung Lobe, Open Approach

0B9J30Z Drainage of Left Lower Lung Lobe with Drainage Device, Percutaneous Approach

0B9J3ZX Drainage of Left Lower Lung Lobe, Percutaneous Approach, Diagnostic

0B9J3ZZ Drainage of Left Lower Lung Lobe, Percutaneous Approach

0B9J40Z Drainage of Left Lower Lung Lobe with Drainage Device, Percutaneous Endoscopic Approach

0B9J4ZX Drainage of Left Lower Lung Lobe, Percutaneous Endoscopic Approach, Diagnostic

0B9J4ZZ Drainage of Left Lower Lung Lobe, Percutaneous Endoscopic Approach

0B9J70Z Drainage of Left Lower Lung Lobe with Drainage Device, Via Natural or Artificial Opening

0B9J7ZX Drainage of Left Lower Lung Lobe, Via Natural or Artificial Opening, Diagnostic

0B9J7ZZ Drainage of Left Lower Lung Lobe, Via Natural or Artificial Opening

0B9J80Z Drainage of Left Lower Lung Lobe with Drainage Device, Via Natural or Artificial Opening Endoscopic

0B9J8ZX Drainage of Left Lower Lung Lobe, Via Natural or Artificial Opening Endoscopic, Diagnostic

0B9J8ZZ Drainage of Left Lower Lung Lobe, Via Natural or Artificial Opening Endoscopic

0B9K00Z Drainage of Right Lung with Drainage Device, Open Approach

0B9K0ZX Drainage of Right Lung, Open Approach, Diagnostic

0B9K0ZZ Drainage of Right Lung, Open Approach

0B9K30Z Drainage of Right Lung with Drainage Device, Percutaneous Approach

0B9K3ZX Drainage of Right Lung, Percutaneous Approach, Diagnostic

0B9K3ZZ Drainage of Right Lung, Percutaneous Approach

0B9K40Z Drainage of Right Lung with Drainage Device, Percutaneous Endoscopic Approach

0B9K4ZX Drainage of Right Lung, Percutaneous Endoscopic Approach, Diagnostic

0B9K4ZZ Drainage of Right Lung, Percutaneous Endoscopic Approach

0B9K70Z Drainage of Right Lung with Drainage Device, Via Natural or Artificial Opening

0B9K7ZX Drainage of Right Lung, Via Natural or Artificial Opening, Diagnostic

0B9K7ZZ Drainage of Right Lung, Via Natural or Artificial Opening

0B9K80Z Drainage of Right Lung with Drainage Device, Via Natural or Artificial Opening Endoscopic

0B9K8ZX Drainage of Right Lung, Via Natural or Artificial Opening Endoscopic, Diagnostic

0B9K8ZZ Drainage of Right Lung, Via Natural or Artificial Opening Endoscopic

0B9L00Z Drainage of Left Lung with Drainage Device, Open Approach

0B9L0ZX Drainage of Left Lung, Open Approach, Diagnostic

0B9L0ZZ Drainage of Left Lung, Open Approach

0B9L30Z Drainage of Left Lung with Drainage Device, Percutaneous Approach

0B9L3ZX Drainage of Left Lung, Percutaneous Approach, Diagnostic

0B9L3ZZ Drainage of Left Lung, Percutaneous Approach

0B9L40Z Drainage of Left Lung with Drainage Device, Percutaneous Endoscopic Approach

0B9L4ZX Drainage of Left Lung, Percutaneous Endoscopic Approach, Diagnostic

0B9L4ZZ Drainage of Left Lung, Percutaneous Endoscopic Approach

0B9L70Z Drainage of Left Lung with Drainage Device, Via Natural or Artificial Opening

0B9L7ZX Drainage of Left Lung, Via Natural or Artificial Opening, Diagnostic

0B9L7ZZ Drainage of Left Lung, Via Natural or Artificial Opening

0B9L80Z Drainage of Left Lung with Drainage Device, Via Natural or Artificial Opening Endoscopic

0B9L8ZX Drainage of Left Lung, Via Natural or Artificial Opening Endoscopic, Diagnostic

0B9L8ZZ Drainage of Left Lung, Via Natural or Artificial Opening Endoscopic

0B9M00Z Drainage of Bilateral Lungs with Drainage Device, Open Approach

0B9M0ZX Drainage of Bilateral Lungs, Open Approach, Diagnostic

0B9M0ZZ Drainage of Bilateral Lungs, Open Approach

0B9M30Z Drainage of Bilateral Lungs with Drainage Device, Percutaneous Approach

0B9M3ZX Drainage of Bilateral Lungs, Percutaneous Approach, Diagnostic

0B9M3ZZ Drainage of Bilateral Lungs, Percutaneous Approach

0B9M40Z Drainage of Bilateral Lungs with Drainage Device, Percutaneous Endoscopic Approach

0B9M4ZX Drainage of Bilateral Lungs, Percutaneous Endoscopic Approach, Diagnostic

0B9M4ZZ Drainage of Bilateral Lungs, Percutaneous Endoscopic Approach

0B9M70Z Drainage of Bilateral Lungs with Drainage Device, Via Natural or Artificial Opening

0B9M7ZX Drainage of Bilateral Lungs, Via Natural or Artificial Opening, Diagnostic

0B9M7ZZ Drainage of Bilateral Lungs, Via Natural or Artificial Opening

0B9M80Z Drainage of Bilateral Lungs with Drainage Device, Via Natural or Artificial Opening Endoscopic

0B9M8ZX Drainage of Bilateral Lungs, Via Natural or Artificial Opening Endoscopic, Diagnostic

0B9M8ZZ Drainage of Bilateral Lungs, Via Natural or Artificial Opening Endoscopic

0B9N00Z Drainage of Right Pleura with Drainage Device, Open Approach

0B9N0ZX Drainage of Right Pleura, Open Approach Diagnostic

0B9N0ZZ Drainage of Right Pleura, Open Approach

0B9N30Z Drainage of Right Pleura with Drainage Device, Percutaneous Approach

0B9N3ZX Drainage of Right Pleura, Percutaneous Approach, Diagnostic

0B9N3ZZ Drainage of Right Pleura, Percutaneous Approach

0B9N40Z Drainage of Right Pleura with Drainage Device, Percutaneous Endoscopic Approach

0B9N4ZX Drainage of Right Pleura, Percutaneous Endoscopic Approach, Diagnostic

0B9N4ZZ Drainage of Right Pleura, Percutaneous Endoscopic Approach

0B9P00Z Drainage of Left Pleura with Drainage Device, Open Approach

0B9P0ZX Drainage of Left Pleura, Open Approach Diagnostic

0B9P0ZZ Drainage of Left Pleura, Open Approach

0B9P30Z Drainage of Left Pleura with Drainage Device, Percutaneous Approach

0B9P3ZX Drainage of Left Pleura, Percutaneous Approach, Diagnostic

0B9P3ZZ Drainage of Left Pleura, Percutaneous Approach

0B9P40Z Drainage of Left Pleura with Drainage Device, Percutaneous Endoscopic Approach

0B9P4ZX Drainage of Left Pleura, Percutaneous Endoscopic Approach, Diagnostic

0B9P4ZZ Drainage of Left Pleura, Percutaneous Endoscopic Approach

0B9R00Z Drainage of Right Diaphragm with Drainage Device, Open Approach

0B9R0ZX Drainage of Right Diaphragm, Open Approach, Diagnostic

0B9R0ZZ Drainage of Right Diaphragm, Open Approach

0B9R30Z Drainage of Right Diaphragm with Drainage Device, Percutaneous Approach

0B9R3ZX Drainage of Right Diaphragm, Percutaneous Approach, Diagnostic

0B9R3ZZ Drainage of Right Diaphragm, Percutaneous Approach

0B9R40Z Drainage of Right Diaphragm with Drainage Device, Percutaneous Endoscopic Approach

0B9R4ZX Drainage of Right Diaphragm, Percutaneous Endoscopic Approach, Diagnostic

0B9R4ZZ Drainage of Right Diaphragm, Percutaneous Endoscopic Approach

0B9S00Z Drainage of Left Diaphragm with Drainage Device, Open Approach

0B9S0ZX Drainage of Left Diaphragm, Open Approach, Diagnostic

0B9S0ZZ Drainage of Left Diaphragm, Open Approach

0B9S30Z Drainage of Left Diaphragm with Drainage Device, Percutaneous Approach

0B9S3ZX Drainage of Left Diaphragm, Percutaneous Approach, Diagnostic

0B9S3ZZ Drainage of Left Diaphragm, Percutaneous Approach

...40Z	Drainage of Left Diaphragm with Drainage Device, Percutaneous Endoscopic Approach	**0B9S4ZX**	Drainage of Left Diaphragm, Percutaneous Endoscopic Approach, Diagnostic	**0B9S4ZZ**	Drainage of Left Diaphragm, Percutaneous Endoscopic Approach

B – Respiratory System, Excision

iew Coding Guidelines B3.4a and B3.4b

iew Coding Guideline B3.8

..10ZX Excision of Trachea, Open Approach, Diagnostic

..10ZZ Excision of Trachea, Open Approach
  AHA CC: 1Q, 2015, 15-16

..13ZX Excision of Trachea, Percutaneous Approach, Diagnostic

..13ZZ Excision of Trachea, Percutaneous Approach

..14ZX Excision of Trachea, Percutaneous Endoscopic Approach, Diagnostic

..14ZZ Excision of Trachea, Percutaneous Endoscopic Approach

..17ZX Excision of Trachea, Via Natural or Artificial Opening, Diagnostic

..17ZZ Excision of Trachea, Via Natural or Artificial Opening

..18ZX Excision of Trachea, Via Natural or Artificial Opening Endoscopic, Diagnostic

..18ZZ Excision of Trachea, Via Natural or Artificial Opening Endoscopic

..20ZX Excision of Carina, Open Approach, Diagnostic

..20ZZ Excision of Carina, Open Approach

..23ZX Excision of Carina, Percutaneous Approach, Diagnostic

..23ZZ Excision of Carina, Percutaneous Approach

..24ZX Excision of Carina, Percutaneous Endoscopic Approach, Diagnostic

..24ZZ Excision of Carina, Percutaneous Endoscopic Approach

..27ZX Excision of Carina, Via Natural or Artificial Opening, Diagnostic

..27ZZ Excision of Carina, Via Natural or Artificial Opening

..28ZX Excision of Carina, Via Natural or Artificial Opening Endoscopic, Diagnostic

..28ZZ Excision of Carina, Via Natural or Artificial Opening Endoscopic

.B30ZX Excision of Right Main Bronchus, Open Approach, Diagnostic

.B30ZZ Excision of Right Main Bronchus, Open Approach

.B33ZX Excision of Right Main Bronchus, Percutaneous Approach, Diagnostic

.B33ZZ Excision of Right Main Bronchus, Percutaneous Approach

.B34ZX Excision of Right Main Bronchus, Percutaneous Endoscopic Approach, Diagnostic

.B34ZZ Excision of Right Main Bronchus, Percutaneous Endoscopic Approach

.B37ZX Excision of Right Main Bronchus, Via Natural or Artificial Opening, Diagnostic

.B37ZZ Excision of Right Main Bronchus, Via Natural or Artificial Opening

.B38ZX Excision of Right Main Bronchus, Via Natural or Artificial Opening Endoscopic, Diagnostic

.B38ZZ Excision of Right Main Bronchus, Via Natural or Artificial Opening Endoscopic

.B40ZX Excision of Right Upper Lobe Bronchus, Open Approach, Diagnostic

.B40ZZ Excision of Right Upper Lobe Bronchus, Open Approach

.B43ZX Excision of Right Upper Lobe Bronchus, Percutaneous Approach, Diagnostic

0BB43ZZ Excision of Right Upper Lobe Bronchus, Percutaneous Approach

0BB44ZX Excision of Right Upper Lobe Bronchus, Percutaneous Endoscopic Approach, Diagnostic

0BB44ZZ Excision of Right Upper Lobe Bronchus, Percutaneous Endoscopic Approach

0BB47ZX Excision of Right Upper Lobe Bronchus, Via Natural or Artificial Opening, Diagnostic

0BB47ZZ Excision of Right Upper Lobe Bronchus, Via Natural or Artificial Opening

0BB48ZX Excision of Right Upper Lobe Bronchus, Via Natural or Artificial Opening Endoscopic, Diagnostic

0BB48ZZ Excision of Right Upper Lobe Bronchus, Via Natural or Artificial Opening Endoscopic

0BB50ZX Excision of Right Middle Lobe Bronchus, Open Approach, Diagnostic

0BB50ZZ Excision of Right Middle Lobe Bronchus, Open Approach

0BB53ZX Excision of Right Middle Lobe Bronchus, Percutaneous Approach, Diagnostic

0BB53ZZ Excision of Right Middle Lobe Bronchus, Percutaneous Approach

0BB54ZX Excision of Right Middle Lobe Bronchus, Percutaneous Endoscopic Approach, Diagnostic

0BB54ZZ Excision of Right Middle Lobe Bronchus, Percutaneous Endoscopic Approach

0BB57ZX Excision of Right Middle Lobe Bronchus, Via Natural or Artificial Opening, Diagnostic

0BB57ZZ Excision of Right Middle Lobe Bronchus, Via Natural or Artificial Opening

0BB58ZX Excision of Right Middle Lobe Bronchus, Via Natural or Artificial Opening Endoscopic, Diagnostic

0BB58ZZ Excision of Right Middle Lobe Bronchus, Via Natural or Artificial Opening Endoscopic

0BB60ZX Excision of Right Lower Lobe Bronchus, Open Approach, Diagnostic

0BB60ZZ Excision of Right Lower Lobe Bronchus, Open Approach

0BB63ZX Excision of Right Lower Lobe Bronchus, Percutaneous Approach, Diagnostic

0BB63ZZ Excision of Right Lower Lobe Bronchus, Percutaneous Approach

0BB64ZX Excision of Right Lower Lobe Bronchus, Percutaneous Endoscopic Approach, Diagnostic

0BB64ZZ Excision of Right Lower Lobe Bronchus, Percutaneous Endoscopic Approach

0BB67ZX Excision of Right Lower Lobe Bronchus, Via Natural or Artificial Opening, Diagnostic

0BB67ZZ Excision of Right Lower Lobe Bronchus, Via Natural or Artificial Opening

0BB68ZX Excision of Right Lower Lobe Bronchus, Via Natural or Artificial Opening Endoscopic, Diagnostic

0BB68ZZ Excision of Right Lower Lobe Bronchus, Via Natural or Artificial Opening Endoscopic

0BB70ZX Excision of Left Main Bronchus, Open Approach, Diagnostic

0BB70ZZ Excision of Left Main Bronchus, Open Approach

0BB73ZX Excision of Left Main Bronchus, Percutaneous Approach, Diagnostic

0BB73ZZ Excision of Left Main Bronchus, Percutaneous Approach

0BB74ZX Excision of Left Main Bronchus, Percutaneous Endoscopic Approach, Diagnostic

0BB74ZZ Excision of Left Main Bronchus, Percutaneous Endoscopic Approach

0BB77ZX Excision of Left Main Bronchus, Via Natural or Artificial Opening, Diagnostic

0BB77ZZ Excision of Left Main Bronchus, Via Natural or Artificial Opening

0BB78ZX Excision of Left Main Bronchus, Via Natural or Artificial Opening Endoscopic, Diagnostic

0BB78ZZ Excision of Left Main Bronchus, Via Natural or Artificial Opening Endoscopic

0BB80ZX Excision of Left Upper Lobe Bronchus, Open Approach, Diagnostic

0BB80ZZ Excision of Left Upper Lobe Bronchus, Open Approach

0BB83ZX Excision of Left Upper Lobe Bronchus, Percutaneous Approach, Diagnostic

0BB83ZZ Excision of Left Upper Lobe Bronchus, Percutaneous Approach

0BB84ZX Excision of Left Upper Lobe Bronchus, Percutaneous Endoscopic Approach, Diagnostic

0BB84ZZ Excision of Left Upper Lobe Bronchus, Percutaneous Endoscopic Approach

0BB87ZX Excision of Left Upper Lobe Bronchus, Via Natural or Artificial Opening, Diagnostic

0BB87ZZ Excision of Left Upper Lobe Bronchus, Via Natural or Artificial Opening

0BB88ZX Excision of Left Upper Lobe Bronchus, Via Natural or Artificial Opening Endoscopic, Diagnostic

0BB88ZZ Excision of Left Upper Lobe Bronchus, Via Natural or Artificial Opening Endoscopic

0BB90ZX Excision of Lingula Bronchus, Open Approach, Diagnostic

0BB90ZZ Excision of Lingula Bronchus, Open Approach

0BB93ZX Excision of Lingula Bronchus, Percutaneous Approach, Diagnostic

0BB93ZZ Excision of Lingula Bronchus, Percutaneous Approach

0BB94ZX Excision of Lingula Bronchus, Percutaneous Endoscopic Approach, Diagnostic

0BB94ZZ Excision of Lingula Bronchus, Percutaneous Endoscopic Approach

0BB97ZX Excision of Lingula Bronchus, Via Natural or Artificial Opening, Diagnostic

0BB97ZZ Excision of Lingula Bronchus, Via Natural or Artificial Opening

0BB98ZX Excision of Lingula Bronchus, Via Natural or Artificial Opening Endoscopic, Diagnostic

Female-only	♂ Male-only	▲ Limited Coverage	● Non-OR	▥ HAC-associated procedure	▲ Non-covered procedures	➕ Combination

0BB98ZZ Excision of Lingula Bronchus, Via Natural or Artificial Opening Endoscopic

0BBB0ZX Excision of Left Lower Lobe Bronchus, Open Approach, Diagnostic

0BBB0ZZ Excision of Left Lower Lobe Bronchus, Open Approach

0BBB3ZX Excision of Left Lower Lobe Bronchus, Percutaneous Approach, Diagnostic

0BBB3ZZ Excision of Left Lower Lobe Bronchus, Percutaneous Approach

0BBB4ZX Excision of Left Lower Lobe Bronchus, Percutaneous Endoscopic Approach, Diagnostic

0BBB4ZZ Excision of Left Lower Lobe Bronchus, Percutaneous Endoscopic Approach

0BBB7ZX Excision of Left Lower Lobe Bronchus, Via Natural or Artificial Opening, Diagnostic

0BBB7ZZ Excision of Left Lower Lobe Bronchus, Via Natural or Artificial Opening

0BBB8ZX Excision of Left Lower Lobe Bronchus, Via Natural or Artificial Opening Endoscopic, Diagnostic

0BBB8ZZ Excision of Left Lower Lobe Bronchus, Via Natural or Artificial Opening Endoscopic

0BBC0ZX Excision of Right Upper Lung Lobe, Open Approach, Diagnostic

0BBC0ZZ Excision of Right Upper Lung Lobe, Open Approach

0BBC3ZX Excision of Right Upper Lung Lobe, Percutaneous Approach, Diagnostic

0BBC3ZZ Excision of Right Upper Lung Lobe, Percutaneous Approach

0BBC4ZX Excision of Right Upper Lung Lobe, Percutaneous Endoscopic Approach, Diagnostic

0BBC4ZZ Excision of Right Upper Lung Lobe, Percutaneous Endoscopic Approach

0BBC7ZX Excision of Right Upper Lung Lobe, Via Natural or Artificial Opening, Diagnostic

0BBC7ZZ Excision of Right Upper Lung Lobe, Via Natural or Artificial Opening

0BBC8ZX Excision of Right Upper Lung Lobe, Via Natural or Artificial Opening Endoscopic, Diagnostic

0BBC8ZZ Excision of Right Upper Lung Lobe, Via Natural or Artificial Opening Endoscopic

0BBD0ZX Excision of Right Middle Lung Lobe, Open Approach, Diagnostic

0BBD0ZZ Excision of Right Middle Lung Lobe, Open Approach

0BBD3ZX Excision of Right Middle Lung Lobe, Percutaneous Approach, Diagnostic

0BBD3ZZ Excision of Right Middle Lung Lobe, Percutaneous Approach

0BBD4ZX Excision of Right Middle Lung Lobe, Percutaneous Endoscopic Approach, Diagnostic

0BBD4ZZ Excision of Right Middle Lung Lobe, Percutaneous Endoscopic Approach

0BBD7ZX Excision of Right Middle Lung Lobe, Via Natural or Artificial Opening, Diagnostic

0BBD7ZZ Excision of Right Middle Lung Lobe, Via Natural or Artificial Opening

0BBD8ZX Excision of Right Middle Lung Lobe, Via Natural or Artificial Opening Endoscopic, Diagnostic

0BBD8ZZ Excision of Right Middle Lung Lobe, Via Natural or Artificial Opening Endoscopic

0BBF0ZX Excision of Right Lower Lung Lobe, Open Approach, Diagnostic

0BBF0ZZ Excision of Right Lower Lung Lobe, Open Approach

0BBF3ZX Excision of Right Lower Lung Lobe, Percutaneous Approach, Diagnostic

0BBF3ZZ Excision of Right Lower Lung Lobe, Percutaneous Approach

0BBF4ZX Excision of Right Lower Lung Lobe, Percutaneous Endoscopic Approach, Diagnostic

0BBF4ZZ Excision of Right Lower Lung Lobe, Percutaneous Endoscopic Approach

0BBF7ZX Excision of Right Lower Lung Lobe, Via Natural or Artificial Opening, Diagnostic

0BBF7ZZ Excision of Right Lower Lung Lobe, Via Natural or Artificial Opening

0BBF8ZX Excision of Right Lower Lung Lobe, Via Natural or Artificial Opening Endoscopic, Diagnostic

0BBF8ZZ Excision of Right Lower Lung Lobe, Via Natural or Artificial Opening Endoscopic

0BBG0ZX Excision of Left Upper Lung Lobe, Open Approach, Diagnostic

0BBG0ZZ Excision of Left Upper Lung Lobe, Open Approach

0BBG3ZX Excision of Left Upper Lung Lobe, Percutaneous Approach, Diagnostic

0BBG3ZZ Excision of Left Upper Lung Lobe, Percutaneous Approach

0BBG4ZX Excision of Left Upper Lung Lobe, Percutaneous Endoscopic Approach, Diagnostic

0BBG4ZZ Excision of Left Upper Lung Lobe, Percutaneous Endoscopic Approach

0BBG7ZX Excision of Left Upper Lung Lobe, Via Natural or Artificial Opening, Diagnostic

0BBG7ZZ Excision of Left Upper Lung Lobe, Via Natural or Artificial Opening

0BBG8ZX Excision of Left Upper Lung Lobe, Via Natural or Artificial Opening Endoscopic, Diagnostic

0BBG8ZZ Excision of Left Upper Lung Lobe, Via Natural or Artificial Opening Endoscopic

0BBH0ZX Excision of Lung Lingula, Open Approach, Diagnostic

0BBH0ZZ Excision of Lung Lingula, Open Approach

0BBH3ZX Excision of Lung Lingula, Percutaneous Approach, Diagnostic

0BBH3ZZ Excision of Lung Lingula, Percutaneous Approach

0BBH4ZX Excision of Lung Lingula, Percutaneous Endoscopic Approach, Diagnostic

0BBH4ZZ Excision of Lung Lingula, Percutaneous Endoscopic Approach

0BBH7ZX Excision of Lung Lingula, Via Natural or Artificial Opening, Diagnostic

0BBH7ZZ Excision of Lung Lingula, Via Natural or Artificial Opening

0BBH8ZX Excision of Lung Lingula, Via Natural or Artificial Opening Endoscopic, Diagnostic

0BBH8ZZ Excision of Lung Lingula, Via Natural or Artificial Opening Endoscopic

0BBJ0ZX Excision of Left Lower Lung Lobe, Open Approach, Diagnostic

0BBJ0ZZ Excision of Left Lower Lung Lobe, Open Approach

0BBJ3ZX Excision of Left Lower Lung Lobe, Percutaneous Approach, Diagnostic

0BBJ3ZZ Excision of Left Lower Lung Lobe, Percutaneous Approach

0BBJ4ZX Excision of Left Lower Lung Lobe, Percutaneous Endoscopic Approach, Diagnostic

0BBJ4ZZ Excision of Left Lower Lung Lobe, Percutaneous Endoscopic Approach

0BBJ7ZX Excision of Left Lower Lung Lobe, Via Natural or Artificial Opening, Diagnostic

0BBJ7ZZ Excision of Left Lower Lung Lobe, Via Natural or Artificial Opening

0BBJ8ZX Excision of Left Lower Lung Lobe, Via Natural or Artificial Opening Endoscopic, Diagnostic

0BBJ8ZZ Excision of Left Lower Lung Lobe, Via Natural or Artificial Opening Endosco

0BBK0ZX Excision of Right Lung, Open Approa Diagnostic

0BBK0ZZ Excision of Right Lung, Open Approa

0BBK3ZX Excision of Right Lung, Percutaneous Approach, Diagnostic

0BBK3ZZ Excision of Right Lung, Percutaneous Approach

0BBK4ZX Excision of Right Lung, Percutaneous Endoscopic Approach, Diagnostic

0BBK4ZZ Excision of Right Lung, Percutaneous Endoscopic Approach

0BBK7ZX Excision of Right Lung, Via Natural or Artificial Opening, Diagnostic

0BBK7ZZ Excision of Right Lung, Via Natural or Artificial Opening

0BBK8ZX Excision of Right Lung, Via Natural or Artificial Opening Endoscopic, Diagno

AHA CC: 1Q, 2014, 20-21

0BBK8ZZ Excision of Right Lung, Via Natural or Artificial Opening Endoscopic

0BBL0ZX Excision of Left Lung, Open Approach Diagnostic

0BBL0ZZ Excision of Left Lung, Open Approach

0BBL3ZX Excision of Left Lung, Percutaneous Approach, Diagnostic

0BBL3ZZ Excision of Left Lung, Percutaneous Approach

0BBL4ZX Excision of Left Lung, Percutaneous Endoscopic Approach, Diagnostic

0BBL4ZZ Excision of Left Lung, Percutaneous Endoscopic Approach

0BBL7ZX Excision of Left Lung, Via Natural or Artificial Opening, Diagnostic

0BBL7ZZ Excision of Left Lung, Via Natural or Artificial Opening

0BBL8ZX Excision of Left Lung, Via Natural or Artificial Opening Endoscopic, Diagnos

0BBL8ZZ Excision of Left Lung, Via Natural or Artificial Opening Endoscopic

0BBM0ZX Excision of Bilateral Lungs, Open Approach, Diagnostic

0BBM0ZZ Excision of Bilateral Lungs, Open Approach

0BBM3ZX Excision of Bilateral Lungs, Percutaneo Approach, Diagnostic

0BBM3ZZ Excision of Bilateral Lungs, Percutaneo Approach

0BBM4ZX Excision of Bilateral Lungs, Percutaneo Endoscopic Approach, Diagnostic

0BBM4ZZ Excision of Bilateral Lungs, Percutaneo Endoscopic Approach

0BBM7ZX Excision of Bilateral Lungs, Via Natural Artificial Opening, Diagnostic

0BBM7ZZ Excision of Bilateral Lungs, Via Natural Artificial Opening

0BBM8ZX Excision of Bilateral Lungs, Via Natural Artificial Opening Endoscopic, Diagnos

0BBM8ZZ Excision of Bilateral Lungs, Via Natural Artificial Opening Endoscopic

0BBN0ZX Excision of Right Pleura, Open Approac Diagnostic

0BBN0ZZ Excision of Right Pleura, Open Approac

0BBN3ZX Excision of Right Pleura, Percutaneous Approach, Diagnostic

0BBN3ZZ Excision of Right Pleura, Percutaneous Approach

0BBN4ZX Excision of Right Pleura, Percutaneous Endoscopic Approach, Diagnostic

0BBN4ZZ Excision of Right Pleura, Percutaneous Endoscopic Approach

0BBP0ZX Excision of Left Pleura, Open Approach, Diagnostic

0BBP0ZZ Excision of Left Pleura, Open Approach

0BBP3ZX Excision of Left Pleura, Percutaneous Approach, Diagnostic

3P3ZZ	Excision of Left Pleura, Percutaneous Approach
3P4ZX	Excision of Left Pleura, Percutaneous Endoscopic Approach, Diagnostic
3P4ZZ	Excision of Left Pleura, Percutaneous Endoscopic Approach
3R0ZX	Excision of Right Diaphragm, Open Approach, Diagnostic
3R0ZZ	Excision of Right Diaphragm, Open Approach

0BBR3ZX	Excision of Right Diaphragm, Percutaneous Approach, Diagnostic
0BBR3ZZ	Excision of Right Diaphragm, Percutaneous Approach
0BBR4ZX	Excision of Right Diaphragm, Percutaneous Endoscopic Approach, Diagnostic
0BBR4ZZ	Excision of Right Diaphragm, Percutaneous Endoscopic Approach
0BBS0ZX	Excision of Left Diaphragm, Open Approach, Diagnostic

0BBS0ZZ	Excision of Left Diaphragm, Open Approach
0BBS3ZX	Excision of Left Diaphragm, Percutaneous Approach, Diagnostic
0BBS3ZZ	Excision of Left Diaphragm, Percutaneous Approach
0BBS4ZX	Excision of Left Diaphragm, Percutaneous Endoscopic Approach, Diagnostic
0BBS4ZZ	Excision of Left Diaphragm, Percutaneous Endoscopic Approach

°C – Respiratory System, Extirpation

C10ZZ	Extirpation of Matter from Trachea, Open Approach
C13ZZ	Extirpation of Matter from Trachea, Percutaneous Approach
C14ZZ	Extirpation of Matter from Trachea, Percutaneous Endoscopic Approach
C17ZZ	Extirpation of Matter from Trachea, Via Natural or Artificial Opening
C18ZZ	Extirpation of Matter from Trachea, Via Natural or Artificial Opening Endoscopic
C20ZZ	Extirpation of Matter from Carina, Open Approach
C23ZZ	Extirpation of Matter from Carina, Percutaneous Approach
C24ZZ	Extirpation of Matter from Carina, Percutaneous Endoscopic Approach
C27ZZ	Extirpation of Matter from Carina, Via Natural or Artificial Opening
C28ZZ	Extirpation of Matter from Carina, Via Natural or Artificial Opening Endoscopic
C30ZZ	Extirpation of Matter from Right Main Bronchus, Open Approach
C33ZZ	Extirpation of Matter from Right Main Bronchus, Percutaneous Approach
C34ZZ	Extirpation of Matter from Right Main Bronchus, Percutaneous Endoscopic Approach
C37ZZ	Extirpation of Matter from Right Main Bronchus, Via Natural or Artificial Opening
C38ZZ	Extirpation of Matter from Right Main Bronchus, Via Natural or Artificial Opening Endoscopic
C40ZZ	Extirpation of Matter from Right Upper Lobe Bronchus, Open Approach
C43ZZ	Extirpation of Matter from Right Upper Lobe Bronchus, Percutaneous Approach
C44ZZ	Extirpation of Matter from Right Upper Lobe Bronchus, Percutaneous Endoscopic Approach
C47ZZ	Extirpation of Matter from Right Upper Lobe Bronchus, Via Natural or Artificial Opening
C48ZZ	Extirpation of Matter from Right Upper Lobe Bronchus, Via Natural or Artificial Opening Endoscopic
C50ZZ	Extirpation of Matter from Right Middle Lobe Bronchus, Open Approach
C53ZZ	Extirpation of Matter from Right Middle Lobe Bronchus, Percutaneous Approach
C54ZZ	Extirpation of Matter from Right Middle Lobe Bronchus, Percutaneous Endoscopic Approach
C57ZZ	Extirpation of Matter from Right Middle Lobe Bronchus, Via Natural or Artificial Opening
C58ZZ	Extirpation of Matter from Right Middle Lobe Bronchus, Via Natural or Artificial Opening Endoscopic
C60ZZ	Extirpation of Matter from Right Lower Lobe Bronchus, Open Approach
C63ZZ	Extirpation of Matter from Right Lower Lobe Bronchus, Percutaneous Approach

0BC64ZZ	Extirpation of Matter from Right Lower Lobe Bronchus, Percutaneous Endoscopic Approach
0BC67ZZ	Extirpation of Matter from Right Lower Lobe Bronchus, Via Natural or Artificial Opening
0BC68ZZ	Extirpation of Matter from Right Lower Lobe Bronchus, Via Natural or Artificial Opening Endoscopic
0BC70ZZ	Extirpation of Matter from Left Main Bronchus, Open Approach
0BC73ZZ	Extirpation of Matter from Left Main Bronchus, Percutaneous Approach
0BC74ZZ	Extirpation of Matter from Left Main Bronchus, Percutaneous Endoscopic Approach
0BC77ZZ	Extirpation of Matter from Left Main Bronchus, Via Natural or Artificial Opening
0BC78ZZ	Extirpation of Matter from Left Main Bronchus, Via Natural or Artificial Opening Endoscopic
0BC80ZZ	Extirpation of Matter from Left Upper Lobe Bronchus, Open Approach
0BC83ZZ	Extirpation of Matter from Left Upper Lobe Bronchus, Percutaneous Approach
0BC84ZZ	Extirpation of Matter from Left Upper Lobe Bronchus, Percutaneous Endoscopic Approach
0BC87ZZ	Extirpation of Matter from Left Upper Lobe Bronchus, Via Natural or Artificial Opening
0BC88ZZ	Extirpation of Matter from Left Upper Lobe Bronchus, Via Natural or Artificial Opening Endoscopic
0BC90ZZ	Extirpation of Matter from Lingula Bronchus, Open Approach
0BC93ZZ	Extirpation of Matter from Lingula Bronchus, Percutaneous Approach
0BC94ZZ	Extirpation of Matter from Lingula Bronchus, Percutaneous Endoscopic Approach
0BC97ZZ	Extirpation of Matter from Lingula Bronchus, Via Natural or Artificial Opening
0BC98ZZ	Extirpation of Matter from Lingula Bronchus, Via Natural or Artificial Opening Endoscopic
0BCB0ZZ	Extirpation of Matter from Left Lower Lobe Bronchus, Open Approach
0BCB3ZZ	Extirpation of Matter from Left Lower Lobe Bronchus, Percutaneous Approach
0BCB4ZZ	Extirpation of Matter from Left Lower Lobe Bronchus, Percutaneous Endoscopic Approach
0BCB7ZZ	Extirpation of Matter from Left Lower Lobe Bronchus, Via Natural or Artificial Opening
0BCB8ZZ	Extirpation of Matter from Left Lower Lobe Bronchus, Via Natural or Artificial Opening Endoscopic
0BCC0ZZ	Extirpation of Matter from Right Upper Lung Lobe, Open Approach

0BCC3ZZ	Extirpation of Matter from Right Upper Lung Lobe, Percutaneous Approach
0BCC4ZZ	Extirpation of Matter from Right Upper Lung Lobe, Percutaneous Endoscopic Approach
0BCC7ZZ	Extirpation of Matter from Right Upper Lung Lobe, Via Natural or Artificial Opening
0BCC8ZZ	Extirpation of Matter from Right Upper Lung Lobe, Via Natural or Artificial Opening Endoscopic
0BCD0ZZ	Extirpation of Matter from Right Middle Lung Lobe, Open Approach
0BCD3ZZ	Extirpation of Matter from Right Middle Lung Lobe, Percutaneous Approach
0BCD4ZZ	Extirpation of Matter from Right Middle Lung Lobe, Percutaneous Endoscopic Approach
0BCD7ZZ	Extirpation of Matter from Right Middle Lung Lobe, Via Natural or Artificial Opening
0BCD8ZZ	Extirpation of Matter from Right Middle Lung Lobe, Via Natural or Artificial Opening Endoscopic
0BCF0ZZ	Extirpation of Matter from Right Lower Lung Lobe, Open Approach
0BCF3ZZ	Extirpation of Matter from Right Lower Lung Lobe, Percutaneous Approach
0BCF4ZZ	Extirpation of Matter from Right Lower Lung Lobe, Percutaneous Endoscopic Approach
0BCF7ZZ	Extirpation of Matter from Right Lower Lung Lobe, Via Natural or Artificial Opening
0BCF8ZZ	Extirpation of Matter from Right Lower Lung Lobe, Via Natural or Artificial Opening Endoscopic
0BCG0ZZ	Extirpation of Matter from Left Upper Lung Lobe, Open Approach
0BCG3ZZ	Extirpation of Matter from Left Upper Lung Lobe, Percutaneous Approach
0BCG4ZZ	Extirpation of Matter from Left Upper Lung Lobe, Percutaneous Endoscopic Approach
0BCG7ZZ	Extirpation of Matter from Left Upper Lung Lobe, Via Natural or Artificial Opening
0BCG8ZZ	Extirpation of Matter from Left Upper Lung Lobe, Via Natural or Artificial Opening Endoscopic
0BCH0ZZ	Extirpation of Matter from Lung Lingula, Open Approach
0BCH3ZZ	Extirpation of Matter from Lung Lingula, Percutaneous Approach
0BCH4ZZ	Extirpation of Matter from Lung Lingula, Percutaneous Endoscopic Approach
0BCH7ZZ	Extirpation of Matter from Lung Lingula, Via Natural or Artificial Opening
0BCH8ZZ	Extirpation of Matter from Lung Lingula, Via Natural or Artificial Opening Endoscopic
0BCJ0ZZ	Extirpation of Matter from Left Lower Lung Lobe, Open Approach

Female-only   ♂ Male-only   ▲ Limited Coverage   ● Non-OR   ■ HAC-associated procedure   ▲ Non-covered procedures   ✛ Combination

0BCJ3ZZ Extirpation of Matter from Left Lower Lung Lobe, Percutaneous Approach

0BCJ4ZZ Extirpation of Matter from Left Lower Lung Lobe, Percutaneous Endoscopic Approach

0BCJ7ZZ Extirpation of Matter from Left Lower Lung Lobe, Via Natural or Artificial Opening

0BCJ8ZZ Extirpation of Matter from Left Lower Lung Lobe, Via Natural or Artificial Opening Endoscopic

0BCK0ZZ Extirpation of Matter from Right Lung, Open Approach

0BCK3ZZ Extirpation of Matter from Right Lung, Percutaneous Approach

0BCK4ZZ Extirpation of Matter from Right Lung, Percutaneous Endoscopic Approach

0BCK7ZZ Extirpation of Matter from Right Lung, Via Natural or Artificial Opening

0BCK8ZZ Extirpation of Matter from Right Lung, Via Natural or Artificial Opening Endoscopic

0BCL0ZZ Extirpation of Matter from Left Lung, Open Approach

0BCL3ZZ Extirpation of Matter from Left Lung, Percutaneous Approach

0BCL4ZZ Extirpation of Matter from Left Lung, Percutaneous Endoscopic Approach

0BCL7ZZ Extirpation of Matter from Left Lung, Via Natural or Artificial Opening

0BCL8ZZ Extirpation of Matter from Left Lung, Via Natural or Artificial Opening Endoscopic

0BCM0ZZ Extirpation of Matter from Bilateral Lungs, Open Approach

0BCM3ZZ Extirpation of Matter from Bilateral Lungs, Percutaneous Approach

0BCM4ZZ Extirpation of Matter from Bilateral Lungs, Percutaneous Endoscopic Approach

0BCM7ZZ Extirpation of Matter from Bilateral Lungs, Via Natural or Artificial Opening

0BCM8ZZ Extirpation of Matter from Bilateral Lungs, Via Natural or Artificial Opening Endoscopic

0BCN0ZZ Extirpation of Matter from Right Pleura, Open Approach

0BCN3ZZ Extirpation of Matter from Right Pleura, Percutaneous Approach

0BCN4ZZ Extirpation of Matter from Right Pleura, Percutaneous Endoscopic Approach

0BCP0ZZ Extirpation of Matter from Left Pleura, Open Approach

0BCP3ZZ Extirpation of Matter from Left Pleura, Percutaneous Approach

0BCP4ZZ Extirpation of Matter from Left Pleura, Percutaneous Endoscopic Approach

0BCR0ZZ Extirpation of Matter from Right Diaphragm, Open Approach

0BCR3ZZ Extirpation of Matter from Right Diaphragm, Percutaneous Approach

0BCR4ZZ Extirpation of Matter from Right Diaphragm, Percutaneous Endoscopic Approach

0BCS0ZZ Extirpation of Matter from Left Diaphragm, Open Approach

0BCS3ZZ Extirpation of Matter from Left Diaphragm, Percutaneous Approach

0BCS4ZZ Extirpation of Matter from Left Diaphragm, Percutaneous Endoscopic Approach

0BD – Respiratory System, Extraction

Review Coding Guidelines B3.4a and B3.4b

0BDN0ZX Extraction of Right Pleura, Open Approach, Diagnostic

0BDN0ZZ Extraction of Right Pleura, Open Approach

0BDN3ZX Extraction of Right Pleura, Percutaneous Approach, Diagnostic

0BDN3ZZ Extraction of Right Pleura, Percutaneous Approach

0BDN4ZX Extraction of Right Pleura, Percutaneous Endoscopic Approach, Diagnostic

0BDN4ZZ Extraction of Right Pleura, Percutaneous Endoscopic Approach

0BDP0ZX Extraction of Left Pleura, Open Approach, Diagnostic

0BDP0ZZ Extraction of Left Pleura, Open Approach

0BDP3ZX Extraction of Left Pleura, Percutaneous Approach, Diagnostic

0BDP3ZZ Extraction of Left Pleura, Percutaneous Approach

0BDP4ZX Extraction of Left Pleura, Percutaneous Endoscopic Approach, Diagnostic

0BDP4ZZ Extraction of Left Pleura, Percutaneous Endoscopic Approach

0BF – Respiratory System, Fragmentation

0BF10ZZ Fragmentation in Trachea, Open Approach

0BF13ZZ Fragmentation in Trachea, Percutaneous Approach

0BF14ZZ Fragmentation in Trachea, Percutaneous Endoscopic Approach

0BF17ZZ Fragmentation in Trachea, Via Natural or Artificial Opening

0BF18ZZ Fragmentation in Trachea, Via Natural or Artificial Opening Endoscopic

▲ 0BF1XZZ Fragmentation in Trachea, External Approach

0BF20ZZ Fragmentation in Carina, Open Approach

0BF23ZZ Fragmentation in Carina, Percutaneous Approach

0BF24ZZ Fragmentation in Carina, Percutaneous Endoscopic Approach

0BF27ZZ Fragmentation in Carina, Via Natural or Artificial Opening

0BF28ZZ Fragmentation in Carina, Via Natural or Artificial Opening Endoscopic

▲ 0BF2XZZ Fragmentation in Carina, External Approach

0BF30ZZ Fragmentation in Right Main Bronchus, Open Approach

0BF33ZZ Fragmentation in Right Main Bronchus, Percutaneous Approach

0BF34ZZ Fragmentation in Right Main Bronchus, Percutaneous Endoscopic Approach

0BF37ZZ Fragmentation in Right Main Bronchus, Via Natural or Artificial Opening

0BF38ZZ Fragmentation in Right Main Bronchus, Via Natural or Artificial Opening Endoscopic

▲ 0BF3XZZ Fragmentation in Right Main Bronchus, External Approach

0BF40ZZ Fragmentation in Right Upper Lobe Bronchus, Open Approach

0BF43ZZ Fragmentation in Right Upper Lobe Bronchus, Percutaneous Approach

0BF44ZZ Fragmentation in Right Upper Lobe Bronchus, Percutaneous Endoscopic Approach

0BF47ZZ Fragmentation in Right Upper Lobe Bronchus, Via Natural or Artificial Opening

0BF48ZZ Fragmentation in Right Upper Lobe Bronchus, Via Natural or Artificial Opening Endoscopic

▲ 0BF4XZZ Fragmentation in Right Upper Lobe Bronchus, External Approach

0BF50ZZ Fragmentation in Right Middle Lobe Bronchus, Open Approach

0BF53ZZ Fragmentation in Right Middle Lobe Bronchus, Percutaneous Approach

0BF54ZZ Fragmentation in Right Middle Lobe Bronchus, Percutaneous Endoscopic Approach

0BF57ZZ Fragmentation in Right Middle Lobe Bronchus, Via Natural or Artificial Opening

0BF58ZZ Fragmentation in Right Middle Lobe Bronchus, Via Natural or Artificial Opening Endoscopic

▲ 0BF5XZZ Fragmentation in Right Middle Lobe Bronchus, External Approach

0BF60ZZ Fragmentation in Right Lower Lobe Bronchus, Open Approach

0BF63ZZ Fragmentation in Right Lower Lobe Bronchus, Percutaneous Approach

0BF64ZZ Fragmentation in Right Lower Lobe Bronchus, Percutaneous Endoscopic Approach

0BF67ZZ Fragmentation in Right Lower Lobe Bronchus, Via Natural or Artificial Opening

0BF68ZZ Fragmentation in Right Lower Lobe Bronchus, Via Natural or Artificial Opening Endoscopic

▲ 0BF6XZZ Fragmentation in Right Lower Lobe Bronchus, External Approach

0BF70ZZ Fragmentation in Left Main Bronchus, Open Approach

0BF73ZZ Fragmentation in Left Main Bronchus, Percutaneous Approach

0BF74ZZ Fragmentation in Left Main Bronchus, Percutaneous Endoscopic Approach

0BF77ZZ Fragmentation in Left Main Bronchus, Via Natural or Artificial Opening

0BF78ZZ Fragmentation in Left Main Bronchus, Via Natural or Artificial Opening Endoscopic

▲ 0BF7XZZ Fragmentation in Left Main Bronchus, External Approach

0BF80ZZ Fragmentation in Left Upper Lobe Bronchus, Open Approach

0BF83ZZ Fragmentation in Left Upper Lobe Bronchus, Percutaneous Approach

0BF84ZZ Fragmentation in Left Upper Lobe Bronchus, Percutaneous Endoscopic Approach

0BF87ZZ Fragmentation in Left Upper Lobe Bronchus, Via Natural or Artificial Opening

0BF88ZZ Fragmentation in Left Upper Lobe Bronchus, Via Natural or Artificial Opening Endoscopic

▲ 0BF8XZZ Fragmentation in Left Upper Lobe Bronchus, External Approach

0BF90ZZ Fragmentation in Lingula Bronchus, Open Approach

♀ Female-only   ♂ Male-only   ▲ Limited Coverage   ● Non-OR   ▩ HAC-associated procedure   ▲ Non-covered procedures   ✚ Combination

F93ZZ Fragmentation in Lingula Bronchus, Percutaneous Approach

F94ZZ Fragmentation in Lingula Bronchus, Percutaneous Endoscopic Approach

F97ZZ Fragmentation in Lingula Bronchus, Via Natural or Artificial Opening

F98ZZ Fragmentation in Lingula Bronchus, Via Natural or Artificial Opening Endoscopic

▲ 0BF9XZZ Fragmentation in Lingula Bronchus, External Approach

0BFB0ZZ Fragmentation in Left Lower Lobe Bronchus, Open Approach

0BFB3ZZ Fragmentation in Left Lower Lobe Bronchus, Percutaneous Approach

0BFB4ZZ Fragmentation in Left Lower Lobe Bronchus, Percutaneous Endoscopic Approach

0BFB7ZZ Fragmentation in Left Lower Lobe Bronchus, Via Natural or Artificial Opening

0BFB8ZZ Fragmentation in Left Lower Lobe Bronchus, Via Natural or Artificial Opening Endoscopic

▲ 0BFBXZZ Fragmentation in Left Lower Lobe Bronchus, External Approach

3H – Respiratory System, Insertion

H001Z Insertion of Radioactive Element into Tracheobronchial Tree, Open Approach

H002Z Insertion of Monitoring Device into Tracheobronchial Tree, Open Approach

H003Z Insertion of Infusion Device into Tracheobronchial Tree, Open Approach

H00DZ Insertion of Intraluminal Device into Tracheobronchial Tree, Open Approach

H031Z Insertion of Radioactive Element into Tracheobronchial Tree, Percutaneous Approach

H032Z Insertion of Monitoring Device into Tracheobronchial Tree, Percutaneous Approach

H033Z Insertion of Infusion Device into Tracheobronchial Tree, Percutaneous Approach

H03DZ Insertion of Intraluminal Device into Tracheobronchial Tree, Percutaneous Approach

H041Z Insertion of Radioactive Element into Tracheobronchial Tree, Percutaneous Endoscopic Approach

H042Z Insertion of Monitoring Device into Tracheobronchial Tree, Percutaneous Endoscopic Approach

H043Z Insertion of Infusion Device into Tracheobronchial Tree, Percutaneous Endoscopic Approach

H04DZ Insertion of Intraluminal Device into Tracheobronchial Tree, Percutaneous Endoscopic Approach

H071Z Insertion of Radioactive Element into Tracheobronchial Tree, Via Natural or Artificial Opening

H072Z Insertion of Monitoring Device into Tracheobronchial Tree, Via Natural or Artificial Opening

H073Z Insertion of Infusion Device into Tracheobronchial Tree, Via Natural or Artificial Opening

H07DZ Insertion of Intraluminal Device into Tracheobronchial Tree, Via Natural or Artificial Opening

H081Z Insertion of Radioactive Element into Tracheobronchial Tree, Via Natural or Artificial Opening Endoscopic

H082Z Insertion of Monitoring Device into Tracheobronchial Tree, Via Natural or Artificial Opening Endoscopic

H083Z Insertion of Infusion Device into Tracheobronchial Tree, Via Natural or Artificial Opening Endoscopic

H08DZ Insertion of Intraluminal Device into Tracheobronchial Tree, Via Natural or Artificial Opening Endoscopic

BH102Z Insertion of Monitoring Device into Trachea, Open Approach

BH10DZ Insertion of Intraluminal Device into Trachea, Open Approach

BH13DZ Insertion of Intraluminal Device into Trachea, Percutaneous Approach

BH13EZ Insertion of Endotracheal Airway into Trachea, Percutaneous Approach

0BH14DZ Insertion of Intraluminal Device into Trachea, Percutaneous Endoscopic Approach

0BH172Z Insertion of Monitoring Device into Trachea, Via Natural or Artificial Opening

0BH17DZ Insertion of Intraluminal Device into Trachea, Via Natural or Artificial Opening

0BH17EZ Insertion of Endotracheal Airway into Trachea, Via Natural or Artificial Opening
AHA CC: 4Q, 2014, 3-15

0BH182Z Insertion of Monitoring Device into Trachea, Via Natural or Artificial Opening Endoscopic

0BH18DZ Insertion of Intraluminal Device into Trachea, Via Natural or Artificial Opening Endoscopic

0BH18EZ Insertion of Endotracheal Airway into Trachea, Via Natural or Artificial Opening Endoscopic
AHA CC: 4Q, 2014, 3-15

0BH30GZ Insertion of Endobronchial Valve into Right Main Bronchus, Open Approach

0BH33GZ Insertion of Endobronchial Valve into Right Main Bronchus, Percutaneous Approach

0BH34GZ Insertion of Endobronchial Valve into Right Main Bronchus, Percutaneous Endoscopic Approach

0BH37GZ Insertion of Endobronchial Valve into Right Main Bronchus, Via Natural or Artificial Opening

0BH38GZ Insertion of Endobronchial Valve into Right Main Bronchus, Via Natural or Artificial Opening Endoscopic

0BH40GZ Insertion of Endobronchial Valve into Right Upper Lobe Bronchus, Open Approach

0BH43GZ Insertion of Endobronchial Valve into Right Upper Lobe Bronchus, Percutaneous Approach

0BH44GZ Insertion of Endobronchial Valve into Right Upper Lobe Bronchus, Percutaneous Endoscopic Approach

0BH47GZ Insertion of Endobronchial Valve into Right Upper Lobe Bronchus, Via Natural or Artificial Opening

0BH48GZ Insertion of Endobronchial Valve into Right Upper Lobe Bronchus, Via Natural or Artificial Opening Endoscopic

0BH50GZ Insertion of Endobronchial Valve into Right Middle Lobe Bronchus, Open Approach

0BH53GZ Insertion of Endobronchial Valve into Right Middle Lobe Bronchus, Percutaneous Approach

0BH54GZ Insertion of Endobronchial Valve into Right Middle Lobe Bronchus, Percutaneous Endoscopic Approach

0BH57GZ Insertion of Endobronchial Valve into Right Middle Lobe Bronchus, Via Natural or Artificial Opening

0BH58GZ Insertion of Endobronchial Valve into Right Middle Lobe Bronchus, Via Natural or Artificial Opening Endoscopic

0BH60GZ Insertion of Endobronchial Valve into Right Lower Lobe Bronchus, Open Approach

0BH63GZ Insertion of Endobronchial Valve into Right Lower Lobe Bronchus, Percutaneous Approach

0BH64GZ Insertion of Endobronchial Valve into Right Lower Lobe Bronchus, Percutaneous Endoscopic Approach

0BH67GZ Insertion of Endobronchial Valve into Right Lower Lobe Bronchus, Via Natural or Artificial Opening

0BH68GZ Insertion of Endobronchial Valve into Right Lower Lobe Bronchus, Via Natural or Artificial Opening Endoscopic

0BH70GZ Insertion of Endobronchial Valve into Left Main Bronchus, Open Approach

0BH73GZ Insertion of Endobronchial Valve into Left Main Bronchus, Percutaneous Approach

0BH74GZ Insertion of Endobronchial Valve into Left Main Bronchus, Percutaneous Endoscopic Approach

0BH77GZ Insertion of Endobronchial Valve into Left Main Bronchus, Via Natural or Artificial Opening

0BH78GZ Insertion of Endobronchial Valve into Left Main Bronchus, Via Natural or Artificial Opening Endoscopic

0BH80GZ Insertion of Endobronchial Valve into Left Upper Lobe Bronchus, Open Approach

0BH83GZ Insertion of Endobronchial Valve into Left Upper Lobe Bronchus, Percutaneous Approach

0BH84GZ Insertion of Endobronchial Valve into Left Upper Lobe Bronchus, Percutaneous Endoscopic Approach

0BH87GZ Insertion of Endobronchial Valve into Left Upper Lobe Bronchus, Via Natural or Artificial Opening

0BH88GZ Insertion of Endobronchial Valve into Left Upper Lobe Bronchus, Via Natural or Artificial Opening Endoscopic

0BH90GZ Insertion of Endobronchial Valve into Lingula Bronchus, Open Approach

0BH93GZ Insertion of Endobronchial Valve into Lingula Bronchus, Percutaneous Approach

0BH94GZ Insertion of Endobronchial Valve into Lingula Bronchus, Percutaneous Endoscopic Approach

0BH97GZ Insertion of Endobronchial Valve into Lingula Bronchus, Via Natural or Artificial Opening

0BH98GZ Insertion of Endobronchial Valve into Lingula Bronchus, Via Natural or Artificial Opening Endoscopic

0BHB0GZ Insertion of Endobronchial Valve into Left Lower Lobe Bronchus, Open Approach

0BHB3GZ Insertion of Endobronchial Valve into Left Lower Lobe Bronchus, Percutaneous Approach

0BHB4GZ Insertion of Endobronchial Valve into Left Lower Lobe Bronchus, Percutaneous Endoscopic Approach

0BHB7GZ Insertion of Endobronchial Valve into Left Lower Lobe Bronchus, Via Natural or Artificial Opening

0BHB8GZ Insertion of Endobronchial Valve into Left Lower Lobe Bronchus, Via Natural or Artificial Opening Endoscopic

0BHK01Z Insertion of Radioactive Element into Right Lung, Open Approach

0BHK02Z Insertion of Monitoring Device into Right Lung, Open Approach

0BHK03Z Insertion of Infusion Device into Right Lung, Open Approach

0BHK31Z Insertion of Radioactive Element into Right Lung, Percutaneous Approach

0BHK32Z Insertion of Monitoring Device into Right Lung, Percutaneous Approach

0BHK33Z Insertion of Infusion Device into Right Lung, Percutaneous Approach

0BHK41Z Insertion of Radioactive Element into Right Lung, Percutaneous Endoscopic Approach

0BHK42Z Insertion of Monitoring Device into Right Lung, Percutaneous Endoscopic Approach

0BHK43Z Insertion of Infusion Device into Right Lung, Percutaneous Endoscopic Approach

0BHK71Z Insertion of Radioactive Element into Right Lung, Via Natural or Artificial Opening

0BHK72Z Insertion of Monitoring Device into Right Lung, Via Natural or Artificial Opening

0BHK73Z Insertion of Infusion Device into Right Lung, Via Natural or Artificial Opening

0BHK81Z Insertion of Radioactive Element into Right Lung, Via Natural or Artificial Opening Endoscopic

0BHK82Z Insertion of Monitoring Device into Right Lung, Via Natural or Artificial Opening Endoscopic

0BHK83Z Insertion of Infusion Device into Right Lung, Via Natural or Artificial Opening Endoscopic

0BHL01Z Insertion of Radioactive Element into Left Lung, Open Approach

0BHL02Z Insertion of Monitoring Device into Left Lung, Open Approach

0BHL03Z Insertion of Infusion Device into Left Lung, Open Approach

0BHL31Z Insertion of Radioactive Element into Left Lung, Percutaneous Approach

0BHL32Z Insertion of Monitoring Device into Left Lung, Percutaneous Approach

0BHL33Z Insertion of Infusion Device into Left Lung, Percutaneous Approach

0BHL41Z Insertion of Radioactive Element into Left Lung, Percutaneous Endoscopic Approach

0BHL42Z Insertion of Monitoring Device into Left Lung, Percutaneous Endoscopic Approach

0BHL43Z Insertion of Infusion Device into Left Lung, Percutaneous Endoscopic Approach

0BHL71Z Insertion of Radioactive Element into Left Lung, Via Natural or Artificial Opening

0BHL72Z Insertion of Monitoring Device into Left Lung, Via Natural or Artificial Opening

0BHL73Z Insertion of Infusion Device into Left Lung, Via Natural or Artificial Opening

0BHL81Z Insertion of Radioactive Element into Left Lung, Via Natural or Artificial Opening Endoscopic

0BHL82Z Insertion of Monitoring Device into Left Lung, Via Natural or Artificial Opening Endoscopic

0BHL83Z Insertion of Infusion Device into Left Lung, Via Natural or Artificial Opening Endoscopic

0BHR02Z Insertion of Monitoring Device into Right Diaphragm, Open Approach

0BHR0MZ Insertion of Diaphragmatic Pacemaker Lead into Right Diaphragm, Open Approach

0BHR32Z Insertion of Monitoring Device into Right Diaphragm, Percutaneous Approach

0BHR3MZ Insertion of Diaphragmatic Pacemaker Lead into Right Diaphragm, Percutaneo Approach

0BHR42Z Insertion of Monitoring Device into Right Diaphragm, Percutaneous Endoscopic Approach

0BHR4MZ Insertion of Diaphragmatic Pacemaker Lead into Right Diaphragm, Percutaneo Endoscopic Approach

0BHS02Z Insertion of Monitoring Device into Left Diaphragm, Open Approach

0BHS0MZ Insertion of Diaphragmatic Pacemaker Lead into Left Diaphragm, Open Approach

0BHS32Z Insertion of Monitoring Device into Left Diaphragm, Percutaneous Approach

0BHS3MZ Insertion of Diaphragmatic Pacemaker Lead into Left Diaphragm, Percutaneous Approach

0BHS42Z Insertion of Monitoring Device into Left Diaphragm, Percutaneous Endoscopic Approach

0BHS4MZ Insertion of Diaphragmatic Pacemaker Lead into Left Diaphragm, Percutaneous Endoscopic Approach

0BJ – Respiratory System, Inspection

Review Coding Guidelines B3.11a, B3.11b and B3.11c

0BJ00ZZ Inspection of Tracheobronchial Tree, Open Approach

0BJ03ZZ Inspection of Tracheobronchial Tree, Percutaneous Approach

0BJ04ZZ Inspection of Tracheobronchial Tree, Percutaneous Endoscopic Approach

0BJ07ZZ Inspection of Tracheobronchial Tree, Via Natural or Artificial Opening

0BJ08ZZ Inspection of Tracheobronchial Tree, Via Natural or Artificial Opening Endoscopic

0BJ0XZZ Inspection of Tracheobronchial Tree, External Approach

0BJ10ZZ Inspection of Trachea, Open Approach

0BJ13ZZ Inspection of Trachea, Percutaneous Approach

0BJ14ZZ Inspection of Trachea, Percutaneous Endoscopic Approach

0BJ17ZZ Inspection of Trachea, Via Natural or Artificial Opening

0BJ18ZZ Inspection of Trachea, Via Natural or Artificial Opening Endoscopic

0BJ1XZZ Inspection of Trachea, External Approach

0BJK0ZZ Inspection of Right Lung, Open Approach

0BJK3ZZ Inspection of Right Lung, Percutaneous Approach

0BJK4ZZ Inspection of Right Lung, Percutaneous Endoscopic Approach

0BJK7ZZ Inspection of Right Lung, Via Natural or Artificial Opening

0BJK8ZZ Inspection of Right Lung, Via Natural or Artificial Opening Endoscopic

0BJKXZZ Inspection of Right Lung, External Approach

0BJL0ZZ Inspection of Left Lung, Open Approach

0BJL3ZZ Inspection of Left Lung, Percutaneous Approach

0BJL4ZZ Inspection of Left Lung, Percutaneous Endoscopic Approach

0BJL7ZZ Inspection of Left Lung, Via Natural or Artificial Opening

0BJL8ZZ Inspection of Left Lung, Via Natural or Artificial Opening Endoscopic

AHA CC: 1Q, 2014, 20

0BJLXZZ Inspection of Left Lung, External Approach

0BJQ0ZZ Inspection of Pleura, Open Approach

0BJQ3ZZ Inspection of Pleura, Percutaneous Approach

0BJQ4ZZ Inspection of Pleura, Percutaneous Endoscopic Approach

0BJQ7ZZ Inspection of Pleura, Via Natural or Artificial Opening

0BJQ8ZZ Inspection of Pleura, Via Natural or Artificial Opening Endoscopic

0BJQXZZ Inspection of Pleura, External Approach

0BJT0ZZ Inspection of Diaphragm, Open Approach

0BJT3ZZ Inspection of Diaphragm, Percutaneous Approach

0BJT4ZZ Inspection of Diaphragm, Percutaneous Endoscopic Approach

0BJT7ZZ Inspection of Diaphragm, Via Natural or Artificial Opening

0BJT8ZZ Inspection of Diaphragm, Via Natural or Artificial Opening Endoscopic

0BJTXZZ Inspection of Diaphragm, External Approach

0BL – Respiratory System, Occlusion

0BL10CZ Occlusion of Trachea with Extraluminal Device, Open Approach

0BL10DZ Occlusion of Trachea with Intraluminal Device, Open Approach

0BL10ZZ Occlusion of Trachea, Open Approach

0BL13CZ Occlusion of Trachea with Extraluminal Device, Percutaneous Approach

0BL13DZ Occlusion of Trachea with Intraluminal Device, Percutaneous Approach

0BL13ZZ Occlusion of Trachea, Percutaneous Approach

0BL14CZ Occlusion of Trachea with Extraluminal Device, Percutaneous Endoscopic Approach

0BL14DZ Occlusion of Trachea with Intraluminal Device, Percutaneous Endoscopic Approach

0BL14ZZ Occlusion of Trachea, Percutaneous Endoscopic Approach

0BL17DZ Occlusion of Trachea with Intraluminal Device, Via Natural or Artificial Opening

0BL17ZZ Occlusion of Trachea, Via Natural or Artificial Opening

0BL18DZ Occlusion of Trachea with Intraluminal Device, Via Natural or Artificial Opening Endoscopic

0BL18ZZ Occlusion of Trachea, Via Natural or Artificial Opening Endoscopic

 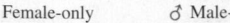

L20CZ Occlusion of Carina with Extraluminal Device, Open Approach
L20DZ Occlusion of Carina with Intraluminal Device, Open Approach
L20ZZ Occlusion of Carina, Open Approach
L23CZ Occlusion of Carina with Extraluminal Device, Percutaneous Approach
L23DZ Occlusion of Carina with Intraluminal Device, Percutaneous Approach
L23ZZ Occlusion of Carina, Percutaneous Approach
L24CZ Occlusion of Carina with Extraluminal Device, Percutaneous Endoscopic Approach
L24DZ Occlusion of Carina with Intraluminal Device, Percutaneous Endoscopic Approach
L24ZZ Occlusion of Carina, Percutaneous Endoscopic Approach
L27DZ Occlusion of Carina with Intraluminal Device, Via Natural or Artificial Opening
L27ZZ Occlusion of Carina, Via Natural or Artificial Opening
L28DZ Occlusion of Carina with Intraluminal Device, Via Natural or Artificial Opening Endoscopic
L28ZZ Occlusion of Carina, Via Natural or Artificial Opening Endoscopic
L30CZ Occlusion of Right Main Bronchus with Extraluminal Device, Open Approach
L30DZ Occlusion of Right Main Bronchus with Intraluminal Device, Open Approach
L30ZZ Occlusion of Right Main Bronchus, Open Approach
L33CZ Occlusion of Right Main Bronchus with Extraluminal Device, Percutaneous Approach
L33DZ Occlusion of Right Main Bronchus with Intraluminal Device, Percutaneous Approach
L33ZZ Occlusion of Right Main Bronchus, Percutaneous Approach
L34CZ Occlusion of Right Main Bronchus with Extraluminal Device, Percutaneous Endoscopic Approach
L34DZ Occlusion of Right Main Bronchus with Intraluminal Device, Percutaneous Endoscopic Approach
L34ZZ Occlusion of Right Main Bronchus, Percutaneous Endoscopic Approach
L37DZ Occlusion of Right Main Bronchus with Intraluminal Device, Via Natural or Artificial Opening
L37ZZ Occlusion of Right Main Bronchus, Via Natural or Artificial Opening
L38DZ Occlusion of Right Main Bronchus with Intraluminal Device, Via Natural or Artificial Opening Endoscopic
L38ZZ Occlusion of Right Main Bronchus, Via Natural or Artificial Opening Endoscopic
BL40CZ Occlusion of Right Upper Lobe Bronchus with Extraluminal Device, Open Approach
BL40DZ Occlusion of Right Upper Lobe Bronchus with Intraluminal Device, Open Approach
BL40ZZ Occlusion of Right Upper Lobe Bronchus, Open Approach
BL43CZ Occlusion of Right Upper Lobe Bronchus with Extraluminal Device, Percutaneous Approach
BL43DZ Occlusion of Right Upper Lobe Bronchus with Intraluminal Device, Percutaneous Approach
BL43ZZ Occlusion of Right Upper Lobe Bronchus, Percutaneous Approach
BL44CZ Occlusion of Right Upper Lobe Bronchus with Extraluminal Device, Percutaneous Endoscopic Approach

0BL44DZ Occlusion of Right Upper Lobe Bronchus with Intraluminal Device, Percutaneous Endoscopic Approach
0BL44ZZ Occlusion of Right Upper Lobe Bronchus, Percutaneous Endoscopic Approach
0BL47DZ Occlusion of Right Upper Lobe Bronchus with Intraluminal Device, Via Natural or Artificial Opening
0BL47ZZ Occlusion of Right Upper Lobe Bronchus, Via Natural or Artificial Opening
0BL48DZ Occlusion of Right Upper Lobe Bronchus with Intraluminal Device, Via Natural or Artificial Opening Endoscopic
0BL48ZZ Occlusion of Right Upper Lobe Bronchus, Via Natural or Artificial Opening Endoscopic
0BL50CZ Occlusion of Right Middle Lobe Bronchus with Extraluminal Device, Open Approach
0BL50DZ Occlusion of Right Middle Lobe Bronchus with Intraluminal Device, Open Approach
0BL50ZZ Occlusion of Right Middle Lobe Bronchus, Open Approach
0BL53CZ Occlusion of Right Middle Lobe Bronchus with Extraluminal Device, Percutaneous Approach
0BL53DZ Occlusion of Right Middle Lobe Bronchus with Intraluminal Device, Percutaneous Approach
0BL53ZZ Occlusion of Right Middle Lobe Bronchus, Percutaneous Approach
0BL54CZ Occlusion of Right Middle Lobe Bronchus with Extraluminal Device, Percutaneous Endoscopic Approach
0BL54DZ Occlusion of Right Middle Lobe Bronchus with Intraluminal Device, Percutaneous Endoscopic Approach
0BL54ZZ Occlusion of Right Middle Lobe Bronchus, Percutaneous Endoscopic Approach
0BL57DZ Occlusion of Right Middle Lobe Bronchus with Intraluminal Device, Via Natural or Artificial Opening
0BL57ZZ Occlusion of Right Middle Lobe Bronchus, Via Natural or Artificial Opening
0BL58DZ Occlusion of Right Middle Lobe Bronchus with Intraluminal Device, Via Natural or Artificial Opening Endoscopic
0BL58ZZ Occlusion of Right Middle Lobe Bronchus, Via Natural or Artificial Opening Endoscopic
0BL60CZ Occlusion of Right Lower Lobe Bronchus with Extraluminal Device, Open Approach
0BL60DZ Occlusion of Right Lower Lobe Bronchus with Intraluminal Device, Open Approach
0BL60ZZ Occlusion of Right Lower Lobe Bronchus, Open Approach
0BL63CZ Occlusion of Right Lower Lobe Bronchus with Extraluminal Device, Percutaneous Approach
0BL63DZ Occlusion of Right Lower Lobe Bronchus with Intraluminal Device, Percutaneous Approach
0BL63ZZ Occlusion of Right Lower Lobe Bronchus, Percutaneous Approach
0BL64CZ Occlusion of Right Lower Lobe Bronchus with Extraluminal Device, Percutaneous Endoscopic Approach
0BL64DZ Occlusion of Right Lower Lobe Bronchus with Intraluminal Device, Percutaneous Endoscopic Approach
0BL64ZZ Occlusion of Right Lower Lobe Bronchus, Percutaneous Endoscopic Approach
0BL67DZ Occlusion of Right Lower Lobe Bronchus with Intraluminal Device, Via Natural or Artificial Opening

0BL67ZZ Occlusion of Right Lower Lobe Bronchus, Via Natural or Artificial Opening
0BL68DZ Occlusion of Right Lower Lobe Bronchus with Intraluminal Device, Via Natural or Artificial Opening Endoscopic
0BL68ZZ Occlusion of Right Lower Lobe Bronchus, Via Natural or Artificial Opening Endoscopic
0BL70CZ Occlusion of Left Main Bronchus with Extraluminal Device, Open Approach
0BL70DZ Occlusion of Left Main Bronchus with Intraluminal Device, Open Approach
0BL70ZZ Occlusion of Left Main Bronchus, Open Approach
0BL73CZ Occlusion of Left Main Bronchus with Extraluminal Device, Percutaneous Approach
0BL73DZ Occlusion of Left Main Bronchus with Intraluminal Device, Percutaneous Approach
0BL73ZZ Occlusion of Left Main Bronchus, Percutaneous Approach
0BL74CZ Occlusion of Left Main Bronchus with Extraluminal Device, Percutaneous Endoscopic Approach
0BL74DZ Occlusion of Left Main Bronchus with Intraluminal Device, Percutaneous Endoscopic Approach
0BL74ZZ Occlusion of Left Main Bronchus, Percutaneous Endoscopic Approach
0BL77DZ Occlusion of Left Main Bronchus with Intraluminal Device, Via Natural or Artificial Opening
0BL77ZZ Occlusion of Left Main Bronchus, Via Natural or Artificial Opening
0BL78DZ Occlusion of Left Main Bronchus with Intraluminal Device, Via Natural or Artificial Opening Endoscopic
0BL78ZZ Occlusion of Left Main Bronchus, Via Natural or Artificial Opening Endoscopic
0BL80CZ Occlusion of Left Upper Lobe Bronchus with Extraluminal Device, Open Approach
0BL80DZ Occlusion of Left Upper Lobe Bronchus with Intraluminal Device, Open Approach
0BL80ZZ Occlusion of Left Upper Lobe Bronchus, Open Approach
0BL83CZ Occlusion of Left Upper Lobe Bronchus with Extraluminal Device, Percutaneous Approach
0BL83DZ Occlusion of Left Upper Lobe Bronchus with Intraluminal Device, Percutaneous Approach
0BL83ZZ Occlusion of Left Upper Lobe Bronchus, Percutaneous Approach
0BL84CZ Occlusion of Left Upper Lobe Bronchus with Extraluminal Device, Percutaneous Endoscopic Approach
0BL84DZ Occlusion of Left Upper Lobe Bronchus with Intraluminal Device, Percutaneous Endoscopic Approach
0BL84ZZ Occlusion of Left Upper Lobe Bronchus, Percutaneous Endoscopic Approach
0BL87DZ Occlusion of Left Upper Lobe Bronchus with Intraluminal Device, Via Natural or Artificial Opening
0BL87ZZ Occlusion of Left Upper Lobe Bronchus, Via Natural or Artificial Opening
0BL88DZ Occlusion of Left Upper Lobe Bronchus with Intraluminal Device, Via Natural or Artificial Opening Endoscopic
0BL88ZZ Occlusion of Left Upper Lobe Bronchus, Via Natural or Artificial Opening Endoscopic
0BL90CZ Occlusion of Lingula Bronchus with Extraluminal Device, Open Approach
0BL90DZ Occlusion of Lingula Bronchus with Intraluminal Device, Open Approach

♀ Female-only   ♂ Male-only   ▲ Limited Coverage   ● Non-OR   ▰ HAC-associated procedure   ▲ Non-covered procedures   ✛ Combination

0BL90ZZ	Occlusion of Lingula Bronchus, Open Approach	
0BL93CZ	Occlusion of Lingula Bronchus with Extraluminal Device, Percutaneous Approach	
0BL93DZ	Occlusion of Lingula Bronchus with Intraluminal Device, Percutaneous Approach	
0BL93ZZ	Occlusion of Lingula Bronchus, Percutaneous Approach	
0BL94CZ	Occlusion of Lingula Bronchus with Extraluminal Device, Percutaneous Endoscopic Approach	
0BL94DZ	Occlusion of Lingula Bronchus with Intraluminal Device, Percutaneous Endoscopic Approach	
0BL94ZZ	Occlusion of Lingula Bronchus, Percutaneous Endoscopic Approach	
0BL97DZ	Occlusion of Lingula Bronchus with Intraluminal Device, Via Natural or Artificial Opening	

0BL97ZZ	Occlusion of Lingula Bronchus, Via Natural or Artificial Opening
0BL98DZ	Occlusion of Lingula Bronchus with Intraluminal Device, Via Natural or Artificial Opening Endoscopic
0BL98ZZ	Occlusion of Lingula Bronchus, Via Natural or Artificial Opening Endoscopic
0BLB0CZ	Occlusion of Left Lower Lobe Bronchus with Extraluminal Device, Open Approach
0BLB0DZ	Occlusion of Left Lower Lobe Bronchus with Intraluminal Device, Open Approach
0BLB0ZZ	Occlusion of Left Lower Lobe Bronchus, Open Approach
0BLB3CZ	Occlusion of Left Lower Lobe Bronchus with Extraluminal Device, Percutaneous Approach
0BLB3DZ	Occlusion of Left Lower Lobe Bronchus with Intraluminal Device, Percutaneous Approach
0BLB3ZZ	Occlusion of Left Lower Lobe Bronchus, Percutaneous Approach

0BLB4CZ	Occlusion of Left Lower Lobe Bronchus with Extraluminal Device, Percutaneous Endoscopic Approach
0BLB4DZ	Occlusion of Left Lower Lobe Bronchus with Intraluminal Device, Percutaneous Endoscopic Approach
0BLB4ZZ	Occlusion of Left Lower Lobe Bronchus Percutaneous Endoscopic Approach
0BLB7DZ	Occlusion of Left Lower Lobe Bronchus with Intraluminal Device, Via Natural or Artificial Opening
0BLB7ZZ	Occlusion of Left Lower Lobe Bronchus Via Natural or Artificial Opening
0BLB8DZ	Occlusion of Left Lower Lobe Bronchus with Intraluminal Device, Via Natural or Artificial Opening Endoscopic
0BLB8ZZ	Occlusion of Left Lower Lobe Bronchus Via Natural or Artificial Opening Endoscopic

0BM – Respiratory System, Reattachment

0BM10ZZ	Reattachment of Trachea, Open Approach
0BM20ZZ	Reattachment of Carina, Open Approach
0BM30ZZ	Reattachment of Right Main Bronchus, Open Approach
0BM40ZZ	Reattachment of Right Upper Lobe Bronchus, Open Approach
0BM50ZZ	Reattachment of Right Middle Lobe Bronchus, Open Approach
0BM60ZZ	Reattachment of Right Lower Lobe Bronchus, Open Approach
0BM70ZZ	Reattachment of Left Main Bronchus, Open Approach
0BM80ZZ	Reattachment of Left Upper Lobe Bronchus, Open Approach

0BM90ZZ	Reattachment of Lingula Bronchus, Open Approach
0BMB0ZZ	Reattachment of Left Lower Lobe Bronchus, Open Approach
0BMC0ZZ	Reattachment of Right Upper Lung Lobe, Open Approach
0BMD0ZZ	Reattachment of Right Middle Lung Lobe, Open Approach
0BMF0ZZ	Reattachment of Right Lower Lung Lobe, Open Approach
0BMG0ZZ	Reattachment of Left Upper Lung Lobe, Open Approach
0BMH0ZZ	Reattachment of Lung Lingula, Open Approach

0BMJ0ZZ	Reattachment of Left Lower Lung Lobe, Open Approach
0BMK0ZZ	Reattachment of Right Lung, Open Approach
0BML0ZZ	Reattachment of Left Lung, Open Approach
0BMR0ZZ	Reattachment of Right Diaphragm, Open Approach
0BMS0ZZ	Reattachment of Left Diaphragm, Open Approach

0BN – Respiratory System, Release

Review Coding Guidelines B3.13 and B3.14

0BN10ZZ	Release Trachea, Open Approach
0BN13ZZ	Release Trachea, Percutaneous Approach
0BN14ZZ	Release Trachea, Percutaneous Endoscopic Approach
0BN17ZZ	Release Trachea, Via Natural or Artificial Opening
0BN18ZZ	Release Trachea, Via Natural or Artificial Opening Endoscopic
0BN20ZZ	Release Carina, Open Approach
0BN23ZZ	Release Carina, Percutaneous Approach
0BN24ZZ	Release Carina, Percutaneous Endoscopic Approach
0BN27ZZ	Release Carina, Via Natural or Artificial Opening
0BN28ZZ	Release Carina, Via Natural or Artificial Opening Endoscopic
0BN30ZZ	Release Right Main Bronchus, Open Approach
0BN33ZZ	Release Right Main Bronchus, Percutaneous Approach
0BN34ZZ	Release Right Main Bronchus, Percutaneous Endoscopic Approach
0BN37ZZ	Release Right Main Bronchus, Via Natural or Artificial Opening
0BN38ZZ	Release Right Main Bronchus, Via Natural or Artificial Opening Endoscopic
0BN40ZZ	Release Right Upper Lobe Bronchus, Open Approach
0BN43ZZ	Release Right Upper Lobe Bronchus, Percutaneous Approach
0BN44ZZ	Release Right Upper Lobe Bronchus, Percutaneous Endoscopic Approach
0BN47ZZ	Release Right Upper Lobe Bronchus, Via Natural or Artificial Opening

0BN48ZZ	Release Right Upper Lobe Bronchus, Via Natural or Artificial Opening Endoscopic
0BN50ZZ	Release Right Middle Lobe Bronchus, Open Approach
0BN53ZZ	Release Right Middle Lobe Bronchus, Percutaneous Approach
0BN54ZZ	Release Right Middle Lobe Bronchus, Percutaneous Endoscopic Approach
0BN57ZZ	Release Right Middle Lobe Bronchus, Via Natural or Artificial Opening
0BN58ZZ	Release Right Middle Lobe Bronchus, Via Natural or Artificial Opening Endoscopic
0BN60ZZ	Release Right Lower Lobe Bronchus, Open Approach
0BN63ZZ	Release Right Lower Lobe Bronchus, Percutaneous Approach
0BN64ZZ	Release Right Lower Lobe Bronchus, Percutaneous Endoscopic Approach
0BN67ZZ	Release Right Lower Lobe Bronchus, Via Natural or Artificial Opening
0BN68ZZ	Release Right Lower Lobe Bronchus, Via Natural or Artificial Opening Endoscopic
0BN70ZZ	Release Left Main Bronchus, Open Approach
0BN73ZZ	Release Left Main Bronchus, Percutaneous Approach
0BN74ZZ	Release Left Main Bronchus, Percutaneous Endoscopic Approach
0BN77ZZ	Release Left Main Bronchus, Via Natural or Artificial Opening
0BN78ZZ	Release Left Main Bronchus, Via Natural or Artificial Opening Endoscopic
0BN80ZZ	Release Left Upper Lobe Bronchus, Open Approach

0BN83ZZ	Release Left Upper Lobe Bronchus, Percutaneous Approach
0BN84ZZ	Release Left Upper Lobe Bronchus, Percutaneous Endoscopic Approach
0BN87ZZ	Release Left Upper Lobe Bronchus, Via Natural or Artificial Opening
0BN88ZZ	Release Left Upper Lobe Bronchus, Via Natural or Artificial Opening Endoscopic
0BN90ZZ	Release Lingula Bronchus, Open Approach
0BN93ZZ	Release Lingula Bronchus, Percutaneous Approach
0BN94ZZ	Release Lingula Bronchus, Percutaneous Endoscopic Approach
0BN97ZZ	Release Lingula Bronchus, Via Natural or Artificial Opening
0BN98ZZ	Release Lingula Bronchus, Via Natural or Artificial Opening Endoscopic
0BNB0ZZ	Release Left Lower Lobe Bronchus, Open Approach
0BNB3ZZ	Release Left Lower Lobe Bronchus, Percutaneous Approach
0BNB4ZZ	Release Left Lower Lobe Bronchus, Percutaneous Endoscopic Approach
0BNB7ZZ	Release Left Lower Lobe Bronchus, Via Natural or Artificial Opening
0BNB8ZZ	Release Left Lower Lobe Bronchus, Via Natural or Artificial Opening Endoscopic
0BNC0ZZ	Release Right Upper Lung Lobe, Open Approach
0BNC3ZZ	Release Right Upper Lung Lobe, Percutaneous Approach
0BNC4ZZ	Release Right Upper Lung Lobe, Percutaneous Endoscopic Approach

C7ZZ	Release Right Upper Lung Lobe, Via Natural or Artificial Opening	**0BNG8ZZ** Release Left Upper Lung Lobe, Via Natural or Artificial Opening Endoscopic
C8ZZ	Release Right Upper Lung Lobe, Via Natural or Artificial Opening Endoscopic	**0BNH0ZZ** Release Lung Lingula, Open Approach

C7ZZ Release Right Upper Lung Lobe, Via Natural or Artificial Opening

C8ZZ Release Right Upper Lung Lobe, Via Natural or Artificial Opening Endoscopic

D0ZZ Release Right Middle Lung Lobe, Open Approach

D3ZZ Release Right Middle Lung Lobe, Percutaneous Approach

D4ZZ Release Right Middle Lung Lobe, Percutaneous Endoscopic Approach

D7ZZ Release Right Middle Lung Lobe, Via Natural or Artificial Opening

D8ZZ Release Right Middle Lung Lobe, Via Natural or Artificial Opening Endoscopic

F0ZZ Release Right Lower Lung Lobe, Open Approach

F3ZZ Release Right Lower Lung Lobe, Percutaneous Approach

F4ZZ Release Right Lower Lung Lobe, Percutaneous Endoscopic Approach

F7ZZ Release Right Lower Lung Lobe, Via Natural or Artificial Opening

F8ZZ Release Right Lower Lung Lobe, Via Natural or Artificial Opening Endoscopic

G0ZZ Release Left Upper Lung Lobe, Open Approach

G3ZZ Release Left Upper Lung Lobe, Percutaneous Approach

G4ZZ Release Left Upper Lung Lobe, Percutaneous Endoscopic Approach

G7ZZ Release Left Upper Lung Lobe, Via Natural or Artificial Opening

0BNG8ZZ Release Left Upper Lung Lobe, Via Natural or Artificial Opening Endoscopic

0BNH0ZZ Release Lung Lingula, Open Approach

0BNH3ZZ Release Lung Lingula, Percutaneous Approach

0BNH4ZZ Release Lung Lingula, Percutaneous Endoscopic Approach

0BNH7ZZ Release Lung Lingula, Via Natural or Artificial Opening

0BNH8ZZ Release Lung Lingula, Via Natural or Artificial Opening Endoscopic

0BNJ0ZZ Release Left Lower Lung Lobe, Open Approach

0BNJ3ZZ Release Left Lower Lung Lobe, Percutaneous Approach

0BNJ4ZZ Release Left Lower Lung Lobe, Percutaneous Endoscopic Approach

0BNJ7ZZ Release Left Lower Lung Lobe, Via Natural or Artificial Opening

0BNJ8ZZ Release Left Lower Lung Lobe, Via Natural or Artificial Opening Endoscopic

0BNK0ZZ Release Right Lung, Open Approach

0BNK3ZZ Release Right Lung, Percutaneous Approach

0BNK4ZZ Release Right Lung, Percutaneous Endoscopic Approach

0BNK7ZZ Release Right Lung, Via Natural or Artificial Opening

0BNK8ZZ Release Right Lung, Via Natural or Artificial Opening Endoscopic

0BNL0ZZ Release Left Lung, Open Approach

0BNL3ZZ Release Left Lung, Percutaneous Approach

0BNL4ZZ Release Left Lung, Percutaneous Endoscopic Approach

0BNL7ZZ Release Left Lung, Via Natural or Artificial Opening

0BNL8ZZ Release Left Lung, Via Natural or Artificial Opening Endoscopic

0BNM0ZZ Release Bilateral Lungs, Open Approach

0BNM3ZZ Release Bilateral Lungs, Percutaneous Approach

0BNM4ZZ Release Bilateral Lungs, Percutaneous Endoscopic Approach

0BNM7ZZ Release Bilateral Lungs, Via Natural or Artificial Opening

0BNM8ZZ Release Bilateral Lungs, Via Natural or Artificial Opening Endoscopic

0BNN0ZZ Release Right Pleura, Open Approach

0BNN3ZZ Release Right Pleura, Percutaneous Approach

0BNN4ZZ Release Right Pleura, Percutaneous Endoscopic Approach

0BNP0ZZ Release Left Pleura, Open Approach

0BNP3ZZ Release Left Pleura, Percutaneous Approach

0BNP4ZZ Release Left Pleura, Percutaneous Endoscopic Approach

0BNR0ZZ Release Right Diaphragm, Open Approach

0BNR3ZZ Release Right Diaphragm, Percutaneous Approach

0BNR4ZZ Release Right Diaphragm, Percutaneous Endoscopic Approach

0BNS0ZZ Release Left Diaphragm, Open Approach

0BNS3ZZ Release Left Diaphragm, Percutaneous Approach

0BNS4ZZ Release Left Diaphragm, Percutaneous Endoscopic Approach

P – Respiratory System, Removal

view Coding Guideline B6.1c

P000Z Removal of Drainage Device from Tracheobronchial Tree, Open Approach

P001Z Removal of Radioactive Element from Tracheobronchial Tree, Open Approach

P002Z Removal of Monitoring Device from Tracheobronchial Tree, Open Approach

P003Z Removal of Infusion Device from Tracheobronchial Tree, Open Approach

P007Z Removal of Autologous Tissue Substitute from Tracheobronchial Tree, Open Approach

P00CZ Removal of Extraluminal Device from Tracheobronchial Tree, Open Approach

P00DZ Removal of Intraluminal Device from Tracheobronchial Tree, Open Approach

P00JZ Removal of Synthetic Substitute from Tracheobronchial Tree, Open Approach

P00KZ Removal of Nonautologous Tissue Substitute from Tracheobronchial Tree, Open Approach

P030Z Removal of Drainage Device from Tracheobronchial Tree, Percutaneous Approach

P031Z Removal of Radioactive Element from Tracheobronchial Tree, Percutaneous Approach

P032Z Removal of Monitoring Device from Tracheobronchial Tree, Percutaneous Approach

P033Z Removal of Infusion Device from Tracheobronchial Tree, Percutaneous Approach

P037Z Removal of Autologous Tissue Substitute from Tracheobronchial Tree, Percutaneous Approach

0BP03CZ Removal of Extraluminal Device from Tracheobronchial Tree, Percutaneous Approach

0BP03DZ Removal of Intraluminal Device from Tracheobronchial Tree, Percutaneous Approach

0BP03JZ Removal of Synthetic Substitute from Tracheobronchial Tree, Percutaneous Approach

0BP03KZ Removal of Nonautologous Tissue Substitute from Tracheobronchial Tree, Percutaneous Approach

0BP040Z Removal of Drainage Device from Tracheobronchial Tree, Percutaneous Endoscopic Approach

0BP041Z Removal of Radioactive Element from Tracheobronchial Tree, Percutaneous Endoscopic Approach

0BP042Z Removal of Monitoring Device from Tracheobronchial Tree, Percutaneous Endoscopic Approach

0BP043Z Removal of Infusion Device from Tracheobronchial Tree, Percutaneous Endoscopic Approach

0BP047Z Removal of Autologous Tissue Substitute from Tracheobronchial Tree, Percutaneous Endoscopic Approach

0BP04CZ Removal of Extraluminal Device from Tracheobronchial Tree, Percutaneous Endoscopic Approach

0BP04DZ Removal of Intraluminal Device from Tracheobronchial Tree, Percutaneous Endoscopic Approach

0BP04JZ Removal of Synthetic Substitute from Tracheobronchial Tree, Percutaneous Endoscopic Approach

0BP04KZ Removal of Nonautologous Tissue Substitute from Tracheobronchial Tree, Percutaneous Endoscopic Approach

0BP070Z Removal of Drainage Device from Tracheobronchial Tree, Via Natural or Artificial Opening

0BP071Z Removal of Radioactive Element from Tracheobronchial Tree, Via Natural or Artificial Opening

0BP072Z Removal of Monitoring Device from Tracheobronchial Tree, Via Natural or Artificial Opening

0BP073Z Removal of Infusion Device from Tracheobronchial Tree, Via Natural or Artificial Opening

0BP077Z Removal of Autologous Tissue Substitute from Tracheobronchial Tree, Via Natural or Artificial Opening

0BP07CZ Removal of Extraluminal Device from Tracheobronchial Tree, Via Natural or Artificial Opening

0BP07DZ Removal of Intraluminal Device from Tracheobronchial Tree, Via Natural or Artificial Opening

0BP07JZ Removal of Synthetic Substitute from Tracheobronchial Tree, Via Natural or Artificial Opening

0BP07KZ Removal of Nonautologous Tissue Substitute from Tracheobronchial Tree, Via Natural or Artificial Opening

0BP080Z Removal of Drainage Device from Tracheobronchial Tree, Via Natural or Artificial Opening Endoscopic

0BP081Z Removal of Radioactive Element from Tracheobronchial Tree, Via Natural or Artificial Opening Endoscopic

481

0BP082Z Removal of Monitoring Device from Tracheobronchial Tree, Via Natural or Artificial Opening Endoscopic

0BP083Z Removal of Infusion Device from Tracheobronchial Tree, Via Natural or Artificial Opening Endoscopic

0BP087Z Removal of Autologous Tissue Substitute from Tracheobronchial Tree, Via Natural or Artificial Opening Endoscopic

0BP08CZ Removal of Extraluminal Device from Tracheobronchial Tree, Via Natural or Artificial Opening Endoscopic

0BP08DZ Removal of Intraluminal Device from Tracheobronchial Tree, Via Natural or Artificial Opening Endoscopic

0BP08JZ Removal of Synthetic Substitute from Tracheobronchial Tree, Via Natural or Artificial Opening Endoscopic

0BP08KZ Removal of Nonautologous Tissue Substitute from Tracheobronchial Tree, Via Natural or Artificial Opening Endoscopic

0BP0X0Z Removal of Drainage Device from Tracheobronchial Tree, External Approach

0BP0X1Z Removal of Radioactive Element from Tracheobronchial Tree, External Approach

0BP0X2Z Removal of Monitoring Device from Tracheobronchial Tree, External Approach

0BP0X3Z Removal of Infusion Device from Tracheobronchial Tree, External Approach

0BP0XDZ Removal of Intraluminal Device from Tracheobronchial Tree, External Approach

0BP100Z Removal of Drainage Device from Trachea, Open Approach

0BP102Z Removal of Monitoring Device from Trachea, Open Approach

0BP107Z Removal of Autologous Tissue Substitute from Trachea, Open Approach

0BP10CZ Removal of Extraluminal Device from Trachea, Open Approach

0BP10DZ Removal of Intraluminal Device from Trachea, Open Approach

0BP10FZ Removal of Tracheostomy Device from Trachea, Open Approach

0BP10JZ Removal of Synthetic Substitute from Trachea, Open Approach

0BP10KZ Removal of Nonautologous Tissue Substitute from Trachea, Open Approach

0BP130Z Removal of Drainage Device from Trachea, Percutaneous Approach

0BP132Z Removal of Monitoring Device from Trachea, Percutaneous Approach

0BP137Z Removal of Autologous Tissue Substitute from Trachea, Percutaneous Approach

0BP13CZ Removal of Extraluminal Device from Trachea, Percutaneous Approach

0BP13DZ Removal of Intraluminal Device from Trachea, Percutaneous Approach

0BP13FZ Removal of Tracheostomy Device from Trachea, Percutaneous Approach

0BP13JZ Removal of Synthetic Substitute from Trachea, Percutaneous Approach

0BP13KZ Removal of Nonautologous Tissue Substitute from Trachea, Percutaneous Approach

0BP140Z Removal of Drainage Device from Trachea, Percutaneous Endoscopic Approach

0BP142Z Removal of Monitoring Device from Trachea, Percutaneous Endoscopic Approach

0BP147Z Removal of Autologous Tissue Substitute from Trachea, Percutaneous Endoscopic Approach

0BP14CZ Removal of Extraluminal Device from Trachea, Percutaneous Endoscopic Approach

0BP14DZ Removal of Intraluminal Device from Trachea, Percutaneous Endoscopic Approach

0BP14FZ Removal of Tracheostomy Device from Trachea, Percutaneous Endoscopic Approach

0BP14JZ Removal of Synthetic Substitute from Trachea, Percutaneous Endoscopic Approach

0BP14KZ Removal of Nonautologous Tissue Substitute from Trachea, Percutaneous Endoscopic Approach

0BP170Z Removal of Drainage Device from Trachea, Via Natural or Artificial Opening

0BP172Z Removal of Monitoring Device from Trachea, Via Natural or Artificial Opening

0BP177Z Removal of Autologous Tissue Substitute from Trachea, Via Natural or Artificial Opening

0BP17CZ Removal of Extraluminal Device from Trachea, Via Natural or Artificial Opening

0BP17DZ Removal of Intraluminal Device from Trachea, Via Natural or Artificial Opening

0BP17FZ Removal of Tracheostomy Device from Trachea, Via Natural or Artificial Opening

0BP17JZ Removal of Synthetic Substitute from Trachea, Via Natural or Artificial Opening

0BP17KZ Removal of Nonautologous Tissue Substitute from Trachea, Via Natural or Artificial Opening

0BP180Z Removal of Drainage Device from Trachea, Via Natural or Artificial Opening Endoscopic

0BP182Z Removal of Monitoring Device from Trachea, Via Natural or Artificial Opening Endoscopic

0BP187Z Removal of Autologous Tissue Substitute from Trachea, Via Natural or Artificial Opening Endoscopic

0BP18CZ Removal of Extraluminal Device from Trachea, Via Natural or Artificial Opening Endoscopic

0BP18DZ Removal of Intraluminal Device from Trachea, Via Natural or Artificial Opening Endoscopic

0BP18FZ Removal of Tracheostomy Device from Trachea, Via Natural or Artificial Opening Endoscopic

0BP18JZ Removal of Synthetic Substitute from Trachea, Via Natural or Artificial Opening Endoscopic

0BP18KZ Removal of Nonautologous Tissue Substitute from Trachea, Via Natural or Artificial Opening Endoscopic

0BP1X0Z Removal of Drainage Device from Trachea, External Approach

0BP1X2Z Removal of Monitoring Device from Trachea, External Approach

0BP1XDZ Removal of Intraluminal Device from Trachea, External Approach

0BP1XFZ Removal of Tracheostomy Device from Trachea, External Approach

0BPK00Z Removal of Drainage Device from Right Lung, Open Approach

0BPK01Z Removal of Radioactive Element from Right Lung, Open Approach

0BPK02Z Removal of Monitoring Device from Right Lung, Open Approach

0BPK03Z Removal of Infusion Device from Right Lung, Open Approach

0BPK30Z Removal of Drainage Device from Right Lung, Percutaneous Approach

0BPK31Z Removal of Radioactive Element from Right Lung, Percutaneous Approach

0BPK32Z Removal of Monitoring Device from Right Lung, Percutaneous Approach

0BPK33Z Removal of Infusion Device from Right Lung, Percutaneous Approach

0BPK40Z Removal of Drainage Device from Right Lung, Percutaneous Endoscopic Approach

0BPK41Z Removal of Radioactive Element from Right Lung, Percutaneous Endoscopic Approach

0BPK42Z Removal of Monitoring Device from Right Lung, Percutaneous Endoscopic Approach

0BPK43Z Removal of Infusion Device from Right Lung, Percutaneous Endoscopic Approach

0BPK70Z Removal of Drainage Device from Right Lung, Via Natural or Artificial Opening

0BPK71Z Removal of Radioactive Element from Right Lung, Via Natural or Artificial Opening

0BPK72Z Removal of Monitoring Device from Right Lung, Via Natural or Artificial Opening

0BPK73Z Removal of Infusion Device from Right Lung, Via Natural or Artificial Opening

0BPK80Z Removal of Drainage Device from Right Lung, Via Natural or Artificial Opening Endoscopic

0BPK81Z Removal of Radioactive Element from Right Lung, Via Natural or Artificial Opening Endoscopic

0BPK82Z Removal of Monitoring Device from Right Lung, Via Natural or Artificial Opening Endoscopic

0BPK83Z Removal of Infusion Device from Right Lung, Via Natural or Artificial Opening Endoscopic

0BPKX0Z Removal of Drainage Device from Right Lung, External Approach

0BPKX1Z Removal of Radioactive Element from Right Lung, External Approach

0BPKX2Z Removal of Monitoring Device from Right Lung, External Approach

0BPKX3Z Removal of Infusion Device from Right Lung, External Approach

0BPL00Z Removal of Drainage Device from Left Lung, Open Approach

0BPL01Z Removal of Radioactive Element from Left Lung, Open Approach

0BPL02Z Removal of Monitoring Device from Left Lung, Open Approach

0BPL03Z Removal of Infusion Device from Left Lung, Open Approach

0BPL30Z Removal of Drainage Device from Left Lung, Percutaneous Approach

0BPL31Z Removal of Radioactive Element from Left Lung, Percutaneous Approach

0BPL32Z Removal of Monitoring Device from Left Lung, Percutaneous Approach

0BPL33Z Removal of Infusion Device from Left Lung, Percutaneous Approach

0BPL40Z Removal of Drainage Device from Left Lung, Percutaneous Endoscopic Approach

0BPL41Z Removal of Radioactive Element from Left Lung, Percutaneous Endoscopic Approach

0BPL42Z Removal of Monitoring Device from Left Lung, Percutaneous Endoscopic Approach

0BPL43Z Removal of Infusion Device from Left Lung, Percutaneous Endoscopic Approach

0BPL70Z Removal of Drainage Device from Left Lung, Via Natural or Artificial Opening

0BPL71Z Removal of Radioactive Element from Left Lung, Via Natural or Artificial Opening

0BPL72Z Removal of Monitoring Device from Left Lung, Via Natural or Artificial Opening

0BPL73Z Removal of Infusion Device from Left Lung, Via Natural or Artificial Opening

0BPL80Z Removal of Drainage Device from Left Lung, Via Natural or Artificial Opening Endoscopic

L81Z Removal of Radioactive Element from Left Lung, Via Natural or Artificial Opening Endoscopic
L82Z Removal of Monitoring Device from Left Lung, Via Natural or Artificial Opening Endoscopic
L83Z Removal of Infusion Device from Left Lung, Via Natural or Artificial Opening Endoscopic
LX0Z Removal of Drainage Device from Left Lung, External Approach
LX1Z Removal of Radioactive Element from Left Lung, External Approach
LX2Z Removal of Monitoring Device from Left Lung, External Approach
LX3Z Removal of Infusion Device from Left Lung, External Approach
Q00Z Removal of Drainage Device from Pleura, Open Approach
Q01Z Removal of Radioactive Element from Pleura, Open Approach
Q02Z Removal of Monitoring Device from Pleura, Open Approach
Q30Z Removal of Drainage Device from Pleura, Percutaneous Approach
Q31Z Removal of Radioactive Element from Pleura, Percutaneous Approach
Q32Z Removal of Monitoring Device from Pleura, Percutaneous Approach
Q40Z Removal of Drainage Device from Pleura, Percutaneous Endoscopic Approach
Q41Z Removal of Radioactive Element from Pleura, Percutaneous Endoscopic Approach
Q42Z Removal of Monitoring Device from Pleura, Percutaneous Endoscopic Approach
Q70Z Removal of Drainage Device from Pleura, Via Natural or Artificial Opening
Q71Z Removal of Radioactive Element from Pleura, Via Natural or Artificial Opening
Q72Z Removal of Monitoring Device from Pleura, Via Natural or Artificial Opening
Q80Z Removal of Drainage Device from Pleura, Via Natural or Artificial Opening Endoscopic
Q81Z Removal of Radioactive Element from Pleura, Via Natural or Artificial Opening Endoscopic

0BPQ82Z Removal of Monitoring Device from Pleura, Via Natural or Artificial Opening Endoscopic
0BPQX0Z Removal of Drainage Device from Pleura, External Approach
0BPQX1Z Removal of Radioactive Element from Pleura, External Approach
0BPQX2Z Removal of Monitoring Device from Pleura, External Approach
0BPT00Z Removal of Drainage Device from Diaphragm, Open Approach
0BPT02Z Removal of Monitoring Device from Diaphragm, Open Approach
0BPT07Z Removal of Autologous Tissue Substitute from Diaphragm, Open Approach
0BPT0JZ Removal of Synthetic Substitute from Diaphragm, Open Approach
0BPT0KZ Removal of Nonautologous Tissue Substitute from Diaphragm, Open Approach
0BPT0MZ Removal of Diaphragmatic Pacemaker Lead from Diaphragm, Open Approach
0BPT30Z Removal of Drainage Device from Diaphragm, Percutaneous Approach
0BPT32Z Removal of Monitoring Device from Diaphragm, Percutaneous Approach
0BPT37Z Removal of Autologous Tissue Substitute from Diaphragm, Percutaneous Approach
0BPT3JZ Removal of Synthetic Substitute from Diaphragm, Percutaneous Approach
0BPT3KZ Removal of Nonautologous Tissue Substitute from Diaphragm, Percutaneous Approach
0BPT3MZ Removal of Diaphragmatic Pacemaker Lead from Diaphragm, Percutaneous Approach
0BPT40Z Removal of Drainage Device from Diaphragm, Percutaneous Endoscopic Approach
0BPT42Z Removal of Monitoring Device from Diaphragm, Percutaneous Endoscopic Approach
0BPT47Z Removal of Autologous Tissue Substitute from Diaphragm, Percutaneous Endoscopic Approach
0BPT4JZ Removal of Synthetic Substitute from Diaphragm, Percutaneous Endoscopic Approach

0BPT4KZ Removal of Nonautologous Tissue Substitute from Diaphragm, Percutaneous Endoscopic Approach
0BPT4MZ Removal of Diaphragmatic Pacemaker Lead from Diaphragm, Percutaneous Endoscopic Approach
0BPT70Z Removal of Drainage Device from Diaphragm, Via Natural or Artificial Opening
0BPT72Z Removal of Monitoring Device from Diaphragm, Via Natural or Artificial Opening
0BPT77Z Removal of Autologous Tissue Substitute from Diaphragm, Via Natural or Artificial Opening
0BPT7JZ Removal of Synthetic Substitute from Diaphragm, Via Natural or Artificial Opening
0BPT7KZ Removal of Nonautologous Tissue Substitute from Diaphragm, Via Natural or Artificial Opening
0BPT7MZ Removal of Diaphragmatic Pacemaker Lead from Diaphragm, Via Natural or Artificial Opening
0BPT80Z Removal of Drainage Device from Diaphragm, Via Natural or Artificial Opening Endoscopic
0BPT82Z Removal of Monitoring Device from Diaphragm, Via Natural or Artificial Opening Endoscopic
0BPT87Z Removal of Autologous Tissue Substitute from Diaphragm, Via Natural or Artificial Opening Endoscopic
0BPT8JZ Removal of Synthetic Substitute from Diaphragm, Via Natural or Artificial Opening Endoscopic
0BPT8KZ Removal of Nonautologous Tissue Substitute from Diaphragm, Via Natural or Artificial Opening Endoscopic
0BPT8MZ Removal of Diaphragmatic Pacemaker Lead from Diaphragm, Via Natural or Artificial Opening Endoscopic
0BPTX0Z Removal of Drainage Device from Diaphragm, External Approach
0BPTX2Z Removal of Monitoring Device from Diaphragm, External Approach
0BPTXMZ Removal of Diaphragmatic Pacemaker Lead from Diaphragm, External Approach

Q – Respiratory System, Repair

Q10ZZ Repair Trachea, Open Approach
Q13ZZ Repair Trachea, Percutaneous Approach
Q14ZZ Repair Trachea, Percutaneous Endoscopic Approach
Q17ZZ Repair Trachea, Via Natural or Artificial Opening
Q18ZZ Repair Trachea, Via Natural or Artificial Opening Endoscopic
Q20ZZ Repair Carina, Open Approach
Q23ZZ Repair Carina, Percutaneous Approach
Q24ZZ Repair Carina, Percutaneous Endoscopic Approach
Q27ZZ Repair Carina, Via Natural or Artificial Opening
Q28ZZ Repair Carina, Via Natural or Artificial Opening Endoscopic
Q30ZZ Repair Right Main Bronchus, Open Approach
Q33ZZ Repair Right Main Bronchus, Percutaneous Approach
Q34ZZ Repair Right Main Bronchus, Percutaneous Endoscopic Approach
Q37ZZ Repair Right Main Bronchus, Via Natural or Artificial Opening

0BQ38ZZ Repair Right Main Bronchus, Via Natural or Artificial Opening Endoscopic
0BQ40ZZ Repair Right Upper Lobe Bronchus, Open Approach
0BQ43ZZ Repair Right Upper Lobe Bronchus, Percutaneous Approach
0BQ44ZZ Repair Right Upper Lobe Bronchus, Percutaneous Endoscopic Approach
0BQ47ZZ Repair Right Upper Lobe Bronchus, Via Natural or Artificial Opening
0BQ48ZZ Repair Right Upper Lobe Bronchus, Via Natural or Artificial Opening Endoscopic
0BQ50ZZ Repair Right Middle Lobe Bronchus, Open Approach
0BQ53ZZ Repair Right Middle Lobe Bronchus, Percutaneous Approach
0BQ54ZZ Repair Right Middle Lobe Bronchus, Percutaneous Endoscopic Approach
0BQ57ZZ Repair Right Middle Lobe Bronchus, Via Natural or Artificial Opening
0BQ58ZZ Repair Right Middle Lobe Bronchus, Via Natural or Artificial Opening Endoscopic
0BQ60ZZ Repair Right Lower Lobe Bronchus, Open Approach

0BQ63ZZ Repair Right Lower Lobe Bronchus, Percutaneous Approach
0BQ64ZZ Repair Right Lower Lobe Bronchus, Percutaneous Endoscopic Approach
0BQ67ZZ Repair Right Lower Lobe Bronchus, Via Natural or Artificial Opening
0BQ68ZZ Repair Right Lower Lobe Bronchus, Via Natural or Artificial Opening Endoscopic
0BQ70ZZ Repair Left Main Bronchus, Open Approach
0BQ73ZZ Repair Left Main Bronchus, Percutaneous Approach
0BQ74ZZ Repair Left Main Bronchus, Percutaneous Endoscopic Approach
0BQ77ZZ Repair Left Main Bronchus, Via Natural or Artificial Opening
0BQ78ZZ Repair Left Main Bronchus, Via Natural or Artificial Opening Endoscopic
0BQ80ZZ Repair Left Upper Lobe Bronchus, Open Approach
0BQ83ZZ Repair Left Upper Lobe Bronchus, Percutaneous Approach

0BQ84ZZ	Repair Left Upper Lobe Bronchus, Percutaneous Endoscopic Approach	0BQD8ZZ	Repair Right Middle Lung Lobe, Via Natural or Artificial Opening Endoscopic	0BQK4ZZ	Repair Right Lung, Percutaneous Endoscopic Approach
0BQ87ZZ	Repair Left Upper Lobe Bronchus, Via Natural or Artificial Opening	0BQF0ZZ	Repair Right Lower Lung Lobe, Open Approach	0BQK7ZZ	Repair Right Lung, Via Natural or Artificial Opening
0BQ88ZZ	Repair Left Upper Lobe Bronchus, Via Natural or Artificial Opening Endoscopic	0BQF3ZZ	Repair Right Lower Lung Lobe, Percutaneous Approach	0BQK8ZZ	Repair Right Lung, Via Natural or Artificial Opening Endoscopic
0BQ90ZZ	Repair Lingula Bronchus, Open Approach	0BQF4ZZ	Repair Right Lower Lung Lobe, Percutaneous Endoscopic Approach	0BQL0ZZ	Repair Left Lung, Open Approach
0BQ93ZZ	Repair Lingula Bronchus, Percutaneous Approach			0BQL3ZZ	Repair Left Lung, Percutaneous Appro...
0BQ94ZZ	Repair Lingula Bronchus, Percutaneous Endoscopic Approach	0BQF7ZZ	Repair Right Lower Lung Lobe, Via Natural or Artificial Opening	0BQL4ZZ	Repair Left Lung, Percutaneous Endoscopic Approach
0BQ97ZZ	Repair Lingula Bronchus, Via Natural or Artificial Opening	0BQF8ZZ	Repair Right Lower Lung Lobe, Via Natural or Artificial Opening Endoscopic	0BQL7ZZ	Repair Left Lung, Via Natural or Artifi... Opening
0BQ98ZZ	Repair Lingula Bronchus, Via Natural or Artificial Opening Endoscopic	0BQG0ZZ	Repair Left Upper Lung Lobe, Open Approach	0BQL8ZZ	Repair Left Lung, Via Natural or Artifi... Opening Endoscopic
0BQB0ZZ	Repair Left Lower Lobe Bronchus, Open Approach	0BQG3ZZ	Repair Left Upper Lung Lobe, Percutaneous Approach	0BQM0ZZ	Repair Bilateral Lungs, Open Approach
0BQB3ZZ	Repair Left Lower Lobe Bronchus, Percutaneous Approach	0BQG4ZZ	Repair Left Upper Lung Lobe, Percutaneous Endoscopic Approach	0BQM3ZZ	Repair Bilateral Lungs, Percutaneous Approach
0BQB4ZZ	Repair Left Lower Lobe Bronchus, Percutaneous Endoscopic Approach	0BQG7ZZ	Repair Left Upper Lung Lobe, Via Natural or Artificial Opening	0BQM4ZZ	Repair Bilateral Lungs, Percutaneous Endoscopic Approach
0BQB7ZZ	Repair Left Lower Lobe Bronchus, Via Natural or Artificial Opening	0BQG8ZZ	Repair Left Upper Lung Lobe, Via Natural or Artificial Opening Endoscopic	0BQM7ZZ	Repair Bilateral Lungs, Via Natural or Artificial Opening
0BQB8ZZ	Repair Left Lower Lobe Bronchus, Via Natural or Artificial Opening Endoscopic	0BQH0ZZ	Repair Lung Lingula, Open Approach	0BQM8ZZ	Repair Bilateral Lungs, Via Natural or Artificial Opening Endoscopic
0BQC0ZZ	Repair Right Upper Lung Lobe, Open Approach	0BQH3ZZ	Repair Lung Lingula, Percutaneous Approach	0BQN0ZZ	Repair Right Pleura, Open Approach
0BQC3ZZ	Repair Right Upper Lung Lobe, Percutaneous Approach	0BQH4ZZ	Repair Lung Lingula, Percutaneous Endoscopic Approach	0BQN3ZZ	Repair Right Pleura, Percutaneous Approach
0BQC4ZZ	Repair Right Upper Lung Lobe, Percutaneous Endoscopic Approach	0BQH7ZZ	Repair Lung Lingula, Via Natural or Artificial Opening	0BQN4ZZ	Repair Right Pleura, Percutaneous Endoscopic Approach
0BQC7ZZ	Repair Right Upper Lung Lobe, Via Natural or Artificial Opening	0BQH8ZZ	Repair Lung Lingula, Via Natural or Artificial Opening Endoscopic	0BQP0ZZ	Repair Left Pleura, Open Approach
0BQC8ZZ	Repair Right Upper Lung Lobe, Via Natural or Artificial Opening Endoscopic	0BQJ0ZZ	Repair Left Lower Lung Lobe, Open Approach	0BQP3ZZ	Repair Left Pleura, Percutaneous Approach
0BQD0ZZ	Repair Right Middle Lung Lobe, Open Approach	0BQJ3ZZ	Repair Left Lower Lung Lobe, Percutaneous Approach	0BQP4ZZ	Repair Left Pleura, Percutaneous Endoscopic Approach
0BQD3ZZ	Repair Right Middle Lung Lobe, Percutaneous Approach	0BQJ4ZZ	Repair Left Lower Lung Lobe, Percutaneous Endoscopic Approach	0BQR0ZZ	Repair Right Diaphragm, Open Approa...
0BQD4ZZ	Repair Right Middle Lung Lobe, Percutaneous Endoscopic Approach	0BQJ7ZZ	Repair Left Lower Lung Lobe, Via Natural or Artificial Opening	0BQR3ZZ	Repair Right Diaphragm, Percutaneous Approach
0BQD7ZZ	Repair Right Middle Lung Lobe, Via Natural or Artificial Opening	0BQJ8ZZ	Repair Left Lower Lung Lobe, Via Natural or Artificial Opening Endoscopic	0BQR4ZZ	Repair Right Diaphragm, Percutaneous Endoscopic Approach
		0BQK0ZZ	Repair Right Lung, Open Approach		*AHA CC: 3Q, 2014, 28*
		0BQK3ZZ	Repair Right Lung, Percutaneous Approach	0BQS0ZZ	Repair Left Diaphragm, Open Approach
				0BQS3ZZ	Repair Left Diaphragm, Percutaneous Approach
				0BQS4ZZ	Repair Left Diaphragm, Percutaneous Endoscopic Approach
					AHA CC: 3Q, 2014, 28

0BS – Respiratory System, Reposition

0BS10ZZ	Reposition Trachea, Open Approach	0BS80ZZ	Reposition Left Upper Lobe Bronchus, Open Approach	0BSG0ZZ	Reposition Left Upper Lung Lobe, Open Approach
0BS20ZZ	Reposition Carina, Open Approach	0BS90ZZ	Reposition Lingula Bronchus, Open Approach	0BSH0ZZ	Reposition Lung Lingula, Open Approac...
0BS30ZZ	Reposition Right Main Bronchus, Open Approach	0BSB0ZZ	Reposition Left Lower Lobe Bronchus, Open Approach	0BSJ0ZZ	Reposition Left Lower Lung Lobe, Ope... Approach
0BS40ZZ	Reposition Right Upper Lobe Bronchus, Open Approach	0BSC0ZZ	Reposition Right Upper Lung Lobe, Open Approach	0BSK0ZZ	Reposition Right Lung, Open Approach
0BS50ZZ	Reposition Right Middle Lobe Bronchus, Open Approach	0BSD0ZZ	Reposition Right Middle Lung Lobe, Open Approach	0BSL0ZZ	Reposition Left Lung, Open Approach
0BS60ZZ	Reposition Right Lower Lobe Bronchus, Open Approach	0BSF0ZZ	Reposition Right Lower Lung Lobe, Open Approach	0BSR0ZZ	Reposition Right Diaphragm, Open Approach
0BS70ZZ	Reposition Left Main Bronchus, Open Approach			0BSS0ZZ	Reposition Left Diaphragm, Open Approach

0BT – Respiratory System, Resection

Review Coding Guideline B3.8

0BT10ZZ	Resection of Trachea, Open Approach	0BT44ZZ	Resection of Right Upper Lobe Bronchus, Percutaneous Endoscopic Approach	0BT70ZZ	Resection of Left Main Bronchus, Open Approach
0BT14ZZ	Resection of Trachea, Percutaneous Endoscopic Approach	0BT50ZZ	Resection of Right Middle Lobe Bronchus, Open Approach	0BT74ZZ	Resection of Left Main Bronchus, Percutaneous Endoscopic Approach
0BT20ZZ	Resection of Carina, Open Approach	0BT54ZZ	Resection of Right Middle Lobe Bronchus, Percutaneous Endoscopic Approach	0BT80ZZ	Resection of Left Upper Lobe Bronchus, Open Approach
0BT24ZZ	Resection of Carina, Percutaneous Endoscopic Approach			0BT84ZZ	Resection of Left Upper Lobe Bronchus, Percutaneous Endoscopic Approach
0BT30ZZ	Resection of Right Main Bronchus, Open Approach	0BT60ZZ	Resection of Right Lower Lobe Bronchus, Open Approach	0BT90ZZ	Resection of Lingula Bronchus, Open Approach
0BT34ZZ	Resection of Right Main Bronchus, Percutaneous Endoscopic Approach	0BT64ZZ	Resection of Right Lower Lobe Bronchus, Percutaneous Endoscopic Approach	0BT94ZZ	Resection of Lingula Bronchus, Percutaneous Endoscopic Approach
0BT40ZZ	Resection of Right Upper Lobe Bronchus, Open Approach				

B0ZZ	Resection of Left Lower Lobe Bronchus, Open Approach	0BTG0ZZ	Resection of Left Upper Lung Lobe, Open Approach	0BTL4ZZ	Resection of Left Lung, Percutaneous Endoscopic Approach

'B4ZZ   Resection of Left Lower Lobe Bronchus, Percutaneous Endoscopic Approach

C0ZZ   Resection of Right Upper Lung Lobe, Open Approach

'C4ZZ   Resection of Right Upper Lung Lobe, Percutaneous Endoscopic Approach

'D0ZZ   Resection of Right Middle Lung Lobe, Open Approach

'D4ZZ   Resection of Right Middle Lung Lobe, Percutaneous Endoscopic Approach

'F0ZZ   Resection of Right Lower Lung Lobe, Open Approach

'F4ZZ   Resection of Right Lower Lung Lobe, Percutaneous Endoscopic Approach

0BTG0ZZ   Resection of Left Upper Lung Lobe, Open Approach

0BTG4ZZ   Resection of Left Upper Lung Lobe, Percutaneous Endoscopic Approach

0BTH0ZZ   Resection of Lung Lingula, Open Approach

0BTH4ZZ   Resection of Lung Lingula, Percutaneous Endoscopic Approach

0BTJ0ZZ   Resection of Left Lower Lung Lobe, Open Approach

0BTJ4ZZ   Resection of Left Lower Lung Lobe, Percutaneous Endoscopic Approach

0BTK0ZZ   Resection of Right Lung, Open Approach

0BTK4ZZ   Resection of Right Lung, Percutaneous Endoscopic Approach

0BTL0ZZ   Resection of Left Lung, Open Approach

0BTL4ZZ   Resection of Left Lung, Percutaneous Endoscopic Approach

0BTM0ZZ   Resection of Bilateral Lungs, Open Approach

0BTM4ZZ   Resection of Bilateral Lungs, Percutaneous Endoscopic Approach

0BTR0ZZ   Resection of Right Diaphragm, Open Approach

0BTR4ZZ   Resection of Right Diaphragm, Percutaneous Endoscopic Approach

0BTS0ZZ   Resection of Left Diaphragm, Open Approach

0BTS4ZZ   Resection of Left Diaphragm, Percutaneous Endoscopic Approach

U – Respiratory System, Supplement

J107Z   Supplement Trachea with Autologous Tissue Substitute, Open Approach

J10JZ   Supplement Trachea with Synthetic Substitute, Open Approach

J10KZ   Supplement Trachea with Nonautologous Tissue Substitute, Open Approach

J147Z   Supplement Trachea with Autologous Tissue Substitute, Percutaneous Endoscopic Approach

J14JZ   Supplement Trachea with Synthetic Substitute, Percutaneous Endoscopic Approach

J14KZ   Supplement Trachea with Nonautologous Tissue Substitute, Percutaneous Endoscopic Approach

U207Z   Supplement Carina with Autologous Tissue Substitute, Open Approach

U20JZ   Supplement Carina with Synthetic Substitute, Open Approach

U20KZ   Supplement Carina with Nonautologous Tissue Substitute, Open Approach

U247Z   Supplement Carina with Autologous Tissue Substitute, Percutaneous Endoscopic Approach

U24JZ   Supplement Carina with Synthetic Substitute, Percutaneous Endoscopic Approach

U24KZ   Supplement Carina with Nonautologous Tissue Substitute, Percutaneous Endoscopic Approach

U307Z   Supplement Right Main Bronchus with Autologous Tissue Substitute, Open Approach

     AHA CC: 1Q, 2015, 28-29

U30JZ   Supplement Right Main Bronchus with Synthetic Substitute, Open Approach

U30KZ   Supplement Right Main Bronchus with Nonautologous Tissue Substitute, Open Approach

U347Z   Supplement Right Main Bronchus with Autologous Tissue Substitute, Percutaneous Endoscopic Approach

U34JZ   Supplement Right Main Bronchus with Synthetic Substitute, Percutaneous Endoscopic Approach

U34KZ   Supplement Right Main Bronchus with Nonautologous Tissue Substitute, Percutaneous Endoscopic Approach

U407Z   Supplement Right Upper Lobe Bronchus with Autologous Tissue Substitute, Open Approach

U40JZ   Supplement Right Upper Lobe Bronchus with Synthetic Substitute, Open Approach

U40KZ   Supplement Right Upper Lobe Bronchus with Nonautologous Tissue Substitute, Open Approach

U447Z   Supplement Right Upper Lobe Bronchus with Autologous Tissue Substitute, Percutaneous Endoscopic Approach

0BU44JZ   Supplement Right Upper Lobe Bronchus with Synthetic Substitute, Percutaneous Endoscopic Approach

0BU44KZ   Supplement Right Upper Lobe Bronchus with Nonautologous Tissue Substitute, Percutaneous Endoscopic Approach

0BU507Z   Supplement Right Middle Lobe Bronchus with Autologous Tissue Substitute, Open Approach

0BU50JZ   Supplement Right Middle Lobe Bronchus with Synthetic Substitute, Open Approach

0BU50KZ   Supplement Right Middle Lobe Bronchus with Nonautologous Tissue Substitute, Open Approach

0BU547Z   Supplement Right Middle Lobe Bronchus with Autologous Tissue Substitute, Percutaneous Endoscopic Approach

0BU54JZ   Supplement Right Middle Lobe Bronchus with Synthetic Substitute, Percutaneous Endoscopic Approach

0BU54KZ   Supplement Right Middle Lobe Bronchus with Nonautologous Tissue Substitute, Percutaneous Endoscopic Approach

0BU607Z   Supplement Right Lower Lobe Bronchus with Autologous Tissue Substitute, Open Approach

0BU60JZ   Supplement Right Lower Lobe Bronchus with Synthetic Substitute, Open Approach

0BU60KZ   Supplement Right Lower Lobe Bronchus with Nonautologous Tissue Substitute, Open Approach

0BU647Z   Supplement Right Lower Lobe Bronchus with Autologous Tissue Substitute, Percutaneous Endoscopic Approach

0BU64JZ   Supplement Right Lower Lobe Bronchus with Synthetic Substitute, Percutaneous Endoscopic Approach

0BU64KZ   Supplement Right Lower Lobe Bronchus with Nonautologous Tissue Substitute, Percutaneous Endoscopic Approach

0BU707Z   Supplement Left Main Bronchus with Autologous Tissue Substitute, Open Approach

0BU70JZ   Supplement Left Main Bronchus with Synthetic Substitute, Open Approach

0BU70KZ   Supplement Left Main Bronchus with Nonautologous Tissue Substitute, Open Approach

0BU747Z   Supplement Left Main Bronchus with Autologous Tissue Substitute, Percutaneous Endoscopic Approach

0BU74JZ   Supplement Left Main Bronchus with Synthetic Substitute, Percutaneous Endoscopic Approach

0BU74KZ   Supplement Left Main Bronchus with Nonautologous Tissue Substitute, Percutaneous Endoscopic Approach

0BU807Z   Supplement Left Upper Lobe Bronchus with Autologous Tissue Substitute, Open Approach

0BU80JZ   Supplement Left Upper Lobe Bronchus with Synthetic Substitute, Open Approach

0BU80KZ   Supplement Left Upper Lobe Bronchus with Nonautologous Tissue Substitute, Open Approach

0BU847Z   Supplement Left Upper Lobe Bronchus with Autologous Tissue Substitute, Percutaneous Endoscopic Approach

0BU84JZ   Supplement Left Upper Lobe Bronchus with Synthetic Substitute, Percutaneous Endoscopic Approach

0BU84KZ   Supplement Left Upper Lobe Bronchus with Nonautologous Tissue Substitute, Percutaneous Endoscopic Approach

0BU907Z   Supplement Lingula Bronchus with Autologous Tissue Substitute, Open Approach

0BU90JZ   Supplement Lingula Bronchus with Synthetic Substitute, Open Approach

0BU90KZ   Supplement Lingula Bronchus with Nonautologous Tissue Substitute, Open Approach

0BU947Z   Supplement Lingula Bronchus with Autologous Tissue Substitute, Percutaneous Endoscopic Approach

0BU94JZ   Supplement Lingula Bronchus with Synthetic Substitute, Percutaneous Endoscopic Approach

0BU94KZ   Supplement Lingula Bronchus with Nonautologous Tissue Substitute, Percutaneous Endoscopic Approach

0BUB07Z   Supplement Left Lower Lobe Bronchus with Autologous Tissue Substitute, Open Approach

0BUB0JZ   Supplement Left Lower Lobe Bronchus with Synthetic Substitute, Open Approach

0BUB0KZ   Supplement Left Lower Lobe Bronchus with Nonautologous Tissue Substitute, Open Approach

0BUB47Z   Supplement Left Lower Lobe Bronchus with Autologous Tissue Substitute, Percutaneous Endoscopic Approach

0BUB4JZ   Supplement Left Lower Lobe Bronchus with Synthetic Substitute, Percutaneous Endoscopic Approach

0BUB4KZ   Supplement Left Lower Lobe Bronchus with Nonautologous Tissue Substitute, Percutaneous Endoscopic Approach

0BUR07Z   Supplement Right Diaphragm with Autologous Tissue Substitute, Open Approach

0BUR0JZ   Supplement Right Diaphragm with Synthetic Substitute, Open Approach

485

0BUR0KZ Supplement Right Diaphragm with Nonautologous Tissue Substitute, Open Approach

0BUR47Z Supplement Right Diaphragm with Autologous Tissue Substitute, Percutaneous Endoscopic Approach

0BUR4JZ Supplement Right Diaphragm with Synthetic Substitute, Percutaneous Endoscopic Approach

0BUR4KZ Supplement Right Diaphragm with Nonautologous Tissue Substitute, Percutaneous Endoscopic Approach

0BUS07Z Supplement Left Diaphragm with Autologous Tissue Substitute, Open Approach

0BUS0JZ Supplement Left Diaphragm with Synthetic Substitute, Open Approach

0BUS0KZ Supplement Left Diaphragm with Nonautologous Tissue Substitute, Open Approach

0BUS47Z Supplement Left Diaphragm with Autologous Tissue Substitute, Percutaneous Endoscopic Approach

0BUS4JZ Supplement Left Diaphragm with Synthetic Substitute, Percutaneous Endoscopic Approach

0BUS4KZ Supplement Left Diaphragm with Nonautologous Tissue Substitute, Percutaneous Endoscopic Approach

0BV – Respiratory System, Restriction

0BV10CZ Restriction of Trachea with Extraluminal Device, Open Approach

0BV10DZ Restriction of Trachea with Intraluminal Device, Open Approach

0BV10ZZ Restriction of Trachea, Open Approach

0BV13CZ Restriction of Trachea with Extraluminal Device, Percutaneous Approach

0BV13DZ Restriction of Trachea with Intraluminal Device, Percutaneous Approach

0BV13ZZ Restriction of Trachea, Percutaneous Approach

0BV14CZ Restriction of Trachea with Extraluminal Device, Percutaneous Endoscopic Approach

0BV14DZ Restriction of Trachea with Intraluminal Device, Percutaneous Endoscopic Approach

0BV14ZZ Restriction of Trachea, Percutaneous Endoscopic Approach

0BV17DZ Restriction of Trachea with Intraluminal Device, Via Natural or Artificial Opening

0BV17ZZ Restriction of Trachea, Via Natural or Artificial Opening

0BV18DZ Restriction of Trachea with Intraluminal Device, Via Natural or Artificial Opening Endoscopic

0BV18ZZ Restriction of Trachea, Via Natural or Artificial Opening Endoscopic

0BV20CZ Restriction of Carina with Extraluminal Device, Open Approach

0BV20DZ Restriction of Carina with Intraluminal Device, Open Approach

0BV20ZZ Restriction of Carina, Open Approach

0BV23CZ Restriction of Carina with Extraluminal Device, Percutaneous Approach

0BV23DZ Restriction of Carina with Intraluminal Device, Percutaneous Approach

0BV23ZZ Restriction of Carina, Percutaneous Approach

0BV24CZ Restriction of Carina with Extraluminal Device, Percutaneous Endoscopic Approach

0BV24DZ Restriction of Carina with Intraluminal Device, Percutaneous Endoscopic Approach

0BV24ZZ Restriction of Carina, Percutaneous Endoscopic Approach

0BV27DZ Restriction of Carina with Intraluminal Device, Via Natural or Artificial Opening

0BV27ZZ Restriction of Carina, Via Natural or Artificial Opening

0BV28DZ Restriction of Carina with Intraluminal Device, Via Natural or Artificial Opening Endoscopic

0BV28ZZ Restriction of Carina, Via Natural or Artificial Opening Endoscopic

0BV30CZ Restriction of Right Main Bronchus with Extraluminal Device, Open Approach

0BV30DZ Restriction of Right Main Bronchus with Intraluminal Device, Open Approach

0BV30ZZ Restriction of Right Main Bronchus, Open Approach

0BV33CZ Restriction of Right Main Bronchus with Extraluminal Device, Percutaneous Approach

0BV33DZ Restriction of Right Main Bronchus with Intraluminal Device, Percutaneous Approach

0BV33ZZ Restriction of Right Main Bronchus, Percutaneous Approach

0BV34CZ Restriction of Right Main Bronchus with Extraluminal Device, Percutaneous Endoscopic Approach

0BV34DZ Restriction of Right Main Bronchus with Intraluminal Device, Percutaneous Endoscopic Approach

0BV34ZZ Restriction of Right Main Bronchus, Percutaneous Endoscopic Approach

0BV37DZ Restriction of Right Main Bronchus with Intraluminal Device, Via Natural or Artificial Opening

0BV37ZZ Restriction of Right Main Bronchus, Via Natural or Artificial Opening

0BV38DZ Restriction of Right Main Bronchus with Intraluminal Device, Via Natural or Artificial Opening Endoscopic

0BV38ZZ Restriction of Right Main Bronchus, Via Natural or Artificial Opening Endoscopic

0BV40CZ Restriction of Right Upper Lobe Bronchus with Extraluminal Device, Open Approach

0BV40DZ Restriction of Right Upper Lobe Bronchus with Intraluminal Device, Open Approach

0BV40ZZ Restriction of Right Upper Lobe Bronchus, Open Approach

0BV43CZ Restriction of Right Upper Lobe Bronchus with Extraluminal Device, Percutaneous Approach

0BV43DZ Restriction of Right Upper Lobe Bronchus with Intraluminal Device, Percutaneous Approach

0BV43ZZ Restriction of Right Upper Lobe Bronchus, Percutaneous Approach

0BV44CZ Restriction of Right Upper Lobe Bronchus with Extraluminal Device, Percutaneous Endoscopic Approach

0BV44DZ Restriction of Right Upper Lobe Bronchus with Intraluminal Device, Percutaneous Endoscopic Approach

0BV44ZZ Restriction of Right Upper Lobe Bronchus, Percutaneous Endoscopic Approach

0BV47DZ Restriction of Right Upper Lobe Bronchus with Intraluminal Device, Via Natural or Artificial Opening

0BV47ZZ Restriction of Right Upper Lobe Bronchus, Via Natural or Artificial Opening

0BV48DZ Restriction of Right Upper Lobe Bronchus with Intraluminal Device, Via Natural or Artificial Opening Endoscopic

0BV48ZZ Restriction of Right Upper Lobe Bronchus, Via Natural or Artificial Opening Endoscopic

0BV50CZ Restriction of Right Middle Lobe Bronchus with Extraluminal Device, Open Approach

0BV50DZ Restriction of Right Middle Lobe Bronchus with Intraluminal Device, Open Approach

0BV50ZZ Restriction of Right Middle Lobe Bronchus, Open Approach

0BV53CZ Restriction of Right Middle Lobe Bronchus with Extraluminal Device, Percutaneous Approach

0BV53DZ Restriction of Right Middle Lobe Bronchus with Intraluminal Device, Percutaneous Approach

0BV53ZZ Restriction of Right Middle Lobe Bronchus, Percutaneous Approach

0BV54CZ Restriction of Right Middle Lobe Bronchus with Extraluminal Device, Percutaneous Endoscopic Approach

0BV54DZ Restriction of Right Middle Lobe Bronchus with Intraluminal Device, Percutaneous Endoscopic Approach

0BV54ZZ Restriction of Right Middle Lobe Bronchus, Percutaneous Endoscopic Approach

0BV57DZ Restriction of Right Middle Lobe Bronchus with Intraluminal Device, Via Natural or Artificial Opening

0BV57ZZ Restriction of Right Middle Lobe Bronchus, Via Natural or Artificial Opening

0BV58DZ Restriction of Right Middle Lobe Bronchus with Intraluminal Device, Via Natural or Artificial Opening Endoscopic

0BV58ZZ Restriction of Right Middle Lobe Bronchus, Via Natural or Artificial Opening Endoscopic

0BV60CZ Restriction of Right Lower Lobe Bronchus with Extraluminal Device, Open Approach

0BV60DZ Restriction of Right Lower Lobe Bronchus with Intraluminal Device, Open Approach

0BV60ZZ Restriction of Right Lower Lobe Bronchus, Open Approach

0BV63CZ Restriction of Right Lower Lobe Bronchus with Extraluminal Device, Percutaneous Approach

0BV63DZ Restriction of Right Lower Lobe Bronchus with Intraluminal Device, Percutaneous Approach

0BV63ZZ Restriction of Right Lower Lobe Bronchus, Percutaneous Approach

0BV64CZ Restriction of Right Lower Lobe Bronchus with Extraluminal Device, Percutaneous Endoscopic Approach

0BV64DZ Restriction of Right Lower Lobe Bronchus with Intraluminal Device, Percutaneous Endoscopic Approach

0BV64ZZ Restriction of Right Lower Lobe Bronchus, Percutaneous Endoscopic Approach

67DZ Restriction of Right Lower Lobe Bronchus with Intraluminal Device, Via Natural or Artificial Opening

67ZZ Restriction of Right Lower Lobe Bronchus, Via Natural or Artificial Opening

68DZ Restriction of Right Lower Lobe Bronchus with Intraluminal Device, Via Natural or Artificial Opening Endoscopic

68ZZ Restriction of Right Lower Lobe Bronchus, Via Natural or Artificial Opening Endoscopic

70CZ Restriction of Left Main Bronchus with Extraluminal Device, Open Approach

70DZ Restriction of Left Main Bronchus with Intraluminal Device, Open Approach

70ZZ Restriction of Left Main Bronchus, Open Approach

73CZ Restriction of Left Main Bronchus with Extraluminal Device, Percutaneous Approach

73DZ Restriction of Left Main Bronchus with Intraluminal Device, Percutaneous Approach

73ZZ Restriction of Left Main Bronchus, Percutaneous Approach

74CZ Restriction of Left Main Bronchus with Extraluminal Device, Percutaneous Endoscopic Approach

74DZ Restriction of Left Main Bronchus with Intraluminal Device, Percutaneous Endoscopic Approach

74ZZ Restriction of Left Main Bronchus, Percutaneous Endoscopic Approach

77DZ Restriction of Left Main Bronchus with Intraluminal Device, Via Natural or Artificial Opening

77ZZ Restriction of Left Main Bronchus, Via Natural or Artificial Opening

78DZ Restriction of Left Main Bronchus with Intraluminal Device, Via Natural or Artificial Opening Endoscopic

78ZZ Restriction of Left Main Bronchus, Via Natural or Artificial Opening Endoscopic

80CZ Restriction of Left Upper Lobe Bronchus with Extraluminal Device, Open Approach

80DZ Restriction of Left Upper Lobe Bronchus with Intraluminal Device, Open Approach

80ZZ Restriction of Left Upper Lobe Bronchus, Open Approach

0BV83CZ Restriction of Left Upper Lobe Bronchus with Extraluminal Device, Percutaneous Approach

0BV83DZ Restriction of Left Upper Lobe Bronchus with Intraluminal Device, Percutaneous Approach

0BV83ZZ Restriction of Left Upper Lobe Bronchus, Percutaneous Approach

0BV84CZ Restriction of Left Upper Lobe Bronchus with Extraluminal Device, Percutaneous Endoscopic Approach

0BV84DZ Restriction of Left Upper Lobe Bronchus with Intraluminal Device, Percutaneous Endoscopic Approach

0BV84ZZ Restriction of Left Upper Lobe Bronchus, Percutaneous Endoscopic Approach

0BV87DZ Restriction of Left Upper Lobe Bronchus with Intraluminal Device, Via Natural or Artificial Opening

0BV87ZZ Restriction of Left Upper Lobe Bronchus, Via Natural or Artificial Opening

0BV88DZ Restriction of Left Upper Lobe Bronchus with Intraluminal Device, Via Natural or Artificial Opening Endoscopic

0BV88ZZ Restriction of Left Upper Lobe Bronchus, Via Natural or Artificial Opening Endoscopic

0BV90CZ Restriction of Lingula Bronchus with Extraluminal Device, Open Approach

0BV90DZ Restriction of Lingula Bronchus with Intraluminal Device, Open Approach

0BV90ZZ Restriction of Lingula Bronchus, Open Approach

0BV93CZ Restriction of Lingula Bronchus with Extraluminal Device, Percutaneous Approach

0BV93DZ Restriction of Lingula Bronchus with Intraluminal Device, Percutaneous Approach

0BV93ZZ Restriction of Lingula Bronchus, Percutaneous Approach

0BV94CZ Restriction of Lingula Bronchus with Extraluminal Device, Percutaneous Endoscopic Approach

0BV94DZ Restriction of Lingula Bronchus with Intraluminal Device, Percutaneous Endoscopic Approach

0BV94ZZ Restriction of Lingula Bronchus, Percutaneous Endoscopic Approach

0BV97DZ Restriction of Lingula Bronchus with Intraluminal Device, Via Natural or Artificial Opening

0BV97ZZ Restriction of Lingula Bronchus, Via Natural or Artificial Opening

0BV98DZ Restriction of Lingula Bronchus with Intraluminal Device, Via Natural or Artificial Opening Endoscopic

0BV98ZZ Restriction of Lingula Bronchus, Via Natural or Artificial Opening Endoscopic

0BVB0CZ Restriction of Left Lower Lobe Bronchus with Extraluminal Device, Open Approach

0BVB0DZ Restriction of Left Lower Lobe Bronchus with Intraluminal Device, Open Approach

0BVB0ZZ Restriction of Left Lower Lobe Bronchus, Open Approach

0BVB3CZ Restriction of Left Lower Lobe Bronchus with Extraluminal Device, Percutaneous Approach

0BVB3DZ Restriction of Left Lower Lobe Bronchus with Intraluminal Device, Percutaneous Approach

0BVB3ZZ Restriction of Left Lower Lobe Bronchus, Percutaneous Approach

0BVB4CZ Restriction of Left Lower Lobe Bronchus with Extraluminal Device, Percutaneous Endoscopic Approach

0BVB4DZ Restriction of Left Lower Lobe Bronchus with Intraluminal Device, Percutaneous Endoscopic Approach

0BVB4ZZ Restriction of Left Lower Lobe Bronchus, Percutaneous Endoscopic Approach

0BVB7DZ Restriction of Left Lower Lobe Bronchus with Intraluminal Device, Via Natural or Artificial Opening

0BVB7ZZ Restriction of Left Lower Lobe Bronchus, Via Natural or Artificial Opening

0BVB8DZ Restriction of Left Lower Lobe Bronchus with Intraluminal Device, Via Natural or Artificial Opening Endoscopic

0BVB8ZZ Restriction of Left Lower Lobe Bronchus, Via Natural or Artificial Opening Endoscopic

BW – Respiratory System, Revision

view Coding Guideline B6.1c

W000Z Revision of Drainage Device in Tracheobronchial Tree, Open Approach

W002Z Revision of Monitoring Device in Tracheobronchial Tree, Open Approach

W003Z Revision of Infusion Device in Tracheobronchial Tree, Open Approach

W007Z Revision of Autologous Tissue Substitute in Tracheobronchial Tree, Open Approach

W00CZ Revision of Extraluminal Device in Tracheobronchial Tree, Open Approach

W00DZ Revision of Intraluminal Device in Tracheobronchial Tree, Open Approach

W00JZ Revision of Synthetic Substitute in Tracheobronchial Tree, Open Approach

W00KZ Revision of Nonautologous Tissue Substitute in Tracheobronchial Tree, Open Approach

W030Z Revision of Drainage Device in Tracheobronchial Tree, Percutaneous Approach

0BW032Z Revision of Monitoring Device in Tracheobronchial Tree, Percutaneous Approach

0BW033Z Revision of Infusion Device in Tracheobronchial Tree, Percutaneous Approach

0BW037Z Revision of Autologous Tissue Substitute in Tracheobronchial Tree, Percutaneous Approach

0BW03CZ Revision of Extraluminal Device in Tracheobronchial Tree, Percutaneous Approach

0BW03DZ Revision of Intraluminal Device in Tracheobronchial Tree, Percutaneous Approach

0BW03JZ Revision of Synthetic Substitute in Tracheobronchial Tree, Percutaneous Approach

0BW03KZ Revision of Nonautologous Tissue Substitute in Tracheobronchial Tree, Percutaneous Approach

0BW040Z Revision of Drainage Device in Tracheobronchial Tree, Percutaneous Endoscopic Approach

0BW042Z Revision of Monitoring Device in Tracheobronchial Tree, Percutaneous Endoscopic Approach

0BW043Z Revision of Infusion Device in Tracheobronchial Tree, Percutaneous Endoscopic Approach

0BW047Z Revision of Autologous Tissue Substitute in Tracheobronchial Tree, Percutaneous Endoscopic Approach

0BW04CZ Revision of Extraluminal Device in Tracheobronchial Tree, Percutaneous Endoscopic Approach

0BW04DZ Revision of Intraluminal Device in Tracheobronchial Tree, Percutaneous Endoscopic Approach

0BW04JZ Revision of Synthetic Substitute in Tracheobronchial Tree, Percutaneous Endoscopic Approach

♀ Female-only   ♂ Male-only   ▲ Limited Coverage   ● Non-OR   ▩ HAC-associated procedure   ▲ Non-covered procedures   ＋ Combination

0BW04KZ Revision of Nonautologous Tissue Substitute in Tracheobronchial Tree, Percutaneous Endoscopic Approach

0BW070Z Revision of Drainage Device in Tracheobronchial Tree, Via Natural or Artificial Opening

0BW072Z Revision of Monitoring Device in Tracheobronchial Tree, Via Natural or Artificial Opening

0BW073Z Revision of Infusion Device in Tracheobronchial Tree, Via Natural or Artificial Opening

0BW077Z Revision of Autologous Tissue Substitute in Tracheobronchial Tree, Via Natural or Artificial Opening

0BW07CZ Revision of Extraluminal Device in Tracheobronchial Tree, Via Natural or Artificial Opening

0BW07DZ Revision of Intraluminal Device in Tracheobronchial Tree, Via Natural or Artificial Opening

0BW07JZ Revision of Synthetic Substitute in Tracheobronchial Tree, Via Natural or Artificial Opening

0BW07KZ Revision of Nonautologous Tissue Substitute in Tracheobronchial Tree, Via Natural or Artificial Opening

0BW080Z Revision of Drainage Device in Tracheobronchial Tree, Via Natural or Artificial Opening Endoscopic

0BW082Z Revision of Monitoring Device in Tracheobronchial Tree, Via Natural or Artificial Opening Endoscopic

0BW083Z Revision of Infusion Device in Tracheobronchial Tree, Via Natural or Artificial Opening Endoscopic

0BW087Z Revision of Autologous Tissue Substitute in Tracheobronchial Tree, Via Natural or Artificial Opening Endoscopic

0BW08CZ Revision of Extraluminal Device in Tracheobronchial Tree, Via Natural or Artificial Opening Endoscopic

0BW08DZ Revision of Intraluminal Device in Tracheobronchial Tree, Via Natural or Artificial Opening Endoscopic

0BW08JZ Revision of Synthetic Substitute in Tracheobronchial Tree, Via Natural or Artificial Opening Endoscopic

0BW08KZ Revision of Nonautologous Tissue Substitute in Tracheobronchial Tree, Via Natural or Artificial Opening Endoscopic

0BW0X0Z Revision of Drainage Device in Tracheobronchial Tree, External Approach

0BW0X2Z Revision of Monitoring Device in Tracheobronchial Tree, External Approach

0BW0X3Z Revision of Infusion Device in Tracheobronchial Tree, External Approach

0BW0X7Z Revision of Autologous Tissue Substitute in Tracheobronchial Tree, External Approach

0BW0XCZ Revision of Extraluminal Device in Tracheobronchial Tree, External Approach

0BW0XDZ Revision of Intraluminal Device in Tracheobronchial Tree, External Approach

0BW0XJZ Revision of Synthetic Substitute in Tracheobronchial Tree, External Approach

0BW0XKZ Revision of Nonautologous Tissue Substitute in Tracheobronchial Tree, External Approach

0BW100Z Revision of Drainage Device in Trachea, Open Approach

0BW102Z Revision of Monitoring Device in Trachea, Open Approach

0BW107Z Revision of Autologous Tissue Substitute in Trachea, Open Approach

0BW10CZ Revision of Extraluminal Device in Trachea, Open Approach

0BW10DZ Revision of Intraluminal Device in Trachea, Open Approach

0BW10FZ Revision of Tracheostomy Device in Trachea, Open Approach

0BW10JZ Revision of Synthetic Substitute in Trachea, Open Approach

0BW10KZ Revision of Nonautologous Tissue Substitute in Trachea, Open Approach

0BW130Z Revision of Drainage Device in Trachea, Percutaneous Approach

0BW132Z Revision of Monitoring Device in Trachea, Percutaneous Approach

0BW137Z Revision of Autologous Tissue Substitute in Trachea, Percutaneous Approach

0BW13CZ Revision of Extraluminal Device in Trachea, Percutaneous Approach

0BW13DZ Revision of Intraluminal Device in Trachea, Percutaneous Approach

0BW13FZ Revision of Tracheostomy Device in Trachea, Percutaneous Approach

0BW13JZ Revision of Synthetic Substitute in Trachea, Percutaneous Approach

0BW13KZ Revision of Nonautologous Tissue Substitute in Trachea, Percutaneous Approach

0BW140Z Revision of Drainage Device in Trachea, Percutaneous Endoscopic Approach

0BW142Z Revision of Monitoring Device in Trachea, Percutaneous Endoscopic Approach

0BW147Z Revision of Autologous Tissue Substitute in Trachea, Percutaneous Endoscopic Approach

0BW14CZ Revision of Extraluminal Device in Trachea, Percutaneous Endoscopic Approach

0BW14DZ Revision of Intraluminal Device in Trachea, Percutaneous Endoscopic Approach

0BW14FZ Revision of Tracheostomy Device in Trachea, Percutaneous Endoscopic Approach

0BW14JZ Revision of Synthetic Substitute in Trachea, Percutaneous Endoscopic Approach

0BW14KZ Revision of Nonautologous Tissue Substitute in Trachea, Percutaneous Endoscopic Approach

0BW170Z Revision of Drainage Device in Trachea, Via Natural or Artificial Opening

0BW172Z Revision of Monitoring Device in Trachea, Via Natural or Artificial Opening

0BW177Z Revision of Autologous Tissue Substitute in Trachea, Via Natural or Artificial Opening

0BW17CZ Revision of Extraluminal Device in Trachea, Via Natural or Artificial Opening

0BW17DZ Revision of Intraluminal Device in Trachea, Via Natural or Artificial Opening

0BW17FZ Revision of Tracheostomy Device in Trachea, Via Natural or Artificial Opening

0BW17JZ Revision of Synthetic Substitute in Trachea, Via Natural or Artificial Opening

0BW17KZ Revision of Nonautologous Tissue Substitute in Trachea, Via Natural or Artificial Opening

0BW180Z Revision of Drainage Device in Trachea, Via Natural or Artificial Opening Endoscopic

0BW182Z Revision of Monitoring Device in Trachea, Via Natural or Artificial Opening Endoscopic

0BW187Z Revision of Autologous Tissue Substitute in Trachea, Via Natural or Artificial Opening Endoscopic

0BW18CZ Revision of Extraluminal Device in Trachea, Via Natural or Artificial Opening Endoscopic

0BW18DZ Revision of Intraluminal Device in Trachea, Via Natural or Artificial Opening Endoscopic

0BW18FZ Revision of Tracheostomy Device in Trachea, Via Natural or Artificial Opening Endoscopic

0BW18JZ Revision of Synthetic Substitute in Trachea, Via Natural or Artificial Opening Endoscopic

0BW18KZ Revision of Nonautologous Tissue Substitute in Trachea, Via Natural or Artificial Opening Endoscopic

0BW1X0Z Revision of Drainage Device in Trachea, External Approach

0BW1X2Z Revision of Monitoring Device in Trachea, External Approach

0BW1X7Z Revision of Autologous Tissue Substitute in Trachea, External Approach

0BW1XCZ Revision of Extraluminal Device in Trachea, External Approach

0BW1XDZ Revision of Intraluminal Device in Trachea, External Approach

0BW1XFZ Revision of Tracheostomy Device in Trachea, External Approach

0BW1XJZ Revision of Synthetic Substitute in Trachea, External Approach

0BW1XKZ Revision of Nonautologous Tissue Substitute in Trachea, External Approach

0BWK00Z Revision of Drainage Device in Right Lung, Open Approach

0BWK02Z Revision of Monitoring Device in Right Lung, Open Approach

0BWK03Z Revision of Infusion Device in Right Lung, Open Approach

0BWK30Z Revision of Drainage Device in Right Lung, Percutaneous Approach

0BWK32Z Revision of Monitoring Device in Right Lung, Percutaneous Approach

0BWK33Z Revision of Infusion Device in Right Lung, Percutaneous Approach

0BWK40Z Revision of Drainage Device in Right Lung, Percutaneous Endoscopic Approach

0BWK42Z Revision of Monitoring Device in Right Lung, Percutaneous Endoscopic Approach

0BWK43Z Revision of Infusion Device in Right Lung, Percutaneous Endoscopic Approach

0BWK70Z Revision of Drainage Device in Right Lung, Via Natural or Artificial Opening

0BWK72Z Revision of Monitoring Device in Right Lung, Via Natural or Artificial Opening

0BWK73Z Revision of Infusion Device in Right Lung, Via Natural or Artificial Opening

0BWK80Z Revision of Drainage Device in Right Lung, Via Natural or Artificial Opening Endoscopic

WK82Z Revision of Monitoring Device in Right Lung, Via Natural or Artificial Opening Endoscopic

WK83Z Revision of Infusion Device in Right Lung, Via Natural or Artificial Opening Endoscopic

WKX0Z Revision of Drainage Device in Right Lung, External Approach

WKX2Z Revision of Monitoring Device in Right Lung, External Approach

WKX3Z Revision of Infusion Device in Right Lung, External Approach

WL00Z Revision of Drainage Device in Left Lung, Open Approach

WL02Z Revision of Monitoring Device in Left Lung, Open Approach

WL03Z Revision of Infusion Device in Left Lung, Open Approach

WL30Z Revision of Drainage Device in Left Lung, Percutaneous Approach

WL32Z Revision of Monitoring Device in Left Lung, Percutaneous Approach

WL33Z Revision of Infusion Device in Left Lung, Percutaneous Approach

WL40Z Revision of Drainage Device in Left Lung, Percutaneous Endoscopic Approach

WL42Z Revision of Monitoring Device in Left Lung, Percutaneous Endoscopic Approach

WL43Z Revision of Infusion Device in Left Lung, Percutaneous Endoscopic Approach

WL70Z Revision of Drainage Device in Left Lung, Via Natural or Artificial Opening

WL72Z Revision of Monitoring Device in Left Lung, Via Natural or Artificial Opening

WL73Z Revision of Infusion Device in Left Lung, Via Natural or Artificial Opening

WL80Z Revision of Drainage Device in Left Lung, Via Natural or Artificial Opening Endoscopic

WL82Z Revision of Monitoring Device in Left Lung, Via Natural or Artificial Opening Endoscopic

WL83Z Revision of Infusion Device in Left Lung, Via Natural or Artificial Opening Endoscopic

WLX0Z Revision of Drainage Device in Left Lung, External Approach

WLX2Z Revision of Monitoring Device in Left Lung, External Approach

WLX3Z Revision of Infusion Device in Left Lung, External Approach

WQ00Z Revision of Drainage Device in Pleura, Open Approach

0BWQ02Z Revision of Monitoring Device in Pleura, Open Approach

0BWQ30Z Revision of Drainage Device in Pleura, Percutaneous Approach

0BWQ32Z Revision of Monitoring Device in Pleura, Percutaneous Approach

0BWQ40Z Revision of Drainage Device in Pleura, Percutaneous Endoscopic Approach

0BWQ42Z Revision of Monitoring Device in Pleura, Percutaneous Endoscopic Approach

0BWQ70Z Revision of Drainage Device in Pleura, Via Natural or Artificial Opening

0BWQ72Z Revision of Monitoring Device in Pleura, Via Natural or Artificial Opening

0BWQ80Z Revision of Drainage Device in Pleura, Via Natural or Artificial Opening Endoscopic

0BWQ82Z Revision of Monitoring Device in Pleura, Via Natural or Artificial Opening Endoscopic

0BWQX0Z Revision of Drainage Device in Pleura, External Approach

0BWQX2Z Revision of Monitoring Device in Pleura, External Approach

0BWT00Z Revision of Drainage Device in Diaphragm, Open Approach

0BWT02Z Revision of Monitoring Device in Diaphragm, Open Approach

0BWT07Z Revision of Autologous Tissue Substitute in Diaphragm, Open Approach

0BWT0JZ Revision of Synthetic Substitute in Diaphragm, Open Approach

0BWT0KZ Revision of Nonautologous Tissue Substitute in Diaphragm, Open Approach

0BWT0MZ Revision of Diaphragmatic Pacemaker Lead in Diaphragm, Open Approach

0BWT30Z Revision of Drainage Device in Diaphragm, Percutaneous Approach

0BWT32Z Revision of Monitoring Device in Diaphragm, Percutaneous Approach

0BWT37Z Revision of Autologous Tissue Substitute in Diaphragm, Percutaneous Approach

0BWT3JZ Revision of Synthetic Substitute in Diaphragm, Percutaneous Approach

0BWT3KZ Revision of Nonautologous Tissue Substitute in Diaphragm, Percutaneous Approach

0BWT3MZ Revision of Diaphragmatic Pacemaker Lead in Diaphragm, Percutaneous Approach

0BWT40Z Revision of Drainage Device in Diaphragm, Percutaneous Endoscopic Approach

0BWT42Z Revision of Monitoring Device in Diaphragm, Percutaneous Endoscopic Approach

0BWT47Z Revision of Autologous Tissue Substitute in Diaphragm, Percutaneous Endoscopic Approach

0BWT4JZ Revision of Synthetic Substitute in Diaphragm, Percutaneous Endoscopic Approach

0BWT4KZ Revision of Nonautologous Tissue Substitute in Diaphragm, Percutaneous Endoscopic Approach

0BWT4MZ Revision of Diaphragmatic Pacemaker Lead in Diaphragm, Percutaneous Endoscopic Approach

0BWT70Z Revision of Drainage Device in Diaphragm, Via Natural or Artificial Opening

0BWT72Z Revision of Monitoring Device in Diaphragm, Via Natural or Artificial Opening

0BWT77Z Revision of Autologous Tissue Substitute in Diaphragm, Via Natural or Artificial Opening

0BWT7JZ Revision of Synthetic Substitute in Diaphragm, Via Natural or Artificial Opening

0BWT7KZ Revision of Nonautologous Tissue Substitute in Diaphragm, Via Natural or Artificial Opening

0BWT7MZ Revision of Diaphragmatic Pacemaker Lead in Diaphragm, Via Natural or Artificial Opening

0BWT80Z Revision of Drainage Device in Diaphragm, Via Natural or Artificial Opening Endoscopic

0BWT82Z Revision of Monitoring Device in Diaphragm, Via Natural or Artificial Opening Endoscopic

0BWT87Z Revision of Autologous Tissue Substitute in Diaphragm, Via Natural or Artificial Opening Endoscopic

0BWT8JZ Revision of Synthetic Substitute in Diaphragm, Via Natural or Artificial Opening Endoscopic

0BWT8KZ Revision of Nonautologous Tissue Substitute in Diaphragm, Via Natural or Artificial Opening Endoscopic

0BWT8MZ Revision of Diaphragmatic Pacemaker Lead in Diaphragm, Via Natural or Artificial Opening Endoscopic

0BWTX0Z Revision of Drainage Device in Diaphragm, External Approach

0BWTX2Z Revision of Monitoring Device in Diaphragm, External Approach

0BWTX7Z Revision of Autologous Tissue Substitute in Diaphragm, External Approach

0BWTXJZ Revision of Synthetic Substitute in Diaphragm, External Approach

0BWTXKZ Revision of Nonautologous Tissue Substitute in Diaphragm, External Approach

0BWTXMZ Revision of Diaphragmatic Pacemaker Lead in Diaphragm, External Approach

BY – Respiratory System, Transplantation

Review Coding Guideline B3.16

0BYC0Z0 Transplantation of Right Upper Lung Lobe, Allogeneic, Open Approach

0BYC0Z1 Transplantation of Right Upper Lung Lobe, Syngeneic, Open Approach

0BYC0Z2 Transplantation of Right Upper Lung Lobe, Zooplastic, Open Approach

0BYD0Z0 Transplantation of Right Middle Lung Lobe, Allogeneic, Open Approach

0BYD0Z1 Transplantation of Right Middle Lung Lobe, Syngeneic, Open Approach

▲ **0BYD0Z2** Transplantation of Right Middle Lung Lobe, Zooplastic, Open Approach

▲ **0BYF0Z0** Transplantation of Right Lower Lung Lobe, Allogeneic, Open Approach

▲ **0BYF0Z1** Transplantation of Right Lower Lung Lobe, Syngeneic, Open Approach

▲ **0BYF0Z2** Transplantation of Right Lower Lung Lobe, Zooplastic, Open Approach

▲ **0BYG0Z0** Transplantation of Left Upper Lung Lobe, Allogeneic, Open Approach

▲ **0BYG0Z1** Transplantation of Left Upper Lung Lobe, Syngeneic, Open Approach

▲ **0BYG0Z2** Transplantation of Left Upper Lung Lobe, Zooplastic, Open Approach

▲ **0BYH0Z0** Transplantation of Lung Lingula, Allogeneic, Open Approach

▲ **0BYH0Z1** Transplantation of Lung Lingula, Syngeneic, Open Approach

▲ **0BYH0Z2** Transplantation of Lung Lingula, Zooplastic, Open Approach

| Female-only | ♂ Male-only | ▲ Limited Coverage | ● Non-OR | HAC-associated procedure | ▲ Non-covered procedures | + Combination |

▲ **0BYJ0Z0** Transplantation of Left Lower Lung Lobe, Allogeneic, Open Approach

▲ **0BYJ0Z1** Transplantation of Left Lower Lung Lobe, Syngeneic, Open Approach

▲ **0BYJ0Z2** Transplantation of Left Lower Lung Lobe, Zooplastic, Open Approach

▲ **0BYK0Z0** Transplantation of Right Lung, Allogeneic, Open Approach

▲ **0BYK0Z1** Transplantation of Right Lung, Syngeneic, Open Approach

▲ **0BYK0Z2** Transplantation of Right Lung, Zooplastic, Open Approach

▲ **0BYL0Z0** Transplantation of Left Lung, Allogeneic, Open Approach

▲ **0BYL0Z1** Transplantation of Left Lung, Syngeneic, Open Approach

▲ **0BYL0Z2** Transplantation of Left Lung, Zooplastic Open Approach

▲ **0BYM0Z0** Transplantation of Bilateral Lungs, Allogeneic, Open Approach

▲ **0BYM0Z1** Transplantation of Bilateral Lungs, Syngeneic, Open Approach

▲ **0BYM0Z2** Transplantation of Bilateral Lungs, Zooplastic, Open Approach

♀ Female-only　　♂ Male-only　　▲ Limited Coverage　　● Non-OR　　▦ HAC-associated procedure　　▲ Non-covered procedures　　✚ Combination

Oral Cavity

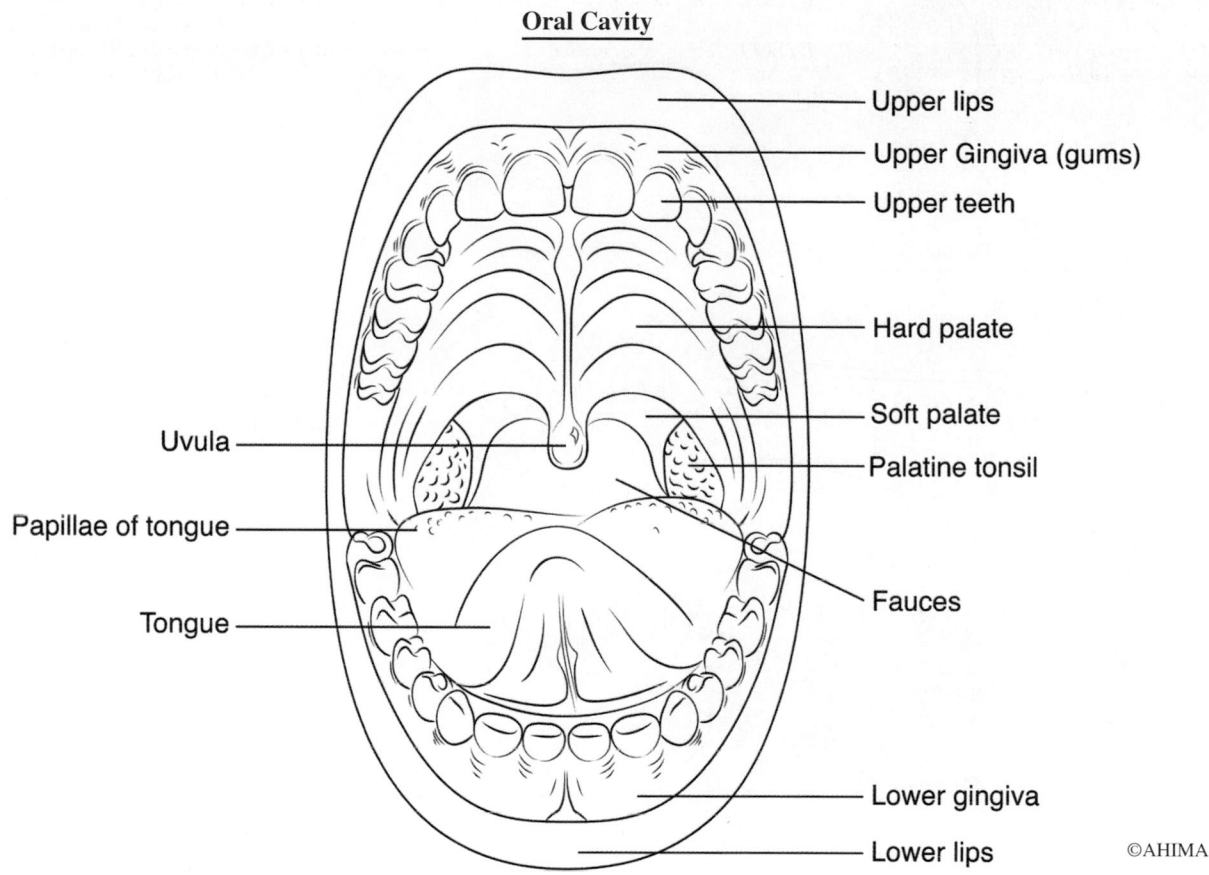

Upper lips

Upper Gingiva (gums)

Upper teeth

Hard palate

Soft palate

Uvula

Palatine tonsil

Papillae of tongue

Fauces

Tongue

Lower gingiva

Lower lips

©AHIMA

Glands of the Oral Cavity

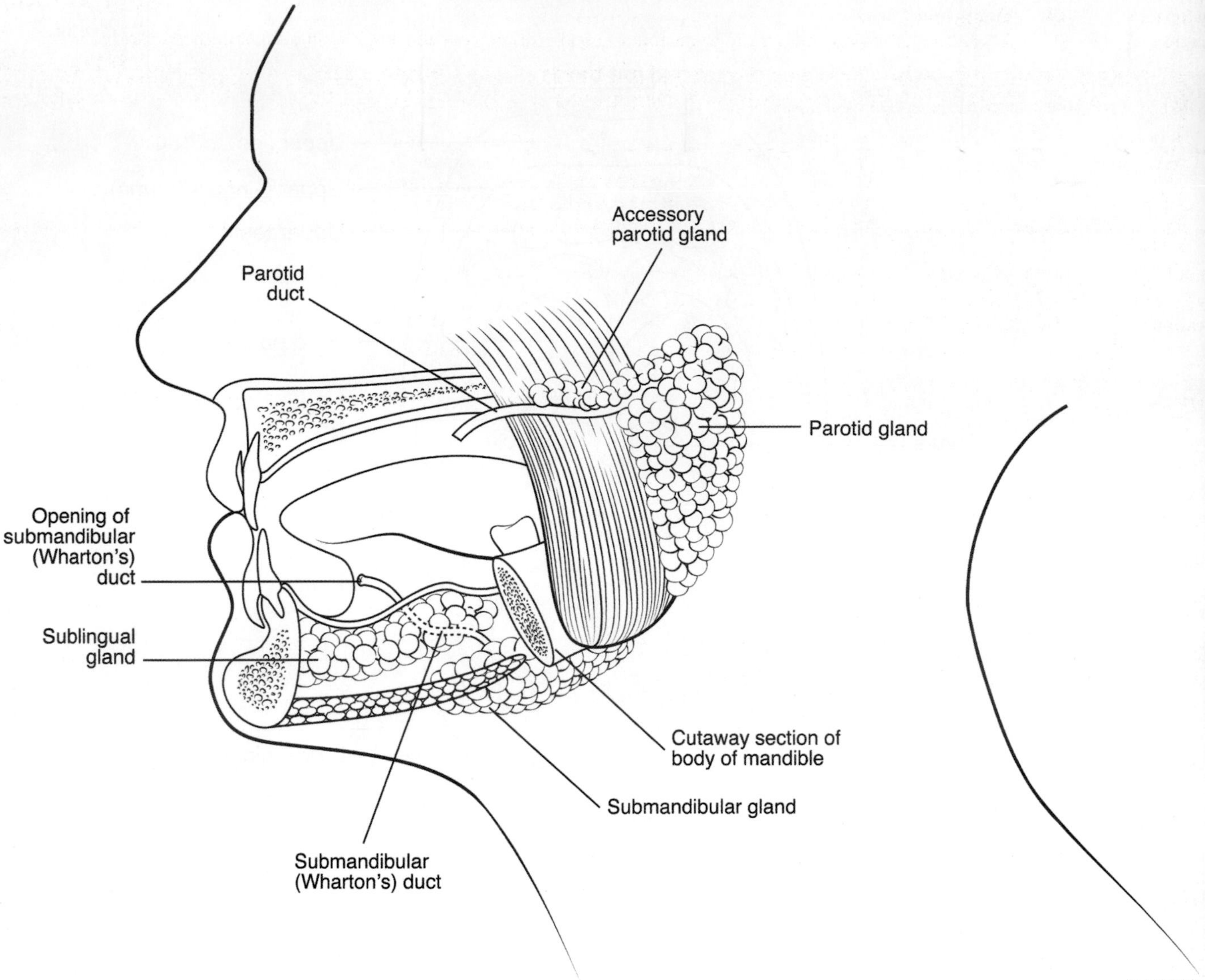

Accessory
parotid gland

Parotid
duct

Parotid gland

Opening of
submandibular
(Wharton's)
duct

Sublingual
gland

Cutaway section of
body of mandible

Submandibular gland

Submandibular
(Wharton's) duct

©AHIMA

Throat

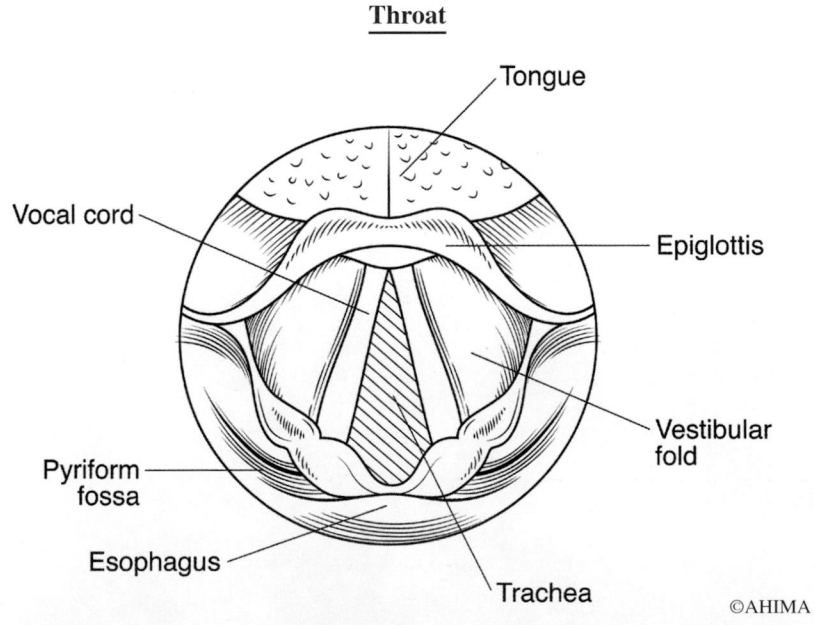

Tongue

Vocal cord

Epiglottis

Pyriform
fossa

Vestibular
fold

Esophagus

Trachea

©AHIMA

ion	0	**Medical and Surgical**
y System	C	**Mouth and Throat**
ration	0	**Alteration:** Modifying the anatomic structure of a body part without affecting the function of the body part

Body Part (4th)	Approach (5th)	Device (6th)	Qualifier (7th)
Upper Lip Lower Lip	**X** External	**7** Autologous Tissue Substitute **J** Synthetic Substitute **K** Nonautologous Tissue Substitute **Z** No Device	**Z** No Qualifier

tion	0	**Medical and Surgical**
dy System	C	**Mouth and Throat**
eration	2	**Change:** Taking out or off a device from a body part and putting back an identical or similar device in or on the same body part without cutting or puncturing the skin or a mucous membrane

Body Part (4th)	Approach (5th)	Device (6th)	Qualifier (7th)
Salivary Gland Larynx Mouth and Throat	**X** External	**0** Drainage Device **Y** Other Device	**Z** No Qualifier

tion	0	**Medical and Surgical**
dy System	C	**Mouth and Throat**
eration	5	**Destruction:** Physical eradication of all or a portion of a body part by the direct use of energy, force, or a destructive agent

Body Part (4th)	Approach (5th)	Device (6th)	Qualifier (7th)
Upper Lip Lower Lip Hard Palate Soft Palate Buccal Mucosa Upper Gingiva Lower Gingiva Tongue Uvula Tonsils Adenoids	**0** Open **3** Percutaneous **X** External	**Z** No Device	**Z** No Qualifier
B Parotid Gland, Right Parotid Gland, Left Parotid Duct, Right C Parotid Duct, Left D Sublingual Gland, Right F Sublingual Gland, Left G Submaxillary Gland, Right H Submaxillary Gland, Left J Minor Salivary Gland	**0** Open **3** Percutaneous	**Z** No Device	**Z** No Qualifier
M Pharynx R Epiglottis S Larynx T Vocal Cord, Right V Vocal Cord, Left	**0** Open **3** Percutaneous **4** Percutaneous Endoscopic **7** Via Natural or Artificial Opening **8** Via Natural or Artificial Opening Endoscopic	**Z** No Device	**Z** No Qualifier
W Upper Tooth X Lower Tooth	**0** Open **X** External	**Z** No Device	**0** Single **1** Multiple **2** All

Section 0 **Medical and Surgical**
Body System C **Mouth and Throat**
Operation 7 **Dilation:** Expanding an orifice or the lumen of a tubular body part

Body Part (4th)	Approach (5th)	Device (6th)	Qualifier (7th)
B Parotid Duct, Right C Parotid Duct, Left	0 Open 3 Percutaneous 7 Via Natural or Artificial Opening	D Intraluminal Device Z No Device	Z No Qualifier
M Pharynx	7 Via Natural or Artificial Opening 8 Via Natural or Artificial Opening Endoscopic	D Intraluminal Device Z No Device	Z No Qualifier
S Larynx	0 Open 3 Percutaneous 4 Percutaneous Endoscopic 7 Via Natural or Artificial Opening 8 Via Natural or Artificial Opening Endoscopic	D Intraluminal Device Z No Device	Z No Qualifier

Section 0 **Medical and Surgical**
Body System C **Mouth and Throat**
Operation 9 **Drainage:** Taking or letting out fluids and/or gases from a body part

Body Part (4th)	Approach (5th)	Device (6th)	Qualifier (7th)
0 Upper Lip 1 Lower Lip 2 Hard Palate 3 Soft Palate 4 Buccal Mucosa 5 Upper Gingiva 6 Lower Gingiva 7 Tongue N Uvula P Tonsils Q Adenoids	0 Open 3 Percutaneous X External	0 Drainage Device	Z No Qualifier
0 Upper Lip 1 Lower Lip 2 Hard Palate 3 Soft Palate 4 Buccal Mucosa 5 Upper Gingiva 6 Lower Gingiva 7 Tongue N Uvula P Tonsils Q Adenoids	0 Open 3 Percutaneous X External	Z No Device	X Diagnostic Z No Qualifier
8 Parotid Gland, Right 9 Parotid Gland, Left B Parotid Duct, Right C Parotid Duct, Left D Sublingual Gland, Right F Sublingual Gland, Left G Submaxillary Gland, Right H Submaxillary Gland, Left J Minor Salivary Gland	0 Open 3 Percutaneous	0 Drainage Device	Z No Qualifier
8 Parotid Gland, Right 9 Parotid Gland, Left B Parotid Duct, Right C Parotid Duct, Left	0 Open 3 Percutaneous	Z No Device	X Diagnostic Z No Qualifier

Continued →

Section | 0 | Medical and Surgical
Body System | C | Mouth and Throat
Operation | 9 | **Drainage:** Taking or letting out fluids and/or gases from a body part

Body Part (4th)	Approach (5th)	Device (6th)	Qualifier (7th)
Pharynx Epiglottis Larynx Vocal Cord, Right Vocal Cord, Left	0 Open 3 Percutaneous 4 Percutaneous Endoscopic 7 Via Natural or Artificial Opening 8 Via Natural or Artificial Opening Endoscopic	0 Drainage Device	Z No Qualifier
Pharynx Epiglottis Larynx Vocal Cord, Right Vocal Cord, Left	0 Open 3 Percutaneous 4 Percutaneous Endoscopic 7 Via Natural or Artificial Opening 8 Via Natural or Artificial Opening Endoscopic	Z No Device	X Diagnostic Z No Qualifier
Upper Tooth Lower Tooth	0 Open X External	0 Drainage Device Z No Device	0 Single 1 Multiple 2 All

Section | 0 | Medical and Surgical
Body System | C | Mouth and Throat
Operation | B | **Excision:** Cutting out or off, without replacement, a portion of a body part

Body Part (4th)	Approach (5th)	Device (6th)	Qualifier (7th)
Upper Lip Lower Lip Hard Palate Soft Palate Buccal Mucosa Upper Gingiva Lower Gingiva Tongue Uvula Tonsils Adenoids	0 Open 3 Percutaneous X External	Z No Device	X Diagnostic Z No Qualifier
Parotid Gland, Right Parotid Gland, Left Parotid Duct, Right Parotid Duct, Left Sublingual Gland, Right Sublingual Gland, Left Submaxillary Gland, Right Submaxillary Gland, Left Minor Salivary Gland	0 Open 3 Percutaneous	Z No Device	X Diagnostic Z No Qualifier
Pharynx Epiglottis Larynx Vocal Cord, Right Vocal Cord, Left	0 Open 3 Percutaneous 4 Percutaneous Endoscopic 7 Via Natural or Artificial Opening 8 Via Natural or Artificial Opening Endoscopic	Z No Device	X Diagnostic Z No Qualifier
Upper Tooth Lower Tooth	0 Open X External	Z No Device	0 Single 1 Multiple 2 All

Section	0	Medical and Surgical
Body System	C	Mouth and Throat
Operation	C	Extirpation: Taking or cutting out solid matter from a body part

Body Part (4th)	Approach (5th)	Device (6th)	Qualifier (7th)
0 Upper Lip 1 Lower Lip 2 Hard Palate 3 Soft Palate 4 Buccal Mucosa 5 Upper Gingiva 6 Lower Gingiva 7 Tongue N Uvula P Tonsils Q Adenoids	0 Open 3 Percutaneous X External	Z No Device	Z No Qualifier
8 Parotid Gland, Right 9 Parotid Gland, Left B Parotid Duct, Right C Parotid Duct, Left D Sublingual Gland, Right F Sublingual Gland, Left G Submaxillary Gland, Right H Submaxillary Gland, Left J Minor Salivary Gland	0 Open 3 Percutaneous	Z No Device	Z No Qualifier
M Pharynx R Epiglottis S Larynx T Vocal Cord, Right V Vocal Cord, Left	0 Open 3 Percutaneous 4 Percutaneous Endoscopic 7 Via Natural or Artificial Opening 8 Via Natural or Artificial Opening Endoscopic	Z No Device	Z No Qualifier
W Upper Tooth X Lower Tooth	0 Open X External	Z No Device	0 Single 1 Multiple 2 All

Section	0	Medical and Surgical
Body System	C	Mouth and Throat
Operation	D	Extraction: Pulling or stripping out or off all or a portion of a body part by the use of force

Body Part (4th)	Approach (5th)	Device (6th)	Qualifier (7th)
T Vocal Cord, Right V Vocal Cord, Left	0 Open 3 Percutaneous 4 Percutaneous Endoscopic 7 Via Natural or Artificial Opening 8 Via Natural or Artificial Opening Endoscopic	Z No Device	Z No Qualifier
W Upper Tooth X Lower Tooth	X External	Z No Device	0 Single 1 Multiple 2 All

Section	0	Medical and Surgical
Body System	C	Mouth and Throat
Operation	F	Fragmentation: Breaking solid matter in a body part into pieces

Body Part (4th)	Approach (5th)	Device (6th)	Qualifier (7th)
B Parotid Duct, Right C Parotid Duct, Left	0 Open 3 Percutaneous 7 Via Natural or Artificial Opening X External	Z No Device	Z No Qualifier

	0	Medical and Surgical
...ion		
...y System	C	Mouth and Throat
...ration	H	**Insertion:** Putting in a nonbiological appliance that monitors, assists, performs, or prevents a physiological function but does not physically take the place of a body part

Body Part (4th)	Approach (5th)	Device (6th)	Qualifier (7th)
Tongue	0 Open 3 Percutaneous X External	1 Radioactive Element	Z No Qualifier
Mouth and Throat	7 Via Natural or Artificial Opening 8 Via Natural or Artificial Opening Endoscopic	B Intraluminal Device, Airway	Z No Qualifier

	0	Medical and Surgical
...tion		
...dy System	C	Mouth and Throat
...eration	J	**Inspection:** Visually and/or manually exploring a body part

Body Part (4th)	Approach (5th)	Device (6th)	Qualifier (7th)
SalivaryGland	0 Open 3 Percutaneous X External	Z No Device	Z No Qualifier
Larynx Mouth and Throat	0 Open 3 Percutaneous 4 Percutaneous Endoscopic 7 Via Natural or Artificial Opening 8 Via Natural or Artificial Opening Endoscopic X External	Z No Device	Z No Qualifier

	0	Medical and Surgical
...tion		
...dy System	C	Mouth and Throat
...eration	L	**Occlusion:** Completely closing an orifice or the lumen of a tubular body part

Body Part (4th)	Approach (5th)	Device (6th)	Qualifier (7th)
B Parotid Duct, Right C Parotid Duct, Left	0 Open 3 Percutaneous 4 Percutaneous Endoscopic	C Extraluminal Device D Intraluminal Device Z No Device	Z No Qualifier
B Parotid Duct, Right C Parotid Duct, Left	7 Via Natural or Artificial Opening 8 Via Natural or Artificial Opening Endoscopic	D Intraluminal Device Z No Device	Z No Qualifier

	0	Medical and Surgical
...tion		
...dy System	C	Mouth and Throat
...eration	M	**Reattachment:** Putting back in or on all or a portion of a separated body part to its normal location or other suitable location

Body Part (4th)	Approach (5th)	Device (6th)	Qualifier (7th)
0 Upper Lip 1 Lower Lip 3 Soft Palate 7 Tongue N Uvula	0 Open	Z No Device	Z No Qualifier
W Upper Tooth X Lower Tooth	0 Open X External	Z No Device	0 Single 1 Multiple 2 All

Section	0	Medical and Surgical
Body System	C	Mouth and Throat
Operation	N	Release: Freeing a body part from an abnormal physical constraint by cutting or by the use of force

Body Part (4th)	Approach (5th)	Device (6th)	Qualifier (7th)
0 Upper Lip 1 Lower Lip 2 Hard Palate 3 Soft Palate 4 Buccal Mucosa 5 Upper Gingiva 6 Lower Gingiva 7 Tongue N Uvula P Tonsils Q Adenoids	0 Open 3 Percutaneous X External	Z No Device	Z No Qualifier
8 Parotid Gland, Right 9 Parotid Gland, Left B Parotid Duct, Right C Parotid Duct, Left D Sublingual Gland, Right F Sublingual Gland, Left G Submaxillary Gland, Right H Submaxillary Gland, Left J Minor Salivary Gland	0 Open 3 Percutaneous	Z No Device	Z No Qualifier
M Pharynx R Epiglottis S Larynx T Vocal Cord, Right V Vocal Cord, Left	0 Open 3 Percutaneous 4 Percutaneous Endoscopic 7 Via Natural or Artificial Opening 8 Via Natural or Artificial Opening Endoscopic	Z No Device	Z No Qualifier
W Upper Tooth X Lower Tooth	0 Open X External	Z No Device	0 Single 1 Multiple 2 All

Section	0	Medical and Surgical
Body System	C	Mouth and Throat
Operation	P	Removal: Taking out or off a device from a body part

Body Part (4th)	Approach (5th)	Device (6th)	Qualifier (7th)
A Salivary Gland	0 Open 3 Percutaneous	0 Drainage Device C Extraluminal Device	Z No Qualifier
Y Mouth and Throat	0 Open 3 Percutaneous 7 Via Natural or Artificial Opening 8 Via Natural or Artificial Opening Endoscopic X External	0 Drainage Device 1 Radioactive Element 7 Autologous Tissue Substitute D Intraluminal Device J Synthetic Substitute K Nonautologous Tissue Substitute	Z No Qualifier

tion	0	**Medical and Surgical**
y System	C	**Mouth and Throat**
ration	Q	**Repair:** Restoring, to the extent possible, a body part to its normal anatomic structure and function

Body Part (4th)	Approach (5th)	Device (6th)	Qualifier (7th)
Upper Lip Lower Lip Hard Palate Soft Palate Buccal Mucosa Upper Gingiva Lower Gingiva Tongue Uvula Tonsils Adenoids	0 Open 3 Percutaneous X External	Z No Device	Z No Qualifier
Parotid Gland, Right Parotid Gland, Left Parotid Duct, Right Parotid Duct, Left Sublingual Gland, Right Sublingual Gland, Left Submaxillary Gland, Right Submaxillary Gland, Left Minor Salivary Gland	0 Open 3 Percutaneous	Z No Device	Z No Qualifier
Pharynx Epiglottis Larynx Vocal Cord, Right Vocal Cord, Left	0 Open 3 Percutaneous 4 Percutaneous Endoscopic 7 Via Natural or Artificial Opening 8 Via Natural or Artificial Opening Endoscopic	Z No Device	Z No Qualifier
Upper Tooth Lower Tooth	0 Open X External	Z No Device	0 Single 1 Multiple 2 All

tion	0	**Medical and Surgical**
dy System	C	**Mouth and Throat**
eration	R	**Replacement:** Putting in or on biological or synthetic material that physically takes the place and/or function of all or a portion of a body part

Body Part (4th)	Approach (5th)	Device (6th)	Qualifier (7th)
Upper Lip Lower Lip Hard Palate Soft Palate Buccal Mucosa Upper Gingiva Lower Gingiva Tongue Uvula	0 Open 3 Percutaneous X External	7 Autologous Tissue Substitute J Synthetic Substitute K Nonautologous Tissue Substitute	Z No Qualifier
Parotid Duct, Right Parotid Duct, Left	0 Open 3 Percutaneous	7 Autologous Tissue Substitute J Synthetic Substitute K Nonautologous Tissue Substitute	Z No Qualifier
Pharynx Epiglottis Larynx Vocal Cord, Right Vocal Cord, Left	0 Open 7 Via Natural or Artificial Opening 8 Via Natural or Artificial Opening Endoscopic	7 Autologous Tissue Substitute J Synthetic Substitute K Nonautologous Tissue Substitute	Z No Qualifier
Upper Tooth Lower Tooth	0 Open X External	7 Autologous Tissue Substitute J Synthetic Substitute K Nonautologous Tissue Substitute	0 Single 1 Multiple 2 All

Section 0 **Medical and Surgical**
Body System C **Mouth and Throat**
Operation S **Reposition:** Moving to its normal location, or other suitable location, all or a portion of a body part

Body Part (4th)	Approach (5th)	Device (6th)	Qualifier (7th)
0 Upper Lip 1 Lower Lip 2 Hard Palate 3 Soft Palate 7 Tongue N Uvula	0 Open X External	Z No Device	Z No Qualifier
B Parotid Duct, Right C Parotid Duct, Left	0 Open 3 Percutaneous	Z No Device	Z No Qualifier
R Epiglottis T Vocal Cord, Right V Vocal Cord, Left	0 Open 7 Via Natural or Artificial Opening 8 Via Natural or Artificial Opening Endoscopic	Z No Device	Z No Qualifier
W Upper Tooth X Lower Tooth	0 Open X External	5 External Fixation Device Z No Device	0 Single 1 Multiple 2 All

Section 0 **Medical and Surgical**
Body System C **Mouth and Throat**
Operation T **Resection:** Cutting out or off, without replacement, all of a body part

Body Part (4th)	Approach (5th)	Device (6th)	Qualifier (7th)
0 Upper Lip 1 Lower Lip 2 Hard Palate 3 Soft Palate 7 Tongue N Uvula P Tonsils Q Adenoids	0 Open X External	Z No Device	Z No Qualifier
8 Parotid Gland, Right 9 Parotid Gland, Left B Parotid Duct, Right C Parotid Duct, Left D Sublingual Gland, Right F Sublingual Gland, Left G Submaxillary Gland, Right H Submaxillary Gland, Left J Minor Salivary Gland	0 Open	Z No Device	Z No Qualifier
M Pharynx R Epiglottis S Larynx T Vocal Cord, Right V Vocal Cord, Left	0 Open 4 Percutaneous Endoscopic 7 Via Natural or Artificial Opening 8 Via Natural or Artificial Opening Endoscopic	Z No Device	Z No Qualifier
W Upper Tooth X Lower Tooth	0 Open	Z No Device	0 Single 1 Multiple 2 All

Section	0	Medical and Surgical
Body System	C	Mouth and Throat
Operation	U	Supplement: Putting in or on biological or synthetic material that physically reinforces and/or augments the function of a portion of a body part

Body Part (4th)	Approach (5th)	Device (6th)	Qualifier (7th)
Upper Lip Lower Lip Hard Palate Soft Palate Buccal Mucosa Upper Gingiva Lower Gingiva Tongue Uvula	0 Open 3 Percutaneous X External	7 Autologous Tissue Substitute J Synthetic Substitute K Nonautologous Tissue Substitute	Z No Qualifier
Pharynx Epiglottis Larynx Vocal Cord, Right Vocal Cord, Left	0 Open 7 Via Natural or Artificial Opening 8 Via Natural or Artificial Opening Endoscopic	7 Autologous Tissue Substitute J Synthetic Substitute K Nonautologous Tissue Substitute	Z No Qualifier

Section	0	Medical and Surgical
Body System	C	Mouth and Throat
Operation	V	Restriction: Partially closing an orifice or the lumen of a tubular body part

Body Part (4th)	Approach (5th)	Device (6th)	Qualifier (7th)
Parotid Duct, Right Parotid Duct, Left	0 Open 3 Percutaneous	C Extraluminal Device D Intraluminal Device Z No Device	Z No Qualifier
Parotid Duct, Right Parotid Duct, Left	7 Via Natural or Artificial Opening 8 Via Natural or Artificial Opening Endoscopic	D Intraluminal Device Z No Device	Z No Qualifier

Section	0	Medical and Surgical
Body System	C	Mouth and Throat
Operation	W	Revision: Correcting, to the extent possible, a portion of a malfunctioning device or the position of a displaced device

Body Part (4th)	Approach (5th)	Device (6th)	Qualifier (7th)
Salivary Gland	0 Open 3 Percutaneous X External	0 Drainage Device C Extraluminal Device	Z No Qualifier
Larynx	0 Open 3 Percutaneous 7 Via Natural or Artificial Opening 8 Via Natural or Artificial Opening Endoscopic X External	0 Drainage Device 7 Autologous Tissue Substitute D Intraluminal Device J Synthetic Substitute K Nonautologous Tissue Substitute	Z No Qualifier
Mouth and Throat	0 Open 3 Percutaneous 7 Via Natural or Artificial Opening 8 Via Natural or Artificial Opening Endoscopic X External	0 Drainage Device 1 Radioactive Element 7 Autologous Tissue Substitute D Intraluminal Device J Synthetic Substitute K Nonautologous Tissue Substitute	Z No Qualifier

Section	0	Medical and Surgical
Body System	C	Mouth and Throat
Operation	X	**Transfer:** Moving, without taking out, all or a portion of a body part to another location to take over the function of all or portion of a body part

Body Part (4th)	Approach (5th)	Device (6th)	Qualifier (7th)
0 Upper Lip 1 Lower Lip 3 Soft Palate 4 Buccal Mucosa 5 Upper Gingiva 6 Lower Gingiva 7 Tongue	0 Open X External	Z No Device	Z No Qualifier

Mouth and Throat Code Listing 0C0–0CX

0C0 – Mouth and Throat, Alteration

0C00X7Z Alteration of Upper Lip with Autologous Tissue Substitute, External Approach
0C00XJZ Alteration of Upper Lip with Synthetic Substitute, External Approach
0C00XKZ Alteration of Upper Lip with Nonautologous Tissue Substitute, External Approach

0C00XZZ Alteration of Upper Lip, External Approach
0C01X7Z Alteration of Lower Lip with Autologous Tissue Substitute, External Approach
0C01XJZ Alteration of Lower Lip with Synthetic Substitute, External Approach

0C01XKZ Alteration of Lower Lip with Nonautologous Tissue Substitute, Exte Approach
0C01XZZ Alteration of Lower Lip, External Approach

0C2 – Mouth and Throat, Change

Review Coding Guideline B6.1c

0C2AX0Z Change Drainage Device in Salivary Gland, External Approach
0C2AXYZ Change Other Device in Salivary Gland, External Approach

0C2SX0Z Change Drainage Device in Larynx, External Approach
0C2SXYZ Change Other Device in Larynx, External Approach

0C2YX0Z Change Drainage Device in Mouth and Throat, External Approach
0C2YXYZ Change Other Device in Mouth and Throat, External Approach

0C5 – Mouth and Throat, Destruction

0C500ZZ Destruction of Upper Lip, Open Approach
0C503ZZ Destruction of Upper Lip, Percutaneous Approach
0C50XZZ Destruction of Upper Lip, External Approach
0C510ZZ Destruction of Lower Lip, Open Approach
0C513ZZ Destruction of Lower Lip, Percutaneous Approach
0C51XZZ Destruction of Lower Lip, External Approach
0C520ZZ Destruction of Hard Palate, Open Approach
0C523ZZ Destruction of Hard Palate, Percutaneous Approach
0C52XZZ Destruction of Hard Palate, External Approach
0C530ZZ Destruction of Soft Palate, Open Approach
0C533ZZ Destruction of Soft Palate, Percutaneous Approach
0C53XZZ Destruction of Soft Palate, External Approach
0C540ZZ Destruction of Buccal Mucosa, Open Approach
0C543ZZ Destruction of Buccal Mucosa, Percutaneous Approach
0C54XZZ Destruction of Buccal Mucosa, External Approach
0C550ZZ Destruction of Upper Gingiva, Open Approach
0C553ZZ Destruction of Upper Gingiva, Percutaneous Approach
0C55XZZ Destruction of Upper Gingiva, External Approach
0C560ZZ Destruction of Lower Gingiva, Open Approach

0C563ZZ Destruction of Lower Gingiva, Percutaneous Approach
0C56XZZ Destruction of Lower Gingiva, External Approach
0C570ZZ Destruction of Tongue, Open Approach
0C573ZZ Destruction of Tongue, Percutaneous Approach
0C57XZZ Destruction of Tongue, External Approach
0C580ZZ Destruction of Right Parotid Gland, Open Approach
0C583ZZ Destruction of Right Parotid Gland, Percutaneous Approach
0C590ZZ Destruction of Left Parotid Gland, Open Approach
0C593ZZ Destruction of Left Parotid Gland, Percutaneous Approach
0C5B0ZZ Destruction of Right Parotid Duct, Open Approach
0C5B3ZZ Destruction of Right Parotid Duct, Percutaneous Approach
0C5C0ZZ Destruction of Left Parotid Duct, Open Approach
0C5C3ZZ Destruction of Left Parotid Duct, Percutaneous Approach
0C5D0ZZ Destruction of Right Sublingual Gland, Open Approach
0C5D3ZZ Destruction of Right Sublingual Gland, Percutaneous Approach
0C5F0ZZ Destruction of Left Sublingual Gland, Open Approach
0C5F3ZZ Destruction of Left Sublingual Gland, Percutaneous Approach
0C5G0ZZ Destruction of Right Submaxillary Gland, Open Approach
0C5G3ZZ Destruction of Right Submaxillary Gland, Percutaneous Approach

0C5H0ZZ Destruction of Left Submaxillary Glan Open Approach
0C5H3ZZ Destruction of Left Submaxillary Glan Percutaneous Approach
0C5J0ZZ Destruction of Minor Salivary Gland, Open Approach
0C5J3ZZ Destruction of Minor Salivary Gland, Percutaneous Approach
0C5M0ZZ Destruction of Pharynx, Open Approac
0C5M3ZZ Destruction of Pharynx, Percutaneous Approach
0C5M4ZZ Destruction of Pharynx, Percutaneous Endoscopic Approach
0C5M7ZZ Destruction of Pharynx, Via Natural or Artificial Opening
0C5M8ZZ Destruction of Pharynx, Via Natural or Artificial Opening Endoscopic
0C5N0ZZ Destruction of Uvula, Open Approach
0C5N3ZZ Destruction of Uvula, Percutaneous Approach
0C5NXZZ Destruction of Uvula, External Approac
0C5P0ZZ Destruction of Tonsils, Open Approach
0C5P3ZZ Destruction of Tonsils, Percutaneous Approach
0C5PXZZ Destruction of Tonsils, External Approach
0C5Q0ZZ Destruction of Adenoids, Open Approac
0C5Q3ZZ Destruction of Adenoids, Percutaneous Approach
0C5QXZZ Destruction of Adenoids, External Approach
0C5R0ZZ Destruction of Epiglottis, Open Approac
0C5R3ZZ Destruction of Epiglottis, Percutaneous Approach
0C5R4ZZ Destruction of Epiglottis, Percutaneous Endoscopic Approach

♀ Female-only   ♂ Male-only   ▲ Limited Coverage   ● Non-OR   HAC HAC-associated procedure   ▲ Non-covered procedures   + Combina

R7ZZ Destruction of Epiglottis, Via Natural or Artificial Opening
R8ZZ Destruction of Epiglottis, Via Natural or Artificial Opening Endoscopic
S0ZZ Destruction of Larynx, Open Approach
S3ZZ Destruction of Larynx, Percutaneous Approach
S4ZZ Destruction of Larynx, Percutaneous Endoscopic Approach
S7ZZ Destruction of Larynx, Via Natural or Artificial Opening
S8ZZ Destruction of Larynx, Via Natural or Artificial Opening Endoscopic
T0ZZ Destruction of Right Vocal Cord, Open Approach
T3ZZ Destruction of Right Vocal Cord, Percutaneous Approach
T4ZZ Destruction of Right Vocal Cord, Percutaneous Endoscopic Approach

0C5T7ZZ Destruction of Right Vocal Cord, Via Natural or Artificial Opening
0C5T8ZZ Destruction of Right Vocal Cord, Via Natural or Artificial Opening Endoscopic
0C5V0ZZ Destruction of Left Vocal Cord, Open Approach
0C5V3ZZ Destruction of Left Vocal Cord, Percutaneous Approach
0C5V4ZZ Destruction of Left Vocal Cord, Percutaneous Endoscopic Approach
0C5V7ZZ Destruction of Left Vocal Cord, Via Natural or Artificial Opening
0C5V8ZZ Destruction of Left Vocal Cord, Via Natural or Artificial Opening Endoscopic
0C5W0Z0 Destruction of Upper Tooth, Single, Open Approach
0C5W0Z1 Destruction of Upper Tooth, Multiple, Open Approach
0C5W0Z2 Destruction of Upper Tooth, All, Open Approach

0C5WXZ0 Destruction of Upper Tooth, Single, External Approach
0C5WXZ1 Destruction of Upper Tooth, Multiple, External Approach
0C5WXZ2 Destruction of Upper Tooth, All, External Approach
0C5X0Z0 Destruction of Lower Tooth, Single, Open Approach
0C5X0Z1 Destruction of Lower Tooth, Multiple, Open Approach
0C5X0Z2 Destruction of Lower Tooth, All, Open Approach
0C5XXZ0 Destruction of Lower Tooth, Single, External Approach
0C5XXZ1 Destruction of Lower Tooth, Multiple, External Approach
0C5XXZ2 Destruction of Lower Tooth, All, External Approach

7 – Mouth and Throat, Dilation

B0DZ Dilation of Right Parotid Duct with Intraluminal Device, Open Approach
B0ZZ Dilation of Right Parotid Duct, Open Approach
B3DZ Dilation of Right Parotid Duct with Intraluminal Device, Percutaneous Approach
B3ZZ Dilation of Right Parotid Duct, Percutaneous Approach
B7DZ Dilation of Right Parotid Duct with Intraluminal Device, Via Natural or Artificial Opening
B7ZZ Dilation of Right Parotid Duct, Via Natural or Artificial Opening
C0DZ Dilation of Left Parotid Duct with Intraluminal Device, Open Approach
C0ZZ Dilation of Left Parotid Duct, Open Approach
C3DZ Dilation of Left Parotid Duct with Intraluminal Device, Percutaneous Approach

0C7C3ZZ Dilation of Left Parotid Duct, Percutaneous Approach
0C7C7DZ Dilation of Left Parotid Duct with Intraluminal Device, Via Natural or Artificial Opening
0C7C7ZZ Dilation of Left Parotid Duct, Via Natural or Artificial Opening
0C7M7DZ Dilation of Pharynx with Intraluminal Device, Via Natural or Artificial Opening
0C7M7ZZ Dilation of Pharynx, Via Natural or Artificial Opening
0C7M8DZ Dilation of Pharynx with Intraluminal Device, Via Natural or Artificial Opening Endoscopic
0C7M8ZZ Dilation of Pharynx, Via Natural or Artificial Opening Endoscopic
0C7S0DZ Dilation of Larynx with Intraluminal Device, Open Approach
0C7S0ZZ Dilation of Larynx, Open Approach

0C7S3DZ Dilation of Larynx with Intraluminal Device, Percutaneous Approach
0C7S3ZZ Dilation of Larynx, Percutaneous Approach
0C7S4DZ Dilation of Larynx with Intraluminal Device, Percutaneous Endoscopic Approach
0C7S4ZZ Dilation of Larynx, Percutaneous Endoscopic Approach
0C7S7DZ Dilation of Larynx with Intraluminal Device, Via Natural or Artificial Opening
0C7S7ZZ Dilation of Larynx, Via Natural or Artificial Opening
0C7S8DZ Dilation of Larynx with Intraluminal Device, Via Natural or Artificial Opening Endoscopic
0C7S8ZZ Dilation of Larynx, Via Natural or Artificial Opening Endoscopic

9 – Mouth and Throat, Drainage

view Coding Guidelines B3.4a and B3.4b

view Coding Guideline B6.2

9000Z Drainage of Upper Lip with Drainage Device, Open Approach
9000ZX Drainage of Upper Lip, Open Approach, Diagnostic
9000ZZ Drainage of Upper Lip, Open Approach
9030Z Drainage of Upper Lip with Drainage Device, Percutaneous Approach
903ZX Drainage of Upper Lip, Percutaneous Approach, Diagnostic
903ZZ Drainage of Upper Lip, Percutaneous Approach
90X0Z Drainage of Upper Lip with Drainage Device, External Approach
90XZX Drainage of Upper Lip, External Approach, Diagnostic
90XZZ Drainage of Upper Lip, External Approach
9100Z Drainage of Lower Lip with Drainage Device, Open Approach
910ZX Drainage of Lower Lip, Open Approach, Diagnostic
910ZZ Drainage of Lower Lip, Open Approach
9130Z Drainage of Lower Lip with Drainage Device, Percutaneous Approach
913ZX Drainage of Lower Lip, Percutaneous Approach, Diagnostic

0C913ZZ Drainage of Lower Lip, Percutaneous Approach
0C91X0Z Drainage of Lower Lip with Drainage Device, External Approach
0C91XZX Drainage of Lower Lip, External Approach, Diagnostic
0C91XZZ Drainage of Lower Lip, External Approach
0C9200Z Drainage of Hard Palate with Drainage Device, Open Approach
0C920ZX Drainage of Hard Palate, Open Approach, Diagnostic
0C920ZZ Drainage of Hard Palate, Open Approach
0C9230Z Drainage of Hard Palate with Drainage Device, Percutaneous Approach
0C923ZX Drainage of Hard Palate, Percutaneous Approach, Diagnostic
0C923ZZ Drainage of Hard Palate, Percutaneous Approach
0C92X0Z Drainage of Hard Palate with Drainage Device, External Approach
0C92XZX Drainage of Hard Palate, External Approach, Diagnostic
0C92XZZ Drainage of Hard Palate, External Approach
0C9300Z Drainage of Soft Palate with Drainage Device, Open Approach

0C930ZX Drainage of Soft Palate, Open Approach, Diagnostic
0C930ZZ Drainage of Soft Palate, Open Approach
0C9330Z Drainage of Soft Palate with Drainage Device, Percutaneous Approach
0C933ZX Drainage of Soft Palate, Percutaneous Approach, Diagnostic
0C933ZZ Drainage of Soft Palate, Percutaneous Approach
0C93X0Z Drainage of Soft Palate with Drainage Device, External Approach
0C93XZX Drainage of Soft Palate, External Approach, Diagnostic
0C93XZZ Drainage of Soft Palate, External Approach
0C9400Z Drainage of Buccal Mucosa with Drainage Device, Open Approach
0C940ZX Drainage of Buccal Mucosa, Open Approach, Diagnostic
0C940ZZ Drainage of Buccal Mucosa, Open Approach
0C9430Z Drainage of Buccal Mucosa with Drainage Device, Percutaneous Approach
0C943ZX Drainage of Buccal Mucosa, Percutaneous Approach, Diagnostic

♀ Female-only ♂ Male-only ▲ Limited Coverage ● Non-OR ▦ HAC-associated procedure ▲ Non-covered procedures ✚ Combination

0C943ZZ Drainage of Buccal Mucosa, Percutaneous Approach

0C94X0Z Drainage of Buccal Mucosa with Drainage Device, External Approach

0C94XZX Drainage of Buccal Mucosa, External Approach, Diagnostic

0C94XZZ Drainage of Buccal Mucosa, External Approach

0C9500Z Drainage of Upper Gingiva with Drainage Device, Open Approach

0C950ZX Drainage of Upper Gingiva, Open Approach, Diagnostic

0C950ZZ Drainage of Upper Gingiva, Open Approach

0C9530Z Drainage of Upper Gingiva with Drainage Device, Percutaneous Approach

0C953ZX Drainage of Upper Gingiva, Percutaneous Approach, Diagnostic

0C953ZZ Drainage of Upper Gingiva, Percutaneous Approach

0C95X0Z Drainage of Upper Gingiva with Drainage Device, External Approach

0C95XZX Drainage of Upper Gingiva, External Approach, Diagnostic

0C95XZZ Drainage of Upper Gingiva, External Approach

0C9600Z Drainage of Lower Gingiva with Drainage Device, Open Approach

0C960ZX Drainage of Lower Gingiva, Open Approach, Diagnostic

0C960ZZ Drainage of Lower Gingiva, Open Approach

0C9630Z Drainage of Lower Gingiva with Drainage Device, Percutaneous Approach

0C963ZX Drainage of Lower Gingiva, Percutaneous Approach, Diagnostic

0C963ZZ Drainage of Lower Gingiva, Percutaneous Approach

0C96X0Z Drainage of Lower Gingiva with Drainage Device, External Approach

0C96XZX Drainage of Lower Gingiva, External Approach, Diagnostic

0C96XZZ Drainage of Lower Gingiva, External Approach

0C9700Z Drainage of Tongue with Drainage Device, Open Approach

0C970ZX Drainage of Tongue, Open Approach, Diagnostic

0C970ZZ Drainage of Tongue, Open Approach

0C9730Z Drainage of Tongue with Drainage Device, Percutaneous Approach

0C973ZX Drainage of Tongue, Percutaneous Approach, Diagnostic

0C973ZZ Drainage of Tongue, Percutaneous Approach

0C97X0Z Drainage of Tongue with Drainage Device, External Approach

0C97XZX Drainage of Tongue, External Approach, Diagnostic

0C97XZZ Drainage of Tongue, External Approach

0C9800Z Drainage of Right Parotid Gland with Drainage Device, Open Approach

0C980ZX Drainage of Right Parotid Gland, Open Approach, Diagnostic

0C980ZZ Drainage of Right Parotid Gland, Open Approach

0C9830Z Drainage of Right Parotid Gland with Drainage Device, Percutaneous Approach

0C983ZX Drainage of Right Parotid Gland, Percutaneous Approach, Diagnostic

0C983ZZ Drainage of Right Parotid Gland, Percutaneous Approach

0C9900Z Drainage of Left Parotid Gland with Drainage Device, Open Approach

0C990ZX Drainage of Left Parotid Gland, Open Approach, Diagnostic

0C990ZZ Drainage of Left Parotid Gland, Open Approach

0C9930Z Drainage of Left Parotid Gland with Drainage Device, Percutaneous Approach

0C993ZX Drainage of Left Parotid Gland, Percutaneous Approach, Diagnostic

0C993ZZ Drainage of Left Parotid Gland, Percutaneous Approach

0C9B00Z Drainage of Right Parotid Duct with Drainage Device, Open Approach

0C9B0ZX Drainage of Right Parotid Duct, Open Approach, Diagnostic

0C9B0ZZ Drainage of Right Parotid Duct, Open Approach

0C9B30Z Drainage of Right Parotid Duct with Drainage Device, Percutaneous Approach

0C9B3ZX Drainage of Right Parotid Duct, Percutaneous Approach, Diagnostic

0C9B3ZZ Drainage of Right Parotid Duct, Percutaneous Approach

0C9C00Z Drainage of Left Parotid Duct with Drainage Device, Open Approach

0C9C0ZX Drainage of Left Parotid Duct, Open Approach, Diagnostic

0C9C0ZZ Drainage of Left Parotid Duct, Open Approach

0C9C30Z Drainage of Left Parotid Duct with Drainage Device, Percutaneous Approach

0C9C3ZX Drainage of Left Parotid Duct, Percutaneous Approach, Diagnostic

0C9C3ZZ Drainage of Left Parotid Duct, Percutaneous Approach

0C9D00Z Drainage of Right Sublingual Gland with Drainage Device, Open Approach

0C9D0ZX Drainage of Right Sublingual Gland, Open Approach, Diagnostic

0C9D0ZZ Drainage of Right Sublingual Gland, Open Approach

0C9D30Z Drainage of Right Sublingual Gland with Drainage Device, Percutaneous Approach

0C9D3ZX Drainage of Right Sublingual Gland, Percutaneous Approach, Diagnostic

0C9D3ZZ Drainage of Right Sublingual Gland, Percutaneous Approach

0C9F00Z Drainage of Left Sublingual Gland with Drainage Device, Open Approach

0C9F0ZX Drainage of Left Sublingual Gland, Open Approach, Diagnostic

0C9F0ZZ Drainage of Left Sublingual Gland, Open Approach

0C9F30Z Drainage of Left Sublingual Gland with Drainage Device, Percutaneous Approach

0C9F3ZX Drainage of Left Sublingual Gland, Percutaneous Approach, Diagnostic

0C9F3ZZ Drainage of Left Sublingual Gland, Percutaneous Approach

0C9G00Z Drainage of Right Submaxillary Gland with Drainage Device, Open Approach

0C9G0ZX Drainage of Right Submaxillary Gland, Open Approach, Diagnostic

0C9G0ZZ Drainage of Right Submaxillary Gland, Open Approach

0C9G30Z Drainage of Right Submaxillary Gland with Drainage Device, Percutaneous Approach

0C9G3ZX Drainage of Right Submaxillary Gland, Percutaneous Approach, Diagnostic

0C9G3ZZ Drainage of Right Submaxillary Gland, Percutaneous Approach

0C9H00Z Drainage of Left Submaxillary Gland with Drainage Device, Open Approach

0C9H0ZX Drainage of Left Submaxillary Gland, Open Approach, Diagnostic

0C9H0ZZ Drainage of Left Submaxillary Gland, Open Approach

0C9H30Z Drainage of Left Submaxillary Gland with Drainage Device, Percutaneous Approach

0C9H3ZX Drainage of Left Submaxillary Gland, Percutaneous Approach, Diagnostic

0C9H3ZZ Drainage of Left Submaxillary Gland, Percutaneous Approach

0C9J00Z Drainage of Minor Salivary Gland with Drainage Device, Open Approach

0C9J0ZX Drainage of Minor Salivary Gland, Open Approach, Diagnostic

0C9J0ZZ Drainage of Minor Salivary Gland, Open Approach

0C9J30Z Drainage of Minor Salivary Gland with Drainage Device, Percutaneous Approach

0C9J3ZX Drainage of Minor Salivary Gland, Percutaneous Approach, Diagnostic

0C9J3ZZ Drainage of Minor Salivary Gland, Percutaneous Approach

0C9M00Z Drainage of Pharynx with Drainage Device, Open Approach

0C9M0ZX Drainage of Pharynx, Open Approach, Diagnostic

0C9M0ZZ Drainage of Pharynx, Open Approach

0C9M30Z Drainage of Pharynx with Drainage Device, Percutaneous Approach

0C9M3ZX Drainage of Pharynx, Percutaneous Approach, Diagnostic

0C9M3ZZ Drainage of Pharynx, Percutaneous Approach

0C9M40Z Drainage of Pharynx with Drainage Device, Percutaneous Endoscopic Approach

0C9M4ZX Drainage of Pharynx, Percutaneous Endoscopic Approach, Diagnostic

0C9M4ZZ Drainage of Pharynx, Percutaneous Endoscopic Approach

0C9M70Z Drainage of Pharynx with Drainage Device, Via Natural or Artificial Opening

0C9M7ZX Drainage of Pharynx, Via Natural or Artificial Opening, Diagnostic

0C9M7ZZ Drainage of Pharynx, Via Natural or Artificial Opening

0C9M80Z Drainage of Pharynx with Drainage Device, Via Natural or Artificial Opening Endoscopic

0C9M8ZX Drainage of Pharynx, Via Natural or Artificial Opening Endoscopic, Diagnostic

0C9M8ZZ Drainage of Pharynx, Via Natural or Artificial Opening Endoscopic

0C9N00Z Drainage of Uvula with Drainage Device, Open Approach

0C9N0ZX Drainage of Uvula, Open Approach, Diagnostic

0C9N0ZZ Drainage of Uvula, Open Approach

0C9N30Z Drainage of Uvula with Drainage Device, Percutaneous Approach

0C9N3ZX Drainage of Uvula, Percutaneous Approach, Diagnostic

0C9N3ZZ Drainage of Uvula, Percutaneous Approach

0C9NX0Z Drainage of Uvula with Drainage Device, External Approach

0C9NXZX Drainage of Uvula, External Approach, Diagnostic

0C9NXZZ Drainage of Uvula, External Approach

0C9P00Z Drainage of Tonsils with Drainage Device, Open Approach

0C9P0ZX Drainage of Tonsils, Open Approach, Diagnostic

0C9P0ZZ Drainage of Tonsils, Open Approach

0C9P30Z Drainage of Tonsils with Drainage Device, Percutaneous Approach

0C9P3ZX Drainage of Tonsils, Percutaneous Approach, Diagnostic

0C9P3ZZ Drainage of Tonsils, Percutaneous Approach

0C9PX0Z Drainage of Tonsils with Drainage Device, External Approach

0C9PXZX Drainage of Tonsils, External Approach, Diagnostic

♀ Female-only   ♂ Male-only   ▲ Limited Coverage   ● Non-OR   ▦ HAC-associated procedure   ▲ Non-covered procedures   ✛ Combinati

⬤XZZ	Drainage of Tonsils, External Approach
⬤00Z	Drainage of Adenoids with Drainage Device, Open Approach
⬤0ZX	Drainage of Adenoids, Open Approach, Diagnostic
⬤0ZZ	Drainage of Adenoids, Open Approach
⬤30Z	Drainage of Adenoids with Drainage Device, Percutaneous Approach
⬤3ZX	Drainage of Adenoids, Percutaneous Approach, Diagnostic
⬤3ZZ	Drainage of Adenoids, Percutaneous Approach
⬤X0Z	Drainage of Adenoids with Drainage Device, External Approach
⬤XZX	Drainage of Adenoids, External Approach, Diagnostic
⬤XZZ	Drainage of Adenoids, External Approach
⬤R00Z	Drainage of Epiglottis with Drainage Device, Open Approach
⬤R0ZX	Drainage of Epiglottis, Open Approach, Diagnostic
⬤R0ZZ	Drainage of Epiglottis, Open Approach
⬤R30Z	Drainage of Epiglottis with Drainage Device, Percutaneous Approach
⬤R3ZX	Drainage of Epiglottis, Percutaneous Approach, Diagnostic
⬤R3ZZ	Drainage of Epiglottis, Percutaneous Approach
⬤R40Z	Drainage of Epiglottis with Drainage Device, Percutaneous Endoscopic Approach
⬤R4ZX	Drainage of Epiglottis, Percutaneous Endoscopic Approach, Diagnostic
⬤R4ZZ	Drainage of Epiglottis, Percutaneous Endoscopic Approach
⬤R70Z	Drainage of Epiglottis with Drainage Device, Via Natural or Artificial Opening
⬤R7ZX	Drainage of Epiglottis, Via Natural or Artificial Opening, Diagnostic
⬤R7ZZ	Drainage of Epiglottis, Via Natural or Artificial Opening
⬤R80Z	Drainage of Epiglottis with Drainage Device, Via Natural or Artificial Opening Endoscopic
⬤R8ZX	Drainage of Epiglottis, Via Natural or Artificial Opening Endoscopic, Diagnostic
⬤R8ZZ	Drainage of Epiglottis, Via Natural or Artificial Opening Endoscopic
⬤S00Z	Drainage of Larynx with Drainage Device, Open Approach
⬤S0ZX	Drainage of Larynx, Open Approach, Diagnostic
⬤S0ZZ	Drainage of Larynx, Open Approach
⬤S30Z	Drainage of Larynx with Drainage Device, Percutaneous Approach
⬤S3ZX	Drainage of Larynx, Percutaneous Approach, Diagnostic
⬤S3ZZ	Drainage of Larynx, Percutaneous Approach
⬤S40Z	Drainage of Larynx with Drainage Device, Percutaneous Endoscopic Approach
⬤S4ZX	Drainage of Larynx, Percutaneous Endoscopic Approach, Diagnostic
⬤S4ZZ	Drainage of Larynx, Percutaneous Endoscopic Approach
0C9S70Z	Drainage of Larynx with Drainage Device, Via Natural or Artificial Opening
0C9S7ZX	Drainage of Larynx, Via Natural or Artificial Opening, Diagnostic
0C9S7ZZ	Drainage of Larynx, Via Natural or Artificial Opening
0C9S80Z	Drainage of Larynx with Drainage Device, Via Natural or Artificial Opening Endoscopic
0C9S8ZX	Drainage of Larynx, Via Natural or Artificial Opening Endoscopic, Diagnostic
0C9S8ZZ	Drainage of Larynx, Via Natural or Artificial Opening Endoscopic
0C9T00Z	Drainage of Right Vocal Cord with Drainage Device, Open Approach
0C9T0ZX	Drainage of Right Vocal Cord, Open Approach, Diagnostic
0C9T0ZZ	Drainage of Right Vocal Cord, Open Approach
0C9T30Z	Drainage of Right Vocal Cord with Drainage Device, Percutaneous Approach
0C9T3ZX	Drainage of Right Vocal Cord, Percutaneous Approach, Diagnostic
0C9T3ZZ	Drainage of Right Vocal Cord, Percutaneous Approach
0C9T40Z	Drainage of Right Vocal Cord with Drainage Device, Percutaneous Endoscopic Approach
0C9T4ZX	Drainage of Right Vocal Cord, Percutaneous Endoscopic Approach, Diagnostic
0C9T4ZZ	Drainage of Right Vocal Cord, Percutaneous Endoscopic Approach
0C9T70Z	Drainage of Right Vocal Cord with Drainage Device, Via Natural or Artificial Opening
0C9T7ZX	Drainage of Right Vocal Cord, Via Natural or Artificial Opening, Diagnostic
0C9T7ZZ	Drainage of Right Vocal Cord, Via Natural or Artificial Opening
0C9T80Z	Drainage of Right Vocal Cord with Drainage Device, Via Natural or Artificial Opening Endoscopic
0C9T8ZX	Drainage of Right Vocal Cord, Via Natural or Artificial Opening Endoscopic, Diagnostic
0C9T8ZZ	Drainage of Right Vocal Cord, Via Natural or Artificial Opening Endoscopic
0C9V00Z	Drainage of Left Vocal Cord with Drainage Device, Open Approach
0C9V0ZX	Drainage of Left Vocal Cord, Open Approach, Diagnostic
0C9V0ZZ	Drainage of Left Vocal Cord, Open Approach
0C9V30Z	Drainage of Left Vocal Cord with Drainage Device, Percutaneous Approach
0C9V3ZX	Drainage of Left Vocal Cord, Percutaneous Approach, Diagnostic
0C9V3ZZ	Drainage of Left Vocal Cord, Percutaneous Approach
0C9V40Z	Drainage of Left Vocal Cord with Drainage Device, Percutaneous Endoscopic Approach
0C9V4ZX	Drainage of Left Vocal Cord, Percutaneous Endoscopic Approach, Diagnostic
0C9V4ZZ	Drainage of Left Vocal Cord, Percutaneous Endoscopic Approach
0C9V70Z	Drainage of Left Vocal Cord with Drainage Device, Via Natural or Artificial Opening
0C9V7ZX	Drainage of Left Vocal Cord, Via Natural or Artificial Opening, Diagnostic
0C9V7ZZ	Drainage of Left Vocal Cord, Via Natural or Artificial Opening
0C9V80Z	Drainage of Left Vocal Cord with Drainage Device, Via Natural or Artificial Opening Endoscopic
0C9V8ZX	Drainage of Left Vocal Cord, Via Natural or Artificial Opening Endoscopic, Diagnostic
0C9V8ZZ	Drainage of Left Vocal Cord, Via Natural or Artificial Opening Endoscopic
0C9W000	Drainage of Upper Tooth with Drainage Device, Open Approach, Single
0C9W001	Drainage of Upper Tooth with Drainage Device, Open Approach, Multiple
0C9W002	Drainage of Upper Tooth with Drainage Device, Open Approach, All
0C9W0Z0	Drainage of Upper Tooth, Open Approach, Single
0C9W0Z1	Drainage of Upper Tooth, Open Approach, Multiple
0C9W0Z2	Drainage of Upper Tooth, Open Approach, All
0C9WX00	Drainage of Upper Tooth with Drainage Device, External Approach, Single
0C9WX01	Drainage of Upper Tooth with Drainage Device, External Approach, Multiple
0C9WX02	Drainage of Upper Tooth with Drainage Device, External Approach, All
0C9WXZ0	Drainage of Upper Tooth, External Approach, Single
0C9WXZ1	Drainage of Upper Tooth, External Approach, Multiple
0C9WXZ2	Drainage of Upper Tooth, External Approach, All
0C9X000	Drainage of Lower Tooth with Drainage Device, Open Approach, Single
0C9X001	Drainage of Lower Tooth with Drainage Device, Open Approach, Multiple
0C9X002	Drainage of Lower Tooth with Drainage Device, Open Approach, All
0C9X0Z0	Drainage of Lower Tooth, Open Approach, Single
0C9X0Z1	Drainage of Lower Tooth, Open Approach, Multiple
0C9X0Z2	Drainage of Lower Tooth, Open Approach, All
0C9XX00	Drainage of Lower Tooth with Drainage Device, External Approach, Single
0C9XX01	Drainage of Lower Tooth with Drainage Device, External Approach, Multiple
0C9XX02	Drainage of Lower Tooth with Drainage Device, External Approach, All
0C9XXZ0	Drainage of Lower Tooth, External Approach, Single
0C9XXZ1	Drainage of Lower Tooth, External Approach, Multiple
0C9XXZ2	Drainage of Lower Tooth, External Approach, All

0CB – Mouth and Throat, Excision

Review Coding Guidelines B3.4a and B3.4b

Review Coding Guideline B3.8

⬤B00ZX	Excision of Upper Lip, Open Approach, Diagnostic
⬤B00ZZ	Excision of Upper Lip, Open Approach
⬤B03ZX	Excision of Upper Lip, Percutaneous Approach, Diagnostic
0CB03ZZ	Excision of Upper Lip, Percutaneous Approach
0CB0XZX	Excision of Upper Lip, External Approach, Diagnostic
0CB0XZZ	Excision of Upper Lip, External Approach
0CB10ZX	Excision of Lower Lip, Open Approach, Diagnostic
0CB10ZZ	Excision of Lower Lip, Open Approach
0CB13ZX	Excision of Lower Lip, Percutaneous Approach, Diagnostic

| ♀ Female-only | ♂ Male-only | ▲ Limited Coverage | ⬤ Non-OR | ▥ HAC-associated procedure | ▲ Non-covered procedures | ✚ Combination |

0CB13ZZ	Excision of Lower Lip, Percutaneous Approach
0CB1XZX	Excision of Lower Lip, External Approach, Diagnostic
0CB1XZZ	Excision of Lower Lip, External Approach
0CB20ZX	Excision of Hard Palate, Open Approach, Diagnostic
0CB20ZZ	Excision of Hard Palate, Open Approach
0CB23ZX	Excision of Hard Palate, Percutaneous Approach, Diagnostic
0CB23ZZ	Excision of Hard Palate, Percutaneous Approach
0CB2XZX	Excision of Hard Palate, External Approach, Diagnostic
0CB2XZZ	Excision of Hard Palate, External Approach
0CB30ZX	Excision of Soft Palate, Open Approach, Diagnostic
0CB30ZZ	Excision of Soft Palate, Open Approach
0CB33ZX	Excision of Soft Palate, Percutaneous Approach, Diagnostic
0CB33ZZ	Excision of Soft Palate, Percutaneous Approach
0CB3XZX	Excision of Soft Palate, External Approach, Diagnostic
0CB3XZZ	Excision of Soft Palate, External Approach
0CB40ZX	Excision of Buccal Mucosa, Open Approach, Diagnostic
0CB40ZZ	Excision of Buccal Mucosa, Open Approach
0CB43ZX	Excision of Buccal Mucosa, Percutaneous Approach, Diagnostic
0CB43ZZ	Excision of Buccal Mucosa, Percutaneous Approach
0CB4XZX	Excision of Buccal Mucosa, External Approach, Diagnostic
0CB4XZZ	Excision of Buccal Mucosa, External Approach
0CB50ZX	Excision of Upper Gingiva, Open Approach, Diagnostic
0CB50ZZ	Excision of Upper Gingiva, Open Approach
0CB53ZX	Excision of Upper Gingiva, Percutaneous Approach, Diagnostic
0CB53ZZ	Excision of Upper Gingiva, Percutaneous Approach
0CB5XZX	Excision of Upper Gingiva, External Approach, Diagnostic
0CB5XZZ	Excision of Upper Gingiva, External Approach
0CB60ZX	Excision of Lower Gingiva, Open Approach, Diagnostic
0CB60ZZ	Excision of Lower Gingiva, Open Approach
0CB63ZX	Excision of Lower Gingiva, Percutaneous Approach, Diagnostic
0CB63ZZ	Excision of Lower Gingiva, Percutaneous Approach
0CB6XZX	Excision of Lower Gingiva, External Approach, Diagnostic
0CB6XZZ	Excision of Lower Gingiva, External Approach
0CB70ZX	Excision of Tongue, Open Approach, Diagnostic
0CB70ZZ	Excision of Tongue, Open Approach
0CB73ZX	Excision of Tongue, Percutaneous Approach, Diagnostic
0CB73ZZ	Excision of Tongue, Percutaneous Approach
0CB7XZX	Excision of Tongue, External Approach, Diagnostic
0CB7XZZ	Excision of Tongue, External Approach
0CB80ZX	Excision of Right Parotid Gland, Open Approach, Diagnostic
0CB80ZZ	Excision of Right Parotid Gland, Open Approach

AHA CC: 3Q, 2014, 21-22

0CB83ZX	Excision of Right Parotid Gland, Percutaneous Approach, Diagnostic
0CB83ZZ	Excision of Right Parotid Gland, Percutaneous Approach
0CB90ZX	Excision of Left Parotid Gland, Open Approach, Diagnostic
0CB90ZZ	Excision of Left Parotid Gland, Open Approach
0CB93ZX	Excision of Left Parotid Gland, Percutaneous Approach, Diagnostic
0CB93ZZ	Excision of Left Parotid Gland, Percutaneous Approach
0CBB0ZX	Excision of Right Parotid Duct, Open Approach, Diagnostic
0CBB0ZZ	Excision of Right Parotid Duct, Open Approach
0CBB3ZX	Excision of Right Parotid Duct, Percutaneous Approach, Diagnostic
0CBB3ZZ	Excision of Right Parotid Duct, Percutaneous Approach
0CBC0ZX	Excision of Left Parotid Duct, Open Approach, Diagnostic
0CBC0ZZ	Excision of Left Parotid Duct, Open Approach
0CBC3ZX	Excision of Left Parotid Duct, Percutaneous Approach, Diagnostic
0CBC3ZZ	Excision of Left Parotid Duct, Percutaneous Approach
0CBD0ZX	Excision of Right Sublingual Gland, Open Approach, Diagnostic
0CBD0ZZ	Excision of Right Sublingual Gland, Open Approach
0CBD3ZX	Excision of Right Sublingual Gland, Percutaneous Approach, Diagnostic
0CBD3ZZ	Excision of Right Sublingual Gland, Percutaneous Approach
0CBF0ZX	Excision of Left Sublingual Gland, Open Approach, Diagnostic
0CBF0ZZ	Excision of Left Sublingual Gland, Open Approach
0CBF3ZX	Excision of Left Sublingual Gland, Percutaneous Approach, Diagnostic
0CBF3ZZ	Excision of Left Sublingual Gland, Percutaneous Approach
0CBG0ZX	Excision of Right Submaxillary Gland, Open Approach, Diagnostic
0CBG0ZZ	Excision of Right Submaxillary Gland, Open Approach
0CBG3ZX	Excision of Right Submaxillary Gland, Percutaneous Approach, Diagnostic
0CBG3ZZ	Excision of Right Submaxillary Gland, Percutaneous Approach
0CBH0ZX	Excision of Left Submaxillary Gland, Open Approach, Diagnostic
0CBH0ZZ	Excision of Left Submaxillary Gland, Open Approach
0CBH3ZX	Excision of Left Submaxillary Gland, Percutaneous Approach, Diagnostic
0CBH3ZZ	Excision of Left Submaxillary Gland, Percutaneous Approach
0CBJ0ZX	Excision of Minor Salivary Gland, Open Approach, Diagnostic
0CBJ0ZZ	Excision of Minor Salivary Gland, Open Approach
0CBJ3ZX	Excision of Minor Salivary Gland, Percutaneous Approach, Diagnostic
0CBJ3ZZ	Excision of Minor Salivary Gland, Percutaneous Approach
0CBM0ZX	Excision of Pharynx, Open Approach, Diagnostic
0CBM0ZZ	Excision of Pharynx, Open Approach
0CBM3ZX	Excision of Pharynx, Percutaneous Approach, Diagnostic
0CBM3ZZ	Excision of Pharynx, Percutaneous Approach
0CBM4ZX	Excision of Pharynx, Percutaneous Endoscopic Approach, Diagnostic

0CBM4ZZ	Excision of Pharynx, Percutaneous Endoscopic Approach
0CBM7ZX	Excision of Pharynx, Via Natural or Artificial Opening, Diagnostic
0CBM7ZZ	Excision of Pharynx, Via Natural or Artificial Opening
0CBM8ZX	Excision of Pharynx, Via Natural or Artificial Opening Endoscopic, Diagr
0CBM8ZZ	Excision of Pharynx, Via Natural or Artificial Opening Endoscopic
0CBN0ZX	Excision of Uvula, Open Approach, Diagnostic
0CBN0ZZ	Excision of Uvula, Open Approach
0CBN3ZX	Excision of Uvula, Percutaneous Approach, Diagnostic
0CBN3ZZ	Excision of Uvula, Percutaneous App
0CBNXZX	Excision of Uvula, External Approach Diagnostic
0CBNXZZ	Excision of Uvula, External Approach
0CBP0ZX	Excision of Tonsils, Open Approach, Diagnostic
0CBP0ZZ	Excision of Tonsils, Open Approach
0CBP3ZX	Excision of Tonsils, Percutaneous Approach, Diagnostic
0CBP3ZZ	Excision of Tonsils, Percutaneous Approach
0CBPXZX	Excision of Tonsils, External Approac Diagnostic
0CBPXZZ	Excision of Tonsils, External Approac
0CBQ0ZX	Excision of Adenoids, Open Approach Diagnostic
0CBQ0ZZ	Excision of Adenoids, Open Approach
0CBQ3ZX	Excision of Adenoids, Percutaneous Approach, Diagnostic
0CBQ3ZZ	Excision of Adenoids, Percutaneous Approach
0CBQXZX	Excision of Adenoids, External Approz Diagnostic
0CBQXZZ	Excision of Adenoids, External Approz
0CBR0ZX	Excision of Epiglottis, Open Approach Diagnostic
0CBR0ZZ	Excision of Epiglottis, Open Approach
0CBR3ZX	Excision of Epiglottis, Percutaneous Approach, Diagnostic
0CBR3ZZ	Excision of Epiglottis, Percutaneous Approach
0CBR4ZX	Excision of Epiglottis, Percutaneous Endoscopic Approach, Diagnostic
0CBR4ZZ	Excision of Epiglottis, Percutaneous Endoscopic Approach
0CBR7ZX	Excision of Epiglottis, Via Natural or Artificial Opening, Diagnostic
0CBR7ZZ	Excision of Epiglottis, Via Natural or Artificial Opening
0CBR8ZX	Excision of Epiglottis, Via Natural or Artificial Opening Endoscopic, Diagno
0CBR8ZZ	Excision of Epiglottis, Via Natural or Artificial Opening Endoscopic
0CBS0ZX	Excision of Larynx, Open Approach, Diagnostic
0CBS0ZZ	Excision of Larynx, Open Approach
0CBS3ZX	Excision of Larynx, Percutaneous Approach, Diagnostic
0CBS3ZZ	Excision of Larynx, Percutaneous Approach
0CBS4ZX	Excision of Larynx, Percutaneous Endoscopic Approach, Diagnostic
0CBS4ZZ	Excision of Larynx, Percutaneous Endoscopic Approach
0CBS7ZX	Excision of Larynx, Via Natural or Artificial Opening, Diagnostic
0CBS7ZZ	Excision of Larynx, Via Natural or Artificial Opening
0CBS8ZX	Excision of Larynx, Via Natural or Artificial Opening Endoscopic, Diagnos
0CBS8ZZ	Excision of Larynx, Via Natural or Artificial Opening Endoscopic

♀ Female-only   ♂ Male-only   ▲ Limited Coverage   ● Non-OR   ▬ HAC-associated procedure   ▲ Non-covered procedures   ✛ Combinat

0CBT0ZX Excision of Right Vocal Cord, Open Approach, Diagnostic
0CBT0ZZ Excision of Right Vocal Cord, Open Approach
0CBT3ZX Excision of Right Vocal Cord, Percutaneous Approach, Diagnostic
0CBT3ZZ Excision of Right Vocal Cord, Percutaneous Approach
0CBT4ZX Excision of Right Vocal Cord, Percutaneous Endoscopic Approach, Diagnostic
0CBT4ZZ Excision of Right Vocal Cord, Percutaneous Endoscopic Approach
0CBT7ZX Excision of Right Vocal Cord, Via Natural or Artificial Opening, Diagnostic
0CBT7ZZ Excision of Right Vocal Cord, Via Natural or Artificial Opening
0CBT8ZX Excision of Right Vocal Cord, Via Natural or Artificial Opening Endoscopic, Diagnostic
0CBT8ZZ Excision of Right Vocal Cord, Via Natural or Artificial Opening Endoscopic

0CBV0ZX Excision of Left Vocal Cord, Open Approach, Diagnostic
0CBV0ZZ Excision of Left Vocal Cord, Open Approach
0CBV3ZX Excision of Left Vocal Cord, Percutaneous Approach, Diagnostic
0CBV3ZZ Excision of Left Vocal Cord, Percutaneous Approach
0CBV4ZX Excision of Left Vocal Cord, Percutaneous Endoscopic Approach, Diagnostic
0CBV4ZZ Excision of Left Vocal Cord, Percutaneous Endoscopic Approach
0CBV7ZX Excision of Left Vocal Cord, Via Natural or Artificial Opening, Diagnostic
0CBV7ZZ Excision of Left Vocal Cord, Via Natural or Artificial Opening
0CBV8ZX Excision of Left Vocal Cord, Via Natural or Artificial Opening Endoscopic, Diagnostic
0CBV8ZZ Excision of Left Vocal Cord, Via Natural or Artificial Opening Endoscopic
0CBW0Z0 Excision of Upper Tooth, Open Approach, Single

0CBW0Z1 Excision of Upper Tooth, Open Approach, Multiple
0CBW0Z2 Excision of Upper Tooth, Open Approach, All
0CBWXZ0 Excision of Upper Tooth, External Approach, Single
0CBWXZ1 Excision of Upper Tooth, External Approach, Multiple
0CBWXZ2 Excision of Upper Tooth, External Approach, All
0CBX0Z0 Excision of Lower Tooth, Open Approach, Single
0CBX0Z1 Excision of Lower Tooth, Open Approach, Multiple
0CBX0Z2 Excision of Lower Tooth, Open Approach, All
0CBXXZ0 Excision of Lower Tooth, External Approach, Single
0CBXXZ1 Excision of Lower Tooth, External Approach, Multiple
0CBXXZ2 Excision of Lower Tooth, External Approach, All

0CC – Mouth and Throat, Extirpation

0CC00ZZ Extirpation of Matter from Upper Lip, Open Approach
0CC03ZZ Extirpation of Matter from Upper Lip, Percutaneous Approach
0CC0XZZ Extirpation of Matter from Upper Lip, External Approach
0CC10ZZ Extirpation of Matter from Lower Lip, Open Approach
0CC13ZZ Extirpation of Matter from Lower Lip, Percutaneous Approach
0CC1XZZ Extirpation of Matter from Lower Lip, External Approach
0CC20ZZ Extirpation of Matter from Hard Palate, Open Approach
0CC23ZZ Extirpation of Matter from Hard Palate, Percutaneous Approach
0CC2XZZ Extirpation of Matter from Hard Palate, External Approach
0CC30ZZ Extirpation of Matter from Soft Palate, Open Approach
0CC33ZZ Extirpation of Matter from Soft Palate, Percutaneous Approach
0CC3XZZ Extirpation of Matter from Soft Palate, External Approach
0CC40ZZ Extirpation of Matter from Buccal Mucosa, Open Approach
0CC43ZZ Extirpation of Matter from Buccal Mucosa, Percutaneous Approach
0CC4XZZ Extirpation of Matter from Buccal Mucosa, External Approach
0CC50ZZ Extirpation of Matter from Upper Gingiva, Open Approach
0CC53ZZ Extirpation of Matter from Upper Gingiva, Percutaneous Approach
0CC5XZZ Extirpation of Matter from Upper Gingiva, External Approach
0CC60ZZ Extirpation of Matter from Lower Gingiva, Open Approach
0CC63ZZ Extirpation of Matter from Lower Gingiva, Percutaneous Approach
0CC6XZZ Extirpation of Matter from Lower Gingiva, External Approach
0CC70ZZ Extirpation of Matter from Tongue, Open Approach
0CC73ZZ Extirpation of Matter from Tongue, Percutaneous Approach
0CC7XZZ Extirpation of Matter from Tongue, External Approach
0CC80ZZ Extirpation of Matter from Right Parotid Gland, Open Approach

0CC83ZZ Extirpation of Matter from Right Parotid Gland, Percutaneous Approach
0CC90ZZ Extirpation of Matter from Left Parotid Gland, Open Approach
0CC93ZZ Extirpation of Matter from Left Parotid Gland, Percutaneous Approach
0CCB0ZZ Extirpation of Matter from Right Parotid Duct, Open Approach
0CCB3ZZ Extirpation of Matter from Right Parotid Duct, Percutaneous Approach
0CCC0ZZ Extirpation of Matter from Left Parotid Duct, Open Approach
0CCC3ZZ Extirpation of Matter from Left Parotid Duct, Percutaneous Approach
0CCD0ZZ Extirpation of Matter from Right Sublingual Gland, Open Approach
0CCD3ZZ Extirpation of Matter from Right Sublingual Gland, Percutaneous Approach
0CCF0ZZ Extirpation of Matter from Left Sublingual Gland, Open Approach
0CCF3ZZ Extirpation of Matter from Left Sublingual Gland, Percutaneous Approach
0CCG0ZZ Extirpation of Matter from Right Submaxillary Gland, Open Approach
0CCG3ZZ Extirpation of Matter from Right Submaxillary Gland, Percutaneous Approach
0CCH0ZZ Extirpation of Matter from Left Submaxillary Gland, Open Approach
0CCH3ZZ Extirpation of Matter from Left Submaxillary Gland, Percutaneous Approach
0CCJ0ZZ Extirpation of Matter from Minor Salivary Gland, Open Approach
0CCJ3ZZ Extirpation of Matter from Minor Salivary Gland, Percutaneous Approach
0CCM0ZZ Extirpation of Matter from Pharynx, Open Approach
0CCM3ZZ Extirpation of Matter from Pharynx, Percutaneous Approach
0CCM4ZZ Extirpation of Matter from Pharynx, Percutaneous Endoscopic Approach
0CCM7ZZ Extirpation of Matter from Pharynx, Via Natural or Artificial Opening
0CCM8ZZ Extirpation of Matter from Pharynx, Via Natural or Artificial Opening Endoscopic
0CCN0ZZ Extirpation of Matter from Uvula, Open Approach
0CCN3ZZ Extirpation of Matter from Uvula, Percutaneous Approach

0CCNXZZ Extirpation of Matter from Uvula, External Approach
0CCP0ZZ Extirpation of Matter from Tonsils, Open Approach
0CCP3ZZ Extirpation of Matter from Tonsils, Percutaneous Approach
0CCPXZZ Extirpation of Matter from Tonsils, External Approach
0CCQ0ZZ Extirpation of Matter from Adenoids, Open Approach
0CCQ3ZZ Extirpation of Matter from Adenoids, Percutaneous Approach
0CCQXZZ Extirpation of Matter from Adenoids, External Approach
0CCR0ZZ Extirpation of Matter from Epiglottis, Open Approach
0CCR3ZZ Extirpation of Matter from Epiglottis, Percutaneous Approach
0CCR4ZZ Extirpation of Matter from Epiglottis, Percutaneous Endoscopic Approach
0CCR7ZZ Extirpation of Matter from Epiglottis, Via Natural or Artificial Opening
0CCR8ZZ Extirpation of Matter from Epiglottis, Via Natural or Artificial Opening Endoscopic
0CCS0ZZ Extirpation of Matter from Larynx, Open Approach
0CCS3ZZ Extirpation of Matter from Larynx, Percutaneous Approach
0CCS4ZZ Extirpation of Matter from Larynx, Percutaneous Endoscopic Approach
0CCS7ZZ Extirpation of Matter from Larynx, Via Natural or Artificial Opening
0CCS8ZZ Extirpation of Matter from Larynx, Via Natural or Artificial Opening Endoscopic
0CCT0ZZ Extirpation of Matter from Right Vocal Cord, Open Approach
0CCT3ZZ Extirpation of Matter from Right Vocal Cord, Percutaneous Approach
0CCT4ZZ Extirpation of Matter from Right Vocal Cord, Percutaneous Endoscopic Approach
0CCT7ZZ Extirpation of Matter from Right Vocal Cord, Via Natural or Artificial Opening
0CCT8ZZ Extirpation of Matter from Right Vocal Cord, Via Natural or Artificial Opening Endoscopic
0CCV0ZZ Extirpation of Matter from Left Vocal Cord, Open Approach
0CCV3ZZ Extirpation of Matter from Left Vocal Cord, Percutaneous Approach

♀ Female-only	♂ Male-only	▲ Limited Coverage	● Non-OR	HAC HAC-associated procedure	▲ Non-covered procedures	✚ Combination

0CCV4ZZ	Extirpation of Matter from Left Vocal Cord, Percutaneous Endoscopic Approach	**0CCW0Z2**	Extirpation of Matter from Upper Tooth, All, Open Approach	**0CCX0Z2**	Extirpation of Matter from Lower To All, Open Approach
0CCV7ZZ	Extirpation of Matter from Left Vocal Cord, Via Natural or Artificial Opening	**0CCWXZ0**	Extirpation of Matter from Upper Tooth, Single, External Approach	**0CCXXZ0**	Extirpation of Matter from Lower To Single, External Approach
0CCV8ZZ	Extirpation of Matter from Left Vocal Cord, Via Natural or Artificial Opening Endoscopic	**0CCWXZ1**	Extirpation of Matter from Upper Tooth, Multiple, External Approach	**0CCXXZ1**	Extirpation of Matter from Lower To Multiple, External Approach
0CCW0Z0	Extirpation of Matter from Upper Tooth, Single, Open Approach	**0CCWXZ2**	Extirpation of Matter from Upper Tooth, All, External Approach	**0CCXXZ2**	Extirpation of Matter from Lower To All, External Approach
0CCW0Z1	Extirpation of Matter from Upper Tooth, Multiple, Open Approach	**0CCX0Z0**	Extirpation of Matter from Lower Tooth, Single, Open Approach		
		0CCX0Z1	Extirpation of Matter from Lower Tooth, Multiple, Open Approach		

0CD – Mouth and Throat, Extraction

0CDT0ZZ	Extraction of Right Vocal Cord, Open Approach	**0CDV3ZZ**	Extraction of Left Vocal Cord, Percutaneous Approach	**0CDWXZ2**	Extraction of Upper Tooth, All, Exter Approach
0CDT3ZZ	Extraction of Right Vocal Cord, Percutaneous Approach	**0CDV4ZZ**	Extraction of Left Vocal Cord, Percutaneous Endoscopic Approach	**0CDXXZ0**	Extraction of Lower Tooth, Single, External Approach
0CDT4ZZ	Extraction of Right Vocal Cord, Percutaneous Endoscopic Approach	**0CDV7ZZ**	Extraction of Left Vocal Cord, Via Natural or Artificial Opening	**0CDXXZ1**	Extraction of Lower Tooth, Multiple, External Approach
0CDT7ZZ	Extraction of Right Vocal Cord, Via Natural or Artificial Opening	**0CDV8ZZ**	Extraction of Left Vocal Cord, Via Natural or Artificial Opening Endoscopic	**0CDXXZ2**	Extraction of Lower Tooth, All, Exter Approach
0CDT8ZZ	Extraction of Right Vocal Cord, Via Natural or Artificial Opening Endoscopic	**0CDWXZ0**	Extraction of Upper Tooth, Single, External Approach		
0CDV0ZZ	Extraction of Left Vocal Cord, Open Approach	**0CDWXZ1**	Extraction of Upper Tooth, Multiple, External Approach		

0CF – Mouth and Throat, Fragmentation

0CFB0ZZ	Fragmentation in Right Parotid Duct, Open Approach	▲ **0CFBXZZ**	Fragmentation in Right Parotid Duct, External Approach	**0CFC7ZZ**	Fragmentation in Left Parotid Duct, V Natural or Artificial Opening
0CFB3ZZ	Fragmentation in Right Parotid Duct, Percutaneous Approach	**0CFC0ZZ**	Fragmentation in Left Parotid Duct, Open Approach	▲ **0CFCXZZ**	Fragmentation in Left Parotid Duct, External Approach
0CFB7ZZ	Fragmentation in Right Parotid Duct, Via Natural or Artificial Opening	**0CFC3ZZ**	Fragmentation in Left Parotid Duct, Percutaneous Approach		

0CH – Mouth and Throat, Insertion

0CH701Z	Insertion of Radioactive Element into Tongue, Open Approach	**0CH7X1Z**	Insertion of Radioactive Element into Tongue, External Approach	**0CHY8BZ**	Insertion of Airway into Mouth and Throat, Via Natural or Artificial Open Endoscopic
0CH731Z	Insertion of Radioactive Element into Tongue, Percutaneous Approach	**0CHY7BZ**	Insertion of Airway into Mouth and Throat, Via Natural or Artificial Opening		

0CJ – Mouth and Throat, Inspection

Review Coding Guidelines B3.11a, B3.11b and B3.11c

0CJA0ZZ	Inspection of Salivary Gland, Open Approach	**0CJS4ZZ**	Inspection of Larynx, Percutaneous Endoscopic Approach	**0CJY3ZZ**	Inspection of Mouth and Throat, Percutaneous Approach
0CJA3ZZ	Inspection of Salivary Gland, Percutaneous Approach	**0CJS7ZZ**	Inspection of Larynx, Via Natural or Artificial Opening	**0CJY4ZZ**	Inspection of Mouth and Throat, Percutaneous Endoscopic Approach
0CJAXZZ	Inspection of Salivary Gland, External Approach	**0CJS8ZZ**	Inspection of Larynx, Via Natural or Artificial Opening Endoscopic	**0CJY7ZZ**	Inspection of Mouth and Throat, Via Natural or Artificial Opening
0CJS0ZZ	Inspection of Larynx, Open Approach	**0CJSXZZ**	Inspection of Larynx, External Approach	**0CJY8ZZ**	Inspection of Mouth and Throat, Via Natural or Artificial Opening Endoscop
0CJS3ZZ	Inspection of Larynx, Percutaneous Approach	**0CJY0ZZ**	Inspection of Mouth and Throat, Open Approach	**0CJYXZZ**	Inspection of Mouth and Throat, Exter Approach

0CL – Mouth and Throat, Occlusion

0CLB0CZ	Occlusion of Right Parotid Duct with Extraluminal Device, Open Approach	**0CLB4CZ**	Occlusion of Right Parotid Duct with Extraluminal Device, Percutaneous Endoscopic Approach	**0CLB8ZZ**	Occlusion of Right Parotid Duct, Via Natural or Artificial Opening Endoscopic
0CLB0DZ	Occlusion of Right Parotid Duct with Intraluminal Device, Open Approach	**0CLB4DZ**	Occlusion of Right Parotid Duct with Intraluminal Device, Percutaneous Endoscopic Approach	**0CLC0CZ**	Occlusion of Left Parotid Duct with Extraluminal Device, Open Approach
0CLB0ZZ	Occlusion of Right Parotid Duct, Open Approach	**0CLB4ZZ**	Occlusion of Right Parotid Duct, Percutaneous Endoscopic Approach	**0CLC0DZ**	Occlusion of Left Parotid Duct with Intraluminal Device, Open Approach
0CLB3CZ	Occlusion of Right Parotid Duct with Extraluminal Device, Percutaneous Approach	**0CLB7DZ**	Occlusion of Right Parotid Duct with Intraluminal Device, Via Natural or Artificial Opening	**0CLC0ZZ**	Occlusion of Left Parotid Duct, Open Approach
0CLB3DZ	Occlusion of Right Parotid Duct with Intraluminal Device, Percutaneous Approach	**0CLB7ZZ**	Occlusion of Right Parotid Duct, Via Natural or Artificial Opening	**0CLC3CZ**	Occlusion of Left Parotid Duct with Extraluminal Device, Percutaneous Approach
0CLB3ZZ	Occlusion of Right Parotid Duct, Percutaneous Approach	**0CLB8DZ**	Occlusion of Right Parotid Duct with Intraluminal Device, Via Natural or Artificial Opening Endoscopic	**0CLC3DZ**	Occlusion of Left Parotid Duct with Intraluminal Device, Percutaneous Approach

C3ZZ   Occlusion of Left Parotid Duct, Percutaneous Approach

C4CZ   Occlusion of Left Parotid Duct with Extraluminal Device, Percutaneous Endoscopic Approach

C4DZ   Occlusion of Left Parotid Duct with Intraluminal Device, Percutaneous Endoscopic Approach

0CLC4ZZ   Occlusion of Left Parotid Duct, Percutaneous Endoscopic Approach

0CLC7DZ   Occlusion of Left Parotid Duct with Intraluminal Device, Via Natural or Artificial Opening

0CLC7ZZ   Occlusion of Left Parotid Duct, Via Natural or Artificial Opening

0CLC8DZ   Occlusion of Left Parotid Duct with Intraluminal Device, Via Natural or Artificial Opening Endoscopic

0CLC8ZZ   Occlusion of Left Parotid Duct, Via Natural or Artificial Opening Endoscopic

M – Mouth and Throat, Reattachment

M00ZZ   Reattachment of Upper Lip, Open Approach

M10ZZ   Reattachment of Lower Lip, Open Approach

M30ZZ   Reattachment of Soft Palate, Open Approach

M70ZZ   Reattachment of Tongue, Open Approach

MN0ZZ   Reattachment of Uvula, Open Approach

MW0Z0   Reattachment of Upper Tooth, Single, Open Approach

0CMW0Z1   Reattachment of Upper Tooth, Multiple, Open Approach

0CMW0Z2   Reattachment of Upper Tooth, All, Open Approach

0CMWXZ0   Reattachment of Upper Tooth, Single, External Approach

0CMWXZ1   Reattachment of Upper Tooth, Multiple, External Approach

0CMWXZ2   Reattachment of Upper Tooth, All, External Approach

0CMX0Z0   Reattachment of Lower Tooth, Single, Open Approach

0CMX0Z1   Reattachment of Lower Tooth, Multiple, Open Approach

0CMX0Z2   Reattachment of Lower Tooth, All, Open Approach

0CMXXZ0   Reattachment of Lower Tooth, Single, External Approach

0CMXXZ1   Reattachment of Lower Tooth, Multiple, External Approach

0CMXXZ2   Reattachment of Lower Tooth, All, External Approach

N – Mouth and Throat, Release

Review Coding Guidelines B3.13 and B3.14

N00ZZ   Release Upper Lip, Open Approach

N03ZZ   Release Upper Lip, Percutaneous Approach

N0XZZ   Release Upper Lip, External Approach

N10ZZ   Release Lower Lip, Open Approach

N13ZZ   Release Lower Lip, Percutaneous Approach

N1XZZ   Release Lower Lip, External Approach

N20ZZ   Release Hard Palate, Open Approach

N23ZZ   Release Hard Palate, Percutaneous Approach

N2XZZ   Release Hard Palate, External Approach

N30ZZ   Release Soft Palate, Open Approach

N33ZZ   Release Soft Palate, Percutaneous Approach

N3XZZ   Release Soft Palate, External Approach

N40ZZ   Release Buccal Mucosa, Open Approach

N43ZZ   Release Buccal Mucosa, Percutaneous Approach

N4XZZ   Release Buccal Mucosa, External Approach

N50ZZ   Release Upper Gingiva, Open Approach

N53ZZ   Release Upper Gingiva, Percutaneous Approach

N5XZZ   Release Upper Gingiva, External Approach

N60ZZ   Release Lower Gingiva, Open Approach

N63ZZ   Release Lower Gingiva, Percutaneous Approach

N6XZZ   Release Lower Gingiva, External Approach

N70ZZ   Release Tongue, Open Approach

N73ZZ   Release Tongue, Percutaneous Approach

N7XZZ   Release Tongue, External Approach

N80ZZ   Release Right Parotid Gland, Open Approach

N83ZZ   Release Right Parotid Gland, Percutaneous Approach

N90ZZ   Release Left Parotid Gland, Open Approach

N93ZZ   Release Left Parotid Gland, Percutaneous Approach

NB0ZZ   Release Right Parotid Duct, Open Approach

NB3ZZ   Release Right Parotid Duct, Percutaneous Approach

0CNC0ZZ   Release Left Parotid Duct, Open Approach

0CNC3ZZ   Release Left Parotid Duct, Percutaneous Approach

0CND0ZZ   Release Right Sublingual Gland, Open Approach

0CND3ZZ   Release Right Sublingual Gland, Percutaneous Approach

0CNF0ZZ   Release Left Sublingual Gland, Open Approach

0CNF3ZZ   Release Left Sublingual Gland, Percutaneous Approach

0CNG0ZZ   Release Right Submaxillary Gland, Open Approach

0CNG3ZZ   Release Right Submaxillary Gland, Percutaneous Approach

0CNH0ZZ   Release Left Submaxillary Gland, Open Approach

0CNH3ZZ   Release Left Submaxillary Gland, Percutaneous Approach

0CNJ0ZZ   Release Minor Salivary Gland, Open Approach

0CNJ3ZZ   Release Minor Salivary Gland, Percutaneous Approach

0CNM0ZZ   Release Pharynx, Open Approach

0CNM3ZZ   Release Pharynx, Percutaneous Approach

0CNM4ZZ   Release Pharynx, Percutaneous Endoscopic Approach

0CNM7ZZ   Release Pharynx, Via Natural or Artificial Opening

0CNM8ZZ   Release Pharynx, Via Natural or Artificial Opening Endoscopic

0CNN0ZZ   Release Uvula, Open Approach

0CNN3ZZ   Release Uvula, Percutaneous Approach

0CNNXZZ   Release Uvula, External Approach

0CNP0ZZ   Release Tonsils, Open Approach

0CNP3ZZ   Release Tonsils, Percutaneous Approach

0CNPXZZ   Release Tonsils, External Approach

0CNQ0ZZ   Release Adenoids, Open Approach

0CNQ3ZZ   Release Adenoids, Percutaneous Approach

0CNQXZZ   Release Adenoids, External Approach

0CNR0ZZ   Release Epiglottis, Open Approach

0CNR3ZZ   Release Epiglottis, Percutaneous Approach

0CNR4ZZ   Release Epiglottis, Percutaneous Endoscopic Approach

0CNR7ZZ   Release Epiglottis, Via Natural or Artificial Opening

0CNR8ZZ   Release Epiglottis, Via Natural or Artificial Opening Endoscopic

0CNS0ZZ   Release Larynx, Open Approach

0CNS3ZZ   Release Larynx, Percutaneous Approach

0CNS4ZZ   Release Larynx, Percutaneous Endoscopic Approach

0CNS7ZZ   Release Larynx, Via Natural or Artificial Opening

0CNS8ZZ   Release Larynx, Via Natural or Artificial Opening Endoscopic

0CNT0ZZ   Release Right Vocal Cord, Open Approach

0CNT3ZZ   Release Right Vocal Cord, Percutaneous Approach

0CNT4ZZ   Release Right Vocal Cord, Percutaneous Endoscopic Approach

0CNT7ZZ   Release Right Vocal Cord, Via Natural or Artificial Opening

0CNT8ZZ   Release Right Vocal Cord, Via Natural or Artificial Opening Endoscopic

0CNV0ZZ   Release Left Vocal Cord, Open Approach

0CNV3ZZ   Release Left Vocal Cord, Percutaneous Approach

0CNV4ZZ   Release Left Vocal Cord, Percutaneous Endoscopic Approach

0CNV7ZZ   Release Left Vocal Cord, Via Natural or Artificial Opening

0CNV8ZZ   Release Left Vocal Cord, Via Natural or Artificial Opening Endoscopic

0CNW0Z0   Release Upper Tooth, Single, Open Approach

0CNW0Z1   Release Upper Tooth, Multiple, Open Approach

0CNW0Z2   Release Upper Tooth, All, Open Approach

0CNWXZ0   Release Upper Tooth, Single, External Approach

0CNWXZ1   Release Upper Tooth, Multiple, External Approach

0CNWXZ2   Release Upper Tooth, All, External Approach

♀ Female-only   ♂ Male-only   ▲ Limited Coverage   ● Non-OR   ▧ HAC-associated procedure   ▲ Non-covered procedures   ✚ Combination

0CNX0Z0	Release Lower Tooth, Single, Open Approach	
0CNX0Z1	Release Lower Tooth, Multiple, Open Approach	

0CNX0Z2 Release Lower Tooth, All, Open Approach

0CNXXZ0 Release Lower Tooth, Single, External Approach

0CNXXZ1 Release Lower Tooth, Multiple, Exte Approach

0CNXXZ2 Release Lower Tooth, All, External Approach

0CP – Mouth and Throat, Removal

Review Coding Guideline B6.1c

0CPA00Z Removal of Drainage Device from Salivary Gland, Open Approach

0CPA0CZ Removal of Extraluminal Device from Salivary Gland, Open Approach

0CPA30Z Removal of Drainage Device from Salivary Gland, Percutaneous Approach

0CPA3CZ Removal of Extraluminal Device from Salivary Gland, Percutaneous Approach

0CPS00Z Removal of Drainage Device from Larynx, Open Approach

0CPS07Z Removal of Autologous Tissue Substitute from Larynx, Open Approach

0CPS0DZ Removal of Intraluminal Device from Larynx, Open Approach

0CPS0JZ Removal of Synthetic Substitute from Larynx, Open Approach

0CPS0KZ Removal of Nonautologous Tissue Substitute from Larynx, Open Approach

0CPS30Z Removal of Drainage Device from Larynx, Percutaneous Approach

0CPS37Z Removal of Autologous Tissue Substitute from Larynx, Percutaneous Approach

0CPS3DZ Removal of Intraluminal Device from Larynx, Percutaneous Approach

0CPS3JZ Removal of Synthetic Substitute from Larynx, Percutaneous Approach

0CPS3KZ Removal of Nonautologous Tissue Substitute from Larynx, Percutaneous Approach

0CPS70Z Removal of Drainage Device from Larynx, Via Natural or Artificial Opening

0CPS77Z Removal of Autologous Tissue Substitute from Larynx, Via Natural or Artificial Opening

0CPS7DZ Removal of Intraluminal Device from Larynx, Via Natural or Artificial Opening

0CPS7JZ Removal of Synthetic Substitute from Larynx, Via Natural or Artificial Opening

0CPS7KZ Removal of Nonautologous Tissue Substitute from Larynx, Via Natural or Artificial Opening

0CPS80Z Removal of Drainage Device from Larynx, Via Natural or Artificial Opening Endoscopic

0CPS87Z Removal of Autologous Tissue Substitute from Larynx, Via Natural or Artificial Opening Endoscopic

0CPS8DZ Removal of Intraluminal Device from Larynx, Via Natural or Artificial Opening Endoscopic

0CPS8JZ Removal of Synthetic Substitute from Larynx, Via Natural or Artificial Opening Endoscopic

0CPS8KZ Removal of Nonautologous Tissue Substitute from Larynx, Via Natural or Artificial Opening Endoscopic

0CPSX0Z Removal of Drainage Device from Larynx, External Approach

0CPSX7Z Removal of Autologous Tissue Substitute from Larynx, External Approach

0CPSXDZ Removal of Intraluminal Device from Larynx, External Approach

0CPSXJZ Removal of Synthetic Substitute from Larynx, External Approach

0CPSXKZ Removal of Nonautologous Tissue Substitute from Larynx, External Approach

0CPY00Z Removal of Drainage Device from Mouth and Throat, Open Approach

0CPY01Z Removal of Radioactive Element from Mouth and Throat, Open Approach

0CPY07Z Removal of Autologous Tissue Substitute from Mouth and Throat, Open Approach

0CPY0DZ Removal of Intraluminal Device from Mouth and Throat, Open Approach

0CPY0JZ Removal of Synthetic Substitute from Mouth and Throat, Open Approach

0CPY0KZ Removal of Nonautologous Tissue Substitute from Mouth and Throat, Open Approach

0CPY30Z Removal of Drainage Device from Mouth and Throat, Percutaneous Approach

0CPY31Z Removal of Radioactive Element from Mouth and Throat, Percutaneous Approach

0CPY37Z Removal of Autologous Tissue Substitute from Mouth and Throat, Percutaneous Approach

0CPY3DZ Removal of Intraluminal Device from Mouth and Throat, Percutaneous Approach

0CPY3JZ Removal of Synthetic Substitute from Mouth and Throat, Percutaneous Approach

0CPY3KZ Removal of Nonautologous Tissue Substitute from Mouth and Throat, Percutaneous Approach

0CPY70Z Removal of Drainage Device from Mouth and Throat, Via Natural or Artificial Opening

0CPY71Z Removal of Radioactive Element from Mouth and Throat, Via Natural or Artificial Opening

0CPY77Z Removal of Autologous Tissue Substit from Mouth and Throat, Via Natural o Artificial Opening

0CPY7DZ Removal of Intraluminal Device from Mouth and Throat, Via Natural or Artificial Opening

0CPY7JZ Removal of Synthetic Substitute from Mouth and Throat, Via Natural or Artificial Opening

0CPY7KZ Removal of Nonautologous Tissue Substitute from Mouth and Throat, Via Natural or Artificial Opening

0CPY80Z Removal of Drainage Device from Mo and Throat, Via Natural or Artificial Opening Endoscopic

0CPY81Z Removal of Radioactive Element from Mouth and Throat, Via Natural or Artificial Opening Endoscopic

0CPY87Z Removal of Autologous Tissue Substit from Mouth and Throat, Via Natural or Artificial Opening Endoscopic

0CPY8DZ Removal of Intraluminal Device from Mouth and Throat, Via Natural or Artificial Opening Endoscopic

0CPY8JZ Removal of Synthetic Substitute from Mouth and Throat, Via Natural or Artificial Opening Endoscopic

0CPY8KZ Removal of Nonautologous Tissue Substitute from Mouth and Throat, Via Natural or Artificial Opening Endoscopic

0CPYX0Z Removal of Drainage Device from Mo and Throat, External Approach

0CPYX1Z Removal of Radioactive Element from Mouth and Throat, External Approach

0CPYX7Z Removal of Autologous Tissue Substitu from Mouth and Throat, External Approach

0CPYXDZ Removal of Intraluminal Device from Mouth and Throat, External Approach

0CPYXJZ Removal of Synthetic Substitute from Mouth and Throat, External Approach

0CPYXKZ Removal of Nonautologous Tissue Substitute from Mouth and Throat, External Approach

0CQ – Mouth and Throat, Repair

0CQ00ZZ Repair Upper Lip, Open Approach

0CQ03ZZ Repair Upper Lip, Percutaneous Approach

0CQ0XZZ Repair Upper Lip, External Approach

0CQ10ZZ Repair Lower Lip, Open Approach

0CQ13ZZ Repair Lower Lip, Percutaneous Approach

0CQ1XZZ Repair Lower Lip, External Approach

0CQ20ZZ Repair Hard Palate, Open Approach

0CQ23ZZ Repair Hard Palate, Percutaneous Approach

0CQ2XZZ Repair Hard Palate, External Approach

0CQ30ZZ Repair Soft Palate, Open Approach

0CQ33ZZ Repair Soft Palate, Percutaneous Approach

0CQ3XZZ Repair Soft Palate, External Approach

0CQ40ZZ Repair Buccal Mucosa, Open Approach

0CQ43ZZ Repair Buccal Mucosa, Percutaneous Approach

0CQ4XZZ Repair Buccal Mucosa, External Approach

0CQ50ZZ Repair Upper Gingiva, Open Approach

0CQ53ZZ Repair Upper Gingiva, Percutaneous Approach

0CQ5XZZ Repair Upper Gingiva, External Approach

0CQ60ZZ Repair Lower Gingiva, Open Approach

0CQ63ZZ Repair Lower Gingiva, Percutaneous Approach

0CQ6XZZ Repair Lower Gingiva, External Approach

0CQ70ZZ Repair Tongue, Open Approach

0CQ73ZZ Repair Tongue, Percutaneous Approach

0CQ7XZZ Repair Tongue, External Approach

0CQ80ZZ Repair Right Parotid Gland, Open Approach

0CQ83ZZ Repair Right Parotid Gland, Percutaneo Approach

0CQ90ZZ Repair Left Parotid Gland, Open Approach

0CQ93ZZ Repair Left Parotid Gland, Percutaneous Approach

0CQB0ZZ Repair Right Parotid Duct, Open Approach

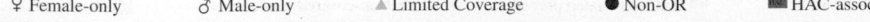

♀ Female-only   ♂ Male-only   ▲ Limited Coverage   ● Non-OR   ▰▰ HAC-associated procedure   ▲ Non-covered procedures   ✚ Combinati

B3ZZ	Repair Right Parotid Duct, Percutaneous Approach
C0ZZ	Repair Left Parotid Duct, Open Approach
C3ZZ	Repair Left Parotid Duct, Percutaneous Approach
D0ZZ	Repair Right Sublingual Gland, Open Approach
D3ZZ	Repair Right Sublingual Gland, Percutaneous Approach
F0ZZ	Repair Left Sublingual Gland, Open Approach
F3ZZ	Repair Left Sublingual Gland, Percutaneous Approach
G0ZZ	Repair Right Submaxillary Gland, Open Approach
G3ZZ	Repair Right Submaxillary Gland, Percutaneous Approach
H0ZZ	Repair Left Submaxillary Gland, Open Approach
H3ZZ	Repair Left Submaxillary Gland, Percutaneous Approach
J0ZZ	Repair Minor Salivary Gland, Open Approach
J3ZZ	Repair Minor Salivary Gland, Percutaneous Approach
M0ZZ	Repair Pharynx, Open Approach
M3ZZ	Repair Pharynx, Percutaneous Approach
M4ZZ	Repair Pharynx, Percutaneous Endoscopic Approach
M7ZZ	Repair Pharynx, Via Natural or Artificial Opening
M8ZZ	Repair Pharynx, Via Natural or Artificial Opening Endoscopic
N0ZZ	Repair Uvula, Open Approach

0CQN3ZZ	Repair Uvula, Percutaneous Approach
0CQNXZZ	Repair Uvula, External Approach
0CQP0ZZ	Repair Tonsils, Open Approach
0CQP3ZZ	Repair Tonsils, Percutaneous Approach
0CQPXZZ	Repair Tonsils, External Approach
0CQQ0ZZ	Repair Adenoids, Open Approach
0CQQ3ZZ	Repair Adenoids, Percutaneous Approach
0CQQXZZ	Repair Adenoids, External Approach
0CQR0ZZ	Repair Epiglottis, Open Approach
0CQR3ZZ	Repair Epiglottis, Percutaneous Approach
0CQR4ZZ	Repair Epiglottis, Percutaneous Endoscopic Approach
0CQR7ZZ	Repair Epiglottis, Via Natural or Artificial Opening
0CQR8ZZ	Repair Epiglottis, Via Natural or Artificial Opening Endoscopic
0CQS0ZZ	Repair Larynx, Open Approach
0CQS3ZZ	Repair Larynx, Percutaneous Approach
0CQS4ZZ	Repair Larynx, Percutaneous Endoscopic Approach
0CQS7ZZ	Repair Larynx, Via Natural or Artificial Opening
0CQS8ZZ	Repair Larynx, Via Natural or Artificial Opening Endoscopic
0CQT0ZZ	Repair Right Vocal Cord, Open Approach
0CQT3ZZ	Repair Right Vocal Cord, Percutaneous Approach
0CQT4ZZ	Repair Right Vocal Cord, Percutaneous Endoscopic Approach
0CQT7ZZ	Repair Right Vocal Cord, Via Natural or Artificial Opening
0CQT8ZZ	Repair Right Vocal Cord, Via Natural or Artificial Opening Endoscopic
0CQV0ZZ	Repair Left Vocal Cord, Open Approach

0CQV3ZZ	Repair Left Vocal Cord, Percutaneous Approach
0CQV4ZZ	Repair Left Vocal Cord, Percutaneous Endoscopic Approach
0CQV7ZZ	Repair Left Vocal Cord, Via Natural or Artificial Opening
0CQV8ZZ	Repair Left Vocal Cord, Via Natural or Artificial Opening Endoscopic
0CQW0Z0	Repair of Upper Tooth, Single, Open Approach
0CQW0Z1	Repair of Upper Tooth, Multiple, Open Approach
0CQW0Z2	Repair of Upper Tooth, All, Open Approach
0CQWXZ0	Repair of Upper Tooth, Single, External Approach
0CQWXZ1	Repair of Upper Tooth, Multiple, External Approach
0CQWXZ2	Repair of Upper Tooth, All, External Approach
0CQX0Z0	Repair of Lower Tooth, Single, Open Approach
0CQX0Z1	Repair of Lower Tooth, Multiple, Open Approach
0CQX0Z2	Repair of Lower Tooth, All, Open Approach
0CQXXZ0	Repair of Lower Tooth, Single, External Approach
0CQXXZ1	Repair of Lower Tooth, Multiple, External Approach
0CQXXZ2	Repair of Lower Tooth, All, External Approach

0CR – Mouth and Throat, Replacement

R007Z	Replacement of Upper Lip with Autologous Tissue Substitute, Open Approach
R00JZ	Replacement of Upper Lip with Synthetic Substitute, Open Approach
R00KZ	Replacement of Upper Lip with Nonautologous Tissue Substitute, Open Approach
R037Z	Replacement of Upper Lip with Autologous Tissue Substitute, Percutaneous Approach
R03JZ	Replacement of Upper Lip with Synthetic Substitute, Percutaneous Approach
R03KZ	Replacement of Upper Lip with Nonautologous Tissue Substitute, Percutaneous Approach
R0X7Z	Replacement of Upper Lip with Autologous Tissue Substitute, External Approach
R0XJZ	Replacement of Upper Lip with Synthetic Substitute, External Approach
R0XKZ	Replacement of Upper Lip with Nonautologous Tissue Substitute, External Approach
R107Z	Replacement of Lower Lip with Autologous Tissue Substitute, Open Approach
R10JZ	Replacement of Lower Lip with Synthetic Substitute, Open Approach
R10KZ	Replacement of Lower Lip with Nonautologous Tissue Substitute, Open Approach
R137Z	Replacement of Lower Lip with Autologous Tissue Substitute, Percutaneous Approach
R13JZ	Replacement of Lower Lip with Synthetic Substitute, Percutaneous Approach

0CR13KZ	Replacement of Lower Lip with Nonautologous Tissue Substitute, Percutaneous Approach
0CR1X7Z	Replacement of Lower Lip with Autologous Tissue Substitute, External Approach
0CR1XJZ	Replacement of Lower Lip with Synthetic Substitute, External Approach
0CR1XKZ	Replacement of Lower Lip with Nonautologous Tissue Substitute, External Approach
0CR207Z	Replacement of Hard Palate with Autologous Tissue Substitute, Open Approach
0CR20JZ	Replacement of Hard Palate with Synthetic Substitute, Open Approach
0CR20KZ	Replacement of Hard Palate with Nonautologous Tissue Substitute, Open Approach
0CR237Z	Replacement of Hard Palate with Autologous Tissue Substitute, Percutaneous Approach
0CR23JZ	Replacement of Hard Palate with Synthetic Substitute, Percutaneous Approach
0CR23KZ	Replacement of Hard Palate with Nonautologous Tissue Substitute, Percutaneous Approach
0CR2X7Z	Replacement of Hard Palate with Autologous Tissue Substitute, External Approach
0CR2XJZ	Replacement of Hard Palate with Synthetic Substitute, External Approach
0CR2XKZ	Replacement of Hard Palate with Nonautologous Tissue Substitute, External Approach
0CR307Z	Replacement of Soft Palate with Autologous Tissue Substitute, Open Approach

0CR30JZ	Replacement of Soft Palate with Synthetic Substitute, Open Approach
0CR30KZ	Replacement of Soft Palate with Nonautologous Tissue Substitute, Open Approach
0CR337Z	Replacement of Soft Palate with Autologous Tissue Substitute, Percutaneous Approach
0CR33JZ	Replacement of Soft Palate with Synthetic Substitute, Percutaneous Approach
0CR33KZ	Replacement of Soft Palate with Nonautologous Tissue Substitute, Percutaneous Approach
0CR3X7Z	Replacement of Soft Palate with Autologous Tissue Substitute, External Approach
0CR3XJZ	Replacement of Soft Palate with Synthetic Substitute, External Approach
	AHA CC: 3Q, 2014, 25
0CR3XKZ	Replacement of Soft Palate with Nonautologous Tissue Substitute, External Approach
0CR407Z	Replacement of Buccal Mucosa with Autologous Tissue Substitute, Open Approach
0CR40JZ	Replacement of Buccal Mucosa with Synthetic Substitute, Open Approach
0CR40KZ	Replacement of Buccal Mucosa with Nonautologous Tissue Substitute, Open Approach
0CR437Z	Replacement of Buccal Mucosa with Autologous Tissue Substitute, Percutaneous Approach
0CR43JZ	Replacement of Buccal Mucosa with Synthetic Substitute, Percutaneous Approach
0CR43KZ	Replacement of Buccal Mucosa with Nonautologous Tissue Substitute, Percutaneous Approach

Female-only   ♂ Male-only   ▲ Limited Coverage   ● Non-OR   ▣ HAC-associated procedure   ▲ Non-covered procedures   ✚ Combination

0CR4X7Z Replacement of Buccal Mucosa with Autologous Tissue Substitute, External Approach

0CR4XJZ Replacement of Buccal Mucosa with Synthetic Substitute, External Approach

0CR4XKZ Replacement of Buccal Mucosa with Nonautologous Tissue Substitute, External Approach
AHA CC: 2Q, 2014, 5-6

0CR507Z Replacement of Upper Gingiva with Autologous Tissue Substitute, Open Approach

0CR50JZ Replacement of Upper Gingiva with Synthetic Substitute, Open Approach

0CR50KZ Replacement of Upper Gingiva with Nonautologous Tissue Substitute, Open Approach

0CR537Z Replacement of Upper Gingiva with Autologous Tissue Substitute, Percutaneous Approach

0CR53JZ Replacement of Upper Gingiva with Synthetic Substitute, Percutaneous Approach

0CR53KZ Replacement of Upper Gingiva with Nonautologous Tissue Substitute, Percutaneous Approach

0CR5X7Z Replacement of Upper Gingiva with Autologous Tissue Substitute, External Approach

0CR5XJZ Replacement of Upper Gingiva with Synthetic Substitute, External Approach

0CR5XKZ Replacement of Upper Gingiva with Nonautologous Tissue Substitute, External Approach

0CR607Z Replacement of Lower Gingiva with Autologous Tissue Substitute, Open Approach

0CR60JZ Replacement of Lower Gingiva with Synthetic Substitute, Open Approach

0CR60KZ Replacement of Lower Gingiva with Nonautologous Tissue Substitute, Open Approach

0CR637Z Replacement of Lower Gingiva with Autologous Tissue Substitute, Percutaneous Approach

0CR63JZ Replacement of Lower Gingiva with Synthetic Substitute, Percutaneous Approach

0CR63KZ Replacement of Lower Gingiva with Nonautologous Tissue Substitute, Percutaneous Approach

0CR6X7Z Replacement of Lower Gingiva with Autologous Tissue Substitute, External Approach

0CR6XJZ Replacement of Lower Gingiva with Synthetic Substitute, External Approach

0CR6XKZ Replacement of Lower Gingiva with Nonautologous Tissue Substitute, External Approach

0CR707Z Replacement of Tongue with Autologous Tissue Substitute, Open Approach

0CR70JZ Replacement of Tongue with Synthetic Substitute, Open Approach

0CR70KZ Replacement of Tongue with Nonautologous Tissue Substitute, Open Approach

0CR737Z Replacement of Tongue with Autologous Tissue Substitute, Percutaneous Approach

0CR73JZ Replacement of Tongue with Synthetic Substitute, Percutaneous Approach

0CR73KZ Replacement of Tongue with Nonautologous Tissue Substitute, Percutaneous Approach

0CR7X7Z Replacement of Tongue with Autologous Tissue Substitute, External Approach

0CR7XJZ Replacement of Tongue with Synthetic Substitute, External Approach

0CR7XKZ Replacement of Tongue with Nonautologous Tissue Substitute, External Approach

0CRB07Z Replacement of Right Parotid Duct with Autologous Tissue Substitute, Open Approach

0CRB0JZ Replacement of Right Parotid Duct with Synthetic Substitute, Open Approach

0CRB0KZ Replacement of Right Parotid Duct with Nonautologous Tissue Substitute, Open Approach

0CRB37Z Replacement of Right Parotid Duct with Autologous Tissue Substitute, Percutaneous Approach

0CRB3JZ Replacement of Right Parotid Duct with Synthetic Substitute, Percutaneous Approach

0CRB3KZ Replacement of Right Parotid Duct with Nonautologous Tissue Substitute, Percutaneous Approach

0CRC07Z Replacement of Left Parotid Duct with Autologous Tissue Substitute, Open Approach

0CRC0JZ Replacement of Left Parotid Duct with Synthetic Substitute, Open Approach

0CRC0KZ Replacement of Left Parotid Duct with Nonautologous Tissue Substitute, Open Approach

0CRC37Z Replacement of Left Parotid Duct with Autologous Tissue Substitute, Percutaneous Approach

0CRC3JZ Replacement of Left Parotid Duct with Synthetic Substitute, Percutaneous Approach

0CRC3KZ Replacement of Left Parotid Duct with Nonautologous Tissue Substitute, Percutaneous Approach

0CRM07Z Replacement of Pharynx with Autologous Tissue Substitute, Open Approach

0CRM0JZ Replacement of Pharynx with Synthetic Substitute, Open Approach

0CRM0KZ Replacement of Pharynx with Nonautologous Tissue Substitute, Open Approach

0CRM77Z Replacement of Pharynx with Autologous Tissue Substitute, Via Natural or Artificial Opening

0CRM7JZ Replacement of Pharynx with Synthetic Substitute, Via Natural or Artificial Opening

0CRM7KZ Replacement of Pharynx with Nonautologous Tissue Substitute, Via Natural or Artificial Opening

0CRM87Z Replacement of Pharynx with Autologous Tissue Substitute, Via Natural or Artificial Opening Endoscopic

0CRM8JZ Replacement of Pharynx with Synthetic Substitute, Via Natural or Artificial Opening Endoscopic

0CRM8KZ Replacement of Pharynx with Nonautologous Tissue Substitute, Via Natural or Artificial Opening Endoscopic

0CRN07Z Replacement of Uvula with Autologous Tissue Substitute, Open Approach

0CRN0JZ Replacement of Uvula with Synthetic Substitute, Open Approach

0CRN0KZ Replacement of Uvula with Nonautologous Tissue Substitute, Open Approach

0CRN37Z Replacement of Uvula with Autologous Tissue Substitute, Percutaneous Approach

0CRN3JZ Replacement of Uvula with Synthetic Substitute, Percutaneous Approach

0CRN3KZ Replacement of Uvula with Nonautologous Tissue Substitute, Percutaneous Approach

0CRNX7Z Replacement of Uvula with Autologous Tissue Substitute, External Approach

0CRNXJZ Replacement of Uvula with Synthetic Substitute, External Approach

0CRNXKZ Replacement of Uvula with Nonautologous Tissue Substitute, External Approach

0CRR07Z Replacement of Epiglottis with Autologous Tissue Substitute, Open Approach

0CRR0JZ Replacement of Epiglottis with Synthetic Substitute, Open Approach

0CRR0KZ Replacement of Epiglottis with Nonautologous Tissue Substitute, Open Approach

0CRR77Z Replacement of Epiglottis with Autologous Tissue Substitute, Via Natural or Artificial Opening

0CRR7JZ Replacement of Epiglottis with Synthetic Substitute, Via Natural or Artificial Opening

0CRR7KZ Replacement of Epiglottis with Nonautologous Tissue Substitute, Via Natural or Artificial Opening

0CRR87Z Replacement of Epiglottis with Autologous Tissue Substitute, Via Natural or Artificial Opening Endoscopic

0CRR8JZ Replacement of Epiglottis with Synthetic Substitute, Via Natural or Artificial Opening Endoscopic

0CRR8KZ Replacement of Epiglottis with Nonautologous Tissue Substitute, Via Natural or Artificial Opening Endoscopic

0CRS07Z Replacement of Larynx with Autologous Tissue Substitute, Open Approach

0CRS0JZ Replacement of Larynx with Synthetic Substitute, Open Approach

0CRS0KZ Replacement of Larynx with Nonautologous Tissue Substitute, Open Approach

0CRS77Z Replacement of Larynx with Autologous Tissue Substitute, Via Natural or Artificial Opening

0CRS7JZ Replacement of Larynx with Synthetic Substitute, Via Natural or Artificial Opening

0CRS7KZ Replacement of Larynx with Nonautologous Tissue Substitute, Via Natural or Artificial Opening

0CRS87Z Replacement of Larynx with Autologous Tissue Substitute, Via Natural or Artificial Opening Endoscopic

0CRS8JZ Replacement of Larynx with Synthetic Substitute, Via Natural or Artificial Opening Endoscopic

0CRS8KZ Replacement of Larynx with Nonautologous Tissue Substitute, Via Natural or Artificial Opening Endoscopic

0CRT07Z Replacement of Right Vocal Cord with Autologous Tissue Substitute, Open Approach

0CRT0JZ Replacement of Right Vocal Cord with Synthetic Substitute, Open Approach

0CRT0KZ Replacement of Right Vocal Cord with Nonautologous Tissue Substitute, Open Approach

0CRT77Z Replacement of Right Vocal Cord with Autologous Tissue Substitute, Via Natural or Artificial Opening

T7JZ	Replacement of Right Vocal Cord with Synthetic Substitute, Via Natural or Artificial Opening
T7KZ	Replacement of Right Vocal Cord with Nonautologous Tissue Substitute, Via Natural or Artificial Opening
T87Z	Replacement of Right Vocal Cord with Autologous Tissue Substitute, Via Natural or Artificial Opening Endoscopic
T8JZ	Replacement of Right Vocal Cord with Synthetic Substitute, Via Natural or Artificial Opening Endoscopic
T8KZ	Replacement of Right Vocal Cord with Nonautologous Tissue Substitute, Via Natural or Artificial Opening Endoscopic
V07Z	Replacement of Left Vocal Cord with Autologous Tissue Substitute, Open Approach
V0JZ	Replacement of Left Vocal Cord with Synthetic Substitute, Open Approach
V0KZ	Replacement of Left Vocal Cord with Nonautologous Tissue Substitute, Open Approach
V77Z	Replacement of Left Vocal Cord with Autologous Tissue Substitute, Via Natural or Artificial Opening
V7JZ	Replacement of Left Vocal Cord with Synthetic Substitute, Via Natural or Artificial Opening
V7KZ	Replacement of Left Vocal Cord with Nonautologous Tissue Substitute, Via Natural or Artificial Opening
V87Z	Replacement of Left Vocal Cord with Autologous Tissue Substitute, Via Natural or Artificial Opening Endoscopic
V8JZ	Replacement of Left Vocal Cord with Synthetic Substitute, Via Natural or Artificial Opening Endoscopic
V8KZ	Replacement of Left Vocal Cord with Nonautologous Tissue Substitute, Via Natural or Artificial Opening Endoscopic
RW070	Replacement of Upper Tooth, Single, with Autologous Tissue Substitute, Open Approach
RW071	Replacement of Upper Tooth, Multiple, with Autologous Tissue Substitute, Open Approach
0CRW072	Replacement of Upper Tooth, All, with Autologous Tissue Substitute, Open Approach
0CRW0J0	Replacement of Upper Tooth, Single, with Synthetic Substitute, Open Approach
0CRW0J1	Replacement of Upper Tooth, Multiple, with Synthetic Substitute, Open Approach
0CRW0J2	Replacement of Upper Tooth, All, with Synthetic Substitute, Open Approach
0CRW0K0	Replacement of Upper Tooth, Single, with Nonautologous Tissue Substitute, Open Approach
0CRW0K1	Replacement of Upper Tooth, Multiple, with Nonautologous Tissue Substitute, Open Approach
0CRW0K2	Replacement of Upper Tooth, All, with Nonautologous Tissue Substitute, Open Approach
0CRWX70	Replacement of Upper Tooth, Single, with Autologous Tissue Substitute, External Approach
0CRWX71	Replacement of Upper Tooth, Multiple, with Autologous Tissue Substitute, External Approach
0CRWX72	Replacement of Upper Tooth, All, with Autologous Tissue Substitute, External Approach
0CRWXJ0	Replacement of Upper Tooth, Single, with Synthetic Substitute, External Approach
0CRWXJ1	Replacement of Upper Tooth, Multiple, with Synthetic Substitute, External Approach
0CRWXJ2	Replacement of Upper Tooth, All, with Synthetic Substitute, External Approach
0CRWXK0	Replacement of Upper Tooth, Single, with Nonautologous Tissue Substitute, External Approach
0CRWXK1	Replacement of Upper Tooth, Multiple, with Nonautologous Tissue Substitute, External Approach
0CRWXK2	Replacement of Upper Tooth, All, with Nonautologous Tissue Substitute, External Approach
0CRX070	Replacement of Lower Tooth, Single, with Autologous Tissue Substitute, Open Approach
0CRX071	Replacement of Lower Tooth, Multiple, with Autologous Tissue Substitute, Open Approach
0CRX072	Replacement of Lower Tooth, All, with Autologous Tissue Substitute, Open Approach
0CRX0J0	Replacement of Lower Tooth, Single, with Synthetic Substitute, Open Approach
0CRX0J1	Replacement of Lower Tooth, Multiple, with Synthetic Substitute, Open Approach
0CRX0J2	Replacement of Lower Tooth, All, with Synthetic Substitute, Open Approach
0CRX0K0	Replacement of Lower Tooth, Single, with Nonautologous Tissue Substitute, Open Approach
0CRX0K1	Replacement of Lower Tooth, Multiple, with Nonautologous Tissue Substitute, Open Approach
0CRX0K2	Replacement of Lower Tooth, All, with Nonautologous Tissue Substitute, Open Approach
0CRXX70	Replacement of Lower Tooth, Single, with Autologous Tissue Substitute, External Approach
0CRXX71	Replacement of Lower Tooth, Multiple, with Autologous Tissue Substitute, External Approach
0CRXX72	Replacement of Lower Tooth, All, with Autologous Tissue Substitute, External Approach
0CRXXJ0	Replacement of Lower Tooth, Single, with Synthetic Substitute, External Approach
0CRXXJ1	Replacement of Lower Tooth, Multiple, with Synthetic Substitute, External Approach
0CRXXJ2	Replacement of Lower Tooth, All, with Synthetic Substitute, External Approach
0CRXXK0	Replacement of Lower Tooth, Single, with Nonautologous Tissue Substitute, External Approach
0CRXXK1	Replacement of Lower Tooth, Multiple, with Nonautologous Tissue Substitute, External Approach
0CRXXK2	Replacement of Lower Tooth, All, with Nonautologous Tissue Substitute, External Approach

S – Mouth and Throat, Reposition

S00ZZ	Reposition Upper Lip, Open Approach
S0XZZ	Reposition Upper Lip, External Approach
S10ZZ	Reposition Lower Lip, Open Approach
S1XZZ	Reposition Lower Lip, External Approach
S20ZZ	Reposition Hard Palate, Open Approach
S2XZZ	Reposition Hard Palate, External Approach
S30ZZ	Reposition Soft Palate, Open Approach
S3XZZ	Reposition Soft Palate, External Approach
S70ZZ	Reposition Tongue, Open Approach
S7XZZ	Reposition Tongue, External Approach
SB0ZZ	Reposition Right Parotid Duct, Open Approach
SB3ZZ	Reposition Right Parotid Duct, Percutaneous Approach
SC0ZZ	Reposition Left Parotid Duct, Open Approach
SC3ZZ	Reposition Left Parotid Duct, Percutaneous Approach
SN0ZZ	Reposition Uvula, Open Approach
SNXZZ	Reposition Uvula, External Approach
SR0ZZ	Reposition Epiglottis, Open Approach
0CSR7ZZ	Reposition Epiglottis, Via Natural or Artificial Opening
0CSR8ZZ	Reposition Epiglottis, Via Natural or Artificial Opening Endoscopic
0CST0ZZ	Reposition Right Vocal Cord, Open Approach
0CST7ZZ	Reposition Right Vocal Cord, Via Natural or Artificial Opening
0CST8ZZ	Reposition Right Vocal Cord, Via Natural or Artificial Opening Endoscopic
0CSV0ZZ	Reposition Left Vocal Cord, Open Approach
0CSV7ZZ	Reposition Left Vocal Cord, Via Natural or Artificial Opening
0CSV8ZZ	Reposition Left Vocal Cord, Via Natural or Artificial Opening Endoscopic
0CSW050	Reposition Upper Tooth with External Fixation Device, Single, Open Approach
0CSW051	Reposition Upper Tooth with External Fixation Device, Multiple, Open Approach
0CSW052	Reposition Upper Tooth with External Fixation Device, All, Open Approach
0CSW0Z0	Reposition Upper Tooth, Single, Open Approach
0CSW0Z1	Reposition Upper Tooth, Multiple, Open Approach
0CSW0Z2	Reposition Upper Tooth, All, Open Approach
0CSWX50	Reposition Upper Tooth, Single, with External Fixation Device, External Approach
0CSWX51	Reposition Upper Tooth, Multiple, with External Fixation Device, External Approach
0CSWX52	Reposition Upper Tooth, All, with External Fixation Device, External Approach
0CSWXZ0	Reposition Upper Tooth, Single, External Approach
0CSWXZ1	Reposition Upper Tooth, Multiple, External Approach
0CSWXZ2	Reposition Upper Tooth, All, External Approach
0CSX050	Reposition Lower Tooth with External Fixation Device, Single, Open Approach

0CSX051 Reposition Lower Tooth with External Fixation Device, Multiple, Open Approach	**0CSX0Z2** Reposition Lower Tooth, All, Open Approach	**0CSXX52** Reposition Lower Tooth, All, with External Fixation Device, External Approach
0CSX052 Reposition Lower Tooth with External Fixation Device, All, Open Approach	**0CSXX50** Reposition Lower Tooth, Single, with External Fixation Device, External Approach	**0CSXXZ0** Reposition Lower Tooth, Single, Ext Approach
0CSX0Z0 Reposition Lower Tooth, Single, Open Approach	**0CSXX51** Reposition Lower Tooth, Multiple, with External Fixation Device, External Approach	**0CSXXZ1** Reposition Lower Tooth, Multiple, External Approach
0CSX0Z1 Reposition Lower Tooth, Multiple, Open Approach		**0CSXXZ2** Reposition Lower Tooth, All, Externa Approach

0CT – Mouth and Throat, Resection

Review Coding Guideline B3.8

0CT00ZZ Resection of Upper Lip, Open Approach	**0CTJ0ZZ** Resection of Minor Salivary Gland, Open Approach	**0CTT0ZZ** Resection of Right Vocal Cord, Open Approach
0CT0XZZ Resection of Upper Lip, External Approach	**0CTM0ZZ** Resection of Pharynx, Open Approach	**0CTT4ZZ** Resection of Right Vocal Cord, Percutaneous Endoscopic Approach
0CT10ZZ Resection of Lower Lip, Open Approach	**0CTM4ZZ** Resection of Pharynx, Percutaneous Endoscopic Approach	**0CTT7ZZ** Resection of Right Vocal Cord, Via Natural or Artificial Opening
0CT1XZZ Resection of Lower Lip, External Approach	**0CTM7ZZ** Resection of Pharynx, Via Natural or Artificial Opening	**0CTT8ZZ** Resection of Right Vocal Cord, Via Natural or Artificial Opening Endosce
0CT20ZZ Resection of Hard Palate, Open Approach	**0CTM8ZZ** Resection of Pharynx, Via Natural or Artificial Opening Endoscopic	**0CTV0ZZ** Resection of Left Vocal Cord, Open Approach
0CT2XZZ Resection of Hard Palate, External Approach	**0CTN0ZZ** Resection of Uvula, Open Approach	**0CTV4ZZ** Resection of Left Vocal Cord, Percutaneous Endoscopic Approach
0CT30ZZ Resection of Soft Palate, Open Approach	**0CTNXZZ** Resection of Uvula, External Approach	**0CTV7ZZ** Resection of Left Vocal Cord, Via Nat or Artificial Opening
0CT3XZZ Resection of Soft Palate, External Approach	**0CTP0ZZ** Resection of Tonsils, Open Approach	**0CTV8ZZ** Resection of Left Vocal Cord, Via Nat or Artificial Opening Endoscopic
0CT70ZZ Resection of Tongue, Open Approach	**0CTPXZZ** Resection of Tonsils, External Approach	
0CT7XZZ Resection of Tongue, External Approach	**0CTQ0ZZ** Resection of Adenoids, Open Approach	**0CTW0Z0** Resection of Upper Tooth, Single, Op Approach
0CT80ZZ Resection of Right Parotid Gland, Open Approach	**0CTQXZZ** Resection of Adenoids, External Approach	**0CTW0Z1** Resection of Upper Tooth, Multiple, Open Approach
0CT90ZZ Resection of Left Parotid Gland, Open Approach	**0CTR0ZZ** Resection of Epiglottis, Open Approach	*AHA CC: 3Q, 2014, 23-24*
0CTB0ZZ Resection of Right Parotid Duct, Open Approach	**0CTR4ZZ** Resection of Epiglottis, Percutaneous Endoscopic Approach	**0CTW0Z2** Resection of Upper Tooth, All, Open Approach
0CTC0ZZ Resection of Left Parotid Duct, Open Approach	**0CTR7ZZ** Resection of Epiglottis, Via Natural or Artificial Opening	**0CTX0Z0** Resection of Lower Tooth, Single, Op Approach
0CTD0ZZ Resection of Right Sublingual Gland, Open Approach	**0CTR8ZZ** Resection of Epiglottis, Via Natural or Artificial Opening Endoscopic	**0CTX0Z1** Resection of Lower Tooth, Multiple, Open Approach
0CTF0ZZ Resection of Left Sublingual Gland, Open Approach	**0CTS0ZZ** Resection of Larynx, Open Approach	*AHA CC: 3Q, 2014, 23-24*
0CTG0ZZ Resection of Right Submaxillary Gland, Open Approach	**0CTS4ZZ** Resection of Larynx, Percutaneous Endoscopic Approach	**0CTX0Z2** Resection of Lower Tooth, All, Open Approach
0CTH0ZZ Resection of Left Submaxillary Gland, Open Approach	**0CTS7ZZ** Resection of Larynx, Via Natural or Artificial Opening	
	0CTS8ZZ Resection of Larynx, Via Natural or Artificial Opening Endoscopic	

0CU – Mouth and Throat, Supplement

0CU007Z Supplement Upper Lip with Autologous Tissue Substitute, Open Approach	**0CU137Z** Supplement Lower Lip with Autologous Tissue Substitute, Percutaneous Approach	**0CU23KZ** Supplement Hard Palate with Nonautologous Tissue Substitute, Percutaneous Approach
0CU00JZ Supplement Upper Lip with Synthetic Substitute, Open Approach	**0CU13JZ** Supplement Lower Lip with Synthetic Substitute, Percutaneous Approach	**0CU2X7Z** Supplement Hard Palate with Autolog Tissue Substitute, External Approach
0CU00KZ Supplement Upper Lip with Nonautologous Tissue Substitute, Open Approach	**0CU13KZ** Supplement Lower Lip with Nonautologous Tissue Substitute, Percutaneous Approach	**0CU2XJZ** Supplement Hard Palate with Syntheti Substitute, External Approach
0CU037Z Supplement Upper Lip with Autologous Tissue Substitute, Percutaneous Approach	**0CU1X7Z** Supplement Lower Lip with Autologous Tissue Substitute, External Approach	**0CU2XKZ** Supplement Hard Palate with Nonautologous Tissue Substitute, External Approach
0CU03JZ Supplement Upper Lip with Synthetic Substitute, Percutaneous Approach	**0CU1XJZ** Supplement Lower Lip with Synthetic Substitute, External Approach	**0CU307Z** Supplement Soft Palate with Autologo Tissue Substitute, Open Approach
0CU03KZ Supplement Upper Lip with Nonautologous Tissue Substitute, Percutaneous Approach	**0CU1XKZ** Supplement Lower Lip with Nonautologous Tissue Substitute, External Approach	**0CU30JZ** Supplement Soft Palate with Synthetic Substitute, Open Approach
0CU0X7Z Supplement Upper Lip with Autologous Tissue Substitute, External Approach	**0CU207Z** Supplement Hard Palate with Autologous Tissue Substitute, Open Approach	**0CU30KZ** Supplement Soft Palate with Nonautologous Tissue Substitute, Ope Approach
0CU0XJZ Supplement Upper Lip with Synthetic Substitute, External Approach	**0CU20JZ** Supplement Hard Palate with Synthetic Substitute, Open Approach	**0CU337Z** Supplement Soft Palate with Autologo Tissue Substitute, Percutaneous Approach
0CU0XKZ Supplement Upper Lip with Nonautologous Tissue Substitute, External Approach	**0CU20KZ** Supplement Hard Palate with Nonautologous Tissue Substitute, Open Approach	**0CU33JZ** Supplement Soft Palate with Synthetic Substitute, Percutaneous Approach
0CU107Z Supplement Lower Lip with Autologous Tissue Substitute, Open Approach	**0CU237Z** Supplement Hard Palate with Autologous Tissue Substitute, Percutaneous Approach	**0CU33KZ** Supplement Soft Palate with Nonautologous Tissue Substitute, Percutaneous Approach
0CU10JZ Supplement Lower Lip with Synthetic Substitute, Open Approach	**0CU23JZ** Supplement Hard Palate with Synthetic Substitute, Percutaneous Approach	**0CU3X7Z** Supplement Soft Palate with Autolgou Tissue Substitute, External Approach
0CU10KZ Supplement Lower Lip with Nonautologous Tissue Substitute, Open Approach		**0CU3XJZ** Supplement Soft Palate with Synthetic Substitute, External Approach

♀ Female-only   ♂ Male-only   ▲ Limited Coverage   ● Non-OR   ▨ HAC-associated procedure   ▲ Non-covered procedures   ✚ Combinat

3XKZ	Supplement Soft Palate with Nonautologous Tissue Substitute, External Approach
407Z	Supplement Buccal Mucosa with Autologous Tissue Substitute, Open Approach
40JZ	Supplement Buccal Mucosa with Synthetic Substitute, Open Approach
40KZ	Supplement Buccal Mucosa with Nonautologous Tissue Substitute, Open Approach
437Z	Supplement Buccal Mucosa with Autologous Tissue Substitute, Percutaneous Approach
43JZ	Supplement Buccal Mucosa with Synthetic Substitute, Percutaneous Approach
43KZ	Supplement Buccal Mucosa with Nonautologous Tissue Substitute, Percutaneous Approach
4X7Z	Supplement Buccal Mucosa with Autologous Tissue Substitute, External Approach
4XJZ	Supplement Buccal Mucosa with Synthetic Substitute, External Approach
4XKZ	Supplement Buccal Mucosa with Nonautologous Tissue Substitute, External Approach
U507Z	Supplement Upper Gingiva with Autologous Tissue Substitute, Open Approach
U50JZ	Supplement Upper Gingiva with Synthetic Substitute, Open Approach
U50KZ	Supplement Upper Gingiva with Nonautologous Tissue Substitute, Open Approach
U537Z	Supplement Upper Gingiva with Autologous Tissue Substitute, Percutaneous Approach
U53JZ	Supplement Upper Gingiva with Synthetic Substitute, Percutaneous Approach
U53KZ	Supplement Upper Gingiva with Nonautologous Tissue Substitute, Percutaneous Approach
U5X7Z	Supplement Upper Gingiva with Autologous Tissue Substitute, External Approach
U5XJZ	Supplement Upper Gingiva with Synthetic Substitute, External Approach
U5XKZ	Supplement Upper Gingiva with Nonautologous Tissue Substitute, External Approach
U607Z	Supplement Lower Gingiva with Autologous Tissue Substitute, Open Approach
U60JZ	Supplement Lower Gingiva with Synthetic Substitute, Open Approach
U60KZ	Supplement Lower Gingiva with Nonautologous Tissue Substitute, Open Approach
U637Z	Supplement Lower Gingiva with Autologous Tissue Substitute, Percutaneous Approach
U63JZ	Supplement Lower Gingiva with Synthetic Substitute, Percutaneous Approach
U63KZ	Supplement Lower Gingiva with Nonautologous Tissue Substitute, Percutaneous Approach
U6X7Z	Supplement Lower Gingiva with Autologous Tissue Substitute, External Approach
U6XJZ	Supplement Lower Gingiva with Synthetic Substitute, External Approach
0CU6XKZ	Supplement Lower Gingiva with Nonautologous Tissue Substitute, External Approach
0CU707Z	Supplement Tongue with Autologous Tissue Substitute, Open Approach
0CU70JZ	Supplement Tongue with Synthetic Substitute, Open Approach
0CU70KZ	Supplement Tongue with Nonautologous Tissue Substitute, Open Approach
0CU737Z	Supplement Tongue with Autologous Tissue Substitute, Percutaneous Approach
0CU73JZ	Supplement Tongue with Synthetic Substitute, Percutaneous Approach
0CU73KZ	Supplement Tongue with Nonautologous Tissue Substitute, Percutaneous Approach
0CU7X7Z	Supplement Tongue with Autologous Tissue Substitute, External Approach
0CU7XJZ	Supplement Tongue with Synthetic Substitute, External Approach
0CU7XKZ	Supplement Tongue with Nonautologous Tissue Substitute, External Approach
0CUM07Z	Supplement Pharynx with Autologous Tissue Substitute, Open Approach
0CUM0JZ	Supplement Pharynx with Synthetic Substitute, Open Approach
0CUM0KZ	Supplement Pharynx with Nonautologous Tissue Substitute, Open Approach
0CUM77Z	Supplement Pharynx with Autologous Tissue Substitute, Via Natural or Artificial Opening
0CUM7JZ	Supplement Pharynx with Synthetic Substitute, Via Natural or Artificial Opening
0CUM7KZ	Supplement Pharynx with Nonautologous Tissue Substitute, Via Natural or Artificial Opening
0CUM87Z	Supplement Pharynx with Autologous Tissue Substitute, Via Natural or Artificial Opening Endoscopic
0CUM8JZ	Supplement Pharynx with Synthetic Substitute, Via Natural or Artificial Opening Endoscopic
0CUM8KZ	Supplement Pharynx with Nonautologous Tissue Substitute, Via Natural or Artificial Opening Endoscopic
0CUN07Z	Supplement Uvula with Autologous Tissue Substitute, Open Approach
0CUN0JZ	Supplement Uvula with Synthetic Substitute, Open Approach
0CUN0KZ	Supplement Uvula with Nonautologous Tissue Substitute, Open Approach
0CUN37Z	Supplement Uvula with Autologous Tissue Substitute, Percutaneous Approach
0CUN3JZ	Supplement Uvula with Synthetic Substitute, Percutaneous Approach
0CUN3KZ	Supplement Uvula with Nonautologous Tissue Substitute, Percutaneous Approach
0CUNX7Z	Supplement Uvula with Autologous Tissue Substitute, External Approach
0CUNXJZ	Supplement Uvula with Synthetic Substitute, External Approach
0CUNXKZ	Supplement Uvula with Nonautologous Tissue Substitute, External Approach
0CUR07Z	Supplement Epiglottis with Autologous Tissue Substitute, Open Approach
0CUR0JZ	Supplement Epiglottis with Synthetic Substitute, Open Approach
0CUR0KZ	Supplement Epiglottis with Nonautologous Tissue Substitute, Open Approach
0CUR77Z	Supplement Epiglottis with Autologous Tissue Substitute, Via Natural or Artificial Opening
0CUR7JZ	Supplement Epiglottis with Synthetic Substitute, Via Natural or Artificial Opening
0CUR7KZ	Supplement Epiglottis with Nonautologous Tissue Substitute, Via Natural or Artificial Opening
0CUR87Z	Supplement Epiglottis with Autologous Tissue Substitute, Via Natural or Artificial Opening Endoscopic
0CUR8JZ	Supplement Epiglottis with Synthetic Substitute, Via Natural or Artificial Opening Endoscopic
0CUR8KZ	Supplement Epiglottis with Nonautologous Tissue Substitute, Via Natural or Artificial Opening Endoscopic
0CUS07Z	Supplement Larynx with Autologous Tissue Substitute, Open Approach
0CUS0JZ	Supplement Larynx with Synthetic Substitute, Open Approach
0CUS0KZ	Supplement Larynx with Nonautologous Tissue Substitute, Open Approach
0CUS77Z	Supplement Larynx with Autologous Tissue Substitute, Via Natural or Artificial Opening
0CUS7JZ	Supplement Larynx with Synthetic Substitute, Via Natural or Artificial Opening
0CUS7KZ	Supplement Larynx with Nonautologous Tissue Substitute, Via Natural or Artificial Opening
0CUS87Z	Supplement Larynx with Autologous Tissue Substitute, Via Natural or Artificial Opening Endoscopic
0CUS8JZ	Supplement Larynx with Synthetic Substitute, Via Natural or Artificial Opening Endoscopic
0CUS8KZ	Supplement Larynx with Nonautologous Tissue Substitute, Via Natural or Artificial Opening Endoscopic
0CUT07Z	Supplement Right Vocal Cord with Autologous Tissue Substitute, Open Approach
0CUT0JZ	Supplement Right Vocal Cord with Synthetic Substitute, Open Approach
0CUT0KZ	Supplement Right Vocal Cord with Nonautologous Tissue Substitute, Open Approach
0CUT77Z	Supplement Right Vocal Cord with Autologous Tissue Substitute, Via Natural or Artificial Opening
0CUT7JZ	Supplement Right Vocal Cord with Synthetic Substitute, Via Natural or Artificial Opening
0CUT7KZ	Supplement Right Vocal Cord with Nonautologous Tissue Substitute, Via Natural or Artificial Opening
0CUT87Z	Supplement Right Vocal Cord with Autologous Tissue Substitute, Via Natural or Artificial Opening Endoscopic
0CUT8JZ	Supplement Right Vocal Cord with Synthetic Substitute, Via Natural or Artificial Opening Endoscopic
0CUT8KZ	Supplement Right Vocal Cord with Nonautologous Tissue Substitute, Via Natural or Artificial Opening Endoscopic
0CUV07Z	Supplement Left Vocal Cord with Autologous Tissue Substitute, Open Approach
0CUV0JZ	Supplement Left Vocal Cord with Synthetic Substitute, Open Approach
0CUV0KZ	Supplement Left Vocal Cord with Nonautologous Tissue Substitute, Open Approach
0CUV77Z	Supplement Left Vocal Cord with Autologous Tissue Substitute, Via Natural or Artificial Opening

♀ Female-only   ♂ Male-only   ▲ Limited Coverage   ● Non-OR   ▩ HAC-associated procedure   ▲ Non-covered procedures   ✛ Combination

0CUV7JZ	Supplement Left Vocal Cord with Synthetic Substitute, Via Natural or Artificial Opening
0CUV7KZ	Supplement Left Vocal Cord with Nonautologous Tissue Substitute, Via Natural or Artificial Opening
0CUV87Z	Supplement Left Vocal Cord with Autologous Tissue Substitute, Via Natural or Artificial Opening Endoscopic
0CUV8JZ	Supplement Left Vocal Cord with Synthetic Substitute, Via Natural or Artificial Opening Endoscopic
0CUV8KZ	Supplement Left Vocal Cord with Nonautologous Tissue Substitute, Via Natural or Artificial Opening Endosc

0CV – Mouth and Throat, Restriction

0CVB0CZ	Restriction of Right Parotid Duct with Extraluminal Device, Open Approach
0CVB0DZ	Restriction of Right Parotid Duct with Intraluminal Device, Open Approach
0CVB0ZZ	Restriction of Right Parotid Duct, Open Approach
0CVB3CZ	Restriction of Right Parotid Duct with Extraluminal Device, Percutaneous Approach
0CVB3DZ	Restriction of Right Parotid Duct with Intraluminal Device, Percutaneous Approach
0CVB3ZZ	Restriction of Right Parotid Duct, Percutaneous Approach
0CVB7DZ	Restriction of Right Parotid Duct with Intraluminal Device, Via Natural or Artificial Opening
0CVB7ZZ	Restriction of Right Parotid Duct, Via Natural or Artificial Opening
0CVB8DZ	Restriction of Right Parotid Duct with Intraluminal Device, Via Natural or Artificial Opening Endoscopic
0CVB8ZZ	Restriction of Right Parotid Duct, Via Natural or Artificial Opening Endoscopic
0CVC0CZ	Restriction of Left Parotid Duct with Extraluminal Device, Open Approach
0CVC0DZ	Restriction of Left Parotid Duct with Intraluminal Device, Open Approach
0CVC0ZZ	Restriction of Left Parotid Duct, Open Approach
0CVC3CZ	Restriction of Left Parotid Duct with Extraluminal Device, Percutaneous Approach
0CVC3DZ	Restriction of Left Parotid Duct with Intraluminal Device, Percutaneous Approach
0CVC3ZZ	Restriction of Left Parotid Duct, Percutaneous Approach
0CVC7DZ	Restriction of Left Parotid Duct with Intraluminal Device, Via Natural or Artificial Opening
0CVC7ZZ	Restriction of Left Parotid Duct, Via Natural or Artificial Opening
0CVC8DZ	Restriction of Left Parotid Duct with Intraluminal Device, Via Natural or Artificial Opening Endoscopic
0CVC8ZZ	Restriction of Left Parotid Duct, Via Natural or Artificial Opening Endosc

0CW – Mouth and Throat, Revision

Review Coding Guideline B6.1c

0CWA00Z	Revision of Drainage Device in Salivary Gland, Open Approach
0CWA0CZ	Revision of Extraluminal Device in Salivary Gland, Open Approach
0CWA30Z	Revision of Drainage Device in Salivary Gland, Percutaneous Approach
0CWA3CZ	Revision of Extraluminal Device in Salivary Gland, Percutaneous Approach
0CWAX0Z	Revision of Drainage Device in Salivary Gland, External Approach
0CWAXCZ	Revision of Extraluminal Device in Salivary Gland, External Approach
0CWS00Z	Revision of Drainage Device in Larynx, Open Approach
0CWS07Z	Revision of Autologous Tissue Substitute in Larynx, Open Approach
0CWS0DZ	Revision of Intraluminal Device in Larynx, Open Approach
0CWS0JZ	Revision of Synthetic Substitute in Larynx, Open Approach
0CWS0KZ	Revision of Nonautologous Tissue Substitute in Larynx, Open Approach
0CWS30Z	Revision of Drainage Device in Larynx, Percutaneous Approach
0CWS37Z	Revision of Autologous Tissue Substitute in Larynx, Percutaneous Approach
0CWS3DZ	Revision of Intraluminal Device in Larynx, Percutaneous Approach
0CWS3JZ	Revision of Synthetic Substitute in Larynx, Percutaneous Approach
0CWS3KZ	Revision of Nonautologous Tissue Substitute in Larynx, Percutaneous Approach
0CWS70Z	Revision of Drainage Device in Larynx, Via Natural or Artificial Opening
0CWS77Z	Revision of Autologous Tissue Substitute in Larynx, Via Natural or Artificial Opening
0CWS7DZ	Revision of Intraluminal Device in Larynx, Via Natural or Artificial Opening
0CWS7JZ	Revision of Synthetic Substitute in Larynx, Via Natural or Artificial Opening
0CWS7KZ	Revision of Nonautologous Tissue Substitute in Larynx, Via Natural or Artificial Opening
0CWS80Z	Revision of Drainage Device in Larynx, Via Natural or Artificial Opening Endoscopic
0CWS87Z	Revision of Autologous Tissue Substitute in Larynx, Via Natural or Artificial Opening Endoscopic
0CWS8DZ	Revision of Intraluminal Device in Larynx, Via Natural or Artificial Opening Endoscopic
0CWS8JZ	Revision of Synthetic Substitute in Larynx, Via Natural or Artificial Opening Endoscopic
0CWS8KZ	Revision of Nonautologous Tissue Substitute in Larynx, Via Natural or Artificial Opening Endoscopic
0CWSX0Z	Revision of Drainage Device in Larynx, External Approach
0CWSX7Z	Revision of Autologous Tissue Substitute in Larynx, External Approach
0CWSXDZ	Revision of Intraluminal Device in Larynx, External Approach
0CWSXJZ	Revision of Synthetic Substitute in Larynx, External Approach
0CWSXKZ	Revision of Nonautologous Tissue Substitute in Larynx, External Approach
0CWY00Z	Revision of Drainage Device in Mouth and Throat, Open Approach
0CWY01Z	Revision of Radioactive Element in Mouth and Throat, Open Approach
0CWY07Z	Revision of Autologous Tissue Substitute in Mouth and Throat, Open Approach
0CWY0DZ	Revision of Intraluminal Device in Mouth and Throat, Open Approach
0CWY0JZ	Revision of Synthetic Substitute in Mouth and Throat, Open Approach
0CWY0KZ	Revision of Nonautologous Tissue Substitute in Mouth and Throat, Open Approach
0CWY30Z	Revision of Drainage Device in Mouth and Throat, Percutaneous Approach
0CWY31Z	Revision of Radioactive Element in Mouth and Throat, Percutaneous Approach
0CWY37Z	Revision of Autologous Tissue Substitute in Mouth and Throat, Percutaneous Approach
0CWY3DZ	Revision of Intraluminal Device in Mouth and Throat, Percutaneous Approach
0CWY3JZ	Revision of Synthetic Substitute in Mouth and Throat, Percutaneous Approach
0CWY3KZ	Revision of Nonautologous Tissue Substitute in Mouth and Throat, Percutaneous Approach
0CWY70Z	Revision of Drainage Device in Mouth and Throat, Via Natural or Artificial Opening
0CWY71Z	Revision of Radioactive Element in Mouth and Throat, Via Natural or Artificial Opening
0CWY77Z	Revision of Autologous Tissue Substitute in Mouth and Throat, Via Natural or Artificial Opening
0CWY7DZ	Revision of Intraluminal Device in Mouth and Throat, Via Natural or Artificial Opening
0CWY7JZ	Revision of Synthetic Substitute in Mouth and Throat, Via Natural or Artificial Opening
0CWY7KZ	Revision of Nonautologous Tissue Substitute in Mouth and Throat, Via Natural or Artificial Opening
0CWY80Z	Revision of Drainage Device in Mouth and Throat, Via Natural or Artificial Opening Endoscopic
0CWY81Z	Revision of Radioactive Element in Mouth and Throat, Via Natural or Artificial Opening Endoscopic
0CWY87Z	Revision of Autologous Tissue Substitute in Mouth and Throat, Via Natural or Artificial Opening Endoscopic
0CWY8DZ	Revision of Intraluminal Device in Mouth and Throat, Via Natural or Artificial Opening Endoscopic

Y8JZ	Revision of Synthetic Substitute in Mouth and Throat, Via Natural or Artificial Opening Endoscopic	0CWYX0Z	Revision of Drainage Device in Mouth and Throat, External Approach	0CWYXDZ	Revision of Intraluminal Device in Mouth and Throat, External Approach
Y8KZ	Revision of Nonautologous Tissue Substitute in Mouth and Throat, Via Natural or Artificial Opening Endoscopic	0CWYX1Z	Revision of Radioactive Element in Mouth and Throat, External Approach	0CWYXJZ	Revision of Synthetic Substitute in Mouth and Throat, External Approach
		0CWYX7Z	Revision of Autologous Tissue Substitute in Mouth and Throat, External Approach	0CWYXKZ	Revision of Nonautologous Tissue Substitute in Mouth and Throat, External Approach

X – Mouth and Throat, Transfer

00ZZ	Transfer Upper Lip, Open Approach	0CX40ZZ	Transfer Buccal Mucosa, Open Approach	0CX60ZZ	Transfer Lower Gingiva, Open Approach
0XZZ	Transfer Upper Lip, External Approach	0CX4XZZ	Transfer Buccal Mucosa, External Approach	0CX6XZZ	Transfer Lower Gingiva, External Approach
10ZZ	Transfer Lower Lip, Open Approach	0CX50ZZ	Transfer Upper Gingiva, Open Approach	0CX70ZZ	Transfer Tongue, Open Approach
1XZZ	Transfer Lower Lip, External Approach	0CX5XZZ	Transfer Upper Gingiva, External Approach	0CX7XZZ	Transfer Tongue, External Approach
30ZZ	Transfer Soft Palate, Open Approach				
3XZZ	Transfer Soft Palate, External Approach				

| Female-only | ♂ Male-only | ▲ Limited Coverage | ● Non-OR | HAC-associated procedure | ▲ Non-covered procedures | + Combination |

Upper Gastrointestinal System

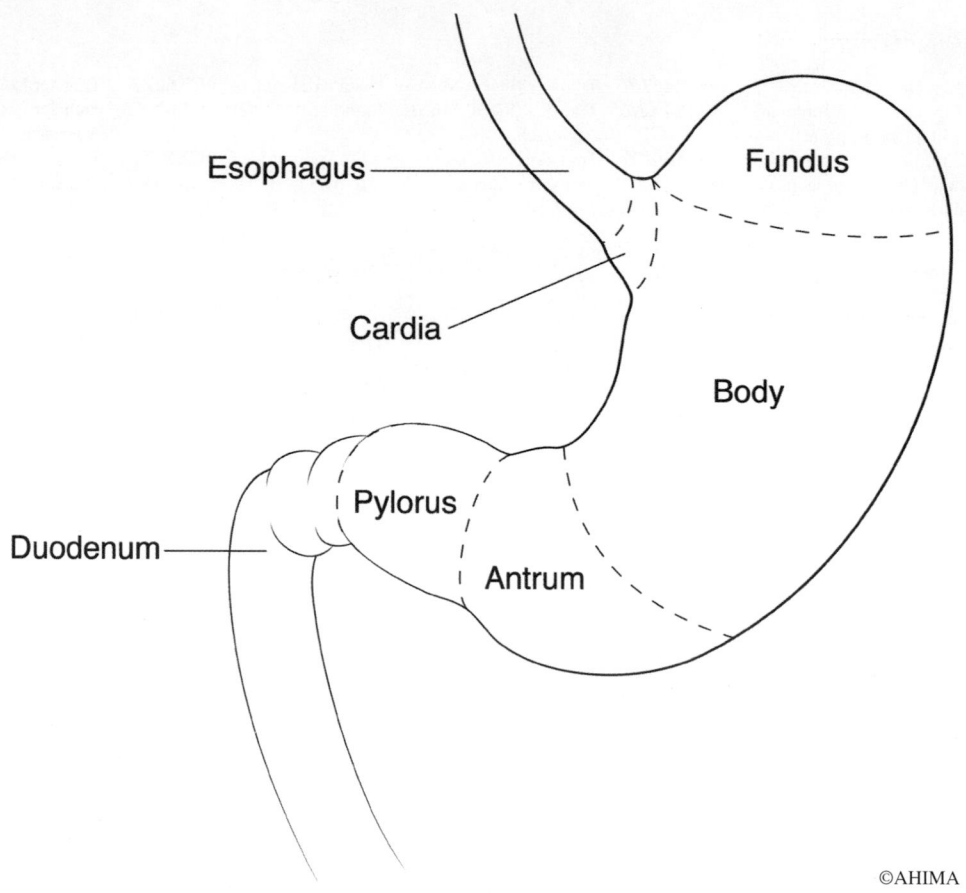

Esophagus

Fundus

Cardia

Body

Pylorus

Duodenum

Antrum

©AHIMA

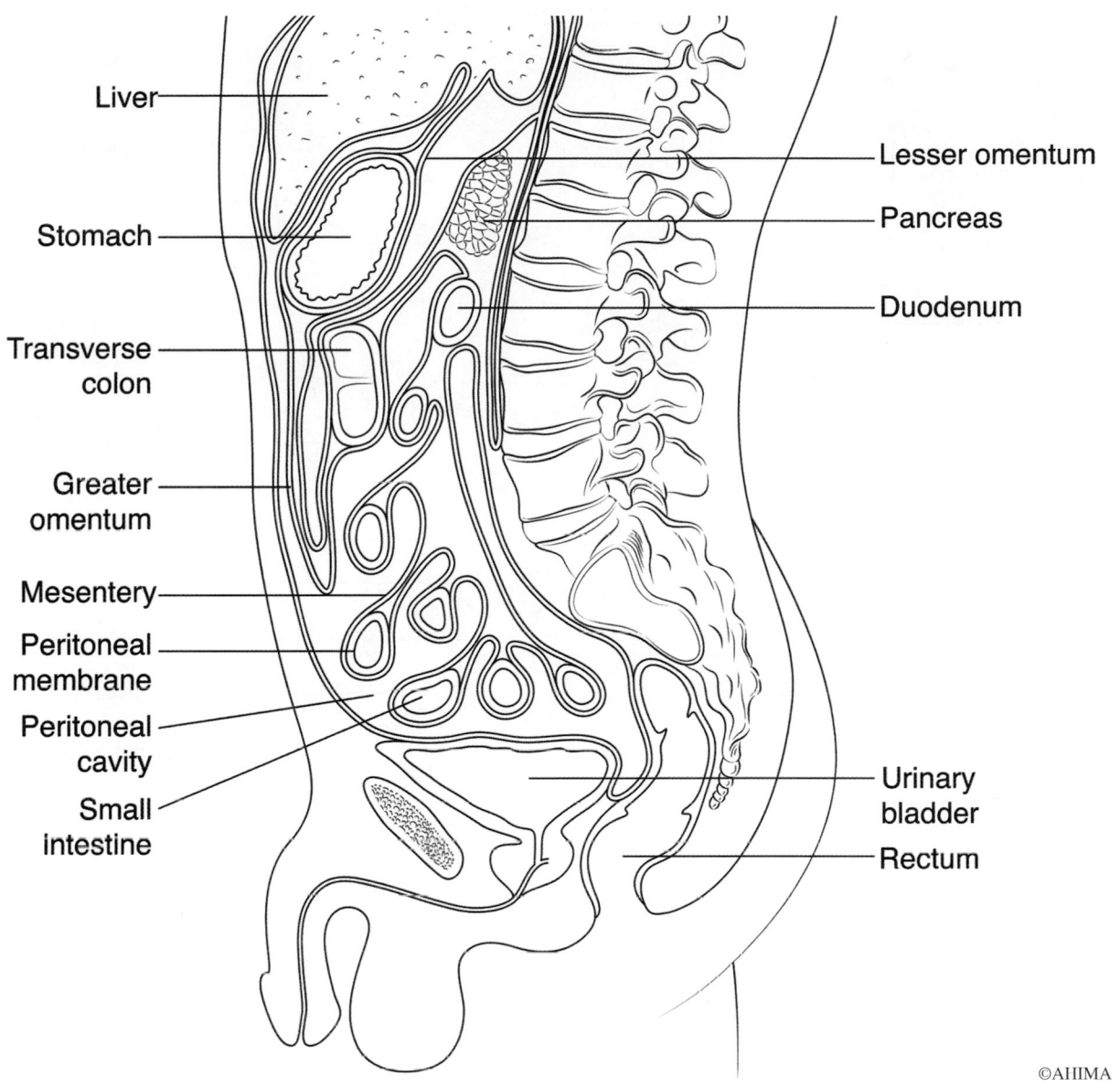

Liver

Stomach

Transverse
colon

Greater
omentum

Mesentery

Peritoneal
membrane

Peritoneal
cavity

Small
intestine

Lesser omentum

Pancreas

Duodenum

Urinary
bladder

Rectum

©AHIMA

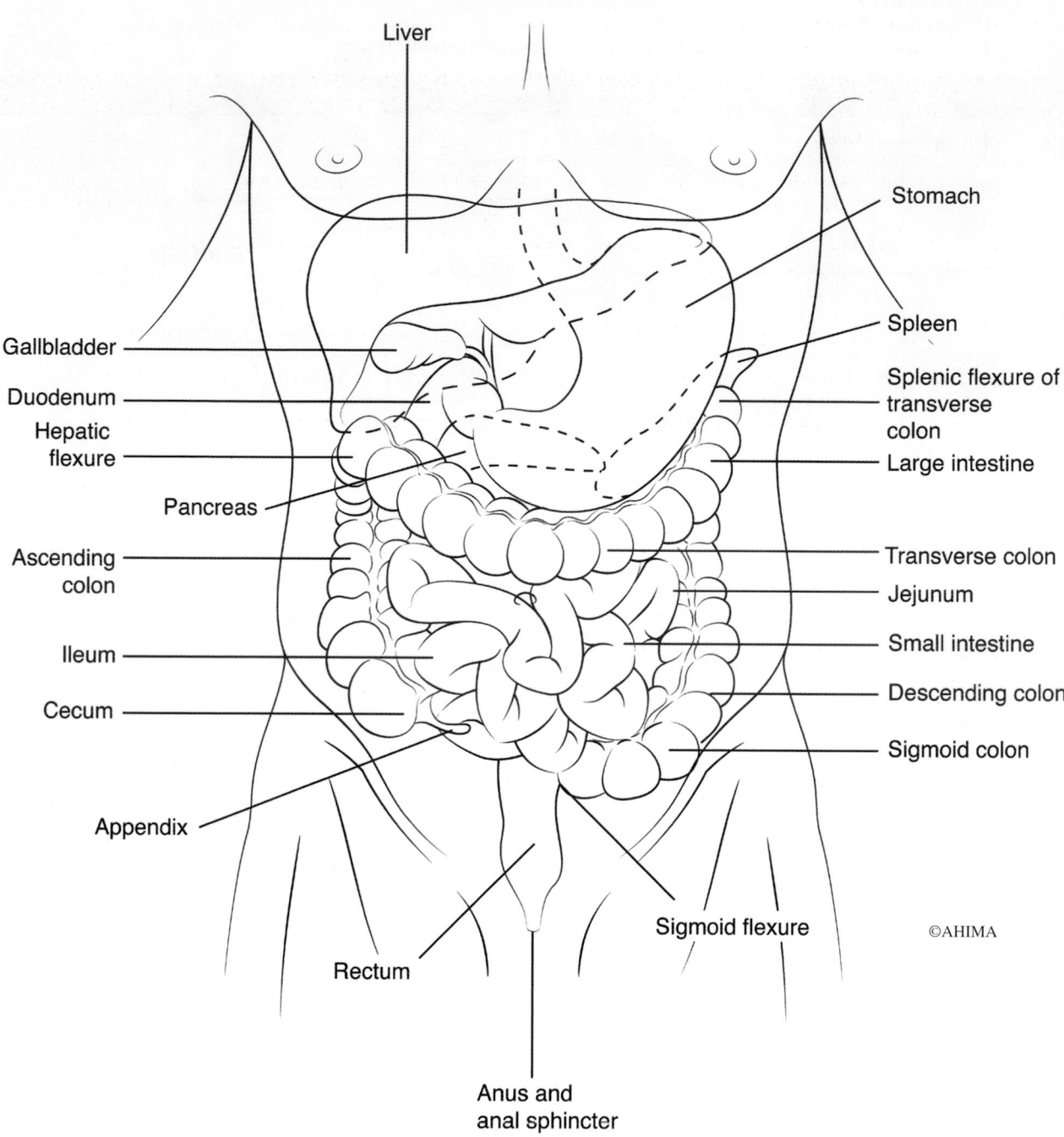

Liver

Stomach

Gallbladder

Spleen

Duodenum

Splenic flexure of
transverse
colon

Hepatic
flexure

Large intestine

Pancreas

Ascending
colon

Transverse colon

Jejunum

Ileum

Small intestine

Cecum

Descending colon

Sigmoid colon

Appendix

©AHIMA

Sigmoid flexure

Rectum

Anus and
anal sphincter

tion | 0 | **Medical and Surgical**
ly System | D | **Gastrointestinal System**
eration | 1 | **Bypass:** Altering the route of passage of the contents of a tubular body part

Body Part (4th)	Approach (5th)	Device (6th)	Qualifier (7th)
Esophagus, Upper Esophagus, Middle Esophagus, Lower Esophagus	0 Open 4 Percutaneous Endoscopic 8 Via Natural or Artificial Opening Endoscopic	7 Autologous Tissue Substitute J Synthetic Substitute K Nonautologous Tissue Substitute Z No Device	4 Cutaneous 6 Stomach 9 Duodenum A Jejunum B Ileum
Esophagus, Upper Esophagus, Middle Esophagus, Lower Esophagus	3 Percutaneous	J Synthetic Substitute	4 Cutaneous
Stomach Duodenum	0 Open 4 Percutaneous Endoscopic 8 Via Natural or Artificial Opening Endoscopic	7 Autologous Tissue Substitute J Synthetic Substitute K Nonautologous Tissue Substitute Z No Device	4 Cutaneous 9 Duodenum A Jejunum B Ileum L Transverse Colon
Stomach Duodenum	3 Percutaneous	J Synthetic Substitute	4 Cutaneous
Jejunum	0 Open 4 Percutaneous Endoscopic 8 Via Natural or Artificial Opening Endoscopic	7 Autologous Tissue Substitute J Synthetic Substitute K Nonautologous Tissue Substitute Z No Device	4 Cutaneous A Jejunum B Ileum H Cecum K Ascending Colon L Transverse Colon M Descending Colon N Sigmoid Colon P Rectum Q Anus
Jejunum	3 Percutaneous	J Synthetic Substitute	4 Cutaneous
Ileum	0 Open 4 Percutaneous Endoscopic 8 Via Natural or Artificial Opening Endoscopic	7 Autologous Tissue Substitute J Synthetic Substitute K Nonautologous Tissue Substitute Z No Device	4 Cutaneous B Ileum H Cecum K Ascending Colon L Transverse Colon M Descending Colon N Sigmoid Colon P Rectum Q Anus
Ileum	3 Percutaneous	J Synthetic Substitute	4 Cutaneous
Cecum	0 Open 4 Percutaneous Endoscopic 8 Via Natural or Artificial Opening Endoscopic	7 Autologous Tissue Substitute J Synthetic Substitute K Nonautologous Tissue Substitute Z No Device	4 Cutaneous H Cecum K Ascending Colon L Transverse Colon M Descending Colon N Sigmoid Colon P Rectum
Cecum	3 Percutaneous	J Synthetic Substitute	4 Cutaneous
Ascending Colon	0 Open 4 Percutaneous Endoscopic 8 Via Natural or Artificial Opening Endoscopic	7 Autologous Tissue Substitute J Synthetic Substitute K Nonautologous Tissue Substitute Z No Device	4 Cutaneous K Ascending Colon L Transverse Colon M Descending Colon N Sigmoid Colon P Rectum
Ascending Colon	3 Percutaneous	J Synthetic Substitute	4 Cutaneous

Continued →

Section	0	Medical and Surgical
Body System	D	Gastrointestinal System
Operation	1	Bypass: Altering the route of passage of the contents of a tubular body part

Body Part (4th)	Approach (5th)	Device (6th)	Qualifier (7th)
L Transverse Colon	0 Open 4 Percutaneous Endoscopic 8 Via Natural or Artificial Opening Endoscopic	7 Autologous Tissue Substitute J Synthetic Substitute K Nonautologous Tissue Substitute Z No Device	4 Cutaneous L Transverse Colon M Descending Colon N Sigmoid Colon P Rectum
L Transverse Colon	3 Percutaneous	J Synthetic Substitute	4 Cutaneous
M Descending Colon	0 Open 4 Percutaneous Endoscopic 8 Via Natural or Artificial Opening Endoscopic	7 Autologous Tissue Substitute J Synthetic Substitute K Nonautologous Tissue Substitute Z No Device	4 Cutaneous M Descending Colon N Sigmoid Colon P Rectum
M Descending Colon	3 Percutaneous	J Synthetic Substitute	4 Cutaneous
N Sigmoid Colon	0 Open 4 Percutaneous Endoscopic 8 Via Natural or Artificial Opening Endoscopic	7 Autologous Tissue Substitute J Synthetic Substitute K Nonautologous Tissue Substitute Z No Device	4 Cutaneous N Sigmoid Colon P Rectum
N Sigmoid Colon	3 Percutaneous	J Synthetic Substitute	4 Cutaneous

Section	0	Medical and Surgical
Body System	D	Gastrointestinal System
Operation	2	Change: Taking out or off a device from a body part and putting back an identical or similar device in or on the same body part without cutting or puncturing the skin or a mucous membrane

Body Part (4th)	Approach (5th)	Device (6th)	Qualifier (7th)
0 Upper Intestinal Tract D Lower Intestinal Tract	X External	0 Drainage Device U Feeding Device Y Other Device	Z No Qualifier
U Omentum V Mesentery W Peritoneum	X External	0 Drainage Device Y Other Device	Z No Qualifier

tion	0	Medical and Surgical
ly System	D	Gastrointestinal System
eration	5	**Destruction:** Physical eradication of all or a portion of a body part by the direct use of energy, force, or a destructive agent

Body Part (4th)	Approach (5th)	Device (6th)	Qualifier (7th)
Esophagus, Upper Esophagus, Middle Esophagus, Lower Esophagogastric Junction Esophagus Stomach Stomach, Pylorus Small Intestine Duodenum Jejunum Ileum Ileocecal Valve Large Intestine Large Intestine, Right Large Intestine, Left Cecum Appendix Ascending Colon Transverse Colon M Descending Colon N Sigmoid Colon Rectum	0 Open 3 Percutaneous 4 Percutaneous Endoscopic 7 Via Natural or Artificial Opening 8 Via Natural or Artificial Opening Endoscopic	Z No Device	Z No Qualifier
Q Anus	0 Open 3 Percutaneous 4 Percutaneous Endoscopic 7 Via Natural or Artificial Opening 8 Via Natural or Artificial Opening Endoscopic X External	Z No Device	Z No Qualifier
R Anal Sphincter S Greater Omentum T Lesser Omentum V Mesentery W Peritoneum	0 Open 3 Percutaneous 4 Percutaneous Endoscopic	Z No Device	Z No Qualifier

ction	0	Medical and Surgical
dy System	D	Gastrointestinal System
peration	7	**Dilation:** Expanding an orifice or the lumen of a tubular body part

Body Part (4th)	Approach (5th)	Device (6th)	Qualifier (7th)
1 Esophagus, Upper 2 Esophagus, Middle 3 Esophagus, Lower 4 Esophagogastric Junction 5 Esophagus 6 Stomach 7 Stomach, Pylorus 8 Small Intestine 9 Duodenum A Jejunum B Ileum C Ileocecal Valve E Large Intestine F Large Intestine, Right G Large Intestine, Left H Cecum K Ascending Colon L Transverse Colon M Descending Colon N Sigmoid Colon P Rectum Q Anus	0 Open 3 Percutaneous 4 Percutaneous Endoscopic 7 Via Natural or Artificial Opening 8 Via Natural or Artificial Opening Endoscopic	D Intraluminal Device Z No Device	Z No Qualifier

Section	0	Medical and Surgical
Body System	D	Gastrointestinal System
Operation	8	**Division:** Cutting into a body part, without draining fluids and/or gases from the body part, in order to separate or transect a body part

Body Part (4th)	Approach (5th)	Device (6th)	Qualifier (7th)
4 Esophagogastric Junction 7 Stomach, Pylorus	0 Open 3 Percutaneous 4 Percutaneous Endoscopic 7 Via Natural or Artificial Opening 8 Via Natural or Artificial Opening Endoscopic	Z No Device	Z No Qualifier
R Anal Sphincter	0 Open 3 Percutaneous	Z No Device	Z No Qualifier

Section	0	Medical and Surgical
Body System	D	Gastrointestinal System
Operation	9	**Drainage:** Taking or letting out fluids and/or gases from a body part

Body Part (4th)	Approach (5th)	Device (6th)	Qualifier (7th)
1 Esophagus, Upper 2 Esophagus, Middle 3 Esophagus, Lower 4 Esophagogastric Junction 5 Esophagus 6 Stomach 7 Stomach, Pylorus 8 Small Intestine 9 Duodenum A Jejunum B Ileum C Ileocecal Valve E Large Intestine F Large Intestine, Right G Large Intestine, Left H Cecum J Appendix K Ascending Colon L Transverse Colon M Descending Colon N Sigmoid Colon P Rectum	0 Open 3 Percutaneous 4 Percutaneous Endoscopic 7 Via Natural or Artificial Opening 8 Via Natural or Artificial Opening Endoscopic	0 Drainage Device	Z No Qualifier
1 Esophagus, Upper 2 Esophagus, Middle 3 Esophagus, Lower 4 Esophagogastric Junction 5 Esophagus 6 Stomach 7 Stomach, Pylorus 8 Small Intestine 9 Duodenum A Jejunum B Ileum C Ileocecal Valve E Large Intestine F Large Intestine, Right G Large Intestine, Left H Cecum J Appendix K Ascending Colon L Transverse Colon M Descending Colon N Sigmoid Colon P Rectum	0 Open 3 Percutaneous 4 Percutaneous Endoscopic 7 Via Natural or Artificial Opening 8 Via Natural or Artificial Opening Endoscopic	Z No Device	X Diagnostic Z No Qualifier

Continued →

Section	0	**Medical and Surgical**	
Body System	D	**Gastrointestinal System**	
Operation	9	**Drainage:** Taking or letting out fluids and/or gases from a body part	

Body Part (4th)	Approach (5th)	Device (6th)	Qualifier (7th)
Q Anus	0 Open 3 Percutaneous 4 Percutaneous Endoscopic 7 Via Natural or Artificial Opening 8 Via Natural or Artificial Opening Endoscopic X External	0 Drainage Device	Z No Qualifier
Q Anus	0 Open 3 Percutaneous 4 Percutaneous Endoscopic 7 Via Natural or Artificial Opening 8 Via Natural or Artificial Opening Endoscopic X External	Z No Device	X Diagnostic Z No Qualifier
R Anal Sphincter S Greater Omentum T Lesser Omentum V Mesentery W Peritoneum	0 Open 3 Percutaneous 4 Percutaneous Endoscopic	0 Drainage Device	Z No Qualifier
R Anal Sphincter S Greater Omentum T Lesser Omentum V Mesentery W Peritoneum	0 Open 3 Percutaneous 4 Percutaneous Endoscopic	Z No Device	X Diagnostic Z No Qualifier

Section	0	**Medical and Surgical**	
Body System	D	**Gastrointestinal System**	
Operation	B	**Excision:** Cutting out or off, without replacement, a portion of a body part	

Body Part (4th)	Approach (5th)	Device (6th)	Qualifier (7th)
1 Esophagus, Upper 2 Esophagus, Middle 3 Esophagus, Lower 4 Esophagogastric Junction 5 Esophagus 7 Stomach, Pylorus 8 Small Intestine 9 Duodenum A Jejunum B Ileum C Ileocecal Valve E Large Intestine F Large Intestine, Right G Large Intestine, Left H Cecum J Appendix K Ascending Colon L Transverse Colon M Descending Colon N Sigmoid Colon P Rectum	0 Open 3 Percutaneous 4 Percutaneous Endoscopic 7 Via Natural or Artificial Opening 8 Via Natural or Artificial Opening Endoscopic	Z No Device	X Diagnostic Z No Qualifier
6 Stomach	0 Open 3 Percutaneous 4 Percutaneous Endoscopic 7 Via Natural or Artificial Opening 8 Via Natural or Artificial Opening Endoscopic	Z No Device	3 Vertical X Diagnostic Z No Qualifier

Continued →

Section	0	Medical and Surgical
Body System	D	Gastrointestinal System
Operation	B	**Excision:** Cutting out or off, without replacement, a portion of a body part

Body Part (4th)	Approach (5th)	Device (6th)	Qualifier (7th)
Q Anus	0 Open 3 Percutaneous 4 Percutaneous Endoscopic 7 Via Natural or Artificial Opening 8 Via Natural or Artificial Opening Endoscopic X External	Z No Device	X Diagnostic Z No Qualifier
R Anal Sphincter S Greater Omentum T Lesser Omentum V Mesentery W Peritoneum	0 Open 3 Percutaneous 4 Percutaneous Endoscopic	Z No Device	X Diagnostic Z No Qualifier

Section	0	Medical and Surgical
Body System	D	Gastrointestinal System
Operation	C	**Extirpation:** Taking or cutting out solid matter from a body part

Body Part (4th)	Approach (5th)	Device (6th)	Qualifier (7th)
1 Esophagus, Upper 2 Esophagus, Middle 3 Esophagus, Lower 4 Esophagogastric Junction 5 Esophagus 6 Stomach 7 Stomach, Pylorus 8 Small Intestine 9 Duodenum A Jejunum B Ileum C Ileocecal Valve E Large Intestine F Large Intestine, Right G Large Intestine, Left H Cecum J Appendix K Ascending Colon L Transverse Colon M Descending Colon N Sigmoid Colon P Rectum	0 Open 3 Percutaneous 4 Percutaneous Endoscopic 7 Via Natural or Artificial Opening 8 Via Natural or Artificial Opening Endoscopic	Z No Device	Z No Qualifier
Q Anus	0 Open 3 Percutaneous 4 Percutaneous Endoscopic 7 Via Natural or Artificial Opening 8 Via Natural or Artificial Opening Endoscopic X External	Z No Device	Z No Qualifier
R Anal Sphincter S Greater Omentum T Lesser Omentum V Mesentery W Peritoneum	0 Open 3 Percutaneous 4 Percutaneous Endoscopic	Z No Device	Z No Qualifier

tion	0	Medical and Surgical
dy System	D	Gastrointestinal System
eration	F	Fragmentation: Breaking solid matter in a body part into pieces

Body Part (4th)	Approach (5th)	Device (6th)	Qualifier (7th)
Esophagus Stomach Small Intestine Duodenum Jejunum Ileum Large Intestine Large Intestine, Right Large Intestine, Left Cecum Appendix Ascending Colon Transverse Colon Descending Colon Sigmoid Colon Rectum Anus	0 Open 3 Percutaneous 4 Percutaneous Endoscopic 7 Via Natural or Artificial Opening 8 Via Natural or Artificial Opening Endoscopic X External	Z No Device	Z No Qualifier

tion	0	Medical and Surgical
dy System	D	Gastrointestinal System
eration	H	Insertion: Putting in a nonbiological appliance that monitors, assists, performs, or prevents a physiological function but does not physically take the place of a body part

Body Part (4th)	Approach (5th)	Device (6th)	Qualifier (7th)
Esophagus	0 Open 3 Percutaneous 4 Percutaneous Endoscopic	1 Radioactive Element 2 Monitoring Device 3 Infusion Device D Intraluminal Device U Feeding Device	Z No Qualifier
Esophagus	7 Via Natural or Artificial Opening 8 Via Natural or Artificial Opening Endoscopic	1 Radioactive Element 2 Monitoring Device 3 Infusion Device B Intraluminal Device, Airway D Intraluminal Device U Feeding Device	Z No Qualifier
Stomach	0 Open 3 Percutaneous 4 Percutaneous Endoscopic	2 Monitoring Device 3 Infusion Device D Intraluminal Device M Stimulator Lead U Feeding Device	Z No Qualifier
Stomach	7 Via Natural or Artificial Opening 8 Via Natural or Artificial Opening Endoscopic	2 Monitoring Device 3 Infusion Device D Intraluminal Device U Feeding Device	Z No Qualifier
Small Intestine Duodenum Jejunum Ileum	0 Open 3 Percutaneous 4 Percutaneous Endoscopic 7 Via Natural or Artificial Opening 8 Via Natural or Artificial Opening Endoscopic	2 Monitoring Device 3 Infusion Device D Intraluminal Device U Feeding Device	Z No Qualifier
Large Intestine	0 Open 3 Percutaneous 4 Percutaneous Endoscopic 7 Via Natural or Artificial Opening 8 Via Natural or Artificial Opening Endoscopic	D Intraluminal Device	Z No Qualifier

Continued →

Section	0	Medical and Surgical
Body System	D	Gastrointestinal System
Operation	H	**Insertion:** Putting in a nonbiological appliance that monitors, assists, performs, or prevents a physiological function but does not physically take the place of a body part

Body Part (4th)	Approach (5th)	Device (6th)	Qualifier (7th)
P Rectum	0 Open 3 Percutaneous 4 Percutaneous Endoscopic 7 Via Natural or Artificial Opening 8 Via Natural or Artificial Opening Endoscopic	1 Radioactive Element D Intraluminal Device	Z No Qualifier
Q Anus	0 Open 3 Percutaneous 4 Percutaneous Endoscopic	D Intraluminal Device L Artificial Sphincter	Z No Qualifier
Q Anus	7 Via Natural or Artificial Opening 8 Via Natural or Artificial Opening Endoscopic	D Intraluminal Device	Z No Qualifier
R Anal Sphincter	0 Open 3 Percutaneous 4 Percutaneous Endoscopic	M Stimulator Lead	Z No Qualifier

Section	0	Medical and Surgical
Body System	D	Gastrointestinal System
Operation	J	**Inspection:** Visually and/or manually exploring a body part

Body Part (4th)	Approach (5th)	Device (6th)	Qualifier (7th)
0 Upper Intestinal Tract 6 Stomach D Lower Intestinal Tract	0 Open 3 Percutaneous 4 Percutaneous Endoscopic 7 Via Natural or Artificial Opening 8 Via Natural or Artificial Opening Endoscopic X External	Z No Device	Z No Qualifier
U Omentum V Mesentery W Peritoneum	0 Open 3 Percutaneous 4 Percutaneous Endoscopic X External	Z No Device	Z No Qualifier

Section	0	Medical and Surgical
Body System	D	Gastrointestinal System
Operation	L	**Occlusion:** Completely closing an orifice or the lumen of a tubular body part

Body Part (4th)	Approach (5th)	Device (6th)	Qualifier (7th)
1 Esophagus, Upper 2 Esophagus, Middle 3 Esophagus, Lower 4 Esophagogastric Junction 5 Esophagus 6 Stomach 7 Stomach, Pylorus 8 Small Intestine 9 Duodenum A Jejunum B Ileum C Ileocecal Valve E Large Intestine F Large Intestine, Right G Large Intestine, Left H Cecum K Ascending Colon L Transverse Colon M Descending Colon N Sigmoid Colon P Rectum	0 Open 3 Percutaneous 4 Percutaneous Endoscopic	C Extraluminal Device D Intraluminal Device Z No Device	Z No Qualifier

Continued —

ction	0	Medical and Surgical
dy System	D	Gastrointestinal System
eration	L	**Occlusion:** Completely closing an orifice or the lumen of a tubular body part

Body Part (4th)	Approach (5th)	Device (6th)	Qualifier (7th)
Esophagus, Upper Esophagus, Middle Esophagus, Lower Esophagogastric Junction Esophagus Stomach Stomach, Pylorus Small Intestine Duodenum A Jejunum B Ileum C Ileocecal Valve E Large Intestine F Large Intestine, Right G Large Intestine, Left H Cecum K Ascending Colon L Transverse Colon M Descending Colon N Sigmoid Colon P Rectum	7 Via Natural or Artificial Opening 8 Via Natural or Artificial Opening Endoscopic	D Intraluminal Device Z No Device	Z No Qualifier
Q Anus	0 Open 3 Percutaneous 4 Percutaneous Endoscopic X External	C Extraluminal Device D Intraluminal Device Z No Device	Z No Qualifier
Q Anus	7 Via Natural or Artificial Opening 8 Via Natural or Artificial Opening Endoscopic	D Intraluminal Device Z No Device	Z No Qualifier

ection	0	Medical and Surgical
ody System	D	Gastrointestinal System
eration	M	**Reattachment:** Putting back in or on all or a portion of a separated body part to its normal location or other suitable location

Body Part (4th)	Approach (5th)	Device (6th)	Qualifier (7th)
5 Esophagus 6 Stomach 8 Small Intestine 9 Duodenum A Jejunum B Ileum E Large Intestine F Large Intestine, Right G Large Intestine, Left H Cecum K Ascending Colon L Transverse Colon M Descending Colon N Sigmoid Colon P Rectum	0 Open 4 Percutaneous Endoscopic	Z No Device	Z No Qualifier

Section	0	Medical and Surgical
Body System	D	Gastrointestinal System
Operation	N	Release: Freeing a body part from an abnormal physical constraint by cutting or by the use of force

Body Part (4th)	Approach (5th)	Device (6th)	Qualifier (7th)
1 Esophagus, Upper 2 Esophagus, Middle 3 Esophagus, Lower 4 Esophagogastric Junction 5 Esophagus 6 Stomach 7 Stomach, Pylorus 8 Small Intestine 9 Duodenum A Jejunum B Ileum C Ileocecal Valve E Large Intestine F Large Intestine, Right G Large Intestine, Left H Cecum J Appendix K Ascending Colon L Transverse Colon M Descending Colon N Sigmoid Colon P Rectum	0 Open 3 Percutaneous 4 Percutaneous Endoscopic 7 Via Natural or Artificial Opening 8 Via Natural or Artificial Opening Endoscopic	Z No Device	Z No Qualifier
Q Anus	0 Open 3 Percutaneous 4 Percutaneous Endoscopic 7 Via Natural or Artificial Opening 8 Via Natural or Artificial Opening Endoscopic X External	Z No Device	Z No Qualifier
R Anal Sphincter S Greater Omentum T Lesser Omentum V Mesentery W Peritoneum	0 Open 3 Percutaneous 4 Percutaneous Endoscopic	Z No Device	Z No Qualifier

Section	0	Medical and Surgical
Body System	D	Gastrointestinal System
Operation	P	Removal: Taking out or off a device from a body part

Body Part (4th)	Approach (5th)	Device (6th)	Qualifier (7th)
0 Upper Intestinal Tract D Lower Intestinal Tract	0 Open 3 Percutaneous 4 Percutaneous Endoscopic 7 Via Natural or Artificial Opening 8 Via Natural or Artificial Opening Endoscopic	0 Drainage Device 2 Monitoring Device 3 Infusion Device 7 Autologous Tissue Substitute C Extraluminal Device D Intraluminal Device J Synthetic Substitute K Nonautologous Tissue Substitute U Feeding Device	Z No Qualifier
0 Upper Intestinal Tract D Lower Intestinal Tract	X External	0 Drainage Device 2 Monitoring Device 3 Infusion Device D Intraluminal Device U Feeding Device	Z No Qualifier
5 Esophagus	0 Open 3 Percutaneous 4 Percutaneous Endoscopic	1 Radioactive Element 2 Monitoring Device 3 Infusion Device U Feeding Device	Z No Qualifier

Continued →

tion	0	Medical and Surgical
ly System	D	Gastrointestinal System
eration	P	**Removal:** Taking out or off a device from a body part

Body Part (4ᵗʰ)	Approach (5ᵗʰ)	Device (6ᵗʰ)	Qualifier (7ᵗʰ)
Esophagus	7 Via Natural or Artificial Opening 8 Via Natural or Artificial Opening Endoscopic	1 Radioactive Element D Intraluminal Device	Z No Qualifier
Esophagus	X External	1 Radioactive Element 2 Monitoring Device 3 Infusion Device D Intraluminal Device U Feeding Device	Z No Qualifier
Stomach	0 Open 3 Percutaneous 4 Percutaneous Endoscopic	0 Drainage Device 2 Monitoring Device 3 Infusion Device 7 Autologous Tissue Substitute C Extraluminal Device D Intraluminal Device J Synthetic Substitute K Nonautologous Tissue Substitute M Stimulator Lead U Feeding Device	Z No Qualifier
Stomach	7 Via Natural or Artificial Opening 8 Via Natural or Artificial Opening Endoscopic	0 Drainage Device 2 Monitoring Device 3 Infusion Device 7 Autologous Tissue Substitute C Extraluminal Device D Intraluminal Device J Synthetic Substitute K Nonautologous Tissue Substitute U Feeding Device	Z No Qualifier
Stomach	X External	0 Drainage Device 2 Monitoring Device 3 Infusion Device D Intraluminal Device U Feeding Device	Z No Qualifier
P Rectum	0 Open 3 Percutaneous 4 Percutaneous Endoscopic 7 Via Natural or Artificial Opening 8 Via Natural or Artificial Opening Endoscopic X External	1 Radioactive Element	Z No Qualifier
Q Anus	0 Open 3 Percutaneous 4 Percutaneous Endoscopic 7 Via Natural or Artificial Opening 8 Via Natural or Artificial Opening Endoscopic	L Artificial Sphincter	Z No Qualifier
R Anal Sphincter	0 Open 3 Percutaneous 4 Percutaneous Endoscopic	M Stimulator Lead	Z No Qualifier
U Omentum V Mesentery W Peritoneum	0 Open 3 Percutaneous 4 Percutaneous Endoscopic	0 Drainage Device 1 Radioactive Element 7 Autologous Tissue Substitute J Synthetic Substitute K Nonautologous Tissue Substitute	Z No Qualifier

Section	0	Medical and Surgical
Body System	D	Gastrointestinal System
Operation	Q	**Repair:** Restoring, to the extent possible, a body part to its normal anatomic structure and function

Body Part (4th)	Approach (5th)	Device (6th)	Qualifier (7th)
1 Esophagus, Upper 2 Esophagus, Middle 3 Esophagus, Lower 4 Esophagogastric Junction 5 Esophagus 6 Stomach 7 Stomach, Pylorus 8 Small Intestine 9 Duodenum A Jejunum B Ileum C Ileocecal Valve E Large Intestine F Large Intestine, Right G Large Intestine, Left H Cecum J Appendix K Ascending Colon L Transverse Colon M Descending Colon N Sigmoid Colon P Rectum	0 Open 3 Percutaneous 4 Percutaneous Endoscopic 7 Via Natural or Artificial Opening 8 Via Natural or Artificial Opening Endoscopic	Z No Device	Z No Qualifier
Q Anus	0 Open 3 Percutaneous 4 Percutaneous Endoscopic 7 Via Natural or Artificial Opening 8 Via Natural or Artificial Opening Endoscopic X External	Z No Device	Z No Qualifier
R Anal Sphincter S Greater Omentum T Lesser Omentum V Mesentery W Peritoneum	0 Open 3 Percutaneous 4 Percutaneous Endoscopic	Z No Device	Z No Qualifier

Section	0	Medical and Surgical
Body System	D	Gastrointestinal System
Operation	R	**Replacement:** Putting in or on biological or synthetic material that physically takes the place and/or function of all or a portion of a body part

Body Part (4th)	Approach (5th)	Device (6th)	Qualifier (7th)
5 Esophagus	0 Open 4 Percutaneous Endoscopic 7 Via Natural or Artificial Opening 8 Via Natural or Artificial Opening Endoscopic	7 Autologous Tissue Substitute J Synthetic Substitute K Nonautologous Tissue Substitute	Z No Qualifier
R Anal Sphincter S Greater Omentum T Lesser Omentum V Mesentery W Peritoneum	0 Open 4 Percutaneous Endoscopic	7 Autologous Tissue Substitute J Synthetic Substitute K Nonautologous Tissue Substitute	Z No Qualifier

Section | 0 | Medical and Surgical
Body System | D | Gastrointestinal System
Operation | S | Reposition: Moving to its normal location, or other suitable location, all or a portion of a body part

Body Part (4th)	Approach (5th)	Device (6th)	Qualifier (7th)
Esophagus Stomach Duodenum Jejunum Ileum Cecum Ascending Colon Transverse Colon Descending Colon Sigmoid Colon Rectum Anus	0 Open 4 Percutaneous Endoscopic 7 Via Natural or Artificial Opening 8 Via Natural or Artificial Opening Endoscopic X External	Z No Device	Z No Qualifier

Section | 0 | Medical and Surgical
Body System | D | Gastrointestinal System
Operation | T | Resection: Cutting out or off, without replacement, all of a body part

Body Part (4th)	Approach (5th)	Device (6th)	Qualifier (7th)
1 Esophagus, Upper 2 Esophagus, Middle 3 Esophagus, Lower 4 Esophagogastric Junction 5 Esophagus 6 Stomach 7 Stomach, Pylorus 8 Small Intestine 9 Duodenum A Jejunum B Ileum C Ileocecal Valve E Large Intestine F Large Intestine, Right G Large Intestine, Left H Cecum J Appendix K Ascending Colon L Transverse Colon M Descending Colon N Sigmoid Colon P Rectum Q Anus	0 Open 4 Percutaneous Endoscopic 7 Via Natural or Artificial Opening 8 Via Natural or Artificial Opening Endoscopic	Z No Device	Z No Qualifier
R Anal Sphincter S Greater Omentum T Lesser Omentum	0 Open 4 Percutaneous Endoscopic	Z No Device	Z No Qualifier

Section	0	Medical and Surgical
Body System	D	Gastrointestinal System
Operation	U	Supplement: Putting in or on biological or synthetic material that physically reinforces and/or augments the function of a portion of a body part

Body Part (4th)	Approach (5th)	Device (6th)	Qualifier (7th)
1 Esophagus, Upper 2 Esophagus, Middle 3 Esophagus, Lower 4 Esophagogastric Junction 5 Esophagus 6 Stomach 7 Stomach, Pylorus 8 Small Intestine 9 Duodenum A Jejunum B Ileum C Ileocecal Valve E Large Intestine F Large Intestine, Right G Large Intestine, Left H Cecum K Ascending Colon L Transverse Colon M Descending Colon N Sigmoid Colon P Rectum	0 Open 4 Percutaneous Endoscopic 7 Via Natural or Artificial Opening 8 Via Natural or Artificial Opening Endoscopic	7 Autologous Tissue Substitute J Synthetic Substitute K Nonautologous Tissue Substitute	Z No Qualifier
Q Anus	0 Open 4 Percutaneous Endoscopic 7 Via Natural or Artificial Opening 8 Via Natural or Artificial Opening Endoscopic X External	7 Autologous Tissue Substitute J Synthetic Substitute K Nonautologous Tissue Substitute	Z No Qualifier
R Anal Sphincter S Greater Omentum T Lesser Omentum V Mesentery W Peritoneum	0 Open 4 Percutaneous Endoscopic	7 Autologous Tissue Substitute J Synthetic Substitute K Nonautologous Tissue Substitute	Z No Qualifier

Section	0	Medical and Surgical
Body System	D	Gastrointestinal System
Operation	V	Restriction: Partially closing an orifice or the lumen of a tubular body part

Body Part (4th)	Approach (5th)	Device (6th)	Qualifier (7th)
1 Esophagus, Upper 2 Esophagus, Middle 3 Esophagus, Lower 4 Esophagogastric Junction 5 Esophagus 6 Stomach 7 Stomach, Pylorus 8 Small Intestine 9 Duodenum A Jejunum B Ileum C Ileocecal Valve E Large Intestine F Large Intestine, Right G Large Intestine, Left H Cecum K Ascending Colon L Transverse Colon M Descending Colon N Sigmoid Colon P Rectum	0 Open 3 Percutaneous 4 Percutaneous Endoscopic	C Extraluminal Device D Intraluminal Device Z No Device	Z No Qualifier

Continued →

Section	0	Medical and Surgical
Body System	D	Gastrointestinal System
Operation	V	Restriction: Partially closing an orifice or the lumen of a tubular body part

Body Part (4ᵗʰ)	Approach (5ᵗʰ)	Device (6ᵗʰ)	Qualifier (7ᵗʰ)
1 Esophagus, Upper 2 Esophagus, Middle 3 Esophagus, Lower 4 Esophagogastric Junction 5 Esophagus 6 Stomach 7 Stomach, Pylorus 8 Small Intestine 9 Duodenum A Jejunum B Ileum C Ileocecal Valve E Large Intestine F Large Intestine, Right G Large Intestine, Left H Cecum K Ascending Colon L Transverse Colon M Descending Colon N Sigmoid Colon P Rectum	7 Via Natural or Artificial Opening 8 Via Natural or Artificial Opening Endoscopic	D Intraluminal Device Z No Device	Z No Qualifier
Q Anus	0 Open 3 Percutaneous 4 Percutaneous Endoscopic X External	C Extraluminal Device D Intraluminal Device Z No Device	Z No Qualifier
Q Anus	7 Via Natural or Artificial Opening 8 Via Natural or Artificial Opening Endoscopic	D Intraluminal Device Z No Device	Z No Qualifier

Section	0	Medical and Surgical
Body System	D	Gastrointestinal System
Operation	W	Revision: Correcting, to the extent possible, a portion of a malfunctioning device or the position of a displaced device

Body Part (4ᵗʰ)	Approach (5ᵗʰ)	Device (6ᵗʰ)	Qualifier (7ᵗʰ)
0 Upper Intestinal Tract D Lower Intestinal Tract	0 Open 3 Percutaneous 4 Percutaneous Endoscopic 7 Via Natural or Artificial Opening 8 Via Natural or Artificial Opening Endoscopic X External	0 Drainage Device 2 Monitoring Device 3 Infusion Device 7 Autologous Tissue Substitute C Extraluminal Device D Intraluminal Device J Synthetic Substitute K Nonautologous Tissue Substitute U Feeding Device	Z No Qualifier
5 Esophagus	7 Via Natural or Artificial Opening 8 Via Natural or Artificial Opening Endoscopic X External	D Intraluminal Device	Z No Qualifier
6 Stomach	0 Open 3 Percutaneous 4 Percutaneous Endoscopic	0 Drainage Device 2 Monitoring Device 3 Infusion Device 7 Autologous Tissue Substitute C Extraluminal Device D Intraluminal Device J Synthetic Substitute K Nonautologous Tissue Substitute M Stimulator Lead U Feeding Device	Z No Qualifier

Continued →

Section   **0**   **Medical and Surgical**
Body System   **D**   **Gastrointestinal System**
Operation   **W**   **Revision:** Correcting, to the extent possible, a portion of a malfunctioning device or the position of a displaced device

Body Part (4th)	Approach (5th)	Device (6th)	Qualifier (7th)
6 Stomach	7 Via Natural or Artificial Opening 8 Via Natural or Artificial Opening Endoscopic X External	0 Drainage Device 2 Monitoring Device 3 Infusion Device 7 Autologous Tissue Substitute C Extraluminal Device D Intraluminal Device J Synthetic Substitute K Nonautologous Tissue Substitute U Feeding Device	Z No Qualifier
8 Small Intestine E Large Intestine	0 Open 4 Percutaneous Endoscopic 7 Via Natural or Artificial Opening 8 Via Natural or Artificial Opening Endoscopic	7 Autologous Tissue Substitute J Synthetic Substitute K Nonautologous Tissue Substitute	Z No Qualifier
Q Anus	0 Open 3 Percutaneous 4 Percutaneous Endoscopic 7 Via Natural or Artificial Opening 8 Via Natural or Artificial Opening Endoscopic	L Artificial Sphincter	Z No Qualifier
R Anal Sphincter	0 Open 3 Percutaneous 4 Percutaneous Endoscopic	M Stimulator Lead	Z No Qualifier
U Omentum V Mesentery W Peritoneum	0 Open 3 Percutaneous 4 Percutaneous Endoscopic	0 Drainage Device 7 Autologous Tissue Substitute J Synthetic Substitute K Nonautologous Tissue Substitute	Z No Qualifier

Section   **0**   **Medical and Surgical**
Body System   **D**   **Gastrointestinal System**
Operation   **X**   **Transfer:** Moving, without taking out, all or a portion of a body part to another location to take over the function of all or a portion of a body part

Body Part (4th)	Approach (5th)	Device (6th)	Qualifier (7th)
6 Stomach 8 Small Intestine E Large Intestine	0 Open 4 Percutaneous Endoscopic	Z No Device	5 Esophagus

Section   **0**   **Medical and Surgical**
Body System   **D**   **Gastrointestinal System**
Operation   **Y**   **Transplantation:** Putting in or on all or a portion of a living body part taken from another individual or animal to physically take the place and/or function of all or a portion of a similar body part

Body Part (4th)	Approach (5th)	Device (6th)	Qualifier (7th)
5 Esophagus 6 Stomach 8 Small Intestine E Large Intestine	0 Open	Z No Device	0 Allogeneic 1 Syngeneic 2 Zooplastic

iew Coding Guideline B4.8

1 – Gastrointestinal System, Bypass

iew Coding Guideline B3.6a

1074	Bypass Upper Esophagus to Cutaneous with Autologous Tissue Substitute, Open Approach	0D114J4	Bypass Upper Esophagus to Cutaneous with Synthetic Substitute, Percutaneous Endoscopic Approach	0D118K4	Bypass Upper Esophagus to Cutaneous with Nonautologous Tissue Substitute, Via Natural or Artificial Opening Endoscopic
1076	Bypass Upper Esophagus to Stomach with Autologous Tissue Substitute, Open Approach	0D114J6	Bypass Upper Esophagus to Stomach with Synthetic Substitute, Percutaneous Endoscopic Approach	0D118K6	Bypass Upper Esophagus to Stomach with Nonautologous Tissue Substitute, Via Natural or Artificial Opening Endoscopic
1079	Bypass Upper Esophagus to Duodenum with Autologous Tissue Substitute, Open Approach	0D114J9	Bypass Upper Esophagus to Duodenum with Synthetic Substitute, Percutaneous Endoscopic Approach	0D118K9	Bypass Upper Esophagus to Duodenum with Nonautologous Tissue Substitute, Via Natural or Artificial Opening Endoscopic
107A	Bypass Upper Esophagus to Jejunum with Autologous Tissue Substitute, Open Approach	0D114JA	Bypass Upper Esophagus to Jejunum with Synthetic Substitute, Percutaneous Endoscopic Approach	0D118KA	Bypass Upper Esophagus to Jejunum with Nonautologous Tissue Substitute, Via Natural or Artificial Opening Endoscopic
107B	Bypass Upper Esophagus to Ileum with Autologous Tissue Substitute, Open Approach	0D114JB	Bypass Upper Esophagus to Ileum with Synthetic Substitute, Percutaneous Endoscopic Approach	0D118KB	Bypass Upper Esophagus to Ileum with Nonautologous Tissue Substitute, Via Natural or Artificial Opening Endoscopic
110J4	Bypass Upper Esophagus to Cutaneous with Synthetic Substitute, Open Approach	0D114K4	Bypass Upper Esophagus to Cutaneous with Nonautologous Tissue Substitute, Percutaneous Endoscopic Approach	0D118Z4	Bypass Upper Esophagus to Cutaneous, Via Natural or Artificial Opening Endoscopic
110J6	Bypass Upper Esophagus to Stomach with Synthetic Substitute, Open Approach	0D114K6	Bypass Upper Esophagus to Stomach with Nonautologous Tissue Substitute, Percutaneous Endoscopic Approach	0D118Z6	Bypass Upper Esophagus to Stomach, Via Natural or Artificial Opening Endoscopic
110J9	Bypass Upper Esophagus to Duodenum with Synthetic Substitute, Open Approach	0D114K9	Bypass Upper Esophagus to Duodenum with Nonautologous Tissue Substitute, Percutaneous Endoscopic Approach	0D118Z9	Bypass Upper Esophagus to Duodenum, Via Natural or Artificial Opening Endoscopic
110JA	Bypass Upper Esophagus to Jejunum with Synthetic Substitute, Open Approach	0D114KA	Bypass Upper Esophagus to Jejunum with Nonautologous Tissue Substitute, Percutaneous Endoscopic Approach	0D118ZA	Bypass Upper Esophagus to Jejunum, Via Natural or Artificial Opening Endoscopic
110JB	Bypass Upper Esophagus to Ileum with Synthetic Substitute, Open Approach	0D114KB	Bypass Upper Esophagus to Ileum with Nonautologous Tissue Substitute, Percutaneous Endoscopic Approach	0D118ZB	Bypass Upper Esophagus to Ileum, Via Natural or Artificial Opening Endoscopic
110K4	Bypass Upper Esophagus to Cutaneous with Nonautologous Tissue Substitute, Open Approach	0D114Z4	Bypass Upper Esophagus to Cutaneous, Percutaneous Endoscopic Approach	0D12074	Bypass Middle Esophagus to Cutaneous with Autologous Tissue Substitute, Open Approach
110K6	Bypass Upper Esophagus to Stomach with Nonautologous Tissue Substitute, Open Approach	0D114Z6	Bypass Upper Esophagus to Stomach, Percutaneous Endoscopic Approach	0D12076	Bypass Middle Esophagus to Stomach with Autologous Tissue Substitute, Open Approach
110K9	Bypass Upper Esophagus to Duodenum with Nonautologous Tissue Substitute, Open Approach	0D114Z9	Bypass Upper Esophagus to Duodenum, Percutaneous Endoscopic Approach	0D12079	Bypass Middle Esophagus to Duodenum with Autologous Tissue Substitute, Open Approach
110KA	Bypass Upper Esophagus to Jejunum with Nonautologous Tissue Substitute, Open Approach	0D114ZA	Bypass Upper Esophagus to Jejunum, Percutaneous Endoscopic Approach	0D1207A	Bypass Middle Esophagus to Jejunum with Autologous Tissue Substitute, Open Approach
110KB	Bypass Upper Esophagus to Ileum with Nonautologous Tissue Substitute, Open Approach	0D114ZB	Bypass Upper Esophagus to Ileum, Percutaneous Endoscopic Approach	0D1207B	Bypass Middle Esophagus to Ileum with Autologous Tissue Substitute, Open Approach
110Z4	Bypass Upper Esophagus to Cutaneous, Open Approach	0D11874	Bypass Upper Esophagus to Cutaneous with Autologous Tissue Substitute, Via Natural or Artificial Opening Endoscopic	0D120J4	Bypass Middle Esophagus to Cutaneous with Synthetic Substitute, Open Approach
110Z6	Bypass Upper Esophagus to Stomach, Open Approach	0D11876	Bypass Upper Esophagus to Stomach with Autologous Tissue Substitute, Via Natural or Artificial Opening Endoscopic	0D120J6	Bypass Middle Esophagus to Stomach with Synthetic Substitute, Open Approach
110Z9	Bypass Upper Esophagus to Duodenum, Open Approach	0D11879	Bypass Upper Esophagus to Duodenum with Autologous Tissue Substitute, Via Natural or Artificial Opening Endoscopic	0D120J9	Bypass Middle Esophagus to Duodenum with Synthetic Substitute, Open Approach
110ZA	Bypass Upper Esophagus to Jejunum, Open Approach	0D1187A	Bypass Upper Esophagus to Jejunum with Autologous Tissue Substitute, Via Natural or Artificial Opening Endoscopic	0D120JA	Bypass Middle Esophagus to Jejunum with Synthetic Substitute, Open Approach
110ZB	Bypass Upper Esophagus to Ileum, Open Approach	0D1187B	Bypass Upper Esophagus to Ileum with Autologous Tissue Substitute, Via Natural or Artificial Opening Endoscopic	0D120JB	Bypass Middle Esophagus to Ileum with Synthetic Substitute, Open Approach
113J4	Bypass Upper Esophagus to Cutaneous with Synthetic Substitute, Percutaneous Approach	0D118J4	Bypass Upper Esophagus to Cutaneous with Synthetic Substitute, Via Natural or Artificial Opening Endoscopic	0D120K4	Bypass Middle Esophagus to Cutaneous with Nonautologous Tissue Substitute, Open Approach
11474	Bypass Upper Esophagus to Cutaneous with Autologous Tissue Substitute, Percutaneous Endoscopic Approach	0D118J6	Bypass Upper Esophagus to Stomach with Synthetic Substitute, Via Natural or Artificial Opening Endoscopic	0D120K6	Bypass Middle Esophagus to Stomach with Nonautologous Tissue Substitute, Open Approach
11476	Bypass Upper Esophagus to Stomach with Autologous Tissue Substitute, Percutaneous Endoscopic Approach	0D118J9	Bypass Upper Esophagus to Duodenum with Synthetic Substitute, Via Natural or Artificial Opening Endoscopic	0D120K9	Bypass Middle Esophagus to Duodenum with Nonautologous Tissue Substitute, Open Approach
11479	Bypass Upper Esophagus to Duodenum with Autologous Tissue Substitute, Percutaneous Endoscopic Approach	0D118JA	Bypass Upper Esophagus to Jejunum with Synthetic Substitute, Via Natural or Artificial Opening Endoscopic	0D120KA	Bypass Middle Esophagus to Jejunum with Nonautologous Tissue Substitute, Open Approach
1147A	Bypass Upper Esophagus to Jejunum with Autologous Tissue Substitute, Percutaneous Endoscopic Approach	0D118JB	Bypass Upper Esophagus to Ileum with Synthetic Substitute, Via Natural or Artificial Opening Endoscopic	0D120KB	Bypass Middle Esophagus to Ileum with Nonautologous Tissue Substitute, Open Approach
1147B	Bypass Upper Esophagus to Ileum with Autologous Tissue Substitute, Percutaneous Endoscopic Approach			0D120Z4	Bypass Middle Esophagus to Cutaneous, Open Approach

Female-only	♂ Male-only	▲ Limited Coverage	● Non-OR	▨ HAC-associated procedure	▲ Non-covered procedures	✛ Combination

0D120Z6 Bypass Middle Esophagus to Stomach, Open Approach

0D120Z9 Bypass Middle Esophagus to Duodenum, Open Approach

0D120ZA Bypass Middle Esophagus to Jejunum, Open Approach

0D120ZB Bypass Middle Esophagus to Ileum, Open Approach

0D123J4 Bypass Middle Esophagus to Cutaneous with Synthetic Substitute, Percutaneous Approach

0D12474 Bypass Middle Esophagus to Cutaneous with Autologous Tissue Substitute, Percutaneous Endoscopic Approach

0D12476 Bypass Middle Esophagus to Stomach with Autologous Tissue Substitute, Percutaneous Endoscopic Approach

0D12479 Bypass Middle Esophagus to Duodenum with Autologous Tissue Substitute, Percutaneous Endoscopic Approach

0D1247A Bypass Middle Esophagus to Jejunum with Autologous Tissue Substitute, Percutaneous Endoscopic Approach

0D1247B Bypass Middle Esophagus to Ileum with Autologous Tissue Substitute, Percutaneous Endoscopic Approach

0D124J4 Bypass Middle Esophagus to Cutaneous with Synthetic Substitute, Percutaneous Endoscopic Approach

0D124J6 Bypass Middle Esophagus to Stomach with Synthetic Substitute, Percutaneous Endoscopic Approach

0D124J9 Bypass Middle Esophagus to Duodenum with Synthetic Substitute, Percutaneous Endoscopic Approach

0D124JA Bypass Middle Esophagus to Jejunum with Synthetic Substitute, Percutaneous Endoscopic Approach

0D124JB Bypass Middle Esophagus to Ileum with Synthetic Substitute, Percutaneous Endoscopic Approach

0D124K4 Bypass Middle Esophagus to Cutaneous with Nonautologous Tissue Substitute, Percutaneous Endoscopic Approach

0D124K6 Bypass Middle Esophagus to Stomach with Nonautologous Tissue Substitute, Percutaneous Endoscopic Approach

0D124K9 Bypass Middle Esophagus to Duodenum with Nonautologous Tissue Substitute, Percutaneous Endoscopic Approach

0D124KA Bypass Middle Esophagus to Jejunum with Nonautologous Tissue Substitute, Percutaneous Endoscopic Approach

0D124KB Bypass Middle Esophagus to Ileum with Nonautologous Tissue Substitute, Percutaneous Endoscopic Approach

0D124Z4 Bypass Middle Esophagus to Cutaneous, Percutaneous Endoscopic Approach

0D124Z6 Bypass Middle Esophagus to Stomach, Percutaneous Endoscopic Approach

0D124Z9 Bypass Middle Esophagus to Duodenum, Percutaneous Endoscopic Approach

0D124ZA Bypass Middle Esophagus to Jejunum, Percutaneous Endoscopic Approach

0D124ZB Bypass Middle Esophagus to Ileum, Percutaneous Endoscopic Approach

0D12874 Bypass Middle Esophagus to Cutaneous with Autologous Tissue Substitute, Via Natural or Artificial Opening Endoscopic

0D12876 Bypass Middle Esophagus to Stomach with Autologous Tissue Substitute, Via Natural or Artificial Opening Endoscopic

0D12879 Bypass Middle Esophagus to Duodenum with Autologous Tissue Substitute, Via Natural or Artificial Opening Endoscopic

0D1287A Bypass Middle Esophagus to Jejunum with Autologous Tissue Substitute, Via Natural or Artificial Opening Endoscopic

0D1287B Bypass Middle Esophagus to Ileum with Autologous Tissue Substitute, Via Natural or Artificial Opening Endoscopic

0D128J4 Bypass Middle Esophagus to Cutaneous with Synthetic Substitute, Via Natural or Artificial Opening Endoscopic

0D128J6 Bypass Middle Esophagus to Stomach with Synthetic Substitute, Via Natural or Artificial Opening Endoscopic

0D128J9 Bypass Middle Esophagus to Duodenum with Synthetic Substitute, Via Natural or Artificial Opening Endoscopic

0D128JA Bypass Middle Esophagus to Jejunum with Synthetic Substitute, Via Natural or Artificial Opening Endoscopic

0D128JB Bypass Middle Esophagus to Ileum with Synthetic Substitute, Via Natural or Artificial Opening Endoscopic

0D128K4 Bypass Middle Esophagus to Cutaneous with Nonautologous Tissue Substitute, Via Natural or Artificial Opening Endoscopic

0D128K6 Bypass Middle Esophagus to Stomach with Nonautologous Tissue Substitute, Via Natural or Artificial Opening Endoscopic

0D128K9 Bypass Middle Esophagus to Duodenum with Nonautologous Tissue Substitute, Via Natural or Artificial Opening Endoscopic

0D128KA Bypass Middle Esophagus to Jejunum with Nonautologous Tissue Substitute, Via Natural or Artificial Opening Endoscopic

0D128KB Bypass Middle Esophagus to Ileum with Nonautologous Tissue Substitute, Via Natural or Artificial Opening Endoscopic

0D128Z4 Bypass Middle Esophagus to Cutaneous, Via Natural or Artificial Opening Endoscopic

0D128Z6 Bypass Middle Esophagus to Stomach, Via Natural or Artificial Opening Endoscopic

0D128Z9 Bypass Middle Esophagus to Duodenum, Via Natural or Artificial Opening Endoscopic

0D128ZA Bypass Middle Esophagus to Jejunum, Via Natural or Artificial Opening Endoscopic

0D128ZB Bypass Middle Esophagus to Ileum, Via Natural or Artificial Opening Endoscopic

0D13074 Bypass Lower Esophagus to Cutaneous with Autologous Tissue Substitute, Open Approach

0D13076 Bypass Lower Esophagus to Stomach with Autologous Tissue Substitute, Open Approach

0D13079 Bypass Lower Esophagus to Duodenum with Autologous Tissue Substitute, Open Approach

0D1307A Bypass Lower Esophagus to Jejunum with Autologous Tissue Substitute, Open Approach

0D1307B Bypass Lower Esophagus to Ileum with Autologous Tissue Substitute, Open Approach

0D130J4 Bypass Lower Esophagus to Cutaneous with Synthetic Substitute, Open Approach

0D130J6 Bypass Lower Esophagus to Stomach with Synthetic Substitute, Open Approach

0D130J9 Bypass Lower Esophagus to Duodenum with Synthetic Substitute, Open Approach

0D130JA Bypass Lower Esophagus to Jejunum with Synthetic Substitute, Open Approach

0D130JB Bypass Lower Esophagus to Ileum with Synthetic Substitute, Open Approach

0D130K4 Bypass Lower Esophagus to Cutaneous with Nonautologous Tissue Substitute, Open Approach

0D130K6 Bypass Lower Esophagus to Stomach with Nonautologous Tissue Substitute, Open Approach

0D130K9 Bypass Lower Esophagus to Duodenum with Nonautologous Tissue Substitute, Open Approach

0D130KA Bypass Lower Esophagus to Jejunum with Nonautologous Tissue Substitute, Open Approach

0D130KB Bypass Lower Esophagus to Ileum with Nonautologous Tissue Substitute, Open Approach

0D130Z4 Bypass Lower Esophagus to Cutaneous, Open Approach

0D130Z6 Bypass Lower Esophagus to Stomach, Open Approach

0D130Z9 Bypass Lower Esophagus to Duodenum, Open Approach

0D130ZA Bypass Lower Esophagus to Jejunum, Open Approach

0D130ZB Bypass Lower Esophagus to Ileum, Open Approach

0D133J4 Bypass Lower Esophagus to Cutaneous with Synthetic Substitute, Percutaneous Approach

0D13474 Bypass Lower Esophagus to Cutaneous with Autologous Tissue Substitute, Percutaneous Endoscopic Approach

0D13476 Bypass Lower Esophagus to Stomach with Autologous Tissue Substitute, Percutaneous Endoscopic Approach

0D13479 Bypass Lower Esophagus to Duodenum with Autologous Tissue Substitute, Percutaneous Endoscopic Approach

0D1347A Bypass Lower Esophagus to Jejunum with Autologous Tissue Substitute, Percutaneous Endoscopic Approach

0D1347B Bypass Lower Esophagus to Ileum with Autologous Tissue Substitute, Percutaneous Endoscopic Approach

0D134J4 Bypass Lower Esophagus to Cutaneous with Synthetic Substitute, Percutaneous Endoscopic Approach

0D134J6 Bypass Lower Esophagus to Stomach with Synthetic Substitute, Percutaneous Endoscopic Approach

0D134J9 Bypass Lower Esophagus to Duodenum with Synthetic Substitute, Percutaneous Endoscopic Approach

0D134JA Bypass Lower Esophagus to Jejunum with Synthetic Substitute, Percutaneous Endoscopic Approach

0D134JB Bypass Lower Esophagus to Ileum with Synthetic Substitute, Percutaneous Endoscopic Approach

0D134K4 Bypass Lower Esophagus to Cutaneous with Nonautologous Tissue Substitute, Percutaneous Endoscopic Approach

0D134K6 Bypass Lower Esophagus to Stomach with Nonautologous Tissue Substitute, Percutaneous Endoscopic Approach

0D134K9 Bypass Lower Esophagus to Duodenum with Nonautologous Tissue Substitute, Percutaneous Endoscopic Approach

0D134KA Bypass Lower Esophagus to Jejunum with Nonautologous Tissue Substitute, Percutaneous Endoscopic Approach

0D134KB Bypass Lower Esophagus to Ileum with Nonautologous Tissue Substitute, Percutaneous Endoscopic Approach

0D134Z4 Bypass Lower Esophagus to Cutaneous, Percutaneous Endoscopic Approach

0D134Z6 Bypass Lower Esophagus to Stomach, Percutaneous Endoscopic Approach

0D134Z9 Bypass Lower Esophagus to Duodenum, Percutaneous Endoscopic Approach

0D134ZA Bypass Lower Esophagus to Jejunum, Percutaneous Endoscopic Approach

0D134ZB Bypass Lower Esophagus to Ileum, Percutaneous Endoscopic Approach

13874	Bypass Lower Esophagus to Cutaneous with Autologous Tissue Substitute, Via Natural or Artificial Opening Endoscopic
13876	Bypass Lower Esophagus to Stomach with Autologous Tissue Substitute, Via Natural or Artificial Opening Endoscopic
13879	Bypass Lower Esophagus to Duodenum with Autologous Tissue Substitute, Via Natural or Artificial Opening Endoscopic
1387A	Bypass Lower Esophagus to Jejunum with Autologous Tissue Substitute, Via Natural or Artificial Opening Endoscopic
1387B	Bypass Lower Esophagus to Ileum with Autologous Tissue Substitute, Via Natural or Artificial Opening Endoscopic
138J4	Bypass Lower Esophagus to Cutaneous with Synthetic Substitute, Via Natural or Artificial Opening Endoscopic
138J6	Bypass Lower Esophagus to Stomach with Synthetic Substitute, Via Natural or Artificial Opening Endoscopic
138J9	Bypass Lower Esophagus to Duodenum with Synthetic Substitute, Via Natural or Artificial Opening Endoscopic
138JA	Bypass Lower Esophagus to Jejunum with Synthetic Substitute, Via Natural or Artificial Opening Endoscopic
138JB	Bypass Lower Esophagus to Ileum with Synthetic Substitute, Via Natural or Artificial Opening Endoscopic
138K4	Bypass Lower Esophagus to Cutaneous with Nonautologous Tissue Substitute, Via Natural or Artificial Opening Endoscopic
138K6	Bypass Lower Esophagus to Stomach with Nonautologous Tissue Substitute, Via Natural or Artificial Opening Endoscopic
138K9	Bypass Lower Esophagus to Duodenum with Nonautologous Tissue Substitute, Via Natural or Artificial Opening Endoscopic
138KA	Bypass Lower Esophagus to Jejunum with Nonautologous Tissue Substitute, Via Natural or Artificial Opening Endoscopic
138KB	Bypass Lower Esophagus to Ileum with Nonautologous Tissue Substitute, Via Natural or Artificial Opening Endoscopic
138Z4	Bypass Lower Esophagus to Cutaneous, Via Natural or Artificial Opening Endoscopic
138Z6	Bypass Lower Esophagus to Stomach, Via Natural or Artificial Opening Endoscopic
138Z9	Bypass Lower Esophagus to Duodenum, Via Natural or Artificial Opening Endoscopic
D138ZA	Bypass Lower Esophagus to Jejunum, Via Natural or Artificial Opening Endoscopic
D138ZB	Bypass Lower Esophagus to Ileum, Via Natural or Artificial Opening Endoscopic
D15074	Bypass Esophagus to Cutaneous with Autologous Tissue Substitute, Open Approach
D15076	Bypass Esophagus to Stomach with Autologous Tissue Substitute, Open Approach
D15079	Bypass Esophagus to Duodenum with Autologous Tissue Substitute, Open Approach
D1507A	Bypass Esophagus to Jejunum with Autologous Tissue Substitute, Open Approach
D1507B	Bypass Esophagus to Ileum with Autologous Tissue Substitute, Open Approach
D150J4	Bypass Esophagus to Cutaneous with Synthetic Substitute, Open Approach
D150J6	Bypass Esophagus to Stomach with Synthetic Substitute, Open Approach
0D150J9	Bypass Esophagus to Duodenum with Synthetic Substitute, Open Approach
0D150JA	Bypass Esophagus to Jejunum with Synthetic Substitute, Open Approach
0D150JB	Bypass Esophagus to Ileum with Synthetic Substitute, Open Approach
0D150K4	Bypass Esophagus to Cutaneous with Nonautologous Tissue Substitute, Open Approach
0D150K6	Bypass Esophagus to Stomach with Nonautologous Tissue Substitute, Open Approach
0D150K9	Bypass Esophagus to Duodenum with Nonautologous Tissue Substitute, Open Approach
0D150KA	Bypass Esophagus to Jejunum with Nonautologous Tissue Substitute, Open Approach
0D150KB	Bypass Esophagus to Ileum with Nonautologous Tissue Substitute, Open Approach
0D150Z4	Bypass Esophagus to Cutaneous, Open Approach
0D150Z6	Bypass Esophagus to Stomach, Open Approach
0D150Z9	Bypass Esophagus to Duodenum, Open Approach
0D150ZA	Bypass Esophagus to Jejunum, Open Approach
0D150ZB	Bypass Esophagus to Ileum, Open Approach
0D153J4	Bypass Esophagus to Cutaneous with Synthetic Substitute, Percutaneous Approach
0D15474	Bypass Esophagus to Cutaneous with Autologous Tissue Substitute, Percutaneous Endoscopic Approach
0D15476	Bypass Esophagus to Stomach with Autologous Tissue Substitute, Percutaneous Endoscopic Approach
0D15479	Bypass Esophagus to Duodenum with Autologous Tissue Substitute, Percutaneous Endoscopic Approach
0D1547A	Bypass Esophagus to Jejunum with Autologous Tissue Substitute, Percutaneous Endoscopic Approach
0D1547B	Bypass Esophagus to Ileum with Autologous Tissue Substitute, Percutaneous Endoscopic Approach
0D154J4	Bypass Esophagus to Cutaneous with Synthetic Substitute, Percutaneous Endoscopic Approach
0D154J6	Bypass Esophagus to Stomach with Synthetic Substitute, Percutaneous Endoscopic Approach
0D154J9	Bypass Esophagus to Duodenum with Synthetic Substitute, Percutaneous Endoscopic Approach
0D154JA	Bypass Esophagus to Jejunum with Synthetic Substitute, Percutaneous Endoscopic Approach
0D154JB	Bypass Esophagus to Ileum with Synthetic Substitute, Percutaneous Endoscopic Approach
0D154K4	Bypass Esophagus to Cutaneous with Nonautologous Tissue Substitute, Percutaneous Endoscopic Approach
0D154K6	Bypass Esophagus to Stomach with Nonautologous Tissue Substitute, Percutaneous Endoscopic Approach
0D154K9	Bypass Esophagus to Duodenum with Nonautologous Tissue Substitute, Percutaneous Endoscopic Approach
0D154KA	Bypass Esophagus to Jejunum with Nonautologous Tissue Substitute, Percutaneous Endoscopic Approach
0D154KB	Bypass Esophagus to Ileum with Nonautologous Tissue Substitute, Percutaneous Endoscopic Approach
0D154Z4	Bypass Esophagus to Cutaneous, Percutaneous Endoscopic Approach
0D154Z6	Bypass Esophagus to Stomach, Percutaneous Endoscopic Approach
0D154Z9	Bypass Esophagus to Duodenum, Percutaneous Endoscopic Approach
0D154ZA	Bypass Esophagus to Jejunum, Percutaneous Endoscopic Approach
0D154ZB	Bypass Esophagus to Ileum, Percutaneous Endoscopic Approach
0D15874	Bypass Esophagus to Cutaneous with Autologous Tissue Substitute, Via Natural or Artificial Opening Endoscopic
0D15876	Bypass Esophagus to Stomach with Autologous Tissue Substitute, Via Natural or Artificial Opening Endoscopic
0D15879	Bypass Esophagus to Duodenum with Autologous Tissue Substitute, Via Natural or Artificial Opening Endoscopic
0D1587A	Bypass Esophagus to Jejunum with Autologous Tissue Substitute, Via Natural or Artificial Opening Endoscopic
0D1587B	Bypass Esophagus to Ileum with Autologous Tissue Substitute, Via Natural or Artificial Opening Endoscopic
0D158J4	Bypass Esophagus to Cutaneous with Synthetic Substitute, Via Natural or Artificial Opening Endoscopic
0D158J6	Bypass Esophagus to Stomach with Synthetic Substitute, Via Natural or Artificial Opening Endoscopic
0D158J9	Bypass Esophagus to Duodenum with Synthetic Substitute, Via Natural or Artificial Opening Endoscopic
0D158JA	Bypass Esophagus to Jejunum with Synthetic Substitute, Via Natural or Artificial Opening Endoscopic
0D158JB	Bypass Esophagus to Ileum with Synthetic Substitute, Via Natural or Artificial Opening Endoscopic
0D158K4	Bypass Esophagus to Cutaneous with Nonautologous Tissue Substitute, Via Natural or Artificial Opening Endoscopic
0D158K6	Bypass Esophagus to Stomach with Nonautologous Tissue Substitute, Via Natural or Artificial Opening Endoscopic
0D158K9	Bypass Esophagus to Duodenum with Nonautologous Tissue Substitute, Via Natural or Artificial Opening Endoscopic
0D158KA	Bypass Esophagus to Jejunum with Nonautologous Tissue Substitute, Via Natural or Artificial Opening Endoscopic
0D158KB	Bypass Esophagus to Ileum with Nonautologous Tissue Substitute, Via Natural or Artificial Opening Endoscopic
0D158Z4	Bypass Esophagus to Cutaneous, Via Natural or Artificial Opening Endoscopic
0D158Z6	Bypass Esophagus to Stomach, Via Natural or Artificial Opening Endoscopic
0D158Z9	Bypass Esophagus to Duodenum, Via Natural or Artificial Opening Endoscopic
0D158ZA	Bypass Esophagus to Jejunum, Via Natural or Artificial Opening Endoscopic
0D158ZB	Bypass Esophagus to Ileum, Via Natural or Artificial Opening Endoscopic
0D16074	Bypass Stomach to Cutaneous with Autologous Tissue Substitute, Open Approach
0D16079	Bypass Stomach to Duodenum with Autologous Tissue Substitute, Open Approach
■■■	When reported with principal diagnosis code K66.01 and secondary diagnosis code K68.11, K95.01, K95.81 or T81.4XXA

♀ Female-only   ♂ Male-only   ▲ Limited Coverage   ● Non-OR   ■■■ HAC-associated procedure   ▲ Non-covered procedures   ✚ Combination

0D1607A Bypass Stomach to Jejunum with Autologous Tissue Substitute, Open Approach

0D1607B Bypass Stomach to Ileum with Autologous Tissue Substitute, Open Approach

When reported with principal diagnosis code K66.01 and secondary diagnosis code K68.11, K95.01, K95.81 or T81.4XXA

0D1607L Bypass Stomach to Transverse Colon with Autologous Tissue Substitute, Open Approach

When reported with principal diagnosis code K66.01 and secondary diagnosis code K68.11, K95.01, K95.81 or T81.4XXA

0D160J4 Bypass Stomach to Cutaneous with Synthetic Substitute, Open Approach

0D160J9 Bypass Stomach to Duodenum with Synthetic Substitute, Open Approach

When reported with principal diagnosis code K66.01 and secondary diagnosis code K68.11, K95.01, K95.81 or T81.4XXA

0D160JA Bypass Stomach to Jejunum with Synthetic Substitute, Open Approach

When reported with principal diagnosis code K66.01 and secondary diagnosis code K68.11, K95.01, K95.81 or T81.4XXA

0D160JB Bypass Stomach to Ileum with Synthetic Substitute, Open Approach

When reported with principal diagnosis code K66.01 and secondary diagnosis code K68.11, K95.01, K95.81 or T81.4XXA

0D160JL Bypass Stomach to Transverse Colon with Synthetic Substitute, Open Approach

When reported with principal diagnosis code K66.01 and secondary diagnosis code K68.11, K95.01, K95.81 or T81.4XXA

0D160K4 Bypass Stomach to Cutaneous with Nonautologous Tissue Substitute, Open Approach

0D160K9 Bypass Stomach to Duodenum with Nonautologous Tissue Substitute, Open Approach

When reported with principal diagnosis code K66.01 and secondary diagnosis code K68.11, K95.01, K95.81 or T81.4XXA

0D160KA Bypass Stomach to Jejunum with Nonautologous Tissue Substitute, Open Approach

When reported with principal diagnosis code K66.01 and secondary diagnosis code K68.11, K95.01, K95.81 or T81.4XXA

0D160KB Bypass Stomach to Ileum with Nonautologous Tissue Substitute, Open Approach

When reported with principal diagnosis code K66.01 and secondary diagnosis code K68.11, K95.01, K95.81 or T81.4XXA

0D160KL Bypass Stomach to Transverse Colon with Nonautologous Tissue Substitute, Open Approach

When reported with principal diagnosis code K66.01 and secondary diagnosis code K68.11, K95.01, K95.81 or T81.4XXA

0D160Z4 Bypass Stomach to Cutaneous, Open Approach

0D160Z9 Bypass Stomach to Duodenum, Open Approach

When reported with principal diagnosis code K66.01 and secondary diagnosis code K68.11, K95.81 or T81.4XXA

0D160ZA Bypass Stomach to Jejunum, Open Approach

When reported with principal diagnosis code K66.01 and secondary diagnosis code K68.11, K95.01, K95.81 or T81.4XXA

0D160ZB Bypass Stomach to Ileum, Open Approach

When reported with principal diagnosis code K66.01 and secondary diagnosis code K68.11, K95.01, K95.81 or T81.4XXA

0D160ZL Bypass Stomach to Transverse Colon, Open Approach

When reported with principal diagnosis code K66.01 and secondary diagnosis code K68.11, K95.01, K95.81 or T81.4XXA

0D163J4 Bypass Stomach to Cutaneous with Synthetic Substitute, Percutaneous Approach

0D16474 Bypass Stomach to Cutaneous with Autologous Tissue Substitute, Percutaneous Endoscopic Approach

0D16479 Bypass Stomach to Duodenum with Autologous Tissue Substitute, Percutaneous Endoscopic Approach

When reported with principal diagnosis code K66.01 and secondary diagnosis code K68.11, K95.01, K95.81 or T81.4XXA

0D1647A Bypass Stomach to Jejunum with Autologous Tissue Substitute, Percutaneous Endoscopic Approach

When reported with principal diagnosis code K66.01 and secondary diagnosis code K68.11, K95.01, K95.81 or T81.4XXA

0D1647B Bypass Stomach to Ileum with Autologous Tissue Substitute, Percutaneous Endoscopic Approach

When reported with principal diagnosis code K66.01 and secondary diagnosis code K68.11, K95.01, K95.81 or T81.4XXA

0D1647L Bypass Stomach to Transverse Colon with Autologous Tissue Substitute, Percutaneous Endoscopic Approach

When reported with principal diagnosis code K66.01 and secondary diagnosis code K68.11, K95.01, K95.81 or T81.4XXA

0D164J4 Bypass Stomach to Cutaneous with Synthetic Substitute, Percutaneous Endoscopic Approach

0D164J9 Bypass Stomach to Duodenum with Synthetic Substitute, Percutaneous Endoscopic Approach

When reported with principal diagnosis code K66.01 and secondary diagnosis code K68.11, K95.01, K95.81 or T81.4XXA

0D164JA Bypass Stomach to Jejunum with Synthetic Substitute, Percutaneous Endoscopic Approach

When reported with principal diagnosis code K66.01 and secondary diagnosis code K68.11, K95.01, K95.81 or T81.4XXA

0D164JB Bypass Stomach to Ileum with Synthetic Substitute, Percutaneous Endoscopic Approach

When reported with principal diagnosis code K66.01 and secondary diagnosis code K68.11, K95.01, K95.81 or T81.4XXA

0D164JL Bypass Stomach to Transverse Colon with Synthetic Substitute, Percutaneous Endoscopic Approach

When reported with principal diagnosis code K66.01 and secondary diagnosis code K68.11, K95.01, K95.81 or T81.4XXA

0D164K4 Bypass Stomach to Cutaneous with Nonautologous Tissue Substitute, Percutaneous Endoscopic Approach

0D164K9 Bypass Stomach to Duodenum with Nonautologous Tissue Substitute, Percutaneous Endoscopic Approach

When reported with principal diagnosis code K66.01 and secondary diagnosis code K68.11, K95.01, K95.81 or T81.4XXA

0D164KA Bypass Stomach to Jejunum with Nonautologous Tissue Substitute, Percutaneous Endoscopic Approach

When reported with principal diagnosis code K66.01 and secondary diagnosis code K68.11, K95.01, K95.81 or T81.4XXA

0D164KB Bypass Stomach to Ileum with Nonautologous Tissue Substitute, Percutaneous Endoscopic Approach

When reported with principal diagnosis code K66.01 and secondary diagnosis code K68.11, K95.01, K95.81 or T81.4XXA

0D164KL Bypass Stomach to Transverse Colon with Nonautologous Tissue Substitute, Percutaneous Endoscopic Approach

When reported with principal diagnosis code K66.01 and secondary diagnosis code K68.11, K95.01, K95.81 or T81.4XXA

0D164Z4 Bypass Stomach to Cutaneous, Percutaneous Endoscopic Approach

0D164Z9 Bypass Stomach to Duodenum, Percutaneous Endoscopic Approach

When reported with principal diagnosis code K66.01 and secondary diagnosis code K68.11, K95.01, K95.81 or T81.4XXA

0D164ZA Bypass Stomach to Jejunum, Percutaneous Endoscopic Approach

When reported with principal diagnosis code K66.01 and secondary diagnosis code K68.11, K95.01, K95.81 or T81.4XXA

0D164ZB Bypass Stomach to Ileum, Percutaneous Endoscopic Approach

When reported with principal diagnosis code K66.01 and secondary diagnosis code K68.11, K95.01, K95.81 or T81.4XXA

0D164ZL Bypass Stomach to Transverse Colon, Percutaneous Endoscopic Approach

0D16874 Bypass Stomach to Cutaneous with Autologous Tissue Substitute, Via Natural or Artificial Opening Endoscopic

0D16879 Bypass Stomach to Duodenum with Autologous Tissue Substitute, Via Natural or Artificial Opening Endoscopic

When reported with principal diagnosis code K66.01 and secondary diagnosis code K68.11, K95.01, K95.81 or T81.4XXA

♀ Female-only   ♂ Male-only   ▲ Limited Coverage   ● Non-OR   ▪ HAC-associated procedure   ▲ Non-covered procedures   ✚ Combination

687A Bypass Stomach to Jejunum with Autologous Tissue Substitute, Via Natural or Artificial Opening Endoscopic

When reported with principal diagnosis code K68.11, K95.01, K95.81 or T81.4XXA

687B Bypass Stomach to Ileum with Autologous Tissue Substitute, Via Natural or Artificial Opening Endoscopic

When reported with principal diagnosis code K66.01 and secondary diagnosis code K68.11, K95.01, K95.81 or T81.4XXA

687L Bypass Stomach to Transverse Colon with Autologous Tissue Substitute, Via Natural or Artificial Opening Endoscopic

When reported with principal diagnosis code K66.01 and secondary diagnosis code K68.11, K95.01, K95.81 or T81.4XXA

168J4 Bypass Stomach to Cutaneous with Synthetic Substitute, Via Natural or Artificial Opening Endoscopic

168J9 Bypass Stomach to Duodenum with Synthetic Substitute, Via Natural or Artificial Opening Endoscopic

When reported with principal diagnosis code K66.01 and secondary diagnosis code K68.11, K95.01, K95.81 or T81.4XXA

168JA Bypass Stomach to Jejunum with Synthetic Substitute, Via Natural or Artificial Opening Endoscopic

When reported with principal diagnosis code K66.01 and secondary diagnosis code K68.11, K95.01, K95.81 or T81.4XXA

168JB Bypass Stomach to Ileum with Synthetic Substitute, Via Natural or Artificial Opening Endoscopic

When reported with principal diagnosis code K66.01 and secondary diagnosis code K68.11, K95.01, K95.81 or T81.4XXA

168JL Bypass Stomach to Transverse Colon with Synthetic Substitute, Via Natural or Artificial Opening Endoscopic

When reported with principal diagnosis code K66.01 and secondary diagnosis code K68.11, K95.01, K95.81 or T81.4XXA

168K4 Bypass Stomach to Cutaneous with Nonautologous Tissue Substitute, Via Natural or Artificial Opening Endoscopic

168K9 Bypass Stomach to Duodenum with Nonautologous Tissue Substitute, Via Natural or Artificial Opening Endoscopic

When reported with principal diagnosis code K66.01 and secondary diagnosis code K68.11, K95.01, K95.81 or T81.4XXA

0168KA Bypass Stomach to Jejunum with Nonautologous Tissue Substitute, Via Natural or Artificial Opening Endoscopic

When reported with principal diagnosis code K66.01 and secondary diagnosis code K68.11, K95.01, K95.81 or T81.4XXA

0168KB Bypass Stomach to Ileum with Nonautologous Tissue Substitute, Via Natural or Artificial Opening Endoscopic

0168KL Bypass Stomach to Transverse Colon with Nonautologous Tissue Substitute, Via Natural or Artificial Opening Endoscopic

When reported with principal diagnosis code K66.01 and secondary diagnosis code K68.11, K95.01, K95.81 or T81.4XXA

0D168Z4 Bypass Stomach to Cutaneous, Via Natural or Artificial Opening Endoscopic

0D168Z9 Bypass Stomach to Duodenum, Via Natural or Artificial Opening Endoscopic

When reported with principal diagnosis code K66.01 and secondary diagnosis code K68.11, K95.01, K95.81 or T81.4XXA

0D168ZA Bypass Stomach to Jejunum, Via Natural or Artificial Opening Endoscopic

When reported with principal diagnosis code K66.01 and secondary diagnosis code K68.11, K95.01, K95.81 or T81.4XXA

0D168ZB Bypass Stomach to Ileum, Via Natural or Artificial Opening Endoscopic

When reported with principal diagnosis code K66.01 and secondary diagnosis code K68.11, K95.01, K95.81 or T81.4XXA

0D168ZL Bypass Stomach to Transverse Colon, Via Natural or Artificial Opening Endoscopic

When reported with principal diagnosis code K66.01 and secondary diagnosis code K68.11, K95.01, K95.81 or T81.4XXA

0D19074 Bypass Duodenum to Cutaneous with Autologous Tissue Substitute, Open Approach

0D19079 Bypass Duodenum to Duodenum with Autologous Tissue Substitute, Open Approach

0D1907A Bypass Duodenum to Jejunum with Autologous Tissue Substitute, Open Approach

0D1907B Bypass Duodenum to Ileum with Autologous Tissue Substitute, Open Approach

0D1907L Bypass Duodenum to Transverse Colon with Autologous Tissue Substitute, Open Approach

0D190J4 Bypass Duodenum to Cutaneous with Synthetic Substitute, Open Approach

0D190J9 Bypass Duodenum to Duodenum with Synthetic Substitute, Open Approach

0D190JA Bypass Duodenum to Jejunum with Synthetic Substitute, Open Approach

0D190JB Bypass Duodenum to Ileum with Synthetic Substitute, Open Approach

0D190JL Bypass Duodenum to Transverse Colon with Synthetic Substitute, Open Approach

0D190K4 Bypass Duodenum to Cutaneous with Nonautologous Tissue Substitute, Open Approach

0D190K9 Bypass Duodenum to Duodenum with Nonautologous Tissue Substitute, Open Approach

0D190KA Bypass Duodenum to Jejunum with Nonautologous Tissue Substitute, Open Approach

0D190KB Bypass Duodenum to Ileum with Nonautologous Tissue Substitute, Open Approach

0D190KL Bypass Duodenum to Transverse Colon with Nonautologous Tissue Substitute, Open Approach

0D190Z4 Bypass Duodenum to Cutaneous, Open Approach

0D190Z9 Bypass Duodenum to Duodenum, Open Approach

0D190ZA Bypass Duodenum to Jejunum, Open Approach

0D190ZB Bypass Duodenum to Ileum, Open Approach

0D190ZL Bypass Duodenum to Transverse Colon, Open Approach

0D193J4 Bypass Duodenum to Cutaneous with Synthetic Substitute, Percutaneous Approach

0D19474 Bypass Duodenum to Cutaneous with Autologous Tissue Substitute, Percutaneous Endoscopic Approach

0D19479 Bypass Duodenum to Duodenum with Autologous Tissue Substitute, Percutaneous Endoscopic Approach

0D1947A Bypass Duodenum to Jejunum with Autologous Tissue Substitute, Percutaneous Endoscopic Approach

0D1947B Bypass Duodenum to Ileum with Autologous Tissue Substitute, Percutaneous Endoscopic Approach

0D1947L Bypass Duodenum to Transverse Colon with Autologous Tissue Substitute, Percutaneous Endoscopic Approach

0D194J4 Bypass Duodenum to Cutaneous with Synthetic Substitute, Percutaneous Endoscopic Approach

0D194J9 Bypass Duodenum to Duodenum with Synthetic Substitute, Percutaneous Endoscopic Approach

0D194JA Bypass Duodenum to Jejunum with Synthetic Substitute, Percutaneous Endoscopic Approach

0D194JB Bypass Duodenum to Ileum with Synthetic Substitute, Percutaneous Endoscopic Approach

0D194JL Bypass Duodenum to Transverse Colon with Synthetic Substitute, Percutaneous Endoscopic Approach

0D194K4 Bypass Duodenum to Cutaneous with Nonautologous Tissue Substitute, Percutaneous Endoscopic Approach

0D194K9 Bypass Duodenum to Duodenum with Nonautologous Tissue Substitute, Percutaneous Endoscopic Approach

0D194KA Bypass Duodenum to Jejunum with Nonautologous Tissue Substitute, Percutaneous Endoscopic Approach

0D194KB Bypass Duodenum to Ileum with Nonautologous Tissue Substitute, Percutaneous Endoscopic Approach

0D194KL Bypass Duodenum to Transverse Colon with Nonautologous Tissue Substitute, Percutaneous Endoscopic Approach

0D194Z4 Bypass Duodenum to Cutaneous, Percutaneous Endoscopic Approach

0D194Z9 Bypass Duodenum to Duodenum, Percutaneous Endoscopic Approach

0D194ZA Bypass Duodenum to Jejunum, Percutaneous Endoscopic Approach

0D194ZB Bypass Duodenum to Ileum, Percutaneous Endoscopic Approach

0D194ZL Bypass Duodenum to Transverse Colon, Percutaneous Endoscopic Approach

0D19874 Bypass Duodenum to Cutaneous with Autologous Tissue Substitute, Via Natural or Artificial Opening Endoscopic

0D19879 Bypass Duodenum to Duodenum with Autologous Tissue Substitute, Via Natural or Artificial Opening Endoscopic

0D1987A Bypass Duodenum to Jejunum with Autologous Tissue Substitute, Via Natural or Artificial Opening Endoscopic

0D1987B Bypass Duodenum to Ileum with Autologous Tissue Substitute, Via Natural or Artificial Opening Endoscopic

0D1987L Bypass Duodenum to Transverse Colon with Autologous Tissue Substitute, Via Natural or Artificial Opening Endoscopic

0D198J4 Bypass Duodenum to Cutaneous with Synthetic Substitute, Via Natural or Artificial Opening Endoscopic

541

Female-only ♂ Male-only ▲ Limited Coverage ● Non-OR ▓ HAC-associated procedure ▲ Non-covered procedures ✚ Combination

0D198J9 Bypass Duodenum to Duodenum with Synthetic Substitute, Via Natural or Artificial Opening Endoscopic

0D198JA Bypass Duodenum to Jejunum with Synthetic Substitute, Via Natural or Artificial Opening Endoscopic

0D198JB Bypass Duodenum to Ileum with Synthetic Substitute, Via Natural or Artificial Opening Endoscopic

0D198JL Bypass Duodenum to Transverse Colon with Synthetic Substitute, Via Natural or Artificial Opening Endoscopic

0D198K4 Bypass Duodenum to Cutaneous with Nonautologous Tissue Substitute, Via Natural or Artificial Opening Endoscopic

0D198K9 Bypass Duodenum to Duodenum with Nonautologous Tissue Substitute, Via Natural or Artificial Opening Endoscopic

0D198KA Bypass Duodenum to Jejunum with Nonautologous Tissue Substitute, Via Natural or Artificial Opening Endoscopic

0D198KB Bypass Duodenum to Ileum with Nonautologous Tissue Substitute, Via Natural or Artificial Opening Endoscopic

0D198KL Bypass Duodenum to Transverse Colon with Nonautologous Tissue Substitute, Via Natural or Artificial Opening Endoscopic

0D198Z4 Bypass Duodenum to Cutaneous, Via Natural or Artificial Opening Endoscopic

0D198Z9 Bypass Duodenum to Duodenum, Via Natural or Artificial Opening Endoscopic

0D198ZA Bypass Duodenum to Jejunum, Via Natural or Artificial Opening Endoscopic

0D198ZB Bypass Duodenum to Ileum, Via Natural or Artificial Opening Endoscopic

0D198ZL Bypass Duodenum to Transverse Colon, Via Natural or Artificial Opening Endoscopic

0D1A074 Bypass Jejunum to Cutaneous with Autologous Tissue Substitute, Open Approach

0D1A07A Bypass Jejunum to Jejunum with Autologous Tissue Substitute, Open Approach

0D1A07B Bypass Jejunum to Ileum with Autologous Tissue Substitute, Open Approach

0D1A07H Bypass Jejunum to Cecum with Autologous Tissue Substitute, Open Approach

0D1A07K Bypass Jejunum to Ascending Colon with Autologous Tissue Substitute, Open Approach

0D1A07L Bypass Jejunum to Transverse Colon with Autologous Tissue Substitute, Open Approach

0D1A07M Bypass Jejunum to Descending Colon with Autologous Tissue Substitute, Open Approach

0D1A07N Bypass Jejunum to Sigmoid Colon with Autologous Tissue Substitute, Open Approach

0D1A07P Bypass Jejunum to Rectum with Autologous Tissue Substitute, Open Approach

0D1A07Q Bypass Jejunum to Anus with Autologous Tissue Substitute, Open Approach

0D1A0J4 Bypass Jejunum to Cutaneous with Synthetic Substitute, Open Approach

0D1A0JA Bypass Jejunum to Jejunum with Synthetic Substitute, Open Approach

0D1A0JB Bypass Jejunum to Ileum with Synthetic Substitute, Open Approach

0D1A0JH Bypass Jejunum to Cecum with Synthetic Substitute, Open Approach

0D1A0JK Bypass Jejunum to Ascending Colon with Synthetic Substitute, Open Approach

0D1A0JL Bypass Jejunum to Transverse Colon with Synthetic Substitute, Open Approach

0D1A0JM Bypass Jejunum to Descending Colon with Synthetic Substitute, Open Approach

0D1A0JN Bypass Jejunum to Sigmoid Colon with Synthetic Substitute, Open Approach

0D1A0JP Bypass Jejunum to Rectum with Synthetic Substitute, Open Approach

0D1A0JQ Bypass Jejunum to Anus with Synthetic Substitute, Open Approach

0D1A0K4 Bypass Jejunum to Cutaneous with Nonautologous Tissue Substitute, Open Approach

0D1A0KA Bypass Jejunum to Jejunum with Nonautologous Tissue Substitute, Open Approach

0D1A0KB Bypass Jejunum to Ileum with Nonautologous Tissue Substitute, Open Approach

0D1A0KH Bypass Jejunum to Cecum with Nonautologous Tissue Substitute, Open Approach

0D1A0KK Bypass Jejunum to Ascending Colon with Nonautologous Tissue Substitute, Open Approach

0D1A0KL Bypass Jejunum to Transverse Colon with Nonautologous Tissue Substitute, Open Approach

0D1A0KM Bypass Jejunum to Descending Colon with Nonautologous Tissue Substitute, Open Approach

0D1A0KN Bypass Jejunum to Sigmoid Colon with Nonautologous Tissue Substitute, Open Approach

0D1A0KP Bypass Jejunum to Rectum with Nonautologous Tissue Substitute, Open Approach

0D1A0KQ Bypass Jejunum to Anus with Nonautologous Tissue Substitute, Open Approach

0D1A0Z4 Bypass Jejunum to Cutaneous, Open Approach

0D1A0ZA Bypass Jejunum to Jejunum, Open Approach

0D1A0ZB Bypass Jejunum to Ileum, Open Approach

0D1A0ZH Bypass Jejunum to Cecum, Open Approach

0D1A0ZK Bypass Jejunum to Ascending Colon, Open Approach

0D1A0ZL Bypass Jejunum to Transverse Colon, Open Approach

0D1A0ZM Bypass Jejunum to Descending Colon, Open Approach

0D1A0ZN Bypass Jejunum to Sigmoid Colon, Open Approach

0D1A0ZP Bypass Jejunum to Rectum, Open Approach

0D1A0ZQ Bypass Jejunum to Anus, Open Approach

0D1A3J4 Bypass Jejunum to Cutaneous with Synthetic Substitute, Percutaneous Approach

0D1A474 Bypass Jejunum to Cutaneous with Autologous Tissue Substitute, Percutaneous Endoscopic Approach

0D1A47A Bypass Jejunum to Jejunum with Autologous Tissue Substitute, Percutaneous Endoscopic Approach

0D1A47B Bypass Jejunum to Ileum with Autologous Tissue Substitute, Percutaneous Endoscopic Approach

0D1A47H Bypass Jejunum to Cecum with Autologous Tissue Substitute, Percutaneous Endoscopic Approach

0D1A47K Bypass Jejunum to Ascending Colon with Autologous Tissue Substitute, Percutaneous Endoscopic Approach

0D1A47L Bypass Jejunum to Transverse Colon with Autologous Tissue Substitute, Percutaneous Endoscopic Approach

0D1A47M Bypass Jejunum to Descending Colon with Autologous Tissue Substitute, Percutaneous Endoscopic Approach

0D1A47N Bypass Jejunum to Sigmoid Colon with Autologous Tissue Substitute, Percutaneous Endoscopic Approach

0D1A47P Bypass Jejunum to Rectum with Autologous Tissue Substitute, Percutaneous Endoscopic Approach

0D1A47Q Bypass Jejunum to Anus with Autologous Tissue Substitute, Percutaneous Endoscopic Approach

0D1A4J4 Bypass Jejunum to Cutaneous with Synthetic Substitute, Percutaneous Endoscopic Approach

0D1A4JA Bypass Jejunum to Jejunum with Synthetic Substitute, Percutaneous Endoscopic Approach

0D1A4JB Bypass Jejunum to Ileum with Synthetic Substitute, Percutaneous Endoscopic Approach

0D1A4JH Bypass Jejunum to Cecum with Synthetic Substitute, Percutaneous Endoscopic Approach

0D1A4JK Bypass Jejunum to Ascending Colon with Synthetic Substitute, Percutaneous Endoscopic Approach

0D1A4JL Bypass Jejunum to Transverse Colon with Synthetic Substitute, Percutaneous Endoscopic Approach

0D1A4JM Bypass Jejunum to Descending Colon with Synthetic Substitute, Percutaneous Endoscopic Approach

0D1A4JN Bypass Jejunum to Sigmoid Colon with Synthetic Substitute, Percutaneous Endoscopic Approach

0D1A4JP Bypass Jejunum to Rectum with Synthetic Substitute, Percutaneous Endoscopic Approach

0D1A4JQ Bypass Jejunum to Anus with Synthetic Substitute, Percutaneous Endoscopic Approach

0D1A4K4 Bypass Jejunum to Cutaneous with Nonautologous Tissue Substitute, Percutaneous Endoscopic Approach

0D1A4KA Bypass Jejunum to Jejunum with Nonautologous Tissue Substitute, Percutaneous Endoscopic Approach

0D1A4KB Bypass Jejunum to Ileum with Nonautologous Tissue Substitute, Percutaneous Endoscopic Approach

0D1A4KH Bypass Jejunum to Cecum with Nonautologous Tissue Substitute, Percutaneous Endoscopic Approach

0D1A4KK Bypass Jejunum to Ascending Colon with Nonautologous Tissue Substitute, Percutaneous Endoscopic Approach

0D1A4KL Bypass Jejunum to Transverse Colon with Nonautologous Tissue Substitute, Percutaneous Endoscopic Approach

0D1A4KM Bypass Jejunum to Descending Colon with Nonautologous Tissue Substitute, Percutaneous Endoscopic Approach

0D1A4KN Bypass Jejunum to Sigmoid Colon with Nonautologous Tissue Substitute, Percutaneous Endoscopic Approach

0D1A4KP Bypass Jejunum to Rectum with Nonautologous Tissue Substitute, Percutaneous Endoscopic Approach

♀ Female-only   ♂ Male-only   ▲ Limited Coverage   ● Non-OR   ▬ HAC-associated procedure   ▲ Non-covered procedures   ✚ Combinatio

1A4KQ Bypass Jejunum to Anus with Nonautologous Tissue Substitute, Percutaneous Endoscopic Approach

1A4Z4 Bypass Jejunum to Cutaneous, Percutaneous Endoscopic Approach

1A4ZA Bypass Jejunum to Jejunum, Percutaneous Endoscopic Approach

1A4ZB Bypass Jejunum to Ileum, Percutaneous Endoscopic Approach

1A4ZH Bypass Jejunum to Cecum, Percutaneous Endoscopic Approach

1A4ZK Bypass Jejunum to Ascending Colon, Percutaneous Endoscopic Approach

1A4ZL Bypass Jejunum to Transverse Colon, Percutaneous Endoscopic Approach

1A4ZM Bypass Jejunum to Descending Colon, Percutaneous Endoscopic Approach

1A4ZN Bypass Jejunum to Sigmoid Colon, Percutaneous Endoscopic Approach

1A4ZP Bypass Jejunum to Rectum, Percutaneous Endoscopic Approach

1A4ZQ Bypass Jejunum to Anus, Percutaneous Endoscopic Approach

1A874 Bypass Jejunum to Cutaneous with Autologous Tissue Substitute, Via Natural or Artificial Opening Endoscopic

1A87A Bypass Jejunum to Jejunum with Autologous Tissue Substitute, Via Natural or Artificial Opening Endoscopic

1A87B Bypass Jejunum to Ileum with Autologous Tissue Substitute, Via Natural or Artificial Opening Endoscopic

1A87H Bypass Jejunum to Cecum with Autologous Tissue Substitute, Via Natural or Artificial Opening Endoscopic

1A87K Bypass Jejunum to Ascending Colon with Autologous Tissue Substitute, Via Natural or Artificial Opening Endoscopic

1A87L Bypass Jejunum to Transverse Colon with Autologous Tissue Substitute, Via Natural or Artificial Opening Endoscopic

1A87M Bypass Jejunum to Descending Colon with Autologous Tissue Substitute, Via Natural or Artificial Opening Endoscopic

1A87N Bypass Jejunum to Sigmoid Colon with Autologous Tissue Substitute, Via Natural or Artificial Opening Endoscopic

1A87P Bypass Jejunum to Rectum with Autologous Tissue Substitute, Via Natural or Artificial Opening Endoscopic

1A87Q Bypass Jejunum to Anus with Autologous Tissue Substitute, Via Natural or Artificial Opening Endoscopic

1A8J4 Bypass Jejunum to Cutaneous with Synthetic Substitute, Via Natural or Artificial Opening Endoscopic

1A8JA Bypass Jejunum to Jejunum with Synthetic Substitute, Via Natural or Artificial Opening Endoscopic

1A8JB Bypass Jejunum to Ileum with Synthetic Substitute, Via Natural or Artificial Opening Endoscopic

1A8JH Bypass Jejunum to Cecum with Synthetic Substitute, Via Natural or Artificial Opening Endoscopic

1A8JK Bypass Jejunum to Ascending Colon with Synthetic Substitute, Via Natural or Artificial Opening Endoscopic

1A8JL Bypass Jejunum to Transverse Colon with Synthetic Substitute, Via Natural or Artificial Opening Endoscopic

1A8JM Bypass Jejunum to Descending Colon with Synthetic Substitute, Via Natural or Artificial Opening Endoscopic

0D1A8JN Bypass Jejunum to Sigmoid Colon with Synthetic Substitute, Via Natural or Artificial Opening Endoscopic

0D1A8JP Bypass Jejunum to Rectum with Synthetic Substitute, Via Natural or Artificial Opening Endoscopic

0D1A8JQ Bypass Jejunum to Anus with Synthetic Substitute, Via Natural or Artificial Opening Endoscopic

0D1A8K4 Bypass Jejunum to Cutaneous with Nonautologous Tissue Substitute, Via Natural or Artificial Opening Endoscopic

0D1A8KA Bypass Jejunum to Jejunum with Nonautologous Tissue Substitute, Via Natural or Artificial Opening Endoscopic

0D1A8KB Bypass Jejunum to Ileum with Nonautologous Tissue Substitute, Via Natural or Artificial Opening Endoscopic

0D1A8KH Bypass Jejunum to Cecum with Nonautologous Tissue Substitute, Via Natural or Artificial Opening Endoscopic

0D1A8KK Bypass Jejunum to Ascending Colon with Nonautologous Tissue Substitute, Via Natural or Artificial Opening Endoscopic

0D1A8KL Bypass Jejunum to Transverse Colon with Nonautologous Tissue Substitute, Via Natural or Artificial Opening Endoscopic

0D1A8KM Bypass Jejunum to Descending Colon with Nonautologous Tissue Substitute, Via Natural or Artificial Opening Endoscopic

0D1A8KN Bypass Jejunum to Sigmoid Colon with Nonautologous Tissue Substitute, Via Natural or Artificial Opening Endoscopic

0D1A8KP Bypass Jejunum to Rectum with Nonautologous Tissue Substitute, Via Natural or Artificial Opening Endoscopic

0D1A8KQ Bypass Jejunum to Anus with Nonautologous Tissue Substitute, Via Natural or Artificial Opening Endoscopic

0D1A8Z4 Bypass Jejunum to Cutaneous, Via Natural or Artificial Opening Endoscopic

0D1A8ZA Bypass Jejunum to Jejunum, Via Natural or Artificial Opening Endoscopic

0D1A8ZB Bypass Jejunum to Ileum, Via Natural or Artificial Opening Endoscopic

0D1A8ZH Bypass Jejunum to Cecum, Via Natural or Artificial Opening Endoscopic

0D1A8ZK Bypass Jejunum to Ascending Colon, Via Natural or Artificial Opening Endoscopic

0D1A8ZL Bypass Jejunum to Transverse Colon, Via Natural or Artificial Opening Endoscopic

0D1A8ZM Bypass Jejunum to Descending Colon, Via Natural or Artificial Opening Endoscopic

0D1A8ZN Bypass Jejunum to Sigmoid Colon, Via Natural or Artificial Opening Endoscopic

0D1A8ZP Bypass Jejunum to Rectum, Via Natural or Artificial Opening Endoscopic

0D1A8ZQ Bypass Jejunum to Anus, Via Natural or Artificial Opening Endoscopic

0D1B074 Bypass Ileum to Cutaneous with Autologous Tissue Substitute, Open Approach

0D1B07B Bypass Ileum to Ileum with Autologous Tissue Substitute, Open Approach

0D1B07H Bypass Ileum to Cecum with Autologous Tissue Substitute, Open Approach

0D1B07K Bypass Ileum to Ascending Colon with Autologous Tissue Substitute, Open Approach

0D1B07L Bypass Ileum to Transverse Colon with Autologous Tissue Substitute, Open Approach

0D1B07M Bypass Ileum to Descending Colon with Autologous Tissue Substitute, Open Approach

0D1B07N Bypass Ileum to Sigmoid Colon with Autologous Tissue Substitute, Open Approach

0D1B07P Bypass Ileum to Rectum with Autologous Tissue Substitute, Open Approach

0D1B07Q Bypass Ileum to Anus with Autologous Tissue Substitute, Open Approach

0D1B0J4 Bypass Ileum to Cutaneous with Synthetic Substitute, Open Approach

0D1B0JB Bypass Ileum to Ileum with Synthetic Substitute, Open Approach

0D1B0JH Bypass Ileum to Cecum with Synthetic Substitute, Open Approach

0D1B0JK Bypass Ileum to Ascending Colon with Synthetic Substitute, Open Approach

0D1B0JL Bypass Ileum to Transverse Colon with Synthetic Substitute, Open Approach

0D1B0JM Bypass Ileum to Descending Colon with Synthetic Substitute, Open Approach

0D1B0JN Bypass Ileum to Sigmoid Colon with Synthetic Substitute, Open Approach

0D1B0JP Bypass Ileum to Rectum with Synthetic Substitute, Open Approach

0D1B0JQ Bypass Ileum to Anus with Synthetic Substitute, Open Approach

0D1B0K4 Bypass Ileum to Cutaneous with Nonautologous Tissue Substitute, Open Approach

0D1B0KB Bypass Ileum to Ileum with Nonautologous Tissue Substitute, Open Approach

0D1B0KH Bypass Ileum to Cecum with Nonautologous Tissue Substitute, Open Approach

0D1B0KK Bypass Ileum to Ascending Colon with Nonautologous Tissue Substitute, Open Approach

0D1B0KL Bypass Ileum to Transverse Colon with Nonautologous Tissue Substitute, Open Approach

0D1B0KM Bypass Ileum to Descending Colon with Nonautologous Tissue Substitute, Open Approach

0D1B0KN Bypass Ileum to Sigmoid Colon with Nonautologous Tissue Substitute, Open Approach

0D1B0KP Bypass Ileum to Rectum with Nonautologous Tissue Substitute, Open Approach

0D1B0KQ Bypass Ileum to Anus with Nonautologous Tissue Substitute, Open Approach

0D1B0Z4 Bypass Ileum to Cutaneous, Open Approach

0D1B0ZB Bypass Ileum to Ileum, Open Approach

0D1B0ZH Bypass Ileum to Cecum, Open Approach

0D1B0ZK Bypass Ileum to Ascending Colon, Open Approach

0D1B0ZL Bypass Ileum to Transverse Colon, Open Approach

0D1B0ZM Bypass Ileum to Descending Colon, Open Approach

0D1B0ZN Bypass Ileum to Sigmoid Colon, Open Approach

0D1B0ZP Bypass Ileum to Rectum, Open Approach

0D1B0ZQ Bypass Ileum to Anus, Open Approach

0D1B3J4 Bypass Ileum to Cutaneous with Synthetic Substitute, Percutaneous Approach

0D1B474 Bypass Ileum to Cutaneous with Autologous Tissue Substitute, Percutaneous Endoscopic Approach

0D1B47B Bypass Ileum to Ileum with Autologous Tissue Substitute, Percutaneous Endoscopic Approach

♀ Female-only   ♂ Male-only   ▲ Limited Coverage   ● Non-OR   ▣ HAC-associated procedure   ▲ Non-covered procedures   ✚ Combination

0D1B47H Bypass Ileum to Cecum with Autologous Tissue Substitute, Percutaneous Endoscopic Approach

0D1B47K Bypass Ileum to Ascending Colon with Autologous Tissue Substitute, Percutaneous Endoscopic Approach

0D1B47L Bypass Ileum to Transverse Colon with Autologous Tissue Substitute, Percutaneous Endoscopic Approach

0D1B47M Bypass Ileum to Descending Colon with Autologous Tissue Substitute, Percutaneous Endoscopic Approach

0D1B47N Bypass Ileum to Sigmoid Colon with Autologous Tissue Substitute, Percutaneous Endoscopic Approach

0D1B47P Bypass Ileum to Rectum with Autologous Tissue Substitute, Percutaneous Endoscopic Approach

0D1B47Q Bypass Ileum to Anus with Autologous Tissue Substitute, Percutaneous Endoscopic Approach

0D1B4J4 Bypass Ileum to Cutaneous with Synthetic Substitute, Percutaneous Endoscopic Approach

0D1B4JB Bypass Ileum to Ileum with Synthetic Substitute, Percutaneous Endoscopic Approach

0D1B4JH Bypass Ileum to Cecum with Synthetic Substitute, Percutaneous Endoscopic Approach

0D1B4JK Bypass Ileum to Ascending Colon with Synthetic Substitute, Percutaneous Endoscopic Approach

0D1B4JL Bypass Ileum to Transverse Colon with Synthetic Substitute, Percutaneous Endoscopic Approach

0D1B4JM Bypass Ileum to Descending Colon with Synthetic Substitute, Percutaneous Endoscopic Approach

0D1B4JN Bypass Ileum to Sigmoid Colon with Synthetic Substitute, Percutaneous Endoscopic Approach

0D1B4JP Bypass Ileum to Rectum with Synthetic Substitute, Percutaneous Endoscopic Approach

0D1B4JQ Bypass Ileum to Anus with Synthetic Substitute, Percutaneous Endoscopic Approach

0D1B4K4 Bypass Ileum to Cutaneous with Nonautologous Tissue Substitute, Percutaneous Endoscopic Approach

0D1B4KB Bypass Ileum to Ileum with Nonautologous Tissue Substitute, Percutaneous Endoscopic Approach

0D1B4KH Bypass Ileum to Cecum with Nonautologous Tissue Substitute, Percutaneous Endoscopic Approach

0D1B4KK Bypass Ileum to Ascending Colon with Nonautologous Tissue Substitute, Percutaneous Endoscopic Approach

0D1B4KL Bypass Ileum to Transverse Colon with Nonautologous Tissue Substitute, Percutaneous Endoscopic Approach

0D1B4KM Bypass Ileum to Descending Colon with Nonautologous Tissue Substitute, Percutaneous Endoscopic Approach

0D1B4KN Bypass Ileum to Sigmoid Colon with Nonautologous Tissue Substitute, Percutaneous Endoscopic Approach

0D1B4KP Bypass Ileum to Rectum with Nonautologous Tissue Substitute, Percutaneous Endoscopic Approach

0D1B4KQ Bypass Ileum to Anus with Nonautologous Tissue Substitute, Percutaneous Endoscopic Approach

0D1B4Z4 Bypass Ileum to Cutaneous, Percutaneous Endoscopic Approach

0D1B4ZB Bypass Ileum to Ileum, Percutaneous Endoscopic Approach

0D1B4ZH Bypass Ileum to Cecum, Percutaneous Endoscopic Approach

0D1B4ZK Bypass Ileum to Ascending Colon, Percutaneous Endoscopic Approach

0D1B4ZL Bypass Ileum to Transverse Colon, Percutaneous Endoscopic Approach

0D1B4ZM Bypass Ileum to Descending Colon, Percutaneous Endoscopic Approach

0D1B4ZN Bypass Ileum to Sigmoid Colon, Percutaneous Endoscopic Approach

0D1B4ZP Bypass Ileum to Rectum, Percutaneous Endoscopic Approach

0D1B4ZQ Bypass Ileum to Anus, Percutaneous Endoscopic Approach

0D1B874 Bypass Ileum to Cutaneous with Autologous Tissue Substitute, Via Natural or Artificial Opening Endoscopic

0D1B87B Bypass Ileum to Ileum with Autologous Tissue Substitute, Via Natural or Artificial Opening Endoscopic

0D1B87H Bypass Ileum to Cecum with Autologous Tissue Substitute, Via Natural or Artificial Opening Endoscopic

0D1B87K Bypass Ileum to Ascending Colon with Autologous Tissue Substitute, Via Natural or Artificial Opening Endoscopic

0D1B87L Bypass Ileum to Transverse Colon with Autologous Tissue Substitute, Via Natural or Artificial Opening Endoscopic

0D1B87M Bypass Ileum to Descending Colon with Autologous Tissue Substitute, Via Natural or Artificial Opening Endoscopic

0D1B87N Bypass Ileum to Sigmoid Colon with Autologous Tissue Substitute, Via Natural or Artificial Opening Endoscopic

0D1B87P Bypass Ileum to Rectum with Autologous Tissue Substitute, Via Natural or Artificial Opening Endoscopic

0D1B87Q Bypass Ileum to Anus with Autologous Tissue Substitute, Via Natural or Artificial Opening Endoscopic

0D1B8J4 Bypass Ileum to Cutaneous with Synthetic Substitute, Via Natural or Artificial Opening Endoscopic

0D1B8JB Bypass Ileum to Ileum with Synthetic Substitute, Via Natural or Artificial Opening Endoscopic

0D1B8JH Bypass Ileum to Cecum with Synthetic Substitute, Via Natural or Artificial Opening Endoscopic

0D1B8JK Bypass Ileum to Ascending Colon with Synthetic Substitute, Via Natural or Artificial Opening Endoscopic

0D1B8JL Bypass Ileum to Transverse Colon with Synthetic Substitute, Via Natural or Artificial Opening Endoscopic

0D1B8JM Bypass Ileum to Descending Colon with Synthetic Substitute, Via Natural or Artificial Opening Endoscopic

0D1B8JN Bypass Ileum to Sigmoid Colon with Synthetic Substitute, Via Natural or Artificial Opening Endoscopic

0D1B8JP Bypass Ileum to Rectum with Synthetic Substitute, Via Natural or Artificial Opening Endoscopic

0D1B8JQ Bypass Ileum to Anus with Synthetic Substitute, Via Natural or Artificial Opening Endoscopic

0D1B8K4 Bypass Ileum to Cutaneous with Nonautologous Tissue Substitute, Via Natural or Artificial Opening Endoscopic

0D1B8KB Bypass Ileum to Ileum with Nonautologous Tissue Substitute, Via Natural or Artificial Opening Endoscopic

0D1B8KH Bypass Ileum to Cecum with Nonautologous Tissue Substitute, Via Natural or Artificial Opening Endoscopic

0D1B8KK Bypass Ileum to Ascending Colon with Nonautologous Tissue Substitute, Via Natural or Artificial Opening Endoscopic

0D1B8KL Bypass Ileum to Transverse Colon with Nonautologous Tissue Substitute, Via Natural or Artificial Opening Endoscopic

0D1B8KM Bypass Ileum to Descending Colon with Nonautologous Tissue Substitute, Via Natural or Artificial Opening Endoscopic

0D1B8KN Bypass Ileum to Sigmoid Colon with Nonautologous Tissue Substitute, Via Natural or Artificial Opening Endoscopic

0D1B8KP Bypass Ileum to Rectum with Nonautologous Tissue Substitute, Via Natural or Artificial Opening Endoscopic

0D1B8KQ Bypass Ileum to Anus with Nonautologous Tissue Substitute, Via Natural or Artificial Opening Endoscopic

0D1B8Z4 Bypass Ileum to Cutaneous, Via Natural or Artificial Opening Endoscopic

0D1B8ZB Bypass Ileum to Ileum, Via Natural or Artificial Opening Endoscopic

0D1B8ZH Bypass Ileum to Cecum, Via Natural or Artificial Opening Endoscopic

0D1B8ZK Bypass Ileum to Ascending Colon, Via Natural or Artificial Opening Endoscopic

0D1B8ZL Bypass Ileum to Transverse Colon, Via Natural or Artificial Opening Endoscopic

0D1B8ZM Bypass Ileum to Descending Colon, Via Natural or Artificial Opening Endoscopic

0D1B8ZN Bypass Ileum to Sigmoid Colon, Via Natural or Artificial Opening Endoscopic

0D1B8ZP Bypass Ileum to Rectum, Via Natural or Artificial Opening Endoscopic

0D1B8ZQ Bypass Ileum to Anus, Via Natural or Artificial Opening Endoscopic

0D1H074 Bypass Cecum to Cutaneous with Autologous Tissue Substitute, Open Approach

0D1H07H Bypass Cecum to Cecum with Autologous Tissue Substitute, Open Approach

0D1H07K Bypass Cecum to Ascending Colon with Autologous Tissue Substitute, Open Approach

0D1H07L Bypass Cecum to Transverse Colon with Autologous Tissue Substitute, Open Approach

0D1H07M Bypass Cecum to Descending Colon with Autologous Tissue Substitute, Open Approach

0D1H07N Bypass Cecum to Sigmoid Colon with Autologous Tissue Substitute, Open Approach

0D1H07P Bypass Cecum to Rectum with Autologous Tissue Substitute, Open Approach

0D1H0J4 Bypass Cecum to Cutaneous with Synthetic Substitute, Open Approach

0D1H0JH Bypass Cecum to Cecum with Synthetic Substitute, Open Approach

0D1H0JK Bypass Cecum to Ascending Colon with Synthetic Substitute, Open Approach

0D1H0JL Bypass Cecum to Transverse Colon with Synthetic Substitute, Open Approach

0D1H0JM Bypass Cecum to Descending Colon with Synthetic Substitute, Open Approach

0D1H0JN Bypass Cecum to Sigmoid Colon with Synthetic Substitute, Open Approach

0D1H0JP Bypass Cecum to Rectum with Synthetic Substitute, Open Approach

0D1H0K4 Bypass Cecum to Cutaneous with Nonautologous Tissue Substitute, Open Approach

0D1H0KH Bypass Cecum to Cecum with Nonautologous Tissue Substitute, Open Approach

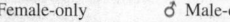

♀ Female-only ♂ Male-only ▲ Limited Coverage ● Non-OR ▒ HAC-associated procedure ▲ Non-covered procedures ✚ Combination

H0KK Bypass Cecum to Ascending Colon with Nonautologous Tissue Substitute, Open Approach

H0KL Bypass Cecum to Transverse Colon with Nonautologous Tissue Substitute, Open Approach

H0KM Bypass Cecum to Descending Colon with Nonautologous Tissue Substitute, Open Approach

H0KN Bypass Cecum to Sigmoid Colon with Nonautologous Tissue Substitute, Open Approach

H0KP Bypass Cecum to Rectum with Nonautologous Tissue Substitute, Open Approach

H0Z4 Bypass Cecum to Cutaneous, Open Approach

H0ZH Bypass Cecum to Cecum, Open Approach

H0ZK Bypass Cecum to Ascending Colon, Open Approach

H0ZL Bypass Cecum to Transverse Colon, Open Approach

H0ZM Bypass Cecum to Descending Colon, Open Approach

H0ZN Bypass Cecum to Sigmoid Colon, Open Approach

H0ZP Bypass Cecum to Rectum, Open Approach

H3J4 Bypass Cecum to Cutaneous with Synthetic Substitute, Percutaneous Approach

H474 Bypass Cecum to Cutaneous with Autologous Tissue Substitute, Percutaneous Endoscopic Approach

H47H Bypass Cecum to Cecum with Autologous Tissue Substitute, Percutaneous Endoscopic Approach

H47K Bypass Cecum to Ascending Colon with Autologous Tissue Substitute, Percutaneous Endoscopic Approach

1H47L Bypass Cecum to Transverse Colon with Autologous Tissue Substitute, Percutaneous Endoscopic Approach

1H47M Bypass Cecum to Descending Colon with Autologous Tissue Substitute, Percutaneous Endoscopic Approach

1H47N Bypass Cecum to Sigmoid Colon with Autologous Tissue Substitute, Percutaneous Endoscopic Approach

1H47P Bypass Cecum to Rectum with Autologous Tissue Substitute, Percutaneous Endoscopic Approach

1H4J4 Bypass Cecum to Cutaneous with Synthetic Substitute, Percutaneous Endoscopic Approach

1H4JH Bypass Cecum to Cecum with Synthetic Substitute, Percutaneous Endoscopic Approach

1H4JK Bypass Cecum to Ascending Colon with Synthetic Substitute, Percutaneous Endoscopic Approach

1H4JL Bypass Cecum to Transverse Colon with Synthetic Substitute, Percutaneous Endoscopic Approach

1H4JM Bypass Cecum to Descending Colon with Synthetic Substitute, Percutaneous Endoscopic Approach

1H4JN Bypass Cecum to Sigmoid Colon with Synthetic Substitute, Percutaneous Endoscopic Approach

1H4JP Bypass Cecum to Rectum with Synthetic Substitute, Percutaneous Endoscopic Approach

1H4K4 Bypass Cecum to Cutaneous with Nonautologous Tissue Substitute, Percutaneous Endoscopic Approach

1H4KH Bypass Cecum to Cecum with Nonautologous Tissue Substitute, Percutaneous Endoscopic Approach

0D1H4KK Bypass Cecum to Ascending Colon with Nonautologous Tissue Substitute, Percutaneous Endoscopic Approach

0D1H4KL Bypass Cecum to Transverse Colon with Nonautologous Tissue Substitute, Percutaneous Endoscopic Approach

0D1H4KM Bypass Cecum to Descending Colon with Nonautologous Tissue Substitute, Percutaneous Endoscopic Approach

0D1H4KN Bypass Cecum to Sigmoid Colon with Nonautologous Tissue Substitute, Percutaneous Endoscopic Approach

0D1H4KP Bypass Cecum to Rectum with Nonautologous Tissue Substitute, Percutaneous Endoscopic Approach

0D1H4Z4 Bypass Cecum to Cutaneous, Percutaneous Endoscopic Approach

0D1H4ZH Bypass Cecum to Cecum, Percutaneous Endoscopic Approach

0D1H4ZK Bypass Cecum to Ascending Colon, Percutaneous Endoscopic Approach

0D1H4ZL Bypass Cecum to Transverse Colon, Percutaneous Endoscopic Approach

0D1H4ZM Bypass Cecum to Descending Colon, Percutaneous Endoscopic Approach

0D1H4ZN Bypass Cecum to Sigmoid Colon, Percutaneous Endoscopic Approach

0D1H4ZP Bypass Cecum to Rectum, Percutaneous Endoscopic Approach

0D1H874 Bypass Cecum to Cutaneous with Autologous Tissue Substitute, Via Natural or Artificial Opening Endoscopic

0D1H87H Bypass Cecum to Cecum with Autologous Tissue Substitute, Via Natural or Artificial Opening Endoscopic

0D1H87K Bypass Cecum to Ascending Colon with Autologous Tissue Substitute, Via Natural or Artificial Opening Endoscopic

0D1H87L Bypass Cecum to Transverse Colon with Autologous Tissue Substitute, Via Natural or Artificial Opening Endoscopic

0D1H87M Bypass Cecum to Descending Colon with Autologous Tissue Substitute, Via Natural or Artificial Opening Endoscopic

0D1H87N Bypass Cecum to Sigmoid Colon with Autologous Tissue Substitute, Via Natural or Artificial Opening Endoscopic

0D1H87P Bypass Cecum to Rectum with Autologous Tissue Substitute, Via Natural or Artificial Opening Endoscopic

0D1H8J4 Bypass Cecum to Cutaneous with Synthetic Substitute, Via Natural or Artificial Opening Endoscopic

0D1H8JH Bypass Cecum to Cecum with Synthetic Substitute, Via Natural or Artificial Opening Endoscopic

0D1H8JK Bypass Cecum to Ascending Colon with Synthetic Substitute, Via Natural or Artificial Opening Endoscopic

0D1H8JL Bypass Cecum to Transverse Colon with Synthetic Substitute, Via Natural or Artificial Opening Endoscopic

0D1H8JM Bypass Cecum to Descending Colon with Synthetic Substitute, Via Natural or Artificial Opening Endoscopic

0D1H8JN Bypass Cecum to Sigmoid Colon with Synthetic Substitute, Via Natural or Artificial Opening Endoscopic

0D1H8JP Bypass Cecum to Rectum with Synthetic Substitute, Via Natural or Artificial Opening Endoscopic

0D1H8K4 Bypass Cecum to Cutaneous with Nonautologous Tissue Substitute, Via Natural or Artificial Opening Endoscopic

0D1H8KH Bypass Cecum to Cecum with Nonautologous Tissue Substitute, Via Natural or Artificial Opening Endoscopic

0D1H8KK Bypass Cecum to Ascending Colon with Nonautologous Tissue Substitute, Via Natural or Artificial Opening Endoscopic

0D1H8KL Bypass Cecum to Transverse Colon with Nonautologous Tissue Substitute, Via Natural or Artificial Opening Endoscopic

0D1H8KM Bypass Cecum to Descending Colon with Nonautologous Tissue Substitute, Via Natural or Artificial Opening Endoscopic

0D1H8KN Bypass Cecum to Sigmoid Colon with Nonautologous Tissue Substitute, Via Natural or Artificial Opening Endoscopic

0D1H8KP Bypass Cecum to Rectum with Nonautologous Tissue Substitute, Via Natural or Artificial Opening Endoscopic

0D1H8Z4 Bypass Cecum to Cutaneous, Via Natural or Artificial Opening Endoscopic

0D1H8ZH Bypass Cecum to Cecum, Via Natural or Artificial Opening Endoscopic

0D1H8ZK Bypass Cecum to Ascending Colon, Via Natural or Artificial Opening Endoscopic

0D1H8ZL Bypass Cecum to Transverse Colon, Via Natural or Artificial Opening Endoscopic

0D1H8ZM Bypass Cecum to Descending Colon, Via Natural or Artificial Opening Endoscopic

0D1H8ZN Bypass Cecum to Sigmoid Colon, Via Natural or Artificial Opening Endoscopic

0D1H8ZP Bypass Cecum to Rectum, Via Natural or Artificial Opening Endoscopic

0D1K074 Bypass Ascending Colon to Cutaneous with Autologous Tissue Substitute, Open Approach

0D1K07K Bypass Ascending Colon to Ascending Colon with Autologous Tissue Substitute, Open Approach

0D1K07L Bypass Ascending Colon to Transverse Colon with Autologous Tissue Substitute, Open Approach

0D1K07M Bypass Ascending Colon to Descending Colon with Autologous Tissue Substitute, Open Approach

0D1K07N Bypass Ascending Colon to Sigmoid Colon with Autologous Tissue Substitute, Open Approach

0D1K07P Bypass Ascending Colon to Rectum with Autologous Tissue Substitute, Open Approach

0D1K0J4 Bypass Ascending Colon to Cutaneous with Synthetic Substitute, Open Approach

0D1K0JK Bypass Ascending Colon to Ascending Colon with Synthetic Substitute, Open Approach

0D1K0JL Bypass Ascending Colon to Transverse Colon with Synthetic Substitute, Open Approach

0D1K0JM Bypass Ascending Colon to Descending Colon with Synthetic Substitute, Open Approach

0D1K0JN Bypass Ascending Colon to Sigmoid Colon with Synthetic Substitute, Open Approach

0D1K0JP Bypass Ascending Colon to Rectum with Synthetic Substitute, Open Approach

0D1K0K4 Bypass Ascending Colon to Cutaneous with Nonautologous Tissue Substitute, Open Approach

0D1K0KK Bypass Ascending Colon to Ascending Colon with Nonautologous Tissue Substitute, Open Approach

0D1K0KL Bypass Ascending Colon to Transverse Colon with Nonautologous Tissue Substitute, Open Approach

0D1K0KM Bypass Ascending Colon to Descending Colon with Nonautologous Tissue Substitute, Open Approach

0D1K0KN Bypass Ascending Colon to Sigmoid Colon with Nonautologous Tissue Substitute, Open Approach

0D1K0KP Bypass Ascending Colon to Rectum with Nonautologous Tissue Substitute, Open Approach

0D1K0Z4 Bypass Ascending Colon to Cutaneous, Open Approach

0D1K0ZK Bypass Ascending Colon to Ascending Colon, Open Approach

0D1K0ZL Bypass Ascending Colon to Transverse Colon, Open Approach

0D1K0ZM Bypass Ascending Colon to Descending Colon, Open Approach

0D1K0ZN Bypass Ascending Colon to Sigmoid Colon, Open Approach

0D1K0ZP Bypass Ascending Colon to Rectum, Open Approach

0D1K3J4 Bypass Ascending Colon to Cutaneous with Synthetic Substitute, Percutaneous Approach

0D1K474 Bypass Ascending Colon to Cutaneous with Autologous Tissue Substitute, Percutaneous Endoscopic Approach

0D1K47K Bypass Ascending Colon to Ascending Colon with Autologous Tissue Substitute, Percutaneous Endoscopic Approach

0D1K47L Bypass Ascending Colon to Transverse Colon with Autologous Tissue Substitute, Percutaneous Endoscopic Approach

0D1K47M Bypass Ascending Colon to Descending Colon with Autologous Tissue Substitute, Percutaneous Endoscopic Approach

0D1K47N Bypass Ascending Colon to Sigmoid Colon with Autologous Tissue Substitute, Percutaneous Endoscopic Approach

0D1K47P Bypass Ascending Colon to Rectum with Autologous Tissue Substitute, Percutaneous Endoscopic Approach

0D1K4J4 Bypass Ascending Colon to Cutaneous with Synthetic Substitute, Percutaneous Endoscopic Approach

0D1K4JK Bypass Ascending Colon to Ascending Colon with Synthetic Substitute, Percutaneous Endoscopic Approach

0D1K4JL Bypass Ascending Colon to Transverse Colon with Synthetic Substitute, Percutaneous Endoscopic Approach

0D1K4JM Bypass Ascending Colon to Descending Colon with Synthetic Substitute, Percutaneous Endoscopic Approach

0D1K4JN Bypass Ascending Colon to Sigmoid Colon with Synthetic Substitute, Percutaneous Endoscopic Approach

0D1K4JP Bypass Ascending Colon to Rectum with Synthetic Substitute, Percutaneous Endoscopic Approach

0D1K4K4 Bypass Ascending Colon to Cutaneous with Nonautologous Tissue Substitute, Percutaneous Endoscopic Approach

0D1K4KK Bypass Ascending Colon to Ascending Colon with Nonautologous Tissue Substitute, Percutaneous Endoscopic Approach

0D1K4KL Bypass Ascending Colon to Transverse Colon with Nonautologous Tissue Substitute, Percutaneous Endoscopic Approach

0D1K4KM Bypass Ascending Colon to Descending Colon with Nonautologous Tissue Substitute, Percutaneous Endoscopic Approach

0D1K4KN Bypass Ascending Colon to Sigmoid Colon with Nonautologous Tissue Substitute, Percutaneous Endoscopic Approach

0D1K4KP Bypass Ascending Colon to Rectum with Nonautologous Tissue Substitute, Percutaneous Endoscopic Approach

0D1K4Z4 Bypass Ascending Colon to Cutaneous, Percutaneous Endoscopic Approach

0D1K4ZK Bypass Ascending Colon to Ascending Colon, Percutaneous Endoscopic Approach

0D1K4ZL Bypass Ascending Colon to Transverse Colon, Percutaneous Endoscopic Approach

0D1K4ZM Bypass Ascending Colon to Descending Colon, Percutaneous Endoscopic Approach

0D1K4ZN Bypass Ascending Colon to Sigmoid Colon, Percutaneous Endoscopic Approach

0D1K4ZP Bypass Ascending Colon to Rectum, Percutaneous Endoscopic Approach

0D1K874 Bypass Ascending Colon to Cutaneous with Autologous Tissue Substitute, Via Natural or Artificial Opening Endoscopic

0D1K87K Bypass Ascending Colon to Ascending Colon with Autologous Tissue Substitute, Via Natural or Artificial Opening Endoscopic

0D1K87L Bypass Ascending Colon to Transverse Colon with Autologous Tissue Substitute, Via Natural or Artificial Opening Endoscopic

0D1K87M Bypass Ascending Colon to Descending Colon with Autologous Tissue Substitute, Via Natural or Artificial Opening Endoscopic

0D1K87N Bypass Ascending Colon to Sigmoid Colon with Autologous Tissue Substitute, Via Natural or Artificial Opening Endoscopic

0D1K87P Bypass Ascending Colon to Rectum with Autologous Tissue Substitute, Via Natural or Artificial Opening Endoscopic

0D1K8J4 Bypass Ascending Colon to Cutaneous with Synthetic Substitute, Via Natural or Artificial Opening Endoscopic

0D1K8JK Bypass Ascending Colon to Ascending Colon with Synthetic Substitute, Via Natural or Artificial Opening Endoscopic

0D1K8JL Bypass Ascending Colon to Transverse Colon with Synthetic Substitute, Via Natural or Artificial Opening Endoscopic

0D1K8JM Bypass Ascending Colon to Descending Colon with Synthetic Substitute, Via Natural or Artificial Opening Endoscopic

0D1K8JN Bypass Ascending Colon to Sigmoid Colon with Synthetic Substitute, Via Natural or Artificial Opening Endoscopic

0D1K8JP Bypass Ascending Colon to Rectum with Synthetic Substitute, Via Natural or Artificial Opening Endoscopic

0D1K8K4 Bypass Ascending Colon to Cutaneous with Nonautologous Tissue Substitute, Via Natural or Artificial Opening Endoscopic

0D1K8KK Bypass Ascending Colon to Ascending Colon with Nonautologous Tissue Substitute, Via Natural or Artificial Opening Endoscopic

0D1K8KL Bypass Ascending Colon to Transverse Colon with Nonautologous Tissue Substitute, Via Natural or Artificial Opening Endoscopic

0D1K8KM Bypass Ascending Colon to Descending Colon with Nonautologous Tissue Substitute, Via Natural or Artificial Opening Endoscopic

0D1K8KN Bypass Ascending Colon to Sigmoid Colon with Nonautologous Tissue Substitute, Via Natural or Artificial Opening Endoscopic

0D1K8KP Bypass Ascending Colon to Rectum with Nonautologous Tissue Substitute, Via Natural or Artificial Opening Endoscopic

0D1K8Z4 Bypass Ascending Colon to Cutaneous Via Natural or Artificial Opening Endoscopic

0D1K8ZK Bypass Ascending Colon to Ascending Colon, Via Natural or Artificial Opening Endoscopic

0D1K8ZL Bypass Ascending Colon to Transverse Colon, Via Natural or Artificial Opening Endoscopic

0D1K8ZM Bypass Ascending Colon to Descending Colon, Via Natural or Artificial Opening Endoscopic

0D1K8ZN Bypass Ascending Colon to Sigmoid Colon, Via Natural or Artificial Opening Endoscopic

0D1K8ZP Bypass Ascending Colon to Rectum, Via Natural or Artificial Opening Endoscopic

0D1L074 Bypass Transverse Colon to Cutaneous with Autologous Tissue Substitute, Open Approach

0D1L07L Bypass Transverse Colon to Transverse Colon with Autologous Tissue Substitute, Open Approach

0D1L07M Bypass Transverse Colon to Descending Colon with Autologous Tissue Substitute, Open Approach

0D1L07N Bypass Transverse Colon to Sigmoid Colon with Autologous Tissue Substitute, Open Approach

0D1L07P Bypass Transverse Colon to Rectum with Autologous Tissue Substitute, Open Approach

0D1L0J4 Bypass Transverse Colon to Cutaneous with Synthetic Substitute, Open Approach

0D1L0JL Bypass Transverse Colon to Transverse Colon with Synthetic Substitute, Open Approach

0D1L0JM Bypass Transverse Colon to Descending Colon with Synthetic Substitute, Open Approach

0D1L0JN Bypass Transverse Colon to Sigmoid Colon with Synthetic Substitute, Open Approach

0D1L0JP Bypass Transverse Colon to Rectum with Synthetic Substitute, Open Approach

0D1L0K4 Bypass Transverse Colon to Cutaneous with Nonautologous Tissue Substitute, Open Approach

0D1L0KL Bypass Transverse Colon to Transverse Colon with Nonautologous Tissue Substitute, Open Approach

0D1L0KM Bypass Transverse Colon to Descending Colon with Nonautologous Tissue Substitute, Open Approach

0D1L0KN Bypass Transverse Colon to Sigmoid Colon with Nonautologous Tissue Substitute, Open Approach

0D1L0KP Bypass Transverse Colon to Rectum with Nonautologous Tissue Substitute, Open Approach

0D1L0Z4 Bypass Transverse Colon to Cutaneous, Open Approach

0D1L0ZL Bypass Transverse Colon to Transverse Colon, Open Approach

0D1L0ZM Bypass Transverse Colon to Descending Colon, Open Approach

0D1L0ZN Bypass Transverse Colon to Sigmoid Colon, Open Approach

0D1L0ZP Bypass Transverse Colon to Rectum, Open Approach

0D1L3J4 Bypass Transverse Colon to Cutaneous with Synthetic Substitute, Percutaneous Approach

0D1L474 Bypass Transverse Colon to Cutaneous with Autologous Tissue Substitute, Percutaneous Endoscopic Approach

L47L Bypass Transverse Colon to Transverse Colon with Autologous Tissue Substitute, Percutaneous Endoscopic Approach

L47M Bypass Transverse Colon to Descending Colon with Autologous Tissue Substitute, Percutaneous Endoscopic Approach

L47N Bypass Transverse Colon to Sigmoid Colon with Autologous Tissue Substitute, Percutaneous Endoscopic Approach

L47P Bypass Transverse Colon to Rectum with Autologous Tissue Substitute, Percutaneous Endoscopic Approach

L4J4 Bypass Transverse Colon to Cutaneous with Synthetic Substitute, Percutaneous Endoscopic Approach

L4JL Bypass Transverse Colon to Transverse Colon with Synthetic Substitute, Percutaneous Endoscopic Approach

1L4JM Bypass Transverse Colon to Descending Colon with Synthetic Substitute, Percutaneous Endoscopic Approach

1L4JN Bypass Transverse Colon to Sigmoid Colon with Synthetic Substitute, Percutaneous Endoscopic Approach

1L4JP Bypass Transverse Colon to Rectum with Synthetic Substitute, Percutaneous Endoscopic Approach

1L4K4 Bypass Transverse Colon to Cutaneous with Nonautologous Tissue Substitute, Percutaneous Endoscopic Approach

1L4KL Bypass Transverse Colon to Transverse Colon with Nonautologous Tissue Substitute, Percutaneous Endoscopic Approach

1L4KM Bypass Transverse Colon to Descending Colon with Nonautologous Tissue Substitute, Percutaneous Endoscopic Approach

1L4KN Bypass Transverse Colon to Sigmoid Colon with Nonautologous Tissue Substitute, Percutaneous Endoscopic Approach

1L4KP Bypass Transverse Colon to Rectum with Nonautologous Tissue Substitute, Percutaneous Endoscopic Approach

1L4Z4 Bypass Transverse Colon to Cutaneous, Percutaneous Endoscopic Approach

1L4ZL Bypass Transverse Colon to Transverse Colon, Percutaneous Endoscopic Approach

1L4ZM Bypass Transverse Colon to Descending Colon, Percutaneous Endoscopic Approach

1L4ZN Bypass Transverse Colon to Sigmoid Colon, Percutaneous Endoscopic Approach

1L4ZP Bypass Transverse Colon to Rectum, Percutaneous Endoscopic Approach

1L874 Bypass Transverse Colon to Cutaneous with Autologous Tissue Substitute, Via Natural or Artificial Opening Endoscopic

1L87L Bypass Transverse Colon to Transverse Colon with Autologous Tissue Substitute, Via Natural or Artificial Opening Endoscopic

1L87M Bypass Transverse Colon to Descending Colon with Autologous Tissue Substitute, Via Natural or Artificial Opening Endoscopic

1L87N Bypass Transverse Colon to Sigmoid Colon with Autologous Tissue Substitute, Via Natural or Artificial Opening Endoscopic

1L87P Bypass Transverse Colon to Rectum with Autologous Tissue Substitute, Via Natural or Artificial Opening Endoscopic

0D1L8J4 Bypass Transverse Colon to Cutaneous with Synthetic Substitute, Via Natural or Artificial Opening Endoscopic

0D1L8JL Bypass Transverse Colon to Transverse Colon with Synthetic Substitute, Via Natural or Artificial Opening Endoscopic

0D1L8JM Bypass Transverse Colon to Descending Colon with Synthetic Substitute, Via Natural or Artificial Opening Endoscopic

0D1L8JN Bypass Transverse Colon to Sigmoid Colon with Synthetic Substitute, Via Natural or Artificial Opening Endoscopic

0D1L8JP Bypass Transverse Colon to Rectum with Synthetic Substitute, Via Natural or Artificial Opening Endoscopic

0D1L8K4 Bypass Transverse Colon to Cutaneous with Nonautologous Tissue Substitute, Via Natural or Artificial Opening Endoscopic

0D1L8KL Bypass Transverse Colon to Transverse Colon with Nonautologous Tissue Substitute, Via Natural or Artificial Opening Endoscopic

0D1L8KM Bypass Transverse Colon to Descending Colon with Nonautologous Tissue Substitute, Via Natural or Artificial Opening Endoscopic

0D1L8KN Bypass Transverse Colon to Sigmoid Colon with Nonautologous Tissue Substitute, Via Natural or Artificial Opening Endoscopic

0D1L8KP Bypass Transverse Colon to Rectum with Nonautologous Tissue Substitute, Via Natural or Artificial Opening Endoscopic

0D1L8Z4 Bypass Transverse Colon to Cutaneous, Via Natural or Artificial Opening Endoscopic

0D1L8ZL Bypass Transverse Colon to Transverse Colon, Via Natural or Artificial Opening Endoscopic

0D1L8ZM Bypass Transverse Colon to Descending Colon, Via Natural or Artificial Opening Endoscopic

0D1L8ZN Bypass Transverse Colon to Sigmoid Colon, Via Natural or Artificial Opening Endoscopic

0D1L8ZP Bypass Transverse Colon to Rectum, Via Natural or Artificial Opening Endoscopic

0D1M074 Bypass Descending Colon to Cutaneous with Autologous Tissue Substitute, Open Approach

0D1M07M Bypass Descending Colon to Descending Colon with Autologous Tissue Substitute, Open Approach

0D1M07N Bypass Descending Colon to Sigmoid Colon with Autologous Tissue Substitute, Open Approach

0D1M07P Bypass Descending Colon to Rectum with Autologous Tissue Substitute, Open Approach

0D1M0J4 Bypass Descending Colon to Cutaneous with Synthetic Substitute, Open Approach

0D1M0JM Bypass Descending Colon to Descending Colon with Synthetic Substitute, Open Approach

0D1M0JN Bypass Descending Colon to Sigmoid Colon with Synthetic Substitute, Open Approach

0D1M0JP Bypass Descending Colon to Rectum with Synthetic Substitute, Open Approach

0D1M0K4 Bypass Descending Colon to Cutaneous with Nonautologous Tissue Substitute, Open Approach

0D1M0KM Bypass Descending Colon to Descending Colon with Nonautologous Tissue Substitute, Open Approach

0D1M0KN Bypass Descending Colon to Sigmoid Colon with Nonautologous Tissue Substitute, Open Approach

0D1M0KP Bypass Descending Colon to Rectum with Nonautologous Tissue Substitute, Open Approach

0D1M0Z4 Bypass Descending Colon to Cutaneous, Open Approach

0D1M0ZM Bypass Descending Colon to Descending Colon, Open Approach

0D1M0ZN Bypass Descending Colon to Sigmoid Colon, Open Approach

0D1M0ZP Bypass Descending Colon to Rectum, Open Approach

0D1M3J4 Bypass Descending Colon to Cutaneous with Synthetic Substitute, Percutaneous Approach

0D1M474 Bypass Descending Colon to Cutaneous with Autologous Tissue Substitute, Percutaneous Endoscopic Approach

0D1M47M Bypass Descending Colon to Descending Colon with Autologous Tissue Substitute, Percutaneous Endoscopic Approach

0D1M47N Bypass Descending Colon to Sigmoid Colon with Autologous Tissue Substitute, Percutaneous Endoscopic Approach

0D1M47P Bypass Descending Colon to Rectum with Autologous Tissue Substitute, Percutaneous Endoscopic Approach

0D1M4J4 Bypass Descending Colon to Cutaneous with Synthetic Substitute, Percutaneous Endoscopic Approach

0D1M4JM Bypass Descending Colon to Descending Colon with Synthetic Substitute, Percutaneous Endoscopic Approach

0D1M4JN Bypass Descending Colon to Sigmoid Colon with Synthetic Substitute, Percutaneous Endoscopic Approach

0D1M4JP Bypass Descending Colon to Rectum with Synthetic Substitute, Percutaneous Endoscopic Approach

0D1M4K4 Bypass Descending Colon to Cutaneous with Nonautologous Tissue Substitute, Percutaneous Endoscopic Approach

0D1M4KM Bypass Descending Colon to Descending Colon with Nonautologous Tissue Substitute, Percutaneous Endoscopic Approach

0D1M4KN Bypass Descending Colon to Sigmoid Colon with Nonautologous Tissue Substitute, Percutaneous Endoscopic Approach

0D1M4KP Bypass Descending Colon to Rectum with Nonautologous Tissue Substitute, Percutaneous Endoscopic Approach

0D1M4Z4 Bypass Descending Colon to Cutaneous, Percutaneous Endoscopic Approach

0D1M4ZM Bypass Descending Colon to Descending Colon, Percutaneous Endoscopic Approach

0D1M4ZN Bypass Descending Colon to Sigmoid Colon, Percutaneous Endoscopic Approach

0D1M4ZP Bypass Descending Colon to Rectum, Percutaneous Endoscopic Approach

0D1M874 Bypass Descending Colon to Cutaneous with Autologous Tissue Substitute, Via Natural or Artificial Opening Endoscopic

0D1M87M Bypass Descending Colon to Descending Colon with Autologous Tissue Substitute, Via Natural or Artificial Opening Endoscopic

0D1M87N Bypass Descending Colon to Sigmoid Colon with Autologous Tissue Substitute, Via Natural or Artificial Opening Endoscopic

Female-only   ♂ Male-only   ▲ Limited Coverage   ● Non-OR   ▬ HAC-associated procedure   ▲ Non-covered procedures   ✚ Combination

0D1M87P	Bypass Descending Colon to Rectum with Autologous Tissue Substitute, Via Natural or Artificial Opening Endoscopic	0D1N07P	Bypass Sigmoid Colon to Rectum with Autologous Tissue Substitute, Open Approach	0D1N4KN	Bypass Sigmoid Colon to Sigmoid Co with Nonautologous Tissue Substitute Percutaneous Endoscopic Approach
0D1M8J4	Bypass Descending Colon to Cutaneous with Synthetic Substitute, Via Natural or Artificial Opening Endoscopic	0D1N0J4	Bypass Sigmoid Colon to Cutaneous with Synthetic Substitute, Open Approach	0D1N4KP	Bypass Sigmoid Colon to Rectum with Nonautologous Tissue Substitute Percutaneous Endoscopic Approach
0D1M8JM	Bypass Descending Colon to Descending Colon with Synthetic Substitute, Via Natural or Artificial Opening Endoscopic	0D1N0JN	Bypass Sigmoid Colon to Sigmoid Colon with Synthetic Substitute, Open Approach	0D1N4Z4	Bypass Sigmoid Colon to Cutaneous, Percutaneous Endoscopic Approach
0D1M8JN	Bypass Descending Colon to Sigmoid Colon with Synthetic Substitute, Via Natural or Artificial Opening Endoscopic	0D1N0JP	Bypass Sigmoid Colon to Rectum with Synthetic Substitute, Open Approach	0D1N4ZN	Bypass Sigmoid Colon to Sigmoid Colon, Percutaneous Endoscopic Approach
0D1M8JP	Bypass Descending Colon to Rectum with Synthetic Substitute, Via Natural or Artificial Opening Endoscopic	0D1N0K4	Bypass Sigmoid Colon to Cutaneous with Nonautologous Tissue Substitute, Open Approach	0D1N4ZP	Bypass Sigmoid Colon to Rectum, Percutaneous Endoscopic Approach
0D1M8K4	Bypass Descending Colon to Cutaneous with Nonautologous Tissue Substitute, Via Natural or Artificial Opening Endoscopic	0D1N0KN	Bypass Sigmoid Colon to Sigmoid Colon with Nonautologous Tissue Substitute, Open Approach	0D1N874	Bypass Sigmoid Colon to Cutaneous with Autologous Tissue Substitute, Via Natural or Artificial Opening Endosco
0D1M8KM	Bypass Descending Colon to Descending Colon with Nonautologous Tissue Substitute, Via Natural or Artificial Opening Endoscopic	0D1N0KP	Bypass Sigmoid Colon to Rectum with Nonautologous Tissue Substitute, Open Approach	0D1N87N	Bypass Sigmoid Colon to Sigmoid Co with Autologous Tissue Substitute, Vi Natural or Artificial Opening Endosco
0D1M8KN	Bypass Descending Colon to Sigmoid Colon with Nonautologous Tissue Substitute, Via Natural or Artificial Opening Endoscopic	0D1N0Z4	Bypass Sigmoid Colon to Cutaneous, Open Approach *AHA CC: 4Q, 2014, 41-42*	0D1N87P	Bypass Sigmoid Colon to Rectum with Autologous Tissue Substitute, Via Natural or Artificial Opening Endosco
0D1M8KP	Bypass Descending Colon to Rectum with Nonautologous Tissue Substitute, Via Natural or Artificial Opening Endoscopic	0D1N0ZN	Bypass Sigmoid Colon to Sigmoid Colon, Open Approach	0D1N8J4	Bypass Sigmoid Colon to Cutaneous with Synthetic Substitute, Via Natural Artificial Opening Endoscopic
0D1M8Z4	Bypass Descending Colon to Cutaneous, Via Natural or Artificial Opening Endoscopic	0D1N0ZP	Bypass Sigmoid Colon to Rectum, Open Approach	0D1N8JN	Bypass Sigmoid Colon to Sigmoid Co with Synthetic Substitute, Via Natural Artificial Opening Endoscopic
0D1M8ZM	Bypass Descending Colon to Descending Colon, Via Natural or Artificial Opening Endoscopic	0D1N3J4	Bypass Sigmoid Colon to Cutaneous with Synthetic Substitute, Percutaneous Approach	0D1N8JP	Bypass Sigmoid Colon to Rectum with Synthetic Substitute, Via Natural or Artificial Opening Endoscopic
0D1M8ZN	Bypass Descending Colon to Sigmoid Colon, Via Natural or Artificial Opening Endoscopic	0D1N474	Bypass Sigmoid Colon to Cutaneous with Autologous Tissue Substitute, Percutaneous Endoscopic Approach	0D1N8K4	Bypass Sigmoid Colon to Cutaneous w Nonautologous Tissue Substitute, Via Natural or Artificial Opening Endoscop
0D1M8ZP	Bypass Descending Colon to Rectum, Via Natural or Artificial Opening Endoscopic	0D1N47N	Bypass Sigmoid Colon to Sigmoid Colon with Autologous Tissue Substitute, Percutaneous Endoscopic Approach	0D1N8KN	Bypass Sigmoid Colon to Sigmoid Col with Nonautologous Tissue Substitute, Via Natural or Artificial Opening Endoscopic
0D1N074	Bypass Sigmoid Colon to Cutaneous with Autologous Tissue Substitute, Open Approach	0D1N47P	Bypass Sigmoid Colon to Rectum with Autologous Tissue Substitute, Percutaneous Endoscopic Approach	0D1N8KP	Bypass Sigmoid Colon to Rectum with Nonautologous Tissue Substitute, Via Natural or Artificial Opening Endoscop
0D1N07N	Bypass Sigmoid Colon to Sigmoid Colon with Autologous Tissue Substitute, Open Approach	0D1N4J4	Bypass Sigmoid Colon to Cutaneous with Synthetic Substitute, Percutaneous Endoscopic Approach	0D1N8Z4	Bypass Sigmoid Colon to Cutaneous, V Natural or Artificial Opening Endoscop
		0D1N4JN	Bypass Sigmoid Colon to Sigmoid Colon with Synthetic Substitute, Percutaneous Endoscopic Approach	0D1N8ZN	Bypass Sigmoid Colon to Sigmoid Colon, Via Natural or Artificial Openin Endoscopic
		0D1N4JP	Bypass Sigmoid Colon to Rectum with Synthetic Substitute, Percutaneous Endoscopic Approach	0D1N8ZP	Bypass Sigmoid Colon to Rectum, Via Natural or Artificial Opening Endoscop
		0D1N4K4	Bypass Sigmoid Colon to Cutaneous with Nonautologous Tissue Substitute, Percutaneous Endoscopic Approach		

0D2 – Gastrointestinal System, Change

Review Coding Guideline B6.1c

0D20X0Z	Change Drainage Device in Upper Intestinal Tract, External Approach	0D2DXUZ	Change Feeding Device in Lower Intestinal Tract, External Approach	0D2VX0Z	Change Drainage Device in Mesentery, External Approach
0D20XUZ	Change Feeding Device in Upper Intestinal Tract, External Approach	0D2DXYZ	Change Other Device in Lower Intestinal Tract, External Approach	0D2VXYZ	Change Other Device in Mesentery, External Approach
0D20XYZ	Change Other Device in Upper Intestinal Tract, External Approach	0D2UX0Z	Change Drainage Device in Omentum, External Approach	0D2WX0Z	Change Drainage Device in Peritoneum External Approach
0D2DX0Z	Change Drainage Device in Lower Intestinal Tract, External Approach	0D2UXYZ	Change Other Device in Omentum, External Approach	0D2WXYZ	Change Other Device in Peritoneum, External Approach

0D5 – Gastrointestinal System, Destruction

0D510ZZ	Destruction of Upper Esophagus, Open Approach	0D520ZZ	Destruction of Middle Esophagus, Open Approach	0D530ZZ	Destruction of Lower Esophagus, Open Approach
0D513ZZ	Destruction of Upper Esophagus, Percutaneous Approach	0D523ZZ	Destruction of Middle Esophagus, Percutaneous Approach	0D533ZZ	Destruction of Lower Esophagus, Percutaneous Approach
0D514ZZ	Destruction of Upper Esophagus, Percutaneous Endoscopic Approach	0D524ZZ	Destruction of Middle Esophagus, Percutaneous Endoscopic Approach	0D534ZZ	Destruction of Lower Esophagus, Percutaneous Endoscopic Approach
0D517ZZ	Destruction of Upper Esophagus, Via Natural or Artificial Opening	0D527ZZ	Destruction of Middle Esophagus, Via Natural or Artificial Opening	0D537ZZ	Destruction of Lower Esophagus, Via Natural or Artificial Opening
0D518ZZ	Destruction of Upper Esophagus, Via Natural or Artificial Opening Endoscopic	0D528ZZ	Destruction of Middle Esophagus, Via Natural or Artificial Opening Endoscopic	0D538ZZ	Destruction of Lower Esophagus, Via Natural or Artificial Opening Endoscopic

♀ Female-only   ♂ Male-only   ▲ Limited Coverage   ● Non-OR   ▦ HAC-associated procedure   ▲ Non-covered procedures   ✛ Combinatio

40ZZ	Destruction of Esophagogastric Junction, Open Approach
43ZZ	Destruction of Esophagogastric Junction, Percutaneous Approach
44ZZ	Destruction of Esophagogastric Junction, Percutaneous Endoscopic Approach
47ZZ	Destruction of Esophagogastric Junction, Via Natural or Artificial Opening
48ZZ	Destruction of Esophagogastric Junction, Via Natural or Artificial Opening Endoscopic
50ZZ	Destruction of Esophagus, Open Approach
53ZZ	Destruction of Esophagus, Percutaneous Approach
54ZZ	Destruction of Esophagus, Percutaneous Endoscopic Approach
57ZZ	Destruction of Esophagus, Via Natural or Artificial Opening
58ZZ	Destruction of Esophagus, Via Natural or Artificial Opening Endoscopic
60ZZ	Destruction of Stomach, Open Approach
63ZZ	Destruction of Stomach, Percutaneous Approach
64ZZ	Destruction of Stomach, Percutaneous Endoscopic Approach
67ZZ	Destruction of Stomach, Via Natural or Artificial Opening
68ZZ	Destruction of Stomach, Via Natural or Artificial Opening Endoscopic
70ZZ	Destruction of Stomach, Pylorus, Open Approach
73ZZ	Destruction of Stomach, Pylorus, Percutaneous Approach
74ZZ	Destruction of Stomach, Pylorus, Percutaneous Endoscopic Approach
77ZZ	Destruction of Stomach, Pylorus, Via Natural or Artificial Opening
78ZZ	Destruction of Stomach, Pylorus, Via Natural or Artificial Opening Endoscopic
80ZZ	Destruction of Small Intestine, Open Approach
83ZZ	Destruction of Small Intestine, Percutaneous Approach
84ZZ	Destruction of Small Intestine, Percutaneous Endoscopic Approach
87ZZ	Destruction of Small Intestine, Via Natural or Artificial Opening
88ZZ	Destruction of Small Intestine, Via Natural or Artificial Opening Endoscopic
90ZZ	Destruction of Duodenum, Open Approach
93ZZ	Destruction of Duodenum, Percutaneous Approach
94ZZ	Destruction of Duodenum, Percutaneous Endoscopic Approach
97ZZ	Destruction of Duodenum, Via Natural or Artificial Opening
98ZZ	Destruction of Duodenum, Via Natural or Artificial Opening Endoscopic
05A0ZZ	Destruction of Jejunum, Open Approach
05A3ZZ	Destruction of Jejunum, Percutaneous Approach
05A4ZZ	Destruction of Jejunum, Percutaneous Endoscopic Approach
05A7ZZ	Destruction of Jejunum, Via Natural or Artificial Opening
05A8ZZ	Destruction of Jejunum, Via Natural or Artificial Opening Endoscopic
05B0ZZ	Destruction of Ileum, Open Approach
05B3ZZ	Destruction of Ileum, Percutaneous Approach
05B4ZZ	Destruction of Ileum, Percutaneous Endoscopic Approach
05B7ZZ	Destruction of Ileum, Via Natural or Artificial Opening

0D5B8ZZ	Destruction of Ileum, Via Natural or Artificial Opening Endoscopic
0D5C0ZZ	Destruction of Ileocecal Valve, Open Approach
0D5C3ZZ	Destruction of Ileocecal Valve, Percutaneous Approach
0D5C4ZZ	Destruction of Ileocecal Valve, Percutaneous Endoscopic Approach
0D5C7ZZ	Destruction of Ileocecal Valve, Via Natural or Artificial Opening
0D5C8ZZ	Destruction of Ileocecal Valve, Via Natural or Artificial Opening Endoscopic
0D5E0ZZ	Destruction of Large Intestine, Open Approach
0D5E3ZZ	Destruction of Large Intestine, Percutaneous Approach
0D5E4ZZ	Destruction of Large Intestine, Percutaneous Endoscopic Approach
0D5E7ZZ	Destruction of Large Intestine, Via Natural or Artificial Opening
0D5E8ZZ	Destruction of Large Intestine, Via Natural or Artificial Opening Endoscopic
0D5F0ZZ	Destruction of Right Large Intestine, Open Approach
0D5F3ZZ	Destruction of Right Large Intestine, Percutaneous Approach
0D5F4ZZ	Destruction of Right Large Intestine, Percutaneous Endoscopic Approach
0D5F7ZZ	Destruction of Right Large Intestine, Via Natural or Artificial Opening
0D5F8ZZ	Destruction of Right Large Intestine, Via Natural or Artificial Opening Endoscopic
0D5G0ZZ	Destruction of Left Large Intestine, Open Approach
0D5G3ZZ	Destruction of Left Large Intestine, Percutaneous Approach
0D5G4ZZ	Destruction of Left Large Intestine, Percutaneous Endoscopic Approach
0D5G7ZZ	Destruction of Left Large Intestine, Via Natural or Artificial Opening
0D5G8ZZ	Destruction of Left Large Intestine, Via Natural or Artificial Opening Endoscopic
0D5H0ZZ	Destruction of Cecum, Open Approach
0D5H3ZZ	Destruction of Cecum, Percutaneous Approach
0D5H4ZZ	Destruction of Cecum, Percutaneous Endoscopic Approach
0D5H7ZZ	Destruction of Cecum, Via Natural or Artificial Opening
0D5H8ZZ	Destruction of Cecum, Via Natural or Artificial Opening Endoscopic
0D5J0ZZ	Destruction of Appendix, Open Approach
0D5J3ZZ	Destruction of Appendix, Percutaneous Approach
0D5J4ZZ	Destruction of Appendix, Percutaneous Endoscopic Approach
0D5J7ZZ	Destruction of Appendix, Via Natural or Artificial Opening
0D5J8ZZ	Destruction of Appendix, Via Natural or Artificial Opening Endoscopic
0D5K0ZZ	Destruction of Ascending Colon, Open Approach
0D5K3ZZ	Destruction of Ascending Colon, Percutaneous Approach
0D5K4ZZ	Destruction of Ascending Colon, Percutaneous Endoscopic Approach
0D5K7ZZ	Destruction of Ascending Colon, Via Natural or Artificial Opening
0D5K8ZZ	Destruction of Ascending Colon, Via Natural or Artificial Opening Endoscopic
0D5L0ZZ	Destruction of Transverse Colon, Open Approach
0D5L3ZZ	Destruction of Transverse Colon, Percutaneous Approach
0D5L4ZZ	Destruction of Transverse Colon, Percutaneous Endoscopic Approach

0D5L7ZZ	Destruction of Transverse Colon, Via Natural or Artificial Opening
0D5L8ZZ	Destruction of Transverse Colon, Via Natural or Artificial Opening Endoscopic
0D5M0ZZ	Destruction of Descending Colon, Open Approach
0D5M3ZZ	Destruction of Descending Colon, Percutaneous Approach
0D5M4ZZ	Destruction of Descending Colon, Percutaneous Endoscopic Approach
0D5M7ZZ	Destruction of Descending Colon, Via Natural or Artificial Opening
0D5M8ZZ	Destruction of Descending Colon, Via Natural or Artificial Opening Endoscopic
0D5N0ZZ	Destruction of Sigmoid Colon, Open Approach
0D5N3ZZ	Destruction of Sigmoid Colon, Percutaneous Approach
0D5N4ZZ	Destruction of Sigmoid Colon, Percutaneous Endoscopic Approach
0D5N7ZZ	Destruction of Sigmoid Colon, Via Natural or Artificial Opening
0D5N8ZZ	Destruction of Sigmoid Colon, Via Natural or Artificial Opening Endoscopic
0D5P0ZZ	Destruction of Rectum, Open Approach
0D5P3ZZ	Destruction of Rectum, Percutaneous Approach
0D5P4ZZ	Destruction of Rectum, Percutaneous Endoscopic Approach
0D5P7ZZ	Destruction of Rectum, Via Natural or Artificial Opening
0D5P8ZZ	Destruction of Rectum, Via Natural or Artificial Opening Endoscopic
0D5Q0ZZ	Destruction of Anus, Open Approach
0D5Q3ZZ	Destruction of Anus, Percutaneous Approach
0D5Q4ZZ	Destruction of Anus, Percutaneous Endoscopic Approach
0D5Q7ZZ	Destruction of Anus, Via Natural or Artificial Opening
0D5Q8ZZ	Destruction of Anus, Via Natural or Artificial Opening Endoscopic
0D5QXZZ	Destruction of Anus, External Approach
0D5R0ZZ	Destruction of Anal Sphincter, Open Approach
0D5R3ZZ	Destruction of Anal Sphincter, Percutaneous Approach
0D5R4ZZ	Destruction of Anal Sphincter, Percutaneous Endoscopic Approach
0D5S0ZZ	Destruction of Greater Omentum, Open Approach
0D5S3ZZ	Destruction of Greater Omentum, Percutaneous Approach
0D5S4ZZ	Destruction of Greater Omentum, Percutaneous Endoscopic Approach
0D5T0ZZ	Destruction of Lesser Omentum, Open Approach
0D5T3ZZ	Destruction of Lesser Omentum, Percutaneous Approach
0D5T4ZZ	Destruction of Lesser Omentum, Percutaneous Endoscopic Approach
0D5V0ZZ	Destruction of Mesentery, Open Approach
0D5V3ZZ	Destruction of Mesentery, Percutaneous Approach
0D5V4ZZ	Destruction of Mesentery, Percutaneous Endoscopic Approach
0D5W0ZZ	Destruction of Peritoneum, Open Approach
0D5W3ZZ	Destruction of Peritoneum, Percutaneous Approach
0D5W4ZZ	Destruction of Peritoneum, Percutaneous Endoscopic Approach

---

Female-only	♂ Male-only	▲ Limited Coverage	● Non-OR	▧ HAC-associated procedure
▲ Non-covered procedures			✚ Combination	

0D710DZ Dilation of Upper Esophagus with Intraluminal Device, Open Approach

0D710ZZ Dilation of Upper Esophagus, Open Approach

0D713DZ Dilation of Upper Esophagus with Intraluminal Device, Percutaneous Approach

0D713ZZ Dilation of Upper Esophagus, Percutaneous Approach

0D714DZ Dilation of Upper Esophagus with Intraluminal Device, Percutaneous Endoscopic Approach

0D714ZZ Dilation of Upper Esophagus, Percutaneous Endoscopic Approach

0D717DZ Dilation of Upper Esophagus with Intraluminal Device, Via Natural or Artificial Opening

0D717ZZ Dilation of Upper Esophagus, Via Natural or Artificial Opening

0D718DZ Dilation of Upper Esophagus with Intraluminal Device, Via Natural or Artificial Opening Endoscopic

0D718ZZ Dilation of Upper Esophagus, Via Natural or Artificial Opening Endoscopic

0D720DZ Dilation of Middle Esophagus with Intraluminal Device, Open Approach

0D720ZZ Dilation of Middle Esophagus, Open Approach

0D723DZ Dilation of Middle Esophagus with Intraluminal Device, Percutaneous Approach

0D723ZZ Dilation of Middle Esophagus, Percutaneous Approach

0D724DZ Dilation of Middle Esophagus with Intraluminal Device, Percutaneous Endoscopic Approach

0D724ZZ Dilation of Middle Esophagus, Percutaneous Endoscopic Approach

0D727DZ Dilation of Middle Esophagus with Intraluminal Device, Via Natural or Artificial Opening

0D727ZZ Dilation of Middle Esophagus, Via Natural or Artificial Opening

0D728DZ Dilation of Middle Esophagus with Intraluminal Device, Via Natural or Artificial Opening Endoscopic

0D728ZZ Dilation of Middle Esophagus, Via Natural or Artificial Opening Endoscopic

0D730DZ Dilation of Lower Esophagus with Intraluminal Device, Open Approach

0D730ZZ Dilation of Lower Esophagus, Open Approach

0D733DZ Dilation of Lower Esophagus with Intraluminal Device, Percutaneous Approach

0D733ZZ Dilation of Lower Esophagus, Percutaneous Approach

0D734DZ Dilation of Lower Esophagus with Intraluminal Device, Percutaneous Endoscopic Approach

0D734ZZ Dilation of Lower Esophagus, Percutaneous Endoscopic Approach

0D737DZ Dilation of Lower Esophagus with Intraluminal Device, Via Natural or Artificial Opening

0D737ZZ Dilation of Lower Esophagus, Via Natural or Artificial Opening

0D738DZ Dilation of Lower Esophagus with Intraluminal Device, Via Natural or Artificial Opening Endoscopic

0D738ZZ Dilation of Lower Esophagus, Via Natural or Artificial Opening Endoscopic

0D740DZ Dilation of Esophagogastric Junction with Intraluminal Device, Open Approach

0D740ZZ Dilation of Esophagogastric Junction, Open Approach

0D743DZ Dilation of Esophagogastric Junction with Intraluminal Device, Percutaneous Approach

0D743ZZ Dilation of Esophagogastric Junction, Percutaneous Approach

0D744DZ Dilation of Esophagogastric Junction with Intraluminal Device, Percutaneous Endoscopic Approach

0D744ZZ Dilation of Esophagogastric Junction, Percutaneous Endoscopic Approach

0D747DZ Dilation of Esophagogastric Junction with Intraluminal Device, Via Natural or Artificial Opening

0D747ZZ Dilation of Esophagogastric Junction, Via Natural or Artificial Opening

0D748DZ Dilation of Esophagogastric Junction with Intraluminal Device, Via Natural or Artificial Opening Endoscopic

0D748ZZ Dilation of Esophagogastric Junction, Via Natural or Artificial Opening Endoscopic

0D750DZ Dilation of Esophagus with Intraluminal Device, Open Approach

0D750ZZ Dilation of Esophagus, Open Approach

0D753DZ Dilation of Esophagus with Intraluminal Device, Percutaneous Approach

0D753ZZ Dilation of Esophagus, Percutaneous Approach

0D754DZ Dilation of Esophagus with Intraluminal Device, Percutaneous Endoscopic Approach

0D754ZZ Dilation of Esophagus, Percutaneous Endoscopic Approach

0D757DZ Dilation of Esophagus with Intraluminal Device, Via Natural or Artificial Opening

0D757ZZ Dilation of Esophagus, Via Natural or Artificial Opening

0D758DZ Dilation of Esophagus with Intraluminal Device, Via Natural or Artificial Opening Endoscopic

0D758ZZ Dilation of Esophagus, Via Natural or Artificial Opening Endoscopic

0D760DZ Dilation of Stomach with Intraluminal Device, Open Approach

0D760ZZ Dilation of Stomach, Open Approach

0D763DZ Dilation of Stomach with Intraluminal Device, Percutaneous Approach

0D763ZZ Dilation of Stomach, Percutaneous Approach

0D764DZ Dilation of Stomach with Intraluminal Device, Percutaneous Endoscopic Approach

0D764ZZ Dilation of Stomach, Percutaneous Endoscopic Approach

0D767DZ Dilation of Stomach with Intraluminal Device, Via Natural or Artificial Opening

0D767ZZ Dilation of Stomach, Via Natural or Artificial Opening

0D768DZ Dilation of Stomach with Intraluminal Device, Via Natural or Artificial Opening Endoscopic

0D768ZZ Dilation of Stomach, Via Natural or Artificial Opening Endoscopic

AHA CC: 4Q, 2014, 40

0D770DZ Dilation of Stomach, Pylorus with Intraluminal Device, Open Approach

0D770ZZ Dilation of Stomach, Pylorus, Open Approach

0D773DZ Dilation of Stomach, Pylorus with Intraluminal Device, Percutaneous Approach

0D773ZZ Dilation of Stomach, Pylorus, Percutaneous Approach

0D774DZ Dilation of Stomach, Pylorus with Intraluminal Device, Percutaneous Endoscopic Approach

0D774ZZ Dilation of Stomach, Pylorus, Percutaneous Endoscopic Approach

0D777DZ Dilation of Stomach, Pylorus with Intraluminal Device, Via Natural or Artificial Opening

0D777ZZ Dilation of Stomach, Pylorus, Via Natural or Artificial Opening

0D778DZ Dilation of Stomach, Pylorus with Intraluminal Device, Via Natural or Artificial Opening Endoscopic

● **0D778ZZ** Dilation of Stomach, Pylorus, Via Natural or Artificial Opening Endoscopic

0D780DZ Dilation of Small Intestine with Intraluminal Device, Open Approach

0D780ZZ Dilation of Small Intestine, Open Approach

0D783DZ Dilation of Small Intestine with Intraluminal Device, Percutaneous Approach

0D783ZZ Dilation of Small Intestine, Percutaneous Approach

0D784DZ Dilation of Small Intestine with Intraluminal Device, Percutaneous Endoscopic Approach

0D784ZZ Dilation of Small Intestine, Percutaneous Endoscopic Approach

0D787DZ Dilation of Small Intestine with Intraluminal Device, Via Natural or Artificial Opening

0D787ZZ Dilation of Small Intestine, Via Natural or Artificial Opening

0D788DZ Dilation of Small Intestine with Intraluminal Device, Via Natural or Artificial Opening Endoscopic

0D788ZZ Dilation of Small Intestine, Via Natural or Artificial Opening Endoscopic

0D790DZ Dilation of Duodenum with Intraluminal Device, Open Approach

0D790ZZ Dilation of Duodenum, Open Approach

0D793DZ Dilation of Duodenum with Intraluminal Device, Percutaneous Approach

0D793ZZ Dilation of Duodenum, Percutaneous Approach

0D794DZ Dilation of Duodenum with Intraluminal Device, Percutaneous Endoscopic Approach

0D794ZZ Dilation of Duodenum, Percutaneous Endoscopic Approach

0D797DZ Dilation of Duodenum with Intraluminal Device, Via Natural or Artificial Opening

0D797ZZ Dilation of Duodenum, Via Natural or Artificial Opening

0D798DZ Dilation of Duodenum with Intraluminal Device, Via Natural or Artificial Opening Endoscopic

0D798ZZ Dilation of Duodenum, Via Natural or Artificial Opening Endoscopic

0D7A0DZ Dilation of Jejunum with Intraluminal Device, Open Approach

0D7A0ZZ Dilation of Jejunum, Open Approach

0D7A3DZ Dilation of Jejunum with Intraluminal Device, Percutaneous Approach

0D7A3ZZ Dilation of Jejunum, Percutaneous Approach

0D7A4DZ Dilation of Jejunum with Intraluminal Device, Percutaneous Endoscopic Approach

0D7A4ZZ Dilation of Jejunum, Percutaneous Endoscopic Approach

0D7A7DZ Dilation of Jejunum with Intraluminal Device, Via Natural or Artificial Opening

0D7A7ZZ Dilation of Jejunum, Via Natural or Artificial Opening

0D7A8DZ Dilation of Jejunum with Intraluminal Device, Via Natural or Artificial Opening Endoscopic

A8ZZ Dilation of Jejunum, Via Natural or Artificial Opening Endoscopic
AHA CC: 4Q, 2014, 40

B0DZ Dilation of Ileum with Intraluminal Device, Open Approach

B0ZZ Dilation of Ileum, Open Approach

B3DZ Dilation of Ileum with Intraluminal Device, Percutaneous Approach

B3ZZ Dilation of Ileum, Percutaneous Approach

B4DZ Dilation of Ileum with Intraluminal Device, Percutaneous Endoscopic Approach

B4ZZ Dilation of Ileum, Percutaneous Endoscopic Approach

B7DZ Dilation of Ileum with Intraluminal Device, Via Natural or Artificial Opening

B7ZZ Dilation of Ileum, Via Natural or Artificial Opening

B8DZ Dilation of Ileum with Intraluminal Device, Via Natural or Artificial Opening Endoscopic

B8ZZ Dilation of Ileum, Via Natural or Artificial Opening Endoscopic

C0DZ Dilation of Ileocecal Valve with Intraluminal Device, Open Approach

C0ZZ Dilation of Ileocecal Valve, Open Approach

C3DZ Dilation of Ileocecal Valve with Intraluminal Device, Percutaneous Approach

C3ZZ Dilation of Ileocecal Valve, Percutaneous Approach

C4DZ Dilation of Ileocecal Valve with Intraluminal Device, Percutaneous Endoscopic Approach

C4ZZ Dilation of Ileocecal Valve, Percutaneous Endoscopic Approach

C7DZ Dilation of Ileocecal Valve with Intraluminal Device, Via Natural or Artificial Opening

C7ZZ Dilation of Ileocecal Valve, Via Natural or Artificial Opening

C8DZ Dilation of Ileocecal Valve with Intraluminal Device, Via Natural or Artificial Opening Endoscopic

C8ZZ Dilation of Ileocecal Valve, Via Natural or Artificial Opening Endoscopic

7E0DZ Dilation of Large Intestine with Intraluminal Device, Open Approach

7E0ZZ Dilation of Large Intestine, Open Approach

7E3DZ Dilation of Large Intestine with Intraluminal Device, Percutaneous Approach

7E3ZZ Dilation of Large Intestine, Percutaneous Approach

7E4DZ Dilation of Large Intestine with Intraluminal Device, Percutaneous Endoscopic Approach

7E4ZZ Dilation of Large Intestine, Percutaneous Endoscopic Approach

7E7DZ Dilation of Large Intestine with Intraluminal Device, Via Natural or Artificial Opening

7E7ZZ Dilation of Large Intestine, Via Natural or Artificial Opening

7E8DZ Dilation of Large Intestine with Intraluminal Device, Via Natural or Artificial Opening Endoscopic

7E8ZZ Dilation of Large Intestine, Via Natural or Artificial Opening Endoscopic

7F0DZ Dilation of Right Large Intestine with Intraluminal Device, Open Approach

7F0ZZ Dilation of Right Large Intestine, Open Approach

7F3DZ Dilation of Right Large Intestine with Intraluminal Device, Percutaneous Approach

0D7F3ZZ Dilation of Right Large Intestine, Percutaneous Approach

0D7F4DZ Dilation of Right Large Intestine with Intraluminal Device, Percutaneous Endoscopic Approach

0D7F4ZZ Dilation of Right Large Intestine, Percutaneous Endoscopic Approach

0D7F7DZ Dilation of Right Large Intestine with Intraluminal Device, Via Natural or Artificial Opening

0D7F7ZZ Dilation of Right Large Intestine, Via Natural or Artificial Opening

0D7F8DZ Dilation of Right Large Intestine with Intraluminal Device, Via Natural or Artificial Opening Endoscopic

0D7F8ZZ Dilation of Right Large Intestine, Via Natural or Artificial Opening Endoscopic

0D7G0DZ Dilation of Left Large Intestine with Intraluminal Device, Open Approach

0D7G0ZZ Dilation of Left Large Intestine, Open Approach

0D7G3DZ Dilation of Left Large Intestine with Intraluminal Device, Percutaneous Approach

0D7G3ZZ Dilation of Left Large Intestine, Percutaneous Approach

0D7G4DZ Dilation of Left Large Intestine with Intraluminal Device, Percutaneous Endoscopic Approach

0D7G4ZZ Dilation of Left Large Intestine, Percutaneous Endoscopic Approach

0D7G7DZ Dilation of Left Large Intestine with Intraluminal Device, Via Natural or Artificial Opening

0D7G7ZZ Dilation of Left Large Intestine, Via Natural or Artificial Opening

0D7G8DZ Dilation of Left Large Intestine with Intraluminal Device, Via Natural or Artificial Opening Endoscopic

0D7G8ZZ Dilation of Left Large Intestine, Via Natural or Artificial Opening Endoscopic

0D7H0DZ Dilation of Cecum with Intraluminal Device, Open Approach

0D7H0ZZ Dilation of Cecum, Open Approach

0D7H3DZ Dilation of Cecum with Intraluminal Device, Percutaneous Approach

0D7H3ZZ Dilation of Cecum, Percutaneous Approach

0D7H4DZ Dilation of Cecum with Intraluminal Device, Percutaneous Endoscopic Approach

0D7H4ZZ Dilation of Cecum, Percutaneous Endoscopic Approach

0D7H7DZ Dilation of Cecum with Intraluminal Device, Via Natural or Artificial Opening

0D7H7ZZ Dilation of Cecum, Via Natural or Artificial Opening

0D7H8DZ Dilation of Cecum with Intraluminal Device, Via Natural or Artificial Opening Endoscopic

0D7H8ZZ Dilation of Cecum, Via Natural or Artificial Opening Endoscopic

0D7K0DZ Dilation of Ascending Colon with Intraluminal Device, Open Approach

0D7K0ZZ Dilation of Ascending Colon, Open Approach

0D7K3DZ Dilation of Ascending Colon with Intraluminal Device, Percutaneous Approach

0D7K3ZZ Dilation of Ascending Colon, Percutaneous Approach

0D7K4DZ Dilation of Ascending Colon with Intraluminal Device, Percutaneous Endoscopic Approach

0D7K4ZZ Dilation of Ascending Colon, Percutaneous Endoscopic Approach

0D7K7DZ Dilation of Ascending Colon with Intraluminal Device, Via Natural or Artificial Opening

0D7K7ZZ Dilation of Ascending Colon, Via Natural or Artificial Opening

0D7K8DZ Dilation of Ascending Colon with Intraluminal Device, Via Natural or Artificial Opening Endoscopic

0D7K8ZZ Dilation of Ascending Colon, Via Natural or Artificial Opening Endoscopic

0D7L0DZ Dilation of Transverse Colon with Intraluminal Device, Open Approach

0D7L0ZZ Dilation of Transverse Colon, Open Approach

0D7L3DZ Dilation of Transverse Colon with Intraluminal Device, Percutaneous Approach

0D7L3ZZ Dilation of Transverse Colon, Percutaneous Approach

0D7L4DZ Dilation of Transverse Colon with Intraluminal Device, Percutaneous Endoscopic Approach

0D7L4ZZ Dilation of Transverse Colon, Percutaneous Endoscopic Approach

0D7L7DZ Dilation of Transverse Colon with Intraluminal Device, Via Natural or Artificial Opening

0D7L7ZZ Dilation of Transverse Colon, Via Natural or Artificial Opening

0D7L8DZ Dilation of Transverse Colon with Intraluminal Device, Via Natural or Artificial Opening Endoscopic

0D7L8ZZ Dilation of Transverse Colon, Via Natural or Artificial Opening Endoscopic

0D7M0DZ Dilation of Descending Colon with Intraluminal Device, Open Approach

0D7M0ZZ Dilation of Descending Colon, Open Approach

0D7M3DZ Dilation of Descending Colon with Intraluminal Device, Percutaneous Approach

0D7M3ZZ Dilation of Descending Colon, Percutaneous Approach

0D7M4DZ Dilation of Descending Colon with Intraluminal Device, Percutaneous Endoscopic Approach

0D7M4ZZ Dilation of Descending Colon, Percutaneous Endoscopic Approach

0D7M7DZ Dilation of Descending Colon with Intraluminal Device, Via Natural or Artificial Opening

0D7M7ZZ Dilation of Descending Colon, Via Natural or Artificial Opening

0D7M8DZ Dilation of Descending Colon with Intraluminal Device, Via Natural or Artificial Opening Endoscopic

0D7M8ZZ Dilation of Descending Colon, Via Natural or Artificial Opening Endoscopic

0D7N0DZ Dilation of Sigmoid Colon with Intraluminal Device, Open Approach

0D7N0ZZ Dilation of Sigmoid Colon, Open Approach

0D7N3DZ Dilation of Sigmoid Colon with Intraluminal Device, Percutaneous Approach

0D7N3ZZ Dilation of Sigmoid Colon, Percutaneous Approach

0D7N4DZ Dilation of Sigmoid Colon with Intraluminal Device, Percutaneous Endoscopic Approach

0D7N4ZZ Dilation of Sigmoid Colon, Percutaneous Endoscopic Approach

Female-only   ♂ Male-only   ▲ Limited Coverage   ● Non-OR   ▨ HAC-associated procedure   ▲ Non-covered procedures   ✚ Combination

0D7N7DZ	Dilation of Sigmoid Colon with Intraluminal Device, Via Natural or Artificial Opening
0D7N7ZZ	Dilation of Sigmoid Colon, Via Natural or Artificial Opening
0D7N8DZ	Dilation of Sigmoid Colon with Intraluminal Device, Via Natural or Artificial Opening Endoscopic
0D7N8ZZ	Dilation of Sigmoid Colon, Via Natural or Artificial Opening Endoscopic
0D7P0DZ	Dilation of Rectum with Intraluminal Device, Open Approach
0D7P0ZZ	Dilation of Rectum, Open Approach
0D7P3DZ	Dilation of Rectum with Intraluminal Device, Percutaneous Approach
0D7P3ZZ	Dilation of Rectum, Percutaneous Approach
0D7P4DZ	Dilation of Rectum with Intraluminal Device, Percutaneous Endoscopic Approach
0D7P4ZZ	Dilation of Rectum, Percutaneous Endoscopic Approach
0D7P7DZ	Dilation of Rectum with Intraluminal Device, Via Natural or Artificial Opening
0D7P7ZZ	Dilation of Rectum, Via Natural or Artificial Opening
0D7P8DZ	Dilation of Rectum with Intraluminal Device, Via Natural or Artificial Opening Endoscopic
0D7P8ZZ	Dilation of Rectum, Via Natural or Artificial Opening Endoscopic
0D7Q0DZ	Dilation of Anus with Intraluminal Device, Open Approach
0D7Q0ZZ	Dilation of Anus, Open Approach
0D7Q3DZ	Dilation of Anus with Intraluminal Device, Percutaneous Approach
0D7Q3ZZ	Dilation of Anus, Percutaneous Appro⟨...⟩
0D7Q4DZ	Dilation of Anus with Intraluminal Device, Percutaneous Endoscopic Approach
0D7Q4ZZ	Dilation of Anus, Percutaneous Endoscopic Approach
0D7Q7DZ	Dilation of Anus with Intraluminal Device, Via Natural or Artificial Open⟨...⟩
0D7Q7ZZ	Dilation of Anus, Via Natural or Artif⟨...⟩ Opening
0D7Q8DZ	Dilation of Anus with Intraluminal Device, Via Natural or Artificial Open⟨...⟩ Endoscopic
0D7Q8ZZ	Dilation of Anus, Via Natural or Artifi⟨...⟩ Opening Endoscopic

0D8 – Gastrointestinal System, Division

Review Coding Guideline B3.14

0D840ZZ	Division of Esophagogastric Junction, Open Approach
0D843ZZ	Division of Esophagogastric Junction, Percutaneous Approach
0D844ZZ	Division of Esophagogastric Junction, Percutaneous Endoscopic Approach
0D847ZZ	Division of Esophagogastric Junction, Via Natural or Artificial Opening
0D848ZZ	Division of Esophagogastric Junction, Via Natural or Artificial Opening Endoscopic
0D870ZZ	Division of Stomach, Pylorus, Open Approach
0D873ZZ	Division of Stomach, Pylorus, Percutaneous Approach
0D874ZZ	Division of Stomach, Pylorus, Percutaneous Endoscopic Approach
0D877ZZ	Division of Stomach, Pylorus, Via Nat⟨...⟩ or Artificial Opening
0D878ZZ	Division of Stomach, Pylorus, Via Nat⟨...⟩ or Artificial Opening Endoscopic
0D8R0ZZ	Division of Anal Sphincter, Open Approach
0D8R3ZZ	Division of Anal Sphincter, Percutane⟨...⟩ Approach

0D9 – Gastrointestinal System, Drainage

Review Coding Guidelines B3.4a and B3.4b

Review Coding Guideline B6.2

0D9100Z	Drainage of Upper Esophagus with Drainage Device, Open Approach
0D910ZX	Drainage of Upper Esophagus, Open Approach, Diagnostic
0D910ZZ	Drainage of Upper Esophagus, Open Approach
0D9130Z	Drainage of Upper Esophagus with Drainage Device, Percutaneous Approach
0D913ZX	Drainage of Upper Esophagus, Percutaneous Approach, Diagnostic
0D913ZZ	Drainage of Upper Esophagus, Percutaneous Approach
0D9140Z	Drainage of Upper Esophagus with Drainage Device, Percutaneous Endoscopic Approach
0D914ZX	Drainage of Upper Esophagus, Percutaneous Endoscopic Approach, Diagnostic
0D914ZZ	Drainage of Upper Esophagus, Percutaneous Endoscopic Approach
0D9170Z	Drainage of Upper Esophagus with Drainage Device, Via Natural or Artificial Opening
0D917ZX	Drainage of Upper Esophagus, Via Natural or Artificial Opening, Diagnostic
0D917ZZ	Drainage of Upper Esophagus, Via Natural or Artificial Opening
0D9180Z	Drainage of Upper Esophagus with Drainage Device, Via Natural or Artificial Opening Endoscopic
0D918ZX	Drainage of Upper Esophagus, Via Natural or Artificial Opening Endoscopic, Diagnostic
0D918ZZ	Drainage of Upper Esophagus, Via Natural or Artificial Opening Endoscopic
0D9200Z	Drainage of Middle Esophagus with Drainage Device, Open Approach
0D920ZX	Drainage of Middle Esophagus, Open Approach, Diagnostic
0D920ZZ	Drainage of Middle Esophagus, Open Approach
0D9230Z	Drainage of Middle Esophagus with Drainage Device, Percutaneous Approach
0D923ZX	Drainage of Middle Esophagus, Percutaneous Approach, Diagnostic
0D923ZZ	Drainage of Middle Esophagus, Percutaneous Approach
0D9240Z	Drainage of Middle Esophagus with Drainage Device, Percutaneous Endoscopic Approach
0D924ZX	Drainage of Middle Esophagus, Percutaneous Endoscopic Approach, Diagnostic
0D924ZZ	Drainage of Middle Esophagus, Percutaneous Endoscopic Approach
0D9270Z	Drainage of Middle Esophagus with Drainage Device, Via Natural or Artificial Opening
0D927ZX	Drainage of Middle Esophagus, Via Natural or Artificial Opening, Diagnostic
0D927ZZ	Drainage of Middle Esophagus, Via Natural or Artificial Opening
0D9280Z	Drainage of Middle Esophagus with Drainage Device, Via Natural or Artificial Opening Endoscopic
0D928ZX	Drainage of Middle Esophagus, Via Natural or Artificial Opening Endoscopic, Diagnostic
0D928ZZ	Drainage of Middle Esophagus, Via Natural or Artificial Opening Endoscopic
0D9300Z	Drainage of Lower Esophagus with Drainage Device, Open Approach
0D930ZX	Drainage of Lower Esophagus, Open Approach, Diagnostic
0D930ZZ	Drainage of Lower Esophagus, Open Approach
0D9330Z	Drainage of Lower Esophagus with Drainage Device, Percutaneous Approa⟨...⟩
0D933ZX	Drainage of Lower Esophagus, Percutaneous Approach, Diagnostic
0D933ZZ	Drainage of Lower Esophagus, Percutaneous Approach
0D9340Z	Drainage of Lower Esophagus with Drainage Device, Percutaneous Endoscopic Approach
0D934ZX	Drainage of Lower Esophagus, Percutaneous Endoscopic Approach, Diagnostic
0D934ZZ	Drainage of Lower Esophagus, Percutaneous Endoscopic Approach
0D9370Z	Drainage of Lower Esophagus with Drainage Device, Via Natural or Artifici⟨...⟩ Opening
0D937ZX	Drainage of Lower Esophagus, Via Natural or Artificial Opening, Diagnosti⟨...⟩
0D937ZZ	Drainage of Lower Esophagus, Via Natural or Artificial Opening
0D9380Z	Drainage of Lower Esophagus with Drainage Device, Via Natural or Artifici⟨...⟩ Opening Endoscopic
0D938ZX	Drainage of Lower Esophagus, Via Natural or Artificial Opening Endoscopi⟨...⟩ Diagnostic
0D938ZZ	Drainage of Lower Esophagus, Via Natural or Artificial Opening Endoscopic
0D9400Z	Drainage of Esophagogastric Junction with Drainage Device, Open Approach
0D940ZX	Drainage of Esophagogastric Junction, Open Approach, Diagnostic
0D940ZZ	Drainage of Esophagogastric Junction, Open Approach
0D9430Z	Drainage of Esophagogastric Junction with Drainage Device, Percutaneous Approach

 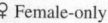

43ZX	Drainage of Esophagogastric Junction, Percutaneous Approach, Diagnostic
43ZZ	Drainage of Esophagogastric Junction, Percutaneous Approach
440Z	Drainage of Esophagogastric Junction with Drainage Device, Percutaneous Endoscopic Approach
44ZX	Drainage of Esophagogastric Junction, Percutaneous Endoscopic Approach, Diagnostic
44ZZ	Drainage of Esophagogastric Junction, Percutaneous Endoscopic Approach
470Z	Drainage of Esophagogastric Junction with Drainage Device, Via Natural or Artificial Opening
947ZX	Drainage of Esophagogastric Junction, Via Natural or Artificial Opening, Diagnostic
947ZZ	Drainage of Esophagogastric Junction, Via Natural or Artificial Opening
480Z	Drainage of Esophagogastric Junction with Drainage Device, Via Natural or Artificial Opening Endoscopic
948ZX	Drainage of Esophagogastric Junction, Via Natural or Artificial Opening Endoscopic, Diagnostic
948ZZ	Drainage of Esophagogastric Junction, Via Natural or Artificial Opening Endoscopic
9500Z	Drainage of Esophagus with Drainage Device, Open Approach
950ZX	Drainage of Esophagus, Open Approach, Diagnostic
950ZZ	Drainage of Esophagus, Open Approach
9530Z	Drainage of Esophagus with Drainage Device, Percutaneous Approach
953ZX	Drainage of Esophagus, Percutaneous Approach, Diagnostic
953ZZ	Drainage of Esophagus, Percutaneous Approach
9540Z	Drainage of Esophagus with Drainage Device, Percutaneous Endoscopic Approach
954ZX	Drainage of Esophagus, Percutaneous Endoscopic Approach, Diagnostic
954ZZ	Drainage of Esophagus, Percutaneous Endoscopic Approach
9570Z	Drainage of Esophagus with Drainage Device, Via Natural or Artificial Opening
957ZX	Drainage of Esophagus, Via Natural or Artificial Opening, Diagnostic
957ZZ	Drainage of Esophagus, Via Natural or Artificial Opening
9580Z	Drainage of Esophagus with Drainage Device, Via Natural or Artificial Opening Endoscopic
958ZX	Drainage of Esophagus, Via Natural or Artificial Opening Endoscopic, Diagnostic
958ZZ	Drainage of Esophagus, Via Natural or Artificial Opening Endoscopic
9600Z	Drainage of Stomach with Drainage Device, Open Approach
960ZX	Drainage of Stomach, Open Approach, Diagnostic
960ZZ	Drainage of Stomach, Open Approach
9630Z	Drainage of Stomach with Drainage Device, Percutaneous Approach
963ZX	Drainage of Stomach, Percutaneous Approach, Diagnostic
963ZZ	Drainage of Stomach, Percutaneous Approach
9640Z	Drainage of Stomach with Drainage Device, Percutaneous Endoscopic Approach
964ZX	Drainage of Stomach, Percutaneous Endoscopic Approach, Diagnostic
0D964ZZ	Drainage of Stomach, Percutaneous Endoscopic Approach
0D9670Z	Drainage of Stomach with Drainage Device, Via Natural or Artificial Opening
0D967ZX	Drainage of Stomach, Via Natural or Artificial Opening, Diagnostic
0D967ZZ	Drainage of Stomach, Via Natural or Artificial Opening
0D9680Z	Drainage of Stomach with Drainage Device, Via Natural or Artificial Opening Endoscopic
0D968ZX	Drainage of Stomach, Via Natural or Artificial Opening Endoscopic, Diagnostic
0D968ZZ	Drainage of Stomach, Via Natural or Artificial Opening Endoscopic
0D9700Z	Drainage of Stomach, Pylorus with Drainage Device, Open Approach
0D970ZX	Drainage of Stomach, Pylorus, Open Approach, Diagnostic
0D970ZZ	Drainage of Stomach, Pylorus, Open Approach
0D9730Z	Drainage of Stomach, Pylorus with Drainage Device, Percutaneous Approach
0D973ZX	Drainage of Stomach, Pylorus, Percutaneous Approach, Diagnostic
0D973ZZ	Drainage of Stomach, Pylorus, Percutaneous Approach
0D9740Z	Drainage of Stomach, Pylorus with Drainage Device, Percutaneous Endoscopic Approach
0D974ZX	Drainage of Stomach, Pylorus, Percutaneous Endoscopic Approach, Diagnostic
0D974ZZ	Drainage of Stomach, Pylorus, Percutaneous Endoscopic Approach
0D9770Z	Drainage of Stomach, Pylorus with Drainage Device, Via Natural or Artificial Opening
0D977ZX	Drainage of Stomach, Pylorus, Via Natural or Artificial Opening, Diagnostic
0D977ZZ	Drainage of Stomach, Pylorus, Via Natural or Artificial Opening
0D9780Z	Drainage of Stomach, Pylorus with Drainage Device, Via Natural or Artificial Opening Endoscopic
0D978ZX	Drainage of Stomach, Pylorus, Via Natural or Artificial Opening Endoscopic, Diagnostic
0D978ZZ	Drainage of Stomach, Pylorus, Via Natural or Artificial Opening Endoscopic
0D9800Z	Drainage of Small Intestine with Drainage Device, Open Approach
0D980ZX	Drainage of Small Intestine, Open Approach, Diagnostic
0D980ZZ	Drainage of Small Intestine, Open Approach
0D9830Z	Drainage of Small Intestine with Drainage Device, Percutaneous Approach
0D983ZX	Drainage of Small Intestine, Percutaneous Approach, Diagnostic
0D983ZZ	Drainage of Small Intestine, Percutaneous Approach
0D9840Z	Drainage of Small Intestine with Drainage Device, Percutaneous Endoscopic Approach
0D984ZX	Drainage of Small Intestine, Percutaneous Endoscopic Approach, Diagnostic
0D984ZZ	Drainage of Small Intestine, Percutaneous Endoscopic Approach
0D9870Z	Drainage of Small Intestine with Drainage Device, Via Natural or Artificial Opening
0D987ZX	Drainage of Small Intestine, Via Natural or Artificial Opening, Diagnostic
0D987ZZ	Drainage of Small Intestine, Via Natural or Artificial Opening
0D9880Z	Drainage of Small Intestine with Drainage Device, Via Natural or Artificial Opening Endoscopic
0D988ZX	Drainage of Small Intestine, Via Natural or Artificial Opening Endoscopic, Diagnostic
0D988ZZ	Drainage of Small Intestine, Via Natural or Artificial Opening Endoscopic
0D9900Z	Drainage of Duodenum with Drainage Device, Open Approach
0D990ZX	Drainage of Duodenum, Open Approach, Diagnostic
0D990ZZ	Drainage of Duodenum, Open Approach
0D9930Z	Drainage of Duodenum with Drainage Device, Percutaneous Approach
0D993ZX	Drainage of Duodenum, Percutaneous Approach, Diagnostic
0D993ZZ	Drainage of Duodenum, Percutaneous Approach
0D9940Z	Drainage of Duodenum with Drainage Device, Percutaneous Endoscopic Approach
0D994ZX	Drainage of Duodenum, Percutaneous Endoscopic Approach, Diagnostic
0D994ZZ	Drainage of Duodenum, Percutaneous Endoscopic Approach
0D9970Z	Drainage of Duodenum with Drainage Device, Via Natural or Artificial Opening
0D997ZX	Drainage of Duodenum, Via Natural or Artificial Opening, Diagnostic
0D997ZZ	Drainage of Duodenum, Via Natural or Artificial Opening
0D9980Z	Drainage of Duodenum with Drainage Device, Via Natural or Artificial Opening Endoscopic
0D998ZX	Drainage of Duodenum, Via Natural or Artificial Opening Endoscopic, Diagnostic
0D998ZZ	Drainage of Duodenum, Via Natural or Artificial Opening Endoscopic
0D9A00Z	Drainage of Jejunum with Drainage Device, Open Approach
0D9A0ZX	Drainage of Jejunum, Open Approach, Diagnostic
0D9A0ZZ	Drainage of Jejunum, Open Approach
0D9A30Z	Drainage of Jejunum with Drainage Device, Percutaneous Approach
0D9A3ZX	Drainage of Jejunum, Percutaneous Approach, Diagnostic
0D9A3ZZ	Drainage of Jejunum, Percutaneous Approach
0D9A40Z	Drainage of Jejunum with Drainage Device, Percutaneous Endoscopic Approach
0D9A4ZX	Drainage of Jejunum, Percutaneous Endoscopic Approach, Diagnostic
0D9A4ZZ	Drainage of Jejunum, Percutaneous Endoscopic Approach
0D9A70Z	Drainage of Jejunum with Drainage Device, Via Natural or Artificial Opening
0D9A7ZX	Drainage of Jejunum, Via Natural or Artificial Opening, Diagnostic
0D9A7ZZ	Drainage of Jejunum, Via Natural or Artificial Opening
0D9A80Z	Drainage of Jejunum with Drainage Device, Via Natural or Artificial Opening Endoscopic
0D9A8ZX	Drainage of Jejunum, Via Natural or Artificial Opening Endoscopic, Diagnostic
0D9A8ZZ	Drainage of Jejunum, Via Natural or Artificial Opening Endoscopic
0D9B00Z	Drainage of Ileum with Drainage Device, Open Approach
0D9B0ZX	Drainage of Ileum, Open Approach, Diagnostic
0D9B0ZZ	Drainage of Ileum, Open Approach
0D9B30Z	Drainage of Ileum with Drainage Device, Percutaneous Approach

Female-only   ♂ Male-only   ▲ Limited Coverage   ● Non-OR   ▬ HAC-associated procedure   ▲ Non-covered procedures   + Combination

0D9B3ZX	Drainage of Ileum, Percutaneous Approach, Diagnostic
0D9B3ZZ	Drainage of Ileum, Percutaneous Approach
0D9B40Z	Drainage of Ileum with Drainage Device, Percutaneous Endoscopic Approach
0D9B4ZX	Drainage of Ileum, Percutaneous Endoscopic Approach, Diagnostic
0D9B4ZZ	Drainage of Ileum, Percutaneous Endoscopic Approach
0D9B70Z	Drainage of Ileum with Drainage Device, Via Natural or Artificial Opening
0D9B7ZX	Drainage of Ileum, Via Natural or Artificial Opening, Diagnostic
0D9B7ZZ	Drainage of Ileum, Via Natural or Artificial Opening
0D9B80Z	Drainage of Ileum with Drainage Device, Via Natural or Artificial Opening Endoscopic
0D9B8ZX	Drainage of Ileum, Via Natural or Artificial Opening Endoscopic, Diagnostic
0D9B8ZZ	Drainage of Ileum, Via Natural or Artificial Opening Endoscopic
0D9C00Z	Drainage of Ileocecal Valve with Drainage Device, Open Approach
0D9C0ZX	Drainage of Ileocecal Valve, Open Approach, Diagnostic
0D9C0ZZ	Drainage of Ileocecal Valve, Open Approach
0D9C30Z	Drainage of Ileocecal Valve with Drainage Device, Percutaneous Approach
0D9C3ZX	Drainage of Ileocecal Valve, Percutaneous Approach, Diagnostic
0D9C3ZZ	Drainage of Ileocecal Valve, Percutaneous Approach
0D9C40Z	Drainage of Ileocecal Valve with Drainage Device, Percutaneous Endoscopic Approach
0D9C4ZX	Drainage of Ileocecal Valve, Percutaneous Endoscopic Approach, Diagnostic
0D9C4ZZ	Drainage of Ileocecal Valve, Percutaneous Endoscopic Approach
0D9C70Z	Drainage of Ileocecal Valve with Drainage Device, Via Natural or Artificial Opening
0D9C7ZX	Drainage of Ileocecal Valve, Via Natural or Artificial Opening, Diagnostic
0D9C7ZZ	Drainage of Ileocecal Valve, Via Natural or Artificial Opening
0D9C80Z	Drainage of Ileocecal Valve with Drainage Device, Via Natural or Artificial Opening Endoscopic
0D9C8ZX	Drainage of Ileocecal Valve, Via Natural or Artificial Opening Endoscopic, Diagnostic
0D9C8ZZ	Drainage of Ileocecal Valve, Via Natural or Artificial Opening Endoscopic
0D9E00Z	Drainage of Large Intestine with Drainage Device, Open Approach
0D9E0ZX	Drainage of Large Intestine, Open Approach, Diagnostic
0D9E0ZZ	Drainage of Large Intestine, Open Approach
0D9E30Z	Drainage of Large Intestine with Drainage Device, Percutaneous Approach
0D9E3ZX	Drainage of Large Intestine, Percutaneous Approach, Diagnostic
0D9E3ZZ	Drainage of Large Intestine, Percutaneous Approach
0D9E40Z	Drainage of Large Intestine with Drainage Device, Percutaneous Endoscopic Approach
0D9E4ZX	Drainage of Large Intestine, Percutaneous Endoscopic Approach, Diagnostic
0D9E4ZZ	Drainage of Large Intestine, Percutaneous Endoscopic Approach
0D9E70Z	Drainage of Large Intestine with Drainage Device, Via Natural or Artificial Opening
0D9E7ZX	Drainage of Large Intestine, Via Natural or Artificial Opening, Diagnostic
0D9E7ZZ	Drainage of Large Intestine, Via Natural or Artificial Opening
0D9E80Z	Drainage of Large Intestine with Drainage Device, Via Natural or Artificial Opening Endoscopic
0D9E8ZX	Drainage of Large Intestine, Via Natural or Artificial Opening Endoscopic, Diagnostic
0D9E8ZZ	Drainage of Large Intestine, Via Natural or Artificial Opening Endoscopic
0D9F00Z	Drainage of Right Large Intestine with Drainage Device, Open Approach
0D9F0ZX	Drainage of Right Large Intestine, Open Approach, Diagnostic
0D9F0ZZ	Drainage of Right Large Intestine, Open Approach
0D9F30Z	Drainage of Right Large Intestine with Drainage Device, Percutaneous Approach
0D9F3ZX	Drainage of Right Large Intestine, Percutaneous Approach, Diagnostic
0D9F3ZZ	Drainage of Right Large Intestine, Percutaneous Approach
0D9F40Z	Drainage of Right Large Intestine with Drainage Device, Percutaneous Endoscopic Approach
0D9F4ZX	Drainage of Right Large Intestine, Percutaneous Endoscopic Approach, Diagnostic
0D9F4ZZ	Drainage of Right Large Intestine, Percutaneous Endoscopic Approach
0D9F70Z	Drainage of Right Large Intestine with Drainage Device, Via Natural or Artificial Opening
0D9F7ZX	Drainage of Right Large Intestine, Via Natural or Artificial Opening, Diagnostic
0D9F7ZZ	Drainage of Right Large Intestine, Via Natural or Artificial Opening
0D9F80Z	Drainage of Right Large Intestine with Drainage Device, Via Natural or Artificial Opening Endoscopic
0D9F8ZX	Drainage of Right Large Intestine, Via Natural or Artificial Opening Endoscopic, Diagnostic
0D9F8ZZ	Drainage of Right Large Intestine, Via Natural or Artificial Opening Endoscopic
0D9G00Z	Drainage of Left Large Intestine with Drainage Device, Open Approach
0D9G0ZX	Drainage of Left Large Intestine, Open Approach, Diagnostic
0D9G0ZZ	Drainage of Left Large Intestine, Open Approach
0D9G30Z	Drainage of Left Large Intestine with Drainage Device, Percutaneous Approach
0D9G3ZX	Drainage of Left Large Intestine, Percutaneous Approach, Diagnostic
0D9G3ZZ	Drainage of Left Large Intestine, Percutaneous Approach
0D9G40Z	Drainage of Left Large Intestine with Drainage Device, Percutaneous Endoscopic Approach
0D9G4ZX	Drainage of Left Large Intestine, Percutaneous Endoscopic Approach, Diagnostic
0D9G4ZZ	Drainage of Left Large Intestine, Percutaneous Endoscopic Approach
0D9G70Z	Drainage of Left Large Intestine with Drainage Device, Via Natural or Artificial Opening
0D9G7ZX	Drainage of Left Large Intestine, Via Natural or Artificial Opening, Diagnostic
0D9G7ZZ	Drainage of Left Large Intestine, Via Natural or Artificial Opening
0D9G80Z	Drainage of Left Large Intestine with Drainage Device, Via Natural or Artificial Opening Endoscopic
0D9G8ZX	Drainage of Left Large Intestine, Via Natural or Artificial Opening Endoscopic Diagnostic
0D9G8ZZ	Drainage of Left Large Intestine, Via Natural or Artificial Opening Endoscopic
0D9H00Z	Drainage of Cecum with Drainage Device, Open Approach
0D9H0ZX	Drainage of Cecum, Open Approach, Diagnostic
0D9H0ZZ	Drainage of Cecum, Open Approach
0D9H30Z	Drainage of Cecum with Drainage Device, Percutaneous Approach
0D9H3ZX	Drainage of Cecum, Percutaneous Approach, Diagnostic
0D9H3ZZ	Drainage of Cecum, Percutaneous Approach
0D9H40Z	Drainage of Cecum with Drainage Device, Percutaneous Endoscopic Approach
0D9H4ZX	Drainage of Cecum, Percutaneous Endoscopic Approach, Diagnostic
0D9H4ZZ	Drainage of Cecum, Percutaneous Endoscopic Approach
0D9H70Z	Drainage of Cecum with Drainage Device, Via Natural or Artificial Opening
0D9H7ZX	Drainage of Cecum, Via Natural or Artificial Opening, Diagnostic
0D9H7ZZ	Drainage of Cecum, Via Natural or Artificial Opening
0D9H80Z	Drainage of Cecum with Drainage Device, Via Natural or Artificial Opening Endoscopic
0D9H8ZX	Drainage of Cecum, Via Natural or Artificial Opening Endoscopic, Diagnostic
0D9H8ZZ	Drainage of Cecum, Via Natural or Artificial Opening Endoscopic
0D9J00Z	Drainage of Appendix with Drainage Device, Open Approach
0D9J0ZX	Drainage of Appendix, Open Approach, Diagnostic
0D9J0ZZ	Drainage of Appendix, Open Approach
0D9J30Z	Drainage of Appendix with Drainage Device, Percutaneous Approach
0D9J3ZX	Drainage of Appendix, Percutaneous Approach, Diagnostic
0D9J3ZZ	Drainage of Appendix, Percutaneous Approach
0D9J40Z	Drainage of Appendix with Drainage Device, Percutaneous Endoscopic Approach
0D9J4ZX	Drainage of Appendix, Percutaneous Endoscopic Approach, Diagnostic
0D9J4ZZ	Drainage of Appendix, Percutaneous Endoscopic Approach
0D9J70Z	Drainage of Appendix with Drainage Device, Via Natural or Artificial Opening
0D9J7ZX	Drainage of Appendix, Via Natural or Artificial Opening, Diagnostic
0D9J7ZZ	Drainage of Appendix, Via Natural or Artificial Opening
0D9J80Z	Drainage of Appendix with Drainage Device, Via Natural or Artificial Opening Endoscopic
0D9J8ZX	Drainage of Appendix, Via Natural or Artificial Opening Endoscopic, Diagnostic
0D9J8ZZ	Drainage of Appendix, Via Natural or Artificial Opening Endoscopic
0D9K00Z	Drainage of Ascending Colon with Drainage Device, Open Approach
0D9K0ZX	Drainage of Ascending Colon, Open Approach, Diagnostic
0D9K0ZZ	Drainage of Ascending Colon, Open Approach
0D9K30Z	Drainage of Ascending Colon with Drainage Device, Percutaneous Approach
0D9K3ZX	Drainage of Ascending Colon, Percutaneous Approach, Diagnostic

♀ Female-only   ♂ Male-only   ▲ Limited Coverage   ● Non-OR   ▨▨▨ HAC-associated procedure   ▲ Non-covered procedures   ✚ Combination

0D9K3ZZ Drainage of Ascending Colon, Percutaneous Approach

0D9K40Z Drainage of Ascending Colon with Drainage Device, Percutaneous Endoscopic Approach

0D9K4ZX Drainage of Ascending Colon, Percutaneous Endoscopic Approach, Diagnostic

0D9K4ZZ Drainage of Ascending Colon, Percutaneous Endoscopic Approach

0D9K70Z Drainage of Ascending Colon with Drainage Device, Via Natural or Artificial Opening

0D9K7ZX Drainage of Ascending Colon, Via Natural or Artificial Opening, Diagnostic

0D9K7ZZ Drainage of Ascending Colon, Via Natural or Artificial Opening

0D9K80Z Drainage of Ascending Colon with Drainage Device, Via Natural or Artificial Opening Endoscopic

0D9K8ZX Drainage of Ascending Colon, Via Natural or Artificial Opening Endoscopic, Diagnostic

0D9K8ZZ Drainage of Ascending Colon, Via Natural or Artificial Opening Endoscopic

0D9L00Z Drainage of Transverse Colon with Drainage Device, Open Approach

0D9L0ZX Drainage of Transverse Colon, Open Approach, Diagnostic

0D9L0ZZ Drainage of Transverse Colon, Open Approach

0D9L30Z Drainage of Transverse Colon with Drainage Device, Percutaneous Approach

0D9L3ZX Drainage of Transverse Colon, Percutaneous Approach, Diagnostic

0D9L3ZZ Drainage of Transverse Colon, Percutaneous Approach

0D9L40Z Drainage of Transverse Colon with Drainage Device, Percutaneous Endoscopic Approach

0D9L4ZX Drainage of Transverse Colon, Percutaneous Endoscopic Approach, Diagnostic

0D9L4ZZ Drainage of Transverse Colon, Percutaneous Endoscopic Approach

0D9L70Z Drainage of Transverse Colon with Drainage Device, Via Natural or Artificial Opening

0D9L7ZX Drainage of Transverse Colon, Via Natural or Artificial Opening, Diagnostic

0D9L7ZZ Drainage of Transverse Colon, Via Natural or Artificial Opening

0D9L80Z Drainage of Transverse Colon with Drainage Device, Via Natural or Artificial Opening Endoscopic

0D9L8ZX Drainage of Transverse Colon, Via Natural or Artificial Opening Endoscopic, Diagnostic

0D9L8ZZ Drainage of Transverse Colon, Via Natural or Artificial Opening Endoscopic

0D9M00Z Drainage of Descending Colon with Drainage Device, Open Approach

0D9M0ZX Drainage of Descending Colon, Open Approach, Diagnostic

0D9M0ZZ Drainage of Descending Colon, Open Approach

0D9M30Z Drainage of Descending Colon with Drainage Device, Percutaneous Approach

0D9M3ZX Drainage of Descending Colon, Percutaneous Approach, Diagnostic

0D9M3ZZ Drainage of Descending Colon, Percutaneous Approach

0D9M40Z Drainage of Descending Colon with Drainage Device, Percutaneous Endoscopic Approach

0D9M4ZX Drainage of Descending Colon, Percutaneous Endoscopic Approach, Diagnostic

0D9M4ZZ Drainage of Descending Colon, Percutaneous Endoscopic Approach

0D9M70Z Drainage of Descending Colon with Drainage Device, Via Natural or Artificial Opening

0D9M7ZX Drainage of Descending Colon, Via Natural or Artificial Opening, Diagnostic

0D9M7ZZ Drainage of Descending Colon, Via Natural or Artificial Opening

0D9M80Z Drainage of Descending Colon with Drainage Device, Via Natural or Artificial Opening Endoscopic

0D9M8ZX Drainage of Descending Colon, Via Natural or Artificial Opening Endoscopic, Diagnostic

0D9M8ZZ Drainage of Descending Colon, Via Natural or Artificial Opening Endoscopic

0D9N00Z Drainage of Sigmoid Colon with Drainage Device, Open Approach

0D9N0ZX Drainage of Sigmoid Colon, Open Approach, Diagnostic

0D9N0ZZ Drainage of Sigmoid Colon, Open Approach

0D9N30Z Drainage of Sigmoid Colon with Drainage Device, Percutaneous Approach

0D9N3ZX Drainage of Sigmoid Colon, Percutaneous Approach, Diagnostic

0D9N3ZZ Drainage of Sigmoid Colon, Percutaneous Approach

0D9N40Z Drainage of Sigmoid Colon with Drainage Device, Percutaneous Endoscopic Approach

0D9N4ZX Drainage of Sigmoid Colon, Percutaneous Endoscopic Approach, Diagnostic

0D9N4ZZ Drainage of Sigmoid Colon, Percutaneous Endoscopic Approach

0D9N70Z Drainage of Sigmoid Colon with Drainage Device, Via Natural or Artificial Opening

0D9N7ZX Drainage of Sigmoid Colon, Via Natural or Artificial Opening, Diagnostic

0D9N7ZZ Drainage of Sigmoid Colon, Via Natural or Artificial Opening

0D9N80Z Drainage of Sigmoid Colon with Drainage Device, Via Natural or Artificial Opening Endoscopic

0D9N8ZX Drainage of Sigmoid Colon, Via Natural or Artificial Opening Endoscopic, Diagnostic

0D9N8ZZ Drainage of Sigmoid Colon, Via Natural or Artificial Opening Endoscopic

0D9P00Z Drainage of Rectum with Drainage Device, Open Approach

0D9P0ZX Drainage of Rectum, Open Approach, Diagnostic

0D9P0ZZ Drainage of Rectum, Open Approach

0D9P30Z Drainage of Rectum with Drainage Device, Percutaneous Approach

0D9P3ZX Drainage of Rectum, Percutaneous Approach, Diagnostic

0D9P3ZZ Drainage of Rectum, Percutaneous Approach

0D9P40Z Drainage of Rectum with Drainage Device, Percutaneous Endoscopic Approach

0D9P4ZX Drainage of Rectum, Percutaneous Endoscopic Approach, Diagnostic

0D9P4ZZ Drainage of Rectum, Percutaneous Endoscopic Approach

0D9P70Z Drainage of Rectum with Drainage Device, Via Natural or Artificial Opening

0D9P7ZX Drainage of Rectum, Via Natural or Artificial Opening, Diagnostic

0D9P7ZZ Drainage of Rectum, Via Natural or Artificial Opening

0D9P80Z Drainage of Rectum with Drainage Device, Via Natural or Artificial Opening Endoscopic

0D9P8ZX Drainage of Rectum, Via Natural or Artificial Opening Endoscopic, Diagnostic

0D9P8ZZ Drainage of Rectum, Via Natural or Artificial Opening Endoscopic

0D9Q00Z Drainage of Anus with Drainage Device, Open Approach

0D9Q0ZX Drainage of Anus, Open Approach, Diagnostic

0D9Q0ZZ Drainage of Anus, Open Approach

0D9Q30Z Drainage of Anus with Drainage Device, Percutaneous Approach

0D9Q3ZX Drainage of Anus, Percutaneous Approach, Diagnostic

0D9Q3ZZ Drainage of Anus, Percutaneous Approach

0D9Q40Z Drainage of Anus with Drainage Device, Percutaneous Endoscopic Approach

0D9Q4ZX Drainage of Anus, Percutaneous Endoscopic Approach, Diagnostic

0D9Q4ZZ Drainage of Anus, Percutaneous Endoscopic Approach

0D9Q70Z Drainage of Anus with Drainage Device, Via Natural or Artificial Opening

0D9Q7ZX Drainage of Anus, Via Natural or Artificial Opening, Diagnostic

0D9Q7ZZ Drainage of Anus, Via Natural or Artificial Opening

0D9Q80Z Drainage of Anus with Drainage Device, Via Natural or Artificial Opening Endoscopic

0D9Q8ZX Drainage of Anus, Via Natural or Artificial Opening Endoscopic, Diagnostic

0D9Q8ZZ Drainage of Anus, Via Natural or Artificial Opening Endoscopic

0D9QX0Z Drainage of Anus with Drainage Device, External Approach

0D9QXZX Drainage of Anus, External Approach, Diagnostic

0D9QXZZ Drainage of Anus, External Approach

0D9R00Z Drainage of Anal Sphincter with Drainage Device, Open Approach

0D9R0ZX Drainage of Anal Sphincter, Open Approach, Diagnostic

0D9R0ZZ Drainage of Anal Sphincter, Open Approach

0D9R30Z Drainage of Anal Sphincter with Drainage Device, Percutaneous Approach

0D9R3ZX Drainage of Anal Sphincter, Percutaneous Approach, Diagnostic

0D9R3ZZ Drainage of Anal Sphincter, Percutaneous Approach

0D9R40Z Drainage of Anal Sphincter with Drainage Device, Percutaneous Endoscopic Approach

0D9R4ZX Drainage of Anal Sphincter, Percutaneous Endoscopic Approach, Diagnostic

0D9R4ZZ Drainage of Anal Sphincter, Percutaneous Endoscopic Approach

0D9S00Z Drainage of Greater Omentum with Drainage Device, Open Approach

0D9S0ZX Drainage of Greater Omentum, Open Approach, Diagnostic

0D9S0ZZ Drainage of Greater Omentum, Open Approach

0D9S30Z Drainage of Greater Omentum with Drainage Device, Percutaneous Approach

0D9S3ZX Drainage of Greater Omentum, Percutaneous Approach, Diagnostic

0D9S3ZZ Drainage of Greater Omentum, Percutaneous Approach

0D9S40Z Drainage of Greater Omentum with Drainage Device, Percutaneous Endoscopic Approach

♀ Female-only   ♂ Male-only   ▲ Limited Coverage   ● Non-OR   ▨ HAC-associated procedure   ▲ Non-covered procedures   ✛ Combination

0D9S4ZX	Drainage of Greater Omentum, Percutaneous Endoscopic Approach, Diagnostic	
0D9S4ZZ	Drainage of Greater Omentum, Percutaneous Endoscopic Approach	
0D9T00Z	Drainage of Lesser Omentum with Drainage Device, Open Approach	
0D9T0ZX	Drainage of Lesser Omentum, Open Approach, Diagnostic	
0D9T0ZZ	Drainage of Lesser Omentum, Open Approach	
0D9T30Z	Drainage of Lesser Omentum with Drainage Device, Percutaneous Approach	
0D9T3ZX	Drainage of Lesser Omentum, Percutaneous Approach, Diagnostic	
0D9T3ZZ	Drainage of Lesser Omentum, Percutaneous Approach	
0D9T40Z	Drainage of Lesser Omentum with Drainage Device, Percutaneous Endoscopic Approach	

0D9T4ZX	Drainage of Lesser Omentum, Percutaneous Endoscopic Approach, Diagnostic
0D9T4ZZ	Drainage of Lesser Omentum, Percutaneous Endoscopic Approach
0D9V00Z	Drainage of Mesentery with Drainage Device, Open Approach
0D9V0ZX	Drainage of Mesentery, Open Approach, Diagnostic
0D9V0ZZ	Drainage of Mesentery, Open Approach
0D9V30Z	Drainage of Mesentery with Drainage Device, Percutaneous Approach
0D9V3ZX	Drainage of Mesentery, Percutaneous Approach, Diagnostic
0D9V3ZZ	Drainage of Mesentery, Percutaneous Approach
0D9V40Z	Drainage of Mesentery with Drainage Device, Percutaneous Endoscopic Approach
0D9V4ZX	Drainage of Mesentery, Percutaneous Endoscopic Approach, Diagnostic

0D9V4ZZ	Drainage of Mesentery, Percutaneous Endoscopic Approach
0D9W00Z	Drainage of Peritoneum with Drainage Device, Open Approach
0D9W0ZX	Drainage of Peritoneum, Open Approach, Diagnostic
0D9W0ZZ	Drainage of Peritoneum, Open Approach
0D9W30Z	Drainage of Peritoneum with Drainage Device, Percutaneous Approach
0D9W3ZX	Drainage of Peritoneum, Percutaneous Approach, Diagnostic
0D9W3ZZ	Drainage of Peritoneum, Percutaneous Approach
0D9W40Z	Drainage of Peritoneum with Drainage Device, Percutaneous Endoscopic Approach
0D9W4ZX	Drainage of Peritoneum, Percutaneous Endoscopic Approach, Diagnostic
0D9W4ZZ	Drainage of Peritoneum, Percutaneous Endoscopic Approach

0DB – Gastrointestinal System, Excision

Review Coding Guidelines B3.4a and B3.4b

Review Coding Guideline B3.8

0DB10ZX	Excision of Upper Esophagus, Open Approach, Diagnostic
0DB10ZZ	Excision of Upper Esophagus, Open Approach
0DB13ZX	Excision of Upper Esophagus, Percutaneous Approach, Diagnostic
0DB13ZZ	Excision of Upper Esophagus, Percutaneous Approach
0DB14ZX	Excision of Upper Esophagus, Percutaneous Endoscopic Approach, Diagnostic
0DB14ZZ	Excision of Upper Esophagus, Percutaneous Endoscopic Approach
0DB17ZX	Excision of Upper Esophagus, Via Natural or Artificial Opening, Diagnostic
0DB17ZZ	Excision of Upper Esophagus, Via Natural or Artificial Opening
0DB18ZX	Excision of Upper Esophagus, Via Natural or Artificial Opening Endoscopic, Diagnostic
0DB18ZZ	Excision of Upper Esophagus, Via Natural or Artificial Opening Endoscopic
0DB20ZX	Excision of Middle Esophagus, Open Approach, Diagnostic
0DB20ZZ	Excision of Middle Esophagus, Open Approach
0DB23ZX	Excision of Middle Esophagus, Percutaneous Approach, Diagnostic
0DB23ZZ	Excision of Middle Esophagus, Percutaneous Approach
0DB24ZX	Excision of Middle Esophagus, Percutaneous Endoscopic Approach, Diagnostic
0DB24ZZ	Excision of Middle Esophagus, Percutaneous Endoscopic Approach
0DB27ZX	Excision of Middle Esophagus, Via Natural or Artificial Opening, Diagnostic
0DB27ZZ	Excision of Middle Esophagus, Via Natural or Artificial Opening
0DB28ZX	Excision of Middle Esophagus, Via Natural or Artificial Opening Endoscopic, Diagnostic
0DB28ZZ	Excision of Middle Esophagus, Via Natural or Artificial Opening Endoscopic
0DB30ZX	Excision of Lower Esophagus, Open Approach, Diagnostic

0DB30ZZ	Excision of Lower Esophagus, Open Approach
0DB33ZX	Excision of Lower Esophagus, Percutaneous Approach, Diagnostic
0DB33ZZ	Excision of Lower Esophagus, Percutaneous Approach
0DB34ZX	Excision of Lower Esophagus, Percutaneous Endoscopic Approach, Diagnostic
0DB34ZZ	Excision of Lower Esophagus, Percutaneous Endoscopic Approach
0DB37ZX	Excision of Lower Esophagus, Via Natural or Artificial Opening, Diagnostic
0DB37ZZ	Excision of Lower Esophagus, Via Natural or Artificial Opening
0DB38ZX	Excision of Lower Esophagus, Via Natural or Artificial Opening Endoscopic, Diagnostic
0DB38ZZ	Excision of Lower Esophagus, Via Natural or Artificial Opening Endoscopic
0DB40ZX	Excision of Esophagogastric Junction, Open Approach, Diagnostic
0DB40ZZ	Excision of Esophagogastric Junction, Open Approach
0DB43ZX	Excision of Esophagogastric Junction, Percutaneous Approach, Diagnostic
0DB43ZZ	Excision of Esophagogastric Junction, Percutaneous Approach
0DB44ZX	Excision of Esophagogastric Junction, Percutaneous Endoscopic Approach, Diagnostic
0DB44ZZ	Excision of Esophagogastric Junction, Percutaneous Endoscopic Approach
0DB47ZX	Excision of Esophagogastric Junction, Via Natural or Artificial Opening, Diagnostic
0DB47ZZ	Excision of Esophagogastric Junction, Via Natural or Artificial Opening
0DB48ZX	Excision of Esophagogastric Junction, Via Natural or Artificial Opening Endoscopic, Diagnostic
0DB48ZZ	Excision of Esophagogastric Junction, Via Natural or Artificial Opening Endoscopic
0DB50ZX	Excision of Esophagus, Open Approach, Diagnostic
0DB50ZZ	Excision of Esophagus, Open Approach
0DB53ZX	Excision of Esophagus, Percutaneous Approach, Diagnostic
0DB53ZZ	Excision of Esophagus, Percutaneous Approach

0DB54ZX	Excision of Esophagus, Percutaneous Endoscopic Approach, Diagnostic
0DB54ZZ	Excision of Esophagus, Percutaneous Endoscopic Approach
0DB57ZX	Excision of Esophagus, Via Natural or Artificial Opening, Diagnostic
0DB57ZZ	Excision of Esophagus, Via Natural or Artificial Opening
0DB58ZX	Excision of Esophagus, Via Natural or Artificial Opening Endoscopic, Diagno...
0DB58ZZ	Excision of Esophagus, Via Natural or Artificial Opening Endoscopic
0DB60Z3	Excision of Stomach, Open Approach, Vertical
0DB60ZX	Excision of Stomach, Open Approach, Diagnostic
0DB60ZZ	Excision of Stomach, Open Approach
0DB63Z3	Excision of Stomach, Percutaneous Approach, Vertical
0DB63ZX	Excision of Stomach, Percutaneous Approach, Diagnostic
0DB63ZZ	Excision of Stomach, Percutaneous Approach
0DB64Z3	Excision of Stomach, Percutaneous Endoscopic Approach, Vertical
0DB64ZX	Excision of Stomach, Percutaneous Endoscopic Approach, Diagnostic
0DB64ZZ	Excision of Stomach, Percutaneous Endoscopic Approach
0DB67Z3	Excision of Stomach, Via Natural or Artificial Opening, Vertical
0DB67ZX	Excision of Stomach, Via Natural or Artificial Opening, Diagnostic
0DB67ZZ	Excision of Stomach, Via Natural or Artificial Opening
0DB68Z3	Excision of Stomach, Via Natural or Artificial Opening Endoscopic, Vertical
0DB68ZX	Excision of Stomach, Via Natural or Artificial Opening Endoscopic, Diagnos...
0DB68ZZ	Excision of Stomach, Via Natural or Artificial Opening Endoscopic
0DB70ZX	Excision of Stomach, Pylorus, Open Approach, Diagnostic
0DB70ZZ	Excision of Stomach, Pylorus, Open Approach
0DB73ZX	Excision of Stomach, Pylorus, Percutaneous Approach, Diagnostic
0DB73ZZ	Excision of Stomach, Pylorus, Percutaneous Approach

♀ Female-only   ♂ Male-only   ▲ Limited Coverage   ● Non-OR   ▰▰ HAC-associated procedure   ▲ Non-covered procedures   ➕ Combinati...

74ZX	Excision of Stomach, Pylorus, Percutaneous Endoscopic Approach, Diagnostic	
74ZZ	Excision of Stomach, Pylorus, Percutaneous Endoscopic Approach	
77ZX	Excision of Stomach, Pylorus, Via Natural or Artificial Opening, Diagnostic	
77ZZ	Excision of Stomach, Pylorus, Via Natural or Artificial Opening	
78ZX	Excision of Stomach, Pylorus, Via Natural or Artificial Opening Endoscopic, Diagnostic	
78ZZ	Excision of Stomach, Pylorus, Via Natural or Artificial Opening Endoscopic	
80ZX	Excision of Small Intestine, Open Approach, Diagnostic	
80ZZ	Excision of Small Intestine, Open Approach	
83ZX	Excision of Small Intestine, Percutaneous Approach, Diagnostic	
83ZZ	Excision of Small Intestine, Percutaneous Approach	
84ZX	Excision of Small Intestine, Percutaneous Endoscopic Approach, Diagnostic	
84ZZ	Excision of Small Intestine, Percutaneous Endoscopic Approach	
87ZX	Excision of Small Intestine, Via Natural or Artificial Opening, Diagnostic	
87ZZ	Excision of Small Intestine, Via Natural or Artificial Opening	
88ZX	Excision of Small Intestine, Via Natural or Artificial Opening Endoscopic, Diagnostic	
88ZZ	Excision of Small Intestine, Via Natural or Artificial Opening Endoscopic	
90ZX	Excision of Duodenum, Open Approach, Diagnostic	
90ZZ	Excision of Duodenum, Open Approach	

AHA CC: 3Q, 2014, 32-33

93ZX	Excision of Duodenum, Percutaneous Approach, Diagnostic
93ZZ	Excision of Duodenum, Percutaneous Approach
94ZX	Excision of Duodenum, Percutaneous Endoscopic Approach, Diagnostic
94ZZ	Excision of Duodenum, Percutaneous Endoscopic Approach
97ZX	Excision of Duodenum, Via Natural or Artificial Opening, Diagnostic
97ZZ	Excision of Duodenum, Via Natural or Artificial Opening
98ZX	Excision of Duodenum, Via Natural or Artificial Opening Endoscopic, Diagnostic
98ZZ	Excision of Duodenum, Via Natural or Artificial Opening Endoscopic
BA0ZX	Excision of Jejunum, Open Approach, Diagnostic
BA0ZZ	Excision of Jejunum, Open Approach
BA3ZX	Excision of Jejunum, Percutaneous Approach, Diagnostic
BA3ZZ	Excision of Jejunum, Percutaneous Approach
BA4ZX	Excision of Jejunum, Percutaneous Endoscopic Approach, Diagnostic
BA4ZZ	Excision of Jejunum, Percutaneous Endoscopic Approach
BA7ZX	Excision of Jejunum, Via Natural or Artificial Opening, Diagnostic
BA7ZZ	Excision of Jejunum, Via Natural or Artificial Opening
BA8ZX	Excision of Jejunum, Via Natural or Artificial Opening Endoscopic, Diagnostic
BA8ZZ	Excision of Jejunum, Via Natural or Artificial Opening Endoscopic
BB0ZX	Excision of Ileum, Open Approach, Diagnostic
BB0ZZ	Excision of Ileum, Open Approach

AHA CC: 3Q, 2014, 28-29

0DBB3ZX	Excision of Ileum, Percutaneous Approach, Diagnostic
0DBB3ZZ	Excision of Ileum, Percutaneous Approach
0DBB4ZX	Excision of Ileum, Percutaneous Endoscopic Approach, Diagnostic
0DBB4ZZ	Excision of Ileum, Percutaneous Endoscopic Approach
0DBB7ZX	Excision of Ileum, Via Natural or Artificial Opening, Diagnostic
0DBB7ZZ	Excision of Ileum, Via Natural or Artificial Opening
0DBB8ZX	Excision of Ileum, Via Natural or Artificial Opening Endoscopic, Diagnostic
0DBB8ZZ	Excision of Ileum, Via Natural or Artificial Opening Endoscopic
0DBC0ZX	Excision of Ileocecal Valve, Open Approach, Diagnostic
0DBC0ZZ	Excision of Ileocecal Valve, Open Approach
0DBC3ZX	Excision of Ileocecal Valve, Percutaneous Approach, Diagnostic
0DBC3ZZ	Excision of Ileocecal Valve, Percutaneous Approach
0DBC4ZX	Excision of Ileocecal Valve, Percutaneous Endoscopic Approach, Diagnostic
0DBC4ZZ	Excision of Ileocecal Valve, Percutaneous Endoscopic Approach
0DBC7ZX	Excision of Ileocecal Valve, Via Natural or Artificial Opening, Diagnostic
0DBC7ZZ	Excision of Ileocecal Valve, Via Natural or Artificial Opening
0DBC8ZX	Excision of Ileocecal Valve, Via Natural or Artificial Opening Endoscopic, Diagnostic
0DBC8ZZ	Excision of Ileocecal Valve, Via Natural or Artificial Opening Endoscopic
0DBE0ZX	Excision of Large Intestine, Open Approach, Diagnostic
0DBE0ZZ	Excision of Large Intestine, Open Approach
0DBE3ZX	Excision of Large Intestine, Percutaneous Approach, Diagnostic
0DBE3ZZ	Excision of Large Intestine, Percutaneous Approach
0DBE4ZX	Excision of Large Intestine, Percutaneous Endoscopic Approach, Diagnostic
0DBE4ZZ	Excision of Large Intestine, Percutaneous Endoscopic Approach
0DBE7ZX	Excision of Large Intestine, Via Natural or Artificial Opening, Diagnostic
0DBE7ZZ	Excision of Large Intestine, Via Natural or Artificial Opening
0DBE8ZX	Excision of Large Intestine, Via Natural or Artificial Opening Endoscopic, Diagnostic
0DBE8ZZ	Excision of Large Intestine, Via Natural or Artificial Opening Endoscopic
0DBF0ZX	Excision of Right Large Intestine, Open Approach, Diagnostic
0DBF0ZZ	Excision of Right Large Intestine, Open Approach
0DBF3ZX	Excision of Right Large Intestine, Percutaneous Approach, Diagnostic
0DBF3ZZ	Excision of Right Large Intestine, Percutaneous Approach
0DBF4ZX	Excision of Right Large Intestine, Percutaneous Endoscopic Approach, Diagnostic
0DBF4ZZ	Excision of Right Large Intestine, Percutaneous Endoscopic Approach
0DBF7ZX	Excision of Right Large Intestine, Via Natural or Artificial Opening, Diagnostic
0DBF7ZZ	Excision of Right Large Intestine, Via Natural or Artificial Opening
0DBF8ZX	Excision of Right Large Intestine, Via Natural or Artificial Opening Endoscopic, Diagnostic

0DBF8ZZ	Excision of Right Large Intestine, Via Natural or Artificial Opening Endoscopic
0DBG0ZX	Excision of Left Large Intestine, Open Approach, Diagnostic
0DBG0ZZ	Excision of Left Large Intestine, Open Approach
0DBG3ZX	Excision of Left Large Intestine, Percutaneous Approach, Diagnostic
0DBG3ZZ	Excision of Left Large Intestine, Percutaneous Approach
0DBG4ZX	Excision of Left Large Intestine, Percutaneous Endoscopic Approach, Diagnostic
0DBG4ZZ	Excision of Left Large Intestine, Percutaneous Endoscopic Approach
0DBG7ZX	Excision of Left Large Intestine, Via Natural or Artificial Opening, Diagnostic
0DBG7ZZ	Excision of Left Large Intestine, Via Natural or Artificial Opening
0DBG8ZX	Excision of Left Large Intestine, Via Natural or Artificial Opening Endoscopic, Diagnostic
0DBG8ZZ	Excision of Left Large Intestine, Via Natural or Artificial Opening Endoscopic
0DBH0ZX	Excision of Cecum, Open Approach, Diagnostic
0DBH0ZZ	Excision of Cecum, Open Approach
0DBH3ZX	Excision of Cecum, Percutaneous Approach, Diagnostic
0DBH3ZZ	Excision of Cecum, Percutaneous Approach
0DBH4ZX	Excision of Cecum, Percutaneous Endoscopic Approach, Diagnostic
0DBH4ZZ	Excision of Cecum, Percutaneous Endoscopic Approach
0DBH7ZX	Excision of Cecum, Via Natural or Artificial Opening, Diagnostic
0DBH7ZZ	Excision of Cecum, Via Natural or Artificial Opening
0DBH8ZX	Excision of Cecum, Via Natural or Artificial Opening Endoscopic, Diagnostic
0DBH8ZZ	Excision of Cecum, Via Natural or Artificial Opening Endoscopic
0DBJ0ZX	Excision of Appendix, Open Approach, Diagnostic
0DBJ0ZZ	Excision of Appendix, Open Approach
0DBJ3ZX	Excision of Appendix, Percutaneous Approach, Diagnostic
0DBJ3ZZ	Excision of Appendix, Percutaneous Approach
0DBJ4ZX	Excision of Appendix, Percutaneous Endoscopic Approach, Diagnostic
0DBJ4ZZ	Excision of Appendix, Percutaneous Endoscopic Approach
0DBJ7ZX	Excision of Appendix, Via Natural or Artificial Opening, Diagnostic
0DBJ7ZZ	Excision of Appendix, Via Natural or Artificial Opening
0DBJ8ZX	Excision of Appendix, Via Natural or Artificial Opening Endoscopic, Diagnostic
0DBJ8ZZ	Excision of Appendix, Via Natural or Artificial Opening Endoscopic
0DBK0ZX	Excision of Ascending Colon, Open Approach, Diagnostic
0DBK0ZZ	Excision of Ascending Colon, Open Approach
0DBK3ZX	Excision of Ascending Colon, Percutaneous Approach, Diagnostic
0DBK3ZZ	Excision of Ascending Colon, Percutaneous Approach
0DBK4ZX	Excision of Ascending Colon, Percutaneous Endoscopic Approach, Diagnostic

Female-only   ♂ Male-only   ▲ Limited Coverage   ● Non-OR   ▬ HAC-associated procedure   ▲ Non-covered procedures   ✛ Combination

0DBK4ZZ	Excision of Ascending Colon, Percutaneous Endoscopic Approach	**0DBN3ZX**	Excision of Sigmoid Colon, Percutaneous Approach, Diagnostic	**0DBR0ZZ**	Excision of Anal Sphincter, Open Approach
0DBK7ZX	Excision of Ascending Colon, Via Natural or Artificial Opening, Diagnostic	**0DBN3ZZ**	Excision of Sigmoid Colon, Percutaneous Approach	**0DBR3ZX**	Excision of Anal Sphincter, Percutaneous Approach, Diagnostic
0DBK7ZZ	Excision of Ascending Colon, Via Natural or Artificial Opening	**0DBN4ZX**	Excision of Sigmoid Colon, Percutaneous Endoscopic Approach, Diagnostic	**0DBR3ZZ**	Excision of Anal Sphincter, Percutaneous Approach
0DBK8ZX	Excision of Ascending Colon, Via Natural or Artificial Opening Endoscopic, Diagnostic	**0DBN4ZZ**	Excision of Sigmoid Colon, Percutaneous Endoscopic Approach	**0DBR4ZX**	Excision of Anal Sphincter, Percutaneous Endoscopic Approach, Diagnostic
0DBK8ZZ	Excision of Ascending Colon, Via Natural or Artificial Opening Endoscopic	**0DBN7ZX**	Excision of Sigmoid Colon, Via Natural or Artificial Opening, Diagnostic	**0DBR4ZZ**	Excision of Anal Sphincter, Percutaneous Endoscopic Approach
0DBL0ZX	Excision of Transverse Colon, Open Approach, Diagnostic	**0DBN7ZZ**	Excision of Sigmoid Colon, Via Natural or Artificial Opening	**0DBS0ZX**	Excision of Greater Omentum, Open Approach, Diagnostic
0DBL0ZZ	Excision of Transverse Colon, Open Approach	**0DBN8ZX**	Excision of Sigmoid Colon, Via Natural or Artificial Opening Endoscopic, Diagnostic	**0DBS0ZZ**	Excision of Greater Omentum, Open Approach
0DBL3ZX	Excision of Transverse Colon, Percutaneous Approach, Diagnostic	**0DBN8ZZ**	Excision of Sigmoid Colon, Via Natural or Artificial Opening Endoscopic	**0DBS3ZX**	Excision of Greater Omentum, Percutaneous Approach, Diagnostic
0DBL3ZZ	Excision of Transverse Colon, Percutaneous Approach	**0DBP0ZX**	Excision of Rectum, Open Approach, Diagnostic	**0DBS3ZZ**	Excision of Greater Omentum, Percutaneous Approach
0DBL4ZX	Excision of Transverse Colon, Percutaneous Endoscopic Approach, Diagnostic	**0DBP0ZZ**	Excision of Rectum, Open Approach	**0DBS4ZX**	Excision of Greater Omentum, Percutaneous Endoscopic Approach, Diagnostic
0DBL4ZZ	Excision of Transverse Colon, Percutaneous Endoscopic Approach	**0DBP3ZX**	Excision of Rectum, Percutaneous Approach, Diagnostic		
		0DBP3ZZ	Excision of Rectum, Percutaneous Approach	**0DBS4ZZ**	Excision of Greater Omentum, Percutaneous Endoscopic Approach
0DBL7ZX	Excision of Transverse Colon, Via Natural or Artificial Opening, Diagnostic	**0DBP4ZX**	Excision of Rectum, Percutaneous Endoscopic Approach, Diagnostic	**0DBT0ZX**	Excision of Lesser Omentum, Open Approach, Diagnostic
0DBL7ZZ	Excision of Transverse Colon, Via Natural or Artificial Opening	**0DBP4ZZ**	Excision of Rectum, Percutaneous Endoscopic Approach	**0DBT0ZZ**	Excision of Lesser Omentum, Open Approach
0DBL8ZX	Excision of Transverse Colon, Via Natural or Artificial Opening Endoscopic, Diagnostic	**0DBP7ZX**	Excision of Rectum, Via Natural or Artificial Opening, Diagnostic	**0DBT3ZX**	Excision of Lesser Omentum, Percutaneous Approach, Diagnostic
		0DBP7ZZ	Excision of Rectum, Via Natural or Artificial Opening	**0DBT3ZZ**	Excision of Lesser Omentum, Percutaneous Approach
0DBL8ZZ	Excision of Transverse Colon, Via Natural or Artificial Opening Endoscopic	**0DBP8ZX**	Excision of Rectum, Via Natural or Artificial Opening Endoscopic, Diagnostic	**0DBT4ZX**	Excision of Lesser Omentum, Percutaneous Endoscopic Approach, Diagnostic
0DBM0ZX	Excision of Descending Colon, Open Approach, Diagnostic	**0DBP8ZZ**	Excision of Rectum, Via Natural or Artificial Opening Endoscopic	**0DBT4ZZ**	Excision of Lesser Omentum, Percutaneous Endoscopic Approach
0DBM0ZZ	Excision of Descending Colon, Open Approach	**0DBQ0ZX**	Excision of Anus, Open Approach, Diagnostic	**0DBV0ZX**	Excision of Mesentery, Open Approach, Diagnostic
0DBM3ZX	Excision of Descending Colon, Percutaneous Approach, Diagnostic	**0DBQ0ZZ**	Excision of Anus, Open Approach	**0DBV0ZZ**	Excision of Mesentery, Open Approach
0DBM3ZZ	Excision of Descending Colon, Percutaneous Approach	**0DBQ3ZX**	Excision of Anus, Percutaneous Approach, Diagnostic	**0DBV3ZX**	Excision of Mesentery, Percutaneous Approach, Diagnostic
0DBM4ZX	Excision of Descending Colon, Percutaneous Endoscopic Approach, Diagnostic	**0DBQ3ZZ**	Excision of Anus, Percutaneous Approach	**0DBV3ZZ**	Excision of Mesentery, Percutaneous Approach
		0DBQ4ZX	Excision of Anus, Percutaneous Endoscopic Approach, Diagnostic	**0DBV4ZX**	Excision of Mesentery, Percutaneous Endoscopic Approach, Diagnostic
0DBM4ZZ	Excision of Descending Colon, Percutaneous Endoscopic Approach	**0DBQ4ZZ**	Excision of Anus, Percutaneous Endoscopic Approach	**0DBV4ZZ**	Excision of Mesentery, Percutaneous Endoscopic Approach
0DBM7ZX	Excision of Descending Colon, Via Natural or Artificial Opening, Diagnostic	**0DBQ7ZX**	Excision of Anus, Via Natural or Artificial Opening, Diagnostic	**0DBW0ZX**	Excision of Peritoneum, Open Approach, Diagnostic
0DBM7ZZ	Excision of Descending Colon, Via Natural or Artificial Opening	**0DBQ7ZZ**	Excision of Anus, Via Natural or Artificial Opening	**0DBW0ZZ**	Excision of Peritoneum, Open Approach
0DBM8ZX	Excision of Descending Colon, Via Natural or Artificial Opening Endoscopic, Diagnostic	**0DBQ8ZX**	Excision of Anus, Via Natural or Artificial Opening Endoscopic, Diagnostic	**0DBW3ZX**	Excision of Peritoneum, Percutaneous Approach, Diagnostic
		0DBQ8ZZ	Excision of Anus, Via Natural or Artificial Opening Endoscopic	**0DBW3ZZ**	Excision of Peritoneum, Percutaneous Approach
0DBM8ZZ	Excision of Descending Colon, Via Natural or Artificial Opening Endoscopic	**0DBQXZX**	Excision of Anus, External Approach, Diagnostic	**0DBW4ZX**	Excision of Peritoneum, Percutaneous Endoscopic Approach, Diagnostic
0DBN0ZX	Excision of Sigmoid Colon, Open Approach, Diagnostic	**0DBQXZZ**	Excision of Anus, External Approach	**0DBW4ZZ**	Excision of Peritoneum, Percutaneous Endoscopic Approach
0DBN0ZZ	Excision of Sigmoid Colon, Open Approach	**0DBR0ZX**	Excision of Anal Sphincter, Open Approach, Diagnostic		
	AHA CC: 4Q, 2014, 40-41				

0DC – Gastrointestinal System, Extirpation

0DC10ZZ	Extirpation of Matter from Upper Esophagus, Open Approach	**0DC20ZZ**	Extirpation of Matter from Middle Esophagus, Open Approach	**0DC30ZZ**	Extirpation of Matter from Lower Esophagus, Open Approach
0DC13ZZ	Extirpation of Matter from Upper Esophagus, Percutaneous Approach	**0DC23ZZ**	Extirpation of Matter from Middle Esophagus, Percutaneous Approach	**0DC33ZZ**	Extirpation of Matter from Lower Esophagus, Percutaneous Approach
0DC14ZZ	Extirpation of Matter from Upper Esophagus, Percutaneous Endoscopic Approach	**0DC24ZZ**	Extirpation of Matter from Middle Esophagus, Percutaneous Endoscopic Approach	**0DC34ZZ**	Extirpation of Matter from Lower Esophagus, Percutaneous Endoscopic Approach
0DC17ZZ	Extirpation of Matter from Upper Esophagus, Via Natural or Artificial Opening	**0DC27ZZ**	Extirpation of Matter from Middle Esophagus, Via Natural or Artificial Opening	**0DC37ZZ**	Extirpation of Matter from Lower Esophagus, Via Natural or Artificial Opening
0DC18ZZ	Extirpation of Matter from Upper Esophagus, Via Natural or Artificial Opening Endoscopic	**0DC28ZZ**	Extirpation of Matter from Middle Esophagus, Via Natural or Artificial Opening Endoscopic	**0DC38ZZ**	Extirpation of Matter from Lower Esophagus, Via Natural or Artificial Opening Endoscopic

♀ Female-only   ♂ Male-only   ▲ Limited Coverage   ● Non-OR   ▥ HAC-associated procedure   ▲ Non-covered procedures   ✚ Combinat

40ZZ	Extirpation of Matter from Esophagogastric Junction, Open Approach
43ZZ	Extirpation of Matter from Esophagogastric Junction, Percutaneous Approach
44ZZ	Extirpation of Matter from Esophagogastric Junction, Percutaneous Endoscopic Approach
47ZZ	Extirpation of Matter from Esophagogastric Junction, Via Natural or Artificial Opening
48ZZ	Extirpation of Matter from Esophagogastric Junction, Via Natural or Artificial Opening Endoscopic
50ZZ	Extirpation of Matter from Esophagus, Open Approach
53ZZ	Extirpation of Matter from Esophagus, Percutaneous Approach
54ZZ	Extirpation of Matter from Esophagus, Percutaneous Endoscopic Approach
57ZZ	Extirpation of Matter from Esophagus, Via Natural or Artificial Opening
58ZZ	Extirpation of Matter from Esophagus, Via Natural or Artificial Opening Endoscopic
60ZZ	Extirpation of Matter from Stomach, Open Approach
63ZZ	Extirpation of Matter from Stomach, Percutaneous Approach
64ZZ	Extirpation of Matter from Stomach, Percutaneous Endoscopic Approach
67ZZ	Extirpation of Matter from Stomach, Via Natural or Artificial Opening
68ZZ	Extirpation of Matter from Stomach, Via Natural or Artificial Opening Endoscopic
70ZZ	Extirpation of Matter from Stomach, Pylorus, Open Approach
73ZZ	Extirpation of Matter from Stomach, Pylorus, Percutaneous Approach
74ZZ	Extirpation of Matter from Stomach, Pylorus, Percutaneous Endoscopic Approach
77ZZ	Extirpation of Matter from Stomach, Pylorus, Via Natural or Artificial Opening
78ZZ	Extirpation of Matter from Stomach, Pylorus, Via Natural or Artificial Opening Endoscopic
C80ZZ	Extirpation of Matter from Small Intestine, Open Approach
C83ZZ	Extirpation of Matter from Small Intestine, Percutaneous Approach
C84ZZ	Extirpation of Matter from Small Intestine, Percutaneous Endoscopic Approach
C87ZZ	Extirpation of Matter from Small Intestine, Via Natural or Artificial Opening
C88ZZ	Extirpation of Matter from Small Intestine, Via Natural or Artificial Opening Endoscopic
C90ZZ	Extirpation of Matter from Duodenum, Open Approach
C93ZZ	Extirpation of Matter from Duodenum, Percutaneous Approach
C94ZZ	Extirpation of Matter from Duodenum, Percutaneous Endoscopic Approach
C97ZZ	Extirpation of Matter from Duodenum, Via Natural or Artificial Opening
C98ZZ	Extirpation of Matter from Duodenum, Via Natural or Artificial Opening Endoscopic
CA0ZZ	Extirpation of Matter from Jejunum, Open Approach
CA3ZZ	Extirpation of Matter from Jejunum, Percutaneous Approach
0DCA4ZZ	Extirpation of Matter from Jejunum, Percutaneous Endoscopic Approach
0DCA7ZZ	Extirpation of Matter from Jejunum, Via Natural or Artificial Opening
0DCA8ZZ	Extirpation of Matter from Jejunum, Via Natural or Artificial Opening Endoscopic
0DCB0ZZ	Extirpation of Matter from Ileum, Open Approach
0DCB3ZZ	Extirpation of Matter from Ileum, Percutaneous Approach
0DCB4ZZ	Extirpation of Matter from Ileum, Percutaneous Endoscopic Approach
0DCB7ZZ	Extirpation of Matter from Ileum, Via Natural or Artificial Opening
0DCB8ZZ	Extirpation of Matter from Ileum, Via Natural or Artificial Opening Endoscopic
0DCC0ZZ	Extirpation of Matter from Ileocecal Valve, Open Approach
0DCC3ZZ	Extirpation of Matter from Ileocecal Valve, Percutaneous Approach
0DCC4ZZ	Extirpation of Matter from Ileocecal Valve, Percutaneous Endoscopic Approach
0DCC7ZZ	Extirpation of Matter from Ileocecal Valve, Via Natural or Artificial Opening
0DCC8ZZ	Extirpation of Matter from Ileocecal Valve, Via Natural or Artificial Opening Endoscopic
0DCE0ZZ	Extirpation of Matter from Large Intestine, Open Approach
0DCE3ZZ	Extirpation of Matter from Large Intestine, Percutaneous Approach
0DCE4ZZ	Extirpation of Matter from Large Intestine, Percutaneous Endoscopic Approach
0DCE7ZZ	Extirpation of Matter from Large Intestine, Via Natural or Artificial Opening
0DCE8ZZ	Extirpation of Matter from Large Intestine, Via Natural or Artificial Opening Endoscopic
0DCF0ZZ	Extirpation of Matter from Right Large Intestine, Open Approach
0DCF3ZZ	Extirpation of Matter from Right Large Intestine, Percutaneous Approach
0DCF4ZZ	Extirpation of Matter from Right Large Intestine, Percutaneous Endoscopic Approach
0DCF7ZZ	Extirpation of Matter from Right Large Intestine, Via Natural or Artificial Opening
0DCF8ZZ	Extirpation of Matter from Right Large Intestine, Via Natural or Artificial Opening Endoscopic
0DCG0ZZ	Extirpation of Matter from Left Large Intestine, Open Approach
0DCG3ZZ	Extirpation of Matter from Left Large Intestine, Percutaneous Approach
0DCG4ZZ	Extirpation of Matter from Left Large Intestine, Percutaneous Endoscopic Approach
0DCG7ZZ	Extirpation of Matter from Left Large Intestine, Via Natural or Artificial Opening
0DCG8ZZ	Extirpation of Matter from Left Large Intestine, Via Natural or Artificial Opening Endoscopic
0DCH0ZZ	Extirpation of Matter from Cecum, Open Approach
0DCH3ZZ	Extirpation of Matter from Cecum, Percutaneous Approach
0DCH4ZZ	Extirpation of Matter from Cecum, Percutaneous Endoscopic Approach
0DCH7ZZ	Extirpation of Matter from Cecum, Via Natural or Artificial Opening
0DCH8ZZ	Extirpation of Matter from Cecum, Via Natural or Artificial Opening Endoscopic
0DCJ0ZZ	Extirpation of Matter from Appendix, Open Approach
0DCJ3ZZ	Extirpation of Matter from Appendix, Percutaneous Approach
0DCJ4ZZ	Extirpation of Matter from Appendix, Percutaneous Endoscopic Approach
0DCJ7ZZ	Extirpation of Matter from Appendix, Via Natural or Artificial Opening
0DCJ8ZZ	Extirpation of Matter from Appendix, Via Natural or Artificial Opening Endoscopic
0DCK0ZZ	Extirpation of Matter from Ascending Colon, Open Approach
0DCK3ZZ	Extirpation of Matter from Ascending Colon, Percutaneous Approach
0DCK4ZZ	Extirpation of Matter from Ascending Colon, Percutaneous Endoscopic Approach
0DCK7ZZ	Extirpation of Matter from Ascending Colon, Via Natural or Artificial Opening
0DCK8ZZ	Extirpation of Matter from Ascending Colon, Via Natural or Artificial Opening Endoscopic
0DCL0ZZ	Extirpation of Matter from Transverse Colon, Open Approach
0DCL3ZZ	Extirpation of Matter from Transverse Colon, Percutaneous Approach
0DCL4ZZ	Extirpation of Matter from Transverse Colon, Percutaneous Endoscopic Approach
0DCL7ZZ	Extirpation of Matter from Transverse Colon, Via Natural or Artificial Opening
0DCL8ZZ	Extirpation of Matter from Transverse Colon, Via Natural or Artificial Opening Endoscopic
0DCM0ZZ	Extirpation of Matter from Descending Colon, Open Approach
0DCM3ZZ	Extirpation of Matter from Descending Colon, Percutaneous Approach
0DCM4ZZ	Extirpation of Matter from Descending Colon, Percutaneous Endoscopic Approach
0DCM7ZZ	Extirpation of Matter from Descending Colon, Via Natural or Artificial Opening
0DCM8ZZ	Extirpation of Matter from Descending Colon, Via Natural or Artificial Opening Endoscopic
0DCN0ZZ	Extirpation of Matter from Sigmoid Colon, Open Approach
0DCN3ZZ	Extirpation of Matter from Sigmoid Colon, Percutaneous Approach
0DCN4ZZ	Extirpation of Matter from Sigmoid Colon, Percutaneous Endoscopic Approach
0DCN7ZZ	Extirpation of Matter from Sigmoid Colon, Via Natural or Artificial Opening
0DCN8ZZ	Extirpation of Matter from Sigmoid Colon, Via Natural or Artificial Opening Endoscopic
0DCP0ZZ	Extirpation of Matter from Rectum, Open Approach
0DCP3ZZ	Extirpation of Matter from Rectum, Percutaneous Approach
0DCP4ZZ	Extirpation of Matter from Rectum, Percutaneous Endoscopic Approach
0DCP7ZZ	Extirpation of Matter from Rectum, Via Natural or Artificial Opening
0DCP8ZZ	Extirpation of Matter from Rectum, Via Natural or Artificial Opening Endoscopic
0DCQ0ZZ	Extirpation of Matter from Anus, Open Approach
0DCQ3ZZ	Extirpation of Matter from Anus, Percutaneous Approach
0DCQ4ZZ	Extirpation of Matter from Anus, Percutaneous Endoscopic Approach

0DCQ7ZZ	Extirpation of Matter from Anus, Via Natural or Artificial Opening	0DCS0ZZ	Extirpation of Matter from Greater Omentum, Open Approach	0DCV0ZZ	Extirpation of Matter from Mesenter Open Approach
0DCQ8ZZ	Extirpation of Matter from Anus, Via Natural or Artificial Opening Endoscopic	0DCS3ZZ	Extirpation of Matter from Greater Omentum, Percutaneous Approach	0DCV3ZZ	Extirpation of Matter from Mesenter Percutaneous Approach
0DCQXZZ	Extirpation of Matter from Anus, External Approach	0DCS4ZZ	Extirpation of Matter from Greater Omentum, Percutaneous Endoscopic Approach	0DCV4ZZ	Extirpation of Matter from Mesenter Percutaneous Endoscopic Approach
0DCR0ZZ	Extirpation of Matter from Anal Sphincter, Open Approach	0DCT0ZZ	Extirpation of Matter from Lesser Omentum, Open Approach	0DCW0ZZ	Extirpation of Matter from Peritoneu Open Approach
0DCR3ZZ	Extirpation of Matter from Anal Sphincter, Percutaneous Approach	0DCT3ZZ	Extirpation of Matter from Lesser Omentum, Percutaneous Approach	0DCW3ZZ	Extirpation of Matter from Peritoneu Percutaneous Approach
0DCR4ZZ	Extirpation of Matter from Anal Sphincter, Percutaneous Endoscopic Approach	0DCT4ZZ	Extirpation of Matter from Lesser Omentum, Percutaneous Endoscopic Approach	0DCW4ZZ	Extirpation of Matter from Peritoneu Percutaneous Endoscopic Approach

0DF – Gastrointestinal System, Fragmentation

0DF50ZZ	Fragmentation in Esophagus, Open Approach	0DFB0ZZ	Fragmentation in Ileum, Open Approach	0DFJ0ZZ	Fragmentation in Appendix, Open Approach
0DF53ZZ	Fragmentation in Esophagus, Percutaneous Approach	0DFB3ZZ	Fragmentation in Ileum, Percutaneous Approach	0DFJ3ZZ	Fragmentation in Appendix, Percutaneous Approach
0DF54ZZ	Fragmentation in Esophagus, Percutaneous Endoscopic Approach	0DFB4ZZ	Fragmentation in Ileum, Percutaneous Endoscopic Approach	0DFJ4ZZ	Fragmentation in Appendix, Percutaneous Endoscopic Approach
0DF57ZZ	Fragmentation in Esophagus, Via Natural or Artificial Opening	0DFB7ZZ	Fragmentation in Ileum, Via Natural or Artificial Opening	0DFJ7ZZ	Fragmentation in Appendix, Via Natu or Artificial Opening
0DF58ZZ	Fragmentation in Esophagus, Via Natural or Artificial Opening Endoscopic	0DFB8ZZ	Fragmentation in Ileum, Via Natural or Artificial Opening Endoscopic	0DFJ8ZZ	Fragmentation in Appendix, Via Natu or Artificial Opening Endoscopic
▲ 0DF5XZZ	Fragmentation in Esophagus, External Approach	▲ 0DFBXZZ	Fragmentation in Ileum, External Approach	▲ 0DFJXZZ	Fragmentation in Appendix, External Approach
0DF60ZZ	Fragmentation in Stomach, Open Approach	0DFE0ZZ	Fragmentation in Large Intestine, Open Approach	0DFK0ZZ	Fragmentation in Ascending Colon, C Approach
0DF63ZZ	Fragmentation in Stomach, Percutaneous Approach	0DFE3ZZ	Fragmentation in Large Intestine, Percutaneous Approach	0DFK3ZZ	Fragmentation in Ascending Colon, Percutaneous Approach
0DF64ZZ	Fragmentation in Stomach, Percutaneous Endoscopic Approach	0DFE4ZZ	Fragmentation in Large Intestine, Percutaneous Endoscopic Approach	0DFK4ZZ	Fragmentation in Ascending Colon, Percutaneous Endoscopic Approach
0DF67ZZ	Fragmentation in Stomach, Via Natural or Artificial Opening	0DFE7ZZ	Fragmentation in Large Intestine, Via Natural or Artificial Opening	0DFK7ZZ	Fragmentation in Ascending Colon, V Natural or Artificial Opening
0DF68ZZ	Fragmentation in Stomach, Via Natural or Artificial Opening Endoscopic	0DFE8ZZ	Fragmentation in Large Intestine, Via Natural or Artificial Opening Endoscopic	0DFK8ZZ	Fragmentation in Ascending Colon, V Natural or Artificial Opening Endosco
▲ 0DF6XZZ	Fragmentation in Stomach, External Approach	▲ 0DFEXZZ	Fragmentation in Large Intestine, External Approach	▲ 0DFKXZZ	Fragmentation in Ascending Colon, External Approach
0DF80ZZ	Fragmentation in Small Intestine, Open Approach	0DFF0ZZ	Fragmentation in Right Large Intestine, Open Approach	0DFL0ZZ	Fragmentation in Transverse Colon, Open Approach
0DF83ZZ	Fragmentation in Small Intestine, Percutaneous Approach	0DFF3ZZ	Fragmentation in Right Large Intestine, Percutaneous Approach	0DFL3ZZ	Fragmentation in Transverse Colon, Percutaneous Approach
0DF84ZZ	Fragmentation in Small Intestine, Percutaneous Endoscopic Approach	0DFF4ZZ	Fragmentation in Right Large Intestine, Percutaneous Endoscopic Approach	0DFL4ZZ	Fragmentation in Transverse Colon, Percutaneous Endoscopic Approach
0DF87ZZ	Fragmentation in Small Intestine, Via Natural or Artificial Opening	0DFF7ZZ	Fragmentation in Right Large Intestine, Via Natural or Artificial Opening	0DFL7ZZ	Fragmentation in Transverse Colon, V Natural or Artificial Opening
0DF88ZZ	Fragmentation in Small Intestine, Via Natural or Artificial Opening Endoscopic	0DFF8ZZ	Fragmentation in Right Large Intestine, Via Natural or Artificial Opening Endoscopic	0DFL8ZZ	Fragmentation in Transverse Colon, V Natural or Artificial Opening Endosco
▲ 0DF8XZZ	Fragmentation in Small Intestine, External Approach	▲ 0DFFXZZ	Fragmentation in Right Large Intestine, External Approach	▲ 0DFLXZZ	Fragmentation in Transverse Colon, External Approach
0DF90ZZ	Fragmentation in Duodenum, Open Approach	0DFG0ZZ	Fragmentation in Left Large Intestine, Open Approach	0DFM0ZZ	Fragmentation in Descending Colon, Open Approach
0DF93ZZ	Fragmentation in Duodenum, Percutaneous Approach	0DFG3ZZ	Fragmentation in Left Large Intestine, Percutaneous Approach	0DFM3ZZ	Fragmentation in Descending Colon, Percutaneous Approach
0DF94ZZ	Fragmentation in Duodenum, Percutaneous Endoscopic Approach	0DFG4ZZ	Fragmentation in Left Large Intestine, Percutaneous Endoscopic Approach	0DFM4ZZ	Fragmentation in Descending Colon, Percutaneous Endoscopic Approach
0DF97ZZ	Fragmentation in Duodenum, Via Natural or Artificial Opening	0DFG7ZZ	Fragmentation in Left Large Intestine, Via Natural or Artificial Opening	0DFM7ZZ	Fragmentation in Descending Colon, V Natural or Artificial Opening
0DF98ZZ	Fragmentation in Duodenum, Via Natural or Artificial Opening Endoscopic	0DFG8ZZ	Fragmentation in Left Large Intestine, Via Natural or Artificial Opening Endoscopic	0DFM8ZZ	Fragmentation in Descending Colon, V Natural or Artificial Opening Endosco
▲ 0DF9XZZ	Fragmentation in Duodenum, External Approach	▲ 0DFGXZZ	Fragmentation in Left Large Intestine, External Approach	▲ 0DFMXZZ	Fragmentation in Descending Colon, External Approach
0DFA0ZZ	Fragmentation in Jejunum, Open Approach	0DFH0ZZ	Fragmentation in Cecum, Open Approach	0DFN0ZZ	Fragmentation in Sigmoid Colon, Ope Approach
0DFA3ZZ	Fragmentation in Jejunum, Percutaneous Approach	0DFH3ZZ	Fragmentation in Cecum, Percutaneous Approach	0DFN3ZZ	Fragmentation in Sigmoid Colon, Percutaneous Approach
0DFA4ZZ	Fragmentation in Jejunum, Percutaneous Endoscopic Approach	0DFH4ZZ	Fragmentation in Cecum, Percutaneous Endoscopic Approach	0DFN4ZZ	Fragmentation in Sigmoid Colon, Percutaneous Endoscopic Approach
0DFA7ZZ	Fragmentation in Jejunum, Via Natural or Artificial Opening	0DFH7ZZ	Fragmentation in Cecum, Via Natural or Artificial Opening	0DFN7ZZ	Fragmentation in Sigmoid Colon, Via Natural or Artificial Opening
0DFA8ZZ	Fragmentation in Jejunum, Via Natural or Artificial Opening Endoscopic	0DFH8ZZ	Fragmentation in Cecum, Via Natural or Artificial Opening Endoscopic	0DFN8ZZ	Fragmentation in Sigmoid Colon, Via Natural or Artificial Opening Endoscop
▲ 0DFAXZZ	Fragmentation in Jejunum, External Approach	▲ 0DFHXZZ	Fragmentation in Cecum, External Approach	▲ 0DFNXZZ	Fragmentation in Sigmoid Colon, External Approach

| ♀ Female-only | ♂ Male-only | ▲ Limited Coverage | ● Non-OR | ▨ HAC-associated procedure | ▲ Non-covered procedures | ✚ Combinati |

P0ZZ	Fragmentation in Rectum, Open Approach	0DFP8ZZ	Fragmentation in Rectum, Via Natural or Artificial Opening Endoscopic	0DFQ4ZZ	Fragmentation in Anus, Percutaneous Endoscopic Approach

P0ZZ Fragmentation in Rectum, Open Approach
P3ZZ Fragmentation in Rectum, Percutaneous Approach
P4ZZ Fragmentation in Rectum, Percutaneous Endoscopic Approach
P7ZZ Fragmentation in Rectum, Via Natural or Artificial Opening

0DFP8ZZ Fragmentation in Rectum, Via Natural or Artificial Opening Endoscopic
▲ **0DFPXZZ** Fragmentation in Rectum, External Approach
0DFQ0ZZ Fragmentation in Anus, Open Approach
0DFQ3ZZ Fragmentation in Anus, Percutaneous Approach

0DFQ4ZZ Fragmentation in Anus, Percutaneous Endoscopic Approach
0DFQ7ZZ Fragmentation in Anus, Via Natural or Artificial Opening
0DFQ8ZZ Fragmentation in Anus, Via Natural or Artificial Opening Endoscopic
▲ **0DFQXZZ** Fragmentation in Anus, External Approach

H – Gastrointestinal System, Insertion

H501Z Insertion of Radioactive Element into Esophagus, Open Approach
H502Z Insertion of Monitoring Device into Esophagus, Open Approach
H503Z Insertion of Infusion Device into Esophagus, Open Approach
H50DZ Insertion of Intraluminal Device into Esophagus, Open Approach
H50UZ Insertion of Feeding Device into Esophagus, Open Approach
H531Z Insertion of Radioactive Element into Esophagus, Percutaneous Approach
H532Z Insertion of Monitoring Device into Esophagus, Percutaneous Approach
H533Z Insertion of Infusion Device into Esophagus, Percutaneous Approach
H53DZ Insertion of Intraluminal Device into Esophagus, Percutaneous Approach
H53UZ Insertion of Feeding Device into Esophagus, Percutaneous Approach
H541Z Insertion of Radioactive Element into Esophagus, Percutaneous Endoscopic Approach
H542Z Insertion of Monitoring Device into Esophagus, Percutaneous Endoscopic Approach
H543Z Insertion of Infusion Device into Esophagus, Percutaneous Endoscopic Approach
H54DZ Insertion of Intraluminal Device into Esophagus, Percutaneous Endoscopic Approach
H54UZ Insertion of Feeding Device into Esophagus, Percutaneous Endoscopic Approach
H571Z Insertion of Radioactive Element into Esophagus, Via Natural or Artificial Opening
H572Z Insertion of Monitoring Device into Esophagus, Via Natural or Artificial Opening
H573Z Insertion of Infusion Device into Esophagus, Via Natural or Artificial Opening
H57BZ Insertion of Airway into Esophagus, Via Natural or Artificial Opening
H57DZ Insertion of Intraluminal Device into Esophagus, Via Natural or Artificial Opening
H57UZ Insertion of Feeding Device into Esophagus, Via Natural or Artificial Opening
H581Z Insertion of Radioactive Element into Esophagus, Via Natural or Artificial Opening Endoscopic
H582Z Insertion of Monitoring Device into Esophagus, Via Natural or Artificial Opening Endoscopic
H583Z Insertion of Infusion Device into Esophagus, Via Natural or Artificial Opening Endoscopic
H58BZ Insertion of Airway into Esophagus, Via Natural or Artificial Opening Endoscopic
H58DZ Insertion of Intraluminal Device into Esophagus, Via Natural or Artificial Opening Endoscopic

0DH58UZ Insertion of Feeding Device into Esophagus, Via Natural or Artificial Opening Endoscopic
0DH602Z Insertion of Monitoring Device into Stomach, Open Approach
0DH603Z Insertion of Infusion Device into Stomach, Open Approach
0DH60DZ Insertion of Intraluminal Device into Stomach, Open Approach
0DH60MZ Insertion of Stimulator Lead into Stomach, Open Approach
0DH60UZ Insertion of Feeding Device into Stomach, Open Approach
0DH632Z Insertion of Monitoring Device into Stomach, Percutaneous Approach
0DH633Z Insertion of Infusion Device into Stomach, Percutaneous Approach
0DH63DZ Insertion of Intraluminal Device into Stomach, Percutaneous Approach
0DH63MZ Insertion of Stimulator Lead into Stomach, Percutaneous Approach
0DH63UZ Insertion of Feeding Device into Stomach, Percutaneous Approach
AHA CC: 4Q, 2013, 117
0DH642Z Insertion of Monitoring Device into Stomach, Percutaneous Endoscopic Approach
0DH643Z Insertion of Infusion Device into Stomach, Percutaneous Endoscopic Approach
0DH64DZ Insertion of Intraluminal Device into Stomach, Percutaneous Endoscopic Approach
0DH64MZ Insertion of Stimulator Lead into Stomach, Percutaneous Endoscopic Approach
0DH64UZ Insertion of Feeding Device into Stomach, Percutaneous Endoscopic Approach
0DH672Z Insertion of Monitoring Device into Stomach, Via Natural or Artificial Opening
0DH673Z Insertion of Infusion Device into Stomach, Via Natural or Artificial Opening
0DH67DZ Insertion of Intraluminal Device into Stomach, Via Natural or Artificial Opening
● **0DH67UZ** Insertion of Feeding Device into Stomach, Via Natural or Artificial Opening
0DH682Z Insertion of Monitoring Device into Stomach, Via Natural or Artificial Opening Endoscopic
0DH683Z Insertion of Infusion Device into Stomach, Via Natural or Artificial Opening Endoscopic
0DH68DZ Insertion of Intraluminal Device into Stomach, Via Natural or Artificial Opening Endoscopic
● **0DH68UZ** Insertion of Feeding Device into Stomach, Via Natural or Artificial Opening Endoscopic
0DH802Z Insertion of Monitoring Device into Small Intestine, Open Approach

0DH803Z Insertion of Infusion Device into Small Intestine, Open Approach
0DH80DZ Insertion of Intraluminal Device into Small Intestine, Open Approach
0DH80UZ Insertion of Feeding Device into Small Intestine, Open Approach
0DH832Z Insertion of Monitoring Device into Small Intestine, Percutaneous Approach
0DH833Z Insertion of Infusion Device into Small Intestine, Percutaneous Approach
0DH83DZ Insertion of Intraluminal Device into Small Intestine, Percutaneous Approach
0DH83UZ Insertion of Feeding Device into Small Intestine, Percutaneous Approach
0DH842Z Insertion of Monitoring Device into Small Intestine, Percutaneous Endoscopic Approach
0DH843Z Insertion of Infusion Device into Small Intestine, Percutaneous Endoscopic Approach
0DH84DZ Insertion of Intraluminal Device into Small Intestine, Percutaneous Endoscopic Approach
0DH84UZ Insertion of Feeding Device into Small Intestine, Percutaneous Endoscopic Approach
0DH872Z Insertion of Monitoring Device into Small Intestine, Via Natural or Artificial Opening
0DH873Z Insertion of Infusion Device into Small Intestine, Via Natural or Artificial Opening
0DH87DZ Insertion of Intraluminal Device into Small Intestine, Via Natural or Artificial Opening
0DH87UZ Insertion of Feeding Device into Small Intestine, Via Natural or Artificial Opening
0DH882Z Insertion of Monitoring Device into Small Intestine, Via Natural or Artificial Opening Endoscopic
0DH883Z Insertion of Infusion Device into Small Intestine, Via Natural or Artificial Opening Endoscopic
0DH88DZ Insertion of Intraluminal Device into Small Intestine, Via Natural or Artificial Opening Endoscopic
0DH88UZ Insertion of Feeding Device into Small Intestine, Via Natural or Artificial Opening Endoscopic
0DH902Z Insertion of Monitoring Device into Duodenum, Open Approach
0DH903Z Insertion of Infusion Device into Duodenum, Open Approach
0DH90DZ Insertion of Intraluminal Device into Duodenum, Open Approach
0DH90UZ Insertion of Feeding Device into Duodenum, Open Approach
0DH932Z Insertion of Monitoring Device into Duodenum, Percutaneous Approach
0DH933Z Insertion of Infusion Device into Duodenum, Percutaneous Approach
0DH93DZ Insertion of Intraluminal Device into Duodenum, Percutaneous Approach

561

0DH93UZ	Insertion of Feeding Device into Duodenum, Percutaneous Approach	
0DH942Z	Insertion of Monitoring Device into Duodenum, Percutaneous Endoscopic Approach	
0DH943Z	Insertion of Infusion Device into Duodenum, Percutaneous Endoscopic Approach	
0DH94DZ	Insertion of Intraluminal Device into Duodenum, Percutaneous Endoscopic Approach	
0DH94UZ	Insertion of Feeding Device into Duodenum, Percutaneous Endoscopic Approach	
0DH972Z	Insertion of Monitoring Device into Duodenum, Via Natural or Artificial Opening	
0DH973Z	Insertion of Infusion Device into Duodenum, Via Natural or Artificial Opening	
0DH97DZ	Insertion of Intraluminal Device into Duodenum, Via Natural or Artificial Opening	
0DH97UZ	Insertion of Feeding Device into Duodenum, Via Natural or Artificial Opening	
0DH982Z	Insertion of Monitoring Device into Duodenum, Via Natural or Artificial Opening Endoscopic	
0DH983Z	Insertion of Infusion Device into Duodenum, Via Natural or Artificial Opening Endoscopic	
0DH98DZ	Insertion of Intraluminal Device into Duodenum, Via Natural or Artificial Opening Endoscopic	
0DH98UZ	Insertion of Feeding Device into Duodenum, Via Natural or Artificial Opening Endoscopic	
0DHA02Z	Insertion of Monitoring Device into Jejunum, Open Approach	
0DHA03Z	Insertion of Infusion Device into Jejunum, Open Approach	
0DHA0DZ	Insertion of Intraluminal Device into Jejunum, Open Approach	
0DHA0UZ	Insertion of Feeding Device into Jejunum, Open Approach	
0DHA32Z	Insertion of Monitoring Device into Jejunum, Percutaneous Approach	
0DHA33Z	Insertion of Infusion Device into Jejunum, Percutaneous Approach	
0DHA3DZ	Insertion of Intraluminal Device into Jejunum, Percutaneous Approach	
0DHA3UZ	Insertion of Feeding Device into Jejunum, Percutaneous Approach	
0DHA42Z	Insertion of Monitoring Device into Jejunum, Percutaneous Endoscopic Approach	
0DHA43Z	Insertion of Infusion Device into Jejunum, Percutaneous Endoscopic Approach	
0DHA4DZ	Insertion of Intraluminal Device into Jejunum, Percutaneous Endoscopic Approach	
0DHA4UZ	Insertion of Feeding Device into Jejunum, Percutaneous Endoscopic Approach	

0DHA72Z	Insertion of Monitoring Device into Jejunum, Via Natural or Artificial Opening
0DHA73Z	Insertion of Infusion Device into Jejunum, Via Natural or Artificial Opening
0DHA7DZ	Insertion of Intraluminal Device into Jejunum, Via Natural or Artificial Opening
0DHA7UZ	Insertion of Feeding Device into Jejunum, Via Natural or Artificial Opening
0DHA82Z	Insertion of Monitoring Device into Jejunum, Via Natural or Artificial Opening Endoscopic
0DHA83Z	Insertion of Infusion Device into Jejunum, Via Natural or Artificial Opening Endoscopic
0DHA8DZ	Insertion of Intraluminal Device into Jejunum, Via Natural or Artificial Opening Endoscopic
0DHA8UZ	Insertion of Feeding Device into Jejunum, Via Natural or Artificial Opening Endoscopic
0DHB02Z	Insertion of Monitoring Device into Ileum, Open Approach
0DHB03Z	Insertion of Infusion Device into Ileum, Open Approach
0DHB0DZ	Insertion of Intraluminal Device into Ileum, Open Approach
0DHB0UZ	Insertion of Feeding Device into Ileum, Open Approach
0DHB32Z	Insertion of Monitoring Device into Ileum, Percutaneous Approach
0DHB33Z	Insertion of Infusion Device into Ileum, Percutaneous Approach
0DHB3DZ	Insertion of Intraluminal Device into Ileum, Percutaneous Approach
0DHB3UZ	Insertion of Feeding Device into Ileum, Percutaneous Approach
0DHB42Z	Insertion of Monitoring Device into Ileum, Percutaneous Endoscopic Approach
0DHB43Z	Insertion of Infusion Device into Ileum, Percutaneous Endoscopic Approach
0DHB4DZ	Insertion of Intraluminal Device into Ileum, Percutaneous Endoscopic Approach
0DHB4UZ	Insertion of Feeding Device into Ileum, Percutaneous Endoscopic Approach
0DHB72Z	Insertion of Monitoring Device into Ileum, Via Natural or Artificial Opening
0DHB73Z	Insertion of Infusion Device into Ileum, Via Natural or Artificial Opening
0DHB7DZ	Insertion of Intraluminal Device into Ileum, Via Natural or Artificial Opening
0DHB7UZ	Insertion of Feeding Device into Ileum, Via Natural or Artificial Opening
0DHB82Z	Insertion of Monitoring Device into Ileum, Via Natural or Artificial Opening Endoscopic
0DHB83Z	Insertion of Infusion Device into Ileum, Via Natural or Artificial Opening Endoscopic
0DHB8DZ	Insertion of Intraluminal Device into Ileum, Via Natural or Artificial Opening Endoscopic

0DHB8UZ	Insertion of Feeding Device into Ileum, Via Natural or Artificial Opening Endoscopic
0DHE0DZ	Insertion of Intraluminal Device into Large Intestine, Open Approach
0DHE3DZ	Insertion of Intraluminal Device into Large Intestine, Percutaneous Approach
0DHE4DZ	Insertion of Intraluminal Device into Large Intestine, Percutaneous Endoscopic Approach
0DHE7DZ	Insertion of Intraluminal Device into Large Intestine, Via Natural or Artificial Opening
0DHE8DZ	Insertion of Intraluminal Device into Large Intestine, Via Natural or Artificial Opening Endoscopic
0DHP01Z	Insertion of Radioactive Element into Rectum, Open Approach
0DHP0DZ	Insertion of Intraluminal Device into Rectum, Open Approach
0DHP31Z	Insertion of Radioactive Element into Rectum, Percutaneous Approach
0DHP3DZ	Insertion of Intraluminal Device into Rectum, Percutaneous Approach
0DHP41Z	Insertion of Radioactive Element into Rectum, Percutaneous Endoscopic Approach
0DHP4DZ	Insertion of Intraluminal Device into Rectum, Percutaneous Endoscopic Approach
0DHP71Z	Insertion of Radioactive Element into Rectum, Via Natural or Artificial Opening
0DHP7DZ	Insertion of Intraluminal Device into Rectum, Via Natural or Artificial Opening
0DHP81Z	Insertion of Radioactive Element into Rectum, Via Natural or Artificial Opening Endoscopic
0DHP8DZ	Insertion of Intraluminal Device into Rectum, Via Natural or Artificial Opening Endoscopic
0DHQ0DZ	Insertion of Intraluminal Device into Anus, Open Approach
0DHQ0LZ	Insertion of Artificial Sphincter into Anus, Open Approach
0DHQ3DZ	Insertion of Intraluminal Device into Anus, Percutaneous Approach
0DHQ3LZ	Insertion of Artificial Sphincter into Anus, Percutaneous Approach
0DHQ4DZ	Insertion of Intraluminal Device into Anus, Percutaneous Endoscopic Approach
0DHQ4LZ	Insertion of Artificial Sphincter into Anus, Percutaneous Endoscopic Approach
0DHQ7DZ	Insertion of Intraluminal Device into Anus, Via Natural or Artificial Opening
0DHQ8DZ	Insertion of Intraluminal Device into Anus, Via Natural or Artificial Opening Endoscopic
0DHR0MZ	Insertion of Stimulator Lead into Anal Sphincter, Open Approach
0DHR3MZ	Insertion of Stimulator Lead into Anal Sphincter, Percutaneous Approach
0DHR4MZ	Insertion of Stimulator Lead into Anal Sphincter, Percutaneous Endoscopic Approach

0DJ – Gastrointestinal System, Inspection

Review Coding Guidelines B3.11a, B3.11b and B3.11c

0DJ00ZZ	Inspection of Upper Intestinal Tract, Open Approach	
0DJ03ZZ	Inspection of Upper Intestinal Tract, Percutaneous Approach	

0DJ04ZZ	Inspection of Upper Intestinal Tract, Percutaneous Endoscopic Approach
0DJ07ZZ	Inspection of Upper Intestinal Tract, Via Natural or Artificial Opening

0DJ08ZZ	Inspection of Upper Intestinal Tract, Via Natural or Artificial Opening Endoscopic
0DJ0XZZ	Inspection of Upper Intestinal Tract, External Approach

60ZZ	Inspection of Stomach, Open Approach
63ZZ	Inspection of Stomach, Percutaneous Approach
64ZZ	Inspection of Stomach, Percutaneous Endoscopic Approach
67ZZ	Inspection of Stomach, Via Natural or Artificial Opening
68ZZ	Inspection of Stomach, Via Natural or Artificial Opening Endoscopic
6XZZ	Inspection of Stomach, External Approach
D0ZZ	Inspection of Lower Intestinal Tract, Open Approach
D3ZZ	Inspection of Lower Intestinal Tract, Percutaneous Approach
0DJD4ZZ	Inspection of Lower Intestinal Tract, Percutaneous Endoscopic Approach
0DJD7ZZ	Inspection of Lower Intestinal Tract, Via Natural or Artificial Opening
0DJD8ZZ	Inspection of Lower Intestinal Tract, Via Natural or Artificial Opening Endoscopic
0DJDXZZ	Inspection of Lower Intestinal Tract, External Approach
0DJU0ZZ	Inspection of Omentum, Open Approach
0DJU3ZZ	Inspection of Omentum, Percutaneous Approach
0DJU4ZZ	Inspection of Omentum, Percutaneous Endoscopic Approach
0DJUXZZ	Inspection of Omentum, External Approach
0DJV0ZZ	Inspection of Mesentery, Open Approach
0DJV3ZZ	Inspection of Mesentery, Percutaneous Approach
0DJV4ZZ	Inspection of Mesentery, Percutaneous Endoscopic Approach
0DJVXZZ	Inspection of Mesentery, External Approach
0DJW0ZZ	Inspection of Peritoneum, Open Approach
0DJW3ZZ	Inspection of Peritoneum, Percutaneous Approach
0DJW4ZZ	Inspection of Peritoneum, Percutaneous Endoscopic Approach
0DJWXZZ	Inspection of Peritoneum, External Approach

L – Gastrointestinal System, Occlusion

10CZ	Occlusion of Upper Esophagus with Extraluminal Device, Open Approach
10DZ	Occlusion of Upper Esophagus with Intraluminal Device, Open Approach
10ZZ	Occlusion of Upper Esophagus, Open Approach
13CZ	Occlusion of Upper Esophagus with Extraluminal Device, Percutaneous Approach
13DZ	Occlusion of Upper Esophagus with Intraluminal Device, Percutaneous Approach
13ZZ	Occlusion of Upper Esophagus, Percutaneous Approach
14CZ	Occlusion of Upper Esophagus with Extraluminal Device, Percutaneous Endoscopic Approach
14DZ	Occlusion of Upper Esophagus with Intraluminal Device, Percutaneous Endoscopic Approach
14ZZ	Occlusion of Upper Esophagus, Percutaneous Endoscopic Approach
17DZ	Occlusion of Upper Esophagus with Intraluminal Device, Via Natural or Artificial Opening
17ZZ	Occlusion of Upper Esophagus, Via Natural or Artificial Opening
18DZ	Occlusion of Upper Esophagus with Intraluminal Device, Via Natural or Artificial Opening Endoscopic
18ZZ	Occlusion of Upper Esophagus, Via Natural or Artificial Opening Endoscopic
20CZ	Occlusion of Middle Esophagus with Extraluminal Device, Open Approach
20DZ	Occlusion of Middle Esophagus with Intraluminal Device, Open Approach
20ZZ	Occlusion of Middle Esophagus, Open Approach
23CZ	Occlusion of Middle Esophagus with Extraluminal Device, Percutaneous Approach
23DZ	Occlusion of Middle Esophagus with Intraluminal Device, Percutaneous Approach
23ZZ	Occlusion of Middle Esophagus, Percutaneous Approach
24CZ	Occlusion of Middle Esophagus with Extraluminal Device, Percutaneous Endoscopic Approach
24DZ	Occlusion of Middle Esophagus with Intraluminal Device, Percutaneous Endoscopic Approach
24ZZ	Occlusion of Middle Esophagus, Percutaneous Endoscopic Approach
27DZ	Occlusion of Middle Esophagus with Intraluminal Device, Via Natural or Artificial Opening

0DL27ZZ	Occlusion of Middle Esophagus, Via Natural or Artificial Opening
0DL28DZ	Occlusion of Middle Esophagus with Intraluminal Device, Via Natural or Artificial Opening Endoscopic
0DL28ZZ	Occlusion of Middle Esophagus, Via Natural or Artificial Opening Endoscopic
0DL30CZ	Occlusion of Lower Esophagus with Extraluminal Device, Open Approach
0DL30DZ	Occlusion of Lower Esophagus with Intraluminal Device, Open Approach
0DL30ZZ	Occlusion of Lower Esophagus, Open Approach
0DL33CZ	Occlusion of Lower Esophagus with Extraluminal Device, Percutaneous Approach
0DL33DZ	Occlusion of Lower Esophagus with Intraluminal Device, Percutaneous Approach
0DL33ZZ	Occlusion of Lower Esophagus, Percutaneous Approach
0DL34CZ	Occlusion of Lower Esophagus with Extraluminal Device, Percutaneous Endoscopic Approach
0DL34DZ	Occlusion of Lower Esophagus with Intraluminal Device, Percutaneous Endoscopic Approach
0DL34ZZ	Occlusion of Lower Esophagus, Percutaneous Endoscopic Approach
0DL37DZ	Occlusion of Lower Esophagus with Intraluminal Device, Via Natural or Artificial Opening
0DL37ZZ	Occlusion of Lower Esophagus, Via Natural or Artificial Opening
0DL38DZ	Occlusion of Lower Esophagus with Intraluminal Device, Via Natural or Artificial Opening Endoscopic
0DL38ZZ	Occlusion of Lower Esophagus, Via Natural or Artificial Opening Endoscopic
0DL40CZ	Occlusion of Esophagogastric Junction with Extraluminal Device, Open Approach
0DL40DZ	Occlusion of Esophagogastric Junction with Intraluminal Device, Open Approach
0DL40ZZ	Occlusion of Esophagogastric Junction, Open Approach
0DL43CZ	Occlusion of Esophagogastric Junction with Extraluminal Device, Percutaneous Approach
0DL43DZ	Occlusion of Esophagogastric Junction with Intraluminal Device, Percutaneous Approach
0DL43ZZ	Occlusion of Esophagogastric Junction, Percutaneous Approach

0DL44CZ	Occlusion of Esophagogastric Junction with Extraluminal Device, Percutaneous Endoscopic Approach
0DL44DZ	Occlusion of Esophagogastric Junction with Intraluminal Device, Percutaneous Endoscopic Approach
0DL44ZZ	Occlusion of Esophagogastric Junction, Percutaneous Endoscopic Approach
0DL47DZ	Occlusion of Esophagogastric Junction with Intraluminal Device, Via Natural or Artificial Opening
0DL47ZZ	Occlusion of Esophagogastric Junction, Via Natural or Artificial Opening
0DL48DZ	Occlusion of Esophagogastric Junction with Intraluminal Device, Via Natural or Artificial Opening Endoscopic
0DL48ZZ	Occlusion of Esophagogastric Junction, Via Natural or Artificial Opening Endoscopic
0DL50CZ	Occlusion of Esophagus with Extraluminal Device, Open Approach
0DL50DZ	Occlusion of Esophagus with Intraluminal Device, Open Approach
0DL50ZZ	Occlusion of Esophagus, Open Approach
0DL53CZ	Occlusion of Esophagus with Extraluminal Device, Percutaneous Approach
0DL53DZ	Occlusion of Esophagus with Intraluminal Device, Percutaneous Approach
0DL53ZZ	Occlusion of Esophagus, Percutaneous Approach
0DL54CZ	Occlusion of Esophagus with Extraluminal Device, Percutaneous Endoscopic Approach
0DL54DZ	Occlusion of Esophagus with Intraluminal Device, Percutaneous Endoscopic Approach
0DL54ZZ	Occlusion of Esophagus, Percutaneous Endoscopic Approach
0DL57DZ	Occlusion of Esophagus with Intraluminal Device, Via Natural or Artificial Opening
0DL57ZZ	Occlusion of Esophagus, Via Natural or Artificial Opening
0DL58DZ	Occlusion of Esophagus with Intraluminal Device, Via Natural or Artificial Opening Endoscopic
0DL58ZZ	Occlusion of Esophagus, Via Natural or Artificial Opening Endoscopic
0DL60CZ	Occlusion of Stomach with Extraluminal Device, Open Approach
0DL60DZ	Occlusion of Stomach with Intraluminal Device, Open Approach
0DL60ZZ	Occlusion of Stomach, Open Approach
0DL63CZ	Occlusion of Stomach with Extraluminal Device, Percutaneous Approach

Female-only   ♂ Male-only   ▲ Limited Coverage   ● Non-OR   HAC-associated procedure   ▲ Non-covered procedures   ✚ Combination

0DL63DZ Occlusion of Stomach with Intraluminal Device, Percutaneous Approach

0DL63ZZ Occlusion of Stomach, Percutaneous Approach

0DL64CZ Occlusion of Stomach with Extraluminal Device, Percutaneous Endoscopic Approach

0DL64DZ Occlusion of Stomach with Intraluminal Device, Percutaneous Endoscopic Approach

0DL64ZZ Occlusion of Stomach, Percutaneous Endoscopic Approach

0DL67DZ Occlusion of Stomach with Intraluminal Device, Via Natural or Artificial Opening

0DL67ZZ Occlusion of Stomach, Via Natural or Artificial Opening

0DL68DZ Occlusion of Stomach with Intraluminal Device, Via Natural or Artificial Opening Endoscopic

0DL68ZZ Occlusion of Stomach, Via Natural or Artificial Opening Endoscopic

0DL70CZ Occlusion of Stomach, Pylorus with Extraluminal Device, Open Approach

0DL70DZ Occlusion of Stomach, Pylorus with Intraluminal Device, Open Approach

0DL70ZZ Occlusion of Stomach, Pylorus, Open Approach

0DL73CZ Occlusion of Stomach, Pylorus with Extraluminal Device, Percutaneous Approach

0DL73DZ Occlusion of Stomach, Pylorus with Intraluminal Device, Percutaneous Approach

0DL73ZZ Occlusion of Stomach, Pylorus, Percutaneous Approach

0DL74CZ Occlusion of Stomach, Pylorus with Extraluminal Device, Percutaneous Endoscopic Approach

0DL74DZ Occlusion of Stomach, Pylorus with Intraluminal Device, Percutaneous Endoscopic Approach

0DL74ZZ Occlusion of Stomach, Pylorus, Percutaneous Endoscopic Approach

0DL77DZ Occlusion of Stomach, Pylorus with Intraluminal Device, Via Natural or Artificial Opening

0DL77ZZ Occlusion of Stomach, Pylorus, Via Natural or Artificial Opening

0DL78DZ Occlusion of Stomach, Pylorus with Intraluminal Device, Via Natural or Artificial Opening Endoscopic

0DL78ZZ Occlusion of Stomach, Pylorus, Via Natural or Artificial Opening Endoscopic

0DL80CZ Occlusion of Small Intestine with Extraluminal Device, Open Approach

0DL80DZ Occlusion of Small Intestine with Intraluminal Device, Open Approach

0DL80ZZ Occlusion of Small Intestine, Open Approach

0DL83CZ Occlusion of Small Intestine with Extraluminal Device, Percutaneous Approach

0DL83DZ Occlusion of Small Intestine with Intraluminal Device, Percutaneous Approach

0DL83ZZ Occlusion of Small Intestine, Percutaneous Approach

0DL84CZ Occlusion of Small Intestine with Extraluminal Device, Percutaneous Endoscopic Approach

0DL84DZ Occlusion of Small Intestine with Intraluminal Device, Percutaneous Endoscopic Approach

0DL84ZZ Occlusion of Small Intestine, Percutaneous Endoscopic Approach

0DL87DZ Occlusion of Small Intestine with Intraluminal Device, Via Natural or Artificial Opening

0DL87ZZ Occlusion of Small Intestine, Via Natural or Artificial Opening

0DL88DZ Occlusion of Small Intestine with Intraluminal Device, Via Natural or Artificial Opening Endoscopic

0DL88ZZ Occlusion of Small Intestine, Via Natural or Artificial Opening Endoscopic

0DL90CZ Occlusion of Duodenum with Extraluminal Device, Open Approach

0DL90DZ Occlusion of Duodenum with Intraluminal Device, Open Approach

0DL90ZZ Occlusion of Duodenum, Open Approach

0DL93CZ Occlusion of Duodenum with Extraluminal Device, Percutaneous Approach

0DL93DZ Occlusion of Duodenum with Intraluminal Device, Percutaneous Approach

0DL93ZZ Occlusion of Duodenum, Percutaneous Approach

0DL94CZ Occlusion of Duodenum with Extraluminal Device, Percutaneous Endoscopic Approach

0DL94DZ Occlusion of Duodenum with Intraluminal Device, Percutaneous Endoscopic Approach

0DL94ZZ Occlusion of Duodenum, Percutaneous Endoscopic Approach

0DL97DZ Occlusion of Duodenum with Intraluminal Device, Via Natural or Artificial Opening

0DL97ZZ Occlusion of Duodenum, Via Natural or Artificial Opening

0DL98DZ Occlusion of Duodenum with Intraluminal Device, Via Natural or Artificial Opening Endoscopic

0DL98ZZ Occlusion of Duodenum, Via Natural or Artificial Opening Endoscopic

0DLA0CZ Occlusion of Jejunum with Extraluminal Device, Open Approach

0DLA0DZ Occlusion of Jejunum with Intraluminal Device, Open Approach

0DLA0ZZ Occlusion of Jejunum, Open Approach

0DLA3CZ Occlusion of Jejunum with Extraluminal Device, Percutaneous Approach

0DLA3DZ Occlusion of Jejunum with Intraluminal Device, Percutaneous Approach

0DLA3ZZ Occlusion of Jejunum, Percutaneous Approach

0DLA4CZ Occlusion of Jejunum with Extraluminal Device, Percutaneous Endoscopic Approach

0DLA4DZ Occlusion of Jejunum with Intraluminal Device, Percutaneous Endoscopic Approach

0DLA4ZZ Occlusion of Jejunum, Percutaneous Endoscopic Approach

0DLA7DZ Occlusion of Jejunum with Intraluminal Device, Via Natural or Artificial Opening

0DLA7ZZ Occlusion of Jejunum, Via Natural or Artificial Opening

0DLA8DZ Occlusion of Jejunum with Intraluminal Device, Via Natural or Artificial Opening Endoscopic

0DLA8ZZ Occlusion of Jejunum, Via Natural or Artificial Opening Endoscopic

0DLB0CZ Occlusion of Ileum with Extraluminal Device, Open Approach

0DLB0DZ Occlusion of Ileum with Intraluminal Device, Open Approach

0DLB0ZZ Occlusion of Ileum, Open Approach

0DLB3CZ Occlusion of Ileum with Extraluminal Device, Percutaneous Approach

0DLB3DZ Occlusion of Ileum with Intraluminal Device, Percutaneous Approach

0DLB3ZZ Occlusion of Ileum, Percutaneous Approach

0DLB4CZ Occlusion of Ileum with Extraluminal Device, Percutaneous Endoscopic Approach

0DLB4DZ Occlusion of Ileum with Intraluminal Device, Percutaneous Endoscopic Approach

0DLB4ZZ Occlusion of Ileum, Percutaneous Endoscopic Approach

0DLB7DZ Occlusion of Ileum with Intraluminal Device, Via Natural or Artificial Opening

0DLB7ZZ Occlusion of Ileum, Via Natural or Artificial Opening

0DLB8DZ Occlusion of Ileum with Intraluminal Device, Via Natural or Artificial Opening Endoscopic

0DLB8ZZ Occlusion of Ileum, Via Natural or Artificial Opening Endoscopic

0DLC0CZ Occlusion of Ileocecal Valve with Extraluminal Device, Open Approach

0DLC0DZ Occlusion of Ileocecal Valve with Intraluminal Device, Open Approach

0DLC0ZZ Occlusion of Ileocecal Valve, Open Approach

0DLC3CZ Occlusion of Ileocecal Valve with Extraluminal Device, Percutaneous Approach

0DLC3DZ Occlusion of Ileocecal Valve with Intraluminal Device, Percutaneous Approach

0DLC3ZZ Occlusion of Ileocecal Valve, Percutaneous Approach

0DLC4CZ Occlusion of Ileocecal Valve with Extraluminal Device, Percutaneous Endoscopic Approach

0DLC4DZ Occlusion of Ileocecal Valve with Intraluminal Device, Percutaneous Endoscopic Approach

0DLC4ZZ Occlusion of Ileocecal Valve, Percutaneous Endoscopic Approach

0DLC7DZ Occlusion of Ileocecal Valve with Intraluminal Device, Via Natural or Artificial Opening

0DLC7ZZ Occlusion of Ileocecal Valve, Via Natural or Artificial Opening

0DLC8DZ Occlusion of Ileocecal Valve with Intraluminal Device, Via Natural or Artificial Opening Endoscopic

0DLC8ZZ Occlusion of Ileocecal Valve, Via Natural or Artificial Opening Endoscopic

0DLE0CZ Occlusion of Large Intestine with Extraluminal Device, Open Approach

0DLE0DZ Occlusion of Large Intestine with Intraluminal Device, Open Approach

0DLE0ZZ Occlusion of Large Intestine, Open Approach

0DLE3CZ Occlusion of Large Intestine with Extraluminal Device, Percutaneous Approach

0DLE3DZ Occlusion of Large Intestine with Intraluminal Device, Percutaneous Approach

0DLE3ZZ Occlusion of Large Intestine, Percutaneous Approach

0DLE4CZ Occlusion of Large Intestine with Extraluminal Device, Percutaneous Endoscopic Approach

0DLE4DZ Occlusion of Large Intestine with Intraluminal Device, Percutaneous Endoscopic Approach

0DLE4ZZ Occlusion of Large Intestine, Percutaneous Endoscopic Approach

E7DZ	Occlusion of Large Intestine with Intraluminal Device, Via Natural or Artificial Opening
E7ZZ	Occlusion of Large Intestine, Via Natural or Artificial Opening
E8DZ	Occlusion of Large Intestine with Intraluminal Device, Via Natural or Artificial Opening Endoscopic
E8ZZ	Occlusion of Large Intestine, Via Natural or Artificial Opening Endoscopic
F0CZ	Occlusion of Right Large Intestine with Extraluminal Device, Open Approach
F0DZ	Occlusion of Right Large Intestine with Intraluminal Device, Open Approach
F0ZZ	Occlusion of Right Large Intestine, Open Approach
F3CZ	Occlusion of Right Large Intestine with Extraluminal Device, Percutaneous Approach
F3DZ	Occlusion of Right Large Intestine with Intraluminal Device, Percutaneous Approach
F3ZZ	Occlusion of Right Large Intestine, Percutaneous Approach
F4CZ	Occlusion of Right Large Intestine with Extraluminal Device, Percutaneous Endoscopic Approach
F4DZ	Occlusion of Right Large Intestine with Intraluminal Device, Percutaneous Endoscopic Approach
F4ZZ	Occlusion of Right Large Intestine, Percutaneous Endoscopic Approach
F7DZ	Occlusion of Right Large Intestine with Intraluminal Device, Via Natural or Artificial Opening
F7ZZ	Occlusion of Right Large Intestine, Via Natural or Artificial Opening
F8DZ	Occlusion of Right Large Intestine with Intraluminal Device, Via Natural or Artificial Opening Endoscopic
F8ZZ	Occlusion of Right Large Intestine, Via Natural or Artificial Opening Endoscopic
G0CZ	Occlusion of Left Large Intestine with Extraluminal Device, Open Approach
G0DZ	Occlusion of Left Large Intestine with Intraluminal Device, Open Approach
G0ZZ	Occlusion of Left Large Intestine, Open Approach
G3CZ	Occlusion of Left Large Intestine with Extraluminal Device, Percutaneous Approach
G3DZ	Occlusion of Left Large Intestine with Intraluminal Device, Percutaneous Approach
G3ZZ	Occlusion of Left Large Intestine, Percutaneous Approach
G4CZ	Occlusion of Left Large Intestine with Extraluminal Device, Percutaneous Endoscopic Approach
G4DZ	Occlusion of Left Large Intestine with Intraluminal Device, Percutaneous Endoscopic Approach
G4ZZ	Occlusion of Left Large Intestine, Percutaneous Endoscopic Approach
G7DZ	Occlusion of Left Large Intestine with Intraluminal Device, Via Natural or Artificial Opening
G7ZZ	Occlusion of Left Large Intestine, Via Natural or Artificial Opening
G8DZ	Occlusion of Left Large Intestine with Intraluminal Device, Via Natural or Artificial Opening Endoscopic
G8ZZ	Occlusion of Left Large Intestine, Via Natural or Artificial Opening Endoscopic
LH0CZ	Occlusion of Cecum with Extraluminal Device, Open Approach

0DLH0DZ	Occlusion of Cecum with Intraluminal Device, Open Approach
0DLH0ZZ	Occlusion of Cecum, Open Approach
0DLH3CZ	Occlusion of Cecum with Extraluminal Device, Percutaneous Approach
0DLH3DZ	Occlusion of Cecum with Intraluminal Device, Percutaneous Approach
0DLH3ZZ	Occlusion of Cecum, Percutaneous Approach
0DLH4CZ	Occlusion of Cecum with Extraluminal Device, Percutaneous Endoscopic Approach
0DLH4DZ	Occlusion of Cecum with Intraluminal Device, Percutaneous Endoscopic Approach
0DLH4ZZ	Occlusion of Cecum, Percutaneous Endoscopic Approach
0DLH7DZ	Occlusion of Cecum with Intraluminal Device, Via Natural or Artificial Opening
0DLH7ZZ	Occlusion of Cecum, Via Natural or Artificial Opening
0DLH8DZ	Occlusion of Cecum with Intraluminal Device, Via Natural or Artificial Opening Endoscopic
0DLH8ZZ	Occlusion of Cecum, Via Natural or Artificial Opening Endoscopic
0DLK0CZ	Occlusion of Ascending Colon with Extraluminal Device, Open Approach
0DLK0DZ	Occlusion of Ascending Colon with Intraluminal Device, Open Approach
0DLK0ZZ	Occlusion of Ascending Colon, Open Approach
0DLK3CZ	Occlusion of Ascending Colon with Extraluminal Device, Percutaneous Approach
0DLK3DZ	Occlusion of Ascending Colon with Intraluminal Device, Percutaneous Approach
0DLK3ZZ	Occlusion of Ascending Colon, Percutaneous Approach
0DLK4CZ	Occlusion of Ascending Colon with Extraluminal Device, Percutaneous Endoscopic Approach
0DLK4DZ	Occlusion of Ascending Colon with Intraluminal Device, Percutaneous Endoscopic Approach
0DLK4ZZ	Occlusion of Ascending Colon, Percutaneous Endoscopic Approach
0DLK7DZ	Occlusion of Ascending Colon with Intraluminal Device, Via Natural or Artificial Opening
0DLK7ZZ	Occlusion of Ascending Colon, Via Natural or Artificial Opening
0DLK8DZ	Occlusion of Ascending Colon with Intraluminal Device, Via Natural or Artificial Opening Endoscopic
0DLK8ZZ	Occlusion of Ascending Colon, Via Natural or Artificial Opening Endoscopic
0DLL0CZ	Occlusion of Transverse Colon with Extraluminal Device, Open Approach
0DLL0DZ	Occlusion of Transverse Colon with Intraluminal Device, Open Approach
0DLL0ZZ	Occlusion of Transverse Colon, Open Approach
0DLL3CZ	Occlusion of Transverse Colon with Extraluminal Device, Percutaneous Approach
0DLL3DZ	Occlusion of Transverse Colon with Intraluminal Device, Percutaneous Approach
0DLL3ZZ	Occlusion of Transverse Colon, Percutaneous Approach
0DLL4CZ	Occlusion of Transverse Colon with Extraluminal Device, Percutaneous Endoscopic Approach

0DLL4DZ	Occlusion of Transverse Colon with Intraluminal Device, Percutaneous Endoscopic Approach
0DLL4ZZ	Occlusion of Transverse Colon, Percutaneous Endoscopic Approach
0DLL7DZ	Occlusion of Transverse Colon with Intraluminal Device, Via Natural or Artificial Opening
0DLL7ZZ	Occlusion of Transverse Colon, Via Natural or Artificial Opening
0DLL8DZ	Occlusion of Transverse Colon with Intraluminal Device, Via Natural or Artificial Opening Endoscopic
0DLL8ZZ	Occlusion of Transverse Colon, Via Natural or Artificial Opening Endoscopic
0DLM0CZ	Occlusion of Descending Colon with Extraluminal Device, Open Approach
0DLM0DZ	Occlusion of Descending Colon with Intraluminal Device, Open Approach
0DLM0ZZ	Occlusion of Descending Colon, Open Approach
0DLM3CZ	Occlusion of Descending Colon with Extraluminal Device, Percutaneous Approach
0DLM3DZ	Occlusion of Descending Colon with Intraluminal Device, Percutaneous Approach
0DLM3ZZ	Occlusion of Descending Colon, Percutaneous Approach
0DLM4CZ	Occlusion of Descending Colon with Extraluminal Device, Percutaneous Endoscopic Approach
0DLM4DZ	Occlusion of Descending Colon with Intraluminal Device, Percutaneous Endoscopic Approach
0DLM4ZZ	Occlusion of Descending Colon, Percutaneous Endoscopic Approach
0DLM7DZ	Occlusion of Descending Colon with Intraluminal Device, Via Natural or Artificial Opening
0DLM7ZZ	Occlusion of Descending Colon, Via Natural or Artificial Opening
0DLM8DZ	Occlusion of Descending Colon with Intraluminal Device, Via Natural or Artificial Opening Endoscopic
0DLM8ZZ	Occlusion of Descending Colon, Via Natural or Artificial Opening Endoscopic
0DLN0CZ	Occlusion of Sigmoid Colon with Extraluminal Device, Open Approach
0DLN0DZ	Occlusion of Sigmoid Colon with Intraluminal Device, Open Approach
0DLN0ZZ	Occlusion of Sigmoid Colon, Open Approach
0DLN3CZ	Occlusion of Sigmoid Colon with Extraluminal Device, Percutaneous Approach
0DLN3DZ	Occlusion of Sigmoid Colon with Intraluminal Device, Percutaneous Approach
0DLN3ZZ	Occlusion of Sigmoid Colon, Percutaneous Approach
0DLN4CZ	Occlusion of Sigmoid Colon with Extraluminal Device, Percutaneous Endoscopic Approach
0DLN4DZ	Occlusion of Sigmoid Colon with Intraluminal Device, Percutaneous Endoscopic Approach
0DLN4ZZ	Occlusion of Sigmoid Colon, Percutaneous Endoscopic Approach
0DLN7DZ	Occlusion of Sigmoid Colon with Intraluminal Device, Via Natural or Artificial Opening
0DLN7ZZ	Occlusion of Sigmoid Colon, Via Natural or Artificial Opening
0DLN8DZ	Occlusion of Sigmoid Colon with Intraluminal Device, Via Natural or Artificial Opening Endoscopic

Female-only   ♂ Male-only   ▲ Limited Coverage   ● Non-OR   ▧ HAC-associated procedure   ▲ Non-covered procedures   ✚ Combination

0DLN8ZZ Occlusion of Sigmoid Colon, Via Natural or Artificial Opening Endoscopic	**0DLP7DZ** Occlusion of Rectum with Intraluminal Device, Via Natural or Artificial Opening	**0DLQ4CZ** Occlusion of Anus with Extraluminal Device, Percutaneous Endoscopic Approach
0DLP0CZ Occlusion of Rectum with Extraluminal Device, Open Approach	**0DLP7ZZ** Occlusion of Rectum, Via Natural or Artificial Opening	**0DLQ4DZ** Occlusion of Anus with Intraluminal Device, Percutaneous Endoscopic Approach
0DLP0DZ Occlusion of Rectum with Intraluminal Device, Open Approach	**0DLP8DZ** Occlusion of Rectum with Intraluminal Device, Via Natural or Artificial Opening Endoscopic	**0DLQ4ZZ** Occlusion of Anus, Percutaneous Endoscopic Approach
0DLP0ZZ Occlusion of Rectum, Open Approach		**0DLQ7DZ** Occlusion of Anus with Intraluminal Device, Via Natural or Artificial Oper
0DLP3CZ Occlusion of Rectum with Extraluminal Device, Percutaneous Approach	**0DLP8ZZ** Occlusion of Rectum, Via Natural or Artificial Opening Endoscopic	**0DLQ7ZZ** Occlusion of Anus, Via Natural or Artificial Opening
0DLP3DZ Occlusion of Rectum with Intraluminal Device, Percutaneous Approach	**0DLQ0CZ** Occlusion of Anus with Extraluminal Device, Open Approach	**0DLQ8DZ** Occlusion of Anus with Intraluminal Device, Via Natural or Artificial Oper Endoscopic
0DLP3ZZ Occlusion of Rectum, Percutaneous Approach	**0DLQ0DZ** Occlusion of Anus with Intraluminal Device, Open Approach	**0DLQ8ZZ** Occlusion of Anus, Via Natural or Artificial Opening Endoscopic
0DLP4CZ Occlusion of Rectum with Extraluminal Device, Percutaneous Endoscopic Approach	**0DLQ0ZZ** Occlusion of Anus, Open Approach	**0DLQXCZ** Occlusion of Anus with Extraluminal Device, External Approach
	0DLQ3CZ Occlusion of Anus with Extraluminal Device, Percutaneous Approach	**0DLQXDZ** Occlusion of Anus with Intraluminal Device, External Approach
0DLP4DZ Occlusion of Rectum with Intraluminal Device, Percutaneous Endoscopic Approach	**0DLQ3DZ** Occlusion of Anus with Intraluminal Device, Percutaneous Approach	**0DLQXZZ** Occlusion of Anus, External Approach
0DLP4ZZ Occlusion of Rectum, Percutaneous Endoscopic Approach	**0DLQ3ZZ** Occlusion of Anus, Percutaneous Approach	

0DM – Gastrointestinal System, Reattachment

0DM50ZZ Reattachment of Esophagus, Open Approach	**0DMB0ZZ** Reattachment of Ileum, Open Approach	**0DMK4ZZ** Reattachment of Ascending Colon, Percutaneous Endoscopic Approach
0DM54ZZ Reattachment of Esophagus, Percutaneous Endoscopic Approach	**0DMB4ZZ** Reattachment of Ileum, Percutaneous Endoscopic Approach	**0DML0ZZ** Reattachment of Transverse Colon, O Approach
0DM60ZZ Reattachment of Stomach, Open Approach	**0DME0ZZ** Reattachment of Large Intestine, Open Approach	**0DML4ZZ** Reattachment of Transverse Colon, Percutaneous Endoscopic Approach
0DM64ZZ Reattachment of Stomach, Percutaneous Endoscopic Approach	**0DME4ZZ** Reattachment of Large Intestine, Percutaneous Endoscopic Approach	**0DMM0ZZ** Reattachment of Descending Colon, Open Approach
0DM80ZZ Reattachment of Small Intestine, Open Approach	**0DMF0ZZ** Reattachment of Right Large Intestine, Open Approach	**0DMM4ZZ** Reattachment of Descending Colon, Percutaneous Endoscopic Approach
0DM84ZZ Reattachment of Small Intestine, Percutaneous Endoscopic Approach	**0DMF4ZZ** Reattachment of Right Large Intestine, Percutaneous Endoscopic Approach	**0DMN0ZZ** Reattachment of Sigmoid Colon, Ope Approach
0DM90ZZ Reattachment of Duodenum, Open Approach	**0DMG0ZZ** Reattachment of Left Large Intestine, Open Approach	**0DMN4ZZ** Reattachment of Sigmoid Colon, Percutaneous Endoscopic Approach
0DM94ZZ Reattachment of Duodenum, Percutaneous Endoscopic Approach	**0DMG4ZZ** Reattachment of Left Large Intestine, Percutaneous Endoscopic Approach	**0DMP0ZZ** Reattachment of Rectum, Open Appro
0DMA0ZZ Reattachment of Jejunum, Open Approach	**0DMH0ZZ** Reattachment of Cecum, Open Approach	**0DMP4ZZ** Reattachment of Rectum, Percutaneou Endoscopic Approach
0DMA4ZZ Reattachment of Jejunum, Percutaneous Endoscopic Approach	**0DMH4ZZ** Reattachment of Cecum, Percutaneous Endoscopic Approach	
	0DMK0ZZ Reattachment of Ascending Colon, Open Approach	

0DN – Gastrointestinal System, Release

Review Coding Guideline B3.13

Review Coding Guideline B3.14

0DN10ZZ Release Upper Esophagus, Open Approach	**0DN34ZZ** Release Lower Esophagus, Percutaneous Endoscopic Approach	**0DN58ZZ** Release Esophagus, Via Natural or Artificial Opening Endoscopic
0DN13ZZ Release Upper Esophagus, Percutaneous Approach	**0DN37ZZ** Release Lower Esophagus, Via Natural or Artificial Opening	**0DN60ZZ** Release Stomach, Open Approach
0DN14ZZ Release Upper Esophagus, Percutaneous Endoscopic Approach	**0DN38ZZ** Release Lower Esophagus, Via Natural or Artificial Opening Endoscopic	**0DN63ZZ** Release Stomach, Percutaneous Approa
		0DN64ZZ Release Stomach, Percutaneous Endoscopic Approach
0DN17ZZ Release Upper Esophagus, Via Natural or Artificial Opening	**0DN40ZZ** Release Esophagogastric Junction, Open Approach	**0DN67ZZ** Release Stomach, Via Natural or Artific Opening
0DN18ZZ Release Upper Esophagus, Via Natural or Artificial Opening Endoscopic	**0DN43ZZ** Release Esophagogastric Junction, Percutaneous Approach	**0DN68ZZ** Release Stomach, Via Natural or Artific Opening Endoscopic
0DN20ZZ Release Middle Esophagus, Open Approach	**0DN44ZZ** Release Esophagogastric Junction, Percutaneous Endoscopic Approach	**0DN70ZZ** Release Stomach, Pylorus, Open Approach
0DN23ZZ Release Middle Esophagus, Percutaneous Approach	**0DN47ZZ** Release Esophagogastric Junction, Via Natural or Artificial Opening	**0DN73ZZ** Release Stomach, Pylorus, Percutaneou Approach
0DN24ZZ Release Middle Esophagus, Percutaneous Endoscopic Approach	**0DN48ZZ** Release Esophagogastric Junction, Via Natural or Artificial Opening Endoscopic	**0DN74ZZ** Release Stomach, Pylorus, Percutaneou Endoscopic Approach
0DN27ZZ Release Middle Esophagus, Via Natural or Artificial Opening	**0DN50ZZ** Release Esophagus, Open Approach	**0DN77ZZ** Release Stomach, Pylorus, Via Natural Artificial Opening
0DN28ZZ Release Middle Esophagus, Via Natural or Artificial Opening Endoscopic	**0DN53ZZ** Release Esophagus, Percutaneous Approach	**0DN78ZZ** Release Stomach, Pylorus, Via Natural o Artificial Opening Endoscopic
0DN30ZZ Release Lower Esophagus, Open Approach	**0DN54ZZ** Release Esophagus, Percutaneous Endoscopic Approach	**0DN80ZZ** Release Small Intestine, Open Approach
0DN33ZZ Release Lower Esophagus, Percutaneous Approach	**0DN57ZZ** Release Esophagus, Via Natural or Artificial Opening	**0DN83ZZ** Release Small Intestine, Percutaneous Approach
		0DN84ZZ Release Small Intestine, Percutaneous Endoscopic Approach

Code	Description	Code	Description	Code	Description
87ZZ	Release Small Intestine, Via Natural or Artificial Opening	0DNG0ZZ	Release Left Large Intestine, Open Approach	0DNN0ZZ	Release Sigmoid Colon, Open Approach
88ZZ	Release Small Intestine, Via Natural or Artificial Opening Endoscopic	0DNG3ZZ	Release Left Large Intestine, Percutaneous Approach	0DNN3ZZ	Release Sigmoid Colon, Percutaneous Approach
90ZZ	Release Duodenum, Open Approach	0DNG4ZZ	Release Left Large Intestine, Percutaneous Endoscopic Approach	0DNN4ZZ	Release Sigmoid Colon, Percutaneous Endoscopic Approach
93ZZ	Release Duodenum, Percutaneous Approach	0DNG7ZZ	Release Left Large Intestine, Via Natural or Artificial Opening	0DNN7ZZ	Release Sigmoid Colon, Via Natural or Artificial Opening
94ZZ	Release Duodenum, Percutaneous Endoscopic Approach	0DNG8ZZ	Release Left Large Intestine, Via Natural or Artificial Opening Endoscopic	0DNN8ZZ	Release Sigmoid Colon, Via Natural or Artificial Opening Endoscopic
97ZZ	Release Duodenum, Via Natural or Artificial Opening	0DNH0ZZ	Release Cecum, Open Approach	0DNP0ZZ	Release Rectum, Open Approach
98ZZ	Release Duodenum, Via Natural or Artificial Opening Endoscopic	0DNH3ZZ	Release Cecum, Percutaneous Approach	0DNP3ZZ	Release Rectum, Percutaneous Approach
A0ZZ	Release Jejunum, Open Approach	0DNH4ZZ	Release Cecum, Percutaneous Endoscopic Approach	0DNP4ZZ	Release Rectum, Percutaneous Endoscopic Approach
A3ZZ	Release Jejunum, Percutaneous Approach	0DNH7ZZ	Release Cecum, Via Natural or Artificial Opening	0DNP7ZZ	Release Rectum, Via Natural or Artificial Opening
A4ZZ	Release Jejunum, Percutaneous Endoscopic Approach	0DNH8ZZ	Release Cecum, Via Natural or Artificial Opening Endoscopic	0DNP8ZZ	Release Rectum, Via Natural or Artificial Opening Endoscopic
A7ZZ	Release Jejunum, Via Natural or Artificial Opening	0DNJ0ZZ	Release Appendix, Open Approach	0DNQ0ZZ	Release Anus, Open Approach
A8ZZ	Release Jejunum, Via Natural or Artificial Opening Endoscopic	0DNJ3ZZ	Release Appendix, Percutaneous Approach	0DNQ3ZZ	Release Anus, Percutaneous Approach
B0ZZ	Release Ileum, Open Approach	0DNJ4ZZ	Release Appendix, Percutaneous Endoscopic Approach	0DNQ4ZZ	Release Anus, Percutaneous Endoscopic Approach
B3ZZ	Release Ileum, Percutaneous Approach	0DNJ7ZZ	Release Appendix, Via Natural or Artificial Opening	0DNQ7ZZ	Release Anus, Via Natural or Artificial Opening
B4ZZ	Release Ileum, Percutaneous Endoscopic Approach	0DNJ8ZZ	Release Appendix, Via Natural or Artificial Opening Endoscopic	0DNQ8ZZ	Release Anus, Via Natural or Artificial Opening Endoscopic
B7ZZ	Release Ileum, Via Natural or Artificial Opening	0DNK0ZZ	Release Ascending Colon, Open Approach	0DNQXZZ	Release Anus, External Approach
B8ZZ	Release Ileum, Via Natural or Artificial Opening Endoscopic	0DNK3ZZ	Release Ascending Colon, Percutaneous Approach	0DNR0ZZ	Release Anal Sphincter, Open Approach
C0ZZ	Release Ileocecal Valve, Open Approach	0DNK4ZZ	Release Ascending Colon, Percutaneous Endoscopic Approach	0DNR3ZZ	Release Anal Sphincter, Percutaneous Approach
C3ZZ	Release Ileocecal Valve, Percutaneous Approach	0DNK7ZZ	Release Ascending Colon, Via Natural or Artificial Opening	0DNR4ZZ	Release Anal Sphincter, Percutaneous Endoscopic Approach
C4ZZ	Release Ileocecal Valve, Percutaneous Endoscopic Approach	0DNK8ZZ	Release Ascending Colon, Via Natural or Artificial Opening Endoscopic	0DNS0ZZ	Release Greater Omentum, Open Approach
C7ZZ	Release Ileocecal Valve, Via Natural or Artificial Opening	0DNL0ZZ	Release Transverse Colon, Open Approach	0DNS3ZZ	Release Greater Omentum, Percutaneous Approach
C8ZZ	Release Ileocecal Valve, Via Natural or Artificial Opening Endoscopic	0DNL3ZZ	Release Transverse Colon, Percutaneous Approach	0DNS4ZZ	Release Greater Omentum, Percutaneous Endoscopic Approach
E0ZZ	Release Large Intestine, Open Approach	0DNL4ZZ	Release Transverse Colon, Percutaneous Endoscopic Approach	0DNT0ZZ	Release Lesser Omentum, Open Approach
E3ZZ	Release Large Intestine, Percutaneous Approach	0DNL7ZZ	Release Transverse Colon, Via Natural or Artificial Opening	0DNT3ZZ	Release Lesser Omentum, Percutaneous Approach
E4ZZ	Release Large Intestine, Percutaneous Endoscopic Approach	0DNL8ZZ	Release Transverse Colon, Via Natural or Artificial Opening Endoscopic	0DNT4ZZ	Release Lesser Omentum, Percutaneous Endoscopic Approach
E7ZZ	Release Large Intestine, Via Natural or Artificial Opening	0DNM0ZZ	Release Descending Colon, Open Approach	0DNV0ZZ	Release Mesentery, Open Approach
E8ZZ	Release Large Intestine, Via Natural or Artificial Opening Endoscopic	0DNM3ZZ	Release Descending Colon, Percutaneous Approach	0DNV3ZZ	Release Mesentery, Percutaneous Approach
F0ZZ	Release Right Large Intestine, Open Approach	0DNM4ZZ	Release Descending Colon, Percutaneous Endoscopic Approach	0DNV4ZZ	Release Mesentery, Percutaneous Endoscopic Approach
F3ZZ	Release Right Large Intestine, Percutaneous Approach	0DNM7ZZ	Release Descending Colon, Via Natural or Artificial Opening	0DNW0ZZ	Release Peritoneum, Open Approach
F4ZZ	Release Right Large Intestine, Percutaneous Endoscopic Approach	0DNM8ZZ	Release Descending Colon, Via Natural or Artificial Opening Endoscopic	0DNW3ZZ	Release Peritoneum, Percutaneous Approach
F7ZZ	Release Right Large Intestine, Via Natural or Artificial Opening			0DNW4ZZ	Release Peritoneum, Percutaneous Endoscopic Approach
F8ZZ	Release Right Large Intestine, Via Natural or Artificial Opening Endoscopic				

0DP – Gastrointestinal System, Removal

Review Coding Guideline B6.1c

Code	Description	Code	Description	Code	Description
0DP000Z	Removal of Drainage Device from Upper Intestinal Tract, Open Approach	0DP00KZ	Removal of Nonautologous Tissue Substitute from Upper Intestinal Tract, Open Approach	0DP03CZ	Removal of Extraluminal Device from Upper Intestinal Tract, Percutaneous Approach
0DP002Z	Removal of Monitoring Device from Upper Intestinal Tract, Open Approach	0DP00UZ	Removal of Feeding Device from Upper Intestinal Tract, Open Approach	0DP03DZ	Removal of Intraluminal Device from Upper Intestinal Tract, Percutaneous Approach
0DP003Z	Removal of Infusion Device from Upper Intestinal Tract, Open Approach	0DP030Z	Removal of Drainage Device from Upper Intestinal Tract, Percutaneous Approach	0DP03JZ	Removal of Synthetic Substitute from Upper Intestinal Tract, Percutaneous Approach
0DP007Z	Removal of Autologous Tissue Substitute from Upper Intestinal Tract, Open Approach	0DP032Z	Removal of Monitoring Device from Upper Intestinal Tract, Percutaneous Approach	0DP03KZ	Removal of Nonautologous Tissue Substitute from Upper Intestinal Tract, Percutaneous Approach
0DP00CZ	Removal of Extraluminal Device from Upper Intestinal Tract, Open Approach	0DP033Z	Removal of Infusion Device from Upper Intestinal Tract, Percutaneous Approach	0DP03UZ	Removal of Feeding Device from Upper Intestinal Tract, Percutaneous Approach
0DP00DZ	Removal of Intraluminal Device from Upper Intestinal Tract, Open Approach	0DP037Z	Removal of Autologous Tissue Substitute from Upper Intestinal Tract, Percutaneous Approach		
0DP00JZ	Removal of Synthetic Substitute from Upper Intestinal Tract, Open Approach				

| ♀ Female-only | ♂ Male-only | ▲ Limited Coverage | ● Non-OR | ▨ HAC-associated procedure | ▲ Non-covered procedures | ✚ Combination |

0DP040Z Removal of Drainage Device from Upper Intestinal Tract, Percutaneous Endoscopic Approach

0DP042Z Removal of Monitoring Device from Upper Intestinal Tract, Percutaneous Endoscopic Approach

0DP043Z Removal of Infusion Device from Upper Intestinal Tract, Percutaneous Endoscopic Approach

0DP047Z Removal of Autologous Tissue Substitute from Upper Intestinal Tract, Percutaneous Endoscopic Approach

0DP04CZ Removal of Extraluminal Device from Upper Intestinal Tract, Percutaneous Endoscopic Approach

0DP04DZ Removal of Intraluminal Device from Upper Intestinal Tract, Percutaneous Endoscopic Approach

0DP04JZ Removal of Synthetic Substitute from Upper Intestinal Tract, Percutaneous Endoscopic Approach

0DP04KZ Removal of Nonautologous Tissue Substitute from Upper Intestinal Tract, Percutaneous Endoscopic Approach

0DP04UZ Removal of Feeding Device from Upper Intestinal Tract, Percutaneous Endoscopic Approach

0DP070Z Removal of Drainage Device from Upper Intestinal Tract, Via Natural or Artificial Opening

0DP072Z Removal of Monitoring Device from Upper Intestinal Tract, Via Natural or Artificial Opening

0DP073Z Removal of Infusion Device from Upper Intestinal Tract, Via Natural or Artificial Opening

0DP077Z Removal of Autologous Tissue Substitute from Upper Intestinal Tract, Via Natural or Artificial Opening

0DP07CZ Removal of Extraluminal Device from Upper Intestinal Tract, Via Natural or Artificial Opening

0DP07DZ Removal of Intraluminal Device from Upper Intestinal Tract, Via Natural or Artificial Opening

0DP07JZ Removal of Synthetic Substitute from Upper Intestinal Tract, Via Natural or Artificial Opening

0DP07KZ Removal of Nonautologous Tissue Substitute from Upper Intestinal Tract, Via Natural or Artificial Opening

0DP07UZ Removal of Feeding Device from Upper Intestinal Tract, Via Natural or Artificial Opening

0DP080Z Removal of Drainage Device from Upper Intestinal Tract, Via Natural or Artificial Opening Endoscopic

0DP082Z Removal of Monitoring Device from Upper Intestinal Tract, Via Natural or Artificial Opening Endoscopic

0DP083Z Removal of Infusion Device from Upper Intestinal Tract, Via Natural or Artificial Opening Endoscopic

0DP087Z Removal of Autologous Tissue Substitute from Upper Intestinal Tract, Via Natural or Artificial Opening Endoscopic

0DP08CZ Removal of Extraluminal Device from Upper Intestinal Tract, Via Natural or Artificial Opening Endoscopic

0DP08DZ Removal of Intraluminal Device from Upper Intestinal Tract, Via Natural or Artificial Opening Endoscopic

0DP08JZ Removal of Synthetic Substitute from Upper Intestinal Tract, Via Natural or Artificial Opening Endoscopic

0DP08KZ Removal of Nonautologous Tissue Substitute from Upper Intestinal Tract, Via Natural or Artificial Opening Endoscopic

0DP08UZ Removal of Feeding Device from Upper Intestinal Tract, Via Natural or Artificial Opening Endoscopic

0DP0X0Z Removal of Drainage Device from Upper Intestinal Tract, External Approach

0DP0X2Z Removal of Monitoring Device from Upper Intestinal Tract, External Approach

0DP0X3Z Removal of Infusion Device from Upper Intestinal Tract, External Approach

0DP0XDZ Removal of Intraluminal Device from Upper Intestinal Tract, External Approach

0DP0XUZ Removal of Feeding Device from Upper Intestinal Tract, External Approach

0DP501Z Removal of Radioactive Element from Esophagus, Open Approach

0DP502Z Removal of Monitoring Device from Esophagus, Open Approach

0DP503Z Removal of Infusion Device from Esophagus, Open Approach

0DP50UZ Removal of Feeding Device from Esophagus, Open Approach

0DP531Z Removal of Radioactive Element from Esophagus, Percutaneous Approach

0DP532Z Removal of Monitoring Device from Esophagus, Percutaneous Approach

0DP533Z Removal of Infusion Device from Esophagus, Percutaneous Approach

0DP53UZ Removal of Feeding Device from Esophagus, Percutaneous Approach

0DP541Z Removal of Radioactive Element from Esophagus, Percutaneous Endoscopic Approach

0DP542Z Removal of Monitoring Device from Esophagus, Percutaneous Endoscopic Approach

0DP543Z Removal of Infusion Device from Esophagus, Percutaneous Endoscopic Approach

0DP54UZ Removal of Feeding Device from Esophagus, Percutaneous Endoscopic Approach

0DP571Z Removal of Radioactive Element from Esophagus, Via Natural or Artificial Opening

0DP57DZ Removal of Intraluminal Device from Esophagus, Via Natural or Artificial Opening

0DP581Z Removal of Radioactive Element from Esophagus, Via Natural or Artificial Opening Endoscopic

0DP58DZ Removal of Intraluminal Device from Esophagus, Via Natural or Artificial Opening Endoscopic

0DP5X1Z Removal of Radioactive Element from Esophagus, External Approach

0DP5X2Z Removal of Monitoring Device from Esophagus, External Approach

0DP5X3Z Removal of Infusion Device from Esophagus, External Approach

0DP5XDZ Removal of Intraluminal Device from Esophagus, External Approach

0DP5XUZ Removal of Feeding Device from Esophagus, External Approach

0DP600Z Removal of Drainage Device from Stomach, Open Approach

0DP602Z Removal of Monitoring Device from Stomach, Open Approach

0DP603Z Removal of Infusion Device from Stomach, Open Approach

0DP607Z Removal of Autologous Tissue Substitute from Stomach, Open Approach

0DP60CZ Removal of Extraluminal Device from Stomach, Open Approach

0DP60DZ Removal of Intraluminal Device from Stomach, Open Approach

0DP60JZ Removal of Synthetic Substitute from Stomach, Open Approach

0DP60KZ Removal of Nonautologous Tissue Substitute from Stomach, Open Appro...

0DP60MZ Removal of Stimulator Lead from Stomach, Open Approach

0DP60UZ Removal of Feeding Device from Stomach, Open Approach

0DP630Z Removal of Drainage Device from Stomach, Percutaneous Approach

0DP632Z Removal of Monitoring Device from Stomach, Percutaneous Approach

0DP633Z Removal of Infusion Device from Stomach, Percutaneous Approach

0DP637Z Removal of Autologous Tissue Substitu... from Stomach, Percutaneous Approach

0DP63CZ Removal of Extraluminal Device from Stomach, Percutaneous Approach

0DP63DZ Removal of Intraluminal Device from Stomach, Percutaneous Approach

0DP63JZ Removal of Synthetic Substitute from Stomach, Percutaneous Approach

0DP63KZ Removal of Nonautologous Tissue Substitute from Stomach, Percutaneous Approach

0DP63MZ Removal of Stimulator Lead from Stomach, Percutaneous Approach

0DP63UZ Removal of Feeding Device from Stomach, Percutaneous Approach

0DP640Z Removal of Drainage Device from Stomach, Percutaneous Endoscopic Approach

0DP642Z Removal of Monitoring Device from Stomach, Percutaneous Endoscopic Approach

0DP643Z Removal of Infusion Device from Stomach, Percutaneous Endoscopic Approach

0DP647Z Removal of Autologous Tissue Substitu... from Stomach, Percutaneous Endoscop... Approach

0DP64CZ Removal of Extraluminal Device from Stomach, Percutaneous Endoscopic Approach

0DP64DZ Removal of Intraluminal Device from Stomach, Percutaneous Endoscopic Approach

0DP64JZ Removal of Synthetic Substitute from Stomach, Percutaneous Endoscopic Approach

0DP64KZ Removal of Nonautologous Tissue Substitute from Stomach, Percutaneous Endoscopic Approach

0DP64MZ Removal of Stimulator Lead from Stomach, Percutaneous Endoscopic Approach

0DP64UZ Removal of Feeding Device from Stomach, Percutaneous Endoscopic Approach

0DP670Z Removal of Drainage Device from Stomach, Via Natural or Artificial Opening

0DP672Z Removal of Monitoring Device from Stomach, Via Natural or Artificial Openi...

0DP673Z Removal of Infusion Device from Stomach, Via Natural or Artificial Openi...

0DP677Z Removal of Autologous Tissue Substitut... from Stomach, Via Natural or Artificial Opening

0DP67CZ Removal of Extraluminal Device from Stomach, Via Natural or Artificial Openi...

0DP67DZ Removal of Intraluminal Device from Stomach, Via Natural or Artificial Openi...

♀ Female-only   ♂ Male-only   ▲ Limited Coverage   ● Non-OR   ▨ HAC-associated procedure   ▲ Non-covered procedures   ➕ Combinat...

..7JZ Removal of Synthetic Substitute from Stomach, Via Natural or Artificial Opening

..7KZ Removal of Nonautologous Tissue Substitute from Stomach, Via Natural or Artificial Opening

..7UZ Removal of Feeding Device from Stomach, Via Natural or Artificial Opening

..80Z Removal of Drainage Device from Stomach, Via Natural or Artificial Opening Endoscopic

..682Z Removal of Monitoring Device from Stomach, Via Natural or Artificial Opening Endoscopic

..683Z Removal of Infusion Device from Stomach, Via Natural or Artificial Opening Endoscopic

..687Z Removal of Autologous Tissue Substitute from Stomach, Via Natural or Artificial Opening Endoscopic

..68CZ Removal of Extraluminal Device from Stomach, Via Natural or Artificial Opening Endoscopic

..68DZ Removal of Intraluminal Device from Stomach, Via Natural or Artificial Opening Endoscopic

..68JZ Removal of Synthetic Substitute from Stomach, Via Natural or Artificial Opening Endoscopic

..68KZ Removal of Nonautologous Tissue Substitute from Stomach, Via Natural or Artificial Opening Endoscopic

..68UZ Removal of Feeding Device from Stomach, Via Natural or Artificial Opening Endoscopic

..6X0Z Removal of Drainage Device from Stomach, External Approach

..6X2Z Removal of Monitoring Device from Stomach, External Approach

..6X3Z Removal of Infusion Device from Stomach, External Approach

..6XDZ Removal of Intraluminal Device from Stomach, External Approach

..6XUZ Removal of Feeding Device from Stomach, External Approach

..D00Z Removal of Drainage Device from Lower Intestinal Tract, Open Approach

..D02Z Removal of Monitoring Device from Lower Intestinal Tract, Open Approach

..D03Z Removal of Infusion Device from Lower Intestinal Tract, Open Approach

..D07Z Removal of Autologous Tissue Substitute from Lower Intestinal Tract, Open Approach

..D0CZ Removal of Extraluminal Device from Lower Intestinal Tract, Open Approach

..D0DZ Removal of Intraluminal Device from Lower Intestinal Tract, Open Approach

..D0JZ Removal of Synthetic Substitute from Lower Intestinal Tract, Open Approach

..D0KZ Removal of Nonautologous Tissue Substitute from Lower Intestinal Tract, Open Approach

..D0UZ Removal of Feeding Device from Lower Intestinal Tract, Open Approach

..D30Z Removal of Drainage Device from Lower Intestinal Tract, Percutaneous Approach

..D32Z Removal of Monitoring Device from Lower Intestinal Tract, Percutaneous Approach

..D33Z Removal of Infusion Device from Lower Intestinal Tract, Percutaneous Approach

..D37Z Removal of Autologous Tissue Substitute from Lower Intestinal Tract, Percutaneous Approach

..D3CZ Removal of Extraluminal Device from Lower Intestinal Tract, Percutaneous Approach

0DPD3DZ Removal of Intraluminal Device from Lower Intestinal Tract, Percutaneous Approach

0DPD3JZ Removal of Synthetic Substitute from Lower Intestinal Tract, Percutaneous Approach

0DPD3KZ Removal of Nonautologous Tissue Substitute from Lower Intestinal Tract, Percutaneous Approach

0DPD3UZ Removal of Feeding Device from Lower Intestinal Tract, Percutaneous Approach

0DPD40Z Removal of Drainage Device from Lower Intestinal Tract, Percutaneous Endoscopic Approach

0DPD42Z Removal of Monitoring Device from Lower Intestinal Tract, Percutaneous Endoscopic Approach

0DPD43Z Removal of Infusion Device from Lower Intestinal Tract, Percutaneous Endoscopic Approach

0DPD47Z Removal of Autologous Tissue Substitute from Lower Intestinal Tract, Percutaneous Endoscopic Approach

0DPD4CZ Removal of Extraluminal Device from Lower Intestinal Tract, Percutaneous Endoscopic Approach

0DPD4DZ Removal of Intraluminal Device from Lower Intestinal Tract, Percutaneous Endoscopic Approach

0DPD4JZ Removal of Synthetic Substitute from Lower Intestinal Tract, Percutaneous Endoscopic Approach

0DPD4KZ Removal of Nonautologous Tissue Substitute from Lower Intestinal Tract, Percutaneous Endoscopic Approach

0DPD4UZ Removal of Feeding Device from Lower Intestinal Tract, Percutaneous Endoscopic Approach

0DPD70Z Removal of Drainage Device from Lower Intestinal Tract, Via Natural or Artificial Opening

0DPD72Z Removal of Monitoring Device from Lower Intestinal Tract, Via Natural or Artificial Opening

0DPD73Z Removal of Infusion Device from Lower Intestinal Tract, Via Natural or Artificial Opening

0DPD77Z Removal of Autologous Tissue Substitute from Lower Intestinal Tract, Via Natural or Artificial Opening

0DPD7CZ Removal of Extraluminal Device from Lower Intestinal Tract, Via Natural or Artificial Opening

0DPD7DZ Removal of Intraluminal Device from Lower Intestinal Tract, Via Natural or Artificial Opening

0DPD7JZ Removal of Synthetic Substitute from Lower Intestinal Tract, Via Natural or Artificial Opening

0DPD7KZ Removal of Nonautologous Tissue Substitute from Lower Intestinal Tract, Via Natural or Artificial Opening

0DPD7UZ Removal of Feeding Device from Lower Intestinal Tract, Via Natural or Artificial Opening

0DPD80Z Removal of Drainage Device from Lower Intestinal Tract, Via Natural or Artificial Opening Endoscopic

0DPD82Z Removal of Monitoring Device from Lower Intestinal Tract, Via Natural or Artificial Opening Endoscopic

0DPD83Z Removal of Infusion Device from Lower Intestinal Tract, Via Natural or Artificial Opening Endoscopic

0DPD87Z Removal of Autologous Tissue Substitute from Lower Intestinal Tract, Via Natural or Artificial Opening Endoscopic

0DPD8CZ Removal of Extraluminal Device from Lower Intestinal Tract, Via Natural or Artificial Opening Endoscopic

0DPD8DZ Removal of Intraluminal Device from Lower Intestinal Tract, Via Natural or Artificial Opening Endoscopic

0DPD8JZ Removal of Synthetic Substitute from Lower Intestinal Tract, Via Natural or Artificial Opening Endoscopic

0DPD8KZ Removal of Nonautologous Tissue Substitute from Lower Intestinal Tract, Via Natural or Artificial Opening Endoscopic

0DPD8UZ Removal of Feeding Device from Lower Intestinal Tract, Via Natural or Artificial Opening Endoscopic

0DPDX0Z Removal of Drainage Device from Lower Intestinal Tract, External Approach

0DPDX2Z Removal of Monitoring Device from Lower Intestinal Tract, External Approach

0DPDX3Z Removal of Infusion Device from Lower Intestinal Tract, External Approach

0DPDXDZ Removal of Intraluminal Device from Lower Intestinal Tract, External Approach

0DPDXUZ Removal of Feeding Device from Lower Intestinal Tract, External Approach

0DPP01Z Removal of Radioactive Element from Rectum, Open Approach

0DPP31Z Removal of Radioactive Element from Rectum, Percutaneous Approach

0DPP41Z Removal of Radioactive Element from Rectum, Percutaneous Endoscopic Approach

0DPP71Z Removal of Radioactive Element from Rectum, Via Natural or Artificial Opening

0DPP81Z Removal of Radioactive Element from Rectum, Via Natural or Artificial Opening Endoscopic

0DPPX1Z Removal of Radioactive Element from Rectum, External Approach

0DPQ0LZ Removal of Artificial Sphincter from Anus, Open Approach

0DPQ3LZ Removal of Artificial Sphincter from Anus, Percutaneous Approach

0DPQ4LZ Removal of Artificial Sphincter from Anus, Percutaneous Endoscopic Approach

0DPQ7LZ Removal of Artificial Sphincter from Anus, Via Natural or Artificial Opening

0DPQ8LZ Removal of Artificial Sphincter from Anus, Via Natural or Artificial Opening Endoscopic

0DPR0MZ Removal of Stimulator Lead from Anal Sphincter, Open Approach

0DPR3MZ Removal of Stimulator Lead from Anal Sphincter, Percutaneous Approach

0DPR4MZ Removal of Stimulator Lead from Anal Sphincter, Percutaneous Endoscopic Approach

0DPU00Z Removal of Drainage Device from Omentum, Open Approach

0DPU01Z Removal of Radioactive Element from Omentum, Open Approach

0DPU07Z Removal of Autologous Tissue Substitute from Omentum, Open Approach

0DPU0JZ Removal of Synthetic Substitute from Omentum, Open Approach

0DPU0KZ Removal of Nonautologous Tissue Substitute from Omentum, Open Approach

0DPU30Z Removal of Drainage Device from Omentum, Percutaneous Approach

0DPU31Z Removal of Radioactive Element from Omentum, Percutaneous Approach

0DPU37Z Removal of Autologous Tissue Substitute from Omentum, Percutaneous Approach

0DPU3JZ Removal of Synthetic Substitute from Omentum, Percutaneous Approach

0DPU3KZ Removal of Nonautologous Tissue Substitute from Omentum, Percutaneous Approach

0DPU40Z Removal of Drainage Device from Omentum, Percutaneous Endoscopic Approach

0DPU41Z Removal of Radioactive Element from Omentum, Percutaneous Endoscopic Approach

0DPU47Z Removal of Autologous Tissue Substitute from Omentum, Percutaneous Endoscopic Approach

0DPU4JZ Removal of Synthetic Substitute from Omentum, Percutaneous Endoscopic Approach

0DPU4KZ Removal of Nonautologous Tissue Substitute from Omentum, Percutaneous Endoscopic Approach

0DPV00Z Removal of Drainage Device from Mesentery, Open Approach

0DPV01Z Removal of Radioactive Element from Mesentery, Open Approach

0DPV07Z Removal of Autologous Tissue Substitute from Mesentery, Open Approach

0DPV0JZ Removal of Synthetic Substitute from Mesentery, Open Approach

0DPV0KZ Removal of Nonautologous Tissue Substitute from Mesentery, Open Approach

0DPV30Z Removal of Drainage Device from Mesentery, Percutaneous Approach

0DPV31Z Removal of Radioactive Element from Mesentery, Percutaneous Approach

0DPV37Z Removal of Autologous Tissue Substitute from Mesentery, Percutaneous Approach

0DPV3JZ Removal of Synthetic Substitute from Mesentery, Percutaneous Approach

0DPV3KZ Removal of Nonautologous Tissue Substitute from Mesentery, Percutaneous Approach

0DPV40Z Removal of Drainage Device from Mesentery, Percutaneous Endoscopic Approach

0DPV41Z Removal of Radioactive Element from Mesentery, Percutaneous Endoscopic Approach

0DPV47Z Removal of Autologous Tissue Substitute from Mesentery, Percutaneous Endoscopic Approach

0DPV4JZ Removal of Synthetic Substitute from Mesentery, Percutaneous Endoscopic Approach

0DPV4KZ Removal of Nonautologous Tissue Substitute from Mesentery, Percutaneous Endoscopic Approach

0DPW00Z Removal of Drainage Device from Peritoneum, Open Approach

0DPW01Z Removal of Radioactive Element from Peritoneum, Open Approach

0DPW07Z Removal of Autologous Tissue Substitute from Peritoneum, Open Approach

0DPW0JZ Removal of Synthetic Substitute from Peritoneum, Open Approach

0DPW0KZ Removal of Nonautologous Tissue Substitute from Peritoneum, Open Approach

0DPW30Z Removal of Drainage Device from Peritoneum, Percutaneous Appr

0DPW31Z Removal of Radioactive Element from Peritoneum, Percutaneous Approach

0DPW37Z Removal of Autologous Tissue Substi from Peritoneum, Percutaneous Appr

0DPW3JZ Removal of Synthetic Substitute from Peritoneum, Percutaneous Appr

0DPW3KZ Removal of Nonautologous Tissue Substitute from Peritoneum, Percutan Approach

0DPW40Z Removal of Drainage Device from Peritoneum, Percutaneous Endoscopi Approach

0DPW41Z Removal of Radioactive Element from Peritoneum, Percutaneous Endoscopi Approach

0DPW47Z Removal of Autologous Tissue Substi from Peritoneum, Percutaneous Endoscopic Approach

0DPW4JZ Removal of Synthetic Substitute from Peritoneum, Percutaneous Endoscopi Approach

0DPW4KZ Removal of Nonautologous Tissue Substitute from Peritoneum, Percutane Endoscopic Approach

0DQ – Gastrointestinal System, Repair

0DQ10ZZ Repair Upper Esophagus, Open Approach

0DQ13ZZ Repair Upper Esophagus, Percutaneous Approach

0DQ14ZZ Repair Upper Esophagus, Percutaneous Endoscopic Approach

0DQ17ZZ Repair Upper Esophagus, Via Natural or Artificial Opening

0DQ18ZZ Repair Upper Esophagus, Via Natural or Artificial Opening Endoscopic

0DQ20ZZ Repair Middle Esophagus, Open Approach

0DQ23ZZ Repair Middle Esophagus, Percutaneous Approach

0DQ24ZZ Repair Middle Esophagus, Percutaneous Endoscopic Approach

0DQ27ZZ Repair Middle Esophagus, Via Natural or Artificial Opening

0DQ28ZZ Repair Middle Esophagus, Via Natural or Artificial Opening Endoscopic

0DQ30ZZ Repair Lower Esophagus, Open Approach

0DQ33ZZ Repair Lower Esophagus, Percutaneous Approach

0DQ34ZZ Repair Lower Esophagus, Percutaneous Endoscopic Approach

0DQ37ZZ Repair Lower Esophagus, Via Natural or Artificial Opening

0DQ38ZZ Repair Lower Esophagus, Via Natural or Artificial Opening Endoscopic

0DQ40ZZ Repair Esophagogastric Junction, Open Approach

0DQ43ZZ Repair Esophagogastric Junction, Percutaneous Approach

0DQ44ZZ Repair Esophagogastric Junction, Percutaneous Endoscopic Approach

0DQ47ZZ Repair Esophagogastric Junction, Via Natural or Artificial Opening

0DQ48ZZ Repair Esophagogastric Junction, Via Natural or Artificial Opening Endoscopic

0DQ50ZZ Repair Esophagus, Open Approach

0DQ53ZZ Repair Esophagus, Percutaneous Approach

0DQ54ZZ Repair Esophagus, Percutaneous Endoscopic Approach

0DQ57ZZ Repair Esophagus, Via Natural or Artificial Opening

0DQ58ZZ Repair Esophagus, Via Natural or Artificial Opening Endoscopic

0DQ60ZZ Repair Stomach, Open Approach

0DQ63ZZ Repair Stomach, Percutaneous Approach

0DQ64ZZ Repair Stomach, Percutaneous Endoscopic Approach

0DQ67ZZ Repair Stomach, Via Natural or Artificial Opening

0DQ68ZZ Repair Stomach, Via Natural or Artificial Opening Endoscopic

0DQ70ZZ Repair Stomach, Pylorus, Open Approach

0DQ73ZZ Repair Stomach, Pylorus, Percutaneous Approach

0DQ74ZZ Repair Stomach, Pylorus, Percutaneous Endoscopic Approach

0DQ77ZZ Repair Stomach, Pylorus, Via Natural or Artificial Opening

0DQ78ZZ Repair Stomach, Pylorus, Via Natural or Artificial Opening Endoscopic

0DQ80ZZ Repair Small Intestine, Open Approach
    + Ileostomy takedown when performed with code 0WQFXZ2, Repair of abdominal wall, stoma, external approach.

0DQ83ZZ Repair Small Intestine, Percutaneous Approach

0DQ84ZZ Repair Small Intestine, Percutaneous Endoscopic Approach

0DQ87ZZ Repair Small Intestine, Via Natural or Artificial Opening

0DQ88ZZ Repair Small Intestine, Via Natural or Artificial Opening Endoscopic

0DQ90ZZ Repair Duodenum, Open Approach
    + Duodenostomy takedown when performed with code 0WQFXZ2, Repair of abdominal wall, stoma, external approach.

0DQ93ZZ Repair Duodenum, Percutaneous Approach

0DQ94ZZ Repair Duodenum, Percutaneous Endoscopic Approach

0DQ97ZZ Repair Duodenum, Via Natural or Artificial Opening

0DQ98ZZ Repair Duodenum, Via Natural or Artificial Opening Endoscopic
    AHA CC: 4Q, 2014, 20

0DQA0ZZ Repair Jejunum, Open Approach
    + Jejunostomy takedown when perform with code 0WQFXZ2, Repair of abdominal wall, stoma, external approach.

0DQA3ZZ Repair Jejunum, Percutaneous Approa

0DQA4ZZ Repair Jejunum, Percutaneous Endoscopic Approach

0DQA7ZZ Repair Jejunum, Via Natural or Artific Opening

0DQA8ZZ Repair Jejunum, Via Natural or Artific Opening Endoscopic

0DQB0ZZ Repair Ileum, Open Approach
    + Ileostomy takedown when performed with code 0WQFXZ2, Repair of abdominal wall, stoma, external approach.

0DQB3ZZ Repair Ileum, Percutaneous Approach

0DQB4ZZ Repair Ileum, Percutaneous Endoscop Approach

0DQB7ZZ Repair Ileum, Via Natural or Artificial Opening

0DQB8ZZ Repair Ileum, Via Natural or Artificial Opening Endoscopic

0DQC0ZZ Repair Ileocecal Valve, Open Approac

0DQC3ZZ Repair Ileocecal Valve, Percutaneous Approach

0DQC4ZZ Repair Ileocecal Valve, Percutaneous Endoscopic Approach

0DQC7ZZ Repair Ileocecal Valve, Via Natural or Artificial Opening

0DQC8ZZ Repair Ileocecal Valve, Via Natural or Artificial Opening Endoscopic

0DQE0ZZ Repair Large Intestine, Open Approach
    + Colostomy takedown when performed with code 0WQFXZ2, Repair of abdominal wall, stoma, external approach.

0DQE3ZZ Repair Large Intestine, Percutaneous Approach

0DQE4ZZ Repair Large Intestine, Percutaneous Endoscopic Approach

0DQE7ZZ Repair Large Intestine, Via Natural or Artificial Opening

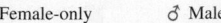

E8ZZ Repair Large Intestine, Via Natural or Artificial Opening Endoscopic

F0ZZ Repair Right Large Intestine, Open Approach

+ Colostomy takedown when performed with code 0WQFXZ2, Repair of abdominal wall, stoma, external approach.

F3ZZ Repair Right Large Intestine, Percutaneous Approach

F4ZZ Repair Right Large Intestine, Percutaneous Endoscopic Approach

F7ZZ Repair Right Large Intestine, Via Natural or Artificial Opening

F8ZZ Repair Right Large Intestine, Via Natural or Artificial Opening Endoscopic

G0ZZ Repair Left Large Intestine, Open Approach

+ Colostomy takedown when performed with code 0WQFXZ2, Repair of abdominal wall, stoma, external approach.

G3ZZ Repair Left Large Intestine, Percutaneous Approach

G4ZZ Repair Left Large Intestine, Percutaneous Endoscopic Approach

G7ZZ Repair Left Large Intestine, Via Natural or Artificial Opening

G8ZZ Repair Left Large Intestine, Via Natural or Artificial Opening Endoscopic

H0ZZ Repair Cecum, Open Approach

+ Cecostomy takedown when performed with code 0WQFXZ2, Repair of abdominal wall, stoma, external approach.

H3ZZ Repair Cecum, Percutaneous Approach

H4ZZ Repair Cecum, Percutaneous Endoscopic Approach

H7ZZ Repair Cecum, Via Natural or Artificial Opening

H8ZZ Repair Cecum, Via Natural or Artificial Opening Endoscopic

J0ZZ Repair Appendix, Open Approach

J3ZZ Repair Appendix, Percutaneous Approach

J4ZZ Repair Appendix, Percutaneous Endoscopic Approach

J7ZZ Repair Appendix, Via Natural or Artificial Opening

J8ZZ Repair Appendix, Via Natural or Artificial Opening Endoscopic

K0ZZ Repair Ascending Colon, Open Approach

+ Colostomy takedown when performed with code 0WQFXZ2, Repair of abdominal wall, stoma, external approach.

0DQK3ZZ Repair Ascending Colon, Percutaneous Approach

0DQK4ZZ Repair Ascending Colon, Percutaneous Endoscopic Approach

0DQK7ZZ Repair Ascending Colon, Via Natural or Artificial Opening

0DQK8ZZ Repair Ascending Colon, Via Natural or Artificial Opening Endoscopic

0DQL0ZZ Repair Transverse Colon, Open Approach

+ Colostomy takedown when performed with code 0WQFXZ2, Repair of abdominal wall, stoma, external approach.

0DQL3ZZ Repair Transverse Colon, Percutaneous Approach

0DQL4ZZ Repair Transverse Colon, Percutaneous Endoscopic Approach

0DQL7ZZ Repair Transverse Colon, Via Natural or Artificial Opening

0DQL8ZZ Repair Transverse Colon, Via Natural or Artificial Opening Endoscopic

0DQM0ZZ Repair Descending Colon, Open Approach

+ Colostomy takedown when performed with code 0WQFXZ2, Repair of abdominal wall, stoma, external approach.

0DQM3ZZ Repair Descending Colon, Percutaneous Approach

0DQM4ZZ Repair Descending Colon, Percutaneous Endoscopic Approach

0DQM7ZZ Repair Descending Colon, Via Natural or Artificial Opening

0DQM8ZZ Repair Descending Colon, Via Natural or Artificial Opening Endoscopic

0DQN0ZZ Repair Sigmoid Colon, Open Approach

+ Colostomy takedown when performed with code 0WQFXZ2, Repair of abdominal wall, stoma, external approach.

0DQN3ZZ Repair Sigmoid Colon, Percutaneous Approach

0DQN4ZZ Repair Sigmoid Colon, Percutaneous Endoscopic Approach

0DQN7ZZ Repair Sigmoid Colon, Via Natural or Artificial Opening

0DQN8ZZ Repair Sigmoid Colon, Via Natural or Artificial Opening Endoscopic

0DQP0ZZ Repair Rectum, Open Approach

0DQP3ZZ Repair Rectum, Percutaneous Approach

0DQP4ZZ Repair Rectum, Percutaneous Endoscopic Approach

0DQP7ZZ Repair Rectum, Via Natural or Artificial Opening

0DQP8ZZ Repair Rectum, Via Natural or Artificial Opening Endoscopic

0DQQ0ZZ Repair Anus, Open Approach

0DQQ3ZZ Repair Anus, Percutaneous Approach

0DQQ4ZZ Repair Anus, Percutaneous Endoscopic Approach

0DQQ7ZZ Repair Anus, Via Natural or Artificial Opening

0DQQ8ZZ Repair Anus, Via Natural or Artificial Opening Endoscopic

0DQQXZZ Repair Anus, External Approach

0DQR0ZZ Repair Anal Sphincter, Open Approach

0DQR3ZZ Repair Anal Sphincter, Percutaneous Approach

0DQR4ZZ Repair Anal Sphincter, Percutaneous Endoscopic Approach

0DQS0ZZ Repair Greater Omentum, Open Approach

0DQS3ZZ Repair Greater Omentum, Percutaneous Approach

0DQS4ZZ Repair Greater Omentum, Percutaneous Endoscopic Approach

0DQT0ZZ Repair Lesser Omentum, Open Approach

0DQT3ZZ Repair Lesser Omentum, Percutaneous Approach

0DQT4ZZ Repair Lesser Omentum, Percutaneous Endoscopic Approach

0DQV0ZZ Repair Mesentery, Open Approach

0DQV3ZZ Repair Mesentery, Percutaneous Approach

0DQV4ZZ Repair Mesentery, Percutaneous Endoscopic Approach

0DQW0ZZ Repair Peritoneum, Open Approach

0DQW3ZZ Repair Peritoneum, Percutaneous Approach

0DQW4ZZ Repair Peritoneum, Percutaneous Endoscopic Approach

R – Gastrointestinal System, Replacement

R507Z Replacement of Esophagus with Autologous Tissue Substitute, Open Approach

R50JZ Replacement of Esophagus with Synthetic Substitute, Open Approach

R50KZ Replacement of Esophagus with Nonautologous Tissue Substitute, Open Approach

R547Z Replacement of Esophagus with Autologous Tissue Substitute, Percutaneous Endoscopic Approach

R54JZ Replacement of Esophagus with Synthetic Substitute, Percutaneous Endoscopic Approach

R54KZ Replacement of Esophagus with Nonautologous Tissue Substitute, Percutaneous Endoscopic Approach

R577Z Replacement of Esophagus with Autologous Tissue Substitute, Via Natural or Artificial Opening

R57JZ Replacement of Esophagus with Synthetic Substitute, Via Natural or Artificial Opening

R57KZ Replacement of Esophagus with Nonautologous Tissue Substitute, Via Natural or Artificial Opening

0DR587Z Replacement of Esophagus with Autologous Tissue Substitute, Via Natural or Artificial Opening Endoscopic

0DR58JZ Replacement of Esophagus with Synthetic Substitute, Via Natural or Artificial Opening Endoscopic

0DR58KZ Replacement of Esophagus with Nonautologous Tissue Substitute, Via Natural or Artificial Opening Endoscopic

0DRR07Z Replacement of Anal Sphincter with Autologous Tissue Substitute, Open Approach

0DRR0JZ Replacement of Anal Sphincter with Synthetic Substitute, Open Approach

0DRR0KZ Replacement of Anal Sphincter with Nonautologous Tissue Substitute, Open Approach

0DRR47Z Replacement of Anal Sphincter with Autologous Tissue Substitute, Percutaneous Endoscopic Approach

0DRR4JZ Replacement of Anal Sphincter with Synthetic Substitute, Percutaneous Endoscopic Approach

0DRR4KZ Replacement of Anal Sphincter with Nonautologous Tissue Substitute, Percutaneous Endoscopic Approach

0DRS07Z Replacement of Greater Omentum with Autologous Tissue Substitute, Open Approach

0DRS0JZ Replacement of Greater Omentum with Synthetic Substitute, Open Approach

0DRS0KZ Replacement of Greater Omentum with Nonautologous Tissue Substitute, Open Approach

0DRS47Z Replacement of Greater Omentum with Autologous Tissue Substitute, Percutaneous Endoscopic Approach

0DRS4JZ Replacement of Greater Omentum with Synthetic Substitute, Percutaneous Endoscopic Approach

0DRS4KZ Replacement of Greater Omentum with Nonautologous Tissue Substitute, Percutaneous Endoscopic Approach

0DRT07Z Replacement of Lesser Omentum with Autologous Tissue Substitute, Open Approach

0DRT0JZ Replacement of Lesser Omentum with Synthetic Substitute, Open Approach

0DRT0KZ Replacement of Lesser Omentum with Nonautologous Tissue Substitute, Open Approach	**0DRV0KZ** Replacement of Mesentery with Nonautologous Tissue Substitute, Open Approach	**0DRW0KZ** Replacement of Peritoneum with Nonautologous Tissue Substitute, Open Approach
0DRT47Z Replacement of Lesser Omentum with Autologous Tissue Substitute, Percutaneous Endoscopic Approach	**0DRV47Z** Replacement of Mesentery with Autologous Tissue Substitute, Percutaneous Endoscopic Approach	**0DRW47Z** Replacement of Peritoneum with Autologous Tissue Substitute, Percutaneous Endoscopic Approach
0DRT4JZ Replacement of Lesser Omentum with Synthetic Substitute, Percutaneous Endoscopic Approach	**0DRV4JZ** Replacement of Mesentery with Synthetic Substitute, Percutaneous Endoscopic Approach	**0DRW4JZ** Replacement of Peritoneum with Synthetic Substitute, Percutaneous Endoscopic Approach
0DRT4KZ Replacement of Lesser Omentum with Nonautologous Tissue Substitute, Percutaneous Endoscopic Approach	**0DRV4KZ** Replacement of Mesentery with Nonautologous Tissue Substitute, Percutaneous Endoscopic Approach	**0DRW4KZ** Replacement of Peritoneum with Nonautologous Tissue Substitute, Percutaneous Endoscopic Approach
0DRV07Z Replacement of Mesentery with Autologous Tissue Substitute, Open Approach	**0DRW07Z** Replacement of Peritoneum with Autologous Tissue Substitute, Open Approach	
0DRV0JZ Replacement of Mesentery with Synthetic Substitute, Open Approach	**0DRW0JZ** Replacement of Peritoneum with Synthetic Substitute, Open Approach	

0DS – Gastrointestinal System, Reposition

0DS50ZZ Reposition Esophagus, Open Approach	**0DSB4ZZ** Reposition Ileum, Percutaneous Endoscopic Approach	**0DSM0ZZ** Reposition Descending Colon, Open Approach
0DS54ZZ Reposition Esophagus, Percutaneous Endoscopic Approach	**0DSB7ZZ** Reposition Ileum, Via Natural or Artificial Opening	**0DSM4ZZ** Reposition Descending Colon, Percutaneous Endoscopic Approach
0DS57ZZ Reposition Esophagus, Via Natural or Artificial Opening	**0DSB8ZZ** Reposition Ileum, Via Natural or Artificial Opening Endoscopic	**0DSM7ZZ** Reposition Descending Colon, Via Natural or Artificial Opening
0DS58ZZ Reposition Esophagus, Via Natural or Artificial Opening Endoscopic	**0DSBXZZ** Reposition Ileum, External Approach	**0DSM8ZZ** Reposition Descending Colon, Via Natural or Artificial Opening Endoscopic
0DS5XZZ Reposition Esophagus, External Approach	**0DSH0ZZ** Reposition Cecum, Open Approach	**0DSMXZZ** Reposition Descending Colon, External Approach
0DS60ZZ Reposition Stomach, Open Approach	**0DSH4ZZ** Reposition Cecum, Percutaneous Endoscopic Approach	**0DSN0ZZ** Reposition Sigmoid Colon, Open Approach
0DS64ZZ Reposition Stomach, Percutaneous Endoscopic Approach	**0DSH7ZZ** Reposition Cecum, Via Natural or Artificial Opening	**0DSN4ZZ** Reposition Sigmoid Colon, Percutaneous Endoscopic Approach
0DS67ZZ Reposition Stomach, Via Natural or Artificial Opening	**0DSH8ZZ** Reposition Cecum, Via Natural or Artificial Opening Endoscopic	**0DSN7ZZ** Reposition Sigmoid Colon, Via Natural Artificial Opening
0DS68ZZ Reposition Stomach, Via Natural or Artificial Opening Endoscopic	**0DSHXZZ** Reposition Cecum, External Approach	**0DSN8ZZ** Reposition Sigmoid Colon, Via Natural Artificial Opening Endoscopic
● **0DS6XZZ** Reposition Stomach, External Approach	**0DSK0ZZ** Reposition Ascending Colon, Open Approach	**0DSNXZZ** Reposition Sigmoid Colon, External Approach
0DS90ZZ Reposition Duodenum, Open Approach	**0DSK4ZZ** Reposition Ascending Colon, Percutaneous Endoscopic Approach	**0DSP0ZZ** Reposition Rectum, Open Approach
0DS94ZZ Reposition Duodenum, Percutaneous Endoscopic Approach	**0DSK7ZZ** Reposition Ascending Colon, Via Natural or Artificial Opening	**0DSP4ZZ** Reposition Rectum, Percutaneous Endoscopic Approach
0DS97ZZ Reposition Duodenum, Via Natural or Artificial Opening	**0DSK8ZZ** Reposition Ascending Colon, Via Natural or Artificial Opening Endoscopic	**0DSP7ZZ** Reposition Rectum, Via Natural or Artificial Opening
0DS98ZZ Reposition Duodenum, Via Natural or Artificial Opening Endoscopic	**0DSKXZZ** Reposition Ascending Colon, External Approach	**0DSP8ZZ** Reposition Rectum, Via Natural or Artificial Opening Endoscopic
0DS9XZZ Reposition Duodenum, External Approach	**0DSL0ZZ** Reposition Transverse Colon, Open Approach	**0DSPXZZ** Reposition Rectum, External Approach
0DSA0ZZ Reposition Jejunum, Open Approach	**0DSL4ZZ** Reposition Transverse Colon, Percutaneous Endoscopic Approach	**0DSQ0ZZ** Reposition Anus, Open Approach
0DSA4ZZ Reposition Jejunum, Percutaneous Endoscopic Approach	**0DSL7ZZ** Reposition Transverse Colon, Via Natural or Artificial Opening	**0DSQ4ZZ** Reposition Anus, Percutaneous Endoscopic Approach
0DSA7ZZ Reposition Jejunum, Via Natural or Artificial Opening	**0DSL8ZZ** Reposition Transverse Colon, Via Natural or Artificial Opening Endoscopic	**0DSQ7ZZ** Reposition Anus, Via Natural or Artificial Opening
0DSA8ZZ Reposition Jejunum, Via Natural or Artificial Opening Endoscopic	**0DSLXZZ** Reposition Transverse Colon, External Approach	**0DSQ8ZZ** Reposition Anus, Via Natural or Artificial Opening Endoscopic
0DSAXZZ Reposition Jejunum, External Approach		**0DSQXZZ** Reposition Anus, External Approach
0DSB0ZZ Reposition Ileum, Open Approach		

0DT – Gastrointestinal System, Resection

Review Coding Guideline B3.8

0DT10ZZ Resection of Upper Esophagus, Open Approach	**0DT28ZZ** Resection of Middle Esophagus, Via Natural or Artificial Opening Endoscopic	**0DT47ZZ** Resection of Esophagogastric Junction, Via Natural or Artificial Opening
0DT14ZZ Resection of Upper Esophagus, Percutaneous Endoscopic Approach	**0DT30ZZ** Resection of Lower Esophagus, Open Approach	**0DT48ZZ** Resection of Esophagogastric Junction Via Natural or Artificial Opening Endoscopic
0DT17ZZ Resection of Upper Esophagus, Via Natural or Artificial Opening	**0DT34ZZ** Resection of Lower Esophagus, Percutaneous Endoscopic Approach	**0DT50ZZ** Resection of Esophagus, Open Approach
0DT18ZZ Resection of Upper Esophagus, Via Natural or Artificial Opening Endoscopic	**0DT37ZZ** Resection of Lower Esophagus, Via Natural or Artificial Opening	**0DT54ZZ** Resection of Esophagus, Percutaneous Endoscopic Approach
0DT20ZZ Resection of Middle Esophagus, Open Approach	**0DT38ZZ** Resection of Lower Esophagus, Via Natural or Artificial Opening Endoscopic	**0DT57ZZ** Resection of Esophagus, Via Natural or Artificial Opening
0DT24ZZ Resection of Middle Esophagus, Percutaneous Endoscopic Approach	**0DT40ZZ** Resection of Esophagogastric Junction, Open Approach	**0DT58ZZ** Resection of Esophagus, Via Natural or Artificial Opening Endoscopic
0DT27ZZ Resection of Middle Esophagus, Via Natural or Artificial Opening	**0DT44ZZ** Resection of Esophagogastric Junction, Percutaneous Endoscopic Approach	**0DT60ZZ** Resection of Stomach, Open Approach

0DT64ZZ–0DU28KZ

‘64ZZ	Resection of Stomach, Percutaneous Endoscopic Approach	
‘67ZZ	Resection of Stomach, Via Natural or Artificial Opening	
‘68ZZ	Resection of Stomach, Via Natural or Artificial Opening Endoscopic	
‘70ZZ	Resection of Stomach, Pylorus, Open Approach	
‘74ZZ	Resection of Stomach, Pylorus, Percutaneous Endoscopic Approach	
‘77ZZ	Resection of Stomach, Pylorus, Via Natural or Artificial Opening	
‘78ZZ	Resection of Stomach, Pylorus, Via Natural or Artificial Opening Endoscopic	

T80ZZ Resection of Small Intestine, Open Approach

T84ZZ Resection of Small Intestine, Percutaneous Endoscopic Approach

T87ZZ Resection of Small Intestine, Via Natural or Artificial Opening

T88ZZ Resection of Small Intestine, Via Natural or Artificial Opening Endoscopic

T90ZZ Resection of Duodenum, Open Approach

+ Pancreaticododenectomy when reported with Resection of the pancreas. *See table 0FT to construct the Resection code.*

T94ZZ Resection of Duodenum, Percutaneous Endoscopic Approach

T97ZZ Resection of Duodenum, Via Natural or Artificial Opening

T98ZZ Resection of Duodenum, Via Natural or Artificial Opening Endoscopic

TA0ZZ Resection of Jejunum, Open Approach

TA4ZZ Resection of Jejunum, Percutaneous Endoscopic Approach

TA7ZZ Resection of Jejunum, Via Natural or Artificial Opening

TA8ZZ Resection of Jejunum, Via Natural or Artificial Opening Endoscopic

TB0ZZ Resection of Ileum, Open Approach

TB4ZZ Resection of Ileum, Percutaneous Endoscopic Approach

TB7ZZ Resection of Ileum, Via Natural or Artificial Opening

TB8ZZ Resection of Ileum, Via Natural or Artificial Opening Endoscopic

TC0ZZ Resection of Ileocecal Valve, Open Approach

TC4ZZ Resection of Ileocecal Valve, Percutaneous Endoscopic Approach

TC7ZZ Resection of Ileocecal Valve, Via Natural or Artificial Opening

0DTC8ZZ Resection of Ileocecal Valve, Via Natural or Artificial Opening Endoscopic

0DTE0ZZ Resection of Large Intestine, Open Approach

0DTE4ZZ Resection of Large Intestine, Percutaneous Endoscopic Approach

0DTE7ZZ Resection of Large Intestine, Via Natural or Artificial Opening

0DTE8ZZ Resection of Large Intestine, Via Natural or Artificial Opening Endoscopic

0DTF0ZZ Resection of Right Large Intestine, Open Approach
AHA CC: 3Q, 2014, 6-7; 4Q, 2014, 42-43

0DTF4ZZ Resection of Right Large Intestine, Percutaneous Endoscopic Approach

0DTF7ZZ Resection of Right Large Intestine, Via Natural or Artificial Opening

0DTF8ZZ Resection of Right Large Intestine, Via Natural or Artificial Opening Endoscopic

0DTG0ZZ Resection of Left Large Intestine, Open Approach

0DTG4ZZ Resection of Left Large Intestine, Percutaneous Endoscopic Approach

0DTG7ZZ Resection of Left Large Intestine, Via Natural or Artificial Opening

0DTG8ZZ Resection of Left Large Intestine, Via Natural or Artificial Opening Endoscopic

0DTH0ZZ Resection of Cecum, Open Approach
AHA CC: 3Q, 2014, 6

0DTH4ZZ Resection of Cecum, Percutaneous Endoscopic Approach

0DTH7ZZ Resection of Cecum, Via Natural or Artificial Opening

0DTH8ZZ Resection of Cecum, Via Natural or Artificial Opening Endoscopic

0DTJ0ZZ Resection of Appendix, Open Approach

0DTJ4ZZ Resection of Appendix, Percutaneous Endoscopic Approach

0DTJ7ZZ Resection of Appendix, Via Natural or Artificial Opening

0DTJ8ZZ Resection of Appendix, Via Natural or Artificial Opening Endoscopic

0DTK0ZZ Resection of Ascending Colon, Open Approach

0DTK4ZZ Resection of Ascending Colon, Percutaneous Endoscopic Approach

0DTK7ZZ Resection of Ascending Colon, Via Natural or Artificial Opening

0DTK8ZZ Resection of Ascending Colon, Via Natural or Artificial Opening Endoscopic

0DTL0ZZ Resection of Transverse Colon, Open Approach

0DTL4ZZ Resection of Transverse Colon, Percutaneous Endoscopic Approach

0DTL7ZZ Resection of Transverse Colon, Via Natural or Artificial Opening

0DTL8ZZ Resection of Transverse Colon, Via Natural or Artificial Opening Endoscopic

0DTM0ZZ Resection of Descending Colon, Open Approach

0DTM4ZZ Resection of Descending Colon, Percutaneous Endoscopic Approach

0DTM7ZZ Resection of Descending Colon, Via Natural or Artificial Opening

0DTM8ZZ Resection of Descending Colon, Via Natural or Artificial Opening Endoscopic

0DTN0ZZ Resection of Sigmoid Colon, Open Approach

0DTN4ZZ Resection of Sigmoid Colon, Percutaneous Endoscopic Approach

0DTN7ZZ Resection of Sigmoid Colon, Via Natural or Artificial Opening

0DTN8ZZ Resection of Sigmoid Colon, Via Natural or Artificial Opening Endoscopic

0DTP0ZZ Resection of Rectum, Open Approach
AHA CC: 4Q, 2014, 40-41

0DTP4ZZ Resection of Rectum, Percutaneous Endoscopic Approach

0DTP7ZZ Resection of Rectum, Via Natural or Artificial Opening

0DTP8ZZ Resection of Rectum, Via Natural or Artificial Opening Endoscopic

0DTQ0ZZ Resection of Anus, Open Approach
AHA CC: 4Q, 2014, 40-41

0DTQ4ZZ Resection of Anus, Percutaneous Endoscopic Approach

0DTQ7ZZ Resection of Anus, Via Natural or Artificial Opening

0DTQ8ZZ Resection of Anus, Via Natural or Artificial Opening Endoscopic

0DTR0ZZ Resection of Anal Sphincter, Open Approach

0DTR4ZZ Resection of Anal Sphincter, Percutaneous Endoscopic Approach

0DTS0ZZ Resection of Greater Omentum, Open Approach

0DTS4ZZ Resection of Greater Omentum, Percutaneous Endoscopic Approach

0DTT0ZZ Resection of Lesser Omentum, Open Approach

0DTT4ZZ Resection of Lesser Omentum, Percutaneous Endoscopic Approach

)U – Gastrointestinal System, Supplement

U107Z Supplement Upper Esophagus with Autologous Tissue Substitute, Open Approach

U10JZ Supplement Upper Esophagus with Synthetic Substitute, Open Approach

U10KZ Supplement Upper Esophagus with Nonautologous Tissue Substitute, Open Approach

U147Z Supplement Upper Esophagus with Autologous Tissue Substitute, Percutaneous Endoscopic Approach

U14JZ Supplement Upper Esophagus with Synthetic Substitute, Percutaneous Endoscopic Approach

U14KZ Supplement Upper Esophagus with Nonautologous Tissue Substitute, Percutaneous Endoscopic Approach

U177Z Supplement Upper Esophagus with Autologous Tissue Substitute, Via Natural or Artificial Opening

U17JZ Supplement Upper Esophagus with Synthetic Substitute, Via Natural or Artificial Opening

0DU17KZ Supplement Upper Esophagus with Nonautologous Tissue Substitute, Via Natural or Artificial Opening

0DU187Z Supplement Upper Esophagus with Autologous Tissue Substitute, Via Natural or Artificial Opening Endoscopic

0DU18JZ Supplement Upper Esophagus with Synthetic Substitute, Via Natural or Artificial Opening Endoscopic

0DU18KZ Supplement Upper Esophagus with Nonautologous Tissue Substitute, Via Natural or Artificial Opening Endoscopic

0DU207Z Supplement Middle Esophagus with Autologous Tissue Substitute, Open Approach

0DU20JZ Supplement Middle Esophagus with Synthetic Substitute, Open Approach

0DU20KZ Supplement Middle Esophagus with Nonautologous Tissue Substitute, Open Approach

0DU247Z Supplement Middle Esophagus with Autologous Tissue Substitute, Percutaneous Endoscopic Approach

0DU24JZ Supplement Middle Esophagus with Synthetic Substitute, Percutaneous Endoscopic Approach

0DU24KZ Supplement Middle Esophagus with Nonautologous Tissue Substitute, Percutaneous Endoscopic Approach

0DU277Z Supplement Middle Esophagus with Autologous Tissue Substitute, Via Natural or Artificial Opening

0DU27JZ Supplement Middle Esophagus with Synthetic Substitute, Via Natural or Artificial Opening

0DU27KZ Supplement Middle Esophagus with Nonautologous Tissue Substitute, Via Natural or Artificial Opening

0DU287Z Supplement Middle Esophagus with Autologous Tissue Substitute, Via Natural or Artificial Opening Endoscopic

0DU28JZ Supplement Middle Esophagus with Synthetic Substitute, Via Natural or Artificial Opening Endoscopic

0DU28KZ Supplement Middle Esophagus with Nonautologous Tissue Substitute, Via Natural or Artificial Opening Endoscopic

Female-only   ♂ Male-only   ▲ Limited Coverage   ● Non-OR   ▨ HAC-associated procedure   ▲ Non-covered procedures   ✚ Combination

0DU307Z   Supplement Lower Esophagus with Autologous Tissue Substitute, Open Approach

0DU30JZ   Supplement Lower Esophagus with Synthetic Substitute, Open Approach

0DU30KZ   Supplement Lower Esophagus with Nonautologous Tissue Substitute, Open Approach

0DU347Z   Supplement Lower Esophagus with Autologous Tissue Substitute, Percutaneous Endoscopic Approach

0DU34JZ   Supplement Lower Esophagus with Synthetic Substitute, Percutaneous Endoscopic Approach

0DU34KZ   Supplement Lower Esophagus with Nonautologous Tissue Substitute, Percutaneous Endoscopic Approach

0DU377Z   Supplement Lower Esophagus with Autologous Tissue Substitute, Via Natural or Artificial Opening

0DU37JZ   Supplement Lower Esophagus with Synthetic Substitute, Via Natural or Artificial Opening

0DU37KZ   Supplement Lower Esophagus with Nonautologous Tissue Substitute, Via Natural or Artificial Opening

0DU387Z   Supplement Lower Esophagus with Autologous Tissue Substitute, Via Natural or Artificial Opening Endoscopic

0DU38JZ   Supplement Lower Esophagus with Synthetic Substitute, Via Natural or Artificial Opening Endoscopic

0DU38KZ   Supplement Lower Esophagus with Nonautologous Tissue Substitute, Via Natural or Artificial Opening Endoscopic

0DU407Z   Supplement Esophagogastric Junction with Autologous Tissue Substitute, Open Approach

0DU40JZ   Supplement Esophagogastric Junction with Synthetic Substitute, Open Approach

0DU40KZ   Supplement Esophagogastric Junction with Nonautologous Tissue Substitute, Open Approach

0DU447Z   Supplement Esophagogastric Junction with Autologous Tissue Substitute, Percutaneous Endoscopic Approach

0DU44JZ   Supplement Esophagogastric Junction with Synthetic Substitute, Percutaneous Endoscopic Approach

0DU44KZ   Supplement Esophagogastric Junction with Nonautologous Tissue Substitute, Percutaneous Endoscopic Approach

0DU477Z   Supplement Esophagogastric Junction with Autologous Tissue Substitute, Via Natural or Artificial Opening

0DU47JZ   Supplement Esophagogastric Junction with Synthetic Substitute, Via Natural or Artificial Opening

0DU47KZ   Supplement Esophagogastric Junction with Nonautologous Tissue Substitute, Via Natural or Artificial Opening

0DU487Z   Supplement Esophagogastric Junction with Autologous Tissue Substitute, Via Natural or Artificial Opening Endoscopic

0DU48JZ   Supplement Esophagogastric Junction with Synthetic Substitute, Via Natural or Artificial Opening Endoscopic

0DU48KZ   Supplement Esophagogastric Junction with Nonautologous Tissue Substitute, Via Natural or Artificial Opening Endoscopic

0DU507Z   Supplement Esophagus with Autologous Tissue Substitute, Open Approach

0DU50JZ   Supplement Esophagus with Synthetic Substitute, Open Approach

0DU50KZ   Supplement Esophagus with Nonautologous Tissue Substitute, Open Approach

0DU547Z   Supplement Esophagus with Autologous Tissue Substitute, Percutaneous Endoscopic Approach

0DU54JZ   Supplement Esophagus with Synthetic Substitute, Percutaneous Endoscopic Approach

0DU54KZ   Supplement Esophagus with Nonautologous Tissue Substitute, Percutaneous Endoscopic Approach

0DU577Z   Supplement Esophagus with Autologous Tissue Substitute, Via Natural or Artificial Opening

0DU57JZ   Supplement Esophagus with Synthetic Substitute, Via Natural or Artificial Opening

0DU57KZ   Supplement Esophagus with Nonautologous Tissue Substitute, Via Natural or Artificial Opening

0DU587Z   Supplement Esophagus with Autologous Tissue Substitute, Via Natural or Artificial Opening Endoscopic

0DU58JZ   Supplement Esophagus with Synthetic Substitute, Via Natural or Artificial Opening Endoscopic

0DU58KZ   Supplement Esophagus with Nonautologous Tissue Substitute, Via Natural or Artificial Opening Endoscopic

0DU607Z   Supplement Stomach with Autologous Tissue Substitute, Open Approach

0DU60JZ   Supplement Stomach with Synthetic Substitute, Open Approach

0DU60KZ   Supplement Stomach with Nonautologous Tissue Substitute, Open Approach

0DU647Z   Supplement Stomach with Autologous Tissue Substitute, Percutaneous Endoscopic Approach

0DU64JZ   Supplement Stomach with Synthetic Substitute, Percutaneous Endoscopic Approach

0DU64KZ   Supplement Stomach with Nonautologous Tissue Substitute, Percutaneous Endoscopic Approach

0DU677Z   Supplement Stomach with Autologous Tissue Substitute, Via Natural or Artificial Opening

0DU67JZ   Supplement Stomach with Synthetic Substitute, Via Natural or Artificial Opening

0DU67KZ   Supplement Stomach with Nonautologous Tissue Substitute, Via Natural or Artificial Opening

0DU687Z   Supplement Stomach with Autologous Tissue Substitute, Via Natural or Artificial Opening Endoscopic

0DU68JZ   Supplement Stomach with Synthetic Substitute, Via Natural or Artificial Opening Endoscopic

0DU68KZ   Supplement Stomach with Nonautologous Tissue Substitute, Via Natural or Artificial Opening Endoscopic

0DU707Z   Supplement Stomach, Pylorus with Autologous Tissue Substitute, Open Approach

0DU70JZ   Supplement Stomach, Pylorus with Synthetic Substitute, Open Approach

0DU70KZ   Supplement Stomach, Pylorus with Nonautologous Tissue Substitute, Open Approach

0DU747Z   Supplement Stomach, Pylorus with Autologous Tissue Substitute, Percutaneous Endoscopic Approach

0DU74JZ   Supplement Stomach, Pylorus with Synthetic Substitute, Percutaneous Endoscopic Approach

0DU74KZ   Supplement Stomach, Pylorus with Nonautologous Tissue Substitute, Percutaneous Endoscopic Approach

0DU777Z   Supplement Stomach, Pylorus with Autologous Tissue Substitute, Via Natural or Artificial Opening

0DU77JZ   Supplement Stomach, Pylorus with Synthetic Substitute, Via Natural or Artificial Opening

0DU77KZ   Supplement Stomach, Pylorus with Nonautologous Tissue Substitute, Via Natural or Artificial Opening

0DU787Z   Supplement Stomach, Pylorus with Autologous Tissue Substitute, Via Natural or Artificial Opening Endoscopic

0DU78JZ   Supplement Stomach, Pylorus with Synthetic Substitute, Via Natural or Artificial Opening Endoscopic

0DU78KZ   Supplement Stomach, Pylorus with Nonautologous Tissue Substitute, Via Natural or Artificial Opening Endoscopic

0DU807Z   Supplement Small Intestine with Autologous Tissue Substitute, Open Approach

0DU80JZ   Supplement Small Intestine with Synthetic Substitute, Open Approach

0DU80KZ   Supplement Small Intestine with Nonautologous Tissue Substitute, Open Approach

0DU847Z   Supplement Small Intestine with Autologous Tissue Substitute, Percutaneous Endoscopic Approach

0DU84JZ   Supplement Small Intestine with Synthetic Substitute, Percutaneous Endoscopic Approach

0DU84KZ   Supplement Small Intestine with Nonautologous Tissue Substitute, Percutaneous Endoscopic Approach

0DU877Z   Supplement Small Intestine with Autologous Tissue Substitute, Via Natural or Artificial Opening

0DU87JZ   Supplement Small Intestine with Synthetic Substitute, Via Natural or Artificial Opening

0DU87KZ   Supplement Small Intestine with Nonautologous Tissue Substitute, Via Natural or Artificial Opening

0DU887Z   Supplement Small Intestine with Autologous Tissue Substitute, Via Natural or Artificial Opening Endoscopic

0DU88JZ   Supplement Small Intestine with Synthetic Substitute, Via Natural or Artificial Opening Endoscopic

0DU88KZ   Supplement Small Intestine with Nonautologous Tissue Substitute, Via Natural or Artificial Opening Endoscopic

0DU907Z   Supplement Duodenum with Autologous Tissue Substitute, Open Approach

0DU90JZ   Supplement Duodenum with Synthetic Substitute, Open Approach

0DU90KZ   Supplement Duodenum with Nonautologous Tissue Substitute, Open Approach

0DU947Z   Supplement Duodenum with Autologous Tissue Substitute, Percutaneous Endoscopic Approach

0DU94JZ   Supplement Duodenum with Synthetic Substitute, Percutaneous Endoscopic Approach

0DU94KZ   Supplement Duodenum with Nonautologous Tissue Substitute, Percutaneous Endoscopic Approach

♀ Female-only   ♂ Male-only   ▲ Limited Coverage   ● Non-OR   ▦ HAC-associated procedure   ▲ Non-covered procedures   ✚ Combination

0DU977Z	Supplement Duodenum with Autologous Tissue Substitute, Via Natural or Artificial Opening
0DU97JZ	Supplement Duodenum with Synthetic Substitute, Via Natural or Artificial Opening
0DU97KZ	Supplement Duodenum with Nonautologous Tissue Substitute, Via Natural or Artificial Opening
0DU987Z	Supplement Duodenum with Autologous Tissue Substitute, Via Natural or Artificial Opening Endoscopic
0DU98JZ	Supplement Duodenum with Synthetic Substitute, Via Natural or Artificial Opening Endoscopic
0DU98KZ	Supplement Duodenum with Nonautologous Tissue Substitute, Via Natural or Artificial Opening Endoscopic
0DUA07Z	Supplement Jejunum with Autologous Tissue Substitute, Open Approach
0DUA0JZ	Supplement Jejunum with Synthetic Substitute, Open Approach
0DUA0KZ	Supplement Jejunum with Nonautologous Tissue Substitute, Open Approach
0DUA47Z	Supplement Jejunum with Autologous Tissue Substitute, Percutaneous Endoscopic Approach
0DUA4JZ	Supplement Jejunum with Synthetic Substitute, Percutaneous Endoscopic Approach
0DUA4KZ	Supplement Jejunum with Nonautologous Tissue Substitute, Percutaneous Endoscopic Approach
0DUA77Z	Supplement Jejunum with Autologous Tissue Substitute, Via Natural or Artificial Opening
0DUA7JZ	Supplement Jejunum with Synthetic Substitute, Via Natural or Artificial Opening
0DUA7KZ	Supplement Jejunum with Nonautologous Tissue Substitute, Via Natural or Artificial Opening
0DUA87Z	Supplement Jejunum with Autologous Tissue Substitute, Via Natural or Artificial Opening Endoscopic
0DUA8JZ	Supplement Jejunum with Synthetic Substitute, Via Natural or Artificial Opening Endoscopic
0DUA8KZ	Supplement Jejunum with Nonautologous Tissue Substitute, Via Natural or Artificial Opening Endoscopic
0DUB07Z	Supplement Ileum with Autologous Tissue Substitute, Open Approach
0DUB0JZ	Supplement Ileum with Synthetic Substitute, Open Approach
0DUB0KZ	Supplement Ileum with Nonautologous Tissue Substitute, Open Approach
0DUB47Z	Supplement Ileum with Autologous Tissue Substitute, Percutaneous Endoscopic Approach
0DUB4JZ	Supplement Ileum with Synthetic Substitute, Percutaneous Endoscopic Approach
0DUB4KZ	Supplement Ileum with Nonautologous Tissue Substitute, Percutaneous Endoscopic Approach
0DUB77Z	Supplement Ileum with Autologous Tissue Substitute, Via Natural or Artificial Opening
0DUB7JZ	Supplement Ileum with Synthetic Substitute, Via Natural or Artificial Opening
0DUB7KZ	Supplement Ileum with Nonautologous Tissue Substitute, Via Natural or Artificial Opening
0DUB87Z	Supplement Ileum with Autologous Tissue Substitute, Via Natural or Artificial Opening Endoscopic
0DUB8JZ	Supplement Ileum with Synthetic Substitute, Via Natural or Artificial Opening Endoscopic
0DUB8KZ	Supplement Ileum with Nonautologous Tissue Substitute, Via Natural or Artificial Opening Endoscopic
0DUC07Z	Supplement Ileocecal Valve with Autologous Tissue Substitute, Open Approach
0DUC0JZ	Supplement Ileocecal Valve with Synthetic Substitute, Open Approach
0DUC0KZ	Supplement Ileocecal Valve with Nonautologous Tissue Substitute, Open Approach
0DUC47Z	Supplement Ileocecal Valve with Autologous Tissue Substitute, Percutaneous Endoscopic Approach
0DUC4JZ	Supplement Ileocecal Valve with Synthetic Substitute, Percutaneous Endoscopic Approach
0DUC4KZ	Supplement Ileocecal Valve with Nonautologous Tissue Substitute, Percutaneous Endoscopic Approach
0DUC77Z	Supplement Ileocecal Valve with Autologous Tissue Substitute, Via Natural or Artificial Opening
0DUC7JZ	Supplement Ileocecal Valve with Synthetic Substitute, Via Natural or Artificial Opening
0DUC7KZ	Supplement Ileocecal Valve with Nonautologous Tissue Substitute, Via Natural or Artificial Opening
0DUC87Z	Supplement Ileocecal Valve with Autologous Tissue Substitute, Via Natural or Artificial Opening Endoscopic
0DUC8JZ	Supplement Ileocecal Valve with Synthetic Substitute, Via Natural or Artificial Opening Endoscopic
0DUC8KZ	Supplement Ileocecal Valve with Nonautologous Tissue Substitute, Via Natural or Artificial Opening Endoscopic
0DUE07Z	Supplement Large Intestine with Autologous Tissue Substitute, Open Approach
0DUE0JZ	Supplement Large Intestine with Synthetic Substitute, Open Approach
0DUE0KZ	Supplement Large Intestine with Nonautologous Tissue Substitute, Open Approach
0DUE47Z	Supplement Large Intestine with Autologous Tissue Substitute, Percutaneous Endoscopic Approach
0DUE4JZ	Supplement Large Intestine with Synthetic Substitute, Percutaneous Endoscopic Approach
0DUE4KZ	Supplement Large Intestine with Nonautologous Tissue Substitute, Percutaneous Endoscopic Approach
0DUE77Z	Supplement Large Intestine with Autologous Tissue Substitute, Via Natural or Artificial Opening
0DUE7JZ	Supplement Large Intestine with Synthetic Substitute, Via Natural or Artificial Opening
0DUE7KZ	Supplement Large Intestine with Nonautologous Tissue Substitute, Via Natural or Artificial Opening
0DUE87Z	Supplement Large Intestine with Autologous Tissue Substitute, Via Natural or Artificial Opening Endoscopic
0DUE8JZ	Supplement Large Intestine with Synthetic Substitute, Via Natural or Artificial Opening Endoscopic
0DUE8KZ	Supplement Large Intestine with Nonautologous Tissue Substitute, Via Natural or Artificial Opening Endoscopic
0DUF07Z	Supplement Right Large Intestine with Autologous Tissue Substitute, Open Approach
0DUF0JZ	Supplement Right Large Intestine with Synthetic Substitute, Open Approach
0DUF0KZ	Supplement Right Large Intestine with Nonautologous Tissue Substitute, Open Approach
0DUF47Z	Supplement Right Large Intestine with Autologous Tissue Substitute, Percutaneous Endoscopic Approach
0DUF4JZ	Supplement Right Large Intestine with Synthetic Substitute, Percutaneous Endoscopic Approach
0DUF4KZ	Supplement Right Large Intestine with Nonautologous Tissue Substitute, Percutaneous Endoscopic Approach
0DUF77Z	Supplement Right Large Intestine with Autologous Tissue Substitute, Via Natural or Artificial Opening
0DUF7JZ	Supplement Right Large Intestine with Synthetic Substitute, Via Natural or Artificial Opening
0DUF7KZ	Supplement Right Large Intestine with Nonautologous Tissue Substitute, Via Natural or Artificial Opening
0DUF87Z	Supplement Right Large Intestine with Autologous Tissue Substitute, Via Natural or Artificial Opening Endoscopic
0DUF8JZ	Supplement Right Large Intestine with Synthetic Substitute, Via Natural or Artificial Opening Endoscopic
0DUF8KZ	Supplement Right Large Intestine with Nonautologous Tissue Substitute, Via Natural or Artificial Opening Endoscopic
0DUG07Z	Supplement Left Large Intestine with Autologous Tissue Substitute, Open Approach
0DUG0JZ	Supplement Left Large Intestine with Synthetic Substitute, Open Approach
0DUG0KZ	Supplement Left Large Intestine with Nonautologous Tissue Substitute, Open Approach
0DUG47Z	Supplement Left Large Intestine with Autologous Tissue Substitute, Percutaneous Endoscopic Approach
0DUG4JZ	Supplement Left Large Intestine with Synthetic Substitute, Percutaneous Endoscopic Approach
0DUG4KZ	Supplement Left Large Intestine with Nonautologous Tissue Substitute, Percutaneous Endoscopic Approach
0DUG77Z	Supplement Left Large Intestine with Autologous Tissue Substitute, Via Natural or Artificial Opening
0DUG7JZ	Supplement Left Large Intestine with Synthetic Substitute, Via Natural or Artificial Opening
0DUG7KZ	Supplement Left Large Intestine with Nonautologous Tissue Substitute, Via Natural or Artificial Opening
0DUG87Z	Supplement Left Large Intestine with Autologous Tissue Substitute, Via Natural or Artificial Opening Endoscopic
0DUG8JZ	Supplement Left Large Intestine with Synthetic Substitute, Via Natural or Artificial Opening Endoscopic
0DUG8KZ	Supplement Left Large Intestine with Nonautologous Tissue Substitute, Via Natural or Artificial Opening Endoscopic
0DUH07Z	Supplement Cecum with Autologous Tissue Substitute, Open Approach
0DUH0JZ	Supplement Cecum with Synthetic Substitute, Open Approach

♀ Female-only   ♂ Male-only   ▲ Limited Coverage   ● Non-OR   ▦ HAC-associated procedure   ▲ Non-covered procedures   ✚ Combination

0DUH0KZ Supplement Cecum with Nonautologous Tissue Substitute, Open Approach
0DUH47Z Supplement Cecum with Autologous Tissue Substitute, Percutaneous Endoscopic Approach
0DUH4JZ Supplement Cecum with Synthetic Substitute, Percutaneous Endoscopic Approach
0DUH4KZ Supplement Cecum with Nonautologous Tissue Substitute, Percutaneous Endoscopic Approach
0DUH77Z Supplement Cecum with Autologous Tissue Substitute, Via Natural or Artificial Opening
0DUH7JZ Supplement Cecum with Synthetic Substitute, Via Natural or Artificial Opening
0DUH7KZ Supplement Cecum with Nonautologous Tissue Substitute, Via Natural or Artificial Opening
0DUH87Z Supplement Cecum with Autologous Tissue Substitute, Via Natural or Artificial Opening Endoscopic
0DUH8JZ Supplement Cecum with Synthetic Substitute, Via Natural or Artificial Opening Endoscopic
0DUH8KZ Supplement Cecum with Nonautologous Tissue Substitute, Via Natural or Artificial Opening Endoscopic
0DUK07Z Supplement Ascending Colon with Autologous Tissue Substitute, Open Approach
0DUK0JZ Supplement Ascending Colon with Synthetic Substitute, Open Approach
0DUK0KZ Supplement Ascending Colon with Nonautologous Tissue Substitute, Open Approach
0DUK47Z Supplement Ascending Colon with Autologous Tissue Substitute, Percutaneous Endoscopic Approach
0DUK4JZ Supplement Ascending Colon with Synthetic Substitute, Percutaneous Endoscopic Approach
0DUK4KZ Supplement Ascending Colon with Nonautologous Tissue Substitute, Percutaneous Endoscopic Approach
0DUK77Z Supplement Ascending Colon with Autologous Tissue Substitute, Via Natural or Artificial Opening
0DUK7JZ Supplement Ascending Colon with Synthetic Substitute, Via Natural or Artificial Opening
0DUK7KZ Supplement Ascending Colon with Nonautologous Tissue Substitute, Via Natural or Artificial Opening
0DUK87Z Supplement Ascending Colon with Autologous Tissue Substitute, Via Natural or Artificial Opening Endoscopic
0DUK8JZ Supplement Ascending Colon with Synthetic Substitute, Via Natural or Artificial Opening Endoscopic
0DUK8KZ Supplement Ascending Colon with Nonautologous Tissue Substitute, Via Natural or Artificial Opening Endoscopic
0DUL07Z Supplement Transverse Colon with Autologous Tissue Substitute, Open Approach
0DUL0JZ Supplement Transverse Colon with Synthetic Substitute, Open Approach
0DUL0KZ Supplement Transverse Colon with Nonautologous Tissue Substitute, Open Approach
0DUL47Z Supplement Transverse Colon with Autologous Tissue Substitute, Percutaneous Endoscopic Approach

0DUL4JZ Supplement Transverse Colon with Synthetic Substitute, Percutaneous Endoscopic Approach
0DUL4KZ Supplement Transverse Colon with Nonautologous Tissue Substitute, Percutaneous Endoscopic Approach
0DUL77Z Supplement Transverse Colon with Autologous Tissue Substitute, Via Natural or Artificial Opening
0DUL7JZ Supplement Transverse Colon with Synthetic Substitute, Via Natural or Artificial Opening
0DUL7KZ Supplement Transverse Colon with Nonautologous Tissue Substitute, Via Natural or Artificial Opening
0DUL87Z Supplement Transverse Colon with Autologous Tissue Substitute, Via Natural or Artificial Opening Endoscopic
0DUL8JZ Supplement Transverse Colon with Synthetic Substitute, Via Natural or Artificial Opening Endoscopic
0DUL8KZ Supplement Transverse Colon with Nonautologous Tissue Substitute, Via Natural or Artificial Opening Endoscopic
0DUM07Z Supplement Descending Colon with Autologous Tissue Substitute, Open Approach
0DUM0JZ Supplement Descending Colon with Synthetic Substitute, Open Approach
0DUM0KZ Supplement Descending Colon with Nonautologous Tissue Substitute, Open Approach
0DUM47Z Supplement Descending Colon with Autologous Tissue Substitute, Percutaneous Endoscopic Approach
0DUM4JZ Supplement Descending Colon with Synthetic Substitute, Percutaneous Endoscopic Approach
0DUM4KZ Supplement Descending Colon with Nonautologous Tissue Substitute, Percutaneous Endoscopic Approach
0DUM77Z Supplement Descending Colon with Autologous Tissue Substitute, Via Natural or Artificial Opening
0DUM7JZ Supplement Descending Colon with Synthetic Substitute, Via Natural or Artificial Opening
0DUM7KZ Supplement Descending Colon with Nonautologous Tissue Substitute, Via Natural or Artificial Opening
0DUM87Z Supplement Descending Colon with Autologous Tissue Substitute, Via Natural or Artificial Opening Endoscopic
0DUM8JZ Supplement Descending Colon with Synthetic Substitute, Via Natural or Artificial Opening Endoscopic
0DUM8KZ Supplement Descending Colon with Nonautologous Tissue Substitute, Via Natural or Artificial Opening Endoscopic
0DUN07Z Supplement Sigmoid Colon with Autologous Tissue Substitute, Open Approach
0DUN0JZ Supplement Sigmoid Colon with Synthetic Substitute, Open Approach
0DUN0KZ Supplement Sigmoid Colon with Nonautologous Tissue Substitute, Open Approach
0DUN47Z Supplement Sigmoid Colon with Autologous Tissue Substitute, Percutaneous Endoscopic Approach
0DUN4JZ Supplement Sigmoid Colon with Synthetic Substitute, Percutaneous Endoscopic Approach
0DUN4KZ Supplement Sigmoid Colon with Nonautologous Tissue Substitute, Percutaneous Endoscopic Approach

0DUN77Z Supplement Sigmoid Colon with Autologous Tissue Substitute, Via Natural or Artificial Opening
0DUN7JZ Supplement Sigmoid Colon with Synthetic Substitute, Via Natural or Artificial Opening
0DUN7KZ Supplement Sigmoid Colon with Nonautologous Tissue Substitute, Via Natural or Artificial Opening
0DUN87Z Supplement Sigmoid Colon with Autologous Tissue Substitute, Via Natural or Artificial Opening Endoscopic
0DUN8JZ Supplement Sigmoid Colon with Synthetic Substitute, Via Natural or Artificial Opening Endoscopic
0DUN8KZ Supplement Sigmoid Colon with Nonautologous Tissue Substitute, Via Natural or Artificial Opening Endoscopic
0DUP07Z Supplement Rectum with Autologous Tissue Substitute, Open Approach
0DUP0JZ Supplement Rectum with Synthetic Substitute, Open Approach
0DUP0KZ Supplement Rectum with Nonautologous Tissue Substitute, Open Approach
0DUP47Z Supplement Rectum with Autologous Tissue Substitute, Percutaneous Endoscopic Approach
0DUP4JZ Supplement Rectum with Synthetic Substitute, Percutaneous Endoscopic Approach
0DUP4KZ Supplement Rectum with Nonautologous Tissue Substitute, Percutaneous Endoscopic Approach
0DUP77Z Supplement Rectum with Autologous Tissue Substitute, Via Natural or Artificial Opening
0DUP7JZ Supplement Rectum with Synthetic Substitute, Via Natural or Artificial Opening
0DUP7KZ Supplement Rectum with Nonautologous Tissue Substitute, Via Natural or Artificial Opening
0DUP87Z Supplement Rectum with Autologous Tissue Substitute, Via Natural or Artificial Opening Endoscopic
0DUP8JZ Supplement Rectum with Synthetic Substitute, Via Natural or Artificial Opening Endoscopic
0DUP8KZ Supplement Rectum with Nonautologous Tissue Substitute, Via Natural or Artificial Opening Endoscopic
0DUQ07Z Supplement Anus with Autologous Tissue Substitute, Open Approach
0DUQ0JZ Supplement Anus with Synthetic Substitute, Open Approach
0DUQ0KZ Supplement Anus with Nonautologous Tissue Substitute, Open Approach
0DUQ47Z Supplement Anus with Autologous Tissue Substitute, Percutaneous Endoscopic Approach
0DUQ4JZ Supplement Anus with Synthetic Substitute, Percutaneous Endoscopic Approach
0DUQ4KZ Supplement Anus with Nonautologous Tissue Substitute, Percutaneous Endoscopic Approach
0DUQ77Z Supplement Anus with Autologous Tissue Substitute, Via Natural or Artificial Opening
0DUQ7JZ Supplement Anus with Synthetic Substitute, Via Natural or Artificial Opening
0DUQ7KZ Supplement Anus with Nonautologous Tissue Substitute, Via Natural or Artificial Opening

♀ Female-only   ♂ Male-only   ▲ Limited Coverage   ● Non-OR   ▦ HAC-associated procedure   ▲ Non-covered procedures   ✚ Combinati

Q87Z Supplement Anus with Autologous Tissue Substitute, Via Natural or Artificial Opening Endoscopic

Q8JZ Supplement Anus with Synthetic Substitute, Via Natural or Artificial Opening Endoscopic

Q8KZ Supplement Anus with Nonautologous Tissue Substitute, Via Natural or Artificial Opening Endoscopic

QX7Z Supplement Anus with Autologous Tissue Substitute, External Approach

QXJZ Supplement Anus with Synthetic Substitute, External Approach

QXKZ Supplement Anus with Nonautologous Tissue Substitute, External Approach

R07Z Supplement Anal Sphincter with Autologous Tissue Substitute, Open Approach

R0JZ Supplement Anal Sphincter with Synthetic Substitute, Open Approach

R0KZ Supplement Anal Sphincter with Nonautologous Tissue Substitute, Open Approach

R47Z Supplement Anal Sphincter with Autologous Tissue Substitute, Percutaneous Endoscopic Approach

R4JZ Supplement Anal Sphincter with Synthetic Substitute, Percutaneous Endoscopic Approach

R4KZ Supplement Anal Sphincter with Nonautologous Tissue Substitute, Percutaneous Endoscopic Approach

S07Z Supplement Greater Omentum with Autologous Tissue Substitute, Open Approach

0DUS0JZ Supplement Greater Omentum with Synthetic Substitute, Open Approach

0DUS0KZ Supplement Greater Omentum with Nonautologous Tissue Substitute, Open Approach

0DUS47Z Supplement Greater Omentum with Autologous Tissue Substitute, Percutaneous Endoscopic Approach

0DUS4JZ Supplement Greater Omentum with Synthetic Substitute, Percutaneous Endoscopic Approach

0DUS4KZ Supplement Greater Omentum with Nonautologous Tissue Substitute, Percutaneous Endoscopic Approach

0DUT07Z Supplement Lesser Omentum with Autologous Tissue Substitute, Open Approach

0DUT0JZ Supplement Lesser Omentum with Synthetic Substitute, Open Approach

0DUT0KZ Supplement Lesser Omentum with Nonautologous Tissue Substitute, Open Approach

0DUT47Z Supplement Lesser Omentum with Autologous Tissue Substitute, Percutaneous Endoscopic Approach

0DUT4JZ Supplement Lesser Omentum with Synthetic Substitute, Percutaneous Endoscopic Approach

0DUT4KZ Supplement Lesser Omentum with Nonautologous Tissue Substitute, Percutaneous Endoscopic Approach

0DUV07Z Supplement Mesentery with Autologous Tissue Substitute, Open Approach

0DUV0JZ Supplement Mesentery with Synthetic Substitute, Open Approach

0DUV0KZ Supplement Mesentery with Nonautologous Tissue Substitute, Open Approach

0DUV47Z Supplement Mesentery with Autologous Tissue Substitute, Percutaneous Endoscopic Approach

0DUV4JZ Supplement Mesentery with Synthetic Substitute, Percutaneous Endoscopic Approach

0DUV4KZ Supplement Mesentery with Nonautologous Tissue Substitute, Percutaneous Endoscopic Approach

0DUW07Z Supplement Peritoneum with Autologous Tissue Substitute, Open Approach

0DUW0JZ Supplement Peritoneum with Synthetic Substitute, Open Approach

0DUW0KZ Supplement Peritoneum with Nonautologous Tissue Substitute, Open Approach

0DUW47Z Supplement Peritoneum with Autologous Tissue Substitute, Percutaneous Endoscopic Approach

0DUW4JZ Supplement Peritoneum with Synthetic Substitute, Percutaneous Endoscopic Approach

0DUW4KZ Supplement Peritoneum with Nonautologous Tissue Substitute, Percutaneous Endoscopic Approach

V – Gastrointestinal System, Restriction

10CZ Restriction of Upper Esophagus with Extraluminal Device, Open Approach

10DZ Restriction of Upper Esophagus with Intraluminal Device, Open Approach

10ZZ Restriction of Upper Esophagus, Open Approach

13CZ Restriction of Upper Esophagus with Extraluminal Device, Percutaneous Approach

13DZ Restriction of Upper Esophagus with Intraluminal Device, Percutaneous Approach

13ZZ Restriction of Upper Esophagus, Percutaneous Approach

14CZ Restriction of Upper Esophagus with Extraluminal Device, Percutaneous Endoscopic Approach

14DZ Restriction of Upper Esophagus with Intraluminal Device, Percutaneous Endoscopic Approach

14ZZ Restriction of Upper Esophagus, Percutaneous Endoscopic Approach

17DZ Restriction of Upper Esophagus with Intraluminal Device, Via Natural or Artificial Opening

17ZZ Restriction of Upper Esophagus, Via Natural or Artificial Opening

18DZ Restriction of Upper Esophagus with Intraluminal Device, Via Natural or Artificial Opening Endoscopic

18ZZ Restriction of Upper Esophagus, Via Natural or Artificial Opening Endoscopic

20CZ Restriction of Middle Esophagus with Extraluminal Device, Open Approach

20DZ Restriction of Middle Esophagus with Intraluminal Device, Open Approach

0DV20ZZ Restriction of Middle Esophagus, Open Approach

0DV23CZ Restriction of Middle Esophagus with Extraluminal Device, Percutaneous Approach

0DV23DZ Restriction of Middle Esophagus with Intraluminal Device, Percutaneous Approach

0DV23ZZ Restriction of Middle Esophagus, Percutaneous Approach

0DV24CZ Restriction of Middle Esophagus with Extraluminal Device, Percutaneous Endoscopic Approach

0DV24DZ Restriction of Middle Esophagus with Intraluminal Device, Percutaneous Endoscopic Approach

0DV24ZZ Restriction of Middle Esophagus, Percutaneous Endoscopic Approach

0DV27DZ Restriction of Middle Esophagus with Intraluminal Device, Via Natural or Artificial Opening

0DV27ZZ Restriction of Middle Esophagus, Via Natural or Artificial Opening

0DV28DZ Restriction of Middle Esophagus with Intraluminal Device, Via Natural or Artificial Opening Endoscopic

0DV28ZZ Restriction of Middle Esophagus, Via Natural or Artificial Opening Endoscopic

0DV30CZ Restriction of Lower Esophagus with Extraluminal Device, Open Approach

0DV30DZ Restriction of Lower Esophagus with Intraluminal Device, Open Approach

0DV30ZZ Restriction of Lower Esophagus, Open Approach

0DV33CZ Restriction of Lower Esophagus with Extraluminal Device, Percutaneous Approach

0DV33DZ Restriction of Lower Esophagus with Intraluminal Device, Percutaneous Approach

0DV33ZZ Restriction of Lower Esophagus, Percutaneous Approach

0DV34CZ Restriction of Lower Esophagus with Extraluminal Device, Percutaneous Endoscopic Approach

0DV34DZ Restriction of Lower Esophagus with Intraluminal Device, Percutaneous Endoscopic Approach

0DV34ZZ Restriction of Lower Esophagus, Percutaneous Endoscopic Approach

0DV37DZ Restriction of Lower Esophagus with Intraluminal Device, Via Natural or Artificial Opening

0DV37ZZ Restriction of Lower Esophagus, Via Natural or Artificial Opening

0DV38DZ Restriction of Lower Esophagus with Intraluminal Device, Via Natural or Artificial Opening Endoscopic

0DV38ZZ Restriction of Lower Esophagus, Via Natural or Artificial Opening Endoscopic

0DV40CZ Restriction of Esophagogastric Junction with Extraluminal Device, Open Approach

0DV40DZ Restriction of Esophagogastric Junction with Intraluminal Device, Open Approach

0DV40ZZ Restriction of Esophagogastric Junction, Open Approach

0DV43CZ Restriction of Esophagogastric Junction with Extraluminal Device, Percutaneous Approach

0DV43DZ Restriction of Esophagogastric Junction with Intraluminal Device, Percutaneous Approach

0DV43ZZ Restriction of Esophagogastric Junction, Percutaneous Approach

0DV44CZ Restriction of Esophagogastric Junction with Extraluminal Device, Percutaneous Endoscopic Approach

0DV44DZ Restriction of Esophagogastric Junction with Intraluminal Device, Percutaneous Endoscopic Approach

0DV44ZZ Restriction of Esophagogastric Junction, Percutaneous Endoscopic Approach
AHA CC: 3Q, 2014, 28

0DV47DZ Restriction of Esophagogastric Junction with Intraluminal Device, Via Natural or Artificial Opening

0DV47ZZ Restriction of Esophagogastric Junction, Via Natural or Artificial Opening

0DV48DZ Restriction of Esophagogastric Junction with Intraluminal Device, Via Natural or Artificial Opening Endoscopic

0DV48ZZ Restriction of Esophagogastric Junction, Via Natural or Artificial Opening Endoscopic

0DV50CZ Restriction of Esophagus with Extraluminal Device, Open Approach

0DV50DZ Restriction of Esophagus with Intraluminal Device, Open Approach

0DV50ZZ Restriction of Esophagus, Open Approach

0DV53CZ Restriction of Esophagus with Extraluminal Device, Percutaneous Approach

0DV53DZ Restriction of Esophagus with Intraluminal Device, Percutaneous Approach

0DV53ZZ Restriction of Esophagus, Percutaneous Approach

0DV54CZ Restriction of Esophagus with Extraluminal Device, Percutaneous Endoscopic Approach

0DV54DZ Restriction of Esophagus with Intraluminal Device, Percutaneous Endoscopic Approach

0DV54ZZ Restriction of Esophagus, Percutaneous Endoscopic Approach

0DV57DZ Restriction of Esophagus with Intraluminal Device, Via Natural or Artificial Opening

0DV57ZZ Restriction of Esophagus, Via Natural or Artificial Opening

0DV58DZ Restriction of Esophagus with Intraluminal Device, Via Natural or Artificial Opening Endoscopic

0DV58ZZ Restriction of Esophagus, Via Natural or Artificial Opening Endoscopic

0DV60CZ Restriction of Stomach with Extraluminal Device, Open Approach

0DV60DZ Restriction of Stomach with Intraluminal Device, Open Approach

0DV60ZZ Restriction of Stomach, Open Approach

0DV63CZ Restriction of Stomach with Extraluminal Device, Percutaneous Approach

0DV63DZ Restriction of Stomach with Intraluminal Device, Percutaneous Approach

0DV63ZZ Restriction of Stomach, Percutaneous Approach

0DV64CZ Restriction of Stomach with Extraluminal Device, Percutaneous Endoscopic Approach
    ▪ When reported with principal diagnosis code K66.01 and secondary diagnosis code K68.11, K95.01, K95.81 or T81.4XXA

0DV64DZ Restriction of Stomach with Intraluminal Device, Percutaneous Endoscopic Approach

0DV64ZZ Restriction of Stomach, Percutaneous Endoscopic Approach

▲ **0DV67DZ** Restriction of Stomach with Intraluminal Device, Via Natural or Artificial Opening

0DV67ZZ Restriction of Stomach, Via Natural or Artificial Opening

▲ **0DV68DZ** Restriction of Stomach with Intraluminal Device, Via Natural or Artificial Opening Endoscopic

0DV68ZZ Restriction of Stomach, Via Natural or Artificial Opening Endoscopic

0DV70CZ Restriction of Stomach, Pylorus with Extraluminal Device, Open Approach

0DV70DZ Restriction of Stomach, Pylorus with Intraluminal Device, Open Approach

0DV70ZZ Restriction of Stomach, Pylorus, Open Approach

0DV73CZ Restriction of Stomach, Pylorus with Extraluminal Device, Percutaneous Approach

0DV73DZ Restriction of Stomach, Pylorus with Intraluminal Device, Percutaneous Approach

0DV73ZZ Restriction of Stomach, Pylorus, Percutaneous Approach

0DV74CZ Restriction of Stomach, Pylorus with Extraluminal Device, Percutaneous Endoscopic Approach

0DV74DZ Restriction of Stomach, Pylorus with Intraluminal Device, Percutaneous Endoscopic Approach

0DV74ZZ Restriction of Stomach, Pylorus, Percutaneous Endoscopic Approach

0DV77DZ Restriction of Stomach, Pylorus with Intraluminal Device, Via Natural or Artificial Opening

0DV77ZZ Restriction of Stomach, Pylorus, Via Natural or Artificial Opening

0DV78DZ Restriction of Stomach, Pylorus with Intraluminal Device, Via Natural or Artificial Opening Endoscopic

0DV78ZZ Restriction of Stomach, Pylorus, Via Natural or Artificial Opening Endoscopic

0DV80CZ Restriction of Small Intestine with Extraluminal Device, Open Approach

0DV80DZ Restriction of Small Intestine with Intraluminal Device, Open Approach

0DV80ZZ Restriction of Small Intestine, Open Approach

0DV83CZ Restriction of Small Intestine with Extraluminal Device, Percutaneous Approach

0DV83DZ Restriction of Small Intestine with Intraluminal Device, Percutaneous Approach

0DV83ZZ Restriction of Small Intestine, Percutaneous Approach

0DV84CZ Restriction of Small Intestine with Extraluminal Device, Percutaneous Endoscopic Approach

0DV84DZ Restriction of Small Intestine with Intraluminal Device, Percutaneous Endoscopic Approach

0DV84ZZ Restriction of Small Intestine, Percutaneous Endoscopic Approach

0DV87DZ Restriction of Small Intestine with Intraluminal Device, Via Natural or Artificial Opening

0DV87ZZ Restriction of Small Intestine, Via Natural or Artificial Opening

0DV88DZ Restriction of Small Intestine with Intraluminal Device, Via Natural or Artificial Opening Endoscopic

0DV88ZZ Restriction of Small Intestine, Via Natural or Artificial Opening Endoscopic

0DV90CZ Restriction of Duodenum with Extraluminal Device, Open Approach

0DV90DZ Restriction of Duodenum with Intraluminal Device, Open Approach

0DV90ZZ Restriction of Duodenum, Open Approach

0DV93CZ Restriction of Duodenum with Extraluminal Device, Percutaneous Approach

0DV93DZ Restriction of Duodenum with Intraluminal Device, Percutaneous Approach

0DV93ZZ Restriction of Duodenum, Percutaneous Approach

0DV94CZ Restriction of Duodenum with Extraluminal Device, Percutaneous Endoscopic Approach

0DV94DZ Restriction of Duodenum with Intraluminal Device, Percutaneous Endoscopic Approach

0DV94ZZ Restriction of Duodenum, Percutaneous Endoscopic Approach

0DV97DZ Restriction of Duodenum with Intraluminal Device, Via Natural or Artificial Opening

0DV97ZZ Restriction of Duodenum, Via Natural or Artificial Opening

0DV98DZ Restriction of Duodenum with Intraluminal Device, Via Natural or Artificial Opening Endoscopic

0DV98ZZ Restriction of Duodenum, Via Natural or Artificial Opening Endoscopic

0DVA0CZ Restriction of Jejunum with Extraluminal Device, Open Approach

0DVA0DZ Restriction of Jejunum with Intraluminal Device, Open Approach

0DVA0ZZ Restriction of Jejunum, Open Approach

0DVA3CZ Restriction of Jejunum with Extraluminal Device, Percutaneous Approach

0DVA3DZ Restriction of Jejunum with Intraluminal Device, Percutaneous Approach

0DVA3ZZ Restriction of Jejunum, Percutaneous Approach

0DVA4CZ Restriction of Jejunum with Extraluminal Device, Percutaneous Endoscopic Approach

0DVA4DZ Restriction of Jejunum with Intraluminal Device, Percutaneous Endoscopic Approach

0DVA4ZZ Restriction of Jejunum, Percutaneous Endoscopic Approach

0DVA7DZ Restriction of Jejunum with Intraluminal Device, Via Natural or Artificial Opening

0DVA7ZZ Restriction of Jejunum, Via Natural or Artificial Opening

0DVA8DZ Restriction of Jejunum with Intraluminal Device, Via Natural or Artificial Opening Endoscopic

0DVA8ZZ Restriction of Jejunum, Via Natural or Artificial Opening Endoscopic

0DVB0CZ Restriction of Ileum with Extraluminal Device, Open Approach

0DVB0DZ Restriction of Ileum with Intraluminal Device, Open Approach

0DVB0ZZ Restriction of Ileum, Open Approach

0DVB3CZ Restriction of Ileum with Extraluminal Device, Percutaneous Approach

0DVB3DZ Restriction of Ileum with Intraluminal Device, Percutaneous Approach

0DVB3ZZ Restriction of Ileum, Percutaneous Approach

0DVB4CZ Restriction of Ileum with Extraluminal Device, Percutaneous Endoscopic Approach

0DVB4DZ Restriction of Ileum with Intraluminal Device, Percutaneous Endoscopic Approach

♀ Female-only   ♂ Male-only   ▲ Limited Coverage   ● Non-OR   ▨ HAC-associated procedure   ▲ Non-covered procedures   ✛ Combinat

B4ZZ	Restriction of Ileum, Percutaneous Endoscopic Approach	**0DVF0CZ**	Restriction of Right Large Intestine with Extraluminal Device, Open Approach	**0DVH4CZ**	Restriction of Cecum with Extraluminal Device, Percutaneous Endoscopic Approach
B7DZ	Restriction of Ileum with Intraluminal Device, Via Natural or Artificial Opening	**0DVF0DZ**	Restriction of Right Large Intestine with Intraluminal Device, Open Approach	**0DVH4DZ**	Restriction of Cecum with Intraluminal Device, Percutaneous Endoscopic Approach
B7ZZ	Restriction of Ileum, Via Natural or Artificial Opening	**0DVF0ZZ**	Restriction of Right Large Intestine, Open Approach	**0DVH4ZZ**	Restriction of Cecum, Percutaneous Endoscopic Approach
B8DZ	Restriction of Ileum with Intraluminal Device, Via Natural or Artificial Opening Endoscopic	**0DVF3CZ**	Restriction of Right Large Intestine with Extraluminal Device, Percutaneous Approach	**0DVH7DZ**	Restriction of Cecum with Intraluminal Device, Via Natural or Artificial Opening
B8ZZ	Restriction of Ileum, Via Natural or Artificial Opening Endoscopic	**0DVF3DZ**	Restriction of Right Large Intestine with Intraluminal Device, Percutaneous Approach	**0DVH7ZZ**	Restriction of Cecum, Via Natural or Artificial Opening
C0CZ	Restriction of Ileocecal Valve with Extraluminal Device, Open Approach	**0DVF3ZZ**	Restriction of Right Large Intestine, Percutaneous Approach	**0DVH8DZ**	Restriction of Cecum with Intraluminal Device, Via Natural or Artificial Opening Endoscopic
C0DZ	Restriction of Ileocecal Valve with Intraluminal Device, Open Approach	**0DVF4CZ**	Restriction of Right Large Intestine with Extraluminal Device, Percutaneous Endoscopic Approach	**0DVH8ZZ**	Restriction of Cecum, Via Natural or Artificial Opening Endoscopic
C0ZZ	Restriction of Ileocecal Valve, Open Approach	**0DVF4DZ**	Restriction of Right Large Intestine with Intraluminal Device, Percutaneous Endoscopic Approach	**0DVK0CZ**	Restriction of Ascending Colon with Extraluminal Device, Open Approach
C3CZ	Restriction of Ileocecal Valve with Extraluminal Device, Percutaneous Approach	**0DVF4ZZ**	Restriction of Right Large Intestine, Percutaneous Endoscopic Approach	**0DVK0DZ**	Restriction of Ascending Colon with Intraluminal Device, Open Approach
C3DZ	Restriction of Ileocecal Valve with Intraluminal Device, Percutaneous Approach	**0DVF7DZ**	Restriction of Right Large Intestine with Intraluminal Device, Via Natural or Artificial Opening	**0DVK0ZZ**	Restriction of Ascending Colon, Open Approach
C3ZZ	Restriction of Ileocecal Valve, Percutaneous Approach	**0DVF7ZZ**	Restriction of Right Large Intestine, Via Natural or Artificial Opening	**0DVK3CZ**	Restriction of Ascending Colon with Extraluminal Device, Percutaneous Approach
C4CZ	Restriction of Ileocecal Valve with Extraluminal Device, Percutaneous Endoscopic Approach	**0DVF8DZ**	Restriction of Right Large Intestine with Intraluminal Device, Via Natural or Artificial Opening Endoscopic	**0DVK3DZ**	Restriction of Ascending Colon with Intraluminal Device, Percutaneous Approach
C4DZ	Restriction of Ileocecal Valve with Intraluminal Device, Percutaneous Endoscopic Approach	**0DVF8ZZ**	Restriction of Right Large Intestine, Via Natural or Artificial Opening Endoscopic	**0DVK3ZZ**	Restriction of Ascending Colon, Percutaneous Approach
C4ZZ	Restriction of Ileocecal Valve, Percutaneous Endoscopic Approach	**0DVG0CZ**	Restriction of Left Large Intestine with Extraluminal Device, Open Approach	**0DVK4CZ**	Restriction of Ascending Colon with Extraluminal Device, Percutaneous Endoscopic Approach
C7DZ	Restriction of Ileocecal Valve with Intraluminal Device, Via Natural or Artificial Opening	**0DVG0DZ**	Restriction of Left Large Intestine with Intraluminal Device, Open Approach	**0DVK4DZ**	Restriction of Ascending Colon with Intraluminal Device, Percutaneous Endoscopic Approach
C7ZZ	Restriction of Ileocecal Valve, Via Natural or Artificial Opening	**0DVG0ZZ**	Restriction of Left Large Intestine, Open Approach	**0DVK4ZZ**	Restriction of Ascending Colon, Percutaneous Endoscopic Approach
C8DZ	Restriction of Ileocecal Valve with Intraluminal Device, Via Natural or Artificial Opening Endoscopic	**0DVG3CZ**	Restriction of Left Large Intestine with Extraluminal Device, Percutaneous Approach	**0DVK7DZ**	Restriction of Ascending Colon with Intraluminal Device, Via Natural or Artificial Opening
C8ZZ	Restriction of Ileocecal Valve, Via Natural or Artificial Opening Endoscopic	**0DVG3DZ**	Restriction of Left Large Intestine with Intraluminal Device, Percutaneous Approach	**0DVK7ZZ**	Restriction of Ascending Colon, Via Natural or Artificial Opening
E0CZ	Restriction of Large Intestine with Extraluminal Device, Open Approach	**0DVG3ZZ**	Restriction of Left Large Intestine, Percutaneous Approach	**0DVK8DZ**	Restriction of Ascending Colon with Intraluminal Device, Via Natural or Artificial Opening Endoscopic
E0DZ	Restriction of Large Intestine with Intraluminal Device, Open Approach	**0DVG4CZ**	Restriction of Left Large Intestine with Extraluminal Device, Percutaneous Endoscopic Approach	**0DVK8ZZ**	Restriction of Ascending Colon, Via Natural or Artificial Opening Endoscopic
E0ZZ	Restriction of Large Intestine, Open Approach	**0DVG4DZ**	Restriction of Left Large Intestine with Intraluminal Device, Percutaneous Endoscopic Approach	**0DVL0CZ**	Restriction of Transverse Colon with Extraluminal Device, Open Approach
E3CZ	Restriction of Large Intestine with Extraluminal Device, Percutaneous Approach	**0DVG4ZZ**	Restriction of Left Large Intestine, Percutaneous Endoscopic Approach	**0DVL0DZ**	Restriction of Transverse Colon with Intraluminal Device, Open Approach
E3DZ	Restriction of Large Intestine with Intraluminal Device, Percutaneous Approach	**0DVG7DZ**	Restriction of Left Large Intestine with Intraluminal Device, Via Natural or Artificial Opening	**0DVL0ZZ**	Restriction of Transverse Colon, Open Approach
E3ZZ	Restriction of Large Intestine, Percutaneous Approach	**0DVG7ZZ**	Restriction of Left Large Intestine, Via Natural or Artificial Opening	**0DVL3CZ**	Restriction of Transverse Colon with Extraluminal Device, Percutaneous Approach
E4CZ	Restriction of Large Intestine with Extraluminal Device, Percutaneous Endoscopic Approach	**0DVG8DZ**	Restriction of Left Large Intestine with Intraluminal Device, Via Natural or Artificial Opening Endoscopic	**0DVL3DZ**	Restriction of Transverse Colon with Intraluminal Device, Percutaneous Approach
E4DZ	Restriction of Large Intestine with Intraluminal Device, Percutaneous Endoscopic Approach	**0DVG8ZZ**	Restriction of Left Large Intestine, Via Natural or Artificial Opening Endoscopic	**0DVL3ZZ**	Restriction of Transverse Colon, Percutaneous Approach
E4ZZ	Restriction of Large Intestine, Percutaneous Endoscopic Approach	**0DVH0CZ**	Restriction of Cecum with Extraluminal Device, Open Approach	**0DVL4CZ**	Restriction of Transverse Colon with Extraluminal Device, Percutaneous Endoscopic Approach
E7DZ	Restriction of Large Intestine with Intraluminal Device, Via Natural or Artificial Opening	**0DVH0DZ**	Restriction of Cecum with Intraluminal Device, Open Approach	**0DVL4DZ**	Restriction of Transverse Colon with Intraluminal Device, Percutaneous Endoscopic Approach
E7ZZ	Restriction of Large Intestine, Via Natural or Artificial Opening	**0DVH0ZZ**	Restriction of Cecum, Open Approach	**0DVL4ZZ**	Restriction of Transverse Colon, Percutaneous Endoscopic Approach
E8DZ	Restriction of Large Intestine with Intraluminal Device, Via Natural or Artificial Opening Endoscopic	**0DVH3CZ**	Restriction of Cecum with Extraluminal Device, Percutaneous Approach	**0DVL7DZ**	Restriction of Transverse Colon with Intraluminal Device, Via Natural or Artificial Opening
E8ZZ	Restriction of Large Intestine, Via Natural or Artificial Opening Endoscopic	**0DVH3DZ**	Restriction of Cecum with Intraluminal Device, Percutaneous Approach		
		0DVH3ZZ	Restriction of Cecum, Percutaneous Approach		

Female-only	♂ Male-only	▲ Limited Coverage	● Non-OR	▦ HAC-associated procedure	▲ Non-covered procedures	✚ Combination

0DVL7ZZ   Restriction of Transverse Colon, Via Natural or Artificial Opening

0DVL8DZ   Restriction of Transverse Colon with Intraluminal Device, Via Natural or Artificial Opening Endoscopic

0DVL8ZZ   Restriction of Transverse Colon, Via Natural or Artificial Opening Endoscopic

0DVM0CZ   Restriction of Descending Colon with Extraluminal Device, Open Approach

0DVM0DZ   Restriction of Descending Colon with Intraluminal Device, Open Approach

0DVM0ZZ   Restriction of Descending Colon, Open Approach

0DVM3CZ   Restriction of Descending Colon with Extraluminal Device, Percutaneous Approach

0DVM3DZ   Restriction of Descending Colon with Intraluminal Device, Percutaneous Approach

0DVM3ZZ   Restriction of Descending Colon, Percutaneous Approach

0DVM4CZ   Restriction of Descending Colon with Extraluminal Device, Percutaneous Endoscopic Approach

0DVM4DZ   Restriction of Descending Colon with Intraluminal Device, Percutaneous Endoscopic Approach

0DVM4ZZ   Restriction of Descending Colon, Percutaneous Endoscopic Approach

0DVM7DZ   Restriction of Descending Colon with Intraluminal Device, Via Natural or Artificial Opening

0DVM7ZZ   Restriction of Descending Colon, Via Natural or Artificial Opening

0DVM8DZ   Restriction of Descending Colon with Intraluminal Device, Via Natural or Artificial Opening Endoscopic

0DVM8ZZ   Restriction of Descending Colon, Via Natural or Artificial Opening Endoscopic

0DVN0CZ   Restriction of Sigmoid Colon with Extraluminal Device, Open Approach

0DVN0DZ   Restriction of Sigmoid Colon with Intraluminal Device, Open Approach

0DVN0ZZ   Restriction of Sigmoid Colon, Open Approach

0DVN3CZ   Restriction of Sigmoid Colon with Extraluminal Device, Percutaneous Approach

0DVN3DZ   Restriction of Sigmoid Colon with Intraluminal Device, Percutaneous Approach

0DVN3ZZ   Restriction of Sigmoid Colon, Percutaneous Approach

0DVN4CZ   Restriction of Sigmoid Colon with Extraluminal Device, Percutaneous Endoscopic Approach

0DVN4DZ   Restriction of Sigmoid Colon with Intraluminal Device, Percutaneous Endoscopic Approach

0DVN4ZZ   Restriction of Sigmoid Colon, Percutaneous Endoscopic Approach

0DVN7DZ   Restriction of Sigmoid Colon with Intraluminal Device, Via Natural or Artificial Opening

0DVN7ZZ   Restriction of Sigmoid Colon, Via Natural or Artificial Opening

0DVN8DZ   Restriction of Sigmoid Colon with Intraluminal Device, Via Natural or Artificial Opening Endoscopic

0DVN8ZZ   Restriction of Sigmoid Colon, Via Natural or Artificial Opening Endoscopic

0DVP0CZ   Restriction of Rectum with Extraluminal Device, Open Approach

0DVP0DZ   Restriction of Rectum with Intraluminal Device, Open Approach

0DVP0ZZ   Restriction of Rectum, Open Approach

0DVP3CZ   Restriction of Rectum with Extraluminal Device, Percutaneous Approach

0DVP3DZ   Restriction of Rectum with Intraluminal Device, Percutaneous Approach

0DVP3ZZ   Restriction of Rectum, Percutaneous Approach

0DVP4CZ   Restriction of Rectum with Extraluminal Device, Percutaneous Endoscopic Approach

0DVP4DZ   Restriction of Rectum with Intraluminal Device, Percutaneous Endoscopic Approach

0DVP4ZZ   Restriction of Rectum, Percutaneous Endoscopic Approach

0DVP7DZ   Restriction of Rectum with Intraluminal Device, Via Natural or Artificial Opening

0DVP7ZZ   Restriction of Rectum, Via Natural or Artificial Opening

0DVP8DZ   Restriction of Rectum with Intraluminal Device, Via Natural or Artificial Opening Endoscopic

0DVP8ZZ   Restriction of Rectum, Via Natural or Artificial Opening Endoscopic

0DVQ0CZ   Restriction of Anus with Extraluminal Device, Open Approach

0DVQ0DZ   Restriction of Anus with Intraluminal Device, Open Approach

0DVQ0ZZ   Restriction of Anus, Open Approach

0DVQ3CZ   Restriction of Anus with Extraluminal Device, Percutaneous Approach

0DVQ3DZ   Restriction of Anus with Intraluminal Device, Percutaneous Approach

0DVQ3ZZ   Restriction of Anus, Percutaneous Approach

0DVQ4CZ   Restriction of Anus with Extraluminal Device, Percutaneous Endoscopic Approach

0DVQ4DZ   Restriction of Anus with Intraluminal Device, Percutaneous Endoscopic Approach

0DVQ4ZZ   Restriction of Anus, Percutaneous Endoscopic Approach

0DVQ7DZ   Restriction of Anus with Intraluminal Device, Via Natural or Artificial Opening

0DVQ7ZZ   Restriction of Anus, Via Natural or Artificial Opening

0DVQ8DZ   Restriction of Anus with Intraluminal Device, Via Natural or Artificial Opening Endoscopic

0DVQ8ZZ   Restriction of Anus, Via Natural or Artificial Opening Endoscopic

0DVQXCZ   Restriction of Anus with Extraluminal Device, External Approach

0DVQXDZ   Restriction of Anus with Intraluminal Device, External Approach

0DVQXZZ   Restriction of Anus, External Approach

0DW – Gastrointestinal System, Revision

Review Coding Guideline B6.1c

0DW000Z   Revision of Drainage Device in Upper Intestinal Tract, Open Approach

0DW002Z   Revision of Monitoring Device in Upper Intestinal Tract, Open Approach

0DW003Z   Revision of Infusion Device in Upper Intestinal Tract, Open Approach

0DW007Z   Revision of Autologous Tissue Substitute in Upper Intestinal Tract, Open Approach

0DW00CZ   Revision of Extraluminal Device in Upper Intestinal Tract, Open Approach

0DW00DZ   Revision of Intraluminal Device in Upper Intestinal Tract, Open Approach

0DW00JZ   Revision of Synthetic Substitute in Upper Intestinal Tract, Open Approach

0DW00KZ   Revision of Nonautologous Tissue Substitute in Upper Intestinal Tract, Open Approach

0DW00UZ   Revision of Feeding Device in Upper Intestinal Tract, Open Approach

0DW030Z   Revision of Drainage Device in Upper Intestinal Tract, Percutaneous Approach

0DW032Z   Revision of Monitoring Device in Upper Intestinal Tract, Percutaneous Approach

0DW033Z   Revision of Infusion Device in Upper Intestinal Tract, Percutaneous Approach

0DW037Z   Revision of Autologous Tissue Substitute in Upper Intestinal Tract, Percutaneous Approach

0DW03CZ   Revision of Extraluminal Device in Upper Intestinal Tract, Percutaneous Approach

0DW03DZ   Revision of Intraluminal Device in Upper Intestinal Tract, Percutaneous Approach

0DW03JZ   Revision of Synthetic Substitute in Upper Intestinal Tract, Percutaneous Approach

0DW03KZ   Revision of Nonautologous Tissue Substitute in Upper Intestinal Tract, Percutaneous Approach

0DW03UZ   Revision of Feeding Device in Upper Intestinal Tract, Percutaneous Approach

0DW040Z   Revision of Drainage Device in Upper Intestinal Tract, Percutaneous Endoscopic Approach

0DW042Z   Revision of Monitoring Device in Upper Intestinal Tract, Percutaneous Endoscopic Approach

0DW043Z   Revision of Infusion Device in Upper Intestinal Tract, Percutaneous Endoscopic Approach

0DW047Z   Revision of Autologous Tissue Substitute in Upper Intestinal Tract, Percutaneous Endoscopic Approach

0DW04CZ   Revision of Extraluminal Device in Upper Intestinal Tract, Percutaneous Endoscopic Approach

0DW04DZ   Revision of Intraluminal Device in Upper Intestinal Tract, Percutaneous Endoscopic Approach

0DW04JZ   Revision of Synthetic Substitute in Upper Intestinal Tract, Percutaneous Endoscopic Approach

0DW04KZ   Revision of Nonautologous Tissue Substitute in Upper Intestinal Tract, Percutaneous Endoscopic Approach

0DW04UZ   Revision of Feeding Device in Upper Intestinal Tract, Percutaneous Endoscopic Approach

0DW070Z   Revision of Drainage Device in Upper Intestinal Tract, Via Natural or Artificial Opening

0DW072Z	Revision of Monitoring Device in Upper Intestinal Tract, Via Natural or Artificial Opening
0DW073Z	Revision of Infusion Device in Upper Intestinal Tract, Via Natural or Artificial Opening
0DW077Z	Revision of Autologous Tissue Substitute in Upper Intestinal Tract, Via Natural or Artificial Opening
0DW07CZ	Revision of Extraluminal Device in Upper Intestinal Tract, Via Natural or Artificial Opening
0DW07DZ	Revision of Intraluminal Device in Upper Intestinal Tract, Via Natural or Artificial Opening
0DW07JZ	Revision of Synthetic Substitute in Upper Intestinal Tract, Via Natural or Artificial Opening
0DW07KZ	Revision of Nonautologous Tissue Substitute in Upper Intestinal Tract, Via Natural or Artificial Opening
0DW07UZ	Revision of Feeding Device in Upper Intestinal Tract, Via Natural or Artificial Opening
0DW080Z	Revision of Drainage Device in Upper Intestinal Tract, Via Natural or Artificial Opening Endoscopic
0DW082Z	Revision of Monitoring Device in Upper Intestinal Tract, Via Natural or Artificial Opening Endoscopic
0DW083Z	Revision of Infusion Device in Upper Intestinal Tract, Via Natural or Artificial Opening Endoscopic
0DW087Z	Revision of Autologous Tissue Substitute in Upper Intestinal Tract, Via Natural or Artificial Opening Endoscopic
0DW08CZ	Revision of Extraluminal Device in Upper Intestinal Tract, Via Natural or Artificial Opening Endoscopic
0DW08DZ	Revision of Intraluminal Device in Upper Intestinal Tract, Via Natural or Artificial Opening Endoscopic
0DW08JZ	Revision of Synthetic Substitute in Upper Intestinal Tract, Via Natural or Artificial Opening Endoscopic
0DW08KZ	Revision of Nonautologous Tissue Substitute in Upper Intestinal Tract, Via Natural or Artificial Opening Endoscopic
0DW08UZ	Revision of Feeding Device in Upper Intestinal Tract, Via Natural or Artificial Opening Endoscopic
0DW0X0Z	Revision of Drainage Device in Upper Intestinal Tract, External Approach
0DW0X2Z	Revision of Monitoring Device in Upper Intestinal Tract, External Approach
0DW0X3Z	Revision of Infusion Device in Upper Intestinal Tract, External Approach
0DW0X7Z	Revision of Autologous Tissue Substitute in Upper Intestinal Tract, External Approach
0DW0XCZ	Revision of Extraluminal Device in Upper Intestinal Tract, External Approach
0DW0XDZ	Revision of Intraluminal Device in Upper Intestinal Tract, External Approach
0DW0XJZ	Revision of Synthetic Substitute in Upper Intestinal Tract, External Approach
0DW0XKZ	Revision of Nonautologous Tissue Substitute in Upper Intestinal Tract, External Approach
0DW0XUZ	Revision of Feeding Device in Upper Intestinal Tract, External Approach
0DW57DZ	Revision of Intraluminal Device in Esophagus, Via Natural or Artificial Opening
0DW58DZ	Revision of Intraluminal Device in Esophagus, Via Natural or Artificial Opening Endoscopic
0DW5XDZ	Revision of Intraluminal Device in Esophagus, External Approach
0DW600Z	Revision of Drainage Device in Stomach, Open Approach
0DW602Z	Revision of Monitoring Device in Stomach, Open Approach
0DW603Z	Revision of Infusion Device in Stomach, Open Approach
0DW607Z	Revision of Autologous Tissue Substitute in Stomach, Open Approach
0DW60CZ	Revision of Extraluminal Device in Stomach, Open Approach
0DW60DZ	Revision of Intraluminal Device in Stomach, Open Approach
0DW60JZ	Revision of Synthetic Substitute in Stomach, Open Approach
0DW60KZ	Revision of Nonautologous Tissue Substitute in Stomach, Open Approach
0DW60MZ	Revision of Stimulator Lead in Stomach, Open Approach
0DW60UZ	Revision of Feeding Device in Stomach, Open Approach
0DW630Z	Revision of Drainage Device in Stomach, Percutaneous Approach
0DW632Z	Revision of Monitoring Device in Stomach, Percutaneous Approach
0DW633Z	Revision of Infusion Device in Stomach, Percutaneous Approach
0DW637Z	Revision of Autologous Tissue Substitute in Stomach, Percutaneous Approach
0DW63CZ	Revision of Extraluminal Device in Stomach, Percutaneous Approach
0DW63DZ	Revision of Intraluminal Device in Stomach, Percutaneous Approach
0DW63JZ	Revision of Synthetic Substitute in Stomach, Percutaneous Approach
0DW63KZ	Revision of Nonautologous Tissue Substitute in Stomach, Percutaneous Approach
0DW63MZ	Revision of Stimulator Lead in Stomach, Percutaneous Approach
0DW63UZ	Revision of Feeding Device in Stomach, Percutaneous Approach
0DW640Z	Revision of Drainage Device in Stomach, Percutaneous Endoscopic Approach
0DW642Z	Revision of Monitoring Device in Stomach, Percutaneous Endoscopic Approach
0DW643Z	Revision of Infusion Device in Stomach, Percutaneous Endoscopic Approach
0DW647Z	Revision of Autologous Tissue Substitute in Stomach, Percutaneous Endoscopic Approach
0DW64CZ	Revision of Extraluminal Device in Stomach, Percutaneous Endoscopic Approach
0DW64DZ	Revision of Intraluminal Device in Stomach, Percutaneous Endoscopic Approach
0DW64JZ	Revision of Synthetic Substitute in Stomach, Percutaneous Endoscopic Approach
0DW64KZ	Revision of Nonautologous Tissue Substitute in Stomach, Percutaneous Endoscopic Approach
0DW64MZ	Revision of Stimulator Lead in Stomach, Percutaneous Endoscopic Approach
0DW64UZ	Revision of Feeding Device in Stomach, Percutaneous Endoscopic Approach
0DW670Z	Revision of Drainage Device in Stomach, Via Natural or Artificial Opening
0DW672Z	Revision of Monitoring Device in Stomach, Via Natural or Artificial Opening
0DW673Z	Revision of Infusion Device in Stomach, Via Natural or Artificial Opening
0DW677Z	Revision of Autologous Tissue Substitute in Stomach, Via Natural or Artificial Opening
0DW67CZ	Revision of Extraluminal Device in Stomach, Via Natural or Artificial Opening
0DW67DZ	Revision of Intraluminal Device in Stomach, Via Natural or Artificial Opening
0DW67JZ	Revision of Synthetic Substitute in Stomach, Via Natural or Artificial Opening
0DW67KZ	Revision of Nonautologous Tissue Substitute in Stomach, Via Natural or Artificial Opening
0DW67UZ	Revision of Feeding Device in Stomach, Via Natural or Artificial Opening
0DW680Z	Revision of Drainage Device in Stomach, Via Natural or Artificial Opening Endoscopic
0DW682Z	Revision of Monitoring Device in Stomach, Via Natural or Artificial Opening Endoscopic
0DW683Z	Revision of Infusion Device in Stomach, Via Natural or Artificial Opening Endoscopic
0DW687Z	Revision of Autologous Tissue Substitute in Stomach, Via Natural or Artificial Opening Endoscopic
0DW68CZ	Revision of Extraluminal Device in Stomach, Via Natural or Artificial Opening Endoscopic
0DW68DZ	Revision of Intraluminal Device in Stomach, Via Natural or Artificial Opening Endoscopic
0DW68JZ	Revision of Synthetic Substitute in Stomach, Via Natural or Artificial Opening Endoscopic
0DW68KZ	Revision of Nonautologous Tissue Substitute in Stomach, Via Natural or Artificial Opening Endoscopic
0DW68UZ	Revision of Feeding Device in Stomach, Via Natural or Artificial Opening Endoscopic
0DW6X0Z	Revision of Drainage Device in Stomach, External Approach
0DW6X2Z	Revision of Monitoring Device in Stomach, External Approach
0DW6X3Z	Revision of Infusion Device in Stomach, External Approach
0DW6X7Z	Revision of Autologous Tissue Substitute in Stomach, External Approach
0DW6XCZ	Revision of Extraluminal Device in Stomach, External Approach
0DW6XDZ	Revision of Intraluminal Device in Stomach, External Approach
0DW6XJZ	Revision of Synthetic Substitute in Stomach, External Approach
0DW6XKZ	Revision of Nonautologous Tissue Substitute in Stomach, External Approach
0DW6XUZ	Revision of Feeding Device in Stomach, External Approach
0DW807Z	Revision of Autologous Tissue Substitute in Small Intestine, Open Approach
0DW80JZ	Revision of Synthetic Substitute in Small Intestine, Open Approach
0DW80KZ	Revision of Nonautologous Tissue Substitute in Small Intestine, Open Approach
0DW847Z	Revision of Autologous Tissue Substitute in Small Intestine, Percutaneous Endoscopic Approach

0DW84JZ Revision of Synthetic Substitute in Small Intestine, Percutaneous Endoscopic Approach

0DW84KZ Revision of Nonautologous Tissue Substitute in Small Intestine, Percutaneous Endoscopic Approach

0DW877Z Revision of Autologous Tissue Substitute in Small Intestine, Via Natural or Artificial Opening

0DW87JZ Revision of Synthetic Substitute in Small Intestine, Via Natural or Artificial Opening

0DW87KZ Revision of Nonautologous Tissue Substitute in Small Intestine, Via Natural or Artificial Opening

0DW887Z Revision of Autologous Tissue Substitute in Small Intestine, Via Natural or Artificial Opening Endoscopic

0DW88JZ Revision of Synthetic Substitute in Small Intestine, Via Natural or Artificial Opening Endoscopic

0DW88KZ Revision of Nonautologous Tissue Substitute in Small Intestine, Via Natural or Artificial Opening Endoscopic

0DWD00Z Revision of Drainage Device in Lower Intestinal Tract, Open Approach

0DWD02Z Revision of Monitoring Device in Lower Intestinal Tract, Open Approach

0DWD03Z Revision of Infusion Device in Lower Intestinal Tract, Open Approach

0DWD07Z Revision of Autologous Tissue Substitute in Lower Intestinal Tract, Open Approach

0DWD0CZ Revision of Extraluminal Device in Lower Intestinal Tract, Open Approach

0DWD0DZ Revision of Intraluminal Device in Lower Intestinal Tract, Open Approach

0DWD0JZ Revision of Synthetic Substitute in Lower Intestinal Tract, Open Approach

0DWD0KZ Revision of Nonautologous Tissue Substitute in Lower Intestinal Tract, Open Approach

0DWD0UZ Revision of Feeding Device in Lower Intestinal Tract, Open Approach

0DWD30Z Revision of Drainage Device in Lower Intestinal Tract, Percutaneous Approach

0DWD32Z Revision of Monitoring Device in Lower Intestinal Tract, Percutaneous Approach

0DWD33Z Revision of Infusion Device in Lower Intestinal Tract, Percutaneous Approach

0DWD37Z Revision of Autologous Tissue Substitute in Lower Intestinal Tract, Percutaneous Approach

0DWD3CZ Revision of Extraluminal Device in Lower Intestinal Tract, Percutaneous Approach

0DWD3DZ Revision of Intraluminal Device in Lower Intestinal Tract, Percutaneous Approach

0DWD3JZ Revision of Synthetic Substitute in Lower Intestinal Tract, Percutaneous Approach

0DWD3KZ Revision of Nonautologous Tissue Substitute in Lower Intestinal Tract, Percutaneous Approach

0DWD3UZ Revision of Feeding Device in Lower Intestinal Tract, Percutaneous Approach

0DWD40Z Revision of Drainage Device in Lower Intestinal Tract, Percutaneous Endoscopic Approach

0DWD42Z Revision of Monitoring Device in Lower Intestinal Tract, Percutaneous Endoscopic Approach

0DWD43Z Revision of Infusion Device in Lower Intestinal Tract, Percutaneous Endoscopic Approach

0DWD47Z Revision of Autologous Tissue Substitute in Lower Intestinal Tract, Percutaneous Endoscopic Approach

0DWD4CZ Revision of Extraluminal Device in Lower Intestinal Tract, Percutaneous Endoscopic Approach

0DWD4DZ Revision of Intraluminal Device in Lower Intestinal Tract, Percutaneous Endoscopic Approach

0DWD4JZ Revision of Synthetic Substitute in Lower Intestinal Tract, Percutaneous Endoscopic Approach

0DWD4KZ Revision of Nonautologous Tissue Substitute in Lower Intestinal Tract, Percutaneous Endoscopic Approach

0DWD4UZ Revision of Feeding Device in Lower Intestinal Tract, Percutaneous Endoscopic Approach

0DWD70Z Revision of Drainage Device in Lower Intestinal Tract, Via Natural or Artificial Opening

0DWD72Z Revision of Monitoring Device in Lower Intestinal Tract, Via Natural or Artificial Opening

0DWD73Z Revision of Infusion Device in Lower Intestinal Tract, Via Natural or Artificial Opening

0DWD77Z Revision of Autologous Tissue Substitute in Lower Intestinal Tract, Via Natural or Artificial Opening

0DWD7CZ Revision of Extraluminal Device in Lower Intestinal Tract, Via Natural or Artificial Opening

0DWD7DZ Revision of Intraluminal Device in Lower Intestinal Tract, Via Natural or Artificial Opening

0DWD7JZ Revision of Synthetic Substitute in Lower Intestinal Tract, Via Natural or Artificial Opening

0DWD7KZ Revision of Nonautologous Tissue Substitute in Lower Intestinal Tract, Via Natural or Artificial Opening

0DWD7UZ Revision of Feeding Device in Lower Intestinal Tract, Via Natural or Artificial Opening

0DWD80Z Revision of Drainage Device in Lower Intestinal Tract, Via Natural or Artificial Opening Endoscopic

0DWD82Z Revision of Monitoring Device in Lower Intestinal Tract, Via Natural or Artificial Opening Endoscopic

0DWD83Z Revision of Infusion Device in Lower Intestinal Tract, Via Natural or Artificial Opening Endoscopic

0DWD87Z Revision of Autologous Tissue Substitute in Lower Intestinal Tract, Via Natural or Artificial Opening Endoscopic

0DWD8CZ Revision of Extraluminal Device in Lower Intestinal Tract, Via Natural or Artificial Opening Endoscopic

0DWD8DZ Revision of Intraluminal Device in Lower Intestinal Tract, Via Natural or Artificial Opening Endoscopic

0DWD8JZ Revision of Synthetic Substitute in Lower Intestinal Tract, Via Natural or Artificial Opening Endoscopic

0DWD8KZ Revision of Nonautologous Tissue Substitute in Lower Intestinal Tract, Via Natural or Artificial Opening Endoscopic

0DWD8UZ Revision of Feeding Device in Lower Intestinal Tract, Via Natural or Artificial Opening Endoscopic

0DWDX0Z Revision of Drainage Device in Lower Intestinal Tract, External Approach

0DWDX2Z Revision of Monitoring Device in Lower Intestinal Tract, External Approach

0DWDX3Z Revision of Infusion Device in Lower Intestinal Tract, External Approach

0DWDX7Z Revision of Autologous Tissue Substitute in Lower Intestinal Tract, External Approach

0DWDXCZ Revision of Extraluminal Device in Lower Intestinal Tract, External Approach

0DWDXDZ Revision of Intraluminal Device in Lower Intestinal Tract, External Approach

0DWDXJZ Revision of Synthetic Substitute in Lower Intestinal Tract, External Approach

0DWDXKZ Revision of Nonautologous Tissue Substitute in Lower Intestinal Tract, External Approach

0DWDXUZ Revision of Feeding Device in Lower Intestinal Tract, External Approach

0DWE07Z Revision of Autologous Tissue Substitute in Large Intestine, Open Approach

0DWE0JZ Revision of Synthetic Substitute in Large Intestine, Open Approach

0DWE0KZ Revision of Nonautologous Tissue Substitute in Large Intestine, Open Approach

0DWE47Z Revision of Autologous Tissue Substitute in Large Intestine, Percutaneous Endoscopic Approach

0DWE4JZ Revision of Synthetic Substitute in Large Intestine, Percutaneous Endoscopic Approach

0DWE4KZ Revision of Nonautologous Tissue Substitute in Large Intestine, Percutaneous Endoscopic Approach

0DWE77Z Revision of Autologous Tissue Substitute in Large Intestine, Via Natural or Artificial Opening

0DWE7JZ Revision of Synthetic Substitute in Large Intestine, Via Natural or Artificial Opening

0DWE7KZ Revision of Nonautologous Tissue Substitute in Large Intestine, Via Natural or Artificial Opening

0DWE87Z Revision of Autologous Tissue Substitute in Large Intestine, Via Natural or Artificial Opening Endoscopic

0DWE8JZ Revision of Synthetic Substitute in Large Intestine, Via Natural or Artificial Opening Endoscopic

0DWE8KZ Revision of Nonautologous Tissue Substitute in Large Intestine, Via Natural or Artificial Opening Endoscopic

0DWQ0LZ Revision of Artificial Sphincter in Anus, Open Approach

0DWQ3LZ Revision of Artificial Sphincter in Anus, Percutaneous Approach

0DWQ4LZ Revision of Artificial Sphincter in Anus, Percutaneous Endoscopic Approach

0DWQ7LZ Revision of Artificial Sphincter in Anus, Via Natural or Artificial Opening

0DWQ8LZ Revision of Artificial Sphincter in Anus, Via Natural or Artificial Opening Endoscopic

0DWR0MZ Revision of Stimulator Lead in Anal Sphincter, Open Approach

0DWR3MZ Revision of Stimulator Lead in Anal Sphincter, Percutaneous Approach

0DWR4MZ Revision of Stimulator Lead in Anal Sphincter, Percutaneous Endoscopic Approach

0DWU00Z Revision of Drainage Device in Omentum, Open Approach

0DWU07Z Revision of Autologous Tissue Substitute in Omentum, Open Approach

U0JZ	Revision of Synthetic Substitute in Omentum, Open Approach	**0DWV0JZ**	Revision of Synthetic Substitute in Mesentery, Open Approach	**0DWW07Z**	Revision of Autologous Tissue Substitute in Peritoneum, Open Approach

U0JZ Revision of Synthetic Substitute in Omentum, Open Approach

U0KZ Revision of Nonautologous Tissue Substitute in Omentum, Open Approach

U30Z Revision of Drainage Device in Omentum, Percutaneous Approach

U37Z Revision of Autologous Tissue Substitute in Omentum, Percutaneous Approach

U3JZ Revision of Synthetic Substitute in Omentum, Percutaneous Approach

U3KZ Revision of Nonautologous Tissue Substitute in Omentum, Percutaneous Approach

U40Z Revision of Drainage Device in Omentum, Percutaneous Endoscopic Approach

U47Z Revision of Autologous Tissue Substitute in Omentum, Percutaneous Endoscopic Approach

U4JZ Revision of Synthetic Substitute in Omentum, Percutaneous Endoscopic Approach

U4KZ Revision of Nonautologous Tissue Substitute in Omentum, Percutaneous Endoscopic Approach

VV00Z Revision of Drainage Device in Mesentery, Open Approach

VV07Z Revision of Autologous Tissue Substitute in Mesentery, Open Approach

0DWV0JZ Revision of Synthetic Substitute in Mesentery, Open Approach

0DWV0KZ Revision of Nonautologous Tissue Substitute in Mesentery, Open Approach

0DWV30Z Revision of Drainage Device in Mesentery, Percutaneous Approach

0DWV37Z Revision of Autologous Tissue Substitute in Mesentery, Percutaneous Approach

0DWV3JZ Revision of Synthetic Substitute in Mesentery, Percutaneous Approach

0DWV3KZ Revision of Nonautologous Tissue Substitute in Mesentery, Percutaneous Approach

0DWV40Z Revision of Drainage Device in Mesentery, Percutaneous Endoscopic Approach

0DWV47Z Revision of Autologous Tissue Substitute in Mesentery, Percutaneous Endoscopic Approach

0DWV4JZ Revision of Synthetic Substitute in Mesentery, Percutaneous Endoscopic Approach

0DWV4KZ Revision of Nonautologous Tissue Substitute in Mesentery, Percutaneous Endoscopic Approach

0DWW00Z Revision of Drainage Device in Peritoneum, Open Approach

0DWW07Z Revision of Autologous Tissue Substitute in Peritoneum, Open Approach

0DWW0JZ Revision of Synthetic Substitute in Peritoneum, Open Approach

0DWW0KZ Revision of Nonautologous Tissue Substitute in Peritoneum, Open Approach

0DWW30Z Revision of Drainage Device in Peritoneum, Percutaneous Approach

0DWW37Z Revision of Autologous Tissue Substitute in Peritoneum, Percutaneous Approach

0DWW3JZ Revision of Synthetic Substitute in Peritoneum, Percutaneous Approach

0DWW3KZ Revision of Nonautologous Tissue Substitute in Peritoneum, Percutaneous Approach

0DWW40Z Revision of Drainage Device in Peritoneum, Percutaneous Endoscopic Approach

0DWW47Z Revision of Autologous Tissue Substitute in Peritoneum, Percutaneous Endoscopic Approach

0DWW4JZ Revision of Synthetic Substitute in Peritoneum, Percutaneous Endoscopic Approach

0DWW4KZ Revision of Nonautologous Tissue Substitute in Peritoneum, Percutaneous Endoscopic Approach

X – Gastrointestinal System, Transfer

X60Z5 Transfer Stomach to Esophagus, Open Approach

X64Z5 Transfer Stomach to Esophagus, Percutaneous Endoscopic Approach

0DX80Z5 Transfer Small Intestine to Esophagus, Open Approach

0DX84Z5 Transfer Small Intestine to Esophagus, Percutaneous Endoscopic Approach

0DXE0Z5 Transfer Large Intestine to Esophagus, Open Approach

0DXE4Z5 Transfer Large Intestine to Esophagus, Percutaneous Endoscopic Approach

Y – Gastrointestinal System, Transplantation

view Coding Guideline B3.16

Y50Z0 Transplantation of Esophagus, Allogeneic, Open Approach

Y50Z1 Transplantation of Esophagus, Syngeneic, Open Approach

Y50Z2 Transplantation of Esophagus, Zooplastic, Open Approach

Y60Z0 Transplantation of Stomach, Allogeneic, Open Approach

0DY60Z1 Transplantation of Stomach, Syngeneic, Open Approach

0DY60Z2 Transplantation of Stomach, Zooplastic, Open Approach

▲ **0DY80Z0** Transplantation of Small Intestine, Allogeneic, Open Approach

▲ **0DY80Z1** Transplantation of Small Intestine, Syngeneic, Open Approach

▲ **0DY80Z2** Transplantation of Small Intestine, Zooplastic, Open Approach

▲ **0DYE0Z0** Transplantation of Large Intestine, Allogeneic, Open Approach

▲ **0DYE0Z1** Transplantation of Large Intestine, Syngeneic, Open Approach`

▲ **0DYE0Z2** Transplantation of Large Intestine, Zooplastic, Open Approach

♀ Female-only   ♂ Male-only   ▲ Limited Coverage   ● Non-OR   ▦ HAC-associated procedure   ▲ Non-covered procedures   ✚ Combination

Hepatobiliary System and Pancreas

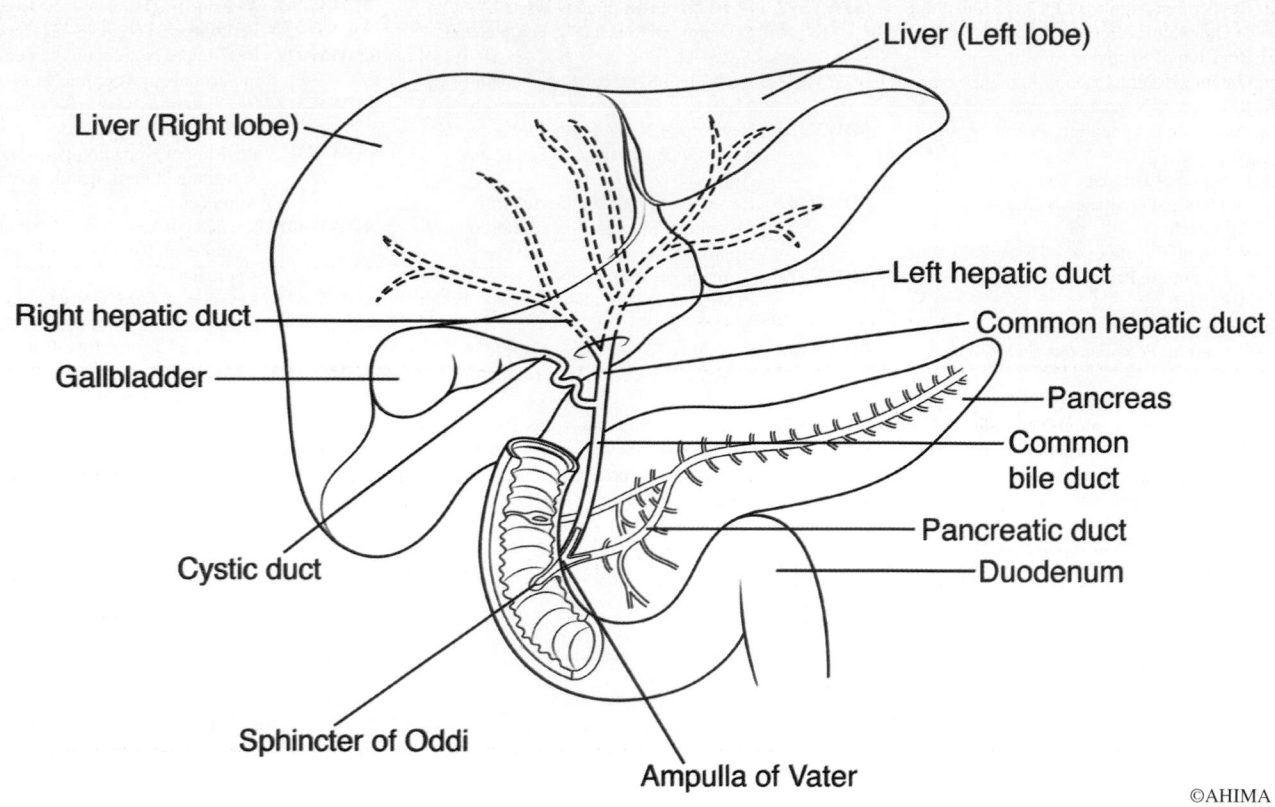

Liver (Left lobe)

Liver (Right lobe)

Left hepatic duct

Right hepatic duct

Common hepatic duct

Gallbladder

Pancreas

Common bile duct

Cystic duct

Pancreatic duct

Duodenum

Sphincter of Oddi

Ampulla of Vater

©AHIMA

ction	0	Medical and Surgical
dy System	F	Hepatobiliary System and Pancreas
eration	1	**Bypass:** Altering the route of passage of the contents of a tubular body part

Body Part (4th)	Approach (5th)	Device (6th)	Qualifier (7th)
Gallbladder Hepatic Duct, Right Hepatic Duct, Left Cystic Duct Common Bile Duct	0 Open 4 Percutaneous Endoscopic	D Intraluminal Device Z No Device	3 Duodenum 4 Stomach 5 Hepatic Duct, Right 6 Hepatic Duct, Left 7 Hepatic Duct, Caudate 8 Cystic Duct 9 Common Bile Duct B Small Intestine
Pancreatic Duct Pancreatic Duct, Accessory G Pancreas	0 Open 4 Percutaneous Endoscopic	D Intraluminal Device Z No Device	3 Duodenum B Small Intestine C Large Intestine

ction	0	Medical and Surgical
dy System	F	Hepatobiliary System and Pancreas
eration	2	**Change:** Taking out or off a device from a body part and putting back an identical or similar device in or on the same body part without cutting or puncturing the skin or a mucous membrane

Body Part (4th)	Approach (5th)	Device (6th)	Qualifier (7th)
Liver 4 Gallbladder B Hepatobiliary Duct D Pancreatic Duct G Pancreas	X External	0 Drainage Device Y Other Device	Z No Qualifier

ction	0	Medical and Surgical
dy System	F	Hepatobiliary System and Pancreas
eration	5	**Destruction:** Physical eradication of all or a portion of a body part by the direct use of energy, force, or a destructive agent

Body Part (4th)	Approach (5th)	Device (6th)	Qualifier (7th)
0 Liver 1 Liver, Right Lobe 2 Liver, Left Lobe 4 Gallbladder G Pancreas	0 Open 3 Percutaneous 4 Percutaneous Endoscopic	Z No Device	Z No Qualifier
5 Hepatic Duct, Right 6 Hepatic Duct, Left 8 Cystic Duct 9 Common Bile Duct C Ampulla of Vater D Pancreatic Duct F Pancreatic Duct, Accessory	0 Open 3 Percutaneous 4 Percutaneous Endoscopic 7 Via Natural or Artificial Opening 8 Via Natural or Artificial Opening Endoscopic	Z No Device	Z No Qualifier

ction	0	Medical and Surgical
dy System	F	Hepatobiliary System and Pancreas
eration	7	**Dilation:** Expanding an orifice or the lumen of a tubular body part

Body Part (4th)	Approach (5th)	Device (6th)	Qualifier (7th)
5 Hepatic Duct, Right 6 Hepatic Duct, Left 8 Cystic Duct 9 Common Bile Duct C Ampulla of Vater D Pancreatic Duct F Pancreatic Duct, Accessory	0 Open 3 Percutaneous 4 Percutaneous Endoscopic 7 Via Natural or Artificial Opening 8 Via Natural or Artificial Opening Endoscopic	D Intraluminal Device Z No Device	Z No Qualifier

Section	0	Medical and Surgical
Body System	F	Hepatobiliary System and Pancreas
Operation	8	Division: Cutting into a body part, without draining fluids and/or gases from the body part, in order to separate or transect a body part

Body Part (4th)	Approach (5th)	Device (6th)	Qualifier (7th)
G Pancreas	0 Open 3 Percutaneous 4 Percutaneous Endoscopic	Z No Device	Z No Qualifier

Section	0	Medical and Surgical
Body System	F	Hepatobiliary System and Pancreas
Operation	9	Drainage: Taking or letting out fluids and/or gases from a body part

Body Part (4th)	Approach (5th)	Device (6th)	Qualifier (7th)
0 Liver 1 Liver, Right Lobe 2 Liver, Left Lobe 4 Gallbladder G Pancreas	0 Open 3 Percutaneous 4 Percutaneous Endoscopic	0 Drainage Device	Z No Qualifier
0 Liver 1 Liver, Right Lobe 2 Liver, Left Lobe 4 Gallbladder G Pancreas	0 Open 3 Percutaneous 4 Percutaneous Endoscopic	Z No Device	X Diagnostic Z No Qualifier
5 Hepatic Duct, Right 6 Hepatic Duct, Left 8 Cystic Duct 9 Common Bile Duct C Ampulla of Vater D Pancreatic Duct F Pancreatic Duct, Accessory	0 Open 3 Percutaneous 4 Percutaneous Endoscopic 7 Via Natural or Artificial Opening 8 Via Natural or Artificial Opening Endoscopic	0 Drainage Device	Z No Qualifier
5 Hepatic Duct, Right 6 Hepatic Duct, Left 8 Cystic Duct 9 Common Bile Duct C Ampulla of Vater D Pancreatic Duct F Pancreatic Duct, Accessory	0 Open 3 Percutaneous 4 Percutaneous Endoscopic 7 Via Natural or Artificial Opening 8 Via Natural or Artificial Opening Endoscopic	Z No Device	X Diagnostic Z No Qualifier

Section	0	Medical and Surgical
Body System	F	Hepatobiliary System and Pancreas
Operation	B	Excision: Cutting out or off, without replacement, a portion of a body part

Body Part (4th)	Approach (5th)	Device (6th)	Qualifier (7th)
0 Liver 1 Liver, Right Lobe 2 Liver, Left Lobe 4 Gallbladder G Pancreas	0 Open 3 Percutaneous 4 Percutaneous Endoscopic	Z No Device	X Diagnostic Z No Qualifier
5 Hepatic Duct, Right 6 Hepatic Duct, Left 8 Cystic Duct 9 Common Bile Duct C Ampulla of Vater D Pancreatic Duct F Pancreatic Duct, Accessory	0 Open 3 Percutaneous 4 Percutaneous Endoscopic 7 Via Natural or Artificial Opening 8 Via Natural or Artificial Opening Endoscopic	Z No Device	X Diagnostic Z No Qualifier

Section	0	Medical and Surgical
Body System	F	Hepatobiliary System and Pancreas
Operation	C	Extirpation: Taking or cutting out solid matter from a body part

Body Part (4th)	Approach (5th)	Device (6th)	Qualifier (7th)
0 Liver 1 Liver, Right Lobe 2 Liver, Left Lobe 4 Gallbladder G Pancreas	0 Open 3 Percutaneous 4 Percutaneous Endoscopic	Z No Device	Z No Qualifier
5 Hepatic Duct, Right 6 Hepatic Duct, Left 8 Cystic Duct 9 Common Bile Duct C Ampulla of Vater D Pancreatic Duct F Pancreatic Duct, Accessory	0 Open 3 Percutaneous 4 Percutaneous Endoscopic 7 Via Natural or Artificial Opening 8 Via Natural or Artificial Opening Endoscopic	Z No Device	Z No Qualifier

Section	0	Medical and Surgical
Body System	F	Hepatobiliary System and Pancreas
Operation	F	Fragmentation: Breaking solid matter in a body part into pieces

Body Part (4th)	Approach (5th)	Device (6th)	Qualifier (7th)
4 Gallbladder 5 Hepatic Duct, Right 6 Hepatic Duct, Left 8 Cystic Duct 9 Common Bile Duct C Ampulla of Vater D Pancreatic Duct F Pancreatic Duct, Accessory	0 Open 3 Percutaneous 4 Percutaneous Endoscopic 7 Via Natural or Artificial Opening 8 Via Natural or Artificial Opening Endoscopic X External	Z No Device	Z No Qualifier

Section	0	Medical and Surgical
Body System	F	Hepatobiliary System and Pancreas
Operation	H	Insertion: Putting in a nonbiological appliance that monitors, assists, performs, or prevents a physiological function but does not physically take the place of a body part

Body Part (4th)	Approach (5th)	Device (6th)	Qualifier (7th)
0 Liver 1 Liver, Right Lobe 2 Liver, Left Lobe 4 Gallbladder G Pancreas	0 Open 3 Percutaneous 4 Percutaneous Endoscopic	2 Monitoring Device 3 Infusion Device	Z No Qualifier
B Hepatobiliary Duct D Pancreatic Duct	0 Open 3 Percutaneous 4 Percutaneous Endoscopic 7 Via Natural or Artificial Opening 8 Via Natural or Artificial Opening Endoscopic	1 Radioactive Element 2 Monitoring Device 3 Infusion Device D Intraluminal Device	Z No Qualifier

Section	0	Medical and Surgical
Body System	F	Hepatobiliary System and Pancreas
Operation	J	Inspection: Visually and/or manually exploring a body part

Body Part (4th)	Approach (5th)	Device (6th)	Qualifier (7th)
0 Liver 4 Gallbladder G Pancreas	0 Open 3 Percutaneous 4 Percutaneous Endoscopic X External	Z No Device	Z No Qualifier

Continued →

Section	0	Medical and Surgical
Body System	F	Hepatobiliary System and Pancreas
Operation	J	Inspection: Visually and/or manually exploring a body part

Body Part (4th)	Approach (5th)	Device (6th)	Qualifier (7th)
B Hepatobiliary Duct D Pancreatic Duct	0 Open 3 Percutaneous 4 Percutaneous Endoscopic 7 Via Natural or Artificial Opening 8 Via Natural or Artificial Opening Endoscopic	Z No Device	Z No Qualifier

Section	0	Medical and Surgical
Body System	F	Hepatobiliary System and Pancreas
Operation	L	Occlusion: Completely closing an orifice or the lumen of a tubular body part

Body Part (4th)	Approach (5th)	Device (6th)	Qualifier (7th)
5 Hepatic Duct, Right 6 Hepatic Duct, Left 8 Cystic Duct 9 Common Bile Duct C Ampulla of Vater D Pancreatic Duct F Pancreatic Duct, Accessory	0 Open 3 Percutaneous 4 Percutaneous Endoscopic	C Extraluminal Device D Intraluminal Device Z No Device	Z No Qualifier
5 Hepatic Duct, Right 6 Hepatic Duct, Left 8 Cystic Duct 9 Common Bile Duct C Ampulla of Vater D Pancreatic Duct F Pancreatic Duct, Accessory	7 Via Natural or Artificial Opening 8 Via Natural or Artificial Opening Endoscopic	D Intraluminal Device Z No Device	Z No Qualifier

Section	0	Medical and Surgical
Body System	F	Hepatobiliary System and Pancreas
Operation	M	Reattachment: Putting back in or on all or a portion of a separated body part to its normal location or other suitable location

Body Part (4th)	Approach (5th)	Device (6th)	Qualifier (7th)
0 Liver 1 Liver, Right Lobe 2 Liver, Left Lobe 4 Gallbladder 5 Hepatic Duct, Right 6 Hepatic Duct, Left 8 Cystic Duct 9 Common Bile Duct C Ampulla of Vater D Pancreatic Duct F Pancreatic Duct, Accessory G Pancreas	0 Open 4 Percutaneous Endoscopic	Z No Device	Z No Qualifier

Section	0	Medical and Surgical
Body System	F	Hepatobiliary System and Pancreas
Operation	N	Release: Freeing a body part from an abnormal physical constraint by cutting or by the use of force

Body Part (4th)	Approach (5th)	Device (6th)	Qualifier (7th)
0 Liver 1 Liver, Right Lobe 2 Liver, Left Lobe 4 Gallbladder G Pancreas	0 Open 3 Percutaneous 4 Percutaneous Endoscopic	Z No Device	Z No Qualifier

Continued →

Section 0 **Medical and Surgical**
Body System F **Hepatobiliary System and Pancreas**
Operation N **Release:** Freeing a body part from an abnormal physical constraint by cutting or by the use of force

Body Part (4ᵗʰ)	Approach (5ᵗʰ)	Device (6ᵗʰ)	Qualifier (7ᵗʰ)
Hepatic Duct, Right Hepatic Duct, Left Cystic Duct Common Bile Duct Ampulla of Vater Pancreatic Duct Pancreatic Duct, Accessory	**0** Open **3** Percutaneous **4** Percutaneous Endoscopic **7** Via Natural or Artificial Opening **8** Via Natural or Artificial Opening Endoscopic	**Z** No Device	**Z** No Qualifier

Section 0 **Medical and Surgical**
Body System F **Hepatobiliary System and Pancreas**
Operation P **Removal:** Taking out or off a device from a body part

Body Part (4ᵗʰ)	Approach (5ᵗʰ)	Device (6ᵗʰ)	Qualifier (7ᵗʰ)
Liver	**0** Open **3** Percutaneous **4** Percutaneous Endoscopic **X** External	**0** Drainage Device **2** Monitoring Device **3** Infusion Device	**Z** No Qualifier
Gallbladder Pancreas	**0** Open **3** Percutaneous **4** Percutaneous Endoscopic **X** External	**0** Drainage Device **2** Monitoring Device **3** Infusion Device **D** Intraluminal Device	**Z** No Qualifier
Hepatobiliary Duct Pancreatic Duct	**0** Open **3** Percutaneous **4** Percutaneous Endoscopic **7** Via Natural or Artificial Opening **8** Via Natural or Artificial Opening Endoscopic	**0** Drainage Device **1** Radioactive Element **2** Monitoring Device **3** Infusion Device **7** Autologous Tissue Substitute **C** Extraluminal Device **D** Intraluminal Device **J** Synthetic Substitute **K** Nonautologous Tissue Substitute	**Z** No Qualifier
Hepatobiliary Duct Pancreatic Duct	**X** External	**0** Drainage Device **1** Radioactive Element **2** Monitoring Device **3** Infusion Device **D** Intraluminal Device	**Z** No Qualifier

Section 0 **Medical and Surgical**
Body System F **Hepatobiliary System and Pancreas**
Operation Q **Repair:** Restoring, to the extent possible, a body part to its normal anatomic structure and function

Body Part (4ᵗʰ)	Approach (5ᵗʰ)	Device (6ᵗʰ)	Qualifier (7ᵗʰ)
Liver Liver, Right Lobe Liver, Left Lobe Gallbladder Pancreas	**0** Open **3** Percutaneous **4** Percutaneous Endoscopic	**Z** No Device	**Z** No Qualifier
Hepatic Duct, Right Hepatic Duct, Left Cystic Duct Common Bile Duct Ampulla of Vater Pancreatic Duct Pancreatic Duct, Accessory	**0** Open **3** Percutaneous **4** Percutaneous Endoscopic **7** Via Natural or Artificial Opening **8** Via Natural or Artificial Opening Endoscopic	**Z** No Device	**Z** No Qualifier

Section	0	Medical and Surgical
Body System	F	Hepatobiliary System and Pancreas
Operation	R	Replacement: Putting in or on biological or synthetic material that physically takes the place and/or function of all or a portion of a body part

Body Part (4th)	Approach (5th)	Device (6th)	Qualifier (7th)
5 Hepatic Duct, Right 6 Hepatic Duct, Left 8 Cystic Duct 9 Common Bile Duct C Ampulla of Vater D Pancreatic Duct F Pancreatic Duct, Accessory	0 Open 4 Percutaneous Endoscopic	7 Autologous Tissue Substitute J Synthetic Substitute K Nonautologous Tissue Substitute	Z No Qualifier

Section	0	Medical and Surgical
Body System	F	Hepatobiliary System and Pancreas
Operation	S	Reposition: Moving to its normal location, or other suitable location, all or a portion of a body part

Body Part (4th)	Approach (5th)	Device (6th)	Qualifier (7th)
0 Liver 4 Gallbladder 5 Hepatic Duct, Right 6 Hepatic Duct, Left 8 Cystic Duct 9 Common Bile Duct C Ampulla of Vater D Pancreatic Duct F Pancreatic Duct, Accessory G Pancreas	0 Open 4 Percutaneous Endoscopic	Z No Device	Z No Qualifier

Section	0	Medical and Surgical
Body System	F	Hepatobiliary System and Pancreas
Operation	T	Resection: Cutting out or off, without replacement, all of a body part

Body Part (4th)	Approach (5th)	Device (6th)	Qualifier (7th)
0 Liver 1 Liver, Right Lobe 2 Liver, Left Lobe 4 Gallbladder G Pancreas	0 Open 4 Percutaneous Endoscopic	Z No Device	Z No Qualifier
5 Hepatic Duct, Right 6 Hepatic Duct, Left 8 Cystic Duct 9 Common Bile Duct C Ampulla of Vater D Pancreatic Duct F Pancreatic Duct, Accessory	0 Open 4 Percutaneous Endoscopic 7 Via Natural or Artificial Opening 8 Via Natural or Artificial Opening Endoscopic	Z No Device	Z No Qualifier

Section	0	Medical and Surgical
Body System	F	Hepatobiliary System and Pancreas
Operation	U	Supplement: Putting in or on biological or synthetic material that physically reinforces and/or augments the function of a portion of a body part

Body Part (4th)	Approach (5th)	Device (6th)	Qualifier (7th)
5 Hepatic Duct, Right 6 Hepatic Duct, Left 8 Cystic Duct 9 Common Bile Duct C Ampulla of Vater D Pancreatic Duct F Pancreatic Duct, Accessory	0 Open 3 Percutaneous 4 Percutaneous Endoscopic	7 Autologous Tissue Substitute J Synthetic Substitute K Nonautologous Tissue Substitute	Z No Qualifier

Section	0	Medical and Surgical	
Body System	F	Hepatobiliary System and Pancreas	
Operation	V	**Restriction:** Partially closing an orifice or the lumen of a tubular body part	

Body Part (4th)	Approach (5th)	Device (6th)	Qualifier (7th)
Hepatic Duct, Right Hepatic Duct, Left Cystic Duct Common Bile Duct Ampulla of Vater Pancreatic Duct Pancreatic Duct, Accessory	0 Open 3 Percutaneous 4 Percutaneous Endoscopic	C Extraluminal Device D Intraluminal Device Z No Device	Z No Qualifier
Hepatic Duct, Right Hepatic Duct, Left Cystic Duct Common Bile Duct Ampulla of Vater Pancreatic Duct Pancreatic Duct, Accessory	7 Via Natural or Artificial Opening 8 Via Natural or Artificial Opening Endoscopic	D Intraluminal Device Z No Device	Z No Qualifier

Section	0	Medical and Surgical	
Body System	F	Hepatobiliary System and Pancreas	
Operation	W	**Revision:** Correcting, to the extent possible, a portion of a malfunctioning device or the position of a displaced device	

Body Part (4th)	Approach (5th)	Device (6th)	Qualifier (7th)
Liver	0 Open 3 Percutaneous 4 Percutaneous Endoscopic X External	0 Drainage Device 2 Monitoring Device 3 Infusion Device	Z No Qualifier
Gallbladder Pancreas	0 Open 3 Percutaneous 4 Percutaneous Endoscopic X External	0 Drainage Device 2 Monitoring Device 3 Infusion Device D Intraluminal Device	Z No Qualifier
Hepatobiliary Duct Pancreatic Duct	0 Open 3 Percutaneous 4 Percutaneous Endoscopic 7 Via Natural or Artificial Opening 8 Via Natural or Artificial Opening Endoscopic X External	0 Drainage Device 2 Monitoring Device 3 Infusion Device 7 Autologous Tissue Substitute C Extraluminal Device D Intraluminal Device J Synthetic Substitute K Nonautologous Tissue Substitute	Z No Qualifier

Section	0	Medical and Surgical	
Body System	F	Hepatobiliary System and Pancreas	
Operation	Y	**Transplantation:** Putting in or on all or a portion of a living body part taken from another individual or animal to physically take the place and/or function of all or a portion of a similar body part	

Body Part (4th)	Approach (5th)	Device (6th)	Qualifier (7th)
Liver Pancreas	0 Open	Z No Device	0 Allogeneic 1 Syngeneic 2 Zooplastic

Hepatobiliary System and Pancreas Code Listing 0F1–0FY

0F1 – Hepatobiliary System and Pancreas, Bypass

Review Coding Guideline B3.6a

0F140D3 Bypass Gallbladder to Duodenum with Intraluminal Device, Open Approach

0F140D4 Bypass Gallbladder to Stomach with Intraluminal Device, Open Approach

0F140D5 Bypass Gallbladder to Right Hepatic Duct with Intraluminal Device, Open Approach

0F140D6 Bypass Gallbladder to Left Hepatic Duct with Intraluminal Device, Open Approach

0F140D7 Bypass Gallbladder to Caudate Hepatic Duct with Intraluminal Device, Open Approach

0F140D8 Bypass Gallbladder to Cystic Duct with Intraluminal Device, Open Approach

0F140D9 Bypass Gallbladder to Common Bile Duct with Intraluminal Device, Open Approach

0F140DB Bypass Gallbladder to Small Intestine with Intraluminal Device, Open Approach

0F140Z3 Bypass Gallbladder to Duodenum, Open Approach

Female-only	♂ Male-only	▲ Limited Coverage	● Non-OR	▬ HAC-associated procedure	▲ Non-covered procedures	✚ Combination

0F140Z4	Bypass Gallbladder to Stomach, Open Approach
0F140Z5	Bypass Gallbladder to Right Hepatic Duct, Open Approach
0F140Z6	Bypass Gallbladder to Left Hepatic Duct, Open Approach
0F140Z7	Bypass Gallbladder to Caudate Hepatic Duct, Open Approach
0F140Z8	Bypass Gallbladder to Cystic Duct, Open Approach
0F140Z9	Bypass Gallbladder to Common Bile Duct, Open Approach
0F140ZB	Bypass Gallbladder to Small Intestine, Open Approach
0F144D3	Bypass Gallbladder to Duodenum with Intraluminal Device, Percutaneous Endoscopic Approach
0F144D4	Bypass Gallbladder to Stomach with Intraluminal Device, Percutaneous Endoscopic Approach
0F144D5	Bypass Gallbladder to Right Hepatic Duct with Intraluminal Device, Percutaneous Endoscopic Approach
0F144D6	Bypass Gallbladder to Left Hepatic Duct with Intraluminal Device, Percutaneous Endoscopic Approach
0F144D7	Bypass Gallbladder to Caudate Hepatic Duct with Intraluminal Device, Percutaneous Endoscopic Approach
0F144D8	Bypass Gallbladder to Cystic Duct with Intraluminal Device, Percutaneous Endoscopic Approach
0F144D9	Bypass Gallbladder to Common Bile Duct with Intraluminal Device, Percutaneous Endoscopic Approach
0F144DB	Bypass Gallbladder to Small Intestine with Intraluminal Device, Percutaneous Endoscopic Approach
0F144Z3	Bypass Gallbladder to Duodenum, Percutaneous Endoscopic Approach
0F144Z4	Bypass Gallbladder to Stomach, Percutaneous Endoscopic Approach
0F144Z5	Bypass Gallbladder to Right Hepatic Duct, Percutaneous Endoscopic Approach
0F144Z6	Bypass Gallbladder to Left Hepatic Duct, Percutaneous Endoscopic Approach
0F144Z7	Bypass Gallbladder to Caudate Hepatic Duct, Percutaneous Endoscopic Approach
0F144Z8	Bypass Gallbladder to Cystic Duct, Percutaneous Endoscopic Approach
0F144Z9	Bypass Gallbladder to Common Bile Duct, Percutaneous Endoscopic Approach
0F144ZB	Bypass Gallbladder to Small Intestine, Percutaneous Endoscopic Approach
0F150D3	Bypass Right Hepatic Duct to Duodenum with Intraluminal Device, Open Approach
0F150D4	Bypass Right Hepatic Duct to Stomach with Intraluminal Device, Open Approach
0F150D5	Bypass Right Hepatic Duct to Right Hepatic Duct with Intraluminal Device, Open Approach
0F150D6	Bypass Right Hepatic Duct to Left Hepatic Duct with Intraluminal Device, Open Approach
0F150D7	Bypass Right Hepatic Duct to Caudate Hepatic Duct with Intraluminal Device, Open Approach
0F150D8	Bypass Right Hepatic Duct to Cystic Duct with Intraluminal Device, Open Approach
0F150D9	Bypass Right Hepatic Duct to Common Bile Duct with Intraluminal Device, Open Approach
0F150DB	Bypass Right Hepatic Duct to Small Intestine with Intraluminal Device, Open Approach
0F150Z3	Bypass Right Hepatic Duct to Duodenum, Open Approach
0F150Z4	Bypass Right Hepatic Duct to Stomach, Open Approach
0F150Z5	Bypass Right Hepatic Duct to Right Hepatic Duct, Open Approach
0F150Z6	Bypass Right Hepatic Duct to Left Hepatic Duct, Open Approach
0F150Z7	Bypass Right Hepatic Duct to Caudate Hepatic Duct, Open Approach
0F150Z8	Bypass Right Hepatic Duct to Cystic Duct, Open Approach
0F150Z9	Bypass Right Hepatic Duct to Common Bile Duct, Open Approach
0F150ZB	Bypass Right Hepatic Duct to Small Intestine, Open Approach
0F154D3	Bypass Right Hepatic Duct to Duodenum with Intraluminal Device, Percutaneous Endoscopic Approach
0F154D4	Bypass Right Hepatic Duct to Stomach with Intraluminal Device, Percutaneous Endoscopic Approach
0F154D5	Bypass Right Hepatic Duct to Right Hepatic Duct with Intraluminal Device, Percutaneous Endoscopic Approach
0F154D6	Bypass Right Hepatic Duct to Left Hepatic Duct with Intraluminal Device, Percutaneous Endoscopic Approach
0F154D7	Bypass Right Hepatic Duct to Caudate Hepatic Duct with Intraluminal Device, Percutaneous Endoscopic Approach
0F154D8	Bypass Right Hepatic Duct to Cystic Duct with Intraluminal Device, Percutaneous Endoscopic Approach
0F154D9	Bypass Right Hepatic Duct to Common Bile Duct with Intraluminal Device, Percutaneous Endoscopic Approach
0F154DB	Bypass Right Hepatic Duct to Small Intestine with Intraluminal Device, Percutaneous Endoscopic Approach
0F154Z3	Bypass Right Hepatic Duct to Duodenum, Percutaneous Endoscopic Approach
0F154Z4	Bypass Right Hepatic Duct to Stomach, Percutaneous Endoscopic Approach
0F154Z5	Bypass Right Hepatic Duct to Right Hepatic Duct, Percutaneous Endoscopic Approach
0F154Z6	Bypass Right Hepatic Duct to Left Hepatic Duct, Percutaneous Endoscopic Approach
0F154Z7	Bypass Right Hepatic Duct to Caudate Hepatic Duct, Percutaneous Endoscopic Approach
0F154Z8	Bypass Right Hepatic Duct to Cystic Duct, Percutaneous Endoscopic Approach
0F154Z9	Bypass Right Hepatic Duct to Common Bile Duct, Percutaneous Endoscopic Approach
0F154ZB	Bypass Right Hepatic Duct to Small Intestine, Percutaneous Endoscopic Approach
0F160D3	Bypass Left Hepatic Duct to Duodenum with Intraluminal Device, Open Approach
0F160D4	Bypass Left Hepatic Duct to Stomach with Intraluminal Device, Open Approach
0F160D5	Bypass Left Hepatic Duct to Right Hepatic Duct with Intraluminal Device, Open Approach
0F160D6	Bypass Left Hepatic Duct to Left Hepatic Duct with Intraluminal Device, Open Approach
0F160D7	Bypass Left Hepatic Duct to Caudate Hepatic Duct with Intraluminal Device, Open Approach
0F160D8	Bypass Left Hepatic Duct to Cystic Duct with Intraluminal Device, Open Approach
0F160D9	Bypass Left Hepatic Duct to Common Bile Duct with Intraluminal Device, Open Approach
0F160DB	Bypass Left Hepatic Duct to Small Intestine with Intraluminal Device, Open Approach
0F160Z3	Bypass Left Hepatic Duct to Duodenum, Open Approach
0F160Z4	Bypass Left Hepatic Duct to Stomach, Open Approach
0F160Z5	Bypass Left Hepatic Duct to Right Hepatic Duct, Open Approach
0F160Z6	Bypass Left Hepatic Duct to Left Hepatic Duct, Open Approach
0F160Z7	Bypass Left Hepatic Duct to Caudate Hepatic Duct, Open Approach
0F160Z8	Bypass Left Hepatic Duct to Cystic Duct, Open Approach
0F160Z9	Bypass Left Hepatic Duct to Common Bile Duct, Open Approach
0F160ZB	Bypass Left Hepatic Duct to Small Intestine, Open Approach
0F164D3	Bypass Left Hepatic Duct to Duodenum with Intraluminal Device, Percutaneous Endoscopic Approach
0F164D4	Bypass Left Hepatic Duct to Stomach with Intraluminal Device, Percutaneous Endoscopic Approach
0F164D5	Bypass Left Hepatic Duct to Right Hepatic Duct with Intraluminal Device, Percutaneous Endoscopic Approach
0F164D6	Bypass Left Hepatic Duct to Left Hepatic Duct with Intraluminal Device, Percutaneous Endoscopic Approach
0F164D7	Bypass Left Hepatic Duct to Caudate Hepatic Duct with Intraluminal Device, Percutaneous Endoscopic Approach
0F164D8	Bypass Left Hepatic Duct to Cystic Duct with Intraluminal Device, Percutaneous Endoscopic Approach
0F164D9	Bypass Left Hepatic Duct to Common Bile Duct with Intraluminal Device, Percutaneous Endoscopic Approach
0F164DB	Bypass Left Hepatic Duct to Small Intestine with Intraluminal Device, Percutaneous Endoscopic Approach
0F164Z3	Bypass Left Hepatic Duct to Duodenum, Percutaneous Endoscopic Approach
0F164Z4	Bypass Left Hepatic Duct to Stomach, Percutaneous Endoscopic Approach
0F164Z5	Bypass Left Hepatic Duct to Right Hepatic Duct, Percutaneous Endoscopic Approach
0F164Z6	Bypass Left Hepatic Duct to Left Hepatic Duct, Percutaneous Endoscopic Approach
0F164Z7	Bypass Left Hepatic Duct to Caudate Hepatic Duct, Percutaneous Endoscopic Approach
0F164Z8	Bypass Left Hepatic Duct to Cystic Duct, Percutaneous Endoscopic Approach
0F164Z9	Bypass Left Hepatic Duct to Common Bile Duct, Percutaneous Endoscopic Approach
0F164ZB	Bypass Left Hepatic Duct to Small Intestine, Percutaneous Endoscopic Approach
0F180D3	Bypass Cystic Duct to Duodenum with Intraluminal Device, Open Approach
0F180D4	Bypass Cystic Duct to Stomach with Intraluminal Device, Open Approach
0F180D5	Bypass Cystic Duct to Right Hepatic Duct with Intraluminal Device, Open Approach
0F180D6	Bypass Cystic Duct to Left Hepatic Duct with Intraluminal Device, Open Approach
0F180D7	Bypass Cystic Duct to Caudate Hepatic Duct with Intraluminal Device, Open Approach

♀ Female-only   ♂ Male-only   ▲ Limited Coverage   ● Non-OR   ▦ HAC-associated procedure   ▲ Non-covered procedures   ✛ Combination

180D8 Bypass Cystic Duct to Cystic Duct with Intraluminal Device, Open Approach

180D9 Bypass Cystic Duct to Common Bile Duct with Intraluminal Device, Open Approach

180DB Bypass Cystic Duct to Small Intestine with Intraluminal Device, Open Approach

180Z3 Bypass Cystic Duct to Duodenum, Open Approach

180Z4 Bypass Cystic Duct to Stomach, Open Approach

180Z5 Bypass Cystic Duct to Right Hepatic Duct, Open Approach

180Z6 Bypass Cystic Duct to Left Hepatic Duct, Open Approach

180Z7 Bypass Cystic Duct to Caudate Hepatic Duct, Open Approach

180Z8 Bypass Cystic Duct to Cystic Duct, Open Approach

180Z9 Bypass Cystic Duct to Common Bile Duct, Open Approach

180ZB Bypass Cystic Duct to Small Intestine, Open Approach

184D3 Bypass Cystic Duct to Duodenum with Intraluminal Device, Percutaneous Endoscopic Approach

184D4 Bypass Cystic Duct to Stomach with Intraluminal Device, Percutaneous Endoscopic Approach

184D5 Bypass Cystic Duct to Right Hepatic Duct with Intraluminal Device, Percutaneous Endoscopic Approach

184D6 Bypass Cystic Duct to Left Hepatic Duct with Intraluminal Device, Percutaneous Endoscopic Approach

184D7 Bypass Cystic Duct to Caudate Hepatic Duct with Intraluminal Device, Percutaneous Endoscopic Approach

184D8 Bypass Cystic Duct to Cystic Duct with Intraluminal Device, Percutaneous Endoscopic Approach

184D9 Bypass Cystic Duct to Common Bile Duct with Intraluminal Device, Percutaneous Endoscopic Approach

184DB Bypass Cystic Duct to Small Intestine with Intraluminal Device, Percutaneous Endoscopic Approach

184Z3 Bypass Cystic Duct to Duodenum, Percutaneous Endoscopic Approach

184Z4 Bypass Cystic Duct to Stomach, Percutaneous Endoscopic Approach

184Z5 Bypass Cystic Duct to Right Hepatic Duct, Percutaneous Endoscopic Approach

184Z6 Bypass Cystic Duct to Left Hepatic Duct, Percutaneous Endoscopic Approach

184Z7 Bypass Cystic Duct to Caudate Hepatic Duct, Percutaneous Endoscopic Approach

184Z8 Bypass Cystic Duct to Cystic Duct, Percutaneous Endoscopic Approach

184Z9 Bypass Cystic Duct to Common Bile Duct, Percutaneous Endoscopic Approach

184ZB Bypass Cystic Duct to Small Intestine, Percutaneous Endoscopic Approach

190D3 Bypass Common Bile Duct to Duodenum with Intraluminal Device, Open Approach

190D4 Bypass Common Bile Duct to Stomach with Intraluminal Device, Open Approach

190D5 Bypass Common Bile Duct to Right Hepatic Duct with Intraluminal Device, Open Approach

190D6 Bypass Common Bile Duct to Left Hepatic Duct with Intraluminal Device, Open Approach

190D7 Bypass Common Bile Duct to Caudate Hepatic Duct with Intraluminal Device, Open Approach

190D8 Bypass Common Bile Duct to Cystic Duct with Intraluminal Device, Open Approach

0F190D9 Bypass Common Bile Duct to Common Bile Duct with Intraluminal Device, Open Approach

0F190DB Bypass Common Bile Duct to Small Intestine with Intraluminal Device, Open Approach

0F190Z3 Bypass Common Bile Duct to Duodenum, Open Approach

0F190Z4 Bypass Common Bile Duct to Stomach, Open Approach

0F190Z5 Bypass Common Bile Duct to Right Hepatic Duct, Open Approach

0F190Z6 Bypass Common Bile Duct to Left Hepatic Duct, Open Approach

0F190Z7 Bypass Common Bile Duct to Caudate Hepatic Duct, Open Approach

0F190Z8 Bypass Common Bile Duct to Cystic Duct, Open Approach

0F190Z9 Bypass Common Bile Duct to Common Bile Duct, Open Approach

0F190ZB Bypass Common Bile Duct to Small Intestine, Open Approach

0F194D3 Bypass Common Bile Duct to Duodenum with Intraluminal Device, Percutaneous Endoscopic Approach

0F194D4 Bypass Common Bile Duct to Stomach with Intraluminal Device, Percutaneous Endoscopic Approach

0F194D5 Bypass Common Bile Duct to Right Hepatic Duct with Intraluminal Device, Percutaneous Endoscopic Approach

0F194D6 Bypass Common Bile Duct to Left Hepatic Duct with Intraluminal Device, Percutaneous Endoscopic Approach

0F194D7 Bypass Common Bile Duct to Caudate Hepatic Duct with Intraluminal Device, Percutaneous Endoscopic Approach

0F194D8 Bypass Common Bile Duct to Cystic Duct with Intraluminal Device, Percutaneous Endoscopic Approach

0F194D9 Bypass Common Bile Duct to Common Bile Duct with Intraluminal Device, Percutaneous Endoscopic Approach

0F194DB Bypass Common Bile Duct to Small Intestine with Intraluminal Device, Percutaneous Endoscopic Approach

0F194Z3 Bypass Common Bile Duct to Duodenum, Percutaneous Endoscopic Approach

0F194Z4 Bypass Common Bile Duct to Stomach, Percutaneous Endoscopic Approach

0F194Z5 Bypass Common Bile Duct to Right Hepatic Duct, Percutaneous Endoscopic Approach

0F194Z6 Bypass Common Bile Duct to Left Hepatic Duct, Percutaneous Endoscopic Approach

0F194Z7 Bypass Common Bile Duct to Caudate Hepatic Duct, Percutaneous Endoscopic Approach

0F194Z8 Bypass Common Bile Duct to Cystic Duct, Percutaneous Endoscopic Approach

0F194Z9 Bypass Common Bile Duct to Common Bile Duct, Percutaneous Endoscopic Approach

0F194ZB Bypass Common Bile Duct to Small Intestine, Percutaneous Endoscopic Approach

0F1D0D3 Bypass Pancreatic Duct to Duodenum with Intraluminal Device, Open Approach

0F1D0DB Bypass Pancreatic Duct to Small Intestine with Intraluminal Device, Open Approach

0F1D0DC Bypass Pancreatic Duct to Large Intestine with Intraluminal Device, Open Approach

0F1D0Z3 Bypass Pancreatic Duct to Duodenum, Open Approach

0F1D0ZB Bypass Pancreatic Duct to Small Intestine, Open Approach

0F1D0ZC Bypass Pancreatic Duct to Large Intestine, Open Approach

0F1D4D3 Bypass Pancreatic Duct to Duodenum with Intraluminal Device, Percutaneous Endoscopic Approach

0F1D4DB Bypass Pancreatic Duct to Small Intestine with Intraluminal Device, Percutaneous Endoscopic Approach

0F1D4DC Bypass Pancreatic Duct to Large Intestine with Intraluminal Device, Percutaneous Endoscopic Approach

0F1D4Z3 Bypass Pancreatic Duct to Duodenum, Percutaneous Endoscopic Approach

0F1D4ZB Bypass Pancreatic Duct to Small Intestine, Percutaneous Endoscopic Approach

0F1D4ZC Bypass Pancreatic Duct to Large Intestine, Percutaneous Endoscopic Approach

0F1F0D3 Bypass Accessory Pancreatic Duct to Duodenum with Intraluminal Device, Open Approach

0F1F0DB Bypass Accessory Pancreatic Duct to Small Intestine with Intraluminal Device, Open Approach

0F1F0DC Bypass Accessory Pancreatic Duct to Large Intestine with Intraluminal Device, Open Approach

0F1F0Z3 Bypass Accessory Pancreatic Duct to Duodenum, Open Approach

0F1F0ZB Bypass Accessory Pancreatic Duct to Small Intestine, Open Approach

0F1F0ZC Bypass Accessory Pancreatic Duct to Large Intestine, Open Approach

0F1F4D3 Bypass Accessory Pancreatic Duct to Duodenum with Intraluminal Device, Percutaneous Endoscopic Approach

0F1F4DB Bypass Accessory Pancreatic Duct to Small Intestine with Intraluminal Device, Percutaneous Endoscopic Approach

0F1F4DC Bypass Accessory Pancreatic Duct to Large Intestine with Intraluminal Device, Percutaneous Endoscopic Approach

0F1F4Z3 Bypass Accessory Pancreatic Duct to Duodenum, Percutaneous Endoscopic Approach

0F1F4ZB Bypass Accessory Pancreatic Duct to Small Intestine, Percutaneous Endoscopic Approach

0F1F4ZC Bypass Accessory Pancreatic Duct to Large Intestine, Percutaneous Endoscopic Approach

0F1G0D3 Bypass Pancreas to Duodenum with Intraluminal Device, Open Approach

0F1G0DB Bypass Pancreas to Small Intestine with Intraluminal Device, Open Approach

0F1G0DC Bypass Pancreas to Large Intestine with Intraluminal Device, Open Approach

0F1G0Z3 Bypass Pancreas to Duodenum, Open Approach

0F1G0ZB Bypass Pancreas to Small Intestine, Open Approach

0F1G0ZC Bypass Pancreas to Large Intestine, Open Approach

0F1G4D3 Bypass Pancreas to Duodenum with Intraluminal Device, Percutaneous Endoscopic Approach

0F1G4DB Bypass Pancreas to Small Intestine with Intraluminal Device, Percutaneous Endoscopic Approach

0F1G4DC Bypass Pancreas to Large Intestine with Intraluminal Device, Percutaneous Endoscopic Approach

0F1G4Z3 Bypass Pancreas to Duodenum, Percutaneous Endoscopic Approach

0F1G4ZB Bypass Pancreas to Small Intestine, Percutaneous Endoscopic Approach

0F1G4ZC Bypass Pancreas to Large Intestine, Percutaneous Endoscopic Approach

Female-only   ♂ Male-only   ▲ Limited Coverage   ● Non-OR   ▥ HAC-associated procedure   ▲ Non-covered procedures   ✚ Combination

0F2 – Hepatobiliary System and Pancreas, Change

Review Coding Guideline B6.1c

0F20X0Z	Change Drainage Device in Liver, External Approach	**0F2BX0Z**	Change Drainage Device in Hepatobiliary Duct, External Approach	**0F2GX0Z**	Change Drainage Device in Pancreas, External Approach
0F20XYZ	Change Other Device in Liver, External Approach	**0F2BXYZ**	Change Other Device in Hepatobiliary Duct, External Approach	**0F2GXYZ**	Change Other Device in Pancreas, External Approach
0F24X0Z	Change Drainage Device in Gallbladder, External Approach	**0F2DX0Z**	Change Drainage Device in Pancreatic Duct, External Approach		
0F24XYZ	Change Other Device in Gallbladder, External Approach	**0F2DXYZ**	Change Other Device in Pancreatic Duct, External Approach		

0F5 – Hepatobiliary System and Pancreas, Destruction

0F500ZZ	Destruction of Liver, Open Approach	**0F560ZZ**	Destruction of Left Hepatic Duct, Open Approach	**0F5C4ZZ**	Destruction of Ampulla of Vater, Percutaneous Endoscopic Approach
0F503ZZ	Destruction of Liver, Percutaneous Approach	**0F563ZZ**	Destruction of Left Hepatic Duct, Percutaneous Approach	**0F5C7ZZ**	Destruction of Ampulla of Vater, Via Natural or Artificial Opening
0F504ZZ	Destruction of Liver, Percutaneous Endoscopic Approach	**0F564ZZ**	Destruction of Left Hepatic Duct, Percutaneous Endoscopic Approach	**0F5C8ZZ**	Destruction of Ampulla of Vater, Via Natural or Artificial Opening Endoscopic
0F510ZZ	Destruction of Right Lobe Liver, Open Approach	**0F567ZZ**	Destruction of Left Hepatic Duct, Via Natural or Artificial Opening	**0F5D0ZZ**	Destruction of Pancreatic Duct, Open Approach
0F513ZZ	Destruction of Right Lobe Liver, Percutaneous Approach	**0F568ZZ**	Destruction of Left Hepatic Duct, Via Natural or Artificial Opening Endoscopic	**0F5D3ZZ**	Destruction of Pancreatic Duct, Percutaneous Approach
0F514ZZ	Destruction of Right Lobe Liver, Percutaneous Endoscopic Approach	**0F580ZZ**	Destruction of Cystic Duct, Open Approach	**0F5D4ZZ**	Destruction of Pancreatic Duct, Percutaneous Endoscopic Approach
0F520ZZ	Destruction of Left Lobe Liver, Open Approach	**0F583ZZ**	Destruction of Cystic Duct, Percutaneous Approach	**0F5D7ZZ**	Destruction of Pancreatic Duct, Via Natural or Artificial Opening
0F523ZZ	Destruction of Left Lobe Liver, Percutaneous Approach	**0F584ZZ**	Destruction of Cystic Duct, Percutaneous Endoscopic Approach	**0F5D8ZZ**	Destruction of Pancreatic Duct, Via Natural or Artificial Opening Endoscopi
0F524ZZ	Destruction of Left Lobe Liver, Percutaneous Endoscopic Approach	**0F587ZZ**	Destruction of Cystic Duct, Via Natural or Artificial Opening	**0F5F0ZZ**	Destruction of Accessory Pancreatic Du Open Approach
0F540ZZ	Destruction of Gallbladder, Open Approach	**0F588ZZ**	Destruction of Cystic Duct, Via Natural or Artificial Opening Endoscopic	**0F5F3ZZ**	Destruction of Accessory Pancreatic Du Percutaneous Approach
0F543ZZ	Destruction of Gallbladder, Percutaneous Approach	**0F590ZZ**	Destruction of Common Bile Duct, Open Approach	**0F5F4ZZ**	Destruction of Accessory Pancreatic Du Percutaneous Endoscopic Approach
0F544ZZ	Destruction of Gallbladder, Percutaneous Endoscopic Approach	**0F593ZZ**	Destruction of Common Bile Duct, Percutaneous Approach	**0F5F7ZZ**	Destruction of Accessory Pancreatic Du Via Natural or Artificial Opening
0F550ZZ	Destruction of Right Hepatic Duct, Open Approach	**0F594ZZ**	Destruction of Common Bile Duct, Percutaneous Endoscopic Approach	**0F5F8ZZ**	Destruction of Accessory Pancreatic Duct, Via Natural or Artificial Opening Endoscopic
0F553ZZ	Destruction of Right Hepatic Duct, Percutaneous Approach	**0F597ZZ**	Destruction of Common Bile Duct, Via Natural or Artificial Opening	**0F5G0ZZ**	Destruction of Pancreas, Open Approach
0F554ZZ	Destruction of Right Hepatic Duct, Percutaneous Endoscopic Approach	**0F598ZZ**	Destruction of Common Bile Duct, Via Natural or Artificial Opening Endoscopic	**0F5G3ZZ**	Destruction of Pancreas, Percutaneous Approach
0F557ZZ	Destruction of Right Hepatic Duct, Via Natural or Artificial Opening	**0F5C0ZZ**	Destruction of Ampulla of Vater, Open Approach	**0F5G4ZZ**	Destruction of Pancreas, Percutaneous Endoscopic Approach
0F558ZZ	Destruction of Right Hepatic Duct, Via Natural or Artificial Opening Endoscopic	**0F5C3ZZ**	Destruction of Ampulla of Vater, Percutaneous Approach		

0F7 – Hepatobiliary System and Pancreas, Dilation

0F750DZ	Dilation of Right Hepatic Duct with Intraluminal Device, Open Approach	**0F760ZZ**	Dilation of Left Hepatic Duct, Open Approach	**0F783DZ**	Dilation of Cystic Duct with Intralumina Device, Percutaneous Approach
0F750ZZ	Dilation of Right Hepatic Duct, Open Approach	**0F763DZ**	Dilation of Left Hepatic Duct with Intraluminal Device, Percutaneous Approach	**0F783ZZ**	Dilation of Cystic Duct, Percutaneous Approach
0F753DZ	Dilation of Right Hepatic Duct with Intraluminal Device, Percutaneous Approach	**0F763ZZ**	Dilation of Left Hepatic Duct, Percutaneous Approach	**0F784DZ**	Dilation of Cystic Duct with Intralumina Device, Percutaneous Endoscopic Approach
0F753ZZ	Dilation of Right Hepatic Duct, Percutaneous Approach	**0F764DZ**	Dilation of Left Hepatic Duct with Intraluminal Device, Percutaneous Endoscopic Approach	**0F784ZZ**	Dilation of Cystic Duct, Percutaneous Endoscopic Approach
0F754DZ	Dilation of Right Hepatic Duct with Intraluminal Device, Percutaneous Endoscopic Approach	**0F764ZZ**	Dilation of Left Hepatic Duct, Percutaneous Endoscopic Approach	● **0F787DZ**	Dilation of Cystic Duct with Intraluminal Device, Via Natural or Artificial Opening
0F754ZZ	Dilation of Right Hepatic Duct, Percutaneous Endoscopic Approach	● **0F767DZ**	Dilation of Left Hepatic Duct with Intraluminal Device, Via Natural or Artificial Opening	**0F787ZZ**	Dilation of Cystic Duct, Via Natural or Artificial Opening
● **0F757DZ**	Dilation of Right Hepatic Duct with Intraluminal Device, Via Natural or Artificial Opening	**0F767ZZ**	Dilation of Left Hepatic Duct, Via Natural or Artificial Opening	● **0F788DZ**	Dilation of Cystic Duct with Intraluminal Device, Via Natural or Artificial Opening Endoscopic
0F757ZZ	Dilation of Right Hepatic Duct, Via Natural or Artificial Opening	● **0F768DZ**	Dilation of Left Hepatic Duct with Intraluminal Device, Via Natural or Artificial Opening Endoscopic	**0F788ZZ**	Dilation of Cystic Duct, Via Natural or Artificial Opening Endoscopic
● **0F758DZ**	Dilation of Right Hepatic Duct with Intraluminal Device, Via Natural or Artificial Opening Endoscopic	**0F768ZZ**	Dilation of Left Hepatic Duct, Via Natural or Artificial Opening Endoscopic	**0F790DZ**	Dilation of Common Bile Duct with Intraluminal Device, Open Approach
0F758ZZ	Dilation of Right Hepatic Duct, Via Natural or Artificial Opening Endoscopic	**0F780DZ**	Dilation of Cystic Duct with Intraluminal Device, Open Approach	**0F790ZZ**	Dilation of Common Bile Duct, Open Approach
0F760DZ	Dilation of Left Hepatic Duct with Intraluminal Device, Open Approach	**0F780ZZ**	Dilation of Cystic Duct, Open Approach	**0F793DZ**	Dilation of Common Bile Duct with Intraluminal Device, Percutaneous Approach

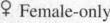

♀ Female-only   ♂ Male-only   ▲ Limited Coverage   ● Non-OR   ▉ HAC-associated procedure   ▲ Non-covered procedures   ✚ Combinati

793ZZ Dilation of Common Bile Duct, Percutaneous Approach

794DZ Dilation of Common Bile Duct with Intraluminal Device, Percutaneous Endoscopic Approach

794ZZ Dilation of Common Bile Duct, Percutaneous Endoscopic Approach

F797DZ Dilation of Common Bile Duct with Intraluminal Device, Via Natural or Artificial Opening

797ZZ Dilation of Common Bile Duct, Via Natural or Artificial Opening

F798DZ Dilation of Common Bile Duct with Intraluminal Device, Via Natural or Artificial Opening Endoscopic
AHA CC: 3Q, 2014, 15-16

798ZZ Dilation of Common Bile Duct, Via Natural or Artificial Opening Endoscopic

7C0DZ Dilation of Ampulla of Vater with Intraluminal Device, Open Approach

7C0ZZ Dilation of Ampulla of Vater, Open Approach

7C3DZ Dilation of Ampulla of Vater with Intraluminal Device, Percutaneous Approach

7C3ZZ Dilation of Ampulla of Vater, Percutaneous Approach

7C4DZ Dilation of Ampulla of Vater with Intraluminal Device, Percutaneous Endoscopic Approach

7C4ZZ Dilation of Ampulla of Vater, Percutaneous Endoscopic Approach

0F7C7DZ Dilation of Ampulla of Vater with Intraluminal Device, Via Natural or Artificial Opening

0F7C7ZZ Dilation of Ampulla of Vater, Via Natural or Artificial Opening

0F7C8DZ Dilation of Ampulla of Vater with Intraluminal Device, Via Natural or Artificial Opening Endoscopic

0F7C8ZZ Dilation of Ampulla of Vater, Via Natural or Artificial Opening Endoscopic

0F7D0DZ Dilation of Pancreatic Duct with Intraluminal Device, Open Approach

0F7D0ZZ Dilation of Pancreatic Duct, Open Approach

0F7D3DZ Dilation of Pancreatic Duct with Intraluminal Device, Percutaneous Approach

0F7D3ZZ Dilation of Pancreatic Duct, Percutaneous Approach

0F7D4DZ Dilation of Pancreatic Duct with Intraluminal Device, Percutaneous Endoscopic Approach

0F7D4ZZ Dilation of Pancreatic Duct, Percutaneous Endoscopic Approach

● 0F7D7DZ Dilation of Pancreatic Duct with Intraluminal Device, Via Natural or Artificial Opening

0F7D7ZZ Dilation of Pancreatic Duct, Via Natural or Artificial Opening

● 0F7D8DZ Dilation of Pancreatic Duct with Intraluminal Device, Via Natural or Artificial Opening Endoscopic

0F7D8ZZ Dilation of Pancreatic Duct, Via Natural or Artificial Opening Endoscopic

0F7F0DZ Dilation of Accessory Pancreatic Duct with Intraluminal Device, Open Approach

0F7F0ZZ Dilation of Accessory Pancreatic Duct, Open Approach

0F7F3DZ Dilation of Accessory Pancreatic Duct with Intraluminal Device, Percutaneous Approach

0F7F3ZZ Dilation of Accessory Pancreatic Duct, Percutaneous Approach

0F7F4DZ Dilation of Accessory Pancreatic Duct with Intraluminal Device, Percutaneous Endoscopic Approach

0F7F4ZZ Dilation of Accessory Pancreatic Duct, Percutaneous Endoscopic Approach

0F7F7DZ Dilation of Accessory Pancreatic Duct with Intraluminal Device, Via Natural or Artificial Opening

0F7F7ZZ Dilation of Accessory Pancreatic Duct, Via Natural or Artificial Opening

0F7F8DZ Dilation of Accessory Pancreatic Duct with Intraluminal Device, Via Natural or Artificial Opening Endoscopic

0F7F8ZZ Dilation of Accessory Pancreatic Duct, Via Natural or Artificial Opening Endoscopic

0F8 – Hepatobiliary System and Pancreas, Division

Review Coding Guideline B3.14

0F8G0ZZ Division of Pancreas, Open Approach

0F8G3ZZ Division of Pancreas, Percutaneous Approach

0F8G4ZZ Division of Pancreas, Percutaneous Endoscopic Approach

0F9 – Hepatobiliary System and Pancreas, Drainage

Review Coding Guidelines B3.4a and B3.4b

Review Coding Guideline B6.2

F9000Z Drainage of Liver with Drainage Device, Open Approach

F900ZX Drainage of Liver, Open Approach, Diagnostic

F900ZZ Drainage of Liver, Open Approach

F9030Z Drainage of Liver with Drainage Device, Percutaneous Approach

F903ZX Drainage of Liver, Percutaneous Approach, Diagnostic

F903ZZ Drainage of Liver, Percutaneous Approach

F9040Z Drainage of Liver with Drainage Device, Percutaneous Endoscopic Approach

F904ZX Drainage of Liver, Percutaneous Endoscopic Approach, Diagnostic

F904ZZ Drainage of Liver, Percutaneous Endoscopic Approach

F9100Z Drainage of Right Lobe Liver with Drainage Device, Open Approach

F910ZX Drainage of Right Lobe Liver, Open Approach, Diagnostic

F910ZZ Drainage of Right Lobe Liver, Open Approach

F9130Z Drainage of Right Lobe Liver with Drainage Device, Percutaneous Approach

F913ZX Drainage of Right Lobe Liver, Percutaneous Approach, Diagnostic

F913ZZ Drainage of Right Lobe Liver, Percutaneous Approach

F9140Z Drainage of Right Lobe Liver with Drainage Device, Percutaneous Endoscopic Approach

0F914ZX Drainage of Right Lobe Liver, Percutaneous Endoscopic Approach, Diagnostic

0F914ZZ Drainage of Right Lobe Liver, Percutaneous Endoscopic Approach

0F9200Z Drainage of Left Lobe Liver with Drainage Device, Open Approach

0F920ZX Drainage of Left Lobe Liver, Open Approach, Diagnostic

0F920ZZ Drainage of Left Lobe Liver, Open Approach

0F9230Z Drainage of Left Lobe Liver with Drainage Device, Percutaneous Approach

0F923ZX Drainage of Left Lobe Liver, Percutaneous Approach, Diagnostic

0F923ZZ Drainage of Left Lobe Liver, Percutaneous Approach

0F9240Z Drainage of Left Lobe Liver with Drainage Device, Percutaneous Endoscopic Approach

0F924ZX Drainage of Left Lobe Liver, Percutaneous Endoscopic Approach, Diagnostic

0F924ZZ Drainage of Left Lobe Liver, Percutaneous Endoscopic Approach

0F9400Z Drainage of Gallbladder with Drainage Device, Open Approach

0F940ZX Drainage of Gallbladder, Open Approach, Diagnostic

0F940ZZ Drainage of Gallbladder, Open Approach

0F9430Z Drainage of Gallbladder with Drainage Device, Percutaneous Approach

0F943ZX Drainage of Gallbladder, Percutaneous Approach, Diagnostic

0F943ZZ Drainage of Gallbladder, Percutaneous Approach

0F9440Z Drainage of Gallbladder with Drainage Device, Percutaneous Endoscopic Approach

0F944ZX Drainage of Gallbladder, Percutaneous Endoscopic Approach, Diagnostic

0F944ZZ Drainage of Gallbladder, Percutaneous Endoscopic Approach

0F9500Z Drainage of Right Hepatic Duct with Drainage Device, Open Approach

0F950ZX Drainage of Right Hepatic Duct, Open Approach, Diagnostic

0F950ZZ Drainage of Right Hepatic Duct, Open Approach

0F9530Z Drainage of Right Hepatic Duct with Drainage Device, Percutaneous Approach

0F953ZX Drainage of Right Hepatic Duct, Percutaneous Approach, Diagnostic

0F953ZZ Drainage of Right Hepatic Duct, Percutaneous Approach

0F9540Z Drainage of Right Hepatic Duct with Drainage Device, Percutaneous Endoscopic Approach

0F954ZX Drainage of Right Hepatic Duct, Percutaneous Endoscopic Approach, Diagnostic

0F954ZZ Drainage of Right Hepatic Duct, Percutaneous Endoscopic Approach

0F9570Z Drainage of Right Hepatic Duct with Drainage Device, Via Natural or Artificial Opening

0F957ZX Drainage of Right Hepatic Duct, Via Natural or Artificial Opening, Diagnostic

♀ Female-only ♂ Male-only ▲ Limited Coverage ● Non-OR ▬ HAC-associated procedure ▲ Non-covered procedures ✚ Combination

0F957ZZ	Drainage of Right Hepatic Duct, Via Natural or Artificial Opening
0F9580Z	Drainage of Right Hepatic Duct with Drainage Device, Via Natural or Artificial Opening Endoscopic
0F958ZX	Drainage of Right Hepatic Duct, Via Natural or Artificial Opening Endoscopic, Diagnostic
0F958ZZ	Drainage of Right Hepatic Duct, Via Natural or Artificial Opening Endoscopic
0F9600Z	Drainage of Left Hepatic Duct with Drainage Device, Open Approach
0F960ZX	Drainage of Left Hepatic Duct, Open Approach, Diagnostic
0F960ZZ	Drainage of Left Hepatic Duct, Open Approach
0F9630Z	Drainage of Left Hepatic Duct with Drainage Device, Percutaneous Approach
	AHA CC: 1Q, 2015, 32
0F963ZX	Drainage of Left Hepatic Duct, Percutaneous Approach, Diagnostic
0F963ZZ	Drainage of Left Hepatic Duct, Percutaneous Approach
0F9640Z	Drainage of Left Hepatic Duct with Drainage Device, Percutaneous Endoscopic Approach
0F964ZX	Drainage of Left Hepatic Duct, Percutaneous Endoscopic Approach, Diagnostic
0F964ZZ	Drainage of Left Hepatic Duct, Percutaneous Endoscopic Approach
0F9670Z	Drainage of Left Hepatic Duct with Drainage Device, Via Natural or Artificial Opening
0F967ZX	Drainage of Left Hepatic Duct, Via Natural or Artificial Opening, Diagnostic
0F967ZZ	Drainage of Left Hepatic Duct, Via Natural or Artificial Opening
0F9680Z	Drainage of Left Hepatic Duct with Drainage Device, Via Natural or Artificial Opening Endoscopic
0F968ZX	Drainage of Left Hepatic Duct, Via Natural or Artificial Opening Endoscopic, Diagnostic
0F968ZZ	Drainage of Left Hepatic Duct, Via Natural or Artificial Opening Endoscopic
0F9800Z	Drainage of Cystic Duct with Drainage Device, Open Approach
0F980ZX	Drainage of Cystic Duct, Open Approach, Diagnostic
0F980ZZ	Drainage of Cystic Duct, Open Approach
0F9830Z	Drainage of Cystic Duct with Drainage Device, Percutaneous Approach
0F983ZX	Drainage of Cystic Duct, Percutaneous Approach, Diagnostic
0F983ZZ	Drainage of Cystic Duct, Percutaneous Approach
0F9840Z	Drainage of Cystic Duct with Drainage Device, Percutaneous Endoscopic Approach
0F984ZX	Drainage of Cystic Duct, Percutaneous Endoscopic Approach, Diagnostic
0F984ZZ	Drainage of Cystic Duct, Percutaneous Endoscopic Approach
0F9870Z	Drainage of Cystic Duct with Drainage Device, Via Natural or Artificial Opening
0F987ZX	Drainage of Cystic Duct, Via Natural or Artificial Opening, Diagnostic
0F987ZZ	Drainage of Cystic Duct, Via Natural or Artificial Opening
0F9880Z	Drainage of Cystic Duct with Drainage Device, Via Natural or Artificial Opening Endoscopic
0F988ZX	Drainage of Cystic Duct, Via Natural or Artificial Opening Endoscopic, Diagnostic
0F988ZZ	Drainage of Cystic Duct, Via Natural or Artificial Opening Endoscopic
0F9900Z	Drainage of Common Bile Duct with Drainage Device, Open Approach

0F990ZX	Drainage of Common Bile Duct, Open Approach, Diagnostic
0F990ZZ	Drainage of Common Bile Duct, Open Approach
0F9930Z	Drainage of Common Bile Duct with Drainage Device, Percutaneous Approach
0F993ZX	Drainage of Common Bile Duct, Percutaneous Approach, Diagnostic
0F993ZZ	Drainage of Common Bile Duct, Percutaneous Approach
0F9940Z	Drainage of Common Bile Duct with Drainage Device, Percutaneous Endoscopic Approach
0F994ZX	Drainage of Common Bile Duct, Percutaneous Endoscopic Approach, Diagnostic
0F994ZZ	Drainage of Common Bile Duct, Percutaneous Endoscopic Approach
0F9970Z	Drainage of Common Bile Duct with Drainage Device, Via Natural or Artificial Opening
0F997ZX	Drainage of Common Bile Duct, Via Natural or Artificial Opening, Diagnostic
0F997ZZ	Drainage of Common Bile Duct, Via Natural or Artificial Opening
0F9980Z	Drainage of Common Bile Duct with Drainage Device, Via Natural or Artificial Opening Endoscopic
0F998ZX	Drainage of Common Bile Duct, Via Natural or Artificial Opening Endoscopic, Diagnostic
0F998ZZ	Drainage of Common Bile Duct, Via Natural or Artificial Opening Endoscopic
0F9C00Z	Drainage of Ampulla of Vater with Drainage Device, Open Approach
0F9C0ZX	Drainage of Ampulla of Vater, Open Approach, Diagnostic
0F9C0ZZ	Drainage of Ampulla of Vater, Open Approach
0F9C30Z	Drainage of Ampulla of Vater with Drainage Device, Percutaneous Approach
0F9C3ZX	Drainage of Ampulla of Vater, Percutaneous Approach, Diagnostic
0F9C3ZZ	Drainage of Ampulla of Vater, Percutaneous Approach
0F9C40Z	Drainage of Ampulla of Vater with Drainage Device, Percutaneous Endoscopic Approach
0F9C4ZX	Drainage of Ampulla of Vater, Percutaneous Endoscopic Approach, Diagnostic
0F9C4ZZ	Drainage of Ampulla of Vater, Percutaneous Endoscopic Approach
0F9C70Z	Drainage of Ampulla of Vater with Drainage Device, Via Natural or Artificial Opening
0F9C7ZX	Drainage of Ampulla of Vater, Via Natural or Artificial Opening, Diagnostic
0F9C7ZZ	Drainage of Ampulla of Vater, Via Natural or Artificial Opening
0F9C80Z	Drainage of Ampulla of Vater with Drainage Device, Via Natural or Artificial Opening Endoscopic
0F9C8ZX	Drainage of Ampulla of Vater, Via Natural or Artificial Opening Endoscopic, Diagnostic
0F9C8ZZ	Drainage of Ampulla of Vater, Via Natural or Artificial Opening Endoscopic
0F9D00Z	Drainage of Pancreatic Duct with Drainage Device, Open Approach
0F9D0ZX	Drainage of Pancreatic Duct, Open Approach, Diagnostic
0F9D0ZZ	Drainage of Pancreatic Duct, Open Approach
0F9D30Z	Drainage of Pancreatic Duct with Drainage Device, Percutaneous Approach
0F9D3ZX	Drainage of Pancreatic Duct, Percutaneous Approach, Diagnostic

0F9D3ZZ	Drainage of Pancreatic Duct, Percutaneous Approach
0F9D40Z	Drainage of Pancreatic Duct with Drainage Device, Percutaneous Endoscopic Approach
0F9D4ZX	Drainage of Pancreatic Duct, Percutaneous Endoscopic Approach, Diagnostic
0F9D4ZZ	Drainage of Pancreatic Duct, Percutaneous Endoscopic Approach
0F9D70Z	Drainage of Pancreatic Duct with Drainage Device, Via Natural or Artificial Opening
0F9D7ZX	Drainage of Pancreatic Duct, Via Natural or Artificial Opening, Diagnostic
0F9D7ZZ	Drainage of Pancreatic Duct, Via Natural or Artificial Opening
0F9D80Z	Drainage of Pancreatic Duct with Drainage Device, Via Natural or Artificial Opening Endoscopic
0F9D8ZX	Drainage of Pancreatic Duct, Via Natural or Artificial Opening Endoscopic, Diagnostic
0F9D8ZZ	Drainage of Pancreatic Duct, Via Natural or Artificial Opening Endoscopic
0F9F00Z	Drainage of Accessory Pancreatic Duct with Drainage Device, Open Approach
0F9F0ZX	Drainage of Accessory Pancreatic Duct, Open Approach, Diagnostic
0F9F0ZZ	Drainage of Accessory Pancreatic Duct, Open Approach
0F9F30Z	Drainage of Accessory Pancreatic Duct with Drainage Device, Percutaneous Approach
0F9F3ZX	Drainage of Accessory Pancreatic Duct, Percutaneous Approach, Diagnostic
0F9F3ZZ	Drainage of Accessory Pancreatic Duct, Percutaneous Approach
0F9F40Z	Drainage of Accessory Pancreatic Duct with Drainage Device, Percutaneous Endoscopic Approach
0F9F4ZX	Drainage of Accessory Pancreatic Duct, Percutaneous Endoscopic Approach, Diagnostic
0F9F4ZZ	Drainage of Accessory Pancreatic Duct, Percutaneous Endoscopic Approach
0F9F70Z	Drainage of Accessory Pancreatic Duct with Drainage Device, Via Natural or Artificial Opening
0F9F7ZX	Drainage of Accessory Pancreatic Duct, Via Natural or Artificial Opening, Diagnostic
0F9F7ZZ	Drainage of Accessory Pancreatic Duct, Via Natural or Artificial Opening
0F9F80Z	Drainage of Accessory Pancreatic Duct with Drainage Device, Via Natural or Artificial Opening Endoscopic
0F9F8ZX	Drainage of Accessory Pancreatic Duct, Via Natural or Artificial Opening Endoscopic, Diagnostic
0F9F8ZZ	Drainage of Accessory Pancreatic Duct, Via Natural or Artificial Opening Endoscopic
0F9G00Z	Drainage of Pancreas with Drainage Device, Open Approach
0F9G0ZX	Drainage of Pancreas, Open Approach, Diagnostic
0F9G0ZZ	Drainage of Pancreas, Open Approach
0F9G30Z	Drainage of Pancreas with Drainage Device, Percutaneous Approach
0F9G3ZX	Drainage of Pancreas, Percutaneous Approach, Diagnostic
0F9G3ZZ	Drainage of Pancreas, Percutaneous Approach
0F9G40Z	Drainage of Pancreas with Drainage Device, Percutaneous Endoscopic Approach
	AHA CC: 3Q, 2014, 15-16
0F9G4ZX	Drainage of Pancreas, Percutaneous Endoscopic Approach, Diagnostic
0F9G4ZZ	Drainage of Pancreas, Percutaneous Endoscopic Approach

---

♀ Female-only   ♂ Male-only   ▲ Limited Coverage   ● Non-OR   ▨ HAC-associated procedure   ▲ Non-covered procedures   ✚ Combinatio

view Coding Guidelines B3.4a and B3.4b

view Coding Guideline B3.8

B00ZX Excision of Liver, Open Approach, Diagnostic	**0FB60ZZ** Excision of Left Hepatic Duct, Open Approach	**0FBC4ZX** Excision of Ampulla of Vater, Percutaneous Endoscopic Approach, Diagnostic
B00ZZ Excision of Liver, Open Approach	**0FB63ZX** Excision of Left Hepatic Duct, Percutaneous Approach, Diagnostic	**0FBC4ZZ** Excision of Ampulla of Vater, Percutaneous Endoscopic Approach
B03ZX Excision of Liver, Percutaneous Approach, Diagnostic	**0FB63ZZ** Excision of Left Hepatic Duct, Percutaneous Approach	**0FBC7ZX** Excision of Ampulla of Vater, Via Natural or Artificial Opening, Diagnostic
B03ZZ Excision of Liver, Percutaneous Approach	**0FB64ZX** Excision of Left Hepatic Duct, Percutaneous Endoscopic Approach, Diagnostic	**0FBC7ZZ** Excision of Ampulla of Vater, Via Natural or Artificial Opening
B04ZX Excision of Liver, Percutaneous Endoscopic Approach, Diagnostic	**0FB64ZZ** Excision of Left Hepatic Duct, Percutaneous Endoscopic Approach	**0FBC8ZX** Excision of Ampulla of Vater, Via Natural or Artificial Opening Endoscopic, Diagnostic
B04ZZ Excision of Liver, Percutaneous Endoscopic Approach	**0FB67ZX** Excision of Left Hepatic Duct, Via Natural or Artificial Opening, Diagnostic	**0FBC8ZZ** Excision of Ampulla of Vater, Via Natural or Artificial Opening Endoscopic
B10ZX Excision of Right Lobe Liver, Open Approach, Diagnostic	**0FB67ZZ** Excision of Left Hepatic Duct, Via Natural or Artificial Opening	**0FBD0ZX** Excision of Pancreatic Duct, Open Approach, Diagnostic
B10ZZ Excision of Right Lobe Liver, Open Approach	**0FB68ZX** Excision of Left Hepatic Duct, Via Natural or Artificial Opening Endoscopic, Diagnostic	**0FBD0ZZ** Excision of Pancreatic Duct, Open Approach
B13ZX Excision of Right Lobe Liver, Percutaneous Approach, Diagnostic	**0FB68ZZ** Excision of Left Hepatic Duct, Via Natural or Artificial Opening Endoscopic	**0FBD3ZX** Excision of Pancreatic Duct, Percutaneous Approach, Diagnostic
B13ZZ Excision of Right Lobe Liver, Percutaneous Approach	**0FB80ZX** Excision of Cystic Duct, Open Approach, Diagnostic	**0FBD3ZZ** Excision of Pancreatic Duct, Percutaneous Approach
B14ZX Excision of Right Lobe Liver, Percutaneous Endoscopic Approach, Diagnostic	**0FB80ZZ** Excision of Cystic Duct, Open Approach	**0FBD4ZX** Excision of Pancreatic Duct, Percutaneous Endoscopic Approach, Diagnostic
B14ZZ Excision of Right Lobe Liver, Percutaneous Endoscopic Approach	**0FB83ZX** Excision of Cystic Duct, Percutaneous Approach, Diagnostic	**0FBD4ZZ** Excision of Pancreatic Duct, Percutaneous Endoscopic Approach
B20ZX Excision of Left Lobe Liver, Open Approach, Diagnostic	**0FB83ZZ** Excision of Cystic Duct, Percutaneous Approach	**0FBD7ZX** Excision of Pancreatic Duct, Via Natural or Artificial Opening, Diagnostic
B20ZZ Excision of Left Lobe Liver, Open Approach	**0FB84ZX** Excision of Cystic Duct, Percutaneous Endoscopic Approach, Diagnostic	**0FBD7ZZ** Excision of Pancreatic Duct, Via Natural or Artificial Opening
B23ZX Excision of Left Lobe Liver, Percutaneous Approach, Diagnostic	**0FB84ZZ** Excision of Cystic Duct, Percutaneous Endoscopic Approach	**0FBD8ZX** Excision of Pancreatic Duct, Via Natural or Artificial Opening Endoscopic, Diagnostic
B23ZZ Excision of Left Lobe Liver, Percutaneous Approach	**0FB87ZX** Excision of Cystic Duct, Via Natural or Artificial Opening, Diagnostic	**0FBD8ZZ** Excision of Pancreatic Duct, Via Natural or Artificial Opening Endoscopic
B24ZX Excision of Left Lobe Liver, Percutaneous Endoscopic Approach, Diagnostic	**0FB87ZZ** Excision of Cystic Duct, Via Natural or Artificial Opening	**0FBF0ZX** Excision of Accessory Pancreatic Duct, Open Approach, Diagnostic
B24ZZ Excision of Left Lobe Liver, Percutaneous Endoscopic Approach	**0FB88ZX** Excision of Cystic Duct, Via Natural or Artificial Opening Endoscopic, Diagnostic	**0FBF0ZZ** Excision of Accessory Pancreatic Duct, Open Approach
B40ZX Excision of Gallbladder, Open Approach, Diagnostic	**0FB88ZZ** Excision of Cystic Duct, Via Natural or Artificial Opening Endoscopic	**0FBF3ZX** Excision of Accessory Pancreatic Duct, Percutaneous Approach, Diagnostic
B40ZZ Excision of Gallbladder, Open Approach	**0FB90ZX** Excision of Common Bile Duct, Open Approach, Diagnostic	**0FBF3ZZ** Excision of Accessory Pancreatic Duct, Percutaneous Approach
B43ZX Excision of Gallbladder, Percutaneous Approach, Diagnostic	**0FB90ZZ** Excision of Common Bile Duct, Open Approach	**0FBF4ZX** Excision of Accessory Pancreatic Duct, Percutaneous Endoscopic Approach, Diagnostic
B43ZZ Excision of Gallbladder, Percutaneous Approach	**0FB93ZX** Excision of Common Bile Duct, Percutaneous Approach, Diagnostic	**0FBF4ZZ** Excision of Accessory Pancreatic Duct, Percutaneous Endoscopic Approach
B44ZX Excision of Gallbladder, Percutaneous Endoscopic Approach, Diagnostic	**0FB93ZZ** Excision of Common Bile Duct, Percutaneous Approach	**0FBF7ZX** Excision of Accessory Pancreatic Duct, Via Natural or Artificial Opening, Diagnostic
B44ZZ Excision of Gallbladder, Percutaneous Endoscopic Approach	**0FB94ZX** Excision of Common Bile Duct, Percutaneous Endoscopic Approach, Diagnostic	**0FBF7ZZ** Excision of Accessory Pancreatic Duct, Via Natural or Artificial Opening
B50ZX Excision of Right Hepatic Duct, Open Approach, Diagnostic	**0FB94ZZ** Excision of Common Bile Duct, Percutaneous Endoscopic Approach	**0FBF8ZX** Excision of Accessory Pancreatic Duct, Via Natural or Artificial Opening Endoscopic, Diagnostic
B50ZZ Excision of Right Hepatic Duct, Open Approach	**0FB97ZX** Excision of Common Bile Duct, Via Natural or Artificial Opening, Diagnostic	**0FBF8ZZ** Excision of Accessory Pancreatic Duct, Via Natural or Artificial Opening Endoscopic
FB53ZX Excision of Right Hepatic Duct, Percutaneous Approach, Diagnostic	**0FB97ZZ** Excision of Common Bile Duct, Via Natural or Artificial Opening	**0FBG0ZX** Excision of Pancreas, Open Approach, Diagnostic
B53ZZ Excision of Right Hepatic Duct, Percutaneous Approach	**0FB98ZX** Excision of Common Bile Duct, Via Natural or Artificial Opening Endoscopic, Diagnostic	**0FBG0ZZ** Excision of Pancreas, Open Approach
FB54ZX Excision of Right Hepatic Duct, Percutaneous Endoscopic Approach, Diagnostic	**0FB98ZZ** Excision of Common Bile Duct, Via Natural or Artificial Opening Endoscopic	*AHA CC: 3Q, 2014, 32-33*
FB54ZZ Excision of Right Hepatic Duct, Percutaneous Endoscopic Approach	**0FBC0ZX** Excision of Ampulla of Vater, Open Approach, Diagnostic	**0FBG3ZX** Excision of Pancreas, Percutaneous Approach, Diagnostic
FB57ZX Excision of Right Hepatic Duct, Via Natural or Artificial Opening, Diagnostic	**0FBC0ZZ** Excision of Ampulla of Vater, Open Approach	**0FBG3ZZ** Excision of Pancreas, Percutaneous Approach
FB57ZZ Excision of Right Hepatic Duct, Via Natural or Artificial Opening	**0FBC3ZX** Excision of Ampulla of Vater, Percutaneous Approach, Diagnostic	**0FBG4ZX** Excision of Pancreas, Percutaneous Endoscopic Approach, Diagnostic
FB58ZX Excision of Right Hepatic Duct, Via Natural or Artificial Opening Endoscopic, Diagnostic	**0FBC3ZZ** Excision of Ampulla of Vater, Percutaneous Approach	**0FBG4ZZ** Excision of Pancreas, Percutaneous Endoscopic Approach
FB58ZZ Excision of Right Hepatic Duct, Via Natural or Artificial Opening Endoscopic		
FB60ZX Excision of Left Hepatic Duct, Open Approach, Diagnostic		

♀ Female-only   ♂ Male-only   ▲ Limited Coverage   ● Non-OR   ▨ HAC-associated procedure   ▲ Non-covered procedures   ✛ Combination

0FC – Hepatobiliary System and Pancreas, Extirpation

0FC00ZZ Extirpation of Matter from Liver, Open Approach

0FC03ZZ Extirpation of Matter from Liver, Percutaneous Approach

0FC04ZZ Extirpation of Matter from Liver, Percutaneous Endoscopic Approach

0FC10ZZ Extirpation of Matter from Right Lobe Liver, Open Approach

0FC13ZZ Extirpation of Matter from Right Lobe Liver, Percutaneous Approach

0FC14ZZ Extirpation of Matter from Right Lobe Liver, Percutaneous Endoscopic Approach

0FC20ZZ Extirpation of Matter from Left Lobe Liver, Open Approach

0FC23ZZ Extirpation of Matter from Left Lobe Liver, Percutaneous Approach

0FC24ZZ Extirpation of Matter from Left Lobe Liver, Percutaneous Endoscopic Approach

0FC40ZZ Extirpation of Matter from Gallbladder, Open Approach

0FC43ZZ Extirpation of Matter from Gallbladder, Percutaneous Approach

0FC44ZZ Extirpation of Matter from Gallbladder, Percutaneous Endoscopic Approach

0FC50ZZ Extirpation of Matter from Right Hepatic Duct, Open Approach

0FC53ZZ Extirpation of Matter from Right Hepatic Duct, Percutaneous Approach

0FC54ZZ Extirpation of Matter from Right Hepatic Duct, Percutaneous Endoscopic Approach

0FC57ZZ Extirpation of Matter from Right Hepatic Duct, Via Natural or Artificial Opening

0FC58ZZ Extirpation of Matter from Right Hepatic Duct, Via Natural or Artificial Opening Endoscopic

0FC60ZZ Extirpation of Matter from Left Hepatic Duct, Open Approach

0FC63ZZ Extirpation of Matter from Left Hepatic Duct, Percutaneous Approach

0FC64ZZ Extirpation of Matter from Left Hepatic Duct, Percutaneous Endoscopic Approach

0FC67ZZ Extirpation of Matter from Left Hepatic Duct, Via Natural or Artificial Opening

0FC68ZZ Extirpation of Matter from Left Hepatic Duct, Via Natural or Artificial Opening Endoscopic

0FC80ZZ Extirpation of Matter from Cystic Duct, Open Approach

0FC83ZZ Extirpation of Matter from Cystic Duct, Percutaneous Approach

0FC84ZZ Extirpation of Matter from Cystic Duct, Percutaneous Endoscopic Approach

0FC87ZZ Extirpation of Matter from Cystic Duct, Via Natural or Artificial Opening

0FC88ZZ Extirpation of Matter from Cystic Duct, Via Natural or Artificial Opening Endoscopic

0FC90ZZ Extirpation of Matter from Common Bile Duct, Open Approach

0FC93ZZ Extirpation of Matter from Common Bile Duct, Percutaneous Approach

0FC94ZZ Extirpation of Matter from Common Bile Duct, Percutaneous Endoscopic Approach

0FC97ZZ Extirpation of Matter from Common Bile Duct, Via Natural or Artificial Opening

0FC98ZZ Extirpation of Matter from Common Bile Duct, Via Natural or Artificial Opening Endoscopic

0FCC0ZZ Extirpation of Matter from Ampulla of Vater, Open Approach

0FCC3ZZ Extirpation of Matter from Ampulla of Vater, Percutaneous Approach

0FCC4ZZ Extirpation of Matter from Ampulla of Vater, Percutaneous Endoscopic Approach

0FCC7ZZ Extirpation of Matter from Ampulla of Vater, Via Natural or Artificial Opening

0FCC8ZZ Extirpation of Matter from Ampulla of Vater, Via Natural or Artificial Opening Endoscopic

0FCD0ZZ Extirpation of Matter from Pancreatic Duct, Open Approach

0FCD3ZZ Extirpation of Matter from Pancreatic Duct, Percutaneous Approach

0FCD4ZZ Extirpation of Matter from Pancreatic Duct, Percutaneous Endoscopic Approach

0FCD7ZZ Extirpation of Matter from Pancreatic Duct, Via Natural or Artificial Opening

0FCD8ZZ Extirpation of Matter from Pancreatic Duct, Via Natural or Artificial Opening Endoscopic

0FCF0ZZ Extirpation of Matter from Accessory Pancreatic Duct, Open Approach

0FCF3ZZ Extirpation of Matter from Accessory Pancreatic Duct, Percutaneous Approach

0FCF4ZZ Extirpation of Matter from Accessory Pancreatic Duct, Percutaneous Endoscopic Approach

0FCF7ZZ Extirpation of Matter from Accessory Pancreatic Duct, Via Natural or Artificial Opening

0FCF8ZZ Extirpation of Matter from Accessory Pancreatic Duct, Via Natural or Artificial Opening Endoscopic

0FCG0ZZ Extirpation of Matter from Pancreas, Open Approach

0FCG3ZZ Extirpation of Matter from Pancreas, Percutaneous Approach

0FCG4ZZ Extirpation of Matter from Pancreas, Percutaneous Endoscopic Approach

0FF – Hepatobiliary System and Pancreas, Fragmentation

0FF40ZZ Fragmentation in Gallbladder, Open Approach

0FF43ZZ Fragmentation in Gallbladder, Percutaneous Approach

0FF44ZZ Fragmentation in Gallbladder, Percutaneous Endoscopic Approach

0FF47ZZ Fragmentation in Gallbladder, Via Natural or Artificial Opening

0FF48ZZ Fragmentation in Gallbladder, Via Natural or Artificial Opening Endoscopic

▲ 0FF4XZZ Fragmentation in Gallbladder, External Approach

0FF50ZZ Fragmentation in Right Hepatic Duct, Open Approach

0FF53ZZ Fragmentation in Right Hepatic Duct, Percutaneous Approach

0FF54ZZ Fragmentation in Right Hepatic Duct, Percutaneous Endoscopic Approach

0FF57ZZ Fragmentation in Right Hepatic Duct, Via Natural or Artificial Opening

0FF58ZZ Fragmentation in Right Hepatic Duct, Via Natural or Artificial Opening Endoscopic

▲ 0FF5XZZ Fragmentation in Right Hepatic Duct, External Approach

0FF60ZZ Fragmentation in Left Hepatic Duct, Open Approach

0FF63ZZ Fragmentation in Left Hepatic Duct, Percutaneous Approach

0FF64ZZ Fragmentation in Left Hepatic Duct, Percutaneous Endoscopic Approach

0FF67ZZ Fragmentation in Left Hepatic Duct, Via Natural or Artificial Opening

0FF68ZZ Fragmentation in Left Hepatic Duct, Via Natural or Artificial Opening Endoscopic

▲ 0FF6XZZ Fragmentation in Left Hepatic Duct, External Approach

0FF80ZZ Fragmentation in Cystic Duct, Open Approach

0FF83ZZ Fragmentation in Cystic Duct, Percutaneous Approach

0FF84ZZ Fragmentation in Cystic Duct, Percutaneous Endoscopic Approach

0FF87ZZ Fragmentation in Cystic Duct, Via Natural or Artificial Opening

0FF88ZZ Fragmentation in Cystic Duct, Via Natural or Artificial Opening Endoscopic

▲ 0FF8XZZ Fragmentation in Cystic Duct, External Approach

0FF90ZZ Fragmentation in Common Bile Duct, Open Approach

0FF93ZZ Fragmentation in Common Bile Duct, Percutaneous Approach

0FF94ZZ Fragmentation in Common Bile Duct, Percutaneous Endoscopic Approach

0FF97ZZ Fragmentation in Common Bile Duct, Via Natural or Artificial Opening

0FF98ZZ Fragmentation in Common Bile Duct, Via Natural or Artificial Opening Endoscopic

▲ 0FF9XZZ Fragmentation in Common Bile Duct, External Approach

0FFC0ZZ Fragmentation in Ampulla of Vater, Open Approach

0FFC3ZZ Fragmentation in Ampulla of Vater, Percutaneous Approach

0FFC4ZZ Fragmentation in Ampulla of Vater, Percutaneous Endoscopic Approach

0FFC7ZZ Fragmentation in Ampulla of Vater, Via Natural or Artificial Opening

0FFC8ZZ Fragmentation in Ampulla of Vater, Via Natural or Artificial Opening Endoscopic

▲ 0FFCXZZ Fragmentation in Ampulla of Vater, External Approach

0FFD0ZZ Fragmentation in Pancreatic Duct, Open Approach

0FFD3ZZ Fragmentation in Pancreatic Duct, Percutaneous Approach

0FFD4ZZ Fragmentation in Pancreatic Duct, Percutaneous Endoscopic Approach

0FFD7ZZ Fragmentation in Pancreatic Duct, Via Natural or Artificial Opening

0FFD8ZZ Fragmentation in Pancreatic Duct, Via Natural or Artificial Opening Endoscopic

▲ 0FFDXZZ Fragmentation in Pancreatic Duct, External Approach

0FFF0ZZ Fragmentation in Accessory Pancreatic Duct, Open Approach

0FFF3ZZ Fragmentation in Accessory Pancreatic Duct, Percutaneous Approach

0FFF4ZZ Fragmentation in Accessory Pancreatic Duct, Percutaneous Endoscopic Approach

0FFF7ZZ Fragmentation in Accessory Pancreatic Duct, Via Natural or Artificial Opening

0FFF8ZZ Fragmentation in Accessory Pancreatic Duct, Via Natural or Artificial Opening Endoscopic

▲ 0FFFXZZ Fragmentation in Accessory Pancreatic Duct, External Approach

♀ Female-only   ♂ Male-only   ▲ Limited Coverage   ● Non-OR   HAC HAC-associated procedure   ▲ Non-covered procedures   + Combination

FH – Hepatobiliary System and Pancreas, Insertion

H002Z   Insertion of Monitoring Device into Liver, Open Approach

H003Z   Insertion of Infusion Device into Liver, Open Approach

H032Z   Insertion of Monitoring Device into Liver, Percutaneous Approach

H033Z   Insertion of Infusion Device into Liver, Percutaneous Approach

H042Z   Insertion of Monitoring Device into Liver, Percutaneous Endoscopic Approach

H043Z   Insertion of Infusion Device into Liver, Percutaneous Endoscopic Approach

H102Z   Insertion of Monitoring Device into Right Lobe Liver, Open Approach

H103Z   Insertion of Infusion Device into Right Lobe Liver, Open Approach

H132Z   Insertion of Monitoring Device into Right Lobe Liver, Percutaneous Approach

H133Z   Insertion of Infusion Device into Right Lobe Liver, Percutaneous Approach

H142Z   Insertion of Monitoring Device into Right Lobe Liver, Percutaneous Endoscopic Approach

H143Z   Insertion of Infusion Device into Right Lobe Liver, Percutaneous Endoscopic Approach

H202Z   Insertion of Monitoring Device into Left Lobe Liver, Open Approach

H203Z   Insertion of Infusion Device into Left Lobe Liver, Open Approach

H232Z   Insertion of Monitoring Device into Left Lobe Liver, Percutaneous Approach

H233Z   Insertion of Infusion Device into Left Lobe Liver, Percutaneous Approach

H242Z   Insertion of Monitoring Device into Left Lobe Liver, Percutaneous Endoscopic Approach

H243Z   Insertion of Infusion Device into Left Lobe Liver, Percutaneous Endoscopic Approach

H402Z   Insertion of Monitoring Device into Gallbladder, Open Approach

H403Z   Insertion of Infusion Device into Gallbladder, Open Approach

H432Z   Insertion of Monitoring Device into Gallbladder, Percutaneous Approach

H433Z   Insertion of Infusion Device into Gallbladder, Percutaneous Approach

H442Z   Insertion of Monitoring Device into Gallbladder, Percutaneous Endoscopic Approach

H443Z   Insertion of Infusion Device into Gallbladder, Percutaneous Endoscopic Approach

HB01Z   Insertion of Radioactive Element into Hepatobiliary Duct, Open Approach

HB02Z   Insertion of Monitoring Device into Hepatobiliary Duct, Open Approach

0FHB03Z   Insertion of Infusion Device into Hepatobiliary Duct, Open Approach

0FHB0DZ   Insertion of Intraluminal Device into Hepatobiliary Duct, Open Approach

0FHB31Z   Insertion of Radioactive Element into Hepatobiliary Duct, Percutaneous Approach

0FHB32Z   Insertion of Monitoring Device into Hepatobiliary Duct, Percutaneous Approach

0FHB33Z   Insertion of Infusion Device into Hepatobiliary Duct, Percutaneous Approach

0FHB3DZ   Insertion of Intraluminal Device into Hepatobiliary Duct, Percutaneous Approach

0FHB41Z   Insertion of Radioactive Element into Hepatobiliary Duct, Percutaneous Endoscopic Approach

0FHB42Z   Insertion of Monitoring Device into Hepatobiliary Duct, Percutaneous Endoscopic Approach

0FHB43Z   Insertion of Infusion Device into Hepatobiliary Duct, Percutaneous Endoscopic Approach

0FHB4DZ   Insertion of Intraluminal Device into Hepatobiliary Duct, Percutaneous Endoscopic Approach

0FHB71Z   Insertion of Radioactive Element into Hepatobiliary Duct, Via Natural or Artificial Opening

0FHB72Z   Insertion of Monitoring Device into Hepatobiliary Duct, Via Natural or Artificial Opening

0FHB73Z   Insertion of Infusion Device into Hepatobiliary Duct, Via Natural or Artificial Opening

0FHB7DZ   Insertion of Intraluminal Device into Hepatobiliary Duct, Via Natural or Artificial Opening

0FHB81Z   Insertion of Radioactive Element into Hepatobiliary Duct, Via Natural or Artificial Opening Endoscopic

0FHB82Z   Insertion of Monitoring Device into Hepatobiliary Duct, Via Natural or Artificial Opening Endoscopic

0FHB83Z   Insertion of Infusion Device into Hepatobiliary Duct, Via Natural or Artificial Opening Endoscopic

● 0FHB8DZ   Insertion of Intraluminal Device into Hepatobiliary Duct, Via Natural or Artificial Opening Endoscopic

0FHD01Z   Insertion of Radioactive Element into Pancreatic Duct, Open Approach

0FHD02Z   Insertion of Monitoring Device into Pancreatic Duct, Open Approach

0FHD03Z   Insertion of Infusion Device into Pancreatic Duct, Open Approach

0FHD0DZ   Insertion of Intraluminal Device into Pancreatic Duct, Open Approach

0FHD31Z   Insertion of Radioactive Element into Pancreatic Duct, Percutaneous Approach

0FHD32Z   Insertion of Monitoring Device into Pancreatic Duct, Percutaneous Approach

0FHD33Z   Insertion of Infusion Device into Pancreatic Duct, Percutaneous Approach

0FHD3DZ   Insertion of Intraluminal Device into Pancreatic Duct, Percutaneous Approach

0FHD41Z   Insertion of Radioactive Element into Pancreatic Duct, Percutaneous Endoscopic Approach

0FHD42Z   Insertion of Monitoring Device into Pancreatic Duct, Percutaneous Endoscopic Approach

0FHD43Z   Insertion of Infusion Device into Pancreatic Duct, Percutaneous Endoscopic Approach

0FHD4DZ   Insertion of Intraluminal Device into Pancreatic Duct, Percutaneous Endoscopic Approach

0FHD71Z   Insertion of Radioactive Element into Pancreatic Duct, Via Natural or Artificial Opening

0FHD72Z   Insertion of Monitoring Device into Pancreatic Duct, Via Natural or Artificial Opening

0FHD73Z   Insertion of Infusion Device into Pancreatic Duct, Via Natural or Artificial Opening

0FHD7DZ   Insertion of Intraluminal Device into Pancreatic Duct, Via Natural or Artificial Opening

0FHD81Z   Insertion of Radioactive Element into Pancreatic Duct, Via Natural or Artificial Opening Endoscopic

0FHD82Z   Insertion of Monitoring Device into Pancreatic Duct, Via Natural or Artificial Opening Endoscopic

0FHD83Z   Insertion of Infusion Device into Pancreatic Duct, Via Natural or Artificial Opening Endoscopic

0FHD8DZ   Insertion of Intraluminal Device into Pancreatic Duct, Via Natural or Artificial Opening Endoscopic

0FHG02Z   Insertion of Monitoring Device into Pancreas, Open Approach

0FHG03Z   Insertion of Infusion Device into Pancreas, Open Approach

0FHG32Z   Insertion of Monitoring Device into Pancreas, Percutaneous Approach

0FHG33Z   Insertion of Infusion Device into Pancreas, Percutaneous Approach

0FHG42Z   Insertion of Monitoring Device into Pancreas, Percutaneous Endoscopic Approach

0FHG43Z   Insertion of Infusion Device into Pancreas, Percutaneous Endoscopic Approach

FJ – Hepatobiliary System and Pancreas, Inspection

eview Coding Guidelines B3.11a, B3.11b and B3.11c

FJ00ZZ   Inspection of Liver, Open Approach

FJ03ZZ   Inspection of Liver, Percutaneous Approach

FJ04ZZ   Inspection of Liver, Percutaneous Endoscopic Approach

FJ0XZZ   Inspection of Liver, External Approach

FJ40ZZ   Inspection of Gallbladder, Open Approach

FJ43ZZ   Inspection of Gallbladder, Percutaneous Approach

FJ44ZZ   Inspection of Gallbladder, Percutaneous Endoscopic Approach

FJ4XZZ   Inspection of Gallbladder, External Approach

0FJB0ZZ   Inspection of Hepatobiliary Duct, Open Approach

0FJB3ZZ   Inspection of Hepatobiliary Duct, Percutaneous Approach

0FJB4ZZ   Inspection of Hepatobiliary Duct, Percutaneous Endoscopic Approach

0FJB7ZZ   Inspection of Hepatobiliary Duct, Via Natural or Artificial Opening

0FJB8ZZ   Inspection of Hepatobiliary Duct, Via Natural or Artificial Opening Endoscopic

0FJD0ZZ   Inspection of Pancreatic Duct, Open Approach

0FJD3ZZ   Inspection of Pancreatic Duct, Percutaneous Approach

0FJD4ZZ   Inspection of Pancreatic Duct, Percutaneous Endoscopic Approach

0FJD7ZZ   Inspection of Pancreatic Duct, Via Natural or Artificial Opening

0FJD8ZZ   Inspection of Pancreatic Duct, Via Natural or Artificial Opening Endoscopic

0FJG0ZZ   Inspection of Pancreas, Open Approach

0FJG3ZZ   Inspection of Pancreas, Percutaneous Approach

0FJG4ZZ   Inspection of Pancreas, Percutaneous Endoscopic Approach

0FJGXZZ   Inspection of Pancreas, External Approach

0FL50CZ Occlusion of Right Hepatic Duct with Extraluminal Device, Open Approach

0FL50DZ Occlusion of Right Hepatic Duct with Intraluminal Device, Open Approach

0FL50ZZ Occlusion of Right Hepatic Duct, Open Approach

0FL53CZ Occlusion of Right Hepatic Duct with Extraluminal Device, Percutaneous Approach

0FL53DZ Occlusion of Right Hepatic Duct with Intraluminal Device, Percutaneous Approach

0FL53ZZ Occlusion of Right Hepatic Duct, Percutaneous Approach

0FL54CZ Occlusion of Right Hepatic Duct with Extraluminal Device, Percutaneous Endoscopic Approach

0FL54DZ Occlusion of Right Hepatic Duct with Intraluminal Device, Percutaneous Endoscopic Approach

0FL54ZZ Occlusion of Right Hepatic Duct, Percutaneous Endoscopic Approach

0FL57DZ Occlusion of Right Hepatic Duct with Intraluminal Device, Via Natural or Artificial Opening

0FL57ZZ Occlusion of Right Hepatic Duct, Via Natural or Artificial Opening

0FL58DZ Occlusion of Right Hepatic Duct with Intraluminal Device, Via Natural or Artificial Opening Endoscopic

0FL58ZZ Occlusion of Right Hepatic Duct, Via Natural or Artificial Opening Endoscopic

0FL60CZ Occlusion of Left Hepatic Duct with Extraluminal Device, Open Approach

0FL60DZ Occlusion of Left Hepatic Duct with Intraluminal Device, Open Approach

0FL60ZZ Occlusion of Left Hepatic Duct, Open Approach

0FL63CZ Occlusion of Left Hepatic Duct with Extraluminal Device, Percutaneous Approach

0FL63DZ Occlusion of Left Hepatic Duct with Intraluminal Device, Percutaneous Approach

0FL63ZZ Occlusion of Left Hepatic Duct, Percutaneous Approach

0FL64CZ Occlusion of Left Hepatic Duct with Extraluminal Device, Percutaneous Endoscopic Approach

0FL64DZ Occlusion of Left Hepatic Duct with Intraluminal Device, Percutaneous Endoscopic Approach

0FL64ZZ Occlusion of Left Hepatic Duct, Percutaneous Endoscopic Approach

0FL67DZ Occlusion of Left Hepatic Duct with Intraluminal Device, Via Natural or Artificial Opening

0FL67ZZ Occlusion of Left Hepatic Duct, Via Natural or Artificial Opening

0FL68DZ Occlusion of Left Hepatic Duct with Intraluminal Device, Via Natural or Artificial Opening Endoscopic

0FL68ZZ Occlusion of Left Hepatic Duct, Via Natural or Artificial Opening Endoscopic

0FL80CZ Occlusion of Cystic Duct with Extraluminal Device, Open Approach

0FL80DZ Occlusion of Cystic Duct with Intraluminal Device, Open Approach

0FL80ZZ Occlusion of Cystic Duct, Open Approach

0FL83CZ Occlusion of Cystic Duct with Extraluminal Device, Percutaneous Hepproach

0FL83DZ Occlusion of Cystic Duct with Intraluminal Device, Percutaneous Approach

0FL83ZZ Occlusion of Cystic Duct, Percutaneous Approach

0FL84CZ Occlusion of Cystic Duct with Extraluminal Device, Percutaneous Endoscopic Approach

0FL84DZ Occlusion of Cystic Duct with Intraluminal Device, Percutaneous Endoscopic Approach

0FL84ZZ Occlusion of Cystic Duct, Percutaneous Endoscopic Approach

0FL87DZ Occlusion of Cystic Duct with Intraluminal Device, Via Natural or Artificial Opening

0FL87ZZ Occlusion of Cystic Duct, Via Natural or Artificial Opening

0FL88DZ Occlusion of Cystic Duct with Intraluminal Device, Via Natural or Artificial Opening Endoscopic

0FL88ZZ Occlusion of Cystic Duct, Via Natural or Artificial Opening Endoscopic

0FL90CZ Occlusion of Common Bile Duct with Extraluminal Device, Open Approach

0FL90DZ Occlusion of Common Bile Duct with Intraluminal Device, Open Approach

0FL90ZZ Occlusion of Common Bile Duct, Open Approach

0FL93CZ Occlusion of Common Bile Duct with Extraluminal Device, Percutaneous Approach

0FL93DZ Occlusion of Common Bile Duct with Intraluminal Device, Percutaneous Approach

0FL93ZZ Occlusion of Common Bile Duct, Percutaneous Approach

0FL94CZ Occlusion of Common Bile Duct with Extraluminal Device, Percutaneous Endoscopic Approach

0FL94DZ Occlusion of Common Bile Duct with Intraluminal Device, Percutaneous Endoscopic Approach

0FL94ZZ Occlusion of Common Bile Duct, Percutaneous Endoscopic Approach

0FL97DZ Occlusion of Common Bile Duct with Intraluminal Device, Via Natural or Artificial Opening

0FL97ZZ Occlusion of Common Bile Duct, Via Natural or Artificial Opening

0FL98DZ Occlusion of Common Bile Duct with Intraluminal Device, Via Natural or Artificial Opening Endoscopic

0FL98ZZ Occlusion of Common Bile Duct, Via Natural or Artificial Opening Endoscopic

0FLC0CZ Occlusion of Ampulla of Vater with Extraluminal Device, Open Approach

0FLC0DZ Occlusion of Ampulla of Vater with Intraluminal Device, Open Approach

0FLC0ZZ Occlusion of Ampulla of Vater, Open Approach

0FLC3CZ Occlusion of Ampulla of Vater with Extraluminal Device, Percutaneous Approach

0FLC3DZ Occlusion of Ampulla of Vater with Intraluminal Device, Percutaneous Approach

0FLC3ZZ Occlusion of Ampulla of Vater, Percutaneous Approach

0FLC4CZ Occlusion of Ampulla of Vater with Extraluminal Device, Percutaneous Endoscopic Approach

0FLC4DZ Occlusion of Ampulla of Vater with Intraluminal Device, Percutaneous Endoscopic Approach

0FLC4ZZ Occlusion of Ampulla of Vater, Percutaneous Endoscopic Approach

0FLC7DZ Occlusion of Ampulla of Vater with Intraluminal Device, Via Natural or Artificial Opening

0FLC7ZZ Occlusion of Ampulla of Vater, Via Natural or Artificial Opening

0FLC8DZ Occlusion of Ampulla of Vater with Intraluminal Device, Via Natural or Artificial Opening Endoscopic

0FLC8ZZ Occlusion of Ampulla of Vater, Via Natural or Artificial Opening Endoscopic

0FLD0CZ Occlusion of Pancreatic Duct with Extraluminal Device, Open Approach

0FLD0DZ Occlusion of Pancreatic Duct with Intraluminal Device, Open Approach

0FLD0ZZ Occlusion of Pancreatic Duct, Open Approach

0FLD3CZ Occlusion of Pancreatic Duct with Extraluminal Device, Percutaneous Approach

0FLD3DZ Occlusion of Pancreatic Duct with Intraluminal Device, Percutaneous Approach

0FLD3ZZ Occlusion of Pancreatic Duct, Percutaneous Approach

0FLD4CZ Occlusion of Pancreatic Duct with Extraluminal Device, Percutaneous Endoscopic Approach

0FLD4DZ Occlusion of Pancreatic Duct with Intraluminal Device, Percutaneous Endoscopic Approach

0FLD4ZZ Occlusion of Pancreatic Duct, Percutaneous Endoscopic Approach

0FLD7DZ Occlusion of Pancreatic Duct with Intraluminal Device, Via Natural or Artificial Opening

0FLD7ZZ Occlusion of Pancreatic Duct, Via Natural or Artificial Opening

0FLD8DZ Occlusion of Pancreatic Duct with Intraluminal Device, Via Natural or Artificial Opening Endoscopic

0FLD8ZZ Occlusion of Pancreatic Duct, Via Natural or Artificial Opening Endoscopic

0FLF0CZ Occlusion of Accessory Pancreatic Duct with Extraluminal Device, Open Approach

0FLF0DZ Occlusion of Accessory Pancreatic Duct with Intraluminal Device, Open Approach

0FLF0ZZ Occlusion of Accessory Pancreatic Duct, Open Approach

0FLF3CZ Occlusion of Accessory Pancreatic Duct with Extraluminal Device, Percutaneous Approach

0FLF3DZ Occlusion of Accessory Pancreatic Duct with Intraluminal Device, Percutaneous Approach

0FLF3ZZ Occlusion of Accessory Pancreatic Duct, Percutaneous Approach

0FLF4CZ Occlusion of Accessory Pancreatic Duct with Extraluminal Device, Percutaneous Endoscopic Approach

0FLF4DZ Occlusion of Accessory Pancreatic Duct with Intraluminal Device, Percutaneous Endoscopic Approach

0FLF4ZZ Occlusion of Accessory Pancreatic Duct, Percutaneous Endoscopic Approach

0FLF7DZ Occlusion of Accessory Pancreatic Duct with Intraluminal Device, Via Natural or Artificial Opening

0FLF7ZZ Occlusion of Accessory Pancreatic Duct, Via Natural or Artificial Opening

0FLF8DZ Occlusion of Accessory Pancreatic Duct with Intraluminal Device, Via Natural or Artificial Opening Endoscopic

0FLF8ZZ Occlusion of Accessory Pancreatic Duct, Via Natural or Artificial Opening Endoscopic

0FM – Hepatobiliary System and Pancreas, Reattachment

0FM00ZZ Reattachment of Liver, Open Approach	**0FM50ZZ** Reattachment of Right Hepatic Duct, Open Approach	**0FMC0ZZ** Reattachment of Ampulla of Vater, Open Approach
0FM04ZZ Reattachment of Liver, Percutaneous Endoscopic Approach	**0FM54ZZ** Reattachment of Right Hepatic Duct, Percutaneous Endoscopic Approach	**0FMC4ZZ** Reattachment of Ampulla of Vater, Percutaneous Endoscopic Approach
0FM10ZZ Reattachment of Right Lobe Liver, Open Approach	**0FM60ZZ** Reattachment of Left Hepatic Duct, Open Approach	**0FMD0ZZ** Reattachment of Pancreatic Duct, Open Approach
0FM14ZZ Reattachment of Right Lobe Liver, Percutaneous Endoscopic Approach	**0FM64ZZ** Reattachment of Left Hepatic Duct, Percutaneous Endoscopic Approach	**0FMD4ZZ** Reattachment of Pancreatic Duct, Percutaneous Endoscopic Approach
0FM20ZZ Reattachment of Left Lobe Liver, Open Approach	**0FM80ZZ** Reattachment of Cystic Duct, Open Approach	**0FMF0ZZ** Reattachment of Accessory Pancreatic Duct, Open Approach
0FM24ZZ Reattachment of Left Lobe Liver, Percutaneous Endoscopic Approach	**0FM84ZZ** Reattachment of Cystic Duct, Percutaneous Endoscopic Approach	**0FMF4ZZ** Reattachment of Accessory Pancreatic Duct, Percutaneous Endoscopic Approach
0FM40ZZ Reattachment of Gallbladder, Open Approach	**0FM90ZZ** Reattachment of Common Bile Duct, Open Approach	**0FMG0ZZ** Reattachment of Pancreas, Open Approach
0FM44ZZ Reattachment of Gallbladder, Percutaneous Endoscopic Approach	**0FM94ZZ** Reattachment of Common Bile Duct, Percutaneous Endoscopic Approach	**0FMG4ZZ** Reattachment of Pancreas, Percutaneous Endoscopic Approach

0FN – Hepatobiliary System and Pancreas, Release

Review Coding Guideline B3.13

Review Coding Guideline B3.14

0FN00ZZ Release Liver, Open Approach	**0FN63ZZ** Release Left Hepatic Duct, Percutaneous Approach	**0FNC4ZZ** Release Ampulla of Vater, Percutaneous Endoscopic Approach
0FN03ZZ Release Liver, Percutaneous Approach	**0FN64ZZ** Release Left Hepatic Duct, Percutaneous Endoscopic Approach	**0FNC7ZZ** Release Ampulla of Vater, Via Natural or Artificial Opening
0FN04ZZ Release Liver, Percutaneous Endoscopic Approach	**0FN67ZZ** Release Left Hepatic Duct, Via Natural or Artificial Opening	**0FNC8ZZ** Release Ampulla of Vater, Via Natural or Artificial Opening Endoscopic
0FN10ZZ Release Right Lobe Liver, Open Approach	**0FN68ZZ** Release Left Hepatic Duct, Via Natural or Artificial Opening Endoscopic	**0FND0ZZ** Release Pancreatic Duct, Open Approach
0FN13ZZ Release Right Lobe Liver, Percutaneous Approach	**0FN80ZZ** Release Cystic Duct, Open Approach	**0FND3ZZ** Release Pancreatic Duct, Percutaneous Approach
0FN14ZZ Release Right Lobe Liver, Percutaneous Endoscopic Approach	**0FN83ZZ** Release Cystic Duct, Percutaneous Approach	**0FND4ZZ** Release Pancreatic Duct, Percutaneous Endoscopic Approach
0FN20ZZ Release Left Lobe Liver, Open Approach	**0FN84ZZ** Release Cystic Duct, Percutaneous Endoscopic Approach	**0FND7ZZ** Release Pancreatic Duct, Via Natural or Artificial Opening
0FN23ZZ Release Left Lobe Liver, Percutaneous Approach	**0FN87ZZ** Release Cystic Duct, Via Natural or Artificial Opening	**0FND8ZZ** Release Pancreatic Duct, Via Natural or Artificial Opening Endoscopic
0FN24ZZ Release Left Lobe Liver, Percutaneous Endoscopic Approach	**0FN88ZZ** Release Cystic Duct, Via Natural or Artificial Opening Endoscopic	**0FNF0ZZ** Release Accessory Pancreatic Duct, Open Approach
0FN40ZZ Release Gallbladder, Open Approach	**0FN90ZZ** Release Common Bile Duct, Open Approach	**0FNF3ZZ** Release Accessory Pancreatic Duct, Percutaneous Approach
0FN43ZZ Release Gallbladder, Percutaneous Approach	**0FN93ZZ** Release Common Bile Duct, Percutaneous Approach	**0FNF4ZZ** Release Accessory Pancreatic Duct, Percutaneous Endoscopic Approach
0FN44ZZ Release Gallbladder, Percutaneous Endoscopic Approach	**0FN94ZZ** Release Common Bile Duct, Percutaneous Endoscopic Approach	**0FNF7ZZ** Release Accessory Pancreatic Duct, Via Natural or Artificial Opening
0FN50ZZ Release Right Hepatic Duct, Open Approach	**0FN97ZZ** Release Common Bile Duct, Via Natural or Artificial Opening	**0FNF8ZZ** Release Accessory Pancreatic Duct, Via Natural or Artificial Opening Endoscopic
0FN53ZZ Release Right Hepatic Duct, Percutaneous Approach	**0FN98ZZ** Release Common Bile Duct, Via Natural or Artificial Opening Endoscopic	**0FNG0ZZ** Release Pancreas, Open Approach
0FN54ZZ Release Right Hepatic Duct, Percutaneous Endoscopic Approach	**0FNC0ZZ** Release Ampulla of Vater, Open Approach	**0FNG3ZZ** Release Pancreas, Percutaneous Approach
0FN57ZZ Release Right Hepatic Duct, Via Natural or Artificial Opening	**0FNC3ZZ** Release Ampulla of Vater, Percutaneous Approach	**0FNG4ZZ** Release Pancreas, Percutaneous Endoscopic Approach
0FN58ZZ Release Right Hepatic Duct, Via Natural or Artificial Opening Endoscopic		
0FN60ZZ Release Left Hepatic Duct, Open Approach		

0FP – Hepatobiliary System and Pancreas, Removal

Review Coding Guideline B6.1c

0FP000Z Removal of Drainage Device from Liver, Open Approach	**0FP043Z** Removal of Infusion Device from Liver, Percutaneous Endoscopic Approach	**0FP430Z** Removal of Drainage Device from Gallbladder, Percutaneous Approach
0FP002Z Removal of Monitoring Device from Liver, Open Approach	**0FP0X0Z** Removal of Drainage Device from Liver, External Approach	**0FP432Z** Removal of Monitoring Device from Gallbladder, Percutaneous Approach
0FP003Z Removal of Infusion Device from Liver, Open Approach	**0FP0X2Z** Removal of Monitoring Device from Liver, External Approach	**0FP433Z** Removal of Infusion Device from Gallbladder, Percutaneous Approach
0FP030Z Removal of Drainage Device from Liver, Percutaneous Approach	**0FP0X3Z** Removal of Infusion Device from Liver, External Approach	**0FP43DZ** Removal of Intraluminal Device from Gallbladder, Percutaneous Approach
0FP032Z Removal of Monitoring Device from Liver, Percutaneous Approach	**0FP400Z** Removal of Drainage Device from Gallbladder, Open Approach	**0FP440Z** Removal of Drainage Device from Gallbladder, Percutaneous Endoscopic Approach
0FP033Z Removal of Infusion Device from Liver, Percutaneous Approach	**0FP402Z** Removal of Monitoring Device from Gallbladder, Open Approach	**0FP442Z** Removal of Monitoring Device from Gallbladder, Percutaneous Endoscopic Approach
0FP040Z Removal of Drainage Device from Liver, Percutaneous Endoscopic Approach	**0FP403Z** Removal of Infusion Device from Gallbladder, Open Approach	**0FP443Z** Removal of Infusion Device from Gallbladder, Percutaneous Endoscopic Approach
0FP042Z Removal of Monitoring Device from Liver, Percutaneous Endoscopic Approach	**0FP40DZ** Removal of Intraluminal Device from Gallbladder, Open Approach	

♀ Female-only   ♂ Male-only   ▲ Limited Coverage   ● Non-OR   ▩ HAC-associated procedure   ▲ Non-covered procedures   ✚ Combination

0FP44DZ Removal of Intraluminal Device from Gallbladder, Percutaneous Endoscopic Approach

0FP4X0Z Removal of Drainage Device from Gallbladder, External Approach

0FP4X2Z Removal of Monitoring Device from Gallbladder, External Approach

0FP4X3Z Removal of Infusion Device from Gallbladder, External Approach

0FP4XDZ Removal of Intraluminal Device from Gallbladder, External Approach

0FPB00Z Removal of Drainage Device from Hepatobiliary Duct, Open Approach

0FPB01Z Removal of Radioactive Element from Hepatobiliary Duct, Open Approach

0FPB02Z Removal of Monitoring Device from Hepatobiliary Duct, Open Approach

0FPB03Z Removal of Infusion Device from Hepatobiliary Duct, Open Approach

0FPB07Z Removal of Autologous Tissue Substitute from Hepatobiliary Duct, Open Approach

0FPB0CZ Removal of Extraluminal Device from Hepatobiliary Duct, Open Approach

0FPB0DZ Removal of Intraluminal Device from Hepatobiliary Duct, Open Approach

0FPB0JZ Removal of Synthetic Substitute from Hepatobiliary Duct, Open Approach

0FPB0KZ Removal of Nonautologous Tissue Substitute from Hepatobiliary Duct, Open Approach

0FPB30Z Removal of Drainage Device from Hepatobiliary Duct, Percutaneous Approach

0FPB31Z Removal of Radioactive Element from Hepatobiliary Duct, Percutaneous Approach

0FPB32Z Removal of Monitoring Device from Hepatobiliary Duct, Percutaneous Approach

0FPB33Z Removal of Infusion Device from Hepatobiliary Duct, Percutaneous Approach

0FPB37Z Removal of Autologous Tissue Substitute from Hepatobiliary Duct, Percutaneous Approach

0FPB3CZ Removal of Extraluminal Device from Hepatobiliary Duct, Percutaneous Approach

0FPB3DZ Removal of Intraluminal Device from Hepatobiliary Duct, Percutaneous Approach

0FPB3JZ Removal of Synthetic Substitute from Hepatobiliary Duct, Percutaneous Approach

0FPB3KZ Removal of Nonautologous Tissue Substitute from Hepatobiliary Duct, Percutaneous Approach

0FPB40Z Removal of Drainage Device from Hepatobiliary Duct, Percutaneous Endoscopic Approach

0FPB41Z Removal of Radioactive Element from Hepatobiliary Duct, Percutaneous Endoscopic Approach

0FPB42Z Removal of Monitoring Device from Hepatobiliary Duct, Percutaneous Endoscopic Approach

0FPB43Z Removal of Infusion Device from Hepatobiliary Duct, Percutaneous Endoscopic Approach

0FPB47Z Removal of Autologous Tissue Substitute from Hepatobiliary Duct, Percutaneous Endoscopic Approach

0FPB4CZ Removal of Extraluminal Device from Hepatobiliary Duct, Percutaneous Endoscopic Approach

0FPB4DZ Removal of Intraluminal Device from Hepatobiliary Duct, Percutaneous Endoscopic Approach

0FPB4JZ Removal of Synthetic Substitute from Hepatobiliary Duct, Percutaneous Endoscopic Approach

0FPB4KZ Removal of Nonautologous Tissue Substitute from Hepatobiliary Duct, Percutaneous Endoscopic Approach

0FPB70Z Removal of Drainage Device from Hepatobiliary Duct, Via Natural or Artificial Opening

0FPB71Z Removal of Radioactive Element from Hepatobiliary Duct, Via Natural or Artificial Opening

0FPB72Z Removal of Monitoring Device from Hepatobiliary Duct, Via Natural or Artificial Opening

0FPB73Z Removal of Infusion Device from Hepatobiliary Duct, Via Natural or Artificial Opening

0FPB77Z Removal of Autologous Tissue Substitute from Hepatobiliary Duct, Via Natural or Artificial Opening

0FPB7CZ Removal of Extraluminal Device from Hepatobiliary Duct, Via Natural or Artificial Opening

0FPB7DZ Removal of Intraluminal Device from Hepatobiliary Duct, Via Natural or Artificial Opening

0FPB7JZ Removal of Synthetic Substitute from Hepatobiliary Duct, Via Natural or Artificial Opening

0FPB7KZ Removal of Nonautologous Tissue Substitute from Hepatobiliary Duct, Via Natural or Artificial Opening

0FPB80Z Removal of Drainage Device from Hepatobiliary Duct, Via Natural or Artificial Opening Endoscopic

0FPB81Z Removal of Radioactive Element from Hepatobiliary Duct, Via Natural or Artificial Opening Endoscopic

0FPB82Z Removal of Monitoring Device from Hepatobiliary Duct, Via Natural or Artificial Opening Endoscopic

0FPB83Z Removal of Infusion Device from Hepatobiliary Duct, Via Natural or Artificial Opening Endoscopic

0FPB87Z Removal of Autologous Tissue Substitute from Hepatobiliary Duct, Via Natural or Artificial Opening Endoscopic

0FPB8CZ Removal of Extraluminal Device from Hepatobiliary Duct, Via Natural or Artificial Opening Endoscopic

0FPB8DZ Removal of Intraluminal Device from Hepatobiliary Duct, Via Natural or Artificial Opening Endoscopic

0FPB8JZ Removal of Synthetic Substitute from Hepatobiliary Duct, Via Natural or Artificial Opening Endoscopic

0FPB8KZ Removal of Nonautologous Tissue Substitute from Hepatobiliary Duct, Via Natural or Artificial Opening Endoscopic

0FPBX0Z Removal of Drainage Device from Hepatobiliary Duct, External Approach

0FPBX1Z Removal of Radioactive Element from Hepatobiliary Duct, External Approach

0FPBX2Z Removal of Monitoring Device from Hepatobiliary Duct, External Approach

0FPBX3Z Removal of Infusion Device from Hepatobiliary Duct, External Approach

● **0FPBXDZ** Removal of Intraluminal Device from Hepatobiliary Duct, External Approach

0FPD00Z Removal of Drainage Device from Pancreatic Duct, Open Approach

0FPD01Z Removal of Radioactive Element from Pancreatic Duct, Open Approach

0FPD02Z Removal of Monitoring Device from Pancreatic Duct, Open Approach

0FPD03Z Removal of Infusion Device from Pancreatic Duct, Open Approach

0FPD07Z Removal of Autologous Tissue Substitute from Pancreatic Duct, Open Approach

0FPD0CZ Removal of Extraluminal Device from Pancreatic Duct, Open Approach

0FPD0DZ Removal of Intraluminal Device from Pancreatic Duct, Open Approach

0FPD0JZ Removal of Synthetic Substitute from Pancreatic Duct, Open Approach

0FPD0KZ Removal of Nonautologous Tissue Substitute from Pancreatic Duct, Open Approach

0FPD30Z Removal of Drainage Device from Pancreatic Duct, Percutaneous Approach

0FPD31Z Removal of Radioactive Element from Pancreatic Duct, Percutaneous Approach

0FPD32Z Removal of Monitoring Device from Pancreatic Duct, Percutaneous Approach

0FPD33Z Removal of Infusion Device from Pancreatic Duct, Percutaneous Approach

0FPD37Z Removal of Autologous Tissue Substitute from Pancreatic Duct, Percutaneous Approach

0FPD3CZ Removal of Extraluminal Device from Pancreatic Duct, Percutaneous Approach

0FPD3DZ Removal of Intraluminal Device from Pancreatic Duct, Percutaneous Approach

0FPD3JZ Removal of Synthetic Substitute from Pancreatic Duct, Percutaneous Approach

0FPD3KZ Removal of Nonautologous Tissue Substitute from Pancreatic Duct, Percutaneous Approach

0FPD40Z Removal of Drainage Device from Pancreatic Duct, Percutaneous Endoscopic Approach

0FPD41Z Removal of Radioactive Element from Pancreatic Duct, Percutaneous Endoscopic Approach

0FPD42Z Removal of Monitoring Device from Pancreatic Duct, Percutaneous Endoscopic Approach

0FPD43Z Removal of Infusion Device from Pancreatic Duct, Percutaneous Endoscopic Approach

0FPD47Z Removal of Autologous Tissue Substitute from Pancreatic Duct, Percutaneous Endoscopic Approach

0FPD4CZ Removal of Extraluminal Device from Pancreatic Duct, Percutaneous Endoscopic Approach

0FPD4DZ Removal of Intraluminal Device from Pancreatic Duct, Percutaneous Endoscopic Approach

0FPD4JZ Removal of Synthetic Substitute from Pancreatic Duct, Percutaneous Endoscopic Approach

0FPD4KZ Removal of Nonautologous Tissue Substitute from Pancreatic Duct, Percutaneous Endoscopic Approach

0FPD70Z Removal of Drainage Device from Pancreatic Duct, Via Natural or Artificial Opening

0FPD71Z Removal of Radioactive Element from Pancreatic Duct, Via Natural or Artificial Opening

0FPD72Z Removal of Monitoring Device from Pancreatic Duct, Via Natural or Artificial Opening

0FPD73Z Removal of Infusion Device from Pancreatic Duct, Via Natural or Artificial Opening

0FPD77Z Removal of Autologous Tissue Substitute from Pancreatic Duct, Via Natural or Artificial Opening

0FPD7CZ Removal of Extraluminal Device from Pancreatic Duct, Via Natural or Artificial Opening

Code	Description

0FPD7DZ   Removal of Intraluminal Device from Pancreatic Duct, Via Natural or Artificial Opening

0FPD7JZ   Removal of Synthetic Substitute from Pancreatic Duct, Via Natural or Artificial Opening

0FPD7KZ   Removal of Nonautologous Tissue Substitute from Pancreatic Duct, Via Natural or Artificial Opening

0FPD80Z   Removal of Drainage Device from Pancreatic Duct, Via Natural or Artificial Opening Endoscopic

0FPD81Z   Removal of Radioactive Element from Pancreatic Duct, Via Natural or Artificial Opening Endoscopic

0FPD82Z   Removal of Monitoring Device from Pancreatic Duct, Via Natural or Artificial Opening Endoscopic

0FPD83Z   Removal of Infusion Device from Pancreatic Duct, Via Natural or Artificial Opening Endoscopic

0FPD87Z   Removal of Autologous Tissue Substitute from Pancreatic Duct, Via Natural or Artificial Opening Endoscopic

0FPD8CZ   Removal of Extraluminal Device from Pancreatic Duct, Via Natural or Artificial Opening Endoscopic

0FPD8DZ   Removal of Intraluminal Device from Pancreatic Duct, Via Natural or Artificial Opening Endoscopic

0FPD8JZ   Removal of Synthetic Substitute from Pancreatic Duct, Via Natural or Artificial Opening Endoscopic

0FPD8KZ   Removal of Nonautologous Tissue Substitute from Pancreatic Duct, Via Natural or Artificial Opening Endoscopic

0FPDX0Z   Removal of Drainage Device from Pancreatic Duct, External Approach

0FPDX1Z   Removal of Radioactive Element from Pancreatic Duct, External Approach

0FPDX2Z   Removal of Monitoring Device from Pancreatic Duct, External Approach

0FPDX3Z   Removal of Infusion Device from Pancreatic Duct, External Approach

● 0FPDXDZ   Removal of Intraluminal Device from Pancreatic Duct, External Approach

0FPG00Z   Removal of Drainage Device from Pancreas, Open Approach

0FPG02Z   Removal of Monitoring Device from Pancreas, Open Approach

0FPG03Z   Removal of Infusion Device from Pancreas, Open Approach

0FPG0DZ   Removal of Intraluminal Device from Pancreas, Open Approach

0FPG30Z   Removal of Drainage Device from Pancreas, Percutaneous Approach

0FPG32Z   Removal of Monitoring Device from Pancreas, Percutaneous Approach

0FPG33Z   Removal of Infusion Device from Pancreas, Percutaneous Approach

0FPG3DZ   Removal of Intraluminal Device from Pancreas, Percutaneous Approach

0FPG40Z   Removal of Drainage Device from Pancreas, Percutaneous Endoscopic Approach

0FPG42Z   Removal of Monitoring Device from Pancreas, Percutaneous Endoscopic Approach

0FPG43Z   Removal of Infusion Device from Pancreas, Percutaneous Endoscopic Approach

0FPG4DZ   Removal of Intraluminal Device from Pancreas, Percutaneous Endoscopic Approach

0FPGX0Z   Removal of Drainage Device from Pancreas, External Approach

0FPGX2Z   Removal of Monitoring Device from Pancreas, External Approach

0FPGX3Z   Removal of Infusion Device from Pancreas, External Approach

0FPGXDZ   Removal of Intraluminal Device from Pancreas, External Approach

0FQ – Hepatobiliary System and Pancreas, Repair

0FQ00ZZ   Repair Liver, Open Approach
    AHA CC: 4Q, 2013, 109-111

0FQ03ZZ   Repair Liver, Percutaneous Approach

0FQ04ZZ   Repair Liver, Percutaneous Endoscopic Approach

0FQ10ZZ   Repair Right Lobe Liver, Open Approach

0FQ13ZZ   Repair Right Lobe Liver, Percutaneous Approach

0FQ14ZZ   Repair Right Lobe Liver, Percutaneous Endoscopic Approach

0FQ20ZZ   Repair Left Lobe Liver, Open Approach

0FQ23ZZ   Repair Left Lobe Liver, Percutaneous Approach

0FQ24ZZ   Repair Left Lobe Liver, Percutaneous Endoscopic Approach

0FQ40ZZ   Repair Gallbladder, Open Approach

0FQ43ZZ   Repair Gallbladder, Percutaneous Approach

0FQ44ZZ   Repair Gallbladder, Percutaneous Endoscopic Approach

0FQ50ZZ   Repair Right Hepatic Duct, Open Approach

0FQ53ZZ   Repair Right Hepatic Duct, Percutaneous Approach

0FQ54ZZ   Repair Right Hepatic Duct, Percutaneous Endoscopic Approach

0FQ57ZZ   Repair Right Hepatic Duct, Via Natural or Artificial Opening

0FQ58ZZ   Repair Right Hepatic Duct, Via Natural or Artificial Opening Endoscopic

0FQ60ZZ   Repair Left Hepatic Duct, Open Approach

0FQ63ZZ   Repair Left Hepatic Duct, Percutaneous Approach

0FQ64ZZ   Repair Left Hepatic Duct, Percutaneous Endoscopic Approach

0FQ67ZZ   Repair Left Hepatic Duct, Via Natural or Artificial Opening

0FQ68ZZ   Repair Left Hepatic Duct, Via Natural or Artificial Opening Endoscopic

0FQ80ZZ   Repair Cystic Duct, Open Approach

0FQ83ZZ   Repair Cystic Duct, Percutaneous Approach

0FQ84ZZ   Repair Cystic Duct, Percutaneous Endoscopic Approach

0FQ87ZZ   Repair Cystic Duct, Via Natural or Artificial Opening

0FQ88ZZ   Repair Cystic Duct, Via Natural or Artificial Opening Endoscopic

0FQ90ZZ   Repair Common Bile Duct, Open Approach

0FQ93ZZ   Repair Common Bile Duct, Percutaneous Approach

0FQ94ZZ   Repair Common Bile Duct, Percutaneous Endoscopic Approach

0FQ97ZZ   Repair Common Bile Duct, Via Natural or Artificial Opening

0FQ98ZZ   Repair Common Bile Duct, Via Natural or Artificial Opening Endoscopic

0FQC0ZZ   Repair Ampulla of Vater, Open Approach

0FQC3ZZ   Repair Ampulla of Vater, Percutaneous Approach

0FQC4ZZ   Repair Ampulla of Vater, Percutaneous Endoscopic Approach

0FQC7ZZ   Repair Ampulla of Vater, Via Natural or Artificial Opening

0FQC8ZZ   Repair Ampulla of Vater, Via Natural or Artificial Opening Endoscopic

0FQD0ZZ   Repair Pancreatic Duct, Open Approach

0FQD3ZZ   Repair Pancreatic Duct, Percutaneous Approach

0FQD4ZZ   Repair Pancreatic Duct, Percutaneous Endoscopic Approach

0FQD7ZZ   Repair Pancreatic Duct, Via Natural or Artificial Opening

0FQD8ZZ   Repair Pancreatic Duct, Via Natural or Artificial Opening Endoscopic

0FQF0ZZ   Repair Accessory Pancreatic Duct, Open Approach

0FQF3ZZ   Repair Accessory Pancreatic Duct, Percutaneous Approach

0FQF4ZZ   Repair Accessory Pancreatic Duct, Percutaneous Endoscopic Approach

0FQF7ZZ   Repair Accessory Pancreatic Duct, Via Natural or Artificial Opening

0FQF8ZZ   Repair Accessory Pancreatic Duct, Via Natural or Artificial Opening Endoscopic

0FQG0ZZ   Repair Pancreas, Open Approach

0FQG3ZZ   Repair Pancreas, Percutaneous Approach

0FQG4ZZ   Repair Pancreas, Percutaneous Endoscopic Approach

0FR – Hepatobiliary System and Pancreas, Replacement

0FR507Z   Replacement of Right Hepatic Duct with Autologous Tissue Substitute, Open Approach

0FR50JZ   Replacement of Right Hepatic Duct with Synthetic Substitute, Open Approach

0FR50KZ   Replacement of Right Hepatic Duct with Nonautologous Tissue Substitute, Open Approach

0FR547Z   Replacement of Right Hepatic Duct with Autologous Tissue Substitute, Percutaneous Endoscopic Approach

0FR54JZ   Replacement of Right Hepatic Duct with Synthetic Substitute, Percutaneous Endoscopic Approach

0FR54KZ   Replacement of Right Hepatic Duct with Nonautologous Tissue Substitute, Percutaneous Endoscopic Approach

0FR607Z   Replacement of Left Hepatic Duct with Autologous Tissue Substitute, Open Approach

0FR60JZ   Replacement of Left Hepatic Duct with Synthetic Substitute, Open Approach

0FR60KZ   Replacement of Left Hepatic Duct with Nonautologous Tissue Substitute, Open Approach

0FR647Z   Replacement of Left Hepatic Duct with Autologous Tissue Substitute, Percutaneous Endoscopic Approach

0FR64JZ   Replacement of Left Hepatic Duct with Synthetic Substitute, Percutaneous Endoscopic Approach

0FR64KZ   Replacement of Left Hepatic Duct with Nonautologous Tissue Substitute, Percutaneous Endoscopic Approach

| Female-only | ♂ Male-only | ▲ Limited Coverage | ● Non-OR | ▥ HAC-associated procedure | ▲ Non-covered procedures | ✚ Combination |

0FR807Z Replacement of Cystic Duct with Autologous Tissue Substitute, Open Approach

0FR80JZ Replacement of Cystic Duct with Synthetic Substitute, Open Approach

0FR80KZ Replacement of Cystic Duct with Nonautologous Tissue Substitute, Open Approach

0FR847Z Replacement of Cystic Duct with Autologous Tissue Substitute, Percutaneous Endoscopic Approach

0FR84JZ Replacement of Cystic Duct with Synthetic Substitute, Percutaneous Endoscopic Approach

0FR84KZ Replacement of Cystic Duct with Nonautologous Tissue Substitute, Percutaneous Endoscopic Approach

0FR907Z Replacement of Common Bile Duct with Autologous Tissue Substitute, Open Approach

0FR90JZ Replacement of Common Bile Duct with Synthetic Substitute, Open Approach

0FR90KZ Replacement of Common Bile Duct with Nonautologous Tissue Substitute, Open Approach

0FR947Z Replacement of Common Bile Duct with Autologous Tissue Substitute, Percutaneous Endoscopic Approach

0FR94JZ Replacement of Common Bile Duct with Synthetic Substitute, Percutaneous Endoscopic Approach

0FR94KZ Replacement of Common Bile Duct with Nonautologous Tissue Substitute, Percutaneous Endoscopic Approach

0FRC07Z Replacement of Ampulla of Vater with Autologous Tissue Substitute, Open Approach

0FRC0JZ Replacement of Ampulla of Vater with Synthetic Substitute, Open Approach

0FRC0KZ Replacement of Ampulla of Vater with Nonautologous Tissue Substitute, Open Approach

0FRC47Z Replacement of Ampulla of Vater with Autologous Tissue Substitute, Percutaneous Endoscopic Approach

0FRC4JZ Replacement of Ampulla of Vater with Synthetic Substitute, Percutaneous Endoscopic Approach

0FRC4KZ Replacement of Ampulla of Vater with Nonautologous Tissue Substitute, Percutaneous Endoscopic Approach

0FRD07Z Replacement of Pancreatic Duct with Autologous Tissue Substitute, Open Approach

0FRD0JZ Replacement of Pancreatic Duct with Synthetic Substitute, Open Approach

0FRD0KZ Replacement of Pancreatic Duct with Nonautologous Tissue Substitute, Open Approach

0FRD47Z Replacement of Pancreatic Duct with Autologous Tissue Substitute, Percutaneous Endoscopic Approach

0FRD4JZ Replacement of Pancreatic Duct with Synthetic Substitute, Percutaneous Endoscopic Approach

0FRD4KZ Replacement of Pancreatic Duct with Nonautologous Tissue Substitute, Percutaneous Endoscopic Approach

0FRF07Z Replacement of Accessory Pancreatic Duct with Autologous Tissue Substitute, Open Approach

0FRF0JZ Replacement of Accessory Pancreatic Duct with Synthetic Substitute, Open Approach

0FRF0KZ Replacement of Accessory Pancreatic Duct with Nonautologous Tissue Substitute, Open Approach

0FRF47Z Replacement of Accessory Pancreatic Duct with Autologous Tissue Substitute, Percutaneous Endoscopic Approach

0FRF4JZ Replacement of Accessory Pancreatic Duct with Synthetic Substitute, Percutaneous Endoscopic Approach

0FRF4KZ Replacement of Accessory Pancreatic Duct with Nonautologous Tissue Substitute, Percutaneous Endoscopic Approach

0FS – Hepatobiliary System and Pancreas, Reposition

0FS00ZZ Reposition Liver, Open Approach

0FS04ZZ Reposition Liver, Percutaneous Endoscopic Approach

0FS40ZZ Reposition Gallbladder, Open Approach

0FS44ZZ Reposition Gallbladder, Percutaneous Endoscopic Approach

0FS50ZZ Reposition Right Hepatic Duct, Open Approach

0FS54ZZ Reposition Right Hepatic Duct, Percutaneous Endoscopic Approach

0FS60ZZ Reposition Left Hepatic Duct, Open Approach

0FS64ZZ Reposition Left Hepatic Duct, Percutaneous Endoscopic Approach

0FS80ZZ Reposition Cystic Duct, Open Approach

0FS84ZZ Reposition Cystic Duct, Percutaneous Endoscopic Approach

0FS90ZZ Reposition Common Bile Duct, Open Approach

0FS94ZZ Reposition Common Bile Duct, Percutaneous Endoscopic Approach

0FSC0ZZ Reposition Ampulla of Vater, Open Approach

0FSC4ZZ Reposition Ampulla of Vater, Percutaneous Endoscopic Approach

0FSD0ZZ Reposition Pancreatic Duct, Open Approach

0FSD4ZZ Reposition Pancreatic Duct, Percutaneous Endoscopic Approach

0FSF0ZZ Reposition Accessory Pancreatic Duct, Open Approach

0FSF4ZZ Reposition Accessory Pancreatic Duct, Percutaneous Endoscopic Approach

0FSG0ZZ Reposition Pancreas, Open Approach

0FSG4ZZ Reposition Pancreas, Percutaneous Endoscopic Approach

0FT – Hepatobiliary System and Pancreas, Resection

Review Coding Guideline B3.8

0FT00ZZ Resection of Liver, Open Approach
AHA CC: 4Q, 2012, 99-101

0FT04ZZ Resection of Liver, Percutaneous Endoscopic Approach

0FT10ZZ Resection of Right Lobe Liver, Open Approach

0FT14ZZ Resection of Right Lobe Liver, Percutaneous Endoscopic Approach

0FT20ZZ Resection of Left Lobe Liver, Open Approach

0FT24ZZ Resection of Left Lobe Liver, Percutaneous Endoscopic Approach

0FT40ZZ Resection of Gallbladder, Open Approach

0FT44ZZ Resection of Gallbladder, Percutaneous Endoscopic Approach

0FT50ZZ Resection of Right Hepatic Duct, Open Approach

0FT54ZZ Resection of Right Hepatic Duct, Percutaneous Endoscopic Approach

0FT57ZZ Resection of Right Hepatic Duct, Via Natural or Artificial Opening

0FT58ZZ Resection of Right Hepatic Duct, Via Natural or Artificial Opening Endoscopic

0FT60ZZ Resection of Left Hepatic Duct, Open Approach

0FT64ZZ Resection of Left Hepatic Duct, Percutaneous Endoscopic Approach

0FT67ZZ Resection of Left Hepatic Duct, Via Natural or Artificial Opening

0FT68ZZ Resection of Left Hepatic Duct, Via Natural or Artificial Opening Endoscopic

0FT80ZZ Resection of Cystic Duct, Open Approach

0FT84ZZ Resection of Cystic Duct, Percutaneous Endoscopic Approach

0FT87ZZ Resection of Cystic Duct, Via Natural or Artificial Opening

0FT88ZZ Resection of Cystic Duct, Via Natural or Artificial Opening Endoscopic

0FT90ZZ Resection of Common Bile Duct, Open Approach

0FT94ZZ Resection of Common Bile Duct, Percutaneous Endoscopic Approach

0FT97ZZ Resection of Common Bile Duct, Via Natural or Artificial Opening

0FT98ZZ Resection of Common Bile Duct, Via Natural or Artificial Opening Endoscopic

0FTC0ZZ Resection of Ampulla of Vater, Open Approach

0FTC4ZZ Resection of Ampulla of Vater, Percutaneous Endoscopic Approach

0FTC7ZZ Resection of Ampulla of Vater, Via Natural or Artificial Opening

0FTC8ZZ Resection of Ampulla of Vater, Via Natural or Artificial Opening Endoscopic

0FTD0ZZ Resection of Pancreatic Duct, Open Approach

0FTD4ZZ Resection of Pancreatic Duct, Percutaneous Endoscopic Approach

0FTD7ZZ Resection of Pancreatic Duct, Via Natural or Artificial Opening

0FTD8ZZ Resection of Pancreatic Duct, Via Natural or Artificial Opening Endoscopic

0FTF0ZZ Resection of Accessory Pancreatic Duct, Open Approach

0FTF4ZZ Resection of Accessory Pancreatic Duct, Percutaneous Endoscopic Approach

0FTF7ZZ Resection of Accessory Pancreatic Duct, Via Natural or Artificial Opening

0FTF8ZZ Resection of Accessory Pancreatic Duct, Via Natural or Artificial Opening Endoscopic

0FTG0ZZ Resection of Pancreas, Open Approach

0FTG4ZZ Resection of Pancreas, Percutaneous Endoscopic Approach

♀ Female-only   ♂ Male-only   ▲ Limited Coverage   ● Non-OR   ▨ HAC-associated procedure   ▲ Non-covered procedures   ✚ Combination

U – Hepatobiliary System and Pancreas, Supplement

J507Z Supplement Right Hepatic Duct with Autologous Tissue Substitute, Open Approach

J50JZ Supplement Right Hepatic Duct with Synthetic Substitute, Open Approach

J50KZ Supplement Right Hepatic Duct with Nonautologous Tissue Substitute, Open Approach

J537Z Supplement Right Hepatic Duct with Autologous Tissue Substitute, Percutaneous Approach

U53JZ Supplement Right Hepatic Duct with Synthetic Substitute, Percutaneous Approach

U53KZ Supplement Right Hepatic Duct with Nonautologous Tissue Substitute, Percutaneous Approach

U547Z Supplement Right Hepatic Duct with Autologous Tissue Substitute, Percutaneous Endoscopic Approach

U54JZ Supplement Right Hepatic Duct with Synthetic Substitute, Percutaneous Endoscopic Approach

U54KZ Supplement Right Hepatic Duct with Nonautologous Tissue Substitute, Percutaneous Endoscopic Approach

U607Z Supplement Left Hepatic Duct with Autologous Tissue Substitute, Open Approach

U60JZ Supplement Left Hepatic Duct with Synthetic Substitute, Open Approach

U60KZ Supplement Left Hepatic Duct with Nonautologous Tissue Substitute, Open Approach

U637Z Supplement Left Hepatic Duct with Autologous Tissue Substitute, Percutaneous Approach

U63JZ Supplement Left Hepatic Duct with Synthetic Substitute, Percutaneous Approach

U63KZ Supplement Left Hepatic Duct with Nonautologous Tissue Substitute, Percutaneous Approach

U647Z Supplement Left Hepatic Duct with Autologous Tissue Substitute, Percutaneous Endoscopic Approach

U64JZ Supplement Left Hepatic Duct with Synthetic Substitute, Percutaneous Endoscopic Approach

U64KZ Supplement Left Hepatic Duct with Nonautologous Tissue Substitute, Percutaneous Endoscopic Approach

U807Z Supplement Cystic Duct with Autologous Tissue Substitute, Open Approach

U80JZ Supplement Cystic Duct with Synthetic Substitute, Open Approach

U80KZ Supplement Cystic Duct with Nonautologous Tissue Substitute, Open Approach

0FU837Z Supplement Cystic Duct with Autologous Tissue Substitute, Percutaneous Approach

0FU83JZ Supplement Cystic Duct with Synthetic Substitute, Percutaneous Approach

0FU83KZ Supplement Cystic Duct with Nonautologous Tissue Substitute, Percutaneous Approach

0FU847Z Supplement Cystic Duct with Autologous Tissue Substitute, Percutaneous Endoscopic Approach

0FU84JZ Supplement Cystic Duct with Synthetic Substitute, Percutaneous Endoscopic Approach

0FU84KZ Supplement Cystic Duct with Nonautologous Tissue Substitute, Percutaneous Endoscopic Approach

0FU907Z Supplement Common Bile Duct with Autologous Tissue Substitute, Open Approach

0FU90JZ Supplement Common Bile Duct with Synthetic Substitute, Open Approach

0FU90KZ Supplement Common Bile Duct with Nonautologous Tissue Substitute, Open Approach

0FU937Z Supplement Common Bile Duct with Autologous Tissue Substitute, Percutaneous Approach

0FU93JZ Supplement Common Bile Duct with Synthetic Substitute, Percutaneous Approach

0FU93KZ Supplement Common Bile Duct with Nonautologous Tissue Substitute, Percutaneous Approach

0FU947Z Supplement Common Bile Duct with Autologous Tissue Substitute, Percutaneous Endoscopic Approach

0FU94JZ Supplement Common Bile Duct with Synthetic Substitute, Percutaneous Endoscopic Approach

0FU94KZ Supplement Common Bile Duct with Nonautologous Tissue Substitute, Percutaneous Endoscopic Approach

0FUC07Z Supplement Ampulla of Vater with Autologous Tissue Substitute, Open Approach

0FUC0JZ Supplement Ampulla of Vater with Synthetic Substitute, Open Approach

0FUC0KZ Supplement Ampulla of Vater with Nonautologous Tissue Substitute, Open Approach

0FUC37Z Supplement Ampulla of Vater with Autologous Tissue Substitute, Percutaneous Approach

0FUC3JZ Supplement Ampulla of Vater with Synthetic Substitute, Percutaneous Approach

0FUC3KZ Supplement Ampulla of Vater with Nonautologous Tissue Substitute, Percutaneous Approach

0FUC47Z Supplement Ampulla of Vater with Autologous Tissue Substitute, Percutaneous Endoscopic Approach

0FUC4JZ Supplement Ampulla of Vater with Synthetic Substitute, Percutaneous Endoscopic Approach

0FUC4KZ Supplement Ampulla of Vater with Nonautologous Tissue Substitute, Percutaneous Endoscopic Approach

0FUD07Z Supplement Pancreatic Duct with Autologous Tissue Substitute, Open Approach

0FUD0JZ Supplement Pancreatic Duct with Synthetic Substitute, Open Approach

0FUD0KZ Supplement Pancreatic Duct with Nonautologous Tissue Substitute, Open Approach

0FUD37Z Supplement Pancreatic Duct with Autologous Tissue Substitute, Percutaneous Approach

0FUD3JZ Supplement Pancreatic Duct with Synthetic Substitute, Percutaneous Approach

0FUD3KZ Supplement Pancreatic Duct with Nonautologous Tissue Substitute, Percutaneous Approach

0FUD47Z Supplement Pancreatic Duct with Autologous Tissue Substitute, Percutaneous Endoscopic Approach

0FUD4JZ Supplement Pancreatic Duct with Synthetic Substitute, Percutaneous Endoscopic Approach

0FUD4KZ Supplement Pancreatic Duct with Nonautologous Tissue Substitute, Percutaneous Endoscopic Approach

0FUF07Z Supplement Accessory Pancreatic Duct with Autologous Tissue Substitute, Open Approach

0FUF0JZ Supplement Accessory Pancreatic Duct with Synthetic Substitute, Open Approach

0FUF0KZ Supplement Accessory Pancreatic Duct with Nonautologous Tissue Substitute, Open Approach

0FUF37Z Supplement Accessory Pancreatic Duct with Autologous Tissue Substitute, Percutaneous Approach

0FUF3JZ Supplement Accessory Pancreatic Duct with Synthetic Substitute, Percutaneous Approach

0FUF3KZ Supplement Accessory Pancreatic Duct with Nonautologous Tissue Substitute, Percutaneous Approach

0FUF47Z Supplement Accessory Pancreatic Duct with Autologous Tissue Substitute, Percutaneous Endoscopic Approach

0FUF4JZ Supplement Accessory Pancreatic Duct with Synthetic Substitute, Percutaneous Endoscopic Approach

0FUF4KZ Supplement Accessory Pancreatic Duct with Nonautologous Tissue Substitute, Percutaneous Endoscopic Approach

FV – Hepatobiliary System and Pancreas, Restriction

FV50CZ Restriction of Right Hepatic Duct with Extraluminal Device, Open Approach

FV50DZ Restriction of Right Hepatic Duct with Intraluminal Device, Open Approach

FV50ZZ Restriction of Right Hepatic Duct, Open Approach

FV53CZ Restriction of Right Hepatic Duct with Extraluminal Device, Percutaneous Approach

FV53DZ Restriction of Right Hepatic Duct with Intraluminal Device, Percutaneous Approach

0FV53ZZ Restriction of Right Hepatic Duct, Percutaneous Approach

0FV54CZ Restriction of Right Hepatic Duct with Extraluminal Device, Percutaneous Endoscopic Approach

0FV54DZ Restriction of Right Hepatic Duct with Intraluminal Device, Percutaneous Endoscopic Approach

0FV54ZZ Restriction of Right Hepatic Duct, Percutaneous Endoscopic Approach

0FV57DZ Restriction of Right Hepatic Duct with Intraluminal Device, Via Natural or Artificial Opening

0FV57ZZ Restriction of Right Hepatic Duct, Via Natural or Artificial Opening

0FV58DZ Restriction of Right Hepatic Duct with Intraluminal Device, Via Natural or Artificial Opening Endoscopic

0FV58ZZ Restriction of Right Hepatic Duct, Via Natural or Artificial Opening Endoscopic

0FV60CZ Restriction of Left Hepatic Duct with Extraluminal Device, Open Approach

♀ Female-only   ♂ Male-only   ▲ Limited Coverage   ● Non-OR   ▦ HAC-associated procedure   ▲ Non-covered procedures   ✚ Combination

0FV60DZ Restriction of Left Hepatic Duct with Intraluminal Device, Open Approach

0FV60ZZ Restriction of Left Hepatic Duct, Open Approach

0FV63CZ Restriction of Left Hepatic Duct with Extraluminal Device, Percutaneous Approach

0FV63DZ Restriction of Left Hepatic Duct with Intraluminal Device, Percutaneous Approach

0FV63ZZ Restriction of Left Hepatic Duct, Percutaneous Approach

0FV64CZ Restriction of Left Hepatic Duct with Extraluminal Device, Percutaneous Endoscopic Approach

0FV64DZ Restriction of Left Hepatic Duct with Intraluminal Device, Percutaneous Endoscopic Approach

0FV64ZZ Restriction of Left Hepatic Duct, Percutaneous Endoscopic Approach

0FV67DZ Restriction of Left Hepatic Duct with Intraluminal Device, Via Natural or Artificial Opening

0FV67ZZ Restriction of Left Hepatic Duct, Via Natural or Artificial Opening

0FV68DZ Restriction of Left Hepatic Duct with Intraluminal Device, Via Natural or Artificial Opening Endoscopic

0FV68ZZ Restriction of Left Hepatic Duct, Via Natural or Artificial Opening Endoscopic

0FV80CZ Restriction of Cystic Duct with Extraluminal Device, Open Approach

0FV80DZ Restriction of Cystic Duct with Intraluminal Device, Open Approach

0FV80ZZ Restriction of Cystic Duct, Open Approach

0FV83CZ Restriction of Cystic Duct with Extraluminal Device, Percutaneous Approach

0FV83DZ Restriction of Cystic Duct with Intraluminal Device, Percutaneous Approach

0FV83ZZ Restriction of Cystic Duct, Percutaneous Approach

0FV84CZ Restriction of Cystic Duct with Extraluminal Device, Percutaneous Endoscopic Approach

0FV84DZ Restriction of Cystic Duct with Intraluminal Device, Percutaneous Endoscopic Approach

0FV84ZZ Restriction of Cystic Duct, Percutaneous Endoscopic Approach

0FV87DZ Restriction of Cystic Duct with Intraluminal Device, Via Natural or Artificial Opening

0FV87ZZ Restriction of Cystic Duct, Via Natural or Artificial Opening

0FV88DZ Restriction of Cystic Duct with Intraluminal Device, Via Natural or Artificial Opening Endoscopic

0FV88ZZ Restriction of Cystic Duct, Via Natural or Artificial Opening Endoscopic

0FV90CZ Restriction of Common Bile Duct with Extraluminal Device, Open Approach

0FV90DZ Restriction of Common Bile Duct with Intraluminal Device, Open Approach

0FV90ZZ Restriction of Common Bile Duct, Open Approach

0FV93CZ Restriction of Common Bile Duct with Extraluminal Device, Percutaneous Approach

0FV93DZ Restriction of Common Bile Duct with Intraluminal Device, Percutaneous Approach

0FV93ZZ Restriction of Common Bile Duct, Percutaneous Approach

0FV94CZ Restriction of Common Bile Duct with Extraluminal Device, Percutaneous Endoscopic Approach

0FV94DZ Restriction of Common Bile Duct with Intraluminal Device, Percutaneous Endoscopic Approach

0FV94ZZ Restriction of Common Bile Duct, Percutaneous Endoscopic Approach

0FV97DZ Restriction of Common Bile Duct with Intraluminal Device, Via Natural or Artificial Opening

0FV97ZZ Restriction of Common Bile Duct, Via Natural or Artificial Opening

0FV98DZ Restriction of Common Bile Duct with Intraluminal Device, Via Natural or Artificial Opening Endoscopic

0FV98ZZ Restriction of Common Bile Duct, Via Natural or Artificial Opening Endoscopic

0FVC0CZ Restriction of Ampulla of Vater with Extraluminal Device, Open Approach

0FVC0DZ Restriction of Ampulla of Vater with Intraluminal Device, Open Approach

0FVC0ZZ Restriction of Ampulla of Vater, Open Approach

0FVC3CZ Restriction of Ampulla of Vater with Extraluminal Device, Percutaneous Approach

0FVC3DZ Restriction of Ampulla of Vater with Intraluminal Device, Percutaneous Approach

0FVC3ZZ Restriction of Ampulla of Vater, Percutaneous Approach

0FVC4CZ Restriction of Ampulla of Vater with Extraluminal Device, Percutaneous Endoscopic Approach

0FVC4DZ Restriction of Ampulla of Vater with Intraluminal Device, Percutaneous Endoscopic Approach

0FVC4ZZ Restriction of Ampulla of Vater, Percutaneous Endoscopic Approach

0FVC7DZ Restriction of Ampulla of Vater with Intraluminal Device, Via Natural or Artificial Opening

0FVC7ZZ Restriction of Ampulla of Vater, Via Natural or Artificial Opening

0FVC8DZ Restriction of Ampulla of Vater with Intraluminal Device, Via Natural or Artificial Opening Endoscopic

0FVC8ZZ Restriction of Ampulla of Vater, Via Natural or Artificial Opening Endoscopic

0FVD0CZ Restriction of Pancreatic Duct with Extraluminal Device, Open Approach

0FVD0DZ Restriction of Pancreatic Duct with Intraluminal Device, Open Approach

0FVD0ZZ Restriction of Pancreatic Duct, Open Approach

0FVD3CZ Restriction of Pancreatic Duct with Extraluminal Device, Percutaneous Approach

0FVD3DZ Restriction of Pancreatic Duct with Intraluminal Device, Percutaneous Approach

0FVD3ZZ Restriction of Pancreatic Duct, Percutaneous Approach

0FVD4CZ Restriction of Pancreatic Duct with Extraluminal Device, Percutaneous Endoscopic Approach

0FVD4DZ Restriction of Pancreatic Duct with Intraluminal Device, Percutaneous Endoscopic Approach

0FVD4ZZ Restriction of Pancreatic Duct, Percutaneous Endoscopic Approach

0FVD7DZ Restriction of Pancreatic Duct with Intraluminal Device, Via Natural or Artificial Opening

0FVD7ZZ Restriction of Pancreatic Duct, Via Natural or Artificial Opening

0FVD8DZ Restriction of Pancreatic Duct with Intraluminal Device, Via Natural or Artificial Opening Endoscopic

0FVD8ZZ Restriction of Pancreatic Duct, Via Natural or Artificial Opening Endoscopic

0FVF0CZ Restriction of Accessory Pancreatic Duct with Extraluminal Device, Open Approach

0FVF0DZ Restriction of Accessory Pancreatic Duct with Intraluminal Device, Open Approach

0FVF0ZZ Restriction of Accessory Pancreatic Duct, Open Approach

0FVF3CZ Restriction of Accessory Pancreatic Duct with Extraluminal Device, Percutaneous Approach

0FVF3DZ Restriction of Accessory Pancreatic Duct with Intraluminal Device, Percutaneous Approach

0FVF3ZZ Restriction of Accessory Pancreatic Duct, Percutaneous Approach

0FVF4CZ Restriction of Accessory Pancreatic Duct with Extraluminal Device, Percutaneous Endoscopic Approach

0FVF4DZ Restriction of Accessory Pancreatic Duct with Intraluminal Device, Percutaneous Endoscopic Approach

0FVF4ZZ Restriction of Accessory Pancreatic Duct, Percutaneous Endoscopic Approach

0FVF7DZ Restriction of Accessory Pancreatic Duct with Intraluminal Device, Via Natural or Artificial Opening

0FVF7ZZ Restriction of Accessory Pancreatic Duct Via Natural or Artificial Opening

0FVF8DZ Restriction of Accessory Pancreatic Duct with Intraluminal Device, Via Natural or Artificial Opening Endoscopic

0FVF8ZZ Restriction of Accessory Pancreatic Duct, Via Natural or Artificial Opening Endoscopic

0FW – Hepatobiliary System and Pancreas, Revision

Review Coding Guideline B6.1c

0FW000Z Revision of Drainage Device in Liver, Open Approach

0FW002Z Revision of Monitoring Device in Liver, Open Approach

0FW003Z Revision of Infusion Device in Liver, Open Approach

0FW030Z Revision of Drainage Device in Liver, Percutaneous Approach

0FW032Z Revision of Monitoring Device in Liver, Percutaneous Approach

0FW033Z Revision of Infusion Device in Liver, Percutaneous Approach

0FW040Z Revision of Drainage Device in Liver, Percutaneous Endoscopic Approach

0FW042Z Revision of Monitoring Device in Liver, Percutaneous Endoscopic Approach

0FW043Z Revision of Infusion Device in Liver, Percutaneous Endoscopic Approach

0FW0X0Z Revision of Drainage Device in Liver, External Approach

0FW0X2Z Revision of Monitoring Device in Liver, External Approach

0FW0X3Z Revision of Infusion Device in Liver, External Approach

♀ Female-only ♂ Male-only ▲ Limited Coverage ● Non-OR ▨ HAC-associated procedure ▲ Non-covered procedures ✛ Combination

0FW400Z Revision of Drainage Device in Gallbladder, Open Approach

0FW402Z Revision of Monitoring Device in Gallbladder, Open Approach

0FW403Z Revision of Infusion Device in Gallbladder, Open Approach

0FW40DZ Revision of Intraluminal Device in Gallbladder, Open Approach

0FW430Z Revision of Drainage Device in Gallbladder, Percutaneous Approach

0FW432Z Revision of Monitoring Device in Gallbladder, Percutaneous Approach

0FW433Z Revision of Infusion Device in Gallbladder, Percutaneous Approach

0FW43DZ Revision of Intraluminal Device in Gallbladder, Percutaneous Approach

0FW440Z Revision of Drainage Device in Gallbladder, Percutaneous Endoscopic Approach

0FW442Z Revision of Monitoring Device in Gallbladder, Percutaneous Endoscopic Approach

0FW443Z Revision of Infusion Device in Gallbladder, Percutaneous Endoscopic Approach

0FW44DZ Revision of Intraluminal Device in Gallbladder, Percutaneous Endoscopic Approach

0FW4X0Z Revision of Drainage Device in Gallbladder, External Approach

0FW4X2Z Revision of Monitoring Device in Gallbladder, External Approach

0FW4X3Z Revision of Infusion Device in Gallbladder, External Approach

0FW4XDZ Revision of Intraluminal Device in Gallbladder, External Approach

0FWB00Z Revision of Drainage Device in Hepatobiliary Duct, Open Approach

0FWB02Z Revision of Monitoring Device in Hepatobiliary Duct, Open Approach

0FWB03Z Revision of Infusion Device in Hepatobiliary Duct, Open Approach

0FWB07Z Revision of Autologous Tissue Substitute in Hepatobiliary Duct, Open Approach

0FWB0CZ Revision of Extraluminal Device in Hepatobiliary Duct, Open Approach

0FWB0DZ Revision of Intraluminal Device in Hepatobiliary Duct, Open Approach

0FWB0JZ Revision of Synthetic Substitute in Hepatobiliary Duct, Open Approach

0FWB0KZ Revision of Nonautologous Tissue Substitute in Hepatobiliary Duct, Open Approach

0FWB30Z Revision of Drainage Device in Hepatobiliary Duct, Percutaneous Approach

0FWB32Z Revision of Monitoring Device in Hepatobiliary Duct, Percutaneous Approach

0FWB33Z Revision of Infusion Device in Hepatobiliary Duct, Percutaneous Approach

0FWB37Z Revision of Autologous Tissue Substitute in Hepatobiliary Duct, Percutaneous Approach

0FWB3CZ Revision of Extraluminal Device in Hepatobiliary Duct, Percutaneous Approach

0FWB3DZ Revision of Intraluminal Device in Hepatobiliary Duct, Percutaneous Approach

0FWB3JZ Revision of Synthetic Substitute in Hepatobiliary Duct, Percutaneous Approach

0FWB3KZ Revision of Nonautologous Tissue Substitute in Hepatobiliary Duct, Percutaneous Approach

0FWB40Z Revision of Drainage Device in Hepatobiliary Duct, Percutaneous Endoscopic Approach

0FWB42Z Revision of Monitoring Device in Hepatobiliary Duct, Percutaneous Endoscopic Approach

0FWB43Z Revision of Infusion Device in Hepatobiliary Duct, Percutaneous Endoscopic Approach

0FWB47Z Revision of Autologous Tissue Substitute in Hepatobiliary Duct, Percutaneous Endoscopic Approach

0FWB4CZ Revision of Extraluminal Device in Hepatobiliary Duct, Percutaneous Endoscopic Approach

0FWB4DZ Revision of Intraluminal Device in Hepatobiliary Duct, Percutaneous Endoscopic Approach

0FWB4JZ Revision of Synthetic Substitute in Hepatobiliary Duct, Percutaneous Endoscopic Approach

0FWB4KZ Revision of Nonautologous Tissue Substitute in Hepatobiliary Duct, Percutaneous Endoscopic Approach

0FWB70Z Revision of Drainage Device in Hepatobiliary Duct, Via Natural or Artificial Opening

0FWB72Z Revision of Monitoring Device in Hepatobiliary Duct, Via Natural or Artificial Opening

0FWB73Z Revision of Infusion Device in Hepatobiliary Duct, Via Natural or Artificial Opening

0FWB77Z Revision of Autologous Tissue Substitute in Hepatobiliary Duct, Via Natural or Artificial Opening

0FWB7CZ Revision of Extraluminal Device in Hepatobiliary Duct, Via Natural or Artificial Opening

0FWB7DZ Revision of Intraluminal Device in Hepatobiliary Duct, Via Natural or Artificial Opening

0FWB7JZ Revision of Synthetic Substitute in Hepatobiliary Duct, Via Natural or Artificial Opening

0FWB7KZ Revision of Nonautologous Tissue Substitute in Hepatobiliary Duct, Via Natural or Artificial Opening

0FWB80Z Revision of Drainage Device in Hepatobiliary Duct, Via Natural or Artificial Opening Endoscopic

0FWB82Z Revision of Monitoring Device in Hepatobiliary Duct, Via Natural or Artificial Opening Endoscopic

0FWB83Z Revision of Infusion Device in Hepatobiliary Duct, Via Natural or Artificial Opening Endoscopic

0FWB87Z Revision of Autologous Tissue Substitute in Hepatobiliary Duct, Via Natural or Artificial Opening Endoscopic

0FWB8CZ Revision of Extraluminal Device in Hepatobiliary Duct, Via Natural or Artificial Opening Endoscopic

0FWB8DZ Revision of Intraluminal Device in Hepatobiliary Duct, Via Natural or Artificial Opening Endoscopic

0FWB8JZ Revision of Synthetic Substitute in Hepatobiliary Duct, Via Natural or Artificial Opening Endoscopic

0FWB8KZ Revision of Nonautologous Tissue Substitute in Hepatobiliary Duct, Via Natural or Artificial Opening Endoscopic

0FWBX0Z Revision of Drainage Device in Hepatobiliary Duct, External Approach

0FWBX2Z Revision of Monitoring Device in Hepatobiliary Duct, External Approach

0FWBX3Z Revision of Infusion Device in Hepatobiliary Duct, External Approach

0FWBX7Z Revision of Autologous Tissue Substitute in Hepatobiliary Duct, External Approach

0FWBXCZ Revision of Extraluminal Device in Hepatobiliary Duct, External Approach

0FWBXDZ Revision of Intraluminal Device in Hepatobiliary Duct, External Approach

0FWBXJZ Revision of Synthetic Substitute in Hepatobiliary Duct, External Approach

0FWBXKZ Revision of Nonautologous Tissue Substitute in Hepatobiliary Duct, External Approach

0FWD00Z Revision of Drainage Device in Pancreatic Duct, Open Approach

0FWD02Z Revision of Monitoring Device in Pancreatic Duct, Open Approach

0FWD03Z Revision of Infusion Device in Pancreatic Duct, Open Approach

0FWD07Z Revision of Autologous Tissue Substitute in Pancreatic Duct, Open Approach

0FWD0CZ Revision of Extraluminal Device in Pancreatic Duct, Open Approach

0FWD0DZ Revision of Intraluminal Device in Pancreatic Duct, Open Approach

0FWD0JZ Revision of Synthetic Substitute in Pancreatic Duct, Open Approach

0FWD0KZ Revision of Nonautologous Tissue Substitute in Pancreatic Duct, Open Approach

0FWD30Z Revision of Drainage Device in Pancreatic Duct, Percutaneous Approach

0FWD32Z Revision of Monitoring Device in Pancreatic Duct, Percutaneous Approach

0FWD33Z Revision of Infusion Device in Pancreatic Duct, Percutaneous Approach

0FWD37Z Revision of Autologous Tissue Substitute in Pancreatic Duct, Percutaneous Approach

0FWD3CZ Revision of Extraluminal Device in Pancreatic Duct, Percutaneous Approach

0FWD3DZ Revision of Intraluminal Device in Pancreatic Duct, Percutaneous Approach

0FWD3JZ Revision of Synthetic Substitute in Pancreatic Duct, Percutaneous Approach

0FWD3KZ Revision of Nonautologous Tissue Substitute in Pancreatic Duct, Percutaneous Approach

0FWD40Z Revision of Drainage Device in Pancreatic Duct, Percutaneous Endoscopic Approach

0FWD42Z Revision of Monitoring Device in Pancreatic Duct, Percutaneous Endoscopic Approach

0FWD43Z Revision of Infusion Device in Pancreatic Duct, Percutaneous Endoscopic Approach

0FWD47Z Revision of Autologous Tissue Substitute in Pancreatic Duct, Percutaneous Endoscopic Approach

0FWD4CZ Revision of Extraluminal Device in Pancreatic Duct, Percutaneous Endoscopic Approach

0FWD4DZ Revision of Intraluminal Device in Pancreatic Duct, Percutaneous Endoscopic Approach

0FWD4JZ Revision of Synthetic Substitute in Pancreatic Duct, Percutaneous Endoscopic Approach

0FWD4KZ Revision of Nonautologous Tissue Substitute in Pancreatic Duct, Percutaneous Endoscopic Approach

0FWD70Z Revision of Drainage Device in Pancreatic Duct, Via Natural or Artificial Opening

0FWD72Z Revision of Monitoring Device in Pancreatic Duct, Via Natural or Artificial Opening

0FWD73Z Revision of Infusion Device in Pancreatic Duct, Via Natural or Artificial Opening

0FWD77Z	Revision of Autologous Tissue Substitute in Pancreatic Duct, Via Natural or Artificial Opening
0FWD7CZ	Revision of Extraluminal Device in Pancreatic Duct, Via Natural or Artificial Opening
0FWD7DZ	Revision of Intraluminal Device in Pancreatic Duct, Via Natural or Artificial Opening
0FWD7JZ	Revision of Synthetic Substitute in Pancreatic Duct, Via Natural or Artificial Opening
0FWD7KZ	Revision of Nonautologous Tissue Substitute in Pancreatic Duct, Via Natural or Artificial Opening
0FWD80Z	Revision of Drainage Device in Pancreatic Duct, Via Natural or Artificial Opening Endoscopic
0FWD82Z	Revision of Monitoring Device in Pancreatic Duct, Via Natural or Artificial Opening Endoscopic
0FWD83Z	Revision of Infusion Device in Pancreatic Duct, Via Natural or Artificial Opening Endoscopic
0FWD87Z	Revision of Autologous Tissue Substitute in Pancreatic Duct, Via Natural or Artificial Opening Endoscopic
0FWD8CZ	Revision of Extraluminal Device in Pancreatic Duct, Via Natural or Artificial Opening Endoscopic

0FWD8DZ	Revision of Intraluminal Device in Pancreatic Duct, Via Natural or Artificial Opening Endoscopic
0FWD8JZ	Revision of Synthetic Substitute in Pancreatic Duct, Via Natural or Artificial Opening Endoscopic
0FWD8KZ	Revision of Nonautologous Tissue Substitute in Pancreatic Duct, Via Natural or Artificial Opening Endoscopic
0FWDX0Z	Revision of Drainage Device in Pancreatic Duct, External Approach
0FWDX2Z	Revision of Monitoring Device in Pancreatic Duct, External Approach
0FWDX3Z	Revision of Infusion Device in Pancreatic Duct, External Approach
0FWDX7Z	Revision of Autologous Tissue Substitute in Pancreatic Duct, External Approach
0FWDXCZ	Revision of Extraluminal Device in Pancreatic Duct, External Approach
0FWDXDZ	Revision of Intraluminal Device in Pancreatic Duct, External Approach
0FWDXJZ	Revision of Synthetic Substitute in Pancreatic Duct, External Approach
0FWDXKZ	Revision of Nonautologous Tissue Substitute in Pancreatic Duct, External Approach
0FWG00Z	Revision of Drainage Device in Pancreas, Open Approach
0FWG02Z	Revision of Monitoring Device in Pancreas, Open Approach

0FWG03Z	Revision of Infusion Device in Pancreas, Open Approach
0FWG0DZ	Revision of Intraluminal Device in Pancreas, Open Approach
0FWG30Z	Revision of Drainage Device in Pancreas, Percutaneous Approach
0FWG32Z	Revision of Monitoring Device in Pancreas, Percutaneous Approach
0FWG33Z	Revision of Infusion Device in Pancreas, Percutaneous Approach
0FWG3DZ	Revision of Intraluminal Device in Pancreas, Percutaneous Approach
0FWG40Z	Revision of Drainage Device in Pancreas, Percutaneous Endoscopic Approach
0FWG42Z	Revision of Monitoring Device in Pancreas, Percutaneous Endoscopic Approach
0FWG43Z	Revision of Infusion Device in Pancreas, Percutaneous Endoscopic Approach
0FWG4DZ	Revision of Intraluminal Device in Pancreas, Percutaneous Endoscopic Approach
0FWGX0Z	Revision of Drainage Device in Pancreas, External Approach
0FWGX2Z	Revision of Monitoring Device in Pancreas, External Approach
0FWGX3Z	Revision of Infusion Device in Pancreas, External Approach
0FWGXDZ	Revision of Intraluminal Device in Pancreas, External Approach

0FY – Hepatobiliary System and Pancreas, Transplantation

Review Coding Guideline B3.16

△ **0FY00Z0** Transplantation of Liver, Allogeneic, Open Approach
AHA CC: 4Q, 2012, 99-101; 3Q, 2014, 13-14

△ **0FY00Z1** Transplantation of Liver, Syngeneic, Open Approach

△ **0FY00Z2** Transplantation of Liver, Zooplastic, Open Approach

△ **0FYG0Z0** Transplantation of Pancreas, Allogeneic, Open Approach

▲ *When reported without an associated kidney transplant code (0TY00Z0, 0TY00Z1, 0TY00Z2, 0TY10Z0, 0TY10Z1 or 0TY10Z2) and without one of the following diagnosis codes E10.10-E10.9, E89.1*

△ **0FYG0Z1** Transplantation of Pancreas, Syngeneic, Open Approah

▲ *When reported without an associated kidney transplant code (0TY00Z0, 0TY00Z1, 0TY00Z2, 0TY10Z0, 0TY10Z1 or 0TY10Z2) and without one of the following diagnosis codes E10.10-E10.9, E89.1*

▲ **0FYG0Z2** Transplantation of Pancreas, Zooplastic, Open Approach

Endocrine System

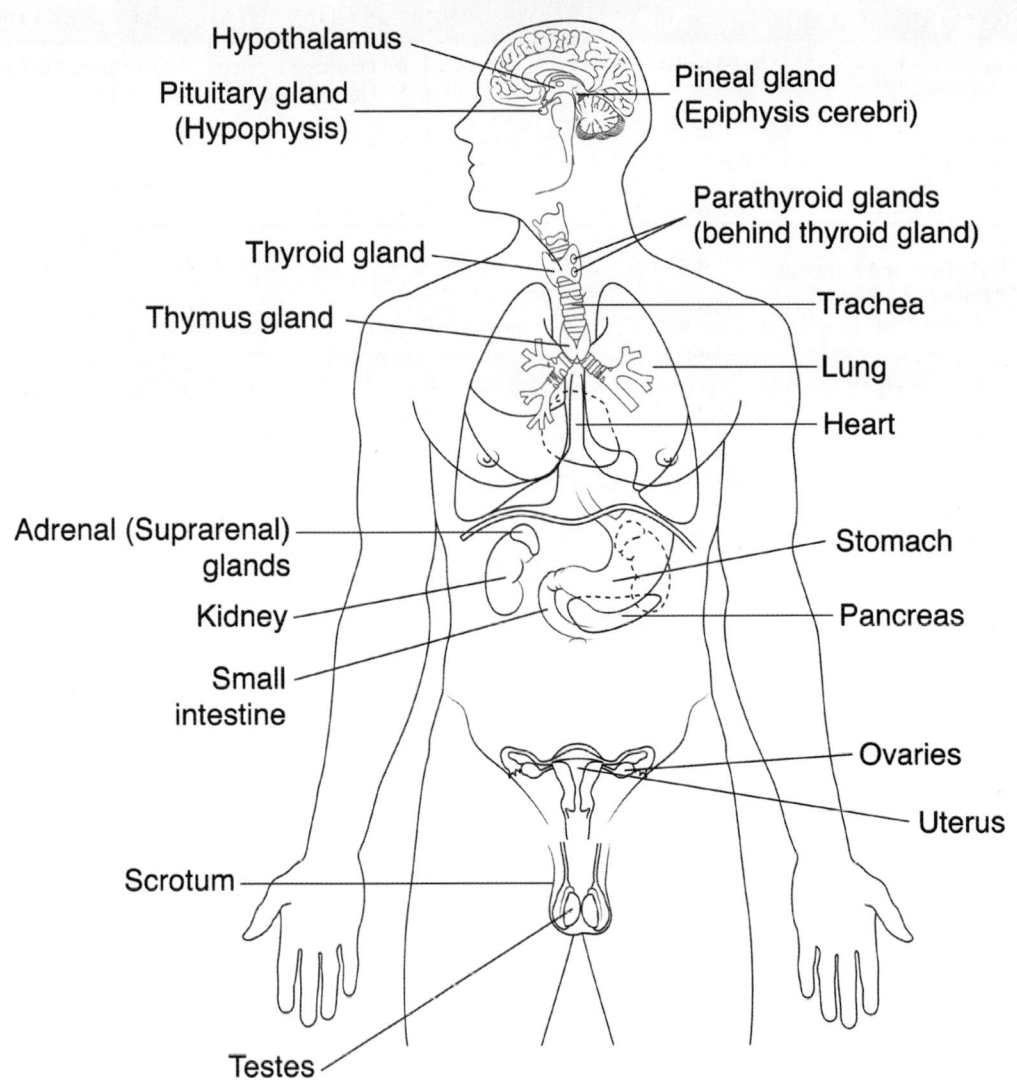

Hypothalamus

Pituitary gland
(Hypophysis)

Pineal gland
(Epiphysis cerebri)

Parathyroid glands
(behind thyroid gland)

Thyroid gland

Thymus gland

Trachea

Lung

Heart

Adrenal (Suprarenal)
glands

Kidney

Small
intestine

Stomach

Pancreas

Ovaries

Uterus

Scrotum

Testes

©AHIMA

Endocrine System Tables 0G2–0GW

Section	0	Medical and Surgical
Body System	G	Endocrine System
Operation	2	**Change:** Taking out or off a device from a body part and putting back an identical or similar device in or on the same body part without cutting or puncturing the skin or a mucous membrane

Body Part (4th)	Approach (5th)	Device (6th)	Qualifier (7th)
0 Pituitary Gland 1 Pineal Body 5 Adrenal Gland K Thyroid Gland R Parathyroid Gland S Endocrine Gland	X External	0 Drainage Device Y Other Device	Z No Qualifier

Section	0	Medical and Surgical
Body System	G	Endocrine System
Operation	5	**Destruction:** Physical eradication of all or a portion of a body part by the direct use of energy, force, or a destructive agent

Body Part (4th)	Approach (5th)	Device (6th)	Qualifier (7th)
0 Pituitary Gland 1 Pineal Body 2 Adrenal Gland, Left 3 Adrenal Gland, Right 4 Adrenal Glands, Bilateral 6 Carotid Body, Left 7 Carotid Body, Right 8 Carotid Bodies, Bilateral 9 Para-aortic Body B Coccygeal Glomus C Glomus Jugulare D Aortic Body F Paraganglion Extremity G Thyroid Gland Lobe, Left H Thyroid Gland Lobe, Right K Thyroid Gland L Superior Parathyroid Gland, Right M Superior Parathyroid Gland, Left N Inferior Parathyroid Gland, Right P Inferior Parathyroid Gland, Left Q Parathyroid Glands, Multiple R Parathyroid Gland	0 Open 3 Percutaneous 4 Percutaneous Endoscopic	Z No Device	Z No Qualifier

Section	0	Medical and Surgical
Body System	G	Endocrine System
Operation	8	**Division:** Cutting into a body part, without draining fluids and/or gases from the body part, in order to separate or transect a body part

Body Part (4th)	Approach (5th)	Device (6th)	Qualifier (7th)
0 Pituitary Gland J Thyroid Gland Isthmus	0 Open 3 Percutaneous 4 Percutaneous Endoscopic	Z No Device	Z No Qualifier

ion	0	Medical and Surgical
y System	G	Endocrine System
ration	9	**Drainage:** Taking or letting out fluids and/or gases from a body part

Body Part (4th)	Approach (5th)	Device (6th)	Qualifier (7th)
Pituitary Gland Pineal Body Adrenal Gland, Left Adrenal Gland, Right Adrenal Glands, Bilateral Carotid Body, Left Carotid Body, Right Carotid Bodies, Bilateral Para-aortic Body Coccygeal Glomus Glomus Jugulare Aortic Body Paraganglion Extremity Thyroid Gland Lobe, Left Thyroid Gland Lobe, Right Thyroid Gland Superior Parathyroid Gland, Right Superior Parathyroid Gland, Left Inferior Parathyroid Gland, Right Inferior Parathyroid Gland, Left Parathyroid Glands, Multiple Parathyroid Gland	**0** Open **3** Percutaneous **4** Percutaneous Endoscopic	**0** Drainage Device	**Z** No Qualifier
Pituitary Gland Pineal Body Adrenal Gland, Left Adrenal Gland, Right Adrenal Glands, Bilateral Carotid Body, Left Carotid Body, Right Carotid Bodies, Bilateral Para-aortic Body Coccygcal Glomus Glomus Jugulare Aortic Body Paraganglion Extremity Thyroid Gland Lobe, Left Thyroid Gland Lobe, Right Thyroid Gland Superior Parathyroid Gland, Right Superior Parathyroid Gland, Left Inferior Parathyroid Gland, Right Inferior Parathyroid Gland, Left Parathyroid Glands, Multiple Parathyroid Gland	**0** Open **3** Percutaneous **4** Percutaneous Endoscopic	**Z** No Device	**X** Diagnostic **Z** No Qualifier

Section	0	Medical and Surgical
Body System	G	Endocrine System
Operation	B	Excision: Cutting out or off, without replacement, a portion of a body part

Body Part (4th)	Approach (5th)	Device (6th)	Qualifier (7th)
0 Pituitary Gland	0 Open	Z No Device	X Diagnostic
1 Pineal Body	3 Percutaneous		Z No Qualifier
2 Adrenal Gland, Left	4 Percutaneous Endoscopic		
3 Adrenal Gland, Right			
4 Adrenal Glands, Bilateral			
6 Carotid Body, Left			
7 Carotid Body, Right			
8 Carotid Bodies, Bilateral			
9 Para-aortic Body			
B Coccygeal Glomus			
C Glomus Jugulare			
D Aortic Body			
F Paraganglion Extremity			
G Thyroid Gland Lobe, Left			
H Thyroid Gland Lobe, Right			
L Superior Parathyroid Gland, Right			
M Superior Parathyroid Gland, Left			
N Inferior Parathyroid Gland, Right			
P Inferior Parathyroid Gland, Left			
Q Parathyroid Glands, Multiple			
R Parathyroid Gland			

Section	0	Medical and Surgical
Body System	G	Endocrine System
Operation	C	Extirpation: Taking or cutting out solid matter from a body part

Body Part (4th)	Approach (5th)	Device (6th)	Qualifier (7th)
0 Pituitary Gland	0 Open	Z No Device	Z No Qualifier
1 Pineal Body	3 Percutaneous		
2 Adrenal Gland, Left	4 Percutaneous Endoscopic		
3 Adrenal Gland, Right			
4 Adrenal Glands, Bilateral			
6 Carotid Body, Left			
7 Carotid Body, Right			
8 Carotid Bodies, Bilateral			
9 Para-aortic Body			
B Coccygeal Glomus			
C Glomus Jugulare			
D Aortic Body			
F Paraganglion Extremity			
G Thyroid Gland Lobe, Left			
H Thyroid Gland Lobe, Right			
K Thyroid Gland			
L Superior Parathyroid Gland, Right			
M Superior Parathyroid Gland, Left			
N Inferior Parathyroid Gland, Right			
P Inferior Parathyroid Gland, Left			
Q Parathyroid Glands, Multiple			
R Parathyroid Gland			

Section	0	Medical and Surgical
Body System	G	Endocrine System
Operation	H	Insertion: Putting in a nonbiological appliance that monitors, assists, performs, or prevents a physiological function but does not physically take the place of a body part

Body Part (4th)	Approach (5th)	Device (6th)	Qualifier (7th)
S Endocrine Gland	0 Open	2 Monitoring Device	Z No Qualifier
	3 Percutaneous	3 Infusion Device	
	4 Percutaneous Endoscopic		

tion	0	Medical and Surgical
y System	G	Endocrine System
ration	J	**Inspection:** Visually and/or manually exploring a body part

Body Part (4th)	Approach (5th)	Device (6th)	Qualifier (7th)
Pituitary Gland Pineal Body Adrenal Gland Thyroid Gland Parathyroid Gland Endocrine Gland	0 Open 3 Percutaneous 4 Percutaneous Endoscopic	Z No Device	Z No Qualifier

tion	0	Medical and Surgical
y System	G	Endocrine System
eration	M	**Reattachment:** Putting back in or on all or a portion of a separated body part to its normal location or other suitable location

Body Part (4th)	Approach (5th)	Device (6th)	Qualifier (7th)
Adrenal Gland, Left Adrenal Gland, Right Thyroid Gland Lobe, Left Thyroid Gland Lobe, Right Superior Parathyroid Gland, Right Superior Parathyroid Gland, Left Inferior Parathyroid Gland, Right Inferior Parathyroid Gland, Left Parathyroid Glands, Multiple Parathyroid Gland	0 Open 4 Percutaneous Endoscopic	Z No Device	Z No Qualifier

tion	0	Medical and Surgical
dy System	G	Endocrine System
eration	N	**Release:** Freeing a body part from an abnormal physical constraint by cutting or by the use of force

Body Part (4th)	Approach (5th)	Device (6th)	Qualifier (7th)
Pituitary Gland Pineal Body Adrenal Gland, Left Adrenal Gland, Right Adrenal Glands, Bilateral Carotid Body, Left Carotid Body, Right Carotid Bodies, Bilateral Para-aortic Body Coccygeal Glomus Glomus Jugulare Aortic Body Paraganglion Extremity Thyroid Gland Lobe, Left Thyroid Gland Lobe, Right Thyroid Gland Superior Parathyroid Gland, Right Superior Parathyroid Gland, Left Inferior Parathyroid Gland, Right Inferior Parathyroid Gland, Left Parathyroid Glands, Multiple Parathyroid Gland	0 Open 3 Percutaneous 4 Percutaneous Endoscopic	Z No Device	Z No Qualifier

Section	0	Medical and Surgical
Body System	G	Endocrine System
Operation	P	Removal: Taking out or off a device from a body part

Body Part (4th)	Approach (5th)	Device (6th)	Qualifier (7th)
0 Pituitary Gland 1 Pineal Body 5 Adrenal Gland K Thyroid Gland R Parathyroid Gland	0 Open 3 Percutaneous 4 Percutaneous Endoscopic X External	0 Drainage Device	Z No Qualifier
S Endocrine Gland	0 Open 3 Percutaneous 4 Percutaneous Endoscopic X External	0 Drainage Device 2 Monitoring Device 3 Infusion Device	Z No Qualifier

Section	0	Medical and Surgical
Body System	G	Endocrine System
Operation	Q	Repair: Restoring, to the extent possible, a body part to its normal anatomic structure and function

Body Part (4th)	Approach (5th)	Device (6th)	Qualifier (7th)
0 Pituitary Gland 1 Pineal Body 2 Adrenal Gland, Left 3 Adrenal Gland, Right 4 Adrenal Glands, Bilateral 6 Carotid Body, Left 7 Carotid Body, Right 8 Carotid Bodies, Bilateral 9 Para-aortic Body B Coccygeal Glomus C Glomus Jugulare D Aortic Body F Paraganglion Extremity G Thyroid Gland Lobe, Left H Thyroid Gland Lobe, Right J Thyroid Gland Isthmus K Thyroid Gland L Superior Parathyroid Gland, Right M Superior Parathyroid Gland, Left N Inferior Parathyroid Gland, Right P Inferior Parathyroid Gland, Left Q Parathyroid Glands, Multiple R Parathyroid Gland	0 Open 3 Percutaneous 4 Percutaneous Endoscopic	Z No Device	Z No Qualifier

Section	0	Medical and Surgical
Body System	G	Endocrine System
Operation	S	Reposition: Moving to its normal location, or other suitable location, all or a portion of a body part

Body Part (4th)	Approach (5th)	Device (6th)	Qualifier (7th)
2 Adrenal Gland, Left 3 Adrenal Gland, Right G Thyroid Gland Lobe, Left H Thyroid Gland Lobe, Right L Superior Parathyroid Gland, Right M Superior Parathyroid Gland, Left N Inferior Parathyroid Gland, Right P Inferior Parathyroid Gland, Left Q Parathyroid Glands, Multiple R Parathyroid Gland	0 Open 4 Percutaneous Endoscopic	Z No Device	Z No Qualifier

tion	0	**Medical and Surgical**		
dy System	G	**Endocrine System**		
eration	T	**Resection:** Cutting out or off, without replacement, all of a body part		

Body Part (4ᵗʰ)	Approach (5ᵗʰ)	Device (6ᵗʰ)	Qualifier (7ᵗʰ)
Pituitary Gland Pineal Body Adrenal Gland, Left Adrenal Gland, Right Adrenal Glands, Bilateral Carotid Body, Left Carotid Body, Right Carotid Bodies, Bilateral Para-aortic Body Coccygeal Glomus Glomus Jugulare Aortic Body Paraganglion Extremity Thyroid Gland Lobe, Left Thyroid Gland Lobe, Right Thyroid Gland Superior Parathyroid Gland, Right Superior Parathyroid Gland, Left Inferior Parathyroid Gland, Right Inferior Parathyroid Gland, Left Parathyroid Glands, Multiple Parathyroid Gland	0 Open 4 Percutaneous Endoscopic	Z No Device	Z No Qualifier

tion	0	**Medical and Surgical**		
dy System	G	**Endocrine System**		
eration	W	**Revision:** Correcting, to the extent possible, a portion of a malfunctioning device or the position of a displaced device		

Body Part (4ᵗʰ)	Approach (5ᵗʰ)	Device (6ᵗʰ)	Qualifier (7ᵗʰ)
Pituitary Gland Pineal Body Adrenal Gland Thyroid Gland Parathyroid Gland	0 Open 3 Percutaneous 4 Percutaneous Endoscopic X External	0 Drainage Device	Z No Qualifier
Endocrine Gland	0 Open 3 Percutaneous 4 Percutaneous Endoscopic X External	0 Drainage Device 2 Monitoring Device 3 Infusion Device	Z No Qualifier

ndocrine System Code Listing 0G2–0GW

G2 – Endocrine System, Change

eview Coding Guideline B6.1c

620X0Z Change Drainage Device in Pituitary Gland, External Approach	0G25X0Z Change Drainage Device in Adrenal Gland, External Approach	0G2RX0Z Change Drainage Device in Parathyroid Gland, External Approach
620XYZ Change Other Device in Pituitary Gland, External Approach	0G25XYZ Change Other Device in Adrenal Gland, External Approach	0G2RXYZ Change Other Device in Parathyroid Gland, External Approach
621X0Z Change Drainage Device in Pineal Body, External Approach	0G2KX0Z Change Drainage Device in Thyroid Gland, External Approach	0G2SX0Z Change Drainage Device in Endocrine Gland, External Approach
621XYZ Change Other Device in Pineal Body, External Approach	0G2KXYZ Change Other Device in Thyroid Gland, External Approach	0G2SXYZ Change Other Device in Endocrine Gland, External Approach

G5 – Endocrine System, Destruction

6500ZZ Destruction of Pituitary Gland, Open Approach	0G513ZZ Destruction of Pineal Body, Percutaneous Approach	0G524ZZ Destruction of Left Adrenal Gland, Percutaneous Endoscopic Approach
6503ZZ Destruction of Pituitary Gland, Percutaneous Approach	0G514ZZ Destruction of Pineal Body, Percutaneous Endoscopic Approach	0G530ZZ Destruction of Right Adrenal Gland, Open Approach
6504ZZ Destruction of Pituitary Gland, Percutaneous Endoscopic Approach	0G520ZZ Destruction of Left Adrenal Gland, Open Approach	0G533ZZ Destruction of Right Adrenal Gland, Percutaneous Approach
6510ZZ Destruction of Pineal Body, Open Approach	0G523ZZ Destruction of Left Adrenal Gland, Percutaneous Approach	0G534ZZ Destruction of Right Adrenal Gland, Percutaneous Endoscopic Approach

0G540ZZ	Destruction of Bilateral Adrenal Glands, Open Approach	0G5C3ZZ	Destruction of Glomus Jugulare, Percutaneous Approach	0G5L4ZZ	Destruction of Right Superior Parathyroid Gland, Percutaneous Endoscopic Approach
0G543ZZ	Destruction of Bilateral Adrenal Glands, Percutaneous Approach	0G5C4ZZ	Destruction of Glomus Jugulare, Percutaneous Endoscopic Approach	0G5M0ZZ	Destruction of Left Superior Parathyroid Gland, Open Approach
0G544ZZ	Destruction of Bilateral Adrenal Glands, Percutaneous Endoscopic Approach	0G5D0ZZ	Destruction of Aortic Body, Open Approach	0G5M3ZZ	Destruction of Left Superior Parathyroid Gland, Percutaneous Approach
0G560ZZ	Destruction of Left Carotid Body, Open Approach	0G5D3ZZ	Destruction of Aortic Body, Percutaneous Approach	0G5M4ZZ	Destruction of Left Superior Parathyroid Gland, Percutaneous Endoscopic Approach
0G563ZZ	Destruction of Left Carotid Body, Percutaneous Approach	0G5D4ZZ	Destruction of Aortic Body, Percutaneous Endoscopic Approach	0G5N0ZZ	Destruction of Right Inferior Parathyroid Gland, Open Approach
0G564ZZ	Destruction of Left Carotid Body, Percutaneous Endoscopic Approach	0G5F0ZZ	Destruction of Paraganglion Extremity, Open Approach	0G5N3ZZ	Destruction of Right Inferior Parathyroid Gland, Percutaneous Approach
0G570ZZ	Destruction of Right Carotid Body, Open Approach	0G5F3ZZ	Destruction of Paraganglion Extremity, Percutaneous Approach	0G5N4ZZ	Destruction of Right Inferior Parathyroid Gland, Percutaneous Endoscopic Approach
0G573ZZ	Destruction of Right Carotid Body, Percutaneous Approach	0G5F4ZZ	Destruction of Paraganglion Extremity, Percutaneous Endoscopic Approach	0G5P0ZZ	Destruction of Left Inferior Parathyroid Gland, Open Approach
0G574ZZ	Destruction of Right Carotid Body, Percutaneous Endoscopic Approach	0G5G0ZZ	Destruction of Left Thyroid Gland Lobe, Open Approach	0G5P3ZZ	Destruction of Left Inferior Parathyroid Gland, Percutaneous Approach
0G580ZZ	Destruction of Bilateral Carotid Bodies, Open Approach	0G5G3ZZ	Destruction of Left Thyroid Gland Lobe, Percutaneous Approach	0G5P4ZZ	Destruction of Left Inferior Parathyroid Gland, Percutaneous Endoscopic Approach
0G583ZZ	Destruction of Bilateral Carotid Bodies, Percutaneous Approach	0G5G4ZZ	Destruction of Left Thyroid Gland Lobe, Percutaneous Endoscopic Approach	0G5Q0ZZ	Destruction of Multiple Parathyroid Glands, Open Approach
0G584ZZ	Destruction of Bilateral Carotid Bodies, Percutaneous Endoscopic Approach	0G5H0ZZ	Destruction of Right Thyroid Gland Lobe, Open Approach	0G5Q3ZZ	Destruction of Multiple Parathyroid Glands, Percutaneous Approach
0G590ZZ	Destruction of Para-aortic Body, Open Approach	0G5H3ZZ	Destruction of Right Thyroid Gland Lobe, Percutaneous Approach	0G5Q4ZZ	Destruction of Multiple Parathyroid Glands, Percutaneous Endoscopic Approach
0G593ZZ	Destruction of Para-aortic Body, Percutaneous Approach	0G5H4ZZ	Destruction of Right Thyroid Gland Lobe, Percutaneous Endoscopic Approach	0G5R0ZZ	Destruction of Parathyroid Gland, Open Approach
0G594ZZ	Destruction of Para-aortic Body, Percutaneous Endoscopic Approach	0G5K0ZZ	Destruction of Thyroid Gland, Open Approach	0G5R3ZZ	Destruction of Parathyroid Gland, Percutaneous Approach
0G5B0ZZ	Destruction of Coccygeal Glomus, Open Approach	0G5K3ZZ	Destruction of Thyroid Gland, Percutaneous Approach	0G5R4ZZ	Destruction of Parathyroid Gland, Percutaneous Endoscopic Approach
0G5B3ZZ	Destruction of Coccygeal Glomus, Percutaneous Approach	0G5K4ZZ	Destruction of Thyroid Gland, Percutaneous Endoscopic Approach		
0G5B4ZZ	Destruction of Coccygeal Glomus, Percutaneous Endoscopic Approach	0G5L0ZZ	Destruction of Right Superior Parathyroid Gland, Open Approach		
0G5C0ZZ	Destruction of Glomus Jugulare, Open Approach	0G5L3ZZ	Destruction of Right Superior Parathyroid Gland, Percutaneous Approach		

0G8 – Endocrine System, Division

Review Coding Guideline B3.14

0G800ZZ	Division of Pituitary Gland, Open Approach	0G804ZZ	Division of Pituitary Gland, Percutaneous Endoscopic Approach	0G8J3ZZ	Division of Thyroid Gland Isthmus, Percutaneous Approach
0G803ZZ	Division of Pituitary Gland, Percutaneous Approach	0G8J0ZZ	Division of Thyroid Gland Isthmus, Open Approach	0G8J4ZZ	Division of Thyroid Gland Isthmus, Percutaneous Endoscopic Approach

0G9 – Endocrine System, Drainage

Review Coding Guidelines B3.4a and B3.4b

Review Coding Guideline B6.2

0G9000Z	Drainage of Pituitary Gland with Drainage Device, Open Approach	0G9130Z	Drainage of Pineal Body with Drainage Device, Percutaneous Approach	0G923ZZ	Drainage of Left Adrenal Gland, Percutaneous Approach
0G900ZX	Drainage of Pituitary Gland, Open Approach, Diagnostic	0G913ZX	Drainage of Pineal Body, Percutaneous Approach, Diagnostic	0G9240Z	Drainage of Left Adrenal Gland with Drainage Device, Percutaneous Endoscopic Approach
0G900ZZ	Drainage of Pituitary Gland, Open Approach	0G913ZZ	Drainage of Pineal Body, Percutaneous Approach	0G924ZX	Drainage of Left Adrenal Gland, Percutaneous Endoscopic Approach, Diagnostic
0G9030Z	Drainage of Pituitary Gland with Drainage Device, Percutaneous Approach	0G9140Z	Drainage of Pineal Body with Drainage Device, Percutaneous Endoscopic Approach	0G924ZZ	Drainage of Left Adrenal Gland, Percutaneous Endoscopic Approach
0G903ZX	Drainage of Pituitary Gland, Percutaneous Approach, Diagnostic	0G914ZX	Drainage of Pineal Body, Percutaneous Endoscopic Approach, Diagnostic	0G9300Z	Drainage of Right Adrenal Gland with Drainage Device, Open Approach
0G903ZZ	Drainage of Pituitary Gland, Percutaneous Approach	0G914ZZ	Drainage of Pineal Body, Percutaneous Endoscopic Approach	0G930ZX	Drainage of Right Adrenal Gland, Open Approach, Diagnostic
0G9040Z	Drainage of Pituitary Gland with Drainage Device, Percutaneous Endoscopic Approach	0G9200Z	Drainage of Left Adrenal Gland with Drainage Device, Open Approach	0G930ZZ	Drainage of Right Adrenal Gland, Open Approach
0G904ZX	Drainage of Pituitary Gland, Percutaneous Endoscopic Approach, Diagnostic	0G920ZX	Drainage of Left Adrenal Gland, Open Approach, Diagnostic	0G9330Z	Drainage of Right Adrenal Gland with Drainage Device, Percutaneous Approach
0G904ZZ	Drainage of Pituitary Gland, Percutaneous Endoscopic Approach	0G920ZZ	Drainage of Left Adrenal Gland, Open Approach	0G933ZX	Drainage of Right Adrenal Gland, Percutaneous Approach, Diagnostic
0G9100Z	Drainage of Pineal Body with Drainage Device, Open Approach	0G9230Z	Drainage of Left Adrenal Gland with Drainage Device, Percutaneous Approach	0G933ZZ	Drainage of Right Adrenal Gland, Percutaneous Approach
0G910ZX	Drainage of Pineal Body, Open Approach, Diagnostic	0G923ZX	Drainage of Left Adrenal Gland, Percutaneous Approach, Diagnostic		
0G910ZZ	Drainage of Pineal Body, Open Approach				

♀ Female-only   ♂ Male-only   ▲ Limited Coverage   ● Non-OR   ▦ HAC-associated procedure   ▲ Non-covered procedures   ✚ Combination

340Z Drainage of Right Adrenal Gland with Drainage Device, Percutaneous Endoscopic Approach

34ZX Drainage of Right Adrenal Gland, Percutaneous Endoscopic Approach, Diagnostic

34ZZ Drainage of Right Adrenal Gland, Percutaneous Endoscopic Approach

400Z Drainage of Bilateral Adrenal Glands with Drainage Device, Open Approach

40ZX Drainage of Bilateral Adrenal Glands, Open Approach, Diagnostic

40ZZ Drainage of Bilateral Adrenal Glands, Open Approach

430Z Drainage of Bilateral Adrenal Glands with Drainage Device, Percutaneous Approach

43ZX Drainage of Bilateral Adrenal Glands, Percutaneous Approach, Diagnostic

43ZZ Drainage of Bilateral Adrenal Glands, Percutaneous Approach

440Z Drainage of Bilateral Adrenal Glands with Drainage Device, Percutaneous Endoscopic Approach

44ZX Drainage of Bilateral Adrenal Glands, Percutaneous Endoscopic Approach, Diagnostic

44ZZ Drainage of Bilateral Adrenal Glands, Percutaneous Endoscopic Approach

9600Z Drainage of Left Carotid Body with Drainage Device, Open Approach

960ZX Drainage of Left Carotid Body, Open Approach, Diagnostic

960ZZ Drainage of Left Carotid Body, Open Approach

9630Z Drainage of Left Carotid Body with Drainage Device, Percutaneous Approach

963ZX Drainage of Left Carotid Body, Percutaneous Approach, Diagnostic

963ZZ Drainage of Left Carotid Body, Percutaneous Approach

9640Z Drainage of Left Carotid Body with Drainage Device, Percutaneous Endoscopic Approach

964ZX Drainage of Left Carotid Body, Percutaneous Endoscopic Approach, Diagnostic

964ZZ Drainage of Left Carotid Body, Percutaneous Endoscopic Approach

9700Z Drainage of Right Carotid Body with Drainage Device, Open Approach

970ZX Drainage of Right Carotid Body, Open Approach, Diagnostic

970ZZ Drainage of Right Carotid Body, Open Approach

9730Z Drainage of Right Carotid Body with Drainage Device, Percutaneous Approach

973ZX Drainage of Right Carotid Body, Percutaneous Approach, Diagnostic

973ZZ Drainage of Right Carotid Body, Percutaneous Approach

9740Z Drainage of Right Carotid Body with Drainage Device, Percutaneous Endoscopic Approach

974ZX Drainage of Right Carotid Body, Percutaneous Endoscopic Approach, Diagnostic

974ZZ Drainage of Right Carotid Body, Percutaneous Endoscopic Approach

9800Z Drainage of Bilateral Carotid Bodies with Drainage Device, Open Approach

980ZX Drainage of Bilateral Carotid Bodies, Open Approach, Diagnostic

980ZZ Drainage of Bilateral Carotid Bodies, Open Approach

9830Z Drainage of Bilateral Carotid Bodies with Drainage Device, Percutaneous Approach

0G983ZX Drainage of Bilateral Carotid Bodies, Percutaneous Approach, Diagnostic

0G983ZZ Drainage of Bilateral Carotid Bodies, Percutaneous Approach

0G9840Z Drainage of Bilateral Carotid Bodies with Drainage Device, Percutaneous Endoscopic Approach

0G984ZX Drainage of Bilateral Carotid Bodies, Percutaneous Endoscopic Approach, Diagnostic

0G984ZZ Drainage of Bilateral Carotid Bodies, Percutaneous Endoscopic Approach

0G9900Z Drainage of Para-aortic Body with Drainage Device, Open Approach

0G990ZX Drainage of Para-aortic Body, Open Approach, Diagnostic

0G990ZZ Drainage of Para-aortic Body, Open Approach

0G9930Z Drainage of Para-aortic Body with Drainage Device, Percutaneous Approach

0G993ZX Drainage of Para-aortic Body, Percutaneous Approach, Diagnostic

0G993ZZ Drainage of Para-aortic Body, Percutaneous Approach

0G9940Z Drainage of Para-aortic Body with Drainage Device, Percutaneous Endoscopic Approach

0G994ZX Drainage of Para-aortic Body, Percutaneous Endoscopic Approach, Diagnostic

0G994ZZ Drainage of Para-aortic Body, Percutaneous Endoscopic Approach

0G9B00Z Drainage of Coccygeal Glomus with Drainage Device, Open Approach

0G9B0ZX Drainage of Coccygeal Glomus, Open Approach, Diagnostic

0G9B0ZZ Drainage of Coccygeal Glomus, Open Approach

0G9B30Z Drainage of Coccygeal Glomus with Drainage Device, Percutaneous Approach

0G9B3ZX Drainage of Coccygeal Glomus, Percutaneous Approach, Diagnostic

0G9B3ZZ Drainage of Coccygeal Glomus, Percutaneous Approach

0G9B40Z Drainage of Coccygeal Glomus with Drainage Device, Percutaneous Endoscopic Approach

0G9B4ZX Drainage of Coccygeal Glomus, Percutaneous Endoscopic Approach, Diagnostic

0G9B4ZZ Drainage of Coccygeal Glomus, Percutaneous Endoscopic Approach

0G9C00Z Drainage of Glomus Jugulare with Drainage Device, Open Approach

0G9C0ZX Drainage of Glomus Jugulare, Open Approach, Diagnostic

0G9C0ZZ Drainage of Glomus Jugulare, Open Approach

0G9C30Z Drainage of Glomus Jugulare with Drainage Device, Percutaneous Approach

0G9C3ZX Drainage of Glomus Jugulare, Percutaneous Approach, Diagnostic

0G9C3ZZ Drainage of Glomus Jugulare, Percutaneous Approach

0G9C40Z Drainage of Glomus Jugulare with Drainage Device, Percutaneous Endoscopic Approach

0G9C4ZX Drainage of Glomus Jugulare, Percutaneous Endoscopic Approach, Diagnostic

0G9C4ZZ Drainage of Glomus Jugulare, Percutaneous Endoscopic Approach

0G9D00Z Drainage of Aortic Body with Drainage Device, Open Approach

0G9D0ZX Drainage of Aortic Body, Open Approach, Diagnostic

0G9D0ZZ Drainage of Aortic Body, Open Approach

0G9D30Z Drainage of Aortic Body with Drainage Device, Percutaneous Approach

0G9D3ZX Drainage of Aortic Body, Percutaneous Approach, Diagnostic

0G9D3ZZ Drainage of Aortic Body, Percutaneous Approach

0G9D40Z Drainage of Aortic Body with Drainage Device, Percutaneous Endoscopic Approach

0G9D4ZX Drainage of Aortic Body, Percutaneous Endoscopic Approach, Diagnostic

0G9D4ZZ Drainage of Aortic Body, Percutaneous Endoscopic Approach

0G9F00Z Drainage of Paraganglion Extremity with Drainage Device, Open Approach

0G9F0ZX Drainage of Paraganglion Extremity, Open Approach, Diagnostic

0G9F0ZZ Drainage of Paraganglion Extremity, Open Approach

0G9F30Z Drainage of Paraganglion Extremity with Drainage Device, Percutaneous Approach

0G9F3ZX Drainage of Paraganglion Extremity, Percutaneous Approach, Diagnostic

0G9F3ZZ Drainage of Paraganglion Extremity, Percutaneous Approach

0G9F40Z Drainage of Paraganglion Extremity with Drainage Device, Percutaneous Endoscopic Approach

0G9F4ZX Drainage of Paraganglion Extremity, Percutaneous Endoscopic Approach, Diagnostic

0G9F4ZZ Drainage of Paraganglion Extremity, Percutaneous Endoscopic Approach

0G9G00Z Drainage of Left Thyroid Gland Lobe with Drainage Device, Open Approach

0G9G0ZX Drainage of Left Thyroid Gland Lobe, Open Approach, Diagnostic

0G9G0ZZ Drainage of Left Thyroid Gland Lobe, Open Approach

0G9G30Z Drainage of Left Thyroid Gland Lobe with Drainage Device, Percutaneous Approach

0G9G3ZX Drainage of Left Thyroid Gland Lobe, Percutaneous Approach, Diagnostic

0G9G3ZZ Drainage of Left Thyroid Gland Lobe, Percutaneous Approach

0G9G40Z Drainage of Left Thyroid Gland Lobe with Drainage Device, Percutaneous Endoscopic Approach

0G9G4ZX Drainage of Left Thyroid Gland Lobe, Percutaneous Endoscopic Approach, Diagnostic

0G9G4ZZ Drainage of Left Thyroid Gland Lobe, Percutaneous Endoscopic Approach

0G9H00Z Drainage of Right Thyroid Gland Lobe with Drainage Device, Open Approach

0G9H0ZX Drainage of Right Thyroid Gland Lobe, Open Approach, Diagnostic

0G9H0ZZ Drainage of Right Thyroid Gland Lobe, Open Approach

0G9H30Z Drainage of Right Thyroid Gland Lobe with Drainage Device, Percutaneous Approach

0G9H3ZX Drainage of Right Thyroid Gland Lobe, Percutaneous Approach, Diagnostic

0G9H3ZZ Drainage of Right Thyroid Gland Lobe, Percutaneous Approach

0G9H40Z Drainage of Right Thyroid Gland Lobe with Drainage Device, Percutaneous Endoscopic Approach

0G9H4ZX Drainage of Right Thyroid Gland Lobe, Percutaneous Endoscopic Approach, Diagnostic

0G9H4ZZ Drainage of Right Thyroid Gland Lobe, Percutaneous Endoscopic Approach

0G9K00Z Drainage of Thyroid Gland with Drainage Device, Open Approach

617

0G9K0ZX	Drainage of Thyroid Gland, Open Approach, Diagnostic	**0G9M3ZX**	Drainage of Left Superior Parathyroid Gland, Percutaneous Approach, Diagnostic	**0G9P40Z**	Drainage of Left Inferior Parathyroid Gland with Drainage Device, Percutaneous Endoscopic Approach
0G9K0ZZ	Drainage of Thyroid Gland, Open Approach	**0G9M3ZZ**	Drainage of Left Superior Parathyroid Gland, Percutaneous Approach	**0G9P4ZX**	Drainage of Left Inferior Parathyroid Gland, Percutaneous Endoscopic Approach, Diagnostic
0G9K30Z	Drainage of Thyroid Gland with Drainage Device, Percutaneous Approach	**0G9M40Z**	Drainage of Left Superior Parathyroid Gland with Drainage Device, Percutaneous Endoscopic Approach	**0G9P4ZZ**	Drainage of Left Inferior Parathyroid Gland, Percutaneous Endoscopic Approach
0G9K3ZX	Drainage of Thyroid Gland, Percutaneous Approach, Diagnostic	**0G9M4ZX**	Drainage of Left Superior Parathyroid Gland, Percutaneous Endoscopic Approach, Diagnostic	**0G9Q00Z**	Drainage of Multiple Parathyroid Glands with Drainage Device, Open Approach
0G9K3ZZ	Drainage of Thyroid Gland, Percutaneous Approach	**0G9M4ZZ**	Drainage of Left Superior Parathyroid Gland, Percutaneous Endoscopic Approach	**0G9Q0ZX**	Drainage of Multiple Parathyroid Glands, Open Approach, Diagnostic
0G9K40Z	Drainage of Thyroid Gland with Drainage Device, Percutaneous Endoscopic Approach	**0G9N00Z**	Drainage of Right Inferior Parathyroid Gland with Drainage Device, Open Approach	**0G9Q0ZZ**	Drainage of Multiple Parathyroid Glands, Open Approach
0G9K4ZX	Drainage of Thyroid Gland, Percutaneous Endoscopic Approach, Diagnostic	**0G9N0ZX**	Drainage of Right Inferior Parathyroid Gland, Open Approach, Diagnostic	**0G9Q30Z**	Drainage of Multiple Parathyroid Glands with Drainage Device, Percutaneous Approach
0G9K4ZZ	Drainage of Thyroid Gland, Percutaneous Endoscopic Approach	**0G9N0ZZ**	Drainage of Right Inferior Parathyroid Gland, Open Approach	**0G9Q3ZX**	Drainage of Multiple Parathyroid Glands, Percutaneous Approach, Diagnostic
0G9L00Z	Drainage of Right Superior Parathyroid Gland with Drainage Device, Open Approach	**0G9N30Z**	Drainage of Right Inferior Parathyroid Gland with Drainage Device, Percutaneous Approach	**0G9Q3ZZ**	Drainage of Multiple Parathyroid Glands, Percutaneous Approach
0G9L0ZX	Drainage of Right Superior Parathyroid Gland, Open Approach, Diagnostic	**0G9N3ZX**	Drainage of Right Inferior Parathyroid Gland, Percutaneous Approach, Diagnostic	**0G9Q4ZX**	Drainage of Multiple Parathyroid Glands, Percutaneous Endoscopic Approach, Diagnostic
0G9L0ZZ	Drainage of Right Superior Parathyroid Gland, Open Approach	**0G9N3ZZ**	Drainage of Right Inferior Parathyroid Gland, Percutaneous Approach	**0G9Q4ZZ**	Drainage of Multiple Parathyroid Glands, Percutaneous Endoscopic Approach
0G9L30Z	Drainage of Right Superior Parathyroid Gland with Drainage Device, Percutaneous Approach	**0G9N40Z**	Drainage of Right Inferior Parathyroid Gland with Drainage Device, Percutaneous Endoscopic Approach	**0G9R00Z**	Drainage of Parathyroid Gland with Drainage Device, Open Approach
0G9L3ZX	Drainage of Right Superior Parathyroid Gland, Percutaneous Approach, Diagnostic	**0G9N4ZX**	Drainage of Right Inferior Parathyroid Gland, Percutaneous Endoscopic Approach, Diagnostic	**0G9R0ZX**	Drainage of Parathyroid Gland, Open Approach, Diagnostic
0G9L3ZZ	Drainage of Right Superior Parathyroid Gland, Percutaneous Approach	**0G9N4ZZ**	Drainage of Right Inferior Parathyroid Gland, Percutaneous Endoscopic Approach	**0G9R0ZZ**	Drainage of Parathyroid Gland, Open Approach
0G9L40Z	Drainage of Right Superior Parathyroid Gland with Drainage Device, Percutaneous Endoscopic Approach	**0G9P00Z**	Drainage of Left Inferior Parathyroid Gland with Drainage Device, Open Approach	**0G9R30Z**	Drainage of Parathyroid Gland with Drainage Device, Percutaneous Approach
0G9L4ZX	Drainage of Right Superior Parathyroid Gland, Percutaneous Endoscopic Approach, Diagnostic	**0G9P0ZX**	Drainage of Left Inferior Parathyroid Gland, Open Approach, Diagnostic	**0G9R3ZX**	Drainage of Parathyroid Gland, Percutaneous Approach, Diagnostic
0G9L4ZZ	Drainage of Right Superior Parathyroid Gland, Percutaneous Endoscopic Approach	**0G9P0ZZ**	Drainage of Left Inferior Parathyroid Gland, Open Approach	**0G9R3ZZ**	Drainage of Parathyroid Gland, Percutaneous Approach
0G9M00Z	Drainage of Left Superior Parathyroid Gland with Drainage Device, Open Approach	**0G9P30Z**	Drainage of Left Inferior Parathyroid Gland with Drainage Device, Percutaneous Approach	**0G9R40Z**	Drainage of Parathyroid Gland with Drainage Device, Percutaneous Endoscopic Approach
0G9M0ZX	Drainage of Left Superior Parathyroid Gland, Open Approach, Diagnostic	**0G9P3ZX**	Drainage of Left Inferior Parathyroid Gland, Percutaneous Approach, Diagnostic	**0G9R4ZX**	Drainage of Parathyroid Gland, Percutaneous Endoscopic Approach, Diagnostic
0G9M0ZZ	Drainage of Left Superior Parathyroid Gland, Open Approach	**0G9P3ZZ**	Drainage of Left Inferior Parathyroid Gland, Percutaneous Approach	**0G9R4ZZ**	Drainage of Parathyroid Gland, Percutaneous Endoscopic Approach
0G9M30Z	Drainage of Left Superior Parathyroid Gland with Drainage Device, Percutaneous Approach				

0GB – Endocrine System, Excision

Review Coding Guidelines B3.4a and B3.4b

Review Coding Guideline B3.8

0GB00ZX	Excision of Pituitary Gland, Open Approach, Diagnostic	**0GB14ZZ**	Excision of Pineal Body, Percutaneous Endoscopic Approach	**0GB33ZZ**	Excision of Right Adrenal Gland, Percutaneous Approach
0GB00ZZ	Excision of Pituitary Gland, Open Approach *AHA CC: 3Q, 2014, 22-23*	**0GB20ZX**	Excision of Left Adrenal Gland, Open Approach, Diagnostic	**0GB34ZX**	Excision of Right Adrenal Gland, Percutaneous Endoscopic Approach, Diagnostic
0GB03ZX	Excision of Pituitary Gland, Percutaneous Approach, Diagnostic	**0GB20ZZ**	Excision of Left Adrenal Gland, Open Approach	**0GB34ZZ**	Excision of Right Adrenal Gland, Percutaneous Endoscopic Approach
0GB03ZZ	Excision of Pituitary Gland, Percutaneous Approach	**0GB23ZX**	Excision of Left Adrenal Gland, Percutaneous Approach, Diagnostic	**0GB40ZX**	Excision of Bilateral Adrenal Glands, Open Approach, Diagnostic
0GB04ZX	Excision of Pituitary Gland, Percutaneous Endoscopic Approach, Diagnostic	**0GB23ZZ**	Excision of Left Adrenal Gland, Percutaneous Approach	**0GB40ZZ**	Excision of Bilateral Adrenal Glands, Open Approach
0GB04ZZ	Excision of Pituitary Gland, Percutaneous Endoscopic Approach	**0GB24ZX**	Excision of Left Adrenal Gland, Percutaneous Endoscopic Approach, Diagnostic	**0GB43ZX**	Excision of Bilateral Adrenal Glands, Percutaneous Approach, Diagnostic
0GB10ZX	Excision of Pineal Body, Open Approach, Diagnostic	**0GB24ZZ**	Excision of Left Adrenal Gland, Percutaneous Endoscopic Approach	**0GB43ZZ**	Excision of Bilateral Adrenal Glands, Percutaneous Approach
0GB10ZZ	Excision of Pineal Body, Open Approach	**0GB30ZX**	Excision of Right Adrenal Gland, Open Approach, Diagnostic	**0GB44ZX**	Excision of Bilateral Adrenal Glands, Percutaneous Endoscopic Approach, Diagnostic
0GB13ZX	Excision of Pineal Body, Percutaneous Approach, Diagnostic	**0GB30ZZ**	Excision of Right Adrenal Gland, Open Approach	**0GB44ZZ**	Excision of Bilateral Adrenal Glands, Percutaneous Endoscopic Approach
0GB13ZZ	Excision of Pineal Body, Percutaneous Approach	**0GB33ZX**	Excision of Right Adrenal Gland, Percutaneous Approach, Diagnostic		
0GB14ZX	Excision of Pineal Body, Percutaneous Endoscopic Approach, Diagnostic				

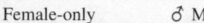 ♀ Female-only   ♂ Male-only   ▲ Limited Coverage   ● Non-OR   HAC HAC-associated procedure   ▲ Non-covered procedures   + Combination

60ZX	Excision of Left Carotid Body, Open Approach, Diagnostic
60ZZ	Excision of Left Carotid Body, Open Approach
63ZX	Excision of Left Carotid Body, Percutaneous Approach, Diagnostic
63ZZ	Excision of Left Carotid Body, Percutaneous Approach
64ZX	Excision of Left Carotid Body, Percutaneous Endoscopic Approach, Diagnostic
64ZZ	Excision of Left Carotid Body, Percutaneous Endoscopic Approach
70ZX	Excision of Right Carotid Body, Open Approach, Diagnostic
70ZZ	Excision of Right Carotid Body, Open Approach
73ZX	Excision of Right Carotid Body, Percutaneous Approach, Diagnostic
73ZZ	Excision of Right Carotid Body, Percutaneous Approach
374ZX	Excision of Right Carotid Body, Percutaneous Endoscopic Approach, Diagnostic
374ZZ	Excision of Right Carotid Body, Percutaneous Endoscopic Approach
80ZX	Excision of Bilateral Carotid Bodies, Open Approach, Diagnostic
80ZZ	Excision of Bilateral Carotid Bodies, Open Approach
83ZX	Excision of Bilateral Carotid Bodies, Percutaneous Approach, Diagnostic
83ZZ	Excision of Bilateral Carotid Bodies, Percutaneous Approach
B84ZX	Excision of Bilateral Carotid Bodies, Percutaneous Endoscopic Approach, Diagnostic
B84ZZ	Excision of Bilateral Carotid Bodies, Percutaneous Endoscopic Approach
B90ZX	Excision of Para-aortic Body, Open Approach, Diagnostic
B90ZZ	Excision of Para-aortic Body, Open Approach
B93ZX	Excision of Para-aortic Body, Percutaneous Approach, Diagnostic
B93ZZ	Excision of Para-aortic Body, Percutaneous Approach
B94ZX	Excision of Para-aortic Body, Percutaneous Endoscopic Approach, Diagnostic
B94ZZ	Excision of Para-aortic Body, Percutaneous Endoscopic Approach
BB0ZX	Excision of Coccygeal Glomus, Open Approach, Diagnostic
BB0ZZ	Excision of Coccygeal Glomus, Open Approach
BB3ZX	Excision of Coccygeal Glomus, Percutaneous Approach, Diagnostic
BB3ZZ	Excision of Coccygeal Glomus, Percutaneous Approach
BB4ZX	Excision of Coccygeal Glomus, Percutaneous Endoscopic Approach, Diagnostic
BB4ZZ	Excision of Coccygeal Glomus, Percutaneous Endoscopic Approach
BC0ZX	Excision of Glomus Jugulare, Open Approach, Diagnostic
BC0ZZ	Excision of Glomus Jugulare, Open Approach
BC3ZX	Excision of Glomus Jugulare, Percutaneous Approach, Diagnostic

0GBC3ZZ	Excision of Glomus Jugulare, Percutaneous Approach
0GBC4ZX	Excision of Glomus Jugulare, Percutaneous Endoscopic Approach, Diagnostic
0GBC4ZZ	Excision of Glomus Jugulare, Percutaneous Endoscopic Approach
0GBD0ZX	Excision of Aortic Body, Open Approach, Diagnostic
0GBD0ZZ	Excision of Aortic Body, Open Approach
0GBD3ZX	Excision of Aortic Body, Percutaneous Approach, Diagnostic
0GBD3ZZ	Excision of Aortic Body, Percutaneous Approach
0GBD4ZX	Excision of Aortic Body, Percutaneous Endoscopic Approach, Diagnostic
0GBD4ZZ	Excision of Aortic Body, Percutaneous Endoscopic Approach
0GBF0ZX	Excision of Paraganglion Extremity, Open Approach, Diagnostic
0GBF0ZZ	Excision of Paraganglion Extremity, Open Approach
0GBF3ZX	Excision of Paraganglion Extremity, Percutaneous Approach, Diagnostic
0GBF3ZZ	Excision of Paraganglion Extremity, Percutaneous Approach
0GBF4ZX	Excision of Paraganglion Extremity, Percutaneous Endoscopic Approach, Diagnostic
0GBF4ZZ	Excision of Paraganglion Extremity, Percutaneous Endoscopic Approach
0GBG0ZX	Excision of Left Thyroid Gland Lobe, Open Approach, Diagnostic
0GBG0ZZ	Excision of Left Thyroid Gland Lobe, Open Approach
0GBG3ZX	Excision of Left Thyroid Gland Lobe, Percutaneous Approach, Diagnostic
0GBG3ZZ	Excision of Left Thyroid Gland Lobe, Percutaneous Approach
0GBG4ZX	Excision of Left Thyroid Gland Lobe, Percutaneous Endoscopic Approach, Diagnostic
0GBG4ZZ	Excision of Left Thyroid Gland Lobe, Percutaneous Endoscopic Approach
0GBH0ZX	Excision of Right Thyroid Gland Lobe, Open Approach, Diagnostic
0GBH0ZZ	Excision of Right Thyroid Gland Lobe, Open Approach
0GBH3ZX	Excision of Right Thyroid Gland Lobe, Percutaneous Approach, Diagnostic
0GBH3ZZ	Excision of Right Thyroid Gland Lobe, Percutaneous Approach
0GBH4ZX	Excision of Right Thyroid Gland Lobe, Percutaneous Endoscopic Approach, Diagnostic
0GBH4ZZ	Excision of Right Thyroid Gland Lobe, Percutaneous Endoscopic Approach
0GBL0ZX	Excision of Right Superior Parathyroid Gland, Open Approach, Diagnostic
0GBL0ZZ	Excision of Right Superior Parathyroid Gland, Open Approach
0GBL3ZX	Excision of Right Superior Parathyroid Gland, Percutaneous Approach, Diagnostic
0GBL3ZZ	Excision of Right Superior Parathyroid Gland, Percutaneous Approach
0GBL4ZX	Excision of Right Superior Parathyroid Gland, Percutaneous Endoscopic Approach, Diagnostic
0GBL4ZZ	Excision of Right Superior Parathyroid Gland, Percutaneous Endoscopic Approach

0GBM0ZX	Excision of Left Superior Parathyroid Gland, Open Approach, Diagnostic
0GBM0ZZ	Excision of Left Superior Parathyroid Gland, Open Approach
0GBM3ZX	Excision of Left Superior Parathyroid Gland, Percutaneous Approach, Diagnostic
0GBM3ZZ	Excision of Left Superior Parathyroid Gland, Percutaneous Approach
0GBM4ZX	Excision of Left Superior Parathyroid Gland, Percutaneous Endoscopic Approach, Diagnostic
0GBM4ZZ	Excision of Left Superior Parathyroid Gland, Percutaneous Endoscopic Approach
0GBN0ZX	Excision of Right Inferior Parathyroid Gland, Open Approach, Diagnostic
0GBN0ZZ	Excision of Right Inferior Parathyroid Gland, Open Approach
0GBN3ZX	Excision of Right Inferior Parathyroid Gland, Percutaneous Approach, Diagnostic
0GBN3ZZ	Excision of Right Inferior Parathyroid Gland, Percutaneous Approach
0GBN4ZX	Excision of Right Inferior Parathyroid Gland, Percutaneous Endoscopic Approach, Diagnostic
0GBN4ZZ	Excision of Right Inferior Parathyroid Gland, Percutaneous Endoscopic Approach
0GBP0ZX	Excision of Left Inferior Parathyroid Gland, Open Approach, Diagnostic
0GBP0ZZ	Excision of Left Inferior Parathyroid Gland, Open Approach
0GBP3ZX	Excision of Left Inferior Parathyroid Gland, Percutaneous Approach, Diagnostic
0GBP3ZZ	Excision of Left Inferior Parathyroid Gland, Percutaneous Approach
0GBP4ZX	Excision of Left Inferior Parathyroid Gland, Percutaneous Endoscopic Approach, Diagnostic
0GBP4ZZ	Excision of Left Inferior Parathyroid Gland, Percutaneous Endoscopic Approach
0GBQ0ZX	Excision of Multiple Parathyroid Glands, Open Approach, Diagnostic
0GBQ0ZZ	Excision of Multiple Parathyroid Glands, Open Approach
0GBQ3ZX	Excision of Multiple Parathyroid Glands, Percutaneous Approach, Diagnostic
0GBQ3ZZ	Excision of Multiple Parathyroid Glands, Percutaneous Approach
0GBQ4ZX	Excision of Multiple Parathyroid Glands, Percutaneous Endoscopic Approach, Diagnostic
0GBQ4ZZ	Excision of Multiple Parathyroid Glands, Percutaneous Endoscopic Approach
0GBR0ZX	Excision of Parathyroid Gland, Open Approach, Diagnostic
0GBR0ZZ	Excision of Parathyroid Gland, Open Approach
0GBR3ZX	Excision of Parathyroid Gland, Percutaneous Approach, Diagnostic
0GBR3ZZ	Excision of Parathyroid Gland, Percutaneous Approach
0GBR4ZX	Excision of Parathyroid Gland, Percutaneous Endoscopic Approach, Diagnostic
0GBR4ZZ	Excision of Parathyroid Gland, Percutaneous Endoscopic Approach

GC – Endocrine System, Extirpation

GC00ZZ	Extirpation of Matter from Pituitary Gland, Open Approach
GC03ZZ	Extirpation of Matter from Pituitary Gland, Percutaneous Approach

0GC04ZZ	Extirpation of Matter from Pituitary Gland, Percutaneous Endoscopic Approach

0GC10ZZ	Extirpation of Matter from Pineal Body, Open Approach
0GC13ZZ	Extirpation of Matter from Pineal Body, Percutaneous Approach

619

Female-only	♂ Male-only	▲ Limited Coverage	● Non-OR	▦ HAC-associated procedure	▲ Non-covered procedures	⊞ Combination

0GC14ZZ Extirpation of Matter from Pineal Body, Percutaneous Endoscopic Approach

0GC20ZZ Extirpation of Matter from Left Adrenal Gland, Open Approach

0GC23ZZ Extirpation of Matter from Left Adrenal Gland, Percutaneous Approach

0GC24ZZ Extirpation of Matter from Left Adrenal Gland, Percutaneous Endoscopic Approach

0GC30ZZ Extirpation of Matter from Right Adrenal Gland, Open Approach

0GC33ZZ Extirpation of Matter from Right Adrenal Gland, Percutaneous Approach

0GC34ZZ Extirpation of Matter from Right Adrenal Gland, Percutaneous Endoscopic Approach

0GC40ZZ Extirpation of Matter from Bilateral Adrenal Glands, Open Approach

0GC43ZZ Extirpation of Matter from Bilateral Adrenal Glands, Percutaneous Approach

0GC44ZZ Extirpation of Matter from Bilateral Adrenal Glands, Percutaneous Endoscopic Approach

0GC60ZZ Extirpation of Matter from Left Carotid Body, Open Approach

0GC63ZZ Extirpation of Matter from Left Carotid Body, Percutaneous Approach

0GC64ZZ Extirpation of Matter from Left Carotid Body, Percutaneous Endoscopic Approach

0GC70ZZ Extirpation of Matter from Right Carotid Body, Open Approach

0GC73ZZ Extirpation of Matter from Right Carotid Body, Percutaneous Approach

0GC74ZZ Extirpation of Matter from Right Carotid Body, Percutaneous Endoscopic Approach

0GC80ZZ Extirpation of Matter from Bilateral Carotid Bodies, Open Approach

0GC83ZZ Extirpation of Matter from Bilateral Carotid Bodies, Percutaneous Approach

0GC84ZZ Extirpation of Matter from Bilateral Carotid Bodies, Percutaneous Endoscopic Approach

0GC90ZZ Extirpation of Matter from Para-aortic Body, Open Approach

0GC93ZZ Extirpation of Matter from Para-aortic Body, Percutaneous Approach

0GC94ZZ Extirpation of Matter from Para-aortic Body, Percutaneous Endoscopic Approach

0GCB0ZZ Extirpation of Matter from Coccygeal Glomus, Open Approach

0GCB3ZZ Extirpation of Matter from Coccygeal Glomus, Percutaneous Approach

0GCB4ZZ Extirpation of Matter from Coccygeal Glomus, Percutaneous Endoscopic Approach

0GCC0ZZ Extirpation of Matter from Glomus Jugulare, Open Approach

0GCC3ZZ Extirpation of Matter from Glomus Jugulare, Percutaneous Approach

0GCC4ZZ Extirpation of Matter from Glomus Jugulare, Percutaneous Endoscopic Approach

0GCD0ZZ Extirpation of Matter from Aortic Body, Open Approach

0GCD3ZZ Extirpation of Matter from Aortic Body, Percutaneous Approach

0GCD4ZZ Extirpation of Matter from Aortic Body, Percutaneous Endoscopic Approach

0GCF0ZZ Extirpation of Matter from Paraganglion Extremity, Open Approach

0GCF3ZZ Extirpation of Matter from Paraganglion Extremity, Percutaneous Approach

0GCF4ZZ Extirpation of Matter from Paraganglion Extremity, Percutaneous Endoscopic Approach

0GCG0ZZ Extirpation of Matter from Left Thyroid Gland Lobe, Open Approach

0GCG3ZZ Extirpation of Matter from Left Thyroid Gland Lobe, Percutaneous Approach

0GCG4ZZ Extirpation of Matter from Left Thyroid Gland Lobe, Percutaneous Endoscopic Approach

0GCH0ZZ Extirpation of Matter from Right Thyroid Gland Lobe, Open Approach

0GCH3ZZ Extirpation of Matter from Right Thyroid Gland Lobe, Percutaneous Approach

0GCH4ZZ Extirpation of Matter from Right Thyroid Gland Lobe, Percutaneous Endoscopic Approach

0GCK0ZZ Extirpation of Matter from Thyroid Gland, Open Approach

0GCK3ZZ Extirpation of Matter from Thyroid Gland, Percutaneous Approach

0GCK4ZZ Extirpation of Matter from Thyroid Gland, Percutaneous Endoscopic Approach

0GCL0ZZ Extirpation of Matter from Right Supe[r] Parathyroid Gland, Open Approach

0GCL3ZZ Extirpation of Matter from Right Supe[r] Parathyroid Gland, Percutaneous Approach

0GCL4ZZ Extirpation of Matter from Right Supe[r] Parathyroid Gland, Percutaneous Endoscopic Approach

0GCM0ZZ Extirpation of Matter from Left Superi[or] Parathyroid Gland, Open Approach

0GCM3ZZ Extirpation of Matter from Left Superi[or] Parathyroid Gland, Percutaneous Approach

0GCM4ZZ Extirpation of Matter from Left Superi[or] Parathyroid Gland, Percutaneous Endoscopic Approach

0GCN0ZZ Extirpation of Matter from Right Inferi[or] Parathyroid Gland, Open Approach

0GCN3ZZ Extirpation of Matter from Right Inferi[or] Parathyroid Gland, Percutaneous Approach

0GCN4ZZ Extirpation of Matter from Right Inferi[or] Parathyroid Gland, Percutaneous Endoscopic Approach

0GCP0ZZ Extirpation of Matter from Left Inferior Parathyroid Gland, Open Approach

0GCP3ZZ Extirpation of Matter from Left Inferior Parathyroid Gland, Percutaneous Approach

0GCP4ZZ Extirpation of Matter from Left Inferior Parathyroid Gland, Percutaneous Endoscopic Approach

0GCQ0ZZ Extirpation of Matter from Multiple Parathyroid Glands, Open Approach

0GCQ3ZZ Extirpation of Matter from Multiple Parathyroid Glands, Percutaneous Approach

0GCQ4ZZ Extirpation of Matter from Multiple Parathyroid Glands, Percutaneous Endoscopic Approach

0GCR0ZZ Extirpation of Matter from Parathyroid Gland, Open Approach

0GCR3ZZ Extirpation of Matter from Parathyroid Gland, Percutaneous Approach

0GCR4ZZ Extirpation of Matter from Parathyroid Gland, Percutaneous Endoscopic Approach

0GH – Endocrine System, Insertion

0GHS02Z Insertion of Monitoring Device into Endocrine Gland, Open Approach

0GHS03Z Insertion of Infusion Device into Endocrine Gland, Open Approach

0GHS32Z Insertion of Monitoring Device into Endocrine Gland, Percutaneous Approach

0GHS33Z Insertion of Infusion Device into Endocrine Gland, Percutaneous Approach

0GHS42Z Insertion of Monitoring Device into Endocrine Gland, Percutaneous Endoscopic Approach

0GHS43Z Insertion of Infusion Device into Endocrine Gland, Percutaneous Endoscopic Approach

0GJ – Endocrine System, Inspection

Review Coding Guidelines B3.11a, B3.11b and B3.11c

0GJ00ZZ Inspection of Pituitary Gland, Open Approach

0GJ03ZZ Inspection of Pituitary Gland, Percutaneous Approach

0GJ04ZZ Inspection of Pituitary Gland, Percutaneous Endoscopic Approach

0GJ10ZZ Inspection of Pineal Body, Open Approach

0GJ13ZZ Inspection of Pineal Body, Percutaneous Approach

0GJ14ZZ Inspection of Pineal Body, Percutaneous Endoscopic Approach

0GJ50ZZ Inspection of Adrenal Gland, Open Approach

0GJ53ZZ Inspection of Adrenal Gland, Percutaneous Approach

0GJ54ZZ Inspection of Adrenal Gland, Percutaneous Endoscopic Approach

0GJK0ZZ Inspection of Thyroid Gland, Open Approach

0GJK3ZZ Inspection of Thyroid Gland, Percutaneous Approach

0GJK4ZZ Inspection of Thyroid Gland, Percutaneous Endoscopic Approach

0GJR0ZZ Inspection of Parathyroid Gland, Open Approach

0GJR3ZZ Inspection of Parathyroid Gland, Percutaneous Approach

0GJR4ZZ Inspection of Parathyroid Gland, Percutaneous Endoscopic Approach

0GJS0ZZ Inspection of Endocrine Gland, Open Approach

0GJS3ZZ Inspection of Endocrine Gland, Percutaneous Approach

0GJS4ZZ Inspection of Endocrine Gland, Percutaneous Endoscopic Approach

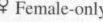

♀ Female-only   ♂ Male-only   ▲ Limited Coverage   ● Non-OR   ▥ HAC-associated procedure   ▲ Non-covered procedures   ✛ Combinati[on]

M – Endocrine System, Reattachment

120ZZ	Reattachment of Left Adrenal Gland, Open Approach
124ZZ	Reattachment of Left Adrenal Gland, Percutaneous Endoscopic Approach
130ZZ	Reattachment of Right Adrenal Gland, Open Approach
134ZZ	Reattachment of Right Adrenal Gland, Percutaneous Endoscopic Approach
1G0ZZ	Reattachment of Left Thyroid Gland Lobe, Open Approach
1G4ZZ	Reattachment of Left Thyroid Gland Lobe, Percutaneous Endoscopic Approach
1H0ZZ	Reattachment of Right Thyroid Gland Lobe, Open Approach

0GMH4ZZ	Reattachment of Right Thyroid Gland Lobe, Percutaneous Endoscopic Approach
0GML0ZZ	Reattachment of Right Superior Parathyroid Gland, Open Approach
0GML4ZZ	Reattachment of Right Superior Parathyroid Gland, Percutaneous Endoscopic Approach
0GMM0ZZ	Reattachment of Left Superior Parathyroid Gland, Open Approach
0GMM4ZZ	Reattachment of Left Superior Parathyroid Gland, Percutaneous Endoscopic Approach
0GMN0ZZ	Reattachment of Right Inferior Parathyroid Gland, Open Approach

0GMN4ZZ	Reattachment of Right Inferior Parathyroid Gland, Percutaneous Endoscopic Approach
0GMP0ZZ	Reattachment of Left Inferior Parathyroid Gland, Open Approach
0GMP4ZZ	Reattachment of Left Inferior Parathyroid Gland, Percutaneous Endoscopic Approach
0GMQ0ZZ	Reattachment of Multiple Parathyroid Glands, Open Approach
0GMQ4ZZ	Reattachment of Multiple Parathyroid Glands, Percutaneous Endoscopic Approach
0GMR0ZZ	Reattachment of Parathyroid Gland, Open Approach
0GMR4ZZ	Reattachment of Parathyroid Gland, Percutaneous Endoscopic Approach

N – Endocrine System, Release

Review Coding Guideline B3.13

Review Coding Guideline B3.14

N00ZZ	Release Pituitary Gland, Open Approach
N03ZZ	Release Pituitary Gland, Percutaneous Approach
N04ZZ	Release Pituitary Gland, Percutaneous Endoscopic Approach
N10ZZ	Release Pineal Body, Open Approach
N13ZZ	Release Pineal Body, Percutaneous Approach
N14ZZ	Release Pineal Body, Percutaneous Endoscopic Approach
N20ZZ	Release Left Adrenal Gland, Open Approach
N23ZZ	Release Left Adrenal Gland, Percutaneous Approach
N24ZZ	Release Left Adrenal Gland, Percutaneous Endoscopic Approach
N30ZZ	Release Right Adrenal Gland, Open Approach
N33ZZ	Release Right Adrenal Gland, Percutaneous Approach
N34ZZ	Release Right Adrenal Gland, Percutaneous Endoscopic Approach
N40ZZ	Release Bilateral Adrenal Glands, Open Approach
N43ZZ	Release Bilateral Adrenal Glands, Percutaneous Approach
N44ZZ	Release Bilateral Adrenal Glands, Percutaneous Endoscopic Approach
N60ZZ	Release Left Carotid Body, Open Approach
N63ZZ	Release Left Carotid Body, Percutaneous Approach
N64ZZ	Release Left Carotid Body, Percutaneous Endoscopic Approach
N70ZZ	Release Right Carotid Body, Open Approach
N73ZZ	Release Right Carotid Body, Percutaneous Approach
N74ZZ	Release Right Carotid Body, Percutaneous Endoscopic Approach

0GN80ZZ	Release Bilateral Carotid Bodies, Open Approach
0GN83ZZ	Release Bilateral Carotid Bodies, Percutaneous Approach
0GN84ZZ	Release Bilateral Carotid Bodies, Percutaneous Endoscopic Approach
0GN90ZZ	Release Para-aortic Body, Open Approach
0GN93ZZ	Release Para-aortic Body, Percutaneous Approach
0GN94ZZ	Release Para-aortic Body, Percutaneous Endoscopic Approach
0GNB0ZZ	Release Coccygeal Glomus, Open Approach
0GNB3ZZ	Release Coccygeal Glomus, Percutaneous Approach
0GNB4ZZ	Release Coccygeal Glomus, Percutaneous Endoscopic Approach
0GNC0ZZ	Release Glomus Jugulare, Open Approach
0GNC3ZZ	Release Glomus Jugulare, Percutaneous Approach
0GNC4ZZ	Release Glomus Jugulare, Percutaneous Endoscopic Approach
0GND0ZZ	Release Aortic Body, Open Approach
0GND3ZZ	Release Aortic Body, Percutaneous Approach
0GND4ZZ	Release Aortic Body, Percutaneous Endoscopic Approach
0GNF0ZZ	Release Paraganglion Extremity, Open Approach
0GNF3ZZ	Release Paraganglion Extremity, Percutaneous Approach
0GNF4ZZ	Release Paraganglion Extremity, Percutaneous Endoscopic Approach
0GNG0ZZ	Release Left Thyroid Gland Lobe, Open Approach
0GNG3ZZ	Release Left Thyroid Gland Lobe, Percutaneous Approach
0GNG4ZZ	Release Left Thyroid Gland Lobe, Percutaneous Endoscopic Approach
0GNH0ZZ	Release Right Thyroid Gland Lobe, Open Approach
0GNH3ZZ	Release Right Thyroid Gland Lobe, Percutaneous Approach

0GNH4ZZ	Release Right Thyroid Gland Lobe, Percutaneous Endoscopic Approach
0GNK0ZZ	Release Thyroid Gland, Open Approach
0GNK3ZZ	Release Thyroid Gland, Percutaneous Approach
0GNK4ZZ	Release Thyroid Gland, Percutaneous Endoscopic Approach
0GNL0ZZ	Release Right Superior Parathyroid Gland, Open Approach
0GNL3ZZ	Release Right Superior Parathyroid Gland, Percutaneous Approach
0GNL4ZZ	Release Right Superior Parathyroid Gland, Percutaneous Endoscopic Approach
0GNM0ZZ	Release Left Superior Parathyroid Gland, Open Approach
0GNM3ZZ	Release Left Superior Parathyroid Gland, Percutaneous Approach
0GNM4ZZ	Release Left Superior Parathyroid Gland, Percutaneous Endoscopic Approach
0GNN0ZZ	Release Right Inferior Parathyroid Gland, Open Approach
0GNN3ZZ	Release Right Inferior Parathyroid Gland, Percutaneous Approach
0GNN4ZZ	Release Right Inferior Parathyroid Gland, Percutaneous Endoscopic Approach
0GNP0ZZ	Release Left Inferior Parathyroid Gland, Open Approach
0GNP3ZZ	Release Left Inferior Parathyroid Gland, Percutaneous Approach
0GNP4ZZ	Release Left Inferior Parathyroid Gland, Percutaneous Endoscopic Approach
0GNQ0ZZ	Release Multiple Parathyroid Glands, Open Approach
0GNQ3ZZ	Release Multiple Parathyroid Glands, Percutaneous Approach
0GNQ4ZZ	Release Multiple Parathyroid Glands, Percutaneous Endoscopic Approach
0GNR0ZZ	Release Parathyroid Gland, Open Approach
0GNR3ZZ	Release Parathyroid Gland, Percutaneous Approach
0GNR4ZZ	Release Parathyroid Gland, Percutaneous Endoscopic Approach

P – Endocrine System, Removal

Review Coding Guideline B6.1c

P000Z	Removal of Drainage Device from Pituitary Gland, Open Approach
P030Z	Removal of Drainage Device from Pituitary Gland, Percutaneous Approach

0GP040Z	Removal of Drainage Device from Pituitary Gland, Percutaneous Endoscopic Approach

0GP0X0Z	Removal of Drainage Device from Pituitary Gland, External Approach
0GP100Z	Removal of Drainage Device from Pineal Body, Open Approach

---

Female-only   ♂ Male-only   ▲ Limited Coverage   ● Non-OR   ▦ HAC-associated procedure   ▲ Non-covered procedures   ✚ Combination

0GP130Z Removal of Drainage Device from Pineal Body, Percutaneous Approach
0GP140Z Removal of Drainage Device from Pineal Body, Percutaneous Endoscopic Approach
0GP1X0Z Removal of Drainage Device from Pineal Body, External Approach
0GP500Z Removal of Drainage Device from Adrenal Gland, Open Approach
0GP530Z Removal of Drainage Device from Adrenal Gland, Percutaneous Approach
0GP540Z Removal of Drainage Device from Adrenal Gland, Percutaneous Endoscopic Approach
0GP5X0Z Removal of Drainage Device from Adrenal Gland, External Approach
0GPK00Z Removal of Drainage Device from Thyroid Gland, Open Approach
0GPK30Z Removal of Drainage Device from Thyroid Gland, Percutaneous Approach
0GPK40Z Removal of Drainage Device from Thyroid Gland, Percutaneous Endoscopic Approach
0GPKX0Z Removal of Drainage Device from Thyroid Gland, External Approach
0GPR00Z Removal of Drainage Device from Parathyroid Gland, Open Approach
0GPR30Z Removal of Drainage Device from Parathyroid Gland, Percutaneous Approach
0GPR40Z Removal of Drainage Device from Parathyroid Gland, Percutaneous Endoscopic Approach
0GPRX0Z Removal of Drainage Device from Parathyroid Gland, External Approach
0GPS00Z Removal of Drainage Device from Endocrine Gland, Open Approach
0GPS02Z Removal of Monitoring Device from Endocrine Gland, Open Approach
0GPS03Z Removal of Infusion Device from Endocrine Gland, Open Approach
0GPS30Z Removal of Drainage Device from Endocrine Gland, Percutaneous Appro
0GPS32Z Removal of Monitoring Device from Endocrine Gland, Percutaneous Appro
0GPS33Z Removal of Infusion Device from Endocrine Gland, Percutaneous Appro
0GPS40Z Removal of Drainage Device from Endocrine Gland, Percutaneous Endoscopic Approach
0GPS42Z Removal of Monitoring Device from Endocrine Gland, Percutaneous Endoscopic Approach
0GPS43Z Removal of Infusion Device from Endocrine Gland, Percutaneous Endoscopic Approach
0GPSX0Z Removal of Drainage Device from Endocrine Gland, External Approach
0GPSX2Z Removal of Monitoring Device from Endocrine Gland, External Approach
0GPSX3Z Removal of Infusion Device from Endocrine Gland, External Approach

0GQ – Endocrine System, Repair

0GQ00ZZ Repair Pituitary Gland, Open Approach
0GQ03ZZ Repair Pituitary Gland, Percutaneous Approach
0GQ04ZZ Repair Pituitary Gland, Percutaneous Endoscopic Approach
0GQ10ZZ Repair Pineal Body, Open Approach
0GQ13ZZ Repair Pineal Body, Percutaneous Approach
0GQ14ZZ Repair Pineal Body, Percutaneous Endoscopic Approach
0GQ20ZZ Repair Left Adrenal Gland, Open Approach
0GQ23ZZ Repair Left Adrenal Gland, Percutaneous Approach
0GQ24ZZ Repair Left Adrenal Gland, Percutaneous Endoscopic Approach
0GQ30ZZ Repair Right Adrenal Gland, Open Approach
0GQ33ZZ Repair Right Adrenal Gland, Percutaneous Approach
0GQ34ZZ Repair Right Adrenal Gland, Percutaneous Endoscopic Approach
0GQ40ZZ Repair Bilateral Adrenal Glands, Open Approach
0GQ43ZZ Repair Bilateral Adrenal Glands, Percutaneous Approach
0GQ44ZZ Repair Bilateral Adrenal Glands, Percutaneous Endoscopic Approach
0GQ60ZZ Repair Left Carotid Body, Open Approach
0GQ63ZZ Repair Left Carotid Body, Percutaneous Approach
0GQ64ZZ Repair Left Carotid Body, Percutaneous Endoscopic Approach
0GQ70ZZ Repair Right Carotid Body, Open Approach
0GQ73ZZ Repair Right Carotid Body, Percutaneous Approach
0GQ74ZZ Repair Right Carotid Body, Percutaneous Endoscopic Approach
0GQ80ZZ Repair Bilateral Carotid Bodies, Open Approach
0GQ83ZZ Repair Bilateral Carotid Bodies, Percutaneous Approach
0GQ84ZZ Repair Bilateral Carotid Bodies, Percutaneous Endoscopic Approach
0GQ90ZZ Repair Para-aortic Body, Open Approach
0GQ93ZZ Repair Para-aortic Body, Percutaneous Approach
0GQ94ZZ Repair Para-aortic Body, Percutaneous Endoscopic Approach
0GQB0ZZ Repair Coccygeal Glomus, Open Approach
0GQB3ZZ Repair Coccygeal Glomus, Percutaneous Approach
0GQB4ZZ Repair Coccygeal Glomus, Percutaneous Endoscopic Approach
0GQC0ZZ Repair Glomus Jugulare, Open Approach
0GQC3ZZ Repair Glomus Jugulare, Percutaneous Approach
0GQC4ZZ Repair Glomus Jugulare, Percutaneous Endoscopic Approach
0GQD0ZZ Repair Aortic Body, Open Approach
0GQD3ZZ Repair Aortic Body, Percutaneous Approach
0GQD4ZZ Repair Aortic Body, Percutaneous Endoscopic Approach
0GQF0ZZ Repair Paraganglion Extremity, Open Approach
0GQF3ZZ Repair Paraganglion Extremity, Percutaneous Approach
0GQF4ZZ Repair Paraganglion Extremity, Percutaneous Endoscopic Approach
0GQG0ZZ Repair Left Thyroid Gland Lobe, Open Approach
0GQG3ZZ Repair Left Thyroid Gland Lobe, Percutaneous Approach
0GQG4ZZ Repair Left Thyroid Gland Lobe, Percutaneous Endoscopic Approach
0GQH0ZZ Repair Right Thyroid Gland Lobe, Open Approach
0GQH3ZZ Repair Right Thyroid Gland Lobe, Percutaneous Approach
0GQH4ZZ Repair Right Thyroid Gland Lobe, Percutaneous Endoscopic Approach
0GQJ0ZZ Repair Thyroid Gland Isthmus, Open Approach
0GQJ3ZZ Repair Thyroid Gland Isthmus, Percutaneous Approach
0GQJ4ZZ Repair Thyroid Gland Isthmus, Percutaneous Endoscopic Approach
0GQK0ZZ Repair Thyroid Gland, Open Approach
0GQK3ZZ Repair Thyroid Gland, Percutaneous Approach
0GQK4ZZ Repair Thyroid Gland, Percutaneous Endoscopic Approach
0GQL0ZZ Repair Right Superior Parathyroid Gla Open Approach
0GQL3ZZ Repair Right Superior Parathyroid Gla Percutaneous Approach
0GQL4ZZ Repair Right Superior Parathyroid Gla Percutaneous Endoscopic Approach
0GQM0ZZ Repair Left Superior Parathyroid Glan Open Approach
0GQM3ZZ Repair Left Superior Parathyroid Glan Percutaneous Approach
0GQM4ZZ Repair Left Superior Parathyroid Glan Percutaneous Endoscopic Approach
0GQN0ZZ Repair Right Inferior Parathyroid Glan Open Approach
0GQN3ZZ Repair Right Inferior Parathyroid Glan Percutaneous Approach
0GQN4ZZ Repair Right Inferior Parathyroid Glan Percutaneous Endoscopic Approach
0GQP0ZZ Repair Left Inferior Parathyroid Gland, Open Approach
0GQP3ZZ Repair Left Inferior Parathyroid Gland, Percutaneous Approach
0GQP4ZZ Repair Left Inferior Parathyroid Gland, Percutaneous Endoscopic Approach
0GQQ0ZZ Repair Multiple Parathyroid Glands, O Approach
0GQQ3ZZ Repair Multiple Parathyroid Glands, Percutaneous Approach
0GQQ4ZZ Repair Multiple Parathyroid Glands, Percutaneous Endoscopic Approach
0GQR0ZZ Repair Parathyroid Gland, Open Appro
0GQR3ZZ Repair Parathyroid Gland, Percutaneous Approach
0GQR4ZZ Repair Parathyroid Gland, Percutaneous Endoscopic Approach

0GS – Endocrine System, Reposition

0GS20ZZ Reposition Left Adrenal Gland, Open Approach
0GS24ZZ Reposition Left Adrenal Gland, Percutaneous Endoscopic Approach
0GS30ZZ Reposition Right Adrenal Gland, Open Approach
0GS34ZZ Reposition Right Adrenal Gland, Percutaneous Endoscopic Approach
0GSG0ZZ Reposition Left Thyroid Gland Lobe, Open Approach
0GSG4ZZ Reposition Left Thyroid Gland Lobe, Percutaneous Endoscopic Approach
0GSH0ZZ Reposition Right Thyroid Gland Lobe, Open Approach
0GSH4ZZ Reposition Right Thyroid Gland Lobe, Percutaneous Endoscopic Approach
0GSL0ZZ Reposition Right Superior Parathyroid Gland, Open Approach

♀ Female-only   ♂ Male-only   ▲ Limited Coverage   ● Non-OR   ▨ HAC-associated procedure   ▲ Non-covered procedures   ✚ Combina

L4ZZ Reposition Right Superior Parathyroid Gland, Percutaneous Endoscopic Approach

M0ZZ Reposition Left Superior Parathyroid Gland, Open Approach

M4ZZ Reposition Left Superior Parathyroid Gland, Percutaneous Endoscopic Approach

N0ZZ Reposition Right Inferior Parathyroid Gland, Open Approach

0GSN4ZZ Reposition Right Inferior Parathyroid Gland, Percutaneous Endoscopic Approach

0GSP0ZZ Reposition Left Inferior Parathyroid Gland, Open Approach

0GSP4ZZ Reposition Left Inferior Parathyroid Gland, Percutaneous Endoscopic Approach

0GSQ0ZZ Reposition Multiple Parathyroid Glands, Open Approach

0GSQ4ZZ Reposition Multiple Parathyroid Glands, Percutaneous Endoscopic Approach

0GSR0ZZ Reposition Parathyroid Gland, Open Approach

0GSR4ZZ Reposition Parathyroid Gland, Percutaneous Endoscopic Approach

T – Endocrine System, Resection

iew Coding Guideline B3.8

00ZZ Resection of Pituitary Gland, Open Approach

04ZZ Resection of Pituitary Gland, Percutaneous Endoscopic Approach

10ZZ Resection of Pineal Body, Open Approach

14ZZ Resection of Pineal Body, Percutaneous Endoscopic Approach

20ZZ Resection of Left Adrenal Gland, Open Approach

24ZZ Resection of Left Adrenal Gland, Percutaneous Endoscopic Approach

30ZZ Resection of Right Adrenal Gland, Open Approach

34ZZ Resection of Right Adrenal Gland, Percutaneous Endoscopic Approach

40ZZ Resection of Bilateral Adrenal Glands, Open Approach

44ZZ Resection of Bilateral Adrenal Glands, Percutaneous Endoscopic Approach

60ZZ Resection of Left Carotid Body, Open Approach

64ZZ Resection of Left Carotid Body, Percutaneous Endoscopic Approach

70ZZ Resection of Right Carotid Body, Open Approach

74ZZ Resection of Right Carotid Body, Percutaneous Endoscopic Approach

80ZZ Resection of Bilateral Carotid Bodies, Open Approach

84ZZ Resection of Bilateral Carotid Bodies, Percutaneous Endoscopic Approach

0GT90ZZ Resection of Para-aortic Body, Open Approach

0GT94ZZ Resection of Para-aortic Body, Percutaneous Endoscopic Approach

0GTB0ZZ Resection of Coccygeal Glomus, Open Approach

0GTB4ZZ Resection of Coccygeal Glomus, Percutaneous Endoscopic Approach

0GTC0ZZ Resection of Glomus Jugulare, Open Approach

0GTC4ZZ Resection of Glomus Jugulare, Percutaneous Endoscopic Approach

0GTD0ZZ Resection of Aortic Body, Open Approach

0GTD4ZZ Resection of Aortic Body, Percutaneous Endoscopic Approach

0GTF0ZZ Resection of Paraganglion Extremity, Open Approach

0GTF4ZZ Resection of Paraganglion Extremity, Percutaneous Endoscopic Approach

0GTG0ZZ Resection of Left Thyroid Gland Lobe, Open Approach

0GTG4ZZ Resection of Left Thyroid Gland Lobe, Percutaneous Endoscopic Approach

0GTH0ZZ Resection of Right Thyroid Gland Lobe, Open Approach

0GTH4ZZ Resection of Right Thyroid Gland Lobe, Percutaneous Endoscopic Approach

0GTK0ZZ Resection of Thyroid Gland, Open Approach

0GTK4ZZ Resection of Thyroid Gland, Percutaneous Endoscopic Approach

0GTL0ZZ Resection of Right Superior Parathyroid Gland, Open Approach

0GTL4ZZ Resection of Right Superior Parathyroid Gland, Percutaneous Endoscopic Approach

0GTM0ZZ Resection of Left Superior Parathyroid Gland, Open Approach

0GTM4ZZ Resection of Left Superior Parathyroid Gland, Percutaneous Endoscopic Approach

0GTN0ZZ Resection of Right Inferior Parathyroid Gland, Open Approach

0GTN4ZZ Resection of Right Inferior Parathyroid Gland, Percutaneous Endoscopic Approach

0GTP0ZZ Resection of Left Inferior Parathyroid Gland, Open Approach

0GTP4ZZ Resection of Left Inferior Parathyroid Gland, Percutaneous Endoscopic Approach

0GTQ0ZZ Resection of Multiple Parathyroid Glands, Open Approach

0GTQ4ZZ Resection of Multiple Parathyroid Glands, Percutaneous Endoscopic Approach

0GTR0ZZ Resection of Parathyroid Gland, Open Approach

0GTR4ZZ Resection of Parathyroid Gland, Percutaneous Endoscopic Approach

W – Endocrine System, Revision

iew Coding Guideline B6.1c

W000Z Revision of Drainage Device in Pituitary Gland, Open Approach

W030Z Revision of Drainage Device in Pituitary Gland, Percutaneous Approach

W040Z Revision of Drainage Device in Pituitary Gland, Percutaneous Endoscopic Approach

W0X0Z Revision of Drainage Device in Pituitary Gland, External Approach

W100Z Revision of Drainage Device in Pineal Body, Open Approach

W130Z Revision of Drainage Device in Pineal Body, Percutaneous Approach

W140Z Revision of Drainage Device in Pineal Body, Percutaneous Endoscopic Approach

W1X0Z Revision of Drainage Device in Pineal Body, External Approach

W500Z Revision of Drainage Device in Adrenal Gland, Open Approach

W530Z Revision of Drainage Device in Adrenal Gland, Percutaneous Approach

W540Z Revision of Drainage Device in Adrenal Gland, Percutaneous Endoscopic Approach

0GW5X0Z Revision of Drainage Device in Adrenal Gland, External Approach

0GWK00Z Revision of Drainage Device in Thyroid Gland, Open Approach

0GWK30Z Revision of Drainage Device in Thyroid Gland, Percutaneous Approach

0GWK40Z Revision of Drainage Device in Thyroid Gland, Percutaneous Endoscopic Approach

0GWKX0Z Revision of Drainage Device in Thyroid Gland, External Approach

0GWR00Z Revision of Drainage Device in Parathyroid Gland, Open Approach

0GWR30Z Revision of Drainage Device in Parathyroid Gland, Percutaneous Approach

0GWR40Z Revision of Drainage Device in Parathyroid Gland, Percutaneous Endoscopic Approach

0GWRX0Z Revision of Drainage Device in Parathyroid Gland, External Approach

0GWS00Z Revision of Drainage Device in Endocrine Gland, Open Approach

0GWS02Z Revision of Monitoring Device in Endocrine Gland, Open Approach

0GWS03Z Revision of Infusion Device in Endocrine Gland, Open Approach

0GWS30Z Revision of Drainage Device in Endocrine Gland, Percutaneous Approach

0GWS32Z Revision of Monitoring Device in Endocrine Gland, Percutaneous Approach

0GWS33Z Revision of Infusion Device in Endocrine Gland, Percutaneous Approach

0GWS40Z Revision of Drainage Device in Endocrine Gland, Percutaneous Endoscopic Approach

0GWS42Z Revision of Monitoring Device in Endocrine Gland, Percutaneous Endoscopic Approach

0GWS43Z Revision of Infusion Device in Endocrine Gland, Percutaneous Endoscopic Approach

0GWSX0Z Revision of Drainage Device in Endocrine Gland, External Approach

0GWSX2Z Revision of Monitoring Device in Endocrine Gland, External Approach

0GWSX3Z Revision of Infusion Device in Endocrine Gland, External Approach

Skin and Subcutaneous Tissue

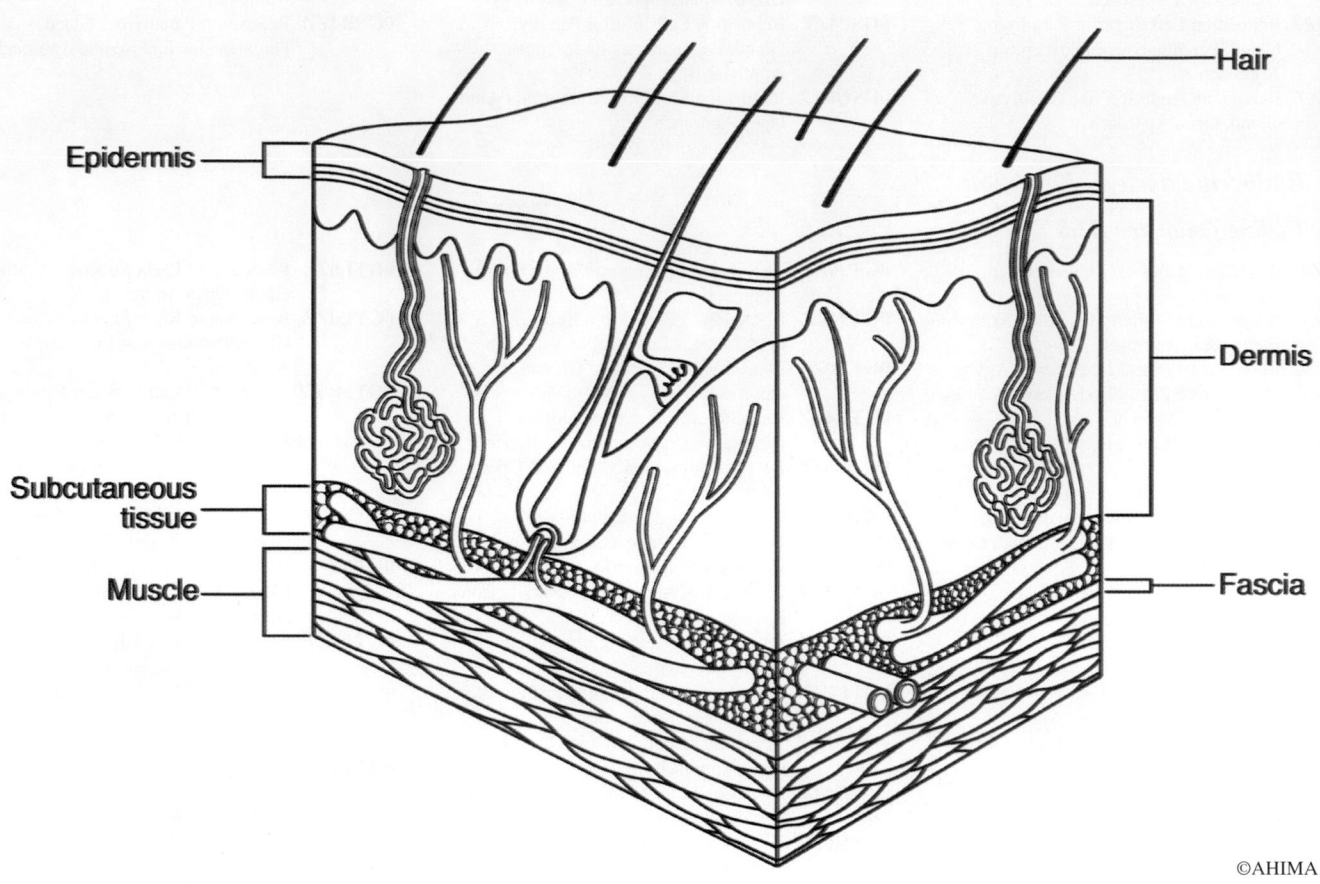

Epidermis

Subcutaneous tissue

Muscle

Hair

Dermis

Fascia

©AHIMA

Breast

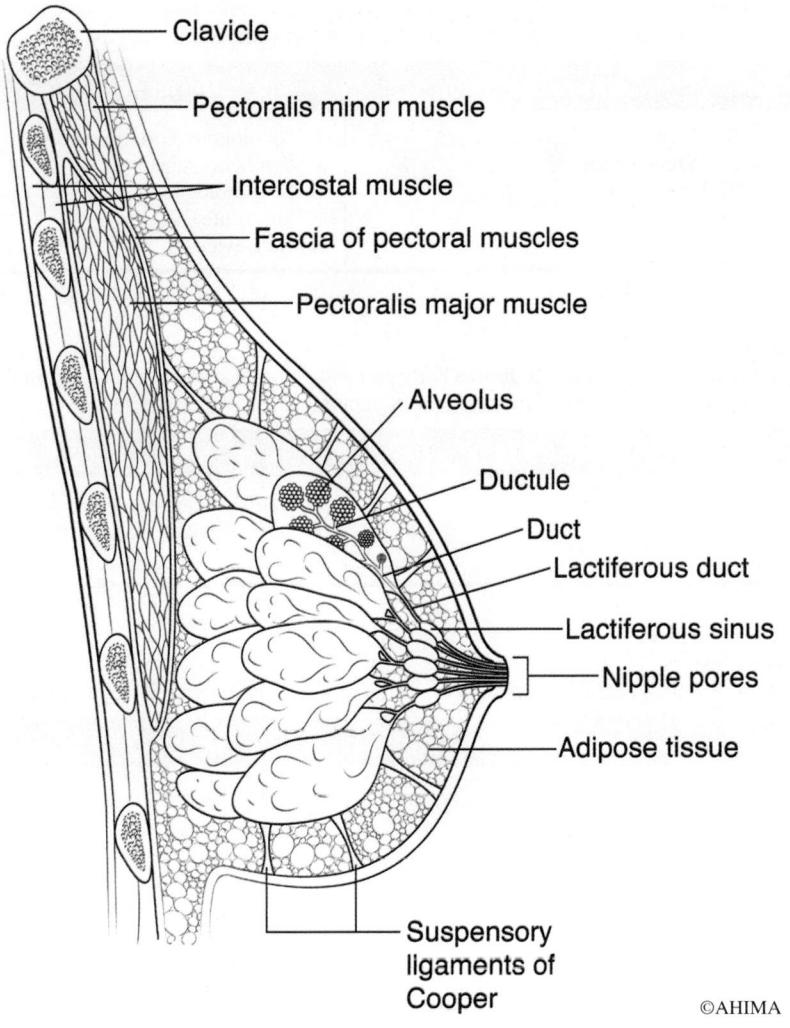

- Clavicle
- Pectoralis minor muscle
- Intercostal muscle
- Fascia of pectoral muscles
- Pectoralis major muscle
- Alveolus
- Ductule
- Duct
- Lactiferous duct
- Lactiferous sinus
- Nipple pores
- Adipose tissue
- Suspensory ligaments of Cooper

©AHIMA

Nail Bed

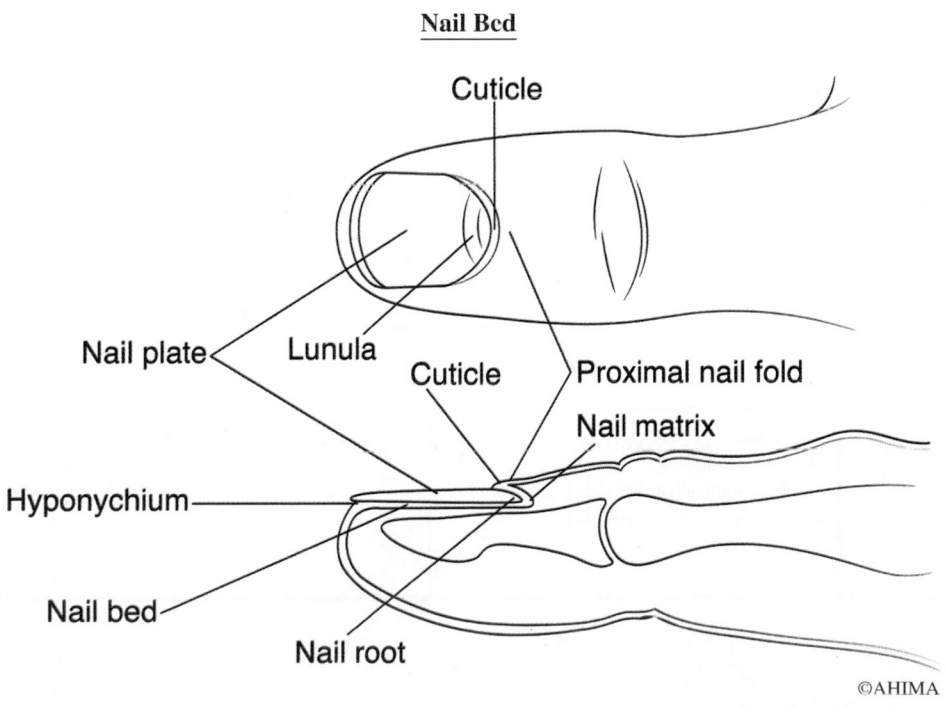

- Cuticle
- Nail plate
- Lunula
- Cuticle
- Proximal nail fold
- Nail matrix
- Hyponychium
- Nail bed
- Nail root

©AHIMA

Skin and Breast Tables 0H0–0HX

Section	0	Medical and Surgical
Body System	H	Skin and Breast
Operation	0	Alteration: Modifying the anatomic structure of a body part without affecting the function of the body part

Body Part (4th)	Approach (5th)	Device (6th)	Qualifier (7th)
T Breast, Right U Breast, Left V Breast, Bilateral	0 Open 3 Percutaneous X External	7 Autologous Tissue Substitute J Synthetic Substitute K Nonautologous Tissue Substitute Z No Device	Z No Qualifier

Section	0	Medical and Surgical
Body System	H	Skin and Breast
Operation	2	Change: Taking out or off a device from a body part and putting back an identical or similar device in or on the same body part without cutting or puncturing the skin or a mucous membrane

Body Part (4th)	Approach (5th)	Device (6th)	Qualifier (7th)
P Skin T Breast, Right U Breast, Left	X External	0 Drainage Device Y Other Device	Z No Qualifier

Section	0	Medical and Surgical
Body System	H	Skin and Breast
Operation	5	Destruction: Physical eradication of all or a portion of a body part by the direct use of energy, force, or a destructive agent

Body Part (4th)	Approach (5th)	Device (6th)	Qualifier (7th)
0 Skin, Scalp 1 Skin, Face 2 Skin, Right Ear 3 Skin, Left Ear 4 Skin, Neck 5 Skin, Chest 6 Skin, Back 7 Skin, Abdomen 8 Skin, Buttock 9 Skin, Perineum A Skin, Genitalia B Skin, Right Upper Arm C Skin, Left Upper Arm D Skin, Right Lower Arm E Skin, Left Lower Arm F Skin, Right Hand G Skin, Left Hand H Skin, Right Upper Leg J Skin, Left Upper Leg K Skin, Right Lower Leg L Skin, Left Lower Leg M Skin, Right Foot N Skin, Left Foot	X External	Z No Device	D Multiple Z No Qualifier
Q Finger Nail R Toe Nail	X External	Z No Device	Z No Qualifier
T Breast, Right U Breast, Left V Breast, Bilateral W Nipple, Right X Nipple, Left	0 Open 3 Percutaneous 7 Via Natural or Artificial Opening 8 Via Natural or Artificial Opening Endoscopic X External	Z No Device	Z No Qualifier

Section 0 Medical and Surgical
Body System H Skin and Breast
Operation 8 **Division:** Cutting into a body part, without draining fluids and/or gases from the body part, in order to separate or transect a body part

Body Part (4ᵗʰ)	Approach (5ᵗʰ)	Device (6ᵗʰ)	Qualifier (7ᵗʰ)
Skin, Scalp	X External	Z No Device	Z No Qualifier
Skin, Face			
Skin, Right Ear			
Skin, Left Ear			
Skin, Neck			
Skin, Chest			
Skin, Back			
Skin, Abdomen			
Skin, Buttock			
Skin, Perineum			
Skin, Genitalia			
Skin, Right Upper Arm			
Skin, Left Upper Arm			
Skin, Right Lower Arm			
Skin, Left Lower Arm			
Skin, Right Hand			
Skin, Left Hand			
Skin, Right Upper Leg			
Skin, Left Upper Leg			
Skin, Right Lower Leg			
Skin, Left Lower Leg			
Skin, Right Foot			
Skin, Left Foot			

Section 0 Medical and Surgical
Body System H Skin and Breast
Operation 9 **Drainage:** Taking or letting out fluids and/or gases from a body part

Body Part (4ᵗʰ)	Approach (5ᵗʰ)	Device (6ᵗʰ)	Qualifier (7ᵗʰ)
Skin, Scalp	X External	0 Drainage Device	Z No Qualifier
Skin, Face			
Skin, Right Ear			
Skin, Left Ear			
Skin, Neck			
Skin, Chest			
Skin, Back			
Skin, Abdomen			
Skin, Buttock			
Skin, Perineum			
Skin, Genitalia			
Skin, Right Upper Arm			
Skin, Left Upper Arm			
Skin, Right Lower Arm			
Skin, Left Lower Arm			
Skin, Right Hand			
Skin, Left Hand			
Skin, Right Upper Leg			
Skin, Left Upper Leg			
Skin, Right Lower Leg			
Skin, Left Lower Leg			
Skin, Right Foot			
Skin, Left Foot			
Finger Nail			
Toe Nail			

Continued →

Section   0   **Medical and Surgical**
Body System   H   **Skin and Breast**
Operation   9   **Drainage:** Taking or letting out fluids and/or gases from a body part

Body Part (4th)	Approach (5th)	Device (6th)	Qualifier (7th)
0 Skin, Scalp 1 Skin, Face 2 Skin, Right Ear 3 Skin, Left Ear 4 Skin, Neck 5 Skin, Chest 6 Skin, Back 7 Skin, Abdomen 8 Skin, Buttock 9 Skin, Perineum A Skin, Genitalia B Skin, Right Upper Arm C Skin, Left Upper Arm D Skin, Right Lower Arm E Skin, Left Lower Arm F Skin, Right Hand G Skin, Left Hand H Skin, Right Upper Leg J Skin, Left Upper Leg K Skin, Right Lower Leg L Skin, Left Lower Leg M Skin, Right Foot N Skin, Left Foot Q Finger Nail R Toe Nail	X External	Z No Device	X Diagnostic Z No Qualifier
T Breast, Right U Breast, Left V Breast, Bilateral W Nipple, Right X Nipple, Left	0 Open 3 Percutaneous 7 Via Natural or Artificial Opening 8 Via Natural or Artificial Opening Endoscopic X External	0 Drainage Device	Z No Qualifier
T Breast, Right U Breast, Left V Breast, Bilateral W Nipple, Right X Nipple, Left	0 Open 3 Percutaneous 7 Via Natural or Artificial Opening 8 Via Natural or Artificial Opening Endoscopic X External	Z No Device	X Diagnostic Z No Qualifier

tion	**0**	**Medical and Surgical**
y System	**H**	**Skin and Breast**
eration	**B**	**Excision:** Cutting out or off, without replacement, a portion of a body part

Body Part (4th)	Approach (5th)	Device (6th)	Qualifier (7th)
Skin, Scalp Skin, Face Skin, Right Ear Skin, Left Ear Skin, Neck Skin, Chest Skin, Back Skin, Abdomen Skin, Buttock Skin, Perineum Skin, Genitalia Skin, Right Upper Arm Skin, Left Upper Arm Skin, Right Lower Arm Skin, Left Lower Arm Skin, Right Hand Skin, Left Hand Skin, Right Upper Leg Skin, Left Upper Leg Skin, Right Lower Leg Skin, Left Lower Leg Skin, Right Foot Skin, Left Foot Finger Nail Toe Nail	**X** External	**Z** No Device	**X** Diagnostic **Z** No Qualifier
Breast, Right Breast, Left Breast, Bilateral Nipple, Right Nipple, Left Supernumerary Breast	**0** Open **3** Percutaneous **7** Via Natural or Artificial Opening **8** Via Natural or Artificial Opening Endoscopic **X** External	**Z** No Device	**X** Diagnostic **Z** No Qualifier

Section	0	Medical and Surgical
Body System	H	Skin and Breast
Operation	C	Extirpation: Taking or cutting out solid matter from a body part

Body Part (4th)	Approach (5th)	Device (6th)	Qualifier (7th)
0 Skin, Scalp 1 Skin, Face 2 Skin, Right Ear 3 Skin, Left Ear 4 Skin, Neck 5 Skin, Chest 6 Skin, Back 7 Skin, Abdomen 8 Skin, Buttock 9 Skin, Perineum A Skin, Genitalia B Skin, Right Upper Arm C Skin, Left Upper Arm D Skin, Right Lower Arm E Skin, Left Lower Arm F Skin, Right Hand G Skin, Left Hand H Skin, Right Upper Leg J Skin, Left Upper Leg K Skin, Right Lower Leg L Skin, Left Lower Leg M Skin, Right Foot N Skin, Left Foot Q Finger Nail R Toe Nail	X External	Z No Device	Z No Qualifier
T Breast, Right U Breast, Left V Breast, Bilateral W Nipple, Right X Nipple, Left	0 Open 3 Percutaneous 7 Via Natural or Artificial Opening 8 Via Natural or Artificial Opening Endoscopic X External	Z No Device	Z No Qualifier

Section	0	Medical and Surgical
Body System	H	Skin and Breast
Operation	D	**Extraction:** Pulling or stripping out or off all or a portion of a body part by the use of force

Body Part (4th)	Approach (5th)	Device (6th)	Qualifier (7th)
Skin, Scalp Skin, Face Skin, Right Ear Skin, Left Ear Skin, Neck Skin, Chest Skin, Back Skin, Abdomen Skin, Buttock Skin, Perineum Skin, Genitalia Skin, Right Upper Arm Skin, Left Upper Arm Skin, Right Lower Arm Skin, Left Lower Arm Skin, Right Hand Skin, Left Hand Skin, Right Upper Leg Skin, Left Upper Leg Skin, Right Lower Leg Skin, Left Lower Leg Skin, Right Foot Skin, Left Foot Finger Nail Toe Nail Hair	**X** External	**Z** No Device	**Z** No Qualifier

Section	0	Medical and Surgical
Body System	H	Skin and Breast
Operation	H	**Insertion:** Putting in a nonbiological appliance that monitors, assists, performs, or prevents a physiological function but does not physically take the place of a body part

Body Part (4th)	Approach (5th)	Device (6th)	Qualifier (7th)
T Breast, Right U Breast, Left V Breast, Bilateral W Nipple, Right X Nipple, Left	**0** Open **3** Percutaneous **7** Via Natural or Artificial Opening **8** Via Natural or Artificial Opening Endoscopic	**1** Radioactive Element **N** Tissue Expander	**Z** No Qualifier
T Breast, Right U Breast, Left V Breast, Bilateral W Nipple, Right X Nipple, Left	**X** External	**1** Radioactive Element	**Z** No Qualifier

Section	0	Medical and Surgical
Body System	H	Skin and Breast
Operation	J	**Inspection:** Visually and/or manually exploring a body part

Body Part (4th)	Approach (5th)	Device (6th)	Qualifier (7th)
P Skin Q Finger Nail R Toe Nail	**X** External	**Z** No Device	**Z** No Qualifier
T Breast, Right U Breast, Left	**0** Open **3** Percutaneous **7** Via Natural or Artificial Opening **8** Via Natural or Artificial Opening Endoscopic **X** External	**Z** No Device	**Z** No Qualifier

Section	0	Medical and Surgical
Body System	H	Skin and Breast
Operation	M	**Reattachment:** Putting back in or on all or a portion of a separated body part to its normal location or other suitable locatio

Body Part (4th)	Approach (5th)	Device (6th)	Qualifier (7th)
0 Skin, Scalp 1 Skin, Face 2 Skin, Right Ear 3 Skin, Left Ear 4 Skin, Neck 5 Skin, Chest 6 Skin, Back 7 Skin, Abdomen 8 Skin, Buttock 9 Skin, Perineum A Skin, Genitalia B Skin, Right Upper Arm C Skin, Left Upper Arm D Skin, Right Lower Arm E Skin, Left Lower Arm F Skin, Right Hand G Skin, Left Hand H Skin, Right Upper Leg J Skin, Left Upper Leg K Skin, Right Lower Leg L Skin, Left Lower Leg M Skin, Right Foot N Skin, Left Foot T Breast, Right U Breast, Left V Breast, Bilateral W Nipple, Right X Nipple, Left	X External	Z No Device	Z No Qualifier

Section	0	Medical and Surgical
Body System	H	Skin and Breast
Operation	N	**Release:** Freeing a body part from an abnormal physical constraint by cutting or by the use of force

Body Part (4th)	Approach (5th)	Device (6th)	Qualifier (7th)
0 Skin, Scalp 1 Skin, Face 2 Skin, Right Ear 3 Skin, Left Ear 4 Skin, Neck 5 Skin, Chest 6 Skin, Back 7 Skin, Abdomen 8 Skin, Buttock 9 Skin, Perineum A Skin, Genitalia B Skin, Right Upper Arm C Skin, Left Upper Arm D Skin, Right Lower Arm E Skin, Left Lower Arm F Skin, Right Hand G Skin, Left Hand H Skin, Right Upper Leg J Skin, Left Upper Leg	X External	Z No Device	Z No Qualifier

Continued —

Section 0 **Medical and Surgical**
Body System H **Skin and Breast**
Operation N **Release:** Freeing a body part from an abnormal physical constraint by cutting or by the use of force

Body Part (4th)	Approach (5th)	Device (6th)	Qualifier (7th)
Skin, Right Lower Leg Skin, Left Lower Leg Skin, Right Foot Skin, Left Foot Finger Nail Toe Nail Breast, Right Breast, Left Breast, Bilateral Nipple, Right Nipple, Left	0 Open 3 Percutaneous 7 Via Natural or Artificial Opening 8 Via Natural or Artificial Opening Endoscopic X External	Z No Device	Z No Qualifier

Section 0 **Medical and Surgical**
Body System H **Skin and Breast**
Operation P **Removal:** Taking out or off a device from a body part

Body Part (4th)	Approach (5th)	Device (6th)	Qualifier (7th)
Skin Finger Nail Toe Nail	X External	0 Drainage Device 7 Autologous Tissue Substitute J Synthetic Substitute K Nonautologous Tissue Substitute	Z No Qualifier
Hair	X External	7 Autologous Tissue Substitute J Synthetic Substitute K Nonautologous Tissue Substitute	Z No Qualifier
Breast, Right Breast, Left	0 Open 3 Percutaneous 7 Via Natural or Artificial Opening 8 Via Natural or Artificial Opening Endoscopic	0 Drainage Device 1 Radioactive Element 7 Autologous Tissue Substitute J Synthetic Substitute K Nonautologous Tissue Substitute N Tissue Expander	Z No Qualifier
Breast, Right Breast, Left	X External	0 Drainage Device 1 Radioactive Element 7 Autologous Tissue Substitute J Synthetic Substitute K Nonautologous Tissue Substitute	Z No Qualifier

Section   **0**   **Medical and Surgical**
Body System   **H**   **Skin and Breast**
Operation   **Q**   **Repair:** Restoring, to the extent possible, a body part to its normal anatomic structure and function

Body Part (4ᵗʰ)	Approach (5ᵗʰ)	Device (6ᵗʰ)	Qualifier (7ᵗʰ)
0 Skin, Scalp 1 Skin, Face 2 Skin, Right Ear 3 Skin, Left Ear 4 Skin, Neck 5 Skin, Chest 6 Skin, Back 7 Skin, Abdomen 8 Skin, Buttock 9 Skin, Perineum A Skin, Genitalia B Skin, Right Upper Arm C Skin, Left Upper Arm D Skin, Right Lower Arm E Skin, Left Lower Arm F Skin, Right Hand G Skin, Left Hand H Skin, Right Upper Leg J Skin, Left Upper Leg K Skin, Right Lower Leg L Skin, Left Lower Leg M Skin, Right Foot N Skin, Left Foot Q Finger Nail R Toe Nail	X External	Z No Device	Z No Qualifier
T Breast, Right U Breast, Left V Breast, Bilateral W Nipple, Right X Nipple, Left Y Supernumerary Breast	0 Open 3 Percutaneous 7 Via Natural or Artificial Opening 8 Via Natural or Artificial Opening Endoscopic X External	Z No Device	Z No Qualifier

Section   **0**   **Medical and Surgical**
Body System   **H**   **Skin and Breast**
Operation   **R**   **Replacement:** Putting in or on biological or synthetic material that physically takes the place and/or function of all or a portion of a body part

Body Part (4ᵗʰ)	Approach (5ᵗʰ)	Device (6ᵗʰ)	Qualifier (7ᵗʰ)
0 Skin, Scalp 1 Skin, Face 2 Skin, Right Ear 3 Skin, Left Ear 4 Skin, Neck 5 Skin, Chest 6 Skin, Back 7 Skin, Abdomen 8 Skin, Buttock 9 Skin, Perineum A Skin, Genitalia B Skin, Right Upper Arm C Skin, Left Upper Arm D Skin, Right Lower Arm E Skin, Left Lower Arm F Skin, Right Hand G Skin, Left Hand H Skin, Right Upper Leg J Skin, Left Upper Leg K Skin, Right Lower Leg L Skin, Left Lower Leg M Skin, Right Foot N Skin, Left Foot	X External	7 Autologous Tissue Substitute K Nonautologous Tissue Substitute	3 Full Thickness 4 Partial Thickness

Continued –

on	0	**Medical and Surgical**
System	H	**Skin and Breast**
ation	R	**Replacement:** Putting in or on biological or synthetic material that physically takes the place and/or function of all or a portion of a body part

Body Part (4th)	Approach (5th)	Device (6th)	Qualifier (7th)
Skin, Scalp Skin, Face Skin, Right Ear Skin, Left Ear Skin, Neck Skin, Chest Skin, Back Skin, Abdomen Skin, Buttock Skin, Perineum Skin, Genitalia Skin, Right Upper Arm Skin, Left Upper Arm Skin, Right Lower Arm Skin, Left Lower Arm Skin, Right Hand Skin, Left Hand Skin, Right Upper Leg Skin, Left Upper Leg Skin, Right Lower Leg Skin, Left Lower Leg Skin, Right Foot Skin, Left Foot	**X** External	**J** Synthetic Substitute	**3** Full Thickness **4** Partial Thickness **Z** No Qualifier
Finger Nail Toe Nail Hair	**X** External	**7** Autologous Tissue Substitute **J** Synthetic Substitute **K** Nonautologous Tissue Substitute	**Z** No Qualifier
Breast, Right Breast, Left Breast, Bilateral	**0** Open	**7** Autologous Tissue Substitute	**5** Latissimus Dorsi Myocutaneous Flap **6** Transverse Rectus Abdominis Myocutaneous Flap **7** Deep Inferior Epigastric Artery Perforator Flap **8** Superficial Inferior Epigastric Artery Flap **9** Gluteal Artery Perforator Flap **Z** No Qualifier
Breast, Right Breast, Left Breast, Bilateral	**0** Open	**J** Synthetic Substitute **K** Nonautologous Tissue Substitute	**Z** No Qualifier
Breast, Right Breast, Left Breast, Bilateral	**3** Percutaneous **X** External	**7** Autologous Tissue Substitute **J** Synthetic Substitute **K** Nonautologous Tissue Substitute	**Z** No Qualifier
Nipple, Right Nipple, Left	**0** Open **3** Percutaneous **X** External	**7** Autologous Tissue Substitute **J** Synthetic Substitute **K** Nonautologous Tissue Substitute	**Z** No Qualifier

tion	0	**Medical and Surgical**
ly System	H	**Skin and Breast**
eration	S	**Reposition:** Moving to its normal location, or other suitable location, all or a portion of a body part

Body Part (4th)	Approach (5th)	Device (6th)	Qualifier (7th)
Hair Nipple, Right Nipple, Left	**X** External	**Z** No Device	**Z** No Qualifier
Breast, Right Breast, Left Breast, Bilateral	**0** Open	**Z** No Device	**Z** No Qualifier

Section	0	Medical and Surgical
Body System	H	Skin and Breast
Operation	T	**Resection:** Cutting out or off, without replacement, all of a body part

Body Part (4th)	Approach (5th)	Device (6th)	Qualifier (7th)
Q Finger Nail R Toe Nail W Nipple, Right X Nipple, Left	X External	Z No Device	Z No Qualifier
T Breast, Right U Breast, Left V Breast, Bilateral Y Supernumerary Breast	0 Open	Z No Device	Z No Qualifier

Section	0	Medical and Surgical
Body System	H	Skin and Breast
Operation	U	**Supplement:** Putting in or on biological or synthetic material that physically reinforces and/or augments the function of a portion of a body part

Body Part (4th)	Approach (5th)	Device (6th)	Qualifier (7th)
T Breast, Right U Breast, Left V Breast, Bilateral W Nipple, Right X Nipple, Left	0 Open 3 Percutaneous 7 Via Natural or Artificial Opening 8 Via Natural or Artificial Opening Endoscopic X External	7 Autologous Tissue Substitute J Synthetic Substitute K Nonautologous Tissue Substitute	Z No Qualifier

Section	0	Medical and Surgical
Body System	H	Skin and Breast
Operation	W	**Revision:** Correcting, to the extent possible, a portion of a malfunctioning device or the position of a displaced device

Body Part (4th)	Approach (5th)	Device (6th)	Qualifier (7th)
P Skin Q Finger Nail R Toe Nail	X External	0 Drainage Device 7 Autologous Tissue Substitute J Synthetic Substitute K Nonautologous Tissue Substitute	Z No Qualifier
S Hair	X External	7 Autologous Tissue Substitute J Synthetic Substitute K Nonautologous Tissue Substitute	Z No Qualifier
T Breast, Right U Breast, Left	0 Open 3 Percutaneous 7 Via Natural or Artificial Opening 8 Via Natural or Artificial Opening Endoscopic	0 Drainage Device 7 Autologous Tissue Substitute J Synthetic Substitute K Nonautologous Tissue Substitute N Tissue Expander	Z No Qualifier
T Breast, Right U Breast, Left	X External	0 Drainage Device 7 Autologous Tissue Substitute J Synthetic Substitute K Nonautologous Tissue Substitute	Z No Qualifier

	0	Medical and Surgical
...tion		
...dy System	H	Skin and Breast
...eration	X	Transfer: Moving, without taking out, all or a portion of a body part to another location to take over the function of all or a portion of a body part

Body Part (4th)	Approach (5th)	Device (6th)	Qualifier (7th)
◢ Skin, Scalp Skin, Face ◢ Skin, Right Ear ◢ Skin, Left Ear ◢ Skin, Neck ◢ Skin, Chest ◢ Skin, Back ◢ Skin, Abdomen ◢ Skin, Buttock ◢ Skin, Perineum ◢ Skin, Genitalia ◢ Skin, Right Upper Arm ◢ Skin, Left Upper Arm ◢ Skin, Right Lower Arm ◢ Skin, Left Lower Arm ◢ Skin, Right Hand ◢ Skin, Left Hand ◢ Skin, Right Upper Leg ◢ Skin, Left Upper Leg ◢ Skin, Right Lower Leg ◢ Skin, Left Lower Leg ◢ Skin, Right Foot ◢ Skin, Left Foot	X External	Z No Device	Z No Qualifier

...kin and Breast Code Listing 0H0–0HX

...0 – Skin and Breast, Alteration

...0T07Z Alteration of Right Breast with Autologous Tissue Substitute, Open Approach

...0T0JZ Alteration of Right Breast with Synthetic Substitute, Open Approach

...0T0KZ Alteration of Right Breast with Nonautologous Tissue Substitute, Open Approach

...0T0ZZ Alteration of Right Breast, Open Approach

...0T37Z Alteration of Right Breast with Autologous Tissue Substitute, Percutaneous Approach

...0T3JZ Alteration of Right Breast with Synthetic Substitute, Percutaneous Approach

...0T3KZ Alteration of Right Breast with Nonautologous Tissue Substitute, Percutaneous Approach

...0T3ZZ Alteration of Right Breast, Percutaneous Approach

...0TX7Z Alteration of Right Breast with Autologous Tissue Substitute, External Approach

...0TXJZ Alteration of Right Breast with Synthetic Substitute, External Approach

...0TXKZ Alteration of Right Breast with Nonautologous Tissue Substitute, External Approach

...0TXZZ Alteration of Right Breast, External Approach

0H0U07Z Alteration of Left Breast with Autologous Tissue Substitute, Open Approach

0H0U0JZ Alteration of Left Breast with Synthetic Substitute, Open Approach

0H0U0KZ Alteration of Left Breast with Nonautologous Tissue Substitute, Open Approach

0H0U0ZZ Alteration of Left Breast, Open Approach

0H0U37Z Alteration of Left Breast with Autologous Tissue Substitute, Percutaneous Approach

0H0U3JZ Alteration of Left Breast with Synthetic Substitute, Percutaneous Approach

0H0U3KZ Alteration of Left Breast with Nonautologous Tissue Substitute, Percutaneous Approach

0H0U3ZZ Alteration of Left Breast, Percutaneous Approach

0H0UX7Z Alteration of Left Breast with Autologous Tissue Substitute, External Approach

0H0UXJZ Alteration of Left Breast with Synthetic Substitute, External Approach

0H0UXKZ Alteration of Left Breast with Nonautologous Tissue Substitute, External Approach

0H0UXZZ Alteration of Left Breast, External Approach

0H0V07Z Alteration of Bilateral Breast with Autologous Tissue Substitute, Open Approach

0H0V0JZ Alteration of Bilateral Breast with Synthetic Substitute, Open Approach

0H0V0KZ Alteration of Bilateral Breast with Nonautologous Tissue Substitute, Open Approach

0H0V0ZZ Alteration of Bilateral Breast, Open Approach

0H0V37Z Alteration of Bilateral Breast with Autologous Tissue Substitute, Percutaneous Approach

0H0V3JZ Alteration of Bilateral Breast with Synthetic Substitute, Percutaneous Approach

0H0V3KZ Alteration of Bilateral Breast with Nonautologous Tissue Substitute, Percutaneous Approach

0H0V3ZZ Alteration of Bilateral Breast, Percutaneous Approach

0H0VX7Z Alteration of Bilateral Breast with Autologous Tissue Substitute, External Approach

0H0VXJZ Alteration of Bilateral Breast with Synthetic Substitute, External Approach

0H0VXKZ Alteration of Bilateral Breast with Nonautologous Tissue Substitute, External Approach

0H0VXZZ Alteration of Bilateral Breast, External Approach

...H2 – Skin and Breast, Change

...eview Coding Guideline B6.1c

...2PX0Z Change Drainage Device in Skin, External Approach

...2PXYZ Change Other Device in Skin, External Approach

0H2TX0Z Change Drainage Device in Right Breast, External Approach

0H2TXYZ Change Other Device in Right Breast, External Approach

0H2UX0Z Change Drainage Device in Left Breast, External Approach

0H2UXYZ Change Other Device in Left Breast, External Approach

♀ Female-only	♂ Male-only	▲ Limited Coverage	● Non-OR	▥ HAC-associated procedure	▲ Non-covered procedures	✚ Combination

0H5 – Skin and Breast, Destruction

- **0H50XZD** Destruction of Scalp Skin, Multiple, External Approach
- **0H50XZZ** Destruction of Scalp Skin, External Approach
- **0H51XZD** Destruction of Face Skin, Multiple, External Approach
- **0H51XZZ** Destruction of Face Skin, External Approach
- **0H52XZD** Destruction of Right Ear Skin, Multiple, External Approach
- **0H52XZZ** Destruction of Right Ear Skin, External Approach
- **0H53XZD** Destruction of Left Ear Skin, Multiple, External Approach
- **0H53XZZ** Destruction of Left Ear Skin, External Approach
- **0H54XZD** Destruction of Neck Skin, Multiple, External Approach
- **0H54XZZ** Destruction of Neck Skin, External Approach
- **0H55XZD** Destruction of Chest Skin, Multiple, External Approach
- **0H55XZZ** Destruction of Chest Skin, External Approach
- **0H56XZD** Destruction of Back Skin, Multiple, External Approach
- **0H56XZZ** Destruction of Back Skin, External Approach
- **0H57XZD** Destruction of Abdomen Skin, Multiple, External Approach
- **0H57XZZ** Destruction of Abdomen Skin, External Approach
- **0H58XZD** Destruction of Buttock Skin, Multiple, External Approach
- **0H58XZZ** Destruction of Buttock Skin, External Approach
- **0H59XZD** Destruction of Perineum Skin, Multiple, External Approach
- **0H59XZZ** Destruction of Perineum Skin, External Approach
- **0H5AXZD** Destruction of Genitalia Skin, Multiple, External Approach
- **0H5AXZZ** Destruction of Genitalia Skin, External Approach
- **0H5BXZD** Destruction of Right Upper Arm Skin, Multiple, External Approach
- **0H5BXZZ** Destruction of Right Upper Arm Skin, External Approach
- **0H5CXZD** Destruction of Left Upper Arm Skin, Multiple, External Approach

- **0H5CXZZ** Destruction of Left Upper Arm Skin, External Approach
- **0H5DXZD** Destruction of Right Lower Arm Skin, Multiple, External Approach
- **0H5DXZZ** Destruction of Right Lower Arm Skin, External Approach
- **0H5EXZD** Destruction of Left Lower Arm Skin, Multiple, External Approach
- **0H5EXZZ** Destruction of Left Lower Arm Skin, External Approach
- **0H5FXZD** Destruction of Right Hand Skin, Multiple, External Approach
- **0H5FXZZ** Destruction of Right Hand Skin, External Approach
- **0H5GXZD** Destruction of Left Hand Skin, Multiple, External Approach
- **0H5GXZZ** Destruction of Left Hand Skin, External Approach
- **0H5HXZD** Destruction of Right Upper Leg Skin, Multiple, External Approach
- **0H5HXZZ** Destruction of Right Upper Leg Skin, External Approach
- **0H5JXZD** Destruction of Left Upper Leg Skin, Multiple, External Approach
- **0H5JXZZ** Destruction of Left Upper Leg Skin, External Approach
- **0H5KXZD** Destruction of Right Lower Leg Skin, Multiple, External Approach
- **0H5KXZZ** Destruction of Right Lower Leg Skin, External Approach
- **0H5LXZD** Destruction of Left Lower Leg Skin, Multiple, External Approach
- **0H5LXZZ** Destruction of Left Lower Leg Skin, External Approach
- **0H5MXZD** Destruction of Right Foot Skin, Multiple, External Approach
- **0H5MXZZ** Destruction of Right Foot Skin, External Approach
- **0H5NXZD** Destruction of Left Foot Skin, Multiple, External Approach
- **0H5NXZZ** Destruction of Left Foot Skin, External Approach
- **0H5QXZZ** Destruction of Finger Nail, External Approach
- **0H5RXZZ** Destruction of Toe Nail, External Approach
- **0H5T0ZZ** Destruction of Right Breast, Open Approach
- **0H5T3ZZ** Destruction of Right Breast, Percutaneous Approach

0H5T7ZZ Destruction of Right Breast, Via Natural or Artificial Opening
0H5T8ZZ Destruction of Right Breast, Via Natural or Artificial Opening Endoscopic
0H5TXZZ Destruction of Right Breast, External Approach
0H5U0ZZ Destruction of Left Breast, Open Approach
0H5U3ZZ Destruction of Left Breast, Percutaneous Approach
0H5U7ZZ Destruction of Left Breast, Via Natural Artificial Opening
0H5U8ZZ Destruction of Left Breast, Via Natural Artificial Opening Endoscopic
0H5UXZZ Destruction of Left Breast, External Approach
0H5V0ZZ Destruction of Bilateral Breast, Open Approach
0H5V3ZZ Destruction of Bilateral Breast, Percutaneous Approach
0H5V7ZZ Destruction of Bilateral Breast, Via Natural or Artificial Opening
0H5V8ZZ Destruction of Bilateral Breast, Via Natural or Artificial Opening Endoscopic
0H5VXZZ Destruction of Bilateral Breast, External Approach
0H5W0ZZ Destruction of Right Nipple, Open Approach
0H5W3ZZ Destruction of Right Nipple, Percutaneous Approach
0H5W7ZZ Destruction of Right Nipple, Via Natural or Artificial Opening
0H5W8ZZ Destruction of Right Nipple, Via Natural or Artificial Opening Endoscopic
0H5WXZZ Destruction of Right Nipple, External Approach
0H5X0ZZ Destruction of Left Nipple, Open Approach
0H5X3ZZ Destruction of Left Nipple, Percutaneous Approach
0H5X7ZZ Destruction of Left Nipple, Via Natural Artificial Opening
0H5X8ZZ Destruction of Left Nipple, Via Natural Artificial Opening Endoscopic
0H5XXZZ Destruction of Left Nipple, External Approach

0H8 – Skin and Breast, Division

Review Coding Guideline B3.14

0H80XZZ Division of Scalp Skin, External Approach
0H81XZZ Division of Face Skin, External Approach
0H82XZZ Division of Right Ear Skin, External Approach
0H83XZZ Division of Left Ear Skin, External Approach
0H84XZZ Division of Neck Skin, External Approach
0H85XZZ Division of Chest Skin, External Approach
0H86XZZ Division of Back Skin, External Approach
0H87XZZ Division of Abdomen Skin, External Approach

0H88XZZ Division of Buttock Skin, External Approach
0H89XZZ Division of Perineum Skin, External Approach
0H8AXZZ Division of Genitalia Skin, External Approach
0H8BXZZ Division of Right Upper Arm Skin, External Approach
0H8CXZZ Division of Left Upper Arm Skin, External Approach
0H8DXZZ Division of Right Lower Arm Skin, External Approach
0H8EXZZ Division of Left Lower Arm Skin, External Approach
0H8FXZZ Division of Right Hand Skin, External Approach

0H8GXZZ Division of Left Hand Skin, External Approach
0H8HXZZ Division of Right Upper Leg Skin, External Approach
0H8JXZZ Division of Left Upper Leg Skin, Exter Approach
0H8KXZZ Division of Right Lower Leg Skin, External Approach
0H8LXZZ Division of Left Lower Leg Skin, External Approach
0H8MXZZ Division of Right Foot Skin, External Approach
0H8NXZZ Division of Left Foot Skin, External Approach

♀ Female-only   ♂ Male-only   ▲ Limited Coverage   ● Non-OR   ▦ HAC-associated procedure   ▲ Non-covered procedures   + Combinat

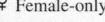

view Coding Guidelines B3.4a and B3.4b

view Coding Guideline B6.2

90X0Z	Drainage of Scalp Skin with Drainage Device, External Approach	
90XZX	Drainage of Scalp Skin, External Approach, Diagnostic	
90XZZ	Drainage of Scalp Skin, External Approach	
91X0Z	Drainage of Face Skin with Drainage Device, External Approach	
91XZX	Drainage of Face Skin, External Approach, Diagnostic	
91XZZ	Drainage of Face Skin, External Approach	
92X0Z	Drainage of Right Ear Skin with Drainage Device, External Approach	
92XZX	Drainage of Right Ear Skin, External Approach, Diagnostic	
92XZZ	Drainage of Right Ear Skin, External Approach	
93X0Z	Drainage of Left Ear Skin with Drainage Device, External Approach	
93XZX	Drainage of Left Ear Skin, External Approach, Diagnostic	
93XZZ	Drainage of Left Ear Skin, External Approach	
94X0Z	Drainage of Neck Skin with Drainage Device, External Approach	
94XZX	Drainage of Neck Skin, External Approach, Diagnostic	
94XZZ	Drainage of Neck Skin, External Approach	
95X0Z	Drainage of Chest Skin with Drainage Device, External Approach	
95XZX	Drainage of Chest Skin, External Approach, Diagnostic	
95XZZ	Drainage of Chest Skin, External Approach	
96X0Z	Drainage of Back Skin with Drainage Device, External Approach	
96XZX	Drainage of Back Skin, External Approach, Diagnostic	
96XZZ	Drainage of Back Skin, External Approach	
97X0Z	Drainage of Abdomen Skin with Drainage Device, External Approach	
97XZX	Drainage of Abdomen Skin, External Approach, Diagnostic	
97XZZ	Drainage of Abdomen Skin, External Approach	
98X0Z	Drainage of Buttock Skin with Drainage Device, External Approach	
98XZX	Drainage of Buttock Skin, External Approach, Diagnostic	
98XZZ	Drainage of Buttock Skin, External Approach	
99X0Z	Drainage of Perineum Skin with Drainage Device, External Approach	
99XZX	Drainage of Perineum Skin, External Approach, Diagnostic	
99XZZ	Drainage of Perineum Skin, External Approach	
9AX0Z	Drainage of Genitalia Skin with Drainage Device, External Approach	
9AXZX	Drainage of Genitalia Skin, External Approach, Diagnostic	
9AXZZ	Drainage of Genitalia Skin, External Approach	
9BX0Z	Drainage of Right Upper Arm Skin with Drainage Device, External Approach	
9BXZX	Drainage of Right Upper Arm Skin, External Approach, Diagnostic	
9BXZZ	Drainage of Right Upper Arm Skin, External Approach	

0H9CX0Z	Drainage of Left Upper Arm Skin with Drainage Device, External Approach	
0H9CXZX	Drainage of Left Upper Arm Skin, External Approach, Diagnostic	
0H9CXZZ	Drainage of Left Upper Arm Skin, External Approach	
0H9DX0Z	Drainage of Right Lower Arm Skin with Drainage Device, External Approach	
0H9DXZX	Drainage of Right Lower Arm Skin, External Approach, Diagnostic	
0H9DXZZ	Drainage of Right Lower Arm Skin, External Approach	
0H9EX0Z	Drainage of Left Lower Arm Skin with Drainage Device, External Approach	
0H9EXZX	Drainage of Left Lower Arm Skin, External Approach, Diagnostic	
0H9EXZZ	Drainage of Left Lower Arm Skin, External Approach	
0H9FX0Z	Drainage of Right Hand Skin with Drainage Device, External Approach	
0H9FXZX	Drainage of Right Hand Skin, External Approach, Diagnostic	
0H9FXZZ	Drainage of Right Hand Skin, External Approach	
0H9GX0Z	Drainage of Left Hand Skin with Drainage Device, External Approach	
0H9GXZX	Drainage of Left Hand Skin, External Approach, Diagnostic	
0H9GXZZ	Drainage of Left Hand Skin, External Approach	
0H9HX0Z	Drainage of Right Upper Leg Skin with Drainage Device, External Approach	
0H9HXZX	Drainage of Right Upper Leg Skin, External Approach, Diagnostic	
0H9HXZZ	Drainage of Right Upper Leg Skin, External Approach	
0H9JX0Z	Drainage of Left Upper Leg Skin with Drainage Device, External Approach	
0H9JXZX	Drainage of Left Upper Leg Skin, External Approach, Diagnostic	
0H9JXZZ	Drainage of Left Upper Leg Skin, External Approach	
0H9KX0Z	Drainage of Right Lower Leg Skin with Drainage Device, External Approach	
0H9KXZX	Drainage of Right Lower Leg Skin, External Approach, Diagnostic	
0H9KXZZ	Drainage of Right Lower Leg Skin, External Approach	
0H9LX0Z	Drainage of Left Lower Leg Skin with Drainage Device, External Approach	
0H9LXZX	Drainage of Left Lower Leg Skin, External Approach, Diagnostic	
0H9LXZZ	Drainage of Left Lower Leg Skin, External Approach	
0H9MX0Z	Drainage of Right Foot Skin with Drainage Device, External Approach	
0H9MXZX	Drainage of Right Foot Skin, External Approach, Diagnostic	
0H9MXZZ	Drainage of Right Foot Skin, External Approach	
0H9NX0Z	Drainage of Left Foot Skin with Drainage Device, External Approach	
0H9NXZX	Drainage of Left Foot Skin, External Approach, Diagnostic	
0H9NXZZ	Drainage of Left Foot Skin, External Approach	
0H9QX0Z	Drainage of Finger Nail with Drainage Device, External Approach	
0H9QXZX	Drainage of Finger Nail, External Approach, Diagnostic	
0H9QXZZ	Drainage of Finger Nail, External Approach	

0H9RX0Z	Drainage of Toe Nail with Drainage Device, External Approach	
0H9RXZX	Drainage of Toe Nail, External Approach, Diagnostic	
0H9RXZZ	Drainage of Toe Nail, External Approach	
0H9T00Z	Drainage of Right Breast with Drainage Device, Open Approach	
0H9T0ZX	Drainage of Right Breast, Open Approach, Diagnostic	
0H9T0ZZ	Drainage of Right Breast, Open Approach	
0H9T30Z	Drainage of Right Breast with Drainage Device, Percutaneous Approach	
0H9T3ZX	Drainage of Right Breast, Percutaneous Approach, Diagnostic	
0H9T3ZZ	Drainage of Right Breast, Percutaneous Approach	
0H9T70Z	Drainage of Right Breast with Drainage Device, Via Natural or Artificial Opening	
0H9T7ZX	Drainage of Right Breast, Via Natural or Artificial Opening, Diagnostic	
0H9T7ZZ	Drainage of Right Breast, Via Natural or Artificial Opening	
0H9T80Z	Drainage of Right Breast with Drainage Device, Via Natural or Artificial Opening Endoscopic	
0H9T8ZX	Drainage of Right Breast, Via Natural or Artificial Opening Endoscopic, Diagnostic	
0H9T8ZZ	Drainage of Right Breast, Via Natural or Artificial Opening Endoscopic	
0H9TX0Z	Drainage of Right Breast with Drainage Device, External Approach	
0H9TXZX	Drainage of Right Breast, External Approach, Diagnostic	
0H9TXZZ	Drainage of Right Breast, External Approach	
0H9U00Z	Drainage of Left Breast with Drainage Device, Open Approach	
0H9U0ZX	Drainage of Left Breast, Open Approach, Diagnostic	
0H9U0ZZ	Drainage of Left Breast, Open Approach	
0H9U30Z	Drainage of Left Breast with Drainage Device, Percutaneous Approach	
0H9U3ZX	Drainage of Left Breast, Percutaneous Approach, Diagnostic	
0H9U3ZZ	Drainage of Left Breast, Percutaneous Approach	
0H9U70Z	Drainage of Left Breast with Drainage Device, Via Natural or Artificial Opening	
0H9U7ZX	Drainage of Left Breast, Via Natural or Artificial Opening, Diagnostic	
0H9U7ZZ	Drainage of Left Breast, Via Natural or Artificial Opening	
0H9U80Z	Drainage of Left Breast with Drainage Device, Via Natural or Artificial Opening Endoscopic	
0H9U8ZX	Drainage of Left Breast, Via Natural or Artificial Opening Endoscopic, Diagnostic	
0H9U8ZZ	Drainage of Left Breast, Via Natural or Artificial Opening Endoscopic	
0H9UX0Z	Drainage of Left Breast with Drainage Device, External Approach	
0H9UXZX	Drainage of Left Breast, External Approach, Diagnostic	
0H9UXZZ	Drainage of Left Breast, External Approach	
0H9V00Z	Drainage of Bilateral Breast with Drainage Device, Open Approach	
0H9V0ZX	Drainage of Bilateral Breast, Open Approach, Diagnostic	

♀ Female-only   ♂ Male-only   ▲ Limited Coverage   ● Non-OR   ▨ HAC-associated procedure   ▲ Non-covered procedures   ✚ Combination

0H9V0ZZ	Drainage of Bilateral Breast, Open Approach	0H9W0ZX	Drainage of Right Nipple, Open Approach, Diagnostic	0H9X00Z	Drainage of Left Nipple with Drainage Device, Open Approach
0H9V30Z	Drainage of Bilateral Breast with Drainage Device, Percutaneous Approach	0H9W0ZZ	Drainage of Right Nipple, Open Approach	0H9X0ZX	Drainage of Left Nipple, Open Approach, Diagnostic
0H9V3ZX	Drainage of Bilateral Breast, Percutaneous Approach, Diagnostic	0H9W30Z	Drainage of Right Nipple with Drainage Device, Percutaneous Approach	0H9X0ZZ	Drainage of Left Nipple, Open Approach
0H9V3ZZ	Drainage of Bilateral Breast, Percutaneous Approach	0H9W3ZX	Drainage of Right Nipple, Percutaneous Approach, Diagnostic	0H9X30Z	Drainage of Left Nipple with Drainage Device, Percutaneous Approach
0H9V70Z	Drainage of Bilateral Breast with Drainage Device, Via Natural or Artificial Opening	0H9W3ZZ	Drainage of Right Nipple, Percutaneous Approach	0H9X3ZX	Drainage of Left Nipple, Percutaneous Approach, Diagnostic
0H9V7ZX	Drainage of Bilateral Breast, Via Natural or Artificial Opening, Diagnostic	0H9W70Z	Drainage of Right Nipple with Drainage Device, Via Natural or Artificial Opening	0H9X3ZZ	Drainage of Left Nipple, Percutaneous Approach
0H9V7ZZ	Drainage of Bilateral Breast, Via Natural or Artificial Opening	0H9W7ZX	Drainage of Right Nipple, Via Natural or Artificial Opening, Diagnostic	0H9X70Z	Drainage of Left Nipple with Drainage Device, Via Natural or Artificial Opening
0H9V80Z	Drainage of Bilateral Breast with Drainage Device, Via Natural or Artificial Opening Endoscopic	0H9W7ZZ	Drainage of Right Nipple, Via Natural or Artificial Opening	0H9X7ZX	Drainage of Left Nipple, Via Natural or Artificial Opening, Diagnostic
0H9V8ZX	Drainage of Bilateral Breast, Via Natural or Artificial Opening Endoscopic, Diagnostic	0H9W80Z	Drainage of Right Nipple with Drainage Device, Via Natural or Artificial Opening Endoscopic	0H9X7ZZ	Drainage of Left Nipple, Via Natural or Artificial Opening
0H9V8ZZ	Drainage of Bilateral Breast, Via Natural or Artificial Opening Endoscopic	0H9W8ZX	Drainage of Right Nipple, Via Natural or Artificial Opening Endoscopic, Diagnostic	0H9X80Z	Drainage of Left Nipple with Drainage Device, Via Natural or Artificial Opening Endoscopic
0H9VX0Z	Drainage of Bilateral Breast with Drainage Device, External Approach	0H9W8ZZ	Drainage of Right Nipple, Via Natural or Artificial Opening Endoscopic	0H9X8ZX	Drainage of Left Nipple, Via Natural or Artificial Opening Endoscopic, Diagnostic
0H9VXZX	Drainage of Bilateral Breast, External Approach, Diagnostic	0H9WX0Z	Drainage of Right Nipple with Drainage Device, External Approach	0H9X8ZZ	Drainage of Left Nipple, Via Natural or Artificial Opening Endoscopic
0H9VXZZ	Drainage of Bilateral Breast, External Approach	0H9WXZX	Drainage of Right Nipple, External Approach, Diagnostic	0H9XX0Z	Drainage of Left Nipple with Drainage Device, External Approach
0H9W00Z	Drainage of Right Nipple with Drainage Device, Open Approach	0H9WXZZ	Drainage of Right Nipple, External Approach	0H9XXZX	Drainage of Left Nipple, External Approach, Diagnostic
				0H9XXZZ	Drainage of Left Nipple, External Approach

0HB – Skin and Breast, Excision

Review Coding Guidelines 3B.4a and 3B.4b

Review Coding Guideline B3.5

Review Coding Guideline B3.8

0HB0XZX	Excision of Scalp Skin, External Approach, Diagnostic	● 0HB9XZZ	Excision of Perineum Skin, External Approach	0HBKXZX	Excision of Right Lower Leg Skin, External Approach, Diagnostic
0HB0XZZ	Excision of Scalp Skin, External Approach	0HBAXZX	Excision of Genitalia Skin, External Approach, Diagnostic	0HBKXZZ	Excision of Right Lower Leg Skin, External Approach
0HB1XZX	Excision of Face Skin, External Approach, Diagnostic	0HBAXZZ	Excision of Genitalia Skin, External Approach	0HBLXZX	Excision of Left Lower Leg Skin, External Approach, Diagnostic
0HB1XZZ	Excision of Face Skin, External Approach	0HBBXZX	Excision of Right Upper Arm Skin, External Approach, Diagnostic	0HBLXZZ	Excision of Left Lower Leg Skin, External Approach
0HB2XZX	Excision of Right Ear Skin, External Approach, Diagnostic	0HBBXZZ	Excision of Right Upper Arm Skin, External Approach	0HBMXZX	Excision of Right Foot Skin, External Approach, Diagnostic
0HB2XZZ	Excision of Right Ear Skin, External Approach	0HBCXZX	Excision of Left Upper Arm Skin, External Approach, Diagnostic	0HBMXZZ	Excision of Right Foot Skin, External Approach
0HB3XZX	Excision of Left Ear Skin, External Approach, Diagnostic	0HBCXZZ	Excision of Left Upper Arm Skin, External Approach	0HBNXZX	Excision of Left Foot Skin, External Approach, Diagnostic
0HB3XZZ	Excision of Left Ear Skin, External Approach	0HBDXZX	Excision of Right Lower Arm Skin, External Approach, Diagnostic	0HBNXZZ	Excision of Left Foot Skin, External Approach
0HB4XZX	Excision of Neck Skin, External Approach, Diagnostic	0HBDXZZ	Excision of Right Lower Arm Skin, External Approach	0HBQXZX	Excision of Finger Nail, External Approach, Diagnostic
0HB4XZZ	Excision of Neck Skin, External Approach	0HBEXZX	Excision of Left Lower Arm Skin, External Approach, Diagnostic	0HBQXZZ	Excision of Finger Nail, External Approach
0HB5XZX	Excision of Chest Skin, External Approach, Diagnostic	0HBEXZZ	Excision of Left Lower Arm Skin, External Approach	0HBRXZX	Excision of Toe Nail, External Approach, Diagnostic
0HB5XZZ	Excision of Chest Skin, External Approach	0HBFXZX	Excision of Right Hand Skin, External Approach, Diagnostic	0HBRXZZ	Excision of Toe Nail, External Approach
0HB6XZX	Excision of Back Skin, External Approach, Diagnostic	0HBFXZZ	Excision of Right Hand Skin, External Approach	0HBT0ZX	Excision of Right Breast, Open Approach, Diagnostic
0HB6XZZ	Excision of Back Skin, External Approach	0HBGXZX	Excision of Left Hand Skin, External Approach, Diagnostic	0HBT0ZZ	Excision of Right Breast, Open Approach
0HB7XZX	Excision of Abdomen Skin, External Approach, Diagnostic	0HBGXZZ	Excision of Left Hand Skin, External Approach	0HBT3ZX	Excision of Right Breast, Percutaneous Approach, Diagnostic
0HB7XZZ	Excision of Abdomen Skin, External Approach	0HBHXZX	Excision of Right Upper Leg Skin, External Approach, Diagnostic	0HBT3ZZ	Excision of Right Breast, Percutaneous Approach
0HB8XZX	Excision of Buttock Skin, External Approach, Diagnostic	0HBHXZZ	Excision of Right Upper Leg Skin, External Approach	0HBT7ZX	Excision of Right Breast, Via Natural or Artificial Opening, Diagnostic
0HB8XZZ	Excision of Buttock Skin, External Approach	0HBJXZX	Excision of Left Upper Leg Skin, External Approach, Diagnostic	0HBT7ZZ	Excision of Right Breast, Via Natural or Artificial Opening
0HB9XZX	Excision of Perineum Skin, External Approach, Diagnostic	0HBJXZZ	Excision of Left Upper Leg Skin, External Approach	0HBT8ZX	Excision of Right Breast, Via Natural or Artificial Opening Endoscopic, Diagnostic

♀ Female-only   ♂ Male-only   ▲ Limited Coverage   ● Non-OR   HAC HAC-associated procedure   ▲ Non-covered procedures   ＋ Combinat

0HBT8ZZ	Excision of Right Breast, Via Natural or Artificial Opening Endoscopic	0HBV7ZZ	Excision of Bilateral Breast, Via Natural or Artificial Opening	0HBX3ZZ	Excision of Left Nipple, Percutaneous Approach
0HBTXZX	Excision of Right Breast, External Approach, Diagnostic	0HBV8ZX	Excision of Bilateral Breast, Via Natural or Artificial Opening Endoscopic, Diagnostic	0HBX7ZX	Excision of Left Nipple, Via Natural or Artificial Opening, Diagnostic
0HBTXZZ	Excision of Right Breast, External Approach	0HBV8ZZ	Excision of Bilateral Breast, Via Natural or Artificial Opening Endoscopic	0HBX7ZZ	Excision of Left Nipple, Via Natural or Artificial Opening
0HBU0ZX	Excision of Left Breast, Open Approach, Diagnostic	0HBVXZX	Excision of Bilateral Breast, External Approach, Diagnostic	0HBX8ZX	Excision of Left Nipple, Via Natural or Artificial Opening Endoscopic, Diagnostic
0HBU0ZZ	Excision of Left Breast, Open Approach	0HBVXZZ	Excision of Bilateral Breast, External Approach	0HBX8ZZ	Excision of Left Nipple, Via Natural or Artificial Opening Endoscopic
0HBU3ZX	Excision of Left Breast, Percutaneous Approach, Diagnostic	0HBW0ZX	Excision of Right Nipple, Open Approach, Diagnostic	0HBXXZX	Excision of Left Nipple, External Approach, Diagnostic
0HBU3ZZ	Excision of Left Breast, Percutaneous Approach	0HBW0ZZ	Excision of Right Nipple, Open Approach	0HBXXZZ	Excision of Left Nipple, External Approach
0HBU7ZX	Excision of Left Breast, Via Natural or Artificial Opening, Diagnostic	0HBW3ZX	Excision of Right Nipple, Percutaneous Approach, Diagnostic	0HBY0ZX	Excision of Supernumerary Breast, Open Approach, Diagnostic
0HBU7ZZ	Excision of Left Breast, Via Natural or Artificial Opening	0HBW3ZZ	Excision of Right Nipple, Percutaneous Approach	0HBY0ZZ	Excision of Supernumerary Breast, Open Approach
0HBU8ZX	Excision of Left Breast, Via Natural or Artificial Opening Endoscopic, Diagnostic	0HBW7ZX	Excision of Right Nipple, Via Natural or Artificial Opening, Diagnostic	0HBY3ZX	Excision of Supernumerary Breast, Percutaneous Approach, Diagnostic
0HBU8ZZ	Excision of Left Breast, Via Natural or Artificial Opening Endoscopic	0HBW7ZZ	Excision of Right Nipple, Via Natural or Artificial Opening	0HBY3ZZ	Excision of Supernumerary Breast, Percutaneous Approach
0HBUXZX	Excision of Left Breast, External Approach, Diagnostic	0HBW8ZX	Excision of Right Nipple, Via Natural or Artificial Opening Endoscopic, Diagnostic	0HBY7ZX	Excision of Supernumerary Breast, Via Natural or Artificial Opening, Diagnostic
0HBUXZZ	Excision of Left Breast, External Approach	0HBW8ZZ	Excision of Right Nipple, Via Natural or Artificial Opening Endoscopic	0HBY7ZZ	Excision of Supernumerary Breast, Via Natural or Artificial Opening
0HBV0ZX	Excision of Bilateral Breast, Open Approach, Diagnostic	0HBWXZX	Excision of Right Nipple, External Approach, Diagnostic	0HBY8ZX	Excision of Supernumerary Breast, Via Natural or Artificial Opening Endoscopic, Diagnostic
0HBV0ZZ	Excision of Bilateral Breast, Open Approach	0HBWXZZ	Excision of Right Nipple, External Approach	0HBY8ZZ	Excision of Supernumerary Breast, Via Natural or Artificial Opening Endoscopic
0HBV3ZX	Excision of Bilateral Breast, Percutaneous Approach, Diagnostic	0HBX0ZX	Excision of Left Nipple, Open Approach, Diagnostic	0HBYXZX	Excision of Supernumerary Breast, External Approach, Diagnostic
0HBV3ZZ	Excision of Bilateral Breast, Percutaneous Approach	0HBX0ZZ	Excision of Left Nipple, Open Approach	0HBYXZZ	Excision of Supernumerary Breast, External Approach
0HBV7ZX	Excision of Bilateral Breast, Via Natural or Artificial Opening, Diagnostic	0HBX3ZX	Excision of Left Nipple, Percutaneous Approach, Diagnostic		

0HC – Skin and Breast, Extirpation

0HC0XZZ	Extirpation of Matter from Scalp Skin, External Approach	0HCJXZZ	Extirpation of Matter from Left Upper Leg Skin, External Approach	0HCV0ZZ	Extirpation of Matter from Bilateral Breast, Open Approach
0HC1XZZ	Extirpation of Matter from Face Skin, External Approach	0HCKXZZ	Extirpation of Matter from Right Lower Leg Skin, External Approach	0HCV3ZZ	Extirpation of Matter from Bilateral Breast, Percutaneous Approach
0HC2XZZ	Extirpation of Matter from Right Ear Skin, External Approach	0HCLXZZ	Extirpation of Matter from Left Lower Leg Skin, External Approach	0HCV7ZZ	Extirpation of Matter from Bilateral Breast, Via Natural or Artificial Opening
0HC3XZZ	Extirpation of Matter from Left Ear Skin, External Approach	0HCMXZZ	Extirpation of Matter from Right Foot Skin, External Approach	0HCV8ZZ	Extirpation of Matter from Bilateral Breast, Via Natural or Artificial Opening Endoscopic
0HC4XZZ	Extirpation of Matter from Neck Skin, External Approach	0HCNXZZ	Extirpation of Matter from Left Foot Skin, External Approach	0HCVXZZ	Extirpation of Matter from Bilateral Breast, External Approach
0HC5XZZ	Extirpation of Matter from Chest Skin, External Approach	0HCQXZZ	Extirpation of Matter from Finger Nail, External Approach	0HCW0ZZ	Extirpation of Matter from Right Nipple, Open Approach
0HC6XZZ	Extirpation of Matter from Back Skin, External Approach	0HCRXZZ	Extirpation of Matter from Toe Nail, External Approach	0HCW3ZZ	Extirpation of Matter from Right Nipple, Percutaneous Approach
0HC7XZZ	Extirpation of Matter from Abdomen Skin, External Approach	0HCT0ZZ	Extirpation of Matter from Right Breast, Open Approach	0HCW7ZZ	Extirpation of Matter from Right Nipple, Via Natural or Artificial Opening
0HC8XZZ	Extirpation of Matter from Buttock Skin, External Approach	0HCT3ZZ	Extirpation of Matter from Right Breast, Percutaneous Approach	0HCW8ZZ	Extirpation of Matter from Right Nipple, Via Natural or Artificial Opening Endoscopic
0HC9XZZ	Extirpation of Matter from Perineum Skin, External Approach	0HCT7ZZ	Extirpation of Matter from Right Breast, Via Natural or Artificial Opening	0HCWXZZ	Extirpation of Matter from Right Nipple, External Approach
0HCAXZZ	Extirpation of Matter from Genitalia Skin, External Approach	0HCT8ZZ	Extirpation of Matter from Right Breast, Via Natural or Artificial Opening Endoscopic	0HCX0ZZ	Extirpation of Matter from Left Nipple, Open Approach
0HCBXZZ	Extirpation of Matter from Right Upper Arm Skin, External Approach	0HCTXZZ	Extirpation of Matter from Right Breast, External Approach	0HCX3ZZ	Extirpation of Matter from Left Nipple, Percutaneous Approach
0HCCXZZ	Extirpation of Matter from Left Upper Arm Skin, External Approach	0HCU0ZZ	Extirpation of Matter from Left Breast, Open Approach	0HCX7ZZ	Extirpation of Matter from Left Nipple, Via Natural or Artificial Opening
0HCDXZZ	Extirpation of Matter from Right Lower Arm Skin, External Approach	0HCU3ZZ	Extirpation of Matter from Left Breast, Percutaneous Approach	0HCX8ZZ	Extirpation of Matter from Left Nipple, Via Natural or Artificial Opening Endoscopic
0HCEXZZ	Extirpation of Matter from Left Lower Arm Skin, External Approach	0HCU7ZZ	Extirpation of Matter from Left Breast, Via Natural or Artificial Opening	0HCXXZZ	Extirpation of Matter from Left Nipple, External Approach
0HCFXZZ	Extirpation of Matter from Right Hand Skin, External Approach	0HCU8ZZ	Extirpation of Matter from Left Breast, Via Natural or Artificial Opening Endoscopic		
0HCGXZZ	Extirpation of Matter from Left Hand Skin, External Approach	0HCUXZZ	Extirpation of Matter from Left Breast, External Approach		
0HCHXZZ	Extirpation of Matter from Right Upper Leg Skin, External Approach				

♀ Female-only   ♂ Male-only   ▲ Limited Coverage   ● Non-OR   ▥ HAC-associated procedure   ▲ Non-covered procedures   ✚ Combination

0HD – Skin and Breast, Extraction

0HD0XZZ	Extraction of Scalp Skin, External Approach	**0HD9XZZ**	Extraction of Perineum Skin, External Approach
0HD1XZZ	Extraction of Face Skin, External Approach	**0HDAXZZ**	Extraction of Genitalia Skin, External Approach
0HD2XZZ	Extraction of Right Ear Skin, External Approach	**0HDBXZZ**	Extraction of Right Upper Arm Skin, External Approach

0HD0XZZ Extraction of Scalp Skin, External Approach
0HD1XZZ Extraction of Face Skin, External Approach
0HD2XZZ Extraction of Right Ear Skin, External Approach
0HD3XZZ Extraction of Left Ear Skin, External Approach
0HD4XZZ Extraction of Neck Skin, External Approach
0HD5XZZ Extraction of Chest Skin, External Approach
0HD6XZZ Extraction of Back Skin, External Approach
0HD7XZZ Extraction of Abdomen Skin, External Approach
0HD8XZZ Extraction of Buttock Skin, External Approach

0HD9XZZ Extraction of Perineum Skin, External Approach
0HDAXZZ Extraction of Genitalia Skin, External Approach
0HDBXZZ Extraction of Right Upper Arm Skin, External Approach
0HDCXZZ Extraction of Left Upper Arm Skin, External Approach
0HDDXZZ Extraction of Right Lower Arm Skin, External Approach
0HDEXZZ Extraction of Left Lower Arm Skin, External Approach
0HDFXZZ Extraction of Right Hand Skin, External Approach
0HDGXZZ Extraction of Left Hand Skin, External Approach
0HDHXZZ Extraction of Right Upper Leg Skin, External Approach

0HDJXZZ Extraction of Left Upper Leg Skin, External Approach
0HDKXZZ Extraction of Right Lower Leg Skin, External Approach
0HDLXZZ Extraction of Left Lower Leg Skin, External Approach
0HDMXZZ Extraction of Right Foot Skin, External Approach
0HDNXZZ Extraction of Left Foot Skin, External Approach
0HDQXZZ Extraction of Finger Nail, External Approach
0HDRXZZ Extraction of Toe Nail, External Approach
0HDSXZZ Extraction of Hair, External Approach

0HH – Skin and Breast, Insertion

0HHT01Z Insertion of Radioactive Element into Right Breast, Open Approach
0HHT0NZ Insertion of Tissue Expander into Right Breast, Open Approach
0HHT31Z Insertion of Radioactive Element into Right Breast, Percutaneous Approach
0HHT3NZ Insertion of Tissue Expander into Right Breast, Percutaneous Approach
0HHT71Z Insertion of Radioactive Element into Right Breast, Via Natural or Artificial Opening
0HHT7NZ Insertion of Tissue Expander into Right Breast, Via Natural or Artificial Opening
0HHT81Z Insertion of Radioactive Element into Right Breast, Via Natural or Artificial Opening Endoscopic
0HHT8NZ Insertion of Tissue Expander into Right Breast, Via Natural or Artificial Opening Endoscopic
0HHTX1Z Insertion of Radioactive Element into Right Breast, External Approach
0HHU01Z Insertion of Radioactive Element into Left Breast, Open Approach
0HHU0NZ Insertion of Tissue Expander into Left Breast, Open Approach
AHA CC: 4Q, 2013, 107
0HHU31Z Insertion of Radioactive Element into Left Breast, Percutaneous Approach
0HHU3NZ Insertion of Tissue Expander into Left Breast, Percutaneous Approach
0HHU71Z Insertion of Radioactive Element into Left Breast, Via Natural or Artificial Opening
0HHU7NZ Insertion of Tissue Expander into Left Breast, Via Natural or Artificial Opening
0HHU81Z Insertion of Radioactive Element into Left Breast, Via Natural or Artificial Opening Endoscopic

0HHU8NZ Insertion of Tissue Expander into Left Breast, Via Natural or Artificial Opening Endoscopic
0HHUX1Z Insertion of Radioactive Element into Left Breast, External Approach
0HHV01Z Insertion of Radioactive Element into Bilateral Breast, Open Approach
0HHV0NZ Insertion of Tissue Expander into Bilateral Breast, Open Approach
AHA CC: 2Q, 2014, 12
0HHV31Z Insertion of Radioactive Element into Bilateral Breast, Percutaneous Approach
0HHV3NZ Insertion of Tissue Expander into Bilateral Breast, Percutaneous Approach
0HHV71Z Insertion of Radioactive Element into Bilateral Breast, Via Natural or Artificial Opening
0HHV7NZ Insertion of Tissue Expander into Bilateral Breast, Via Natural or Artificial Opening
0HHV81Z Insertion of Radioactive Element into Bilateral Breast, Via Natural or Artificial Opening Endoscopic
0HHV8NZ Insertion of Tissue Expander into Bilateral Breast, Via Natural or Artificial Opening Endoscopic
0HHVX1Z Insertion of Radioactive Element into Bilateral Breast, External Approach
0HHW01Z Insertion of Radioactive Element into Right Nipple, Open Approach
0HHW0NZ Insertion of Tissue Expander into Right Nipple, Open Approach
0HHW31Z Insertion of Radioactive Element into Right Nipple, Percutaneous Approach
0HHW3NZ Insertion of Tissue Expander into Right Nipple, Percutaneous Approach

0HHW71Z Insertion of Radioactive Element into Right Nipple, Via Natural or Artificial Opening
0HHW7NZ Insertion of Tissue Expander into Right Nipple, Via Natural or Artificial Opening
0HHW81Z Insertion of Radioactive Element into Right Nipple, Via Natural or Artificial Opening Endoscopic
0HHW8NZ Insertion of Tissue Expander into Right Nipple, Via Natural or Artificial Opening Endoscopic
0HHWX1Z Insertion of Radioactive Element into Right Nipple, External Approach
0HHX01Z Insertion of Radioactive Element into Left Nipple, Open Approach
0HHX0NZ Insertion of Tissue Expander into Left Nipple, Open Approach
0HHX31Z Insertion of Radioactive Element into Left Nipple, Percutaneous Approach
0HHX3NZ Insertion of Tissue Expander into Left Nipple, Percutaneous Approach
0HHX71Z Insertion of Radioactive Element into Left Nipple, Via Natural or Artificial Opening
0HHX7NZ Insertion of Tissue Expander into Left Nipple, Via Natural or Artificial Opening
0HHX81Z Insertion of Radioactive Element into Left Nipple, Via Natural or Artificial Opening Endoscopic
0HHX8NZ Insertion of Tissue Expander into Left Nipple, Via Natural or Artificial Opening Endoscopic
0HHXX1Z Insertion of Radioactive Element into Left Nipple, External Approach

0HJ – Skin and Breast, Inspection

Review Coding Guideline B3.5

Review Coding Guidelines B3.11a, B3.11b and B3.11c

0HJPXZZ Inspection of Skin, External Approach
0HJQXZZ Inspection of Finger Nail, External Approach
0HJRXZZ Inspection of Toe Nail, External Approach
0HJT0ZZ Inspection of Right Breast, Open Approach
0HJT3ZZ Inspection of Right Breast, Percutaneous Approach

0HJT7ZZ Inspection of Right Breast, Via Natural or Artificial Opening
0HJT8ZZ Inspection of Right Breast, Via Natural or Artificial Opening Endoscopic
0HJTXZZ Inspection of Right Breast, External Approach
0HJU0ZZ Inspection of Left Breast, Open Approach

0HJU3ZZ Inspection of Left Breast, Percutaneous Approach
0HJU7ZZ Inspection of Left Breast, Via Natural or Artificial Opening
0HJU8ZZ Inspection of Left Breast, Via Natural or Artificial Opening Endoscopic
0HJUXZZ Inspection of Left Breast, External Approach

♀ Female-only   ♂ Male-only   ▲ Limited Coverage   ● Non-OR   ▬ HAC-associated procedure   ▲ Non-covered procedures   ✚ Combinat

M – Skin and Breast, Reattachment

M0XZZ	Reattachment of Scalp Skin, External Approach	0HMAXZZ Reattachment of Genitalia Skin, External Approach
M1XZZ	Reattachment of Face Skin, External Approach	0HMBXZZ Reattachment of Right Upper Arm Skin, External Approach
M2XZZ	Reattachment of Right Ear Skin, External Approach	0HMCXZZ Reattachment of Left Upper Arm Skin, External Approach

0HMLXZZ Reattachment of Left Lower Leg Skin, External Approach
0HMMXZZ Reattachment of Right Foot Skin, External Approach
0HMNXZZ Reattachment of Left Foot Skin, External Approach

M3XZZ Reattachment of Left Ear Skin, External Approach
0HMDXZZ Reattachment of Right Lower Arm Skin, External Approach
0HMTXZZ Reattachment of Right Breast, External Approach

M4XZZ Reattachment of Neck Skin, External Approach
0HMEXZZ Reattachment of Left Lower Arm Skin, External Approach
0HMUXZZ Reattachment of Left Breast, External Approach

M5XZZ Reattachment of Chest Skin, External Approach
0HMFXZZ Reattachment of Right Hand Skin, External Approach
0HMVXZZ Reattachment of Bilateral Breast, External Approach

M6XZZ Reattachment of Back Skin, External Approach
0HMGXZZ Reattachment of Left Hand Skin, External Approach
0HMWXZZ Reattachment of Right Nipple, External Approach

M7XZZ Reattachment of Abdomen Skin, External Approach
0HMHXZZ Reattachment of Right Upper Leg Skin, External Approach
0HMXXZZ Reattachment of Left Nipple, External Approach

M8XZZ Reattachment of Buttock Skin, External Approach
0HMJXZZ Reattachment of Left Upper Leg Skin, External Approach

M9XZZ Reattachment of Perineum Skin, External Approach
0HMKXZZ Reattachment of Right Lower Leg Skin, External Approach

N – Skin and Breast, Release

view Coding Guideline B3.13

view Coding Guideline B3.14

N0XZZ Release Scalp Skin, External Approach
N1XZZ Release Face Skin, External Approach
N2XZZ Release Right Ear Skin, External Approach
N3XZZ Release Left Ear Skin, External Approach
N4XZZ Release Neck Skin, External Approach
N5XZZ Release Chest Skin, External Approach
N6XZZ Release Back Skin, External Approach
N7XZZ Release Abdomen Skin, External Approach
N8XZZ Release Buttock Skin, External Approach
N9XZZ Release Perineum Skin, External Approach
NAXZZ Release Genitalia Skin, External Approach
NBXZZ Release Right Upper Arm Skin, External Approach
NCXZZ Release Left Upper Arm Skin, External Approach
NDXZZ Release Right Lower Arm Skin, External Approach
NEXZZ Release Left Lower Arm Skin, External Approach
NFXZZ Release Right Hand Skin, External Approach
NGXZZ Release Left Hand Skin, External Approach

0HNHXZZ Release Right Upper Leg Skin, External Approach
0HNJXZZ Release Left Upper Leg Skin, External Approach
0HNKXZZ Release Right Lower Leg Skin, External Approach
0HNLXZZ Release Left Lower Leg Skin, External Approach
0HNMXZZ Release Right Foot Skin, External Approach
0HNNXZZ Release Left Foot Skin, External Approach
0HNQXZZ Release Finger Nail, External Approach
0HNRXZZ Release Toe Nail, External Approach
0HNT0ZZ Release Right Breast, Open Approach
0HNT3ZZ Release Right Breast, Percutaneous Approach
0HNT7ZZ Release Right Breast, Via Natural or Artificial Opening
0HNT8ZZ Release Right Breast, Via Natural or Artificial Opening Endoscopic
0HNTXZZ Release Right Breast, External Approach
0HNU0ZZ Release Left Breast, Open Approach
0HNU3ZZ Release Left Breast, Percutaneous Approach
0HNU7ZZ Release Left Breast, Via Natural or Artificial Opening

0HNU8ZZ Release Left Breast, Via Natural or Artificial Opening Endoscopic
0HNUXZZ Release Left Breast, External Approach
0HNV0ZZ Release Bilateral Breast, Open Approach
0HNV3ZZ Release Bilateral Breast, Percutaneous Approach
0HNV7ZZ Release Bilateral Breast, Via Natural or Artificial Opening
0HNV8ZZ Release Bilateral Breast, Via Natural or Artificial Opening Endoscopic
0HNVXZZ Release Bilateral Breast, External Approach
0HNW0ZZ Release Right Nipple, Open Approach
0HNW3ZZ Release Right Nipple, Percutaneous Approach
0HNW7ZZ Release Right Nipple, Via Natural or Artificial Opening
0HNW8ZZ Release Right Nipple, Via Natural or Artificial Opening Endoscopic
0HNWXZZ Release Right Nipple, External Approach
0HNX0ZZ Release Left Nipple, Open Approach
0HNX3ZZ Release Left Nipple, Percutaneous Approach
0HNX7ZZ Release Left Nipple, Via Natural or Artificial Opening
0HNX8ZZ Release Left Nipple, Via Natural or Artificial Opening Endoscopic
0HNXXZZ Release Left Nipple, External Approach

P – Skin and Breast, Removal

view Coding Guideline B6.1c

PPX0Z Removal of Drainage Device from Skin, External Approach
PPX7Z Removal of Autologous Tissue Substitute from Skin, External Approach
PPXJZ Removal of Synthetic Substitute from Skin, External Approach
PPXKZ Removal of Nonautologous Tissue Substitute from Skin, External Approach
PQX0Z Removal of Drainage Device from Finger Nail, External Approach
PQX7Z Removal of Autologous Tissue Substitute from Finger Nail, External Approach
PQXJZ Removal of Synthetic Substitute from Finger Nail, External Approach

0HPQXKZ Removal of Nonautologous Tissue Substitute from Finger Nail, External Approach
0HPRX0Z Removal of Drainage Device from Toe Nail, External Approach
0HPRX7Z Removal of Autologous Tissue Substitute from Toe Nail, External Approach
0HPRXJZ Removal of Synthetic Substitute from Toe Nail, External Approach
0HPRXKZ Removal of Nonautologous Tissue Substitute from Toe Nail, External Approach
0HPSX7Z Removal of Autologous Tissue Substitute from Hair, External Approach

0HPSXJZ Removal of Synthetic Substitute from Hair, External Approach
0HPSXKZ Removal of Nonautologous Tissue Substitute from Hair, External Approach
0HPT00Z Removal of Drainage Device from Right Breast, Open Approach
0HPT01Z Removal of Radioactive Element from Right Breast, Open Approach
0HPT07Z Removal of Autologous Tissue Substitute from Right Breast, Open Approach
0HPT0JZ Removal of Synthetic Substitute from Right Breast, Open Approach
0HPT0KZ Removal of Nonautologous Tissue Substitute from Right Breast, Open Approach

| Female-only | ♂ Male-only | ▲ Limited Coverage | ● Non-OR | HAC HAC-associated procedure | ▲ Non-covered procedures | + Combination |

0HPT0NZ Removal of Tissue Expander from Right Breast, Open Approach

0HPT30Z Removal of Drainage Device from Right Breast, Percutaneous Approach

0HPT31Z Removal of Radioactive Element from Right Breast, Percutaneous Approach

0HPT37Z Removal of Autologous Tissue Substitute from Right Breast, Percutaneous Approach

0HPT3JZ Removal of Synthetic Substitute from Right Breast, Percutaneous Approach

0HPT3KZ Removal of Nonautologous Tissue Substitute from Right Breast, Percutaneous Approach

0HPT3NZ Removal of Tissue Expander from Right Breast, Percutaneous Approach

0HPT70Z Removal of Drainage Device from Right Breast, Via Natural or Artificial Opening

0HPT71Z Removal of Radioactive Element from Right Breast, Via Natural or Artificial Opening

0HPT77Z Removal of Autologous Tissue Substitute from Right Breast, Via Natural or Artificial Opening

0HPT7JZ Removal of Synthetic Substitute from Right Breast, Via Natural or Artificial Opening

0HPT7KZ Removal of Nonautologous Tissue Substitute from Right Breast, Via Natural or Artificial Opening

0HPT7NZ Removal of Tissue Expander from Right Breast, Via Natural or Artificial Opening

0HPT80Z Removal of Drainage Device from Right Breast, Via Natural or Artificial Opening Endoscopic

0HPT81Z Removal of Radioactive Element from Right Breast, Via Natural or Artificial Opening Endoscopic

0HPT87Z Removal of Autologous Tissue Substitute from Right Breast, Via Natural or Artificial Opening Endoscopic

0HPT8JZ Removal of Synthetic Substitute from Right Breast, Via Natural or Artificial Opening Endoscopic

0HPT8KZ Removal of Nonautologous Tissue Substitute from Right Breast, Via Natural or Artificial Opening Endoscopic

0HPT8NZ Removal of Tissue Expander from Right Breast, Via Natural or Artificial Opening Endoscopic

0HPTX0Z Removal of Drainage Device from Right Breast, External Approach

0HPTX1Z Removal of Radioactive Element from Right Breast, External Approach

0HPTX7Z Removal of Autologous Tissue Substitute from Right Breast, External Approach

0HPTXJZ Removal of Synthetic Substitute from Right Breast, External Approach

0HPTXKZ Removal of Nonautologous Tissue Substitute from Right Breast, External Approach

0HPU00Z Removal of Drainage Device from Left Breast, Open Approach

0HPU01Z Removal of Radioactive Element from Left Breast, Open Approach

0HPU07Z Removal of Autologous Tissue Substitute from Left Breast, Open Approach

0HPU0JZ Removal of Synthetic Substitute from Left Breast, Open Approach

0HPU0KZ Removal of Nonautologous Tissue Substitute from Left Breast, Open Approach

0HPU0NZ Removal of Tissue Expander from Left Breast, Open Approach

0HPU30Z Removal of Drainage Device from Left Breast, Percutaneous Approach

0HPU31Z Removal of Radioactive Element from Left Breast, Percutaneous Approach

0HPU37Z Removal of Autologous Tissue Substitute from Left Breast, Percutaneous Approach

0HPU3JZ Removal of Synthetic Substitute from Left Breast, Percutaneous Approach

0HPU3KZ Removal of Nonautologous Tissue Substitute from Left Breast, Percutaneous Approach

0HPU3NZ Removal of Tissue Expander from Left Breast, Percutaneous Approach

0HPU70Z Removal of Drainage Device from Left Breast, Via Natural or Artificial Opening

0HPU71Z Removal of Radioactive Element from Left Breast, Via Natural or Artificial Opening

0HPU77Z Removal of Autologous Tissue Substitute from Left Breast, Via Natural or Artificial Opening

0HPU7JZ Removal of Synthetic Substitute from Left Breast, Via Natural or Artificial Opening

0HPU7KZ Removal of Nonautologous Tissue Substitute from Left Breast, Via Natural or Artificial Opening

0HPU7NZ Removal of Tissue Expander from Left Breast, Via Natural or Artificial Opening

0HPU80Z Removal of Drainage Device from Left Breast, Via Natural or Artificial Opening Endoscopic

0HPU81Z Removal of Radioactive Element from Left Breast, Via Natural or Artificial Opening Endoscopic

0HPU87Z Removal of Autologous Tissue Substitute from Left Breast, Via Natural or Artificial Opening Endoscopic

0HPU8JZ Removal of Synthetic Substitute from Left Breast, Via Natural or Artificial Opening Endoscopic

0HPU8KZ Removal of Nonautologous Tissue Substitute from Left Breast, Via Natural or Artificial Opening Endoscopic

0HPU8NZ Removal of Tissue Expander from Left Breast, Via Natural or Artificial Opening Endoscopic

0HPUX0Z Removal of Drainage Device from Left Breast, External Approach

0HPUX1Z Removal of Radioactive Element from Left Breast, External Approach

0HPUX7Z Removal of Autologous Tissue Substitute from Left Breast, External Approach

0HPUXJZ Removal of Synthetic Substitute from Left Breast, External Approach

0HPUXKZ Removal of Nonautologous Tissue Substitute from Left Breast, External Approach

0HQ – Skin and Breast, Repair

Review Coding Guideline B3.5

0HQ0XZZ Repair Scalp Skin, External Approach

0HQ1XZZ Repair Face Skin, External Approach

0HQ2XZZ Repair Right Ear Skin, External Approach

0HQ3XZZ Repair Left Ear Skin, External Approach

0HQ4XZZ Repair Neck Skin, External Approach

0HQ5XZZ Repair Chest Skin, External Approach

0HQ6XZZ Repair Back Skin, External Approach

0HQ7XZZ Repair Abdomen Skin, External Approach

0HQ8XZZ Repair Buttock Skin, External Approach

● **0HQ9XZZ** Repair Perineum Skin, External Approach

0HQAXZZ Repair Genitalia Skin, External Approach

0HQBXZZ Repair Right Upper Arm Skin, External Approach

0HQCXZZ Repair Left Upper Arm Skin, External Approach

0HQDXZZ Repair Right Lower Arm Skin, External Approach

0HQEXZZ Repair Left Lower Arm Skin, External Approach

AHA CC: 4Q, 2014, 31-32

0HQFXZZ Repair Right Hand Skin, External Approach

0HQGXZZ Repair Left Hand Skin, External Approach

0HQHXZZ Repair Right Upper Leg Skin, External Approach

0HQJXZZ Repair Left Upper Leg Skin, External Approach

0HQKXZZ Repair Right Lower Leg Skin, External Approach

0HQLXZZ Repair Left Lower Leg Skin, External Approach

0HQMXZZ Repair Right Foot Skin, External Approach

0HQNXZZ Repair Left Foot Skin, External Approach

0HQQXZZ Repair Finger Nail, External Approach

0HQRXZZ Repair Toe Nail, External Approach

0HQT0ZZ Repair Right Breast, Open Approach

0HQT3ZZ Repair Right Breast, Percutaneous Approach

0HQT7ZZ Repair Right Breast, Via Natural or Artificial Opening

0HQT8ZZ Repair Right Breast, Via Natural or Artificial Opening Endoscopic

0HQTXZZ Repair Right Breast, External Approach

0HQU0ZZ Repair Left Breast, Open Approach

0HQU3ZZ Repair Left Breast, Percutaneous Approach

0HQU7ZZ Repair Left Breast, Via Natural or Artificial Opening

0HQU8ZZ Repair Left Breast, Via Natural or Artificial Opening Endoscopic

0HQUXZZ Repair Left Breast, External Approach

0HQV0ZZ Repair Bilateral Breast, Open Approach

0HQV3ZZ Repair Bilateral Breast, Percutaneous Approach

0HQV7ZZ Repair Bilateral Breast, Via Natural or Artificial Opening

0HQV8ZZ Repair Bilateral Breast, Via Natural or Artificial Opening Endoscopic

0HQVXZZ Repair Bilateral Breast, External Approach

0HQW0ZZ Repair Right Nipple, Open Approach

0HQW3ZZ Repair Right Nipple, Percutaneous Approach

0HQW7ZZ Repair Right Nipple, Via Natural or Artificial Opening

0HQW8ZZ Repair Right Nipple, Via Natural or Artificial Opening Endoscopic

0HQWXZZ Repair Right Nipple, External Approach

0HQX0ZZ Repair Left Nipple, Open Approach

0HQX3ZZ Repair Left Nipple, Percutaneous Approach

0HQX7ZZ Repair Left Nipple, Via Natural or Artificial Opening

0HQX8ZZ Repair Left Nipple, Via Natural or Artificial Opening Endoscopic

♀ Female-only   ♂ Male-only   ▲ Limited Coverage   ● Non-OR   ■ HAC-associated procedure   ▲ Non-covered procedures   ✛ Combination

QXXZZ Repair Left Nipple, External Approach

QY0ZZ Repair Supernumerary Breast, Open Approach

0HQY3ZZ Repair Supernumerary Breast, Percutaneous Approach

0HQY7ZZ Repair Supernumerary Breast, Via Natural or Artificial Opening

0HQY8ZZ Repair Supernumerary Breast, Via Natural or Artificial Opening Endoscopic

0HQYXZZ Repair Supernumerary Breast, External Approach

R – Skin and Breast, Replacement

R0X73 Replacement of Scalp Skin with Autologous Tissue Substitute, Full Thickness, External Approach

R0X74 Replacement of Scalp Skin with Autologous Tissue Substitute, Partial Thickness, External Approach

R0XJ3 Replacement of Scalp Skin with Synthetic Substitute, Full Thickness, External Approach

R0XJ4 Replacement of Scalp Skin with Synthetic Substitute, Partial Thickness, External Approach

R0XJZ Replacement of Scalp Skin with Synthetic Substitute, External Approach

R0XK3 Replacement of Scalp Skin with Nonautologous Tissue Substitute, Full Thickness, External Approach

R0XK4 Replacement of Scalp Skin with Nonautologous Tissue Substitute, Partial Thickness, External Approach

R1X73 Replacement of Face Skin with Autologous Tissue Substitute, Full Thickness, External Approach

R1X74 Replacement of Face Skin with Autologous Tissue Substitute, Partial Thickness, External Approach

R1XJ3 Replacement of Face Skin with Synthetic Substitute, Full Thickness, External Approach

R1XJ4 Replacement of Face Skin with Synthetic Substitute, Partial Thickness, External Approach

R1XJZ Replacement of Face Skin with Synthetic Substitute, External Approach

R1XK3 Replacement of Face Skin with Nonautologous Tissue Substitute, Full Thickness, External Approach

R1XK4 Replacement of Face Skin with Nonautologous Tissue Substitute, Partial Thickness, External Approach

R2X73 Replacement of Right Ear Skin with Autologous Tissue Substitute, Full Thickness, External Approach

R2X74 Replacement of Right Ear Skin with Autologous Tissue Substitute, Partial Thickness, External Approach

R2XJ3 Replacement of Right Ear Skin with Synthetic Substitute, Full Thickness, External Approach

R2XJ4 Replacement of Right Ear Skin with Synthetic Substitute, Partial Thickness, External Approach

R2XJZ Replacement of Right Ear Skin with Synthetic Substitute, External Approach

R2XK3 Replacement of Right Ear Skin with Nonautologous Tissue Substitute, Full Thickness, External Approach

R2XK4 Replacement of Right Ear Skin with Nonautologous Tissue Substitute, Partial Thickness, External Approach

R3X73 Replacement of Left Ear Skin with Autologous Tissue Substitute, Full Thickness, External Approach

R3X74 Replacement of Left Ear Skin with Autologous Tissue Substitute, Partial Thickness, External Approach

R3XJ3 Replacement of Left Ear Skin with Synthetic Substitute, Full Thickness, External Approach

0HR3XJ4 Replacement of Left Ear Skin with Synthetic Substitute, Partial Thickness, External Approach

0HR3XJZ Replacement of Left Ear Skin with Synthetic Substitute, External Approach

0HR3XK3 Replacement of Left Ear Skin with Nonautologous Tissue Substitute, Full Thickness, External Approach

0HR3XK4 Replacement of Left Ear Skin with Nonautologous Tissue Substitute, Partial Thickness, External Approach

0HR4X73 Replacement of Neck Skin with Autologous Tissue Substitute, Full Thickness, External Approach

0HR4X74 Replacement of Neck Skin with Autologous Tissue Substitute, Partial Thickness, External Approach

0HR4XJ3 Replacement of Neck Skin with Synthetic Substitute, Full Thickness, External Approach

0HR4XJ4 Replacement of Neck Skin with Synthetic Substitute, Partial Thickness, External Approach

0HR4XJZ Replacement of Neck Skin with Synthetic Substitute, External Approach

0HR4XK3 Replacement of Neck Skin with Nonautologous Tissue Substitute, Full Thickness, External Approach

0HR4XK4 Replacement of Neck Skin with Nonautologous Tissue Substitute, Partial Thickness, External Approach

0HR5X73 Replacement of Chest Skin with Autologous Tissue Substitute, Full Thickness, External Approach

0HR5X74 Replacement of Chest Skin with Autologous Tissue Substitute, Partial Thickness, External Approach

0HR5XJ3 Replacement of Chest Skin with Synthetic Substitute, Full Thickness, External Approach

0HR5XJ4 Replacement of Chest Skin with Synthetic Substitute, Partial Thickness, External Approach

0HR5XJZ Replacement of Chest Skin with Synthetic Substitute, External Approach

0HR5XK3 Replacement of Chest Skin with Nonautologous Tissue Substitute, Full Thickness, External Approach

0HR5XK4 Replacement of Chest Skin with Nonautologous Tissue Substitute, Partial Thickness, External Approach

0HR6X73 Replacement of Back Skin with Autologous Tissue Substitute, Full Thickness, External Approach

0HR6X74 Replacement of Back Skin with Autologous Tissue Substitute, Partial Thickness, External Approach

0HR6XJ3 Replacement of Back Skin with Synthetic Substitute, Full Thickness, External Approach

0HR6XJ4 Replacement of Back Skin with Synthetic Substitute, Partial Thickness, External Approach

0HR6XJZ Replacement of Back Skin with Synthetic Substitute, External Approach

0HR6XK3 Replacement of Back Skin with Nonautologous Tissue Substitute, Full Thickness, External Approach

0HR6XK4 Replacement of Back Skin with Nonautologous Tissue Substitute, Partial Thickness, External Approach

0HR7X73 Replacement of Abdomen Skin with Autologous Tissue Substitute, Full Thickness, External Approach

0HR7X74 Replacement of Abdomen Skin with Autologous Tissue Substitute, Partial Thickness, External Approach

0HR7XJ3 Replacement of Abdomen Skin with Synthetic Substitute, Full Thickness, External Approach

0HR7XJ4 Replacement of Abdomen Skin with Synthetic Substitute, Partial Thickness, External Approach

0HR7XJZ Replacement of Abdomen Skin with Synthetic Substitute, External Approach

0HR7XK3 Replacement of Abdomen Skin with Nonautologous Tissue Substitute, Full Thickness, External Approach

0HR7XK4 Replacement of Abdomen Skin with Nonautologous Tissue Substitute, Partial Thickness, External Approach

0HR8X73 Replacement of Buttock Skin with Autologous Tissue Substitute, Full Thickness, External Approach

0HR8X74 Replacement of Buttock Skin with Autologous Tissue Substitute, Partial Thickness, External Approach

0HR8XJ3 Replacement of Buttock Skin with Synthetic Substitute, Full Thickness, External Approach

0HR8XJ4 Replacement of Buttock Skin with Synthetic Substitute, Partial Thickness, External Approach

0HR8XJZ Replacement of Buttock Skin with Synthetic Substitute, External Approach

0HR8XK3 Replacement of Buttock Skin with Nonautologous Tissue Substitute, Full Thickness, External Approach

0HR8XK4 Replacement of Buttock Skin with Nonautologous Tissue Substitute, Partial Thickness, External Approach

0HR9X73 Replacement of Perineum Skin with Autologous Tissue Substitute, Full Thickness, External Approach

0HR9X74 Replacement of Perineum Skin with Autologous Tissue Substitute, Partial Thickness, External Approach

0HR9XJ3 Replacement of Perineum Skin with Synthetic Substitute, Full Thickness, External Approach

0HR9XJ4 Replacement of Perineum Skin with Synthetic Substitute, Partial Thickness, External Approach

0HR9XJZ Replacement of Perineum Skin with Synthetic Substitute, External Approach

0HR9XK3 Replacement of Perineum Skin with Nonautologous Tissue Substitute, Full Thickness, External Approach

0HR9XK4 Replacement of Perineum Skin with Nonautologous Tissue Substitute, Partial Thickness, External Approach

0HRAX73 Replacement of Genitalia Skin with Autologous Tissue Substitute, Full Thickness, External Approach

0HRAX74 Replacement of Genitalia Skin with Autologous Tissue Substitute, Partial Thickness, External Approach

0HRAXJ3 Replacement of Genitalia Skin with Synthetic Substitute, Full Thickness, External Approach

♀ Female-only ♂ Male-only ▲ Limited Coverage ● Non-OR ■ HAC-associated procedure ▲ Non-covered procedures ✛ Combination

0HRAXJ4 Replacement of Genitalia Skin with Synthetic Substitute, Partial Thickness, External Approach

0HRAXJZ Replacement of Genitalia Skin with Synthetic Substitute, External Approach

0HRAXK3 Replacement of Genitalia Skin with Nonautologous Tissue Substitute, Full Thickness, External Approach

0HRAXK4 Replacement of Genitalia Skin with Nonautologous Tissue Substitute, Partial Thickness, External Approach

0HRBX73 Replacement of Right Upper Arm Skin with Autologous Tissue Substitute, Full Thickness, External Approach

0HRBX74 Replacement of Right Upper Arm Skin with Autologous Tissue Substitute, Partial Thickness, External Approach

0HRBXJ3 Replacement of Right Upper Arm Skin with Synthetic Substitute, Full Thickness, External Approach

0HRBXJ4 Replacement of Right Upper Arm Skin with Synthetic Substitute, Partial Thickness, External Approach

0HRBXJZ Replacement of Right Upper Arm Skin with Synthetic Substitute, External Approach

0HRBXK3 Replacement of Right Upper Arm Skin with Nonautologous Tissue Substitute, Full Thickness, External Approach

0HRBXK4 Replacement of Right Upper Arm Skin with Nonautologous Tissue Substitute, Partial Thickness, External Approach

0HRCX73 Replacement of Left Upper Arm Skin with Autologous Tissue Substitute, Full Thickness, External Approach

0HRCX74 Replacement of Left Upper Arm Skin with Autologous Tissue Substitute, Partial Thickness, External Approach

0HRCXJ3 Replacement of Left Upper Arm Skin with Synthetic Substitute, Full Thickness, External Approach

0HRCXJ4 Replacement of Left Upper Arm Skin with Synthetic Substitute, Partial Thickness, External Approach

0HRCXJZ Replacement of Left Upper Arm Skin with Synthetic Substitute, External Approach

0HRCXK3 Replacement of Left Upper Arm Skin with Nonautologous Tissue Substitute, Full Thickness, External Approach

0HRCXK4 Replacement of Left Upper Arm Skin with Nonautologous Tissue Substitute, Partial Thickness, External Approach

0HRDX73 Replacement of Right Lower Arm Skin with Autologous Tissue Substitute, Full Thickness, External Approach

0HRDX74 Replacement of Right Lower Arm Skin with Autologous Tissue Substitute, Partial Thickness, External Approach

0HRDXJ3 Replacement of Right Lower Arm Skin with Synthetic Substitute, Full Thickness, External Approach

0HRDXJ4 Replacement of Right Lower Arm Skin with Synthetic Substitute, Partial Thickness, External Approach

0HRDXJZ Replacement of Right Lower Arm Skin with Synthetic Substitute, External Approach

0HRDXK3 Replacement of Right Lower Arm Skin with Nonautologous Tissue Substitute, Full Thickness, External Approach

0HRDXK4 Replacement of Right Lower Arm Skin with Nonautologous Tissue Substitute, Partial Thickness, External Approach

0HREX73 Replacement of Left Lower Arm Skin with Autologous Tissue Substitute, Full Thickness, External Approach

0HREX74 Replacement of Left Lower Arm Skin with Autologous Tissue Substitute, Partial Thickness, External Approach

0HREXJ3 Replacement of Left Lower Arm Skin with Synthetic Substitute, Full Thickness, External Approach

0HREXJ4 Replacement of Left Lower Arm Skin with Synthetic Substitute, Partial Thickness, External Approach

0HREXJZ Replacement of Left Lower Arm Skin with Synthetic Substitute, External Approach

0HREXK3 Replacement of Left Lower Arm Skin with Nonautologous Tissue Substitute, Full Thickness, External Approach

0HREXK4 Replacement of Left Lower Arm Skin with Nonautologous Tissue Substitute, Partial Thickness, External Approach

0HRFX73 Replacement of Right Hand Skin with Autologous Tissue Substitute, Full Thickness, External Approach

0HRFX74 Replacement of Right Hand Skin with Autologous Tissue Substitute, Partial Thickness, External Approach

0HRFXJ3 Replacement of Right Hand Skin with Synthetic Substitute, Full Thickness, External Approach

0HRFXJ4 Replacement of Right Hand Skin with Synthetic Substitute, Partial Thickness, External Approach

0HRFXJZ Replacement of Right Hand Skin with Synthetic Substitute, External Approach

0HRFXK3 Replacement of Right Hand Skin with Nonautologous Tissue Substitute, Full Thickness, External Approach

0HRFXK4 Replacement of Right Hand Skin with Nonautologous Tissue Substitute, Partial Thickness, External Approach

0HRGX73 Replacement of Left Hand Skin with Autologous Tissue Substitute, Full Thickness, External Approach

0HRGX74 Replacement of Left Hand Skin with Autologous Tissue Substitute, Partial Thickness, External Approach

0HRGXJ3 Replacement of Left Hand Skin with Synthetic Substitute, Full Thickness, External Approach

0HRGXJ4 Replacement of Left Hand Skin with Synthetic Substitute, Partial Thickness, External Approach

0HRGXJZ Replacement of Left Hand Skin with Synthetic Substitute, External Approach

0HRGXK3 Replacement of Left Hand Skin with Nonautologous Tissue Substitute, Full Thickness, External Approach

0HRGXK4 Replacement of Left Hand Skin with Nonautologous Tissue Substitute, Partial Thickness, External Approach

0HRHX73 Replacement of Right Upper Leg Skin with Autologous Tissue Substitute, Full Thickness, External Approach

0HRHX74 Replacement of Right Upper Leg Skin with Autologous Tissue Substitute, Partial Thickness, External Approach

0HRHXJ3 Replacement of Right Upper Leg Skin with Synthetic Substitute, Full Thickness, External Approach

0HRHXJ4 Replacement of Right Upper Leg Skin with Synthetic Substitute, Partial Thickness, External Approach

0HRHXJZ Replacement of Right Upper Leg Skin with Synthetic Substitute, External Approach

0HRHXK3 Replacement of Right Upper Leg Skin with Nonautologous Tissue Substitute, Full Thickness, External Approach

0HRHXK4 Replacement of Right Upper Leg Skin with Nonautologous Tissue Substitute, Partial Thickness, External Approach

0HRJX73 Replacement of Left Upper Leg Skin with Autologous Tissue Substitute, Full Thickness, External Approach

0HRJX74 Replacement of Left Upper Leg Skin with Autologous Tissue Substitute, Partial Thickness, External Approach

0HRJXJ3 Replacement of Left Upper Leg Skin with Synthetic Substitute, Full Thickness, External Approach

0HRJXJ4 Replacement of Left Upper Leg Skin with Synthetic Substitute, Partial Thickness, External Approach

0HRJXJZ Replacement of Left Upper Leg Skin with Synthetic Substitute, External Approach

0HRJXK3 Replacement of Left Upper Leg Skin with Nonautologous Tissue Substitute, Full Thickness, External Approach

0HRJXK4 Replacement of Left Upper Leg Skin with Nonautologous Tissue Substitute, Partial Thickness, External Approach

0HRKX73 Replacement of Right Lower Leg Skin with Autologous Tissue Substitute, Full Thickness, External Approach

0HRKX74 Replacement of Right Lower Leg Skin with Autologous Tissue Substitute, Partial Thickness, External Approach

0HRKXJ3 Replacement of Right Lower Leg Skin with Synthetic Substitute, Full Thickness, External Approach

0HRKXJ4 Replacement of Right Lower Leg Skin with Synthetic Substitute, Partial Thickness, External Approach

0HRKXJZ Replacement of Right Lower Leg Skin with Synthetic Substitute, External Approach

0HRKXK3 Replacement of Right Lower Leg Skin with Nonautologous Tissue Substitute, Full Thickness, External Approach

0HRKXK4 Replacement of Right Lower Leg Skin with Nonautologous Tissue Substitute, Partial Thickness, External Approach

0HRLX73 Replacement of Left Lower Leg Skin with Autologous Tissue Substitute, Full Thickness, External Approach

0HRLX74 Replacement of Left Lower Leg Skin with Autologous Tissue Substitute, Partial Thickness, External Approach

0HRLXJ3 Replacement of Left Lower Leg Skin with Synthetic Substitute, Full Thickness, External Approach

0HRLXJ4 Replacement of Left Lower Leg Skin with Synthetic Substitute, Partial Thickness, External Approach

0HRLXJZ Replacement of Left Lower Leg Skin with Synthetic Substitute, External Approach

0HRLXK3 Replacement of Left Lower Leg Skin with Nonautologous Tissue Substitute, Full Thickness, External Approach

0HRLXK4 Replacement of Left Lower Leg Skin with Nonautologous Tissue Substitute, Partial Thickness, External Approach

0HRMX73 Replacement of Right Foot Skin with Autologous Tissue Substitute, Full Thickness, External Approach

0HRMX74 Replacement of Right Foot Skin with Autologous Tissue Substitute, Partial Thickness, External Approach

0HRMXJ3 Replacement of Right Foot Skin with Synthetic Substitute, Full Thickness, External Approach

RMXJ4 Replacement of Right Foot Skin with Synthetic Substitute, Partial Thickness, External Approach

RMXJZ Replacement of Right Foot Skin with Synthetic Substitute, External Approach

RMXK3 Replacement of Right Foot Skin with Nonautologous Tissue Substitute, Full Thickness, External Approach

RMXK4 Replacement of Right Foot Skin with Nonautologous Tissue Substitute, Partial Thickness, External Approach

RNX73 Replacement of Left Foot Skin with Autologous Tissue Substitute, Full Thickness, External Approach

RNX74 Replacement of Left Foot Skin with Autologous Tissue Substitute, Partial Thickness, External Approach

RNXJ3 Replacement of Left Foot Skin with Synthetic Substitute, Full Thickness, External Approach

RNXJ4 Replacement of Left Foot Skin with Synthetic Substitute, Partial Thickness, External Approach

RNXJZ Replacement of Left Foot Skin with Synthetic Substitute, External Approach

RNXK3 Replacement of Left Foot Skin with Nonautologous Tissue Substitute, Full Thickness, External Approach

AHA CC: 3Q, 2014, 14-15

RNXK4 Replacement of Left Foot Skin with Nonautologous Tissue Substitute, Partial Thickness, External Approach

RQX7Z Replacement of Finger Nail with Autologous Tissue Substitute, External Approach

RQXJZ Replacement of Finger Nail with Synthetic Substitute, External Approach

RQXKZ Replacement of Finger Nail with Nonautologous Tissue Substitute, External Approach

RRX7Z Replacement of Toe Nail with Autologous Tissue Substitute, External Approach

RRXJZ Replacement of Toe Nail with Synthetic Substitute, External Approach

RRXKZ Replacement of Toe Nail with Nonautologous Tissue Substitute, External Approach

RSX7Z Replacement of Hair with Autologous Tissue Substitute, External Approach

RSXJZ Replacement of Hair with Synthetic Substitute, External Approach

RSXKZ Replacement of Hair with Nonautologous Tissue Substitute, External Approach

RT075 Replacement of Right Breast using Latissimus Dorsi Myocutaneous Flap, Open Approach

RT076 Replacement of Right Breast using Transverse Rectus Abdominis Myocutaneous Flap, Open Approach

RT077 Replacement of Right Breast using Deep Inferior Epigastric Artery Perforator Flap, Open Approach

RT078 Replacement of Right Breast using Superficial Inferior Epigastric Artery Flap, Open Approach

RT079 Replacement of Right Breast using Gluteal Artery Perforator Flap, Open Approach

RT07Z Replacement of Right Breast with Autologous Tissue Substitute, Open Approach

RT0JZ Replacement of Right Breast with Synthetic Substitute, Open Approach

RT0KZ Replacement of Right Breast with Nonautologous Tissue Substitute, Open Approach

RT37Z Replacement of Right Breast with Autologous Tissue Substitute, Percutaneous Approach

➕ Breast replacement when reported with Extraction of subcutaneous tissue and fascia (4th characters 6,7,8,9,L or M). *See table 0JD to construct the Extraction code.*

0HRT3JZ Replacement of Right Breast with Synthetic Substitute, Percutaneous Approach

0HRT3KZ Replacement of Right Breast with Nonautologous Tissue Substitute, Percutaneous Approach

0HRTX7Z Replacement of Right Breast with Autologous Tissue Substitute, External Approach

0HRTXJZ Replacement of Right Breast with Synthetic Substitute, External Approach

0HRTXKZ Replacement of Right Breast with Nonautologous Tissue Substitute, External Approach

0HRU075 Replacement of Left Breast using Latissimus Dorsi Myocutaneous Flap, Open Approach

0HRU076 Replacement of Left Breast using Transverse Rectus Abdominis Myocutaneous Flap, Open Approach

0HRU077 Replacement of Left Breast using Deep Inferior Epigastric Artery Perforator Flap, Open Approach

0HRU078 Replacement of Left Breast using Superficial Inferior Epigastric Artery Flap, Open Approach

0HRU079 Replacement of Left Breast using Gluteal Artery Perforator Flap, Open Approach

0HRU07Z Replacement of Left Breast with Autologous Tissue Substitute, Open Approach

0HRU0JZ Replacement of Left Breast with Synthetic Substitute, Open Approach

0HRU0KZ Replacement of Left Breast with Nonautologous Tissue Substitute, Open Approach

0HRU37Z Replacement of Left Breast with Autologous Tissue Substitute, Percutaneous Approach

0HRU3JZ Replacement of Left Breast with Synthetic Substitute, Percutaneous Approach

➕ Breast replacement when reported with Extraction of subcutaneous tissue and fascia (4th characters 6,7,8,9,L or M). *See table 0JD to construct the Extraction code.*

0HRU3KZ Replacement of Left Breast with Nonautologous Tissue Substitute, Percutaneous Approach

0HRUX7Z Replacement of Left Breast with Autologous Tissue Substitute, External Approach

0HRUXJZ Replacement of Left Breast with Synthetic Substitute, External Approach

0HRUXKZ Replacement of Left Breast with Nonautologous Tissue Substitute, External Approach

0HRV075 Replacement of Bilateral Breast using Latissimus Dorsi Myocutaneous Flap, Open Approach

0HRV076 Replacement of Bilateral Breast using Transverse Rectus Abdominis Myocutaneous Flap, Open Approach

0HRV077 Replacement of Bilateral Breast using Deep Inferior Epigastric Artery Perforator Flap, Open Approach

0HRV078 Replacement of Bilateral Breast using Superficial Inferior Epigastric Artery Flap, Open Approach

0HRV079 Replacement of Bilateral Breast using Gluteal Artery Perforator Flap, Open Approach

0HRV07Z Replacement of Bilateral Breast with Autologous Tissue Substitute, Open Approach

0HRV0JZ Replacement of Bilateral Breast with Synthetic Substitute, Open Approach

0HRV0KZ Replacement of Bilateral Breast with Nonautologous Tissue Substitute, Open Approach

0HRV37Z Replacement of Bilateral Breast with Autologous Tissue Substitute, Percutaneous Approach

➕ Breast replacement when reported with Extraction of subcutaneous tissue and fascia (4th characters 6,7,8,9,L or M). *See table 0JD to construct the Extraction code.*

0HRV3JZ Replacement of Bilateral Breast with Synthetic Substitute, Percutaneous Approach

0HRV3KZ Replacement of Bilateral Breast with Nonautologous Tissue Substitute, Percutaneous Approach

0HRVX7Z Replacement of Bilateral Breast with Autologous Tissue Substitute, External Approach

0HRVXJZ Replacement of Bilateral Breast with Synthetic Substitute, External Approach

0HRVXKZ Replacement of Bilateral Breast with Nonautologous Tissue Substitute, External Approach

0HRW07Z Replacement of Right Nipple with Autologous Tissue Substitute, Open Approach

0HRW0JZ Replacement of Right Nipple with Synthetic Substitute, Open Approach

0HRW0KZ Replacement of Right Nipple with Nonautologous Tissue Substitute, Open Approach

0HRW37Z Replacement of Right Nipple with Autologous Tissue Substitute, Percutaneous Approach

0HRW3JZ Replacement of Right Nipple with Synthetic Substitute, Percutaneous Approach

0HRW3KZ Replacement of Right Nipple with Nonautologous Tissue Substitute, Percutaneous Approach

0HRWX7Z Replacement of Right Nipple with Autologous Tissue Substitute, External Approach

0HRWXJZ Replacement of Right Nipple with Synthetic Substitute, External Approach

0HRWXKZ Replacement of Right Nipple with Nonautologous Tissue Substitute, External Approach

0HRX07Z Replacement of Left Nipple with Autologous Tissue Substitute, Open Approach

0HRX0JZ Replacement of Left Nipple with Synthetic Substitute, Open Approach

0HRX0KZ Replacement of Left Nipple with Nonautologous Tissue Substitute, Open Approach

0HRX37Z Replacement of Left Nipple with Autologous Tissue Substitute, Percutaneous Approach

0HRX3JZ Replacement of Left Nipple with Synthetic Substitute, Percutaneous Approach

0HRX3KZ Replacement of Left Nipple with Nonautologous Tissue Substitute, Percutaneous Approach

0HRXX7Z Replacement of Left Nipple with Autologous Tissue Substitute, External Approach

0HRXXJZ Replacement of Left Nipple with Synthetic Substitute, External Approach

0HRXXKZ Replacement of Left Nipple with Nonautologous Tissue Substitute, External Approach

0HS – Skin and Breast, Reposition

0HSSXZZ	Reposition Hair, External Approach	
0HST0ZZ	Reposition Right Breast, Open Approach	
0HSU0ZZ	Reposition Left Breast, Open Approach	

0HSV0ZZ	Reposition Bilateral Breast, Open Approach
0HSWXZZ	Reposition Right Nipple, External Approach

0HSXXZZ	Reposition Left Nipple, External Approach

0HT – Skin and Breast, Resection

Review Coding Guideline B3.8

0HTQXZZ	Resection of Finger Nail, External Approach	
0HTRXZZ	Resection of Toe Nail, External Approach	
0HTT0ZZ	Resection of Right Breast, Open Approach	
	AHA CC: 4Q, 2014, 34	

0HTU0ZZ	Resection of Left Breast, Open Approach
0HTV0ZZ	Resection of Bilateral Breast, Open Approach
0HTWXZZ	Resection of Right Nipple, External Approach

0HTXXZZ	Resection of Left Nipple, External Approach
0HTY0ZZ	Resection of Supernumerary Breast, Open Approach

0HU – Skin and Breast, Supplement

0HUT07Z	Supplement Right Breast with Autologous Tissue Substitute, Open Approach
0HUT0JZ	Supplement Right Breast with Synthetic Substitute, Open Approach
0HUT0KZ	Supplement Right Breast with Nonautologous Tissue Substitute, Open Approach
0HUT37Z	Supplement Right Breast with Autologous Tissue Substitute, Percutaneous Approach
0HUT3JZ	Supplement Right Breast with Synthetic Substitute, Percutaneous Approach
0HUT3KZ	Supplement Right Breast with Nonautologous Tissue Substitute, Percutaneous Approach
0HUT77Z	Supplement Right Breast with Autologous Tissue Substitute, Via Natural or Artificial Opening
0HUT7JZ	Supplement Right Breast with Synthetic Substitute, Via Natural or Artificial Opening
0HUT7KZ	Supplement Right Breast with Nonautologous Tissue Substitute, Via Natural or Artificial Opening
0HUT87Z	Supplement Right Breast with Autologous Tissue Substitute, Via Natural or Artificial Opening Endoscopic
0HUT8JZ	Supplement Right Breast with Synthetic Substitute, Via Natural or Artificial Opening Endoscopic
0HUT8KZ	Supplement Right Breast with Nonautologous Tissue Substitute, Via Natural or Artificial Opening Endoscopic
0HUTX7Z	Supplement Right Breast with Autologous Tissue Substitute, External Approach
0HUTXJZ	Supplement Right Breast with Synthetic Substitute, External Approach
0HUTXKZ	Supplement Right Breast with Nonautologous Tissue Substitute, External Approach
0HUU07Z	Supplement Left Breast with Autologous Tissue Substitute, Open Approach
0HUU0JZ	Supplement Left Breast with Synthetic Substitute, Open Approach
0HUU0KZ	Supplement Left Breast with Nonautologous Tissue Substitute, Open Approach
0HUU37Z	Supplement Left Breast with Autologous Tissue Substitute, Percutaneous Approach
0HUU3JZ	Supplement Left Breast with Synthetic Substitute, Percutaneous Approach
0HUU3KZ	Supplement Left Breast with Nonautologous Tissue Substitute, Percutaneous Approach

0HUU77Z	Supplement Left Breast with Autologous Tissue Substitute, Via Natural or Artificial Opening
0HUU7JZ	Supplement Left Breast with Synthetic Substitute, Via Natural or Artificial Opening
0HUU7KZ	Supplement Left Breast with Nonautologous Tissue Substitute, Via Natural or Artificial Opening
0HUU87Z	Supplement Left Breast with Autologous Tissue Substitute, Via Natural or Artificial Opening Endoscopic
0HUU8JZ	Supplement Left Breast with Synthetic Substitute, Via Natural or Artificial Opening Endoscopic
0HUU8KZ	Supplement Left Breast with Nonautologous Tissue Substitute, Via Natural or Artificial Opening Endoscopic
0HUUX7Z	Supplement Left Breast with Autologous Tissue Substitute, External Approach
0HUUXJZ	Supplement Left Breast with Synthetic Substitute, External Approach
0HUUXKZ	Supplement Left Breast with Nonautologous Tissue Substitute, External Approach
0HUV07Z	Supplement Bilateral Breast with Autologous Tissue Substitute, Open Approach
0HUV0JZ	Supplement Bilateral Breast with Synthetic Substitute, Open Approach
0HUV0KZ	Supplement Bilateral Breast with Nonautologous Tissue Substitute, Open Approach
0HUV37Z	Supplement Bilateral Breast with Autologous Tissue Substitute, Percutaneous Approach
0HUV3JZ	Supplement Bilateral Breast with Synthetic Substitute, Percutaneous Approach
0HUV3KZ	Supplement Bilateral Breast with Nonautologous Tissue Substitute, Percutaneous Approach
0HUV77Z	Supplement Bilateral Breast with Autologous Tissue Substitute, Via Natural or Artificial Opening
0HUV7JZ	Supplement Bilateral Breast with Synthetic Substitute, Via Natural or Artificial Opening
0HUV7KZ	Supplement Bilateral Breast with Nonautologous Tissue Substitute, Via Natural or Artificial Opening
0HUV87Z	Supplement Bilateral Breast with Autologous Tissue Substitute, Via Natural or Artificial Opening Endoscopic
0HUV8JZ	Supplement Bilateral Breast with Synthetic Substitute, Via Natural or Artificial Opening Endoscopic

0HUV8KZ	Supplement Bilateral Breast with Nonautologous Tissue Substitute, Via Natural or Artificial Opening Endoscopic
0HUVX7Z	Supplement Bilateral Breast with Autologous Tissue Substitute, External Approach
0HUVXJZ	Supplement Bilateral Breast with Synthetic Substitute, External Approach
0HUVXKZ	Supplement Bilateral Breast with Nonautologous Tissue Substitute, External Approach
0HUW07Z	Supplement Right Nipple with Autologous Tissue Substitute, Open Approach
0HUW0JZ	Supplement Right Nipple with Synthetic Substitute, Open Approach
0HUW0KZ	Supplement Right Nipple with Nonautologous Tissue Substitute, Open Approach
0HUW37Z	Supplement Right Nipple with Autologous Tissue Substitute, Percutaneous Approach
0HUW3JZ	Supplement Right Nipple with Synthetic Substitute, Percutaneous Approach
0HUW3KZ	Supplement Right Nipple with Nonautologous Tissue Substitute, Percutaneous Approach
0HUW77Z	Supplement Right Nipple with Autologous Tissue Substitute, Via Natural or Artificial Opening
0HUW7JZ	Supplement Right Nipple with Synthetic Substitute, Via Natural or Artificial Opening
0HUW7KZ	Supplement Right Nipple with Nonautologous Tissue Substitute, Via Natural or Artificial Opening
0HUW87Z	Supplement Right Nipple with Autologous Tissue Substitute, Via Natural or Artificial Opening Endoscopic
0HUW8JZ	Supplement Right Nipple with Synthetic Substitute, Via Natural or Artificial Opening Endoscopic
0HUW8KZ	Supplement Right Nipple with Nonautologous Tissue Substitute, Via Natural or Artificial Opening Endoscopic
0HUWX7Z	Supplement Right Nipple with Autologous Tissue Substitute, External Approach
0HUWXJZ	Supplement Right Nipple with Synthetic Substitute, External Approach
0HUWXKZ	Supplement Right Nipple with Nonautologous Tissue Substitute, External Approach
0HUX07Z	Supplement Left Nipple with Autologous Tissue Substitute, Open Approach
0HUX0JZ	Supplement Left Nipple with Synthetic Substitute, Open Approach

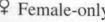 Female-only   ♂ Male-only   ▲ Limited Coverage   ● Non-OR   ▨ HAC-associated procedure   ▲ Non-covered procedures   + Combinati

UX0KZ   Supplement Left Nipple with Nonautologous Tissue Substitute, Open Approach

UX37Z   Supplement Left Nipple with Autologous Tissue Substitute, Percutaneous Approach

UX3JZ   Supplement Left Nipple with Synthetic Substitute, Percutaneous Approach

UX3KZ   Supplement Left Nipple with Nonautologous Tissue Substitute, Percutaneous Approach

UX77Z   Supplement Left Nipple with Autologous Tissue Substitute, Via Natural or Artificial Opening

0HUX7JZ   Supplement Left Nipple with Synthetic Substitute, Via Natural or Artificial Opening

0HUX7KZ   Supplement Left Nipple with Nonautologous Tissue Substitute, Via Natural or Artificial Opening

0HUX87Z   Supplement Left Nipple with Autologous Tissue Substitute, Via Natural or Artificial Opening Endoscopic

0HUX8JZ   Supplement Left Nipple with Synthetic Substitute, Via Natural or Artificial Opening Endoscopic

0HUX8KZ   Supplement Left Nipple with Nonautologous Tissue Substitute, Via Natural or Artificial Opening Endoscopic

0HUXX7Z   Supplement Left Nipple with Autologous Tissue Substitute, External Approach

0HUXXJZ   Supplement Left Nipple with Synthetic Substitute, External Approach

0HUXXKZ   Supplement Left Nipple with Nonautologous Tissue Substitute, External Approach

IW – Skin and Breast, Revision

view Coding Guideline B6.1c

WPX0Z   Revision of Drainage Device in Skin, External Approach

WPX7Z   Revision of Autologous Tissue Substitute in Skin, External Approach

WPXJZ   Revision of Synthetic Substitute in Skin, External Approach

WPXKZ   Revision of Nonautologous Tissue Substitute in Skin, External Approach

WQX0Z   Revision of Drainage Device in Finger Nail, External Approach

WQX7Z   Revision of Autologous Tissue Substitute in Finger Nail, External Approach

WQXJZ   Revision of Synthetic Substitute in Finger Nail, External Approach

WQXKZ   Revision of Nonautologous Tissue Substitute in Finger Nail, External Approach

WRX0Z   Revision of Drainage Device in Toe Nail, External Approach

WRX7Z   Revision of Autologous Tissue Substitute in Toe Nail, External Approach

WRXJZ   Revision of Synthetic Substitute in Toe Nail, External Approach

WRXKZ   Revision of Nonautologous Tissue Substitute in Toe Nail, External Approach

WSX7Z   Revision of Autologous Tissue Substitute in Hair, External Approach

WSXJZ   Revision of Synthetic Substitute in Hair, External Approach

WSXKZ   Revision of Nonautologous Tissue Substitute in Hair, External Approach

WT00Z   Revision of Drainage Device in Right Breast, Open Approach

WT07Z   Revision of Autologous Tissue Substitute in Right Breast, Open Approach

WT0JZ   Revision of Synthetic Substitute in Right Breast, Open Approach

WT0KZ   Revision of Nonautologous Tissue Substitute in Right Breast, Open Approach

WT0NZ   Revision of Tissue Expander in Right Breast, Open Approach

WT30Z   Revision of Drainage Device in Right Breast, Percutaneous Approach

WT37Z   Revision of Autologous Tissue Substitute in Right Breast, Percutaneous Approach

WT3JZ   Revision of Synthetic Substitute in Right Breast, Percutaneous Approach

0HWT3KZ   Revision of Nonautologous Tissue Substitute in Right Breast, Percutaneous Approach

0HWT3NZ   Revision of Tissue Expander in Right Breast, Percutaneous Approach

0HWT70Z   Revision of Drainage Device in Right Breast, Via Natural or Artificial Opening

0HWT77Z   Revision of Autologous Tissue Substitute in Right Breast, Via Natural or Artificial Opening

0HWT7JZ   Revision of Synthetic Substitute in Right Breast, Via Natural or Artificial Opening

0HWT7KZ   Revision of Nonautologous Tissue Substitute in Right Breast, Via Natural or Artificial Opening

0HWT7NZ   Revision of Tissue Expander in Right Breast, Via Natural or Artificial Opening

0HWT80Z   Revision of Drainage Device in Right Breast, Via Natural or Artificial Opening Endoscopic

0HWT87Z   Revision of Autologous Tissue Substitute in Right Breast, Via Natural or Artificial Opening Endoscopic

0HWT8JZ   Revision of Synthetic Substitute in Right Breast, Via Natural or Artificial Opening Endoscopic

0HWT8KZ   Revision of Nonautologous Tissue Substitute in Right Breast, Via Natural or Artificial Opening Endoscopic

0HWT8NZ   Revision of Tissue Expander in Right Breast, Via Natural or Artificial Opening Endoscopic

0HWTX0Z   Revision of Drainage Device in Right Breast, External Approach

0HWTX7Z   Revision of Autologous Tissue Substitute in Right Breast, External Approach

0HWTXJZ   Revision of Synthetic Substitute in Right Breast, External Approach

0HWTXKZ   Revision of Nonautologous Tissue Substitute in Right Breast, External Approach

0HWU00Z   Revision of Drainage Device in Left Breast, Open Approach

0HWU07Z   Revision of Autologous Tissue Substitute in Left Breast, Open Approach

0HWU0JZ   Revision of Synthetic Substitute in Left Breast, Open Approach

0HWU0KZ   Revision of Nonautologous Tissue Substitute in Left Breast, Open Approach

0HWU0NZ   Revision of Tissue Expander in Left Breast, Open Approach

0HWU30Z   Revision of Drainage Device in Left Breast, Percutaneous Approach

0HWU37Z   Revision of Autologous Tissue Substitute in Left Breast, Percutaneous Approach

0HWU3JZ   Revision of Synthetic Substitute in Left Breast, Percutaneous Approach

0HWU3KZ   Revision of Nonautologous Tissue Substitute in Left Breast, Percutaneous Approach

0HWU3NZ   Revision of Tissue Expander in Left Breast, Percutaneous Approach

0HWU70Z   Revision of Drainage Device in Left Breast, Via Natural or Artificial Opening

0HWU77Z   Revision of Autologous Tissue Substitute in Left Breast, Via Natural or Artificial Opening

0HWU7JZ   Revision of Synthetic Substitute in Left Breast, Via Natural or Artificial Opening

0HWU7KZ   Revision of Nonautologous Tissue Substitute in Left Breast, Via Natural or Artificial Opening

0HWU7NZ   Revision of Tissue Expander in Left Breast, Via Natural or Artificial Opening

0HWU80Z   Revision of Drainage Device in Left Breast, Via Natural or Artificial Opening Endoscopic

0HWU87Z   Revision of Autologous Tissue Substitute in Left Breast, Via Natural or Artificial Opening Endoscopic

0HWU8JZ   Revision of Synthetic Substitute in Left Breast, Via Natural or Artificial Opening Endoscopic

0HWU8KZ   Revision of Nonautologous Tissue Substitute in Left Breast, Via Natural or Artificial Opening Endoscopic

0HWU8NZ   Revision of Tissue Expander in Left Breast, Via Natural or Artificial Opening Endoscopic

0HWUX0Z   Revision of Drainage Device in Left Breast, External Approach

0HWUX7Z   Revision of Autologous Tissue Substitute in Left Breast, External Approach

0HWUXJZ   Revision of Synthetic Substitute in Left Breast, External Approach

0HWUXKZ   Revision of Nonautologous Tissue Substitute in Left Breast, External Approach

HX – Skin and Breast, Transfer

HX0XZZ   Transfer Scalp Skin, External Approach

HX1XZZ   Transfer Face Skin, External Approach

0HX2XZZ   Transfer Right Ear Skin, External Approach

0HX3XZZ   Transfer Left Ear Skin, External Approach

Female-only   ♂ Male-only   ▲ Limited Coverage   ● Non-OR   ▩ HAC-associated procedure   ▲ Non-covered procedures   ✚ Combination

0HX4XZZ Transfer Neck Skin, External Approach

0HX5XZZ Transfer Chest Skin, External Approach

0HX6XZZ Transfer Back Skin, External Approach

0HX7XZZ Transfer Abdomen Skin, External Approach

0HX8XZZ Transfer Buttock Skin, External Approach

0HX9XZZ Transfer Perineum Skin, External Approach

0HXAXZZ Transfer Genitalia Skin, External Approach

0HXBXZZ Transfer Right Upper Arm Skin, External Approach

0HXCXZZ Transfer Left Upper Arm Skin, External Approach

0HXDXZZ Transfer Right Lower Arm Skin, External Approach

0HXEXZZ Transfer Left Lower Arm Skin, External Approach

0HXFXZZ Transfer Right Hand Skin, External Approach

0HXGXZZ Transfer Left Hand Skin, External Approach

0HXHXZZ Transfer Right Upper Leg Skin, External Approach

0HXJXZZ Transfer Left Upper Leg Skin, External Approach

0HXKXZZ Transfer Right Lower Leg Skin, External Approach

0HXLXZZ Transfer Left Lower Leg Skin, External Approach

0HXMXZZ Transfer Right Foot Skin, External Approach

0HXNXZZ Transfer Left Foot Skin, External Approach

Subcutaneous Tissue and Fascia

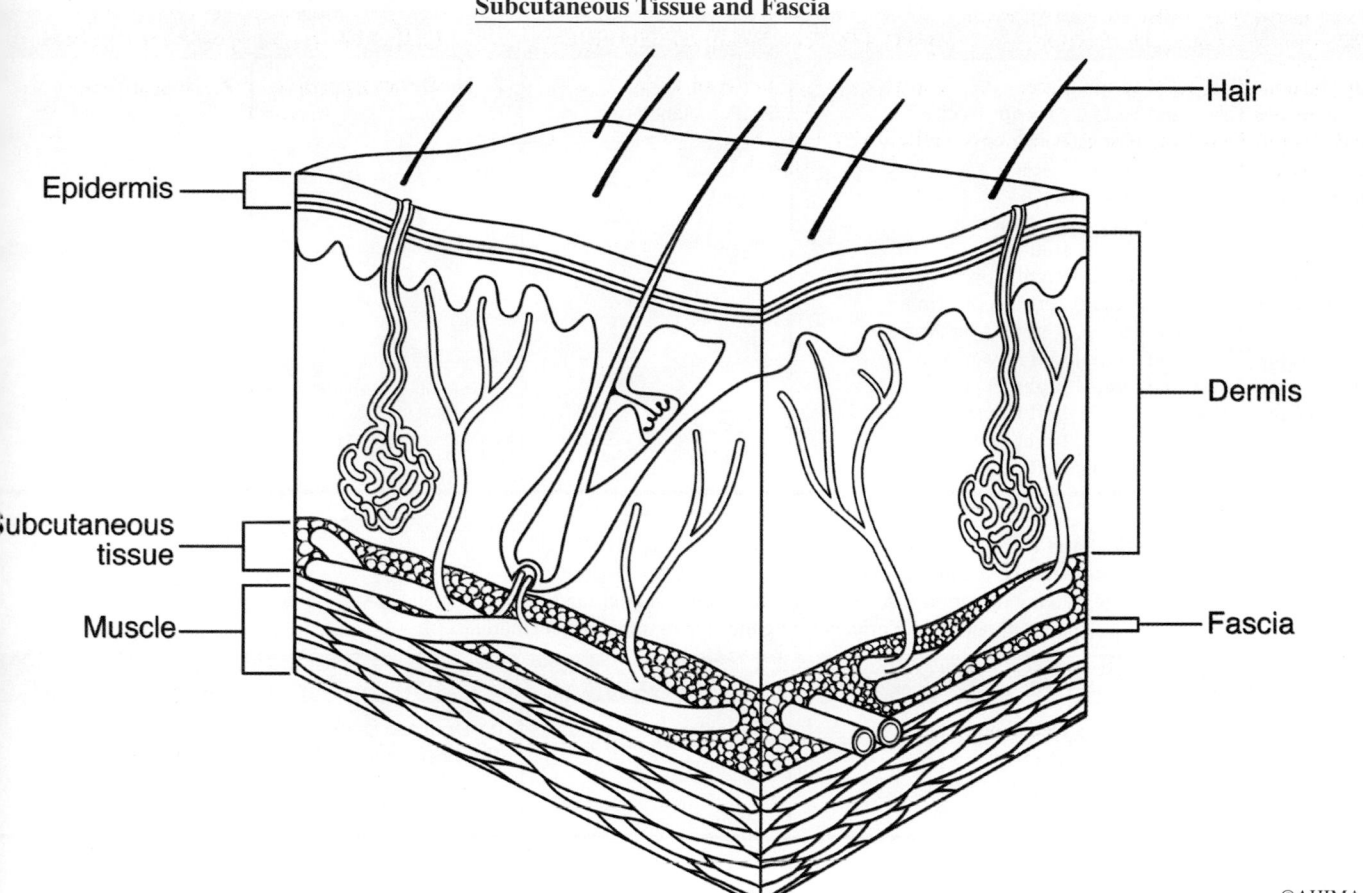

Epidermis

Hair

Dermis

Subcutaneous tissue

Muscle

Fascia

©AHIMA

Subcutaneous Tissue and Fascia Tables 0J0–0JX

Section	0	Medical and Surgical
Body System	J	Subcutaneous Tissue and Fascia
Operation	0	Alteration: Modifying the anatomic structure of a body part without affecting the function of the body part

Body Part (4th)	Approach (5th)	Device (6th)	Qualifier (7th)
1 Subcutaneous Tissue and Fascia, Face 4 Subcutaneous Tissue and Fascia, Anterior Neck 5 Subcutaneous Tissue and Fascia, Posterior Neck 6 Subcutaneous Tissue and Fascia, Chest 7 Subcutaneous Tissue and Fascia, Back 8 Subcutaneous Tissue and Fascia, Abdomen 9 Subcutaneous Tissue and Fascia, Buttock D Subcutaneous Tissue and Fascia, Right Upper Arm F Subcutaneous Tissue and Fascia, Left Upper Arm G Subcutaneous Tissue and Fascia, Right Lower Arm H Subcutaneous Tissue and Fascia, Left Lower Arm L Subcutaneous Tissue and Fascia, Right Upper Leg M Subcutaneous Tissue and Fascia, Left Upper Leg N Subcutaneous Tissue and Fascia, Right Lower Leg P Subcutaneous Tissue and Fascia, Left Lower Leg	0 Open 3 Percutaneous	Z No Device	Z No Qualifier

Section	0	Medical and Surgical
Body System	J	Subcutaneous Tissue and Fascia
Operation	2	Change: Taking out or off a device from a body part and putting back an identical or similar device in or on the same body part without cutting or puncturing the skin or a mucous membrane

Body Part (4th)	Approach (5th)	Device (6th)	Qualifier (7th)
S Subcutaneous Tissue and Fascia, Head and Neck T Subcutaneous Tissue and Fascia, Trunk V Subcutaneous Tissue and Fascia, Upper Extremity W Subcutaneous Tissue and Fascia, Lower Extremity	X External	0 Drainage Device Y Other Device	Z No Qualifier

Section	0	Medical and Surgical
Body System	J	Subcutaneous Tissue and Fascia
Operation	5	Destruction: Physical eradication of all or a portion of a body part by the direct use of energy, force, or a destructive agent

Body Part (4th)	Approach (5th)	Device (6th)	Qualifier (7th)
0 Subcutaneous Tissue and Fascia, Scalp 1 Subcutaneous Tissue and Fascia, Face 4 Subcutaneous Tissue and Fascia, Anterior Neck 5 Subcutaneous Tissue and Fascia, Posterior Neck 6 Subcutaneous Tissue and Fascia, Chest 7 Subcutaneous Tissue and Fascia, Back 8 Subcutaneous Tissue and Fascia, Abdomen 9 Subcutaneous Tissue and Fascia, Buttock B Subcutaneous Tissue and Fascia, Perineum C Subcutaneous Tissue and Fascia, Pelvic Region D Subcutaneous Tissue and Fascia, Right Upper Arm F Subcutaneous Tissue and Fascia, Left Upper Arm G Subcutaneous Tissue and Fascia, Right Lower Arm H Subcutaneous Tissue and Fascia, Left Lower Arm J Subcutaneous Tissue and Fascia, Right Hand K Subcutaneous Tissue and Fascia, Left Hand L Subcutaneous Tissue and Fascia, Right Upper Leg M Subcutaneous Tissue and Fascia, Left Upper Leg N Subcutaneous Tissue and Fascia, Right Lower Leg P Subcutaneous Tissue and Fascia, Left Lower Leg Q Subcutaneous Tissue and Fascia, Right Foot R Subcutaneous Tissue and Fascia, Left Foot	0 Open 3 Percutaneous	Z No Device	Z No Qualifier

Section 0 Medical and Surgical
Body System J Subcutaneous Tissue and Fascia
Operation 8 **Division:** Cutting into a body part, without draining fluids and/or gases from the body part, in order to separate or transect a body part

Body Part (4th)	Approach (5th)	Device (6th)	Qualifier (7th)
0 Subcutaneous Tissue and Fascia, Scalp	0 Open	Z No Device	Z No Qualifier
1 Subcutaneous Tissue and Fascia, Face	3 Percutaneous		
4 Subcutaneous Tissue and Fascia, Anterior Neck			
5 Subcutaneous Tissue and Fascia, Posterior Neck			
6 Subcutaneous Tissue and Fascia, Chest			
7 Subcutaneous Tissue and Fascia, Back			
8 Subcutaneous Tissue and Fascia, Abdomen			
9 Subcutaneous Tissue and Fascia, Buttock			
B Subcutaneous Tissue and Fascia, Perineum			
C Subcutaneous Tissue and Fascia, Pelvic Region			
D Subcutaneous Tissue and Fascia, Right Upper Arm			
F Subcutaneous Tissue and Fascia, Left Upper Arm			
G Subcutaneous Tissue and Fascia, Right Lower Arm			
H Subcutaneous Tissue and Fascia, Left Lower Arm			
J Subcutaneous Tissue and Fascia, Right Hand			
K Subcutaneous Tissue and Fascia, Left Hand			
L Subcutaneous Tissue and Fascia, Right Upper Leg			
M Subcutaneous Tissue and Fascia, Left Upper Leg			
N Subcutaneous Tissue and Fascia, Right Lower Leg			
P Subcutaneous Tissue and Fascia, Left Lower Leg			
Q Subcutaneous Tissue and Fascia, Right Foot			
R Subcutaneous Tissue and Fascia, Left Foot			
S Subcutaneous Tissue and Fascia, Head and Neck			
T Subcutaneous Tissue and Fascia, Trunk			
V Subcutaneous Tissue and Fascia, Upper Extremity			
W Subcutaneous Tissue and Fascia, Lower Extremity			

Section 0 Medical and Surgical
Body System J Subcutaneous Tissue and Fascia
Operation 9 **Drainage:** Taking or letting out fluids and/or gases from a body part

Body Part (4th)	Approach (5th)	Device (6th)	Qualifier (7th)
0 Subcutaneous Tissue and Fascia, Scalp	0 Open	0 Drainage Device	Z No Qualifier
1 Subcutaneous Tissue and Fascia, Face	3 Percutaneous		
4 Subcutaneous Tissue and Fascia, Anterior Neck			
5 Subcutaneous Tissue and Fascia, Posterior Neck			
6 Subcutaneous Tissue and Fascia, Chest			
7 Subcutaneous Tissue and Fascia, Back			
8 Subcutaneous Tissue and Fascia, Abdomen			
9 Subcutaneous Tissue and Fascia, Buttock			
B Subcutaneous Tissue and Fascia, Perineum			
C Subcutaneous Tissue and Fascia, Pelvic Region			
D Subcutaneous Tissue and Fascia, Right Upper Arm			
F Subcutaneous Tissue and Fascia, Left Upper Arm			
G Subcutaneous Tissue and Fascia, Right Lower Arm			
H Subcutaneous Tissue and Fascia, Left Lower Arm			
J Subcutaneous Tissue and Fascia, Right Hand			
K Subcutaneous Tissue and Fascia, Left Hand			
L Subcutaneous Tissue and Fascia, Right Upper Leg			
M Subcutaneous Tissue and Fascia, Left Upper Leg			
N Subcutaneous Tissue and Fascia, Right Lower Leg			
P Subcutaneous Tissue and Fascia, Left Lower Leg			
Q Subcutaneous Tissue and Fascia, Right Foot			
R Subcutaneous Tissue and Fascia, Left Foot			

Continued →

Medical and Surgical, Subcutaneous Tissue and Fascia Tables

Section	0	Medical and Surgical
Body System	J	Subcutaneous Tissue and Fascia
Operation	9	Drainage: Taking or letting out fluids and/or gases from a body part

Body Part (4ᵗʰ)	Approach (5ᵗʰ)	Device (6ᵗʰ)	Qualifier (7ᵗʰ)
0 Subcutaneous Tissue and Fascia, Scalp 1 Subcutaneous Tissue and Fascia, Face 4 Subcutaneous Tissue and Fascia, Anterior Neck 5 Subcutaneous Tissue and Fascia, Posterior Neck 6 Subcutaneous Tissue and Fascia, Chest 7 Subcutaneous Tissue and Fascia, Back 8 Subcutaneous Tissue and Fascia, Abdomen 9 Subcutaneous Tissue and Fascia, Buttock B Subcutaneous Tissue and Fascia, Perineum C Subcutaneous Tissue and Fascia, Pelvic Region D Subcutaneous Tissue and Fascia, Right Upper Arm F Subcutaneous Tissue and Fascia, Left Upper Arm G Subcutaneous Tissue and Fascia, Right Lower Arm H Subcutaneous Tissue and Fascia, Left Lower Arm J Subcutaneous Tissue and Fascia, Right Hand K Subcutaneous Tissue and Fascia, Left Hand L Subcutaneous Tissue and Fascia, Right Upper Leg M Subcutaneous Tissue and Fascia, Left Upper Leg N Subcutaneous Tissue and Fascia, Right Lower Leg P Subcutaneous Tissue and Fascia, Left Lower Leg Q Subcutaneous Tissue and Fascia, Right Foot R Subcutaneous Tissue and Fascia, Left Foot	0 Open 3 Percutaneous	Z No Device	X Diagnostic Z No Qualifier

Section	0	Medical and Surgical
Body System	J	Subcutaneous Tissue and Fascia
Operation	B	Excision: Cutting out or off, without replacement, a portion of a body part

Body Part (4ᵗʰ)	Approach (5ᵗʰ)	Device (6ᵗʰ)	Qualifier (7ᵗʰ)
0 Subcutaneous Tissue and Fascia, Scalp 1 Subcutaneous Tissue and Fascia, Face 4 Subcutaneous Tissue and Fascia, Anterior Neck 5 Subcutaneous Tissue and Fascia, Posterior Neck 6 Subcutaneous Tissue and Fascia, Chest 7 Subcutaneous Tissue and Fascia, Back 8 Subcutaneous Tissue and Fascia, Abdomen 9 Subcutaneous Tissue and Fascia, Buttock B Subcutaneous Tissue and Fascia, Perineum C Subcutaneous Tissue and Fascia, Pelvic Region D Subcutaneous Tissue and Fascia, Right Upper Arm F Subcutaneous Tissue and Fascia, Left Upper Arm G Subcutaneous Tissue and Fascia, Right Lower Arm H Subcutaneous Tissue and Fascia, Left Lower Arm J Subcutaneous Tissue and Fascia, Right Hand K Subcutaneous Tissue and Fascia, Left Hand L Subcutaneous Tissue and Fascia, Right Upper Leg M Subcutaneous Tissue and Fascia, Left Upper Leg N Subcutaneous Tissue and Fascia, Right Lower Leg P Subcutaneous Tissue and Fascia, Left Lower Leg Q Subcutaneous Tissue and Fascia, Right Foot R Subcutaneous Tissue and Fascia, Left Foot	0 Open 3 Percutaneous	Z No Device	X Diagnostic Z No Qualifier

Section	0	Medical and Surgical
Body System	J	Subcutaneous Tissue and Fascia
Operation	C	Extirpation: Taking or cutting out solid matter from a body part

Body Part (4th)	Approach (5th)	Device (6th)	Qualifier (7th)
0 Subcutaneous Tissue and Fascia, Scalp	0 Open	Z No Device	Z No Qualifier
1 Subcutaneous Tissue and Fascia, Face	3 Percutaneous		
4 Subcutaneous Tissue and Fascia, Anterior Neck			
5 Subcutaneous Tissue and Fascia, Posterior Neck			
6 Subcutaneous Tissue and Fascia, Chest			
7 Subcutaneous Tissue and Fascia, Back			
8 Subcutaneous Tissue and Fascia, Abdomen			
9 Subcutaneous Tissue and Fascia, Buttock			
B Subcutaneous Tissue and Fascia, Perineum			
C Subcutaneous Tissue and Fascia, Pelvic Region			
D Subcutaneous Tissue and Fascia, Right Upper Arm			
F Subcutaneous Tissue and Fascia, Left Upper Arm			
G Subcutaneous Tissue and Fascia, Right Lower Arm			
H Subcutaneous Tissue and Fascia, Left Lower Arm			
J Subcutaneous Tissue and Fascia, Right Hand			
K Subcutaneous Tissue and Fascia, Left Hand			
L Subcutaneous Tissue and Fascia, Right Upper Leg			
M Subcutaneous Tissue and Fascia, Left Upper Leg			
N Subcutaneous Tissue and Fascia, Right Lower Leg			
P Subcutaneous Tissue and Fascia, Left Lower Leg			
Q Subcutaneous Tissue and Fascia, Right Foot			
R Subcutaneous Tissue and Fascia, Left Foot			

Section	0	Medical and Surgical
Body System	J	Subcutaneous Tissue and Fascia
Operation	D	Extraction: Pulling or stripping out or off all or a portion of a body part by the use of force

Body Part (4th)	Approach (5th)	Device (6th)	Qualifier (7th)
0 Subcutaneous Tissue and Fascia, Scalp	0 Open	Z No Device	Z No Qualifier
1 Subcutaneous Tissue and Fascia, Face	3 Percutaneous		
4 Subcutaneous Tissue and Fascia, Anterior Neck			
5 Subcutaneous Tissue and Fascia, Posterior Neck			
6 Subcutaneous Tissue and Fascia, Chest			
7 Subcutaneous Tissue and Fascia, Back			
8 Subcutaneous Tissue and Fascia, Abdomen			
9 Subcutaneous Tissue and Fascia, Buttock			
B Subcutaneous Tissue and Fascia, Perineum			
C Subcutaneous Tissue and Fascia, Pelvic Region			
D Subcutaneous Tissue and Fascia, Right Upper Arm			
F Subcutaneous Tissue and Fascia, Left Upper Arm			
G Subcutaneous Tissue and Fascia, Right Lower Arm			
H Subcutaneous Tissue and Fascia, Left Lower Arm			
J Subcutaneous Tissue and Fascia, Right Hand			
K Subcutaneous Tissue and Fascia, Left Hand			
L Subcutaneous Tissue and Fascia, Right Upper Leg			
M Subcutaneous Tissue and Fascia, Left Upper Leg			
N Subcutaneous Tissue and Fascia, Right Lower Leg			
P Subcutaneous Tissue and Fascia, Left Lower Leg			
Q Subcutaneous Tissue and Fascia, Right Foot			
R Subcutaneous Tissue and Fascia, Left Foot			

Section	0	Medical and Surgical
Body System	J	Subcutaneous Tissue and Fascia
Operation	H	Insertion: Putting in a nonbiological appliance that monitors, assists, performs, or prevents a physiological function but does not physically take the place of a body part

Body Part (4th)	Approach (5th)	Device (6th)	Qualifier (7th)
0 Subcutaneous Tissue and Fascia, Scalp 1 Subcutaneous Tissue and Fascia, Face 4 Subcutaneous Tissue and Fascia, Anterior Neck 5 Subcutaneous Tissue and Fascia, Posterior Neck 9 Subcutaneous Tissue and Fascia, Buttock B Subcutaneous Tissue and Fascia, Perineum C Subcutaneous Tissue and Fascia, Pelvic Region J Subcutaneous Tissue and Fascia, Right Hand K Subcutaneous Tissue and Fascia, Left Hand Q Subcutaneous Tissue and Fascia, Right Foot R Subcutaneous Tissue and Fascia, Left Foot	0 Open 3 Percutaneous	N Tissue Expander	Z No Qualifier
6 Subcutaneous Tissue and Fascia, Chest 8 Subcutaneous Tissue and Fascia, Abdomen	0 Open 3 Percutaneous	0 Monitoring Device, Hemodynamic 2 Monitoring Device 4 Pacemaker, Single Chamber 5 Pacemaker, Single Chamber Rate Responsive 6 Pacemaker, Dual Chamber 7 Cardiac Resynchronization Pacemaker Pulse Generator 8 Defibrillator Generator 9 Cardiac Resynchronization Defibrillator Pulse Generator A Contractility Modulation Device B Stimulator Generator, Single Array C Stimulator Generator, Single Array Rechargeable D Stimulator Generator, Multiple Array E Stimulator Generator, Multiple Array Rechargeable H Contraceptive Device M Stimulator Generator N Tissue Expander P Cardiac Rhythm Related Device V Infusion Device, Pump W Vascular Access Device, Reservoir X Vascular Access Device	Z No Qualifier
7 Subcutaneous Tissue and Fascia, Back	0 Open 3 Percutaneous	B Stimulator Generator, Single Array C Stimulator Generator, Single Array Rechargeable D Stimulator Generator, Multiple Array E Stimulator Generator, Multiple Array Rechargeable M Stimulator Generator N Tissue Expander V Infusion Device, Pump	Z No Qualifier
D Subcutaneous Tissue and Fascia, Right Upper Arm F Subcutaneous Tissue and Fascia, Left Upper Arm G Subcutaneous Tissue and Fascia, Right Lower Arm H Subcutaneous Tissue and Fascia, Left Lower Arm L Subcutaneous Tissue and Fascia, Right Upper Leg M Subcutaneous Tissue and Fascia, Left Upper Leg N Subcutaneous Tissue and Fascia, Right Lower Leg P Subcutaneous Tissue and Fascia, Left Lower Leg	0 Open 3 Percutaneous	H Contraceptive Device N Tissue Expander V Infusion Device, Pump W Vascular Access Device, Reservoir X Vascular Access Device	Z No Qualifier
S Subcutaneous Tissue and Fascia, Head and Neck V Subcutaneous Tissue and Fascia, Upper Extremity W Subcutaneous Tissue and Fascia, Lower Extremity	0 Open 3 Percutaneous	1 Radioactive Element 3 Infusion Device	Z No Qualifier
T Subcutaneous Tissue and Fascia, Trunk	0 Open 3 Percutaneous	1 Radioactive Element 3 Infusion Device V Infusion Device, Pump	Z No Qualifier

Section	0	Medical and Surgical
Body System	J	Subcutaneous Tissue and Fascia
Operation	J	**Inspection:** Visually and/or manually exploring a body part

Body Part (4th)	Approach (5th)	Device (6th)	Qualifier (7th)
Subcutaneous Tissue and Fascia, Head and Neck Subcutaneous Tissue and Fascia, Trunk Subcutaneous Tissue and Fascia, Upper Extremity Subcutaneous Tissue and Fascia, Lower Extremity	0 Open 3 Percutaneous X External	Z No Device	Z No Qualifier

Section	0	Medical and Surgical
Body System	J	Subcutaneous Tissue and Fascia
Operation	N	**Release:** Freeing a body part from an abnormal physical constraint by cutting or by the use of force

Body Part (4th)	Approach (5th)	Device (6th)	Qualifier (7th)
Subcutaneous Tissue and Fascia, Scalp Subcutaneous Tissue and Fascia, Face Subcutaneous Tissue and Fascia, Anterior Neck Subcutaneous Tissue and Fascia, Posterior Neck Subcutaneous Tissue and Fascia, Chest Subcutaneous Tissue and Fascia, Back Subcutaneous Tissue and Fascia, Abdomen Subcutaneous Tissue and Fascia, Buttock Subcutaneous Tissue and Fascia, Perineum Subcutaneous Tissue and Fascia, Pelvic Region Subcutaneous Tissue and Fascia, Right Upper Arm Subcutaneous Tissue and Fascia, Left Upper Arm Subcutaneous Tissue and Fascia, Right Lower Arm Subcutaneous Tissue and Fascia, Left Lower Arm Subcutaneous Tissue and Fascia, Right Hand Subcutaneous Tissue and Fascia, Left Hand Subcutaneous Tissue and Fascia, Right Upper Leg Subcutaneous Tissue and Fascia, Left Upper Leg Subcutaneous Tissue and Fascia, Right Lower Leg Subcutaneous Tissue and Fascia, Left Lower Leg Subcutaneous Tissue and Fascia, Right Foot Subcutaneous Tissue and Fascia, Left Foot	0 Open 3 Percutaneous X External	Z No Device	Z No Qualifier

Section	0	Medical and Surgical
Body System	J	Subcutaneous Tissue and Fascia
Operation	P	**Removal:** Taking out or off a device from a body part

Body Part (4th)	Approach (5th)	Device (6th)	Qualifier (7th)
S Subcutaneous Tissue and Fascia, Head and Neck	0 Open 3 Percutaneous	0 Drainage Device 1 Radioactive Element 3 Infusion Device 7 Autologous Tissue Substitute J Synthetic Substitute K Nonautologous Tissue Substitute N Tissue Expander	Z No Qualifier
S Subcutaneous Tissue and Fascia, Head and Neck	X External	0 Drainage Device 1 Radioactive Element 3 Infusion Device	Z No Qualifier

Continued →

Section 0 **Medical and Surgical**
Body System J **Subcutaneous Tissue and Fascia**
Operation P **Removal:** Taking out or off a device from a body part

Body Part (4th)	Approach (5th)	Device (6th)	Qualifier (7th)
T Subcutaneous Tissue and Fascia, Trunk	**0** Open **3** Percutaneous	**0** Drainage Device **1** Radioactive Element **2** Monitoring Device **3** Infusion Device **7** Autologous Tissue Substitute **H** Contraceptive Device **J** Synthetic Substitute **K** Nonautologous Tissue Substitute **M** Stimulator Generator **N** Tissue Expander **P** Cardiac Rhythm Related Device **V** Infusion Device, Pump **W** Vascular Access Device, Reservoir **X** Vascular Access Device	**Z** No Qualifier
T Subcutaneous Tissue and Fascia, Trunk	**X** External	**0** Drainage Device **1** Radioactive Element **2** Monitoring Device **3** Infusion Device **H** Contraceptive Device **V** Infusion Device, Pump **X** Vascular Access Device	**Z** No Qualifier
V Subcutaneous Tissue and Fascia, Upper Extremity **W** Subcutaneous Tissue and Fascia, Lower Extremity	**0** Open **3** Percutaneous	**0** Drainage Device **1** Radioactive Element **3** Infusion Device **7** Autologous Tissue Substitute **H** Contraceptive Device **J** Synthetic Substitute **K** Nonautologous Tissue Substitute **N** Tissue Expander **V** Infusion Device, Pump **W** Vascular Access Device, Reservoir **X** Vascular Access Device	**Z** No Qualifier
V Subcutaneous Tissue and Fascia, Upper Extremity **W** Subcutaneous Tissue and Fascia, Lower Extremity	**X** External	**0** Drainage Device **1** Radioactive Element **3** Infusion Device **H** Contraceptive Device **V** Infusion Device, Pump **X** Vascular Access Device	**Z** No Qualifier

Section	0	Medical and Surgical
Body System	J	Subcutaneous Tissue and Fascia
Operation	Q	Repair: Restoring, to the extent possible, a body part to its normal anatomic structure and function

Body Part (4th)	Approach (5th)	Device (6th)	Qualifier (7th)
0 Subcutaneous Tissue and Fascia, Scalp 1 Subcutaneous Tissue and Fascia, Face 4 Subcutaneous Tissue and Fascia, Anterior Neck 5 Subcutaneous Tissue and Fascia, Posterior Neck 6 Subcutaneous Tissue and Fascia, Chest 7 Subcutaneous Tissue and Fascia, Back 8 Subcutaneous Tissue and Fascia, Abdomen 9 Subcutaneous Tissue and Fascia, Buttock B Subcutaneous Tissue and Fascia, Perineum C Subcutaneous Tissue and Fascia, Pelvic Region D Subcutaneous Tissue and Fascia, Right Upper Arm F Subcutaneous Tissue and Fascia, Left Upper Arm G Subcutaneous Tissue and Fascia, Right Lower Arm H Subcutaneous Tissue and Fascia, Left Lower Arm J Subcutaneous Tissue and Fascia, Right Hand K Subcutaneous Tissue and Fascia, Left Hand L Subcutaneous Tissue and Fascia, Right Upper Leg M Subcutaneous Tissue and Fascia, Left Upper Leg N Subcutaneous Tissue and Fascia, Right Lower Leg P Subcutaneous Tissue and Fascia, Left Lower Leg Q Subcutaneous Tissue and Fascia, Right Foot R Subcutaneous Tissue and Fascia, Left Foot	0 Open 3 Percutaneous	Z No Device	Z No Qualifier

Section	0	Medical and Surgical
Body System	J	Subcutaneous Tissue and Fascia
Operation	R	Replacement: Putting in or on biological or synthetic material that physically takes the place and/or function of all or a portion of a body part

Body Part (4th)	Approach (5th)	Device (6th)	Qualifier (7th)
0 Subcutaneous Tissue and Fascia, Scalp 1 Subcutaneous Tissue and Fascia, Face 4 Subcutaneous Tissue and Fascia, Anterior Neck 5 Subcutaneous Tissue and Fascia, Posterior Neck 6 Subcutaneous Tissue and Fascia, Chest 7 Subcutaneous Tissue and Fascia, Back 8 Subcutaneous Tissue and Fascia, Abdomen 9 Subcutaneous Tissue and Fascia, Buttock B Subcutaneous Tissue and Fascia, Perineum C Subcutaneous Tissue and Fascia, Pelvic Region D Subcutaneous Tissue and Fascia, Right Upper Arm F Subcutaneous Tissue and Fascia, Left Upper Arm G Subcutaneous Tissue and Fascia, Right Lower Arm H Subcutaneous Tissue and Fascia, Left Lower Arm J Subcutaneous Tissue and Fascia, Right Hand K Subcutaneous Tissue and Fascia, Left Hand L Subcutaneous Tissue and Fascia, Right Upper Leg M Subcutaneous Tissue and Fascia, Left Upper Leg N Subcutaneous Tissue and Fascia, Right Lower Leg P Subcutaneous Tissue and Fascia, Left Lower Leg Q Subcutaneous Tissue and Fascia, Right Foot R Subcutaneous Tissue and Fascia, Left Foot	0 Open 3 Percutaneous	7 Autologous Tissue Substitute J Synthetic Substitute K Nonautologous Tissue Substitute	Z No Qualifier

Section	0	Medical and Surgical
Body System	J	Subcutaneous Tissue and Fascia
Operation	U	Supplement: Putting in or on biological or synthetic material that physically reinforces and/or augments the function of a portion of a body part

Body Part (4th)	Approach (5th)	Device (6th)	Qualifier (7th)
0 Subcutaneous Tissue and Fascia, Scalp 1 Subcutaneous Tissue and Fascia, Face 4 Subcutaneous Tissue and Fascia, Anterior Neck 5 Subcutaneous Tissue and Fascia, Posterior Neck 6 Subcutaneous Tissue and Fascia, Chest 7 Subcutaneous Tissue and Fascia, Back 8 Subcutaneous Tissue and Fascia, Abdomen 9 Subcutaneous Tissue and Fascia, Buttock B Subcutaneous Tissue and Fascia, Perineum C Subcutaneous Tissue and Fascia, Pelvic Region D Subcutaneous Tissue and Fascia, Right Upper Arm F Subcutaneous Tissue and Fascia, Left Upper Arm G Subcutaneous Tissue and Fascia, Right Lower Arm H Subcutaneous Tissue and Fascia, Left Lower Arm J Subcutaneous Tissue and Fascia, Right Hand K Subcutaneous Tissue and Fascia, Left Hand L Subcutaneous Tissue and Fascia, Right Upper Leg M Subcutaneous Tissue and Fascia, Left Upper Leg N Subcutaneous Tissue and Fascia, Right Lower Leg P Subcutaneous Tissue and Fascia, Left Lower Leg Q Subcutaneous Tissue and Fascia, Right Foot R Subcutaneous Tissue and Fascia, Left Foot	0 Open 3 Percutaneous	7 Autologous Tissue Substitute J Synthetic Substitute K Nonautologous Tissue Substitute	Z No Qualifier

Section	0	Medical and Surgical
Body System	J	Subcutaneous Tissue and Fascia
Operation	W	Revision: Correcting, to the extent possible, a portion of a malfunctioning device or the position of a displaced device

Body Part (4th)	Approach (5th)	Device (6th)	Qualifier (7th)
S Subcutaneous Tissue and Fascia, Head and Neck	0 Open 3 Percutaneous X External	0 Drainage Device 3 Infusion Device 7 Autologous Tissue Substitute J Synthetic Substitute K Nonautologous Tissue Substitute N Tissue Expander	Z No Qualifier
T Subcutaneous Tissue and Fascia, Trunk	0 Open 3 Percutaneous X External	0 Drainage Device 2 Monitoring Device 3 Infusion Device 7 Autologous Tissue Substitute H Contraceptive Device J Synthetic Substitute K Nonautologous Tissue Substitute M Stimulator Generator N Tissue Expander P Cardiac Rhythm Related Device V Infusion Device, Pump W Vascular Access Device, Reservoir X Vascular Access Device	Z No Qualifier
V Subcutaneous Tissue and Fascia, Upper Extremity W Subcutaneous Tissue and Fascia, Lower Extremity	0 Open 3 Percutaneous X External	0 Drainage Device 3 Infusion Device 7 Autologous Tissue Substitute H Contraceptive Device J Synthetic Substitute K Nonautologous Tissue Substitute N Tissue Expander V Infusion Device, Pump W Vascular Access Device, Reservoir X Vascular Access Device	Z No Qualifier

Section	0	Medical and Surgical
Body System	J	Subcutaneous Tissue and Fascia
Operation	X	**Transfer:** Moving, without taking out, all or a portion of a body part to another location to take over the function of all or a portion of a body part

Body Part (4th)	Approach (5th)	Device (6th)	Qualifier (7th)
0 Subcutaneous Tissue and Fascia, Scalp 1 Subcutaneous Tissue and Fascia, Face 4 Subcutaneous Tissue and Fascia, Anterior Neck 5 Subcutaneous Tissue and Fascia, Posterior Neck 6 Subcutaneous Tissue and Fascia, Chest 7 Subcutaneous Tissue and Fascia, Back 8 Subcutaneous Tissue and Fascia, Abdomen 9 Subcutaneous Tissue and Fascia, Buttock B Subcutaneous Tissue and Fascia, Perineum C Subcutaneous Tissue and Fascia, Pelvic Region D Subcutaneous Tissue and Fascia, Right Upper Arm F Subcutaneous Tissue and Fascia, Left Upper Arm G Subcutaneous Tissue and Fascia, Right Lower Arm H Subcutaneous Tissue and Fascia, Left Lower Arm J Subcutaneous Tissue and Fascia, Right Hand K Subcutaneous Tissue and Fascia, Left Hand L Subcutaneous Tissue and Fascia, Right Upper Leg M Subcutaneous Tissue and Fascia, Left Upper Leg N Subcutaneous Tissue and Fascia, Right Lower Leg P Subcutaneous Tissue and Fascia, Left Lower Leg Q Subcutaneous Tissue and Fascia, Right Foot R Subcutaneous Tissue and Fascia, Left Foot	0 Open 3 Percutaneous	Z No Device	B Skin and Subcutaneous Tissue C Skin, Subcutaneous Tissue and Fascia Z No Qualifier

Subcutaneous Tissue and Fascia Code Listing 0J0–0JX

Review Coding Guideline B4.5

Review Coding Guideline B4.6

0J0 – Subcutaneous Tissue and Fascia, Alteration

0J010ZZ Alteration of Face Subcutaneous Tissue and Fascia, Open Approach

0J013ZZ Alteration of Face Subcutaneous Tissue and Fascia, Percutaneous Approach

0J040ZZ Alteration of Anterior Neck Subcutaneous Tissue and Fascia, Open Approach

0J043ZZ Alteration of Anterior Neck Subcutaneous Tissue and Fascia, Percutaneous Approach

0J050ZZ Alteration of Posterior Neck Subcutaneous Tissue and Fascia, Open Approach

0J053ZZ Alteration of Posterior Neck Subcutaneous Tissue and Fascia, Percutaneous Approach

0J060ZZ Alteration of Chest Subcutaneous Tissue and Fascia, Open Approach

0J063ZZ Alteration of Chest Subcutaneous Tissue and Fascia, Percutaneous Approach

0J070ZZ Alteration of Back Subcutaneous Tissue and Fascia, Open Approach

0J073ZZ Alteration of Back Subcutaneous Tissue and Fascia, Percutaneous Approach

0J080ZZ Alteration of Abdomen Subcutaneous Tissue and Fascia, Open Approach

0J083ZZ Alteration of Abdomen Subcutaneous Tissue and Fascia, Percutaneous Approach

0J090ZZ Alteration of Buttock Subcutaneous Tissue and Fascia, Open Approach

0J093ZZ Alteration of Buttock Subcutaneous Tissue and Fascia, Percutaneous Approach

0J0D0ZZ Alteration of Right Upper Arm Subcutaneous Tissue and Fascia, Open Approach

0J0D3ZZ Alteration of Right Upper Arm Subcutaneous Tissue and Fascia, Percutaneous Approach

0J0F0ZZ Alteration of Left Upper Arm Subcutaneous Tissue and Fascia, Open Approach

0J0F3ZZ Alteration of Left Upper Arm Subcutaneous Tissue and Fascia, Percutaneous Approach

0J0G0ZZ Alteration of Right Lower Arm Subcutaneous Tissue and Fascia, Open Approach

0J0G3ZZ Alteration of Right Lower Arm Subcutaneous Tissue and Fascia, Percutaneous Approach

0J0H0ZZ Alteration of Left Lower Arm Subcutaneous Tissue and Fascia, Open Approach

0J0H3ZZ Alteration of Left Lower Arm Subcutaneous Tissue and Fascia, Percutaneous Approach

0J0L0ZZ Alteration of Right Upper Leg Subcutaneous Tissue and Fascia, Open Approach

0J0L3ZZ Alteration of Right Upper Leg Subcutaneous Tissue and Fascia, Percutaneous Approach

0J0M0ZZ Alteration of Left Upper Leg Subcutaneous Tissue and Fascia, Open Approach

0J0M3ZZ Alteration of Left Upper Leg Subcutaneous Tissue and Fascia, Percutaneous Approach

0J0N0ZZ Alteration of Right Lower Leg Subcutaneous Tissue and Fascia, Open Approach

0J0N3ZZ Alteration of Right Lower Leg Subcutaneous Tissue and Fascia, Percutaneous Approach

0J0P0ZZ Alteration of Left Lower Leg Subcutaneous Tissue and Fascia, Open Approach

0J0P3ZZ Alteration of Left Lower Leg Subcutaneous Tissue and Fascia, Percutaneous Approach

0J2 – Subcutaneous Tissue and Fascia, Change

Review Coding Guideline B6.1c

0J2SX0Z Change Drainage Device in Head and Neck Subcutaneous Tissue and Fascia, External Approach

0J2SXYZ Change Other Device in Head and Neck Subcutaneous Tissue and Fascia, External Approach

0J2TX0Z Change Drainage Device in Trunk Subcutaneous Tissue and Fascia, External Approach

0J2TXYZ Change Other Device in Trunk Subcutaneous Tissue and Fascia, External Approach

0J2VX0Z Change Drainage Device in Upper Extremity Subcutaneous Tissue and Fascia, External Approach

0J2VXYZ Change Other Device in Upper Extremity Subcutaneous Tissue and Fascia, External Approach

| ♀ Female-only | ♂ Male-only | ▲ Limited Coverage | ● Non-OR | ▬ HAC-associated procedure | ▲ Non-covered procedures | ✚ Combination |

| 0J2WX0Z | Change Drainage Device in Lower Extremity Subcutaneous Tissue and Fascia, External Approach | 0J2WXYZ | Change Other Device in Lower Extremity Subcutaneous Tissue and Fascia, External Approach |

0J5 – Subcutaneous Tissue and Fascia, Destruction

● 0J500ZZ Destruction of Scalp Subcutaneous Tissue and Fascia, Open Approach
● 0J503ZZ Destruction of Scalp Subcutaneous Tissue and Fascia, Percutaneous Approach
● 0J510ZZ Destruction of Face Subcutaneous Tissue and Fascia, Open Approach
● 0J513ZZ Destruction of Face Subcutaneous Tissue and Fascia, Percutaneous Approach
● 0J540ZZ Destruction of Anterior Neck Subcutaneous Tissue and Fascia, Open Approach
● 0J543ZZ Destruction of Anterior Neck Subcutaneous Tissue and Fascia, Percutaneous Approach
● 0J550ZZ Destruction of Posterior Neck Subcutaneous Tissue and Fascia, Open Approach
● 0J553ZZ Destruction of Posterior Neck Subcutaneous Tissue and Fascia, Percutaneous Approach
● 0J560ZZ Destruction of Chest Subcutaneous Tissue and Fascia, Open Approach
● 0J563ZZ Destruction of Chest Subcutaneous Tissue and Fascia, Percutaneous Approach
● 0J570ZZ Destruction of Back Subcutaneous Tissue and Fascia, Open Approach
● 0J573ZZ Destruction of Back Subcutaneous Tissue and Fascia, Percutaneous Approach
● 0J580ZZ Destruction of Abdomen Subcutaneous Tissue and Fascia, Open Approach
● 0J583ZZ Destruction of Abdomen Subcutaneous Tissue and Fascia, Percutaneous Approach
● 0J590ZZ Destruction of Buttock Subcutaneous Tissue and Fascia, Open Approach
● 0J593ZZ Destruction of Buttock Subcutaneous Tissue and Fascia, Percutaneous Approach
● 0J5B0ZZ Destruction of Perineum Subcutaneous Tissue and Fascia, Open Approach

● 0J5B3ZZ Destruction of Perineum Subcutaneous Tissue and Fascia, Percutaneous Approach
● 0J5C0ZZ Destruction of Pelvic Region Subcutaneous Tissue and Fascia, Open Approach
● 0J5C3ZZ Destruction of Pelvic Region Subcutaneous Tissue and Fascia, Percutaneous Approach
● 0J5D0ZZ Destruction of Right Upper Arm Subcutaneous Tissue and Fascia, Open Approach
● 0J5D3ZZ Destruction of Right Upper Arm Subcutaneous Tissue and Fascia, Percutaneous Approach
● 0J5F0ZZ Destruction of Left Upper Arm Subcutaneous Tissue and Fascia, Open Approach
● 0J5F3ZZ Destruction of Left Upper Arm Subcutaneous Tissue and Fascia, Percutaneous Approach
● 0J5G0ZZ Destruction of Right Lower Arm Subcutaneous Tissue and Fascia, Open Approach
● 0J5G3ZZ Destruction of Right Lower Arm Subcutaneous Tissue and Fascia, Percutaneous Approach
● 0J5H0ZZ Destruction of Left Lower Arm Subcutaneous Tissue and Fascia, Open Approach
● 0J5H3ZZ Destruction of Left Lower Arm Subcutaneous Tissue and Fascia, Percutaneous Approach
● 0J5J0ZZ Destruction of Right Hand Subcutaneous Tissue and Fascia, Open Approach
● 0J5J3ZZ Destruction of Right Hand Subcutaneous Tissue and Fascia, Percutaneous Approach

● 0J5K0ZZ Destruction of Left Hand Subcutaneous Tissue and Fascia, Open Approach
● 0J5K3ZZ Destruction of Left Hand Subcutaneous Tissue and Fascia, Percutaneous Approa
● 0J5L0ZZ Destruction of Right Upper Leg Subcutaneous Tissue and Fascia, Open Approach
● 0J5L3ZZ Destruction of Right Upper Leg Subcutaneous Tissue and Fascia, Percutaneous Approach
● 0J5M0ZZ Destruction of Left Upper Leg Subcutaneous Tissue and Fascia, Open Approach
● 0J5M3ZZ Destruction of Left Upper Leg Subcutaneous Tissue and Fascia, Percutaneous Approach
● 0J5N0ZZ Destruction of Right Lower Leg Subcutaneous Tissue and Fascia, Open Approach
● 0J5N3ZZ Destruction of Right Lower Leg Subcutaneous Tissue and Fascia, Percutaneous Approach
● 0J5P0ZZ Destruction of Left Lower Leg Subcutaneous Tissue and Fascia, Open Approach
● 0J5P3ZZ Destruction of Left Lower Leg Subcutaneous Tissue and Fascia, Percutaneous Approach
● 0J5Q0ZZ Destruction of Right Foot Subcutaneous Tissue and Fascia, Open Approach
● 0J5Q3ZZ Destruction of Right Foot Subcutaneous Tissue and Fascia, Percutaneous Approac
● 0J5R0ZZ Destruction of Left Foot Subcutaneous Tissue and Fascia, Open Approach
● 0J5R3ZZ Destruction of Left Foot Subcutaneous Tissue and Fascia, Percutaneous Approac

0J8 – Subcutaneous Tissue and Fascia, Division

Review Coding Guideline B3.14

0J800ZZ Division of Scalp Subcutaneous Tissue and Fascia, Open Approach
0J803ZZ Division of Scalp Subcutaneous Tissue and Fascia, Percutaneous Approach
0J810ZZ Division of Face Subcutaneous Tissue and Fascia, Open Approach
0J813ZZ Division of Face Subcutaneous Tissue and Fascia, Percutaneous Approach
0J840ZZ Division of Anterior Neck Subcutaneous Tissue and Fascia, Open Approach
0J843ZZ Division of Anterior Neck Subcutaneous Tissue and Fascia, Percutaneous Approach
0J850ZZ Division of Posterior Neck Subcutaneous Tissue and Fascia, Open Approach
0J853ZZ Division of Posterior Neck Subcutaneous Tissue and Fascia, Percutaneous Approach
0J860ZZ Division of Chest Subcutaneous Tissue and Fascia, Open Approach
0J863ZZ Division of Chest Subcutaneous Tissue and Fascia, Percutaneous Approach
0J870ZZ Division of Back Subcutaneous Tissue and Fascia, Open Approach
0J873ZZ Division of Back Subcutaneous Tissue and Fascia, Percutaneous Approach
0J880ZZ Division of Abdomen Subcutaneous Tissue and Fascia, Open Approach
0J883ZZ Division of Abdomen Subcutaneous Tissue and Fascia, Percutaneous Approach

0J890ZZ Division of Buttock Subcutaneous Tissue and Fascia, Open Approach
0J893ZZ Division of Buttock Subcutaneous Tissue and Fascia, Percutaneous Approach
0J8B0ZZ Division of Perineum Subcutaneous Tissue and Fascia, Open Approach
0J8B3ZZ Division of Perineum Subcutaneous Tissue and Fascia, Percutaneous Approach
0J8C0ZZ Division of Pelvic Region Subcutaneous Tissue and Fascia, Open Approach
0J8C3ZZ Division of Pelvic Region Subcutaneous Tissue and Fascia, Percutaneous Approach
0J8D0ZZ Division of Right Upper Arm Subcutaneous Tissue and Fascia, Open Approach
0J8D3ZZ Division of Right Upper Arm Subcutaneous Tissue and Fascia, Percutaneous Approach
0J8F0ZZ Division of Left Upper Arm Subcutaneous Tissue and Fascia, Open Approach
0J8F3ZZ Division of Left Upper Arm Subcutaneous Tissue and Fascia, Percutaneous Approach
0J8G0ZZ Division of Right Lower Arm Subcutaneous Tissue and Fascia, Open Approach
0J8G3ZZ Division of Right Lower Arm Subcutaneous Tissue and Fascia, Percutaneous Approach

0J8H0ZZ Division of Left Lower Arm Subcutaneou Tissue and Fascia, Open Approach
0J8H3ZZ Division of Left Lower Arm Subcutaneou Tissue and Fascia, Percutaneous Approach
0J8J0ZZ Division of Right Hand Subcutaneous Tissue and Fascia, Open Approach
0J8J3ZZ Division of Right Hand Subcutaneous Tissue and Fascia, Percutaneous Approach
0J8K0ZZ Division of Left Hand Subcutaneous Tissue and Fascia, Open Approach
0J8K3ZZ Division of Left Hand Subcutaneous Tissue and Fascia, Percutaneous Approach
0J8L0ZZ Division of Right Upper Leg Subcutaneous Tissue and Fascia, Open Approach
0J8L3ZZ Division of Right Upper Leg Subcutaneous Tissue and Fascia, Percutaneous Approach
0J8M0ZZ Division of Left Upper Leg Subcutaneous Tissue and Fascia, Open Approach
0J8M3ZZ Division of Left Upper Leg Subcutaneous Tissue and Fascia, Percutaneous Approach
0J8N0ZZ Division of Right Lower Leg Subcutaneous Tissue and Fascia, Open Approach
0J8N3ZZ Division of Right Lower Leg Subcutaneous Tissue and Fascia, Percutaneous Approach

♀ Female-only   ♂ Male-only   ▲ Limited Coverage   ● Non-OR   ▨ HAC-associated procedure   ▲ Non-covered procedures   ✚ Combination

P0ZZ	Division of Left Lower Leg Subcutaneous Tissue and Fascia, Open Approach	0J8R3ZZ	Division of Left Foot Subcutaneous Tissue and Fascia, Percutaneous Approach	0J8V0ZZ	Division of Upper Extremity Subcutaneous Tissue and Fascia, Open Approach
P3ZZ	Division of Left Lower Leg Subcutaneous Tissue and Fascia, Percutaneous Approach	0J8S0ZZ	Division of Head and Neck Subcutaneous Tissue and Fascia, Open Approach	0J8V3ZZ	Division of Upper Extremity Subcutaneous Tissue and Fascia, Percutaneous Approach
Q0ZZ	Division of Right Foot Subcutaneous Tissue and Fascia, Open Approach	0J8S3ZZ	Division of Head and Neck Subcutaneous Tissue and Fascia, Percutaneous Approach	0J8W0ZZ	Division of Lower Extremity Subcutaneous Tissue and Fascia, Open Approach
Q3ZZ	Division of Right Foot Subcutaneous Tissue and Fascia, Percutaneous Approach	0J8T0ZZ	Division of Trunk Subcutaneous Tissue and Fascia, Open Approach	0J8W3ZZ	Division of Lower Extremity Subcutaneous Tissue and Fascia, Percutaneous Approach
R0ZZ	Division of Left Foot Subcutaneous Tissue and Fascia, Open Approach	0J8T3ZZ	Division of Trunk Subcutaneous Tissue and Fascia, Percutaneous Approach		

9 – Subcutaneous Tissue and Fascia, Drainage

view Coding Guidelines B3.4a and B3.4b

view Coding Guideline B6.2

000Z	Drainage of Scalp Subcutaneous Tissue and Fascia with Drainage Device, Open Approach	0J9600Z	Drainage of Chest Subcutaneous Tissue and Fascia with Drainage Device, Open Approach	0J9B00Z	Drainage of Perineum Subcutaneous Tissue and Fascia with Drainage Device, Open Approach
00ZX	Drainage of Scalp Subcutaneous Tissue and Fascia, Open Approach, Diagnostic	0J960ZX	Drainage of Chest Subcutaneous Tissue and Fascia, Open Approach, Diagnostic	0J9B0ZX	Drainage of Perineum Subcutaneous Tissue and Fascia, Open Approach, Diagnostic
00ZZ	Drainage of Scalp Subcutaneous Tissue and Fascia, Open Approach	0J960ZZ	Drainage of Chest Subcutaneous Tissue and Fascia, Open Approach	0J9B0ZZ	Drainage of Perineum Subcutaneous Tissue and Fascia, Open Approach
030Z	Drainage of Scalp Subcutaneous Tissue and Fascia with Drainage Device, Percutaneous Approach	0J9630Z	Drainage of Chest Subcutaneous Tissue and Fascia with Drainage Device, Percutaneous Approach	0J9B30Z	Drainage of Perineum Subcutaneous Tissue and Fascia with Drainage Device, Percutaneous Approach
03ZX	Drainage of Scalp Subcutaneous Tissue and Fascia, Percutaneous Approach, Diagnostic	0J963ZX	Drainage of Chest Subcutaneous Tissue and Fascia, Percutaneous Approach, Diagnostic	0J9B3ZX	Drainage of Perineum Subcutaneous Tissue and Fascia, Percutaneous Approach, Diagnostic
03ZZ	Drainage of Scalp Subcutaneous Tissue and Fascia, Percutaneous Approach	0J963ZZ	Drainage of Chest Subcutaneous Tissue and Fascia, Percutaneous Approach	0J9B3ZZ	Drainage of Perineum Subcutaneous Tissue and Fascia, Percutaneous Approach
0100Z	Drainage of Face Subcutaneous Tissue and Fascia with Drainage Device, Open Approach	0J9700Z	Drainage of Back Subcutaneous Tissue and Fascia with Drainage Device, Open Approach	0J9C00Z	Drainage of Pelvic Region Subcutaneous Tissue and Fascia with Drainage Device, Open Approach
010ZX	Drainage of Face Subcutaneous Tissue and Fascia, Open Approach, Diagnostic	0J970ZX	Drainage of Back Subcutaneous Tissue and Fascia, Open Approach, Diagnostic	0J9C0ZX	Drainage of Pelvic Region Subcutaneous Tissue and Fascia, Open Approach, Diagnostic
010ZZ	Drainage of Face Subcutaneous Tissue and Fascia, Open Approach	0J970ZZ	Drainage of Back Subcutaneous Tissue and Fascia, Open Approach	0J9C0ZZ	Drainage of Pelvic Region Subcutaneous Tissue and Fascia, Open Approach
9130Z	Drainage of Face Subcutaneous Tissue and Fascia with Drainage Device, Percutaneous Approach	0J9730Z	Drainage of Back Subcutaneous Tissue and Fascia with Drainage Device, Percutaneous Approach	0J9C30Z	Drainage of Pelvic Region Subcutaneous Tissue and Fascia with Drainage Device, Percutaneous Approach
913ZX	Drainage of Face Subcutaneous Tissue and Fascia, Percutaneous Approach, Diagnostic	0J973ZX	Drainage of Back Subcutaneous Tissue and Fascia, Percutaneous Approach, Diagnostic	0J9C3ZX	Drainage of Pelvic Region Subcutaneous Tissue and Fascia, Percutaneous Approach, Diagnostic
913ZZ	Drainage of Face Subcutaneous Tissue and Fascia, Percutaneous Approach	0J973ZZ	Drainage of Back Subcutaneous Tissue and Fascia, Percutaneous Approach	0J9C3ZZ	Drainage of Pelvic Region Subcutaneous Tissue and Fascia, Percutaneous Approach
9400Z	Drainage of Anterior Neck Subcutaneous Tissue and Fascia with Drainage Device, Open Approach	0J9800Z	Drainage of Abdomen Subcutaneous Tissue and Fascia with Drainage Device, Open Approach	0J9D00Z	Drainage of Right Upper Arm Subcutaneous Tissue and Fascia with Drainage Device, Open Approach
940ZX	Drainage of Anterior Neck Subcutaneous Tissue and Fascia, Open Approach, Diagnostic	0J980ZX	Drainage of Abdomen Subcutaneous Tissue and Fascia, Open Approach, Diagnostic	0J9D0ZX	Drainage of Right Upper Arm Subcutaneous Tissue and Fascia, Open Approach, Diagnostic
940ZZ	Drainage of Anterior Neck Subcutaneous Tissue and Fascia, Open Approach	0J980ZZ	Drainage of Abdomen Subcutaneous Tissue and Fascia, Open Approach	0J9D0ZZ	Drainage of Right Upper Arm Subcutaneous Tissue and Fascia, Open Approach
9430Z	Drainage of Anterior Neck Subcutaneous Tissue and Fascia with Drainage Device, Percutaneous Approach	0J9830Z	Drainage of Abdomen Subcutaneous Tissue and Fascia with Drainage Device, Percutaneous Approach	0J9D30Z	Drainage of Right Upper Arm Subcutaneous Tissue and Fascia with Drainage Device, Percutaneous Approach
943ZX	Drainage of Anterior Neck Subcutaneous Tissue and Fascia, Percutaneous Approach, Diagnostic	0J983ZX	Drainage of Abdomen Subcutaneous Tissue and Fascia, Percutaneous Approach, Diagnostic	0J9D3ZX	Drainage of Right Upper Arm Subcutaneous Tissue and Fascia, Percutaneous Approach, Diagnostic
943ZZ	Drainage of Anterior Neck Subcutaneous Tissue and Fascia, Percutaneous Approach	0J983ZZ	Drainage of Abdomen Subcutaneous Tissue and Fascia, Percutaneous Approach	0J9D3ZZ	Drainage of Right Upper Arm Subcutaneous Tissue and Fascia, Percutaneous Approach
9500Z	Drainage of Posterior Neck Subcutaneous Tissue and Fascia with Drainage Device, Open Approach	0J9900Z	Drainage of Buttock Subcutaneous Tissue and Fascia with Drainage Device, Open Approach	0J9F00Z	Drainage of Left Upper Arm Subcutaneous Tissue and Fascia with Drainage Device, Open Approach
950ZX	Drainage of Posterior Neck Subcutaneous Tissue and Fascia, Open Approach, Diagnostic	0J990ZX	Drainage of Buttock Subcutaneous Tissue and Fascia, Open Approach, Diagnostic	0J9F0ZX	Drainage of Left Upper Arm Subcutaneous Tissue and Fascia, Open Approach, Diagnostic
J950ZZ	Drainage of Posterior Neck Subcutaneous Tissue and Fascia, Open Approach	0J990ZZ	Drainage of Buttock Subcutaneous Tissue and Fascia, Open Approach	0J9F0ZZ	Drainage of Left Upper Arm Subcutaneous Tissue and Fascia, Open Approach
J9530Z	Drainage of Posterior Neck Subcutaneous Tissue and Fascia with Drainage Device, Percutaneous Approach	0J9930Z	Drainage of Buttock Subcutaneous Tissue and Fascia with Drainage Device, Percutaneous Approach	0J9F30Z	Drainage of Left Upper Arm Subcutaneous Tissue and Fascia with Drainage Device, Percutaneous Approach
J953ZX	Drainage of Posterior Neck Subcutaneous Tissue and Fascia, Percutaneous Approach, Diagnostic	0J993ZX	Drainage of Buttock Subcutaneous Tissue and Fascia, Percutaneous Approach, Diagnostic		
J953ZZ	Drainage of Posterior Neck Subcutaneous Tissue and Fascia, Percutaneous Approach	0J993ZZ	Drainage of Buttock Subcutaneous Tissue and Fascia, Percutaneous Approach		

Female-only	♂ Male-only	▲ Limited Coverage	● Non-OR	▩ HAC-associated procedure	▲ Non-covered procedures	✛ Combination

0J9F3ZX	Drainage of Left Upper Arm Subcutaneous Tissue and Fascia, Percutaneous Approach, Diagnostic	**0J9K00Z**	Drainage of Left Hand Subcutaneous Tissue and Fascia with Drainage Device, Open Approach	**0J9N30Z**	Drainage of Right Lower Leg Subcutaneous Tissue and Fascia with Drainage Device, Percutaneous Approach
0J9F3ZZ	Drainage of Left Upper Arm Subcutaneous Tissue and Fascia, Percutaneous Approach	**0J9K0ZX**	Drainage of Left Hand Subcutaneous Tissue and Fascia, Open Approach, Diagnostic	**0J9N3ZX**	Drainage of Right Lower Leg Subcutaneous Tissue and Fascia, Percutaneous Approach, Diagnostic
0J9G00Z	Drainage of Right Lower Arm Subcutaneous Tissue and Fascia with Drainage Device, Open Approach	**0J9K0ZZ**	Drainage of Left Hand Subcutaneous Tissue and Fascia, Open Approach	**0J9N3ZZ**	Drainage of Right Lower Leg Subcutaneous Tissue and Fascia, Percutaneous Approach
0J9G0ZX	Drainage of Right Lower Arm Subcutaneous Tissue and Fascia, Open Approach, Diagnostic	**0J9K30Z**	Drainage of Left Hand Subcutaneous Tissue and Fascia with Drainage Device, Percutaneous Approach	**0J9P00Z**	Drainage of Left Lower Leg Subcutaneous Tissue and Fascia with Drainage Device, Open Approach
0J9G0ZZ	Drainage of Right Lower Arm Subcutaneous Tissue and Fascia, Open Approach	**0J9K3ZX**	Drainage of Left Hand Subcutaneous Tissue and Fascia, Percutaneous Approach, Diagnostic	**0J9P0ZX**	Drainage of Left Lower Leg Subcutaneous Tissue and Fascia, Open Approach, Diagnostic
0J9G30Z	Drainage of Right Lower Arm Subcutaneous Tissue and Fascia with Drainage Device, Percutaneous Approach	● **0J9K3ZZ**	Drainage of Left Hand Subcutaneous Tissue and Fascia, Percutaneous Approach	**0J9P0ZZ**	Drainage of Left Lower Leg Subcutaneous Tissue and Fascia, Open Approach
0J9G3ZX	Drainage of Right Lower Arm Subcutaneous Tissue and Fascia, Percutaneous Approach, Diagnostic	**0J9L00Z**	Drainage of Right Upper Leg Subcutaneous Tissue and Fascia with Drainage Device, Open Approach	**0J9P30Z**	Drainage of Left Lower Leg Subcutaneous Tissue and Fascia with Drainage Device, Percutaneous Approach
0J9G3ZZ	Drainage of Right Lower Arm Subcutaneous Tissue and Fascia, Percutaneous Approach	**0J9L0ZX**	Drainage of Right Upper Leg Subcutaneous Tissue and Fascia, Open Approach, Diagnostic	**0J9P3ZX**	Drainage of Left Lower Leg Subcutaneous Tissue and Fascia, Percutaneous Approach, Diagnostic
0J9H00Z	Drainage of Left Lower Arm Subcutaneous Tissue and Fascia with Drainage Device, Open Approach	**0J9L0ZZ**	Drainage of Right Upper Leg Subcutaneous Tissue and Fascia, Open Approach	**0J9P3ZZ**	Drainage of Left Lower Leg Subcutaneous Tissue and Fascia, Percutaneous Approach
0J9H0ZX	Drainage of Left Lower Arm Subcutaneous Tissue and Fascia, Open Approach, Diagnostic	**0J9L30Z**	Drainage of Right Upper Leg Subcutaneous Tissue and Fascia with Drainage Device, Percutaneous Approach	**0J9Q00Z**	Drainage of Right Foot Subcutaneous Tissue and Fascia with Drainage Device, Open Approach
0J9H0ZZ	Drainage of Left Lower Arm Subcutaneous Tissue and Fascia, Open Approach	**0J9L3ZX**	Drainage of Right Upper Leg Subcutaneous Tissue and Fascia, Percutaneous Approach, Diagnostic	**0J9Q0ZX**	Drainage of Right Foot Subcutaneous Tissue and Fascia, Open Approach, Diagnostic
0J9H30Z	Drainage of Left Lower Arm Subcutaneous Tissue and Fascia with Drainage Device, Percutaneous Approach	**0J9L3ZZ**	Drainage of Right Upper Leg Subcutaneous Tissue and Fascia, Percutaneous Approach	**0J9Q0ZZ**	Drainage of Right Foot Subcutaneous Tissue and Fascia, Open Approach
0J9H3ZX	Drainage of Left Lower Arm Subcutaneous Tissue and Fascia, Percutaneous Approach, Diagnostic	**0J9M00Z**	Drainage of Left Upper Leg Subcutaneous Tissue and Fascia with Drainage Device, Open Approach	**0J9Q30Z**	Drainage of Right Foot Subcutaneous Tissue and Fascia with Drainage Device, Percutaneous Approach
0J9H3ZZ	Drainage of Left Lower Arm Subcutaneous Tissue and Fascia, Percutaneous Approach	**0J9M0ZX**	Drainage of Left Upper Leg Subcutaneous Tissue and Fascia, Open Approach, Diagnostic	**0J9Q3ZX**	Drainage of Right Foot Subcutaneous Tissue and Fascia, Percutaneous Approach, Diagnostic
0J9J00Z	Drainage of Right Hand Subcutaneous Tissue and Fascia with Drainage Device, Open Approach	**0J9M0ZZ**	Drainage of Left Upper Leg Subcutaneous Tissue and Fascia, Open Approach	**0J9Q3ZZ**	Drainage of Right Foot Subcutaneous Tissue and Fascia, Percutaneous Approach
0J9J0ZX	Drainage of Right Hand Subcutaneous Tissue and Fascia, Open Approach, Diagnostic	**0J9M30Z**	Drainage of Left Upper Leg Subcutaneous Tissue and Fascia with Drainage Device, Percutaneous Approach	**0J9R00Z**	Drainage of Left Foot Subcutaneous Tissue and Fascia with Drainage Device, Open Approach
0J9J0ZZ	Drainage of Right Hand Subcutaneous Tissue and Fascia, Open Approach	**0J9M3ZX**	Drainage of Left Upper Leg Subcutaneous Tissue and Fascia, Percutaneous Approach, Diagnostic	**0J9R0ZX**	Drainage of Left Foot Subcutaneous Tissue and Fascia, Open Approach, Diagnostic
0J9J30Z	Drainage of Right Hand Subcutaneous Tissue and Fascia with Drainage Device, Percutaneous Approach	**0J9M3ZZ**	Drainage of Left Upper Leg Subcutaneous Tissue and Fascia, Percutaneous Approach	**0J9R0ZZ**	Drainage of Left Foot Subcutaneous Tissue and Fascia, Open Approach
0J9J3ZX	Drainage of Right Hand Subcutaneous Tissue and Fascia, Percutaneous Approach, Diagnostic	**0J9N00Z**	Drainage of Right Lower Leg Subcutaneous Tissue and Fascia with Drainage Device, Open Approach	**0J9R30Z**	Drainage of Left Foot Subcutaneous Tissue and Fascia with Drainage Device, Percutaneous Approach
● **0J9J3ZZ**	Drainage of Right Hand Subcutaneous Tissue and Fascia, Percutaneous Approach	**0J9N0ZX**	Drainage of Right Lower Leg Subcutaneous Tissue and Fascia, Open Approach, Diagnostic	**0J9R3ZX**	Drainage of Left Foot Subcutaneous Tissue and Fascia, Percutaneous Approach, Diagnostic
		0J9N0ZZ	Drainage of Right Lower Leg Subcutaneous Tissue and Fascia, Open Approach	**0J9R3ZZ**	Drainage of Left Foot Subcutaneous Tissue and Fascia, Percutaneous Approach

0JB – Subcutaneous Tissue and Fascia, Excision

Review Coding Guidelines B3.4a and B3.4b

Review Coding Guideline B3.5

Review Coding Guideline B3.8

0JB00ZX	Excision of Scalp Subcutaneous Tissue and Fascia, Open Approach, Diagnostic	**0JB10ZZ**	Excision of Face Subcutaneous Tissue and Fascia, Open Approach	**0JB43ZX**	Excision of Anterior Neck Subcutaneous Tissue and Fascia, Percutaneous Approach, Diagnostic
0JB00ZZ	Excision of Scalp Subcutaneous Tissue and Fascia, Open Approach	**0JB13ZX**	Excision of Face Subcutaneous Tissue and Fascia, Percutaneous Approach, Diagnostic	**0JB43ZZ**	Excision of Anterior Neck Subcutaneous Tissue and Fascia, Percutaneous Approach
0JB03ZX	Excision of Scalp Subcutaneous Tissue and Fascia, Percutaneous Approach, Diagnostic	**0JB13ZZ**	Excision of Face Subcutaneous Tissue and Fascia, Percutaneous Approach	**0JB50ZX**	Excision of Posterior Neck Subcutaneous Tissue and Fascia, Open Approach, Diagnostic
0JB03ZZ	Excision of Scalp Subcutaneous Tissue and Fascia, Percutaneous Approach	**0JB40ZX**	Excision of Anterior Neck Subcutaneous Tissue and Fascia, Open Approach, Diagnostic	**0JB50ZZ**	Excision of Posterior Neck Subcutaneous Tissue and Fascia, Open Approach
0JB10ZX	Excision of Face Subcutaneous Tissue and Fascia, Open Approach, Diagnostic	**0JB40ZZ**	Excision of Anterior Neck Subcutaneous Tissue and Fascia, Open Approach		

♀ Female-only   ♂ Male-only   ▲ Limited Coverage   ● Non-OR   ▦ HAC-associated procedure   ▲ Non-covered procedures   + Combination

B53ZX	Excision of Posterior Neck Subcutaneous Tissue and Fascia, Percutaneous Approach, Diagnostic	
B53ZZ	Excision of Posterior Neck Subcutaneous Tissue and Fascia, Percutaneous Approach	
B60ZX	Excision of Chest Subcutaneous Tissue and Fascia, Open Approach, Diagnostic	
B60ZZ	Excision of Chest Subcutaneous Tissue and Fascia, Open Approach	
B63ZX	Excision of Chest Subcutaneous Tissue and Fascia, Percutaneous Approach, Diagnostic	
B63ZZ	Excision of Chest Subcutaneous Tissue and Fascia, Percutaneous Approach	
JB70ZX	Excision of Back Subcutaneous Tissue and Fascia, Open Approach, Diagnostic	
JB70ZZ	Excision of Back Subcutaneous Tissue and Fascia, Open Approach	
JB73ZX	Excision of Back Subcutaneous Tissue and Fascia, Percutaneous Approach, Diagnostic	
JB73ZZ	Excision of Back Subcutaneous Tissue and Fascia, Percutaneous Approach	
JB80ZX	Excision of Abdomen Subcutaneous Tissue and Fascia, Open Approach, Diagnostic	
JB80ZZ	Excision of Abdomen Subcutaneous Tissue and Fascia, Open Approach
	AHA CC: 3Q, 2014, 22-23; 4Q, 2014, 39-40	
JB83ZX	Excision of Abdomen Subcutaneous Tissue and Fascia, Percutaneous Approach, Diagnostic	
JB83ZZ	Excision of Abdomen Subcutaneous Tissue and Fascia, Percutaneous Approach	
JB90ZX	Excision of Buttock Subcutaneous Tissue and Fascia, Open Approach, Diagnostic	
JB90ZZ	Excision of Buttock Subcutaneous Tissue and Fascia, Open Approach	
JB93ZX	Excision of Buttock Subcutaneous Tissue and Fascia, Percutaneous Approach, Diagnostic	
JB93ZZ	Excision of Buttock Subcutaneous Tissue and Fascia, Percutaneous Approach	
JBB0ZX	Excision of Perineum Subcutaneous Tissue and Fascia, Open Approach, Diagnostic	
JBB0ZZ	Excision of Perineum Subcutaneous Tissue and Fascia, Open Approach
	AHA CC: 1Q, 2015, 29-30	
JBB3ZX	Excision of Perineum Subcutaneous Tissue and Fascia, Percutaneous Approach, Diagnostic	
0JBB3ZZ	Excision of Perineum Subcutaneous Tissue and Fascia, Percutaneous Approach	
0JBC0ZX	Excision of Pelvic Region Subcutaneous Tissue and Fascia, Open Approach, Diagnostic	
0JBC0ZZ	Excision of Pelvic Region Subcutaneous Tissue and Fascia, Open Approach	
0JBC3ZX	Excision of Pelvic Region Subcutaneous Tissue and Fascia, Percutaneous Approach, Diagnostic	
0JBC3ZZ	Excision of Pelvic Region Subcutaneous Tissue and Fascia, Percutaneous Approach	
0JBD0ZX	Excision of Right Upper Arm Subcutaneous Tissue and Fascia, Open Approach, Diagnostic	

0JBD0ZZ	Excision of Right Upper Arm Subcutaneous Tissue and Fascia, Open Approach
0JBD3ZX	Excision of Right Upper Arm Subcutaneous Tissue and Fascia, Percutaneous Approach, Diagnostic
0JBD3ZZ	Excision of Right Upper Arm Subcutaneous Tissue and Fascia, Percutaneous Approach
0JBF0ZX	Excision of Left Upper Arm Subcutaneous Tissue and Fascia, Open Approach, Diagnostic
0JBF0ZZ	Excision of Left Upper Arm Subcutaneous Tissue and Fascia, Open Approach
0JBF3ZX	Excision of Left Upper Arm Subcutaneous Tissue and Fascia, Percutaneous Approach, Diagnostic
0JBF3ZZ	Excision of Left Upper Arm Subcutaneous Tissue and Fascia, Percutaneous Approach
0JBG0ZX	Excision of Right Lower Arm Subcutaneous Tissue and Fascia, Open Approach, Diagnostic
0JBG0ZZ	Excision of Right Lower Arm Subcutaneous Tissue and Fascia, Open Approach
0JBG3ZX	Excision of Right Lower Arm Subcutaneous Tissue and Fascia, Percutaneous Approach, Diagnostic
0JBG3ZZ	Excision of Right Lower Arm Subcutaneous Tissue and Fascia, Percutaneous Approach
0JBH0ZX	Excision of Left Lower Arm Subcutaneous Tissue and Fascia, Open Approach, Diagnostic
0JBH0ZZ	Excision of Left Lower Arm Subcutaneous Tissue and Fascia, Open Approach
0JBH3ZX	Excision of Left Lower Arm Subcutaneous Tissue and Fascia, Percutaneous Approach, Diagnostic
0JBH3ZZ	Excision of Left Lower Arm Subcutaneous Tissue and Fascia, Percutaneous Approach
0JBJ0ZX	Excision of Right Hand Subcutaneous Tissue and Fascia, Open Approach, Diagnostic
0JBJ0ZZ	Excision of Right Hand Subcutaneous Tissue and Fascia, Open Approach
0JBJ3ZX	Excision of Right Hand Subcutaneous Tissue and Fascia, Percutaneous Approach, Diagnostic
0JBJ3ZZ	Excision of Right Hand Subcutaneous Tissue and Fascia, Percutaneous Approach
0JBK0ZX	Excision of Left Hand Subcutaneous Tissue and Fascia, Open Approach, Diagnostic
0JBK0ZZ	Excision of Left Hand Subcutaneous Tissue and Fascia, Open Approach
0JBK3ZX	Excision of Left Hand Subcutaneous Tissue and Fascia, Percutaneous Approach, Diagnostic
0JBK3ZZ	Excision of Left Hand Subcutaneous Tissue and Fascia, Percutaneous Approach
0JBL0ZX	Excision of Right Upper Leg Subcutaneous Tissue and Fascia, Open Approach, Diagnostic

0JBL0ZZ	Excision of Right Upper Leg Subcutaneous Tissue and Fascia, Open Approach
0JBL3ZX	Excision of Right Upper Leg Subcutaneous Tissue and Fascia, Percutaneous Approach, Diagnostic
0JBL3ZZ	Excision of Right Upper Leg Subcutaneous Tissue and Fascia, Percutaneous Approach
0JBM0ZX	Excision of Left Upper Leg Subcutaneous Tissue and Fascia, Open Approach, Diagnostic
0JBM0ZZ	Excision of Left Upper Leg Subcutaneous Tissue and Fascia, Open Approach
0JBM3ZX	Excision of Left Upper Leg Subcutaneous Tissue and Fascia, Percutaneous Approach, Diagnostic
0JBM3ZZ	Excision of Left Upper Leg Subcutaneous Tissue and Fascia, Percutaneous Approach
0JBN0ZX	Excision of Right Lower Leg Subcutaneous Tissue and Fascia, Open Approach, Diagnostic
0JBN0ZZ	Excision of Right Lower Leg Subcutaneous Tissue and Fascia, Open Approach
0JBN3ZX	Excision of Right Lower Leg Subcutaneous Tissue and Fascia, Percutaneous Approach, Diagnostic
0JBN3ZZ	Excision of Right Lower Leg Subcutaneous Tissue and Fascia, Percutaneous Approach
0JBP0ZX	Excision of Left Lower Leg Subcutaneous Tissue and Fascia, Open Approach, Diagnostic
0JBP0ZZ	Excision of Left Lower Leg Subcutaneous Tissue and Fascia, Open Approach
0JBP3ZX	Excision of Left Lower Leg Subcutaneous Tissue and Fascia, Percutaneous Approach, Diagnostic
0JBP3ZZ	Excision of Left Lower Leg Subcutaneous Tissue and Fascia, Percutaneous Approach
0JBQ0ZX	Excision of Right Foot Subcutaneous Tissue and Fascia, Open Approach, Diagnostic
0JBQ0ZZ	Excision of Right Foot Subcutaneous Tissue and Fascia, Open Approach
0JBQ3ZX	Excision of Right Foot Subcutaneous Tissue and Fascia, Percutaneous Approach, Diagnostic
0JBQ3ZZ	Excision of Right Foot Subcutaneous Tissue and Fascia, Percutaneous Approach
0JBR0ZX	Excision of Left Foot Subcutaneous Tissue and Fascia, Open Approach, Diagnostic
0JBR0ZZ	Excision of Left Foot Subcutaneous Tissue and Fascia, Open Approach
0JBR3ZX	Excision of Left Foot Subcutaneous Tissue and Fascia, Percutaneous Approach, Diagnostic
0JBR3ZZ	Excision of Left Foot Subcutaneous Tissue and Fascia, Percutaneous Approach

0JC – Subcutaneous Tissue and Fascia, Extirpation

0JC00ZZ	Extirpation of Matter from Scalp Subcutaneous Tissue and Fascia, Open Approach	
0JC03ZZ	Extirpation of Matter from Scalp Subcutaneous Tissue and Fascia, Percutaneous Approach	
0JC10ZZ	Extirpation of Matter from Face Subcutaneous Tissue and Fascia, Open Approach	
0JC13ZZ	Extirpation of Matter from Face Subcutaneous Tissue and Fascia, Percutaneous Approach	
0JC40ZZ	Extirpation of Matter from Anterior Neck Subcutaneous Tissue and Fascia, Open Approach	
0JC43ZZ	Extirpation of Matter from Anterior Neck Subcutaneous Tissue and Fascia, Percutaneous Approach	
0JC50ZZ	Extirpation of Matter from Posterior Neck Subcutaneous Tissue and Fascia, Open Approach	
0JC53ZZ	Extirpation of Matter from Posterior Neck Subcutaneous Tissue and Fascia, Percutaneous Approach	
0JC60ZZ	Extirpation of Matter from Chest Subcutaneous Tissue and Fascia, Open Approach	

♀ Female-only   ♂ Male-only   ▲ Limited Coverage   ● Non-OR   ▥ HAC-associated procedure   ▲ Non-covered procedures   ✚ Combination

0JC63ZZ Extirpation of Matter from Chest Subcutaneous Tissue and Fascia, Percutaneous Approach

0JC70ZZ Extirpation of Matter from Back Subcutaneous Tissue and Fascia, Open Approach

0JC73ZZ Extirpation of Matter from Back Subcutaneous Tissue and Fascia, Percutaneous Approach

0JC80ZZ Extirpation of Matter from Abdomen Subcutaneous Tissue and Fascia, Open Approach

0JC83ZZ Extirpation of Matter from Abdomen Subcutaneous Tissue and Fascia, Percutaneous Approach

0JC90ZZ Extirpation of Matter from Buttock Subcutaneous Tissue and Fascia, Open Approach

0JC93ZZ Extirpation of Matter from Buttock Subcutaneous Tissue and Fascia, Percutaneous Approach

0JCB0ZZ Extirpation of Matter from Perineum Subcutaneous Tissue and Fascia, Open Approach

0JCB3ZZ Extirpation of Matter from Perineum Subcutaneous Tissue and Fascia, Percutaneous Approach

0JCC0ZZ Extirpation of Matter from Pelvic Region Subcutaneous Tissue and Fascia, Open Approach

0JCC3ZZ Extirpation of Matter from Pelvic Region Subcutaneous Tissue and Fascia, Percutaneous Approach

0JCD0ZZ Extirpation of Matter from Right Upper Arm Subcutaneous Tissue and Fascia, Open Approach

0JCD3ZZ Extirpation of Matter from Right Upper Arm Subcutaneous Tissue and Fascia, Percutaneous Approach

0JCF0ZZ Extirpation of Matter from Left Upper Arm Subcutaneous Tissue and Fascia, Open Approach

0JCF3ZZ Extirpation of Matter from Left Upper Arm Subcutaneous Tissue and Fascia, Percutaneous Approach

0JCG0ZZ Extirpation of Matter from Right Lower Arm Subcutaneous Tissue and Fascia, Open Approach

0JCG3ZZ Extirpation of Matter from Right Lower Arm Subcutaneous Tissue and Fascia, Percutaneous Approach

0JCH0ZZ Extirpation of Matter from Left Lower Arm Subcutaneous Tissue and Fascia, Open Approach

0JCH3ZZ Extirpation of Matter from Left Lower Arm Subcutaneous Tissue and Fascia, Percutaneous Approach

0JCJ0ZZ Extirpation of Matter from Right Hand Subcutaneous Tissue and Fascia, Open Approach

0JCJ3ZZ Extirpation of Matter from Right Hand Subcutaneous Tissue and Fascia, Percutaneous Approach

0JCK0ZZ Extirpation of Matter from Left Hand Subcutaneous Tissue and Fascia, Open Approach

0JCK3ZZ Extirpation of Matter from Left Hand Subcutaneous Tissue and Fascia, Percutaneous Approach

0JCL0ZZ Extirpation of Matter from Right Upper Leg Subcutaneous Tissue and Fascia, Open Approach

0JCL3ZZ Extirpation of Matter from Right Upper Leg Subcutaneous Tissue and Fascia, Percutaneous Approach

0JCM0ZZ Extirpation of Matter from Left Upper Leg Subcutaneous Tissue and Fascia, Open Approach

0JCM3ZZ Extirpation of Matter from Left Upper Leg Subcutaneous Tissue and Fascia, Percutaneous Approach

0JCN0ZZ Extirpation of Matter from Right Lower Leg Subcutaneous Tissue and Fascia, Open Approach

0JCN3ZZ Extirpation of Matter from Right Lower Leg Subcutaneous Tissue and Fascia, Percutaneous Approach

0JCP0ZZ Extirpation of Matter from Left Lower Leg Subcutaneous Tissue and Fascia, Open Approach

0JCP3ZZ Extirpation of Matter from Left Lower Leg Subcutaneous Tissue and Fascia, Percutaneous Approach

0JCQ0ZZ Extirpation of Matter from Right Foot Subcutaneous Tissue and Fascia, Open Approach

0JCQ3ZZ Extirpation of Matter from Right Foot Subcutaneous Tissue and Fascia, Percutaneous Approach

0JCR0ZZ Extirpation of Matter from Left Foot Subcutaneous Tissue and Fascia, Open Approach

0JCR3ZZ Extirpation of Matter from Left Foot Subcutaneous Tissue and Fascia, Percutaneous Approach

0JD – Subcutaneous Tissue and Fascia, Extraction

0JD00ZZ Extraction of Scalp Subcutaneous Tissue and Fascia, Open Approach

0JD03ZZ Extraction of Scalp Subcutaneous Tissue and Fascia, Percutaneous Approach

0JD10ZZ Extraction of Face Subcutaneous Tissue and Fascia, Open Approach

0JD13ZZ Extraction of Face Subcutaneous Tissue and Fascia, Percutaneous Approach

0JD40ZZ Extraction of Anterior Neck Subcutaneous Tissue and Fascia, Open Approach

0JD43ZZ Extraction of Anterior Neck Subcutaneous Tissue and Fascia, Percutaneous Approach

0JD50ZZ Extraction of Posterior Neck Subcutaneous Tissue and Fascia, Open Approach

0JD53ZZ Extraction of Posterior Neck Subcutaneous Tissue and Fascia, Percutaneous Approach

0JD60ZZ Extraction of Chest Subcutaneous Tissue and Fascia, Open Approach

0JD63ZZ Extraction of Chest Subcutaneous Tissue and Fascia, Percutaneous Approach

0JD70ZZ Extraction of Back Subcutaneous Tissue and Fascia, Open Approach

0JD73ZZ Extraction of Back Subcutaneous Tissue and Fascia, Percutaneous Approach

0JD80ZZ Extraction of Abdomen Subcutaneous Tissue and Fascia, Open Approach

0JD83ZZ Extraction of Abdomen Subcutaneous Tissue and Fascia, Percutaneous Approach

0JD90ZZ Extraction of Buttock Subcutaneous Tissue and Fascia, Open Approach

0JD93ZZ Extraction of Buttock Subcutaneous Tissue and Fascia, Percutaneous Approach

0JDB0ZZ Extraction of Perineum Subcutaneous Tissue and Fascia, Open Approach

0JDB3ZZ Extraction of Perineum Subcutaneous Tissue and Fascia, Percutaneous Approach

0JDC0ZZ Extraction of Pelvic Region Subcutaneous Tissue and Fascia, Open Approach

AHA CC: 1Q, 2015, 23

0JDC3ZZ Extraction of Pelvic Region Subcutaneous Tissue and Fascia, Percutaneous Approach

0JDD0ZZ Extraction of Right Upper Arm Subcutaneous Tissue and Fascia, Open Approach

0JDD3ZZ Extraction of Right Upper Arm Subcutaneous Tissue and Fascia, Percutaneous Approach

0JDF0ZZ Extraction of Left Upper Arm Subcutaneous Tissue and Fascia, Open Approach

0JDF3ZZ Extraction of Left Upper Arm Subcutaneous Tissue and Fascia, Percutaneous Approach

0JDG0ZZ Extraction of Right Lower Arm Subcutaneous Tissue and Fascia, Open Approach

0JDG3ZZ Extraction of Right Lower Arm Subcutaneous Tissue and Fascia, Percutaneous Approach

0JDH0ZZ Extraction of Left Lower Arm Subcutaneous Tissue and Fascia, Open Approach

0JDH3ZZ Extraction of Left Lower Arm Subcutaneous Tissue and Fascia, Percutaneous Approach

0JDJ0ZZ Extraction of Right Hand Subcutaneous Tissue and Fascia, Open Approach

0JDJ3ZZ Extraction of Right Hand Subcutaneous Tissue and Fascia, Percutaneous Approach

0JDK0ZZ Extraction of Left Hand Subcutaneous Tissue and Fascia, Open Approach

0JDK3ZZ Extraction of Left Hand Subcutaneous Tissue and Fascia, Percutaneous Approach

0JDL0ZZ Extraction of Right Upper Leg Subcutaneous Tissue and Fascia, Open Approach

0JDL3ZZ Extraction of Right Upper Leg Subcutaneous Tissue and Fascia, Percutaneous Approach

0JDM0ZZ Extraction of Left Upper Leg Subcutaneous Tissue and Fascia, Open Approach

0JDM3ZZ Extraction of Left Upper Leg Subcutaneous Tissue and Fascia, Percutaneous Approach

0JDN0ZZ Extraction of Right Lower Leg Subcutaneous Tissue and Fascia, Open Approach

0JDN3ZZ Extraction of Right Lower Leg Subcutaneous Tissue and Fascia, Percutaneous Approach

0JDP0ZZ Extraction of Left Lower Leg Subcutaneous Tissue and Fascia, Open Approach

0JDP3ZZ Extraction of Left Lower Leg Subcutaneous Tissue and Fascia, Percutaneous Approach

0JDQ0ZZ Extraction of Right Foot Subcutaneous Tissue and Fascia, Open Approach

0JDQ3ZZ Extraction of Right Foot Subcutaneous Tissue and Fascia, Percutaneous Approach

0JDR0ZZ Extraction of Left Foot Subcutaneous Tissue and Fascia, Open Approach

0JDR3ZZ Extraction of Left Foot Subcutaneous Tissue and Fascia, Percutaneous Approach

H00NZ Insertion of Tissue Expander into Scalp Subcutaneous Tissue and Fascia, Open Approach

H03NZ Insertion of Tissue Expander into Scalp Subcutaneous Tissue and Fascia, Percutaneous Approach

H10NZ Insertion of Tissue Expander into Face Subcutaneous Tissue and Fascia, Open Approach

H13NZ Insertion of Tissue Expander into Face Subcutaneous Tissue and Fascia, Percutaneous Approach

H40NZ Insertion of Tissue Expander into Anterior Neck Subcutaneous Tissue and Fascia, Open Approach

H43NZ Insertion of Tissue Expander into Anterior Neck Subcutaneous Tissue and Fascia, Percutaneous Approach

H50NZ Insertion of Tissue Expander into Posterior Neck Subcutaneous Tissue and Fascia, Open Approach

H53NZ Insertion of Tissue Expander into Posterior Neck Subcutaneous Tissue and Fascia, Percutaneous Approach

H600Z Insertion of Hemodynamic Monitoring Device into Chest Subcutaneous Tissue and Fascia, Open Approach

0JH602Z Insertion of Monitoring Device into Chest Subcutaneous Tissue and Fascia, Open Approach

0JH604Z Insertion of Pacemaker, Single Chamber into Chest Subcutaneous Tissue and Fascia, Open Approach

⊞ With a secondary diagnosis code of K68.11, T81.4XXA, T82.6XXA, T82.7XXA

➕ Pacemaker device when reported with an Insertion of a cardiac lead (6th character J or M) into the coronary vein, atrium, ventricle or pericardium (4th characters 4, 6, 7, K, L and N). *See table 02H to construct the Insertion code.* When a device is replaced, also report the Removal of the cardiac rhythm device (6th character P) from the trunk subcutaneous tissue and fascia. *See table 0JP to construct the Removal code.* When a cardiac lead is replaced, also report the Removal of the cardiac lead (6th character M) from the heart. *See table 02P to construct the Removal code.*

0JH605Z Insertion of Pacemaker, Single Chamber Rate Responsive into Chest Subcutaneous Tissue and Fascia, Open Approach

⊞ With a secondary diagnosis code of K68.11, T81.4XXA, T82.6XXA, T82.7XXA

➕ Pacemaker device when reported with an Insertion of a cardiac lead (6th character J or M) into the coronary vein, atrium, ventricle or pericardium (4th characters 4, 6, 7, K, L and N). *See table 02H to construct the Insertion code.* When a device is replaced, also report the Removal of the cardiac rhythm device (6th character P) from the trunk subcutaneous tissue and fascia. *See table 0JP to construct the Removal code.* When a cardiac lead is replaced, also report the Removal of the cardiac lead (6th character M) from the heart. *See table 02P to construct the Removal code.*

0JH606Z Insertion of Pacemaker, Dual Chamber into Chest Subcutaneous Tissue and Fascia, Open Approach

⊞ With a secondary diagnosis code of K68.11, T81.4XXA, T82.6XXA, T82.7XXA

Pacemaker device when reported with an Insertion of a cardiac lead (6th character J or M) into the coronary vein, atrium, ventricle or pericardium (4th characters 4, 6, 7, K, L and N). *See table 02H to construct the Insertion code.* When a device is replaced, also report the Removal of the cardiac rhythm device (6th character P) from the trunk subcutaneous tissue and fascia. *See table 0JP to construct the Removal code.* When a cardiac lead is replaced, also report the Removal of the cardiac lead (6th character M) from the heart. *See table 02P to construct the Removal code.*

0JH607Z Insertion of Cardiac Resynchronization Pacemaker Pulse Generator into Chest Subcutaneous Tissue and Fascia, Open Approach

⊞ With a secondary diagnosis code of K68.11, T81.4XXA, T82.6XXA, T82.7XXA

➕ Pacemaker device when reported with an Insertion of a cardiac lead (6th character J or M) into the coronary vein, atrium, ventricle or pericardium (4th characters 4, 6, 7, K, L and N). *See table 02H to construct the Insertion code.* When a cardiac lead is replaced, also report the Removal of the cardiac lead (6th character M) from the heart. *See table 02P to construct the Removal code.*

0JH608Z Insertion of Defibrillator Generator into Chest Subcutaneous Tissue and Fascia, Open Approach

AHA CC: 4Q, 2012, 104-106

⊞ With a secondary diagnosis code of K68.11, T81.4XXA, T82.6XXA, T82.7XXA

➕ Cardioverter-Defibrillator lead(s)/ generator when reported with Insertion of a defibrillator cardiac lead (6th character K) into the coronary vein, atrium, or ventricle. Also applicable with Insertion of pacemaker cardiac lead, defibrillator cardiac lead or cardiac lead (6th characters J, K, M) into the pericardium. *See table 02H to construct the Insertion code.*

0JH609Z Insertion of Cardiac Resynchronization Defibrillator Pulse Generator into Chest Subcutaneous Tissue and Fascia, Open Approach

⊞ With a secondary diagnosis code of K68.11, T81.4XXA, T82.6XXA, T82.7XXA

➕ Cardioverter-Defibrillator lead(s)/ generator when reported with Insertion of a defibrillator cardiac lead (6th character K) into the atrium, or ventricle. Also applicable with Insertion of pacemaker cardiac lead, defibrillator cardiac lead or cardiac lead (6th characters J, K, M) into the coronary vein or pericardium. *See table 02H to construct the Insertion code.*

0JH60AZ Insertion of Contractility Modulation Device into Chest Subcutaneous Tissue and Fascia, Open Approach

➕ Cardioverter-Defibrillator lead(s)/ generator when reported with Insertion of a cardiac lead (6th character M) into the left ventricle. *See table 02H to construct the Insertion code.*

0JH60BZ Insertion of Single Array Stimulator Generator into Chest Subcutaneous Tissue and Fascia, Open Approach

➕ Neurotransmitter/Neurostimulator when reported with an Insertion of a neurostimulator lead (6th character M) into the cranial nerve, spinal canal or spinal cord. *See table 00H to construct the Insertion code.* Also applicable when reported with Insertion of neurostimulator lead (6th character M) into the peripheral nerve. *See table 01H to construct the Insertion code.* Also applicable when reported with Insertion of a stimulator lead (6th character M) into the stomach. *See table 0DH to construct the Insertion code.*

0JH60CZ Insertion of Single Array Rechargeable Stimulator Generator into Chest Subcutaneous Tissue and Fascia, Open Approach

➕ Neurotransmitter/Neurostimulator when reported with an Insertion of a neurostimulator lead (6th character M) into the cranial nerve, spinal canal or spinal cord. *See table 00H to construct the Insertion code.* Also applicable when reported with Insertion of neurostimulator lead (6th character M) into the peripheral nerve. *See table 01H to construct the Insertion code.* Also applicable when reported with Insertion of a stimulator lead (6th character M) into the stomach. *See table 0DH to construct the Insertion code.*

0JH60DZ Insertion of Multiple Array Stimulator Generator into Chest Subcutaneous Tissue and Fascia, Open Approach

➕ Major brain device implant when reported with an Insertion of a neurostimulator lead (6th character M) into the brain or cerebral ventricle. *See table 00H to construct the Insertion code.*

➕ Neurotransmitter/Neurostimulator when reported with an Insertion of a neurostimulator lead (6th character M) into the cranial nerve, spinal canal or spinal cord. *See table 00H to construct the Insertion code.* Also applicable when reported with Insertion of neurostimulator lead (6th character M) into the peripheral nerve. *See table 01H to construct the Insertion code.* Also applicable when reported with Insertion of a stimulator lead (6th character M) into the stomach. *See table 0DH to construct the Insertion code.*

0JH60EZ Insertion of Multiple Array Rechargeable Stimulator Generator into Chest Subcutaneous Tissue and Fascia, Open Approach

➕ Major brain device implant when reported with an Insertion of a neurostimulator lead (6th character M) into the brain or cerebral ventricle. *See table 00H to construct the Insertion code.*

➕ Neurotransmitter/Neurostimulator when reported with an Insertion of a neurostimulator lead (6th character M) into the cranial nerve, spinal canal or spinal cord. *See table 00H to construct the Insertion code.* Also applicable when reported with Insertion of neurostimulator lead (6th character M) into the peripheral nerve. *See table 01H to construct the Insertion code.* Also applicable when reported with Insertion of a stimulator lead (6th character M) into the stomach. *See table 0DH to construct the Insertion code.*

● **0JH60HZ** Insertion of Contraceptive Device into Chest Subcutaneous Tissue and Fascia, Open Approach

0JH60MZ Insertion of Stimulator Generator into Chest Subcutaneous Tissue and Fascia, Open Approach

0JH60NZ Insertion of Tissue Expander into Chest Subcutaneous Tissue and Fascia, Open Approach

0JH60PZ Insertion of Cardiac Rhythm Related Device into Chest Subcutaneous Tissue and Fascia, Open Approach

AHA CC: 4Q, 2012, 104-106

[HAC] With a secondary diagnosis code of K68.11, T81.4XXA, T82.6XXA, T82.7XXA

[+] Pacemaker device when reported with an Insertion of a cardiac lead (6th character J or M) into the coronary vein, atrium, ventricle or pericardium (4th characters 4, 6, 7, K, L and N). *See table 02H to construct the Insertion code.* When a cardiac lead is replaced, also report the Removal of the cardiac lead (6th character M) from the heart. *See table 02P to construct the Removal code.*

0JH60VZ Insertion of Infusion Pump into Chest Subcutaneous Tissue and Fascia, Open Approach

● **0JH60WZ** Insertion of Reservoir into Chest Subcutaneous Tissue and Fascia, Open Approach

● **0JH60XZ** Insertion of Vascular Access Device into Chest Subcutaneous Tissue and Fascia, Open Approach

0JH630Z Insertion of Hemodynamic Monitoring Device into Chest Subcutaneous Tissue and Fascia, Percutaneous Approach

● **0JH632Z** Insertion of Monitoring Device into Chest Subcutaneous Tissue and Fascia, Percutaneous Approach

● **0JH634Z** Insertion of Pacemaker, Single Chamber into Chest Subcutaneous Tissue and Fascia, Percutaneous Approach

[HAC] With a secondary diagnosis code of K68.11, T81.4XXA, T82.6XXA, T82.7XXA

[+] Pacemaker device when reported with an Insertion of a cardiac lead (6th character J or M) into the coronary vein, atrium, ventricle or pericardium (4th characters 4, 6, 7, K, L and N). *See table 02H to construct the Insertion code.* When a device is replaced, also report the Removal of the cardiac rhythm device (6th character P) from the trunk subcutaneous tissue and fascia. *See table 0JP to construct the Removal code.* When a cardiac lead is replaced, also report the Removal of the cardiac lead (6th character M) from the heart. *See table 02P to construct the Removal code.*

● **0JH635Z** Insertion of Pacemaker, Single Chamber Rate Responsive into Chest Subcutaneous Tissue and Fascia, Percutaneous Approach

[HAC] With a secondary diagnosis code of K68.11, T81.4XXA, T82.6XXA, T82.7XXA

[+] Pacemaker device when reported with an Insertion of a cardiac lead (6th character J or M) into the coronary vein, atrium, ventricle or pericardium (4th characters 4, 6, 7, K, L and N). *See table 02H to construct the Insertion code.* When a device is replaced, also report the Removal of the cardiac rhythm device (6th character P) from the trunk subcutaneous tissue and fascia. *See table 0JP to construct the Removal code.* When a cardiac lead is replaced, also report the Removal of the cardiac lead (6th character M) from the heart. *See table 02P to construct the Removal code.*

● **0JH636Z** Insertion of Pacemaker, Dual Chamber into Chest Subcutaneous Tissue and Fascia, Percutaneous Approach

[HAC] With a secondary diagnosis code of K68.11, T81.4XXA, T82.6XXA, T82.7XXA

[+] Pacemaker device when reported with an Insertion of a cardiac lead (6th character J or M) into the coronary vein, atrium, ventricle or pericardium (4th characters 4, 6, 7, K, L and N). *See table 02H to construct the Insertion code.* When a device is replaced, also report the Removal of the cardiac rhythm device (6th character P) from the trunk subcutaneous tissue and fascia. *See table 0JP to construct the Removal code.* When a cardiac lead is replaced, also report the Removal of the cardiac lead (6th character M) from the heart. *See table 02P to construct the Removal code.*

0JH637Z Insertion of Cardiac Resynchronization Pacemaker Pulse Generator into Chest Subcutaneous Tissue and Fascia, Percutaneous Approach

[HAC] With a secondary diagnosis code of K68.11, T81.4XXA, T82.6XXA, T82.7XXA

[+] Pacemaker device when reported with an Insertion of a cardiac lead (6th character J or M) into the coronary vein, atrium, ventricle or pericardium (4th characters 4, 6, 7, K, L and N). *See table 02H to construct the Insertion code.* When a cardiac lead is replaced, also report the Removal of the cardiac lead (6th character M) from the heart. *See table 02P to construct the Removal code.*

0JH638Z Insertion of Defibrillator Generator into Chest Subcutaneous Tissue and Fascia, Percutaneous Approach

[HAC] With a secondary diagnosis code of K68.11, T81.4XXA, T82.6XXA, T82.7XXA

[+] Cardioverter-Defibrillator lead(s)/ generator when reported with Insertion of a defibrillator cardiac lead (6th character K) into the coronary vein, atrium, or ventricle. Also applicable with Insertion of pacemaker cardiac lead, defibrillator cardiac lead or cardiac lead (6th characters J, K, M) into the pericardium. *See table 02H to construct the Insertion code.*

0JH639Z Insertion of Cardiac Resynchronization Defibrillator Pulse Generator into Chest Subcutaneous Tissue and Fascia, Percutaneous Approach

[HAC] With a secondary diagnosis code of K68.11, T81.4XXA, T82.6XXA, T82.7XXA

[+] Cardioverter-Defibrillator lead(s)/ generator when reported with Insertion of a defibrillator cardiac lead (6th character K) into the atrium, or ventricle. Also applicable with Insertion of pacemaker cardiac lead, defibrillator cardiac lead or cardiac lead (6th characters J, K, M) into the coronary vein or pericardium. *See table 02H to construct the Insertion code.*

0JH63AZ Insertion of Contractility Modulation Device into Chest Subcutaneous Tissue and Fascia, Percutaneous Approach

[+] Cardioverter-Defibrillator lead(s)/ generator when reported with Insertion of a cardiac lead (6th character M) into the

left ventricle. *See table 02H to construct the Insertion code.*

0JH63BZ Insertion of Single Array Stimulator Generator into Chest Subcutaneous Tiss and Fascia, Percutaneous Approach

[+] Neurotransmitter/Neurostimulator when reported with an Insertion of a neurostimulator lead (6th character M) into the cranial nerve, spinal canal or spinal cord. *See table 00H to construct the Insertion code.* Also applicable when reported with Insertion of neurostimulato lead (6th character M) into the periphera nerve. *See table 01H to construct the Insertion code.* Also applicable when reported with Insertion of a stimulator le (6th character M) into the stomach. *See table 0DH to construct the Insertion cod*

0JH63CZ Insertion of Single Array Rechargeable Stimulator Generator into Chest Subcutaneous Tissue and Fascia, Percutaneous Approach

[+] Neurotransmitter/Neurostimulator when reported with an Insertion of a neurostimulator lead (6th character M) into the cranial nerve, spinal canal or spinal cord. *See table 00H to construct the Insertion code.* Also applicable when reported with Insertion of neurostimulato lead (6th character M) into the peripheral nerve. *See table 01H to construct the Insertion code.* Also applicable when reported with Insertion of a stimulator lea (6th character M) into the stomach. *See table 0DH to construct the Insertion code*

0JH63DZ Insertion of Multiple Array Stimulator Generator into Chest Subcutaneous Tissu and Fascia, Percutaneous Approach

[+] Major brain device implant when reporte with an Insertion of a neurostimulator lea (6th character M) into the brain or cerebr ventricle. *See table 00H to construct the Insertion code.*

[+] Neurotransmitter/Neurostimulator when reported with an Insertion of a neurostimulator lead (6th character M) into the cranial nerve, spinal canal or spinal cord. *See table 00H to construct the Insertion code.* Also applicable when reported with Insertion of neurostimulator lead (6th character M) into the peripheral nerve. *See table 01H to construct the Insertion code.* Also applicable when reported with Insertion of a stimulator lea (6th character M) into the stomach. *See table 0DH to construct the Insertion code.*

0JH63EZ Insertion of Multiple Array Rechargeable Stimulator Generator into Chest Subcutaneous Tissue and Fascia, Percutaneous Approach

[+] Major brain device implant when reported with an Insertion of a neurostimulator lead (6th character M) into the brain or cerebral ventricle. *See table 00H to construct the Insertion code.*

[+] Neurotransmitter/Neurostimulator when reported with an Insertion of a neurostimulator lead (6th character M) into the cranial nerve, spinal canal or spinal cord. *See table 00H to construct the Insertion code.* Also applicable when reported with Insertion of neurostimulator lead (6th character M) into the peripheral nerve. *See table 01H to construct the Insertion code.* Also applicable when reported with Insertion of a stimulator lead (6th character M) into the stomach. *See table 0DH to construct the Insertion code.*

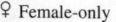

♀ Female-only ♂ Male-only ▲ Limited Coverage ● Non-OR [HAC] HAC-associated procedure ▲ Non-covered procedures [+] Combination

0JH63HZ Insertion of Contraceptive Device into Chest Subcutaneous Tissue and Fascia, Percutaneous Approach

0JH63MZ Insertion of Stimulator Generator into Chest Subcutaneous Tissue and Fascia, Percutaneous Approach

0JH63NZ Insertion of Tissue Expander into Chest Subcutaneous Tissue and Fascia, Percutaneous Approach

0JH63PZ Insertion of Cardiac Rhythm Related Device into Chest Subcutaneous Tissue and Fascia, Percutaneous Approach

◾ With a secondary diagnosis code of K68.11, T81.4XXA, T82.6XXA, T82.7XXA

⊞ Pacemaker device when reported with an Insertion of a cardiac lead (6th character J or M) into the coronary vein, atrium, ventricle or pericardium (4th characters 4, 6, 7, K, L and N). *See table 02H to construct the Insertion code.* When a cardiac lead is replaced, also report the Removal of the cardiac lead (6th character M) from the heart. *See table 02P to construct the Removal code.*

0JH63VZ Insertion of Infusion Pump into Chest Subcutaneous Tissue and Fascia, Percutaneous Approach

0JH63WZ Insertion of Reservoir into Chest Subcutaneous Tissue and Fascia, Percutaneous Approach

0JH63XZ Insertion of Vascular Access Device into Chest Subcutaneous Tissue and Fascia, Percutaneous Approach

AHA CC: 4Q, 2013, 116-117

◾ With secondary diagnosis code J95.811

0JH70BZ Insertion of Single Array Stimulator Generator into Back Subcutaneous Tissue and Fascia, Open Approach

⊞ Neurotransmitter/Neurostimulator when reported with an Insertion of a neurostimulator lead (6th character M) into the cranial nerve, spinal canal or spinal cord. *See table 00H to construct the Insertion code.* Also applicable when reported with Insertion of neurostimulator lead (6th character M) into the peripheral nerve. *See table 01H to construct the Insertion code.* Also applicable when reported with Insertion of a stimulator lead (6th character M) into the stomach. *See table 0DH to construct the Insertion code.*

0JH70CZ Insertion of Single Array Rechargeable Stimulator Generator into Back Subcutaneous Tissue and Fascia, Open Approach

⊞ Neurotransmitter/Neurostimulator when reported with an Insertion of a neurostimulator lead (6th character M) into the cranial nerve, spinal canal or spinal cord. *See table 00H to construct the Insertion code.* Also applicable when reported with Insertion of neurostimulator lead (6th character M) into the peripheral nerve. *See table 01H to construct the Insertion code.* Also applicable when reported with Insertion of a stimulator lead (6th character M) into the stomach. *See table 0DH to construct the Insertion code.*

0JH70DZ Insertion of Multiple Array Stimulator Generator into Back Subcutaneous Tissue and Fascia, Open Approach

⊞ Major brain device implant when reported with an Insertion of a neurostimulator lead (6th character M) into the brain or cerebral ventricle. *See table 00H to construct the Insertion code.*

⊞ Neurotransmitter/Neurostimulator when reported with an Insertion of a neurostimulator lead (6th character M) into the cranial nerve, spinal canal or spinal cord. *See table 00H to construct the Insertion code.* Also applicable when reported with Insertion of neurostimulator lead (6th character M) into the peripheral nerve. *See table 01H to construct the Insertion code.* Also applicable when reported with Insertion of a stimulator lead (6th character M) into the stomach. *See table 0DH to construct the Insertion code.*

0JH70EZ Insertion of Multiple Array Rechargeable Stimulator Generator into Back Subcutaneous Tissue and Fascia, Open Approach

⊞ Major brain device implant when reported with an Insertion of a neurostimulator lead (6th character M) into the brain or cerebral ventricle. *See table 00H to construct the Insertion code.*

⊞ Neurotransmitter/Neurostimulator when reported with an Insertion of a neurostimulator lead (6th character M) into the cranial nerve, spinal canal or spinal cord. *See table 00H to construct the Insertion code.* Also applicable when reported with Insertion of neurostimulator lead (6th character M) into the peripheral nerve. *See table 01H to construct the Insertion code.* Also applicable when reported with Insertion of a stimulator lead (6th character M) into the stomach. *See table 0DH to construct the Insertion code.*

▲ **0JH70MZ** Insertion of Stimulator Generator into Back Subcutaneous Tissue and Fascia, Open Approach

0JH70NZ Insertion of Tissue Expander into Back Subcutaneous Tissue and Fascia, Open Approach

0JH70VZ Insertion of Infusion Pump into Back Subcutaneous Tissue and Fascia, Open Approach

0JH73BZ Insertion of Single Array Stimulator Generator into Back Subcutaneous Tissue and Fascia, Percutaneous Approach

⊞ Neurotransmitter/Neurostimulator when reported with an Insertion of a neurostimulator lead (6th character M) into the cranial nerve, spinal canal or spinal cord. *See table 00H to construct the Insertion code.* Also applicable when reported with Insertion of neurostimulator lead (6th character M) into the peripheral nerve. *See table 01H to construct the Insertion code.* Also applicable when reported with Insertion of a stimulator lead (6th character M) into the stomach. *See table 0DH to construct the Insertion code.*

0JH73CZ Insertion of Single Array Rechargeable Stimulator Generator into Back Subcutaneous Tissue and Fascia, Percutaneous Approach

⊞ Neurotransmitter/Neurostimulator when reported with an Insertion of a neurostimulator lead (6th character M) into the cranial nerve, spinal canal or spinal cord. *See table 00H to construct the Insertion code.* Also applicable when reported with Insertion of neurostimulator lead (6th character M) into the peripheral

nerve. *See table 01H to construct the Insertion code.* Also applicable when reported with Insertion of a stimulator lead (6th character M) into the stomach. *See table 0DH to construct the Insertion code.*

0JH73DZ Insertion of Multiple Array Stimulator Generator into Back Subcutaneous Tissue and Fascia, Percutaneous Approach

⊞ Major brain device implant when reported with an Insertion of a neurostimulator lead (6th character M) into the brain or cerebral ventricle. *See table 00H to construct the Insertion code.*

⊞ Neurotransmitter/Neurostimulator when reported with an Insertion of a neurostimulator lead (6th character M) into the cranial nerve, spinal canal or spinal cord. *See table 00H to construct the Insertion code.* Also applicable when reported with Insertion of neurostimulator lead (6th character M) into the peripheral nerve. *See table 01H to construct the Insertion code.* Also applicable when reported with Insertion of a stimulator lead (6th character M) into the stomach. *See table 0DH to construct the Insertion code.*

0JH73EZ Insertion of Multiple Array Rechargeable Stimulator Generator into Back Subcutaneous Tissue and Fascia, Percutaneous Approach

⊞ Major brain device implant when reported with an Insertion of a neurostimulator lead (6th character M) into the brain or cerebral ventricle. *See table 00H to construct the Insertion code.*

⊞ Neurotransmitter/Neurostimulator when reported with an Insertion of a neurostimulator lead (6th character M) into the cranial nerve, spinal canal or spinal cord. *See table 00H to construct the Insertion code.* Also applicable when reported with Insertion of neurostimulator lead (6th character M) into the peripheral nerve. *See table 01H to construct the Insertion code.* Also applicable when reported with Insertion of a stimulator lead (6th character M) into the stomach. *See table 0DH to construct the Insertion code.*

▲ **0JH73MZ** Insertion of Stimulator Generator into Back Subcutaneous Tissue and Fascia, Percutaneous Approach

0JH73NZ Insertion of Tissue Expander into Back Subcutaneous Tissue and Fascia, Percutaneous Approach

0JH73VZ Insertion of Infusion Pump into Back Subcutaneous Tissue and Fascia, Percutaneous Approach

0JH800Z Insertion of Hemodynamic Monitoring Device into Abdomen Subcutaneous Tissue and Fascia, Open Approach

● **0JH802Z** Insertion of Monitoring Device into Abdomen Subcutaneous Tissue and Fascia, Open Approach

● **0JH804Z** Insertion of Pacemaker, Single Chamber into Abdomen Subcutaneous Tissue and Fascia, Open Approach

◾ With a secondary diagnosis code of K68.11, T81.4XXA, T82.6XXA, T82.7XXA

⊞ Pacemaker device when reported with an Insertion of a cardiac lead (6th character J or M) into the coronary vein, atrium, ventricle or pericardium (4th characters 4, 6, 7, K, L and N). *See table 02H to construct the Insertion code.* When a device is replaced, also report the

Note continued

Female-only   ♂ Male-only   ▲ Limited Coverage   ● Non-OR   ◾ HAC-associated procedure   ▲ Non-covered procedures   ⊞ Combination

Continued note

Removal of the cardiac rhythm device (6th character P) from the trunk subcutaneous tissue and fascia. *See table 0JP to construct the Removal code.* When a cardiac lead is replaced, also report the Removal of the cardiac lead (6th character M) from the heart. *See table 02P to construct the Removal code.*

● **0JH805Z** Insertion of Pacemaker, Single Chamber Rate Responsive into Abdomen Subcutaneous Tissue and Fascia, Open Approach

　　HAC With a secondary diagnosis code of K68.11, T81.4XXA, T82.6XXA, T82.7XXA

　　+ Pacemaker device when reported with an Insertion of a cardiac lead (6th character J or M) into the coronary vein, atrium, ventricle or pericardium (4th characters 4, 6, 7, K, L and N). *See table 02H to construct the Insertion code.* When a device is replaced, also report the Removal of the cardiac rhythm device (6th character P) from the trunk subcutaneous tissue and fascia. *See table 0JP to construct the Removal code.* When a cardiac lead is replaced, also report the Removal of the cardiac lead (6th character M) from the heart. *See table 02P to construct the Removal code.*

● **0JH806Z** Insertion of Pacemaker, Dual Chamber into Abdomen Subcutaneous Tissue and Fascia, Open Approach

　　HAC With a secondary diagnosis code of K68.11, T81.4XXA, T82.6XXA, T82.7XXA

　　+ Pacemaker device when reported with an Insertion of a cardiac lead (6th character J or M) into the coronary vein, atrium, ventricle or pericardium (4th characters 4, 6, 7, K, L and N). *See table 02H to construct the Insertion code.* When a device is replaced, also report the Removal of the cardiac rhythm device (6th character P) from the trunk subcutaneous tissue and fascia. *See table 0JP to construct the Removal code.* When a cardiac lead is replaced, also report the Removal of the cardiac lead (6th character M) from the heart. *See table 02P to construct the Removal code.*

0JH807Z Insertion of Cardiac Resynchronization Pacemaker Pulse Generator into Abdomen Subcutaneous Tissue and Fascia, Open Approach

　　HAC With a secondary diagnosis code of K68.11, T81.4XXA, T82.6XXA, T82.7XXA

　　+ Pacemaker device when reported with an Insertion of a cardiac lead (6th character J or M) into the coronary vein, atrium, ventricle or pericardium (4th characters 4, 6, 7, K, L and N). *See table 02H to construct the Insertion code.* When a cardiac lead is replaced, also report the Removal of the cardiac lead (6th character M) from the heart. *See table 02P to construct the Removal code.*

0JH808Z Insertion of Defibrillator Generator into Abdomen Subcutaneous Tissue and Fascia, Open Approach

　　HAC With a secondary diagnosis code of K68.11, T81.4XXA, T82.6XXA, T82.7XXA

　　+ Cardioverter-Defibrillator lead(s)/ generator when reported with Insertion of

a defibrillator cardiac lead (6th character K) into the coronary vein, atrium, or ventricle. Also applicable with Insertion of pacemaker cardiac lead, defibrillator cardiac lead or cardiac lead (6th characters J, K, M) into the pericardium. *See table 02H to construct the Insertion code.*

0JH809Z Insertion of Cardiac Resynchronization Defibrillator Pulse Generator into Abdomen Subcutaneous Tissue and Fascia, Open Approach

　　HAC With a secondary diagnosis code of K68.11, T81.4XXA, T82.6XXA, T82.7XXA

　　+ Cardioverter-Defibrillator lead(s)/ generator when reported with Insertion of a defibrillator cardiac lead (6th character K) into the atrium, or ventricle. Also applicable with Insertion of pacemaker cardiac lead, defibrillator cardiac lead or cardiac lead (6th characters J, K, M) into the coronary vein or pericardium. *See table 02H to construct the Insertion code.*

0JH80AZ Insertion of Contractility Modulation Device into Abdomen Subcutaneous Tissue and Fascia, Open Approach

　　+ Cardioverter-Defibrillator lead(s)/ generator when reported with Insertion of a cardiac lead (6th character M) into the left ventricle. *See table 02H to construct the Insertion code.*

0JH80BZ Insertion of Single Array Stimulator Generator into Abdomen Subcutaneous Tissue and Fascia, Open Approach

　　+ Neurotransmitter/Neurostimulator when reported with an Insertion of a neurostimulator lead (6th character M) into the cranial nerve, spinal canal or spinal cord. *See table 00H to construct the Insertion code.* Also applicable when reported with Insertion of neurostimulator lead (6th character M) into the peripheral nerve. *See table 01H to construct the Insertion code.* Also applicable when reported with Insertion of a stimulator lead (6th character M) into the stomach. *See table 0DH to construct the Insertion code.*

0JH80CZ Insertion of Single Array Rechargeable Stimulator Generator into Abdomen Subcutaneous Tissue and Fascia, Open Approach

　　+ Neurotransmitter/Neurostimulator when reported with an Insertion of a neurostimulator lead (6th character M) into the cranial nerve, spinal canal or spinal cord. *See table 00H to construct the Insertion code.* Also applicable when reported with Insertion of neurostimulator lead (6th character M) into the peripheral nerve. *See table 01H to construct the Insertion code.* Also applicable when reported with Insertion of a stimulator lead (6th character M) into the stomach. *See table 0DH to construct the Insertion code.*

0JH80DZ Insertion of Multiple Array Stimulator Generator into Abdomen Subcutaneous Tissue and Fascia, Open Approach

　　+ Major brain device implant when reported with an Insertion of a neurostimulator lead (6th character M) into the brain or cerebral ventricle. *See table 00H to construct the Insertion code.*

　　+ Neurotransmitter/Neurostimulator when reported with an Insertion of a neurostimulator lead (6th character M)

into the cranial nerve, spinal canal or spinal cord. *See table 00H to construct the Insertion code.* Also applicable when reported with Insertion of neurostimulator lead (6th character M) into the peripheral nerve. *See table 01H to construct the Insertion code.* Also applicable when reported with Insertion of a stimulator lead (6th character M) into the stomach. *See table 0DH to construct the Insertion code.*

0JH80EZ Insertion of Multiple Array Rechargeable Stimulator Generator into Abdomen Subcutaneous Tissue and Fascia, Open Approach

　　+ Major brain device implant when reported with an Insertion of a neurostimulator lead (6th character M) into the brain or cerebral ventricle. *See table 00H to construct the Insertion code.*

　　+ Neurotransmitter/Neurostimulator when reported with an Insertion of a neurostimulator lead (6th character M) into the cranial nerve, spinal canal or spinal cord. *See table 00H to construct the Insertion code.* Also applicable when reported with Insertion of neurostimulator lead (6th character M) into the peripheral nerve. *See table 01H to construct the Insertion code.* Also applicable when reported with Insertion of a stimulator lead (6th character M) into the stomach. *See table 0DH to construct the Insertion code.*

● **0JH80HZ** Insertion of Contraceptive Device into Abdomen Subcutaneous Tissue and Fascia, Open Approach

▲ **0JH80MZ** Insertion of Stimulator Generator into Abdomen Subcutaneous Tissue and Fascia, Open Approach

0JH80NZ Insertion of Tissue Expander into Abdomen Subcutaneous Tissue and Fascia, Open Approach

0JH80PZ Insertion of Cardiac Rhythm Related Device into Abdomen Subcutaneous Tissue and Fascia, Open Approach

　　HAC With a secondary diagnosis code of K68.11, T81.4XXA, T82.6XXA, T82.7XXA

　　+ Pacemaker device when reported with an Insertion of a cardiac lead (6th character J or M) into the coronary vein, atrium, ventricle or pericardium (4th characters 4, 6, 7, K, L and N). *See table 02H to construct the Insertion code.* When a cardiac lead is replaced, also report the Removal of the cardiac lead (6th character M) from the heart. *See table 02P to construct the Removal code.*

0JH80VZ Insertion of Infusion Pump into Abdomen Subcutaneous Tissue and Fascia, Open Approach

　　AHA CC: 3Q, 2014, 19-20

● **0JH80WZ** Insertion of Reservoir into Abdomen Subcutaneous Tissue and Fascia, Open Approach

● **0JH80XZ** Insertion of Vascular Access Device into Abdomen Subcutaneous Tissue and Fascia, Open Approach

0JH830Z Insertion of Hemodynamic Monitoring Device into Abdomen Subcutaneous Tissue and Fascia, Percutaneous Approach

● **0JH832Z** Insertion of Monitoring Device into Abdomen Subcutaneous Tissue and Fascia, Percutaneous Approach

1834Z Insertion of Pacemaker, Single Chamber into Abdomen Subcutaneous Tissue and Fascia, Percutaneous Approach

▪ With a secondary diagnosis code of K68.11, T81.4XXA, T82.6XXA, T82.7XXA

➕ Pacemaker device when reported with an Insertion of a cardiac lead (6th character J or M) into the coronary vein, atrium, ventricle or pericardium (4th characters 4, 6, 7, K, L and N). *See table 02H to construct the Insertion code. When a device is replaced, also report the Removal of the cardiac rhythm device (6th character P) from the trunk subcutaneous tissue and fascia. See table 0JP to construct the Removal code. When a cardiac lead is replaced, also report the Removal of the cardiac lead (6th character M) from the heart. See table 02P to construct the Removal code.*

H835Z Insertion of Pacemaker, Single Chamber Rate Responsive into Abdomen Subcutaneous Tissue and Fascia, Percutaneous Approach

▪ With a secondary diagnosis code of K68.11, T81.4XXA, T82.6XXA, T82.7XXA

➕ Pacemaker device when reported with an Insertion of a cardiac lead (6th character J or M) into the coronary vein, atrium, ventricle or pericardium (4th characters 4, 6, 7, K, L and N). *See table 02H to construct the Insertion code. When a device is replaced, also report the Removal of the cardiac rhythm device (6th character P) from the trunk subcutaneous tissue and fascia. See table 0JP to construct the Removal code. When a cardiac lead is replaced, also report the Removal of the cardiac lead (6th character M) from the heart. See table 02P to construct the Removal code.*

H836Z Insertion of Pacemaker, Dual Chamber into Abdomen Subcutaneous Tissue and Fascia, Percutaneous Approach

▪ With a secondary diagnosis code of K68.11, T81.4XXA, T82.6XXA, T82.7XXA

➕ Pacemaker device when reported with an Insertion of a cardiac lead (6th character J or M) into the coronary vein, atrium, ventricle or pericardium (4th characters 4, 6, 7, K, L and N). *See table 02H to construct the Insertion code. When a device is replaced, also report the Removal of the cardiac rhythm device (6th character P) from the trunk subcutaneous tissue and fascia. See table 0JP to construct the Removal code. When a cardiac lead is replaced, also report the Removal of the cardiac lead (6th character M) from the heart. See table 02P to construct the Removal code.*

H837Z Insertion of Cardiac Resynchronization Pacemaker Pulse Generator into Abdomen Subcutaneous Tissue and Fascia, Percutaneous Approach

▪ With a secondary diagnosis code of K68.11, T81.4XXA, T82.6XXA, T82.7XXA

➕ Pacemaker device when reported with an Insertion of a cardiac lead (6th character J or M) into the coronary vein, atrium, ventricle or pericardium (4th characters 4, 6, 7, K, L and N). *See table 02H to construct the Insertion code. When a cardiac lead is replaced, also report the*

Removal of the cardiac lead (6th character M) from the heart. *See table 02P to construct the Removal code.*

0JH838Z Insertion of Defibrillator Generator into Abdomen Subcutaneous Tissue and Fascia, Percutaneous Approach

▪ With a secondary diagnosis code of K68.11, T81.4XXA, T82.6XXA, T82.7XXA

➕ Cardioverter-Defibrillator lead(s)/generator when reported with Insertion of a defibrillator cardiac lead (6th character K) into the coronary vein, atrium, or ventricle. Also applicable with Insertion of pacemaker cardiac lead, defibrillator cardiac lead or cardiac lead (6th characters J, K, M) into the pericardium. *See table 02H to construct the Insertion code.*

0JH839Z Insertion of Cardiac Resynchronization Defibrillator Pulse Generator into Abdomen Subcutaneous Tissue and Fascia, Percutaneous Approach

▪ With a secondary diagnosis code of K68.11, T81.4XXA, T82.6XXA, T82.7XXA

➕ Cardioverter-Defibrillator lead(s)/generator when reported with Insertion of a defibrillator cardiac lead (6th character K) into the atrium, or ventricle. Also applicable with Insertion of pacemaker cardiac lead, defibrillator cardiac lead or cardiac lead (6th characters J, K, M) into the coronary vein or pericardium. *See table 02H to construct the Insertion code.*

0JH83AZ Insertion of Contractility Modulation Device into Abdomen Subcutaneous Tissue and Fascia, Percutaneous Approach

➕ Cardioverter-Defibrillator lead(s)/generator when reported with Insertion of a cardiac lead (6th character M) into the left ventricle. *See table 02H to construct the Insertion code.*

0JH83BZ Insertion of Single Array Stimulator Generator into Abdomen Subcutaneous Tissue and Fascia, Percutaneous Approach

➕ Neurotransmitter/Neurostimulator when reported with an Insertion of a neurostimulator lead (6th character M) into the cranial nerve, spinal canal or spinal cord. *See table 00H to construct the Insertion code. Also applicable when reported with Insertion of neurostimulator lead (6th character M) into the peripheral nerve. See table 01H to construct the Insertion code. Also applicable when reported with Insertion of a stimulator lead (6th character M) into the stomach. See table 0DH to construct the Insertion code.*

0JH83CZ Insertion of Single Array Rechargeable Stimulator Generator into Abdomen Subcutaneous Tissue and Fascia, Percutaneous Approach

➕ Neurotransmitter/Neurostimulator when reported with an Insertion of a neurostimulator lead (6th character M) into the cranial nerve, spinal canal or spinal cord. *See table 00H to construct the Insertion code. Also applicable when reported with Insertion of neurostimulator lead (6th character M) into the peripheral nerve. See table 01H to construct the Insertion code. Also applicable when reported with Insertion of a stimulator lead (6th character M) into the stomach. See table 0DH to construct the Insertion code.*

0JH83DZ Insertion of Multiple Array Stimulator Generator into Abdomen Subcutaneous Tissue and Fascia, Percutaneous Approach

➕ Major brain device implant when reported with an Insertion of a neurostimulator lead (6th character M) into the brain or cerebral ventricle. *See table 00H to construct the Insertion code.*

➕ Neurotransmitter/Neurostimulator when reported with an Insertion of a neurostimulator lead (6th character M) into the cranial nerve, spinal canal or spinal cord. *See table 00H to construct the Insertion code. Also applicable when reported with Insertion of neurostimulator lead (6th character M) into the peripheral nerve. See table 01H to construct the Insertion code. Also applicable when reported with Insertion of a stimulator lead (6th character M) into the stomach. See table 0DH to construct the Insertion code.*

0JH83EZ Insertion of Multiple Array Rechargeable Stimulator Generator into Abdomen Subcutaneous Tissue and Fascia, Percutaneous Approach

➕ Major brain device implant when reported with an Insertion of a neurostimulator lead (6th character M) into the brain or cerebral ventricle. *See table 00H to construct the Insertion code.*

➕ Neurotransmitter/Neurostimulator when reported with an Insertion of a neurostimulator lead (6th character M) into the cranial nerve, spinal canal or spinal cord. *See table 00H to construct the Insertion code. Also applicable when reported with Insertion of neurostimulator lead (6th character M) into the peripheral nerve. See table 01H to construct the Insertion code. Also applicable when reported with Insertion of a stimulator lead (6th character M) into the stomach. See table 0DH to construct the Insertion code.*

● **0JH83HZ** Insertion of Contraceptive Device into Abdomen Subcutaneous Tissue and Fascia, Percutaneous Approach

▲ **0JH83MZ** Insertion of Stimulator Generator into Abdomen Subcutaneous Tissue and Fascia, Percutaneous Approach

0JH83NZ Insertion of Tissue Expander into Abdomen Subcutaneous Tissue and Fascia, Percutaneous Approach

0JH83PZ Insertion of Cardiac Rhythm Related Device into Abdomen Subcutaneous Tissue and Fascia, Percutaneous Approach

▪ With a secondary diagnosis code of K68.11, T81.4XXA, T82.6XXA, T82.7XXA

➕ Pacemaker device when reported with an Insertion of a cardiac lead (6th character J or M) into the coronary vein, atrium, ventricle or pericardium (4th characters 4, 6, 7, K, L and N). *See table 02H to construct the Insertion code. When a cardiac lead is replaced, also report the Removal of the cardiac lead (6th character M) from the heart. See table 02P to construct the Removal code.*

0JH83VZ Insertion of Infusion Pump into Abdomen Subcutaneous Tissue and Fascia, Percutaneous Approach

● **0JH83WZ** Insertion of Reservoir into Abdomen Subcutaneous Tissue and Fascia, Percutaneous Approach

● **0JH83XZ** Insertion of Vascular Access Device into Abdomen Subcutaneous Tissue and Fascia, Percutaneous Approach

0JH90NZ Insertion of Tissue Expander into Buttock Subcutaneous Tissue and Fascia, Open Approach

♀ Female-only   ♂ Male-only   ▲ Limited Coverage   ● Non-OR   ▪ HAC-associated procedure   ▲ Non-covered procedures   ➕ Combination

0JH93NZ Insertion of Tissue Expander into Buttock Subcutaneous Tissue and Fascia, Percutaneous Approach

0JHB0NZ Insertion of Tissue Expander into Perineum Subcutaneous Tissue and Fascia, Open Approach

0JHB3NZ Insertion of Tissue Expander into Perineum Subcutaneous Tissue and Fascia, Percutaneous Approach

0JHC0NZ Insertion of Tissue Expander into Pelvic Region Subcutaneous Tissue and Fascia, Open Approach

0JHC3NZ Insertion of Tissue Expander into Pelvic Region Subcutaneous Tissue and Fascia, Percutaneous Approach

0JHD0HZ Insertion of Contraceptive Device into Right Upper Arm Subcutaneous Tissue and Fascia, Open Approach

0JHD0NZ Insertion of Tissue Expander into Right Upper Arm Subcutaneous Tissue and Fascia, Open Approach

0JHD0VZ Insertion of Infusion Pump into Right Upper Arm Subcutaneous Tissue and Fascia, Open Approach

● 0JHD0WZ Insertion of Reservoir into Right Upper Arm Subcutaneous Tissue and Fascia, Open Approach

● 0JHD0XZ Insertion of Vascular Access Device into Right Upper Arm Subcutaneous Tissue and Fascia, Open Approach

0JHD3HZ Insertion of Contraceptive Device into Right Upper Arm Subcutaneous Tissue and Fascia, Percutaneous Approach

0JHD3NZ Insertion of Tissue Expander into Right Upper Arm Subcutaneous Tissue and Fascia, Percutaneous Approach

0JHD3VZ Insertion of Infusion Pump into Right Upper Arm Subcutaneous Tissue and Fascia, Percutaneous Approach

● 0JHD3WZ Insertion of Reservoir into Right Upper Arm Subcutaneous Tissue and Fascia, Percutaneous Approach

● 0JHD3XZ Insertion of Vascular Access Device into Right Upper Arm Subcutaneous Tissue and Fascia, Percutaneous Approach

0JHF0HZ Insertion of Contraceptive Device into Left Upper Arm Subcutaneous Tissue and Fascia, Open Approach

0JHF0NZ Insertion of Tissue Expander into Left Upper Arm Subcutaneous Tissue and Fascia, Open Approach

0JHF0VZ Insertion of Infusion Pump into Left Upper Arm Subcutaneous Tissue and Fascia, Open Approach

● 0JHF0WZ Insertion of Reservoir into Left Upper Arm Subcutaneous Tissue and Fascia, Open Approach

● 0JHF0XZ Insertion of Vascular Access Device into Left Upper Arm Subcutaneous Tissue and Fascia, Open Approach

0JHF3HZ Insertion of Contraceptive Device into Left Upper Arm Subcutaneous Tissue and Fascia, Percutaneous Approach

0JHF3NZ Insertion of Tissue Expander into Left Upper Arm Subcutaneous Tissue and Fascia, Percutaneous Approach

0JHF3VZ Insertion of Infusion Pump into Left Upper Arm Subcutaneous Tissue and Fascia, Percutaneous Approach

● 0JHF3WZ Insertion of Reservoir into Left Upper Arm Subcutaneous Tissue and Fascia, Percutaneous Approach

● 0JHF3XZ Insertion of Vascular Access Device into Left Upper Arm Subcutaneous Tissue and Fascia, Percutaneous Approach

0JHG0HZ Insertion of Contraceptive Device into Right Lower Arm Subcutaneous Tissue and Fascia, Open Approach

0JHG0NZ Insertion of Tissue Expander into Right Lower Arm Subcutaneous Tissue and Fascia, Open Approach

0JHG0VZ Insertion of Infusion Pump into Right Lower Arm Subcutaneous Tissue and Fascia, Open Approach

● 0JHG0WZ Insertion of Reservoir into Right Lower Arm Subcutaneous Tissue and Fascia, Open Approach

● 0JHG0XZ Insertion of Vascular Access Device into Right Lower Arm Subcutaneous Tissue and Fascia, Open Approach

0JHG3HZ Insertion of Contraceptive Device into Right Lower Arm Subcutaneous Tissue and Fascia, Percutaneous Approach

0JHG3NZ Insertion of Tissue Expander into Right Lower Arm Subcutaneous Tissue and Fascia, Percutaneous Approach

0JHG3VZ Insertion of Infusion Pump into Right Lower Arm Subcutaneous Tissue and Fascia, Percutaneous Approach

● 0JHG3WZ Insertion of Reservoir into Right Lower Arm Subcutaneous Tissue and Fascia, Percutaneous Approach

● 0JHG3XZ Insertion of Vascular Access Device into Right Lower Arm Subcutaneous Tissue and Fascia, Percutaneous Approach

0JHH0HZ Insertion of Contraceptive Device into Left Lower Arm Subcutaneous Tissue and Fascia, Open Approach

0JHH0NZ Insertion of Tissue Expander into Left Lower Arm Subcutaneous Tissue and Fascia, Open Approach

0JHH0VZ Insertion of Infusion Pump into Left Lower Arm Subcutaneous Tissue and Fascia, Open Approach

● 0JHH0WZ Insertion of Reservoir into Left Lower Arm Subcutaneous Tissue and Fascia, Open Approach

● 0JHH0XZ Insertion of Vascular Access Device into Left Lower Arm Subcutaneous Tissue and Fascia, Open Approach

0JHH3HZ Insertion of Contraceptive Device into Left Lower Arm Subcutaneous Tissue and Fascia, Percutaneous Approach

0JHH3NZ Insertion of Tissue Expander into Left Lower Arm Subcutaneous Tissue and Fascia, Percutaneous Approach

0JHH3VZ Insertion of Infusion Pump into Left Lower Arm Subcutaneous Tissue and Fascia, Percutaneous Approach

● 0JHH3WZ Insertion of Reservoir into Left Lower Arm Subcutaneous Tissue and Fascia, Percutaneous Approach

● 0JHH3XZ Insertion of Vascular Access Device into Left Lower Arm Subcutaneous Tissue and Fascia, Percutaneous Approach

0JHJ0NZ Insertion of Tissue Expander into Right Hand Subcutaneous Tissue and Fascia, Open Approach

0JHJ3NZ Insertion of Tissue Expander into Right Hand Subcutaneous Tissue and Fascia, Percutaneous Approach

0JHK0NZ Insertion of Tissue Expander into Left Hand Subcutaneous Tissue and Fascia, Open Approach

0JHK3NZ Insertion of Tissue Expander into Left Hand Subcutaneous Tissue and Fascia, Percutaneous Approach

0JHL0HZ Insertion of Contraceptive Device into Right Upper Leg Subcutaneous Tissue and Fascia, Open Approach

0JHL0NZ Insertion of Tissue Expander into Right Upper Leg Subcutaneous Tissue and Fascia, Open Approach

0JHL0VZ Insertion of Infusion Pump into Right Upper Leg Subcutaneous Tissue and Fascia, Open Approach

● 0JHL0WZ Insertion of Reservoir into Right Upper Leg Subcutaneous Tissue and Fascia, Open Approach

● 0JHL0XZ Insertion of Vascular Access Device into Right Upper Leg Subcutaneous Tissue and Fascia, Open Approach

0JHL3HZ Insertion of Contraceptive Device into Right Upper Leg Subcutaneous Tissue and Fascia, Percutaneous Approach

0JHL3NZ Insertion of Tissue Expander into Right Upper Leg Subcutaneous Tissue and Fascia, Percutaneous Approach

0JHL3VZ Insertion of Infusion Pump into Right Upper Leg Subcutaneous Tissue and Fascia, Percutaneous Approach

● 0JHL3WZ Insertion of Reservoir into Right Upper Leg Subcutaneous Tissue and Fascia, Percutaneous Approach

● 0JHL3XZ Insertion of Vascular Access Device into Right Upper Leg Subcutaneous Tissue and Fascia, Percutaneous Approach

0JHM0HZ Insertion of Contraceptive Device into Left Upper Leg Subcutaneous Tissue and Fascia, Open Approach

0JHM0NZ Insertion of Tissue Expander into Left Upper Leg Subcutaneous Tissue and Fascia, Open Approach

0JHM0VZ Insertion of Infusion Pump into Left Upper Leg Subcutaneous Tissue and Fascia, Open Approach

● 0JHM0WZ Insertion of Reservoir into Left Upper Leg Subcutaneous Tissue and Fascia, Open Approach

● 0JHM0XZ Insertion of Vascular Access Device into Left Upper Leg Subcutaneous Tissue and Fascia, Open Approach

0JHM3HZ Insertion of Contraceptive Device into Left Upper Leg Subcutaneous Tissue and Fascia, Percutaneous Approach

0JHM3NZ Insertion of Tissue Expander into Left Upper Leg Subcutaneous Tissue and Fascia, Percutaneous Approach

0JHM3VZ Insertion of Infusion Pump into Left Upper Leg Subcutaneous Tissue and Fascia, Percutaneous Approach

● 0JHM3WZ Insertion of Reservoir into Left Upper Leg Subcutaneous Tissue and Fascia, Percutaneous Approach

● 0JHM3XZ Insertion of Vascular Access Device into Left Upper Leg Subcutaneous Tissue and Fascia, Percutaneous Approach

0JHN0HZ Insertion of Contraceptive Device into Right Lower Leg Subcutaneous Tissue and Fascia, Open Approach

0JHN0NZ Insertion of Tissue Expander into Right Lower Leg Subcutaneous Tissue and Fascia, Open Approach

0JHN0VZ Insertion of Infusion Pump into Right Lower Leg Subcutaneous Tissue and Fascia, Open Approach

● 0JHN0WZ Insertion of Reservoir into Right Lower Leg Subcutaneous Tissue and Fascia, Open Approach

● 0JHN0XZ Insertion of Vascular Access Device into Right Lower Leg Subcutaneous Tissue and Fascia, Open Approach

● 0JHN3HZ Insertion of Contraceptive Device into Right Lower Leg Subcutaneous Tissue and Fascia, Percutaneous Approach

0JHN3NZ Insertion of Tissue Expander into Right Lower Leg Subcutaneous Tissue and Fascia, Percutaneous Approach

0JHN3VZ Insertion of Infusion Pump into Right Lower Leg Subcutaneous Tissue and Fascia, Percutaneous Approach

● 0JHN3WZ Insertion of Reservoir into Right Lower Leg Subcutaneous Tissue and Fascia, Percutaneous Approach

♀ Female-only   ♂ Male-only   ▲ Limited Coverage   ● Non-OR   ▥ HAC-associated procedure   ▲ Non-covered procedures   ✚ Combinat

0JHN3XZ Insertion of Vascular Access Device into Right Lower Leg Subcutaneous Tissue and Fascia, Percutaneous Approach	**0JHQ0NZ** Insertion of Tissue Expander into Right Foot Subcutaneous Tissue and Fascia, Open Approach	**0JHT31Z** Insertion of Radioactive Element into Trunk Subcutaneous Tissue and Fascia, Percutaneous Approach
0JHP0HZ Insertion of Contraceptive Device into Left Lower Leg Subcutaneous Tissue and Fascia, Open Approach	**0JHQ3NZ** Insertion of Tissue Expander into Right Foot Subcutaneous Tissue and Fascia, Percutaneous Approach	**0JHT33Z** Insertion of Infusion Device into Trunk Subcutaneous Tissue and Fascia, Percutaneous Approach
0JHP0NZ Insertion of Tissue Expander into Left Lower Leg Subcutaneous Tissue and Fascia, Open Approach	**0JHR0NZ** Insertion of Tissue Expander into Left Foot Subcutaneous Tissue and Fascia, Open Approach	**0JHT3VZ** Insertion of Infusion Pump into Trunk Subcutaneous Tissue and Fascia, Percutaneous Approach
0JHP0VZ Insertion of Infusion Pump into Left Lower Leg Subcutaneous Tissue and Fascia, Open Approach	**0JHR3NZ** Insertion of Tissue Expander into Left Foot Subcutaneous Tissue and Fascia, Percutaneous Approach	**0JHV01Z** Insertion of Radioactive Element into Upper Extremity Subcutaneous Tissue and Fascia, Open Approach
0JHP0WZ Insertion of Reservoir into Left Lower Leg Subcutaneous Tissue and Fascia, Open Approach	**0JHS01Z** Insertion of Radioactive Element into Head and Neck Subcutaneous Tissue and Fascia, Open Approach	**0JHV03Z** Insertion of Infusion Device into Upper Extremity Subcutaneous Tissue and Fascia, Open Approach
0JHP0XZ Insertion of Vascular Access Device into Left Lower Leg Subcutaneous Tissue and Fascia, Open Approach	**0JHS03Z** Insertion of Infusion Device into Head and Neck Subcutaneous Tissue and Fascia, Open Approach	**0JHV31Z** Insertion of Radioactive Element into Upper Extremity Subcutaneous Tissue and Fascia, Percutaneous Approach
0JHP3HZ Insertion of Contraceptive Device into Left Lower Leg Subcutaneous Tissue and Fascia, Percutaneous Approach	**0JHS31Z** Insertion of Radioactive Element into Head and Neck Subcutaneous Tissue and Fascia, Percutaneous Approach	**0JHV33Z** Insertion of Infusion Device into Upper Extremity Subcutaneous Tissue and Fascia, Percutaneous Approach
0JHP3NZ Insertion of Tissue Expander into Left Lower Leg Subcutaneous Tissue and Fascia, Percutaneous Approach	**0JHS33Z** Insertion of Infusion Device into Head and Neck Subcutaneous Tissue and Fascia, Percutaneous Approach	**0JHW01Z** Insertion of Radioactive Element into Lower Extremity Subcutaneous Tissue and Fascia, Open Approach
0JHP3VZ Insertion of Infusion Pump into Left Lower Leg Subcutaneous Tissue and Fascia, Percutaneous Approach	**0JHT01Z** Insertion of Radioactive Element into Trunk Subcutaneous Tissue and Fascia, Open Approach	**0JHW03Z** Insertion of Infusion Device into Lower Extremity Subcutaneous Tissue and Fascia, Open Approach
0JHP3WZ Insertion of Reservoir into Left Lower Leg Subcutaneous Tissue and Fascia, Percutaneous Approach	**0JHT03Z** Insertion of Infusion Device into Trunk Subcutaneous Tissue and Fascia, Open Approach	**0JHW31Z** Insertion of Radioactive Element into Lower Extremity Subcutaneous Tissue and Fascia, Percutaneous Approach
0JHP3XZ Insertion of Vascular Access Device into Left Lower Leg Subcutaneous Tissue and Fascia, Percutaneous Approach	**0JHT0VZ** Insertion of Infusion Pump into Trunk Subcutaneous Tissue and Fascia, Open Approach	**0JHW33Z** Insertion of Infusion Device into Lower Extremity Subcutaneous Tissue and Fascia, Percutaneous Approach

0JJ – Subcutaneous Tissue and Fascia, Inspection

Review Coding Guideline B3.5

Review Coding Guidelines B3.11a, B3.11b and B3.11c

0JJS0ZZ Inspection of Head and Neck Subcutaneous Tissue and Fascia, Open Approach	**0JJT3ZZ** Inspection of Trunk Subcutaneous Tissue and Fascia, Percutaneous Approach	**0JJVXZZ** Inspection of Upper Extremity Subcutaneous Tissue and Fascia, External Approach
0JJS3ZZ Inspection of Head and Neck Subcutaneous Tissue and Fascia, Percutaneous Approach	**0JJTXZZ** Inspection of Trunk Subcutaneous Tissue and Fascia, External Approach	**0JJW0ZZ** Inspection of Lower Extremity Subcutaneous Tissue and Fascia, Open Approach
0JJSXZZ Inspection of Head and Neck Subcutaneous Tissue and Fascia, External Approach	**0JJV0ZZ** Inspection of Upper Extremity Subcutaneous Tissue and Fascia, Open Approach	**0JJW3ZZ** Inspection of Lower Extremity Subcutaneous Tissue and Fascia, Percutaneous Approach
0JJT0ZZ Inspection of Trunk Subcutaneous Tissue and Fascia, Open Approach	**0JJV3ZZ** Inspection of Upper Extremity Subcutaneous Tissue and Fascia, Percutaneous Approach	**0JJWXZZ** Inspection of Lower Extremity Subcutaneous Tissue and Fascia, External Approach

0JN – Subcutaneous Tissue and Fascia, Release

Review Coding Guideline B3.13

Review Coding Guideline B3.14

0JN00ZZ Release Scalp Subcutaneous Tissue and Fascia, Open Approach	**0JN50ZZ** Release Posterior Neck Subcutaneous Tissue and Fascia, Open Approach	**0JN80ZZ** Release Abdomen Subcutaneous Tissue and Fascia, Open Approach
0JN03ZZ Release Scalp Subcutaneous Tissue and Fascia, Percutaneous Approach	**0JN53ZZ** Release Posterior Neck Subcutaneous Tissue and Fascia, Percutaneous Approach	**0JN83ZZ** Release Abdomen Subcutaneous Tissue and Fascia, Percutaneous Approach
0JN0XZZ Release Scalp Subcutaneous Tissue and Fascia, External Approach	**0JN5XZZ** Release Posterior Neck Subcutaneous Tissue and Fascia, External Approach	**0JN8XZZ** Release Abdomen Subcutaneous Tissue and Fascia, External Approach
0JN10ZZ Release Face Subcutaneous Tissue and Fascia, Open Approach	**0JN60ZZ** Release Chest Subcutaneous Tissue and Fascia, Open Approach	**0JN90ZZ** Release Buttock Subcutaneous Tissue and Fascia, Open Approach
0JN13ZZ Release Face Subcutaneous Tissue and Fascia, Percutaneous Approach	**0JN63ZZ** Release Chest Subcutaneous Tissue and Fascia, Percutaneous Approach	**0JN93ZZ** Release Buttock Subcutaneous Tissue and Fascia, Percutaneous Approach
0JN1XZZ Release Face Subcutaneous Tissue and Fascia, External Approach	**0JN6XZZ** Release Chest Subcutaneous Tissue and Fascia, External Approach	**0JN9XZZ** Release Buttock Subcutaneous Tissue and Fascia, External Approach
0JN40ZZ Release Anterior Neck Subcutaneous Tissue and Fascia, Open Approach	**0JN70ZZ** Release Back Subcutaneous Tissue and Fascia, Open Approach	**0JNB0ZZ** Release Perineum Subcutaneous Tissue and Fascia, Open Approach
0JN43ZZ Release Anterior Neck Subcutaneous Tissue and Fascia, Percutaneous Approach	**0JN73ZZ** Release Back Subcutaneous Tissue and Fascia, Percutaneous Approach	**0JNB3ZZ** Release Perineum Subcutaneous Tissue and Fascia, Percutaneous Approach
0JN4XZZ Release Anterior Neck Subcutaneous Tissue and Fascia, External Approach	**0JN7XZZ** Release Back Subcutaneous Tissue and Fascia, External Approach	**0JNBXZZ** Release Perineum Subcutaneous Tissue and Fascia, External Approach

♀ Female-only ♂ Male-only ▲ Limited Coverage ● Non-OR ▧ HAC-associated procedure ▲ Non-covered procedures ✚ Combination

0JNC0ZZ Release Pelvic Region Subcutaneous Tissue and Fascia, Open Approach

0JNC3ZZ Release Pelvic Region Subcutaneous Tissue and Fascia, Percutaneous Approach

0JNCXZZ Release Pelvic Region Subcutaneous Tissue and Fascia, External Approach

0JND0ZZ Release Right Upper Arm Subcutaneous Tissue and Fascia, Open Approach

0JND3ZZ Release Right Upper Arm Subcutaneous Tissue and Fascia, Percutaneous Approach

0JNDXZZ Release Right Upper Arm Subcutaneous Tissue and Fascia, External Approach

0JNF0ZZ Release Left Upper Arm Subcutaneous Tissue and Fascia, Open Approach

0JNF3ZZ Release Left Upper Arm Subcutaneous Tissue and Fascia, Percutaneous Approach

0JNFXZZ Release Left Upper Arm Subcutaneous Tissue and Fascia, External Approach

0JNG0ZZ Release Right Lower Arm Subcutaneous Tissue and Fascia, Open Approach

0JNG3ZZ Release Right Lower Arm Subcutaneous Tissue and Fascia, Percutaneous Approach

0JNGXZZ Release Right Lower Arm Subcutaneous Tissue and Fascia, External Approach

0JNH0ZZ Release Left Lower Arm Subcutaneous Tissue and Fascia, Open Approach

0JNH3ZZ Release Left Lower Arm Subcutaneous Tissue and Fascia, Percutaneous Approach

0JNHXZZ Release Left Lower Arm Subcutaneous Tissue and Fascia, External Approach

0JNJ0ZZ Release Right Hand Subcutaneous Tissue and Fascia, Open Approach

0JNJ3ZZ Release Right Hand Subcutaneous Tissue and Fascia, Percutaneous Approach

0JNJXZZ Release Right Hand Subcutaneous Tissue and Fascia, External Approach

0JNK0ZZ Release Left Hand Subcutaneous Tissue and Fascia, Open Approach

0JNK3ZZ Release Left Hand Subcutaneous Tissue and Fascia, Percutaneous Approach

0JNKXZZ Release Left Hand Subcutaneous Tissue and Fascia, External Approach

0JNL0ZZ Release Right Upper Leg Subcutaneous Tissue and Fascia, Open Approach

0JNL3ZZ Release Right Upper Leg Subcutaneous Tissue and Fascia, Percutaneous Approach

0JNLXZZ Release Right Upper Leg Subcutaneous Tissue and Fascia, External Approach

0JNM0ZZ Release Left Upper Leg Subcutaneous Tissue and Fascia, Open Approach

0JNM3ZZ Release Left Upper Leg Subcutaneous Tissue and Fascia, Percutaneous Approach

0JNMXZZ Release Left Upper Leg Subcutaneous Tissue and Fascia, External Approach

0JNN0ZZ Release Right Lower Leg Subcutaneous Tissue and Fascia, Open Approach

0JNN3ZZ Release Right Lower Leg Subcutaneous Tissue and Fascia, Percutaneous Approach

0JNNXZZ Release Right Lower Leg Subcutaneous Tissue and Fascia, External Approach

0JNP0ZZ Release Left Lower Leg Subcutaneous Tissue and Fascia, Open Approach

0JNP3ZZ Release Left Lower Leg Subcutaneous Tissue and Fascia, Percutaneous Approach

0JNPXZZ Release Left Lower Leg Subcutaneous Tissue and Fascia, External Approach

0JNQ0ZZ Release Right Foot Subcutaneous Tissue and Fascia, Open Approach

0JNQ3ZZ Release Right Foot Subcutaneous Tissue and Fascia, Percutaneous Approach

0JNQXZZ Release Right Foot Subcutaneous Tissue and Fascia, External Approach

0JNR0ZZ Release Left Foot Subcutaneous Tissue and Fascia, Open Approach

0JNR3ZZ Release Left Foot Subcutaneous Tissue and Fascia, Percutaneous Approach

0JNRXZZ Release Left Foot Subcutaneous Tissue and Fascia, External Approach

0JP – Subcutaneous Tissue and Fascia, Removal

Review Coding Guideline B6.1c

0JPS00Z Removal of Drainage Device from Head and Neck Subcutaneous Tissue and Fascia, Open Approach

0JPS01Z Removal of Radioactive Element from Head and Neck Subcutaneous Tissue and Fascia, Open Approach

0JPS03Z Removal of Infusion Device from Head and Neck Subcutaneous Tissue and Fascia, Open Approach

0JPS07Z Removal of Autologous Tissue Substitute from Head and Neck Subcutaneous Tissue and Fascia, Open Approach

0JPS0JZ Removal of Synthetic Substitute from Head and Neck Subcutaneous Tissue and Fascia, Open Approach

0JPS0KZ Removal of Nonautologous Tissue Substitute from Head and Neck Subcutaneous Tissue and Fascia, Open Approach

0JPS0NZ Removal of Tissue Expander from Head and Neck Subcutaneous Tissue and Fascia, Open Approach

0JPS30Z Removal of Drainage Device from Head and Neck Subcutaneous Tissue and Fascia, Percutaneous Approach

0JPS31Z Removal of Radioactive Element from Head and Neck Subcutaneous Tissue and Fascia, Percutaneous Approach

0JPS33Z Removal of Infusion Device from Head and Neck Subcutaneous Tissue and Fascia, Percutaneous Approach

0JPS37Z Removal of Autologous Tissue Substitute from Head and Neck Subcutaneous Tissue and Fascia, Percutaneous Approach

0JPS3JZ Removal of Synthetic Substitute from Head and Neck Subcutaneous Tissue and Fascia, Percutaneous Approach

0JPS3KZ Removal of Nonautologous Tissue Substitute from Head and Neck Subcutaneous Tissue and Fascia, Percutaneous Approach

0JPS3NZ Removal of Tissue Expander from Head and Neck Subcutaneous Tissue and Fascia, Percutaneous Approach

0JPSX0Z Removal of Drainage Device from Head and Neck Subcutaneous Tissue and Fascia, External Approach

0JPSX1Z Removal of Radioactive Element from Head and Neck Subcutaneous Tissue and Fascia, External Approach

0JPSX3Z Removal of Infusion Device from Head and Neck Subcutaneous Tissue and Fascia, External Approach

0JPT00Z Removal of Drainage Device from Trunk Subcutaneous Tissue and Fascia, Open Approach

0JPT01Z Removal of Radioactive Element from Trunk Subcutaneous Tissue and Fascia, Open Approach

0JPT02Z Removal of Monitoring Device from Trunk Subcutaneous Tissue and Fascia, Open Approach

0JPT03Z Removal of Infusion Device from Trunk Subcutaneous Tissue and Fascia, Open Approach

0JPT07Z Removal of Autologous Tissue Substitute from Trunk Subcutaneous Tissue and Fascia, Open Approach

0JPT0HZ Removal of Contraceptive Device from Trunk Subcutaneous Tissue and Fascia, Open Approach

0JPT0JZ Removal of Synthetic Substitute from Trunk Subcutaneous Tissue and Fascia, Open Approach

0JPT0KZ Removal of Nonautologous Tissue Substitute from Trunk Subcutaneous Tissue and Fascia, Open Approach

0JPT0MZ Removal of Stimulator Generator from Trunk Subcutaneous Tissue and Fascia, Open Approach

0JPT0NZ Removal of Tissue Expander from Trunk Subcutaneous Tissue and Fascia, Open Approach
AHA CC: 4Q, 2013, 109-111

0JPT0PZ Removal of Cardiac Rhythm Related Device from Trunk Subcutaneous Tissue and Fascia, Open Approach
AHA CC: 4Q, 2012, 104-106
With a secondary diagnosis code of K68.11, T81.4XXA, T82.6XXA, T82.7XXA

0JPT0VZ Removal of Infusion Pump from Trunk Subcutaneous Tissue and Fascia, Open Approach
AHA CC: 3Q, 2014, 19-20

0JPT0WZ Removal of Reservoir from Trunk Subcutaneous Tissue and Fascia, Open Approach

0JPT0XZ Removal of Vascular Access Device from Trunk Subcutaneous Tissue and Fascia, Open Approach

0JPT30Z Removal of Drainage Device from Trunk Subcutaneous Tissue and Fascia, Percutaneous Approach

0JPT31Z Removal of Radioactive Element from Trunk Subcutaneous Tissue and Fascia, Percutaneous Approach

0JPT32Z Removal of Monitoring Device from Trunk Subcutaneous Tissue and Fascia, Percutaneous Approach

0JPT33Z Removal of Infusion Device from Trunk Subcutaneous Tissue and Fascia, Percutaneous Approach

0JPT37Z Removal of Autologous Tissue Substitute from Trunk Subcutaneous Tissue and Fascia, Percutaneous Approach

0JPT3HZ Removal of Contraceptive Device from Trunk Subcutaneous Tissue and Fascia, Percutaneous Approach

0JPT3JZ Removal of Synthetic Substitute from Trunk Subcutaneous Tissue and Fascia, Percutaneous Approach

0JPT3KZ Removal of Nonautologous Tissue Substitute from Trunk Subcutaneous Tissue and Fascia, Percutaneous Approach

0JPT3MZ Removal of Stimulator Generator from Trunk Subcutaneous Tissue and Fascia, Percutaneous Approach

0JPT3NZ Removal of Tissue Expander from Trunk Subcutaneous Tissue and Fascia, Percutaneous Approach

0JPT3PZ Removal of Cardiac Rhythm Related Device from Trunk Subcutaneous Tissue and Fascia, Percutaneous Approach
With a secondary diagnosis code of K68.11, T81.4XXA, T82.6XXA, T82.7XXA

0JPT3VZ Removal of Infusion Pump from Trunk Subcutaneous Tissue and Fascia, Percutaneous Approach

0JPT3WZ Removal of Reservoir from Trunk Subcutaneous Tissue and Fascia, Percutaneous Approach

♀ Female-only   ♂ Male-only   ▲ Limited Coverage   ● Non-OR   HAC HAC-associated procedure   ▲ Non-covered procedures   ✛ Combination

T3XZ	Removal of Vascular Access Device from Trunk Subcutaneous Tissue and Fascia, Percutaneous Approach	
TX0Z	Removal of Drainage Device from Trunk Subcutaneous Tissue and Fascia, External Approach	
TX1Z	Removal of Radioactive Element from Trunk Subcutaneous Tissue and Fascia, External Approach	
TX2Z	Removal of Monitoring Device from Trunk Subcutaneous Tissue and Fascia, External Approach	
TX3Z	Removal of Infusion Device from Trunk Subcutaneous Tissue and Fascia, External Approach	
TXHZ	Removal of Contraceptive Device from Trunk Subcutaneous Tissue and Fascia, External Approach	
TXVZ	Removal of Infusion Pump from Trunk Subcutaneous Tissue and Fascia, External Approach	
TXXZ	Removal of Vascular Access Device from Trunk Subcutaneous Tissue and Fascia, External Approach	
V00Z	Removal of Drainage Device from Upper Extremity Subcutaneous Tissue and Fascia, Open Approach	
V01Z	Removal of Radioactive Element from Upper Extremity Subcutaneous Tissue and Fascia, Open Approach	
V03Z	Removal of Infusion Device from Upper Extremity Subcutaneous Tissue and Fascia, Open Approach	
V07Z	Removal of Autologous Tissue Substitute from Upper Extremity Subcutaneous Tissue and Fascia, Open Approach	
V0HZ	Removal of Contraceptive Device from Upper Extremity Subcutaneous Tissue and Fascia, Open Approach	
V0JZ	Removal of Synthetic Substitute from Upper Extremity Subcutaneous Tissue and Fascia, Open Approach	
V0KZ	Removal of Nonautologous Tissue Substitute from Upper Extremity Subcutaneous Tissue and Fascia, Open Approach	
V0NZ	Removal of Tissue Expander from Upper Extremity Subcutaneous Tissue and Fascia, Open Approach	
V0VZ	Removal of Infusion Pump from Upper Extremity Subcutaneous Tissue and Fascia, Open Approach	
V0WZ	Removal of Reservoir from Upper Extremity Subcutaneous Tissue and Fascia, Open Approach	
V0XZ	Removal of Vascular Access Device from Upper Extremity Subcutaneous Tissue and Fascia, Open Approach	
V30Z	Removal of Drainage Device from Upper Extremity Subcutaneous Tissue and Fascia, Percutaneous Approach	
V31Z	Removal of Radioactive Element from Upper Extremity Subcutaneous Tissue and Fascia, Percutaneous Approach	
V33Z	Removal of Infusion Device from Upper Extremity Subcutaneous Tissue and Fascia, Percutaneous Approach	

0JPV37Z	Removal of Autologous Tissue Substitute from Upper Extremity Subcutaneous Tissue and Fascia, Percutaneous Approach
0JPV3HZ	Removal of Contraceptive Device from Upper Extremity Subcutaneous Tissue and Fascia, Percutaneous Approach
0JPV3JZ	Removal of Synthetic Substitute from Upper Extremity Subcutaneous Tissue and Fascia, Percutaneous Approach
0JPV3KZ	Removal of Nonautologous Tissue Substitute from Upper Extremity Subcutaneous Tissue and Fascia, Percutaneous Approach
0JPV3NZ	Removal of Tissue Expander from Upper Extremity Subcutaneous Tissue and Fascia, Percutaneous Approach
0JPV3VZ	Removal of Infusion Pump from Upper Extremity Subcutaneous Tissue and Fascia, Percutaneous Approach
0JPV3WZ	Removal of Reservoir from Upper Extremity Subcutaneous Tissue and Fascia, Percutaneous Approach
0JPV3XZ	Removal of Vascular Access Device from Upper Extremity Subcutaneous Tissue and Fascia, Percutaneous Approach
0JPVX0Z	Removal of Drainage Device from Upper Extremity Subcutaneous Tissue and Fascia, External Approach
0JPVX1Z	Removal of Radioactive Element from Upper Extremity Subcutaneous Tissue and Fascia, External Approach
0JPVX3Z	Removal of Infusion Device from Upper Extremity Subcutaneous Tissue and Fascia, External Approach
0JPVXHZ	Removal of Contraceptive Device from Upper Extremity Subcutaneous Tissue and Fascia, External Approach
0JPVXVZ	Removal of Infusion Pump from Upper Extremity Subcutaneous Tissue and Fascia, External Approach
0JPVXXZ	Removal of Vascular Access Device from Upper Extremity Subcutaneous Tissue and Fascia, External Approach
0JPW00Z	Removal of Drainage Device from Lower Extremity Subcutaneous Tissue and Fascia, Open Approach
0JPW01Z	Removal of Radioactive Element from Lower Extremity Subcutaneous Tissue and Fascia, Open Approach
0JPW03Z	Removal of Infusion Device from Lower Extremity Subcutaneous Tissue and Fascia, Open Approach
0JPW07Z	Removal of Autologous Tissue Substitute from Lower Extremity Subcutaneous Tissue and Fascia, Open Approach
0JPW0HZ	Removal of Contraceptive Device from Lower Extremity Subcutaneous Tissue and Fascia, Open Approach
0JPW0JZ	Removal of Synthetic Substitute from Lower Extremity Subcutaneous Tissue and Fascia, Open Approach
0JPW0KZ	Removal of Nonautologous Tissue Substitute from Lower Extremity Subcutaneous Tissue and Fascia, Open Approach

0JPW0NZ	Removal of Tissue Expander from Lower Extremity Subcutaneous Tissue and Fascia, Open Approach
0JPW0VZ	Removal of Infusion Pump from Lower Extremity Subcutaneous Tissue and Fascia, Open Approach
0JPW0WZ	Removal of Reservoir from Lower Extremity Subcutaneous Tissue and Fascia, Open Approach
0JPW0XZ	Removal of Vascular Access Device from Lower Extremity Subcutaneous Tissue and Fascia, Open Approach
0JPW30Z	Removal of Drainage Device from Lower Extremity Subcutaneous Tissue and Fascia, Percutaneous Approach
0JPW31Z	Removal of Radioactive Element from Lower Extremity Subcutaneous Tissue and Fascia, Percutaneous Approach
0JPW33Z	Removal of Infusion Device from Lower Extremity Subcutaneous Tissue and Fascia, Percutaneous Approach
0JPW37Z	Removal of Autologous Tissue Substitute from Lower Extremity Subcutaneous Tissue and Fascia, Percutaneous Approach
0JPW3HZ	Removal of Contraceptive Device from Lower Extremity Subcutaneous Tissue and Fascia, Percutaneous Approach
0JPW3JZ	Removal of Synthetic Substitute from Lower Extremity Subcutaneous Tissue and Fascia, Percutaneous Approach
0JPW3KZ	Removal of Nonautologous Tissue Substitute from Lower Extremity Subcutaneous Tissue and Fascia, Percutaneous Approach
0JPW3NZ	Removal of Tissue Expander from Lower Extremity Subcutaneous Tissue and Fascia, Percutaneous Approach
0JPW3VZ	Removal of Infusion Pump from Lower Extremity Subcutaneous Tissue and Fascia, Percutaneous Approach
0JPW3WZ	Removal of Reservoir from Lower Extremity Subcutaneous Tissue and Fascia, Percutaneous Approach
0JPW3XZ	Removal of Vascular Access Device from Lower Extremity Subcutaneous Tissue and Fascia, Percutaneous Approach
0JPWX0Z	Removal of Drainage Device from Lower Extremity Subcutaneous Tissue and Fascia, External Approach
0JPWX1Z	Removal of Radioactive Element from Lower Extremity Subcutaneous Tissue and Fascia, External Approach
0JPWX3Z	Removal of Infusion Device from Lower Extremity Subcutaneous Tissue and Fascia, External Approach
0JPWXHZ	Removal of Contraceptive Device from Lower Extremity Subcutaneous Tissue and Fascia, External Approach
0JPWXVZ	Removal of Infusion Pump from Lower Extremity Subcutaneous Tissue and Fascia, External Approach
0JPWXXZ	Removal of Vascular Access Device from Lower Extremity Subcutaneous Tissue and Fascia, External Approach

0JQ – Subcutaneous Tissue and Fascia, Repair

Review Coding Guideline B3.5

0JQ00ZZ	Repair Scalp Subcutaneous Tissue and Fascia, Open Approach	
0JQ03ZZ	Repair Scalp Subcutaneous Tissue and Fascia, Percutaneous Approach	
0JQ10ZZ	Repair Face Subcutaneous Tissue and Fascia, Open Approach	

0JQ13ZZ	Repair Face Subcutaneous Tissue and Fascia, Percutaneous Approach
0JQ40ZZ	Repair Anterior Neck Subcutaneous Tissue and Fascia, Open Approach
0JQ43ZZ	Repair Anterior Neck Subcutaneous Tissue and Fascia, Percutaneous Approach

0JQ50ZZ	Repair Posterior Neck Subcutaneous Tissue and Fascia, Open Approach
0JQ53ZZ	Repair Posterior Neck Subcutaneous Tissue and Fascia, Percutaneous Approach
0JQ60ZZ	Repair Chest Subcutaneous Tissue and Fascia, Open Approach

Female-only ♂ Male-only ▲ Limited Coverage ● Non-OR ▦ HAC-associated procedure ▲ Non-covered procedures ✛ Combination

0JQ63ZZ Repair Chest Subcutaneous Tissue and Fascia, Percutaneous Approach

0JQ70ZZ Repair Back Subcutaneous Tissue and Fascia, Open Approach

0JQ73ZZ Repair Back Subcutaneous Tissue and Fascia, Percutaneous Approach

0JQ80ZZ Repair Abdomen Subcutaneous Tissue and Fascia, Open Approach

0JQ83ZZ Repair Abdomen Subcutaneous Tissue and Fascia, Percutaneous Approach

0JQ90ZZ Repair Buttock Subcutaneous Tissue and Fascia, Open Approach

0JQ93ZZ Repair Buttock Subcutaneous Tissue and Fascia, Percutaneous Approach

0JQB0ZZ Repair Perineum Subcutaneous Tissue and Fascia, Open Approach

0JQB3ZZ Repair Perineum Subcutaneous Tissue and Fascia, Percutaneous Approach

0JQC0ZZ Repair Pelvic Region Subcutaneous Tissue and Fascia, Open Approach
AHA CC: 4Q, 2014, 44-45

0JQC3ZZ Repair Pelvic Region Subcutaneous Tissue and Fascia, Percutaneous Approach

0JQD0ZZ Repair Right Upper Arm Subcutaneous Tissue and Fascia, Open Approach

0JQD3ZZ Repair Right Upper Arm Subcutaneous Tissue and Fascia, Percutaneous Approach

0JQF0ZZ Repair Left Upper Arm Subcutaneous Tissue and Fascia, Open Approach

0JQF3ZZ Repair Left Upper Arm Subcutaneous Tissue and Fascia, Percutaneous Approach

0JQG0ZZ Repair Right Lower Arm Subcutaneous Tissue and Fascia, Open Approach

0JQG3ZZ Repair Right Lower Arm Subcutaneous Tissue and Fascia, Percutaneous Approach

0JQH0ZZ Repair Left Lower Arm Subcutaneous Tissue and Fascia, Open Approach

0JQH3ZZ Repair Left Lower Arm Subcutaneous Tissue and Fascia, Percutaneous Approach

0JQJ0ZZ Repair Right Hand Subcutaneous Tissue and Fascia, Open Approach

0JQJ3ZZ Repair Right Hand Subcutaneous Tissue and Fascia, Percutaneous Approach

0JQK0ZZ Repair Left Hand Subcutaneous Tissue and Fascia, Open Approach

0JQK3ZZ Repair Left Hand Subcutaneous Tissue and Fascia, Percutaneous Approach

0JQL0ZZ Repair Right Upper Leg Subcutaneous Tissue and Fascia, Open Approach

0JQL3ZZ Repair Right Upper Leg Subcutaneous Tissue and Fascia, Percutaneous Appro

0JQM0ZZ Repair Left Upper Leg Subcutaneous Tissue and Fascia, Open Approach

0JQM3ZZ Repair Left Upper Leg Subcutaneous Tissue and Fascia, Percutaneous Appro

0JQN0ZZ Repair Right Lower Leg Subcutaneous Tissue and Fascia, Open Approach

0JQN3ZZ Repair Right Lower Leg Subcutaneous Tissue and Fascia, Percutaneous Appro

0JQP0ZZ Repair Left Lower Leg Subcutaneous Tissue and Fascia, Open Approach

0JQP3ZZ Repair Left Lower Leg Subcutaneous Tissue and Fascia, Percutaneous Appro

0JQQ0ZZ Repair Right Foot Subcutaneous Tissue and Fascia, Open Approach

0JQQ3ZZ Repair Right Foot Subcutaneous Tissue and Fascia, Percutaneous Approach

0JQR0ZZ Repair Left Foot Subcutaneous Tissue and Fascia, Open Approach

0JQR3ZZ Repair Left Foot Subcutaneous Tissue and Fascia, Percutaneous Approach

0JR – Subcutaneous Tissue and Fascia, Replacement

0JR007Z Replacement of Scalp Subcutaneous Tissue and Fascia with Autologous Tissue Substitute, Open Approach

0JR00JZ Replacement of Scalp Subcutaneous Tissue and Fascia with Synthetic Substitute, Open Approach

0JR00KZ Replacement of Scalp Subcutaneous Tissue and Fascia with Nonautologous Tissue Substitute, Open Approach

0JR037Z Replacement of Scalp Subcutaneous Tissue and Fascia with Autologous Tissue Substitute, Percutaneous Approach

0JR03JZ Replacement of Scalp Subcutaneous Tissue and Fascia with Synthetic Substitute, Percutaneous Approach

0JR03KZ Replacement of Scalp Subcutaneous Tissue and Fascia with Nonautologous Tissue Substitute, Percutaneous Approach

0JR107Z Replacement of Face Subcutaneous Tissue and Fascia with Autologous Tissue Substitute, Open Approach

0JR10JZ Replacement of Face Subcutaneous Tissue and Fascia with Synthetic Substitute, Open Approach

0JR10KZ Replacement of Face Subcutaneous Tissue and Fascia with Nonautologous Tissue Substitute, Open Approach

0JR137Z Replacement of Face Subcutaneous Tissue and Fascia with Autologous Tissue Substitute, Percutaneous Approach

0JR13JZ Replacement of Face Subcutaneous Tissue and Fascia with Synthetic Substitute, Percutaneous Approach

0JR13KZ Replacement of Face Subcutaneous Tissue and Fascia with Nonautologous Tissue Substitute, Percutaneous Approach

0JR407Z Replacement of Anterior Neck Subcutaneous Tissue and Fascia with Autologous Tissue Substitute, Open Approach

0JR40JZ Replacement of Anterior Neck Subcutaneous Tissue and Fascia with Synthetic Substitute, Open Approach

0JR40KZ Replacement of Anterior Neck Subcutaneous Tissue and Fascia with Nonautologous Tissue Substitute, Open Approach

0JR437Z Replacement of Anterior Neck Subcutaneous Tissue and Fascia with Autologous Tissue Substitute, Percutaneous Approach

0JR43JZ Replacement of Anterior Neck Subcutaneous Tissue and Fascia with Synthetic Substitute, Percutaneous Approach

0JR43KZ Replacement of Anterior Neck Subcutaneous Tissue and Fascia with Nonautologous Tissue Substitute, Percutaneous Approach

0JR507Z Replacement of Posterior Neck Subcutaneous Tissue and Fascia with Autologous Tissue Substitute, Open Approach

0JR50JZ Replacement of Posterior Neck Subcutaneous Tissue and Fascia with Synthetic Substitute, Open Approach

0JR50KZ Replacement of Posterior Neck Subcutaneous Tissue and Fascia with Nonautologous Tissue Substitute, Open Approach

0JR537Z Replacement of Posterior Neck Subcutaneous Tissue and Fascia with Autologous Tissue Substitute, Percutaneous Approach

0JR53JZ Replacement of Posterior Neck Subcutaneous Tissue and Fascia with Synthetic Substitute, Percutaneous Approach

0JR53KZ Replacement of Posterior Neck Subcutaneous Tissue and Fascia with Nonautologous Tissue Substitute, Percutaneous Approach

0JR607Z Replacement of Chest Subcutaneous Tissue and Fascia with Autologous Tissue Substitute, Open Approach

0JR60JZ Replacement of Chest Subcutaneous Tissue and Fascia with Synthetic Substitute, Open Approach

0JR60KZ Replacement of Chest Subcutaneous Tissue and Fascia with Nonautologous Tissue Substitute, Open Approach

0JR637Z Replacement of Chest Subcutaneous Tissue and Fascia with Autologous Tissue Substitute, Percutaneous Approach

0JR63JZ Replacement of Chest Subcutaneous Tissue and Fascia with Synthetic Substitute, Percutaneous Approach

0JR63KZ Replacement of Chest Subcutaneous Tissue and Fascia with Nonautologous Tissue Substitute, Percutaneous Approach

0JR707Z Replacement of Back Subcutaneous Tissue and Fascia with Autologous Tiss Substitute, Open Approach

0JR70JZ Replacement of Back Subcutaneous Tis and Fascia with Synthetic Substitute, O Approach

0JR70KZ Replacement of Back Subcutaneous Tis and Fascia with Nonautologous Tissue Substitute, Open Approach

0JR737Z Replacement of Back Subcutaneous Tissue and Fascia with Autologous Tiss Substitute, Percutaneous Approach

0JR73JZ Replacement of Back Subcutaneous Tis and Fascia with Synthetic Substitute, Percutaneous Approach

0JR73KZ Replacement of Back Subcutaneous Tis and Fascia with Nonautologous Tissue Substitute, Percutaneous Approach

0JR807Z Replacement of Abdomen Subcutaneou Tissue and Fascia with Autologous Tiss Substitute, Open Approach

0JR80JZ Replacement of Abdomen Subcutaneous Tissue and Fascia with Synthetic Substitute, Open Approach

0JR80KZ Replacement of Abdomen Subcutaneous Tissue and Fascia with Nonautologous Tissue Substitute, Open Approach

0JR837Z Replacement of Abdomen Subcutaneous Tissue and Fascia with Autologous Tissu Substitute, Percutaneous Approach

0JR83JZ Replacement of Abdomen Subcutaneous Tissue and Fascia with Synthetic Substitute, Percutaneous Approach

0JR83KZ Replacement of Abdomen Subcutaneous Tissue and Fascia with Nonautologous Tissue Substitute, Percutaneous Approac

0JR907Z Replacement of Buttock Subcutaneous Tissue and Fascia with Autologous Tissu Substitute, Open Approach

0JR90JZ Replacement of Buttock Subcutaneous Tissue and Fascia with Synthetic Substitute, Open Approach

0JR90KZ Replacement of Buttock Subcutaneous Tissue and Fascia with Nonautologous Tissue Substitute, Open Approach

0JR937Z Replacement of Buttock Subcutaneous Tissue and Fascia with Autologous Tissu Substitute, Percutaneous Approach

0JR93JZ Replacement of Buttock Subcutaneous Tissue and Fascia with Synthetic Substitute, Percutaneous Approach

♀ Female-only   ♂ Male-only   ▲ Limited Coverage   ● Non-OR   ▬ HAC-associated procedure   ▲ Non-covered procedures   ✛ Combinati

93KZ	Replacement of Buttock Subcutaneous Tissue and Fascia with Nonautologous Tissue Substitute, Percutaneous Approach
B07Z	Replacement of Perineum Subcutaneous Tissue and Fascia with Autologous Tissue Substitute, Open Approach
B0JZ	Replacement of Perineum Subcutaneous Tissue and Fascia with Synthetic Substitute, Open Approach
B0KZ	Replacement of Perineum Subcutaneous Tissue and Fascia with Nonautologous Tissue Substitute, Open Approach
B37Z	Replacement of Perineum Subcutaneous Tissue and Fascia with Autologous Tissue Substitute, Percutaneous Approach
B3JZ	Replacement of Perineum Subcutaneous Tissue and Fascia with Synthetic Substitute, Percutaneous Approach
B3KZ	Replacement of Perineum Subcutaneous Tissue and Fascia with Nonautologous Tissue Substitute, Percutaneous Approach
C07Z	Replacement of Pelvic Region Subcutaneous Tissue and Fascia with Autologous Tissue Substitute, Open Approach
C0JZ	Replacement of Pelvic Region Subcutaneous Tissue and Fascia with Synthetic Substitute, Open Approach
C0KZ	Replacement of Pelvic Region Subcutaneous Tissue and Fascia with Nonautologous Tissue Substitute, Open Approach
C37Z	Replacement of Pelvic Region Subcutaneous Tissue and Fascia with Autologous Tissue Substitute, Percutaneous Approach
C3JZ	Replacement of Pelvic Region Subcutaneous Tissue and Fascia with Synthetic Substitute, Percutaneous Approach
C3KZ	Replacement of Pelvic Region Subcutaneous Tissue and Fascia with Nonautologous Tissue Substitute, Percutaneous Approach
D07Z	Replacement of Right Upper Arm Subcutaneous Tissue and Fascia with Autologous Tissue Substitute, Open Approach
D0JZ	Replacement of Right Upper Arm Subcutaneous Tissue and Fascia with Synthetic Substitute, Open Approach
D0KZ	Replacement of Right Upper Arm Subcutaneous Tissue and Fascia with Nonautologous Tissue Substitute, Open Approach
D37Z	Replacement of Right Upper Arm Subcutaneous Tissue and Fascia with Autologous Tissue Substitute, Percutaneous Approach
D3JZ	Replacement of Right Upper Arm Subcutaneous Tissue and Fascia with Synthetic Substitute, Percutaneous Approach
D3KZ	Replacement of Right Upper Arm Subcutaneous Tissue and Fascia with Nonautologous Tissue Substitute, Percutaneous Approach
RF07Z	Replacement of Left Upper Arm Subcutaneous Tissue and Fascia with Autologous Tissue Substitute, Open Approach
RF0JZ	Replacement of Left Upper Arm Subcutaneous Tissue and Fascia with Synthetic Substitute, Open Approach
RF0KZ	Replacement of Left Upper Arm Subcutaneous Tissue and Fascia with Nonautologous Tissue Substitute, Open Approach

0JRF37Z	Replacement of Left Upper Arm Subcutaneous Tissue and Fascia with Autologous Tissue Substitute, Percutaneous Approach
0JRF3JZ	Replacement of Left Upper Arm Subcutaneous Tissue and Fascia with Synthetic Substitute, Percutaneous Approach
0JRF3KZ	Replacement of Left Upper Arm Subcutaneous Tissue and Fascia with Nonautologous Tissue Substitute, Percutaneous Approach
0JRG07Z	Replacement of Right Lower Arm Subcutaneous Tissue and Fascia with Autologous Tissue Substitute, Open Approach
0JRG0JZ	Replacement of Right Lower Arm Subcutaneous Tissue and Fascia with Synthetic Substitute, Open Approach
0JRG0KZ	Replacement of Right Lower Arm Subcutaneous Tissue and Fascia with Nonautologous Tissue Substitute, Open Approach
0JRG37Z	Replacement of Right Lower Arm Subcutaneous Tissue and Fascia with Autologous Tissue Substitute, Percutaneous Approach
0JRG3JZ	Replacement of Right Lower Arm Subcutaneous Tissue and Fascia with Synthetic Substitute, Percutaneous Approach
0JRG3KZ	Replacement of Right Lower Arm Subcutaneous Tissue and Fascia with Nonautologous Tissue Substitute, Percutaneous Approach
0JRH07Z	Replacement of Left Lower Arm Subcutaneous Tissue and Fascia with Autologous Tissue Substitute, Open Approach
0JRH0JZ	Replacement of Left Lower Arm Subcutaneous Tissue and Fascia with Synthetic Substitute, Open Approach
0JRH0KZ	Replacement of Left Lower Arm Subcutaneous Tissue and Fascia with Nonautologous Tissue Substitute, Open Approach
0JRH37Z	Replacement of Left Lower Arm Subcutaneous Tissue and Fascia with Autologous Tissue Substitute, Percutaneous Approach
0JRH3JZ	Replacement of Left Lower Arm Subcutaneous Tissue and Fascia with Synthetic Substitute, Percutaneous Approach
0JRH3KZ	Replacement of Left Lower Arm Subcutaneous Tissue and Fascia with Nonautologous Tissue Substitute, Percutaneous Approach
0JRJ07Z	Replacement of Right Hand Subcutaneous Tissue and Fascia with Autologous Tissue Substitute, Open Approach
0JRJ0JZ	Replacement of Right Hand Subcutaneous Tissue and Fascia with Synthetic Substitute, Open Approach
0JRJ0KZ	Replacement of Right Hand Subcutaneous Tissue and Fascia with Nonautologous Tissue Substitute, Open Approach
0JRJ37Z	Replacement of Right Hand Subcutaneous Tissue and Fascia with Autologous Tissue Substitute, Percutaneous Approach
0JRJ3JZ	Replacement of Right Hand Subcutaneous Tissue and Fascia with Synthetic Substitute, Percutaneous Approach
0JRJ3KZ	Replacement of Right Hand Subcutaneous Tissue and Fascia with Nonautologous Tissue Substitute, Percutaneous Approach

0JRK07Z	Replacement of Left Hand Subcutaneous Tissue and Fascia with Autologous Tissue Substitute, Open Approach
0JRK0JZ	Replacement of Left Hand Subcutaneous Tissue and Fascia with Synthetic Substitute, Open Approach
0JRK0KZ	Replacement of Left Hand Subcutaneous Tissue and Fascia with Nonautologous Tissue Substitute, Open Approach
0JRK37Z	Replacement of Left Hand Subcutaneous Tissue and Fascia with Autologous Tissue Substitute, Percutaneous Approach
0JRK3JZ	Replacement of Left Hand Subcutaneous Tissue and Fascia with Synthetic Substitute, Percutaneous Approach
0JRK3KZ	Replacement of Left Hand Subcutaneous Tissue and Fascia with Nonautologous Tissue Substitute, Percutaneous Approach
0JRL07Z	Replacement of Right Upper Leg Subcutaneous Tissue and Fascia with Autologous Tissue Substitute, Open Approach
0JRL0JZ	Replacement of Right Upper Leg Subcutaneous Tissue and Fascia with Synthetic Substitute, Open Approach
0JRL0KZ	Replacement of Right Upper Leg Subcutaneous Tissue and Fascia with Nonautologous Tissue Substitute, Open Approach
0JRL37Z	Replacement of Right Upper Leg Subcutaneous Tissue and Fascia with Autologous Tissue Substitute, Percutaneous Approach
0JRL3JZ	Replacement of Right Upper Leg Subcutaneous Tissue and Fascia with Synthetic Substitute, Percutaneous Approach
0JRL3KZ	Replacement of Right Upper Leg Subcutaneous Tissue and Fascia with Nonautologous Tissue Substitute, Percutaneous Approach
0JRM07Z	Replacement of Left Upper Leg Subcutaneous Tissue and Fascia with Autologous Tissue Substitute, Open Approach
0JRM0JZ	Replacement of Left Upper Leg Subcutaneous Tissue and Fascia with Synthetic Substitute, Open Approach
0JRM0KZ	Replacement of Left Upper Leg Subcutaneous Tissue and Fascia with Nonautologous Tissue Substitute, Open Approach
0JRM37Z	Replacement of Left Upper Leg Subcutaneous Tissue and Fascia with Autologous Tissue Substitute, Percutaneous Approach
0JRM3JZ	Replacement of Left Upper Leg Subcutaneous Tissue and Fascia with Synthetic Substitute, Percutaneous Approach
0JRM3KZ	Replacement of Left Upper Leg Subcutaneous Tissue and Fascia with Nonautologous Tissue Substitute, Percutaneous Approach
0JRN07Z	Replacement of Right Lower Leg Subcutaneous Tissue and Fascia with Autologous Tissue Substitute, Open Approach
0JRN0JZ	Replacement of Right Lower Leg Subcutaneous Tissue and Fascia with Synthetic Substitute, Open Approach
0JRN0KZ	Replacement of Right Lower Leg Subcutaneous Tissue and Fascia with Nonautologous Tissue Substitute, Open Approach

Female-only	♂ Male-only	▲ Limited Coverage	● Non-OR	▰▰ HAC-associated procedure	▲ Non-covered procedures	✚ Combination

0JRN37Z Replacement of Right Lower Leg Subcutaneous Tissue and Fascia with Autologous Tissue Substitute, Percutaneous Approach

0JRN3JZ Replacement of Right Lower Leg Subcutaneous Tissue and Fascia with Synthetic Substitute, Percutaneous Approach

0JRN3KZ Replacement of Right Lower Leg Subcutaneous Tissue and Fascia with Nonautologous Tissue Substitute, Percutaneous Approach

0JRP07Z Replacement of Left Lower Leg Subcutaneous Tissue and Fascia with Autologous Tissue Substitute, Open Approach

0JRP0JZ Replacement of Left Lower Leg Subcutaneous Tissue and Fascia with Synthetic Substitute, Open Approach

0JRP0KZ Replacement of Left Lower Leg Subcutaneous Tissue and Fascia with Nonautologous Tissue Substitute, Open Approach

0JRP37Z Replacement of Left Lower Leg Subcutaneous Tissue and Fascia with Autologous Tissue Substitute, Percutaneous Approach

0JRP3JZ Replacement of Left Lower Leg Subcutaneous Tissue and Fascia with Synthetic Substitute, Percutaneous Approach

0JRP3KZ Replacement of Left Lower Leg Subcutaneous Tissue and Fascia with Nonautologous Tissue Substitute, Percutaneous Approach

0JRQ07Z Replacement of Right Foot Subcutaneous Tissue and Fascia with Autologous Tissue Substitute, Open Approach

0JRQ0JZ Replacement of Right Foot Subcutaneous Tissue and Fascia with Synthetic Substitute, Open Approach

0JRQ0KZ Replacement of Right Foot Subcutaneous Tissue and Fascia with Nonautologous Tissue Substitute, Open Approach

0JRQ37Z Replacement of Right Foot Subcutaneous Tissue and Fascia with Autologous Tissue Substitute, Percutaneous Approach

0JRQ3JZ Replacement of Right Foot Subcutane[ous] Tissue and Fascia with Synthetic Substitute, Percutaneous Approach

0JRQ3KZ Replacement of Right Foot Subcutane[ous] Tissue and Fascia with Nonautologous Tissue Substitute, Percutaneous Appro[ach]

0JRR07Z Replacement of Left Foot Subcutaneous Tissue and Fascia with Autologous Tis[sue] Substitute, Open Approach

0JRR0JZ Replacement of Left Foot Subcutaneou[s] Tissue and Fascia with Synthetic Substitute, Open Approach

0JRR0KZ Replacement of Left Foot Subcutaneou[s] Tissue and Fascia with Nonautologous Tissue Substitute, Open Approach

0JRR37Z Replacement of Left Foot Subcutaneou[s] Tissue and Fascia with Autologous Tis[sue] Substitute, Percutaneous Approach

0JRR3JZ Replacement of Left Foot Subcutaneou[s] Tissue and Fascia with Synthetic Substitute, Percutaneous Approach

0JRR3KZ Replacement of Left Foot Subcutaneou[s] Tissue and Fascia with Nonautologous Tissue Substitute, Percutaneous Appro[ach]

0JU – Subcutaneous Tissue and Fascia, Supplement

0JU007Z Supplement of Scalp Subcutaneous Tissue and Fascia with Autologous Tissue Substitute, Open Approach

0JU00JZ Supplement of Scalp Subcutaneous Tissue and Fascia with Synthetic Substitute, Open Approach

0JU00KZ Supplement of Scalp Subcutaneous Tissue and Fascia with Nonautologous Tissue Substitute, Open Approach

0JU037Z Supplement of Scalp Subcutaneous Tissue and Fascia with Autologous Tissue Substitute, Percutaneous Approach

0JU03JZ Supplement of Scalp Subcutaneous Tissue and Fascia with Synthetic Substitute, Percutaneous Approach

0JU03KZ Supplement of Scalp Subcutaneous Tissue and Fascia with Nonautologous Tissue Substitute, Percutaneous Approach

0JU107Z Supplement of Face Subcutaneous Tissue and Fascia with Autologous Tissue Substitute, Open Approach

0JU10JZ Supplement of Face Subcutaneous Tissue and Fascia with Synthetic Substitute, Open Approach

0JU10KZ Supplement of Face Subcutaneous Tissue and Fascia with Nonautologous Tissue Substitute, Open Approach

0JU137Z Supplement of Face Subcutaneous Tissue and Fascia with Autologous Tissue Substitute, Percutaneous Approach

0JU13JZ Supplement of Face Subcutaneous Tissue and Fascia with Synthetic Substitute, Percutaneous Approach

0JU13KZ Supplement of Face Subcutaneous Tissue and Fascia with Nonautologous Tissue Substitute, Percutaneous Approach

0JU407Z Supplement of Anterior Neck Subcutaneous Tissue and Fascia with Autologous Tissue Substitute, Open Approach

0JU40JZ Supplement of Anterior Neck Subcutaneous Tissue and Fascia with Synthetic Substitute, Open Approach

0JU40KZ Supplement of Anterior Neck Subcutaneous Tissue and Fascia with Nonautologous Tissue Substitute, Open Approach

0JU437Z Supplement of Anterior Neck Subcutaneous Tissue and Fascia with Autologous Tissue Substitute, Percutaneous Approach

0JU43JZ Supplement of Anterior Neck Subcutaneous Tissue and Fascia with Synthetic Substitute, Percutaneous Approach

0JU43KZ Supplement of Anterior Neck Subcutaneous Tissue and Fascia with Nonautologous Tissue Substitute, Percutaneous Approach

0JU507Z Supplement of Posterior Neck Subcutaneous Tissue and Fascia with Autologous Tissue Substitute, Open Approach

0JU50JZ Supplement of Posterior Neck Subcutaneous Tissue and Fascia with Synthetic Substitute, Open Approach

0JU50KZ Supplement of Posterior Neck Subcutaneous Tissue and Fascia with Nonautologous Tissue Substitute, Open Approach

0JU537Z Supplement of Posterior Neck Subcutaneous Tissue and Fascia with Autologous Tissue Substitute, Percutaneous Approach

0JU53JZ Supplement of Posterior Neck Subcutaneous Tissue and Fascia with Synthetic Substitute, Percutaneous Approach

0JU53KZ Supplement of Posterior Neck Subcutaneous Tissue and Fascia with Nonautologous Tissue Substitute, Percutaneous Approach

0JU607Z Supplement of Chest Subcutaneous Tissue and Fascia with Autologous Tissue Substitute, Open Approach

0JU60JZ Supplement of Chest Subcutaneous Tissue and Fascia with Synthetic Substitute, Open Approach

0JU60KZ Supplement of Chest Subcutaneous Tissue and Fascia with Nonautologous Tissue Substitute, Open Approach

0JU637Z Supplement of Chest Subcutaneous Tissue and Fascia with Autologous Tissue Substitute, Percutaneous Approach

0JU63JZ Supplement of Chest Subcutaneous Tissue and Fascia with Synthetic Substitute, Percutaneous Approach

0JU63KZ Supplement of Chest Subcutaneous Tissue and Fascia with Nonautologous Tissue Substitute, Percutaneous Approach

0JU707Z Supplement of Back Subcutaneous Tissue and Fascia with Autologous Tissue Substitute, Open Approach

0JU70JZ Supplement of Back Subcutaneous Tiss[ue] and Fascia with Synthetic Substitute, O[pen] Approach

0JU70KZ Supplement of Back Subcutaneous Tiss[ue] and Fascia with Nonautologous Tissue Substitute, Open Approach

0JU737Z Supplement of Back Subcutaneous Tissue and Fascia with Autologous Tiss[ue] Substitute, Percutaneous Approach

0JU73JZ Supplement of Back Subcutaneous Tiss[ue] and Fascia with Synthetic Substitute, Percutaneous Approach

0JU73KZ Supplement of Back Subcutaneous Tiss[ue] and Fascia with Nonautologous Tissue Substitute, Percutaneous Approach

0JU807Z Supplement of Abdomen Subcutaneous Tissue and Fascia with Autologous Tiss[ue] Substitute, Open Approach

0JU80JZ Supplement of Abdomen Subcutaneous Tissue and Fascia with Synthetic Substitute, Open Approach

0JU80KZ Supplement of Abdomen Subcutaneous Tissue and Fascia with Nonautologous Tissue Substitute, Open Approach

0JU837Z Supplement of Abdomen Subcutaneous Tissue and Fascia with Autologous Tiss[ue] Substitute, Percutaneous Approach

0JU83JZ Supplement of Abdomen Subcutaneous Tissue and Fascia with Synthetic Substitute, Percutaneous Approach

0JU83KZ Supplement of Abdomen Subcutaneous Tissue and Fascia with Nonautologous Tissue Substitute, Percutaneous Approac[h]

0JU907Z Supplement of Buttock Subcutaneous Tissue and Fascia with Autologous Tissu[e] Substitute, Open Approach

0JU90JZ Supplement of Buttock Subcutaneous Tissue and Fascia with Synthetic Substitute, Open Approach

0JU90KZ Supplement of Buttock Subcutaneous Tissue and Fascia with Nonautologous Tissue Substitute, Open Approach

0JU937Z Supplement of Buttock Subcutaneous Tissue and Fascia with Autologous Tissu[e] Substitute, Percutaneous Approach

0JU93JZ Supplement of Buttock Subcutaneous Tissue and Fascia with Synthetic Substitute, Percutaneous Approach

0JU93KZ Supplement of Buttock Subcutaneous Tissue and Fascia with Nonautologous Tissue Substitute, Percutaneous Approac[h]

♀ Female-only   ♂ Male-only   ▲ Limited Coverage   ●Non-OR   ■HAC-associated procedure   ▲Non-covered procedures   ✚ Combinati[on]

0JB07Z   Supplement of Perineum Subcutaneous Tissue and Fascia with Autologous Tissue Substitute, Open Approach

0JB0JZ   Supplement of Perineum Subcutaneous Tissue and Fascia with Synthetic Substitute, Open Approach

0JB0KZ   Supplement of Perineum Subcutaneous Tissue and Fascia with Nonautologous Tissue Substitute, Open Approach

0JB37Z   Supplement of Perineum Subcutaneous Tissue and Fascia with Autologous Tissue Substitute, Percutaneous Approach

0JB3JZ   Supplement of Perineum Subcutaneous Tissue and Fascia with Synthetic Substitute, Percutaneous Approach

0JB3KZ   Supplement of Perineum Subcutaneous Tissue and Fascia with Nonautologous Tissue Substitute, Percutaneous Approach

0JUC07Z   Supplement of Pelvic Region Subcutaneous Tissue and Fascia with Autologous Tissue Substitute, Open Approach

0JUC0JZ   Supplement of Pelvic Region Subcutaneous Tissue and Fascia with Synthetic Substitute, Open Approach

0JUC0KZ   Supplement of Pelvic Region Subcutaneous Tissue and Fascia with Nonautologous Tissue Substitute, Open Approach

0JUC37Z   Supplement of Pelvic Region Subcutaneous Tissue and Fascia with Autologous Tissue Substitute, Percutaneous Approach

0JUC3JZ   Supplement of Pelvic Region Subcutaneous Tissue and Fascia with Synthetic Substitute, Percutaneous Approach

0JUC3KZ   Supplement of Pelvic Region Subcutaneous Tissue and Fascia with Nonautologous Tissue Substitute, Percutaneous Approach

0JUD07Z   Supplement of Right Upper Arm Subcutaneous Tissue and Fascia with Autologous Tissue Substitute, Open Approach

0JUD0JZ   Supplement of Right Upper Arm Subcutaneous Tissue and Fascia with Synthetic Substitute, Open Approach

0JUD0KZ   Supplement of Right Upper Arm Subcutaneous Tissue and Fascia with Nonautologous Tissue Substitute, Open Approach

0JUD37Z   Supplement of Right Upper Arm Subcutaneous Tissue and Fascia with Autologous Tissue Substitute, Percutaneous Approach

0JUD3JZ   Supplement of Right Upper Arm Subcutaneous Tissue and Fascia with Synthetic Substitute, Percutaneous Approach

0JUD3KZ   Supplement of Right Upper Arm Subcutaneous Tissue and Fascia with Nonautologous Tissue Substitute, Percutaneous Approach

0JUF07Z   Supplement of Left Upper Arm Subcutaneous Tissue and Fascia with Autologous Tissue Substitute, Open Approach

0JUF0JZ   Supplement of Left Upper Arm Subcutaneous Tissue and Fascia with Synthetic Substitute, Open Approach

0JUF0KZ   Supplement of Left Upper Arm Subcutaneous Tissue and Fascia with Nonautologous Tissue Substitute, Open Approach

0JUF37Z   Supplement of Left Upper Arm Subcutaneous Tissue and Fascia

with Autologous Tissue Substitute, Percutaneous Approach

0JUF3JZ   Supplement of Left Upper Arm Subcutaneous Tissue and Fascia with Synthetic Substitute, Percutaneous Approach

0JUF3KZ   Supplement of Left Upper Arm Subcutaneous Tissue and Fascia with Nonautologous Tissue Substitute, Percutaneous Approach

0JUG07Z   Supplement of Right Lower Arm Subcutaneous Tissue and Fascia with Autologous Tissue Substitute, Open Approach

0JUG0JZ   Supplement of Right Lower Arm Subcutaneous Tissue and Fascia with Synthetic Substitute, Open Approach

0JUG0KZ   Supplement of Right Lower Arm Subcutaneous Tissue and Fascia with Nonautologous Tissue Substitute, Open Approach

0JUG37Z   Supplement of Right Lower Arm Subcutaneous Tissue and Fascia with Autologous Tissue Substitute, Percutaneous Approach

0JUG3JZ   Supplement of Right Lower Arm Subcutaneous Tissue and Fascia with Synthetic Substitute, Percutaneous Approach

0JUG3KZ   Supplement of Right Lower Arm Subcutaneous Tissue and Fascia with Nonautologous Tissue Substitute, Percutaneous Approach

0JUH07Z   Supplement of Left Lower Arm Subcutaneous Tissue and Fascia with Autologous Tissue Substitute, Open Approach

0JUH0JZ   Supplement of Left Lower Arm Subcutaneous Tissue and Fascia with Synthetic Substitute, Open Approach

0JUH0KZ   Supplement of Left Lower Arm Subcutaneous Tissue and Fascia with Nonautologous Tissue Substitute, Open Approach

0JUH37Z   Supplement of Left Lower Arm Subcutaneous Tissue and Fascia with Autologous Tissue Substitute, Percutaneous Approach

0JUH3JZ   Supplement of Left Lower Arm Subcutaneous Tissue and Fascia with Synthetic Substitute, Percutaneous Approach

0JUH3KZ   Supplement of Left Lower Arm Subcutaneous Tissue and Fascia with Nonautologous Tissue Substitute, Percutaneous Approach

0JUJ07Z   Supplement of Right Hand Subcutaneous Tissue and Fascia with Autologous Tissue Substitute, Open Approach

0JUJ0JZ   Supplement of Right Hand Subcutaneous Tissue and Fascia with Synthetic Substitute, Open Approach

0JUJ0KZ   Supplement of Right Hand Subcutaneous Tissue and Fascia with Nonautologous Tissue Substitute, Open Approach

0JUJ37Z   Supplement of Right Hand Subcutaneous Tissue and Fascia with Autologous Tissue Substitute, Percutaneous Approach

0JUJ3JZ   Supplement of Right Hand Subcutaneous Tissue and Fascia with Synthetic Substitute, Percutaneous Approach

0JUJ3KZ   Supplement of Right Hand Subcutaneous Tissue and Fascia with Nonautologous Tissue Substitute, Percutaneous Approach

0JUK07Z   Supplement of Left Hand Subcutaneous Tissue and Fascia with Autologous Tissue Substitute, Open Approach

0JUK0JZ   Supplement of Left Hand Subcutaneous Tissue and Fascia with Synthetic Substitute, Open Approach

0JUK0KZ   Supplement of Left Hand Subcutaneous Tissue and Fascia with Nonautologous Tissue Substitute, Open Approach

0JUK37Z   Supplement of Left Hand Subcutaneous Tissue and Fascia with Autologous Tissue Substitute, Percutaneous Approach

0JUK3JZ   Supplement of Left Hand Subcutaneous Tissue and Fascia with Synthetic Substitute, Percutaneous Approach

0JUK3KZ   Supplement of Left Hand Subcutaneous Tissue and Fascia with Nonautologous Tissue Substitute, Percutaneous Approach

0JUL07Z   Supplement of Right Upper Leg Subcutaneous Tissue and Fascia with Autologous Tissue Substitute, Open Approach

0JUL0JZ   Supplement of Right Upper Leg Subcutaneous Tissue and Fascia with Synthetic Substitute, Open Approach

0JUL0KZ   Supplement of Right Upper Leg Subcutaneous Tissue and Fascia with Nonautologous Tissue Substitute, Open Approach

0JUL37Z   Supplement of Right Upper Leg Subcutaneous Tissue and Fascia with Autologous Tissue Substitute, Percutaneous Approach

0JUL3JZ   Supplement of Right Upper Leg Subcutaneous Tissue and Fascia with Synthetic Substitute, Percutaneous Approach

0JUL3KZ   Supplement of Right Upper Leg Subcutaneous Tissue and Fascia with Nonautologous Tissue Substitute, Percutaneous Approach

0JUM07Z   Supplement of Left Upper Leg Subcutaneous Tissue and Fascia with Autologous Tissue Substitute, Open Approach

0JUM0JZ   Supplement of Left Upper Leg Subcutaneous Tissue and Fascia with Synthetic Substitute, Open Approach

0JUM0KZ   Supplement of Left Upper Leg Subcutaneous Tissue and Fascia with Nonautologous Tissue Substitute, Open Approach

0JUM37Z   Supplement of Left Upper Leg Subcutaneous Tissue and Fascia with Autologous Tissue Substitute, Percutaneous Approach

0JUM3JZ   Supplement of Left Upper Leg Subcutaneous Tissue and Fascia with Synthetic Substitute, Percutaneous Approach

0JUM3KZ   Supplement of Left Upper Leg Subcutaneous Tissue and Fascia with Nonautologous Tissue Substitute, Percutaneous Approach

0JUN07Z   Supplement of Right Lower Leg Subcutaneous Tissue and Fascia with Autologous Tissue Substitute, Open Approach

0JUN0JZ   Supplement of Right Lower Leg Subcutaneous Tissue and Fascia with Synthetic Substitute, Open Approach

0JUN0KZ   Supplement of Right Lower Leg Subcutaneous Tissue and Fascia with Nonautologous Tissue Substitute, Open Approach

0JUN37Z   Supplement of Right Lower Leg Subcutaneous Tissue and Fascia with Autologous Tissue Substitute, Percutaneous Approach

Female-only   ♂ Male-only   ▲ Limited Coverage   ● Non-OR   ▨ HAC-associated procedure   ▲ Non-covered procedures   ✛ Combination

0JUN3JZ Supplement of Right Lower Leg Subcutaneous Tissue and Fascia with Synthetic Substitute, Percutaneous Approach

0JUN3KZ Supplement of Right Lower Leg Subcutaneous Tissue and Fascia with Nonautologous Tissue Substitute, Percutaneous Approach

0JUP07Z Supplement of Left Lower Leg Subcutaneous Tissue and Fascia with Autologous Tissue Substitute, Open Approach

0JUP0JZ Supplement of Left Lower Leg Subcutaneous Tissue and Fascia with Synthetic Substitute, Open Approach

0JUP0KZ Supplement of Left Lower Leg Subcutaneous Tissue and Fascia with Nonautologous Tissue Substitute, Open Approach

0JUP37Z Supplement of Left Lower Leg Subcutaneous Tissue and Fascia with Autologous Tissue Substitute, Percutaneous Approach

0JUP3JZ Supplement of Left Lower Leg Subcutaneous Tissue and Fascia with Synthetic Substitute, Percutaneous Approach

0JUP3KZ Supplement of Left Lower Leg Subcutaneous Tissue and Fascia with Nonautologous Tissue Substitute, Percutaneous Approach

0JUQ07Z Supplement of Right Foot Subcutaneous Tissue and Fascia with Autologous Tissue Substitute, Open Approach

0JUQ0JZ Supplement of Right Foot Subcutaneous Tissue and Fascia with Synthetic Substitute, Open Approach

0JUQ0KZ Supplement of Right Foot Subcutaneous Tissue and Fascia with Nonautologous Tissue Substitute, Open Approach

0JUQ37Z Supplement of Right Foot Subcutaneous Tissue and Fascia with Autologous Tissue Substitute, Percutaneous Approach

0JUQ3JZ Supplement of Right Foot Subcutaneous Tissue and Fascia with Synthetic Substitute, Percutaneous Approach

0JUQ3KZ Supplement of Right Foot Subcutaneous Tissue and Fascia with Nonautologous Tissue Substitute, Percutaneous Approach

0JUR07Z Supplement of Left Foot Subcutaneous Tissue and Fascia with Autologous Tissue Substitute, Open Approach

0JUR0JZ Supplement of Left Foot Subcutaneous Tissue and Fascia with Synthetic Substitute, Open Approach

0JUR0KZ Supplement of Left Foot Subcutaneous Tissue and Fascia with Nonautologous Tissue Substitute, Open Approach

0JUR37Z Supplement of Left Foot Subcutaneous Tissue and Fascia with Autologous Tissue Substitute, Percutaneous Approach

0JUR3JZ Supplement of Left Foot Subcutaneous Tissue and Fascia with Synthetic Substitute, Percutaneous Approach

0JUR3KZ Supplement of Left Foot Subcutaneous Tissue and Fascia with Nonautologous Tissue Substitute, Percutaneous Approach

0JW – Subcutaneous Tissue and Fascia, Revision

Review Coding Guideline B6.1c

● **0JWS00Z** Revision of Drainage Device in Head and Neck Subcutaneous Tissue and Fascia, Open Approach

● **0JWS03Z** Revision of Infusion Device in Head and Neck Subcutaneous Tissue and Fascia, Open Approach

● **0JWS07Z** Revision of Autologous Tissue Substitute in Head and Neck Subcutaneous Tissue and Fascia, Open Approach

● **0JWS0JZ** Revision of Synthetic Substitute in Head and Neck Subcutaneous Tissue and Fascia, Open Approach

● **0JWS0KZ** Revision of Nonautologous Tissue Substitute in Head and Neck Subcutaneous Tissue and Fascia, Open Approach

● **0JWS0NZ** Revision of Tissue Expander in Head and Neck Subcutaneous Tissue and Fascia, Open Approach

● **0JWS30Z** Revision of Drainage Device in Head and Neck Subcutaneous Tissue and Fascia, Percutaneous Approach

● **0JWS33Z** Revision of Infusion Device in Head and Neck Subcutaneous Tissue and Fascia, Percutaneous Approach

● **0JWS37Z** Revision of Autologous Tissue Substitute in Head and Neck Subcutaneous Tissue and Fascia, Percutaneous Approach

● **0JWS3JZ** Revision of Synthetic Substitute in Head and Neck Subcutaneous Tissue and Fascia, Percutaneous Approach

● **0JWS3KZ** Revision of Nonautologous Tissue Substitute in Head and Neck Subcutaneous Tissue and Fascia, Percutaneous Approach

● **0JWS3NZ** Revision of Tissue Expander in Head and Neck Subcutaneous Tissue and Fascia, Percutaneous Approach

0JWSX0Z Revision of Drainage Device in Head and Neck Subcutaneous Tissue and Fascia, External Approach

0JWSX3Z Revision of Infusion Device in Head and Neck Subcutaneous Tissue and Fascia, External Approach

0JWSX7Z Revision of Autologous Tissue Substitute in Head and Neck Subcutaneous Tissue and Fascia, External Approach

0JWSXJZ Revision of Synthetic Substitute in Head and Neck Subcutaneous Tissue and Fascia, External Approach

0JWSXKZ Revision of Nonautologous Tissue Substitute in Head and Neck Subcutaneous Tissue and Fascia, External Approach

0JWSXNZ Revision of Tissue Expander in Head and Neck Subcutaneous Tissue and Fascia, External Approach

● **0JWT00Z** Revision of Drainage Device in Trunk Subcutaneous Tissue and Fascia, Open Approach

● **0JWT02Z** Revision of Monitoring Device in Trunk Subcutaneous Tissue and Fascia, Open Approach

● **0JWT03Z** Revision of Infusion Device in Trunk Subcutaneous Tissue and Fascia, Open Approach

● **0JWT07Z** Revision of Autologous Tissue Substitute in Trunk Subcutaneous Tissue and Fascia, Open Approach

● **0JWT0HZ** Revision of Contraceptive Device in Trunk Subcutaneous Tissue and Fascia, Open Approach

● **0JWT0JZ** Revision of Synthetic Substitute in Trunk Subcutaneous Tissue and Fascia, Open Approach

● **0JWT0KZ** Revision of Nonautologous Tissue Substitute in Trunk Subcutaneous Tissue and Fascia, Open Approach

0JWT0MZ Revision of Stimulator Generator in Trunk Subcutaneous Tissue and Fascia, Open Approach

● **0JWT0NZ** Revision of Tissue Expander in Trunk Subcutaneous Tissue and Fascia, Open Approach

0JWT0PZ Revision of Cardiac Rhythm Related Device in Trunk Subcutaneous Tissue and Fascia, Open Approach
AHA CC: 4Q, 2012, 104-106
With a secondary diagnosis code of K68.11, T81.4XXA, T82.6XXA, T82.7XXA

● **0JWT0VZ** Revision of Infusion Pump in Trunk Subcutaneous Tissue and Fascia, Open Approach

● **0JWT0WZ** Revision of Reservoir in Trunk Subcutaneous Tissue and Fascia, Open Approach

● **0JWT0XZ** Revision of Vascular Access Device in Trunk Subcutaneous Tissue and Fascia, Open Approach

● **0JWT30Z** Revision of Drainage Device in Trunk Subcutaneous Tissue and Fascia, Percutaneous Approach

● **0JWT32Z** Revision of Monitoring Device in Trunk Subcutaneous Tissue and Fascia, Percutaneous Approach

● **0JWT33Z** Revision of Infusion Device in Trunk Subcutaneous Tissue and Fascia, Percutaneous Approach

● **0JWT37Z** Revision of Autologous Tissue Substitute in Trunk Subcutaneous Tissue and Fascia, Percutaneous Approach

● **0JWT3HZ** Revision of Contraceptive Device in Trunk Subcutaneous Tissue and Fascia, Percutaneous Approach

● **0JWT3JZ** Revision of Synthetic Substitute in Trunk Subcutaneous Tissue and Fascia, Percutaneous Approach

● **0JWT3KZ** Revision of Nonautologous Tissue Substitute in Trunk Subcutaneous Tissue and Fascia, Percutaneous Approach

0JWT3MZ Revision of Stimulator Generator in Trunk Subcutaneous Tissue and Fascia, Percutaneous Approach

● **0JWT3NZ** Revision of Tissue Expander in Trunk Subcutaneous Tissue and Fascia, Percutaneous Approach

0JWT3PZ Revision of Cardiac Rhythm Related Device in Trunk Subcutaneous Tissue and Fascia, Percutaneous Approach
With a secondary diagnosis code of K68.11, T81.4XXA, T82.6XXA, T82.7XXA

● **0JWT3VZ** Revision of Infusion Pump in Trunk Subcutaneous Tissue and Fascia, Percutaneous Approach

● **0JWT3WZ** Revision of Reservoir in Trunk Subcutaneous Tissue and Fascia, Percutaneous Approach

♀ Female-only   ♂ Male-only   ▲ Limited Coverage   ● Non-OR   ▨ HAC-associated procedure   ▲ Non-covered procedures   ✚ Combinatio

...T3XZ Revision of Vascular Access Device in Trunk Subcutaneous Tissue and Fascia, Percutaneous Approach

...TX0Z Revision of Drainage Device in Trunk Subcutaneous Tissue and Fascia, External Approach

...TX2Z Revision of Monitoring Device in Trunk Subcutaneous Tissue and Fascia, External Approach

...TX3Z Revision of Infusion Device in Trunk Subcutaneous Tissue and Fascia, External Approach

...TX7Z Revision of Autologous Tissue Substitute in Trunk Subcutaneous Tissue and Fascia, External Approach

...TXHZ Revision of Contraceptive Device in Trunk Subcutaneous Tissue and Fascia, External Approach

...TXJZ Revision of Synthetic Substitute in Trunk Subcutaneous Tissue and Fascia, External Approach

...TXKZ Revision of Nonautologous Tissue Substitute in Trunk Subcutaneous Tissue and Fascia, External Approach

...TXMZ Revision of Stimulator Generator in Trunk Subcutaneous Tissue and Fascia, External Approach

...TXNZ Revision of Tissue Expander in Trunk Subcutaneous Tissue and Fascia, External Approach

...TXPZ Revision of Cardiac Rhythm Related Device in Trunk Subcutaneous Tissue and Fascia, External Approach

...TXVZ Revision of Infusion Pump in Trunk Subcutaneous Tissue and Fascia, External Approach

...TXWZ Revision of Reservoir in Trunk Subcutaneous Tissue and Fascia, External Approach

...TXXZ Revision of Vascular Access Device in Trunk Subcutaneous Tissue and Fascia, External Approach

...WV00Z Revision of Drainage Device in Upper Extremity Subcutaneous Tissue and Fascia, Open Approach

...WV03Z Revision of Infusion Device in Upper Extremity Subcutaneous Tissue and Fascia, Open Approach

...WV07Z Revision of Autologous Tissue Substitute in Upper Extremity Subcutaneous Tissue and Fascia, Open Approach

...WV0HZ Revision of Contraceptive Device in Upper Extremity Subcutaneous Tissue and Fascia, Open Approach

...WV0JZ Revision of Synthetic Substitute in Upper Extremity Subcutaneous Tissue and Fascia, Open Approach

...WV0KZ Revision of Nonautologous Tissue Substitute in Upper Extremity Subcutaneous Tissue and Fascia, Open Approach

...WV0NZ Revision of Tissue Expander in Upper Extremity Subcutaneous Tissue and Fascia, Open Approach

...WV0VZ Revision of Infusion Pump in Upper Extremity Subcutaneous Tissue and Fascia, Open Approach

...WV0WZ Revision of Reservoir in Upper Extremity Subcutaneous Tissue and Fascia, Open Approach

...WV0XZ Revision of Vascular Access Device in Upper Extremity Subcutaneous Tissue and Fascia, Open Approach

...WV30Z Revision of Drainage Device in Upper Extremity Subcutaneous Tissue and Fascia, Percutaneous Approach

● **0JWV33Z** Revision of Infusion Device in Upper Extremity Subcutaneous Tissue and Fascia, Percutaneous Approach

● **0JWV37Z** Revision of Autologous Tissue Substitute in Upper Extremity Subcutaneous Tissue and Fascia, Percutaneous Approach

● **0JWV3HZ** Revision of Contraceptive Device in Upper Extremity Subcutaneous Tissue and Fascia, Percutaneous Approach

● **0JWV3JZ** Revision of Synthetic Substitute in Upper Extremity Subcutaneous Tissue and Fascia, Percutaneous Approach

● **0JWV3KZ** Revision of Nonautologous Tissue Substitute in Upper Extremity Subcutaneous Tissue and Fascia, Percutaneous Approach

● **0JWV3NZ** Revision of Tissue Expander in Upper Extremity Subcutaneous Tissue and Fascia, Percutaneous Approach

● **0JWV3VZ** Revision of Infusion Pump in Upper Extremity Subcutaneous Tissue and Fascia, Percutaneous Approach

● **0JWV3WZ** Revision of Reservoir in Upper Extremity Subcutaneous Tissue and Fascia, Percutaneous Approach

0JWV3XZ Revision of Vascular Access Device in Upper Extremity Subcutaneous Tissue and Fascia, Percutaneous Approach

0JWVX0Z Revision of Drainage Device in Upper Extremity Subcutaneous Tissue and Fascia, External Approach

0JWVX3Z Revision of Infusion Device in Upper Extremity Subcutaneous Tissue and Fascia, External Approach

0JWVX7Z Revision of Autologous Tissue Substitute in Upper Extremity Subcutaneous Tissue and Fascia, External Approach

0JWVXHZ Revision of Contraceptive Device in Upper Extremity Subcutaneous Tissue and Fascia, External Approach

0JWVXJZ Revision of Synthetic Substitute in Upper Extremity Subcutaneous Tissue and Fascia, External Approach

0JWVXKZ Revision of Nonautologous Tissue Substitute in Upper Extremity Subcutaneous Tissue and Fascia, External Approach

0JWVXNZ Revision of Tissue Expander in Upper Extremity Subcutaneous Tissue and Fascia, External Approach

0JWVXVZ Revision of Infusion Pump in Upper Extremity Subcutaneous Tissue and Fascia, External Approach

0JWVXWZ Revision of Reservoir in Upper Extremity Subcutaneous Tissue and Fascia, External Approach

0JWVXXZ Revision of Vascular Access Device in Upper Extremity Subcutaneous Tissue and Fascia, External Approach

● **0JWW00Z** Revision of Drainage Device in Lower Extremity Subcutaneous Tissue and Fascia, Open Approach

● **0JWW03Z** Revision of Infusion Device in Lower Extremity Subcutaneous Tissue and Fascia, Open Approach

● **0JWW07Z** Revision of Autologous Tissue Substitute in Lower Extremity Subcutaneous Tissue and Fascia, Open Approach

● **0JWW0HZ** Revision of Contraceptive Device in Lower Extremity Subcutaneous Tissue and Fascia, Open Approach

● **0JWW0JZ** Revision of Synthetic Substitute in Lower Extremity Subcutaneous Tissue and Fascia, Open Approach

● **0JWW0KZ** Revision of Nonautologous Tissue Substitute in Lower Extremity Subcutaneous Tissue and Fascia, Open Approach

● **0JWW0NZ** Revision of Tissue Expander in Lower Extremity Subcutaneous Tissue and Fascia, Open Approach

● **0JWW0VZ** Revision of Infusion Pump in Lower Extremity Subcutaneous Tissue and Fascia, Open Approach

● **0JWW0WZ** Revision of Reservoir in Lower Extremity Subcutaneous Tissue and Fascia, Open Approach

● **0JWW0XZ** Revision of Vascular Access Device in Lower Extremity Subcutaneous Tissue and Fascia, Open Approach

● **0JWW30Z** Revision of Drainage Device in Lower Extremity Subcutaneous Tissue and Fascia, Percutaneous Approach

● **0JWW33Z** Revision of Infusion Device in Lower Extremity Subcutaneous Tissue and Fascia, Percutaneous Approach

● **0JWW37Z** Revision of Autologous Tissue Substitute in Lower Extremity Subcutaneous Tissue and Fascia, Percutaneous Approach

● **0JWW3HZ** Revision of Contraceptive Device in Lower Extremity Subcutaneous Tissue and Fascia, Percutaneous Approach

● **0JWW3JZ** Revision of Synthetic Substitute in Lower Extremity Subcutaneous Tissue and Fascia, Percutaneous Approach

● **0JWW3KZ** Revision of Nonautologous Tissue Substitute in Lower Extremity Subcutaneous Tissue and Fascia, Percutaneous Approach

● **0JWW3NZ** Revision of Tissue Expander in Lower Extremity Subcutaneous Tissue and Fascia, Percutaneous Approach

● **0JWW3VZ** Revision of Infusion Pump in Lower Extremity Subcutaneous Tissue and Fascia, Percutaneous Approach

● **0JWW3WZ** Revision of Reservoir in Lower Extremity Subcutaneous Tissue and Fascia, Percutaneous Approach

● **0JWW3XZ** Revision of Vascular Access Device in Lower Extremity Subcutaneous Tissue and Fascia, Percutaneous Approach

0JWWX0Z Revision of Drainage Device in Lower Extremity Subcutaneous Tissue and Fascia, External Approach

0JWWX3Z Revision of Infusion Device in Lower Extremity Subcutaneous Tissue and Fascia, External Approach

0JWWX7Z Revision of Autologous Tissue Substitute in Lower Extremity Subcutaneous Tissue and Fascia, External Approach

0JWWXHZ Revision of Contraceptive Device in Lower Extremity Subcutaneous Tissue and Fascia, External Approach

0JWWXJZ Revision of Synthetic Substitute in Lower Extremity Subcutaneous Tissue and Fascia, External Approach

0JWWXKZ Revision of Nonautologous Tissue Substitute in Lower Extremity Subcutaneous Tissue and Fascia, External Approach

0JWWXNZ Revision of Tissue Expander in Lower Extremity Subcutaneous Tissue and Fascia, External Approach

0JWWXVZ Revision of Infusion Pump in Lower Extremity Subcutaneous Tissue and Fascia, External Approach

0JWWXWZ Revision of Reservoir in Lower Extremity Subcutaneous Tissue and Fascia, External Approach

0JWWXXZ Revision of Vascular Access Device in Lower Extremity Subcutaneous Tissue and Fascia, External Approach

0JX00ZB Transfer Scalp Subcutaneous Tissue and Fascia with Skin and Subcutaneous Tissue, Open Approach

0JX00ZC Transfer Scalp Subcutaneous Tissue and Fascia with Skin, Subcutaneous Tissue and Fascia, Open Approach

0JX00ZZ Transfer Scalp Subcutaneous Tissue and Fascia, Open Approach

0JX03ZB Transfer Scalp Subcutaneous Tissue and Fascia with Skin and Subcutaneous Tissue, Percutaneous Approach

0JX03ZC Transfer Scalp Subcutaneous Tissue and Fascia with Skin, Subcutaneous Tissue and Fascia, Percutaneous Approach

0JX03ZZ Transfer Scalp Subcutaneous Tissue and Fascia, Percutaneous Approach

0JX10ZB Transfer Face Subcutaneous Tissue and Fascia with Skin and Subcutaneous Tissue, Open Approach

0JX10ZC Transfer Face Subcutaneous Tissue and Fascia with Skin, Subcutaneous Tissue and Fascia, Open Approach

0JX10ZZ Transfer Face Subcutaneous Tissue and Fascia, Open Approach

0JX13ZB Transfer Face Subcutaneous Tissue and Fascia with Skin and Subcutaneous Tissue, Percutaneous Approach

0JX13ZC Transfer Face Subcutaneous Tissue and Fascia with Skin, Subcutaneous Tissue and Fascia, Percutaneous Approach

0JX13ZZ Transfer Face Subcutaneous Tissue and Fascia, Percutaneous Approach

0JX40ZB Transfer Anterior Neck Subcutaneous Tissue and Fascia with Skin and Subcutaneous Tissue, Open Approach

0JX40ZC Transfer Anterior Neck Subcutaneous Tissue and Fascia with Skin, Subcutaneous Tissue and Fascia, Open Approach

0JX40ZZ Transfer Anterior Neck Subcutaneous Tissue and Fascia, Open Approach

0JX43ZB Transfer Anterior Neck Subcutaneous Tissue and Fascia with Skin and Subcutaneous Tissue, Percutaneous Approach

0JX43ZC Transfer Anterior Neck Subcutaneous Tissue and Fascia with Skin, Subcutaneous Tissue and Fascia, Percutaneous Approach

0JX43ZZ Transfer Anterior Neck Subcutaneous Tissue and Fascia, Percutaneous Approach

0JX50ZB Transfer Posterior Neck Subcutaneous Tissue and Fascia with Skin and Subcutaneous Tissue, Open Approach

0JX50ZC Transfer Posterior Neck Subcutaneous Tissue and Fascia with Skin, Subcutaneous Tissue and Fascia, Open Approach

0JX50ZZ Transfer Posterior Neck Subcutaneous Tissue and Fascia, Open Approach

0JX53ZB Transfer Posterior Neck Subcutaneous Tissue and Fascia with Skin and Subcutaneous Tissue, Percutaneous Approach

0JX53ZC Transfer Posterior Neck Subcutaneous Tissue and Fascia with Skin, Subcutaneous Tissue and Fascia, Percutaneous Approach

0JX53ZZ Transfer Posterior Neck Subcutaneous Tissue and Fascia, Percutaneous Approach

0JX60ZB Transfer Chest Subcutaneous Tissue and Fascia with Skin and Subcutaneous Tissue, Open Approach
AHA CC: 4Q, 2013, 109-111

0JX60ZC Transfer Chest Subcutaneous Tissue and Fascia with Skin, Subcutaneous Tissue and Fascia, Open Approach

0JX60ZZ Transfer Chest Subcutaneous Tissue and Fascia, Open Approach

0JX63ZB Transfer Chest Subcutaneous Tissue and Fascia with Skin and Subcutaneous Tissue, Percutaneous Approach

0JX63ZC Transfer Chest Subcutaneous Tissue and Fascia with Skin, Subcutaneous Tissue and Fascia, Percutaneous Approach

0JX63ZZ Transfer Chest Subcutaneous Tissue and Fascia, Percutaneous Approach

0JX70ZB Transfer Back Subcutaneous Tissue and Fascia with Skin and Subcutaneous Tissue, Open Approach

0JX70ZC Transfer Back Subcutaneous Tissue and Fascia with Skin, Subcutaneous Tissue and Fascia, Open Approach

0JX70ZZ Transfer Back Subcutaneous Tissue and Fascia, Open Approach

0JX73ZB Transfer Back Subcutaneous Tissue and Fascia with Skin and Subcutaneous Tissue, Percutaneous Approach

0JX73ZC Transfer Back Subcutaneous Tissue and Fascia with Skin, Subcutaneous Tissue and Fascia, Percutaneous Approach

0JX73ZZ Transfer Back Subcutaneous Tissue and Fascia, Percutaneous Approach

0JX80ZB Transfer Abdomen Subcutaneous Tissue and Fascia with Skin and Subcutaneous Tissue, Open Approach
AHA CC: 4Q, 2013, 109-111

0JX80ZC Transfer Abdomen Subcutaneous Tissue and Fascia with Skin, Subcutaneous Tissue and Fascia, Open Approach

0JX80ZZ Transfer Abdomen Subcutaneous Tissue and Fascia, Open Approach

0JX83ZB Transfer Abdomen Subcutaneous Tissue and Fascia with Skin and Subcutaneous Tissue, Percutaneous Approach

0JX83ZC Transfer Abdomen Subcutaneous Tissue and Fascia with Skin, Subcutaneous Tissue and Fascia, Percutaneous Approach

0JX83ZZ Transfer Abdomen Subcutaneous Tissue and Fascia, Percutaneous Approach

0JX90ZB Transfer Buttock Subcutaneous Tissue and Fascia with Skin and Subcutaneous Tissue, Open Approach

0JX90ZC Transfer Buttock Subcutaneous Tissue and Fascia with Skin, Subcutaneous Tissue and Fascia, Open Approach

0JX90ZZ Transfer Buttock Subcutaneous Tissue and Fascia, Open Approach

0JX93ZB Transfer Buttock Subcutaneous Tissue and Fascia with Skin and Subcutaneous Tissue, Percutaneous Approach

0JX93ZC Transfer Buttock Subcutaneous Tissue and Fascia with Skin, Subcutaneous Tissue and Fascia, Percutaneous Approach

0JX93ZZ Transfer Buttock Subcutaneous Tissue and Fascia, Percutaneous Approach

0JXB0ZB Transfer Perineum Subcutaneous Tissue and Fascia with Skin and Subcutaneous Tissue, Open Approach

0JXB0ZC Transfer Perineum Subcutaneous Tissue and Fascia with Skin, Subcutaneous Tissue and Fascia, Open Approach

0JXB0ZZ Transfer Perineum Subcutaneous Tissue and Fascia, Open Approach

0JXB3ZB Transfer Perineum Subcutaneous Tissue and Fascia with Skin and Subcutaneous Tissue, Percutaneous Approach

0JXB3ZC Transfer Perineum Subcutaneous Tissue and Fascia with Skin, Subcutaneous Tissue and Fascia, Percutaneous Approach

0JXB3ZZ Transfer Perineum Subcutaneous Tissue and Fascia, Percutaneous Approach

0JXC0ZB Transfer Pelvic Region Subcutaneous Tissue and Fascia with Skin and Subcutaneous Tissue, Open Approach

0JXC0ZC Transfer Pelvic Region Subcutaneous Tissue and Fascia with Skin, Subcutaneous Tissue and Fascia, Open Approach

0JXC0ZZ Transfer Pelvic Region Subcutaneous Tissue and Fascia, Open Approach

0JXC3ZB Transfer Pelvic Region Subcutaneous Tissue and Fascia with Skin and Subcutaneous Tissue, Percutaneous Approach

0JXC3ZC Transfer Pelvic Region Subcutaneous Tissue and Fascia with Skin, Subcutaneous Tissue and Fascia, Percutaneous Approach

0JXC3ZZ Transfer Pelvic Region Subcutaneous Tissue and Fascia, Percutaneous Approach

0JXD0ZB Transfer Right Upper Arm Subcutaneous Tissue and Fascia with Skin and Subcutaneous Tissue, Open Approach

0JXD0ZC Transfer Right Upper Arm Subcutaneous Tissue and Fascia with Skin, Subcutaneous Tissue and Fascia, Open Approach

0JXD0ZZ Transfer Right Upper Arm Subcutaneous Tissue and Fascia, Open Approach

0JXD3ZB Transfer Right Upper Arm Subcutaneous Tissue and Fascia with Skin and Subcutaneous Tissue, Percutaneous Approach

0JXD3ZC Transfer Right Upper Arm Subcutaneous Tissue and Fascia with Skin, Subcutaneous Tissue and Fascia, Percutaneous Approach

0JXD3ZZ Transfer Right Upper Arm Subcutaneous Tissue and Fascia, Percutaneous Approach

0JXF0ZB Transfer Left Upper Arm Subcutaneous Tissue and Fascia with Skin and Subcutaneous Tissue, Open Approach

0JXF0ZC Transfer Left Upper Arm Subcutaneous Tissue and Fascia with Skin, Subcutaneous Tissue and Fascia, Open Approach

0JXF0ZZ Transfer Left Upper Arm Subcutaneous Tissue and Fascia, Open Approach

0JXF3ZB Transfer Left Upper Arm Subcutaneous Tissue and Fascia with Skin and Subcutaneous Tissue, Percutaneous Approach

0JXF3ZC Transfer Left Upper Arm Subcutaneous Tissue and Fascia with Skin, Subcutaneous Tissue and Fascia, Percutaneous Approach

0JXF3ZZ Transfer Left Upper Arm Subcutaneous Tissue and Fascia with Skin, Subcutaneous Tissue and Fascia, Percutaneous Approach

0JXG0ZB Transfer Right Lower Arm Subcutaneous Tissue and Fascia with Skin and Subcutaneous Tissue, Open Approach

0JXG0ZC Transfer Right Lower Arm Subcutaneous Tissue and Fascia with Skin, Subcutaneous Tissue and Fascia, Open Approach

0JXG0ZZ Transfer Right Lower Arm Subcutaneous Tissue and Fascia, Open Approach

0JXG3ZB Transfer Right Lower Arm Subcutaneous Tissue and Fascia with Skin and Subcutaneous Tissue, Percutaneous Approach

0JXG3ZC Transfer Right Lower Arm Subcutaneous Tissue and Fascia with Skin, Subcutaneous Tissue and Fascia, Percutaneous Approach

0JXG3ZZ Transfer Right Lower Arm Subcutaneous Tissue and Fascia, Percutaneous Approach

0JXH0ZB Transfer Left Lower Arm Subcutaneous Tissue and Fascia with Skin and Subcutaneous Tissue, Open Approach

0JXH0ZC Transfer Left Lower Arm Subcutaneous Tissue and Fascia with Skin, Subcutaneous Tissue and Fascia, Open Approach

0JXH0ZZ Transfer Left Lower Arm Subcutaneous Tissue and Fascia, Open Approach

H3ZB Transfer Left Lower Arm Subcutaneous Tissue and Fascia with Skin and Subcutaneous Tissue, Percutaneous Approach

H3ZC Transfer Left Lower Arm Subcutaneous Tissue and Fascia with Skin, Subcutaneous Tissue and Fascia, Percutaneous Approach

H3ZZ Transfer Left Lower Arm Subcutaneous Tissue and Fascia, Percutaneous Approach

J0ZB Transfer Right Hand Subcutaneous Tissue and Fascia with Skin and Subcutaneous Tissue, Open Approach

J0ZC Transfer Right Hand Subcutaneous Tissue and Fascia with Skin, Subcutaneous Tissue and Fascia, Open Approach

J0ZZ Transfer Right Hand Subcutaneous Tissue and Fascia, Open Approach

J3ZB Transfer Right Hand Subcutaneous Tissue and Fascia with Skin and Subcutaneous Tissue, Percutaneous Approach

J3ZC Transfer Right Hand Subcutaneous Tissue and Fascia with Skin, Subcutaneous Tissue and Fascia, Percutaneous Approach

J3ZZ Transfer Right Hand Subcutaneous Tissue and Fascia, Percutaneous Approach

K0ZB Transfer Left Hand Subcutaneous Tissue and Fascia with Skin and Subcutaneous Tissue, Open Approach

K0ZC Transfer Left Hand Subcutaneous Tissue and Fascia with Skin, Subcutaneous Tissue and Fascia, Open Approach

K0ZZ Transfer Left Hand Subcutaneous Tissue and Fascia, Open Approach

K3ZB Transfer Left Hand Subcutaneous Tissue and Fascia with Skin and Subcutaneous Tissue, Percutaneous Approach

K3ZC Transfer Left Hand Subcutaneous Tissue and Fascia with Skin, Subcutaneous Tissue and Fascia, Percutaneous Approach

K3ZZ Transfer Left Hand Subcutaneous Tissue and Fascia, Percutaneous Approach

L0ZB Transfer Right Upper Leg Subcutaneous Tissue and Fascia with Skin and Subcutaneous Tissue, Open Approach

L0ZC Transfer Right Upper Leg Subcutaneous Tissue and Fascia with Skin, Subcutaneous Tissue and Fascia, Open Approach

L0ZZ Transfer Right Upper Leg Subcutaneous Tissue and Fascia, Open Approach

0JXL3ZB Transfer Right Upper Leg Subcutaneous Tissue and Fascia with Skin and Subcutaneous Tissue, Percutaneous Approach

0JXL3ZC Transfer Right Upper Leg Subcutaneous Tissue and Fascia with Skin, Subcutaneous Tissue and Fascia, Percutaneous Approach

0JXL3ZZ Transfer Right Upper Leg Subcutaneous Tissue and Fascia, Percutaneous Approach

0JXM0ZB Transfer Left Upper Leg Subcutaneous Tissue and Fascia with Skin and Subcutaneous Tissue, Open Approach

0JXM0ZC Transfer Left Upper Leg Subcutaneous Tissue and Fascia with Skin, Subcutaneous Tissue and Fascia, Open Approach

0JXM0ZZ Transfer Left Upper Leg Subcutaneous Tissue and Fascia, Open Approach

0JXM3ZB Transfer Left Upper Leg Subcutaneous Tissue and Fascia with Skin and Subcutaneous Tissue, Percutaneous Approach

0JXM3ZC Transfer Left Upper Leg Subcutaneous Tissue and Fascia with Skin, Subcutaneous Tissue and Fascia, Percutaneous Approach

0JXM3ZZ Transfer Left Upper Leg Subcutaneous Tissue and Fascia, Percutaneous Approach

0JXN0ZB Transfer Right Lower Leg Subcutaneous Tissue and Fascia with Skin and Subcutaneous Tissue, Open Approach

0JXN0ZC Transfer Right Lower Leg Subcutaneous Tissue and Fascia with Skin, Subcutaneous Tissue and Fascia, Open Approach
AHA CC: 3Q, 2014, 18-19

0JXN0ZZ Transfer Right Lower Leg Subcutaneous Tissue and Fascia, Open Approach

0JXN3ZB Transfer Right Lower Leg Subcutaneous Tissue and Fascia with Skin and Subcutaneous Tissue, Percutaneous Approach

0JXN3ZC Transfer Right Lower Leg Subcutaneous Tissue and Fascia with Skin, Subcutaneous Tissue and Fascia, Percutaneous Approach

0JXN3ZZ Transfer Right Lower Leg Subcutaneous Tissue and Fascia, Percutaneous Approach

0JXP0ZB Transfer Left Lower Leg Subcutaneous Tissue and Fascia with Skin and Subcutaneous Tissue, Open Approach

0JXP0ZC Transfer Left Lower Leg Subcutaneous Tissue and Fascia with Skin, Subcutaneous Tissue and Fascia, Open Approach

0JXP0ZZ Transfer Left Lower Leg Subcutaneous Tissue and Fascia, Open Approach

0JXP3ZB Transfer Left Lower Leg Subcutaneous Tissue and Fascia with Skin and Subcutaneous Tissue, Percutaneous Approach

0JXP3ZC Transfer Left Lower Leg Subcutaneous Tissue and Fascia with Skin, Subcutaneous Tissue and Fascia, Percutaneous Approach

0JXP3ZZ Transfer Left Lower Leg Subcutaneous Tissue and Fascia, Percutaneous Approach

0JXQ0ZB Transfer Right Foot Subcutaneous Tissue and Fascia with Skin and Subcutaneous Tissue, Open Approach

0JXQ0ZC Transfer Right Foot Subcutaneous Tissue and Fascia with Skin, Subcutaneous Tissue and Fascia, Open Approach

0JXQ0ZZ Transfer Right Foot Subcutaneous Tissue and Fascia, Open Approach

0JXQ3ZB Transfer Right Foot Subcutaneous Tissue and Fascia with Skin and Subcutaneous Tissue, Percutaneous Approach

0JXQ3ZC Transfer Right Foot Subcutaneous Tissue and Fascia with Skin, Subcutaneous Tissue and Fascia, Percutaneous Approach

0JXQ3ZZ Transfer Right Foot Subcutaneous Tissue and Fascia, Percutaneous Approach

0JXR0ZB Transfer Left Foot Subcutaneous Tissue and Fascia with Skin and Subcutaneous Tissue, Open Approach

0JXR0ZC Transfer Left Foot Subcutaneous Tissue and Fascia with Skin, Subcutaneous Tissue and Fascia, Open Approach

0JXR0ZZ Transfer Left Foot Subcutaneous Tissue and Fascia, Open Approach

0JXR3ZB Transfer Left Foot Subcutaneous Tissue and Fascia with Skin and Subcutaneous Tissue, Percutaneous Approach

0JXR3ZC Transfer Left Foot Subcutaneous Tissue and Fascia with Skin, Subcutaneous Tissue and Fascia, Percutaneous Approach

0JXR3ZZ Transfer Left Foot Subcutaneous Tissue and Fascia, Percutaneous Approach

Female-only　　♂ Male-only　　▲ Limited Coverage　　● Non-OR　　▬ HAC-associated procedure　　▲ Non-covered procedures　　✚ Combination

Muscles

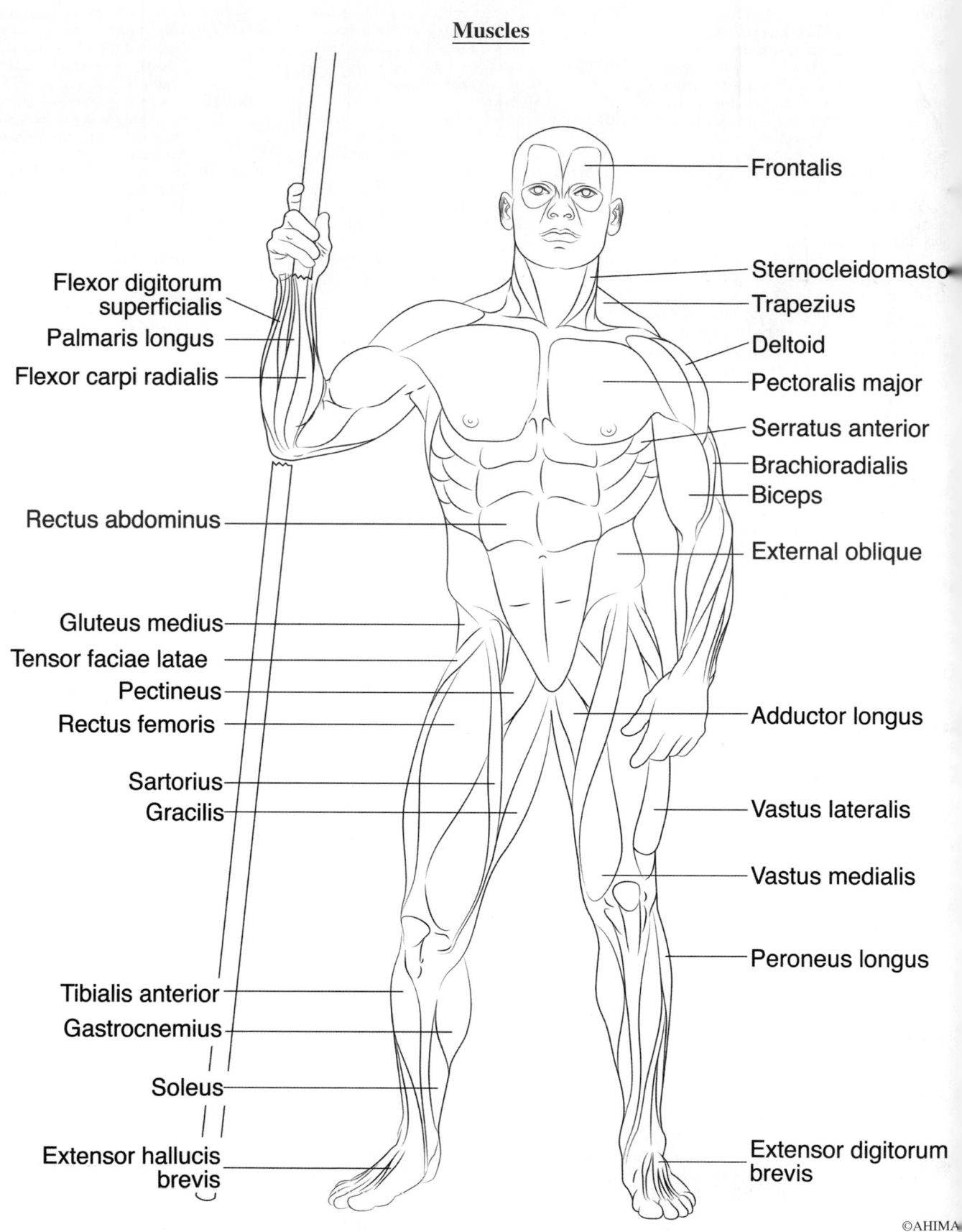

Frontalis

Sternocleidomasto

Trapezius

Deltoid

Pectoralis major

Serratus anterior

Brachioradialis

Biceps

External oblique

Adductor longus

Vastus lateralis

Vastus medialis

Peroneus longus

Extensor digitorum
brevis

Flexor digitorum
superficialis

Palmaris longus

Flexor carpi radialis

Rectus abdominus

Gluteus medius

Tensor faciae latae

Pectineus

Rectus femoris

Sartorius

Gracilis

Tibialis anterior

Gastrocnemius

Soleus

Extensor hallucis
brevis

©AHIMA

Muscles of the Hand

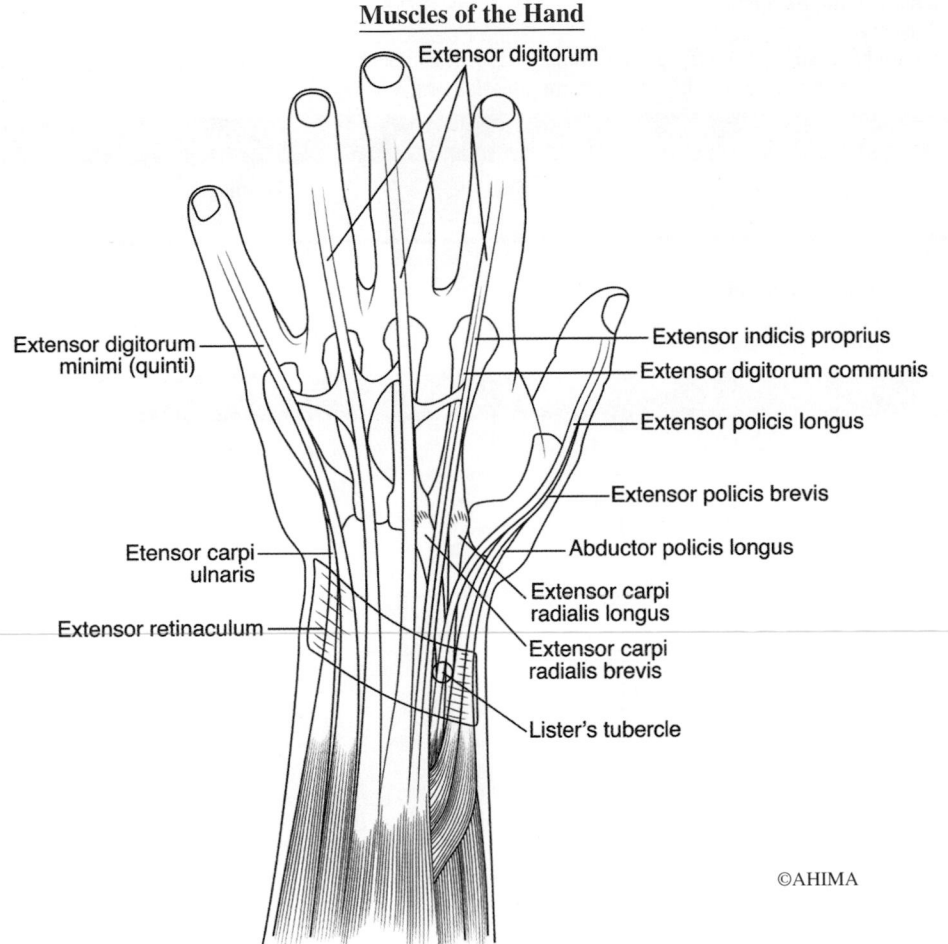

Extensor digitorum

Extensor digitorum minimi (quinti)

Extensor indicis proprius

Extensor digitorum communis

Extensor policis longus

Extensor policis brevis

Abductor policis longus

Etensor carpi ulnaris

Extensor carpi radialis longus

Extensor retinaculum

Extensor carpi radialis brevis

Lister's tubercle

©AHIMA

Muscles of the Foot

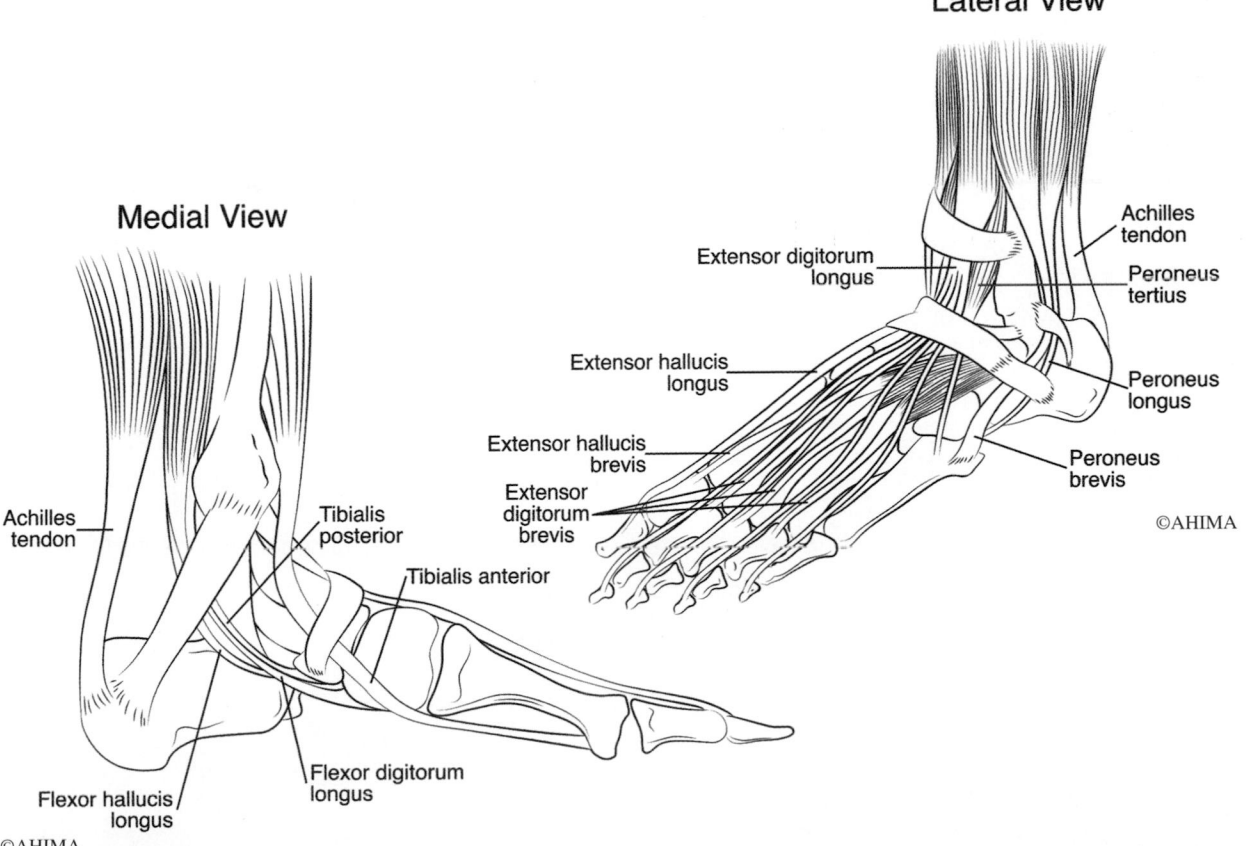

Lateral View

Achilles tendon

Extensor digitorum longus

Peroneus tertius

Peroneus longus

Extensor hallucis longus

Extensor hallucis brevis

Extensor digitorum brevis

Peroneus brevis

©AHIMA

Medial View

Achilles tendon

Tibialis posterior

Tibialis anterior

Flexor hallucis longus

Flexor digitorum longus

©AHIMA

Muscles Tables 0K2–0KX

Section	0	Medical and Surgical
Body System	K	Muscles
Operation	2	**Change:** Taking out or off a device from a body part and putting back an identical or similar device in or on the same body part without cutting or puncturing the skin or a mucous membrane

Body Part (4th)	Approach (5th)	Device (6th)	Qualifier (7th)
X Upper Muscle Y Lower Muscle	X External	0 Drainage Device Y Other Device	Z No Qualifier

Section	0	Medical and Surgical
Body System	K	Muscles
Operation	5	**Destruction:** Physical eradication of all or a portion of a body part by the direct use of energy, force, or a destructive agent

Body Part (4th)	Approach (5th)	Device (6th)	Qualifier (7th)
0 Head Muscle 1 Facial Muscle 2 Neck Muscle, Right 3 Neck Muscle, Left 4 Tongue, Palate, Pharynx Muscle 5 Shoulder Muscle, Right 6 Shoulder Muscle, Left 7 Upper Arm Muscle, Right 8 Upper Arm Muscle, Left 9 Lower Arm and Wrist Muscle, Right B Lower Arm and Wrist Muscle, Left C Hand Muscle, Right D Hand Muscle, Left F Trunk Muscle, Right G Trunk Muscle, Left H Thorax Muscle, Right J Thorax Muscle, Left K Abdomen Muscle, Right L Abdomen Muscle, Left M Perineum Muscle N Hip Muscle, Right P Hip Muscle, Left Q Upper Leg Muscle, Right R Upper Leg Muscle, Left S Lower Leg Muscle, Right T Lower Leg Muscle, Left V Foot Muscle, Right W Foot Muscle, Left	0 Open 3 Percutaneous 4 Percutaneous Endoscopic	Z No Device	Z No Qualifier

ion	0	Medical and Surgical
System	K	Muscles
ration	8	**Division:** Cutting into a body part, without draining fluids and/or gases from the body part, in order to separate or transect a body part

Body Part (4th)	Approach (5th)	Device (6th)	Qualifier (7th)
Head Muscle Facial Muscle Neck Muscle, Right Neck Muscle, Left Tongue, Palate, Pharynx Muscle Shoulder Muscle, Right Shoulder Muscle, Left Upper Arm Muscle, Right Upper Arm Muscle, Left Lower Arm and Wrist Muscle, Right Lower Arm and Wrist Muscle, Left Hand Muscle, Right Hand Muscle, Left Trunk Muscle, Right Trunk Muscle, Left Thorax Muscle, Right Thorax Muscle, Left Abdomen Muscle, Right Abdomen Muscle, Left Perineum Muscle Hip Muscle, Right Hip Muscle, Left Upper Leg Muscle, Right Upper Leg Muscle, Left Lower Leg Muscle, Right Lower Leg Muscle, Left Foot Muscle, Right Foot Muscle, Left	**0** Open **3** Percutaneous **4** Percutaneous Endoscopic	**Z** No Device	**Z** No Qualifier

Section	0	Medical and Surgical
Body System	K	Muscles
Operation	9	**Drainage:** Taking or letting out fluids and/or gases from a body part

Body Part (4th)	Approach (5th)	Device (6th)	Qualifier (7th)
0 Head Muscle 1 Facial Muscle 2 Neck Muscle, Right 3 Neck Muscle, Left 4 Tongue, Palate, Pharynx Muscle 5 Shoulder Muscle, Right 6 Shoulder Muscle, Left 7 Upper Arm Muscle, Right 8 Upper Arm Muscle, Left 9 Lower Arm and Wrist Muscle, Right B Lower Arm and Wrist Muscle, Left C Hand Muscle, Right D Hand Muscle, Left F Trunk Muscle, Right G Trunk Muscle, Left H Thorax Muscle, Right J Thorax Muscle, Left K Abdomen Muscle, Right L Abdomen Muscle, Left M Perineum Muscle N Hip Muscle, Right P Hip Muscle, Left Q Upper Leg Muscle, Right R Upper Leg Muscle, Left S Lower Leg Muscle, Right T Lower Leg Muscle, Left V Foot Muscle, Right W Foot Muscle, Left	0 Open 3 Percutaneous 4 Percutaneous Endoscopic	0 Drainage Device	Z No Qualifier
0 Head Muscle 1 Facial Muscle 2 Neck Muscle, Right 3 Neck Muscle, Left 4 Tongue, Palate, Pharynx Muscle 5 Shoulder Muscle, Right 6 Shoulder Muscle, Left 7 Upper Arm Muscle, Right 8 Upper Arm Muscle, Left 9 Lower Arm and Wrist Muscle, Right B Lower Arm and Wrist Muscle, Left C Hand Muscle, Right D Hand Muscle, Left F Trunk Muscle, Right G Trunk Muscle, Left H Thorax Muscle, Right J Thorax Muscle, Left K Abdomen Muscle, Right L Abdomen Muscle, Left M Perineum Muscle N Hip Muscle, Right P Hip Muscle, Left Q Upper Leg Muscle, Right R Upper Leg Muscle, Left S Lower Leg Muscle, Right T Lower Leg Muscle, Left V Foot Muscle, Right W Foot Muscle, Left	0 Open 3 Percutaneous 4 Percutaneous Endoscopic	Z No Device	X Diagnostic Z No Qualifier

tion	**0**	**Medical and Surgical**	
y System	**K**	**Muscles**	
ration	**B**	**Excision:** Cutting out or off, without replacement, a portion of a body part	

Body Part (4th)	Approach (5th)	Device (6th)	Qualifier (7th)
Head Muscle Facial Muscle Neck Muscle, Right Neck Muscle, Left Tongue, Palate, Pharynx Muscle Shoulder Muscle, Right Shoulder Muscle, Left Upper Arm Muscle, Right Upper Arm Muscle, Left Lower Arm and Wrist Muscle, Right Lower Arm and Wrist Muscle, Left Hand Muscle, Right Hand Muscle, Left Trunk Muscle, Right Trunk Muscle, Left Thorax Muscle, Right Thorax Muscle, Left Abdomen Muscle, Right Abdomen Muscle, Left Perineum Muscle Hip Muscle, Right Hip Muscle, Left Upper Leg Muscle, Right Upper Leg Muscle, Left Lower Leg Muscle, Right Lower Leg Muscle, Left Foot Muscle, Right Foot Muscle, Left	**0** Open **3** Percutaneous **4** Percutaneous Endoscopic	**Z** No Device	**X** Diagnostic **Z** No Qualifier

tion	**0**	**Medical and Surgical**	
dy System	**K**	**Muscles**	
eration	**C**	**Extirpation:** Taking or cutting out solid matter from a body part	

Body Part (4th)	Approach (5th)	Device (6th)	Qualifier (7th)
0 Head Muscle **1** Facial Muscle **2** Neck Muscle, Right **3** Neck Muscle, Left **4** Tongue, Palate, Pharynx Muscle **5** Shoulder Muscle, Right **6** Shoulder Muscle, Left **7** Upper Arm Muscle, Right **8** Upper Arm Muscle, Left **9** Lower Arm and Wrist Muscle, Right **B** Lower Arm and Wrist Muscle, Left **C** Hand Muscle, Right **D** Hand Muscle, Left **F** Trunk Muscle, Right **G** Trunk Muscle, Left **H** Thorax Muscle, Right **J** Thorax Muscle, Left **K** Abdomen Muscle, Right **L** Abdomen Muscle, Left **M** Perineum Muscle **N** Hip Muscle, Right **P** Hip Muscle, Left **Q** Upper Leg Muscle, Right **R** Upper Leg Muscle, Left **S** Lower Leg Muscle, Right **T** Lower Leg Muscle, Left **V** Foot Muscle, Right **W** Foot Muscle, Left	**0** Open **3** Percutaneous **4** Percutaneous Endoscopic	**Z** No Device	**Z** No Qualifier

Section	0	Medical and Surgical
Body System	K	Muscles
Operation	H	Insertion: Putting in a nonbiological appliance that monitors, assists, performs, or prevents a physiological function but do not physically take the place of a body part

Body Part (4th)	Approach (5th)	Device (6th)	Qualifier (7th)
X Upper Muscle Y Lower Muscle	0 Open 3 Percutaneous 4 Percutaneous Endoscopic	M Stimulator Lead	Z No Qualifier

Section	0	Medical and Surgical
Body System	K	Muscles
Operation	J	Inspection: Visually and/or manually exploring a body part

Body Part (4th)	Approach (5th)	Device (6th)	Qualifier (7th)
X Upper Muscle Y Lower Muscle	0 Open 3 Percutaneous 4 Percutaneous Endoscopic X External	Z No Device	Z No Qualifier

Section	0	Medical and Surgical
Body System	K	Muscles
Operation	M	Reattachment: Putting back in or on all or a portion of a separated body part to its normal location or other suitable locatio

Body Part (4th)	Approach (5th)	Device (6th)	Qualifier (7th)
0 Head Muscle 1 Facial Muscle 2 Neck Muscle, Right 3 Neck Muscle, Left 4 Tongue, Palate, Pharynx Muscle 5 Shoulder Muscle, Right 6 Shoulder Muscle, Left 7 Upper Arm Muscle, Right 8 Upper Arm Muscle, Left 9 Lower Arm and Wrist Muscle, Right B Lower Arm and Wrist Muscle, Left C Hand Muscle, Right D Hand Muscle, Left F Trunk Muscle, Right G Trunk Muscle, Left H Thorax Muscle, Right J Thorax Muscle, Left K Abdomen Muscle, Right L Abdomen Muscle, Left M Perineum Muscle N Hip Muscle, Right P Hip Muscle, Left Q Upper Leg Muscle, Right R Upper Leg Muscle, Left S Lower Leg Muscle, Right T Lower Leg Muscle, Left V Foot Muscle, Right W Foot Muscle, Left	0 Open 4 Percutaneous Endoscopic	Z No Device	Z No Qualifier

	0	Medical and Surgical
System	K	Muscles
ration	N	Release: Freeing a body part from an abnormal physical constraint by cutting or by the use of force

Body Part (4th)	Approach (5th)	Device (6th)	Qualifier (7th)
Head Muscle Facial Muscle Neck Muscle, Right Neck Muscle, Left Tongue, Palate, Pharynx Muscle Shoulder Muscle, Right Shoulder Muscle, Left Upper Arm Muscle, Right Upper Arm Muscle, Left Lower Arm and Wrist Muscle, Right Lower Arm and Wrist Muscle, Left Hand Muscle, Right Hand Muscle, Left Trunk Muscle, Right Trunk Muscle, Left Thorax Muscle, Right Thorax Muscle, Left Abdomen Muscle, Right Abdomen Muscle, Left Perineum Muscle Hip Muscle, Right Hip Muscle, Left Upper Leg Muscle, Right Upper Leg Muscle, Left Lower Leg Muscle, Right Lower Leg Muscle, Left Foot Muscle, Right Foot Muscle, Left	0 Open 3 Percutaneous 4 Percutaneous Endoscopic X External	Z No Device	Z No Qualifier

	0	Medical and Surgical
dy System	K	Muscles
eration	P	Removal: Taking out or off a device from a body part

Body Part (4th)	Approach (5th)	Device (6th)	Qualifier (7th)
Upper Muscle Lower Muscle	0 Open 3 Percutaneous 4 Percutaneous Endoscopic	0 Drainage Device 7 Autologous Tissue Substitute J Synthetic Substitute K Nonautologous Tissue Substitute M Stimulator Lead	Z No Qualifier
Upper Muscle Lower Muscle	X External	0 Drainage Device M Stimulator Lead	Z No Qualifier

Section	0	Medical and Surgical
Body System	K	Muscles
Operation	Q	**Repair:** Restoring, to the extent possible, a body part to its normal anatomic structure and function

Body Part (4th)	Approach (5th)	Device (6th)	Qualifier (7th)
0 Head Muscle 1 Facial Muscle 2 Neck Muscle, Right 3 Neck Muscle, Left 4 Tongue, Palate, Pharynx Muscle 5 Shoulder Muscle, Right 6 Shoulder Muscle, Left 7 Upper Arm Muscle, Right 8 Upper Arm Muscle, Left 9 Lower Arm and Wrist Muscle, Right B Lower Arm and Wrist Muscle, Left C Hand Muscle, Right D Hand Muscle, Left F Trunk Muscle, Right G Trunk Muscle, Left H Thorax Muscle, Right J Thorax Muscle, Left K Abdomen Muscle, Right L Abdomen Muscle, Left M Perineum Muscle N Hip Muscle, Right P Hip Muscle, Left Q Upper Leg Muscle, Right R Upper Leg Muscle, Left S Lower Leg Muscle, Right T Lower Leg Muscle, Left V Foot Muscle, Right W Foot Muscle, Left	0 Open 3 Percutaneous 4 Percutaneous Endoscopic	Z No Device	Z No Qualifier

Section	0	Medical and Surgical
Body System	K	Muscles
Operation	S	**Reposition:** Moving to its normal location, or other suitable location, all or a portion of a body part

Body Part (4th)	Approach (5th)	Device (6th)	Qualifier (7th)
0 Head Muscle 1 Facial Muscle 2 Neck Muscle, Right 3 Neck Muscle, Left 4 Tongue, Palate, Pharynx Muscle 5 Shoulder Muscle, Right 6 Shoulder Muscle, Left 7 Upper Arm Muscle, Right 8 Upper Arm Muscle, Left 9 Lower Arm and Wrist Muscle, Right B Lower Arm and Wrist Muscle, Left C Hand Muscle, Right D Hand Muscle, Left F Trunk Muscle, Right G Trunk Muscle, Left H Thorax Muscle, Right J Thorax Muscle, Left K Abdomen Muscle, Right L Abdomen Muscle, Left M Perineum Muscle N Hip Muscle, Right P Hip Muscle, Left Q Upper Leg Muscle, Right R Upper Leg Muscle, Left S Lower Leg Muscle, Right T Lower Leg Muscle, Left V Foot Muscle, Right W Foot Muscle, Left	0 Open 4 Percutaneous Endoscopic	Z No Device	Z No Qualifier

...ion	0	**Medical and Surgical**
...y System	K	**Muscles**
...ration	T	**Resection:** Cutting out or off, without replacement, all of a body part

Body Part (4th)	Approach (5th)	Device (6th)	Qualifier (7th)
Head Muscle Facial Muscle Neck Muscle, Right Neck Muscle, Left Tongue, Palate, Pharynx Muscle Shoulder Muscle, Right Shoulder Muscle, Left Upper Arm Muscle, Right Upper Arm Muscle, Left Lower Arm and Wrist Muscle, Right Lower Arm and Wrist Muscle, Left Hand Muscle, Right Hand Muscle, Left Trunk Muscle, Right Trunk Muscle, Left Thorax Muscle, Right Thorax Muscle, Left Abdomen Muscle, Right Abdomen Muscle, Left Perineum Muscle Hip Muscle, Right Hip Muscle, Left Upper Leg Muscle, Right Upper Leg Muscle, Left Lower Leg Muscle, Right Lower Leg Muscle, Left Foot Muscle, Right Foot Muscle, Left	**0** Open **4** Percutaneous Endoscopic	**Z** No Device	**Z** No Qualifier

...tion	0	**Medical and Surgical**
...dy System	K	**Muscles**
...eration	U	**Supplement:** Putting in or on biological or synthetic material that physically reinforces and/or augments the function of a portion of a body part

Body Part (4th)	Approach (5th)	Device (6th)	Qualifier (7th)
Head Muscle Facial Muscle Neck Muscle, Right Neck Muscle, Left Tongue, Palate, Pharynx Muscle Shoulder Muscle, Right Shoulder Muscle, Left Upper Arm Muscle, Right Upper Arm Muscle, Left Lower Arm and Wrist Muscle, Right Lower Arm and Wrist Muscle, Left Hand Muscle, Right Hand Muscle, Left Trunk Muscle, Right Trunk Muscle, Left Thorax Muscle, Right Thorax Muscle, Left Abdomen Muscle, Right Abdomen Muscle, Left Perineum Muscle Hip Muscle, Right Hip Muscle, Left Upper Leg Muscle, Right Upper Leg Muscle, Left Lower Leg Muscle, Right Lower Leg Muscle, Left Foot Muscle, Right Foot Muscle, Left	**0** Open **4** Percutaneous Endoscopic	**7** Autologous Tissue Substitute **J** Synthetic Substitute **K** Nonautologous Tissue Substitute	**Z** No Qualifier

Section	0	Medical and Surgical
Body System	K	Muscles
Operation	W	Revision: Correcting, to the extent possible, a portion of a malfunctioning device or the position of a displaced device

Body Part (4th)	Approach (5th)	Device (6th)	Qualifier (7th)
X Upper Muscle Y Lower Muscle	0 Open 3 Percutaneous 4 Percutaneous Endoscopic X External	0 Drainage Device 7 Autologous Tissue Substitute J Synthetic Substitute K Nonautologous Tissue Substitute M Stimulator Lead	Z No Qualifier

Section	0	Medical and Surgical
Body System	K	Muscles
Operation	X	Transfer: Moving, without taking out, all or a portion of a body part to another location to take over the function of all or a portion of a body part

Body Part (4th)	Approach (5th)	Device (6th)	Qualifier (7th)
0 Head Muscle 1 Facial Muscle 2 Neck Muscle, Right 3 Neck Muscle, Left 4 Tongue, Palate, Pharynx Muscle 5 Shoulder Muscle, Right 6 Shoulder Muscle, Left 7 Upper Arm Muscle, Right 8 Upper Arm Muscle, Left 9 Lower Arm and Wrist Muscle, Right B Lower Arm and Wrist Muscle, Left C Hand Muscle, Right D Hand Muscle, Left F Trunk Muscle, Right G Trunk Muscle, Left H Thorax Muscle, Right J Thorax Muscle, Left M Perineum Muscle N Hip Muscle, Right P Hip Muscle, Left Q Upper Leg Muscle, Right R Upper Leg Muscle, Left S Lower Leg Muscle, Right T Lower Leg Muscle, Left V Foot Muscle, Right W Foot Muscle, Left	0 Open 4 Percutaneous Endoscopic	Z No Device	0 Skin 1 Subcutaneous Tissue 2 Skin and Subcutaneous Tissue Z No Qualifier
K Abdomen Muscle, Right L Abdomen Muscle, Left	0 Open 4 Percutaneous Endoscopic	Z No Device	0 Skin 1 Subcutaneous Tissue 2 Skin and Subcutaneous Tissue 6 Transverse Rectus Abdominis Myocutaneous Flap Z No Qualifier

Muscles Code Listing 0K2–0KX

0K2 – Muscles, Change

Review Coding Guideline B6.1c

0K2XX0Z Change Drainage Device in Upper Muscle, External Approach
0K2XXYZ Change Other Device in Upper Muscle, External Approach

0K2YX0Z Change Drainage Device in Lower Muscle, External Approach

0K2YXYZ Change Other Device in Lower Muscle, External Approach

0K5 – Muscles, Destruction

0K500ZZ Destruction of Head Muscle, Open Approach
0K503ZZ Destruction of Head Muscle, Percutaneous Approach

0K504ZZ Destruction of Head Muscle, Percutaneous Endoscopic Approach
0K510ZZ Destruction of Facial Muscle, Open Approach

0K513ZZ Destruction of Facial Muscle, Percutaneous Approach
0K514ZZ Destruction of Facial Muscle, Percutaneous Endoscopic Approach

♀ Female-only　　♂ Male-only　　▲ Limited Coverage　　● Non-OR　　▥ HAC-associated procedure　　▲ Non-covered procedures　　+ Combinati

0ZZ Destruction of Right Neck Muscle, Open Approach

3ZZ Destruction of Right Neck Muscle, Percutaneous Approach

4ZZ Destruction of Right Neck Muscle, Percutaneous Endoscopic Approach

0ZZ Destruction of Left Neck Muscle, Open Approach

3ZZ Destruction of Left Neck Muscle, Percutaneous Approach

4ZZ Destruction of Left Neck Muscle, Percutaneous Endoscopic Approach

40ZZ Destruction of Tongue, Palate, Pharynx Muscle, Open Approach

43ZZ Destruction of Tongue, Palate, Pharynx Muscle, Percutaneous Approach

44ZZ Destruction of Tongue, Palate, Pharynx Muscle, Percutaneous Endoscopic Approach

50ZZ Destruction of Right Shoulder Muscle, Open Approach

53ZZ Destruction of Right Shoulder Muscle, Percutaneous Approach

54ZZ Destruction of Right Shoulder Muscle, Percutaneous Endoscopic Approach

60ZZ Destruction of Left Shoulder Muscle, Open Approach

63ZZ Destruction of Left Shoulder Muscle, Percutaneous Approach

64ZZ Destruction of Left Shoulder Muscle, Percutaneous Endoscopic Approach

70ZZ Destruction of Right Upper Arm Muscle, Open Approach

73ZZ Destruction of Right Upper Arm Muscle, Percutaneous Approach

74ZZ Destruction of Right Upper Arm Muscle, Percutaneous Endoscopic Approach

580ZZ Destruction of Left Upper Arm Muscle, Open Approach

583ZZ Destruction of Left Upper Arm Muscle, Percutaneous Approach

584ZZ Destruction of Left Upper Arm Muscle, Percutaneous Endoscopic Approach

590ZZ Destruction of Right Lower Arm and Wrist Muscle, Open Approach

593ZZ Destruction of Right Lower Arm and Wrist Muscle, Percutaneous Approach

594ZZ Destruction of Right Lower Arm and Wrist Muscle, Percutaneous Endoscopic Approach

5B0ZZ Destruction of Left Lower Arm and Wrist Muscle, Open Approach

0K5B3ZZ Destruction of Left Lower Arm and Wrist Muscle, Percutaneous Approach

0K5B4ZZ Destruction of Left Lower Arm and Wrist Muscle, Percutaneous Endoscopic Approach

0K5C0ZZ Destruction of Right Hand Muscle, Open Approach

0K5C3ZZ Destruction of Right Hand Muscle, Percutaneous Approach

0K5C4ZZ Destruction of Right Hand Muscle, Percutaneous Endoscopic Approach

0K5D0ZZ Destruction of Left Hand Muscle, Open Approach

0K5D3ZZ Destruction of Left Hand Muscle, Percutaneous Approach

0K5D4ZZ Destruction of Left Hand Muscle, Percutaneous Endoscopic Approach

0K5F0ZZ Destruction of Right Trunk Muscle, Open Approach

0K5F3ZZ Destruction of Right Trunk Muscle, Percutaneous Approach

0K5F4ZZ Destruction of Right Trunk Muscle, Percutaneous Endoscopic Approach

0K5G0ZZ Destruction of Left Trunk Muscle, Open Approach

0K5G3ZZ Destruction of Left Trunk Muscle, Percutaneous Approach

0K5G4ZZ Destruction of Left Trunk Muscle, Percutaneous Endoscopic Approach

0K5H0ZZ Destruction of Right Thorax Muscle, Open Approach

0K5H3ZZ Destruction of Right Thorax Muscle, Percutaneous Approach

0K5H4ZZ Destruction of Right Thorax Muscle, Percutaneous Endoscopic Approach

0K5J0ZZ Destruction of Left Thorax Muscle, Open Approach

0K5J3ZZ Destruction of Left Thorax Muscle, Percutaneous Approach

0K5J4ZZ Destruction of Left Thorax Muscle, Percutaneous Endoscopic Approach

0K5K0ZZ Destruction of Right Abdomen Muscle, Open Approach

0K5K3ZZ Destruction of Right Abdomen Muscle, Percutaneous Approach

0K5K4ZZ Destruction of Right Abdomen Muscle, Percutaneous Endoscopic Approach

0K5L0ZZ Destruction of Left Abdomen Muscle, Open Approach

0K5L3ZZ Destruction of Left Abdomen Muscle, Percutaneous Approach

0K5L4ZZ Destruction of Left Abdomen Muscle, Percutaneous Endoscopic Approach

0K5M0ZZ Destruction of Perineum Muscle, Open Approach

0K5M3ZZ Destruction of Perineum Muscle, Percutaneous Approach

0K5M4ZZ Destruction of Perineum Muscle, Percutaneous Endoscopic Approach

0K5N0ZZ Destruction of Right Hip Muscle, Open Approach

0K5N3ZZ Destruction of Right Hip Muscle, Percutaneous Approach

0K5N4ZZ Destruction of Right Hip Muscle, Percutaneous Endoscopic Approach

0K5P0ZZ Destruction of Left Hip Muscle, Open Approach

0K5P3ZZ Destruction of Left Hip Muscle, Percutaneous Approach

0K5P4ZZ Destruction of Left Hip Muscle, Percutaneous Endoscopic Approach

0K5Q0ZZ Destruction of Right Upper Leg Muscle, Open Approach

0K5Q3ZZ Destruction of Right Upper Leg Muscle, Percutaneous Approach

0K5Q4ZZ Destruction of Right Upper Leg Muscle, Percutaneous Endoscopic Approach

0K5R0ZZ Destruction of Left Upper Leg Muscle, Open Approach

0K5R3ZZ Destruction of Left Upper Leg Muscle, Percutaneous Approach

0K5R4ZZ Destruction of Left Upper Leg Muscle, Percutaneous Endoscopic Approach

0K5S0ZZ Destruction of Right Lower Leg Muscle, Open Approach

0K5S3ZZ Destruction of Right Lower Leg Muscle, Percutaneous Approach

0K5S4ZZ Destruction of Right Lower Leg Muscle, Percutaneous Endoscopic Approach

0K5T0ZZ Destruction of Left Lower Leg Muscle, Open Approach

0K5T3ZZ Destruction of Left Lower Leg Muscle, Percutaneous Approach

0K5T4ZZ Destruction of Left Lower Leg Muscle, Percutaneous Endoscopic Approach

0K5V0ZZ Destruction of Right Foot Muscle, Open Approach

0K5V3ZZ Destruction of Right Foot Muscle, Percutaneous Approach

0K5V4ZZ Destruction of Right Foot Muscle, Percutaneous Endoscopic Approach

0K5W0ZZ Destruction of Left Foot Muscle, Open Approach

0K5W3ZZ Destruction of Left Foot Muscle, Percutaneous Approach

0K5W4ZZ Destruction of Left Foot Muscle, Percutaneous Endoscopic Approach

K8 – Muscles, Division

view Coding Guideline B3.14

800ZZ Division of Head Muscle, Open Approach

803ZZ Division of Head Muscle, Percutaneous Approach

804ZZ Division of Head Muscle, Percutaneous Endoscopic Approach

810ZZ Division of Facial Muscle, Open Approach

813ZZ Division of Facial Muscle, Percutaneous Approach

814ZZ Division of Facial Muscle, Percutaneous Endoscopic Approach

820ZZ Division of Right Neck Muscle, Open Approach

823ZZ Division of Right Neck Muscle, Percutaneous Approach

824ZZ Division of Right Neck Muscle, Percutaneous Endoscopic Approach

0K830ZZ Division of Left Neck Muscle, Open Approach

0K833ZZ Division of Left Neck Muscle, Percutaneous Approach

0K834ZZ Division of Left Neck Muscle, Percutaneous Endoscopic Approach

0K840ZZ Division of Tongue, Palate, Pharynx Muscle, Open Approach

0K843ZZ Division of Tongue, Palate, Pharynx Muscle, Percutaneous Approach

0K844ZZ Division of Tongue, Palate, Pharynx Muscle, Percutaneous Endoscopic Approach

0K850ZZ Division of Right Shoulder Muscle, Open Approach

0K853ZZ Division of Right Shoulder Muscle, Percutaneous Approach

0K854ZZ Division of Right Shoulder Muscle, Percutaneous Endoscopic Approach

0K860ZZ Division of Left Shoulder Muscle, Open Approach

0K863ZZ Division of Left Shoulder Muscle, Percutaneous Approach

0K864ZZ Division of Left Shoulder Muscle, Percutaneous Endoscopic Approach

0K870ZZ Division of Right Upper Arm Muscle, Open Approach

0K873ZZ Division of Right Upper Arm Muscle, Percutaneous Approach

0K874ZZ Division of Right Upper Arm Muscle, Percutaneous Endoscopic Approach

0K880ZZ Division of Left Upper Arm Muscle, Open Approach

▲ Female-only ♂ Male-only ▲ Limited Coverage ● Non-OR ▨ HAC-associated procedure ▲ Non-covered procedures ✚ Combination

0K883ZZ	Division of Left Upper Arm Muscle, Percutaneous Approach	
0K884ZZ	Division of Left Upper Arm Muscle, Percutaneous Endoscopic Approach	
0K890ZZ	Division of Right Lower Arm and Wrist Muscle, Open Approach	
0K893ZZ	Division of Right Lower Arm and Wrist Muscle, Percutaneous Approach	
0K894ZZ	Division of Right Lower Arm and Wrist Muscle, Percutaneous Endoscopic Approach	
0K8B0ZZ	Division of Left Lower Arm and Wrist Muscle, Open Approach	
0K8B3ZZ	Division of Left Lower Arm and Wrist Muscle, Percutaneous Approach	
0K8B4ZZ	Division of Left Lower Arm and Wrist Muscle, Percutaneous Endoscopic Approach	
0K8C0ZZ	Division of Right Hand Muscle, Open Approach	
0K8C3ZZ	Division of Right Hand Muscle, Percutaneous Approach	
0K8C4ZZ	Division of Right Hand Muscle, Percutaneous Endoscopic Approach	
0K8D0ZZ	Division of Left Hand Muscle, Open Approach	
0K8D3ZZ	Division of Left Hand Muscle, Percutaneous Approach	
0K8D4ZZ	Division of Left Hand Muscle, Percutaneous Endoscopic Approach	
0K8F0ZZ	Division of Right Trunk Muscle, Open Approach	
0K8F3ZZ	Division of Right Trunk Muscle, Percutaneous Approach	
0K8F4ZZ	Division of Right Trunk Muscle, Percutaneous Endoscopic Approach	
0K8G0ZZ	Division of Left Trunk Muscle, Open Approach	
0K8G3ZZ	Division of Left Trunk Muscle, Percutaneous Approach	

0K8G4ZZ	Division of Left Trunk Muscle, Percutaneous Endoscopic Approach
0K8H0ZZ	Division of Right Thorax Muscle, Open Approach
0K8H3ZZ	Division of Right Thorax Muscle, Percutaneous Approach
0K8H4ZZ	Division of Right Thorax Muscle, Percutaneous Endoscopic Approach
0K8J0ZZ	Division of Left Thorax Muscle, Open Approach
0K8J3ZZ	Division of Left Thorax Muscle, Percutaneous Approach
0K8J4ZZ	Division of Left Thorax Muscle, Percutaneous Endoscopic Approach
0K8K0ZZ	Division of Right Abdomen Muscle, Open Approach
0K8K3ZZ	Division of Right Abdomen Muscle, Percutaneous Approach
0K8K4ZZ	Division of Right Abdomen Muscle, Percutaneous Endoscopic Approach
0K8L0ZZ	Division of Left Abdomen Muscle, Open Approach
0K8L3ZZ	Division of Left Abdomen Muscle, Percutaneous Approach
0K8L4ZZ	Division of Left Abdomen Muscle, Percutaneous Endoscopic Approach
0K8M0ZZ	Division of Perineum Muscle, Open Approach
0K8M3ZZ	Division of Perineum Muscle, Percutaneous Approach
0K8M4ZZ	Division of Perineum Muscle, Percutaneous Endoscopic Approach
0K8N0ZZ	Division of Right Hip Muscle, Open Approach
0K8N3ZZ	Division of Right Hip Muscle, Percutaneous Approach
0K8N4ZZ	Division of Right Hip Muscle, Percutaneous Endoscopic Approach
0K8P0ZZ	Division of Left Hip Muscle, Open Approach

0K8P3ZZ	Division of Left Hip Muscle, Percuta... Approach
0K8P4ZZ	Division of Left Hip Muscle, Percuta... Endoscopic Approach
0K8Q0ZZ	Division of Right Upper Leg Muscle, Open Approach
0K8Q3ZZ	Division of Right Upper Leg Muscle, Percutaneous Approach
0K8Q4ZZ	Division of Right Upper Leg Muscle, Percutaneous Endoscopic Approach
0K8R0ZZ	Division of Left Upper Leg Muscle, O... Approach
0K8R3ZZ	Division of Left Upper Leg Muscle, Percutaneous Approach
0K8R4ZZ	Division of Left Upper Leg Muscle, Percutaneous Endoscopic Approach
0K8S0ZZ	Division of Right Lower Leg Muscle, Open Approach
0K8S3ZZ	Division of Right Lower Leg Muscle, Percutaneous Approach
0K8S4ZZ	Division of Right Lower Leg Muscle, Percutaneous Endoscopic Approach
0K8T0ZZ	Division of Left Lower Leg Muscle, O... Approach
0K8T3ZZ	Division of Left Lower Leg Muscle, Percutaneous Approach
0K8T4ZZ	Division of Left Lower Leg Muscle, Percutaneous Endoscopic Approach
0K8V0ZZ	Division of Right Foot Muscle, Open Approach
0K8V3ZZ	Division of Right Foot Muscle, Percutaneous Approach
0K8V4ZZ	Division of Right Foot Muscle, Percutaneous Endoscopic Approach
0K8W0ZZ	Division of Left Foot Muscle, Open Approach
0K8W3ZZ	Division of Left Foot Muscle, Percutaneous Approach
0K8W4ZZ	Division of Left Foot Muscle, Percutaneous Endoscopic Approach

0K9 – Muscles, Drainage

Review Coding Guidelines B3.4a and B3.4b

Review Coding Guideline B6.2

0K9000Z	Drainage of Head Muscle with Drainage Device, Open Approach
0K900ZX	Drainage of Head Muscle, Open Approach, Diagnostic
0K900ZZ	Drainage of Head Muscle, Open Approach
0K9030Z	Drainage of Head Muscle with Drainage Device, Percutaneous Approach
0K903ZX	Drainage of Head Muscle, Percutaneous Approach, Diagnostic
0K903ZZ	Drainage of Head Muscle, Percutaneous Approach
0K9040Z	Drainage of Head Muscle with Drainage Device, Percutaneous Endoscopic Approach
0K904ZX	Drainage of Head Muscle, Percutaneous Endoscopic Approach, Diagnostic
0K904ZZ	Drainage of Head Muscle, Percutaneous Endoscopic Approach
0K9100Z	Drainage of Facial Muscle with Drainage Device, Open Approach
0K910ZX	Drainage of Facial Muscle, Open Approach, Diagnostic
0K910ZZ	Drainage of Facial Muscle, Open Approach
0K9130Z	Drainage of Facial Muscle with Drainage Device, Percutaneous Approach
0K913ZX	Drainage of Facial Muscle, Percutaneous Approach, Diagnostic

0K913ZZ	Drainage of Facial Muscle, Percutaneous Approach
0K9140Z	Drainage of Facial Muscle with Drainage Device, Percutaneous Endoscopic Approach
0K914ZX	Drainage of Facial Muscle, Percutaneous Endoscopic Approach, Diagnostic
0K914ZZ	Drainage of Facial Muscle, Percutaneous Endoscopic Approach
0K9200Z	Drainage of Right Neck Muscle with Drainage Device, Open Approach
0K920ZX	Drainage of Right Neck Muscle, Open Approach, Diagnostic
0K920ZZ	Drainage of Right Neck Muscle, Open Approach
0K9230Z	Drainage of Right Neck Muscle with Drainage Device, Percutaneous Approach
0K923ZX	Drainage of Right Neck Muscle, Percutaneous Approach, Diagnostic
0K923ZZ	Drainage of Right Neck Muscle, Percutancous Approach
0K9240Z	Drainage of Right Neck Muscle with Drainage Device, Percutaneous Endoscopic Approach
0K924ZX	Drainage of Right Neck Muscle, Percutaneous Endoscopic Approach, Diagnostic

0K924ZZ	Drainage of Right Neck Muscle, Percutaneous Endoscopic Approach
0K9300Z	Drainage of Left Neck Muscle with Drainage Device, Open Approach
0K930ZX	Drainage of Left Neck Muscle, Open Approach, Diagnostic
0K930ZZ	Drainage of Left Neck Muscle, Open Approach
0K9330Z	Drainage of Left Neck Muscle with Drainage Device, Percutaneous Approach
0K933ZX	Drainage of Left Neck Muscle, Percutaneous Approach, Diagnostic
0K933ZZ	Drainage of Left Neck Muscle, Percutaneous Approach
0K9340Z	Drainage of Left Neck Muscle with Drainage Device, Percutaneous Endoscopic Approach
0K934ZX	Drainage of Left Neck Muscle, Percutaneous Endoscopic Approach, Diagnostic
0K934ZZ	Drainage of Left Neck Muscle, Percutaneous Endoscopic Approach
0K9400Z	Drainage of Tongue, Palate, Pharynx Muscle with Drainage Device, Open Approach
0K940ZX	Drainage of Tongue, Palate, Pharynx Muscle, Open Approach, Diagnostic

0ZZ Drainage of Tongue, Palate, Pharynx Muscle, Open Approach

30Z Drainage of Tongue, Palate, Pharynx Muscle with Drainage Device, Percutaneous Approach

3ZX Drainage of Tongue, Palate, Pharynx Muscle, Percutaneous Approach, Diagnostic

3ZZ Drainage of Tongue, Palate, Pharynx Muscle, Percutaneous Approach

40Z Drainage of Tongue, Palate, Pharynx Muscle with Drainage Device, Percutaneous Endoscopic Approach

4ZX Drainage of Tongue, Palate, Pharynx Muscle, Percutaneous Endoscopic Approach, Diagnostic

4ZZ Drainage of Tongue, Palate, Pharynx Muscle, Percutaneous Endoscopic Approach

500Z Drainage of Right Shoulder Muscle with Drainage Device, Open Approach

50ZX Drainage of Right Shoulder Muscle, Open Approach, Diagnostic

50ZZ Drainage of Right Shoulder Muscle, Open Approach

530Z Drainage of Right Shoulder Muscle with Drainage Device, Percutaneous Approach

53ZX Drainage of Right Shoulder Muscle, Percutaneous Approach, Diagnostic

53ZZ Drainage of Right Shoulder Muscle, Percutaneous Approach

540Z Drainage of Right Shoulder Muscle with Drainage Device, Percutaneous Endoscopic Approach

54ZX Drainage of Right Shoulder Muscle, Percutaneous Endoscopic Approach, Diagnostic

54ZZ Drainage of Right Shoulder Muscle, Percutaneous Endoscopic Approach

600Z Drainage of Left Shoulder Muscle with Drainage Device, Open Approach

60ZX Drainage of Left Shoulder Muscle, Open Approach, Diagnostic

60ZZ Drainage of Left Shoulder Muscle, Open Approach

630Z Drainage of Left Shoulder Muscle with Drainage Device, Percutaneous Approach

63ZX Drainage of Left Shoulder Muscle, Percutaneous Approach, Diagnostic

63ZZ Drainage of Left Shoulder Muscle, Percutaneous Approach

640Z Drainage of Left Shoulder Muscle with Drainage Device, Percutaneous Endoscopic Approach

64ZX Drainage of Left Shoulder Muscle, Percutaneous Endoscopic Approach, Diagnostic

64ZZ Drainage of Left Shoulder Muscle, Percutaneous Endoscopic Approach

9700Z Drainage of Right Upper Arm Muscle with Drainage Device, Open Approach

970ZX Drainage of Right Upper Arm Muscle, Open Approach, Diagnostic

970ZZ Drainage of Right Upper Arm Muscle, Open Approach

9730Z Drainage of Right Upper Arm Muscle with Drainage Device, Percutaneous Approach

973ZX Drainage of Right Upper Arm Muscle, Percutaneous Approach, Diagnostic

973ZZ Drainage of Right Upper Arm Muscle, Percutaneous Approach

9740Z Drainage of Right Upper Arm Muscle with Drainage Device, Percutaneous Endoscopic Approach

0K974ZX Drainage of Right Upper Arm Muscle, Percutaneous Endoscopic Approach, Diagnostic

0K974ZZ Drainage of Right Upper Arm Muscle, Percutaneous Endoscopic Approach

0K9800Z Drainage of Left Upper Arm Muscle with Drainage Device, Open Approach

0K980ZX Drainage of Left Upper Arm Muscle, Open Approach, Diagnostic

0K980ZZ Drainage of Left Upper Arm Muscle, Open Approach

0K9830Z Drainage of Left Upper Arm Muscle with Drainage Device, Percutaneous Approach

0K983ZX Drainage of Left Upper Arm Muscle, Percutaneous Approach, Diagnostic

0K983ZZ Drainage of Left Upper Arm Muscle, Percutaneous Approach

0K9840Z Drainage of Left Upper Arm Muscle with Drainage Device, Percutaneous Endoscopic Approach

0K984ZX Drainage of Left Upper Arm Muscle, Percutaneous Endoscopic Approach, Diagnostic

0K984ZZ Drainage of Left Upper Arm Muscle, Percutaneous Endoscopic Approach

0K9900Z Drainage of Right Lower Arm and Wrist Muscle with Drainage Device, Open Approach

0K990ZX Drainage of Right Lower Arm and Wrist Muscle, Open Approach, Diagnostic

0K990ZZ Drainage of Right Lower Arm and Wrist Muscle, Open Approach

0K9930Z Drainage of Right Lower Arm and Wrist Muscle with Drainage Device, Percutaneous Approach

0K993ZX Drainage of Right Lower Arm and Wrist Muscle, Percutaneous Approach, Diagnostic

0K993ZZ Drainage of Right Lower Arm and Wrist Muscle, Percutaneous Approach

0K9940Z Drainage of Right Lower Arm and Wrist Muscle with Drainage Device, Percutaneous Endoscopic Approach

0K994ZX Drainage of Right Lower Arm and Wrist Muscle, Percutaneous Endoscopic Approach, Diagnostic

0K994ZZ Drainage of Right Lower Arm and Wrist Muscle, Percutaneous Endoscopic Approach

0K9B00Z Drainage of Left Lower Arm and Wrist Muscle with Drainage Device, Open Approach

0K9B0ZX Drainage of Left Lower Arm and Wrist Muscle, Open Approach, Diagnostic

0K9B0ZZ Drainage of Left Lower Arm and Wrist Muscle, Open Approach

0K9B30Z Drainage of Left Lower Arm and Wrist Muscle with Drainage Device, Percutaneous Approach

0K9B3ZX Drainage of Left Lower Arm and Wrist Muscle, Percutaneous Approach, Diagnostic

0K9B3ZZ Drainage of Left Lower Arm and Wrist Muscle, Percutaneous Approach

0K9B40Z Drainage of Left Lower Arm and Wrist Muscle with Drainage Device, Percutaneous Endoscopic Approach

0K9B4ZX Drainage of Left Lower Arm and Wrist Muscle, Percutaneous Endoscopic Approach, Diagnostic

0K9B4ZZ Drainage of Left Lower Arm and Wrist Muscle, Percutaneous Endoscopic Approach

0K9C00Z Drainage of Right Hand Muscle with Drainage Device, Open Approach

0K9C0ZX Drainage of Right Hand Muscle, Open Approach, Diagnostic

0K9C0ZZ Drainage of Right Hand Muscle, Open Approach

0K9C30Z Drainage of Right Hand Muscle with Drainage Device, Percutaneous Approach

0K9C3ZX Drainage of Right Hand Muscle, Percutaneous Approach, Diagnostic

0K9C3ZZ Drainage of Right Hand Muscle, Percutaneous Approach

0K9C40Z Drainage of Right Hand Muscle with Drainage Device, Percutaneous Endoscopic Approach

0K9C4ZX Drainage of Right Hand Muscle, Percutaneous Endoscopic Approach, Diagnostic

0K9C4ZZ Drainage of Right Hand Muscle, Percutaneous Endoscopic Approach

0K9D00Z Drainage of Left Hand Muscle with Drainage Device, Open Approach

0K9D0ZX Drainage of Left Hand Muscle, Open Approach, Diagnostic

0K9D0ZZ Drainage of Left Hand Muscle, Open Approach

0K9D30Z Drainage of Left Hand Muscle with Drainage Device, Percutaneous Approach

0K9D3ZX Drainage of Left Hand Muscle, Percutaneous Approach, Diagnostic

0K9D3ZZ Drainage of Left Hand Muscle, Percutaneous Approach

0K9D40Z Drainage of Left Hand Muscle with Drainage Device, Percutaneous Endoscopic Approach

0K9D4ZX Drainage of Left Hand Muscle, Percutaneous Endoscopic Approach, Diagnostic

0K9D4ZZ Drainage of Left Hand Muscle, Percutaneous Endoscopic Approach

0K9F00Z Drainage of Right Trunk Muscle with Drainage Device, Open Approach

0K9F0ZX Drainage of Right Trunk Muscle, Open Approach, Diagnostic

0K9F0ZZ Drainage of Right Trunk Muscle, Open Approach

0K9F30Z Drainage of Right Trunk Muscle with Drainage Device, Percutaneous Approach

0K9F3ZX Drainage of Right Trunk Muscle, Percutaneous Approach, Diagnostic

0K9F3ZZ Drainage of Right Trunk Muscle, Percutaneous Approach

0K9F40Z Drainage of Right Trunk Muscle with Drainage Device, Percutaneous Endoscopic Approach

0K9F4ZX Drainage of Right Trunk Muscle, Percutaneous Endoscopic Approach, Diagnostic

0K9F4ZZ Drainage of Right Trunk Muscle, Percutaneous Endoscopic Approach

0K9G00Z Drainage of Left Trunk Muscle with Drainage Device, Open Approach

0K9G0ZX Drainage of Left Trunk Muscle, Open Approach, Diagnostic

0K9G0ZZ Drainage of Left Trunk Muscle, Open Approach

0K9G30Z Drainage of Left Trunk Muscle with Drainage Device, Percutaneous Approach

0K9G3ZX Drainage of Left Trunk Muscle, Percutaneous Approach, Diagnostic

0K9G3ZZ Drainage of Left Trunk Muscle, Percutaneous Approach

0K9G40Z Drainage of Left Trunk Muscle with Drainage Device, Percutaneous Endoscopic Approach

0K9G4ZX Drainage of Left Trunk Muscle, Percutaneous Endoscopic Approach, Diagnostic

| Female-only | ♂ Male-only | ▲ Limited Coverage | ● Non-OR | ▥ HAC-associated procedure | ▲ Non-covered procedures | + Combination |

0K9G4ZZ	Drainage of Left Trunk Muscle, Percutaneous Endoscopic Approach
0K9H00Z	Drainage of Right Thorax Muscle with Drainage Device, Open Approach
0K9H0ZX	Drainage of Right Thorax Muscle, Open Approach, Diagnostic
0K9H0ZZ	Drainage of Right Thorax Muscle, Open Approach
0K9H30Z	Drainage of Right Thorax Muscle with Drainage Device, Percutaneous Approach
0K9H3ZX	Drainage of Right Thorax Muscle, Percutaneous Approach, Diagnostic
0K9H3ZZ	Drainage of Right Thorax Muscle, Percutaneous Approach
0K9H40Z	Drainage of Right Thorax Muscle with Drainage Device, Percutaneous Endoscopic Approach
0K9H4ZX	Drainage of Right Thorax Muscle, Percutaneous Endoscopic Approach, Diagnostic
0K9H4ZZ	Drainage of Right Thorax Muscle, Percutaneous Endoscopic Approach
0K9J00Z	Drainage of Left Thorax Muscle with Drainage Device, Open Approach
0K9J0ZX	Drainage of Left Thorax Muscle, Open Approach, Diagnostic
0K9J0ZZ	Drainage of Left Thorax Muscle, Open Approach
0K9J30Z	Drainage of Left Thorax Muscle with Drainage Device, Percutaneous Approach
0K9J3ZX	Drainage of Left Thorax Muscle, Percutaneous Approach, Diagnostic
0K9J3ZZ	Drainage of Left Thorax Muscle, Percutaneous Approach
0K9J40Z	Drainage of Left Thorax Muscle with Drainage Device, Percutaneous Endoscopic Approach
0K9J4ZX	Drainage of Left Thorax Muscle, Percutaneous Endoscopic Approach, Diagnostic
0K9J4ZZ	Drainage of Left Thorax Muscle, Percutaneous Endoscopic Approach
0K9K00Z	Drainage of Right Abdomen Muscle with Drainage Device, Open Approach
0K9K0ZX	Drainage of Right Abdomen Muscle, Open Approach, Diagnostic
0K9K0ZZ	Drainage of Right Abdomen Muscle, Open Approach
0K9K30Z	Drainage of Right Abdomen Muscle with Drainage Device, Percutaneous Approach
0K9K3ZX	Drainage of Right Abdomen Muscle, Percutaneous Approach, Diagnostic
0K9K3ZZ	Drainage of Right Abdomen Muscle, Percutaneous Approach
0K9K40Z	Drainage of Right Abdomen Muscle with Drainage Device, Percutaneous Endoscopic Approach
0K9K4ZX	Drainage of Right Abdomen Muscle, Percutaneous Endoscopic Approach, Diagnostic
0K9K4ZZ	Drainage of Right Abdomen Muscle, Percutaneous Endoscopic Approach
0K9L00Z	Drainage of Left Abdomen Muscle with Drainage Device, Open Approach
0K9L0ZX	Drainage of Left Abdomen Muscle, Open Approach, Diagnostic
0K9L0ZZ	Drainage of Left Abdomen Muscle, Open Approach
0K9L30Z	Drainage of Left Abdomen Muscle with Drainage Device, Percutaneous Approach
0K9L3ZX	Drainage of Left Abdomen Muscle, Percutaneous Approach, Diagnostic
0K9L3ZZ	Drainage of Left Abdomen Muscle, Percutaneous Approach
0K9L40Z	Drainage of Left Abdomen Muscle with Drainage Device, Percutaneous Endoscopic Approach
0K9L4ZX	Drainage of Left Abdomen Muscle, Percutaneous Endoscopic Approach, Diagnostic
0K9L4ZZ	Drainage of Left Abdomen Muscle, Percutaneous Endoscopic Approach
0K9M00Z	Drainage of Perineum Muscle with Drainage Device, Open Approach
0K9M0ZX	Drainage of Perineum Muscle, Open Approach, Diagnostic
0K9M0ZZ	Drainage of Perineum Muscle, Open Approach
0K9M30Z	Drainage of Perineum Muscle with Drainage Device, Percutaneous Approach
0K9M3ZX	Drainage of Perineum Muscle, Percutaneous Approach, Diagnostic
0K9M3ZZ	Drainage of Perineum Muscle, Percutaneous Approach
0K9M40Z	Drainage of Perineum Muscle with Drainage Device, Percutaneous Endoscopic Approach
0K9M4ZX	Drainage of Perineum Muscle, Percutaneous Endoscopic Approach, Diagnostic
0K9M4ZZ	Drainage of Perineum Muscle, Percutaneous Endoscopic Approach
0K9N00Z	Drainage of Right Hip Muscle with Drainage Device, Open Approach
0K9N0ZX	Drainage of Right Hip Muscle, Open Approach, Diagnostic
0K9N0ZZ	Drainage of Right Hip Muscle, Open Approach
0K9N30Z	Drainage of Right Hip Muscle with Drainage Device, Percutaneous Approach
0K9N3ZX	Drainage of Right Hip Muscle, Percutaneous Approach, Diagnostic
0K9N3ZZ	Drainage of Right Hip Muscle, Percutaneous Approach
0K9N40Z	Drainage of Right Hip Muscle with Drainage Device, Percutaneous Endoscopic Approach
0K9N4ZX	Drainage of Right Hip Muscle, Percutaneous Endoscopic Approach, Diagnostic
0K9N4ZZ	Drainage of Right Hip Muscle, Percutaneous Endoscopic Approach
0K9P00Z	Drainage of Left Hip Muscle with Drainage Device, Open Approach
0K9P0ZX	Drainage of Left Hip Muscle, Open Approach, Diagnostic
0K9P0ZZ	Drainage of Left Hip Muscle, Open Approach
0K9P30Z	Drainage of Left Hip Muscle with Drainage Device, Percutaneous Approach
0K9P3ZX	Drainage of Left Hip Muscle, Percutaneous Approach, Diagnostic
0K9P3ZZ	Drainage of Left Hip Muscle, Percutaneous Approach
0K9P40Z	Drainage of Left Hip Muscle with Drainage Device, Percutaneous Endoscopic Approach
0K9P4ZX	Drainage of Left Hip Muscle, Percutaneous Endoscopic Approach, Diagnostic
0K9P4ZZ	Drainage of Left Hip Muscle, Percutaneous Endoscopic Approach
0K9Q00Z	Drainage of Right Upper Leg Muscle with Drainage Device, Open Approach
0K9Q0ZX	Drainage of Right Upper Leg Muscle, Open Approach, Diagnostic
0K9Q0ZZ	Drainage of Right Upper Leg Muscle, Open Approach
0K9Q30Z	Drainage of Right Upper Leg Muscle with Drainage Device, Percutaneous Approach
0K9Q3ZX	Drainage of Right Upper Leg Muscle, Percutaneous Approach, Diagnostic
0K9Q3ZZ	Drainage of Right Upper Leg Muscle, Percutaneous Approach
0K9Q40Z	Drainage of Right Upper Leg Muscle with Drainage Device, Percutaneous Endoscopic Approach
0K9Q4ZX	Drainage of Right Upper Leg Muscle, Percutaneous Endoscopic Approach, Diagnostic
0K9Q4ZZ	Drainage of Right Upper Leg Muscle, Percutaneous Endoscopic Approach
0K9R00Z	Drainage of Left Upper Leg Muscle with Drainage Device, Open Approach
0K9R0ZX	Drainage of Left Upper Leg Muscle, Open Approach, Diagnostic
0K9R0ZZ	Drainage of Left Upper Leg Muscle, Open Approach
0K9R30Z	Drainage of Left Upper Leg Muscle with Drainage Device, Percutaneous Approach
0K9R3ZX	Drainage of Left Upper Leg Muscle, Percutaneous Approach, Diagnostic
0K9R3ZZ	Drainage of Left Upper Leg Muscle, Percutaneous Approach
0K9R40Z	Drainage of Left Upper Leg Muscle with Drainage Device, Percutaneous Endoscopic Approach
0K9R4ZX	Drainage of Left Upper Leg Muscle, Percutaneous Endoscopic Approach, Diagnostic
0K9R4ZZ	Drainage of Left Upper Leg Muscle, Percutaneous Endoscopic Approach
0K9S00Z	Drainage of Right Lower Leg Muscle with Drainage Device, Open Approach
0K9S0ZX	Drainage of Right Lower Leg Muscle, Open Approach, Diagnostic
0K9S0ZZ	Drainage of Right Lower Leg Muscle, Open Approach
0K9S30Z	Drainage of Right Lower Leg Muscle with Drainage Device, Percutaneous Approach
0K9S3ZX	Drainage of Right Lower Leg Muscle, Percutaneous Approach, Diagnostic
0K9S3ZZ	Drainage of Right Lower Leg Muscle, Percutaneous Approach
0K9S40Z	Drainage of Right Lower Leg Muscle with Drainage Device, Percutaneous Endoscopic Approach
0K9S4ZX	Drainage of Right Lower Leg Muscle, Percutaneous Endoscopic Approach, Diagnostic
0K9S4ZZ	Drainage of Right Lower Leg Muscle, Percutaneous Endoscopic Approach
0K9T00Z	Drainage of Left Lower Leg Muscle with Drainage Device, Open Approach
0K9T0ZX	Drainage of Left Lower Leg Muscle, Open Approach, Diagnostic
0K9T0ZZ	Drainage of Left Lower Leg Muscle, Open Approach
0K9T30Z	Drainage of Left Lower Leg Muscle with Drainage Device, Percutaneous Approach
0K9T3ZX	Drainage of Left Lower Leg Muscle, Percutaneous Approach, Diagnostic
0K9T3ZZ	Drainage of Left Lower Leg Muscle, Percutaneous Approach
0K9T40Z	Drainage of Left Lower Leg Muscle with Drainage Device, Percutaneous Endoscopic Approach
0K9T4ZX	Drainage of Left Lower Leg Muscle, Percutaneous Endoscopic Approach, Diagnostic

4ZZ	Drainage of Left Lower Leg Muscle, Percutaneous Endoscopic Approach
00Z	Drainage of Right Foot Muscle with Drainage Device, Open Approach
0ZX	Drainage of Right Foot Muscle, Open Approach, Diagnostic
0ZZ	Drainage of Right Foot Muscle, Open Approach
30Z	Drainage of Right Foot Muscle with Drainage Device, Percutaneous Approach
3ZX	Drainage of Right Foot Muscle, Percutaneous Approach, Diagnostic
3ZZ	Drainage of Right Foot Muscle, Percutaneous Approach

0K9V40Z	Drainage of Right Foot Muscle with Drainage Device, Percutaneous Endoscopic Approach
0K9V4ZX	Drainage of Right Foot Muscle, Percutaneous Endoscopic Approach, Diagnostic
0K9V4ZZ	Drainage of Right Foot Muscle, Percutaneous Endoscopic Approach
0K9W00Z	Drainage of Left Foot Muscle with Drainage Device, Open Approach
0K9W0ZX	Drainage of Left Foot Muscle, Open Approach, Diagnostic
0K9W0ZZ	Drainage of Left Foot Muscle, Open Approach

0K9W30Z	Drainage of Left Foot Muscle with Drainage Device, Percutaneous Approach
0K9W3ZX	Drainage of Left Foot Muscle, Percutaneous Approach, Diagnostic
0K9W3ZZ	Drainage of Left Foot Muscle, Percutaneous Approach
0K9W40Z	Drainage of Left Foot Muscle with Drainage Device, Percutaneous Endoscopic Approach
0K9W4ZX	Drainage of Left Foot Muscle, Percutaneous Endoscopic Approach, Diagnostic
0K9W4ZZ	Drainage of Left Foot Muscle, Percutaneous Endoscopic Approach

B – Muscles, Excision

New Coding Guidelines B3.4a and B3.4b

New Coding Guideline B3.5

New Coding Guideline B3.8

00ZX	Excision of Head Muscle, Open Approach, Diagnostic
00ZZ	Excision of Head Muscle, Open Approach
03ZX	Excision of Head Muscle, Percutaneous Approach, Diagnostic
03ZZ	Excision of Head Muscle, Percutaneous Approach
04ZX	Excision of Head Muscle, Percutaneous Endoscopic Approach, Diagnostic
04ZZ	Excision of Head Muscle, Percutaneous Endoscopic Approach
10ZX	Excision of Facial Muscle, Open Approach, Diagnostic
10ZZ	Excision of Facial Muscle, Open Approach
13ZX	Excision of Facial Muscle, Percutaneous Approach, Diagnostic
13ZZ	Excision of Facial Muscle, Percutaneous Approach
14ZX	Excision of Facial Muscle, Percutaneous Endoscopic Approach, Diagnostic
14ZZ	Excision of Facial Muscle, Percutaneous Endoscopic Approach
20ZX	Excision of Right Neck Muscle, Open Approach, Diagnostic
20ZZ	Excision of Right Neck Muscle, Open Approach
23ZX	Excision of Right Neck Muscle, Percutaneous Approach, Diagnostic
23ZZ	Excision of Right Neck Muscle, Percutaneous Approach
24ZX	Excision of Right Neck Muscle, Percutaneous Endoscopic Approach, Diagnostic
24ZZ	Excision of Right Neck Muscle, Percutaneous Endoscopic Approach
B30ZX	Excision of Left Neck Muscle, Open Approach, Diagnostic
B30ZZ	Excision of Left Neck Muscle, Open Approach
B33ZX	Excision of Left Neck Muscle, Percutaneous Approach, Diagnostic
B33ZZ	Excision of Left Neck Muscle, Percutaneous Approach
B34ZX	Excision of Left Neck Muscle, Percutaneous Endoscopic Approach, Diagnostic
B34ZZ	Excision of Left Neck Muscle, Percutaneous Endoscopic Approach
B40ZX	Excision of Tongue, Palate, Pharynx Muscle, Open Approach, Diagnostic

0KB40ZZ	Excision of Tongue, Palate, Pharynx Muscle, Open Approach
0KB43ZX	Excision of Tongue, Palate, Pharynx Muscle, Percutaneous Approach, Diagnostic
0KB43ZZ	Excision of Tongue, Palate, Pharynx Muscle, Percutaneous Approach
0KB44ZX	Excision of Tongue, Palate, Pharynx Muscle, Percutaneous Endoscopic Approach, Diagnostic
0KB44ZZ	Excision of Tongue, Palate, Pharynx Muscle, Percutaneous Endoscopic Approach
0KB50ZX	Excision of Right Shoulder Muscle, Open Approach, Diagnostic
0KB50ZZ	Excision of Right Shoulder Muscle, Open Approach
0KB53ZX	Excision of Right Shoulder Muscle, Percutaneous Approach, Diagnostic
0KB53ZZ	Excision of Right Shoulder Muscle, Percutaneous Approach
0KB54ZX	Excision of Right Shoulder Muscle, Percutaneous Endoscopic Approach, Diagnostic
0KB54ZZ	Excision of Right Shoulder Muscle, Percutaneous Endoscopic Approach
0KB60ZX	Excision of Left Shoulder Muscle, Open Approach, Diagnostic
0KB60ZZ	Excision of Left Shoulder Muscle, Open Approach
0KB63ZX	Excision of Left Shoulder Muscle, Percutaneous Approach, Diagnostic
0KB63ZZ	Excision of Left Shoulder Muscle, Percutaneous Approach
0KB64ZX	Excision of Left Shoulder Muscle, Percutaneous Endoscopic Approach, Diagnostic
0KB64ZZ	Excision of Left Shoulder Muscle, Percutaneous Endoscopic Approach
0KB70ZX	Excision of Right Upper Arm Muscle, Open Approach, Diagnostic
0KB70ZZ	Excision of Right Upper Arm Muscle, Open Approach
0KB73ZX	Excision of Right Upper Arm Muscle, Percutaneous Approach, Diagnostic
0KB73ZZ	Excision of Right Upper Arm Muscle, Percutaneous Approach
0KB74ZX	Excision of Right Upper Arm Muscle, Percutaneous Endoscopic Approach, Diagnostic
0KB74ZZ	Excision of Right Upper Arm Muscle, Percutaneous Endoscopic Approach

0KB80ZX	Excision of Left Upper Arm Muscle, Open Approach, Diagnostic
0KB80ZZ	Excision of Left Upper Arm Muscle, Open Approach
0KB83ZX	Excision of Left Upper Arm Muscle, Percutaneous Approach, Diagnostic
0KB83ZZ	Excision of Left Upper Arm Muscle, Percutaneous Approach
0KB84ZX	Excision of Left Upper Arm Muscle, Percutaneous Endoscopic Approach, Diagnostic
0KB84ZZ	Excision of Left Upper Arm Muscle, Percutaneous Endoscopic Approach
0KB90ZX	Excision of Right Lower Arm and Wrist Muscle, Open Approach, Diagnostic
0KB90ZZ	Excision of Right Lower Arm and Wrist Muscle, Open Approach
0KB93ZX	Excision of Right Lower Arm and Wrist Muscle, Percutaneous Approach, Diagnostic
0KB93ZZ	Excision of Right Lower Arm and Wrist Muscle, Percutaneous Approach
0KB94ZX	Excision of Right Lower Arm and Wrist Muscle, Percutaneous Endoscopic Approach, Diagnostic
0KB94ZZ	Excision of Right Lower Arm and Wrist Muscle, Percutaneous Endoscopic Approach
0KBB0ZX	Excision of Left Lower Arm and Wrist Muscle, Open Approach, Diagnostic
0KBB0ZZ	Excision of Left Lower Arm and Wrist Muscle, Open Approach
0KBB3ZX	Excision of Left Lower Arm and Wrist Muscle, Percutaneous Approach, Diagnostic
0KBB3ZZ	Excision of Left Lower Arm and Wrist Muscle, Percutaneous Approach
0KBB4ZX	Excision of Left Lower Arm and Wrist Muscle, Percutaneous Endoscopic Approach, Diagnostic
0KBB4ZZ	Excision of Left Lower Arm and Wrist Muscle, Percutaneous Endoscopic Approach
0KBC0ZX	Excision of Right Hand Muscle, Open Approach, Diagnostic
0KBC0ZZ	Excision of Right Hand Muscle, Open Approach
0KBC3ZX	Excision of Right Hand Muscle, Percutaneous Approach, Diagnostic
0KBC3ZZ	Excision of Right Hand Muscle, Percutaneous Approach

Female-only   ♂ Male-only   ▲ Limited Coverage   ● Non-OR   ▦ HAC-associated procedure   ▲ Non-covered procedures   ✚ Combination

0KBC4ZX Excision of Right Hand Muscle, Percutaneous Endoscopic Approach, Diagnostic

0KBC4ZZ Excision of Right Hand Muscle, Percutaneous Endoscopic Approach

0KBD0ZX Excision of Left Hand Muscle, Open Approach, Diagnostic

0KBD0ZZ Excision of Left Hand Muscle, Open Approach

0KBD3ZX Excision of Left Hand Muscle, Percutaneous Approach, Diagnostic

0KBD3ZZ Excision of Left Hand Muscle, Percutaneous Approach

0KBD4ZX Excision of Left Hand Muscle, Percutaneous Endoscopic Approach, Diagnostic

0KBD4ZZ Excision of Left Hand Muscle, Percutaneous Endoscopic Approach

0KBF0ZX Excision of Right Trunk Muscle, Open Approach, Diagnostic

0KBF0ZZ Excision of Right Trunk Muscle, Open Approach

0KBF3ZX Excision of Right Trunk Muscle, Percutaneous Approach, Diagnostic

0KBF3ZZ Excision of Right Trunk Muscle, Percutaneous Approach

0KBF4ZX Excision of Right Trunk Muscle, Percutaneous Endoscopic Approach, Diagnostic

0KBF4ZZ Excision of Right Trunk Muscle, Percutaneous Endoscopic Approach

0KBG0ZX Excision of Left Trunk Muscle, Open Approach, Diagnostic

0KBG0ZZ Excision of Left Trunk Muscle, Open Approach

0KBG3ZX Excision of Left Trunk Muscle, Percutaneous Approach, Diagnostic

0KBG3ZZ Excision of Left Trunk Muscle, Percutaneous Approach

0KBG4ZX Excision of Left Trunk Muscle, Percutaneous Endoscopic Approach, Diagnostic

0KBG4ZZ Excision of Left Trunk Muscle, Percutaneous Endoscopic Approach

0KBH0ZX Excision of Right Thorax Muscle, Open Approach, Diagnostic

0KBH0ZZ Excision of Right Thorax Muscle, Open Approach

0KBH3ZX Excision of Right Thorax Muscle, Percutaneous Approach, Diagnostic

0KBH3ZZ Excision of Right Thorax Muscle, Percutaneous Approach

0KBH4ZX Excision of Right Thorax Muscle, Percutaneous Endoscopic Approach, Diagnostic

0KBH4ZZ Excision of Right Thorax Muscle, Percutaneous Endoscopic Approach

0KBJ0ZX Excision of Left Thorax Muscle, Open Approach, Diagnostic

0KBJ0ZZ Excision of Left Thorax Muscle, Open Approach

0KBJ3ZX Excision of Left Thorax Muscle, Percutaneous Approach, Diagnostic

0KBJ3ZZ Excision of Left Thorax Muscle, Percutaneous Approach

0KBJ4ZX Excision of Left Thorax Muscle, Percutaneous Endoscopic Approach, Diagnostic

0KBJ4ZZ Excision of Left Thorax Muscle, Percutaneous Endoscopic Approach

0KBK0ZX Excision of Right Abdomen Muscle, Open Approach, Diagnostic

0KBK0ZZ Excision of Right Abdomen Muscle, Open Approach

0KBK3ZX Excision of Right Abdomen Muscle, Percutaneous Approach, Diagnostic

0KBK3ZZ Excision of Right Abdomen Muscle, Percutaneous Approach

0KBK4ZX Excision of Right Abdomen Muscle, Percutaneous Endoscopic Approach, Diagnostic

0KBK4ZZ Excision of Right Abdomen Muscle, Percutaneous Endoscopic Approach

0KBL0ZX Excision of Left Abdomen Muscle, Open Approach, Diagnostic

0KBL0ZZ Excision of Left Abdomen Muscle, Open Approach

0KBL3ZX Excision of Left Abdomen Muscle, Percutaneous Approach, Diagnostic

0KBL3ZZ Excision of Left Abdomen Muscle, Percutaneous Approach

0KBL4ZX Excision of Left Abdomen Muscle, Percutaneous Endoscopic Approach, Diagnostic

0KBL4ZZ Excision of Left Abdomen Muscle, Percutaneous Endoscopic Approach

0KBM0ZX Excision of Perineum Muscle, Open Approach, Diagnostic

0KBM0ZZ Excision of Perineum Muscle, Open Approach

0KBM3ZX Excision of Perineum Muscle, Percutaneous Approach, Diagnostic

0KBM3ZZ Excision of Perineum Muscle, Percutaneous Approach

0KBM4ZX Excision of Perineum Muscle, Percutaneous Endoscopic Approach, Diagnostic

0KBM4ZZ Excision of Perineum Muscle, Percutaneous Endoscopic Approach

0KBN0ZX Excision of Right Hip Muscle, Open Approach, Diagnostic

0KBN0ZZ Excision of Right Hip Muscle, Open Approach

0KBN3ZX Excision of Right Hip Muscle, Percutaneous Approach, Diagnostic

0KBN3ZZ Excision of Right Hip Muscle, Percutaneous Approach

0KBN4ZX Excision of Right Hip Muscle, Percutaneous Endoscopic Approach, Diagnostic

0KBN4ZZ Excision of Right Hip Muscle, Percutaneous Endoscopic Approach

0KBP0ZX Excision of Left Hip Muscle, Open Approach, Diagnostic

0KBP0ZZ Excision of Left Hip Muscle, Open Approach

0KBP3ZX Excision of Left Hip Muscle, Percutaneous Approach, Diagnostic

0KBP3ZZ Excision of Left Hip Muscle, Percutaneous Approach

0KBP4ZX Excision of Left Hip Muscle, Percutaneous Endoscopic Approach, Diagnostic

0KBP4ZZ Excision of Left Hip Muscle, Percutaneous Endoscopic Approach

0KBQ0ZX Excision of Right Upper Leg Muscle, Open Approach, Diagnostic

0KBQ0ZZ Excision of Right Upper Leg Muscle, Open Approach

0KBQ3ZX Excision of Right Upper Leg Muscle, Percutaneous Approach, Diagnostic

0KBQ3ZZ Excision of Right Upper Leg Muscle, Percutaneous Approach

0KBQ4ZX Excision of Right Upper Leg Muscle, Percutaneous Endoscopic Approach, Diagnostic

0KBQ4ZZ Excision of Right Upper Leg Muscle, Percutaneous Endoscopic Approach

0KBR0ZX Excision of Left Upper Leg Muscle, Approach, Diagnostic

0KBR0ZZ Excision of Left Upper Leg Muscle, Approach

0KBR3ZX Excision of Left Upper Leg Muscle, Percutaneous Approach, Diagnostic

0KBR3ZZ Excision of Left Upper Leg Muscle, Percutaneous Approach

0KBR4ZX Excision of Left Upper Leg Muscle, Percutaneous Endoscopic Approach, Diagnostic

0KBR4ZZ Excision of Left Upper Leg Muscle, Percutaneous Endoscopic Approach

0KBS0ZX Excision of Right Lower Leg Muscle, Open Approach, Diagnostic

0KBS0ZZ Excision of Right Lower Leg Muscle, Open Approach

0KBS3ZX Excision of Right Lower Leg Muscle, Percutaneous Approach, Diagnostic

0KBS3ZZ Excision of Right Lower Leg Muscle, Percutaneous Approach

0KBS4ZX Excision of Right Lower Leg Muscle, Percutaneous Endoscopic Approach, Diagnostic

0KBS4ZZ Excision of Right Lower Leg Muscle, Percutaneous Endoscopic Approach

0KBT0ZX Excision of Left Lower Leg Muscle, Approach, Diagnostic

0KBT0ZZ Excision of Left Lower Leg Muscle, Approach

0KBT3ZX Excision of Left Lower Leg Muscle, Percutaneous Approach, Diagnostic

0KBT3ZZ Excision of Left Lower Leg Muscle, Percutaneous Approach

0KBT4ZX Excision of Left Lower Leg Muscle, Percutaneous Endoscopic Approach, Diagnostic

0KBT4ZZ Excision of Left Lower Leg Muscle, Percutaneous Endoscopic Approach

0KBV0ZX Excision of Right Foot Muscle, Open Approach, Diagnostic

0KBV0ZZ Excision of Right Foot Muscle, Open Approach

0KBV3ZX Excision of Right Foot Muscle, Percutaneous Approach, Diagnostic

0KBV3ZZ Excision of Right Foot Muscle, Percutaneous Approach

0KBV4ZX Excision of Right Foot Muscle, Percutaneous Endoscopic Approach, Diagnostic

0KBV4ZZ Excision of Right Foot Muscle, Percutaneous Endoscopic Approach

0KBW0ZX Excision of Left Foot Muscle, Open Approach, Diagnostic

0KBW0ZZ Excision of Left Foot Muscle, Open Approach

0KBW3ZX Excision of Left Foot Muscle, Percutaneous Approach, Diagnostic

0KBW3ZZ Excision of Left Foot Muscle, Percutaneous Approach

0KBW4ZX Excision of Left Foot Muscle, Percutaneous Endoscopic Approach, Diagnostic

0KBW4ZZ Excision of Left Foot Muscle, Percutaneous Endoscopic Approach

0KC – Muscles, Extirpation

0KC00ZZ Extirpation of Matter from Head Muscle, Open Approach

0KC03ZZ Extirpation of Matter from Head Muscle, Percutaneous Approach

0KC04ZZ Extirpation of Matter from Head Muscle, Percutaneous Endoscopic Approach

C10ZZ Extirpation of Matter from Facial Muscle, Open Approach
C13ZZ Extirpation of Matter from Facial Muscle, Percutaneous Approach
C14ZZ Extirpation of Matter from Facial Muscle, Percutaneous Endoscopic Approach
C20ZZ Extirpation of Matter from Right Neck Muscle, Open Approach
C23ZZ Extirpation of Matter from Right Neck Muscle, Percutaneous Approach
C24ZZ Extirpation of Matter from Right Neck Muscle, Percutaneous Endoscopic Approach
C30ZZ Extirpation of Matter from Left Neck Muscle, Open Approach
C33ZZ Extirpation of Matter from Left Neck Muscle, Percutaneous Approach
C34ZZ Extirpation of Matter from Left Neck Muscle, Percutaneous Endoscopic Approach
C40ZZ Extirpation of Matter from Tongue, Palate, Pharynx Muscle, Open Approach
C43ZZ Extirpation of Matter from Tongue, Palate, Pharynx Muscle, Percutaneous Approach
C44ZZ Extirpation of Matter from Tongue, Palate, Pharynx Muscle, Percutaneous Endoscopic Approach
C50ZZ Extirpation of Matter from Right Shoulder Muscle, Open Approach
C53ZZ Extirpation of Matter from Right Shoulder Muscle, Percutaneous Approach
C54ZZ Extirpation of Matter from Right Shoulder Muscle, Percutaneous Endoscopic Approach
C60ZZ Extirpation of Matter from Left Shoulder Muscle, Open Approach
C63ZZ Extirpation of Matter from Left Shoulder Muscle, Percutaneous Approach
C64ZZ Extirpation of Matter from Left Shoulder Muscle, Percutaneous Endoscopic Approach
C70ZZ Extirpation of Matter from Right Upper Arm Muscle, Open Approach
C73ZZ Extirpation of Matter from Right Upper Arm Muscle, Percutaneous Approach
C74ZZ Extirpation of Matter from Right Upper Arm Muscle, Percutaneous Endoscopic Approach
C80ZZ Extirpation of Matter from Left Upper Arm Muscle, Open Approach
C83ZZ Extirpation of Matter from Left Upper Arm Muscle, Percutaneous Approach
C84ZZ Extirpation of Matter from Left Upper Arm Muscle, Percutaneous Endoscopic Approach
C90ZZ Extirpation of Matter from Right Lower Arm and Wrist Muscle, Open Approach
C93ZZ Extirpation of Matter from Right Lower Arm and Wrist Muscle, Percutaneous Approach

0KC94ZZ Extirpation of Matter from Right Lower Arm and Wrist Muscle, Percutaneous Endoscopic Approach
0KCB0ZZ Extirpation of Matter from Left Lower Arm and Wrist Muscle, Open Approach
0KCB3ZZ Extirpation of Matter from Left Lower Arm and Wrist Muscle, Percutaneous Approach
0KCB4ZZ Extirpation of Matter from Left Lower Arm and Wrist Muscle, Percutaneous Endoscopic Approach
0KCC0ZZ Extirpation of Matter from Right Hand Muscle, Open Approach
0KCC3ZZ Extirpation of Matter from Right Hand Muscle, Percutaneous Approach
0KCC4ZZ Extirpation of Matter from Right Hand Muscle, Percutaneous Endoscopic Approach
0KCD0ZZ Extirpation of Matter from Left Hand Muscle, Open Approach
0KCD3ZZ Extirpation of Matter from Left Hand Muscle, Percutaneous Approach
0KCD4ZZ Extirpation of Matter from Left Hand Muscle, Percutaneous Endoscopic Approach
0KCF0ZZ Extirpation of Matter from Right Trunk Muscle, Open Approach
0KCF3ZZ Extirpation of Matter from Right Trunk Muscle, Percutaneous Approach
0KCF4ZZ Extirpation of Matter from Right Trunk Muscle, Percutaneous Endoscopic Approach
0KCG0ZZ Extirpation of Matter from Left Trunk Muscle, Open Approach
0KCG3ZZ Extirpation of Matter from Left Trunk Muscle, Percutaneous Approach
0KCG4ZZ Extirpation of Matter from Left Trunk Muscle, Percutaneous Endoscopic Approach
0KCH0ZZ Extirpation of Matter from Right Thorax Muscle, Open Approach
0KCH3ZZ Extirpation of Matter from Right Thorax Muscle, Percutaneous Approach
0KCH4ZZ Extirpation of Matter from Right Thorax Muscle, Percutaneous Endoscopic Approach
0KCJ0ZZ Extirpation of Matter from Left Thorax Muscle, Open Approach
0KCJ3ZZ Extirpation of Matter from Left Thorax Muscle, Percutaneous Approach
0KCJ4ZZ Extirpation of Matter from Left Thorax Muscle, Percutaneous Endoscopic Approach
0KCK0ZZ Extirpation of Matter from Right Abdomen Muscle, Open Approach
0KCK3ZZ Extirpation of Matter from Right Abdomen Muscle, Percutaneous Approach
0KCK4ZZ Extirpation of Matter from Right Abdomen Muscle, Percutaneous Endoscopic Approach
0KCL0ZZ Extirpation of Matter from Left Abdomen Muscle, Open Approach
0KCL3ZZ Extirpation of Matter from Left Abdomen Muscle, Percutaneous Approach
0KCL4ZZ Extirpation of Matter from Left Abdomen Muscle, Percutaneous Endoscopic Approach

0KCM0ZZ Extirpation of Matter from Perineum Muscle, Open Approach
0KCM3ZZ Extirpation of Matter from Perineum Muscle, Percutaneous Approach
0KCM4ZZ Extirpation of Matter from Perineum Muscle, Percutaneous Endoscopic Approach
0KCN0ZZ Extirpation of Matter from Right Hip Muscle, Open Approach
0KCN3ZZ Extirpation of Matter from Right Hip Muscle, Percutaneous Approach
0KCN4ZZ Extirpation of Matter from Right Hip Muscle, Percutaneous Endoscopic Approach
0KCP0ZZ Extirpation of Matter from Left Hip Muscle, Open Approach
0KCP3ZZ Extirpation of Matter from Left Hip Muscle, Percutaneous Approach
0KCP4ZZ Extirpation of Matter from Left Hip Muscle, Percutaneous Endoscopic Approach
0KCQ0ZZ Extirpation of Matter from Right Upper Leg Muscle, Open Approach
0KCQ3ZZ Extirpation of Matter from Right Upper Leg Muscle, Percutaneous Approach
0KCQ4ZZ Extirpation of Matter from Right Upper Leg Muscle, Percutaneous Endoscopic Approach
0KCR0ZZ Extirpation of Matter from Left Upper Leg Muscle, Open Approach
0KCR3ZZ Extirpation of Matter from Left Upper Leg Muscle, Percutaneous Approach
0KCR4ZZ Extirpation of Matter from Left Upper Leg Muscle, Percutaneous Endoscopic Approach
0KCS0ZZ Extirpation of Matter from Right Lower Leg Muscle, Open Approach
0KCS3ZZ Extirpation of Matter from Right Lower Leg Muscle, Percutaneous Approach
0KCS4ZZ Extirpation of Matter from Right Lower Leg Muscle, Percutaneous Endoscopic Approach
0KCT0ZZ Extirpation of Matter from Left Lower Leg Muscle, Open Approach
0KCT3ZZ Extirpation of Matter from Left Lower Leg Muscle, Percutaneous Approach
0KCT4ZZ Extirpation of Matter from Left Lower Leg Muscle, Percutaneous Endoscopic Approach
0KCV0ZZ Extirpation of Matter from Right Foot Muscle, Open Approach
0KCV3ZZ Extirpation of Matter from Right Foot Muscle, Percutaneous Approach
0KCV4ZZ Extirpation of Matter from Right Foot Muscle, Percutaneous Endoscopic Approach
0KCW0ZZ Extirpation of Matter from Left Foot Muscle, Open Approach
0KCW3ZZ Extirpation of Matter from Left Foot Muscle, Percutaneous Approach
0KCW4ZZ Extirpation of Matter from Left Foot Muscle, Percutaneous Endoscopic Approach

KH – Muscles, Insertion

KHX0MZ Insertion of Stimulator Lead into Upper Muscle, Open Approach
KHX3MZ Insertion of Stimulator Lead into Upper Muscle, Percutaneous Approach

0KHX4MZ Insertion of Stimulator Lead into Upper Muscle, Percutaneous Endoscopic Approach
0KHY0MZ Insertion of Stimulator Lead into Lower Muscle, Open Approach

0KHY3MZ Insertion of Stimulator Lead into Lower Muscle, Percutaneous Approach
0KHY4MZ Insertion of Stimulator Lead into Lower Muscle, Percutaneous Endoscopic Approach

♀ Female-only   ♂ Male-only   ▲ Limited Coverage   ● Non-OR   ▥ HAC-associated procedure   ▲ Non-covered procedures   ✛ Combination

0KJ – Muscles, Inspection

Review Coding Guideline B3.5

Review Coding Guidelines B3.11a, B3.11b and B3.11c

0KJX0ZZ	Inspection of Upper Muscle, Open Approach
0KJX3ZZ	Inspection of Upper Muscle, Percutaneous Approach
0KJX4ZZ	Inspection of Upper Muscle, Percutaneous Endoscopic Approach
0KJXXZZ	Inspection of Upper Muscle, External Approach
0KJY0ZZ	Inspection of Lower Muscle, Open Approach
0KJY3ZZ	Inspection of Lower Muscle, Percutaneous Approach
0KJY4ZZ	Inspection of Lower Muscle, Percutane Endoscopic Approach
0KJYXZZ	Inspection of Lower Muscle, External Approach

0KM – Muscles, Reattachment

0KM00ZZ	Reattachment of Head Muscle, Open Approach
0KM04ZZ	Reattachment of Head Muscle, Percutaneous Endoscopic Approach
0KM10ZZ	Reattachment of Facial Muscle, Open Approach
0KM14ZZ	Reattachment of Facial Muscle, Percutaneous Endoscopic Approach
0KM20ZZ	Reattachment of Right Neck Muscle, Open Approach
0KM24ZZ	Reattachment of Right Neck Muscle, Percutaneous Endoscopic Approach
0KM30ZZ	Reattachment of Left Neck Muscle, Open Approach
0KM34ZZ	Reattachment of Left Neck Muscle, Percutaneous Endoscopic Approach
0KM40ZZ	Reattachment of Tongue, Palate, Pharynx Muscle, Open Approach
0KM44ZZ	Reattachment of Tongue, Palate, Pharynx Muscle, Percutaneous Endoscopic Approach
0KM50ZZ	Reattachment of Right Shoulder Muscle, Open Approach
0KM54ZZ	Reattachment of Right Shoulder Muscle, Percutaneous Endoscopic Approach
0KM60ZZ	Reattachment of Left Shoulder Muscle, Open Approach
0KM64ZZ	Reattachment of Left Shoulder Muscle, Percutaneous Endoscopic Approach
0KM70ZZ	Reattachment of Right Upper Arm Muscle, Open Approach
0KM74ZZ	Reattachment of Right Upper Arm Muscle, Percutaneous Endoscopic Approach
0KM80ZZ	Reattachment of Left Upper Arm Muscle, Open Approach
0KM84ZZ	Reattachment of Left Upper Arm Muscle, Percutaneous Endoscopic Approach
0KM90ZZ	Reattachment of Right Lower Arm and Wrist Muscle, Open Approach
0KM94ZZ	Reattachment of Right Lower Arm and Wrist Muscle, Percutaneous Endoscopic Approach
0KMB0ZZ	Reattachment of Left Lower Arm and Wrist Muscle, Open Approach
0KMB4ZZ	Reattachment of Left Lower Arm and Wrist Muscle, Percutaneous Endoscopic Approach
0KMC0ZZ	Reattachment of Right Hand Muscle, Open Approach
0KMC4ZZ	Reattachment of Right Hand Muscle, Percutaneous Endoscopic Approach
0KMD0ZZ	Reattachment of Left Hand Muscle, Open Approach
0KMD4ZZ	Reattachment of Left Hand Muscle, Percutaneous Endoscopic Approach
0KMF0ZZ	Reattachment of Right Trunk Muscle, Open Approach
0KMF4ZZ	Reattachment of Right Trunk Muscle, Percutaneous Endoscopic Approach
0KMG0ZZ	Reattachment of Left Trunk Muscle, Open Approach
0KMG4ZZ	Reattachment of Left Trunk Muscle, Percutaneous Endoscopic Approach
0KMH0ZZ	Reattachment of Right Thorax Muscle, Open Approach
0KMH4ZZ	Reattachment of Right Thorax Muscle, Percutaneous Endoscopic Approach
0KMJ0ZZ	Reattachment of Left Thorax Muscle, Open Approach
0KMJ4ZZ	Reattachment of Left Thorax Muscle, Percutaneous Endoscopic Approach
0KMK0ZZ	Reattachment of Right Abdomen Muscle, Open Approach
0KMK4ZZ	Reattachment of Right Abdomen Muscle, Percutaneous Endoscopic Approach
0KML0ZZ	Reattachment of Left Abdomen Muscle, Open Approach
0KML4ZZ	Reattachment of Left Abdomen Muscle, Percutaneous Endoscopic Approach
0KMM0ZZ	Reattachment of Perineum Muscle, Op Approach
0KMM4ZZ	Reattachment of Perineum Muscle, Percutaneous Endoscopic Approach
0KMN0ZZ	Reattachment of Right Hip Muscle, Op Approach
0KMN4ZZ	Reattachment of Right Hip Muscle, Percutaneous Endoscopic Approach
0KMP0ZZ	Reattachment of Left Hip Muscle, Ope Approach
0KMP4ZZ	Reattachment of Left Hip Muscle, Percutaneous Endoscopic Approach
0KMQ0ZZ	Reattachment of Right Upper Leg Muscle, Open Approach
0KMQ4ZZ	Reattachment of Right Upper Leg Muscle, Percutaneous Endoscopic Approach
0KMR0ZZ	Reattachment of Left Upper Leg Musc Open Approach
0KMR4ZZ	Reattachment of Left Upper Leg Musc Percutaneous Endoscopic Approach
0KMS0ZZ	Reattachment of Right Lower Leg Muscle, Open Approach
0KMS4ZZ	Reattachment of Right Lower Leg Muscle, Percutaneous Endoscopic Approach
0KMT0ZZ	Reattachment of Left Lower Leg Musc Open Approach
0KMT4ZZ	Reattachment of Left Lower Leg Musc Percutaneous Endoscopic Approach
0KMV0ZZ	Reattachment of Right Foot Muscle, Open Approach
0KMV4ZZ	Reattachment of Right Foot Muscle, Percutaneous Endoscopic Approach
0KMW0ZZ	Reattachment of Left Foot Muscle, Op Approach
0KMW4ZZ	Reattachment of Left Foot Muscle, Percutaneous Endoscopic Approach

0KN – Muscles, Release

Review Coding Guideline B3.13

Review Coding Guideline B3.14

0KN00ZZ	Release Head Muscle, Open Approach
0KN03ZZ	Release Head Muscle, Percutaneous Approach
0KN04ZZ	Release Head Muscle, Percutaneous Endoscopic Approach
0KN0XZZ	Release Head Muscle, External Approach
0KN10ZZ	Release Facial Muscle, Open Approach
0KN13ZZ	Release Facial Muscle, Percutaneous Approach
0KN14ZZ	Release Facial Muscle, Percutaneous Endoscopic Approach
0KN1XZZ	Release Facial Muscle, External Approach
0KN20ZZ	Release Right Neck Muscle, Open Approach
0KN23ZZ	Release Right Neck Muscle, Percutaneous Approach
0KN24ZZ	Release Right Neck Muscle, Percutaneous Endoscopic Approach
0KN2XZZ	Release Right Neck Muscle, External Approach
0KN30ZZ	Release Left Neck Muscle, Open Approach
0KN33ZZ	Release Left Neck Muscle, Percutaneous Approach
0KN34ZZ	Release Left Neck Muscle, Percutaneous Endoscopic Approach
0KN3XZZ	Release Left Neck Muscle, External Approach
0KN40ZZ	Release Tongue, Palate, Pharynx Muscle, Open Approach
0KN43ZZ	Release Tongue, Palate, Pharynx Muscle, Percutaneous Approach
0KN44ZZ	Release Tongue, Palate, Pharynx Muscle, Percutaneous Endoscopic Approach
0KN4XZZ	Release Tongue, Palate, Pharynx Muscle, External Approach
0KN50ZZ	Release Right Shoulder Muscle, Open Approach
0KN53ZZ	Release Right Shoulder Muscle, Percutaneous Approach
0KN54ZZ	Release Right Shoulder Muscle, Percutaneous Endoscopic Approach
0KN5XZZ	Release Right Shoulder Muscle, External Approach

♀ Female-only   ♂ Male-only   ▲ Limited Coverage   ● Non-OR   ▨ HAC-associated procedure   ▲ Non-covered procedures   ✚ Combinati

60ZZ	Release Left Shoulder Muscle, Open Approach	0KNF3ZZ	Release Right Trunk Muscle, Percutaneous Approach	0KNN4ZZ	Release Right Hip Muscle, Percutaneous Endoscopic Approach
63ZZ	Release Left Shoulder Muscle, Percutaneous Approach	0KNF4ZZ	Release Right Trunk Muscle, Percutaneous Endoscopic Approach	0KNNXZZ	Release Right Hip Muscle, External Approach
64ZZ	Release Left Shoulder Muscle, Percutaneous Endoscopic Approach	0KNFXZZ	Release Right Trunk Muscle, External Approach	0KNP0ZZ	Release Left Hip Muscle, Open Approach
6XZZ	Release Left Shoulder Muscle, External Approach	0KNG0ZZ	Release Left Trunk Muscle, Open Approach	0KNP3ZZ	Release Left Hip Muscle, Percutaneous Approach
70ZZ	Release Right Upper Arm Muscle, Open Approach	0KNG3ZZ	Release Left Trunk Muscle, Percutaneous Approach	0KNP4ZZ	Release Left Hip Muscle, Percutaneous Endoscopic Approach
73ZZ	Release Right Upper Arm Muscle, Percutaneous Approach	0KNG4ZZ	Release Left Trunk Muscle, Percutaneous Endoscopic Approach	0KNPXZZ	Release Left Hip Muscle, External Approach
74ZZ	Release Right Upper Arm Muscle, Percutaneous Endoscopic Approach	0KNGXZZ	Release Left Trunk Muscle, External Approach	0KNQ0ZZ	Release Right Upper Leg Muscle, Open Approach
7XZZ	Release Right Upper Arm Muscle, External Approach	0KNH0ZZ	Release Right Thorax Muscle, Open Approach	0KNQ3ZZ	Release Right Upper Leg Muscle, Percutaneous Approach
80ZZ	Release Left Upper Arm Muscle, Open Approach	0KNH3ZZ	Release Right Thorax Muscle, Percutaneous Approach	0KNQ4ZZ	Release Right Upper Leg Muscle, Percutaneous Endoscopic Approach
83ZZ	Release Left Upper Arm Muscle, Percutaneous Approach	0KNH4ZZ	Release Right Thorax Muscle, Percutaneous Endoscopic Approach	0KNQXZZ	Release Right Upper Leg Muscle, External Approach
84ZZ	Release Left Upper Arm Muscle, Percutaneous Endoscopic Approach	0KNHXZZ	Release Right Thorax Muscle, External Approach	0KNR0ZZ	Release Left Upper Leg Muscle, Open Approach
8XZZ	Release Left Upper Arm Muscle, External Approach	0KNJ0ZZ	Release Left Thorax Muscle, Open Approach	0KNR3ZZ	Release Left Upper Leg Muscle, Percutaneous Approach
90ZZ	Release Right Lower Arm and Wrist Muscle, Open Approach	0KNJ3ZZ	Release Left Thorax Muscle, Percutaneous Approach	0KNR4ZZ	Release Left Upper Leg Muscle, Percutaneous Endoscopic Approach
93ZZ	Release Right Lower Arm and Wrist Muscle, Percutaneous Approach	0KNJ4ZZ	Release Left Thorax Muscle, Percutaneous Endoscopic Approach	0KNRXZZ	Release Left Upper Leg Muscle, External Approach
94ZZ	Release Right Lower Arm and Wrist Muscle, Percutaneous Endoscopic Approach	0KNJXZZ	Release Left Thorax Muscle, External Approach	0KNS0ZZ	Release Right Lower Leg Muscle, Open Approach
9XZZ	Release Right Lower Arm and Wrist Muscle, External Approach	0KNK0ZZ	Release Right Abdomen Muscle, Open Approach	0KNS3ZZ	Release Right Lower Leg Muscle, Percutaneous Approach
		AHA CC: 4Q, 2014, 39-40	0KNS4ZZ	Release Right Lower Leg Muscle, Percutaneous Endoscopic Approach
NB0ZZ	Release Left Lower Arm and Wrist Muscle, Open Approach	0KNK3ZZ	Release Right Abdomen Muscle, Percutaneous Approach	0KNSXZZ	Release Right Lower Leg Muscle, External Approach
NB3ZZ	Release Left Lower Arm and Wrist Muscle, Percutaneous Approach	0KNK4ZZ	Release Right Abdomen Muscle, Percutaneous Endoscopic Approach	0KNT0ZZ	Release Left Lower Leg Muscle, Open Approach
NB4ZZ	Release Left Lower Arm and Wrist Muscle, Percutaneous Endoscopic Approach	0KNKXZZ	Release Right Abdomen Muscle, External Approach	0KNT3ZZ	Release Left Lower Leg Muscle, Percutaneous Approach
NBXZZ	Release Left Lower Arm and Wrist Muscle, External Approach	0KNL0ZZ	Release Left Abdomen Muscle, Open Approach	0KNT4ZZ	Release Left Lower Leg Muscle, Percutaneous Endoscopic Approach
		AHA CC: 4Q, 2014, 39-40	0KNTXZZ	Release Left Lower Leg Muscle, External Approach
NC0ZZ	Release Right Hand Muscle, Open Approach	0KNL3ZZ	Release Left Abdomen Muscle, Percutaneous Approach	0KNV0ZZ	Release Right Foot Muscle, Open Approach
NC3ZZ	Release Right Hand Muscle, Percutaneous Approach	0KNL4ZZ	Release Left Abdomen Muscle, Percutaneous Endoscopic Approach	0KNV3ZZ	Release Right Foot Muscle, Percutaneous Approach
NC4ZZ	Release Right Hand Muscle, Percutaneous Endoscopic Approach	0KNLXZZ	Release Left Abdomen Muscle, External Approach	0KNV4ZZ	Release Right Foot Muscle, Percutaneous Endoscopic Approach
NCXZZ	Release Right Hand Muscle, External Approach	0KNM0ZZ	Release Perineum Muscle, Open Approach	0KNVXZZ	Release Right Foot Muscle, External Approach
ND0ZZ	Release Left Hand Muscle, Open Approach	0KNM3ZZ	Release Perineum Muscle, Percutaneous Approach	0KNW0ZZ	Release Left Foot Muscle, Open Approach
ND3ZZ	Release Left Hand Muscle, Percutaneous Approach	0KNM4ZZ	Release Perineum Muscle, Percutaneous Endoscopic Approach	0KNW3ZZ	Release Left Foot Muscle, Percutaneous Approach
ND4ZZ	Release Left Hand Muscle, Percutaneous Endoscopic Approach	0KNMXZZ	Release Perineum Muscle, External Approach	0KNW4ZZ	Release Left Foot Muscle, Percutaneous Endoscopic Approach
NDXZZ	Release Left Hand Muscle, External Approach	0KNN0ZZ	Release Right Hip Muscle, Open Approach	0KNWXZZ	Release Left Foot Muscle, External Approach
NF0ZZ	Release Right Trunk Muscle, Open Approach	0KNN3ZZ	Release Right Hip Muscle, Percutaneous Approach		

KP – Muscles, Removal

view Coding Guideline B6.1c

PX00Z	Removal of Drainage Device from Upper Muscle, Open Approach	0KPX30Z	Removal of Drainage Device from Upper Muscle, Percutaneous Approach	0KPX40Z	Removal of Drainage Device from Upper Muscle, Percutaneous Endoscopic Approach
PX07Z	Removal of Autologous Tissue Substitute from Upper Muscle, Open Approach	0KPX37Z	Removal of Autologous Tissue Substitute from Upper Muscle, Percutaneous Approach	0KPX47Z	Removal of Autologous Tissue Substitute from Upper Muscle, Percutaneous Endoscopic Approach
PX0JZ	Removal of Synthetic Substitute from Upper Muscle, Open Approach	0KPX3JZ	Removal of Synthetic Substitute from Upper Muscle, Percutaneous Approach	0KPX4JZ	Removal of Synthetic Substitute from Upper Muscle, Percutaneous Endoscopic Approach
PX0KZ	Removal of Nonautologous Tissue Substitute from Upper Muscle, Open Approach	0KPX3KZ	Removal of Nonautologous Tissue Substitute from Upper Muscle, Percutaneous Approach	0KPX4KZ	Removal of Nonautologous Tissue Substitute from Upper Muscle, Percutaneous Endoscopic Approach
PX0MZ	Removal of Stimulator Lead from Upper Muscle, Open Approach	0KPX3MZ	Removal of Stimulator Lead from Upper Muscle, Percutaneous Approach		

Female-only	♂ Male-only	▲ Limited Coverage	● Non-OR	HAC-associated procedure	▲ Non-covered procedures	+ Combination

0KPX4MZ	Removal of Stimulator Lead from Upper Muscle, Percutaneous Endoscopic Approach	0KPY0MZ	Removal of Stimulator Lead from Lower Muscle, Open Approach	0KPY47Z	Removal of Autologous Tissue Substitute from Lower Muscle, Percutaneous Endoscopic Approach
0KPXX0Z	Removal of Drainage Device from Upper Muscle, External Approach	0KPY30Z	Removal of Drainage Device from Lower Muscle, Percutaneous Approach	0KPY4JZ	Removal of Synthetic Substitute from Lower Muscle, Percutaneous Endoscopic Approach
0KPXXMZ	Removal of Stimulator Lead from Upper Muscle, External Approach	0KPY37Z	Removal of Autologous Tissue Substitute from Lower Muscle, Percutaneous Approach	0KPY4KZ	Removal of Nonautologous Tissue Substitute from Lower Muscle, Percutaneous Endoscopic Approach
0KPY00Z	Removal of Drainage Device from Lower Muscle, Open Approach	0KPY3JZ	Removal of Synthetic Substitute from Lower Muscle, Percutaneous Approach	0KPY4MZ	Removal of Stimulator Lead from Lower Muscle, Percutaneous Endoscopic Approach
0KPY07Z	Removal of Autologous Tissue Substitute from Lower Muscle, Open Approach	0KPY3KZ	Removal of Nonautologous Tissue Substitute from Lower Muscle, Percutaneous Approach	0KPYX0Z	Removal of Drainage Device from Lower Muscle, External Approach
0KPY0JZ	Removal of Synthetic Substitute from Lower Muscle, Open Approach	0KPY3MZ	Removal of Stimulator Lead from Lower Muscle, Percutaneous Approach	0KPYXMZ	Removal of Stimulator Lead from Lower Muscle, External Approach
0KPY0KZ	Removal of Nonautologous Tissue Substitute from Lower Muscle, Open Approach	0KPY40Z	Removal of Drainage Device from Lower Muscle, Percutaneous Endoscopic Approach		

0KQ – Muscles, Repair

Review Coding Guideline B3.5

0KQ00ZZ	Repair Head Muscle, Open Approach	0KQ94ZZ	Repair Right Lower Arm and Wrist Muscle, Percutaneous Endoscopic Approach	0KQL4ZZ	Repair Left Abdomen Muscle, Percutaneous Endoscopic Approach
0KQ03ZZ	Repair Head Muscle, Percutaneous Approach	0KQB0ZZ	Repair Left Lower Arm and Wrist Muscle, Open Approach	0KQM0ZZ	Repair Perineum Muscle, Open Approach
0KQ04ZZ	Repair Head Muscle, Percutaneous Endoscopic Approach	0KQB3ZZ	Repair Left Lower Arm and Wrist Muscle, Percutaneous Approach		*AHA CC: 4Q, 2013, 120*
0KQ10ZZ	Repair Facial Muscle, Open Approach	0KQB4ZZ	Repair Left Lower Arm and Wrist Muscle, Percutaneous Endoscopic Approach	0KQM3ZZ	Repair Perineum Muscle, Percutaneous Approach
0KQ13ZZ	Repair Facial Muscle, Percutaneous Approach	0KQC0ZZ	Repair Right Hand Muscle, Open Approach	0KQM4ZZ	Repair Perineum Muscle, Percutaneous Endoscopic Approach
0KQ14ZZ	Repair Facial Muscle, Percutaneous Endoscopic Approach	0KQC3ZZ	Repair Right Hand Muscle, Percutaneous Approach	0KQN0ZZ	Repair Right Hip Muscle, Open Approach
0KQ20ZZ	Repair Right Neck Muscle, Open Approach	0KQC4ZZ	Repair Right Hand Muscle, Percutaneous Endoscopic Approach	0KQN3ZZ	Repair Right Hip Muscle, Percutaneous Approach
0KQ23ZZ	Repair Right Neck Muscle, Percutaneous Approach	0KQD0ZZ	Repair Left Hand Muscle, Open Approach	0KQN4ZZ	Repair Right Hip Muscle, Percutaneous Endoscopic Approach
0KQ24ZZ	Repair Right Neck Muscle, Percutaneous Endoscopic Approach	0KQD3ZZ	Repair Left Hand Muscle, Percutaneous Approach	0KQP0ZZ	Repair Left Hip Muscle, Open Approach
0KQ30ZZ	Repair Left Neck Muscle, Open Approach	0KQD4ZZ	Repair Left Hand Muscle, Percutaneous Endoscopic Approach	0KQP3ZZ	Repair Left Hip Muscle, Percutaneous Approach
0KQ33ZZ	Repair Left Neck Muscle, Percutaneous Approach	0KQF0ZZ	Repair Right Trunk Muscle, Open Approach	0KQP4ZZ	Repair Left Hip Muscle, Percutaneous Endoscopic Approach
0KQ34ZZ	Repair Left Neck Muscle, Percutaneous Endoscopic Approach	0KQF3ZZ	Repair Right Trunk Muscle, Percutaneous Approach	0KQQ0ZZ	Repair Right Upper Leg Muscle, Open Approach
0KQ40ZZ	Repair Tongue, Palate, Pharynx Muscle, Open Approach	0KQF4ZZ	Repair Right Trunk Muscle, Percutaneous Endoscopic Approach	0KQQ3ZZ	Repair Right Upper Leg Muscle, Percutaneous Approach
0KQ43ZZ	Repair Tongue, Palate, Pharynx Muscle, Percutaneous Approach	0KQG0ZZ	Repair Left Trunk Muscle, Open Approach	0KQQ4ZZ	Repair Right Upper Leg Muscle, Percutaneous Endoscopic Approach
0KQ44ZZ	Repair Tongue, Palate, Pharynx Muscle, Percutaneous Endoscopic Approach	0KQG3ZZ	Repair Left Trunk Muscle, Percutaneous Approach	0KQR0ZZ	Repair Left Upper Leg Muscle, Open Approach
0KQ50ZZ	Repair Right Shoulder Muscle, Open Approach	0KQG4ZZ	Repair Left Trunk Muscle, Percutaneous Endoscopic Approach	0KQR3ZZ	Repair Left Upper Leg Muscle, Percutaneous Approach
0KQ53ZZ	Repair Right Shoulder Muscle, Percutaneous Approach	0KQH0ZZ	Repair Right Thorax Muscle, Open Approach	0KQR4ZZ	Repair Left Upper Leg Muscle, Percutaneous Endoscopic Approach
0KQ54ZZ	Repair Right Shoulder Muscle, Percutaneous Endoscopic Approach	0KQH3ZZ	Repair Right Thorax Muscle, Percutaneous Approach	0KQS0ZZ	Repair Right Lower Leg Muscle, Open Approach
0KQ60ZZ	Repair Left Shoulder Muscle, Open Approach	0KQH4ZZ	Repair Right Thorax Muscle, Percutaneous Endoscopic Approach	0KQS3ZZ	Repair Right Lower Leg Muscle, Percutaneous Approach
0KQ63ZZ	Repair Left Shoulder Muscle, Percutaneous Approach	0KQJ0ZZ	Repair Left Thorax Muscle, Open Approach	0KQS4ZZ	Repair Right Lower Leg Muscle, Percutaneous Endoscopic Approach
0KQ64ZZ	Repair Left Shoulder Muscle, Percutaneous Endoscopic Approach	0KQJ3ZZ	Repair Left Thorax Muscle, Percutaneous Approach	0KQT0ZZ	Repair Left Lower Leg Muscle, Open Approach
0KQ70ZZ	Repair Right Upper Arm Muscle, Open Approach	0KQJ4ZZ	Repair Left Thorax Muscle, Percutaneous Endoscopic Approach	0KQT3ZZ	Repair Left Lower Leg Muscle, Percutaneous Approach
0KQ73ZZ	Repair Right Upper Arm Muscle, Percutaneous Approach	0KQK0ZZ	Repair Right Abdomen Muscle, Open Approach	0KQT4ZZ	Repair Left Lower Leg Muscle, Percutaneous Endoscopic Approach
0KQ74ZZ	Repair Right Upper Arm Muscle, Percutaneous Endoscopic Approach	0KQK3ZZ	Repair Right Abdomen Muscle, Percutaneous Approach	0KQV0ZZ	Repair Right Foot Muscle, Open Approach
0KQ80ZZ	Repair Left Upper Arm Muscle, Open Approach	0KQK4ZZ	Repair Right Abdomen Muscle, Percutaneous Endoscopic Approach	0KQV3ZZ	Repair Right Foot Muscle, Percutaneous Approach
0KQ83ZZ	Repair Left Upper Arm Muscle, Percutaneous Approach	0KQL0ZZ	Repair Left Abdomen Muscle, Open Approach	0KQV4ZZ	Repair Right Foot Muscle, Percutaneous Endoscopic Approach
0KQ84ZZ	Repair Left Upper Arm Muscle, Percutaneous Endoscopic Approach	0KQL3ZZ	Repair Left Abdomen Muscle, Percutaneous Approach	0KQW0ZZ	Repair Left Foot Muscle, Open Approach
0KQ90ZZ	Repair Right Lower Arm and Wrist Muscle, Open Approach			0KQW3ZZ	Repair Left Foot Muscle, Percutaneous Approach
0KQ93ZZ	Repair Right Lower Arm and Wrist Muscle, Percutaneous Approach			0KQW4ZZ	Repair Left Foot Muscle, Percutaneous Endoscopic Approach

♀ Female-only   ♂ Male-only   ▲ Limited Coverage   ● Non-OR   ▦ HAC-associated procedure   ▲ Non-covered procedures   ＋ Combinati

0KS – Muscles, Reposition

0KS00ZZ	Reposition Head Muscle, Open Approach	0KS94ZZ	Reposition Right Lower Arm and Wrist Muscle, Percutaneous Endoscopic Approach	0KSL4ZZ	Reposition Left Abdomen Muscle, Percutaneous Endoscopic Approach
0KS04ZZ	Reposition Head Muscle, Percutaneous Endoscopic Approach	0KSB0ZZ	Reposition Left Lower Arm and Wrist Muscle, Open Approach	0KSM0ZZ	Reposition Perineum Muscle, Open Approach
0KS10ZZ	Reposition Facial Muscle, Open Approach	0KSB4ZZ	Reposition Left Lower Arm and Wrist Muscle, Percutaneous Endoscopic Approach	0KSM4ZZ	Reposition Perineum Muscle, Percutaneous Endoscopic Approach
0KS14ZZ	Reposition Facial Muscle, Percutaneous Endoscopic Approach	0KSC0ZZ	Reposition Right Hand Muscle, Open Approach	0KSN0ZZ	Reposition Right Hip Muscle, Open Approach
0KS20ZZ	Reposition Right Neck Muscle, Open Approach	0KSC4ZZ	Reposition Right Hand Muscle, Percutaneous Endoscopic Approach	0KSN4ZZ	Reposition Right Hip Muscle, Percutaneous Endoscopic Approach
0KS24ZZ	Reposition Right Neck Muscle, Percutaneous Endoscopic Approach	0KSD0ZZ	Reposition Left Hand Muscle, Open Approach	0KSP0ZZ	Reposition Left Hip Muscle, Open Approach
0KS30ZZ	Reposition Left Neck Muscle, Open Approach	0KSD4ZZ	Reposition Left Hand Muscle, Percutaneous Endoscopic Approach	0KSP4ZZ	Reposition Left Hip Muscle, Percutaneous Endoscopic Approach
0KS34ZZ	Reposition Left Neck Muscle, Percutaneous Endoscopic Approach	0KSF0ZZ	Reposition Right Trunk Muscle, Open Approach	0KSQ0ZZ	Reposition Right Upper Leg Muscle, Open Approach
0KS40ZZ	Reposition Tongue, Palate, Pharynx Muscle, Open Approach	0KSF4ZZ	Reposition Right Trunk Muscle, Percutaneous Endoscopic Approach	0KSQ4ZZ	Reposition Right Upper Leg Muscle, Percutaneous Endoscopic Approach
0KS44ZZ	Reposition Tongue, Palate, Pharynx Muscle, Percutaneous Endoscopic Approach	0KSG0ZZ	Reposition Left Trunk Muscle, Open Approach	0KSR0ZZ	Reposition Left Upper Leg Muscle, Open Approach
0KS50ZZ	Reposition Right Shoulder Muscle, Open Approach	0KSG4ZZ	Reposition Left Trunk Muscle, Percutaneous Endoscopic Approach	0KSR4ZZ	Reposition Left Upper Leg Muscle, Percutaneous Endoscopic Approach
0KS54ZZ	Reposition Right Shoulder Muscle, Percutaneous Endoscopic Approach	0KSH0ZZ	Reposition Right Thorax Muscle, Open Approach	0KSS0ZZ	Reposition Right Lower Leg Muscle, Open Approach
0KS60ZZ	Reposition Left Shoulder Muscle, Open Approach	0KSH4ZZ	Reposition Right Thorax Muscle, Percutaneous Endoscopic Approach	0KSS4ZZ	Reposition Right Lower Leg Muscle, Percutaneous Endoscopic Approach
0KS64ZZ	Reposition Left Shoulder Muscle, Percutaneous Endoscopic Approach	0KSJ0ZZ	Reposition Left Thorax Muscle, Open Approach	0KST0ZZ	Reposition Left Lower Leg Muscle, Open Approach
0KS70ZZ	Reposition Right Upper Arm Muscle, Open Approach	0KSJ4ZZ	Reposition Left Thorax Muscle, Percutaneous Endoscopic Approach	0KST4ZZ	Reposition Left Lower Leg Muscle, Percutaneous Endoscopic Approach
0KS74ZZ	Reposition Right Upper Arm Muscle, Percutaneous Endoscopic Approach	0KSK0ZZ	Reposition Right Abdomen Muscle, Open Approach	0KSV0ZZ	Reposition Right Foot Muscle, Open Approach
0KS80ZZ	Reposition Left Upper Arm Muscle, Open Approach	0KSK4ZZ	Reposition Right Abdomen Muscle, Percutaneous Endoscopic Approach	0KSV4ZZ	Reposition Right Foot Muscle, Percutaneous Endoscopic Approach
0KS84ZZ	Reposition Left Upper Arm Muscle, Percutaneous Endoscopic Approach	0KSL0ZZ	Reposition Left Abdomen Muscle, Open Approach	0KSW0ZZ	Reposition Left Foot Muscle, Open Approach
0KS90ZZ	Reposition Right Lower Arm and Wrist Muscle, Open Approach			0KSW4ZZ	Reposition Left Foot Muscle, Percutaneous Endoscopic Approach

0KT – Muscles, Resection

Review Coding Guideline B3.8

0KT00ZZ	Resection of Head Muscle, Open Approach	0KT74ZZ	Resection of Right Upper Arm Muscle, Percutaneous Endoscopic Approach	0KTH0ZZ	Resection of Right Thorax Muscle, Open Approach
0KT04ZZ	Resection of Head Muscle, Percutaneous Endoscopic Approach	0KT80ZZ	Resection of Left Upper Arm Muscle, Open Approach	0KTH4ZZ	Resection of Right Thorax Muscle, Percutaneous Endoscopic Approach
0KT10ZZ	Resection of Facial Muscle, Open Approach	0KT84ZZ	Resection of Left Upper Arm Muscle, Percutaneous Endoscopic Approach	0KTJ0ZZ	Resection of Left Thorax Muscle, Open Approach
0KT14ZZ	Resection of Facial Muscle, Percutaneous Endoscopic Approach	0KT90ZZ	Resection of Right Lower Arm and Wrist Muscle, Open Approach	0KTJ4ZZ	Resection of Left Thorax Muscle, Percutaneous Endoscopic Approach
0KT20ZZ	Resection of Right Neck Muscle, Open Approach	0KT94ZZ	Resection of Right Lower Arm and Wrist Muscle, Percutaneous Endoscopic Approach	0KTK0ZZ	Resection of Right Abdomen Muscle, Open Approach
0KT24ZZ	Resection of Right Neck Muscle, Percutaneous Endoscopic Approach	0KTB0ZZ	Resection of Left Lower Arm and Wrist Muscle, Open Approach	0KTK4ZZ	Resection of Right Abdomen Muscle, Percutaneous Endoscopic Approach
0KT30ZZ	Resection of Left Neck Muscle, Open Approach	0KTB4ZZ	Resection of Left Lower Arm and Wrist Muscle, Percutaneous Endoscopic Approach	0KTL0ZZ	Resection of Left Abdomen Muscle, Open Approach
0KT34ZZ	Resection of Left Neck Muscle, Percutaneous Endoscopic Approach	0KTC0ZZ	Resection of Right Hand Muscle, Open Approach	0KTL4ZZ	Resection of Left Abdomen Muscle, Percutaneous Endoscopic Approach
0KT40ZZ	Resection of Tongue, Palate, Pharynx Muscle, Open Approach	0KTC4ZZ	Resection of Right Hand Muscle, Percutaneous Endoscopic Approach	0KTM0ZZ	Resection of Perineum Muscle, Open Approach
0KT44ZZ	Resection of Tongue, Palate, Pharynx Muscle, Percutaneous Endoscopic Approach	0KTD0ZZ	Resection of Left Hand Muscle, Open Approach		*AHA CC: 4Q, 2014, 40-41; 1Q, 2015, 38*
0KT50ZZ	Resection of Right Shoulder Muscle, Open Approach	0KTD4ZZ	Resection of Left Hand Muscle, Percutaneous Endoscopic Approach	0KTM4ZZ	Resection of Perineum Muscle, Percutaneous Endoscopic Approach
0KT54ZZ	Resection of Right Shoulder Muscle, Percutaneous Endoscopic Approach	0KTF0ZZ	Resection of Right Trunk Muscle, Open Approach	0KTN0ZZ	Resection of Right Hip Muscle, Open Approach
0KT60ZZ	Resection of Left Shoulder Muscle, Open Approach	0KTF4ZZ	Resection of Right Trunk Muscle, Percutaneous Endoscopic Approach	0KTN4ZZ	Resection of Right Hip Muscle, Percutaneous Endoscopic Approach
0KT64ZZ	Resection of Left Shoulder Muscle, Percutaneous Endoscopic Approach	0KTG0ZZ	Resection of Left Trunk Muscle, Open Approach	0KTP0ZZ	Resection of Left Hip Muscle, Open Approach
0KT70ZZ	Resection of Right Upper Arm Muscle, Open Approach	0KTG4ZZ	Resection of Left Trunk Muscle, Percutaneous Endoscopic Approach	0KTP4ZZ	Resection of Left Hip Muscle, Percutaneous Endoscopic Approach
				0KTQ0ZZ	Resection of Right Upper Leg Muscle, Open Approach

Female-only	♂ Male-only	▲ Limited Coverage	● Non-OR
▨ HAC-associated procedure	▲ Non-covered procedures	➕ Combination	

0KTQ4ZZ Resection of Right Upper Leg Muscle, Percutaneous Endoscopic Approach

0KTR0ZZ Resection of Left Upper Leg Muscle, Open Approach

0KTR4ZZ Resection of Left Upper Leg Muscle, Percutaneous Endoscopic Approach

0KTS0ZZ Resection of Right Lower Leg Muscle, Open Approach

0KTS4ZZ Resection of Right Lower Leg Muscle, Percutaneous Endoscopic Approach

0KTT0ZZ Resection of Left Lower Leg Muscle, Open Approach

0KTT4ZZ Resection of Left Lower Leg Muscle, Percutaneous Endoscopic Approach

0KTV0ZZ Resection of Right Foot Muscle, Open Approach

0KTV4ZZ Resection of Right Foot Muscle, Percutaneous Endoscopic Approach

0KTW0ZZ Resection of Left Foot Muscle, Open Approach

0KTW4ZZ Resection of Left Foot Muscle, Percutaneous Endoscopic Approach

0KU – Muscles, Supplement

0KU007Z Supplement Head Muscle with Autologous Tissue Substitute, Open Approach

0KU00JZ Supplement Head Muscle with Synthetic Substitute, Open Approach

0KU00KZ Supplement Head Muscle with Nonautologous Tissue Substitute, Open Approach

0KU047Z Supplement Head Muscle with Autologous Tissue Substitute, Percutaneous Endoscopic Approach

0KU04JZ Supplement Head Muscle with Synthetic Substitute, Percutaneous Endoscopic Approach

0KU04KZ Supplement Head Muscle with Nonautologous Tissue Substitute, Percutaneous Endoscopic Approach

0KU107Z Supplement Facial Muscle with Autologous Tissue Substitute, Open Approach

0KU10JZ Supplement Facial Muscle with Synthetic Substitute, Open Approach

0KU10KZ Supplement Facial Muscle with Nonautologous Tissue Substitute, Open Approach

0KU147Z Supplement Facial Muscle with Autologous Tissue Substitute, Percutaneous Endoscopic Approach

0KU14JZ Supplement Facial Muscle with Synthetic Substitute, Percutaneous Endoscopic Approach

0KU14KZ Supplement Facial Muscle with Nonautologous Tissue Substitute, Percutaneous Endoscopic Approach

0KU207Z Supplement Right Neck Muscle with Autologous Tissue Substitute, Open Approach

0KU20JZ Supplement Right Neck Muscle with Synthetic Substitute, Open Approach

0KU20KZ Supplement Right Neck Muscle with Nonautologous Tissue Substitute, Open Approach

0KU247Z Supplement Right Neck Muscle with Autologous Tissue Substitute, Percutaneous Endoscopic Approach

0KU24JZ Supplement Right Neck Muscle with Synthetic Substitute, Percutaneous Endoscopic Approach

0KU24KZ Supplement Right Neck Muscle with Nonautologous Tissue Substitute, Percutaneous Endoscopic Approach

0KU307Z Supplement Left Neck Muscle with Autologous Tissue Substitute, Open Approach

0KU30JZ Supplement Left Neck Muscle with Synthetic Substitute, Open Approach

0KU30KZ Supplement Left Neck Muscle with Nonautologous Tissue Substitute, Open Approach

0KU347Z Supplement Left Neck Muscle with Autologous Tissue Substitute, Percutaneous Endoscopic Approach

0KU34JZ Supplement Left Neck Muscle with Synthetic Substitute, Percutaneous Endoscopic Approach

0KU34KZ Supplement Left Neck Muscle with Nonautologous Tissue Substitute, Percutaneous Endoscopic Approach

0KU407Z Supplement Tongue, Palate, Pharynx Muscle with Autologous Tissue Substitute, Open Approach

0KU40JZ Supplement Tongue, Palate, Pharynx Muscle with Synthetic Substitute, Open Approach

0KU40KZ Supplement Tongue, Palate, Pharynx Muscle with Nonautologous Tissue Substitute, Open Approach

0KU447Z Supplement Tongue, Palate, Pharynx Muscle with Autologous Tissue Substitute, Percutaneous Endoscopic Approach

0KU44JZ Supplement Tongue, Palate, Pharynx Muscle with Synthetic Substitute, Percutaneous Endoscopic Approach

0KU44KZ Supplement Tongue, Palate, Pharynx Muscle with Nonautologous Tissue Substitute, Percutaneous Endoscopic Approach

0KU507Z Supplement Right Shoulder Muscle with Autologous Tissue Substitute, Open Approach

0KU50JZ Supplement Right Shoulder Muscle with Synthetic Substitute, Open Approach

0KU50KZ Supplement Right Shoulder Muscle with Nonautologous Tissue Substitute, Open Approach

0KU547Z Supplement Right Shoulder Muscle with Autologous Tissue Substitute, Percutaneous Endoscopic Approach

0KU54JZ Supplement Right Shoulder Muscle with Synthetic Substitute, Percutaneous Endoscopic Approach

0KU54KZ Supplement Right Shoulder Muscle with Nonautologous Tissue Substitute, Percutaneous Endoscopic Approach

0KU607Z Supplement Left Shoulder Muscle with Autologous Tissue Substitute, Open Approach

0KU60JZ Supplement Left Shoulder Muscle with Synthetic Substitute, Open Approach

0KU60KZ Supplement Left Shoulder Muscle with Nonautologous Tissue Substitute, Open Approach

0KU647Z Supplement Left Shoulder Muscle with Autologous Tissue Substitute, Percutaneous Endoscopic Approach

0KU64JZ Supplement Left Shoulder Muscle with Synthetic Substitute, Percutaneous Endoscopic Approach

0KU64KZ Supplement Left Shoulder Muscle with Nonautologous Tissue Substitute, Percutaneous Endoscopic Approach

0KU707Z Supplement Right Upper Arm Muscle with Autologous Tissue Substitute, Open Approach

0KU70JZ Supplement Right Upper Arm Muscle with Synthetic Substitute, Open Approach

0KU70KZ Supplement Right Upper Arm Muscle with Nonautologous Tissue Substitute, Open Approach

0KU747Z Supplement Right Upper Arm Muscle with Autologous Tissue Substitute, Percutaneous Endoscopic Approach

0KU74JZ Supplement Right Upper Arm Muscle with Synthetic Substitute, Percutaneous Endoscopic Approach

0KU74KZ Supplement Right Upper Arm Muscle with Nonautologous Tissue Substitute, Percutaneous Endoscopic Approach

0KU807Z Supplement Left Upper Arm Muscle with Autologous Tissue Substitute, Open Approach

0KU80JZ Supplement Left Upper Arm Muscle with Synthetic Substitute, Open Approach

0KU80KZ Supplement Left Upper Arm Muscle with Nonautologous Tissue Substitute, Open Approach

0KU847Z Supplement Left Upper Arm Muscle with Autologous Tissue Substitute, Percutaneous Endoscopic Approach

0KU84JZ Supplement Left Upper Arm Muscle with Synthetic Substitute, Percutaneous Endoscopic Approach

0KU84KZ Supplement Left Upper Arm Muscle with Nonautologous Tissue Substitute, Percutaneous Endoscopic Approach

0KU907Z Supplement Right Lower Arm and Wrist Muscle with Autologous Tissue Substitute, Open Approach

0KU90JZ Supplement Right Lower Arm and Wrist Muscle with Synthetic Substitute, Open Approach

0KU90KZ Supplement Right Lower Arm and Wrist Muscle with Nonautologous Tissue Substitute, Open Approach

0KU947Z Supplement Right Lower Arm and Wrist Muscle with Autologous Tissue Substitute, Percutaneous Endoscopic Approach

0KU94JZ Supplement Right Lower Arm and Wrist Muscle with Synthetic Substitute, Percutaneous Endoscopic Approach

0KU94KZ Supplement Right Lower Arm and Wrist Muscle with Nonautologous Tissue Substitute, Percutaneous Endoscopic Approach

0KUB07Z Supplement Left Lower Arm and Wrist Muscle with Autologous Tissue Substitute, Open Approach

0KUB0JZ Supplement Left Lower Arm and Wrist Muscle with Synthetic Substitute, Open Approach

0KUB0KZ Supplement Left Lower Arm and Wrist Muscle with Nonautologous Tissue Substitute, Open Approach

0KUB47Z Supplement Left Lower Arm and Wrist Muscle with Autologous Tissue Substitute, Percutaneous Endoscopic Approach

0KUB4JZ Supplement Left Lower Arm and Wrist Muscle with Synthetic Substitute, Percutaneous Endoscopic Approach

0KUB4KZ Supplement Left Lower Arm and Wrist Muscle with Nonautologous Tissue Substitute, Percutaneous Endoscopic Approach

JC07Z	Supplement Right Hand Muscle with Autologous Tissue Substitute, Open Approach
JC0JZ	Supplement Right Hand Muscle with Synthetic Substitute, Open Approach
JC0KZ	Supplement Right Hand Muscle with Nonautologous Tissue Substitute, Open Approach
JC47Z	Supplement Right Hand Muscle with Autologous Tissue Substitute, Percutaneous Endoscopic Approach
JC4JZ	Supplement Right Hand Muscle with Synthetic Substitute, Percutaneous Endoscopic Approach
JC4KZ	Supplement Right Hand Muscle with Nonautologous Tissue Substitute, Percutaneous Endoscopic Approach
UD07Z	Supplement Left Hand Muscle with Autologous Tissue Substitute, Open Approach
UD0JZ	Supplement Left Hand Muscle with Synthetic Substitute, Open Approach
UD0KZ	Supplement Left Hand Muscle with Nonautologous Tissue Substitute, Open Approach
UD47Z	Supplement Left Hand Muscle with Autologous Tissue Substitute, Percutaneous Endoscopic Approach
UD4JZ	Supplement Left Hand Muscle with Synthetic Substitute, Percutaneous Endoscopic Approach
UD4KZ	Supplement Left Hand Muscle with Nonautologous Tissue Substitute, Percutaneous Endoscopic Approach
UF07Z	Supplement Right Trunk Muscle with Autologous Tissue Substitute, Open Approach
UF0JZ	Supplement Right Trunk Muscle with Synthetic Substitute, Open Approach
UF0KZ	Supplement Right Trunk Muscle with Nonautologous Tissue Substitute, Open Approach
UF47Z	Supplement Right Trunk Muscle with Autologous Tissue Substitute, Percutaneous Endoscopic Approach
UF4JZ	Supplement Right Trunk Muscle with Synthetic Substitute, Percutaneous Endoscopic Approach
UF4KZ	Supplement Right Trunk Muscle with Nonautologous Tissue Substitute, Percutaneous Endoscopic Approach
UG07Z	Supplement Left Trunk Muscle with Autologous Tissue Substitute, Open Approach
UG0JZ	Supplement Left Trunk Muscle with Synthetic Substitute, Open Approach
UG0KZ	Supplement Left Trunk Muscle with Nonautologous Tissue Substitute, Open Approach
UG47Z	Supplement Left Trunk Muscle with Autologous Tissue Substitute, Percutaneous Endoscopic Approach
UG4JZ	Supplement Left Trunk Muscle with Synthetic Substitute, Percutaneous Endoscopic Approach
UG4KZ	Supplement Left Trunk Muscle with Nonautologous Tissue Substitute, Percutaneous Endoscopic Approach
UH07Z	Supplement Right Thorax Muscle with Autologous Tissue Substitute, Open Approach
UH0JZ	Supplement Right Thorax Muscle with Synthetic Substitute, Open Approach

0KUH0KZ	Supplement Right Thorax Muscle with Nonautologous Tissue Substitute, Open Approach
0KUH47Z	Supplement Right Thorax Muscle with Autologous Tissue Substitute, Percutaneous Endoscopic Approach
0KUH4JZ	Supplement Right Thorax Muscle with Synthetic Substitute, Percutaneous Endoscopic Approach
0KUH4KZ	Supplement Right Thorax Muscle with Nonautologous Tissue Substitute, Percutaneous Endoscopic Approach
0KUJ07Z	Supplement Left Thorax Muscle with Autologous Tissue Substitute, Open Approach
0KUJ0JZ	Supplement Left Thorax Muscle with Synthetic Substitute, Open Approach
0KUJ0KZ	Supplement Left Thorax Muscle with Nonautologous Tissue Substitute, Open Approach
0KUJ47Z	Supplement Left Thorax Muscle with Autologous Tissue Substitute, Percutaneous Endoscopic Approach
0KUJ4JZ	Supplement Left Thorax Muscle with Synthetic Substitute, Percutaneous Endoscopic Approach
0KUJ4KZ	Supplement Left Thorax Muscle with Nonautologous Tissue Substitute, Percutaneous Endoscopic Approach
0KUK07Z	Supplement Right Abdomen Muscle with Autologous Tissue Substitute, Open Approach
0KUK0JZ	Supplement Right Abdomen Muscle with Synthetic Substitute, Open Approach
0KUK0KZ	Supplement Right Abdomen Muscle with Nonautologous Tissue Substitute, Open Approach
0KUK47Z	Supplement Right Abdomen Muscle with Autologous Tissue Substitute, Percutaneous Endoscopic Approach
0KUK4JZ	Supplement Right Abdomen Muscle with Synthetic Substitute, Percutaneous Endoscopic Approach
0KUK4KZ	Supplement Right Abdomen Muscle with Nonautologous Tissue Substitute, Percutaneous Endoscopic Approach
0KUL07Z	Supplement Left Abdomen Muscle with Autologous Tissue Substitute, Open Approach
0KUL0JZ	Supplement Left Abdomen Muscle with Synthetic Substitute, Open Approach
0KUL0KZ	Supplement Left Abdomen Muscle with Nonautologous Tissue Substitute, Open Approach
0KUL47Z	Supplement Left Abdomen Muscle with Autologous Tissue Substitute, Percutaneous Endoscopic Approach
0KUL4JZ	Supplement Left Abdomen Muscle with Synthetic Substitute, Percutaneous Endoscopic Approach
0KUL4KZ	Supplement Left Abdomen Muscle with Nonautologous Tissue Substitute, Percutaneous Endoscopic Approach
0KUM07Z	Supplement Perineum Muscle with Autologous Tissue Substitute, Open Approach
0KUM0JZ	Supplement Perineum Muscle with Synthetic Substitute, Open Approach
0KUM0KZ	Supplement Perineum Muscle with Nonautologous Tissue Substitute, Open Approach
0KUM47Z	Supplement Perineum Muscle with Autologous Tissue Substitute, Percutaneous Endoscopic Approach
0KUM4JZ	Supplement Perineum Muscle with Synthetic Substitute, Percutaneous Endoscopic Approach

0KUM4KZ	Supplement Perineum Muscle with Nonautologous Tissue Substitute, Percutaneous Endoscopic Approach
0KUN07Z	Supplement Right Hip Muscle with Autologous Tissue Substitute, Open Approach
0KUN0JZ	Supplement Right Hip Muscle with Synthetic Substitute, Open Approach
0KUN0KZ	Supplement Right Hip Muscle with Nonautologous Tissue Substitute, Open Approach
0KUN47Z	Supplement Right Hip Muscle with Autologous Tissue Substitute, Percutaneous Endoscopic Approach
0KUN4JZ	Supplement Right Hip Muscle with Synthetic Substitute, Percutaneous Endoscopic Approach
0KUN4KZ	Supplement Right Hip Muscle with Nonautologous Tissue Substitute, Percutaneous Endoscopic Approach
0KUP07Z	Supplement Left Hip Muscle with Autologous Tissue Substitute, Open Approach
0KUP0JZ	Supplement Left Hip Muscle with Synthetic Substitute, Open Approach
0KUP0KZ	Supplement Left Hip Muscle with Nonautologous Tissue Substitute, Open Approach
0KUP47Z	Supplement Left Hip Muscle with Autologous Tissue Substitute, Percutaneous Endoscopic Approach
0KUP4JZ	Supplement Left Hip Muscle with Synthetic Substitute, Percutaneous Endoscopic Approach
0KUP4KZ	Supplement Left Hip Muscle with Nonautologous Tissue Substitute, Percutaneous Endoscopic Approach
0KUQ07Z	Supplement Right Upper Leg Muscle with Autologous Tissue Substitute, Open Approach
0KUQ0JZ	Supplement Right Upper Leg Muscle with Synthetic Substitute, Open Approach
0KUQ0KZ	Supplement Right Upper Leg Muscle with Nonautologous Tissue Substitute, Open Approach
0KUQ47Z	Supplement Right Upper Leg Muscle with Autologous Tissue Substitute, Percutaneous Endoscopic Approach
0KUQ4JZ	Supplement Right Upper Leg Muscle with Synthetic Substitute, Percutaneous Endoscopic Approach
0KUQ4KZ	Supplement Right Upper Leg Muscle with Nonautologous Tissue Substitute, Percutaneous Endoscopic Approach
0KUR07Z	Supplement Left Upper Leg Muscle with Autologous Tissue Substitute, Open Approach
0KUR0JZ	Supplement Left Upper Leg Muscle with Synthetic Substitute, Open Approach
0KUR0KZ	Supplement Left Upper Leg Muscle with Nonautologous Tissue Substitute, Open Approach
0KUR47Z	Supplement Left Upper Leg Muscle with Autologous Tissue Substitute, Percutaneous Endoscopic Approach
0KUR4JZ	Supplement Left Upper Leg Muscle with Synthetic Substitute, Percutaneous Endoscopic Approach
0KUR4KZ	Supplement Left Upper Leg Muscle with Nonautologous Tissue Substitute, Percutaneous Endoscopic Approach
0KUS07Z	Supplement Right Lower Leg Muscle with Autologous Tissue Substitute, Open Approach

707

0KUS0JZ   Supplement Right Lower Leg Muscle with Synthetic Substitute, Open Approach

0KUS0KZ   Supplement Right Lower Leg Muscle with Nonautologous Tissue Substitute, Open Approach

0KUS47Z   Supplement Right Lower Leg Muscle with Autologous Tissue Substitute, Percutaneous Endoscopic Approach

0KUS4JZ   Supplement Right Lower Leg Muscle with Synthetic Substitute, Percutaneous Endoscopic Approach

0KUS4KZ   Supplement Right Lower Leg Muscle with Nonautologous Tissue Substitute, Percutaneous Endoscopic Approach

0KUT07Z   Supplement Left Lower Leg Muscle with Autologous Tissue Substitute, Open Approach

0KUT0JZ   Supplement Left Lower Leg Muscle with Synthetic Substitute, Open Approach

0KUT0KZ   Supplement Left Lower Leg Muscle with Nonautologous Tissue Substitute, Open Approach

0KUT47Z   Supplement Left Lower Leg Muscle with Autologous Tissue Substitute, Percutaneous Endoscopic Approach

0KUT4JZ   Supplement Left Lower Leg Muscle with Synthetic Substitute, Percutaneous Endoscopic Approach

0KUT4KZ   Supplement Left Lower Leg Muscle with Nonautologous Tissue Substitute, Percutaneous Endoscopic Approach

0KUV07Z   Supplement Right Foot Muscle with Autologous Tissue Substitute, Open Approach

0KUV0JZ   Supplement Right Foot Muscle with Synthetic Substitute, Open Approach

0KUV0KZ   Supplement Right Foot Muscle with Nonautologous Tissue Substitute, Open Approach

0KUV47Z   Supplement Right Foot Muscle with Autologous Tissue Substitute, Percutaneous Endoscopic Approach

0KUV4JZ   Supplement Right Foot Muscle with Synthetic Substitute, Percutaneous Endoscopic Approach

0KUV4KZ   Supplement Right Foot Muscle with Nonautologous Tissue Substitute, Percutaneous Endoscopic Approach

0KUW07Z   Supplement Left Foot Muscle with Autologous Tissue Substitute, Open Approach

0KUW0JZ   Supplement Left Foot Muscle with Synthetic Substitute, Open Approach

0KUW0KZ   Supplement Left Foot Muscle with Nonautologous Tissue Substitute, Ope Approach

0KUW47Z   Supplement Left Foot Muscle with Autologous Tissue Substitute, Percutaneous Endoscopic Approach

0KUW4JZ   Supplement Left Foot Muscle with Synthetic Substitute, Percutaneous Endoscopic Approach

0KUW4KZ   Supplement Left Foot Muscle with Nonautologous Tissue Substitute, Percutaneous Endoscopic Approach

0KW – Muscles, Revision

Review Coding Guideline B6.1c

0KWX00Z   Revision of Drainage Device in Upper Muscle, Open Approach

0KWX07Z   Revision of Autologous Tissue Substitute in Upper Muscle, Open Approach

0KWX0JZ   Revision of Synthetic Substitute in Upper Muscle, Open Approach

0KWX0KZ   Revision of Nonautologous Tissue Substitute in Upper Muscle, Open Approach

0KWX0MZ   Revision of Stimulator Lead in Upper Muscle, Open Approach

0KWX30Z   Revision of Drainage Device in Upper Muscle, Percutaneous Approach

0KWX37Z   Revision of Autologous Tissue Substitute in Upper Muscle, Percutaneous Approach

0KWX3JZ   Revision of Synthetic Substitute in Upper Muscle, Percutaneous Approach

0KWX3KZ   Revision of Nonautologous Tissue Substitute in Upper Muscle, Percutaneous Approach

0KWX3MZ   Revision of Stimulator Lead in Upper Muscle, Percutaneous Approach

0KWX40Z   Revision of Drainage Device in Upper Muscle, Percutaneous Endoscopic Approach

0KWX47Z   Revision of Autologous Tissue Substitute in Upper Muscle, Percutaneous Endoscopic Approach

0KWX4JZ   Revision of Synthetic Substitute in Upper Muscle, Percutaneous Endoscopic Approach

0KWX4KZ   Revision of Nonautologous Tissue Substitute in Upper Muscle, Percutaneous Endoscopic Approach

0KWX4MZ   Revision of Stimulator Lead in Upper Muscle, Percutaneous Endoscopic Approach

0KWXX0Z   Revision of Drainage Device in Upper Muscle, External Approach

0KWXX7Z   Revision of Autologous Tissue Substitute in Upper Muscle, External Approach

0KWXXJZ   Revision of Synthetic Substitute in Upper Muscle, External Approach

0KWXXKZ   Revision of Nonautologous Tissue Substitute in Upper Muscle, External Approach

0KWXXMZ   Revision of Stimulator Lead in Upper Muscle, External Approach

0KWY00Z   Revision of Drainage Device in Lower Muscle, Open Approach

0KWY07Z   Revision of Autologous Tissue Substitute in Lower Muscle, Open Approach

0KWY0JZ   Revision of Synthetic Substitute in Lower Muscle, Open Approach

0KWY0KZ   Revision of Nonautologous Tissue Substitute in Lower Muscle, Open Approach

0KWY0MZ   Revision of Stimulator Lead in Lower Muscle, Open Approach

0KWY30Z   Revision of Drainage Device in Lower Muscle, Percutaneous Approach

0KWY37Z   Revision of Autologous Tissue Substitute in Lower Muscle, Percutaneous Approach

0KWY3JZ   Revision of Synthetic Substitute in Lower Muscle, Percutaneous Approac

0KWY3KZ   Revision of Nonautologous Tissue Substitute in Lower Muscle, Percutaneous Approach

0KWY3MZ   Revision of Stimulator Lead in Lower Muscle, Percutaneous Approach

0KWY40Z   Revision of Drainage Device in Lower Muscle, Percutaneous Endoscopic Approach

0KWY47Z   Revision of Autologous Tissue Substitute in Lower Muscle, Percutaneous Endoscopic Approach

0KWY4JZ   Revision of Synthetic Substitute in Lower Muscle, Percutaneous Endoscopic Approach

0KWY4KZ   Revision of Nonautologous Tissue Substitute in Lower Muscle, Percutaneous Endoscopic Approach

0KWY4MZ   Revision of Stimulator Lead in Lower Muscle, Percutaneous Endoscopic Approach

0KWYX0Z   Revision of Drainage Device in Lower Muscle, External Approach

0KWYX7Z   Revision of Autologous Tissue Substitute in Lower Muscle, External Approach

0KWYXJZ   Revision of Synthetic Substitute in Lower Muscle, External Approach

0KWYXKZ   Revision of Nonautologous Tissue Substitute in Lower Muscle, External Approach

0KWYXMZ   Revision of Stimulator Lead in Lower Muscle, External Approach

0KX – Muscles, Transfer

0KX00Z0   Transfer Head Muscle with Skin, Open Approach

0KX00Z1   Transfer Head Muscle with Subcutaneous Tissue, Open Approach

0KX00Z2   Transfer Head Muscle with Skin and Subcutaneous Tissue, Open Approach

0KX00ZZ   Transfer Head Muscle, Open Approach

0KX04Z0   Transfer Head Muscle with Skin, Percutaneous Endoscopic Approach

0KX04Z1   Transfer Head Muscle with Subcutaneous Tissue, Percutaneous Endoscopic Approach

0KX04Z2   Transfer Head Muscle with Skin and Subcutaneous Tissue, Percutaneous Endoscopic Approach

0KX04ZZ   Transfer Head Muscle, Percutaneous Endoscopic Approach

0KX10Z0   Transfer Facial Muscle with Skin, Open Approach

0KX10Z1   Transfer Facial Muscle with Subcutaneous Tissue, Open Approach

0KX10Z2   Transfer Facial Muscle with Skin and Subcutaneous Tissue, Open Approach

0KX10ZZ   Transfer Facial Muscle, Open Approach

0KX14Z0   Transfer Facial Muscle with Skin, Percutaneous Endoscopic Approach

0KX14Z1   Transfer Facial Muscle with Subcutaneous Tissue, Percutaneous Endoscopic Approach

0KX14Z2   Transfer Facial Muscle with Skin and Subcutaneous Tissue, Percutaneous Endoscopic Approach

0KX14ZZ   Transfer Facial Muscle, Percutaneous Endoscopic Approach

0KX20Z0   Transfer Right Neck Muscle with Skin, Open Approach

X20Z1	Transfer Right Neck Muscle with Subcutaneous Tissue, Open Approach
X20Z2	Transfer Right Neck Muscle with Skin and Subcutaneous Tissue, Open Approach
X20ZZ	Transfer Right Neck Muscle, Open Approach
X24Z0	Transfer Right Neck Muscle with Skin, Percutaneous Endoscopic Approach
X24Z1	Transfer Right Neck Muscle with Subcutaneous Tissue, Percutaneous Endoscopic Approach
X24Z2	Transfer Right Neck Muscle with Skin and Subcutaneous Tissue, Percutaneous Endoscopic Approach
X24ZZ	Transfer Right Neck Muscle, Percutaneous Endoscopic Approach
X30Z0	Transfer Left Neck Muscle with Skin, Open Approach
X30Z1	Transfer Left Neck Muscle with Subcutaneous Tissue, Open Approach
X30Z2	Transfer Left Neck Muscle with Skin and Subcutaneous Tissue, Open Approach
X30ZZ	Transfer Left Neck Muscle, Open Approach
X34Z0	Transfer Left Neck Muscle with Skin, Percutaneous Endoscopic Approach
X34Z1	Transfer Left Neck Muscle with Subcutaneous Tissue, Percutaneous Endoscopic Approach
X34Z2	Transfer Left Neck Muscle with Skin and Subcutaneous Tissue, Percutaneous Endoscopic Approach
X34ZZ	Transfer Left Neck Muscle, Percutaneous Endoscopic Approach
X40Z0	Transfer Tongue, Palate, Pharynx Muscle with Skin, Open Approach
X40Z1	Transfer Tongue, Palate, Pharynx Muscle with Subcutaneous Tissue, Open Approach
X40Z2	Transfer Tongue, Palate, Pharynx Muscle with Skin and Subcutaneous Tissue, Open Approach
X40ZZ	Transfer Tongue, Palate, Pharynx Muscle, Open Approach
X44Z0	Transfer Tongue, Palate, Pharynx Muscle with Skin, Percutaneous Endoscopic Approach
X44Z1	Transfer Tongue, Palate, Pharynx Muscle with Subcutaneous Tissue, Percutaneous Endoscopic Approach
X44Z2	Transfer Tongue, Palate, Pharynx Muscle with Skin and Subcutaneous Tissue, Percutaneous Endoscopic Approach
X44ZZ	Transfer Tongue, Palate, Pharynx Muscle, Percutaneous Endoscopic Approach
X50Z0	Transfer Right Shoulder Muscle with Skin, Open Approach
X50Z1	Transfer Right Shoulder Muscle with Subcutaneous Tissue, Open Approach
X50Z2	Transfer Right Shoulder Muscle with Skin and Subcutaneous Tissue, Open Approach
X50ZZ	Transfer Right Shoulder Muscle, Open Approach
X54Z0	Transfer Right Shoulder Muscle with Skin, Percutaneous Endoscopic Approach
X54Z1	Transfer Right Shoulder Muscle with Subcutaneous Tissue, Percutaneous Endoscopic Approach
X54Z2	Transfer Right Shoulder Muscle with Skin and Subcutaneous Tissue, Percutaneous Endoscopic Approach
KX54ZZ	Transfer Right Shoulder Muscle, Percutaneous Endoscopic Approach
KX60Z0	Transfer Left Shoulder Muscle with Skin, Open Approach
KX60Z1	Transfer Left Shoulder Muscle with Subcutaneous Tissue, Open Approach
0KX60Z2	Transfer Left Shoulder Muscle with Skin and Subcutaneous Tissue, Open Approach
0KX60ZZ	Transfer Left Shoulder Muscle, Open Approach
0KX64Z0	Transfer Left Shoulder Muscle with Skin, Percutaneous Endoscopic Approach
0KX64Z1	Transfer Left Shoulder Muscle with Subcutaneous Tissue, Percutaneous Endoscopic Approach
0KX64Z2	Transfer Left Shoulder Muscle with Skin and Subcutaneous Tissue, Percutaneous Endoscopic Approach
0KX64ZZ	Transfer Left Shoulder Muscle, Percutaneous Endoscopic Approach
0KX70Z0	Transfer Right Upper Arm Muscle with Skin, Open Approach
0KX70Z1	Transfer Right Upper Arm Muscle with Subcutaneous Tissue, Open Approach
0KX70Z2	Transfer Right Upper Arm Muscle with Skin and Subcutaneous Tissue, Open Approach
0KX70ZZ	Transfer Right Upper Arm Muscle, Open Approach
0KX74Z0	Transfer Right Upper Arm Muscle with Skin, Percutaneous Endoscopic Approach
0KX74Z1	Transfer Right Upper Arm Muscle with Subcutaneous Tissue, Percutaneous Endoscopic Approach
0KX74Z2	Transfer Right Upper Arm Muscle with Skin and Subcutaneous Tissue, Percutaneous Endoscopic Approach
0KX74ZZ	Transfer Right Upper Arm Muscle, Percutaneous Endoscopic Approach
0KX80Z0	Transfer Left Upper Arm Muscle with Skin, Open Approach
0KX80Z1	Transfer Left Upper Arm Muscle with Subcutaneous Tissue, Open Approach
0KX80Z2	Transfer Left Upper Arm Muscle with Skin and Subcutaneous Tissue, Open Approach
0KX80ZZ	Transfer Left Upper Arm Muscle, Open Approach
0KX84Z0	Transfer Left Upper Arm Muscle with Skin, Percutaneous Endoscopic Approach
0KX84Z1	Transfer Left Upper Arm Muscle with Subcutaneous Tissue, Percutaneous Endoscopic Approach
0KX84Z2	Transfer Left Upper Arm Muscle with Skin and Subcutaneous Tissue, Percutaneous Endoscopic Approach
0KX84ZZ	Transfer Left Upper Arm Muscle, Percutaneous Endoscopic Approach
0KX90Z0	Transfer Right Lower Arm and Wrist Muscle with Skin, Open Approach
0KX90Z1	Transfer Right Lower Arm and Wrist Muscle with Subcutaneous Tissue, Open Approach
0KX90Z2	Transfer Right Lower Arm and Wrist Muscle with Skin and Subcutaneous Tissue, Open Approach
0KX90ZZ	Transfer Right Lower Arm and Wrist Muscle, Open Approach
0KX94Z0	Transfer Right Lower Arm and Wrist Muscle with Skin, Percutaneous Endoscopic Approach
0KX94Z1	Transfer Right Lower Arm and Wrist Muscle with Subcutaneous Tissue, Percutaneous Endoscopic Approach
0KX94Z2	Transfer Right Lower Arm and Wrist Muscle with Skin and Subcutaneous Tissue, Percutaneous Endoscopic Approach
0KX94ZZ	Transfer Right Lower Arm and Wrist Muscle, Percutaneous Endoscopic Approach
0KXB0Z0	Transfer Left Lower Arm and Wrist Muscle with Skin, Open Approach
0KXB0Z1	Transfer Left Lower Arm and Wrist Muscle with Subcutaneous Tissue, Open Approach
0KXB0Z2	Transfer Left Lower Arm and Wrist Muscle with Skin and Subcutaneous Tissue, Open Approach
0KXB0ZZ	Transfer Left Lower Arm and Wrist Muscle, Open Approach
0KXB4Z0	Transfer Left Lower Arm and Wrist Muscle with Skin, Percutaneous Endoscopic Approach
0KXB4Z1	Transfer Left Lower Arm and Wrist Muscle with Subcutaneous Tissue, Percutaneous Endoscopic Approach
0KXB4Z2	Transfer Left Lower Arm and Wrist Muscle with Skin and Subcutaneous Tissue, Percutaneous Endoscopic Approach
0KXB4ZZ	Transfer Left Lower Arm and Wrist Muscle, Percutaneous Endoscopic Approach
0KXC0Z0	Transfer Right Hand Muscle with Skin, Open Approach
0KXC0Z1	Transfer Right Hand Muscle with Subcutaneous Tissue, Open Approach
0KXC0Z2	Transfer Right Hand Muscle with Skin and Subcutaneous Tissue, Open Approach
0KXC0ZZ	Transfer Right Hand Muscle, Open Approach
0KXC4Z0	Transfer Right Hand Muscle with Skin, Percutaneous Endoscopic Approach
0KXC4Z1	Transfer Right Hand Muscle with Subcutaneous Tissue, Percutaneous Endoscopic Approach
0KXC4Z2	Transfer Right Hand Muscle with Skin and Subcutaneous Tissue, Percutaneous Endoscopic Approach
0KXC4ZZ	Transfer Right Hand Muscle, Percutaneous Endoscopic Approach
0KXD0Z0	Transfer Left Hand Muscle with Skin, Open Approach
0KXD0Z1	Transfer Left Hand Muscle with Subcutaneous Tissue, Open Approach
0KXD0Z2	Transfer Left Hand Muscle with Skin and Subcutaneous Tissue, Open Approach
0KXD0ZZ	Transfer Left Hand Muscle, Open Approach
0KXD4Z0	Transfer Left Hand Muscle with Skin, Percutaneous Endoscopic Approach
0KXD4Z1	Transfer Left Hand Muscle with Subcutaneous Tissue, Percutaneous Endoscopic Approach
0KXD4Z2	Transfer Left Hand Muscle with Skin and Subcutaneous Tissue, Percutaneous Endoscopic Approach
0KXD4ZZ	Transfer Left Hand Muscle, Percutaneous Endoscopic Approach
0KXF0Z0	Transfer Right Trunk Muscle with Skin, Open Approach
0KXF0Z1	Transfer Right Trunk Muscle with Subcutaneous Tissue, Open Approach
0KXF0Z2	Transfer Right Trunk Muscle with Skin and Subcutaneous Tissue, Open Approach

AHA CC: 2Q, 2014, 12

0KXF0ZZ	Transfer Right Trunk Muscle, Open Approach
0KXF4Z0	Transfer Right Trunk Muscle with Skin, Percutaneous Endoscopic Approach
0KXF4Z1	Transfer Right Trunk Muscle with Subcutaneous Tissue, Percutaneous Endoscopic Approach
0KXF4Z2	Transfer Right Trunk Muscle with Skin and Subcutaneous Tissue, Percutaneous Endoscopic Approach

Female-only   ♂ Male-only   ▲ Limited Coverage   ● Non-OR   ▦ HAC-associated procedure   ▲ Non-covered procedures   ✚ Combination

0KXF4ZZ Transfer Right Trunk Muscle, Percutaneous Endoscopic Approach

0KXG0Z0 Transfer Left Trunk Muscle with Skin, Open Approach

0KXG0Z1 Transfer Left Trunk Muscle with Subcutaneous Tissue, Open Approach

0KXG0Z2 Transfer Left Trunk Muscle with Skin and Subcutaneous Tissue, Open Approach

0KXG0ZZ Transfer Left Trunk Muscle, Open Approach

0KXG4Z0 Transfer Left Trunk Muscle with Skin, Percutaneous Endoscopic Approach

0KXG4Z1 Transfer Left Trunk Muscle with Subcutaneous Tissue, Percutaneous Endoscopic Approach

0KXG4Z2 Transfer Left Trunk Muscle with Skin and Subcutaneous Tissue, Percutaneous Endoscopic Approach

0KXG4ZZ Transfer Left Trunk Muscle, Percutaneous Endoscopic Approach

0KXH0Z0 Transfer Right Thorax Muscle with Skin, Open Approach

0KXH0Z1 Transfer Right Thorax Muscle with Subcutaneous Tissue, Open Approach

0KXH0Z2 Transfer Right Thorax Muscle with Skin and Subcutaneous Tissue, Open Approach

0KXH0ZZ Transfer Right Thorax Muscle, Open Approach

0KXH4Z0 Transfer Right Thorax Muscle with Skin, Percutaneous Endoscopic Approach

0KXH4Z1 Transfer Right Thorax Muscle with Subcutaneous Tissue, Percutaneous Endoscopic Approach

0KXH4Z2 Transfer Right Thorax Muscle with Skin and Subcutaneous Tissue, Percutaneous Endoscopic Approach

0KXH4ZZ Transfer Right Thorax Muscle, Percutaneous Endoscopic Approach

0KXJ0Z0 Transfer Left Thorax Muscle with Skin, Open Approach

0KXJ0Z1 Transfer Left Thorax Muscle with Subcutaneous Tissue, Open Approach

0KXJ0Z2 Transfer Left Thorax Muscle with Skin and Subcutaneous Tissue, Open Approach

0KXJ0ZZ Transfer Left Thorax Muscle, Open Approach

0KXJ4Z0 Transfer Left Thorax Muscle with Skin, Percutaneous Endoscopic Approach

0KXJ4Z1 Transfer Left Thorax Muscle with Subcutaneous Tissue, Percutaneous Endoscopic Approach

0KXJ4Z2 Transfer Left Thorax Muscle with Skin and Subcutaneous Tissue, Percutaneous Endoscopic Approach

0KXJ4ZZ Transfer Left Thorax Muscle, Percutaneous Endoscopic Approach

0KXK0Z0 Transfer Right Abdomen Muscle with Skin, Open Approach

0KXK0Z1 Transfer Right Abdomen Muscle with Subcutaneous Tissue, Open Approach

0KXK0Z2 Transfer Right Abdomen Muscle with Skin and Subcutaneous Tissue, Open Approach

0KXK0Z6 Transfer Right Abdomen Muscle, Transverse Rectus Abdominis Myocutaneous Flap, Open Approach
AHA CC: 4Q, 2014, 41

0KXK0ZZ Transfer Right Abdomen Muscle, Open Approach

0KXK4Z0 Transfer Right Abdomen Muscle with Skin, Percutaneous Endoscopic Approach

0KXK4Z1 Transfer Right Abdomen Muscle with Subcutaneous Tissue, Percutaneous Endoscopic Approach

0KXK4Z2 Transfer Right Abdomen Muscle with Skin and Subcutaneous Tissue, Percutaneous Endoscopic Approach

0KXK4Z6 Transfer Right Abdomen Muscle, Transverse Rectus Abdominis Myocutaneous Flap, Percutaneous Endoscopic Approach

0KXK4ZZ Transfer Right Abdomen Muscle, Percutaneous Endoscopic Approach

0KXL0Z0 Transfer Left Abdomen Muscle with Skin, Open Approach

0KXL0Z1 Transfer Left Abdomen Muscle with Subcutaneous Tissue, Open Approach

0KXL0Z2 Transfer Left Abdomen Muscle with Skin and Subcutaneous Tissue, Open Approach

0KXL0Z6 Transfer Left Abdomen Muscle, Transverse Rectus Abdominis Myocutaneous Flap, Open Approach
AHA CC: 2Q, 2014, 10-11

0KXL0ZZ Transfer Left Abdomen Muscle, Open Approach

0KXL4Z0 Transfer Left Abdomen Muscle with Skin, Percutaneous Endoscopic Approach

0KXL4Z1 Transfer Left Abdomen Muscle with Subcutaneous Tissue, Percutaneous Endoscopic Approach

0KXL4Z2 Transfer Left Abdomen Muscle with Skin and Subcutaneous Tissue, Percutaneous Endoscopic Approach

0KXL4Z6 Transfer Left Abdomen Muscle, Transverse Rectus Abdominis Myocutaneous Flap, Percutaneous Endoscopic Approach

0KXL4ZZ Transfer Left Abdomen Muscle, Percutaneous Endoscopic Approach

0KXM0Z0 Transfer Perineum Muscle with Skin, Open Approach

0KXM0Z1 Transfer Perineum Muscle with Subcutaneous Tissue, Open Approach

0KXM0Z2 Transfer Perineum Muscle with Skin and Subcutaneous Tissue, Open Approach

0KXM0ZZ Transfer Perineum Muscle, Open Approach

0KXM4Z0 Transfer Perineum Muscle with Skin, Percutaneous Endoscopic Approach

0KXM4Z1 Transfer Perineum Muscle with Subcutaneous Tissue, Percutaneous Endoscopic Approach

0KXM4Z2 Transfer Perineum Muscle with Skin and Subcutaneous Tissue, Percutaneous Endoscopic Approach

0KXM4ZZ Transfer Perineum Muscle, Percutaneous Endoscopic Approach

0KXN0Z0 Transfer Right Hip Muscle with Skin, Open Approach

0KXN0Z1 Transfer Right Hip Muscle with Subcutaneous Tissue, Open Approach

0KXN0Z2 Transfer Right Hip Muscle with Skin and Subcutaneous Tissue, Open Approach

0KXN0ZZ Transfer Right Hip Muscle, Open Approach

0KXN4Z0 Transfer Right Hip Muscle with Skin, Percutaneous Endoscopic Approach

0KXN4Z1 Transfer Right Hip Muscle with Subcutaneous Tissue, Percutaneous Endoscopic Approach

0KXN4Z2 Transfer Right Hip Muscle with Skin and Subcutaneous Tissue, Percutaneous Endoscopic Approach

0KXN4ZZ Transfer Right Hip Muscle, Percutaneous Endoscopic Approach

0KXP0Z0 Transfer Left Hip Muscle with Skin, Open Approach

0KXP0Z1 Transfer Left Hip Muscle with Subcutaneous Tissue, Open Approach

0KXP0Z2 Transfer Left Hip Muscle with Skin and Subcutaneous Tissue, Open Approach

0KXP0ZZ Transfer Left Hip Muscle, Open Approach

0KXP4Z0 Transfer Left Hip Muscle with Skin, Percutaneous Endoscopic Approach

0KXP4Z1 Transfer Left Hip Muscle with Subcutaneous Tissue, Percutaneous Endoscopic Approach

0KXP4Z2 Transfer Left Hip Muscle with Skin and Subcutaneous Tissue, Percutaneous Endoscopic Approach

0KXP4ZZ Transfer Left Hip Muscle, Percutaneous Endoscopic Approach

0KXQ0Z0 Transfer Right Upper Leg Muscle with Skin, Open Approach

0KXQ0Z1 Transfer Right Upper Leg Muscle with Subcutaneous Tissue, Open Approach

0KXQ0Z2 Transfer Right Upper Leg Muscle with Skin and Subcutaneous Tissue, Open Approach

0KXQ0ZZ Transfer Right Upper Leg Muscle, Open Approach

0KXQ4Z0 Transfer Right Upper Leg Muscle with Skin, Percutaneous Endoscopic Approach

0KXQ4Z1 Transfer Right Upper Leg Muscle with Subcutaneous Tissue, Percutaneous Endoscopic Approach

0KXQ4Z2 Transfer Right Upper Leg Muscle with Skin and Subcutaneous Tissue, Percutaneous Endoscopic Approach

0KXQ4ZZ Transfer Right Upper Leg Muscle, Percutaneous Endoscopic Approach

0KXR0Z0 Transfer Left Upper Leg Muscle with Skin, Open Approach

0KXR0Z1 Transfer Left Upper Leg Muscle with Subcutaneous Tissue, Open Approach

0KXR0Z2 Transfer Left Upper Leg Muscle with Skin and Subcutaneous Tissue, Open Approach

0KXR0ZZ Transfer Left Upper Leg Muscle, Open Approach

0KXR4Z0 Transfer Left Upper Leg Muscle with Skin, Percutaneous Endoscopic Approach

0KXR4Z1 Transfer Left Upper Leg Muscle with Subcutaneous Tissue, Percutaneous Endoscopic Approach

0KXR4Z2 Transfer Left Upper Leg Muscle with Skin and Subcutaneous Tissue, Percutaneous Endoscopic Approach

0KXR4ZZ Transfer Left Upper Leg Muscle, Percutaneous Endoscopic Approach

0KXS0Z0 Transfer Right Lower Leg Muscle with Skin, Open Approach

0KXS0Z1 Transfer Right Lower Leg Muscle with Subcutaneous Tissue, Open Approach

0KXS0Z2 Transfer Right Lower Leg Muscle with Skin and Subcutaneous Tissue, Open Approach

0KXS0ZZ Transfer Right Lower Leg Muscle, Open Approach

0KXS4Z0 Transfer Right Lower Leg Muscle with Skin, Percutaneous Endoscopic Approach

0KXS4Z1 Transfer Right Lower Leg Muscle with Subcutaneous Tissue, Percutaneous Endoscopic Approach

0KXS4Z2 Transfer Right Lower Leg Muscle with Skin and Subcutaneous Tissue, Percutaneous Endoscopic Approach

0KXS4ZZ Transfer Right Lower Leg Muscle, Percutaneous Endoscopic Approach

0KXT0Z0 Transfer Left Lower Leg Muscle with Skin, Open Approach

0KXT0Z1 Transfer Left Lower Leg Muscle with Subcutaneous Tissue, Open Approach

XT0Z2   Transfer Left Lower Leg Muscle with Skin and Subcutaneous Tissue, Open Approach

XT0ZZ   Transfer Left Lower Leg Muscle, Open Approach

XT4Z0   Transfer Left Lower Leg Muscle with Skin, Percutaneous Endoscopic Approach

XT4Z1   Transfer Left Lower Leg Muscle with Subcutaneous Tissue, Percutaneous Endoscopic Approach

XT4Z2   Transfer Left Lower Leg Muscle with Skin and Subcutaneous Tissue, Percutaneous Endoscopic Approach

XT4ZZ   Transfer Left Lower Leg Muscle, Percutaneous Endoscopic Approach

XV0Z0   Transfer Right Foot Muscle with Skin, Open Approach

0KXV0Z1   Transfer Right Foot Muscle with Subcutaneous Tissue, Open Approach

0KXV0Z2   Transfer Right Foot Muscle with Skin and Subcutaneous Tissue, Open Approach

0KXV0ZZ   Transfer Right Foot Muscle, Open Approach

0KXV4Z0   Transfer Right Foot Muscle with Skin, Percutaneous Endoscopic Approach

0KXV4Z1   Transfer Right Foot Muscle with Subcutaneous Tissue, Percutaneous Endoscopic Approach

0KXV4Z2   Transfer Right Foot Muscle with Skin and Subcutaneous Tissue, Percutaneous Endoscopic Approach

0KXV4ZZ   Transfer Right Foot Muscle, Percutaneous Endoscopic Approach

0KXW0Z0   Transfer Left Foot Muscle with Skin, Open Approach

0KXW0Z1   Transfer Left Foot Muscle with Subcutaneous Tissue, Open Approach

0KXW0Z2   Transfer Left Foot Muscle with Skin and Subcutaneous Tissue, Open Approach

0KXW0ZZ   Transfer Left Foot Muscle, Open Approach

0KXW4Z0   Transfer Left Foot Muscle with Skin, Percutaneous Endoscopic Approach

0KXW4Z1   Transfer Left Foot Muscle with Subcutaneous Tissue, Percutaneous Endoscopic Approach

0KXW4Z2   Transfer Left Foot Muscle with Skin and Subcutaneous Tissue, Percutaneous Endoscopic Approach

0KXW4ZZ   Transfer Left Foot Muscle, Percutaneous Endoscopic Approach

♀ Female-only   ♂ Male-only   ▲ Limited Coverage   ● Non-OR   ▦ HAC-associated procedure   ▲ Non-covered procedures   ✚ Combination

Shoulder Tendons and Ligaments

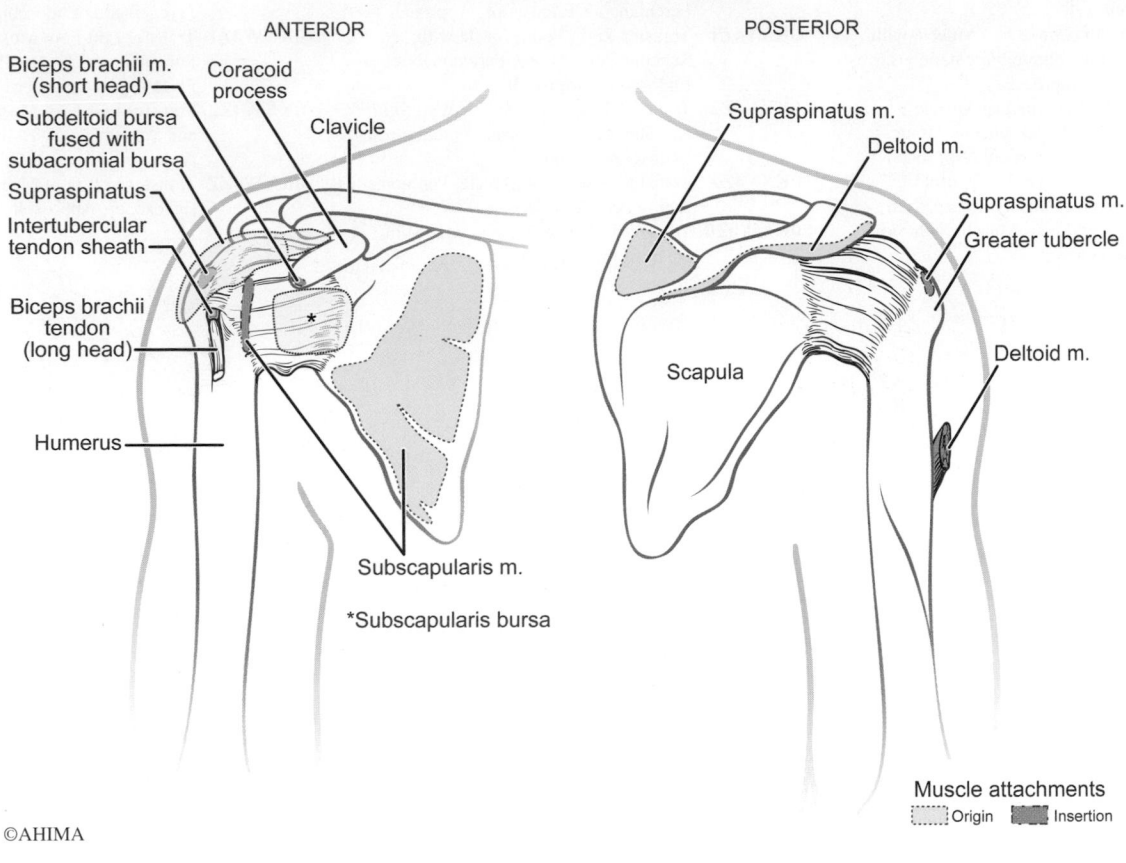

ANTERIOR

Biceps brachii m.
(short head)
Coracoid
process
Clavicle
Subdeltoid bursa
fused with
subacromial bursa
Supraspinatus
Intertubercular
tendon sheath
Biceps brachii
tendon
(long head)
Humerus
Subscapularis m.

*Subscapularis bursa

POSTERIOR

Supraspinatus m.
Deltoid m.
Supraspinatus m.
Greater tubercle
Deltoid m.
Scapula

©AHIMA

Muscle attachments
Origin   Insertion

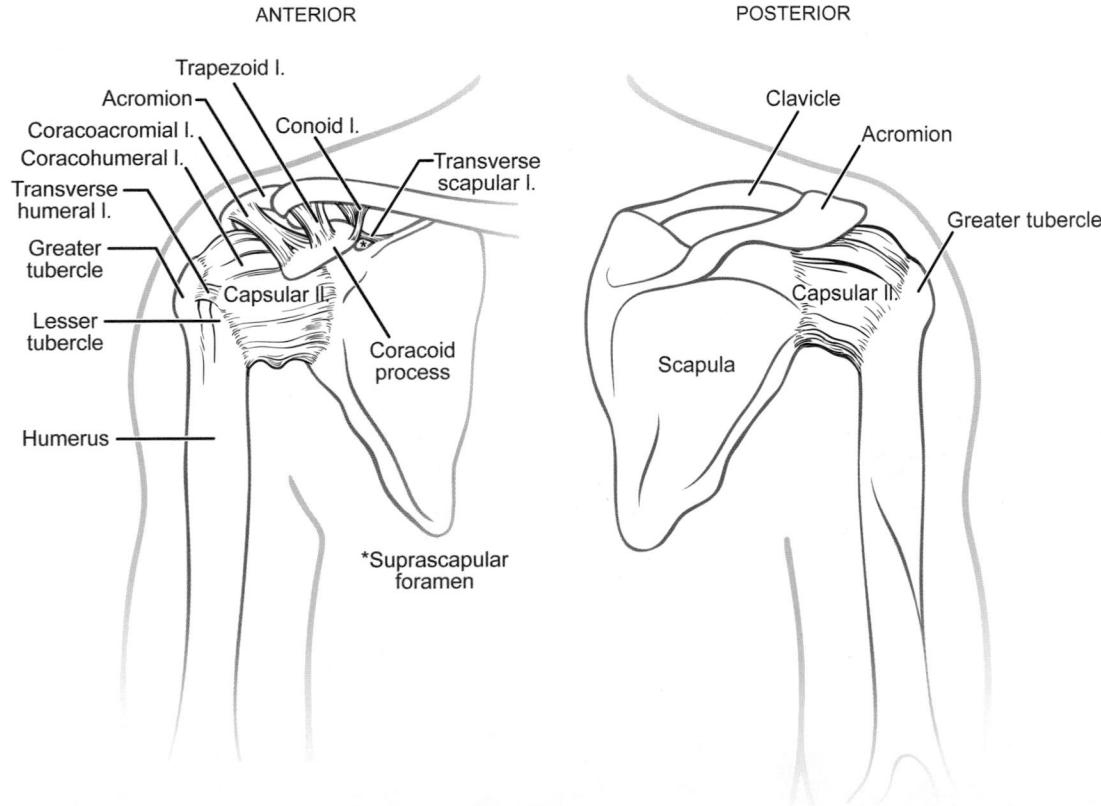

ANTERIOR

Trapezoid l.
Acromion
Coracoacromial l.
Coracohumeral l.
Conoid l.
Transverse
humeral l.
Transverse
scapular l.
Greater
tubercle
Capsular l.
Lesser
tubercle
Humerus
Coracoid
process

*Suprascapular
foramen

POSTERIOR

Clavicle
Acromion
Greater tubercle
Capsular l.
Scapula

©AHIMA

Hip Tendons and Ligaments

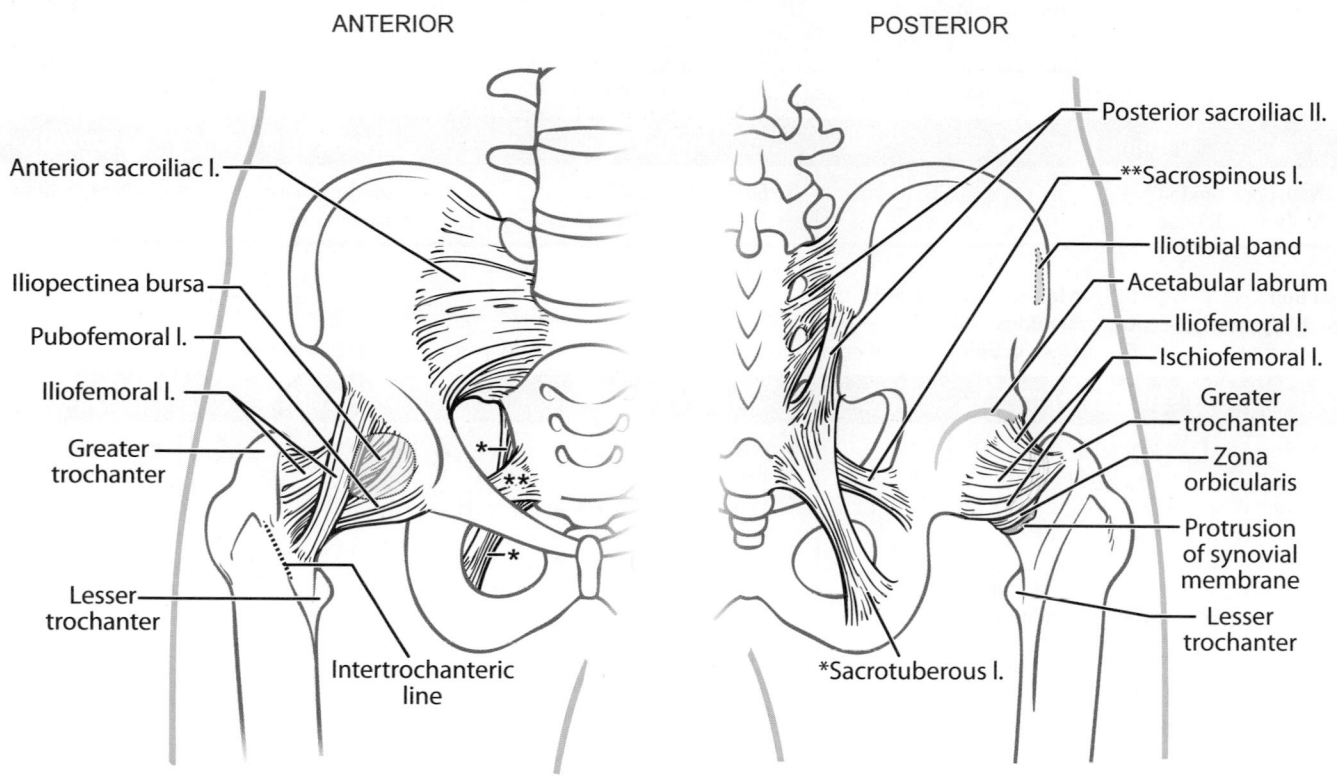

ANTERIOR

- Anterior sacroiliac l.
- Iliopectinea bursa
- Pubofemoral l.
- Iliofemoral l.
- Greater trochanter
- Lesser trochanter
- Intertrochanteric line
- *
- **
- *

POSTERIOR

- Posterior sacroiliac ll.
- **Sacrospinous l.
- Iliotibial band
- Acetabular labrum
- Iliofemoral l.
- Ischiofemoral l.
- Greater trochanter
- Zona orbicularis
- Protrusion of synovial membrane
- Lesser trochanter
- *Sacrotuberous l.

©AHIMA

Knee Tendons and Ligaments

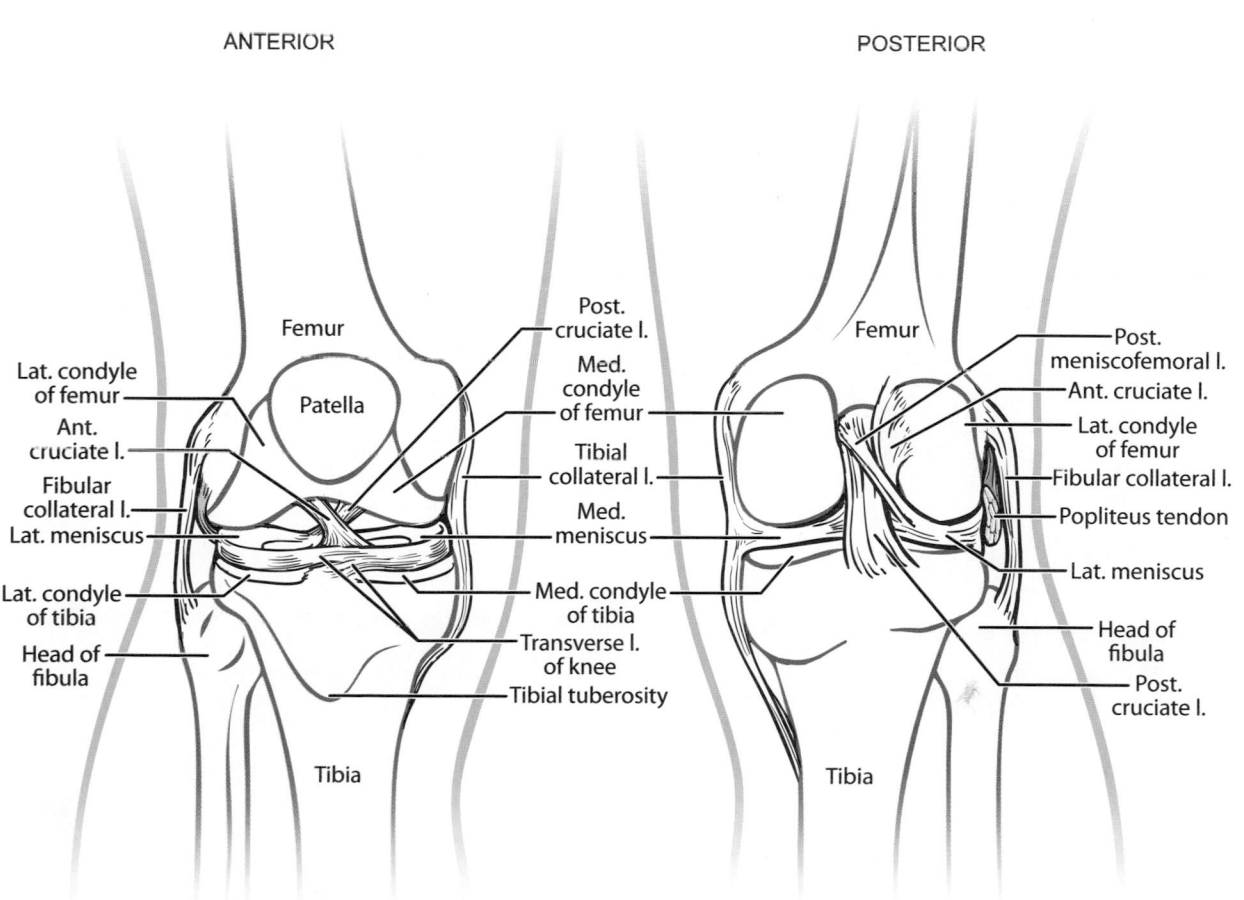

ANTERIOR

- Femur
- Patella
- Lat. condyle of femur
- Ant. cruciate l.
- Fibular collateral l.
- Lat. meniscus
- Lat. condyle of tibia
- Head of fibula
- Tibia
- Post. cruciate l.
- Med. condyle of femur
- Tibial collateral l.
- Med. meniscus
- Med. condyle of tibia
- Transverse l. of knee
- Tibial tuberosity

POSTERIOR

- Femur
- Post. meniscofemoral l.
- Ant. cruciate l.
- Lat. condyle of femur
- Fibular collateral l.
- Popliteus tendon
- Lat. meniscus
- Head of fibula
- Post. cruciate l.
- Tibia

©AHIMA

Tendons Tables 0L2–0LX

Section	0	Medical and Surgical
Body System	L	Tendons
Operation	2	**Change:** Taking out or off a device from a body part and putting back an identical or similar device in or on the same body part without cutting or puncturing the skin or a mucous membrane

Body Part (4th)	Approach (5th)	Device (6th)	Qualifier (7th)
X Upper Tendon Y Lower Tendon	X External	0 Drainage Device Y Other Device	Z No Qualifier

Section	0	Medical and Surgical
Body System	L	Tendons
Operation	5	**Destruction:** Physical eradication of all or a portion of a body part by the direct use of energy, force, or a destructive agent

Body Part (4th)	Approach (5th)	Device (6th)	Qualifier (7th)
0 Head and Neck Tendon 1 Shoulder Tendon, Right 2 Shoulder Tendon, Left 3 Upper Arm Tendon, Right 4 Upper Arm Tendon, Left 5 Lower Arm and Wrist Tendon, Right 6 Lower Arm and Wrist Tendon, Left 7 Hand Tendon, Right 8 Hand Tendon, Left 9 Trunk Tendon, Right B Trunk Tendon, Left C Thorax Tendon, Right D Thorax Tendon, Left F Abdomen Tendon, Right G Abdomen Tendon, Left H Perineum Tendon J Hip Tendon, Right K Hip Tendon, Left L Upper Leg Tendon, Right M Upper Leg Tendon, Left N Lower Leg Tendon, Right P Lower Leg Tendon, Left Q Knee Tendon, Right R Knee Tendon, Left S Ankle Tendon, Right T Ankle Tendon, Left V Foot Tendon, Right W Foot Tendon, Left	0 Open 3 Percutaneous 4 Percutaneous Endoscopic	Z No Device	Z No Qualifier

Section	0	Medical and Surgical
Body System	L	Tendons
Operation	8	**Division:** Cutting into a body part, without draining fluids and/or gases from the body part, in order to separate or transect a body part

Body Part (4th)	Approach (5th)	Device (6th)	Qualifier (7th)
0 Head and Neck Tendon	0 Open	Z No Device	Z No Qualifier
1 Shoulder Tendon, Right	3 Percutaneous		
2 Shoulder Tendon, Left	4 Percutaneous Endoscopic		
3 Upper Arm Tendon, Right			
4 Upper Arm Tendon, Left			
5 Lower Arm and Wrist Tendon, Right			
6 Lower Arm and Wrist Tendon, Left			
7 Hand Tendon, Right			
8 Hand Tendon, Left			
9 Trunk Tendon, Right			
B Trunk Tendon, Left			
C Thorax Tendon, Right			
D Thorax Tendon, Left			
F Abdomen Tendon, Right			
G Abdomen Tendon, Left			
H Perineum Tendon			
J Hip Tendon, Right			
K Hip Tendon, Left			
L Upper Leg Tendon, Right			
M Upper Leg Tendon, Left			
N Lower Leg Tendon, Right			
P Lower Leg Tendon, Left			
Q Knee Tendon, Right			
R Knee Tendon, Left			
S Ankle Tendon, Right			
T Ankle Tendon, Left			
V Foot Tendon, Right			
W Foot Tendon, Left			

Section	0	Medical and Surgical
Body System	L	Tendons
Operation	9	**Drainage:** Taking or letting out fluids and/or gases from a body part

Body Part (4th)	Approach (5th)	Device (6th)	Qualifier (7th)
0 Head and Neck Tendon	0 Open	0 Drainage Device	Z No Qualifier
1 Shoulder Tendon, Right	3 Percutaneous		
2 Shoulder Tendon, Left	4 Percutaneous Endoscopic		
3 Upper Arm Tendon, Right			
4 Upper Arm Tendon, Left			
5 Lower Arm and Wrist Tendon, Right			
6 Lower Arm and Wrist Tendon, Left			
7 Hand Tendon, Right			
8 Hand Tendon, Left			
9 Trunk Tendon, Right			
B Trunk Tendon, Left			
C Thorax Tendon, Right			
D Thorax Tendon, Left			
F Abdomen Tendon, Right			
G Abdomen Tendon, Left			
H Perineum Tendon			
J Hip Tendon, Right			
K Hip Tendon, Left			
L Upper Leg Tendon, Right			
M Upper Leg Tendon, Left			
N Lower Leg Tendon, Right			
P Lower Leg Tendon, Left			
Q Knee Tendon, Right			
R Knee Tendon, Left			
S Ankle Tendon, Right			
T Ankle Tendon, Left			
V Foot Tendon, Right			
W Foot Tendon, Left			

Continued →

Section	0	Medical and Surgical
Body System	L	Tendons
Operation	9	**Drainage:** Taking or letting out fluids and/or gases from a body part

Body Part (4th)	Approach (5th)	Device (6th)	Qualifier (7th)
0 Head and Neck Tendon 1 Shoulder Tendon, Right 2 Shoulder Tendon, Left 3 Upper Arm Tendon, Right 4 Upper Arm Tendon, Left 5 Lower Arm and Wrist Tendon, Right 6 Lower Arm and Wrist Tendon, Left 7 Hand Tendon, Right 8 Hand Tendon, Left 9 Trunk Tendon, Right B Trunk Tendon, Left C Thorax Tendon, Right D Thorax Tendon, Left F Abdomen Tendon, Right G Abdomen Tendon, Left H Perineum Tendon J Hip Tendon, Right K Hip Tendon, Left L Upper Leg Tendon, Right M Upper Leg Tendon, Left N Lower Leg Tendon, Right P Lower Leg Tendon, Left Q Knee Tendon, Right R Knee Tendon, Left S Ankle Tendon, Right T Ankle Tendon, Left V Foot Tendon, Right W Foot Tendon, Left	0 Open 3 Percutaneous 4 Percutaneous Endoscopic	Z No Device	X Diagnostic Z No Qualifier

Section	0	Medical and Surgical
Body System	L	Tendons
Operation	B	**Excision:** Cutting out or off, without replacement, a portion of a body part

Body Part (4th)	Approach (5th)	Device (6th)	Qualifier (7th)
0 Head and Neck Tendon 1 Shoulder Tendon, Right 2 Shoulder Tendon, Left 3 Upper Arm Tendon, Right 4 Upper Arm Tendon, Left 5 Lower Arm and Wrist Tendon, Right 6 Lower Arm and Wrist Tendon, Left 7 Hand Tendon, Right 8 Hand Tendon, Left 9 Trunk Tendon, Right B Trunk Tendon, Left C Thorax Tendon, Right D Thorax Tendon, Left F Abdomen Tendon, Right G Abdomen Tendon, Left H Perineum Tendon J Hip Tendon, Right K Hip Tendon, Left L Upper Leg Tendon, Right M Upper Leg Tendon, Left N Lower Leg Tendon, Right P Lower Leg Tendon, Left Q Knee Tendon, Right R Knee Tendon, Left S Ankle Tendon, Right T Ankle Tendon, Left V Foot Tendon, Right W Foot Tendon, Left	0 Open 3 Percutaneous 4 Percutaneous Endoscopic	Z No Device	X Diagnostic Z No Qualifier

tion	**0**	**Medical and Surgical**	
y System	**L**	**Tendons**	
eration	**C**	**Extirpation:** Taking or cutting out solid matter from a body part	

Body Part (4th)	Approach (5th)	Device (6th)	Qualifier (7th)
Head and Neck Tendon Shoulder Tendon, Right Shoulder Tendon, Left Upper Arm Tendon, Right Upper Arm Tendon, Left Lower Arm and Wrist Tendon, Right Lower Arm and Wrist Tendon, Left Hand Tendon, Right Hand Tendon, Left Trunk Tendon, Right Trunk Tendon, Left Thorax Tendon, Right Thorax Tendon, Left Abdomen Tendon, Right Abdomen Tendon, Left Perineum Tendon Hip Tendon, Right Hip Tendon, Left Upper Leg Tendon, Right Upper Leg Tendon, Left Lower Leg Tendon, Right Lower Leg Tendon, Left Knee Tendon, Right Knee Tendon, Left Ankle Tendon, Right Ankle Tendon, Left Foot Tendon, Right Foot Tendon, Left	**0** Open **3** Percutaneous **4** Percutaneous Endoscopic	**Z** No Device	**Z** No Qualifier

tion	**0**	**Medical and Surgical**	
dy System	**L**	**Tendons**	
eration	**J**	**Inspection:** Visually and/or manually exploring a body part	

Body Part (4th)	Approach (5th)	Device (6th)	Qualifier (7th)
Upper Tendon Lower Tendon	**0** Open **3** Percutaneous **4** Percutaneous Endoscopic **X** External	**Z** No Device	**Z** No Qualifier

Section   **0**   **Medical and Surgical**
Body System   **L**   **Tendons**
Operation   **M**   **Reattachment:** Putting back in or on all or a portion of a separated body part to its normal location or other suitable locatio

Body Part (4ᵗʰ)	Approach (5ᵗʰ)	Device (6ᵗʰ)	Qualifier (7ᵗʰ)
0 Head and Neck Tendon	0 Open	Z No Device	Z No Qualifier
1 Shoulder Tendon, Right	4 Percutaneous Endoscopic		
2 Shoulder Tendon, Left			
3 Upper Arm Tendon, Right			
4 Upper Arm Tendon, Left			
5 Lower Arm and Wrist Tendon, Right			
6 Lower Arm and Wrist Tendon, Left			
7 Hand Tendon, Right			
8 Hand Tendon, Left			
9 Trunk Tendon, Right			
B Trunk Tendon, Left			
C Thorax Tendon, Right			
D Thorax Tendon, Left			
F Abdomen Tendon, Right			
G Abdomen Tendon, Left			
H Perineum Tendon			
J Hip Tendon, Right			
K Hip Tendon, Left			
L Upper Leg Tendon, Right			
M Upper Leg Tendon, Left			
N Lower Leg Tendon, Right			
P Lower Leg Tendon, Left			
Q Knee Tendon, Right			
R Knee Tendon, Left			
S Ankle Tendon, Right			
T Ankle Tendon, Left			
V Foot Tendon, Right			
W Foot Tendon, Left			

Section   **0**   **Medical and Surgical**
Body System   **L**   **Tendons**
Operation   **N**   **Release:** Freeing a body part from an abnormal physical constraint by cutting or by the use of force

Body Part (4ᵗʰ)	Approach (5ᵗʰ)	Device (6ᵗʰ)	Qualifier (7ᵗʰ)
0 Head and Neck Tendon	0 Open	Z No Device	Z No Qualifier
1 Shoulder Tendon, Right	3 Percutaneous		
2 Shoulder Tendon, Left	4 Percutaneous Endoscopic		
3 Upper Arm Tendon, Right	X External		
4 Upper Arm Tendon, Left			
5 Lower Arm and Wrist Tendon, Right			
6 Lower Arm and Wrist Tendon, Left			
7 Hand Tendon, Right			
8 Hand Tendon, Left			
9 Trunk Tendon, Right			
B Trunk Tendon, Left			
C Thorax Tendon, Right			
D Thorax Tendon, Left			
F Abdomen Tendon, Right			
G Abdomen Tendon, Left			
H Perineum Tendon			
J Hip Tendon, Right			
K Hip Tendon, Left			
L Upper Leg Tendon, Right			
M Upper Leg Tendon, Left			
N Lower Leg Tendon, Right			
P Lower Leg Tendon, Left			
Q Knee Tendon, Right			
R Knee Tendon, Left			
S Ankle Tendon, Right			
T Ankle Tendon, Left			
V Foot Tendon, Right			
W Foot Tendon, Left			

Section 0 **Medical and Surgical**
Body System L **Tendons**
Operation P **Removal:** Taking out or off a device from a body part

Body Part (4th)	Approach (5th)	Device (6th)	Qualifier (7th)
Upper Tendon Lower Tendon	0 Open 3 Percutaneous 4 Percutaneous Endoscopic	0 Drainage Device 7 Autologous Tissue Substitute J Synthetic Substitute K Nonautologous Tissue Substitute	Z No Qualifier
Upper Tendon Lower Tendon	X External	0 Drainage Device	Z No Qualifier

Section 0 **Medical and Surgical**
Body System L **Tendons**
Operation Q **Repair:** Restoring, to the extent possible, a body part to its normal anatomic structure and function

Body Part (4th)	Approach (5th)	Device (6th)	Qualifier (7th)
Head and Neck Tendon Shoulder Tendon, Right Shoulder Tendon, Left Upper Arm Tendon, Right Upper Arm Tendon, Left Lower Arm and Wrist Tendon, Right Lower Arm and Wrist Tendon, Left Hand Tendon, Right Hand Tendon, Left Trunk Tendon, Right Trunk Tendon, Left Thorax Tendon, Right Thorax Tendon, Left Abdomen Tendon, Right Abdomen Tendon, Left Perineum Tendon Hip Tendon, Right Hip Tendon, Left Upper Leg Tendon, Right Upper Leg Tendon, Left Lower Leg Tendon, Right Lower Leg Tendon, Left Knee Tendon, Right Knee Tendon, Left Ankle Tendon, Right Ankle Tendon, Left Foot Tendon, Right Foot Tendon, Left	0 Open 3 Percutaneous 4 Percutaneous Endoscopic	Z No Device	Z No Qualifier

Section   0   **Medical and Surgical**
Body System   L   **Tendons**
Operation   R   **Replacement:** Putting in or on biological or synthetic material that physically takes the place and/or function of all or a portion of a body part

Body Part (4ᵗʰ)	Approach (5ᵗʰ)	Device (6ᵗʰ)	Qualifier (7ᵗʰ)
0 Head and Neck Tendon	0 Open	7 Autologous Tissue Substitute	Z No Qualifier
1 Shoulder Tendon, Right	4 Percutaneous	J Synthetic Substitute	
2 Shoulder Tendon, Left	Endoscopic	K Nonautologous Tissue Substitute	
3 Upper Arm Tendon, Right			
4 Upper Arm Tendon, Left			
5 Lower Arm and Wrist Tendon, Right			
6 Lower Arm and Wrist Tendon, Left			
7 Hand Tendon, Right			
8 Hand Tendon, Left			
9 Trunk Tendon, Right			
B Trunk Tendon, Left			
C Thorax Tendon, Right			
D Thorax Tendon, Left			
F Abdomen Tendon, Right			
G Abdomen Tendon, Left			
H Perineum Tendon			
J Hip Tendon, Right			
K Hip Tendon, Left			
L Upper Leg Tendon, Right			
M Upper Leg Tendon, Left			
N Lower Leg Tendon, Right			
P Lower Leg Tendon, Left			
Q Knee Tendon, Right			
R Knee Tendon, Left			
S Ankle Tendon, Right			
T Ankle Tendon, Left			
V Foot Tendon, Right			
W Foot Tendon, Left			

Section   0   **Medical and Surgical**
Body System   L   **Tendons**
Operation   S   **Reposition:** Moving to its normal location, or other suitable location, all or a portion of a body part

Body Part (4ᵗʰ)	Approach (5ᵗʰ)	Device (6ᵗʰ)	Qualifier (7ᵗʰ)
0 Head and Neck Tendon	0 Open	Z No Device	Z No Qualifier
1 Shoulder Tendon, Right	4 Percutaneous Endoscopic		
2 Shoulder Tendon, Left			
3 Upper Arm Tendon, Right			
4 Upper Arm Tendon, Left			
5 Lower Arm and Wrist Tendon, Right			
6 Lower Arm and Wrist Tendon, Left			
7 Hand Tendon, Right			
8 Hand Tendon, Left			
9 Trunk Tendon, Right			
B Trunk Tendon, Left			
C Thorax Tendon, Right			
D Thorax Tendon, Left			
F Abdomen Tendon, Right			
G Abdomen Tendon, Left			
H Perineum Tendon			
J Hip Tendon, Right			
K Hip Tendon, Left			
L Upper Leg Tendon, Right			
M Upper Leg Tendon, Left			
N Lower Leg Tendon, Right			
P Lower Leg Tendon, Left			
Q Knee Tendon, Right			
R Knee Tendon, Left			
S Ankle Tendon, Right			
T Ankle Tendon, Left			
V Foot Tendon, Right			
W Foot Tendon, Left			

Section | 0 | Medical and Surgical
Body System | L | Tendons
Operation | T | **Resection:** Cutting out or off, without replacement, all of a body part

Body Part (4th)	Approach (5th)	Device (6th)	Qualifier (7th)
Head and Neck Tendon Shoulder Tendon, Right Shoulder Tendon, Left Upper Arm Tendon, Right Upper Arm Tendon, Left Lower Arm and Wrist Tendon, Right Lower Arm and Wrist Tendon, Left Hand Tendon, Right Hand Tendon, Left Trunk Tendon, Right Trunk Tendon, Left Thorax Tendon, Right Thorax Tendon, Left Abdomen Tendon, Right Abdomen Tendon, Left Perineum Tendon Hip Tendon, Right Hip Tendon, Left Upper Leg Tendon, Right Upper Leg Tendon, Left Lower Leg Tendon, Right Lower Leg Tendon, Left Knee Tendon, Right Knee Tendon, Left Ankle Tendon, Right Ankle Tendon, Left Foot Tendon, Right Foot Tendon, Left	**0** Open **4** Percutaneous Endoscopic	**Z** No Device	**Z** No Qualifier

Section | 0 | Medical and Surgical
Body System | L | Tendons
Operation | U | **Supplement:** Putting in or on biological or synthetic material that physically reinforces and/or augments the function of a portion of a body part

Body Part (4th)	Approach (5th)	Device (6th)	Qualifier (7th)
0 Head and Neck Tendon 1 Shoulder Tendon, Right 2 Shoulder Tendon, Left 3 Upper Arm Tendon, Right 4 Upper Arm Tendon, Left 5 Lower Arm and Wrist Tendon, Right 6 Lower Arm and Wrist Tendon, Left 7 Hand Tendon, Right 8 Hand Tendon, Left 9 Trunk Tendon, Right B Trunk Tendon, Left C Thorax Tendon, Right D Thorax Tendon, Left F Abdomen Tendon, Right G Abdomen Tendon, Left H Perineum Tendon J Hip Tendon, Right K Hip Tendon, Left L Upper Leg Tendon, Right M Upper Leg Tendon, Left N Lower Leg Tendon, Right P Lower Leg Tendon, Left Q Knee Tendon, Right R Knee Tendon, Left S Ankle Tendon, Right T Ankle Tendon, Left V Foot Tendon, Right W Foot Tendon, Left	**0** Open **4** Percutaneous Endoscopic	**7** Autologous Tissue Substitute **J** Synthetic Substitute **K** Nonautologous Tissue Substitute	**Z** No Qualifier

721

Section	0	Medical and Surgical
Body System	L	Tendons
Operation	W	**Revision:** Correcting, to the extent possible, a portion of a malfunctioning device or the position of a displaced device

Body Part (4th)	Approach (5th)	Device (6th)	Qualifier (7th)
X Upper Tendon Y Lower Tendon	0 Open 3 Percutaneous 4 Percutaneous Endoscopic X External	0 Drainage Device 7 Autologous Tissue Substitute J Synthetic Substitute K Nonautologous Tissue Substitute	Z No Qualifier

Section	0	Medical and Surgical
Body System	L	Tendons
Operation	X	**Transfer:** Moving, without taking out, all or a portion of a body part to another location to take over the function of all or a portion of a body part

Body Part (4th)	Approach (5th)	Device (6th)	Qualifier (7th)
0 Head and Neck Tendon 1 Shoulder Tendon, Right 2 Shoulder Tendon, Left 3 Upper Arm Tendon, Right 4 Upper Arm Tendon, Left 5 Lower Arm and Wrist Tendon, Right 6 Lower Arm and Wrist Tendon, Left 7 Hand Tendon, Right 8 Hand Tendon, Left 9 Trunk Tendon, Right B Trunk Tendon, Left C Thorax Tendon, Right D Thorax Tendon, Left F Abdomen Tendon, Right G Abdomen Tendon, Left H Perineum Tendon J Hip Tendon, Right K Hip Tendon, Left L Upper Leg Tendon, Right M Upper Leg Tendon, Left N Lower Leg Tendon, Right P Lower Leg Tendon, Left Q Knee Tendon, Right R Knee Tendon, Left S Ankle Tendon, Right T Ankle Tendon, Left V Foot Tendon, Right W Foot Tendon, Left	0 Open 4 Percutaneous Endoscopic	Z No Device	Z No Qualifier

Tendons Code Listing 0L2–0LX

Review Coding Guideline B4.5

0L2 – Tendons, Change

Review Coding Guideline B6.1c

0L2XX0Z Change Drainage Device in Upper Tendon, External Approach
0L2XXYZ Change Other Device in Upper Tendon, External Approach

0L2YX0Z Change Drainage Device in Lower Tendon, External Approach

0L2YXYZ Change Other Device in Lower Tendon, External Approach

0L5 – Tendons, Destruction

0L500ZZ Destruction of Head and Neck Tendon, Open Approach
0L503ZZ Destruction of Head and Neck Tendon, Percutaneous Approach
0L504ZZ Destruction of Head and Neck Tendon, Percutaneous Endoscopic Approach
0L510ZZ Destruction of Right Shoulder Tendon, Open Approach
0L513ZZ Destruction of Right Shoulder Tendon, Percutaneous Approach

0L514ZZ Destruction of Right Shoulder Tendon, Percutaneous Endoscopic Approach
0L520ZZ Destruction of Left Shoulder Tendon, Open Approach
0L523ZZ Destruction of Left Shoulder Tendon, Percutaneous Approach
0L524ZZ Destruction of Left Shoulder Tendon, Percutaneous Endoscopic Approach

0L530ZZ Destruction of Right Upper Arm Tendon, Open Approach
0L533ZZ Destruction of Right Upper Arm Tendon, Percutaneous Approach
0L534ZZ Destruction of Right Upper Arm Tendon, Percutaneous Endoscopic Approach
0L540ZZ Destruction of Left Upper Arm Tendon, Open Approach
0L543ZZ Destruction of Left Upper Arm Tendon, Percutaneous Approach

♀ Female-only   ♂ Male-only   ▲ Limited Coverage   ● Non-OR   ▨ HAC-associated procedure   ▲ Non-covered procedures   ✚ Combinatio

544ZZ	Destruction of Left Upper Arm Tendon, Percutaneous Endoscopic Approach	
550ZZ	Destruction of Right Lower Arm and Wrist Tendon, Open Approach	
553ZZ	Destruction of Right Lower Arm and Wrist Tendon, Percutaneous Approach	
554ZZ	Destruction of Right Lower Arm and Wrist Tendon, Percutaneous Endoscopic Approach	
560ZZ	Destruction of Left Lower Arm and Wrist Tendon, Open Approach	
563ZZ	Destruction of Left Lower Arm and Wrist Tendon, Percutaneous Approach	
564ZZ	Destruction of Left Lower Arm and Wrist Tendon, Percutaneous Endoscopic Approach	
570ZZ	Destruction of Right Hand Tendon, Open Approach	
573ZZ	Destruction of Right Hand Tendon, Percutaneous Approach	
574ZZ	Destruction of Right Hand Tendon, Percutaneous Endoscopic Approach	
580ZZ	Destruction of Left Hand Tendon, Open Approach	
583ZZ	Destruction of Left Hand Tendon, Percutaneous Approach	
584ZZ	Destruction of Left Hand Tendon, Percutaneous Endoscopic Approach	
590ZZ	Destruction of Right Trunk Tendon, Open Approach	
593ZZ	Destruction of Right Trunk Tendon, Percutaneous Approach	
594ZZ	Destruction of Right Trunk Tendon, Percutaneous Endoscopic Approach	
5B0ZZ	Destruction of Left Trunk Tendon, Open Approach	
5B3ZZ	Destruction of Left Trunk Tendon, Percutaneous Approach	
5B4ZZ	Destruction of Left Trunk Tendon, Percutaneous Endoscopic Approach	
5C0ZZ	Destruction of Right Thorax Tendon, Open Approach	
5C3ZZ	Destruction of Right Thorax Tendon, Percutaneous Approach	
5C4ZZ	Destruction of Right Thorax Tendon, Percutaneous Endoscopic Approach	
5D0ZZ	Destruction of Left Thorax Tendon, Open Approach	

0L5D3ZZ	Destruction of Left Thorax Tendon, Percutaneous Approach	
0L5D4ZZ	Destruction of Left Thorax Tendon, Percutaneous Endoscopic Approach	
0L5F0ZZ	Destruction of Right Abdomen Tendon, Open Approach	
0L5F3ZZ	Destruction of Right Abdomen Tendon, Percutaneous Approach	
0L5F4ZZ	Destruction of Right Abdomen Tendon, Percutaneous Endoscopic Approach	
0L5G0ZZ	Destruction of Left Abdomen Tendon, Open Approach	
0L5G3ZZ	Destruction of Left Abdomen Tendon, Percutaneous Approach	
0L5G4ZZ	Destruction of Left Abdomen Tendon, Percutaneous Endoscopic Approach	
0L5H0ZZ	Destruction of Perineum Tendon, Open Approach	
0L5H3ZZ	Destruction of Perineum Tendon, Percutaneous Approach	
0L5H4ZZ	Destruction of Perineum Tendon, Percutaneous Endoscopic Approach	
0L5J0ZZ	Destruction of Right Hip Tendon, Open Approach	
0L5J3ZZ	Destruction of Right Hip Tendon, Percutaneous Approach	
0L5J4ZZ	Destruction of Right Hip Tendon, Percutaneous Endoscopic Approach	
0L5K0ZZ	Destruction of Left Hip Tendon, Open Approach	
0L5K3ZZ	Destruction of Left Hip Tendon, Percutaneous Approach	
0L5K4ZZ	Destruction of Left Hip Tendon, Percutaneous Endoscopic Approach	
0L5L0ZZ	Destruction of Right Upper Leg Tendon, Open Approach	
0L5L3ZZ	Destruction of Right Upper Leg Tendon, Percutaneous Approach	
0L5L4ZZ	Destruction of Right Upper Leg Tendon, Percutaneous Endoscopic Approach	
0L5M0ZZ	Destruction of Left Upper Leg Tendon, Open Approach	
0L5M3ZZ	Destruction of Left Upper Leg Tendon, Percutaneous Approach	
0L5M4ZZ	Destruction of Left Upper Leg Tendon, Percutaneous Endoscopic Approach	

0L5N0ZZ	Destruction of Right Lower Leg Tendon, Open Approach	
0L5N3ZZ	Destruction of Right Lower Leg Tendon, Percutaneous Approach	
0L5N4ZZ	Destruction of Right Lower Leg Tendon, Percutaneous Endoscopic Approach	
0L5P0ZZ	Destruction of Left Lower Leg Tendon, Open Approach	
0L5P3ZZ	Destruction of Left Lower Leg Tendon, Percutaneous Approach	
0L5P4ZZ	Destruction of Left Lower Leg Tendon, Percutaneous Endoscopic Approach	
0L5Q0ZZ	Destruction of Right Knee Tendon, Open Approach	
0L5Q3ZZ	Destruction of Right Knee Tendon, Percutaneous Approach	
0L5Q4ZZ	Destruction of Right Knee Tendon, Percutaneous Endoscopic Approach	
0L5R0ZZ	Destruction of Left Knee Tendon, Open Approach	
0L5R3ZZ	Destruction of Left Knee Tendon, Percutaneous Approach	
0L5R4ZZ	Destruction of Left Knee Tendon, Percutaneous Endoscopic Approach	
0L5S0ZZ	Destruction of Right Ankle Tendon, Open Approach	
0L5S3ZZ	Destruction of Right Ankle Tendon, Percutaneous Approach	
0L5S4ZZ	Destruction of Right Ankle Tendon, Percutaneous Endoscopic Approach	
0L5T0ZZ	Destruction of Left Ankle Tendon, Open Approach	
0L5T3ZZ	Destruction of Left Ankle Tendon, Percutaneous Approach	
0L5T4ZZ	Destruction of Left Ankle Tendon, Percutaneous Endoscopic Approach	
0L5V0ZZ	Destruction of Right Foot Tendon, Open Approach	
0L5V3ZZ	Destruction of Right Foot Tendon, Percutaneous Approach	
0L5V4ZZ	Destruction of Right Foot Tendon, Percutaneous Endoscopic Approach	
0L5W0ZZ	Destruction of Left Foot Tendon, Open Approach	
0L5W3ZZ	Destruction of Left Foot Tendon, Percutaneous Approach	
0L5W4ZZ	Destruction of Left Foot Tendon, Percutaneous Endoscopic Approach	

L8 – Tendons, Division

Review Coding Guideline B3.14

L800ZZ	Division of Head and Neck Tendon, Open Approach	
L803ZZ	Division of Head and Neck Tendon, Percutaneous Approach	
L804ZZ	Division of Head and Neck Tendon, Percutaneous Endoscopic Approach	
L810ZZ	Division of Right Shoulder Tendon, Open Approach	
L813ZZ	Division of Right Shoulder Tendon, Percutaneous Approach	
L814ZZ	Division of Right Shoulder Tendon, Percutaneous Endoscopic Approach	
L820ZZ	Division of Left Shoulder Tendon, Open Approach	
L823ZZ	Division of Left Shoulder Tendon, Percutaneous Approach	
L824ZZ	Division of Left Shoulder Tendon, Percutaneous Endoscopic Approach	
L830ZZ	Division of Right Upper Arm Tendon, Open Approach	
L833ZZ	Division of Right Upper Arm Tendon, Percutaneous Approach	

0L834ZZ	Division of Right Upper Arm Tendon, Percutaneous Endoscopic Approach	
0L840ZZ	Division of Left Upper Arm Tendon, Open Approach	
0L843ZZ	Division of Left Upper Arm Tendon, Percutaneous Approach	
0L844ZZ	Division of Left Upper Arm Tendon, Percutaneous Endoscopic Approach	
0L850ZZ	Division of Right Lower Arm and Wrist Tendon, Open Approach	
0L853ZZ	Division of Right Lower Arm and Wrist Tendon, Percutaneous Approach	
0L854ZZ	Division of Right Lower Arm and Wrist Tendon, Percutaneous Endoscopic Approach	
0L860ZZ	Division of Left Lower Arm and Wrist Tendon, Open Approach	
0L863ZZ	Division of Left Lower Arm and Wrist Tendon, Percutaneous Approach	
0L864ZZ	Division of Left Lower Arm and Wrist Tendon, Percutaneous Endoscopic Approach	

0L870ZZ	Division of Right Hand Tendon, Open Approach	
0L873ZZ	Division of Right Hand Tendon, Percutaneous Approach	
0L874ZZ	Division of Right Hand Tendon, Percutaneous Endoscopic Approach	
0L880ZZ	Division of Left Hand Tendon, Open Approach	
0L883ZZ	Division of Left Hand Tendon, Percutaneous Approach	
0L884ZZ	Division of Left Hand Tendon, Percutaneous Endoscopic Approach	
0L890ZZ	Division of Right Trunk Tendon, Open Approach	
0L893ZZ	Division of Right Trunk Tendon, Percutaneous Approach	
0L894ZZ	Division of Right Trunk Tendon, Percutaneous Endoscopic Approach	
0L8B0ZZ	Division of Left Trunk Tendon, Open Approach	
0L8B3ZZ	Division of Left Trunk Tendon, Percutaneous Approach	

♀ Female-only	♂ Male-only	▲ Limited Coverage	● Non-OR	▦ HAC-associated procedure	▲ Non-covered procedures	✚ Combination

0L8B4ZZ Division of Left Trunk Tendon, Percutaneous Endoscopic Approach

0L8C0ZZ Division of Right Thorax Tendon, Open Approach

0L8C3ZZ Division of Right Thorax Tendon, Percutaneous Approach

0L8C4ZZ Division of Right Thorax Tendon, Percutaneous Endoscopic Approach

0L8D0ZZ Division of Left Thorax Tendon, Open Approach

0L8D3ZZ Division of Left Thorax Tendon, Percutaneous Approach

0L8D4ZZ Division of Left Thorax Tendon, Percutaneous Endoscopic Approach

0L8F0ZZ Division of Right Abdomen Tendon, Open Approach

0L8F3ZZ Division of Right Abdomen Tendon, Percutaneous Approach

0L8F4ZZ Division of Right Abdomen Tendon, Percutaneous Endoscopic Approach

0L8G0ZZ Division of Left Abdomen Tendon, Open Approach

0L8G3ZZ Division of Left Abdomen Tendon, Percutaneous Approach

0L8G4ZZ Division of Left Abdomen Tendon, Percutaneous Endoscopic Approach

0L8H0ZZ Division of Perineum Tendon, Open Approach

0L8H3ZZ Division of Perineum Tendon, Percutaneous Approach

0L8H4ZZ Division of Perineum Tendon, Percutaneous Endoscopic Approach

0L8J0ZZ Division of Right Hip Tendon, Open Approach

0L8J3ZZ Division of Right Hip Tendon, Percutaneous Approach

0L8J4ZZ Division of Right Hip Tendon, Percutaneous Endoscopic Approach

0L8K0ZZ Division of Left Hip Tendon, Open Approach

0L8K3ZZ Division of Left Hip Tendon, Percutaneous Approach

0L8K4ZZ Division of Left Hip Tendon, Percutaneous Endoscopic Approach

0L8L0ZZ Division of Right Upper Leg Tendon, Open Approach

0L8L3ZZ Division of Right Upper Leg Tendon, Percutaneous Approach

0L8L4ZZ Division of Right Upper Leg Tendon, Percutaneous Endoscopic Approach

0L8M0ZZ Division of Left Upper Leg Tendon, Open Approach

0L8M3ZZ Division of Left Upper Leg Tendon, Percutaneous Approach

0L8M4ZZ Division of Left Upper Leg Tendon, Percutaneous Endoscopic Approach

0L8N0ZZ Division of Right Lower Leg Tendon, Open Approach

0L8N3ZZ Division of Right Lower Leg Tendon, Percutaneous Approach

0L8N4ZZ Division of Right Lower Leg Tendon, Percutaneous Endoscopic Approach

0L8P0ZZ Division of Left Lower Leg Tendon, Open Approach

0L8P3ZZ Division of Left Lower Leg Tendon, Percutaneous Approach

0L8P4ZZ Division of Left Lower Leg Tendon, Percutaneous Endoscopic Approach

0L8Q0ZZ Division of Right Knee Tendon, Open Approach

0L8Q3ZZ Division of Right Knee Tendon, Percutaneous Approach

0L8Q4ZZ Division of Right Knee Tendon, Percutaneous Endoscopic Approach

0L8R0ZZ Division of Left Knee Tendon, Open Approach

0L8R3ZZ Division of Left Knee Tendon, Percutaneous Approach

0L8R4ZZ Division of Left Knee Tendon, Percutaneous Endoscopic Approach

0L8S0ZZ Division of Right Ankle Tendon, Open Approach

0L8S3ZZ Division of Right Ankle Tendon, Percutaneous Approach

0L8S4ZZ Division of Right Ankle Tendon, Percutaneous Endoscopic Approach

0L8T0ZZ Division of Left Ankle Tendon, Open Approach

0L8T3ZZ Division of Left Ankle Tendon, Percutaneous Approach

0L8T4ZZ Division of Left Ankle Tendon, Percutaneous Endoscopic Approach

0L8V0ZZ Division of Right Foot Tendon, Open Approach

0L8V3ZZ Division of Right Foot Tendon, Percutaneous Approach

0L8V4ZZ Division of Right Foot Tendon, Percutaneous Endoscopic Approach

0L8W0ZZ Division of Left Foot Tendon, Open Approach

0L8W3ZZ Division of Left Foot Tendon, Percutaneous Approach

0L8W4ZZ Division of Left Foot Tendon, Percutaneous Endoscopic Approach

0L9 – Tendons, Drainage

Review Coding Guidelines B3.4a and B3.4b

Review Coding Guideline B6.2

0L9000Z Drainage of Head and Neck Tendon with Drainage Device, Open Approach

0L900ZX Drainage of Head and Neck Tendon, Open Approach, Diagnostic

0L900ZZ Drainage of Head and Neck Tendon, Open Approach

0L9030Z Drainage of Head and Neck Tendon with Drainage Device, Percutaneous Approach

0L903ZX Drainage of Head and Neck Tendon, Percutaneous Approach, Diagnostic

0L903ZZ Drainage of Head and Neck Tendon, Percutaneous Approach

0L9040Z Drainage of Head and Neck Tendon with Drainage Device, Percutaneous Endoscopic Approach

0L904ZX Drainage of Head and Neck Tendon, Percutaneous Endoscopic Approach, Diagnostic

0L904ZZ Drainage of Head and Neck Tendon, Percutaneous Endoscopic Approach

0L9100Z Drainage of Right Shoulder Tendon with Drainage Device, Open Approach

0L910ZX Drainage of Right Shoulder Tendon, Open Approach, Diagnostic

0L910ZZ Drainage of Right Shoulder Tendon, Open Approach

0L9130Z Drainage of Right Shoulder Tendon with Drainage Device, Percutaneous Approach

0L913ZX Drainage of Right Shoulder Tendon, Percutaneous Approach, Diagnostic

0L913ZZ Drainage of Right Shoulder Tendon, Percutaneous Approach

0L9140Z Drainage of Right Shoulder Tendon with Drainage Device, Percutaneous Endoscopic Approach

0L914ZX Drainage of Right Shoulder Tendon, Percutaneous Endoscopic Approach, Diagnostic

0L914ZZ Drainage of Right Shoulder Tendon, Percutaneous Endoscopic Approach

0L9200Z Drainage of Left Shoulder Tendon with Drainage Device, Open Approach

0L920ZX Drainage of Left Shoulder Tendon, Open Approach, Diagnostic

0L920ZZ Drainage of Left Shoulder Tendon, Open Approach

0L9230Z Drainage of Left Shoulder Tendon with Drainage Device, Percutaneous Approach

0L923ZX Drainage of Left Shoulder Tendon, Percutaneous Approach, Diagnostic

0L923ZZ Drainage of Left Shoulder Tendon, Percutaneous Approach

0L9240Z Drainage of Left Shoulder Tendon with Drainage Device, Percutaneous Endoscopic Approach

0L924ZX Drainage of Left Shoulder Tendon, Percutaneous Endoscopic Approach, Diagnostic

0L924ZZ Drainage of Left Shoulder Tendon, Percutaneous Endoscopic Approach

0L9300Z Drainage of Right Upper Arm Tendon with Drainage Device, Open Approach

0L930ZX Drainage of Right Upper Arm Tendon, Open Approach, Diagnostic

0L930ZZ Drainage of Right Upper Arm Tendon, Open Approach

0L9330Z Drainage of Right Upper Arm Tendon with Drainage Device, Percutaneous Approach

0L933ZX Drainage of Right Upper Arm Tendon, Percutaneous Approach, Diagnostic

0L933ZZ Drainage of Right Upper Arm Tendon, Percutaneous Approach

0L9340Z Drainage of Right Upper Arm Tendon with Drainage Device, Percutaneous Endoscopic Approach

0L934ZX Drainage of Right Upper Arm Tendon, Percutaneous Endoscopic Approach, Diagnostic

0L934ZZ Drainage of Right Upper Arm Tendon, Percutaneous Endoscopic Approach

0L9400Z Drainage of Left Upper Arm Tendon with Drainage Device, Open Approach

0L940ZX Drainage of Left Upper Arm Tendon, Open Approach, Diagnostic

0L940ZZ Drainage of Left Upper Arm Tendon, Open Approach

0L9430Z Drainage of Left Upper Arm Tendon with Drainage Device, Percutaneous Approach

0L943ZX Drainage of Left Upper Arm Tendon, Percutaneous Approach, Diagnostic

0L943ZZ Drainage of Left Upper Arm Tendon, Percutaneous Approach

0L9440Z Drainage of Left Upper Arm Tendon with Drainage Device, Percutaneous Endoscopic Approach

0L944ZX Drainage of Left Upper Arm Tendon, Percutaneous Endoscopic Approach, Diagnostic

0L944ZZ Drainage of Left Upper Arm Tendon, Percutaneous Endoscopic Approach

9500Z Drainage of Right Lower Arm and Wrist Tendon with Drainage Device, Open Approach

950ZX Drainage of Right Lower Arm and Wrist Tendon, Open Approach, Diagnostic

950ZZ Drainage of Right Lower Arm and Wrist Tendon, Open Approach

9530Z Drainage of Right Lower Arm and Wrist Tendon with Drainage Device, Percutaneous Approach

953ZX Drainage of Right Lower Arm and Wrist Tendon, Percutaneous Approach, Diagnostic

953ZZ Drainage of Right Lower Arm and Wrist Tendon, Percutaneous Approach

9540Z Drainage of Right Lower Arm and Wrist Tendon with Drainage Device, Percutaneous Endoscopic Approach

954ZX Drainage of Right Lower Arm and Wrist Tendon, Percutaneous Endoscopic Approach, Diagnostic

954ZZ Drainage of Right Lower Arm and Wrist Tendon, Percutaneous Endoscopic Approach

9600Z Drainage of Left Lower Arm and Wrist Tendon with Drainage Device, Open Approach

960ZX Drainage of Left Lower Arm and Wrist Tendon, Open Approach, Diagnostic

960ZZ Drainage of Left Lower Arm and Wrist Tendon, Open Approach

9630Z Drainage of Left Lower Arm and Wrist Tendon with Drainage Device, Percutaneous Approach

963ZX Drainage of Left Lower Arm and Wrist Tendon, Percutaneous Approach, Diagnostic

963ZZ Drainage of Left Lower Arm and Wrist Tendon, Percutaneous Approach

9640Z Drainage of Left Lower Arm and Wrist Tendon with Drainage Device, Percutaneous Endoscopic Approach

964ZX Drainage of Left Lower Arm and Wrist Tendon, Percutaneous Endoscopic Approach, Diagnostic

964ZZ Drainage of Left Lower Arm and Wrist Tendon, Percutaneous Endoscopic Approach

9700Z Drainage of Right Hand Tendon with Drainage Device, Open Approach

970ZX Drainage of Right Hand Tendon, Open Approach, Diagnostic

970ZZ Drainage of Right Hand Tendon, Open Approach

9730Z Drainage of Right Hand Tendon with Drainage Device, Percutaneous Approach

973ZX Drainage of Right Hand Tendon, Percutaneous Approach, Diagnostic

L973ZZ Drainage of Right Hand Tendon, Percutaneous Approach

9740Z Drainage of Right Hand Tendon with Drainage Device, Percutaneous Endoscopic Approach

974ZX Drainage of Right Hand Tendon, Percutaneous Endoscopic Approach, Diagnostic

974ZZ Drainage of Right Hand Tendon, Percutaneous Endoscopic Approach

L9800Z Drainage of Left Hand Tendon with Drainage Device, Open Approach

L980ZX Drainage of Left Hand Tendon, Open Approach, Diagnostic

L980ZZ Drainage of Left Hand Tendon, Open Approach

L9830Z Drainage of Left Hand Tendon with Drainage Device, Percutaneous Approach

0L983ZX Drainage of Left Hand Tendon, Percutaneous Approach, Diagnostic

0L983ZZ Drainage of Left Hand Tendon, Percutaneous Approach

0L9840Z Drainage of Left Hand Tendon with Drainage Device, Percutaneous Endoscopic Approach

0L984ZX Drainage of Left Hand Tendon, Percutaneous Endoscopic Approach, Diagnostic

0L984ZZ Drainage of Left Hand Tendon, Percutaneous Endoscopic Approach

0L9900Z Drainage of Right Trunk Tendon with Drainage Device, Open Approach

0L990ZX Drainage of Right Trunk Tendon, Open Approach, Diagnostic

0L990ZZ Drainage of Right Trunk Tendon, Open Approach

0L9930Z Drainage of Right Trunk Tendon with Drainage Device, Percutaneous Approach

0L993ZX Drainage of Right Trunk Tendon, Percutaneous Approach, Diagnostic

0L993ZZ Drainage of Right Trunk Tendon, Percutaneous Approach

0L9940Z Drainage of Right Trunk Tendon with Drainage Device, Percutaneous Endoscopic Approach

0L994ZX Drainage of Right Trunk Tendon, Percutaneous Endoscopic Approach, Diagnostic

0L994ZZ Drainage of Right Trunk Tendon, Percutaneous Endoscopic Approach

0L9B00Z Drainage of Left Trunk Tendon with Drainage Device, Open Approach

0L9B0ZX Drainage of Left Trunk Tendon, Open Approach, Diagnostic

0L9B0ZZ Drainage of Left Trunk Tendon, Open Approach

0L9B30Z Drainage of Left Trunk Tendon with Drainage Device, Percutaneous Approach

0L9B3ZX Drainage of Left Trunk Tendon, Percutaneous Approach, Diagnostic

0L9B3ZZ Drainage of Left Trunk Tendon, Percutaneous Approach

0L9B40Z Drainage of Left Trunk Tendon with Drainage Device, Percutaneous Endoscopic Approach

0L9B4ZX Drainage of Left Trunk Tendon, Percutaneous Endoscopic Approach, Diagnostic

0L9B4ZZ Drainage of Left Trunk Tendon, Percutaneous Endoscopic Approach

0L9C00Z Drainage of Right Thorax Tendon with Drainage Device, Open Approach

0L9C0ZX Drainage of Right Thorax Tendon, Open Approach, Diagnostic

0L9C0ZZ Drainage of Right Thorax Tendon, Open Approach

0L9C30Z Drainage of Right Thorax Tendon with Drainage Device, Percutaneous Approach

0L9C3ZX Drainage of Right Thorax Tendon, Percutaneous Approach, Diagnostic

0L9C3ZZ Drainage of Right Thorax Tendon, Percutaneous Approach

0L9C40Z Drainage of Right Thorax Tendon with Drainage Device, Percutaneous Endoscopic Approach

0L9C4ZX Drainage of Right Thorax Tendon, Percutaneous Endoscopic Approach, Diagnostic

0L9C4ZZ Drainage of Right Thorax Tendon, Percutaneous Endoscopic Approach

0L9D00Z Drainage of Left Thorax Tendon with Drainage Device, Open Approach

0L9D0ZX Drainage of Left Thorax Tendon, Open Approach, Diagnostic

0L9D0ZZ Drainage of Left Thorax Tendon, Open Approach

0L9D30Z Drainage of Left Thorax Tendon with Drainage Device, Percutaneous Approach

0L9D3ZX Drainage of Left Thorax Tendon, Percutaneous Approach, Diagnostic

0L9D3ZZ Drainage of Left Thorax Tendon, Percutaneous Approach

0L9D40Z Drainage of Left Thorax Tendon with Drainage Device, Percutaneous Endoscopic Approach

0L9D4ZX Drainage of Left Thorax Tendon, Percutaneous Endoscopic Approach, Diagnostic

0L9D4ZZ Drainage of Left Thorax Tendon, Percutaneous Endoscopic Approach

0L9F00Z Drainage of Right Abdomen Tendon with Drainage Device, Open Approach

0L9F0ZX Drainage of Right Abdomen Tendon, Open Approach, Diagnostic

0L9F0ZZ Drainage of Right Abdomen Tendon, Open Approach

0L9F30Z Drainage of Right Abdomen Tendon with Drainage Device, Percutaneous Approach

0L9F3ZX Drainage of Right Abdomen Tendon, Percutaneous Approach, Diagnostic

0L9F3ZZ Drainage of Right Abdomen Tendon, Percutaneous Approach

0L9F40Z Drainage of Right Abdomen Tendon with Drainage Device, Percutaneous Endoscopic Approach

0L9F4ZX Drainage of Right Abdomen Tendon, Percutaneous Endoscopic Approach, Diagnostic

0L9F4ZZ Drainage of Right Abdomen Tendon, Percutaneous Endoscopic Approach

0L9G00Z Drainage of Left Abdomen Tendon with Drainage Device, Open Approach

0L9G0ZX Drainage of Left Abdomen Tendon, Open Approach, Diagnostic

0L9G0ZZ Drainage of Left Abdomen Tendon, Open Approach

0L9G30Z Drainage of Left Abdomen Tendon with Drainage Device, Percutaneous Approach

0L9G3ZX Drainage of Left Abdomen Tendon, Percutaneous Approach, Diagnostic

0L9G3ZZ Drainage of Left Abdomen Tendon, Percutaneous Approach

0L9G40Z Drainage of Left Abdomen Tendon with Drainage Device, Percutaneous Endoscopic Approach

0L9G4ZX Drainage of Left Abdomen Tendon, Percutaneous Endoscopic Approach, Diagnostic

0L9G4ZZ Drainage of Left Abdomen Tendon, Percutaneous Endoscopic Approach

0L9H00Z Drainage of Perineum Tendon with Drainage Device, Open Approach

0L9H0ZX Drainage of Perineum Tendon, Open Approach, Diagnostic

0L9H0ZZ Drainage of Perineum Tendon, Open Approach

0L9H30Z Drainage of Perineum Tendon with Drainage Device, Percutaneous Approach

0L9H3ZX Drainage of Perineum Tendon, Percutaneous Approach, Diagnostic

0L9H3ZZ Drainage of Perineum Tendon, Percutaneous Approach

0L9H40Z Drainage of Perineum Tendon with Drainage Device, Percutaneous Endoscopic Approach

0L9H4ZX Drainage of Perineum Tendon, Percutaneous Endoscopic Approach, Diagnostic

0L9H4ZZ Drainage of Perineum Tendon, Percutaneous Endoscopic Approach

0L9J00Z Drainage of Right Hip Tendon with Drainage Device, Open Approach

0L9J0ZX Drainage of Right Hip Tendon, Open Approach, Diagnostic

0L9J0ZZ Drainage of Right Hip Tendon, Open Approach

0L9J30Z Drainage of Right Hip Tendon with Drainage Device, Percutaneous Approach

0L9J3ZX Drainage of Right Hip Tendon, Percutaneous Approach, Diagnostic

0L9J3ZZ Drainage of Right Hip Tendon, Percutaneous Approach

0L9J40Z Drainage of Right Hip Tendon with Drainage Device, Percutaneous Endoscopic Approach

0L9J4ZX Drainage of Right Hip Tendon, Percutaneous Endoscopic Approach, Diagnostic

0L9J4ZZ Drainage of Right Hip Tendon, Percutaneous Endoscopic Approach

0L9K00Z Drainage of Left Hip Tendon with Drainage Device, Open Approach

0L9K0ZX Drainage of Left Hip Tendon, Open Approach, Diagnostic

0L9K0ZZ Drainage of Left Hip Tendon, Open Approach

0L9K30Z Drainage of Left Hip Tendon with Drainage Device, Percutaneous Approach

0L9K3ZX Drainage of Left Hip Tendon, Percutaneous Approach, Diagnostic

0L9K3ZZ Drainage of Left Hip Tendon, Percutaneous Approach

0L9K40Z Drainage of Left Hip Tendon with Drainage Device, Percutaneous Endoscopic Approach

0L9K4ZX Drainage of Left Hip Tendon, Percutaneous Endoscopic Approach, Diagnostic

0L9K4ZZ Drainage of Left Hip Tendon, Percutaneous Endoscopic Approach

0L9L00Z Drainage of Right Upper Leg Tendon with Drainage Device, Open Approach

0L9L0ZX Drainage of Right Upper Leg Tendon, Open Approach, Diagnostic

0L9L0ZZ Drainage of Right Upper Leg Tendon, Open Approach

0L9L30Z Drainage of Right Upper Leg Tendon with Drainage Device, Percutaneous Approach

0L9L3ZX Drainage of Right Upper Leg Tendon, Percutaneous Approach, Diagnostic

0L9L3ZZ Drainage of Right Upper Leg Tendon, Percutaneous Approach

0L9L40Z Drainage of Right Upper Leg Tendon with Drainage Device, Percutaneous Endoscopic Approach

0L9L4ZX Drainage of Right Upper Leg Tendon, Percutaneous Endoscopic Approach, Diagnostic

0L9L4ZZ Drainage of Right Upper Leg Tendon, Percutaneous Endoscopic Approach

0L9M00Z Drainage of Left Upper Leg Tendon with Drainage Device, Open Approach

0L9M0ZX Drainage of Left Upper Leg Tendon, Open Approach, Diagnostic

0L9M0ZZ Drainage of Left Upper Leg Tendon, Open Approach

0L9M30Z Drainage of Left Upper Leg Tendon with Drainage Device, Percutaneous Approach

0L9M3ZX Drainage of Left Upper Leg Tendon, Percutaneous Approach, Diagnostic

0L9M3ZZ Drainage of Left Upper Leg Tendon, Percutaneous Approach

0L9M40Z Drainage of Left Upper Leg Tendon with Drainage Device, Percutaneous Endoscopic Approach

0L9M4ZX Drainage of Left Upper Leg Tendon, Percutaneous Endoscopic Approach, Diagnostic

0L9M4ZZ Drainage of Left Upper Leg Tendon, Percutaneous Endoscopic Approach

0L9N00Z Drainage of Right Lower Leg Tendon with Drainage Device, Open Approach

0L9N0ZX Drainage of Right Lower Leg Tendon, Open Approach, Diagnostic

0L9N0ZZ Drainage of Right Lower Leg Tendon, Open Approach

0L9N30Z Drainage of Right Lower Leg Tendon with Drainage Device, Percutaneous Approach

0L9N3ZX Drainage of Right Lower Leg Tendon, Percutaneous Approach, Diagnostic

0L9N3ZZ Drainage of Right Lower Leg Tendon, Percutaneous Approach

0L9N40Z Drainage of Right Lower Leg Tendon with Drainage Device, Percutaneous Endoscopic Approach

0L9N4ZX Drainage of Right Lower Leg Tendon, Percutaneous Endoscopic Approach, Diagnostic

0L9N4ZZ Drainage of Right Lower Leg Tendon, Percutaneous Endoscopic Approach

0L9P00Z Drainage of Left Lower Leg Tendon with Drainage Device, Open Approach

0L9P0ZX Drainage of Left Lower Leg Tendon, Open Approach, Diagnostic

0L9P0ZZ Drainage of Left Lower Leg Tendon, Open Approach

0L9P30Z Drainage of Left Lower Leg Tendon with Drainage Device, Percutaneous Approach

0L9P3ZX Drainage of Left Lower Leg Tendon, Percutaneous Approach, Diagnostic

0L9P3ZZ Drainage of Left Lower Leg Tendon, Percutaneous Approach

0L9P40Z Drainage of Left Lower Leg Tendon with Drainage Device, Percutaneous Endoscopic Approach

0L9P4ZX Drainage of Left Lower Leg Tendon, Percutaneous Endoscopic Approach, Diagnostic

0L9P4ZZ Drainage of Left Lower Leg Tendon, Percutaneous Endoscopic Approach

0L9Q00Z Drainage of Right Knee Tendon with Drainage Device, Open Approach

0L9Q0ZX Drainage of Right Knee Tendon, Open Approach, Diagnostic

0L9Q0ZZ Drainage of Right Knee Tendon, Open Approach

0L9Q30Z Drainage of Right Knee Tendon with Drainage Device, Percutaneous Approach

0L9Q3ZX Drainage of Right Knee Tendon, Percutaneous Approach, Diagnostic

0L9Q3ZZ Drainage of Right Knee Tendon, Percutaneous Approach

0L9Q40Z Drainage of Right Knee Tendon with Drainage Device, Percutaneous Endoscopic Approach

0L9Q4ZX Drainage of Right Knee Tendon, Percutaneous Endoscopic Approach, Diagnostic

0L9Q4ZZ Drainage of Right Knee Tendon, Percutaneous Endoscopic Approach

0L9R00Z Drainage of Left Knee Tendon with Drainage Device, Open Approach

0L9R0ZX Drainage of Left Knee Tendon, Open Approach, Diagnostic

0L9R0ZZ Drainage of Left Knee Tendon, Open Approach

0L9R30Z Drainage of Left Knee Tendon with Drainage Device, Percutaneous Approach

0L9R3ZX Drainage of Left Knee Tendon, Percutaneous Approach, Diagnostic

0L9R3ZZ Drainage of Left Knee Tendon, Percutaneous Approach

0L9R40Z Drainage of Left Knee Tendon with Drainage Device, Percutaneous Endoscopic Approach

0L9R4ZX Drainage of Left Knee Tendon, Percutaneous Endoscopic Approach, Diagnostic

0L9R4ZZ Drainage of Left Knee Tendon, Percutaneous Endoscopic Approach

0L9S00Z Drainage of Right Ankle Tendon with Drainage Device, Open Approach

0L9S0ZX Drainage of Right Ankle Tendon, Open Approach, Diagnostic

0L9S0ZZ Drainage of Right Ankle Tendon, Open Approach

0L9S30Z Drainage of Right Ankle Tendon with Drainage Device, Percutaneous Approach

0L9S3ZX Drainage of Right Ankle Tendon, Percutaneous Approach, Diagnostic

0L9S3ZZ Drainage of Right Ankle Tendon, Percutaneous Approach

0L9S40Z Drainage of Right Ankle Tendon with Drainage Device, Percutaneous Endoscopic Approach

0L9S4ZX Drainage of Right Ankle Tendon, Percutaneous Endoscopic Approach, Diagnostic

0L9S4ZZ Drainage of Right Ankle Tendon, Percutaneous Endoscopic Approach

0L9T00Z Drainage of Left Ankle Tendon with Drainage Device, Open Approach

0L9T0ZX Drainage of Left Ankle Tendon, Open Approach, Diagnostic

0L9T0ZZ Drainage of Left Ankle Tendon, Open Approach

0L9T30Z Drainage of Left Ankle Tendon with Drainage Device, Percutaneous Approach

0L9T3ZX Drainage of Left Ankle Tendon, Percutaneous Approach, Diagnostic

0L9T3ZZ Drainage of Left Ankle Tendon, Percutaneous Approach

0L9T40Z Drainage of Left Ankle Tendon with Drainage Device, Percutaneous Endoscopic Approach

0L9T4ZX Drainage of Left Ankle Tendon, Percutaneous Endoscopic Approach, Diagnostic

0L9T4ZZ Drainage of Left Ankle Tendon, Percutaneous Endoscopic Approach

0L9V00Z Drainage of Right Foot Tendon with Drainage Device, Open Approach

0L9V0ZX Drainage of Right Foot Tendon, Open Approach, Diagnostic

0L9V0ZZ Drainage of Right Foot Tendon, Open Approach

0L9V30Z Drainage of Right Foot Tendon with Drainage Device, Percutaneous Approach

0L9V3ZX Drainage of Right Foot Tendon, Percutaneous Approach, Diagnostic

0L9V3ZZ Drainage of Right Foot Tendon, Percutaneous Approach

0L9V40Z Drainage of Right Foot Tendon with Drainage Device, Percutaneous Endoscopic Approach

0L9V4ZX Drainage of Right Foot Tendon, Percutaneous Endoscopic Approach, Diagnostic

0L9V4ZZ Drainage of Right Foot Tendon, Percutaneous Endoscopic Approach

0L9W00Z Drainage of Left Foot Tendon with Drainage Device, Open Approach

0L9W0ZX Drainage of Left Foot Tendon, Open Approach, Diagnostic

0L9W0ZZ Drainage of Left Foot Tendon, Open Approach

0L9W30Z Drainage of Left Foot Tendon with Drainage Device, Percutaneous Approach

9W3ZX   Drainage of Left Foot Tendon, Percutaneous Approach, Diagnostic
9W3ZZ   Drainage of Left Foot Tendon, Percutaneous Approach

0L9W40Z   Drainage of Left Foot Tendon with Drainage Device, Percutaneous Endoscopic Approach

0L9W4ZX   Drainage of Left Foot Tendon, Percutaneous Endoscopic Approach, Diagnostic
0L9W4ZZ   Drainage of Left Foot Tendon, Percutaneous Endoscopic Approach

B – Tendons, Excision

view Coding Guidelines B3.4a and B3.4b

view Coding Guideline B3.5

view Coding Guideline B3.8

B00ZX   Excision of Head and Neck Tendon, Open Approach, Diagnostic
B00ZZ   Excision of Head and Neck Tendon, Open Approach
B03ZX   Excision of Head and Neck Tendon, Percutaneous Approach, Diagnostic
B03ZZ   Excision of Head and Neck Tendon, Percutaneous Approach
B04ZX   Excision of Head and Neck Tendon, Percutaneous Endoscopic Approach, Diagnostic
B04ZZ   Excision of Head and Neck Tendon, Percutaneous Endoscopic Approach
B10ZX   Excision of Right Shoulder Tendon, Open Approach, Diagnostic
B10ZZ   Excision of Right Shoulder Tendon, Open Approach
B13ZX   Excision of Right Shoulder Tendon, Percutaneous Approach, Diagnostic
B13ZZ   Excision of Right Shoulder Tendon, Percutaneous Approach
B14ZX   Excision of Right Shoulder Tendon, Percutaneous Endoscopic Approach, Diagnostic
B14ZZ   Excision of Right Shoulder Tendon, Percutaneous Endoscopic Approach
B20ZX   Excision of Left Shoulder Tendon, Open Approach, Diagnostic
B20ZZ   Excision of Left Shoulder Tendon, Open Approach
B23ZX   Excision of Left Shoulder Tendon, Percutaneous Approach, Diagnostic
B23ZZ   Excision of Left Shoulder Tendon, Percutaneous Approach
LB24ZX   Excision of Left Shoulder Tendon, Percutaneous Endoscopic Approach, Diagnostic
LB24ZZ   Excision of Left Shoulder Tendon, Percutaneous Endoscopic Approach
LB30ZX   Excision of Right Upper Arm Tendon, Open Approach, Diagnostic
LB30ZZ   Excision of Right Upper Arm Tendon, Open Approach
LB33ZX   Excision of Right Upper Arm Tendon, Percutaneous Approach, Diagnostic
LB33ZZ   Excision of Right Upper Arm Tendon, Percutaneous Approach
LB34ZX   Excision of Right Upper Arm Tendon, Percutaneous Endoscopic Approach, Diagnostic
LB34ZZ   Excision of Right Upper Arm Tendon, Percutaneous Endoscopic Approach
LB40ZX   Excision of Left Upper Arm Tendon, Open Approach, Diagnostic
LB40ZZ   Excision of Left Upper Arm Tendon, Open Approach
LB43ZX   Excision of Left Upper Arm Tendon, Percutaneous Approach, Diagnostic
LB43ZZ   Excision of Left Upper Arm Tendon, Percutaneous Approach

0LB44ZX   Excision of Left Upper Arm Tendon, Percutaneous Endoscopic Approach, Diagnostic
0LB44ZZ   Excision of Left Upper Arm Tendon, Percutaneous Endoscopic Approach
0LB50ZX   Excision of Right Lower Arm and Wrist Tendon, Open Approach, Diagnostic
0LB50ZZ   Excision of Right Lower Arm and Wrist Tendon, Open Approach
0LB53ZX   Excision of Right Lower Arm and Wrist Tendon, Percutaneous Approach, Diagnostic
0LB53ZZ   Excision of Right Lower Arm and Wrist Tendon, Percutaneous Approach
0LB54ZX   Excision of Right Lower Arm and Wrist Tendon, Percutaneous Endoscopic Approach, Diagnostic
0LB54ZZ   Excision of Right Lower Arm and Wrist Tendon, Percutaneous Endoscopic Approach
0LB60ZX   Excision of Left Lower Arm and Wrist Tendon, Open Approach, Diagnostic
0LB60ZZ   Excision of Left Lower Arm and Wrist Tendon, Open Approach
0LB63ZX   Excision of Left Lower Arm and Wrist Tendon, Percutaneous Approach, Diagnostic
0LB63ZZ   Excision of Left Lower Arm and Wrist Tendon, Percutaneous Approach
0LB64ZX   Excision of Left Lower Arm and Wrist Tendon, Percutaneous Endoscopic Approach, Diagnostic
0LB64ZZ   Excision of Left Lower Arm and Wrist Tendon, Percutaneous Endoscopic Approach
0LB70ZX   Excision of Right Hand Tendon, Open Approach, Diagnostic
0LB70ZZ   Excision of Right Hand Tendon, Open Approach
0LB73ZX   Excision of Right Hand Tendon, Percutaneous Approach, Diagnostic
0LB73ZZ   Excision of Right Hand Tendon, Percutaneous Approach
0LB74ZX   Excision of Right Hand Tendon, Percutaneous Endoscopic Approach, Diagnostic
0LB74ZZ   Excision of Right Hand Tendon, Percutaneous Endoscopic Approach
0LB80ZX   Excision of Left Hand Tendon, Open Approach, Diagnostic
0LB80ZZ   Excision of Left Hand Tendon, Open Approach
0LB83ZX   Excision of Left Hand Tendon, Percutaneous Approach, Diagnostic
0LB83ZZ   Excision of Left Hand Tendon, Percutaneous Approach
0LB84ZX   Excision of Left Hand Tendon, Percutaneous Endoscopic Approach, Diagnostic
0LB84ZZ   Excision of Left Hand Tendon, Percutaneous Endoscopic Approach
0LB90ZX   Excision of Right Trunk Tendon, Open Approach, Diagnostic

0LB90ZZ   Excision of Right Trunk Tendon, Open Approach
0LB93ZX   Excision of Right Trunk Tendon, Percutaneous Approach, Diagnostic
0LB93ZZ   Excision of Right Trunk Tendon, Percutaneous Approach
0LB94ZX   Excision of Right Trunk Tendon, Percutaneous Endoscopic Approach, Diagnostic
0LB94ZZ   Excision of Right Trunk Tendon, Percutaneous Endoscopic Approach
0LBB0ZX   Excision of Left Trunk Tendon, Open Approach, Diagnostic
0LBB0ZZ   Excision of Left Trunk Tendon, Open Approach
0LBB3ZX   Excision of Left Trunk Tendon, Percutaneous Approach, Diagnostic
0LBB3ZZ   Excision of Left Trunk Tendon, Percutaneous Approach
0LBB4ZX   Excision of Left Trunk Tendon, Percutaneous Endoscopic Approach, Diagnostic
0LBB4ZZ   Excision of Left Trunk Tendon, Percutaneous Endoscopic Approach
0LBC0ZX   Excision of Right Thorax Tendon, Open Approach, Diagnostic
0LBC0ZZ   Excision of Right Thorax Tendon, Open Approach
0LBC3ZX   Excision of Right Thorax Tendon, Percutaneous Approach, Diagnostic
0LBC3ZZ   Excision of Right Thorax Tendon, Percutaneous Approach
0LBC4ZX   Excision of Right Thorax Tendon, Percutaneous Endoscopic Approach, Diagnostic
0LBC4ZZ   Excision of Right Thorax Tendon, Percutaneous Endoscopic Approach
0LBD0ZX   Excision of Left Thorax Tendon, Open Approach, Diagnostic
0LBD0ZZ   Excision of Left Thorax Tendon, Open Approach
0LBD3ZX   Excision of Left Thorax Tendon, Percutaneous Approach, Diagnostic
0LBD3ZZ   Excision of Left Thorax Tendon, Percutaneous Approach
0LBD4ZX   Excision of Left Thorax Tendon, Percutaneous Endoscopic Approach, Diagnostic
0LBD4ZZ   Excision of Left Thorax Tendon, Percutaneous Endoscopic Approach
0LBF0ZX   Excision of Right Abdomen Tendon, Open Approach, Diagnostic
0LBF0ZZ   Excision of Right Abdomen Tendon, Open Approach
0LBF3ZX   Excision of Right Abdomen Tendon, Percutaneous Approach, Diagnostic
0LBF3ZZ   Excision of Right Abdomen Tendon, Percutaneous Approach
0LBF4ZX   Excision of Right Abdomen Tendon, Percutaneous Endoscopic Approach, Diagnostic
0LBF4ZZ   Excision of Right Abdomen Tendon, Percutaneous Endoscopic Approach

Female-only   ♂ Male-only   ▲ Limited Coverage   ● Non-OR   ▨ HAC-associated procedure   ▲ Non-covered procedures   + Combination

0LBG0ZX Excision of Left Abdomen Tendon, Open Approach, Diagnostic
0LBG0ZZ Excision of Left Abdomen Tendon, Open Approach
0LBG3ZX Excision of Left Abdomen Tendon, Percutaneous Approach, Diagnostic
0LBG3ZZ Excision of Left Abdomen Tendon, Percutaneous Approach
0LBG4ZX Excision of Left Abdomen Tendon, Percutaneous Endoscopic Approach, Diagnostic
0LBG4ZZ Excision of Left Abdomen Tendon, Percutaneous Endoscopic Approach
0LBH0ZX Excision of Perineum Tendon, Open Approach, Diagnostic
0LBH0ZZ Excision of Perineum Tendon, Open Approach
0LBH3ZX Excision of Perineum Tendon, Percutaneous Approach, Diagnostic
0LBH3ZZ Excision of Perineum Tendon, Percutaneous Approach
0LBH4ZX Excision of Perineum Tendon, Percutaneous Endoscopic Approach, Diagnostic
0LBH4ZZ Excision of Perineum Tendon, Percutaneous Endoscopic Approach
0LBJ0ZX Excision of Right Hip Tendon, Open Approach, Diagnostic
0LBJ0ZZ Excision of Right Hip Tendon, Open Approach
0LBJ3ZX Excision of Right Hip Tendon, Percutaneous Approach, Diagnostic
0LBJ3ZZ Excision of Right Hip Tendon, Percutaneous Approach
0LBJ4ZX Excision of Right Hip Tendon, Percutaneous Endoscopic Approach, Diagnostic
0LBJ4ZZ Excision of Right Hip Tendon, Percutaneous Endoscopic Approach
0LBK0ZX Excision of Left Hip Tendon, Open Approach, Diagnostic
0LBK0ZZ Excision of Left Hip Tendon, Open Approach
0LBK3ZX Excision of Left Hip Tendon, Percutaneous Approach, Diagnostic
0LBK3ZZ Excision of Left Hip Tendon, Percutaneous Approach
0LBK4ZX Excision of Left Hip Tendon, Percutaneous Endoscopic Approach, Diagnostic
0LBK4ZZ Excision of Left Hip Tendon, Percutaneous Endoscopic Approach
0LBL0ZX Excision of Right Upper Leg Tendon, Open Approach, Diagnostic
0LBL0ZZ Excision of Right Upper Leg Tendon, Open Approach
0LBL3ZX Excision of Right Upper Leg Tendon, Percutaneous Approach, Diagnostic
0LBL3ZZ Excision of Right Upper Leg Tendon, Percutaneous Approach

0LBL4ZX Excision of Right Upper Leg Tendon, Percutaneous Endoscopic Approach, Diagnostic
0LBL4ZZ Excision of Right Upper Leg Tendon, Percutaneous Endoscopic Approach
0LBM0ZX Excision of Left Upper Leg Tendon, Open Approach, Diagnostic
0LBM0ZZ Excision of Left Upper Leg Tendon, Open Approach
0LBM3ZX Excision of Left Upper Leg Tendon, Percutaneous Approach, Diagnostic
0LBM3ZZ Excision of Left Upper Leg Tendon, Percutaneous Approach
0LBM4ZX Excision of Left Upper Leg Tendon, Percutaneous Endoscopic Approach, Diagnostic
0LBM4ZZ Excision of Left Upper Leg Tendon, Percutaneous Endoscopic Approach
0LBN0ZX Excision of Right Lower Leg Tendon, Open Approach, Diagnostic
0LBN0ZZ Excision of Right Lower Leg Tendon, Open Approach
0LBN3ZX Excision of Right Lower Leg Tendon, Percutaneous Approach, Diagnostic
0LBN3ZZ Excision of Right Lower Leg Tendon, Percutaneous Approach
0LBN4ZX Excision of Right Lower Leg Tendon, Percutaneous Endoscopic Approach, Diagnostic
0LBN4ZZ Excision of Right Lower Leg Tendon, Percutaneous Endoscopic Approach
0LBP0ZX Excision of Left Lower Leg Tendon, Open Approach, Diagnostic
0LBP0ZZ Excision of Left Lower Leg Tendon, Open Approach
  AHA CC: 3Q, 2014, 18-19
0LBP3ZX Excision of Left Lower Leg Tendon, Percutaneous Approach, Diagnostic
0LBP3ZZ Excision of Left Lower Leg Tendon, Percutaneous Approach
0LBP4ZX Excision of Left Lower Leg Tendon, Percutaneous Endoscopic Approach, Diagnostic
0LBP4ZZ Excision of Left Lower Leg Tendon, Percutaneous Endoscopic Approach
0LBQ0ZX Excision of Right Knee Tendon, Open Approach, Diagnostic
0LBQ0ZZ Excision of Right Knee Tendon, Open Approach
0LBQ3ZX Excision of Right Knee Tendon, Percutaneous Approach, Diagnostic
0LBQ3ZZ Excision of Right Knee Tendon, Percutaneous Approach
0LBQ4ZX Excision of Right Knee Tendon, Percutaneous Endoscopic Approach, Diagnostic
0LBQ4ZZ Excision of Right Knee Tendon, Percutaneous Endoscopic Approach
0LBR0ZX Excision of Left Knee Tendon, Open Approach, Diagnostic
0LBR0ZZ Excision of Left Knee Tendon, Open Approach

0LBR3ZX Excision of Left Knee Tendon, Percutaneous Approach, Diagnostic
0LBR3ZZ Excision of Left Knee Tendon, Percutaneous Approach
0LBR4ZX Excision of Left Knee Tendon, Percutaneous Endoscopic Approach, Diagnostic
0LBR4ZZ Excision of Left Knee Tendon, Percutaneous Endoscopic Approach
0LBS0ZX Excision of Right Ankle Tendon, Open Approach, Diagnostic
0LBS0ZZ Excision of Right Ankle Tendon, Open Approach
0LBS3ZX Excision of Right Ankle Tendon, Percutaneous Approach, Diagnostic
0LBS3ZZ Excision of Right Ankle Tendon, Percutaneous Approach
0LBS4ZX Excision of Right Ankle Tendon, Percutaneous Endoscopic Approach, Diagnostic
0LBS4ZZ Excision of Right Ankle Tendon, Percutaneous Endoscopic Approach
0LBT0ZX Excision of Left Ankle Tendon, Open Approach, Diagnostic
0LBT0ZZ Excision of Left Ankle Tendon, Open Approach
  AHA CC: 3Q, 2014, 14-15
0LBT3ZX Excision of Left Ankle Tendon, Percutaneous Approach, Diagnostic
0LBT3ZZ Excision of Left Ankle Tendon, Percutaneous Approach
0LBT4ZX Excision of Left Ankle Tendon, Percutaneous Endoscopic Approach, Diagnostic
0LBT4ZZ Excision of Left Ankle Tendon, Percutaneous Endoscopic Approach
0LBV0ZX Excision of Right Foot Tendon, Open Approach, Diagnostic
0LBV0ZZ Excision of Right Foot Tendon, Open Approach
0LBV3ZX Excision of Right Foot Tendon, Percutaneous Approach, Diagnostic
0LBV3ZZ Excision of Right Foot Tendon, Percutaneous Approach
0LBV4ZX Excision of Right Foot Tendon, Percutaneous Endoscopic Approach, Diagnostic
0LBV4ZZ Excision of Right Foot Tendon, Percutaneous Endoscopic Approach
0LBW0ZX Excision of Left Foot Tendon, Open Approach, Diagnostic
0LBW0ZZ Excision of Left Foot Tendon, Open Approach
0LBW3ZX Excision of Left Foot Tendon, Percutaneous Approach, Diagnostic
0LBW3ZZ Excision of Left Foot Tendon, Percutaneous Approach
0LBW4ZX Excision of Left Foot Tendon, Percutaneous Endoscopic Approach, Diagnostic
0LBW4ZZ Excision of Left Foot Tendon, Percutaneous Endoscopic Approach

0LC – Tendons, Extirpation

0LC00ZZ Extirpation of Matter from Head and Neck Tendon, Open Approach
0LC03ZZ Extirpation of Matter from Head and Neck Tendon, Percutaneous Approach
0LC04ZZ Extirpation of Matter from Head and Neck Tendon, Percutaneous Endoscopic Approach
0LC10ZZ Extirpation of Matter from Right Shoulder Tendon, Open Approach
0LC13ZZ Extirpation of Matter from Right Shoulder Tendon, Percutaneous Approach

0LC14ZZ Extirpation of Matter from Right Shoulder Tendon, Percutaneous Endoscopic Approach
0LC20ZZ Extirpation of Matter from Left Shoulder Tendon, Open Approach
0LC23ZZ Extirpation of Matter from Left Shoulder Tendon, Percutaneous Approach
0LC24ZZ Extirpation of Matter from Left Shoulder Tendon, Percutaneous Endoscopic Approach

0LC30ZZ Extirpation of Matter from Right Upper Arm Tendon, Open Approach
0LC33ZZ Extirpation of Matter from Right Upper Arm Tendon, Percutaneous Approach
0LC34ZZ Extirpation of Matter from Right Upper Arm Tendon, Percutaneous Endoscopic Approach
0LC40ZZ Extirpation of Matter from Left Upper Arm Tendon, Open Approach
0LC43ZZ Extirpation of Matter from Left Upper Arm Tendon, Percutaneous Approach

♀ Female-only　　♂ Male-only　　▲ Limited Coverage　　● Non-OR　　■ HAC-associated procedure　　▲ Non-covered procedures　　✛ Combination

44ZZ Extirpation of Matter from Left Upper Arm Tendon, Percutaneous Endoscopic Approach

50ZZ Extirpation of Matter from Right Lower Arm and Wrist Tendon, Open Approach

53ZZ Extirpation of Matter from Right Lower Arm and Wrist Tendon, Percutaneous Approach

54ZZ Extirpation of Matter from Right Lower Arm and Wrist Tendon, Percutaneous Endoscopic Approach

60ZZ Extirpation of Matter from Left Lower Arm and Wrist Tendon, Open Approach

63ZZ Extirpation of Matter from Left Lower Arm and Wrist Tendon, Percutaneous Approach

C64ZZ Extirpation of Matter from Left Lower Arm and Wrist Tendon, Percutaneous Endoscopic Approach

C70ZZ Extirpation of Matter from Right Hand Tendon, Open Approach

C73ZZ Extirpation of Matter from Right Hand Tendon, Percutaneous Approach

C74ZZ Extirpation of Matter from Right Hand Tendon, Percutaneous Endoscopic Approach

C80ZZ Extirpation of Matter from Left Hand Tendon, Open Approach

C83ZZ Extirpation of Matter from Left Hand Tendon, Percutaneous Approach

C84ZZ Extirpation of Matter from Left Hand Tendon, Percutaneous Endoscopic Approach

C90ZZ Extirpation of Matter from Right Trunk Tendon, Open Approach

C93ZZ Extirpation of Matter from Right Trunk Tendon, Percutaneous Approach

C94ZZ Extirpation of Matter from Right Trunk Tendon, Percutaneous Endoscopic Approach

CB0ZZ Extirpation of Matter from Left Trunk Tendon, Open Approach

CB3ZZ Extirpation of Matter from Left Trunk Tendon, Percutaneous Approach

CB4ZZ Extirpation of Matter from Left Trunk Tendon, Percutaneous Endoscopic Approach

CC0ZZ Extirpation of Matter from Right Thorax Tendon, Open Approach

CC3ZZ Extirpation of Matter from Right Thorax Tendon, Percutaneous Approach

CC4ZZ Extirpation of Matter from Right Thorax Tendon, Percutaneous Endoscopic Approach

CD0ZZ Extirpation of Matter from Left Thorax Tendon, Open Approach

0LCD3ZZ Extirpation of Matter from Left Thorax Tendon, Percutaneous Approach

0LCD4ZZ Extirpation of Matter from Left Thorax Tendon, Percutaneous Endoscopic Approach

0LCF0ZZ Extirpation of Matter from Right Abdomen Tendon, Open Approach

0LCF3ZZ Extirpation of Matter from Right Abdomen Tendon, Percutaneous Approach

0LCF4ZZ Extirpation of Matter from Right Abdomen Tendon, Percutaneous Endoscopic Approach

0LCG0ZZ Extirpation of Matter from Left Abdomen Tendon, Open Approach

0LCG3ZZ Extirpation of Matter from Left Abdomen Tendon, Percutaneous Approach

0LCG4ZZ Extirpation of Matter from Left Abdomen Tendon, Percutaneous Endoscopic Approach

0LCH0ZZ Extirpation of Matter from Perineum Tendon, Open Approach

0LCH3ZZ Extirpation of Matter from Perineum Tendon, Percutaneous Approach

0LCH4ZZ Extirpation of Matter from Perineum Tendon, Percutaneous Endoscopic Approach

0LCJ0ZZ Extirpation of Matter from Right Hip Tendon, Open Approach

0LCJ3ZZ Extirpation of Matter from Right Hip Tendon, Percutaneous Approach

0LCJ4ZZ Extirpation of Matter from Right Hip Tendon, Percutaneous Endoscopic Approach

0LCK0ZZ Extirpation of Matter from Left Hip Tendon, Open Approach

0LCK3ZZ Extirpation of Matter from Left Hip Tendon, Percutaneous Approach

0LCK4ZZ Extirpation of Matter from Left Hip Tendon, Percutaneous Endoscopic Approach

0LCL0ZZ Extirpation of Matter from Right Upper Leg Tendon, Open Approach

0LCL3ZZ Extirpation of Matter from Right Upper Leg Tendon, Percutaneous Approach

0LCL4ZZ Extirpation of Matter from Right Upper Leg Tendon, Percutaneous Endoscopic Approach

0LCM0ZZ Extirpation of Matter from Left Upper Leg Tendon, Open Approach

0LCM3ZZ Extirpation of Matter from Left Upper Leg Tendon, Percutaneous Approach

0LCM4ZZ Extirpation of Matter from Left Upper Leg Tendon, Percutaneous Endoscopic Approach

0LCN0ZZ Extirpation of Matter from Right Lower Leg Tendon, Open Approach

0LCN3ZZ Extirpation of Matter from Right Lower Leg Tendon, Percutaneous Approach

0LCN4ZZ Extirpation of Matter from Right Lower Leg Tendon, Percutaneous Endoscopic Approach

0LCP0ZZ Extirpation of Matter from Left Lower Leg Tendon, Open Approach

0LCP3ZZ Extirpation of Matter from Left Lower Leg Tendon, Percutaneous Approach

0LCP4ZZ Extirpation of Matter from Left Lower Leg Tendon, Percutaneous Endoscopic Approach

0LCQ0ZZ Extirpation of Matter from Right Knee Tendon, Open Approach

0LCQ3ZZ Extirpation of Matter from Right Knee Tendon, Percutaneous Approach

0LCQ4ZZ Extirpation of Matter from Right Knee Tendon, Percutaneous Endoscopic Approach

0LCR0ZZ Extirpation of Matter from Left Knee Tendon, Open Approach

0LCR3ZZ Extirpation of Matter from Left Knee Tendon, Percutaneous Approach

0LCR4ZZ Extirpation of Matter from Left Knee Tendon, Percutaneous Endoscopic Approach

0LCS0ZZ Extirpation of Matter from Right Ankle Tendon, Open Approach

0LCS3ZZ Extirpation of Matter from Right Ankle Tendon, Percutaneous Approach

0LCS4ZZ Extirpation of Matter from Right Ankle Tendon, Percutaneous Endoscopic Approach

0LCT0ZZ Extirpation of Matter from Left Ankle Tendon, Open Approach

0LCT3ZZ Extirpation of Matter from Left Ankle Tendon, Percutaneous Approach

0LCT4ZZ Extirpation of Matter from Left Ankle Tendon, Percutaneous Endoscopic Approach

0LCV0ZZ Extirpation of Matter from Right Foot Tendon, Open Approach

0LCV3ZZ Extirpation of Matter from Right Foot Tendon, Percutaneous Approach

0LCV4ZZ Extirpation of Matter from Right Foot Tendon, Percutaneous Endoscopic Approach

0LCW0ZZ Extirpation of Matter from Left Foot Tendon, Open Approach

0LCW3ZZ Extirpation of Matter from Left Foot Tendon, Percutaneous Approach

0LCW4ZZ Extirpation of Matter from Left Foot Tendon, Percutaneous Endoscopic Approach

LJ – Tendons, Inspection

eview Coding Guidelines B3.5

eview Coding Guidelines B3.11a, B3.11b and B3.11c

LJX0ZZ Inspection of Upper Tendon, Open Approach

LJX3ZZ Inspection of Upper Tendon, Percutaneous Approach

LJX4ZZ Inspection of Upper Tendon, Percutaneous Endoscopic Approach

0LJXXZZ Inspection of Upper Tendon, External Approach

0LJY0ZZ Inspection of Lower Tendon, Open Approach

0LJY3ZZ Inspection of Lower Tendon, Percutaneous Approach

0LJY4ZZ Inspection of Lower Tendon, Percutaneous Endoscopic Approach

0LJYXZZ Inspection of Lower Tendon, External Approach

LM – Tendons, Reattachment

LM00ZZ Reattachment of Head and Neck Tendon, Open Approach

LM04ZZ Reattachment of Head and Neck Tendon, Percutaneous Endoscopic Approach

0LM10ZZ Reattachment of Right Shoulder Tendon, Open Approach

0LM14ZZ Reattachment of Right Shoulder Tendon, Percutaneous Endoscopic Approach

0LM20ZZ Reattachment of Left Shoulder Tendon, Open Approach

0LM24ZZ Reattachment of Left Shoulder Tendon, Percutaneous Endoscopic Approach

Female-only   ♂ Male-only   ▲ Limited Coverage   ● Non-OR   ■ HAC-associated procedure   ▲ Non-covered procedures   + Combination

0LM30ZZ Reattachment of Right Upper Arm Tendon, Open Approach

0LM34ZZ Reattachment of Right Upper Arm Tendon, Percutaneous Endoscopic Approach

0LM40ZZ Reattachment of Left Upper Arm Tendon, Open Approach

0LM44ZZ Reattachment of Left Upper Arm Tendon, Percutaneous Endoscopic Approach

0LM50ZZ Reattachment of Right Lower Arm and Wrist Tendon, Open Approach

0LM54ZZ Reattachment of Right Lower Arm and Wrist Tendon, Percutaneous Endoscopic Approach

0LM60ZZ Reattachment of Left Lower Arm and Wrist Tendon, Open Approach

0LM64ZZ Reattachment of Left Lower Arm and Wrist Tendon, Percutaneous Endoscopic Approach

0LM70ZZ Reattachment of Right Hand Tendon, Open Approach

0LM74ZZ Reattachment of Right Hand Tendon, Percutaneous Endoscopic Approach

0LM80ZZ Reattachment of Left Hand Tendon, Open Approach

0LM84ZZ Reattachment of Left Hand Tendon, Percutaneous Endoscopic Approach

0LM90ZZ Reattachment of Right Trunk Tendon, Open Approach

0LM94ZZ Reattachment of Right Trunk Tendon, Percutaneous Endoscopic Approach

0LMB0ZZ Reattachment of Left Trunk Tendon, Open Approach

0LMB4ZZ Reattachment of Left Trunk Tendon, Percutaneous Endoscopic Approach

0LMC0ZZ Reattachment of Right Thorax Tendon, Open Approach

0LMC4ZZ Reattachment of Right Thorax Tendon, Percutaneous Endoscopic Approach

0LMD0ZZ Reattachment of Left Thorax Tendon, Open Approach

0LMD4ZZ Reattachment of Left Thorax Tendon, Percutaneous Endoscopic Approach

0LMF0ZZ Reattachment of Right Abdomen Tendon, Open Approach

0LMF4ZZ Reattachment of Right Abdomen Tendon, Percutaneous Endoscopic Approach

0LMG0ZZ Reattachment of Left Abdomen Tendon, Open Approach

0LMG4ZZ Reattachment of Left Abdomen Tendon, Percutaneous Endoscopic Approach

0LMH0ZZ Reattachment of Perineum Tendon, Open Approach

0LMH4ZZ Reattachment of Perineum Tendon, Percutaneous Endoscopic Approach

0LMJ0ZZ Reattachment of Right Hip Tendon, Open Approach

0LMJ4ZZ Reattachment of Right Hip Tendon, Percutaneous Endoscopic Approach

0LMK0ZZ Reattachment of Left Hip Tendon, Open Approach

0LMK4ZZ Reattachment of Left Hip Tendon, Percutaneous Endoscopic Approach

0LML0ZZ Reattachment of Right Upper Leg Tendon, Open Approach

0LML4ZZ Reattachment of Right Upper Leg Tendon, Percutaneous Endoscopic Approach

0LMM0ZZ Reattachment of Left Upper Leg Tendon, Open Approach

0LMM4ZZ Reattachment of Left Upper Leg Tendon, Percutaneous Endoscopic Approach

0LMN0ZZ Reattachment of Right Lower Leg Tendon, Open Approach

0LMN4ZZ Reattachment of Right Lower Leg Tendon, Percutaneous Endoscopic Approach

0LMP0ZZ Reattachment of Left Lower Leg Tendon, Open Approach

0LMP4ZZ Reattachment of Left Lower Leg Tendon, Percutaneous Endoscopic Approach

0LMQ0ZZ Reattachment of Right Knee Tendon, Open Approach

0LMQ4ZZ Reattachment of Right Knee Tendon, Percutaneous Endoscopic Approach

0LMR0ZZ Reattachment of Left Knee Tendon, Open Approach

0LMR4ZZ Reattachment of Left Knee Tendon, Percutaneous Endoscopic Approach

0LMS0ZZ Reattachment of Right Ankle Tendon, Open Approach

0LMS4ZZ Reattachment of Right Ankle Tendon, Percutaneous Endoscopic Approach

0LMT0ZZ Reattachment of Left Ankle Tendon, Open Approach

0LMT4ZZ Reattachment of Left Ankle Tendon, Percutaneous Endoscopic Approach

0LMV0ZZ Reattachment of Right Foot Tendon, Open Approach

0LMV4ZZ Reattachment of Right Foot Tendon, Percutaneous Endoscopic Approach

0LMW0ZZ Reattachment of Left Foot Tendon, Open Approach

0LMW4ZZ Reattachment of Left Foot Tendon, Percutaneous Endoscopic Approach

0LN – Tendons, Release

Review Coding Guideline B3.13

Review Coding Guideline B3.14

0LN00ZZ Release Head and Neck Tendon, Open Approach

0LN03ZZ Release Head and Neck Tendon, Percutaneous Approach

0LN04ZZ Release Head and Neck Tendon, Percutaneous Endoscopic Approach

0LN0XZZ Release Head and Neck Tendon, External Approach

0LN10ZZ Release Right Shoulder Tendon, Open Approach

0LN13ZZ Release Right Shoulder Tendon, Percutaneous Approach

0LN14ZZ Release Right Shoulder Tendon, Percutaneous Endoscopic Approach

0LN1XZZ Release Right Shoulder Tendon, External Approach

0LN20ZZ Release Left Shoulder Tendon, Open Approach

0LN23ZZ Release Left Shoulder Tendon, Percutaneous Approach

0LN24ZZ Release Left Shoulder Tendon, Percutaneous Endoscopic Approach

0LN2XZZ Release Left Shoulder Tendon, External Approach

0LN30ZZ Release Right Upper Arm Tendon, Open Approach

0LN33ZZ Release Right Upper Arm Tendon, Percutaneous Approach

0LN34ZZ Release Right Upper Arm Tendon, Percutaneous Endoscopic Approach

0LN3XZZ Release Right Upper Arm Tendon, External Approach

0LN40ZZ Release Left Upper Arm Tendon, Open Approach

0LN43ZZ Release Left Upper Arm Tendon, Percutaneous Approach

0LN44ZZ Release Left Upper Arm Tendon, Percutaneous Endoscopic Approach

0LN4XZZ Release Left Upper Arm Tendon, External Approach

0LN50ZZ Release Right Lower Arm and Wrist Tendon, Open Approach

0LN53ZZ Release Right Lower Arm and Wrist Tendon, Percutaneous Approach

0LN54ZZ Release Right Lower Arm and Wrist Tendon, Percutaneous Endoscopic Approach

0LN5XZZ Release Right Lower Arm and Wrist Tendon, External Approach

0LN60ZZ Release Left Lower Arm and Wrist Tendon, Open Approach

0LN63ZZ Release Left Lower Arm and Wrist Tendon, Percutaneous Approach

0LN64ZZ Release Left Lower Arm and Wrist Tendon, Percutaneous Endoscopic Approach

0LN6XZZ Release Left Lower Arm and Wrist Tendon, External Approach

0LN70ZZ Release Right Hand Tendon, Open Approach

0LN73ZZ Release Right Hand Tendon, Percutaneous Approach

0LN74ZZ Release Right Hand Tendon, Percutaneous Endoscopic Approach

0LN7XZZ Release Right Hand Tendon, External Approach

0LN80ZZ Release Left Hand Tendon, Open Approach

0LN83ZZ Release Left Hand Tendon, Percutaneous Approach

0LN84ZZ Release Left Hand Tendon, Percutaneous Endoscopic Approach

0LN8XZZ Release Left Hand Tendon, External Approach

0LN90ZZ Release Right Trunk Tendon, Open Approach

0LN93ZZ Release Right Trunk Tendon, Percutaneous Approach

0LN94ZZ Release Right Trunk Tendon, Percutaneous Endoscopic Approach

0LN9XZZ Release Right Trunk Tendon, External Approach

0LNB0ZZ Release Left Trunk Tendon, Open Approach

0LNB3ZZ Release Left Trunk Tendon, Percutaneous Approach

0LNB4ZZ Release Left Trunk Tendon, Percutaneous Endoscopic Approach

0LNBXZZ Release Left Trunk Tendon, External Approach

♀ Female-only   ♂ Male-only   ▲ Limited Coverage   ● Non-OR   ▨ HAC-associated procedure   ▲ Non-covered procedures   ✚ Combination

NC0ZZ	Release Right Thorax Tendon, Open Approach	0LNJ4ZZ	Release Right Hip Tendon, Percutaneous Endoscopic Approach	0LNQ3ZZ	Release Right Knee Tendon, Percutaneous Approach

NC0ZZ Release Right Thorax Tendon, Open Approach

NC3ZZ Release Right Thorax Tendon, Percutaneous Approach

NC4ZZ Release Right Thorax Tendon, Percutaneous Endoscopic Approach

NCXZZ Release Right Thorax Tendon, External Approach

ND0ZZ Release Left Thorax Tendon, Open Approach

ND3ZZ Release Left Thorax Tendon, Percutaneous Approach

ND4ZZ Release Left Thorax Tendon, Percutaneous Endoscopic Approach

NDXZZ Release Left Thorax Tendon, External Approach

NF0ZZ Release Right Abdomen Tendon, Open Approach

NF3ZZ Release Right Abdomen Tendon, Percutaneous Approach

NF4ZZ Release Right Abdomen Tendon, Percutaneous Endoscopic Approach

NFXZZ Release Right Abdomen Tendon, External Approach

NG0ZZ Release Left Abdomen Tendon, Open Approach

NG3ZZ Release Left Abdomen Tendon, Percutaneous Approach

NG4ZZ Release Left Abdomen Tendon, Percutaneous Endoscopic Approach

NGXZZ Release Left Abdomen Tendon, External Approach

NH0ZZ Release Perineum Tendon, Open Approach

NH3ZZ Release Perineum Tendon, Percutaneous Approach

NH4ZZ Release Perineum Tendon, Percutaneous Endoscopic Approach

NHXZZ Release Perineum Tendon, External Approach

NJ0ZZ Release Right Hip Tendon, Open Approach

NJ3ZZ Release Right Hip Tendon, Percutaneous Approach

0LNJ4ZZ Release Right Hip Tendon, Percutaneous Endoscopic Approach

0LNJXZZ Release Right Hip Tendon, External Approach

0LNK0ZZ Release Left Hip Tendon, Open Approach

0LNK3ZZ Release Left Hip Tendon, Percutaneous Approach

0LNK4ZZ Release Left Hip Tendon, Percutaneous Endoscopic Approach

0LNKXZZ Release Left Hip Tendon, External Approach

0LNL0ZZ Release Right Upper Leg Tendon, Open Approach

0LNL3ZZ Release Right Upper Leg Tendon, Percutaneous Approach

0LNL4ZZ Release Right Upper Leg Tendon, Percutaneous Endoscopic Approach

0LNLXZZ Release Right Upper Leg Tendon, External Approach

0LNM0ZZ Release Left Upper Leg Tendon, Open Approach

0LNM3ZZ Release Left Upper Leg Tendon, Percutaneous Approach

0LNM4ZZ Release Left Upper Leg Tendon, Percutaneous Endoscopic Approach

0LNMXZZ Release Left Upper Leg Tendon, External Approach

0LNN0ZZ Release Right Lower Leg Tendon, Open Approach

0LNN3ZZ Release Right Lower Leg Tendon, Percutaneous Approach

0LNN4ZZ Release Right Lower Leg Tendon, Percutaneous Endoscopic Approach

0LNNXZZ Release Right Lower Leg Tendon, External Approach

0LNP0ZZ Release Left Lower Leg Tendon, Open Approach

0LNP3ZZ Release Left Lower Leg Tendon, Percutaneous Approach

0LNP4ZZ Release Left Lower Leg Tendon, Percutaneous Endoscopic Approach

0LNPXZZ Release Left Lower Leg Tendon, External Approach

0LNQ0ZZ Release Right Knee Tendon, Open Approach

0LNQ3ZZ Release Right Knee Tendon, Percutaneous Approach

0LNQ4ZZ Release Right Knee Tendon, Percutaneous Endoscopic Approach

0LNQXZZ Release Right Knee Tendon, External Approach

0LNR0ZZ Release Left Knee Tendon, Open Approach

0LNR3ZZ Release Left Knee Tendon, Percutaneous Approach

0LNR4ZZ Release Left Knee Tendon, Percutaneous Endoscopic Approach

0LNRXZZ Release Left Knee Tendon, External Approach

0LNS0ZZ Release Right Ankle Tendon, Open Approach

0LNS3ZZ Release Right Ankle Tendon, Percutaneous Approach

0LNS4ZZ Release Right Ankle Tendon, Percutaneous Endoscopic Approach

0LNSXZZ Release Right Ankle Tendon, External Approach

0LNT0ZZ Release Left Ankle Tendon, Open Approach

0LNT3ZZ Release Left Ankle Tendon, Percutaneous Approach

0LNT4ZZ Release Left Ankle Tendon, Percutaneous Endoscopic Approach

0LNTXZZ Release Left Ankle Tendon, External Approach

0LNV0ZZ Release Right Foot Tendon, Open Approach

0LNV3ZZ Release Right Foot Tendon, Percutaneous Approach

0LNV4ZZ Release Right Foot Tendon, Percutaneous Endoscopic Approach

0LNVXZZ Release Right Foot Tendon, External Approach

0LNW0ZZ Release Left Foot Tendon, Open Approach

0LNW3ZZ Release Left Foot Tendon, Percutaneous Approach

0LNW4ZZ Release Left Foot Tendon, Percutaneous Endoscopic Approach

0LNWXZZ Release Left Foot Tendon, External Approach

LP – Tendons, Removal

eview Coding Guideline B6.1c

LPX00Z Removal of Drainage Device from Upper Tendon, Open Approach

LPX07Z Removal of Autologous Tissue Substitute from Upper Tendon, Open Approach

LPX0JZ Removal of Synthetic Substitute from Upper Tendon, Open Approach

LPX0KZ Removal of Nonautologous Tissue Substitute from Upper Tendon, Open Approach

LPX30Z Removal of Drainage Device from Upper Tendon, Percutaneous Approach

LPX37Z Removal of Autologous Tissue Substitute from Upper Tendon, Percutaneous Approach

LPX3JZ Removal of Synthetic Substitute from Upper Tendon, Percutaneous Approach

LPX3KZ Removal of Nonautologous Tissue Substitute from Upper Tendon, Percutaneous Approach

LPX40Z Removal of Drainage Device from Upper Tendon, Percutaneous Endoscopic Approach

0LPX47Z Removal of Autologous Tissue Substitute from Upper Tendon, Percutaneous Endoscopic Approach

0LPX4JZ Removal of Synthetic Substitute from Upper Tendon, Percutaneous Endoscopic Approach

0LPX4KZ Removal of Nonautologous Tissue Substitute from Upper Tendon, Percutaneous Endoscopic Approach

0LPXX0Z Removal of Drainage Device from Upper Tendon, External Approach

0LPY00Z Removal of Drainage Device from Lower Tendon, Open Approach

0LPY07Z Removal of Autologous Tissue Substitute from Lower Tendon, Open Approach

0LPY0JZ Removal of Synthetic Substitute from Lower Tendon, Open Approach

0LPY0KZ Removal of Nonautologous Tissue Substitute from Lower Tendon, Open Approach

0LPY30Z Removal of Drainage Device from Lower Tendon, Percutaneous Approach

0LPY37Z Removal of Autologous Tissue Substitute from Lower Tendon, Percutaneous Approach

0LPY3JZ Removal of Synthetic Substitute from Lower Tendon, Percutaneous Approach

0LPY3KZ Removal of Nonautologous Tissue Substitute from Lower Tendon, Percutaneous Approach

0LPY40Z Removal of Drainage Device from Lower Tendon, Percutaneous Endoscopic Approach

0LPY47Z Removal of Autologous Tissue Substitute from Lower Tendon, Percutaneous Endoscopic Approach

0LPY4JZ Removal of Synthetic Substitute from Lower Tendon, Percutaneous Endoscopic Approach

0LPY4KZ Removal of Nonautologous Tissue Substitute from Lower Tendon, Percutaneous Endoscopic Approach

0LPYX0Z Removal of Drainage Device from Lower Tendon, External Approach

Female-only   ♂ Male-only   ▲ Limited Coverage   ● Non-OR   ▦ HAC-associated procedure   ▲ Non-covered procedures   ✚ Combination

0LQ – Tendons, Repair

Review Coding Guideline B3.5

0LQ00ZZ	Repair Head and Neck Tendon, Open Approach
0LQ03ZZ	Repair Head and Neck Tendon, Percutaneous Approach
0LQ04ZZ	Repair Head and Neck Tendon, Percutaneous Endoscopic Approach
0LQ10ZZ	Repair Right Shoulder Tendon, Open Approach
0LQ13ZZ	Repair Right Shoulder Tendon, Percutaneous Approach
0LQ14ZZ	Repair Right Shoulder Tendon, Percutaneous Endoscopic Approach
	AHA CC: 3Q, 2013, 20-22
0LQ20ZZ	Repair Left Shoulder Tendon, Open Approach
0LQ23ZZ	Repair Left Shoulder Tendon, Percutaneous Approach
0LQ24ZZ	Repair Left Shoulder Tendon, Percutaneous Endoscopic Approach
0LQ30ZZ	Repair Right Upper Arm Tendon, Open Approach
0LQ33ZZ	Repair Right Upper Arm Tendon, Percutaneous Approach
0LQ34ZZ	Repair Right Upper Arm Tendon, Percutaneous Endoscopic Approach
0LQ40ZZ	Repair Left Upper Arm Tendon, Open Approach
0LQ43ZZ	Repair Left Upper Arm Tendon, Percutaneous Approach
0LQ44ZZ	Repair Left Upper Arm Tendon, Percutaneous Endoscopic Approach
0LQ50ZZ	Repair Right Lower Arm and Wrist Tendon, Open Approach
0LQ53ZZ	Repair Right Lower Arm and Wrist Tendon, Percutaneous Approach
0LQ54ZZ	Repair Right Lower Arm and Wrist Tendon, Percutaneous Endoscopic Approach
0LQ60ZZ	Repair Left Lower Arm and Wrist Tendon, Open Approach
0LQ63ZZ	Repair Left Lower Arm and Wrist Tendon, Percutaneous Approach
0LQ64ZZ	Repair Left Lower Arm and Wrist Tendon, Percutaneous Endoscopic Approach
0LQ70ZZ	Repair Right Hand Tendon, Open Approach
0LQ73ZZ	Repair Right Hand Tendon, Percutaneous Approach
0LQ74ZZ	Repair Right Hand Tendon, Percutaneous Endoscopic Approach
0LQ80ZZ	Repair Left Hand Tendon, Open Approach
0LQ83ZZ	Repair Left Hand Tendon, Percutaneous Approach
0LQ84ZZ	Repair Left Hand Tendon, Percutaneous Endoscopic Approach
0LQ90ZZ	Repair Right Trunk Tendon, Open Approach
0LQ93ZZ	Repair Right Trunk Tendon, Percutaneous Approach
0LQ94ZZ	Repair Right Trunk Tendon, Percutaneous Endoscopic Approach
0LQB0ZZ	Repair Left Trunk Tendon, Open Approach
0LQB3ZZ	Repair Left Trunk Tendon, Percutaneous Approach
0LQB4ZZ	Repair Left Trunk Tendon, Percutaneous Endoscopic Approach
0LQC0ZZ	Repair Right Thorax Tendon, Open Approach
0LQC3ZZ	Repair Right Thorax Tendon, Percutaneous Approach
0LQC4ZZ	Repair Right Thorax Tendon, Percutaneous Endoscopic Approach
0LQD0ZZ	Repair Left Thorax Tendon, Open Approach
0LQD3ZZ	Repair Left Thorax Tendon, Percutaneous Approach
0LQD4ZZ	Repair Left Thorax Tendon, Percutaneous Endoscopic Approach
0LQF0ZZ	Repair Right Abdomen Tendon, Open Approach
0LQF3ZZ	Repair Right Abdomen Tendon, Percutaneous Approach
0LQF4ZZ	Repair Right Abdomen Tendon, Percutaneous Endoscopic Approach
0LQG0ZZ	Repair Left Abdomen Tendon, Open Approach
0LQG3ZZ	Repair Left Abdomen Tendon, Percutaneous Approach
0LQG4ZZ	Repair Left Abdomen Tendon, Percutaneous Endoscopic Approach
0LQH0ZZ	Repair Perineum Tendon, Open Approach
0LQH3ZZ	Repair Perineum Tendon, Percutaneous Approach
0LQH4ZZ	Repair Perineum Tendon, Percutaneous Endoscopic Approach
0LQJ0ZZ	Repair Right Hip Tendon, Open Approach
0LQJ3ZZ	Repair Right Hip Tendon, Percutaneous Approach
0LQJ4ZZ	Repair Right Hip Tendon, Percutaneous Endoscopic Approach
0LQK0ZZ	Repair Left Hip Tendon, Open Approach
0LQK3ZZ	Repair Left Hip Tendon, Percutaneous Approach
0LQK4ZZ	Repair Left Hip Tendon, Percutaneous Endoscopic Approach
0LQL0ZZ	Repair Right Upper Leg Tendon, Open Approach
0LQL3ZZ	Repair Right Upper Leg Tendon, Percutaneous Approach
0LQL4ZZ	Repair Right Upper Leg Tendon, Percutaneous Endoscopic Approach
0LQM0ZZ	Repair Left Upper Leg Tendon, Open Approach
0LQM3ZZ	Repair Left Upper Leg Tendon, Percutaneous Approach
0LQM4ZZ	Repair Left Upper Leg Tendon, Percutaneous Endoscopic Approach
0LQN0ZZ	Repair Right Lower Leg Tendon, Open Approach
0LQN3ZZ	Repair Right Lower Leg Tendon, Percutaneous Approach
0LQN4ZZ	Repair Right Lower Leg Tendon, Percutaneous Endoscopic Approach
0LQP0ZZ	Repair Left Lower Leg Tendon, Open Approach
0LQP3ZZ	Repair Left Lower Leg Tendon, Percutaneous Approach
0LQP4ZZ	Repair Left Lower Leg Tendon, Percutaneous Endoscopic Approach
0LQQ0ZZ	Repair Right Knee Tendon, Open Approach
0LQQ3ZZ	Repair Right Knee Tendon, Percutaneous Approach
0LQQ4ZZ	Repair Right Knee Tendon, Percutaneous Endoscopic Approach
0LQR0ZZ	Repair Left Knee Tendon, Open Approach
0LQR3ZZ	Repair Left Knee Tendon, Percutaneous Approach
0LQR4ZZ	Repair Left Knee Tendon, Percutaneous Endoscopic Approach
0LQS0ZZ	Repair Right Ankle Tendon, Open Approach
0LQS3ZZ	Repair Right Ankle Tendon, Percutaneous Approach
0LQS4ZZ	Repair Right Ankle Tendon, Percutaneous Endoscopic Approach
0LQT0ZZ	Repair Left Ankle Tendon, Open Approach
0LQT3ZZ	Repair Left Ankle Tendon, Percutaneous Approach
0LQT4ZZ	Repair Left Ankle Tendon, Percutaneous Endoscopic Approach
0LQV0ZZ	Repair Right Foot Tendon, Open Approach
0LQV3ZZ	Repair Right Foot Tendon, Percutaneous Approach
0LQV4ZZ	Repair Right Foot Tendon, Percutaneous Endoscopic Approach
0LQW0ZZ	Repair Left Foot Tendon, Open Approach
0LQW3ZZ	Repair Left Foot Tendon, Percutaneous Approach
0LQW4ZZ	Repair Left Foot Tendon, Percutaneous Endoscopic Approach

0LR – Tendons, Replacement

0LR007Z	Replacement of Head and Neck Tendon with Autologous Tissue Substitute, Open Approach
0LR00JZ	Replacement of Head and Neck Tendon with Synthetic Substitute, Open Approach
0LR00KZ	Replacement of Head and Neck Tendon with Nonautologous Tissue Substitute, Open Approach
0LR047Z	Replacement of Head and Neck Tendon with Autologous Tissue Substitute, Percutaneous Endoscopic Approach
0LR04JZ	Replacement of Head and Neck Tendon with Synthetic Substitute, Percutaneous Endoscopic Approach
0LR04KZ	Replacement of Head and Neck Tendon with Nonautologous Tissue Substitute, Percutaneous Endoscopic Approach
0LR107Z	Replacement of Right Shoulder Tendon with Autologous Tissue Substitute, Open Approach
0LR10JZ	Replacement of Right Shoulder Tendon with Synthetic Substitute, Open Approach
0LR10KZ	Replacement of Right Shoulder Tendon with Nonautologous Tissue Substitute, Open Approach
0LR147Z	Replacement of Right Shoulder Tendon with Autologous Tissue Substitute, Percutaneous Endoscopic Approach
0LR14JZ	Replacement of Right Shoulder Tendon with Synthetic Substitute, Percutaneous Endoscopic Approach
0LR14KZ	Replacement of Right Shoulder Tendon with Nonautologous Tissue Substitute, Percutaneous Endoscopic Approach

R207Z	Replacement of Left Shoulder Tendon with Autologous Tissue Substitute, Open Approach
R20JZ	Replacement of Left Shoulder Tendon with Synthetic Substitute, Open Approach
R20KZ	Replacement of Left Shoulder Tendon with Nonautologous Tissue Substitute, Open Approach
R247Z	Replacement of Left Shoulder Tendon with Autologous Tissue Substitute, Percutaneous Endoscopic Approach
R24JZ	Replacement of Left Shoulder Tendon with Synthetic Substitute, Percutaneous Endoscopic Approach
R24KZ	Replacement of Left Shoulder Tendon with Nonautologous Tissue Substitute, Percutaneous Endoscopic Approach
R307Z	Replacement of Right Upper Arm Tendon with Autologous Tissue Substitute, Open Approach
R30JZ	Replacement of Right Upper Arm Tendon with Synthetic Substitute, Open Approach
R30KZ	Replacement of Right Upper Arm Tendon with Nonautologous Tissue Substitute, Open Approach
R347Z	Replacement of Right Upper Arm Tendon with Autologous Tissue Substitute, Percutaneous Endoscopic Approach
R34JZ	Replacement of Right Upper Arm Tendon with Synthetic Substitute, Percutaneous Endoscopic Approach
R34KZ	Replacement of Right Upper Arm Tendon with Nonautologous Tissue Substitute, Percutaneous Endoscopic Approach
R407Z	Replacement of Left Upper Arm Tendon with Autologous Tissue Substitute, Open Approach
R40JZ	Replacement of Left Upper Arm Tendon with Synthetic Substitute, Open Approach
R40KZ	Replacement of Left Upper Arm Tendon with Nonautologous Tissue Substitute, Open Approach
R447Z	Replacement of Left Upper Arm Tendon with Autologous Tissue Substitute, Percutaneous Endoscopic Approach
R44JZ	Replacement of Left Upper Arm Tendon with Synthetic Substitute, Percutaneous Endoscopic Approach
LR44KZ	Replacement of Left Upper Arm Tendon with Nonautologous Tissue Substitute, Percutaneous Endoscopic Approach
LR507Z	Replacement of Right Lower Arm and Wrist Tendon with Autologous Tissue Substitute, Open Approach
LR50JZ	Replacement of Right Lower Arm and Wrist Tendon with Synthetic Substitute, Open Approach
LR50KZ	Replacement of Right Lower Arm and Wrist Tendon with Nonautologous Tissue Substitute, Open Approach
LR547Z	Replacement of Right Lower Arm and Wrist Tendon with Autologous Tissue Substitute, Percutaneous Endoscopic Approach
LR54JZ	Replacement of Right Lower Arm and Wrist Tendon with Synthetic Substitute, Percutaneous Endoscopic Approach
LR54KZ	Replacement of Right Lower Arm and Wrist Tendon with Nonautologous Tissue Substitute, Percutaneous Endoscopic Approach
0LR607Z	Replacement of Left Lower Arm and Wrist Tendon with Autologous Tissue Substitute, Open Approach
0LR60JZ	Replacement of Left Lower Arm and Wrist Tendon with Synthetic Substitute, Open Approach

0LR60KZ	Replacement of Left Lower Arm and Wrist Tendon with Nonautologous Tissue Substitute, Open Approach
0LR647Z	Replacement of Left Lower Arm and Wrist Tendon with Autologous Tissue Substitute, Percutaneous Endoscopic Approach
0LR64JZ	Replacement of Left Lower Arm and Wrist Tendon with Synthetic Substitute, Percutaneous Endoscopic Approach
0LR64KZ	Replacement of Left Lower Arm and Wrist Tendon with Nonautologous Tissue Substitute, Percutaneous Endoscopic Approach
0LR707Z	Replacement of Right Hand Tendon with Autologous Tissue Substitute, Open Approach
0LR70JZ	Replacement of Right Hand Tendon with Synthetic Substitute, Open Approach
0LR70KZ	Replacement of Right Hand Tendon with Nonautologous Tissue Substitute, Open Approach
0LR747Z	Replacement of Right Hand Tendon with Autologous Tissue Substitute, Percutaneous Endoscopic Approach
0LR74JZ	Replacement of Right Hand Tendon with Synthetic Substitute, Percutaneous Endoscopic Approach
0LR74KZ	Replacement of Right Hand Tendon with Nonautologous Tissue Substitute, Percutaneous Endoscopic Approach
0LR807Z	Replacement of Left Hand Tendon with Autologous Tissue Substitute, Open Approach
0LR80JZ	Replacement of Left Hand Tendon with Synthetic Substitute, Open Approach
0LR80KZ	Replacement of Left Hand Tendon with Nonautologous Tissue Substitute, Open Approach
0LR847Z	Replacement of Left Hand Tendon with Autologous Tissue Substitute, Percutaneous Endoscopic Approach
0LR84JZ	Replacement of Left Hand Tendon with Synthetic Substitute, Percutaneous Endoscopic Approach
0LR84KZ	Replacement of Left Hand Tendon with Nonautologous Tissue Substitute, Percutaneous Endoscopic Approach
0LR907Z	Replacement of Right Trunk Tendon with Autologous Tissue Substitute, Open Approach
0LR90JZ	Replacement of Right Trunk Tendon with Synthetic Substitute, Open Approach
0LR90KZ	Replacement of Right Trunk Tendon with Nonautologous Tissue Substitute, Open Approach
0LR947Z	Replacement of Right Trunk Tendon with Autologous Tissue Substitute, Percutaneous Endoscopic Approach
0LR94JZ	Replacement of Right Trunk Tendon with Synthetic Substitute, Percutaneous Endoscopic Approach
0LR94KZ	Replacement of Right Trunk Tendon with Nonautologous Tissue Substitute, Percutaneous Endoscopic Approach
0LRB07Z	Replacement of Left Trunk Tendon with Autologous Tissue Substitute, Open Approach
0LRB0JZ	Replacement of Left Trunk Tendon with Synthetic Substitute, Open Approach
0LRB0KZ	Replacement of Left Trunk Tendon with Nonautologous Tissue Substitute, Open Approach
0LRB47Z	Replacement of Left Trunk Tendon with Autologous Tissue Substitute, Percutaneous Endoscopic Approach

0LRB4JZ	Replacement of Left Trunk Tendon with Synthetic Substitute, Percutaneous Endoscopic Approach
0LRB4KZ	Replacement of Left Trunk Tendon with Nonautologous Tissue Substitute, Percutaneous Endoscopic Approach
0LRC07Z	Replacement of Right Thorax Tendon with Autologous Tissue Substitute, Open Approach
0LRC0JZ	Replacement of Right Thorax Tendon with Synthetic Substitute, Open Approach
0LRC0KZ	Replacement of Right Thorax Tendon with Nonautologous Tissue Substitute, Open Approach
0LRC47Z	Replacement of Right Thorax Tendon with Autologous Tissue Substitute, Percutaneous Endoscopic Approach
0LRC4JZ	Replacement of Right Thorax Tendon with Synthetic Substitute, Percutaneous Endoscopic Approach
0LRC4KZ	Replacement of Right Thorax Tendon with Nonautologous Tissue Substitute, Percutaneous Endoscopic Approach
0LRD07Z	Replacement of Left Thorax Tendon with Autologous Tissue Substitute, Open Approach
0LRD0JZ	Replacement of Left Thorax Tendon with Synthetic Substitute, Open Approach
0LRD0KZ	Replacement of Left Thorax Tendon with Nonautologous Tissue Substitute, Open Approach
0LRD47Z	Replacement of Left Thorax Tendon with Autologous Tissue Substitute, Percutaneous Endoscopic Approach
0LRD4JZ	Replacement of Left Thorax Tendon with Synthetic Substitute, Percutaneous Endoscopic Approach
0LRD4KZ	Replacement of Left Thorax Tendon with Nonautologous Tissue Substitute, Percutaneous Endoscopic Approach
0LRF07Z	Replacement of Right Abdomen Tendon with Autologous Tissue Substitute, Open Approach
0LRF0JZ	Replacement of Right Abdomen Tendon with Synthetic Substitute, Open Approach
0LRF0KZ	Replacement of Right Abdomen Tendon with Nonautologous Tissue Substitute, Open Approach
0LRF47Z	Replacement of Right Abdomen Tendon with Autologous Tissue Substitute, Percutaneous Endoscopic Approach
0LRF4JZ	Replacement of Right Abdomen Tendon with Synthetic Substitute, Percutaneous Endoscopic Approach
0LRF4KZ	Replacement of Right Abdomen Tendon with Nonautologous Tissue Substitute, Percutaneous Endoscopic Approach
0LRG07Z	Replacement of Left Abdomen Tendon with Autologous Tissue Substitute, Open Approach
0LRG0JZ	Replacement of Left Abdomen Tendon with Synthetic Substitute, Open Approach
0LRG0KZ	Replacement of Left Abdomen Tendon with Nonautologous Tissue Substitute, Open Approach
0LRG47Z	Replacement of Left Abdomen Tendon with Autologous Tissue Substitute, Percutaneous Endoscopic Approach
0LRG4JZ	Replacement of Left Abdomen Tendon with Synthetic Substitute, Percutaneous Endoscopic Approach
0LRG4KZ	Replacement of Left Abdomen Tendon with Nonautologous Tissue Substitute, Percutaneous Endoscopic Approach

733

0LRH07Z Replacement of Perineum Tendon with Autologous Tissue Substitute, Open Approach

0LRH0JZ Replacement of Perineum Tendon with Synthetic Substitute, Open Approach

0LRH0KZ Replacement of Perineum Tendon with Nonautologous Tissue Substitute, Open Approach

0LRH47Z Replacement of Perineum Tendon with Autologous Tissue Substitute, Percutaneous Endoscopic Approach

0LRH4JZ Replacement of Perineum Tendon with Synthetic Substitute, Percutaneous Endoscopic Approach

0LRH4KZ Replacement of Perineum Tendon with Nonautologous Tissue Substitute, Percutaneous Endoscopic Approach

0LRJ07Z Replacement of Right Hip Tendon with Autologous Tissue Substitute, Open Approach

0LRJ0JZ Replacement of Right Hip Tendon with Synthetic Substitute, Open Approach

0LRJ0KZ Replacement of Right Hip Tendon with Nonautologous Tissue Substitute, Open Approach

0LRJ47Z Replacement of Right Hip Tendon with Autologous Tissue Substitute, Percutaneous Endoscopic Approach

0LRJ4JZ Replacement of Right Hip Tendon with Synthetic Substitute, Percutaneous Endoscopic Approach

0LRJ4KZ Replacement of Right Hip Tendon with Nonautologous Tissue Substitute, Percutaneous Endoscopic Approach

0LRK07Z Replacement of Left Hip Tendon with Autologous Tissue Substitute, Open Approach

0LRK0JZ Replacement of Left Hip Tendon with Synthetic Substitute, Open Approach

0LRK0KZ Replacement of Left Hip Tendon with Nonautologous Tissue Substitute, Open Approach

0LRK47Z Replacement of Left Hip Tendon with Autologous Tissue Substitute, Percutaneous Endoscopic Approach

0LRK4JZ Replacement of Left Hip Tendon with Synthetic Substitute, Percutaneous Endoscopic Approach

0LRK4KZ Replacement of Left Hip Tendon with Nonautologous Tissue Substitute, Percutaneous Endoscopic Approach

0LRL07Z Replacement of Right Upper Leg Tendon with Autologous Tissue Substitute, Open Approach

0LRL0JZ Replacement of Right Upper Leg Tendon with Synthetic Substitute, Open Approach

0LRL0KZ Replacement of Right Upper Leg Tendon with Nonautologous Tissue Substitute, Open Approach

0LRL47Z Replacement of Right Upper Leg Tendon with Autologous Tissue Substitute, Percutaneous Endoscopic Approach

0LRL4JZ Replacement of Right Upper Leg Tendon with Synthetic Substitute, Percutaneous Endoscopic Approach

0LRL4KZ Replacement of Right Upper Leg Tendon with Nonautologous Tissue Substitute, Percutaneous Endoscopic Approach

0LRM07Z Replacement of Left Upper Leg Tendon with Autologous Tissue Substitute, Open Approach

0LRM0JZ Replacement of Left Upper Leg Tendon with Synthetic Substitute, Open Approach

0LRM0KZ Replacement of Left Upper Leg Tendon with Nonautologous Tissue Substitute, Open Approach

0LRM47Z Replacement of Left Upper Leg Tendon with Autologous Tissue Substitute, Percutaneous Endoscopic Approach

0LRM4JZ Replacement of Left Upper Leg Tendon with Synthetic Substitute, Percutaneous Endoscopic Approach

0LRM4KZ Replacement of Left Upper Leg Tendon with Nonautologous Tissue Substitute, Percutaneous Endoscopic Approach

0LRN07Z Replacement of Right Lower Leg Tendon with Autologous Tissue Substitute, Open Approach

0LRN0JZ Replacement of Right Lower Leg Tendon with Synthetic Substitute, Open Approach

0LRN0KZ Replacement of Right Lower Leg Tendon with Nonautologous Tissue Substitute, Open Approach

0LRN47Z Replacement of Right Lower Leg Tendon with Autologous Tissue Substitute, Percutaneous Endoscopic Approach

0LRN4JZ Replacement of Right Lower Leg Tendon with Synthetic Substitute, Percutaneous Endoscopic Approach

0LRN4KZ Replacement of Right Lower Leg Tendon with Nonautologous Tissue Substitute, Percutaneous Endoscopic Approach

0LRP07Z Replacement of Left Lower Leg Tendon with Autologous Tissue Substitute, Open Approach

0LRP0JZ Replacement of Left Lower Leg Tendon with Synthetic Substitute, Open Approach

0LRP0KZ Replacement of Left Lower Leg Tendon with Nonautologous Tissue Substitute, Open Approach

0LRP47Z Replacement of Left Lower Leg Tendon with Autologous Tissue Substitute, Percutaneous Endoscopic Approach

0LRP4JZ Replacement of Left Lower Leg Tendon with Synthetic Substitute, Percutaneous Endoscopic Approach

0LRP4KZ Replacement of Left Lower Leg Tendon with Nonautologous Tissue Substitute, Percutaneous Endoscopic Approach

0LRQ07Z Replacement of Right Knee Tendon with Autologous Tissue Substitute, Open Approach

0LRQ0JZ Replacement of Right Knee Tendon with Synthetic Substitute, Open Approach

0LRQ0KZ Replacement of Right Knee Tendon with Nonautologous Tissue Substitute, Open Approach

0LRQ47Z Replacement of Right Knee Tendon with Autologous Tissue Substitute, Percutaneous Endoscopic Approach

0LRQ4JZ Replacement of Right Knee Tendon with Synthetic Substitute, Percutaneous Endoscopic Approach

0LRQ4KZ Replacement of Right Knee Tendon with Nonautologous Tissue Substitute, Percutaneous Endoscopic Approach

0LRR07Z Replacement of Left Knee Tendon with Autologous Tissue Substitute, Open Approach

0LRR0JZ Replacement of Left Knee Tendon with Synthetic Substitute, Open Approach

0LRR0KZ Replacement of Left Knee Tendon with Nonautologous Tissue Substitute, Open Approach

0LRR47Z Replacement of Left Knee Tendon with Autologous Tissue Substitute, Percutaneous Endoscopic Approach

0LRR4JZ Replacement of Left Knee Tendon with Synthetic Substitute, Percutaneous Endoscopic Approach

0LRR4KZ Replacement of Left Knee Tendon with Nonautologous Tissue Substitute, Percutaneous Endoscopic Approach

0LRS07Z Replacement of Right Ankle Tendon with Autologous Tissue Substitute, Open Approach

0LRS0JZ Replacement of Right Ankle Tendon with Synthetic Substitute, Open Approach

0LRS0KZ Replacement of Right Ankle Tendon with Nonautologous Tissue Substitute, Open Approach

0LRS47Z Replacement of Right Ankle Tendon with Autologous Tissue Substitute, Percutaneous Endoscopic Approach

0LRS4JZ Replacement of Right Ankle Tendon with Synthetic Substitute, Percutaneous Endoscopic Approach

0LRS4KZ Replacement of Right Ankle Tendon with Nonautologous Tissue Substitute, Percutaneous Endoscopic Approach

0LRT07Z Replacement of Left Ankle Tendon with Autologous Tissue Substitute, Open Approach

0LRT0JZ Replacement of Left Ankle Tendon with Synthetic Substitute, Open Approach

0LRT0KZ Replacement of Left Ankle Tendon with Nonautologous Tissue Substitute, Open Approach

0LRT47Z Replacement of Left Ankle Tendon with Autologous Tissue Substitute, Percutaneous Endoscopic Approach

0LRT4JZ Replacement of Left Ankle Tendon with Synthetic Substitute, Percutaneous Endoscopic Approach

0LRT4KZ Replacement of Left Ankle Tendon with Nonautologous Tissue Substitute, Percutaneous Endoscopic Approach

0LRV07Z Replacement of Right Foot Tendon with Autologous Tissue Substitute, Open Approach

0LRV0JZ Replacement of Right Foot Tendon with Synthetic Substitute, Open Approach

0LRV0KZ Replacement of Right Foot Tendon with Nonautologous Tissue Substitute, Open Approach

0LRV47Z Replacement of Right Foot Tendon with Autologous Tissue Substitute, Percutaneous Endoscopic Approach

0LRV4JZ Replacement of Right Foot Tendon with Synthetic Substitute, Percutaneous Endoscopic Approach

0LRV4KZ Replacement of Right Foot Tendon with Nonautologous Tissue Substitute, Percutaneous Endoscopic Approach

0LRW07Z Replacement of Left Foot Tendon with Autologous Tissue Substitute, Open Approach

0LRW0JZ Replacement of Left Foot Tendon with Synthetic Substitute, Open Approach

0LRW0KZ Replacement of Left Foot Tendon with Nonautologous Tissue Substitute, Open Approach

0LRW47Z Replacement of Left Foot Tendon with Autologous Tissue Substitute, Percutaneous Endoscopic Approach

0LRW4JZ Replacement of Left Foot Tendon with Synthetic Substitute, Percutaneous Endoscopic Approach

0LRW4KZ Replacement of Left Foot Tendon with Nonautologous Tissue Substitute, Percutaneous Endoscopic Approach

.S – Tendons, Reposition

S00ZZ	Reposition Head and Neck Tendon, Open Approach	**0LS90ZZ**	Reposition Right Trunk Tendon, Open Approach	**0LSL4ZZ**	Reposition Right Upper Leg Tendon, Percutaneous Endoscopic Approach
S04ZZ	Reposition Head and Neck Tendon, Percutaneous Endoscopic Approach	**0LS94ZZ**	Reposition Right Trunk Tendon, Percutaneous Endoscopic Approach	**0LSM0ZZ**	Reposition Left Upper Leg Tendon, Open Approach
S10ZZ	Reposition Right Shoulder Tendon, Open Approach	**0LSB0ZZ**	Reposition Left Trunk Tendon, Open Approach	**0LSM4ZZ**	Reposition Left Upper Leg Tendon, Percutaneous Endoscopic Approach
S14ZZ	Reposition Right Shoulder Tendon, Percutaneous Endoscopic Approach	**0LSB4ZZ**	Reposition Left Trunk Tendon, Percutaneous Endoscopic Approach	**0LSN0ZZ**	Reposition Right Lower Leg Tendon, Open Approach
S20ZZ	Reposition Left Shoulder Tendon, Open Approach	**0LSC0ZZ**	Reposition Right Thorax Tendon, Open Approach	**0LSN4ZZ**	Reposition Right Lower Leg Tendon, Percutaneous Endoscopic Approach
S24ZZ	Reposition Left Shoulder Tendon, Percutaneous Endoscopic Approach	**0LSC4ZZ**	Reposition Right Thorax Tendon, Percutaneous Endoscopic Approach	**0LSP0ZZ**	Reposition Left Lower Leg Tendon, Open Approach
S30ZZ	Reposition Right Upper Arm Tendon, Open Approach	**0LSD0ZZ**	Reposition Left Thorax Tendon, Open Approach	**0LSP4ZZ**	Reposition Left Lower Leg Tendon, Percutaneous Endoscopic Approach
S34ZZ	Reposition Right Upper Arm Tendon, Percutaneous Endoscopic Approach	**0LSD4ZZ**	Reposition Left Thorax Tendon, Percutaneous Endoscopic Approach	**0LSQ0ZZ**	Reposition Right Knee Tendon, Open Approach
S40ZZ	Reposition Left Upper Arm Tendon, Open Approach	**0LSF0ZZ**	Reposition Right Abdomen Tendon, Open Approach	**0LSQ4ZZ**	Reposition Right Knee Tendon, Percutaneous Endoscopic Approach
S44ZZ	Reposition Left Upper Arm Tendon, Percutaneous Endoscopic Approach	**0LSF4ZZ**	Reposition Right Abdomen Tendon, Percutaneous Endoscopic Approach	**0LSR0ZZ**	Reposition Left Knee Tendon, Open Approach
S50ZZ	Reposition Right Lower Arm and Wrist Tendon, Open Approach	**0LSG0ZZ**	Reposition Left Abdomen Tendon, Open Approach	**0LSR4ZZ**	Reposition Left Knee Tendon, Percutaneous Endoscopic Approach
S54ZZ	Reposition Right Lower Arm and Wrist Tendon, Percutaneous Endoscopic Approach	**0LSG4ZZ**	Reposition Left Abdomen Tendon, Percutaneous Endoscopic Approach	**0LSS0ZZ**	Reposition Right Ankle Tendon, Open Approach
S60ZZ	Reposition Left Lower Arm and Wrist Tendon, Open Approach	**0LSH0ZZ**	Reposition Perineum Tendon, Open Approach	**0LSS4ZZ**	Reposition Right Ankle Tendon, Percutaneous Endoscopic Approach
S64ZZ	Reposition Left Lower Arm and Wrist Tendon, Percutaneous Endoscopic Approach	**0LSH4ZZ**	Reposition Perineum Tendon, Percutaneous Endoscopic Approach	**0LST0ZZ**	Reposition Left Ankle Tendon, Open Approach
S70ZZ	Reposition Right Hand Tendon, Open Approach	**0LSJ0ZZ**	Reposition Right Hip Tendon, Open Approach	**0LST4ZZ**	Reposition Left Ankle Tendon, Percutaneous Endoscopic Approach
S74ZZ	Reposition Right Hand Tendon, Percutaneous Endoscopic Approach	**0LSJ4ZZ**	Reposition Right Hip Tendon, Percutaneous Endoscopic Approach	**0LSV0ZZ**	Reposition Right Foot Tendon, Open Approach
S80ZZ	Reposition Left Hand Tendon, Open Approach	**0LSK0ZZ**	Reposition Left Hip Tendon, Open Approach	**0LSV4ZZ**	Reposition Right Foot Tendon, Percutaneous Endoscopic Approach
S84ZZ	Reposition Left Hand Tendon, Percutaneous Endoscopic Approach	**0LSK4ZZ**	Reposition Left Hip Tendon, Percutaneous Endoscopic Approach	**0LSW0ZZ**	Reposition Left Foot Tendon, Open Approach
		0LSL0ZZ	Reposition Right Upper Leg Tendon, Open Approach	**0LSW4ZZ**	Reposition Left Foot Tendon, Percutaneous Endoscopic Approach

LT – Tendons, Resection

eview Coding Guideline B3.8

LT00ZZ	Resection of Head and Neck Tendon, Open Approach	**0LT74ZZ**	Resection of Right Hand Tendon, Percutaneous Endoscopic Approach	**0LTH4ZZ**	Resection of Perineum Tendon, Percutaneous Endoscopic Approach
LT04ZZ	Resection of Head and Neck Tendon, Percutaneous Endoscopic Approach	**0LT80ZZ**	Resection of Left Hand Tendon, Open Approach	**0LTJ0ZZ**	Resection of Right Hip Tendon, Open Approach
LT10ZZ	Resection of Right Shoulder Tendon, Open Approach	**0LT84ZZ**	Resection of Left Hand Tendon, Percutaneous Endoscopic Approach	**0LTJ4ZZ**	Resection of Right Hip Tendon, Percutaneous Endoscopic Approach
LT14ZZ	Resection of Right Shoulder Tendon, Percutaneous Endoscopic Approach	**0LT90ZZ**	Resection of Right Trunk Tendon, Open Approach	**0LTK0ZZ**	Resection of Left Hip Tendon, Open Approach
LT20ZZ	Resection of Left Shoulder Tendon, Open Approach	**0LT94ZZ**	Resection of Right Trunk Tendon, Percutaneous Endoscopic Approach	**0LTK4ZZ**	Resection of Left Hip Tendon, Percutaneous Endoscopic Approach
LT24ZZ	Resection of Left Shoulder Tendon, Percutaneous Endoscopic Approach	**0LTB0ZZ**	Resection of Left Trunk Tendon, Open Approach	**0LTL0ZZ**	Resection of Right Upper Leg Tendon, Open Approach
LT30ZZ	Resection of Right Upper Arm Tendon, Open Approach	**0LTB4ZZ**	Resection of Left Trunk Tendon, Percutaneous Endoscopic Approach	**0LTL4ZZ**	Resection of Right Upper Leg Tendon, Percutaneous Endoscopic Approach
LT34ZZ	Resection of Right Upper Arm Tendon, Percutaneous Endoscopic Approach	**0LTC0ZZ**	Resection of Right Thorax Tendon, Open Approach	**0LTM0ZZ**	Resection of Left Upper Leg Tendon, Open Approach
LT40ZZ	Resection of Left Upper Arm Tendon, Open Approach	**0LTC4ZZ**	Resection of Right Thorax Tendon, Percutaneous Endoscopic Approach	**0LTM4ZZ**	Resection of Left Upper Leg Tendon, Percutaneous Endoscopic Approach
LT44ZZ	Resection of Left Upper Arm Tendon, Percutaneous Endoscopic Approach	**0LTD0ZZ**	Resection of Left Thorax Tendon, Open Approach	**0LTN0ZZ**	Resection of Right Lower Leg Tendon, Open Approach
LT50ZZ	Resection of Right Lower Arm and Wrist Tendon, Open Approach	**0LTD4ZZ**	Resection of Left Thorax Tendon, Percutaneous Endoscopic Approach	**0LTN4ZZ**	Resection of Right Lower Leg Tendon, Percutaneous Endoscopic Approach
LT54ZZ	Resection of Right Lower Arm and Wrist Tendon, Percutaneous Endoscopic Approach	**0LTF0ZZ**	Resection of Right Abdomen Tendon, Open Approach	**0LTP0ZZ**	Resection of Left Lower Leg Tendon, Open Approach
LT60ZZ	Resection of Left Lower Arm and Wrist Tendon, Open Approach	**0LTF4ZZ**	Resection of Right Abdomen Tendon, Percutaneous Endoscopic Approach	**0LTP4ZZ**	Resection of Left Lower Leg Tendon, Percutaneous Endoscopic Approach
LT64ZZ	Resection of Left Lower Arm and Wrist Tendon, Percutaneous Endoscopic Approach	**0LTG0ZZ**	Resection of Left Abdomen Tendon, Open Approach	**0LTQ0ZZ**	Resection of Right Knee Tendon, Open Approach
LT70ZZ	Resection of Right Hand Tendon, Open Approach	**0LTG4ZZ**	Resection of Left Abdomen Tendon, Percutaneous Endoscopic Approach	**0LTQ4ZZ**	Resection of Right Knee Tendon, Percutaneous Endoscopic Approach
		0LTH0ZZ	Resection of Perineum Tendon, Open Approach		

| ♀ Female-only | ♂ Male-only | ▲ Limited Coverage | ● Non-OR | ▨ HAC-associated procedure | ▲ Non-covered procedures | ✚ Combination |

0LTR0ZZ Resection of Left Knee Tendon, Open Approach

0LTR4ZZ Resection of Left Knee Tendon, Percutaneous Endoscopic Approach

0LTS0ZZ Resection of Right Ankle Tendon, Open Approach

0LTS4ZZ Resection of Right Ankle Tendon, Percutaneous Endoscopic Approach

0LTT0ZZ Resection of Left Ankle Tendon, Open Approach

0LTT4ZZ Resection of Left Ankle Tendon, Percutaneous Endoscopic Approach

0LTV0ZZ Resection of Right Foot Tendon, Open Approach

0LTV4ZZ Resection of Right Foot Tendon, Percutaneous Endoscopic Approach

0LTW0ZZ Resection of Left Foot Tendon, Open Approach

0LTW4ZZ Resection of Left Foot Tendon, Percutaneous Endoscopic Approach

0LU – Tendons, Supplement

0LU007Z Supplement Head and Neck Tendon with Autologous Tissue Substitute, Open Approach

0LU00JZ Supplement Head and Neck Tendon with Synthetic Substitute, Open Approach

0LU00KZ Supplement Head and Neck Tendon with Nonautologous Tissue Substitute, Open Approach

0LU047Z Supplement Head and Neck Tendon with Autologous Tissue Substitute, Percutaneous Endoscopic Approach

0LU04JZ Supplement Head and Neck Tendon with Synthetic Substitute, Percutaneous Endoscopic Approach

0LU04KZ Supplement Head and Neck Tendon with Nonautologous Tissue Substitute, Percutaneous Endoscopic Approach

0LU107Z Supplement Right Shoulder Tendon with Autologous Tissue Substitute, Open Approach

0LU10JZ Supplement Right Shoulder Tendon with Synthetic Substitute, Open Approach

0LU10KZ Supplement Right Shoulder Tendon with Nonautologous Tissue Substitute, Open Approach

0LU147Z Supplement Right Shoulder Tendon with Autologous Tissue Substitute, Percutaneous Endoscopic Approach

0LU14JZ Supplement Right Shoulder Tendon with Synthetic Substitute, Percutaneous Endoscopic Approach

0LU14KZ Supplement Right Shoulder Tendon with Nonautologous Tissue Substitute, Percutaneous Endoscopic Approach

0LU207Z Supplement Left Shoulder Tendon with Autologous Tissue Substitute, Open Approach

0LU20JZ Supplement Left Shoulder Tendon with Synthetic Substitute, Open Approach

0LU20KZ Supplement Left Shoulder Tendon with Nonautologous Tissue Substitute, Open Approach

0LU247Z Supplement Left Shoulder Tendon with Autologous Tissue Substitute, Percutaneous Endoscopic Approach

0LU24JZ Supplement Left Shoulder Tendon with Synthetic Substitute, Percutaneous Endoscopic Approach

0LU24KZ Supplement Left Shoulder Tendon with Nonautologous Tissue Substitute, Percutaneous Endoscopic Approach

0LU307Z Supplement Right Upper Arm Tendon with Autologous Tissue Substitute, Open Approach

0LU30JZ Supplement Right Upper Arm Tendon with Synthetic Substitute, Open Approach

0LU30KZ Supplement Right Upper Arm Tendon with Nonautologous Tissue Substitute, Open Approach

0LU347Z Supplement Right Upper Arm Tendon with Autologous Tissue Substitute, Percutaneous Endoscopic Approach

0LU34JZ Supplement Right Upper Arm Tendon with Synthetic Substitute, Percutaneous Endoscopic Approach

0LU34KZ Supplement Right Upper Arm Tendon with Nonautologous Tissue Substitute, Percutaneous Endoscopic Approach

0LU407Z Supplement Left Upper Arm Tendon with Autologous Tissue Substitute, Open Approach

0LU40JZ Supplement Left Upper Arm Tendon with Synthetic Substitute, Open Approach

0LU40KZ Supplement Left Upper Arm Tendon with Nonautologous Tissue Substitute, Open Approach

0LU447Z Supplement Left Upper Arm Tendon with Autologous Tissue Substitute, Percutaneous Endoscopic Approach

0LU44JZ Supplement Left Upper Arm Tendon with Synthetic Substitute, Percutaneous Endoscopic Approach

0LU44KZ Supplement Left Upper Arm Tendon with Nonautologous Tissue Substitute, Percutaneous Endoscopic Approach

0LU507Z Supplement Right Lower Arm and Wrist Tendon with Autologous Tissue Substitute, Open Approach

0LU50JZ Supplement Right Lower Arm and Wrist Tendon with Synthetic Substitute, Open Approach

0LU50KZ Supplement Right Lower Arm and Wrist Tendon with Nonautologous Tissue Substitute, Open Approach

0LU547Z Supplement Right Lower Arm and Wrist Tendon with Autologous Tissue Substitute, Percutaneous Endoscopic Approach

0LU54JZ Supplement Right Lower Arm and Wrist Tendon with Synthetic Substitute, Percutaneous Endoscopic Approach

0LU54KZ Supplement Right Lower Arm and Wrist Tendon with Nonautologous Tissue Substitute, Percutaneous Endoscopic Approach

0LU607Z Supplement Left Lower Arm and Wrist Tendon with Autologous Tissue Substitute, Open Approach

0LU60JZ Supplement Left Lower Arm and Wrist Tendon with Synthetic Substitute, Open Approach

0LU60KZ Supplement Left Lower Arm and Wrist Tendon with Nonautologous Tissue Substitute, Open Approach

0LU647Z Supplement Left Lower Arm and Wrist Tendon with Autologous Tissue Substitute, Percutaneous Endoscopic Approach

0LU64JZ Supplement Left Lower Arm and Wrist Tendon with Synthetic Substitute, Percutaneous Endoscopic Approach

0LU64KZ Supplement Left Lower Arm and Wrist Tendon with Nonautologous Tissue Substitute, Percutaneous Endoscopic Approach

0LU707Z Supplement Right Hand Tendon with Autologous Tissue Substitute, Open Approach

0LU70JZ Supplement Right Hand Tendon with Synthetic Substitute, Open Approach

0LU70KZ Supplement Right Hand Tendon with Nonautologous Tissue Substitute, Open Approach

0LU747Z Supplement Right Hand Tendon with Autologous Tissue Substitute, Percutaneous Endoscopic Approach

0LU74JZ Supplement Right Hand Tendon with Synthetic Substitute, Percutaneous Endoscopic Approach

0LU74KZ Supplement Right Hand Tendon with Nonautologous Tissue Substitute, Percutaneous Endoscopic Approach

0LU807Z Supplement Left Hand Tendon with Autologous Tissue Substitute, Open Approach

0LU80JZ Supplement Left Hand Tendon with Synthetic Substitute, Open Approach

0LU80KZ Supplement Left Hand Tendon with Nonautologous Tissue Substitute, Open Approach

0LU847Z Supplement Left Hand Tendon with Autologous Tissue Substitute, Percutaneous Endoscopic Approach

0LU84JZ Supplement Left Hand Tendon with Synthetic Substitute, Percutaneous Endoscopic Approach

0LU84KZ Supplement Left Hand Tendon with Nonautologous Tissue Substitute, Percutaneous Endoscopic Approach

0LU907Z Supplement Right Trunk Tendon with Autologous Tissue Substitute, Open Approach

0LU90JZ Supplement Right Trunk Tendon with Synthetic Substitute, Open Approach

0LU90KZ Supplement Right Trunk Tendon with Nonautologous Tissue Substitute, Open Approach

0LU947Z Supplement Right Trunk Tendon with Autologous Tissue Substitute, Percutaneous Endoscopic Approach

0LU94JZ Supplement Right Trunk Tendon with Synthetic Substitute, Percutaneous Endoscopic Approach

0LU94KZ Supplement Right Trunk Tendon with Nonautologous Tissue Substitute, Percutaneous Endoscopic Approach

0LUB07Z Supplement Left Trunk Tendon with Autologous Tissue Substitute, Open Approach

0LUB0JZ Supplement Left Trunk Tendon with Synthetic Substitute, Open Approach

0LUB0KZ Supplement Left Trunk Tendon with Nonautologous Tissue Substitute, Open Approach

0LUB47Z Supplement Left Trunk Tendon with Autologous Tissue Substitute, Percutaneous Endoscopic Approach

0LUB4JZ Supplement Left Trunk Tendon with Synthetic Substitute, Percutaneous Endoscopic Approach

0LUB4KZ Supplement Left Trunk Tendon with Nonautologous Tissue Substitute, Percutaneous Endoscopic Approach

0LUC07Z Supplement Right Thorax Tendon with Autologous Tissue Substitute, Open Approach

0LUC0JZ Supplement Right Thorax Tendon with Synthetic Substitute, Open Approach

0LUC0KZ Supplement Right Thorax Tendon with Nonautologous Tissue Substitute, Open Approach

0LUC47Z Supplement Right Thorax Tendon with Autologous Tissue Substitute, Percutaneous Endoscopic Approach

0LUC4JZ Supplement Right Thorax Tendon with Synthetic Substitute, Percutaneous Endoscopic Approach

0LUC4KZ Supplement Right Thorax Tendon with Nonautologous Tissue Substitute, Percutaneous Endoscopic Approach

0LUD07Z Supplement Left Thorax Tendon with Autologous Tissue Substitute, Open Approach

0LUD0JZ Supplement Left Thorax Tendon with Synthetic Substitute, Open Approach

0LUD0KZ Supplement Left Thorax Tendon with Nonautologous Tissue Substitute, Open Approach

0LUD47Z Supplement Left Thorax Tendon with Autologous Tissue Substitute, Percutaneous Endoscopic Approach

0LUD4JZ Supplement Left Thorax Tendon with Synthetic Substitute, Percutaneous Endoscopic Approach

0LUD4KZ Supplement Left Thorax Tendon with Nonautologous Tissue Substitute, Percutaneous Endoscopic Approach

0LUF07Z Supplement Right Abdomen Tendon with Autologous Tissue Substitute, Open Approach

0LUF0JZ Supplement Right Abdomen Tendon with Synthetic Substitute, Open Approach

0LUF0KZ Supplement Right Abdomen Tendon with Nonautologous Tissue Substitute, Open Approach

0LUF47Z Supplement Right Abdomen Tendon with Autologous Tissue Substitute, Percutaneous Endoscopic Approach

0LUF4JZ Supplement Right Abdomen Tendon with Synthetic Substitute, Percutaneous Endoscopic Approach

0LUF4KZ Supplement Right Abdomen Tendon with Nonautologous Tissue Substitute, Percutaneous Endoscopic Approach

0LUG07Z Supplement Left Abdomen Tendon with Autologous Tissue Substitute, Open Approach

0LUG0JZ Supplement Left Abdomen Tendon with Synthetic Substitute, Open Approach

0LUG0KZ Supplement Left Abdomen Tendon with Nonautologous Tissue Substitute, Open Approach

0LUG47Z Supplement Left Abdomen Tendon with Autologous Tissue Substitute, Percutaneous Endoscopic Approach

0LUG4JZ Supplement Left Abdomen Tendon with Synthetic Substitute, Percutaneous Endoscopic Approach

0LUG4KZ Supplement Left Abdomen Tendon with Nonautologous Tissue Substitute, Percutaneous Endoscopic Approach

0LUH07Z Supplement Perineum Tendon with Autologous Tissue Substitute, Open Approach

0LUH0JZ Supplement Perineum Tendon with Synthetic Substitute, Open Approach

0LUH0KZ Supplement Perineum Tendon with Nonautologous Tissue Substitute, Open Approach

0LUH47Z Supplement Perineum Tendon with Autologous Tissue Substitute, Percutaneous Endoscopic Approach

0LUH4JZ Supplement Perineum Tendon with Synthetic Substitute, Percutaneous Endoscopic Approach

0LUH4KZ Supplement Perineum Tendon with Nonautologous Tissue Substitute, Percutaneous Endoscopic Approach

0LUJ07Z Supplement Right Hip Tendon with Autologous Tissue Substitute, Open Approach

0LUJ0JZ Supplement Right Hip Tendon with Synthetic Substitute, Open Approach

0LUJ0KZ Supplement Right Hip Tendon with Nonautologous Tissue Substitute, Open Approach

0LUJ47Z Supplement Right Hip Tendon with Autologous Tissue Substitute, Percutaneous Endoscopic Approach

0LUJ4JZ Supplement Right Hip Tendon with Synthetic Substitute, Percutaneous Endoscopic Approach

0LUJ4KZ Supplement Right Hip Tendon with Nonautologous Tissue Substitute, Percutaneous Endoscopic Approach

0LUK07Z Supplement Left Hip Tendon with Autologous Tissue Substitute, Open Approach

0LUK0JZ Supplement Left Hip Tendon with Synthetic Substitute, Open Approach

0LUK0KZ Supplement Left Hip Tendon with Nonautologous Tissue Substitute, Open Approach

0LUK47Z Supplement Left Hip Tendon with Autologous Tissue Substitute, Percutaneous Endoscopic Approach

0LUK4JZ Supplement Left Hip Tendon with Synthetic Substitute, Percutaneous Endoscopic Approach

0LUK4KZ Supplement Left Hip Tendon with Nonautologous Tissue Substitute, Percutaneous Endoscopic Approach

0LUL07Z Supplement Right Upper Leg Tendon with Autologous Tissue Substitute, Open Approach

0LUL0JZ Supplement Right Upper Leg Tendon with Synthetic Substitute, Open Approach

0LUL0KZ Supplement Right Upper Leg Tendon with Nonautologous Tissue Substitute, Open Approach

0LUL47Z Supplement Right Upper Leg Tendon with Autologous Tissue Substitute, Percutaneous Endoscopic Approach

0LUL4JZ Supplement Right Upper Leg Tendon with Synthetic Substitute, Percutaneous Endoscopic Approach

0LUL4KZ Supplement Right Upper Leg Tendon with Nonautologous Tissue Substitute, Percutaneous Endoscopic Approach

0LUM07Z Supplement Left Upper Leg Tendon with Autologous Tissue Substitute, Open Approach

0LUM0JZ Supplement Left Upper Leg Tendon with Synthetic Substitute, Open Approach

0LUM0KZ Supplement Left Upper Leg Tendon with Nonautologous Tissue Substitute, Open Approach

0LUM47Z Supplement Left Upper Leg Tendon with Autologous Tissue Substitute, Percutaneous Endoscopic Approach

0LUM4JZ Supplement Left Upper Leg Tendon with Synthetic Substitute, Percutaneous Endoscopic Approach

0LUM4KZ Supplement Left Upper Leg Tendon with Nonautologous Tissue Substitute, Percutaneous Endoscopic Approach

0LUN07Z Supplement Right Lower Leg Tendon with Autologous Tissue Substitute, Open Approach

0LUN0JZ Supplement Right Lower Leg Tendon with Synthetic Substitute, Open Approach

0LUN0KZ Supplement Right Lower Leg Tendon with Nonautologous Tissue Substitute, Open Approach

0LUN47Z Supplement Right Lower Leg Tendon with Autologous Tissue Substitute, Percutaneous Endoscopic Approach

0LUN4JZ Supplement Right Lower Leg Tendon with Synthetic Substitute, Percutaneous Endoscopic Approach

0LUN4KZ Supplement Right Lower Leg Tendon with Nonautologous Tissue Substitute, Percutaneous Endoscopic Approach

0LUP07Z Supplement Left Lower Leg Tendon with Autologous Tissue Substitute, Open Approach

0LUP0JZ Supplement Left Lower Leg Tendon with Synthetic Substitute, Open Approach

0LUP0KZ Supplement Left Lower Leg Tendon with Nonautologous Tissue Substitute, Open Approach

0LUP47Z Supplement Left Lower Leg Tendon with Autologous Tissue Substitute, Percutaneous Endoscopic Approach

0LUP4JZ Supplement Left Lower Leg Tendon with Synthetic Substitute, Percutaneous Endoscopic Approach

0LUP4KZ Supplement Left Lower Leg Tendon with Nonautologous Tissue Substitute, Percutaneous Endoscopic Approach

0LUQ07Z Supplement Right Knee Tendon with Autologous Tissue Substitute, Open Approach

0LUQ0JZ Supplement Right Knee Tendon with Synthetic Substitute, Open Approach

0LUQ0KZ Supplement Right Knee Tendon with Nonautologous Tissue Substitute, Open Approach

0LUQ47Z Supplement Right Knee Tendon with Autologous Tissue Substitute, Percutaneous Endoscopic Approach

0LUQ4JZ Supplement Right Knee Tendon with Synthetic Substitute, Percutaneous Endoscopic Approach

0LUQ4KZ Supplement Right Knee Tendon with Nonautologous Tissue Substitute, Percutaneous Endoscopic Approach

0LUR07Z Supplement Left Knee Tendon with Autologous Tissue Substitute, Open Approach

0LUR0JZ Supplement Left Knee Tendon with Synthetic Substitute, Open Approach

0LUR0KZ Supplement Left Knee Tendon with Nonautologous Tissue Substitute, Open Approach

0LUR47Z Supplement Left Knee Tendon with Autologous Tissue Substitute, Percutaneous Endoscopic Approach

0LUR4JZ Supplement Left Knee Tendon with Synthetic Substitute, Percutaneous Endoscopic Approach

0LUR4KZ Supplement Left Knee Tendon with Nonautologous Tissue Substitute, Percutaneous Endoscopic Approach

0LUS07Z Supplement Right Ankle Tendon with Autologous Tissue Substitute, Open Approach

0LUS0JZ Supplement Right Ankle Tendon with Synthetic Substitute, Open Approach

0LUS0KZ Supplement Right Ankle Tendon with Nonautologous Tissue Substitute, Open Approach

0LUS47Z Supplement Right Ankle Tendon with Autologous Tissue Substitute, Percutaneous Endoscopic Approach

0LUS4JZ Supplement Right Ankle Tendon with Synthetic Substitute, Percutaneous Endoscopic Approach

0LUS4KZ Supplement Right Ankle Tendon with Nonautologous Tissue Substitute, Percutaneous Endoscopic Approach

0LUT07Z Supplement Left Ankle Tendon with Autologous Tissue Substitute, Open Approach

0LUT0JZ Supplement Left Ankle Tendon with Synthetic Substitute, Open Approach

0LUT0KZ Supplement Left Ankle Tendon with Nonautologous Tissue Substitute, Open Approach

0LUT47Z Supplement Left Ankle Tendon with Autologous Tissue Substitute, Percutaneous Endoscopic Approach

0LUT4JZ Supplement Left Ankle Tendon with Synthetic Substitute, Percutaneous Endoscopic Approach

0LUT4KZ Supplement Left Ankle Tendon with Nonautologous Tissue Substitute, Percutaneous Endoscopic Approach

0LUV07Z Supplement Right Foot Tendon with Autologous Tissue Substitute, Open Approach

0LUV0JZ Supplement Right Foot Tendon with Synthetic Substitute, Open Approach

0LUV0KZ Supplement Right Foot Tendon with Nonautologous Tissue Substitute, Open Approach

0LUV47Z Supplement Right Foot Tendon with Autologous Tissue Substitute, Percutaneous Endoscopic Approach

0LUV4JZ Supplement Right Foot Tendon with Synthetic Substitute, Percutaneous Endoscopic Approach

0LUV4KZ Supplement Right Foot Tendon with Nonautologous Tissue Substitute, Percutaneous Endoscopic Approach

0LUW07Z Supplement Left Foot Tendon with Autologous Tissue Substitute, Open Approach

0LUW0JZ Supplement Left Foot Tendon with Synthetic Substitute, Open Approach

0LUW0KZ Supplement Left Foot Tendon with Nonautologous Tissue Substitute, Ope Approach

0LUW47Z Supplement Left Foot Tendon with Autologous Tissue Substitute, Percutaneous Endoscopic Approach

0LUW4JZ Supplement Left Foot Tendon with Synthetic Substitute, Percutaneous Endoscopic Approach

0LUW4KZ Supplement Left Foot Tendon with Nonautologous Tissue Substitute, Percutaneous Endoscopic Approach

0LW – Tendons, Revision

Review Coding Guideline B6.1c

0LWX00Z Revision of Drainage Device in Upper Tendon, Open Approach

0LWX07Z Revision of Autologous Tissue Substitute in Upper Tendon, Open Approach

0LWX0JZ Revision of Synthetic Substitute in Upper Tendon, Open Approach

0LWX0KZ Revision of Nonautologous Tissue Substitute in Upper Tendon, Open Approach

0LWX30Z Revision of Drainage Device in Upper Tendon, Percutaneous Approach

0LWX37Z Revision of Autologous Tissue Substitute in Upper Tendon, Percutaneous Approach

0LWX3JZ Revision of Synthetic Substitute in Upper Tendon, Percutaneous Approach

0LWX3KZ Revision of Nonautologous Tissue Substitute in Upper Tendon, Percutaneous Approach

0LWX40Z Revision of Drainage Device in Upper Tendon, Percutaneous Endoscopic Approach

0LWX47Z Revision of Autologous Tissue Substitute in Upper Tendon, Percutaneous Endoscopic Approach

0LWX4JZ Revision of Synthetic Substitute in Upper Tendon, Percutaneous Endoscopic Approach

0LWX4KZ Revision of Nonautologous Tissue Substitute in Upper Tendon, Percutaneous Endoscopic Approach

0LWXX0Z Revision of Drainage Device in Upper Tendon, External Approach

0LWXX7Z Revision of Autologous Tissue Substitute in Upper Tendon, External Approach

0LWXXJZ Revision of Synthetic Substitute in Upper Tendon, External Approach

0LWXXKZ Revision of Nonautologous Tissue Substitute in Upper Tendon, External Approach

0LWY00Z Revision of Drainage Device in Lower Tendon, Open Approach

0LWY07Z Revision of Autologous Tissue Substitute in Lower Tendon, Open Approach

0LWY0JZ Revision of Synthetic Substitute in Lower Tendon, Open Approach

0LWY0KZ Revision of Nonautologous Tissue Substitute in Lower Tendon, Open Approach

0LWY30Z Revision of Drainage Device in Lower Tendon, Percutaneous Approach

0LWY37Z Revision of Autologous Tissue Substitute in Lower Tendon, Percutaneous Approach

0LWY3JZ Revision of Synthetic Substitute in Lower Tendon, Percutaneous Approach

0LWY3KZ Revision of Nonautologous Tissue Substitute in Lower Tendon, Percutaneous Approach

0LWY40Z Revision of Drainage Device in Lower Tendon, Percutaneous Endoscopic Approach

0LWY47Z Revision of Autologous Tissue Substitu in Lower Tendon, Percutaneous Endoscopic Approach

0LWY4JZ Revision of Synthetic Substitute in Lower Tendon, Percutaneous Endoscop Approach

0LWY4KZ Revision of Nonautologous Tissue Substitute in Lower Tendon, Percutaneous Endoscopic Approach

0LWYX0Z Revision of Drainage Device in Lower Tendon, External Approach

0LWYX7Z Revision of Autologous Tissue Substitu in Lower Tendon, External Approach

0LWYXJZ Revision of Synthetic Substitute in Lower Tendon, External Approach

0LWYXKZ Revision of Nonautologous Tissue Substitute in Lower Tendon, External Approach

0LX – Tendons, Transfer

0LX00ZZ Transfer Head and Neck Tendon, Open Approach

0LX04ZZ Transfer Head and Neck Tendon, Percutaneous Endoscopic Approach

0LX10ZZ Transfer Right Shoulder Tendon, Open Approach

0LX14ZZ Transfer Right Shoulder Tendon, Percutaneous Endoscopic Approach

0LX20ZZ Transfer Left Shoulder Tendon, Open Approach

0LX24ZZ Transfer Left Shoulder Tendon, Percutaneous Endoscopic Approach

0LX30ZZ Transfer Right Upper Arm Tendon, Open Approach

0LX34ZZ Transfer Right Upper Arm Tendon, Percutaneous Endoscopic Approach

0LX40ZZ Transfer Left Upper Arm Tendon, Open Approach

0LX44ZZ Transfer Left Upper Arm Tendon, Percutaneous Endoscopic Approach

0LX50ZZ Transfer Right Lower Arm and Wrist Tendon, Open Approach

0LX54ZZ Transfer Right Lower Arm and Wrist Tendon, Percutaneous Endoscopic Approach

0LX60ZZ Transfer Left Lower Arm and Wrist Tendon, Open Approach

0LX64ZZ Transfer Left Lower Arm and Wrist Tendon, Percutaneous Endoscopic Approach

0LX70ZZ Transfer Right Hand Tendon, Open Approach

0LX74ZZ Transfer Right Hand Tendon, Percutaneous Endoscopic Approach

0LX80ZZ Transfer Left Hand Tendon, Open Approach

0LX84ZZ Transfer Left Hand Tendon, Percutaneous Endoscopic Approach

0LX90ZZ Transfer Right Trunk Tendon, Open Approach

0LX94ZZ Transfer Right Trunk Tendon, Percutaneous Endoscopic Approach

0LXB0ZZ Transfer Left Trunk Tendon, Open Approach

0LXB4ZZ Transfer Left Trunk Tendon, Percutaneou Endoscopic Approach

0LXC0ZZ Transfer Right Thorax Tendon, Open Approach

0LXC4ZZ Transfer Right Thorax Tendon, Percutaneous Endoscopic Approach

0LXD0ZZ Transfer Left Thorax Tendon, Open Approach

0LXD4ZZ Transfer Left Thorax Tendon, Percutaneous Endoscopic Approach

0LXF0ZZ Transfer Right Abdomen Tendon, Open Approach

0LXF4ZZ Transfer Right Abdomen Tendon, Percutaneous Endoscopic Approach

0LXG0ZZ Transfer Left Abdomen Tendon, Open Approach

0LXG4ZZ Transfer Left Abdomen Tendon, Percutaneous Endoscopic Approach

0LXH0ZZ Transfer Perineum Tendon, Open Approach

0LXH4ZZ Transfer Perineum Tendon, Percutaneous Endoscopic Approach

XJ0ZZ Transfer Right Hip Tendon, Open Approach

XJ4ZZ Transfer Right Hip Tendon, Percutaneous Endoscopic Approach

XK0ZZ Transfer Left Hip Tendon, Open Approach

XK4ZZ Transfer Left Hip Tendon, Percutaneous Endoscopic Approach

XL0ZZ Transfer Right Upper Leg Tendon, Open Approach

XL4ZZ Transfer Right Upper Leg Tendon, Percutaneous Endoscopic Approach

XM0ZZ Transfer Left Upper Leg Tendon, Open Approach

XM4ZZ Transfer Left Upper Leg Tendon, Percutaneous Endoscopic Approach

0LXN0ZZ Transfer Right Lower Leg Tendon, Open Approach

0LXN4ZZ Transfer Right Lower Leg Tendon, Percutaneous Endoscopic Approach

0LXP0ZZ Transfer Left Lower Leg Tendon, Open Approach

0LXP4ZZ Transfer Left Lower Leg Tendon, Percutaneous Endoscopic Approach

0LXQ0ZZ Transfer Right Knee Tendon, Open Approach

0LXQ4ZZ Transfer Right Knee Tendon, Percutaneous Endoscopic Approach

0LXR0ZZ Transfer Left Knee Tendon, Open Approach

0LXR4ZZ Transfer Left Knee Tendon, Percutaneous Endoscopic Approach

0LXS0ZZ Transfer Right Ankle Tendon, Open Approach

0LXS4ZZ Transfer Right Ankle Tendon, Percutaneous Endoscopic Approach

0LXT0ZZ Transfer Left Ankle Tendon, Open Approach

0LXT4ZZ Transfer Left Ankle Tendon, Percutaneous Endoscopic Approach

0LXV0ZZ Transfer Right Foot Tendon, Open Approach

0LXV4ZZ Transfer Right Foot Tendon, Percutaneous Endoscopic Approach

0LXW0ZZ Transfer Left Foot Tendon, Open Approach

0LXW4ZZ Transfer Left Foot Tendon, Percutaneous Endoscopic Approach

Bursa of the Knee

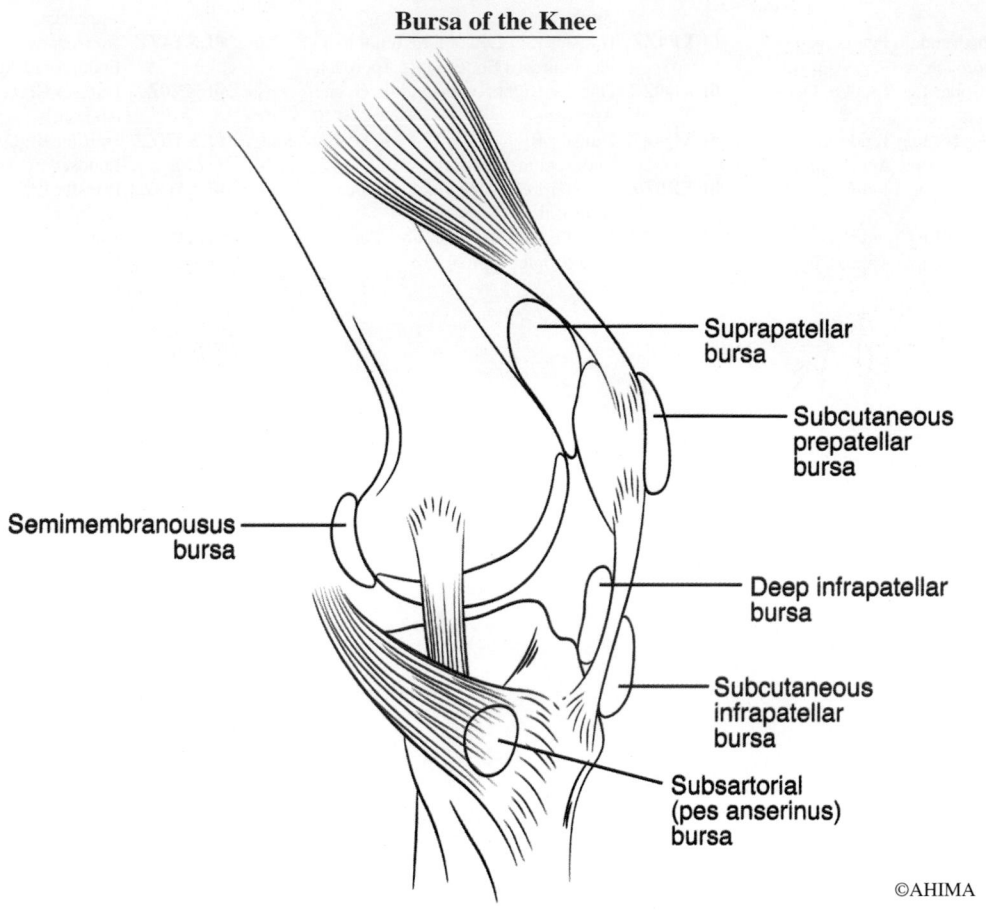

Suprapatellar
bursa

Subcutaneous
prepatellar
bursa

Semimembranousus
bursa

Deep infrapatellar
bursa

Subcutaneous
infrapatellar
bursa

Subsartorial
(pes anserinus)
bursa

©AHIMA

Ligaments of the Knee

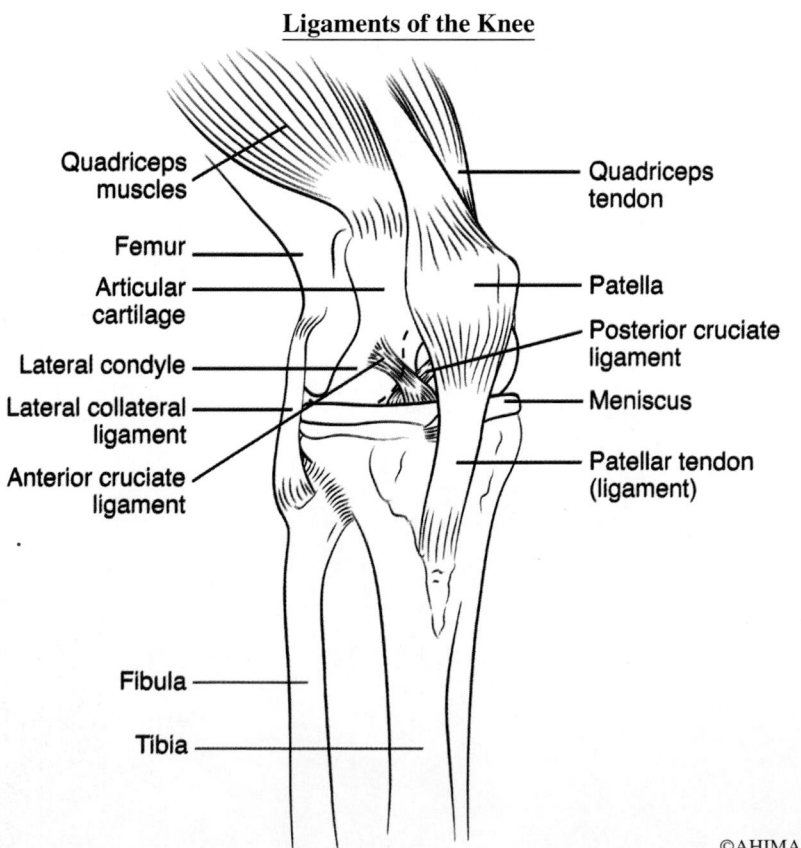

Quadriceps
muscles

Femur

Articular
cartilage

Lateral condyle

Lateral collateral
ligament

Anterior cruciate
ligament

Quadriceps
tendon

Patella

Posterior cruciate
ligament

Meniscus

Patellar tendon
(ligament)

Fibula

Tibia

©AHIMA

Shoulder Tendons and Ligaments

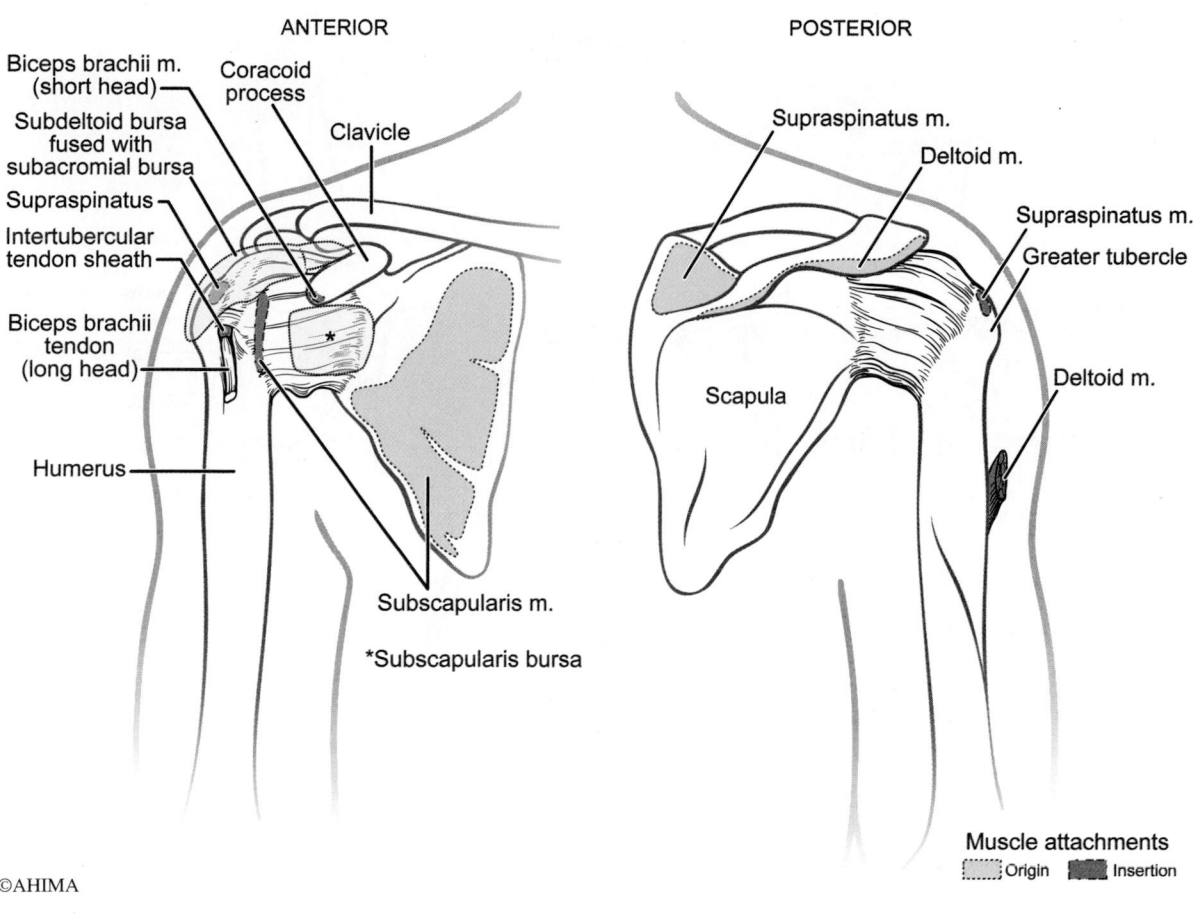

ANTERIOR

- Biceps brachii m. (short head)
- Subdeltoid bursa fused with subacromial bursa
- Supraspinatus
- Intertubercular tendon sheath
- Biceps brachii tendon (long head)
- Humerus
- Coracoid process
- Clavicle
- Subscapularis m.
- *Subscapularis bursa

©AHIMA

POSTERIOR

- Supraspinatus m.
- Deltoid m.
- Supraspinatus m.
- Greater tubercle
- Scapula
- Deltoid m.

Muscle attachments
- Origin
- Insertion

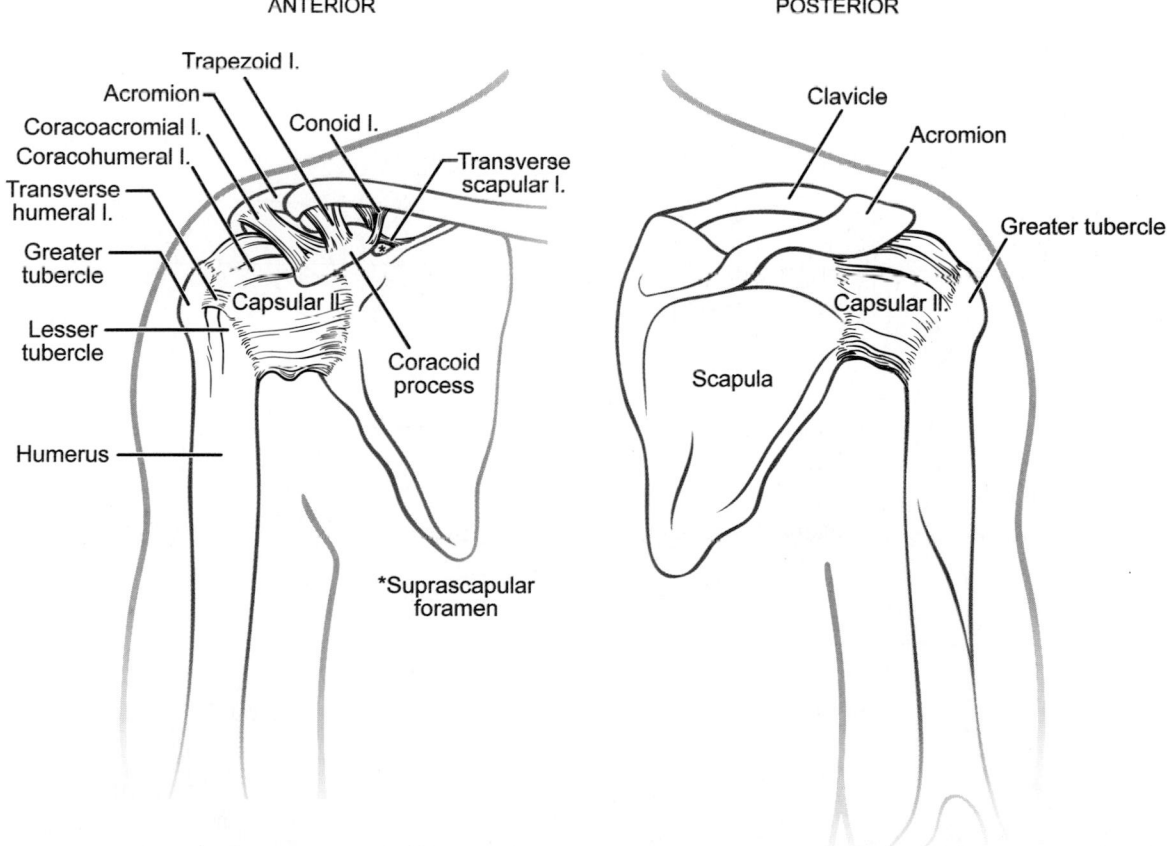

ANTERIOR

- Trapezoid l.
- Acromion
- Coracoacromial l.
- Coracohumeral l.
- Transverse humeral l.
- Greater tubercle
- Lesser tubercle
- Humerus
- Conoid l.
- Transverse scapular l.
- Capsular l.
- Coracoid process
- *Suprascapular foramen

©AHIMA

POSTERIOR

- Clavicle
- Acromion
- Greater tubercle
- Capsular l.
- Scapula

Knee Tendons and Ligaments

ANTERIOR

POSTERIOR

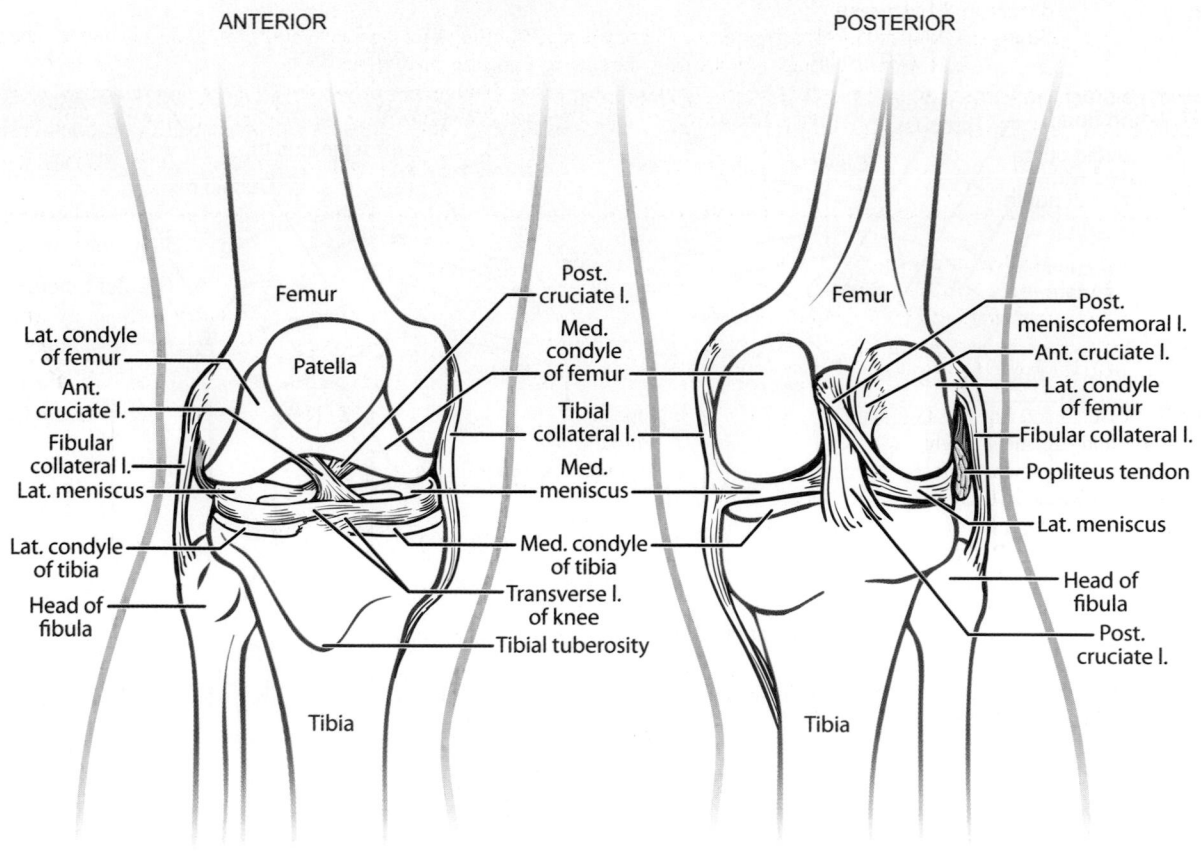

Lat. condyle of femur
Ant. cruciate l.
Fibular collateral l.
Lat. meniscus
Lat. condyle of tibia
Head of fibula

Femur
Patella

Post. cruciate l.
Med. condyle of femur
Tibial collateral l.
Med. meniscus
Med. condyle of tibia
Transverse l. of knee
Tibial tuberosity

Tibia

Femur

Post. meniscofemoral l.
Ant. cruciate l.
Lat. condyle of femur
Fibular collateral l.
Popliteus tendon
Lat. meniscus
Head of fibula
Post. cruciate l.

Tibia

©AHIMA

Hip Tendons and Ligaments

ANTERIOR

POSTERIOR

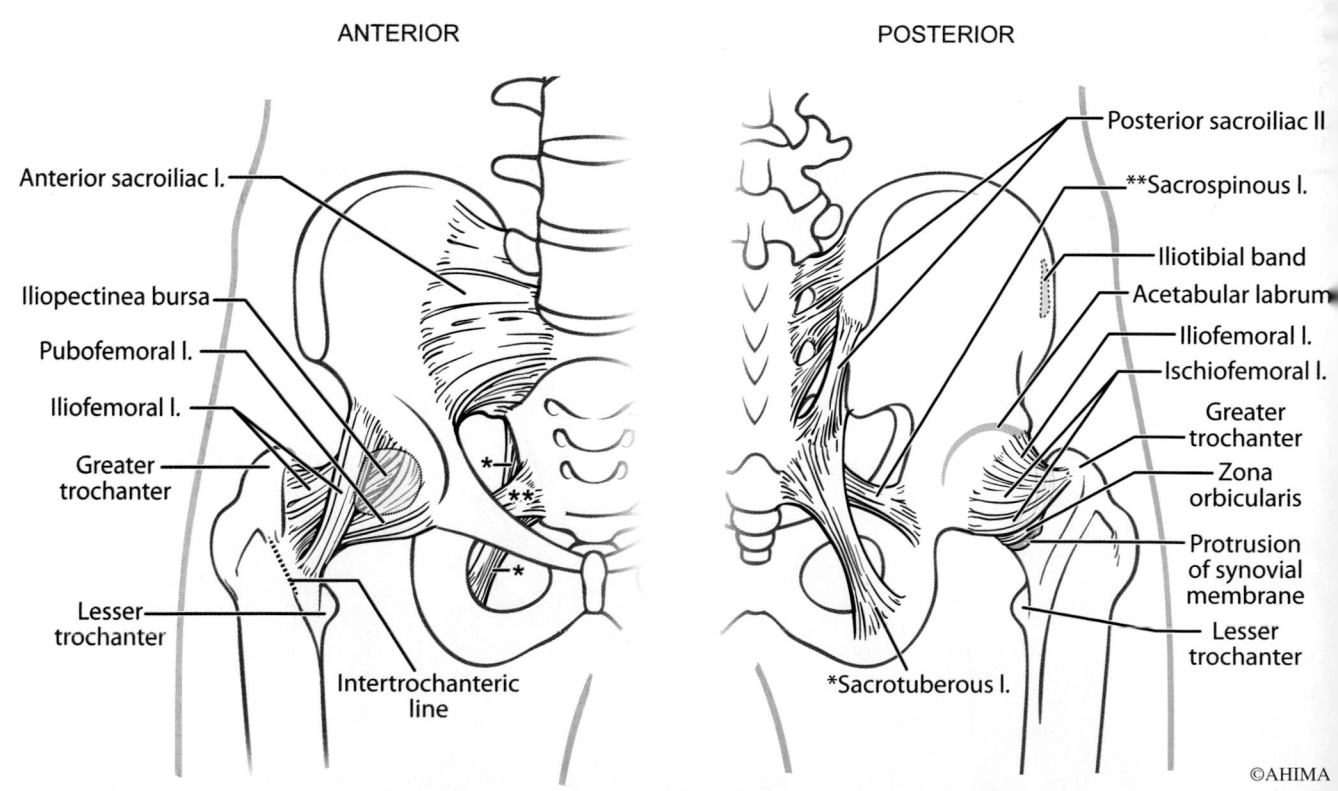

Anterior sacroiliac l.
Iliopectinea bursa
Pubofemoral l.
Iliofemoral l.
Greater trochanter
Lesser trochanter
Intertrochanteric line

Posterior sacroiliac ll
**Sacrospinous l.
Iliotibial band
Acetabular labrum
Iliofemoral l.
Ischiofemoral l.
Greater trochanter
Zona orbicularis
Protrusion of synovial membrane
Lesser trochanter
*Sacrotuberous l.

©AHIMA

Section   **0**   **Medical and Surgical**
Body System   **M**   **Bursae and Ligaments**
Operation   **2**   **Change:** Taking out or off a device from a body part and putting back an identical or similar device in or on the same body part without cutting or puncturing the skin or a mucous membrane

Body Part (4th)	Approach (5th)	Device (6th)	Qualifier (7th)
X Upper Bursa and Ligament Y Lower Bursa and Ligament	X External	0 Drainage Device Y Other Device	Z No Qualifier

Section   **0**   **Medical and Surgical**
Body System   **M**   **Bursae and Ligaments**
Operation   **5**   **Destruction:** Physical eradication of all or a portion of a body part by the direct use of energy, force, or a destructive agent

Body Part (4th)	Approach (5th)	Device (6th)	Qualifier (7th)
0 Head and Neck Bursa and Ligament 1 Shoulder Bursa and Ligament, Right 2 Shoulder Bursa and Ligament, Left 3 Elbow Bursa and Ligament, Right 4 Elbow Bursa and Ligament, Left 5 Wrist Bursa and Ligament, Right 6 Wrist Bursa and Ligament, Left 7 Hand Bursa and Ligament, Right 8 Hand Bursa and Ligament, Left 9 Upper Extremity Bursa and Ligament, Right B Upper Extremity Bursa and Ligament, Left C Trunk Bursa and Ligament, Right D Trunk Bursa and Ligament, Left F Thorax Bursa and Ligament, Right G Thorax Bursa and Ligament, Left H Abdomen Bursa and Ligament, Right J Abdomen Bursa and Ligament, Left K Perineum Bursa and Ligament L Hip Bursa and Ligament, Right M Hip Bursa and Ligament, Left N Knee Bursa and Ligament, Right P Knee Bursa and Ligament, Left Q Ankle Bursa and Ligament, Right R Ankle Bursa and Ligament, Left S Foot Bursa and Ligament, Right T Foot Bursa and Ligament, Left V Lower Extremity Bursa and Ligament, Right W Lower Extremity Bursa and Ligament, Left	0 Open 3 Percutaneous 4 Percutaneous Endoscopic	Z No Device	Z No Qualifier

Section	0	Medical and Surgical
Body System	M	Bursae and Ligaments
Operation	8	**Division:** Cutting into a body part, without draining fluids and/or gases from the body part, in order to separate or transect a body part

Body Part (4th)	Approach (5th)	Device (6th)	Qualifier (7th)
0 Head and Neck Bursa and Ligament	0 Open	Z No Device	Z No Qualifier
1 Shoulder Bursa and Ligament, Right	3 Percutaneous		
2 Shoulder Bursa and Ligament, Left	4 Percutaneous Endoscopic		
3 Elbow Bursa and Ligament, Right			
4 Elbow Bursa and Ligament, Left			
5 Wrist Bursa and Ligament, Right			
6 Wrist Bursa and Ligament, Left			
7 Hand Bursa and Ligament, Right			
8 Hand Bursa and Ligament, Left			
9 Upper Extremity Bursa and Ligament, Right			
B Upper Extremity Bursa and Ligament, Left			
C Trunk Bursa and Ligament, Right			
D Trunk Bursa and Ligament, Left			
F Thorax Bursa and Ligament, Right			
G Thorax Bursa and Ligament, Left			
H Abdomen Bursa and Ligament, Right			
J Abdomen Bursa and Ligament, Left			
K Perineum Bursa and Ligament			
L Hip Bursa and Ligament, Right			
M Hip Bursa and Ligament, Left			
N Knee Bursa and Ligament, Right			
P Knee Bursa and Ligament, Left			
Q Ankle Bursa and Ligament, Right			
R Ankle Bursa and Ligament, Left			
S Foot Bursa and Ligament, Right			
T Foot Bursa and Ligament, Left			
V Lower Extremity Bursa and Ligament, Right			
W Lower Extremity Bursa and Ligament, Left			

Section	0	Medical and Surgical
Body System	M	Bursae and Ligaments
Operation	9	**Drainage:** Taking or letting out fluids and/or gases from a body part

Body Part (4th)	Approach (5th)	Device (6th)	Qualifier (7th)
0 Head and Neck Bursa and Ligament	0 Open	0 Drainage Device	Z No Qualifier
1 Shoulder Bursa and Ligament, Right	3 Percutaneous		
2 Shoulder Bursa and Ligament, Left	4 Percutaneous Endoscopic		
3 Elbow Bursa and Ligament, Right			
4 Elbow Bursa and Ligament, Left			
5 Wrist Bursa and Ligament, Right			
6 Wrist Bursa and Ligament, Left			
7 Hand Bursa and Ligament, Right			
8 Hand Bursa and Ligament, Left			
9 Upper Extremity Bursa and Ligament, Right			
B Upper Extremity Bursa and Ligament, Left			
C Trunk Bursa and Ligament, Right			
D Trunk Bursa and Ligament, Left			
F Thorax Bursa and Ligament, Right			
G Thorax Bursa and Ligament, Left			
H Abdomen Bursa and Ligament, Right			
J Abdomen Bursa and Ligament, Left			
K Perineum Bursa and Ligament			
L Hip Bursa and Ligament, Right			
M Hip Bursa and Ligament, Left			
N Knee Bursa and Ligament, Right			
P Knee Bursa and Ligament, Left			
Q Ankle Bursa and Ligament, Right			
R Ankle Bursa and Ligament, Left			
S Foot Bursa and Ligament, Right			
T Foot Bursa and Ligament, Left			
V Lower Extremity Bursa and Ligament, Right			
W Lower Extremity Bursa and Ligament, Left			

Continued →

Section 0 **Medical and Surgical**
Body System M **Bursae and Ligaments**
Operation 9 **Drainage:** Taking or letting out fluids and/or gases from a body part

Body Part (4th)	Approach (5th)	Device (6th)	Qualifier (7th)
0 Head and Neck Bursa and Ligament	0 Open	Z No Device	X Diagnostic
1 Shoulder Bursa and Ligament, Right	3 Percutaneous		Z No Qualifier
2 Shoulder Bursa and Ligament, Left	4 Percutaneous Endoscopic		
3 Elbow Bursa and Ligament, Right			
4 Elbow Bursa and Ligament, Left			
5 Wrist Bursa and Ligament, Right			
6 Wrist Bursa and Ligament, Left			
7 Hand Bursa and Ligament, Right			
8 Hand Bursa and Ligament, Left			
9 Upper Extremity Bursa and Ligament, Right			
B Upper Extremity Bursa and Ligament, Left			
C Trunk Bursa and Ligament, Right			
D Trunk Bursa and Ligament, Left			
F Thorax Bursa and Ligament, Right			
G Thorax Bursa and Ligament, Left			
H Abdomen Bursa and Ligament, Right			
J Abdomen Bursa and Ligament, Left			
K Perineum Bursa and Ligament			
L Hip Bursa and Ligament, Right			
M Hip Bursa and Ligament, Left			
N Knee Bursa and Ligament, Right			
P Knee Bursa and Ligament, Left			
Q Ankle Bursa and Ligament, Right			
R Ankle Bursa and Ligament, Left			
S Foot Bursa and Ligament, Right			
T Foot Bursa and Ligament, Left			
V Lower Extremity Bursa and Ligament, Right			
W Lower Extremity Bursa and Ligament, Left			

Section 0 **Medical and Surgical**
Body System M **Bursae and Ligaments**
Operation B **Excision:** Cutting out or off, without replacement, a portion of a body part

Body Part (4th)	Approach (5th)	Device (6th)	Qualifier (7th)
0 Head and Neck Bursa and Ligament	0 Open	Z No Device	X Diagnostic
1 Shoulder Bursa and Ligament, Right	3 Percutaneous		Z No Qualifier
2 Shoulder Bursa and Ligament, Left	4 Percutaneous Endoscopic		
3 Elbow Bursa and Ligament, Right			
4 Elbow Bursa and Ligament, Left			
5 Wrist Bursa and Ligament, Right			
6 Wrist Bursa and Ligament, Left			
7 Hand Bursa and Ligament, Right			
8 Hand Bursa and Ligament, Left			
9 Upper Extremity Bursa and Ligament, Right			
B Upper Extremity Bursa and Ligament, Left			
C Trunk Bursa and Ligament, Right			
D Trunk Bursa and Ligament, Left			
F Thorax Bursa and Ligament, Right			
G Thorax Bursa and Ligament, Left			
H Abdomen Bursa and Ligament, Right			
J Abdomen Bursa and Ligament, Left			
K Perineum Bursa and Ligament			
L Hip Bursa and Ligament, Right			
M Hip Bursa and Ligament, Left			
N Knee Bursa and Ligament, Right			
P Knee Bursa and Ligament, Left			
Q Ankle Bursa and Ligament, Right			
R Ankle Bursa and Ligament, Left			
S Foot Bursa and Ligament, Right			
T Foot Bursa and Ligament, Left			
V Lower Extremity Bursa and Ligament, Right			
W Lower Extremity Bursa and Ligament, Left			

Section	0	Medical and Surgical
Body System	M	Bursae and Ligaments
Operation	C	Extirpation: Taking or cutting out solid matter from a body part

Body Part (4th)	Approach (5th)	Device (6th)	Qualifier (7th)
0 Head and Neck Bursa and Ligament 1 Shoulder Bursa and Ligament, Right 2 Shoulder Bursa and Ligament, Left 3 Elbow Bursa and Ligament, Right 4 Elbow Bursa and Ligament, Left 5 Wrist Bursa and Ligament, Right 6 Wrist Bursa and Ligament, Left 7 Hand Bursa and Ligament, Right 8 Hand Bursa and Ligament, Left 9 Upper Extremity Bursa and Ligament, Right B Upper Extremity Bursa and Ligament, Left C Trunk Bursa and Ligament, Right D Trunk Bursa and Ligament, Left F Thorax Bursa and Ligament, Right G Thorax Bursa and Ligament, Left H Abdomen Bursa and Ligament, Right J Abdomen Bursa and Ligament, Left K Perineum Bursa and Ligament L Hip Bursa and Ligament, Right M Hip Bursa and Ligament, Left N Knee Bursa and Ligament, Right P Knee Bursa and Ligament, Left Q Ankle Bursa and Ligament, Right R Ankle Bursa and Ligament, Left S Foot Bursa and Ligament, Right T Foot Bursa and Ligament, Left V Lower Extremity Bursa and Ligament, Right W Lower Extremity Bursa and Ligament, Left	0 Open 3 Percutaneous 4 Percutaneous Endoscopic	Z No Device	Z No Qualifier

Section	0	Medical and Surgical
Body System	M	Bursae and Ligaments
Operation	D	Extraction: Pulling or stripping out or off all or a portion of a body part by the use of force

Body Part (4th)	Approach (5th)	Device (6th)	Qualifier (7th)
0 Head and Neck Bursa and Ligament 1 Shoulder Bursa and Ligament, Right 2 Shoulder Bursa and Ligament, Left 3 Elbow Bursa and Ligament, Right 4 Elbow Bursa and Ligament, Left 5 Wrist Bursa and Ligament, Right 6 Wrist Bursa and Ligament, Left 7 Hand Bursa and Ligament, Right 8 Hand Bursa and Ligament, Left 9 Upper Extremity Bursa and Ligament, Right B Upper Extremity Bursa and Ligament, Left C Trunk Bursa and Ligament, Right D Trunk Bursa and Ligament, Left F Thorax Bursa and Ligament, Right G Thorax Bursa and Ligament, Left H Abdomen Bursa and Ligament, Right J Abdomen Bursa and Ligament, Left K Perineum Bursa and Ligament L Hip Bursa and Ligament, Right M Hip Bursa and Ligament, Left N Knee Bursa and Ligament, Right P Knee Bursa and Ligament, Left Q Ankle Bursa and Ligament, Right R Ankle Bursa and Ligament, Left S Foot Bursa and Ligament, Right T Foot Bursa and Ligament, Left V Lower Extremity Bursa and Ligament, Right W Lower Extremity Bursa and Ligament, Left	0 Open 3 Percutaneous 4 Percutaneous Endoscopic	Z No Device	Z No Qualifier

Section	0	Medical and Surgical
Body System	M	Bursae and Ligaments
Operation	J	Inspection: Visually and/or manually exploring a body part

Body Part (4th)	Approach (5th)	Device (6th)	Qualifier (7th)
X Upper Bursa and Ligament Y Lower Bursa and Ligament	0 Open 3 Percutaneous 4 Percutaneous Endoscopic X External	Z No Device	Z No Qualifier

Section	0	Medical and Surgical
Body System	M	Bursae and Ligaments
Operation	M	Reattachment: Putting back in or on all or a portion of a separated body part to its normal location or other suitable location

Body Part (4th)	Approach (5th)	Device (6th)	Qualifier (7th)
0 Head and Neck Bursa and Ligament 1 Shoulder Bursa and Ligament, Right 2 Shoulder Bursa and Ligament, Left 3 Elbow Bursa and Ligament, Right 4 Elbow Bursa and Ligament, Left 5 Wrist Bursa and Ligament, Right 6 Wrist Bursa and Ligament, Left 7 Hand Bursa and Ligament, Right 8 Hand Bursa and Ligament, Left 9 Upper Extremity Bursa and Ligament, Right B Upper Extremity Bursa and Ligament, Left C Trunk Bursa and Ligament, Right D Trunk Bursa and Ligament, Left F Thorax Bursa and Ligament, Right G Thorax Bursa and Ligament, Left H Abdomen Bursa and Ligament, Right J Abdomen Bursa and Ligament, Left K Perineum Bursa and Ligament L Hip Bursa and Ligament, Right M Hip Bursa and Ligament, Left N Knee Bursa and Ligament, Right P Knee Bursa and Ligament, Left Q Ankle Bursa and Ligament, Right R Ankle Bursa and Ligament, Left S Foot Bursa and Ligament, Right T Foot Bursa and Ligament, Left V Lower Extremity Bursa and Ligament, Right W Lower Extremity Bursa and Ligament, Left	0 Open 4 Percutaneous Endoscopic	Z No Device	Z No Qualifier

Section	0	Medical and Surgical
Body System	M	Bursae and Ligaments
Operation	N	Release: Freeing a body part from an abnormal physical constraint by cutting or by the use of force

Body Part (4th)	Approach (5th)	Device (6th)	Qualifier (7th)
0 Head and Neck Bursa and Ligament	0 Open	Z No Device	Z No Qualifier
1 Shoulder Bursa and Ligament, Right	3 Percutaneous		
2 Shoulder Bursa and Ligament, Left	4 Percutaneous Endoscopic		
3 Elbow Bursa and Ligament, Right	X External		
4 Elbow Bursa and Ligament, Left			
5 Wrist Bursa and Ligament, Right			
6 Wrist Bursa and Ligament, Left			
7 Hand Bursa and Ligament, Right			
8 Hand Bursa and Ligament, Left			
9 Upper Extremity Bursa and Ligament, Right			
B Upper Extremity Bursa and Ligament, Left			
C Trunk Bursa and Ligament, Right			
D Trunk Bursa and Ligament, Left			
F Thorax Bursa and Ligament, Right			
G Thorax Bursa and Ligament, Left			
H Abdomen Bursa and Ligament, Right			
J Abdomen Bursa and Ligament, Left			
K Perineum Bursa and Ligament			
L Hip Bursa and Ligament, Right			
M Hip Bursa and Ligament, Left			
N Knee Bursa and Ligament, Right			
P Knee Bursa and Ligament, Left			
Q Ankle Bursa and Ligament, Right			
R Ankle Bursa and Ligament, Left			
S Foot Bursa and Ligament, Right			
T Foot Bursa and Ligament, Left			
V Lower Extremity Bursa and Ligament, Right			
W Lower Extremity Bursa and Ligament, Left			

Section	0	Medical and Surgical
Body System	M	Bursae and Ligaments
Operation	P	Removal: Taking out or off a device from a body part

Body Part (4th)	Approach (5th)	Device (6th)	Qualifier (7th)
X Upper Bursa and Ligament	0 Open	0 Drainage Device	Z No Qualifier
Y Lower Bursa and Ligament	3 Percutaneous	7 Autologous Tissue Substitute	
	4 Percutaneous Endoscopic	J Synthetic Substitute	
		K Nonautologous Tissue Substitute	
X Upper Bursa and Ligament	X External	0 Drainage Device	Z No Qualifier
Y Lower Bursa and Ligament			

Section 0 Medical and Surgical
Body System M Bursae and Ligaments
Operation Q **Repair:** Restoring, to the extent possible, a body part to its normal anatomic structure and function

Body Part (4th)	Approach (5th)	Device (6th)	Qualifier (7th)
Head and Neck Bursa and Ligament Shoulder Bursa and Ligament, Right Shoulder Bursa and Ligament, Left Elbow Bursa and Ligament, Right Elbow Bursa and Ligament, Left Wrist Bursa and Ligament, Right Wrist Bursa and Ligament, Left Hand Bursa and Ligament, Right Hand Bursa and Ligament, Left Upper Extremity Bursa and Ligament, Right Upper Extremity Bursa and Ligament, Left Trunk Bursa and Ligament, Right Trunk Bursa and Ligament, Left Thorax Bursa and Ligament, Right Thorax Bursa and Ligament, Left Abdomen Bursa and Ligament, Right Abdomen Bursa and Ligament, Left Perineum Bursa and Ligament Hip Bursa and Ligament, Right Hip Bursa and Ligament, Left Knee Bursa and Ligament, Right Knee Bursa and Ligament, Left Ankle Bursa and Ligament, Right Ankle Bursa and Ligament, Left Foot Bursa and Ligament, Right Foot Bursa and Ligament, Left Lower Extremity Bursa and Ligament, Right Lower Extremity Bursa and Ligament, Left	**0** Open **3** Percutaneous **4** Percutaneous Endoscopic	**Z** No Device	**Z** No Qualifier

Section 0 Medical and Surgical
Body System M Bursae and Ligaments
Operation S **Reposition:** Moving to its normal location, or other suitable location, all or a portion of a body part

Body Part (4th)	Approach (5th)	Device (6th)	Qualifier (7th)
Head and Neck Bursa and Ligament Shoulder Bursa and Ligament, Right Shoulder Bursa and Ligament, Left Elbow Bursa and Ligament, Right Elbow Bursa and Ligament, Left Wrist Bursa and Ligament, Right Wrist Bursa and Ligament, Left Hand Bursa and Ligament, Right Hand Bursa and Ligament, Left Upper Extremity Bursa and Ligament, Right Upper Extremity Bursa and Ligament, Left Trunk Bursa and Ligament, Right Trunk Bursa and Ligament, Left Thorax Bursa and Ligament, Right Thorax Bursa and Ligament, Left Abdomen Bursa and Ligament, Right Abdomen Bursa and Ligament, Left Perineum Bursa and Ligament Hip Bursa and Ligament, Right Hip Bursa and Ligament, Left Knee Bursa and Ligament, Right Knee Bursa and Ligament, Left Ankle Bursa and Ligament, Right Ankle Bursa and Ligament, Left Foot Bursa and Ligament, Right Foot Bursa and Ligament, Left Lower Extremity Bursa and Ligament, Right Lower Extremity Bursa and Ligament, Left	**0** Open **4** Percutaneous Endoscopic	**Z** No Device	**Z** No Qualifier

Section   **0**   **Medical and Surgical**
Body System   **M**   **Bursae and Ligaments**
Operation   **T**   **Resection:** Cutting out or off, without replacement, all of a body part

Body Part (4th)	Approach (5th)	Device (6th)	Qualifier (7th)
0 Head and Neck Bursa and Ligament	0 Open	Z No Device	Z No Qualifier
1 Shoulder Bursa and Ligament, Right	4 Percutaneous Endoscopic		
2 Shoulder Bursa and Ligament, Left			
3 Elbow Bursa and Ligament, Right			
4 Elbow Bursa and Ligament, Left			
5 Wrist Bursa and Ligament, Right			
6 Wrist Bursa and Ligament, Left			
7 Hand Bursa and Ligament, Right			
8 Hand Bursa and Ligament, Left			
9 Upper Extremity Bursa and Ligament, Right			
B Upper Extremity Bursa and Ligament, Left			
C Trunk Bursa and Ligament, Right			
D Trunk Bursa and Ligament, Left			
F Thorax Bursa and Ligament, Right			
G Thorax Bursa and Ligament, Left			
H Abdomen Bursa and Ligament, Right			
J Abdomen Bursa and Ligament, Left			
K Perineum Bursa and Ligament			
L Hip Bursa and Ligament, Right			
M Hip Bursa and Ligament, Left			
N Knee Bursa and Ligament, Right			
P Knee Bursa and Ligament, Left			
Q Ankle Bursa and Ligament, Right			
R Ankle Bursa and Ligament, Left			
S Foot Bursa and Ligament, Right			
T Foot Bursa and Ligament, Left			
V Lower Extremity Bursa and Ligament, Right			
W Lower Extremity Bursa and Ligament, Left			

Section   **0**   **Medical and Surgical**
Body System   **M**   **Bursae and Ligaments**
Operation   **U**   **Supplement:** Putting in or on biological or synthetic material that physically reinforces and/or augments the function of a portion of a body part

Body Part (4th)	Approach (5th)	Device (6th)	Qualifier (7th)
0 Head and Neck Bursa and Ligament	0 Open	7 Autologous Tissue Substitute	Z No Qualifier
1 Shoulder Bursa and Ligament, Right	4 Percutaneous Endoscopic	J Synthetic Substitute	
2 Shoulder Bursa and Ligament, Left		K Nonautologous Tissue Substitute	
3 Elbow Bursa and Ligament, Right			
4 Elbow Bursa and Ligament, Left			
5 Wrist Bursa and Ligament, Right			
6 Wrist Bursa and Ligament, Left			
7 Hand Bursa and Ligament, Right			
8 Hand Bursa and Ligament, Left			
9 Upper Extremity Bursa and Ligament, Right			
B Upper Extremity Bursa and Ligament, Left			
C Trunk Bursa and Ligament, Right			
D Trunk Bursa and Ligament, Left			
F Thorax Bursa and Ligament, Right			
G Thorax Bursa and Ligament, Left			
H Abdomen Bursa and Ligament, Right			
J Abdomen Bursa and Ligament, Left			
K Perineum Bursa and Ligament			
L Hip Bursa and Ligament, Right			
M Hip Bursa and Ligament, Left			
N Knee Bursa and Ligament, Right			
P Knee Bursa and Ligament, Left			
Q Ankle Bursa and Ligament, Right			
R Ankle Bursa and Ligament, Left			
S Foot Bursa and Ligament, Right			
T Foot Bursa and Ligament, Left			
V Lower Extremity Bursa and Ligament, Right			
W Lower Extremity Bursa and Ligament, Left			

tion	0	Medical and Surgical
ly System	M	Bursae and Ligaments
eration	W	**Revision:** Correcting, to the extent possible, a portion of a malfunctioning device or the position of a displaced device

Body Part (4ᵗʰ)	Approach (5ᵗʰ)	Device (6ᵗʰ)	Qualifier (7ᵗʰ)
Upper Bursa and Ligament Lower Bursa and Ligament	0 Open 3 Percutaneous 4 Percutaneous Endoscopic X External	0 Drainage Device 7 Autologous Tissue Substitute J Synthetic Substitute K Nonautologous Tissue Substitute	Z No Qualifier

tion	0	Medical and Surgical
ly System	M	Bursae and Ligaments
eration	X	**Transfer:** Moving, without taking out, all or a portion of a body part to another location to take over the function of all or a portion of a body part

Body Part (4ᵗʰ)	Approach (5ᵗʰ)	Device (6ᵗʰ)	Qualifier (7ᵗʰ)
Head and Neck Bursa and Ligament Shoulder Bursa and Ligament, Right Shoulder Bursa and Ligament, Left Elbow Bursa and Ligament, Right Elbow Bursa and Ligament, Left Wrist Bursa and Ligament, Right Wrist Bursa and Ligament, Left Hand Bursa and Ligament, Right Hand Bursa and Ligament, Left Upper Extremity Bursa and Ligament, Right Upper Extremity Bursa and Ligament, Left Trunk Bursa and Ligament, Right Trunk Bursa and Ligament, Left Thorax Bursa and Ligament, Right Thorax Bursa and Ligament, Left Abdomen Bursa and Ligament, Right Abdomen Bursa and Ligament, Left Perineum Bursa and Ligament Hip Bursa and Ligament, Right Hip Bursa and Ligament, Left Knee Bursa and Ligament, Right Knee Bursa and Ligament, Left Ankle Bursa and Ligament, Right Ankle Bursa and Ligament, Left Foot Bursa and Ligament, Right Foot Bursa and Ligament, Left Lower Extremity Bursa and Ligament, Right Lower Extremity Bursa and Ligament, Left	0 Open 4 Percutaneous Endoscopic	Z No Device	Z No Qualifier

ursae and Ligaments Code Listing 0M2–0MX

eview Coding Guideline B4.5

M2 – Bursae and Ligaments, Change

M2XX0Z Change Drainage Device in Upper Bursa and Ligament, External Approach

M2XXYZ Change Other Device in Upper Bursa and Ligament, External Approach

0M2YX0Z Change Drainage Device in Lower Bursa and Ligament, External Approach

0M2YXYZ Change Other Device in Lower Bursa and Ligament, External Approach

M5 – Bursae and Ligaments, Destruction

eview Coding Guideline B6.1c

M500ZZ Destruction of Head and Neck Bursa and Ligament, Open Approach

M503ZZ Destruction of Head and Neck Bursa and Ligament, Percutaneous Approach

0M504ZZ Destruction of Head and Neck Bursa and Ligament, Percutaneous Endoscopic Approach

0M510ZZ Destruction of Right Shoulder Bursa and Ligament, Open Approach

0M513ZZ Destruction of Right Shoulder Bursa and Ligament, Percutaneous Approach

0M514ZZ Destruction of Right Shoulder Bursa and Ligament, Percutaneous Endoscopic Approach

Female-only	♂ Male-only	▲ Limited Coverage	● Non-OR	▨ HAC-associated procedure	▲ Non-covered procedures	+ Combination

0M520ZZ	Destruction of Left Shoulder Bursa and Ligament, Open Approach
0M523ZZ	Destruction of Left Shoulder Bursa and Ligament, Percutaneous Approach
0M524ZZ	Destruction of Left Shoulder Bursa and Ligament, Percutaneous Endoscopic Approach
0M530ZZ	Destruction of Right Elbow Bursa and Ligament, Open Approach
0M533ZZ	Destruction of Right Elbow Bursa and Ligament, Percutaneous Approach
0M534ZZ	Destruction of Right Elbow Bursa and Ligament, Percutaneous Endoscopic Approach
0M540ZZ	Destruction of Left Elbow Bursa and Ligament, Open Approach
0M543ZZ	Destruction of Left Elbow Bursa and Ligament, Percutaneous Approach
0M544ZZ	Destruction of Left Elbow Bursa and Ligament, Percutaneous Endoscopic Approach
0M550ZZ	Destruction of Right Wrist Bursa and Ligament, Open Approach
0M553ZZ	Destruction of Right Wrist Bursa and Ligament, Percutaneous Approach
0M554ZZ	Destruction of Right Wrist Bursa and Ligament, Percutaneous Endoscopic Approach
0M560ZZ	Destruction of Left Wrist Bursa and Ligament, Open Approach
0M563ZZ	Destruction of Left Wrist Bursa and Ligament, Percutaneous Approach
0M564ZZ	Destruction of Left Wrist Bursa and Ligament, Percutaneous Endoscopic Approach
0M570ZZ	Destruction of Right Hand Bursa and Ligament, Open Approach
0M573ZZ	Destruction of Right Hand Bursa and Ligament, Percutaneous Approach
0M574ZZ	Destruction of Right Hand Bursa and Ligament, Percutaneous Endoscopic Approach
0M580ZZ	Destruction of Left Hand Bursa and Ligament, Open Approach
0M583ZZ	Destruction of Left Hand Bursa and Ligament, Percutaneous Approach
0M584ZZ	Destruction of Left Hand Bursa and Ligament, Percutaneous Endoscopic Approach
0M590ZZ	Destruction of Right Upper Extremity Bursa and Ligament, Open Approach
0M593ZZ	Destruction of Right Upper Extremity Bursa and Ligament, Percutaneous Approach
0M594ZZ	Destruction of Right Upper Extremity Bursa and Ligament, Percutaneous Endoscopic Approach
0M5B0ZZ	Destruction of Left Upper Extremity Bursa and Ligament, Open Approach
0M5B3ZZ	Destruction of Left Upper Extremity Bursa and Ligament, Percutaneous Approach

0M5B4ZZ	Destruction of Left Upper Extremity Bursa and Ligament, Percutaneous Endoscopic Approach
0M5C0ZZ	Destruction of Right Trunk Bursa and Ligament, Open Approach
0M5C3ZZ	Destruction of Right Trunk Bursa and Ligament, Percutaneous Approach
0M5C4ZZ	Destruction of Right Trunk Bursa and Ligament, Percutaneous Endoscopic Approach
0M5D0ZZ	Destruction of Left Trunk Bursa and Ligament, Open Approach
0M5D3ZZ	Destruction of Left Trunk Bursa and Ligament, Percutaneous Approach
0M5D4ZZ	Destruction of Left Trunk Bursa and Ligament, Percutaneous Endoscopic Approach
0M5F0ZZ	Destruction of Right Thorax Bursa and Ligament, Open Approach
0M5F3ZZ	Destruction of Right Thorax Bursa and Ligament, Percutaneous Approach
0M5F4ZZ	Destruction of Right Thorax Bursa and Ligament, Percutaneous Endoscopic Approach
0M5G0ZZ	Destruction of Left Thorax Bursa and Ligament, Open Approach
0M5G3ZZ	Destruction of Left Thorax Bursa and Ligament, Percutaneous Approach
0M5G4ZZ	Destruction of Left Thorax Bursa and Ligament, Percutaneous Endoscopic Approach
0M5H0ZZ	Destruction of Right Abdomen Bursa and Ligament, Open Approach
0M5H3ZZ	Destruction of Right Abdomen Bursa and Ligament, Percutaneous Approach
0M5H4ZZ	Destruction of Right Abdomen Bursa and Ligament, Percutaneous Endoscopic Approach
0M5J0ZZ	Destruction of Left Abdomen Bursa and Ligament, Open Approach
0M5J3ZZ	Destruction of Left Abdomen Bursa and Ligament, Percutaneous Approach
0M5J4ZZ	Destruction of Left Abdomen Bursa and Ligament, Percutaneous Endoscopic Approach
0M5K0ZZ	Destruction of Perineum Bursa and Ligament, Open Approach
0M5K3ZZ	Destruction of Perineum Bursa and Ligament, Percutaneous Approach
0M5K4ZZ	Destruction of Perineum Bursa and Ligament, Percutaneous Endoscopic Approach
0M5L0ZZ	Destruction of Right Hip Bursa and Ligament, Open Approach
0M5L3ZZ	Destruction of Right Hip Bursa and Ligament, Percutaneous Approach
0M5L4ZZ	Destruction of Right Hip Bursa and Ligament, Percutaneous Endoscopic Approach
0M5M0ZZ	Destruction of Left Hip Bursa and Ligament, Open Approach
0M5M3ZZ	Destruction of Left Hip Bursa and Ligament, Percutaneous Approach

0M5M4ZZ	Destruction of Left Hip Bursa and Ligament, Percutaneous Endoscopic Approach
0M5N0ZZ	Destruction of Right Knee Bursa and Ligament, Open Approach
0M5N3ZZ	Destruction of Right Knee Bursa and Ligament, Percutaneous Approach
0M5N4ZZ	Destruction of Right Knee Bursa and Ligament, Percutaneous Endoscopic Approach
0M5P0ZZ	Destruction of Left Knee Bursa and Ligament, Open Approach
0M5P3ZZ	Destruction of Left Knee Bursa and Ligament, Percutaneous Approach
0M5P4ZZ	Destruction of Left Knee Bursa and Ligament, Percutaneous Endoscopic Approach
0M5Q0ZZ	Destruction of Right Ankle Bursa and Ligament, Open Approach
0M5Q3ZZ	Destruction of Right Ankle Bursa and Ligament, Percutaneous Approach
0M5Q4ZZ	Destruction of Right Ankle Bursa and Ligament, Percutaneous Endoscopic Approach
0M5R0ZZ	Destruction of Left Ankle Bursa and Ligament, Open Approach
0M5R3ZZ	Destruction of Left Ankle Bursa and Ligament, Percutaneous Approach
0M5R4ZZ	Destruction of Left Ankle Bursa and Ligament, Percutaneous Endoscopic Approach
0M5S0ZZ	Destruction of Right Foot Bursa and Ligament, Open Approach
0M5S3ZZ	Destruction of Right Foot Bursa and Ligament, Percutaneous Approach
0M5S4ZZ	Destruction of Right Foot Bursa and Ligament, Percutaneous Endoscopic Approach
0M5T0ZZ	Destruction of Left Foot Bursa and Ligament, Open Approach
0M5T3ZZ	Destruction of Left Foot Bursa and Ligament, Percutaneous Approach
0M5T4ZZ	Destruction of Left Foot Bursa and Ligament, Percutaneous Endoscopic Approach
0M5V0ZZ	Destruction of Right Lower Extremity Bursa and Ligament, Open Approach
0M5V3ZZ	Destruction of Right Lower Extremity Bursa and Ligament, Percutaneous Approach
0M5V4ZZ	Destruction of Right Lower Extremity Bursa and Ligament, Percutaneous Endoscopic Approach
0M5W0ZZ	Destruction of Left Lower Extremity Bursa and Ligament, Open Approach
0M5W3ZZ	Destruction of Left Lower Extremity Bursa and Ligament, Percutaneous Approach
0M5W4ZZ	Destruction of Left Lower Extremity Bursa and Ligament, Percutaneous Endoscopic Approach

0M8 – Bursae and Ligaments, Division

Review Coding Guideline B3.14

0M800ZZ	Division of Head and Neck Bursa and Ligament, Open Approach
0M803ZZ	Division of Head and Neck Bursa and Ligament, Percutaneous Approach
0M804ZZ	Division of Head and Neck Bursa and Ligament, Percutaneous Endoscopic Approach

0M810ZZ	Division of Right Shoulder Bursa and Ligament, Open Approach
0M813ZZ	Division of Right Shoulder Bursa and Ligament, Percutaneous Approach
0M814ZZ	Division of Right Shoulder Bursa and Ligament, Percutaneous Endoscopic Approach

0M820ZZ	Division of Left Shoulder Bursa and Ligament, Open Approach
0M823ZZ	Division of Left Shoulder Bursa and Ligament, Percutaneous Approach
0M824ZZ	Division of Left Shoulder Bursa and Ligament, Percutaneous Endoscopic Approach

♀ Female-only   ♂ Male-only   ▲ Limited Coverage   ● Non-OR   ▦ HAC-associated procedure   ▲ Non-covered procedures   ✚ Combinatic

30ZZ Division of Right Elbow Bursa and Ligament, Open Approach	**0M8C3ZZ** Division of Right Trunk Bursa and Ligament, Percutaneous Approach	**0M8M4ZZ** Division of Left Hip Bursa and Ligament, Percutaneous Endoscopic Approach
33ZZ Division of Right Elbow Bursa and Ligament, Percutaneous Approach	**0M8C4ZZ** Division of Right Trunk Bursa and Ligament, Percutaneous Endoscopic Approach	**0M8N0ZZ** Division of Right Knee Bursa and Ligament, Open Approach
34ZZ Division of Right Elbow Bursa and Ligament, Percutaneous Endoscopic Approach	**0M8D0ZZ** Division of Left Trunk Bursa and Ligament, Open Approach	**0M8N3ZZ** Division of Right Knee Bursa and Ligament, Percutaneous Approach
40ZZ Division of Left Elbow Bursa and Ligament, Open Approach	**0M8D3ZZ** Division of Left Trunk Bursa and Ligament, Percutaneous Approach	**0M8N4ZZ** Division of Right Knee Bursa and Ligament, Percutaneous Endoscopic Approach
43ZZ Division of Left Elbow Bursa and Ligament, Percutaneous Approach	**0M8D4ZZ** Division of Left Trunk Bursa and Ligament, Percutaneous Endoscopic Approach	**0M8P0ZZ** Division of Left Knee Bursa and Ligament, Open Approach
44ZZ Division of Left Elbow Bursa and Ligament, Percutaneous Endoscopic Approach	**0M8F0ZZ** Division of Right Thorax Bursa and Ligament, Open Approach	**0M8P3ZZ** Division of Left Knee Bursa and Ligament, Percutaneous Approach
50ZZ Division of Right Wrist Bursa and Ligament, Open Approach	**0M8F3ZZ** Division of Right Thorax Bursa and Ligament, Percutaneous Approach	**0M8P4ZZ** Division of Left Knee Bursa and Ligament, Percutaneous Endoscopic Approach
53ZZ Division of Right Wrist Bursa and Ligament, Percutaneous Approach	**0M8F4ZZ** Division of Right Thorax Bursa and Ligament, Percutaneous Endoscopic Approach	**0M8Q0ZZ** Division of Right Ankle Bursa and Ligament, Open Approach
54ZZ Division of Right Wrist Bursa and Ligament, Percutaneous Endoscopic Approach	**0M8G0ZZ** Division of Left Thorax Bursa and Ligament, Open Approach	**0M8Q3ZZ** Division of Right Ankle Bursa and Ligament, Percutaneous Approach
60ZZ Division of Left Wrist Bursa and Ligament, Open Approach	**0M8G3ZZ** Division of Left Thorax Bursa and Ligament, Percutaneous Approach	**0M8Q4ZZ** Division of Right Ankle Bursa and Ligament, Percutaneous Endoscopic Approach
63ZZ Division of Left Wrist Bursa and Ligament, Percutaneous Approach	**0M8G4ZZ** Division of Left Thorax Bursa and Ligament, Percutaneous Endoscopic Approach	**0M8R0ZZ** Division of Left Ankle Bursa and Ligament, Open Approach
64ZZ Division of Left Wrist Bursa and Ligament, Percutaneous Endoscopic Approach	**0M8H0ZZ** Division of Right Abdomen Bursa and Ligament, Open Approach	**0M8R3ZZ** Division of Left Ankle Bursa and Ligament, Percutaneous Approach
70ZZ Division of Right Hand Bursa and Ligament, Open Approach	**0M8H3ZZ** Division of Right Abdomen Bursa and Ligament, Percutaneous Approach	**0M8R4ZZ** Division of Left Ankle Bursa and Ligament, Percutaneous Endoscopic Approach
73ZZ Division of Right Hand Bursa and Ligament, Percutaneous Approach	**0M8H4ZZ** Division of Right Abdomen Bursa and Ligament, Percutaneous Endoscopic Approach	**0M8S0ZZ** Division of Right Foot Bursa and Ligament, Open Approach
74ZZ Division of Right Hand Bursa and Ligament, Percutaneous Endoscopic Approach	**0M8J0ZZ** Division of Left Abdomen Bursa and Ligament, Open Approach	**0M8S3ZZ** Division of Right Foot Bursa and Ligament, Percutaneous Approach
80ZZ Division of Left Hand Bursa and Ligament, Open Approach	**0M8J3ZZ** Division of Left Abdomen Bursa and Ligament, Percutaneous Approach	**0M8S4ZZ** Division of Right Foot Bursa and Ligament, Percutaneous Endoscopic Approach
83ZZ Division of Left Hand Bursa and Ligament, Percutaneous Approach	**0M8J4ZZ** Division of Left Abdomen Bursa and Ligament, Percutaneous Endoscopic Approach	**0M8T0ZZ** Division of Left Foot Bursa and Ligament, Open Approach
84ZZ Division of Left Hand Bursa and Ligament, Percutaneous Endoscopic Approach	**0M8K0ZZ** Division of Perineum Bursa and Ligament, Open Approach	**0M8T3ZZ** Division of Left Foot Bursa and Ligament, Percutaneous Approach
90ZZ Division of Right Upper Extremity Bursa and Ligament, Open Approach	**0M8K3ZZ** Division of Perineum Bursa and Ligament, Percutaneous Approach	**0M8T4ZZ** Division of Left Foot Bursa and Ligament, Percutaneous Endoscopic Approach
93ZZ Division of Right Upper Extremity Bursa and Ligament, Percutaneous Approach	**0M8K4ZZ** Division of Perineum Bursa and Ligament, Percutaneous Endoscopic Approach	**0M8V0ZZ** Division of Right Lower Extremity Bursa and Ligament, Open Approach
94ZZ Division of Right Upper Extremity Bursa and Ligament, Percutaneous Endoscopic Approach	**0M8L0ZZ** Division of Right Hip Bursa and Ligament, Open Approach	**0M8V3ZZ** Division of Right Lower Extremity Bursa and Ligament, Percutaneous Approach
8B0ZZ Division of Left Upper Extremity Bursa and Ligament, Open Approach	**0M8L3ZZ** Division of Right Hip Bursa and Ligament, Percutaneous Approach	**0M8V4ZZ** Division of Right Lower Extremity Bursa and Ligament, Percutaneous Endoscopic Approach
8B3ZZ Division of Left Upper Extremity Bursa and Ligament, Percutaneous Approach	**0M8L4ZZ** Division of Right Hip Bursa and Ligament, Percutaneous Endoscopic Approach	**0M8W0ZZ** Division of Left Lower Extremity Bursa and Ligament, Open Approach
8B4ZZ Division of Left Upper Extremity Bursa and Ligament, Percutaneous Endoscopic Approach	**0M8M0ZZ** Division of Left Hip Bursa and Ligament, Open Approach	**0M8W3ZZ** Division of Left Lower Extremity Bursa and Ligament, Percutaneous Approach
8C0ZZ Division of Right Trunk Bursa and Ligament, Open Approach	**0M8M3ZZ** Division of Left Hip Bursa and Ligament, Percutaneous Approach	**0M8W4ZZ** Division of Left Lower Extremity Bursa and Ligament, Percutaneous Endoscopic Approach

9 – Bursae and Ligaments, Drainage

view Coding Guidelines B3.4a and B3.4b

view Coding Guideline B6.2

9000Z Drainage of Head and Neck Bursa and Ligament with Drainage Device, Open Approach	**0M9030Z** Drainage of Head and Neck Bursa and Ligament with Drainage Device, Percutaneous Approach	**0M9040Z** Drainage of Head and Neck Bursa and Ligament with Drainage Device, Percutaneous Endoscopic Approach
900ZX Drainage of Head and Neck Bursa and Ligament, Open Approach, Diagnostic	**0M903ZX** Drainage of Head and Neck Bursa and Ligament, Percutaneous Approach, Diagnostic	**0M904ZX** Drainage of Head and Neck Bursa and Ligament, Percutaneous Endoscopic Approach, Diagnostic
900ZZ Drainage of Head and Neck Bursa and Ligament, Open Approach	**0M903ZZ** Drainage of Head and Neck Bursa and Ligament, Percutaneous Approach	**0M904ZZ** Drainage of Head and Neck Bursa and Ligament, Percutaneous Endoscopic Approach

0M9100Z   Drainage of Right Shoulder Bursa and Ligament with Drainage Device, Open Approach

0M910ZX   Drainage of Right Shoulder Bursa and Ligament, Open Approach, Diagnostic

0M910ZZ   Drainage of Right Shoulder Bursa and Ligament, Open Approach

0M9130Z   Drainage of Right Shoulder Bursa and Ligament with Drainage Device, Percutaneous Approach

0M913ZX   Drainage of Right Shoulder Bursa and Ligament, Percutaneous Approach, Diagnostic

0M913ZZ   Drainage of Right Shoulder Bursa and Ligament, Percutaneous Approach

0M9140Z   Drainage of Right Shoulder Bursa and Ligament with Drainage Device, Percutaneous Endoscopic Approach

0M914ZX   Drainage of Right Shoulder Bursa and Ligament, Percutaneous Endoscopic Approach, Diagnostic

0M914ZZ   Drainage of Right Shoulder Bursa and Ligament, Percutaneous Endoscopic Approach

0M9200Z   Drainage of Left Shoulder Bursa and Ligament with Drainage Device, Open Approach

0M920ZX   Drainage of Left Shoulder Bursa and Ligament, Open Approach, Diagnostic

0M920ZZ   Drainage of Left Shoulder Bursa and Ligament, Open Approach

0M9230Z   Drainage of Left Shoulder Bursa and Ligament with Drainage Device, Percutaneous Approach

0M923ZX   Drainage of Left Shoulder Bursa and Ligament, Percutaneous Approach, Diagnostic

0M923ZZ   Drainage of Left Shoulder Bursa and Ligament, Percutaneous Approach

0M9240Z   Drainage of Left Shoulder Bursa and Ligament with Drainage Device, Percutaneous Endoscopic Approach

0M924ZX   Drainage of Left Shoulder Bursa and Ligament, Percutaneous Endoscopic Approach, Diagnostic

0M924ZZ   Drainage of Left Shoulder Bursa and Ligament, Percutaneous Endoscopic Approach

0M9300Z   Drainage of Right Elbow Bursa and Ligament with Drainage Device, Open Approach

0M930ZX   Drainage of Right Elbow Bursa and Ligament, Open Approach, Diagnostic

0M930ZZ   Drainage of Right Elbow Bursa and Ligament, Open Approach

0M9330Z   Drainage of Right Elbow Bursa and Ligament with Drainage Device, Percutaneous Approach

0M933ZX   Drainage of Right Elbow Bursa and Ligament, Percutaneous Approach, Diagnostic

0M933ZZ   Drainage of Right Elbow Bursa and Ligament, Percutaneous Approach

0M9340Z   Drainage of Right Elbow Bursa and Ligament with Drainage Device, Percutaneous Endoscopic Approach

0M934ZX   Drainage of Right Elbow Bursa and Ligament, Percutaneous Endoscopic Approach, Diagnostic

0M934ZZ   Drainage of Right Elbow Bursa and Ligament, Percutaneous Endoscopic Approach

0M9400Z   Drainage of Left Elbow Bursa and Ligament with Drainage Device, Open Approach

0M940ZX   Drainage of Left Elbow Bursa and Ligament, Open Approach, Diagnostic

0M940ZZ   Drainage of Left Elbow Bursa and Ligament, Open Approach

0M9430Z   Drainage of Left Elbow Bursa and Ligament with Drainage Device, Percutaneous Approach

0M943ZX   Drainage of Left Elbow Bursa and Ligament, Percutaneous Approach, Diagnostic

0M943ZZ   Drainage of Left Elbow Bursa and Ligament, Percutaneous Approach

0M9440Z   Drainage of Left Elbow Bursa and Ligament with Drainage Device, Percutaneous Endoscopic Approach

0M944ZX   Drainage of Left Elbow Bursa and Ligament, Percutaneous Endoscopic Approach, Diagnostic

0M944ZZ   Drainage of Left Elbow Bursa and Ligament, Percutaneous Endoscopic Approach

0M9500Z   Drainage of Right Wrist Bursa and Ligament with Drainage Device, Open Approach

0M950ZX   Drainage of Right Wrist Bursa and Ligament, Open Approach, Diagnostic

0M950ZZ   Drainage of Right Wrist Bursa and Ligament, Open Approach

0M9530Z   Drainage of Right Wrist Bursa and Ligament with Drainage Device, Percutaneous Approach

0M953ZX   Drainage of Right Wrist Bursa and Ligament, Percutaneous Approach, Diagnostic

0M953ZZ   Drainage of Right Wrist Bursa and Ligament, Percutaneous Approach

0M9540Z   Drainage of Right Wrist Bursa and Ligament with Drainage Device, Percutaneous Endoscopic Approach

0M954ZX   Drainage of Right Wrist Bursa and Ligament, Percutaneous Endoscopic Approach, Diagnostic

0M954ZZ   Drainage of Right Wrist Bursa and Ligament, Percutaneous Endoscopic Approach

0M9600Z   Drainage of Left Wrist Bursa and Ligament with Drainage Device, Open Approach

0M960ZX   Drainage of Left Wrist Bursa and Ligament, Open Approach, Diagnostic

0M960ZZ   Drainage of Left Wrist Bursa and Ligament, Open Approach

0M9630Z   Drainage of Left Wrist Bursa and Ligament with Drainage Device, Percutaneous Approach

0M963ZX   Drainage of Left Wrist Bursa and Ligament, Percutaneous Approach, Diagnostic

0M963ZZ   Drainage of Left Wrist Bursa and Ligament, Percutaneous Approach

0M9640Z   Drainage of Left Wrist Bursa and Ligament with Drainage Device, Percutaneous Endoscopic Approach

0M964ZX   Drainage of Left Wrist Bursa and Ligament, Percutaneous Endoscopic Approach, Diagnostic

0M964ZZ   Drainage of Left Wrist Bursa and Ligament, Percutaneous Endoscopic Approach

0M9700Z   Drainage of Right Hand Bursa and Ligament with Drainage Device, Open Approach

0M970ZX   Drainage of Right Hand Bursa and Ligament, Open Approach, Diagnostic

0M970ZZ   Drainage of Right Hand Bursa and Ligament, Open Approach

0M9730Z   Drainage of Right Hand Bursa and Ligament with Drainage Device, Percutaneous Approach

0M973ZX   Drainage of Right Hand Bursa and Ligament, Percutaneous Approach, Diagnostic

0M973ZZ   Drainage of Right Hand Bursa and Ligament, Percutaneous Approach

0M9740Z   Drainage of Right Hand Bursa and Ligament with Drainage Device, Percutaneous Endoscopic Approach

0M974ZX   Drainage of Right Hand Bursa and Ligament, Percutaneous Endoscopic Approach, Diagnostic

0M974ZZ   Drainage of Right Hand Bursa and Ligament, Percutaneous Endoscopic Approach

0M9800Z   Drainage of Left Hand Bursa and Ligament with Drainage Device, Open Approach

0M980ZX   Drainage of Left Hand Bursa and Ligament, Open Approach, Diagnostic

0M980ZZ   Drainage of Left Hand Bursa and Ligament, Open Approach

0M9830Z   Drainage of Left Hand Bursa and Ligament with Drainage Device, Percutaneous Approach

0M983ZX   Drainage of Left Hand Bursa and Ligament, Percutaneous Approach, Diagnostic

0M983ZZ   Drainage of Left Hand Bursa and Ligament, Percutaneous Approach

0M9840Z   Drainage of Left Hand Bursa and Ligament with Drainage Device, Percutaneous Endoscopic Approach

0M984ZX   Drainage of Left Hand Bursa and Ligament, Percutaneous Endoscopic Approach, Diagnostic

0M984ZZ   Drainage of Left Hand Bursa and Ligament, Percutaneous Endoscopic Approach

0M9900Z   Drainage of Right Upper Extremity Bursa and Ligament with Drainage Device, Open Approach

0M990ZX   Drainage of Right Upper Extremity Bursa and Ligament, Open Approach, Diagnostic

0M990ZZ   Drainage of Right Upper Extremity Bursa and Ligament, Open Approach

0M9930Z   Drainage of Right Upper Extremity Bursa and Ligament with Drainage Device, Percutaneous Approach

0M993ZX   Drainage of Right Upper Extremity Bursa and Ligament, Percutaneous Approach, Diagnostic

0M993ZZ   Drainage of Right Upper Extremity Bursa and Ligament, Percutaneous Approach

0M9940Z   Drainage of Right Upper Extremity Bursa and Ligament with Drainage Device, Percutaneous Endoscopic Approach

0M994ZX   Drainage of Right Upper Extremity Bursa and Ligament, Percutaneous Endoscopic Approach, Diagnostic

0M994ZZ   Drainage of Right Upper Extremity Bursa and Ligament, Percutaneous Endoscopic Approach

0M9B00Z   Drainage of Left Upper Extremity Bursa and Ligament with Drainage Device, Open Approach

0M9B0ZX   Drainage of Left Upper Extremity Bursa and Ligament, Open Approach, Diagnostic

0M9B0ZZ   Drainage of Left Upper Extremity Bursa and Ligament, Open Approach

0M9B30Z   Drainage of Left Upper Extremity Bursa and Ligament with Drainage Device, Percutaneous Approach

B3ZX Drainage of Left Upper Extremity Bursa and Ligament, Percutaneous Approach, Diagnostic

B3ZZ Drainage of Left Upper Extremity Bursa and Ligament, Percutaneous Approach

B40Z Drainage of Left Upper Extremity Bursa and Ligament with Drainage Device, Percutaneous Endoscopic Approach

B4ZX Drainage of Left Upper Extremity Bursa and Ligament, Percutaneous Endoscopic Approach, Diagnostic

B4ZZ Drainage of Left Upper Extremity Bursa and Ligament, Percutaneous Endoscopic Approach

C00Z Drainage of Right Trunk Bursa and Ligament with Drainage Device, Open Approach

C0ZX Drainage of Right Trunk Bursa and Ligament, Open Approach, Diagnostic

C0ZZ Drainage of Right Trunk Bursa and Ligament, Open Approach

C30Z Drainage of Right Trunk Bursa and Ligament with Drainage Device, Percutaneous Approach

C3ZX Drainage of Right Trunk Bursa and Ligament, Percutaneous Approach, Diagnostic

C3ZZ Drainage of Right Trunk Bursa and Ligament, Percutaneous Approach

C40Z Drainage of Right Trunk Bursa and Ligament with Drainage Device, Percutaneous Endoscopic Approach

C4ZX Drainage of Right Trunk Bursa and Ligament, Percutaneous Endoscopic Approach, Diagnostic

C4ZZ Drainage of Right Trunk Bursa and Ligament, Percutaneous Endoscopic Approach

9D00Z Drainage of Left Trunk Bursa and Ligament with Drainage Device, Open Approach

9D0ZX Drainage of Left Trunk Bursa and Ligament, Open Approach, Diagnostic

9D0ZZ Drainage of Left Trunk Bursa and Ligament, Open Approach

9D30Z Drainage of Left Trunk Bursa and Ligament with Drainage Device, Percutaneous Approach

9D3ZX Drainage of Left Trunk Bursa and Ligament, Percutaneous Approach, Diagnostic

9D3ZZ Drainage of Left Trunk Bursa and Ligament, Percutaneous Approach

9D40Z Drainage of Left Trunk Bursa and Ligament with Drainage Device, Percutaneous Endoscopic Approach

9D4ZX Drainage of Left Trunk Bursa and Ligament, Percutaneous Endoscopic Approach, Diagnostic

9D4ZZ Drainage of Left Trunk Bursa and Ligament, Percutaneous Endoscopic Approach

9F00Z Drainage of Right Thorax Bursa and Ligament with Drainage Device, Open Approach

9F0ZX Drainage of Right Thorax Bursa and Ligament, Open Approach, Diagnostic

9F0ZZ Drainage of Right Thorax Bursa and Ligament, Open Approach

9F30Z Drainage of Right Thorax Bursa and Ligament with Drainage Device, Percutaneous Approach

9F3ZX Drainage of Right Thorax Bursa and Ligament, Percutaneous Approach, Diagnostic

9F3ZZ Drainage of Right Thorax Bursa and Ligament, Percutaneous Approach

0M9F40Z Drainage of Right Thorax Bursa and Ligament with Drainage Device, Percutaneous Endoscopic Approach

0M9F4ZX Drainage of Right Thorax Bursa and Ligament, Percutaneous Endoscopic Approach, Diagnostic

0M9F4ZZ Drainage of Right Thorax Bursa and Ligament, Percutaneous Endoscopic Approach

0M9G00Z Drainage of Left Thorax Bursa and Ligament with Drainage Device, Open Approach

0M9G0ZX Drainage of Left Thorax Bursa and Ligament, Open Approach, Diagnostic

0M9G0ZZ Drainage of Left Thorax Bursa and Ligament, Open Approach

0M9G30Z Drainage of Left Thorax Bursa and Ligament with Drainage Device, Percutaneous Approach

0M9G3ZX Drainage of Left Thorax Bursa and Ligament, Percutaneous Approach, Diagnostic

0M9G3ZZ Drainage of Left Thorax Bursa and Ligament, Percutaneous Approach

0M9G40Z Drainage of Left Thorax Bursa and Ligament with Drainage Device, Percutaneous Endoscopic Approach

0M9G4ZX Drainage of Left Thorax Bursa and Ligament, Percutaneous Endoscopic Approach, Diagnostic

0M9G4ZZ Drainage of Left Thorax Bursa and Ligament, Percutaneous Endoscopic Approach

0M9H00Z Drainage of Right Abdomen Bursa and Ligament with Drainage Device, Open Approach

0M9H0ZX Drainage of Right Abdomen Bursa and Ligament, Open Approach, Diagnostic

0M9H0ZZ Drainage of Right Abdomen Bursa and Ligament, Open Approach

0M9H30Z Drainage of Right Abdomen Bursa and Ligament with Drainage Device, Percutaneous Approach

0M9H3ZX Drainage of Right Abdomen Bursa and Ligament, Percutaneous Approach, Diagnostic

0M9H3ZZ Drainage of Right Abdomen Bursa and Ligament, Percutaneous Approach

0M9H40Z Drainage of Right Abdomen Bursa and Ligament with Drainage Device, Percutaneous Endoscopic Approach

0M9H4ZX Drainage of Right Abdomen Bursa and Ligament, Percutaneous Endoscopic Approach, Diagnostic

0M9H4ZZ Drainage of Right Abdomen Bursa and Ligament, Percutaneous Endoscopic Approach

0M9J00Z Drainage of Left Abdomen Bursa and Ligament with Drainage Device, Open Approach

0M9J0ZX Drainage of Left Abdomen Bursa and Ligament, Open Approach, Diagnostic

0M9J0ZZ Drainage of Left Abdomen Bursa and Ligament, Open Approach

0M9J30Z Drainage of Left Abdomen Bursa and Ligament with Drainage Device, Percutaneous Approach

0M9J3ZX Drainage of Left Abdomen Bursa and Ligament, Percutaneous Approach, Diagnostic

0M9J3ZZ Drainage of Left Abdomen Bursa and Ligament, Percutaneous Approach

0M9J40Z Drainage of Left Abdomen Bursa and Ligament with Drainage Device, Percutaneous Endoscopic Approach

0M9J4ZX Drainage of Left Abdomen Bursa and Ligament, Percutaneous Endoscopic Approach, Diagnostic

0M9J4ZZ Drainage of Left Abdomen Bursa and Ligament, Percutaneous Endoscopic Approach

0M9K00Z Drainage of Perineum Bursa and Ligament with Drainage Device, Open Approach

0M9K0ZX Drainage of Perineum Bursa and Ligament, Open Approach, Diagnostic

0M9K0ZZ Drainage of Perineum Bursa and Ligament, Open Approach

0M9K30Z Drainage of Perineum Bursa and Ligament with Drainage Device, Percutaneous Approach

0M9K3ZX Drainage of Perineum Bursa and Ligament, Percutaneous Approach, Diagnostic

0M9K3ZZ Drainage of Perineum Bursa and Ligament, Percutaneous Approach

0M9K40Z Drainage of Perineum Bursa and Ligament with Drainage Device, Percutaneous Endoscopic Approach

0M9K4ZX Drainage of Perineum Bursa and Ligament, Percutaneous Endoscopic Approach, Diagnostic

0M9K4ZZ Drainage of Perineum Bursa and Ligament, Percutaneous Endoscopic Approach

0M9L00Z Drainage of Right Hip Bursa and Ligament with Drainage Device, Open Approach

0M9L0ZX Drainage of Right Hip Bursa and Ligament, Open Approach, Diagnostic

0M9L0ZZ Drainage of Right Hip Bursa and Ligament, Open Approach

0M9L30Z Drainage of Right Hip Bursa and Ligament with Drainage Device, Percutaneous Approach

0M9L3ZX Drainage of Right Hip Bursa and Ligament, Percutaneous Approach, Diagnostic

0M9L3ZZ Drainage of Right Hip Bursa and Ligament, Percutaneous Approach

0M9L40Z Drainage of Right Hip Bursa and Ligament with Drainage Device, Percutaneous Endoscopic Approach

0M9L4ZX Drainage of Right Hip Bursa and Ligament, Percutaneous Endoscopic Approach, Diagnostic

0M9L4ZZ Drainage of Right Hip Bursa and Ligament, Percutaneous Endoscopic Approach

0M9M00Z Drainage of Left Hip Bursa and Ligament with Drainage Device, Open Approach

0M9M0ZX Drainage of Left Hip Bursa and Ligament, Open Approach, Diagnostic

0M9M0ZZ Drainage of Left Hip Bursa and Ligament, Open Approach

0M9M30Z Drainage of Left Hip Bursa and Ligament with Drainage Device, Percutaneous Approach

0M9M3ZX Drainage of Left Hip Bursa and Ligament, Percutaneous Approach, Diagnostic

0M9M3ZZ Drainage of Left Hip Bursa and Ligament, Percutaneous Approach

0M9M40Z Drainage of Left Hip Bursa and Ligament with Drainage Device, Percutaneous Endoscopic Approach

0M9M4ZX Drainage of Left Hip Bursa and Ligament, Percutaneous Endoscopic Approach, Diagnostic

0M9M4ZZ Drainage of Left Hip Bursa and Ligament, Percutaneous Endoscopic Approach

Female-only   ♂ Male-only   ▲ Limited Coverage   ● Non-OR   ▥ HAC-associated procedure   ▲ Non-covered procedures   ✚ Combination

0M9N00Z   Drainage of Right Knee Bursa and Ligament with Drainage Device, Open Approach

0M9N0ZX   Drainage of Right Knee Bursa and Ligament, Open Approach, Diagnostic

0M9N0ZZ   Drainage of Right Knee Bursa and Ligament, Open Approach

0M9N30Z   Drainage of Right Knee Bursa and Ligament with Drainage Device, Percutaneous Approach

0M9N3ZX   Drainage of Right Knee Bursa and Ligament, Percutaneous Approach, Diagnostic

0M9N3ZZ   Drainage of Right Knee Bursa and Ligament, Percutaneous Approach

0M9N40Z   Drainage of Right Knee Bursa and Ligament with Drainage Device, Percutaneous Endoscopic Approach

0M9N4ZX   Drainage of Right Knee Bursa and Ligament, Percutaneous Endoscopic Approach, Diagnostic

0M9N4ZZ   Drainage of Right Knee Bursa and Ligament, Percutaneous Endoscopic Approach

0M9P00Z   Drainage of Left Knee Bursa and Ligament with Drainage Device, Open Approach

0M9P0ZX   Drainage of Left Knee Bursa and Ligament, Open Approach, Diagnostic

0M9P0ZZ   Drainage of Left Knee Bursa and Ligament, Open Approach

0M9P30Z   Drainage of Left Knee Bursa and Ligament with Drainage Device, Percutaneous Approach

0M9P3ZX   Drainage of Left Knee Bursa and Ligament, Percutaneous Approach, Diagnostic

0M9P3ZZ   Drainage of Left Knee Bursa and Ligament, Percutaneous Approach

0M9P40Z   Drainage of Left Knee Bursa and Ligament with Drainage Device, Percutaneous Endoscopic Approach

0M9P4ZX   Drainage of Left Knee Bursa and Ligament, Percutaneous Endoscopic Approach, Diagnostic

0M9P4ZZ   Drainage of Left Knee Bursa and Ligament, Percutaneous Endoscopic Approach

0M9Q00Z   Drainage of Right Ankle Bursa and Ligament with Drainage Device, Open Approach

0M9Q0ZX   Drainage of Right Ankle Bursa and Ligament, Open Approach, Diagnostic

0M9Q0ZZ   Drainage of Right Ankle Bursa and Ligament, Open Approach

0M9Q30Z   Drainage of Right Ankle Bursa and Ligament with Drainage Device, Percutaneous Approach

0M9Q3ZX   Drainage of Right Ankle Bursa and Ligament, Percutaneous Approach, Diagnostic

0M9Q3ZZ   Drainage of Right Ankle Bursa and Ligament, Percutaneous Approach

0M9Q40Z   Drainage of Right Ankle Bursa and Ligament with Drainage Device, Percutaneous Endoscopic Approach

0M9Q4ZX   Drainage of Right Ankle Bursa and Ligament, Percutaneous Endoscopic Approach, Diagnostic

0M9Q4ZZ   Drainage of Right Ankle Bursa and Ligament, Percutaneous Endoscopic Approach

0M9R00Z   Drainage of Left Ankle Bursa and Ligament with Drainage Device, Open Approach

0M9R0ZX   Drainage of Left Ankle Bursa and Ligament, Open Approach, Diagnostic

0M9R0ZZ   Drainage of Left Ankle Bursa and Ligament, Open Approach

0M9R30Z   Drainage of Left Ankle Bursa and Ligament with Drainage Device, Percutaneous Approach

0M9R3ZX   Drainage of Left Ankle Bursa and Ligament, Percutaneous Approach, Diagnostic

0M9R3ZZ   Drainage of Left Ankle Bursa and Ligament, Percutaneous Approach

0M9R40Z   Drainage of Left Ankle Bursa and Ligament with Drainage Device, Percutaneous Endoscopic Approach

0M9R4ZX   Drainage of Left Ankle Bursa and Ligament, Percutaneous Endoscopic Approach, Diagnostic

0M9R4ZZ   Drainage of Left Ankle Bursa and Ligament, Percutaneous Endoscopic Approach

0M9S00Z   Drainage of Right Foot Bursa and Ligament with Drainage Device, Open Approach

0M9S0ZX   Drainage of Right Foot Bursa and Ligament, Open Approach, Diagnostic

0M9S0ZZ   Drainage of Right Foot Bursa and Ligament, Open Approach

0M9S30Z   Drainage of Right Foot Bursa and Ligament with Drainage Device, Percutaneous Approach

0M9S3ZX   Drainage of Right Foot Bursa and Ligament, Percutaneous Approach, Diagnostic

0M9S3ZZ   Drainage of Right Foot Bursa and Ligament, Percutaneous Approach

0M9S40Z   Drainage of Right Foot Bursa and Ligament with Drainage Device, Percutaneous Endoscopic Approach

0M9S4ZX   Drainage of Right Foot Bursa and Ligament, Percutaneous Endoscopic Approach, Diagnostic

0M9S4ZZ   Drainage of Right Foot Bursa and Ligament, Percutaneous Endoscopic Approach

0M9T00Z   Drainage of Left Foot Bursa and Ligament with Drainage Device, Open Approach

0M9T0ZX   Drainage of Left Foot Bursa and Ligament, Open Approach, Diagnostic

0M9T0ZZ   Drainage of Left Foot Bursa and Ligament, Open Approach

0M9T30Z   Drainage of Left Foot Bursa and Ligament with Drainage Device, Percutaneous Approach

0M9T3ZX   Drainage of Left Foot Bursa and Ligament, Percutaneous Approach, Diagnostic

0M9T3ZZ   Drainage of Left Foot Bursa and Ligament, Percutaneous Approach

0M9T40Z   Drainage of Left Foot Bursa and Ligament with Drainage Device, Percutaneous Endoscopic Approach

0M9T4ZX   Drainage of Left Foot Bursa and Ligament, Percutaneous Endoscopic Approach, Diagnostic

0M9T4ZZ   Drainage of Left Foot Bursa and Ligament, Percutaneous Endoscopic Approach

0M9V00Z   Drainage of Right Lower Extremity Bursa and Ligament with Drainage Device, Open Approach

0M9V0ZX   Drainage of Right Lower Extremity Bursa and Ligament, Open Approach, Diagnostic

0M9V0ZZ   Drainage of Right Lower Extremity Bursa and Ligament, Open Approach

0M9V30Z   Drainage of Right Lower Extremity Bursa and Ligament with Drainage Device, Percutaneous Approach

0M9V3ZX   Drainage of Right Lower Extremity Bursa and Ligament, Percutaneous Approach, Diagnostic

0M9V3ZZ   Drainage of Right Lower Extremity Bursa and Ligament, Percutaneous Approach

0M9V40Z   Drainage of Right Lower Extremity Bursa and Ligament with Drainage Device, Percutaneous Endoscopic Approach

0M9V4ZX   Drainage of Right Lower Extremity Bursa and Ligament, Percutaneous Endoscopic Approach, Diagnostic

0M9V4ZZ   Drainage of Right Lower Extremity Bursa and Ligament, Percutaneous Endoscopic Approach

0M9W00Z   Drainage of Left Lower Extremity Bursa and Ligament with Drainage Device, Open Approach

0M9W0ZX   Drainage of Left Lower Extremity Bursa and Ligament, Open Approach, Diagnostic

0M9W0ZZ   Drainage of Left Lower Extremity Bursa and Ligament, Open Approach

0M9W30Z   Drainage of Left Lower Extremity Bursa and Ligament with Drainage Device, Percutaneous Approach

0M9W3ZX   Drainage of Left Lower Extremity Bursa and Ligament, Percutaneous Approach, Diagnostic

0M9W3ZZ   Drainage of Left Lower Extremity Bursa and Ligament, Percutaneous Approach

0M9W40Z   Drainage of Left Lower Extremity Bursa and Ligament with Drainage Device, Percutaneous Endoscopic Approach

0M9W4ZX   Drainage of Left Lower Extremity Bursa and Ligament, Percutaneous Endoscopic Approach, Diagnostic

0M9W4ZZ   Drainage of Left Lower Extremity Bursa and Ligament, Percutaneous Endoscopic Approach

0MB – Bursae and Ligaments, Excision

Review Coding Guidelines B3.4a and B3.4b

Review Coding Guideline B3.5

Review Coding Guideline B3.8

0MB00ZX   Excision of Head and Neck Bursa and Ligament, Open Approach, Diagnostic

0MB00ZZ   Excision of Head and Neck Bursa and Ligament, Open Approach

0MB03ZX   Excision of Head and Neck Bursa and Ligament, Percutaneous Approach, Diagnostic

03ZZ	Excision of Head and Neck Bursa and Ligament, Percutaneous Approach
04ZX	Excision of Head and Neck Bursa and Ligament, Percutaneous Endoscopic Approach, Diagnostic
04ZZ	Excision of Head and Neck Bursa and Ligament, Percutaneous Endoscopic Approach
10ZX	Excision of Right Shoulder Bursa and Ligament, Open Approach, Diagnostic
10ZZ	Excision of Right Shoulder Bursa and Ligament, Open Approach
13ZX	Excision of Right Shoulder Bursa and Ligament, Percutaneous Approach, Diagnostic
13ZZ	Excision of Right Shoulder Bursa and Ligament, Percutaneous Approach
14ZX	Excision of Right Shoulder Bursa and Ligament, Percutaneous Endoscopic Approach, Diagnostic
14ZZ	Excision of Right Shoulder Bursa and Ligament, Percutaneous Endoscopic Approach
20ZX	Excision of Left Shoulder Bursa and Ligament, Open Approach, Diagnostic
20ZZ	Excision of Left Shoulder Bursa and Ligament, Open Approach
23ZX	Excision of Left Shoulder Bursa and Ligament, Percutaneous Approach, Diagnostic
23ZZ	Excision of Left Shoulder Bursa and Ligament, Percutaneous Approach
24ZX	Excision of Left Shoulder Bursa and Ligament, Percutaneous Endoscopic Approach, Diagnostic
24ZZ	Excision of Left Shoulder Bursa and Ligament, Percutaneous Endoscopic Approach
B30ZX	Excision of Right Elbow Bursa and Ligament, Open Approach, Diagnostic
B30ZZ	Excision of Right Elbow Bursa and Ligament, Open Approach
B33ZX	Excision of Right Elbow Bursa and Ligament, Percutaneous Approach, Diagnostic
B33ZZ	Excision of Right Elbow Bursa and Ligament, Percutaneous Approach
B34ZX	Excision of Right Elbow Bursa and Ligament, Percutaneous Endoscopic Approach, Diagnostic
B34ZZ	Excision of Right Elbow Bursa and Ligament, Percutaneous Endoscopic Approach
B40ZX	Excision of Left Elbow Bursa and Ligament, Open Approach, Diagnostic
B40ZZ	Excision of Left Elbow Bursa and Ligament, Open Approach
B43ZX	Excision of Left Elbow Bursa and Ligament, Percutaneous Approach, Diagnostic
B43ZZ	Excision of Left Elbow Bursa and Ligament, Percutaneous Approach
B44ZX	Excision of Left Elbow Bursa and Ligament, Percutaneous Endoscopic Approach, Diagnostic
B44ZZ	Excision of Left Elbow Bursa and Ligament, Percutaneous Endoscopic Approach
B50ZX	Excision of Right Wrist Bursa and Ligament, Open Approach, Diagnostic
B50ZZ	Excision of Right Wrist Bursa and Ligament, Open Approach
B53ZX	Excision of Right Wrist Bursa and Ligament, Percutaneous Approach, Diagnostic
B53ZZ	Excision of Right Wrist Bursa and Ligament, Percutaneous Approach

0MB54ZX	Excision of Right Wrist Bursa and Ligament, Percutaneous Endoscopic Approach, Diagnostic
0MB54ZZ	Excision of Right Wrist Bursa and Ligament, Percutaneous Endoscopic Approach
0MB60ZX	Excision of Left Wrist Bursa and Ligament, Open Approach, Diagnostic
0MB60ZZ	Excision of Left Wrist Bursa and Ligament, Open Approach
0MB63ZX	Excision of Left Wrist Bursa and Ligament, Percutaneous Approach, Diagnostic
0MB63ZZ	Excision of Left Wrist Bursa and Ligament, Percutaneous Approach
0MB64ZX	Excision of Left Wrist Bursa and Ligament, Percutaneous Endoscopic Approach, Diagnostic
0MB64ZZ	Excision of Left Wrist Bursa and Ligament, Percutaneous Endoscopic Approach
0MB70ZX	Excision of Right Hand Bursa and Ligament, Open Approach, Diagnostic
0MB70ZZ	Excision of Right Hand Bursa and Ligament, Open Approach
0MB73ZX	Excision of Right Hand Bursa and Ligament, Percutaneous Approach, Diagnostic
0MB73ZZ	Excision of Right Hand Bursa and Ligament, Percutaneous Approach
0MB74ZX	Excision of Right Hand Bursa and Ligament, Percutaneous Endoscopic Approach, Diagnostic
0MB74ZZ	Excision of Right Hand Bursa and Ligament, Percutaneous Endoscopic Approach
0MB80ZX	Excision of Left Hand Bursa and Ligament, Open Approach, Diagnostic
0MB80ZZ	Excision of Left Hand Bursa and Ligament, Open Approach
0MB83ZX	Excision of Left Hand Bursa and Ligament, Percutaneous Approach, Diagnostic
0MB83ZZ	Excision of Left Hand Bursa and Ligament, Percutaneous Approach
0MB84ZX	Excision of Left Hand Bursa and Ligament, Percutaneous Endoscopic Approach, Diagnostic
0MB84ZZ	Excision of Left Hand Bursa and Ligament, Percutaneous Endoscopic Approach
0MB90ZX	Excision of Right Upper Extremity Bursa and Ligament, Open Approach, Diagnostic
0MB90ZZ	Excision of Right Upper Extremity Bursa and Ligament, Open Approach
0MB93ZX	Excision of Right Upper Extremity Bursa and Ligament, Percutaneous Approach, Diagnostic
0MB93ZZ	Excision of Right Upper Extremity Bursa and Ligament, Percutaneous Approach
0MB94ZX	Excision of Right Upper Extremity Bursa and Ligament, Percutaneous Endoscopic Approach, Diagnostic
0MB94ZZ	Excision of Right Upper Extremity Bursa and Ligament, Percutaneous Endoscopic Approach
0MBB0ZX	Excision of Left Upper Extremity Bursa and Ligament, Open Approach, Diagnostic
0MBB0ZZ	Excision of Left Upper Extremity Bursa and Ligament, Open Approach
0MBB3ZX	Excision of Left Upper Extremity Bursa and Ligament, Percutaneous Approach, Diagnostic

0MBB3ZZ	Excision of Left Upper Extremity Bursa and Ligament, Percutaneous Approach
0MBB4ZX	Excision of Left Upper Extremity Bursa and Ligament, Percutaneous Endoscopic Approach, Diagnostic
0MBB4ZZ	Excision of Left Upper Extremity Bursa and Ligament, Percutaneous Endoscopic Approach
0MBC0ZX	Excision of Right Trunk Bursa and Ligament, Open Approach, Diagnostic
0MBC0ZZ	Excision of Right Trunk Bursa and Ligament, Open Approach
0MBC3ZX	Excision of Right Trunk Bursa and Ligament, Percutaneous Approach, Diagnostic
0MBC3ZZ	Excision of Right Trunk Bursa and Ligament, Percutaneous Approach
0MBC4ZX	Excision of Right Trunk Bursa and Ligament, Percutaneous Endoscopic Approach, Diagnostic
0MBC4ZZ	Excision of Right Trunk Bursa and Ligament, Percutaneous Endoscopic Approach
0MBD0ZX	Excision of Left Trunk Bursa and Ligament, Open Approach, Diagnostic
0MBD0ZZ	Excision of Left Trunk Bursa and Ligament, Open Approach
0MBD3ZX	Excision of Left Trunk Bursa and Ligament, Percutaneous Approach, Diagnostic
0MBD3ZZ	Excision of Left Trunk Bursa and Ligament, Percutaneous Approach
0MBD4ZX	Excision of Left Trunk Bursa and Ligament, Percutaneous Endoscopic Approach, Diagnostic
0MBD4ZZ	Excision of Left Trunk Bursa and Ligament, Percutaneous Endoscopic Approach
0MBF0ZX	Excision of Right Thorax Bursa and Ligament, Open Approach, Diagnostic
0MBF0ZZ	Excision of Right Thorax Bursa and Ligament, Open Approach
0MBF3ZX	Excision of Right Thorax Bursa and Ligament, Percutaneous Approach, Diagnostic
0MBF3ZZ	Excision of Right Thorax Bursa and Ligament, Percutaneous Approach
0MBF4ZX	Excision of Right Thorax Bursa and Ligament, Percutaneous Endoscopic Approach, Diagnostic
0MBF4ZZ	Excision of Right Thorax Bursa and Ligament, Percutaneous Endoscopic Approach
0MBG0ZX	Excision of Left Thorax Bursa and Ligament, Open Approach, Diagnostic
0MBG0ZZ	Excision of Left Thorax Bursa and Ligament, Open Approach
0MBG3ZX	Excision of Left Thorax Bursa and Ligament, Percutaneous Approach, Diagnostic
0MBG3ZZ	Excision of Left Thorax Bursa and Ligament, Percutaneous Approach
0MBG4ZX	Excision of Left Thorax Bursa and Ligament, Percutaneous Endoscopic Approach, Diagnostic
0MBG4ZZ	Excision of Left Thorax Bursa and Ligament, Percutaneous Endoscopic Approach
0MBH0ZX	Excision of Right Abdomen Bursa and Ligament, Open Approach, Diagnostic
0MBH0ZZ	Excision of Right Abdomen Bursa and Ligament, Open Approach
0MBH3ZX	Excision of Right Abdomen Bursa and Ligament, Percutaneous Approach, Diagnostic
0MBH3ZZ	Excision of Right Abdomen Bursa and Ligament, Percutaneous Approach

♀ Female-only	♂ Male-only	▲ Limited Coverage	● Non-OR	▥ HAC-associated procedure	▲ Non-covered procedures	✛ Combination

0MBH4ZX	Excision of Right Abdomen Bursa and Ligament, Percutaneous Endoscopic Approach, Diagnostic	**0MBM4ZZ**	Excision of Left Hip Bursa and Ligament, Percutaneous Endoscopic Approach	**0MBS0ZX**	Excision of Right Foot Bursa and Ligament, Open Approach, Diagnost
0MBH4ZZ	Excision of Right Abdomen Bursa and Ligament, Percutaneous Endoscopic Approach	**0MBN0ZX**	Excision of Right Knee Bursa and Ligament, Open Approach, Diagnostic	**0MBS0ZZ**	Excision of Right Foot Bursa and Ligament, Open Approach
0MBJ0ZX	Excision of Left Abdomen Bursa and Ligament, Open Approach, Diagnostic	**0MBN0ZZ**	Excision of Right Knee Bursa and Ligament, Open Approach	**0MBS3ZX**	Excision of Right Foot Bursa and Ligament, Percutaneous Approach, Diagnostic
0MBJ0ZZ	Excision of Left Abdomen Bursa and Ligament, Open Approach	**0MBN3ZX**	Excision of Right Knee Bursa and Ligament, Percutaneous Approach, Diagnostic	**0MBS3ZZ**	Excision of Right Foot Bursa and Ligament, Percutaneous Approach
0MBJ3ZX	Excision of Left Abdomen Bursa and Ligament, Percutaneous Approach, Diagnostic	**0MBN3ZZ**	Excision of Right Knee Bursa and Ligament, Percutaneous Approach	**0MBS4ZX**	Excision of Right Foot Bursa and Ligament, Percutaneous Endoscopic Approach, Diagnostic
0MBJ3ZZ	Excision of Left Abdomen Bursa and Ligament, Percutaneous Approach	**0MBN4ZX**	Excision of Right Knee Bursa and Ligament, Percutaneous Endoscopic Approach, Diagnostic	**0MBS4ZZ**	Excision of Right Foot Bursa and Ligament, Percutaneous Endoscopic Approach
0MBJ4ZX	Excision of Left Abdomen Bursa and Ligament, Percutaneous Endoscopic Approach, Diagnostic	**0MBN4ZZ**	Excision of Right Knee Bursa and Ligament, Percutaneous Endoscopic Approach	**0MBT0ZX**	Excision of Left Foot Bursa and Ligament, Open Approach, Diagnost
0MBJ4ZZ	Excision of Left Abdomen Bursa and Ligament, Percutaneous Endoscopic Approach	**0MBP0ZX**	Excision of Left Knee Bursa and Ligament, Open Approach, Diagnostic	**0MBT0ZZ**	Excision of Left Foot Bursa and Ligament, Open Approach
0MBK0ZX	Excision of Perineum Bursa and Ligament, Open Approach, Diagnostic	**0MBP0ZZ**	Excision of Left Knee Bursa and Ligament, Open Approach	**0MBT3ZX**	Excision of Left Foot Bursa and Ligament, Percutaneous Approach, Diagnostic
0MBK0ZZ	Excision of Perineum Bursa and Ligament, Open Approach	**0MBP3ZX**	Excision of Left Knee Bursa and Ligament, Percutaneous Approach, Diagnostic	**0MBT3ZZ**	Excision of Left Foot Bursa and Ligament, Percutaneous Approac
0MBK3ZX	Excision of Perineum Bursa and Ligament, Percutaneous Approach, Diagnostic	**0MBP3ZZ**	Excision of Left Knee Bursa and Ligament, Percutaneous Approach	**0MBT4ZX**	Excision of Left Foot Bursa and Ligament, Percutaneous Endoscopic Approach, Diagnostic
0MBK3ZZ	Excision of Perineum Bursa and Ligament, Percutaneous Approach	**0MBP4ZX**	Excision of Left Knee Bursa and Ligament, Percutaneous Endoscopic Approach, Diagnostic	**0MBT4ZZ**	Excision of Left Foot Bursa and Ligament, Percutaneous Endoscopic Approach
0MBK4ZX	Excision of Perineum Bursa and Ligament, Percutaneous Endoscopic Approach, Diagnostic	**0MBP4ZZ**	Excision of Left Knee Bursa and Ligament, Percutaneous Endoscopic Approach	**0MBV0ZX**	Excision of Right Lower Extremity Bursa and Ligament, Open Approach Diagnostic
0MBK4ZZ	Excision of Perineum Bursa and Ligament, Percutaneous Endoscopic Approach	**0MBQ0ZX**	Excision of Right Ankle Bursa and Ligament, Open Approach, Diagnostic	**0MBV0ZZ**	Excision of Right Lower Extremity B and Ligament, Open Approach
0MBL0ZX	Excision of Right Hip Bursa and Ligament, Open Approach, Diagnostic	**0MBQ0ZZ**	Excision of Right Ankle Bursa and Ligament, Open Approach	**0MBV3ZX**	Excision of Right Lower Extremity B and Ligament, Percutaneous Approach Diagnostic
0MBL0ZZ	Excision of Right Hip Bursa and Ligament, Open Approach	**0MBQ3ZX**	Excision of Right Ankle Bursa and Ligament, Percutaneous Approach, Diagnostic	**0MBV3ZZ**	Excision of Right Lower Extremity B and Ligament, Percutaneous Approach
0MBL3ZX	Excision of Right Hip Bursa and Ligament, Percutaneous Approach, Diagnostic	**0MBQ3ZZ**	Excision of Right Ankle Bursa and Ligament, Percutaneous Approach	**0MBV4ZX**	Excision of Right Lower Extremity B and Ligament, Percutaneous Endosco Approach, Diagnostic
0MBL3ZZ	Excision of Right Hip Bursa and Ligament, Percutaneous Approach	**0MBQ4ZX**	Excision of Right Ankle Bursa and Ligament, Percutaneous Endoscopic Approach, Diagnostic	**0MBV4ZZ**	Excision of Right Lower Extremity B and Ligament, Percutaneous Endosco Approach
0MBL4ZX	Excision of Right Hip Bursa and Ligament, Percutaneous Endoscopic Approach, Diagnostic	**0MBQ4ZZ**	Excision of Right Ankle Bursa and Ligament, Percutaneous Endoscopic Approach	**0MBW0ZX**	Excision of Left Lower Extremity Bursa and Ligament, Open Approach, Diagnostic
0MBL4ZZ	Excision of Right Hip Bursa and Ligament, Percutaneous Endoscopic Approach	**0MBR0ZX**	Excision of Left Ankle Bursa and Ligament, Open Approach, Diagnostic	**0MBW0ZZ**	Excision of Left Lower Extremity Bur and Ligament, Open Approach
0MBM0ZX	Excision of Left Hip Bursa and Ligament, Open Approach, Diagnostic	**0MBR0ZZ**	Excision of Left Ankle Bursa and Ligament, Open Approach	**0MBW3ZX**	Excision of Left Lower Extremity Bur and Ligament, Percutaneous Approach Diagnostic
0MBM0ZZ	Excision of Left Hip Bursa and Ligament, Open Approach	**0MBR3ZX**	Excision of Left Ankle Bursa and Ligament, Percutaneous Approach, Diagnostic	**0MBW3ZZ**	Excision of Left Lower Extremity Bur and Ligament, Percutaneous Approach
0MBM3ZX	Excision of Left Hip Bursa and Ligament, Percutaneous Approach, Diagnostic	**0MBR3ZZ**	Excision of Left Ankle Bursa and Ligament, Percutaneous Approach	**0MBW4ZX**	Excision of Left Lower Extremity Bur and Ligament, Percutaneous Endoscop Approach, Diagnostic
0MBM3ZZ	Excision of Left Hip Bursa and Ligament, Percutaneous Approach	**0MBR4ZX**	Excision of Left Ankle Bursa and Ligament, Percutaneous Endoscopic Approach, Diagnostic	**0MBW4ZZ**	Excision of Left Lower Extremity Bur and Ligament, Percutaneous Endoscop Approach
0MBM4ZX	Excision of Left Hip Bursa and Ligament, Percutaneous Endoscopic Approach, Diagnostic	**0MBR4ZZ**	Excision of Left Ankle Bursa and Ligament, Percutaneous Endoscopic Approach		

0MC – Bursae and Ligaments, Extirpation

0MC00ZZ	Extirpation of Matter from Head and Neck Bursa and Ligament, Open Approach	**0MC13ZZ**	Extirpation of Matter from Right Shoulder Bursa and Ligament, Percutaneous Approach	**0MC24ZZ**	Extirpation of Matter from Left Should Bursa and Ligament, Percutaneous Endoscopic Approach
0MC03ZZ	Extirpation of Matter from Head and Neck Bursa and Ligament, Percutaneous Approach	**0MC14ZZ**	Extirpation of Matter from Right Shoulder Bursa and Ligament, Percutaneous Endoscopic Approach	**0MC30ZZ**	Extirpation of Matter from Right Elbow Bursa and Ligament, Open Approach
0MC04ZZ	Extirpation of Matter from Head and Neck Bursa and Ligament, Percutaneous Endoscopic Approach	**0MC20ZZ**	Extirpation of Matter from Left Shoulder Bursa and Ligament, Open Approach	**0MC33ZZ**	Extirpation of Matter from Right Elbow Bursa and Ligament, Percutaneous Approach
0MC10ZZ	Extirpation of Matter from Right Shoulder Bursa and Ligament, Open Approach	**0MC23ZZ**	Extirpation of Matter from Left Shoulder Bursa and Ligament, Percutaneous Approach	**0MC34ZZ**	Extirpation of Matter from Right Elbow Bursa and Ligament, Percutaneous Endoscopic Approach

♀ Female-only   ♂ Male-only   ▲ Limited Coverage   ● Non-OR   ▬ HAC-associated procedure   ▲ Non-covered procedures   ✚ Combinat

...40ZZ	Extirpation of Matter from Left Elbow Bursa and Ligament, Open Approach
...43ZZ	Extirpation of Matter from Left Elbow Bursa and Ligament, Percutaneous Approach
...44ZZ	Extirpation of Matter from Left Elbow Bursa and Ligament, Percutaneous Endoscopic Approach
...50ZZ	Extirpation of Matter from Right Wrist Bursa and Ligament, Open Approach
...53ZZ	Extirpation of Matter from Right Wrist Bursa and Ligament, Percutaneous Approach
...54ZZ	Extirpation of Matter from Right Wrist Bursa and Ligament, Percutaneous Endoscopic Approach
...60ZZ	Extirpation of Matter from Left Wrist Bursa and Ligament, Open Approach
...63ZZ	Extirpation of Matter from Left Wrist Bursa and Ligament, Percutaneous Approach
...64ZZ	Extirpation of Matter from Left Wrist Bursa and Ligament, Percutaneous Endoscopic Approach
...70ZZ	Extirpation of Matter from Right Hand Bursa and Ligament, Open Approach
...73ZZ	Extirpation of Matter from Right Hand Bursa and Ligament, Percutaneous Approach
...74ZZ	Extirpation of Matter from Right Hand Bursa and Ligament, Percutaneous Endoscopic Approach
...80ZZ	Extirpation of Matter from Left Hand Bursa and Ligament, Open Approach
...83ZZ	Extirpation of Matter from Left Hand Bursa and Ligament, Percutaneous Approach
...84ZZ	Extirpation of Matter from Left Hand Bursa and Ligament, Percutaneous Endoscopic Approach
...90ZZ	Extirpation of Matter from Right Upper Extremity Bursa and Ligament, Open Approach
...93ZZ	Extirpation of Matter from Right Upper Extremity Bursa and Ligament, Percutaneous Approach
...94ZZ	Extirpation of Matter from Right Upper Extremity Bursa and Ligament, Percutaneous Endoscopic Approach
...B0ZZ	Extirpation of Matter from Left Upper Extremity Bursa and Ligament, Open Approach
...B3ZZ	Extirpation of Matter from Left Upper Extremity Bursa and Ligament, Percutaneous Approach
...B4ZZ	Extirpation of Matter from Left Upper Extremity Bursa and Ligament, Percutaneous Endoscopic Approach
...C0ZZ	Extirpation of Matter from Right Trunk Bursa and Ligament, Open Approach
...C3ZZ	Extirpation of Matter from Right Trunk Bursa and Ligament, Percutaneous Approach
...C4ZZ	Extirpation of Matter from Right Trunk Bursa and Ligament, Percutaneous Endoscopic Approach

0MCD0ZZ	Extirpation of Matter from Left Trunk Bursa and Ligament, Open Approach
0MCD3ZZ	Extirpation of Matter from Left Trunk Bursa and Ligament, Percutaneous Approach
0MCD4ZZ	Extirpation of Matter from Left Trunk Bursa and Ligament, Percutaneous Endoscopic Approach
0MCF0ZZ	Extirpation of Matter from Right Thorax Bursa and Ligament, Open Approach
0MCF3ZZ	Extirpation of Matter from Right Thorax Bursa and Ligament, Percutaneous Approach
0MCF4ZZ	Extirpation of Matter from Right Thorax Bursa and Ligament, Percutaneous Endoscopic Approach
0MCG0ZZ	Extirpation of Matter from Left Thorax Bursa and Ligament, Open Approach
0MCG3ZZ	Extirpation of Matter from Left Thorax Bursa and Ligament, Percutaneous Approach
0MCG4ZZ	Extirpation of Matter from Left Thorax Bursa and Ligament, Percutaneous Endoscopic Approach
0MCH0ZZ	Extirpation of Matter from Right Abdomen Bursa and Ligament, Open Approach
0MCH3ZZ	Extirpation of Matter from Right Abdomen Bursa and Ligament, Percutaneous Approach
0MCH4ZZ	Extirpation of Matter from Right Abdomen Bursa and Ligament, Percutaneous Endoscopic Approach
0MCJ0ZZ	Extirpation of Matter from Left Abdomen Bursa and Ligament, Open Approach
0MCJ3ZZ	Extirpation of Matter from Left Abdomen Bursa and Ligament, Percutaneous Approach
0MCJ4ZZ	Extirpation of Matter from Left Abdomen Bursa and Ligament, Percutaneous Endoscopic Approach
0MCK0ZZ	Extirpation of Matter from Perineum Bursa and Ligament, Open Approach
0MCK3ZZ	Extirpation of Matter from Perineum Bursa and Ligament, Percutaneous Approach
0MCK4ZZ	Extirpation of Matter from Perineum Bursa and Ligament, Percutaneous Endoscopic Approach
0MCL0ZZ	Extirpation of Matter from Right Hip Bursa and Ligament, Open Approach
0MCL3ZZ	Extirpation of Matter from Right Hip Bursa and Ligament, Percutaneous Approach
0MCL4ZZ	Extirpation of Matter from Right Hip Bursa and Ligament, Percutaneous Endoscopic Approach
0MCM0ZZ	Extirpation of Matter from Left Hip Bursa and Ligament, Open Approach
0MCM3ZZ	Extirpation of Matter from Left Hip Bursa and Ligament, Percutaneous Approach
0MCM4ZZ	Extirpation of Matter from Left Hip Bursa and Ligament, Percutaneous Endoscopic Approach
0MCN0ZZ	Extirpation of Matter from Right Knee Bursa and Ligament, Open Approach

0MCN3ZZ	Extirpation of Matter from Right Knee Bursa and Ligament, Percutaneous Approach
0MCN4ZZ	Extirpation of Matter from Right Knee Bursa and Ligament, Percutaneous Endoscopic Approach
0MCP0ZZ	Extirpation of Matter from Left Knee Bursa and Ligament, Open Approach
0MCP3ZZ	Extirpation of Matter from Left Knee Bursa and Ligament, Percutaneous Approach
0MCP4ZZ	Extirpation of Matter from Left Knee Bursa and Ligament, Percutaneous Endoscopic Approach
0MCQ0ZZ	Extirpation of Matter from Right Ankle Bursa and Ligament, Open Approach
0MCQ3ZZ	Extirpation of Matter from Right Ankle Bursa and Ligament, Percutaneous Approach
0MCQ4ZZ	Extirpation of Matter from Right Ankle Bursa and Ligament, Percutaneous Endoscopic Approach
0MCR0ZZ	Extirpation of Matter from Left Ankle Bursa and Ligament, Open Approach
0MCR3ZZ	Extirpation of Matter from Left Ankle Bursa and Ligament, Percutaneous Approach
0MCR4ZZ	Extirpation of Matter from Left Ankle Bursa and Ligament, Percutaneous Endoscopic Approach
0MCS0ZZ	Extirpation of Matter from Right Foot Bursa and Ligament, Open Approach
0MCS3ZZ	Extirpation of Matter from Right Foot Bursa and Ligament, Percutaneous Approach
0MCS4ZZ	Extirpation of Matter from Right Foot Bursa and Ligament, Percutaneous Endoscopic Approach
0MCT0ZZ	Extirpation of Matter from Left Foot Bursa and Ligament, Open Approach
0MCT3ZZ	Extirpation of Matter from Left Foot Bursa and Ligament, Percutaneous Approach
0MCT4ZZ	Extirpation of Matter from Left Foot Bursa and Ligament, Percutaneous Endoscopic Approach
0MCV0ZZ	Extirpation of Matter from Right Lower Extremity Bursa and Ligament, Open Approach
0MCV3ZZ	Extirpation of Matter from Right Lower Extremity Bursa and Ligament, Percutaneous Approach
0MCV4ZZ	Extirpation of Matter from Right Lower Extremity Bursa and Ligament, Percutaneous Endoscopic Approach
0MCW0ZZ	Extirpation of Matter from Left Lower Extremity Bursa and Ligament, Open Approach
0MCW3ZZ	Extirpation of Matter from Left Lower Extremity Bursa and Ligament, Percutaneous Approach
0MCW4ZZ	Extirpation of Matter from Left Lower Extremity Bursa and Ligament, Percutaneous Endoscopic Approach

0MD – Bursae and Ligaments, Extraction

0MD00ZZ	Extraction of Head and Neck Bursa and Ligament, Open Approach
0MD03ZZ	Extraction of Head and Neck Bursa and Ligament, Percutaneous Approach
0MD04ZZ	Extraction of Head and Neck Bursa and Ligament, Percutaneous Endoscopic Approach
0MD10ZZ	Extraction of Right Shoulder Bursa and Ligament, Open Approach
0MD13ZZ	Extraction of Right Shoulder Bursa and Ligament, Percutaneous Approach
0MD14ZZ	Extraction of Right Shoulder Bursa and Ligament, Percutaneous Endoscopic Approach
0MD20ZZ	Extraction of Left Shoulder Bursa and Ligament, Open Approach
0MD23ZZ	Extraction of Left Shoulder Bursa and Ligament, Percutaneous Approach
0MD24ZZ	Extraction of Left Shoulder Bursa and Ligament, Percutaneous Endoscopic Approach

0MD30ZZ	Extraction of Right Elbow Bursa and Ligament, Open Approach	
0MD33ZZ	Extraction of Right Elbow Bursa and Ligament, Percutaneous Approach	
0MD34ZZ	Extraction of Right Elbow Bursa and Ligament, Percutaneous Endoscopic Approach	
0MD40ZZ	Extraction of Left Elbow Bursa and Ligament, Open Approach	
0MD43ZZ	Extraction of Left Elbow Bursa and Ligament, Percutaneous Approach	
0MD44ZZ	Extraction of Left Elbow Bursa and Ligament, Percutaneous Endoscopic Approach	
0MD50ZZ	Extraction of Right Wrist Bursa and Ligament, Open Approach	
0MD53ZZ	Extraction of Right Wrist Bursa and Ligament, Percutaneous Approach	
0MD54ZZ	Extraction of Right Wrist Bursa and Ligament, Percutaneous Endoscopic Approach	
0MD60ZZ	Extraction of Left Wrist Bursa and Ligament, Open Approach	
0MD63ZZ	Extraction of Left Wrist Bursa and Ligament, Percutaneous Approach	
0MD64ZZ	Extraction of Left Wrist Bursa and Ligament, Percutaneous Endoscopic Approach	
0MD70ZZ	Extraction of Right Hand Bursa and Ligament, Open Approach	
0MD73ZZ	Extraction of Right Hand Bursa and Ligament, Percutaneous Approach	
0MD74ZZ	Extraction of Right Hand Bursa and Ligament, Percutaneous Endoscopic Approach	
0MD80ZZ	Extraction of Left Hand Bursa and Ligament, Open Approach	
0MD83ZZ	Extraction of Left Hand Bursa and Ligament, Percutaneous Approach	
0MD84ZZ	Extraction of Left Hand Bursa and Ligament, Percutaneous Endoscopic Approach	
0MD90ZZ	Extraction of Right Upper Extremity Bursa and Ligament, Open Approach	
0MD93ZZ	Extraction of Right Upper Extremity Bursa and Ligament, Percutaneous Approach	
0MD94ZZ	Extraction of Right Upper Extremity Bursa and Ligament, Percutaneous Endoscopic Approach	
0MDB0ZZ	Extraction of Left Upper Extremity Bursa and Ligament, Open Approach	
0MDB3ZZ	Extraction of Left Upper Extremity Bursa and Ligament, Percutaneous Approach	
0MDB4ZZ	Extraction of Left Upper Extremity Bursa and Ligament, Percutaneous Endoscopic Approach	
0MDC0ZZ	Extraction of Right Trunk Bursa and Ligament, Open Approach	
0MDC3ZZ	Extraction of Right Trunk Bursa and Ligament, Percutaneous Approach	
0MDC4ZZ	Extraction of Right Trunk Bursa and Ligament, Percutaneous Endoscopic Approach	
0MDD0ZZ	Extraction of Left Trunk Bursa and Ligament, Open Approach	
0MDD3ZZ	Extraction of Left Trunk Bursa and Ligament, Percutaneous Approach	
0MDD4ZZ	Extraction of Left Trunk Bursa and Ligament, Percutaneous Endoscopic Approach	
0MDF0ZZ	Extraction of Right Thorax Bursa and Ligament, Open Approach	
0MDF3ZZ	Extraction of Right Thorax Bursa and Ligament, Percutaneous Approach	
0MDF4ZZ	Extraction of Right Thorax Bursa and Ligament, Percutaneous Endoscopic Approach	
0MDG0ZZ	Extraction of Left Thorax Bursa and Ligament, Open Approach	
0MDG3ZZ	Extraction of Left Thorax Bursa and Ligament, Percutaneous Approach	
0MDG4ZZ	Extraction of Left Thorax Bursa and Ligament, Percutaneous Endoscopic Approach	
0MDH0ZZ	Extraction of Right Abdomen Bursa and Ligament, Open Approach	
0MDH3ZZ	Extraction of Right Abdomen Bursa and Ligament, Percutaneous Approach	
0MDH4ZZ	Extraction of Right Abdomen Bursa and Ligament, Percutaneous Endoscopic Approach	
0MDJ0ZZ	Extraction of Left Abdomen Bursa and Ligament, Open Approach	
0MDJ3ZZ	Extraction of Left Abdomen Bursa and Ligament, Percutaneous Approach	
0MDJ4ZZ	Extraction of Left Abdomen Bursa and Ligament, Percutaneous Endoscopic Approach	
0MDK0ZZ	Extraction of Perineum Bursa and Ligament, Open Approach	
0MDK3ZZ	Extraction of Perineum Bursa and Ligament, Percutaneous Approach	
0MDK4ZZ	Extraction of Perineum Bursa and Ligament, Percutaneous Endoscopic Approach	
0MDL0ZZ	Extraction of Right Hip Bursa and Ligament, Open Approach	
0MDL3ZZ	Extraction of Right Hip Bursa and Ligament, Percutaneous Approach	
0MDL4ZZ	Extraction of Right Hip Bursa and Ligament, Percutaneous Endoscopic Approach	
0MDM0ZZ	Extraction of Left Hip Bursa and Ligament, Open Approach	
0MDM3ZZ	Extraction of Left Hip Bursa and Ligament, Percutaneous Approach	
0MDM4ZZ	Extraction of Left Hip Bursa and Ligament, Percutaneous Endoscopic Approach	
0MDN0ZZ	Extraction of Right Knee Bursa and Ligament, Open Approach	
0MDN3ZZ	Extraction of Right Knee Bursa and Ligament, Percutaneous Approach	
0MDN4ZZ	Extraction of Right Knee Bursa and Ligament, Percutaneous Endoscopic Approach	
0MDP0ZZ	Extraction of Left Knee Bursa and Ligament, Open Approach	
0MDP3ZZ	Extraction of Left Knee Bursa and Ligament, Percutaneous Approach	
0MDP4ZZ	Extraction of Left Knee Bursa and Ligament, Percutaneous Endoscopic Approach	
0MDQ0ZZ	Extraction of Right Ankle Bursa and Ligament, Open Approach	
0MDQ3ZZ	Extraction of Right Ankle Bursa and Ligament, Percutaneous Approach	
0MDQ4ZZ	Extraction of Right Ankle Bursa and Ligament, Percutaneous Endoscopic Approach	
0MDR0ZZ	Extraction of Left Ankle Bursa and Ligament, Open Approach	
0MDR3ZZ	Extraction of Left Ankle Bursa and Ligament, Percutaneous Approach	
0MDR4ZZ	Extraction of Left Ankle Bursa and Ligament, Percutaneous Endoscopic Approach	
0MDS0ZZ	Extraction of Right Foot Bursa and Ligament, Open Approach	
0MDS3ZZ	Extraction of Right Foot Bursa and Ligament, Percutaneous Approach	
0MDS4ZZ	Extraction of Right Foot Bursa and Ligament, Percutaneous Endoscopic Approach	
0MDT0ZZ	Extraction of Left Foot Bursa and Ligament, Open Approach	
0MDT3ZZ	Extraction of Left Foot Bursa and Ligament, Percutaneous Approach	
0MDT4ZZ	Extraction of Left Foot Bursa and Ligament, Percutaneous Endoscopic Approach	
0MDV0ZZ	Extraction of Right Lower Extremity Bursa and Ligament, Open Approach	
0MDV3ZZ	Extraction of Right Lower Extremity Bursa and Ligament, Percutaneous Approach	
0MDV4ZZ	Extraction of Right Lower Extremity Bursa and Ligament, Percutaneous Endoscopic Approach	
0MDW0ZZ	Extraction of Left Lower Extremity Bursa and Ligament, Open Approach	
0MDW3ZZ	Extraction of Left Lower Extremity Bursa and Ligament, Percutaneous Approach	
0MDW4ZZ	Extraction of Left Lower Extremity Bursa and Ligament, Percutaneous Endoscopic Approach	

0MJ – Bursae and Ligaments, Inspection

Review Coding Guideline B3.5

Review Coding Guidelines B3.11a, B3.11b and B3.11c

0MJX0ZZ	Inspection of Upper Bursa and Ligament, Open Approach	
0MJX3ZZ	Inspection of Upper Bursa and Ligament, Percutaneous Approach	
0MJX4ZZ	Inspection of Upper Bursa and Ligament, Percutaneous Endoscopic Approach	
0MJXXZZ	Inspection of Upper Bursa and Ligament, External Approach	
0MJY0ZZ	Inspection of Lower Bursa and Ligament, Open Approach	
0MJY3ZZ	Inspection of Lower Bursa and Ligament, Percutaneous Approach	
0MJY4ZZ	Inspection of Lower Bursa and Ligament, Percutaneous Endoscopic Approach	
0MJYXZZ	Inspection of Lower Bursa and Ligament, External Approach	

0M – Bursae and Ligaments, Reattachment

0MM00ZZ	Reattachment of Head and Neck Bursa and Ligament, Open Approach	**0MM94ZZ**	Reattachment of Right Upper Extremity Bursa and Ligament, Percutaneous Endoscopic Approach	**0MMM0ZZ**	Reattachment of Left Hip Bursa and Ligament, Open Approach

0MM00ZZ Reattachment of Head and Neck Bursa and Ligament, Open Approach

0MM04ZZ Reattachment of Head and Neck Bursa and Ligament, Percutaneous Endoscopic Approach

0MM10ZZ Reattachment of Right Shoulder Bursa and Ligament, Open Approach

0MM14ZZ Reattachment of Right Shoulder Bursa and Ligament, Percutaneous Endoscopic Approach

AHA CC: 3Q, 2013, 20-22

0MM20ZZ Reattachment of Left Shoulder Bursa and Ligament, Open Approach

0MM24ZZ Reattachment of Left Shoulder Bursa and Ligament, Percutaneous Endoscopic Approach

0MM30ZZ Reattachment of Right Elbow Bursa and Ligament, Open Approach

0MM34ZZ Reattachment of Right Elbow Bursa and Ligament, Percutaneous Endoscopic Approach

0MM40ZZ Reattachment of Left Elbow Bursa and Ligament, Open Approach

0MM44ZZ Reattachment of Left Elbow Bursa and Ligament, Percutaneous Endoscopic Approach

0MM50ZZ Reattachment of Right Wrist Bursa and Ligament, Open Approach

0MM54ZZ Reattachment of Right Wrist Bursa and Ligament, Percutaneous Endoscopic Approach

0MM60ZZ Reattachment of Left Wrist Bursa and Ligament, Open Approach

0MM64ZZ Reattachment of Left Wrist Bursa and Ligament, Percutaneous Endoscopic Approach

0MM70ZZ Reattachment of Right Hand Bursa and Ligament, Open Approach

0MM74ZZ Reattachment of Right Hand Bursa and Ligament, Percutaneous Endoscopic Approach

0MM80ZZ Reattachment of Left Hand Bursa and Ligament, Open Approach

0MM84ZZ Reattachment of Left Hand Bursa and Ligament, Percutaneous Endoscopic Approach

0MM90ZZ Reattachment of Right Upper Extremity Bursa and Ligament, Open Approach

0MM94ZZ Reattachment of Right Upper Extremity Bursa and Ligament, Percutaneous Endoscopic Approach

0MMB0ZZ Reattachment of Left Upper Extremity Bursa and Ligament, Open Approach

0MMB4ZZ Reattachment of Left Upper Extremity Bursa and Ligament, Percutaneous Endoscopic Approach

0MMC0ZZ Reattachment of Right Trunk Bursa and Ligament, Open Approach

0MMC4ZZ Reattachment of Right Trunk Bursa and Ligament, Percutaneous Endoscopic Approach

0MMD0ZZ Reattachment of Left Trunk Bursa and Ligament, Open Approach

0MMD4ZZ Reattachment of Left Trunk Bursa and Ligament, Percutaneous Endoscopic Approach

0MMF0ZZ Reattachment of Right Thorax Bursa and Ligament, Open Approach

0MMF4ZZ Reattachment of Right Thorax Bursa and Ligament, Percutaneous Endoscopic Approach

0MMG0ZZ Reattachment of Left Thorax Bursa and Ligament, Open Approach

0MMG4ZZ Reattachment of Left Thorax Bursa and Ligament, Percutaneous Endoscopic Approach

0MMH0ZZ Reattachment of Right Abdomen Bursa and Ligament, Open Approach

0MMH4ZZ Reattachment of Right Abdomen Bursa and Ligament, Percutaneous Endoscopic Approach

0MMJ0ZZ Reattachment of Left Abdomen Bursa and Ligament, Open Approach

0MMJ4ZZ Reattachment of Left Abdomen Bursa and Ligament, Percutaneous Endoscopic Approach

0MMK0ZZ Reattachment of Perineum Bursa and Ligament, Open Approach

0MMK4ZZ Reattachment of Perineum Bursa and Ligament, Percutaneous Endoscopic Approach

0MML0ZZ Reattachment of Right Hip Bursa and Ligament, Open Approach

0MML4ZZ Reattachment of Right Hip Bursa and Ligament, Percutaneous Endoscopic Approach

0MMM0ZZ Reattachment of Left Hip Bursa and Ligament, Open Approach

0MMM4ZZ Reattachment of Left Hip Bursa and Ligament, Percutaneous Endoscopic Approach

0MMN0ZZ Reattachment of Right Knee Bursa and Ligament, Open Approach

0MMN4ZZ Reattachment of Right Knee Bursa and Ligament, Percutaneous Endoscopic Approach

0MMP0ZZ Reattachment of Left Knee Bursa and Ligament, Open Approach

0MMP4ZZ Reattachment of Left Knee Bursa and Ligament, Percutaneous Endoscopic Approach

0MMQ0ZZ Reattachment of Right Ankle Bursa and Ligament, Open Approach

0MMQ4ZZ Reattachment of Right Ankle Bursa and Ligament, Percutaneous Endoscopic Approach

0MMR0ZZ Reattachment of Left Ankle Bursa and Ligament, Open Approach

0MMR4ZZ Reattachment of Left Ankle Bursa and Ligament, Percutaneous Endoscopic Approach

0MMS0ZZ Reattachment of Right Foot Bursa and Ligament, Open Approach

0MMS4ZZ Reattachment of Right Foot Bursa and Ligament, Percutaneous Endoscopic Approach

0MMT0ZZ Reattachment of Left Foot Bursa and Ligament, Open Approach

0MMT4ZZ Reattachment of Left Foot Bursa and Ligament, Percutaneous Endoscopic Approach

0MMV0ZZ Reattachment of Right Lower Extremity Bursa and Ligament, Open Approach

0MMV4ZZ Reattachment of Right Lower Extremity Bursa and Ligament, Percutaneous Endoscopic Approach

0MMW0ZZ Reattachment of Left Lower Extremity Bursa and Ligament, Open Approach

0MMW4ZZ Reattachment of Left Lower Extremity Bursa and Ligament, Percutaneous Endoscopic Approach

0N – Bursae and Ligaments, Release

view Coding Guideline B3.13

view Coding Guideline B3.14

0MN00ZZ Release Head and Neck Bursa and Ligament, Open Approach

0MN03ZZ Release Head and Neck Bursa and Ligament, Percutaneous Approach

0MN04ZZ Release Head and Neck Bursa and Ligament, Percutaneous Endoscopic Approach

0MN0XZZ Release Head and Neck Bursa and Ligament, External Approach

0MN10ZZ Release Right Shoulder Bursa and Ligament, Open Approach

0MN13ZZ Release Right Shoulder Bursa and Ligament, Percutaneous Approach

0MN14ZZ Release Right Shoulder Bursa and Ligament, Percutaneous Endoscopic Approach

0MN1XZZ Release Right Shoulder Bursa and Ligament, External Approach

0MN20ZZ Release Left Shoulder Bursa and Ligament, Open Approach

0MN23ZZ Release Left Shoulder Bursa and Ligament, Percutaneous Approach

0MN24ZZ Release Left Shoulder Bursa and Ligament, Percutaneous Endoscopic Approach

0MN2XZZ Release Left Shoulder Bursa and Ligament, External Approach

0MN30ZZ Release Right Elbow Bursa and Ligament, Open Approach

0MN33ZZ Release Right Elbow Bursa and Ligament, Percutaneous Approach

0MN34ZZ Release Right Elbow Bursa and Ligament, Percutaneous Endoscopic Approach

0MN3XZZ Release Right Elbow Bursa and Ligament, External Approach

0MN40ZZ Release Left Elbow Bursa and Ligament, Open Approach

0MN43ZZ Release Left Elbow Bursa and Ligament, Percutaneous Approach

0MN44ZZ Release Left Elbow Bursa and Ligament, Percutaneous Endoscopic Approach

0MN4XZZ Release Left Elbow Bursa and Ligament, External Approach

0MN50ZZ Release Right Wrist Bursa and Ligament, Open Approach

0MN53ZZ Release Right Wrist Bursa and Ligament, Percutaneous Approach

0MN54ZZ Release Right Wrist Bursa and Ligament, Percutaneous Endoscopic Approach

0MN5XZZ Release Right Wrist Bursa and Ligament, External Approach

0MN60ZZ Release Left Wrist Bursa and Ligament, Open Approach

Female-only   ♂ Male-only   ▲ Limited Coverage   ● Non-OR   ▨ HAC-associated procedure   ▲ Non-covered procedures   ✚ Combination

0MN63ZZ Release Left Wrist Bursa and Ligament, Percutaneous Approach

0MN64ZZ Release Left Wrist Bursa and Ligament, Percutaneous Endoscopic Approach

0MN6XZZ Release Left Wrist Bursa and Ligament, External Approach

0MN70ZZ Release Right Hand Bursa and Ligament, Open Approach

0MN73ZZ Release Right Hand Bursa and Ligament, Percutaneous Approach

0MN74ZZ Release Right Hand Bursa and Ligament, Percutaneous Endoscopic Approach

0MN7XZZ Release Right Hand Bursa and Ligament, External Approach

0MN80ZZ Release Left Hand Bursa and Ligament, Open Approach

0MN83ZZ Release Left Hand Bursa and Ligament, Percutaneous Approach

0MN84ZZ Release Left Hand Bursa and Ligament, Percutaneous Endoscopic Approach

0MN8XZZ Release Left Hand Bursa and Ligament, External Approach

0MN90ZZ Release Right Upper Extremity Bursa and Ligament, Open Approach

0MN93ZZ Release Right Upper Extremity Bursa and Ligament, Percutaneous Approach

0MN94ZZ Release Right Upper Extremity Bursa and Ligament, Percutaneous Endoscopic Approach

0MN9XZZ Release Right Upper Extremity Bursa and Ligament, External Approach

0MNB0ZZ Release Left Upper Extremity Bursa and Ligament, Open Approach

0MNB3ZZ Release Left Upper Extremity Bursa and Ligament, Percutaneous Approach

0MNB4ZZ Release Left Upper Extremity Bursa and Ligament, Percutaneous Endoscopic Approach

0MNBXZZ Release Left Upper Extremity Bursa and Ligament, External Approach

0MNC0ZZ Release Right Trunk Bursa and Ligament, Open Approach

0MNC3ZZ Release Right Trunk Bursa and Ligament, Percutaneous Approach

0MNC4ZZ Release Right Trunk Bursa and Ligament, Percutaneous Endoscopic Approach

0MNCXZZ Release Right Trunk Bursa and Ligament, External Approach

0MND0ZZ Release Left Trunk Bursa and Ligament, Open Approach

0MND3ZZ Release Left Trunk Bursa and Ligament, Percutaneous Approach

0MND4ZZ Release Left Trunk Bursa and Ligament, Percutaneous Endoscopic Approach

0MNDXZZ Release Left Trunk Bursa and Ligament, External Approach

0MNF0ZZ Release Right Thorax Bursa and Ligament, Open Approach

0MNF3ZZ Release Right Thorax Bursa and Ligament, Percutaneous Approach

0MNF4ZZ Release Right Thorax Bursa and Ligament, Percutaneous Endoscopic Approach

0MNFXZZ Release Right Thorax Bursa and Ligament, External Approach

0MNG0ZZ Release Left Thorax Bursa and Ligament, Open Approach

0MNG3ZZ Release Left Thorax Bursa and Ligament, Percutaneous Approach

0MNG4ZZ Release Left Thorax Bursa and Ligament, Percutaneous Endoscopic Approach

0MNGXZZ Release Left Thorax Bursa and Ligament, External Approach

0MNH0ZZ Release Right Abdomen Bursa and Ligament, Open Approach

0MNH3ZZ Release Right Abdomen Bursa and Ligament, Percutaneous Approach

0MNH4ZZ Release Right Abdomen Bursa and Ligament, Percutaneous Endoscopic Approach

0MNHXZZ Release Right Abdomen Bursa and Ligament, External Approach

0MNJ0ZZ Release Left Abdomen Bursa and Ligament, Open Approach

0MNJ3ZZ Release Left Abdomen Bursa and Ligament, Percutaneous Approach

0MNJ4ZZ Release Left Abdomen Bursa and Ligament, Percutaneous Endoscopic Approach

0MNJXZZ Release Left Abdomen Bursa and Ligament, External Approach

0MNK0ZZ Release Perineum Bursa and Ligament, Open Approach

0MNK3ZZ Release Perineum Bursa and Ligament, Percutaneous Approach

0MNK4ZZ Release Perineum Bursa and Ligament, Percutaneous Endoscopic Approach

0MNKXZZ Release Perineum Bursa and Ligament, External Approach

0MNL0ZZ Release Right Hip Bursa and Ligament, Open Approach

0MNL3ZZ Release Right Hip Bursa and Ligament, Percutaneous Approach

0MNL4ZZ Release Right Hip Bursa and Ligament, Percutaneous Endoscopic Approach

0MNLXZZ Release Right Hip Bursa and Ligament, External Approach

0MNM0ZZ Release Left Hip Bursa and Ligament, Open Approach

0MNM3ZZ Release Left Hip Bursa and Ligament, Percutaneous Approach

0MNM4ZZ Release Left Hip Bursa and Ligament, Percutaneous Endoscopic Approach

0MNMXZZ Release Left Hip Bursa and Ligament, External Approach

0MNN0ZZ Release Right Knee Bursa and Ligament, Open Approach

0MNN3ZZ Release Right Knee Bursa and Ligament, Percutaneous Approach

0MNN4ZZ Release Right Knee Bursa and Ligament, Percutaneous Endoscopic Approach

0MNNXZZ Release Right Knee Bursa and Ligament, External Approach

0MNP0ZZ Release Left Knee Bursa and Ligam[ent], Open Approach

0MNP3ZZ Release Left Knee Bursa and Ligam[ent], Percutaneous Approach

0MNP4ZZ Release Left Knee Bursa and Ligam[ent], Percutaneous Endoscopic Approach

0MNPXZZ Release Left Knee Bursa and Ligam[ent], External Approach

0MNQ0ZZ Release Right Ankle Bursa and Ligament, Open Approach

0MNQ3ZZ Release Right Ankle Bursa and Ligament, Percutaneous Approach

0MNQ4ZZ Release Right Ankle Bursa and Ligament, Percutaneous Endoscopic Approach

0MNQXZZ Release Right Ankle Bursa and Ligament, External Approach

0MNR0ZZ Release Left Ankle Bursa and Ligam[ent], Open Approach

0MNR3ZZ Release Left Ankle Bursa and Ligam[ent], Percutaneous Approach

0MNR4ZZ Release Left Ankle Bursa and Ligam[ent], Percutaneous Endoscopic Approach

0MNRXZZ Release Left Ankle Bursa and Ligam[ent], External Approach

0MNS0ZZ Release Right Foot Bursa and Ligam[ent], Open Approach

0MNS3ZZ Release Right Foot Bursa and Ligam[ent], Percutaneous Approach

0MNS4ZZ Release Right Foot Bursa and Ligam[ent], Percutaneous Endoscopic Approach

0MNSXZZ Release Right Foot Bursa and Ligam[ent], External Approach

0MNT0ZZ Release Left Foot Bursa and Ligamer[t], Open Approach

0MNT3ZZ Release Left Foot Bursa and Ligamer[t], Percutaneous Approach

0MNT4ZZ Release Left Foot Bursa and Ligamer[t], Percutaneous Endoscopic Approach

0MNTXZZ Release Left Foot Bursa and Ligamer[t], External Approach

0MNV0ZZ Release Right Lower Extremity Burs[a] and Ligament, Open Approach

0MNV3ZZ Release Right Lower Extremity Burs[a] and Ligament, Percutaneous Approach

0MNV4ZZ Release Right Lower Extremity Burs[a] and Ligament, Percutaneous Endosco[pic] Approach

0MNVXZZ Release Right Lower Extremity Burs[a] and Ligament, External Approach

0MNW0ZZ Release Left Lower Extremity Bursa a[nd] Ligament, Open Approach

0MNW3ZZ Release Left Lower Extremity Bursa a[nd] Ligament, Percutaneous Approach

0MNW4ZZ Release Left Lower Extremity Bursa a[nd] Ligament, Percutaneous Endosco[pic] Approach

0MNWXZZ Release Left Lower Extremity Bursa and Ligament, External Approa[ch]

0MP – Bursae and Ligaments, Removal

Review Coding Guideline B6.1c

0MPX00Z Removal of Drainage Device from Upper Bursa and Ligament, Open Approach

0MPX07Z Removal of Autologous Tissue Substitute from Upper Bursa and Ligament, Open Approach

0MPX0JZ Removal of Synthetic Substitute from Upper Bursa and Ligament, Open Approach

0MPX0KZ Removal of Nonautologous Tissue Substitute from Upper Bursa and Ligament, Open Approach

0MPX30Z Removal of Drainage Device from Upper Bursa and Ligament, Percutaneous Approach

0MPX37Z Removal of Autologous Tissue Substitute from Upper Bursa and Ligament, Percutaneous Approach

0MPX3JZ Removal of Synthetic Substitute from Upper Bursa and Ligament, Percutaneo[us] Approach

0MPX3KZ Removal of Nonautologous Tissue Substitute from Upper Bursa an[d] Ligament, Percutaneous Approach

0MPX40Z Removal of Drainage Device from Upp[er] Bursa and Ligament, Percutaneous Endoscopic Approach

X47Z Removal of Autologous Tissue Substitute from Upper Bursa and Ligament, Percutaneous Endoscopic Approach

X4JZ Removal of Synthetic Substitute from Upper Bursa and Ligament, Percutaneous Endoscopic Approach

X4KZ Removal of Nonautologous Tissue Substitute from Upper Bursa and Ligament, Percutaneous Endoscopic Approach

XX0Z Removal of Drainage Device from Upper Bursa and Ligament, External Approach

Y00Z Removal of Drainage Device from Lower Bursa and Ligament, Open Approach

Y07Z Removal of Autologous Tissue Substitute from Lower Bursa and Ligament, Open Approach

0MPY0JZ Removal of Synthetic Substitute from Lower Bursa and Ligament, Open Approach

0MPY0KZ Removal of Nonautologous Tissue Substitute from Lower Bursa and Ligament, Open Approach

0MPY30Z Removal of Drainage Device from Lower Bursa and Ligament, Percutaneous Approach

0MPY37Z Removal of Autologous Tissue Substitute from Lower Bursa and Ligament, Percutaneous Approach

0MPY3JZ Removal of Synthetic Substitute from Lower Bursa and Ligament, Percutaneous Approach

0MPY3KZ Removal of Nonautologous Tissue Substitute from Lower Bursa and Ligament, Percutaneous Approach

0MPY40Z Removal of Drainage Device from Lower Bursa and Ligament, Percutaneous Endoscopic Approach

0MPY47Z Removal of Autologous Tissue Substitute from Lower Bursa and Ligament, Percutaneous Endoscopic Approach

0MPY4JZ Removal of Synthetic Substitute from Lower Bursa and Ligament, Percutaneous Endoscopic Approach

0MPY4KZ Removal of Nonautologous Tissue Substitute from Lower Bursa and Ligament, Percutaneous Endoscopic Approach

0MPYX0Z Removal of Drainage Device from Lower Bursa and Ligament, External Approach

Q – Bursae and Ligaments, Repair

iew Coding Guideline B3.5

00ZZ Repair Head and Neck Bursa and Ligament, Open Approach
AHA CC: 3Q, 2014, 9

03ZZ Repair Head and Neck Bursa and Ligament, Percutaneous Approach

04ZZ Repair Head and Neck Bursa and Ligament, Percutaneous Endoscopic Approach

10ZZ Repair Right Shoulder Bursa and Ligament, Open Approach

13ZZ Repair Right Shoulder Bursa and Ligament, Percutaneous Approach

14ZZ Repair Right Shoulder Bursa and Ligament, Percutaneous Endoscopic Approach

20ZZ Repair Left Shoulder Bursa and Ligament, Open Approach

23ZZ Repair Left Shoulder Bursa and Ligament, Percutaneous Approach

24ZZ Repair Left Shoulder Bursa and Ligament, Percutaneous Endoscopic Approach

30ZZ Repair Right Elbow Bursa and Ligament, Open Approach

33ZZ Repair Right Elbow Bursa and Ligament, Percutaneous Approach

34ZZ Repair Right Elbow Bursa and Ligament, Percutaneous Endoscopic Approach

40ZZ Repair Left Elbow Bursa and Ligament, Open Approach

43ZZ Repair Left Elbow Bursa and Ligament, Percutaneous Approach

44ZZ Repair Left Elbow Bursa and Ligament, Percutaneous Endoscopic Approach

50ZZ Repair Right Wrist Bursa and Ligament, Open Approach

53ZZ Repair Right Wrist Bursa and Ligament, Percutaneous Approach

54ZZ Repair Right Wrist Bursa and Ligament, Percutaneous Endoscopic Approach

60ZZ Repair Left Wrist Bursa and Ligament, Open Approach

63ZZ Repair Left Wrist Bursa and Ligament, Percutaneous Approach

64ZZ Repair Left Wrist Bursa and Ligament, Percutaneous Endoscopic Approach

70ZZ Repair Right Hand Bursa and Ligament, Open Approach

73ZZ Repair Right Hand Bursa and Ligament, Percutaneous Approach

74ZZ Repair Right Hand Bursa and Ligament, Percutaneous Endoscopic Approach

0MQ80ZZ Repair Left Hand Bursa and Ligament, Open Approach

0MQ83ZZ Repair Left Hand Bursa and Ligament, Percutaneous Approach

0MQ84ZZ Repair Left Hand Bursa and Ligament, Percutaneous Endoscopic Approach

0MQ90ZZ Repair Right Upper Extremity Bursa and Ligament, Open Approach

0MQ93ZZ Repair Right Upper Extremity Bursa and Ligament, Percutaneous Approach

0MQ94ZZ Repair Right Upper Extremity Bursa and Ligament, Percutaneous Endoscopic Approach

0MQB0ZZ Repair Left Upper Extremity Bursa and Ligament, Open Approach

0MQB3ZZ Repair Left Upper Extremity Bursa and Ligament, Percutaneous Approach

0MQB4ZZ Repair Left Upper Extremity Bursa and Ligament, Percutaneous Endoscopic Approach

0MQC0ZZ Repair Right Trunk Bursa and Ligament, Open Approach

0MQC3ZZ Repair Right Trunk Bursa and Ligament, Percutaneous Approach

0MQC4ZZ Repair Right Trunk Bursa and Ligament, Percutaneous Endoscopic Approach

0MQD0ZZ Repair Left Trunk Bursa and Ligament, Open Approach

0MQD3ZZ Repair Left Trunk Bursa and Ligament, Percutaneous Approach

0MQD4ZZ Repair Left Trunk Bursa and Ligament, Percutaneous Endoscopic Approach

0MQF0ZZ Repair Right Thorax Bursa and Ligament, Open Approach

0MQF3ZZ Repair Right Thorax Bursa and Ligament, Percutaneous Approach

0MQF4ZZ Repair Right Thorax Bursa and Ligament, Percutaneous Endoscopic Approach

0MQG0ZZ Repair Left Thorax Bursa and Ligament, Open Approach

0MQG3ZZ Repair Left Thorax Bursa and Ligament, Percutaneous Approach

0MQG4ZZ Repair Left Thorax Bursa and Ligament, Percutaneous Endoscopic Approach

0MQH0ZZ Repair Right Abdomen Bursa and Ligament, Open Approach

0MQH3ZZ Repair Right Abdomen Bursa and Ligament, Percutaneous Approach

0MQH4ZZ Repair Right Abdomen Bursa and Ligament, Percutaneous Endoscopic Approach

0MQJ0ZZ Repair Left Abdomen Bursa and Ligament, Open Approach

0MQJ3ZZ Repair Left Abdomen Bursa and Ligament, Percutaneous Approach

0MQJ4ZZ Repair Left Abdomen Bursa and Ligament, Percutaneous Endoscopic Approach

0MQK0ZZ Repair Perineum Bursa and Ligament, Open Approach

0MQK3ZZ Repair Perineum Bursa and Ligament, Percutaneous Approach

0MQK4ZZ Repair Perineum Bursa and Ligament, Percutaneous Endoscopic Approach

0MQL0ZZ Repair Right Hip Bursa and Ligament, Open Approach

0MQL3ZZ Repair Right Hip Bursa and Ligament, Percutaneous Approach

0MQL4ZZ Repair Right Hip Bursa and Ligament, Percutaneous Endoscopic Approach

0MQM0ZZ Repair Left Hip Bursa and Ligament, Open Approach

0MQM3ZZ Repair Left Hip Bursa and Ligament, Percutaneous Approach

0MQM4ZZ Repair Left Hip Bursa and Ligament, Percutaneous Endoscopic Approach

0MQN0ZZ Repair Right Knee Bursa and Ligament, Open Approach

0MQN3ZZ Repair Right Knee Bursa and Ligament, Percutaneous Approach

0MQN4ZZ Repair Right Knee Bursa and Ligament, Percutaneous Endoscopic Approach

0MQP0ZZ Repair Left Knee Bursa and Ligament, Open Approach

0MQP3ZZ Repair Left Knee Bursa and Ligament, Percutaneous Approach

0MQP4ZZ Repair Left Knee Bursa and Ligament, Percutaneous Endoscopic Approach

0MQQ0ZZ Repair Right Ankle Bursa and Ligament, Open Approach

0MQQ3ZZ Repair Right Ankle Bursa and Ligament, Percutaneous Approach

0MQQ4ZZ Repair Right Ankle Bursa and Ligament, Percutaneous Endoscopic Approach

0MQR0ZZ Repair Left Ankle Bursa and Ligament, Open Approach

0MQR3ZZ Repair Left Ankle Bursa and Ligament, Percutaneous Approach

0MQR4ZZ Repair Left Ankle Bursa and Ligament, Percutaneous Endoscopic Approach

0MQS0ZZ Repair Right Foot Bursa and Ligament, Open Approach

emale-only   ♂ Male-only   ▲ Limited Coverage   ● Non-OR   ▰▰ HAC-associated procedure   ▲ Non-covered procedures   ➕ Combination

0MQS3ZZ	Repair Right Foot Bursa and Ligament, Percutaneous Approach	**0MQT4ZZ**	Repair Left Foot Bursa and Ligament, Percutaneous Endoscopic Approach	**0MQW0ZZ**	Repair Left Lower Extremity Bursa Ligament, Open Approach
0MQS4ZZ	Repair Right Foot Bursa and Ligament, Percutaneous Endoscopic Approach	**0MQV0ZZ**	Repair Right Lower Extremity Bursa and Ligament, Open Approach	**0MQW3ZZ**	Repair Left Lower Extremity Bursa Ligament, Percutaneous Approach
0MQT0ZZ	Repair Left Foot Bursa and Ligament, Open Approach	**0MQV3ZZ**	Repair Right Lower Extremity Bursa and Ligament, Percutaneous Approach	**0MQW4ZZ**	Repair Left Lower Extremity Bursa Ligament, Percutaneous Endoscopi Approach
0MQT3ZZ	Repair Left Foot Bursa and Ligament, Percutaneous Approach	**0MQV4ZZ**	Repair Right Lower Extremity Bursa and Ligament, Percutaneous Endoscopic Approach		

0MS – Bursae and Ligaments, Reposition

0MS00ZZ	Reposition Head and Neck Bursa and Ligament, Open Approach	**0MS90ZZ**	Reposition Right Upper Extremity Bursa and Ligament, Open Approach	**0MSL4ZZ**	Reposition Right Hip Bursa and Ligament, Percutaneous Endoscopic Approach
0MS04ZZ	Reposition Head and Neck Bursa and Ligament, Percutaneous Endoscopic Approach	**0MS94ZZ**	Reposition Right Upper Extremity Bursa and Ligament, Percutaneous Endoscopic Approach	**0MSM0ZZ**	Reposition Left Hip Bursa and Ligam Open Approach
0MS10ZZ	Reposition Right Shoulder Bursa and Ligament, Open Approach	**0MSB0ZZ**	Reposition Left Upper Extremity Bursa and Ligament, Open Approach	**0MSM4ZZ**	Reposition Left Hip Bursa and Ligam Percutaneous Endoscopic Approach
0MS14ZZ	Reposition Right Shoulder Bursa and Ligament, Percutaneous Endoscopic Approach	**0MSB4ZZ**	Reposition Left Upper Extremity Bursa and Ligament, Percutaneous Endoscopic Approach	**0MSN0ZZ**	Reposition Right Knee Bursa and Ligament, Open Approach
0MS20ZZ	Reposition Left Shoulder Bursa and Ligament, Open Approach	**0MSC0ZZ**	Reposition Right Trunk Bursa and Ligament, Open Approach	**0MSN4ZZ**	Reposition Right Knee Bursa and Ligament, Percutaneous Endoscopic Approach
0MS24ZZ	Reposition Left Shoulder Bursa and Ligament, Percutaneous Endoscopic Approach	**0MSC4ZZ**	Reposition Right Trunk Bursa and Ligament, Percutaneous Endoscopic Approach	**0MSP0ZZ**	Reposition Left Knee Bursa and Ligament, Open Approach
0MS30ZZ	Reposition Right Elbow Bursa and Ligament, Open Approach	**0MSD0ZZ**	Reposition Left Trunk Bursa and Ligament, Open Approach	**0MSP4ZZ**	Reposition Left Knee Bursa and Ligament, Percutaneous Endoscopic Approach
0MS34ZZ	Reposition Right Elbow Bursa and Ligament, Percutaneous Endoscopic Approach	**0MSD4ZZ**	Reposition Left Trunk Bursa and Ligament, Percutaneous Endoscopic Approach	**0MSQ0ZZ**	Reposition Right Ankle Bursa and Ligament, Open Approach
0MS40ZZ	Reposition Left Elbow Bursa and Ligament, Open Approach	**0MSF0ZZ**	Reposition Right Thorax Bursa and Ligament, Open Approach	**0MSQ4ZZ**	Reposition Right Ankle Bursa and Ligament, Percutaneous Endoscopic Approach
0MS44ZZ	Reposition Left Elbow Bursa and Ligament, Percutaneous Endoscopic Approach	**0MSF4ZZ**	Reposition Right Thorax Bursa and Ligament, Percutaneous Endoscopic Approach	**0MSR0ZZ**	Reposition Left Ankle Bursa and Ligament, Open Approach
0MS50ZZ	Reposition Right Wrist Bursa and Ligament, Open Approach	**0MSG0ZZ**	Reposition Left Thorax Bursa and Ligament, Open Approach	**0MSR4ZZ**	Reposition Left Ankle Bursa and Ligament, Percutaneous Endoscopic Approach
0MS54ZZ	Reposition Right Wrist Bursa and Ligament, Percutaneous Endoscopic Approach	**0MSG4ZZ**	Reposition Left Thorax Bursa and Ligament, Percutaneous Endoscopic Approach	**0MSS0ZZ**	Reposition Right Foot Bursa and Ligament, Open Approach
0MS60ZZ	Reposition Left Wrist Bursa and Ligament, Open Approach	**0MSH0ZZ**	Reposition Right Abdomen Bursa and Ligament, Open Approach	**0MSS4ZZ**	Reposition Right Foot Bursa and Ligament, Percutaneous Endoscopic Approach
0MS64ZZ	Reposition Left Wrist Bursa and Ligament, Percutaneous Endoscopic Approach	**0MSH4ZZ**	Reposition Right Abdomen Bursa and Ligament, Percutaneous Endoscopic Approach	**0MST0ZZ**	Reposition Left Foot Bursa and Ligament, Open Approach
0MS70ZZ	Reposition Right Hand Bursa and Ligament, Open Approach	**0MSJ0ZZ**	Reposition Left Abdomen Bursa and Ligament, Open Approach	**0MST4ZZ**	Reposition Left Foot Bursa and Ligament, Percutaneous Endoscopic Approach
0MS74ZZ	Reposition Right Hand Bursa and Ligament, Percutaneous Endoscopic Approach	**0MSJ4ZZ**	Reposition Left Abdomen Bursa and Ligament, Percutaneous Endoscopic Approach	**0MSV0ZZ**	Reposition Right Lower Extremity Bu and Ligament, Open Approach
0MS80ZZ	Reposition Left Hand Bursa and Ligament, Open Approach	**0MSK0ZZ**	Reposition Perineum Bursa and Ligament, Open Approach	**0MSV4ZZ**	Reposition Right Lower Extremity Bu and Ligament, Percutaneous Endosco Approach
0MS84ZZ	Reposition Left Hand Bursa and Ligament, Percutaneous Endoscopic Approach	**0MSK4ZZ**	Reposition Perineum Bursa and Ligament, Percutaneous Endoscopic Approach	**0MSW0ZZ**	Reposition Left Lower Extremity Bur and Ligament, Open Approach
		0MSL0ZZ	Reposition Right Hip Bursa and Ligament, Open Approach	**0MSW4ZZ**	Reposition Left Lower Extremity Burs and Ligament, Percutaneous Endosco Approach

0MT – Bursae and Ligaments, Resection

Review Coding Guideline B3.8

0MT00ZZ	Resection of Head and Neck Bursa and Ligament, Open Approach	**0MT24ZZ**	Resection of Left Shoulder Bursa and Ligament, Percutaneous Endoscopic Approach	**0MT50ZZ**	Resection of Right Wrist Bursa and Ligament, Open Approach
0MT04ZZ	Resection of Head and Neck Bursa and Ligament, Percutaneous Endoscopic Approach	**0MT30ZZ**	Resection of Right Elbow Bursa and Ligament, Open Approach	**0MT54ZZ**	Resection of Right Wrist Bursa and Ligament, Percutaneous Endoscopic Approach
0MT10ZZ	Resection of Right Shoulder Bursa and Ligament, Open Approach	**0MT34ZZ**	Resection of Right Elbow Bursa and Ligament, Percutaneous Endoscopic Approach	**0MT60ZZ**	Resection of Left Wrist Bursa and Ligament, Open Approach
0MT14ZZ	Resection of Right Shoulder Bursa and Ligament, Percutaneous Endoscopic Approach	**0MT40ZZ**	Resection of Left Elbow Bursa and Ligament, Open Approach	**0MT64ZZ**	Resection of Left Wrist Bursa and Ligament, Percutaneous Endoscopic Approach
0MT20ZZ	Resection of Left Shoulder Bursa and Ligament, Open Approach	**0MT44ZZ**	Resection of Left Elbow Bursa and Ligament, Percutaneous Endoscopic Approach	**0MT70ZZ**	Resection of Right Hand Bursa and Ligament, Open Approach

♀ Female-only	♂ Male-only	▲ Limited Coverage	● Non-OR	▩ HAC-associated procedure	▲ Non-covered procedures	✛ Combinat

T74ZZ Resection of Right Hand Bursa and Ligament, Percutaneous Endoscopic Approach	**0MTG4ZZ** Resection of Left Thorax Bursa and Ligament, Percutaneous Endoscopic Approach	**0MTP4ZZ** Resection of Left Knee Bursa and Ligament, Percutaneous Endoscopic Approach
T80ZZ Resection of Left Hand Bursa and Ligament, Open Approach	**0MTH0ZZ** Resection of Right Abdomen Bursa and Ligament, Open Approach	**0MTQ0ZZ** Resection of Right Ankle Bursa and Ligament, Open Approach
T84ZZ Resection of Left Hand Bursa and Ligament, Percutaneous Endoscopic Approach	**0MTH4ZZ** Resection of Right Abdomen Bursa and Ligament, Percutaneous Endoscopic Approach	**0MTQ4ZZ** Resection of Right Ankle Bursa and Ligament, Percutaneous Endoscopic Approach
T90ZZ Resection of Right Upper Extremity Bursa and Ligament, Open Approach	**0MTJ0ZZ** Resection of Left Abdomen Bursa and Ligament, Open Approach	**0MTR0ZZ** Resection of Left Ankle Bursa and Ligament, Open Approach
T94ZZ Resection of Right Upper Extremity Bursa and Ligament, Percutaneous Endoscopic Approach	**0MTJ4ZZ** Resection of Left Abdomen Bursa and Ligament, Percutaneous Endoscopic Approach	**0MTR4ZZ** Resection of Left Ankle Bursa and Ligament, Percutaneous Endoscopic Approach
TB0ZZ Resection of Left Upper Extremity Bursa and Ligament, Open Approach	**0MTK0ZZ** Resection of Perineum Bursa and Ligament, Open Approach	**0MTS0ZZ** Resection of Right Foot Bursa and Ligament, Open Approach
TB4ZZ Resection of Left Upper Extremity Bursa and Ligament, Percutaneous Endoscopic Approach	**0MTK4ZZ** Resection of Perineum Bursa and Ligament, Percutaneous Endoscopic Approach	**0MTS4ZZ** Resection of Right Foot Bursa and Ligament, Percutaneous Endoscopic Approach
TC0ZZ Resection of Right Trunk Bursa and Ligament, Open Approach	**0MTL0ZZ** Resection of Right Hip Bursa and Ligament, Open Approach	**0MTT0ZZ** Resection of Left Foot Bursa and Ligament, Open Approach
TC4ZZ Resection of Right Trunk Bursa and Ligament, Percutaneous Endoscopic Approach	**0MTL4ZZ** Resection of Right Hip Bursa and Ligament, Percutaneous Endoscopic Approach	**0MTT4ZZ** Resection of Left Foot Bursa and Ligament, Percutaneous Endoscopic Approach
TD0ZZ Resection of Left Trunk Bursa and Ligament, Open Approach	**0MTM0ZZ** Resection of Left Hip Bursa and Ligament, Open Approach	**0MTV0ZZ** Resection of Right Lower Extremity Bursa and Ligament, Open Approach
TD4ZZ Resection of Left Trunk Bursa and Ligament, Percutaneous Endoscopic Approach	**0MTM4ZZ** Resection of Left Hip Bursa and Ligament, Percutaneous Endoscopic Approach	**0MTV4ZZ** Resection of Right Lower Extremity Bursa and Ligament, Percutaneous Endoscopic Approach
TF0ZZ Resection of Right Thorax Bursa and Ligament, Open Approach	**0MTN0ZZ** Resection of Right Knee Bursa and Ligament, Open Approach	**0MTW0ZZ** Resection of Left Lower Extremity Bursa and Ligament, Open Approach
TF4ZZ Resection of Right Thorax Bursa and Ligament, Percutaneous Endoscopic Approach	**0MTN4ZZ** Resection of Right Knee Bursa and Ligament, Percutaneous Endoscopic Approach	**0MTW4ZZ** Resection of Left Lower Extremity Bursa and Ligament, Percutaneous Endoscopic Approach
TG0ZZ Resection of Left Thorax Bursa and Ligament, Open Approach	**0MTP0ZZ** Resection of Left Knee Bursa and Ligament, Open Approach	

1U – Bursae and Ligaments, Supplement

U007Z Supplement Head and Neck Bursa and Ligament with Autologous Tissue Substitute, Open Approach	Substitute, Percutaneous Endoscopic Approach	**0MU34KZ** Supplement Right Elbow Bursa and Ligament with Nonautologous Tissue Substitute, Percutaneous Endoscopic Approach
U00JZ Supplement Head and Neck Bursa and Ligament with Synthetic Substitute, Open Approach	**0MU207Z** Supplement Left Shoulder Bursa and Ligament with Autologous Tissue Substitute, Open Approach	**0MU407Z** Supplement Left Elbow Bursa and Ligament with Autologous Tissue Substitute, Open Approach
U00KZ Supplement Head and Neck Bursa and Ligament with Nonautologous Tissue Substitute, Open Approach	**0MU20JZ** Supplement Left Shoulder Bursa and Ligament with Synthetic Substitute, Open Approach	**0MU40JZ** Supplement Left Elbow Bursa and Ligament with Synthetic Substitute, Open Approach
U047Z Supplement Head and Neck Bursa and Ligament with Autologous Tissue Substitute, Percutaneous Endoscopic Approach	**0MU20KZ** Supplement Left Shoulder Bursa and Ligament with Nonautologous Tissue Substitute, Open Approach	**0MU40KZ** Supplement Left Elbow Bursa and Ligament with Nonautologous Tissue Substitute, Open Approach
U04JZ Supplement Head and Neck Bursa and Ligament with Synthetic Substitute, Percutaneous Endoscopic Approach	**0MU247Z** Supplement Left Shoulder Bursa and Ligament with Autologous Tissue Substitute, Percutaneous Endoscopic Approach	**0MU447Z** Supplement Left Elbow Bursa and Ligament with Autologous Tissue Substitute, Percutaneous Endoscopic Approach
U04KZ Supplement Head and Neck Bursa and Ligament with Nonautologous Tissue Substitute, Percutaneous Endoscopic Approach	**0MU24JZ** Supplement Left Shoulder Bursa and Ligament with Synthetic Substitute, Percutaneous Endoscopic Approach	**0MU44JZ** Supplement Left Elbow Bursa and Ligament with Synthetic Substitute, Percutaneous Endoscopic Approach
U107Z Supplement Right Shoulder Bursa and Ligament with Autologous Tissue Substitute, Open Approach	**0MU24KZ** Supplement Left Shoulder Bursa and Ligament with Nonautologous Tissue Substitute, Percutaneous Endoscopic Approach	**0MU44KZ** Supplement Left Elbow Bursa and Ligament with Nonautologous Tissue Substitute, Percutaneous Endoscopic Approach
U10JZ Supplement Right Shoulder Bursa and Ligament with Synthetic Substitute, Open Approach	**0MU307Z** Supplement Right Elbow Bursa and Ligament with Autologous Tissue Substitute, Open Approach	**0MU507Z** Supplement Right Wrist Bursa and Ligament with Autologous Tissue Substitute, Open Approach
U10KZ Supplement Right Shoulder Bursa and Ligament with Nonautologous Tissue Substitute, Open Approach	**0MU30JZ** Supplement Right Elbow Bursa and Ligament with Synthetic Substitute, Open Approach	**0MU50JZ** Supplement Right Wrist Bursa and Ligament with Synthetic Substitute, Open Approach
U147Z Supplement Right Shoulder Bursa and Ligament with Autologous Tissue Substitute, Percutaneous Endoscopic Approach	**0MU30KZ** Supplement Right Elbow Bursa and Ligament with Nonautologous Tissue Substitute, Open Approach	**0MU50KZ** Supplement Right Wrist Bursa and Ligament with Nonautologous Tissue Substitute, Open Approach
U14JZ Supplement Right Shoulder Bursa and Ligament with Synthetic Substitute, Percutaneous Endoscopic Approach	**0MU347Z** Supplement Right Elbow Bursa and Ligament with Autologous Tissue Substitute, Percutaneous Endoscopic Approach	**0MU547Z** Supplement Right Wrist Bursa and Ligament with Autologous Tissue Substitute, Percutaneous Endoscopic Approach
U14KZ Supplement Right Shoulder Bursa and Ligament with Nonautologous Tissue	**0MU34JZ** Supplement Right Elbow Bursa and Ligament with Synthetic Substitute, Percutaneous Endoscopic Approach	

Female-only	♂ Male-only	▲ Limited Coverage	● Non-OR	▰ HAC-associated procedure	▲ Non-covered procedures	✚ Combination

0MU54JZ	Supplement Right Wrist Bursa and Ligament with Synthetic Substitute, Percutaneous Endoscopic Approach
0MU54KZ	Supplement Right Wrist Bursa and Ligament with Nonautologous Tissue Substitute, Percutaneous Endoscopic Approach
0MU607Z	Supplement Left Wrist Bursa and Ligament with Autologous Tissue Substitute, Open Approach
0MU60JZ	Supplement Left Wrist Bursa and Ligament with Synthetic Substitute, Open Approach
0MU60KZ	Supplement Left Wrist Bursa and Ligament with Nonautologous Tissue Substitute, Open Approach
0MU647Z	Supplement Left Wrist Bursa and Ligament with Autologous Tissue Substitute, Percutaneous Endoscopic Approach
0MU64JZ	Supplement Left Wrist Bursa and Ligament with Synthetic Substitute, Percutaneous Endoscopic Approach
0MU64KZ	Supplement Left Wrist Bursa and Ligament with Nonautologous Tissue Substitute, Percutaneous Endoscopic Approach
0MU707Z	Supplement Right Hand Bursa and Ligament with Autologous Tissue Substitute, Open Approach
0MU70JZ	Supplement Right Hand Bursa and Ligament with Synthetic Substitute, Open Approach
0MU70KZ	Supplement Right Hand Bursa and Ligament with Nonautologous Tissue Substitute, Open Approach
0MU747Z	Supplement Right Hand Bursa and Ligament with Autologous Tissue Substitute, Percutaneous Endoscopic Approach
0MU74JZ	Supplement Right Hand Bursa and Ligament with Synthetic Substitute, Percutaneous Endoscopic Approach
0MU74KZ	Supplement Right Hand Bursa and Ligament with Nonautologous Tissue Substitute, Percutaneous Endoscopic Approach
0MU807Z	Supplement Left Hand Bursa and Ligament with Autologous Tissue Substitute, Open Approach
0MU80JZ	Supplement Left Hand Bursa and Ligament with Synthetic Substitute, Open Approach
0MU80KZ	Supplement Left Hand Bursa and Ligament with Nonautologous Tissue Substitute, Open Approach
0MU847Z	Supplement Left Hand Bursa and Ligament with Autologous Tissue Substitute, Percutaneous Endoscopic Approach
0MU84JZ	Supplement Left Hand Bursa and Ligament with Synthetic Substitute, Percutaneous Endoscopic Approach
0MU84KZ	Supplement Left Hand Bursa and Ligament with Nonautologous Tissue Substitute, Percutaneous Endoscopic Approach
0MU907Z	Supplement Right Upper Extremity Bursa and Ligament with Autologous Tissue Substitute, Open Approach
0MU90JZ	Supplement Right Upper Extremity Bursa and Ligament with Synthetic Substitute, Open Approach
0MU90KZ	Supplement Right Upper Extremity Bursa and Ligament with Nonautologous Tissue Substitute, Open Approach
0MU947Z	Supplement Right Upper Extremity Bursa and Ligament with Autologous Tissue Substitute, Percutaneous Endoscopic Approach
0MU94JZ	Supplement Right Upper Extremity Bursa and Ligament with Synthetic Substitute, Percutaneous Endoscopic Approach
0MU94KZ	Supplement Right Upper Extremity Bursa and Ligament with Nonautologous Tissue Substitute, Percutaneous Endoscopic Approach
0MUB07Z	Supplement Left Upper Extremity Bursa and Ligament with Autologous Tissue Substitute, Open Approach
0MUB0JZ	Supplement Left Upper Extremity Bursa and Ligament with Synthetic Substitute, Open Approach
0MUB0KZ	Supplement Left Upper Extremity Bursa and Ligament with Nonautologous Tissue Substitute, Open Approach
0MUB47Z	Supplement Left Upper Extremity Bursa and Ligament with Autologous Tissue Substitute, Percutaneous Endoscopic Approach
0MUB4JZ	Supplement Left Upper Extremity Bursa and Ligament with Synthetic Substitute, Percutaneous Endoscopic Approach
0MUB4KZ	Supplement Left Upper Extremity Bursa and Ligament with Nonautologous Tissue Substitute, Percutaneous Endoscopic Approach
0MUC07Z	Supplement Right Trunk Bursa and Ligament with Autologous Tissue Substitute, Open Approach
0MUC0JZ	Supplement Right Trunk Bursa and Ligament with Synthetic Substitute, Open Approach
0MUC0KZ	Supplement Right Trunk Bursa and Ligament with Nonautologous Tissue Substitute, Open Approach
0MUC47Z	Supplement Right Trunk Bursa and Ligament with Autologous Tissue Substitute, Percutaneous Endoscopic Approach
0MUC4JZ	Supplement Right Trunk Bursa and Ligament with Synthetic Substitute, Percutaneous Endoscopic Approach
0MUC4KZ	Supplement Right Trunk Bursa and Ligament with Nonautologous Tissue Substitute, Percutaneous Endoscopic Approach
0MUD07Z	Supplement Left Trunk Bursa and Ligament with Autologous Tissue Substitute, Open Approach
0MUD0JZ	Supplement Left Trunk Bursa and Ligament with Synthetic Substitute, Open Approach
0MUD0KZ	Supplement Left Trunk Bursa and Ligament with Nonautologous Tissue Substitute, Open Approach
0MUD47Z	Supplement Left Trunk Bursa and Ligament with Autologous Tissue Substitute, Percutaneous Endoscopic Approach
0MUD4JZ	Supplement Left Trunk Bursa and Ligament with Synthetic Substitute, Percutaneous Endoscopic Approach
0MUD4KZ	Supplement Left Trunk Bursa and Ligament with Nonautologous Tissue Substitute, Percutaneous Endoscopic Approach
0MUF07Z	Supplement Right Thorax Bursa and Ligament with Autologous Tissue Substitute, Open Approach
0MUF0JZ	Supplement Right Thorax Bursa and Ligament with Synthetic Substitute, Open Approach
0MUF0KZ	Supplement Right Thorax Bursa and Ligament with Nonautologous Tissue Substitute, Open Approach
0MUF47Z	Supplement Right Thorax Bursa and Ligament with Autologous Tissue Substitute, Percutaneous Endoscopic Approach
0MUF4JZ	Supplement Right Thorax Bursa and Ligament with Synthetic Substitute, Percutaneous Endoscopic Approach
0MUF4KZ	Supplement Right Thorax Bursa and Ligament with Nonautologous Tissue Substitute, Percutaneous Endoscopic Approach
0MUG07Z	Supplement Left Thorax Bursa and Ligament with Autologous Tissue Substitute, Open Approach
0MUG0JZ	Supplement Left Thorax Bursa and Ligament with Synthetic Substitute, Open Approach
0MUG0KZ	Supplement Left Thorax Bursa and Ligament with Nonautologous Tissue Substitute, Open Approach
0MUG47Z	Supplement Left Thorax Bursa and Ligament with Autologous Tissue Substitute, Percutaneous Endoscopic Approach
0MUG4JZ	Supplement Left Thorax Bursa and Ligament with Synthetic Substitute, Percutaneous Endoscopic Approach
0MUG4KZ	Supplement Left Thorax Bursa and Ligament with Nonautologous Tissue Substitute, Percutaneous Endoscopic Approach
0MUH07Z	Supplement Right Abdomen Bursa and Ligament with Autologous Tissue Substitute, Open Approach
0MUH0JZ	Supplement Right Abdomen Bursa and Ligament with Synthetic Substitute, Open Approach
0MUH0KZ	Supplement Right Abdomen Bursa and Ligament with Nonautologous Tissue Substitute, Open Approach
0MUH47Z	Supplement Right Abdomen Bursa and Ligament with Autologous Tissue Substitute, Percutaneous Endoscopic Approach
0MUH4JZ	Supplement Right Abdomen Bursa and Ligament with Synthetic Substitute, Percutaneous Endoscopic Approach
0MUH4KZ	Supplement Right Abdomen Bursa and Ligament with Nonautologous Tissue Substitute, Percutaneous Endoscopic Approach
0MUJ07Z	Supplement Left Abdomen Bursa and Ligament with Autologous Tissue Substitute, Open Approach
0MUJ0JZ	Supplement Left Abdomen Bursa and Ligament with Synthetic Substitute, Open Approach
0MUJ0KZ	Supplement Left Abdomen Bursa and Ligament with Nonautologous Tissue Substitute, Open Approach
0MUJ47Z	Supplement Left Abdomen Bursa and Ligament with Autologous Tissue Substitute, Percutaneous Endoscopic Approach
0MUJ4JZ	Supplement Left Abdomen Bursa and Ligament with Synthetic Substitute, Percutaneous Endoscopic Approach
0MUJ4KZ	Supplement Left Abdomen Bursa and Ligament with Nonautologous Tissue Substitute, Percutaneous Endoscopic Approach

♀ Female-only   ♂ Male-only   ▲ Limited Coverage   ● Non-OR   ▨ HAC-associated procedure   ▲ Non-covered procedures   ✛ Combinati

K07Z	Supplement Perineum Bursa and Ligament with Autologous Tissue Substitute, Open Approach
K0JZ	Supplement Perineum Bursa and Ligament with Synthetic Substitute, Open Approach
K0KZ	Supplement Perineum Bursa and Ligament with Nonautologous Tissue Substitute, Open Approach
K47Z	Supplement Perineum Bursa and Ligament with Autologous Tissue Substitute, Percutaneous Endoscopic Approach
K4JZ	Supplement Perineum Bursa and Ligament with Synthetic Substitute, Percutaneous Endoscopic Approach
K4KZ	Supplement Perineum Bursa and Ligament with Nonautologous Tissue Substitute, Percutaneous Endoscopic Approach
L07Z	Supplement Right Hip Bursa and Ligament with Autologous Tissue Substitute, Open Approach
L0JZ	Supplement Right Hip Bursa and Ligament with Synthetic Substitute, Open Approach
L0KZ	Supplement Right Hip Bursa and Ligament with Nonautologous Tissue Substitute, Open Approach
L47Z	Supplement Right Hip Bursa and Ligament with Autologous Tissue Substitute, Percutaneous Endoscopic Approach
L4JZ	Supplement Right Hip Bursa and Ligament with Synthetic Substitute, Percutaneous Endoscopic Approach
L4KZ	Supplement Right Hip Bursa and Ligament with Nonautologous Tissue Substitute, Percutaneous Endoscopic Approach
M07Z	Supplement Left Hip Bursa and Ligament with Autologous Tissue Substitute, Open Approach
M0JZ	Supplement Left Hip Bursa and Ligament with Synthetic Substitute, Open Approach
M0KZ	Supplement Left Hip Bursa and Ligament with Nonautologous Tissue Substitute, Open Approach
M47Z	Supplement Left Hip Bursa and Ligament with Autologous Tissue Substitute, Percutaneous Endoscopic Approach
M4JZ	Supplement Left Hip Bursa and Ligament with Synthetic Substitute, Percutaneous Endoscopic Approach
M4KZ	Supplement Left Hip Bursa and Ligament with Nonautologous Tissue Substitute, Percutaneous Endoscopic Approach
N07Z	Supplement Right Knee Bursa and Ligament with Autologous Tissue Substitute, Open Approach
N0JZ	Supplement Right Knee Bursa and Ligament with Synthetic Substitute, Open Approach
N0KZ	Supplement Right Knee Bursa and Ligament with Nonautologous Tissue Substitute, Open Approach
N47Z	Supplement Right Knee Bursa and Ligament with Autologous Tissue Substitute, Percutaneous Endoscopic Approach
0MUN4JZ	Supplement Right Knee Bursa and Ligament with Synthetic Substitute, Percutaneous Endoscopic Approach
0MUN4KZ	Supplement Right Knee Bursa and Ligament with Nonautologous Tissue Substitute, Percutaneous Endoscopic Approach
0MUP07Z	Supplement Left Knee Bursa and Ligament with Autologous Tissue Substitute, Open Approach
0MUP0JZ	Supplement Left Knee Bursa and Ligament with Synthetic Substitute, Open Approach
0MUP0KZ	Supplement Left Knee Bursa and Ligament with Nonautologous Tissue Substitute, Open Approach
0MUP47Z	Supplement Left Knee Bursa and Ligament with Autologous Tissue Substitute, Percutaneous Endoscopic Approach
0MUP4JZ	Supplement Left Knee Bursa and Ligament with Synthetic Substitute, Percutaneous Endoscopic Approach
0MUP4KZ	Supplement Left Knee Bursa and Ligament with Nonautologous Tissue Substitute, Percutaneous Endoscopic Approach
0MUQ07Z	Supplement Right Ankle Bursa and Ligament with Autologous Tissue Substitute, Open Approach
0MUQ0JZ	Supplement Right Ankle Bursa and Ligament with Synthetic Substitute, Open Approach
0MUQ0KZ	Supplement Right Ankle Bursa and Ligament with Nonautologous Tissue Substitute, Open Approach
0MUQ47Z	Supplement Right Ankle Bursa and Ligament with Autologous Tissue Substitute, Percutaneous Endoscopic Approach
0MUQ4JZ	Supplement Right Ankle Bursa and Ligament with Synthetic Substitute, Percutaneous Endoscopic Approach
0MUQ4KZ	Supplement Right Ankle Bursa and Ligament with Nonautologous Tissue Substitute, Percutaneous Endoscopic Approach
0MUR07Z	Supplement Left Ankle Bursa and Ligament with Autologous Tissue Substitute, Open Approach
0MUR0JZ	Supplement Left Ankle Bursa and Ligament with Synthetic Substitute, Open Approach
0MUR0KZ	Supplement Left Ankle Bursa and Ligament with Nonautologous Tissue Substitute, Open Approach
0MUR47Z	Supplement Left Ankle Bursa and Ligament with Autologous Tissue Substitute, Percutaneous Endoscopic Approach
0MUR4JZ	Supplement Left Ankle Bursa and Ligament with Synthetic Substitute, Percutaneous Endoscopic Approach
0MUR4KZ	Supplement Left Ankle Bursa and Ligament with Nonautologous Tissue Substitute, Percutaneous Endoscopic Approach
0MUS07Z	Supplement Right Foot Bursa and Ligament with Autologous Tissue Substitute, Open Approach
0MUS0JZ	Supplement Right Foot Bursa and Ligament with Synthetic Substitute, Open Approach
0MUS0KZ	Supplement Right Foot Bursa and Ligament with Nonautologous Tissue Substitute, Open Approach
0MUS47Z	Supplement Right Foot Bursa and Ligament with Autologous Tissue Substitute, Percutaneous Endoscopic Approach
0MUS4JZ	Supplement Right Foot Bursa and Ligament with Synthetic Substitute, Percutaneous Endoscopic Approach
0MUS4KZ	Supplement Right Foot Bursa and Ligament with Nonautologous Tissue Substitute, Percutaneous Endoscopic Approach
0MUT07Z	Supplement Left Foot Bursa and Ligament with Autologous Tissue Substitute, Open Approach
0MUT0JZ	Supplement Left Foot Bursa and Ligament with Synthetic Substitute, Open Approach
0MUT0KZ	Supplement Left Foot Bursa and Ligament with Nonautologous Tissue Substitute, Open Approach
0MUT47Z	Supplement Left Foot Bursa and Ligament with Autologous Tissue Substitute, Percutaneous Endoscopic Approach
0MUT4JZ	Supplement Left Foot Bursa and Ligament with Synthetic Substitute, Percutaneous Endoscopic Approach
0MUT4KZ	Supplement Left Foot Bursa and Ligament with Nonautologous Tissue Substitute, Percutaneous Endoscopic Approach
0MUV07Z	Supplement Right Lower Extremity Bursa and Ligament with Autologous Tissue Substitute, Open Approach
0MUV0JZ	Supplement Right Lower Extremity Bursa and Ligament with Synthetic Substitute, Open Approach
0MUV0KZ	Supplement Right Lower Extremity Bursa and Ligament with Nonautologous Tissue Substitute, Open Approach
0MUV47Z	Supplement Right Lower Extremity Bursa and Ligament with Autologous Tissue Substitute, Percutaneous Endoscopic Approach
0MUV4JZ	Supplement Right Lower Extremity Bursa and Ligament with Synthetic Substitute, Percutaneous Endoscopic Approach
0MUV4KZ	Supplement Right Lower Extremity Bursa and Ligament with Nonautologous Tissue Substitute, Percutaneous Endoscopic Approach
0MUW07Z	Supplement Left Lower Extremity Bursa and Ligament with Autologous Tissue Substitute, Open Approach
0MUW0JZ	Supplement Left Lower Extremity Bursa and Ligament with Synthetic Substitute, Open Approach
0MUW0KZ	Supplement Left Lower Extremity Bursa and Ligament with Nonautologous Tissue Substitute, Open Approach
0MUW47Z	Supplement Left Lower Extremity Bursa and Ligament with Autologous Tissue Substitute, Percutaneous Endoscopic Approach
0MUW4JZ	Supplement Left Lower Extremity Bursa and Ligament with Synthetic Substitute, Percutaneous Endoscopic Approach
0MUW4KZ	Supplement Left Lower Extremity Bursa and Ligament with Nonautologous Tissue Substitute, Percutaneous Endoscopic Approach

♀ Female-only ♂ Male-only ▲ Limited Coverage ● Non-OR ▬ HAC-associated procedure ▲ Non-covered procedures ✚ Combination

0MW – Bursae and Ligaments, Revision

Review Coding Guideline B6.1c

0MWX00Z Revision of Drainage Device in Upper Bursa and Ligament, Open Approach

0MWX07Z Revision of Autologous Tissue Substitute in Upper Bursa and Ligament, Open Approach

0MWX0JZ Revision of Synthetic Substitute in Upper Bursa and Ligament, Open Approach

0MWX0KZ Revision of Nonautologous Tissue Substitute in Upper Bursa and Ligament, Open Approach

0MWX30Z Revision of Drainage Device in Upper Bursa and Ligament, Percutaneous Approach

0MWX37Z Revision of Autologous Tissue Substitute in Upper Bursa and Ligament, Percutaneous Approach

0MWX3JZ Revision of Synthetic Substitute in Upper Bursa and Ligament, Percutaneous Approach

0MWX3KZ Revision of Nonautologous Tissue Substitute in Upper Bursa and Ligament, Percutaneous Approach

0MWX40Z Revision of Drainage Device in Upper Bursa and Ligament, Percutaneous Endoscopic Approach

0MWX47Z Revision of Autologous Tissue Substitute in Upper Bursa and Ligament, Percutaneous Endoscopic Approach

0MWX4JZ Revision of Synthetic Substitute in Upper Bursa and Ligament, Percutaneous Endoscopic Approach

0MWX4KZ Revision of Nonautologous Tissue Substitute in Upper Bursa and Ligament, Percutaneous Endoscopic Approach

0MWXX0Z Revision of Drainage Device in Upper Bursa and Ligament, External Approach

0MWXX7Z Revision of Autologous Tissue Substitute in Upper Bursa and Ligament, External Approach

0MWXXJZ Revision of Synthetic Substitute in Upper Bursa and Ligament, External Approach

0MWXXKZ Revision of Nonautologous Tissue Substitute in Upper Bursa and Ligament, External Approach

0MWY00Z Revision of Drainage Device in Lower Bursa and Ligament, Open Approach

0MWY07Z Revision of Autologous Tissue Substitute in Lower Bursa and Ligament, Open Approach

0MWY0JZ Revision of Synthetic Substitute in Lower Bursa and Ligament, Open Approach

0MWY0KZ Revision of Nonautologous Tissue Substitute in Lower Bursa and Ligament, Open Approach

0MWY30Z Revision of Drainage Device in Lower Bursa and Ligament, Percutaneous Approach

0MWY37Z Revision of Autologous Tissue Substitute in Lower Bursa and Ligament, Percutaneous Approach

0MWY3JZ Revision of Synthetic Substitute in Lower Bursa and Ligament, Percutaneous Approach

0MWY3KZ Revision of Nonautologous Tissue Substitute in Lower Bursa and Ligament, Percutaneous Approach

0MWY40Z Revision of Drainage Device in Lower Bursa and Ligament, Percutaneous Endoscopic Approach

0MWY47Z Revision of Autologous Tissue Substitute in Lower Bursa and Ligament, Percutaneous Endoscopic Approach

0MWY4JZ Revision of Synthetic Substitute in Lower Bursa and Ligament, Percutaneous Endoscopic Approach

0MWY4KZ Revision of Nonautologous Tissue Substitute in Lower Bursa and Ligament, Percutaneous Endoscopic Approach

0MWYX0Z Revision of Drainage Device in Lower Bursa and Ligament, External Approach

0MWYX7Z Revision of Autologous Tissue Substitute in Lower Bursa and Ligament, External Approach

0MWYXJZ Revision of Synthetic Substitute in Lower Bursa and Ligament, External Approach

0MWYXKZ Revision of Nonautologous Tissue Substitute in Lower Bursa and Ligament, External Approach

0MX – Bursae and Ligaments, Transfer

0MX00ZZ Transfer Head and Neck Bursa and Ligament, Open Approach

0MX04ZZ Transfer Head and Neck Bursa and Ligament, Percutaneous Endoscopic Approach

0MX10ZZ Transfer Right Shoulder Bursa and Ligament, Open Approach

0MX14ZZ Transfer Right Shoulder Bursa and Ligament, Percutaneous Endoscopic Approach

0MX20ZZ Transfer Left Shoulder Bursa and Ligament, Open Approach

0MX24ZZ Transfer Left Shoulder Bursa and Ligament, Percutaneous Endoscopic Approach

0MX30ZZ Transfer Right Elbow Bursa and Ligament, Open Approach

0MX34ZZ Transfer Right Elbow Bursa and Ligament, Percutaneous Endoscopic Approach

0MX40ZZ Transfer Left Elbow Bursa and Ligament, Open Approach

0MX44ZZ Transfer Left Elbow Bursa and Ligament, Percutaneous Endoscopic Approach

0MX50ZZ Transfer Right Wrist Bursa and Ligament, Open Approach

0MX54ZZ Transfer Right Wrist Bursa and Ligament, Percutaneous Endoscopic Approach

0MX60ZZ Transfer Left Wrist Bursa and Ligament, Open Approach

0MX64ZZ Transfer Left Wrist Bursa and Ligament, Percutaneous Endoscopic Approach

0MX70ZZ Transfer Right Hand Bursa and Ligament, Open Approach

0MX74ZZ Transfer Right Hand Bursa and Ligament, Percutaneous Endoscopic Approach

0MX80ZZ Transfer Left Hand Bursa and Ligament, Open Approach

0MX84ZZ Transfer Left Hand Bursa and Ligament, Percutaneous Endoscopic Approach

0MX90ZZ Transfer Right Upper Extremity Bursa and Ligament, Open Approach

0MX94ZZ Transfer Right Upper Extremity Bursa and Ligament, Percutaneous Endoscopic Approach

0MXB0ZZ Transfer Left Upper Extremity Bursa and Ligament, Open Approach

0MXB4ZZ Transfer Left Upper Extremity Bursa and Ligament, Percutaneous Endoscopic Approach

0MXC0ZZ Transfer Right Trunk Bursa and Ligament, Open Approach

0MXC4ZZ Transfer Right Trunk Bursa and Ligament, Percutaneous Endoscopic Approach

0MXD0ZZ Transfer Left Trunk Bursa and Ligament, Open Approach

0MXD4ZZ Transfer Left Trunk Bursa and Ligament, Percutaneous Endoscopic Approach

0MXF0ZZ Transfer Right Thorax Bursa and Ligament, Open Approach

0MXF4ZZ Transfer Right Thorax Bursa and Ligament, Percutaneous Endoscopic Approach

0MXG0ZZ Transfer Left Thorax Bursa and Ligament, Open Approach

0MXG4ZZ Transfer Left Thorax Bursa and Ligament, Percutaneous Endoscopic Approach

0MXH0ZZ Transfer Right Abdomen Bursa and Ligament, Open Approach

0MXH4ZZ Transfer Right Abdomen Bursa and Ligament, Percutaneous Endoscopic Approach

0MXJ0ZZ Transfer Left Abdomen Bursa and Ligament, Open Approach

0MXJ4ZZ Transfer Left Abdomen Bursa and Ligament, Percutaneous Endoscopic Approach

0MXK0ZZ Transfer Perineum Bursa and Ligament, Open Approach

0MXK4ZZ Transfer Perineum Bursa and Ligament, Percutaneous Endoscopic Approach

0MXL0ZZ Transfer Right Hip Bursa and Ligament, Open Approach

0MXL4ZZ Transfer Right Hip Bursa and Ligament, Percutaneous Endoscopic Approach

0MXM0ZZ Transfer Left Hip Bursa and Ligament, Open Approach

0MXM4ZZ Transfer Left Hip Bursa and Ligament, Percutaneous Endoscopic Approach

0MXN0ZZ Transfer Right Knee Bursa and Ligament, Open Approach

0MXN4ZZ Transfer Right Knee Bursa and Ligament, Percutaneous Endoscopic Approach

0MXP0ZZ Transfer Left Knee Bursa and Ligament, Open Approach

0MXP4ZZ Transfer Left Knee Bursa and Ligament, Percutaneous Endoscopic Approach

0MXQ0ZZ Transfer Right Ankle Bursa and Ligament, Open Approach

0MXQ4ZZ Transfer Right Ankle Bursa and Ligament, Percutaneous Endoscopic Approach

0MXR0ZZ Transfer Left Ankle Bursa and Ligament, Open Approach

0MXR4ZZ Transfer Left Ankle Bursa and Ligament, Percutaneous Endoscopic Approach

XS0ZZ Transfer Right Foot Bursa and Ligament, Open Approach

XS4ZZ Transfer Right Foot Bursa and Ligament, Percutaneous Endoscopic Approach

XT0ZZ Transfer Left Foot Bursa and Ligament, Open Approach

0MXT4ZZ Transfer Left Foot Bursa and Ligament, Percutaneous Endoscopic Approach

0MXV0ZZ Transfer Right Lower Extremity Bursa and Ligament, Open Approach

0MXV4ZZ Transfer Right Lower Extremity Bursa and Ligament, Percutaneous Endoscopic Approach

0MXW0ZZ Transfer Left Lower Extremity Bursa and Ligament, Open Approach

0MXW4ZZ Transfer Left Lower Extremity Bursa and Ligament, Percutaneous Endoscopic Approach

Female-only   ♂ Male-only   ▲ Limited Coverage   ● Non-OR   HAC-associated procedure   ▲ Non-covered procedures   ✚ Combination

Head and Facial Bones

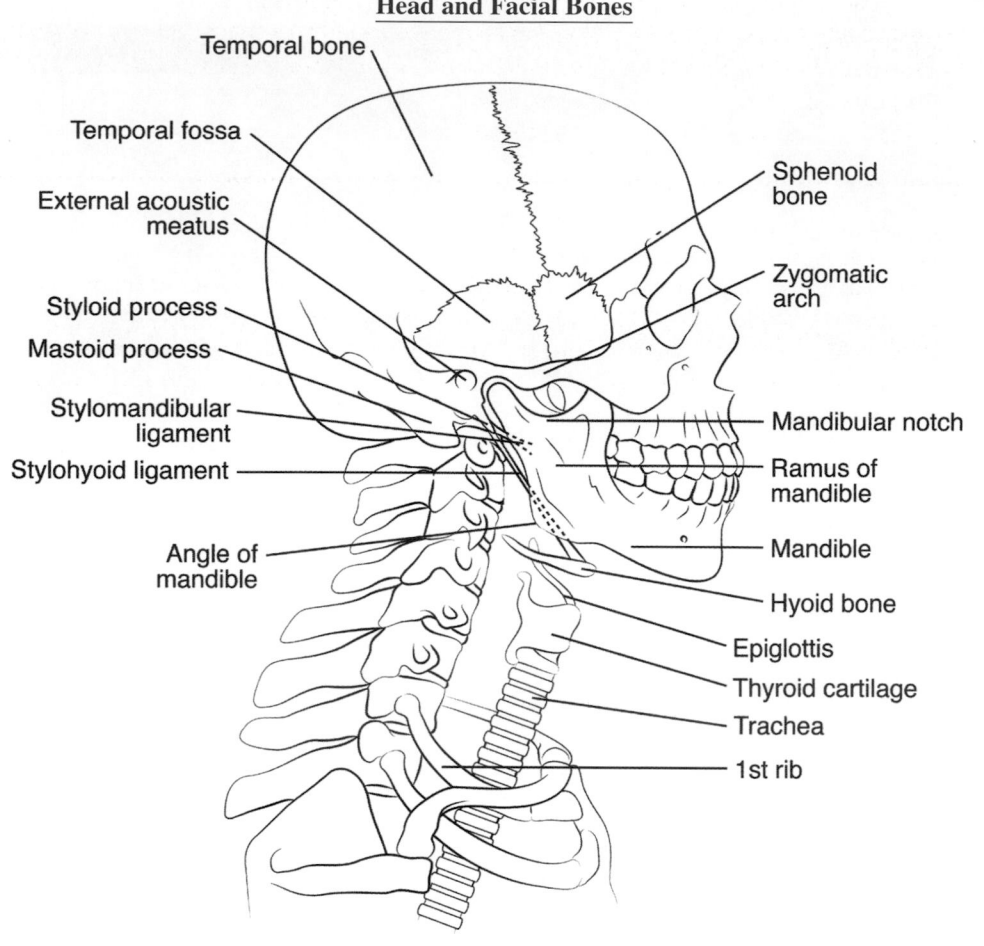

Temporal bone

Temporal fossa

External acoustic meatus

Styloid process

Mastoid process

Stylomandibular ligament

Stylohyoid ligament

Angle of mandible

Sphenoid bone

Zygomatic arch

Mandibular notch

Ramus of mandible

Mandible

Hyoid bone

Epiglottis

Thyroid cartilage

Trachea

1st rib

©AHIMA

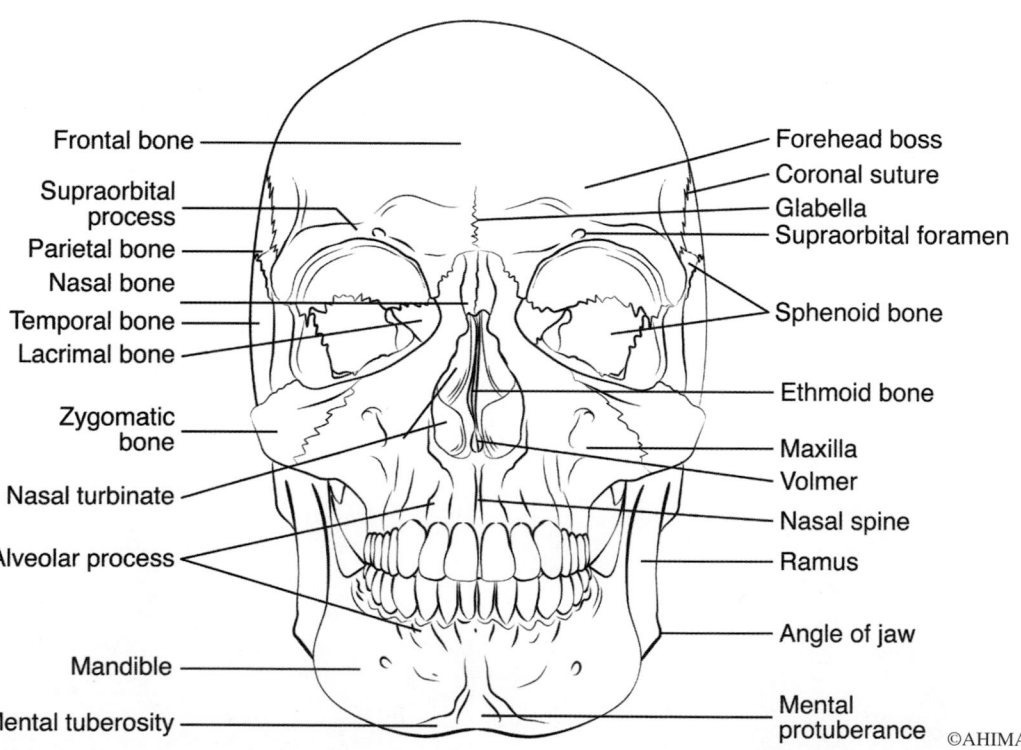

Frontal bone

Supraorbital process

Parietal bone

Nasal bone

Temporal bone

Lacrimal bone

Zygomatic bone

Nasal turbinate

Alveolar process

Mandible

Mental tuberosity

Forehead boss

Coronal suture

Glabella

Supraorbital foramen

Sphenoid bone

Ethmoid bone

Maxilla

Volmer

Nasal spine

Ramus

Angle of jaw

Mental protuberance

©AHIMA

tion	0	**Medical and Surgical**	
ly System	N	**Head and Facial Bones**	
eration	2	**Change:** Taking out or off a device from a body part and putting back an identical or similar device in or on the same body part without cutting or puncturing the skin or a mucous membrane	

Body Part (4th)	Approach (5th)	Device (6th)	Qualifier (7th)
Skull Nasal Bone Facial Bone	**X** External	**0** Drainage Device **Y** Other Device	**Z** No Qualifier

tion	0	**Medical and Surgical**	
ly System	N	**Head and Facial Bones**	
eration	5	**Destruction:** Physical eradication of all or a portion of a body part by the direct use of energy, force, or a destructive agent	

Body Part (4th)	Approach (5th)	Device (6th)	Qualifier (7th)
Skull Frontal Bone, Right Frontal Bone, Left Parietal Bone, Right Parietal Bone, Left Temporal Bone, Right Temporal Bone, Left Occipital Bone, Right Occipital Bone, Left Nasal Bone Sphenoid Bone, Right Sphenoid Bone, Left Ethmoid Bone, Right Ethmoid Bone, Left Lacrimal Bone, Right Lacrimal Bone, Left Palatine Bone, Right Palatine Bone, Left Zygomatic Bone, Right Zygomatic Bone, Left Orbit, Right Orbit, Left Maxilla, Right Maxilla, Left Mandible, Right Mandible, Left Hyoid Bone	**0** Open **3** Percutaneous **4** Percutaneous Endoscopic	**Z** No Device	**Z** No Qualifier

Section	0	Medical and Surgical
Body System	N	Head and Facial Bones
Operation	8	**Division:** Cutting into a body part, without draining fluids and/or gases from the body part, in order to separate or transect body part

Body Part (4th)	Approach (5th)	Device (6th)	Qualifier (7th)
0 Skull	0 Open	Z No Device	Z No Qualifier
1 Frontal Bone, Right	3 Percutaneous		
2 Frontal Bone, Left	4 Percutaneous Endoscopic		
3 Parietal Bone, Right			
4 Parietal Bone, Left			
5 Temporal Bone, Right			
6 Temporal Bone, Left			
7 Occipital Bone, Right			
8 Occipital Bone, Left			
B Nasal Bone			
C Sphenoid Bone, Right			
D Sphenoid Bone, Left			
F Ethmoid Bone, Right			
G Ethmoid Bone, Left			
H Lacrimal Bone, Right			
J Lacrimal Bone, Left			
K Palatine Bone, Right			
L Palatine Bone, Left			
M Zygomatic Bone, Right			
N Zygomatic Bone, Left			
P Orbit, Right			
Q Orbit, Left			
R Maxilla, Right			
S Maxilla, Left			
T Mandible, Right			
V Mandible, Left			
X Hyoid Bone			

Section	0	Medical and Surgical
Body System	N	Head and Facial Bones
Operation	9	**Drainage:** Taking or letting out fluids and/or gases from a body part

Body Part (4th)	Approach (5th)	Device (6th)	Qualifier (7th)
0 Skull	0 Open	0 Drainage Device	Z No Qualifier
1 Frontal Bone, Right	3 Percutaneous		
2 Frontal Bone, Left	4 Percutaneous Endoscopic		
3 Parietal Bone, Right			
4 Parietal Bone, Left			
5 Temporal Bone, Right			
6 Temporal Bone, Left			
7 Occipital Bone, Right			
8 Occipital Bone, Left			
B Nasal Bone			
C Sphenoid Bone, Right			
D Sphenoid Bone, Left			
F Ethmoid Bone, Right			
G Ethmoid Bone, Left			
H Lacrimal Bone, Right			
J Lacrimal Bone, Left			
K Palatine Bone, Right			
L Palatine Bone, Left			
M Zygomatic Bone, Right			
N Zygomatic Bone, Left			
P Orbit, Right			
Q Orbit, Left			
R Maxilla, Right			
S Maxilla, Left			
T Mandible, Right			
V Mandible, Left			
X Hyoid Bone			

Continued →

Section 0 **Medical and Surgical**
Body System N **Head and Facial Bones**
Operation 9 **Drainage:** Taking or letting out fluids and/or gases from a body part

Body Part (4th)	Approach (5th)	Device (6th)	Qualifier (7th)
Skull	0 Open	Z No Device	X Diagnostic
Frontal Bone, Right	3 Percutaneous		Z No Qualifier
Frontal Bone, Left	4 Percutaneous Endoscopic		
Parietal Bone, Right			
Parietal Bone, Left			
Temporal Bone, Right			
Temporal Bone, Left			
Occipital Bone, Right			
Occipital Bone, Left			
Nasal Bone			
Sphenoid Bone, Right			
Sphenoid Bone, Left			
Ethmoid Bone, Right			
Ethmoid Bone, Left			
Lacrimal Bone, Right			
Lacrimal Bone, Left			
Palatine Bone, Right			
Palatine Bone, Left			
Zygomatic Bone, Right			
Zygomatic Bone, Left			
Orbit, Right			
Orbit, Left			
Maxilla, Right			
Maxilla, Left			
Mandible, Right			
Mandible, Left			
Hyoid Bone			

Section 0 **Medical and Surgical**
Body System N **Head and Facial Bones**
Operation B **Excision:** Cutting out or off, without replacement, a portion of a body part

Body Part (4th)	Approach (5th)	Device (6th)	Qualifier (7th)
0 Skull	0 Open	Z No Device	X Diagnostic
1 Frontal Bone, Right	3 Percutaneous		Z No Qualifier
2 Frontal Bone, Left	4 Percutaneous Endoscopic		
3 Parietal Bone, Right			
4 Parietal Bone, Left			
5 Temporal Bone, Right			
6 Temporal Bone, Left			
7 Occipital Bone, Right			
8 Occipital Bone, Left			
B Nasal Bone			
C Sphenoid Bone, Right			
D Sphenoid Bone, Left			
F Ethmoid Bone, Right			
G Ethmoid Bone, Left			
H Lacrimal Bone, Right			
J Lacrimal Bone, Left			
K Palatine Bone, Right			
L Palatine Bone, Left			
M Zygomatic Bone, Right			
N Zygomatic Bone, Left			
P Orbit, Right			
Q Orbit, Left			
R Maxilla, Right			
S Maxilla, Left			
T Mandible, Right			
V Mandible, Left			
X Hyoid Bone			

Section	0	Medical and Surgical
Body System	N	Head and Facial Bones
Operation	C	Extirpation: Taking or cutting out solid matter from a body part

Body Part (4th)	Approach (5th)	Device (6th)	Qualifier (7th)
1 Frontal Bone, Right 2 Frontal Bone, Left 3 Parietal Bone, Right 4 Parietal Bone, Left 5 Temporal Bone, Right 6 Temporal Bone, Left 7 Occipital Bone, Right 8 Occipital Bone, Left B Nasal Bone C Sphenoid Bone, Right D Sphenoid Bone, Left F Ethmoid Bone, Right G Ethmoid Bone, Left H Lacrimal Bone, Right J Lacrimal Bone, Left K Palatine Bone, Right L Palatine Bone, Left M Zygomatic Bone, Right N Zygomatic Bone, Left P Orbit, Right Q Orbit, Left R Maxilla, Right S Maxilla, Left T Mandible, Right V Mandible, Left X Hyoid Bone	0 Open 3 Percutaneous 4 Percutaneous Endoscopic	Z No Device	Z No Qualifier

Section	0	Medical and Surgical
Body System	N	Head and Facial Bones
Operation	H	Insertion: Putting in a nonbiological appliance that monitors, assists, performs, or prevents a physiological function but doe not physically take the place of a body part

Body Part (4th)	Approach (5th)	Device (6th)	Qualifier (7th)
0 Skull	0 Open	4 Internal Fixation Device 5 External Fixation Device M Bone Growth Stimulator N Neurostimulator Generator	Z No Qualifier
0 Skull	3 Percutaneous 4 Percutaneous Endoscopic	4 Internal Fixation Device 5 External Fixation Device M Bone Growth Stimulator	Z No Qualifier
1 Frontal Bone, Right 2 Frontal Bone, Left 3 Parietal Bone, Right 4 Parietal Bone, Left 7 Occipital Bone, Right 8 Occipital Bone, Left C Sphenoid Bone, Right D Sphenoid Bone, Left F Ethmoid Bone, Right G Ethmoid Bone, Left H Lacrimal Bone, Right J Lacrimal Bone, Left K Palatine Bone, Right L Palatine Bone, Left M Zygomatic Bone, Right N Zygomatic Bone, Left P Orbit, Right Q Orbit, Left X Hyoid Bone	0 Open 3 Percutaneous 4 Percutaneous Endoscopic	4 Internal Fixation Device	Z No Qualifier

Continued →

Section | 0 | Medical and Surgical
Body System | N | Head and Facial Bones
Operation | H | **Insertion:** Putting in a nonbiological appliance that monitors, assists, performs, or prevents a physiological function but does not physically take the place of a body part

Body Part (4th)	Approach (5th)	Device (6th)	Qualifier (7th)
Temporal Bone, Right Temporal Bone, Left	0 Open 3 Percutaneous 4 Percutaneous Endoscopic	4 Internal Fixation Device S Hearing Device	Z No Qualifier
Nasal Bone	0 Open 3 Percutaneous 4 Percutaneous Endoscopic	4 Internal Fixation Device M Bone Growth Stimulator	Z No Qualifier
Maxilla, Right Maxilla, Left Mandible, Right Mandible, Left	0 Open 3 Percutaneous 4 Percutaneous Endoscopic	4 Internal Fixation Device 5 External Fixation Device	Z No Qualifier
Facial Bone	0 Open 3 Percutaneous 4 Percutaneous Endoscopic	M Bone Growth Stimulator	Z No Qualifier

Section | 0 | Medical and Surgical
Body System | N | Head and Facial Bones
Operation | J | **Inspection:** Visually and/or manually exploring a body part

Body Part (4th)	Approach (5th)	Device (6th)	Qualifier (7th)
Skull Nasal Bone Facial Bone	0 Open 3 Percutaneous 4 Percutaneous Endoscopic X External	Z No Device	Z No Qualifier

Section | 0 | Medical and Surgical
Body System | N | Head and Facial Bones
Operation | N | **Release:** Freeing a body part from an abnormal physical constraint by cutting or by the use of force

Body Part (4th)	Approach (5th)	Device (6th)	Qualifier (7th)
1 Frontal Bone, Right 2 Frontal Bone, Left 3 Parietal Bone, Right 4 Parietal Bone, Left 5 Temporal Bone, Right 6 Temporal Bone, Left 7 Occipital Bone, Right 8 Occipital Bone, Left B Nasal Bone C Sphenoid Bone, Right D Sphenoid Bone, Left F Ethmoid Bone, Right G Ethmoid Bone, Left H Lacrimal Bone, Right J Lacrimal Bone, Left K Palatine Bone, Right L Palatine Bone, Left M Zygomatic Bone, Right N Zygomatic Bone, Left P Orbit, Right Q Orbit, Left R Maxilla, Right S Maxilla, Left T Mandible, Right V Mandible, Left X Hyoid Bone	0 Open 3 Percutaneous 4 Percutaneous Endoscopic	Z No Device	Z No Qualifier

Section	0	Medical and Surgical
Body System	N	Head and Facial Bones
Operation	P	Removal: Taking out or off a device from a body part

Body Part (4ᵗʰ)	Approach (5ᵗʰ)	Device (6ᵗʰ)	Qualifier (7ᵗʰ)
0 Skull	0 Open	0 Drainage Device 4 Internal Fixation Device 5 External Fixation Device 7 Autologous Tissue Substitute J Synthetic Substitute K Nonautologous Tissue Substitute M Bone Growth Stimulator N Neurostimulator Generator S Hearing Device	Z No Qualifier
0 Skull	3 Percutaneous 4 Percutaneous Endoscopic	0 Drainage Device 4 Internal Fixation Device 5 External Fixation Device 7 Autologous Tissue Substitute J Synthetic Substitute K Nonautologous Tissue Substitute M Bone Growth Stimulator S Hearing Device	Z No Qualifier
0 Skull	X External	0 Drainage Device 4 Internal Fixation Device 5 External Fixation Device M Bone Growth Stimulator S Hearing Device	Z No Qualifier
B Nasal Bone W Facial Bone	0 Open 3 Percutaneous 4 Percutaneous Endoscopic	0 Drainage Device 4 Internal Fixation Device 7 Autologous Tissue Substitute J Synthetic Substitute K Nonautologous Tissue Substitute M Bone Growth Stimulator	Z No Qualifier
B Nasal Bone W Facial Bone	X External	0 Drainage Device 4 Internal Fixation Device M Bone Growth Stimulator	Z No Qualifier

Section 0 **Medical and Surgical**
Body System N **Head and Facial Bones**
Operation Q **Repair:** Restoring, to the extent possible, a body part to its normal anatomic structure and function

Body Part (4th)	Approach (5th)	Device (6th)	Qualifier (7th)
Skull Frontal Bone, Right Frontal Bone, Left Parietal Bone, Right Parietal Bone, Left Temporal Bone, Right Temporal Bone, Left Occipital Bone, Right Occipital Bone, Left Nasal Bone Sphenoid Bone, Right Sphenoid Bone, Left Ethmoid Bone, Right Ethmoid Bone, Left Lacrimal Bone, Right Lacrimal Bone, Left Palatine Bone, Right Palatine Bone, Left Zygomatic Bone, Right Zygomatic Bone, Left Orbit, Right Orbit, Left Maxilla, Right Maxilla, Left Mandible, Right Mandible, Left Hyoid Bone	**0** Open **3** Percutaneous **4** Percutaneous Endoscopic **X** External	**Z** No Device	**Z** No Qualifier

Section 0 **Medical and Surgical**
Body System N **Head and Facial Bones**
Operation R **Replacement:** Putting in or on biological or synthetic material that physically takes the place and/or function of all or a portion of a body part

Body Part (4th)	Approach (5th)	Device (6th)	Qualifier (7th)
Skull Frontal Bone, Right Frontal Bone, Left Parietal Bone, Right Parietal Bone, Left Temporal Bone, Right Temporal Bone, Left Occipital Bone, Right Occipital Bone, Left Nasal Bone Sphenoid Bone, Right Sphenoid Bone, Left Ethmoid Bone, Right Ethmoid Bone, Left Lacrimal Bone, Right Lacrimal Bone, Left Palatine Bone, Right Palatine Bone, Left Zygomatic Bone, Right Zygomatic Bone, Left Orbit, Right Orbit, Left Maxilla, Right Maxilla, Left Mandible, Right Mandible, Left Hyoid Bone	**0** Open **3** Percutaneous **4** Percutaneous Endoscopic	**7** Autologous Tissue Substitute **J** Synthetic Substitute **K** Nonautologous Tissue Substitute	**Z** No Qualifier

Section   0   **Medical and Surgical**
Body System   N   **Head and Facial Bones**
Operation   S   **Reposition:** Moving to its normal location, or other suitable location, all or a portion of a body part

Body Part (4ᵗʰ)	Approach (5ᵗʰ)	Device (6ᵗʰ)	Qualifier (7ᵗʰ)
0 Skull **R** Maxilla, Right **S** Maxilla, Left **T** Mandible, Right **V** Mandible, Left	**0** Open **3** Percutaneous **4** Percutaneous Endoscopic	**4** Internal Fixation Device **5** External Fixation Device **Z** No Device	**Z** No Qualifier
0 Skull **R** Maxilla, Right **S** Maxilla, Left **T** Mandible, Right **V** Mandible, Left	**X** External	**Z** No Device	**Z** No Qualifier
1 Frontal Bone, Right **2** Frontal Bone, Left **3** Parietal Bone, Right **4** Parietal Bone, Left **5** Temporal Bone, Right **6** Temporal Bone, Left **7** Occipital Bone, Right **8** Occipital Bone, Left **B** Nasal Bone **C** Sphenoid Bone, Right **D** Sphenoid Bone, Left **F** Ethmoid Bone, Right **G** Ethmoid Bone, Left **H** Lacrimal Bone, Right **J** Lacrimal Bone, Left **K** Palatine Bone, Right **L** Palatine Bone, Left **M** Zygomatic Bone, Right **N** Zygomatic Bone, Left **P** Orbit, Right **Q** Orbit, Left **X** Hyoid Bone	**0** Open **3** Percutaneous **4** Percutaneous Endoscopic	**4** Internal Fixation Device **Z** No Device	**Z** No Qualifier
1 Frontal Bone, Right **2** Frontal Bone, Left **3** Parietal Bone, Right **4** Parietal Bone, Left **5** Temporal Bone, Right **6** Temporal Bone, Left **7** Occipital Bone, Right **8** Occipital Bone, Left **B** Nasal Bone **C** Sphenoid Bone, Right **D** Sphenoid Bone, Left **F** Ethmoid Bone, Right **G** Ethmoid Bone, Left **H** Lacrimal Bone, Right **J** Lacrimal Bone, Left **K** Palatine Bone, Right **L** Palatine Bone, Left **M** Zygomatic Bone, Right **N** Zygomatic Bone, Left **P** Orbit, Right **Q** Orbit, Left **X** Hyoid Bone	**X** External	**Z** No Device	**Z** No Qualifier

tion 0 **Medical and Surgical**
dy System N **Head and Facial Bones**
eration T **Resection:** Cutting out or off, without replacement, all of a body part

Body Part (4th)	Approach (5th)	Device (6th)	Qualifier (7th)
Frontal Bone, Right Frontal Bone, Left Parietal Bone, Right Parietal Bone, Left Temporal Bone, Right Temporal Bone, Left Occipital Bone, Right Occipital Bone, Left Nasal Bone Sphenoid Bone, Right Sphenoid Bone, Left Ethmoid Bone, Right Ethmoid Bone, Left Lacrimal Bone, Right Lacrimal Bone, Left Palatine Bone, Right Palatine Bone, Left Zygomatic Bone, Right Zygomatic Bone, Left Orbit, Right Orbit, Left Maxilla, Right Maxilla, Left Mandible, Right Mandible, Left Hyoid Bone	0 Open	Z No Device	Z No Qualifier

ction 0 **Medical and Surgical**
dy System N **Head and Facial Bones**
eration U **Supplement:** Putting in or on biological or synthetic material that physically reinforces and/or augments the function of a portion of a body part

Body Part (4th)	Approach (5th)	Device (6th)	Qualifier (7th)
0 Skull 1 Frontal Bone, Right 2 Frontal Bone, Left 3 Parietal Bone, Right 4 Parietal Bone, Left 5 Temporal Bone, Right 6 Temporal Bone, Left 7 Occipital Bone, Right 8 Occipital Bone, Left B Nasal Bone C Sphenoid Bone, Right D Sphenoid Bone, Left F Ethmoid Bone, Right G Ethmoid Bone, Left H Lacrimal Bone, Right J Lacrimal Bone, Left K Palatine Bone, Right L Palatine Bone, Left M Zygomatic Bone, Right N Zygomatic Bone, Left P Orbit, Right Q Orbit, Left R Maxilla, Right S Maxilla, Left T Mandible, Right V Mandible, Left X Hyoid Bone	0 Open 3 Percutaneous 4 Percutaneous Endoscopic	7 Autologous Tissue Substitute J Synthetic Substitute K Nonautologous Tissue Substitute	Z No Qualifier

Section	0	Medical and Surgical
Body System	N	Head and Facial Bones
Operation	W	Revision: Correcting, to the extent possible, a portion of a malfunctioning device or the position of a displaced device

Body Part (4th)	Approach (5th)	Device (6th)	Qualifier (7th)
0 Skull	0 Open	0 Drainage Device 4 Internal Fixation Device 5 External Fixation Device 7 Autologous Tissue Substitute J Synthetic Substitute K Nonautologous Tissue Substitute M Bone Growth Stimulator N Neurostimulator Generator S Hearing Device	Z No Qualifier
0 Skull	3 Percutaneous 4 Percutaneous Endoscopic X External	0 Drainage Device 4 Internal Fixation Device 5 External Fixation Device 7 Autologous Tissue Substitute J Synthetic Substitute K Nonautologous Tissue Substitute M Bone Growth Stimulator S Hearing Device	Z No Qualifier
B Nasal Bone W Facial Bone	0 Open 3 Percutaneous 4 Percutaneous Endoscopic X External	0 Drainage Device 4 Internal Fixation Device 7 Autologous Tissue Substitute J Synthetic Substitute K Nonautologous Tissue Substitute M Bone Growth Stimulator	Z No Qualifier

Head and Facial Bones Code Listing 0N2–0NW

0N2 – Head and Facial Bones, Change

Review Coding Guideline B6.1c

0N20X0Z Change Drainage Device in Skull, External Approach
0N20XYZ Change Other Device in Skull, External Approach

0N2BX0Z Change Drainage Device in Nasal Bone, External Approach
0N2BXYZ Change Other Device in Nasal Bone, External Approach

0N2WX0Z Change Drainage Device in Facial Bone, External Approach
0N2WXYZ Change Other Device in Facial Bone, External Approach

0N5 – Head and Facial Bones, Destruction

0N500ZZ Destruction of Skull, Open Approach
0N503ZZ Destruction of Skull, Percutaneous Approach
0N504ZZ Destruction of Skull, Percutaneous Endoscopic Approach
0N510ZZ Destruction of Right Frontal Bone, Open Approach
0N513ZZ Destruction of Right Frontal Bone, Percutaneous Approach
0N514ZZ Destruction of Right Frontal Bone, Percutaneous Endoscopic Approach
0N520ZZ Destruction of Left Frontal Bone, Open Approach
0N523ZZ Destruction of Left Frontal Bone, Percutaneous Approach
0N524ZZ Destruction of Left Frontal Bone, Percutaneous Endoscopic Approach
0N530ZZ Destruction of Right Parietal Bone, Open Approach
0N533ZZ Destruction of Right Parietal Bone, Percutaneous Approach
0N534ZZ Destruction of Right Parietal Bone, Percutaneous Endoscopic Approach
0N540ZZ Destruction of Left Parietal Bone, Open Approach
0N543ZZ Destruction of Left Parietal Bone, Percutaneous Approach

0N544ZZ Destruction of Left Parietal Bone, Percutaneous Endoscopic Approach
0N550ZZ Destruction of Right Temporal Bone, Open Approach
0N553ZZ Destruction of Right Temporal Bone, Percutaneous Approach
0N554ZZ Destruction of Right Temporal Bone, Percutaneous Endoscopic Approach
0N560ZZ Destruction of Left Temporal Bone, Open Approach
0N563ZZ Destruction of Left Temporal Bone, Percutaneous Approach
0N564ZZ Destruction of Left Temporal Bone, Percutaneous Endoscopic Approach
0N570ZZ Destruction of Right Occipital Bone, Open Approach
0N573ZZ Destruction of Right Occipital Bone, Percutaneous Approach
0N574ZZ Destruction of Right Occipital Bone, Percutaneous Endoscopic Approach
0N580ZZ Destruction of Left Occipital Bone, Open Approach
0N583ZZ Destruction of Left Occipital Bone, Percutaneous Approach
0N584ZZ Destruction of Left Occipital Bone, Percutaneous Endoscopic Approach
0N5B0ZZ Destruction of Nasal Bone, Open Approach

0N5B3ZZ Destruction of Nasal Bone, Percutaneous Approach
0N5B4ZZ Destruction of Nasal Bone, Percutaneous Endoscopic Approach
0N5C0ZZ Destruction of Right Sphenoid Bone, Open Approach
0N5C3ZZ Destruction of Right Sphenoid Bone, Percutaneous Approach
0N5C4ZZ Destruction of Right Sphenoid Bone, Percutaneous Endoscopic Approach
0N5D0ZZ Destruction of Left Sphenoid Bone, Open Approach
0N5D3ZZ Destruction of Left Sphenoid Bone, Percutaneous Approach
0N5D4ZZ Destruction of Left Sphenoid Bone, Percutaneous Endoscopic Approach
0N5F0ZZ Destruction of Right Ethmoid Bone, Open Approach
0N5F3ZZ Destruction of Right Ethmoid Bone, Percutaneous Approach
0N5F4ZZ Destruction of Right Ethmoid Bone, Percutaneous Endoscopic Approach
0N5G0ZZ Destruction of Left Ethmoid Bone, Open Approach
0N5G3ZZ Destruction of Left Ethmoid Bone, Percutaneous Approach
0N5G4ZZ Destruction of Left Ethmoid Bone, Percutaneous Endoscopic Approach

5H0ZZ Destruction of Right Lacrimal Bone, Open Approach

5H3ZZ Destruction of Right Lacrimal Bone, Percutaneous Approach

5H4ZZ Destruction of Right Lacrimal Bone, Percutaneous Endoscopic Approach

5J0ZZ Destruction of Left Lacrimal Bone, Open Approach

5J3ZZ Destruction of Left Lacrimal Bone, Percutaneous Approach

5J4ZZ Destruction of Left Lacrimal Bone, Percutaneous Endoscopic Approach

5K0ZZ Destruction of Right Palatine Bone, Open Approach

5K3ZZ Destruction of Right Palatine Bone, Percutaneous Approach

5K4ZZ Destruction of Right Palatine Bone, Percutaneous Endoscopic Approach

5L0ZZ Destruction of Left Palatine Bone, Open Approach

5L3ZZ Destruction of Left Palatine Bone, Percutaneous Approach

5L4ZZ Destruction of Left Palatine Bone, Percutaneous Endoscopic Approach

5M0ZZ Destruction of Right Zygomatic Bone, Open Approach

0N5M3ZZ Destruction of Right Zygomatic Bone, Percutaneous Approach

0N5M4ZZ Destruction of Right Zygomatic Bone, Percutaneous Endoscopic Approach

0N5N0ZZ Destruction of Left Zygomatic Bone, Open Approach

0N5N3ZZ Destruction of Left Zygomatic Bone, Percutaneous Approach

0N5N4ZZ Destruction of Left Zygomatic Bone, Percutaneous Endoscopic Approach

0N5P0ZZ Destruction of Right Orbit, Open Approach

0N5P3ZZ Destruction of Right Orbit, Percutaneous Approach

0N5P4ZZ Destruction of Right Orbit, Percutaneous Endoscopic Approach

0N5Q0ZZ Destruction of Left Orbit, Open Approach

0N5Q3ZZ Destruction of Left Orbit, Percutaneous Approach

0N5Q4ZZ Destruction of Left Orbit, Percutaneous Endoscopic Approach

0N5R0ZZ Destruction of Right Maxilla, Open Approach

0N5R3ZZ Destruction of Right Maxilla, Percutaneous Approach

0N5R4ZZ Destruction of Right Maxilla, Percutaneous Endoscopic Approach

0N5S0ZZ Destruction of Left Maxilla, Open Approach

0N5S3ZZ Destruction of Left Maxilla, Percutaneous Approach

0N5S4ZZ Destruction of Left Maxilla, Percutaneous Endoscopic Approach

0N5T0ZZ Destruction of Right Mandible, Open Approach

0N5T3ZZ Destruction of Right Mandible, Percutaneous Approach

0N5T4ZZ Destruction of Right Mandible, Percutaneous Endoscopic Approach

0N5V0ZZ Destruction of Left Mandible, Open Approach

0N5V3ZZ Destruction of Left Mandible, Percutaneous Approach

0N5V4ZZ Destruction of Left Mandible, Percutaneous Endoscopic Approach

0N5X0ZZ Destruction of Hyoid Bone, Open Approach

0N5X3ZZ Destruction of Hyoid Bone, Percutaneous Approach

0N5X4ZZ Destruction of Hyoid Bone, Percutaneous Endoscopic Approach

N8 – Head and Facial Bones, Division

eview Coding Guideline B3.14

N800ZZ Division of Skull, Open Approach

N803ZZ Division of Skull, Percutaneous Approach

N804ZZ Division of Skull, Percutaneous Endoscopic Approach

N810ZZ Division of Right Frontal Bone, Open Approach

N813ZZ Division of Right Frontal Bone, Percutaneous Approach

N814ZZ Division of Right Frontal Bone, Percutaneous Endoscopic Approach

N820ZZ Division of Left Frontal Bone, Open Approach

N823ZZ Division of Left Frontal Bone, Percutaneous Approach

N824ZZ Division of Left Frontal Bone, Percutaneous Endoscopic Approach

N830ZZ Division of Right Parietal Bone, Open Approach

N833ZZ Division of Right Parietal Bone, Percutaneous Approach

N834ZZ Division of Right Parietal Bone, Percutaneous Endoscopic Approach

N840ZZ Division of Left Parietal Bone, Open Approach

N843ZZ Division of Left Parietal Bone, Percutaneous Approach

N844ZZ Division of Left Parietal Bone, Percutaneous Endoscopic Approach

N850ZZ Division of Right Temporal Bone, Open Approach

N853ZZ Division of Right Temporal Bone, Percutaneous Approach

N854ZZ Division of Right Temporal Bone, Percutaneous Endoscopic Approach

N860ZZ Division of Left Temporal Bone, Open Approach

N863ZZ Division of Left Temporal Bone, Percutaneous Approach

N864ZZ Division of Left Temporal Bone, Percutaneous Endoscopic Approach

N870ZZ Division of Right Occipital Bone, Open Approach

N873ZZ Division of Right Occipital Bone, Percutaneous Approach

N874ZZ Division of Right Occipital Bone, Percutaneous Endoscopic Approach

0N880ZZ Division of Left Occipital Bone, Open Approach

0N883ZZ Division of Left Occipital Bone, Percutaneous Approach

0N884ZZ Division of Left Occipital Bone, Percutaneous Endoscopic Approach

0N8B0ZZ Division of Nasal Bone, Open Approach

0N8B3ZZ Division of Nasal Bone, Percutaneous Approach

0N8B4ZZ Division of Nasal Bone, Percutaneous Endoscopic Approach

0N8C0ZZ Division of Right Sphenoid Bone, Open Approach

0N8C3ZZ Division of Right Sphenoid Bone, Percutaneous Approach

0N8C4ZZ Division of Right Sphenoid Bone, Percutaneous Endoscopic Approach

0N8D0ZZ Division of Left Sphenoid Bone, Open Approach

0N8D3ZZ Division of Left Sphenoid Bone, Percutaneous Approach

0N8D4ZZ Division of Left Sphenoid Bone, Percutaneous Endoscopic Approach

0N8F0ZZ Division of Right Ethmoid Bone, Open Approach

0N8F3ZZ Division of Right Ethmoid Bone, Percutaneous Approach

0N8F4ZZ Division of Right Ethmoid Bone, Percutaneous Endoscopic Approach

0N8G0ZZ Division of Left Ethmoid Bone, Open Approach

0N8G3ZZ Division of Left Ethmoid Bone, Percutaneous Approach

0N8G4ZZ Division of Left Ethmoid Bone, Percutaneous Endoscopic Approach

0N8H0ZZ Division of Right Lacrimal Bone, Open Approach

0N8H3ZZ Division of Right Lacrimal Bone, Percutaneous Approach

0N8H4ZZ Division of Right Lacrimal Bone, Percutaneous Endoscopic Approach

0N8J0ZZ Division of Left Lacrimal Bone, Open Approach

0N8J3ZZ Division of Left Lacrimal Bone, Percutaneous Approach

0N8J4ZZ Division of Left Lacrimal Bone, Percutaneous Endoscopic Approach

0N8K0ZZ Division of Right Palatine Bone, Open Approach

0N8K3ZZ Division of Right Palatine Bone, Percutaneous Approach

0N8K4ZZ Division of Right Palatine Bone, Percutaneous Endoscopic Approach

0N8L0ZZ Division of Left Palatine Bone, Open Approach

0N8L3ZZ Division of Left Palatine Bone, Percutaneous Approach

0N8L4ZZ Division of Left Palatine Bone, Percutaneous Endoscopic Approach

0N8M0ZZ Division of Right Zygomatic Bone, Open Approach

0N8M3ZZ Division of Right Zygomatic Bone, Percutaneous Approach

0N8M4ZZ Division of Right Zygomatic Bone, Percutaneous Endoscopic Approach

0N8N0ZZ Division of Left Zygomatic Bone, Open Approach

0N8N3ZZ Division of Left Zygomatic Bone, Percutaneous Approach

0N8N4ZZ Division of Left Zygomatic Bone, Percutaneous Endoscopic Approach

0N8P0ZZ Division of Right Orbit, Open Approach

0N8P3ZZ Division of Right Orbit, Percutaneous Approach

0N8P4ZZ Division of Right Orbit, Percutaneous Endoscopic Approach

0N8Q0ZZ Division of Left Orbit, Open Approach

0N8Q3ZZ Division of Left Orbit, Percutaneous Approach

0N8Q4ZZ Division of Left Orbit, Percutaneous Endoscopic Approach

0N8R0ZZ Division of Right Maxilla, Open Approach

0N8R3ZZ Division of Right Maxilla, Percutaneous Approach

0N8R4ZZ Division of Right Maxilla, Percutaneous Endoscopic Approach

0N8S0ZZ Division of Left Maxilla, Open Approach

0N8S3ZZ Division of Left Maxilla, Percutaneous Approach

0N8S4ZZ Division of Left Maxilla, Percutaneous Endoscopic Approach

♀ Female-only ♂ Male-only ▲ Limited Coverage ● Non-OR ▬ HAC-associated procedure ▲ Non-covered procedures ➕ Combination

0N8T0ZZ Division of Right Mandible, Open Approach	**0N8V0ZZ** Division of Left Mandible, Open Approach	**0N8X0ZZ** Division of Hyoid Bone, Open Approach
0N8T3ZZ Division of Right Mandible, Percutaneous Approach	**0N8V3ZZ** Division of Left Mandible, Percutaneous Approach	**0N8X3ZZ** Division of Hyoid Bone, Percutaneous Approach
0N8T4ZZ Division of Right Mandible, Percutaneous Endoscopic Approach	**0N8V4ZZ** Division of Left Mandible, Percutaneous Endoscopic Approach	**0N8X4ZZ** Division of Hyoid Bone, Percutaneous Endoscopic Approach

0N9 – Head and Facial Bones, Drainage

Review Coding Guidelines B3.4a and B3.4b

Review Coding Guideline B6.2

0N9000Z Drainage of Skull with Drainage Device, Open Approach	**0N933ZX** Drainage of Right Parietal Bone, Percutaneous Approach, Diagnostic	**0N963ZZ** Drainage of Left Temporal Bone, Percutaneous Approach
0N900ZX Drainage of Skull, Open Approach, Diagnostic	**0N933ZZ** Drainage of Right Parietal Bone, Percutaneous Approach	**0N9640Z** Drainage of Left Temporal Bone with Drainage Device, Percutaneous Endoscopic Approach
0N900ZZ Drainage of Skull, Open Approach	**0N9340Z** Drainage of Right Parietal Bone with Drainage Device, Percutaneous Endoscopic Approach	**0N964ZX** Drainage of Left Temporal Bone, Percutaneous Endoscopic Approach, Diagnostic
0N9030Z Drainage of Skull with Drainage Device, Percutaneous Approach	**0N934ZX** Drainage of Right Parietal Bone, Percutaneous Endoscopic Approach, Diagnostic	**0N964ZZ** Drainage of Left Temporal Bone, Percutaneous Endoscopic Approach
0N903ZX Drainage of Skull, Percutaneous Approach, Diagnostic	**0N934ZZ** Drainage of Right Parietal Bone, Percutaneous Endoscopic Approach	**0N9700Z** Drainage of Right Occipital Bone with Drainage Device, Open Approach
0N903ZZ Drainage of Skull, Percutaneous Approach	**0N9400Z** Drainage of Left Parietal Bone with Drainage Device, Open Approach	**0N970ZX** Drainage of Right Occipital Bone, Open Approach, Diagnostic
0N9040Z Drainage of Skull with Drainage Device, Percutaneous Endoscopic Approach	**0N940ZX** Drainage of Left Parietal Bone, Open Approach, Diagnostic	**0N970ZZ** Drainage of Right Occipital Bone, Open Approach
0N904ZX Drainage of Skull, Percutaneous Endoscopic Approach, Diagnostic	**0N940ZZ** Drainage of Left Parietal Bone, Open Approach	**0N9730Z** Drainage of Right Occipital Bone with Drainage Device, Percutaneous Approach
0N904ZZ Drainage of Skull, Percutaneous Endoscopic Approach	**0N9430Z** Drainage of Left Parietal Bone with Drainage Device, Percutaneous Approach	**0N973ZX** Drainage of Right Occipital Bone, Percutaneous Approach, Diagnostic
0N9100Z Drainage of Right Frontal Bone with Drainage Device, Open Approach	**0N943ZX** Drainage of Left Parietal Bone, Percutaneous Approach, Diagnostic	**0N973ZZ** Drainage of Right Occipital Bone, Percutaneous Approach
0N910ZX Drainage of Right Frontal Bone, Open Approach, Diagnostic	**0N943ZZ** Drainage of Left Parietal Bone, Percutaneous Approach	**0N9740Z** Drainage of Right Occipital Bone with Drainage Device, Percutaneous Endoscopic Approach
0N910ZZ Drainage of Right Frontal Bone, Open Approach	**0N9440Z** Drainage of Left Parietal Bone with Drainage Device, Percutaneous Endoscopic Approach	**0N974ZX** Drainage of Right Occipital Bone, Percutaneous Endoscopic Approach, Diagnostic
0N9130Z Drainage of Right Frontal Bone with Drainage Device, Percutaneous Approach	**0N944ZX** Drainage of Left Parietal Bone, Percutaneous Endoscopic Approach, Diagnostic	**0N974ZZ** Drainage of Right Occipital Bone, Percutaneous Endoscopic Approach
0N913ZX Drainage of Right Frontal Bone, Percutaneous Approach, Diagnostic	**0N944ZZ** Drainage of Left Parietal Bone, Percutaneous Endoscopic Approach	**0N9800Z** Drainage of Left Occipital Bone with Drainage Device, Open Approach
0N913ZZ Drainage of Right Frontal Bone, Percutaneous Approach	**0N9500Z** Drainage of Right Temporal Bone with Drainage Device, Open Approach	**0N980ZX** Drainage of Left Occipital Bone, Open Approach, Diagnostic
0N9140Z Drainage of Right Frontal Bone with Drainage Device, Percutaneous Endoscopic Approach	**0N950ZX** Drainage of Right Temporal Bone, Open Approach, Diagnostic	**0N980ZZ** Drainage of Left Occipital Bone, Open Approach
0N914ZX Drainage of Right Frontal Bone, Percutaneous Endoscopic Approach, Diagnostic	**0N950ZZ** Drainage of Right Temporal Bone, Open Approach	**0N9830Z** Drainage of Left Occipital Bone with Drainage Device, Percutaneous Approach
0N914ZZ Drainage of Right Frontal Bone, Percutaneous Endoscopic Approach	**0N9530Z** Drainage of Right Temporal Bone with Drainage Device, Percutaneous Approach	**0N983ZX** Drainage of Left Occipital Bone, Percutaneous Approach, Diagnostic
0N9200Z Drainage of Left Frontal Bone with Drainage Device, Open Approach	**0N953ZX** Drainage of Right Temporal Bone, Percutaneous Approach, Diagnostic	**0N983ZZ** Drainage of Left Occipital Bone, Percutaneous Approach
0N920ZX Drainage of Left Frontal Bone, Open Approach, Diagnostic	**0N953ZZ** Drainage of Right Temporal Bone, Percutaneous Approach	**0N9840Z** Drainage of Left Occipital Bone with Drainage Device, Percutaneous Endoscopic Approach
0N920ZZ Drainage of Left Frontal Bone, Open Approach	**0N9540Z** Drainage of Right Temporal Bone with Drainage Device, Percutaneous Endoscopic Approach	**0N984ZX** Drainage of Left Occipital Bone, Percutaneous Endoscopic Approach, Diagnostic
0N9230Z Drainage of Left Frontal Bone with Drainage Device, Percutaneous Approach	**0N954ZX** Drainage of Right Temporal Bone, Percutaneous Endoscopic Approach, Diagnostic	**0N984ZZ** Drainage of Left Occipital Bone, Percutaneous Endoscopic Approach
0N923ZX Drainage of Left Frontal Bone, Percutaneous Approach, Diagnostic	**0N954ZZ** Drainage of Right Temporal Bone, Percutaneous Endoscopic Approach	**0N9B00Z** Drainage of Nasal Bone with Drainage Device, Open Approach
0N923ZZ Drainage of Left Frontal Bone, Percutaneous Approach	**0N9600Z** Drainage of Left Temporal Bone with Drainage Device, Open Approach	**0N9B0ZX** Drainage of Nasal Bone, Open Approach, Diagnostic
0N9240Z Drainage of Left Frontal Bone with Drainage Device, Percutaneous Endoscopic Approach	**0N960ZX** Drainage of Left Temporal Bone, Open Approach, Diagnostic	**0N9B0ZZ** Drainage of Nasal Bone, Open Approach
0N924ZX Drainage of Left Frontal Bone, Percutaneous Endoscopic Approach, Diagnostic	**0N960ZZ** Drainage of Left Temporal Bone, Open Approach	**0N9B30Z** Drainage of Nasal Bone with Drainage Device, Percutaneous Approach
0N924ZZ Drainage of Left Frontal Bone, Percutaneous Endoscopic Approach	**0N9630Z** Drainage of Left Temporal Bone with Drainage Device, Percutaneous Approach	**0N9B3ZX** Drainage of Nasal Bone, Percutaneous Approach, Diagnostic
0N9300Z Drainage of Right Parietal Bone with Drainage Device, Open Approach	**0N963ZX** Drainage of Left Temporal Bone, Percutaneous Approach, Diagnostic	**0N9B3ZZ** Drainage of Nasal Bone, Percutaneous Approach
0N930ZX Drainage of Right Parietal Bone, Open Approach, Diagnostic		**0N9B40Z** Drainage of Nasal Bone with Drainage Device, Percutaneous Endoscopic Approach
0N930ZZ Drainage of Right Parietal Bone, Open Approach		
0N9330Z Drainage of Right Parietal Bone with Drainage Device, Percutaneous Approach		

B4ZX   Drainage of Nasal Bone, Percutaneous Endoscopic Approach, Diagnostic

B4ZZ   Drainage of Nasal Bone, Percutaneous Endoscopic Approach

C00Z   Drainage of Right Sphenoid Bone with Drainage Device, Open Approach

C0ZX   Drainage of Right Sphenoid Bone, Open Approach, Diagnostic

C0ZZ   Drainage of Right Sphenoid Bone, Open Approach

C30Z   Drainage of Right Sphenoid Bone with Drainage Device, Percutaneous Approach

C3ZX   Drainage of Right Sphenoid Bone, Percutaneous Approach, Diagnostic

C3ZZ   Drainage of Right Sphenoid Bone, Percutaneous Approach

C40Z   Drainage of Right Sphenoid Bone with Drainage Device, Percutaneous Endoscopic Approach

C4ZX   Drainage of Right Sphenoid Bone, Percutaneous Endoscopic Approach, Diagnostic

C4ZZ   Drainage of Right Sphenoid Bone, Percutaneous Endoscopic Approach

D00Z   Drainage of Left Sphenoid Bone with Drainage Device, Open Approach

D0ZX   Drainage of Left Sphenoid Bone, Open Approach, Diagnostic

D0ZZ   Drainage of Left Sphenoid Bone, Open Approach

D30Z   Drainage of Left Sphenoid Bone with Drainage Device, Percutaneous Approach

D3ZX   Drainage of Left Sphenoid Bone, Percutaneous Approach, Diagnostic

D3ZZ   Drainage of Left Sphenoid Bone, Percutaneous Approach

D40Z   Drainage of Left Sphenoid Bone with Drainage Device, Percutaneous Endoscopic Approach

D4ZX   Drainage of Left Sphenoid Bone, Percutaneous Endoscopic Approach, Diagnostic

D4ZZ   Drainage of Left Sphenoid Bone, Percutaneous Endoscopic Approach

9F00Z   Drainage of Right Ethmoid Bone with Drainage Device, Open Approach

9F0ZX   Drainage of Right Ethmoid Bone, Open Approach, Diagnostic

9F0ZZ   Drainage of Right Ethmoid Bone, Open Approach

9F30Z   Drainage of Right Ethmoid Bone with Drainage Device, Percutaneous Approach

9F3ZX   Drainage of Right Ethmoid Bone, Percutaneous Approach, Diagnostic

9F3ZZ   Drainage of Right Ethmoid Bone, Percutaneous Approach

9F40Z   Drainage of Right Ethmoid Bone with Drainage Device, Percutaneous Endoscopic Approach

9F4ZX   Drainage of Right Ethmoid Bone, Percutaneous Endoscopic Approach, Diagnostic

9F4ZZ   Drainage of Right Ethmoid Bone, Percutaneous Endoscopic Approach

9G00Z   Drainage of Left Ethmoid Bone with Drainage Device, Open Approach

9G0ZX   Drainage of Left Ethmoid Bone, Open Approach, Diagnostic

9G0ZZ   Drainage of Left Ethmoid Bone, Open Approach

9G30Z   Drainage of Left Ethmoid Bone with Drainage Device, Percutaneous Approach

9G3ZX   Drainage of Left Ethmoid Bone, Percutaneous Approach, Diagnostic

9G3ZZ   Drainage of Left Ethmoid Bone, Percutaneous Approach

0N9G40Z   Drainage of Left Ethmoid Bone with Drainage Device, Percutaneous Endoscopic Approach

0N9G4ZX   Drainage of Left Ethmoid Bone, Percutaneous Endoscopic Approach, Diagnostic

0N9G4ZZ   Drainage of Left Ethmoid Bone, Percutaneous Endoscopic Approach

0N9H00Z   Drainage of Right Lacrimal Bone with Drainage Device, Open Approach

0N9H0ZX   Drainage of Right Lacrimal Bone, Open Approach, Diagnostic

0N9H0ZZ   Drainage of Right Lacrimal Bone, Open Approach

0N9H30Z   Drainage of Right Lacrimal Bone with Drainage Device, Percutaneous Approach

0N9H3ZX   Drainage of Right Lacrimal Bone, Percutaneous Approach, Diagnostic

0N9H3ZZ   Drainage of Right Lacrimal Bone, Percutaneous Approach

0N9H40Z   Drainage of Right Lacrimal Bone with Drainage Device, Percutaneous Endoscopic Approach

0N9H4ZX   Drainage of Right Lacrimal Bone, Percutaneous Endoscopic Approach, Diagnostic

0N9H4ZZ   Drainage of Right Lacrimal Bone, Percutaneous Endoscopic Approach

0N9J00Z   Drainage of Left Lacrimal Bone with Drainage Device, Open Approach

0N9J0ZX   Drainage of Left Lacrimal Bone, Open Approach, Diagnostic

0N9J0ZZ   Drainage of Left Lacrimal Bone, Open Approach

0N9J30Z   Drainage of Left Lacrimal Bone with Drainage Device, Percutaneous Approach

0N9J3ZX   Drainage of Left Lacrimal Bone, Percutaneous Approach, Diagnostic

0N9J3ZZ   Drainage of Left Lacrimal Bone, Percutaneous Approach

0N9J40Z   Drainage of Left Lacrimal Bone with Drainage Device, Percutaneous Endoscopic Approach

0N9J4ZX   Drainage of Left Lacrimal Bone, Percutaneous Endoscopic Approach, Diagnostic

0N9J4ZZ   Drainage of Left Lacrimal Bone, Percutaneous Endoscopic Approach

0N9K00Z   Drainage of Right Palatine Bone with Drainage Device, Open Approach

0N9K0ZX   Drainage of Right Palatine Bone, Open Approach, Diagnostic

0N9K0ZZ   Drainage of Right Palatine Bone, Open Approach

0N9K30Z   Drainage of Right Palatine Bone with Drainage Device, Percutaneous Approach

0N9K3ZX   Drainage of Right Palatine Bone, Percutaneous Approach, Diagnostic

0N9K3ZZ   Drainage of Right Palatine Bone, Percutaneous Approach

0N9K40Z   Drainage of Right Palatine Bone with Drainage Device, Percutaneous Endoscopic Approach

0N9K4ZX   Drainage of Right Palatine Bone, Percutaneous Endoscopic Approach, Diagnostic

0N9K4ZZ   Drainage of Right Palatine Bone, Percutaneous Endoscopic Approach

0N9L00Z   Drainage of Left Palatine Bone with Drainage Device, Open Approach

0N9L0ZX   Drainage of Left Palatine Bone, Open Approach, Diagnostic

0N9L0ZZ   Drainage of Left Palatine Bone, Open Approach

0N9L30Z   Drainage of Left Palatine Bone with Drainage Device, Percutaneous Approach

0N9L3ZX   Drainage of Left Palatine Bone, Percutaneous Approach, Diagnostic

0N9L3ZZ   Drainage of Left Palatine Bone, Percutaneous Approach

0N9L40Z   Drainage of Left Palatine Bone with Drainage Device, Percutaneous Endoscopic Approach

0N9L4ZX   Drainage of Left Palatine Bone, Percutaneous Endoscopic Approach, Diagnostic

0N9L4ZZ   Drainage of Left Palatine Bone, Percutaneous Endoscopic Approach

0N9M00Z   Drainage of Right Zygomatic Bone with Drainage Device, Open Approach

0N9M0ZX   Drainage of Right Zygomatic Bone, Open Approach, Diagnostic

0N9M0ZZ   Drainage of Right Zygomatic Bone, Open Approach

0N9M30Z   Drainage of Right Zygomatic Bone with Drainage Device, Percutaneous Approach

0N9M3ZX   Drainage of Right Zygomatic Bone, Percutaneous Approach, Diagnostic

0N9M3ZZ   Drainage of Right Zygomatic Bone, Percutaneous Approach

0N9M40Z   Drainage of Right Zygomatic Bone with Drainage Device, Percutaneous Endoscopic Approach

0N9M4ZX   Drainage of Right Zygomatic Bone, Percutaneous Endoscopic Approach, Diagnostic

0N9M4ZZ   Drainage of Right Zygomatic Bone, Percutaneous Endoscopic Approach

0N9N00Z   Drainage of Left Zygomatic Bone with Drainage Device, Open Approach

0N9N0ZX   Drainage of Left Zygomatic Bone, Open Approach, Diagnostic

0N9N0ZZ   Drainage of Left Zygomatic Bone, Open Approach

0N9N30Z   Drainage of Left Zygomatic Bone with Drainage Device, Percutaneous Approach

0N9N3ZX   Drainage of Left Zygomatic Bone, Percutaneous Approach, Diagnostic

0N9N3ZZ   Drainage of Left Zygomatic Bone, Percutaneous Approach

0N9N40Z   Drainage of Left Zygomatic Bone with Drainage Device, Percutaneous Endoscopic Approach

0N9N4ZX   Drainage of Left Zygomatic Bone, Percutaneous Endoscopic Approach, Diagnostic

0N9N4ZZ   Drainage of Left Zygomatic Bone, Percutaneous Endoscopic Approach

0N9P00Z   Drainage of Right Orbit with Drainage Device, Open Approach

0N9P0ZX   Drainage of Right Orbit, Open Approach, Diagnostic

0N9P0ZZ   Drainage of Right Orbit, Open Approach

0N9P30Z   Drainage of Right Orbit with Drainage Device, Percutaneous Approach

0N9P3ZX   Drainage of Right Orbit, Percutaneous Approach, Diagnostic

0N9P3ZZ   Drainage of Right Orbit, Percutaneous Approach

0N9P40Z   Drainage of Right Orbit with Drainage Device, Percutaneous Endoscopic Approach

0N9P4ZX   Drainage of Right Orbit, Percutaneous Endoscopic Approach, Diagnostic

0N9P4ZZ   Drainage of Right Orbit, Percutaneous Endoscopic Approach

0N9Q00Z   Drainage of Left Orbit with Drainage Device, Open Approach

0N9Q0ZX   Drainage of Left Orbit, Open Approach, Diagnostic

0N9Q0ZZ   Drainage of Left Orbit, Open Approach

0N9Q30Z   Drainage of Left Orbit with Drainage Device, Percutaneous Approach

Female-only   ♂ Male-only   ▲ Limited Coverage   ● Non-OR   ▦ HAC-associated procedure   ▲ Non-covered procedures   + Combination

0N9Q3ZX	Drainage of Left Orbit, Percutaneous Approach, Diagnostic
0N9Q3ZZ	Drainage of Left Orbit, Percutaneous Approach
0N9Q40Z	Drainage of Left Orbit with Drainage Device, Percutaneous Endoscopic Approach
0N9Q4ZX	Drainage of Left Orbit, Percutaneous Endoscopic Approach, Diagnostic
0N9Q4ZZ	Drainage of Left Orbit, Percutaneous Endoscopic Approach
0N9R00Z	Drainage of Right Maxilla with Drainage Device, Open Approach
0N9R0ZX	Drainage of Right Maxilla, Open Approach, Diagnostic
0N9R0ZZ	Drainage of Right Maxilla, Open Approach
0N9R30Z	Drainage of Right Maxilla with Drainage Device, Percutaneous Approach
0N9R3ZX	Drainage of Right Maxilla, Percutaneous Approach, Diagnostic
0N9R3ZZ	Drainage of Right Maxilla, Percutaneous Approach
0N9R40Z	Drainage of Right Maxilla with Drainage Device, Percutaneous Endoscopic Approach
0N9R4ZX	Drainage of Right Maxilla, Percutaneous Endoscopic Approach, Diagnostic
0N9R4ZZ	Drainage of Right Maxilla, Percutaneous Endoscopic Approach
0N9S00Z	Drainage of Left Maxilla with Drainage Device, Open Approach
0N9S0ZX	Drainage of Left Maxilla, Open Approach, Diagnostic
0N9S0ZZ	Drainage of Left Maxilla, Open Approach
0N9S30Z	Drainage of Left Maxilla with Drainage Device, Percutaneous Approach
0N9S3ZX	Drainage of Left Maxilla, Percutaneous Approach, Diagnostic
0N9S3ZZ	Drainage of Left Maxilla, Percutaneous Approach
0N9S40Z	Drainage of Left Maxilla with Drainage Device, Percutaneous Endoscopic Approach
0N9S4ZX	Drainage of Left Maxilla, Percutaneous Endoscopic Approach, Diagnostic
0N9S4ZZ	Drainage of Left Maxilla, Percutaneous Endoscopic Approach
0N9T00Z	Drainage of Right Mandible with Drainage Device, Open Approach
0N9T0ZX	Drainage of Right Mandible, Open Approach, Diagnostic
0N9T0ZZ	Drainage of Right Mandible, Open Approach
0N9T30Z	Drainage of Right Mandible with Drainage Device, Percutaneous Approach
0N9T3ZX	Drainage of Right Mandible, Percutaneous Approach, Diagnostic
0N9T3ZZ	Drainage of Right Mandible, Percutaneous Approach
0N9T40Z	Drainage of Right Mandible with Drainage Device, Percutaneous Endoscopic Approach
0N9T4ZX	Drainage of Right Mandible, Percutaneous Endoscopic Approach, Diagnostic
0N9T4ZZ	Drainage of Right Mandible, Percutaneous Endoscopic Approach
0N9V00Z	Drainage of Left Mandible with Drainage Device, Open Approach
0N9V0ZX	Drainage of Left Mandible, Open Approach, Diagnostic
0N9V0ZZ	Drainage of Left Mandible, Open Approach
0N9V30Z	Drainage of Left Mandible with Drainage Device, Percutaneous Approach
0N9V3ZX	Drainage of Left Mandible, Percutaneous Approach, Diagnostic
0N9V3ZZ	Drainage of Left Mandible, Percutaneous Approach
0N9V40Z	Drainage of Left Mandible with Drainage Device, Percutaneous Endoscopic Approach
0N9V4ZX	Drainage of Left Mandible, Percutaneous Endoscopic Approach, Diagnostic
0N9V4ZZ	Drainage of Left Mandible, Percutaneous Endoscopic Approach
0N9X00Z	Drainage of Hyoid Bone with Drainage Device, Open Approach
0N9X0ZX	Drainage of Hyoid Bone, Open Approach, Diagnostic
0N9X0ZZ	Drainage of Hyoid Bone, Open Approach
0N9X30Z	Drainage of Hyoid Bone with Drainage Device, Percutaneous Approach
0N9X3ZX	Drainage of Hyoid Bone, Percutaneous Approach, Diagnostic
0N9X3ZZ	Drainage of Hyoid Bone, Percutaneous Approach
0N9X40Z	Drainage of Hyoid Bone with Drainage Device, Percutaneous Endoscopic Approach
0N9X4ZX	Drainage of Hyoid Bone, Percutaneous Endoscopic Approach, Diagnostic
0N9X4ZZ	Drainage of Hyoid Bone, Percutaneous Endoscopic Approach

0NB – Head and Facial Bones, Excision

Review Coding Guidelines B3.4a and B3.4b

Review Coding Guideline B3.5

Review Coding Guideline B3.8

0NB00ZX	Excision of Skull, Open Approach, Diagnostic
0NB00ZZ	Excision of Skull, Open Approach
0NB03ZX	Excision of Skull, Percutaneous Approach, Diagnostic
0NB03ZZ	Excision of Skull, Percutaneous Approach
0NB04ZX	Excision of Skull, Percutaneous Endoscopic Approach, Diagnostic
0NB04ZZ	Excision of Skull, Percutaneous Endoscopic Approach
0NB10ZX	Excision of Right Frontal Bone, Open Approach, Diagnostic
0NB10ZZ	Excision of Right Frontal Bone, Open Approach
0NB13ZX	Excision of Right Frontal Bone, Percutaneous Approach, Diagnostic
0NB13ZZ	Excision of Right Frontal Bone, Percutaneous Approach
0NB14ZX	Excision of Right Frontal Bone, Percutaneous Endoscopic Approach, Diagnostic
0NB14ZZ	Excision of Right Frontal Bone, Percutaneous Endoscopic Approach
0NB20ZX	Excision of Left Frontal Bone, Open Approach, Diagnostic
0NB20ZZ	Excision of Left Frontal Bone, Open Approach
0NB23ZX	Excision of Left Frontal Bone, Percutaneous Approach, Diagnostic
0NB23ZZ	Excision of Left Frontal Bone, Percutaneous Approach
0NB24ZX	Excision of Left Frontal Bone, Percutaneous Endoscopic Approach, Diagnostic
0NB24ZZ	Excision of Left Frontal Bone, Percutaneous Endoscopic Approach
0NB30ZX	Excision of Right Parietal Bone, Open Approach, Diagnostic
0NB30ZZ	Excision of Right Parietal Bone, Open Approach
0NB33ZX	Excision of Right Parietal Bone, Percutaneous Approach, Diagnostic
0NB33ZZ	Excision of Right Parietal Bone, Percutaneous Approach
0NB34ZX	Excision of Right Parietal Bone, Percutaneous Endoscopic Approach, Diagnostic
0NB34ZZ	Excision of Right Parietal Bone, Percutaneous Endoscopic Approach
0NB40ZX	Excision of Left Parietal Bone, Open Approach, Diagnostic
0NB40ZZ	Excision of Left Parietal Bone, Open Approach
0NB43ZX	Excision of Left Parietal Bone, Percutaneous Approach, Diagnostic
0NB43ZZ	Excision of Left Parietal Bone, Percutaneous Approach
0NB44ZX	Excision of Left Parietal Bone, Percutaneous Endoscopic Approach, Diagnostic
0NB44ZZ	Excision of Left Parietal Bone, Percutaneous Endoscopic Approach
0NB50ZX	Excision of Right Temporal Bone, Open Approach, Diagnostic
0NB50ZZ	Excision of Right Temporal Bone, Open Approach
0NB53ZX	Excision of Right Temporal Bone, Percutaneous Approach, Diagnostic
0NB53ZZ	Excision of Right Temporal Bone, Percutaneous Approach
0NB54ZX	Excision of Right Temporal Bone, Percutaneous Endoscopic Approach, Diagnostic
0NB54ZZ	Excision of Right Temporal Bone, Percutaneous Endoscopic Approach
0NB60ZX	Excision of Left Temporal Bone, Open Approach, Diagnostic
0NB60ZZ	Excision of Left Temporal Bone, Open Approach
0NB63ZX	Excision of Left Temporal Bone, Percutaneous Approach, Diagnostic
0NB63ZZ	Excision of Left Temporal Bone, Percutaneous Approach
0NB64ZX	Excision of Left Temporal Bone, Percutaneous Endoscopic Approach, Diagnostic
0NB64ZZ	Excision of Left Temporal Bone, Percutaneous Endoscopic Approach
0NB70ZX	Excision of Right Occipital Bone, Open Approach, Diagnostic
0NB70ZZ	Excision of Right Occipital Bone, Open Approach
0NB73ZX	Excision of Right Occipital Bone, Percutaneous Approach, Diagnostic
0NB73ZZ	Excision of Right Occipital Bone, Percutaneous Approach
0NB74ZX	Excision of Right Occipital Bone, Percutaneous Endoscopic Approach, Diagnostic
0NB74ZZ	Excision of Right Occipital Bone, Percutaneous Endoscopic Approach

80ZX Excision of Left Occipital Bone, Open Approach, Diagnostic

80ZZ Excision of Left Occipital Bone, Open Approach

83ZX Excision of Left Occipital Bone, Percutaneous Approach, Diagnostic

83ZZ Excision of Left Occipital Bone, Percutaneous Approach

84ZX Excision of Left Occipital Bone, Percutaneous Endoscopic Approach, Diagnostic

84ZZ Excision of Left Occipital Bone, Percutaneous Endoscopic Approach

BB0ZX Excision of Nasal Bone, Open Approach, Diagnostic

BB0ZZ Excision of Nasal Bone, Open Approach

BB3ZX Excision of Nasal Bone, Percutaneous Approach, Diagnostic

BB3ZZ Excision of Nasal Bone, Percutaneous Approach

BB4ZX Excision of Nasal Bone, Percutaneous Endoscopic Approach, Diagnostic

BB4ZZ Excision of Nasal Bone, Percutaneous Endoscopic Approach

BC0ZX Excision of Right Sphenoid Bone, Open Approach, Diagnostic

BC0ZZ Excision of Right Sphenoid Bone, Open Approach

BC3ZX Excision of Right Sphenoid Bone, Percutaneous Approach, Diagnostic

BC3ZZ Excision of Right Sphenoid Bone, Percutaneous Approach

BC4ZX Excision of Right Sphenoid Bone, Percutaneous Endoscopic Approach, Diagnostic

BC4ZZ Excision of Right Sphenoid Bone, Percutaneous Endoscopic Approach

BD0ZX Excision of Left Sphenoid Bone, Open Approach, Diagnostic

BD0ZZ Excision of Left Sphenoid Bone, Open Approach

BD3ZX Excision of Left Sphenoid Bone, Percutaneous Approach, Diagnostic

BD3ZZ Excision of Left Sphenoid Bone, Percutaneous Approach

BD4ZX Excision of Left Sphenoid Bone, Percutaneous Endoscopic Approach, Diagnostic

BD4ZZ Excision of Left Sphenoid Bone, Percutaneous Endoscopic Approach

BF0ZX Excision of Right Ethmoid Bone, Open Approach, Diagnostic

BF0ZZ Excision of Right Ethmoid Bone, Open Approach

BF3ZX Excision of Right Ethmoid Bone, Percutaneous Approach, Diagnostic

BF3ZZ Excision of Right Ethmoid Bone, Percutaneous Approach

BF4ZX Excision of Right Ethmoid Bone, Percutaneous Endoscopic Approach, Diagnostic

BF4ZZ Excision of Right Ethmoid Bone, Percutaneous Endoscopic Approach

NBG0ZX Excision of Left Ethmoid Bone, Open Approach, Diagnostic

NBG0ZZ Excision of Left Ethmoid Bone, Open Approach

NBG3ZX Excision of Left Ethmoid Bone, Percutaneous Approach, Diagnostic

NBG3ZZ Excision of Left Ethmoid Bone, Percutaneous Approach

NBG4ZX Excision of Left Ethmoid Bone, Percutaneous Endoscopic Approach, Diagnostic

NBG4ZZ Excision of Left Ethmoid Bone, Percutaneous Endoscopic Approach

NBH0ZX Excision of Right Lacrimal Bone, Open Approach, Diagnostic

0NBH0ZZ Excision of Right Lacrimal Bone, Open Approach

0NBH3ZX Excision of Right Lacrimal Bone, Percutaneous Approach, Diagnostic

0NBH3ZZ Excision of Right Lacrimal Bone, Percutaneous Approach

0NBH4ZX Excision of Right Lacrimal Bone, Percutaneous Endoscopic Approach, Diagnostic

0NBH4ZZ Excision of Right Lacrimal Bone, Percutaneous Endoscopic Approach

0NBJ0ZX Excision of Left Lacrimal Bone, Open Approach, Diagnostic

0NBJ0ZZ Excision of Left Lacrimal Bone, Open Approach

0NBJ3ZX Excision of Left Lacrimal Bone, Percutaneous Approach, Diagnostic

0NBJ3ZZ Excision of Left Lacrimal Bone, Percutaneous Approach

0NBJ4ZX Excision of Left Lacrimal Bone, Percutaneous Endoscopic Approach, Diagnostic

0NBJ4ZZ Excision of Left Lacrimal Bone, Percutaneous Endoscopic Approach

0NBK0ZX Excision of Right Palatine Bone, Open Approach, Diagnostic

0NBK0ZZ Excision of Right Palatine Bone, Open Approach

0NBK3ZX Excision of Right Palatine Bone, Percutaneous Approach, Diagnostic

0NBK3ZZ Excision of Right Palatine Bone, Percutaneous Approach

0NBK4ZX Excision of Right Palatine Bone, Percutaneous Endoscopic Approach, Diagnostic

0NBK4ZZ Excision of Right Palatine Bone, Percutaneous Endoscopic Approach

0NBL0ZX Excision of Left Palatine Bone, Open Approach, Diagnostic

0NBL0ZZ Excision of Left Palatine Bone, Open Approach

0NBL3ZX Excision of Left Palatine Bone, Percutaneous Approach, Diagnostic

0NBL3ZZ Excision of Left Palatine Bone, Percutaneous Approach

0NBL4ZX Excision of Left Palatine Bone, Percutaneous Endoscopic Approach, Diagnostic

0NBL4ZZ Excision of Left Palatine Bone, Percutaneous Endoscopic Approach

0NBM0ZX Excision of Right Zygomatic Bone, Open Approach, Diagnostic

0NBM0ZZ Excision of Right Zygomatic Bone, Open Approach

0NBM3ZX Excision of Right Zygomatic Bone, Percutaneous Approach, Diagnostic

0NBM3ZZ Excision of Right Zygomatic Bone, Percutaneous Approach

0NBM4ZX Excision of Right Zygomatic Bone, Percutaneous Endoscopic Approach, Diagnostic

0NBM4ZZ Excision of Right Zygomatic Bone, Percutaneous Endoscopic Approach

0NBN0ZX Excision of Left Zygomatic Bone, Open Approach, Diagnostic

0NBN0ZZ Excision of Left Zygomatic Bone, Open Approach

0NBN3ZX Excision of Left Zygomatic Bone, Percutaneous Approach, Diagnostic

0NBN3ZZ Excision of Left Zygomatic Bone, Percutaneous Approach

0NBN4ZX Excision of Left Zygomatic Bone, Percutaneous Endoscopic Approach, Diagnostic

0NBN4ZZ Excision of Left Zygomatic Bone, Percutaneous Endoscopic Approach

0NBP0ZX Excision of Right Orbit, Open Approach, Diagnostic

0NBP0ZZ Excision of Right Orbit, Open Approach

0NBP3ZX Excision of Right Orbit, Percutaneous Approach, Diagnostic

0NBP3ZZ Excision of Right Orbit, Percutaneous Approach

0NBP4ZX Excision of Right Orbit, Percutaneous Endoscopic Approach, Diagnostic

0NBP4ZZ Excision of Right Orbit, Percutaneous Endoscopic Approach

0NBQ0ZX Excision of Left Orbit, Open Approach, Diagnostic

0NBQ0ZZ Excision of Left Orbit, Open Approach

0NBQ3ZX Excision of Left Orbit, Percutaneous Approach, Diagnostic

0NBQ3ZZ Excision of Left Orbit, Percutaneous Approach

0NBQ4ZX Excision of Left Orbit, Percutaneous Endoscopic Approach, Diagnostic

0NBQ4ZZ Excision of Left Orbit, Percutaneous Endoscopic Approach

0NBR0ZX Excision of Right Maxilla, Open Approach, Diagnostic

0NBR0ZZ Excision of Right Maxilla, Open Approach

0NBR3ZX Excision of Right Maxilla, Percutaneous Approach, Diagnostic

0NBR3ZZ Excision of Right Maxilla, Percutaneous Approach

0NBR4ZX Excision of Right Maxilla, Percutaneous Endoscopic Approach, Diagnostic

0NBR4ZZ Excision of Right Maxilla, Percutaneous Endoscopic Approach

0NBS0ZX Excision of Left Maxilla, Open Approach, Diagnostic

0NBS0ZZ Excision of Left Maxilla, Open Approach

0NBS3ZX Excision of Left Maxilla, Percutaneous Approach, Diagnostic

0NBS3ZZ Excision of Left Maxilla, Percutaneous Approach

0NBS4ZX Excision of Left Maxilla, Percutaneous Endoscopic Approach, Diagnostic

0NBS4ZZ Excision of Left Maxilla, Percutaneous Endoscopic Approach

0NBT0ZX Excision of Right Mandible, Open Approach, Diagnostic

0NBT0ZZ Excision of Right Mandible, Open Approach

0NBT3ZX Excision of Right Mandible, Percutaneous Approach, Diagnostic

0NBT3ZZ Excision of Right Mandible, Percutaneous Approach

0NBT4ZX Excision of Right Mandible, Percutaneous Endoscopic Approach, Diagnostic

0NBT4ZZ Excision of Right Mandible, Percutaneous Endoscopic Approach

0NBV0ZX Excision of Left Mandible, Open Approach, Diagnostic

0NBV0ZZ Excision of Left Mandible, Open Approach

0NBV3ZX Excision of Left Mandible, Percutaneous Approach, Diagnostic

0NBV3ZZ Excision of Left Mandible, Percutaneous Approach

0NBV4ZX Excision of Left Mandible, Percutaneous Endoscopic Approach, Diagnostic

0NBV4ZZ Excision of Left Mandible, Percutaneous Endoscopic Approach

0NBX0ZX Excision of Hyoid Bone, Open Approach, Diagnostic

0NBX0ZZ Excision of Hyoid Bone, Open Approach

0NBX3ZX Excision of Hyoid Bone, Percutaneous Approach, Diagnostic

0NBX3ZZ Excision of Hyoid Bone, Percutaneous Approach

0NBX4ZX Excision of Hyoid Bone, Percutaneous Endoscopic Approach, Diagnostic

0NBX4ZZ Excision of Hyoid Bone, Percutaneous Endoscopic Approach

0NBH0ZX Excision of Right Lacrimal Bone, Open Approach, Diagnostic

0NBP0ZX Excision of Right Orbit, Open Approach, Diagnostic

785

♀ Female-only   ♂ Male-only   ▲ Limited Coverage   ● Non-OR   ▨ HAC-associated procedure   ▲ Non-covered procedures   ➕ Combination

0NC – Head and Facial Bones, Extirpation

0NC10ZZ Extirpation of Matter from Right Frontal Bone, Open Approach

0NC13ZZ Extirpation of Matter from Right Frontal Bone, Percutaneous Approach

0NC14ZZ Extirpation of Matter from Right Frontal Bone, Percutaneous Endoscopic Approach

0NC20ZZ Extirpation of Matter from Left Frontal Bone, Open Approach

0NC23ZZ Extirpation of Matter from Left Frontal Bone, Percutaneous Approach

0NC24ZZ Extirpation of Matter from Left Frontal Bone, Percutaneous Endoscopic Approach

0NC30ZZ Extirpation of Matter from Right Parietal Bone, Open Approach

0NC33ZZ Extirpation of Matter from Right Parietal Bone, Percutaneous Approach

0NC34ZZ Extirpation of Matter from Right Parietal Bone, Percutaneous Endoscopic Approach

0NC40ZZ Extirpation of Matter from Left Parietal Bone, Open Approach

0NC43ZZ Extirpation of Matter from Left Parietal Bone, Percutaneous Approach

0NC44ZZ Extirpation of Matter from Left Parietal Bone, Percutaneous Endoscopic Approach

0NC50ZZ Extirpation of Matter from Right Temporal Bone, Open Approach

0NC53ZZ Extirpation of Matter from Right Temporal Bone, Percutaneous Approach

0NC54ZZ Extirpation of Matter from Right Temporal Bone, Percutaneous Endoscopic Approach

0NC60ZZ Extirpation of Matter from Left Temporal Bone, Open Approach

0NC63ZZ Extirpation of Matter from Left Temporal Bone, Percutaneous Approach

0NC64ZZ Extirpation of Matter from Left Temporal Bone, Percutaneous Endoscopic Approach

0NC70ZZ Extirpation of Matter from Right Occipital Bone, Open Approach

0NC73ZZ Extirpation of Matter from Right Occipital Bone, Percutaneous Approach

0NC74ZZ Extirpation of Matter from Right Occipital Bone, Percutaneous Endoscopic Approach

0NC80ZZ Extirpation of Matter from Left Occipital Bone, Open Approach

0NC83ZZ Extirpation of Matter from Left Occipital Bone, Percutaneous Approach

0NC84ZZ Extirpation of Matter from Left Occipital Bone, Percutaneous Endoscopic Approach

0NCB0ZZ Extirpation of Matter from Nasal Bone, Open Approach

0NCB3ZZ Extirpation of Matter from Nasal Bone, Percutaneous Approach

0NCB4ZZ Extirpation of Matter from Nasal Bone, Percutaneous Endoscopic Approach

0NCC0ZZ Extirpation of Matter from Right Sphenoid Bone, Open Approach

0NCC3ZZ Extirpation of Matter from Right Sphenoid Bone, Percutaneous Approach

0NCC4ZZ Extirpation of Matter from Right Sphenoid Bone, Percutaneous Endoscopic Approach

0NCD0ZZ Extirpation of Matter from Left Sphenoid Bone, Open Approach

0NCD3ZZ Extirpation of Matter from Left Sphenoid Bone, Percutaneous Approach

0NCD4ZZ Extirpation of Matter from Left Sphenoid Bone, Percutaneous Endoscopic Approach

0NCF0ZZ Extirpation of Matter from Right Ethmoid Bone, Open Approach

0NCF3ZZ Extirpation of Matter from Right Ethmoid Bone, Percutaneous Approach

0NCF4ZZ Extirpation of Matter from Right Ethmoid Bone, Percutaneous Endoscopic Approach

0NCG0ZZ Extirpation of Matter from Left Ethmoid Bone, Open Approach

0NCG3ZZ Extirpation of Matter from Left Ethmoid Bone, Percutaneous Approach

0NCG4ZZ Extirpation of Matter from Left Ethmoid Bone, Percutaneous Endoscopic Approach

0NCH0ZZ Extirpation of Matter from Right Lacrimal Bone, Open Approach

0NCH3ZZ Extirpation of Matter from Right Lacrimal Bone, Percutaneous Approach

0NCH4ZZ Extirpation of Matter from Right Lacrimal Bone, Percutaneous Endoscopic Approach

0NCJ0ZZ Extirpation of Matter from Left Lacrimal Bone, Open Approach

0NCJ3ZZ Extirpation of Matter from Left Lacrimal Bone, Percutaneous Approach

0NCJ4ZZ Extirpation of Matter from Left Lacrimal Bone, Percutaneous Endoscopic Approach

0NCK0ZZ Extirpation of Matter from Right Palatine Bone, Open Approach

0NCK3ZZ Extirpation of Matter from Right Palatine Bone, Percutaneous Approach

0NCK4ZZ Extirpation of Matter from Right Palatine Bone, Percutaneous Endoscopic Approach

0NCL0ZZ Extirpation of Matter from Left Palatine Bone, Open Approach

0NCL3ZZ Extirpation of Matter from Left Palatine Bone, Percutaneous Approach

0NCL4ZZ Extirpation of Matter from Left Palatine Bone, Percutaneous Endoscopic Approach

0NCM0ZZ Extirpation of Matter from Right Zygomatic Bone, Open Approach

0NCM3ZZ Extirpation of Matter from Right Zygomatic Bone, Percutaneous Appro...

0NCM4ZZ Extirpation of Matter from Right Zygomatic Bone, Percutaneous Endoscopic Approach

0NCN0ZZ Extirpation of Matter from Left Zygomatic Bone, Open Approach

0NCN3ZZ Extirpation of Matter from Left Zygomatic Bone, Percutaneous Appro...

0NCN4ZZ Extirpation of Matter from Left Zygomatic Bone, Percutaneous Endoscopic Approach

0NCP0ZZ Extirpation of Matter from Right Orbit Open Approach

0NCP3ZZ Extirpation of Matter from Right Orbit Percutaneous Approach

0NCP4ZZ Extirpation of Matter from Right Orbit Percutaneous Endoscopic Approach

0NCQ0ZZ Extirpation of Matter from Left Orbit, Open Approach

0NCQ3ZZ Extirpation of Matter from Left Orbit, Percutaneous Approach

0NCQ4ZZ Extirpation of Matter from Left Orbit, Percutaneous Endoscopic Appro...

0NCR0ZZ Extirpation of Matter from Right Maxil... Open Approach

0NCR3ZZ Extirpation of Matter from Right Maxil... Percutaneous Approach

0NCR4ZZ Extirpation of Matter from Right Maxil... Percutaneous Endoscopic Approach

0NCS0ZZ Extirpation of Matter from Left Maxilla... Open Approach

0NCS3ZZ Extirpation of Matter from Left Maxilla... Percutaneous Approach

0NCS4ZZ Extirpation of Matter from Left Maxilla... Percutaneous Endoscopic Approach

0NCT0ZZ Extirpation of Matter from Right Mandible, Open Approach

0NCT3ZZ Extirpation of Matter from Right Mandible, Percutaneous Approach

0NCT4ZZ Extirpation of Matter from Right Mandib... Percutaneous Endoscopic Approach

0NCV0ZZ Extirpation of Matter from Left Mandib... Open Approach

0NCV3ZZ Extirpation of Matter from Left Mandib... Percutaneous Approach

0NCV4ZZ Extirpation of Matter from Left Mandib... Percutaneous Endoscopic Approach

0NCX0ZZ Extirpation of Matter from Hyoid Bone, Open Approach

0NCX3ZZ Extirpation of Matter from Hyoid Bone, Percutaneous Approach

0NCX4ZZ Extirpation of Matter from Hyoid Bone, Percutaneous Endoscopic Approach

0NH – Head and Facial Bones, Insertion

0NH004Z Insertion of Internal Fixation Device into Skull, Open Approach

0NH005Z Insertion of External Fixation Device into Skull, Open Approach

0NH00MZ Insertion of Bone Growth Stimulator into Skull, Open Approach

0NH00NZ Insertion of Neurostimulator Generator into Skull, Open Approach

➕ Major brain device implant when reported with an Insertion of a neurostimulator lead (6th character M) into the brain or cerebral ventricle. See table 00H to construct the Insertion code.

0NH034Z Insertion of Internal Fixation Device into Skull, Percutaneous Approach

0NH035Z Insertion of External Fixation Device into Skull, Percutaneous Approach

0NH03MZ Insertion of Bone Growth Stimulator into Skull, Percutaneous Approach

0NH044Z Insertion of Internal Fixation Device into Skull, Percutaneous Endoscopic Approach

0NH045Z Insertion of External Fixation Device into Skull, Percutaneous Endoscopic Approach

0NH04MZ Insertion of Bone Growth Stimulator into Skull, Percutaneous Endoscopic Approach

0NH104Z Insertion of Internal Fixation Device into Right Frontal Bone, Open Approach

0NH134Z Insertion of Internal Fixation Device into Right Frontal Bone, Percutaneous Approach

0NH144Z Insertion of Internal Fixation Device into Right Frontal Bone, Percutaneous Endoscopic Approach

0NH204Z Insertion of Internal Fixation Device into Left Frontal Bone, Open Approach

0NH234Z Insertion of Internal Fixation Device into Left Frontal Bone, Percutaneous Approach

0NH244Z Insertion of Internal Fixation Device into Left Frontal Bone, Percutaneous Endoscopic Approach

0NH304Z Insertion of Internal Fixation Device into Right Parietal Bone, Open Approach

0NH334Z Insertion of Internal Fixation Device into Right Parietal Bone, Percutaneous Approach

0NH344Z Insertion of Internal Fixation Device into Right Parietal Bone, Percutaneous Endoscopic Approach

0NH404Z Insertion of Internal Fixation Device into Left Parietal Bone, Open Approach

0NH434Z Insertion of Internal Fixation Device into Left Parietal Bone, Percutaneous Approach

♀ Female-only   ♂ Male-only   ▲ Limited Coverage   ● Non-OR   ▨ HAC-associated procedure   ▲ Non-covered procedures   ➕ Combinatio...

0NH444Z Insertion of Internal Fixation Device into Left Parietal Bone, Percutaneous Endoscopic Approach
0NH504Z Insertion of Internal Fixation Device into Right Temporal Bone, Open Approach
0NH50SZ Insertion of Hearing Device into Right Temporal Bone, Open Approach
0NH534Z Insertion of Internal Fixation Device into Right Temporal Bone, Percutaneous Approach
0NH53SZ Insertion of Hearing Device into Right Temporal Bone, Percutaneous Approach
0NH544Z Insertion of Internal Fixation Device into Right Temporal Bone, Percutaneous Endoscopic Approach
0NH54SZ Insertion of Hearing Device into Right Temporal Bone, Percutaneous Endoscopic Approach
0NH604Z Insertion of Internal Fixation Device into Left Temporal Bone, Open Approach
0NH60SZ Insertion of Hearing Device into Left Temporal Bone, Open Approach
0NH634Z Insertion of Internal Fixation Device into Left Temporal Bone, Percutaneous Approach
0NH63SZ Insertion of Hearing Device into Left Temporal Bone, Percutaneous Approach
0NH644Z Insertion of Internal Fixation Device into Left Temporal Bone, Percutaneous Endoscopic Approach
0NH64SZ Insertion of Hearing Device into Left Temporal Bone, Percutaneous Endoscopic Approach
0NH704Z Insertion of Internal Fixation Device into Right Occipital Bone, Open Approach
0NH734Z Insertion of Internal Fixation Device into Right Occipital Bone, Percutaneous Approach
0NH744Z Insertion of Internal Fixation Device into Right Occipital Bone, Percutaneous Endoscopic Approach
0NH804Z Insertion of Internal Fixation Device into Left Occipital Bone, Open Approach
0NH834Z Insertion of Internal Fixation Device into Left Occipital Bone, Percutaneous Approach
0NH844Z Insertion of Internal Fixation Device into Left Occipital Bone, Percutaneous Endoscopic Approach
0NHB04Z Insertion of Internal Fixation Device into Nasal Bone, Open Approach
0NHB0MZ Insertion of Bone Growth Stimulator into Nasal Bone, Open Approach
0NHB34Z Insertion of Internal Fixation Device into Nasal Bone, Percutaneous Approach
0NHB3MZ Insertion of Bone Growth Stimulator into Nasal Bone, Percutaneous Approach
0NHB44Z Insertion of Internal Fixation Device into Nasal Bone, Percutaneous Endoscopic Approach
0NHB4MZ Insertion of Bone Growth Stimulator into Nasal Bone, Percutaneous Endoscopic Approach
0NHC04Z Insertion of Internal Fixation Device into Right Sphenoid Bone, Open Approach
0NHC34Z Insertion of Internal Fixation Device into Right Sphenoid Bone, Percutaneous Approach
0NHC44Z Insertion of Internal Fixation Device into Right Sphenoid Bone, Percutaneous Endoscopic Approach
0NHD04Z Insertion of Internal Fixation Device into Left Sphenoid Bone, Open Approach
0NHD34Z Insertion of Internal Fixation Device into Left Sphenoid Bone, Percutaneous Approach

0NHD44Z Insertion of Internal Fixation Device into Left Sphenoid Bone, Percutaneous Endoscopic Approach
0NHF04Z Insertion of Internal Fixation Device into Right Ethmoid Bone, Open Approach
0NHF34Z Insertion of Internal Fixation Device into Right Ethmoid Bone, Percutaneous Approach
0NHF44Z Insertion of Internal Fixation Device into Right Ethmoid Bone, Percutaneous Endoscopic Approach
0NHG04Z Insertion of Internal Fixation Device into Left Ethmoid Bone, Open Approach
0NHG34Z Insertion of Internal Fixation Device into Left Ethmoid Bone, Percutaneous Approach
0NHG44Z Insertion of Internal Fixation Device into Left Ethmoid Bone, Percutaneous Endoscopic Approach
0NHH04Z Insertion of Internal Fixation Device into Right Lacrimal Bone, Open Approach
0NHH34Z Insertion of Internal Fixation Device into Right Lacrimal Bone, Percutaneous Approach
0NHH44Z Insertion of Internal Fixation Device into Right Lacrimal Bone, Percutaneous Endoscopic Approach
0NHJ04Z Insertion of Internal Fixation Device into Left Lacrimal Bone, Open Approach
0NHJ34Z Insertion of Internal Fixation Device into Left Lacrimal Bone, Percutaneous Approach
0NHJ44Z Insertion of Internal Fixation Device into Left Lacrimal Bone, Percutaneous Endoscopic Approach
0NHK04Z Insertion of Internal Fixation Device into Right Palatine Bone, Open Approach
0NHK34Z Insertion of Internal Fixation Device into Right Palatine Bone, Percutaneous Approach
0NHK44Z Insertion of Internal Fixation Device into Right Palatine Bone, Percutaneous Endoscopic Approach
0NHL04Z Insertion of Internal Fixation Device into Left Palatine Bone, Open Approach
0NHL34Z Insertion of Internal Fixation Device into Left Palatine Bone, Percutaneous Approach
0NHL44Z Insertion of Internal Fixation Device into Left Palatine Bone, Percutaneous Endoscopic Approach
0NHM04Z Insertion of Internal Fixation Device into Right Zygomatic Bone, Open Approach
0NHM34Z Insertion of Internal Fixation Device into Right Zygomatic Bone, Percutaneous Approach
0NHM44Z Insertion of Internal Fixation Device into Right Zygomatic Bone, Percutaneous Endoscopic Approach
0NHN04Z Insertion of Internal Fixation Device into Left Zygomatic Bone, Open Approach
0NHN34Z Insertion of Internal Fixation Device into Left Zygomatic Bone, Percutaneous Approach
0NHN44Z Insertion of Internal Fixation Device into Left Zygomatic Bone, Percutaneous Endoscopic Approach
0NHP04Z Insertion of Internal Fixation Device into Right Orbit, Open Approach
0NHP34Z Insertion of Internal Fixation Device into Right Orbit, Percutaneous Approach
0NHP44Z Insertion of Internal Fixation Device into Right Orbit, Percutaneous Endoscopic Approach
0NHQ04Z Insertion of Internal Fixation Device into Left Orbit, Open Approach

0NHQ34Z Insertion of Internal Fixation Device into Left Orbit, Percutaneous Approach
0NHQ44Z Insertion of Internal Fixation Device into Left Orbit, Percutaneous Endoscopic Approach
0NHR04Z Insertion of Internal Fixation Device into Right Maxilla, Open Approach
0NHR05Z Insertion of External Fixation Device into Right Maxilla, Open Approach
0NHR34Z Insertion of Internal Fixation Device into Right Maxilla, Percutaneous Approach
0NHR35Z Insertion of External Fixation Device into Right Maxilla, Percutaneous Approach
0NHR44Z Insertion of Internal Fixation Device into Right Maxilla, Percutaneous Endoscopic Approach
0NHR45Z Insertion of External Fixation Device into Right Maxilla, Percutaneous Endoscopic Approach
0NHS04Z Insertion of Internal Fixation Device into Left Maxilla, Open Approach
0NHS05Z Insertion of External Fixation Device into Left Maxilla, Open Approach
0NHS34Z Insertion of Internal Fixation Device into Left Maxilla, Percutaneous Approach
0NHS35Z Insertion of External Fixation Device into Left Maxilla, Percutaneous Approach
0NHS44Z Insertion of Internal Fixation Device into Left Maxilla, Percutaneous Endoscopic Approach
0NHS45Z Insertion of External Fixation Device into Left Maxilla, Percutaneous Endoscopic Approach
0NHT04Z Insertion of Internal Fixation Device into Right Mandible, Open Approach
0NHT05Z Insertion of External Fixation Device into Right Mandible, Open Approach
0NHT34Z Insertion of Internal Fixation Device into Right Mandible, Percutaneous Approach
0NHT35Z Insertion of External Fixation Device into Right Mandible, Percutaneous Approach
0NHT44Z Insertion of Internal Fixation Device into Right Mandible, Percutaneous Endoscopic Approach
0NHT45Z Insertion of External Fixation Device into Right Mandible, Percutaneous Endoscopic Approach
0NHV04Z Insertion of Internal Fixation Device into Left Mandible, Open Approach
0NHV05Z Insertion of External Fixation Device into Left Mandible, Open Approach
0NHV34Z Insertion of Internal Fixation Device into Left Mandible, Percutaneous Approach
0NHV35Z Insertion of External Fixation Device into Left Mandible, Percutaneous Approach
0NHV44Z Insertion of Internal Fixation Device into Left Mandible, Percutaneous Endoscopic Approach
0NHV45Z Insertion of External Fixation Device into Left Mandible, Percutaneous Endoscopic Approach
0NHW0MZ Insertion of Bone Growth Stimulator into Facial Bone, Open Approach
0NHW3MZ Insertion of Bone Growth Stimulator into Facial Bone, Percutaneous Approach
0NHW4MZ Insertion of Bone Growth Stimulator into Facial Bone, Percutaneous Endoscopic Approach
0NHX04Z Insertion of Internal Fixation Device into Hyoid Bone, Open Approach
0NHX34Z Insertion of Internal Fixation Device into Hyoid Bone, Percutaneous Approach
0NHX44Z Insertion of Internal Fixation Device into Hyoid Bone, Percutaneous Endoscopic Approach

♀ Female-only   ♂ Male-only   ▲ Limited Coverage   ● Non-OR   ▤ HAC-associated procedure   ▲ Non-covered procedures   + Combination

0NJ – Head and Facial Bones, Inspection

Review Coding Guideline B3.5

Review Coding Guidelines B3.11a, B3.11b and B3.11c

0NJ00ZZ Inspection of Skull, Open Approach
0NJ03ZZ Inspection of Skull, Percutaneous Approach
0NJ04ZZ Inspection of Skull, Percutaneous Endoscopic Approach
0NJ0XZZ Inspection of Skull, External Approach
0NJB0ZZ Inspection of Nasal Bone, Open Approach

0NJB3ZZ Inspection of Nasal Bone, Percutaneous Approach
0NJB4ZZ Inspection of Nasal Bone, Percutaneous Endoscopic Approach
0NJBXZZ Inspection of Nasal Bone, External Approach
0NJW0ZZ Inspection of Facial Bone, Open Approach

0NJW3ZZ Inspection of Facial Bone, Percutaneous Approach
0NJW4ZZ Inspection of Facial Bone, Percutaneous Endoscopic Approach
0NJWXZZ Inspection of Facial Bone, External Approach

0NN – Head and Facial Bones, Release

Review Coding Guideline B3.13

Review Coding Guideline B3.14

0NN10ZZ Release Right Frontal Bone, Open Approach
0NN13ZZ Release Right Frontal Bone, Percutaneous Approach
0NN14ZZ Release Right Frontal Bone, Percutaneous Endoscopic Approach
0NN20ZZ Release Left Frontal Bone, Open Approach
0NN23ZZ Release Left Frontal Bone, Percutaneous Approach
0NN24ZZ Release Left Frontal Bone, Percutaneous Endoscopic Approach
0NN30ZZ Release Right Parietal Bone, Open Approach
0NN33ZZ Release Right Parietal Bone, Percutaneous Approach
0NN34ZZ Release Right Parietal Bone, Percutaneous Endoscopic Approach
0NN40ZZ Release Left Parietal Bone, Open Approach
0NN43ZZ Release Left Parietal Bone, Percutaneous Approach
0NN44ZZ Release Left Parietal Bone, Percutaneous Endoscopic Approach
0NN50ZZ Release Right Temporal Bone, Open Approach
0NN53ZZ Release Right Temporal Bone, Percutaneous Approach
0NN54ZZ Release Right Temporal Bone, Percutaneous Endoscopic Approach
0NN60ZZ Release Left Temporal Bone, Open Approach
0NN63ZZ Release Left Temporal Bone, Percutaneous Approach
0NN64ZZ Release Left Temporal Bone, Percutaneous Endoscopic Approach
0NN70ZZ Release Right Occipital Bone, Open Approach
0NN73ZZ Release Right Occipital Bone, Percutaneous Approach
0NN74ZZ Release Right Occipital Bone, Percutaneous Endoscopic Approach
0NN80ZZ Release Left Occipital Bone, Open Approach
0NN83ZZ Release Left Occipital Bone, Percutaneous Approach
0NN84ZZ Release Left Occipital Bone, Percutaneous Endoscopic Approach
0NNB0ZZ Release Nasal Bone, Open Approach
0NNB3ZZ Release Nasal Bone, Percutaneous Approach

0NNB4ZZ Release Nasal Bone, Percutaneous Endoscopic Approach
0NNC0ZZ Release Right Sphenoid Bone, Open Approach
0NNC3ZZ Release Right Sphenoid Bone, Percutaneous Approach
0NNC4ZZ Release Right Sphenoid Bone, Percutaneous Endoscopic Approach
0NND0ZZ Release Left Sphenoid Bone, Open Approach
0NND3ZZ Release Left Sphenoid Bone, Percutaneous Approach
0NND4ZZ Release Left Sphenoid Bone, Percutaneous Endoscopic Approach
0NNF0ZZ Release Right Ethmoid Bone, Open Approach
0NNF3ZZ Release Right Ethmoid Bone, Percutaneous Approach
0NNF4ZZ Release Right Ethmoid Bone, Percutaneous Endoscopic Approach
0NNG0ZZ Release Left Ethmoid Bone, Open Approach
0NNG3ZZ Release Left Ethmoid Bone, Percutaneous Approach
0NNG4ZZ Release Left Ethmoid Bone, Percutaneous Endoscopic Approach
0NNH0ZZ Release Right Lacrimal Bone, Open Approach
0NNH3ZZ Release Right Lacrimal Bone, Percutaneous Approach
0NNH4ZZ Release Right Lacrimal Bone, Percutaneous Endoscopic Approach
0NNJ0ZZ Release Left Lacrimal Bone, Open Approach
0NNJ3ZZ Release Left Lacrimal Bone, Percutaneous Approach
0NNJ4ZZ Release Left Lacrimal Bone, Percutaneous Endoscopic Approach
0NNK0ZZ Release Right Palatine Bone, Open Approach
0NNK3ZZ Release Right Palatine Bone, Percutaneous Approach
0NNK4ZZ Release Right Palatine Bone, Percutaneous Endoscopic Approach
0NNL0ZZ Release Left Palatine Bone, Open Approach
0NNL3ZZ Release Left Palatine Bone, Percutaneous Approach

0NNL4ZZ Release Left Palatine Bone, Percutaneous Endoscopic Approach
0NNM0ZZ Release Right Zygomatic Bone, Open Approach
0NNM3ZZ Release Right Zygomatic Bone, Percutaneous Approach
0NNM4ZZ Release Right Zygomatic Bone, Percutaneous Endoscopic Approach
0NNN0ZZ Release Left Zygomatic Bone, Open Approach
0NNN3ZZ Release Left Zygomatic Bone, Percutaneous Approach
0NNN4ZZ Release Left Zygomatic Bone, Percutaneous Endoscopic Approach
0NNP0ZZ Release Right Orbit, Open Approach
0NNP3ZZ Release Right Orbit, Percutaneous Approach
0NNP4ZZ Release Right Orbit, Percutaneous Endoscopic Approach
0NNQ0ZZ Release Left Orbit, Open Approach
0NNQ3ZZ Release Left Orbit, Percutaneous Approach
0NNQ4ZZ Release Left Orbit, Percutaneous Endoscopic Approach
0NNR0ZZ Release Right Maxilla, Open Approach
0NNR3ZZ Release Right Maxilla, Percutaneous Approach
0NNR4ZZ Release Right Maxilla, Percutaneous Endoscopic Approach
0NNS0ZZ Release Left Maxilla, Open Approach
0NNS3ZZ Release Left Maxilla, Percutaneous Approach
0NNS4ZZ Release Left Maxilla, Percutaneous Endoscopic Approach
0NNT0ZZ Release Right Mandible, Open Approach
0NNT3ZZ Release Right Mandible, Percutaneous Approach
0NNT4ZZ Release Right Mandible, Percutaneous Endoscopic Approach
0NNV0ZZ Release Left Mandible, Open Approach
0NNV3ZZ Release Left Mandible, Percutaneous Approach
0NNV4ZZ Release Left Mandible, Percutaneous Endoscopic Approach
0NNX0ZZ Release Hyoid Bone, Open Approach
0NNX3ZZ Release Hyoid Bone, Percutaneous Approach
0NNX4ZZ Release Hyoid Bone, Percutaneous Endoscopic Approach

0NP – Head and Facial Bones, Removal

Review Coding Guideline B6.1c

0NP000Z Removal of Drainage Device from Skull, Open Approach

0NP004Z Removal of Internal Fixation Device from Skull, Open Approach

0NP005Z Removal of External Fixation Device from Skull, Open Approach

♀ Female-only   ♂ Male-only   ▲ Limited Coverage   ● Non-OR   ▧ HAC-associated procedure   ▲ Non-covered procedures   ✚ Combinatio

Code	Description	Code	Description	Code	Description
007Z	Removal of Autologous Tissue Substitute from Skull, Open Approach	0NP0X4Z	Removal of Internal Fixation Device from Skull, External Approach	0NPBXMZ	Removal of Bone Growth Stimulator from Nasal Bone, External Approach
00JZ	Removal of Synthetic Substitute from Skull, Open Approach	0NP0X5Z	Removal of External Fixation Device from Skull, External Approach	0NPW00Z	Removal of Drainage Device from Facial Bone, Open Approach
00KZ	Removal of Nonautologous Tissue Substitute from Skull, Open Approach	0NP0XMZ	Removal of Bone Growth Stimulator from Skull, External Approach	0NPW04Z	Removal of Internal Fixation Device from Facial Bone, Open Approach
00MZ	Removal of Bone Growth Stimulator from Skull, Open Approach	0NP0XSZ	Removal of Hearing Device from Skull, External Approach	0NPW07Z	Removal of Autologous Tissue Substitute from Facial Bone, Open Approach
00NZ	Removal of Neurostimulator Generator from Skull, Open Approach	0NPB00Z	Removal of Drainage Device from Nasal Bone, Open Approach	0NPW0JZ	Removal of Synthetic Substitute from Facial Bone, Open Approach
00SZ	Removal of Hearing Device from Skull, Open Approach	0NPB04Z	Removal of Internal Fixation Device from Nasal Bone, Open Approach	0NPW0KZ	Removal of Nonautologous Tissue Substitute from Facial Bone, Open Approach
030Z	Removal of Drainage Device from Skull, Percutaneous Approach	0NPB07Z	Removal of Autologous Tissue Substitute from Nasal Bone, Open Approach	0NPW0MZ	Removal of Bone Growth Stimulator from Facial Bone, Open Approach
034Z	Removal of Internal Fixation Device from Skull, Percutaneous Approach	0NPB0JZ	Removal of Synthetic Substitute from Nasal Bone, Open Approach	0NPW30Z	Removal of Drainage Device from Facial Bone, Percutaneous Approach
035Z	Removal of External Fixation Device from Skull, Percutaneous Approach	0NPB0KZ	Removal of Nonautologous Tissue Substitute from Nasal Bone, Open Approach	0NPW34Z	Removal of Internal Fixation Device from Facial Bone, Percutaneous Approach
037Z	Removal of Autologous Tissue Substitute from Skull, Percutaneous Approach	0NPB0MZ	Removal of Bone Growth Stimulator from Nasal Bone, Open Approach	0NPW37Z	Removal of Autologous Tissue Substitute from Facial Bone, Percutaneous Approach
03JZ	Removal of Synthetic Substitute from Skull, Percutaneous Approach	0NPB30Z	Removal of Drainage Device from Nasal Bone, Percutaneous Approach	0NPW3JZ	Removal of Synthetic Substitute from Facial Bone, Percutaneous Approach
03KZ	Removal of Nonautologous Tissue Substitute from Skull, Percutaneous Approach	0NPB34Z	Removal of Internal Fixation Device from Nasal Bone, Percutaneous Approach	0NPW3KZ	Removal of Nonautologous Tissue Substitute from Facial Bone, Percutaneous Approach
03MZ	Removal of Bone Growth Stimulator from Skull, Percutaneous Approach	0NPB37Z	Removal of Autologous Tissue Substitute from Nasal Bone, Percutaneous Approach	0NPW3MZ	Removal of Bone Growth Stimulator from Facial Bone, Percutaneous Approach
P03SZ	Removal of Hearing Device from Skull, Percutaneous Approach	0NPB3JZ	Removal of Synthetic Substitute from Nasal Bone, Percutaneous Approach		
P040Z	Removal of Drainage Device from Skull, Percutaneous Endoscopic Approach	0NPB3KZ	Removal of Nonautologous Tissue Substitute from Nasal Bone, Percutaneous Approach	0NPW40Z	Removal of Drainage Device from Facial Bone, Percutaneous Endoscopic Approach
P044Z	Removal of Internal Fixation Device from Skull, Percutaneous Endoscopic Approach	0NPB3MZ	Removal of Bone Growth Stimulator from Nasal Bone, Percutaneous Approach	0NPW44Z	Removal of Internal Fixation Device from Facial Bone, Percutaneous Endoscopic Approach
P045Z	Removal of External Fixation Device from Skull, Percutaneous Endoscopic Approach	0NPB40Z	Removal of Drainage Device from Nasal Bone, Percutaneous Endoscopic Approach	0NPW47Z	Removal of Autologous Tissue Substitute from Facial Bone, Percutaneous Endoscopic Approach
P047Z	Removal of Autologous Tissue Substitute from Skull, Percutaneous Endoscopic Approach	0NPB44Z	Removal of Internal Fixation Device from Nasal Bone, Percutaneous Endoscopic Approach	0NPW4JZ	Removal of Synthetic Substitute from Facial Bone, Percutaneous Endoscopic Approach
P04JZ	Removal of Synthetic Substitute from Skull, Percutaneous Endoscopic Approach	0NPB47Z	Removal of Autologous Tissue Substitute from Nasal Bone, Percutaneous Endoscopic Approach	0NPW4KZ	Removal of Nonautologous Tissue Substitute from Facial Bone, Percutaneous Endoscopic Approach
P04KZ	Removal of Nonautologous Tissue Substitute from Skull, Percutaneous Endoscopic Approach	0NPB4JZ	Removal of Synthetic Substitute from Nasal Bone, Percutaneous Endoscopic Approach	0NPW4MZ	Removal of Bone Growth Stimulator from Facial Bone, Percutaneous Endoscopic Approach
P04MZ	Removal of Bone Growth Stimulator from Skull, Percutaneous Endoscopic Approach	0NPB4KZ	Removal of Nonautologous Tissue Substitute from Nasal Bone, Percutaneous Endoscopic Approach	0NPWX0Z	Removal of Drainage Device from Facial Bone, External Approach
P04SZ	Removal of Hearing Device from Skull, Percutaneous Endoscopic Approach	0NPB4MZ	Removal of Bone Growth Stimulator from Nasal Bone, Percutaneous Endoscopic Approach	0NPWX4Z	Removal of Internal Fixation Device from Facial Bone, External Approach
P0X0Z	Removal of Drainage Device from Skull, External Approach	0NPBX0Z	Removal of Drainage Device from Nasal Bone, External Approach	0NPWXMZ	Removal of Bone Growth Stimulator from Facial Bone, External Approach
		0NPBX4Z	Removal of Internal Fixation Device from Nasal Bone, External Approach		

0NQ – Head and Facial Bones, Repair

Review Coding Guideline B3.5

Code	Description	Code	Description	Code	Description
0NQ00ZZ	Repair Skull, Open Approach	0NQ24ZZ	Repair Left Frontal Bone, Percutaneous Endoscopic Approach	0NQ44ZZ	Repair Left Parietal Bone, Percutaneous Endoscopic Approach
0NQ03ZZ	Repair Skull, Percutaneous Approach	0NQ2XZZ	Repair Left Frontal Bone, External Approach	0NQ4XZZ	Repair Left Parietal Bone, External Approach
0NQ04ZZ	Repair Skull, Percutaneous Endoscopic Approach	0NQ30ZZ	Repair Right Parietal Bone, Open Approach	0NQ50ZZ	Repair Right Temporal Bone, Open Approach
0NQ0XZZ	Repair Skull, External Approach	0NQ33ZZ	Repair Right Parietal Bone, Percutaneous Approach	0NQ53ZZ	Repair Right Temporal Bone, Percutaneous Approach
0NQ10ZZ	Repair Right Frontal Bone, Open Approach	0NQ34ZZ	Repair Right Parietal Bone, Percutaneous Endoscopic Approach	0NQ54ZZ	Repair Right Temporal Bone, Percutaneous Endoscopic Approach
0NQ13ZZ	Repair Right Frontal Bone, Percutaneous Approach	0NQ3XZZ	Repair Right Parietal Bone, External Approach		
0NQ14ZZ	Repair Right Frontal Bone, Percutaneous Endoscopic Approach	0NQ40ZZ	Repair Left Parietal Bone, Open Approach	0NQ5XZZ	Repair Right Temporal Bone, External Approach
0NQ1XZZ	Repair Right Frontal Bone, External Approach	0NQ43ZZ	Repair Left Parietal Bone, Percutaneous Approach	0NQ60ZZ	Repair Left Temporal Bone, Open Approach
0NQ20ZZ	Repair Left Frontal Bone, Open Approach				
0NQ23ZZ	Repair Left Frontal Bone, Percutaneous Approach				

♀ Female-only	♂ Male-only	▲ Limited Coverage	● Non-OR	■ HAC-associated procedure	▲ Non-covered procedures	✚ Combination

0NQ63ZZ   Repair Left Temporal Bone, Percutaneous Approach

0NQ64ZZ   Repair Left Temporal Bone, Percutaneous Endoscopic Approach

0NQ6XZZ   Repair Left Temporal Bone, External Approach

0NQ70ZZ   Repair Right Occipital Bone, Open Approach

0NQ73ZZ   Repair Right Occipital Bone, Percutaneous Approach

0NQ74ZZ   Repair Right Occipital Bone, Percutaneous Endoscopic Approach

0NQ7XZZ   Repair Right Occipital Bone, External Approach

0NQ80ZZ   Repair Left Occipital Bone, Open Approach

0NQ83ZZ   Repair Left Occipital Bone, Percutaneous Approach

0NQ84ZZ   Repair Left Occipital Bone, Percutaneous Endoscopic Approach

0NQ8XZZ   Repair Left Occipital Bone, External Approach

0NQB0ZZ   Repair Nasal Bone, Open Approach

0NQB3ZZ   Repair Nasal Bone, Percutaneous Approach

0NQB4ZZ   Repair Nasal Bone, Percutaneous Endoscopic Approach

0NQBXZZ   Repair Nasal Bone, External Approach

0NQC0ZZ   Repair Right Sphenoid Bone, Open Approach

0NQC3ZZ   Repair Right Sphenoid Bone, Percutaneous Approach

0NQC4ZZ   Repair Right Sphenoid Bone, Percutaneous Endoscopic Approach

0NQCXZZ   Repair Right Sphenoid Bone, External Approach

0NQD0ZZ   Repair Left Sphenoid Bone, Open Approach

0NQD3ZZ   Repair Left Sphenoid Bone, Percutaneous Approach

0NQD4ZZ   Repair Left Sphenoid Bone, Percutaneous Endoscopic Approach

0NQDXZZ   Repair Left Sphenoid Bone, External Approach

0NQF0ZZ   Repair Right Ethmoid Bone, Open Approach

0NQF3ZZ   Repair Right Ethmoid Bone, Percutaneous Approach

0NQF4ZZ   Repair Right Ethmoid Bone, Percutaneous Endoscopic Approach

0NQFXZZ   Repair Right Ethmoid Bone, External Approach

0NQG0ZZ   Repair Left Ethmoid Bone, Open Approach

0NQG3ZZ   Repair Left Ethmoid Bone, Percutaneous Approach

0NQG4ZZ   Repair Left Ethmoid Bone, Percutaneous Endoscopic Approach

0NQGXZZ   Repair Left Ethmoid Bone, External Approach

0NQH0ZZ   Repair Right Lacrimal Bone, Open Approach

0NQH3ZZ   Repair Right Lacrimal Bone, Percutaneous Approach

0NQH4ZZ   Repair Right Lacrimal Bone, Percutaneous Endoscopic Approach

0NQHXZZ   Repair Right Lacrimal Bone, External Approach

0NQJ0ZZ   Repair Left Lacrimal Bone, Open Approach

0NQJ3ZZ   Repair Left Lacrimal Bone, Percutaneous Approach

0NQJ4ZZ   Repair Left Lacrimal Bone, Percutaneous Endoscopic Approach

0NQJXZZ   Repair Left Lacrimal Bone, External Approach

0NQK0ZZ   Repair Right Palatine Bone, Open Approach

0NQK3ZZ   Repair Right Palatine Bone, Percutaneous Approach

0NQK4ZZ   Repair Right Palatine Bone, Percutaneous Endoscopic Approach

0NQKXZZ   Repair Right Palatine Bone, External Approach

0NQL0ZZ   Repair Left Palatine Bone, Open Approach

0NQL3ZZ   Repair Left Palatine Bone, Percutaneous Approach

0NQL4ZZ   Repair Left Palatine Bone, Percutaneous Endoscopic Approach

0NQLXZZ   Repair Left Palatine Bone, External Approach

0NQM0ZZ   Repair Right Zygomatic Bone, Open Approach

0NQM3ZZ   Repair Right Zygomatic Bone, Percutaneous Approach

0NQM4ZZ   Repair Right Zygomatic Bone, Percutaneous Endoscopic Approach

0NQMXZZ   Repair Right Zygomatic Bone, External Approach

0NQN0ZZ   Repair Left Zygomatic Bone, Open Approach

0NQN3ZZ   Repair Left Zygomatic Bone, Percutaneous Approach

0NQN4ZZ   Repair Left Zygomatic Bone, Percutaneous Endoscopic Approach

0NQNXZZ   Repair Left Zygomatic Bone, External Approach

0NQP0ZZ   Repair Right Orbit, Open Approach

0NQP3ZZ   Repair Right Orbit, Percutaneous Approach

0NQP4ZZ   Repair Right Orbit, Percutaneous Endoscopic Approach

0NQPXZZ   Repair Right Orbit, External Approach

0NQQ0ZZ   Repair Left Orbit, Open Approach

0NQQ3ZZ   Repair Left Orbit, Percutaneous Approach

0NQQ4ZZ   Repair Left Orbit, Percutaneous Endoscopic Approach

0NQQXZZ   Repair Left Orbit, External Approach

0NQR0ZZ   Repair Right Maxilla, Open Approach

0NQR3ZZ   Repair Right Maxilla, Percutaneous Approach

0NQR4ZZ   Repair Right Maxilla, Percutaneous Endoscopic Approach

0NQRXZZ   Repair Right Maxilla, External Approach

0NQS0ZZ   Repair Left Maxilla, Open Approach

0NQS3ZZ   Repair Left Maxilla, Percutaneous Approach

0NQS4ZZ   Repair Left Maxilla, Percutaneous Endoscopic Approach

0NQSXZZ   Repair Left Maxilla, External Approach

0NQT0ZZ   Repair Right Mandible, Open Approach

0NQT3ZZ   Repair Right Mandible, Percutaneous Approach

0NQT4ZZ   Repair Right Mandible, Percutaneous Endoscopic Approach

0NQTXZZ   Repair Right Mandible, External Approach

0NQV0ZZ   Repair Left Mandible, Open Approach

0NQV3ZZ   Repair Left Mandible, Percutaneous Approach

0NQV4ZZ   Repair Left Mandible, Percutaneous Endoscopic Approach

0NQVXZZ   Repair Left Mandible, External Approach

0NQX0ZZ   Repair Hyoid Bone, Open Approach

0NQX3ZZ   Repair Hyoid Bone, Percutaneous Approach

0NQX4ZZ   Repair Hyoid Bone, Percutaneous Endoscopic Approach

0NQXXZZ   Repair Hyoid Bone, External Approach

0NR – Head and Facial Bones, Replacement

0NR007Z   Replacement of Skull with Autologous Tissue Substitute, Open Approach

0NR00JZ   Replacement of Skull with Synthetic Substitute, Open Approach

AHA CC: 3Q, 2014, 7-8

0NR00KZ   Replacement of Skull with Nonautologous Tissue Substitute, Open Approach

0NR037Z   Replacement of Skull with Autologous Tissue Substitute, Percutaneous Approach

0NR03JZ   Replacement of Skull with Synthetic Substitute, Percutaneous Approach

0NR03KZ   Replacement of Skull with Nonautologous Tissue Substitute, Percutaneous Approach

0NR047Z   Replacement of Skull with Autologous Tissue Substitute, Percutaneous Endoscopic Approach

0NR04JZ   Replacement of Skull with Synthetic Substitute, Percutaneous Endoscopic Approach

0NR04KZ   Replacement of Skull with Nonautologous Tissue Substitute, Percutaneous Endoscopic Approach

0NR107Z   Replacement of Right Frontal Bone with Autologous Tissue Substitute, Open Approach

0NR10JZ   Replacement of Right Frontal Bone with Synthetic Substitute, Open Approach

0NR10KZ   Replacement of Right Frontal Bone with Nonautologous Tissue Substitute, Open Approach

0NR137Z   Replacement of Right Frontal Bone with Autologous Tissue Substitute, Percutaneous Approach

0NR13JZ   Replacement of Right Frontal Bone with Synthetic Substitute, Percutaneous Approach

0NR13KZ   Replacement of Right Frontal Bone with Nonautologous Tissue Substitute, Percutaneous Approach

0NR147Z   Replacement of Right Frontal Bone with Autologous Tissue Substitute, Percutaneous Endoscopic Approach

0NR14JZ   Replacement of Right Frontal Bone with Synthetic Substitute, Percutaneous Endoscopic Approach

0NR14KZ   Replacement of Right Frontal Bone with Nonautologous Tissue Substitute, Percutaneous Endoscopic Approach

0NR207Z   Replacement of Left Frontal Bone with Autologous Tissue Substitute, Open Approach

0NR20JZ   Replacement of Left Frontal Bone with Synthetic Substitute, Open Approach

0NR20KZ   Replacement of Left Frontal Bone with Nonautologous Tissue Substitute, Open Approach

0NR237Z   Replacement of Left Frontal Bone with Autologous Tissue Substitute, Percutaneous Approach

0NR23JZ   Replacement of Left Frontal Bone with Synthetic Substitute, Percutaneous Approach

0NR23KZ   Replacement of Left Frontal Bone with Nonautologous Tissue Substitute, Percutaneous Approach

0NR247Z   Replacement of Left Frontal Bone with Autologous Tissue Substitute, Percutaneous Endoscopic Approach

0NR24JZ	Replacement of Left Frontal Bone with Synthetic Substitute, Percutaneous Endoscopic Approach
0NR24KZ	Replacement of Left Frontal Bone with Nonautologous Tissue Substitute, Percutaneous Endoscopic Approach
0NR307Z	Replacement of Right Parietal Bone with Autologous Tissue Substitute, Open Approach
0NR30JZ	Replacement of Right Parietal Bone with Synthetic Substitute, Open Approach
0NR30KZ	Replacement of Right Parietal Bone with Nonautologous Tissue Substitute, Open Approach
0NR337Z	Replacement of Right Parietal Bone with Autologous Tissue Substitute, Percutaneous Approach
0NR33JZ	Replacement of Right Parietal Bone with Synthetic Substitute, Percutaneous Approach
0NR33KZ	Replacement of Right Parietal Bone with Nonautologous Tissue Substitute, Percutaneous Approach
0NR347Z	Replacement of Right Parietal Bone with Autologous Tissue Substitute, Percutaneous Endoscopic Approach
0NR34JZ	Replacement of Right Parietal Bone with Synthetic Substitute, Percutaneous Endoscopic Approach
0NR34KZ	Replacement of Right Parietal Bone with Nonautologous Tissue Substitute, Percutaneous Endoscopic Approach
0NR407Z	Replacement of Left Parietal Bone with Autologous Tissue Substitute, Open Approach
0NR40JZ	Replacement of Left Parietal Bone with Synthetic Substitute, Open Approach
0NR40KZ	Replacement of Left Parietal Bone with Nonautologous Tissue Substitute, Open Approach
0NR437Z	Replacement of Left Parietal Bone with Autologous Tissue Substitute, Percutaneous Approach
0NR43JZ	Replacement of Left Parietal Bone with Synthetic Substitute, Percutaneous Approach
0NR43KZ	Replacement of Left Parietal Bone with Nonautologous Tissue Substitute, Percutaneous Approach
0NR447Z	Replacement of Left Parietal Bone with Autologous Tissue Substitute, Percutaneous Endoscopic Approach
0NR44JZ	Replacement of Left Parietal Bone with Synthetic Substitute, Percutaneous Endoscopic Approach
0NR44KZ	Replacement of Left Parietal Bone with Nonautologous Tissue Substitute, Percutaneous Endoscopic Approach
0NR507Z	Replacement of Right Temporal Bone with Autologous Tissue Substitute, Open Approach
0NR50JZ	Replacement of Right Temporal Bone with Synthetic Substitute, Open Approach
0NR50KZ	Replacement of Right Temporal Bone with Nonautologous Tissue Substitute, Open Approach
0NR537Z	Replacement of Right Temporal Bone with Autologous Tissue Substitute, Percutaneous Approach
0NR53JZ	Replacement of Right Temporal Bone with Synthetic Substitute, Percutaneous Approach
0NR53KZ	Replacement of Right Temporal Bone with Nonautologous Tissue Substitute, Percutaneous Approach
0NR547Z	Replacement of Right Temporal Bone with Autologous Tissue Substitute, Percutaneous Endoscopic Approach
0NR54JZ	Replacement of Right Temporal Bone with Synthetic Substitute, Percutaneous Endoscopic Approach
0NR54KZ	Replacement of Right Temporal Bone with Nonautologous Tissue Substitute, Percutaneous Endoscopic Approach
0NR607Z	Replacement of Left Temporal Bone with Autologous Tissue Substitute, Open Approach
0NR60JZ	Replacement of Left Temporal Bone with Synthetic Substitute, Open Approach
0NR60KZ	Replacement of Left Temporal Bone with Nonautologous Tissue Substitute, Open Approach
0NR637Z	Replacement of Left Temporal Bone with Autologous Tissue Substitute, Percutaneous Approach
0NR63JZ	Replacement of Left Temporal Bone with Synthetic Substitute, Percutaneous Approach
0NR63KZ	Replacement of Left Temporal Bone with Nonautologous Tissue Substitute, Percutaneous Approach
0NR647Z	Replacement of Left Temporal Bone with Autologous Tissue Substitute, Percutaneous Endoscopic Approach
0NR64JZ	Replacement of Left Temporal Bone with Synthetic Substitute, Percutaneous Endoscopic Approach
0NR64KZ	Replacement of Left Temporal Bone with Nonautologous Tissue Substitute, Percutaneous Endoscopic Approach
0NR707Z	Replacement of Right Occipital Bone with Autologous Tissue Substitute, Open Approach
0NR70JZ	Replacement of Right Occipital Bone with Synthetic Substitute, Open Approach
0NR70KZ	Replacement of Right Occipital Bone with Nonautologous Tissue Substitute, Open Approach
0NR737Z	Replacement of Right Occipital Bone with Autologous Tissue Substitute, Percutaneous Approach
0NR73JZ	Replacement of Right Occipital Bone with Synthetic Substitute, Percutaneous Approach
0NR73KZ	Replacement of Right Occipital Bone with Nonautologous Tissue Substitute, Percutaneous Approach
0NR747Z	Replacement of Right Occipital Bone with Autologous Tissue Substitute, Percutaneous Endoscopic Approach
0NR74JZ	Replacement of Right Occipital Bone with Synthetic Substitute, Percutaneous Endoscopic Approach
0NR74KZ	Replacement of Right Occipital Bone with Nonautologous Tissue Substitute, Percutaneous Endoscopic Approach
0NR807Z	Replacement of Left Occipital Bone with Autologous Tissue Substitute, Open Approach
0NR80JZ	Replacement of Left Occipital Bone with Synthetic Substitute, Open Approach
0NR80KZ	Replacement of Left Occipital Bone with Nonautologous Tissue Substitute, Open Approach
0NR837Z	Replacement of Left Occipital Bone with Autologous Tissue Substitute, Percutaneous Approach
0NR83JZ	Replacement of Left Occipital Bone with Synthetic Substitute, Percutaneous Approach
0NR83KZ	Replacement of Left Occipital Bone with Nonautologous Tissue Substitute, Percutaneous Approach
0NR847Z	Replacement of Left Occipital Bone with Autologous Tissue Substitute, Percutaneous Endoscopic Approach
0NR84JZ	Replacement of Left Occipital Bone with Synthetic Substitute, Percutaneous Endoscopic Approach
0NR84KZ	Replacement of Left Occipital Bone with Nonautologous Tissue Substitute, Percutaneous Endoscopic Approach
0NRB07Z	Replacement of Nasal Bone with Autologous Tissue Substitute, Open Approach
0NRB0JZ	Replacement of Nasal Bone with Synthetic Substitute, Open Approach
0NRB0KZ	Replacement of Nasal Bone with Nonautologous Tissue Substitute, Open Approach
0NRB37Z	Replacement of Nasal Bone with Autologous Tissue Substitute, Percutaneous Approach
0NRB3JZ	Replacement of Nasal Bone with Synthetic Substitute, Percutaneous Approach
0NRB3KZ	Replacement of Nasal Bone with Nonautologous Tissue Substitute, Percutaneous Approach
0NRB47Z	Replacement of Nasal Bone with Autologous Tissue Substitute, Percutaneous Endoscopic Approach
0NRB4JZ	Replacement of Nasal Bone with Synthetic Substitute, Percutaneous Endoscopic Approach
0NRB4KZ	Replacement of Nasal Bone with Nonautologous Tissue Substitute, Percutaneous Endoscopic Approach
0NRC07Z	Replacement of Right Sphenoid Bone with Autologous Tissue Substitute, Open Approach
0NRC0JZ	Replacement of Right Sphenoid Bone with Synthetic Substitute, Open Approach
0NRC0KZ	Replacement of Right Sphenoid Bone with Nonautologous Tissue Substitute, Open Approach
0NRC37Z	Replacement of Right Sphenoid Bone with Autologous Tissue Substitute, Percutaneous Approach
0NRC3JZ	Replacement of Right Sphenoid Bone with Synthetic Substitute, Percutaneous Approach
0NRC3KZ	Replacement of Right Sphenoid Bone with Nonautologous Tissue Substitute, Percutaneous Approach
0NRC47Z	Replacement of Right Sphenoid Bone with Autologous Tissue Substitute, Percutaneous Endoscopic Approach
0NRC4JZ	Replacement of Right Sphenoid Bone with Synthetic Substitute, Percutaneous Endoscopic Approach
0NRC4KZ	Replacement of Right Sphenoid Bone with Nonautologous Tissue Substitute, Percutaneous Endoscopic Approach
0NRD07Z	Replacement of Left Sphenoid Bone with Autologous Tissue Substitute, Open Approach
0NRD0JZ	Replacement of Left Sphenoid Bone with Synthetic Substitute, Open Approach
0NRD0KZ	Replacement of Left Sphenoid Bone with Nonautologous Tissue Substitute, Open Approach
0NRD37Z	Replacement of Left Sphenoid Bone with Autologous Tissue Substitute, Percutaneous Approach
0NRD3JZ	Replacement of Left Sphenoid Bone with Synthetic Substitute, Percutaneous Approach
0NRD3KZ	Replacement of Left Sphenoid Bone with Nonautologous Tissue Substitute, Percutaneous Approach
0NRD47Z	Replacement of Left Sphenoid Bone with Autologous Tissue Substitute, Percutaneous Endoscopic Approach

0NRD4JZ Replacement of Left Sphenoid Bone with Synthetic Substitute, Percutaneous Endoscopic Approach

0NRD4KZ Replacement of Left Sphenoid Bone with Nonautologous Tissue Substitute, Percutaneous Endoscopic Approach

0NRF07Z Replacement of Right Ethmoid Bone with Autologous Tissue Substitute, Open Approach

0NRF0JZ Replacement of Right Ethmoid Bone with Synthetic Substitute, Open Approach

0NRF0KZ Replacement of Right Ethmoid Bone with Nonautologous Tissue Substitute, Open Approach

0NRF37Z Replacement of Right Ethmoid Bone with Autologous Tissue Substitute, Percutaneous Approach

0NRF3JZ Replacement of Right Ethmoid Bone with Synthetic Substitute, Percutaneous Approach

0NRF3KZ Replacement of Right Ethmoid Bone with Nonautologous Tissue Substitute, Percutaneous Approach

0NRF47Z Replacement of Right Ethmoid Bone with Autologous Tissue Substitute, Percutaneous Endoscopic Approach

0NRF4JZ Replacement of Right Ethmoid Bone with Synthetic Substitute, Percutaneous Endoscopic Approach

0NRF4KZ Replacement of Right Ethmoid Bone with Nonautologous Tissue Substitute, Percutaneous Endoscopic Approach

0NRG07Z Replacement of Left Ethmoid Bone with Autologous Tissue Substitute, Open Approach

0NRG0JZ Replacement of Left Ethmoid Bone with Synthetic Substitute, Open Approach

0NRG0KZ Replacement of Left Ethmoid Bone with Nonautologous Tissue Substitute, Open Approach

0NRG37Z Replacement of Left Ethmoid Bone with Autologous Tissue Substitute, Percutaneous Approach

0NRG3JZ Replacement of Left Ethmoid Bone with Synthetic Substitute, Percutaneous Approach

0NRG3KZ Replacement of Left Ethmoid Bone with Nonautologous Tissue Substitute, Percutaneous Approach

0NRG47Z Replacement of Left Ethmoid Bone with Autologous Tissue Substitute, Percutaneous Endoscopic Approach

0NRG4JZ Replacement of Left Ethmoid Bone with Synthetic Substitute, Percutaneous Endoscopic Approach

0NRG4KZ Replacement of Left Ethmoid Bone with Nonautologous Tissue Substitute, Percutaneous Endoscopic Approach

0NRH07Z Replacement of Right Lacrimal Bone with Autologous Tissue Substitute, Open Approach

0NRH0JZ Replacement of Right Lacrimal Bone with Synthetic Substitute, Open Approach

0NRH0KZ Replacement of Right Lacrimal Bone with Nonautologous Tissue Substitute, Open Approach

0NRH37Z Replacement of Right Lacrimal Bone with Autologous Tissue Substitute, Percutaneous Approach

0NRH3JZ Replacement of Right Lacrimal Bone with Synthetic Substitute, Percutaneous Approach

0NRH3KZ Replacement of Right Lacrimal Bone with Nonautologous Tissue Substitute, Percutaneous Approach

0NRH47Z Replacement of Right Lacrimal Bone with Autologous Tissue Substitute, Percutaneous Endoscopic Approach

0NRH4JZ Replacement of Right Lacrimal Bone with Synthetic Substitute, Percutaneous Endoscopic Approach

0NRH4KZ Replacement of Right Lacrimal Bone with Nonautologous Tissue Substitute, Percutaneous Endoscopic Approach

0NRJ07Z Replacement of Left Lacrimal Bone with Autologous Tissue Substitute, Open Approach

0NRJ0JZ Replacement of Left Lacrimal Bone with Synthetic Substitute, Open Approach

0NRJ0KZ Replacement of Left Lacrimal Bone with Nonautologous Tissue Substitute, Open Approach

0NRJ37Z Replacement of Left Lacrimal Bone with Autologous Tissue Substitute, Percutaneous Approach

0NRJ3JZ Replacement of Left Lacrimal Bone with Synthetic Substitute, Percutaneous Approach

0NRJ3KZ Replacement of Left Lacrimal Bone with Nonautologous Tissue Substitute, Percutaneous Approach

0NRJ47Z Replacement of Left Lacrimal Bone with Autologous Tissue Substitute, Percutaneous Endoscopic Approach

0NRJ4JZ Replacement of Left Lacrimal Bone with Synthetic Substitute, Percutaneous Endoscopic Approach

0NRJ4KZ Replacement of Left Lacrimal Bone with Nonautologous Tissue Substitute, Percutaneous Endoscopic Approach

0NRK07Z Replacement of Right Palatine Bone with Autologous Tissue Substitute, Open Approach

0NRK0JZ Replacement of Right Palatine Bone with Synthetic Substitute, Open Approach

0NRK0KZ Replacement of Right Palatine Bone with Nonautologous Tissue Substitute, Open Approach

0NRK37Z Replacement of Right Palatine Bone with Autologous Tissue Substitute, Percutaneous Approach

0NRK3JZ Replacement of Right Palatine Bone with Synthetic Substitute, Percutaneous Approach

0NRK3KZ Replacement of Right Palatine Bone with Nonautologous Tissue Substitute, Percutaneous Approach

0NRK47Z Replacement of Right Palatine Bone with Autologous Tissue Substitute, Percutaneous Endoscopic Approach

0NRK4JZ Replacement of Right Palatine Bone with Synthetic Substitute, Percutaneous Endoscopic Approach

0NRK4KZ Replacement of Right Palatine Bone with Nonautologous Tissue Substitute, Percutaneous Endoscopic Approach

0NRL07Z Replacement of Left Palatine Bone with Autologous Tissue Substitute, Open Approach

0NRL0JZ Replacement of Left Palatine Bone with Synthetic Substitute, Open Approach

0NRL0KZ Replacement of Left Palatine Bone with Nonautologous Tissue Substitute, Open Approach

0NRL37Z Replacement of Left Palatine Bone with Autologous Tissue Substitute, Percutaneous Approach

0NRL3JZ Replacement of Left Palatine Bone with Synthetic Substitute, Percutaneous Approach

0NRL3KZ Replacement of Left Palatine Bone with Nonautologous Tissue Substitute, Percutaneous Approach

0NRL47Z Replacement of Left Palatine Bone with Autologous Tissue Substitute, Percutaneous Endoscopic Approach

0NRL4JZ Replacement of Left Palatine Bone with Synthetic Substitute, Percutaneous Endoscopic Approach

0NRL4KZ Replacement of Left Palatine Bone with Nonautologous Tissue Substitute, Percutaneous Endoscopic Approach

0NRM07Z Replacement of Right Zygomatic Bone with Autologous Tissue Substitute, Open Approach

0NRM0JZ Replacement of Right Zygomatic Bone with Synthetic Substitute, Open Approach

0NRM0KZ Replacement of Right Zygomatic Bone with Nonautologous Tissue Substitute, Open Approach

0NRM37Z Replacement of Right Zygomatic Bone with Autologous Tissue Substitute, Percutaneous Approach

0NRM3JZ Replacement of Right Zygomatic Bone with Synthetic Substitute, Percutaneous Approach

0NRM3KZ Replacement of Right Zygomatic Bone with Nonautologous Tissue Substitute, Percutaneous Approach

0NRM47Z Replacement of Right Zygomatic Bone with Autologous Tissue Substitute, Percutaneous Endoscopic Approach

0NRM4JZ Replacement of Right Zygomatic Bone with Synthetic Substitute, Percutaneous Endoscopic Approach

0NRM4KZ Replacement of Right Zygomatic Bone with Nonautologous Tissue Substitute, Percutaneous Endoscopic Approach

0NRN07Z Replacement of Left Zygomatic Bone with Autologous Tissue Substitute, Open Approach

0NRN0JZ Replacement of Left Zygomatic Bone with Synthetic Substitute, Open Approach

0NRN0KZ Replacement of Left Zygomatic Bone with Nonautologous Tissue Substitute, Open Approach

0NRN37Z Replacement of Left Zygomatic Bone with Autologous Tissue Substitute, Percutaneous Approach

0NRN3JZ Replacement of Left Zygomatic Bone with Synthetic Substitute, Percutaneous Approach

0NRN3KZ Replacement of Left Zygomatic Bone with Nonautologous Tissue Substitute, Percutaneous Approach

0NRN47Z Replacement of Left Zygomatic Bone with Autologous Tissue Substitute, Percutaneous Endoscopic Approach

0NRN4JZ Replacement of Left Zygomatic Bone with Synthetic Substitute, Percutaneous Endoscopic Approach

0NRN4KZ Replacement of Left Zygomatic Bone with Nonautologous Tissue Substitute, Percutaneous Endoscopic Approach

0NRP07Z Replacement of Right Orbit with Autologous Tissue Substitute, Open Approach

0NRP0JZ Replacement of Right Orbit with Synthetic Substitute, Open Approach

0NRP0KZ Replacement of Right Orbit with Nonautologous Tissue Substitute, Open Approach

0NRP37Z Replacement of Right Orbit with Autologous Tissue Substitute, Percutaneous Approach

0NRP3JZ Replacement of Right Orbit with Synthetic Substitute, Percutaneous Approach

0NRP3KZ Replacement of Right Orbit with Nonautologous Tissue Substitute, Percutaneous Approach

♀ Female-only   ♂ Male-only   ▲ Limited Coverage   ● Non-OR   █ HAC-associated procedure   ▲ Non-covered procedures   ✚ Combination

RP47Z	Replacement of Right Orbit with Autologous Tissue Substitute, Percutaneous Endoscopic Approach	
RP4JZ	Replacement of Right Orbit with Synthetic Substitute, Percutaneous Endoscopic Approach	
RP4KZ	Replacement of Right Orbit with Nonautologous Tissue Substitute, Percutaneous Endoscopic Approach	
RQ07Z	Replacement of Left Orbit with Autologous Tissue Substitute, Open Approach	
RQ0JZ	Replacement of Left Orbit with Synthetic Substitute, Open Approach	
RQ0KZ	Replacement of Left Orbit with Nonautologous Tissue Substitute, Open Approach	
RQ37Z	Replacement of Left Orbit with Autologous Tissue Substitute, Percutaneous Approach	
RQ3JZ	Replacement of Left Orbit with Synthetic Substitute, Percutaneous Approach	
RQ3KZ	Replacement of Left Orbit with Nonautologous Tissue Substitute, Percutaneous Approach	
RQ47Z	Replacement of Left Orbit with Autologous Tissue Substitute, Percutaneous Endoscopic Approach	
RQ4JZ	Replacement of Left Orbit with Synthetic Substitute, Percutaneous Endoscopic Approach	
RQ4KZ	Replacement of Left Orbit with Nonautologous Tissue Substitute, Percutaneous Endoscopic Approach	
RR07Z	Replacement of Right Maxilla with Autologous Tissue Substitute, Open Approach	
RR0JZ	Replacement of Right Maxilla with Synthetic Substitute, Open Approach	
RR0KZ	Replacement of Right Maxilla with Nonautologous Tissue Substitute, Open Approach	
RR37Z	Replacement of Right Maxilla with Autologous Tissue Substitute, Percutaneous Approach	
RR3JZ	Replacement of Right Maxilla with Synthetic Substitute, Percutaneous Approach	
RR3KZ	Replacement of Right Maxilla with Nonautologous Tissue Substitute, Percutaneous Approach	
RR47Z	Replacement of Right Maxilla with Autologous Tissue Substitute, Percutaneous Endoscopic Approach	

0NRR4JZ	Replacement of Right Maxilla with Synthetic Substitute, Percutaneous Endoscopic Approach
0NRR4KZ	Replacement of Right Maxilla with Nonautologous Tissue Substitute, Percutaneous Endoscopic Approach
0NRS07Z	Replacement of Left Maxilla with Autologous Tissue Substitute, Open Approach
0NRS0JZ	Replacement of Left Maxilla with Synthetic Substitute, Open Approach
0NRS0KZ	Replacement of Left Maxilla with Nonautologous Tissue Substitute, Open Approach
0NRS37Z	Replacement of Left Maxilla with Autologous Tissue Substitute, Percutaneous Approach
0NRS3JZ	Replacement of Left Maxilla with Synthetic Substitute, Percutaneous Approach
0NRS3KZ	Replacement of Left Maxilla with Nonautologous Tissue Substitute, Percutaneous Approach
0NRS47Z	Replacement of Left Maxilla with Autologous Tissue Substitute, Percutaneous Endoscopic Approach
0NRS4JZ	Replacement of Left Maxilla with Synthetic Substitute, Percutaneous Endoscopic Approach
0NRS4KZ	Replacement of Left Maxilla with Nonautologous Tissue Substitute, Percutaneous Endoscopic Approach
0NRT07Z	Replacement of Right Mandible with Autologous Tissue Substitute, Open Approach
0NRT0JZ	Replacement of Right Mandible with Synthetic Substitute, Open Approach
0NRT0KZ	Replacement of Right Mandible with Nonautologous Tissue Substitute, Open Approach
0NRT37Z	Replacement of Right Mandible with Autologous Tissue Substitute, Percutaneous Approach
0NRT3JZ	Replacement of Right Mandible with Synthetic Substitute, Percutaneous Approach
0NRT3KZ	Replacement of Right Mandible with Nonautologous Tissue Substitute, Percutaneous Approach
0NRT47Z	Replacement of Right Mandible with Autologous Tissue Substitute, Percutaneous Endoscopic Approach
0NRT4JZ	Replacement of Right Mandible with Synthetic Substitute, Percutaneous Endoscopic Approach

0NRT4KZ	Replacement of Right Mandible with Nonautologous Tissue Substitute, Percutaneous Endoscopic Approach
0NRV07Z	Replacement of Left Mandible with Autologous Tissue Substitute, Open Approach
0NRV0JZ	Replacement of Left Mandible with Synthetic Substitute, Open Approach
0NRV0KZ	Replacement of Left Mandible with Nonautologous Tissue Substitute, Open Approach
0NRV37Z	Replacement of Left Mandible with Autologous Tissue Substitute, Percutaneous Approach
0NRV3JZ	Replacement of Left Mandible with Synthetic Substitute, Percutaneous Approach
0NRV3KZ	Replacement of Left Mandible with Nonautologous Tissue Substitute, Percutaneous Approach
0NRV47Z	Replacement of Left Mandible with Autologous Tissue Substitute, Percutaneous Endoscopic Approach
0NRV4JZ	Replacement of Left Mandible with Synthetic Substitute, Percutaneous Endoscopic Approach
0NRV4KZ	Replacement of Left Mandible with Nonautologous Tissue Substitute, Percutaneous Endoscopic Approach
0NRX07Z	Replacement of Hyoid Bone with Autologous Tissue Substitute, Open Approach
0NRX0JZ	Replacement of Hyoid Bone with Synthetic Substitute, Open Approach
0NRX0KZ	Replacement of Hyoid Bone with Nonautologous Tissue Substitute, Open Approach
0NRX37Z	Replacement of Hyoid Bone with Autologous Tissue Substitute, Percutaneous Approach
0NRX3JZ	Replacement of Hyoid Bone with Synthetic Substitute, Percutaneous Approach
0NRX3KZ	Replacement of Hyoid Bone with Nonautologous Tissue Substitute, Percutaneous Approach
0NRX47Z	Replacement of Hyoid Bone with Autologous Tissue Substitute, Percutaneous Endoscopic Approach
0NRX4JZ	Replacement of Hyoid Bone with Synthetic Substitute, Percutaneous Endoscopic Approach
0NRX4KZ	Replacement of Hyoid Bone with Nonautologous Tissue Substitute, Percutaneous Endoscopic Approach

NS – Head and Facial Bones, Reposition

eview Coding Guideline B3.15

NS004Z	Reposition Skull with Internal Fixation Device, Open Approach
NS005Z	Reposition Skull with External Fixation Device, Open Approach
	AHA CC: 3Q, 2013, 24-25
NS00ZZ	Reposition Skull, Open Approach
NS034Z	Reposition Skull with Internal Fixation Device, Percutaneous Approach
NS035Z	Reposition Skull with External Fixation Device, Percutaneous Approach
NS03ZZ	Reposition Skull, Percutaneous Approach
NS044Z	Reposition Skull with Internal Fixation Device, Percutaneous Endoscopic Approach
NS045Z	Reposition Skull with External Fixation Device, Percutaneous Endoscopic Approach

0NS04ZZ	Reposition Skull, Percutaneous Endoscopic Approach
0NS0XZZ	Reposition Skull, External Approach
0NS104Z	Reposition Right Frontal Bone with Internal Fixation Device, Open Approach
	AHA CC: 3Q, 2013, 25
0NS10ZZ	Reposition Right Frontal Bone, Open Approach
0NS134Z	Reposition Right Frontal Bone with Internal Fixation Device, Percutaneous Approach
0NS13ZZ	Reposition Right Frontal Bone, Percutaneous Approach
0NS144Z	Reposition Right Frontal Bone with Internal Fixation Device, Percutaneous Endoscopic Approach

0NS14ZZ	Reposition Right Frontal Bone, Percutaneous Endoscopic Approach
0NS1XZZ	Reposition Right Frontal Bone, External Approach
0NS204Z	Reposition Left Frontal Bone with Internal Fixation Device, Open Approach
0NS20ZZ	Reposition Left Frontal Bone, Open Approach
0NS234Z	Reposition Left Frontal Bone with Internal Fixation Device, Percutaneous Approach
0NS23ZZ	Reposition Left Frontal Bone, Percutaneous Approach
0NS244Z	Reposition Left Frontal Bone with Internal Fixation Device, Percutaneous Endoscopic Approach
0NS24ZZ	Reposition Left Frontal Bone, Percutaneous Endoscopic Approach

♀ Female-only	♂ Male-only	▲ Limited Coverage	● Non-OR	▨ HAC-associated procedure	▲ Non-covered procedures	+ Combination

0NS2XZZ Reposition Left Frontal Bone, External Approach

0NS304Z Reposition Right Parietal Bone with Internal Fixation Device, Open Approach

0NS30ZZ Reposition Right Parietal Bone, Open Approach

0NS334Z Reposition Right Parietal Bone with Internal Fixation Device, Percutaneous Approach

0NS33ZZ Reposition Right Parietal Bone, Percutaneous Approach

0NS344Z Reposition Right Parietal Bone with Internal Fixation Device, Percutaneous Endoscopic Approach

0NS34ZZ Reposition Right Parietal Bone, Percutaneous Endoscopic Approach

0NS3XZZ Reposition Right Parietal Bone, External Approach

0NS404Z Reposition Left Parietal Bone with Internal Fixation Device, Open Approach

0NS40ZZ Reposition Left Parietal Bone, Open Approach

0NS434Z Reposition Left Parietal Bone with Internal Fixation Device, Percutaneous Approach

0NS43ZZ Reposition Left Parietal Bone, Percutaneous Approach

0NS444Z Reposition Left Parietal Bone with Internal Fixation Device, Percutaneous Endoscopic Approach

0NS44ZZ Reposition Left Parietal Bone, Percutaneous Endoscopic Approach

0NS4XZZ Reposition Left Parietal Bone, External Approach

0NS504Z Reposition Right Temporal Bone with Internal Fixation Device, Open Approach

0NS50ZZ Reposition Right Temporal Bone, Open Approach

0NS534Z Reposition Right Temporal Bone with Internal Fixation Device, Percutaneous Approach

0NS53ZZ Reposition Right Temporal Bone, Percutaneous Approach

0NS544Z Reposition Right Temporal Bone with Internal Fixation Device, Percutaneous Endoscopic Approach

0NS54ZZ Reposition Right Temporal Bone, Percutaneous Endoscopic Approach

0NS5XZZ Reposition Right Temporal Bone, External Approach

0NS604Z Reposition Left Temporal Bone with Internal Fixation Device, Open Approach

0NS60ZZ Reposition Left Temporal Bone, Open Approach

0NS634Z Reposition Left Temporal Bone with Internal Fixation Device, Percutaneous Approach

0NS63ZZ Reposition Left Temporal Bone, Percutaneous Approach

0NS644Z Reposition Left Temporal Bone with Internal Fixation Device, Percutaneous Endoscopic Approach

0NS64ZZ Reposition Left Temporal Bone, Percutaneous Endoscopic Approach

0NS6XZZ Reposition Left Temporal Bone, External Approach

0NS704Z Reposition Right Occipital Bone with Internal Fixation Device, Open Approach

0NS70ZZ Reposition Right Occipital Bone, Open Approach

0NS734Z Reposition Right Occipital Bone with Internal Fixation Device, Percutaneous Approach

0NS73ZZ Reposition Right Occipital Bone, Percutaneous Approach

0NS744Z Reposition Right Occipital Bone with Internal Fixation Device, Percutaneous Endoscopic Approach

0NS74ZZ Reposition Right Occipital Bone, Percutaneous Endoscopic Approach

0NS7XZZ Reposition Right Occipital Bone, External Approach

0NS804Z Reposition Left Occipital Bone with Internal Fixation Device, Open Approach

0NS80ZZ Reposition Left Occipital Bone, Open Approach

0NS834Z Reposition Left Occipital Bone with Internal Fixation Device, Percutaneous Approach

0NS83ZZ Reposition Left Occipital Bone, Percutaneous Approach

0NS844Z Reposition Left Occipital Bone with Internal Fixation Device, Percutaneous Endoscopic Approach

0NS84ZZ Reposition Left Occipital Bone, Percutaneous Endoscopic Approach

0NS8XZZ Reposition Left Occipital Bone, External Approach

0NSB04Z Reposition Nasal Bone with Internal Fixation Device, Open Approach

0NSB0ZZ Reposition Nasal Bone, Open Approach

0NSB34Z Reposition Nasal Bone with Internal Fixation Device, Percutaneous Approach

0NSB3ZZ Reposition Nasal Bone, Percutaneous Approach

0NSB44Z Reposition Nasal Bone with Internal Fixation Device, Percutaneous Endoscopic Approach

0NSB4ZZ Reposition Nasal Bone, Percutaneous Endoscopic Approach

0NSBXZZ Reposition Nasal Bone, External Approach

0NSC04Z Reposition Right Sphenoid Bone with Internal Fixation Device, Open Approach

0NSC0ZZ Reposition Right Sphenoid Bone, Open Approach

0NSC34Z Reposition Right Sphenoid Bone with Internal Fixation Device, Percutaneous Approach

0NSC3ZZ Reposition Right Sphenoid Bone, Percutaneous Approach

0NSC44Z Reposition Right Sphenoid Bone with Internal Fixation Device, Percutaneous Endoscopic Approach

0NSC4ZZ Reposition Right Sphenoid Bone, Percutaneous Endoscopic Approach

0NSCXZZ Reposition Right Sphenoid Bone, External Approach

0NSD04Z Reposition Left Sphenoid Bone with Internal Fixation Device, Open Approach

0NSD0ZZ Reposition Left Sphenoid Bone, Open Approach

0NSD34Z Reposition Left Sphenoid Bone with Internal Fixation Device, Percutaneous Approach

0NSD3ZZ Reposition Left Sphenoid Bone, Percutaneous Approach

0NSD44Z Reposition Left Sphenoid Bone with Internal Fixation Device, Percutaneous Endoscopic Approach

0NSD4ZZ Reposition Left Sphenoid Bone, Percutaneous Endoscopic Approach

0NSDXZZ Reposition Left Sphenoid Bone, External Approach

0NSF04Z Reposition Right Ethmoid Bone with Internal Fixation Device, Open Approach

0NSF0ZZ Reposition Right Ethmoid Bone, Open Approach

0NSF34Z Reposition Right Ethmoid Bone with Internal Fixation Device, Percutaneous Approach

0NSF3ZZ Reposition Right Ethmoid Bone, Percutaneous Approach

0NSF44Z Reposition Right Ethmoid Bone with Internal Fixation Device, Percutaneous Endoscopic Approach

0NSF4ZZ Reposition Right Ethmoid Bone, Percutaneous Endoscopic Approach

0NSFXZZ Reposition Right Ethmoid Bone, External Approach

0NSG04Z Reposition Left Ethmoid Bone with Internal Fixation Device, Open Approach

0NSG0ZZ Reposition Left Ethmoid Bone, Open Approach

0NSG34Z Reposition Left Ethmoid Bone with Internal Fixation Device, Percutaneous Approach

0NSG3ZZ Reposition Left Ethmoid Bone, Percutaneous Approach

0NSG44Z Reposition Left Ethmoid Bone with Internal Fixation Device, Percutaneous Endoscopic Approach

0NSG4ZZ Reposition Left Ethmoid Bone, Percutaneous Endoscopic Approach

0NSGXZZ Reposition Left Ethmoid Bone, External Approach

0NSH04Z Reposition Right Lacrimal Bone with Internal Fixation Device, Open Approach

0NSH0ZZ Reposition Right Lacrimal Bone, Open Approach

0NSH34Z Reposition Right Lacrimal Bone with Internal Fixation Device, Percutaneous Approach

0NSH3ZZ Reposition Right Lacrimal Bone, Percutaneous Approach

0NSH44Z Reposition Right Lacrimal Bone with Internal Fixation Device, Percutaneous Endoscopic Approach

0NSH4ZZ Reposition Right Lacrimal Bone, Percutaneous Endoscopic Approach

0NSHXZZ Reposition Right Lacrimal Bone, External Approach

0NSJ04Z Reposition Left Lacrimal Bone with Internal Fixation Device, Open Approach

0NSJ0ZZ Reposition Left Lacrimal Bone, Open Approach

0NSJ34Z Reposition Left Lacrimal Bone with Internal Fixation Device, Percutaneous Approach

0NSJ3ZZ Reposition Left Lacrimal Bone, Percutaneous Approach

0NSJ44Z Reposition Left Lacrimal Bone with Internal Fixation Device, Percutaneous Endoscopic Approach

0NSJ4ZZ Reposition Left Lacrimal Bone, Percutaneous Endoscopic Approach

0NSJXZZ Reposition Left Lacrimal Bone, External Approach

0NSK04Z Reposition Right Palatine Bone with Internal Fixation Device, Open Approach

0NSK0ZZ Reposition Right Palatine Bone, Open Approach

0NSK34Z Reposition Right Palatine Bone with Internal Fixation Device, Percutaneous Approach

0NSK3ZZ Reposition Right Palatine Bone, Percutaneous Approach

0NSK44Z Reposition Right Palatine Bone with Internal Fixation Device, Percutaneous Endoscopic Approach

♀ Female-only   ♂ Male-only   ▲ Limited Coverage   ● Non-OR   ▦ HAC-associated procedure   ▲ Non-covered procedures   ✚ Combination

SK4ZZ Reposition Right Palatine Bone, Percutaneous Endoscopic Approach

SKXZZ Reposition Right Palatine Bone, External Approach

SL04Z Reposition Left Palatine Bone with Internal Fixation Device, Open Approach

SL0ZZ Reposition Left Palatine Bone, Open Approach

SL34Z Reposition Left Palatine Bone with Internal Fixation Device, Percutaneous Approach

SL3ZZ Reposition Left Palatine Bone, Percutaneous Approach

SL44Z Reposition Left Palatine Bone with Internal Fixation Device, Percutaneous Endoscopic Approach

SL4ZZ Reposition Left Palatine Bone, Percutaneous Endoscopic Approach

SLXZZ Reposition Left Palatine Bone, External Approach

SM04Z Reposition Right Zygomatic Bone with Internal Fixation Device, Open Approach

SM0ZZ Reposition Right Zygomatic Bone, Open Approach

SM34Z Reposition Right Zygomatic Bone with Internal Fixation Device, Percutaneous Approach

SM3ZZ Reposition Right Zygomatic Bone, Percutaneous Approach

SM44Z Reposition Right Zygomatic Bone with Internal Fixation Device, Percutaneous Endoscopic Approach

SM4ZZ Reposition Right Zygomatic Bone, Percutaneous Endoscopic Approach

SMXZZ Reposition Right Zygomatic Bone, External Approach

SN04Z Reposition Left Zygomatic Bone with Internal Fixation Device, Open Approach

SN0ZZ Reposition Left Zygomatic Bone, Open Approach

SN34Z Reposition Left Zygomatic Bone with Internal Fixation Device, Percutaneous Approach

SN3ZZ Reposition Left Zygomatic Bone, Percutaneous Approach

SN44Z Reposition Left Zygomatic Bone with Internal Fixation Device, Percutaneous Endoscopic Approach

SN4ZZ Reposition Left Zygomatic Bone, Percutaneous Endoscopic Approach

SNXZZ Reposition Left Zygomatic Bone, External Approach

NSP04Z Reposition Right Orbit with Internal Fixation Device, Open Approach

NSP0ZZ Reposition Right Orbit, Open Approach

NSP34Z Reposition Right Orbit with Internal Fixation Device, Percutaneous Approach

NSP3ZZ Reposition Right Orbit, Percutaneous Approach

0NSP44Z Reposition Right Orbit with Internal Fixation Device, Percutaneous Endoscopic Approach

0NSP4ZZ Reposition Right Orbit, Percutaneous Endoscopic Approach

0NSPXZZ Reposition Right Orbit, External Approach

0NSQ04Z Reposition Left Orbit with Internal Fixation Device, Open Approach

0NSQ0ZZ Reposition Left Orbit, Open Approach

0NSQ34Z Reposition Left Orbit with Internal Fixation Device, Percutaneous Approach

0NSQ3ZZ Reposition Left Orbit, Percutaneous Approach

0NSQ44Z Reposition Left Orbit with Internal Fixation Device, Percutaneous Endoscopic Approach

0NSQ4ZZ Reposition Left Orbit, Percutaneous Endoscopic Approach

0NSQXZZ Reposition Left Orbit, External Approach

0NSR04Z Reposition Right Maxilla with Internal Fixation Device, Open Approach
AHA CC: 3Q, 2014, 23-24

0NSR05Z Reposition Right Maxilla with External Fixation Device, Open Approach

0NSR0ZZ Reposition Right Maxilla, Open Approach

0NSR34Z Reposition Right Maxilla with Internal Fixation Device, Percutaneous Approach

0NSR35Z Reposition Right Maxilla with External Fixation Device, Percutaneous Approach

0NSR3ZZ Reposition Right Maxilla, Percutaneous Approach

0NSR44Z Reposition Right Maxilla with Internal Fixation Device, Percutaneous Endoscopic Approach

0NSR45Z Reposition Right Maxilla with External Fixation Device, Percutaneous Endoscopic Approach

0NSR4ZZ Reposition Right Maxilla, Percutaneous Endoscopic Approach

0NSRXZZ Reposition Right Maxilla, External Approach

0NSS04Z Reposition Left Maxilla with Internal Fixation Device, Open Approach
AHA CC: 3Q, 2014, 23-24

0NSS05Z Reposition Left Maxilla with External Fixation Device, Open Approach

0NSS0ZZ Reposition Left Maxilla, Open Approach

0NSS34Z Reposition Left Maxilla with Internal Fixation Device, Percutaneous Approach

0NSS35Z Reposition Left Maxilla with External Fixation Device, Percutaneous Approach

0NSS3ZZ Reposition Left Maxilla, Percutaneous Approach

0NSS44Z Reposition Left Maxilla with Internal Fixation Device, Percutaneous Endoscopic Approach

0NSS45Z Reposition Left Maxilla with External Fixation Device, Percutaneous Endoscopic Approach

0NSS4ZZ Reposition Left Maxilla, Percutaneous Endoscopic Approach

0NSSXZZ Reposition Left Maxilla, External Approach

0NST04Z Reposition Right Mandible with Internal Fixation Device, Open Approach

0NST05Z Reposition Right Mandible with External Fixation Device, Open Approach

0NST0ZZ Reposition Right Mandible, Open Approach

0NST34Z Reposition Right Mandible with Internal Fixation Device, Percutaneous Approach

0NST35Z Reposition Right Mandible with External Fixation Device, Percutaneous Approach

0NST3ZZ Reposition Right Mandible, Percutaneous Approach

0NST44Z Reposition Right Mandible with Internal Fixation Device, Percutaneous Endoscopic Approach

0NST45Z Reposition Right Mandible with External Fixation Device, Percutaneous Endoscopic Approach

0NST4ZZ Reposition Right Mandible, Percutaneous Endoscopic Approach

0NSTXZZ Reposition Right Mandible, External Approach

0NSV04Z Reposition Left Mandible with Internal Fixation Device, Open Approach

0NSV05Z Reposition Left Mandible with External Fixation Device, Open Approach

0NSV0ZZ Reposition Left Mandible, Open Approach

0NSV34Z Reposition Left Mandible with Internal Fixation Device, Percutaneous Approach

0NSV35Z Reposition Left Mandible with External Fixation Device, Percutaneous Approach

0NSV3ZZ Reposition Left Mandible, Percutaneous Approach

0NSV44Z Reposition Left Mandible with Internal Fixation Device, Percutaneous Endoscopic Approach

0NSV45Z Reposition Left Mandible with External Fixation Device, Percutaneous Endoscopic Approach

0NSV4ZZ Reposition Left Mandible, Percutaneous Endoscopic Approach

0NSVXZZ Reposition Left Mandible, External Approach

0NSX04Z Reposition Hyoid Bone with Internal Fixation Device, Open Approach

0NSX0ZZ Reposition Hyoid Bone, Open Approach

0NSX34Z Reposition Hyoid Bone with Internal Fixation Device, Percutaneous Approach

0NSX3ZZ Reposition Hyoid Bone, Percutaneous Approach

0NSX44Z Reposition Hyoid Bone with Internal Fixation Device, Percutaneous Endoscopic Approach

0NSX4ZZ Reposition Hyoid Bone, Percutaneous Endoscopic Approach

0NSXXZZ Reposition Hyoid Bone, External Approach

0NT – Head and Facial Bones, Resection

Review Coding Guideline B3.8

0NT10ZZ Resection of Right Frontal Bone, Open Approach

0NT20ZZ Resection of Left Frontal Bone, Open Approach

0NT30ZZ Resection of Right Parietal Bone, Open Approach

0NT40ZZ Resection of Left Parietal Bone, Open Approach

0NT50ZZ Resection of Right Temporal Bone, Open Approach

0NT60ZZ Resection of Left Temporal Bone, Open Approach

0NT70ZZ Resection of Right Occipital Bone, Open Approach

0NT80ZZ Resection of Left Occipital Bone, Open Approach

0NTB0ZZ Resection of Nasal Bone, Open Approach

0NTC0ZZ Resection of Right Sphenoid Bone, Open Approach

0NTD0ZZ Resection of Left Sphenoid Bone, Open Approach

0NTF0ZZ Resection of Right Ethmoid Bone, Open Approach

0NTG0ZZ Resection of Left Ethmoid Bone, Open Approach

0NTH0ZZ Resection of Right Lacrimal Bone, Open Approach

0NTJ0ZZ Resection of Left Lacrimal Bone, Open Approach

0NTK0ZZ Resection of Right Palatine Bone, Open Approach

0NTL0ZZ Resection of Left Palatine Bone, Open Approach

0NTM0ZZ Resection of Right Zygomatic Bone, Open Approach

♀ Female-only   ♂ Male-only   ▲ Limited Coverage   ● Non-OR   ▬ HAC-associated procedure   ▲ Non-covered procedures   ✚ Combination

0NTN0ZZ   Resection of Left Zygomatic Bone, Open Approach
0NTP0ZZ   Resection of Right Orbit, Open Approach
0NTQ0ZZ   Resection of Left Orbit, Open Approach

0NTR0ZZ   Resection of Right Maxilla, Open Approach
0NTS0ZZ   Resection of Left Maxilla, Open Approach

0NTT0ZZ   Resection of Right Mandible, Open Approach
0NTV0ZZ   Resection of Left Mandible, Open Approach
0NTX0ZZ   Resection of Hyoid Bone, Open Approa

0NU – Head and Facial Bones, Supplement

0NU007Z   Supplement Skull with Autologous Tissue Substitute, Open Approach
0NU00JZ   Supplement Skull with Synthetic Substitute, Open Approach
          AHA CC: 3Q, 2013, 24-25
0NU00KZ   Supplement Skull with Nonautologous Tissue Substitute, Open Approach
0NU037Z   Supplement Skull with Autologous Tissue Substitute, Percutaneous Approach
0NU03JZ   Supplement Skull with Synthetic Substitute, Percutaneous Approach
0NU03KZ   Supplement Skull with Nonautologous Tissue Substitute, Percutaneous Approach
0NU047Z   Supplement Skull with Autologous Tissue Substitute, Percutaneous Endoscopic Approach
0NU04JZ   Supplement Skull with Synthetic Substitute, Percutaneous Endoscopic Approach
0NU04KZ   Supplement Skull with Nonautologous Tissue Substitute, Percutaneous Endoscopic Approach
0NU107Z   Supplement Right Frontal Bone with Autologous Tissue Substitute, Open Approach
0NU10JZ   Supplement Right Frontal Bone with Synthetic Substitute, Open Approach
0NU10KZ   Supplement Right Frontal Bone with Nonautologous Tissue Substitute, Open Approach
0NU137Z   Supplement Right Frontal Bone with Autologous Tissue Substitute, Percutaneous Approach
0NU13JZ   Supplement Right Frontal Bone with Synthetic Substitute, Percutaneous Approach
0NU13KZ   Supplement Right Frontal Bone with Nonautologous Tissue Substitute, Percutaneous Approach
0NU147Z   Supplement Right Frontal Bone with Autologous Tissue Substitute, Percutaneous Endoscopic Approach
0NU14JZ   Supplement Right Frontal Bone with Synthetic Substitute, Percutaneous Endoscopic Approach
0NU14KZ   Supplement Right Frontal Bone with Nonautologous Tissue Substitute, Percutaneous Endoscopic Approach
0NU207Z   Supplement Left Frontal Bone with Autologous Tissue Substitute, Open Approach
0NU20JZ   Supplement Left Frontal Bone with Synthetic Substitute, Open Approach
0NU20KZ   Supplement Left Frontal Bone with Nonautologous Tissue Substitute, Open Approach
0NU237Z   Supplement Left Frontal Bone with Autologous Tissue Substitute, Percutaneous Approach
0NU23JZ   Supplement Left Frontal Bone with Synthetic Substitute, Percutaneous Approach
0NU23KZ   Supplement Left Frontal Bone with Nonautologous Tissue Substitute, Percutaneous Approach
0NU247Z   Supplement Left Frontal Bone with Autologous Tissue Substitute, Percutaneous Endoscopic Approach

0NU24JZ   Supplement Left Frontal Bone with Synthetic Substitute, Percutaneous Endoscopic Approach
0NU24KZ   Supplement Left Frontal Bone with Nonautologous Tissue Substitute, Percutaneous Endoscopic Approach
0NU307Z   Supplement Right Parietal Bone with Autologous Tissue Substitute, Open Approach
0NU30JZ   Supplement Right Parietal Bone with Synthetic Substitute, Open Approach
0NU30KZ   Supplement Right Parietal Bone with Nonautologous Tissue Substitute, Open Approach
0NU337Z   Supplement Right Parietal Bone with Autologous Tissue Substitute, Percutaneous Approach
0NU33JZ   Supplement Right Parietal Bone with Synthetic Substitute, Percutaneous Approach
0NU33KZ   Supplement Right Parietal Bone with Nonautologous Tissue Substitute, Percutaneous Approach
0NU347Z   Supplement Right Parietal Bone with Autologous Tissue Substitute, Percutaneous Endoscopic Approach
0NU34JZ   Supplement Right Parietal Bone with Synthetic Substitute, Percutaneous Endoscopic Approach
0NU34KZ   Supplement Right Parietal Bone with Nonautologous Tissue Substitute, Percutaneous Endoscopic Approach
0NU407Z   Supplement Left Parietal Bone with Autologous Tissue Substitute, Open Approach
0NU40JZ   Supplement Left Parietal Bone with Synthetic Substitute, Open Approach
0NU40KZ   Supplement Left Parietal Bone with Nonautologous Tissue Substitute, Open Approach
0NU437Z   Supplement Left Parietal Bone with Autologous Tissue Substitute, Percutaneous Approach
0NU43JZ   Supplement Left Parietal Bone with Synthetic Substitute, Percutaneous Approach
0NU43KZ   Supplement Left Parietal Bone with Nonautologous Tissue Substitute, Percutaneous Approach
0NU447Z   Supplement Left Parietal Bone with Autologous Tissue Substitute, Percutaneous Endoscopic Approach
0NU44JZ   Supplement Left Parietal Bone with Synthetic Substitute, Percutaneous Endoscopic Approach
0NU44KZ   Supplement Left Parietal Bone with Nonautologous Tissue Substitute, Percutaneous Endoscopic Approach
0NU507Z   Supplement Right Temporal Bone with Autologous Tissue Substitute, Open Approach
0NU50JZ   Supplement Right Temporal Bone with Synthetic Substitute, Open Approach
0NU50KZ   Supplement Right Temporal Bone with Nonautologous Tissue Substitute, Open Approach
0NU537Z   Supplement Right Temporal Bone with Autologous Tissue Substitute, Percutaneous Approach

0NU53JZ   Supplement Right Temporal Bone with Synthetic Substitute, Percutaneous Approach
0NU53KZ   Supplement Right Temporal Bone with Nonautologous Tissue Substitute, Percutaneous Approach
0NU547Z   Supplement Right Temporal Bone with Autologous Tissue Substitute, Percutaneous Endoscopic Approach
0NU54JZ   Supplement Right Temporal Bone with Synthetic Substitute, Percutaneous Endoscopic Approach
0NU54KZ   Supplement Right Temporal Bone with Nonautologous Tissue Substitute, Percutaneous Endoscopic Approach
0NU607Z   Supplement Left Temporal Bone with Autologous Tissue Substitute, Open Approach
0NU60JZ   Supplement Left Temporal Bone with Synthetic Substitute, Open Approach
0NU60KZ   Supplement Left Temporal Bone with Nonautologous Tissue Substitute, Open Approach
0NU637Z   Supplement Left Temporal Bone with Autologous Tissue Substitute, Percutaneous Approach
0NU63JZ   Supplement Left Temporal Bone with Synthetic Substitute, Percutaneous Approach
0NU63KZ   Supplement Left Temporal Bone with Nonautologous Tissue Substitute, Percutaneous Approach
0NU647Z   Supplement Left Temporal Bone with Autologous Tissue Substitute, Percutaneous Endoscopic Approach
0NU64JZ   Supplement Left Temporal Bone with Synthetic Substitute, Percutaneous Endoscopic Approach
0NU64KZ   Supplement Left Temporal Bone with Nonautologous Tissue Substitute, Percutaneous Endoscopic Approach
0NU707Z   Supplement Right Occipital Bone with Autologous Tissue Substitute, Open Approach
0NU70JZ   Supplement Right Occipital Bone with Synthetic Substitute, Open Approach
0NU70KZ   Supplement Right Occipital Bone with Nonautologous Tissue Substitute, Open Approach
0NU737Z   Supplement Right Occipital Bone with Autologous Tissue Substitute, Percutaneous Approach
0NU73JZ   Supplement Right Occipital Bone with Synthetic Substitute, Percutaneous Approach
0NU73KZ   Supplement Right Occipital Bone with Nonautologous Tissue Substitute, Percutaneous Approach
0NU747Z   Supplement Right Occipital Bone with Autologous Tissue Substitute, Percutaneous Endoscopic Approach
0NU74JZ   Supplement Right Occipital Bone with Synthetic Substitute, Percutaneous Endoscopic Approach
0NU74KZ   Supplement Right Occipital Bone with Nonautologous Tissue Substitute, Percutaneous Endoscopic Approach

U807Z	Supplement Left Occipital Bone with Autologous Tissue Substitute, Open Approach
U80JZ	Supplement Left Occipital Bone with Synthetic Substitute, Open Approach
U80KZ	Supplement Left Occipital Bone with Nonautologous Tissue Substitute, Open Approach
U837Z	Supplement Left Occipital Bone with Autologous Tissue Substitute, Percutaneous Approach
U83JZ	Supplement Left Occipital Bone with Synthetic Substitute, Percutaneous Approach
U83KZ	Supplement Left Occipital Bone with Nonautologous Tissue Substitute, Percutaneous Approach
U847Z	Supplement Left Occipital Bone with Autologous Tissue Substitute, Percutaneous Endoscopic Approach
U84JZ	Supplement Left Occipital Bone with Synthetic Substitute, Percutaneous Endoscopic Approach
U84KZ	Supplement Left Occipital Bone with Nonautologous Tissue Substitute, Percutaneous Endoscopic Approach
UB07Z	Supplement Nasal Bone with Autologous Tissue Substitute, Open Approach
UB0JZ	Supplement Nasal Bone with Synthetic Substitute, Open Approach
UB0KZ	Supplement Nasal Bone with Nonautologous Tissue Substitute, Open Approach
UB37Z	Supplement Nasal Bone with Autologous Tissue Substitute, Percutaneous Approach
UB3JZ	Supplement Nasal Bone with Synthetic Substitute, Percutaneous Approach
UB3KZ	Supplement Nasal Bone with Nonautologous Tissue Substitute, Percutaneous Approach
UB47Z	Supplement Nasal Bone with Autologous Tissue Substitute, Percutaneous Endoscopic Approach
UB4JZ	Supplement Nasal Bone with Synthetic Substitute, Percutaneous Endoscopic Approach
UB4KZ	Supplement Nasal Bone with Nonautologous Tissue Substitute, Percutaneous Endoscopic Approach
UC07Z	Supplement Right Sphenoid Bone with Autologous Tissue Substitute, Open Approach
UC0JZ	Supplement Right Sphenoid Bone with Synthetic Substitute, Open Approach
UC0KZ	Supplement Right Sphenoid Bone with Nonautologous Tissue Substitute, Open Approach
UC37Z	Supplement Right Sphenoid Bone with Autologous Tissue Substitute, Percutaneous Approach
UC3JZ	Supplement Right Sphenoid Bone with Synthetic Substitute, Percutaneous Approach
UC3KZ	Supplement Right Sphenoid Bone with Nonautologous Tissue Substitute, Percutaneous Approach
UC47Z	Supplement Right Sphenoid Bone with Autologous Tissue Substitute, Percutaneous Endoscopic Approach
UC4JZ	Supplement Right Sphenoid Bone with Synthetic Substitute, Percutaneous Endoscopic Approach
UC4KZ	Supplement Right Sphenoid Bone with Nonautologous Tissue Substitute, Percutaneous Endoscopic Approach

0NUD07Z	Supplement Left Sphenoid Bone with Autologous Tissue Substitute, Open Approach
0NUD0JZ	Supplement Left Sphenoid Bone with Synthetic Substitute, Open Approach
0NUD0KZ	Supplement Left Sphenoid Bone with Nonautologous Tissue Substitute, Open Approach
0NUD37Z	Supplement Left Sphenoid Bone with Autologous Tissue Substitute, Percutaneous Approach
0NUD3JZ	Supplement Left Sphenoid Bone with Synthetic Substitute, Percutaneous Approach
0NUD3KZ	Supplement Left Sphenoid Bone with Nonautologous Tissue Substitute, Percutaneous Approach
0NUD47Z	Supplement Left Sphenoid Bone with Autologous Tissue Substitute, Percutaneous Endoscopic Approach
0NUD4JZ	Supplement Left Sphenoid Bone with Synthetic Substitute, Percutaneous Endoscopic Approach
0NUD4KZ	Supplement Left Sphenoid Bone with Nonautologous Tissue Substitute, Percutaneous Endoscopic Approach
0NUF07Z	Supplement Right Ethmoid Bone with Autologous Tissue Substitute, Open Approach
0NUF0JZ	Supplement Right Ethmoid Bone with Synthetic Substitute, Open Approach
0NUF0KZ	Supplement Right Ethmoid Bone with Nonautologous Tissue Substitute, Open Approach
0NUF37Z	Supplement Right Ethmoid Bone with Autologous Tissue Substitute, Percutaneous Approach
0NUF3JZ	Supplement Right Ethmoid Bone with Synthetic Substitute, Percutaneous Approach
0NUF3KZ	Supplement Right Ethmoid Bone with Nonautologous Tissue Substitute, Percutaneous Approach
0NUF47Z	Supplement Right Ethmoid Bone with Autologous Tissue Substitute, Percutaneous Endoscopic Approach
0NUF4JZ	Supplement Right Ethmoid Bone with Synthetic Substitute, Percutaneous Endoscopic Approach
0NUF4KZ	Supplement Right Ethmoid Bone with Nonautologous Tissue Substitute, Percutaneous Endoscopic Approach
0NUG07Z	Supplement Left Ethmoid Bone with Autologous Tissue Substitute, Open Approach
0NUG0JZ	Supplement Left Ethmoid Bone with Synthetic Substitute, Open Approach
0NUG0KZ	Supplement Left Ethmoid Bone with Nonautologous Tissue Substitute, Open Approach
0NUG37Z	Supplement Left Ethmoid Bone with Autologous Tissue Substitute, Percutaneous Approach
0NUG3JZ	Supplement Left Ethmoid Bone with Synthetic Substitute, Percutaneous Approach
0NUG3KZ	Supplement Left Ethmoid Bone with Nonautologous Tissue Substitute, Percutaneous Approach
0NUG47Z	Supplement Left Ethmoid Bone with Autologous Tissue Substitute, Percutaneous Endoscopic Approach
0NUG4JZ	Supplement Left Ethmoid Bone with Synthetic Substitute, Percutaneous Endoscopic Approach

0NUG4KZ	Supplement Left Ethmoid Bone with Nonautologous Tissue Substitute, Percutaneous Endoscopic Approach
0NUH07Z	Supplement Right Lacrimal Bone with Autologous Tissue Substitute, Open Approach
0NUH0JZ	Supplement Right Lacrimal Bone with Synthetic Substitute, Open Approach
0NUH0KZ	Supplement Right Lacrimal Bone with Nonautologous Tissue Substitute, Open Approach
0NUH37Z	Supplement Right Lacrimal Bone with Autologous Tissue Substitute, Percutaneous Approach
0NUH3JZ	Supplement Right Lacrimal Bone with Synthetic Substitute, Percutaneous Approach
0NUH3KZ	Supplement Right Lacrimal Bone with Nonautologous Tissue Substitute, Percutaneous Approach
0NUH47Z	Supplement Right Lacrimal Bone with Autologous Tissue Substitute, Percutaneous Endoscopic Approach
0NUH4JZ	Supplement Right Lacrimal Bone with Synthetic Substitute, Percutaneous Endoscopic Approach
0NUH4KZ	Supplement Right Lacrimal Bone with Nonautologous Tissue Substitute, Percutaneous Endoscopic Approach
0NUJ07Z	Supplement Left Lacrimal Bone with Autologous Tissue Substitute, Open Approach
0NUJ0JZ	Supplement Left Lacrimal Bone with Synthetic Substitute, Open Approach
0NUJ0KZ	Supplement Left Lacrimal Bone with Nonautologous Tissue Substitute, Open Approach
0NUJ37Z	Supplement Left Lacrimal Bone with Autologous Tissue Substitute, Percutaneous Approach
0NUJ3JZ	Supplement Left Lacrimal Bone with Synthetic Substitute, Percutaneous Approach
0NUJ3KZ	Supplement Left Lacrimal Bone with Nonautologous Tissue Substitute, Percutaneous Approach
0NUJ47Z	Supplement Left Lacrimal Bone with Autologous Tissue Substitute, Percutaneous Endoscopic Approach
0NUJ4JZ	Supplement Left Lacrimal Bone with Synthetic Substitute, Percutaneous Endoscopic Approach
0NUJ4KZ	Supplement Left Lacrimal Bone with Nonautologous Tissue Substitute, Percutaneous Endoscopic Approach
0NUK07Z	Supplement Right Palatine Bone with Autologous Tissue Substitute, Open Approach
0NUK0JZ	Supplement Right Palatine Bone with Synthetic Substitute, Open Approach
0NUK0KZ	Supplement Right Palatine Bone with Nonautologous Tissue Substitute, Open Approach
0NUK37Z	Supplement Right Palatine Bone with Autologous Tissue Substitute, Percutaneous Approach
0NUK3JZ	Supplement Right Palatine Bone with Synthetic Substitute, Percutaneous Approach
0NUK3KZ	Supplement Right Palatine Bone with Nonautologous Tissue Substitute, Percutaneous Approach
0NUK47Z	Supplement Right Palatine Bone with Autologous Tissue Substitute, Percutaneous Endoscopic Approach

Female-only	♂ Male-only	▲ Limited Coverage	● Non-OR	▦ HAC-associated procedure	▲ Non-covered procedures

Combination

0NUK4JZ   Supplement Right Palatine Bone with Synthetic Substitute, Percutaneous Endoscopic Approach
0NUK4KZ   Supplement Right Palatine Bone with Nonautologous Tissue Substitute, Percutaneous Endoscopic Approach
0NUL07Z   Supplement Left Palatine Bone with Autologous Tissue Substitute, Open Approach
0NUL0JZ   Supplement Left Palatine Bone with Synthetic Substitute, Open Approach
0NUL0KZ   Supplement Left Palatine Bone with Nonautologous Tissue Substitute, Open Approach
0NUL37Z   Supplement Left Palatine Bone with Autologous Tissue Substitute, Percutaneous Approach
0NUL3JZ   Supplement Left Palatine Bone with Synthetic Substitute, Percutaneous Approach
0NUL3KZ   Supplement Left Palatine Bone with Nonautologous Tissue Substitute, Percutaneous Approach
0NUL47Z   Supplement Left Palatine Bone with Autologous Tissue Substitute, Percutaneous Endoscopic Approach
0NUL4JZ   Supplement Left Palatine Bone with Synthetic Substitute, Percutaneous Endoscopic Approach
0NUL4KZ   Supplement Left Palatine Bone with Nonautologous Tissue Substitute, Percutaneous Endoscopic Approach
0NUM07Z   Supplement Right Zygomatic Bone with Autologous Tissue Substitute, Open Approach
0NUM0JZ   Supplement Right Zygomatic Bone with Synthetic Substitute, Open Approach
0NUM0KZ   Supplement Right Zygomatic Bone with Nonautologous Tissue Substitute, Open Approach
0NUM37Z   Supplement Right Zygomatic Bone with Autologous Tissue Substitute, Percutaneous Approach
0NUM3JZ   Supplement Right Zygomatic Bone with Synthetic Substitute, Percutaneous Approach
0NUM3KZ   Supplement Right Zygomatic Bone with Nonautologous Tissue Substitute, Percutaneous Approach
0NUM47Z   Supplement Right Zygomatic Bone with Autologous Tissue Substitute, Percutaneous Endoscopic Approach
0NUM4JZ   Supplement Right Zygomatic Bone with Synthetic Substitute, Percutaneous Endoscopic Approach
0NUM4KZ   Supplement Right Zygomatic Bone with Nonautologous Tissue Substitute, Percutaneous Endoscopic Approach
0NUN07Z   Supplement Left Zygomatic Bone with Autologous Tissue Substitute, Open Approach
0NUN0JZ   Supplement Left Zygomatic Bone with Synthetic Substitute, Open Approach
0NUN0KZ   Supplement Left Zygomatic Bone with Nonautologous Tissue Substitute, Open Approach
0NUN37Z   Supplement Left Zygomatic Bone with Autologous Tissue Substitute, Percutaneous Approach
0NUN3JZ   Supplement Left Zygomatic Bone with Synthetic Substitute, Percutaneous Approach
0NUN3KZ   Supplement Left Zygomatic Bone with Nonautologous Tissue Substitute, Percutaneous Approach
0NUN47Z   Supplement Left Zygomatic Bone with Autologous Tissue Substitute, Percutaneous Endoscopic Approach

0NUN4JZ   Supplement Left Zygomatic Bone with Synthetic Substitute, Percutaneous Endoscopic Approach
0NUN4KZ   Supplement Left Zygomatic Bone with Nonautologous Tissue Substitute, Percutaneous Endoscopic Approach
0NUP07Z   Supplement Right Orbit with Autologous Tissue Substitute, Open Approach
0NUP0JZ   Supplement Right Orbit with Synthetic Substitute, Open Approach
0NUP0KZ   Supplement Right Orbit with Nonautologous Tissue Substitute, Open Approach
0NUP37Z   Supplement Right Orbit with Autologous Tissue Substitute, Percutaneous Approach
0NUP3JZ   Supplement Right Orbit with Synthetic Substitute, Percutaneous Approach
0NUP3KZ   Supplement Right Orbit with Nonautologous Tissue Substitute, Percutaneous Approach
0NUP47Z   Supplement Right Orbit with Autologous Tissue Substitute, Percutaneous Endoscopic Approach
0NUP4JZ   Supplement Right Orbit with Synthetic Substitute, Percutaneous Endoscopic Approach
0NUP4KZ   Supplement Right Orbit with Nonautologous Tissue Substitute, Percutaneous Endoscopic Approach
0NUQ07Z   Supplement Left Orbit with Autologous Tissue Substitute, Open Approach
0NUQ0JZ   Supplement Left Orbit with Synthetic Substitute, Open Approach
0NUQ0KZ   Supplement Left Orbit with Nonautologous Tissue Substitute, Open Approach
0NUQ37Z   Supplement Left Orbit with Autologous Tissue Substitute, Percutaneous Approach
0NUQ3JZ   Supplement Left Orbit with Synthetic Substitute, Percutaneous Approach
0NUQ3KZ   Supplement Left Orbit with Nonautologous Tissue Substitute, Percutaneous Approach
0NUQ47Z   Supplement Left Orbit with Autologous Tissue Substitute, Percutaneous Endoscopic Approach
0NUQ4JZ   Supplement Left Orbit with Synthetic Substitute, Percutaneous Endoscopic Approach
0NUQ4KZ   Supplement Left Orbit with Nonautologous Tissue Substitute, Percutaneous Endoscopic Approach
0NUR07Z   Supplement Right Maxilla with Autologous Tissue Substitute, Open Approach
0NUR0JZ   Supplement Right Maxilla with Synthetic Substitute, Open Approach
0NUR0KZ   Supplement Right Maxilla with Nonautologous Tissue Substitute, Open Approach
0NUR37Z   Supplement Right Maxilla with Autologous Tissue Substitute, Percutaneous Approach
0NUR3JZ   Supplement Right Maxilla with Synthetic Substitute, Percutaneous Approach
0NUR3KZ   Supplement Right Maxilla with Nonautologous Tissue Substitute, Percutaneous Approach
0NUR47Z   Supplement Right Maxilla with Autologous Tissue Substitute, Percutaneous Endoscopic Approach
0NUR4JZ   Supplement Right Maxilla with Synthetic Substitute, Percutaneous Endoscopic Approach
0NUR4KZ   Supplement Right Maxilla with Nonautologous Tissue Substitute, Percutaneous Endoscopic Approach

0NUS07Z   Supplement Left Maxilla with Autologous Tissue Substitute, Open Approach
0NUS0JZ   Supplement Left Maxilla with Synthetic Substitute, Open Approach
0NUS0KZ   Supplement Left Maxilla with Nonautologous Tissue Substitute, Open Approach
0NUS37Z   Supplement Left Maxilla with Autologous Tissue Substitute, Percutaneous Approach
0NUS3JZ   Supplement Left Maxilla with Synthetic Substitute, Percutaneous Approach
0NUS3KZ   Supplement Left Maxilla with Nonautologous Tissue Substitute, Percutaneous Approach
0NUS47Z   Supplement Left Maxilla with Autologous Tissue Substitute, Percutaneous Endoscopic Approach
0NUS4JZ   Supplement Left Maxilla with Synthetic Substitute, Percutaneous Endoscopic Approach
0NUS4KZ   Supplement Left Maxilla with Nonautologous Tissue Substitute, Percutaneous Endoscopic Approach
0NUT07Z   Supplement Right Mandible with Autologous Tissue Substitute, Open Approach
0NUT0JZ   Supplement Right Mandible with Synthetic Substitute, Open Approach
0NUT0KZ   Supplement Right Mandible with Nonautologous Tissue Substitute, Open Approach
0NUT37Z   Supplement Right Mandible with Autologous Tissue Substitute, Percutaneous Approach
0NUT3JZ   Supplement Right Mandible with Synthetic Substitute, Percutaneous Approach
0NUT3KZ   Supplement Right Mandible with Nonautologous Tissue Substitute, Percutaneous Approach
0NUT47Z   Supplement Right Mandible with Autologous Tissue Substitute, Percutaneous Endoscopic Approach
0NUT4JZ   Supplement Right Mandible with Synthetic Substitute, Percutaneous Endoscopic Approach
0NUT4KZ   Supplement Right Mandible with Nonautologous Tissue Substitute, Percutaneous Endoscopic Approach
0NUV07Z   Supplement Left Mandible with Autologous Tissue Substitute, Open Approach
0NUV0JZ   Supplement Left Mandible with Synthetic Substitute, Open Approach
0NUV0KZ   Supplement Left Mandible with Nonautologous Tissue Substitute, Open Approach
0NUV37Z   Supplement Left Mandible with Autologous Tissue Substitute, Percutaneous Approach
0NUV3JZ   Supplement Left Mandible with Synthetic Substitute, Percutaneous Approach
0NUV3KZ   Supplement Left Mandible with Nonautologous Tissue Substitute, Percutaneous Approach
0NUV47Z   Supplement Left Mandible with Autologous Tissue Substitute, Percutaneous Endoscopic Approach
0NUV4JZ   Supplement Left Mandible with Synthetic Substitute, Percutaneous Endoscopic Approach
0NUV4KZ   Supplement Left Mandible with Nonautologous Tissue Substitute, Percutaneous Endoscopic Approach
0NUX07Z   Supplement Hyoid Bone with Autologous Tissue Substitute, Open Approach

0NUX0JZ Supplement Hyoid Bone with Synthetic Substitute, Open Approach
0NUX0KZ Supplement Hyoid Bone with Nonautologous Tissue Substitute, Open Approach
0NUX37Z Supplement Hyoid Bone with Autologous Tissue Substitute, Percutaneous Approach

0NUX3JZ Supplement Hyoid Bone with Synthetic Substitute, Percutaneous Approach
0NUX3KZ Supplement Hyoid Bone with Nonautologous Tissue Substitute, Percutaneous Approach
0NUX47Z Supplement Hyoid Bone with Autologous Tissue Substitute, Percutaneous Endoscopic Approach

0NUX4JZ Supplement Hyoid Bone with Synthetic Substitute, Percutaneous Endoscopic Approach
0NUX4KZ Supplement Hyoid Bone with Nonautologous Tissue Substitute, Percutaneous Endoscopic Approach

0NW – Head and Facial Bones, Revision

Review Coding Guideline B6.1c

0NW000Z Revision of Drainage Device in Skull, Open Approach
0NW004Z Revision of Internal Fixation Device in Skull, Open Approach
0NW005Z Revision of External Fixation Device in Skull, Open Approach
0NW007Z Revision of Autologous Tissue Substitute in Skull, Open Approach
0NW00JZ Revision of Synthetic Substitute in Skull, Open Approach
0NW00KZ Revision of Nonautologous Tissue Substitute in Skull, Open Approach
0NW00MZ Revision of Bone Growth Stimulator in Skull, Open Approach
0NW00NZ Revision of Neurostimulator Generator in Skull, Open Approach
0NW00SZ Revision of Hearing Device in Skull, Open Approach
0NW030Z Revision of Drainage Device in Skull, Percutaneous Approach
0NW034Z Revision of Internal Fixation Device in Skull, Percutaneous Approach
0NW035Z Revision of External Fixation Device in Skull, Percutaneous Approach
0NW037Z Revision of Autologous Tissue Substitute in Skull, Percutaneous Approach
0NW03JZ Revision of Synthetic Substitute in Skull, Percutaneous Approach
0NW03KZ Revision of Nonautologous Tissue Substitute in Skull, Percutaneous Approach
0NW03MZ Revision of Bone Growth Stimulator in Skull, Percutaneous Approach
0NW03SZ Revision of Hearing Device in Skull, Percutaneous Approach
0NW040Z Revision of Drainage Device in Skull, Percutaneous Endoscopic Approach
0NW044Z Revision of Internal Fixation Device in Skull, Percutaneous Endoscopic Approach
0NW045Z Revision of External Fixation Device in Skull, Percutaneous Endoscopic Approach
0NW047Z Revision of Autologous Tissue Substitute in Skull, Percutaneous Endoscopic Approach
0NW04JZ Revision of Synthetic Substitute in Skull, Percutaneous Endoscopic Approach
0NW04KZ Revision of Nonautologous Tissue Substitute in Skull, Percutaneous Endoscopic Approach
0NW04MZ Revision of Bone Growth Stimulator in Skull, Percutaneous Endoscopic Approach
0NW04SZ Revision of Hearing Device in Skull, Percutaneous Endoscopic Approach
0NW0X0Z Revision of Drainage Device in Skull, External Approach
0NW0X4Z Revision of Internal Fixation Device in Skull, External Approach
0NW0X5Z Revision of External Fixation Device in Skull, External Approach
0NW0X7Z Revision of Autologous Tissue Substitute in Skull, External Approach

0NW0XJZ Revision of Synthetic Substitute in Skull, External Approach
0NW0XKZ Revision of Nonautologous Tissue Substitute in Skull, External Approach
0NW0XMZ Revision of Bone Growth Stimulator in Skull, External Approach
0NW0XSZ Revision of Hearing Device in Skull, External Approach
0NWB00Z Revision of Drainage Device in Nasal Bone, Open Approach
0NWB04Z Revision of Internal Fixation Device in Nasal Bone, Open Approach
0NWB07Z Revision of Autologous Tissue Substitute in Nasal Bone, Open Approach
0NWB0JZ Revision of Synthetic Substitute in Nasal Bone, Open Approach
0NWB0KZ Revision of Nonautologous Tissue Substitute in Nasal Bone, Open Approach
0NWB0MZ Revision of Bone Growth Stimulator in Nasal Bone, Open Approach
0NWB30Z Revision of Drainage Device in Nasal Bone, Percutaneous Approach
0NWB34Z Revision of Internal Fixation Device in Nasal Bone, Percutaneous Approach
0NWB37Z Revision of Autologous Tissue Substitute in Nasal Bone, Percutaneous Approach
0NWB3JZ Revision of Synthetic Substitute in Nasal Bone, Percutaneous Approach
0NWB3KZ Revision of Nonautologous Tissue Substitute in Nasal Bone, Percutaneous Approach
0NWB3MZ Revision of Bone Growth Stimulator in Nasal Bone, Percutaneous Approach
0NWB40Z Revision of Drainage Device in Nasal Bone, Percutaneous Endoscopic Approach
0NWB44Z Revision of Internal Fixation Device in Nasal Bone, Percutaneous Endoscopic Approach
0NWB47Z Revision of Autologous Tissue Substitute in Nasal Bone, Percutaneous Endoscopic Approach
0NWB4JZ Revision of Synthetic Substitute in Nasal Bone, Percutaneous Endoscopic Approach
0NWB4KZ Revision of Nonautologous Tissue Substitute in Nasal Bone, Percutaneous Endoscopic Approach
0NWB4MZ Revision of Bone Growth Stimulator in Nasal Bone, Percutaneous Endoscopic Approach
0NWBX0Z Revision of Drainage Device in Nasal Bone, External Approach
0NWBX4Z Revision of Internal Fixation Device in Nasal Bone, External Approach
0NWBX7Z Revision of Autologous Tissue Substitute in Nasal Bone, External Approach
0NWBXJZ Revision of Synthetic Substitute in Nasal Bone, External Approach
0NWBXKZ Revision of Nonautologous Tissue Substitute in Nasal Bone, External Approach

0NWBXMZ Revision of Bone Growth Stimulator in Nasal Bone, External Approach
0NWW00Z Revision of Drainage Device in Facial Bone, Open Approach
0NWW04Z Revision of Internal Fixation Device in Facial Bone, Open Approach
0NWW07Z Revision of Autologous Tissue Substitute in Facial Bone, Open Approach
0NWW0JZ Revision of Synthetic Substitute in Facial Bone, Open Approach
0NWW0KZ Revision of Nonautologous Tissue Substitute in Facial Bone, Open Approach
0NWW0MZ Revision of Bone Growth Stimulator in Facial Bone, Open Approach
0NWW30Z Revision of Drainage Device in Facial Bone, Percutaneous Approach
0NWW34Z Revision of Internal Fixation Device in Facial Bone, Percutaneous Approach
0NWW37Z Revision of Autologous Tissue Substitute in Facial Bone, Percutaneous Approach
0NWW3JZ Revision of Synthetic Substitute in Facial Bone, Percutaneous Approach
0NWW3KZ Revision of Nonautologous Tissue Substitute in Facial Bone, Percutaneous Approach
0NWW3MZ Revision of Bone Growth Stimulator in Facial Bone, Percutaneous Approach
0NWW40Z Revision of Drainage Device in Facial Bone, Percutaneous Endoscopic Approach
0NWW44Z Revision of Internal Fixation Device in Facial Bone, Percutaneous Endoscopic Approach
0NWW47Z Revision of Autologous Tissue Substitute in Facial Bone, Percutaneous Endoscopic Approach
0NWW4JZ Revision of Synthetic Substitute in Facial Bone, Percutaneous Endoscopic Approach
0NWW4KZ Revision of Nonautologous Tissue Substitute in Facial Bone, Percutaneous Endoscopic Approach
0NWW4MZ Revision of Bone Growth Stimulator in Facial Bone, Percutaneous Endoscopic Approach
0NWWX0Z Revision of Drainage Device in Facial Bone, External Approach
0NWWX4Z Revision of Internal Fixation Device in Facial Bone, External Approach
0NWWX7Z Revision of Autologous Tissue Substitute in Facial Bone, External Approach
0NWWXJZ Revision of Synthetic Substitute in Facial Bone, External Approach
0NWWXKZ Revision of Nonautologous Tissue Substitute in Facial Bone, External Approach
0NWWXMZ Revision of Bone Growth Stimulator in Facial Bone, External Approach

♀ Female-only   ♂ Male-only   ▲ Limited Coverage   ● Non-OR   ▬ HAC-associated procedure   ▲ Non-covered procedures   ✚ Combination

Bones - Front and Back Views

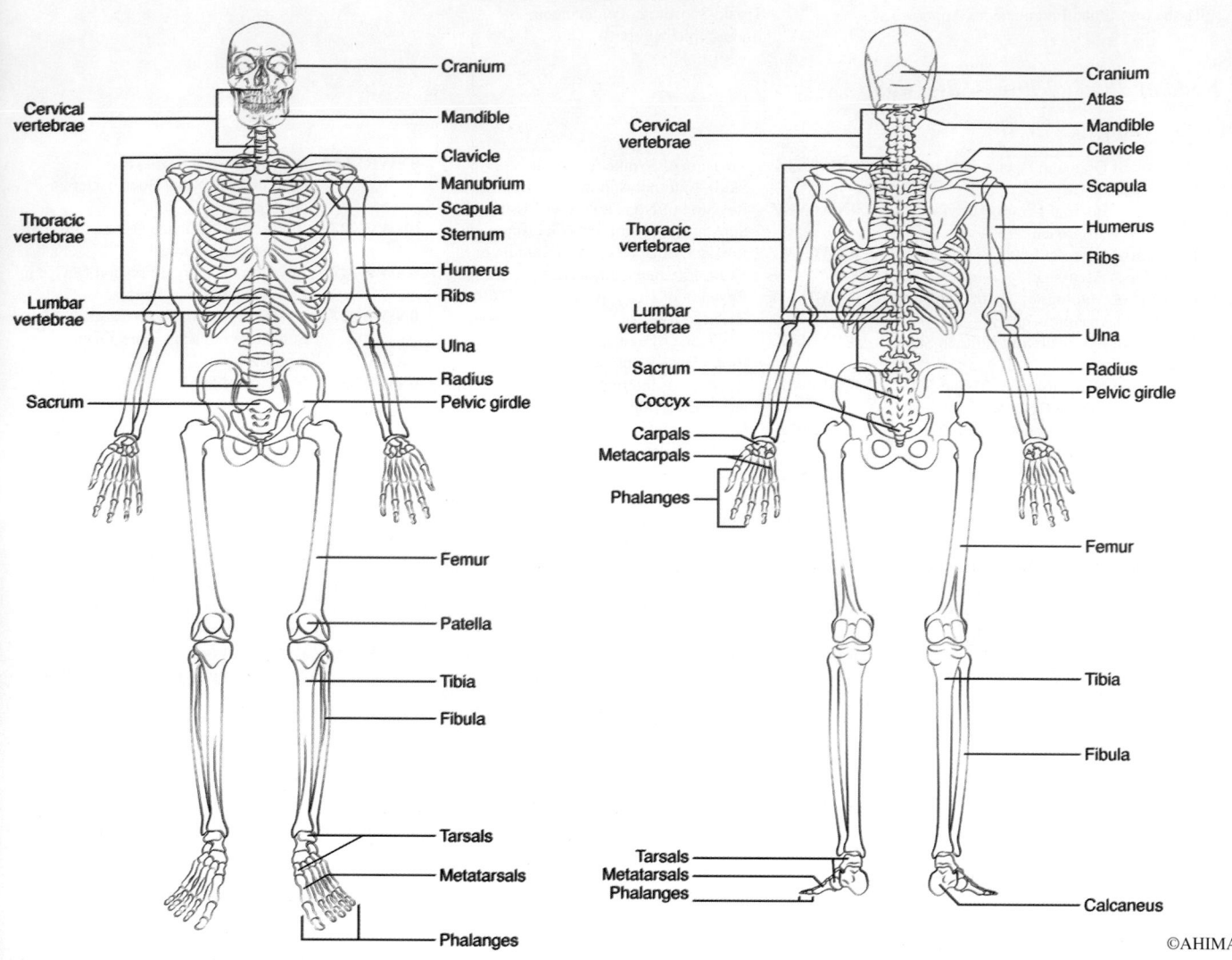

©AHIMA

Vertebrae

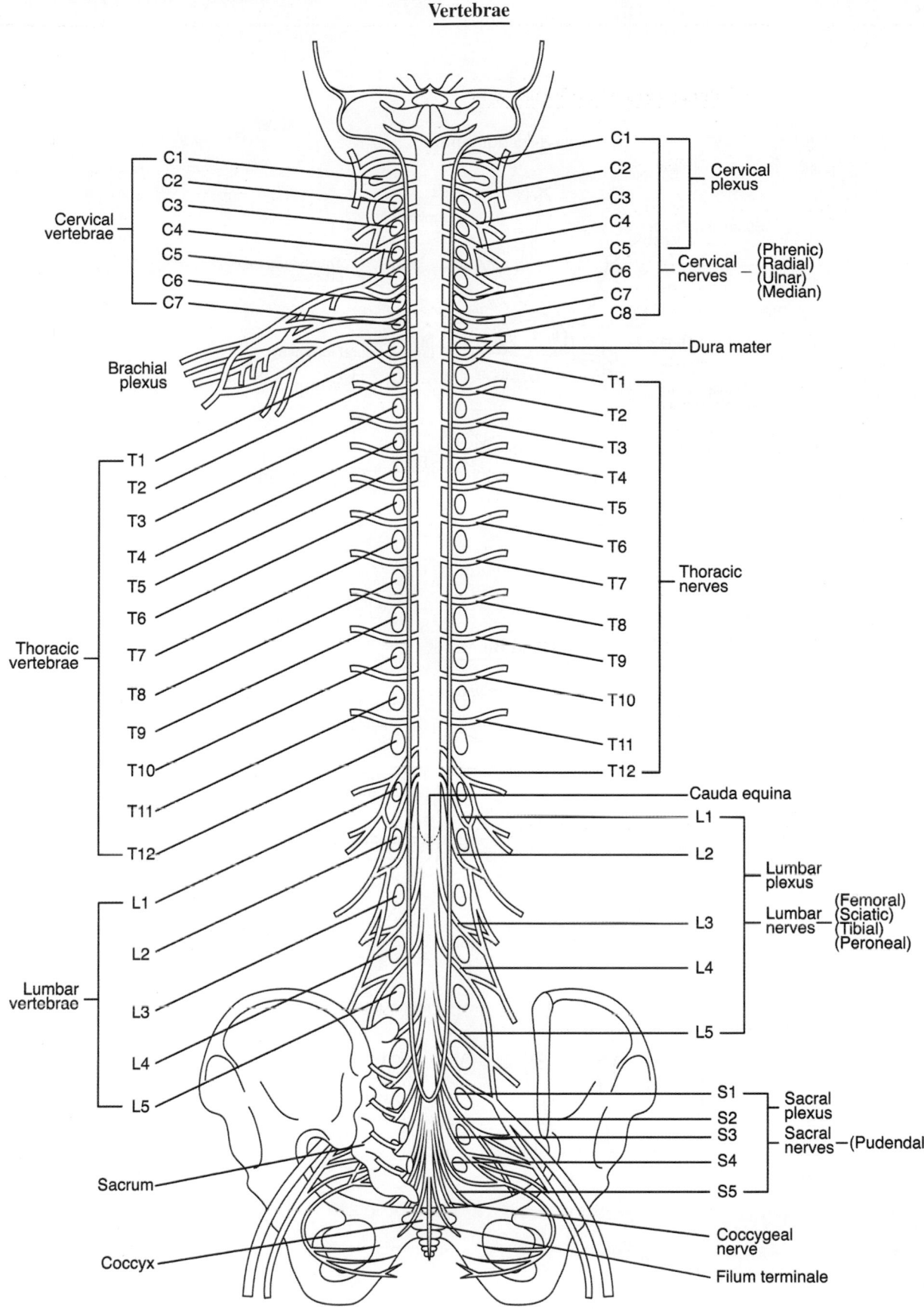

Cervical vertebrae — C1, C2, C3, C4, C5, C6, C7

C1, C2, C3, C4 — Cervical plexus

C5, C6, C7, C8 — Cervical nerves — (Phrenic) (Radial) (Ulnar) (Median)

Brachial plexus

Dura mater

Thoracic vertebrae — T1, T2, T3, T4, T5, T6, T7, T8, T9, T10, T11, T12

T1, T2, T3, T4, T5, T6, T7, T8, T9, T10, T11, T12 — Thoracic nerves

Cauda equina

Lumbar vertebrae — L1, L2, L3, L4, L5

L1, L2 — Lumbar plexus

L3 — Lumbar nerves — (Femoral) (Sciatic) (Tibial) (Peroneal)

L4, L5

S1, S2 — Sacral plexus

S3 — Sacral nerves — (Pudendal)

S4, S5

Sacrum

Coccyx

Coccygeal nerve

Filum terminale

Cross-section Spine

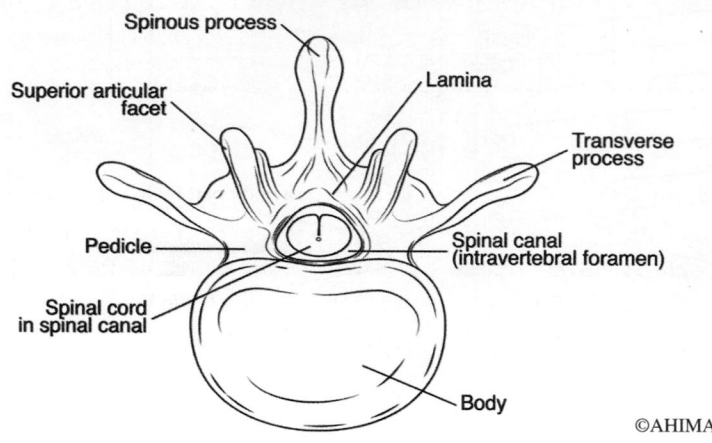

Spinous process

Superior articular facet

Lamina

Transverse process

Pedicle

Spinal canal (intravertebral foramen)

Spinal cord in spinal canal

Body

©AHIMA

Hand Bones

Ulna

Radius

Lunate (semilunar)

Scaphoid (navicular)

Triangular (triquetrum)

Capitate

Carpals

Pisiform

Trapezoid (lesser multangular)

Hamate (unciform)

Trapezium (greater multangular)

Carpals

Metacarpals

1

5 4 3 2

Phalanges

Proimal phalanx

Middle phalanx

Distal phalanx

©AHIMA

Upper Bones Tables 0P2–0PW

Section	0	Medical and Surgical
Body System	P	Upper Bones
Operation	2	**Change:** Taking out or off a device from a body part and putting back an identical or similar device in or on the same body part without cutting or puncturing the skin or a mucous membrane

Body Part (4th)	Approach (5th)	Device (6th)	Qualifier (7th)
Y Upper Bone	X External	0 Drainage Device Y Other Device	Z No Qualifier

Section	0	Medical and Surgical
Body System	P	Upper Bones
Operation	5	**Destruction:** Physical eradication of all or a portion of a body part by the direct use of energy, force, or a destructive agent

Body Part (4th)	Approach (5th)	Device (6th)	Qualifier (7th)
0 Sternum 1 Rib, Right 2 Rib, Left 3 Cervical Vertebra 4 Thoracic Vertebra 5 Scapula, Right 6 Scapula, Left 7 Glenoid Cavity, Right 8 Glenoid Cavity, Left 9 Clavicle, Right B Clavicle, Left C Humeral Head, Right D Humeral Head, Left F Humeral Shaft, Right G Humeral Shaft, Left H Radius, Right J Radius, Left K Ulna, Right L Ulna, Left M Carpal, Right N Carpal, Left P Metacarpal, Right Q Metacarpal, Left R Thumb Phalanx, Right S Thumb Phalanx, Left T Finger Phalanx, Right V Finger Phalanx, Left	0 Open 3 Percutaneous 4 Percutaneous Endoscopic	Z No Device	Z No Qualifier

Section	0	Medical and Surgical
Body System	P	Upper Bones
Operation	8	**Division:** Cutting into a body part, without draining fluids and/or gases from the body part, in order to separate or transect a body part

Body Part (4ᵗʰ)	Approach (5ᵗʰ)	Device (6ᵗʰ)	Qualifier (7ᵗʰ)
0 Sternum	0 Open	Z No Device	Z No Qualifier
1 Rib, Right	3 Percutaneous		
2 Rib, Left	4 Percutaneous Endoscopic		
3 Cervical Vertebra			
4 Thoracic Vertebra			
5 Scapula, Right			
6 Scapula, Left			
7 Glenoid Cavity, Right			
8 Glenoid Cavity, Left			
9 Clavicle, Right			
B Clavicle, Left			
C Humeral Head, Right			
D Humeral Head, Left			
F Humeral Shaft, Right			
G Humeral Shaft, Left			
H Radius, Right			
J Radius, Left			
K Ulna, Right			
L Ulna, Left			
M Carpal, Right			
N Carpal, Left			
P Metacarpal, Right			
Q Metacarpal, Left			
R Thumb Phalanx, Right			
S Thumb Phalanx, Left			
T Finger Phalanx, Right			
V Finger Phalanx, Left			

Section	0	Medical and Surgical
Body System	P	Upper Bones
Operation	9	**Drainage:** Taking or letting out fluids and/or gases from a body part

Body Part (4ᵗʰ)	Approach (5ᵗʰ)	Device (6ᵗʰ)	Qualifier (7ᵗʰ)
0 Sternum	0 Open	0 Drainage Device	Z No Qualifier
1 Rib, Right	3 Percutaneous		
2 Rib, Left	4 Percutaneous Endoscopic		
3 Cervical Vertebra			
4 Thoracic Vertebra			
5 Scapula, Right			
6 Scapula, Left			
7 Glenoid Cavity, Right			
8 Glenoid Cavity, Left			
9 Clavicle, Right			
B Clavicle, Left			
C Humeral Head, Right			
D Humeral Head, Left			
F Humeral Shaft, Right			
G Humeral Shaft, Left			
H Radius, Right			
J Radius, Left			
K Ulna, Right			
L Ulna, Left			
M Carpal, Right			
N Carpal, Left			
P Metacarpal, Right			
Q Metacarpal, Left			
R Thumb Phalanx, Right			
S Thumb Phalanx, Left			
T Finger Phalanx, Right			
V Finger Phalanx, Left			

Continued →

Section	0	Medical and Surgical
Body System	P	Upper Bones
Operation	9	Drainage: Taking or letting out fluids and/or gases from a body part

Body Part (4th)	Approach (5th)	Device (6th)	Qualifier (7th)
0 Sternum	0 Open	Z No Device	X Diagnostic
1 Rib, Right	3 Percutaneous		Z No Qualifier
2 Rib, Left	4 Percutaneous Endoscopic		
3 Cervical Vertebra			
4 Thoracic Vertebra			
5 Scapula, Right			
6 Scapula, Left			
7 Glenoid Cavity, Right			
8 Glenoid Cavity, Left			
9 Clavicle, Right			
B Clavicle, Left			
C Humeral Head, Right			
D Humeral Head, Left			
F Humeral Shaft, Right			
G Humeral Shaft, Left			
H Radius, Right			
J Radius, Left			
K Ulna, Right			
L Ulna, Left			
M Carpal, Right			
N Carpal, Left			
P Metacarpal, Right			
Q Metacarpal, Left			
R Thumb Phalanx, Right			
S Thumb Phalanx, Left			
T Finger Phalanx, Right			
V Finger Phalanx, Left			

Section	0	Medical and Surgical
Body System	P	Upper Bones
Operation	B	Excision: Cutting out or off, without replacement, a portion of a body part

Body Part (4th)	Approach (5th)	Device (6th)	Qualifier (7th)
0 Sternum	0 Open	Z No Device	X Diagnostic
1 Rib, Right	3 Percutaneous		Z No Qualifier
2 Rib, Left	4 Percutaneous Endoscopic		
3 Cervical Vertebra			
4 Thoracic Vertebra			
5 Scapula, Right			
6 Scapula, Left			
7 Glenoid Cavity, Right			
8 Glenoid Cavity, Left			
9 Clavicle, Right			
B Clavicle, Left			
C Humeral Head, Right			
D Humeral Head, Left			
F Humeral Shaft, Right			
G Humeral Shaft, Left			
H Radius, Right			
J Radius, Left			
K Ulna, Right			
L Ulna, Left			
M Carpal, Right			
N Carpal, Left			
P Metacarpal, Right			
Q Metacarpal, Left			
R Thumb Phalanx, Right			
S Thumb Phalanx, Left			
T Finger Phalanx, Right			
V Finger Phalanx, Left			

Section   0   **Medical and Surgical**
Body System   P   **Upper Bones**
Operation   C   **Extirpation:** Taking or cutting out solid matter from a body part

Body Part (4th)	Approach (5th)	Device (6th)	Qualifier (7th)
0 Sternum 1 Rib, Right 2 Rib, Left 3 Cervical Vertebra 4 Thoracic Vertebra 5 Scapula, Right 6 Scapula, Left 7 Glenoid Cavity, Right 8 Glenoid Cavity, Left 9 Clavicle, Right B Clavicle, Left C Humeral Head, Right D Humeral Head, Left F Humeral Shaft, Right G Humeral Shaft, Left H Radius, Right J Radius, Left K Ulna, Right L Ulna, Left M Carpal, Right N Carpal, Left P Metacarpal, Right Q Metacarpal, Left R Thumb Phalanx, Right S Thumb Phalanx, Left T Finger Phalanx, Right V Finger Phalanx, Left	0 Open 3 Percutaneous 4 Percutaneous Endoscopic	Z No Device	Z No Qualifier

Section   0   **Medical and Surgical**
Body System   P   **Upper Bones**
Operation   H   **Insertion:** Putting in a nonbiological appliance that monitors, assists, performs, or prevents a physiological function but does not physically take the place of a body part

Body Part (4th)	Approach (5th)	Device (6th)	Qualifier (7th)
0 Sternum	0 Open 3 Percutaneous 4 Percutaneous Endoscopic	0 Internal Fixation Device, Rigid Plate 4 Internal Fixation Device	Z No Qualifier
1 Rib, Right 2 Rib, Left 3 Cervical Vertebra 4 Thoracic Vertebra 5 Scapula, Right 6 Scapula, Left 7 Glenoid Cavity, Right 8 Glenoid Cavity, Left 9 Clavicle, Right B Clavicle, Left	0 Open 3 Percutaneous 4 Percutaneous Endoscopic	4 Internal Fixation Device	Z No Qualifier
C Humeral Head, Right D Humeral Head, Left F Humeral Shaft, Right G Humeral Shaft, Left H Radius, Right J Radius, Left K Ulna, Right L Ulna, Left	0 Open 3 Percutaneous 4 Percutaneous Endoscopic	4 Internal Fixation Device 5 External Fixation Device 6 Internal Fixation Device, Intramedullary 8 External Fixation Device, Limb Lengthening B External Fixation Device, Monoplanar C External Fixation Device, Ring D External Fixation Device, Hybrid	Z No Qualifier

Continued →

Section 0 Medical and Surgical
Body System P Upper Bones
Operation H Insertion: Putting in a nonbiological appliance that monitors, assists, performs, or prevents a physiological function but does not physically take the place of a body part

Body Part (4th)	Approach (5th)	Device (6th)	Qualifier (7th)
M Carpal, Right N Carpal, Left P Metacarpal, Right Q Metacarpal, Left R Thumb Phalanx, Right S Thumb Phalanx, Left T Finger Phalanx, Right V Finger Phalanx, Left	0 Open 3 Percutaneous 4 Percutaneous Endoscopic	4 Internal Fixation Device 5 External Fixation Device	Z No Qualifier
Y Upper Bone	0 Open 3 Percutaneous 4 Percutaneous Endoscopic	M Bone Growth Stimulator	Z No Qualifier

Section 0 Medical and Surgical
Body System P Upper Bones
Operation J Inspection: Visually and/or manually exploring a body part

Body Part (4th)	Approach (5th)	Device (6th)	Qualifier (7th)
Y Upper Bone	0 Open 3 Percutaneous 4 Percutaneous Endoscopic X External	Z No Device	Z No Qualifier

Section 0 Medical and Surgical
Body System P Upper Bones
Operation N Release: Freeing a body part from an abnormal physical constraint by cutting or by the use of force

Body Part (4th)	Approach (5th)	Device (6th)	Qualifier (7th)
0 Sternum 1 Rib, Right 2 Rib, Left 3 Cervical Vertebra 4 Thoracic Vertebra 5 Scapula, Right 6 Scapula, Left 7 Glenoid Cavity, Right 8 Glenoid Cavity, Left 9 Clavicle, Right B Clavicle, Left C Humeral Head, Right D Humeral Head, Left F Humeral Shaft, Right G Humeral Shaft, Left H Radius, Right J Radius, Left K Ulna, Right L Ulna, Left M Carpal, Right N Carpal, Left P Metacarpal, Right Q Metacarpal, Left R Thumb Phalanx, Right S Thumb Phalanx, Left T Finger Phalanx, Right V Finger Phalanx, Left	0 Open 3 Percutaneous 4 Percutaneous Endoscopic	Z No Device	Z No Qualifier

Section 0 Medical and Surgical
Body System P Upper Bones
Operation P Removal: Taking out or off a device from a body part

Body Part (4th)	Approach (5th)	Device (6th)	Qualifier (7th)
0 Sternum 1 Rib, Right 2 Rib, Left 3 Cervical Vertebra 4 Thoracic Vertebra 5 Scapula, Right 6 Scapula, Left 7 Glenoid Cavity, Right 8 Glenoid Cavity, Left 9 Clavicle, Right B Clavicle, Left	0 Open 3 Percutaneous 4 Percutaneous Endoscopic	4 Internal Fixation Device 7 Autologous Tissue Substitute J Synthetic Substitute K Nonautologous Tissue Substitute	Z No Qualifier
0 Sternum 1 Rib, Right 2 Rib, Left 3 Cervical Vertebra 4 Thoracic Vertebra 5 Scapula, Right 6 Scapula, Left 7 Glenoid Cavity, Right 8 Glenoid Cavity, Left 9 Clavicle, Right B Clavicle, Left	X External	4 Internal Fixation Device	Z No Qualifier
C Humeral Head, Right D Humeral Head, Left F Humeral Shaft, Right G Humeral Shaft, Left H Radius, Right J Radius, Left K Ulna, Right L Ulna, Left M Carpal, Right N Carpal, Left P Metacarpal, Right Q Metacarpal, Left R Thumb Phalanx, Right S Thumb Phalanx, Left T Finger Phalanx, Right V Finger Phalanx, Left	0 Open 3 Percutaneous 4 Percutaneous Endoscopic	4 Internal Fixation Device 5 External Fixation Device 7 Autologous Tissue Substitute J Synthetic Substitute K Nonautologous Tissue Substitute	Z No Qualifier
C Humeral Head, Right D Humeral Head, Left F Humeral Shaft, Right G Humeral Shaft, Left H Radius, Right J Radius, Left K Ulna, Right L Ulna, Left M Carpal, Right N Carpal, Left P Metacarpal, Right Q Metacarpal, Left R Thumb Phalanx, Right S Thumb Phalanx, Left T Finger Phalanx, Right V Finger Phalanx, Left	X External	4 Internal Fixation Device 5 External Fixation Device	Z No Qualifier
Y Upper Bone	0 Open 3 Percutaneous 4 Percutaneous Endoscopic X External	0 Drainage Device M Bone Growth Stimulator	Z No Qualifier

Section   0   Medical and Surgical
Body System   P   Upper Bones
Operation   Q   **Repair:** Restoring, to the extent possible, a body part to its normal anatomic structure and function

Body Part (4th)	Approach (5th)	Device (6th)	Qualifier (7th)
0 Sternum	0 Open	Z No Device	Z No Qualifier
1 Rib, Right	3 Percutaneous		
2 Rib, Left	4 Percutaneous Endoscopic		
3 Cervical Vertebra	X External		
4 Thoracic Vertebra			
5 Scapula, Right			
6 Scapula, Left			
7 Glenoid Cavity, Right			
8 Glenoid Cavity, Left			
9 Clavicle, Right			
B Clavicle, Left			
C Humeral Head, Right			
D Humeral Head, Left			
F Humeral Shaft, Right			
G Humeral Shaft, Left			
H Radius, Right			
J Radius, Left			
K Ulna, Right			
L Ulna, Left			
M Carpal, Right			
N Carpal, Left			
P Metacarpal, Right			
Q Metacarpal, Left			
R Thumb Phalanx, Right			
S Thumb Phalanx, Left			
T Finger Phalanx, Right			
V Finger Phalanx, Left			

Section   0   Medical and Surgical
Body System   P   Upper Bones
Operation   R   **Replacement:** Putting in or on biological or synthetic material that physically takes the place and/or function of all or a portion of a body part

Body Part (4th)	Approach (5th)	Device (6th)	Qualifier (7th)
0 Sternum	0 Open	7 Autologous Tissue Substitute	Z No Qualifier
1 Rib, Right	3 Percutaneous	J Synthetic Substitute	
2 Rib, Left	4 Percutaneous Endoscopic	K Nonautologous Tissue Substitute	
3 Cervical Vertebra			
4 Thoracic Vertebra			
5 Scapula, Right			
6 Scapula, Left			
7 Glenoid Cavity, Right			
8 Glenoid Cavity, Left			
9 Clavicle, Right			
B Clavicle, Left			
C Humeral Head, Right			
D Humeral Head, Left			
F Humeral Shaft, Right			
G Humeral Shaft, Left			
H Radius, Right			
J Radius, Left			
K Ulna, Right			
L Ulna, Left			
M Carpal, Right			
N Carpal, Left			
P Metacarpal, Right			
Q Metacarpal, Left			
R Thumb Phalanx, Right			
S Thumb Phalanx, Left			
T Finger Phalanx, Right			
V Finger Phalanx, Left			

Section	0	Medical and Surgical
Body System	P	Upper Bones
Operation	S	Reposition: Moving to its normal location, or other suitable location, all or a portion of a body part

Body Part (4th)	Approach (5th)	Device (6th)	Qualifier (7th)
0 Sternum	0 Open 3 Percutaneous 4 Percutaneous Endoscopic	0 Internal Fixation Device, Rigid Plate 4 Internal Fixation Device Z No Device	Z No Qualifier
0 Sternum	X External	Z No Device	Z No Qualifier
1 Rib, Right 2 Rib, Left 3 Cervical Vertebra 4 Thoracic Vertebra 5 Scapula, Right 6 Scapula, Left 7 Glenoid Cavity, Right 8 Glenoid Cavity, Left 9 Clavicle, Right B Clavicle, Left	0 Open 3 Percutaneous 4 Percutaneous Endoscopic	4 Internal Fixation Device Z No Device	Z No Qualifier
1 Rib, Right 2 Rib, Left 3 Cervical Vertebra 4 Thoracic Vertebra 5 Scapula, Right 6 Scapula, Left 7 Glenoid Cavity, Right 8 Glenoid Cavity, Left 9 Clavicle, Right B Clavicle, Left	X External	Z No Device	Z No Qualifier
C Humeral Head, Right D Humeral Head, Left F Humeral Shaft, Right G Humeral Shaft, Left H Radius, Right J Radius, Left K Ulna, Right L Ulna, Left	0 Open 3 Percutaneous 4 Percutaneous Endoscopic	4 Internal Fixation Device 5 External Fixation Device 6 Internal Fixation Device, Intramedullary B External Fixation Device, Monoplanar C External Fixation Device, Ring D External Fixation Device, Hybrid Z No Device	Z No Qualifier
C Humeral Head, Right D Humeral Head, Left F Humeral Shaft, Right G Humeral Shaft, Left H Radius, Right J Radius, Left K Ulna, Right L Ulna, Left	X External	Z No Device	Z No Qualifier
M Carpal, Right N Carpal, Left P Metacarpal, Right Q Metacarpal, Left R Thumb Phalanx, Right S Thumb Phalanx, Left T Finger Phalanx, Right V Finger Phalanx, Left	0 Open 3 Percutaneous 4 Percutaneous Endoscopic	4 Internal Fixation Device 5 External Fixation Device Z No Device	Z No Qualifier
M Carpal, Right N Carpal, Left P Metacarpal, Right Q Metacarpal, Left R Thumb Phalanx, Right S Thumb Phalanx, Left T Finger Phalanx, Right V Finger Phalanx, Left	X External	Z No Device	Z No Qualifier

tion	0	Medical and Surgical
dy System	P	Upper Bones
eration	T	Resection: Cutting out or off, without replacement, all of a body part

Body Part (4th)	Approach (5th)	Device (6th)	Qualifier (7th)
Sternum Rib, Right Rib, Left Scapula, Right Scapula, Left Glenoid Cavity, Right Glenoid Cavity, Left Clavicle, Right Clavicle, Left Humeral Head, Right Humeral Head, Left Humeral Shaft, Right Humeral Shaft, Left Radius, Right Radius, Left Ulna, Right Ulna, Left Carpal, Right Carpal, Left Metacarpal, Right Metacarpal, Left Thumb Phalanx, Right Thumb Phalanx, Left Finger Phalanx, Right Finger Phalanx, Left	0 Open	Z No Device	Z No Qualifier

ction	0	Medical and Surgical
dy System	P	Upper Bones
eration	U	Supplement: Putting in or on biological or synthetic material that physically reinforces and/or augments the function of a portion of a body part

Body Part (4th)	Approach (5th)	Device (6th)	Qualifier (7th)
Sternum Rib, Right Rib, Left Cervical Vertebra Thoracic Vertebra Scapula, Right Scapula, Left Glenoid Cavity, Right Glenoid Cavity, Left Clavicle, Right Clavicle, Left Humeral Head, Right Humeral Head, Left Humeral Shaft, Right Humeral Shaft, Left Radius, Right Radius, Left Ulna, Right Ulna, Left Carpal, Right Carpal, Left Metacarpal, Right Metacarpal, Left Thumb Phalanx, Right Thumb Phalanx, Left Finger Phalanx, Right Finger Phalanx, Left	0 Open 3 Percutaneous 4 Percutaneous Endoscopic	7 Autologous Tissue Substitute J Synthetic Substitute K Nonautologous Tissue Substitute	Z No Qualifier

Section   0   Medical and Surgical
Body System   P   Upper Bones
Operation   W   **Revision:** Correcting, to the extent possible, a portion of a malfunctioning device or the position of a displaced device

Body Part (4th)	Approach (5th)	Device (6th)	Qualifier (7th)
0 Sternum 1 Rib, Right 2 Rib, Left 3 Cervical Vertebra 4 Thoracic Vertebra 5 Scapula, Right 6 Scapula, Left 7 Glenoid Cavity, Right 8 Glenoid Cavity, Left 9 Clavicle, Right B Clavicle, Left	0 Open 3 Percutaneous 4 Percutaneous Endoscopic X External	4 Internal Fixation Device 7 Autologous Tissue Substitute J Synthetic Substitute K Nonautologous Tissue Substitute	Z No Qualifier
C Humeral Head, Right D Humeral Head, Left F Humeral Shaft, Right G Humeral Shaft, Left H Radius, Right J Radius, Left K Ulna, Right L Ulna, Left M Carpal, Right N Carpal, Left P Metacarpal, Right Q Metacarpal, Left R Thumb Phalanx, Right S Thumb Phalanx, Left T Finger Phalanx, Right V Finger Phalanx, Left	0 Open 3 Percutaneous 4 Percutaneous Endoscopic X External	4 Internal Fixation Device 5 External Fixation Device 7 Autologous Tissue Substitute J Synthetic Substitute K Nonautologous Tissue Substitute	Z No Qualifier
Y Upper Bone	0 Open 3 Percutaneous 4 Percutaneous Endoscopic X External	0 Drainage Device M Bone Growth Stimulator	Z No Qualifier

Upper Bones Code Listing 0P2–0PW

0P2 – Upper Bones, Change

Review Coding Guideline B6.1c

0P2YX0Z Change Drainage Device in Upper Bone,
         External Approach

0P2YXYZ Change Other Device in Upper Bone,
         External Approach

0P5 – Upper Bones, Destruction

0P500ZZ Destruction of Sternum, Open Approach
0P503ZZ Destruction of Sternum, Percutaneous
         Approach
0P504ZZ Destruction of Sternum, Percutaneous
         Endoscopic Approach
0P510ZZ Destruction of Right Rib, Open Approach
0P513ZZ Destruction of Right Rib, Percutaneous
         Approach
0P514ZZ Destruction of Right Rib, Percutaneous
         Endoscopic Approach
0P520ZZ Destruction of Left Rib, Open Approach
0P523ZZ Destruction of Left Rib, Percutaneous
         Approach
0P524ZZ Destruction of Left Rib, Percutaneous
         Endoscopic Approach
0P530ZZ Destruction of Cervical Vertebra, Open
         Approach
0P533ZZ Destruction of Cervical Vertebra,
         Percutaneous Approach

0P534ZZ Destruction of Cervical Vertebra,
         Percutaneous Endoscopic Approach
0P540ZZ Destruction of Thoracic Vertebra, Open
         Approach
0P543ZZ Destruction of Thoracic Vertebra,
         Percutaneous Approach
0P544ZZ Destruction of Thoracic Vertebra,
         Percutaneous Endoscopic Approach
0P550ZZ Destruction of Right Scapula, Open
         Approach
0P553ZZ Destruction of Right Scapula,
         Percutaneous Approach
0P554ZZ Destruction of Right Scapula,
         Percutaneous Endoscopic
         Approach
0P560ZZ Destruction of Left Scapula, Open
         Approach
0P563ZZ Destruction of Left Scapula, Percutaneous
         Approach

0P564ZZ Destruction of Left Scapula, Percutaneo
         Endoscopic Approach
0P570ZZ Destruction of Right Glenoid Cavity, Op
         Approach
0P573ZZ Destruction of Right Glenoid Cavity,
         Percutaneous Approach
0P574ZZ Destruction of Right Glenoid
         Cavity, Percutaneous Endoscopic
         Approach
0P580ZZ Destruction of Left Glenoid Cavity, Ope
         Approach
0P583ZZ Destruction of Left Glenoid Cavity,
         Percutaneous Approach
0P584ZZ Destruction of Left Glenoid Cavity,
         Percutaneous Endoscopic Approach
0P590ZZ Destruction of Right Clavicle, Open
         Approach
0P593ZZ Destruction of Right Clavicle,
         Percutaneous Approach

♀ Female-only   ♂ Male-only   ▲ Limited Coverage   ● Non-OR   ■ HAC-associated procedure   ▲ Non-covered procedures   ✚ Combinati

⁀94ZZ	Destruction of Right Clavicle, Percutaneous Endoscopic Approach	
⁀B0ZZ	Destruction of Left Clavicle, Open Approach	
⁀B3ZZ	Destruction of Left Clavicle, Percutaneous Approach	
⁀B4ZZ	Destruction of Left Clavicle, Percutaneous Endoscopic Approach	
⁀C0ZZ	Destruction of Right Humeral Head, Open Approach	
⁀C3ZZ	Destruction of Right Humeral Head, Percutaneous Approach	
⁀C4ZZ	Destruction of Right Humeral Head, Percutaneous Endoscopic Approach	
⁀D0ZZ	Destruction of Left Humeral Head, Open Approach	
⁀D3ZZ	Destruction of Left Humeral Head, Percutaneous Approach	
⁀D4ZZ	Destruction of Left Humeral Head, Percutaneous Endoscopic Approach	
⁀F0ZZ	Destruction of Right Humeral Shaft, Open Approach	
⁀F3ZZ	Destruction of Right Humeral Shaft, Percutaneous Approach	
⁀F4ZZ	Destruction of Right Humeral Shaft, Percutaneous Endoscopic Approach	
⁀G0ZZ	Destruction of Left Humeral Shaft, Open Approach	
⁀G3ZZ	Destruction of Left Humeral Shaft, Percutaneous Approach	
⁀G4ZZ	Destruction of Left Humeral Shaft, Percutaneous Endoscopic Approach	
⁀H0ZZ	Destruction of Right Radius, Open Approach	

0P5H3ZZ	Destruction of Right Radius, Percutaneous Approach
0P5H4ZZ	Destruction of Right Radius, Percutaneous Endoscopic Approach
0P5J0ZZ	Destruction of Left Radius, Open Approach
0P5J3ZZ	Destruction of Left Radius, Percutaneous Approach
0P5J4ZZ	Destruction of Left Radius, Percutaneous Endoscopic Approach
0P5K0ZZ	Destruction of Right Ulna, Open Approach
0P5K3ZZ	Destruction of Right Ulna, Percutaneous Approach
0P5K4ZZ	Destruction of Right Ulna, Percutaneous Endoscopic Approach
0P5L0ZZ	Destruction of Left Ulna, Open Approach
0P5L3ZZ	Destruction of Left Ulna, Percutaneous Approach
0P5L4ZZ	Destruction of Left Ulna, Percutaneous Endoscopic Approach
0P5M0ZZ	Destruction of Right Carpal, Open Approach
0P5M3ZZ	Destruction of Right Carpal, Percutaneous Approach
0P5M4ZZ	Destruction of Right Carpal, Percutaneous Endoscopic Approach
0P5N0ZZ	Destruction of Left Carpal, Open Approach
0P5N3ZZ	Destruction of Left Carpal, Percutaneous Approach
0P5N4ZZ	Destruction of Left Carpal, Percutaneous Endoscopic Approach
0P5P0ZZ	Destruction of Right Metacarpal, Open Approach

0P5P3ZZ	Destruction of Right Metacarpal, Percutaneous Approach
0P5P4ZZ	Destruction of Right Metacarpal, Percutaneous Endoscopic Approach
0P5Q0ZZ	Destruction of Left Metacarpal, Open Approach
0P5Q3ZZ	Destruction of Left Metacarpal, Percutaneous Approach
0P5Q4ZZ	Destruction of Left Metacarpal, Percutaneous Endoscopic Approach
0P5R0ZZ	Destruction of Right Thumb Phalanx, Open Approach
0P5R3ZZ	Destruction of Right Thumb Phalanx, Percutaneous Approach
0P5R4ZZ	Destruction of Right Thumb Phalanx, Percutaneous Endoscopic Approach
0P5S0ZZ	Destruction of Left Thumb Phalanx, Open Approach
0P5S3ZZ	Destruction of Left Thumb Phalanx, Percutaneous Approach
0P5S4ZZ	Destruction of Left Thumb Phalanx, Percutaneous Endoscopic Approach
0P5T0ZZ	Destruction of Right Finger Phalanx, Open Approach
0P5T3ZZ	Destruction of Right Finger Phalanx, Percutaneous Approach
0P5T4ZZ	Destruction of Right Finger Phalanx, Percutaneous Endoscopic Approach
0P5V0ZZ	Destruction of Left Finger Phalanx, Open Approach
0P5V3ZZ	Destruction of Left Finger Phalanx, Percutaneous Approach
0P5V4ZZ	Destruction of Left Finger Phalanx, Percutaneous Endoscopic Approach

⁀8 – Upper Bones, Division

⁀view Coding Guideline B3.14

⁀800ZZ	Division of Sternum, Open Approach
⁀803ZZ	Division of Sternum, Percutaneous Approach
⁀804ZZ	Division of Sternum, Percutaneous Endoscopic Approach
⁀810ZZ	Division of Right Rib, Open Approach
⁀813ZZ	Division of Right Rib, Percutaneous Approach
⁀814ZZ	Division of Right Rib, Percutaneous Endoscopic Approach
⁀820ZZ	Division of Left Rib, Open Approach
⁀823ZZ	Division of Left Rib, Percutaneous Approach
⁀824ZZ	Division of Left Rib, Percutaneous Endoscopic Approach
⁀830ZZ	Division of Cervical Vertebra, Open Approach
⁀833ZZ	Division of Cervical Vertebra, Percutaneous Approach
⁀834ZZ	Division of Cervical Vertebra, Percutaneous Endoscopic Approach
⁀840ZZ	Division of Thoracic Vertebra, Open Approach
⁀843ZZ	Division of Thoracic Vertebra, Percutaneous Approach
⁀844ZZ	Division of Thoracic Vertebra, Percutaneous Endoscopic Approach
⁀850ZZ	Division of Right Scapula, Open Approach
⁀853ZZ	Division of Right Scapula, Percutaneous Approach
⁀854ZZ	Division of Right Scapula, Percutaneous Endoscopic Approach
⁀860ZZ	Division of Left Scapula, Open Approach
⁀863ZZ	Division of Left Scapula, Percutaneous Approach
⁀864ZZ	Division of Left Scapula, Percutaneous Endoscopic Approach
⁀870ZZ	Division of Right Glenoid Cavity, Open Approach

0P873ZZ	Division of Right Glenoid Cavity, Percutaneous Approach
0P874ZZ	Division of Right Glenoid Cavity, Percutaneous Endoscopic Approach
0P880ZZ	Division of Left Glenoid Cavity, Open Approach
0P883ZZ	Division of Left Glenoid Cavity, Percutaneous Approach
0P884ZZ	Division of Left Glenoid Cavity, Percutaneous Endoscopic Approach
0P890ZZ	Division of Right Clavicle, Open Approach
0P893ZZ	Division of Right Clavicle, Percutaneous Approach
0P894ZZ	Division of Right Clavicle, Percutaneous Endoscopic Approach
0P8B0ZZ	Division of Left Clavicle, Open Approach
0P8B3ZZ	Division of Left Clavicle, Percutaneous Approach
0P8B4ZZ	Division of Left Clavicle, Percutaneous Endoscopic Approach
0P8C0ZZ	Division of Right Humeral Head, Open Approach
0P8C3ZZ	Division of Right Humeral Head, Percutaneous Approach
0P8C4ZZ	Division of Right Humeral Head, Percutaneous Endoscopic Approach
0P8D0ZZ	Division of Left Humeral Head, Open Approach
0P8D3ZZ	Division of Left Humeral Head, Percutaneous Approach
0P8D4ZZ	Division of Left Humeral Head, Percutaneous Endoscopic Approach
0P8F0ZZ	Division of Right Humeral Shaft, Open Approach
0P8F3ZZ	Division of Right Humeral Shaft, Percutaneous Approach

0P8F4ZZ	Division of Right Humeral Shaft, Percutaneous Endoscopic Approach
0P8G0ZZ	Division of Left Humeral Shaft, Open Approach
0P8G3ZZ	Division of Left Humeral Shaft, Percutaneous Approach
0P8G4ZZ	Division of Left Humeral Shaft, Percutaneous Endoscopic Approach
0P8H0ZZ	Division of Right Radius, Open Approach
0P8H3ZZ	Division of Right Radius, Percutaneous Approach
0P8H4ZZ	Division of Right Radius, Percutaneous Endoscopic Approach
0P8J0ZZ	Division of Left Radius, Open Approach
0P8J3ZZ	Division of Left Radius, Percutaneous Approach
0P8J4ZZ	Division of Left Radius, Percutaneous Endoscopic Approach
0P8K0ZZ	Division of Right Ulna, Open Approach
0P8K3ZZ	Division of Right Ulna, Percutaneous Approach
0P8K4ZZ	Division of Right Ulna, Percutaneous Endoscopic Approach
0P8L0ZZ	Division of Left Ulna, Open Approach
0P8L3ZZ	Division of Left Ulna, Percutaneous Approach
0P8L4ZZ	Division of Left Ulna, Percutaneous Endoscopic Approach
0P8M0ZZ	Division of Right Carpal, Open Approach
0P8M3ZZ	Division of Right Carpal, Percutaneous Approach
0P8M4ZZ	Division of Right Carpal, Percutaneous Endoscopic Approach
0P8N0ZZ	Division of Left Carpal, Open Approach
0P8N3ZZ	Division of Left Carpal, Percutaneous Approach
0P8N4ZZ	Division of Left Carpal, Percutaneous Endoscopic Approach

Female-only	♂ Male-only	▲ Limited Coverage	● Non-OR	■ HAC-associated procedure	▲ Non-covered procedures	✚ Combination

0P8P0ZZ Division of Right Metacarpal, Open Approach	**0P8R0ZZ** Division of Right Thumb Phalanx, Open Approach	**0P8T0ZZ** Division of Right Finger Phalanx, Open Approach
0P8P3ZZ Division of Right Metacarpal, Percutaneous Approach	**0P8R3ZZ** Division of Right Thumb Phalanx, Percutaneous Approach	**0P8T3ZZ** Division of Right Finger Phalanx, Percutaneous Approach
0P8P4ZZ Division of Right Metacarpal, Percutaneous Endoscopic Approach	**0P8R4ZZ** Division of Right Thumb Phalanx, Percutaneous Endoscopic Approach	**0P8T4ZZ** Division of Right Finger Phalanx, Percutaneous Endoscopic Approach
0P8Q0ZZ Division of Left Metacarpal, Open Approach	**0P8S0ZZ** Division of Left Thumb Phalanx, Open Approach	**0P8V0ZZ** Division of Left Finger Phalanx, Open Approach
0P8Q3ZZ Division of Left Metacarpal, Percutaneous Approach	**0P8S3ZZ** Division of Left Thumb Phalanx, Percutaneous Approach	**0P8V3ZZ** Division of Left Finger Phalanx, Percutaneous Approach
0P8Q4ZZ Division of Left Metacarpal, Percutaneous Endoscopic Approach	**0P8S4ZZ** Division of Left Thumb Phalanx, Percutaneous Endoscopic Approach	**0P8V4ZZ** Division of Left Finger Phalanx, Percutaneous Endoscopic Approach

0P9 – Upper Bones, Drainage

Review Coding Guidelines B3.4a and B3.4b

Review Coding Guideline B6.2

0P9000Z Drainage of Sternum with Drainage Device, Open Approach	**0P930ZZ** Drainage of Cervical Vertebra, Open Approach	**0P960ZX** Drainage of Left Scapula, Open Approach, Diagnostic
0P900ZX Drainage of Sternum, Open Approach, Diagnostic	**0P9330Z** Drainage of Cervical Vertebra with Drainage Device, Percutaneous Approach	**0P960ZZ** Drainage of Left Scapula, Open Approach
0P900ZZ Drainage of Sternum, Open Approach	**0P933ZX** Drainage of Cervical Vertebra, Percutaneous Approach, Diagnostic	**0P9630Z** Drainage of Left Scapula with Drainage Device, Percutaneous Approach
0P9030Z Drainage of Sternum with Drainage Device, Percutaneous Approach	**0P933ZZ** Drainage of Cervical Vertebra, Percutaneous Approach	**0P963ZX** Drainage of Left Scapula, Percutaneous Approach, Diagnostic
0P903ZX Drainage of Sternum, Percutaneous Approach, Diagnostic	**0P9340Z** Drainage of Cervical Vertebra with Drainage Device, Percutaneous Endoscopic Approach	**0P963ZZ** Drainage of Left Scapula, Percutaneous Approach
0P903ZZ Drainage of Sternum, Percutaneous Approach	**0P934ZX** Drainage of Cervical Vertebra, Percutaneous Endoscopic Approach, Diagnostic	**0P9640Z** Drainage of Left Scapula with Drainage Device, Percutaneous Endoscopic Approach
0P9040Z Drainage of Sternum with Drainage Device, Percutaneous Endoscopic Approach	**0P934ZZ** Drainage of Cervical Vertebra, Percutaneous Endoscopic Approach	**0P964ZX** Drainage of Left Scapula, Percutaneous Endoscopic Approach, Diagnostic
0P904ZX Drainage of Sternum, Percutaneous Endoscopic Approach, Diagnostic	**0P9400Z** Drainage of Thoracic Vertebra with Drainage Device, Open Approach	**0P964ZZ** Drainage of Left Scapula, Percutaneous Endoscopic Approach
0P904ZZ Drainage of Sternum, Percutaneous Endoscopic Approach	**0P940ZX** Drainage of Thoracic Vertebra, Open Approach, Diagnostic	**0P9700Z** Drainage of Right Glenoid Cavity with Drainage Device, Open Approach
0P9100Z Drainage of Right Rib with Drainage Device, Open Approach	**0P940ZZ** Drainage of Thoracic Vertebra, Open Approach	**0P970ZX** Drainage of Right Glenoid Cavity, Open Approach, Diagnostic
0P910ZX Drainage of Right Rib, Open Approach, Diagnostic	**0P9430Z** Drainage of Thoracic Vertebra with Drainage Device, Percutaneous Approach	**0P970ZZ** Drainage of Right Glenoid Cavity, Open Approach
0P910ZZ Drainage of Right Rib, Open Approach	**0P943ZX** Drainage of Thoracic Vertebra, Percutaneous Approach, Diagnostic	**0P9730Z** Drainage of Right Glenoid Cavity with Drainage Device, Percutaneous Approach
0P9130Z Drainage of Right Rib with Drainage Device, Percutaneous Approach	**0P943ZZ** Drainage of Thoracic Vertebra, Percutaneous Approach	**0P973ZX** Drainage of Right Glenoid Cavity, Percutaneous Approach, Diagnostic
0P913ZX Drainage of Right Rib, Percutaneous Approach, Diagnostic	**0P9440Z** Drainage of Thoracic Vertebra with Drainage Device, Percutaneous Endoscopic Approach	**0P973ZZ** Drainage of Right Glenoid Cavity, Percutaneous Approach
0P913ZZ Drainage of Right Rib, Percutaneous Approach	**0P944ZX** Drainage of Thoracic Vertebra, Percutaneous Endoscopic Approach, Diagnostic	**0P9740Z** Drainage of Right Glenoid Cavity with Drainage Device, Percutaneous Endoscopic Approach
0P9140Z Drainage of Right Rib with Drainage Device, Percutaneous Endoscopic Approach	**0P944ZZ** Drainage of Thoracic Vertebra, Percutaneous Endoscopic Approach	**0P974ZX** Drainage of Right Glenoid Cavity, Percutaneous Endoscopic Approach, Diagnostic
0P914ZX Drainage of Right Rib, Percutaneous Endoscopic Approach, Diagnostic	**0P9500Z** Drainage of Right Scapula with Drainage Device, Open Approach	**0P974ZZ** Drainage of Right Glenoid Cavity, Percutaneous Endoscopic Approach
0P914ZZ Drainage of Right Rib, Percutaneous Endoscopic Approach	**0P950ZX** Drainage of Right Scapula, Open Approach, Diagnostic	**0P9800Z** Drainage of Left Glenoid Cavity with Drainage Device, Open Approach
0P9200Z Drainage of Left Rib with Drainage Device, Open Approach	**0P950ZZ** Drainage of Right Scapula, Open Approach	**0P980ZX** Drainage of Left Glenoid Cavity, Open Approach, Diagnostic
0P920ZX Drainage of Left Rib, Open Approach, Diagnostic	**0P9530Z** Drainage of Right Scapula with Drainage Device, Percutaneous Approach	**0P980ZZ** Drainage of Left Glenoid Cavity, Open Approach
0P920ZZ Drainage of Left Rib, Open Approach	**0P953ZX** Drainage of Right Scapula, Percutaneous Approach, Diagnostic	**0P9830Z** Drainage of Left Glenoid Cavity with Drainage Device, Percutaneous Approach
0P9230Z Drainage of Left Rib with Drainage Device, Percutaneous Approach	**0P953ZZ** Drainage of Right Scapula, Percutaneous Approach	**0P983ZX** Drainage of Left Glenoid Cavity, Percutaneous Approach, Diagnostic
0P923ZX Drainage of Left Rib, Percutaneous Approach, Diagnostic	**0P9540Z** Drainage of Right Scapula with Drainage Device, Percutaneous Endoscopic Approach	**0P983ZZ** Drainage of Left Glenoid Cavity, Percutaneous Approach
0P923ZZ Drainage of Left Rib, Percutaneous Approach	**0P954ZX** Drainage of Right Scapula, Percutaneous Endoscopic Approach, Diagnostic	**0P9840Z** Drainage of Left Glenoid Cavity with Drainage Device, Percutaneous Endoscopic Approach
0P9240Z Drainage of Left Rib with Drainage Device, Percutaneous Endoscopic Approach	**0P954ZZ** Drainage of Right Scapula, Percutaneous Endoscopic Approach	**0P984ZX** Drainage of Left Glenoid Cavity, Percutaneous Endoscopic Approach, Diagnostic
0P924ZX Drainage of Left Rib, Percutaneous Endoscopic Approach, Diagnostic	**0P9600Z** Drainage of Left Scapula with Drainage Device, Open Approach	**0P984ZZ** Drainage of Left Glenoid Cavity, Percutaneous Endoscopic Approach
0P924ZZ Drainage of Left Rib, Percutaneous Endoscopic Approach		**0P9900Z** Drainage of Right Clavicle with Drainage Device, Open Approach
0P9300Z Drainage of Cervical Vertebra with Drainage Device, Open Approach		
0P930ZX Drainage of Cervical Vertebra, Open Approach, Diagnostic		

814

♀ Female-only	♂ Male-only	▲ Limited Coverage	● Non-OR	◨ HAC-associated procedure	▲ Non-covered procedures	✚ Combination

990ZX	Drainage of Right Clavicle, Open Approach, Diagnostic
990ZZ	Drainage of Right Clavicle, Open Approach
9930Z	Drainage of Right Clavicle with Drainage Device, Percutaneous Approach
993ZX	Drainage of Right Clavicle, Percutaneous Approach, Diagnostic
993ZZ	Drainage of Right Clavicle, Percutaneous Approach
9940Z	Drainage of Right Clavicle with Drainage Device, Percutaneous Endoscopic Approach
994ZX	Drainage of Right Clavicle, Percutaneous Endoscopic Approach, Diagnostic
994ZZ	Drainage of Right Clavicle, Percutaneous Endoscopic Approach
9B00Z	Drainage of Left Clavicle with Drainage Device, Open Approach
9B0ZX	Drainage of Left Clavicle, Open Approach, Diagnostic
9B0ZZ	Drainage of Left Clavicle, Open Approach
9B30Z	Drainage of Left Clavicle with Drainage Device, Percutaneous Approach
9B3ZX	Drainage of Left Clavicle, Percutaneous Approach, Diagnostic
9B3ZZ	Drainage of Left Clavicle, Percutaneous Approach
9B40Z	Drainage of Left Clavicle with Drainage Device, Percutaneous Endoscopic Approach
9B4ZX	Drainage of Left Clavicle, Percutaneous Endoscopic Approach, Diagnostic
9B4ZZ	Drainage of Left Clavicle, Percutaneous Endoscopic Approach
9C00Z	Drainage of Right Humeral Head with Drainage Device, Open Approach
9C0ZX	Drainage of Right Humeral Head, Open Approach, Diagnostic
9C0ZZ	Drainage of Right Humeral Head, Open Approach
9C30Z	Drainage of Right Humeral Head with Drainage Device, Percutaneous Approach
9C3ZX	Drainage of Right Humeral Head, Percutaneous Approach, Diagnostic
9C3ZZ	Drainage of Right Humeral Head, Percutaneous Approach
9C40Z	Drainage of Right Humeral Head with Drainage Device, Percutaneous Endoscopic Approach
9C4ZX	Drainage of Right Humeral Head, Percutaneous Endoscopic Approach, Diagnostic
9C4ZZ	Drainage of Right Humeral Head, Percutaneous Endoscopic Approach
9D00Z	Drainage of Left Humeral Head with Drainage Device, Open Approach
9D0ZX	Drainage of Left Humeral Head, Open Approach, Diagnostic
9D0ZZ	Drainage of Left Humeral Head, Open Approach
9D30Z	Drainage of Left Humeral Head with Drainage Device, Percutaneous Approach
9D3ZX	Drainage of Left Humeral Head, Percutaneous Approach, Diagnostic
9D3ZZ	Drainage of Left Humeral Head, Percutaneous Approach
9D40Z	Drainage of Left Humeral Head with Drainage Device, Percutaneous Endoscopic Approach
9D4ZX	Drainage of Left Humeral Head, Percutaneous Endoscopic Approach, Diagnostic
9D4ZZ	Drainage of Left Humeral Head, Percutaneous Endoscopic Approach
9F00Z	Drainage of Right Humeral Shaft with Drainage Device, Open Approach
0P9F0ZX	Drainage of Right Humeral Shaft, Open Approach, Diagnostic
0P9F0ZZ	Drainage of Right Humeral Shaft, Open Approach
0P9F30Z	Drainage of Right Humeral Shaft with Drainage Device, Percutaneous Approach
0P9F3ZX	Drainage of Right Humeral Shaft, Percutaneous Approach, Diagnostic
0P9F3ZZ	Drainage of Right Humeral Shaft, Percutaneous Approach
0P9F40Z	Drainage of Right Humeral Shaft with Drainage Device, Percutaneous Endoscopic Approach
0P9F4ZX	Drainage of Right Humeral Shaft, Percutaneous Endoscopic Approach, Diagnostic
0P9F4ZZ	Drainage of Right Humeral Shaft, Percutaneous Endoscopic Approach
0P9G00Z	Drainage of Left Humeral Shaft with Drainage Device, Open Approach
0P9G0ZX	Drainage of Left Humeral Shaft, Open Approach, Diagnostic
0P9G0ZZ	Drainage of Left Humeral Shaft, Open Approach
0P9G30Z	Drainage of Left Humeral Shaft with Drainage Device, Percutaneous Approach
0P9G3ZX	Drainage of Left Humeral Shaft, Percutaneous Approach, Diagnostic
0P9G3ZZ	Drainage of Left Humeral Shaft, Percutaneous Approach
0P9G40Z	Drainage of Left Humeral Shaft with Drainage Device, Percutaneous Endoscopic Approach
0P9G4ZX	Drainage of Left Humeral Shaft, Percutaneous Endoscopic Approach, Diagnostic
0P9G4ZZ	Drainage of Left Humeral Shaft, Percutaneous Endoscopic Approach
0P9H00Z	Drainage of Right Radius with Drainage Device, Open Approach
0P9H0ZX	Drainage of Right Radius, Open Approach, Diagnostic
0P9H0ZZ	Drainage of Right Radius, Open Approach
0P9H30Z	Drainage of Right Radius with Drainage Device, Percutaneous Approach
0P9H3ZX	Drainage of Right Radius, Percutaneous Approach, Diagnostic
0P9H3ZZ	Drainage of Right Radius, Percutaneous Approach
0P9H40Z	Drainage of Right Radius with Drainage Device, Percutaneous Endoscopic Approach
0P9H4ZX	Drainage of Right Radius, Percutaneous Endoscopic Approach, Diagnostic
0P9H4ZZ	Drainage of Right Radius, Percutaneous Endoscopic Approach
0P9J00Z	Drainage of Left Radius with Drainage Device, Open Approach
0P9J0ZX	Drainage of Left Radius, Open Approach, Diagnostic
0P9J0ZZ	Drainage of Left Radius, Open Approach
0P9J30Z	Drainage of Left Radius with Drainage Device, Percutaneous Approach
0P9J3ZX	Drainage of Left Radius, Percutaneous Approach, Diagnostic
0P9J3ZZ	Drainage of Left Radius, Percutaneous Approach
0P9J40Z	Drainage of Left Radius with Drainage Device, Percutaneous Endoscopic Approach
0P9J4ZX	Drainage of Left Radius, Percutaneous Endoscopic Approach, Diagnostic
0P9J4ZZ	Drainage of Left Radius, Percutaneous Endoscopic Approach
0P9K00Z	Drainage of Right Ulna with Drainage Device, Open Approach
0P9K0ZX	Drainage of Right Ulna, Open Approach, Diagnostic
0P9K0ZZ	Drainage of Right Ulna, Open Approach
0P9K30Z	Drainage of Right Ulna with Drainage Device, Percutaneous Approach
0P9K3ZX	Drainage of Right Ulna, Percutaneous Approach, Diagnostic
0P9K3ZZ	Drainage of Right Ulna, Percutaneous Approach
0P9K40Z	Drainage of Right Ulna with Drainage Device, Percutaneous Endoscopic Approach
0P9K4ZX	Drainage of Right Ulna, Percutaneous Endoscopic Approach, Diagnostic
0P9K4ZZ	Drainage of Right Ulna, Percutaneous Endoscopic Approach
0P9L00Z	Drainage of Left Ulna with Drainage Device, Open Approach
0P9L0ZX	Drainage of Left Ulna, Open Approach, Diagnostic
0P9L0ZZ	Drainage of Left Ulna, Open Approach
0P9L30Z	Drainage of Left Ulna with Drainage Device, Percutaneous Approach
0P9L3ZX	Drainage of Left Ulna, Percutaneous Approach, Diagnostic
0P9L3ZZ	Drainage of Left Ulna, Percutaneous Approach
0P9L40Z	Drainage of Left Ulna with Drainage Device, Percutaneous Endoscopic Approach
0P9L4ZX	Drainage of Left Ulna, Percutaneous Endoscopic Approach, Diagnostic
0P9L4ZZ	Drainage of Left Ulna, Percutaneous Endoscopic Approach
0P9M00Z	Drainage of Right Carpal with Drainage Device, Open Approach
0P9M0ZX	Drainage of Right Carpal, Open Approach, Diagnostic
0P9M0ZZ	Drainage of Right Carpal, Open Approach
0P9M30Z	Drainage of Right Carpal with Drainage Device, Percutaneous Approach
0P9M3ZX	Drainage of Right Carpal, Percutaneous Approach, Diagnostic
0P9M3ZZ	Drainage of Right Carpal, Percutaneous Approach
0P9M40Z	Drainage of Right Carpal with Drainage Device, Percutaneous Endoscopic Approach
0P9M4ZX	Drainage of Right Carpal, Percutaneous Endoscopic Approach, Diagnostic
0P9M4ZZ	Drainage of Right Carpal, Percutaneous Endoscopic Approach
0P9N00Z	Drainage of Left Carpal with Drainage Device, Open Approach
0P9N0ZX	Drainage of Left Carpal, Open Approach, Diagnostic
0P9N0ZZ	Drainage of Left Carpal, Open Approach
0P9N30Z	Drainage of Left Carpal with Drainage Device, Percutaneous Approach
0P9N3ZX	Drainage of Left Carpal, Percutaneous Approach, Diagnostic
0P9N3ZZ	Drainage of Left Carpal, Percutaneous Approach
0P9N40Z	Drainage of Left Carpal with Drainage Device, Percutaneous Endoscopic Approach
0P9N4ZX	Drainage of Left Carpal, Percutaneous Endoscopic Approach, Diagnostic
0P9N4ZZ	Drainage of Left Carpal, Percutaneous Endoscopic Approach
0P9P00Z	Drainage of Right Metacarpal with Drainage Device, Open Approach
0P9P0ZX	Drainage of Right Metacarpal, Open Approach, Diagnostic
0P9P0ZZ	Drainage of Right Metacarpal, Open Approach

♀ Female-only ♂ Male-only · ▲ Limited Coverage ● Non-OR ▬ HAC-associated procedure ▲ Non-covered procedures ✚ Combination

0P9P30Z Drainage of Right Metacarpal with Drainage Device, Percutaneous Approach

0P9P3ZX Drainage of Right Metacarpal, Percutaneous Approach, Diagnostic

0P9P3ZZ Drainage of Right Metacarpal, Percutaneous Approach

0P9P40Z Drainage of Right Metacarpal with Drainage Device, Percutaneous Endoscopic Approach

0P9P4ZX Drainage of Right Metacarpal, Percutaneous Endoscopic Approach, Diagnostic

0P9P4ZZ Drainage of Right Metacarpal, Percutaneous Endoscopic Approach

0P9Q00Z Drainage of Left Metacarpal with Drainage Device, Open Approach

0P9Q0ZX Drainage of Left Metacarpal, Open Approach, Diagnostic

0P9Q0ZZ Drainage of Left Metacarpal, Open Approach

0P9Q30Z Drainage of Left Metacarpal with Drainage Device, Percutaneous Approach

0P9Q3ZX Drainage of Left Metacarpal, Percutaneous Approach, Diagnostic

0P9Q3ZZ Drainage of Left Metacarpal, Percutaneous Approach

0P9Q40Z Drainage of Left Metacarpal with Drainage Device, Percutaneous Endoscopic Approach

0P9Q4ZX Drainage of Left Metacarpal, Percutaneous Endoscopic Approach, Diagnostic

0P9Q4ZZ Drainage of Left Metacarpal, Percutaneous Endoscopic Approach

0P9R00Z Drainage of Right Thumb Phalanx with Drainage Device, Open Approach

0P9R0ZX Drainage of Right Thumb Phalanx, Open Approach, Diagnostic

0P9R0ZZ Drainage of Right Thumb Phalanx, Open Approach

0P9R30Z Drainage of Right Thumb Phalanx with Drainage Device, Percutaneous Approach

0P9R3ZX Drainage of Right Thumb Phalanx, Percutaneous Approach, Diagnostic

0P9R3ZZ Drainage of Right Thumb Phalanx, Percutaneous Approach

0P9R40Z Drainage of Right Thumb Phalanx with Drainage Device, Percutaneous Endoscopic Approach

0P9R4ZX Drainage of Right Thumb Phalanx, Percutaneous Endoscopic Approach, Diagnostic

0P9R4ZZ Drainage of Right Thumb Phalanx, Percutaneous Endoscopic Approach

0P9S00Z Drainage of Left Thumb Phalanx with Drainage Device, Open Approach

0P9S0ZX Drainage of Left Thumb Phalanx, Open Approach, Diagnostic

0P9S0ZZ Drainage of Left Thumb Phalanx, Open Approach

0P9S30Z Drainage of Left Thumb Phalanx with Drainage Device, Percutaneous Approach

0P9S3ZX Drainage of Left Thumb Phalanx, Percutaneous Approach, Diagnostic

0P9S3ZZ Drainage of Left Thumb Phalanx, Percutaneous Approach

0P9S40Z Drainage of Left Thumb Phalanx with Drainage Device, Percutaneous Endoscopic Approach

0P9S4ZX Drainage of Left Thumb Phalanx, Percutaneous Endoscopic Approach, Diagnostic

0P9S4ZZ Drainage of Left Thumb Phalanx, Percutaneous Endoscopic Approach

0P9T00Z Drainage of Right Finger Phalanx with Drainage Device, Open Approach

0P9T0ZX Drainage of Right Finger Phalanx, Open Approach, Diagnostic

0P9T0ZZ Drainage of Right Finger Phalanx, Open Approach

0P9T30Z Drainage of Right Finger Phalanx with Drainage Device, Percutaneous Approach

0P9T3ZX Drainage of Right Finger Phalanx, Percutaneous Approach, Diagnostic

0P9T3ZZ Drainage of Right Finger Phalanx, Percutaneous Approach

0P9T40Z Drainage of Right Finger Phalanx with Drainage Device, Percutaneous Endoscopic Approach

0P9T4ZX Drainage of Right Finger Phalanx, Percutaneous Endoscopic Approach, Diagnostic

0P9T4ZZ Drainage of Right Finger Phalanx, Percutaneous Endoscopic Approach

0P9V00Z Drainage of Left Finger Phalanx with Drainage Device, Open Approach

0P9V0ZX Drainage of Left Finger Phalanx, Open Approach, Diagnostic

0P9V0ZZ Drainage of Left Finger Phalanx, Open Approach

0P9V30Z Drainage of Left Finger Phalanx with Drainage Device, Percutaneous Approach

0P9V3ZX Drainage of Left Finger Phalanx, Percutaneous Approach, Diagnostic

0P9V3ZZ Drainage of Left Finger Phalanx, Percutaneous Approach

0P9V40Z Drainage of Left Finger Phalanx with Drainage Device, Percutaneous Endoscopic Approach

0P9V4ZX Drainage of Left Finger Phalanx, Percutaneous Endoscopic Approach, Diagnostic

0P9V4ZZ Drainage of Left Finger Phalanx, Percutaneous Endoscopic Approach

0PB – Upper Bones, Excision

Review Coding Guideline B3.5

Review Coding Guidelines B3.4a and B3.4b

Review Coding Guideline B3.8

0PB00ZX Excision of Sternum, Open Approach, Diagnostic

0PB00ZZ Excision of Sternum, Open Approach

0PB03ZX Excision of Sternum, Percutaneous Approach, Diagnostic

0PB03ZZ Excision of Sternum, Percutaneous Approach

0PB04ZX Excision of Sternum, Percutaneous Endoscopic Approach, Diagnostic

0PB04ZZ Excision of Sternum, Percutaneous Endoscopic Approach

0PB10ZX Excision of Right Rib, Open Approach, Diagnostic

0PB10ZZ Excision of Right Rib, Open Approach
AHA CC: 4Q, 2012, 101-102; 4Q, 2013, 109-111

0PB13ZX Excision of Right Rib, Percutaneous Approach, Diagnostic

0PB13ZZ Excision of Right Rib, Percutaneous Approach

0PB14ZX Excision of Right Rib, Percutaneous Endoscopic Approach, Diagnostic

0PB14ZZ Excision of Right Rib, Percutaneous Endoscopic Approach

0PB20ZX Excision of Left Rib, Open Approach, Diagnostic

0PB20ZZ Excision of Left Rib, Open Approach
AHA CC: 4Q, 2013, 109-111

0PB23ZX Excision of Left Rib, Percutaneous Approach, Diagnostic

0PB23ZZ Excision of Left Rib, Percutaneous Approach

0PB24ZX Excision of Left Rib, Percutaneous Endoscopic Approach, Diagnostic

0PB24ZZ Excision of Left Rib, Percutaneous Endoscopic Approach

0PB30ZX Excision of Cervical Vertebra, Open Approach, Diagnostic

0PB30ZZ Excision of Cervical Vertebra, Open Approach

0PB33ZX Excision of Cervical Vertebra, Percutaneous Approach, Diagnostic

0PB33ZZ Excision of Cervical Vertebra, Percutaneous Approach

0PB34ZX Excision of Cervical Vertebra, Percutaneous Endoscopic Approach, Diagnostic

0PB34ZZ Excision of Cervical Vertebra, Percutaneous Endoscopic Approach

0PB40ZX Excision of Thoracic Vertebra, Open Approach, Diagnostic

0PB40ZZ Excision of Thoracic Vertebra, Open Approach

0PB43ZX Excision of Thoracic Vertebra, Percutaneous Approach, Diagnostic

0PB43ZZ Excision of Thoracic Vertebra, Percutaneous Approach

0PB44ZX Excision of Thoracic Vertebra, Percutaneous Endoscopic Approach, Diagnostic

0PB44ZZ Excision of Thoracic Vertebra, Percutaneous Endoscopic Approach

0PB50ZX Excision of Right Scapula, Open Approach, Diagnostic

0PB50ZZ Excision of Right Scapula, Open Approach

0PB53ZX Excision of Right Scapula, Percutaneous Approach, Diagnostic

0PB53ZZ Excision of Right Scapula, Percutaneous Approach

0PB54ZX Excision of Right Scapula, Percutaneous Endoscopic Approach, Diagnostic

0PB54ZZ Excision of Right Scapula, Percutaneous Endoscopic Approach
AHA CC: 3Q, 2013, 20-22

0PB60ZX Excision of Left Scapula, Open Approach, Diagnostic

0PB60ZZ Excision of Left Scapula, Open Approach

0PB63ZX Excision of Left Scapula, Percutaneous Approach, Diagnostic

0PB63ZZ Excision of Left Scapula, Percutaneous Approach

0PB64ZX Excision of Left Scapula, Percutaneous Endoscopic Approach, Diagnostic

0PB64ZZ Excision of Left Scapula, Percutaneous Endoscopic Approach

0PB70ZX Excision of Right Glenoid Cavity, Open Approach, Diagnostic

0PB70ZZ Excision of Right Glenoid Cavity, Open Approach

0PB73ZX Excision of Right Glenoid Cavity, Percutaneous Approach, Diagnostic

♀ Female-only   ♂ Male-only   ▲ Limited Coverage   ● Non-OR   ▦ HAC-associated procedure   ▲ Non-covered procedures   ✚ Combination

73ZZ Excision of Right Glenoid Cavity, Percutaneous Approach

74ZX Excision of Right Glenoid Cavity, Percutaneous Endoscopic Approach, Diagnostic

74ZZ Excision of Right Glenoid Cavity, Percutaneous Endoscopic Approach

80ZX Excision of Left Glenoid Cavity, Open Approach, Diagnostic

80ZZ Excision of Left Glenoid Cavity, Open Approach

83ZX Excision of Left Glenoid Cavity, Percutaneous Approach, Diagnostic

83ZZ Excision of Left Glenoid Cavity, Percutaneous Approach

84ZX Excision of Left Glenoid Cavity, Percutaneous Endoscopic Approach, Diagnostic

84ZZ Excision of Left Glenoid Cavity, Percutaneous Endoscopic Approach

90ZX Excision of Right Clavicle, Open Approach, Diagnostic

90ZZ Excision of Right Clavicle, Open Approach

93ZX Excision of Right Clavicle, Percutaneous Approach, Diagnostic

93ZZ Excision of Right Clavicle, Percutaneous Approach

94ZX Excision of Right Clavicle, Percutaneous Endoscopic Approach, Diagnostic

94ZZ Excision of Right Clavicle, Percutaneous Endoscopic Approach

3B0ZX Excision of Left Clavicle, Open Approach, Diagnostic

3B0ZZ Excision of Left Clavicle, Open Approach

3B3ZX Excision of Left Clavicle, Percutaneous Approach, Diagnostic

3B3ZZ Excision of Left Clavicle, Percutaneous Approach

3B4ZX Excision of Left Clavicle, Percutaneous Endoscopic Approach, Diagnostic

3B4ZZ Excision of Left Clavicle, Percutaneous Endoscopic Approach

BC0ZX Excision of Right Humeral Head, Open Approach, Diagnostic

BC0ZZ Excision of Right Humeral Head, Open Approach

BC3ZX Excision of Right Humeral Head, Percutaneous Approach, Diagnostic

BC3ZZ Excision of Right Humeral Head, Percutaneous Approach

BC4ZX Excision of Right Humeral Head, Percutaneous Endoscopic Approach, Diagnostic

BC4ZZ Excision of Right Humeral Head, Percutaneous Endoscopic Approach

BD0ZX Excision of Left Humeral Head, Open Approach, Diagnostic

BD0ZZ Excision of Left Humeral Head, Open Approach

BD3ZX Excision of Left Humeral Head, Percutaneous Approach, Diagnostic

BD3ZZ Excision of Left Humeral Head, Percutaneous Approach

BD4ZX Excision of Left Humeral Head, Percutaneous Endoscopic Approach, Diagnostic

BD4ZZ Excision of Left Humeral Head, Percutaneous Endoscopic Approach

BF0ZX Excision of Right Humeral Shaft, Open Approach, Diagnostic

BF0ZZ Excision of Right Humeral Shaft, Open Approach

BF3ZX Excision of Right Humeral Shaft, Percutaneous Approach, Diagnostic

BF3ZZ Excision of Right Humeral Shaft, Percutaneous Approach

0PBF4ZX Excision of Right Humeral Shaft, Percutaneous Endoscopic Approach, Diagnostic

0PBF4ZZ Excision of Right Humeral Shaft, Percutaneous Endoscopic Approach

0PBG0ZX Excision of Left Humeral Shaft, Open Approach, Diagnostic

0PBG0ZZ Excision of Left Humeral Shaft, Open Approach

0PBG3ZX Excision of Left Humeral Shaft, Percutaneous Approach, Diagnostic

0PBG3ZZ Excision of Left Humeral Shaft, Percutaneous Approach

0PBG4ZX Excision of Left Humeral Shaft, Percutaneous Endoscopic Approach, Diagnostic

0PBG4ZZ Excision of Left Humeral Shaft, Percutaneous Endoscopic Approach

0PBH0ZX Excision of Right Radius, Open Approach, Diagnostic

0PBH0ZZ Excision of Right Radius, Open Approach

0PBH3ZX Excision of Right Radius, Percutaneous Approach, Diagnostic

0PBH3ZZ Excision of Right Radius, Percutaneous Approach

0PBH4ZX Excision of Right Radius, Percutaneous Endoscopic Approach, Diagnostic

0PBH4ZZ Excision of Right Radius, Percutaneous Endoscopic Approach

0PBJ0ZX Excision of Left Radius, Open Approach, Diagnostic

0PBJ0ZZ Excision of Left Radius, Open Approach

0PBJ3ZX Excision of Left Radius, Percutaneous Approach, Diagnostic

0PBJ3ZZ Excision of Left Radius, Percutaneous Approach

0PBJ4ZX Excision of Left Radius, Percutaneous Endoscopic Approach, Diagnostic

0PBJ4ZZ Excision of Left Radius, Percutaneous Endoscopic Approach

0PBK0ZX Excision of Right Ulna, Open Approach, Diagnostic

0PBK0ZZ Excision of Right Ulna, Open Approach

0PBK3ZX Excision of Right Ulna, Percutaneous Approach, Diagnostic

0PBK3ZZ Excision of Right Ulna, Percutaneous Approach

0PBK4ZX Excision of Right Ulna, Percutaneous Endoscopic Approach, Diagnostic

0PBK4ZZ Excision of Right Ulna, Percutaneous Endoscopic Approach

0PBL0ZX Excision of Left Ulna, Open Approach, Diagnostic

0PBL0ZZ Excision of Left Ulna, Open Approach

0PBL3ZX Excision of Left Ulna, Percutaneous Approach, Diagnostic

0PBL3ZZ Excision of Left Ulna, Percutaneous Approach

0PBL4ZX Excision of Left Ulna, Percutaneous Endoscopic Approach, Diagnostic

0PBL4ZZ Excision of Left Ulna, Percutaneous Endoscopic Approach

0PBM0ZX Excision of Right Carpal, Open Approach, Diagnostic

0PBM0ZZ Excision of Right Carpal, Open Approach

0PBM3ZX Excision of Right Carpal, Percutaneous Approach, Diagnostic

0PBM3ZZ Excision of Right Carpal, Percutaneous Approach

0PBM4ZX Excision of Right Carpal, Percutaneous Endoscopic Approach, Diagnostic

0PBM4ZZ Excision of Right Carpal, Percutaneous Endoscopic Approach

0PBN0ZX Excision of Left Carpal, Open Approach, Diagnostic

0PBN0ZZ Excision of Left Carpal, Open Approach

0PBN3ZX Excision of Left Carpal, Percutaneous Approach, Diagnostic

0PBN3ZZ Excision of Left Carpal, Percutaneous Approach

0PBN4ZX Excision of Left Carpal, Percutaneous Endoscopic Approach, Diagnostic

0PBN4ZZ Excision of Left Carpal, Percutaneous Endoscopic Approach

0PBP0ZX Excision of Right Metacarpal, Open Approach, Diagnostic

0PBP0ZZ Excision of Right Metacarpal, Open Approach

0PBP3ZX Excision of Right Metacarpal, Percutaneous Approach, Diagnostic

0PBP3ZZ Excision of Right Metacarpal, Percutaneous Approach

0PBP4ZX Excision of Right Metacarpal, Percutaneous Endoscopic Approach, Diagnostic

0PBP4ZZ Excision of Right Metacarpal, Percutaneous Endoscopic Approach

0PBQ0ZX Excision of Left Metacarpal, Open Approach, Diagnostic

0PBQ0ZZ Excision of Left Metacarpal, Open Approach

0PBQ3ZX Excision of Left Metacarpal, Percutaneous Approach, Diagnostic

0PBQ3ZZ Excision of Left Metacarpal, Percutaneous Approach

0PBQ4ZX Excision of Left Metacarpal, Percutaneous Endoscopic Approach, Diagnostic

0PBQ4ZZ Excision of Left Metacarpal, Percutaneous Endoscopic Approach

0PBR0ZX Excision of Right Thumb Phalanx, Open Approach, Diagnostic

0PBR0ZZ Excision of Right Thumb Phalanx, Open Approach

0PBR3ZX Excision of Right Thumb Phalanx, Percutaneous Approach, Diagnostic

0PBR3ZZ Excision of Right Thumb Phalanx, Percutaneous Approach

0PBR4ZX Excision of Right Thumb Phalanx, Percutaneous Endoscopic Approach, Diagnostic

0PBR4ZZ Excision of Right Thumb Phalanx, Percutaneous Endoscopic Approach

0PBS0ZX Excision of Left Thumb Phalanx, Open Approach, Diagnostic

0PBS0ZZ Excision of Left Thumb Phalanx, Open Approach

0PBS3ZX Excision of Left Thumb Phalanx, Percutaneous Approach, Diagnostic

0PBS3ZZ Excision of Left Thumb Phalanx, Percutaneous Approach

0PBS4ZX Excision of Left Thumb Phalanx, Percutaneous Endoscopic Approach, Diagnostic

0PBS4ZZ Excision of Left Thumb Phalanx, Percutaneous Endoscopic Approach

0PBT0ZX Excision of Right Finger Phalanx, Open Approach, Diagnostic

0PBT0ZZ Excision of Right Finger Phalanx, Open Approach

0PBT3ZX Excision of Right Finger Phalanx, Percutaneous Approach, Diagnostic

0PBT3ZZ Excision of Right Finger Phalanx, Percutaneous Approach

0PBT4ZX Excision of Right Finger Phalanx, Percutaneous Endoscopic Approach, Diagnostic

0PBT4ZZ Excision of Right Finger Phalanx, Percutaneous Endoscopic Approach

0PBV0ZX Excision of Left Finger Phalanx, Open Approach, Diagnostic

0PBV0ZZ Excision of Left Finger Phalanx, Open Approach

0PBV3ZX Excision of Left Finger Phalanx, Percutaneous Approach, Diagnostic

0PBV3ZZ Excision of Left Finger Phalanx, Percutaneous Approach	**0PBV4ZX** Excision of Left Finger Phalanx, Percutaneous Endoscopic Approach, Diagnostic	**0PBV4ZZ** Excision of Left Finger Phalanx, Percutaneous Endoscopic Approach

0PC – Upper Bones, Extirpation

0PC00ZZ Extirpation of Matter from Sternum, Open Approach	**0PC90ZZ** Extirpation of Matter from Right Clavicle, Open Approach	**0PCL4ZZ** Extirpation of Matter from Left Ulna, Percutaneous Endoscopic Approach
0PC03ZZ Extirpation of Matter from Sternum, Percutaneous Approach	**0PC93ZZ** Extirpation of Matter from Right Clavicle, Percutaneous Approach	**0PCM0ZZ** Extirpation of Matter from Right Carpal, Open Approach
0PC04ZZ Extirpation of Matter from Sternum, Percutaneous Endoscopic Approach	**0PC94ZZ** Extirpation of Matter from Right Clavicle, Percutaneous Endoscopic Approach	**0PCM3ZZ** Extirpation of Matter from Right Carpal, Percutaneous Approach
0PC10ZZ Extirpation of Matter from Right Rib, Open Approach	**0PCB0ZZ** Extirpation of Matter from Left Clavicle, Open Approach	**0PCM4ZZ** Extirpation of Matter from Right Carpal, Percutaneous Endoscopic Approach
0PC13ZZ Extirpation of Matter from Right Rib, Percutaneous Approach	**0PCB3ZZ** Extirpation of Matter from Left Clavicle, Percutaneous Approach	**0PCN0ZZ** Extirpation of Matter from Left Carpal, Open Approach
0PC14ZZ Extirpation of Matter from Right Rib, Percutaneous Endoscopic Approach	**0PCB4ZZ** Extirpation of Matter from Left Clavicle, Percutaneous Endoscopic Approach	**0PCN3ZZ** Extirpation of Matter from Left Carpal, Percutaneous Approach
0PC20ZZ Extirpation of Matter from Left Rib, Open Approach	**0PCC0ZZ** Extirpation of Matter from Right Humeral Head, Open Approach	**0PCN4ZZ** Extirpation of Matter from Left Carpal, Percutaneous Endoscopic Approach
0PC23ZZ Extirpation of Matter from Left Rib, Percutaneous Approach	**0PCC3ZZ** Extirpation of Matter from Right Humeral Head, Percutaneous Approach	**0PCP0ZZ** Extirpation of Matter from Right Metacarpal, Open Approach
0PC24ZZ Extirpation of Matter from Left Rib, Percutaneous Endoscopic Approach	**0PCC4ZZ** Extirpation of Matter from Right Humeral Head, Percutaneous Endoscopic Approach	**0PCP3ZZ** Extirpation of Matter from Right Metacarpal, Percutaneous Approach
0PC30ZZ Extirpation of Matter from Cervical Vertebra, Open Approach	**0PCD0ZZ** Extirpation of Matter from Left Humeral Head, Open Approach	**0PCP4ZZ** Extirpation of Matter from Right Metacarpal, Percutaneous Endoscopic Approach
0PC33ZZ Extirpation of Matter from Cervical Vertebra, Percutaneous Approach	**0PCD3ZZ** Extirpation of Matter from Left Humeral Head, Percutaneous Approach	**0PCQ0ZZ** Extirpation of Matter from Left Metacarpal, Open Approach
0PC34ZZ Extirpation of Matter from Cervical Vertebra, Percutaneous Endoscopic Approach	**0PCD4ZZ** Extirpation of Matter from Left Humeral Head, Percutaneous Endoscopic Approach	**0PCQ3ZZ** Extirpation of Matter from Left Metacarpal, Percutaneous Approach
0PC40ZZ Extirpation of Matter from Thoracic Vertebra, Open Approach	**0PCF0ZZ** Extirpation of Matter from Right Humeral Shaft, Open Approach	**0PCQ4ZZ** Extirpation of Matter from Left Metacarpal, Percutaneous Endoscopic Approach
0PC43ZZ Extirpation of Matter from Thoracic Vertebra, Percutaneous Approach	**0PCF3ZZ** Extirpation of Matter from Right Humeral Shaft, Percutaneous Approach	**0PCR0ZZ** Extirpation of Matter from Right Thumb Phalanx, Open Approach
0PC44ZZ Extirpation of Matter from Thoracic Vertebra, Percutaneous Endoscopic Approach	**0PCF4ZZ** Extirpation of Matter from Right Humeral Shaft, Percutaneous Endoscopic Approach	**0PCR3ZZ** Extirpation of Matter from Right Thumb Phalanx, Percutaneous Approach
0PC50ZZ Extirpation of Matter from Right Scapula, Open Approach	**0PCG0ZZ** Extirpation of Matter from Left Humeral Shaft, Open Approach	**0PCR4ZZ** Extirpation of Matter from Right Thumb Phalanx, Percutaneous Endoscopic Approach
0PC53ZZ Extirpation of Matter from Right Scapula, Percutaneous Approach	**0PCG3ZZ** Extirpation of Matter from Left Humeral Shaft, Percutaneous Approach	**0PCS0ZZ** Extirpation of Matter from Left Thumb Phalanx, Open Approach
0PC54ZZ Extirpation of Matter from Right Scapula, Percutaneous Endoscopic Approach	**0PCG4ZZ** Extirpation of Matter from Left Humeral Shaft, Percutaneous Endoscopic Approach	**0PCS3ZZ** Extirpation of Matter from Left Thumb Phalanx, Percutaneous Approach
0PC60ZZ Extirpation of Matter from Left Scapula, Open Approach	**0PCH0ZZ** Extirpation of Matter from Right Radius, Open Approach	**0PCS4ZZ** Extirpation of Matter from Left Thumb Phalanx, Percutaneous Endoscopic Approach
0PC63ZZ Extirpation of Matter from Left Scapula, Percutaneous Approach	**0PCH3ZZ** Extirpation of Matter from Right Radius, Percutaneous Approach	**0PCT0ZZ** Extirpation of Matter from Right Finger Phalanx, Open Approach
0PC64ZZ Extirpation of Matter from Left Scapula, Percutaneous Endoscopic Approach	**0PCH4ZZ** Extirpation of Matter from Right Radius, Percutaneous Endoscopic Approach	**0PCT3ZZ** Extirpation of Matter from Right Finger Phalanx, Percutaneous Approach
0PC70ZZ Extirpation of Matter from Right Glenoid Cavity, Open Approach	**0PCJ0ZZ** Extirpation of Matter from Left Radius, Open Approach	**0PCT4ZZ** Extirpation of Matter from Right Finger Phalanx, Percutaneous Endoscopic Approach
0PC73ZZ Extirpation of Matter from Right Glenoid Cavity, Percutaneous Approach	**0PCJ3ZZ** Extirpation of Matter from Left Radius, Percutaneous Approach	**0PCV0ZZ** Extirpation of Matter from Left Finger Phalanx, Open Approach
0PC74ZZ Extirpation of Matter from Right Glenoid Cavity, Percutaneous Endoscopic Approach	**0PCJ4ZZ** Extirpation of Matter from Left Radius, Percutaneous Endoscopic Approach	**0PCV3ZZ** Extirpation of Matter from Left Finger Phalanx, Percutaneous Approach
0PC80ZZ Extirpation of Matter from Left Glenoid Cavity, Open Approach	**0PCK0ZZ** Extirpation of Matter from Right Ulna, Open Approach	**0PCV4ZZ** Extirpation of Matter from Left Finger Phalanx, Percutaneous Endoscopic Approach
0PC83ZZ Extirpation of Matter from Left Glenoid Cavity, Percutaneous Approach	**0PCK3ZZ** Extirpation of Matter from Right Ulna, Percutaneous Approach	
0PC84ZZ Extirpation of Matter from Left Glenoid Cavity, Percutaneous Endoscopic Approach	**0PCK4ZZ** Extirpation of Matter from Right Ulna, Percutaneous Endoscopic Approach	
	0PCL0ZZ Extirpation of Matter from Left Ulna, Open Approach	
	0PCL3ZZ Extirpation of Matter from Left Ulna, Percutaneous Approach	

0PH – Upper Bones, Insertion

0PH000Z Insertion of Rigid Plate Internal Fixation Device into Sternum, Open Approach	**0PH040Z** Insertion of Rigid Plate Internal Fixation Device into Sternum, Percutaneous Endoscopic Approach	**0PH134Z** Insertion of Internal Fixation Device into Right Rib, Percutaneous Approach
0PH004Z Insertion of Internal Fixation Device into Sternum, Open Approach	**0PH044Z** Insertion of Internal Fixation Device into Sternum, Percutaneous Endoscopic Approach	**0PH144Z** Insertion of Internal Fixation Device into Right Rib, Percutaneous Endoscopic Approach
0PH030Z Insertion of Rigid Plate Internal Fixation Device into Sternum, Percutaneous Approach	**0PH104Z** Insertion of Internal Fixation Device into Right Rib, Open Approach	**0PH204Z** Insertion of Internal Fixation Device into Left Rib, Open Approach
0PH034Z Insertion of Internal Fixation Device into Sternum, Percutaneous Approach		**0PH234Z** Insertion of Internal Fixation Device into Left Rib, Percutaneous Approach

1244Z Insertion of Internal Fixation Device into Left Rib, Percutaneous Endoscopic Approach

1304Z Insertion of Internal Fixation Device into Cervical Vertebra, Open Approach

1334Z Insertion of Internal Fixation Device into Cervical Vertebra, Percutaneous Approach

1344Z Insertion of Internal Fixation Device into Cervical Vertebra, Percutaneous Endoscopic Approach

1404Z Insertion of Internal Fixation Device into Thoracic Vertebra, Open Approach
AHA CC: 4Q, 2014, 28-29

1434Z Insertion of Internal Fixation Device into Thoracic Vertebra, Percutaneous Approach

1444Z Insertion of Internal Fixation Device into Thoracic Vertebra, Percutaneous Endoscopic Approach

1504Z Insertion of Internal Fixation Device into Right Scapula, Open Approach

1534Z Insertion of Internal Fixation Device into Right Scapula, Percutaneous Approach

1544Z Insertion of Internal Fixation Device into Right Scapula, Percutaneous Endoscopic Approach

1604Z Insertion of Internal Fixation Device into Left Scapula, Open Approach

1634Z Insertion of Internal Fixation Device into Left Scapula, Percutaneous Approach

1644Z Insertion of Internal Fixation Device into Left Scapula, Percutaneous Endoscopic Approach

H704Z Insertion of Internal Fixation Device into Right Glenoid Cavity, Open Approach

H734Z Insertion of Internal Fixation Device into Right Glenoid Cavity, Percutaneous Approach

H744Z Insertion of Internal Fixation Device into Right Glenoid Cavity, Percutaneous Endoscopic Approach

H804Z Insertion of Internal Fixation Device into Left Glenoid Cavity, Open Approach

H834Z Insertion of Internal Fixation Device into Left Glenoid Cavity, Percutaneous Approach

H844Z Insertion of Internal Fixation Device into Left Glenoid Cavity, Percutaneous Endoscopic Approach

H904Z Insertion of Internal Fixation Device into Right Clavicle, Open Approach

H934Z Insertion of Internal Fixation Device into Right Clavicle, Percutaneous Approach

H944Z Insertion of Internal Fixation Device into Right Clavicle, Percutaneous Endoscopic Approach

HB04Z Insertion of Internal Fixation Device into Left Clavicle, Open Approach

HB34Z Insertion of Internal Fixation Device into Left Clavicle, Percutaneous Approach

HB44Z Insertion of Internal Fixation Device into Left Clavicle, Percutaneous Endoscopic Approach

HC04Z Insertion of Internal Fixation Device into Right Humeral Head, Open Approach

HC05Z Insertion of External Fixation Device into Right Humeral Head, Open Approach

HC06Z Insertion of Intramedullary Internal Fixation Device into Right Humeral Head, Open Approach

HC08Z Insertion of Limb Lengthening External Fixation Device into Right Humeral Head, Open Approach

HC0BZ Insertion of Monoplanar External Fixation Device into Right Humeral Head, Open Approach

HC0CZ Insertion of Ring External Fixation Device into Right Humeral Head, Open Approach

0PHC0DZ Insertion of Hybrid External Fixation Device into Right Humeral Head, Open Approach

0PHC34Z Insertion of Internal Fixation Device into Right Humeral Head, Percutaneous Approach

0PHC35Z Insertion of External Fixation Device into Right Humeral Head, Percutaneous Approach

0PHC36Z Insertion of Intramedullary Internal Fixation Device into Right Humeral Head, Percutaneous Approach

0PHC38Z Insertion of Limb Lengthening External Fixation Device into Right Humeral Head, Percutaneous Approach

0PHC3BZ Insertion of Monoplanar External Fixation Device into Right Humeral Head, Percutaneous Approach

0PHC3CZ Insertion of Ring External Fixation Device into Right Humeral Head, Percutaneous Approach

0PHC3DZ Insertion of Hybrid External Fixation Device into Right Humeral Head, Percutaneous Approach

0PHC44Z Insertion of Internal Fixation Device into Right Humeral Head, Percutaneous Endoscopic Approach

0PHC45Z Insertion of External Fixation Device into Right Humeral Head, Percutaneous Endoscopic Approach

0PHC46Z Insertion of Intramedullary Internal Fixation Device into Right Humeral Head, Percutaneous Endoscopic Approach

0PHC48Z Insertion of Limb Lengthening External Fixation Device into Right Humeral Head, Percutaneous Endoscopic Approach

0PHC4BZ Insertion of Monoplanar External Fixation Device into Right Humeral Head, Percutaneous Endoscopic Approach

0PHC4CZ Insertion of Ring External Fixation Device into Right Humeral Head, Percutaneous Endoscopic Approach

0PHC4DZ Insertion of Hybrid External Fixation Device into Right Humeral Head, Percutaneous Endoscopic Approach

0PHD04Z Insertion of Internal Fixation Device into Left Humeral Head, Open Approach

0PHD05Z Insertion of External Fixation Device into Left Humeral Head, Open Approach

0PHD06Z Insertion of Intramedullary Internal Fixation Device into Left Humeral Head, Open Approach

0PHD08Z Insertion of Limb Lengthening External Fixation Device into Left Humeral Head, Open Approach

0PHD0BZ Insertion of Monoplanar External Fixation Device into Left Humeral Head, Open Approach

0PHD0CZ Insertion of Ring External Fixation Device into Left Humeral Head, Open Approach

0PHD0DZ Insertion of Hybrid External Fixation Device into Left Humeral Head, Open Approach

0PHD34Z Insertion of Internal Fixation Device into Left Humeral Head, Percutaneous Approach

0PHD35Z Insertion of External Fixation Device into Left Humeral Head, Percutaneous Approach

0PHD36Z Insertion of Intramedullary Internal Fixation Device into Left Humeral Head, Percutaneous Approach

0PHD38Z Insertion of Limb Lengthening External Fixation Device into Left Humeral Head, Percutaneous Approach

0PHD3BZ Insertion of Monoplanar External Fixation Device into Left Humeral Head, Percutaneous Approach

0PHD3CZ Insertion of Ring External Fixation Device into Left Humeral Head, Percutaneous Approach

0PHD3DZ Insertion of Hybrid External Fixation Device into Left Humeral Head, Percutaneous Approach

0PHD44Z Insertion of Internal Fixation Device into Left Humeral Head, Percutaneous Endoscopic Approach

0PHD45Z Insertion of External Fixation Device into Left Humeral Head, Percutaneous Endoscopic Approach

0PHD46Z Insertion of Intramedullary Internal Fixation Device into Left Humeral Head, Percutaneous Endoscopic Approach

0PHD48Z Insertion of Limb Lengthening External Fixation Device into Left Humeral Head, Percutaneous Endoscopic Approach

0PHD4BZ Insertion of Monoplanar External Fixation Device into Left Humeral Head, Percutaneous Endoscopic Approach

0PHD4CZ Insertion of Ring External Fixation Device into Left Humeral Head, Percutaneous Endoscopic Approach

0PHD4DZ Insertion of Hybrid External Fixation Device into Left Humeral Head, Percutaneous Endoscopic Approach

0PHF04Z Insertion of Internal Fixation Device into Right Humeral Shaft, Open Approach

0PHF05Z Insertion of External Fixation Device into Right Humeral Shaft, Open Approach

0PHF06Z Insertion of Intramedullary Internal Fixation Device into Right Humeral Shaft, Open Approach

0PHF08Z Insertion of Limb Lengthening External Fixation Device into Right Humeral Shaft, Open Approach

0PHF0BZ Insertion of Monoplanar External Fixation Device into Right Humeral Shaft, Open Approach

0PHF0CZ Insertion of Ring External Fixation Device into Right Humeral Shaft, Open Approach

0PHF0DZ Insertion of Hybrid External Fixation Device into Right Humeral Shaft, Open Approach

0PHF34Z Insertion of Internal Fixation Device into Right Humeral Shaft, Percutaneous Approach

0PHF35Z Insertion of External Fixation Device into Right Humeral Shaft, Percutaneous Approach

0PHF36Z Insertion of Intramedullary Internal Fixation Device into Right Humeral Shaft, Percutaneous Approach

0PHF38Z Insertion of Limb Lengthening External Fixation Device into Right Humeral Shaft, Percutaneous Approach

0PHF3BZ Insertion of Monoplanar External Fixation Device into Right Humeral Shaft, Percutaneous Approach

0PHF3CZ Insertion of Ring External Fixation Device into Right Humeral Shaft, Percutaneous Approach

0PHF3DZ Insertion of Hybrid External Fixation Device into Right Humeral Shaft, Percutaneous Approach

0PHF44Z Insertion of Internal Fixation Device into Right Humeral Shaft, Percutaneous Endoscopic Approach

0PHF45Z Insertion of External Fixation Device into Right Humeral Shaft, Percutaneous Endoscopic Approach

---

Female-only ♂ Male-only ▲ Limited Coverage ● Non-OR ▇ HAC-associated procedure ▲ Non-covered procedures ✚ Combination

0PHF46Z Insertion of Intramedullary Internal Fixation Device into Right Humeral Shaft, Percutaneous Endoscopic Approach

0PHF48Z Insertion of Limb Lengthening External Fixation Device into Right Humeral Shaft, Percutaneous Endoscopic Approach

0PHF4BZ Insertion of Monoplanar External Fixation Device into Right Humeral Shaft, Percutaneous Endoscopic Approach

0PHF4CZ Insertion of Ring External Fixation Device into Right Humeral Shaft, Percutaneous Endoscopic Approach

0PHF4DZ Insertion of Hybrid External Fixation Device into Right Humeral Shaft, Percutaneous Endoscopic Approach

0PHG04Z Insertion of Internal Fixation Device into Left Humeral Shaft, Open Approach

0PHG05Z Insertion of External Fixation Device into Left Humeral Shaft, Open Approach

0PHG06Z Insertion of Intramedullary Internal Fixation Device into Left Humeral Shaft, Open Approach

0PHG08Z Insertion of Limb Lengthening External Fixation Device into Left Humeral Shaft, Open Approach

0PHG0BZ Insertion of Monoplanar External Fixation Device into Left Humeral Shaft, Open Approach

0PHG0CZ Insertion of Ring External Fixation Device into Left Humeral Shaft, Open Approach

0PHG0DZ Insertion of Hybrid External Fixation Device into Left Humeral Shaft, Open Approach

0PHG34Z Insertion of Internal Fixation Device into Left Humeral Shaft, Percutaneous Approach

0PHG35Z Insertion of External Fixation Device into Left Humeral Shaft, Percutaneous Approach

0PHG36Z Insertion of Intramedullary Internal Fixation Device into Left Humeral Shaft, Percutaneous Approach

0PHG38Z Insertion of Limb Lengthening External Fixation Device into Left Humeral Shaft, Percutaneous Approach

0PHG3BZ Insertion of Monoplanar External Fixation Device into Left Humeral Shaft, Percutaneous Approach

0PHG3CZ Insertion of Ring External Fixation Device into Left Humeral Shaft, Percutaneous Approach

0PHG3DZ Insertion of Hybrid External Fixation Device into Left Humeral Shaft, Percutaneous Approach

0PHG44Z Insertion of Internal Fixation Device into Left Humeral Shaft, Percutaneous Endoscopic Approach

0PHG45Z Insertion of External Fixation Device into Left Humeral Shaft, Percutaneous Endoscopic Approach

0PHG46Z Insertion of Intramedullary Internal Fixation Device into Left Humeral Shaft, Percutaneous Endoscopic Approach

0PHG48Z Insertion of Limb Lengthening External Fixation Device into Left Humeral Shaft, Percutaneous Endoscopic Approach

0PHG4BZ Insertion of Monoplanar External Fixation Device into Left Humeral Shaft, Percutaneous Endoscopic Approach

0PHG4CZ Insertion of Ring External Fixation Device into Left Humeral Shaft, Percutaneous Endoscopic Approach

0PHG4DZ Insertion of Hybrid External Fixation Device into Left Humeral Shaft, Percutaneous Endoscopic Approach

0PHH04Z Insertion of Internal Fixation Device into Right Radius, Open Approach

0PHH05Z Insertion of External Fixation Device into Right Radius, Open Approach

0PHH06Z Insertion of Intramedullary Internal Fixation Device into Right Radius, Open Approach

0PHH08Z Insertion of Limb Lengthening External Fixation Device into Right Radius, Open Approach

0PHH0BZ Insertion of Monoplanar External Fixation Device into Right Radius, Open Approach

0PHH0CZ Insertion of Ring External Fixation Device into Right Radius, Open Approach

0PHH0DZ Insertion of Hybrid External Fixation Device into Right Radius, Open Approach

0PHH34Z Insertion of Internal Fixation Device into Right Radius, Percutaneous Approach

0PHH35Z Insertion of External Fixation Device into Right Radius, Percutaneous Approach

0PHH36Z Insertion of Intramedullary Internal Fixation Device into Right Radius, Percutaneous Approach

0PHH38Z Insertion of Limb Lengthening External Fixation Device into Right Radius, Percutaneous Approach

0PHH3BZ Insertion of Monoplanar External Fixation Device into Right Radius, Percutaneous Approach

0PHH3CZ Insertion of Ring External Fixation Device into Right Radius, Percutaneous Approach

0PHH3DZ Insertion of Hybrid External Fixation Device into Right Radius, Percutaneous Approach

0PHH44Z Insertion of Internal Fixation Device into Right Radius, Percutaneous Endoscopic Approach

0PHH45Z Insertion of External Fixation Device into Right Radius, Percutaneous Endoscopic Approach

0PHH46Z Insertion of Intramedullary Internal Fixation Device into Right Radius, Percutaneous Endoscopic Approach

0PHH48Z Insertion of Limb Lengthening External Fixation Device into Right Radius, Percutaneous Endoscopic Approach

0PHH4BZ Insertion of Monoplanar External Fixation Device into Right Radius, Percutaneous Endoscopic Approach

0PHH4CZ Insertion of Ring External Fixation Device into Right Radius, Percutaneous Endoscopic Approach

0PHH4DZ Insertion of Hybrid External Fixation Device into Right Radius, Percutaneous Endoscopic Approach

0PHJ04Z Insertion of Internal Fixation Device into Left Radius, Open Approach

0PHJ05Z Insertion of External Fixation Device into Left Radius, Open Approach

0PHJ06Z Insertion of Intramedullary Internal Fixation Device into Left Radius, Open Approach

0PHJ08Z Insertion of Limb Lengthening External Fixation Device into Left Radius, Open Approach

0PHJ0BZ Insertion of Monoplanar External Fixation Device into Left Radius, Open Approach

0PHJ0CZ Insertion of Ring External Fixation Device into Left Radius, Open Approach

0PHJ0DZ Insertion of Hybrid External Fixation Device into Left Radius, Open Approach

0PHJ34Z Insertion of Internal Fixation Device into Left Radius, Percutaneous Approach

0PHJ35Z Insertion of External Fixation Device into Left Radius, Percutaneous Approach

0PHJ36Z Insertion of Intramedullary Internal Fixation Device into Left Radius, Percutaneous Approach

0PHJ38Z Insertion of Limb Lengthening External Fixation Device into Left Radius, Percutaneous Approach

0PHJ3BZ Insertion of Monoplanar External Fixation Device into Left Radius, Percutaneous Approach

0PHJ3CZ Insertion of Ring External Fixation Device into Left Radius, Percutaneous Approach

0PHJ3DZ Insertion of Hybrid External Fixation Device into Left Radius, Percutaneous Approach

0PHJ44Z Insertion of Internal Fixation Device into Left Radius, Percutaneous Endoscopic Approach

0PHJ45Z Insertion of External Fixation Device into Left Radius, Percutaneous Endoscopic Approach

0PHJ46Z Insertion of Intramedullary Internal Fixation Device into Left Radius, Percutaneous Endoscopic Approach

0PHJ48Z Insertion of Limb Lengthening External Fixation Device into Left Radius, Percutaneous Endoscopic Approach

0PHJ4BZ Insertion of Monoplanar External Fixation Device into Left Radius, Percutaneous Endoscopic Approach

0PHJ4CZ Insertion of Ring External Fixation Device into Left Radius, Percutaneous Endoscopic Approach

0PHJ4DZ Insertion of Hybrid External Fixation Device into Left Radius, Percutaneous Endoscopic Approach

0PHK04Z Insertion of Internal Fixation Device into Right Ulna, Open Approach

0PHK05Z Insertion of External Fixation Device into Right Ulna, Open Approach

0PHK06Z Insertion of Intramedullary Internal Fixation Device into Right Ulna, Open Approach

0PHK08Z Insertion of Limb Lengthening External Fixation Device into Right Ulna, Open Approach

0PHK0BZ Insertion of Monoplanar External Fixation Device into Right Ulna, Open Approach

0PHK0CZ Insertion of Ring External Fixation Device into Right Ulna, Open Approach

0PHK0DZ Insertion of Hybrid External Fixation Device into Right Ulna, Open Approach

0PHK34Z Insertion of Internal Fixation Device into Right Ulna, Percutaneous Approach

0PHK35Z Insertion of External Fixation Device into Right Ulna, Percutaneous Approach

0PHK36Z Insertion of Intramedullary Internal Fixation Device into Right Ulna, Percutaneous Approach

0PHK38Z Insertion of Limb Lengthening External Fixation Device into Right Ulna, Percutaneous Approach

0PHK3BZ Insertion of Monoplanar External Fixation Device into Right Ulna, Percutaneous Approach

0PHK3CZ Insertion of Ring External Fixation Device into Right Ulna, Percutaneous Approach

0PHK3DZ Insertion of Hybrid External Fixation Device into Right Ulna, Percutaneous Approach

0PHK44Z Insertion of Internal Fixation Device into Right Ulna, Percutaneous Endoscopic Approach

0PHK45Z Insertion of External Fixation Device into Right Ulna, Percutaneous Endoscopic Approach

0PHK46Z Insertion of Intramedullary Internal Fixation Device into Right Ulna, Percutaneous Endoscopic Approach

0PHK48Z Insertion of Limb Lengthening External Fixation Device into Right Ulna, Percutaneous Endoscopic Approach

0PHK4BZ Insertion of Monoplanar External Fixation Device into Right Ulna, Percutaneous Endoscopic Approach

0PHK4CZ Insertion of Ring External Fixation Device into Right Ulna, Percutaneous Endoscopic Approach

0PHK4DZ Insertion of Hybrid External Fixation Device into Right Ulna, Percutaneous Endoscopic Approach

0PHL04Z Insertion of Internal Fixation Device into Left Ulna, Open Approach

0PHL05Z Insertion of External Fixation Device into Left Ulna, Open Approach

0PHL06Z Insertion of Intramedullary Internal Fixation Device into Left Ulna, Open Approach

0PHL08Z Insertion of Limb Lengthening External Fixation Device into Left Ulna, Open Approach

0PHL0BZ Insertion of Monoplanar External Fixation Device into Left Ulna, Open Approach

0PHL0CZ Insertion of Ring External Fixation Device into Left Ulna, Open Approach

0PHL0DZ Insertion of Hybrid External Fixation Device into Left Ulna, Open Approach

0PHL34Z Insertion of Internal Fixation Device into Left Ulna, Percutaneous Approach

0PHL35Z Insertion of External Fixation Device into Left Ulna, Percutaneous Approach

0PHL36Z Insertion of Intramedullary Internal Fixation Device into Left Ulna, Percutaneous Approach

0PHL38Z Insertion of Limb Lengthening External Fixation Device into Left Ulna, Percutaneous Approach

0PHL3BZ Insertion of Monoplanar External Fixation Device into Left Ulna, Percutaneous Approach

0PHL3CZ Insertion of Ring External Fixation Device into Left Ulna, Percutaneous Approach

0PHL3DZ Insertion of Hybrid External Fixation Device into Left Ulna, Percutaneous Approach

0PHL44Z Insertion of Internal Fixation Device into Left Ulna, Percutaneous Endoscopic Approach

0PHL45Z Insertion of External Fixation Device into Left Ulna, Percutaneous Endoscopic Approach

0PHL46Z Insertion of Intramedullary Internal Fixation Device into Left Ulna, Percutaneous Endoscopic Approach

0PHL48Z Insertion of Limb Lengthening External Fixation Device into Left Ulna, Percutaneous Endoscopic Approach

0PHL4BZ Insertion of Monoplanar External Fixation Device into Left Ulna, Percutaneous Endoscopic Approach

0PHL4CZ Insertion of Ring External Fixation Device into Left Ulna, Percutaneous Endoscopic Approach

0PHL4DZ Insertion of Hybrid External Fixation Device into Left Ulna, Percutaneous Endoscopic Approach

0PHM04Z Insertion of Internal Fixation Device into Right Carpal, Open Approach

0PHM05Z Insertion of External Fixation Device into Right Carpal, Open Approach

0PHM34Z Insertion of Internal Fixation Device into Right Carpal, Percutaneous Approach

0PHM35Z Insertion of External Fixation Device into Right Carpal, Percutaneous Approach

0PHM44Z Insertion of Internal Fixation Device into Right Carpal, Percutaneous Endoscopic Approach

0PHM45Z Insertion of External Fixation Device into Right Carpal, Percutaneous Endoscopic Approach

0PHN04Z Insertion of Internal Fixation Device into Left Carpal, Open Approach

0PHN05Z Insertion of External Fixation Device into Left Carpal, Open Approach

0PHN34Z Insertion of Internal Fixation Device into Left Carpal, Percutaneous Approach

0PHN35Z Insertion of External Fixation Device into Left Carpal, Percutaneous Approach

0PHN44Z Insertion of Internal Fixation Device into Left Carpal, Percutaneous Endoscopic Approach

0PHN45Z Insertion of External Fixation Device into Left Carpal, Percutaneous Endoscopic Approach

0PHP04Z Insertion of Internal Fixation Device into Right Metacarpal, Open Approach

0PHP05Z Insertion of External Fixation Device into Right Metacarpal, Open Approach

0PHP34Z Insertion of Internal Fixation Device into Right Metacarpal, Percutaneous Approach

0PHP35Z Insertion of External Fixation Device into Right Metacarpal, Percutaneous Approach

0PHP44Z Insertion of Internal Fixation Device into Right Metacarpal, Percutaneous Endoscopic Approach

0PHP45Z Insertion of External Fixation Device into Right Metacarpal, Percutaneous Endoscopic Approach

0PHQ04Z Insertion of Internal Fixation Device into Left Metacarpal, Open Approach

0PHQ05Z Insertion of External Fixation Device into Left Metacarpal, Open Approach

0PHQ34Z Insertion of Internal Fixation Device into Left Metacarpal, Percutaneous Approach

0PHQ35Z Insertion of External Fixation Device into Left Metacarpal, Percutaneous Approach

0PHQ44Z Insertion of Internal Fixation Device into Left Metacarpal, Percutaneous Endoscopic Approach

0PHQ45Z Insertion of External Fixation Device into Left Metacarpal, Percutaneous Endoscopic Approach

0PHR04Z Insertion of Internal Fixation Device into Right Thumb Phalanx, Open Approach

0PHR05Z Insertion of External Fixation Device into Right Thumb Phalanx, Open Approach

0PHR34Z Insertion of Internal Fixation Device into Right Thumb Phalanx, Percutaneous Approach

0PHR35Z Insertion of External Fixation Device into Right Thumb Phalanx, Percutaneous Approach

0PHR44Z Insertion of Internal Fixation Device into Right Thumb Phalanx, Percutaneous Endoscopic Approach

0PHR45Z Insertion of External Fixation Device into Right Thumb Phalanx, Percutaneous Endoscopic Approach

0PHS04Z Insertion of Internal Fixation Device into Left Thumb Phalanx, Open Approach

0PHS05Z Insertion of External Fixation Device into Left Thumb Phalanx, Open Approach

0PHS34Z Insertion of Internal Fixation Device into Left Thumb Phalanx, Percutaneous Approach

0PHS35Z Insertion of External Fixation Device into Left Thumb Phalanx, Percutaneous Approach

0PHS44Z Insertion of Internal Fixation Device into Left Thumb Phalanx, Percutaneous Endoscopic Approach

0PHS45Z Insertion of External Fixation Device into Left Thumb Phalanx, Percutaneous Endoscopic Approach

0PHT04Z Insertion of Internal Fixation Device into Right Finger Phalanx, Open Approach

0PHT05Z Insertion of External Fixation Device into Right Finger Phalanx, Open Approach

0PHT34Z Insertion of Internal Fixation Device into Right Finger Phalanx, Percutaneous Approach

0PHT35Z Insertion of External Fixation Device into Right Finger Phalanx, Percutaneous Approach

0PHT44Z Insertion of Internal Fixation Device into Right Finger Phalanx, Percutaneous Endoscopic Approach

0PHT45Z Insertion of External Fixation Device into Right Finger Phalanx, Percutaneous Endoscopic Approach

0PHV04Z Insertion of Internal Fixation Device into Left Finger Phalanx, Open Approach

0PHV05Z Insertion of External Fixation Device into Left Finger Phalanx, Open Approach

0PHV34Z Insertion of Internal Fixation Device into Left Finger Phalanx, Percutaneous Approach

0PHV35Z Insertion of External Fixation Device into Left Finger Phalanx, Percutaneous Approach

0PHV44Z Insertion of Internal Fixation Device into Left Finger Phalanx, Percutaneous Endoscopic Approach

0PHV45Z Insertion of External Fixation Device into Left Finger Phalanx, Percutaneous Endoscopic Approach

0PHY0MZ Insertion of Bone Growth Stimulator into Upper Bone, Open Approach

0PHY3MZ Insertion of Bone Growth Stimulator into Upper Bone, Percutaneous Approach

0PHY4MZ Insertion of Bone Growth Stimulator into Upper Bone, Percutaneous Endoscopic Approach

0PJ – Upper Bones, Inspection

Review Coding Guideline B3.5

Review Coding Guidelines B3.11a, B3.11b and B3.11c

0PJY0ZZ Inspection of Upper Bone, Open Approach

0PJY3ZZ Inspection of Upper Bone, Percutaneous Approach

0PJY4ZZ Inspection of Upper Bone, Percutaneous Endoscopic Approach

0PJYXZZ Inspection of Upper Bone, External Approach

Female-only   ♂ Male-only   ▲ Limited Coverage   ● Non-OR   ▦ HAC-associated procedure   ▲ Non-covered procedures   ✛ Combination

0PN – Upper Bones, Release

Review Coding Guideline B3.13

Review Coding Guideline B3.14

0PN00ZZ	Release Sternum, Open Approach
0PN03ZZ	Release Sternum, Percutaneous Approach
0PN04ZZ	Release Sternum, Percutaneous Endoscopic Approach
0PN10ZZ	Release Right Rib, Open Approach
0PN13ZZ	Release Right Rib, Percutaneous Approach
0PN14ZZ	Release Right Rib, Percutaneous Endoscopic Approach
0PN20ZZ	Release Left Rib, Open Approach
0PN23ZZ	Release Left Rib, Percutaneous Approach
0PN24ZZ	Release Left Rib, Percutaneous Endoscopic Approach
0PN30ZZ	Release Cervical Vertebra, Open Approach
0PN33ZZ	Release Cervical Vertebra, Percutaneous Approach
0PN34ZZ	Release Cervical Vertebra, Percutaneous Endoscopic Approach
0PN40ZZ	Release Thoracic Vertebra, Open Approach
0PN43ZZ	Release Thoracic Vertebra, Percutaneous Approach
0PN44ZZ	Release Thoracic Vertebra, Percutaneous Endoscopic Approach
0PN50ZZ	Release Right Scapula, Open Approach
0PN53ZZ	Release Right Scapula, Percutaneous Approach
0PN54ZZ	Release Right Scapula, Percutaneous Endoscopic Approach
0PN60ZZ	Release Left Scapula, Open Approach
0PN63ZZ	Release Left Scapula, Percutaneous Approach
0PN64ZZ	Release Left Scapula, Percutaneous Endoscopic Approach
0PN70ZZ	Release Right Glenoid Cavity, Open Approach
0PN73ZZ	Release Right Glenoid Cavity, Percutaneous Approach
0PN74ZZ	Release Right Glenoid Cavity, Percutaneous Endoscopic Approach
0PN80ZZ	Release Left Glenoid Cavity, Open Approach
0PN83ZZ	Release Left Glenoid Cavity, Percutaneous Approach
0PN84ZZ	Release Left Glenoid Cavity, Percutaneous Endoscopic Approach
0PN90ZZ	Release Right Clavicle, Open Approach
0PN93ZZ	Release Right Clavicle, Percutaneous Approach
0PN94ZZ	Release Right Clavicle, Percutaneous Endoscopic Approach
0PNB0ZZ	Release Left Clavicle, Open Approach
0PNB3ZZ	Release Left Clavicle, Percutaneous Approach
0PNB4ZZ	Release Left Clavicle, Percutaneous Endoscopic Approach
0PNC0ZZ	Release Right Humeral Head, Open Approach
0PNC3ZZ	Release Right Humeral Head, Percutaneous Approach
0PNC4ZZ	Release Right Humeral Head, Percutaneous Endoscopic Approach
0PND0ZZ	Release Left Humeral Head, Open Approach
0PND3ZZ	Release Left Humeral Head, Percutaneous Approach
0PND4ZZ	Release Left Humeral Head, Percutaneous Endoscopic Approach
0PNF0ZZ	Release Right Humeral Shaft, Open Approach
0PNF3ZZ	Release Right Humeral Shaft, Percutaneous Approach
0PNF4ZZ	Release Right Humeral Shaft, Percutaneous Endoscopic Approach
0PNG0ZZ	Release Left Humeral Shaft, Open Approach
0PNG3ZZ	Release Left Humeral Shaft, Percutaneous Approach
0PNG4ZZ	Release Left Humeral Shaft, Percutaneous Endoscopic Approach
0PNH0ZZ	Release Right Radius, Open Approach
0PNH3ZZ	Release Right Radius, Percutaneous Approach
0PNH4ZZ	Release Right Radius, Percutaneous Endoscopic Approach
0PNJ0ZZ	Release Left Radius, Open Approach
0PNJ3ZZ	Release Left Radius, Percutaneous Approach
0PNJ4ZZ	Release Left Radius, Percutaneous Endoscopic Approach
0PNK0ZZ	Release Right Ulna, Open Approach
0PNK3ZZ	Release Right Ulna, Percutaneous Approach
0PNK4ZZ	Release Right Ulna, Percutaneous Endoscopic Approach
0PNL0ZZ	Release Left Ulna, Open Approach
0PNL3ZZ	Release Left Ulna, Percutaneous Approach
0PNL4ZZ	Release Left Ulna, Percutaneous Endoscopic Approach
0PNM0ZZ	Release Right Carpal, Open Approach
0PNM3ZZ	Release Right Carpal, Percutaneous Approach
0PNM4ZZ	Release Right Carpal, Percutaneous Endoscopic Approach
0PNN0ZZ	Release Left Carpal, Open Approach
0PNN3ZZ	Release Left Carpal, Percutaneous Approach
0PNN4ZZ	Release Left Carpal, Percutaneous Endoscopic Approach
0PNP0ZZ	Release Right Metacarpal, Open Approach
0PNP3ZZ	Release Right Metacarpal, Percutaneous Approach
0PNP4ZZ	Release Right Metacarpal, Percutaneous Endoscopic Approach
0PNQ0ZZ	Release Left Metacarpal, Open Approach
0PNQ3ZZ	Release Left Metacarpal, Percutaneous Approach
0PNQ4ZZ	Release Left Metacarpal, Percutaneous Endoscopic Approach
0PNR0ZZ	Release Right Thumb Phalanx, Open Approach
0PNR3ZZ	Release Right Thumb Phalanx, Percutaneous Approach
0PNR4ZZ	Release Right Thumb Phalanx, Percutaneous Endoscopic Approach
0PNS0ZZ	Release Left Thumb Phalanx, Open Approach
0PNS3ZZ	Release Left Thumb Phalanx, Percutaneous Approach
0PNS4ZZ	Release Left Thumb Phalanx, Percutaneous Endoscopic Approach
0PNT0ZZ	Release Right Finger Phalanx, Open Approach
0PNT3ZZ	Release Right Finger Phalanx, Percutaneous Approach
0PNT4ZZ	Release Right Finger Phalanx, Percutaneous Endoscopic Approach
0PNV0ZZ	Release Left Finger Phalanx, Open Approach
0PNV3ZZ	Release Left Finger Phalanx, Percutaneous Approach
0PNV4ZZ	Release Left Finger Phalanx, Percutaneous Endoscopic Approach

0PP – Upper Bones, Removal

Review Coding Guideline B6.1c

0PP004Z	Removal of Internal Fixation Device from Sternum, Open Approach
0PP007Z	Removal of Autologous Tissue Substitute from Sternum, Open Approach
0PP00JZ	Removal of Synthetic Substitute from Sternum, Open Approach
0PP00KZ	Removal of Nonautologous Tissue Substitute from Sternum, Open Approach
0PP034Z	Removal of Internal Fixation Device from Sternum, Percutaneous Approach
0PP037Z	Removal of Autologous Tissue Substitute from Sternum, Percutaneous Approach
0PP03JZ	Removal of Synthetic Substitute from Sternum, Percutaneous Approach
0PP03KZ	Removal of Nonautologous Tissue Substitute from Sternum, Percutaneous Approach
0PP044Z	Removal of Internal Fixation Device from Sternum, Percutaneous Endoscopic Approach
0PP047Z	Removal of Autologous Tissue Substitute from Sternum, Percutaneous Endoscopic Approach
0PP04JZ	Removal of Synthetic Substitute from Sternum, Percutaneous Endoscopic Approach
0PP04KZ	Removal of Nonautologous Tissue Substitute from Sternum, Percutaneous Endoscopic Approach
0PP0X4Z	Removal of Internal Fixation Device from Sternum, External Approach
0PP104Z	Removal of Internal Fixation Device from Right Rib, Open Approach
0PP107Z	Removal of Autologous Tissue Substitute from Right Rib, Open Approach
0PP10JZ	Removal of Synthetic Substitute from Right Rib, Open Approach
0PP10KZ	Removal of Nonautologous Tissue Substitute from Right Rib, Open Approach
0PP134Z	Removal of Internal Fixation Device from Right Rib, Percutaneous Approach
0PP137Z	Removal of Autologous Tissue Substitute from Right Rib, Percutaneous Approach
0PP13JZ	Removal of Synthetic Substitute from Right Rib, Percutaneous Approach
0PP13KZ	Removal of Nonautologous Tissue Substitute from Right Rib, Percutaneous Approach
0PP144Z	Removal of Internal Fixation Device from Right Rib, Percutaneous Endoscopic Approach
0PP147Z	Removal of Autologous Tissue Substitute from Right Rib, Percutaneous Endoscopic Approach

♀ Female-only   ♂ Male-only   ▲ Limited Coverage   ● Non-OR   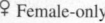 HAC-associated procedure   ▲ Non-covered procedures   ✚ Combinati

14JZ Removal of Synthetic Substitute from Right Rib, Percutaneous Endoscopic Approach

14KZ Removal of Nonautologous Tissue Substitute from Right Rib, Percutaneous Endoscopic Approach

1X4Z Removal of Internal Fixation Device from Right Rib, External Approach

204Z Removal of Internal Fixation Device from Left Rib, Open Approach

207Z Removal of Autologous Tissue Substitute from Left Rib, Open Approach

20JZ Removal of Synthetic Substitute from Left Rib, Open Approach

20KZ Removal of Nonautologous Tissue Substitute from Left Rib, Open Approach

234Z Removal of Internal Fixation Device from Left Rib, Percutaneous Approach

237Z Removal of Autologous Tissue Substitute from Left Rib, Percutaneous Approach

23JZ Removal of Synthetic Substitute from Left Rib, Percutaneous Approach

23KZ Removal of Nonautologous Tissue Substitute from Left Rib, Percutaneous Approach

244Z Removal of Internal Fixation Device from Left Rib, Percutaneous Endoscopic Approach

247Z Removal of Autologous Tissue Substitute from Left Rib, Percutaneous Endoscopic Approach

24JZ Removal of Synthetic Substitute from Left Rib, Percutaneous Endoscopic Approach

24KZ Removal of Nonautologous Tissue Substitute from Left Rib, Percutaneous Endoscopic Approach

2X4Z Removal of Internal Fixation Device from Left Rib, External Approach

304Z Removal of Internal Fixation Device from Cervical Vertebra, Open Approach

307Z Removal of Autologous Tissue Substitute from Cervical Vertebra, Open Approach

30JZ Removal of Synthetic Substitute from Cervical Vertebra, Open Approach

30KZ Removal of Nonautologous Tissue Substitute from Cervical Vertebra, Open Approach

334Z Removal of Internal Fixation Device from Cervical Vertebra, Percutaneous Approach

337Z Removal of Autologous Tissue Substitute from Cervical Vertebra, Percutaneous Approach

33JZ Removal of Synthetic Substitute from Cervical Vertebra, Percutaneous Approach

33KZ Removal of Nonautologous Tissue Substitute from Cervical Vertebra, Percutaneous Approach

344Z Removal of Internal Fixation Device from Cervical Vertebra, Percutaneous Endoscopic Approach

347Z Removal of Autologous Tissue Substitute from Cervical Vertebra, Percutaneous Endoscopic Approach

34JZ Removal of Synthetic Substitute from Cervical Vertebra, Percutaneous Endoscopic Approach

34KZ Removal of Nonautologous Tissue Substitute from Cervical Vertebra, Percutaneous Endoscopic Approach

3X4Z Removal of Internal Fixation Device from Cervical Vertebra, External Approach

P404Z Removal of Internal Fixation Device from Thoracic Vertebra, Open Approach

AHA CC: 4Q, 2014, 28-29

P407Z Removal of Autologous Tissue Substitute from Thoracic Vertebra, Open Approach

P40JZ Removal of Synthetic Substitute from Thoracic Vertebra, Open Approach

0PP40KZ Removal of Nonautologous Tissue Substitute from Thoracic Vertebra, Open Approach

0PP434Z Removal of Internal Fixation Device from Thoracic Vertebra, Percutaneous Approach

0PP437Z Removal of Autologous Tissue Substitute from Thoracic Vertebra, Percutaneous Approach

0PP43JZ Removal of Synthetic Substitute from Thoracic Vertebra, Percutaneous Approach

0PP43KZ Removal of Nonautologous Tissue Substitute from Thoracic Vertebra, Percutaneous Approach

0PP444Z Removal of Internal Fixation Device from Thoracic Vertebra, Percutaneous Endoscopic Approach

0PP447Z Removal of Autologous Tissue Substitute from Thoracic Vertebra, Percutaneous Endoscopic Approach

0PP44JZ Removal of Synthetic Substitute from Thoracic Vertebra, Percutaneous Endoscopic Approach

0PP44KZ Removal of Nonautologous Tissue Substitute from Thoracic Vertebra, Percutaneous Endoscopic Approach

0PP4X4Z Removal of Internal Fixation Device from Thoracic Vertebra, External Approach

0PP504Z Removal of Internal Fixation Device from Right Scapula, Open Approach

0PP507Z Removal of Autologous Tissue Substitute from Right Scapula, Open Approach

0PP50JZ Removal of Synthetic Substitute from Right Scapula, Open Approach

0PP50KZ Removal of Nonautologous Tissue Substitute from Right Scapula, Open Approach

0PP534Z Removal of Internal Fixation Device from Right Scapula, Percutaneous Approach

0PP537Z Removal of Autologous Tissue Substitute from Right Scapula, Percutaneous Approach

0PP53JZ Removal of Synthetic Substitute from Right Scapula, Percutaneous Approach

0PP53KZ Removal of Nonautologous Tissue Substitute from Right Scapula, Percutaneous Approach

0PP544Z Removal of Internal Fixation Device from Right Scapula, Percutaneous Endoscopic Approach

0PP547Z Removal of Autologous Tissue Substitute from Right Scapula, Percutaneous Endoscopic Approach

0PP54JZ Removal of Synthetic Substitute from Right Scapula, Percutaneous Endoscopic Approach

0PP54KZ Removal of Nonautologous Tissue Substitute from Right Scapula, Percutaneous Endoscopic Approach

0PP5X4Z Removal of Internal Fixation Device from Right Scapula, External Approach

0PP604Z Removal of Internal Fixation Device from Left Scapula, Open Approach

0PP607Z Removal of Autologous Tissue Substitute from Left Scapula, Open Approach

0PP60JZ Removal of Synthetic Substitute from Left Scapula, Open Approach

0PP60KZ Removal of Nonautologous Tissue Substitute from Left Scapula, Open Approach

0PP634Z Removal of Internal Fixation Device from Left Scapula, Percutaneous Approach

0PP637Z Removal of Autologous Tissue Substitute from Left Scapula, Percutaneous Approach

0PP63JZ Removal of Synthetic Substitute from Left Scapula, Percutaneous Approach

0PP63KZ Removal of Nonautologous Tissue Substitute from Left Scapula, Percutaneous Approach

0PP644Z Removal of Internal Fixation Device from Left Scapula, Percutaneous Endoscopic Approach

0PP647Z Removal of Autologous Tissue Substitute from Left Scapula, Percutaneous Endoscopic Approach

0PP64JZ Removal of Synthetic Substitute from Left Scapula, Percutaneous Endoscopic Approach

0PP64KZ Removal of Nonautologous Tissue Substitute from Left Scapula, Percutaneous Endoscopic Approach

0PP6X4Z Removal of Internal Fixation Device from Left Scapula, External Approach

0PP704Z Removal of Internal Fixation Device from Right Glenoid Cavity, Open Approach

0PP707Z Removal of Autologous Tissue Substitute from Right Glenoid Cavity, Open Approach

0PP70JZ Removal of Synthetic Substitute from Right Glenoid Cavity, Open Approach

0PP70KZ Removal of Nonautologous Tissue Substitute from Right Glenoid Cavity, Open Approach

0PP734Z Removal of Internal Fixation Device from Right Glenoid Cavity, Percutaneous Approach

0PP737Z Removal of Autologous Tissue Substitute from Right Glenoid Cavity, Percutaneous Approach

0PP73JZ Removal of Synthetic Substitute from Right Glenoid Cavity, Percutaneous Approach

0PP73KZ Removal of Nonautologous Tissue Substitute from Right Glenoid Cavity, Percutaneous Approach

0PP744Z Removal of Internal Fixation Device from Right Glenoid Cavity, Percutaneous Endoscopic Approach

0PP747Z Removal of Autologous Tissue Substitute from Right Glenoid Cavity, Percutaneous Endoscopic Approach

0PP74JZ Removal of Synthetic Substitute from Right Glenoid Cavity, Percutaneous Endoscopic Approach

0PP74KZ Removal of Nonautologous Tissue Substitute from Right Glenoid Cavity, Percutaneous Endoscopic Approach

0PP7X4Z Removal of Internal Fixation Device from Right Glenoid Cavity, External Approach

0PP804Z Removal of Internal Fixation Device from Left Glenoid Cavity, Open Approach

0PP807Z Removal of Autologous Tissue Substitute from Left Glenoid Cavity, Open Approach

0PP80JZ Removal of Synthetic Substitute from Left Glenoid Cavity, Open Approach

0PP80KZ Removal of Nonautologous Tissue Substitute from Left Glenoid Cavity, Open Approach

0PP834Z Removal of Internal Fixation Device from Left Glenoid Cavity, Percutaneous Approach

0PP837Z Removal of Autologous Tissue Substitute from Left Glenoid Cavity, Percutaneous Approach

0PP83JZ Removal of Synthetic Substitute from Left Glenoid Cavity, Percutaneous Approach

0PP83KZ Removal of Nonautologous Tissue Substitute from Left Glenoid Cavity, Percutaneous Approach

0PP844Z Removal of Internal Fixation Device from Left Glenoid Cavity, Percutaneous Endoscopic Approach

0PP847Z Removal of Autologous Tissue Substitute from Left Glenoid Cavity, Percutaneous Endoscopic Approach

0PP84JZ Removal of Synthetic Substitute from Left Glenoid Cavity, Percutaneous Endoscopic Approach

0PP84KZ Removal of Nonautologous Tissue Substitute from Left Glenoid Cavity, Percutaneous Endoscopic Approach

0PP8X4Z Removal of Internal Fixation Device from Left Glenoid Cavity, External Approach

0PP904Z Removal of Internal Fixation Device from Right Clavicle, Open Approach

0PP907Z Removal of Autologous Tissue Substitute from Right Clavicle, Open Approach

0PP90JZ Removal of Synthetic Substitute from Right Clavicle, Open Approach

0PP90KZ Removal of Nonautologous Tissue Substitute from Right Clavicle, Open Approach

0PP934Z Removal of Internal Fixation Device from Right Clavicle, Percutaneous Approach

0PP937Z Removal of Autologous Tissue Substitute from Right Clavicle, Percutaneous Approach

0PP93JZ Removal of Synthetic Substitute from Right Clavicle, Percutaneous Approach

0PP93KZ Removal of Nonautologous Tissue Substitute from Right Clavicle, Percutaneous Approach

0PP944Z Removal of Internal Fixation Device from Right Clavicle, Percutaneous Endoscopic Approach

0PP947Z Removal of Autologous Tissue Substitute from Right Clavicle, Percutaneous Endoscopic Approach

0PP94JZ Removal of Synthetic Substitute from Right Clavicle, Percutaneous Endoscopic Approach

0PP94KZ Removal of Nonautologous Tissue Substitute from Right Clavicle, Percutaneous Endoscopic Approach

0PP9X4Z Removal of Internal Fixation Device from Right Clavicle, External Approach

0PPB04Z Removal of Internal Fixation Device from Left Clavicle, Open Approach

0PPB07Z Removal of Autologous Tissue Substitute from Left Clavicle, Open Approach

0PPB0JZ Removal of Synthetic Substitute from Left Clavicle, Open Approach

0PPB0KZ Removal of Nonautologous Tissue Substitute from Left Clavicle, Open Approach

0PPB34Z Removal of Internal Fixation Device from Left Clavicle, Percutaneous Approach

0PPB37Z Removal of Autologous Tissue Substitute from Left Clavicle, Percutaneous Approach

0PPB3JZ Removal of Synthetic Substitute from Left Clavicle, Percutaneous Approach

0PPB3KZ Removal of Nonautologous Tissue Substitute from Left Clavicle, Percutaneous Approach

0PPB44Z Removal of Internal Fixation Device from Left Clavicle, Percutaneous Endoscopic Approach

0PPB47Z Removal of Autologous Tissue Substitute from Left Clavicle, Percutaneous Endoscopic Approach

0PPB4JZ Removal of Synthetic Substitute from Left Clavicle, Percutaneous Endoscopic Approach

0PPB4KZ Removal of Nonautologous Tissue Substitute from Left Clavicle, Percutaneous Endoscopic Approach

0PPBX4Z Removal of Internal Fixation Device from Left Clavicle, External Approach

0PPC04Z Removal of Internal Fixation Device from Right Humeral Head, Open Approach

0PPC05Z Removal of External Fixation Device from Right Humeral Head, Open Approach

0PPC07Z Removal of Autologous Tissue Substitute from Right Humeral Head, Open Approach

0PPC0JZ Removal of Synthetic Substitute from Right Humeral Head, Open Approach

0PPC0KZ Removal of Nonautologous Tissue Substitute from Right Humeral Head, Open Approach

0PPC34Z Removal of Internal Fixation Device from Right Humeral Head, Percutaneous Approach

0PPC35Z Removal of External Fixation Device from Right Humeral Head, Percutaneous Approach

0PPC37Z Removal of Autologous Tissue Substitute from Right Humeral Head, Percutaneous Approach

0PPC3JZ Removal of Synthetic Substitute from Right Humeral Head, Percutaneous Approach

0PPC3KZ Removal of Nonautologous Tissue Substitute from Right Humeral Head, Percutaneous Approach

0PPC44Z Removal of Internal Fixation Device from Right Humeral Head, Percutaneous Endoscopic Approach

0PPC45Z Removal of External Fixation Device from Right Humeral Head, Percutaneous Endoscopic Approach

0PPC47Z Removal of Autologous Tissue Substitute from Right Humeral Head, Percutaneous Endoscopic Approach

0PPC4JZ Removal of Synthetic Substitute from Right Humeral Head, Percutaneous Endoscopic Approach

0PPC4KZ Removal of Nonautologous Tissue Substitute from Right Humeral Head, Percutaneous Endoscopic Approach

0PPCX4Z Removal of Internal Fixation Device from Right Humeral Head, External Approach

0PPCX5Z Removal of External Fixation Device from Right Humeral Head, External Approach

0PPD04Z Removal of Internal Fixation Device from Left Humeral Head, Open Approach

0PPD05Z Removal of External Fixation Device from Left Humeral Head, Open Approach

0PPD07Z Removal of Autologous Tissue Substitute from Left Humeral Head, Open Approach

0PPD0JZ Removal of Synthetic Substitute from Left Humeral Head, Open Approach

0PPD0KZ Removal of Nonautologous Tissue Substitute from Left Humeral Head, Open Approach

0PPD34Z Removal of Internal Fixation Device from Left Humeral Head, Percutaneous Approach

0PPD35Z Removal of External Fixation Device from Left Humeral Head, Percutaneous Approach

0PPD37Z Removal of Autologous Tissue Substitute from Left Humeral Head, Percutaneous Approach

0PPD3JZ Removal of Synthetic Substitute from Left Humeral Head, Percutaneous Approach

0PPD3KZ Removal of Nonautologous Tissue Substitute from Left Humeral Head, Percutaneous Approach

0PPD44Z Removal of Internal Fixation Device from Left Humeral Head, Percutaneous Endoscopic Approach

0PPD45Z Removal of External Fixation Device from Left Humeral Head, Percutaneous Endoscopic Approach

0PPD47Z Removal of Autologous Tissue Substitute from Left Humeral Head, Percutaneous Endoscopic Approach

0PPD4JZ Removal of Synthetic Substitute from Left Humeral Head, Percutaneous Endoscopic Approach

0PPD4KZ Removal of Nonautologous Tissue Substitute from Left Humeral Head, Percutaneous Endoscopic Approach

0PPDX4Z Removal of Internal Fixation Device from Left Humeral Head, External Approach

0PPDX5Z Removal of External Fixation Device from Left Humeral Head, External Approach

0PPF04Z Removal of Internal Fixation Device from Right Humeral Shaft, Open Approach

0PPF05Z Removal of External Fixation Device from Right Humeral Shaft, Open Approach

0PPF07Z Removal of Autologous Tissue Substitute from Right Humeral Shaft, Open Approach

0PPF0JZ Removal of Synthetic Substitute from Right Humeral Shaft, Open Approach

0PPF0KZ Removal of Nonautologous Tissue Substitute from Right Humeral Shaft, Open Approach

0PPF34Z Removal of Internal Fixation Device from Right Humeral Shaft, Percutaneous Approach

0PPF35Z Removal of External Fixation Device from Right Humeral Shaft, Percutaneous Approach

0PPF37Z Removal of Autologous Tissue Substitute from Right Humeral Shaft, Percutaneous Approach

0PPF3JZ Removal of Synthetic Substitute from Right Humeral Shaft, Percutaneous Approach

0PPF3KZ Removal of Nonautologous Tissue Substitute from Right Humeral Shaft, Percutaneous Approach

0PPF44Z Removal of Internal Fixation Device from Right Humeral Shaft, Percutaneous Endoscopic Approach

0PPF45Z Removal of External Fixation Device from Right Humeral Shaft, Percutaneous Endoscopic Approach

0PPF47Z Removal of Autologous Tissue Substitute from Right Humeral Shaft, Percutaneous Endoscopic Approach

0PPF4JZ Removal of Synthetic Substitute from Right Humeral Shaft, Percutaneous Endoscopic Approach

0PPF4KZ Removal of Nonautologous Tissue Substitute from Right Humeral Shaft, Percutaneous Endoscopic Approach

0PPFX4Z Removal of Internal Fixation Device from Right Humeral Shaft, External Approach

0PPFX5Z Removal of External Fixation Device from Right Humeral Shaft, External Approach

0PPG04Z Removal of Internal Fixation Device from Left Humeral Shaft, Open Approach

0PPG05Z Removal of External Fixation Device from Left Humeral Shaft, Open Approach

0PPG07Z Removal of Autologous Tissue Substitute from Left Humeral Shaft, Open Approach

0PPG0JZ Removal of Synthetic Substitute from Left Humeral Shaft, Open Approach

0PPG0KZ Removal of Nonautologous Tissue Substitute from Left Humeral Shaft, Open Approach

0PPG34Z Removal of Internal Fixation Device from Left Humeral Shaft, Percutaneous Approach

♀ Female-only   ♂ Male-only   ▲ Limited Coverage   ● Non-OR   ▦ HAC-associated procedure   ▲ Non-covered procedures   ✚ Combinat

'G35Z Removal of External Fixation Device from Left Humeral Shaft, Percutaneous Approach	**0PPJ07Z** Removal of Autologous Tissue Substitute from Left Radius, Open Approach	**0PPKX5Z** Removal of External Fixation Device from Right Ulna, External Approach
'G37Z Removal of Autologous Tissue Substitute from Left Humeral Shaft, Percutaneous Approach	**0PPJ0JZ** Removal of Synthetic Substitute from Left Radius, Open Approach	**0PPL04Z** Removal of Internal Fixation Device from Left Ulna, Open Approach
'G3JZ Removal of Synthetic Substitute from Left Humeral Shaft, Percutaneous Approach	**0PPJ0KZ** Removal of Nonautologous Tissue Substitute from Left Radius, Open Approach	**0PPL05Z** Removal of External Fixation Device from Left Ulna, Open Approach
'G3KZ Removal of Nonautologous Tissue Substitute from Left Humeral Shaft, Percutaneous Approach	**0PPJ34Z** Removal of Internal Fixation Device from Left Radius, Percutaneous Approach	**0PPL07Z** Removal of Autologous Tissue Substitute from Left Ulna, Open Approach
'G44Z Removal of Internal Fixation Device from Left Humeral Shaft, Percutaneous Endoscopic Approach	**0PPJ35Z** Removal of External Fixation Device from Left Radius, Percutaneous Approach	**0PPL0JZ** Removal of Synthetic Substitute from Left Ulna, Open Approach
'G45Z Removal of External Fixation Device from Left Humeral Shaft, Percutaneous Endoscopic Approach	**0PPJ37Z** Removal of Autologous Tissue Substitute from Left Radius, Percutaneous Approach	**0PPL0KZ** Removal of Nonautologous Tissue Substitute from Left Ulna, Open Approach
'G47Z Removal of Autologous Tissue Substitute from Left Humeral Shaft, Percutaneous Endoscopic Approach	**0PPJ3JZ** Removal of Synthetic Substitute from Left Radius, Percutaneous Approach	**0PPL34Z** Removal of Internal Fixation Device from Left Ulna, Percutaneous Approach
'G4JZ Removal of Synthetic Substitute from Left Humeral Shaft, Percutaneous Endoscopic Approach	**0PPJ3KZ** Removal of Nonautologous Tissue Substitute from Left Radius, Percutaneous Approach	**0PPL35Z** Removal of External Fixation Device from Left Ulna, Percutaneous Approach
'G4KZ Removal of Nonautologous Tissue Substitute from Left Humeral Shaft, Percutaneous Endoscopic Approach	**0PPJ44Z** Removal of Internal Fixation Device from Left Radius, Percutaneous Endoscopic Approach	**0PPL37Z** Removal of Autologous Tissue Substitute from Left Ulna, Percutaneous Approach
'GX4Z Removal of Internal Fixation Device from Left Humeral Shaft, External Approach	**0PPJ45Z** Removal of External Fixation Device from Left Radius, Percutaneous Endoscopic Approach	**0PPL3JZ** Removal of Synthetic Substitute from Left Ulna, Percutaneous Approach
'GX5Z Removal of External Fixation Device from Left Humeral Shaft, External Approach	**0PPJ47Z** Removal of Autologous Tissue Substitute from Left Radius, Percutaneous Endoscopic Approach	**0PPL3KZ** Removal of Nonautologous Tissue Substitute from Left Ulna, Percutaneous Approach
'PH04Z Removal of Internal Fixation Device from Right Radius, Open Approach	**0PPJ4JZ** Removal of Synthetic Substitute from Left Radius, Percutaneous Endoscopic Approach	**0PPL44Z** Removal of Internal Fixation Device from Left Ulna, Percutaneous Endoscopic Approach
'PH05Z Removal of External Fixation Device from Right Radius, Open Approach	**0PPJ4KZ** Removal of Nonautologous Tissue Substitute from Left Radius, Percutaneous Endoscopic Approach	**0PPL45Z** Removal of External Fixation Device from Left Ulna, Percutaneous Endoscopic Approach
'PH07Z Removal of Autologous Tissue Substitute from Right Radius, Open Approach	**0PPJX4Z** Removal of Internal Fixation Device from Left Radius, External Approach	**0PPL47Z** Removal of Autologous Tissue Substitute from Left Ulna, Percutaneous Endoscopic Approach
'PH0JZ Removal of Synthetic Substitute from Right Radius, Open Approach	**0PPJX5Z** Removal of External Fixation Device from Left Radius, External Approach	**0PPL4JZ** Removal of Synthetic Substitute from Left Ulna, Percutaneous Endoscopic Approach
'PH0KZ Removal of Nonautologous Tissue Substitute from Right Radius, Open Approach	**0PPK04Z** Removal of Internal Fixation Device from Right Ulna, Open Approach	**0PPL4KZ** Removal of Nonautologous Tissue Substitute from Left Ulna, Percutaneous Endoscopic Approach
'PH34Z Removal of Internal Fixation Device from Right Radius, Percutaneous Approach	**0PPK05Z** Removal of External Fixation Device from Right Ulna, Open Approach	**0PPLX4Z** Removal of Internal Fixation Device from Left Ulna, External Approach
'PH35Z Removal of External Fixation Device from Right Radius, Percutaneous Approach	**0PPK07Z** Removal of Autologous Tissue Substitute from Right Ulna, Open Approach	**0PPLX5Z** Removal of External Fixation Device from Left Ulna, External Approach
'PH37Z Removal of Autologous Tissue Substitute from Right Radius, Percutaneous Approach	**0PPK0JZ** Removal of Synthetic Substitute from Right Ulna, Open Approach	**0PPM04Z** Removal of Internal Fixation Device from Right Carpal, Open Approach
'PH3JZ Removal of Synthetic Substitute from Right Radius, Percutaneous Approach	**0PPK0KZ** Removal of Nonautologous Tissue Substitute from Right Ulna, Open Approach	**0PPM05Z** Removal of External Fixation Device from Right Carpal, Open Approach
'PH3KZ Removal of Nonautologous Tissue Substitute from Right Radius, Percutaneous Approach	**0PPK34Z** Removal of Internal Fixation Device from Right Ulna, Percutaneous Approach	**0PPM07Z** Removal of Autologous Tissue Substitute from Right Carpal, Open Approach
'PH44Z Removal of Internal Fixation Device from Right Radius, Percutaneous Endoscopic Approach	**0PPK35Z** Removal of External Fixation Device from Right Ulna, Percutaneous Approach	**0PPM0JZ** Removal of Synthetic Substitute from Right Carpal, Open Approach
'PH45Z Removal of External Fixation Device from Right Radius, Percutaneous Endoscopic Approach	**0PPK37Z** Removal of Autologous Tissue Substitute from Right Ulna, Percutaneous Approach	**0PPM0KZ** Removal of Nonautologous Tissue Substitute from Right Carpal, Open Approach
'PH47Z Removal of Autologous Tissue Substitute from Right Radius, Percutaneous Endoscopic Approach	**0PPK3JZ** Removal of Synthetic Substitute from Right Ulna, Percutaneous Approach	**0PPM34Z** Removal of Internal Fixation Device from Right Carpal, Percutaneous Approach
'PH4JZ Removal of Synthetic Substitute from Right Radius, Percutaneous Endoscopic Approach	**0PPK3KZ** Removal of Nonautologous Tissue Substitute from Right Ulna, Percutaneous Approach	**0PPM35Z** Removal of External Fixation Device from Right Carpal, Percutaneous Approach
'PH4KZ Removal of Nonautologous Tissue Substitute from Right Radius, Percutaneous Endoscopic Approach	**0PPK44Z** Removal of Internal Fixation Device from Right Ulna, Percutaneous Endoscopic Approach	**0PPM37Z** Removal of Autologous Tissue Substitute from Right Carpal, Percutaneous Approach
'PHX4Z Removal of Internal Fixation Device from Right Radius, External Approach	**0PPK45Z** Removal of External Fixation Device from Right Ulna, Percutaneous Endoscopic Approach	**0PPM3JZ** Removal of Synthetic Substitute from Right Carpal, Percutaneous Approach
'PHX5Z Removal of External Fixation Device from Right Radius, External Approach	**0PPK47Z** Removal of Autologous Tissue Substitute from Right Ulna, Percutaneous Endoscopic Approach	**0PPM3KZ** Removal of Nonautologous Tissue Substitute from Right Carpal, Percutaneous Approach
'PJ04Z Removal of Internal Fixation Device from Left Radius, Open Approach	**0PPK4JZ** Removal of Synthetic Substitute from Right Ulna, Percutaneous Endoscopic Approach	**0PPM44Z** Removal of Internal Fixation Device from Right Carpal, Percutaneous Endoscopic Approach
'PJ05Z Removal of External Fixation Device from Left Radius, Open Approach	**0PPK4KZ** Removal of Nonautologous Tissue Substitute from Right Ulna, Percutaneous Endoscopic Approach	**0PPM45Z** Removal of External Fixation Device from Right Carpal, Percutaneous Endoscopic Approach
	0PPKX4Z Removal of Internal Fixation Device from Right Ulna, External Approach	**0PPM47Z** Removal of Autologous Tissue Substitute from Right Carpal, Percutaneous Endoscopic Approach
		0PPM4JZ Removal of Synthetic Substitute from Right Carpal, Percutaneous Endoscopic Approach

Female-only	♂ Male-only	▲ Limited Coverage	● Non-OR	▨ HAC-associated procedure	▲ Non-covered procedures	➕ Combination

0PPM4KZ Removal of Nonautologous Tissue Substitute from Right Carpal, Percutaneous Endoscopic Approach

0PPMX4Z Removal of Internal Fixation Device from Right Carpal, External Approach

0PPMX5Z Removal of External Fixation Device from Right Carpal, External Approach

0PPN04Z Removal of Internal Fixation Device from Left Carpal, Open Approach

0PPN05Z Removal of External Fixation Device from Left Carpal, Open Approach

0PPN07Z Removal of Autologous Tissue Substitute from Left Carpal, Open Approach

0PPN0JZ Removal of Synthetic Substitute from Left Carpal, Open Approach

0PPN0KZ Removal of Nonautologous Tissue Substitute from Left Carpal, Open Approach

0PPN34Z Removal of Internal Fixation Device from Left Carpal, Percutaneous Approach

0PPN35Z Removal of External Fixation Device from Left Carpal, Percutaneous Approach

0PPN37Z Removal of Autologous Tissue Substitute from Left Carpal, Percutaneous Approach

0PPN3JZ Removal of Synthetic Substitute from Left Carpal, Percutaneous Approach

0PPN3KZ Removal of Nonautologous Tissue Substitute from Left Carpal, Percutaneous Approach

0PPN44Z Removal of Internal Fixation Device from Left Carpal, Percutaneous Endoscopic Approach

0PPN45Z Removal of External Fixation Device from Left Carpal, Percutaneous Endoscopic Approach

0PPN47Z Removal of Autologous Tissue Substitute from Left Carpal, Percutaneous Endoscopic Approach

0PPN4JZ Removal of Synthetic Substitute from Left Carpal, Percutaneous Endoscopic Approach

0PPN4KZ Removal of Nonautologous Tissue Substitute from Left Carpal, Percutaneous Endoscopic Approach

0PPNX4Z Removal of Internal Fixation Device from Left Carpal, External Approach

0PPNX5Z Removal of External Fixation Device from Left Carpal, External Approach

0PPP04Z Removal of Internal Fixation Device from Right Metacarpal, Open Approach

0PPP05Z Removal of External Fixation Device from Right Metacarpal, Open Approach

0PPP07Z Removal of Autologous Tissue Substitute from Right Metacarpal, Open Approach

0PPP0JZ Removal of Synthetic Substitute from Right Metacarpal, Open Approach

0PPP0KZ Removal of Nonautologous Tissue Substitute from Right Metacarpal, Open Approach

0PPP34Z Removal of Internal Fixation Device from Right Metacarpal, Percutaneous Approach

0PPP35Z Removal of External Fixation Device from Right Metacarpal, Percutaneous Approach

0PPP37Z Removal of Autologous Tissue Substitute from Right Metacarpal, Percutaneous Approach

0PPP3JZ Removal of Synthetic Substitute from Right Metacarpal, Percutaneous Approach

0PPP3KZ Removal of Nonautologous Tissue Substitute from Right Metacarpal, Percutaneous Approach

0PPP44Z Removal of Internal Fixation Device from Right Metacarpal, Percutaneous Endoscopic Approach

0PPP45Z Removal of External Fixation Device from Right Metacarpal, Percutaneous Endoscopic Approach

0PPP47Z Removal of Autologous Tissue Substitute from Right Metacarpal, Percutaneous Endoscopic Approach

0PPP4JZ Removal of Synthetic Substitute from Right Metacarpal, Percutaneous Endoscopic Approach

0PPP4KZ Removal of Nonautologous Tissue Substitute from Right Metacarpal, Percutaneous Endoscopic Approach

0PPPX4Z Removal of Internal Fixation Device from Right Metacarpal, External Approach

0PPPX5Z Removal of External Fixation Device from Right Metacarpal, External Approach

0PPQ04Z Removal of Internal Fixation Device from Left Metacarpal, Open Approach

0PPQ05Z Removal of External Fixation Device from Left Metacarpal, Open Approach

0PPQ07Z Removal of Autologous Tissue Substitute from Left Metacarpal, Open Approach

0PPQ0JZ Removal of Synthetic Substitute from Left Metacarpal, Open Approach

0PPQ0KZ Removal of Nonautologous Tissue Substitute from Left Metacarpal, Open Approach

0PPQ34Z Removal of Internal Fixation Device from Left Metacarpal, Percutaneous Approach

0PPQ35Z Removal of External Fixation Device from Left Metacarpal, Percutaneous Approach

0PPQ37Z Removal of Autologous Tissue Substitute from Left Metacarpal, Percutaneous Approach

0PPQ3JZ Removal of Synthetic Substitute from Left Metacarpal, Percutaneous Approach

0PPQ3KZ Removal of Nonautologous Tissue Substitute from Left Metacarpal, Percutaneous Approach

0PPQ44Z Removal of Internal Fixation Device from Left Metacarpal, Percutaneous Endoscopic Approach

0PPQ45Z Removal of External Fixation Device from Left Metacarpal, Percutaneous Endoscopic Approach

0PPQ47Z Removal of Autologous Tissue Substitute from Left Metacarpal, Percutaneous Endoscopic Approach

0PPQ4JZ Removal of Synthetic Substitute from Left Metacarpal, Percutaneous Endoscopic Approach

0PPQ4KZ Removal of Nonautologous Tissue Substitute from Left Metacarpal, Percutaneous Endoscopic Approach

0PPQX4Z Removal of Internal Fixation Device from Left Metacarpal, External Approach

0PPQX5Z Removal of External Fixation Device from Left Metacarpal, External Approach

0PPR04Z Removal of Internal Fixation Device from Right Thumb Phalanx, Open Approach

0PPR05Z Removal of External Fixation Device from Right Thumb Phalanx, Open Approach

0PPR07Z Removal of Autologous Tissue Substitute from Right Thumb Phalanx, Open Approach

0PPR0JZ Removal of Synthetic Substitute from Right Thumb Phalanx, Open Approach

0PPR0KZ Removal of Nonautologous Tissue Substitute from Right Thumb Phalanx, Open Approach

0PPR34Z Removal of Internal Fixation Device from Right Thumb Phalanx, Percutaneous Approach

0PPR35Z Removal of External Fixation Device from Right Thumb Phalanx, Percutaneous Approach

0PPR37Z Removal of Autologous Tissue Substitute from Right Thumb Phalanx, Percutaneous Approach

0PPR3JZ Removal of Synthetic Substitute from Right Thumb Phalanx, Percutaneous Approach

0PPR3KZ Removal of Nonautologous Tissue Substitute from Right Thumb Phalanx, Percutaneous Approach

0PPR44Z Removal of Internal Fixation Device from Right Thumb Phalanx, Percutaneous Endoscopic Approach

0PPR45Z Removal of External Fixation Device from Right Thumb Phalanx, Percutaneous Endoscopic Approach

0PPR47Z Removal of Autologous Tissue Substitute from Right Thumb Phalanx, Percutaneous Endoscopic Approach

0PPR4JZ Removal of Synthetic Substitute from Right Thumb Phalanx, Percutaneous Endoscopic Approach

0PPR4KZ Removal of Nonautologous Tissue Substitute from Right Thumb Phalanx, Percutaneous Endoscopic Approach

0PPRX4Z Removal of Internal Fixation Device from Right Thumb Phalanx, External Approach

0PPRX5Z Removal of External Fixation Device from Right Thumb Phalanx, External Approach

0PPS04Z Removal of Internal Fixation Device from Left Thumb Phalanx, Open Approach

0PPS05Z Removal of External Fixation Device from Left Thumb Phalanx, Open Approach

0PPS07Z Removal of Autologous Tissue Substitute from Left Thumb Phalanx, Open Approach

0PPS0JZ Removal of Synthetic Substitute from Left Thumb Phalanx, Open Approach

0PPS0KZ Removal of Nonautologous Tissue Substitute from Left Thumb Phalanx, Open Approach

0PPS34Z Removal of Internal Fixation Device from Left Thumb Phalanx, Percutaneous Approach

0PPS35Z Removal of External Fixation Device from Left Thumb Phalanx, Percutaneous Approach

0PPS37Z Removal of Autologous Tissue Substitute from Left Thumb Phalanx, Percutaneous Approach

0PPS3JZ Removal of Synthetic Substitute from Left Thumb Phalanx, Percutaneous Approach

0PPS3KZ Removal of Nonautologous Tissue Substitute from Left Thumb Phalanx, Percutaneous Approach

0PPS44Z Removal of Internal Fixation Device from Left Thumb Phalanx, Percutaneous Endoscopic Approach

0PPS45Z Removal of External Fixation Device from Left Thumb Phalanx, Percutaneous Endoscopic Approach

0PPS47Z Removal of Autologous Tissue Substitute from Left Thumb Phalanx, Percutaneous Endoscopic Approach

0PPS4JZ Removal of Synthetic Substitute from Left Thumb Phalanx, Percutaneous Endoscopic Approach

0PPS4KZ Removal of Nonautologous Tissue Substitute from Left Thumb Phalanx, Percutaneous Endoscopic Approach

0PPSX4Z Removal of Internal Fixation Device from Left Thumb Phalanx, External Approach

0PPSX5Z Removal of External Fixation Device from Left Thumb Phalanx, External Approach

0PPT04Z Removal of Internal Fixation Device from Right Finger Phalanx, Open Approach

T05Z Removal of External Fixation Device from Right Finger Phalanx, Open Approach

T07Z Removal of Autologous Tissue Substitute from Right Finger Phalanx, Open Approach

T0JZ Removal of Synthetic Substitute from Right Finger Phalanx, Open Approach

T0KZ Removal of Nonautologous Tissue Substitute from Right Finger Phalanx, Open Approach

T34Z Removal of Internal Fixation Device from Right Finger Phalanx, Percutaneous Approach

T35Z Removal of External Fixation Device from Right Finger Phalanx, Percutaneous Approach

T37Z Removal of Autologous Tissue Substitute from Right Finger Phalanx, Percutaneous Approach

T3JZ Removal of Synthetic Substitute from Right Finger Phalanx, Percutaneous Approach

T3KZ Removal of Nonautologous Tissue Substitute from Right Finger Phalanx, Percutaneous Approach

T44Z Removal of Internal Fixation Device from Right Finger Phalanx, Percutaneous Endoscopic Approach

T45Z Removal of External Fixation Device from Right Finger Phalanx, Percutaneous Endoscopic Approach

T47Z Removal of Autologous Tissue Substitute from Right Finger Phalanx, Percutaneous Endoscopic Approach

T4JZ Removal of Synthetic Substitute from Right Finger Phalanx, Percutaneous Endoscopic Approach

0PPT4KZ Removal of Nonautologous Tissue Substitute from Right Finger Phalanx, Percutaneous Endoscopic Approach

0PPTX4Z Removal of Internal Fixation Device from Right Finger Phalanx, External Approach

0PPTX5Z Removal of External Fixation Device from Right Finger Phalanx, External Approach

0PPV04Z Removal of Internal Fixation Device from Left Finger Phalanx, Open Approach

0PPV05Z Removal of External Fixation Device from Left Finger Phalanx, Open Approach

0PPV07Z Removal of Autologous Tissue Substitute from Left Finger Phalanx, Open Approach

0PPV0JZ Removal of Synthetic Substitute from Left Finger Phalanx, Open Approach

0PPV0KZ Removal of Nonautologous Tissue Substitute from Left Finger Phalanx, Open Approach

0PPV34Z Removal of Internal Fixation Device from Left Finger Phalanx, Percutaneous Approach

0PPV35Z Removal of External Fixation Device from Left Finger Phalanx, Percutaneous Approach

0PPV37Z Removal of Autologous Tissue Substitute from Left Finger Phalanx, Percutaneous Approach

0PPV3JZ Removal of Synthetic Substitute from Left Finger Phalanx, Percutaneous Approach

0PPV3KZ Removal of Nonautologous Tissue Substitute from Left Finger Phalanx, Percutaneous Approach

0PPV44Z Removal of Internal Fixation Device from Left Finger Phalanx, Percutaneous Endoscopic Approach

0PPV45Z Removal of External Fixation Device from Left Finger Phalanx, Percutaneous Endoscopic Approach

0PPV47Z Removal of Autologous Tissue Substitute from Left Finger Phalanx, Percutaneous Endoscopic Approach

0PPV4JZ Removal of Synthetic Substitute from Left Finger Phalanx, Percutaneous Endoscopic Approach

0PPV4KZ Removal of Nonautologous Tissue Substitute from Left Finger Phalanx, Percutaneous Endoscopic Approach

0PPVX4Z Removal of Internal Fixation Device from Left Finger Phalanx, External Approach

0PPVX5Z Removal of External Fixation Device from Left Finger Phalanx, External Approach

0PPY00Z Removal of Drainage Device from Upper Bone, Open Approach

0PPY0MZ Removal of Bone Growth Stimulator from Upper Bone, Open Approach

0PPY30Z Removal of Drainage Device from Upper Bone, Percutaneous Approach

0PPY3MZ Removal of Bone Growth Stimulator from Upper Bone, Percutaneous Approach

0PPY40Z Removal of Drainage Device from Upper Bone, Percutaneous Endoscopic Approach

0PPY4MZ Removal of Bone Growth Stimulator from Upper Bone, Percutaneous Endoscopic Approach

0PPYX0Z Removal of Drainage Device from Upper Bone, External Approach

0PPYXMZ Removal of Bone Growth Stimulator from Upper Bone, External Approach

Q – Upper Bones, Repair

Review Coding Guideline B3.5

00ZZ Repair Sternum, Open Approach

03ZZ Repair Sternum, Percutaneous Approach

04ZZ Repair Sternum, Percutaneous Endoscopic Approach

0XZZ Repair Sternum, External Approach

Q10ZZ Repair Right Rib, Open Approach

Q13ZZ Repair Right Rib, Percutaneous Approach

Q14ZZ Repair Right Rib, Percutaneous Endoscopic Approach

Q1XZZ Repair Right Rib, External Approach

Q20ZZ Repair Left Rib, Open Approach

Q23ZZ Repair Left Rib, Percutaneous Approach

Q24ZZ Repair Left Rib, Percutaneous Endoscopic Approach

Q2XZZ Repair Left Rib, External Approach

Q30ZZ Repair Cervical Vertebra, Open Approach

Q33ZZ Repair Cervical Vertebra, Percutaneous Approach

Q34ZZ Repair Cervical Vertebra, Percutaneous Endoscopic Approach

Q3XZZ Repair Cervical Vertebra, External Approach

Q40ZZ Repair Thoracic Vertebra, Open Approach

Q43ZZ Repair Thoracic Vertebra, Percutaneous Approach

Q44ZZ Repair Thoracic Vertebra, Percutaneous Endoscopic Approach

Q4XZZ Repair Thoracic Vertebra, External Approach

Q50ZZ Repair Right Scapula, Open Approach

Q53ZZ Repair Right Scapula, Percutaneous Approach

Q54ZZ Repair Right Scapula, Percutaneous Endoscopic Approach

Q5XZZ Repair Right Scapula, External Approach

0PQ60ZZ Repair Left Scapula, Open Approach

0PQ63ZZ Repair Left Scapula, Percutaneous Approach

0PQ64ZZ Repair Left Scapula, Percutaneous Endoscopic Approach

0PQ6XZZ Repair Left Scapula, External Approach

0PQ70ZZ Repair Right Glenoid Cavity, Open Approach

0PQ73ZZ Repair Right Glenoid Cavity, Percutaneous Approach

0PQ74ZZ Repair Right Glenoid Cavity, Percutaneous Endoscopic Approach

0PQ7XZZ Repair Right Glenoid Cavity, External Approach

0PQ80ZZ Repair Left Glenoid Cavity, Open Approach

0PQ83ZZ Repair Left Glenoid Cavity, Percutaneous Approach

0PQ84ZZ Repair Left Glenoid Cavity, Percutaneous Endoscopic Approach

0PQ8XZZ Repair Left Glenoid Cavity, External Approach

0PQ90ZZ Repair Right Clavicle, Open Approach

0PQ93ZZ Repair Right Clavicle, Percutaneous Approach

0PQ94ZZ Repair Right Clavicle, Percutaneous Endoscopic Approach

0PQ9XZZ Repair Right Clavicle, External Approach

0PQB0ZZ Repair Left Clavicle, Open Approach

0PQB3ZZ Repair Left Clavicle, Percutaneous Approach

0PQB4ZZ Repair Left Clavicle, Percutaneous Endoscopic Approach

0PQBXZZ Repair Left Clavicle, External Approach

0PQC0ZZ Repair Right Humeral Head, Open Approach

0PQC3ZZ Repair Right Humeral Head, Percutaneous Approach

0PQC4ZZ Repair Right Humeral Head, Percutaneous Endoscopic Approach

0PQCXZZ Repair Right Humeral Head, External Approach

0PQD0ZZ Repair Left Humeral Head, Open Approach

0PQD3ZZ Repair Left Humeral Head, Percutaneous Approach

0PQD4ZZ Repair Left Humeral Head, Percutaneous Endoscopic Approach

0PQDXZZ Repair Left Humeral Head, External Approach

0PQF0ZZ Repair Right Humeral Shaft, Open Approach

0PQF3ZZ Repair Right Humeral Shaft, Percutaneous Approach

0PQF4ZZ Repair Right Humeral Shaft, Percutaneous Endoscopic Approach

0PQFXZZ Repair Right Humeral Shaft, External Approach

0PQG0ZZ Repair Left Humeral Shaft, Open Approach

0PQG3ZZ Repair Left Humeral Shaft, Percutaneous Approach

0PQG4ZZ Repair Left Humeral Shaft, Percutaneous Endoscopic Approach

0PQGXZZ Repair Left Humeral Shaft, External Approach

0PQH0ZZ Repair Right Radius, Open Approach

0PQH3ZZ Repair Right Radius, Percutaneous Approach

Female-only   ♂ Male-only   ▲ Limited Coverage   ● Non-OR   ▨ HAC-associated procedure   ▲ Non-covered procedures   ✛ Combination

0PQH4ZZ	Repair Right Radius, Percutaneous Endoscopic Approach	
0PQHXZZ	Repair Right Radius, External Approach	
0PQJ0ZZ	Repair Left Radius, Open Approach	
0PQJ3ZZ	Repair Left Radius, Percutaneous Approach	
0PQJ4ZZ	Repair Left Radius, Percutaneous Endoscopic Approach	
0PQJXZZ	Repair Left Radius, External Approach	
0PQK0ZZ	Repair Right Ulna, Open Approach	
0PQK3ZZ	Repair Right Ulna, Percutaneous Approach	
0PQK4ZZ	Repair Right Ulna, Percutaneous Endoscopic Approach	
0PQKXZZ	Repair Right Ulna, External Approach	
0PQL0ZZ	Repair Left Ulna, Open Approach	
0PQL3ZZ	Repair Left Ulna, Percutaneous Approach	
0PQL4ZZ	Repair Left Ulna, Percutaneous Endoscopic Approach	
0PQLXZZ	Repair Left Ulna, External Approach	
0PQM0ZZ	Repair Right Carpal, Open Approach	
0PQM3ZZ	Repair Right Carpal, Percutaneous Approach	
0PQM4ZZ	Repair Right Carpal, Percutaneous Endoscopic Approach	
0PQMXZZ	Repair Right Carpal, External Approach	

0PQN0ZZ	Repair Left Carpal, Open Approach
0PQN3ZZ	Repair Left Carpal, Percutaneous Approach
0PQN4ZZ	Repair Left Carpal, Percutaneous Endoscopic Approach
0PQNXZZ	Repair Left Carpal, External Approach
0PQP0ZZ	Repair Right Metacarpal, Open Approach
0PQP3ZZ	Repair Right Metacarpal, Percutaneous Approach
0PQP4ZZ	Repair Right Metacarpal, Percutaneous Endoscopic Approach
0PQPXZZ	Repair Right Metacarpal, External Approach
0PQQ0ZZ	Repair Left Metacarpal, Open Approach
0PQQ3ZZ	Repair Left Metacarpal, Percutaneous Approach
0PQQ4ZZ	Repair Left Metacarpal, Percutaneous Endoscopic Approach
0PQQXZZ	Repair Left Metacarpal, External Approach
0PQR0ZZ	Repair Right Thumb Phalanx, Open Approach
0PQR3ZZ	Repair Right Thumb Phalanx, Percutaneous Approach
0PQR4ZZ	Repair Right Thumb Phalanx, Percutaneous Endoscopic Approach

0PQRXZZ	Repair Right Thumb Phalanx, External Approach
0PQS0ZZ	Repair Left Thumb Phalanx, Open Approach
0PQS3ZZ	Repair Left Thumb Phalanx, Percutaneous Approach
0PQS4ZZ	Repair Left Thumb Phalanx, Percutaneous Endoscopic Approach
0PQSXZZ	Repair Left Thumb Phalanx, External Approach
0PQT0ZZ	Repair Right Finger Phalanx, Open Approach
0PQT3ZZ	Repair Right Finger Phalanx, Percutaneous Approach
0PQT4ZZ	Repair Right Finger Phalanx, Percutaneous Endoscopic Approach
0PQTXZZ	Repair Right Finger Phalanx, External Approach
0PQV0ZZ	Repair Left Finger Phalanx, Open Approach
0PQV3ZZ	Repair Left Finger Phalanx, Percutaneous Approach
0PQV4ZZ	Repair Left Finger Phalanx, Percutaneous Endoscopic Approach
0PQVXZZ	Repair Left Finger Phalanx, External Approach

0PR – Upper Bones, Replacement

0PR007Z	Replacement of Sternum with Autologous Tissue Substitute, Open Approach
0PR00JZ	Replacement of Sternum with Synthetic Substitute, Open Approach
0PR00KZ	Replacement of Sternum with Nonautologous Tissue Substitute, Open Approach
0PR037Z	Replacement of Sternum with Autologous Tissue Substitute, Percutaneous Approach
0PR03JZ	Replacement of Sternum with Synthetic Substitute, Percutaneous Approach
0PR03KZ	Replacement of Sternum with Nonautologous Tissue Substitute, Percutaneous Approach
0PR047Z	Replacement of Sternum with Autologous Tissue Substitute, Percutaneous Endoscopic Approach
0PR04JZ	Replacement of Sternum with Synthetic Substitute, Percutaneous Endoscopic Approach
0PR04KZ	Replacement of Sternum with Nonautologous Tissue Substitute, Percutaneous Endoscopic Approach
0PR107Z	Replacement of Right Rib with Autologous Tissue Substitute, Open Approach
0PR10JZ	Replacement of Right Rib with Synthetic Substitute, Open Approach
0PR10KZ	Replacement of Right Rib with Nonautologous Tissue Substitute, Open Approach
0PR137Z	Replacement of Right Rib with Autologous Tissue Substitute, Percutaneous Approach
0PR13JZ	Replacement of Right Rib with Synthetic Substitute, Percutaneous Approach
0PR13KZ	Replacement of Right Rib with Nonautologous Tissue Substitute, Percutaneous Approach
0PR147Z	Replacement of Right Rib with Autologous Tissue Substitute, Percutaneous Endoscopic Approach
0PR14JZ	Replacement of Right Rib with Synthetic Substitute, Percutaneous Endoscopic Approach
0PR14KZ	Replacement of Right Rib with Nonautologous Tissue Substitute, Percutaneous Endoscopic Approach

0PR207Z	Replacement of Left Rib with Autologous Tissue Substitute, Open Approach
0PR20JZ	Replacement of Left Rib with Synthetic Substitute, Open Approach
0PR20KZ	Replacement of Left Rib with Nonautologous Tissue Substitute, Open Approach
0PR237Z	Replacement of Left Rib with Autologous Tissue Substitute, Percutaneous Approach
0PR23JZ	Replacement of Left Rib with Synthetic Substitute, Percutaneous Approach
0PR23KZ	Replacement of Left Rib with Nonautologous Tissue Substitute, Percutaneous Approach
0PR247Z	Replacement of Left Rib with Autologous Tissue Substitute, Percutaneous Endoscopic Approach
0PR24JZ	Replacement of Left Rib with Synthetic Substitute, Percutaneous Endoscopic Approach
0PR24KZ	Replacement of Left Rib with Nonautologous Tissue Substitute, Percutaneous Endoscopic Approach
0PR307Z	Replacement of Cervical Vertebra with Autologous Tissue Substitute, Open Approach
0PR30JZ	Replacement of Cervical Vertebra with Synthetic Substitute, Open Approach
0PR30KZ	Replacement of Cervical Vertebra with Nonautologous Tissue Substitute, Open Approach
0PR337Z	Replacement of Cervical Vertebra with Autologous Tissue Substitute, Percutaneous Approach
0PR33JZ	Replacement of Cervical Vertebra with Synthetic Substitute, Percutaneous Approach
0PR33KZ	Replacement of Cervical Vertebra with Nonautologous Tissue Substitute, Percutaneous Approach
0PR347Z	Replacement of Cervical Vertebra with Autologous Tissue Substitute, Percutaneous Endoscopic Approach
0PR34JZ	Replacement of Cervical Vertebra with Synthetic Substitute, Percutaneous Endoscopic Approach
0PR34KZ	Replacement of Cervical Vertebra with Nonautologous Tissue Substitute, Percutaneous Endoscopic Approach

0PR407Z	Replacement of Thoracic Vertebra with Autologous Tissue Substitute, Open Approach
0PR40JZ	Replacement of Thoracic Vertebra with Synthetic Substitute, Open Approach
0PR40KZ	Replacement of Thoracic Vertebra with Nonautologous Tissue Substitute, Open Approach
0PR437Z	Replacement of Thoracic Vertebra with Autologous Tissue Substitute, Percutaneous Approach
0PR43JZ	Replacement of Thoracic Vertebra with Synthetic Substitute, Percutaneous Approach
0PR43KZ	Replacement of Thoracic Vertebra with Nonautologous Tissue Substitute, Percutaneous Approach
0PR447Z	Replacement of Thoracic Vertebra with Autologous Tissue Substitute, Percutaneous Endoscopic Approach
0PR44JZ	Replacement of Thoracic Vertebra with Synthetic Substitute, Percutaneous Endoscopic Approach
0PR44KZ	Replacement of Thoracic Vertebra with Nonautologous Tissue Substitute, Percutaneous Endoscopic Approach
0PR507Z	Replacement of Right Scapula with Autologous Tissue Substitute, Open Approach
0PR50JZ	Replacement of Right Scapula with Synthetic Substitute, Open Approach
0PR50KZ	Replacement of Right Scapula with Nonautologous Tissue Substitute, Open Approach
0PR537Z	Replacement of Right Scapula with Autologous Tissue Substitute, Percutaneous Approach
0PR53JZ	Replacement of Right Scapula with Synthetic Substitute, Percutaneous Approach
0PR53KZ	Replacement of Right Scapula with Nonautologous Tissue Substitute, Percutaneous Approach
0PR547Z	Replacement of Right Scapula with Autologous Tissue Substitute, Percutaneous Endoscopic Approach
0PR54JZ	Replacement of Right Scapula with Synthetic Substitute, Percutaneous Endoscopic Approach

♀ Female-only	♂ Male-only	▲ Limited Coverage	● Non-OR	▦ HAC-associated procedure

▲ Non-covered procedures   ✚ Combinati

54KZ Replacement of Right Scapula with Nonautologous Tissue Substitute, Percutaneous Endoscopic Approach

607Z Replacement of Left Scapula with Autologous Tissue Substitute, Open Approach

50JZ Replacement of Left Scapula with Synthetic Substitute, Open Approach

50KZ Replacement of Left Scapula with Nonautologous Tissue Substitute, Open Approach

537Z Replacement of Left Scapula with Autologous Tissue Substitute, Percutaneous Approach

63JZ Replacement of Left Scapula with Synthetic Substitute, Percutaneous Approach

63KZ Replacement of Left Scapula with Nonautologous Tissue Substitute, Percutaneous Approach

647Z Replacement of Left Scapula with Autologous Tissue Substitute, Percutaneous Endoscopic Approach

64JZ Replacement of Left Scapula with Synthetic Substitute, Percutaneous Endoscopic Approach

64KZ Replacement of Left Scapula with Nonautologous Tissue Substitute, Percutaneous Endoscopic Approach

707Z Replacement of Right Glenoid Cavity with Autologous Tissue Substitute, Open Approach

70JZ Replacement of Right Glenoid Cavity with Synthetic Substitute, Open Approach

70KZ Replacement of Right Glenoid Cavity with Nonautologous Tissue Substitute, Open Approach

737Z Replacement of Right Glenoid Cavity with Autologous Tissue Substitute, Percutaneous Approach

73JZ Replacement of Right Glenoid Cavity with Synthetic Substitute, Percutaneous Approach

73KZ Replacement of Right Glenoid Cavity with Nonautologous Tissue Substitute, Percutaneous Approach

747Z Replacement of Right Glenoid Cavity with Autologous Tissue Substitute, Percutaneous Endoscopic Approach

74JZ Replacement of Right Glenoid Cavity with Synthetic Substitute, Percutaneous Endoscopic Approach

74KZ Replacement of Right Glenoid Cavity with Nonautologous Tissue Substitute, Percutaneous Endoscopic Approach

807Z Replacement of Left Glenoid Cavity with Autologous Tissue Substitute, Open Approach

R80JZ Replacement of Left Glenoid Cavity with Synthetic Substitute, Open Approach

R80KZ Replacement of Left Glenoid Cavity with Nonautologous Tissue Substitute, Open Approach

R837Z Replacement of Left Glenoid Cavity with Autologous Tissue Substitute, Percutaneous Approach

R83JZ Replacement of Left Glenoid Cavity with Synthetic Substitute, Percutaneous Approach

R83KZ Replacement of Left Glenoid Cavity with Nonautologous Tissue Substitute, Percutaneous Approach

R847Z Replacement of Left Glenoid Cavity with Autologous Tissue Substitute, Percutaneous Endoscopic Approach

0PR84JZ Replacement of Left Glenoid Cavity with Synthetic Substitute, Percutaneous Endoscopic Approach

0PR84KZ Replacement of Left Glenoid Cavity with Nonautologous Tissue Substitute, Percutaneous Endoscopic Approach

0PR907Z Replacement of Right Clavicle with Autologous Tissue Substitute, Open Approach

0PR90JZ Replacement of Right Clavicle with Synthetic Substitute, Open Approach

0PR90KZ Replacement of Right Clavicle with Nonautologous Tissue Substitute, Open Approach

0PR937Z Replacement of Right Clavicle with Autologous Tissue Substitute, Percutaneous Approach

0PR93JZ Replacement of Right Clavicle with Synthetic Substitute, Percutaneous Approach

0PR93KZ Replacement of Right Clavicle with Nonautologous Tissue Substitute, Percutaneous Approach

0PR947Z Replacement of Right Clavicle with Autologous Tissue Substitute, Percutaneous Endoscopic Approach

0PR94JZ Replacement of Right Clavicle with Synthetic Substitute, Percutaneous Endoscopic Approach

0PR94KZ Replacement of Right Clavicle with Nonautologous Tissue Substitute, Percutaneous Endoscopic Approach

0PRB07Z Replacement of Left Clavicle with Autologous Tissue Substitute, Open Approach

0PRB0JZ Replacement of Left Clavicle with Synthetic Substitute, Open Approach

0PRB0KZ Replacement of Left Clavicle with Nonautologous Tissue Substitute, Open Approach

0PRB37Z Replacement of Left Clavicle with Autologous Tissue Substitute, Percutaneous Approach

0PRB3JZ Replacement of Left Clavicle with Synthetic Substitute, Percutaneous Approach

0PRB3KZ Replacement of Left Clavicle with Nonautologous Tissue Substitute, Percutaneous Approach

0PRB47Z Replacement of Left Clavicle with Autologous Tissue Substitute, Percutaneous Endoscopic Approach

0PRB4JZ Replacement of Left Clavicle with Synthetic Substitute, Percutaneous Endoscopic Approach

0PRB4KZ Replacement of Left Clavicle with Nonautologous Tissue Substitute, Percutaneous Endoscopic Approach

0PRC07Z Replacement of Right Humeral Head with Autologous Tissue Substitute, Open Approach

0PRC0JZ Replacement of Right Humeral Head with Synthetic Substitute, Open Approach

0PRC0KZ Replacement of Right Humeral Head with Nonautologous Tissue Substitute, Open Approach

0PRC37Z Replacement of Right Humeral Head with Autologous Tissue Substitute, Percutaneous Approach

0PRC3JZ Replacement of Right Humeral Head with Synthetic Substitute, Percutaneous Approach

0PRC3KZ Replacement of Right Humeral Head with Nonautologous Tissue Substitute, Percutaneous Approach

0PRC47Z Replacement of Right Humeral Head with Autologous Tissue Substitute, Percutaneous Endoscopic Approach

0PRC4JZ Replacement of Right Humeral Head with Synthetic Substitute, Percutaneous Endoscopic Approach

0PRC4KZ Replacement of Right Humeral Head with Nonautologous Tissue Substitute, Percutaneous Endoscopic Approach

0PRD07Z Replacement of Left Humeral Head with Autologous Tissue Substitute, Open Approach

0PRD0JZ Replacement of Left Humeral Head with Synthetic Substitute, Open Approach

0PRD0KZ Replacement of Left Humeral Head with Nonautologous Tissue Substitute, Open Approach

0PRD37Z Replacement of Left Humeral Head with Autologous Tissue Substitute, Percutaneous Approach

0PRD3JZ Replacement of Left Humeral Head with Synthetic Substitute, Percutaneous Approach

0PRD3KZ Replacement of Left Humeral Head with Nonautologous Tissue Substitute, Percutaneous Approach

0PRD47Z Replacement of Left Humeral Head with Autologous Tissue Substitute, Percutaneous Endoscopic Approach

0PRD4JZ Replacement of Left Humeral Head with Synthetic Substitute, Percutaneous Endoscopic Approach

0PRD4KZ Replacement of Left Humeral Head with Nonautologous Tissue Substitute, Percutaneous Endoscopic Approach

0PRF07Z Replacement of Right Humeral Shaft with Autologous Tissue Substitute, Open Approach

0PRF0JZ Replacement of Right Humeral Shaft with Synthetic Substitute, Open Approach

0PRF0KZ Replacement of Right Humeral Shaft with Nonautologous Tissue Substitute, Open Approach

0PRF37Z Replacement of Right Humeral Shaft with Autologous Tissue Substitute, Percutaneous Approach

0PRF3JZ Replacement of Right Humeral Shaft with Synthetic Substitute, Percutaneous Approach

0PRF3KZ Replacement of Right Humeral Shaft with Nonautologous Tissue Substitute, Percutaneous Approach

0PRF47Z Replacement of Right Humeral Shaft with Autologous Tissue Substitute, Percutaneous Endoscopic Approach

0PRF4JZ Replacement of Right Humeral Shaft with Synthetic Substitute, Percutaneous Endoscopic Approach

0PRF4KZ Replacement of Right Humeral Shaft with Nonautologous Tissue Substitute, Percutaneous Endoscopic Approach

0PRG07Z Replacement of Left Humeral Shaft with Autologous Tissue Substitute, Open Approach

0PRG0JZ Replacement of Left Humeral Shaft with Synthetic Substitute, Open Approach

0PRG0KZ Replacement of Left Humeral Shaft with Nonautologous Tissue Substitute, Open Approach

0PRG37Z Replacement of Left Humeral Shaft with Autologous Tissue Substitute, Percutaneous Approach

0PRG3JZ Replacement of Left Humeral Shaft with Synthetic Substitute, Percutaneous Approach

0PRG3KZ Replacement of Left Humeral Shaft with Nonautologous Tissue Substitute, Percutaneous Approach

0PRG47Z Replacement of Left Humeral Shaft with Autologous Tissue Substitute, Percutaneous Endoscopic Approach

0PRG4JZ Replacement of Left Humeral Shaft with Synthetic Substitute, Percutaneous Endoscopic Approach

0PRG4KZ Replacement of Left Humeral Shaft with Nonautologous Tissue Substitute, Percutaneous Endoscopic Approach

0PRH07Z Replacement of Right Radius with Autologous Tissue Substitute, Open Approach

0PRH0JZ Replacement of Right Radius with Synthetic Substitute, Open Approach

0PRH0KZ Replacement of Right Radius with Nonautologous Tissue Substitute, Open Approach

0PRH37Z Replacement of Right Radius with Autologous Tissue Substitute, Percutaneous Approach

0PRH3JZ Replacement of Right Radius with Synthetic Substitute, Percutaneous Approach

0PRH3KZ Replacement of Right Radius with Nonautologous Tissue Substitute, Percutaneous Approach

0PRH47Z Replacement of Right Radius with Autologous Tissue Substitute, Percutaneous Endoscopic Approach

0PRH4JZ Replacement of Right Radius with Synthetic Substitute, Percutaneous Endoscopic Approach

0PRH4KZ Replacement of Right Radius with Nonautologous Tissue Substitute, Percutaneous Endoscopic Approach

0PRJ07Z Replacement of Left Radius with Autologous Tissue Substitute, Open Approach

0PRJ0JZ Replacement of Left Radius with Synthetic Substitute, Open Approach

0PRJ0KZ Replacement of Left Radius with Nonautologous Tissue Substitute, Open Approach

0PRJ37Z Replacement of Left Radius with Autologous Tissue Substitute, Percutaneous Approach

0PRJ3JZ Replacement of Left Radius with Synthetic Substitute, Percutaneous Approach

0PRJ3KZ Replacement of Left Radius with Nonautologous Tissue Substitute, Percutaneous Approach

0PRJ47Z Replacement of Left Radius with Autologous Tissue Substitute, Percutaneous Endoscopic Approach

0PRJ4JZ Replacement of Left Radius with Synthetic Substitute, Percutaneous Endoscopic Approach

0PRJ4KZ Replacement of Left Radius with Nonautologous Tissue Substitute, Percutaneous Endoscopic Approach

0PRK07Z Replacement of Right Ulna with Autologous Tissue Substitute, Open Approach

0PRK0JZ Replacement of Right Ulna with Synthetic Substitute, Open Approach

0PRK0KZ Replacement of Right Ulna with Nonautologous Tissue Substitute, Open Approach

0PRK37Z Replacement of Right Ulna with Autologous Tissue Substitute, Percutaneous Approach

0PRK3JZ Replacement of Right Ulna with Synthetic Substitute, Percutaneous Approach

0PRK3KZ Replacement of Right Ulna with Nonautologous Tissue Substitute, Percutaneous Approach

0PRK47Z Replacement of Right Ulna with Autologous Tissue Substitute, Percutaneous Endoscopic Approach

0PRK4JZ Replacement of Right Ulna with Synthetic Substitute, Percutaneous Endoscopic Approach

0PRK4KZ Replacement of Right Ulna with Nonautologous Tissue Substitute, Percutaneous Endoscopic Approach

0PRL07Z Replacement of Left Ulna with Autologous Tissue Substitute, Open Approach

0PRL0JZ Replacement of Left Ulna with Synthetic Substitute, Open Approach

0PRL0KZ Replacement of Left Ulna with Nonautologous Tissue Substitute, Open Approach

0PRL37Z Replacement of Left Ulna with Autologous Tissue Substitute, Percutaneous Approach

0PRL3JZ Replacement of Left Ulna with Synthetic Substitute, Percutaneous Approach

0PRL3KZ Replacement of Left Ulna with Nonautologous Tissue Substitute, Percutaneous Approach

0PRL47Z Replacement of Left Ulna with Autologous Tissue Substitute, Percutaneous Endoscopic Approach

0PRL4JZ Replacement of Left Ulna with Synthetic Substitute, Percutaneous Endoscopic Approach

0PRL4KZ Replacement of Left Ulna with Nonautologous Tissue Substitute, Percutaneous Endoscopic Approach

0PRM07Z Replacement of Right Carpal with Autologous Tissue Substitute, Open Approach

0PRM0JZ Replacement of Right Carpal with Synthetic Substitute, Open Approach

0PRM0KZ Replacement of Right Carpal with Nonautologous Tissue Substitute, Open Approach

0PRM37Z Replacement of Right Carpal with Autologous Tissue Substitute, Percutaneous Approach

0PRM3JZ Replacement of Right Carpal with Synthetic Substitute, Percutaneous Approach

0PRM3KZ Replacement of Right Carpal with Nonautologous Tissue Substitute, Percutaneous Approach

0PRM47Z Replacement of Right Carpal with Autologous Tissue Substitute, Percutaneous Endoscopic Approach

0PRM4JZ Replacement of Right Carpal with Synthetic Substitute, Percutaneous Endoscopic Approach

0PRM4KZ Replacement of Right Carpal with Nonautologous Tissue Substitute, Percutaneous Endoscopic Approach

0PRN07Z Replacement of Left Carpal with Autologous Tissue Substitute, Open Approach

0PRN0JZ Replacement of Left Carpal with Synthetic Substitute, Open Approach

0PRN0KZ Replacement of Left Carpal with Nonautologous Tissue Substitute, Open Approach

0PRN37Z Replacement of Left Carpal with Autologous Tissue Substitute, Percutaneous Approach

0PRN3JZ Replacement of Left Carpal with Synthetic Substitute, Percutaneous Approach

0PRN3KZ Replacement of Left Carpal with Nonautologous Tissue Substitute, Percutaneous Approach

0PRN47Z Replacement of Left Carpal with Autologous Tissue Substitute, Percutaneous Endoscopic Approach

0PRN4JZ Replacement of Left Carpal with Synthetic Substitute, Percutaneous Endoscopic Approach

0PRN4KZ Replacement of Left Carpal with Nonautologous Tissue Substitute, Percutaneous Endoscopic Approach

0PRP07Z Replacement of Right Metacarpal with Autologous Tissue Substitute, Open Approach

0PRP0JZ Replacement of Right Metacarpal with Synthetic Substitute, Open Approach

0PRP0KZ Replacement of Right Metacarpal with Nonautologous Tissue Substitute, Open Approach

0PRP37Z Replacement of Right Metacarpal with Autologous Tissue Substitute, Percutaneous Approach

0PRP3JZ Replacement of Right Metacarpal with Synthetic Substitute, Percutaneous Approach

0PRP3KZ Replacement of Right Metacarpal with Nonautologous Tissue Substitute, Percutaneous Approach

0PRP47Z Replacement of Right Metacarpal with Autologous Tissue Substitute, Percutaneous Endoscopic Approach

0PRP4JZ Replacement of Right Metacarpal with Synthetic Substitute, Percutaneous Endoscopic Approach

0PRP4KZ Replacement of Right Metacarpal with Nonautologous Tissue Substitute, Percutaneous Endoscopic Approach

0PRQ07Z Replacement of Left Metacarpal with Autologous Tissue Substitute, Open Approach

0PRQ0JZ Replacement of Left Metacarpal with Synthetic Substitute, Open Approach

0PRQ0KZ Replacement of Left Metacarpal with Nonautologous Tissue Substitute, Open Approach

0PRQ37Z Replacement of Left Metacarpal with Autologous Tissue Substitute, Percutaneous Approach

0PRQ3JZ Replacement of Left Metacarpal with Synthetic Substitute, Percutaneous Approach

0PRQ3KZ Replacement of Left Metacarpal with Nonautologous Tissue Substitute, Percutaneous Approach

0PRQ47Z Replacement of Left Metacarpal with Autologous Tissue Substitute, Percutaneous Endoscopic Approach

0PRQ4JZ Replacement of Left Metacarpal with Synthetic Substitute, Percutaneous Endoscopic Approach

0PRQ4KZ Replacement of Left Metacarpal with Nonautologous Tissue Substitute, Percutaneous Endoscopic Approach

0PRR07Z Replacement of Right Thumb Phalanx with Autologous Tissue Substitute, Open Approach

0PRR0JZ Replacement of Right Thumb Phalanx with Synthetic Substitute, Open Approach

0PRR0KZ Replacement of Right Thumb Phalanx with Nonautologous Tissue Substitute, Open Approach

0PRR37Z Replacement of Right Thumb Phalanx with Autologous Tissue Substitute, Percutaneous Approach

♀ Female-only   ♂ Male-only   ▲ Limited Coverage   ● Non-OR   ▦ HAC-associated procedure   ▲ Non-covered procedures   ✚ Combinati

0PRR3JZ	Replacement of Right Thumb Phalanx with Synthetic Substitute, Percutaneous Approach
0PRR3KZ	Replacement of Right Thumb Phalanx with Nonautologous Tissue Substitute, Percutaneous Approach
0PRR47Z	Replacement of Right Thumb Phalanx with Autologous Tissue Substitute, Percutaneous Endoscopic Approach
0PRR4JZ	Replacement of Right Thumb Phalanx with Synthetic Substitute, Percutaneous Endoscopic Approach
0PRR4KZ	Replacement of Right Thumb Phalanx with Nonautologous Tissue Substitute, Percutaneous Endoscopic Approach
0PRS07Z	Replacement of Left Thumb Phalanx with Autologous Tissue Substitute, Open Approach
0PRS0JZ	Replacement of Left Thumb Phalanx with Synthetic Substitute, Open Approach
0PRS0KZ	Replacement of Left Thumb Phalanx with Nonautologous Tissue Substitute, Open Approach
0PRS37Z	Replacement of Left Thumb Phalanx with Autologous Tissue Substitute, Percutaneous Approach
0PRS3JZ	Replacement of Left Thumb Phalanx with Synthetic Substitute, Percutaneous Approach
0PRS3KZ	Replacement of Left Thumb Phalanx with Nonautologous Tissue Substitute, Percutaneous Approach
0PRS47Z	Replacement of Left Thumb Phalanx with Autologous Tissue Substitute, Percutaneous Endoscopic Approach
0PRS4JZ	Replacement of Left Thumb Phalanx with Synthetic Substitute, Percutaneous Endoscopic Approach
0PRS4KZ	Replacement of Left Thumb Phalanx with Nonautologous Tissue Substitute, Percutaneous Endoscopic Approach
0PRT07Z	Replacement of Right Finger Phalanx with Autologous Tissue Substitute, Open Approach
0PRT0JZ	Replacement of Right Finger Phalanx with Synthetic Substitute, Open Approach
0PRT0KZ	Replacement of Right Finger Phalanx with Nonautologous Tissue Substitute, Open Approach
0PRT37Z	Replacement of Right Finger Phalanx with Autologous Tissue Substitute, Percutaneous Approach
0PRT3JZ	Replacement of Right Finger Phalanx with Synthetic Substitute, Percutaneous Approach
0PRT3KZ	Replacement of Right Finger Phalanx with Nonautologous Tissue Substitute, Percutaneous Approach
0PRT47Z	Replacement of Right Finger Phalanx with Autologous Tissue Substitute, Percutaneous Endoscopic Approach
0PRT4JZ	Replacement of Right Finger Phalanx with Synthetic Substitute, Percutaneous Endoscopic Approach
0PRT4KZ	Replacement of Right Finger Phalanx with Nonautologous Tissue Substitute, Percutaneous Endoscopic Approach
0PRV07Z	Replacement of Left Finger Phalanx with Autologous Tissue Substitute, Open Approach
0PRV0JZ	Replacement of Left Finger Phalanx with Synthetic Substitute, Open Approach
0PRV0KZ	Replacement of Left Finger Phalanx with Nonautologous Tissue Substitute, Open Approach
0PRV37Z	Replacement of Left Finger Phalanx with Autologous Tissue Substitute, Percutaneous Approach
0PRV3JZ	Replacement of Left Finger Phalanx with Synthetic Substitute, Percutaneous Approach
0PRV3KZ	Replacement of Left Finger Phalanx with Nonautologous Tissue Substitute, Percutaneous Approach
0PRV47Z	Replacement of Left Finger Phalanx with Autologous Tissue Substitute, Percutaneous Endoscopic Approach
0PRV4JZ	Replacement of Left Finger Phalanx with Synthetic Substitute, Percutaneous Endoscopic Approach
0PRV4KZ	Replacement of Left Finger Phalanx with Nonautologous Tissue Substitute, Percutaneous Endoscopic Approach

S – Upper Bones, Reposition

Review Coding Guideline B3.15

0PS000Z	Reposition Sternum with Rigid Plate Internal Fixation Device, Open Approach
0PS004Z	Reposition Sternum with Internal Fixation Device, Open Approach
0PS00ZZ	Reposition Sternum, Open Approach
0PS030Z	Reposition Sternum with Rigid Plate Internal Fixation Device, Percutaneous Approach
0PS034Z	Reposition Sternum with Internal Fixation Device, Percutaneous Approach
0PS03ZZ	Reposition Sternum, Percutaneous Approach
0PS040Z	Reposition Sternum with Rigid Plate Internal Fixation Device, Percutaneous Endoscopic Approach
0PS044Z	Reposition Sternum with Internal Fixation Device, Percutaneous Endoscopic Approach
0PS04ZZ	Reposition Sternum, Percutaneous Endoscopic Approach
0PS0XZZ	Reposition Sternum, External Approach
0PS104Z	Reposition Right Rib with Internal Fixation Device, Open Approach
0PS10ZZ	Reposition Right Rib, Open Approach
0PS134Z	Reposition Right Rib with Internal Fixation Device, Percutaneous Approach
0PS13ZZ	Reposition Right Rib, Percutaneous Approach
0PS144Z	Reposition Right Rib with Internal Fixation Device, Percutaneous Endoscopic Approach
0PS14ZZ	Reposition Right Rib, Percutaneous Endoscopic Approach
0PS1XZZ	Reposition Right Rib, External Approach
0PS204Z	Reposition Left Rib with Internal Fixation Device, Open Approach *AHA CC: 4Q, 2014, 26*
0PS20ZZ	Reposition Left Rib, Open Approach
0PS234Z	Reposition Left Rib with Internal Fixation Device, Percutaneous Approach
0PS23ZZ	Reposition Left Rib, Percutaneous Approach
0PS244Z	Reposition Left Rib with Internal Fixation Device, Percutaneous Endoscopic Approach
0PS24ZZ	Reposition Left Rib, Percutaneous Endoscopic Approach
0PS2XZZ	Reposition Left Rib, External Approach
0PS304Z	Reposition Cervical Vertebra with Internal Fixation Device, Open Approach
0PS30ZZ	Reposition Cervical Vertebra, Open Approach
0PS334Z	Reposition Cervical Vertebra with Internal Fixation Device, Percutaneous Approach
0PS33ZZ	Reposition Cervical Vertebra, Percutaneous Approach

+ *See table 0PU to construct a code for Supplement with synthetic substitute.*

0PS344Z	Reposition Cervical Vertebra with Internal Fixation Device, Percutaneous Endoscopic Approach
0PS34ZZ	Reposition Cervical Vertebra, Percutaneous Endoscopic Approach
0PS3XZZ	Reposition Cervical Vertebra, External Approach
0PS404Z	Reposition Thoracic Vertebra with Internal Fixation Device, Open Approach
0PS40ZZ	Reposition Thoracic Vertebra, Open Approach
0PS434Z	Reposition Thoracic Vertebra with Internal Fixation Device, Percutaneous Approach
0PS43ZZ	Reposition Thoracic Vertebra, Percutaneous Approach

+ *See table 0PU to construct a code for Supplement with synthetic substitute.*

0PS444Z	Reposition Thoracic Vertebra with Internal Fixation Device, Percutaneous Endoscopic Approach
0PS44ZZ	Reposition Thoracic Vertebra, Percutaneous Endoscopic Approach
0PS4XZZ	Reposition Thoracic Vertebra, External Approach
0PS504Z	Reposition Right Scapula with Internal Fixation Device, Open Approach
0PS50ZZ	Reposition Right Scapula, Open Approach
0PS534Z	Reposition Right Scapula with Internal Fixation Device, Percutaneous Approach
0PS53ZZ	Reposition Right Scapula, Percutaneous Approach
0PS544Z	Reposition Right Scapula with Internal Fixation Device, Percutaneous Endoscopic Approach
0PS547Z	Reposition Right Scapula, Percutaneous Endoscopic Approach
0PS5XZZ	Reposition Right Scapula, External Approach
0PS604Z	Reposition Left Scapula with Internal Fixation Device, Open Approach
0PS60ZZ	Reposition Left Scapula, Open Approach
0PS634Z	Reposition Left Scapula with Internal Fixation Device, Percutaneous Approach
0PS63ZZ	Reposition Left Scapula, Percutaneous Approach
0PS644Z	Reposition Left Scapula with Internal Fixation Device, Percutaneous Endoscopic Approach
0PS64ZZ	Reposition Left Scapula, Percutaneous Endoscopic Approach
0PS6XZZ	Reposition Left Scapula, External Approach
0PS704Z	Reposition Right Glenoid Cavity with Internal Fixation Device, Open Approach
0PS70ZZ	Reposition Right Glenoid Cavity, Open Approach
0PS734Z	Reposition Right Glenoid Cavity with Internal Fixation Device, Percutaneous Approach
0PS73ZZ	Reposition Right Glenoid Cavity, Percutaneous Approach
0PS744Z	Reposition Right Glenoid Cavity with Internal Fixation Device, Percutaneous Endoscopic Approach

Female-only   ♂ Male-only   ▲ Limited Coverage   ● Non-OR   ▦ HAC-associated procedure   ▲ Non-covered procedures   ✚ Combination

0PS74ZZ Reposition Right Glenoid Cavity, Percutaneous Endoscopic Approach

0PS7XZZ Reposition Right Glenoid Cavity, External Approach

0PS804Z Reposition Left Glenoid Cavity with Internal Fixation Device, Open Approach

0PS80ZZ Reposition Left Glenoid Cavity, Open Approach

0PS834Z Reposition Left Glenoid Cavity with Internal Fixation Device, Percutaneous Approach

0PS83ZZ Reposition Left Glenoid Cavity, Percutaneous Approach

0PS844Z Reposition Left Glenoid Cavity with Internal Fixation Device, Percutaneous Endoscopic Approach

0PS84ZZ Reposition Left Glenoid Cavity, Percutaneous Endoscopic Approach

0PS8XZZ Reposition Left Glenoid Cavity, External Approach

0PS904Z Reposition Right Clavicle with Internal Fixation Device, Open Approach

0PS90ZZ Reposition Right Clavicle, Open Approach

0PS934Z Reposition Right Clavicle with Internal Fixation Device, Percutaneous Approach

0PS93ZZ Reposition Right Clavicle, Percutaneous Approach

0PS944Z Reposition Right Clavicle with Internal Fixation Device, Percutaneous Endoscopic Approach

0PS94ZZ Reposition Right Clavicle, Percutaneous Endoscopic Approach

0PS9XZZ Reposition Right Clavicle, External Approach

0PSB04Z Reposition Left Clavicle with Internal Fixation Device, Open Approach

0PSB0ZZ Reposition Left Clavicle, Open Approach

0PSB34Z Reposition Left Clavicle with Internal Fixation Device, Percutaneous Approach

0PSB3ZZ Reposition Left Clavicle, Percutaneous Approach

0PSB44Z Reposition Left Clavicle with Internal Fixation Device, Percutaneous Endoscopic Approach

0PSB4ZZ Reposition Left Clavicle, Percutaneous Endoscopic Approach

0PSBXZZ Reposition Left Clavicle, External Approach

0PSC04Z Reposition Right Humeral Head with Internal Fixation Device, Open Approach

0PSC05Z Reposition Right Humeral Head with External Fixation Device, Open Approach

0PSC06Z Reposition Right Humeral Head with Intramedullary Internal Fixation Device, Open Approach

0PSC0BZ Reposition Right Humeral Head with Monoplanar External Fixation Device, Open Approach

0PSC0CZ Reposition Right Humeral Head with Ring External Fixation Device, Open Approach

0PSC0DZ Reposition Right Humeral Head with Hybrid External Fixation Device, Open Approach

0PSC0ZZ Reposition Right Humeral Head, Open Approach

0PSC34Z Reposition Right Humeral Head with Internal Fixation Device, Percutaneous Approach

0PSC35Z Reposition Right Humeral Head with External Fixation Device, Percutaneous Approach

0PSC36Z Reposition Right Humeral Head with Intramedullary Internal Fixation Device, Percutaneous Approach

0PSC3BZ Reposition Right Humeral Head with Monoplanar External Fixation Device, Percutaneous Approach

0PSC3CZ Reposition Right Humeral Head with Ring External Fixation Device, Percutaneous Approach

0PSC3DZ Reposition Right Humeral Head with Hybrid External Fixation Device, Percutaneous Approach

0PSC3ZZ Reposition Right Humeral Head, Percutaneous Approach

0PSC44Z Reposition Right Humeral Head with Internal Fixation Device, Percutaneous Endoscopic Approach

0PSC45Z Reposition Right Humeral Head with External Fixation Device, Percutaneous Endoscopic Approach

0PSC46Z Reposition Right Humeral Head with Intramedullary Internal Fixation Device, Percutaneous Endoscopic Approach

0PSC4BZ Reposition Right Humeral Head with Monoplanar External Fixation Device, Percutaneous Endoscopic Approach

0PSC4CZ Reposition Right Humeral Head with Ring External Fixation Device, Percutaneous Endoscopic Approach

0PSC4DZ Reposition Right Humeral Head with Hybrid External Fixation Device, Percutaneous Endoscopic Approach

0PSC4ZZ Reposition Right Humeral Head, Percutaneous Endoscopic Approach

0PSCXZZ Reposition Right Humeral Head, External Approach

0PSD04Z Reposition Left Humeral Head with Internal Fixation Device, Open Approach

0PSD05Z Reposition Left Humeral Head with External Fixation Device, Open Approach

0PSD06Z Reposition Left Humeral Head with Intramedullary Internal Fixation Device, Open Approach

0PSD0BZ Reposition Left Humeral Head with Monoplanar External Fixation Device, Open Approach

0PSD0CZ Reposition Left Humeral Head with Ring External Fixation Device, Open Approach

0PSD0DZ Reposition Left Humeral Head with Hybrid External Fixation Device, Open Approach

0PSD0ZZ Reposition Left Humeral Head, Open Approach

0PSD34Z Reposition Left Humeral Head with Internal Fixation Device, Percutaneous Approach

0PSD35Z Reposition Left Humeral Head with External Fixation Device, Percutaneous Approach

0PSD36Z Reposition Left Humeral Head with Intramedullary Internal Fixation Device, Percutaneous Approach

0PSD3BZ Reposition Left Humeral Head with Monoplanar External Fixation Device, Percutaneous Approach

0PSD3CZ Reposition Left Humeral Head with Ring External Fixation Device, Percutaneous Approach

0PSD3DZ Reposition Left Humeral Head with Hybrid External Fixation Device, Percutaneous Approach

0PSD3ZZ Reposition Left Humeral Head, Percutaneous Approach

0PSD44Z Reposition Left Humeral Head with Internal Fixation Device, Percutaneous Endoscopic Approach

0PSD45Z Reposition Left Humeral Head with External Fixation Device, Percutaneous Endoscopic Approach

0PSD46Z Reposition Left Humeral Head with Intramedullary Internal Fixation Device, Percutaneous Endoscopic Approach

0PSD4BZ Reposition Left Humeral Head with Monoplanar External Fixation Device, Percutaneous Endoscopic Approach

0PSD4CZ Reposition Left Humeral Head with Ring External Fixation Device, Percutaneous Endoscopic Approach

0PSD4DZ Reposition Left Humeral Head with Hybrid External Fixation Device, Percutaneous Endoscopic Approach

0PSD4ZZ Reposition Left Humeral Head, Percutaneous Endoscopic Approach

0PSDXZZ Reposition Left Humeral Head, External Approach

0PSF04Z Reposition Right Humeral Shaft with Internal Fixation Device, Open Approach

0PSF05Z Reposition Right Humeral Shaft with External Fixation Device, Open Approach

0PSF06Z Reposition Right Humeral Shaft with Intramedullary Internal Fixation Device, Open Approach

0PSF0BZ Reposition Right Humeral Shaft with Monoplanar External Fixation Device, Open Approach

0PSF0CZ Reposition Right Humeral Shaft with Ring External Fixation Device, Open Approach

0PSF0DZ Reposition Right Humeral Shaft with Hybrid External Fixation Device, Open Approach

0PSF0ZZ Reposition Right Humeral Shaft, Open Approach

0PSF34Z Reposition Right Humeral Shaft with Internal Fixation Device, Percutaneous Approach

0PSF35Z Reposition Right Humeral Shaft with External Fixation Device, Percutaneous Approach

0PSF36Z Reposition Right Humeral Shaft with Intramedullary Internal Fixation Device, Percutaneous Approach

0PSF3BZ Reposition Right Humeral Shaft with Monoplanar External Fixation Device, Percutaneous Approach

0PSF3CZ Reposition Right Humeral Shaft with Ring External Fixation Device, Percutaneous Approach

0PSF3DZ Reposition Right Humeral Shaft with Hybrid External Fixation Device, Percutaneous Approach

0PSF3ZZ Reposition Right Humeral Shaft, Percutaneous Approach

0PSF44Z Reposition Right Humeral Shaft with Internal Fixation Device, Percutaneous Endoscopic Approach

0PSF45Z Reposition Right Humeral Shaft with External Fixation Device, Percutaneous Endoscopic Approach

0PSF46Z Reposition Right Humeral Shaft with Intramedullary Internal Fixation Device, Percutaneous Endoscopic Approach

0PSF4BZ Reposition Right Humeral Shaft with Monoplanar External Fixation Device, Percutaneous Endoscopic Approach

0PSF4CZ Reposition Right Humeral Shaft with Ring External Fixation Device, Percutaneous Endoscopic Approach

0PSF4DZ Reposition Right Humeral Shaft with Hybrid External Fixation Device, Percutaneous Endoscopic Approach

0PSF4ZZ Reposition Right Humeral Shaft, Percutaneous Endoscopic Approach

0PSFXZZ Reposition Right Humeral Shaft, External Approach

0PSG04Z Reposition Left Humeral Shaft with Internal Fixation Device, Open Approach

0PSG05Z Reposition Left Humeral Shaft with External Fixation Device, Open Approach

0PSG06Z Reposition Left Humeral Shaft with Intramedullary Internal Fixation Device, Open Approach

0PSG0BZ Reposition Left Humeral Shaft with Monoplanar External Fixation Device, Open Approach

0PSG0CZ Reposition Left Humeral Shaft with Ring External Fixation Device, Open Approach

0PSG0DZ Reposition Left Humeral Shaft with Hybrid External Fixation Device, Open Approach

0PSG0ZZ Reposition Left Humeral Shaft, Open Approach

0PSG34Z Reposition Left Humeral Shaft with Internal Fixation Device, Percutaneous Approach

0PSG35Z Reposition Left Humeral Shaft with External Fixation Device, Percutaneous Approach

0PSG36Z Reposition Left Humeral Shaft with Intramedullary Internal Fixation Device, Percutaneous Approach

0PSG3BZ Reposition Left Humeral Shaft with Monoplanar External Fixation Device, Percutaneous Approach

0PSG3CZ Reposition Left Humeral Shaft with Ring External Fixation Device, Percutaneous Approach

0PSG3DZ Reposition Left Humeral Shaft with Hybrid External Fixation Device, Percutaneous Approach

0PSG3ZZ Reposition Left Humeral Shaft, Percutaneous Approach

0PSG44Z Reposition Left Humeral Shaft with Internal Fixation Device, Percutaneous Endoscopic Approach

0PSG45Z Reposition Left Humeral Shaft with External Fixation Device, Percutaneous Endoscopic Approach

0PSG46Z Reposition Left Humeral Shaft with Intramedullary Internal Fixation Device, Percutaneous Endoscopic Approach

0PSG4BZ Reposition Left Humeral Shaft with Monoplanar External Fixation Device, Percutaneous Endoscopic Approach

0PSG4CZ Reposition Left Humeral Shaft with Ring External Fixation Device, Percutaneous Endoscopic Approach

0PSG4DZ Reposition Left Humeral Shaft with Hybrid External Fixation Device, Percutaneous Endoscopic Approach

0PSG4ZZ Reposition Left Humeral Shaft, Percutaneous Endoscopic Approach

0PSGXZZ Reposition Left Humeral Shaft, External Approach

0PSH04Z Reposition Right Radius with Internal Fixation Device, Open Approach

0PSH05Z Reposition Right Radius with External Fixation Device, Open Approach

0PSH06Z Reposition Right Radius with Intramedullary Internal Fixation Device, Open Approach

0PSH0BZ Reposition Right Radius with Monoplanar External Fixation Device, Open Approach

0PSH0CZ Reposition Right Radius with Ring External Fixation Device, Open Approach

0PSH0DZ Reposition Right Radius with Hybrid External Fixation Device, Open Approach

0PSH0ZZ Reposition Right Radius, Open Approach

0PSH34Z Reposition Right Radius with Internal Fixation Device, Percutaneous Approach

0PSH35Z Reposition Right Radius with External Fixation Device, Percutaneous Approach

0PSH36Z Reposition Right Radius with Intramedullary Internal Fixation Device, Percutaneous Approach

0PSH3BZ Reposition Right Radius with Monoplanar External Fixation Device, Percutaneous Approach

0PSH3CZ Reposition Right Radius with Ring External Fixation Device, Percutaneous Approach

0PSH3DZ Reposition Right Radius with Hybrid External Fixation Device, Percutaneous Approach

0PSH3ZZ Reposition Right Radius, Percutaneous Approach

0PSH44Z Reposition Right Radius with Internal Fixation Device, Percutaneous Endoscopic Approach

0PSH45Z Reposition Right Radius with External Fixation Device, Percutaneous Endoscopic Approach

0PSH46Z Reposition Right Radius with Intramedullary Internal Fixation Device, Percutaneous Endoscopic Approach

0PSH4BZ Reposition Right Radius with Monoplanar External Fixation Device, Percutaneous Endoscopic Approach

0PSH4CZ Reposition Right Radius with Ring External Fixation Device, Percutaneous Endoscopic Approach

0PSH4DZ Reposition Right Radius with Hybrid External Fixation Device, Percutaneous Endoscopic Approach

0PSH4ZZ Reposition Right Radius, Percutaneous Endoscopic Approach

0PSHXZZ Reposition Right Radius, External Approach

0PSJ04Z Reposition Left Radius with Internal Fixation Device, Open Approach

AHA CC: 3Q, 2014, 33-34; 4Q, 2014, 32-33

0PSJ05Z Reposition Left Radius with External Fixation Device, Open Approach

0PSJ06Z Reposition Left Radius with Intramedullary Internal Fixation Device, Open Approach

0PSJ0BZ Reposition Left Radius with Monoplanar External Fixation Device, Open Approach

0PSJ0CZ Reposition Left Radius with Ring External Fixation Device, Open Approach

0PSJ0DZ Reposition Left Radius with Hybrid External Fixation Device, Open Approach

0PSJ0ZZ Reposition Left Radius, Open Approach

0PSJ34Z Reposition Left Radius with Internal Fixation Device, Percutaneous Approach

0PSJ35Z Reposition Left Radius with External Fixation Device, Percutaneous Approach

0PSJ36Z Reposition Left Radius with Intramedullary Internal Fixation Device, Percutaneous Approach

0PSJ3BZ Reposition Left Radius with Monoplanar External Fixation Device, Percutaneous Approach

0PSJ3CZ Reposition Left Radius with Ring External Fixation Device, Percutaneous Approach

0PSJ3DZ Reposition Left Radius with Hybrid External Fixation Device, Percutaneous Approach

0PSJ3ZZ Reposition Left Radius, Percutaneous Approach

0PSJ44Z Reposition Left Radius with Internal Fixation Device, Percutaneous Endoscopic Approach

0PSJ45Z Reposition Left Radius with External Fixation Device, Percutaneous Endoscopic Approach

0PSJ46Z Reposition Left Radius with Intramedullary Internal Fixation Device, Percutaneous Endoscopic Approach

0PSJ4BZ Reposition Left Radius with Monoplanar External Fixation Device, Percutaneous Endoscopic Approach

0PSJ4CZ Reposition Left Radius with Ring External Fixation Device, Percutaneous Endoscopic Approach

0PSJ4DZ Reposition Left Radius with Hybrid External Fixation Device, Percutaneous Endoscopic Approach

0PSJ4ZZ Reposition Left Radius, Percutaneous Endoscopic Approach

0PSJXZZ Reposition Left Radius, External Approach

0PSK04Z Reposition Right Ulna with Internal Fixation Device, Open Approach

0PSK05Z Reposition Right Ulna with External Fixation Device, Open Approach

0PSK06Z Reposition Right Ulna with Intramedullary Internal Fixation Device, Open Approach

0PSK0BZ Reposition Right Ulna with Monoplanar External Fixation Device, Open Approach

0PSK0CZ Reposition Right Ulna with Ring External Fixation Device, Open Approach

0PSK0DZ Reposition Right Ulna with Hybrid External Fixation Device, Open Approach

0PSK0ZZ Reposition Right Ulna, Open Approach

0PSK34Z Reposition Right Ulna with Internal Fixation Device, Percutaneous Approach

0PSK35Z Reposition Right Ulna with External Fixation Device, Percutaneous Approach

0PSK36Z Reposition Right Ulna with Intramedullary Internal Fixation Device, Percutaneous Approach

0PSK3BZ Reposition Right Ulna with Monoplanar External Fixation Device, Percutaneous Approach

0PSK3CZ Reposition Right Ulna with Ring External Fixation Device, Percutaneous Approach

0PSK3DZ Reposition Right Ulna with Hybrid External Fixation Device, Percutaneous Approach

0PSK3ZZ Reposition Right Ulna, Percutaneous Approach

0PSK44Z Reposition Right Ulna with Internal Fixation Device, Percutaneous Endoscopic Approach

0PSK45Z Reposition Right Ulna with External Fixation Device, Percutaneous Endoscopic Approach

0PSK46Z Reposition Right Ulna with Intramedullary Internal Fixation Device, Percutaneous Endoscopic Approach

0PSK4BZ Reposition Right Ulna with Monoplanar External Fixation Device, Percutaneous Endoscopic Approach

0PSK4CZ Reposition Right Ulna with Ring External Fixation Device, Percutaneous Endoscopic Approach

0PSK4DZ Reposition Right Ulna with Hybrid External Fixation Device, Percutaneous Endoscopic Approach

0PSK4ZZ Reposition Right Ulna, Percutaneous Endoscopic Approach

0PSKXZZ Reposition Right Ulna, External Approach

0PSL04Z Reposition Left Ulna with Internal Fixation Device, Open Approach

AHA CC: 4Q, 2014, 32-33

0PSL05Z Reposition Left Ulna with External Fixation Device, Open Approach

0PSL06Z	Reposition Left Ulna with Intramedullary Internal Fixation Device, Open Approach
0PSL0BZ	Reposition Left Ulna with Monoplanar External Fixation Device, Open Approach
0PSL0CZ	Reposition Left Ulna with Ring External Fixation Device, Open Approach
0PSL0DZ	Reposition Left Ulna with Hybrid External Fixation Device, Open Approach
0PSL0ZZ	Reposition Left Ulna, Open Approach
0PSL34Z	Reposition Left Ulna with Internal Fixation Device, Percutaneous Approach
0PSL35Z	Reposition Left Ulna with External Fixation Device, Percutaneous Approach
0PSL36Z	Reposition Left Ulna with Intramedullary Internal Fixation Device, Percutaneous Approach
0PSL3BZ	Reposition Left Ulna with Monoplanar External Fixation Device, Percutaneous Approach
0PSL3CZ	Reposition Left Ulna with Ring External Fixation Device, Percutaneous Approach
0PSL3DZ	Reposition Left Ulna with Hybrid External Fixation Device, Percutaneous Approach
0PSL3ZZ	Reposition Left Ulna, Percutaneous Approach
0PSL44Z	Reposition Left Ulna with Internal Fixation Device, Percutaneous Endoscopic Approach
0PSL45Z	Reposition Left Ulna with External Fixation Device, Percutaneous Endoscopic Approach
0PSL46Z	Reposition Left Ulna with Intramedullary Internal Fixation Device, Percutaneous Endoscopic Approach
0PSL4BZ	Reposition Left Ulna with Monoplanar External Fixation Device, Percutaneous Endoscopic Approach
0PSL4CZ	Reposition Left Ulna with Ring External Fixation Device, Percutaneous Endoscopic Approach
0PSL4DZ	Reposition Left Ulna with Hybrid External Fixation Device, Percutaneous Endoscopic Approach
0PSL4ZZ	Reposition Left Ulna, Percutaneous Endoscopic Approach
0PSLXZZ	Reposition Left Ulna, External Approach
0PSM04Z	Reposition Right Carpal with Internal Fixation Device, Open Approach
0PSM05Z	Reposition Right Carpal with External Fixation Device, Open Approach
0PSM0ZZ	Reposition Right Carpal, Open Approach
0PSM34Z	Reposition Right Carpal with Internal Fixation Device, Percutaneous Approach
0PSM35Z	Reposition Right Carpal with External Fixation Device, Percutaneous Approach
0PSM3ZZ	Reposition Right Carpal, Percutaneous Approach
0PSM44Z	Reposition Right Carpal with Internal Fixation Device, Percutaneous Endoscopic Approach
0PSM45Z	Reposition Right Carpal with External Fixation Device, Percutaneous Endoscopic Approach
0PSM4ZZ	Reposition Right Carpal, Percutaneous Endoscopic Approach
0PSMXZZ	Reposition Right Carpal, External Approach
0PSN04Z	Reposition Left Carpal with Internal Fixation Device, Open Approach
0PSN05Z	Reposition Left Carpal with External Fixation Device, Open Approach
0PSN0ZZ	Reposition Left Carpal, Open Approach
0PSN34Z	Reposition Left Carpal with Internal Fixation Device, Percutaneous Approach
0PSN35Z	Reposition Left Carpal with External Fixation Device, Percutaneous Approach
0PSN3ZZ	Reposition Left Carpal, Percutaneous Approach
0PSN44Z	Reposition Left Carpal with Internal Fixation Device, Percutaneous Endoscopic Approach
0PSN45Z	Reposition Left Carpal with External Fixation Device, Percutaneous Endoscopic Approach
0PSN4ZZ	Reposition Left Carpal, Percutaneous Endoscopic Approach
0PSNXZZ	Reposition Left Carpal, External Approach
0PSP04Z	Reposition Right Metacarpal with Internal Fixation Device, Open Approach
0PSP05Z	Reposition Right Metacarpal with External Fixation Device, Open Approach
0PSP0ZZ	Reposition Right Metacarpal, Open Approach
0PSP34Z	Reposition Right Metacarpal with Internal Fixation Device, Percutaneous Approach
0PSP35Z	Reposition Right Metacarpal with External Fixation Device, Percutaneous Approach
0PSP3ZZ	Reposition Right Metacarpal, Percutaneous Approach
0PSP44Z	Reposition Right Metacarpal with Internal Fixation Device, Percutaneous Endoscopic Approach
0PSP45Z	Reposition Right Metacarpal with External Fixation Device, Percutaneous Endoscopic Approach
0PSP4ZZ	Reposition Right Metacarpal, Percutaneous Endoscopic Approach
0PSPXZZ	Reposition Right Metacarpal, External Approach
0PSQ04Z	Reposition Left Metacarpal with Internal Fixation Device, Open Approach
0PSQ05Z	Reposition Left Metacarpal with External Fixation Device, Open Approach
0PSQ0ZZ	Reposition Left Metacarpal, Open Approach
0PSQ34Z	Reposition Left Metacarpal with Internal Fixation Device, Percutaneous Approach
0PSQ35Z	Reposition Left Metacarpal with External Fixation Device, Percutaneous Approach
0PSQ3ZZ	Reposition Left Metacarpal, Percutaneous Approach
0PSQ44Z	Reposition Left Metacarpal with Internal Fixation Device, Percutaneous Endoscopic Approach
0PSQ45Z	Reposition Left Metacarpal with External Fixation Device, Percutaneous Endoscopic Approach
0PSQ4ZZ	Reposition Left Metacarpal, Percutaneous Endoscopic Approach
0PSQXZZ	Reposition Left Metacarpal, External Approach
0PSR04Z	Reposition Right Thumb Phalanx with Internal Fixation Device, Open Approach
0PSR05Z	Reposition Right Thumb Phalanx with External Fixation Device, Open Approach
0PSR0ZZ	Reposition Right Thumb Phalanx, Open Approach
0PSR34Z	Reposition Right Thumb Phalanx with Internal Fixation Device, Percutaneous Approach
0PSR35Z	Reposition Right Thumb Phalanx with External Fixation Device, Percutaneous Approach
0PSR3ZZ	Reposition Right Thumb Phalanx, Percutaneous Approach
0PSR44Z	Reposition Right Thumb Phalanx with Internal Fixation Device, Percutaneous Endoscopic Approach
0PSR45Z	Reposition Right Thumb Phalanx with External Fixation Device, Percutaneous Endoscopic Approach
0PSR4ZZ	Reposition Right Thumb Phalanx, Percutaneous Endoscopic Approach
0PSRXZZ	Reposition Right Thumb Phalanx, External Approach
0PSS04Z	Reposition Left Thumb Phalanx with Internal Fixation Device, Open Approach
0PSS05Z	Reposition Left Thumb Phalanx with External Fixation Device, Open Approach
0PSS0ZZ	Reposition Left Thumb Phalanx, Open Approach
0PSS34Z	Reposition Left Thumb Phalanx with Internal Fixation Device, Percutaneous Approach
0PSS35Z	Reposition Left Thumb Phalanx with External Fixation Device, Percutaneous Approach
0PSS3ZZ	Reposition Left Thumb Phalanx, Percutaneous Approach
0PSS44Z	Reposition Left Thumb Phalanx with Internal Fixation Device, Percutaneous Endoscopic Approach
0PSS45Z	Reposition Left Thumb Phalanx with External Fixation Device, Percutaneous Endoscopic Approach
0PSS4ZZ	Reposition Left Thumb Phalanx, Percutaneous Endoscopic Approach
0PSSXZZ	Reposition Left Thumb Phalanx, External Approach
0PST04Z	Reposition Right Finger Phalanx with Internal Fixation Device, Open Approach
0PST05Z	Reposition Right Finger Phalanx with External Fixation Device, Open Approach
0PST0ZZ	Reposition Right Finger Phalanx, Open Approach
0PST34Z	Reposition Right Finger Phalanx with Internal Fixation Device, Percutaneous Approach
0PST35Z	Reposition Right Finger Phalanx with External Fixation Device, Percutaneous Approach
0PST3ZZ	Reposition Right Finger Phalanx, Percutaneous Approach
0PST44Z	Reposition Right Finger Phalanx with Internal Fixation Device, Percutaneous Endoscopic Approach
0PST45Z	Reposition Right Finger Phalanx with External Fixation Device, Percutaneous Endoscopic Approach
0PST4ZZ	Reposition Right Finger Phalanx, Percutaneous Endoscopic Approach
0PSTXZZ	Reposition Right Finger Phalanx, External Approach
0PSV04Z	Reposition Left Finger Phalanx with Internal Fixation Device, Open Approach
0PSV05Z	Reposition Left Finger Phalanx with External Fixation Device, Open Approach
0PSV0ZZ	Reposition Left Finger Phalanx, Open Approach
0PSV34Z	Reposition Left Finger Phalanx with Internal Fixation Device, Percutaneous Approach
0PSV35Z	Reposition Left Finger Phalanx with External Fixation Device, Percutaneous Approach
0PSV3ZZ	Reposition Left Finger Phalanx, Percutaneous Approach
0PSV44Z	Reposition Left Finger Phalanx with Internal Fixation Device, Percutaneous Endoscopic Approach
0PSV45Z	Reposition Left Finger Phalanx with External Fixation Device, Percutaneous Endoscopic Approach
0PSV4ZZ	Reposition Left Finger Phalanx, Percutaneous Endoscopic Approach
0PSVXZZ	Reposition Left Finger Phalanx, External Approach

♀ Female-only ♂ Male-only ▲ Limited Coverage ● Non-OR ▨ HAC-associated procedure ▲ Non-covered procedures ✛ Combinatio

T – Upper Bones, Resection

~iew Coding Guideline B3.8

~00ZZ	Resection of Sternum, Open Approach	0PTC0ZZ	Resection of Right Humeral Head, Open Approach	0PTN0ZZ	Resection of Left Carpal, Open Approach
~10ZZ	Resection of Right Rib, Open Approach	0PTD0ZZ	Resection of Left Humeral Head, Open Approach	0PTP0ZZ	Resection of Right Metacarpal, Open Approach
~20ZZ	Resection of Left Rib, Open Approach	0PTF0ZZ	Resection of Right Humeral Shaft, Open Approach	0PTQ0ZZ	Resection of Left Metacarpal, Open Approach
~50ZZ	Resection of Right Scapula, Open Approach	0PTG0ZZ	Resection of Left Humeral Shaft, Open Approach	0PTR0ZZ	Resection of Right Thumb Phalanx, Open Approach
~60ZZ	Resection of Left Scapula, Open Approach	0PTH0ZZ	Resection of Right Radius, Open Approach	0PTS0ZZ	Resection of Left Thumb Phalanx, Open Approach
~70ZZ	Resection of Right Glenoid Cavity, Open Approach	0PTJ0ZZ	Resection of Left Radius, Open Approach	0PTT0ZZ	Resection of Right Finger Phalanx, Open Approach
~80ZZ	Resection of Left Glenoid Cavity, Open Approach	0PTK0ZZ	Resection of Right Ulna, Open Approach	0PTV0ZZ	Resection of Left Finger Phalanx, Open Approach
~90ZZ	Resection of Right Clavicle, Open Approach	0PTL0ZZ	Resection of Left Ulna, Open Approach		
~B0ZZ	Resection of Left Clavicle, Open Approach	0PTM0ZZ	Resection of Right Carpal, Open Approach		

U – Upper Bones, Supplement

J007Z	Supplement Sternum with Autologous Tissue Substitute, Open Approach	0PU23KZ	Supplement Left Rib with Nonautologous Tissue Substitute, Percutaneous Approach	0PU447Z	Supplement Thoracic Vertebra with Autologous Tissue Substitute, Percutaneous Endoscopic Approach
J00JZ	Supplement Sternum with Synthetic Substitute, Open Approach *AHA CC: 4Q, 2013, 109-111*	0PU247Z	Supplement Left Rib with Autologous Tissue Substitute, Percutaneous Endoscopic Approach	0PU44JZ	Supplement Thoracic Vertebra with Synthetic Substitute, Percutaneous Endoscopic Approach
J00KZ	Supplement Sternum with Nonautologous Tissue Substitute, Open Approach	0PU24JZ	Supplement Left Rib with Synthetic Substitute, Percutaneous Endoscopic Approach	0PU44KZ	Supplement Thoracic Vertebra with Nonautologous Tissue Substitute, Percutaneous Endoscopic Approach
J037Z	Supplement Sternum with Autologous Tissue Substitute, Percutaneous Approach	0PU24KZ	Supplement Left Rib with Nonautologous Tissue Substitute, Percutaneous Endoscopic Approach	0PU507Z	Supplement Right Scapula with Autologous Tissue Substitute, Open Approach
J03JZ	Supplement Sternum with Synthetic Substitute, Percutaneous Approach	0PU307Z	Supplement Cervical Vertebra with Autologous Tissue Substitute, Open Approach	0PU50JZ	Supplement Right Scapula with Synthetic Substitute, Open Approach
U03KZ	Supplement Sternum with Nonautologous Tissue Substitute, Percutaneous Approach	0PU30JZ	Supplement Cervical Vertebra with Synthetic Substitute, Open Approach	0PU50KZ	Supplement Right Scapula with Nonautologous Tissue Substitute, Open Approach
U047Z	Supplement Sternum with Autologous Tissue Substitute, Percutaneous Endoscopic Approach	0PU30KZ	Supplement Cervical Vertebra with Nonautologous Tissue Substitute, Open Approach	0PU537Z	Supplement Right Scapula with Autologous Tissue Substitute, Percutaneous Approach
U04JZ	Supplement Sternum with Synthetic Substitute, Percutaneous Endoscopic Approach	0PU337Z	Supplement Cervical Vertebra with Autologous Tissue Substitute, Percutaneous Approach	0PU53JZ	Supplement Right Scapula with Synthetic Substitute, Percutaneous Approach
U04KZ	Supplement Sternum with Nonautologous Tissue Substitute, Percutaneous Endoscopic Approach	0PU33JZ	Supplement Cervical Vertebra with Synthetic Substitute, Percutaneous Approach	0PU53KZ	Supplement Right Scapula with Nonautologous Tissue Substitute, Percutaneous Approach
U107Z	Supplement Right Rib with Autologous Tissue Substitute, Open Approach	0PU33KZ	Supplement Cervical Vertebra with Nonautologous Tissue Substitute, Percutaneous Approach	0PU547Z	Supplement Right Scapula with Autologous Tissue Substitute, Percutaneous Endoscopic Approach
U10JZ	Supplement Right Rib with Synthetic Substitute, Open Approach	0PU347Z	Supplement Cervical Vertebra with Autologous Tissue Substitute, Percutaneous Endoscopic Approach	0PU54JZ	Supplement Right Scapula with Synthetic Substitute, Percutaneous Endoscopic Approach
U10KZ	Supplement Right Rib with Nonautologous Tissue Substitute, Open Approach	0PU34JZ	Supplement Cervical Vertebra with Synthetic Substitute, Percutaneous Endoscopic Approach	0PU54KZ	Supplement Right Scapula with Nonautologous Tissue Substitute, Percutaneous Endoscopic Approach
U137Z	Supplement Right Rib with Autologous Tissue Substitute, Percutaneous Approach	0PU34KZ	Supplement Cervical Vertebra with Nonautologous Tissue Substitute, Percutaneous Endoscopic Approach	0PU607Z	Supplement Left Scapula with Autologous Tissue Substitute, Open Approach
U13JZ	Supplement Right Rib with Synthetic Substitute, Percutaneous Approach	0PU407Z	Supplement Thoracic Vertebra with Autologous Tissue Substitute, Open Approach	0PU60JZ	Supplement Left Scapula with Synthetic Substitute, Open Approach
U13KZ	Supplement Right Rib with Nonautologous Tissue Substitute, Percutaneous Approach	0PU40JZ	Supplement Thoracic Vertebra with Synthetic Substitute, Open Approach	0PU60KZ	Supplement Left Scapula with Nonautologous Tissue Substitute, Open Approach
U147Z	Supplement Right Rib with Autologous Tissue Substitute, Percutaneous Endoscopic Approach	0PU40KZ	Supplement Thoracic Vertebra with Nonautologous Tissue Substitute, Open Approach	0PU637Z	Supplement Left Scapula with Autologous Tissue Substitute, Percutaneous Approach
U14JZ	Supplement Right Rib with Synthetic Substitute, Percutaneous Endoscopic Approach	0PU437Z	Supplement Thoracic Vertebra with Autologous Tissue Substitute, Percutaneous Approach	0PU63JZ	Supplement Left Scapula with Synthetic Substitute, Percutaneous Approach
U14KZ	Supplement Right Rib with Nonautologous Tissue Substitute, Percutaneous Endoscopic Approach	0PU43JZ	Supplement Thoracic Vertebra with Synthetic Substitute, Percutaneous Approach	0PU63KZ	Supplement Left Scapula with Nonautologous Tissue Substitute, Percutaneous Approach
PU207Z	Supplement Left Rib with Autologous Tissue Substitute, Open Approach	0PU43KZ	Supplement Thoracic Vertebra with Nonautologous Tissue Substitute, Percutaneous Approach	0PU647Z	Supplement Left Scapula with Autologous Tissue Substitute, Percutaneous Endoscopic Approach
PU20JZ	Supplement Left Rib with Synthetic Substitute, Open Approach			0PU64JZ	Supplement Left Scapula with Synthetic Substitute, Percutaneous Endoscopic Approach
PU20KZ	Supplement Left Rib with Nonautologous Tissue Substitute, Open Approach				
PU237Z	Supplement Left Rib with Autologous Tissue Substitute, Percutaneous Approach				
PU23JZ	Supplement Left Rib with Synthetic Substitute, Percutaneous Approach				

Female-only	♂ Male-only	▲ Limited Coverage	● Non-OR	▇ HAC-associated procedure	▲ Non-covered procedures	✚ Combination

0PU64KZ Supplement Left Scapula with Nonautologous Tissue Substitute, Percutaneous Endoscopic Approach

0PU707Z Supplement Right Glenoid Cavity with Autologous Tissue Substitute, Open Approach

0PU70JZ Supplement Right Glenoid Cavity with Synthetic Substitute, Open Approach

0PU70KZ Supplement Right Glenoid Cavity with Nonautologous Tissue Substitute, Open Approach

0PU737Z Supplement Right Glenoid Cavity with Autologous Tissue Substitute, Percutaneous Approach

0PU73JZ Supplement Right Glenoid Cavity with Synthetic Substitute, Percutaneous Approach

0PU73KZ Supplement Right Glenoid Cavity with Nonautologous Tissue Substitute, Percutaneous Approach

0PU747Z Supplement Right Glenoid Cavity with Autologous Tissue Substitute, Percutaneous Endoscopic Approach

0PU74JZ Supplement Right Glenoid Cavity with Synthetic Substitute, Percutaneous Endoscopic Approach

0PU74KZ Supplement Right Glenoid Cavity with Nonautologous Tissue Substitute, Percutaneous Endoscopic Approach

0PU807Z Supplement Left Glenoid Cavity with Autologous Tissue Substitute, Open Approach

0PU80JZ Supplement Left Glenoid Cavity with Synthetic Substitute, Open Approach

0PU80KZ Supplement Left Glenoid Cavity with Nonautologous Tissue Substitute, Open Approach

0PU837Z Supplement Left Glenoid Cavity with Autologous Tissue Substitute, Percutaneous Approach

0PU83JZ Supplement Left Glenoid Cavity with Synthetic Substitute, Percutaneous Approach

0PU83KZ Supplement Left Glenoid Cavity with Nonautologous Tissue Substitute, Percutaneous Approach

0PU847Z Supplement Left Glenoid Cavity with Autologous Tissue Substitute, Percutaneous Endoscopic Approach

0PU84JZ Supplement Left Glenoid Cavity with Synthetic Substitute, Percutaneous Endoscopic Approach

0PU84KZ Supplement Left Glenoid Cavity with Nonautologous Tissue Substitute, Percutaneous Endoscopic Approach

0PU907Z Supplement Right Clavicle with Autologous Tissue Substitute, Open Approach

0PU90JZ Supplement Right Clavicle with Synthetic Substitute, Open Approach

0PU90KZ Supplement Right Clavicle with Nonautologous Tissue Substitute, Open Approach

0PU937Z Supplement Right Clavicle with Autologous Tissue Substitute, Percutaneous Approach

0PU93JZ Supplement Right Clavicle with Synthetic Substitute, Percutaneous Approach

0PU93KZ Supplement Right Clavicle with Nonautologous Tissue Substitute, Percutaneous Approach

0PU947Z Supplement Right Clavicle with Autologous Tissue Substitute, Percutaneous Endoscopic Approach

0PU94JZ Supplement Right Clavicle with Synthetic Substitute, Percutaneous Endoscopic Approach

0PU94KZ Supplement Right Clavicle with Nonautologous Tissue Substitute, Percutaneous Endoscopic Approach

0PUB07Z Supplement Left Clavicle with Autologous Tissue Substitute, Open Approach

0PUB0JZ Supplement Left Clavicle with Synthetic Substitute, Open Approach

0PUB0KZ Supplement Left Clavicle with Nonautologous Tissue Substitute, Open Approach

0PUB37Z Supplement Left Clavicle with Autologous Tissue Substitute, Percutaneous Approach

0PUB3JZ Supplement Left Clavicle with Synthetic Substitute, Percutaneous Approach

0PUB3KZ Supplement Left Clavicle with Nonautologous Tissue Substitute, Percutaneous Approach

0PUB47Z Supplement Left Clavicle with Autologous Tissue Substitute, Percutaneous Endoscopic Approach

0PUB4JZ Supplement Left Clavicle with Synthetic Substitute, Percutaneous Endoscopic Approach

0PUB4KZ Supplement Left Clavicle with Nonautologous Tissue Substitute, Percutaneous Endoscopic Approach

0PUC07Z Supplement Right Humeral Head with Autologous Tissue Substitute, Open Approach

0PUC0JZ Supplement Right Humeral Head with Synthetic Substitute, Open Approach

0PUC0KZ Supplement Right Humeral Head with Nonautologous Tissue Substitute, Open Approach

0PUC37Z Supplement Right Humeral Head with Autologous Tissue Substitute, Percutaneous Approach

0PUC3JZ Supplement Right Humeral Head with Synthetic Substitute, Percutaneous Approach

0PUC3KZ Supplement Right Humeral Head with Nonautologous Tissue Substitute, Percutaneous Approach

0PUC47Z Supplement Right Humeral Head with Autologous Tissue Substitute, Percutaneous Endoscopic Approach

0PUC4JZ Supplement Right Humeral Head with Synthetic Substitute, Percutaneous Endoscopic Approach

0PUC4KZ Supplement Right Humeral Head with Nonautologous Tissue Substitute, Percutaneous Endoscopic Approach

0PUD07Z Supplement Left Humeral Head with Autologous Tissue Substitute, Open Approach

0PUD0JZ Supplement Left Humeral Head with Synthetic Substitute, Open Approach

0PUD0KZ Supplement Left Humeral Head with Nonautologous Tissue Substitute, Open Approach

0PUD37Z Supplement Left Humeral Head with Autologous Tissue Substitute, Percutaneous Approach

0PUD3JZ Supplement Left Humeral Head with Synthetic Substitute, Percutaneous Approach

0PUD3KZ Supplement Left Humeral Head with Nonautologous Tissue Substitute, Percutaneous Approach

0PUD47Z Supplement Left Humeral Head with Autologous Tissue Substitute, Percutaneous Endoscopic Approach

0PUD4JZ Supplement Left Humeral Head with Synthetic Substitute, Percutaneous Endoscopic Approach

0PUD4KZ Supplement Left Humeral Head with Nonautologous Tissue Substitute, Percutaneous Endoscopic Approach

0PUF07Z Supplement Right Humeral Shaft with Autologous Tissue Substitute, Open Approach

0PUF0JZ Supplement Right Humeral Shaft with Synthetic Substitute, Open Approach

0PUF0KZ Supplement Right Humeral Shaft with Nonautologous Tissue Substitute, Open Approach

0PUF37Z Supplement Right Humeral Shaft with Autologous Tissue Substitute, Percutaneous Approach

0PUF3JZ Supplement Right Humeral Shaft with Synthetic Substitute, Percutaneous Approach

0PUF3KZ Supplement Right Humeral Shaft with Nonautologous Tissue Substitute, Percutaneous Approach

0PUF47Z Supplement Right Humeral Shaft with Autologous Tissue Substitute, Percutaneous Endoscopic Approach

0PUF4JZ Supplement Right Humeral Shaft with Synthetic Substitute, Percutaneous Endoscopic Approach

0PUF4KZ Supplement Right Humeral Shaft with Nonautologous Tissue Substitute, Percutaneous Endoscopic Approach

0PUG07Z Supplement Left Humeral Shaft with Autologous Tissue Substitute, Open Approach

0PUG0JZ Supplement Left Humeral Shaft with Synthetic Substitute, Open Approach

0PUG0KZ Supplement Left Humeral Shaft with Nonautologous Tissue Substitute, Open Approach

0PUG37Z Supplement Left Humeral Shaft with Autologous Tissue Substitute, Percutaneous Approach

0PUG3JZ Supplement Left Humeral Shaft with Synthetic Substitute, Percutaneous Approach

0PUG3KZ Supplement Left Humeral Shaft with Nonautologous Tissue Substitute, Percutaneous Approach

0PUG47Z Supplement Left Humeral Shaft with Autologous Tissue Substitute, Percutaneous Endoscopic Approach

0PUG4JZ Supplement Left Humeral Shaft with Synthetic Substitute, Percutaneous Endoscopic Approach

0PUG4KZ Supplement Left Humeral Shaft with Nonautologous Tissue Substitute, Percutaneous Endoscopic Approach

0PUH07Z Supplement Right Radius with Autologous Tissue Substitute, Open Approach

0PUH0JZ Supplement Right Radius with Synthetic Substitute, Open Approach

0PUH0KZ Supplement Right Radius with Nonautologous Tissue Substitute, Open Approach

0PUH37Z Supplement Right Radius with Autologous Tissue Substitute, Percutaneous Approach

0PUH3JZ Supplement Right Radius with Synthetic Substitute, Percutaneous Approach

0PUH3KZ Supplement Right Radius with Nonautologous Tissue Substitute, Percutaneous Approach

0PUH47Z Supplement Right Radius with Autologous Tissue Substitute, Percutaneous Endoscopic Approach

0PUH4JZ Supplement Right Radius with Synthetic Substitute, Percutaneous Endoscopic Approach

♀ Female-only   ♂ Male-only   ▲ Limited Coverage   ● Non-OR   ▦ HAC-associated procedure   ▲ Non-covered procedures   ✚ Combinatio

H4KZ	Supplement Right Radius with Nonautologous Tissue Substitute, Percutaneous Endoscopic Approach
J07Z	Supplement Left Radius with Autologous Tissue Substitute, Open Approach
J0JZ	Supplement Left Radius with Synthetic Substitute, Open Approach
J0KZ	Supplement Left Radius with Nonautologous Tissue Substitute, Open Approach
J37Z	Supplement Left Radius with Autologous Tissue Substitute, Percutaneous Approach
J3JZ	Supplement Left Radius with Synthetic Substitute, Percutaneous Approach
J3KZ	Supplement Left Radius with Nonautologous Tissue Substitute, Percutaneous Approach
J47Z	Supplement Left Radius with Autologous Tissue Substitute, Percutaneous Endoscopic Approach
J4JZ	Supplement Left Radius with Synthetic Substitute, Percutaneous Endoscopic Approach
J4KZ	Supplement Left Radius with Nonautologous Tissue Substitute, Percutaneous Endoscopic Approach
UK07Z	Supplement Right Ulna with Autologous Tissue Substitute, Open Approach
UK0JZ	Supplement Right Ulna with Synthetic Substitute, Open Approach
UK0KZ	Supplement Right Ulna with Nonautologous Tissue Substitute, Open Approach
UK37Z	Supplement Right Ulna with Autologous Tissue Substitute, Percutaneous Approach
UK3JZ	Supplement Right Ulna with Synthetic Substitute, Percutaneous Approach
UK3KZ	Supplement Right Ulna with Nonautologous Tissue Substitute, Percutaneous Approach
UK47Z	Supplement Right Ulna with Autologous Tissue Substitute, Percutaneous Endoscopic Approach
UK4JZ	Supplement Right Ulna with Synthetic Substitute, Percutaneous Endoscopic Approach
UK4KZ	Supplement Right Ulna with Nonautologous Tissue Substitute, Percutaneous Endoscopic Approach
UL07Z	Supplement Left Ulna with Autologous Tissue Substitute, Open Approach
UL0JZ	Supplement Left Ulna with Synthetic Substitute, Open Approach
UL0KZ	Supplement Left Ulna with Nonautologous Tissue Substitute, Open Approach
PUL37Z	Supplement Left Ulna with Autologous Tissue Substitute, Percutaneous Approach
PUL3JZ	Supplement Left Ulna with Synthetic Substitute, Percutaneous Approach
PUL3KZ	Supplement Left Ulna with Nonautologous Tissue Substitute, Percutaneous Approach
PUL47Z	Supplement Left Ulna with Autologous Tissue Substitute, Percutaneous Endoscopic Approach
PUL4JZ	Supplement Left Ulna with Synthetic Substitute, Percutaneous Endoscopic Approach
PUL4KZ	Supplement Left Ulna with Nonautologous Tissue Substitute, Percutaneous Endoscopic Approach
PUM07Z	Supplement Right Carpal with Autologous Tissue Substitute, Open Approach

0PUM0JZ	Supplement Right Carpal with Synthetic Substitute, Open Approach
0PUM0KZ	Supplement Right Carpal with Nonautologous Tissue Substitute, Open Approach
0PUM37Z	Supplement Right Carpal with Autologous Tissue Substitute, Percutaneous Approach
0PUM3JZ	Supplement Right Carpal with Synthetic Substitute, Percutaneous Approach
0PUM3KZ	Supplement Right Carpal with Nonautologous Tissue Substitute, Percutaneous Approach
0PUM47Z	Supplement Right Carpal with Autologous Tissue Substitute, Percutaneous Endoscopic Approach
0PUM4JZ	Supplement Right Carpal with Synthetic Substitute, Percutaneous Endoscopic Approach
0PUM4KZ	Supplement Right Carpal with Nonautologous Tissue Substitute, Percutaneous Endoscopic Approach
0PUN07Z	Supplement Left Carpal with Autologous Tissue Substitute, Open Approach
0PUN0JZ	Supplement Left Carpal with Synthetic Substitute, Open Approach
0PUN0KZ	Supplement Left Carpal with Nonautologous Tissue Substitute, Open Approach
0PUN37Z	Supplement Left Carpal with Autologous Tissue Substitute, Percutaneous Approach
0PUN3JZ	Supplement Left Carpal with Synthetic Substitute, Percutaneous Approach
0PUN3KZ	Supplement Left Carpal with Nonautologous Tissue Substitute, Percutaneous Approach
0PUN47Z	Supplement Left Carpal with Autologous Tissue Substitute, Percutaneous Endoscopic Approach
0PUN4JZ	Supplement Left Carpal with Synthetic Substitute, Percutaneous Endoscopic Approach
0PUN4KZ	Supplement Left Carpal with Nonautologous Tissue Substitute, Percutaneous Endoscopic Approach
0PUP07Z	Supplement Right Metacarpal with Autologous Tissue Substitute, Open Approach
0PUP0JZ	Supplement Right Metacarpal with Synthetic Substitute, Open Approach
0PUP0KZ	Supplement Right Metacarpal with Nonautologous Tissue Substitute, Open Approach
0PUP37Z	Supplement Right Metacarpal with Autologous Tissue Substitute, Percutaneous Approach
0PUP3JZ	Supplement Right Metacarpal with Synthetic Substitute, Percutaneous Approach
0PUP3KZ	Supplement Right Metacarpal with Nonautologous Tissue Substitute, Percutaneous Approach
0PUP47Z	Supplement Right Metacarpal with Autologous Tissue Substitute, Percutaneous Endoscopic Approach
0PUP4JZ	Supplement Right Metacarpal with Synthetic Substitute, Percutaneous Endoscopic Approach
0PUP4KZ	Supplement Right Metacarpal with Nonautologous Tissue Substitute, Percutaneous Endoscopic Approach
0PUQ07Z	Supplement Left Metacarpal with Autologous Tissue Substitute, Open Approach
0PUQ0JZ	Supplement Left Metacarpal with Synthetic Substitute, Open Approach

0PUQ0KZ	Supplement Left Metacarpal with Nonautologous Tissue Substitute, Open Approach
0PUQ37Z	Supplement Left Metacarpal with Autologous Tissue Substitute, Percutaneous Approach
0PUQ3JZ	Supplement Left Metacarpal with Synthetic Substitute, Percutaneous Approach
0PUQ3KZ	Supplement Left Metacarpal with Nonautologous Tissue Substitute, Percutaneous Approach
0PUQ47Z	Supplement Left Metacarpal with Autologous Tissue Substitute, Percutaneous Endoscopic Approach
0PUQ4JZ	Supplement Left Metacarpal with Synthetic Substitute, Percutaneous Endoscopic Approach
0PUQ4KZ	Supplement Left Metacarpal with Nonautologous Tissue Substitute, Percutaneous Endoscopic Approach
0PUR07Z	Supplement Right Thumb Phalanx with Autologous Tissue Substitute, Open Approach
0PUR0JZ	Supplement Right Thumb Phalanx with Synthetic Substitute, Open Approach
0PUR0KZ	Supplement Right Thumb Phalanx with Nonautologous Tissue Substitute, Open Approach
0PUR37Z	Supplement Right Thumb Phalanx with Autologous Tissue Substitute, Percutaneous Approach
0PUR3JZ	Supplement Right Thumb Phalanx with Synthetic Substitute, Percutaneous Approach
0PUR3KZ	Supplement Right Thumb Phalanx with Nonautologous Tissue Substitute, Percutaneous Approach
0PUR47Z	Supplement Right Thumb Phalanx with Autologous Tissue Substitute, Percutaneous Endoscopic Approach
0PUR4JZ	Supplement Right Thumb Phalanx with Synthetic Substitute, Percutaneous Endoscopic Approach
0PUR4KZ	Supplement Right Thumb Phalanx with Nonautologous Tissue Substitute, Percutaneous Endoscopic Approach
0PUS07Z	Supplement Left Thumb Phalanx with Autologous Tissue Substitute, Open Approach
0PUS0JZ	Supplement Left Thumb Phalanx with Synthetic Substitute, Open Approach
0PUS0KZ	Supplement Left Thumb Phalanx with Nonautologous Tissue Substitute, Open Approach
0PUS37Z	Supplement Left Thumb Phalanx with Autologous Tissue Substitute, Percutaneous Approach
0PUS3JZ	Supplement Left Thumb Phalanx with Synthetic Substitute, Percutaneous Approach
0PUS3KZ	Supplement Left Thumb Phalanx with Nonautologous Tissue Substitute, Percutaneous Approach
0PUS47Z	Supplement Left Thumb Phalanx with Autologous Tissue Substitute, Percutaneous Endoscopic Approach
0PUS4JZ	Supplement Left Thumb Phalanx with Synthetic Substitute, Percutaneous Endoscopic Approach
0PUS4KZ	Supplement Left Thumb Phalanx with Nonautologous Tissue Substitute, Percutaneous Endoscopic Approach
0PUT07Z	Supplement Right Finger Phalanx with Autologous Tissue Substitute, Open Approach

837

♀ Female-only	♂ Male-only	▲ Limited Coverage	● Non-OR	▨ HAC-associated procedure	▲ Non-covered procedures	✚ Combination

0PUT0JZ	Supplement Right Finger Phalanx with Synthetic Substitute, Open Approach
0PUT0KZ	Supplement Right Finger Phalanx with Nonautologous Tissue Substitute, Open Approach
0PUT37Z	Supplement Right Finger Phalanx with Autologous Tissue Substitute, Percutaneous Approach
0PUT3JZ	Supplement Right Finger Phalanx with Synthetic Substitute, Percutaneous Approach
0PUT3KZ	Supplement Right Finger Phalanx with Nonautologous Tissue Substitute, Percutaneous Approach
0PUT47Z	Supplement Right Finger Phalanx with Autologous Tissue Substitute, Percutaneous Endoscopic Approach

0PUT4JZ	Supplement Right Finger Phalanx with Synthetic Substitute, Percutaneous Endoscopic Approach
0PUT4KZ	Supplement Right Finger Phalanx with Nonautologous Tissue Substitute, Percutaneous Endoscopic Approach
0PUV07Z	Supplement Left Finger Phalanx with Autologous Tissue Substitute, Open Approach
0PUV0JZ	Supplement Left Finger Phalanx with Synthetic Substitute, Open Approach
0PUV0KZ	Supplement Left Finger Phalanx with Nonautologous Tissue Substitute, Open Approach
0PUV37Z	Supplement Left Finger Phalanx with Autologous Tissue Substitute, Percutaneous Approach

0PUV3JZ	Supplement Left Finger Phalanx with Synthetic Substitute, Percutaneous Approach
0PUV3KZ	Supplement Left Finger Phalanx with Nonautologous Tissue Substitute, Percutaneous Approach
0PUV47Z	Supplement Left Finger Phalanx with Autologous Tissue Substitute, Percutaneous Endoscopic Approach
0PUV4JZ	Supplement Left Finger Phalanx with Synthetic Substitute, Percutaneous Endoscopic Approach
0PUV4KZ	Supplement Left Finger Phalanx with Nonautologous Tissue Substitute, Percutaneous Endoscopic Approach

0PW – Upper Bones, Revision

Review Coding Guideline B6.1c

0PW004Z	Revision of Internal Fixation Device in Sternum, Open Approach
0PW007Z	Revision of Autologous Tissue Substitute in Sternum, Open Approach
0PW00JZ	Revision of Synthetic Substitute in Sternum, Open Approach
0PW00KZ	Revision of Nonautologous Tissue Substitute in Sternum, Open Approach
0PW034Z	Revision of Internal Fixation Device in Sternum, Percutaneous Approach
0PW037Z	Revision of Autologous Tissue Substitute in Sternum, Percutaneous Approach
0PW03JZ	Revision of Synthetic Substitute in Sternum, Percutaneous Approach
0PW03KZ	Revision of Nonautologous Tissue Substitute in Sternum, Percutaneous Approach
0PW044Z	Revision of Internal Fixation Device in Sternum, Percutaneous Endoscopic Approach
0PW047Z	Revision of Autologous Tissue Substitute in Sternum, Percutaneous Endoscopic Approach
0PW04JZ	Revision of Synthetic Substitute in Sternum, Percutaneous Endoscopic Approach
0PW04KZ	Revision of Nonautologous Tissue Substitute in Sternum, Percutaneous Endoscopic Approach
0PW0X4Z	Revision of Internal Fixation Device in Sternum, External Approach
0PW0X7Z	Revision of Autologous Tissue Substitute in Sternum, External Approach
0PW0XJZ	Revision of Synthetic Substitute in Sternum, External Approach
0PW0XKZ	Revision of Nonautologous Tissue Substitute in Sternum, External Approach
0PW104Z	Revision of Internal Fixation Device in Right Rib, Open Approach
	AHA CC: 4Q, 2014, 26-27
0PW107Z	Revision of Autologous Tissue Substitute in Right Rib, Open Approach
0PW10JZ	Revision of Synthetic Substitute in Right Rib, Open Approach
0PW10KZ	Revision of Nonautologous Tissue Substitute in Right Rib, Open Approach
0PW134Z	Revision of Internal Fixation Device in Right Rib, Percutaneous Approach
0PW137Z	Revision of Autologous Tissue Substitute in Right Rib, Percutaneous Approach
0PW13JZ	Revision of Synthetic Substitute in Right Rib, Percutaneous Approach
0PW13KZ	Revision of Nonautologous Tissue Substitute in Right Rib, Percutaneous Approach

0PW144Z	Revision of Internal Fixation Device in Right Rib, Percutaneous Endoscopic Approach
0PW147Z	Revision of Autologous Tissue Substitute in Right Rib, Percutaneous Endoscopic Approach
0PW14JZ	Revision of Synthetic Substitute in Right Rib, Percutaneous Endoscopic Approach
0PW14KZ	Revision of Nonautologous Tissue Substitute in Right Rib, Percutaneous Endoscopic Approach
0PW1X4Z	Revision of Internal Fixation Device in Right Rib, External Approach
0PW1X7Z	Revision of Autologous Tissue Substitute in Right Rib, External Approach
0PW1XJZ	Revision of Synthetic Substitute in Right Rib, External Approach
0PW1XKZ	Revision of Nonautologous Tissue Substitute in Right Rib, External Approach
0PW204Z	Revision of Internal Fixation Device in Left Rib, Open Approach
	AHA CC: 4Q, 2014, 26-27
0PW207Z	Revision of Autologous Tissue Substitute in Left Rib, Open Approach
0PW20JZ	Revision of Synthetic Substitute in Left Rib, Open Approach
0PW20KZ	Revision of Nonautologous Tissue Substitute in Left Rib, Open Approach
0PW234Z	Revision of Internal Fixation Device in Left Rib, Percutaneous Approach
0PW237Z	Revision of Autologous Tissue Substitute in Left Rib, Percutaneous Approach
0PW23JZ	Revision of Synthetic Substitute in Left Rib, Percutaneous Approach
0PW23KZ	Revision of Nonautologous Tissue Substitute in Left Rib, Percutaneous Approach
0PW244Z	Revision of Internal Fixation Device in Left Rib, Percutaneous Endoscopic Approach
0PW247Z	Revision of Autologous Tissue Substitute in Left Rib, Percutaneous Endoscopic Approach
0PW24JZ	Revision of Synthetic Substitute in Left Rib, Percutaneous Endoscopic Approach
0PW24KZ	Revision of Nonautologous Tissue Substitute in Left Rib, Percutaneous Endoscopic Approach
0PW2X4Z	Revision of Internal Fixation Device in Left Rib, External Approach
0PW2X7Z	Revision of Autologous Tissue Substitute in Left Rib, External Approach
0PW2XJZ	Revision of Synthetic Substitute in Left Rib, External Approach

0PW2XKZ	Revision of Nonautologous Tissue Substitute in Left Rib, External Approach
0PW304Z	Revision of Internal Fixation Device in Cervical Vertebra, Open Approach
0PW307Z	Revision of Autologous Tissue Substitute in Cervical Vertebra, Open Approach
0PW30JZ	Revision of Synthetic Substitute in Cervical Vertebra, Open Approach
0PW30KZ	Revision of Nonautologous Tissue Substitute in Cervical Vertebra, Open Approach
0PW334Z	Revision of Internal Fixation Device in Cervical Vertebra, Percutaneous Approach
0PW337Z	Revision of Autologous Tissue Substitute in Cervical Vertebra, Percutaneous Approach
0PW33JZ	Revision of Synthetic Substitute in Cervical Vertebra, Percutaneous Approach
0PW33KZ	Revision of Nonautologous Tissue Substitute in Cervical Vertebra, Percutaneous Approach
0PW344Z	Revision of Internal Fixation Device in Cervical Vertebra, Percutaneous Endoscopic Approach
0PW347Z	Revision of Autologous Tissue Substitute in Cervical Vertebra, Percutaneous Endoscopic Approach
0PW34JZ	Revision of Synthetic Substitute in Cervical Vertebra, Percutaneous Endoscopic Approach
0PW34KZ	Revision of Nonautologous Tissue Substitute in Cervical Vertebra, Percutaneous Endoscopic Approach
0PW3X4Z	Revision of Internal Fixation Device in Cervical Vertebra, External Approach
0PW3X7Z	Revision of Autologous Tissue Substitute in Cervical Vertebra, External Approach
0PW3XJZ	Revision of Synthetic Substitute in Cervical Vertebra, External Approach
0PW3XKZ	Revision of Nonautologous Tissue Substitute in Cervical Vertebra, External Approach
0PW404Z	Revision of Internal Fixation Device in Thoracic Vertebra, Open Approach
	AHA CC: 4Q, 2014, 27-28
0PW407Z	Revision of Autologous Tissue Substitute in Thoracic Vertebra, Open Approach
0PW40JZ	Revision of Synthetic Substitute in Thoracic Vertebra, Open Approach
0PW40KZ	Revision of Nonautologous Tissue Substitute in Thoracic Vertebra, Open Approach
0PW434Z	Revision of Internal Fixation Device in Thoracic Vertebra, Percutaneous Approach

♀ Female-only   ♂ Male-only   ▲ Limited Coverage   ● Non-OR   ▨ HAC-associated procedure   ▲ Non-covered procedures   ✚ Combinatio

437Z Revision of Autologous Tissue Substitute in Thoracic Vertebra, Percutaneous Approach

43JZ Revision of Synthetic Substitute in Thoracic Vertebra, Percutaneous Approach

43KZ Revision of Nonautologous Tissue Substitute in Thoracic Vertebra, Percutaneous Approach

444Z Revision of Internal Fixation Device in Thoracic Vertebra, Percutaneous Endoscopic Approach

447Z Revision of Autologous Tissue Substitute in Thoracic Vertebra, Percutaneous Endoscopic Approach

44JZ Revision of Synthetic Substitute in Thoracic Vertebra, Percutaneous Endoscopic Approach

44KZ Revision of Nonautologous Tissue Substitute in Thoracic Vertebra, Percutaneous Endoscopic Approach

4X4Z Revision of Internal Fixation Device in Thoracic Vertebra, External Approach

4X7Z Revision of Autologous Tissue Substitute in Thoracic Vertebra, External Approach

4XJZ Revision of Synthetic Substitute in Thoracic Vertebra, External Approach

4XKZ Revision of Nonautologous Tissue Substitute in Thoracic Vertebra, External Approach

W504Z Revision of Internal Fixation Device in Right Scapula, Open Approach

W507Z Revision of Autologous Tissue Substitute in Right Scapula, Open Approach

W50JZ Revision of Synthetic Substitute in Right Scapula, Open Approach

W50KZ Revision of Nonautologous Tissue Substitute in Right Scapula, Open Approach

W534Z Revision of Internal Fixation Device in Right Scapula, Percutaneous Approach

W537Z Revision of Autologous Tissue Substitute in Right Scapula, Percutaneous Approach

W53JZ Revision of Synthetic Substitute in Right Scapula, Percutaneous Approach

W53KZ Revision of Nonautologous Tissue Substitute in Right Scapula, Percutaneous Approach

W544Z Revision of Internal Fixation Device in Right Scapula, Percutaneous Endoscopic Approach

W547Z Revision of Autologous Tissue Substitute in Right Scapula, Percutaneous Endoscopic Approach

W54JZ Revision of Synthetic Substitute in Right Scapula, Percutaneous Endoscopic Approach

W54KZ Revision of Nonautologous Tissue Substitute in Right Scapula, Percutaneous Endoscopic Approach

W5X4Z Revision of Internal Fixation Device in Right Scapula, External Approach

W5X7Z Revision of Autologous Tissue Substitute in Right Scapula, External Approach

W5XJZ Revision of Synthetic Substitute in Right Scapula, External Approach

W5XKZ Revision of Nonautologous Tissue Substitute in Right Scapula, External Approach

PW604Z Revision of Internal Fixation Device in Left Scapula, Open Approach

PW607Z Revision of Autologous Tissue Substitute in Left Scapula, Open Approach

PW60JZ Revision of Synthetic Substitute in Left Scapula, Open Approach

0PW60KZ Revision of Nonautologous Tissue Substitute in Left Scapula, Open Approach

0PW634Z Revision of Internal Fixation Device in Left Scapula, Percutaneous Approach

0PW637Z Revision of Autologous Tissue Substitute in Left Scapula, Percutaneous Approach

0PW63JZ Revision of Synthetic Substitute in Left Scapula, Percutaneous Approach

0PW63KZ Revision of Nonautologous Tissue Substitute in Left Scapula, Percutaneous Approach

0PW644Z Revision of Internal Fixation Device in Left Scapula, Percutaneous Endoscopic Approach

0PW647Z Revision of Autologous Tissue Substitute in Left Scapula, Percutaneous Endoscopic Approach

0PW64JZ Revision of Synthetic Substitute in Left Scapula, Percutaneous Endoscopic Approach

0PW64KZ Revision of Nonautologous Tissue Substitute in Left Scapula, Percutaneous Endoscopic Approach

0PW6X4Z Revision of Internal Fixation Device in Left Scapula, External Approach

0PW6X7Z Revision of Autologous Tissue Substitute in Left Scapula, External Approach

0PW6XJZ Revision of Synthetic Substitute in Left Scapula, External Approach

0PW6XKZ Revision of Nonautologous Tissue Substitute in Left Scapula, External Approach

0PW704Z Revision of Internal Fixation Device in Right Glenoid Cavity, Open Approach

0PW707Z Revision of Autologous Tissue Substitute in Right Glenoid Cavity, Open Approach

0PW70JZ Revision of Synthetic Substitute in Right Glenoid Cavity, Open Approach

0PW70KZ Revision of Nonautologous Tissue Substitute in Right Glenoid Cavity, Open Approach

0PW734Z Revision of Internal Fixation Device in Right Glenoid Cavity, Percutaneous Approach

0PW737Z Revision of Autologous Tissue Substitute in Right Glenoid Cavity, Percutaneous Approach

0PW73JZ Revision of Synthetic Substitute in Right Glenoid Cavity, Percutaneous Approach

0PW73KZ Revision of Nonautologous Tissue Substitute in Right Glenoid Cavity, Percutaneous Approach

0PW744Z Revision of Internal Fixation Device in Right Glenoid Cavity, Percutaneous Endoscopic Approach

0PW747Z Revision of Autologous Tissue Substitute in Right Glenoid Cavity, Percutaneous Endoscopic Approach

0PW74JZ Revision of Synthetic Substitute in Right Glenoid Cavity, Percutaneous Endoscopic Approach

0PW74KZ Revision of Nonautologous Tissue Substitute in Right Glenoid Cavity, Percutaneous Endoscopic Approach

0PW7X4Z Revision of Internal Fixation Device in Right Glenoid Cavity, External Approach

0PW7X7Z Revision of Autologous Tissue Substitute in Right Glenoid Cavity, External Approach

0PW7XJZ Revision of Synthetic Substitute in Right Glenoid Cavity, External Approach

0PW7XKZ Revision of Nonautologous Tissue Substitute in Right Glenoid Cavity, External Approach

0PW804Z Revision of Internal Fixation Device in Left Glenoid Cavity, Open Approach

0PW807Z Revision of Autologous Tissue Substitute in Left Glenoid Cavity, Open Approach

0PW80JZ Revision of Synthetic Substitute in Left Glenoid Cavity, Open Approach

0PW80KZ Revision of Nonautologous Tissue Substitute in Left Glenoid Cavity, Open Approach

0PW834Z Revision of Internal Fixation Device in Left Glenoid Cavity, Percutaneous Approach

0PW837Z Revision of Autologous Tissue Substitute in Left Glenoid Cavity, Percutaneous Approach

0PW83JZ Revision of Synthetic Substitute in Left Glenoid Cavity, Percutaneous Approach

0PW83KZ Revision of Nonautologous Tissue Substitute in Left Glenoid Cavity, Percutaneous Approach

0PW844Z Revision of Internal Fixation Device in Left Glenoid Cavity, Percutaneous Endoscopic Approach

0PW847Z Revision of Autologous Tissue Substitute in Left Glenoid Cavity, Percutaneous Endoscopic Approach

0PW84JZ Revision of Synthetic Substitute in Left Glenoid Cavity, Percutaneous Endoscopic Approach

0PW84KZ Revision of Nonautologous Tissue Substitute in Left Glenoid Cavity, Percutaneous Endoscopic Approach

0PW8X4Z Revision of Internal Fixation Device in Left Glenoid Cavity, External Approach

0PW8X7Z Revision of Autologous Tissue Substitute in Left Glenoid Cavity, External Approach

0PW8XJZ Revision of Synthetic Substitute in Left Glenoid Cavity, External Approach

0PW8XKZ Revision of Nonautologous Tissue Substitute in Left Glenoid Cavity, External Approach

0PW904Z Revision of Internal Fixation Device in Right Clavicle, Open Approach

0PW907Z Revision of Autologous Tissue Substitute in Right Clavicle, Open Approach

0PW90JZ Revision of Synthetic Substitute in Right Clavicle, Open Approach

0PW90KZ Revision of Nonautologous Tissue Substitute in Right Clavicle, Open Approach

0PW934Z Revision of Internal Fixation Device in Right Clavicle, Percutaneous Approach

0PW937Z Revision of Autologous Tissue Substitute in Right Clavicle, Percutaneous Approach

0PW93JZ Revision of Synthetic Substitute in Right Clavicle, Percutaneous Approach

0PW93KZ Revision of Nonautologous Tissue Substitute in Right Clavicle, Percutaneous Approach

0PW944Z Revision of Internal Fixation Device in Right Clavicle, Percutaneous Endoscopic Approach

0PW947Z Revision of Autologous Tissue Substitute in Right Clavicle, Percutaneous Endoscopic Approach

0PW94JZ Revision of Synthetic Substitute in Right Clavicle, Percutaneous Endoscopic Approach

0PW94KZ Revision of Nonautologous Tissue Substitute in Right Clavicle, Percutaneous Endoscopic Approach

0PW9X4Z Revision of Internal Fixation Device in Right Clavicle, External Approach

0PW9X7Z Revision of Autologous Tissue Substitute in Right Clavicle, External Approach

0PW9XJZ	Revision of Synthetic Substitute in Right Clavicle, External Approach
0PW9XKZ	Revision of Nonautologous Tissue Substitute in Right Clavicle, External Approach
0PWB04Z	Revision of Internal Fixation Device in Left Clavicle, Open Approach
0PWB07Z	Revision of Autologous Tissue Substitute in Left Clavicle, Open Approach
0PWB0JZ	Revision of Synthetic Substitute in Left Clavicle, Open Approach
0PWB0KZ	Revision of Nonautologous Tissue Substitute in Left Clavicle, Open Approach
0PWB34Z	Revision of Internal Fixation Device in Left Clavicle, Percutaneous Approach
0PWB37Z	Revision of Autologous Tissue Substitute in Left Clavicle, Percutaneous Approach
0PWB3JZ	Revision of Synthetic Substitute in Left Clavicle, Percutaneous Approach
0PWB3KZ	Revision of Nonautologous Tissue Substitute in Left Clavicle, Percutaneous Approach
0PWB44Z	Revision of Internal Fixation Device in Left Clavicle, Percutaneous Endoscopic Approach
0PWB47Z	Revision of Autologous Tissue Substitute in Left Clavicle, Percutaneous Endoscopic Approach
0PWB4JZ	Revision of Synthetic Substitute in Left Clavicle, Percutaneous Endoscopic Approach
0PWB4KZ	Revision of Nonautologous Tissue Substitute in Left Clavicle, Percutaneous Endoscopic Approach
0PWBX4Z	Revision of Internal Fixation Device in Left Clavicle, External Approach
0PWBX7Z	Revision of Autologous Tissue Substitute in Left Clavicle, External Approach
0PWBXJZ	Revision of Synthetic Substitute in Left Clavicle, External Approach
0PWBXKZ	Revision of Nonautologous Tissue Substitute in Left Clavicle, External Approach
0PWC04Z	Revision of Internal Fixation Device in Right Humeral Head, Open Approach
0PWC05Z	Revision of External Fixation Device in Right Humeral Head, Open Approach
0PWC07Z	Revision of Autologous Tissue Substitute in Right Humeral Head, Open Approach
0PWC0JZ	Revision of Synthetic Substitute in Right Humeral Head, Open Approach
0PWC0KZ	Revision of Nonautologous Tissue Substitute in Right Humeral Head, Open Approach
0PWC34Z	Revision of Internal Fixation Device in Right Humeral Head, Percutaneous Approach
0PWC35Z	Revision of External Fixation Device in Right Humeral Head, Percutaneous Approach
0PWC37Z	Revision of Autologous Tissue Substitute in Right Humeral Head, Percutaneous Approach
0PWC3JZ	Revision of Synthetic Substitute in Right Humeral Head, Percutaneous Approach
0PWC3KZ	Revision of Nonautologous Tissue Substitute in Right Humeral Head, Percutaneous Approach
0PWC44Z	Revision of Internal Fixation Device in Right Humeral Head, Percutaneous Endoscopic Approach
0PWC45Z	Revision of External Fixation Device in Right Humeral Head, Percutaneous Endoscopic Approach
0PWC47Z	Revision of Autologous Tissue Substitute in Right Humeral Head, Percutaneous Endoscopic Approach
0PWC4JZ	Revision of Synthetic Substitute in Right Humeral Head, Percutaneous Endoscopic Approach
0PWC4KZ	Revision of Nonautologous Tissue Substitute in Right Humeral Head, Percutaneous Endoscopic Approach
0PWCX4Z	Revision of Internal Fixation Device in Right Humeral Head, External Approach
0PWCX5Z	Revision of External Fixation Device in Right Humeral Head, External Approach
0PWCX7Z	Revision of Autologous Tissue Substitute in Right Humeral Head, External Approach
0PWCXJZ	Revision of Synthetic Substitute in Right Humeral Head, External Approach
0PWCXKZ	Revision of Nonautologous Tissue Substitute in Right Humeral Head, External Approach
0PWD04Z	Revision of Internal Fixation Device in Left Humeral Head, Open Approach
0PWD05Z	Revision of External Fixation Device in Left Humeral Head, Open Approach
0PWD07Z	Revision of Autologous Tissue Substitute in Left Humeral Head, Open Approach
0PWD0JZ	Revision of Synthetic Substitute in Left Humeral Head, Open Approach
0PWD0KZ	Revision of Nonautologous Tissue Substitute in Left Humeral Head, Open Approach
0PWD34Z	Revision of Internal Fixation Device in Left Humeral Head, Percutaneous Approach
0PWD35Z	Revision of External Fixation Device in Left Humeral Head, Percutaneous Approach
0PWD37Z	Revision of Autologous Tissue Substitute in Left Humeral Head, Percutaneous Approach
0PWD3JZ	Revision of Synthetic Substitute in Left Humeral Head, Percutaneous Approach
0PWD3KZ	Revision of Nonautologous Tissue Substitute in Left Humeral Head, Percutaneous Approach
0PWD44Z	Revision of Internal Fixation Device in Left Humeral Head, Percutaneous Endoscopic Approach
0PWD45Z	Revision of External Fixation Device in Left Humeral Head, Percutaneous Endoscopic Approach
0PWD47Z	Revision of Autologous Tissue Substitute in Left Humeral Head, Percutaneous Endoscopic Approach
0PWD4JZ	Revision of Synthetic Substitute in Left Humeral Head, Percutaneous Endoscopic Approach
0PWD4KZ	Revision of Nonautologous Tissue Substitute in Left Humeral Head, Percutaneous Endoscopic Approach
0PWDX4Z	Revision of Internal Fixation Device in Left Humeral Head, External Approach
0PWDX5Z	Revision of External Fixation Device in Left Humeral Head, External Approach
0PWDX7Z	Revision of Autologous Tissue Substitute in Left Humeral Head, External Approach
0PWDXJZ	Revision of Synthetic Substitute in Left Humeral Head, External Approach
0PWDXKZ	Revision of Nonautologous Tissue Substitute in Left Humeral Head, External Approach
0PWF04Z	Revision of Internal Fixation Device in Right Humeral Shaft, Open Approach
0PWF05Z	Revision of External Fixation Device in Right Humeral Shaft, Open Approach
0PWF07Z	Revision of Autologous Tissue Substitute in Right Humeral Shaft, Open Approach
0PWF0JZ	Revision of Synthetic Substitute in Right Humeral Shaft, Open Approach
0PWF0KZ	Revision of Nonautologous Tissue Substitute in Right Humeral Shaft, Open Approach
0PWF34Z	Revision of Internal Fixation Device in Right Humeral Shaft, Percutaneous Approach
0PWF35Z	Revision of External Fixation Device in Right Humeral Shaft, Percutaneous Approach
0PWF37Z	Revision of Autologous Tissue Substitute in Right Humeral Shaft, Percutaneous Approach
0PWF3JZ	Revision of Synthetic Substitute in Right Humeral Shaft, Percutaneous Approach
0PWF3KZ	Revision of Nonautologous Tissue Substitute in Right Humeral Shaft, Percutaneous Approach
0PWF44Z	Revision of Internal Fixation Device in Right Humeral Shaft, Percutaneous Endoscopic Approach
0PWF45Z	Revision of External Fixation Device in Right Humeral Shaft, Percutaneous Endoscopic Approach
0PWF47Z	Revision of Autologous Tissue Substitute in Right Humeral Shaft, Percutaneous Endoscopic Approach
0PWF4JZ	Revision of Synthetic Substitute in Right Humeral Shaft, Percutaneous Endoscopic Approach
0PWF4KZ	Revision of Nonautologous Tissue Substitute in Right Humeral Shaft, Percutaneous Endoscopic Approach
0PWFX4Z	Revision of Internal Fixation Device in Right Humeral Shaft, External Approach
0PWFX5Z	Revision of External Fixation Device in Right Humeral Shaft, External Approach
0PWFX7Z	Revision of Autologous Tissue Substitute in Right Humeral Shaft, External Approach
0PWFXJZ	Revision of Synthetic Substitute in Right Humeral Shaft, External Approach
0PWFXKZ	Revision of Nonautologous Tissue Substitute in Right Humeral Shaft, External Approach
0PWG04Z	Revision of Internal Fixation Device in Left Humeral Shaft, Open Approach
0PWG05Z	Revision of External Fixation Device in Left Humeral Shaft, Open Approach
0PWG07Z	Revision of Autologous Tissue Substitute in Left Humeral Shaft, Open Approach
0PWG0JZ	Revision of Synthetic Substitute in Left Humeral Shaft, Open Approach
0PWG0KZ	Revision of Nonautologous Tissue Substitute in Left Humeral Shaft, Open Approach
0PWG34Z	Revision of Internal Fixation Device in Left Humeral Shaft, Percutaneous Approach
0PWG35Z	Revision of External Fixation Device in Left Humeral Shaft, Percutaneous Approach
0PWG37Z	Revision of Autologous Tissue Substitute in Left Humeral Shaft, Percutaneous Approach
0PWG3JZ	Revision of Synthetic Substitute in Left Humeral Shaft, Percutaneous Approach
0PWG3KZ	Revision of Nonautologous Tissue Substitute in Left Humeral Shaft, Percutaneous Approach

0PWG44Z	Revision of Internal Fixation Device in Left Humeral Shaft, Percutaneous Endoscopic Approach
0PWG45Z	Revision of External Fixation Device in Left Humeral Shaft, Percutaneous Endoscopic Approach
0PWG47Z	Revision of Autologous Tissue Substitute in Left Humeral Shaft, Percutaneous Endoscopic Approach
0PWG4JZ	Revision of Synthetic Substitute in Left Humeral Shaft, Percutaneous Endoscopic Approach
0PWG4KZ	Revision of Nonautologous Tissue Substitute in Left Humeral Shaft, Percutaneous Endoscopic Approach
0PWGX4Z	Revision of Internal Fixation Device in Left Humeral Shaft, External Approach
0PWGX5Z	Revision of External Fixation Device in Left Humeral Shaft, External Approach
0PWGX7Z	Revision of Autologous Tissue Substitute in Left Humeral Shaft, External Approach
0PWGXJZ	Revision of Synthetic Substitute in Left Humeral Shaft, External Approach
0PWGXKZ	Revision of Nonautologous Tissue Substitute in Left Humeral Shaft, External Approach
0PWH04Z	Revision of Internal Fixation Device in Right Radius, Open Approach
0PWH05Z	Revision of External Fixation Device in Right Radius, Open Approach
0PWH07Z	Revision of Autologous Tissue Substitute in Right Radius, Open Approach
0PWH0JZ	Revision of Synthetic Substitute in Right Radius, Open Approach
0PWH0KZ	Revision of Nonautologous Tissue Substitute in Right Radius, Open Approach
0PWH34Z	Revision of Internal Fixation Device in Right Radius, Percutaneous Approach
0PWH35Z	Revision of External Fixation Device in Right Radius, Percutaneous Approach
0PWH37Z	Revision of Autologous Tissue Substitute in Right Radius, Percutaneous Approach
0PWH3JZ	Revision of Synthetic Substitute in Right Radius, Percutaneous Approach
0PWH3KZ	Revision of Nonautologous Tissue Substitute in Right Radius, Percutaneous Approach
0PWH44Z	Revision of Internal Fixation Device in Right Radius, Percutaneous Endoscopic Approach
0PWH45Z	Revision of External Fixation Device in Right Radius, Percutaneous Endoscopic Approach
0PWH47Z	Revision of Autologous Tissue Substitute in Right Radius, Percutaneous Endoscopic Approach
0PWH4JZ	Revision of Synthetic Substitute in Right Radius, Percutaneous Endoscopic Approach
0PWH4KZ	Revision of Nonautologous Tissue Substitute in Right Radius, Percutaneous Endoscopic Approach
0PWHX4Z	Revision of Internal Fixation Device in Right Radius, External Approach
0PWHX5Z	Revision of External Fixation Device in Right Radius, External Approach
0PWHX7Z	Revision of Autologous Tissue Substitute in Right Radius, External Approach
0PWHXJZ	Revision of Synthetic Substitute in Right Radius, External Approach
0PWHXKZ	Revision of Nonautologous Tissue Substitute in Right Radius, External Approach
0PWJ04Z	Revision of Internal Fixation Device in Left Radius, Open Approach
0PWJ05Z	Revision of External Fixation Device in Left Radius, Open Approach
0PWJ07Z	Revision of Autologous Tissue Substitute in Left Radius, Open Approach
0PWJ0JZ	Revision of Synthetic Substitute in Left Radius, Open Approach
0PWJ0KZ	Revision of Nonautologous Tissue Substitute in Left Radius, Open Approach
0PWJ34Z	Revision of Internal Fixation Device in Left Radius, Percutaneous Approach
0PWJ35Z	Revision of External Fixation Device in Left Radius, Percutaneous Approach
0PWJ37Z	Revision of Autologous Tissue Substitute in Left Radius, Percutaneous Approach
0PWJ3JZ	Revision of Synthetic Substitute in Left Radius, Percutaneous Approach
0PWJ3KZ	Revision of Nonautologous Tissue Substitute in Left Radius, Percutaneous Approach
0PWJ44Z	Revision of Internal Fixation Device in Left Radius, Percutaneous Endoscopic Approach
0PWJ45Z	Revision of External Fixation Device in Left Radius, Percutaneous Endoscopic Approach
0PWJ47Z	Revision of Autologous Tissue Substitute in Left Radius, Percutaneous Endoscopic Approach
0PWJ4JZ	Revision of Synthetic Substitute in Left Radius, Percutaneous Endoscopic Approach
0PWJ4KZ	Revision of Nonautologous Tissue Substitute in Left Radius, Percutaneous Endoscopic Approach
0PWJX4Z	Revision of Internal Fixation Device in Left Radius, External Approach
0PWJX5Z	Revision of External Fixation Device in Left Radius, External Approach
0PWJX7Z	Revision of Autologous Tissue Substitute in Left Radius, External Approach
0PWJXJZ	Revision of Synthetic Substitute in Left Radius, External Approach
0PWJXKZ	Revision of Nonautologous Tissue Substitute in Left Radius, External Approach
0PWK04Z	Revision of Internal Fixation Device in Right Ulna, Open Approach
0PWK05Z	Revision of External Fixation Device in Right Ulna, Open Approach
0PWK07Z	Revision of Autologous Tissue Substitute in Right Ulna, Open Approach
0PWK0JZ	Revision of Synthetic Substitute in Right Ulna, Open Approach
0PWK0KZ	Revision of Nonautologous Tissue Substitute in Right Ulna, Open Approach
0PWK34Z	Revision of Internal Fixation Device in Right Ulna, Percutaneous Approach
0PWK35Z	Revision of External Fixation Device in Right Ulna, Percutaneous Approach
0PWK37Z	Revision of Autologous Tissue Substitute in Right Ulna, Percutaneous Approach
0PWK3JZ	Revision of Synthetic Substitute in Right Ulna, Percutaneous Approach
0PWK3KZ	Revision of Nonautologous Tissue Substitute in Right Ulna, Percutaneous Approach
0PWK44Z	Revision of Internal Fixation Device in Right Ulna, Percutaneous Endoscopic Approach
0PWK45Z	Revision of External Fixation Device in Right Ulna, Percutaneous Endoscopic Approach
0PWK47Z	Revision of Autologous Tissue Substitute in Right Ulna, Percutaneous Endoscopic Approach
0PWK4JZ	Revision of Synthetic Substitute in Right Ulna, Percutaneous Endoscopic Approach
0PWK4KZ	Revision of Nonautologous Tissue Substitute in Right Ulna, Percutaneous Endoscopic Approach
0PWKX4Z	Revision of Internal Fixation Device in Right Ulna, External Approach
0PWKX5Z	Revision of External Fixation Device in Right Ulna, External Approach
0PWKX7Z	Revision of Autologous Tissue Substitute in Right Ulna, External Approach
0PWKXJZ	Revision of Synthetic Substitute in Right Ulna, External Approach
0PWKXKZ	Revision of Nonautologous Tissue Substitute in Right Ulna, External Approach
0PWL04Z	Revision of Internal Fixation Device in Left Ulna, Open Approach
0PWL05Z	Revision of External Fixation Device in Left Ulna, Open Approach
0PWL07Z	Revision of Autologous Tissue Substitute in Left Ulna, Open Approach
0PWL0JZ	Revision of Synthetic Substitute in Left Ulna, Open Approach
0PWL0KZ	Revision of Nonautologous Tissue Substitute in Left Ulna, Open Approach
0PWL34Z	Revision of Internal Fixation Device in Left Ulna, Percutaneous Approach
0PWL35Z	Revision of External Fixation Device in Left Ulna, Percutaneous Approach
0PWL37Z	Revision of Autologous Tissue Substitute in Left Ulna, Percutaneous Approach
0PWL3JZ	Revision of Synthetic Substitute in Left Ulna, Percutaneous Approach
0PWL3KZ	Revision of Nonautologous Tissue Substitute in Left Ulna, Percutaneous Approach
0PWL44Z	Revision of Internal Fixation Device in Left Ulna, Percutaneous Endoscopic Approach
0PWL45Z	Revision of External Fixation Device in Left Ulna, Percutaneous Endoscopic Approach
0PWL47Z	Revision of Autologous Tissue Substitute in Left Ulna, Percutaneous Endoscopic Approach
0PWL4JZ	Revision of Synthetic Substitute in Left Ulna, Percutaneous Endoscopic Approach
0PWL4KZ	Revision of Nonautologous Tissue Substitute in Left Ulna, Percutaneous Endoscopic Approach
0PWLX4Z	Revision of Internal Fixation Device in Left Ulna, External Approach
0PWLX5Z	Revision of External Fixation Device in Left Ulna, External Approach
0PWLX7Z	Revision of Autologous Tissue Substitute in Left Ulna, External Approach
0PWLXJZ	Revision of Synthetic Substitute in Left Ulna, External Approach
0PWLXKZ	Revision of Nonautologous Tissue Substitute in Left Ulna, External Approach
0PWM04Z	Revision of Internal Fixation Device in Right Carpal, Open Approach
0PWM05Z	Revision of External Fixation Device in Right Carpal, Open Approach
0PWM07Z	Revision of Autologous Tissue Substitute in Right Carpal, Open Approach
0PWM0JZ	Revision of Synthetic Substitute in Right Carpal, Open Approach

Female-only   ♂ Male-only   ▲ Limited Coverage   ● Non-OR   ▨ HAC-associated procedure   ▲ Non-covered procedures   ➕ Combination

0PWM0KZ	Revision of Nonautologous Tissue Substitute in Right Carpal, Open Approach
0PWM34Z	Revision of Internal Fixation Device in Right Carpal, Percutaneous Approach
0PWM35Z	Revision of External Fixation Device in Right Carpal, Percutaneous Approach
0PWM37Z	Revision of Autologous Tissue Substitute in Right Carpal, Percutaneous Approach
0PWM3JZ	Revision of Synthetic Substitute in Right Carpal, Percutaneous Approach
0PWM3KZ	Revision of Nonautologous Tissue Substitute in Right Carpal, Percutaneous Approach
0PWM44Z	Revision of Internal Fixation Device in Right Carpal, Percutaneous Endoscopic Approach
0PWM45Z	Revision of External Fixation Device in Right Carpal, Percutaneous Endoscopic Approach
0PWM47Z	Revision of Autologous Tissue Substitute in Right Carpal, Percutaneous Endoscopic Approach
0PWM4JZ	Revision of Synthetic Substitute in Right Carpal, Percutaneous Endoscopic Approach
0PWM4KZ	Revision of Nonautologous Tissue Substitute in Right Carpal, Percutaneous Endoscopic Approach
0PWMX4Z	Revision of Internal Fixation Device in Right Carpal, External Approach
0PWMX5Z	Revision of External Fixation Device in Right Carpal, External Approach
0PWMX7Z	Revision of Autologous Tissue Substitute in Right Carpal, External Approach
0PWMXJZ	Revision of Synthetic Substitute in Right Carpal, External Approach
0PWMXKZ	Revision of Nonautologous Tissue Substitute in Right Carpal, External Approach
0PWN04Z	Revision of Internal Fixation Device in Left Carpal, Open Approach
0PWN05Z	Revision of External Fixation Device in Left Carpal, Open Approach
0PWN07Z	Revision of Autologous Tissue Substitute in Left Carpal, Open Approach
0PWN0JZ	Revision of Synthetic Substitute in Left Carpal, Open Approach
0PWN0KZ	Revision of Nonautologous Tissue Substitute in Left Carpal, Open Approach
0PWN34Z	Revision of Internal Fixation Device in Left Carpal, Percutaneous Approach
0PWN35Z	Revision of External Fixation Device in Left Carpal, Percutaneous Approach
0PWN37Z	Revision of Autologous Tissue Substitute in Left Carpal, Percutaneous Approach
0PWN3JZ	Revision of Synthetic Substitute in Left Carpal, Percutaneous Approach
0PWN3KZ	Revision of Nonautologous Tissue Substitute in Left Carpal, Percutaneous Approach
0PWN44Z	Revision of Internal Fixation Device in Left Carpal, Percutaneous Endoscopic Approach
0PWN45Z	Revision of External Fixation Device in Left Carpal, Percutaneous Endoscopic Approach
0PWN47Z	Revision of Autologous Tissue Substitute in Left Carpal, Percutaneous Endoscopic Approach
0PWN4JZ	Revision of Synthetic Substitute in Left Carpal, Percutaneous Endoscopic Approach
0PWN4KZ	Revision of Nonautologous Tissue Substitute in Left Carpal, Percutaneous Endoscopic Approach
0PWNX4Z	Revision of Internal Fixation Device in Left Carpal, External Approach
0PWNX5Z	Revision of External Fixation Device in Left Carpal, External Approach
0PWNX7Z	Revision of Autologous Tissue Substitute in Left Carpal, External Approach
0PWNXJZ	Revision of Synthetic Substitute in Left Carpal, External Approach
0PWNXKZ	Revision of Nonautologous Tissue Substitute in Left Carpal, External Approach
0PWP04Z	Revision of Internal Fixation Device in Right Metacarpal, Open Approach
0PWP05Z	Revision of External Fixation Device in Right Metacarpal, Open Approach
0PWP07Z	Revision of Autologous Tissue Substitute in Right Metacarpal, Open Approach
0PWP0JZ	Revision of Synthetic Substitute in Right Metacarpal, Open Approach
0PWP0KZ	Revision of Nonautologous Tissue Substitute in Right Metacarpal, Open Approach
0PWP34Z	Revision of Internal Fixation Device in Right Metacarpal, Percutaneous Approach
0PWP35Z	Revision of External Fixation Device in Right Metacarpal, Percutaneous Approach
0PWP37Z	Revision of Autologous Tissue Substitute in Right Metacarpal, Percutaneous Approach
0PWP3JZ	Revision of Synthetic Substitute in Right Metacarpal, Percutaneous Approach
0PWP3KZ	Revision of Nonautologous Tissue Substitute in Right Metacarpal, Percutaneous Approach
0PWP44Z	Revision of Internal Fixation Device in Right Metacarpal, Percutaneous Endoscopic Approach
0PWP45Z	Revision of External Fixation Device in Right Metacarpal, Percutaneous Endoscopic Approach
0PWP47Z	Revision of Autologous Tissue Substitute in Right Metacarpal, Percutaneous Endoscopic Approach
0PWP4JZ	Revision of Synthetic Substitute in Right Metacarpal, Percutaneous Endoscopic Approach
0PWP4KZ	Revision of Nonautologous Tissue Substitute in Right Metacarpal, Percutaneous Endoscopic Approach
0PWPX4Z	Revision of Internal Fixation Device in Right Metacarpal, External Approach
0PWPX5Z	Revision of External Fixation Device in Right Metacarpal, External Approach
0PWPX7Z	Revision of Autologous Tissue Substitute in Right Metacarpal, External Approach
0PWPXJZ	Revision of Synthetic Substitute in Right Metacarpal, External Approach
0PWPXKZ	Revision of Nonautologous Tissue Substitute in Right Metacarpal, External Approach
0PWQ04Z	Revision of Internal Fixation Device in Left Metacarpal, Open Approach
0PWQ05Z	Revision of External Fixation Device in Left Metacarpal, Open Approach
0PWQ07Z	Revision of Autologous Tissue Substitute in Left Metacarpal, Open Approach
0PWQ0JZ	Revision of Synthetic Substitute in Left Metacarpal, Open Approach
0PWQ0KZ	Revision of Nonautologous Tissue Substitute in Left Metacarpal, Open Approach
0PWQ34Z	Revision of Internal Fixation Device in Left Metacarpal, Percutaneous Approach
0PWQ35Z	Revision of External Fixation Device in Left Metacarpal, Percutaneous Approach
0PWQ37Z	Revision of Autologous Tissue Subst. in Left Metacarpal, Percutaneous Approach
0PWQ3JZ	Revision of Synthetic Substitute in Left Metacarpal, Percutaneous Approach
0PWQ3KZ	Revision of Nonautologous Tissue Substitute in Left Metacarpal, Percutaneous Approach
0PWQ44Z	Revision of Internal Fixation Device in Left Metacarpal, Percutaneous Endoscopic Approach
0PWQ45Z	Revision of External Fixation Device in Left Metacarpal, Percutaneous Endoscopic Approach
0PWQ47Z	Revision of Autologous Tissue Subst. in Left Metacarpal, Percutaneous Endoscopic Approach
0PWQ4JZ	Revision of Synthetic Substitute in Left Metacarpal, Percutaneous Endoscopic Approach
0PWQ4KZ	Revision of Nonautologous Tissue Substitute in Left Metacarpal, Percutaneous Endoscopic Approach
0PWQX4Z	Revision of Internal Fixation Device in Left Metacarpal, External Approach
0PWQX5Z	Revision of External Fixation Device in Left Metacarpal, External Approach
0PWQX7Z	Revision of Autologous Tissue Substit. in Left Metacarpal, External Approach
0PWQXJZ	Revision of Synthetic Substitute in Left Metacarpal, External Approach
0PWQXKZ	Revision of Nonautologous Tissue Substitute in Left Metacarpal, External Approach
0PWR04Z	Revision of Internal Fixation Device in Right Thumb Phalanx, Open Approach
0PWR05Z	Revision of External Fixation Device in Right Thumb Phalanx, Open Approach
0PWR07Z	Revision of Autologous Tissue Substitute in Right Thumb Phalanx, Open Approach
0PWR0JZ	Revision of Synthetic Substitute in Right Thumb Phalanx, Open Approach
0PWR0KZ	Revision of Nonautologous Tissue Substitute in Right Thumb Phalanx, Open Approach
0PWR34Z	Revision of Internal Fixation Device in Right Thumb Phalanx, Percutaneous Approach
0PWR35Z	Revision of External Fixation Device in Right Thumb Phalanx, Percutaneous Approach
0PWR37Z	Revision of Autologous Tissue Substitute in Right Thumb Phalanx, Percutaneous Approach
0PWR3JZ	Revision of Synthetic Substitute in Right Thumb Phalanx, Percutaneous Approach
0PWR3KZ	Revision of Nonautologous Tissue Substitute in Right Thumb Phalanx, Percutaneous Approach
0PWR44Z	Revision of Internal Fixation Device in Right Thumb Phalanx, Percutaneous Endoscopic Approach
0PWR45Z	Revision of External Fixation Device in Right Thumb Phalanx, Percutaneous Endoscopic Approach
0PWR47Z	Revision of Autologous Tissue Substitute in Right Thumb Phalanx, Percutaneous Endoscopic Approach
0PWR4JZ	Revision of Synthetic Substitute in Right Thumb Phalanx, Percutaneous Endoscopic Approach
0PWR4KZ	Revision of Nonautologous Tissue Substitute in Right Thumb Phalanx, Percutaneous Endoscopic Approach

♀ Female-only   ♂ Male-only   ▲ Limited Coverage   ● Non-OR   ▨ HAC-associated procedure   ▲ Non-covered procedures   ✚ Combinati

'RX4Z	Revision of Internal Fixation Device in Right Thumb Phalanx, External Approach
'RX5Z	Revision of External Fixation Device in Right Thumb Phalanx, External Approach
'RX7Z	Revision of Autologous Tissue Substitute in Right Thumb Phalanx, External Approach
'RXJZ	Revision of Synthetic Substitute in Right Thumb Phalanx, External Approach
'RXKZ	Revision of Nonautologous Tissue Substitute in Right Thumb Phalanx, External Approach
'S04Z	Revision of Internal Fixation Device in Left Thumb Phalanx, Open Approach
'S05Z	Revision of External Fixation Device in Left Thumb Phalanx, Open Approach
'S07Z	Revision of Autologous Tissue Substitute in Left Thumb Phalanx, Open Approach
'S0JZ	Revision of Synthetic Substitute in Left Thumb Phalanx, Open Approach
'S0KZ	Revision of Nonautologous Tissue Substitute in Left Thumb Phalanx, Open Approach
'S34Z	Revision of Internal Fixation Device in Left Thumb Phalanx, Percutaneous Approach
'S35Z	Revision of External Fixation Device in Left Thumb Phalanx, Percutaneous Approach
'S37Z	Revision of Autologous Tissue Substitute in Left Thumb Phalanx, Percutaneous Approach
'S3JZ	Revision of Synthetic Substitute in Left Thumb Phalanx, Percutaneous Approach
'S3KZ	Revision of Nonautologous Tissue Substitute in Left Thumb Phalanx, Percutaneous Approach
'S44Z	Revision of Internal Fixation Device in Left Thumb Phalanx, Percutaneous Endoscopic Approach
'S45Z	Revision of External Fixation Device in Left Thumb Phalanx, Percutaneous Endoscopic Approach
'S47Z	Revision of Autologous Tissue Substitute in Left Thumb Phalanx, Percutaneous Endoscopic Approach
'S4JZ	Revision of Synthetic Substitute in Left Thumb Phalanx, Percutaneous Endoscopic Approach
'S4KZ	Revision of Nonautologous Tissue Substitute in Left Thumb Phalanx, Percutaneous Endoscopic Approach
'SX4Z	Revision of Internal Fixation Device in Left Thumb Phalanx, External Approach
'SX5Z	Revision of External Fixation Device in Left Thumb Phalanx, External Approach
'SX7Z	Revision of Autologous Tissue Substitute in Left Thumb Phalanx, External Approach
'SXJZ	Revision of Synthetic Substitute in Left Thumb Phalanx, External Approach

0PWSXKZ	Revision of Nonautologous Tissue Substitute in Left Thumb Phalanx, External Approach
0PWT04Z	Revision of Internal Fixation Device in Right Finger Phalanx, Open Approach
0PWT05Z	Revision of External Fixation Device in Right Finger Phalanx, Open Approach
0PWT07Z	Revision of Autologous Tissue Substitute in Right Finger Phalanx, Open Approach
0PWT0JZ	Revision of Synthetic Substitute in Right Finger Phalanx, Open Approach
0PWT0KZ	Revision of Nonautologous Tissue Substitute in Right Finger Phalanx, Open Approach
0PWT34Z	Revision of Internal Fixation Device in Right Finger Phalanx, Percutaneous Approach
0PWT35Z	Revision of External Fixation Device in Right Finger Phalanx, Percutaneous Approach
0PWT37Z	Revision of Autologous Tissue Substitute in Right Finger Phalanx, Percutaneous Approach
0PWT3JZ	Revision of Synthetic Substitute in Right Finger Phalanx, Percutaneous Approach
0PWT3KZ	Revision of Nonautologous Tissue Substitute in Right Finger Phalanx, Percutaneous Approach
0PWT44Z	Revision of Internal Fixation Device in Right Finger Phalanx, Percutaneous Endoscopic Approach
0PWT45Z	Revision of External Fixation Device in Right Finger Phalanx, Percutaneous Endoscopic Approach
0PWT47Z	Revision of Autologous Tissue Substitute in Right Finger Phalanx, Percutaneous Endoscopic Approach
0PWT4JZ	Revision of Synthetic Substitute in Right Finger Phalanx, Percutaneous Endoscopic Approach
0PWT4KZ	Revision of Nonautologous Tissue Substitute in Right Finger Phalanx, Percutaneous Endoscopic Approach
0PWTX4Z	Revision of Internal Fixation Device in Right Finger Phalanx, External Approach
0PWTX5Z	Revision of External Fixation Device in Right Finger Phalanx, External Approach
0PWTX7Z	Revision of Autologous Tissue Substitute in Right Finger Phalanx, External Approach
0PWTXJZ	Revision of Synthetic Substitute in Right Finger Phalanx, External Approach
0PWTXKZ	Revision of Nonautologous Tissue Substitute in Right Finger Phalanx, External Approach
0PWV04Z	Revision of Internal Fixation Device in Left Finger Phalanx, Open Approach
0PWV05Z	Revision of External Fixation Device in Left Finger Phalanx, Open Approach
0PWV07Z	Revision of Autologous Tissue Substitute in Left Finger Phalanx, Open Approach
0PWV0JZ	Revision of Synthetic Substitute in Left Finger Phalanx, Open Approach

0PWV0KZ	Revision of Nonautologous Tissue Substitute in Left Finger Phalanx, Open Approach
0PWV34Z	Revision of Internal Fixation Device in Left Finger Phalanx, Percutaneous Approach
0PWV35Z	Revision of External Fixation Device in Left Finger Phalanx, Percutaneous Approach
0PWV37Z	Revision of Autologous Tissue Substitute in Left Finger Phalanx, Percutaneous Approach
0PWV3JZ	Revision of Synthetic Substitute in Left Finger Phalanx, Percutaneous Approach
0PWV3KZ	Revision of Nonautologous Tissue Substitute in Left Finger Phalanx, Percutaneous Approach
0PWV44Z	Revision of Internal Fixation Device in Left Finger Phalanx, Percutaneous Endoscopic Approach
0PWV45Z	Revision of External Fixation Device in Left Finger Phalanx, Percutaneous Endoscopic Approach
0PWV47Z	Revision of Autologous Tissue Substitute in Left Finger Phalanx, Percutaneous Endoscopic Approach
0PWV4JZ	Revision of Synthetic Substitute in Left Finger Phalanx, Percutaneous Endoscopic Approach
0PWV4KZ	Revision of Nonautologous Tissue Substitute in Left Finger Phalanx, Percutaneous Endoscopic Approach
0PWVX4Z	Revision of Internal Fixation Device in Left Finger Phalanx, External Approach
0PWVX5Z	Revision of External Fixation Device in Left Finger Phalanx, External Approach
0PWVX7Z	Revision of Autologous Tissue Substitute in Left Finger Phalanx, External Approach
0PWVXJZ	Revision of Synthetic Substitute in Left Finger Phalanx, External Approach
0PWVXKZ	Revision of Nonautologous Tissue Substitute in Left Finger Phalanx, External Approach
0PWY00Z	Revision of Drainage Device in Upper Bone, Open Approach
0PWY0MZ	Revision of Bone Growth Stimulator in Upper Bone, Open Approach
0PWY30Z	Revision of Drainage Device in Upper Bone, Percutaneous Approach
0PWY3MZ	Revision of Bone Growth Stimulator in Upper Bone, Percutaneous Approach
0PWY40Z	Revision of Drainage Device in Upper Bone, Percutaneous Endoscopic Approach
0PWY4MZ	Revision of Bone Growth Stimulator in Upper Bone, Percutaneous Endoscopic Approach
0PWYX0Z	Revision of Drainage Device in Upper Bone, External Approach
0PWYXMZ	Revision of Bone Growth Stimulator in Upper Bone, External Approach

Female-only   ♂ Male-only   ▲ Limited Coverage   ● Non-OR   ▨ HAC-associated procedure   ▲ Non-covered procedures   ✛ Combination

Bones - Front and Back Views

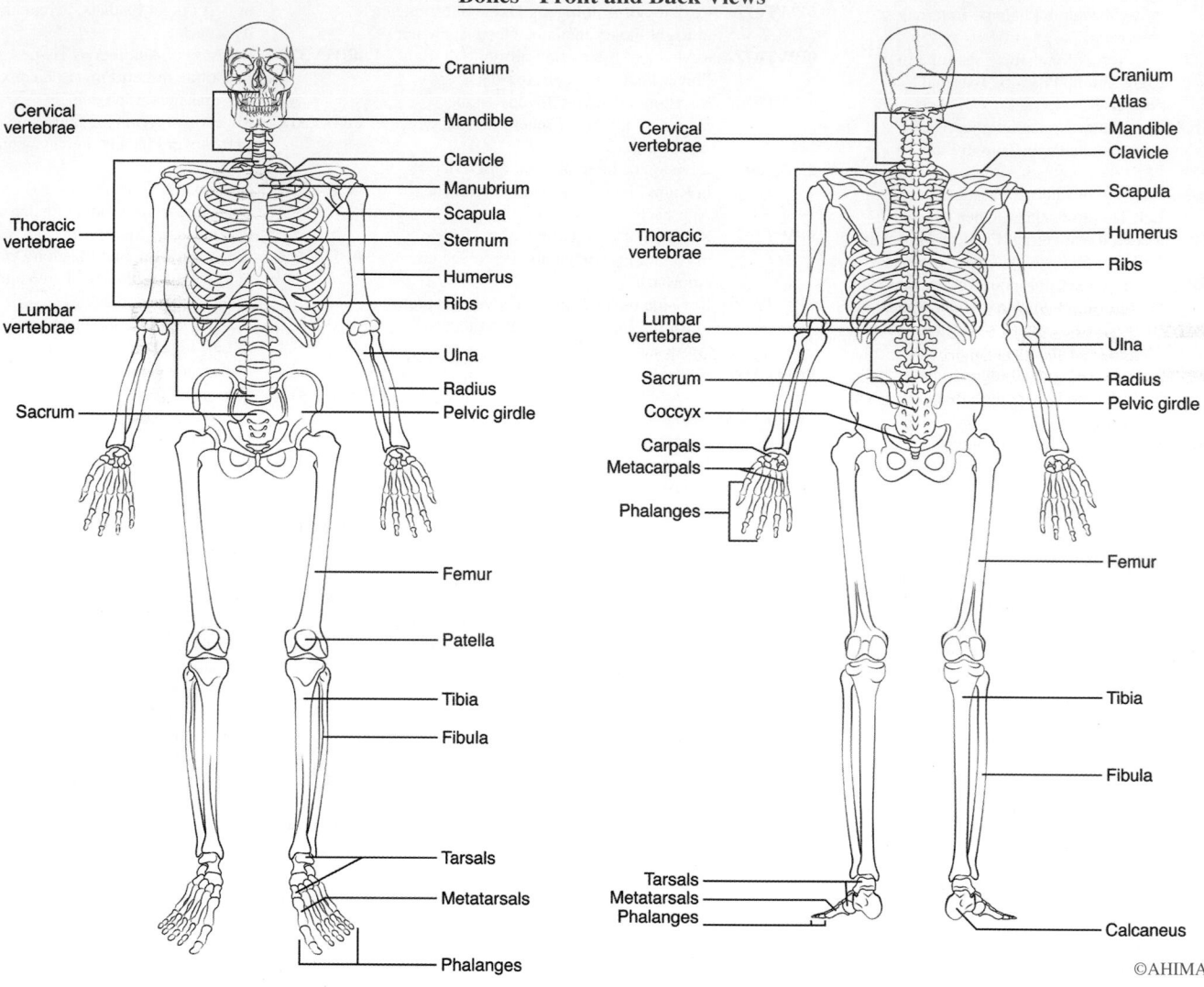

Cranium
Mandible
Clavicle
Manubrium
Scapula
Sternum
Humerus
Ribs
Ulna
Radius
Pelvic girdle
Femur
Patella
Tibia
Fibula
Tarsals
Metatarsals
Phalanges

Cervical vertebrae
Thoracic vertebrae
Lumbar vertebrae
Sacrum

Cranium
Atlas
Mandible
Clavicle
Scapula
Humerus
Ribs
Ulna
Radius
Pelvic girdle
Femur
Tibia
Fibula
Calcaneus

Cervical vertebrae
Thoracic vertebrae
Lumbar vertebrae
Sacrum
Coccyx
Carpals
Metacarpals
Phalanges
Tarsals
Metatarsals
Phalanges

©AHIMA

Vertebrae

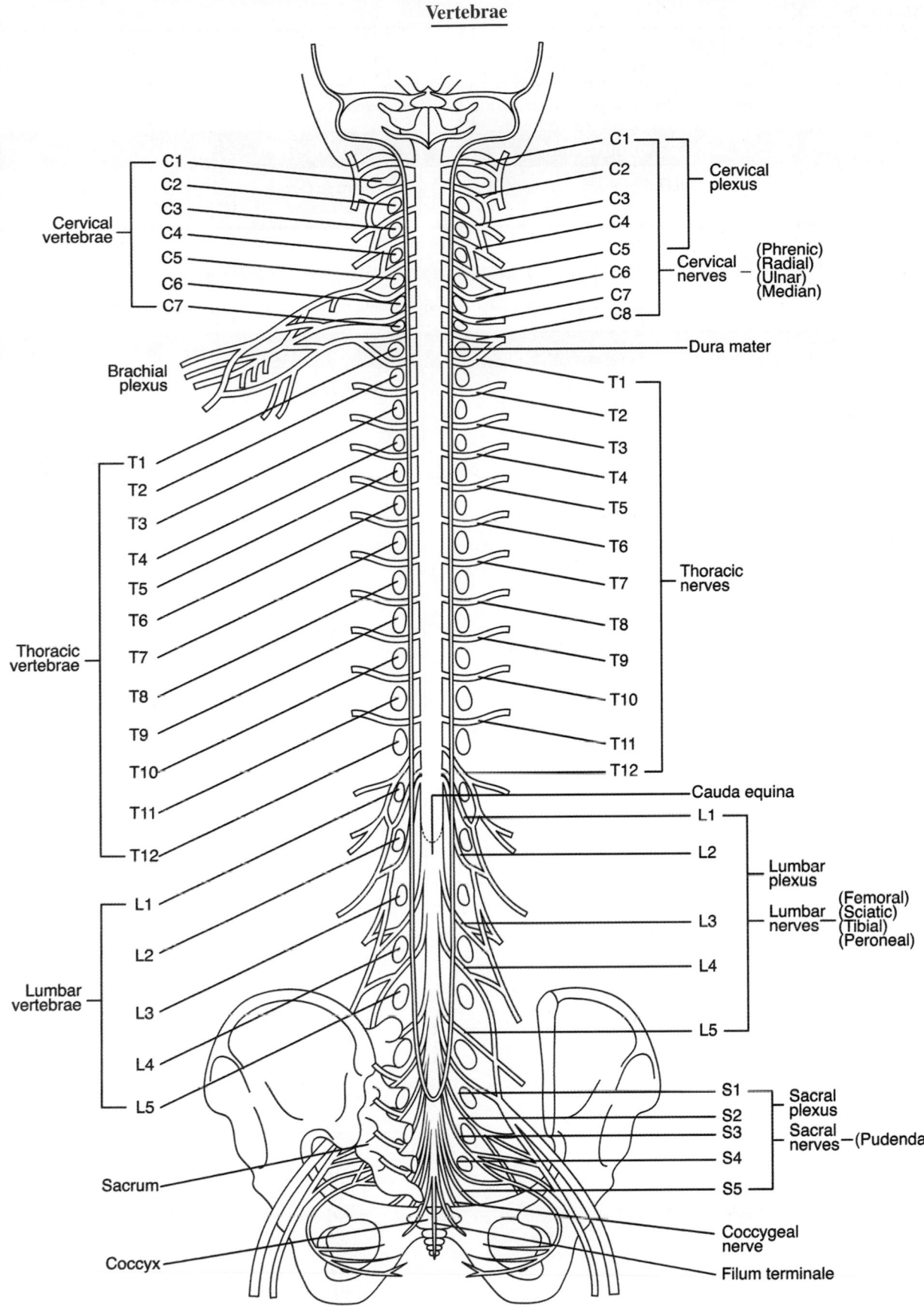

C1
C2
Cervical
vertebrae
C3
C4
C5
C6
C7

C1
C2
C3
C4
C5
C6
C7

Cervical
plexus

Cervical
nerves

(Phrenic)
(Radial)
(Ulnar)
(Median)

C8

Brachial
plexus

Dura mater

T1
T2
T3
T4
T5
T6
T7
T8
T9
T10
T11
T12

T1
T2
T3
T4
T5
T6
T7
T8
T9
T10
T11
T12

Thoracic
vertebrae

Thoracic
nerves

Cauda equina

L1
L2
L3
L4
L5

L1
L2

Lumbar
plexus

L3

Lumbar
nerves

(Femoral)
(Sciatic)
(Tibial)
(Peroneal)

L4

L5

Lumbar
vertebrae

S1
S2
S3
S4
S5

Sacral
plexus

Sacral
nerves

(Pudendal)

Sacrum

Coccygeal
nerve

Coccyx

Filum terminale

Lower Bones Tables 0Q2–0QW

Section	0	Medical and Surgical
Body System	Q	Lower Bones
Operation	2	**Change:** Taking out or off a device from a body part and putting back an identical or similar device in or on the same body part without cutting or puncturing the skin or a mucous membrane

Body Part (4ᵗʰ)	Approach (5ᵗʰ)	Device (6ᵗʰ)	Qualifier (7ᵗʰ)
Y Lower Bone	**X** External	**0** Drainage Device **Y** Other Device	**Z** No Qualifier

Section	0	Medical and Surgical
Body System	Q	Lower Bones
Operation	5	**Destruction:** Physical eradication of all or a portion of a body part by the direct use of energy, force, or a destructive agent

Body Part (4ᵗʰ)	Approach (5ᵗʰ)	Device (6ᵗʰ)	Qualifier (7ᵗʰ)
0 Lumbar Vertebra **1** Sacrum **2** Pelvic Bone, Right **3** Pelvic Bone, Left **4** Acetabulum, Right **5** Acetabulum, Left **6** Upper Femur, Right **7** Upper Femur, Left **8** Femoral Shaft, Right **9** Femoral Shaft, Left **B** Lower Femur, Right **C** Lower Femur, Left **D** Patella, Right **F** Patella, Left **G** Tibia, Right **H** Tibia, Left **J** Fibula, Right **K** Fibula, Left **L** Tarsal, Right **M** Tarsal, Left **N** Metatarsal, Right **P** Metatarsal, Left **Q** Toe Phalanx, Right **R** Toe Phalanx, Left **S** Coccyx	**0** Open **3** Percutaneous **4** Percutaneous Endoscopic	**Z** No Device	**Z** No Qualifier

Section 0 **Medical and Surgical**
Body System Q **Lower Bones**
Operation 8 **Division:** Cutting into a body part, without draining fluids and/or gases from the body part, in order to separate or transect a body part

Body Part (4th)	Approach (5th)	Device (6th)	Qualifier (7th)
Lumbar Vertebra Sacrum Pelvic Bone, Right Pelvic Bone, Left Acetabulum, Right Acetabulum, Left Upper Femur, Right Upper Femur, Left Femoral Shaft, Right Femoral Shaft, Left Lower Femur, Right Lower Femur, Left Patella, Right Patella, Left Tibia, Right Tibia, Left Fibula, Right Fibula, Left Tarsal, Right Tarsal, Left Metatarsal, Right Metatarsal, Left Toe Phalanx, Right Toe Phalanx, Left Coccyx	0 Open 3 Percutaneous 4 Percutaneous Endoscopic	Z No Device	Z No Qualifier

Section 0 **Medical and Surgical**
Body System Q **Lower Bones**
Operation 9 **Drainage:** Taking or letting out fluids and/or gases from a body part

Body Part (4th)	Approach (5th)	Device (6th)	Qualifier (7th)
0 Lumbar Vertebra 1 Sacrum 2 Pelvic Bone, Right 3 Pelvic Bone, Left 4 Acetabulum, Right 5 Acetabulum, Left 6 Upper Femur, Right 7 Upper Femur, Left 8 Femoral Shaft, Right 9 Femoral Shaft, Left B Lower Femur, Right C Lower Femur, Left D Patella, Right F Patella, Left G Tibia, Right H Tibia, Left J Fibula, Right K Fibula, Left L Tarsal, Right M Tarsal, Left N Metatarsal, Right P Metatarsal, Left Q Toe Phalanx, Right R Toe Phalanx, Left S Coccyx	0 Open 3 Percutaneous 4 Percutaneous Endoscopic	0 Drainage Device	Z No Qualifier

Continued →

Section   0   **Medical and Surgical**
Body System   Q   **Lower Bones**
Operation   9   **Drainage:** Taking or letting out fluids and/or gases from a body part

Body Part (4th)	Approach (5th)	Device (6th)	Qualifier (7th)
0 Lumbar Vertebra 1 Sacrum 2 Pelvic Bone, Right 3 Pelvic Bone, Left 4 Acetabulum, Right 5 Acetabulum, Left 6 Upper Femur, Right 7 Upper Femur, Left 8 Femoral Shaft, Right 9 Femoral Shaft, Left B Lower Femur, Right C Lower Femur, Left D Patella, Right F Patella, Left G Tibia, Right H Tibia, Left J Fibula, Right K Fibula, Left L Tarsal, Right M Tarsal, Left N Metatarsal, Right P Metatarsal, Left Q Toe Phalanx, Right R Toe Phalanx, Left S Coccyx	0 Open 3 Percutaneous 4 Percutaneous Endoscopic	Z No Device	X Diagnostic Z No Qualifier

Section   0   **Medical and Surgical**
Body System   Q   **Lower Bones**
Operation   B   **Excision:** Cutting out or off, without replacement, a portion of a body part

Body Part (4th)	Approach (5th)	Device (6th)	Qualifier (7th)
0 Lumbar Vertebra 1 Sacrum 2 Pelvic Bone, Right 3 Pelvic Bone, Left 4 Acetabulum, Right 5 Acetabulum, Left 6 Upper Femur, Right 7 Upper Femur, Left 8 Femoral Shaft, Right 9 Femoral Shaft, Left B Lower Femur, Right C Lower Femur, Left D Patella, Right F Patella, Left G Tibia, Right H Tibia, Left J Fibula, Right K Fibula, Left L Tarsal, Right M Tarsal, Left N Metatarsal, Right P Metatarsal, Left Q Toe Phalanx, Right R Toe Phalanx, Left S Coccyx	0 Open 3 Percutaneous 4 Percutaneous Endoscopic	Z No Device	X Diagnostic Z No Qualifier

Section 0 **Medical and Surgical**
Body System Q **Lower Bones**
Operation C **Extirpation:** Taking or cutting out solid matter from a body part

Body Part (4th)	Approach (5th)	Device (6th)	Qualifier (7th)
Lumbar Vertebra Sacrum Pelvic Bone, Right Pelvic Bone, Left Acetabulum, Right Acetabulum, Left Upper Femur, Right Upper Femur, Left Femoral Shaft, Right Femoral Shaft, Left B Lower Femur, Right C Lower Femur, Left D Patella, Right F Patella, Left G Tibia, Right H Tibia, Left J Fibula, Right K Fibula, Left L Tarsal, Right M Tarsal, Left N Metatarsal, Right P Metatarsal, Left Q Toe Phalanx, Right R Toe Phalanx, Left S Coccyx	0 Open 3 Percutaneous 4 Percutaneous Endoscopic	Z No Device	Z No Qualifier

Section 0 **Medical and Surgical**
Body System Q **Lower Bones**
Operation H **Insertion:** Putting in a nonbiological appliance that monitors, assists, performs, or prevents a physiological function but does not physically take the place of a body part

Body Part (4th)	Approach (5th)	Device (6th)	Qualifier (7th)
0 Lumbar Vertebra 1 Sacrum 2 Pelvic Bone, Right 3 Pelvic Bone, Left 4 Acetabulum, Right 5 Acetabulum, Left D Patella, Right F Patella, Left L Tarsal, Right M Tarsal, Left N Metatarsal, Right P Metatarsal, Left Q Toe Phalanx, Right R Toe Phalanx, Left S Coccyx	0 Open 3 Percutaneous 4 Percutaneous Endoscopic	4 Internal Fixation Device 5 External Fixation Device	Z No Qualifier
6 Upper Femur, Right 7 Upper Femur, Left 8 Femoral Shaft, Right 9 Femoral Shaft, Left B Lower Femur, Right C Lower Femur, Left G Tibia, Right H Tibia, Left J Fibula, Right K Fibula, Left	0 Open 3 Percutaneous 4 Percutaneous Endoscopic	4 Internal Fixation Device 5 External Fixation Device 6 Internal Fixation Device, Intramedullary 8 External Fixation Device, Limb Lengthening B External Fixation Device, Monoplanar C External Fixation Device, Ring D External Fixation Device, Hybrid	Z No Qualifier

Continued →

Section	0	Medical and Surgical
Body System	Q	Lower Bones
Operation	H	Insertion: Putting in a nonbiological appliance that monitors, assists, performs, or prevents a physiological function but do not physically take the place of a body part

Body Part (4ᵗʰ)	Approach (5ᵗʰ)	Device (6ᵗʰ)	Qualifier (7ᵗʰ)
Y Lower Bone	0 Open 3 Percutaneous 4 Percutaneous Endoscopic	M Bone Growth Stimulator	Z No Qualifier

Section	0	Medical and Surgical
Body System	Q	Lower Bones
Operation	J	Inspection: Visually and/or manually exploring a body part

Body Part (4ᵗʰ)	Approach (5ᵗʰ)	Device (6ᵗʰ)	Qualifier (7ᵗʰ)
Y Lower Bone	0 Open 3 Percutaneous 4 Percutaneous Endoscopic X External	Z No Device	Z No Qualifier

Section	0	Medical and Surgical
Body System	Q	Lower Bones
Operation	N	Release: Freeing a body part from an abnormal physical constraint by cutting or by the use of force

Body Part (4ᵗʰ)	Approach (5ᵗʰ)	Device (6ᵗʰ)	Qualifier (7ᵗʰ)
0 Lumbar Vertebra 1 Sacrum 2 Pelvic Bone, Right 3 Pelvic Bone, Left 4 Acetabulum, Right 5 Acetabulum, Left 6 Upper Femur, Right 7 Upper Femur, Left 8 Femoral Shaft, Right 9 Femoral Shaft, Left B Lower Femur, Right C Lower Femur, Left D Patella, Right F Patella, Left G Tibia, Right H Tibia, Left J Fibula, Right K Fibula, Left L Tarsal, Right M Tarsal, Left N Metatarsal, Right P Metatarsal, Left Q Toe Phalanx, Right R Toe Phalanx, Left S Coccyx	0 Open 3 Percutaneous 4 Percutaneous Endoscopic	Z No Device	Z No Qualifier

Section	0	Medical and Surgical
Body System	Q	Lower Bones
Operation	P	Removal: Taking out or off a device from a body part

Body Part (4ᵗʰ)	Approach (5ᵗʰ)	Device (6ᵗʰ)	Qualifier (7ᵗʰ)
0 Lumbar Vertebra 1 Sacrum 4 Acetabulum, Right 5 Acetabulum, Left S Coccyx	0 Open 3 Percutaneous 4 Percutaneous Endoscopic	4 Internal Fixation Device 7 Autologous Tissue Substitute J Synthetic Substitute K Nonautologous Tissue Substitute	Z No Qualifier

Continued →

Section	**0**	**Medical and Surgical**	
Body System	**Q**	**Lower Bones**	
Operation	**P**	**Removal:** Taking out or off a device from a body part	

Body Part (4th)	Approach (5th)	Device (6th)	Qualifier (7th)
Lumbar Vertebra Sacrum Acetabulum, Right Acetabulum, Left Coccyx	**X** External	**4** Internal Fixation Device	**Z** No Qualifier
2 Pelvic Bone, Right **3** Pelvic Bone, Left **5** Upper Femur, Right **7** Upper Femur, Left **8** Femoral Shaft, Right **9** Femoral Shaft, Left **B** Lower Femur, Right **C** Lower Femur, Left **D** Patella, Right **F** Patella, Left **G** Tibia, Right **H** Tibia, Left **J** Fibula, Right **K** Fibula, Left **L** Tarsal, Right **M** Tarsal, Left **N** Metatarsal, Right **P** Metatarsal, Left **Q** Toe Phalanx, Right **R** Toe Phalanx, Left	**0** Open **3** Percutaneous **4** Percutaneous Endoscopic	**4** Internal Fixation Device **5** External Fixation Device **7** Autologous Tissue Substitute **J** Synthetic Substitute **K** Nonautologous Tissue Substitute	**Z** No Qualifier
2 Pelvic Bone, Right **3** Pelvic Bone, Left **6** Upper Femur, Right **7** Upper Femur, Left **8** Femoral Shaft, Right **9** Femoral Shaft, Left **B** Lower Femur, Right **C** Lower Femur, Left **D** Patella, Right **F** Patella, Left **G** Tibia, Right **H** Tibia, Left **J** Fibula, Right **K** Fibula, Left **L** Tarsal, Right **M** Tarsal, Left **N** Metatarsal, Right **P** Metatarsal, Left **Q** Toe Phalanx, Right **R** Toe Phalanx, Left	**X** External	**4** Internal Fixation Device **5** External Fixation Device	**Z** No Qualifier
Y Lower Bone	**0** Open **3** Percutaneous **4** Percutaneous Endoscopic **X** External	**0** Drainage Device **M** Bone Growth Stimulator	**Z** No Qualifier

Section 0 **Medical and Surgical**
Body System Q **Lower Bones**
Operation Q **Repair:** Restoring, to the extent possible, a body part to its normal anatomic structure and function

Body Part (4th)	Approach (5th)	Device (6th)	Qualifier (7th)
0 Lumbar Vertebra	0 Open	Z No Device	Z No Qualifier
1 Sacrum	3 Percutaneous		
2 Pelvic Bone, Right	4 Percutaneous Endoscopic		
3 Pelvic Bone, Left	X External		
4 Acetabulum, Right			
5 Acetabulum, Left			
6 Upper Femur, Right			
7 Upper Femur, Left			
8 Femoral Shaft, Right			
9 Femoral Shaft, Left			
B Lower Femur, Right			
C Lower Femur, Left			
D Patella, Right			
F Patella, Left			
G Tibia, Right			
H Tibia, Left			
J Fibula, Right			
K Fibula, Left			
L Tarsal, Right			
M Tarsal, Left			
N Metatarsal, Right			
P Metatarsal, Left			
Q Toe Phalanx, Right			
R Toe Phalanx, Left			
S Coccyx			

Section 0 **Medical and Surgical**
Body System Q **Lower Bones**
Operation R **Replacement:** Putting in or on biological or synthetic material that physically takes the place and/or function of all or a portion of a body part

Body Part (4th)	Approach (5th)	Device (6th)	Qualifier (7th)
0 Lumbar Vertebra	0 Open	7 Autologous Tissue Substitute	Z No Qualifier
1 Sacrum	3 Percutaneous	J Synthetic Substitute	
2 Pelvic Bone, Right	4 Percutaneous Endoscopic	K Nonautologous Tissue Substitute	
3 Pelvic Bone, Left			
4 Acetabulum, Right			
5 Acetabulum, Left			
6 Upper Femur, Right			
7 Upper Femur, Left			
8 Femoral Shaft, Right			
9 Femoral Shaft, Left			
B Lower Femur, Right			
C Lower Femur, Left			
D Patella, Right			
F Patella, Left			
G Tibia, Right			
H Tibia, Left			
J Fibula, Right			
K Fibula, Left			
L Tarsal, Right			
M Tarsal, Left			
N Metatarsal, Right			
P Metatarsal, Left			
Q Toe Phalanx, Right			
R Toe Phalanx, Left			
S Coccyx			

tion	0	Medical and Surgical	
dy System	Q	Lower Bones	
eration	S	Reposition: Moving to its normal location, or other suitable location, all or a portion of a body part	

Body Part (4th)	Approach (5th)	Device (6th)	Qualifier (7th)
Lumbar Vertebra Sacrum Acetabulum, Right Acetabulum, Left Coccyx	0 Open 3 Percutaneous 4 Percutaneous Endoscopic	4 Internal Fixation Device Z No Device	Z No Qualifier
Lumbar Vertebra Sacrum Acetabulum, Right Acetabulum, Left Coccyx	X External	Z No Device	Z No Qualifier
2 Pelvic Bone, Right 3 Pelvic Bone, Left D Patella, Right F Patella, Left L Tarsal, Right M Tarsal, Left N Metatarsal, Right P Metatarsal, Left Q Toe Phalanx, Right R Toe Phalanx, Left	0 Open 3 Percutaneous 4 Percutaneous Endoscopic	4 Internal Fixation Device 5 External Fixation Device Z No Device	Z No Qualifier
2 Pelvic Bone, Right 3 Pelvic Bone, Left D Patella, Right F Patella, Left L Tarsal, Right M Tarsal, Left N Metatarsal, Right P Metatarsal, Left Q Toe Phalanx, Right R Toe Phalanx, Left	X External	Z No Device	Z No Qualifier
6 Upper Femur, Right 7 Upper Femur, Left 8 Femoral Shaft, Right 9 Femoral Shaft, Left B Lower Femur, Right C Lower Femur, Left G Tibia, Right H Tibia, Left J Fibula, Right K Fibula, Left	0 Open 3 Percutaneous 4 Percutaneous Endoscopic	4 Internal Fixation Device 5 External Fixation Device 6 Internal Fixation Device, Intramedullary B External Fixation Device, Monoplanar C External Fixation Device, Ring D External Fixation Device, Hybrid Z No Device	Z No Qualifier
6 Upper Femur, Right 7 Upper Femur, Left 8 Femoral Shaft, Right 9 Femoral Shaft, Left B Lower Femur, Right C Lower Femur, Left G Tibia, Right H Tibia, Left J Fibula, Right K Fibula, Left	X External	Z No Device	Z No Qualifier

Section	0	Medical and Surgical
Body System	Q	Lower Bones
Operation	T	Resection: Cutting out or off, without replacement, all of a body part

Body Part (4th)	Approach (5th)	Device (6th)	Qualifier (7th)
2 Pelvic Bone, Right	0 Open	Z No Device	Z No Qualifier
3 Pelvic Bone, Left			
4 Acetabulum, Right			
5 Acetabulum, Left			
6 Upper Femur, Right			
7 Upper Femur, Left			
8 Femoral Shaft, Right			
9 Femoral Shaft, Left			
B Lower Femur, Right			
C Lower Femur, Left			
D Patella, Right			
F Patella, Left			
G Tibia, Right			
H Tibia, Left			
J Fibula, Right			
K Fibula, Left			
L Tarsal, Right			
M Tarsal, Left			
N Metatarsal, Right			
P Metatarsal, Left			
Q Toe Phalanx, Right			
R Toe Phalanx, Left			
S Coccyx			

Section	0	Medical and Surgical
Body System	Q	Lower Bones
Operation	U	Supplement: Putting in or on biological or synthetic material that physically reinforces and/or augments the function of a portion of a body part

Body Part (4th)	Approach (5th)	Device (6th)	Qualifier (7th)
0 Lumbar Vertebra	0 Open	7 Autologous Tissue Substitute	Z No Qualifier
1 Sacrum	3 Percutaneous	J Synthetic Substitute	
2 Pelvic Bone, Right	4 Percutaneous Endoscopic	K Nonautologous Tissue Substitute	
3 Pelvic Bone, Left			
4 Acetabulum, Right			
5 Acetabulum, Left			
6 Upper Femur, Right			
7 Upper Femur, Left			
8 Femoral Shaft, Right			
9 Femoral Shaft, Left			
B Lower Femur, Right			
C Lower Femur, Left			
D Patella, Right			
F Patella, Left			
G Tibia, Right			
H Tibia, Left			
J Fibula, Right			
K Fibula, Left			
L Tarsal, Right			
M Tarsal, Left			
N Metatarsal, Right			
P Metatarsal, Left			
Q Toe Phalanx, Right			
R Toe Phalanx, Left			
S Coccyx			

	0	Medical and Surgical
	Q	Lower Bones
	W	**Revision:** Correcting, to the extent possible, a portion of a malfunctioning device or the position of a displaced device

Body Part (4ᵗʰ)	Approach (5ᵗʰ)	Device (6ᵗʰ)	Qualifier (7ᵗʰ)
Lumbar Vertebra Sacrum Acetabulum, Right Acetabulum, Left Coccyx	0 Open 3 Percutaneous 4 Percutaneous Endoscopic X External	4 Internal Fixation Device 7 Autologous Tissue Substitute J Synthetic Substitute K Nonautologous Tissue Substitute	Z No Qualifier
Pelvic Bone, Right Pelvic Bone, Left Upper Femur, Right Upper Femur, Left Femoral Shaft, Right Femoral Shaft, Left Lower Femur, Right Lower Femur, Left Patella, Right Patella, Left Tibia, Right Tibia, Left Fibula, Right Fibula, Left Tarsal, Right Tarsal, Left Metatarsal, Right Metatarsal, Left Toe Phalanx, Right Toe Phalanx, Left	0 Open 3 Percutaneous 4 Percutaneous Endoscopic X External	4 Internal Fixation Device 5 External Fixation Device 7 Autologous Tissue Substitute J Synthetic Substitute K Nonautologous Tissue Substitute	Z No Qualifier
Y Lower Bone	0 Open 3 Percutaneous 4 Percutaneous Endoscopic X External	0 Drainage Device M Bone Growth Stimulator	Z No Qualifier

Lower Bones Code Listing 0Q2–0QW

0Q2 – Lower Bones, Change

Review Coding Guideline B6.1c

0Q2YX0Z Change Drainage Device in Lower Bone, External Approach

0Q2YXYZ Change Other Device in Lower Bone, External Approach

0Q5 – Lower Bones, Destruction

0Q500ZZ Destruction of Lumbar Vertebra, Open Approach

0Q503ZZ Destruction of Lumbar Vertebra, Percutaneous Approach

0Q504ZZ Destruction of Lumbar Vertebra, Percutaneous Endoscopic Approach

0Q510ZZ Destruction of Sacrum, Open Approach

0Q513ZZ Destruction of Sacrum, Percutaneous Approach

0Q514ZZ Destruction of Sacrum, Percutaneous Endoscopic Approach

0Q520ZZ Destruction of Right Pelvic Bone, Open Approach

0Q523ZZ Destruction of Right Pelvic Bone, Percutaneous Approach

0Q524ZZ Destruction of Right Pelvic Bone, Percutaneous Endoscopic Approach

0Q530ZZ Destruction of Left Pelvic Bone, Open Approach

0Q533ZZ Destruction of Left Pelvic Bone, Percutaneous Approach

0Q534ZZ Destruction of Left Pelvic Bone, Percutaneous Endoscopic Approach

0Q540ZZ Destruction of Right Acetabulum, Open Approach

0Q543ZZ Destruction of Right Acetabulum, Percutaneous Approach

0Q544ZZ Destruction of Right Acetabulum, Percutaneous Endoscopic Approach

0Q550ZZ Destruction of Left Acetabulum, Open Approach

0Q553ZZ Destruction of Left Acetabulum, Percutaneous Approach

0Q554ZZ Destruction of Left Acetabulum, Percutaneous Endoscopic Approach

0Q560ZZ Destruction of Right Upper Femur, Open Approach

0Q563ZZ Destruction of Right Upper Femur, Percutaneous Approach

0Q564ZZ Destruction of Right Upper Femur, Percutaneous Endoscopic Approach

0Q570ZZ Destruction of Left Upper Femur, Open Approach

0Q573ZZ Destruction of Left Upper Femur, Percutaneous Approach

0Q574ZZ Destruction of Left Upper Femur, Percutaneous Endoscopic Approach

0Q580ZZ Destruction of Right Femoral Shaft, Open Approach

0Q583ZZ Destruction of Right Femoral Shaft, Percutaneous Approach

0Q584ZZ Destruction of Right Femoral Shaft, Percutaneous Endoscopic Approach

0Q590ZZ Destruction of Left Femoral Shaft, Open Approach

0Q593ZZ Destruction of Left Femoral Shaft, Percutaneous Approach

0Q594ZZ Destruction of Left Femoral Shaft, Percutaneous Endoscopic Approach

0Q5B0ZZ Destruction of Right Lower Femur, Open Approach

0Q5B3ZZ Destruction of Right Lower Femur, Percutaneous Approach

0Q5B4ZZ Destruction of Right Lower Femur, Percutaneous Endoscopic Approach

0Q5C0ZZ Destruction of Left Lower Femur, Open Approach

♀ Female-only   ♂ Male-only   ▲ Limited Coverage   ● Non-OR   ▦ HAC-associated procedure   ▲ Non-covered procedures   ✚ Combination

0Q5C3ZZ Destruction of Left Lower Femur, Percutaneous Approach

0Q5C4ZZ Destruction of Left Lower Femur, Percutaneous Endoscopic Approach

0Q5D0ZZ Destruction of Right Patella, Open Approach

0Q5D3ZZ Destruction of Right Patella, Percutaneous Approach

0Q5D4ZZ Destruction of Right Patella, Percutaneous Endoscopic Approach

0Q5F0ZZ Destruction of Left Patella, Open Approach

0Q5F3ZZ Destruction of Left Patella, Percutaneous Approach

0Q5F4ZZ Destruction of Left Patella, Percutaneous Endoscopic Approach

0Q5G0ZZ Destruction of Right Tibia, Open Approach

0Q5G3ZZ Destruction of Right Tibia, Percutaneous Approach

0Q5G4ZZ Destruction of Right Tibia, Percutaneous Endoscopic Approach

0Q5H0ZZ Destruction of Left Tibia, Open Approach

0Q5H3ZZ Destruction of Left Tibia, Percutaneous Approach

0Q5H4ZZ Destruction of Left Tibia, Percutaneous Endoscopic Approach

0Q5J0ZZ Destruction of Right Fibula, Open Approach

0Q5J3ZZ Destruction of Right Fibula, Percutaneous Approach

0Q5J4ZZ Destruction of Right Fibula, Percutaneous Endoscopic Approach

0Q5K0ZZ Destruction of Left Fibula, Open Approach

0Q5K3ZZ Destruction of Left Fibula, Percutaneous Approach

0Q5K4ZZ Destruction of Left Fibula, Percutaneous Endoscopic Approach

0Q5L0ZZ Destruction of Right Tarsal, Open Approach

0Q5L3ZZ Destruction of Right Tarsal, Percutaneous Approach

0Q5L4ZZ Destruction of Right Tarsal, Percutaneous Endoscopic Approach

0Q5M0ZZ Destruction of Left Tarsal, Open Approach

0Q5M3ZZ Destruction of Left Tarsal, Percutaneous Approach

0Q5M4ZZ Destruction of Left Tarsal, Percutaneous Endoscopic Approach

0Q5N0ZZ Destruction of Right Metatarsal, Open Approach

0Q5N3ZZ Destruction of Right Metatarsal, Percutaneous Approach

0Q5N4ZZ Destruction of Right Metatarsal, Percutaneous Endoscopic Approach

0Q5P0ZZ Destruction of Left Metatarsal, Open Approach

0Q5P3ZZ Destruction of Left Metatarsal, Percutaneous Approach

0Q5P4ZZ Destruction of Left Metatarsal, Percutaneous Endoscopic Approach

0Q5Q0ZZ Destruction of Right Toe Phalanx, Open Approach

0Q5Q3ZZ Destruction of Right Toe Phalanx, Percutaneous Approach

0Q5Q4ZZ Destruction of Right Toe Phalanx, Percutaneous Endoscopic Approach

0Q5R0ZZ Destruction of Left Toe Phalanx, Open Approach

0Q5R3ZZ Destruction of Left Toe Phalanx, Percutaneous Approach

0Q5R4ZZ Destruction of Left Toe Phalanx, Percutaneous Endoscopic Approach

0Q5S0ZZ Destruction of Coccyx, Open Approach

0Q5S3ZZ Destruction of Coccyx, Percutaneous Approach

0Q5S4ZZ Destruction of Coccyx, Percutaneous Endoscopic Approach

0Q8 – Lower Bones, Division

Review Coding Guideline B3.14

0Q800ZZ Division of Lumbar Vertebra, Open Approach

0Q803ZZ Division of Lumbar Vertebra, Percutaneous Approach

0Q804ZZ Division of Lumbar Vertebra, Percutaneous Endoscopic Approach

0Q810ZZ Division of Sacrum, Open Approach

0Q813ZZ Division of Sacrum, Percutaneous Approach

0Q814ZZ Division of Sacrum, Percutaneous Endoscopic Approach

0Q820ZZ Division of Right Pelvic Bone, Open Approach

0Q823ZZ Division of Right Pelvic Bone, Percutaneous Approach

0Q824ZZ Division of Right Pelvic Bone, Percutaneous Endoscopic Approach

0Q830ZZ Division of Left Pelvic Bone, Open Approach

0Q833ZZ Division of Left Pelvic Bone, Percutaneous Approach

0Q834ZZ Division of Left Pelvic Bone, Percutaneous Endoscopic Approach

0Q840ZZ Division of Right Acetabulum, Open Approach

0Q843ZZ Division of Right Acetabulum, Percutaneous Approach

0Q844ZZ Division of Right Acetabulum, Percutaneous Endoscopic Approach

0Q850ZZ Division of Left Acetabulum, Open Approach

0Q853ZZ Division of Left Acetabulum, Percutaneous Approach

0Q854ZZ Division of Left Acetabulum, Percutaneous Endoscopic Approach

0Q860ZZ Division of Right Upper Femur, Open Approach

0Q863ZZ Division of Right Upper Femur, Percutaneous Approach

0Q864ZZ Division of Right Upper Femur, Percutaneous Endoscopic Approach

0Q870ZZ Division of Left Upper Femur, Open Approach

0Q873ZZ Division of Left Upper Femur, Percutaneous Approach

0Q874ZZ Division of Left Upper Femur, Percutaneous Endoscopic Approach

0Q880ZZ Division of Right Femoral Shaft, Open Approach

0Q883ZZ Division of Right Femoral Shaft, Percutaneous Approach

0Q884ZZ Division of Right Femoral Shaft, Percutaneous Endoscopic Approach

0Q890ZZ Division of Left Femoral Shaft, Open Approach

0Q893ZZ Division of Left Femoral Shaft, Percutaneous Approach

0Q894ZZ Division of Left Femoral Shaft, Percutaneous Endoscopic Approach

0Q8B0ZZ Division of Right Lower Femur, Open Approach

0Q8B3ZZ Division of Right Lower Femur, Percutaneous Approach

0Q8B4ZZ Division of Right Lower Femur, Percutaneous Endoscopic Approach

0Q8C0ZZ Division of Left Lower Femur, Open Approach

0Q8C3ZZ Division of Left Lower Femur, Percutaneous Approach

0Q8C4ZZ Division of Left Lower Femur, Percutaneous Endoscopic Approach

0Q8D0ZZ Division of Right Patella, Open Approach

0Q8D3ZZ Division of Right Patella, Percutaneous Approach

0Q8D4ZZ Division of Right Patella, Percutaneous Endoscopic Approach

0Q8F0ZZ Division of Left Patella, Open Approach

0Q8F3ZZ Division of Left Patella, Percutaneous Approach

0Q8F4ZZ Division of Left Patella, Percutaneous Endoscopic Approach

0Q8G0ZZ Division of Right Tibia, Open Approach

0Q8G3ZZ Division of Right Tibia, Percutaneous Approach

0Q8G4ZZ Division of Right Tibia, Percutaneous Endoscopic Approach

0Q8H0ZZ Division of Left Tibia, Open Approach

0Q8H3ZZ Division of Left Tibia, Percutaneous Approach

0Q8H4ZZ Division of Left Tibia, Percutaneous Endoscopic Approach

0Q8J0ZZ Division of Right Fibula, Open Approach

0Q8J3ZZ Division of Right Fibula, Percutaneous Approach

0Q8J4ZZ Division of Right Fibula, Percutaneous Endoscopic Approach

0Q8K0ZZ Division of Left Fibula, Open Approach

0Q8K3ZZ Division of Left Fibula, Percutaneous Approach

0Q8K4ZZ Division of Left Fibula, Percutaneous Endoscopic Approach

0Q8L0ZZ Division of Right Tarsal, Open Approach

0Q8L3ZZ Division of Right Tarsal, Percutaneous Approach

0Q8L4ZZ Division of Right Tarsal, Percutaneous Endoscopic Approach

0Q8M0ZZ Division of Left Tarsal, Open Approach

0Q8M3ZZ Division of Left Tarsal, Percutaneous Approach

0Q8M4ZZ Division of Left Tarsal, Percutaneous Endoscopic Approach

0Q8N0ZZ Division of Right Metatarsal, Open Approach

0Q8N3ZZ Division of Right Metatarsal, Percutaneous Approach

0Q8N4ZZ Division of Right Metatarsal, Percutaneous Endoscopic Approach

0Q8P0ZZ Division of Left Metatarsal, Open Approach

0Q8P3ZZ Division of Left Metatarsal, Percutaneous Approach

0Q8P4ZZ Division of Left Metatarsal, Percutaneous Endoscopic Approach

0Q8Q0ZZ Division of Right Toe Phalanx, Open Approach

0Q8Q3ZZ Division of Right Toe Phalanx, Percutaneous Approach

0Q8Q4ZZ Division of Right Toe Phalanx, Percutaneous Endoscopic Approach

0Q8R0ZZ Division of Left Toe Phalanx, Open Approach

0Q8R3ZZ Division of Left Toe Phalanx, Percutaneous Approach

R4ZZ	Division of Left Toe Phalanx, Percutaneous Endoscopic Approach	
S0ZZ	Division of Coccyx, Open Approach	

0Q8S3ZZ	Division of Coccyx, Percutaneous Approach

0Q8S4ZZ	Division of Coccyx, Percutaneous Endoscopic Approach

9 – Lower Bones, Drainage

view Coding Guidelines B3.4a and B3.4b

view Coding Guideline B6.2

0000Z	Drainage of Lumbar Vertebra with Drainage Device, Open Approach
000ZX	Drainage of Lumbar Vertebra, Open Approach, Diagnostic
000ZZ	Drainage of Lumbar Vertebra, Open Approach
9030Z	Drainage of Lumbar Vertebra with Drainage Device, Percutaneous Approach
903ZX	Drainage of Lumbar Vertebra, Percutaneous Approach, Diagnostic
903ZZ	Drainage of Lumbar Vertebra, Percutaneous Approach
9040Z	Drainage of Lumbar Vertebra with Drainage Device, Percutaneous Endoscopic Approach
904ZX	Drainage of Lumbar Vertebra, Percutaneous Endoscopic Approach, Diagnostic
904ZZ	Drainage of Lumbar Vertebra, Percutaneous Endoscopic Approach
9100Z	Drainage of Sacrum with Drainage Device, Open Approach
910ZX	Drainage of Sacrum, Open Approach, Diagnostic
910ZZ	Drainage of Sacrum, Open Approach
9130Z	Drainage of Sacrum with Drainage Device, Percutaneous Approach
913ZX	Drainage of Sacrum, Percutaneous Approach, Diagnostic
913ZZ	Drainage of Sacrum, Percutaneous Approach
9140Z	Drainage of Sacrum with Drainage Device, Percutaneous Endoscopic Approach
914ZX	Drainage of Sacrum, Percutaneous Endoscopic Approach, Diagnostic
914ZZ	Drainage of Sacrum, Percutaneous Endoscopic Approach
9200Z	Drainage of Right Pelvic Bone with Drainage Device, Open Approach
920ZX	Drainage of Right Pelvic Bone, Open Approach, Diagnostic
920ZZ	Drainage of Right Pelvic Bone, Open Approach
9230Z	Drainage of Right Pelvic Bone with Drainage Device, Percutaneous Approach
Q923ZX	Drainage of Right Pelvic Bone, Percutaneous Approach, Diagnostic
Q923ZZ	Drainage of Right Pelvic Bone, Percutaneous Approach
Q9240Z	Drainage of Right Pelvic Bone with Drainage Device, Percutaneous Endoscopic Approach
Q924ZX	Drainage of Right Pelvic Bone, Percutaneous Endoscopic Approach, Diagnostic
Q924ZZ	Drainage of Right Pelvic Bone, Percutaneous Endoscopic Approach
9300Z	Drainage of Left Pelvic Bone with Drainage Device, Open Approach
930ZX	Drainage of Left Pelvic Bone, Open Approach, Diagnostic
930ZZ	Drainage of Left Pelvic Bone, Open Approach
9330Z	Drainage of Left Pelvic Bone with Drainage Device, Percutaneous Approach

0Q933ZX	Drainage of Left Pelvic Bone, Percutaneous Approach, Diagnostic
0Q933ZZ	Drainage of Left Pelvic Bone, Percutaneous Approach
0Q9340Z	Drainage of Left Pelvic Bone with Drainage Device, Percutaneous Endoscopic Approach
0Q934ZX	Drainage of Left Pelvic Bone, Percutaneous Endoscopic Approach, Diagnostic
0Q934ZZ	Drainage of Left Pelvic Bone, Percutaneous Endoscopic Approach
0Q9400Z	Drainage of Right Acetabulum with Drainage Device, Open Approach
0Q940ZX	Drainage of Right Acetabulum, Open Approach, Diagnostic
0Q940ZZ	Drainage of Right Acetabulum, Open Approach
0Q9430Z	Drainage of Right Acetabulum with Drainage Device, Percutaneous Approach
0Q943ZX	Drainage of Right Acetabulum, Percutaneous Approach, Diagnostic
0Q943ZZ	Drainage of Right Acetabulum, Percutaneous Approach
0Q9440Z	Drainage of Right Acetabulum with Drainage Device, Percutaneous Endoscopic Approach
0Q944ZX	Drainage of Right Acetabulum, Percutaneous Endoscopic Approach, Diagnostic
0Q944ZZ	Drainage of Right Acetabulum, Percutaneous Endoscopic Approach
0Q9500Z	Drainage of Left Acetabulum with Drainage Device, Open Approach
0Q950ZX	Drainage of Left Acetabulum, Open Approach, Diagnostic
0Q950ZZ	Drainage of Left Acetabulum, Open Approach
0Q9530Z	Drainage of Left Acetabulum with Drainage Device, Percutaneous Approach
0Q953ZX	Drainage of Left Acetabulum, Percutaneous Approach, Diagnostic
0Q953ZZ	Drainage of Left Acetabulum, Percutaneous Approach
0Q9540Z	Drainage of Left Acetabulum with Drainage Device, Percutaneous Endoscopic Approach
0Q954ZX	Drainage of Left Acetabulum, Percutaneous Endoscopic Approach, Diagnostic
0Q954ZZ	Drainage of Left Acetabulum, Percutaneous Endoscopic Approach
0Q9600Z	Drainage of Right Upper Femur with Drainage Device, Open Approach
0Q960ZX	Drainage of Right Upper Femur, Open Approach, Diagnostic
0Q960ZZ	Drainage of Right Upper Femur, Open Approach
0Q9630Z	Drainage of Right Upper Femur with Drainage Device, Percutaneous Approach
0Q963ZX	Drainage of Right Upper Femur, Percutaneous Approach, Diagnostic
0Q963ZZ	Drainage of Right Upper Femur, Percutaneous Approach
0Q9640Z	Drainage of Right Upper Femur with Drainage Device, Percutaneous Endoscopic Approach

0Q964ZX	Drainage of Right Upper Femur, Percutaneous Endoscopic Approach, Diagnostic
0Q964ZZ	Drainage of Right Upper Femur, Percutaneous Endoscopic Approach
0Q9700Z	Drainage of Left Upper Femur with Drainage Device, Open Approach
0Q970ZX	Drainage of Left Upper Femur, Open Approach, Diagnostic
0Q970ZZ	Drainage of Left Upper Femur, Open Approach
0Q9730Z	Drainage of Left Upper Femur with Drainage Device, Percutaneous Approach
0Q973ZX	Drainage of Left Upper Femur, Percutaneous Approach, Diagnostic
0Q973ZZ	Drainage of Left Upper Femur, Percutaneous Approach
0Q9740Z	Drainage of Left Upper Femur with Drainage Device, Percutaneous Endoscopic Approach
0Q974ZX	Drainage of Left Upper Femur, Percutaneous Endoscopic Approach, Diagnostic
0Q974ZZ	Drainage of Left Upper Femur, Percutaneous Endoscopic Approach
0Q9800Z	Drainage of Right Femoral Shaft with Drainage Device, Open Approach
0Q980ZX	Drainage of Right Femoral Shaft, Open Approach, Diagnostic
0Q980ZZ	Drainage of Right Femoral Shaft, Open Approach
0Q9830Z	Drainage of Right Femoral Shaft with Drainage Device, Percutaneous Approach
0Q983ZX	Drainage of Right Femoral Shaft, Percutaneous Approach, Diagnostic
0Q983ZZ	Drainage of Right Femoral Shaft, Percutaneous Approach
0Q9840Z	Drainage of Right Femoral Shaft with Drainage Device, Percutaneous Endoscopic Approach
0Q984ZX	Drainage of Right Femoral Shaft, Percutaneous Endoscopic Approach, Diagnostic
0Q984ZZ	Drainage of Right Femoral Shaft, Percutaneous Endoscopic Approach
0Q9900Z	Drainage of Left Femoral Shaft with Drainage Device, Open Approach
0Q990ZX	Drainage of Left Femoral Shaft, Open Approach, Diagnostic
0Q990ZZ	Drainage of Left Femoral Shaft, Open Approach
0Q9930Z	Drainage of Left Femoral Shaft with Drainage Device, Percutaneous Approach
0Q993ZX	Drainage of Left Femoral Shaft, Percutaneous Approach, Diagnostic
0Q993ZZ	Drainage of Left Femoral Shaft, Percutaneous Approach
0Q9940Z	Drainage of Left Femoral Shaft with Drainage Device, Percutaneous Endoscopic Approach
0Q994ZX	Drainage of Left Femoral Shaft, Percutaneous Endoscopic Approach, Diagnostic
0Q994ZZ	Drainage of Left Femoral Shaft, Percutaneous Endoscopic Approach
0Q9B00Z	Drainage of Right Lower Femur with Drainage Device, Open Approach

♀ Female-only   ♂ Male-only   ▲ Limited Coverage   ● Non-OR   ▨ HAC-associated procedure   ▲ Non-covered procedures   ✚ Combination

0Q9B0ZX	Drainage of Right Lower Femur, Open Approach, Diagnostic
0Q9B0ZZ	Drainage of Right Lower Femur, Open Approach
0Q9B30Z	Drainage of Right Lower Femur with Drainage Device, Percutaneous Approach
0Q9B3ZX	Drainage of Right Lower Femur, Percutaneous Approach, Diagnostic
0Q9B3ZZ	Drainage of Right Lower Femur, Percutaneous Approach
0Q9B40Z	Drainage of Right Lower Femur with Drainage Device, Percutaneous Endoscopic Approach
0Q9B4ZX	Drainage of Right Lower Femur, Percutaneous Endoscopic Approach, Diagnostic
0Q9B4ZZ	Drainage of Right Lower Femur, Percutaneous Endoscopic Approach
0Q9C00Z	Drainage of Left Lower Femur with Drainage Device, Open Approach
0Q9C0ZX	Drainage of Left Lower Femur, Open Approach, Diagnostic
0Q9C0ZZ	Drainage of Left Lower Femur, Open Approach
0Q9C30Z	Drainage of Left Lower Femur with Drainage Device, Percutaneous Approach
0Q9C3ZX	Drainage of Left Lower Femur, Percutaneous Approach, Diagnostic
0Q9C3ZZ	Drainage of Left Lower Femur, Percutaneous Approach
0Q9C40Z	Drainage of Left Lower Femur with Drainage Device, Percutaneous Endoscopic Approach
0Q9C4ZX	Drainage of Left Lower Femur, Percutaneous Endoscopic Approach, Diagnostic
0Q9C4ZZ	Drainage of Left Lower Femur, Percutaneous Endoscopic Approach
0Q9D00Z	Drainage of Right Patella with Drainage Device, Open Approach
0Q9D0ZX	Drainage of Right Patella, Open Approach, Diagnostic
0Q9D0ZZ	Drainage of Right Patella, Open Approach
0Q9D30Z	Drainage of Right Patella with Drainage Device, Percutaneous Approach
0Q9D3ZX	Drainage of Right Patella, Percutaneous Approach, Diagnostic
0Q9D3ZZ	Drainage of Right Patella, Percutaneous Approach
0Q9D40Z	Drainage of Right Patella with Drainage Device, Percutaneous Endoscopic Approach
0Q9D4ZX	Drainage of Right Patella, Percutaneous Endoscopic Approach, Diagnostic
0Q9D4ZZ	Drainage of Right Patella, Percutaneous Endoscopic Approach
0Q9F00Z	Drainage of Left Patella with Drainage Device, Open Approach
0Q9F0ZX	Drainage of Left Patella, Open Approach, Diagnostic
0Q9F0ZZ	Drainage of Left Patella, Open Approach
0Q9F30Z	Drainage of Left Patella with Drainage Device, Percutaneous Approach
0Q9F3ZX	Drainage of Left Patella, Percutaneous Approach, Diagnostic
0Q9F3ZZ	Drainage of Left Patella, Percutaneous Approach
0Q9F40Z	Drainage of Left Patella with Drainage Device, Percutaneous Endoscopic Approach
0Q9F4ZX	Drainage of Left Patella, Percutaneous Endoscopic Approach, Diagnostic
0Q9F4ZZ	Drainage of Left Patella, Percutaneous Endoscopic Approach
0Q9G00Z	Drainage of Right Tibia with Drainage Device, Open Approach
0Q9G0ZX	Drainage of Right Tibia, Open Approach, Diagnostic
0Q9G0ZZ	Drainage of Right Tibia, Open Approach
0Q9G30Z	Drainage of Right Tibia with Drainage Device, Percutaneous Approach
0Q9G3ZX	Drainage of Right Tibia, Percutaneous Approach, Diagnostic
0Q9G3ZZ	Drainage of Right Tibia, Percutaneous Approach
0Q9G40Z	Drainage of Right Tibia with Drainage Device, Percutaneous Endoscopic Approach
0Q9G4ZX	Drainage of Right Tibia, Percutaneous Endoscopic Approach, Diagnostic
0Q9G4ZZ	Drainage of Right Tibia, Percutaneous Endoscopic Approach
0Q9H00Z	Drainage of Left Tibia with Drainage Device, Open Approach
0Q9H0ZX	Drainage of Left Tibia, Open Approach, Diagnostic
0Q9H0ZZ	Drainage of Left Tibia, Open Approach
0Q9H30Z	Drainage of Left Tibia with Drainage Device, Percutaneous Approach
0Q9H3ZX	Drainage of Left Tibia, Percutaneous Approach, Diagnostic
0Q9H3ZZ	Drainage of Left Tibia, Percutaneous Approach
0Q9H40Z	Drainage of Left Tibia with Drainage Device, Percutaneous Endoscopic Approach
0Q9H4ZX	Drainage of Left Tibia, Percutaneous Endoscopic Approach, Diagnostic
0Q9H4ZZ	Drainage of Left Tibia, Percutaneous Endoscopic Approach
0Q9J00Z	Drainage of Right Fibula with Drainage Device, Open Approach
0Q9J0ZX	Drainage of Right Fibula, Open Approach, Diagnostic
0Q9J0ZZ	Drainage of Right Fibula, Open Approach
0Q9J30Z	Drainage of Right Fibula with Drainage Device, Percutaneous Approach
0Q9J3ZX	Drainage of Right Fibula, Percutaneous Approach, Diagnostic
0Q9J3ZZ	Drainage of Right Fibula, Percutaneous Approach
0Q9J40Z	Drainage of Right Fibula with Drainage Device, Percutaneous Endoscopic Approach
0Q9J4ZX	Drainage of Right Fibula, Percutaneous Endoscopic Approach, Diagnostic
0Q9J4ZZ	Drainage of Right Fibula, Percutaneous Endoscopic Approach
0Q9K00Z	Drainage of Left Fibula with Drainage Device, Open Approach
0Q9K0ZX	Drainage of Left Fibula, Open Approach, Diagnostic
0Q9K0ZZ	Drainage of Left Fibula, Open Approach
0Q9K30Z	Drainage of Left Fibula with Drainage Device, Percutaneous Approach
0Q9K3ZX	Drainage of Left Fibula, Percutaneous Approach, Diagnostic
0Q9K3ZZ	Drainage of Left Fibula, Percutaneous Approach
0Q9K40Z	Drainage of Left Fibula with Drainage Device, Percutaneous Endoscopic Approach
0Q9K4ZX	Drainage of Left Fibula, Percutaneous Endoscopic Approach, Diagnostic
0Q9K4ZZ	Drainage of Left Fibula, Percutaneous Endoscopic Approach
0Q9L00Z	Drainage of Right Tarsal with Drainage Device, Open Approach
0Q9L0ZX	Drainage of Right Tarsal, Open Approach, Diagnostic
0Q9L0ZZ	Drainage of Right Tarsal, Open Approach
0Q9L30Z	Drainage of Right Tarsal with Drainage Device, Percutaneous Approach
0Q9L3ZX	Drainage of Right Tarsal, Percutaneous Approach, Diagnostic
0Q9L3ZZ	Drainage of Right Tarsal, Percutaneous Approach
0Q9L40Z	Drainage of Right Tarsal with Drainage Device, Percutaneous Endoscopic Approach
0Q9L4ZX	Drainage of Right Tarsal, Percutaneous Endoscopic Approach, Diagnostic
0Q9L4ZZ	Drainage of Right Tarsal, Percutaneous Endoscopic Approach
0Q9M00Z	Drainage of Left Tarsal with Drainage Device, Open Approach
0Q9M0ZX	Drainage of Left Tarsal, Open Approach, Diagnostic
0Q9M0ZZ	Drainage of Left Tarsal, Open Approach
0Q9M30Z	Drainage of Left Tarsal with Drainage Device, Percutaneous Approach
0Q9M3ZX	Drainage of Left Tarsal, Percutaneous Approach, Diagnostic
0Q9M3ZZ	Drainage of Left Tarsal, Percutaneous Approach
0Q9M40Z	Drainage of Left Tarsal with Drainage Device, Percutaneous Endoscopic Approach
0Q9M4ZX	Drainage of Left Tarsal, Percutaneous Endoscopic Approach, Diagnostic
0Q9M4ZZ	Drainage of Left Tarsal, Percutaneous Endoscopic Approach
0Q9N00Z	Drainage of Right Metatarsal with Drainage Device, Open Approach
0Q9N0ZX	Drainage of Right Metatarsal, Open Approach, Diagnostic
0Q9N0ZZ	Drainage of Right Metatarsal, Open Approach
0Q9N30Z	Drainage of Right Metatarsal with Drainage Device, Percutaneous Approach
0Q9N3ZX	Drainage of Right Metatarsal, Percutaneous Approach, Diagnostic
0Q9N3ZZ	Drainage of Right Metatarsal, Percutaneous Approach
0Q9N40Z	Drainage of Right Metatarsal with Drainage Device, Percutaneous Endoscopic Approach
0Q9N4ZX	Drainage of Right Metatarsal, Percutaneous Endoscopic Approach, Diagnostic
0Q9N4ZZ	Drainage of Right Metatarsal, Percutaneous Endoscopic Approach
0Q9P00Z	Drainage of Left Metatarsal with Drainage Device, Open Approach
0Q9P0ZX	Drainage of Left Metatarsal, Open Approach, Diagnostic
0Q9P0ZZ	Drainage of Left Metatarsal, Open Approach
0Q9P30Z	Drainage of Left Metatarsal with Drainage Device, Percutaneous Approach
0Q9P3ZX	Drainage of Left Metatarsal, Percutaneous Approach, Diagnostic
0Q9P3ZZ	Drainage of Left Metatarsal, Percutaneous Approach
0Q9P40Z	Drainage of Left Metatarsal with Drainage Device, Percutaneous Endoscopic Approach
0Q9P4ZX	Drainage of Left Metatarsal, Percutaneous Endoscopic Approach, Diagnostic
0Q9P4ZZ	Drainage of Left Metatarsal, Percutaneous Endoscopic Approach
0Q9Q00Z	Drainage of Right Toe Phalanx with Drainage Device, Open Approach
0Q9Q0ZX	Drainage of Right Toe Phalanx, Open Approach, Diagnostic
0Q9Q0ZZ	Drainage of Right Toe Phalanx, Open Approach
0Q9Q30Z	Drainage of Right Toe Phalanx with Drainage Device, Percutaneous Approach

♀ Female-only ♂ Male-only ▲ Limited Coverage ● Non-OR ▦ HAC-associated procedure ▲ Non-covered procedures ✛ Combination

0Q3ZX Drainage of Right Toe Phalanx, Percutaneous Approach, Diagnostic

Q3ZZ Drainage of Right Toe Phalanx, Percutaneous Approach

Q40Z Drainage of Right Toe Phalanx with Drainage Device, Percutaneous Endoscopic Approach

Q4ZX Drainage of Right Toe Phalanx, Percutaneous Endoscopic Approach, Diagnostic

Q4ZZ Drainage of Right Toe Phalanx, Percutaneous Endoscopic Approach

R00Z Drainage of Left Toe Phalanx with Drainage Device, Open Approach

R0ZX Drainage of Left Toe Phalanx, Open Approach, Diagnostic

R0ZZ Drainage of Left Toe Phalanx, Open Approach

0Q9R30Z Drainage of Left Toe Phalanx with Drainage Device, Percutaneous Approach

0Q9R3ZX Drainage of Left Toe Phalanx, Percutaneous Approach, Diagnostic

0Q9R3ZZ Drainage of Left Toe Phalanx, Percutaneous Approach

0Q9R40Z Drainage of Left Toe Phalanx with Drainage Device, Percutaneous Endoscopic Approach

0Q9R4ZX Drainage of Left Toe Phalanx, Percutaneous Endoscopic Approach, Diagnostic

0Q9R4ZZ Drainage of Left Toe Phalanx, Percutaneous Endoscopic Approach

0Q9S00Z Drainage of Coccyx with Drainage Device, Open Approach

0Q9S0ZX Drainage of Coccyx, Open Approach, Diagnostic

0Q9S0ZZ Drainage of Coccyx, Open Approach

0Q9S30Z Drainage of Coccyx with Drainage Device, Percutaneous Approach

0Q9S3ZX Drainage of Coccyx, Percutaneous Approach, Diagnostic

0Q9S3ZZ Drainage of Coccyx, Percutaneous Approach

0Q9S40Z Drainage of Coccyx with Drainage Device, Percutaneous Endoscopic Approach

0Q9S4ZX Drainage of Coccyx, Percutaneous Endoscopic Approach, Diagnostic

0Q9S4ZZ Drainage of Coccyx, Percutaneous Endoscopic Approach

B – Lower Bones, Excision

view Coding Guidelines B3.4a and B3.4b

view Coding Guideline B3.5

view Coding Guideline B3.8

B00ZX Excision of Lumbar Vertebra, Open Approach, Diagnostic

B00ZZ Excision of Lumbar Vertebra, Open Approach

B03ZX Excision of Lumbar Vertebra, Percutaneous Approach, Diagnostic

B03ZZ Excision of Lumbar Vertebra, Percutaneous Approach

B04ZX Excision of Lumbar Vertebra, Percutaneous Endoscopic Approach, Diagnostic

B04ZZ Excision of Lumbar Vertebra, Percutaneous Endoscopic Approach

QB10ZX Excision of Sacrum, Open Approach, Diagnostic

QB10ZZ Excision of Sacrum, Open Approach

QB13ZX Excision of Sacrum, Percutaneous Approach, Diagnostic

QB13ZZ Excision of Sacrum, Percutaneous Approach

QB14ZX Excision of Sacrum, Percutaneous Endoscopic Approach, Diagnostic

QB14ZZ Excision of Sacrum, Percutaneous Endoscopic Approach

QB20ZX Excision of Right Pelvic Bone, Open Approach, Diagnostic

QB20ZZ Excision of Right Pelvic Bone, Open Approach

AHA CC: 2Q, 2014, 6-7

QB23ZX Excision of Right Pelvic Bone, Percutaneous Approach, Diagnostic

QB23ZZ Excision of Right Pelvic Bone, Percutaneous Approach

QB24ZX Excision of Right Pelvic Bone, Percutaneous Endoscopic Approach, Diagnostic

QB24ZZ Excision of Right Pelvic Bone, Percutaneous Endoscopic Approach

QB30ZX Excision of Left Pelvic Bone, Open Approach, Diagnostic

QB30ZZ Excision of Left Pelvic Bone, Open Approach

QB33ZX Excision of Left Pelvic Bone, Percutaneous Approach, Diagnostic

QB33ZZ Excision of Left Pelvic Bone, Percutaneous Approach

QB34ZX Excision of Left Pelvic Bone, Percutaneous Endoscopic Approach, Diagnostic

QB34ZZ Excision of Left Pelvic Bone, Percutaneous Endoscopic Approach

0QB40ZX Excision of Right Acetabulum, Open Approach, Diagnostic

0QB40ZZ Excision of Right Acetabulum, Open Approach

0QB43ZX Excision of Right Acetabulum, Percutaneous Approach, Diagnostic

0QB43ZZ Excision of Right Acetabulum, Percutaneous Approach

0QB44ZX Excision of Right Acetabulum, Percutaneous Endoscopic Approach, Diagnostic

0QB44ZZ Excision of Right Acetabulum, Percutaneous Endoscopic Approach

0QB50ZX Excision of Left Acetabulum, Open Approach, Diagnostic

0QB50ZZ Excision of Left Acetabulum, Open Approach

0QB53ZX Excision of Left Acetabulum, Percutaneous Approach, Diagnostic

0QB53ZZ Excision of Left Acetabulum, Percutaneous Approach

0QB54ZX Excision of Left Acetabulum, Percutaneous Endoscopic Approach, Diagnostic

0QB54ZZ Excision of Left Acetabulum, Percutaneous Endoscopic Approach

0QB60ZX Excision of Right Upper Femur, Open Approach, Diagnostic

0QB60ZZ Excision of Right Upper Femur, Open Approach

0QB63ZX Excision of Right Upper Femur, Percutaneous Approach, Diagnostic

0QB63ZZ Excision of Right Upper Femur, Percutaneous Approach

0QB64ZX Excision of Right Upper Femur, Percutaneous Endoscopic Approach, Diagnostic

0QB64ZZ Excision of Right Upper Femur, Percutaneous Endoscopic Approach

0QB70ZX Excision of Left Upper Femur, Open Approach, Diagnostic

0QB70ZZ Excision of Left Upper Femur, Open Approach

0QB73ZX Excision of Left Upper Femur, Percutaneous Approach, Diagnostic

0QB73ZZ Excision of Left Upper Femur, Percutaneous Approach

0QB74ZX Excision of Left Upper Femur, Percutaneous Endoscopic Approach, Diagnostic

0QB74ZZ Excision of Left Upper Femur, Percutaneous Endoscopic Approach

AHA CC: 4Q, 2014, 25-26

0QB80ZX Excision of Right Femoral Shaft, Open Approach, Diagnostic

0QB80ZZ Excision of Right Femoral Shaft, Open Approach

0QB83ZX Excision of Right Femoral Shaft, Percutaneous Approach, Diagnostic

0QB83ZZ Excision of Right Femoral Shaft, Percutaneous Approach

0QB84ZX Excision of Right Femoral Shaft, Percutaneous Endoscopic Approach, Diagnostic

0QB84ZZ Excision of Right Femoral Shaft, Percutaneous Endoscopic Approach

0QB90ZX Excision of Left Femoral Shaft, Open Approach, Diagnostic

0QB90ZZ Excision of Left Femoral Shaft, Open Approach

0QB93ZX Excision of Left Femoral Shaft, Percutaneous Approach, Diagnostic

0QB93ZZ Excision of Left Femoral Shaft, Percutaneous Approach

0QB94ZX Excision of Left Femoral Shaft, Percutaneous Endoscopic Approach, Diagnostic

0QB94ZZ Excision of Left Femoral Shaft, Percutaneous Endoscopic Approach

0QBB0ZX Excision of Right Lower Femur, Open Approach, Diagnostic

0QBB0ZZ Excision of Right Lower Femur, Open Approach

0QBB3ZX Excision of Right Lower Femur, Percutaneous Approach, Diagnostic

0QBB3ZZ Excision of Right Lower Femur, Percutaneous Approach

0QBB4ZX Excision of Right Lower Femur, Percutaneous Endoscopic Approach, Diagnostic

0QBB4ZZ Excision of Right Lower Femur, Percutaneous Endoscopic Approach

0QBC0ZX Excision of Left Lower Femur, Open Approach, Diagnostic

0QBC0ZZ Excision of Left Lower Femur, Open Approach

0QBC3ZX Excision of Left Lower Femur, Percutaneous Approach, Diagnostic

0QBC3ZZ Excision of Left Lower Femur, Percutaneous Approach

0QBC4ZX Excision of Left Lower Femur, Percutaneous Endoscopic Approach, Diagnostic
0QBC4ZZ Excision of Left Lower Femur, Percutaneous Endoscopic Approach
0QBD0ZX Excision of Right Patella, Open Approach, Diagnostic
0QBD0ZZ Excision of Right Patella, Open Approach
0QBD3ZX Excision of Right Patella, Percutaneous Approach, Diagnostic
0QBD3ZZ Excision of Right Patella, Percutaneous Approach
0QBD4ZX Excision of Right Patella, Percutaneous Endoscopic Approach, Diagnostic
0QBD4ZZ Excision of Right Patella, Percutaneous Endoscopic Approach
0QBF0ZX Excision of Left Patella, Open Approach, Diagnostic
0QBF0ZZ Excision of Left Patella, Open Approach
0QBF3ZX Excision of Left Patella, Percutaneous Approach, Diagnostic
0QBF3ZZ Excision of Left Patella, Percutaneous Approach
0QBF4ZX Excision of Left Patella, Percutaneous Endoscopic Approach, Diagnostic
0QBF4ZZ Excision of Left Patella, Percutaneous Endoscopic Approach
0QBG0ZX Excision of Right Tibia, Open Approach, Diagnostic
0QBG0ZZ Excision of Right Tibia, Open Approach
0QBG3ZX Excision of Right Tibia, Percutaneous Approach, Diagnostic
0QBG3ZZ Excision of Right Tibia, Percutaneous Approach
0QBG4ZX Excision of Right Tibia, Percutaneous Endoscopic Approach, Diagnostic
0QBG4ZZ Excision of Right Tibia, Percutaneous Endoscopic Approach
0QBH0ZX Excision of Left Tibia, Open Approach, Diagnostic
0QBH0ZZ Excision of Left Tibia, Open Approach
0QBH3ZX Excision of Left Tibia, Percutaneous Approach, Diagnostic
0QBH3ZZ Excision of Left Tibia, Percutaneous Approach
0QBH4ZX Excision of Left Tibia, Percutaneous Endoscopic Approach, Diagnostic
0QBH4ZZ Excision of Left Tibia, Percutaneous Endoscopic Approach
0QBJ0ZX Excision of Right Fibula, Open Approach, Diagnostic
0QBJ0ZZ Excision of Right Fibula, Open Approach

0QBJ3ZX Excision of Right Fibula, Percutaneous Approach, Diagnostic
0QBJ3ZZ Excision of Right Fibula, Percutaneous Approach
0QBJ4ZX Excision of Right Fibula, Percutaneous Endoscopic Approach, Diagnostic
0QBJ4ZZ Excision of Right Fibula, Percutaneous Endoscopic Approach
0QBK0ZX Excision of Left Fibula, Open Approach, Diagnostic
0QBK0ZZ Excision of Left Fibula, Open Approach
  AHA CC: 2Q, 2013, 39-40
0QBK3ZX Excision of Left Fibula, Percutaneous Approach, Diagnostic
0QBK3ZZ Excision of Left Fibula, Percutaneous Approach
0QBK4ZX Excision of Left Fibula, Percutaneous Endoscopic Approach, Diagnostic
0QBK4ZZ Excision of Left Fibula, Percutaneous Endoscopic Approach
0QBL0ZX Excision of Right Tarsal, Open Approach, Diagnostic
0QBL0ZZ Excision of Right Tarsal, Open Approach
0QBL3ZX Excision of Right Tarsal, Percutaneous Approach, Diagnostic
0QBL3ZZ Excision of Right Tarsal, Percutaneous Approach
0QBL4ZX Excision of Right Tarsal, Percutaneous Endoscopic Approach, Diagnostic
0QBL4ZZ Excision of Right Tarsal, Percutaneous Endoscopic Approach
0QBM0ZX Excision of Left Tarsal, Open Approach, Diagnostic
0QBM0ZZ Excision of Left Tarsal, Open Approach
0QBM3ZX Excision of Left Tarsal, Percutaneous Approach, Diagnostic
0QBM3ZZ Excision of Left Tarsal, Percutaneous Approach
0QBM4ZX Excision of Left Tarsal, Percutaneous Endoscopic Approach, Diagnostic
0QBM4ZZ Excision of Left Tarsal, Percutaneous Endoscopic Approach
0QBN0ZX Excision of Right Metatarsal, Open Approach, Diagnostic
0QBN0ZZ Excision of Right Metatarsal, Open Approach
0QBN3ZX Excision of Right Metatarsal, Percutaneous Approach, Diagnostic
0QBN3ZZ Excision of Right Metatarsal, Percutaneous Approach
0QBN4ZX Excision of Right Metatarsal, Percutaneous Endoscopic Approach, Diagnostic

0QBN4ZZ Excision of Right Metatarsal, Percutaneous Endoscopic Approach
0QBP0ZX Excision of Left Metatarsal, Open Approach, Diagnostic
0QBP0ZZ Excision of Left Metatarsal, Open Approach
0QBP3ZX Excision of Left Metatarsal, Percutaneous Approach, Diagnostic
0QBP3ZZ Excision of Left Metatarsal, Percutaneous Approach
0QBP4ZX Excision of Left Metatarsal, Percutaneous Endoscopic Approach, Diagnostic
0QBP4ZZ Excision of Left Metatarsal, Percutaneous Endoscopic Approach
0QBQ0ZX Excision of Right Toe Phalanx, Open Approach, Diagnostic
0QBQ0ZZ Excision of Right Toe Phalanx, Open Approach
0QBQ3ZX Excision of Right Toe Phalanx, Percutaneous Approach, Diagnostic
0QBQ3ZZ Excision of Right Toe Phalanx, Percutaneous Approach
0QBQ4ZX Excision of Right Toe Phalanx, Percutaneous Endoscopic Approach, Diagnostic
0QBQ4ZZ Excision of Right Toe Phalanx, Percutaneous Endoscopic Approach
0QBR0ZX Excision of Left Toe Phalanx, Open Approach, Diagnostic
0QBR0ZZ Excision of Left Toe Phalanx, Open Approach
0QBR3ZX Excision of Left Toe Phalanx, Percutaneous Approach, Diagnostic
0QBR3ZZ Excision of Left Toe Phalanx, Percutaneous Approach
0QBR4ZX Excision of Left Toe Phalanx, Percutaneous Endoscopic Approach, Diagnostic
0QBR4ZZ Excision of Left Toe Phalanx, Percutaneous Endoscopic Approach
0QBS0ZX Excision of Coccyx, Open Approach, Diagnostic
0QBS0ZZ Excision of Coccyx, Open Approach
0QBS3ZX Excision of Coccyx, Percutaneous Approach, Diagnostic
0QBS3ZZ Excision of Coccyx, Percutaneous Approach
0QBS4ZX Excision of Coccyx, Percutaneous Endoscopic Approach, Diagnostic
0QBS4ZZ Excision of Coccyx, Percutaneous Endoscopic Approach

0QC – Lower Bones, Extirpation

0QC00ZZ Extirpation of Matter from Lumbar Vertebra, Open Approach
0QC03ZZ Extirpation of Matter from Lumbar Vertebra, Percutaneous Approach
0QC04ZZ Extirpation of Matter from Lumbar Vertebra, Percutaneous Endoscopic Approach
0QC10ZZ Extirpation of Matter from Sacrum, Open Approach
0QC13ZZ Extirpation of Matter from Sacrum, Percutaneous Approach
0QC14ZZ Extirpation of Matter from Sacrum, Percutaneous Endoscopic Approach
0QC20ZZ Extirpation of Matter from Right Pelvic Bone, Open Approach
0QC23ZZ Extirpation of Matter from Right Pelvic Bone, Percutaneous Approach
0QC24ZZ Extirpation of Matter from Right Pelvic Bone, Percutaneous Endoscopic Approach

0QC30ZZ Extirpation of Matter from Left Pelvic Bone, Open Approach
0QC33ZZ Extirpation of Matter from Left Pelvic Bone, Percutaneous Approach
0QC34ZZ Extirpation of Matter from Left Pelvic Bone, Percutaneous Endoscopic Approach
0QC40ZZ Extirpation of Matter from Right Acetabulum, Open Approach
0QC43ZZ Extirpation of Matter from Right Acetabulum, Percutaneous Approach
0QC44ZZ Extirpation of Matter from Right Acetabulum, Percutaneous Endoscopic Approach
0QC50ZZ Extirpation of Matter from Left Acetabulum, Open Approach
0QC53ZZ Extirpation of Matter from Left Acetabulum, Percutaneous Approach
0QC54ZZ Extirpation of Matter from Left Acetabulum, Percutaneous Endoscopic Approach

0QC60ZZ Extirpation of Matter from Right Upper Femur, Open Approach
0QC63ZZ Extirpation of Matter from Right Upper Femur, Percutaneous Approach
0QC64ZZ Extirpation of Matter from Right Upper Femur, Percutaneous Endoscopic Approach
0QC70ZZ Extirpation of Matter from Left Upper Femur, Open Approach
0QC73ZZ Extirpation of Matter from Left Upper Femur, Percutaneous Approach
0QC74ZZ Extirpation of Matter from Left Upper Femur, Percutaneous Endoscopic Approach
0QC80ZZ Extirpation of Matter from Right Femoral Shaft, Open Approach
0QC83ZZ Extirpation of Matter from Right Femoral Shaft, Percutaneous Approach
0QC84ZZ Extirpation of Matter from Right Femoral Shaft, Percutaneous Endoscopic Approach

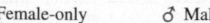

♀ Female-only   ♂ Male-only   ▲ Limited Coverage   ● Non-OR   ▦ HAC-associated procedure   ▲ Non-covered procedures   ✚ Combination

0QC90ZZ	Extirpation of Matter from Left Femoral Shaft, Open Approach	
0QC93ZZ	Extirpation of Matter from Left Femoral Shaft, Percutaneous Approach	
0QC94ZZ	Extirpation of Matter from Left Femoral Shaft, Percutaneous Endoscopic Approach	
0QCB0ZZ	Extirpation of Matter from Right Lower Femur, Open Approach	
0QCB3ZZ	Extirpation of Matter from Right Lower Femur, Percutaneous Approach	
0QCB4ZZ	Extirpation of Matter from Right Lower Femur, Percutaneous Endoscopic Approach	
0QCC0ZZ	Extirpation of Matter from Left Lower Femur, Open Approach	
0QCC3ZZ	Extirpation of Matter from Left Lower Femur, Percutaneous Approach	
0QCC4ZZ	Extirpation of Matter from Left Lower Femur, Percutaneous Endoscopic Approach	
0QCD0ZZ	Extirpation of Matter from Right Patella, Open Approach	
0QCD3ZZ	Extirpation of Matter from Right Patella, Percutaneous Approach	
0QCD4ZZ	Extirpation of Matter from Right Patella, Percutaneous Endoscopic Approach	
0QCF0ZZ	Extirpation of Matter from Left Patella, Open Approach	
0QCF3ZZ	Extirpation of Matter from Left Patella, Percutaneous Approach	
0QCF4ZZ	Extirpation of Matter from Left Patella, Percutaneous Endoscopic Approach	
0QCG0ZZ	Extirpation of Matter from Right Tibia, Open Approach	

0QCG3ZZ	Extirpation of Matter from Right Tibia, Percutaneous Approach
0QCG4ZZ	Extirpation of Matter from Right Tibia, Percutaneous Endoscopic Approach
0QCH0ZZ	Extirpation of Matter from Left Tibia, Open Approach
0QCH3ZZ	Extirpation of Matter from Left Tibia, Percutaneous Approach
0QCH4ZZ	Extirpation of Matter from Left Tibia, Percutaneous Endoscopic Approach
0QCJ0ZZ	Extirpation of Matter from Right Fibula, Open Approach
0QCJ3ZZ	Extirpation of Matter from Right Fibula, Percutaneous Approach
0QCJ4ZZ	Extirpation of Matter from Right Fibula, Percutaneous Endoscopic Approach
0QCK0ZZ	Extirpation of Matter from Left Fibula, Open Approach
0QCK3ZZ	Extirpation of Matter from Left Fibula, Percutaneous Approach
0QCK4ZZ	Extirpation of Matter from Left Fibula, Percutaneous Endoscopic Approach
0QCL0ZZ	Extirpation of Matter from Right Tarsal, Open Approach
0QCL3ZZ	Extirpation of Matter from Right Tarsal, Percutaneous Approach
0QCL4ZZ	Extirpation of Matter from Right Tarsal, Percutaneous Endoscopic Approach
0QCM0ZZ	Extirpation of Matter from Left Tarsal, Open Approach
0QCM3ZZ	Extirpation of Matter from Left Tarsal, Percutaneous Approach
0QCM4ZZ	Extirpation of Matter from Left Tarsal, Percutaneous Endoscopic Approach

0QCN0ZZ	Extirpation of Matter from Right Metatarsal, Open Approach
0QCN3ZZ	Extirpation of Matter from Right Metatarsal, Percutaneous Approach
0QCN4ZZ	Extirpation of Matter from Right Metatarsal, Percutaneous Endoscopic Approach
0QCP0ZZ	Extirpation of Matter from Left Metatarsal, Open Approach
0QCP3ZZ	Extirpation of Matter from Left Metatarsal, Percutaneous Approach
0QCP4ZZ	Extirpation of Matter from Left Metatarsal, Percutaneous Endoscopic Approach
0QCQ0ZZ	Extirpation of Matter from Right Toe Phalanx, Open Approach
0QCQ3ZZ	Extirpation of Matter from Right Toe Phalanx, Percutaneous Approach
0QCQ4ZZ	Extirpation of Matter from Right Toe Phalanx, Percutaneous Endoscopic Approach
0QCR0ZZ	Extirpation of Matter from Left Toe Phalanx, Open Approach
0QCR3ZZ	Extirpation of Matter from Left Toe Phalanx, Percutaneous Approach
0QCR4ZZ	Extirpation of Matter from Left Toe Phalanx, Percutaneous Endoscopic Approach
0QCS0ZZ	Extirpation of Matter from Coccyx, Open Approach
0QCS3ZZ	Extirpation of Matter from Coccyx, Percutaneous Approach
0QCS4ZZ	Extirpation of Matter from Coccyx, Percutaneous Endoscopic Approach

QH – Lower Bones, Insertion

0QH004Z	Insertion of Internal Fixation Device into Lumbar Vertebra, Open Approach
0QH005Z	Insertion of External Fixation Device into Lumbar Vertebra, Open Approach
0QH034Z	Insertion of Internal Fixation Device into Lumbar Vertebra, Percutaneous Approach
0QH035Z	Insertion of External Fixation Device into Lumbar Vertebra, Percutaneous Approach
0QH044Z	Insertion of Internal Fixation Device into Lumbar Vertebra, Percutaneous Endoscopic Approach
0QH045Z	Insertion of External Fixation Device into Lumbar Vertebra, Percutaneous Endoscopic Approach
0QH104Z	Insertion of Internal Fixation Device into Sacrum, Open Approach
0QH105Z	Insertion of External Fixation Device into Sacrum, Open Approach
0QH134Z	Insertion of Internal Fixation Device into Sacrum, Percutaneous Approach
0QH135Z	Insertion of External Fixation Device into Sacrum, Percutaneous Approach
0QH144Z	Insertion of Internal Fixation Device into Sacrum, Percutaneous Endoscopic Approach
0QH145Z	Insertion of External Fixation Device into Sacrum, Percutaneous Endoscopic Approach
0QH204Z	Insertion of Internal Fixation Device into Right Pelvic Bone, Open Approach
0QH205Z	Insertion of External Fixation Device into Right Pelvic Bone, Open Approach
0QH234Z	Insertion of Internal Fixation Device into Right Pelvic Bone, Percutaneous Approach
0QH235Z	Insertion of External Fixation Device into Right Pelvic Bone, Percutaneous Approach

0QH244Z	Insertion of Internal Fixation Device into Right Pelvic Bone, Percutaneous Endoscopic Approach
0QH245Z	Insertion of External Fixation Device into Right Pelvic Bone, Percutaneous Endoscopic Approach
0QH304Z	Insertion of Internal Fixation Device into Left Pelvic Bone, Open Approach
0QH305Z	Insertion of External Fixation Device into Left Pelvic Bone, Open Approach
0QH334Z	Insertion of Internal Fixation Device into Left Pelvic Bone, Percutaneous Approach
0QH335Z	Insertion of External Fixation Device into Left Pelvic Bone, Percutaneous Approach
0QH344Z	Insertion of Internal Fixation Device into Left Pelvic Bone, Percutaneous Endoscopic Approach
0QH345Z	Insertion of External Fixation Device into Left Pelvic Bone, Percutaneous Endoscopic Approach
0QH404Z	Insertion of Internal Fixation Device into Right Acetabulum, Open Approach
0QH405Z	Insertion of External Fixation Device into Right Acetabulum, Open Approach
0QH434Z	Insertion of Internal Fixation Device into Right Acetabulum, Percutaneous Approach
0QH435Z	Insertion of External Fixation Device into Right Acetabulum, Percutaneous Approach
0QH444Z	Insertion of Internal Fixation Device into Right Acetabulum, Percutaneous Endoscopic Approach
0QH445Z	Insertion of External Fixation Device into Right Acetabulum, Percutaneous Endoscopic Approach

0QH504Z	Insertion of Internal Fixation Device into Left Acetabulum, Open Approach
0QH505Z	Insertion of External Fixation Device into Left Acetabulum, Open Approach
0QH534Z	Insertion of Internal Fixation Device into Left Acetabulum, Percutaneous Approach
0QH535Z	Insertion of External Fixation Device into Left Acetabulum, Percutaneous Approach
0QH544Z	Insertion of Internal Fixation Device into Left Acetabulum, Percutaneous Endoscopic Approach
0QH545Z	Insertion of External Fixation Device into Left Acetabulum, Percutaneous Endoscopic Approach
0QH604Z	Insertion of Internal Fixation Device into Right Upper Femur, Open Approach
0QH605Z	Insertion of External Fixation Device into Right Upper Femur, Open Approach
0QH606Z	Insertion of Intramedullary Internal Fixation Device into Right Upper Femur, Open Approach
0QH608Z	Insertion of Limb Lengthening External Fixation Device into Right Upper Femur, Open Approach
0QH60BZ	Insertion of Monoplanar External Fixation Device into Right Upper Femur, Open Approach
0QH60CZ	Insertion of Ring External Fixation Device into Right Upper Femur, Open Approach
0QH60DZ	Insertion of Hybrid External Fixation Device into Right Upper Femur, Open Approach
0QH634Z	Insertion of Internal Fixation Device into Right Upper Femur, Percutaneous Approach

♀ Female-only   ♂ Male-only   ▲ Limited Coverage   ● Non-OR   ▦ HAC-associated procedure   ▲ Non-covered procedures   ✚ Combination

0QH635Z Insertion of External Fixation Device into Right Upper Femur, Percutaneous Approach

0QH636Z Insertion of Intramedullary Internal Fixation Device into Right Upper Femur, Percutaneous Approach

0QH638Z Insertion of Limb Lengthening External Fixation Device into Right Upper Femur, Percutaneous Approach

0QH63BZ Insertion of Monoplanar External Fixation Device into Right Upper Femur, Percutaneous Approach

0QH63CZ Insertion of Ring External Fixation Device into Right Upper Femur, Percutaneous Approach

0QH63DZ Insertion of Hybrid External Fixation Device into Right Upper Femur, Percutaneous Approach

0QH644Z Insertion of Internal Fixation Device into Right Upper Femur, Percutaneous Endoscopic Approach

0QH645Z Insertion of External Fixation Device into Right Upper Femur, Percutaneous Endoscopic Approach

0QH646Z Insertion of Intramedullary Internal Fixation Device into Right Upper Femur, Percutaneous Endoscopic Approach

0QH648Z Insertion of Limb Lengthening External Fixation Device into Right Upper Femur, Percutaneous Endoscopic Approach

0QH64BZ Insertion of Monoplanar External Fixation Device into Right Upper Femur, Percutaneous Endoscopic Approach

0QH64CZ Insertion of Ring External Fixation Device into Right Upper Femur, Percutaneous Endoscopic Approach

0QH64DZ Insertion of Hybrid External Fixation Device into Right Upper Femur, Percutaneous Endoscopic Approach

0QH704Z Insertion of Internal Fixation Device into Left Upper Femur, Open Approach

0QH705Z Insertion of External Fixation Device into Left Upper Femur, Open Approach

0QH706Z Insertion of Intramedullary Internal Fixation Device into Left Upper Femur, Open Approach

0QH708Z Insertion of Limb Lengthening External Fixation Device into Left Upper Femur, Open Approach

0QH70BZ Insertion of Monoplanar External Fixation Device into Left Upper Femur, Open Approach

0QH70CZ Insertion of Ring External Fixation Device into Left Upper Femur, Open Approach

0QH70DZ Insertion of Hybrid External Fixation Device into Left Upper Femur, Open Approach

0QH734Z Insertion of Internal Fixation Device into Left Upper Femur, Percutaneous Approach

0QH735Z Insertion of External Fixation Device into Left Upper Femur, Percutaneous Approach

0QH736Z Insertion of Intramedullary Internal Fixation Device into Left Upper Femur, Percutaneous Approach

0QH738Z Insertion of Limb Lengthening External Fixation Device into Left Upper Femur, Percutaneous Approach

0QH73BZ Insertion of Monoplanar External Fixation Device into Left Upper Femur, Percutaneous Approach

0QH73CZ Insertion of Ring External Fixation Device into Left Upper Femur, Percutaneous Approach

0QH73DZ Insertion of Hybrid External Fixation Device into Left Upper Femur, Percutaneous Approach

0QH744Z Insertion of Internal Fixation Device into Left Upper Femur, Percutaneous Endoscopic Approach

0QH745Z Insertion of External Fixation Device into Left Upper Femur, Percutaneous Endoscopic Approach

0QH746Z Insertion of Intramedullary Internal Fixation Device into Left Upper Femur, Percutaneous Endoscopic Approach

0QH748Z Insertion of Limb Lengthening External Fixation Device into Left Upper Femur, Percutaneous Endoscopic Approach

0QH74BZ Insertion of Monoplanar External Fixation Device into Left Upper Femur, Percutaneous Endoscopic Approach

0QH74CZ Insertion of Ring External Fixation Device into Left Upper Femur, Percutaneous Endoscopic Approach

0QH74DZ Insertion of Hybrid External Fixation Device into Left Upper Femur, Percutaneous Endoscopic Approach

0QH804Z Insertion of Internal Fixation Device into Right Femoral Shaft, Open Approach

0QH805Z Insertion of External Fixation Device into Right Femoral Shaft, Open Approach

0QH806Z Insertion of Intramedullary Internal Fixation Device into Right Femoral Shaft, Open Approach

0QH808Z Insertion of Limb Lengthening External Fixation Device into Right Femoral Shaft, Open Approach

0QH80BZ Insertion of Monoplanar External Fixation Device into Right Femoral Shaft, Open Approach

0QH80CZ Insertion of Ring External Fixation Device into Right Femoral Shaft, Open Approach

0QH80DZ Insertion of Hybrid External Fixation Device into Right Femoral Shaft, Open Approach

0QH834Z Insertion of Internal Fixation Device into Right Femoral Shaft, Percutaneous Approach

0QH835Z Insertion of External Fixation Device into Right Femoral Shaft, Percutaneous Approach

0QH836Z Insertion of Intramedullary Internal Fixation Device into Right Femoral Shaft, Percutaneous Approach

0QH838Z Insertion of Limb Lengthening External Fixation Device into Right Femoral Shaft, Percutaneous Approach

0QH83BZ Insertion of Monoplanar External Fixation Device into Right Femoral Shaft, Percutaneous Approach

0QH83CZ Insertion of Ring External Fixation Device into Right Femoral Shaft, Percutaneous Approach

0QH83DZ Insertion of Hybrid External Fixation Device into Right Femoral Shaft, Percutaneous Approach

0QH844Z Insertion of Internal Fixation Device into Right Femoral Shaft, Percutaneous Endoscopic Approach

0QH845Z Insertion of External Fixation Device into Right Femoral Shaft, Percutaneous Endoscopic Approach

0QH846Z Insertion of Intramedullary Internal Fixation Device into Right Femoral Shaft, Percutaneous Endoscopic Approach

0QH848Z Insertion of Limb Lengthening External Fixation Device into Right Femoral Shaft, Percutaneous Endoscopic Approach

0QH84BZ Insertion of Monoplanar External Fixation Device into Right Femoral Shaft, Percutaneous Endoscopic Approach

0QH84CZ Insertion of Ring External Fixation Device into Right Femoral Shaft, Percutaneous Endoscopic Approach

0QH84DZ Insertion of Hybrid External Fixation Device into Right Femoral Shaft, Percutaneous Endoscopic Approach

0QH904Z Insertion of Internal Fixation Device into Left Femoral Shaft, Open Approach

0QH905Z Insertion of External Fixation Device into Left Femoral Shaft, Open Approach

0QH906Z Insertion of Intramedullary Internal Fixation Device into Left Femoral Shaft, Open Approach

0QH908Z Insertion of Limb Lengthening External Fixation Device into Left Femoral Shaft, Open Approach

0QH90BZ Insertion of Monoplanar External Fixation Device into Left Femoral Shaft, Open Approach

0QH90CZ Insertion of Ring External Fixation Device into Left Femoral Shaft, Open Approach

0QH90DZ Insertion of Hybrid External Fixation Device into Left Femoral Shaft, Open Approach

0QH934Z Insertion of Internal Fixation Device into Left Femoral Shaft, Percutaneous Approach

0QH935Z Insertion of External Fixation Device into Left Femoral Shaft, Percutaneous Approach

0QH936Z Insertion of Intramedullary Internal Fixation Device into Left Femoral Shaft, Percutaneous Approach

0QH938Z Insertion of Limb Lengthening External Fixation Device into Left Femoral Shaft, Percutaneous Approach

0QH93BZ Insertion of Monoplanar External Fixation Device into Left Femoral Shaft, Percutaneous Approach

0QH93CZ Insertion of Ring External Fixation Device into Left Femoral Shaft, Percutaneous Approach

0QH93DZ Insertion of Hybrid External Fixation Device into Left Femoral Shaft, Percutaneous Approach

0QH944Z Insertion of Internal Fixation Device into Left Femoral Shaft, Percutaneous Endoscopic Approach

0QH945Z Insertion of External Fixation Device into Left Femoral Shaft, Percutaneous Endoscopic Approach

0QH946Z Insertion of Intramedullary Internal Fixation Device into Left Femoral Shaft, Percutaneous Endoscopic Approach

0QH948Z Insertion of Limb Lengthening External Fixation Device into Left Femoral Shaft, Percutaneous Endoscopic Approach

0QH94BZ Insertion of Monoplanar External Fixation Device into Left Femoral Shaft, Percutaneous Endoscopic Approach

0QH94CZ Insertion of Ring External Fixation Device into Left Femoral Shaft, Percutaneous Endoscopic Approach

0QH94DZ Insertion of Hybrid External Fixation Device into Left Femoral Shaft, Percutaneous Endoscopic Approach

0QHB04Z Insertion of Internal Fixation Device into Right Lower Femur, Open Approach

0QHB05Z Insertion of External Fixation Device into Right Lower Femur, Open Approach

0QHB06Z Insertion of Intramedullary Internal Fixation Device into Right Lower Femur, Open Approach

0QHB08Z Insertion of Limb Lengthening External Fixation Device into Right Lower Femur, Open Approach

0HB0BZ Insertion of Monoplanar External Fixation Device into Right Lower Femur, Open Approach

0HB0CZ Insertion of Ring External Fixation Device into Right Lower Femur, Open Approach

0HB0DZ Insertion of Hybrid External Fixation Device into Right Lower Femur, Open Approach

0HB34Z Insertion of Internal Fixation Device into Right Lower Femur, Percutaneous Approach

0HB35Z Insertion of External Fixation Device into Right Lower Femur, Percutaneous Approach

0HB36Z Insertion of Intramedullary Internal Fixation Device into Right Lower Femur, Percutaneous Approach

0HB38Z Insertion of Limb Lengthening External Fixation Device into Right Lower Femur, Percutaneous Approach

0HB3BZ Insertion of Monoplanar External Fixation Device into Right Lower Femur, Percutaneous Approach

0HB3CZ Insertion of Ring External Fixation Device into Right Lower Femur, Percutaneous Approach

0HB3DZ Insertion of Hybrid External Fixation Device into Right Lower Femur, Percutaneous Approach

0HB44Z Insertion of Internal Fixation Device into Right Lower Femur, Percutaneous Endoscopic Approach

0HB45Z Insertion of External Fixation Device into Right Lower Femur, Percutaneous Endoscopic Approach

0HB46Z Insertion of Intramedullary Internal Fixation Device into Right Lower Femur, Percutaneous Endoscopic Approach

0HB48Z Insertion of Limb Lengthening External Fixation Device into Right Lower Femur, Percutaneous Endoscopic Approach

0HB4BZ Insertion of Monoplanar External Fixation Device into Right Lower Femur, Percutaneous Endoscopic Approach

0HB4CZ Insertion of Ring External Fixation Device into Right Lower Femur, Percutaneous Endoscopic Approach

0HB4DZ Insertion of Hybrid External Fixation Device into Right Lower Femur, Percutaneous Endoscopic Approach

0QHC04Z Insertion of Internal Fixation Device into Left Lower Femur, Open Approach

0QHC05Z Insertion of External Fixation Device into Left Lower Femur, Open Approach

0QHC06Z Insertion of Intramedullary Internal Fixation Device into Left Lower Femur, Open Approach

0QHC08Z Insertion of Limb Lengthening External Fixation Device into Left Lower Femur, Open Approach

0QHC0BZ Insertion of Monoplanar External Fixation Device into Left Lower Femur, Open Approach

0QHC0CZ Insertion of Ring External Fixation Device into Left Lower Femur, Open Approach

0QHC0DZ Insertion of Hybrid External Fixation Device into Left Lower Femur, Open Approach

0QHC34Z Insertion of Internal Fixation Device into Left Lower Femur, Percutaneous Approach

0QHC35Z Insertion of External Fixation Device into Left Lower Femur, Percutaneous Approach

0QHC36Z Insertion of Intramedullary Internal Fixation Device into Left Lower Femur, Percutaneous Approach

0QHC38Z Insertion of Limb Lengthening External Fixation Device into Left Lower Femur, Percutaneous Approach

0QHC3BZ Insertion of Monoplanar External Fixation Device into Left Lower Femur, Percutaneous Approach

0QHC3CZ Insertion of Ring External Fixation Device into Left Lower Femur, Percutaneous Approach

0QHC3DZ Insertion of Hybrid External Fixation Device into Left Lower Femur, Percutaneous Approach

0QHC44Z Insertion of Internal Fixation Device into Left Lower Femur, Percutaneous Endoscopic Approach

0QHC45Z Insertion of External Fixation Device into Left Lower Femur, Percutaneous Endoscopic Approach

0QHC46Z Insertion of Intramedullary Internal Fixation Device into Left Lower Femur, Percutaneous Endoscopic Approach

0QHC48Z Insertion of Limb Lengthening External Fixation Device into Left Lower Femur, Percutaneous Endoscopic Approach

0QHC4BZ Insertion of Monoplanar External Fixation Device into Left Lower Femur, Percutaneous Endoscopic Approach

0QHC4CZ Insertion of Ring External Fixation Device into Left Lower Femur, Percutaneous Endoscopic Approach

0QHC4DZ Insertion of Hybrid External Fixation Device into Left Lower Femur, Percutaneous Endoscopic Approach

0QHD04Z Insertion of Internal Fixation Device into Right Patella, Open Approach

0QHD05Z Insertion of External Fixation Device into Right Patella, Open Approach

0QHD34Z Insertion of Internal Fixation Device into Right Patella, Percutaneous Approach

0QHD35Z Insertion of External Fixation Device into Right Patella, Percutaneous Approach

0QHD44Z Insertion of Internal Fixation Device into Right Patella, Percutaneous Endoscopic Approach

0QHD45Z Insertion of External Fixation Device into Right Patella, Percutaneous Endoscopic Approach

0QHF04Z Insertion of Internal Fixation Device into Left Patella, Open Approach

0QHF05Z Insertion of External Fixation Device into Left Patella, Open Approach

0QHF34Z Insertion of Internal Fixation Device into Left Patella, Percutaneous Approach

0QHF35Z Insertion of External Fixation Device into Left Patella, Percutaneous Approach

0QHF44Z Insertion of Internal Fixation Device into Left Patella, Percutaneous Endoscopic Approach

0QHF45Z Insertion of External Fixation Device into Left Patella, Percutaneous Endoscopic Approach

0QHG04Z Insertion of Internal Fixation Device into Right Tibia, Open Approach

0QHG05Z Insertion of External Fixation Device into Right Tibia, Open Approach

0QHG06Z Insertion of Intramedullary Internal Fixation Device into Right Tibia, Open Approach

0QHG08Z Insertion of Limb Lengthening External Fixation Device into Right Tibia, Open Approach

0QHG0BZ Insertion of Monoplanar External Fixation Device into Right Tibia, Open Approach

0QHG0CZ Insertion of Ring External Fixation Device into Right Tibia, Open Approach

0QHG0DZ Insertion of Hybrid External Fixation Device into Right Tibia, Open Approach

0QHG34Z Insertion of Internal Fixation Device into Right Tibia, Percutaneous Approach

0QHG35Z Insertion of External Fixation Device into Right Tibia, Percutaneous Approach

0QHG36Z Insertion of Intramedullary Internal Fixation Device into Right Tibia, Percutaneous Approach

0QHG38Z Insertion of Limb Lengthening External Fixation Device into Right Tibia, Percutaneous Approach

0QHG3BZ Insertion of Monoplanar External Fixation Device into Right Tibia, Percutaneous Approach

0QHG3CZ Insertion of Ring External Fixation Device into Right Tibia, Percutaneous Approach

0QHG3DZ Insertion of Hybrid External Fixation Device into Right Tibia, Percutaneous Approach

0QHG44Z Insertion of Internal Fixation Device into Right Tibia, Percutaneous Endoscopic Approach

0QHG45Z Insertion of External Fixation Device into Right Tibia, Percutaneous Endoscopic Approach

0QHG46Z Insertion of Intramedullary Internal Fixation Device into Right Tibia, Percutaneous Endoscopic Approach

0QHG48Z Insertion of Limb Lengthening External Fixation Device into Right Tibia, Percutaneous Endoscopic Approach

0QHG4BZ Insertion of Monoplanar External Fixation Device into Right Tibia, Percutaneous Endoscopic Approach

0QHG4CZ Insertion of Ring External Fixation Device into Right Tibia, Percutaneous Endoscopic Approach

0QHG4DZ Insertion of Hybrid External Fixation Device into Right Tibia, Percutaneous Endoscopic Approach

0QHH04Z Insertion of Internal Fixation Device into Left Tibia, Open Approach

0QHH05Z Insertion of External Fixation Device into Left Tibia, Open Approach

0QHH06Z Insertion of Intramedullary Internal Fixation Device into Left Tibia, Open Approach

0QHH08Z Insertion of Limb Lengthening External Fixation Device into Left Tibia, Open Approach

0QHH0BZ Insertion of Monoplanar External Fixation Device into Left Tibia, Open Approach

0QHH0CZ Insertion of Ring External Fixation Device into Left Tibia, Open Approach

0QHH0DZ Insertion of Hybrid External Fixation Device into Left Tibia, Open Approach

0QHH34Z Insertion of Internal Fixation Device into Left Tibia, Percutaneous Approach

0QHH35Z Insertion of External Fixation Device into Left Tibia, Percutaneous Approach

0QHH36Z Insertion of Intramedullary Internal Fixation Device into Left Tibia, Percutaneous Approach

0QHH38Z Insertion of Limb Lengthening External Fixation Device into Left Tibia, Percutaneous Approach

0QHH3BZ Insertion of Monoplanar External Fixation Device into Left Tibia, Percutaneous Approach

♀ Female-only　　♂ Male-only　　▲ Limited Coverage　　● Non-OR　　▨ HAC-associated procedure　　▲ Non-covered procedures　　✛ Combination

0QHH3CZ	Insertion of Ring External Fixation Device into Left Tibia, Percutaneous Approach	
0QHH3DZ	Insertion of Hybrid External Fixation Device into Left Tibia, Percutaneous Approach	
0QHH44Z	Insertion of Internal Fixation Device into Left Tibia, Percutaneous Endoscopic Approach	
0QHH45Z	Insertion of External Fixation Device into Left Tibia, Percutaneous Endoscopic Approach	
0QHH46Z	Insertion of Intramedullary Internal Fixation Device into Left Tibia, Percutaneous Endoscopic Approach	
0QHH48Z	Insertion of Limb Lengthening External Fixation Device into Left Tibia, Percutaneous Endoscopic Approach	
0QHH4BZ	Insertion of Monoplanar External Fixation Device into Left Tibia, Percutaneous Endoscopic Approach	
0QHH4CZ	Insertion of Ring External Fixation Device into Left Tibia, Percutaneous Endoscopic Approach	
0QHH4DZ	Insertion of Hybrid External Fixation Device into Left Tibia, Percutaneous Endoscopic Approach	
0QHJ04Z	Insertion of Internal Fixation Device into Right Fibula, Open Approach	
0QHJ05Z	Insertion of External Fixation Device into Right Fibula, Open Approach	
0QHJ06Z	Insertion of Intramedullary Internal Fixation Device into Right Fibula, Open Approach	
0QHJ08Z	Insertion of Limb Lengthening External Fixation Device into Right Fibula, Open Approach	
0QHJ0BZ	Insertion of Monoplanar External Fixation Device into Right Fibula, Open Approach	
0QHJ0CZ	Insertion of Ring External Fixation Device into Right Fibula, Open Approach	
0QHJ0DZ	Insertion of Hybrid External Fixation Device into Right Fibula, Open Approach	
0QHJ34Z	Insertion of Internal Fixation Device into Right Fibula, Percutaneous Approach	
0QHJ35Z	Insertion of External Fixation Device into Right Fibula, Percutaneous Approach	
0QHJ36Z	Insertion of Intramedullary Internal Fixation Device into Right Fibula, Percutaneous Approach	
0QHJ38Z	Insertion of Limb Lengthening External Fixation Device into Right Fibula, Percutaneous Approach	
0QHJ3BZ	Insertion of Monoplanar External Fixation Device into Right Fibula, Percutaneous Approach	
0QHJ3CZ	Insertion of Ring External Fixation Device into Right Fibula, Percutaneous Approach	
0QHJ3DZ	Insertion of Hybrid External Fixation Device into Right Fibula, Percutaneous Approach	
0QHJ44Z	Insertion of Internal Fixation Device into Right Fibula, Percutaneous Endoscopic Approach	
0QHJ45Z	Insertion of External Fixation Device into Right Fibula, Percutaneous Endoscopic Approach	
0QHJ46Z	Insertion of Intramedullary Internal Fixation Device into Right Fibula, Percutaneous Endoscopic Approach	
0QHJ48Z	Insertion of Limb Lengthening External Fixation Device into Right Fibula, Percutaneous Endoscopic Approach	

0QHJ4BZ	Insertion of Monoplanar External Fixation Device into Right Fibula, Percutaneous Endoscopic Approach
0QHJ4CZ	Insertion of Ring External Fixation Device into Right Fibula, Percutaneous Endoscopic Approach
0QHJ4DZ	Insertion of Hybrid External Fixation Device into Right Fibula, Percutaneous Endoscopic Approach
0QHK04Z	Insertion of Internal Fixation Device into Left Fibula, Open Approach
0QHK05Z	Insertion of External Fixation Device into Left Fibula, Open Approach
0QHK06Z	Insertion of Intramedullary Internal Fixation Device into Left Fibula, Open Approach
0QHK08Z	Insertion of Limb Lengthening External Fixation Device into Left Fibula, Open Approach
0QHK0BZ	Insertion of Monoplanar External Fixation Device into Left Fibula, Open Approach
0QHK0CZ	Insertion of Ring External Fixation Device into Left Fibula, Open Approach
0QHK0DZ	Insertion of Hybrid External Fixation Device into Left Fibula, Open Approach
0QHK34Z	Insertion of Internal Fixation Device into Left Fibula, Percutaneous Approach
0QHK35Z	Insertion of External Fixation Device into Left Fibula, Percutaneous Approach
0QHK36Z	Insertion of Intramedullary Internal Fixation Device into Left Fibula, Percutaneous Approach
0QHK38Z	Insertion of Limb Lengthening External Fixation Device into Left Fibula, Percutaneous Approach
0QHK3BZ	Insertion of Monoplanar External Fixation Device into Left Fibula, Percutaneous Approach
0QHK3CZ	Insertion of Ring External Fixation Device into Left Fibula, Percutaneous Approach
0QHK3DZ	Insertion of Hybrid External Fixation Device into Left Fibula, Percutaneous Approach
0QHK44Z	Insertion of Internal Fixation Device into Left Fibula, Percutaneous Endoscopic Approach
0QHK45Z	Insertion of External Fixation Device into Left Fibula, Percutaneous Endoscopic Approach
0QHK46Z	Insertion of Intramedullary Internal Fixation Device into Left Fibula, Percutaneous Endoscopic Approach
0QHK48Z	Insertion of Limb Lengthening External Fixation Device into Left Fibula, Percutaneous Endoscopic Approach
0QHK4BZ	Insertion of Monoplanar External Fixation Device into Left Fibula, Percutaneous Endoscopic Approach
0QHK4CZ	Insertion of Ring External Fixation Device into Left Fibula, Percutaneous Endoscopic Approach
0QHK4DZ	Insertion of Hybrid External Fixation Device into Left Fibula, Percutaneous Endoscopic Approach
0QHL04Z	Insertion of Internal Fixation Device into Right Tarsal, Open Approach
0QHL05Z	Insertion of External Fixation Device into Right Tarsal, Open Approach
0QHL34Z	Insertion of Internal Fixation Device into Right Tarsal, Percutaneous Approach
0QHL35Z	Insertion of External Fixation Device into Right Tarsal, Percutaneous Approach
0QHL44Z	Insertion of Internal Fixation Device into Right Tarsal, Percutaneous Endoscopic Approach

0QHL45Z	Insertion of External Fixation Device into Right Tarsal, Percutaneous Endoscopic Approach
0QHM04Z	Insertion of Internal Fixation Device into Left Tarsal, Open Approach
0QHM05Z	Insertion of External Fixation Device into Left Tarsal, Open Approach
0QHM34Z	Insertion of Internal Fixation Device into Left Tarsal, Percutaneous Approach
0QHM35Z	Insertion of External Fixation Device into Left Tarsal, Percutaneous Approach
0QHM44Z	Insertion of Internal Fixation Device into Left Tarsal, Percutaneous Endoscopic Approach
0QHM45Z	Insertion of External Fixation Device into Left Tarsal, Percutaneous Endoscopic Approach
0QHN04Z	Insertion of Internal Fixation Device into Right Metatarsal, Open Approach
0QHN05Z	Insertion of External Fixation Device into Right Metatarsal, Open Approach
0QHN34Z	Insertion of Internal Fixation Device into Right Metatarsal, Percutaneous Approach
0QHN35Z	Insertion of External Fixation Device into Right Metatarsal, Percutaneous Approach
0QHN44Z	Insertion of Internal Fixation Device into Right Metatarsal, Percutaneous Endoscopic Approach
0QHN45Z	Insertion of External Fixation Device into Right Metatarsal, Percutaneous Endoscopic Approach
0QHP04Z	Insertion of Internal Fixation Device into Left Metatarsal, Open Approach
0QHP05Z	Insertion of External Fixation Device into Left Metatarsal, Open Approach
0QHP34Z	Insertion of Internal Fixation Device into Left Metatarsal, Percutaneous Approach
0QHP35Z	Insertion of External Fixation Device into Left Metatarsal, Percutaneous Approach
0QHP44Z	Insertion of Internal Fixation Device into Left Metatarsal, Percutaneous Endoscopic Approach
0QHP45Z	Insertion of External Fixation Device into Left Metatarsal, Percutaneous Endoscopic Approach
0QHQ04Z	Insertion of Internal Fixation Device into Right Toe Phalanx, Open Approach
0QHQ05Z	Insertion of External Fixation Device into Right Toe Phalanx, Open Approach
0QHQ34Z	Insertion of Internal Fixation Device into Right Toe Phalanx, Percutaneous Approach
0QHQ35Z	Insertion of External Fixation Device into Right Toe Phalanx, Percutaneous Approach
0QHQ44Z	Insertion of Internal Fixation Device into Right Toe Phalanx, Percutaneous Endoscopic Approach
0QHQ45Z	Insertion of External Fixation Device into Right Toe Phalanx, Percutaneous Endoscopic Approach
0QHR04Z	Insertion of Internal Fixation Device into Left Toe Phalanx, Open Approach
0QHR05Z	Insertion of External Fixation Device into Left Toe Phalanx, Open Approach
0QHR34Z	Insertion of Internal Fixation Device into Left Toe Phalanx, Percutaneous Approach
0QHR35Z	Insertion of External Fixation Device into Left Toe Phalanx, Percutaneous Approach
0QHR44Z	Insertion of Internal Fixation Device into Left Toe Phalanx, Percutaneous Endoscopic Approach
0QHR45Z	Insertion of External Fixation Device into Left Toe Phalanx, Percutaneous Endoscopic Approach

HS04Z	Insertion of Internal Fixation Device into Coccyx, Open Approach	0QHS44Z	Insertion of Internal Fixation Device into Coccyx, Percutaneous Endoscopic Approach	0QHY3MZ	Insertion of Bone Growth Stimulator into Lower Bone, Percutaneous Approach
HS05Z	Insertion of External Fixation Device into Coccyx, Open Approach			0QHY4MZ	Insertion of Bone Growth Stimulator into Lower Bone, Percutaneous Endoscopic Approach
HS34Z	Insertion of Internal Fixation Device into Coccyx, Percutaneous Approach	0QHS45Z	Insertion of External Fixation Device into Coccyx, Percutaneous Endoscopic Approach		
HS35Z	Insertion of External Fixation Device into Coccyx, Percutaneous Approach	0QHY0MZ	Insertion of Bone Growth Stimulator into Lower Bone, Open Approach		

QJ – Lower Bones, Inspection

Review Coding Guideline B3.5

Review Coding Guidelines B3.11a, B3.11b and B3.11c

QJY0ZZ	Inspection of Lower Bone, Open Approach	0QJY4ZZ	Inspection of Lower Bone, Percutaneous Endoscopic Approach
QJY3ZZ	Inspection of Lower Bone, Percutaneous Approach	0QJYXZZ	Inspection of Lower Bone, External Approach

QN – Lower Bones, Release

Review Coding Guideline B3.13

Review Coding Guideline B3.14

QN00ZZ	Release Lumbar Vertebra, Open Approach	0QN83ZZ	Release Right Femoral Shaft, Percutaneous Approach	0QNJ4ZZ	Release Right Fibula, Percutaneous Endoscopic Approach
QN03ZZ	Release Lumbar Vertebra, Percutaneous Approach	0QN84ZZ	Release Right Femoral Shaft, Percutaneous Endoscopic Approach	0QNK0ZZ	Release Left Fibula, Open Approach
QN04ZZ	Release Lumbar Vertebra, Percutaneous Endoscopic Approach	0QN90ZZ	Release Left Femoral Shaft, Open Approach	0QNK3ZZ	Release Left Fibula, Percutaneous Approach
QN10ZZ	Release Sacrum, Open Approach	0QN93ZZ	Release Left Femoral Shaft, Percutaneous Approach	0QNK4ZZ	Release Left Fibula, Percutaneous Endoscopic Approach
QN13ZZ	Release Sacrum, Percutaneous Approach	0QN94ZZ	Release Left Femoral Shaft, Percutaneous Endoscopic Approach	0QNL0ZZ	Release Right Tarsal, Open Approach
QN14ZZ	Release Sacrum, Percutaneous Endoscopic Approach	0QNB0ZZ	Release Right Lower Femur, Open Approach	0QNL3ZZ	Release Right Tarsal, Percutaneous Approach
QN20ZZ	Release Right Pelvic Bone, Open Approach	0QNB3ZZ	Release Right Lower Femur, Percutaneous Approach	0QNL4ZZ	Release Right Tarsal, Percutaneous Endoscopic Approach
QN23ZZ	Release Right Pelvic Bone, Percutaneous Approach	0QNB4ZZ	Release Right Lower Femur, Percutaneous Endoscopic Approach	0QNM0ZZ	Release Left Tarsal, Open Approach
QN24ZZ	Release Right Pelvic Bone, Percutaneous Endoscopic Approach	0QNC0ZZ	Release Left Lower Femur, Open Approach	0QNM3ZZ	Release Left Tarsal, Percutaneous Approach
QN30ZZ	Release Left Pelvic Bone, Open Approach	0QNC3ZZ	Release Left Lower Femur, Percutaneous Approach	0QNM4ZZ	Release Left Tarsal, Percutaneous Endoscopic Approach
QN33ZZ	Release Left Pelvic Bone, Percutaneous Approach	0QNC4ZZ	Release Left Lower Femur, Percutaneous Endoscopic Approach	0QNN0ZZ	Release Right Metatarsal, Open Approach
QN34ZZ	Release Left Pelvic Bone, Percutaneous Endoscopic Approach	0QND0ZZ	Release Right Patella, Open Approach	0QNN3ZZ	Release Right Metatarsal, Percutaneous Approach
QN40ZZ	Release Right Acetabulum, Open Approach	0QND3ZZ	Release Right Patella, Percutaneous Approach	0QNN4ZZ	Release Right Metatarsal, Percutaneous Endoscopic Approach
QN43ZZ	Release Right Acetabulum, Percutaneous Approach	0QND4ZZ	Release Right Patella, Percutaneous Endoscopic Approach	0QNP0ZZ	Release Left Metatarsal, Open Approach
QN44ZZ	Release Right Acetabulum, Percutaneous Endoscopic Approach	0QNF0ZZ	Release Left Patella, Open Approach	0QNP3ZZ	Release Left Metatarsal, Percutaneous Approach
QN50ZZ	Release Left Acetabulum, Open Approach	0QNF3ZZ	Release Left Patella, Percutaneous Approach	0QNP4ZZ	Release Left Metatarsal, Percutaneous Endoscopic Approach
QN53ZZ	Release Left Acetabulum, Percutaneous Approach	0QNF4ZZ	Release Left Patella, Percutaneous Endoscopic Approach	0QNQ0ZZ	Release Right Toe Phalanx, Open Approach
QN54ZZ	Release Left Acetabulum, Percutaneous Endoscopic Approach	0QNG0ZZ	Release Right Tibia, Open Approach	0QNQ3ZZ	Release Right Toe Phalanx, Percutaneous Approach
QN60ZZ	Release Right Upper Femur, Open Approach	0QNG3ZZ	Release Right Tibia, Percutaneous Approach	0QNQ4ZZ	Release Right Toe Phalanx, Percutaneous Endoscopic Approach
QN63ZZ	Release Right Upper Femur, Percutaneous Approach	0QNG4ZZ	Release Right Tibia, Percutaneous Endoscopic Approach	0QNR0ZZ	Release Left Toe Phalanx, Open Approach
QN64ZZ	Release Right Upper Femur, Percutaneous Endoscopic Approach	0QNH0ZZ	Release Left Tibia, Open Approach	0QNR3ZZ	Release Left Toe Phalanx, Percutaneous Approach
QN70ZZ	Release Left Upper Femur, Open Approach	0QNH3ZZ	Release Left Tibia, Percutaneous Approach	0QNR4ZZ	Release Left Toe Phalanx, Percutaneous Endoscopic Approach
QN73ZZ	Release Left Upper Femur, Percutaneous Approach	0QNH4ZZ	Release Left Tibia, Percutaneous Endoscopic Approach	0QNS0ZZ	Release Coccyx, Open Approach
QN74ZZ	Release Left Upper Femur, Percutaneous Endoscopic Approach	0QNJ0ZZ	Release Right Fibula, Open Approach	0QNS3ZZ	Release Coccyx, Percutaneous Approach
QN80ZZ	Release Right Femoral Shaft, Open Approach	0QNJ3ZZ	Release Right Fibula, Percutaneous Approach	0QNS4ZZ	Release Coccyx, Percutaneous Endoscopic Approach

QP – Lower Bones, Removal

Review Coding Guideline B6.1c

QP004Z	Removal of Internal Fixation Device from Lumbar Vertebra, Open Approach	0QP007Z	Removal of Autologous Tissue Substitute from Lumbar Vertebra, Open Approach	0QP00JZ	Removal of Synthetic Substitute from Lumbar Vertebra, Open Approach

♀ Female-only   ♂ Male-only   ▲ Limited Coverage   ● Non-OR   ■ HAC-associated procedure   ▲ Non-covered procedures   ✚ Combination

0QP00KZ Removal of Nonautologous Tissue Substitute from Lumbar Vertebra, Open Approach

0QP034Z Removal of Internal Fixation Device from Lumbar Vertebra, Percutaneous Approach

0QP037Z Removal of Autologous Tissue Substitute from Lumbar Vertebra, Percutaneous Approach

0QP03JZ Removal of Synthetic Substitute from Lumbar Vertebra, Percutaneous Approach

0QP03KZ Removal of Nonautologous Tissue Substitute from Lumbar Vertebra, Percutaneous Approach

0QP044Z Removal of Internal Fixation Device from Lumbar Vertebra, Percutaneous Endoscopic Approach

0QP047Z Removal of Autologous Tissue Substitute from Lumbar Vertebra, Percutaneous Endoscopic Approach

0QP04JZ Removal of Synthetic Substitute from Lumbar Vertebra, Percutaneous Endoscopic Approach

0QP04KZ Removal of Nonautologous Tissue Substitute from Lumbar Vertebra, Percutaneous Endoscopic Approach

0QP0X4Z Removal of Internal Fixation Device from Lumbar Vertebra, External Approach

0QP104Z Removal of Internal Fixation Device from Sacrum, Open Approach

0QP107Z Removal of Autologous Tissue Substitute from Sacrum, Open Approach

0QP10JZ Removal of Synthetic Substitute from Sacrum, Open Approach

0QP10KZ Removal of Nonautologous Tissue Substitute from Sacrum, Open Approach

0QP134Z Removal of Internal Fixation Device from Sacrum, Percutaneous Approach

0QP137Z Removal of Autologous Tissue Substitute from Sacrum, Percutaneous Approach

0QP13JZ Removal of Synthetic Substitute from Sacrum, Percutaneous Approach

0QP13KZ Removal of Nonautologous Tissue Substitute from Sacrum, Percutaneous Approach

0QP144Z Removal of Internal Fixation Device from Sacrum, Percutaneous Endoscopic Approach

0QP147Z Removal of Autologous Tissue Substitute from Sacrum, Percutaneous Endoscopic Approach

0QP14JZ Removal of Synthetic Substitute from Sacrum, Percutaneous Endoscopic Approach

0QP14KZ Removal of Nonautologous Tissue Substitute from Sacrum, Percutaneous Endoscopic Approach

0QP1X4Z Removal of Internal Fixation Device from Sacrum, External Approach

0QP204Z Removal of Internal Fixation Device from Right Pelvic Bone, Open Approach

0QP205Z Removal of External Fixation Device from Right Pelvic Bone, Open Approach

0QP207Z Removal of Autologous Tissue Substitute from Right Pelvic Bone, Open Approach

0QP20JZ Removal of Synthetic Substitute from Right Pelvic Bone, Open Approach

0QP20KZ Removal of Nonautologous Tissue Substitute from Right Pelvic Bone, Open Approach

0QP234Z Removal of Internal Fixation Device from Right Pelvic Bone, Percutaneous Approach

0QP235Z Removal of External Fixation Device from Right Pelvic Bone, Percutaneous Approach

0QP237Z Removal of Autologous Tissue Substitute from Right Pelvic Bone, Percutaneous Approach

0QP23JZ Removal of Synthetic Substitute from Right Pelvic Bone, Percutaneous Approach

0QP23KZ Removal of Nonautologous Tissue Substitute from Right Pelvic Bone, Percutaneous Approach

0QP244Z Removal of Internal Fixation Device from Right Pelvic Bone, Percutaneous Endoscopic Approach

0QP245Z Removal of External Fixation Device from Right Pelvic Bone, Percutaneous Endoscopic Approach

0QP247Z Removal of Autologous Tissue Substitute from Right Pelvic Bone, Percutaneous Endoscopic Approach

0QP24JZ Removal of Synthetic Substitute from Right Pelvic Bone, Percutaneous Endoscopic Approach

0QP24KZ Removal of Nonautologous Tissue Substitute from Right Pelvic Bone, Percutaneous Endoscopic Approach

0QP2X4Z Removal of Internal Fixation Device from Right Pelvic Bone, External Approach

0QP2X5Z Removal of External Fixation Device from Right Pelvic Bone, External Approach

0QP304Z Removal of Internal Fixation Device from Left Pelvic Bone, Open Approach

0QP305Z Removal of External Fixation Device from Left Pelvic Bone, Open Approach

0QP307Z Removal of Autologous Tissue Substitute from Left Pelvic Bone, Open Approach

0QP30JZ Removal of Synthetic Substitute from Left Pelvic Bone, Open Approach

0QP30KZ Removal of Nonautologous Tissue Substitute from Left Pelvic Bone, Open Approach

0QP334Z Removal of Internal Fixation Device from Left Pelvic Bone, Percutaneous Approach

0QP335Z Removal of External Fixation Device from Left Pelvic Bone, Percutaneous Approach

0QP337Z Removal of Autologous Tissue Substitute from Left Pelvic Bone, Percutaneous Approach

0QP33JZ Removal of Synthetic Substitute from Left Pelvic Bone, Percutaneous Approach

0QP33KZ Removal of Nonautologous Tissue Substitute from Left Pelvic Bone, Percutaneous Approach

0QP344Z Removal of Internal Fixation Device from Left Pelvic Bone, Percutaneous Endoscopic Approach

0QP345Z Removal of External Fixation Device from Left Pelvic Bone, Percutaneous Endoscopic Approach

0QP347Z Removal of Autologous Tissue Substitute from Left Pelvic Bone, Percutaneous Endoscopic Approach

0QP34JZ Removal of Synthetic Substitute from Left Pelvic Bone, Percutaneous Endoscopic Approach

0QP34KZ Removal of Nonautologous Tissue Substitute from Left Pelvic Bone, Percutaneous Endoscopic Approach

0QP3X4Z Removal of Internal Fixation Device from Left Pelvic Bone, External Approach

0QP3X5Z Removal of External Fixation Device from Left Pelvic Bone, External Approach

0QP404Z Removal of Internal Fixation Device from Right Acetabulum, Open Approach

0QP407Z Removal of Autologous Tissue Substitute from Right Acetabulum, Open Approach

0QP40JZ Removal of Synthetic Substitute from Right Acetabulum, Open Approach

0QP40KZ Removal of Nonautologous Tissue Substitute from Right Acetabulum, Open Approach

0QP434Z Removal of Internal Fixation Device from Right Acetabulum, Percutaneous Approach

0QP437Z Removal of Autologous Tissue Substitute from Right Acetabulum, Percutaneous Approach

0QP43JZ Removal of Synthetic Substitute from Right Acetabulum, Percutaneous Approach

0QP43KZ Removal of Nonautologous Tissue Substitute from Right Acetabulum, Percutaneous Approach

0QP444Z Removal of Internal Fixation Device from Right Acetabulum, Percutaneous Endoscopic Approach

0QP447Z Removal of Autologous Tissue Substitute from Right Acetabulum, Percutaneous Endoscopic Approach

0QP44JZ Removal of Synthetic Substitute from Right Acetabulum, Percutaneous Endoscopic Approach

0QP44KZ Removal of Nonautologous Tissue Substitute from Right Acetabulum, Percutaneous Endoscopic Approach

0QP4X4Z Removal of Internal Fixation Device from Right Acetabulum, External Approach

0QP504Z Removal of Internal Fixation Device from Left Acetabulum, Open Approach

0QP507Z Removal of Autologous Tissue Substitute from Left Acetabulum, Open Approach

0QP50JZ Removal of Synthetic Substitute from Left Acetabulum, Open Approach

0QP50KZ Removal of Nonautologous Tissue Substitute from Left Acetabulum, Open Approach

0QP534Z Removal of Internal Fixation Device from Left Acetabulum, Percutaneous Approach

0QP537Z Removal of Autologous Tissue Substitute from Left Acetabulum, Percutaneous Approach

0QP53JZ Removal of Synthetic Substitute from Left Acetabulum, Percutaneous Approach

0QP53KZ Removal of Nonautologous Tissue Substitute from Left Acetabulum, Percutaneous Approach

0QP544Z Removal of Internal Fixation Device from Left Acetabulum, Percutaneous Endoscopic Approach

0QP547Z Removal of Autologous Tissue Substitute from Left Acetabulum, Percutaneous Endoscopic Approach

0QP54JZ Removal of Synthetic Substitute from Left Acetabulum, Percutaneous Endoscopic Approach

0QP54KZ Removal of Nonautologous Tissue Substitute from Left Acetabulum, Percutaneous Endoscopic Approach

0QP5X4Z Removal of Internal Fixation Device from Left Acetabulum, External Approach

0QP604Z Removal of Internal Fixation Device from Right Upper Femur, Open Approach

0QP605Z Removal of External Fixation Device from Right Upper Femur, Open Approach

0QP607Z Removal of Autologous Tissue Substitute from Right Upper Femur, Open Approach

0QP60JZ Removal of Synthetic Substitute from Right Upper Femur, Open Approach

0QP60KZ Removal of Nonautologous Tissue Substitute from Right Upper Femur, Open Approach

0QP634Z Removal of Internal Fixation Device from Right Upper Femur, Percutaneous Approach

P635Z Removal of External Fixation Device from Right Upper Femur, Percutaneous Approach

P637Z Removal of Autologous Tissue Substitute from Right Upper Femur, Percutaneous Approach

P63JZ Removal of Synthetic Substitute from Right Upper Femur, Percutaneous Approach

P63KZ Removal of Nonautologous Tissue Substitute from Right Upper Femur, Percutaneous Approach

P644Z Removal of Internal Fixation Device from Right Upper Femur, Percutaneous Endoscopic Approach

P645Z Removal of External Fixation Device from Right Upper Femur, Percutaneous Endoscopic Approach

P647Z Removal of Autologous Tissue Substitute from Right Upper Femur, Percutaneous Endoscopic Approach

P64JZ Removal of Synthetic Substitute from Right Upper Femur, Percutaneous Endoscopic Approach

P64KZ Removal of Nonautologous Tissue Substitute from Right Upper Femur, Percutaneous Endoscopic Approach

P6X4Z Removal of Internal Fixation Device from Right Upper Femur, External Approach

P6X5Z Removal of External Fixation Device from Right Upper Femur, External Approach

P704Z Removal of Internal Fixation Device from Left Upper Femur, Open Approach

P705Z Removal of External Fixation Device from Left Upper Femur, Open Approach

P707Z Removal of Autologous Tissue Substitute from Left Upper Femur, Open Approach

P70JZ Removal of Synthetic Substitute from Left Upper Femur, Open Approach

P70KZ Removal of Nonautologous Tissue Substitute from Left Upper Femur, Open Approach

P734Z Removal of Internal Fixation Device from Left Upper Femur, Percutaneous Approach

P735Z Removal of External Fixation Device from Left Upper Femur, Percutaneous Approach

P737Z Removal of Autologous Tissue Substitute from Left Upper Femur, Percutaneous Approach

P73JZ Removal of Synthetic Substitute from Left Upper Femur, Percutaneous Approach

P73KZ Removal of Nonautologous Tissue Substitute from Left Upper Femur, Percutaneous Approach

P744Z Removal of Internal Fixation Device from Left Upper Femur, Percutaneous Endoscopic Approach

P745Z Removal of External Fixation Device from Left Upper Femur, Percutaneous Endoscopic Approach

P747Z Removal of Autologous Tissue Substitute from Left Upper Femur, Percutaneous Endoscopic Approach

P74JZ Removal of Synthetic Substitute from Left Upper Femur, Percutaneous Endoscopic Approach

P74KZ Removal of Nonautologous Tissue Substitute from Left Upper Femur, Percutaneous Endoscopic Approach

P7X4Z Removal of Internal Fixation Device from Left Upper Femur, External Approach

P7X5Z Removal of External Fixation Device from Left Upper Femur, External Approach

P804Z Removal of Internal Fixation Device from Right Femoral Shaft, Open Approach

0QP805Z Removal of External Fixation Device from Right Femoral Shaft, Open Approach

0QP807Z Removal of Autologous Tissue Substitute from Right Femoral Shaft, Open Approach

0QP80JZ Removal of Synthetic Substitute from Right Femoral Shaft, Open Approach

0QP80KZ Removal of Nonautologous Tissue Substitute from Right Femoral Shaft, Open Approach

0QP834Z Removal of Internal Fixation Device from Right Femoral Shaft, Percutaneous Approach

0QP835Z Removal of External Fixation Device from Right Femoral Shaft, Percutaneous Approach

0QP837Z Removal of Autologous Tissue Substitute from Right Femoral Shaft, Percutaneous Approach

0QP83JZ Removal of Synthetic Substitute from Right Femoral Shaft, Percutaneous Approach

0QP83KZ Removal of Nonautologous Tissue Substitute from Right Femoral Shaft, Percutaneous Approach

0QP844Z Removal of Internal Fixation Device from Right Femoral Shaft, Percutaneous Endoscopic Approach

0QP845Z Removal of External Fixation Device from Right Femoral Shaft, Percutaneous Endoscopic Approach

0QP847Z Removal of Autologous Tissue Substitute from Right Femoral Shaft, Percutaneous Endoscopic Approach

0QP84JZ Removal of Synthetic Substitute from Right Femoral Shaft, Percutaneous Endoscopic Approach

0QP84KZ Removal of Nonautologous Tissue Substitute from Right Femoral Shaft, Percutaneous Endoscopic Approach

0QP8X4Z Removal of Internal Fixation Device from Right Femoral Shaft, External Approach

0QP8X5Z Removal of External Fixation Device from Right Femoral Shaft, External Approach

0QP904Z Removal of Internal Fixation Device from Left Femoral Shaft, Open Approach

0QP905Z Removal of External Fixation Device from Left Femoral Shaft, Open Approach

0QP907Z Removal of Autologous Tissue Substitute from Left Femoral Shaft, Open Approach

0QP90JZ Removal of Synthetic Substitute from Left Femoral Shaft, Open Approach

0QP90KZ Removal of Nonautologous Tissue Substitute from Left Femoral Shaft, Open Approach

0QP934Z Removal of Internal Fixation Device from Left Femoral Shaft, Percutaneous Approach

0QP935Z Removal of External Fixation Device from Left Femoral Shaft, Percutaneous Approach

0QP937Z Removal of Autologous Tissue Substitute from Left Femoral Shaft, Percutaneous Approach

0QP93JZ Removal of Synthetic Substitute from Left Femoral Shaft, Percutaneous Approach

0QP93KZ Removal of Nonautologous Tissue Substitute from Left Femoral Shaft, Percutaneous Approach

0QP944Z Removal of Internal Fixation Device from Left Femoral Shaft, Percutaneous Endoscopic Approach

0QP945Z Removal of External Fixation Device from Left Femoral Shaft, Percutaneous Endoscopic Approach

0QP947Z Removal of Autologous Tissue Substitute from Left Femoral Shaft, Percutaneous Endoscopic Approach

0QP94JZ Removal of Synthetic Substitute from Left Femoral Shaft, Percutaneous Endoscopic Approach

0QP94KZ Removal of Nonautologous Tissue Substitute from Left Femoral Shaft, Percutaneous Endoscopic Approach

0QP9X4Z Removal of Internal Fixation Device from Left Femoral Shaft, External Approach

0QP9X5Z Removal of External Fixation Device from Left Femoral Shaft, External Approach

0QPB04Z Removal of Internal Fixation Device from Right Lower Femur, Open Approach

0QPB05Z Removal of External Fixation Device from Right Lower Femur, Open Approach

0QPB07Z Removal of Autologous Tissue Substitute from Right Lower Femur, Open Approach

0QPB0JZ Removal of Synthetic Substitute from Right Lower Femur, Open Approach

0QPB0KZ Removal of Nonautologous Tissue Substitute from Right Lower Femur, Open Approach

0QPB34Z Removal of Internal Fixation Device from Right Lower Femur, Percutaneous Approach

0QPB35Z Removal of External Fixation Device from Right Lower Femur, Percutaneous Approach

0QPB37Z Removal of Autologous Tissue Substitute from Right Lower Femur, Percutaneous Approach

0QPB3JZ Removal of Synthetic Substitute from Right Lower Femur, Percutaneous Approach

0QPB3KZ Removal of Nonautologous Tissue Substitute from Right Lower Femur, Percutaneous Approach

0QPB44Z Removal of Internal Fixation Device from Right Lower Femur, Percutaneous Endoscopic Approach

0QPB45Z Removal of External Fixation Device from Right Lower Femur, Percutaneous Endoscopic Approach

0QPB47Z Removal of Autologous Tissue Substitute from Right Lower Femur, Percutaneous Endoscopic Approach

0QPB4JZ Removal of Synthetic Substitute from Right Lower Femur, Percutaneous Endoscopic Approach

0QPB4KZ Removal of Nonautologous Tissue Substitute from Right Lower Femur, Percutaneous Endoscopic Approach

0QPBX4Z Removal of Internal Fixation Device from Right Lower Femur, External Approach

0QPBX5Z Removal of External Fixation Device from Right Lower Femur, External Approach

0QPC04Z Removal of Internal Fixation Device from Left Lower Femur, Open Approach

0QPC05Z Removal of External Fixation Device from Left Lower Femur, Open Approach

0QPC07Z Removal of Autologous Tissue Substitute from Left Lower Femur, Open Approach

0QPC0JZ Removal of Synthetic Substitute from Left Lower Femur, Open Approach

0QPC0KZ Removal of Nonautologous Tissue Substitute from Left Lower Femur, Open Approach

0QPC34Z Removal of Internal Fixation Device from Left Lower Femur, Percutaneous Approach

0QPC35Z Removal of External Fixation Device from Left Lower Femur, Percutaneous Approach

0QPC37Z Removal of Autologous Tissue Substitute from Left Lower Femur, Percutaneous Approach

Female-only   ♂ Male-only   ▲ Limited Coverage   ● Non-OR   ■ HAC-associated procedure   ▲ Non-covered procedures   ✛ Combination

0QPC3JZ Removal of Synthetic Substitute from Left Lower Femur, Percutaneous Approach

0QPC3KZ Removal of Nonautologous Tissue Substitute from Left Lower Femur, Percutaneous Approach

0QPC44Z Removal of Internal Fixation Device from Left Lower Femur, Percutaneous Endoscopic Approach

0QPC45Z Removal of External Fixation Device from Left Lower Femur, Percutaneous Endoscopic Approach

0QPC47Z Removal of Autologous Tissue Substitute from Left Lower Femur, Percutaneous Endoscopic Approach

0QPC4JZ Removal of Synthetic Substitute from Left Lower Femur, Percutaneous Endoscopic Approach

0QPC4KZ Removal of Nonautologous Tissue Substitute from Left Lower Femur, Percutaneous Endoscopic Approach

0QPCX4Z Removal of Internal Fixation Device from Left Lower Femur, External Approach

0QPCX5Z Removal of External Fixation Device from Left Lower Femur, External Approach

0QPD04Z Removal of Internal Fixation Device from Right Patella, Open Approach

0QPD05Z Removal of External Fixation Device from Right Patella, Open Approach

0QPD07Z Removal of Autologous Tissue Substitute from Right Patella, Open Approach

0QPD0JZ Removal of Synthetic Substitute from Right Patella, Open Approach

0QPD0KZ Removal of Nonautologous Tissue Substitute from Right Patella, Open Approach

0QPD34Z Removal of Internal Fixation Device from Right Patella, Percutaneous Approach

0QPD35Z Removal of External Fixation Device from Right Patella, Percutaneous Approach

0QPD37Z Removal of Autologous Tissue Substitute from Right Patella, Percutaneous Approach

0QPD3JZ Removal of Synthetic Substitute from Right Patella, Percutaneous Approach

0QPD3KZ Removal of Nonautologous Tissue Substitute from Right Patella, Percutaneous Approach

0QPD44Z Removal of Internal Fixation Device from Right Patella, Percutaneous Endoscopic Approach

0QPD45Z Removal of External Fixation Device from Right Patella, Percutaneous Endoscopic Approach

0QPD47Z Removal of Autologous Tissue Substitute from Right Patella, Percutaneous Endoscopic Approach

0QPD4JZ Removal of Synthetic Substitute from Right Patella, Percutaneous Endoscopic Approach

0QPD4KZ Removal of Nonautologous Tissue Substitute from Right Patella, Percutaneous Endoscopic Approach

0QPDX4Z Removal of Internal Fixation Device from Right Patella, External Approach

0QPDX5Z Removal of External Fixation Device from Right Patella, External Approach

0QPF04Z Removal of Internal Fixation Device from Left Patella, Open Approach

0QPF05Z Removal of External Fixation Device from Left Patella, Open Approach

0QPF07Z Removal of Autologous Tissue Substitute from Left Patella, Open Approach

0QPF0JZ Removal of Synthetic Substitute from Left Patella, Open Approach

0QPF0KZ Removal of Nonautologous Tissue Substitute from Left Patella, Open Approach

0QPF34Z Removal of Internal Fixation Device from Left Patella, Percutaneous Approach

0QPF35Z Removal of External Fixation Device from Left Patella, Percutaneous Approach

0QPF37Z Removal of Autologous Tissue Substitute from Left Patella, Percutaneous Approach

0QPF3JZ Removal of Synthetic Substitute from Left Patella, Percutaneous Approach

0QPF3KZ Removal of Nonautologous Tissue Substitute from Left Patella, Percutaneous Approach

0QPF44Z Removal of Internal Fixation Device from Left Patella, Percutaneous Endoscopic Approach

0QPF45Z Removal of External Fixation Device from Left Patella, Percutaneous Endoscopic Approach

0QPF47Z Removal of Autologous Tissue Substitute from Left Patella, Percutaneous Endoscopic Approach

0QPF4JZ Removal of Synthetic Substitute from Left Patella, Percutaneous Endoscopic Approach

0QPF4KZ Removal of Nonautologous Tissue Substitute from Left Patella, Percutaneous Endoscopic Approach

0QPFX4Z Removal of Internal Fixation Device from Left Patella, External Approach

0QPFX5Z Removal of External Fixation Device from Left Patella, External Approach

0QPG04Z Removal of Internal Fixation Device from Right Tibia, Open Approach

0QPG05Z Removal of External Fixation Device from Right Tibia, Open Approach

0QPG07Z Removal of Autologous Tissue Substitute from Right Tibia, Open Approach

0QPG0JZ Removal of Synthetic Substitute from Right Tibia, Open Approach

0QPG0KZ Removal of Nonautologous Tissue Substitute from Right Tibia, Open Approach

0QPG34Z Removal of Internal Fixation Device from Right Tibia, Percutaneous Approach

0QPG35Z Removal of External Fixation Device from Right Tibia, Percutaneous Approach

0QPG37Z Removal of Autologous Tissue Substitute from Right Tibia, Percutaneous Approach

0QPG3JZ Removal of Synthetic Substitute from Right Tibia, Percutaneous Approach

0QPG3KZ Removal of Nonautologous Tissue Substitute from Right Tibia, Percutaneous Approach

0QPG44Z Removal of Internal Fixation Device from Right Tibia, Percutaneous Endoscopic Approach

0QPG45Z Removal of External Fixation Device from Right Tibia, Percutaneous Endoscopic Approach

0QPG47Z Removal of Autologous Tissue Substitute from Right Tibia, Percutaneous Endoscopic Approach

0QPG4JZ Removal of Synthetic Substitute from Right Tibia, Percutaneous Endoscopic Approach

0QPG4KZ Removal of Nonautologous Tissue Substitute from Right Tibia, Percutaneous Endoscopic Approach

0QPGX4Z Removal of Internal Fixation Device from Right Tibia, External Approach

0QPGX5Z Removal of External Fixation Device from Right Tibia, External Approach

0QPH04Z Removal of Internal Fixation Device from Left Tibia, Open Approach

0QPH05Z Removal of External Fixation Device from Left Tibia, Open Approach

0QPH07Z Removal of Autologous Tissue Substitute from Left Tibia, Open Approach

0QPH0JZ Removal of Synthetic Substitute from Left Tibia, Open Approach

0QPH0KZ Removal of Nonautologous Tissue Substitute from Left Tibia, Open Approach

0QPH34Z Removal of Internal Fixation Device from Left Tibia, Percutaneous Approach

0QPH35Z Removal of External Fixation Device from Left Tibia, Percutaneous Approach

0QPH37Z Removal of Autologous Tissue Substitute from Left Tibia, Percutaneous Approach

0QPH3JZ Removal of Synthetic Substitute from Left Tibia, Percutaneous Approach

0QPH3KZ Removal of Nonautologous Tissue Substitute from Left Tibia, Percutaneous Approach

0QPH44Z Removal of Internal Fixation Device from Left Tibia, Percutaneous Endoscopic Approach

0QPH45Z Removal of External Fixation Device from Left Tibia, Percutaneous Endoscopic Approach

0QPH47Z Removal of Autologous Tissue Substitute from Left Tibia, Percutaneous Endoscopic Approach

0QPH4JZ Removal of Synthetic Substitute from Left Tibia, Percutaneous Endoscopic Approach

0QPH4KZ Removal of Nonautologous Tissue Substitute from Left Tibia, Percutaneous Endoscopic Approach

0QPHX4Z Removal of Internal Fixation Device from Left Tibia, External Approach

0QPHX5Z Removal of External Fixation Device from Left Tibia, External Approach

0QPJ04Z Removal of Internal Fixation Device from Right Fibula, Open Approach

0QPJ05Z Removal of External Fixation Device from Right Fibula, Open Approach

0QPJ07Z Removal of Autologous Tissue Substitute from Right Fibula, Open Approach

0QPJ0JZ Removal of Synthetic Substitute from Right Fibula, Open Approach

0QPJ0KZ Removal of Nonautologous Tissue Substitute from Right Fibula, Open Approach

0QPJ34Z Removal of Internal Fixation Device from Right Fibula, Percutaneous Approach

0QPJ35Z Removal of External Fixation Device from Right Fibula, Percutaneous Approach

0QPJ37Z Removal of Autologous Tissue Substitute from Right Fibula, Percutaneous Approach

0QPJ3JZ Removal of Synthetic Substitute from Right Fibula, Percutaneous Approach

0QPJ3KZ Removal of Nonautologous Tissue Substitute from Right Fibula, Percutaneous Approach

0QPJ44Z Removal of Internal Fixation Device from Right Fibula, Percutaneous Endoscopic Approach

0QPJ45Z Removal of External Fixation Device from Right Fibula, Percutaneous Endoscopic Approach

0QPJ47Z Removal of Autologous Tissue Substitute from Right Fibula, Percutaneous Endoscopic Approach

PJ4JZ Removal of Synthetic Substitute from Right Fibula, Percutaneous Endoscopic Approach

PJ4KZ Removal of Nonautologous Tissue Substitute from Right Fibula, Percutaneous Endoscopic Approach

PJX4Z Removal of Internal Fixation Device from Right Fibula, External Approach

PJX5Z Removal of External Fixation Device from Right Fibula, External Approach

PK04Z Removal of Internal Fixation Device from Left Fibula, Open Approach

PK05Z Removal of External Fixation Device from Left Fibula, Open Approach

PK07Z Removal of Autologous Tissue Substitute from Left Fibula, Open Approach

PK0JZ Removal of Synthetic Substitute from Left Fibula, Open Approach

PK0KZ Removal of Nonautologous Tissue Substitute from Left Fibula, Open Approach

PK34Z Removal of Internal Fixation Device from Left Fibula, Percutaneous Approach

PK35Z Removal of External Fixation Device from Left Fibula, Percutaneous Approach

PK37Z Removal of Autologous Tissue Substitute from Left Fibula, Percutaneous Approach

PK3JZ Removal of Synthetic Substitute from Left Fibula, Percutaneous Approach

PK3KZ Removal of Nonautologous Tissue Substitute from Left Fibula, Percutaneous Approach

PK44Z Removal of Internal Fixation Device from Left Fibula, Percutaneous Endoscopic Approach

PK45Z Removal of External Fixation Device from Left Fibula, Percutaneous Endoscopic Approach

PK47Z Removal of Autologous Tissue Substitute from Left Fibula, Percutaneous Endoscopic Approach

PK4JZ Removal of Synthetic Substitute from Left Fibula, Percutaneous Endoscopic Approach

PK4KZ Removal of Nonautologous Tissue Substitute from Left Fibula, Percutaneous Endoscopic Approach

PKX4Z Removal of Internal Fixation Device from Left Fibula, External Approach

PKX5Z Removal of External Fixation Device from Left Fibula, External Approach

PL04Z Removal of Internal Fixation Device from Right Tarsal, Open Approach

PL05Z Removal of External Fixation Device from Right Tarsal, Open Approach

PL07Z Removal of Autologous Tissue Substitute from Right Tarsal, Open Approach

PL0JZ Removal of Synthetic Substitute from Right Tarsal, Open Approach

PL0KZ Removal of Nonautologous Tissue Substitute from Right Tarsal, Open Approach

PL34Z Removal of Internal Fixation Device from Right Tarsal, Percutaneous Approach

PL35Z Removal of External Fixation Device from Right Tarsal, Percutaneous Approach

PL37Z Removal of Autologous Tissue Substitute from Right Tarsal, Percutaneous Approach

PL3JZ Removal of Synthetic Substitute from Right Tarsal, Percutaneous Approach

PL3KZ Removal of Nonautologous Tissue Substitute from Right Tarsal, Percutaneous Approach

0QPL44Z Removal of Internal Fixation Device from Right Tarsal, Percutaneous Endoscopic Approach

0QPL45Z Removal of External Fixation Device from Right Tarsal, Percutaneous Endoscopic Approach

0QPL47Z Removal of Autologous Tissue Substitute from Right Tarsal, Percutaneous Endoscopic Approach

0QPL4JZ Removal of Synthetic Substitute from Right Tarsal, Percutaneous Endoscopic Approach

0QPL4KZ Removal of Nonautologous Tissue Substitute from Right Tarsal, Percutaneous Endoscopic Approach

0QPLX4Z Removal of Internal Fixation Device from Right Tarsal, External Approach

0QPLX5Z Removal of External Fixation Device from Right Tarsal, External Approach

0QPM04Z Removal of Internal Fixation Device from Left Tarsal, Open Approach

0QPM05Z Removal of External Fixation Device from Left Tarsal, Open Approach

0QPM07Z Removal of Autologous Tissue Substitute from Left Tarsal, Open Approach

0QPM0JZ Removal of Synthetic Substitute from Left Tarsal, Open Approach

0QPM0KZ Removal of Nonautologous Tissue Substitute from Left Tarsal, Open Approach

0QPM34Z Removal of Internal Fixation Device from Left Tarsal, Percutaneous Approach

0QPM35Z Removal of External Fixation Device from Left Tarsal, Percutaneous Approach

0QPM37Z Removal of Autologous Tissue Substitute from Left Tarsal, Percutaneous Approach

0QPM3JZ Removal of Synthetic Substitute from Left Tarsal, Percutaneous Approach

0QPM3KZ Removal of Nonautologous Tissue Substitute from Left Tarsal, Percutaneous Approach

0QPM44Z Removal of Internal Fixation Device from Left Tarsal, Percutaneous Endoscopic Approach

0QPM45Z Removal of External Fixation Device from Left Tarsal, Percutaneous Endoscopic Approach

0QPM47Z Removal of Autologous Tissue Substitute from Left Tarsal, Percutaneous Endoscopic Approach

0QPM4JZ Removal of Synthetic Substitute from Left Tarsal, Percutaneous Endoscopic Approach

0QPM4KZ Removal of Nonautologous Tissue Substitute from Left Tarsal, Percutaneous Endoscopic Approach

0QPMX4Z Removal of Internal Fixation Device from Left Tarsal, External Approach

0QPMX5Z Removal of External Fixation Device from Left Tarsal, External Approach

0QPN04Z Removal of Internal Fixation Device from Right Metatarsal, Open Approach

0QPN05Z Removal of External Fixation Device from Right Metatarsal, Open Approach

0QPN07Z Removal of Autologous Tissue Substitute from Right Metatarsal, Open Approach

0QPN0JZ Removal of Synthetic Substitute from Right Metatarsal, Open Approach

0QPN0KZ Removal of Nonautologous Tissue Substitute from Right Metatarsal, Open Approach

0QPN34Z Removal of Internal Fixation Device from Right Metatarsal, Percutaneous Approach

0QPN35Z Removal of External Fixation Device from Right Metatarsal, Percutaneous Approach

0QPN37Z Removal of Autologous Tissue Substitute from Right Metatarsal, Percutaneous Approach

0QPN3JZ Removal of Synthetic Substitute from Right Metatarsal, Percutaneous Approach

0QPN3KZ Removal of Nonautologous Tissue Substitute from Right Metatarsal, Percutaneous Approach

0QPN44Z Removal of Internal Fixation Device from Right Metatarsal, Percutaneous Endoscopic Approach

0QPN45Z Removal of External Fixation Device from Right Metatarsal, Percutaneous Endoscopic Approach

0QPN47Z Removal of Autologous Tissue Substitute from Right Metatarsal, Percutaneous Endoscopic Approach

0QPN4JZ Removal of Synthetic Substitute from Right Metatarsal, Percutaneous Endoscopic Approach

0QPN4KZ Removal of Nonautologous Tissue Substitute from Right Metatarsal, Percutaneous Endoscopic Approach

0QPNX4Z Removal of Internal Fixation Device from Right Metatarsal, External Approach

0QPNX5Z Removal of External Fixation Device from Right Metatarsal, External Approach

0QPP04Z Removal of Internal Fixation Device from Left Metatarsal, Open Approach

0QPP05Z Removal of External Fixation Device from Left Metatarsal, Open Approach

0QPP07Z Removal of Autologous Tissue Substitute from Left Metatarsal, Open Approach

0QPP0JZ Removal of Synthetic Substitute from Left Metatarsal, Open Approach

0QPP0KZ Removal of Nonautologous Tissue Substitute from Left Metatarsal, Open Approach

0QPP34Z Removal of Internal Fixation Device from Left Metatarsal, Percutaneous Approach

0QPP35Z Removal of External Fixation Device from Left Metatarsal, Percutaneous Approach

0QPP37Z Removal of Autologous Tissue Substitute from Left Metatarsal, Percutaneous Approach

0QPP3JZ Removal of Synthetic Substitute from Left Metatarsal, Percutaneous Approach

0QPP3KZ Removal of Nonautologous Tissue Substitute from Left Metatarsal, Percutaneous Approach

0QPP44Z Removal of Internal Fixation Device from Left Metatarsal, Percutaneous Endoscopic Approach

0QPP45Z Removal of External Fixation Device from Left Metatarsal, Percutaneous Endoscopic Approach

0QPP47Z Removal of Autologous Tissue Substitute from Left Metatarsal, Percutaneous Endoscopic Approach

0QPP4JZ Removal of Synthetic Substitute from Left Metatarsal, Percutaneous Endoscopic Approach

0QPP4KZ Removal of Nonautologous Tissue Substitute from Left Metatarsal, Percutaneous Endoscopic Approach

0QPPX4Z Removal of Internal Fixation Device from Left Metatarsal, External Approach

0QPPX5Z Removal of External Fixation Device from Left Metatarsal, External Approach

0QPQ04Z Removal of Internal Fixation Device from Right Toe Phalanx, Open Approach

0QPQ05Z Removal of External Fixation Device from Right Toe Phalanx, Open Approach

0QPQ07Z Removal of Autologous Tissue Substitute from Right Toe Phalanx, Open Approach

Female-only   ♂ Male-only   ▲ Limited Coverage   ● Non-OR   ▬ HAC-associated procedure   ▲ Non-covered procedures   + Combination

0QPQ0JZ Removal of Synthetic Substitute from Right Toe Phalanx, Open Approach

0QPQ0KZ Removal of Nonautologous Tissue Substitute from Right Toe Phalanx, Open Approach

0QPQ34Z Removal of Internal Fixation Device from Right Toe Phalanx, Percutaneous Approach

0QPQ35Z Removal of External Fixation Device from Right Toe Phalanx, Percutaneous Approach

0QPQ37Z Removal of Autologous Tissue Substitute from Right Toe Phalanx, Percutaneous Approach

0QPQ3JZ Removal of Synthetic Substitute from Right Toe Phalanx, Percutaneous Approach

0QPQ3KZ Removal of Nonautologous Tissue Substitute from Right Toe Phalanx, Percutaneous Approach

0QPQ44Z Removal of Internal Fixation Device from Right Toe Phalanx, Percutaneous Endoscopic Approach

0QPQ45Z Removal of External Fixation Device from Right Toe Phalanx, Percutaneous Endoscopic Approach

0QPQ47Z Removal of Autologous Tissue Substitute from Right Toe Phalanx, Percutaneous Endoscopic Approach

0QPQ4JZ Removal of Synthetic Substitute from Right Toe Phalanx, Percutaneous Endoscopic Approach

0QPQ4KZ Removal of Nonautologous Tissue Substitute from Right Toe Phalanx, Percutaneous Endoscopic Approach

0QPQX4Z Removal of Internal Fixation Device from Right Toe Phalanx, External Approach

0QPQX5Z Removal of External Fixation Device from Right Toe Phalanx, External Approach

0QPR04Z Removal of Internal Fixation Device from Left Toe Phalanx, Open Approach

0QPR05Z Removal of External Fixation Device from Left Toe Phalanx, Open Approach

0QPR07Z Removal of Autologous Tissue Substitute from Left Toe Phalanx, Open Approach

0QPR0JZ Removal of Synthetic Substitute from Left Toe Phalanx, Open Approach

0QPR0KZ Removal of Nonautologous Tissue Substitute from Left Toe Phalanx, Open Approach

0QPR34Z Removal of Internal Fixation Device from Left Toe Phalanx, Percutaneous Approach

0QPR35Z Removal of External Fixation Device from Left Toe Phalanx, Percutaneous Approach

0QPR37Z Removal of Autologous Tissue Substitute from Left Toe Phalanx, Percutaneous Approach

0QPR3JZ Removal of Synthetic Substitute from Left Toe Phalanx, Percutaneous Approach

0QPR3KZ Removal of Nonautologous Tissue Substitute from Left Toe Phalanx, Percutaneous Approach

0QPR44Z Removal of Internal Fixation Device from Left Toe Phalanx, Percutaneous Endoscopic Approach

0QPR45Z Removal of External Fixation Device from Left Toe Phalanx, Percutaneous Endoscopic Approach

0QPR47Z Removal of Autologous Tissue Substitute from Left Toe Phalanx, Percutaneous Endoscopic Approach

0QPR4JZ Removal of Synthetic Substitute from Left Toe Phalanx, Percutaneous Endoscopic Approach

0QPR4KZ Removal of Nonautologous Tissue Substitute from Left Toe Phalanx, Percutaneous Endoscopic Approach

0QPRX4Z Removal of Internal Fixation Device from Left Toe Phalanx, External Approach

0QPRX5Z Removal of External Fixation Device from Left Toe Phalanx, External Approach

0QPS04Z Removal of Internal Fixation Device from Coccyx, Open Approach

0QPS07Z Removal of Autologous Tissue Substitute from Coccyx, Open Approach

0QPS0JZ Removal of Synthetic Substitute from Coccyx, Open Approach

0QPS0KZ Removal of Nonautologous Tissue Substitute from Coccyx, Open Approach

0QPS34Z Removal of Internal Fixation Device from Coccyx, Percutaneous Approach

0QPS37Z Removal of Autologous Tissue Substitute from Coccyx, Percutaneous Approach

0QPS3JZ Removal of Synthetic Substitute from Coccyx, Percutaneous Approach

0QPS3KZ Removal of Nonautologous Tissue Substitute from Coccyx, Percutaneous Approach

0QPS44Z Removal of Internal Fixation Device from Coccyx, Percutaneous Endoscopic Approach

0QPS47Z Removal of Autologous Tissue Substitute from Coccyx, Percutaneous Endoscopic Approach

0QPS4JZ Removal of Synthetic Substitute from Coccyx, Percutaneous Endoscopic Approach

0QPS4KZ Removal of Nonautologous Tissue Substitute from Coccyx, Percutaneous Endoscopic Approach

0QPSX4Z Removal of Internal Fixation Device from Coccyx, External Approach

0QPY00Z Removal of Drainage Device from Lower Bone, Open Approach

0QPY0MZ Removal of Bone Growth Stimulator from Lower Bone, Open Approach

0QPY30Z Removal of Drainage Device from Lower Bone, Percutaneous Approach

0QPY3MZ Removal of Bone Growth Stimulator from Lower Bone, Percutaneous Approach

0QPY40Z Removal of Drainage Device from Lower Bone, Percutaneous Endoscopic Approach

0QPY4MZ Removal of Bone Growth Stimulator from Lower Bone, Percutaneous Endoscopic Approach

0QPYX0Z Removal of Drainage Device from Lower Bone, External Approach

0QPYXMZ Removal of Bone Growth Stimulator from Lower Bone, External Approach

0QQ – Lower Bones, Repair

Review Coding Guideline B3.5

0QQ00ZZ Repair Lumbar Vertebra, Open Approach

0QQ03ZZ Repair Lumbar Vertebra, Percutaneous Approach

0QQ04ZZ Repair Lumbar Vertebra, Percutaneous Endoscopic Approach

0QQ0XZZ Repair Lumbar Vertebra, External Approach

0QQ10ZZ Repair Sacrum, Open Approach
AHA CC: 3Q, 2014, 24

0QQ13ZZ Repair Sacrum, Percutaneous Approach

0QQ14ZZ Repair Sacrum, Percutaneous Endoscopic Approach

0QQ1XZZ Repair Sacrum, External Approach

0QQ20ZZ Repair Right Pelvic Bone, Open Approach

0QQ23ZZ Repair Right Pelvic Bone, Percutaneous Approach

0QQ24ZZ Repair Right Pelvic Bone, Percutaneous Endoscopic Approach

0QQ2XZZ Repair Right Pelvic Bone, External Approach

0QQ30ZZ Repair Left Pelvic Bone, Open Approach

0QQ33ZZ Repair Left Pelvic Bone, Percutaneous Approach

0QQ34ZZ Repair Left Pelvic Bone, Percutaneous Endoscopic Approach

0QQ3XZZ Repair Left Pelvic Bone, External Approach

0QQ40ZZ Repair Right Acetabulum, Open Approach

0QQ43ZZ Repair Right Acetabulum, Percutaneous Approach

0QQ44ZZ Repair Right Acetabulum, Percutaneous Endoscopic Approach

0QQ4XZZ Repair Right Acetabulum, External Approach

0QQ50ZZ Repair Left Acetabulum, Open Approach

0QQ53ZZ Repair Left Acetabulum, Percutaneous Approach

0QQ54ZZ Repair Left Acetabulum, Percutaneous Endoscopic Approach

0QQ5XZZ Repair Left Acetabulum, External Approach

0QQ60ZZ Repair Right Upper Femur, Open Approach

0QQ63ZZ Repair Right Upper Femur, Percutaneous Approach

0QQ64ZZ Repair Right Upper Femur, Percutaneous Endoscopic Approach

0QQ6XZZ Repair Right Upper Femur, External Approach

0QQ70ZZ Repair Left Upper Femur, Open Approach

0QQ73ZZ Repair Left Upper Femur, Percutaneous Approach

0QQ74ZZ Repair Left Upper Femur, Percutaneous Endoscopic Approach

0QQ7XZZ Repair Left Upper Femur, External Approach

0QQ80ZZ Repair Right Femoral Shaft, Open Approach

0QQ83ZZ Repair Right Femoral Shaft, Percutaneous Approach

0QQ84ZZ Repair Right Femoral Shaft, Percutaneous Endoscopic Approach

0QQ8XZZ Repair Right Femoral Shaft, External Approach

0QQ90ZZ Repair Left Femoral Shaft, Open Approach

0QQ93ZZ Repair Left Femoral Shaft, Percutaneous Approach

0QQ94ZZ Repair Left Femoral Shaft, Percutaneous Endoscopic Approach

0QQ9XZZ Repair Left Femoral Shaft, External Approach

0QQB0ZZ Repair Right Lower Femur, Open Approach

0QQB3ZZ Repair Right Lower Femur, Percutaneous Approach

♀ Female-only　　♂ Male-only　　▲ Limited Coverage　　● Non-OR　　HAC-associated procedure　　▲ Non-covered procedures　　+ Combinatio

0QB4ZZ	Repair Right Lower Femur, Percutaneous Endoscopic Approach
0QBXZZ	Repair Right Lower Femur, External Approach
0QC0ZZ	Repair Left Lower Femur, Open Approach
0QC3ZZ	Repair Left Lower Femur, Percutaneous Approach
0QC4ZZ	Repair Left Lower Femur, Percutaneous Endoscopic Approach
0QCXZZ	Repair Left Lower Femur, External Approach
0QD0ZZ	Repair Right Patella, Open Approach
0QD3ZZ	Repair Right Patella, Percutaneous Approach
0QD4ZZ	Repair Right Patella, Percutaneous Endoscopic Approach
0QDXZZ	Repair Right Patella, External Approach
0QF0ZZ	Repair Left Patella, Open Approach
0QF3ZZ	Repair Left Patella, Percutaneous Approach
0QF4ZZ	Repair Left Patella, Percutaneous Endoscopic Approach
0QFXZZ	Repair Left Patella, External Approach
0QG0ZZ	Repair Right Tibia, Open Approach
0QG3ZZ	Repair Right Tibia, Percutaneous Approach
0QG4ZZ	Repair Right Tibia, Percutaneous Endoscopic Approach
0QGXZZ	Repair Right Tibia, External Approach
0QH0ZZ	Repair Left Tibia, Open Approach

0QQH3ZZ	Repair Left Tibia, Percutaneous Approach
0QQH4ZZ	Repair Left Tibia, Percutaneous Endoscopic Approach
0QQHXZZ	Repair Left Tibia, External Approach
0QQJ0ZZ	Repair Right Fibula, Open Approach
0QQJ3ZZ	Repair Right Fibula, Percutaneous Approach
0QQJ4ZZ	Repair Right Fibula, Percutaneous Endoscopic Approach
0QQJXZZ	Repair Right Fibula, External Approach
0QQK0ZZ	Repair Left Fibula, Open Approach
0QQK3ZZ	Repair Left Fibula, Percutaneous Approach
0QQK4ZZ	Repair Left Fibula, Percutaneous Endoscopic Approach
0QQKXZZ	Repair Left Fibula, External Approach
0QQL0ZZ	Repair Right Tarsal, Open Approach
0QQL3ZZ	Repair Right Tarsal, Percutaneous Approach
0QQL4ZZ	Repair Right Tarsal, Percutaneous Endoscopic Approach
0QQLXZZ	Repair Right Tarsal, External Approach
0QQM0ZZ	Repair Left Tarsal, Open Approach
0QQM3ZZ	Repair Left Tarsal, Percutaneous Approach
0QQM4ZZ	Repair Left Tarsal, Percutaneous Endoscopic Approach
0QQMXZZ	Repair Left Tarsal, External Approach
0QQN0ZZ	Repair Right Metatarsal, Open Approach
0QQN3ZZ	Repair Right Metatarsal, Percutaneous Approach

0QQN4ZZ	Repair Right Metatarsal, Percutaneous Endoscopic Approach
0QQNXZZ	Repair Right Metatarsal, External Approach
0QQP0ZZ	Repair Left Metatarsal, Open Approach
0QQP3ZZ	Repair Left Metatarsal, Percutaneous Approach
0QQP4ZZ	Repair Left Metatarsal, Percutaneous Endoscopic Approach
0QQPXZZ	Repair Left Metatarsal, External Approach
0QQQ0ZZ	Repair Right Toe Phalanx, Open Approach
0QQQ3ZZ	Repair Right Toe Phalanx, Percutaneous Approach
0QQQ4ZZ	Repair Right Toe Phalanx, Percutaneous Endoscopic Approach
0QQQXZZ	Repair Right Toe Phalanx, External Approach
0QQR0ZZ	Repair Left Toe Phalanx, Open Approach
0QQR3ZZ	Repair Left Toe Phalanx, Percutaneous Approach
0QQR4ZZ	Repair Left Toe Phalanx, Percutaneous Endoscopic Approach
0QQRXZZ	Repair Left Toe Phalanx, External Approach
0QQS0ZZ	Repair Coccyx, Open Approach
0QQS3ZZ	Repair Coccyx, Percutaneous Approach
0QQS4ZZ	Repair Coccyx, Percutaneous Endoscopic Approach
0QQSXZZ	Repair Coccyx, External Approach

QR – Lower Bones, Replacement

0QR007Z	Replacement of Lumbar Vertebra with Autologous Tissue Substitute, Open Approach
0QR00JZ	Replacement of Lumbar Vertebra with Synthetic Substitute, Open Approach
0QR00KZ	Replacement of Lumbar Vertebra with Nonautologous Tissue Substitute, Open Approach
0QR037Z	Replacement of Lumbar Vertebra with Autologous Tissue Substitute, Percutaneous Approach
0QR03JZ	Replacement of Lumbar Vertebra with Synthetic Substitute, Percutaneous Approach
0QR03KZ	Replacement of Lumbar Vertebra with Nonautologous Tissue Substitute, Percutaneous Approach
0QR047Z	Replacement of Lumbar Vertebra with Autologous Tissue Substitute, Percutaneous Endoscopic Approach
0QR04JZ	Replacement of Lumbar Vertebra with Synthetic Substitute, Percutaneous Endoscopic Approach
0QR04KZ	Replacement of Lumbar Vertebra with Nonautologous Tissue Substitute, Percutaneous Endoscopic Approach
0QR107Z	Replacement of Sacrum with Autologous Tissue Substitute, Open Approach
0QR10JZ	Replacement of Sacrum with Synthetic Substitute, Open Approach
0QR10KZ	Replacement of Sacrum with Nonautologous Tissue Substitute, Open Approach
0QR137Z	Replacement of Sacrum with Autologous Tissue Substitute, Percutaneous Approach
0QR13JZ	Replacement of Sacrum with Synthetic Substitute, Percutaneous Approach
0QR13KZ	Replacement of Sacrum with Nonautologous Tissue Substitute, Percutaneous Approach

0QR147Z	Replacement of Sacrum with Autologous Tissue Substitute, Percutaneous Endoscopic Approach
0QR14JZ	Replacement of Sacrum with Synthetic Substitute, Percutaneous Endoscopic Approach
0QR14KZ	Replacement of Sacrum with Nonautologous Tissue Substitute, Percutaneous Endoscopic Approach
0QR207Z	Replacement of Right Pelvic Bone with Autologous Tissue Substitute, Open Approach
0QR20JZ	Replacement of Right Pelvic Bone with Synthetic Substitute, Open Approach
0QR20KZ	Replacement of Right Pelvic Bone with Nonautologous Tissue Substitute, Open Approach
0QR237Z	Replacement of Right Pelvic Bone with Autologous Tissue Substitute, Percutaneous Approach
0QR23JZ	Replacement of Right Pelvic Bone with Synthetic Substitute, Percutaneous Approach
0QR23KZ	Replacement of Right Pelvic Bone with Nonautologous Tissue Substitute, Percutaneous Approach
0QR247Z	Replacement of Right Pelvic Bone with Autologous Tissue Substitute, Percutaneous Endoscopic Approach
0QR24JZ	Replacement of Right Pelvic Bone with Synthetic Substitute, Percutaneous Endoscopic Approach
0QR24KZ	Replacement of Right Pelvic Bone with Nonautologous Tissue Substitute, Percutaneous Endoscopic Approach
0QR307Z	Replacement of Left Pelvic Bone with Autologous Tissue Substitute, Open Approach
0QR30JZ	Replacement of Left Pelvic Bone with Synthetic Substitute, Open Approach

0QR30KZ	Replacement of Left Pelvic Bone with Nonautologous Tissue Substitute, Open Approach
0QR337Z	Replacement of Left Pelvic Bone with Autologous Tissue Substitute, Percutaneous Approach
0QR33JZ	Replacement of Left Pelvic Bone with Synthetic Substitute, Percutaneous Approach
0QR33KZ	Replacement of Left Pelvic Bone with Nonautologous Tissue Substitute, Percutaneous Approach
0QR347Z	Replacement of Left Pelvic Bone with Autologous Tissue Substitute, Percutaneous Endoscopic Approach
0QR34JZ	Replacement of Left Pelvic Bone with Synthetic Substitute, Percutaneous Endoscopic Approach
0QR34KZ	Replacement of Left Pelvic Bone with Nonautologous Tissue Substitute, Percutaneous Endoscopic Approach
0QR407Z	Replacement of Right Acetabulum with Autologous Tissue Substitute, Open Approach
0QR40JZ	Replacement of Right Acetabulum with Synthetic Substitute, Open Approach
0QR40KZ	Replacement of Right Acetabulum with Nonautologous Tissue Substitute, Open Approach
0QR437Z	Replacement of Right Acetabulum with Autologous Tissue Substitute, Percutaneous Approach
0QR43JZ	Replacement of Right Acetabulum with Synthetic Substitute, Percutaneous Approach
0QR43KZ	Replacement of Right Acetabulum with Nonautologous Tissue Substitute, Percutaneous Approach
0QR447Z	Replacement of Right Acetabulum with Autologous Tissue Substitute, Percutaneous Endoscopic Approach

Female-only	♂ Male-only	▲ Limited Coverage	● Non-OR	HAC-associated procedure	▲ Non-covered procedures

+ Combination

0QR44JZ Replacement of Right Acetabulum with Synthetic Substitute, Percutaneous Endoscopic Approach

0QR44KZ Replacement of Right Acetabulum with Nonautologous Tissue Substitute, Percutaneous Endoscopic Approach

0QR507Z Replacement of Left Acetabulum with Autologous Tissue Substitute, Open Approach

0QR50JZ Replacement of Left Acetabulum with Synthetic Substitute, Open Approach

0QR50KZ Replacement of Left Acetabulum with Nonautologous Tissue Substitute, Open Approach

0QR537Z Replacement of Left Acetabulum with Autologous Tissue Substitute, Percutaneous Approach

0QR53JZ Replacement of Left Acetabulum with Synthetic Substitute, Percutaneous Approach

0QR53KZ Replacement of Left Acetabulum with Nonautologous Tissue Substitute, Percutaneous Approach

0QR547Z Replacement of Left Acetabulum with Autologous Tissue Substitute, Percutaneous Endoscopic Approach

0QR54JZ Replacement of Left Acetabulum with Synthetic Substitute, Percutaneous Endoscopic Approach

0QR54KZ Replacement of Left Acetabulum with Nonautologous Tissue Substitute, Percutaneous Endoscopic Approach

0QR607Z Replacement of Right Upper Femur with Autologous Tissue Substitute, Open Approach

0QR60JZ Replacement of Right Upper Femur with Synthetic Substitute, Open Approach

0QR60KZ Replacement of Right Upper Femur with Nonautologous Tissue Substitute, Open Approach

0QR637Z Replacement of Right Upper Femur with Autologous Tissue Substitute, Percutaneous Approach

0QR63JZ Replacement of Right Upper Femur with Synthetic Substitute, Percutaneous Approach

0QR63KZ Replacement of Right Upper Femur with Nonautologous Tissue Substitute, Percutaneous Approach

0QR647Z Replacement of Right Upper Femur with Autologous Tissue Substitute, Percutaneous Endoscopic Approach

0QR64JZ Replacement of Right Upper Femur with Synthetic Substitute, Percutaneous Endoscopic Approach

0QR64KZ Replacement of Right Upper Femur with Nonautologous Tissue Substitute, Percutaneous Endoscopic Approach

0QR707Z Replacement of Left Upper Femur with Autologous Tissue Substitute, Open Approach

0QR70JZ Replacement of Left Upper Femur with Synthetic Substitute, Open Approach

0QR70KZ Replacement of Left Upper Femur with Nonautologous Tissue Substitute, Open Approach

0QR737Z Replacement of Left Upper Femur with Autologous Tissue Substitute, Percutaneous Approach

0QR73JZ Replacement of Left Upper Femur with Synthetic Substitute, Percutaneous Approach

0QR73KZ Replacement of Left Upper Femur with Nonautologous Tissue Substitute, Percutaneous Approach

0QR747Z Replacement of Left Upper Femur with Autologous Tissue Substitute, Percutaneous Endoscopic Approach

0QR74JZ Replacement of Left Upper Femur with Synthetic Substitute, Percutaneous Endoscopic Approach

0QR74KZ Replacement of Left Upper Femur with Nonautologous Tissue Substitute, Percutaneous Endoscopic Approach

0QR807Z Replacement of Right Femoral Shaft with Autologous Tissue Substitute, Open Approach

0QR80JZ Replacement of Right Femoral Shaft with Synthetic Substitute, Open Approach

0QR80KZ Replacement of Right Femoral Shaft with Nonautologous Tissue Substitute, Open Approach

0QR837Z Replacement of Right Femoral Shaft with Autologous Tissue Substitute, Percutaneous Approach

0QR83JZ Replacement of Right Femoral Shaft with Synthetic Substitute, Percutaneous Approach

0QR83KZ Replacement of Right Femoral Shaft with Nonautologous Tissue Substitute, Percutaneous Approach

0QR847Z Replacement of Right Femoral Shaft with Autologous Tissue Substitute, Percutaneous Endoscopic Approach

0QR84JZ Replacement of Right Femoral Shaft with Synthetic Substitute, Percutaneous Endoscopic Approach

0QR84KZ Replacement of Right Femoral Shaft with Nonautologous Tissue Substitute, Percutaneous Endoscopic Approach

0QR907Z Replacement of Left Femoral Shaft with Autologous Tissue Substitute, Open Approach

0QR90JZ Replacement of Left Femoral Shaft with Synthetic Substitute, Open Approach

0QR90KZ Replacement of Left Femoral Shaft with Nonautologous Tissue Substitute, Open Approach

0QR937Z Replacement of Left Femoral Shaft with Autologous Tissue Substitute, Percutaneous Approach

0QR93JZ Replacement of Left Femoral Shaft with Synthetic Substitute, Percutaneous Approach

0QR93KZ Replacement of Left Femoral Shaft with Nonautologous Tissue Substitute, Percutaneous Approach

0QR947Z Replacement of Left Femoral Shaft with Autologous Tissue Substitute, Percutaneous Endoscopic Approach

0QR94JZ Replacement of Left Femoral Shaft with Synthetic Substitute, Percutaneous Endoscopic Approach

0QR94KZ Replacement of Left Femoral Shaft with Nonautologous Tissue Substitute, Percutaneous Endoscopic Approach

0QRB07Z Replacement of Right Lower Femur with Autologous Tissue Substitute, Open Approach

0QRB0JZ Replacement of Right Lower Femur with Synthetic Substitute, Open Approach

0QRB0KZ Replacement of Right Lower Femur with Nonautologous Tissue Substitute, Open Approach

0QRB37Z Replacement of Right Lower Femur with Autologous Tissue Substitute, Percutaneous Approach

0QRB3JZ Replacement of Right Lower Femur with Synthetic Substitute, Percutaneous Approach

0QRB3KZ Replacement of Right Lower Femur with Nonautologous Tissue Substitute, Percutaneous Approach

0QRB47Z Replacement of Right Lower Femur with Autologous Tissue Substitute, Percutaneous Endoscopic Approach

0QRB4JZ Replacement of Right Lower Femur with Synthetic Substitute, Percutaneous Endoscopic Approach

0QRB4KZ Replacement of Right Lower Femur with Nonautologous Tissue Substitute, Percutaneous Endoscopic Approach

0QRC07Z Replacement of Left Lower Femur with Autologous Tissue Substitute, Open Approach

0QRC0JZ Replacement of Left Lower Femur with Synthetic Substitute, Open Approach

0QRC0KZ Replacement of Left Lower Femur with Nonautologous Tissue Substitute, Open Approach

0QRC37Z Replacement of Left Lower Femur with Autologous Tissue Substitute, Percutaneous Approach

0QRC3JZ Replacement of Left Lower Femur with Synthetic Substitute, Percutaneous Approach

0QRC3KZ Replacement of Left Lower Femur with Nonautologous Tissue Substitute, Percutaneous Approach

0QRC47Z Replacement of Left Lower Femur with Autologous Tissue Substitute, Percutaneous Endoscopic Approach

0QRC4JZ Replacement of Left Lower Femur with Synthetic Substitute, Percutaneous Endoscopic Approach

0QRC4KZ Replacement of Left Lower Femur with Nonautologous Tissue Substitute, Percutaneous Endoscopic Approach

0QRD07Z Replacement of Right Patella with Autologous Tissue Substitute, Open Approach

0QRD0JZ Replacement of Right Patella with Synthetic Substitute, Open Approach

0QRD0KZ Replacement of Right Patella with Nonautologous Tissue Substitute, Open Approach

0QRD37Z Replacement of Right Patella with Autologous Tissue Substitute, Percutaneous Approach

0QRD3JZ Replacement of Right Patella with Synthetic Substitute, Percutaneous Approach

0QRD3KZ Replacement of Right Patella with Nonautologous Tissue Substitute, Percutaneous Approach

0QRD47Z Replacement of Right Patella with Autologous Tissue Substitute, Percutaneous Endoscopic Approach

0QRD4JZ Replacement of Right Patella with Synthetic Substitute, Percutaneous Endoscopic Approach

0QRD4KZ Replacement of Right Patella with Nonautologous Tissue Substitute, Percutaneous Endoscopic Approach

0QRF07Z Replacement of Left Patella with Autologous Tissue Substitute, Open Approach

0QRF0JZ Replacement of Left Patella with Synthetic Substitute, Open Approach

0QRF0KZ Replacement of Left Patella with Nonautologous Tissue Substitute, Open Approach

0QRF37Z Replacement of Left Patella with Autologous Tissue Substitute, Percutaneous Approach

0QRF3JZ	Replacement of Left Patella with Synthetic Substitute, Percutaneous Approach	**0QRJ3JZ**	Replacement of Right Fibula with Synthetic Substitute, Percutaneous Approach	**0QRM3JZ**	Replacement of Left Tarsal with Synthetic Substitute, Percutaneous Approach

0QRF3JZ Replacement of Left Patella with Synthetic Substitute, Percutaneous Approach

0QRF3KZ Replacement of Left Patella with Nonautologous Tissue Substitute, Percutaneous Approach

0QRF47Z Replacement of Left Patella with Autologous Tissue Substitute, Percutaneous Endoscopic Approach

0QRF4JZ Replacement of Left Patella with Synthetic Substitute, Percutaneous Endoscopic Approach

0QRF4KZ Replacement of Left Patella with Nonautologous Tissue Substitute, Percutaneous Endoscopic Approach

0QRG07Z Replacement of Right Tibia with Autologous Tissue Substitute, Open Approach

0QRG0JZ Replacement of Right Tibia with Synthetic Substitute, Open Approach

0QRG0KZ Replacement of Right Tibia with Nonautologous Tissue Substitute, Open Approach

0QRG37Z Replacement of Right Tibia with Autologous Tissue Substitute, Percutaneous Approach

0QRG3JZ Replacement of Right Tibia with Synthetic Substitute, Percutaneous Approach

0QRG3KZ Replacement of Right Tibia with Nonautologous Tissue Substitute, Percutaneous Approach

0QRG47Z Replacement of Right Tibia with Autologous Tissue Substitute, Percutaneous Endoscopic Approach

0QRG4JZ Replacement of Right Tibia with Synthetic Substitute, Percutaneous Endoscopic Approach

0QRG4KZ Replacement of Right Tibia with Nonautologous Tissue Substitute, Percutaneous Endoscopic Approach

0QRH07Z Replacement of Left Tibia with Autologous Tissue Substitute, Open Approach

0QRH0JZ Replacement of Left Tibia with Synthetic Substitute, Open Approach

0QRH0KZ Replacement of Left Tibia with Nonautologous Tissue Substitute, Open Approach

0QRH37Z Replacement of Left Tibia with Autologous Tissue Substitute, Percutaneous Approach

0QRH3JZ Replacement of Left Tibia with Synthetic Substitute, Percutaneous Approach

0QRH3KZ Replacement of Left Tibia with Nonautologous Tissue Substitute, Percutaneous Approach

0QRH47Z Replacement of Left Tibia with Autologous Tissue Substitute, Percutaneous Endoscopic Approach

0QRH4JZ Replacement of Left Tibia with Synthetic Substitute, Percutaneous Endoscopic Approach

0QRH4KZ Replacement of Left Tibia with Nonautologous Tissue Substitute, Percutaneous Endoscopic Approach

0QRJ07Z Replacement of Right Fibula with Autologous Tissue Substitute, Open Approach

0QRJ0JZ Replacement of Right Fibula with Synthetic Substitute, Open Approach

0QRJ0KZ Replacement of Right Fibula with Nonautologous Tissue Substitute, Open Approach

0QRJ37Z Replacement of Right Fibula with Autologous Tissue Substitute, Percutaneous Approach

0QRJ3JZ Replacement of Right Fibula with Synthetic Substitute, Percutaneous Approach

0QRJ3KZ Replacement of Right Fibula with Nonautologous Tissue Substitute, Percutaneous Approach

0QRJ47Z Replacement of Right Fibula with Autologous Tissue Substitute, Percutaneous Endoscopic Approach

0QRJ4JZ Replacement of Right Fibula with Synthetic Substitute, Percutaneous Endoscopic Approach

0QRJ4KZ Replacement of Right Fibula with Nonautologous Tissue Substitute, Percutaneous Endoscopic Approach

0QRK07Z Replacement of Left Fibula with Autologous Tissue Substitute, Open Approach

0QRK0JZ Replacement of Left Fibula with Synthetic Substitute, Open Approach

0QRK0KZ Replacement of Left Fibula with Nonautologous Tissue Substitute, Open Approach

0QRK37Z Replacement of Left Fibula with Autologous Tissue Substitute, Percutaneous Approach

0QRK3JZ Replacement of Left Fibula with Synthetic Substitute, Percutaneous Approach

0QRK3KZ Replacement of Left Fibula with Nonautologous Tissue Substitute, Percutaneous Approach

0QRK47Z Replacement of Left Fibula with Autologous Tissue Substitute, Percutaneous Endoscopic Approach

0QRK4JZ Replacement of Left Fibula with Synthetic Substitute, Percutaneous Endoscopic Approach

0QRK4KZ Replacement of Left Fibula with Nonautologous Tissue Substitute, Percutaneous Endoscopic Approach

0QRL07Z Replacement of Right Tarsal with Autologous Tissue Substitute, Open Approach

0QRL0JZ Replacement of Right Tarsal with Synthetic Substitute, Open Approach

0QRL0KZ Replacement of Right Tarsal with Nonautologous Tissue Substitute, Open Approach

0QRL37Z Replacement of Right Tarsal with Autologous Tissue Substitute, Percutaneous Approach

0QRL3JZ Replacement of Right Tarsal with Synthetic Substitute, Percutaneous Approach

0QRL3KZ Replacement of Right Tarsal with Nonautologous Tissue Substitute, Percutaneous Approach

0QRL47Z Replacement of Right Tarsal with Autologous Tissue Substitute, Percutaneous Endoscopic Approach

0QRL4JZ Replacement of Right Tarsal with Synthetic Substitute, Percutaneous Endoscopic Approach

0QRL4KZ Replacement of Right Tarsal with Nonautologous Tissue Substitute, Percutaneous Endoscopic Approach

0QRM07Z Replacement of Left Tarsal with Autologous Tissue Substitute, Open Approach

0QRM0JZ Replacement of Left Tarsal with Synthetic Substitute, Open Approach

0QRM0KZ Replacement of Left Tarsal with Nonautologous Tissue Substitute, Open Approach

0QRM37Z Replacement of Left Tarsal with Autologous Tissue Substitute, Percutaneous Approach

0QRM3JZ Replacement of Left Tarsal with Synthetic Substitute, Percutaneous Approach

0QRM3KZ Replacement of Left Tarsal with Nonautologous Tissue Substitute, Percutaneous Approach

0QRM47Z Replacement of Left Tarsal with Autologous Tissue Substitute, Percutaneous Endoscopic Approach

0QRM4JZ Replacement of Left Tarsal with Synthetic Substitute, Percutaneous Endoscopic Approach

0QRM4KZ Replacement of Left Tarsal with Nonautologous Tissue Substitute, Percutaneous Endoscopic Approach

0QRN07Z Replacement of Right Metatarsal with Autologous Tissue Substitute, Open Approach

0QRN0JZ Replacement of Right Metatarsal with Synthetic Substitute, Open Approach

0QRN0KZ Replacement of Right Metatarsal with Nonautologous Tissue Substitute, Open Approach

0QRN37Z Replacement of Right Metatarsal with Autologous Tissue Substitute, Percutaneous Approach

0QRN3JZ Replacement of Right Metatarsal with Synthetic Substitute, Percutaneous Approach

0QRN3KZ Replacement of Right Metatarsal with Nonautologous Tissue Substitute, Percutaneous Approach

0QRN47Z Replacement of Right Metatarsal with Autologous Tissue Substitute, Percutaneous Endoscopic Approach

0QRN4JZ Replacement of Right Metatarsal with Synthetic Substitute, Percutaneous Endoscopic Approach

0QRN4KZ Replacement of Right Metatarsal with Nonautologous Tissue Substitute, Percutaneous Endoscopic Approach

0QRP07Z Replacement of Left Metatarsal with Autologous Tissue Substitute, Open Approach

0QRP0JZ Replacement of Left Metatarsal with Synthetic Substitute, Open Approach

0QRP0KZ Replacement of Left Metatarsal with Nonautologous Tissue Substitute, Open Approach

0QRP37Z Replacement of Left Metatarsal with Autologous Tissue Substitute, Percutaneous Approach

0QRP3JZ Replacement of Left Metatarsal with Synthetic Substitute, Percutaneous Approach

0QRP3KZ Replacement of Left Metatarsal with Nonautologous Tissue Substitute, Percutaneous Approach

0QRP47Z Replacement of Left Metatarsal with Autologous Tissue Substitute, Percutaneous Endoscopic Approach

0QRP4JZ Replacement of Left Metatarsal with Synthetic Substitute, Percutaneous Endoscopic Approach

0QRP4KZ Replacement of Left Metatarsal with Nonautologous Tissue Substitute, Percutaneous Endoscopic Approach

0QRQ07Z Replacement of Right Toe Phalanx with Autologous Tissue Substitute, Open Approach

0QRQ0JZ Replacement of Right Toe Phalanx with Synthetic Substitute, Open Approach

0QRQ0KZ Replacement of Right Toe Phalanx with Nonautologous Tissue Substitute, Open Approach

Female-only	♂ Male-only	▲ Limited Coverage	● Non-OR	▨ HAC-associated procedure	▲ Non-covered procedures	✚ Combination

0QRQ37Z Replacement of Right Toe Phalanx with Autologous Tissue Substitute, Percutaneous Approach

0QRQ3JZ Replacement of Right Toe Phalanx with Synthetic Substitute, Percutaneous Approach

0QRQ3KZ Replacement of Right Toe Phalanx with Nonautologous Tissue Substitute, Percutaneous Approach

0QRQ47Z Replacement of Right Toe Phalanx with Autologous Tissue Substitute, Percutaneous Endoscopic Approach

0QRQ4JZ Replacement of Right Toe Phalanx with Synthetic Substitute, Percutaneous Endoscopic Approach

0QRQ4KZ Replacement of Right Toe Phalanx with Nonautologous Tissue Substitute, Percutaneous Endoscopic Approach

0QRR07Z Replacement of Left Toe Phalanx with Autologous Tissue Substitute, Open Approach

0QRR0JZ Replacement of Left Toe Phalanx with Synthetic Substitute, Open Approach

0QRR0KZ Replacement of Left Toe Phalanx with Nonautologous Tissue Substitute, Open Approach

0QRR37Z Replacement of Left Toe Phalanx with Autologous Tissue Substitute, Percutaneous Approach

0QRR3JZ Replacement of Left Toe Phalanx with Synthetic Substitute, Percutaneous Approach

0QRR3KZ Replacement of Left Toe Phalanx with Nonautologous Tissue Substitute, Percutaneous Approach

0QRR47Z Replacement of Left Toe Phalanx with Autologous Tissue Substitute, Percutaneous Endoscopic Approach

0QRR4JZ Replacement of Left Toe Phalanx with Synthetic Substitute, Percutaneous Endoscopic Approach

0QRR4KZ Replacement of Left Toe Phalanx with Nonautologous Tissue Substitute, Percutaneous Endoscopic Approach

0QRS07Z Replacement of Coccyx with Autologous Tissue Substitute, Open Approach

0QRS0JZ Replacement of Coccyx with Synthetic Substitute, Open Approach

0QRS0KZ Replacement of Coccyx with Nonautologous Tissue Substitute, Open Approach

0QRS37Z Replacement of Coccyx with Autologous Tissue Substitute, Percutaneous Approach

0QRS3JZ Replacement of Coccyx with Synthetic Substitute, Percutaneous Approach

0QRS3KZ Replacement of Coccyx with Nonautologous Tissue Substitute, Percutaneous Approach

0QRS47Z Replacement of Coccyx with Autologous Tissue Substitute, Percutaneous Endoscopic Approach

0QRS4JZ Replacement of Coccyx with Synthetic Substitute, Percutaneous Endoscopic Approach

0QRS4KZ Replacement of Coccyx with Nonautologous Tissue Substitute, Percutaneous Endoscopic Approach

0QS – Lower Bones, Reposition

Review Coding Guideline B3.15

0QS004Z Reposition Lumbar Vertebra with Internal Fixation Device, Open Approach

0QS00ZZ Reposition Lumbar Vertebra, Open Approach

0QS034Z Reposition Lumbar Vertebra with Internal Fixation Device, Percutaneous Approach

0QS03ZZ Reposition Lumbar Vertebra, Percutaneous Approach

➕ *See table 0QU to construct a code for Supplement of with synthetic substitute.*

0QS044Z Reposition Lumbar Vertebra with Internal Fixation Device, Percutaneous Endoscopic Approach

0QS04ZZ Reposition Lumbar Vertebra, Percutaneous Endoscopic Approach

0QS0XZZ Reposition Lumbar Vertebra, External Approach

0QS104Z Reposition Sacrum with Internal Fixation Device, Open Approach

0QS10ZZ Reposition Sacrum, Open Approach

0QS134Z Reposition Sacrum with Internal Fixation Device, Percutaneous Approach

0QS13ZZ Reposition Sacrum, Percutaneous Approach

➕ *See table 0QU to construct a code for Supplement of with synthetic substitute.*

0QS144Z Reposition Sacrum with Internal Fixation Device, Percutaneous Endoscopic Approach

0QS14ZZ Reposition Sacrum, Percutaneous Endoscopic Approach

0QS1XZZ Reposition Sacrum, External Approach

0QS204Z Reposition Right Pelvic Bone with Internal Fixation Device, Open Approach

0QS205Z Reposition Right Pelvic Bone with External Fixation Device, Open Approach

0QS20ZZ Reposition Right Pelvic Bone, Open Approach

0QS234Z Reposition Right Pelvic Bone with Internal Fixation Device, Percutaneous Approach

0QS235Z Reposition Right Pelvic Bone with External Fixation Device, Percutaneous Approach

0QS23ZZ Reposition Right Pelvic Bone, Percutaneous Approach

0QS244Z Reposition Right Pelvic Bone with Internal Fixation Device, Percutaneous Endoscopic Approach

0QS245Z Reposition Right Pelvic Bone with External Fixation Device, Percutaneous Endoscopic Approach

0QS24ZZ Reposition Right Pelvic Bone, Percutaneous Endoscopic Approach

0QS2XZZ Reposition Right Pelvic Bone, External Approach

0QS304Z Reposition Left Pelvic Bone with Internal Fixation Device, Open Approach

0QS305Z Reposition Left Pelvic Bone with External Fixation Device, Open Approach

0QS30ZZ Reposition Left Pelvic Bone, Open Approach

0QS334Z Reposition Left Pelvic Bone with Internal Fixation Device, Percutaneous Approach

0QS335Z Reposition Left Pelvic Bone with External Fixation Device, Percutaneous Approach

0QS33ZZ Reposition Left Pelvic Bone, Percutaneous Approach

0QS344Z Reposition Left Pelvic Bone with Internal Fixation Device, Percutaneous Endoscopic Approach

0QS345Z Reposition Left Pelvic Bone with External Fixation Device, Percutaneous Endoscopic Approach

0QS34ZZ Reposition Left Pelvic Bone, Percutaneous Endoscopic Approach

0QS3XZZ Reposition Left Pelvic Bone, External Approach

0QS404Z Reposition Right Acetabulum with Internal Fixation Device, Open Approach

0QS40ZZ Reposition Right Acetabulum, Open Approach

0QS434Z Reposition Right Acetabulum with Internal Fixation Device, Percutaneous Approach

0QS43ZZ Reposition Right Acetabulum, Percutaneous Approach

0QS444Z Reposition Right Acetabulum with Internal Fixation Device, Percutaneous Endoscopic Approach

0QS44ZZ Reposition Right Acetabulum, Percutaneous Endoscopic Approach

0QS4XZZ Reposition Right Acetabulum, External Approach

0QS504Z Reposition Left Acetabulum with Internal Fixation Device, Open Approach

0QS50ZZ Reposition Left Acetabulum, Open Approach

0QS534Z Reposition Left Acetabulum with Internal Fixation Device, Percutaneous Approach

0QS53ZZ Reposition Left Acetabulum, Percutaneous Approach

0QS544Z Reposition Left Acetabulum with Internal Fixation Device, Percutaneous Endoscopic Approach

0QS54ZZ Reposition Left Acetabulum, Percutaneous Endoscopic Approach

0QS5XZZ Reposition Left Acetabulum, External Approach

0QS604Z Reposition Right Upper Femur with Internal Fixation Device, Open Approach

0QS605Z Reposition Right Upper Femur with External Fixation Device, Open Approach

0QS606Z Reposition Right Upper Femur with Intramedullary Internal Fixation Device, Open Approach

0QS60BZ Reposition Right Upper Femur with Monoplanar External Fixation Device, Open Approach

0QS60CZ Reposition Right Upper Femur with Ring External Fixation Device, Open Approach

0QS60DZ Reposition Right Upper Femur with Hybrid External Fixation Device, Open Approach

0QS60ZZ Reposition Right Upper Femur, Open Approach

0QS634Z Reposition Right Upper Femur with Internal Fixation Device, Percutaneous Approach

0QS635Z Reposition Right Upper Femur with External Fixation Device, Percutaneous Approach

0QS636Z Reposition Right Upper Femur with Intramedullary Internal Fixation Device, Percutaneous Approach

0QS63BZ Reposition Right Upper Femur with Monoplanar External Fixation Device, Percutaneous Approach

0QS63CZ Reposition Right Upper Femur with Ring External Fixation Device, Percutaneous Approach

0QS63DZ Reposition Right Upper Femur with Hybrid External Fixation Device, Percutaneous Approach

0QS63ZZ	Reposition Right Upper Femur, Percutaneous Approach	
0QS644Z	Reposition Right Upper Femur with Internal Fixation Device, Percutaneous Endoscopic Approach	
0QS645Z	Reposition Right Upper Femur with External Fixation Device, Percutaneous Endoscopic Approach	
0QS646Z	Reposition Right Upper Femur with Intramedullary Internal Fixation Device, Percutaneous Endoscopic Approach	
0QS64BZ	Reposition Right Upper Femur with Monoplanar External Fixation Device, Percutaneous Endoscopic Approach	
0QS64CZ	Reposition Right Upper Femur with Ring External Fixation Device, Percutaneous Endoscopic Approach	
0QS64DZ	Reposition Right Upper Femur with Hybrid External Fixation Device, Percutaneous Endoscopic Approach	
0QS64ZZ	Reposition Right Upper Femur, Percutaneous Endoscopic Approach	
0QS6XZZ	Reposition Right Upper Femur, External Approach	
0QS704Z	Reposition Left Upper Femur with Internal Fixation Device, Open Approach	
0QS705Z	Reposition Left Upper Femur with External Fixation Device, Open Approach	
0QS706Z	Reposition Left Upper Femur with Intramedullary Internal Fixation Device, Open Approach	
0QS70BZ	Reposition Left Upper Femur with Monoplanar External Fixation Device, Open Approach	
0QS70CZ	Reposition Left Upper Femur with Ring External Fixation Device, Open Approach	
0QS70DZ	Reposition Left Upper Femur with Hybrid External Fixation Device, Open Approach	
0QS70ZZ	Reposition Left Upper Femur, Open Approach	
0QS734Z	Reposition Left Upper Femur with Internal Fixation Device, Percutaneous Approach	
0QS735Z	Reposition Left Upper Femur with External Fixation Device, Percutaneous Approach	
0QS736Z	Reposition Left Upper Femur with Intramedullary Internal Fixation Device, Percutaneous Approach	
0QS73BZ	Reposition Left Upper Femur with Monoplanar External Fixation Device, Percutaneous Approach	
0QS73CZ	Reposition Left Upper Femur with Ring External Fixation Device, Percutaneous Approach	
0QS73DZ	Reposition Left Upper Femur with Hybrid External Fixation Device, Percutaneous Approach	
0QS73ZZ	Reposition Left Upper Femur, Percutaneous Approach	
0QS744Z	Reposition Left Upper Femur with Internal Fixation Device, Percutaneous Endoscopic Approach	
0QS745Z	Reposition Left Upper Femur with External Fixation Device, Percutaneous Endoscopic Approach	
0QS746Z	Reposition Left Upper Femur with Intramedullary Internal Fixation Device, Percutaneous Endoscopic Approach	
0QS74BZ	Reposition Left Upper Femur with Monoplanar External Fixation Device, Percutaneous Endoscopic Approach	
0QS74CZ	Reposition Left Upper Femur with Ring External Fixation Device, Percutaneous Endoscopic Approach	
0QS74DZ	Reposition Left Upper Femur with Hybrid External Fixation Device, Percutaneous Endoscopic Approach	

0QS74ZZ	Reposition Left Upper Femur, Percutaneous Endoscopic Approach	
0QS7XZZ	Reposition Left Upper Femur, External Approach	
0QS804Z	Reposition Right Femoral Shaft with Internal Fixation Device, Open Approach	
0QS805Z	Reposition Right Femoral Shaft with External Fixation Device, Open Approach	
0QS806Z	Reposition Right Femoral Shaft with Intramedullary Internal Fixation Device, Open Approach	
0QS80BZ	Reposition Right Femoral Shaft with Monoplanar External Fixation Device, Open Approach	
0QS80CZ	Reposition Right Femoral Shaft with Ring External Fixation Device, Open Approach	
0QS80DZ	Reposition Right Femoral Shaft with Hybrid External Fixation Device, Open Approach	
0QS80ZZ	Reposition Right Femoral Shaft, Open Approach	
0QS834Z	Reposition Right Femoral Shaft with Internal Fixation Device, Percutaneous Approach	
0QS835Z	Reposition Right Femoral Shaft with External Fixation Device, Percutaneous Approach	
0QS836Z	Reposition Right Femoral Shaft with Intramedullary Internal Fixation Device, Percutaneous Approach	
0QS83BZ	Reposition Right Femoral Shaft with Monoplanar External Fixation Device, Percutaneous Approach	
0QS83CZ	Reposition Right Femoral Shaft with Ring External Fixation Device, Percutaneous Approach	
0QS83DZ	Reposition Right Femoral Shaft with Hybrid External Fixation Device, Percutaneous Approach	
0QS83ZZ	Reposition Right Femoral Shaft, Percutaneous Approach	
0QS844Z	Reposition Right Femoral Shaft with Internal Fixation Device, Percutaneous Endoscopic Approach	
0QS845Z	Reposition Right Femoral Shaft with External Fixation Device, Percutaneous Endoscopic Approach	
0QS846Z	Reposition Right Femoral Shaft with Intramedullary Internal Fixation Device, Percutaneous Endoscopic Approach	
0QS84BZ	Reposition Right Femoral Shaft with Monoplanar External Fixation Device, Percutaneous Endoscopic Approach	
0QS84CZ	Reposition Right Femoral Shaft with Ring External Fixation Device, Percutaneous Endoscopic Approach	
0QS84DZ	Reposition Right Femoral Shaft with Hybrid External Fixation Device, Percutaneous Endoscopic Approach	
0QS84ZZ	Reposition Right Femoral Shaft, Percutaneous Endoscopic Approach	
0QS8XZZ	Reposition Right Femoral Shaft, External Approach	
0QS904Z	Reposition Left Femoral Shaft with Internal Fixation Device, Open Approach	
0QS905Z	Reposition Left Femoral Shaft with External Fixation Device, Open Approach	
0QS906Z	Reposition Left Femoral Shaft with Intramedullary Internal Fixation Device, Open Approach	
0QS90BZ	Reposition Left Femoral Shaft with Monoplanar External Fixation Device, Open Approach	
0QS90CZ	Reposition Left Femoral Shaft with Ring External Fixation Device, Open Approach	

0QS90DZ	Reposition Left Femoral Shaft with Hybrid External Fixation Device, Open Approach	
0QS90ZZ	Reposition Left Femoral Shaft, Open Approach	
0QS934Z	Reposition Left Femoral Shaft with Internal Fixation Device, Percutaneous Approach	
0QS935Z	Reposition Left Femoral Shaft with External Fixation Device, Percutaneous Approach	
0QS936Z	Reposition Left Femoral Shaft with Intramedullary Internal Fixation Device, Percutaneous Approach	
0QS93BZ	Reposition Left Femoral Shaft with Monoplanar External Fixation Device, Percutaneous Approach	
0QS93CZ	Reposition Left Femoral Shaft with Ring External Fixation Device, Percutaneous Approach	
0QS93DZ	Reposition Left Femoral Shaft with Hybrid External Fixation Device, Percutaneous Approach	
0QS93ZZ	Reposition Left Femoral Shaft, Percutaneous Approach	
0QS944Z	Reposition Left Femoral Shaft with Internal Fixation Device, Percutaneous Endoscopic Approach	
0QS945Z	Reposition Left Femoral Shaft with External Fixation Device, Percutaneous Endoscopic Approach	
0QS946Z	Reposition Left Femoral Shaft with Intramedullary Internal Fixation Device, Percutaneous Endoscopic Approach	
0QS94BZ	Reposition Left Femoral Shaft with Monoplanar External Fixation Device, Percutaneous Endoscopic Approach	
0QS94CZ	Reposition Left Femoral Shaft with Ring External Fixation Device, Percutaneous Endoscopic Approach	
0QS94DZ	Reposition Left Femoral Shaft with Hybrid External Fixation Device, Percutaneous Endoscopic Approach	
0QS94ZZ	Reposition Left Femoral Shaft, Percutaneous Endoscopic Approach	
0QS9XZZ	Reposition Left Femoral Shaft, External Approach	
0QSB04Z	Reposition Right Lower Femur with Internal Fixation Device, Open Approach	
0QSB05Z	Reposition Right Lower Femur with External Fixation Device, Open Approach	
0QSB06Z	Reposition Right Lower Femur with Intramedullary Internal Fixation Device, Open Approach	
0QSB0BZ	Reposition Right Lower Femur with Monoplanar External Fixation Device, Open Approach	
0QSB0CZ	Reposition Right Lower Femur with Ring External Fixation Device, Open Approach	
0QSB0DZ	Reposition Right Lower Femur with Hybrid External Fixation Device, Open Approach	
0QSB0ZZ	Reposition Right Lower Femur, Open Approach	
0QSB34Z	Reposition Right Lower Femur with Internal Fixation Device, Percutaneous Approach	
0QSB35Z	Reposition Right Lower Femur with External Fixation Device, Percutaneous Approach	
0QSB36Z	Reposition Right Lower Femur with Intramedullary Internal Fixation Device, Percutaneous Approach	

Female-only	♂ Male-only	▲ Limited Coverage	● Non-OR	▬▬ HAC-associated procedure	▲ Non-covered procedures	✚ Combination

0QSB3BZ Reposition Right Lower Femur with Monoplanar External Fixation Device, Percutaneous Approach

0QSB3CZ Reposition Right Lower Femur with Ring External Fixation Device, Percutaneous Approach

0QSB3DZ Reposition Right Lower Femur with Hybrid External Fixation Device, Percutaneous Approach

0QSB3ZZ Reposition Right Lower Femur, Percutaneous Approach

0QSB44Z Reposition Right Lower Femur with Internal Fixation Device, Percutaneous Endoscopic Approach

0QSB45Z Reposition Right Lower Femur with External Fixation Device, Percutaneous Endoscopic Approach

0QSB46Z Reposition Right Lower Femur with Intramedullary Internal Fixation Device, Percutaneous Endoscopic Approach

0QSB4BZ Reposition Right Lower Femur with Monoplanar External Fixation Device, Percutaneous Endoscopic Approach

0QSB4CZ Reposition Right Lower Femur with Ring External Fixation Device, Percutaneous Endoscopic Approach

0QSB4DZ Reposition Right Lower Femur with Hybrid External Fixation Device, Percutaneous Endoscopic Approach

0QSB4ZZ Reposition Right Lower Femur, Percutaneous Endoscopic Approach

0QSBXZZ Reposition Right Lower Femur, External Approach

0QSC04Z Reposition Left Lower Femur with Internal Fixation Device, Open Approach
  AHA CC: 4Q, 2014, 31

0QSC05Z Reposition Left Lower Femur with External Fixation Device, Open Approach

0QSC06Z Reposition Left Lower Femur with Intramedullary Internal Fixation Device, Open Approach

0QSC0BZ Reposition Left Lower Femur with Monoplanar External Fixation Device, Open Approach

0QSC0CZ Reposition Left Lower Femur with Ring External Fixation Device, Open Approach

0QSC0DZ Reposition Left Lower Femur with Hybrid External Fixation Device, Open Approach

0QSC0ZZ Reposition Left Lower Femur, Open Approach

0QSC34Z Reposition Left Lower Femur with Internal Fixation Device, Percutaneous Approach

0QSC35Z Reposition Left Lower Femur with External Fixation Device, Percutaneous Approach

0QSC36Z Reposition Left Lower Femur with Intramedullary Internal Fixation Device, Percutaneous Approach

0QSC3BZ Reposition Left Lower Femur with Monoplanar External Fixation Device, Percutaneous Approach

0QSC3CZ Reposition Left Lower Femur with Ring External Fixation Device, Percutaneous Approach

0QSC3DZ Reposition Left Lower Femur with Hybrid External Fixation Device, Percutaneous Approach

0QSC3ZZ Reposition Left Lower Femur, Percutaneous Approach

0QSC44Z Reposition Left Lower Femur with Internal Fixation Device, Percutaneous Endoscopic Approach

0QSC45Z Reposition Left Lower Femur with External Fixation Device, Percutaneous Endoscopic Approach

0QSC46Z Reposition Left Lower Femur with Intramedullary Internal Fixation Device, Percutaneous Endoscopic Approach

0QSC4BZ Reposition Left Lower Femur with Monoplanar External Fixation Device, Percutaneous Endoscopic Approach

0QSC4CZ Reposition Left Lower Femur with Ring External Fixation Device, Percutaneous Endoscopic Approach

0QSC4DZ Reposition Left Lower Femur with Hybrid External Fixation Device, Percutaneous Endoscopic Approach

0QSC4ZZ Reposition Left Lower Femur, Percutaneous Endoscopic Approach

0QSCXZZ Reposition Left Lower Femur, External Approach

0QSD04Z Reposition Right Patella with Internal Fixation Device, Open Approach

0QSD05Z Reposition Right Patella with External Fixation Device, Open Approach

0QSD0ZZ Reposition Right Patella, Open Approach

0QSD34Z Reposition Right Patella with Internal Fixation Device, Percutaneous Approach

0QSD35Z Reposition Right Patella with External Fixation Device, Percutaneous Approach

0QSD3ZZ Reposition Right Patella, Percutaneous Approach

0QSD44Z Reposition Right Patella with Internal Fixation Device, Percutaneous Endoscopic Approach

0QSD45Z Reposition Right Patella with External Fixation Device, Percutaneous Endoscopic Approach

0QSD4ZZ Reposition Right Patella, Percutaneous Endoscopic Approach

0QSDXZZ Reposition Right Patella, External Approach

0QSF04Z Reposition Left Patella with Internal Fixation Device, Open Approach

0QSF05Z Reposition Left Patella with External Fixation Device, Open Approach

0QSF0ZZ Reposition Left Patella, Open Approach

0QSF34Z Reposition Left Patella with Internal Fixation Device, Percutaneous Approach

0QSF35Z Reposition Left Patella with External Fixation Device, Percutaneous Approach

0QSF3ZZ Reposition Left Patella, Percutaneous Approach

0QSF44Z Reposition Left Patella with Internal Fixation Device, Percutaneous Endoscopic Approach

0QSF45Z Reposition Left Patella with External Fixation Device, Percutaneous Endoscopic Approach

0QSF4ZZ Reposition Left Patella, Percutaneous Endoscopic Approach

0QSFXZZ Reposition Left Patella, External Approach

0QSG04Z Reposition Right Tibia with Internal Fixation Device, Open Approach

0QSG05Z Reposition Right Tibia with External Fixation Device, Open Approach

0QSG06Z Reposition Right Tibia with Intramedullary Internal Fixation Device, Open Approach

0QSG0BZ Reposition Right Tibia with Monoplanar External Fixation Device, Open Approach

0QSG0CZ Reposition Right Tibia with Ring External Fixation Device, Open Approach

0QSG0DZ Reposition Right Tibia with Hybrid External Fixation Device, Open Approach

0QSG0ZZ Reposition Right Tibia, Open Approach

0QSG34Z Reposition Right Tibia with Internal Fixation Device, Percutaneous Approach

0QSG35Z Reposition Right Tibia with External Fixation Device, Percutaneous Approach

0QSG36Z Reposition Right Tibia with Intramedullary Internal Fixation Device, Percutaneous Approach

0QSG3BZ Reposition Right Tibia with Monoplanar External Fixation Device, Percutaneous Approach

0QSG3CZ Reposition Right Tibia with Ring External Fixation Device, Percutaneous Approach

0QSG3DZ Reposition Right Tibia with Hybrid External Fixation Device, Percutaneous Approach

0QSG3ZZ Reposition Right Tibia, Percutaneous Approach

0QSG44Z Reposition Right Tibia with Internal Fixation Device, Percutaneous Endoscopic Approach

0QSG45Z Reposition Right Tibia with External Fixation Device, Percutaneous Endoscopic Approach

0QSG46Z Reposition Right Tibia with Intramedullary Internal Fixation Device, Percutaneous Endoscopic Approach

0QSG4BZ Reposition Right Tibia with Monoplanar External Fixation Device, Percutaneous Endoscopic Approach

0QSG4CZ Reposition Right Tibia with Ring External Fixation Device, Percutaneous Endoscopic Approach

0QSG4DZ Reposition Right Tibia with Hybrid External Fixation Device, Percutaneous Endoscopic Approach

0QSG4ZZ Reposition Right Tibia, Percutaneous Endoscopic Approach

0QSGXZZ Reposition Right Tibia, External Approach

0QSH04Z Reposition Left Tibia with Internal Fixation Device, Open Approach
  AHA CC: 4Q, 2014, 30-31

0QSH05Z Reposition Left Tibia with External Fixation Device, Open Approach

0QSH06Z Reposition Left Tibia with Intramedullary Internal Fixation Device, Open Approach

0QSH0BZ Reposition Left Tibia with Monoplanar External Fixation Device, Open Approach

0QSH0CZ Reposition Left Tibia with Ring External Fixation Device, Open Approach

0QSH0DZ Reposition Left Tibia with Hybrid External Fixation Device, Open Approach

0QSH0ZZ Reposition Left Tibia, Open Approach

0QSH34Z Reposition Left Tibia with Internal Fixation Device, Percutaneous Approach

0QSH35Z Reposition Left Tibia with External Fixation Device, Percutaneous Approach

0QSH36Z Reposition Left Tibia with Intramedullary Internal Fixation Device, Percutaneous Approach

0QSH3BZ Reposition Left Tibia with Monoplanar External Fixation Device, Percutaneous Approach

0QSH3CZ Reposition Left Tibia with Ring External Fixation Device, Percutaneous Approach

0QSH3DZ Reposition Left Tibia with Hybrid External Fixation Device, Percutaneous Approach

0QSH3ZZ Reposition Left Tibia, Percutaneous Approach

0QSH44Z Reposition Left Tibia with Internal Fixation Device, Percutaneous Endoscopic Approach

0QSH45Z Reposition Left Tibia with External Fixation Device, Percutaneous Endoscopic Approach

0QSH46Z Reposition Left Tibia with Intramedullary Internal Fixation Device, Percutaneous Endoscopic Approach

0QSH4BZ Reposition Left Tibia with Monoplanar External Fixation Device, Percutaneous Endoscopic Approach

SH4CZ Reposition Left Tibia with Ring External Fixation Device, Percutaneous Endoscopic Approach

SH4DZ Reposition Left Tibia with Hybrid External Fixation Device, Percutaneous Endoscopic Approach

SH4ZZ Reposition Left Tibia, Percutaneous Endoscopic Approach

SHXZZ Reposition Left Tibia, External Approach

SJ04Z Reposition Right Fibula with Internal Fixation Device, Open Approach

SJ05Z Reposition Right Fibula with External Fixation Device, Open Approach

SJ06Z Reposition Right Fibula with Intramedullary Internal Fixation Device, Open Approach

SJ0BZ Reposition Right Fibula with Monoplanar External Fixation Device, Open Approach

SJ0CZ Reposition Right Fibula with Ring External Fixation Device, Open Approach

SJ0DZ Reposition Right Fibula with Hybrid External Fixation Device, Open Approach

SJ0ZZ Reposition Right Fibula, Open Approach

SJ34Z Reposition Right Fibula with Internal Fixation Device, Percutaneous Approach

SJ35Z Reposition Right Fibula with External Fixation Device, Percutaneous Approach

SJ36Z Reposition Right Fibula with Intramedullary Internal Fixation Device, Percutaneous Approach

SJ3BZ Reposition Right Fibula with Monoplanar External Fixation Device, Percutaneous Approach

SJ3CZ Reposition Right Fibula with Ring External Fixation Device, Percutaneous Approach

SJ3DZ Reposition Right Fibula with Hybrid External Fixation Device, Percutaneous Approach

SJ3ZZ Reposition Right Fibula, Percutaneous Approach

SJ44Z Reposition Right Fibula with Internal Fixation Device, Percutaneous Endoscopic Approach

SJ45Z Reposition Right Fibula with External Fixation Device, Percutaneous Endoscopic Approach

SJ46Z Reposition Right Fibula with Intramedullary Internal Fixation Device, Percutaneous Endoscopic Approach

SJ4BZ Reposition Right Fibula with Monoplanar External Fixation Device, Percutaneous Endoscopic Approach

SJ4CZ Reposition Right Fibula with Ring External Fixation Device, Percutaneous Endoscopic Approach

SJ4DZ Reposition Right Fibula with Hybrid External Fixation Device, Percutaneous Endoscopic Approach

SJ4ZZ Reposition Right Fibula, Percutaneous Endoscopic Approach

SJXZZ Reposition Right Fibula, External Approach

SK04Z Reposition Left Fibula with Internal Fixation Device, Open Approach

SK05Z Reposition Left Fibula with External Fixation Device, Open Approach

SK06Z Reposition Left Fibula with Intramedullary Internal Fixation Device, Open Approach

SK0BZ Reposition Left Fibula with Monoplanar External Fixation Device, Open Approach

SK0CZ Reposition Left Fibula with Ring External Fixation Device, Open Approach

SK0DZ Reposition Left Fibula with Hybrid External Fixation Device, Open Approach

0QSK0ZZ Reposition Left Fibula, Open Approach

0QSK34Z Reposition Left Fibula with Internal Fixation Device, Percutaneous Approach

0QSK35Z Reposition Left Fibula with External Fixation Device, Percutaneous Approach

0QSK36Z Reposition Left Fibula with Intramedullary Internal Fixation Device, Percutaneous Approach

0QSK3BZ Reposition Left Fibula with Monoplanar External Fixation Device, Percutaneous Approach

0QSK3CZ Reposition Left Fibula with Ring External Fixation Device, Percutaneous Approach

0QSK3DZ Reposition Left Fibula with Hybrid External Fixation Device, Percutaneous Approach

0QSK3ZZ Reposition Left Fibula, Percutaneous Approach

0QSK44Z Reposition Left Fibula with Internal Fixation Device, Percutaneous Endoscopic Approach

0QSK45Z Reposition Left Fibula with External Fixation Device, Percutaneous Endoscopic Approach

0QSK46Z Reposition Left Fibula with Intramedullary Internal Fixation Device, Percutaneous Endoscopic Approach

0QSK4BZ Reposition Left Fibula with Monoplanar External Fixation Device, Percutaneous Endoscopic Approach

0QSK4CZ Reposition Left Fibula with Ring External Fixation Device, Percutaneous Endoscopic Approach

0QSK4DZ Reposition Left Fibula with Hybrid External Fixation Device, Percutaneous Endoscopic Approach

0QSK4ZZ Reposition Left Fibula, Percutaneous Endoscopic Approach

0QSKXZZ Reposition Left Fibula, External Approach

0QSL04Z Reposition Right Tarsal with Internal Fixation Device, Open Approach

0QSL05Z Reposition Right Tarsal with External Fixation Device, Open Approach

0QSL0ZZ Reposition Right Tarsal, Open Approach

0QSL34Z Reposition Right Tarsal with Internal Fixation Device, Percutaneous Approach

0QSL35Z Reposition Right Tarsal with External Fixation Device, Percutaneous Approach

0QSL3ZZ Reposition Right Tarsal, Percutaneous Approach

0QSL44Z Reposition Right Tarsal with Internal Fixation Device, Percutaneous Endoscopic Approach

0QSL45Z Reposition Right Tarsal with External Fixation Device, Percutaneous Endoscopic Approach

0QSL4ZZ Reposition Right Tarsal, Percutaneous Endoscopic Approach

0QSLXZZ Reposition Right Tarsal, External Approach

0QSM04Z Reposition Left Tarsal with Internal Fixation Device, Open Approach

0QSM05Z Reposition Left Tarsal with External Fixation Device, Open Approach

0QSM0ZZ Reposition Left Tarsal, Open Approach

0QSM34Z Reposition Left Tarsal with Internal Fixation Device, Percutaneous Approach

0QSM35Z Reposition Left Tarsal with External Fixation Device, Percutaneous Approach

0QSM3ZZ Reposition Left Tarsal, Percutaneous Approach

0QSM44Z Reposition Left Tarsal with Internal Fixation Device, Percutaneous Endoscopic Approach

0QSM45Z Reposition Left Tarsal with External Fixation Device, Percutaneous Endoscopic Approach

0QSM4ZZ Reposition Left Tarsal, Percutaneous Endoscopic Approach

0QSMXZZ Reposition Left Tarsal, External Approach

0QSN04Z Reposition Right Metatarsal with Internal Fixation Device, Open Approach

0QSN05Z Reposition Right Metatarsal with External Fixation Device, Open Approach

0QSN0ZZ Reposition Right Metatarsal, Open Approach

0QSN34Z Reposition Right Metatarsal with Internal Fixation Device, Percutaneous Approach

0QSN35Z Reposition Right Metatarsal with External Fixation Device, Percutaneous Approach

0QSN3ZZ Reposition Right Metatarsal, Percutaneous Approach

0QSN44Z Reposition Right Metatarsal with Internal Fixation Device, Percutaneous Endoscopic Approach

0QSN45Z Reposition Right Metatarsal with External Fixation Device, Percutaneous Endoscopic Approach

0QSN4ZZ Reposition Right Metatarsal, Percutaneous Endoscopic Approach

0QSNXZZ Reposition Right Metatarsal, External Approach

0QSP04Z Reposition Left Metatarsal with Internal Fixation Device, Open Approach

0QSP05Z Reposition Left Metatarsal with External Fixation Device, Open Approach

0QSP0ZZ Reposition Left Metatarsal, Open Approach

0QSP34Z Reposition Left Metatarsal with Internal Fixation Device, Percutaneous Approach

0QSP35Z Reposition Left Metatarsal with External Fixation Device, Percutaneous Approach

0QSP3ZZ Reposition Left Metatarsal, Percutaneous Approach

0QSP44Z Reposition Left Metatarsal with Internal Fixation Device, Percutaneous Endoscopic Approach

0QSP45Z Reposition Left Metatarsal with External Fixation Device, Percutaneous Endoscopic Approach

0QSP4ZZ Reposition Left Metatarsal, Percutaneous Endoscopic Approach

0QSPXZZ Reposition Left Metatarsal, External Approach

0QSQ04Z Reposition Right Toe Phalanx with Internal Fixation Device, Open Approach

0QSQ05Z Reposition Right Toe Phalanx with External Fixation Device, Open Approach

0QSQ0ZZ Reposition Right Toe Phalanx, Open Approach

0QSQ34Z Reposition Right Toe Phalanx with Internal Fixation Device, Percutaneous Approach

0QSQ35Z Reposition Right Toe Phalanx with External Fixation Device, Percutaneous Approach

0QSQ3ZZ Reposition Right Toe Phalanx, Percutaneous Approach

0QSQ44Z Reposition Right Toe Phalanx with Internal Fixation Device, Percutaneous Endoscopic Approach

0QSQ45Z Reposition Right Toe Phalanx with External Fixation Device, Percutaneous Endoscopic Approach

0QSQ4ZZ Reposition Right Toe Phalanx, Percutaneous Endoscopic Approach

0QSQXZZ Reposition Right Toe Phalanx, External Approach

0QSR04Z Reposition Left Toe Phalanx with Internal Fixation Device, Open Approach

877

0QSR05Z	Reposition Left Toe Phalanx with External Fixation Device, Open Approach
0QSR0ZZ	Reposition Left Toe Phalanx, Open Approach
0QSR34Z	Reposition Left Toe Phalanx with Internal Fixation Device, Percutaneous Approach
0QSR35Z	Reposition Left Toe Phalanx with External Fixation Device, Percutaneous Approach
0QSR3ZZ	Reposition Left Toe Phalanx, Percutaneous Approach

0QSR44Z	Reposition Left Toe Phalanx with Internal Fixation Device, Percutaneous Endoscopic Approach
0QSR45Z	Reposition Left Toe Phalanx with External Fixation Device, Percutaneous Endoscopic Approach
0QSR4ZZ	Reposition Left Toe Phalanx, Percutaneous Endoscopic Approach
0QSRXZZ	Reposition Left Toe Phalanx, External Approach
0QSS04Z	Reposition Coccyx with Internal Fixation Device, Open Approach
0QSS0ZZ	Reposition Coccyx, Open Approach

0QSS34Z	Reposition Coccyx with Internal Fixation Device, Percutaneous Approach
0QSS3ZZ	Reposition Coccyx, Percutaneous Approach
✚	*See table 0QU to construct a code for Supplement of with synthetic substitute.*
0QSS44Z	Reposition Coccyx with Internal Fixation Device, Percutaneous Endoscopic Approach
0QSS4ZZ	Reposition Coccyx, Percutaneous Endoscopic Approach
0QSSXZZ	Reposition Coccyx, External Approach

0QT – Lower Bones, Resection

Review Coding Guideline B3.8

0QT20ZZ	Resection of Right Pelvic Bone, Open Approach
0QT30ZZ	Resection of Left Pelvic Bone, Open Approach
0QT40ZZ	Resection of Right Acetabulum, Open Approach
0QT50ZZ	Resection of Left Acetabulum, Open Approach
0QT60ZZ	Resection of Right Upper Femur, Open Approach
0QT70ZZ	Resection of Left Upper Femur, Open Approach
0QT80ZZ	Resection of Right Femoral Shaft, Open Approach

0QT90ZZ	Resection of Left Femoral Shaft, Open Approach
0QTB0ZZ	Resection of Right Lower Femur, Open Approach
0QTC0ZZ	Resection of Left Lower Femur, Open Approach
	AHA CC: 4Q, 2014, 30-31
0QTD0ZZ	Resection of Right Patella, Open Approach
0QTF0ZZ	Resection of Left Patella, Open Approach
0QTG0ZZ	Resection of Right Tibia, Open Approach
0QTH0ZZ	Resection of Left Tibia, Open Approach
0QTJ0ZZ	Resection of Right Fibula, Open Approach

0QTK0ZZ	Resection of Left Fibula, Open Approach
0QTL0ZZ	Resection of Right Tarsal, Open Approach
0QTM0ZZ	Resection of Left Tarsal, Open Approach
0QTN0ZZ	Resection of Right Metatarsal, Open Approach
0QTP0ZZ	Resection of Left Metatarsal, Open Approach
0QTQ0ZZ	Resection of Right Toe Phalanx, Open Approach
0QTR0ZZ	Resection of Left Toe Phalanx, Open Approach
0QTS0ZZ	Resection of Coccyx, Open Approach

0QU – Lower Bones, Supplement

0QU007Z	Supplement Lumbar Vertebra with Autologous Tissue Substitute, Open Approach
0QU00JZ	Supplement Lumbar Vertebra with Synthetic Substitute, Open Approach
0QU00KZ	Supplement Lumbar Vertebra with Nonautologous Tissue Substitute, Open Approach
0QU037Z	Supplement Lumbar Vertebra with Autologous Tissue Substitute, Percutaneous Approach
0QU03JZ	Supplement Lumbar Vertebra with Synthetic Substitute, Percutaneous Approach
	AHA CC: 2Q, 2014, 12-13
0QU03KZ	Supplement Lumbar Vertebra with Nonautologous Tissue Substitute, Percutaneous Approach
0QU047Z	Supplement Lumbar Vertebra with Autologous Tissue Substitute, Percutaneous Endoscopic Approach
0QU04JZ	Supplement Lumbar Vertebra with Synthetic Substitute, Percutaneous Endoscopic Approach
0QU04KZ	Supplement Lumbar Vertebra with Nonautologous Tissue Substitute, Percutaneous Endoscopic Approach
0QU107Z	Supplement Sacrum with Autologous Tissue Substitute, Open Approach
0QU10JZ	Supplement Sacrum with Synthetic Substitute, Open Approach
0QU10KZ	Supplement Sacrum with Nonautologous Tissue Substitute, Open Approach
0QU137Z	Supplement Sacrum with Autologous Tissue Substitute, Percutaneous Approach
0QU13JZ	Supplement Sacrum with Synthetic Substitute, Percutaneous Approach
0QU13KZ	Supplement Sacrum with Nonautologous Tissue Substitute, Percutaneous Approach

0QU147Z	Supplement Sacrum with Autologous Tissue Substitute, Percutaneous Endoscopic Approach
0QU14JZ	Supplement Sacrum with Synthetic Substitute, Percutaneous Endoscopic Approach
0QU14KZ	Supplement Sacrum with Nonautologous Tissue Substitute, Percutaneous Endoscopic Approach
0QU207Z	Supplement Right Pelvic Bone with Autologous Tissue Substitute, Open Approach
0QU20JZ	Supplement Right Pelvic Bone with Synthetic Substitute, Open Approach
	AHA CC: 2Q, 2013, 35-36
0QU20KZ	Supplement Right Pelvic Bone with Nonautologous Tissue Substitute, Open Approach
0QU237Z	Supplement Right Pelvic Bone with Autologous Tissue Substitute, Percutaneous Approach
0QU23JZ	Supplement Right Pelvic Bone with Synthetic Substitute, Percutaneous Approach
0QU23KZ	Supplement Right Pelvic Bone with Nonautologous Tissue Substitute, Percutaneous Approach
0QU247Z	Supplement Right Pelvic Bone with Autologous Tissue Substitute, Percutaneous Endoscopic Approach
0QU24JZ	Supplement Right Pelvic Bone with Synthetic Substitute, Percutaneous Endoscopic Approach
0QU24KZ	Supplement Right Pelvic Bone with Nonautologous Tissue Substitute, Percutaneous Endoscopic Approach
0QU307Z	Supplement Left Pelvic Bone with Autologous Tissue Substitute, Open Approach
0QU30JZ	Supplement Left Pelvic Bone with Synthetic Substitute, Open Approach

0QU30KZ	Supplement Left Pelvic Bone with Nonautologous Tissue Substitute, Open Approach
0QU337Z	Supplement Left Pelvic Bone with Autologous Tissue Substitute, Percutaneous Approach
0QU33JZ	Supplement Left Pelvic Bone with Synthetic Substitute, Percutaneous Approach
0QU33KZ	Supplement Left Pelvic Bone with Nonautologous Tissue Substitute, Percutaneous Approach
0QU347Z	Supplement Left Pelvic Bone with Autologous Tissue Substitute, Percutaneous Endoscopic Approach
0QU34JZ	Supplement Left Pelvic Bone with Synthetic Substitute, Percutaneous Endoscopic Approach
0QU34KZ	Supplement Left Pelvic Bone with Nonautologous Tissue Substitute, Percutaneous Endoscopic Approach
0QU407Z	Supplement Right Acetabulum with Autologous Tissue Substitute, Open Approach
0QU40JZ	Supplement Right Acetabulum with Synthetic Substitute, Open Approach
0QU40KZ	Supplement Right Acetabulum with Nonautologous Tissue Substitute, Open Approach
0QU437Z	Supplement Right Acetabulum with Autologous Tissue Substitute, Percutaneous Approach
0QU43JZ	Supplement Right Acetabulum with Synthetic Substitute, Percutaneous Approach
0QU43KZ	Supplement Right Acetabulum with Nonautologous Tissue Substitute, Percutaneous Approach
0QU447Z	Supplement Right Acetabulum with Autologous Tissue Substitute, Percutaneous Endoscopic Approach

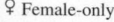

0QU44JZ	Supplement Right Acetabulum with Synthetic Substitute, Percutaneous Endoscopic Approach
0QU44KZ	Supplement Right Acetabulum with Nonautologous Tissue Substitute, Percutaneous Endoscopic Approach
0QU507Z	Supplement Left Acetabulum with Autologous Tissue Substitute, Open Approach
0QU50JZ	Supplement Left Acetabulum with Synthetic Substitute, Open Approach
0QU50KZ	Supplement Left Acetabulum with Nonautologous Tissue Substitute, Open Approach
0QU537Z	Supplement Left Acetabulum with Autologous Tissue Substitute, Percutaneous Approach
0QU53JZ	Supplement Left Acetabulum with Synthetic Substitute, Percutaneous Approach
0QU53KZ	Supplement Left Acetabulum with Nonautologous Tissue Substitute, Percutaneous Approach
0QU547Z	Supplement Left Acetabulum with Autologous Tissue Substitute, Percutaneous Endoscopic Approach
0QU54JZ	Supplement Left Acetabulum with Synthetic Substitute, Percutaneous Endoscopic Approach
0QU54KZ	Supplement Left Acetabulum with Nonautologous Tissue Substitute, Percutaneous Endoscopic Approach
0QU607Z	Supplement Right Upper Femur with Autologous Tissue Substitute, Open Approach
0QU60JZ	Supplement Right Upper Femur with Synthetic Substitute, Open Approach
0QU60KZ	Supplement Right Upper Femur with Nonautologous Tissue Substitute, Open Approach
0QU637Z	Supplement Right Upper Femur with Autologous Tissue Substitute, Percutaneous Approach
0QU63JZ	Supplement Right Upper Femur with Synthetic Substitute, Percutaneous Approach
0QU63KZ	Supplement Right Upper Femur with Nonautologous Tissue Substitute, Percutaneous Approach
0QU647Z	Supplement Right Upper Femur with Autologous Tissue Substitute, Percutaneous Endoscopic Approach
0QU64JZ	Supplement Right Upper Femur with Synthetic Substitute, Percutaneous Endoscopic Approach
0QU64KZ	Supplement Right Upper Femur with Nonautologous Tissue Substitute, Percutaneous Endoscopic Approach
0QU707Z	Supplement Left Upper Femur with Autologous Tissue Substitute, Open Approach
0QU70JZ	Supplement Left Upper Femur with Synthetic Substitute, Open Approach
0QU70KZ	Supplement Left Upper Femur with Nonautologous Tissue Substitute, Open Approach
0QU737Z	Supplement Left Upper Femur with Autologous Tissue Substitute, Percutaneous Approach
0QU73JZ	Supplement Left Upper Femur with Synthetic Substitute, Percutaneous Approach
0QU73KZ	Supplement Left Upper Femur with Nonautologous Tissue Substitute, Percutaneous Approach
0QU747Z	Supplement Left Upper Femur with Autologous Tissue Substitute, Percutaneous Endoscopic Approach

0QU74JZ	Supplement Left Upper Femur with Synthetic Substitute, Percutaneous Endoscopic Approach
0QU74KZ	Supplement Left Upper Femur with Nonautologous Tissue Substitute, Percutaneous Endoscopic Approach
0QU807Z	Supplement Right Femoral Shaft with Autologous Tissue Substitute, Open Approach
0QU80JZ	Supplement Right Femoral Shaft with Synthetic Substitute, Open Approach
0QU80KZ	Supplement Right Femoral Shaft with Nonautologous Tissue Substitute, Open Approach
0QU837Z	Supplement Right Femoral Shaft with Autologous Tissue Substitute, Percutaneous Approach
0QU83JZ	Supplement Right Femoral Shaft with Synthetic Substitute, Percutaneous Approach
0QU83KZ	Supplement Right Femoral Shaft with Nonautologous Tissue Substitute, Percutaneous Approach
0QU847Z	Supplement Right Femoral Shaft with Autologous Tissue Substitute, Percutaneous Endoscopic Approach
0QU84JZ	Supplement Right Femoral Shaft with Synthetic Substitute, Percutaneous Endoscopic Approach
0QU84KZ	Supplement Right Femoral Shaft with Nonautologous Tissue Substitute, Percutaneous Endoscopic Approach
0QU907Z	Supplement Left Femoral Shaft with Autologous Tissue Substitute, Open Approach
0QU90JZ	Supplement Left Femoral Shaft with Synthetic Substitute, Open Approach
0QU90KZ	Supplement Left Femoral Shaft with Nonautologous Tissue Substitute, Open Approach
0QU937Z	Supplement Left Femoral Shaft with Autologous Tissue Substitute, Percutaneous Approach
0QU93JZ	Supplement Left Femoral Shaft with Synthetic Substitute, Percutaneous Approach
0QU93KZ	Supplement Left Femoral Shaft with Nonautologous Tissue Substitute, Percutaneous Approach
0QU947Z	Supplement Left Femoral Shaft with Autologous Tissue Substitute, Percutaneous Endoscopic Approach
0QU94JZ	Supplement Left Femoral Shaft with Synthetic Substitute, Percutaneous Endoscopic Approach
0QU94KZ	Supplement Left Femoral Shaft with Nonautologous Tissue Substitute, Percutaneous Endoscopic Approach
0QUB07Z	Supplement Right Lower Femur with Autologous Tissue Substitute, Open Approach
0QUB0JZ	Supplement Right Lower Femur with Synthetic Substitute, Open Approach
0QUB0KZ	Supplement Right Lower Femur with Nonautologous Tissue Substitute, Open Approach
0QUB37Z	Supplement Right Lower Femur with Autologous Tissue Substitute, Percutaneous Approach
0QUB3JZ	Supplement Right Lower Femur with Synthetic Substitute, Percutaneous Approach
0QUB3KZ	Supplement Right Lower Femur with Nonautologous Tissue Substitute, Percutaneous Approach
0QUB47Z	Supplement Right Lower Femur with Autologous Tissue Substitute, Percutaneous Endoscopic Approach

0QUB4JZ	Supplement Right Lower Femur with Synthetic Substitute, Percutaneous Endoscopic Approach
0QUB4KZ	Supplement Right Lower Femur with Nonautologous Tissue Substitute, Percutaneous Endoscopic Approach
0QUC07Z	Supplement Left Lower Femur with Autologous Tissue Substitute, Open Approach
0QUC0JZ	Supplement Left Lower Femur with Synthetic Substitute, Open Approach
0QUC0KZ	Supplement Left Lower Femur with Nonautologous Tissue Substitute, Open Approach
	AHA CC: 4Q, 2014, 31
0QUC37Z	Supplement Left Lower Femur with Autologous Tissue Substitute, Percutaneous Approach
0QUC3JZ	Supplement Left Lower Femur with Synthetic Substitute, Percutaneous Approach
0QUC3KZ	Supplement Left Lower Femur with Nonautologous Tissue Substitute, Percutaneous Approach
0QUC47Z	Supplement Left Lower Femur with Autologous Tissue Substitute, Percutaneous Endoscopic Approach
0QUC4JZ	Supplement Left Lower Femur with Synthetic Substitute, Percutaneous Endoscopic Approach
0QUC4KZ	Supplement Left Lower Femur with Nonautologous Tissue Substitute, Percutaneous Endoscopic Approach
0QUD07Z	Supplement Right Patella with Autologous Tissue Substitute, Open Approach
0QUD0JZ	Supplement Right Patella with Synthetic Substitute, Open Approach
0QUD0KZ	Supplement Right Patella with Nonautologous Tissue Substitute, Open Approach
0QUD37Z	Supplement Right Patella with Autologous Tissue Substitute, Percutaneous Approach
0QUD3JZ	Supplement Right Patella with Synthetic Substitute, Percutaneous Approach
0QUD3KZ	Supplement Right Patella with Nonautologous Tissue Substitute, Percutaneous Approach
0QUD47Z	Supplement Right Patella with Autologous Tissue Substitute, Percutaneous Endoscopic Approach
0QUD4JZ	Supplement Right Patella with Synthetic Substitute, Percutaneous Endoscopic Approach
0QUD4KZ	Supplement Right Patella with Nonautologous Tissue Substitute, Percutaneous Endoscopic Approach
0QUF07Z	Supplement Left Patella with Autologous Tissue Substitute, Open Approach
0QUF0JZ	Supplement Left Patella with Synthetic Substitute, Open Approach
0QUF0KZ	Supplement Left Patella with Nonautologous Tissue Substitute, Open Approach
0QUF37Z	Supplement Left Patella with Autologous Tissue Substitute, Percutaneous Approach
0QUF3JZ	Supplement Left Patella with Synthetic Substitute, Percutaneous Approach
0QUF3KZ	Supplement Left Patella with Nonautologous Tissue Substitute, Percutaneous Approach
0QUF47Z	Supplement Left Patella with Autologous Tissue Substitute, Percutaneous Endoscopic Approach
0QUF4JZ	Supplement Left Patella with Synthetic Substitute, Percutaneous Endoscopic Approach

Female-only	♂ Male-only	▲ Limited Coverage	● Non-OR	■ HAC-associated procedure	▲ Non-covered procedures	✛ Combination

0QUF4KZ Supplement Left Patella with Nonautologous Tissue Substitute, Percutaneous Endoscopic Approach

0QUG07Z Supplement Right Tibia with Autologous Tissue Substitute, Open Approach

0QUG0JZ Supplement Right Tibia with Synthetic Substitute, Open Approach

0QUG0KZ Supplement Right Tibia with Nonautologous Tissue Substitute, Open Approach

0QUG37Z Supplement Right Tibia with Autologous Tissue Substitute, Percutaneous Approach

0QUG3JZ Supplement Right Tibia with Synthetic Substitute, Percutaneous Approach

0QUG3KZ Supplement Right Tibia with Nonautologous Tissue Substitute, Percutaneous Approach

0QUG47Z Supplement Right Tibia with Autologous Tissue Substitute, Percutaneous Endoscopic Approach

0QUG4JZ Supplement Right Tibia with Synthetic Substitute, Percutaneous Endoscopic Approach

0QUG4KZ Supplement Right Tibia with Nonautologous Tissue Substitute, Percutaneous Endoscopic Approach

0QUH07Z Supplement Left Tibia with Autologous Tissue Substitute, Open Approach

0QUH0JZ Supplement Left Tibia with Synthetic Substitute, Open Approach

0QUH0KZ Supplement Left Tibia with Nonautologous Tissue Substitute, Open Approach

0QUH37Z Supplement Left Tibia with Autologous Tissue Substitute, Percutaneous Approach

0QUH3JZ Supplement Left Tibia with Synthetic Substitute, Percutaneous Approach

0QUH3KZ Supplement Left Tibia with Nonautologous Tissue Substitute, Percutaneous Approach

0QUH47Z Supplement Left Tibia with Autologous Tissue Substitute, Percutaneous Endoscopic Approach

0QUH4JZ Supplement Left Tibia with Synthetic Substitute, Percutaneous Endoscopic Approach

0QUH4KZ Supplement Left Tibia with Nonautologous Tissue Substitute, Percutaneous Endoscopic Approach

0QUJ07Z Supplement Right Fibula with Autologous Tissue Substitute, Open Approach

0QUJ0JZ Supplement Right Fibula with Synthetic Substitute, Open Approach

0QUJ0KZ Supplement Right Fibula with Nonautologous Tissue Substitute, Open Approach

0QUJ37Z Supplement Right Fibula with Autologous Tissue Substitute, Percutaneous Approach

0QUJ3JZ Supplement Right Fibula with Synthetic Substitute, Percutaneous Approach

0QUJ3KZ Supplement Right Fibula with Nonautologous Tissue Substitute, Percutaneous Approach

0QUJ47Z Supplement Right Fibula with Autologous Tissue Substitute, Percutaneous Endoscopic Approach

0QUJ4JZ Supplement Right Fibula with Synthetic Substitute, Percutaneous Endoscopic Approach

0QUJ4KZ Supplement Right Fibula with Nonautologous Tissue Substitute, Percutaneous Endoscopic Approach

0QUK07Z Supplement Left Fibula with Autologous Tissue Substitute, Open Approach

0QUK0JZ Supplement Left Fibula with Synthetic Substitute, Open Approach

0QUK0KZ Supplement Left Fibula with Nonautologous Tissue Substitute, Open Approach

0QUK37Z Supplement Left Fibula with Autologous Tissue Substitute, Percutaneous Approach

0QUK3JZ Supplement Left Fibula with Synthetic Substitute, Percutaneous Approach

0QUK3KZ Supplement Left Fibula with Nonautologous Tissue Substitute, Percutaneous Approach

0QUK47Z Supplement Left Fibula with Autologous Tissue Substitute, Percutaneous Endoscopic Approach

0QUK4JZ Supplement Left Fibula with Synthetic Substitute, Percutaneous Endoscopic Approach

0QUK4KZ Supplement Left Fibula with Nonautologous Tissue Substitute, Percutaneous Endoscopic Approach

0QUL07Z Supplement Right Tarsal with Autologous Tissue Substitute, Open Approach

0QUL0JZ Supplement Right Tarsal with Synthetic Substitute, Open Approach

0QUL0KZ Supplement Right Tarsal with Nonautologous Tissue Substitute, Open Approach

0QUL37Z Supplement Right Tarsal with Autologous Tissue Substitute, Percutaneous Approach

0QUL3JZ Supplement Right Tarsal with Synthetic Substitute, Percutaneous Approach

0QUL3KZ Supplement Right Tarsal with Nonautologous Tissue Substitute, Percutaneous Approach

0QUL47Z Supplement Right Tarsal with Autologous Tissue Substitute, Percutaneous Endoscopic Approach

0QUL4JZ Supplement Right Tarsal with Synthetic Substitute, Percutaneous Endoscopic Approach

0QUL4KZ Supplement Right Tarsal with Nonautologous Tissue Substitute, Percutaneous Endoscopic Approach

0QUM07Z Supplement Left Tarsal with Autologous Tissue Substitute, Open Approach

0QUM0JZ Supplement Left Tarsal with Synthetic Substitute, Open Approach

0QUM0KZ Supplement Left Tarsal with Nonautologous Tissue Substitute, Open Approach

0QUM37Z Supplement Left Tarsal with Autologous Tissue Substitute, Percutaneous Approach

0QUM3JZ Supplement Left Tarsal with Synthetic Substitute, Percutaneous Approach

0QUM3KZ Supplement Left Tarsal with Nonautologous Tissue Substitute, Percutaneous Approach

0QUM47Z Supplement Left Tarsal with Autologous Tissue Substitute, Percutaneous Endoscopic Approach

0QUM4JZ Supplement Left Tarsal with Synthetic Substitute, Percutaneous Endoscopic Approach

0QUM4KZ Supplement Left Tarsal with Nonautologous Tissue Substitute, Percutaneous Endoscopic Approach

0QUN07Z Supplement Right Metatarsal with Autologous Tissue Substitute, Open Approach

0QUN0JZ Supplement Right Metatarsal with Synthetic Substitute, Open Approach

0QUN0KZ Supplement Right Metatarsal with Nonautologous Tissue Substitute, Open Approach

0QUN37Z Supplement Right Metatarsal with Autologous Tissue Substitute, Percutaneous Approach

0QUN3JZ Supplement Right Metatarsal with Synthetic Substitute, Percutaneous Approach

0QUN3KZ Supplement Right Metatarsal with Nonautologous Tissue Substitute, Percutaneous Approach

0QUN47Z Supplement Right Metatarsal with Autologous Tissue Substitute, Percutaneous Endoscopic Approach

0QUN4JZ Supplement Right Metatarsal with Synthetic Substitute, Percutaneous Endoscopic Approach

0QUN4KZ Supplement Right Metatarsal with Nonautologous Tissue Substitute, Percutaneous Endoscopic Approach

0QUP07Z Supplement Left Metatarsal with Autologous Tissue Substitute, Open Approach

0QUP0JZ Supplement Left Metatarsal with Synthetic Substitute, Open Approach

0QUP0KZ Supplement Left Metatarsal with Nonautologous Tissue Substitute, Open Approach

0QUP37Z Supplement Left Metatarsal with Autologous Tissue Substitute, Percutaneous Approach

0QUP3JZ Supplement Left Metatarsal with Synthetic Substitute, Percutaneous Approach

0QUP3KZ Supplement Left Metatarsal with Nonautologous Tissue Substitute, Percutaneous Approach

0QUP47Z Supplement Left Metatarsal with Autologous Tissue Substitute, Percutaneous Endoscopic Approach

0QUP4JZ Supplement Left Metatarsal with Synthetic Substitute, Percutaneous Endoscopic Approach

0QUP4KZ Supplement Left Metatarsal with Nonautologous Tissue Substitute, Percutaneous Endoscopic Approach

0QUQ07Z Supplement Right Toe Phalanx with Autologous Tissue Substitute, Open Approach

0QUQ0JZ Supplement Right Toe Phalanx with Synthetic Substitute, Open Approach

0QUQ0KZ Supplement Right Toe Phalanx with Nonautologous Tissue Substitute, Open Approach

0QUQ37Z Supplement Right Toe Phalanx with Autologous Tissue Substitute, Percutaneous Approach

0QUQ3JZ Supplement Right Toe Phalanx with Synthetic Substitute, Percutaneous Approach

0QUQ3KZ Supplement Right Toe Phalanx with Nonautologous Tissue Substitute, Percutaneous Approach

0QUQ47Z Supplement Right Toe Phalanx with Autologous Tissue Substitute, Percutaneous Endoscopic Approach

0QUQ4JZ Supplement Right Toe Phalanx with Synthetic Substitute, Percutaneous Endoscopic Approach

0QUQ4KZ Supplement Right Toe Phalanx with Nonautologous Tissue Substitute, Percutaneous Endoscopic Approach

0QUR07Z Supplement Left Toe Phalanx with Autologous Tissue Substitute, Open Approach

0QUR0JZ Supplement Left Toe Phalanx with Synthetic Substitute, Open Approach

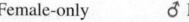

♀ Female-only   ♂ Male-only   ▲ Limited Coverage   ● Non-OR   ▨ HAC-associated procedure   ▲ Non-covered procedures   + Combination

UR0KZ	Supplement Left Toe Phalanx with Nonautologous Tissue Substitute, Open Approach	0QUR4JZ	Supplement Left Toe Phalanx with Synthetic Substitute, Percutaneous Endoscopic Approach	0QUS3JZ	Supplement Coccyx with Synthetic Substitute, Percutaneous Approach

UR0KZ Supplement Left Toe Phalanx with Nonautologous Tissue Substitute, Open Approach

UR37Z Supplement Left Toe Phalanx with Autologous Tissue Substitute, Percutaneous Approach

UR3JZ Supplement Left Toe Phalanx with Synthetic Substitute, Percutaneous Approach

UR3KZ Supplement Left Toe Phalanx with Nonautologous Tissue Substitute, Percutaneous Approach

UR47Z Supplement Left Toe Phalanx with Autologous Tissue Substitute, Percutaneous Endoscopic Approach

0QUR4JZ Supplement Left Toe Phalanx with Synthetic Substitute, Percutaneous Endoscopic Approach

0QUR4KZ Supplement Left Toe Phalanx with Nonautologous Tissue Substitute, Percutaneous Endoscopic Approach

0QUS07Z Supplement Coccyx with Autologous Tissue Substitute, Open Approach

0QUS0JZ Supplement Coccyx with Synthetic Substitute, Open Approach

0QUS0KZ Supplement Coccyx with Nonautologous Tissue Substitute, Open Approach

0QUS37Z Supplement Coccyx with Autologous Tissue Substitute, Percutaneous Approach

0QUS3JZ Supplement Coccyx with Synthetic Substitute, Percutaneous Approach

0QUS3KZ Supplement Coccyx with Nonautologous Tissue Substitute, Percutaneous Approach

0QUS47Z Supplement Coccyx with Autologous Tissue Substitute, Percutaneous Endoscopic Approach

0QUS4JZ Supplement Coccyx with Synthetic Substitute, Percutaneous Endoscopic Approach

0QUS4KZ Supplement Coccyx with Nonautologous Tissue Substitute, Percutaneous Endoscopic Approach

W – Lower Bones, Revision

view Coding Guideline B6.1c

W004Z Revision of Internal Fixation Device in Lumbar Vertebra, Open Approach

W007Z Revision of Autologous Tissue Substitute in Lumbar Vertebra, Open Approach

W00JZ Revision of Synthetic Substitute in Lumbar Vertebra, Open Approach

W00KZ Revision of Nonautologous Tissue Substitute in Lumbar Vertebra, Open Approach

W034Z Revision of Internal Fixation Device in Lumbar Vertebra, Percutaneous Approach

W037Z Revision of Autologous Tissue Substitute in Lumbar Vertebra, Percutaneous Approach

W03JZ Revision of Synthetic Substitute in Lumbar Vertebra, Percutaneous Approach

W03KZ Revision of Nonautologous Tissue Substitute in Lumbar Vertebra, Percutaneous Approach

W044Z Revision of Internal Fixation Device in Lumbar Vertebra, Percutaneous Endoscopic Approach

W047Z Revision of Autologous Tissue Substitute in Lumbar Vertebra, Percutaneous Endoscopic Approach

W04JZ Revision of Synthetic Substitute in Lumbar Vertebra, Percutaneous Endoscopic Approach

W04KZ Revision of Nonautologous Tissue Substitute in Lumbar Vertebra, Percutaneous Endoscopic Approach

W0X4Z Revision of Internal Fixation Device in Lumbar Vertebra, External Approach

W0X7Z Revision of Autologous Tissue Substitute in Lumbar Vertebra, External Approach

W0XJZ Revision of Synthetic Substitute in Lumbar Vertebra, External Approach

W0XKZ Revision of Nonautologous Tissue Substitute in Lumbar Vertebra, External Approach

W104Z Revision of Internal Fixation Device in Sacrum, Open Approach

W107Z Revision of Autologous Tissue Substitute in Sacrum, Open Approach

W10JZ Revision of Synthetic Substitute in Sacrum, Open Approach

W10KZ Revision of Nonautologous Tissue Substitute in Sacrum, Open Approach

W134Z Revision of Internal Fixation Device in Sacrum, Percutaneous Approach

W137Z Revision of Autologous Tissue Substitute in Sacrum, Percutaneous Approach

W13JZ Revision of Synthetic Substitute in Sacrum, Percutaneous Approach

W13KZ Revision of Nonautologous Tissue Substitute in Sacrum, Percutaneous Approach

0QW144Z Revision of Internal Fixation Device in Sacrum, Percutaneous Endoscopic Approach

0QW147Z Revision of Autologous Tissue Substitute in Sacrum, Percutaneous Endoscopic Approach

0QW14JZ Revision of Synthetic Substitute in Sacrum, Percutaneous Endoscopic Approach

0QW14KZ Revision of Nonautologous Tissue Substitute in Sacrum, Percutaneous Endoscopic Approach

0QW1X4Z Revision of Internal Fixation Device in Sacrum, External Approach

0QW1X7Z Revision of Autologous Tissue Substitute in Sacrum, External Approach

0QW1XJZ Revision of Synthetic Substitute in Sacrum, External Approach

0QW1XKZ Revision of Nonautologous Tissue Substitute in Sacrum, External Approach

0QW204Z Revision of Internal Fixation Device in Right Pelvic Bone, Open Approach

0QW205Z Revision of External Fixation Device in Right Pelvic Bone, Open Approach

0QW207Z Revision of Autologous Tissue Substitute in Right Pelvic Bone, Open Approach

0QW20JZ Revision of Synthetic Substitute in Right Pelvic Bone, Open Approach

0QW20KZ Revision of Nonautologous Tissue Substitute in Right Pelvic Bone, Open Approach

0QW234Z Revision of Internal Fixation Device in Right Pelvic Bone, Percutaneous Approach

0QW235Z Revision of External Fixation Device in Right Pelvic Bone, Percutaneous Approach

0QW237Z Revision of Autologous Tissue Substitute in Right Pelvic Bone, Percutaneous Approach

0QW23JZ Revision of Synthetic Substitute in Right Pelvic Bone, Percutaneous Approach

0QW23KZ Revision of Nonautologous Tissue Substitute in Right Pelvic Bone, Percutaneous Approach

0QW244Z Revision of Internal Fixation Device in Right Pelvic Bone, Percutaneous Endoscopic Approach

0QW245Z Revision of External Fixation Device in Right Pelvic Bone, Percutaneous Endoscopic Approach

0QW247Z Revision of Autologous Tissue Substitute in Right Pelvic Bone, Percutaneous Endoscopic Approach

0QW24JZ Revision of Synthetic Substitute in Right Pelvic Bone, Percutaneous Endoscopic Approach

0QW24KZ Revision of Nonautologous Tissue Substitute in Right Pelvic Bone, Percutaneous Endoscopic Approach

0QW2X4Z Revision of Internal Fixation Device in Right Pelvic Bone, External Approach

0QW2X5Z Revision of External Fixation Device in Right Pelvic Bone, External Approach

0QW2X7Z Revision of Autologous Tissue Substitute in Right Pelvic Bone, External Approach

0QW2XJZ Revision of Synthetic Substitute in Right Pelvic Bone, External Approach

0QW2XKZ Revision of Nonautologous Tissue Substitute in Right Pelvic Bone, External Approach

0QW304Z Revision of Internal Fixation Device in Left Pelvic Bone, Open Approach

0QW305Z Revision of External Fixation Device in Left Pelvic Bone, Open Approach

0QW307Z Revision of Autologous Tissue Substitute in Left Pelvic Bone, Open Approach

0QW30JZ Revision of Synthetic Substitute in Left Pelvic Bone, Open Approach

0QW30KZ Revision of Nonautologous Tissue Substitute in Left Pelvic Bone, Open Approach

0QW334Z Revision of Internal Fixation Device in Left Pelvic Bone, Percutaneous Approach

0QW335Z Revision of External Fixation Device in Left Pelvic Bone, Percutaneous Approach

0QW337Z Revision of Autologous Tissue Substitute in Left Pelvic Bone, Percutaneous Approach

0QW33JZ Revision of Synthetic Substitute in Left Pelvic Bone, Percutaneous Approach

0QW33KZ Revision of Nonautologous Tissue Substitute in Left Pelvic Bone, Percutaneous Approach

0QW344Z Revision of Internal Fixation Device in Left Pelvic Bone, Percutaneous Endoscopic Approach

0QW345Z Revision of External Fixation Device in Left Pelvic Bone, Percutaneous Endoscopic Approach

0QW347Z Revision of Autologous Tissue Substitute in Left Pelvic Bone, Percutaneous Endoscopic Approach

0QW34JZ Revision of Synthetic Substitute in Left Pelvic Bone, Percutaneous Endoscopic Approach

0QW34KZ Revision of Nonautologous Tissue Substitute in Left Pelvic Bone, Percutaneous Endoscopic Approach

0QW3X4Z Revision of Internal Fixation Device in Left Pelvic Bone, External Approach

---

Female-only   ♂ Male-only   ▲ Limited Coverage   ● Non-OR   ■ HAC-associated procedure   ▲ Non-covered procedures   ✚ Combination

0QW3X5Z Revision of External Fixation Device in Left Pelvic Bone, External Approach
0QW3X7Z Revision of Autologous Tissue Substitute in Left Pelvic Bone, External Approach
0QW3XJZ Revision of Synthetic Substitute in Left Pelvic Bone, External Approach
0QW3XKZ Revision of Nonautologous Tissue Substitute in Left Pelvic Bone, External Approach
0QW404Z Revision of Internal Fixation Device in Right Acetabulum, Open Approach
0QW407Z Revision of Autologous Tissue Substitute in Right Acetabulum, Open Approach
0QW40JZ Revision of Synthetic Substitute in Right Acetabulum, Open Approach
0QW40KZ Revision of Nonautologous Tissue Substitute in Right Acetabulum, Open Approach
0QW434Z Revision of Internal Fixation Device in Right Acetabulum, Percutaneous Approach
0QW437Z Revision of Autologous Tissue Substitute in Right Acetabulum, Percutaneous Approach
0QW43JZ Revision of Synthetic Substitute in Right Acetabulum, Percutaneous Approach
0QW43KZ Revision of Nonautologous Tissue Substitute in Right Acetabulum, Percutaneous Approach
0QW444Z Revision of Internal Fixation Device in Right Acetabulum, Percutaneous Endoscopic Approach
0QW447Z Revision of Autologous Tissue Substitute in Right Acetabulum, Percutaneous Endoscopic Approach
0QW44JZ Revision of Synthetic Substitute in Right Acetabulum, Percutaneous Endoscopic Approach
0QW44KZ Revision of Nonautologous Tissue Substitute in Right Acetabulum, Percutaneous Endoscopic Approach
0QW4X4Z Revision of Internal Fixation Device in Right Acetabulum, External Approach
0QW4X7Z Revision of Autologous Tissue Substitute in Right Acetabulum, External Approach
0QW4XJZ Revision of Synthetic Substitute in Right Acetabulum, External Approach
0QW4XKZ Revision of Nonautologous Tissue Substitute in Right Acetabulum, External Approach
0QW504Z Revision of Internal Fixation Device in Left Acetabulum, Open Approach
0QW507Z Revision of Autologous Tissue Substitute in Left Acetabulum, Open Approach
0QW50JZ Revision of Synthetic Substitute in Left Acetabulum, Open Approach
0QW50KZ Revision of Nonautologous Tissue Substitute in Left Acetabulum, Open Approach
0QW534Z Revision of Internal Fixation Device in Left Acetabulum, Percutaneous Approach
0QW537Z Revision of Autologous Tissue Substitute in Left Acetabulum, Percutaneous Approach
0QW53JZ Revision of Synthetic Substitute in Left Acetabulum, Percutaneous Approach
0QW53KZ Revision of Nonautologous Tissue Substitute in Left Acetabulum, Percutaneous Approach
0QW544Z Revision of Internal Fixation Device in Left Acetabulum, Percutaneous Endoscopic Approach
0QW547Z Revision of Autologous Tissue Substitute in Left Acetabulum, Percutaneous Endoscopic Approach

0QW54JZ Revision of Synthetic Substitute in Left Acetabulum, Percutaneous Endoscopic Approach
0QW54KZ Revision of Nonautologous Tissue Substitute in Left Acetabulum, Percutaneous Endoscopic Approach
0QW5X4Z Revision of Internal Fixation Device in Left Acetabulum, External Approach
0QW5X7Z Revision of Autologous Tissue Substitute in Left Acetabulum, External Approach
0QW5XJZ Revision of Synthetic Substitute in Left Acetabulum, External Approach
0QW5XKZ Revision of Nonautologous Tissue Substitute in Left Acetabulum, External Approach
0QW604Z Revision of Internal Fixation Device in Right Upper Femur, Open Approach
0QW605Z Revision of External Fixation Device in Right Upper Femur, Open Approach
0QW607Z Revision of Autologous Tissue Substitute in Right Upper Femur, Open Approach
0QW60JZ Revision of Synthetic Substitute in Right Upper Femur, Open Approach
0QW60KZ Revision of Nonautologous Tissue Substitute in Right Upper Femur, Open Approach
0QW634Z Revision of Internal Fixation Device in Right Upper Femur, Percutaneous Approach
0QW635Z Revision of External Fixation Device in Right Upper Femur, Percutaneous Approach
0QW637Z Revision of Autologous Tissue Substitute in Right Upper Femur, Percutaneous Approach
0QW63JZ Revision of Synthetic Substitute in Right Upper Femur, Percutaneous Approach
0QW63KZ Revision of Nonautologous Tissue Substitute in Right Upper Femur, Percutaneous Approach
0QW644Z Revision of Internal Fixation Device in Right Upper Femur, Percutaneous Endoscopic Approach
0QW645Z Revision of External Fixation Device in Right Upper Femur, Percutaneous Endoscopic Approach
0QW647Z Revision of Autologous Tissue Substitute in Right Upper Femur, Percutaneous Endoscopic Approach
0QW64JZ Revision of Synthetic Substitute in Right Upper Femur, Percutaneous Endoscopic Approach
0QW64KZ Revision of Nonautologous Tissue Substitute in Right Upper Femur, Percutaneous Endoscopic Approach
0QW6X4Z Revision of Internal Fixation Device in Right Upper Femur, External Approach
0QW6X5Z Revision of External Fixation Device in Right Upper Femur, External Approach
0QW6X7Z Revision of Autologous Tissue Substitute in Right Upper Femur, External Approach
0QW6XJZ Revision of Synthetic Substitute in Right Upper Femur, External Approach
0QW6XKZ Revision of Nonautologous Tissue Substitute in Right Upper Femur, External Approach
0QW704Z Revision of Internal Fixation Device in Left Upper Femur, Open Approach
0QW705Z Revision of External Fixation Device in Left Upper Femur, Open Approach
0QW707Z Revision of Autologous Tissue Substitute in Left Upper Femur, Open Approach
0QW70JZ Revision of Synthetic Substitute in Left Upper Femur, Open Approach

0QW70KZ Revision of Nonautologous Tissue Substitute in Left Upper Femur, Open Approach
0QW734Z Revision of Internal Fixation Device in Left Upper Femur, Percutaneous Approach
0QW735Z Revision of External Fixation Device in Left Upper Femur, Percutaneous Approach
0QW737Z Revision of Autologous Tissue Substit in Left Upper Femur, Percutaneous Approach
0QW73JZ Revision of Synthetic Substitute in Le Upper Femur, Percutaneous Approach
0QW73KZ Revision of Nonautologous Tissue Substitute in Left Upper Femur, Percutaneous Approach
0QW744Z Revision of Internal Fixation Device in Left Upper Femur, Percutaneous Endoscopic Approach
0QW745Z Revision of External Fixation Device in Left Upper Femur, Percutaneous Endoscopic Approach
0QW747Z Revision of Autologous Tissue Substit in Left Upper Femur, Percutaneous Endoscopic Approach
0QW74JZ Revision of Synthetic Substitute in Lef Upper Femur, Percutaneous Endoscopi Approach
0QW74KZ Revision of Nonautologous Tissue Substitute in Left Upper Femur, Percutaneous Endoscopic Approach
0QW7X4Z Revision of Internal Fixation Device in Left Upper Femur, External Approach
0QW7X5Z Revision of External Fixation Device i Left Upper Femur, External Approach
0QW7X7Z Revision of Autologous Tissue Substit in Left Upper Femur, External Approac
0QW7XJZ Revision of Synthetic Substitute in Lef Upper Femur, External Approach
0QW7XKZ Revision of Nonautologous Tissue Substitute in Left Upper Femur, Extern Approach
0QW804Z Revision of Internal Fixation Device in Right Femoral Shaft, Open Approach
0QW805Z Revision of External Fixation Device i Right Femoral Shaft, Open Approach
0QW807Z Revision of Autologous Tissue Substitu in Right Femoral Shaft, Open Approach
0QW80JZ Revision of Synthetic Substitute in Rig Femoral Shaft, Open Approach
0QW80KZ Revision of Nonautologous Tissue Substitute in Right Femoral Shaft, Ope Approach
0QW834Z Revision of Internal Fixation Device in Right Femoral Shaft, Percutaneous Approach
0QW835Z Revision of External Fixation Device in Right Femoral Shaft, Percutaneous Approach
0QW837Z Revision of Autologous Tissue Substitu in Right Femoral Shaft, Percutaneous Approach
0QW83JZ Revision of Synthetic Substitute in Righ Femoral Shaft, Percutaneous Approach
0QW83KZ Revision of Nonautologous Tissue Substitute in Right Femoral Shaft, Percutaneous Approach
0QW844Z Revision of Internal Fixation Device in Right Femoral Shaft, Percutaneous Endoscopic Approach
0QW845Z Revision of External Fixation Device in Right Femoral Shaft, Percutaneous Endoscopic Approach
0QW847Z Revision of Autologous Tissue Substitut in Right Femoral Shaft, Percutaneous Endoscopic Approach

W84JZ Revision of Synthetic Substitute in Right Femoral Shaft, Percutaneous Endoscopic Approach

W84KZ Revision of Nonautologous Tissue Substitute in Right Femoral Shaft, Percutaneous Endoscopic Approach

W8X4Z Revision of Internal Fixation Device in Right Femoral Shaft, External Approach

W8X5Z Revision of External Fixation Device in Right Femoral Shaft, External Approach

W8X7Z Revision of Autologous Tissue Substitute in Right Femoral Shaft, External Approach

W8XJZ Revision of Synthetic Substitute in Right Femoral Shaft, External Approach

W8XKZ Revision of Nonautologous Tissue Substitute in Right Femoral Shaft, External Approach

W904Z Revision of Internal Fixation Device in Left Femoral Shaft, Open Approach

W905Z Revision of External Fixation Device in Left Femoral Shaft, Open Approach

W907Z Revision of Autologous Tissue Substitute in Left Femoral Shaft, Open Approach

W90JZ Revision of Synthetic Substitute in Left Femoral Shaft, Open Approach

W90KZ Revision of Nonautologous Tissue Substitute in Left Femoral Shaft, Open Approach

W934Z Revision of Internal Fixation Device in Left Femoral Shaft, Percutaneous Approach

W935Z Revision of External Fixation Device in Left Femoral Shaft, Percutaneous Approach

W937Z Revision of Autologous Tissue Substitute in Left Femoral Shaft, Percutaneous Approach

W93JZ Revision of Synthetic Substitute in Left Femoral Shaft, Percutaneous Approach

W93KZ Revision of Nonautologous Tissue Substitute in Left Femoral Shaft, Percutaneous Approach

W944Z Revision of Internal Fixation Device in Left Femoral Shaft, Percutaneous Endoscopic Approach

W945Z Revision of External Fixation Device in Left Femoral Shaft, Percutaneous Endoscopic Approach

W947Z Revision of Autologous Tissue Substitute in Left Femoral Shaft, Percutaneous Endoscopic Approach

W94JZ Revision of Synthetic Substitute in Left Femoral Shaft, Percutaneous Endoscopic Approach

W94KZ Revision of Nonautologous Tissue Substitute in Left Femoral Shaft, Percutaneous Endoscopic Approach

W9X4Z Revision of Internal Fixation Device in Left Femoral Shaft, External Approach

W9X5Z Revision of External Fixation Device in Left Femoral Shaft, External Approach

W9X7Z Revision of Autologous Tissue Substitute in Left Femoral Shaft, External Approach

W9XJZ Revision of Synthetic Substitute in Left Femoral Shaft, External Approach

W9XKZ Revision of Nonautologous Tissue Substitute in Left Femoral Shaft, External Approach

WB04Z Revision of Internal Fixation Device in Right Lower Femur, Open Approach

WB05Z Revision of External Fixation Device in Right Lower Femur, Open Approach

WB07Z Revision of Autologous Tissue Substitute in Right Lower Femur, Open Approach

WB0JZ Revision of Synthetic Substitute in Right Lower Femur, Open Approach

0QWB0KZ Revision of Nonautologous Tissue Substitute in Right Lower Femur, Open Approach

0QWB34Z Revision of Internal Fixation Device in Right Lower Femur, Percutaneous Approach

0QWB35Z Revision of External Fixation Device in Right Lower Femur, Percutaneous Approach

0QWB37Z Revision of Autologous Tissue Substitute in Right Lower Femur, Percutaneous Approach

0QWB3JZ Revision of Synthetic Substitute in Right Lower Femur, Percutaneous Approach

0QWB3KZ Revision of Nonautologous Tissue Substitute in Right Lower Femur, Percutaneous Approach

0QWB44Z Revision of Internal Fixation Device in Right Lower Femur, Percutaneous Endoscopic Approach

0QWB45Z Revision of External Fixation Device in Right Lower Femur, Percutaneous Endoscopic Approach

0QWB47Z Revision of Autologous Tissue Substitute in Right Lower Femur, Percutaneous Endoscopic Approach

0QWB4JZ Revision of Synthetic Substitute in Right Lower Femur, Percutaneous Endoscopic Approach

0QWB4KZ Revision of Nonautologous Tissue Substitute in Right Lower Femur, Percutaneous Endoscopic Approach

0QWBX4Z Revision of Internal Fixation Device in Right Lower Femur, External Approach

0QWBX5Z Revision of External Fixation Device in Right Lower Femur, External Approach

0QWBX7Z Revision of Autologous Tissue Substitute in Right Lower Femur, External Approach

0QWBXJZ Revision of Synthetic Substitute in Right Lower Femur, External Approach

0QWBXKZ Revision of Nonautologous Tissue Substitute in Right Lower Femur, External Approach

0QWC04Z Revision of Internal Fixation Device in Left Lower Femur, Open Approach

0QWC05Z Revision of External Fixation Device in Left Lower Femur, Open Approach

0QWC07Z Revision of Autologous Tissue Substitute in Left Lower Femur, Open Approach

0QWC0JZ Revision of Synthetic Substitute in Left Lower Femur, Open Approach

0QWC0KZ Revision of Nonautologous Tissue Substitute in Left Lower Femur, Open Approach

0QWC34Z Revision of Internal Fixation Device in Left Lower Femur, Percutaneous Approach

0QWC35Z Revision of External Fixation Device in Left Lower Femur, Percutaneous Approach

0QWC37Z Revision of Autologous Tissue Substitute in Left Lower Femur, Percutaneous Approach

0QWC3JZ Revision of Synthetic Substitute in Left Lower Femur, Percutaneous Approach

0QWC3KZ Revision of Nonautologous Tissue Substitute in Left Lower Femur, Percutaneous Approach

0QWC44Z Revision of Internal Fixation Device in Left Lower Femur, Percutaneous Endoscopic Approach

0QWC45Z Revision of External Fixation Device in Left Lower Femur, Percutaneous Endoscopic Approach

0QWC47Z Revision of Autologous Tissue Substitute in Left Lower Femur, Percutaneous Endoscopic Approach

0QWC4JZ Revision of Synthetic Substitute in Left Lower Femur, Percutaneous Endoscopic Approach

0QWC4KZ Revision of Nonautologous Tissue Substitute in Left Lower Femur, Percutaneous Endoscopic Approach

0QWCX4Z Revision of Internal Fixation Device in Left Lower Femur, External Approach

0QWCX5Z Revision of External Fixation Device in Left Lower Femur, External Approach

0QWCX7Z Revision of Autologous Tissue Substitute in Left Lower Femur, External Approach

0QWCXJZ Revision of Synthetic Substitute in Left Lower Femur, External Approach

0QWCXKZ Revision of Nonautologous Tissue Substitute in Left Lower Femur, External Approach

0QWD04Z Revision of Internal Fixation Device in Right Patella, Open Approach

0QWD05Z Revision of External Fixation Device in Right Patella, Open Approach

0QWD07Z Revision of Autologous Tissue Substitute in Right Patella, Open Approach

0QWD0JZ Revision of Synthetic Substitute in Right Patella, Open Approach

0QWD0KZ Revision of Nonautologous Tissue Substitute in Right Patella, Open Approach

0QWD34Z Revision of Internal Fixation Device in Right Patella, Percutaneous Approach

0QWD35Z Revision of External Fixation Device in Right Patella, Percutaneous Approach

0QWD37Z Revision of Autologous Tissue Substitute in Right Patella, Percutaneous Approach

0QWD3JZ Revision of Synthetic Substitute in Right Patella, Percutaneous Approach

0QWD3KZ Revision of Nonautologous Tissue Substitute in Right Patella, Percutaneous Approach

0QWD44Z Revision of Internal Fixation Device in Right Patella, Percutaneous Endoscopic Approach

0QWD45Z Revision of External Fixation Device in Right Patella, Percutaneous Endoscopic Approach

0QWD47Z Revision of Autologous Tissue Substitute in Right Patella, Percutaneous Endoscopic Approach

0QWD4JZ Revision of Synthetic Substitute in Right Patella, Percutaneous Endoscopic Approach

0QWD4KZ Revision of Nonautologous Tissue Substitute in Right Patella, Percutaneous Endoscopic Approach

0QWDX4Z Revision of Internal Fixation Device in Right Patella, External Approach

0QWDX5Z Revision of External Fixation Device in Right Patella, External Approach

0QWDX7Z Revision of Autologous Tissue Substitute in Right Patella, External Approach

0QWDXJZ Revision of Synthetic Substitute in Right Patella, External Approach

0QWDXKZ Revision of Nonautologous Tissue Substitute in Right Patella, External Approach

0QWF04Z Revision of Internal Fixation Device in Left Patella, Open Approach

0QWF05Z Revision of External Fixation Device in Left Patella, Open Approach

Female-only   ♂ Male-only   ▲ Limited Coverage   ● Non-OR   ■ HAC-associated procedure   ▲ Non-covered procedures   ✛ Combination

0QWF07Z	Revision of Autologous Tissue Substitute in Left Patella, Open Approach	
0QWF0JZ	Revision of Synthetic Substitute in Left Patella, Open Approach	
0QWF0KZ	Revision of Nonautologous Tissue Substitute in Left Patella, Open Approach	
0QWF34Z	Revision of Internal Fixation Device in Left Patella, Percutaneous Approach	
0QWF35Z	Revision of External Fixation Device in Left Patella, Percutaneous Approach	
0QWF37Z	Revision of Autologous Tissue Substitute in Left Patella, Percutaneous Approach	
0QWF3JZ	Revision of Synthetic Substitute in Left Patella, Percutaneous Approach	
0QWF3KZ	Revision of Nonautologous Tissue Substitute in Left Patella, Percutaneous Approach	
0QWF44Z	Revision of Internal Fixation Device in Left Patella, Percutaneous Endoscopic Approach	
0QWF45Z	Revision of External Fixation Device in Left Patella, Percutaneous Endoscopic Approach	
0QWF47Z	Revision of Autologous Tissue Substitute in Left Patella, Percutaneous Endoscopic Approach	
0QWF4JZ	Revision of Synthetic Substitute in Left Patella, Percutaneous Endoscopic Approach	
0QWF4KZ	Revision of Nonautologous Tissue Substitute in Left Patella, Percutaneous Endoscopic Approach	
0QWFX4Z	Revision of Internal Fixation Device in Left Patella, External Approach	
0QWFX5Z	Revision of External Fixation Device in Left Patella, External Approach	
0QWFX7Z	Revision of Autologous Tissue Substitute in Left Patella, External Approach	
0QWFXJZ	Revision of Synthetic Substitute in Left Patella, External Approach	
0QWFXKZ	Revision of Nonautologous Tissue Substitute in Left Patella, External Approach	
0QWG04Z	Revision of Internal Fixation Device in Right Tibia, Open Approach	
0QWG05Z	Revision of External Fixation Device in Right Tibia, Open Approach	
0QWG07Z	Revision of Autologous Tissue Substitute in Right Tibia, Open Approach	
0QWG0JZ	Revision of Synthetic Substitute in Right Tibia, Open Approach	
0QWG0KZ	Revision of Nonautologous Tissue Substitute in Right Tibia, Open Approach	
0QWG34Z	Revision of Internal Fixation Device in Right Tibia, Percutaneous Approach	
0QWG35Z	Revision of External Fixation Device in Right Tibia, Percutaneous Approach	
0QWG37Z	Revision of Autologous Tissue Substitute in Right Tibia, Percutaneous Approach	
0QWG3JZ	Revision of Synthetic Substitute in Right Tibia, Percutaneous Approach	
0QWG3KZ	Revision of Nonautologous Tissue Substitute in Right Tibia, Percutaneous Approach	
0QWG44Z	Revision of Internal Fixation Device in Right Tibia, Percutaneous Endoscopic Approach	
0QWG45Z	Revision of External Fixation Device in Right Tibia, Percutaneous Endoscopic Approach	
0QWG47Z	Revision of Autologous Tissue Substitute in Right Tibia, Percutaneous Endoscopic Approach	
0QWG4JZ	Revision of Synthetic Substitute in Right Tibia, Percutaneous Endoscopic Approach	
0QWG4KZ	Revision of Nonautologous Tissue Substitute in Right Tibia, Percutaneous Endoscopic Approach	
0QWGX4Z	Revision of Internal Fixation Device in Right Tibia, External Approach	
0QWGX5Z	Revision of External Fixation Device in Right Tibia, External Approach	
0QWGX7Z	Revision of Autologous Tissue Substitute in Right Tibia, External Approach	
0QWGXJZ	Revision of Synthetic Substitute in Right Tibia, External Approach	
0QWGXKZ	Revision of Nonautologous Tissue Substitute in Right Tibia, External Approach	
0QWH04Z	Revision of Internal Fixation Device in Left Tibia, Open Approach	
0QWH05Z	Revision of External Fixation Device in Left Tibia, Open Approach	
0QWH07Z	Revision of Autologous Tissue Substitute in Left Tibia, Open Approach	
0QWH0JZ	Revision of Synthetic Substitute in Left Tibia, Open Approach	
0QWH0KZ	Revision of Nonautologous Tissue Substitute in Left Tibia, Open Approach	
0QWH34Z	Revision of Internal Fixation Device in Left Tibia, Percutaneous Approach	
0QWH35Z	Revision of External Fixation Device in Left Tibia, Percutaneous Approach	
0QWH37Z	Revision of Autologous Tissue Substitute in Left Tibia, Percutaneous Approach	
0QWH3JZ	Revision of Synthetic Substitute in Left Tibia, Percutaneous Approach	
0QWH3KZ	Revision of Nonautologous Tissue Substitute in Left Tibia, Percutaneous Approach	
0QWH44Z	Revision of Internal Fixation Device in Left Tibia, Percutaneous Endoscopic Approach	
0QWH45Z	Revision of External Fixation Device in Left Tibia, Percutaneous Endoscopic Approach	
0QWH47Z	Revision of Autologous Tissue Substitute in Left Tibia, Percutaneous Endoscopic Approach	
0QWH4JZ	Revision of Synthetic Substitute in Left Tibia, Percutaneous Endoscopic Approach	
0QWH4KZ	Revision of Nonautologous Tissue Substitute in Left Tibia, Percutaneous Endoscopic Approach	
0QWHX4Z	Revision of Internal Fixation Device in Left Tibia, External Approach	
0QWHX5Z	Revision of External Fixation Device in Left Tibia, External Approach	
0QWHX7Z	Revision of Autologous Tissue Substitute in Left Tibia, External Approach	
0QWHXJZ	Revision of Synthetic Substitute in Left Tibia, External Approach	
0QWHXKZ	Revision of Nonautologous Tissue Substitute in Left Tibia, External Approach	
0QWJ04Z	Revision of Internal Fixation Device in Right Fibula, Open Approach	
0QWJ05Z	Revision of External Fixation Device in Right Fibula, Open Approach	
0QWJ07Z	Revision of Autologous Tissue Substitute in Right Fibula, Open Approach	
0QWJ0JZ	Revision of Synthetic Substitute in Right Fibula, Open Approach	
0QWJ0KZ	Revision of Nonautologous Tissue Substitute in Right Fibula, Open Approach	
0QWJ34Z	Revision of Internal Fixation Device in Right Fibula, Percutaneous Approach	
0QWJ35Z	Revision of External Fixation Device in Right Fibula, Percutaneous Approach	
0QWJ37Z	Revision of Autologous Tissue Substitute in Right Fibula, Percutaneous Approach	
0QWJ3JZ	Revision of Synthetic Substitute in Right Fibula, Percutaneous Approach	
0QWJ3KZ	Revision of Nonautologous Tissue Substitute in Right Fibula, Percutaneous Approach	
0QWJ44Z	Revision of Internal Fixation Device in Right Fibula, Percutaneous Endoscopic Approach	
0QWJ45Z	Revision of External Fixation Device in Right Fibula, Percutaneous Endoscopic Approach	
0QWJ47Z	Revision of Autologous Tissue Substitute in Right Fibula, Percutaneous Endoscopic Approach	
0QWJ4JZ	Revision of Synthetic Substitute in Right Fibula, Percutaneous Endoscopic Approach	
0QWJ4KZ	Revision of Nonautologous Tissue Substitute in Right Fibula, Percutaneous Endoscopic Approach	
0QWJX4Z	Revision of Internal Fixation Device in Right Fibula, External Approach	
0QWJX5Z	Revision of External Fixation Device in Right Fibula, External Approach	
0QWJX7Z	Revision of Autologous Tissue Substitute in Right Fibula, External Approach	
0QWJXJZ	Revision of Synthetic Substitute in Right Fibula, External Approach	
0QWJXKZ	Revision of Nonautologous Tissue Substitute in Right Fibula, External Approach	
0QWK04Z	Revision of Internal Fixation Device in Left Fibula, Open Approach	
0QWK05Z	Revision of External Fixation Device in Left Fibula, Open Approach	
0QWK07Z	Revision of Autologous Tissue Substitute in Left Fibula, Open Approach	
0QWK0JZ	Revision of Synthetic Substitute in Left Fibula, Open Approach	
0QWK0KZ	Revision of Nonautologous Tissue Substitute in Left Fibula, Open Approach	
0QWK34Z	Revision of Internal Fixation Device in Left Fibula, Percutaneous Approach	
0QWK35Z	Revision of External Fixation Device in Left Fibula, Percutaneous Approach	
0QWK37Z	Revision of Autologous Tissue Substitute in Left Fibula, Percutaneous Approach	
0QWK3JZ	Revision of Synthetic Substitute in Left Fibula, Percutaneous Approach	
0QWK3KZ	Revision of Nonautologous Tissue Substitute in Left Fibula, Percutaneous Approach	
0QWK44Z	Revision of Internal Fixation Device in Left Fibula, Percutaneous Endoscopic Approach	
0QWK45Z	Revision of External Fixation Device in Left Fibula, Percutaneous Endoscopic Approach	
0QWK47Z	Revision of Autologous Tissue Substitute in Left Fibula, Percutaneous Endoscopic Approach	

0QWK4JZ	Revision of Synthetic Substitute in Left Fibula, Percutaneous Endoscopic Approach
0QWK4KZ	Revision of Nonautologous Tissue Substitute in Left Fibula, Percutaneous Endoscopic Approach
0QWKX4Z	Revision of Internal Fixation Device in Left Fibula, External Approach
0QWKX5Z	Revision of External Fixation Device in Left Fibula, External Approach
0QWKX7Z	Revision of Autologous Tissue Substitute in Left Fibula, External Approach
0QWKXJZ	Revision of Synthetic Substitute in Left Fibula, External Approach
0QWKXKZ	Revision of Nonautologous Tissue Substitute in Left Fibula, External Approach
0QWL04Z	Revision of Internal Fixation Device in Right Tarsal, Open Approach
0QWL05Z	Revision of External Fixation Device in Right Tarsal, Open Approach
0QWL07Z	Revision of Autologous Tissue Substitute in Right Tarsal, Open Approach
0QWL0JZ	Revision of Synthetic Substitute in Right Tarsal, Open Approach
0QWL0KZ	Revision of Nonautologous Tissue Substitute in Right Tarsal, Open Approach
0QWL34Z	Revision of Internal Fixation Device in Right Tarsal, Percutaneous Approach
0QWL35Z	Revision of External Fixation Device in Right Tarsal, Percutaneous Approach
0QWL37Z	Revision of Autologous Tissue Substitute in Right Tarsal, Percutaneous Approach
0QWL3JZ	Revision of Synthetic Substitute in Right Tarsal, Percutaneous Approach
0QWL3KZ	Revision of Nonautologous Tissue Substitute in Right Tarsal, Percutaneous Approach
0QWL44Z	Revision of Internal Fixation Device in Right Tarsal, Percutaneous Endoscopic Approach
0QWL45Z	Revision of External Fixation Device in Right Tarsal, Percutaneous Endoscopic Approach
0QWL47Z	Revision of Autologous Tissue Substitute in Right Tarsal, Percutaneous Endoscopic Approach
0QWL4JZ	Revision of Synthetic Substitute in Right Tarsal, Percutaneous Endoscopic Approach
0QWL4KZ	Revision of Nonautologous Tissue Substitute in Right Tarsal, Percutaneous Endoscopic Approach
0QWLX4Z	Revision of Internal Fixation Device in Right Tarsal, External Approach
0QWLX5Z	Revision of External Fixation Device in Right Tarsal, External Approach
0QWLX7Z	Revision of Autologous Tissue Substitute in Right Tarsal, External Approach
0QWLXJZ	Revision of Synthetic Substitute in Right Tarsal, External Approach
0QWLXKZ	Revision of Nonautologous Tissue Substitute in Right Tarsal, External Approach
0QWM04Z	Revision of Internal Fixation Device in Left Tarsal, Open Approach
0QWM05Z	Revision of External Fixation Device in Left Tarsal, Open Approach
0QWM07Z	Revision of Autologous Tissue Substitute in Left Tarsal, Open Approach
0QWM0JZ	Revision of Synthetic Substitute in Left Tarsal, Open Approach
0QWM0KZ	Revision of Nonautologous Tissue Substitute in Left Tarsal, Open Approach
0QWM34Z	Revision of Internal Fixation Device in Left Tarsal, Percutaneous Approach
0QWM35Z	Revision of External Fixation Device in Left Tarsal, Percutaneous Approach
0QWM37Z	Revision of Autologous Tissue Substitute in Left Tarsal, Percutaneous Approach
0QWM3JZ	Revision of Synthetic Substitute in Left Tarsal, Percutaneous Approach
0QWM3KZ	Revision of Nonautologous Tissue Substitute in Left Tarsal, Percutaneous Approach
0QWM44Z	Revision of Internal Fixation Device in Left Tarsal, Percutaneous Endoscopic Approach
0QWM45Z	Revision of External Fixation Device in Left Tarsal, Percutaneous Endoscopic Approach
0QWM47Z	Revision of Autologous Tissue Substitute in Left Tarsal, Percutaneous Endoscopic Approach
0QWM4JZ	Revision of Synthetic Substitute in Left Tarsal, Percutaneous Endoscopic Approach
0QWM4KZ	Revision of Nonautologous Tissue Substitute in Left Tarsal, Percutaneous Endoscopic Approach
0QWMX4Z	Revision of Internal Fixation Device in Left Tarsal, External Approach
0QWMX5Z	Revision of External Fixation Device in Left Tarsal, External Approach
0QWMX7Z	Revision of Autologous Tissue Substitute in Left Tarsal, External Approach
0QWMXJZ	Revision of Synthetic Substitute in Left Tarsal, External Approach
0QWMXKZ	Revision of Nonautologous Tissue Substitute in Left Tarsal, External Approach
0QWN04Z	Revision of Internal Fixation Device in Right Metatarsal, Open Approach
0QWN05Z	Revision of External Fixation Device in Right Metatarsal, Open Approach
0QWN07Z	Revision of Autologous Tissue Substitute in Right Metatarsal, Open Approach
0QWN0JZ	Revision of Synthetic Substitute in Right Metatarsal, Open Approach
0QWN0KZ	Revision of Nonautologous Tissue Substitute in Right Metatarsal, Open Approach
0QWN34Z	Revision of Internal Fixation Device in Right Metatarsal, Percutaneous Approach
0QWN35Z	Revision of External Fixation Device in Right Metatarsal, Percutaneous Approach
0QWN37Z	Revision of Autologous Tissue Substitute in Right Metatarsal, Percutaneous Approach
0QWN3JZ	Revision of Synthetic Substitute in Right Metatarsal, Percutaneous Approach
0QWN3KZ	Revision of Nonautologous Tissue Substitute in Right Metatarsal, Percutaneous Approach
0QWN44Z	Revision of Internal Fixation Device in Right Metatarsal, Percutaneous Endoscopic Approach
0QWN45Z	Revision of External Fixation Device in Right Metatarsal, Percutaneous Endoscopic Approach
0QWN47Z	Revision of Autologous Tissue Substitute in Right Metatarsal, Percutaneous Endoscopic Approach
0QWN4JZ	Revision of Synthetic Substitute in Right Metatarsal, Percutaneous Endoscopic Approach
0QWN4KZ	Revision of Nonautologous Tissue Substitute in Right Metatarsal, Percutaneous Endoscopic Approach
0QWNX4Z	Revision of Internal Fixation Device in Right Metatarsal, External Approach
0QWNX5Z	Revision of External Fixation Device in Right Metatarsal, External Approach
0QWNX7Z	Revision of Autologous Tissue Substitute in Right Metatarsal, External Approach
0QWNXJZ	Revision of Synthetic Substitute in Right Metatarsal, External Approach
0QWNXKZ	Revision of Nonautologous Tissue Substitute in Right Metatarsal, External Approach
0QWP04Z	Revision of Internal Fixation Device in Left Metatarsal, Open Approach
0QWP05Z	Revision of External Fixation Device in Left Metatarsal, Open Approach
0QWP07Z	Revision of Autologous Tissue Substitute in Left Metatarsal, Open Approach
0QWP0JZ	Revision of Synthetic Substitute in Left Metatarsal, Open Approach
0QWP0KZ	Revision of Nonautologous Tissue Substitute in Left Metatarsal, Open Approach
0QWP34Z	Revision of Internal Fixation Device in Left Metatarsal, Percutaneous Approach
0QWP35Z	Revision of External Fixation Device in Left Metatarsal, Percutaneous Approach
0QWP37Z	Revision of Autologous Tissue Substitute in Left Metatarsal, Percutaneous Approach
0QWP3JZ	Revision of Synthetic Substitute in Left Metatarsal, Percutaneous Approach
0QWP3KZ	Revision of Nonautologous Tissue Substitute in Left Metatarsal, Percutaneous Approach
0QWP44Z	Revision of Internal Fixation Device in Left Metatarsal, Percutaneous Endoscopic Approach
0QWP45Z	Revision of External Fixation Device in Left Metatarsal, Percutaneous Endoscopic Approach
0QWP47Z	Revision of Autologous Tissue Substitute in Left Metatarsal, Percutaneous Endoscopic Approach
0QWP4JZ	Revision of Synthetic Substitute in Left Metatarsal, Percutaneous Endoscopic Approach
0QWP4KZ	Revision of Nonautologous Tissue Substitute in Left Metatarsal, Percutaneous Endoscopic Approach
0QWPX4Z	Revision of Internal Fixation Device in Left Metatarsal, External Approach
0QWPX5Z	Revision of External Fixation Device in Left Metatarsal, External Approach
0QWPX7Z	Revision of Autologous Tissue Substitute in Left Metatarsal, External Approach
0QWPXJZ	Revision of Synthetic Substitute in Left Metatarsal, External Approach
0QWPXKZ	Revision of Nonautologous Tissue Substitute in Left Metatarsal, External Approach
0QWQ04Z	Revision of Internal Fixation Device in Right Toe Phalanx, Open Approach
0QWQ05Z	Revision of External Fixation Device in Right Toe Phalanx, Open Approach

0QWQ07Z	Revision of Autologous Tissue Substitute in Right Toe Phalanx, Open Approach	**0QWR05Z**	Revision of External Fixation Device in Left Toe Phalanx, Open Approach	**0QWS07Z**	Revision of Autologous Tissue Substitute in Coccyx, Open Approach
0QWQ0JZ	Revision of Synthetic Substitute in Right Toe Phalanx, Open Approach	**0QWR07Z**	Revision of Autologous Tissue Substitute in Left Toe Phalanx, Open Approach	**0QWS0JZ**	Revision of Synthetic Substitute in Coccyx, Open Approach
0QWQ0KZ	Revision of Nonautologous Tissue Substitute in Right Toe Phalanx, Open Approach	**0QWR0JZ**	Revision of Synthetic Substitute in Left Toe Phalanx, Open Approach	**0QWS0KZ**	Revision of Nonautologous Tissue Substitute in Coccyx, Open Approach
0QWQ34Z	Revision of Internal Fixation Device in Right Toe Phalanx, Percutaneous Approach	**0QWR0KZ**	Revision of Nonautologous Tissue Substitute in Left Toe Phalanx, Open Approach	**0QWS34Z**	Revision of Internal Fixation Device Coccyx, Percutaneous Approach
0QWQ35Z	Revision of External Fixation Device in Right Toe Phalanx, Percutaneous Approach	**0QWR34Z**	Revision of Internal Fixation Device in Left Toe Phalanx, Percutaneous Approach	**0QWS37Z**	Revision of Autologous Tissue Substitute in Coccyx, Percutaneous Approach
0QWQ37Z	Revision of Autologous Tissue Substitute in Right Toe Phalanx, Percutaneous Approach	**0QWR35Z**	Revision of External Fixation Device in Left Toe Phalanx, Percutaneous Approach	**0QWS3JZ**	Revision of Synthetic Substitute in Coccyx, Percutaneous Approach
0QWQ3JZ	Revision of Synthetic Substitute in Right Toe Phalanx, Percutaneous Approach	**0QWR37Z**	Revision of Autologous Tissue Substitute in Left Toe Phalanx, Percutaneous Approach	**0QWS3KZ**	Revision of Nonautologous Tissue Substitute in Coccyx, Percutaneous Approach
0QWQ3KZ	Revision of Nonautologous Tissue Substitute in Right Toe Phalanx, Percutaneous Approach	**0QWR3JZ**	Revision of Synthetic Substitute in Left Toe Phalanx, Percutaneous Approach	**0QWS44Z**	Revision of Internal Fixation Device in Coccyx, Percutaneous Endoscopic Approach
0QWQ44Z	Revision of Internal Fixation Device in Right Toe Phalanx, Percutaneous Endoscopic Approach	**0QWR3KZ**	Revision of Nonautologous Tissue Substitute in Left Toe Phalanx, Percutaneous Approach	**0QWS47Z**	Revision of Autologous Tissue Substitute in Coccyx, Percutaneous Endoscopic Approach
0QWQ45Z	Revision of External Fixation Device in Right Toe Phalanx, Percutaneous Endoscopic Approach	**0QWR44Z**	Revision of Internal Fixation Device in Left Toe Phalanx, Percutaneous Endoscopic Approach	**0QWS4JZ**	Revision of Synthetic Substitute in Coccyx, Percutaneous Endoscopic Approach
0QWQ47Z	Revision of Autologous Tissue Substitute in Right Toe Phalanx, Percutaneous Endoscopic Approach	**0QWR45Z**	Revision of External Fixation Device in Left Toe Phalanx, Percutaneous Endoscopic Approach	**0QWS4KZ**	Revision of Nonautologous Tissue Substitute in Coccyx, Percutaneous Endoscopic Approach
0QWQ4JZ	Revision of Synthetic Substitute in Right Toe Phalanx, Percutaneous Endoscopic Approach	**0QWR47Z**	Revision of Autologous Tissue Substitute in Left Toe Phalanx, Percutaneous Endoscopic Approach	**0QWSX4Z**	Revision of Internal Fixation Device i Coccyx, External Approach
0QWQ4KZ	Revision of Nonautologous Tissue Substitute in Right Toe Phalanx, Percutaneous Endoscopic Approach	**0QWR4JZ**	Revision of Synthetic Substitute in Left Toe Phalanx, Percutaneous Endoscopic Approach	**0QWSX7Z**	Revision of Autologous Tissue Substitute in Coccyx, External Approa
0QWQX4Z	Revision of Internal Fixation Device in Right Toe Phalanx, External Approach	**0QWR4KZ**	Revision of Nonautologous Tissue Substitute in Left Toe Phalanx, Percutaneous Endoscopic Approach	**0QWSXJZ**	Revision of Synthetic Substitute in Coccyx, External Approach
0QWQX5Z	Revision of External Fixation Device in Right Toe Phalanx, External Approach	**0QWRX4Z**	Revision of Internal Fixation Device in Left Toe Phalanx, External Approach	**0QWSXKZ**	Revision of Nonautologous Tissue Substitute in Coccyx, External Approa
0QWQX7Z	Revision of Autologous Tissue Substitute in Right Toe Phalanx, External Approach	**0QWRX5Z**	Revision of External Fixation Device in Left Toe Phalanx, External Approach	**0QWY00Z**	Revision of Drainage Device in Lowe Bone, Open Approach
0QWQXJZ	Revision of Synthetic Substitute in Right Toe Phalanx, External Approach	**0QWRX7Z**	Revision of Autologous Tissue Substitute in Left Toe Phalanx, External Approach	**0QWY0MZ**	Revision of Bone Growth Stimulator i Lower Bone, Open Approach
0QWQXKZ	Revision of Nonautologous Tissue Substitute in Right Toe Phalanx, External Approach	**0QWRXJZ**	Revision of Synthetic Substitute in Left Toe Phalanx, External Approach	**0QWY30Z**	Revision of Drainage Device in Lowe Bone, Percutaneous Approach
0QWR04Z	Revision of Internal Fixation Device in Left Toe Phalanx, Open Approach	**0QWRXKZ**	Revision of Nonautologous Tissue Substitute in Left Toe Phalanx, External Approach	**0QWY3MZ**	Revision of Bone Growth Stimulator i Lower Bone, Percutaneous Approach
		0QWS04Z	Revision of Internal Fixation Device in Coccyx, Open Approach	**0QWY40Z**	Revision of Drainage Device in Lowe Bone, Percutaneous Endoscopic Approach
				0QWY4MZ	Revision of Bone Growth Stimulator i Lower Bone, Percutaneous Endoscopi Approach
				0QWYX0Z	Revision of Drainage Device in Lowe Bone, External Approach
				0QWYXMZ	Revision of Bone Growth Stimulator i Lower Bone, External Approach

Intervertebral Joint

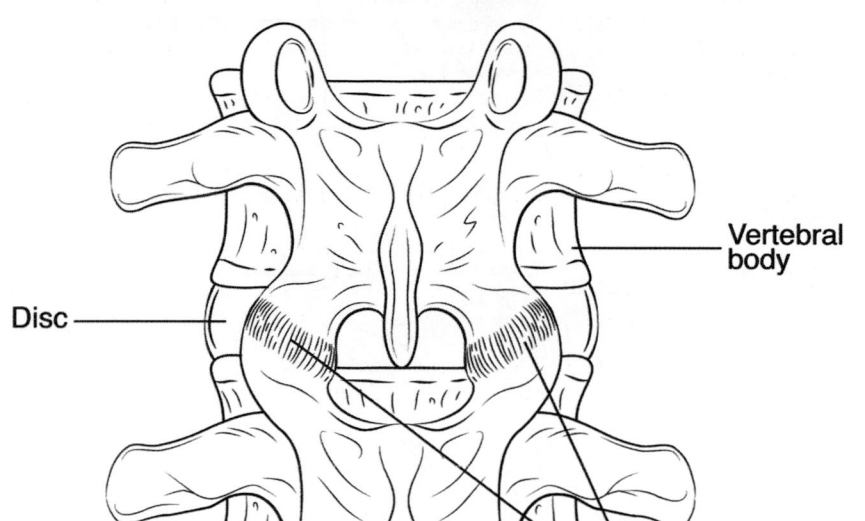

Disc

Vertebral body

Facet joint

©AHIMA

Shoulder

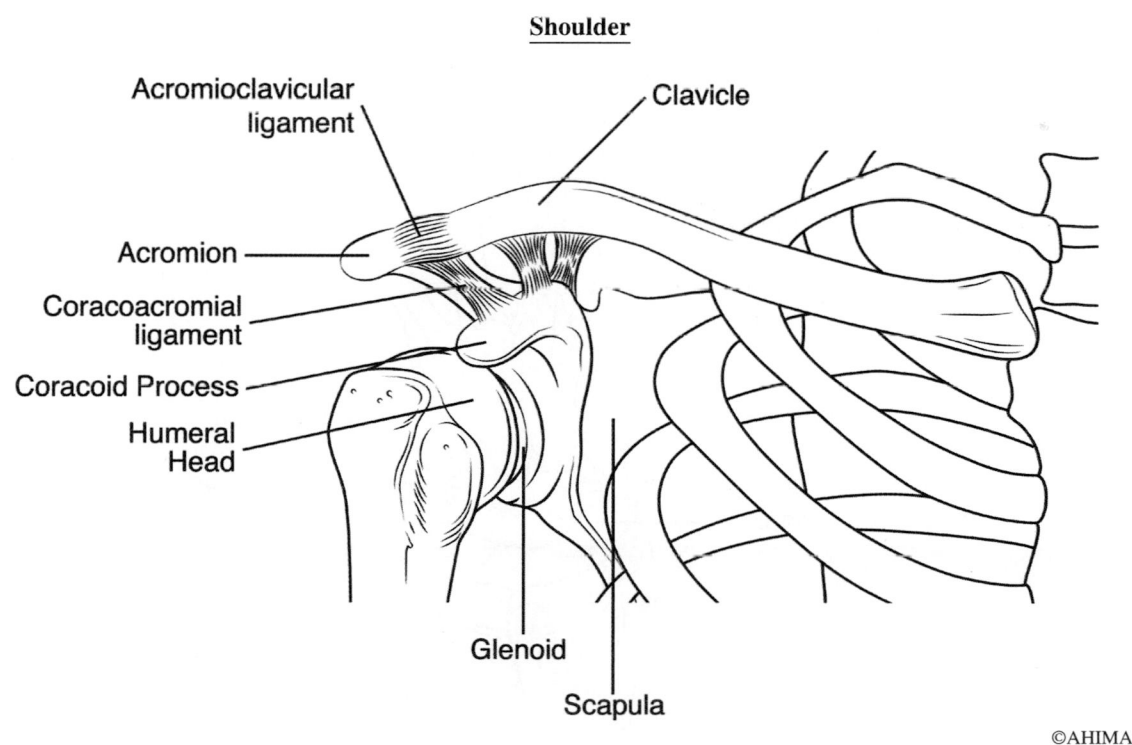

Acromioclavicular ligament

Clavicle

Acromion

Coracoacromial ligament

Coracoid Process

Humeral Head

Glenoid

Scapula

©AHIMA

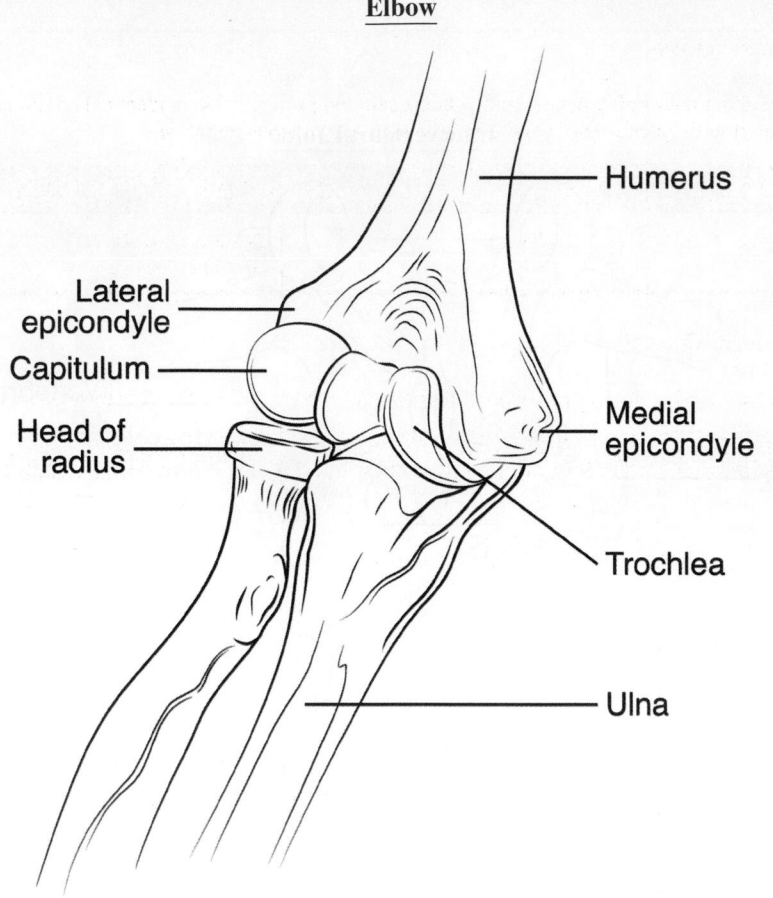

Humerus

Lateral
epicondyle

Capitulum

Head of
radius

Medial
epicondyle

Trochlea

Ulna

©AHIMA

Wrist

Capitate

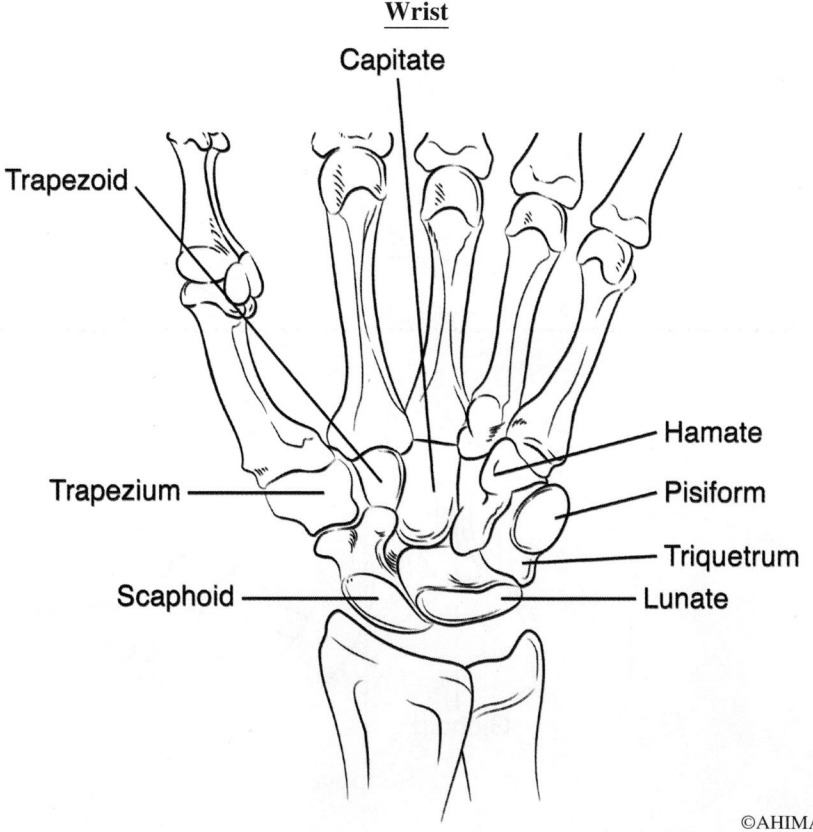

Trapezoid

Trapezium

Scaphoid

Hamate

Pisiform

Triquetrum

Lunate

©AHIMA

	0	Medical and Surgical
tion		
dy System	R	Upper Joints
eration	2	Change: Taking out or off a device from a body part and putting back an identical or similar device in or on the same body part without cutting or puncturing the skin or a mucous membrane

Body Part (4th)	Approach (5th)	Device (6th)	Qualifier (7th)
Upper Joint	X External	0 Drainage Device Y Other Device	Z No Qualifier

	0	Medical and Surgical
tion		
dy System	R	Upper Joints
eration	5	Destruction: Physical eradication of all or a portion of a body part by the direct use of energy, force, or a destructive agent

Body Part (4th)	Approach (5th)	Device (6th)	Qualifier (7th)
Occipital-cervical Joint Cervical Vertebral Joint Cervical Vertebral Disc Cervicothoracic Vertebral Joint Cervicothoracic Vertebral Disc Thoracic Vertebral Joint Thoracic Vertebral Disc Thoracolumbar Vertebral Joint Thoracolumbar Vertebral Disc Temporomandibular Joint, Right Temporomandibular Joint, Left Sternoclavicular Joint, Right Sternoclavicular Joint, Left Acromioclavicular Joint, Right Acromioclavicular Joint, Left Shoulder Joint, Right Shoulder Joint, Left Elbow Joint, Right Elbow Joint, Left Wrist Joint, Right Wrist Joint, Left Carpal Joint, Right Carpal Joint, Left Metacarpocarpal Joint, Right Metacarpocarpal Joint, Left Metacarpophalangeal Joint, Right Metacarpophalangeal Joint, Left Finger Phalangeal Joint, Right Finger Phalangeal Joint, Left	0 Open 3 Percutaneous 4 Percutaneous Endoscopic	Z No Device	Z No Qualifier

Section   0   **Medical and Surgical**
Body System   R   **Upper Joints**
Operation   9   **Drainage:** Taking or letting out fluids and/or gases from a body part

Body Part (4th)	Approach (5th)	Device (6th)	Qualifier (7th)
0 Occipital-cervical Joint 1 Cervical Vertebral Joint 3 Cervical Vertebral Disc 4 Cervicothoracic Vertebral Joint 5 Cervicothoracic Vertebral Disc 6 Thoracic Vertebral Joint 9 Thoracic Vertebral Disc A Thoracolumbar Vertebral Joint B Thoracolumbar Vertebral Disc C Temporomandibular Joint, Right D Temporomandibular Joint, Left E Sternoclavicular Joint, Right F Sternoclavicular Joint, Left G Acromioclavicular Joint, Right H Acromioclavicular Joint, Left J Shoulder Joint, Right K Shoulder Joint, Left L Elbow Joint, Right M Elbow Joint, Left N Wrist Joint, Right P Wrist Joint, Left Q Carpal Joint, Right R Carpal Joint, Left S Metacarpocarpal Joint, Right T Metacarpocarpal Joint, Left U Metacarpophalangeal Joint, Right V Metacarpophalangeal Joint, Left W Finger Phalangeal Joint, Right X Finger Phalangeal Joint, Left	0 Open 3 Percutaneous 4 Percutaneous Endoscopic	0 Drainage Device	Z No Qualifier
0 Occipital-cervical Joint 1 Cervical Vertebral Joint 3 Cervical Vertebral Disc 4 Cervicothoracic Vertebral Joint 5 Cervicothoracic Vertebral Disc 6 Thoracic Vertebral Joint 9 Thoracic Vertebral Disc A Thoracolumbar Vertebral Joint B Thoracolumbar Vertebral Disc C Temporomandibular Joint, Right D Temporomandibular Joint, Left E Sternoclavicular Joint, Right F Sternoclavicular Joint, Left G Acromioclavicular Joint, Right H Acromioclavicular Joint, Left J Shoulder Joint, Right K Shoulder Joint, Left L Elbow Joint, Right M Elbow Joint, Left N Wrist Joint, Right P Wrist Joint, Left Q Carpal Joint, Right R Carpal Joint, Left S Metacarpocarpal Joint, Right T Metacarpocarpal Joint, Left U Metacarpophalangeal Joint, Right V Metacarpophalangeal Joint, Left W Finger Phalangeal Joint, Right X Finger Phalangeal Joint, Left	0 Open 3 Percutaneous 4 Percutaneous Endoscopic	Z No Device	X Diagnostic Z No Qualifier

tion	**0**	**Medical and Surgical**		
ly System	**R**	**Upper Joints**		
eration	**B**	**Excision:** Cutting out or off, without replacement, a portion of a body part		

Body Part (4th)	Approach (5th)	Device (6th)	Qualifier (7th)
Occipital-cervical Joint	**0** Open	**Z** No Device	**X** Diagnostic
Cervical Vertebral Joint	**3** Percutaneous		**Z** No Qualifier
Cervical Vertebral Disc	**4** Percutaneous Endoscopic		
Cervicothoracic Vertebral Joint			
Cervicothoracic Vertebral Disc			
Thoracic Vertebral Joint			
Thoracic Vertebral Disc			
Thoracolumbar Vertebral Joint			
B Thoracolumbar Vertebral Disc			
C Temporomandibular Joint, Right			
D Temporomandibular Joint, Left			
E Sternoclavicular Joint, Right			
F Sternoclavicular Joint, Left			
G Acromioclavicular Joint, Right			
H Acromioclavicular Joint, Left			
Shoulder Joint, Right			
K Shoulder Joint, Left			
L Elbow Joint, Right			
M Elbow Joint, Left			
N Wrist Joint, Right			
P Wrist Joint, Left			
Q Carpal Joint, Right			
R Carpal Joint, Left			
S Metacarpocarpal Joint, Right			
T Metacarpocarpal Joint, Left			
U Metacarpophalangeal Joint, Right			
V Metacarpophalangeal Joint, Left			
W Finger Phalangeal Joint, Right			
X Finger Phalangeal Joint, Left			

Section	0	Medical and Surgical
Body System	R	Upper Joints
Operation	C	Extirpation: Taking or cutting out solid matter from a body part

Body Part (4th)	Approach (5th)	Device (6th)	Qualifier (7th)
0 Occipital-cervical Joint 1 Cervical Vertebral Joint 3 Cervical Vertebral Disc 4 Cervicothoracic Vertebral Joint 5 Cervicothoracic Vertebral Disc 6 Thoracic Vertebral Joint 9 Thoracic Vertebral Disc A Thoracolumbar Vertebral Joint B Thoracolumbar Vertebral Disc C Temporomandibular Joint, Right D Temporomandibular Joint, Left E Sternoclavicular Joint, Right F Sternoclavicular Joint, Left G Acromioclavicular Joint, Right H Acromioclavicular Joint, Left J Shoulder Joint, Right K Shoulder Joint, Left L Elbow Joint, Right M Elbow Joint, Left N Wrist Joint, Right P Wrist Joint, Left Q Carpal Joint, Right R Carpal Joint, Left S Metacarpocarpal Joint, Right T Metacarpocarpal Joint, Left U Metacarpophalangeal Joint, Right V Metacarpophalangeal Joint, Left W Finger Phalangeal Joint, Right X Finger Phalangeal Joint, Left	0 Open 3 Percutaneous 4 Percutaneous Endoscopic	Z No Device	Z No Qualifier

Section	0	Medical and Surgical
Body System	R	Upper Joints
Operation	G	Fusion: Joining together portions of an articular body part rendering the articular body part immobile

Body Part (4th)	Approach (5th)	Device (6th)	Qualifier (7th)
0 Occipital-cervical Joint 1 Cervical Vertebral Joint 2 Cervical Vertebral Joints, 2 or more 4 Cervicothoracic Vertebral Joint 6 Thoracic Vertebral Joint 7 Thoracic Vertebral Joints, 2 to 7 8 Thoracic Vertebral Joints, 8 or more A Thoracolumbar Vertebral Joint	0 Open 3 Percutaneous 4 Percutaneous Endoscopic	7 Autologous Tissue Substitute A Interbody Fusion Device J Synthetic Substitute K Nonautologous Tissue Substitute Z No Device	0 Anterior Approach, Anterior Column 1 Posterior Approach, Posterior Column J Posterior Approach, Anterior Column
C Temporomandibular Joint, Right D Temporomandibular Joint, Left E Sternoclavicular Joint, Right F Sternoclavicular Joint, Left G Acromioclavicular Joint, Right H Acromioclavicular Joint, Left J Shoulder Joint, Right K Shoulder Joint, Left	0 Open 3 Percutaneous 4 Percutaneous Endoscopic	4 Internal Fixation Device 7 Autologous Tissue Substitute J Synthetic Substitute K Nonautologous Tissue Substitute Z No Device	Z No Qualifier

Continued →

tion	0	Medical and Surgical	
y System	R	Upper Joints	
ration	G	Fusion: Joining together portions of an articular body part rendering the articular body part immobile	

Body Part (4th)	Approach (5th)	Device (6th)	Qualifier (7th)
Elbow Joint, Right Elbow Joint, Left Wrist Joint, Right Wrist Joint, Left Carpal Joint, Right Carpal Joint, Left Metacarpocarpal Joint, Right Metacarpocarpal Joint, Left Metacarpophalangeal Joint, Right Metacarpophalangeal Joint, Left Finger Phalangeal Joint, Right Finger Phalangeal Joint, Left	0 Open 3 Percutaneous 4 Percutaneous Endoscopic	4 Internal Fixation Device 5 External Fixation Device 7 Autologous Tissue Substitute J Synthetic Substitute K Nonautologous Tissue Substitute Z No Device	Z No Qualifier

tion	0	Medical and Surgical	
y System	R	Upper Joints	
ration	H	Insertion: Putting in a nonbiological appliance that monitors, assists, performs, or prevents a physiological function but does not physically take the place of a body part	

Body Part (4th)	Approach (5th)	Device (6th)	Qualifier (7th)
Occipital-cervical Joint Cervical Vertebral Joint Cervicothoracic Vertebral Joint Thoracic Vertebral Joint Thoracolumbar Vertebral Joint	0 Open 3 Percutaneous 4 Percutaneous Endoscopic	3 Infusion Device 4 Internal Fixation Device 8 Spacer B Spinal Stabilization Device, Interspinous Process C Spinal Stabilization Device, Pedicle-Based D Spinal Stabilization Device, Facet Replacement	Z No Qualifier
Cervical Vertebral Disc Cervicothoracic Vertebral Disc Thoracic Vertebral Disc Thoracolumbar Vertebral Disc	0 Open 3 Percutaneous 4 Percutaneous Endoscopic	3 Infusion Device	Z No Qualifier
Temporomandibular Joint, Right Temporomandibular Joint, Left Sternoclavicular Joint, Right Sternoclavicular Joint, Left Acromioclavicular Joint, Right Acromioclavicular Joint, Left Shoulder Joint, Right Shoulder Joint, Left	0 Open 3 Percutaneous 4 Percutaneous Endoscopic	3 Infusion Device 4 Internal Fixation Device 8 Spacer	Z No Qualifier
Elbow Joint, Right Elbow Joint, Left Wrist Joint, Right Wrist Joint, Left Carpal Joint, Right Carpal Joint, Left Metacarpocarpal Joint, Right Metacarpocarpal Joint, Left Metacarpophalangeal Joint, Right Metacarpophalangeal Joint, Left Finger Phalangeal Joint, Right Finger Phalangeal Joint, Left	0 Open 3 Percutaneous 4 Percutaneous Endoscopic	3 Infusion Device 4 Internal Fixation Device 5 External Fixation Device 8 Spacer	Z No Qualifier

Section	0	Medical and Surgical
Body System	R	Upper Joints
Operation	J	**Inspection:** Visually and/or manually exploring a body part

Body Part (4th)	Approach (5th)	Device (6th)	Qualifier (7th)
0 Occipital-cervical Joint	0 Open	Z No Device	Z No Qualifier
1 Cervical Vertebral Joint	3 Percutaneous		
3 Cervical Vertebral Disc	4 Percutaneous Endoscopic		
4 Cervicothoracic Vertebral Joint	X External		
5 Cervicothoracic Vertebral Disc			
6 Thoracic Vertebral Joint			
9 Thoracic Vertebral Disc			
A Thoracolumbar Vertebral Joint			
B Thoracolumbar Vertebral Disc			
C Temporomandibular Joint, Right			
D Temporomandibular Joint, Left			
E Sternoclavicular Joint, Right			
F Sternoclavicular Joint, Left			
G Acromioclavicular Joint, Right			
H Acromioclavicular Joint, Left			
J Shoulder Joint, Right			
K Shoulder Joint, Left			
L Elbow Joint, Right			
M Elbow Joint, Left			
N Wrist Joint, Right			
P Wrist Joint, Left			
Q Carpal Joint, Right			
R Carpal Joint, Left			
S Metacarpocarpal Joint, Right			
T Metacarpocarpal Joint, Left			
U Metacarpophalangeal Joint, Right			
V Metacarpophalangeal Joint, Left			
W Finger Phalangeal Joint, Right			
X Finger Phalangeal Joint, Left			

Section	0	Medical and Surgical
Body System	R	Upper Joints
Operation	N	**Release:** Freeing a body part from an abnormal physical constraint by cutting or by the use of force

Body Part (4th)	Approach (5th)	Device (6th)	Qualifier (7th)
0 Occipital-cervical Joint	0 Open	Z No Device	Z No Qualifier
1 Cervical Vertebral Joint	3 Percutaneous		
3 Cervical Vertebral Disc	4 Percutaneous Endoscopic		
4 Cervicothoracic Vertebral Joint	X External		
5 Cervicothoracic Vertebral Disc			
6 Thoracic Vertebral Joint			
9 Thoracic Vertebral Disc			
A Thoracolumbar Vertebral Joint			
B Thoracolumbar Vertebral Disc			
C Temporomandibular Joint, Right			
D Temporomandibular Joint, Left			
E Sternoclavicular Joint, Right			
F Sternoclavicular Joint, Left			
G Acromioclavicular Joint, Right			
H Acromioclavicular Joint, Left			
J Shoulder Joint, Right			
K Shoulder Joint, Left			
L Elbow Joint, Right			
M Elbow Joint, Left			
N Wrist Joint, Right			
P Wrist Joint, Left			
Q Carpal Joint, Right			
R Carpal Joint, Left			
S Metacarpocarpal Joint, Right			
T Metacarpocarpal Joint, Left			
U Metacarpophalangeal Joint, Right			
V Metacarpophalangeal Joint, Left			
W Finger Phalangeal Joint, Right			
X Finger Phalangeal Joint, Left			

	0	Medical and Surgical
	R	Upper Joints
	P	**Removal:** Taking out or off a device from a body part

Body Part (4th)	Approach (5th)	Device (6th)	Qualifier (7th)
Occipital-cervical Joint Cervical Vertebral Joint Cervicothoracic Vertebral Joint Thoracic Vertebral Joint Thoracolumbar Vertebral Joint	0 Open 3 Percutaneous 4 Percutaneous Endoscopic	0 Drainage Device 3 Infusion Device 4 Internal Fixation Device 7 Autologous Tissue Substitute 8 Spacer A Interbody Fusion Device J Synthetic Substitute K Nonautologous Tissue Substitute	Z No Qualifier
Occipital-cervical Joint Cervical Vertebral Joint Cervicothoracic Vertebral Joint Thoracic Vertebral Joint Thoracolumbar Vertebral Joint	X External	0 Drainage Device 3 Infusion Device 4 Internal Fixation Device	Z No Qualifier
Cervical Vertebral Disc Cervicothoracic Vertebral Disc Thoracic Vertebral Disc Thoracolumbar Vertebral Disc	0 Open 3 Percutaneous 4 Percutaneous Endoscopic	0 Drainage Device 3 Infusion Device 7 Autologous Tissue Substitute J Synthetic Substitute K Nonautologous Tissue Substitute	Z No Qualifier
Cervical Vertebral Disc Cervicothoracic Vertebral Disc Thoracic Vertebral Disc Thoracolumbar Vertebral Disc	X External	0 Drainage Device 3 Infusion Device	Z No Qualifier
Temporomandibular Joint, Right Temporomandibular Joint, Left Sternoclavicular Joint, Right Sternoclavicular Joint, Left Acromioclavicular Joint, Right Acromioclavicular Joint, Left Shoulder Joint, Right Shoulder Joint, Left	0 Open 3 Percutaneous 4 Percutaneous Endoscopic	0 Drainage Device 3 Infusion Device 4 Internal Fixation Device 7 Autologous Tissue Substitute 8 Spacer J Synthetic Substitute K Nonautologous Tissue Substitute	Z No Qualifier
Temporomandibular Joint, Right Temporomandibular Joint, Left Sternoclavicular Joint, Right Sternoclavicular Joint, Left Acromioclavicular Joint, Right Acromioclavicular Joint, Left Shoulder Joint, Right Shoulder Joint, Left	X External	0 Drainage Device 3 Infusion Device 4 Internal Fixation Device	Z No Qualifier
Elbow Joint, Right Elbow Joint, Left Wrist Joint, Right Wrist Joint, Left Carpal Joint, Right Carpal Joint, Left Metacarpocarpal Joint, Right Metacarpocarpal Joint, Left Metacarpophalangeal Joint, Right Metacarpophalangeal Joint, Left Finger Phalangeal Joint, Right Finger Phalangeal Joint, Left	0 Open 3 Percutaneous 4 Percutaneous Endoscopic	0 Drainage Device 3 Infusion Device 4 Internal Fixation Device 5 External Fixation Device 7 Autologous Tissue Substitute 8 Spacer J Synthetic Substitute K Nonautologous Tissue Substitute	Z No Qualifier

Continued →

Section 0 Medical and Surgical
Body System R Upper Joints
Operation P Removal: Taking out or off a device from a body part

Body Part (4th)	Approach (5th)	Device (6th)	Qualifier (7th)
L Elbow Joint, Right M Elbow Joint, Left N Wrist Joint, Right P Wrist Joint, Left Q Carpal Joint, Right R Carpal Joint, Left S Metacarpocarpal Joint, Right T Metacarpocarpal Joint, Left U Metacarpophalangeal Joint, Right V Metacarpophalangeal Joint, Left W Finger Phalangeal Joint, Right X Finger Phalangeal Joint, Left	X External	0 Drainage Device 3 Infusion Device 4 Internal Fixation Device 5 External Fixation Device	Z No Qualifier

Section 0 Medical and Surgical
Body System R Upper Joints
Operation Q Repair: Restoring, to the extent possible, a body part to its normal anatomic structure and function

Body Part (4th)	Approach (5th)	Device (6th)	Qualifier (7th)
0 Occipital-cervical Joint 1 Cervical Vertebral Joint 3 Cervical Vertebral Disc 4 Cervicothoracic Vertebral Joint 5 Cervicothoracic Vertebral Disc 6 Thoracic Vertebral Joint 9 Thoracic Vertebral Disc A Thoracolumbar Vertebral Joint B Thoracolumbar Vertebral Disc C Temporomandibular Joint, Right D Temporomandibular Joint, Left E Sternoclavicular Joint, Right F Sternoclavicular Joint, Left G Acromioclavicular Joint, Right H Acromioclavicular Joint, Left J Shoulder Joint, Right K Shoulder Joint, Left L Elbow Joint, Right M Elbow Joint, Left N Wrist Joint, Right P Wrist Joint, Left Q Carpal Joint, Right R Carpal Joint, Left S Metacarpocarpal Joint, Right T Metacarpocarpal Joint, Left U Metacarpophalangeal Joint, Right V Metacarpophalangeal Joint, Left W Finger Phalangeal Joint, Right X Finger Phalangeal Joint, Left	0 Open 3 Percutaneous 4 Percutaneous Endoscopic X External	Z No Device	Z No Qualifier

ion	0	**Medical and Surgical**	
y System	R	**Upper Joints**	
ration	R	**Replacement:** Putting in or on biological or synthetic material that physically takes the place and/or function of all or a portion of a body part	

Body Part (4th)	Approach (5th)	Device (6th)	Qualifier (7th)
Occipital-cervical Joint Cervical Vertebral Joint Cervical Vertebral Disc Cervicothoracic Vertebral Joint Cervicothoracic Vertebral Disc Thoracic Vertebral Joint Thoracic Vertebral Disc Thoracolumbar Vertebral Joint Thoracolumbar Vertebral Disc Temporomandibular Joint, Right Temporomandibular Joint, Left Sternoclavicular Joint, Right Sternoclavicular Joint, Left Acromioclavicular Joint, Right Acromioclavicular Joint, Left Elbow Joint, Right Elbow Joint, Left Wrist Joint, Right Wrist Joint, Left Carpal Joint, Right Carpal Joint, Left Metacarpocarpal Joint, Right Metacarpocarpal Joint, Left Metacarpophalangeal Joint, Right Metacarpophalangeal Joint, Left Finger Phalangeal Joint, Right Finger Phalangeal Joint, Left	0 Open	7 Autologous Tissue Substitute J Synthetic Substitute K Nonautologous Tissue Substitute	Z No Qualifier
Shoulder Joint, Right Shoulder Joint, Left	0 Open	0 Synthetic Substitute, Reverse Ball and Socket 7 Autologous Tissue Substitute K Nonautologous Tissue Substitute	Z No Qualifier
Shoulder Joint, Right Shoulder Joint, Left	0 Open	J Synthetic Substitute	6 Humeral Surface 7 Glenoid Surface Z No Qualifier

ction	0	**Medical and Surgical**	
dy System	R	**Upper Joints**	
eration	S	**Reposition:** Moving to its normal location, or other suitable location, all or a portion of a body part	

Body Part (4th)	Approach (5th)	Device (6th)	Qualifier (7th)
Occipital-cervical Joint Cervical Vertebral Joint Cervicothoracic Vertebral Joint Thoracic Vertebral Joint Thoracolumbar Vertebral Joint Temporomandibular Joint, Right Temporomandibular Joint, Left Sternoclavicular Joint, Right Sternoclavicular Joint, Left Acromioclavicular Joint, Right Acromioclavicular Joint, Left Shoulder Joint, Right Shoulder Joint, Left	0 Open 3 Percutaneous 4 Percutaneous Endoscopic X External	4 Internal Fixation Device Z No Device	Z No Qualifier

Continued →

Section	0	Medical and Surgical
Body System	R	Upper Joints
Operation	S	Reposition: Moving to its normal location, or other suitable location, all or a portion of a body part

Body Part (4th)	Approach (5th)	Device (6th)	Qualifier (7th)
L Elbow Joint, Right	0 Open	4 Internal Fixation Device	Z No Qualifier
M Elbow Joint, Left	3 Percutaneous	5 External Fixation Device	
N Wrist Joint, Right	4 Percutaneous Endoscopic	Z No Device	
P Wrist Joint, Left	X External		
Q Carpal Joint, Right			
R Carpal Joint, Left			
S Metacarpocarpal Joint, Right			
T Metacarpocarpal Joint, Left			
U Metacarpophalangeal Joint, Right			
V Metacarpophalangeal Joint, Left			
W Finger Phalangeal Joint, Right			
X Finger Phalangeal Joint, Left			

Section	0	Medical and Surgical
Body System	R	Upper Joints
Operation	T	Resection: Cutting out or off, without replacement, all of a body part

Body Part (4th)	Approach (5th)	Device (6th)	Qualifier (7th)
3 Cervical Vertebral Disc	0 Open	Z No Device	Z No Qualifier
4 Cervicothoracic Vertebral Joint			
5 Cervicothoracic Vertebral Disc			
9 Thoracic Vertebral Disc			
B Thoracolumbar Vertebral Disc			
C Temporomandibular Joint, Right			
D Temporomandibular Joint, Left			
E Sternoclavicular Joint, Right			
F Sternoclavicular Joint, Left			
G Acromioclavicular Joint, Right			
H Acromioclavicular Joint, Left			
J Shoulder Joint, Right			
K Shoulder Joint, Left			
L Elbow Joint, Right			
M Elbow Joint, Left			
N Wrist Joint, Right			
P Wrist Joint, Left			
Q Carpal Joint, Right			
R Carpal Joint, Left			
S Metacarpocarpal Joint, Right			
T Metacarpocarpal Joint, Left			
U Metacarpophalangeal Joint, Right			
V Metacarpophalangeal Joint, Left			
W Finger Phalangeal Joint, Right			
X Finger Phalangeal Joint, Left			

Section 0 **Medical and Surgical**
Body System R **Upper Joints**
Operation U **Supplement:** Putting in or on biological or synthetic material that physically reinforces and/or augments the function of a portion of a body part

Body Part (4th)	Approach (5th)	Device (6th)	Qualifier (7th)
Occipital-cervical Joint Cervical Vertebral Joint Cervical Vertebral Disc Cervicothoracic Vertebral Joint Cervicothoracic Vertebral Disc Thoracic Vertebral Joint Thoracic Vertebral Disc Thoracolumbar Vertebral Joint Thoracolumbar Vertebral Disc Temporomandibular Joint, Right Temporomandibular Joint, Left Sternoclavicular Joint, Right Sternoclavicular Joint, Left Acromioclavicular Joint, Right Acromioclavicular Joint, Left Shoulder Joint, Right Shoulder Joint, Left Elbow Joint, Right Elbow Joint, Left Wrist Joint, Right Wrist Joint, Left Carpal Joint, Right Carpal Joint, Left Metacarpocarpal Joint, Right Metacarpocarpal Joint, Left Metacarpophalangeal Joint, Right Metacarpophalangeal Joint, Left Finger Phalangeal Joint, Right Finger Phalangeal Joint, Left	0 Open 3 Percutaneous 4 Percutaneous Endoscopic	7 Autologous Tissue Substitute J Synthetic Substitute K Nonautologous Tissue Substitute	Z No Qualifier

Section 0 **Medical and Surgical**
Body System R **Upper Joints**
Operation W **Revision:** Correcting, to the extent possible, a portion of a malfunctioning device or the position of a displaced device

Body Part (4th)	Approach (5th)	Device (6th)	Qualifier (7th)
Occipital-cervical Joint Cervical Vertebral Joint Cervicothoracic Vertebral Joint Thoracic Vertebral Joint Thoracolumbar Vertebral Joint	0 Open 3 Percutaneous 4 Percutaneous Endoscopic X External	0 Drainage Device 3 Infusion Device 4 Internal Fixation Device 7 Autologous Tissue Substitute 8 Spacer A Interbody Fusion Device J Synthetic Substitute K Nonautologous Tissue Substitute	Z No Qualifier
Cervical Vertebral Disc Cervicothoracic Vertebral Disc Thoracic Vertebral Disc Thoracolumbar Vertebral Disc	0 Open 3 Percutaneous 4 Percutaneous Endoscopic X External	0 Drainage Device 3 Infusion Device 7 Autologous Tissue Substitute J Synthetic Substitute K Nonautologous Tissue Substitute	Z No Qualifier
Temporomandibular Joint, Right Temporomandibular Joint, Left Sternoclavicular Joint, Right Sternoclavicular Joint, Left Acromioclavicular Joint, Right Acromioclavicular Joint, Left Shoulder Joint, Right Shoulder Joint, Left	0 Open 3 Percutaneous 4 Percutaneous Endoscopic X External	0 Drainage Device 3 Infusion Device 4 Internal Fixation Device 7 Autologous Tissue Substitute 8 Spacer J Synthetic Substitute K Nonautologous Tissue Substitute	Z No Qualifier

Continued →

Section   **0**   **Medical and Surgical**
Body System   **R**   **Upper Joints**
Operation   **W**   **Revision:** Correcting, to the extent possible, a portion of a malfunctioning device or the position of a displaced device

Body Part (4th)	Approach (5th)	Device (6th)	Qualifier (7th)
L Elbow Joint, Right **M** Elbow Joint, Left **N** Wrist Joint, Right **P** Wrist Joint, Left **Q** Carpal Joint, Right **R** Carpal Joint, Left **S** Metacarpocarpal Joint, Right **T** Metacarpocarpal Joint, Left **U** Metacarpophalangeal Joint, Right **V** Metacarpophalangeal Joint, Left **W** Finger Phalangeal Joint, Right **X** Finger Phalangeal Joint, Left	**0** Open **3** Percutaneous **4** Percutaneous Endoscopic **X** External	**0** Drainage Device **3** Infusion Device **4** Internal Fixation Device **5** External Fixation Device **7** Autologous Tissue Substitute **8** Spacer **J** Synthetic Substitute **K** Nonautologous Tissue Substitute	**Z** No Qualifier

Upper Joints Code Listing 0R2–0RW

Review Coding Guideline B4.5

0R2 – Upper Joints, Change

Review Coding Guideline B6.1c

0R2YX0Z   Change Drainage Device in Upper Joint, External Approach

0R2YXYZ   Change Other Device in Upper Joint, External Approach

0R5 – Upper Joints, Destruction

0R500ZZ Destruction of Occipital-cervical Joint, Open Approach
0R503ZZ Destruction of Occipital-cervical Joint, Percutaneous Approach
0R504ZZ Destruction of Occipital-cervical Joint, Percutaneous Endoscopic Approach
0R510ZZ Destruction of Cervical Vertebral Joint, Open Approach
0R513ZZ Destruction of Cervical Vertebral Joint, Percutaneous Approach
0R514ZZ Destruction of Cervical Vertebral Joint, Percutaneous Endoscopic Approach
0R530ZZ Destruction of Cervical Vertebral Disc, Open Approach
0R533ZZ Destruction of Cervical Vertebral Disc, Percutaneous Approach
0R534ZZ Destruction of Cervical Vertebral Disc, Percutaneous Endoscopic Approach
0R540ZZ Destruction of Cervicothoracic Vertebral Joint, Open Approach
0R543ZZ Destruction of Cervicothoracic Vertebral Joint, Percutaneous Approach
0R544ZZ Destruction of Cervicothoracic Vertebral Joint, Percutaneous Endoscopic Approach
0R550ZZ Destruction of Cervicothoracic Vertebral Disc, Open Approach
0R553ZZ Destruction of Cervicothoracic Vertebral Disc, Percutaneous Approach
0R554ZZ Destruction of Cervicothoracic Vertebral Disc, Percutaneous Endoscopic Approach
0R560ZZ Destruction of Thoracic Vertebral Joint, Open Approach
0R563ZZ Destruction of Thoracic Vertebral Joint, Percutaneous Approach
0R564ZZ Destruction of Thoracic Vertebral Joint, Percutaneous Endoscopic Approach
0R590ZZ Destruction of Thoracic Vertebral Disc, Open Approach
0R593ZZ Destruction of Thoracic Vertebral Disc, Percutaneous Approach

0R594ZZ Destruction of Thoracic Vertebral Disc, Percutaneous Endoscopic Approach
0R5A0ZZ Destruction of Thoracolumbar Vertebral Joint, Open Approach
0R5A3ZZ Destruction of Thoracolumbar Vertebral Joint, Percutaneous Approach
0R5A4ZZ Destruction of Thoracolumbar Vertebral Joint, Percutaneous Endoscopic Approach
0R5B0ZZ Destruction of Thoracolumbar Vertebral Disc, Open Approach
0R5B3ZZ Destruction of Thoracolumbar Vertebral Disc, Percutaneous Approach
0R5B4ZZ Destruction of Thoracolumbar Vertebral Disc, Percutaneous Endoscopic Approach
0R5C0ZZ Destruction of Right Temporomandibular Joint, Open Approach
0R5C3ZZ Destruction of Right Temporomandibular Joint, Percutaneous Approach
0R5C4ZZ Destruction of Right Temporomandibular Joint, Percutaneous Endoscopic Approach
0R5D0ZZ Destruction of Left Temporomandibular Joint, Open Approach
0R5D3ZZ Destruction of Left Temporomandibular Joint, Percutaneous Approach
0R5D4ZZ Destruction of Left Temporomandibular Joint, Percutaneous Endoscopic Approach
0R5E0ZZ Destruction of Right Sternoclavicular Joint, Open Approach
0R5E3ZZ Destruction of Right Sternoclavicular Joint, Percutaneous Approach
0R5E4ZZ Destruction of Right Sternoclavicular Joint, Percutaneous Endoscopic Approach
0R5F0ZZ Destruction of Left Sternoclavicular Joint, Open Approach
0R5F3ZZ Destruction of Left Sternoclavicular Joint, Percutaneous Approach
0R5F4ZZ Destruction of Left Sternoclavicular Joint, Percutaneous Endoscopic Approach
0R5G0ZZ Destruction of Right Acromioclavicular Joint, Open Approach

0R5G3ZZ Destruction of Right Acromioclavicular Joint, Percutaneous Approach
0R5G4ZZ Destruction of Right Acromioclavicular Joint, Percutaneous Endoscopic Approach
0R5H0ZZ Destruction of Left Acromioclavicular Joint, Open Approach
0R5H3ZZ Destruction of Left Acromioclavicular Joint, Percutaneous Approach
0R5H4ZZ Destruction of Left Acromioclavicular Joint, Percutaneous Endoscopic Approach
0R5J0ZZ Destruction of Right Shoulder Joint, Open Approach
0R5J3ZZ Destruction of Right Shoulder Joint, Percutaneous Approach
0R5J4ZZ Destruction of Right Shoulder Joint, Percutaneous Endoscopic Approach
0R5K0ZZ Destruction of Left Shoulder Joint, Open Approach
0R5K3ZZ Destruction of Left Shoulder Joint, Percutaneous Approach
0R5K4ZZ Destruction of Left Shoulder Joint, Percutaneous Endoscopic Approach
0R5L0ZZ Destruction of Right Elbow Joint, Open Approach
0R5L3ZZ Destruction of Right Elbow Joint, Percutaneous Approach
0R5L4ZZ Destruction of Right Elbow Joint, Percutaneous Endoscopic Approach
0R5M0ZZ Destruction of Left Elbow Joint, Open Approach
0R5M3ZZ Destruction of Left Elbow Joint, Percutaneous Approach
0R5M4ZZ Destruction of Left Elbow Joint, Percutaneous Endoscopic Approach
0R5N0ZZ Destruction of Right Wrist Joint, Open Approach
0R5N3ZZ Destruction of Right Wrist Joint, Percutaneous Approach
0R5N4ZZ Destruction of Right Wrist Joint, Percutaneous Endoscopic Approach

Code	Description	Code	Description	Code	Description
0R5P0ZZ	Destruction of Left Wrist Joint, Open Approach	0R5S0ZZ	Destruction of Right Metacarpocarpal Joint, Open Approach	0R5V0ZZ	Destruction of Left Metacarpophalangeal Joint, Open Approach
0R5P3ZZ	Destruction of Left Wrist Joint, Percutaneous Approach	0R5S3ZZ	Destruction of Right Metacarpocarpal Joint, Percutaneous Approach	0R5V3ZZ	Destruction of Left Metacarpophalangeal Joint, Percutaneous Approach
0R5P4ZZ	Destruction of Left Wrist Joint, Percutaneous Endoscopic Approach	0R5S4ZZ	Destruction of Right Metacarpocarpal Joint, Percutaneous Endoscopic Approach	0R5V4ZZ	Destruction of Left Metacarpophalangeal Joint, Percutaneous Endoscopic Approach
0R5Q0ZZ	Destruction of Right Carpal Joint, Open Approach	0R5T0ZZ	Destruction of Left Metacarpocarpal Joint, Open Approach	0R5W0ZZ	Destruction of Right Finger Phalangeal Joint, Open Approach
0R5Q3ZZ	Destruction of Right Carpal Joint, Percutaneous Approach	0R5T3ZZ	Destruction of Left Metacarpocarpal Joint, Percutaneous Approach	0R5W3ZZ	Destruction of Right Finger Phalangeal Joint, Percutaneous Approach
0R5Q4ZZ	Destruction of Right Carpal Joint, Percutaneous Endoscopic Approach	0R5T4ZZ	Destruction of Left Metacarpocarpal Joint, Percutaneous Endoscopic Approach	0R5W4ZZ	Destruction of Right Finger Phalangeal Joint, Percutaneous Endoscopic Approach
0R5R0ZZ	Destruction of Left Carpal Joint, Open Approach	0R5U0ZZ	Destruction of Right Metacarpophalangeal Joint, Open Approach	0R5X0ZZ	Destruction of Left Finger Phalangeal Joint, Open Approach
0R5R3ZZ	Destruction of Left Carpal Joint, Percutaneous Approach	0R5U3ZZ	Destruction of Right Metacarpophalangeal Joint, Percutaneous Approach	0R5X3ZZ	Destruction of Left Finger Phalangeal Joint, Percutaneous Approach
0R5R4ZZ	Destruction of Left Carpal Joint, Percutaneous Endoscopic Approach	0R5U4ZZ	Destruction of Right Metacarpophalangeal Joint, Percutaneous Endoscopic Approach	0R5X4ZZ	Destruction of Left Finger Phalangeal Joint, Percutaneous Endoscopic Approach

0R9 – Upper Joints, Drainage

See Coding Guidelines B3.4a and B3.4b

See Coding Guideline B6.2

Code	Description	Code	Description	Code	Description
0R9000Z	Drainage of Occipital-cervical Joint with Drainage Device, Open Approach	0R9340Z	Drainage of Cervical Vertebral Disc with Drainage Device, Percutaneous Endoscopic Approach	0R9600Z	Drainage of Thoracic Vertebral Joint with Drainage Device, Open Approach
0R900ZX	Drainage of Occipital-cervical Joint, Open Approach, Diagnostic	0R934ZX	Drainage of Cervical Vertebral Disc, Percutaneous Endoscopic Approach, Diagnostic	0R960ZX	Drainage of Thoracic Vertebral Joint, Open Approach, Diagnostic
0R900ZZ	Drainage of Occipital-cervical Joint, Open Approach	0R934ZZ	Drainage of Cervical Vertebral Disc, Percutaneous Endoscopic Approach	0R960ZZ	Drainage of Thoracic Vertebral Joint, Open Approach
0R9030Z	Drainage of Occipital-cervical Joint with Drainage Device, Percutaneous Approach	0R9400Z	Drainage of Cervicothoracic Vertebral Joint with Drainage Device, Open Approach	0R9630Z	Drainage of Thoracic Vertebral Joint with Drainage Device, Percutaneous Approach
0R903ZX	Drainage of Occipital-cervical Joint, Percutaneous Approach, Diagnostic	0R940ZX	Drainage of Cervicothoracic Vertebral Joint, Open Approach, Diagnostic	0R963ZX	Drainage of Thoracic Vertebral Joint, Percutaneous Approach, Diagnostic
0R903ZZ	Drainage of Occipital-cervical Joint, Percutaneous Approach	0R940ZZ	Drainage of Cervicothoracic Vertebral Joint, Open Approach	0R963ZZ	Drainage of Thoracic Vertebral Joint, Percutaneous Approach
0R9040Z	Drainage of Occipital-cervical Joint with Drainage Device, Percutaneous Endoscopic Approach	0R9430Z	Drainage of Cervicothoracic Vertebral Joint with Drainage Device, Percutaneous Approach	0R9640Z	Drainage of Thoracic Vertebral Joint with Drainage Device, Percutaneous Endoscopic Approach
0R904ZX	Drainage of Occipital-cervical Joint, Percutaneous Endoscopic Approach, Diagnostic	0R943ZX	Drainage of Cervicothoracic Vertebral Joint, Percutaneous Approach, Diagnostic	0R964ZX	Drainage of Thoracic Vertebral Joint, Percutaneous Endoscopic Approach, Diagnostic
0R904ZZ	Drainage of Occipital-cervical Joint, Percutaneous Endoscopic Approach	0R943ZZ	Drainage of Cervicothoracic Vertebral Joint, Percutaneous Approach	0R964ZZ	Drainage of Thoracic Vertebral Joint, Percutaneous Endoscopic Approach
0R9100Z	Drainage of Cervical Vertebral Joint with Drainage Device, Open Approach	0R9440Z	Drainage of Cervicothoracic Vertebral Joint with Drainage Device, Percutaneous Endoscopic Approach	0R9900Z	Drainage of Thoracic Vertebral Disc with Drainage Device, Open Approach
0R910ZX	Drainage of Cervical Vertebral Joint, Open Approach, Diagnostic	0R944ZX	Drainage of Cervicothoracic Vertebral Joint, Percutaneous Endoscopic Approach, Diagnostic	0R990ZX	Drainage of Thoracic Vertebral Disc, Open Approach, Diagnostic
0R910ZZ	Drainage of Cervical Vertebral Joint, Open Approach	0R944ZZ	Drainage of Cervicothoracic Vertebral Joint, Percutaneous Endoscopic Approach	0R990ZZ	Drainage of Thoracic Vertebral Disc, Open Approach
0R9130Z	Drainage of Cervical Vertebral Joint with Drainage Device, Percutaneous Approach	0R9500Z	Drainage of Cervicothoracic Vertebral Disc with Drainage Device, Open Approach	0R9930Z	Drainage of Thoracic Vertebral Disc with Drainage Device, Percutaneous Approach
0R913ZX	Drainage of Cervical Vertebral Joint, Percutaneous Approach, Diagnostic	0R950ZX	Drainage of Cervicothoracic Vertebral Disc, Open Approach, Diagnostic	0R993ZX	Drainage of Thoracic Vertebral Disc, Percutaneous Approach, Diagnostic
0R913ZZ	Drainage of Cervical Vertebral Joint, Percutaneous Approach	0R950ZZ	Drainage of Cervicothoracic Vertebral Disc, Open Approach	0R993ZZ	Drainage of Thoracic Vertebral Disc, Percutaneous Approach
0R9140Z	Drainage of Cervical Vertebral Joint with Drainage Device, Percutaneous Endoscopic Approach	0R9530Z	Drainage of Cervicothoracic Vertebral Disc with Drainage Device, Percutaneous Approach	0R9940Z	Drainage of Thoracic Vertebral Disc with Drainage Device, Percutaneous Endoscopic Approach
0R914ZX	Drainage of Cervical Vertebral Joint, Percutaneous Endoscopic Approach, Diagnostic	0R953ZX	Drainage of Cervicothoracic Vertebral Disc, Percutaneous Approach, Diagnostic	0R994ZX	Drainage of Thoracic Vertebral Disc, Percutaneous Endoscopic Approach, Diagnostic
0R914ZZ	Drainage of Cervical Vertebral Joint, Percutaneous Endoscopic Approach	0R953ZZ	Drainage of Cervicothoracic Vertebral Disc, Percutaneous Approach	0R994ZZ	Drainage of Thoracic Vertebral Disc, Percutaneous Endoscopic Approach
0R9300Z	Drainage of Cervical Vertebral Disc with Drainage Device, Open Approach	0R9540Z	Drainage of Cervicothoracic Vertebral Disc with Drainage Device, Percutaneous Endoscopic Approach	0R9A00Z	Drainage of Thoracolumbar Vertebral Joint with Drainage Device, Open Approach
0R930ZX	Drainage of Cervical Vertebral Disc, Open Approach, Diagnostic	0R954ZX	Drainage of Cervicothoracic Vertebral Disc, Percutaneous Endoscopic Approach, Diagnostic	0R9A0ZX	Drainage of Thoracolumbar Vertebral Joint, Open Approach, Diagnostic
0R930ZZ	Drainage of Cervical Vertebral Disc, Open Approach	0R954ZZ	Drainage of Cervicothoracic Vertebral Disc, Percutaneous Endoscopic Approach	0R9A0ZZ	Drainage of Thoracolumbar Vertebral Joint, Open Approach
0R9330Z	Drainage of Cervical Vertebral Disc with Drainage Device, Percutaneous Approach			0R9A30Z	Drainage of Thoracolumbar Vertebral Joint with Drainage Device, Percutaneous Approach
0R933ZX	Drainage of Cervical Vertebral Disc, Percutaneous Approach, Diagnostic			0R9A3ZX	Drainage of Thoracolumbar Vertebral Joint, Percutaneous Approach, Diagnostic
0R933ZZ	Drainage of Cervical Vertebral Disc, Percutaneous Approach				

♀ Female-only   ♂ Male-only   ▲ Limited Coverage   ● Non-OR   ▨ HAC-associated procedure   ▲ Non-covered procedures   ✚ Combination

0R9A3ZZ	Drainage of Thoracolumbar Vertebral Joint, Percutaneous Approach
0R9A40Z	Drainage of Thoracolumbar Vertebral Joint with Drainage Device, Percutaneous Endoscopic Approach
0R9A4ZX	Drainage of Thoracolumbar Vertebral Joint, Percutaneous Endoscopic Approach, Diagnostic
0R9A4ZZ	Drainage of Thoracolumbar Vertebral Joint, Percutaneous Endoscopic Approach
0R9B00Z	Drainage of Thoracolumbar Vertebral Disc with Drainage Device, Open Approach
0R9B0ZX	Drainage of Thoracolumbar Vertebral Disc, Open Approach, Diagnostic
0R9B0ZZ	Drainage of Thoracolumbar Vertebral Disc, Open Approach
0R9B30Z	Drainage of Thoracolumbar Vertebral Disc with Drainage Device, Percutaneous Approach
0R9B3ZX	Drainage of Thoracolumbar Vertebral Disc, Percutaneous Approach, Diagnostic
0R9B3ZZ	Drainage of Thoracolumbar Vertebral Disc, Percutaneous Approach
0R9B40Z	Drainage of Thoracolumbar Vertebral Disc with Drainage Device, Percutaneous Endoscopic Approach
0R9B4ZX	Drainage of Thoracolumbar Vertebral Disc, Percutaneous Endoscopic Approach, Diagnostic
0R9B4ZZ	Drainage of Thoracolumbar Vertebral Disc, Percutaneous Endoscopic Approach
0R9C00Z	Drainage of Right Temporomandibular Joint with Drainage Device, Open Approach
0R9C0ZX	Drainage of Right Temporomandibular Joint, Open Approach, Diagnostic
0R9C0ZZ	Drainage of Right Temporomandibular Joint, Open Approach
0R9C30Z	Drainage of Right Temporomandibular Joint with Drainage Device, Percutaneous Approach
0R9C3ZX	Drainage of Right Temporomandibular Joint, Percutaneous Approach, Diagnostic
0R9C3ZZ	Drainage of Right Temporomandibular Joint, Percutaneous Approach
0R9C40Z	Drainage of Right Temporomandibular Joint with Drainage Device, Percutaneous Endoscopic Approach
0R9C4ZX	Drainage of Right Temporomandibular Joint, Percutaneous Endoscopic Approach, Diagnostic
0R9C4ZZ	Drainage of Right Temporomandibular Joint, Percutaneous Endoscopic Approach
0R9D00Z	Drainage of Left Temporomandibular Joint with Drainage Device, Open Approach
0R9D0ZX	Drainage of Left Temporomandibular Joint, Open Approach, Diagnostic
0R9D0ZZ	Drainage of Left Temporomandibular Joint, Open Approach
0R9D30Z	Drainage of Left Temporomandibular Joint with Drainage Device, Percutaneous Approach
0R9D3ZX	Drainage of Left Temporomandibular Joint, Percutaneous Approach, Diagnostic
0R9D3ZZ	Drainage of Left Temporomandibular Joint, Percutaneous Approach
0R9D40Z	Drainage of Left Temporomandibular Joint with Drainage Device, Percutaneous Endoscopic Approach
0R9D4ZX	Drainage of Left Temporomandibular Joint, Percutaneous Endoscopic Approach, Diagnostic
0R9D4ZZ	Drainage of Left Temporomandibular Joint, Percutaneous Endoscopic Approach

0R9E00Z	Drainage of Right Sternoclavicular Joint with Drainage Device, Open Approach
0R9E0ZX	Drainage of Right Sternoclavicular Joint, Open Approach, Diagnostic
0R9E0ZZ	Drainage of Right Sternoclavicular Joint, Open Approach
0R9E30Z	Drainage of Right Sternoclavicular Joint with Drainage Device, Percutaneous Approach
0R9E3ZX	Drainage of Right Sternoclavicular Joint, Percutaneous Approach, Diagnostic
0R9E3ZZ	Drainage of Right Sternoclavicular Joint, Percutaneous Approach
0R9E40Z	Drainage of Right Sternoclavicular Joint with Drainage Device, Percutaneous Endoscopic Approach
0R9E4ZX	Drainage of Right Sternoclavicular Joint, Percutaneous Endoscopic Approach, Diagnostic
0R9E4ZZ	Drainage of Right Sternoclavicular Joint, Percutaneous Endoscopic Approach
0R9F00Z	Drainage of Left Sternoclavicular Joint with Drainage Device, Open Approach
0R9F0ZX	Drainage of Left Sternoclavicular Joint, Open Approach, Diagnostic
0R9F0ZZ	Drainage of Left Sternoclavicular Joint, Open Approach
0R9F30Z	Drainage of Left Sternoclavicular Joint with Drainage Device, Percutaneous Approach
0R9F3ZX	Drainage of Left Sternoclavicular Joint, Percutaneous Approach, Diagnostic
0R9F3ZZ	Drainage of Left Sternoclavicular Joint, Percutaneous Approach
0R9F40Z	Drainage of Left Sternoclavicular Joint with Drainage Device, Percutaneous Endoscopic Approach
0R9F4ZX	Drainage of Left Sternoclavicular Joint, Percutaneous Endoscopic Approach, Diagnostic
0R9F4ZZ	Drainage of Left Sternoclavicular Joint, Percutaneous Endoscopic Approach
0R9G00Z	Drainage of Right Acromioclavicular Joint with Drainage Device, Open Approach
0R9G0ZX	Drainage of Right Acromioclavicular Joint, Open Approach, Diagnostic
0R9G0ZZ	Drainage of Right Acromioclavicular Joint, Open Approach
0R9G30Z	Drainage of Right Acromioclavicular Joint with Drainage Device, Percutaneous Approach
0R9G3ZX	Drainage of Right Acromioclavicular Joint, Percutaneous Approach, Diagnostic
0R9G3ZZ	Drainage of Right Acromioclavicular Joint, Percutaneous Approach
0R9G40Z	Drainage of Right Acromioclavicular Joint with Drainage Device, Percutaneous Endoscopic Approach
0R9G4ZX	Drainage of Right Acromioclavicular Joint, Percutaneous Endoscopic Approach, Diagnostic
0R9G4ZZ	Drainage of Right Acromioclavicular Joint, Percutaneous Endoscopic Approach
0R9H00Z	Drainage of Left Acromioclavicular Joint with Drainage Device, Open Approach
0R9H0ZX	Drainage of Left Acromioclavicular Joint, Open Approach, Diagnostic
0R9H0ZZ	Drainage of Left Acromioclavicular Joint, Open Approach
0R9H30Z	Drainage of Left Acromioclavicular Joint with Drainage Device, Percutaneous Approach
0R9H3ZX	Drainage of Left Acromioclavicular Joint, Percutaneous Approach, Diagnostic
0R9H3ZZ	Drainage of Left Acromioclavicular Joint, Percutaneous Approach

0R9H40Z	Drainage of Left Acromioclavicular Joint with Drainage Device, Percutaneous Endoscopic Approach
0R9H4ZX	Drainage of Left Acromioclavicular Joint, Percutaneous Endoscopic Approach, Diagnostic
0R9H4ZZ	Drainage of Left Acromioclavicular Joint, Percutaneous Endoscopic Approach
0R9J00Z	Drainage of Right Shoulder Joint with Drainage Device, Open Approach
0R9J0ZX	Drainage of Right Shoulder Joint, Open Approach, Diagnostic
0R9J0ZZ	Drainage of Right Shoulder Joint, Open Approach
0R9J30Z	Drainage of Right Shoulder Joint with Drainage Device, Percutaneous Approach
0R9J3ZX	Drainage of Right Shoulder Joint, Percutaneous Approach, Diagnostic
0R9J3ZZ	Drainage of Right Shoulder Joint, Percutaneous Approach
0R9J40Z	Drainage of Right Shoulder Joint with Drainage Device, Percutaneous Endoscopic Approach
0R9J4ZX	Drainage of Right Shoulder Joint, Percutaneous Endoscopic Approach, Diagnostic
0R9J4ZZ	Drainage of Right Shoulder Joint, Percutaneous Endoscopic Approach
0R9K00Z	Drainage of Left Shoulder Joint with Drainage Device, Open Approach
0R9K0ZX	Drainage of Left Shoulder Joint, Open Approach, Diagnostic
0R9K0ZZ	Drainage of Left Shoulder Joint, Open Approach
0R9K30Z	Drainage of Left Shoulder Joint with Drainage Device, Percutaneous Approach
0R9K3ZX	Drainage of Left Shoulder Joint, Percutaneous Approach, Diagnostic
0R9K3ZZ	Drainage of Left Shoulder Joint, Percutaneous Approach
0R9K40Z	Drainage of Left Shoulder Joint with Drainage Device, Percutaneous Endoscopic Approach
0R9K4ZX	Drainage of Left Shoulder Joint, Percutaneous Endoscopic Approach, Diagnostic
0R9K4ZZ	Drainage of Left Shoulder Joint, Percutaneous Endoscopic Approach
0R9L00Z	Drainage of Right Elbow Joint with Drainage Device, Open Approach
0R9L0ZX	Drainage of Right Elbow Joint, Open Approach, Diagnostic
0R9L0ZZ	Drainage of Right Elbow Joint, Open Approach
0R9L30Z	Drainage of Right Elbow Joint with Drainage Device, Percutaneous Approach
0R9L3ZX	Drainage of Right Elbow Joint, Percutaneous Approach, Diagnostic
0R9L3ZZ	Drainage of Right Elbow Joint, Percutaneous Approach
0R9L40Z	Drainage of Right Elbow Joint with Drainage Device, Percutaneous Endoscopic Approach
0R9L4ZX	Drainage of Right Elbow Joint, Percutaneous Endoscopic Approach, Diagnostic
0R9L4ZZ	Drainage of Right Elbow Joint, Percutaneous Endoscopic Approach
0R9M00Z	Drainage of Left Elbow Joint with Drainage Device, Open Approach
0R9M0ZX	Drainage of Left Elbow Joint, Open Approach, Diagnostic
0R9M0ZZ	Drainage of Left Elbow Joint, Open Approach

M30Z	Drainage of Left Elbow Joint with Drainage Device, Percutaneous Approach
M3ZX	Drainage of Left Elbow Joint, Percutaneous Approach, Diagnostic
M3ZZ	Drainage of Left Elbow Joint, Percutaneous Approach
M40Z	Drainage of Left Elbow Joint with Drainage Device, Percutaneous Endoscopic Approach
M4ZX	Drainage of Left Elbow Joint, Percutaneous Endoscopic Approach, Diagnostic
M4ZZ	Drainage of Left Elbow Joint, Percutaneous Endoscopic Approach
N00Z	Drainage of Right Wrist Joint with Drainage Device, Open Approach
N0ZX	Drainage of Right Wrist Joint, Open Approach, Diagnostic
N0ZZ	Drainage of Right Wrist Joint, Open Approach
N30Z	Drainage of Right Wrist Joint with Drainage Device, Percutaneous Approach
N3ZX	Drainage of Right Wrist Joint, Percutaneous Approach, Diagnostic
N3ZZ	Drainage of Right Wrist Joint, Percutaneous Approach
N40Z	Drainage of Right Wrist Joint with Drainage Device, Percutaneous Endoscopic Approach
N4ZX	Drainage of Right Wrist Joint, Percutaneous Endoscopic Approach, Diagnostic
N4ZZ	Drainage of Right Wrist Joint, Percutaneous Endoscopic Approach
P00Z	Drainage of Left Wrist Joint with Drainage Device, Open Approach
P0ZX	Drainage of Left Wrist Joint, Open Approach, Diagnostic
P0ZZ	Drainage of Left Wrist Joint, Open Approach
P30Z	Drainage of Left Wrist Joint with Drainage Device, Percutaneous Approach
P3ZX	Drainage of Left Wrist Joint, Percutaneous Approach, Diagnostic
P3ZZ	Drainage of Left Wrist Joint, Percutaneous Approach
P40Z	Drainage of Left Wrist Joint with Drainage Device, Percutaneous Endoscopic Approach
P4ZX	Drainage of Left Wrist Joint, Percutaneous Endoscopic Approach, Diagnostic
P4ZZ	Drainage of Left Wrist Joint, Percutaneous Endoscopic Approach
Q00Z	Drainage of Right Carpal Joint with Drainage Device, Open Approach
Q0ZX	Drainage of Right Carpal Joint, Open Approach, Diagnostic
Q0ZZ	Drainage of Right Carpal Joint, Open Approach
Q30Z	Drainage of Right Carpal Joint with Drainage Device, Percutaneous Approach
Q3ZX	Drainage of Right Carpal Joint, Percutaneous Approach, Diagnostic
Q3ZZ	Drainage of Right Carpal Joint, Percutaneous Approach
Q40Z	Drainage of Right Carpal Joint with Drainage Device, Percutaneous Endoscopic Approach
Q4ZX	Drainage of Right Carpal Joint, Percutaneous Endoscopic Approach, Diagnostic
Q4ZZ	Drainage of Right Carpal Joint, Percutaneous Endoscopic Approach

0R9R00Z	Drainage of Left Carpal Joint with Drainage Device, Open Approach
0R9R0ZX	Drainage of Left Carpal Joint, Open Approach, Diagnostic
0R9R0ZZ	Drainage of Left Carpal Joint, Open Approach
0R9R30Z	Drainage of Left Carpal Joint with Drainage Device, Percutaneous Approach
0R9R3ZX	Drainage of Left Carpal Joint, Percutaneous Approach, Diagnostic
0R9R3ZZ	Drainage of Left Carpal Joint, Percutaneous Approach
0R9R40Z	Drainage of Left Carpal Joint with Drainage Device, Percutaneous Endoscopic Approach
0R9R4ZX	Drainage of Left Carpal Joint, Percutaneous Endoscopic Approach, Diagnostic
0R9R4ZZ	Drainage of Left Carpal Joint, Percutaneous Endoscopic Approach
0R9S00Z	Drainage of Right Metacarpocarpal Joint with Drainage Device, Open Approach
0R9S0ZX	Drainage of Right Metacarpocarpal Joint, Open Approach, Diagnostic
0R9S0ZZ	Drainage of Right Metacarpocarpal Joint, Open Approach
0R9S30Z	Drainage of Right Metacarpocarpal Joint with Drainage Device, Percutaneous Approach
0R9S3ZX	Drainage of Right Metacarpocarpal Joint, Percutaneous Approach, Diagnostic
0R9S3ZZ	Drainage of Right Metacarpocarpal Joint, Percutaneous Approach
0R9S40Z	Drainage of Right Metacarpocarpal Joint with Drainage Device, Percutaneous Endoscopic Approach
0R9S4ZX	Drainage of Right Metacarpocarpal Joint, Percutaneous Endoscopic Approach, Diagnostic
0R9S4ZZ	Drainage of Right Metacarpocarpal Joint, Percutaneous Endoscopic Approach
0R9T00Z	Drainage of Left Metacarpocarpal Joint with Drainage Device, Open Approach
0R9T0ZX	Drainage of Left Metacarpocarpal Joint, Open Approach, Diagnostic
0R9T0ZZ	Drainage of Left Metacarpocarpal Joint, Open Approach
0R9T30Z	Drainage of Left Metacarpocarpal Joint with Drainage Device, Percutaneous Approach
0R9T3ZX	Drainage of Left Metacarpocarpal Joint, Percutaneous Approach, Diagnostic
0R9T3ZZ	Drainage of Left Metacarpocarpal Joint, Percutaneous Approach
0R9T40Z	Drainage of Left Metacarpocarpal Joint with Drainage Device, Percutaneous Endoscopic Approach
0R9T4ZX	Drainage of Left Metacarpocarpal Joint, Percutaneous Endoscopic Approach, Diagnostic
0R9T4ZZ	Drainage of Left Metacarpocarpal Joint, Percutaneous Endoscopic Approach
0R9U00Z	Drainage of Right Metacarpophalangeal Joint with Drainage Device, Open Approach
0R9U0ZX	Drainage of Right Metacarpophalangeal Joint, Open Approach, Diagnostic
0R9U0ZZ	Drainage of Right Metacarpophalangeal Joint, Open Approach
0R9U30Z	Drainage of Right Metacarpophalangeal Joint with Drainage Device, Percutaneous Approach
0R9U3ZX	Drainage of Right Metacarpophalangeal Joint, Percutaneous Approach, Diagnostic
0R9U3ZZ	Drainage of Right Metacarpophalangeal Joint, Percutaneous Approach

0R9U40Z	Drainage of Right Metacarpophalangeal Joint with Drainage Device, Percutaneous Endoscopic Approach
0R9U4ZX	Drainage of Right Metacarpophalangeal Joint, Percutaneous Endoscopic Approach, Diagnostic
0R9U4ZZ	Drainage of Right Metacarpophalangeal Joint, Percutaneous Endoscopic Approach
0R9V00Z	Drainage of Left Metacarpophalangeal Joint with Drainage Device, Open Approach
0R9V0ZX	Drainage of Left Metacarpophalangeal Joint, Open Approach, Diagnostic
0R9V0ZZ	Drainage of Left Metacarpophalangeal Joint, Open Approach
0R9V30Z	Drainage of Left Metacarpophalangeal Joint with Drainage Device, Percutaneous Approach
0R9V3ZX	Drainage of Left Metacarpophalangeal Joint, Percutaneous Approach, Diagnostic
0R9V3ZZ	Drainage of Left Metacarpophalangeal Joint, Percutaneous Approach
0R9V40Z	Drainage of Left Metacarpophalangeal Joint with Drainage Device, Percutaneous Endoscopic Approach
0R9V4ZX	Drainage of Left Metacarpophalangeal Joint, Percutaneous Endoscopic Approach, Diagnostic
0R9V4ZZ	Drainage of Left Metacarpophalangeal Joint, Percutaneous Endoscopic Approach
0R9W00Z	Drainage of Right Finger Phalangeal Joint with Drainage Device, Open Approach
0R9W0ZX	Drainage of Right Finger Phalangeal Joint, Open Approach, Diagnostic
0R9W0ZZ	Drainage of Right Finger Phalangeal Joint, Open Approach
0R9W30Z	Drainage of Right Finger Phalangeal Joint with Drainage Device, Percutaneous Approach
0R9W3ZX	Drainage of Right Finger Phalangeal Joint, Percutaneous Approach, Diagnostic
0R9W3ZZ	Drainage of Right Finger Phalangeal Joint, Percutaneous Approach
0R9W40Z	Drainage of Right Finger Phalangeal Joint with Drainage Device, Percutaneous Endoscopic Approach
0R9W4ZX	Drainage of Right Finger Phalangeal Joint, Percutaneous Endoscopic Approach, Diagnostic
0R9W4ZZ	Drainage of Right Finger Phalangeal Joint, Percutaneous Endoscopic Approach
0R9X00Z	Drainage of Left Finger Phalangeal Joint with Drainage Device, Open Approach
0R9X0ZX	Drainage of Left Finger Phalangeal Joint, Open Approach, Diagnostic
0R9X0ZZ	Drainage of Left Finger Phalangeal Joint, Open Approach
0R9X30Z	Drainage of Left Finger Phalangeal Joint with Drainage Device, Percutaneous Approach
0R9X3ZX	Drainage of Left Finger Phalangeal Joint, Percutaneous Approach, Diagnostic
0R9X3ZZ	Drainage of Left Finger Phalangeal Joint, Percutaneous Approach
0R9X40Z	Drainage of Left Finger Phalangeal Joint with Drainage Device, Percutaneous Endoscopic Approach
0R9X4ZX	Drainage of Left Finger Phalangeal Joint, Percutaneous Endoscopic Approach, Diagnostic
0R9X4ZZ	Drainage of Left Finger Phalangeal Joint, Percutaneous Endoscopic Approach

Review Coding Guidelines B3.4a and B3.4b

Review Coding Guideline B3.5

Review Coding Guideline B3.8

Code	Description	Code	Description	Code	Description
0RB00ZX	Excision of Occipital-cervical Joint, Open Approach, Diagnostic	0RB63ZX	Excision of Thoracic Vertebral Joint, Percutaneous Approach, Diagnostic	0RBD4ZX	Excision of Left Temporomandibular Joint, Percutaneous Endoscopic Approach, Diagnostic
0RB00ZZ	Excision of Occipital-cervical Joint, Open Approach	0RB63ZZ	Excision of Thoracic Vertebral Joint, Percutaneous Approach	0RBD4ZZ	Excision of Left Temporomandibular Joint, Percutaneous Endoscopic Approach
0RB03ZX	Excision of Occipital-cervical Joint, Percutaneous Approach, Diagnostic	0RB64ZX	Excision of Thoracic Vertebral Joint, Percutaneous Endoscopic Approach, Diagnostic	0RBE0ZX	Excision of Right Sternoclavicular Joint, Open Approach, Diagnostic
0RB03ZZ	Excision of Occipital-cervical Joint, Percutaneous Approach	0RB64ZZ	Excision of Thoracic Vertebral Joint, Percutaneous Endoscopic Approach	0RBE0ZZ	Excision of Right Sternoclavicular Joint, Open Approach
0RB04ZX	Excision of Occipital-cervical Joint, Percutaneous Endoscopic Approach, Diagnostic	0RB90ZX	Excision of Thoracic Vertebral Disc, Open Approach, Diagnostic	0RBE3ZX	Excision of Right Sternoclavicular Joint, Percutaneous Approach, Diagnostic
0RB04ZZ	Excision of Occipital-cervical Joint, Percutaneous Endoscopic Approach	0RB90ZZ	Excision of Thoracic Vertebral Disc, Open Approach	0RBE3ZZ	Excision of Right Sternoclavicular Joint, Percutaneous Approach
0RB10ZX	Excision of Cervical Vertebral Joint, Open Approach, Diagnostic	0RB93ZX	Excision of Thoracic Vertebral Disc, Percutaneous Approach, Diagnostic	0RBE4ZX	Excision of Right Sternoclavicular Joint, Percutaneous Endoscopic Approach, Diagnostic
0RB10ZZ	Excision of Cervical Vertebral Joint, Open Approach	0RB93ZZ	Excision of Thoracic Vertebral Disc, Percutaneous Approach	0RBE4ZZ	Excision of Right Sternoclavicular Joint, Percutaneous Endoscopic Approach
0RB13ZX	Excision of Cervical Vertebral Joint, Percutaneous Approach, Diagnostic	0RB94ZX	Excision of Thoracic Vertebral Disc, Percutaneous Endoscopic Approach, Diagnostic	0RBF0ZX	Excision of Left Sternoclavicular Joint, Open Approach, Diagnostic
0RB13ZZ	Excision of Cervical Vertebral Joint, Percutaneous Approach	0RB94ZZ	Excision of Thoracic Vertebral Disc, Percutaneous Endoscopic Approach	0RBF0ZZ	Excision of Left Sternoclavicular Joint, Open Approach
0RB14ZX	Excision of Cervical Vertebral Joint, Percutaneous Endoscopic Approach, Diagnostic	0RBA0ZX	Excision of Thoracolumbar Vertebral Joint, Open Approach, Diagnostic	0RBF3ZX	Excision of Left Sternoclavicular Joint, Percutaneous Approach, Diagnostic
0RB14ZZ	Excision of Cervical Vertebral Joint, Percutaneous Endoscopic Approach	0RBA0ZZ	Excision of Thoracolumbar Vertebral Joint, Open Approach	0RBF3ZZ	Excision of Left Sternoclavicular Joint, Percutaneous Approach
0RB30ZX	Excision of Cervical Vertebral Disc, Open Approach, Diagnostic	0RBA3ZX	Excision of Thoracolumbar Vertebral Joint, Percutaneous Approach, Diagnostic	0RBF4ZX	Excision of Left Sternoclavicular Joint, Percutaneous Endoscopic Approach, Diagnostic
0RB30ZZ	Excision of Cervical Vertebral Disc, Open Approach	0RBA3ZZ	Excision of Thoracolumbar Vertebral Joint, Percutaneous Approach	0RBF4ZZ	Excision of Left Sternoclavicular Joint, Percutaneous Endoscopic Approach
0RB33ZX	Excision of Cervical Vertebral Disc, Percutaneous Approach, Diagnostic	0RBA4ZX	Excision of Thoracolumbar Vertebral Joint, Percutaneous Endoscopic Approach, Diagnostic	0RBG0ZX	Excision of Right Acromioclavicular Joint, Open Approach, Diagnostic
0RB33ZZ	Excision of Cervical Vertebral Disc, Percutaneous Approach	0RBA4ZZ	Excision of Thoracolumbar Vertebral Joint, Percutaneous Endoscopic Approach	0RBG0ZZ	Excision of Right Acromioclavicular Joint, Open Approach
0RB34ZX	Excision of Cervical Vertebral Disc, Percutaneous Endoscopic Approach, Diagnostic	0RBB0ZX	Excision of Thoracolumbar Vertebral Disc, Open Approach, Diagnostic	0RBG3ZX	Excision of Right Acromioclavicular Joint, Percutaneous Approach, Diagnos
0RB34ZZ	Excision of Cervical Vertebral Disc, Percutaneous Endoscopic Approach	0RBB0ZZ	Excision of Thoracolumbar Vertebral Disc, Open Approach	0RBG3ZZ	Excision of Right Acromioclavicular Joint, Percutaneous Approach
0RB40ZX	Excision of Cervicothoracic Vertebral Joint, Open Approach, Diagnostic	0RBB3ZX	Excision of Thoracolumbar Vertebral Disc, Percutaneous Approach, Diagnostic	0RBG4ZX	Excision of Right Acromioclavicular Joint, Percutaneous Endoscopic Approach, Diagnostic
0RB40ZZ	Excision of Cervicothoracic Vertebral Joint, Open Approach	0RBB3ZZ	Excision of Thoracolumbar Vertebral Disc, Percutaneous Approach	0RBG4ZZ	Excision of Right Acromioclavicular Joint, Percutaneous Endoscopic Approa
0RB43ZX	Excision of Cervicothoracic Vertebral Joint, Percutaneous Approach, Diagnostic	0RBB4ZX	Excision of Thoracolumbar Vertebral Disc, Percutaneous Endoscopic Approach, Diagnostic	0RBH0ZX	Excision of Left Acromioclavicular Joi Open Approach, Diagnostic
0RB43ZZ	Excision of Cervicothoracic Vertebral Joint, Percutaneous Approach	0RBB4ZZ	Excision of Thoracolumbar Vertebral Disc, Percutaneous Endoscopic Approach	0RBH0ZZ	Excision of Left Acromioclavicular Joi Open Approach
0RB44ZX	Excision of Cervicothoracic Vertebral Joint, Percutaneous Endoscopic Approach, Diagnostic	0RBC0ZX	Excision of Right Temporomandibular Joint, Open Approach, Diagnostic	0RBH3ZX	Excision of Left Acromioclavicular Joi Percutaneous Approach, Diagnostic
0RB44ZZ	Excision of Cervicothoracic Vertebral Joint, Percutaneous Endoscopic Approach	0RBC0ZZ	Excision of Right Temporomandibular Joint, Open Approach	0RBH3ZZ	Excision of Left Acromioclavicular Joi Percutaneous Approach
0RB50ZX	Excision of Cervicothoracic Vertebral Disc, Open Approach, Diagnostic	0RBC3ZX	Excision of Right Temporomandibular Joint, Percutaneous Approach, Diagnostic	0RBH4ZX	Excision of Left Acromioclavicular Joi Percutaneous Endoscopic Approach, Diagnostic
0RB50ZZ	Excision of Cervicothoracic Vertebral Disc, Open Approach	0RBC3ZZ	Excision of Right Temporomandibular Joint, Percutaneous Approach	0RBH4ZZ	Excision of Left Acromioclavicular Joi Percutaneous Endoscopic Approach
0RB53ZX	Excision of Cervicothoracic Vertebral Disc, Percutaneous Approach, Diagnostic	0RBC4ZX	Excision of Right Temporomandibular Joint, Percutaneous Endoscopic Approach, Diagnostic	0RBJ0ZX	Excision of Right Shoulder Joint, Open Approach, Diagnostic
0RB53ZZ	Excision of Cervicothoracic Vertebral Disc, Percutaneous Approach	0RBC4ZZ	Excision of Right Temporomandibular Joint, Percutaneous Endoscopic Approach	0RBJ0ZZ	Excision of Right Shoulder Joint, Open Approach
0RB54ZX	Excision of Cervicothoracic Vertebral Disc, Percutaneous Endoscopic Approach, Diagnostic	0RBD0ZX	Excision of Left Temporomandibular Joint, Open Approach, Diagnostic	0RBJ3ZX	Excision of Right Shoulder Joint, Percutaneous Approach, Diagnostic
0RB54ZZ	Excision of Cervicothoracic Vertebral Disc, Percutaneous Endoscopic Approach	0RBD0ZZ	Excision of Left Temporomandibular Joint, Open Approach	0RBJ3ZZ	Excision of Right Shoulder Joint, Percutaneous Approach
0RB60ZX	Excision of Thoracic Vertebral Joint, Open Approach, Diagnostic	0RBD3ZX	Excision of Left Temporomandibular Joint, Percutaneous Approach, Diagnostic	0RBJ4ZX	Excision of Right Shoulder Joint, Percutaneous Endoscopic Approach, Diagnostic
0RB60ZZ	Excision of Thoracic Vertebral Joint, Open Approach	0RBD3ZZ	Excision of Left Temporomandibular Joint, Percutaneous Approach	0RBJ4ZZ	Excision of Right Shoulder Joint, Percutaneous Endoscopic Approach

♀ Female-only   ♂ Male-only   ▲ Limited Coverage   ● Non-OR   ▦ HAC-associated procedure   ▲ Non-covered procedures   ✚ Combinati

0RBK0ZX	Excision of Left Shoulder Joint, Open Approach, Diagnostic
0RBK0ZZ	Excision of Left Shoulder Joint, Open Approach
0RBK3ZX	Excision of Left Shoulder Joint, Percutaneous Approach, Diagnostic
0RBK3ZZ	Excision of Left Shoulder Joint, Percutaneous Approach
0RBK4ZX	Excision of Left Shoulder Joint, Percutaneous Endoscopic Approach, Diagnostic
0RBK4ZZ	Excision of Left Shoulder Joint, Percutaneous Endoscopic Approach
0RBL0ZX	Excision of Right Elbow Joint, Open Approach, Diagnostic
0RBL0ZZ	Excision of Right Elbow Joint, Open Approach
0RBL3ZX	Excision of Right Elbow Joint, Percutaneous Approach, Diagnostic
0RBL3ZZ	Excision of Right Elbow Joint, Percutaneous Approach
0RBL4ZX	Excision of Right Elbow Joint, Percutaneous Endoscopic Approach, Diagnostic
0RBL4ZZ	Excision of Right Elbow Joint, Percutaneous Endoscopic Approach
0RBM0ZX	Excision of Left Elbow Joint, Open Approach, Diagnostic
0RBM0ZZ	Excision of Left Elbow Joint, Open Approach
0RBM3ZX	Excision of Left Elbow Joint, Percutaneous Approach, Diagnostic
0RBM3ZZ	Excision of Left Elbow Joint, Percutaneous Approach
0RBM4ZX	Excision of Left Elbow Joint, Percutaneous Endoscopic Approach, Diagnostic
0RBM4ZZ	Excision of Left Elbow Joint, Percutaneous Endoscopic Approach
0RBN0ZX	Excision of Right Wrist Joint, Open Approach, Diagnostic
0RBN0ZZ	Excision of Right Wrist Joint, Open Approach
0RBN3ZX	Excision of Right Wrist Joint, Percutaneous Approach, Diagnostic
0RBN3ZZ	Excision of Right Wrist Joint, Percutaneous Approach
0RBN4ZX	Excision of Right Wrist Joint, Percutaneous Endoscopic Approach, Diagnostic
0RBN4ZZ	Excision of Right Wrist Joint, Percutaneous Endoscopic Approach
0RBP0ZX	Excision of Left Wrist Joint, Open Approach, Diagnostic
0RBP0ZZ	Excision of Left Wrist Joint, Open Approach
0RBP3ZX	Excision of Left Wrist Joint, Percutaneous Approach, Diagnostic

0RBP3ZZ	Excision of Left Wrist Joint, Percutaneous Approach
0RBP4ZX	Excision of Left Wrist Joint, Percutaneous Endoscopic Approach, Diagnostic
0RBP4ZZ	Excision of Left Wrist Joint, Percutaneous Endoscopic Approach
0RBQ0ZX	Excision of Right Carpal Joint, Open Approach, Diagnostic
0RBQ0ZZ	Excision of Right Carpal Joint, Open Approach
0RBQ3ZX	Excision of Right Carpal Joint, Percutaneous Approach, Diagnostic
0RBQ3ZZ	Excision of Right Carpal Joint, Percutaneous Approach
0RBQ4ZX	Excision of Right Carpal Joint, Percutaneous Endoscopic Approach, Diagnostic
0RBQ4ZZ	Excision of Right Carpal Joint, Percutaneous Endoscopic Approach
0RBR0ZX	Excision of Left Carpal Joint, Open Approach, Diagnostic
0RBR0ZZ	Excision of Left Carpal Joint, Open Approach
0RBR3ZX	Excision of Left Carpal Joint, Percutaneous Approach, Diagnostic
0RBR3ZZ	Excision of Left Carpal Joint, Percutaneous Approach
0RBR4ZX	Excision of Left Carpal Joint, Percutaneous Endoscopic Approach, Diagnostic
0RBR4ZZ	Excision of Left Carpal Joint, Percutaneous Endoscopic Approach
0RBS0ZX	Excision of Right Metacarpocarpal Joint, Open Approach, Diagnostic
0RBS0ZZ	Excision of Right Metacarpocarpal Joint, Open Approach
0RBS3ZX	Excision of Right Metacarpocarpal Joint, Percutaneous Approach, Diagnostic
0RBS3ZZ	Excision of Right Metacarpocarpal Joint, Percutaneous Approach
0RBS4ZX	Excision of Right Metacarpocarpal Joint, Percutaneous Endoscopic Approach, Diagnostic
0RBS4ZZ	Excision of Right Metacarpocarpal Joint, Percutaneous Endoscopic Approach
0RBT0ZX	Excision of Left Metacarpocarpal Joint, Open Approach, Diagnostic
0RBT0ZZ	Excision of Left Metacarpocarpal Joint, Open Approach
0RBT3ZX	Excision of Left Metacarpocarpal Joint, Percutaneous Approach, Diagnostic
0RBT3ZZ	Excision of Left Metacarpocarpal Joint, Percutaneous Approach
0RBT4ZX	Excision of Left Metacarpocarpal Joint, Percutaneous Endoscopic Approach, Diagnostic
0RBT4ZZ	Excision of Left Metacarpocarpal Joint, Percutaneous Endoscopic Approach

0RBU0ZX	Excision of Right Metacarpophalangeal Joint, Open Approach, Diagnostic
0RBU0ZZ	Excision of Right Metacarpophalangeal Joint, Open Approach
0RBU3ZX	Excision of Right Metacarpophalangeal Joint, Percutaneous Approach, Diagnostic
0RBU3ZZ	Excision of Right Metacarpophalangeal Joint, Percutaneous Approach
0RBU4ZX	Excision of Right Metacarpophalangeal Joint, Percutaneous Endoscopic Approach, Diagnostic
0RBU4ZZ	Excision of Right Metacarpophalangeal Joint, Percutaneous Endoscopic Approach
0RBV0ZX	Excision of Left Metacarpophalangeal Joint, Open Approach, Diagnostic
0RBV0ZZ	Excision of Left Metacarpophalangeal Joint, Open Approach
0RBV3ZX	Excision of Left Metacarpophalangeal Joint, Percutaneous Approach, Diagnostic
0RBV3ZZ	Excision of Left Metacarpophalangeal Joint, Percutaneous Approach
0RBV4ZX	Excision of Left Metacarpophalangeal Joint, Percutaneous Endoscopic Approach, Diagnostic
0RBV4ZZ	Excision of Left Metacarpophalangeal Joint, Percutaneous Endoscopic Approach
0RBW0ZX	Excision of Right Finger Phalangeal Joint, Open Approach, Diagnostic
0RBW0ZZ	Excision of Right Finger Phalangeal Joint, Open Approach
0RBW3ZX	Excision of Right Finger Phalangeal Joint, Percutaneous Approach, Diagnostic
0RBW3ZZ	Excision of Right Finger Phalangeal Joint, Percutaneous Approach
0RBW4ZX	Excision of Right Finger Phalangeal Joint, Percutaneous Endoscopic Approach, Diagnostic
0RBW4ZZ	Excision of Right Finger Phalangeal Joint, Percutaneous Endoscopic Approach
0RBX0ZX	Excision of Left Finger Phalangeal Joint, Open Approach, Diagnostic
0RBX0ZZ	Excision of Left Finger Phalangeal Joint, Open Approach
0RBX3ZX	Excision of Left Finger Phalangeal Joint, Percutaneous Approach, Diagnostic
0RBX3ZZ	Excision of Left Finger Phalangeal Joint, Percutaneous Approach
0RBX4ZX	Excision of Left Finger Phalangeal Joint, Percutaneous Endoscopic Approach, Diagnostic
0RBX4ZZ	Excision of Left Finger Phalangeal Joint, Percutaneous Endoscopic Approach

0RC – Upper Joints, Extirpation

0RC00ZZ	Extirpation of Matter from Occipital-cervical Joint, Open Approach
0RC03ZZ	Extirpation of Matter from Occipital-cervical Joint, Percutaneous Approach
0RC04ZZ	Extirpation of Matter from Occipital-cervical Joint, Percutaneous Endoscopic Approach
0RC10ZZ	Extirpation of Matter from Cervical Vertebral Joint, Open Approach
0RC13ZZ	Extirpation of Matter from Cervical Vertebral Joint, Percutaneous Approach
0RC14ZZ	Extirpation of Matter from Cervical Vertebral Joint, Percutaneous Endoscopic Approach
0RC30ZZ	Extirpation of Matter from Cervical Vertebral Disc, Open Approach

0RC33ZZ	Extirpation of Matter from Cervical Vertebral Disc, Percutaneous Approach
0RC34ZZ	Extirpation of Matter from Cervical Vertebral Disc, Percutaneous Endoscopic Approach
0RC40ZZ	Extirpation of Matter from Cervicothoracic Vertebral Joint, Open Approach
0RC43ZZ	Extirpation of Matter from Cervicothoracic Vertebral Joint, Percutaneous Approach
0RC44ZZ	Extirpation of Matter from Cervicothoracic Vertebral Joint, Percutaneous Endoscopic Approach
0RC50ZZ	Extirpation of Matter from Cervicothoracic Vertebral Disc, Open Approach

0RC53ZZ	Extirpation of Matter from Cervicothoracic Vertebral Disc, Percutaneous Approach
0RC54ZZ	Extirpation of Matter from Cervicothoracic Vertebral Disc, Percutaneous Endoscopic Approach
0RC60ZZ	Extirpation of Matter from Thoracic Vertebral Joint, Open Approach
0RC63ZZ	Extirpation of Matter from Thoracic Vertebral Joint, Percutaneous Approach
0RC64ZZ	Extirpation of Matter from Thoracic Vertebral Joint, Percutaneous Endoscopic Approach
0RC90ZZ	Extirpation of Matter from Thoracic Vertebral Disc, Open Approach
0RC93ZZ	Extirpation of Matter from Thoracic Vertebral Disc, Percutaneous Approach

905

Female-only	♂ Male-only	▲ Limited Coverage	● Non-OR	HAC-associated procedure	▲ Non-covered procedures	+ Combination

0RC94ZZ Extirpation of Matter from Thoracic Vertebral Disc, Percutaneous Endoscopic Approach

0RCA0ZZ Extirpation of Matter from Thoracolumbar Vertebral Joint, Open Approach

0RCA3ZZ Extirpation of Matter from Thoracolumbar Vertebral Joint, Percutaneous Approach

0RCA4ZZ Extirpation of Matter from Thoracolumbar Vertebral Joint, Percutaneous Endoscopic Approach

0RCB0ZZ Extirpation of Matter from Thoracolumbar Vertebral Disc, Open Approach

0RCB3ZZ Extirpation of Matter from Thoracolumbar Vertebral Disc, Percutaneous Approach

0RCB4ZZ Extirpation of Matter from Thoracolumbar Vertebral Disc, Percutaneous Endoscopic Approach

0RCC0ZZ Extirpation of Matter from Right Temporomandibular Joint, Open Approach

0RCC3ZZ Extirpation of Matter from Right Temporomandibular Joint, Percutaneous Approach

0RCC4ZZ Extirpation of Matter from Right Temporomandibular Joint, Percutaneous Endoscopic Approach

0RCD0ZZ Extirpation of Matter from Left Temporomandibular Joint, Open Approach

0RCD3ZZ Extirpation of Matter from Left Temporomandibular Joint, Percutaneous Approach

0RCD4ZZ Extirpation of Matter from Left Temporomandibular Joint, Percutaneous Endoscopic Approach

0RCE0ZZ Extirpation of Matter from Right Sternoclavicular Joint, Open Approach

0RCE3ZZ Extirpation of Matter from Right Sternoclavicular Joint, Percutaneous Approach

0RCE4ZZ Extirpation of Matter from Right Sternoclavicular Joint, Percutaneous Endoscopic Approach

0RCF0ZZ Extirpation of Matter from Left Sternoclavicular Joint, Open Approach

0RCF3ZZ Extirpation of Matter from Left Sternoclavicular Joint, Percutaneous Approach

0RCF4ZZ Extirpation of Matter from Left Sternoclavicular Joint, Percutaneous Endoscopic Approach

0RCG0ZZ Extirpation of Matter from Right Acromioclavicular Joint, Open Approach

0RCG3ZZ Extirpation of Matter from Right Acromioclavicular Joint, Percutaneous Approach

0RCG4ZZ Extirpation of Matter from Right Acromioclavicular Joint, Percutaneous Endoscopic Approach

0RCH0ZZ Extirpation of Matter from Left Acromioclavicular Joint, Open Approach

0RCH3ZZ Extirpation of Matter from Left Acromioclavicular Joint, Percutaneous Approach

0RCH4ZZ Extirpation of Matter from Left Acromioclavicular Joint, Percutaneous Endoscopic Approach

0RCJ0ZZ Extirpation of Matter from Right Shoulder Joint, Open Approach

0RCJ3ZZ Extirpation of Matter from Right Shoulder Joint, Percutaneous Approach

0RCJ4ZZ Extirpation of Matter from Right Shoulder Joint, Percutaneous Endoscopic Approach

0RCK0ZZ Extirpation of Matter from Left Shoulder Joint, Open Approach

0RCK3ZZ Extirpation of Matter from Left Shoulder Joint, Percutaneous Approach

0RCK4ZZ Extirpation of Matter from Left Shoulder Joint, Percutaneous Endoscopic Approach

0RCL0ZZ Extirpation of Matter from Right Elbow Joint, Open Approach

0RCL3ZZ Extirpation of Matter from Right Elbow Joint, Percutaneous Approach

0RCL4ZZ Extirpation of Matter from Right Elbow Joint, Percutaneous Endoscopic Approach

0RCM0ZZ Extirpation of Matter from Left Elbow Joint, Open Approach

0RCM3ZZ Extirpation of Matter from Left Elbow Joint, Percutaneous Approach

0RCM4ZZ Extirpation of Matter from Left Elbow Joint, Percutaneous Endoscopic Approach

0RCN0ZZ Extirpation of Matter from Right Wrist Joint, Open Approach

0RCN3ZZ Extirpation of Matter from Right Wrist Joint, Percutaneous Approach

0RCN4ZZ Extirpation of Matter from Right Wrist Joint, Percutaneous Endoscopic Approach

0RCP0ZZ Extirpation of Matter from Left Wrist Joint, Open Approach

0RCP3ZZ Extirpation of Matter from Left Wrist Joint, Percutaneous Approach

0RCP4ZZ Extirpation of Matter from Left Wrist Joint, Percutaneous Endoscopic Approach

0RCQ0ZZ Extirpation of Matter from Right Carpal Joint, Open Approach

0RCQ3ZZ Extirpation of Matter from Right Carpal Joint, Percutaneous Approach

0RCQ4ZZ Extirpation of Matter from Right Carpal Joint, Percutaneous Endoscopic Approach

0RCR0ZZ Extirpation of Matter from Left Carpal Joint, Open Approach

0RCR3ZZ Extirpation of Matter from Left Carpal Joint, Percutaneous Approach

0RCR4ZZ Extirpation of Matter from Left Carpal Joint, Percutaneous Endoscopic Approach

0RCS0ZZ Extirpation of Matter from Right Metacarpocarpal Joint, Open Approach

0RCS3ZZ Extirpation of Matter from Right Metacarpocarpal Joint, Percutaneous Approach

0RCS4ZZ Extirpation of Matter from Right Metacarpocarpal Joint, Percutaneous Endoscopic Approach

0RCT0ZZ Extirpation of Matter from Left Metacarpocarpal Joint, Open Approach

0RCT3ZZ Extirpation of Matter from Left Metacarpocarpal Joint, Percutaneous Approach

0RCT4ZZ Extirpation of Matter from Left Metacarpocarpal Joint, Percutaneous Endoscopic Approach

0RCU0ZZ Extirpation of Matter from Right Metacarpophalangeal Joint, Open Approach

0RCU3ZZ Extirpation of Matter from Right Metacarpophalangeal Joint, Percutaneous Approach

0RCU4ZZ Extirpation of Matter from Right Metacarpophalangeal Joint, Percutaneous Endoscopic Approach

0RCV0ZZ Extirpation of Matter from Left Metacarpophalangeal Joint, Open Approach

0RCV3ZZ Extirpation of Matter from Left Metacarpophalangeal Joint, Percutaneous Approach

0RCV4ZZ Extirpation of Matter from Left Metacarpophalangeal Joint, Percutaneous Endoscopic Approach

0RCW0ZZ Extirpation of Matter from Right Finger Phalangeal Joint, Open Approach

0RCW3ZZ Extirpation of Matter from Right Finger Phalangeal Joint, Percutaneous Approach

0RCW4ZZ Extirpation of Matter from Right Finger Phalangeal Joint, Percutaneous Endoscopic Approach

0RCX0ZZ Extirpation of Matter from Left Finger Phalangeal Joint, Open Approach

0RCX3ZZ Extirpation of Matter from Left Finger Phalangeal Joint, Percutaneous Approach

0RCX4ZZ Extirpation of Matter from Left Finger Phalangeal Joint, Percutaneous Endoscopic Approach

0RG – Upper Joints, Fusion

For Fusion procedures involving the vertebral joints

Review Coding Guidelines B3.10a, B3.10b and B3.10c

0RG0070 Fusion of Occipital-cervical Joint with Autologous Tissue Substitute, Anterior Approach, Anterior Column, Open Approach

⬛ When reported with secondary diagnosis code T84.60XA, T84.610A, T84.611A, T84.612A, T84.613A, T84.614A, T84.615A, T84.619A, T84.63XA, T84.69XA, T84.7XXA

0RG0071 Fusion of Occipital-cervical Joint with Autologous Tissue Substitute, Posterior Approach, Posterior Column, Open Approach

⬛ When reported with secondary diagnosis code T84.60XA, T84.610A, T84.611A, T84.612A, T84.613A, T84.614A, T84.615A, T84.619A, T84.63XA, T84.69XA, T84.7XXA

0RG007J Fusion of Occipital-cervical Joint with Autologous Tissue Substitute, Posterior Approach, Anterior Column, Open Approach

⬛ When reported with secondary diagnosis code T84.60XA, T84.610A, T84.611A, T84.612A, T84.613A, T84.614A, T84.615A, T84.619A, T84.63XA, T84.69XA, T84.7XXA

0RG00A0 Fusion of Occipital-cervical Joint with Interbody Fusion Device, Anterior Approach, Anterior Column, Open Approach

⬛ When reported with secondary diagnosis code T84.60XA, T84.610A, T84.611A, T84.612A, T84.613A, T84.614A, T84.615A, T84.619A, T84.63XA, T84.69XA, T84.7XXA

0RG00A1 Fusion of Occipital-cervical Joint with Interbody Fusion Device, Posterior Approach, Posterior Column, Open Approach

Note Continue

0RG00A1 Continued Note

▪ When reported with secondary diagnosis code T84.60XA, T84.610A, T84.611A, T84.612A, T84.613A, T84.614A, T84.615A, T84.619A, T84.63XA, T84.69XA, T84.7XXA

00AJ Fusion of Occipital-cervical Joint with Interbody Fusion Device, Posterior Approach, Anterior Column, Open Approach

▪ When reported with secondary diagnosis code T84.60XA, T84.610A, T84.611A, T84.612A, T84.613A, T84.614A, T84.615A, T84.619A, T84.63XA, T84.69XA, T84.7XXA

00J0 Fusion of Occipital-cervical Joint with Synthetic Substitute, Anterior Approach, Anterior Column, Open Approach

▪ When reported with secondary diagnosis code T84.60XA, T84.610A, T84.611A, T84.612A, T84.613A, T84.614A, T84.615A, T84.619A, T84.63XA, T84.69XA, T84.7XXA

00J1 Fusion of Occipital-cervical Joint with Synthetic Substitute, Posterior Approach, Posterior Column, Open Approach

▪ When reported with secondary diagnosis code T84.60XA, T84.610A, T84.611A, T84.612A, T84.613A, T84.614A, T84.615A, T84.619A, T84.63XA, T84.69XA, T84.7XXA

00JJ Fusion of Occipital-cervical Joint with Synthetic Substitute, Posterior Approach, Anterior Column, Open Approach

▪ When reported with secondary diagnosis code T84.60XA, T84.610A, T84.611A, T84.612A, T84.613A, T84.614A, T84.615A, T84.619A, T84.63XA, T84.69XA, T84.7XXA

00K0 Fusion of Occipital-cervical Joint with Nonautologous Tissue Substitute, Anterior Approach, Anterior Column, Open Approach

▪ When reported with secondary diagnosis code T84.60XA, T84.610A, T84.611A, T84.612A, T84.613A, T84.614A, T84.615A, T84.619A, T84.63XA, T84.69XA, T84.7XXA

00K1 Fusion of Occipital-cervical Joint with Nonautologous Tissue Substitute, Posterior Approach, Posterior Column, Open Approach

▪ When reported with secondary diagnosis code T84.60XA, T84.610A, T84.611A, T84.612A, T84.613A, T84.614A, T84.615A, T84.619A, T84.63XA, T84.69XA, T84.7XXA

00KJ Fusion of Occipital-cervical Joint with Nonautologous Tissue Substitute, Posterior Approach, Anterior Column, Open Approach

▪ When reported with secondary diagnosis code T84.60XA, T84.610A, T84.611A, T84.612A, T84.613A, T84.614A, T84.615A, T84.619A, T84.63XA, T84.69XA, T84.7XXA

G00Z0 Fusion of Occipital-cervical Joint, Anterior Approach, Anterior Column, Open Approach

▪ When reported with secondary diagnosis code T84.60XA, T84.610A, T84.611A, T84.612A, T84.613A, T84.614A, T84.615A, T84.619A, T84.63XA, T84.69XA, T84.7XXA

RG00Z1 Fusion of Occipital-cervical Joint, Posterior Approach, Posterior Column, Open Approach

▪ When reported with secondary diagnosis code T84.60XA, T84.610A, T84.611A,

T84.612A, T84.613A, T84.614A, T84.615A, T84.619A, T84.63XA, T84.69XA, T84.7XXA

0RG00ZJ Fusion of Occipital-cervical Joint, Posterior Approach, Anterior Column, Open Approach

▪ When reported with secondary diagnosis code T84.60XA, T84.610A, T84.611A, T84.612A, T84.613A, T84.614A, T84.615A, T84.619A, T84.63XA, T84.69XA, T84.7XXA

0RG0370 Fusion of Occipital-cervical Joint with Autologous Tissue Substitute, Anterior Approach, Anterior Column, Percutaneous Approach

▪ When reported with secondary diagnosis code T84.60XA, T84.610A, T84.611A, T84.612A, T84.613A, T84.614A, T84.615A, T84.619A, T84.63XA, T84.69XA, T84.7XXA

0RG0371 Fusion of Occipital-cervical Joint with Autologous Tissue Substitute, Posterior Approach, Posterior Column, Percutaneous Approach

▪ When reported with secondary diagnosis code T84.60XA, T84.610A, T84.611A, T84.612A, T84.613A, T84.614A, T84.615A, T84.619A, T84.63XA, T84.69XA, T84.7XXA

0RG037J Fusion of Occipital-cervical Joint with Autologous Tissue Substitute, Posterior Approach, Anterior Column, Percutaneous Approach

▪ When reported with secondary diagnosis code T84.60XA, T84.610A, T84.611A, T84.612A, T84.613A, T84.614A, T84.615A, T84.619A, T84.63XA, T84.69XA, T84.7XXA

0RG03A0 Fusion of Occipital-cervical Joint with Interbody Fusion Device, Anterior Approach, Anterior Column, Percutaneous Approach

▪ When reported with secondary diagnosis code T84.60XA, T84.610A, T84.611A, T84.612A, T84.613A, T84.614A, T84.615A, T84.619A, T84.63XA, T84.69XA, T84.7XXA

0RG03A1 Fusion of Occipital-cervical Joint with Interbody Fusion Device, Posterior Approach, Posterior Column, Percutaneous Approach

▪ When reported with secondary diagnosis code T84.60XA, T84.610A, T84.611A, T84.612A, T84.613A, T84.614A, T84.615A, T84.619A, T84.63XA, T84.69XA, T84.7XXA

0RG03AJ Fusion of Occipital-cervical Joint with Interbody Fusion Device, Posterior Approach, Anterior Column, Percutaneous Approach

▪ When reported with secondary diagnosis code T84.60XA, T84.610A, T84.611A, T84.612A, T84.613A, T84.614A, T84.615A, T84.619A, T84.63XA, T84.69XA, T84.7XXA

0RG03J0 Fusion of Occipital-cervical Joint with Synthetic Substitute, Anterior Approach, Anterior Column, Percutaneous Approach

▪ When reported with secondary diagnosis code T84.60XA, T84.610A, T84.611A, T84.612A, T84.613A, T84.614A, T84.615A, T84.619A, T84.63XA, T84.69XA, T84.7XXA

0RG03J1 Fusion of Occipital-cervical Joint with Synthetic Substitute, Posterior Approach, Posterior Column, Percutaneous Approach

▪ When reported with secondary diagnosis code T84.60XA, T84.610A, T84.611A, T84.612A, T84.613A, T84.614A, T84.615A, T84.619A, T84.63XA, T84.69XA, T84.7XXA

0RG03JJ Fusion of Occipital-cervical Joint with Synthetic Substitute, Posterior Approach, Anterior Column, Percutaneous Approach

▪ When reported with secondary diagnosis code T84.60XA, T84.610A, T84.611A, T84.612A, T84.613A, T84.614A, T84.615A, T84.619A, T84.63XA, T84.69XA, T84.7XXA

0RG03K0 Fusion of Occipital-cervical Joint with Nonautologous Tissue Substitute, Anterior Approach, Anterior Column, Percutaneous Approach

▪ When reported with secondary diagnosis code T84.60XA, T84.610A, T84.611A, T84.612A, T84.613A, T84.614A, T84.615A, T84.619A, T84.63XA, T84.69XA, T84.7XXA

0RG03K1 Fusion of Occipital-cervical Joint with Nonautologous Tissue Substitute, Posterior Approach, Posterior Column, Percutaneous Approach

▪ When reported with secondary diagnosis code T84.60XA, T84.610A, T84.611A, T84.612A, T84.613A, T84.614A, T84.615A, T84.619A, T84.63XA, T84.69XA, T84.7XXA

0RG03KJ Fusion of Occipital-cervical Joint with Nonautologous Tissue Substitute, Posterior Approach, Anterior Column, Percutaneous Approach

▪ When reported with secondary diagnosis code T84.60XA, T84.610A, T84.611A, T84.612A, T84.613A, T84.614A, T84.615A, T84.619A, T84.63XA, T84.69XA, T84.7XXA

0RG03Z0 Fusion of Occipital-cervical Joint, Anterior Approach, Anterior Column, Percutaneous Approach

▪ When reported with secondary diagnosis code T84.60XA, T84.610A, T84.611A, T84.612A, T84.613A, T84.614A, T84.615A, T84.619A, T84.63XA, T84.69XA, T84.7XXA

0RG03Z1 Fusion of Occipital-cervical Joint, Posterior Approach, Posterior Column, Percutaneous Approach

▪ When reported with secondary diagnosis code T84.60XA, T84.610A, T84.611A, T84.612A, T84.613A, T84.614A, T84.615A, T84.619A, T84.63XA, T84.69XA, T84.7XXA

0RG03ZJ Fusion of Occipital-cervical Joint, Posterior Approach, Anterior Column, Percutaneous Approach

▪ When reported with secondary diagnosis code T84.60XA, T84.610A, T84.611A, T84.612A, T84.613A, T84.614A, T84.615A, T84.619A, T84.63XA, T84.69XA, T84.7XXA

0RG0470 Fusion of Occipital-cervical Joint with Autologous Tissue Substitute, Anterior Approach, Anterior Column, Percutaneous Endoscopic Approach

▪ When reported with secondary diagnosis code T84.60XA, T84.610A, T84.611A, T84.612A, T84.613A, T84.614A, T84.615A, T84.619A, T84.63XA, T84.69XA, T84.7XXA

0RG0471 Fusion of Occipital-cervical Joint with Autologous Tissue Substitute, Posterior Approach, Posterior Column, Percutaneous Endoscopic Approach

Note Continued

0RG0471 Continued Note

■ When reported with secondary diagnosis code T84.60XA, T84.610A, T84.611A, T84.612A, T84.613A, T84.614A, T84.615A, T84.619A, T84.63XA, T84.69XA, T84.7XXA

0RG047J Fusion of Occipital-cervical Joint with Autologous Tissue Substitute, Posterior Approach, Anterior Column, Percutaneous Endoscopic Approach

■ When reported with secondary diagnosis code T84.60XA, T84.610A, T84.611A, T84.612A, T84.613A, T84.614A, T84.615A, T84.619A, T84.63XA, T84.69XA, T84.7XXA

0RG04A0 Fusion of Occipital-cervical Joint with Interbody Fusion Device, Anterior Approach, Anterior Column, Percutaneous Endoscopic Approach

■ When reported with secondary diagnosis code T84.60XA, T84.610A, T84.611A, T84.612A, T84.613A, T84.614A, T84.615A, T84.619A, T84.63XA, T84.69XA, T84.7XXA

0RG04A1 Fusion of Occipital-cervical Joint with Interbody Fusion Device, Posterior Approach, Posterior Column, Percutaneous Endoscopic Approach

■ When reported with secondary diagnosis code T84.60XA, T84.610A, T84.611A, T84.612A, T84.613A, T84.614A, T84.615A, T84.619A, T84.63XA, T84.69XA, T84.7XXA

0RG04AJ Fusion of Occipital-cervical Joint with Interbody Fusion Device, Posterior Approach, Anterior Column, Percutaneous Endoscopic Approach

■ When reported with secondary diagnosis code T84.60XA, T84.610A, T84.611A, T84.612A, T84.613A, T84.614A, T84.615A, T84.619A, T84.63XA, T84.69XA, T84.7XXA

0RG04J0 Fusion of Occipital-cervical Joint with Synthetic Substitute, Anterior Approach, Anterior Column, Percutaneous Endoscopic Approach

■ When reported with secondary diagnosis code T84.60XA, T84.610A, T84.611A, T84.612A, T84.613A, T84.614A, T84.615A, T84.619A, T84.63XA, T84.69XA, T84.7XXA

0RG04J1 Fusion of Occipital-cervical Joint with Synthetic Substitute, Posterior Approach, Posterior Column, Percutaneous Endoscopic Approach

■ When reported with secondary diagnosis code T84.60XA, T84.610A, T84.611A, T84.612A, T84.613A, T84.614A, T84.615A, T84.619A, T84.63XA, T84.69XA, T84.7XXA

0RG04JJ Fusion of Occipital-cervical Joint with Synthetic Substitute, Posterior Approach, Anterior Column, Percutaneous Endoscopic Approach

■ When reported with secondary diagnosis code T84.60XA, T84.610A, T84.611A, T84.612A, T84.613A, T84.614A, T84.615A, T84.619A, T84.63XA, T84.69XA, T84.7XXA

0RG04K0 Fusion of Occipital-cervical Joint with Nonautologous Tissue Substitute, Anterior Approach, Anterior Column, Percutaneous Endoscopic Approach

■ When reported with secondary diagnosis code T84.60XA, T84.610A, T84.611A, T84.612A, T84.613A, T84.614A, T84.615A, T84.619A, T84.63XA, T84.69XA, T84.7XXA

0RG04K1 Fusion of Occipital-cervical Joint with Nonautologous Tissue Substitute, Posterior Approach, Posterior Column, Percutaneous Endoscopic Approach

■ When reported with secondary diagnosis code T84.60XA, T84.610A, T84.611A, T84.612A, T84.613A, T84.614A, T84.615A, T84.619A, T84.63XA, T84.69XA, T84.7XXA

0RG04KJ Fusion of Occipital-cervical Joint with Nonautologous Tissue Substitute, Posterior Approach, Anterior Column, Percutaneous Endoscopic Approach

■ When reported with secondary diagnosis code T84.60XA, T84.610A, T84.611A, T84.612A, T84.613A, T84.614A, T84.615A, T84.619A, T84.63XA, T84.69XA, T84.7XXA

0RG04Z0 Fusion of Occipital-cervical Joint, Anterior Approach, Anterior Column, Percutaneous Endoscopic Approach

■ When reported with secondary diagnosis code T84.60XA, T84.610A, T84.611A, T84.612A, T84.613A, T84.614A, T84.615A, T84.619A, T84.63XA, T84.69XA, T84.7XXA

0RG04Z1 Fusion of Occipital-cervical Joint, Posterior Approach, Posterior Column, Percutaneous Endoscopic Approach

■ When reported with secondary diagnosis code T84.60XA, T84.610A, T84.611A, T84.612A, T84.613A, T84.614A, T84.615A, T84.619A, T84.63XA, T84.69XA, T84.7XXA

0RG04ZJ Fusion of Occipital-cervical Joint, Posterior Approach, Anterior Column, Percutaneous Endoscopic Approach

■ When reported with secondary diagnosis code T84.60XA, T84.610A, T84.611A, T84.612A, T84.613A, T84.614A, T84.615A, T84.619A, T84.63XA, T84.69XA, T84.7XXA

0RG1070 Fusion of Cervical Vertebral Joint with Autologous Tissue Substitute, Anterior Approach, Anterior Column, Open Approach

■ When reported with secondary diagnosis code T84.60XA, T84.610A, T84.611A, T84.612A, T84.613A, T84.614A, T84.615A, T84.619A, T84.63XA, T84.69XA, T84.7XXA

0RG1071 Fusion of Cervical Vertebral Joint with Autologous Tissue Substitute, Posterior Approach, Posterior Column, Open Approach

■ When reported with secondary diagnosis code T84.60XA, T84.610A, T84.611A, T84.612A, T84.613A, T84.614A, T84.615A, T84.619A, T84.63XA, T84.69XA, T84.7XXA

0RG107J Fusion of Cervical Vertebral Joint with Autologous Tissue Substitute, Posterior Approach, Anterior Column, Open Approach

■ When reported with secondary diagnosis code T84.60XA, T84.610A, T84.611A, T84.612A, T84.613A, T84.614A, T84.615A, T84.619A, T84.63XA, T84.69XA, T84.7XXA

0RG10A0 Fusion of Cervical Vertebral Joint with Interbody Fusion Device, Anterior Approach, Anterior Column, Open Approach

■ When reported with secondary diagnosis code T84.60XA, T84.610A, T84.611A, T84.612A, T84.613A, T84.614A, T84.615A, T84.619A, T84.63XA, T84.69XA, T84.7XXA

0RG10A1 Fusion of Cervical Vertebral Joint with Interbody Fusion Device, Posterior Approach, Posterior Column, Open Approach

■ When reported with secondary diagnos code T84.60XA, T84.610A, T84.611A, T84.612A, T84.613A, T84.614A, T84.615A, T84.619A, T84.63XA, T84.69XA, T84.7XXA

0RG10AJ Fusion of Cervical Vertebral Joint with Interbody Fusion Device, Posterior Approach, Anterior Column, Open Approach

■ When reported with secondary diagnos code T84.60XA, T84.610A, T84.611A, T84.612A, T84.613A, T84.614A, T84.615A, T84.619A, T84.63XA, T84.69XA, T84.7XXA

0RG10J0 Fusion of Cervical Vertebral Joint with Synthetic Substitute, Anterior Approach, Anterior Column, Open Approach

■ When reported with secondary diagnos code T84.60XA, T84.610A, T84.611A, T84.612A, T84.613A, T84.614A, T84.615A, T84.619A, T84.63XA, T84.69XA, T84.7XXA

0RG10J1 Fusion of Cervical Vertebral Joint with Synthetic Substitute, Posterior Approach, Posterior Column, Open Approach

■ When reported with secondary diagnos code T84.60XA, T84.610A, T84.611A, T84.612A, T84.613A, T84.614A, T84.615A, T84.619A, T84.63XA, T84.69XA, T84.7XXA

0RG10JJ Fusion of Cervical Vertebral Joint with Synthetic Substitute, Posterior Approach, Anterior Column, Open Approach

■ When reported with secondary diagnosis code T84.60XA, T84.610A, T84.611A, T84.612A, T84.613A, T84.614A, T84.615A, T84.619A, T84.63XA, T84.69XA, T84.7XXA

0RG10K0 Fusion of Cervical Vertebral Joint with Nonautologous Tissue Substitute, Anter Approach, Anterior Column, Open Approach

■ When reported with secondary diagnosi code T84.60XA, T84.610A, T84.611A, T84.612A, T84.613A, T84.614A, T84.615A, T84.619A, T84.63XA, T84.69XA, T84.7XXA

0RG10K1 Fusion of Cervical Vertebral Joint with Nonautologous Tissue Substitute, Posterior Approach, Posterior Column, Open Approach

■ When reported with secondary diagnosi code T84.60XA, T84.610A, T84.611A, T84.612A, T84.613A, T84.614A, T84.615A, T84.619A, T84.63XA, T84.69XA, T84.7XXA

0RG10KJ Fusion of Cervical Vertebral Joint with Nonautologous Tissue Substitute, Posterior Approach, Anterior Column, Open Approach

■ When reported with secondary diagnosi code T84.60XA, T84.610A, T84.611A, T84.612A, T84.613A, T84.614A, T84.615A, T84.619A, T84.63XA, T84.69XA, T84.7XXA

0RG10Z0 Fusion of Cervical Vertebral Joint, Anterior Approach, Anterior Column, Open Approach

■ When reported with secondary diagnosis code T84.60XA, T84.610A, T84.611A, T84.612A, T84.613A, T84.614A, T84.615A, T84.619A, T84.63XA, T84.69XA, T84.7XXA

♀ Female-only   ♂ Male-only   ▲ Limited Coverage   ● Non-OR   ■ HAC-associated procedure   ▲ Non-covered procedures   ✚ Combinati

0RG10Z1 Fusion of Cervical Vertebral Joint, Posterior Approach, Posterior Column, Open Approach

▣ When reported with secondary diagnosis code T84.60XA, T84.610A, T84.611A, T84.612A, T84.613A, T84.614A, T84.615A, T84.619A, T84.63XA, T84.69XA, T84.7XXA

0RG10ZJ Fusion of Cervical Vertebral Joint, Posterior Approach, Anterior Column, Open Approach

▣ When reported with secondary diagnosis code T84.60XA, T84.610A, T84.611A, T84.612A, T84.613A, T84.614A, T84.615A, T84.619A, T84.63XA, T84.69XA, T84.7XXA

0RG1370 Fusion of Cervical Vertebral Joint with Autologous Tissue Substitute, Anterior Approach, Anterior Column, Percutaneous Approach

▣ When reported with secondary diagnosis code T84.60XA, T84.610A, T84.611A, T84.612A, T84.613A, T84.614A, T84.615A, T84.619A, T84.63XA, T84.69XA, T84.7XXA

0RG1371 Fusion of Cervical Vertebral Joint with Autologous Tissue Substitute, Posterior Approach, Posterior Column, Percutaneous Approach

▣ When reported with secondary diagnosis code T84.60XA, T84.610A, T84.611A, T84.612A, T84.613A, T84.614A, T84.615A, T84.619A, T84.63XA, T84.69XA, T84.7XXA

0RG137J Fusion of Cervical Vertebral Joint with Autologous Tissue Substitute, Posterior Approach, Anterior Column, Percutaneous Approach

▣ When reported with secondary diagnosis code T84.60XA, T84.610A, T84.611A, T84.612A, T84.613A, T84.614A, T84.615A, T84.619A, T84.63XA, T84.69XA, T84.7XXA

0RG13A0 Fusion of Cervical Vertebral Joint with Interbody Fusion Device, Anterior Approach, Anterior Column, Percutaneous Approach

▣ When reported with secondary diagnosis code T84.60XA, T84.610A, T84.611A, T84.612A, T84.613A, T84.614A, T84.615A, T84.619A, T84.63XA, T84.69XA, T84.7XXA

0RG13A1 Fusion of Cervical Vertebral Joint with Interbody Fusion Device, Posterior Approach, Posterior Column, Percutaneous Approach

▣ When reported with secondary diagnosis code T84.60XA, T84.610A, T84.611A, T84.612A, T84.613A, T84.614A, T84.615A, T84.619A, T84.63XA, T84.69XA, T84.7XXA

0RG13AJ Fusion of Cervical Vertebral Joint with Interbody Fusion Device, Posterior Approach, Anterior Column, Percutaneous Approach

▣ When reported with secondary diagnosis code T84.60XA, T84.610A, T84.611A, T84.612A, T84.613A, T84.614A, T84.615A, T84.619A, T84.63XA, T84.69XA, T84.7XXA

0RG13J0 Fusion of Cervical Vertebral Joint with Synthetic Substitute, Anterior Approach, Anterior Column, Percutaneous Approach

▣ When reported with secondary diagnosis code T84.60XA, T84.610A, T84.611A, T84.612A, T84.613A, T84.614A,

T84.615A, T84.619A, T84.63XA, T84.69XA, T84.7XXA

0RG13J1 Fusion of Cervical Vertebral Joint with Synthetic Substitute, Posterior Approach, Posterior Column, Percutaneous Approach

▣ When reported with secondary diagnosis code T84.60XA, T84.610A, T84.611A, T84.612A, T84.613A, T84.614A, T84.615A, T84.619A, T84.63XA, T84.69XA, T84.7XXA

0RG13JJ Fusion of Cervical Vertebral Joint with Synthetic Substitute, Posterior Approach, Anterior Column, Percutaneous Approach

▣ When reported with secondary diagnosis code T84.60XA, T84.610A, T84.611A, T84.612A, T84.613A, T84.614A, T84.615A, T84.619A, T84.63XA, T84.69XA, T84.7XXA

0RG13K0 Fusion of Cervical Vertebral Joint with Nonautologous Tissue Substitute, Anterior Approach, Anterior Column, Percutaneous Approach

▣ When reported with secondary diagnosis code T84.60XA, T84.610A, T84.611A, T84.612A, T84.613A, T84.614A, T84.615A, T84.619A, T84.63XA, T84.69XA, T84.7XXA

0RG13K1 Fusion of Cervical Vertebral Joint with Nonautologous Tissue Substitute, Posterior Approach, Posterior Column, Percutaneous Approach

▣ When reported with secondary diagnosis code T84.60XA, T84.610A, T84.611A, T84.612A, T84.613A, T84.614A, T84.615A, T84.619A, T84.63XA, T84.69XA, T84.7XXA

0RG13KJ Fusion of Cervical Vertebral Joint with Nonautologous Tissue Substitute, Posterior Approach, Anterior Column, Percutaneous Approach

▣ When reported with secondary diagnosis code T84.60XA, T84.610A, T84.611A, T84.612A, T84.613A, T84.614A, T84.615A, T84.619A, T84.63XA, T84.69XA, T84.7XXA

0RG13Z0 Fusion of Cervical Vertebral Joint, Anterior Approach, Anterior Column, Percutaneous Approach

▣ When reported with secondary diagnosis code T84.60XA, T84.610A, T84.611A, T84.612A, T84.613A, T84.614A, T84.615A, T84.619A, T84.63XA, T84.69XA, T84.7XXA

0RG13Z1 Fusion of Cervical Vertebral Joint, Posterior Approach, Posterior Column, Percutaneous Approach

▣ When reported with secondary diagnosis code T84.60XA, T84.610A, T84.611A, T84.612A, T84.613A, T84.614A, T84.615A, T84.619A, T84.63XA, T84.69XA, T84.7XXA

0RG13ZJ Fusion of Cervical Vertebral Joint, Posterior Approach, Anterior Column, Percutaneous Approach

▣ When reported with secondary diagnosis code T84.60XA, T84.610A, T84.611A, T84.612A, T84.613A, T84.614A, T84.615A, T84.619A, T84.63XA, T84.69XA, T84.7XXA

0RG1470 Fusion of Cervical Vertebral Joint with Autologous Tissue Substitute, Anterior Approach, Anterior Column, Percutaneous Endoscopic Approach

▣ When reported with secondary diagnosis code T84.60XA, T84.610A, T84.611A, T84.612A, T84.613A, T84.614A,

T84.615A, T84.619A, T84.63XA, T84.69XA, T84.7XXA

0RG1471 Fusion of Cervical Vertebral Joint with Autologous Tissue Substitute, Posterior Approach, Posterior Column, Percutaneous Endoscopic Approach

▣ When reported with secondary diagnosis code T84.60XA, T84.610A, T84.611A, T84.612A, T84.613A, T84.614A, T84.615A, T84.619A, T84.63XA, T84.69XA, T84.7XXA

0RG147J Fusion of Cervical Vertebral Joint with Autologous Tissue Substitute, Posterior Approach, Anterior Column, Percutaneous Endoscopic Approach

▣ When reported with secondary diagnosis code T84.60XA, T84.610A, T84.611A, T84.612A, T84.613A, T84.614A, T84.615A, T84.619A, T84.63XA, T84.69XA, T84.7XXA

0RG14A0 Fusion of Cervical Vertebral Joint with Interbody Fusion Device, Anterior Approach, Anterior Column, Percutaneous Endoscopic Approach

▣ When reported with secondary diagnosis code T84.60XA, T84.610A, T84.611A, T84.612A, T84.613A, T84.614A, T84.615A, T84.619A, T84.63XA, T84.69XA, T84.7XXA

0RG14A1 Fusion of Cervical Vertebral Joint with Interbody Fusion Device, Posterior Approach, Posterior Column, Percutaneous Endoscopic Approach

▣ When reported with secondary diagnosis code T84.60XA, T84.610A, T84.611A, T84.612A, T84.613A, T84.614A, T84.615A, T84.619A, T84.63XA, T84.69XA, T84.7XXA

0RG14AJ Fusion of Cervical Vertebral Joint with Interbody Fusion Device, Posterior Approach, Anterior Column, Percutaneous Endoscopic Approach

▣ When reported with secondary diagnosis code T84.60XA, T84.610A, T84.611A, T84.612A, T84.613A, T84.614A, T84.615A, T84.619A, T84.63XA, T84.69XA, T84.7XXA

0RG14J0 Fusion of Cervical Vertebral Joint with Synthetic Substitute, Anterior Approach, Anterior Column, Percutaneous Endoscopic Approach

▣ When reported with secondary diagnosis code T84.60XA, T84.610A, T84.611A, T84.612A, T84.613A, T84.614A, T84.615A, T84.619A, T84.63XA, T84.69XA, T84.7XXA

0RG14J1 Fusion of Cervical Vertebral Joint with Synthetic Substitute, Posterior Approach, Posterior Column, Percutaneous Endoscopic Approach

▣ When reported with secondary diagnosis code T84.60XA, T84.610A, T84.611A, T84.612A, T84.613A, T84.614A, T84.615A, T84.619A, T84.63XA, T84.69XA, T84.7XXA

0RG14JJ Fusion of Cervical Vertebral Joint with Synthetic Substitute, Posterior Approach, Anterior Column, Percutaneous Endoscopic Approach

▣ When reported with secondary diagnosis code T84.60XA, T84.610A, T84.611A, T84.612A, T84.613A, T84.614A, T84.615A, T84.619A, T84.63XA, T84.69XA, T84.7XXA

0RG14K0 Fusion of Cervical Vertebral Joint with Nonautologous Tissue Substitute, Anterior Approach, Anterior Column, Percutaneous Endoscopic Approach

Note Continued

♀ Female-only   ♂ Male-only   ▲ Limited Coverage   ● Non-OR   ▣ HAC-associated procedure   ▲ Non-covered procedures   ✛ Combination

0RG14K0 Continued Note

When reported with secondary diagnosis code T84.60XA, T84.610A, T84.611A, T84.612A, T84.613A, T84.614A, T84.615A, T84.619A, T84.63XA, T84.69XA, T84.7XXA

0RG14K1 Fusion of Cervical Vertebral Joint with Nonautologous Tissue Substitute, Posterior Approach, Posterior Column, Percutaneous Endoscopic Approach

When reported with secondary diagnosis code T84.60XA, T84.610A, T84.611A, T84.612A, T84.613A, T84.614A, T84.615A, T84.619A, T84.63XA, T84.69XA, T84.7XXA

0RG14KJ Fusion of Cervical Vertebral Joint with Nonautologous Tissue Substitute, Posterior Approach, Anterior Column, Percutaneous Endoscopic Approach

When reported with secondary diagnosis code T84.60XA, T84.610A, T84.611A, T84.612A, T84.613A, T84.614A, T84.615A, T84.619A, T84.63XA, T84.69XA, T84.7XXA

0RG14Z0 Fusion of Cervical Vertebral Joint, Anterior Approach, Anterior Column, Percutaneous Endoscopic Approach

When reported with secondary diagnosis code T84.60XA, T84.610A, T84.611A, T84.612A, T84.613A, T84.614A, T84.615A, T84.619A, T84.63XA, T84.69XA, T84.7XXA

0RG14Z1 Fusion of Cervical Vertebral Joint, Posterior Approach, Posterior Column, Percutaneous Endoscopic Approach

When reported with secondary diagnosis code T84.60XA, T84.610A, T84.611A, T84.612A, T84.613A, T84.614A, T84.615A, T84.619A, T84.63XA, T84.69XA, T84.7XXA

0RG14ZJ Fusion of Cervical Vertebral Joint, Posterior Approach, Anterior Column, Percutaneous Endoscopic Approach

When reported with secondary diagnosis code T84.60XA, T84.610A, T84.611A, T84.612A, T84.613A, T84.614A, T84.615A, T84.619A, T84.63XA, T84.69XA, T84.7XXA

0RG2070 Fusion of 2 or more Cervical Vertebral Joints with Autologous Tissue Substitute, Anterior Approach, Anterior Column, Open Approach

When reported with secondary diagnosis code T84.60XA, T84.610A, T84.611A, T84.612A, T84.613A, T84.614A, T84.615A, T84.619A, T84.63XA, T84.69XA, T84.7XXA

0RG2071 Fusion of 2 or more Cervical Vertebral Joints with Autologous Tissue Substitute, Posterior Approach, Posterior Column, Open Approach

When reported with secondary diagnosis code T84.60XA, T84.610A, T84.611A, T84.612A, T84.613A, T84.614A, T84.615A, T84.619A, T84.63XA, T84.69XA, T84.7XXA

0RG207J Fusion of 2 or more Cervical Vertebral Joints with Autologous Tissue Substitute, Posterior Approach, Anterior Column, Open Approach

When reported with secondary diagnosis code T84.60XA, T84.610A, T84.611A, T84.612A, T84.613A, T84.614A, T84.615A, T84.619A, T84.63XA, T84.69XA, T84.7XXA

0RG20A0 Fusion of 2 or more Cervical Vertebral Joints with Interbody Fusion Device, Anterior Approach, Anterior Column, Open Approach

When reported with secondary diagnosis code T84.60XA, T84.610A, T84.611A, T84.612A, T84.613A, T84.614A, T84.615A, T84.619A, T84.63XA, T84.69XA, T84.7XXA

0RG20A1 Fusion of 2 or more Cervical Vertebral Joints with Interbody Fusion Device, Posterior Approach, Posterior Column, Open Approach

When reported with secondary diagnosis code T84.60XA, T84.610A, T84.611A, T84.612A, T84.613A, T84.614A, T84.615A, T84.619A, T84.63XA, T84.69XA, T84.7XXA

0RG20AJ Fusion of 2 or more Cervical Vertebral Joints with Interbody Fusion Device, Posterior Approach, Anterior Column, Open Approach

When reported with secondary diagnosis code T84.60XA, T84.610A, T84.611A, T84.612A, T84.613A, T84.614A, T84.615A, T84.619A, T84.63XA, T84.69XA, T84.7XXA

0RG20J0 Fusion of 2 or more Cervical Vertebral Joints with Synthetic Substitute, Anterior Approach, Anterior Column, Open Approach

When reported with secondary diagnosis code T84.60XA, T84.610A, T84.611A, T84.612A, T84.613A, T84.614A, T84.615A, T84.619A, T84.63XA, T84.69XA, T84.7XXA

0RG20J1 Fusion of 2 or more Cervical Vertebral Joints with Synthetic Substitute, Posterior Approach, Posterior Column, Open Approach

When reported with secondary diagnosis code T84.60XA, T84.610A, T84.611A, T84.612A, T84.613A, T84.614A, T84.615A, T84.619A, T84.63XA, T84.69XA, T84.7XXA

0RG20JJ Fusion of 2 or more Cervical Vertebral Joints with Synthetic Substitute, Posterior Approach, Anterior Column, Open Approach

When reported with secondary diagnosis code T84.60XA, T84.610A, T84.611A, T84.612A, T84.613A, T84.614A, T84.615A, T84.619A, T84.63XA, T84.69XA, T84.7XXA

0RG20K0 Fusion of 2 or more Cervical Vertebral Joints with Nonautologous Tissue Substitute, Anterior Approach, Anterior Column, Open Approach

When reported with secondary diagnosis code T84.60XA, T84.610A, T84.611A, T84.612A, T84.613A, T84.614A, T84.615A, T84.619A, T84.63XA, T84.69XA, T84.7XXA

0RG20K1 Fusion of 2 or more Cervical Vertebral Joints with Nonautologous Tissue Substitute, Posterior Approach, Posterior Column, Open Approach

When reported with secondary diagnosis code T84.60XA, T84.610A, T84.611A, T84.612A, T84.613A, T84.614A, T84.615A, T84.619A, T84.63XA, T84.69XA, T84.7XXA

0RG20KJ Fusion of 2 or more Cervical Vertebral Joints with Nonautologous Tissue Substitute, Posterior Approach, Anterior Column, Open Approach

When reported with secondary diagnosis code T84.60XA, T84.610A, T84.611A, T84.612A, T84.613A, T84.614A, T84.615A, T84.619A, T84.63XA, T84.69XA, T84.7XXA

0RG20Z0 Fusion of 2 or more Cervical Vertebral Joints, Anterior Approach, Anterior Column, Open Approach

When reported with secondary diagnosis code T84.60XA, T84.610A, T84.611A, T84.612A, T84.613A, T84.614A, T84.615A, T84.619A, T84.63XA, T84.69XA, T84.7XXA

0RG20Z1 Fusion of 2 or more Cervical Vertebral Joints, Posterior Approach, Posterior Column, Open Approach

When reported with secondary diagnosis code T84.60XA, T84.610A, T84.611A, T84.612A, T84.613A, T84.614A, T84.615A, T84.619A, T84.63XA, T84.69XA, T84.7XXA

0RG20ZJ Fusion of 2 or more Cervical Vertebral Joints, Posterior Approach, Anterior Column, Open Approach

When reported with secondary diagnosis code T84.60XA, T84.610A, T84.611A, T84.612A, T84.613A, T84.614A, T84.615A, T84.619A, T84.63XA, T84.69XA, T84.7XXA

0RG2370 Fusion of 2 or more Cervical Vertebral Joints with Autologous Tissue Substitute, Anterior Approach, Anterior Column, Percutaneous Approach

When reported with secondary diagnosis code T84.60XA, T84.610A, T84.611A, T84.612A, T84.613A, T84.614A, T84.615A, T84.619A, T84.63XA, T84.69XA, T84.7XXA

0RG2371 Fusion of 2 or more Cervical Vertebral Joints with Autologous Tissue Substitute, Posterior Approach, Posterior Column, Percutaneous Approach

When reported with secondary diagnosis code T84.60XA, T84.610A, T84.611A, T84.612A, T84.613A, T84.614A, T84.615A, T84.619A, T84.63XA, T84.69XA, T84.7XXA

0RG237J Fusion of 2 or more Cervical Vertebral Joints with Autologous Tissue Substitute, Posterior Approach, Anterior Column, Percutaneous Approach

When reported with secondary diagnosis code T84.60XA, T84.610A, T84.611A, T84.612A, T84.613A, T84.614A, T84.615A, T84.619A, T84.63XA, T84.69XA, T84.7XXA

0RG23A0 Fusion of 2 or more Cervical Vertebral Joints with Interbody Fusion Device, Anterior Approach, Anterior Column, Percutaneous Approach

When reported with secondary diagnosis code T84.60XA, T84.610A, T84.611A, T84.612A, T84.613A, T84.614A, T84.615A, T84.619A, T84.63XA, T84.69XA, T84.7XXA

0RG23A1 Fusion of 2 or more Cervical Vertebral Joints with Interbody Fusion Device, Posterior Approach, Posterior Column, Percutaneous Approach

When reported with secondary diagnosis code T84.60XA, T84.610A, T84.611A, T84.612A, T84.613A, T84.614A, T84.615A, T84.619A, T84.63XA, T84.69XA, T84.7XXA

0RG23AJ Fusion of 2 or more Cervical Vertebral Joints with Interbody Fusion Device, Posterior Approach, Anterior Column, Percutaneous Approach

Note Continued

RG23AJ Continued Note

- HAC When reported with secondary diagnosis code T84.60XA, T84.610A, T84.611A, T84.612A, T84.613A, T84.614A, T84.615A, T84.619A, T84.63XA, T84.69XA, T84.7XXA

RG23J0 Fusion of 2 or more Cervical Vertebral Joints with Synthetic Substitute, Anterior Approach, Anterior Column, Percutaneous Approach
- HAC When reported with secondary diagnosis code T84.60XA, T84.610A, T84.611A, T84.612A, T84.613A, T84.614A, T84.615A, T84.619A, T84.63XA, T84.69XA, T84.7XXA

RG23J1 Fusion of 2 or more Cervical Vertebral Joints with Synthetic Substitute, Posterior Approach, Posterior Column, Percutaneous Approach
- HAC When reported with secondary diagnosis code T84.60XA, T84.610A, T84.611A, T84.612A, T84.613A, T84.614A, T84.615A, T84.619A, T84.63XA, T84.69XA, T84.7XXA

RG23JJ Fusion of 2 or more Cervical Vertebral Joints with Synthetic Substitute, Posterior Approach, Anterior Column, Percutaneous Approach
- HAC When reported with secondary diagnosis code T84.60XA, T84.610A, T84.611A, T84.612A, T84.613A, T84.614A, T84.615A, T84.619A, T84.63XA, T84.69XA, T84.7XXA

RG23K0 Fusion of 2 or more Cervical Vertebral Joints with Nonautologous Tissue Substitute, Anterior Approach, Anterior Column, Percutaneous Approach
- HAC When reported with secondary diagnosis code T84.60XA, T84.610A, T84.611A, T84.612A, T84.613A, T84.614A, T84.615A, T84.619A, T84.63XA, T84.69XA, T84.7XXA

RG23K1 Fusion of 2 or more Cervical Vertebral Joints with Nonautologous Tissue Substitute, Posterior Approach, Posterior Column, Percutaneous Approach
- HAC When reported with secondary diagnosis code T84.60XA, T84.610A, T84.611A, T84.612A, T84.613A, T84.614A, T84.615A, T84.619A, T84.63XA, T84.69XA, T84.7XXA

RG23KJ Fusion of 2 or more Cervical Vertebral Joints with Nonautologous Tissue Substitute, Posterior Approach, Anterior Column, Percutaneous Approach
- HAC When reported with secondary diagnosis code T84.60XA, T84.610A, T84.611A, T84.612A, T84.613A, T84.614A, T84.615A, T84.619A, T84.63XA, T84.69XA, T84.7XXA

RG23Z0 Fusion of 2 or more Cervical Vertebral Joints, Anterior Approach, Anterior Column, Percutaneous Approach
- HAC When reported with secondary diagnosis code T84.60XA, T84.610A, T84.611A, T84.612A, T84.613A, T84.614A, T84.615A, T84.619A, T84.63XA, T84.69XA, T84.7XXA

RG23Z1 Fusion of 2 or more Cervical Vertebral Joints, Posterior Approach, Posterior Column, Percutaneous Approach
- HAC When reported with secondary diagnosis code T84.60XA, T84.610A, T84.611A, T84.612A, T84.613A, T84.614A, T84.615A, T84.619A, T84.63XA, T84.69XA, T84.7XXA

0RG23ZJ Fusion of 2 or more Cervical Vertebral Joints, Posterior Approach, Anterior Column, Percutaneous Approach
- HAC When reported with secondary diagnosis code T84.60XA, T84.610A, T84.611A, T84.612A, T84.613A, T84.614A, T84.615A, T84.619A, T84.63XA, T84.69XA, T84.7XXA

0RG2470 Fusion of 2 or more Cervical Vertebral Joints with Autologous Tissue Substitute, Anterior Approach, Anterior Column, Percutaneous Endoscopic Approach
- HAC When reported with secondary diagnosis code T84.60XA, T84.610A, T84.611A, T84.612A, T84.613A, T84.614A, T84.615A, T84.619A, T84.63XA, T84.69XA, T84.7XXA

0RG2471 Fusion of 2 or more Cervical Vertebral Joints with Autologous Tissue Substitute, Posterior Approach, Posterior Column, Percutaneous Endoscopic Approach
- HAC When reported with secondary diagnosis code T84.60XA, T84.610A, T84.611A, T84.612A, T84.613A, T84.614A, T84.615A, T84.619A, T84.63XA, T84.69XA, T84.7XXA

0RG247J Fusion of 2 or more Cervical Vertebral Joints with Autologous Tissue Substitute, Posterior Approach, Anterior Column, Percutaneous Endoscopic Approach
- HAC When reported with secondary diagnosis code T84.60XA, T84.610A, T84.611A, T84.612A, T84.613A, T84.614A, T84.615A, T84.619A, T84.63XA, T84.69XA, T84.7XXA

0RG24A0 Fusion of 2 or more Cervical Vertebral Joints with Interbody Fusion Device, Anterior Approach, Anterior Column, Percutaneous Endoscopic Approach
- HAC When reported with secondary diagnosis code T84.60XA, T84.610A, T84.611A, T84.612A, T84.613A, T84.614A, T84.615A, T84.619A, T84.63XA, T84.69XA, T84.7XXA

0RG24A1 Fusion of 2 or more Cervical Vertebral Joints with Interbody Fusion Device, Posterior Approach, Posterior Column, Percutaneous Endoscopic Approach
- HAC When reported with secondary diagnosis code T84.60XA, T84.610A, T84.611A, T84.612A, T84.613A, T84.614A, T84.615A, T84.619A, T84.63XA, T84.69XA, T84.7XXA

0RG24AJ Fusion of 2 or more Cervical Vertebral Joints with Interbody Fusion Device, Posterior Approach, Anterior Column, Percutaneous Endoscopic Approach
- HAC When reported with secondary diagnosis code T84.60XA, T84.610A, T84.611A, T84.612A, T84.613A, T84.614A, T84.615A, T84.619A, T84.63XA, T84.69XA, T84.7XXA

0RG24J0 Fusion of 2 or more Cervical Vertebral Joints with Synthetic Substitute, Anterior Approach, Anterior Column, Percutaneous Endoscopic Approach
- HAC When reported with secondary diagnosis code T84.60XA, T84.610A, T84.611A, T84.612A, T84.613A, T84.614A, T84.615A, T84.619A, T84.63XA, T84.69XA, T84.7XXA

0RG24J1 Fusion of 2 or more Cervical Vertebral Joints with Synthetic Substitute, Posterior Approach, Posterior Column, Percutaneous Endoscopic Approach
- HAC When reported with secondary diagnosis code T84.60XA, T84.610A, T84.611A, T84.612A, T84.613A, T84.614A,

T84.615A, T84.619A, T84.63XA, T84.69XA, T84.7XXA

0RG24JJ Fusion of 2 or more Cervical Vertebral Joints with Synthetic Substitute, Posterior Approach, Anterior Column, Percutaneous Endoscopic Approach
- HAC When reported with secondary diagnosis code T84.60XA, T84.610A, T84.611A, T84.612A, T84.613A, T84.614A, T84.615A, T84.619A, T84.63XA, T84.69XA, T84.7XXA

0RG24K0 Fusion of 2 or more Cervical Vertebral Joints with Nonautologous Tissue Substitute, Anterior Approach, Anterior Column, Percutaneous Endoscopic Approach
- HAC When reported with secondary diagnosis code T84.60XA, T84.610A, T84.611A, T84.612A, T84.613A, T84.614A, T84.615A, T84.619A, T84.63XA, T84.69XA, T84.7XXA

0RG24K1 Fusion of 2 or more Cervical Vertebral Joints with Nonautologous Tissue Substitute, Posterior Approach, Posterior Column, Percutaneous Endoscopic Approach
- HAC When reported with secondary diagnosis code T84.60XA, T84.610A, T84.611A, T84.612A, T84.613A, T84.614A, T84.615A, T84.619A, T84.63XA, T84.69XA, T84.7XXA

0RG24KJ Fusion of 2 or more Cervical Vertebral Joints with Nonautologous Tissue Substitute, Posterior Approach, Anterior Column, Percutaneous Endoscopic Approach
- HAC When reported with secondary diagnosis code T84.60XA, T84.610A, T84.611A, T84.612A, T84.613A, T84.614A, T84.615A, T84.619A, T84.63XA, T84.69XA, T84.7XXA

0RG24Z0 Fusion of 2 or more Cervical Vertebral Joints, Anterior Approach, Anterior Column, Percutaneous Endoscopic Approach
- HAC When reported with secondary diagnosis code T84.60XA, T84.610A, T84.611A, T84.612A, T84.613A, T84.614A, T84.615A, T84.619A, T84.63XA, T84.69XA, T84.7XXA

0RG24Z1 Fusion of 2 or more Cervical Vertebral Joints, Posterior Approach, Posterior Column, Percutaneous Endoscopic Approach
- HAC When reported with secondary diagnosis code T84.60XA, T84.610A, T84.611A, T84.612A, T84.613A, T84.614A, T84.615A, T84.619A, T84.63XA, T84.69XA, T84.7XXA

0RG24ZJ Fusion of 2 or more Cervical Vertebral Joints, Posterior Approach, Anterior Column, Percutaneous Endoscopic Approach
- HAC When reported with secondary diagnosis code T84.60XA, T84.610A, T84.611A, T84.612A, T84.613A, T84.614A, T84.615A, T84.619A, T84.63XA, T84.69XA, T84.7XXA

0RG4070 Fusion of Cervicothoracic Vertebral Joint with Autologous Tissue Substitute, Anterior Approach, Anterior Column, Open Approach
- HAC When reported with secondary diagnosis code T84.60XA, T84.610A, T84.611A, T84.612A, T84.613A, T84.614A, T84.615A, T84.619A, T84.63XA, T84.69XA, T84.7XXA

♀ Female-only   ♂ Male-only   ▲ Limited Coverage   ● Non-OR   HAC HAC-associated procedure   ▲ Non-covered procedures   ✚ Combination

0RG4071 Fusion of Cervicothoracic Vertebral Joint with Autologous Tissue Substitute, Posterior Approach, Posterior Column, Open Approach

HAC When reported with secondary diagnosis code T84.60XA, T84.610A, T84.611A, T84.612A, T84.613A, T84.614A, T84.615A, T84.619A, T84.63XA, T84.69XA, T84.7XXA

0RG407J Fusion of Cervicothoracic Vertebral Joint with Autologous Tissue Substitute, Posterior Approach, Anterior Column, Open Approach

HAC When reported with secondary diagnosis code T84.60XA, T84.610A, T84.611A, T84.612A, T84.613A, T84.614A, T84.615A, T84.619A, T84.63XA, T84.69XA, T84.7XXA

0RG40A0 Fusion of Cervicothoracic Vertebral Joint with Interbody Fusion Device, Anterior Approach, Anterior Column, Open Approach

AHA CC: 1Q, 2013, 29-30; 2Q, 2014, 7-8

HAC When reported with secondary diagnosis code T84.60XA, T84.610A, T84.611A, T84.612A, T84.613A, T84.614A, T84.615A, T84.619A, T84.63XA, T84.69XA, T84.7XXA

0RG40A1 Fusion of Cervicothoracic Vertebral Joint with Interbody Fusion Device, Posterior Approach, Posterior Column, Open Approach

HAC When reported with secondary diagnosis code T84.60XA, T84.610A, T84.611A, T84.612A, T84.613A, T84.614A, T84.615A, T84.619A, T84.63XA, T84.69XA, T84.7XXA

0RG40AJ Fusion of Cervicothoracic Vertebral Joint with Interbody Fusion Device, Posterior Approach, Anterior Column, Open Approach

HAC When reported with secondary diagnosis code T84.60XA, T84.610A, T84.611A, T84.612A, T84.613A, T84.614A, T84.615A, T84.619A, T84.63XA, T84.69XA, T84.7XXA

0RG40J0 Fusion of Cervicothoracic Vertebral Joint with Synthetic Substitute, Anterior Approach, Anterior Column, Open Approach

HAC When reported with secondary diagnosis code T84.60XA, T84.610A, T84.611A, T84.612A, T84.613A, T84.614A, T84.615A, T84.619A, T84.63XA, T84.69XA, T84.7XXA

0RG40J1 Fusion of Cervicothoracic Vertebral Joint with Synthetic Substitute, Posterior Approach, Posterior Column, Open Approach

HAC When reported with secondary diagnosis code T84.60XA, T84.610A, T84.611A, T84.612A, T84.613A, T84.614A, T84.615A, T84.619A, T84.63XA, T84.69XA, T84.7XXA

0RG40JJ Fusion of Cervicothoracic Vertebral Joint with Synthetic Substitute, Posterior Approach, Anterior Column, Open Approach

HAC When reported with secondary diagnosis code T84.60XA, T84.610A, T84.611A, T84.612A, T84.613A, T84.614A, T84.615A, T84.619A, T84.63XA, T84.69XA, T84.7XXA

0RG40K0 Fusion of Cervicothoracic Vertebral Joint with Nonautologous Tissue Substitute, Anterior Approach, Anterior Column, Open Approach

HAC When reported with secondary diagnosis code T84.60XA, T84.610A, T84.611A,

T84.612A, T84.613A, T84.614A, T84.615A, T84.619A, T84.63XA, T84.69XA, T84.7XXA

0RG40K1 Fusion of Cervicothoracic Vertebral Joint with Nonautologous Tissue Substitute, Posterior Approach, Posterior Column, Open Approach

HAC When reported with secondary diagnosis code T84.60XA, T84.610A, T84.611A, T84.612A, T84.613A, T84.614A, T84.615A, T84.619A, T84.63XA, T84.69XA, T84.7XXA

0RG40KJ Fusion of Cervicothoracic Vertebral Joint with Nonautologous Tissue Substitute, Posterior Approach, Anterior Column, Open Approach

HAC When reported with secondary diagnosis code T84.60XA, T84.610A, T84.611A, T84.612A, T84.613A, T84.614A, T84.615A, T84.619A, T84.63XA, T84.69XA, T84.7XXA

0RG40Z0 Fusion of Cervicothoracic Vertebral Joint, Anterior Approach, Anterior Column, Open Approach

HAC When reported with secondary diagnosis code T84.60XA, T84.610A, T84.611A, T84.612A, T84.613A, T84.614A, T84.615A, T84.619A, T84.63XA, T84.69XA, T84.7XXA

0RG40Z1 Fusion of Cervicothoracic Vertebral Joint, Posterior Approach, Posterior Column, Open Approach

HAC When reported with secondary diagnosis code T84.60XA, T84.610A, T84.611A, T84.612A, T84.613A, T84.614A, T84.615A, T84.619A, T84.63XA, T84.69XA, T84.7XXA

0RG40ZJ Fusion of Cervicothoracic Vertebral Joint, Posterior Approach, Anterior Column, Open Approach

HAC When reported with secondary diagnosis code T84.60XA, T84.610A, T84.611A, T84.612A, T84.613A, T84.614A, T84.615A, T84.619A, T84.63XA, T84.69XA, T84.7XXA

0RG4370 Fusion of Cervicothoracic Vertebral Joint with Autologous Tissue Substitute, Anterior Approach, Anterior Column, Percutaneous Approach

HAC When reported with secondary diagnosis code T84.60XA, T84.610A, T84.611A, T84.612A, T84.613A, T84.614A, T84.615A, T84.619A, T84.63XA, T84.69XA, T84.7XXA

0RG4371 Fusion of Cervicothoracic Vertebral Joint with Autologous Tissue Substitute, Posterior Approach, Posterior Column, Percutaneous Approach

HAC When reported with secondary diagnosis code T84.60XA, T84.610A, T84.611A, T84.612A, T84.613A, T84.614A, T84.615A, T84.619A, T84.63XA, T84.69XA, T84.7XXA

0RG437J Fusion of Cervicothoracic Vertebral Joint with Autologous Tissue Substitute, Posterior Approach, Anterior Column, Percutaneous Approach

HAC When reported with secondary diagnosis code T84.60XA, T84.610A, T84.611A, T84.612A, T84.613A, T84.614A, T84.615A, T84.619A, T84.63XA, T84.69XA, T84.7XXA

0RG43A0 Fusion of Cervicothoracic Vertebral Joint with Interbody Fusion Device, Anterior Approach, Anterior Column, Percutaneous Approach

HAC When reported with secondary diagnosis code T84.60XA, T84.610A, T84.611A,

T84.612A, T84.613A, T84.614A, T84.615A, T84.619A, T84.63XA, T84.69XA, T84.7XXA

0RG43A1 Fusion of Cervicothoracic Vertebral Joint with Interbody Fusion Device, Posterior Approach, Posterior Column, Percutaneous Approach

HAC When reported with secondary diagnosis code T84.60XA, T84.610A, T84.611A, T84.612A, T84.613A, T84.614A, T84.615A, T84.619A, T84.63XA, T84.69XA, T84.7XXA

0RG43AJ Fusion of Cervicothoracic Vertebral Joint with Interbody Fusion Device, Posterior Approach, Anterior Column, Percutaneous Approach

HAC When reported with secondary diagnosis code T84.60XA, T84.610A, T84.611A, T84.612A, T84.613A, T84.614A, T84.615A, T84.619A, T84.63XA, T84.69XA, T84.7XXA

0RG43J0 Fusion of Cervicothoracic Vertebral Joint with Synthetic Substitute, Anterior Approach, Anterior Column, Percutaneous Approach

HAC When reported with secondary diagnosis code T84.60XA, T84.610A, T84.611A, T84.612A, T84.613A, T84.614A, T84.615A, T84.619A, T84.63XA, T84.69XA, T84.7XXA

0RG43J1 Fusion of Cervicothoracic Vertebral Joint with Synthetic Substitute, Posterior Approach, Posterior Column, Percutaneous Approach

HAC When reported with secondary diagnosis code T84.60XA, T84.610A, T84.611A, T84.612A, T84.613A, T84.614A, T84.615A, T84.619A, T84.63XA, T84.69XA, T84.7XXA

0RG43JJ Fusion of Cervicothoracic Vertebral Joint with Synthetic Substitute, Posterior Approach, Anterior Column, Percutaneous Approach

HAC When reported with secondary diagnosis code T84.60XA, T84.610A, T84.611A, T84.612A, T84.613A, T84.614A, T84.615A, T84.619A, T84.63XA, T84.69XA, T84.7XXA

0RG43K0 Fusion of Cervicothoracic Vertebral Joint with Nonautologous Tissue Substitute, Anterior Approach, Anterior Column, Percutaneous Approach

HAC When reported with secondary diagnosis code T84.60XA, T84.610A, T84.611A, T84.612A, T84.613A, T84.614A, T84.615A, T84.619A, T84.63XA, T84.69XA, T84.7XXA

0RG43K1 Fusion of Cervicothoracic Vertebral Joint with Nonautologous Tissue Substitute, Posterior Approach, Posterior Column, Percutaneous Approach

HAC When reported with secondary diagnosis code T84.60XA, T84.610A, T84.611A, T84.612A, T84.613A, T84.614A, T84.615A, T84.619A, T84.63XA, T84.69XA, T84.7XXA

0RG43KJ Fusion of Cervicothoracic Vertebral Joint with Nonautologous Tissue Substitute, Posterior Approach, Anterior Column, Percutaneous Approach

HAC When reported with secondary diagnosis code T84.60XA, T84.610A, T84.611A, T84.612A, T84.613A, T84.614A, T84.615A, T84.619A, T84.63XA, T84.69XA, T84.7XXA

G43Z0 Fusion of Cervicothoracic Vertebral Joint, Anterior Approach, Anterior Column, Percutaneous Approach

⬛ When reported with secondary diagnosis code T84.60XA, T84.610A, T84.611A, T84.612A, T84.613A, T84.614A, T84.615A, T84.619A, T84.63XA, T84.69XA, T84.7XXA

RG43Z1 Fusion of Cervicothoracic Vertebral Joint, Posterior Approach, Posterior Column, Percutaneous Approach

⬛ When reported with secondary diagnosis code T84.60XA, T84.610A, T84.611A, T84.612A, T84.613A, T84.614A, T84.615A, T84.619A, T84.63XA, T84.69XA, T84.7XXA

RG43ZJ Fusion of Cervicothoracic Vertebral Joint, Posterior Approach, Anterior Column, Percutaneous Approach

⬛ When reported with secondary diagnosis code T84.60XA, T84.610A, T84.611A, T84.612A, T84.613A, T84.614A, T84.615A, T84.619A, T84.63XA, T84.69XA, T84.7XXA

RG4470 Fusion of Cervicothoracic Vertebral Joint with Autologous Tissue Substitute, Anterior Approach, Anterior Column, Percutaneous Endoscopic Approach

⬛ When reported with secondary diagnosis code T84.60XA, T84.610A, T84.611A, T84.612A, T84.613A, T84.614A, T84.615A, T84.619A, T84.63XA, T84.69XA, T84.7XXA

RG4471 Fusion of Cervicothoracic Vertebral Joint with Autologous Tissue Substitute, Posterior Approach, Posterior Column, Percutaneous Endoscopic Approach

⬛ When reported with secondary diagnosis code T84.60XA, T84.610A, T84.611A, T84.612A, T84.613A, T84.614A, T84.615A, T84.619A, T84.63XA, T84.69XA, T84.7XXA

RG447J Fusion of Cervicothoracic Vertebral Joint with Autologous Tissue Substitute, Posterior Approach, Anterior Column, Percutaneous Endoscopic Approach

⬛ When reported with secondary diagnosis code T84.60XA, T84.610A, T84.611A, T84.612A, T84.613A, T84.614A, T84.615A, T84.619A, T84.63XA, T84.69XA, T84.7XXA

RG44A0 Fusion of Cervicothoracic Vertebral Joint with Interbody Fusion Device, Anterior Approach, Anterior Column, Percutaneous Endoscopic Approach

⬛ When reported with secondary diagnosis code T84.60XA, T84.610A, T84.611A, T84.612A, T84.613A, T84.614A, T84.615A, T84.619A, T84.63XA, T84.69XA, T84.7XXA

0RG44A1 Fusion of Cervicothoracic Vertebral Joint with Interbody Fusion Device, Posterior Approach, Posterior Column, Percutaneous Endoscopic Approach

⬛ When reported with secondary diagnosis code T84.60XA, T84.610A, T84.611A, T84.612A, T84.613A, T84.614A, T84.615A, T84.619A, T84.63XA, T84.69XA, T84.7XXA

0RG44AJ Fusion of Cervicothoracic Vertebral Joint with Interbody Fusion Device, Posterior Approach, Anterior Column, Percutaneous Endoscopic Approach

⬛ When reported with secondary diagnosis code T84.60XA, T84.610A, T84.611A, T84.612A, T84.613A, T84.614A, T84.615A, T84.619A, T84.63XA, T84.69XA, T84.7XXA

0RG44J0 Fusion of Cervicothoracic Vertebral Joint with Synthetic Substitute, Anterior Approach, Anterior Column, Percutaneous Endoscopic Approach

⬛ When reported with secondary diagnosis code T84.60XA, T84.610A, T84.611A, T84.612A, T84.613A, T84.614A, T84.615A, T84.619A, T84.63XA, T84.69XA, T84.7XXA

0RG44J1 Fusion of Cervicothoracic Vertebral Joint with Synthetic Substitute, Posterior Approach, Posterior Column, Percutaneous Endoscopic Approach

⬛ When reported with secondary diagnosis code T84.60XA, T84.610A, T84.611A, T84.612A, T84.613A, T84.614A, T84.615A, T84.619A, T84.63XA, T84.69XA, T84.7XXA

0RG44JJ Fusion of Cervicothoracic Vertebral Joint with Synthetic Substitute, Posterior Approach, Anterior Column, Percutaneous Endoscopic Approach

⬛ When reported with secondary diagnosis code T84.60XA, T84.610A, T84.611A, T84.612A, T84.613A, T84.614A, T84.615A, T84.619A, T84.63XA, T84.69XA, T84.7XXA

0RG44K0 Fusion of Cervicothoracic Vertebral Joint with Nonautologous Tissue Substitute, Anterior Approach, Anterior Column, Percutaneous Endoscopic Approach

⬛ When reported with secondary diagnosis code T84.60XA, T84.610A, T84.611A, T84.612A, T84.613A, T84.614A, T84.615A, T84.619A, T84.63XA, T84.69XA, T84.7XXA

0RG44K1 Fusion of Cervicothoracic Vertebral Joint with Nonautologous Tissue Substitute, Posterior Approach, Posterior Column, Percutaneous Endoscopic Approach

⬛ When reported with secondary diagnosis code T84.60XA, T84.610A, T84.611A, T84.612A, T84.613A, T84.614A, T84.615A, T84.619A, T84.63XA, T84.69XA, T84.7XXA

0RG44KJ Fusion of Cervicothoracic Vertebral Joint with Nonautologous Tissue Substitute, Posterior Approach, Anterior Column, Percutaneous Endoscopic Approach

⬛ When reported with secondary diagnosis code T84.60XA, T84.610A, T84.611A, T84.612A, T84.613A, T84.614A, T84.615A, T84.619A, T84.63XA, T84.69XA, T84.7XXA

0RG44Z0 Fusion of Cervicothoracic Vertebral Joint, Anterior Approach, Anterior Column, Percutaneous Endoscopic Approach

⬛ When reported with secondary diagnosis code T84.60XA, T84.610A, T84.611A, T84.612A, T84.613A, T84.614A, T84.615A, T84.619A, T84.63XA, T84.69XA, T84.7XXA

0RG44Z1 Fusion of Cervicothoracic Vertebral Joint, Posterior Approach, Posterior Column, Percutaneous Endoscopic Approach

⬛ When reported with secondary diagnosis code T84.60XA, T84.610A, T84.611A, T84.612A, T84.613A, T84.614A, T84.615A, T84.619A, T84.63XA, T84.69XA, T84.7XXA

0RG44ZJ Fusion of Cervicothoracic Vertebral Joint, Posterior Approach, Anterior Column, Percutaneous Endoscopic Approach

⬛ When reported with secondary diagnosis code T84.60XA, T84.610A, T84.611A, T84.612A, T84.613A, T84.614A, T84.615A, T84.619A, T84.63XA, T84.69XA, T84.7XXA

0RG6070 Fusion of Thoracic Vertebral Joint with Autologous Tissue Substitute, Anterior Approach, Anterior Column, Open Approach

⬛ When reported with secondary diagnosis code T84.60XA, T84.610A, T84.611A, T84.612A, T84.613A, T84.614A, T84.615A, T84.619A, T84.63XA, T84.69XA, T84.7XXA

0RG6071 Fusion of Thoracic Vertebral Joint with Autologous Tissue Substitute, Posterior Approach, Posterior Column, Open Approach

⬛ When reported with secondary diagnosis code T84.60XA, T84.610A, T84.611A, T84.612A, T84.613A, T84.614A, T84.615A, T84.619A, T84.63XA, T84.69XA, T84.7XXA

0RG607J Fusion of Thoracic Vertebral Joint with Autologous Tissue Substitute, Posterior Approach, Anterior Column, Open Approach

⬛ When reported with secondary diagnosis code T84.60XA, T84.610A, T84.611A, T84.612A, T84.613A, T84.614A, T84.615A, T84.619A, T84.63XA, T84.69XA, T84.7XXA

0RG60A0 Fusion of Thoracic Vertebral Joint with Interbody Fusion Device, Anterior Approach, Anterior Column, Open Approach

⬛ When reported with secondary diagnosis code T84.60XA, T84.610A, T84.611A, T84.612A, T84.613A, T84.614A, T84.615A, T84.619A, T84.63XA, T84.69XA, T84.7XXA

0RG60A1 Fusion of Thoracic Vertebral Joint with Interbody Fusion Device, Posterior Approach, Posterior Column, Open Approach

⬛ When reported with secondary diagnosis code T84.60XA, T84.610A, T84.611A, T84.612A, T84.613A, T84.614A, T84.615A, T84.619A, T84.63XA, T84.69XA, T84.7XXA

0RG60AJ Fusion of Thoracic Vertebral Joint with Interbody Fusion Device, Posterior Approach, Anterior Column, Open Approach

⬛ When reported with secondary diagnosis code T84.60XA, T84.610A, T84.611A, T84.612A, T84.613A, T84.614A, T84.615A, T84.619A, T84.63XA, T84.69XA, T84.7XXA

0RG60J0 Fusion of Thoracic Vertebral Joint with Synthetic Substitute, Anterior Approach, Anterior Column, Open Approach

⬛ When reported with secondary diagnosis code T84.60XA, T84.610A, T84.611A, T84.612A, T84.613A, T84.614A, T84.615A, T84.619A, T84.63XA, T84.69XA, T84.7XXA

0RG60J1 Fusion of Thoracic Vertebral Joint with Synthetic Substitute, Posterior Approach, Posterior Column, Open Approach

⬛ When reported with secondary diagnosis code T84.60XA, T84.610A, T84.611A, T84.612A, T84.613A, T84.614A, T84.615A, T84.619A, T84.63XA, T84.69XA, T84.7XXA

0RG60JJ Fusion of Thoracic Vertebral Joint with Synthetic Substitute, Posterior Approach, Anterior Column, Open Approach

⬛ When reported with secondary diagnosis code T84.60XA, T84.610A, T84.611A, T84.612A, T84.613A, T84.614A, T84.615A, T84.619A, T84.63XA, T84.69XA, T84.7XXA

♀ Female-only ♂ Male-only ▲ Limited Coverage ● Non-OR ⬛ HAC-associated procedure ▲ Non-covered procedures ✚ Combination

0RG60K0 Fusion of Thoracic Vertebral Joint with Nonautologous Tissue Substitute, Anterior Approach, Anterior Column, Open Approach

HAC When reported with secondary diagnosis code T84.60XA, T84.610A, T84.611A, T84.612A, T84.613A, T84.614A, T84.615A, T84.619A, T84.63XA, T84.69XA, T84.7XXA

0RG60K1 Fusion of Thoracic Vertebral Joint with Nonautologous Tissue Substitute, Posterior Approach, Posterior Column, Open Approach

HAC When reported with secondary diagnosis code T84.60XA, T84.610A, T84.611A, T84.612A, T84.613A, T84.614A, T84.615A, T84.619A, T84.63XA, T84.69XA, T84.7XXA

0RG60KJ Fusion of Thoracic Vertebral Joint with Nonautologous Tissue Substitute, Posterior Approach, Anterior Column, Open Approach

HAC When reported with secondary diagnosis code T84.60XA, T84.610A, T84.611A, T84.612A, T84.613A, T84.614A, T84.615A, T84.619A, T84.63XA, T84.69XA, T84.7XXA

0RG60Z0 Fusion of Thoracic Vertebral Joint, Anterior Approach, Anterior Column, Open Approach

HAC When reported with secondary diagnosis code T84.60XA, T84.610A, T84.611A, T84.612A, T84.613A, T84.614A, T84.615A, T84.619A, T84.63XA, T84.69XA, T84.7XXA

0RG60Z1 Fusion of Thoracic Vertebral Joint, Posterior Approach, Posterior Column, Open Approach

HAC When reported with secondary diagnosis code T84.60XA, T84.610A, T84.611A, T84.612A, T84.613A, T84.614A, T84.615A, T84.619A, T84.63XA, T84.69XA, T84.7XXA

0RG60ZJ Fusion of Thoracic Vertebral Joint, Posterior Approach, Anterior Column, Open Approach

HAC When reported with secondary diagnosis code T84.60XA, T84.610A, T84.611A, T84.612A, T84.613A, T84.614A, T84.615A, T84.619A, T84.63XA, T84.69XA, T84.7XXA

0RG6370 Fusion of Thoracic Vertebral Joint with Autologous Tissue Substitute, Anterior Approach, Anterior Column, Percutaneous Approach

HAC When reported with secondary diagnosis code T84.60XA, T84.610A, T84.611A, T84.612A, T84.613A, T84.614A, T84.615A, T84.619A, T84.63XA, T84.69XA, T84.7XXA

0RG6371 Fusion of Thoracic Vertebral Joint with Autologous Tissue Substitute, Posterior Approach, Posterior Column, Percutaneous Approach

HAC When reported with secondary diagnosis code T84.60XA, T84.610A, T84.611A, T84.612A, T84.613A, T84.614A, T84.615A, T84.619A, T84.63XA, T84.69XA, T84.7XXA

0RG637J Fusion of Thoracic Vertebral Joint with Autologous Tissue Substitute, Posterior Approach, Anterior Column, Percutaneous Approach

HAC When reported with secondary diagnosis code T84.60XA, T84.610A, T84.611A, T84.612A, T84.613A, T84.614A, T84.615A, T84.619A, T84.63XA, T84.69XA, T84.7XXA

0RG63A0 Fusion of Thoracic Vertebral Joint with Interbody Fusion Device, Anterior Approach, Anterior Column, Percutaneous Approach

HAC When reported with secondary diagnosis code T84.60XA, T84.610A, T84.611A, T84.612A, T84.613A, T84.614A, T84.615A, T84.619A, T84.63XA, T84.69XA, T84.7XXA

0RG63A1 Fusion of Thoracic Vertebral Joint with Interbody Fusion Device, Posterior Approach, Posterior Column, Percutaneous Approach

HAC When reported with secondary diagnosis code T84.60XA, T84.610A, T84.611A, T84.612A, T84.613A, T84.614A, T84.615A, T84.619A, T84.63XA, T84.69XA, T84.7XXA

0RG63AJ Fusion of Thoracic Vertebral Joint with Interbody Fusion Device, Posterior Approach, Anterior Column, Percutaneous Approach

HAC When reported with secondary diagnosis code T84.60XA, T84.610A, T84.611A, T84.612A, T84.613A, T84.614A, T84.615A, T84.619A, T84.63XA, T84.69XA, T84.7XXA

0RG63J0 Fusion of Thoracic Vertebral Joint with Synthetic Substitute, Anterior Approach, Anterior Column, Percutaneous Approach

HAC When reported with secondary diagnosis code T84.60XA, T84.610A, T84.611A, T84.612A, T84.613A, T84.614A, T84.615A, T84.619A, T84.63XA, T84.69XA, T84.7XXA

0RG63J1 Fusion of Thoracic Vertebral Joint with Synthetic Substitute, Posterior Approach, Posterior Column, Percutaneous Approach

HAC When reported with secondary diagnosis code T84.60XA, T84.610A, T84.611A, T84.612A, T84.613A, T84.614A, T84.615A, T84.619A, T84.63XA, T84.69XA, T84.7XXA

0RG63JJ Fusion of Thoracic Vertebral Joint with Synthetic Substitute, Posterior Approach, Anterior Column, Percutaneous Approach

HAC When reported with secondary diagnosis code T84.60XA, T84.610A, T84.611A, T84.612A, T84.613A, T84.614A, T84.615A, T84.619A, T84.63XA, T84.69XA, T84.7XXA

0RG63K0 Fusion of Thoracic Vertebral Joint with Nonautologous Tissue Substitute, Anterior Approach, Anterior Column, Percutaneous Approach

HAC When reported with secondary diagnosis code T84.60XA, T84.610A, T84.611A, T84.612A, T84.613A, T84.614A, T84.615A, T84.619A, T84.63XA, T84.69XA, T84.7XXA

0RG63K1 Fusion of Thoracic Vertebral Joint with Nonautologous Tissue Substitute, Posterior Approach, Posterior Column, Percutaneous Approach

HAC When reported with secondary diagnosis code T84.60XA, T84.610A, T84.611A, T84.612A, T84.613A, T84.614A, T84.615A, T84.619A, T84.63XA, T84.69XA, T84.7XXA

0RG63KJ Fusion of Thoracic Vertebral Joint with Nonautologous Tissue Substitute, Posterior Approach, Anterior Column, Percutaneous Approach

HAC When reported with secondary diagnosis code T84.60XA, T84.610A, T84.611A, T84.612A, T84.613A, T84.614A, T84.615A, T84.619A, T84.63XA, T84.69XA, T84.7XXA

0RG63Z0 Fusion of Thoracic Vertebral Joint, Anterior Approach, Anterior Column, Percutaneous Approach

HAC When reported with secondary diagnosi code T84.60XA, T84.610A, T84.611A, T84.612A, T84.613A, T84.614A, T84.615A, T84.619A, T84.63XA, T84.69XA, T84.7XXA

0RG63Z1 Fusion of Thoracic Vertebral Joint, Posterior Approach, Posterior Column, Percutaneous Approach

HAC When reported with secondary diagnosis code T84.60XA, T84.610A, T84.611A, T84.612A, T84.613A, T84.614A, T84.615A, T84.619A, T84.63XA, T84.69XA, T84.7XXA

0RG63ZJ Fusion of Thoracic Vertebral Joint, Posterior Approach, Anterior Column, Percutaneous Approach

HAC When reported with secondary diagnosis code T84.60XA, T84.610A, T84.611A, T84.612A, T84.613A, T84.614A, T84.615A, T84.619A, T84.63XA, T84.69XA, T84.7XXA

0RG6470 Fusion of Thoracic Vertebral Joint with Autologous Tissue Substitute, Anterior Approach, Anterior Column, Percutaneo Endoscopic Approach

HAC When reported with secondary diagnosis code T84.60XA, T84.610A, T84.611A, T84.612A, T84.613A, T84.614A, T84.615A, T84.619A, T84.63XA, T84.69XA, T84.7XXA

0RG6471 Fusion of Thoracic Vertebral Joint with Autologous Tissue Substitute, Posterior Approach, Posterior Column, Percutaneous Endoscopic Approach

HAC When reported with secondary diagnosis code T84.60XA, T84.610A, T84.611A, T84.612A, T84.613A, T84.614A, T84.615A, T84.619A, T84.63XA, T84.69XA, T84.7XXA

0RG647J Fusion of Thoracic Vertebral Joint with Autologous Tissue Substitute, Posterior Approach, Anterior Column, Percutaneou Endoscopic Approach

HAC When reported with secondary diagnosis code T84.60XA, T84.610A, T84.611A, T84.612A, T84.613A, T84.614A, T84.615A, T84.619A, T84.63XA, T84.69XA, T84.7XXA

0RG64A0 Fusion of Thoracic Vertebral Joint with Interbody Fusion Device, Anterior Approach, Anterior Column, Percutaneou Endoscopic Approach

HAC When reported with secondary diagnosis code T84.60XA, T84.610A, T84.611A, T84.612A, T84.613A, T84.614A, T84.615A, T84.619A, T84.63XA, T84.69XA, T84.7XXA

0RG64A1 Fusion of Thoracic Vertebral Joint with Interbody Fusion Device, Posterior Approach, Posterior Column, Percutaneous Endoscopic Approach

HAC When reported with secondary diagnosis code T84.60XA, T84.610A, T84.611A, T84.612A, T84.613A, T84.614A, T84.615A, T84.619A, T84.63XA, T84.69XA, T84.7XXA

0RG64AJ Fusion of Thoracic Vertebral Joint with Interbody Fusion Device, Posterior Approach, Anterior Column, Percutaneous Endoscopic Approach

HAC When reported with secondary diagnosis code T84.60XA, T84.610A, T84.611A, T84.612A, T84.613A, T84.614A, T84.615A, T84.619A, T84.63XA, T84.69XA, T84.7XXA

♀ Female-only ♂ Male-only ▲ Limited Coverage ● Non-OR HAC HAC-associated procedure ▲ Non-covered procedures + Combination

G64J0 Fusion of Thoracic Vertebral Joint with Synthetic Substitute, Anterior Approach, Anterior Column, Percutaneous Endoscopic Approach
- HAC When reported with secondary diagnosis code T84.60XA, T84.610A, T84.611A, T84.612A, T84.613A, T84.614A, T84.615A, T84.619A, T84.63XA, T84.69XA, T84.7XXA

G64J1 Fusion of Thoracic Vertebral Joint with Synthetic Substitute, Posterior Approach, Posterior Column, Percutaneous Endoscopic Approach
- HAC When reported with secondary diagnosis code T84.60XA, T84.610A, T84.611A, T84.612A, T84.613A, T84.614A, T84.615A, T84.619A, T84.63XA, T84.69XA, T84.7XXA

G64JJ Fusion of Thoracic Vertebral Joint with Synthetic Substitute, Posterior Approach, Anterior Column, Percutaneous Endoscopic Approach
- HAC When reported with secondary diagnosis code T84.60XA, T84.610A, T84.611A, T84.612A, T84.613A, T84.614A, T84.615A, T84.619A, T84.63XA, T84.69XA, T84.7XXA

G64K0 Fusion of Thoracic Vertebral Joint with Nonautologous Tissue Substitute, Anterior Approach, Anterior Column, Percutaneous Endoscopic Approach
- HAC When reported with secondary diagnosis code T84.60XA, T84.610A, T84.611A, T84.612A, T84.613A, T84.614A, T84.615A, T84.619A, T84.63XA, T84.69XA, T84.7XXA

G64K1 Fusion of Thoracic Vertebral Joint with Nonautologous Tissue Substitute, Posterior Approach, Posterior Column, Percutaneous Endoscopic Approach
- HAC When reported with secondary diagnosis code T84.60XA, T84.610A, T84.611A, T84.612A, T84.613A, T84.614A, T84.615A, T84.619A, T84.63XA, T84.69XA, T84.7XXA

RG64KJ Fusion of Thoracic Vertebral Joint with Nonautologous Tissue Substitute, Posterior Approach, Anterior Column, Percutaneous Endoscopic Approach
- HAC When reported with secondary diagnosis code T84.60XA, T84.610A, T84.611A, T84.612A, T84.613A, T84.614A, T84.615A, T84.619A, T84.63XA, T84.69XA, T84.7XXA

RG64Z0 Fusion of Thoracic Vertebral Joint, Anterior Approach, Anterior Column, Percutaneous Endoscopic Approach
- HAC When reported with secondary diagnosis code T84.60XA, T84.610A, T84.611A, T84.612A, T84.613A, T84.614A, T84.615A, T84.619A, T84.63XA, T84.69XA, T84.7XXA

RG64Z1 Fusion of Thoracic Vertebral Joint, Posterior Approach, Posterior Column, Percutaneous Endoscopic Approach
- HAC When reported with secondary diagnosis code T84.60XA, T84.610A, T84.611A, T84.612A, T84.613A, T84.614A, T84.615A, T84.619A, T84.63XA, T84.69XA, T84.7XXA

0RG64ZJ Fusion of Thoracic Vertebral Joint, Posterior Approach, Anterior Column, Percutaneous Endoscopic Approach
- HAC When reported with secondary diagnosis code T84.60XA, T84.610A, T84.611A, T84.612A, T84.613A, T84.614A, T84.615A, T84.619A, T84.63XA, T84.69XA, T84.7XXA

0RG7070 Fusion of 2 to 7 Thoracic Vertebral Joints with Autologous Tissue Substitute, Anterior Approach, Anterior Column, Open Approach
- HAC When reported with secondary diagnosis code T84.60XA, T84.610A, T84.611A, T84.612A, T84.613A, T84.614A, T84.615A, T84.619A, T84.63XA, T84.69XA, T84.7XXA
- + Fusion of nine or more joints when reported with Fusion of two or more lumbar vertebral joints. *See table 0SG to construct Fusion code.*

0RG7071 Fusion of 2 to 7 Thoracic Vertebral Joints with Autologous Tissue Substitute, Posterior Approach, Posterior Column, Open Approach
  - *AHA CC: 1Q, 2013, 21-23*
- HAC When reported with secondary diagnosis code T84.60XA, T84.610A, T84.611A, T84.612A, T84.613A, T84.614A, T84.615A, T84.619A, T84.63XA, T84.69XA, T84.7XXA
- + Fusion of nine or more joints when reported with Fusion of two or more lumbar vertebral joints. *See table 0SG to construct Fusion code.*

0RG707J Fusion of 2 to 7 Thoracic Vertebral Joints with Autologous Tissue Substitute, Posterior Approach, Anterior Column, Open Approach
- HAC When reported with secondary diagnosis code T84.60XA, T84.610A, T84.611A, T84.612A, T84.613A, T84.614A, T84.615A, T84.619A, T84.63XA, T84.69XA, T84.7XXA
- + Fusion of nine or more joints when reported with Fusion of two or more lumbar vertebral joints. *See table 0SG to construct Fusion code.*

0RG70A0 Fusion of 2 to 7 Thoracic Vertebral Joints with Interbody Fusion Device, Anterior Approach, Anterior Column, Open Approach
- HAC When reported with secondary diagnosis code T84.60XA, T84.610A, T84.611A, T84.612A, T84.613A, T84.614A, T84.615A, T84.619A, T84.63XA, T84.69XA, T84.7XXA
- + Fusion of nine or more joints when reported with Fusion of two or more lumbar vertebral joints. *See table 0SG to construct Fusion code.*

0RG70A1 Fusion of 2 to 7 Thoracic Vertebral Joints with Interbody Fusion Device, Posterior Approach, Posterior Column, Open Approach
- HAC When reported with secondary diagnosis code T84.60XA, T84.610A, T84.611A, T84.612A, T84.613A, T84.614A, T84.615A, T84.619A, T84.63XA, T84.69XA, T84.7XXA
- + Fusion of nine or more joints when reported with Fusion of two or more lumbar vertebral joints. *See table 0SG to construct Fusion code.*

0RG70AJ Fusion of 2 to 7 Thoracic Vertebral Joints with Interbody Fusion Device, Posterior Approach, Anterior Column, Open Approach
- HAC When reported with secondary diagnosis code T84.60XA, T84.610A, T84.611A, T84.612A, T84.613A, T84.614A, T84.615A, T84.619A, T84.63XA, T84.69XA, T84.7XXA
- + Fusion of nine or more joints when reported with Fusion of two or more lumbar vertebral joints. *See table 0SG to construct Fusion code.*

0RG70J0 Fusion of 2 to 7 Thoracic Vertebral Joints with Synthetic Substitute, Anterior Approach, Anterior Column, Open Approach
- HAC When reported with secondary diagnosis code T84.60XA, T84.610A, T84.611A, T84.612A, T84.613A, T84.614A, T84.615A, T84.619A, T84.63XA, T84.69XA, T84.7XXA
- + Fusion of nine or more joints when reported with Fusion of two or more lumbar vertebral joints. *See table 0SG to construct Fusion code.*

0RG70J1 Fusion of 2 to 7 Thoracic Vertebral Joints with Synthetic Substitute, Posterior Approach, Posterior Column, Open Approach
- HAC When reported with secondary diagnosis code T84.60XA, T84.610A, T84.611A, T84.612A, T84.613A, T84.614A, T84.615A, T84.619A, T84.63XA, T84.69XA, T84.7XXA
- + Fusion of nine or more joints when reported with Fusion of two or more lumbar vertebral joints. *See table 0SG to construct Fusion code.*

0RG70JJ Fusion of 2 to 7 Thoracic Vertebral Joints with Synthetic Substitute, Posterior Approach, Anterior Column, Open Approach
- HAC When reported with secondary diagnosis code T84.60XA, T84.610A, T84.611A, T84.612A, T84.613A, T84.614A, T84.615A, T84.619A, T84.63XA, T84.69XA, T84.7XXA
- + Fusion of nine or more joints when reported with Fusion of two or more lumbar vertebral joints. *See table 0SG to construct Fusion code.*

0RG70K0 Fusion of 2 to 7 Thoracic Vertebral Joints with Nonautologous Tissue Substitute, Anterior Approach, Anterior Column, Open Approach
- HAC When reported with secondary diagnosis code T84.60XA, T84.610A, T84.611A, T84.612A, T84.613A, T84.614A, T84.615A, T84.619A, T84.63XA, T84.69XA, T84.7XXA
- + Fusion of nine or more joints when reported with Fusion of two or more lumbar vertebral joints. *See table 0SG to construct Fusion code.*

0RG70K1 Fusion of 2 to 7 Thoracic Vertebral Joints with Nonautologous Tissue Substitute, Posterior Approach, Posterior Column, Open Approach
- HAC When reported with secondary diagnosis code T84.60XA, T84.610A, T84.611A, T84.612A, T84.613A, T84.614A, T84.615A, T84.619A, T84.63XA, T84.69XA, T84.7XXA
- + Fusion of nine or more joints when reported with Fusion of two or more lumbar vertebral joints. *See table 0SG to construct Fusion code.*

0RG70KJ Fusion of 2 to 7 Thoracic Vertebral Joints with Nonautologous Tissue Substitute, Posterior Approach, Anterior Column, Open Approach
- HAC When reported with secondary diagnosis code T84.60XA, T84.610A, T84.611A, T84.612A, T84.613A, T84.614A, T84.615A, T84.619A, T84.63XA, T84.69XA, T84.7XXA
- + Fusion of nine or more joints when reported with Fusion of two or more lumbar vertebral joints. *See table 0SG to construct Fusion code.*

♀ Female-only   ♂ Male-only   ▲ Limited Coverage   ● Non-OR   HAC HAC-associated procedure   ▲ Non-covered procedures   + Combination

0RG70Z0 Fusion of 2 to 7 Thoracic Vertebral Joints, Anterior Approach, Anterior Column, Open Approach
- When reported with secondary diagnosis code T84.60XA, T84.610A, T84.611A, T84.612A, T84.613A, T84.614A, T84.615A, T84.619A, T84.63XA, T84.69XA, T84.7XXA
- + Fusion of nine or more joints when reported with Fusion of two or more lumbar vertebral joints. *See table 0SG to construct Fusion code.*

0RG70Z1 Fusion of 2 to 7 Thoracic Vertebral Joints, Posterior Approach, Posterior Column, Open Approach
- When reported with secondary diagnosis code T84.60XA, T84.610A, T84.611A, T84.612A, T84.613A, T84.614A, T84.615A, T84.619A, T84.63XA, T84.69XA, T84.7XXA
- + Fusion of nine or more joints when reported with Fusion of two or more lumbar vertebral joints. *See table 0SG to construct Fusion code.*

0RG70ZJ Fusion of 2 to 7 Thoracic Vertebral Joints, Posterior Approach, Anterior Column, Open Approach
- When reported with secondary diagnosis code T84.60XA, T84.610A, T84.611A, T84.612A, T84.613A, T84.614A, T84.615A, T84.619A, T84.63XA, T84.69XA, T84.7XXA
- + Fusion of nine or more joints when reported with Fusion of two or more lumbar vertebral joints. *See table 0SG to construct Fusion code.*

0RG7370 Fusion of 2 to 7 Thoracic Vertebral Joints with Autologous Tissue Substitute, Anterior Approach, Anterior Column, Percutaneous Approach
- When reported with secondary diagnosis code T84.60XA, T84.610A, T84.611A, T84.612A, T84.613A, T84.614A, T84.615A, T84.619A, T84.63XA, T84.69XA, T84.7XXA
- + Fusion of nine or more joints when reported with Fusion of two or more lumbar vertebral joints. *See table 0SG to construct Fusion code.*

0RG7371 Fusion of 2 to 7 Thoracic Vertebral Joints with Autologous Tissue Substitute, Posterior Approach, Posterior Column, Percutaneous Approach
- When reported with secondary diagnosis code T84.60XA, T84.610A, T84.611A, T84.612A, T84.613A, T84.614A, T84.615A, T84.619A, T84.63XA, T84.69XA, T84.7XXA
- + Fusion of nine or more joints when reported with Fusion of two or more lumbar vertebral joints. *See table 0SG to construct Fusion code.*

0RG737J Fusion of 2 to 7 Thoracic Vertebral Joints with Autologous Tissue Substitute, Posterior Approach, Anterior Column, Percutaneous Approach
- When reported with secondary diagnosis code T84.60XA, T84.610A, T84.611A, T84.612A, T84.613A, T84.614A, T84.615A, T84.619A, T84.63XA, T84.69XA, T84.7XXA
- + Fusion of nine or more joints when reported with Fusion of two or more lumbar vertebral joints. *See table 0SG to construct Fusion code.*

0RG73A0 Fusion of 2 to 7 Thoracic Vertebral Joints with Interbody Fusion Device, Anterior Approach, Anterior Column, Percutaneous Approach
- When reported with secondary diagnosis code T84.60XA, T84.610A, T84.611A, T84.612A, T84.613A, T84.614A, T84.615A, T84.619A, T84.63XA, T84.69XA, T84.7XXA
- + Fusion of nine or more joints when reported with Fusion of two or more lumbar vertebral joints. *See table 0SG to construct Fusion code.*

0RG73A1 Fusion of 2 to 7 Thoracic Vertebral Joints with Interbody Fusion Device, Posterior Approach, Posterior Column, Percutaneous Approach
- When reported with secondary diagnosis code T84.60XA, T84.610A, T84.611A, T84.612A, T84.613A, T84.614A, T84.615A, T84.619A, T84.63XA, T84.69XA, T84.7XXA
- + Fusion of nine or more joints when reported with Fusion of two or more lumbar vertebral joints. *See table 0SG to construct Fusion code.*

0RG73AJ Fusion of 2 to 7 Thoracic Vertebral Joints with Interbody Fusion Device, Posterior Approach, Anterior Column, Percutaneous Approach
- When reported with secondary diagnosis code T84.60XA, T84.610A, T84.611A, T84.612A, T84.613A, T84.614A, T84.615A, T84.619A, T84.63XA, T84.69XA, T84.7XXA
- + Fusion of nine or more joints when reported with Fusion of two or more lumbar vertebral joints. *See table 0SG to construct Fusion code.*

0RG73J0 Fusion of 2 to 7 Thoracic Vertebral Joints with Synthetic Substitute, Anterior Approach, Anterior Column, Percutaneous Approach
- When reported with secondary diagnosis code T84.60XA, T84.610A, T84.611A, T84.612A, T84.613A, T84.614A, T84.615A, T84.619A, T84.63XA, T84.69XA, T84.7XXA
- + Fusion of nine or more joints when reported with Fusion of two or more lumbar vertebral joints. *See table 0SG to construct Fusion code.*

0RG73J1 Fusion of 2 to 7 Thoracic Vertebral Joints with Synthetic Substitute, Posterior Approach, Posterior Column, Percutaneous Approach
- When reported with secondary diagnosis code T84.60XA, T84.610A, T84.611A, T84.612A, T84.613A, T84.614A, T84.615A, T84.619A, T84.63XA, T84.69XA, T84.7XXA
- + Fusion of nine or more joints when reported with Fusion of two or more lumbar vertebral joints. *See table 0SG to construct Fusion code.*

0RG73JJ Fusion of 2 to 7 Thoracic Vertebral Joints with Synthetic Substitute, Posterior Approach, Anterior Column, Percutaneous Approach
- When reported with secondary diagnosis code T84.60XA, T84.610A, T84.611A, T84.612A, T84.613A, T84.614A, T84.615A, T84.619A, T84.63XA, T84.69XA, T84.7XXA
- + Fusion of nine or more joints when reported with Fusion of two or more lumbar vertebral joints. *See table 0SG to construct Fusion code.*

0RG73K0 Fusion of 2 to 7 Thoracic Vertebral Joints with Nonautologous Tissue Substitute, Anterior Approach, Anterior Column, Percutaneous Approach
- When reported with secondary diagnosis code T84.60XA, T84.610A, T84.611A, T84.612A, T84.613A, T84.614A, T84.615A, T84.619A, T84.63XA, T84.69XA, T84.7XXA
- + Fusion of nine or more joints when reported with Fusion of two or more lumbar vertebral joints. *See table 0SG to construct Fusion code.*

0RG73K1 Fusion of 2 to 7 Thoracic Vertebral Joints with Nonautologous Tissue Substitute, Posterior Approach, Posterior Column, Percutaneous Approach
- When reported with secondary diagnosis code T84.60XA, T84.610A, T84.611A, T84.612A, T84.613A, T84.614A, T84.615A, T84.619A, T84.63XA, T84.69XA, T84.7XXA
- + Fusion of nine or more joints when reported with Fusion of two or more lumbar vertebral joints. *See table 0SG to construct Fusion code.*

0RG73KJ Fusion of 2 to 7 Thoracic Vertebral Joints with Nonautologous Tissue Substitute, Posterior Approach, Anterior Column, Percutaneous Approach
- When reported with secondary diagnosis code T84.60XA, T84.610A, T84.611A, T84.612A, T84.613A, T84.614A, T84.615A, T84.619A, T84.63XA, T84.69XA, T84.7XXA
- + Fusion of nine or more joints when reported with Fusion of two or more lumbar vertebral joints. *See table 0SG to construct Fusion code.*

0RG73Z0 Fusion of 2 to 7 Thoracic Vertebral Joints, Anterior Approach, Anterior Column, Percutaneous Approach
- When reported with secondary diagnosis code T84.60XA, T84.610A, T84.611A, T84.612A, T84.613A, T84.614A, T84.615A, T84.619A, T84.63XA, T84.69XA, T84.7XXA
- + Fusion of nine or more joints when reported with Fusion of two or more lumbar vertebral joints. *See table 0SG to construct Fusion code.*

0RG73Z1 Fusion of 2 to 7 Thoracic Vertebral Joints, Posterior Approach, Posterior Column, Percutaneous Approach
- When reported with secondary diagnosis code T84.60XA, T84.610A, T84.611A, T84.612A, T84.613A, T84.614A, T84.615A, T84.619A, T84.63XA, T84.69XA, T84.7XXA
- + Fusion of nine or more joints when reported with Fusion of two or more lumbar vertebral joints. *See table 0SG to construct Fusion code.*

0RG73ZJ Fusion of 2 to 7 Thoracic Vertebral Joints, Posterior Approach, Anterior Column, Percutaneous Approach
- When reported with secondary diagnosis code T84.60XA, T84.610A, T84.611A, T84.612A, T84.613A, T84.614A, T84.615A, T84.619A, T84.63XA, T84.69XA, T84.7XXA
- + Fusion of nine or more joints when reported with Fusion of two or more lumbar vertebral joints. *See table 0SG to construct Fusion code.*

0RG7470 Fusion of 2 to 7 Thoracic Vertebral Joints with Autologous Tissue Substitute, Anterior Approach, Anterior Column, Percutaneous Endoscopic Approach

Note Continued

♀ Female-only   ♂ Male-only   ▲ Limited Coverage   ● Non-OR   ▨ HAC-associated procedure   ▲ Non-covered procedures   + Combination

0RG7470 Continued Note

When reported with secondary diagnosis code T84.60XA, T84.610A, T84.611A, T84.612A, T84.613A, T84.614A, T84.615A, T84.619A, T84.63XA, T84.69XA, T84.7XXA

+ Fusion of nine or more joints when reported with Fusion of two or more lumbar vertebral joints. *See table 0SG to construct Fusion code.*

0RG7471 Fusion of 2 to 7 Thoracic Vertebral Joints with Autologous Tissue Substitute, Posterior Approach, Posterior Column, Percutaneous Endoscopic Approach

When reported with secondary diagnosis code T84.60XA, T84.610A, T84.611A, T84.612A, T84.613A, T84.614A, T84.615A, T84.619A, T84.63XA, T84.69XA, T84.7XXA

+ Fusion of nine or more joints when reported with Fusion of two or more lumbar vertebral joints. *See table 0SG to construct Fusion code.*

0RG747J Fusion of 2 to 7 Thoracic Vertebral Joints with Autologous Tissue Substitute, Posterior Approach, Anterior Column, Percutaneous Endoscopic Approach

When reported with secondary diagnosis code T84.60XA, T84.610A, T84.611A, T84.612A, T84.613A, T84.614A, T84.615A, T84.619A, T84.63XA, T84.69XA, T84.7XXA

+ Fusion of nine or more joints when reported with Fusion of two or more lumbar vertebral joints. *See table 0SG to construct Fusion code.*

0RG74A0 Fusion of 2 to 7 Thoracic Vertebral Joints with Interbody Fusion Device, Anterior Approach, Anterior Column, Percutaneous Endoscopic Approach

When reported with secondary diagnosis code T84.60XA, T84.610A, T84.611A, T84.612A, T84.613A, T84.614A, T84.615A, T84.619A, T84.63XA, T84.69XA, T84.7XXA

+ Fusion of nine or more joints when reported with Fusion of two or more lumbar vertebral joints. *See table 0SG to construct Fusion code.*

0RG74A1 Fusion of 2 to 7 Thoracic Vertebral Joints with Interbody Fusion Device, Posterior Approach, Posterior Column, Percutaneous Endoscopic Approach

When reported with secondary diagnosis code T84.60XA, T84.610A, T84.611A, T84.612A, T84.613A, T84.614A, T84.615A, T84.619A, T84.63XA, T84.69XA, T84.7XXA

+ Fusion of nine or more joints when reported with Fusion of two or more lumbar vertebral joints. *See table 0SG to construct Fusion code.*

0RG74AJ Fusion of 2 to 7 Thoracic Vertebral Joints with Interbody Fusion Device, Posterior Approach, Anterior Column, Percutaneous Endoscopic Approach

When reported with secondary diagnosis code T84.60XA, T84.610A, T84.611A, T84.612A, T84.613A, T84.614A, T84.615A, T84.619A, T84.63XA, T84.69XA, T84.7XXA

+ Fusion of nine or more joints when reported with Fusion of two or more lumbar vertebral joints. *See table 0SG to construct Fusion code.*

0RG74J0 Fusion of 2 to 7 Thoracic Vertebral Joints with Synthetic Substitute, Anterior Approach, Anterior Column, Percutaneous Endoscopic Approach

When reported with secondary diagnosis code T84.60XA, T84.610A, T84.611A, T84.612A, T84.613A, T84.614A, T84.615A, T84.619A, T84.63XA, T84.69XA, T84.7XXA

+ Fusion of nine or more joints when reported with Fusion of two or more lumbar vertebral joints. *See table 0SG to construct Fusion code.*

0RG74J1 Fusion of 2 to 7 Thoracic Vertebral Joints with Synthetic Substitute, Posterior Approach, Posterior Column, Percutaneous Endoscopic Approach

When reported with secondary diagnosis code T84.60XA, T84.610A, T84.611A, T84.612A, T84.613A, T84.614A, T84.615A, T84.619A, T84.63XA, T84.69XA, T84.7XXA

+ Fusion of nine or more joints when reported with Fusion of two or more lumbar vertebral joints. *See table 0SG to construct Fusion code.*

0RG74JJ Fusion of 2 to 7 Thoracic Vertebral Joints with Synthetic Substitute, Posterior Approach, Anterior Column, Percutaneous Endoscopic Approach

When reported with secondary diagnosis code T84.60XA, T84.610A, T84.611A, T84.612A, T84.613A, T84.614A, T84.615A, T84.619A, T84.63XA, T84.69XA, T84.7XXA

+ Fusion of nine or more joints when reported with Fusion of two or more lumbar vertebral joints. *See table 0SG to construct Fusion code.*

0RG74K0 Fusion of 2 to 7 Thoracic Vertebral Joints with Nonautologous Tissue Substitute, Anterior Approach, Anterior Column, Percutaneous Endoscopic Approach

When reported with secondary diagnosis code T84.60XA, T84.610A, T84.611A, T84.612A, T84.613A, T84.614A, T84.615A, T84.619A, T84.63XA, T84.69XA, T84.7XXA

+ Fusion of nine or more joints when reported with Fusion of two or more lumbar vertebral joints. *See table 0SG to construct Fusion code.*

0RG74K1 Fusion of 2 to 7 Thoracic Vertebral Joints with Nonautologous Tissue Substitute, Posterior Approach, Posterior Column, Percutaneous Endoscopic Approach

When reported with secondary diagnosis code T84.60XA, T84.610A, T84.611A, T84.612A, T84.613A, T84.614A, T84.615A, T84.619A, T84.63XA, T84.69XA, T84.7XXA

+ Fusion of nine or more joints when reported with Fusion of two or more lumbar vertebral joints. *See table 0SG to construct Fusion code.*

0RG74KJ Fusion of 2 to 7 Thoracic Vertebral Joints with Nonautologous Tissue Substitute, Posterior Approach, Anterior Column, Percutaneous Endoscopic Approach

When reported with secondary diagnosis code T84.60XA, T84.610A, T84.611A, T84.612A, T84.613A, T84.614A, T84.615A, T84.619A, T84.63XA, T84.69XA, T84.7XXA

+ Fusion of nine or more joints when reported with Fusion of two or more lumbar vertebral joints. *See table 0SG to construct Fusion code.*

0RG74Z0 Fusion of 2 to 7 Thoracic Vertebral Joints, Anterior Approach, Anterior Column, Percutaneous Endoscopic Approach

When reported with secondary diagnosis code T84.60XA, T84.610A, T84.611A, T84.612A, T84.613A, T84.614A, T84.615A, T84.619A, T84.63XA, T84.69XA, T84.7XXA

+ Fusion of nine or more joints when reported with Fusion of two or more lumbar vertebral joints. *See table 0SG to construct Fusion code.*

0RG74Z1 Fusion of 2 to 7 Thoracic Vertebral Joints, Posterior Approach, Posterior Column, Percutaneous Endoscopic Approach

When reported with secondary diagnosis code T84.60XA, T84.610A, T84.611A, T84.612A, T84.613A, T84.614A, T84.615A, T84.619A, T84.63XA, T84.69XA, T84.7XXA

+ Fusion of nine or more joints when reported with Fusion of two or more lumbar vertebral joints. *See table 0SG to construct Fusion code.*

0RG74ZJ Fusion of 2 to 7 Thoracic Vertebral Joints, Posterior Approach, Anterior Column, Percutaneous Endoscopic Approach

When reported with secondary diagnosis code T84.60XA, T84.610A, T84.611A, T84.612A, T84.613A, T84.614A, T84.615A, T84.619A, T84.63XA, T84.69XA, T84.7XXA

+ Fusion of nine or more joints when reported with Fusion of two or more lumbar vertebral joints. *See table 0SG to construct Fusion code.*

0RG8070 Fusion of 8 or more Thoracic Vertebral Joints with Autologous Tissue Substitute, Anterior Approach, Anterior Column, Open Approach

When reported with secondary diagnosis code T84.60XA, T84.610A, T84.611A, T84.612A, T84.613A, T84.614A, T84.615A, T84.619A, T84.63XA, T84.69XA, T84.7XXA

0RG8071 Fusion of 8 or more Thoracic Vertebral Joints with Autologous Tissue Substitute, Posterior Approach, Posterior Column, Open Approach

When reported with secondary diagnosis code T84.60XA, T84.610A, T84.611A, T84.612A, T84.613A, T84.614A, T84.615A, T84.619A, T84.63XA, T84.69XA, T84.7XXA

0RG807J Fusion of 8 or more Thoracic Vertebral Joints with Autologous Tissue Substitute, Posterior Approach, Anterior Column, Open Approach

When reported with secondary diagnosis code T84.60XA, T84.610A, T84.611A, T84.612A, T84.613A, T84.614A, T84.615A, T84.619A, T84.63XA, T84.69XA, T84.7XXA

0RG80A0 Fusion of 8 or more Thoracic Vertebral Joints with Interbody Fusion Device, Anterior Approach, Anterior Column, Open Approach

When reported with secondary diagnosis code T84.60XA, T84.610A, T84.611A, T84.612A, T84.613A, T84.614A, T84.615A, T84.619A, T84.63XA, T84.69XA, T84.7XXA

0RG80A1 Fusion of 8 or more Thoracic Vertebral Joints with Interbody Fusion Device, Posterior Approach, Posterior Column, Open Approach

Note Continued

♀ Female-only   ♂ Male-only   ▲ Limited Coverage   ● Non-OR   ▨ HAC-associated procedure   ▲ Non-covered procedures   + Combination

0RG80A1 Continued Note

When reported with secondary diagnosis code T84.60XA, T84.610A, T84.611A, T84.612A, T84.613A, T84.614A, T84.615A, T84.619A, T84.63XA, T84.69XA, T84.7XXA

0RG80AJ Fusion of 8 or more Thoracic Vertebral Joints with Interbody Fusion Device, Posterior Approach, Anterior Column, Open Approach

When reported with secondary diagnosis code T84.60XA, T84.610A, T84.611A, T84.612A, T84.613A, T84.614A, T84.615A, T84.619A, T84.63XA, T84.69XA, T84.7XXA

0RG80J0 Fusion of 8 or more Thoracic Vertebral Joints with Synthetic Substitute, Anterior Approach, Anterior Column, Open Approach

When reported with secondary diagnosis code T84.60XA, T84.610A, T84.611A, T84.612A, T84.613A, T84.614A, T84.615A, T84.619A, T84.63XA, T84.69XA, T84.7XXA

0RG80J1 Fusion of 8 or more Thoracic Vertebral Joints with Synthetic Substitute, Posterior Approach, Posterior Column, Open Approach

When reported with secondary diagnosis code T84.60XA, T84.610A, T84.611A, T84.612A, T84.613A, T84.614A, T84.615A, T84.619A, T84.63XA, T84.69XA, T84.7XXA

0RG80JJ Fusion of 8 or more Thoracic Vertebral Joints with Synthetic Substitute, Posterior Approach, Anterior Column, Open Approach

When reported with secondary diagnosis code T84.60XA, T84.610A, T84.611A, T84.612A, T84.613A, T84.614A, T84.615A, T84.619A, T84.63XA, T84.69XA, T84.7XXA

0RG80K0 Fusion of 8 or more Thoracic Vertebral Joints with Nonautologous Tissue Substitute, Anterior Approach, Anterior Column, Open Approach

When reported with secondary diagnosis code T84.60XA, T84.610A, T84.611A, T84.612A, T84.613A, T84.614A, T84.615A, T84.619A, T84.63XA, T84.69XA, T84.7XXA

0RG80K1 Fusion of 8 or more Thoracic Vertebral Joints with Nonautologous Tissue Substitute, Posterior Approach, Posterior Column, Open Approach

When reported with secondary diagnosis code T84.60XA, T84.610A, T84.611A, T84.612A, T84.613A, T84.614A, T84.615A, T84.619A, T84.63XA, T84.69XA, T84.7XXA

0RG80KJ Fusion of 8 or more Thoracic Vertebral Joints with Nonautologous Tissue Substitute, Posterior Approach, Anterior Column, Open Approach

When reported with secondary diagnosis code T84.60XA, T84.610A, T84.611A, T84.612A, T84.613A, T84.614A, T84.615A, T84.619A, T84.63XA, T84.69XA, T84.7XXA

0RG80Z0 Fusion of 8 or more Thoracic Vertebral Joints, Anterior Approach, Anterior Column, Open Approach

When reported with secondary diagnosis code T84.60XA, T84.610A, T84.611A, T84.612A, T84.613A, T84.614A, T84.615A, T84.619A, T84.63XA, T84.69XA, T84.7XXA

0RG80Z1 Fusion of 8 or more Thoracic Vertebral Joints, Posterior Approach, Posterior Column, Open Approach

When reported with secondary diagnosis code T84.60XA, T84.610A, T84.611A, T84.612A, T84.613A, T84.614A, T84.615A, T84.619A, T84.63XA, T84.69XA, T84.7XXA

0RG80ZJ Fusion of 8 or more Thoracic Vertebral Joints, Posterior Approach, Anterior Column, Open Approach

When reported with secondary diagnosis code T84.60XA, T84.610A, T84.611A, T84.612A, T84.613A, T84.614A, T84.615A, T84.619A, T84.63XA, T84.69XA, T84.7XXA

0RG8370 Fusion of 8 or more Thoracic Vertebral Joints with Autologous Tissue Substitute, Anterior Approach, Anterior Column, Percutaneous Approach

When reported with secondary diagnosis code T84.60XA, T84.610A, T84.611A, T84.612A, T84.613A, T84.614A, T84.615A, T84.619A, T84.63XA, T84.69XA, T84.7XXA

0RG8371 Fusion of 8 or more Thoracic Vertebral Joints with Autologous Tissue Substitute, Posterior Approach, Posterior Column, Percutaneous Approach

When reported with secondary diagnosis code T84.60XA, T84.610A, T84.611A, T84.612A, T84.613A, T84.614A, T84.615A, T84.619A, T84.63XA, T84.69XA, T84.7XXA

0RG837J Fusion of 8 or more Thoracic Vertebral Joints with Autologous Tissue Substitute, Posterior Approach, Anterior Column, Percutaneous Approach

When reported with secondary diagnosis code T84.60XA, T84.610A, T84.611A, T84.612A, T84.613A, T84.614A, T84.615A, T84.619A, T84.63XA, T84.69XA, T84.7XXA

0RG83A0 Fusion of 8 or more Thoracic Vertebral Joints with Interbody Fusion Device, Anterior Approach, Anterior Column, Percutaneous Approach

When reported with secondary diagnosis code T84.60XA, T84.610A, T84.611A, T84.612A, T84.613A, T84.614A, T84.615A, T84.619A, T84.63XA, T84.69XA, T84.7XXA

0RG83A1 Fusion of 8 or more Thoracic Vertebral Joints with Interbody Fusion Device, Posterior Approach, Posterior Column, Percutaneous Approach

When reported with secondary diagnosis code T84.60XA, T84.610A, T84.611A, T84.612A, T84.613A, T84.614A, T84.615A, T84.619A, T84.63XA, T84.69XA, T84.7XXA

0RG83AJ Fusion of 8 or more Thoracic Vertebral Joints with Interbody Fusion Device, Posterior Approach, Anterior Column, Percutaneous Approach

When reported with secondary diagnosis code T84.60XA, T84.610A, T84.611A, T84.612A, T84.613A, T84.614A, T84.615A, T84.619A, T84.63XA, T84.69XA, T84.7XXA

0RG83J0 Fusion of 8 or more Thoracic Vertebral Joints with Synthetic Substitute, Anterior Approach, Anterior Column, Percutaneous Approach

When reported with secondary diagnosis code T84.60XA, T84.610A, T84.611A, T84.612A, T84.613A, T84.614A,

T84.615A, T84.619A, T84.63XA, T84.69XA, T84.7XXA

0RG83J1 Fusion of 8 or more Thoracic Vertebral Joints with Synthetic Substitute, Posterior Approach, Posterior Column, Percutaneous Approach

When reported with secondary diagnosis code T84.60XA, T84.610A, T84.611A, T84.612A, T84.613A, T84.614A, T84.615A, T84.619A, T84.63XA, T84.69XA, T84.7XXA

0RG83JJ Fusion of 8 or more Thoracic Vertebral Joints with Synthetic Substitute, Posterior Approach, Anterior Column, Percutaneous Approach

When reported with secondary diagnosis code T84.60XA, T84.610A, T84.611A, T84.612A, T84.613A, T84.614A, T84.615A, T84.619A, T84.63XA, T84.69XA, T84.7XXA

0RG83K0 Fusion of 8 or more Thoracic Vertebral Joints with Nonautologous Tissue Substitute, Anterior Approach, Anterior Column, Percutaneous Approach

When reported with secondary diagnosis code T84.60XA, T84.610A, T84.611A, T84.612A, T84.613A, T84.614A, T84.615A, T84.619A, T84.63XA, T84.69XA, T84.7XXA

0RG83K1 Fusion of 8 or more Thoracic Vertebral Joints with Nonautologous Tissue Substitute, Posterior Approach, Posterior Column, Percutaneous Approach

When reported with secondary diagnosis code T84.60XA, T84.610A, T84.611A, T84.612A, T84.613A, T84.614A, T84.615A, T84.619A, T84.63XA, T84.69XA, T84.7XXA

0RG83KJ Fusion of 8 or more Thoracic Vertebral Joints with Nonautologous Tissue Substitute, Posterior Approach, Anterior Column, Percutaneous Approach

When reported with secondary diagnosis code T84.60XA, T84.610A, T84.611A, T84.612A, T84.613A, T84.614A, T84.615A, T84.619A, T84.63XA, T84.69XA, T84.7XXA

0RG83Z0 Fusion of 8 or more Thoracic Vertebral Joints, Anterior Approach, Anterior Column, Percutaneous Approach

When reported with secondary diagnosis code T84.60XA, T84.610A, T84.611A, T84.612A, T84.613A, T84.614A, T84.615A, T84.619A, T84.63XA, T84.69XA, T84.7XXA

0RG83Z1 Fusion of 8 or more Thoracic Vertebral Joints, Posterior Approach, Posterior Column, Percutaneous Approach

When reported with secondary diagnosis code T84.60XA, T84.610A, T84.611A, T84.612A, T84.613A, T84.614A, T84.615A, T84.619A, T84.63XA, T84.69XA, T84.7XXA

0RG83ZJ Fusion of 8 or more Thoracic Vertebral Joints, Posterior Approach, Anterior Column, Percutaneous Approach

When reported with secondary diagnosis code T84.60XA, T84.610A, T84.611A, T84.612A, T84.613A, T84.614A, T84.615A, T84.619A, T84.63XA, T84.69XA, T84.7XXA

0RG8470 Fusion of 8 or more Thoracic Vertebral Joints with Autologous Tissue Substitute, Anterior Approach, Anterior Column, Percutaneous Endoscopic Approach

Note Continued

0RG8470 Continued Note

- HAC When reported with secondary diagnosis code T84.60XA, T84.610A, T84.611A, T84.612A, T84.613A, T84.614A, T84.615A, T84.619A, T84.63XA, T84.69XA, T84.7XXA

0RG8471 Fusion of 8 or more Thoracic Vertebral Joints with Autologous Tissue Substitute, Posterior Approach, Posterior Column, Percutaneous Endoscopic Approach

- HAC When reported with secondary diagnosis code T84.60XA, T84.610A, T84.611A, T84.612A, T84.613A, T84.614A, T84.615A, T84.619A, T84.63XA, T84.69XA, T84.7XXA

0RG847J Fusion of 8 or more Thoracic Vertebral Joints with Autologous Tissue Substitute, Posterior Approach, Anterior Column, Percutaneous Endoscopic Approach

- HAC When reported with secondary diagnosis code T84.60XA, T84.610A, T84.611A, T84.612A, T84.613A, T84.614A, T84.615A, T84.619A, T84.63XA, T84.69XA, T84.7XXA

0RG84A0 Fusion of 8 or more Thoracic Vertebral Joints with Interbody Fusion Device, Anterior Approach, Anterior Column, Percutaneous Endoscopic Approach

- HAC When reported with secondary diagnosis code T84.60XA, T84.610A, T84.611A, T84.612A, T84.613A, T84.614A, T84.615A, T84.619A, T84.63XA, T84.69XA, T84.7XXA

0RG84A1 Fusion of 8 or more Thoracic Vertebral Joints with Interbody Fusion Device, Posterior Approach, Posterior Column, Percutaneous Endoscopic Approach

- HAC When reported with secondary diagnosis code T84.60XA, T84.610A, T84.611A, T84.612A, T84.613A, T84.614A, T84.615A, T84.619A, T84.63XA, T84.69XA, T84.7XXA

0RG84AJ Fusion of 8 or more Thoracic Vertebral Joints with Interbody Fusion Device, Posterior Approach, Anterior Column, Percutaneous Endoscopic Approach

- HAC When reported with secondary diagnosis code T84.60XA, T84.610A, T84.611A, T84.612A, T84.613A, T84.614A, T84.615A, T84.619A, T84.63XA, T84.69XA, T84.7XXA

0RG84J0 Fusion of 8 or more Thoracic Vertebral Joints with Synthetic Substitute, Anterior Approach, Anterior Column, Percutaneous Endoscopic Approach

- HAC When reported with secondary diagnosis code T84.60XA, T84.610A, T84.611A, T84.612A, T84.613A, T84.614A, T84.615A, T84.619A, T84.63XA, T84.69XA, T84.7XXA

0RG84J1 Fusion of 8 or more Thoracic Vertebral Joints with Synthetic Substitute, Posterior Approach, Posterior Column, Percutaneous Endoscopic Approach

- HAC When reported with secondary diagnosis code T84.60XA, T84.610A, T84.611A, T84.612A, T84.613A, T84.614A, T84.615A, T84.619A, T84.63XA, T84.69XA, T84.7XXA

0RG84JJ Fusion of 8 or more Thoracic Vertebral Joints with Synthetic Substitute, Posterior Approach, Anterior Column, Percutaneous Endoscopic Approach

- HAC When reported with secondary diagnosis code T84.60XA, T84.610A, T84.611A, T84.612A, T84.613A, T84.614A, T84.615A, T84.619A, T84.63XA, T84.69XA, T84.7XXA

0RG84K0 Fusion of 8 or more Thoracic Vertebral Joints with Nonautologous Tissue Substitute, Anterior Approach, Anterior Column, Percutaneous Endoscopic Approach

- HAC When reported with secondary diagnosis code T84.60XA, T84.610A, T84.611A, T84.612A, T84.613A, T84.614A, T84.615A, T84.619A, T84.63XA, T84.69XA, T84.7XXA

0RG84K1 Fusion of 8 or more Thoracic Vertebral Joints with Nonautologous Tissue Substitute, Posterior Approach, Posterior Column, Percutaneous Endoscopic Approach

- HAC When reported with secondary diagnosis code T84.60XA, T84.610A, T84.611A, T84.612A, T84.613A, T84.614A, T84.615A, T84.619A, T84.63XA, T84.69XA, T84.7XXA

0RG84KJ Fusion of 8 or more Thoracic Vertebral Joints with Nonautologous Tissue Substitute, Posterior Approach, Anterior Column, Percutaneous Endoscopic Approach

- HAC When reported with secondary diagnosis code T84.60XA, T84.610A, T84.611A, T84.612A, T84.613A, T84.614A, T84.615A, T84.619A, T84.63XA, T84.69XA, T84.7XXA

0RG84Z0 Fusion of 8 or more Thoracic Vertebral Joints, Anterior Approach, Anterior Column, Percutaneous Endoscopic Approach

- HAC When reported with secondary diagnosis code T84.60XA, T84.610A, T84.611A, T84.612A, T84.613A, T84.614A, T84.615A, T84.619A, T84.63XA, T84.69XA, T84.7XXA

0RG84Z1 Fusion of 8 or more Thoracic Vertebral Joints, Posterior Approach, Posterior Column, Percutaneous Endoscopic Approach

- HAC When reported with secondary diagnosis code T84.60XA, T84.610A, T84.611A, T84.612A, T84.613A, T84.614A, T84.615A, T84.619A, T84.63XA, T84.69XA, T84.7XXA

0RG84ZJ Fusion of 8 or more Thoracic Vertebral Joints, Posterior Approach, Anterior Column, Percutaneous Endoscopic Approach

- HAC When reported with secondary diagnosis code T84.60XA, T84.610A, T84.611A, T84.612A, T84.613A, T84.614A, T84.615A, T84.619A, T84.63XA, T84.69XA, T84.7XXA

0RGA070 Fusion of Thoracolumbar Vertebral Joint with Autologous Tissue Substitute, Anterior Approach, Anterior Column, Open Approach

- HAC When reported with secondary diagnosis code T84.60XA, T84.610A, T84.611A, T84.612A, T84.613A, T84.614A, T84.615A, T84.619A, T84.63XA, T84.69XA, T84.7XXA

0RGA071 Fusion of Thoracolumbar Vertebral Joint with Autologous Tissue Substitute, Posterior Approach, Posterior Column, Open Approach

AHA CC: 1Q, 2013, 21-23

- HAC When reported with secondary diagnosis code T84.60XA, T84.610A, T84.611A, T84.612A, T84.613A, T84.614A, T84.615A, T84.619A, T84.63XA, T84.69XA, T84.7XXA

0RGA07J Fusion of Thoracolumbar Vertebral Joint with Autologous Tissue Substitute, Posterior Approach, Anterior Column, Open Approach

- HAC When reported with secondary diagnosis code T84.60XA, T84.610A, T84.611A, T84.612A, T84.613A, T84.614A, T84.615A, T84.619A, T84.63XA, T84.69XA, T84.7XXA

0RGA0A0 Fusion of Thoracolumbar Vertebral Joint with Interbody Fusion Device, Anterior Approach, Anterior Column, Open Approach

- HAC When reported with secondary diagnosis code T84.60XA, T84.610A, T84.611A, T84.612A, T84.613A, T84.614A, T84.615A, T84.619A, T84.63XA, T84.69XA, T84.7XXA

0RGA0A1 Fusion of Thoracolumbar Vertebral Joint with Interbody Fusion Device, Posterior Approach, Posterior Column, Open Approach

- HAC When reported with secondary diagnosis code T84.60XA, T84.610A, T84.611A, T84.612A, T84.613A, T84.614A, T84.615A, T84.619A, T84.63XA, T84.69XA, T84.7XXA

0RGA0AJ Fusion of Thoracolumbar Vertebral Joint with Interbody Fusion Device, Posterior Approach, Anterior Column, Open Approach

- HAC When reported with secondary diagnosis code T84.60XA, T84.610A, T84.611A, T84.612A, T84.613A, T84.614A, T84.615A, T84.619A, T84.63XA, T84.69XA, T84.7XXA

0RGA0J0 Fusion of Thoracolumbar Vertebral Joint with Synthetic Substitute, Anterior Approach, Anterior Column, Open Approach

- HAC When reported with secondary diagnosis code T84.60XA, T84.610A, T84.611A, T84.612A, T84.613A, T84.614A, T84.615A, T84.619A, T84.63XA, T84.69XA, T84.7XXA

0RGA0J1 Fusion of Thoracolumbar Vertebral Joint with Synthetic Substitute, Posterior Approach, Posterior Column, Open Approach

- HAC When reported with secondary diagnosis code T84.60XA, T84.610A, T84.611A, T84.612A, T84.613A, T84.614A, T84.615A, T84.619A, T84.63XA, T84.69XA, T84.7XXA

0RGA0JJ Fusion of Thoracolumbar Vertebral Joint with Synthetic Substitute, Posterior Approach, Anterior Column, Open Approach

- HAC When reported with secondary diagnosis code T84.60XA, T84.610A, T84.611A, T84.612A, T84.613A, T84.614A, T84.615A, T84.619A, T84.63XA, T84.69XA, T84.7XXA

0RGA0K0 Fusion of Thoracolumbar Vertebral Joint with Nonautologous Tissue Substitute, Anterior Approach, Anterior Column, Open Approach

- HAC When reported with secondary diagnosis code T84.60XA, T84.610A, T84.611A, T84.612A, T84.613A, T84.614A, T84.615A, T84.619A, T84.63XA, T84.69XA, T84.7XXA

0RGA0K1 Fusion of Thoracolumbar Vertebral Joint with Nonautologous Tissue Substitute, Posterior Approach, Posterior Column, Open Approach

Note Continued

♀ Female-only   ♂ Male-only   ▲ Limited Coverage   ● Non-OR   HAC HAC-associated procedure   ▲ Non-covered procedures   ✛ Combination

0RGA0K1 Continued Note

When reported with secondary diagnosis code T84.60XA, T84.610A, T84.611A, T84.612A, T84.613A, T84.614A, T84.615A, T84.619A, T84.63XA, T84.69XA, T84.7XXA

0RGA0KJ Fusion of Thoracolumbar Vertebral Joint with Nonautologous Tissue Substitute, Posterior Approach, Anterior Column, Open Approach

When reported with secondary diagnosis code T84.60XA, T84.610A, T84.611A, T84.612A, T84.613A, T84.614A, T84.615A, T84.619A, T84.63XA, T84.69XA, T84.7XXA

0RGA0Z0 Fusion of Thoracolumbar Vertebral Joint, Anterior Approach, Anterior Column, Open Approach

When reported with secondary diagnosis code T84.60XA, T84.610A, T84.611A, T84.612A, T84.613A, T84.614A, T84.615A, T84.619A, T84.63XA, T84.69XA, T84.7XXA

0RGA0Z1 Fusion of Thoracolumbar Vertebral Joint, Posterior Approach, Posterior Column, Open Approach

When reported with secondary diagnosis code T84.60XA, T84.610A, T84.611A, T84.612A, T84.613A, T84.614A, T84.615A, T84.619A, T84.63XA, T84.69XA, T84.7XXA

0RGA0ZJ Fusion of Thoracolumbar Vertebral Joint, Posterior Approach, Anterior Column, Open Approach

When reported with secondary diagnosis code T84.60XA, T84.610A, T84.611A, T84.612A, T84.613A, T84.614A, T84.615A, T84.619A, T84.63XA, T84.69XA, T84.7XXA

0RGA370 Fusion of Thoracolumbar Vertebral Joint with Autologous Tissue Substitute, Anterior Approach, Anterior Column, Percutaneous Approach

When reported with secondary diagnosis code T84.60XA, T84.610A, T84.611A, T84.612A, T84.613A, T84.614A, T84.615A, T84.619A, T84.63XA, T84.69XA, T84.7XXA

0RGA371 Fusion of Thoracolumbar Vertebral Joint with Autologous Tissue Substitute, Posterior Approach, Posterior Column, Percutaneous Approach

When reported with secondary diagnosis code T84.60XA, T84.610A, T84.611A, T84.612A, T84.613A, T84.614A, T84.615A, T84.619A, T84.63XA, T84.69XA, T84.7XXA

0RGA37J Fusion of Thoracolumbar Vertebral Joint with Autologous Tissue Substitute, Posterior Approach, Anterior Column, Percutaneous Approach

When reported with secondary diagnosis code T84.60XA, T84.610A, T84.611A, T84.612A, T84.613A, T84.614A, T84.615A, T84.619A, T84.63XA, T84.69XA, T84.7XXA

0RGA3A0 Fusion of Thoracolumbar Vertebral Joint with Interbody Fusion Device, Anterior Approach, Anterior Column, Percutaneous Approach

When reported with secondary diagnosis code T84.60XA, T84.610A, T84.611A, T84.612A, T84.613A, T84.614A, T84.615A, T84.619A, T84.63XA, T84.69XA, T84.7XXA

0RGA3A1 Fusion of Thoracolumbar Vertebral Joint with Interbody Fusion Device, Posterior Approach, Posterior Column, Percutaneous Approach

When reported with secondary diagnosis code T84.60XA, T84.610A, T84.611A, T84.612A, T84.613A, T84.614A, T84.615A, T84.619A, T84.63XA, T84.69XA, T84.7XXA

0RGA3AJ Fusion of Thoracolumbar Vertebral Joint with Interbody Fusion Device, Posterior Approach, Anterior Column, Percutaneous Approach

When reported with secondary diagnosis code T84.60XA, T84.610A, T84.611A, T84.612A, T84.613A, T84.614A, T84.615A, T84.619A, T84.63XA, T84.69XA, T84.7XXA

0RGA3J0 Fusion of Thoracolumbar Vertebral Joint with Synthetic Substitute, Anterior Approach, Anterior Column, Percutaneous Approach

When reported with secondary diagnosis code T84.60XA, T84.610A, T84.611A, T84.612A, T84.613A, T84.614A, T84.615A, T84.619A, T84.63XA, T84.69XA, T84.7XXA

0RGA3J1 Fusion of Thoracolumbar Vertebral Joint with Synthetic Substitute, Posterior Approach, Posterior Column, Percutaneous Approach

When reported with secondary diagnosis code T84.60XA, T84.610A, T84.611A, T84.612A, T84.613A, T84.614A, T84.615A, T84.619A, T84.63XA, T84.69XA, T84.7XXA

0RGA3JJ Fusion of Thoracolumbar Vertebral Joint with Synthetic Substitute, Posterior Approach, Anterior Column, Percutaneous Approach

When reported with secondary diagnosis code T84.60XA, T84.610A, T84.611A, T84.612A, T84.613A, T84.614A, T84.615A, T84.619A, T84.63XA, T84.69XA, T84.7XXA

0RGA3K0 Fusion of Thoracolumbar Vertebral Joint with Nonautologous Tissue Substitute, Anterior Approach, Anterior Column, Percutaneous Approach

When reported with secondary diagnosis code T84.60XA, T84.610A, T84.611A, T84.612A, T84.613A, T84.614A, T84.615A, T84.619A, T84.63XA, T84.69XA, T84.7XXA

0RGA3K1 Fusion of Thoracolumbar Vertebral Joint with Nonautologous Tissue Substitute, Posterior Approach, Posterior Column, Percutaneous Approach

When reported with secondary diagnosis code T84.60XA, T84.610A, T84.611A, T84.612A, T84.613A, T84.614A, T84.615A, T84.619A, T84.63XA, T84.69XA, T84.7XXA

0RGA3KJ Fusion of Thoracolumbar Vertebral Joint with Nonautologous Tissue Substitute, Posterior Approach, Anterior Column, Percutaneous Approach

When reported with secondary diagnosis code T84.60XA, T84.610A, T84.611A, T84.612A, T84.613A, T84.614A, T84.615A, T84.619A, T84.63XA, T84.69XA, T84.7XXA

0RGA3Z0 Fusion of Thoracolumbar Vertebral Joint, Anterior Approach, Anterior Column, Percutaneous Approach

When reported with secondary diagnosis code T84.60XA, T84.610A, T84.611A, T84.612A, T84.613A, T84.614A, T84.615A, T84.619A, T84.63XA, T84.69XA, T84.7XXA

0RGA3Z1 Fusion of Thoracolumbar Vertebral Joint, Posterior Approach, Posterior Column, Percutaneous Approach

When reported with secondary diagnosis code T84.60XA, T84.610A, T84.611A, T84.612A, T84.613A, T84.614A, T84.615A, T84.619A, T84.63XA, T84.69XA, T84.7XXA

0RGA3ZJ Fusion of Thoracolumbar Vertebral Joint, Posterior Approach, Anterior Column, Percutaneous Approach

When reported with secondary diagnosis code T84.60XA, T84.610A, T84.611A, T84.612A, T84.613A, T84.614A, T84.615A, T84.619A, T84.63XA, T84.69XA, T84.7XXA

0RGA470 Fusion of Thoracolumbar Vertebral Joint with Autologous Tissue Substitute, Anterior Approach, Anterior Column, Percutaneous Endoscopic Approach

When reported with secondary diagnosis code T84.60XA, T84.610A, T84.611A, T84.612A, T84.613A, T84.614A, T84.615A, T84.619A, T84.63XA, T84.69XA, T84.7XXA

0RGA471 Fusion of Thoracolumbar Vertebral Joint with Autologous Tissue Substitute, Posterior Approach, Posterior Column, Percutaneous Endoscopic Approach

When reported with secondary diagnosis code T84.60XA, T84.610A, T84.611A, T84.612A, T84.613A, T84.614A, T84.615A, T84.619A, T84.63XA, T84.69XA, T84.7XXA

0RGA47J Fusion of Thoracolumbar Vertebral Joint with Autologous Tissue Substitute, Posterior Approach, Anterior Column, Percutaneous Endoscopic Approach

When reported with secondary diagnosis code T84.60XA, T84.610A, T84.611A, T84.612A, T84.613A, T84.614A, T84.615A, T84.619A, T84.63XA, T84.69XA, T84.7XXA

0RGA4A0 Fusion of Thoracolumbar Vertebral Joint with Interbody Fusion Device, Anterior Approach, Anterior Column, Percutaneous Endoscopic Approach

When reported with secondary diagnosis code T84.60XA, T84.610A, T84.611A, T84.612A, T84.613A, T84.614A, T84.615A, T84.619A, T84.63XA, T84.69XA, T84.7XXA

0RGA4A1 Fusion of Thoracolumbar Vertebral Joint with Interbody Fusion Device, Posterior Approach, Posterior Column, Percutaneous Endoscopic Approach

When reported with secondary diagnosis code T84.60XA, T84.610A, T84.611A, T84.612A, T84.613A, T84.614A, T84.615A, T84.619A, T84.63XA, T84.69XA, T84.7XXA

0RGA4AJ Fusion of Thoracolumbar Vertebral Joint with Interbody Fusion Device, Posterior Approach, Anterior Column, Percutaneous Endoscopic Approach

When reported with secondary diagnosis code T84.60XA, T84.610A, T84.611A, T84.612A, T84.613A, T84.614A, T84.615A, T84.619A, T84.63XA, T84.69XA, T84.7XXA

0RGA4J0 Fusion of Thoracolumbar Vertebral Joint with Synthetic Substitute, Anterior Approach, Anterior Column, Percutaneous Endoscopic Approach

Note Continued

0RGA4J0 Continued Note

HAC When reported with secondary diagnosis code T84.60XA, T84.610A, T84.611A, T84.612A, T84.613A, T84.614A, T84.615A, T84.619A, T84.63XA, T84.69XA, T84.7XXA

0RGA4J1 Fusion of Thoracolumbar Vertebral Joint with Synthetic Substitute, Posterior Approach, Posterior Column, Percutaneous Endoscopic Approach

HAC When reported with secondary diagnosis code T84.60XA, T84.610A, T84.611A, T84.612A, T84.613A, T84.614A, T84.615A, T84.619A, T84.63XA, T84.69XA, T84.7XXA

0RGA4JJ Fusion of Thoracolumbar Vertebral Joint with Synthetic Substitute, Posterior Approach, Anterior Column, Percutaneous Endoscopic Approach

HAC When reported with secondary diagnosis code T84.60XA, T84.610A, T84.611A, T84.612A, T84.613A, T84.614A, T84.615A, T84.619A, T84.63XA, T84.69XA, T84.7XXA

0RGA4K0 Fusion of Thoracolumbar Vertebral Joint with Nonautologous Tissue Substitute, Anterior Approach, Anterior Column, Percutaneous Endoscopic Approach

HAC When reported with secondary diagnosis code T84.60XA, T84.610A, T84.611A, T84.612A, T84.613A, T84.614A, T84.615A, T84.619A, T84.63XA, T84.69XA, T84.7XXA

0RGA4K1 Fusion of Thoracolumbar Vertebral Joint with Nonautologous Tissue Substitute, Posterior Approach, Posterior Column, Percutaneous Endoscopic Approach

HAC When reported with secondary diagnosis code T84.60XA, T84.610A, T84.611A, T84.612A, T84.613A, T84.614A, T84.615A, T84.619A, T84.63XA, T84.69XA, T84.7XXA

0RGA4KJ Fusion of Thoracolumbar Vertebral Joint with Nonautologous Tissue Substitute, Posterior Approach, Anterior Column, Percutaneous Endoscopic Approach

HAC When reported with secondary diagnosis code T84.60XA, T84.610A, T84.611A, T84.612A, T84.613A, T84.614A, T84.615A, T84.619A, T84.63XA, T84.69XA, T84.7XXA

0RGA4Z0 Fusion of Thoracolumbar Vertebral Joint, Anterior Approach, Anterior Column, Percutaneous Endoscopic Approach

HAC When reported with secondary diagnosis code T84.60XA, T84.610A, T84.611A, T84.612A, T84.613A, T84.614A, T84.615A, T84.619A, T84.63XA, T84.69XA, T84.7XXA

0RGA4Z1 Fusion of Thoracolumbar Vertebral Joint, Posterior Approach, Posterior Column, Percutaneous Endoscopic Approach

HAC When reported with secondary diagnosis code T84.60XA, T84.610A, T84.611A, T84.612A, T84.613A, T84.614A, T84.615A, T84.619A, T84.63XA, T84.69XA, T84.7XXA

0RGA4ZJ Fusion of Thoracolumbar Vertebral Joint, Posterior Approach, Anterior Column, Percutaneous Endoscopic Approach

HAC When reported with secondary diagnosis code T84.60XA, T84.610A, T84.611A, T84.612A, T84.613A, T84.614A, T84.615A, T84.619A, T84.63XA, T84.69XA, T84.7XXA

0RGC04Z Fusion of Right Temporomandibular Joint with Internal Fixation Device, Open Approach

0RGC07Z Fusion of Right Temporomandibular Joint with Autologous Tissue Substitute, Open Approach

0RGC0JZ Fusion of Right Temporomandibular Joint with Synthetic Substitute, Open Approach

0RGC0KZ Fusion of Right Temporomandibular Joint with Nonautologous Tissue Substitute, Open Approach

0RGC0ZZ Fusion of Right Temporomandibular Joint, Open Approach

0RGC34Z Fusion of Right Temporomandibular Joint with Internal Fixation Device, Percutaneous Approach

0RGC37Z Fusion of Right Temporomandibular Joint with Autologous Tissue Substitute, Percutaneous Approach

0RGC3JZ Fusion of Right Temporomandibular Joint with Synthetic Substitute, Percutaneous Approach

0RGC3KZ Fusion of Right Temporomandibular Joint with Nonautologous Tissue Substitute, Percutaneous Approach

0RGC3ZZ Fusion of Right Temporomandibular Joint, Percutaneous Approach

0RGC44Z Fusion of Right Temporomandibular Joint with Internal Fixation Device, Percutaneous Endoscopic Approach

0RGC47Z Fusion of Right Temporomandibular Joint with Autologous Tissue Substitute, Percutaneous Endoscopic Approach

0RGC4JZ Fusion of Right Temporomandibular Joint with Synthetic Substitute, Percutaneous Endoscopic Approach

0RGC4KZ Fusion of Right Temporomandibular Joint with Nonautologous Tissue Substitute, Percutaneous Endoscopic Approach

0RGC4ZZ Fusion of Right Temporomandibular Joint, Percutaneous Endoscopic Approach

0RGD04Z Fusion of Left Temporomandibular Joint with Internal Fixation Device, Open Approach

0RGD07Z Fusion of Left Temporomandibular Joint with Autologous Tissue Substitute, Open Approach

0RGD0JZ Fusion of Left Temporomandibular Joint with Synthetic Substitute, Open Approach

0RGD0KZ Fusion of Left Temporomandibular Joint with Nonautologous Tissue Substitute, Open Approach

0RGD0ZZ Fusion of Left Temporomandibular Joint, Open Approach

0RGD34Z Fusion of Left Temporomandibular Joint with Internal Fixation Device, Percutaneous Approach

0RGD37Z Fusion of Left Temporomandibular Joint with Autologous Tissue Substitute, Percutaneous Approach

0RGD3JZ Fusion of Left Temporomandibular Joint with Synthetic Substitute, Percutaneous Approach

0RGD3KZ Fusion of Left Temporomandibular Joint with Nonautologous Tissue Substitute, Percutaneous Approach

0RGD3ZZ Fusion of Left Temporomandibular Joint, Percutaneous Approach

0RGD44Z Fusion of Left Temporomandibular Joint with Internal Fixation Device, Percutaneous Endoscopic Approach

0RGD47Z Fusion of Left Temporomandibular Joint with Autologous Tissue Substitute, Percutaneous Endoscopic Approach

0RGD4JZ Fusion of Left Temporomandibular Joint with Synthetic Substitute, Percutaneous Endoscopic Approach

0RGD4KZ Fusion of Left Temporomandibular Joint with Nonautologous Tissue Substitute, Percutaneous Endoscopic Approach

0RGD4ZZ Fusion of Left Temporomandibular Joint, Percutaneous Endoscopic Approach

0RGE04Z Fusion of Right Sternoclavicular Joint with Internal Fixation Device, Open Approach

HAC When reported with secondary diagnosis code T84.60XA, T84.610A, T84.611A, T84.612A, T84.613A, T84.614A, T84.615A, T84.619A, T84.63XA, T84.69XA, T84.7XXA

0RGE07Z Fusion of Right Sternoclavicular Joint with Autologous Tissue Substitute, Open Approach

HAC When reported with secondary diagnosis code T84.60XA, T84.610A, T84.611A, T84.612A, T84.613A, T84.614A, T84.615A, T84.619A, T84.63XA, T84.69XA, T84.7XXA

0RGE0JZ Fusion of Right Sternoclavicular Joint with Synthetic Substitute, Open Approach

HAC When reported with secondary diagnosis code T84.60XA, T84.610A, T84.611A, T84.612A, T84.613A, T84.614A, T84.615A, T84.619A, T84.63XA, T84.69XA, T84.7XXA

0RGE0KZ Fusion of Right Sternoclavicular Joint with Nonautologous Tissue Substitute, Open Approach

HAC When reported with secondary diagnosis code T84.60XA, T84.610A, T84.611A, T84.612A, T84.613A, T84.614A, T84.615A, T84.619A, T84.63XA, T84.69XA, T84.7XXA

0RGE0ZZ Fusion of Right Sternoclavicular Joint, Open Approach

HAC When reported with secondary diagnosis code T84.60XA, T84.610A, T84.611A, T84.612A, T84.613A, T84.614A, T84.615A, T84.619A, T84.63XA, T84.69XA, T84.7XXA

0RGE34Z Fusion of Right Sternoclavicular Joint with Internal Fixation Device, Percutaneous Approach

HAC When reported with secondary diagnosis code T84.60XA, T84.610A, T84.611A, T84.612A, T84.613A, T84.614A, T84.615A, T84.619A, T84.63XA, T84.69XA, T84.7XXA

0RGE37Z Fusion of Right Sternoclavicular Joint with Autologous Tissue Substitute, Percutaneous Approach

HAC When reported with secondary diagnosis code T84.60XA, T84.610A, T84.611A, T84.612A, T84.613A, T84.614A, T84.615A, T84.619A, T84.63XA, T84.69XA, T84.7XXA

0RGE3JZ Fusion of Right Sternoclavicular Joint with Synthetic Substitute, Percutaneous Approach

HAC When reported with secondary diagnosis code T84.60XA, T84.610A, T84.611A, T84.612A, T84.613A, T84.614A, T84.615A, T84.619A, T84.63XA, T84.69XA, T84.7XXA

0RGE3KZ Fusion of Right Sternoclavicular Joint with Nonautologous Tissue Substitute, Percutaneous Approach

HAC When reported with secondary diagnosis code T84.60XA, T84.610A, T84.611A, T84.612A, T84.613A, T84.614A, T84.615A, T84.619A, T84.63XA, T84.69XA, T84.7XXA

921

0RGE3ZZ Fusion of Right Sternoclavicular Joint, Percutaneous Approach

⬛ When reported with secondary diagnosis code T84.60XA, T84.610A, T84.611A, T84.612A, T84.613A, T84.614A, T84.615A, T84.619A, T84.63XA, T84.69XA, T84.7XXA

0RGE44Z Fusion of Right Sternoclavicular Joint with Internal Fixation Device, Percutaneous Endoscopic Approach

⬛ When reported with secondary diagnosis code T84.60XA, T84.610A, T84.611A, T84.612A, T84.613A, T84.614A, T84.615A, T84.619A, T84.63XA, T84.69XA, T84.7XXA

0RGE47Z Fusion of Right Sternoclavicular Joint with Autologous Tissue Substitute, Percutaneous Endoscopic Approach

⬛ When reported with secondary diagnosis code T84.60XA, T84.610A, T84.611A, T84.612A, T84.613A, T84.614A, T84.615A, T84.619A, T84.63XA, T84.69XA, T84.7XXA

0RGE4JZ Fusion of Right Sternoclavicular Joint with Synthetic Substitute, Percutaneous Endoscopic Approach

⬛ When reported with secondary diagnosis code T84.60XA, T84.610A, T84.611A, T84.612A, T84.613A, T84.614A, T84.615A, T84.619A, T84.63XA, T84.69XA, T84.7XXA

0RGE4KZ Fusion of Right Sternoclavicular Joint with Nonautologous Tissue Substitute, Percutaneous Endoscopic Approach

⬛ When reported with secondary diagnosis code T84.60XA, T84.610A, T84.611A, T84.612A, T84.613A, T84.614A, T84.615A, T84.619A, T84.63XA, T84.69XA, T84.7XXA

0RGE4ZZ Fusion of Right Sternoclavicular Joint, Percutaneous Endoscopic Approach

⬛ When reported with secondary diagnosis code T84.60XA, T84.610A, T84.611A, T84.612A, T84.613A, T84.614A, T84.615A, T84.619A, T84.63XA, T84.69XA, T84.7XXA

0RGF04Z Fusion of Left Sternoclavicular Joint with Internal Fixation Device, Open Approach

⬛ When reported with secondary diagnosis code T84.60XA, T84.610A, T84.611A, T84.612A, T84.613A, T84.614A, T84.615A, T84.619A, T84.63XA, T84.69XA, T84.7XXA

0RGF07Z Fusion of Left Sternoclavicular Joint with Autologous Tissue Substitute, Open Approach

⬛ When reported with secondary diagnosis code T84.60XA, T84.610A, T84.611A, T84.612A, T84.613A, T84.614A, T84.615A, T84.619A, T84.63XA, T84.69XA, T84.7XXA

0RGF0JZ Fusion of Left Sternoclavicular Joint with Synthetic Substitute, Open Approach

⬛ When reported with secondary diagnosis code T84.60XA, T84.610A, T84.611A, T84.612A, T84.613A, T84.614A, T84.615A, T84.619A, T84.63XA, T84.69XA, T84.7XXA

0RGF0KZ Fusion of Left Sternoclavicular Joint with Nonautologous Tissue Substitute, Open Approach

⬛ When reported with secondary diagnosis code T84.60XA, T84.610A, T84.611A, T84.612A, T84.613A, T84.614A, T84.615A, T84.619A, T84.63XA, T84.69XA, T84.7XXA

0RGF0ZZ Fusion of Left Sternoclavicular Joint, Open Approach

⬛ When reported with secondary diagnosis code T84.60XA, T84.610A, T84.611A, T84.612A, T84.613A, T84.614A, T84.615A, T84.619A, T84.63XA, T84.69XA, T84.7XXA

0RGF34Z Fusion of Left Sternoclavicular Joint with Internal Fixation Device, Percutaneous Approach

⬛ When reported with secondary diagnosis code T84.60XA, T84.610A, T84.611A, T84.612A, T84.613A, T84.614A, T84.615A, T84.619A, T84.63XA, T84.69XA, T84.7XXA

0RGF37Z Fusion of Left Sternoclavicular Joint with Autologous Tissue Substitute, Percutaneous Approach

⬛ When reported with secondary diagnosis code T84.60XA, T84.610A, T84.611A, T84.612A, T84.613A, T84.614A, T84.615A, T84.619A, T84.63XA, T84.69XA, T84.7XXA

0RGF3JZ Fusion of Left Sternoclavicular Joint with Synthetic Substitute, Percutaneous Approach

⬛ When reported with secondary diagnosis code T84.60XA, T84.610A, T84.611A, T84.612A, T84.613A, T84.614A, T84.615A, T84.619A, T84.63XA, T84.69XA, T84.7XXA

0RGF3KZ Fusion of Left Sternoclavicular Joint with Nonautologous Tissue Substitute, Percutaneous Approach

⬛ When reported with secondary diagnosis code T84.60XA, T84.610A, T84.611A, T84.612A, T84.613A, T84.614A, T84.615A, T84.619A, T84.63XA, T84.69XA, T84.7XXA

0RGF3ZZ Fusion of Left Sternoclavicular Joint, Percutaneous Approach

⬛ When reported with secondary diagnosis code T84.60XA, T84.610A, T84.611A, T84.612A, T84.613A, T84.614A, T84.615A, T84.619A, T84.63XA, T84.69XA, T84.7XXA

0RGF44Z Fusion of Left Sternoclavicular Joint with Internal Fixation Device, Percutaneous Endoscopic Approach

⬛ When reported with secondary diagnosis code T84.60XA, T84.610A, T84.611A, T84.612A, T84.613A, T84.614A, T84.615A, T84.619A, T84.63XA, T84.69XA, T84.7XXA

0RGF47Z Fusion of Left Sternoclavicular Joint with Autologous Tissue Substitute, Percutaneous Endoscopic Approach

⬛ When reported with secondary diagnosis code T84.60XA, T84.610A, T84.611A, T84.612A, T84.613A, T84.614A, T84.615A, T84.619A, T84.63XA, T84.69XA, T84.7XXA

0RGF4JZ Fusion of Left Sternoclavicular Joint with Synthetic Substitute, Percutaneous Endoscopic Approach

⬛ When reported with secondary diagnosis code T84.60XA, T84.610A, T84.611A, T84.612A, T84.613A, T84.614A, T84.615A, T84.619A, T84.63XA, T84.69XA, T84.7XXA

0RGF4KZ Fusion of Left Sternoclavicular Joint with Nonautologous Tissue Substitute, Percutaneous Endoscopic Approach

⬛ When reported with secondary diagnosis code T84.60XA, T84.610A, T84.611A, T84.612A, T84.613A, T84.614A, T84.615A, T84.619A, T84.63XA, T84.69XA, T84.7XXA

0RGF4ZZ Fusion of Left Sternoclavicular Joint, Percutaneous Endoscopic Approach

⬛ When reported with secondary diagnosis code T84.60XA, T84.610A, T84.611A, T84.612A, T84.613A, T84.614A, T84.615A, T84.619A, T84.63XA, T84.69XA, T84.7XXA

0RGG04Z Fusion of Right Acromioclavicular Joint with Internal Fixation Device, Open Approach

⬛ When reported with secondary diagnosis code T84.60XA, T84.610A, T84.611A, T84.612A, T84.613A, T84.614A, T84.615A, T84.619A, T84.63XA, T84.69XA, T84.7XXA

0RGG07Z Fusion of Right Acromioclavicular Joint with Autologous Tissue Substitute, Open Approach

⬛ When reported with secondary diagnosis code T84.60XA, T84.610A, T84.611A, T84.612A, T84.613A, T84.614A, T84.615A, T84.619A, T84.63XA, T84.69XA, T84.7XXA

0RGG0JZ Fusion of Right Acromioclavicular Joint with Synthetic Substitute, Open Approach

⬛ When reported with secondary diagnosis code T84.60XA, T84.610A, T84.611A, T84.612A, T84.613A, T84.614A, T84.615A, T84.619A, T84.63XA, T84.69XA, T84.7XXA

0RGG0KZ Fusion of Right Acromioclavicular Joint with Nonautologous Tissue Substitute, Open Approach

⬛ When reported with secondary diagnosis code T84.60XA, T84.610A, T84.611A, T84.612A, T84.613A, T84.614A, T84.615A, T84.619A, T84.63XA, T84.69XA, T84.7XXA

0RGG0ZZ Fusion of Right Acromioclavicular Joint, Open Approach

⬛ When reported with secondary diagnosis code T84.60XA, T84.610A, T84.611A, T84.612A, T84.613A, T84.614A, T84.615A, T84.619A, T84.63XA, T84.69XA, T84.7XXA

0RGG34Z Fusion of Right Acromioclavicular Joint with Internal Fixation Device, Percutaneous Approach

⬛ When reported with secondary diagnosis code T84.60XA, T84.610A, T84.611A, T84.612A, T84.613A, T84.614A, T84.615A, T84.619A, T84.63XA, T84.69XA, T84.7XXA

0RGG37Z Fusion of Right Acromioclavicular Joint with Autologous Tissue Substitute, Percutaneous Approach

⬛ When reported with secondary diagnosis code T84.60XA, T84.610A, T84.611A, T84.612A, T84.613A, T84.614A, T84.615A, T84.619A, T84.63XA, T84.69XA, T84.7XXA

0RGG3JZ Fusion of Right Acromioclavicular Joint with Synthetic Substitute, Percutaneous Approach

⬛ When reported with secondary diagnosis code T84.60XA, T84.610A, T84.611A, T84.612A, T84.613A, T84.614A, T84.615A, T84.619A, T84.63XA, T84.69XA, T84.7XXA

0RGG3KZ Fusion of Right Acromioclavicular Joint with Nonautologous Tissue Substitute, Percutaneous Approach

⬛ When reported with secondary diagnosis code T84.60XA, T84.610A, T84.611A, T84.612A, T84.613A, T84.614A, T84.615A, T84.619A, T84.63XA, T84.69XA, T84.7XXA

♀ Female-only   ♂ Male-only   ▲ Limited Coverage   ● Non-OR   ⬛ HAC-associated procedure   ▲ Non-covered procedures   ✚ Combination

RGG3ZZ Fusion of Right Acromioclavicular Joint, Percutaneous Approach
- ▣ When reported with secondary diagnosis code T84.60XA, T84.610A, T84.611A, T84.612A, T84.613A, T84.614A, T84.615A, T84.619A, T84.63XA, T84.69XA, T84.7XXA

RGG44Z Fusion of Right Acromioclavicular Joint with Internal Fixation Device, Percutaneous Endoscopic Approach
- ▣ When reported with secondary diagnosis code T84.60XA, T84.610A, T84.611A, T84.612A, T84.613A, T84.614A, T84.615A, T84.619A, T84.63XA, T84.69XA, T84.7XXA

RGG47Z Fusion of Right Acromioclavicular Joint with Autologous Tissue Substitute, Percutaneous Endoscopic Approach
- ▣ When reported with secondary diagnosis code T84.60XA, T84.610A, T84.611A, T84.612A, T84.613A, T84.614A, T84.615A, T84.619A, T84.63XA, T84.69XA, T84.7XXA

RGG4JZ Fusion of Right Acromioclavicular Joint with Synthetic Substitute, Percutaneous Endoscopic Approach
- ▣ When reported with secondary diagnosis code T84.60XA, T84.610A, T84.611A, T84.612A, T84.613A, T84.614A, T84.615A, T84.619A, T84.63XA, T84.69XA, T84.7XXA

RGG4KZ Fusion of Right Acromioclavicular Joint with Nonautologous Tissue Substitute, Percutaneous Endoscopic Approach
- ▣ When reported with secondary diagnosis code T84.60XA, T84.610A, T84.611A, T84.612A, T84.613A, T84.614A, T84.615A, T84.619A, T84.63XA, T84.69XA, T84.7XXA

RGG4ZZ Fusion of Right Acromioclavicular Joint, Percutaneous Endoscopic Approach
- ▣ When reported with secondary diagnosis code T84.60XA, T84.610A, T84.611A, T84.612A, T84.613A, T84.614A, T84.615A, T84.619A, T84.63XA, T84.69XA, T84.7XXA

0RGH04Z Fusion of Left Acromioclavicular Joint with Internal Fixation Device, Open Approach
- ▣ When reported with secondary diagnosis code T84.60XA, T84.610A, T84.611A, T84.612A, T84.613A, T84.614A, T84.615A, T84.619A, T84.63XA, T84.69XA, T84.7XXA

0RGH07Z Fusion of Left Acromioclavicular Joint with Autologous Tissue Substitute, Open Approach
- ▣ When reported with secondary diagnosis code T84.60XA, T84.610A, T84.611A, T84.612A, T84.613A, T84.614A, T84.615A, T84.619A, T84.63XA, T84.69XA, T84.7XXA

0RGH0JZ Fusion of Left Acromioclavicular Joint with Synthetic Substitute, Open Approach
- ▣ When reported with secondary diagnosis code T84.60XA, T84.610A, T84.611A, T84.612A, T84.613A, T84.614A, T84.615A, T84.619A, T84.63XA, T84.69XA, T84.7XXA

0RGH0KZ Fusion of Left Acromioclavicular Joint with Nonautologous Tissue Substitute, Open Approach
- ▣ When reported with secondary diagnosis code T84.60XA, T84.610A, T84.611A, T84.612A, T84.613A, T84.614A, T84.615A, T84.619A, T84.63XA, T84.69XA, T84.7XXA

0RGH0ZZ Fusion of Left Acromioclavicular Joint, Open Approach
- ▣ When reported with secondary diagnosis code T84.60XA, T84.610A, T84.611A, T84.612A, T84.613A, T84.614A, T84.615A, T84.619A, T84.63XA, T84.69XA, T84.7XXA

0RGH34Z Fusion of Left Acromioclavicular Joint with Internal Fixation Device, Percutaneous Approach
- ▣ When reported with secondary diagnosis code T84.60XA, T84.610A, T84.611A, T84.612A, T84.613A, T84.614A, T84.615A, T84.619A, T84.63XA, T84.69XA, T84.7XXA

0RGH37Z Fusion of Left Acromioclavicular Joint with Autologous Tissue Substitute, Percutaneous Approach
- ▣ When reported with secondary diagnosis code T84.60XA, T84.610A, T84.611A, T84.612A, T84.613A, T84.614A, T84.615A, T84.619A, T84.63XA, T84.69XA, T84.7XXA

0RGH3JZ Fusion of Left Acromioclavicular Joint with Synthetic Substitute, Percutaneous Approach
- ▣ When reported with secondary diagnosis code T84.60XA, T84.610A, T84.611A, T84.612A, T84.613A, T84.614A, T84.615A, T84.619A, T84.63XA, T84.69XA, T84.7XXA

0RGH3KZ Fusion of Left Acromioclavicular Joint with Nonautologous Tissue Substitute, Percutaneous Approach
- ▣ When reported with secondary diagnosis code T84.60XA, T84.610A, T84.611A, T84.612A, T84.613A, T84.614A, T84.615A, T84.619A, T84.63XA, T84.69XA, T84.7XXA

0RGH3ZZ Fusion of Left Acromioclavicular Joint, Percutaneous Approach
- ▣ When reported with secondary diagnosis code T84.60XA, T84.610A, T84.611A, T84.612A, T84.613A, T84.614A, T84.615A, T84.619A, T84.63XA, T84.69XA, T84.7XXA

0RGH44Z Fusion of Left Acromioclavicular Joint with Internal Fixation Device, Percutaneous Endoscopic Approach
- ▣ When reported with secondary diagnosis code T84.60XA, T84.610A, T84.611A, T84.612A, T84.613A, T84.614A, T84.615A, T84.619A, T84.63XA, T84.69XA, T84.7XXA

0RGH47Z Fusion of Left Acromioclavicular Joint with Autologous Tissue Substitute, Percutaneous Endoscopic Approach
- ▣ When reported with secondary diagnosis code T84.60XA, T84.610A, T84.611A, T84.612A, T84.613A, T84.614A, T84.615A, T84.619A, T84.63XA, T84.69XA, T84.7XXA

0RGH4JZ Fusion of Left Acromioclavicular Joint with Synthetic Substitute, Percutaneous Endoscopic Approach
- ▣ When reported with secondary diagnosis code T84.60XA, T84.610A, T84.611A, T84.612A, T84.613A, T84.614A, T84.615A, T84.619A, T84.63XA, T84.69XA, T84.7XXA

0RGH4KZ Fusion of Left Acromioclavicular Joint with Nonautologous Tissue Substitute, Percutaneous Endoscopic Approach
- ▣ When reported with secondary diagnosis code T84.60XA, T84.610A, T84.611A, T84.612A, T84.613A, T84.614A, T84.615A, T84.619A, T84.63XA, T84.69XA, T84.7XXA

0RGJ04Z Fusion of Right Shoulder Joint with Internal Fixation Device, Open Approach
- ▣ When reported with secondary diagnosis code T84.60XA, T84.610A, T84.611A, T84.612A, T84.613A, T84.614A, T84.615A, T84.619A, T84.63XA, T84.69XA, T84.7XXA

0RGJ07Z Fusion of Right Shoulder Joint with Autologous Tissue Substitute, Open Approach
- ▣ When reported with secondary diagnosis code T84.60XA, T84.610A, T84.611A, T84.612A, T84.613A, T84.614A, T84.615A, T84.619A, T84.63XA, T84.69XA, T84.7XXA

0RGJ0JZ Fusion of Right Shoulder Joint with Synthetic Substitute, Open Approach
- ▣ When reported with secondary diagnosis code T84.60XA, T84.610A, T84.611A, T84.612A, T84.613A, T84.614A, T84.615A, T84.619A, T84.63XA, T84.69XA, T84.7XXA

0RGJ0KZ Fusion of Right Shoulder Joint with Nonautologous Tissue Substitute, Open Approach
- ▣ When reported with secondary diagnosis code T84.60XA, T84.610A, T84.611A, T84.612A, T84.613A, T84.614A, T84.615A, T84.619A, T84.63XA, T84.69XA, T84.7XXA

0RGJ0ZZ Fusion of Right Shoulder Joint, Open Approach
- ▣ When reported with secondary diagnosis code T84.60XA, T84.610A, T84.611A, T84.612A, T84.613A, T84.614A, T84.615A, T84.619A, T84.63XA, T84.69XA, T84.7XXA

0RGJ34Z Fusion of Right Shoulder Joint with Internal Fixation Device, Percutaneous Approach
- ▣ When reported with secondary diagnosis code T84.60XA, T84.610A, T84.611A, T84.612A, T84.613A, T84.614A, T84.615A, T84.619A, T84.63XA, T84.69XA, T84.7XXA

0RGJ37Z Fusion of Right Shoulder Joint with Autologous Tissue Substitute, Percutaneous Approach
- ▣ When reported with secondary diagnosis code T84.60XA, T84.610A, T84.611A, T84.612A, T84.613A, T84.614A, T84.615A, T84.619A, T84.63XA, T84.69XA, T84.7XXA

0RGJ3JZ Fusion of Right Shoulder Joint with Synthetic Substitute, Percutaneous Approach
- ▣ When reported with secondary diagnosis code T84.60XA, T84.610A, T84.611A, T84.612A, T84.613A, T84.614A, T84.615A, T84.619A, T84.63XA, T84.69XA, T84.7XXA

0RGJ3KZ Fusion of Right Shoulder Joint with Nonautologous Tissue Substitute, Percutaneous Approach
- ▣ When reported with secondary diagnosis code T84.60XA, T84.610A, T84.611A, T84.612A, T84.613A, T84.614A, T84.615A, T84.619A, T84.63XA, T84.69XA, T84.7XXA

♀ Female-only   ♂ Male-only   ▲ Limited Coverage   ● Non-OR   ▣ HAC-associated procedure   ▲ Non-covered procedures   ＋ Combination

0RGJ3ZZ Fusion of Right Shoulder Joint, Percutaneous Approach
- When reported with secondary diagnosis code T84.60XA, T84.610A, T84.611A, T84.612A, T84.613A, T84.614A, T84.615A, T84.619A, T84.63XA, T84.69XA, T84.7XXA

0RGJ44Z Fusion of Right Shoulder Joint with Internal Fixation Device, Percutaneous Endoscopic Approach
- When reported with secondary diagnosis code T84.60XA, T84.610A, T84.611A, T84.612A, T84.613A, T84.614A, T84.615A, T84.619A, T84.63XA, T84.69XA, T84.7XXA

0RGJ47Z Fusion of Right Shoulder Joint with Autologous Tissue Substitute, Percutaneous Endoscopic Approach
- When reported with secondary diagnosis code T84.60XA, T84.610A, T84.611A, T84.612A, T84.613A, T84.614A, T84.615A, T84.619A, T84.63XA, T84.69XA, T84.7XXA

0RGJ4JZ Fusion of Right Shoulder Joint with Synthetic Substitute, Percutaneous Endoscopic Approach
- When reported with secondary diagnosis code T84.60XA, T84.610A, T84.611A, T84.612A, T84.613A, T84.614A, T84.615A, T84.619A, T84.63XA, T84.69XA, T84.7XXA

0RGJ4KZ Fusion of Right Shoulder Joint with Nonautologous Tissue Substitute, Percutaneous Endoscopic Approach
- When reported with secondary diagnosis code T84.60XA, T84.610A, T84.611A, T84.612A, T84.613A, T84.614A, T84.615A, T84.619A, T84.63XA, T84.69XA, T84.7XXA

0RGJ4ZZ Fusion of Right Shoulder Joint, Percutaneous Endoscopic Approach
- When reported with secondary diagnosis code T84.60XA, T84.610A, T84.611A, T84.612A, T84.613A, T84.614A, T84.615A, T84.619A, T84.63XA, T84.69XA, T84.7XXA

0RGK04Z Fusion of Left Shoulder Joint with Internal Fixation Device, Open Approach
- When reported with secondary diagnosis code T84.60XA, T84.610A, T84.611A, T84.612A, T84.613A, T84.614A, T84.615A, T84.619A, T84.63XA, T84.69XA, T84.7XXA

0RGK07Z Fusion of Left Shoulder Joint with Autologous Tissue Substitute, Open Approach
- When reported with secondary diagnosis code T84.60XA, T84.610A, T84.611A, T84.612A, T84.613A, T84.614A, T84.615A, T84.619A, T84.63XA, T84.69XA, T84.7XXA

0RGK0JZ Fusion of Left Shoulder Joint with Synthetic Substitute, Open Approach
- When reported with secondary diagnosis code T84.60XA, T84.610A, T84.611A, T84.612A, T84.613A, T84.614A, T84.615A, T84.619A, T84.63XA, T84.69XA, T84.7XXA

0RGK0KZ Fusion of Left Shoulder Joint with Nonautologous Tissue Substitute, Open Approach
- When reported with secondary diagnosis code T84.60XA, T84.610A, T84.611A, T84.612A, T84.613A, T84.614A, T84.615A, T84.619A, T84.63XA, T84.69XA, T84.7XXA

0RGK0ZZ Fusion of Left Shoulder Joint, Open Approach
- When reported with secondary diagnosis code T84.60XA, T84.610A, T84.611A, T84.612A, T84.613A, T84.614A, T84.615A, T84.619A, T84.63XA, T84.69XA, T84.7XXA

0RGK34Z Fusion of Left Shoulder Joint with Internal Fixation Device, Percutaneous Approach
- When reported with secondary diagnosis code T84.60XA, T84.610A, T84.611A, T84.612A, T84.613A, T84.614A, T84.615A, T84.619A, T84.63XA, T84.69XA, T84.7XXA

0RGK37Z Fusion of Left Shoulder Joint with Autologous Tissue Substitute, Percutaneous Approach
- When reported with secondary diagnosis code T84.60XA, T84.610A, T84.611A, T84.612A, T84.613A, T84.614A, T84.615A, T84.619A, T84.63XA, T84.69XA, T84.7XXA

0RGK3JZ Fusion of Left Shoulder Joint with Synthetic Substitute, Percutaneous Approach
- When reported with secondary diagnosis code T84.60XA, T84.610A, T84.611A, T84.612A, T84.613A, T84.614A, T84.615A, T84.619A, T84.63XA, T84.69XA, T84.7XXA

0RGK3KZ Fusion of Left Shoulder Joint with Nonautologous Tissue Substitute, Percutaneous Approach
- When reported with secondary diagnosis code T84.60XA, T84.610A, T84.611A, T84.612A, T84.613A, T84.614A, T84.615A, T84.619A, T84.63XA, T84.69XA, T84.7XXA

0RGK3ZZ Fusion of Left Shoulder Joint, Percutaneous Approach
- When reported with secondary diagnosis code T84.60XA, T84.610A, T84.611A, T84.612A, T84.613A, T84.614A, T84.615A, T84.619A, T84.63XA, T84.69XA, T84.7XXA

0RGK44Z Fusion of Left Shoulder Joint with Internal Fixation Device, Percutaneous Endoscopic Approach
- When reported with secondary diagnosis code T84.60XA, T84.610A, T84.611A, T84.612A, T84.613A, T84.614A, T84.615A, T84.619A, T84.63XA, T84.69XA, T84.7XXA

0RGK47Z Fusion of Left Shoulder Joint with Autologous Tissue Substitute, Percutaneous Endoscopic Approach
- When reported with secondary diagnosis code T84.60XA, T84.610A, T84.611A, T84.612A, T84.613A, T84.614A, T84.615A, T84.619A, T84.63XA, T84.69XA, T84.7XXA

0RGK4JZ Fusion of Left Shoulder Joint with Synthetic Substitute, Percutaneous Endoscopic Approach
- When reported with secondary diagnosis code T84.60XA, T84.610A, T84.611A, T84.612A, T84.613A, T84.614A, T84.615A, T84.619A, T84.63XA, T84.69XA, T84.7XXA

0RGK4KZ Fusion of Left Shoulder Joint with Nonautologous Tissue Substitute, Percutaneous Endoscopic Approach
- When reported with secondary diagnosis code T84.60XA, T84.610A, T84.611A, T84.612A, T84.613A, T84.614A, T84.615A, T84.619A, T84.63XA, T84.69XA, T84.7XXA

0RGL04Z Fusion of Right Elbow Joint with Internal Fixation Device, Open Approach
- When reported with secondary diagnosis code T84.60XA, T84.610A, T84.611A, T84.612A, T84.613A, T84.614A, T84.615A, T84.619A, T84.63XA, T84.69XA, T84.7XXA

0RGL05Z Fusion of Right Elbow Joint with External Fixation Device, Open Approach
- When reported with secondary diagnosis code T84.60XA, T84.610A, T84.611A, T84.612A, T84.613A, T84.614A, T84.615A, T84.619A, T84.63XA, T84.69XA, T84.7XXA

0RGL07Z Fusion of Right Elbow Joint with Autologous Tissue Substitute, Open Approach
- When reported with secondary diagnosis code T84.60XA, T84.610A, T84.611A, T84.612A, T84.613A, T84.614A, T84.615A, T84.619A, T84.63XA, T84.69XA, T84.7XXA

0RGL0JZ Fusion of Right Elbow Joint with Synthetic Substitute, Open Approach
- When reported with secondary diagnosis code T84.60XA, T84.610A, T84.611A, T84.612A, T84.613A, T84.614A, T84.615A, T84.619A, T84.63XA, T84.69XA, T84.7XXA

0RGL0KZ Fusion of Right Elbow Joint with Nonautologous Tissue Substitute, Open Approach
- When reported with secondary diagnosis code T84.60XA, T84.610A, T84.611A, T84.612A, T84.613A, T84.614A, T84.615A, T84.619A, T84.63XA, T84.69XA, T84.7XXA

0RGL0ZZ Fusion of Right Elbow Joint, Open Approach
- When reported with secondary diagnosis code T84.60XA, T84.610A, T84.611A, T84.612A, T84.613A, T84.614A, T84.615A, T84.619A, T84.63XA, T84.69XA, T84.7XXA

0RGL34Z Fusion of Right Elbow Joint with Internal Fixation Device, Percutaneous Approach
- When reported with secondary diagnosis code T84.60XA, T84.610A, T84.611A, T84.612A, T84.613A, T84.614A, T84.615A, T84.619A, T84.63XA, T84.69XA, T84.7XXA

0RGL35Z Fusion of Right Elbow Joint with External Fixation Device, Percutaneous Approach
- When reported with secondary diagnosis code T84.60XA, T84.610A, T84.611A, T84.612A, T84.613A, T84.614A, T84.615A, T84.619A, T84.63XA, T84.69XA, T84.7XXA

0RGL37Z Fusion of Right Elbow Joint with Autologous Tissue Substitute, Percutaneous Approach
- When reported with secondary diagnosis code T84.60XA, T84.610A, T84.611A, T84.612A, T84.613A, T84.614A, T84.615A, T84.619A, T84.63XA, T84.69XA, T84.7XXA

0RGL3JZ Fusion of Right Elbow Joint with Synthetic Substitute, Percutaneous Approach

Note Continued

♀ Female-only   ♂ Male-only   ▲ Limited Coverage   ● Non-OR   ▦ HAC-associated procedure   ▲ Non-covered procedures   ✚ Combination

GL3JZ Continued Note

- When reported with secondary diagnosis code T84.60XA, T84.610A, T84.611A, T84.612A, T84.613A, T84.614A, T84.615A, T84.619A, T84.63XA, T84.69XA, T84.7XXA

GL3KZ Fusion of Right Elbow Joint with Nonautologous Tissue Substitute, Percutaneous Approach
- When reported with secondary diagnosis code T84.60XA, T84.610A, T84.611A, T84.612A, T84.613A, T84.614A, T84.615A, T84.619A, T84.63XA, T84.69XA, T84.7XXA

GL3ZZ Fusion of Right Elbow Joint, Percutaneous Approach
- When reported with secondary diagnosis code T84.60XA, T84.610A, T84.611A, T84.612A, T84.613A, T84.614A, T84.615A, T84.619A, T84.63XA, T84.69XA, T84.7XXA

GL44Z Fusion of Right Elbow Joint with Internal Fixation Device, Percutaneous Endoscopic Approach
- When reported with secondary diagnosis code T84.60XA, T84.610A, T84.611A, T84.612A, T84.613A, T84.614A, T84.615A, T84.619A, T84.63XA, T84.69XA, T84.7XXA

GL45Z Fusion of Right Elbow Joint with External Fixation Device, Percutaneous Endoscopic Approach
- When reported with secondary diagnosis code T84.60XA, T84.610A, T84.611A, T84.612A, T84.613A, T84.614A, T84.615A, T84.619A, T84.63XA, T84.69XA, T84.7XXA

GL47Z Fusion of Right Elbow Joint with Autologous Tissue Substitute, Percutaneous Endoscopic Approach
- When reported with secondary diagnosis code T84.60XA, T84.610A, T84.611A, T84.612A, T84.613A, T84.614A, T84.615A, T84.619A, T84.63XA, T84.69XA, T84.7XXA

GL4JZ Fusion of Right Elbow Joint with Synthetic Substitute, Percutaneous Endoscopic Approach
- When reported with secondary diagnosis code T84.60XA, T84.610A, T84.611A, T84.612A, T84.613A, T84.614A, T84.615A, T84.619A, T84.63XA, T84.69XA, T84.7XXA

GL4KZ Fusion of Right Elbow Joint with Nonautologous Tissue Substitute, Percutaneous Endoscopic Approach
- When reported with secondary diagnosis code T84.60XA, T84.610A, T84.611A, T84.612A, T84.613A, T84.614A, T84.615A, T84.619A, T84.63XA, T84.69XA, T84.7XXA

GL4ZZ Fusion of Right Elbow Joint, Percutaneous Endoscopic Approach
- When reported with secondary diagnosis code T84.60XA, T84.610A, T84.611A, T84.612A, T84.613A, T84.614A, T84.615A, T84.619A, T84.63XA, T84.69XA, T84.7XXA

RGM04Z Fusion of Left Elbow Joint with Internal Fixation Device, Open Approach
- When reported with secondary diagnosis code T84.60XA, T84.610A, T84.611A, T84.612A, T84.613A, T84.614A, T84.615A, T84.619A, T84.63XA, T84.69XA, T84.7XXA

RGM05Z Fusion of Left Elbow Joint with External Fixation Device, Open Approach
- When reported with secondary diagnosis code T84.60XA, T84.610A, T84.611A,
T84.612A, T84.613A, T84.614A, T84.615A, T84.619A, T84.63XA, T84.69XA, T84.7XXA

0RGM07Z Fusion of Left Elbow Joint with Autologous Tissue Substitute, Open Approach
- When reported with secondary diagnosis code T84.60XA, T84.610A, T84.611A, T84.612A, T84.613A, T84.614A, T84.615A, T84.619A, T84.63XA, T84.69XA, T84.7XXA

0RGM0JZ Fusion of Left Elbow Joint with Synthetic Substitute, Open Approach
- When reported with secondary diagnosis code T84.60XA, T84.610A, T84.611A, T84.612A, T84.613A, T84.614A, T84.615A, T84.619A, T84.63XA, T84.69XA, T84.7XXA

0RGM0KZ Fusion of Left Elbow Joint with Nonautologous Tissue Substitute, Open Approach
- When reported with secondary diagnosis code T84.60XA, T84.610A, T84.611A, T84.612A, T84.613A, T84.614A, T84.615A, T84.619A, T84.63XA, T84.69XA, T84.7XXA

0RGM0ZZ Fusion of Left Elbow Joint, Open Approach
- When reported with secondary diagnosis code T84.60XA, T84.610A, T84.611A, T84.612A, T84.613A, T84.614A, T84.615A, T84.619A, T84.63XA, T84.69XA, T84.7XXA

0RGM34Z Fusion of Left Elbow Joint with Internal Fixation Device, Percutaneous Approach
- When reported with secondary diagnosis code T84.60XA, T84.610A, T84.611A, T84.612A, T84.613A, T84.614A, T84.615A, T84.619A, T84.63XA, T84.69XA, T84.7XXA

0RGM35Z Fusion of Left Elbow Joint with External Fixation Device, Percutaneous Approach
- When reported with secondary diagnosis code T84.60XA, T84.610A, T84.611A, T84.612A, T84.613A, T84.614A, T84.615A, T84.619A, T84.63XA, T84.69XA, T84.7XXA

0RGM37Z Fusion of Left Elbow Joint with Autologous Tissue Substitute, Percutaneous Approach
- When reported with secondary diagnosis code T84.60XA, T84.610A, T84.611A, T84.612A, T84.613A, T84.614A, T84.615A, T84.619A, T84.63XA, T84.69XA, T84.7XXA

0RGM3JZ Fusion of Left Elbow Joint with Synthetic Substitute, Percutaneous Approach
- When reported with secondary diagnosis code T84.60XA, T84.610A, T84.611A, T84.612A, T84.613A, T84.614A, T84.615A, T84.619A, T84.63XA, T84.69XA, T84.7XXA

0RGM3KZ Fusion of Left Elbow Joint with Nonautologous Tissue Substitute, Percutaneous Approach
- When reported with secondary diagnosis code T84.60XA, T84.610A, T84.611A, T84.612A, T84.613A, T84.614A, T84.615A, T84.619A, T84.63XA, T84.69XA, T84.7XXA

0RGM3ZZ Fusion of Left Elbow Joint, Percutaneous Approach
- When reported with secondary diagnosis code T84.60XA, T84.610A, T84.611A,

0RGM44Z Fusion of Left Elbow Joint with Internal Fixation Device, Percutaneous Endoscopic Approach
- When reported with secondary diagnosis code T84.60XA, T84.610A, T84.611A, T84.612A, T84.613A, T84.614A, T84.615A, T84.619A, T84.63XA, T84.69XA, T84.7XXA

0RGM45Z Fusion of Left Elbow Joint with External Fixation Device, Percutaneous Endoscopic Approach
- When reported with secondary diagnosis code T84.60XA, T84.610A, T84.611A, T84.612A, T84.613A, T84.614A, T84.615A, T84.619A, T84.63XA, T84.69XA, T84.7XXA

0RGM47Z Fusion of Left Elbow Joint with Autologous Tissue Substitute, Percutaneous Endoscopic Approach
- When reported with secondary diagnosis code T84.60XA, T84.610A, T84.611A, T84.612A, T84.613A, T84.614A, T84.615A, T84.619A, T84.63XA, T84.69XA, T84.7XXA

0RGM4JZ Fusion of Left Elbow Joint with Synthetic Substitute, Percutaneous Endoscopic Approach
- When reported with secondary diagnosis code T84.60XA, T84.610A, T84.611A, T84.612A, T84.613A, T84.614A, T84.615A, T84.619A, T84.63XA, T84.69XA, T84.7XXA

0RGM4KZ Fusion of Left Elbow Joint with Nonautologous Tissue Substitute, Percutaneous Endoscopic Approach
- When reported with secondary diagnosis code T84.60XA, T84.610A, T84.611A, T84.612A, T84.613A, T84.614A, T84.615A, T84.619A, T84.63XA, T84.69XA, T84.7XXA

0RGM4ZZ Fusion of Left Elbow Joint, Percutaneous Endoscopic Approach
- When reported with secondary diagnosis code T84.60XA, T84.610A, T84.611A, T84.612A, T84.613A, T84.614A, T84.615A, T84.619A, T84.63XA, T84.69XA, T84.7XXA

0RGN04Z Fusion of Right Wrist Joint with Internal Fixation Device, Open Approach

0RGN05Z Fusion of Right Wrist Joint with External Fixation Device, Open Approach

0RGN07Z Fusion of Right Wrist Joint with Autologous Tissue Substitute, Open Approach

0RGN0JZ Fusion of Right Wrist Joint with Synthetic Substitute, Open Approach

0RGN0KZ Fusion of Right Wrist Joint with Nonautologous Tissue Substitute, Open Approach

0RGN0ZZ Fusion of Right Wrist Joint, Open Approach

0RGN34Z Fusion of Right Wrist Joint with Internal Fixation Device, Percutaneous Approach

0RGN35Z Fusion of Right Wrist Joint with External Fixation Device, Percutaneous Approach

0RGN37Z Fusion of Right Wrist Joint with Autologous Tissue Substitute, Percutaneous Approach

0RGN3JZ Fusion of Right Wrist Joint with Synthetic Substitute, Percutaneous Approach

0RGN3KZ Fusion of Right Wrist Joint with Nonautologous Tissue Substitute, Percutaneous Approach

---

♀ Female-only	♂ Male-only	▲ Limited Coverage	● Non-OR	▪ HAC-associated procedure	▲ Non-covered procedures	✛ Combination

0RGN3ZZ Fusion of Right Wrist Joint, Percutaneous Approach	**0RGQ34Z** Fusion of Right Carpal Joint with Internal Fixation Device, Percutaneous Approach	**0RGR4ZZ** Fusion of Left Carpal Joint, Percutaneous Endoscopic Approach
0RGN44Z Fusion of Right Wrist Joint with Internal Fixation Device, Percutaneous Endoscopic Approach	**0RGQ35Z** Fusion of Right Carpal Joint with External Fixation Device, Percutaneous Approach	**0RGS04Z** Fusion of Right Metacarpocarpal Joint with Internal Fixation Device, Open Approach
0RGN45Z Fusion of Right Wrist Joint with External Fixation Device, Percutaneous Endoscopic Approach	**0RGQ37Z** Fusion of Right Carpal Joint with Autologous Tissue Substitute, Percutaneous Approach	**0RGS05Z** Fusion of Right Metacarpocarpal Joint with External Fixation Device, Open Approach
0RGN47Z Fusion of Right Wrist Joint with Autologous Tissue Substitute, Percutaneous Endoscopic Approach	**0RGQ3JZ** Fusion of Right Carpal Joint with Synthetic Substitute, Percutaneous Approach	**0RGS07Z** Fusion of Right Metacarpocarpal Joint with Autologous Tissue Substitute, Open Approach
0RGN4JZ Fusion of Right Wrist Joint with Synthetic Substitute, Percutaneous Endoscopic Approach	**0RGQ3KZ** Fusion of Right Carpal Joint with Nonautologous Tissue Substitute, Percutaneous Approach	**0RGS0JZ** Fusion of Right Metacarpocarpal Joint with Synthetic Substitute, Open Approach
0RGN4KZ Fusion of Right Wrist Joint with Nonautologous Tissue Substitute, Percutaneous Endoscopic Approach	**0RGQ3ZZ** Fusion of Right Carpal Joint, Percutaneous Approach	**0RGS0KZ** Fusion of Right Metacarpocarpal Joint with Nonautologous Tissue Substitute, Open Approach
0RGN4ZZ Fusion of Right Wrist Joint, Percutaneous Endoscopic Approach	**0RGQ44Z** Fusion of Right Carpal Joint with Internal Fixation Device, Percutaneous Endoscopic Approach	**0RGS0ZZ** Fusion of Right Metacarpocarpal Joint, Open Approach
0RGP04Z Fusion of Left Wrist Joint with Internal Fixation Device, Open Approach	**0RGQ45Z** Fusion of Right Carpal Joint with External Fixation Device, Percutaneous Endoscopic Approach	**0RGS34Z** Fusion of Right Metacarpocarpal Joint with Internal Fixation Device, Percutaneous Approach
0RGP05Z Fusion of Left Wrist Joint with External Fixation Device, Open Approach	**0RGQ47Z** Fusion of Right Carpal Joint with Autologous Tissue Substitute, Percutaneous Endoscopic Approach	**0RGS35Z** Fusion of Right Metacarpocarpal Joint with External Fixation Device, Percutaneous Approach
0RGP07Z Fusion of Left Wrist Joint with Autologous Tissue Substitute, Open Approach	**0RGQ4JZ** Fusion of Right Carpal Joint with Synthetic Substitute, Percutaneous Endoscopic Approach	**0RGS37Z** Fusion of Right Metacarpocarpal Joint with Autologous Tissue Substitute, Percutaneous Approach
0RGP0JZ Fusion of Left Wrist Joint with Synthetic Substitute, Open Approach	**0RGQ4KZ** Fusion of Right Carpal Joint with Nonautologous Tissue Substitute, Percutaneous Endoscopic Approach	**0RGS3JZ** Fusion of Right Metacarpocarpal Joint with Synthetic Substitute, Percutaneous Approach
0RGP0KZ Fusion of Left Wrist Joint with Nonautologous Tissue Substitute, Open Approach	**0RGQ4ZZ** Fusion of Right Carpal Joint, Percutaneous Endoscopic Approach	**0RGS3KZ** Fusion of Right Metacarpocarpal Joint with Nonautologous Tissue Substitute, Percutaneous Approach
0RGP0ZZ Fusion of Left Wrist Joint, Open Approach	**0RGR04Z** Fusion of Left Carpal Joint with Internal Fixation Device, Open Approach	**0RGS3ZZ** Fusion of Right Metacarpocarpal Joint, Percutaneous Approach
0RGP34Z Fusion of Left Wrist Joint with Internal Fixation Device, Percutaneous Approach	**0RGR05Z** Fusion of Left Carpal Joint with External Fixation Device, Open Approach	**0RGS44Z** Fusion of Right Metacarpocarpal Joint with Internal Fixation Device, Percutaneous Endoscopic Approach
0RGP35Z Fusion of Left Wrist Joint with External Fixation Device, Percutaneous Approach	**0RGR07Z** Fusion of Left Carpal Joint with Autologous Tissue Substitute, Open Approach	**0RGS45Z** Fusion of Right Metacarpocarpal Joint with External Fixation Device, Percutaneous Endoscopic Approach
0RGP37Z Fusion of Left Wrist Joint with Autologous Tissue Substitute, Percutaneous Approach	**0RGR0JZ** Fusion of Left Carpal Joint with Synthetic Substitute, Open Approach	**0RGS47Z** Fusion of Right Metacarpocarpal Joint with Autologous Tissue Substitute, Percutaneous Endoscopic Approach
0RGP3JZ Fusion of Left Wrist Joint with Synthetic Substitute, Percutaneous Approach	**0RGR0KZ** Fusion of Left Carpal Joint with Nonautologous Tissue Substitute, Open Approach	**0RGS4JZ** Fusion of Right Metacarpocarpal Joint with Synthetic Substitute, Percutaneous Endoscopic Approach
0RGP3KZ Fusion of Left Wrist Joint with Nonautologous Tissue Substitute, Percutaneous Approach	**0RGR0ZZ** Fusion of Left Carpal Joint, Open Approach	**0RGS4KZ** Fusion of Right Metacarpocarpal Joint with Nonautologous Tissue Substitute, Percutaneous Endoscopic Approach
0RGP3ZZ Fusion of Left Wrist Joint, Percutaneous Approach	**0RGR34Z** Fusion of Left Carpal Joint with Internal Fixation Device, Percutaneous Approach	**0RGS4ZZ** Fusion of Right Metacarpocarpal Joint, Percutaneous Endoscopic Approach
0RGP44Z Fusion of Left Wrist Joint with Internal Fixation Device, Percutaneous Endoscopic Approach	**0RGR35Z** Fusion of Left Carpal Joint with External Fixation Device, Percutaneous Approach	**0RGT04Z** Fusion of Left Metacarpocarpal Joint with Internal Fixation Device, Open Approach
0RGP45Z Fusion of Left Wrist Joint with External Fixation Device, Percutaneous Endoscopic Approach	**0RGR37Z** Fusion of Left Carpal Joint with Autologous Tissue Substitute, Percutaneous Approach	**0RGT05Z** Fusion of Left Metacarpocarpal Joint with External Fixation Device, Open Approach
0RGP47Z Fusion of Left Wrist Joint with Autologous Tissue Substitute, Percutaneous Endoscopic Approach	**0RGR3JZ** Fusion of Left Carpal Joint with Synthetic Substitute, Percutaneous Approach	**0RGT07Z** Fusion of Left Metacarpocarpal Joint with Autologous Tissue Substitute, Open Approach
0RGP4JZ Fusion of Left Wrist Joint with Synthetic Substitute, Percutaneous Endoscopic Approach	**0RGR3KZ** Fusion of Left Carpal Joint with Nonautologous Tissue Substitute, Percutaneous Approach	**0RGT0JZ** Fusion of Left Metacarpocarpal Joint with Synthetic Substitute, Open Approach
0RGP4KZ Fusion of Left Wrist Joint with Nonautologous Tissue Substitute, Percutaneous Endoscopic Approach	**0RGR3ZZ** Fusion of Left Carpal Joint, Percutaneous Approach	**0RGT0KZ** Fusion of Left Metacarpocarpal Joint with Nonautologous Tissue Substitute, Open Approach
0RGP4ZZ Fusion of Left Wrist Joint, Percutaneous Endoscopic Approach	**0RGR44Z** Fusion of Left Carpal Joint with Internal Fixation Device, Percutaneous Endoscopic Approach	**0RGT0ZZ** Fusion of Left Metacarpocarpal Joint, Open Approach
0RGQ04Z Fusion of Right Carpal Joint with Internal Fixation Device, Open Approach	**0RGR45Z** Fusion of Left Carpal Joint with External Fixation Device, Percutaneous Endoscopic Approach	**0RGT34Z** Fusion of Left Metacarpocarpal Joint with Internal Fixation Device, Percutaneous Approach
0RGQ05Z Fusion of Right Carpal Joint with External Fixation Device, Open Approach	**0RGR47Z** Fusion of Left Carpal Joint with Autologous Tissue Substitute, Percutaneous Endoscopic Approach	**0RGT35Z** Fusion of Left Metacarpocarpal Joint with External Fixation Device, Percutaneous Approach
0RGQ07Z Fusion of Right Carpal Joint with Autologous Tissue Substitute, Open Approach	**0RGR4JZ** Fusion of Left Carpal Joint with Synthetic Substitute, Percutaneous Endoscopic Approach	**0RGT37Z** Fusion of Left Metacarpocarpal Joint with Autologous Tissue Substitute, Percutaneous Approach
0RGQ0JZ Fusion of Right Carpal Joint with Synthetic Substitute, Open Approach	**0RGR4KZ** Fusion of Left Carpal Joint with Nonautologous Tissue Substitute, Percutaneous Endoscopic Approach	**0RGT3JZ** Fusion of Left Metacarpocarpal Joint with Synthetic Substitute, Percutaneous Approach
0RGQ0KZ Fusion of Right Carpal Joint with Nonautologous Tissue Substitute, Open Approach		
0RGQ0ZZ Fusion of Right Carpal Joint, Open Approach		

♀ Female-only   ♂ Male-only   ▲ Limited Coverage   ● Non-OR   ▬ HAC-associated procedure   ▲ Non-covered procedures   ✚ Combination

GT3KZ Fusion of Left Metacarpocarpal Joint with Nonautologous Tissue Substitute, Percutaneous Approach

GT3ZZ Fusion of Left Metacarpocarpal Joint, Percutaneous Approach

GT44Z Fusion of Left Metacarpocarpal Joint with Internal Fixation Device, Percutaneous Endoscopic Approach

GT45Z Fusion of Left Metacarpocarpal Joint with External Fixation Device, Percutaneous Endoscopic Approach

GT47Z Fusion of Left Metacarpocarpal Joint with Autologous Tissue Substitute, Percutaneous Endoscopic Approach

GT4JZ Fusion of Left Metacarpocarpal Joint with Synthetic Substitute, Percutaneous Endoscopic Approach

GT4KZ Fusion of Left Metacarpocarpal Joint with Nonautologous Tissue Substitute, Percutaneous Endoscopic Approach

GT4ZZ Fusion of Left Metacarpocarpal Joint, Percutaneous Endoscopic Approach

GU04Z Fusion of Right Metacarpophalangeal Joint with Internal Fixation Device, Open Approach

GU05Z Fusion of Right Metacarpophalangeal Joint with External Fixation Device, Open Approach

RGU07Z Fusion of Right Metacarpophalangeal Joint with Autologous Tissue Substitute, Open Approach

RGU0JZ Fusion of Right Metacarpophalangeal Joint with Synthetic Substitute, Open Approach

RGU0KZ Fusion of Right Metacarpophalangeal Joint with Nonautologous Tissue Substitute, Open Approach

RGU0ZZ Fusion of Right Metacarpophalangeal Joint, Open Approach

RGU34Z Fusion of Right Metacarpophalangeal Joint with Internal Fixation Device, Percutaneous Approach

RGU35Z Fusion of Right Metacarpophalangeal Joint with External Fixation Device, Percutaneous Approach

RGU37Z Fusion of Right Metacarpophalangeal Joint with Autologous Tissue Substitute, Percutaneous Approach

RGU3JZ Fusion of Right Metacarpophalangeal Joint with Synthetic Substitute, Percutaneous Approach

RGU3KZ Fusion of Right Metacarpophalangeal Joint with Nonautologous Tissue Substitute, Percutaneous Approach

RGU3ZZ Fusion of Right Metacarpophalangeal Joint, Percutaneous Approach

RGU44Z Fusion of Right Metacarpophalangeal Joint with Internal Fixation Device, Percutaneous Endoscopic Approach

RGU45Z Fusion of Right Metacarpophalangeal Joint with External Fixation Device, Percutaneous Endoscopic Approach

RGU47Z Fusion of Right Metacarpophalangeal Joint with Autologous Tissue Substitute, Percutaneous Endoscopic Approach

RGU4JZ Fusion of Right Metacarpophalangeal Joint with Synthetic Substitute, Percutaneous Endoscopic Approach

RGU4KZ Fusion of Right Metacarpophalangeal Joint with Nonautologous Tissue Substitute, Percutaneous Endoscopic Approach

RGU4ZZ Fusion of Right Metacarpophalangeal Joint, Percutaneous Endoscopic Approach

RGV04Z Fusion of Left Metacarpophalangeal Joint with Internal Fixation Device, Open Approach

0RGV05Z Fusion of Left Metacarpophalangeal Joint with External Fixation Device, Open Approach

0RGV07Z Fusion of Left Metacarpophalangeal Joint with Autologous Tissue Substitute, Open Approach

0RGV0JZ Fusion of Left Metacarpophalangeal Joint with Synthetic Substitute, Open Approach

0RGV0KZ Fusion of Left Metacarpophalangeal Joint with Nonautologous Tissue Substitute, Open Approach

0RGV0ZZ Fusion of Left Metacarpophalangeal Joint, Open Approach

0RGV34Z Fusion of Left Metacarpophalangeal Joint with Internal Fixation Device, Percutaneous Approach

0RGV35Z Fusion of Left Metacarpophalangeal Joint with External Fixation Device, Percutaneous Approach

0RGV37Z Fusion of Left Metacarpophalangeal Joint with Autologous Tissue Substitute, Percutaneous Approach

0RGV3JZ Fusion of Left Metacarpophalangeal Joint with Synthetic Substitute, Percutaneous Approach

0RGV3KZ Fusion of Left Metacarpophalangeal Joint with Nonautologous Tissue Substitute, Percutaneous Approach

0RGV3ZZ Fusion of Left Metacarpophalangeal Joint, Percutaneous Approach

0RGV44Z Fusion of Left Metacarpophalangeal Joint with Internal Fixation Device, Percutaneous Endoscopic Approach

0RGV45Z Fusion of Left Metacarpophalangeal Joint with External Fixation Device, Percutaneous Endoscopic Approach

0RGV47Z Fusion of Left Metacarpophalangeal Joint with Autologous Tissue Substitute, Percutaneous Endoscopic Approach

0RGV4JZ Fusion of Left Metacarpophalangeal Joint with Synthetic Substitute, Percutaneous Endoscopic Approach

0RGV4KZ Fusion of Left Metacarpophalangeal Joint with Nonautologous Tissue Substitute, Percutaneous Endoscopic Approach

0RGV4ZZ Fusion of Left Metacarpophalangeal Joint, Percutaneous Endoscopic Approach

0RGW04Z Fusion of Right Finger Phalangeal Joint with Internal Fixation Device, Open Approach

0RGW05Z Fusion of Right Finger Phalangeal Joint with External Fixation Device, Open Approach

0RGW07Z Fusion of Right Finger Phalangeal Joint with Autologous Tissue Substitute, Open Approach

0RGW0JZ Fusion of Right Finger Phalangeal Joint with Synthetic Substitute, Open Approach

0RGW0KZ Fusion of Right Finger Phalangeal Joint with Nonautologous Tissue Substitute, Open Approach

0RGW0ZZ Fusion of Right Finger Phalangeal Joint, Open Approach

0RGW34Z Fusion of Right Finger Phalangeal Joint with Internal Fixation Device, Percutaneous Approach

0RGW35Z Fusion of Right Finger Phalangeal Joint with External Fixation Device, Percutaneous Approach

0RGW37Z Fusion of Right Finger Phalangeal Joint with Autologous Tissue Substitute, Percutaneous Approach

0RGW3JZ Fusion of Right Finger Phalangeal Joint with Synthetic Substitute, Percutaneous Approach

0RGW3KZ Fusion of Right Finger Phalangeal Joint with Nonautologous Tissue Substitute, Percutaneous Approach

0RGW3ZZ Fusion of Right Finger Phalangeal Joint, Percutaneous Approach

0RGW44Z Fusion of Right Finger Phalangeal Joint with Internal Fixation Device, Percutaneous Endoscopic Approach

0RGW45Z Fusion of Right Finger Phalangeal Joint with External Fixation Device, Percutaneous Endoscopic Approach

0RGW47Z Fusion of Right Finger Phalangeal Joint with Autologous Tissue Substitute, Percutaneous Endoscopic Approach

0RGW4JZ Fusion of Right Finger Phalangeal Joint with Synthetic Substitute, Percutaneous Endoscopic Approach

0RGW4KZ Fusion of Right Finger Phalangeal Joint with Nonautologous Tissue Substitute, Percutaneous Endoscopic Approach

0RGW4ZZ Fusion of Right Finger Phalangeal Joint, Percutaneous Endoscopic Approach

0RGX04Z Fusion of Left Finger Phalangeal Joint with Internal Fixation Device, Open Approach

0RGX05Z Fusion of Left Finger Phalangeal Joint with External Fixation Device, Open Approach

0RGX07Z Fusion of Left Finger Phalangeal Joint with Autologous Tissue Substitute, Open Approach

0RGX0JZ Fusion of Left Finger Phalangeal Joint with Synthetic Substitute, Open Approach

0RGX0KZ Fusion of Left Finger Phalangeal Joint with Nonautologous Tissue Substitute, Open Approach

0RGX0ZZ Fusion of Left Finger Phalangeal Joint, Open Approach

0RGX34Z Fusion of Left Finger Phalangeal Joint with Internal Fixation Device, Percutaneous Approach

0RGX35Z Fusion of Left Finger Phalangeal Joint with External Fixation Device, Percutaneous Approach

0RGX37Z Fusion of Left Finger Phalangeal Joint with Autologous Tissue Substitute, Percutaneous Approach

0RGX3JZ Fusion of Left Finger Phalangeal Joint with Synthetic Substitute, Percutaneous Approach

0RGX3KZ Fusion of Left Finger Phalangeal Joint with Nonautologous Tissue Substitute, Percutaneous Approach

0RGX3ZZ Fusion of Left Finger Phalangeal Joint, Percutaneous Approach

0RGX44Z Fusion of Left Finger Phalangeal Joint with Internal Fixation Device, Percutaneous Endoscopic Approach

0RGX45Z Fusion of Left Finger Phalangeal Joint with External Fixation Device, Percutaneous Endoscopic Approach

0RGX47Z Fusion of Left Finger Phalangeal Joint with Autologous Tissue Substitute, Percutaneous Endoscopic Approach

0RGX4JZ Fusion of Left Finger Phalangeal Joint with Synthetic Substitute, Percutaneous Endoscopic Approach

0RGX4KZ Fusion of Left Finger Phalangeal Joint with Nonautologous Tissue Substitute, Percutaneous Endoscopic Approach

0RGX4ZZ Fusion of Left Finger Phalangeal Joint, Percutaneous Endoscopic Approach

0RH003Z Insertion of Infusion Device into Occipital-cervical Joint, Open Approach

0RH004Z Insertion of Internal Fixation Device into Occipital-cervical Joint, Open Approach

0RH008Z Insertion of Spacer into Occipital-cervical Joint, Open Approach

0RH00BZ Insertion of Interspinous Process Spinal Stabilization Device into Occipital-cervical Joint, Open Approach

0RH00CZ Insertion of Pedicle-Based Spinal Stabilization Device into Occipital-cervical Joint, Open Approach

0RH00DZ Insertion of Facet Replacement Spinal Stabilization Device into Occipital-cervical Joint, Open Approach

0RH033Z Insertion of Infusion Device into Occipital-cervical Joint, Percutaneous Approach

0RH034Z Insertion of Internal Fixation Device into Occipital-cervical Joint, Percutaneous Approach

0RH038Z Insertion of Spacer into Occipital-cervical Joint, Percutaneous Approach

0RH03BZ Insertion of Interspinous Process Spinal Stabilization Device into Occipital-cervical Joint, Percutaneous Approach

0RH03CZ Insertion of Pedicle-Based Spinal Stabilization Device into Occipital-cervical Joint, Percutaneous Approach

0RH03DZ Insertion of Facet Replacement Spinal Stabilization Device into Occipital-cervical Joint, Percutaneous Approach

0RH043Z Insertion of Infusion Device into Occipital-cervical Joint, Percutaneous Endoscopic Approach

0RH044Z Insertion of Internal Fixation Device into Occipital-cervical Joint, Percutaneous Endoscopic Approach

0RH048Z Insertion of Spacer into Occipital-cervical Joint, Percutaneous Endoscopic Approach

0RH04BZ Insertion of Interspinous Process Spinal Stabilization Device into Occipital-cervical Joint, Percutaneous Endoscopic Approach

0RH04CZ Insertion of Pedicle-Based Spinal Stabilization Device into Occipital-cervical Joint, Percutaneous Endoscopic Approach

0RH04DZ Insertion of Facet Replacement Spinal Stabilization Device into Occipital-cervical Joint, Percutaneous Endoscopic Approach

0RH103Z Insertion of Infusion Device into Cervical Vertebral Joint, Open Approach

0RH104Z Insertion of Internal Fixation Device into Cervical Vertebral Joint, Open Approach

0RH108Z Insertion of Spacer into Cervical Vertebral Joint, Open Approach

0RH10BZ Insertion of Interspinous Process Spinal Stabilization Device into Cervical Vertebral Joint, Open Approach

0RH10CZ Insertion of Pedicle-Based Spinal Stabilization Device into Cervical Vertebral Joint, Open Approach

0RH10DZ Insertion of Facet Replacement Spinal Stabilization Device into Cervical Vertebral Joint, Open Approach

0RH133Z Insertion of Infusion Device into Cervical Vertebral Joint, Percutaneous Approach

0RH134Z Insertion of Internal Fixation Device into Cervical Vertebral Joint, Percutaneous Approach

0RH138Z Insertion of Spacer into Cervical Vertebral Joint, Percutaneous Approach

0RH13BZ Insertion of Interspinous Process Spinal Stabilization Device into Cervical Vertebral Joint, Percutaneous Approach

0RH13CZ Insertion of Pedicle-Based Spinal Stabilization Device into Cervical Vertebral Joint, Percutaneous Approach

0RH13DZ Insertion of Facet Replacement Spinal Stabilization Device into Cervical Vertebral Joint, Percutaneous Approach

0RH143Z Insertion of Infusion Device into Cervical Vertebral Joint, Percutaneous Endoscopic Approach

0RH144Z Insertion of Internal Fixation Device into Cervical Vertebral Joint, Percutaneous Endoscopic Approach

0RH148Z Insertion of Spacer into Cervical Vertebral Joint, Percutaneous Endoscopic Approach

0RH14BZ Insertion of Interspinous Process Spinal Stabilization Device into Cervical Vertebral Joint, Percutaneous Endoscopic Approach

0RH14CZ Insertion of Pedicle-Based Spinal Stabilization Device into Cervical Vertebral Joint, Percutaneous Endoscopic Approach

0RH14DZ Insertion of Facet Replacement Spinal Stabilization Device into Cervical Vertebral Joint, Percutaneous Endoscopic Approach

0RH303Z Insertion of Infusion Device into Cervical Vertebral Disc, Open Approach

0RH333Z Insertion of Infusion Device into Cervical Vertebral Disc, Percutaneous Approach

0RH343Z Insertion of Infusion Device into Cervical Vertebral Disc, Percutaneous Endoscopic Approach

0RH403Z Insertion of Infusion Device into Cervicothoracic Vertebral Joint, Open Approach

0RH404Z Insertion of Internal Fixation Device into Cervicothoracic Vertebral Joint, Open Approach

0RH408Z Insertion of Spacer into Cervicothoracic Vertebral Joint, Open Approach

0RH40BZ Insertion of Interspinous Process Spinal Stabilization Device into Cervicothoracic Vertebral Joint, Open Approach

0RH40CZ Insertion of Pedicle-Based Spinal Stabilization Device into Cervicothoracic Vertebral Joint, Open Approach

0RH40DZ Insertion of Facet Replacement Spinal Stabilization Device into Cervicothoracic Vertebral Joint, Open Approach

0RH433Z Insertion of Infusion Device into Cervicothoracic Vertebral Joint, Percutaneous Approach

0RH434Z Insertion of Internal Fixation Device into Cervicothoracic Vertebral Joint, Percutaneous Approach

0RH438Z Insertion of Spacer into Cervicothoracic Vertebral Joint, Percutaneous Approach

0RH43BZ Insertion of Interspinous Process Spinal Stabilization Device into Cervicothoracic Vertebral Joint, Percutaneous Approach

0RH43CZ Insertion of Pedicle-Based Spinal Stabilization Device into Cervicothoracic Vertebral Joint, Percutaneous Approach

0RH43DZ Insertion of Facet Replacement Spinal Stabilization Device into Cervicothoracic Vertebral Joint, Percutaneous Approach

0RH443Z Insertion of Infusion Device into Cervicothoracic Vertebral Joint, Percutaneous Endoscopic Approach

0RH444Z Insertion of Internal Fixation Device into Cervicothoracic Vertebral Joint, Percutaneous Endoscopic Approach

0RH448Z Insertion of Spacer into Cervicothoracic Vertebral Joint, Percutaneous Endoscopic Approach

0RH44BZ Insertion of Interspinous Process Spinal Stabilization Device into Cervicothoracic Vertebral Joint, Percutaneous Endoscopic Approach

0RH44CZ Insertion of Pedicle-Based Spinal Stabilization Device into Cervicothoracic Vertebral Joint, Percutaneous Endoscopic Approach

0RH44DZ Insertion of Facet Replacement Spinal Stabilization Device into Cervicothoracic Vertebral Joint, Percutaneous Endoscopic Approach

0RH503Z Insertion of Infusion Device into Cervicothoracic Vertebral Disc, Open Approach

0RH533Z Insertion of Infusion Device into Cervicothoracic Vertebral Disc, Percutaneous Approach

0RH543Z Insertion of Infusion Device into Cervicothoracic Vertebral Disc, Percutaneous Endoscopic Approach

0RH603Z Insertion of Infusion Device into Thoracic Vertebral Joint, Open Approach

0RH604Z Insertion of Internal Fixation Device into Thoracic Vertebral Joint, Open Approach

0RH608Z Insertion of Spacer into Thoracic Vertebral Joint, Open Approach

0RH60BZ Insertion of Interspinous Process Spinal Stabilization Device into Thoracic Vertebral Joint, Open Approach

0RH60CZ Insertion of Pedicle-Based Spinal Stabilization Device into Thoracic Vertebral Joint, Open Approach

0RH60DZ Insertion of Facet Replacement Spinal Stabilization Device into Thoracic Vertebral Joint, Open Approach

0RH633Z Insertion of Infusion Device into Thoracic Vertebral Joint, Percutaneous Approach

0RH634Z Insertion of Internal Fixation Device into Thoracic Vertebral Joint, Percutaneous Approach

0RH638Z Insertion of Spacer into Thoracic Vertebral Joint, Percutaneous Approach

0RH63BZ Insertion of Interspinous Process Spinal Stabilization Device into Thoracic Vertebral Joint, Percutaneous Approach

0RH63CZ Insertion of Pedicle-Based Spinal Stabilization Device into Thoracic Vertebral Joint, Percutaneous Approach

0RH63DZ Insertion of Facet Replacement Spinal Stabilization Device into Thoracic Vertebral Joint, Percutaneous Approach

0RH643Z Insertion of Infusion Device into Thoracic Vertebral Joint, Percutaneous Endoscopic Approach

0RH644Z Insertion of Internal Fixation Device into Thoracic Vertebral Joint, Percutaneous Endoscopic Approach

0RH648Z Insertion of Spacer into Thoracic Vertebral Joint, Percutaneous Endoscopic Approach

0RH64BZ Insertion of Interspinous Process Spinal Stabilization Device into Thoracic Vertebral Joint, Percutaneous Endoscopic Approach

0RH64CZ Insertion of Pedicle-Based Spinal Stabilization Device into Thoracic Vertebral Joint, Percutaneous Endoscopic Approach

0RH64DZ Insertion of Facet Replacement Spinal Stabilization Device into Thoracic Vertebral Joint, Percutaneous Endoscopic Approach

♀ Female-only   ♂ Male-only   ▲ Limited Coverage   ● Non-OR   ■ HAC-associated procedure   ▲ Non-covered procedures   ✛ Combination

1903Z	Insertion of Infusion Device into Thoracic Vertebral Disc, Open Approach
H933Z	Insertion of Infusion Device into Thoracic Vertebral Disc, Percutaneous Approach
H943Z	Insertion of Infusion Device into Thoracic Vertebral Disc, Percutaneous Endoscopic Approach
HA03Z	Insertion of Infusion Device into Thoracolumbar Vertebral Joint, Open Approach
HA04Z	Insertion of Internal Fixation Device into Thoracolumbar Vertebral Joint, Open Approach
HA08Z	Insertion of Spacer into Thoracolumbar Vertebral Joint, Open Approach
HA0BZ	Insertion of Interspinous Process Spinal Stabilization Device into Thoracolumbar Vertebral Joint, Open Approach
HA0CZ	Insertion of Pedicle-Based Spinal Stabilization Device into Thoracolumbar Vertebral Joint, Open Approach
HA0DZ	Insertion of Facet Replacement Spinal Stabilization Device into Thoracolumbar Vertebral Joint, Open Approach
HA33Z	Insertion of Infusion Device into Thoracolumbar Vertebral Joint, Percutaneous Approach
HA34Z	Insertion of Internal Fixation Device into Thoracolumbar Vertebral Joint, Percutaneous Approach
HA38Z	Insertion of Spacer into Thoracolumbar Vertebral Joint, Percutaneous Approach
HA3BZ	Insertion of Interspinous Process Spinal Stabilization Device into Thoracolumbar Vertebral Joint, Percutaneous Approach
HA3CZ	Insertion of Pedicle-Based Spinal Stabilization Device into Thoracolumbar Vertebral Joint, Percutaneous Approach
HA3DZ	Insertion of Facet Replacement Spinal Stabilization Device into Thoracolumbar Vertebral Joint, Percutaneous Approach
HA43Z	Insertion of Infusion Device into Thoracolumbar Vertebral Joint, Percutaneous Endoscopic Approach
HA44Z	Insertion of Internal Fixation Device into Thoracolumbar Vertebral Joint, Percutaneous Endoscopic Approach
HA48Z	Insertion of Spacer into Thoracolumbar Vertebral Joint, Percutaneous Endoscopic Approach
HA4BZ	Insertion of Interspinous Process Spinal Stabilization Device into Thoracolumbar Vertebral Joint, Percutaneous Endoscopic Approach
HA4CZ	Insertion of Pedicle-Based Spinal Stabilization Device into Thoracolumbar Vertebral Joint, Percutaneous Endoscopic Approach
HA4DZ	Insertion of Facet Replacement Spinal Stabilization Device into Thoracolumbar Vertebral Joint, Percutaneous Endoscopic Approach
RHB03Z	Insertion of Infusion Device into Thoracolumbar Vertebral Disc, Open Approach
RHB33Z	Insertion of Infusion Device into Thoracolumbar Vertebral Disc, Percutaneous Approach
RHB43Z	Insertion of Infusion Device into Thoracolumbar Vertebral Disc, Percutaneous Endoscopic Approach
RHC03Z	Insertion of Infusion Device into Right Temporomandibular Joint, Open Approach
RHC04Z	Insertion of Internal Fixation Device into Right Temporomandibular Joint, Open Approach
0RHC08Z	Insertion of Spacer into Right Temporomandibular Joint, Open Approach
0RHC33Z	Insertion of Infusion Device into Right Temporomandibular Joint, Percutaneous Approach
0RHC34Z	Insertion of Internal Fixation Device into Right Temporomandibular Joint, Percutaneous Approach
0RHC38Z	Insertion of Spacer into Right Temporomandibular Joint, Percutaneous Approach
0RHC43Z	Insertion of Infusion Device into Right Temporomandibular Joint, Percutaneous Endoscopic Approach
0RHC44Z	Insertion of Internal Fixation Device into Right Temporomandibular Joint, Percutaneous Endoscopic Approach
0RHC48Z	Insertion of Spacer into Right Temporomandibular Joint, Percutaneous Endoscopic Approach
0RHD03Z	Insertion of Infusion Device into Left Temporomandibular Joint, Open Approach
0RHD04Z	Insertion of Internal Fixation Device into Left Temporomandibular Joint, Open Approach
0RHD08Z	Insertion of Spacer into Left Temporomandibular Joint, Open Approach
0RHD33Z	Insertion of Infusion Device into Left Temporomandibular Joint, Percutaneous Approach
0RHD34Z	Insertion of Internal Fixation Device into Left Temporomandibular Joint, Percutaneous Approach
0RHD38Z	Insertion of Spacer into Left Temporomandibular Joint, Percutaneous Approach
0RHD43Z	Insertion of Infusion Device into Left Temporomandibular Joint, Percutaneous Endoscopic Approach
0RHD44Z	Insertion of Internal Fixation Device into Left Temporomandibular Joint, Percutaneous Endoscopic Approach
0RHD48Z	Insertion of Spacer into Left Temporomandibular Joint, Percutaneous Endoscopic Approach
0RHE03Z	Insertion of Infusion Device into Right Sternoclavicular Joint, Open Approach
0RHE04Z	Insertion of Internal Fixation Device into Right Sternoclavicular Joint, Open Approach
0RHE08Z	Insertion of Spacer into Right Sternoclavicular Joint, Open Approach
0RHE33Z	Insertion of Infusion Device into Right Sternoclavicular Joint, Percutaneous Approach
0RHE34Z	Insertion of Internal Fixation Device into Right Sternoclavicular Joint, Percutaneous Approach
0RHE38Z	Insertion of Spacer into Right Sternoclavicular Joint, Percutaneous Approach
0RHE43Z	Insertion of Infusion Device into Right Sternoclavicular Joint, Percutaneous Endoscopic Approach
0RHE44Z	Insertion of Internal Fixation Device into Right Sternoclavicular Joint, Percutaneous Endoscopic Approach
0RHE48Z	Insertion of Spacer into Right Sternoclavicular Joint, Percutaneous Endoscopic Approach
0RHF03Z	Insertion of Infusion Device into Left Sternoclavicular Joint, Open Approach
0RHF04Z	Insertion of Internal Fixation Device into Left Sternoclavicular Joint, Open Approach
0RHF08Z	Insertion of Spacer into Left Sternoclavicular Joint, Open Approach
0RHF33Z	Insertion of Infusion Device into Left Sternoclavicular Joint, Percutaneous Approach
0RHF34Z	Insertion of Internal Fixation Device into Left Sternoclavicular Joint, Percutaneous Approach
0RHF38Z	Insertion of Spacer into Left Sternoclavicular Joint, Percutaneous Approach
0RHF43Z	Insertion of Infusion Device into Left Sternoclavicular Joint, Percutaneous Endoscopic Approach
0RHF44Z	Insertion of Internal Fixation Device into Left Sternoclavicular Joint, Percutaneous Endoscopic Approach
0RHF48Z	Insertion of Spacer into Left Sternoclavicular Joint, Percutaneous Endoscopic Approach
0RHG03Z	Insertion of Infusion Device into Right Acromioclavicular Joint, Open Approach
0RHG04Z	Insertion of Internal Fixation Device into Right Acromioclavicular Joint, Open Approach
0RHG08Z	Insertion of Spacer into Right Acromioclavicular Joint, Open Approach
0RHG33Z	Insertion of Infusion Device into Right Acromioclavicular Joint, Percutaneous Approach
0RHG34Z	Insertion of Internal Fixation Device into Right Acromioclavicular Joint, Percutaneous Approach
0RHG38Z	Insertion of Spacer into Right Acromioclavicular Joint, Percutaneous Approach
0RHG43Z	Insertion of Infusion Device into Right Acromioclavicular Joint, Percutaneous Endoscopic Approach
0RHG44Z	Insertion of Internal Fixation Device into Right Acromioclavicular Joint, Percutaneous Endoscopic Approach
0RHG48Z	Insertion of Spacer into Right Acromioclavicular Joint, Percutaneous Endoscopic Approach
0RHH03Z	Insertion of Infusion Device into Left Acromioclavicular Joint, Open Approach
0RHH04Z	Insertion of Internal Fixation Device into Left Acromioclavicular Joint, Open Approach
0RHH08Z	Insertion of Spacer into Left Acromioclavicular Joint, Open Approach
0RHH33Z	Insertion of Infusion Device into Left Acromioclavicular Joint, Percutaneous Approach
0RHH34Z	Insertion of Internal Fixation Device into Left Acromioclavicular Joint, Percutaneous Approach
0RHH38Z	Insertion of Spacer into Left Acromioclavicular Joint, Percutaneous Approach
0RHH43Z	Insertion of Infusion Device into Left Acromioclavicular Joint, Percutaneous Endoscopic Approach
0RHH44Z	Insertion of Internal Fixation Device into Left Acromioclavicular Joint, Percutaneous Endoscopic Approach
0RHH48Z	Insertion of Spacer into Left Acromioclavicular Joint, Percutaneous Endoscopic Approach
0RHJ03Z	Insertion of Infusion Device into Right Shoulder Joint, Open Approach
0RHJ04Z	Insertion of Internal Fixation Device into Right Shoulder Joint, Open Approach
0RHJ08Z	Insertion of Spacer into Right Shoulder Joint, Open Approach
0RHJ33Z	Insertion of Infusion Device into Right Shoulder Joint, Percutaneous Approach

929

Female-only   ♂ Male-only   ▲ Limited Coverage   ● Non-OR   ■ HAC-associated procedure   ▲ Non-covered procedures   ✛ Combination

0RHJ34Z Insertion of Internal Fixation Device into Right Shoulder Joint, Percutaneous Approach

0RHJ38Z Insertion of Spacer into Right Shoulder Joint, Percutaneous Approach

0RHJ43Z Insertion of Infusion Device into Right Shoulder Joint, Percutaneous Endoscopic Approach

0RHJ44Z Insertion of Internal Fixation Device into Right Shoulder Joint, Percutaneous Endoscopic Approach

0RHJ48Z Insertion of Spacer into Right Shoulder Joint, Percutaneous Endoscopic Approach

0RHK03Z Insertion of Infusion Device into Left Shoulder Joint, Open Approach

0RHK04Z Insertion of Internal Fixation Device into Left Shoulder Joint, Open Approach

0RHK08Z Insertion of Spacer into Left Shoulder Joint, Open Approach

0RHK33Z Insertion of Infusion Device into Left Shoulder Joint, Percutaneous Approach

0RHK34Z Insertion of Internal Fixation Device into Left Shoulder Joint, Percutaneous Approach

0RHK38Z Insertion of Spacer into Left Shoulder Joint, Percutaneous Approach

0RHK43Z Insertion of Infusion Device into Left Shoulder Joint, Percutaneous Endoscopic Approach

0RHK44Z Insertion of Internal Fixation Device into Left Shoulder Joint, Percutaneous Endoscopic Approach

0RHK48Z Insertion of Spacer into Left Shoulder Joint, Percutaneous Endoscopic Approach

0RHL03Z Insertion of Infusion Device into Right Elbow Joint, Open Approach

0RHL04Z Insertion of Internal Fixation Device into Right Elbow Joint, Open Approach

0RHL05Z Insertion of External Fixation Device into Right Elbow Joint, Open Approach

0RHL08Z Insertion of Spacer into Right Elbow Joint, Open Approach

0RHL33Z Insertion of Infusion Device into Right Elbow Joint, Percutaneous Approach

0RHL34Z Insertion of Internal Fixation Device into Right Elbow Joint, Percutaneous Approach

0RHL35Z Insertion of External Fixation Device into Right Elbow Joint, Percutaneous Approach

0RHL38Z Insertion of Spacer into Right Elbow Joint, Percutaneous Approach

0RHL43Z Insertion of Infusion Device into Right Elbow Joint, Percutaneous Endoscopic Approach

0RHL44Z Insertion of Internal Fixation Device into Right Elbow Joint, Percutaneous Endoscopic Approach

0RHL45Z Insertion of External Fixation Device into Right Elbow Joint, Percutaneous Endoscopic Approach

0RHL48Z Insertion of Spacer into Right Elbow Joint, Percutaneous Endoscopic Approach

0RHM03Z Insertion of Infusion Device into Left Elbow Joint, Open Approach

0RHM04Z Insertion of Internal Fixation Device into Left Elbow Joint, Open Approach

0RHM05Z Insertion of External Fixation Device into Left Elbow Joint, Open Approach

0RHM08Z Insertion of Spacer into Left Elbow Joint, Open Approach

0RHM33Z Insertion of Infusion Device into Left Elbow Joint, Percutaneous Approach

0RHM34Z Insertion of Internal Fixation Device into Left Elbow Joint, Percutaneous Approach

0RHM35Z Insertion of External Fixation Device into Left Elbow Joint, Percutaneous Approach

0RHM38Z Insertion of Spacer into Left Elbow Joint, Percutaneous Approach

0RHM43Z Insertion of Infusion Device into Left Elbow Joint, Percutaneous Endoscopic Approach

0RHM44Z Insertion of Internal Fixation Device into Left Elbow Joint, Percutaneous Endoscopic Approach

0RHM45Z Insertion of External Fixation Device into Left Elbow Joint, Percutaneous Endoscopic Approach

0RHM48Z Insertion of Spacer into Left Elbow Joint, Percutaneous Endoscopic Approach

0RHN03Z Insertion of Infusion Device into Right Wrist Joint, Open Approach

0RHN04Z Insertion of Internal Fixation Device into Right Wrist Joint, Open Approach

0RHN05Z Insertion of External Fixation Device into Right Wrist Joint, Open Approach

0RHN08Z Insertion of Spacer into Right Wrist Joint, Open Approach

0RHN33Z Insertion of Infusion Device into Right Wrist Joint, Percutaneous Approach

0RHN34Z Insertion of Internal Fixation Device into Right Wrist Joint, Percutaneous Approach

0RHN35Z Insertion of External Fixation Device into Right Wrist Joint, Percutaneous Approach

0RHN38Z Insertion of Spacer into Right Wrist Joint, Percutaneous Approach

0RHN43Z Insertion of Infusion Device into Right Wrist Joint, Percutaneous Endoscopic Approach

0RHN44Z Insertion of Internal Fixation Device into Right Wrist Joint, Percutaneous Endoscopic Approach

0RHN45Z Insertion of External Fixation Device into Right Wrist Joint, Percutaneous Endoscopic Approach

0RHN48Z Insertion of Spacer into Right Wrist Joint, Percutaneous Endoscopic Approach

0RHP03Z Insertion of Infusion Device into Left Wrist Joint, Open Approach

0RHP04Z Insertion of Internal Fixation Device into Left Wrist Joint, Open Approach

0RHP05Z Insertion of External Fixation Device into Left Wrist Joint, Open Approach

0RHP08Z Insertion of Spacer into Left Wrist Joint, Open Approach

0RHP33Z Insertion of Infusion Device into Left Wrist Joint, Percutaneous Approach

0RHP34Z Insertion of Internal Fixation Device into Left Wrist Joint, Percutaneous Approach

0RHP35Z Insertion of External Fixation Device into Left Wrist Joint, Percutaneous Approach

0RHP38Z Insertion of Spacer into Left Wrist Joint, Percutaneous Approach

0RHP43Z Insertion of Infusion Device into Left Wrist Joint, Percutaneous Endoscopic Approach

0RHP44Z Insertion of Internal Fixation Device into Left Wrist Joint, Percutaneous Endoscopic Approach

0RHP45Z Insertion of External Fixation Device into Left Wrist Joint, Percutaneous Endoscopic Approach

0RHP48Z Insertion of Spacer into Left Wrist Joint, Percutaneous Endoscopic Approach

0RHQ03Z Insertion of Infusion Device into Right Carpal Joint, Open Approach

0RHQ04Z Insertion of Internal Fixation Device into Right Carpal Joint, Open Approach

0RHQ05Z Insertion of External Fixation Device into Right Carpal Joint, Open Approach

0RHQ08Z Insertion of Spacer into Right Carpal Joint, Open Approach

0RHQ33Z Insertion of Infusion Device into Right Carpal Joint, Percutaneous Approach

0RHQ34Z Insertion of Internal Fixation Device into Right Carpal Joint, Percutaneous Approach

0RHQ35Z Insertion of External Fixation Device into Right Carpal Joint, Percutaneous Approach

0RHQ38Z Insertion of Spacer into Right Carpal Joint, Percutaneous Approach

0RHQ43Z Insertion of Infusion Device into Right Carpal Joint, Percutaneous Endoscopic Approach

0RHQ44Z Insertion of Internal Fixation Device into Right Carpal Joint, Percutaneous Endoscopic Approach

0RHQ45Z Insertion of External Fixation Device into Right Carpal Joint, Percutaneous Endoscopic Approach

0RHQ48Z Insertion of Spacer into Right Carpal Joint, Percutaneous Endoscopic Approach

0RHR03Z Insertion of Infusion Device into Left Carpal Joint, Open Approach

0RHR04Z Insertion of Internal Fixation Device into Left Carpal Joint, Open Approach

0RHR05Z Insertion of External Fixation Device into Left Carpal Joint, Open Approach

0RHR08Z Insertion of Spacer into Left Carpal Joint, Open Approach

0RHR33Z Insertion of Infusion Device into Left Carpal Joint, Percutaneous Approach

0RHR34Z Insertion of Internal Fixation Device into Left Carpal Joint, Percutaneous Approach

0RHR35Z Insertion of External Fixation Device into Left Carpal Joint, Percutaneous Approach

0RHR38Z Insertion of Spacer into Left Carpal Joint, Percutaneous Approach

0RHR43Z Insertion of Infusion Device into Left Carpal Joint, Percutaneous Endoscopic Approach

0RHR44Z Insertion of Internal Fixation Device into Left Carpal Joint, Percutaneous Endoscopic Approach

0RHR45Z Insertion of External Fixation Device into Left Carpal Joint, Percutaneous Endoscopic Approach

0RHR48Z Insertion of Spacer into Left Carpal Joint, Percutaneous Endoscopic Approach

0RHS03Z Insertion of Infusion Device into Right Metacarpocarpal Joint, Open Approach

0RHS04Z Insertion of Internal Fixation Device into Right Metacarpocarpal Joint, Open Approach

0RHS05Z Insertion of External Fixation Device into Right Metacarpocarpal Joint, Open Approach

0RHS08Z Insertion of Spacer into Right Metacarpocarpal Joint, Open Approach

0RHS33Z Insertion of Infusion Device into Right Metacarpocarpal Joint, Percutaneous Approach

0RHS34Z Insertion of Internal Fixation Device into Right Metacarpocarpal Joint, Percutaneous Approach

0RHS35Z Insertion of External Fixation Device into Right Metacarpocarpal Joint, Percutaneous Approach

0RHS38Z Insertion of Spacer into Right Metacarpocarpal Joint, Percutaneous Approach

0RHS43Z Insertion of Infusion Device into Right Metacarpocarpal Joint, Percutaneous Endoscopic Approach

0RHS44Z Insertion of Internal Fixation Device into Right Metacarpocarpal Joint, Percutaneous Endoscopic Approach

0RHS45Z Insertion of External Fixation Device into Right Metacarpocarpal Joint, Percutaneous Endoscopic Approach

♀ Female-only   ♂ Male-only   ▲ Limited Coverage   ● Non-OR   ⬛ HAC-associated procedure   ▲ Non-covered procedures   ✚ Combination

HS48Z   Insertion of Spacer into Right Metacarpocarpal Joint, Percutaneous Endoscopic Approach

HT03Z   Insertion of Infusion Device into Left Metacarpocarpal Joint, Open Approach

HT04Z   Insertion of Internal Fixation Device into Left Metacarpocarpal Joint, Open Approach

HT05Z   Insertion of External Fixation Device into Left Metacarpocarpal Joint, Open Approach

HT08Z   Insertion of Spacer into Left Metacarpocarpal Joint, Open Approach

HT33Z   Insertion of Infusion Device into Left Metacarpocarpal Joint, Percutaneous Approach

HT34Z   Insertion of Internal Fixation Device into Left Metacarpocarpal Joint, Percutaneous Approach

HT35Z   Insertion of External Fixation Device into Left Metacarpocarpal Joint, Percutaneous Approach

HT38Z   Insertion of Spacer into Left Metacarpocarpal Joint, Percutaneous Approach

HT43Z   Insertion of Infusion Device into Left Metacarpocarpal Joint, Percutaneous Endoscopic Approach

HT44Z   Insertion of Internal Fixation Device into Left Metacarpocarpal Joint, Percutaneous Endoscopic Approach

HT45Z   Insertion of External Fixation Device into Left Metacarpocarpal Joint, Percutaneous Endoscopic Approach

HT48Z   Insertion of Spacer into Left Metacarpocarpal Joint, Percutaneous Endoscopic Approach

RHU03Z   Insertion of Infusion Device into Right Metacarpophalangeal Joint, Open Approach

RHU04Z   Insertion of Internal Fixation Device into Right Metacarpophalangeal Joint, Open Approach

RHU05Z   Insertion of External Fixation Device into Right Metacarpophalangeal Joint, Open Approach

RHU08Z   Insertion of Spacer into Right Metacarpophalangeal Joint, Open Approach

RHU33Z   Insertion of Infusion Device into Right Metacarpophalangeal Joint, Percutaneous Approach

RHU34Z   Insertion of Internal Fixation Device into Right Metacarpophalangeal Joint, Percutaneous Approach

RHU35Z   Insertion of External Fixation Device into Right Metacarpophalangeal Joint, Percutaneous Approach

0RHU38Z   Insertion of Spacer into Right Metacarpophalangeal Joint, Percutaneous Approach

0RHU43Z   Insertion of Infusion Device into Right Metacarpophalangeal Joint, Percutaneous Endoscopic Approach

0RHU44Z   Insertion of Internal Fixation Device into Right Metacarpophalangeal Joint, Percutaneous Endoscopic Approach

0RHU45Z   Insertion of External Fixation Device into Right Metacarpophalangeal Joint, Percutaneous Endoscopic Approach

0RHU48Z   Insertion of Spacer into Right Metacarpophalangeal Joint, Percutaneous Endoscopic Approach

0RHV03Z   Insertion of Infusion Device into Left Metacarpophalangeal Joint, Open Approach

0RHV04Z   Insertion of Internal Fixation Device into Left Metacarpophalangeal Joint, Open Approach

0RHV05Z   Insertion of External Fixation Device into Left Metacarpophalangeal Joint, Open Approach

0RHV08Z   Insertion of Spacer into Left Metacarpophalangeal Joint, Open Approach

0RHV33Z   Insertion of Infusion Device into Left Metacarpophalangeal Joint, Percutaneous Approach

0RHV34Z   Insertion of Internal Fixation Device into Left Metacarpophalangeal Joint, Percutaneous Approach

0RHV35Z   Insertion of External Fixation Device into Left Metacarpophalangeal Joint, Percutaneous Approach

0RHV38Z   Insertion of Spacer into Left Metacarpophalangcal Joint, Percutaneous Approach

0RHV43Z   Insertion of Infusion Device into Left Metacarpophalangeal Joint, Percutaneous Endoscopic Approach

0RHV44Z   Insertion of Internal Fixation Device into Left Metacarpophalangeal Joint, Percutaneous Endoscopic Approach

0RHV45Z   Insertion of External Fixation Device into Left Metacarpophalangeal Joint, Percutaneous Endoscopic Approach

0RHV48Z   Insertion of Spacer into Left Metacarpophalangeal Joint, Percutaneous Endoscopic Approach

0RHW03Z   Insertion of Infusion Device into Right Finger Phalangeal Joint, Open Approach

0RHW04Z   Insertion of Internal Fixation Device into Right Finger Phalangcal Joint, Open Approach

0RHW05Z   Insertion of External Fixation Device into Right Finger Phalangeal Joint, Open Approach

0RHW08Z   Insertion of Spacer into Right Finger Phalangeal Joint, Open Approach

0RHW33Z   Insertion of Infusion Device into Right Finger Phalangeal Joint, Percutaneous Approach

0RHW34Z   Insertion of Internal Fixation Device into Right Finger Phalangeal Joint, Percutaneous Approach

0RHW35Z   Insertion of External Fixation Device into Right Finger Phalangeal Joint, Percutaneous Approach

0RHW38Z   Insertion of Spacer into Right Finger Phalangeal Joint, Percutaneous Approach

0RHW43Z   Insertion of Infusion Device into Right Finger Phalangeal Joint, Percutaneous Endoscopic Approach

0RHW44Z   Insertion of Internal Fixation Device into Right Finger Phalangeal Joint, Percutaneous Endoscopic Approach

0RHW45Z   Insertion of External Fixation Device into Right Finger Phalangeal Joint, Percutaneous Endoscopic Approach

0RHW48Z   Insertion of Spacer into Right Finger Phalangeal Joint, Percutaneous Endoscopic Approach

0RHX03Z   Insertion of Infusion Device into Left Finger Phalangeal Joint, Open Approach

0RHX04Z   Insertion of Internal Fixation Device into Left Finger Phalangeal Joint, Open Approach

0RHX05Z   Insertion of External Fixation Device into Left Finger Phalangeal Joint, Open Approach

0RHX08Z   Insertion of Spacer into Left Finger Phalangeal Joint, Open Approach

0RHX33Z   Insertion of Infusion Device into Left Finger Phalangeal Joint, Percutaneous Approach

0RHX34Z   Insertion of Internal Fixation Device into Left Finger Phalangeal Joint, Percutaneous Approach

0RHX35Z   Insertion of External Fixation Device into Left Finger Phalangeal Joint, Percutaneous Approach

0RHX38Z   Insertion of Spacer into Left Finger Phalangeal Joint, Percutaneous Approach

0RHX43Z   Insertion of Infusion Device into Left Finger Phalangeal Joint, Percutaneous Endoscopic Approach

0RHX44Z   Insertion of Internal Fixation Device into Left Finger Phalangeal Joint, Percutaneous Endoscopic Approach

0RHX45Z   Insertion of External Fixation Device into Left Finger Phalangeal Joint, Percutaneous Endoscopic Approach

0RHX48Z   Insertion of Spacer into Left Finger Phalangeal Joint, Percutaneous Endoscopic Approach

RJ – Upper Joints, Inspection

eview Coding Guideline B3.5

eview Coding Guidelines B3.11a, B3.11b and B3.11c

RJ00ZZ   Inspection of Occipital-cervical Joint, Open Approach

RJ03ZZ   Inspection of Occipital-cervical Joint, Percutaneous Approach

RJ04ZZ   Inspection of Occipital-cervical Joint, Percutaneous Endoscopic Approach

RJ0XZZ   Inspection of Occipital-cervical Joint, External Approach

RJ10ZZ   Inspection of Cervical Vertebral Joint, Open Approach

RJ13ZZ   Inspection of Cervical Vertebral Joint, Percutaneous Approach

0RJ14ZZ   Inspection of Cervical Vertebral Joint, Percutaneous Endoscopic Approach

0RJ1XZZ   Inspection of Cervical Vertebral Joint, External Approach

0RJ30ZZ   Inspection of Cervical Vertebral Disc, Open Approach

0RJ33ZZ   Inspection of Cervical Vertebral Disc, Percutaneous Approach

0RJ34ZZ   Inspection of Cervical Vertebral Disc, Percutaneous Endoscopic Approach

0RJ3XZZ   Inspection of Cervical Vertebral Disc, External Approach

0RJ40ZZ   Inspection of Cervicothoracic Vertebral Joint, Open Approach

0RJ43ZZ   Inspection of Cervicothoracic Vertebral Joint, Percutaneous Approach

0RJ44ZZ   Inspection of Cervicothoracic Vertebral Joint, Percutaneous Endoscopic Approach

0RJ4XZZ   Inspection of Cervicothoracic Vertebral Joint, External Approach

0RJ50ZZ   Inspection of Cervicothoracic Vertebral Disc, Open Approach

0RJ53ZZ   Inspection of Cervicothoracic Vertebral Disc, Percutaneous Approach

Female-only   ♂ Male-only   ▲ Limited Coverage   ● Non-OR   ▦ HAC-associated procedure   ▲ Non-covered procedures   ✛ Combination

Code	Description	Code	Description	Code	Description
0RJ54ZZ	Inspection of Cervicothoracic Vertebral Disc, Percutaneous Endoscopic Approach	0RJFXZZ	Inspection of Left Sternoclavicular Joint, External Approach	0RJQ0ZZ	Inspection of Right Carpal Joint, Open Approach
0RJ5XZZ	Inspection of Cervicothoracic Vertebral Disc, External Approach	0RJG0ZZ	Inspection of Right Acromioclavicular Joint, Open Approach	0RJQ3ZZ	Inspection of Right Carpal Joint, Percutaneous Approach
0RJ60ZZ	Inspection of Thoracic Vertebral Joint, Open Approach	0RJG3ZZ	Inspection of Right Acromioclavicular Joint, Percutaneous Approach	0RJQ4ZZ	Inspection of Right Carpal Joint, Percutaneous Endoscopic Approach
0RJ63ZZ	Inspection of Thoracic Vertebral Joint, Percutaneous Approach	0RJG4ZZ	Inspection of Right Acromioclavicular Joint, Percutaneous Endoscopic Approach	0RJQXZZ	Inspection of Right Carpal Joint, External Approach
0RJ64ZZ	Inspection of Thoracic Vertebral Joint, Percutaneous Endoscopic Approach	0RJGXZZ	Inspection of Right Acromioclavicular Joint, External Approach	0RJR0ZZ	Inspection of Left Carpal Joint, Open Approach
0RJ6XZZ	Inspection of Thoracic Vertebral Joint, External Approach	0RJH0ZZ	Inspection of Left Acromioclavicular Joint, Open Approach	0RJR3ZZ	Inspection of Left Carpal Joint, Percutaneous Approach
0RJ90ZZ	Inspection of Thoracic Vertebral Disc, Open Approach	0RJH3ZZ	Inspection of Left Acromioclavicular Joint, Percutaneous Approach	0RJR4ZZ	Inspection of Left Carpal Joint, Percutaneous Endoscopic Approach
0RJ93ZZ	Inspection of Thoracic Vertebral Disc, Percutaneous Approach	0RJH4ZZ	Inspection of Left Acromioclavicular Joint, Percutaneous Endoscopic Approach	0RJRXZZ	Inspection of Left Carpal Joint, External Approach
0RJ94ZZ	Inspection of Thoracic Vertebral Disc, Percutaneous Endoscopic Approach	0RJHXZZ	Inspection of Left Acromioclavicular Joint, External Approach	0RJS0ZZ	Inspection of Right Metacarpocarpal Joint, Open Approach
0RJ9XZZ	Inspection of Thoracic Vertebral Disc, External Approach	0RJJ0ZZ	Inspection of Right Shoulder Joint, Open Approach	0RJS3ZZ	Inspection of Right Metacarpocarpal Joint, Percutaneous Approach
0RJA0ZZ	Inspection of Thoracolumbar Vertebral Joint, Open Approach	0RJJ3ZZ	Inspection of Right Shoulder Joint, Percutaneous Approach	0RJS4ZZ	Inspection of Right Metacarpocarpal Joint, Percutaneous Endoscopic Approach
0RJA3ZZ	Inspection of Thoracolumbar Vertebral Joint, Percutaneous Approach	0RJJ4ZZ	Inspection of Right Shoulder Joint, Percutaneous Endoscopic Approach	0RJSXZZ	Inspection of Right Metacarpocarpal Joint, External Approach
0RJA4ZZ	Inspection of Thoracolumbar Vertebral Joint, Percutaneous Endoscopic Approach	0RJJXZZ	Inspection of Right Shoulder Joint, External Approach	0RJT0ZZ	Inspection of Left Metacarpocarpal Joint, Open Approach
0RJAXZZ	Inspection of Thoracolumbar Vertebral Joint, External Approach	0RJK0ZZ	Inspection of Left Shoulder Joint, Open Approach	0RJT3ZZ	Inspection of Left Metacarpocarpal Joint, Percutaneous Approach
0RJB0ZZ	Inspection of Thoracolumbar Vertebral Disc, Open Approach	0RJK3ZZ	Inspection of Left Shoulder Joint, Percutaneous Approach	0RJT4ZZ	Inspection of Left Metacarpocarpal Joint, Percutaneous Endoscopic Approach
0RJB3ZZ	Inspection of Thoracolumbar Vertebral Disc, Percutaneous Approach	0RJK4ZZ	Inspection of Left Shoulder Joint, Percutaneous Endoscopic Approach	0RJTXZZ	Inspection of Left Metacarpocarpal Joint, External Approach
0RJB4ZZ	Inspection of Thoracolumbar Vertebral Disc, Percutaneous Endoscopic Approach	0RJKXZZ	Inspection of Left Shoulder Joint, External Approach	0RJU0ZZ	Inspection of Right Metacarpophalangeal Joint, Open Approach
0RJBXZZ	Inspection of Thoracolumbar Vertebral Disc, External Approach	0RJL0ZZ	Inspection of Right Elbow Joint, Open Approach	0RJU3ZZ	Inspection of Right Metacarpophalangeal Joint, Percutaneous Approach
0RJC0ZZ	Inspection of Right Temporomandibular Joint, Open Approach	0RJL3ZZ	Inspection of Right Elbow Joint, Percutaneous Approach	0RJU4ZZ	Inspection of Right Metacarpophalangeal Joint, Percutaneous Endoscopic Approach
0RJC3ZZ	Inspection of Right Temporomandibular Joint, Percutaneous Approach	0RJL4ZZ	Inspection of Right Elbow Joint, Percutaneous Endoscopic Approach	0RJUXZZ	Inspection of Right Metacarpophalangeal Joint, External Approach
0RJC4ZZ	Inspection of Right Temporomandibular Joint, Percutaneous Endoscopic Approach	0RJLXZZ	Inspection of Right Elbow Joint, External Approach	0RJV0ZZ	Inspection of Left Metacarpophalangeal Joint, Open Approach
0RJCXZZ	Inspection of Right Temporomandibular Joint, External Approach	0RJM0ZZ	Inspection of Left Elbow Joint, Open Approach	0RJV3ZZ	Inspection of Left Metacarpophalangeal Joint, Percutaneous Approach
0RJD0ZZ	Inspection of Left Temporomandibular Joint, Open Approach	0RJM3ZZ	Inspection of Left Elbow Joint, Percutaneous Approach	0RJV4ZZ	Inspection of Left Metacarpophalangeal Joint, Percutaneous Endoscopic Approach
0RJD3ZZ	Inspection of Left Temporomandibular Joint, Percutaneous Approach	0RJM4ZZ	Inspection of Left Elbow Joint, Percutaneous Endoscopic Approach	0RJVXZZ	Inspection of Left Metacarpophalangeal Joint, External Approach
0RJD4ZZ	Inspection of Left Temporomandibular Joint, Percutaneous Endoscopic Approach	0RJMXZZ	Inspection of Left Elbow Joint, External Approach	0RJW0ZZ	Inspection of Right Finger Phalangeal Joint, Open Approach
0RJDXZZ	Inspection of Left Temporomandibular Joint, External Approach	0RJN0ZZ	Inspection of Right Wrist Joint, Open Approach	0RJW3ZZ	Inspection of Right Finger Phalangeal Joint, Percutaneous Approach
0RJE0ZZ	Inspection of Right Sternoclavicular Joint, Open Approach	0RJN3ZZ	Inspection of Right Wrist Joint, Percutaneous Approach	0RJW4ZZ	Inspection of Right Finger Phalangeal Joint, Percutaneous Endoscopic Approach
0RJE3ZZ	Inspection of Right Sternoclavicular Joint, Percutaneous Approach	0RJN4ZZ	Inspection of Right Wrist Joint, Percutaneous Endoscopic Approach	0RJWXZZ	Inspection of Right Finger Phalangeal Joint, External Approach
0RJE4ZZ	Inspection of Right Sternoclavicular Joint, Percutaneous Endoscopic Approach	0RJNXZZ	Inspection of Right Wrist Joint, External Approach	0RJX0ZZ	Inspection of Left Finger Phalangeal Joint, Open Approach
0RJEXZZ	Inspection of Right Sternoclavicular Joint, External Approach	0RJP0ZZ	Inspection of Left Wrist Joint, Open Approach	0RJX3ZZ	Inspection of Left Finger Phalangeal Joint, Percutaneous Approach
0RJF0ZZ	Inspection of Left Sternoclavicular Joint, Open Approach	0RJP3ZZ	Inspection of Left Wrist Joint, Percutaneous Approach	0RJX4ZZ	Inspection of Left Finger Phalangeal Joint, Percutaneous Endoscopic Approach
0RJF3ZZ	Inspection of Left Sternoclavicular Joint, Percutaneous Approach	0RJP4ZZ	Inspection of Left Wrist Joint, Percutaneous Endoscopic Approach	0RJXXZZ	Inspection of Left Finger Phalangeal Joint, External Approach
0RJF4ZZ	Inspection of Left Sternoclavicular Joint, Percutaneous Endoscopic Approach	0RJPXZZ	Inspection of Left Wrist Joint, External Approach		

0RN – Upper Joints, Release

Review Coding Guideline B3.13

0RN00ZZ	Release Occipital-cervical Joint, Open Approach	0RN0XZZ	Release Occipital-cervical Joint, External Approach	0RN14ZZ	Release Cervical Vertebral Joint, Percutaneous Endoscopic Approach
0RN03ZZ	Release Occipital-cervical Joint, Percutaneous Approach	0RN10ZZ	Release Cervical Vertebral Joint, Open Approach	0RN1XZZ	Release Cervical Vertebral Joint, External Approach
0RN04ZZ	Release Occipital-cervical Joint, Percutaneous Endoscopic Approach	0RN13ZZ	Release Cervical Vertebral Joint, Percutaneous Approach	0RN30ZZ	Release Cervical Vertebral Disc, Open Approach

N33ZZ	Release Cervical Vertebral Disc, Percutaneous Approach	
N34ZZ	Release Cervical Vertebral Disc, Percutaneous Endoscopic Approach	
N3XZZ	Release Cervical Vertebral Disc, External Approach	
N40ZZ	Release Cervicothoracic Vertebral Joint, Open Approach	
N43ZZ	Release Cervicothoracic Vertebral Joint, Percutaneous Approach	
N44ZZ	Release Cervicothoracic Vertebral Joint, Percutaneous Endoscopic Approach	
N4XZZ	Release Cervicothoracic Vertebral Joint, External Approach	
N50ZZ	Release Cervicothoracic Vertebral Disc, Open Approach	
N53ZZ	Release Cervicothoracic Vertebral Disc, Percutaneous Approach	
N54ZZ	Release Cervicothoracic Vertebral Disc, Percutaneous Endoscopic Approach	
N5XZZ	Release Cervicothoracic Vertebral Disc, External Approach	
N60ZZ	Release Thoracic Vertebral Joint, Open Approach	
N63ZZ	Release Thoracic Vertebral Joint, Percutaneous Approach	
N64ZZ	Release Thoracic Vertebral Joint, Percutaneous Endoscopic Approach	
N6XZZ	Release Thoracic Vertebral Joint, External Approach	
N90ZZ	Release Thoracic Vertebral Disc, Open Approach	
N93ZZ	Release Thoracic Vertebral Disc, Percutaneous Approach	
N94ZZ	Release Thoracic Vertebral Disc, Percutaneous Endoscopic Approach	
N9XZZ	Release Thoracic Vertebral Disc, External Approach	
NA0ZZ	Release Thoracolumbar Vertebral Joint, Open Approach	
NA3ZZ	Release Thoracolumbar Vertebral Joint, Percutaneous Approach	
NA4ZZ	Release Thoracolumbar Vertebral Joint, Percutaneous Endoscopic Approach	
NAXZZ	Release Thoracolumbar Vertebral Joint, External Approach	
NB0ZZ	Release Thoracolumbar Vertebral Disc, Open Approach	
NB3ZZ	Release Thoracolumbar Vertebral Disc, Percutaneous Approach	
NB4ZZ	Release Thoracolumbar Vertebral Disc, Percutaneous Endoscopic Approach	
NBXZZ	Release Thoracolumbar Vertebral Disc, External Approach	
NC0ZZ	Release Right Temporomandibular Joint, Open Approach	
NC3ZZ	Release Right Temporomandibular Joint, Percutaneous Approach	
NC4ZZ	Release Right Temporomandibular Joint, Percutaneous Endoscopic Approach	
NCXZZ	Release Right Temporomandibular Joint, External Approach	
ND0ZZ	Release Left Temporomandibular Joint, Open Approach	
ND3ZZ	Release Left Temporomandibular Joint, Percutaneous Approach	
ND4ZZ	Release Left Temporomandibular Joint, Percutaneous Endoscopic Approach	
NDXZZ	Release Left Temporomandibular Joint, External Approach	

0RNE0ZZ	Release Right Sternoclavicular Joint, Open Approach
0RNE3ZZ	Release Right Sternoclavicular Joint, Percutaneous Approach
0RNE4ZZ	Release Right Sternoclavicular Joint, Percutaneous Endoscopic Approach
0RNEXZZ	Release Right Sternoclavicular Joint, External Approach
0RNF0ZZ	Release Left Sternoclavicular Joint, Open Approach
0RNF3ZZ	Release Left Sternoclavicular Joint, Percutaneous Approach
0RNF4ZZ	Release Left Sternoclavicular Joint, Percutaneous Endoscopic Approach
0RNFXZZ	Release Left Sternoclavicular Joint, External Approach
0RNG0ZZ	Release Right Acromioclavicular Joint, Open Approach
0RNG3ZZ	Release Right Acromioclavicular Joint, Percutaneous Approach
0RNG4ZZ	Release Right Acromioclavicular Joint, Percutaneous Endoscopic Approach
0RNGXZZ	Release Right Acromioclavicular Joint, External Approach
0RNH0ZZ	Release Left Acromioclavicular Joint, Open Approach
0RNH3ZZ	Release Left Acromioclavicular Joint, Percutaneous Approach
0RNH4ZZ	Release Left Acromioclavicular Joint, Percutaneous Endoscopic Approach
0RNHXZZ	Release Left Acromioclavicular Joint, External Approach
0RNJ0ZZ	Release Right Shoulder Joint, Open Approach
0RNJ3ZZ	Release Right Shoulder Joint, Percutaneous Approach
0RNJ4ZZ	Release Right Shoulder Joint, Percutaneous Endoscopic Approach
0RNJXZZ	Release Right Shoulder Joint, External Approach
0RNK0ZZ	Release Left Shoulder Joint, Open Approach
0RNK3ZZ	Release Left Shoulder Joint, Percutaneous Approach
0RNK4ZZ	Release Left Shoulder Joint, Percutaneous Endoscopic Approach
0RNKXZZ	Release Left Shoulder Joint, External Approach
0RNL0ZZ	Release Right Elbow Joint, Open Approach
0RNL3ZZ	Release Right Elbow Joint, Percutaneous Approach
0RNL4ZZ	Release Right Elbow Joint, Percutaneous Endoscopic Approach
0RNLXZZ	Release Right Elbow Joint, External Approach
0RNM0ZZ	Release Left Elbow Joint, Open Approach
0RNM3ZZ	Release Left Elbow Joint, Percutaneous Approach
0RNM4ZZ	Release Left Elbow Joint, Percutaneous Endoscopic Approach
0RNMXZZ	Release Left Elbow Joint, External Approach
0RNN0ZZ	Release Right Wrist Joint, Open Approach
0RNN3ZZ	Release Right Wrist Joint, Percutaneous Approach
0RNN4ZZ	Release Right Wrist Joint, Percutaneous Endoscopic Approach
0RNNXZZ	Release Right Wrist Joint, External Approach

0RNP0ZZ	Release Left Wrist Joint, Open Approach
0RNP3ZZ	Release Left Wrist Joint, Percutaneous Approach
0RNP4ZZ	Release Left Wrist Joint, Percutaneous Endoscopic Approach
0RNPXZZ	Release Left Wrist Joint, External Approach
0RNQ0ZZ	Release Right Carpal Joint, Open Approach
0RNQ3ZZ	Release Right Carpal Joint, Percutaneous Approach
0RNQ4ZZ	Release Right Carpal Joint, Percutaneous Endoscopic Approach
0RNQXZZ	Release Right Carpal Joint, External Approach
0RNR0ZZ	Release Left Carpal Joint, Open Approach
0RNR3ZZ	Release Left Carpal Joint, Percutaneous Approach
0RNR4ZZ	Release Left Carpal Joint, Percutaneous Endoscopic Approach
0RNRXZZ	Release Left Carpal Joint, External Approach
0RNS0ZZ	Release Right Metacarpocarpal Joint, Open Approach
0RNS3ZZ	Release Right Metacarpocarpal Joint, Percutaneous Approach
0RNS4ZZ	Release Right Metacarpocarpal Joint, Percutaneous Endoscopic Approach
0RNSXZZ	Release Right Metacarpocarpal Joint, External Approach
0RNT0ZZ	Release Left Metacarpocarpal Joint, Open Approach
0RNT3ZZ	Release Left Metacarpocarpal Joint, Percutaneous Approach
0RNT4ZZ	Release Left Metacarpocarpal Joint, Percutaneous Endoscopic Approach
0RNTXZZ	Release Left Metacarpocarpal Joint, External Approach
0RNU0ZZ	Release Right Metacarpophalangeal Joint, Open Approach
0RNU3ZZ	Release Right Metacarpophalangeal Joint, Percutaneous Approach
0RNU4ZZ	Release Right Metacarpophalangeal Joint, Percutaneous Endoscopic Approach
0RNUXZZ	Release Right Metacarpophalangeal Joint, External Approach
0RNV0ZZ	Release Left Metacarpophalangeal Joint, Open Approach
0RNV3ZZ	Release Left Metacarpophalangeal Joint, Percutaneous Approach
0RNV4ZZ	Release Left Metacarpophalangeal Joint, Percutaneous Endoscopic Approach
0RNVXZZ	Release Left Metacarpophalangeal Joint, External Approach
0RNW0ZZ	Release Right Finger Phalangeal Joint, Open Approach
0RNW3ZZ	Release Right Finger Phalangeal Joint, Percutaneous Approach
0RNW4ZZ	Release Right Finger Phalangeal Joint, Percutaneous Endoscopic Approach
0RNWXZZ	Release Right Finger Phalangeal Joint, External Approach
0RNX0ZZ	Release Left Finger Phalangeal Joint, Open Approach
0RNX3ZZ	Release Left Finger Phalangeal Joint, Percutaneous Approach
0RNX4ZZ	Release Left Finger Phalangeal Joint, Percutaneous Endoscopic Approach
0RNXXZZ	Release Left Finger Phalangeal Joint, External Approach

0RP – Upper Joints, Removal

Review Coding Guideline B6.1c

RP000Z	Removal of Drainage Device from Occipital-cervical Joint, Open Approach	0RP003Z	Removal of Infusion Device from Occipital-cervical Joint, Open Approach	0RP004Z	Removal of Internal Fixation Device from Occipital-cervical Joint, Open Approach

933

Female-only	♂ Male-only	▲ Limited Coverage	● Non-OR	▥ HAC-associated procedure	▲ Non-covered procedures	➕ Combination

0RP007Z Removal of Autologous Tissue Substitute from Occipital-cervical Joint, Open Approach

0RP008Z Removal of Spacer from Occipital-cervical Joint, Open Approach

0RP00AZ Removal of Interbody Fusion Device from Occipital-cervical Joint, Open Approach

0RP00JZ Removal of Synthetic Substitute from Occipital-cervical Joint, Open Approach

0RP00KZ Removal of Nonautologous Tissue Substitute from Occipital-cervical Joint, Open Approach

0RP030Z Removal of Drainage Device from Occipital-cervical Joint, Percutaneous Approach

0RP033Z Removal of Infusion Device from Occipital-cervical Joint, Percutaneous Approach

0RP034Z Removal of Internal Fixation Device from Occipital-cervical Joint, Percutaneous Approach

0RP037Z Removal of Autologous Tissue Substitute from Occipital-cervical Joint, Percutaneous Approach

0RP038Z Removal of Spacer from Occipital-cervical Joint, Percutaneous Approach

0RP03AZ Removal of Interbody Fusion Device from Occipital-cervical Joint, Percutaneous Approach

0RP03JZ Removal of Synthetic Substitute from Occipital-cervical Joint, Percutaneous Approach

0RP03KZ Removal of Nonautologous Tissue Substitute from Occipital-cervical Joint, Percutaneous Approach

0RP040Z Removal of Drainage Device from Occipital-cervical Joint, Percutaneous Endoscopic Approach

0RP043Z Removal of Infusion Device from Occipital-cervical Joint, Percutaneous Endoscopic Approach

0RP044Z Removal of Internal Fixation Device from Occipital-cervical Joint, Percutaneous Endoscopic Approach

0RP047Z Removal of Autologous Tissue Substitute from Occipital-cervical Joint, Percutaneous Endoscopic Approach

0RP048Z Removal of Spacer from Occipital-cervical Joint, Percutaneous Endoscopic Approach

0RP04AZ Removal of Interbody Fusion Device from Occipital-cervical Joint, Percutaneous Endoscopic Approach

0RP04JZ Removal of Synthetic Substitute from Occipital-cervical Joint, Percutaneous Endoscopic Approach

0RP04KZ Removal of Nonautologous Tissue Substitute from Occipital-cervical Joint, Percutaneous Endoscopic Approach

0RP0X0Z Removal of Drainage Device from Occipital-cervical Joint, External Approach

0RP0X3Z Removal of Infusion Device from Occipital-cervical Joint, External Approach

0RP0X4Z Removal of Internal Fixation Device from Occipital-cervical Joint, External Approach

0RP100Z Removal of Drainage Device from Cervical Vertebral Joint, Open Approach

0RP103Z Removal of Infusion Device from Cervical Vertebral Joint, Open Approach

0RP104Z Removal of Internal Fixation Device from Cervical Vertebral Joint, Open Approach

0RP107Z Removal of Autologous Tissue Substitute from Cervical Vertebral Joint, Open Approach

0RP108Z Removal of Spacer from Cervical Vertebral Joint, Open Approach

0RP10AZ Removal of Interbody Fusion Device from Cervical Vertebral Joint, Open Approach

0RP10JZ Removal of Synthetic Substitute from Cervical Vertebral Joint, Open Approach

0RP10KZ Removal of Nonautologous Tissue Substitute from Cervical Vertebral Joint, Open Approach

0RP130Z Removal of Drainage Device from Cervical Vertebral Joint, Percutaneous Approach

0RP133Z Removal of Infusion Device from Cervical Vertebral Joint, Percutaneous Approach

0RP134Z Removal of Internal Fixation Device from Cervical Vertebral Joint, Percutaneous Approach

0RP137Z Removal of Autologous Tissue Substitute from Cervical Vertebral Joint, Percutaneous Approach

0RP138Z Removal of Spacer from Cervical Vertebral Joint, Percutaneous Approach

0RP13AZ Removal of Interbody Fusion Device from Cervical Vertebral Joint, Percutaneous Approach

0RP13JZ Removal of Synthetic Substitute from Cervical Vertebral Joint, Percutaneous Approach

0RP13KZ Removal of Nonautologous Tissue Substitute from Cervical Vertebral Joint, Percutaneous Approach

0RP140Z Removal of Drainage Device from Cervical Vertebral Joint, Percutaneous Endoscopic Approach

0RP143Z Removal of Infusion Device from Cervical Vertebral Joint, Percutaneous Endoscopic Approach

0RP144Z Removal of Internal Fixation Device from Cervical Vertebral Joint, Percutaneous Endoscopic Approach

0RP147Z Removal of Autologous Tissue Substitute from Cervical Vertebral Joint, Percutaneous Endoscopic Approach

0RP148Z Removal of Spacer from Cervical Vertebral Joint, Percutaneous Endoscopic Approach

0RP14AZ Removal of Interbody Fusion Device from Cervical Vertebral Joint, Percutaneous Endoscopic Approach

0RP14JZ Removal of Synthetic Substitute from Cervical Vertebral Joint, Percutaneous Endoscopic Approach

0RP14KZ Removal of Nonautologous Tissue Substitute from Cervical Vertebral Joint, Percutaneous Endoscopic Approach

0RP1X0Z Removal of Drainage Device from Cervical Vertebral Joint, External Approach

0RP1X3Z Removal of Infusion Device from Cervical Vertebral Joint, External Approach

0RP1X4Z Removal of Internal Fixation Device from Cervical Vertebral Joint, External Approach

0RP300Z Removal of Drainage Device from Cervical Vertebral Disc, Open Approach

0RP303Z Removal of Infusion Device from Cervical Vertebral Disc, Open Approach

0RP307Z Removal of Autologous Tissue Substitute from Cervical Vertebral Disc, Open Approach

0RP30JZ Removal of Synthetic Substitute from Cervical Vertebral Disc, Open Approach

0RP30KZ Removal of Nonautologous Tissue Substitute from Cervical Vertebral Disc, Open Approach

0RP330Z Removal of Drainage Device from Cervical Vertebral Disc, Percutaneous Approach

0RP333Z Removal of Infusion Device from Cervical Vertebral Disc, Percutaneous Approach

0RP337Z Removal of Autologous Tissue Substitute from Cervical Vertebral Disc, Percutaneous Approach

0RP33JZ Removal of Synthetic Substitute from Cervical Vertebral Disc, Percutaneous Approach

0RP33KZ Removal of Nonautologous Tissue Substitute from Cervical Vertebral Disc, Percutaneous Approach

0RP340Z Removal of Drainage Device from Cervical Vertebral Disc, Percutaneous Endoscopic Approach

0RP343Z Removal of Infusion Device from Cervical Vertebral Disc, Percutaneous Endoscopic Approach

0RP347Z Removal of Autologous Tissue Substitute from Cervical Vertebral Disc, Percutaneous Endoscopic Approach

0RP34JZ Removal of Synthetic Substitute from Cervical Vertebral Disc, Percutaneous Endoscopic Approach

0RP34KZ Removal of Nonautologous Tissue Substitute from Cervical Vertebral Disc, Percutaneous Endoscopic Approach

0RP3X0Z Removal of Drainage Device from Cervical Vertebral Disc, External Approach

0RP3X3Z Removal of Infusion Device from Cervical Vertebral Disc, External Approach

0RP400Z Removal of Drainage Device from Cervicothoracic Vertebral Joint, Open Approach

0RP403Z Removal of Infusion Device from Cervicothoracic Vertebral Joint, Open Approach

0RP404Z Removal of Internal Fixation Device from Cervicothoracic Vertebral Joint, Open Approach

0RP407Z Removal of Autologous Tissue Substitute from Cervicothoracic Vertebral Joint, Open Approach

0RP408Z Removal of Spacer from Cervicothoracic Vertebral Joint, Open Approach

0RP40AZ Removal of Interbody Fusion Device from Cervicothoracic Vertebral Joint, Open Approach

0RP40JZ Removal of Synthetic Substitute from Cervicothoracic Vertebral Joint, Open Approach

0RP40KZ Removal of Nonautologous Tissue Substitute from Cervicothoracic Vertebral Joint, Open Approach

0RP430Z Removal of Drainage Device from Cervicothoracic Vertebral Joint, Percutaneous Approach

0RP433Z Removal of Infusion Device from Cervicothoracic Vertebral Joint, Percutaneous Approach

0RP434Z Removal of Internal Fixation Device from Cervicothoracic Vertebral Joint, Percutaneous Approach

0RP437Z Removal of Autologous Tissue Substitute from Cervicothoracic Vertebral Joint, Percutaneous Approach

0RP438Z Removal of Spacer from Cervicothoracic Vertebral Joint, Percutaneous Approach

0RP43AZ Removal of Interbody Fusion Device from Cervicothoracic Vertebral Joint, Percutaneous Approach

0RP43JZ Removal of Synthetic Substitute from Cervicothoracic Vertebral Joint, Percutaneous Approach

0RP43KZ Removal of Nonautologous Tissue Substitute from Cervicothoracic Vertebral Joint, Percutaneous Approach

♀ Female-only   ♂ Male-only   ▲ Limited Coverage   ● Non-OR   ▧ HAC-associated procedure   ▲ Non-covered procedures   ✚ Combination

P440Z Removal of Drainage Device from Cervicothoracic Vertebral Joint, Percutaneous Endoscopic Approach

P443Z Removal of Infusion Device from Cervicothoracic Vertebral Joint, Percutaneous Endoscopic Approach

P444Z Removal of Internal Fixation Device from Cervicothoracic Vertebral Joint, Percutaneous Endoscopic Approach

P447Z Removal of Autologous Tissue Substitute from Cervicothoracic Vertebral Joint, Percutaneous Endoscopic Approach

P448Z Removal of Spacer from Cervicothoracic Vertebral Joint, Percutaneous Endoscopic Approach

P44AZ Removal of Interbody Fusion Device from Cervicothoracic Vertebral Joint, Percutaneous Endoscopic Approach

P44JZ Removal of Synthetic Substitute from Cervicothoracic Vertebral Joint, Percutaneous Endoscopic Approach

P44KZ Removal of Nonautologous Tissue Substitute from Cervicothoracic Vertebral Joint, Percutaneous Endoscopic Approach

P4X0Z Removal of Drainage Device from Cervicothoracic Vertebral Joint, External Approach

P4X3Z Removal of Infusion Device from Cervicothoracic Vertebral Joint, External Approach

P4X4Z Removal of Internal Fixation Device from Cervicothoracic Vertebral Joint, External Approach

P500Z Removal of Drainage Device from Cervicothoracic Vertebral Disc, Open Approach

P503Z Removal of Infusion Device from Cervicothoracic Vertebral Disc, Open Approach

P507Z Removal of Autologous Tissue Substitute from Cervicothoracic Vertebral Disc, Open Approach

P50JZ Removal of Synthetic Substitute from Cervicothoracic Vertebral Disc, Open Approach

P50KZ Removal of Nonautologous Tissue Substitute from Cervicothoracic Vertebral Disc, Open Approach

P530Z Removal of Drainage Device from Cervicothoracic Vertebral Disc, Percutaneous Approach

P533Z Removal of Infusion Device from Cervicothoracic Vertebral Disc, Percutaneous Approach

P537Z Removal of Autologous Tissue Substitute from Cervicothoracic Vertebral Disc, Percutaneous Approach

P53JZ Removal of Synthetic Substitute from Cervicothoracic Vertebral Disc, Percutaneous Approach

P53KZ Removal of Nonautologous Tissue Substitute from Cervicothoracic Vertebral Disc, Percutaneous Approach

P540Z Removal of Drainage Device from Cervicothoracic Vertebral Disc, Percutaneous Endoscopic Approach

P543Z Removal of Infusion Device from Cervicothoracic Vertebral Disc, Percutaneous Endoscopic Approach

P547Z Removal of Autologous Tissue Substitute from Cervicothoracic Vertebral Disc, Percutaneous Endoscopic Approach

P54JZ Removal of Synthetic Substitute from Cervicothoracic Vertebral Disc, Percutaneous Endoscopic Approach

P54KZ Removal of Nonautologous Tissue Substitute from Cervicothoracic Vertebral Disc, Percutaneous Endoscopic Approach

0RP5X0Z Removal of Drainage Device from Cervicothoracic Vertebral Disc, External Approach

0RP5X3Z Removal of Infusion Device from Cervicothoracic Vertebral Disc, External Approach

0RP600Z Removal of Drainage Device from Thoracic Vertebral Joint, Open Approach

0RP603Z Removal of Infusion Device from Thoracic Vertebral Joint, Open Approach

0RP604Z Removal of Internal Fixation Device from Thoracic Vertebral Joint, Open Approach

0RP607Z Removal of Autologous Tissue Substitute from Thoracic Vertebral Joint, Open Approach

0RP608Z Removal of Spacer from Thoracic Vertebral Joint, Open Approach

0RP60AZ Removal of Interbody Fusion Device from Thoracic Vertebral Joint, Open Approach

0RP60JZ Removal of Synthetic Substitute from Thoracic Vertebral Joint, Open Approach

0RP60KZ Removal of Nonautologous Tissue Substitute from Thoracic Vertebral Joint, Open Approach

0RP630Z Removal of Drainage Device from Thoracic Vertebral Joint, Percutaneous Approach

0RP633Z Removal of Infusion Device from Thoracic Vertebral Joint, Percutaneous Approach

0RP634Z Removal of Internal Fixation Device from Thoracic Vertebral Joint, Percutaneous Approach

0RP637Z Removal of Autologous Tissue Substitute from Thoracic Vertebral Joint, Percutaneous Approach

0RP638Z Removal of Spacer from Thoracic Vertebral Joint, Percutaneous Approach

0RP63AZ Removal of Interbody Fusion Device from Thoracic Vertebral Joint, Percutaneous Approach

0RP63JZ Removal of Synthetic Substitute from Thoracic Vertebral Joint, Percutaneous Approach

0RP63KZ Removal of Nonautologous Tissue Substitute from Thoracic Vertebral Joint, Percutaneous Approach

0RP640Z Removal of Drainage Device from Thoracic Vertebral Joint, Percutaneous Endoscopic Approach

0RP643Z Removal of Infusion Device from Thoracic Vertebral Joint, Percutaneous Endoscopic Approach

0RP644Z Removal of Internal Fixation Device from Thoracic Vertebral Joint, Percutaneous Endoscopic Approach

0RP647Z Removal of Autologous Tissue Substitute from Thoracic Vertebral Joint, Percutaneous Endoscopic Approach

0RP648Z Removal of Spacer from Thoracic Vertebral Joint, Percutaneous Endoscopic Approach

0RP64AZ Removal of Interbody Fusion Device from Thoracic Vertebral Joint, Percutaneous Endoscopic Approach

0RP64JZ Removal of Synthetic Substitute from Thoracic Vertebral Joint, Percutaneous Endoscopic Approach

0RP64KZ Removal of Nonautologous Tissue Substitute from Thoracic Vertebral Joint, Percutaneous Endoscopic Approach

0RP6X0Z Removal of Drainage Device from Thoracic Vertebral Joint, External Approach

0RP6X3Z Removal of Infusion Device from Thoracic Vertebral Joint, External Approach

0RP6X4Z Removal of Internal Fixation Device from Thoracic Vertebral Joint, External Approach

0RP900Z Removal of Drainage Device from Thoracic Vertebral Disc, Open Approach

0RP903Z Removal of Infusion Device from Thoracic Vertebral Disc, Open Approach

0RP907Z Removal of Autologous Tissue Substitute from Thoracic Vertebral Disc, Open Approach

0RP90JZ Removal of Synthetic Substitute from Thoracic Vertebral Disc, Open Approach

0RP90KZ Removal of Nonautologous Tissue Substitute from Thoracic Vertebral Disc, Open Approach

0RP930Z Removal of Drainage Device from Thoracic Vertebral Disc, Percutaneous Approach

0RP933Z Removal of Infusion Device from Thoracic Vertebral Disc, Percutaneous Approach

0RP937Z Removal of Autologous Tissue Substitute from Thoracic Vertebral Disc, Percutaneous Approach

0RP93JZ Removal of Synthetic Substitute from Thoracic Vertebral Disc, Percutaneous Approach

0RP93KZ Removal of Nonautologous Tissue Substitute from Thoracic Vertebral Disc, Percutaneous Approach

0RP940Z Removal of Drainage Device from Thoracic Vertebral Disc, Percutaneous Endoscopic Approach

0RP943Z Removal of Infusion Device from Thoracic Vertebral Disc, Percutaneous Endoscopic Approach

0RP947Z Removal of Autologous Tissue Substitute from Thoracic Vertebral Disc, Percutaneous Endoscopic Approach

0RP94JZ Removal of Synthetic Substitute from Thoracic Vertebral Disc, Percutaneous Endoscopic Approach

0RP94KZ Removal of Nonautologous Tissue Substitute from Thoracic Vertebral Disc, Percutaneous Endoscopic Approach

0RP9X0Z Removal of Drainage Device from Thoracic Vertebral Disc, External Approach

0RP9X3Z Removal of Infusion Device from Thoracic Vertebral Disc, External Approach

0RPA00Z Removal of Drainage Device from Thoracolumbar Vertebral Joint, Open Approach

0RPA03Z Removal of Infusion Device from Thoracolumbar Vertebral Joint, Open Approach

0RPA04Z Removal of Internal Fixation Device from Thoracolumbar Vertebral Joint, Open Approach

0RPA07Z Removal of Autologous Tissue Substitute from Thoracolumbar Vertebral Joint, Open Approach

0RPA08Z Removal of Spacer from Thoracolumbar Vertebral Joint, Open Approach

0RPA0AZ Removal of Interbody Fusion Device from Thoracolumbar Vertebral Joint, Open Approach

0RPA0JZ Removal of Synthetic Substitute from Thoracolumbar Vertebral Joint, Open Approach

0RPA0KZ Removal of Nonautologous Tissue Substitute from Thoracolumbar Vertebral Joint, Open Approach

0RPA30Z Removal of Drainage Device from Thoracolumbar Vertebral Joint, Percutaneous Approach

935

0RPA33Z Removal of Infusion Device from Thoracolumbar Vertebral Joint, Percutaneous Approach

0RPA34Z Removal of Internal Fixation Device from Thoracolumbar Vertebral Joint, Percutaneous Approach

0RPA37Z Removal of Autologous Tissue Substitute from Thoracolumbar Vertebral Joint, Percutaneous Approach

0RPA38Z Removal of Spacer from Thoracolumbar Vertebral Joint, Percutaneous Approach

0RPA3AZ Removal of Interbody Fusion Device from Thoracolumbar Vertebral Joint, Percutaneous Approach

0RPA3JZ Removal of Synthetic Substitute from Thoracolumbar Vertebral Joint, Percutaneous Approach

0RPA3KZ Removal of Nonautologous Tissue Substitute from Thoracolumbar Vertebral Joint, Percutaneous Approach

0RPA40Z Removal of Drainage Device from Thoracolumbar Vertebral Joint, Percutaneous Endoscopic Approach

0RPA43Z Removal of Infusion Device from Thoracolumbar Vertebral Joint, Percutaneous Endoscopic Approach

0RPA44Z Removal of Internal Fixation Device from Thoracolumbar Vertebral Joint, Percutaneous Endoscopic Approach

0RPA47Z Removal of Autologous Tissue Substitute from Thoracolumbar Vertebral Joint, Percutaneous Endoscopic Approach

0RPA48Z Removal of Spacer from Thoracolumbar Vertebral Joint, Percutaneous Endoscopic Approach

0RPA4AZ Removal of Interbody Fusion Device from Thoracolumbar Vertebral Joint, Percutaneous Endoscopic Approach

0RPA4JZ Removal of Synthetic Substitute from Thoracolumbar Vertebral Joint, Percutaneous Endoscopic Approach

0RPA4KZ Removal of Nonautologous Tissue Substitute from Thoracolumbar Vertebral Joint, Percutaneous Endoscopic Approach

0RPAX0Z Removal of Drainage Device from Thoracolumbar Vertebral Joint, External Approach

0RPAX3Z Removal of Infusion Device from Thoracolumbar Vertebral Joint, External Approach

0RPAX4Z Removal of Internal Fixation Device from Thoracolumbar Vertebral Joint, External Approach

0RPB00Z Removal of Drainage Device from Thoracolumbar Vertebral Disc, Open Approach

0RPB03Z Removal of Infusion Device from Thoracolumbar Vertebral Disc, Open Approach

0RPB07Z Removal of Autologous Tissue Substitute from Thoracolumbar Vertebral Disc, Open Approach

0RPB0JZ Removal of Synthetic Substitute from Thoracolumbar Vertebral Disc, Open Approach

0RPB0KZ Removal of Nonautologous Tissue Substitute from Thoracolumbar Vertebral Disc, Open Approach

0RPB30Z Removal of Drainage Device from Thoracolumbar Vertebral Disc, Percutaneous Approach

0RPB33Z Removal of Infusion Device from Thoracolumbar Vertebral Disc, Percutaneous Approach

0RPB37Z Removal of Autologous Tissue Substitute from Thoracolumbar Vertebral Disc, Percutaneous Approach

0RPB3JZ Removal of Synthetic Substitute from Thoracolumbar Vertebral Disc, Percutaneous Approach

0RPB3KZ Removal of Nonautologous Tissue Substitute from Thoracolumbar Vertebral Disc, Percutaneous Approach

0RPB40Z Removal of Drainage Device from Thoracolumbar Vertebral Disc, Percutaneous Endoscopic Approach

0RPB43Z Removal of Infusion Device from Thoracolumbar Vertebral Disc, Percutaneous Endoscopic Approach

0RPB47Z Removal of Autologous Tissue Substitute from Thoracolumbar Vertebral Disc, Percutaneous Endoscopic Approach

0RPB4JZ Removal of Synthetic Substitute from Thoracolumbar Vertebral Disc, Percutaneous Endoscopic Approach

0RPB4KZ Removal of Nonautologous Tissue Substitute from Thoracolumbar Vertebral Disc, Percutaneous Endoscopic Approach

0RPBX0Z Removal of Drainage Device from Thoracolumbar Vertebral Disc, External Approach

0RPBX3Z Removal of Infusion Device from Thoracolumbar Vertebral Disc, External Approach

0RPC00Z Removal of Drainage Device from Right Temporomandibular Joint, Open Approach

0RPC03Z Removal of Infusion Device from Right Temporomandibular Joint, Open Approach

0RPC04Z Removal of Internal Fixation Device from Right Temporomandibular Joint, Open Approach

0RPC07Z Removal of Autologous Tissue Substitute from Right Temporomandibular Joint, Open Approach

0RPC08Z Removal of Spacer from Right Temporomandibular Joint, Open Approach

0RPC0JZ Removal of Synthetic Substitute from Right Temporomandibular Joint, Open Approach

0RPC0KZ Removal of Nonautologous Tissue Substitute from Right Temporomandibular Joint, Open Approach

0RPC30Z Removal of Drainage Device from Right Temporomandibular Joint, Percutaneous Approach

0RPC33Z Removal of Infusion Device from Right Temporomandibular Joint, Percutaneous Approach

0RPC34Z Removal of Internal Fixation Device from Right Temporomandibular Joint, Percutaneous Approach

0RPC37Z Removal of Autologous Tissue Substitute from Right Temporomandibular Joint, Percutaneous Approach

0RPC38Z Removal of Spacer from Right Temporomandibular Joint, Percutaneous Approach

0RPC3JZ Removal of Synthetic Substitute from Right Temporomandibular Joint, Percutaneous Approach

0RPC3KZ Removal of Nonautologous Tissue Substitute from Right Temporomandibular Joint, Percutaneous Approach

0RPC40Z Removal of Drainage Device from Right Temporomandibular Joint, Percutaneous Endoscopic Approach

0RPC43Z Removal of Infusion Device from Right Temporomandibular Joint, Percutaneous Endoscopic Approach

0RPC44Z Removal of Internal Fixation Device from Right Temporomandibular Joint, Percutaneous Endoscopic Approach

0RPC47Z Removal of Autologous Tissue Substitute from Right Temporomandibular Joint, Percutaneous Endoscopic Approach

0RPC48Z Removal of Spacer from Right Temporomandibular Joint, Percutaneous Endoscopic Approach

0RPC4JZ Removal of Synthetic Substitute from Right Temporomandibular Joint, Percutaneous Endoscopic Approach

0RPC4KZ Removal of Nonautologous Tissue Substitute from Right Temporomandibular Joint, Percutaneous Endoscopic Approach

0RPCX0Z Removal of Drainage Device from Right Temporomandibular Joint, External Approach

0RPCX3Z Removal of Infusion Device from Right Temporomandibular Joint, External Approach

0RPCX4Z Removal of Internal Fixation Device from Right Temporomandibular Joint, External Approach

0RPD00Z Removal of Drainage Device from Left Temporomandibular Joint, Open Approach

0RPD03Z Removal of Infusion Device from Left Temporomandibular Joint, Open Approach

0RPD04Z Removal of Internal Fixation Device from Left Temporomandibular Joint, Open Approach

0RPD07Z Removal of Autologous Tissue Substitute from Left Temporomandibular Joint, Open Approach

0RPD08Z Removal of Spacer from Left Temporomandibular Joint, Open Approach

0RPD0JZ Removal of Synthetic Substitute from Left Temporomandibular Joint, Open Approach

0RPD0KZ Removal of Nonautologous Tissue Substitute from Left Temporomandibular Joint, Open Approach

0RPD30Z Removal of Drainage Device from Left Temporomandibular Joint, Percutaneous Approach

0RPD33Z Removal of Infusion Device from Left Temporomandibular Joint, Percutaneous Approach

0RPD34Z Removal of Internal Fixation Device from Left Temporomandibular Joint, Percutaneous Approach

0RPD37Z Removal of Autologous Tissue Substitute from Left Temporomandibular Joint, Percutaneous Approach

0RPD38Z Removal of Spacer from Left Temporomandibular Joint, Percutaneous Approach

0RPD3JZ Removal of Synthetic Substitute from Left Temporomandibular Joint, Percutaneous Approach

0RPD3KZ Removal of Nonautologous Tissue Substitute from Left Temporomandibular Joint, Percutaneous Approach

0RPD40Z Removal of Drainage Device from Left Temporomandibular Joint, Percutaneous Endoscopic Approach

0RPD43Z Removal of Infusion Device from Left Temporomandibular Joint, Percutaneous Endoscopic Approach

0RPD44Z Removal of Internal Fixation Device from Left Temporomandibular Joint, Percutaneous Endoscopic Approach

0RPD47Z Removal of Autologous Tissue Substitute from Left Temporomandibular Joint, Percutaneous Endoscopic Approach

0RPD48Z Removal of Spacer from Left Temporomandibular Joint, Percutaneous Endoscopic Approach

♀ Female-only ♂ Male-only ▲ Limited Coverage ● Non-OR ▨ HAC-associated procedure ▲ Non-covered procedures ✛ Combination

0RPD4JZ Removal of Synthetic Substitute from Left Temporomandibular Joint, Percutaneous Endoscopic Approach
0RPD4KZ Removal of Nonautologous Tissue Substitute from Left Temporomandibular Joint, Percutaneous Endoscopic Approach
0RPDX0Z Removal of Drainage Device from Left Temporomandibular Joint, External Approach
0RPDX3Z Removal of Infusion Device from Left Temporomandibular Joint, External Approach
0RPDX4Z Removal of Internal Fixation Device from Left Temporomandibular Joint, External Approach
0RPE00Z Removal of Drainage Device from Right Sternoclavicular Joint, Open Approach
0RPE03Z Removal of Infusion Device from Right Sternoclavicular Joint, Open Approach
0RPE04Z Removal of Internal Fixation Device from Right Sternoclavicular Joint, Open Approach
0RPE07Z Removal of Autologous Tissue Substitute from Right Sternoclavicular Joint, Open Approach
0RPE08Z Removal of Spacer from Right Sternoclavicular Joint, Open Approach
0RPE0JZ Removal of Synthetic Substitute from Right Sternoclavicular Joint, Open Approach
0RPE0KZ Removal of Nonautologous Tissue Substitute from Right Sternoclavicular Joint, Open Approach
0RPE30Z Removal of Drainage Device from Right Sternoclavicular Joint, Percutaneous Approach
0RPE33Z Removal of Infusion Device from Right Sternoclavicular Joint, Percutaneous Approach
0RPE34Z Removal of Internal Fixation Device from Right Sternoclavicular Joint, Percutaneous Approach
0RPE37Z Removal of Autologous Tissue Substitute from Right Sternoclavicular Joint, Percutaneous Approach
0RPE38Z Removal of Spacer from Right Sternoclavicular Joint, Percutaneous Approach
0RPE3JZ Removal of Synthetic Substitute from Right Sternoclavicular Joint, Percutaneous Approach
0RPE3KZ Removal of Nonautologous Tissue Substitute from Right Sternoclavicular Joint, Percutaneous Approach
0RPE40Z Removal of Drainage Device from Right Sternoclavicular Joint, Percutaneous Endoscopic Approach
0RPE43Z Removal of Infusion Device from Right Sternoclavicular Joint, Percutaneous Endoscopic Approach
0RPE44Z Removal of Internal Fixation Device from Right Sternoclavicular Joint, Percutaneous Endoscopic Approach
0RPE47Z Removal of Autologous Tissue Substitute from Right Sternoclavicular Joint, Percutaneous Endoscopic Approach
0RPE48Z Removal of Spacer from Right Sternoclavicular Joint, Percutaneous Endoscopic Approach
0RPE4JZ Removal of Synthetic Substitute from Right Sternoclavicular Joint, Percutaneous Endoscopic Approach
0RPE4KZ Removal of Nonautologous Tissue Substitute from Right Sternoclavicular Joint, Percutaneous Endoscopic Approach
0RPEX0Z Removal of Drainage Device from Right Sternoclavicular Joint, External Approach

0RPEX3Z Removal of Infusion Device from Right Sternoclavicular Joint, External Approach
0RPEX4Z Removal of Internal Fixation Device from Right Sternoclavicular Joint, External Approach
0RPF00Z Removal of Drainage Device from Left Sternoclavicular Joint, Open Approach
0RPF03Z Removal of Infusion Device from Left Sternoclavicular Joint, Open Approach
0RPF04Z Removal of Internal Fixation Device from Left Sternoclavicular Joint, Open Approach
0RPF07Z Removal of Autologous Tissue Substitute from Left Sternoclavicular Joint, Open Approach
0RPF08Z Removal of Spacer from Left Sternoclavicular Joint, Open Approach
0RPF0JZ Removal of Synthetic Substitute from Left Sternoclavicular Joint, Open Approach
0RPF0KZ Removal of Nonautologous Tissue Substitute from Left Sternoclavicular Joint, Open Approach
0RPF30Z Removal of Drainage Device from Left Sternoclavicular Joint, Percutaneous Approach
0RPF33Z Removal of Infusion Device from Left Sternoclavicular Joint, Percutaneous Approach
0RPF34Z Removal of Internal Fixation Device from Left Sternoclavicular Joint, Percutaneous Approach
0RPF37Z Removal of Autologous Tissue Substitute from Left Sternoclavicular Joint, Percutaneous Approach
0RPF38Z Removal of Spacer from Left Sternoclavicular Joint, Percutaneous Approach
0RPF3JZ Removal of Synthetic Substitute from Left Sternoclavicular Joint, Percutaneous Approach
0RPF3KZ Removal of Nonautologous Tissue Substitute from Left Sternoclavicular Joint, Percutaneous Approach
0RPF40Z Removal of Drainage Device from Left Sternoclavicular Joint, Percutaneous Endoscopic Approach
0RPF43Z Removal of Infusion Device from Left Sternoclavicular Joint, Percutaneous Endoscopic Approach
0RPF44Z Removal of Internal Fixation Device from Left Sternoclavicular Joint, Percutaneous Endoscopic Approach
0RPF47Z Removal of Autologous Tissue Substitute from Left Sternoclavicular Joint, Percutaneous Endoscopic Approach
0RPF48Z Removal of Spacer from Left Sternoclavicular Joint, Percutaneous Endoscopic Approach
0RPF4JZ Removal of Synthetic Substitute from Left Sternoclavicular Joint, Percutaneous Endoscopic Approach
0RPF4KZ Removal of Nonautologous Tissue Substitute from Left Sternoclavicular Joint, Percutaneous Endoscopic Approach
0RPFX0Z Removal of Drainage Device from Left Sternoclavicular Joint, External Approach
0RPFX3Z Removal of Infusion Device from Left Sternoclavicular Joint, External Approach
0RPFX4Z Removal of Internal Fixation Device from Left Sternoclavicular Joint, External Approach
0RPG00Z Removal of Drainage Device from Right Acromioclavicular Joint, Open Approach
0RPG03Z Removal of Infusion Device from Right Acromioclavicular Joint, Open Approach

0RPG04Z Removal of Internal Fixation Device from Right Acromioclavicular Joint, Open Approach
0RPG07Z Removal of Autologous Tissue Substitute from Right Acromioclavicular Joint, Open Approach
0RPG08Z Removal of Spacer from Right Acromioclavicular Joint, Open Approach
0RPG0JZ Removal of Synthetic Substitute from Right Acromioclavicular Joint, Open Approach
0RPG0KZ Removal of Nonautologous Tissue Substitute from Right Acromioclavicular Joint, Open Approach
0RPG30Z Removal of Drainage Device from Right Acromioclavicular Joint, Percutaneous Approach
0RPG33Z Removal of Infusion Device from Right Acromioclavicular Joint, Percutaneous Approach
0RPG34Z Removal of Internal Fixation Device from Right Acromioclavicular Joint, Percutaneous Approach
0RPG37Z Removal of Autologous Tissue Substitute from Right Acromioclavicular Joint, Percutaneous Approach
0RPG38Z Removal of Spacer from Right Acromioclavicular Joint, Percutaneous Approach
0RPG3JZ Removal of Synthetic Substitute from Right Acromioclavicular Joint, Percutaneous Approach
0RPG3KZ Removal of Nonautologous Tissue Substitute from Right Acromioclavicular Joint, Percutaneous Approach
0RPG40Z Removal of Drainage Device from Right Acromioclavicular Joint, Percutaneous Endoscopic Approach
0RPG43Z Removal of Infusion Device from Right Acromioclavicular Joint, Percutaneous Endoscopic Approach
0RPG44Z Removal of Internal Fixation Device from Right Acromioclavicular Joint, Percutaneous Endoscopic Approach
0RPG47Z Removal of Autologous Tissue Substitute from Right Acromioclavicular Joint, Percutaneous Endoscopic Approach
0RPG48Z Removal of Spacer from Right Acromioclavicular Joint, Percutaneous Endoscopic Approach
0RPG4JZ Removal of Synthetic Substitute from Right Acromioclavicular Joint, Percutaneous Endoscopic Approach
0RPG4KZ Removal of Nonautologous Tissue Substitute from Right Acromioclavicular Joint, Percutaneous Endoscopic Approach
0RPGX0Z Removal of Drainage Device from Right Acromioclavicular Joint, External Approach
0RPGX3Z Removal of Infusion Device from Right Acromioclavicular Joint, External Approach
0RPGX4Z Removal of Internal Fixation Device from Right Acromioclavicular Joint, External Approach
0RPH00Z Removal of Drainage Device from Left Acromioclavicular Joint, Open Approach
0RPH03Z Removal of Infusion Device from Left Acromioclavicular Joint, Open Approach
0RPH04Z Removal of Internal Fixation Device from Left Acromioclavicular Joint, Open Approach
0RPH07Z Removal of Autologous Tissue Substitute from Left Acromioclavicular Joint, Open Approach
0RPH08Z Removal of Spacer from Left Acromioclavicular Joint, Open Approach

♀ Female-only   ♂ Male-only   ▲ Limited Coverage   ● Non-OR   ▨ HAC-associated procedure   ▲ Non-covered procedures   ✛ Combination

0RPH0JZ Removal of Synthetic Substitute from Left Acromioclavicular Joint, Open Approach

0RPH0KZ Removal of Nonautologous Tissue Substitute from Left Acromioclavicular Joint, Open Approach

0RPH30Z Removal of Drainage Device from Left Acromioclavicular Joint, Percutaneous Approach

0RPH33Z Removal of Infusion Device from Left Acromioclavicular Joint, Percutaneous Approach

0RPH34Z Removal of Internal Fixation Device from Left Acromioclavicular Joint, Percutaneous Approach

0RPH37Z Removal of Autologous Tissue Substitute from Left Acromioclavicular Joint, Percutaneous Approach

0RPH38Z Removal of Spacer from Left Acromioclavicular Joint, Percutaneous Approach

0RPH3JZ Removal of Synthetic Substitute from Left Acromioclavicular Joint, Percutaneous Approach

0RPH3KZ Removal of Nonautologous Tissue Substitute from Left Acromioclavicular Joint, Percutaneous Approach

0RPH40Z Removal of Drainage Device from Left Acromioclavicular Joint, Percutaneous Endoscopic Approach

0RPH43Z Removal of Infusion Device from Left Acromioclavicular Joint, Percutaneous Endoscopic Approach

0RPH44Z Removal of Internal Fixation Device from Left Acromioclavicular Joint, Percutaneous Endoscopic Approach

0RPH47Z Removal of Autologous Tissue Substitute from Left Acromioclavicular Joint, Percutaneous Endoscopic Approach

0RPH48Z Removal of Spacer from Left Acromioclavicular Joint, Percutaneous Endoscopic Approach

0RPH4JZ Removal of Synthetic Substitute from Left Acromioclavicular Joint, Percutaneous Endoscopic Approach

0RPH4KZ Removal of Nonautologous Tissue Substitute from Left Acromioclavicular Joint, Percutaneous Endoscopic Approach

0RPHX0Z Removal of Drainage Device from Left Acromioclavicular Joint, External Approach

0RPHX3Z Removal of Infusion Device from Left Acromioclavicular Joint, External Approach

0RPHX4Z Removal of Internal Fixation Device from Left Acromioclavicular Joint, External Approach

0RPJ00Z Removal of Drainage Device from Right Shoulder Joint, Open Approach

0RPJ03Z Removal of Infusion Device from Right Shoulder Joint, Open Approach

0RPJ04Z Removal of Internal Fixation Device from Right Shoulder Joint, Open Approach

0RPJ07Z Removal of Autologous Tissue Substitute from Right Shoulder Joint, Open Approach

0RPJ08Z Removal of Spacer from Right Shoulder Joint, Open Approach

0RPJ0JZ Removal of Synthetic Substitute from Right Shoulder Joint, Open Approach

0RPJ0KZ Removal of Nonautologous Tissue Substitute from Right Shoulder Joint, Open Approach

0RPJ30Z Removal of Drainage Device from Right Shoulder Joint, Percutaneous Approach

0RPJ33Z Removal of Infusion Device from Right Shoulder Joint, Percutaneous Approach

0RPJ34Z Removal of Internal Fixation Device from Right Shoulder Joint, Percutaneous Approach

0RPJ37Z Removal of Autologous Tissue Substitute from Right Shoulder Joint, Percutaneous Approach

0RPJ38Z Removal of Spacer from Right Shoulder Joint, Percutaneous Approach

0RPJ3JZ Removal of Synthetic Substitute from Right Shoulder Joint, Percutaneous Approach

0RPJ3KZ Removal of Nonautologous Tissue Substitute from Right Shoulder Joint, Percutaneous Approach

0RPJ40Z Removal of Drainage Device from Right Shoulder Joint, Percutaneous Endoscopic Approach

0RPJ43Z Removal of Infusion Device from Right Shoulder Joint, Percutaneous Endoscopic Approach

0RPJ44Z Removal of Internal Fixation Device from Right Shoulder Joint, Percutaneous Endoscopic Approach

0RPJ47Z Removal of Autologous Tissue Substitute from Right Shoulder Joint, Percutaneous Endoscopic Approach

0RPJ48Z Removal of Spacer from Right Shoulder Joint, Percutaneous Endoscopic Approach

0RPJ4JZ Removal of Synthetic Substitute from Right Shoulder Joint, Percutaneous Endoscopic Approach

0RPJ4KZ Removal of Nonautologous Tissue Substitute from Right Shoulder Joint, Percutaneous Endoscopic Approach

0RPJX0Z Removal of Drainage Device from Right Shoulder Joint, External Approach

0RPJX3Z Removal of Infusion Device from Right Shoulder Joint, External Approach

0RPJX4Z Removal of Internal Fixation Device from Right Shoulder Joint, External Approach

0RPK00Z Removal of Drainage Device from Left Shoulder Joint, Open Approach

0RPK03Z Removal of Infusion Device from Left Shoulder Joint, Open Approach

0RPK04Z Removal of Internal Fixation Device from Left Shoulder Joint, Open Approach

0RPK07Z Removal of Autologous Tissue Substitute from Left Shoulder Joint, Open Approach

0RPK08Z Removal of Spacer from Left Shoulder Joint, Open Approach

0RPK0JZ Removal of Synthetic Substitute from Left Shoulder Joint, Open Approach

0RPK0KZ Removal of Nonautologous Tissue Substitute from Left Shoulder Joint, Open Approach

0RPK30Z Removal of Drainage Device from Left Shoulder Joint, Percutaneous Approach

0RPK33Z Removal of Infusion Device from Left Shoulder Joint, Percutaneous Approach

0RPK34Z Removal of Internal Fixation Device from Left Shoulder Joint, Percutaneous Approach

0RPK37Z Removal of Autologous Tissue Substitute from Left Shoulder Joint, Percutaneous Approach

0RPK38Z Removal of Spacer from Left Shoulder Joint, Percutaneous Approach

0RPK3JZ Removal of Synthetic Substitute from Left Shoulder Joint, Percutaneous Approach

0RPK3KZ Removal of Nonautologous Tissue Substitute from Left Shoulder Joint, Percutaneous Approach

0RPK40Z Removal of Drainage Device from Left Shoulder Joint, Percutaneous Endoscopic Approach

0RPK43Z Removal of Infusion Device from Left Shoulder Joint, Percutaneous Endoscopic Approach

0RPK44Z Removal of Internal Fixation Device from Left Shoulder Joint, Percutaneous Endoscopic Approach

0RPK47Z Removal of Autologous Tissue Substitute from Left Shoulder Joint, Percutaneous Endoscopic Approach

0RPK48Z Removal of Spacer from Left Shoulder Joint, Percutaneous Endoscopic Approach

0RPK4JZ Removal of Synthetic Substitute from Left Shoulder Joint, Percutaneous Endoscopic Approach

0RPK4KZ Removal of Nonautologous Tissue Substitute from Left Shoulder Joint, Percutaneous Endoscopic Approach

0RPKX0Z Removal of Drainage Device from Left Shoulder Joint, External Approach

0RPKX3Z Removal of Infusion Device from Left Shoulder Joint, External Approach

0RPKX4Z Removal of Internal Fixation Device from Left Shoulder Joint, External Approach

0RPL00Z Removal of Drainage Device from Right Elbow Joint, Open Approach

0RPL03Z Removal of Infusion Device from Right Elbow Joint, Open Approach

0RPL04Z Removal of Internal Fixation Device from Right Elbow Joint, Open Approach

0RPL05Z Removal of External Fixation Device from Right Elbow Joint, Open Approach

0RPL07Z Removal of Autologous Tissue Substitute from Right Elbow Joint, Open Approach

0RPL08Z Removal of Spacer from Right Elbow Joint, Open Approach

0RPL0JZ Removal of Synthetic Substitute from Right Elbow Joint, Open Approach

0RPL0KZ Removal of Nonautologous Tissue Substitute from Right Elbow Joint, Open Approach

0RPL30Z Removal of Drainage Device from Right Elbow Joint, Percutaneous Approach

0RPL33Z Removal of Infusion Device from Right Elbow Joint, Percutaneous Approach

0RPL34Z Removal of Internal Fixation Device from Right Elbow Joint, Percutaneous Approach

0RPL35Z Removal of External Fixation Device from Right Elbow Joint, Percutaneous Approach

0RPL37Z Removal of Autologous Tissue Substitute from Right Elbow Joint, Percutaneous Approach

0RPL38Z Removal of Spacer from Right Elbow Joint, Percutaneous Approach

0RPL3JZ Removal of Synthetic Substitute from Right Elbow Joint, Percutaneous Approach

0RPL3KZ Removal of Nonautologous Tissue Substitute from Right Elbow Joint, Percutaneous Approach

0RPL40Z Removal of Drainage Device from Right Elbow Joint, Percutaneous Endoscopic Approach

0RPL43Z Removal of Infusion Device from Right Elbow Joint, Percutaneous Endoscopic Approach

0RPL44Z Removal of Internal Fixation Device from Right Elbow Joint, Percutaneous Endoscopic Approach

0RPL45Z Removal of External Fixation Device from Right Elbow Joint, Percutaneous Endoscopic Approach

0RPL47Z Removal of Autologous Tissue Substitute from Right Elbow Joint, Percutaneous Endoscopic Approach

L48Z Removal of Spacer from Right Elbow Joint, Percutaneous Endoscopic Approach	**0RPM4KZ** Removal of Nonautologous Tissue Substitute from Left Elbow Joint, Percutaneous Endoscopic Approach	**0RPNX4Z** Removal of Internal Fixation Device from Right Wrist Joint, External Approach
L4JZ Removal of Synthetic Substitute from Right Elbow Joint, Percutaneous Endoscopic Approach	**0RPMX0Z** Removal of Drainage Device from Left Elbow Joint, External Approach	**0RPNX5Z** Removal of External Fixation Device from Right Wrist Joint, External Approach
L4KZ Removal of Nonautologous Tissue Substitute from Right Elbow Joint, Percutaneous Endoscopic Approach	**0RPMX3Z** Removal of Infusion Device from Left Elbow Joint, External Approach	**0RPP00Z** Removal of Drainage Device from Left Wrist Joint, Open Approach
LX0Z Removal of Drainage Device from Right Elbow Joint, External Approach	**0RPMX4Z** Removal of Internal Fixation Device from Left Elbow Joint, External Approach	**0RPP03Z** Removal of Infusion Device from Left Wrist Joint, Open Approach
LX3Z Removal of Infusion Device from Right Elbow Joint, External Approach	**0RPMX5Z** Removal of External Fixation Device from Left Elbow Joint, External Approach	**0RPP04Z** Removal of Internal Fixation Device from Left Wrist Joint, Open Approach
LX4Z Removal of Internal Fixation Device from Right Elbow Joint, External Approach	**0RPN00Z** Removal of Drainage Device from Right Wrist Joint, Open Approach	**0RPP05Z** Removal of External Fixation Device from Left Wrist Joint, Open Approach
LX5Z Removal of External Fixation Device from Right Elbow Joint, External Approach	**0RPN03Z** Removal of Infusion Device from Right Wrist Joint, Open Approach	**0RPP07Z** Removal of Autologous Tissue Substitute from Left Wrist Joint, Open Approach
PM00Z Removal of Drainage Device from Left Elbow Joint, Open Approach	**0RPN04Z** Removal of Internal Fixation Device from Right Wrist Joint, Open Approach	**0RPP08Z** Removal of Spacer from Left Wrist Joint, Open Approach
PM03Z Removal of Infusion Device from Left Elbow Joint, Open Approach	**0RPN05Z** Removal of External Fixation Device from Right Wrist Joint, Open Approach	**0RPP0JZ** Removal of Synthetic Substitute from Left Wrist Joint, Open Approach
PM04Z Removal of Internal Fixation Device from Left Elbow Joint, Open Approach	**0RPN07Z** Removal of Autologous Tissue Substitute from Right Wrist Joint, Open Approach	**0RPP0KZ** Removal of Nonautologous Tissue Substitute from Left Wrist Joint, Open Approach
PM05Z Removal of External Fixation Device from Left Elbow Joint, Open Approach	**0RPN08Z** Removal of Spacer from Right Wrist Joint, Open Approach	**0RPP30Z** Removal of Drainage Device from Left Wrist Joint, Percutaneous Approach
PM07Z Removal of Autologous Tissue Substitute from Left Elbow Joint, Open Approach	**0RPN0JZ** Removal of Synthetic Substitute from Right Wrist Joint, Open Approach	**0RPP33Z** Removal of Infusion Device from Left Wrist Joint, Percutaneous Approach
PM08Z Removal of Spacer from Left Elbow Joint, Open Approach	**0RPN0KZ** Removal of Nonautologous Tissue Substitute from Right Wrist Joint, Open Approach	**0RPP34Z** Removal of Internal Fixation Device from Left Wrist Joint, Percutaneous Approach
PM0JZ Removal of Synthetic Substitute from Left Elbow Joint, Open Approach	**0RPN30Z** Removal of Drainage Device from Right Wrist Joint, Percutaneous Approach	**0RPP35Z** Removal of External Fixation Device from Left Wrist Joint, Percutaneous Approach
PM0KZ Removal of Nonautologous Tissue Substitute from Left Elbow Joint, Open Approach	**0RPN33Z** Removal of Infusion Device from Right Wrist Joint, Percutaneous Approach	**0RPP37Z** Removal of Autologous Tissue Substitute from Left Wrist Joint, Percutaneous Approach
PM30Z Removal of Drainage Device from Left Elbow Joint, Percutaneous Approach	**0RPN34Z** Removal of Internal Fixation Device from Right Wrist Joint, Percutaneous Approach	**0RPP38Z** Removal of Spacer from Left Wrist Joint, Percutaneous Approach
PM33Z Removal of Infusion Device from Left Elbow Joint, Percutaneous Approach	**0RPN35Z** Removal of External Fixation Device from Right Wrist Joint, Percutaneous Approach	**0RPP3JZ** Removal of Synthetic Substitute from Left Wrist Joint, Percutaneous Approach
PM34Z Removal of Internal Fixation Device from Left Elbow Joint, Percutaneous Approach	**0RPN37Z** Removal of Autologous Tissue Substitute from Right Wrist Joint, Percutaneous Approach	**0RPP3KZ** Removal of Nonautologous Tissue Substitute from Left Wrist Joint, Percutaneous Approach
PM35Z Removal of External Fixation Device from Left Elbow Joint, Percutaneous Approach	**0RPN38Z** Removal of Spacer from Right Wrist Joint, Percutaneous Approach	**0RPP40Z** Removal of Drainage Device from Left Wrist Joint, Percutaneous Endoscopic Approach
PM37Z Removal of Autologous Tissue Substitute from Left Elbow Joint, Percutaneous Approach	**0RPN3JZ** Removal of Synthetic Substitute from Right Wrist Joint, Percutaneous Approach	**0RPP43Z** Removal of Infusion Device from Left Wrist Joint, Percutaneous Endoscopic Approach
PM38Z Removal of Spacer from Left Elbow Joint, Percutaneous Approach	**0RPN3KZ** Removal of Nonautologous Tissue Substitute from Right Wrist Joint, Percutaneous Approach	**0RPP44Z** Removal of Internal Fixation Device from Left Wrist Joint, Percutaneous Endoscopic Approach
PM3JZ Removal of Synthetic Substitute from Left Elbow Joint, Percutaneous Approach	**0RPN40Z** Removal of Drainage Device from Right Wrist Joint, Percutaneous Endoscopic Approach	**0RPP45Z** Removal of External Fixation Device from Left Wrist Joint, Percutaneous Endoscopic Approach
PM3KZ Removal of Nonautologous Tissue Substitute from Left Elbow Joint, Percutaneous Approach	**0RPN43Z** Removal of Infusion Device from Right Wrist Joint, Percutaneous Endoscopic Approach	**0RPP47Z** Removal of Autologous Tissue Substitute from Left Wrist Joint, Percutaneous Endoscopic Approach
PM40Z Removal of Drainage Device from Left Elbow Joint, Percutaneous Endoscopic Approach	**0RPN44Z** Removal of Internal Fixation Device from Right Wrist Joint, Percutaneous Endoscopic Approach	**0RPP48Z** Removal of Spacer from Left Wrist Joint, Percutaneous Endoscopic Approach
PM43Z Removal of Infusion Device from Left Elbow Joint, Percutaneous Endoscopic Approach	**0RPN45Z** Removal of External Fixation Device from Right Wrist Joint, Percutaneous Endoscopic Approach	**0RPP4JZ** Removal of Synthetic Substitute from Left Wrist Joint, Percutaneous Endoscopic Approach
PM44Z Removal of Internal Fixation Device from Left Elbow Joint, Percutaneous Endoscopic Approach	**0RPN47Z** Removal of Autologous Tissue Substitute from Right Wrist Joint, Percutaneous Endoscopic Approach	**0RPP4KZ** Removal of Nonautologous Tissue Substitute from Left Wrist Joint, Percutaneous Endoscopic Approach
PM45Z Removal of External Fixation Device from Left Elbow Joint, Percutaneous Endoscopic Approach	**0RPN48Z** Removal of Spacer from Right Wrist Joint, Percutaneous Endoscopic Approach	**0RPPX0Z** Removal of Drainage Device from Left Wrist Joint, External Approach
PM47Z Removal of Autologous Tissue Substitute from Left Elbow Joint, Percutaneous Endoscopic Approach	**0RPN4JZ** Removal of Synthetic Substitute from Right Wrist Joint, Percutaneous Endoscopic Approach	**0RPPX3Z** Removal of Infusion Device from Left Wrist Joint, External Approach
PM48Z Removal of Spacer from Left Elbow Joint, Percutaneous Endoscopic Approach	**0RPN4KZ** Removal of Nonautologous Tissue Substitute from Right Wrist Joint, Percutaneous Endoscopic Approach	**0RPPX4Z** Removal of Internal Fixation Device from Left Wrist Joint, External Approach
PM4JZ Removal of Synthetic Substitute from Left Elbow Joint, Percutaneous Endoscopic Approach	**0RPNX0Z** Removal of Drainage Device from Right Wrist Joint, External Approach	**0RPPX5Z** Removal of External Fixation Device from Left Wrist Joint, External Approach
	0RPNX3Z Removal of Infusion Device from Right Wrist Joint, External Approach	**0RPQ00Z** Removal of Drainage Device from Right Carpal Joint, Open Approach

939

Female-only   ♂ Male-only   ▲ Limited Coverage   ● Non-OR   ▬ HAC-associated procedure   ▲ Non-covered procedures   ✛ Combination

0RPQ03Z Removal of Infusion Device from Right Carpal Joint, Open Approach

0RPQ04Z Removal of Internal Fixation Device from Right Carpal Joint, Open Approach

0RPQ05Z Removal of External Fixation Device from Right Carpal Joint, Open Approach

0RPQ07Z Removal of Autologous Tissue Substitute from Right Carpal Joint, Open Approach

0RPQ08Z Removal of Spacer from Right Carpal Joint, Open Approach

0RPQ0JZ Removal of Synthetic Substitute from Right Carpal Joint, Open Approach

0RPQ0KZ Removal of Nonautologous Tissue Substitute from Right Carpal Joint, Open Approach

0RPQ30Z Removal of Drainage Device from Right Carpal Joint, Percutaneous Approach

0RPQ33Z Removal of Infusion Device from Right Carpal Joint, Percutaneous Approach

0RPQ34Z Removal of Internal Fixation Device from Right Carpal Joint, Percutaneous Approach

0RPQ35Z Removal of External Fixation Device from Right Carpal Joint, Percutaneous Approach

0RPQ37Z Removal of Autologous Tissue Substitute from Right Carpal Joint, Percutaneous Approach

0RPQ38Z Removal of Spacer from Right Carpal Joint, Percutaneous Approach

0RPQ3JZ Removal of Synthetic Substitute from Right Carpal Joint, Percutaneous Approach

0RPQ3KZ Removal of Nonautologous Tissue Substitute from Right Carpal Joint, Percutaneous Approach

0RPQ40Z Removal of Drainage Device from Right Carpal Joint, Percutaneous Endoscopic Approach

0RPQ43Z Removal of Infusion Device from Right Carpal Joint, Percutaneous Endoscopic Approach

0RPQ44Z Removal of Internal Fixation Device from Right Carpal Joint, Percutaneous Endoscopic Approach

0RPQ45Z Removal of External Fixation Device from Right Carpal Joint, Percutaneous Endoscopic Approach

0RPQ47Z Removal of Autologous Tissue Substitute from Right Carpal Joint, Percutaneous Endoscopic Approach

0RPQ48Z Removal of Spacer from Right Carpal Joint, Percutaneous Endoscopic Approach

0RPQ4JZ Removal of Synthetic Substitute from Right Carpal Joint, Percutaneous Endoscopic Approach

0RPQ4KZ Removal of Nonautologous Tissue Substitute from Right Carpal Joint, Percutaneous Endoscopic Approach

0RPQX0Z Removal of Drainage Device from Right Carpal Joint, External Approach

0RPQX3Z Removal of Infusion Device from Right Carpal Joint, External Approach

0RPQX4Z Removal of Internal Fixation Device from Right Carpal Joint, External Approach

0RPQX5Z Removal of External Fixation Device from Right Carpal Joint, External Approach

0RPR00Z Removal of Drainage Device from Left Carpal Joint, Open Approach

0RPR03Z Removal of Infusion Device from Left Carpal Joint, Open Approach

0RPR04Z Removal of Internal Fixation Device from Left Carpal Joint, Open Approach

0RPR05Z Removal of External Fixation Device from Left Carpal Joint, Open Approach

0RPR07Z Removal of Autologous Tissue Substitute from Left Carpal Joint, Open Approach

0RPR08Z Removal of Spacer from Left Carpal Joint, Open Approach

0RPR0JZ Removal of Synthetic Substitute from Left Carpal Joint, Open Approach

0RPR0KZ Removal of Nonautologous Tissue Substitute from Left Carpal Joint, Open Approach

0RPR30Z Removal of Drainage Device from Left Carpal Joint, Percutaneous Approach

0RPR33Z Removal of Infusion Device from Left Carpal Joint, Percutaneous Approach

0RPR34Z Removal of Internal Fixation Device from Left Carpal Joint, Percutaneous Approach

0RPR35Z Removal of External Fixation Device from Left Carpal Joint, Percutaneous Approach

0RPR37Z Removal of Autologous Tissue Substitute from Left Carpal Joint, Percutaneous Approach

0RPR38Z Removal of Spacer from Left Carpal Joint, Percutaneous Approach

0RPR3JZ Removal of Synthetic Substitute from Left Carpal Joint, Percutaneous Approach

0RPR3KZ Removal of Nonautologous Tissue Substitute from Left Carpal Joint, Percutaneous Approach

0RPR40Z Removal of Drainage Device from Left Carpal Joint, Percutaneous Endoscopic Approach

0RPR43Z Removal of Infusion Device from Left Carpal Joint, Percutaneous Endoscopic Approach

0RPR44Z Removal of Internal Fixation Device from Left Carpal Joint, Percutaneous Endoscopic Approach

0RPR45Z Removal of External Fixation Device from Left Carpal Joint, Percutaneous Endoscopic Approach

0RPR47Z Removal of Autologous Tissue Substitute from Left Carpal Joint, Percutaneous Endoscopic Approach

0RPR48Z Removal of Spacer from Left Carpal Joint, Percutaneous Endoscopic Approach

0RPR4JZ Removal of Synthetic Substitute from Left Carpal Joint, Percutaneous Endoscopic Approach

0RPR4KZ Removal of Nonautologous Tissue Substitute from Left Carpal Joint, Percutaneous Endoscopic Approach

0RPRX0Z Removal of Drainage Device from Left Carpal Joint, External Approach

0RPRX3Z Removal of Infusion Device from Left Carpal Joint, External Approach

0RPRX4Z Removal of Internal Fixation Device from Left Carpal Joint, External Approach

0RPRX5Z Removal of External Fixation Device from Left Carpal Joint, External Approach

0RPS00Z Removal of Drainage Device from Right Metacarpocarpal Joint, Open Approach

0RPS03Z Removal of Infusion Device from Right Metacarpocarpal Joint, Open Approach

0RPS04Z Removal of Internal Fixation Device from Right Metacarpocarpal Joint, Open Approach

0RPS05Z Removal of External Fixation Device from Right Metacarpocarpal Joint, Open Approach

0RPS07Z Removal of Autologous Tissue Substitute from Right Metacarpocarpal Joint, Open Approach

0RPS08Z Removal of Spacer from Right Metacarpocarpal Joint, Open Approach

0RPS0JZ Removal of Synthetic Substitute from Right Metacarpocarpal Joint, Open Approach

0RPS0KZ Removal of Nonautologous Tissue Substitute from Right Metacarpocarpal Joint, Open Approach

0RPS30Z Removal of Drainage Device from Right Metacarpocarpal Joint, Percutaneous Approach

0RPS33Z Removal of Infusion Device from Right Metacarpocarpal Joint, Percutaneous Approach

0RPS34Z Removal of Internal Fixation Device from Right Metacarpocarpal Joint, Percutaneous Approach

0RPS35Z Removal of External Fixation Device from Right Metacarpocarpal Joint, Percutaneous Approach

0RPS37Z Removal of Autologous Tissue Substitute from Right Metacarpocarpal Joint, Percutaneous Approach

0RPS38Z Removal of Spacer from Right Metacarpocarpal Joint, Percutaneous Approach

0RPS3JZ Removal of Synthetic Substitute from Right Metacarpocarpal Joint, Percutaneous Approach

0RPS3KZ Removal of Nonautologous Tissue Substitute from Right Metacarpocarpal Joint, Percutaneous Approach

0RPS40Z Removal of Drainage Device from Right Metacarpocarpal Joint, Percutaneous Endoscopic Approach

0RPS43Z Removal of Infusion Device from Right Metacarpocarpal Joint, Percutaneous Endoscopic Approach

0RPS44Z Removal of Internal Fixation Device from Right Metacarpocarpal Joint, Percutaneous Endoscopic Approach

0RPS45Z Removal of External Fixation Device from Right Metacarpocarpal Joint, Percutaneous Endoscopic Approach

0RPS47Z Removal of Autologous Tissue Substitute from Right Metacarpocarpal Joint, Percutaneous Endoscopic Approach

0RPS48Z Removal of Spacer from Right Metacarpocarpal Joint, Percutaneous Endoscopic Approach

0RPS4JZ Removal of Synthetic Substitute from Right Metacarpocarpal Joint, Percutaneous Endoscopic Approach

0RPS4KZ Removal of Nonautologous Tissue Substitute from Right Metacarpocarpal Joint, Percutaneous Endoscopic Approach

0RPSX0Z Removal of Drainage Device from Right Metacarpocarpal Joint, External Approach

0RPSX3Z Removal of Infusion Device from Right Metacarpocarpal Joint, External Approach

0RPSX4Z Removal of Internal Fixation Device from Right Metacarpocarpal Joint, External Approach

0RPSX5Z Removal of External Fixation Device from Right Metacarpocarpal Joint, External Approach

0RPT00Z Removal of Drainage Device from Left Metacarpocarpal Joint, Open Approach

0RPT03Z Removal of Infusion Device from Left Metacarpocarpal Joint, Open Approach

0RPT04Z Removal of Internal Fixation Device from Left Metacarpocarpal Joint, Open Approach

0RPT05Z Removal of External Fixation Device from Left Metacarpocarpal Joint, Open Approach

0RPT07Z Removal of Autologous Tissue Substitute from Left Metacarpocarpal Joint, Open Approach

0RPT08Z Removal of Spacer from Left Metacarpocarpal Joint, Open Approach

0RPT0JZ Removal of Synthetic Substitute from Left Metacarpocarpal Joint, Open Approach

0RPT0KZ Removal of Nonautologous Tissue Substitute from Left Metacarpocarpal Joint, Open Approach

PT30Z Removal of Drainage Device from Left Metacarpocarpal Joint, Percutaneous Approach

PT33Z Removal of Infusion Device from Left Metacarpocarpal Joint, Percutaneous Approach

PT34Z Removal of Internal Fixation Device from Left Metacarpocarpal Joint, Percutaneous Approach

RPT35Z Removal of External Fixation Device from Left Metacarpocarpal Joint, Percutaneous Approach

RPT37Z Removal of Autologous Tissue Substitute from Left Metacarpocarpal Joint, Percutaneous Approach

RPT38Z Removal of Spacer from Left Metacarpocarpal Joint, Percutaneous Approach

RPT3JZ Removal of Synthetic Substitute from Left Metacarpocarpal Joint, Percutaneous Approach

RPT3KZ Removal of Nonautologous Tissue Substitute from Left Metacarpocarpal Joint, Percutaneous Approach

RPT40Z Removal of Drainage Device from Left Metacarpocarpal Joint, Percutaneous Endoscopic Approach

RPT43Z Removal of Infusion Device from Left Metacarpocarpal Joint, Percutaneous Endoscopic Approach

RPT44Z Removal of Internal Fixation Device from Left Metacarpocarpal Joint, Percutaneous Endoscopic Approach

RPT45Z Removal of External Fixation Device from Left Metacarpocarpal Joint, Percutaneous Endoscopic Approach

RPT47Z Removal of Autologous Tissue Substitute from Left Metacarpocarpal Joint, Percutaneous Endoscopic Approach

RPT48Z Removal of Spacer from Left Metacarpocarpal Joint, Percutaneous Endoscopic Approach

RPT4JZ Removal of Synthetic Substitute from Left Metacarpocarpal Joint, Percutaneous Endoscopic Approach

RPT4KZ Removal of Nonautologous Tissue Substitute from Left Metacarpocarpal Joint, Percutaneous Endoscopic Approach

RPTX0Z Removal of Drainage Device from Left Metacarpocarpal Joint, External Approach

RPTX3Z Removal of Infusion Device from Left Metacarpocarpal Joint, External Approach

RPTX4Z Removal of Internal Fixation Device from Left Metacarpocarpal Joint, External Approach

RPTX5Z Removal of External Fixation Device from Left Metacarpocarpal Joint, External Approach

RPU00Z Removal of Drainage Device from Right Metacarpophalangeal Joint, Open Approach

RPU03Z Removal of Infusion Device from Right Metacarpophalangeal Joint, Open Approach

RPU04Z Removal of Internal Fixation Device from Right Metacarpophalangeal Joint, Open Approach

RPU05Z Removal of External Fixation Device from Right Metacarpophalangeal Joint, Open Approach

0RPU07Z Removal of Autologous Tissue Substitute from Right Metacarpophalangeal Joint, Open Approach

0RPU08Z Removal of Spacer from Right Metacarpophalangeal Joint, Open Approach

0RPU0JZ Removal of Synthetic Substitute from Right Metacarpophalangeal Joint, Open Approach

0RPU0KZ Removal of Nonautologous Tissue Substitute from Right Metacarpophalangeal Joint, Open Approach

0RPU30Z Removal of Drainage Device from Right Metacarpophalangeal Joint, Percutaneous Approach

0RPU33Z Removal of Infusion Device from Right Metacarpophalangeal Joint, Percutaneous Approach

0RPU34Z Removal of Internal Fixation Device from Right Metacarpophalangeal Joint, Percutaneous Approach

0RPU35Z Removal of External Fixation Device from Right Metacarpophalangeal Joint, Percutaneous Approach

0RPU37Z Removal of Autologous Tissue Substitute from Right Metacarpophalangeal Joint, Percutaneous Approach

0RPU38Z Removal of Spacer from Right Metacarpophalangeal Joint, Percutaneous Approach

0RPU3JZ Removal of Synthetic Substitute from Right Metacarpophalangeal Joint, Percutaneous Approach

0RPU3KZ Removal of Nonautologous Tissue Substitute from Right Metacarpophalangeal Joint, Percutaneous Approach

0RPU40Z Removal of Drainage Device from Right Metacarpophalangeal Joint, Percutaneous Endoscopic Approach

0RPU43Z Removal of Infusion Device from Right Metacarpophalangeal Joint, Percutaneous Endoscopic Approach

0RPU44Z Removal of Internal Fixation Device from Right Metacarpophalangeal Joint, Percutaneous Endoscopic Approach

0RPU45Z Removal of External Fixation Device from Right Metacarpophalangeal Joint, Percutaneous Endoscopic Approach

0RPU47Z Removal of Autologous Tissue Substitute from Right Metacarpophalangeal Joint, Percutaneous Endoscopic Approach

0RPU48Z Removal of Spacer from Right Metacarpophalangeal Joint, Percutaneous Endoscopic Approach

0RPU4JZ Removal of Synthetic Substitute from Right Metacarpophalangeal Joint, Percutaneous Endoscopic Approach

0RPU4KZ Removal of Nonautologous Tissue Substitute from Right Metacarpophalangeal Joint, Percutaneous Endoscopic Approach

0RPUX0Z Removal of Drainage Device from Right Metacarpophalangeal Joint, External Approach

0RPUX3Z Removal of Infusion Device from Right Metacarpophalangeal Joint, External Approach

0RPUX4Z Removal of Internal Fixation Device from Right Metacarpophalangeal Joint, External Approach

0RPUX5Z Removal of External Fixation Device from Right Metacarpophalangeal Joint, External Approach

0RPV00Z Removal of Drainage Device from Left Metacarpophalangeal Joint, Open Approach

0RPV03Z Removal of Infusion Device from Left Metacarpophalangeal Joint, Open Approach

0RPV04Z Removal of Internal Fixation Device from Left Metacarpophalangeal Joint, Open Approach

0RPV05Z Removal of External Fixation Device from Left Metacarpophalangeal Joint, Open Approach

0RPV07Z Removal of Autologous Tissue Substitute from Left Metacarpophalangeal Joint, Open Approach

0RPV08Z Removal of Spacer from Left Metacarpophalangeal Joint, Open Approach

0RPV0JZ Removal of Synthetic Substitute from Left Metacarpophalangeal Joint, Open Approach

0RPV0KZ Removal of Nonautologous Tissue Substitute from Left Metacarpophalangeal Joint, Open Approach

0RPV30Z Removal of Drainage Device from Left Metacarpophalangeal Joint, Percutaneous Approach

0RPV33Z Removal of Infusion Device from Left Metacarpophalangeal Joint, Percutaneous Approach

0RPV34Z Removal of Internal Fixation Device from Left Metacarpophalangeal Joint, Percutaneous Approach

0RPV35Z Removal of External Fixation Device from Left Metacarpophalangeal Joint, Percutaneous Approach

0RPV37Z Removal of Autologous Tissue Substitute from Left Metacarpophalangeal Joint, Percutaneous Approach

0RPV38Z Removal of Spacer from Left Metacarpophalangeal Joint, Percutaneous Approach

0RPV3JZ Removal of Synthetic Substitute from Left Metacarpophalangeal Joint, Percutaneous Approach

0RPV3KZ Removal of Nonautologous Tissue Substitute from Left Metacarpophalangeal Joint, Percutaneous Approach

0RPV40Z Removal of Drainage Device from Left Metacarpophalangeal Joint, Percutaneous Endoscopic Approach

0RPV43Z Removal of Infusion Device from Left Metacarpophalangeal Joint, Percutaneous Endoscopic Approach

0RPV44Z Removal of Internal Fixation Device from Left Metacarpophalangeal Joint, Percutaneous Endoscopic Approach

0RPV45Z Removal of External Fixation Device from Left Metacarpophalangeal Joint, Percutaneous Endoscopic Approach

0RPV47Z Removal of Autologous Tissue Substitute from Left Metacarpophalangeal Joint, Percutaneous Endoscopic Approach

0RPV48Z Removal of Spacer from Left Metacarpophalangeal Joint, Percutaneous Endoscopic Approach

0RPV4JZ Removal of Synthetic Substitute from Left Metacarpophalangeal Joint, Percutaneous Endoscopic Approach

0RPV4KZ Removal of Nonautologous Tissue Substitute from Left Metacarpophalangeal Joint, Percutaneous Endoscopic Approach

0RPVX0Z Removal of Drainage Device from Left Metacarpophalangeal Joint, External Approach

0RPVX3Z Removal of Infusion Device from Left Metacarpophalangeal Joint, External Approach

0RPVX4Z Removal of Internal Fixation Device from Left Metacarpophalangeal Joint, External Approach

0RPVX5Z Removal of External Fixation Device from Left Metacarpophalangeal Joint, External Approach

941

0RPW00Z Removal of Drainage Device from Right Finger Phalangeal Joint, Open Approach	**0RPW45Z** Removal of External Fixation Device from Right Finger Phalangeal Joint, Percutaneous Endoscopic Approach	**0RPX34Z** Removal of Internal Fixation Device from Left Finger Phalangeal Joint, Percutaneous Approach
0RPW03Z Removal of Infusion Device from Right Finger Phalangeal Joint, Open Approach	**0RPW47Z** Removal of Autologous Tissue Substitute from Right Finger Phalangeal Joint, Percutaneous Endoscopic Approach	**0RPX35Z** Removal of External Fixation Device from Left Finger Phalangeal Joint, Percutaneous Approach
0RPW04Z Removal of Internal Fixation Device from Right Finger Phalangeal Joint, Open Approach	**0RPW48Z** Removal of Spacer from Right Finger Phalangeal Joint, Percutaneous Endoscopic Approach	**0RPX37Z** Removal of Autologous Tissue Substitu from Left Finger Phalangeal Joint, Percutaneous Approach
0RPW05Z Removal of External Fixation Device from Right Finger Phalangeal Joint, Open Approach	**0RPW4JZ** Removal of Synthetic Substitute from Right Finger Phalangeal Joint, Percutaneous Endoscopic Approach	**0RPX38Z** Removal of Spacer from Left Finger Phalangeal Joint, Percutaneous Approac
0RPW07Z Removal of Autologous Tissue Substitute from Right Finger Phalangeal Joint, Open Approach	**0RPW4KZ** Removal of Nonautologous Tissue Substitute from Right Finger Phalangeal Joint, Percutaneous Endoscopic Approach	**0RPX3JZ** Removal of Synthetic Substitute from Left Finger Phalangeal Joint, Percutaneous Approach
0RPW08Z Removal of Spacer from Right Finger Phalangeal Joint, Open Approach	**0RPWX0Z** Removal of Drainage Device from Right Finger Phalangeal Joint, External Approach	**0RPX3KZ** Removal of Nonautologous Tissue Substitute from Left Finger Phalangeal Joint, Percutaneous Approach
0RPW0JZ Removal of Synthetic Substitute from Right Finger Phalangeal Joint, Open Approach	**0RPWX3Z** Removal of Infusion Device from Right Finger Phalangeal Joint, External Approach	**0RPX40Z** Removal of Drainage Device from Left Finger Phalangeal Joint, Percutaneous Endoscopic Approach
0RPW0KZ Removal of Nonautologous Tissue Substitute from Right Finger Phalangeal Joint, Open Approach	**0RPWX4Z** Removal of Internal Fixation Device from Right Finger Phalangeal Joint, External Approach	**0RPX43Z** Removal of Infusion Device from Left Finger Phalangeal Joint, Percutaneous Endoscopic Approach
0RPW30Z Removal of Drainage Device from Right Finger Phalangeal Joint, Percutaneous Approach	**0RPWX5Z** Removal of External Fixation Device from Right Finger Phalangeal Joint, External Approach	**0RPX44Z** Removal of Internal Fixation Device from Left Finger Phalangeal Joint, Percutaneous Endoscopic Approach
0RPW33Z Removal of Infusion Device from Right Finger Phalangeal Joint, Percutaneous Approach	**0RPX00Z** Removal of Drainage Device from Left Finger Phalangeal Joint, Open Approach	**0RPX45Z** Removal of External Fixation Device from Left Finger Phalangeal Joint, Percutaneous Endoscopic Approach
0RPW34Z Removal of Internal Fixation Device from Right Finger Phalangeal Joint, Percutaneous Approach	**0RPX03Z** Removal of Infusion Device from Left Finger Phalangeal Joint, Open Approach	**0RPX47Z** Removal of Autologous Tissue Substitut from Left Finger Phalangeal Joint, Percutaneous Endoscopic Approach
0RPW35Z Removal of External Fixation Device from Right Finger Phalangeal Joint, Percutaneous Approach	**0RPX04Z** Removal of Internal Fixation Device from Left Finger Phalangeal Joint, Open Approach	**0RPX48Z** Removal of Spacer from Left Finger Phalangeal Joint, Percutaneous Endoscopic Approach
0RPW37Z Removal of Autologous Tissue Substitute from Right Finger Phalangeal Joint, Percutaneous Approach	**0RPX05Z** Removal of External Fixation Device from Left Finger Phalangeal Joint, Open Approach	**0RPX4JZ** Removal of Synthetic Substitute from Left Finger Phalangeal Joint, Percutaneous Endoscopic Approach
0RPW38Z Removal of Spacer from Right Finger Phalangeal Joint, Percutaneous Approach	**0RPX07Z** Removal of Autologous Tissue Substitute from Left Finger Phalangeal Joint, Open Approach	**0RPX4KZ** Removal of Nonautologous Tissue Substitute from Left Finger Phalangeal Joint, Percutaneous Endoscopic Approac
0RPW3JZ Removal of Synthetic Substitute from Right Finger Phalangeal Joint, Percutaneous Approach	**0RPX08Z** Removal of Spacer from Left Finger Phalangeal Joint, Open Approach	**0RPXX0Z** Removal of Drainage Device from Left Finger Phalangeal Joint, External Approach
0RPW3KZ Removal of Nonautologous Tissue Substitute from Right Finger Phalangeal Joint, Percutaneous Approach	**0RPX0JZ** Removal of Synthetic Substitute from Left Finger Phalangeal Joint, Open Approach	**0RPXX3Z** Removal of Infusion Device from Left Finger Phalangeal Joint, External Approach
0RPW40Z Removal of Drainage Device from Right Finger Phalangeal Joint, Percutaneous Endoscopic Approach	**0RPX0KZ** Removal of Nonautologous Tissue Substitute from Left Finger Phalangeal Joint, Open Approach	**0RPXX4Z** Removal of Internal Fixation Device from Left Finger Phalangeal Joint, External Approach
0RPW43Z Removal of Infusion Device from Right Finger Phalangeal Joint, Percutaneous Endoscopic Approach	**0RPX30Z** Removal of Drainage Device from Left Finger Phalangeal Joint, Percutaneous Approach	**0RPXX5Z** Removal of External Fixation Device from Left Finger Phalangeal Joint, External Approach
0RPW44Z Removal of Internal Fixation Device from Right Finger Phalangeal Joint, Percutaneous Endoscopic Approach	**0RPX33Z** Removal of Infusion Device from Left Finger Phalangeal Joint, Percutaneous Approach	

0RQ – Upper Joints, Repair

Review Coding Guideline B3.5

0RQ00ZZ Repair Occipital-cervical Joint, Open Approach	**0RQ30ZZ** Repair Cervical Vertebral Disc, Open Approach	**0RQ50ZZ** Repair Cervicothoracic Vertebral Disc, Open Approach
0RQ03ZZ Repair Occipital-cervical Joint, Percutaneous Approach	**0RQ33ZZ** Repair Cervical Vertebral Disc, Percutaneous Approach	**0RQ53ZZ** Repair Cervicothoracic Vertebral Disc, Percutaneous Approach
0RQ04ZZ Repair Occipital-cervical Joint, Percutaneous Endoscopic Approach	**0RQ34ZZ** Repair Cervical Vertebral Disc, Percutaneous Endoscopic Approach	**0RQ54ZZ** Repair Cervicothoracic Vertebral Disc, Percutaneous Endoscopic Approach
0RQ0XZZ Repair Occipital-cervical Joint, External Approach	**0RQ3XZZ** Repair Cervical Vertebral Disc, External Approach	**0RQ5XZZ** Repair Cervicothoracic Vertebral Disc, External Approach
0RQ10ZZ Repair Cervical Vertebral Joint, Open Approach	**0RQ40ZZ** Repair Cervicothoracic Vertebral Joint, Open Approach	**0RQ60ZZ** Repair Thoracic Vertebral Joint, Open Approach
0RQ13ZZ Repair Cervical Vertebral Joint, Percutaneous Approach	**0RQ43ZZ** Repair Cervicothoracic Vertebral Joint, Percutaneous Approach	**0RQ63ZZ** Repair Thoracic Vertebral Joint, Percutaneous Approach
0RQ14ZZ Repair Cervical Vertebral Joint, Percutaneous Endoscopic Approach	**0RQ44ZZ** Repair Cervicothoracic Vertebral Joint, Percutaneous Endoscopic Approach	**0RQ64ZZ** Repair Thoracic Vertebral Joint, Percutaneous Endoscopic Approach
0RQ1XZZ Repair Cervical Vertebral Joint, External Approach	**0RQ4XZZ** Repair Cervicothoracic Vertebral Joint, External Approach	**0RQ6XZZ** Repair Thoracic Vertebral Joint, External Approach

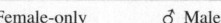

♀ Female-only   ♂ Male-only   ▲ Limited Coverage   ● Non-OR   ■ HAC-associated procedure   ▲ Non-covered procedures   ✚ Combination

RQ90ZZ   Repair Thoracic Vertebral Disc, Open Approach

RQ93ZZ   Repair Thoracic Vertebral Disc, Percutaneous Approach

RQ94ZZ   Repair Thoracic Vertebral Disc, Percutaneous Endoscopic Approach

RQ9XZZ   Repair Thoracic Vertebral Disc, External Approach

RQA0ZZ   Repair Thoracolumbar Vertebral Joint, Open Approach

RQA3ZZ   Repair Thoracolumbar Vertebral Joint, Percutaneous Approach

RQA4ZZ   Repair Thoracolumbar Vertebral Joint, Percutaneous Endoscopic Approach

RQAXZZ   Repair Thoracolumbar Vertebral Joint, External Approach

RQB0ZZ   Repair Thoracolumbar Vertebral Disc, Open Approach

RQB3ZZ   Repair Thoracolumbar Vertebral Disc, Percutaneous Approach

RQB4ZZ   Repair Thoracolumbar Vertebral Disc, Percutaneous Endoscopic Approach

RQBXZZ   Repair Thoracolumbar Vertebral Disc, External Approach

RQC0ZZ   Repair Right Temporomandibular Joint, Open Approach

RQC3ZZ   Repair Right Temporomandibular Joint, Percutaneous Approach

RQC4ZZ   Repair Right Temporomandibular Joint, Percutaneous Endoscopic Approach

RQCXZZ   Repair Right Temporomandibular Joint, External Approach

RQD0ZZ   Repair Left Temporomandibular Joint, Open Approach

RQD3ZZ   Repair Left Temporomandibular Joint, Percutaneous Approach

RQD4ZZ   Repair Left Temporomandibular Joint, Percutaneous Endoscopic Approach

RQDXZZ   Repair Left Temporomandibular Joint, External Approach

RQE0ZZ   Repair Right Sternoclavicular Joint, Open Approach
■ When reported with secondary diagnosis code T84.60XA, T84.610A, T84.611A, T84.612A, T84.613A, T84.614A, T84.615A, T84.619A, T84.63XA, T84.69XA, T84.7XXA

RQE3ZZ   Repair Right Sternoclavicular Joint, Percutaneous Approach
■ When reported with secondary diagnosis code T84.60XA, T84.610A, T84.611A, T84.612A, T84.613A, T84.614A, T84.615A, T84.619A, T84.63XA, T84.69XA, T84.7XXA

RQE4ZZ   Repair Right Sternoclavicular Joint, Percutaneous Endoscopic Approach
■ When reported with secondary diagnosis code T84.60XA, T84.610A, T84.611A, T84.612A, T84.613A, T84.614A, T84.615A, T84.619A, T84.63XA, T84.69XA, T84.7XXA

0RQEXZZ   Repair Right Sternoclavicular Joint, External Approach
■ When reported with secondary diagnosis code T84.60XA, T84.610A, T84.611A, T84.612A, T84.613A, T84.614A, T84.615A, T84.619A, T84.63XA, T84.69XA, T84.7XXA

0RQF0ZZ   Repair Left Sternoclavicular Joint, Open Approach
■ When reported with secondary diagnosis code T84.60XA, T84.610A, T84.611A, T84.612A, T84.613A, T84.614A, T84.615A, T84.619A, T84.63XA, T84.69XA, T84.7XXA

0RQF3ZZ   Repair Left Sternoclavicular Joint, Percutaneous Approach

■ When reported with secondary diagnosis code T84.60XA, T84.610A, T84.611A, T84.612A, T84.613A, T84.614A, T84.615A, T84.619A, T84.63XA, T84.69XA, T84.7XXA

0RQF4ZZ   Repair Left Sternoclavicular Joint, Percutaneous Endoscopic Approach
■ When reported with secondary diagnosis code T84.60XA, T84.610A, T84.611A, T84.612A, T84.613A, T84.614A, T84.615A, T84.619A, T84.63XA, T84.69XA, T84.7XXA

0RQFXZZ   Repair Left Sternoclavicular Joint, External Approach
■ When reported with secondary diagnosis code T84.60XA, T84.610A, T84.611A, T84.612A, T84.613A, T84.614A, T84.615A, T84.619A, T84.63XA, T84.69XA, T84.7XXA

0RQG0ZZ   Repair Right Acromioclavicular Joint, Open Approach
■ When reported with secondary diagnosis code T84.60XA, T84.610A, T84.611A, T84.612A, T84.613A, T84.614A, T84.615A, T84.619A, T84.63XA, T84.69XA, T84.7XXA

0RQG3ZZ   Repair Right Acromioclavicular Joint, Percutaneous Approach
■ When reported with secondary diagnosis code T84.60XA, T84.610A, T84.611A, T84.612A, T84.613A, T84.614A, T84.615A, T84.619A, T84.63XA, T84.69XA, T84.7XXA

0RQG4ZZ   Repair Right Acromioclavicular Joint, Percutaneous Endoscopic Approach
■ When reported with secondary diagnosis code T84.60XA, T84.610A, T84.611A, T84.612A, T84.613A, T84.614A, T84.615A, T84.619A, T84.63XA, T84.69XA, T84.7XXA

0RQGXZZ   Repair Right Acromioclavicular Joint, External Approach
■ When reported with secondary diagnosis code T84.60XA, T84.610A, T84.611A, T84.612A, T84.613A, T84.614A, T84.615A, T84.619A, T84.63XA, T84.69XA, T84.7XXA

0RQH0ZZ   Repair Left Acromioclavicular Joint, Open Approach
■ When reported with secondary diagnosis code T84.60XA, T84.610A, T84.611A, T84.612A, T84.613A, T84.614A, T84.615A, T84.619A, T84.63XA, T84.69XA, T84.7XXA

0RQH3ZZ   Repair Left Acromioclavicular Joint, Percutaneous Approach
■ When reported with secondary diagnosis code T84.60XA, T84.610A, T84.611A, T84.612A, T84.613A, T84.614A, T84.615A, T84.619A, T84.63XA, T84.69XA, T84.7XXA

0RQH4ZZ   Repair Left Acromioclavicular Joint, Percutaneous Endoscopic Approach
■ When reported with secondary diagnosis code T84.60XA, T84.610A, T84.611A, T84.612A, T84.613A, T84.614A, T84.615A, T84.619A, T84.63XA, T84.69XA, T84.7XXA

0RQHXZZ   Repair Left Acromioclavicular Joint, External Approach
■ When reported with secondary diagnosis code T84.60XA, T84.610A, T84.611A, T84.612A, T84.613A, T84.614A, T84.615A, T84.619A, T84.63XA, T84.69XA, T84.7XXA

0RQJ0ZZ   Repair Right Shoulder Joint, Open Approach
■ When reported with secondary diagnosis code T84.60XA, T84.610A, T84.611A, T84.612A, T84.613A, T84.614A, T84.615A, T84.619A, T84.63XA, T84.69XA, T84.7XXA

0RQJ3ZZ   Repair Right Shoulder Joint, Percutaneous Approach
■ When reported with secondary diagnosis code T84.60XA, T84.610A, T84.611A, T84.612A, T84.613A, T84.614A, T84.615A, T84.619A, T84.63XA, T84.69XA, T84.7XXA

0RQJ4ZZ   Repair Right Shoulder Joint, Percutaneous Endoscopic Approach
■ When reported with secondary diagnosis code T84.60XA, T84.610A, T84.611A, T84.612A, T84.613A, T84.614A, T84.615A, T84.619A, T84.63XA, T84.69XA, T84.7XXA

0RQJXZZ   Repair Right Shoulder Joint, External Approach
■ When reported with secondary diagnosis code T84.60XA, T84.610A, T84.611A, T84.612A, T84.613A, T84.614A, T84.615A, T84.619A, T84.63XA, T84.69XA, T84.7XXA

0RQK0ZZ   Repair Left Shoulder Joint, Open Approach
■ When reported with secondary diagnosis code T84.60XA, T84.610A, T84.611A, T84.612A, T84.613A, T84.614A, T84.615A, T84.619A, T84.63XA, T84.69XA, T84.7XXA

0RQK3ZZ   Repair Left Shoulder Joint, Percutaneous Approach
■ When reported with secondary diagnosis code T84.60XA, T84.610A, T84.611A, T84.612A, T84.613A, T84.614A, T84.615A, T84.619A, T84.63XA, T84.69XA, T84.7XXA

0RQK4ZZ   Repair Left Shoulder Joint, Percutaneous Endoscopic Approach
■ When reported with secondary diagnosis code T84.60XA, T84.610A, T84.611A, T84.612A, T84.613A, T84.614A, T84.615A, T84.619A, T84.63XA, T84.69XA, T84.7XXA

0RQKXZZ   Repair Left Shoulder Joint, External Approach
■ When reported with secondary diagnosis code T84.60XA, T84.610A, T84.611A, T84.612A, T84.613A, T84.614A, T84.615A, T84.619A, T84.63XA, T84.69XA, T84.7XXA

0RQL0ZZ   Repair Right Elbow Joint, Open Approach
■ When reported with secondary diagnosis code T84.60XA, T84.610A, T84.611A, T84.612A, T84.613A, T84.614A, T84.615A, T84.619A, T84.63XA, T84.69XA, T84.7XXA

0RQL3ZZ   Repair Right Elbow Joint, Percutaneous Approach
■ When reported with secondary diagnosis code T84.60XA, T84.610A, T84.611A, T84.612A, T84.613A, T84.614A, T84.615A, T84.619A, T84.63XA, T84.69XA, T84.7XXA

0RQL4ZZ   Repair Right Elbow Joint, Percutaneous Endoscopic Approach
■ When reported with secondary diagnosis code T84.60XA, T84.610A, T84.611A, T84.612A, T84.613A, T84.614A, T84.615A, T84.619A, T84.63XA, T84.69XA, T84.7XXA

♀ Female-only   ♂ Male-only   ▲ Limited Coverage   ● Non-OR   ■ HAC-associated procedure   ▲ Non-covered procedures   + Combination

0RQLXZZ Repair Right Elbow Joint, External Approach	**0RQN4ZZ** Repair Right Wrist Joint, Percutaneous Endoscopic Approach	**0RQT4ZZ** Repair Left Metacarpocarpal Joint, Percutaneous Endoscopic Approach
▣ When reported with secondary diagnosis code T84.60XA, T84.610A, T84.611A, T84.612A, T84.613A, T84.614A, T84.615A, T84.619A, T84.63XA, T84.69XA, T84.7XXA	**0RQNXZZ** Repair Right Wrist Joint, External Approach	**0RQTXZZ** Repair Left Metacarpocarpal Joint, External Approach
	0RQP0ZZ Repair Left Wrist Joint, Open Approach	**0RQU0ZZ** Repair Right Metacarpophalangeal Joi Open Approach
0RQM0ZZ Repair Left Elbow Joint, Open Approach	**0RQP3ZZ** Repair Left Wrist Joint, Percutaneous Approach	**0RQU3ZZ** Repair Right Metacarpophalangeal Joi Percutaneous Approach
▣ When reported with secondary diagnosis code T84.60XA, T84.610A, T84.611A, T84.612A, T84.613A, T84.614A, T84.615A, T84.619A, T84.63XA, T84.69XA, T84.7XXA	**0RQP4ZZ** Repair Left Wrist Joint, Percutaneous Endoscopic Approach	**0RQU4ZZ** Repair Right Metacarpophalangeal Joi Percutaneous Endoscopic Approach
	0RQPXZZ Repair Left Wrist Joint, External Approach	**0RQUXZZ** Repair Right Metacarpophalangeal Joi External Approach
0RQM3ZZ Repair Left Elbow Joint, Percutaneous Approach	**0RQQ0ZZ** Repair Right Carpal Joint, Open Approach	**0RQV0ZZ** Repair Left Metacarpophalangeal Joint Open Approach
▣ When reported with secondary diagnosis code T84.60XA, T84.610A, T84.611A, T84.612A, T84.613A, T84.614A, T84.615A, T84.619A, T84.63XA, T84.69XA, T84.7XXA	**0RQQ3ZZ** Repair Right Carpal Joint, Percutaneous Approach	**0RQV3ZZ** Repair Left Metacarpophalangeal Joint Percutaneous Approach
	0RQQ4ZZ Repair Right Carpal Joint, Percutaneous Endoscopic Approach	**0RQV4ZZ** Repair Left Metacarpophalangeal Joint Percutaneous Endoscopic Approach
0RQM4ZZ Repair Left Elbow Joint, Percutaneous Endoscopic Approach	**0RQQXZZ** Repair Right Carpal Joint, External Approach	**0RQVXZZ** Repair Left Metacarpophalangeal Joint External Approach
▣ When reported with secondary diagnosis code T84.60XA, T84.610A, T84.611A, T84.612A, T84.613A, T84.614A, T84.615A, T84.619A, T84.63XA, T84.69XA, T84.7XXA	**0RQR0ZZ** Repair Left Carpal Joint, Open Approach	**0RQW0ZZ** Repair Right Finger Phalangeal Joint, Open Approach
	0RQR3ZZ Repair Left Carpal Joint, Percutaneous Approach	**0RQW3ZZ** Repair Right Finger Phalangeal Joint, Percutaneous Approach
0RQMXZZ Repair Left Elbow Joint, External Approach	**0RQR4ZZ** Repair Left Carpal Joint, Percutaneous Endoscopic Approach	**0RQW4ZZ** Repair Right Finger Phalangeal Joint, Percutaneous Endoscopic Approach
▣ When reported with secondary diagnosis code T84.60XA, T84.610A, T84.611A, T84.612A, T84.613A, T84.614A, T84.615A, T84.619A, T84.63XA, T84.69XA, T84.7XXA	**0RQRXZZ** Repair Left Carpal Joint, External Approach	**0RQWXZZ** Repair Right Finger Phalangeal Joint, External Approach
	0RQS0ZZ Repair Right Metacarpocarpal Joint, Open Approach	**0RQX0ZZ** Repair Left Finger Phalangeal Joint, Open Approach
	0RQS3ZZ Repair Right Metacarpocarpal Joint, Percutaneous Approach	**0RQX3ZZ** Repair Left Finger Phalangeal Joint, Percutaneous Approach
	0RQS4ZZ Repair Right Metacarpocarpal Joint, Percutaneous Endoscopic Approach	**0RQX4ZZ** Repair Left Finger Phalangeal Joint, Percutaneous Endoscopic Approach
0RQN0ZZ Repair Right Wrist Joint, Open Approach	**0RQSXZZ** Repair Right Metacarpocarpal Joint, External Approach	
	0RQT0ZZ Repair Left Metacarpocarpal Joint, Open Approach	**0RQXXZZ** Repair Left Finger Phalangeal Joint, External Approach
0RQN3ZZ Repair Right Wrist Joint, Percutaneous Approach	**0RQT3ZZ** Repair Left Metacarpocarpal Joint, Percutaneous Approach	

0RR – Upper Joints, Replacement

0RR007Z Replacement of Occipital-cervical Joint with Autologous Tissue Substitute, Open Approach	**0RR50JZ** Replacement of Cervicothoracic Vertebral Disc with Synthetic Substitute, Open Approach	**0RRB0KZ** Replacement of Thoracolumbar Vertebra Disc with Nonautologous Tissue Substitute, Open Approach
0RR00JZ Replacement of Occipital-cervical Joint with Synthetic Substitute, Open Approach	**0RR50KZ** Replacement of Cervicothoracic Vertebral Disc with Nonautologous Tissue Substitute, Open Approach	**0RRC07Z** Replacement of Right Temporomandibula Joint with Autologous Tissue Substitute, Open Approach
0RR00KZ Replacement of Occipital-cervical Joint with Nonautologous Tissue Substitute, Open Approach	**0RR607Z** Replacement of Thoracic Vertebral Joint with Autologous Tissue Substitute, Open Approach	**0RRC0JZ** Replacement of Right Temporomandibular Joint with Synthetic Substitute, Open Approach
0RR107Z Replacement of Cervical Vertebral Joint with Autologous Tissue Substitute, Open Approach	**0RR60JZ** Replacement of Thoracic Vertebral Joint with Synthetic Substitute, Open Approach	**0RRC0KZ** Replacement of Right Temporomandibular Joint with Nonautologous Tissue Substitute, Open Approach
0RR10JZ Replacement of Cervical Vertebral Joint with Synthetic Substitute, Open Approach	**0RR60KZ** Replacement of Thoracic Vertebral Joint with Nonautologous Tissue Substitute, Open Approach	**0RRD07Z** Replacement of Left Temporomandibular Joint with Autologous Tissue Substitute, Open Approach
0RR10KZ Replacement of Cervical Vertebral Joint with Nonautologous Tissue Substitute, Open Approach	**0RR907Z** Replacement of Thoracic Vertebral Disc with Autologous Tissue Substitute, Open Approach	**0RRD0JZ** Replacement of Left Temporomandibular Joint with Synthetic Substitute, Open Approach
0RR307Z Replacement of Cervical Vertebral Disc with Autologous Tissue Substitute, Open Approach	**0RR90JZ** Replacement of Thoracic Vertebral Disc with Synthetic Substitute, Open Approach	**0RRD0KZ** Replacement of Left Temporomandibular Joint with Nonautologous Tissue Substitute, Open Approach
0RR30JZ Replacement of Cervical Vertebral Disc with Synthetic Substitute, Open Approach	**0RR90KZ** Replacement of Thoracic Vertebral Disc with Nonautologous Tissue Substitute, Open Approach	**0RRE07Z** Replacement of Right Sternoclavicular Joint with Autologous Tissue Substitute, Open Approach
0RR30KZ Replacement of Cervical Vertebral Disc with Nonautologous Tissue Substitute, Open Approach	**0RRA07Z** Replacement of Thoracolumbar Vertebral Joint with Autologous Tissue Substitute, Open Approach	**0RRE0JZ** Replacement of Right Sternoclavicular Joint with Synthetic Substitute, Open Approach
0RR407Z Replacement of Cervicothoracic Vertebral Joint with Autologous Tissue Substitute, Open Approach	**0RRA0JZ** Replacement of Thoracolumbar Vertebral Joint with Synthetic Substitute, Open Approach	**0RRE0KZ** Replacement of Right Sternoclavicular Joint with Nonautologous Tissue Substitute, Open Approach
0RR40JZ Replacement of Cervicothoracic Vertebral Joint with Synthetic Substitute, Open Approach	**0RRA0KZ** Replacement of Thoracolumbar Vertebral Joint with Nonautologous Tissue Substitute, Open Approach	**0RRF07Z** Replacement of Left Sternoclavicular Joint with Autologous Tissue Substitute, Open Approach
0RR40KZ Replacement of Cervicothoracic Vertebral Joint with Nonautologous Tissue Substitute, Open Approach	**0RRB07Z** Replacement of Thoracolumbar Vertebral Disc with Autologous Tissue Substitute, Open Approach	**0RRF0JZ** Replacement of Left Sternoclavicular Joint with Synthetic Substitute, Open Approach
0RR507Z Replacement of Cervicothoracic Vertebral Disc with Autologous Tissue Substitute, Open Approach	**0RRB0JZ** Replacement of Thoracolumbar Vertebral Disc with Synthetic Substitute, Open Approach	

944

♀ Female-only   ♂ Male-only   ▲ Limited Coverage   ● Non-OR   ▣ HAC-associated procedure   ▲ Non-covered procedures   ✚ Combination

0RRF0KZ Replacement of Left Sternoclavicular Joint with Nonautologous Tissue Substitute, Open Approach

0RRG07Z Replacement of Right Acromioclavicular Joint with Autologous Tissue Substitute, Open Approach

0RRG0JZ Replacement of Right Acromioclavicular Joint with Synthetic Substitute, Open Approach

0RRG0KZ Replacement of Right Acromioclavicular Joint with Nonautologous Tissue Substitute, Open Approach

0RRH07Z Replacement of Left Acromioclavicular Joint with Autologous Tissue Substitute, Open Approach

0RRH0JZ Replacement of Left Acromioclavicular Joint with Synthetic Substitute, Open Approach

0RRH0KZ Replacement of Left Acromioclavicular Joint with Nonautologous Tissue Substitute, Open Approach

0RRJ00Z Replacement of Right Shoulder Joint with Reverse Ball and Socket Synthetic Substitute, Open Approach
AHA CC: 1Q, 2015, 27

0RRJ07Z Replacement of Right Shoulder Joint with Autologous Tissue Substitute, Open Approach

0RRJ0J6 Replacement of Right Shoulder Joint with Synthetic Substitute, Humeral Surface, Open Approach

0RRJ0J7 Replacement of Right Shoulder Joint with Synthetic Substitute, Glenoid Surface, Open Approach

0RRJ0JZ Replacement of Right Shoulder Joint with Synthetic Substitute, Open Approach

0RRJ0KZ Replacement of Right Shoulder Joint with Nonautologous Tissue Substitute, Open Approach

0RRK00Z Replacement of Left Shoulder Joint with Reverse Ball and Socket Synthetic Substitute, Open Approach

0RRK07Z Replacement of Left Shoulder Joint with Autologous Tissue Substitute, Open Approach

0RRK0J6 Replacement of Left Shoulder Joint with Synthetic Substitute, Humeral Surface, Open Approach

0RRK0J7 Replacement of Left Shoulder Joint with Synthetic Substitute, Glenoid Surface, Open Approach

0RRK0JZ Replacement of Left Shoulder Joint with Synthetic Substitute, Open Approach

0RRK0KZ Replacement of Left Shoulder Joint with Nonautologous Tissue Substitute, Open Approach

0RRL07Z Replacement of Right Elbow Joint with Autologous Tissue Substitute, Open Approach

0RRL0JZ Replacement of Right Elbow Joint with Synthetic Substitute, Open Approach

0RRL0KZ Replacement of Right Elbow Joint with Nonautologous Tissue Substitute, Open Approach

0RRM07Z Replacement of Left Elbow Joint with Autologous Tissue Substitute, Open Approach

0RRM0JZ Replacement of Left Elbow Joint with Synthetic Substitute, Open Approach

0RRM0KZ Replacement of Left Elbow Joint with Nonautologous Tissue Substitute, Open Approach

0RRN07Z Replacement of Right Wrist Joint with Autologous Tissue Substitute, Open Approach

0RRN0JZ Replacement of Right Wrist Joint with Synthetic Substitute, Open Approach

0RRN0KZ Replacement of Right Wrist Joint with Nonautologous Tissue Substitute, Open Approach

0RRP07Z Replacement of Left Wrist Joint with Autologous Tissue Substitute, Open Approach

0RRP0JZ Replacement of Left Wrist Joint with Synthetic Substitute, Open Approach

0RRP0KZ Replacement of Left Wrist Joint with Nonautologous Tissue Substitute, Open Approach

0RRQ07Z Replacement of Right Carpal Joint with Autologous Tissue Substitute, Open Approach

0RRQ0JZ Replacement of Right Carpal Joint with Synthetic Substitute, Open Approach

0RRQ0KZ Replacement of Right Carpal Joint with Nonautologous Tissue Substitute, Open Approach

0RRR07Z Replacement of Left Carpal Joint with Autologous Tissue Substitute, Open Approach

0RRR0JZ Replacement of Left Carpal Joint with Synthetic Substitute, Open Approach

0RRR0KZ Replacement of Left Carpal Joint with Nonautologous Tissue Substitute, Open Approach

0RRS07Z Replacement of Right Metacarpocarpal Joint with Autologous Tissue Substitute, Open Approach

0RRS0JZ Replacement of Right Metacarpocarpal Joint with Synthetic Substitute, Open Approach

0RRS0KZ Replacement of Right Metacarpocarpal Joint with Nonautologous Tissue Substitute, Open Approach

0RRT07Z Replacement of Left Metacarpocarpal Joint with Autologous Tissue Substitute, Open Approach

0RRT0JZ Replacement of Left Metacarpocarpal Joint with Synthetic Substitute, Open Approach

0RRT0KZ Replacement of Left Metacarpocarpal Joint with Nonautologous Tissue Substitute, Open Approach

0RRU07Z Replacement of Right Metacarpophalangeal Joint with Autologous Tissue Substitute, Open Approach

0RRU0JZ Replacement of Right Metacarpophalangeal Joint with Synthetic Substitute, Open Approach

0RRU0KZ Replacement of Right Metacarpophalangeal Joint with Nonautologous Tissue Substitute, Open Approach

0RRV07Z Replacement of Left Metacarpophalangeal Joint with Autologous Tissue Substitute, Open Approach

0RRV0JZ Replacement of Left Metacarpophalangeal Joint with Synthetic Substitute, Open Approach

0RRV0KZ Replacement of Left Metacarpophalangeal Joint with Nonautologous Tissue Substitute, Open Approach

0RRW07Z Replacement of Right Finger Phalangeal Joint with Autologous Tissue Substitute, Open Approach

0RRW0JZ Replacement of Right Finger Phalangeal Joint with Synthetic Substitute, Open Approach

0RRW0KZ Replacement of Right Finger Phalangeal Joint with Nonautologous Tissue Substitute, Open Approach

0RRX07Z Replacement of Left Finger Phalangeal Joint with Autologous Tissue Substitute, Open Approach

0RRX0JZ Replacement of Left Finger Phalangeal Joint with Synthetic Substitute, Open Approach

0RRX0KZ Replacement of Left Finger Phalangeal Joint with Nonautologous Tissue Substitute, Open Approach

0RS – Upper Joints, Reposition

0RS004Z Reposition Occipital-cervical Joint with Internal Fixation Device, Open Approach

0RS00ZZ Reposition Occipital-cervical Joint, Open Approach

0RS034Z Reposition Occipital-cervical Joint with Internal Fixation Device, Percutaneous Approach

0RS03ZZ Reposition Occipital-cervical Joint, Percutaneous Approach

0RS044Z Reposition Occipital-cervical Joint with Internal Fixation Device, Percutaneous Endoscopic Approach

0RS04ZZ Reposition Occipital-cervical Joint, Percutaneous Endoscopic Approach

0RS0X4Z Reposition Occipital-cervical Joint with Internal Fixation Device, External Approach

0RS0XZZ Reposition Occipital-cervical Joint, External Approach

0RS104Z Reposition Cervical Vertebral Joint with Internal Fixation Device, Open Approach

0RS10ZZ Reposition Cervical Vertebral Joint, Open Approach

0RS134Z Reposition Cervical Vertebral Joint with Internal Fixation Device, Percutaneous Approach

0RS13ZZ Reposition Cervical Vertebral Joint, Percutaneous Approach

0RS144Z Reposition Cervical Vertebral Joint with Internal Fixation Device, Percutaneous Endoscopic Approach

0RS14ZZ Reposition Cervical Vertebral Joint, Percutaneous Endoscopic Approach

0RS1X4Z Reposition Cervical Vertebral Joint with Internal Fixation Device, External Approach

0RS1XZZ Reposition Cervical Vertebral Joint, External Approach
AHA CC: 2Q, 2013, 39

0RS404Z Reposition Cervicothoracic Vertebral Joint with Internal Fixation Device, Open Approach

0RS40ZZ Reposition Cervicothoracic Vertebral Joint, Open Approach

0RS434Z Reposition Cervicothoracic Vertebral Joint with Internal Fixation Device, Percutaneous Approach

0RS43ZZ Reposition Cervicothoracic Vertebral Joint, Percutaneous Approach

0RS444Z Reposition Cervicothoracic Vertebral Joint with Internal Fixation Device, Percutaneous Endoscopic Approach

0RS44ZZ Reposition Cervicothoracic Vertebral Joint, Percutaneous Endoscopic Approach

0RS4X4Z Reposition Cervicothoracic Vertebral Joint with Internal Fixation Device, External Approach

0RS4XZZ Reposition Cervicothoracic Vertebral Joint, External Approach

♀ Female-only   ♂ Male-only   ▲ Limited Coverage   ● Non-OR   ▦ HAC-associated procedure   ▲ Non-covered procedures   ✚ Combination

0RS604Z Reposition Thoracic Vertebral Joint with Internal Fixation Device, Open Approach

0RS60ZZ Reposition Thoracic Vertebral Joint, Open Approach

0RS634Z Reposition Thoracic Vertebral Joint with Internal Fixation Device, Percutaneous Approach

0RS63ZZ Reposition Thoracic Vertebral Joint, Percutaneous Approach

0RS644Z Reposition Thoracic Vertebral Joint with Internal Fixation Device, Percutaneous Endoscopic Approach

0RS64ZZ Reposition Thoracic Vertebral Joint, Percutaneous Endoscopic Approach

0RS6X4Z Reposition Thoracic Vertebral Joint with Internal Fixation Device, External Approach

0RS6XZZ Reposition Thoracic Vertebral Joint, External Approach

0RSA04Z Reposition Thoracolumbar Vertebral Joint with Internal Fixation Device, Open Approach

0RSA0ZZ Reposition Thoracolumbar Vertebral Joint, Open Approach

0RSA34Z Reposition Thoracolumbar Vertebral Joint with Internal Fixation Device, Percutaneous Approach

0RSA3ZZ Reposition Thoracolumbar Vertebral Joint, Percutaneous Approach

0RSA44Z Reposition Thoracolumbar Vertebral Joint with Internal Fixation Device, Percutaneous Endoscopic Approach

0RSA4ZZ Reposition Thoracolumbar Vertebral Joint, Percutaneous Endoscopic Approach

0RSAX4Z Reposition Thoracolumbar Vertebral Joint with Internal Fixation Device, External Approach

0RSAXZZ Reposition Thoracolumbar Vertebral Joint, External Approach

0RSC04Z Reposition Right Temporomandibular Joint with Internal Fixation Device, Open Approach

0RSC0ZZ Reposition Right Temporomandibular Joint, Open Approach

0RSC34Z Reposition Right Temporomandibular Joint with Internal Fixation Device, Percutaneous Approach

0RSC3ZZ Reposition Right Temporomandibular Joint, Percutaneous Approach

0RSC44Z Reposition Right Temporomandibular Joint with Internal Fixation Device, Percutaneous Endoscopic Approach

0RSC4ZZ Reposition Right Temporomandibular Joint, Percutaneous Endoscopic Approach

0RSCX4Z Reposition Right Temporomandibular Joint with Internal Fixation Device, External Approach

0RSCXZZ Reposition Right Temporomandibular Joint, External Approach

0RSD04Z Reposition Left Temporomandibular Joint with Internal Fixation Device, Open Approach

0RSD0ZZ Reposition Left Temporomandibular Joint, Open Approach

0RSD34Z Reposition Left Temporomandibular Joint with Internal Fixation Device, Percutaneous Approach

0RSD3ZZ Reposition Left Temporomandibular Joint, Percutaneous Approach

0RSD44Z Reposition Left Temporomandibular Joint with Internal Fixation Device, Percutaneous Endoscopic Approach

0RSD4ZZ Reposition Left Temporomandibular Joint, Percutaneous Endoscopic Approach

0RSDX4Z Reposition Left Temporomandibular Joint with Internal Fixation Device, External Approach

0RSDXZZ Reposition Left Temporomandibular Joint, External Approach

0RSE04Z Reposition Right Sternoclavicular Joint with Internal Fixation Device, Open Approach

0RSE0ZZ Reposition Right Sternoclavicular Joint, Open Approach

0RSE34Z Reposition Right Sternoclavicular Joint with Internal Fixation Device, Percutaneous Approach

0RSE3ZZ Reposition Right Sternoclavicular Joint, Percutaneous Approach

0RSE44Z Reposition Right Sternoclavicular Joint with Internal Fixation Device, Percutaneous Endoscopic Approach

0RSE4ZZ Reposition Right Sternoclavicular Joint, Percutaneous Endoscopic Approach

0RSEX4Z Reposition Right Sternoclavicular Joint with Internal Fixation Device, External Approach

0RSEXZZ Reposition Right Sternoclavicular Joint, External Approach

0RSF04Z Reposition Left Sternoclavicular Joint with Internal Fixation Device, Open Approach

0RSF0ZZ Reposition Left Sternoclavicular Joint, Open Approach

0RSF34Z Reposition Left Sternoclavicular Joint with Internal Fixation Device, Percutaneous Approach

0RSF3ZZ Reposition Left Sternoclavicular Joint, Percutaneous Approach

0RSF44Z Reposition Left Sternoclavicular Joint with Internal Fixation Device, Percutaneous Endoscopic Approach

0RSF4ZZ Reposition Left Sternoclavicular Joint, Percutaneous Endoscopic Approach

0RSFX4Z Reposition Left Sternoclavicular Joint with Internal Fixation Device, External Approach

0RSFXZZ Reposition Left Sternoclavicular Joint, External Approach

0RSG04Z Reposition Right Acromioclavicular Joint with Internal Fixation Device, Open Approach

0RSG0ZZ Reposition Right Acromioclavicular Joint, Open Approach

0RSG34Z Reposition Right Acromioclavicular Joint with Internal Fixation Device, Percutaneous Approach

0RSG3ZZ Reposition Right Acromioclavicular Joint, Percutaneous Approach

0RSG44Z Reposition Right Acromioclavicular Joint with Internal Fixation Device, Percutaneous Endoscopic Approach

0RSG4ZZ Reposition Right Acromioclavicular Joint, Percutaneous Endoscopic Approach

0RSGX4Z Reposition Right Acromioclavicular Joint with Internal Fixation Device, External Approach

0RSGXZZ Reposition Right Acromioclavicular Joint, External Approach

0RSH04Z Reposition Left Acromioclavicular Joint with Internal Fixation Device, Open Approach

0RSH0ZZ Reposition Left Acromioclavicular Joint, Open Approach

0RSH34Z Reposition Left Acromioclavicular Joint with Internal Fixation Device, Percutaneous Approach

0RSH3ZZ Reposition Left Acromioclavicular Joint, Percutaneous Approach

0RSH44Z Reposition Left Acromioclavicular Joint with Internal Fixation Device, Percutaneous Endoscopic Approach

0RSH4ZZ Reposition Left Acromioclavicular Joint, Percutaneous Endoscopic Approach

0RSHX4Z Reposition Left Acromioclavicular Joint with Internal Fixation Device, External Approach

0RSHXZZ Reposition Left Acromioclavicular Joint, External Approach

0RSJ04Z Reposition Right Shoulder Joint with Internal Fixation Device, Open Approach

0RSJ0ZZ Reposition Right Shoulder Joint, Open Approach

0RSJ34Z Reposition Right Shoulder Joint with Internal Fixation Device, Percutaneous Approach

0RSJ3ZZ Reposition Right Shoulder Joint, Percutaneous Approach

0RSJ44Z Reposition Right Shoulder Joint with Internal Fixation Device, Percutaneous Endoscopic Approach

0RSJ4ZZ Reposition Right Shoulder Joint, Percutaneous Endoscopic Approach

0RSJX4Z Reposition Right Shoulder Joint with Internal Fixation Device, External Approach

0RSJXZZ Reposition Right Shoulder Joint, External Approach

0RSK04Z Reposition Left Shoulder Joint with Internal Fixation Device, Open Approach

0RSK0ZZ Reposition Left Shoulder Joint, Open Approach

0RSK34Z Reposition Left Shoulder Joint with Internal Fixation Device, Percutaneous Approach

0RSK3ZZ Reposition Left Shoulder Joint, Percutaneous Approach

0RSK44Z Reposition Left Shoulder Joint with Internal Fixation Device, Percutaneous Endoscopic Approach

0RSK4ZZ Reposition Left Shoulder Joint, Percutaneous Endoscopic Approach

0RSKX4Z Reposition Left Shoulder Joint with Internal Fixation Device, External Approach

0RSKXZZ Reposition Left Shoulder Joint, External Approach

0RSL04Z Reposition Right Elbow Joint with Internal Fixation Device, Open Approach

0RSL05Z Reposition Right Elbow Joint with External Fixation Device, Open Approach

0RSL0ZZ Reposition Right Elbow Joint, Open Approach

0RSL34Z Reposition Right Elbow Joint with Internal Fixation Device, Percutaneous Approach

0RSL35Z Reposition Right Elbow Joint with External Fixation Device, Percutaneous Approach

0RSL3ZZ Reposition Right Elbow Joint, Percutaneous Approach

0RSL44Z Reposition Right Elbow Joint with Internal Fixation Device, Percutaneous Endoscopic Approach

0RSL45Z Reposition Right Elbow Joint with External Fixation Device, Percutaneous Endoscopic Approach

0RSL4ZZ Reposition Right Elbow Joint, Percutaneous Endoscopic Approach

0RSLX4Z Reposition Right Elbow Joint with Internal Fixation Device, External Approach

0RSLX5Z Reposition Right Elbow Joint with External Fixation Device, External Approach

0RSLXZZ Reposition Right Elbow Joint, External Approach

0RSM04Z Reposition Left Elbow Joint with Internal Fixation Device, Open Approach

0RSM05Z Reposition Left Elbow Joint with External Fixation Device, Open Approach

0RSM0ZZ Reposition Left Elbow Joint, Open Approach

SM34Z Reposition Left Elbow Joint with Internal Fixation Device, Percutaneous Approach
SM35Z Reposition Left Elbow Joint with External Fixation Device, Percutaneous Approach
SM3ZZ Reposition Left Elbow Joint, Percutaneous Approach
SM44Z Reposition Left Elbow Joint with Internal Fixation Device, Percutaneous Endoscopic Approach
SM45Z Reposition Left Elbow Joint with External Fixation Device, Percutaneous Endoscopic Approach
SM4ZZ Reposition Left Elbow Joint, Percutaneous Endoscopic Approach
RSMX4Z Reposition Left Elbow Joint with Internal Fixation Device, External Approach
RSMX5Z Reposition Left Elbow Joint with External Fixation Device, External Approach
RSMXZZ Reposition Left Elbow Joint, External Approach
RSN04Z Reposition Right Wrist Joint with Internal Fixation Device, Open Approach
RSN05Z Reposition Right Wrist Joint with External Fixation Device, Open Approach
RSN0ZZ Reposition Right Wrist Joint, Open Approach
RSN34Z Reposition Right Wrist Joint with Internal Fixation Device, Percutaneous Approach
RSN35Z Reposition Right Wrist Joint with External Fixation Device, Percutaneous Approach
RSN3ZZ Reposition Right Wrist Joint, Percutaneous Approach
RSN44Z Reposition Right Wrist Joint with Internal Fixation Device, Percutaneous Endoscopic Approach
RSN45Z Reposition Right Wrist Joint with External Fixation Device, Percutaneous Endoscopic Approach
RSN4ZZ Reposition Right Wrist Joint, Percutaneous Endoscopic Approach
RSNX4Z Reposition Right Wrist Joint with Internal Fixation Device, External Approach
RSNX5Z Reposition Right Wrist Joint with External Fixation Device, External Approach
RSNXZZ Reposition Right Wrist Joint, External Approach
RSP04Z Reposition Left Wrist Joint with Internal Fixation Device, Open Approach
RSP05Z Reposition Left Wrist Joint with External Fixation Device, Open Approach
RSP0ZZ Reposition Left Wrist Joint, Open Approach
RSP34Z Reposition Left Wrist Joint with Internal Fixation Device, Percutaneous Approach
RSP35Z Reposition Left Wrist Joint with External Fixation Device, Percutaneous Approach
RSP3ZZ Reposition Left Wrist Joint, Percutaneous Approach
RSP44Z Reposition Left Wrist Joint with Internal Fixation Device, Percutaneous Endoscopic Approach
RSP45Z Reposition Left Wrist Joint with External Fixation Device, Percutaneous Endoscopic Approach
RSP4ZZ Reposition Left Wrist Joint, Percutaneous Endoscopic Approach
RSPX4Z Reposition Left Wrist Joint with Internal Fixation Device, External Approach
RSPX5Z Reposition Left Wrist Joint with External Fixation Device, External Approach
RSPXZZ Reposition Left Wrist Joint, External Approach

AHA CC: 4Q, 2014, 32-33

RSQ04Z Reposition Right Carpal Joint with Internal Fixation Device, Open Approach
RSQ05Z Reposition Right Carpal Joint with External Fixation Device, Open Approach

0RSQ0ZZ Reposition Right Carpal Joint, Open Approach
0RSQ34Z Reposition Right Carpal Joint with Internal Fixation Device, Percutaneous Approach
0RSQ35Z Reposition Right Carpal Joint with External Fixation Device, Percutaneous Approach
0RSQ3ZZ Reposition Right Carpal Joint, Percutaneous Approach
0RSQ44Z Reposition Right Carpal Joint with Internal Fixation Device, Percutaneous Endoscopic Approach
0RSQ45Z Reposition Right Carpal Joint with External Fixation Device, Percutaneous Endoscopic Approach
0RSQ4ZZ Reposition Right Carpal Joint, Percutaneous Endoscopic Approach
0RSQX4Z Reposition Right Carpal Joint with Internal Fixation Device, External Approach
0RSQX5Z Reposition Right Carpal Joint with External Fixation Device, External Approach
0RSQXZZ Reposition Right Carpal Joint, External Approach
0RSR04Z Reposition Left Carpal Joint with Internal Fixation Device, Open Approach

AHA CC: 3Q, 2014, 33-34

0RSR05Z Reposition Left Carpal Joint with External Fixation Device, Open Approach
0RSR0ZZ Reposition Left Carpal Joint, Open Approach
0RSR34Z Reposition Left Carpal Joint with Internal Fixation Device, Percutaneous Approach
0RSR35Z Reposition Left Carpal Joint with External Fixation Device, Percutaneous Approach
0RSR3ZZ Reposition Left Carpal Joint, Percutaneous Approach
0RSR44Z Reposition Left Carpal Joint with Internal Fixation Device, Percutaneous Endoscopic Approach
0RSR45Z Reposition Left Carpal Joint with External Fixation Device, Percutaneous Endoscopic Approach
0RSR4ZZ Reposition Left Carpal Joint, Percutaneous Endoscopic Approach
0RSRX4Z Reposition Left Carpal Joint with Internal Fixation Device, External Approach
0RSRX5Z Reposition Left Carpal Joint with External Fixation Device, External Approach
0RSRXZZ Reposition Left Carpal Joint, External Approach
0RSS04Z Reposition Right Metacarpocarpal Joint with Internal Fixation Device, Open Approach
0RSS05Z Reposition Right Metacarpocarpal Joint with External Fixation Device, Open Approach
0RSS0ZZ Reposition Right Metacarpocarpal Joint, Open Approach
0RSS34Z Reposition Right Metacarpocarpal Joint with Internal Fixation Device, Percutaneous Approach
0RSS35Z Reposition Right Metacarpocarpal Joint with External Fixation Device, Percutaneous Approach
0RSS3ZZ Reposition Right Metacarpocarpal Joint, Percutaneous Approach
0RSS44Z Reposition Right Metacarpocarpal Joint with Internal Fixation Device, Percutaneous Endoscopic Approach
0RSS45Z Reposition Right Metacarpocarpal Joint with External Fixation Device, Percutaneous Endoscopic Approach
0RSS4ZZ Reposition Right Metacarpocarpal Joint, Percutaneous Endoscopic Approach

0RSSX4Z Reposition Right Metacarpocarpal Joint with Internal Fixation Device, External Approach
0RSSX5Z Reposition Right Metacarpocarpal Joint with External Fixation Device, External Approach
0RSSXZZ Reposition Right Metacarpocarpal Joint, External Approach
0RST04Z Reposition Left Metacarpocarpal Joint with Internal Fixation Device, Open Approach
0RST05Z Reposition Left Metacarpocarpal Joint with External Fixation Device, Open Approach
0RST0ZZ Reposition Left Metacarpocarpal Joint, Open Approach
0RST34Z Reposition Left Metacarpocarpal Joint with Internal Fixation Device, Percutaneous Approach
0RST35Z Reposition Left Metacarpocarpal Joint with External Fixation Device, Percutaneous Approach
0RST3ZZ Reposition Left Metacarpocarpal Joint, Percutaneous Approach
0RST44Z Reposition Left Metacarpocarpal Joint with Internal Fixation Device, Percutaneous Endoscopic Approach
0RST45Z Reposition Left Metacarpocarpal Joint with External Fixation Device, Percutaneous Endoscopic Approach
0RST4ZZ Reposition Left Metacarpocarpal Joint, Percutaneous Endoscopic Approach
0RSTX4Z Reposition Left Metacarpocarpal Joint with Internal Fixation Device, External Approach
0RSTX5Z Reposition Left Metacarpocarpal Joint with External Fixation Device, External Approach
0RSTXZZ Reposition Left Metacarpocarpal Joint, External Approach
0RSU04Z Reposition Right Metacarpophalangeal Joint with Internal Fixation Device, Open Approach
0RSU05Z Reposition Right Metacarpophalangeal Joint with External Fixation Device, Open Approach
0RSU0ZZ Reposition Right Metacarpophalangeal Joint, Open Approach
0RSU34Z Reposition Right Metacarpophalangeal Joint with Internal Fixation Device, Percutaneous Approach
0RSU35Z Reposition Right Metacarpophalangeal Joint with External Fixation Device, Percutaneous Approach
0RSU3ZZ Reposition Right Metacarpophalangeal Joint, Percutaneous Approach
0RSU44Z Reposition Right Metacarpophalangeal Joint with Internal Fixation Device, Percutaneous Endoscopic Approach
0RSU45Z Reposition Right Metacarpophalangeal Joint with External Fixation Device, Percutaneous Endoscopic Approach
0RSU4ZZ Reposition Right Metacarpophalangeal Joint, Percutaneous Endoscopic Approach
0RSUX4Z Reposition Right Metacarpophalangeal Joint with Internal Fixation Device, External Approach
0RSUX5Z Reposition Right Metacarpophalangeal Joint with External Fixation Device, External Approach
0RSUXZZ Reposition Right Metacarpophalangeal Joint, External Approach
0RSV04Z Reposition Left Metacarpophalangeal Joint with Internal Fixation Device, Open Approach
0RSV05Z Reposition Left Metacarpophalangeal Joint with External Fixation Device, Open Approach

947

0RSV0ZZ	Reposition Left Metacarpophalangeal Joint, Open Approach	0RSW05Z	Reposition Right Finger Phalangeal Joint with External Fixation Device, Open Approach	0RSX05Z	Reposition Left Finger Phalangeal Joint with External Fixation Device, Open Approach
0RSV34Z	Reposition Left Metacarpophalangeal Joint with Internal Fixation Device, Percutaneous Approach	0RSW0ZZ	Reposition Right Finger Phalangeal Joint, Open Approach	0RSX0ZZ	Reposition Left Finger Phalangeal Joint, Open Approach
0RSV35Z	Reposition Left Metacarpophalangeal Joint with External Fixation Device, Percutaneous Approach	0RSW34Z	Reposition Right Finger Phalangeal Joint with Internal Fixation Device, Percutaneous Approach	0RSX34Z	Reposition Left Finger Phalangeal Joint with Internal Fixation Device, Percutaneous Approach
0RSV3ZZ	Reposition Left Metacarpophalangeal Joint, Percutaneous Approach	0RSW35Z	Reposition Right Finger Phalangeal Joint with External Fixation Device, Percutaneous Approach	0RSX35Z	Reposition Left Finger Phalangeal Joint with External Fixation Device, Percutaneous Approach
0RSV44Z	Reposition Left Metacarpophalangeal Joint with Internal Fixation Device, Percutaneous Endoscopic Approach	0RSW3ZZ	Reposition Right Finger Phalangeal Joint, Percutaneous Approach	0RSX3ZZ	Reposition Left Finger Phalangeal Joint, Percutaneous Approach
0RSV45Z	Reposition Left Metacarpophalangeal Joint with External Fixation Device, Percutaneous Endoscopic Approach	0RSW44Z	Reposition Right Finger Phalangeal Joint with Internal Fixation Device, Percutaneous Endoscopic Approach	0RSX44Z	Reposition Left Finger Phalangeal Joint with Internal Fixation Device, Percutaneous Endoscopic Approach
0RSV4ZZ	Reposition Left Metacarpophalangeal Joint, Percutaneous Endoscopic Approach	0RSW45Z	Reposition Right Finger Phalangeal Joint with External Fixation Device, Percutaneous Endoscopic Approach	0RSX45Z	Reposition Left Finger Phalangeal Joint with External Fixation Device, Percutaneous Endoscopic Approach
0RSVX4Z	Reposition Left Metacarpophalangeal Joint with Internal Fixation Device, External Approach	0RSW4ZZ	Reposition Right Finger Phalangeal Joint, Percutaneous Endoscopic Approach	0RSX4ZZ	Reposition Left Finger Phalangeal Joint, Percutaneous Endoscopic Approach
0RSVX5Z	Reposition Left Metacarpophalangeal Joint with External Fixation Device, External Approach	0RSWX4Z	Reposition Right Finger Phalangeal Joint with Internal Fixation Device, External Approach	0RSXX4Z	Reposition Left Finger Phalangeal Joint with Internal Fixation Device, External Approach
0RSVXZZ	Reposition Left Metacarpophalangeal Joint, External Approach	0RSWX5Z	Reposition Right Finger Phalangeal Joint with External Fixation Device, External Approach	0RSXX5Z	Reposition Left Finger Phalangeal Joint with External Fixation Device, External Approach
0RSW04Z	Reposition Right Finger Phalangeal Joint with Internal Fixation Device, Open Approach	0RSWXZZ	Reposition Right Finger Phalangeal Joint, External Approach	0RSXXZZ	Reposition Left Finger Phalangeal Joint, External Approach
		0RSX04Z	Reposition Left Finger Phalangeal Joint with Internal Fixation Device, Open Approach		

0RT – Upper Joints, Resection

Review Coding Guideline B3.8

0RT30ZZ	Resection of Cervical Vertebral Disc, Open Approach	0RTF0ZZ	Resection of Left Sternoclavicular Joint, Open Approach	0RTQ0ZZ	Resection of Right Carpal Joint, Open Approach
0RT40ZZ	Resection of Cervicothoracic Vertebral Joint, Open Approach	0RTG0ZZ	Resection of Right Acromioclavicular Joint, Open Approach	0RTR0ZZ	Resection of Left Carpal Joint, Open Approach
0RT50ZZ	Resection of Cervicothoracic Vertebral Disc, Open Approach *AHA CC: 2Q, 2014, 7-8*	0RTH0ZZ	Resection of Left Acromioclavicular Joint, Open Approach	0RTS0ZZ	Resection of Right Metacarpocarpal Joint, Open Approach
0RT90ZZ	Resection of Thoracic Vertebral Disc, Open Approach	0RTJ0ZZ	Resection of Right Shoulder Joint, Open Approach	0RTT0ZZ	Resection of Left Metacarpocarpal Joint, Open Approach
0RTB0ZZ	Resection of Thoracolumbar Vertebral Disc, Open Approach	0RTK0ZZ	Resection of Left Shoulder Joint, Open Approach	0RTU0ZZ	Resection of Right Metacarpophalangeal Joint, Open Approach
0RTC0ZZ	Resection of Right Temporomandibular Joint, Open Approach	0RTL0ZZ	Resection of Right Elbow Joint, Open Approach	0RTV0ZZ	Resection of Left Metacarpophalangeal Joint, Open Approach
0RTD0ZZ	Resection of Left Temporomandibular Joint, Open Approach	0RTM0ZZ	Resection of Left Elbow Joint, Open Approach	0RTW0ZZ	Resection of Right Finger Phalangeal Joint, Open Approach
0RTE0ZZ	Resection of Right Sternoclavicular Joint, Open Approach	0RTN0ZZ	Resection of Right Wrist Joint, Open Approach	0RTX0ZZ	Resection of Left Finger Phalangeal Joint, Open Approach
		0RTP0ZZ	Resection of Left Wrist Joint, Open Approach		

0RU – Upper Joints, Supplement

0RU007Z	Supplement Occipital-cervical Joint with Autologous Tissue Substitute, Open Approach	0RU04JZ	Supplement Occipital-cervical Joint with Synthetic Substitute, Percutaneous Endoscopic Approach	0RU13KZ	Supplement Cervical Vertebral Joint with Nonautologous Tissue Substitute, Percutaneous Approach
0RU00JZ	Supplement Occipital-cervical Joint with Synthetic Substitute, Open Approach	0RU04KZ	Supplement Occipital-cervical Joint with Nonautologous Tissue Substitute, Percutaneous Endoscopic Approach	0RU147Z	Supplement Cervical Vertebral Joint with Autologous Tissue Substitute, Percutaneous Endoscopic Approach
0RU00KZ	Supplement Occipital-cervical Joint with Nonautologous Tissue Substitute, Open Approach	0RU107Z	Supplement Cervical Vertebral Joint with Autologous Tissue Substitute, Open Approach	0RU14JZ	Supplement Cervical Vertebral Joint with Synthetic Substitute, Percutaneous Endoscopic Approach
0RU037Z	Supplement Occipital-cervical Joint with Autologous Tissue Substitute, Percutaneous Approach	0RU10JZ	Supplement Cervical Vertebral Joint with Synthetic Substitute, Open Approach	0RU14KZ	Supplement Cervical Vertebral Joint with Nonautologous Tissue Substitute, Percutaneous Endoscopic Approach
0RU03JZ	Supplement Occipital-cervical Joint with Synthetic Substitute, Percutaneous Approach	0RU10KZ	Supplement Cervical Vertebral Joint with Nonautologous Tissue Substitute, Open Approach	0RU307Z	Supplement Cervical Vertebral Disc with Autologous Tissue Substitute, Open Approach
0RU03KZ	Supplement Occipital-cervical Joint with Nonautologous Tissue Substitute, Percutaneous Approach	0RU137Z	Supplement Cervical Vertebral Joint with Autologous Tissue Substitute, Percutaneous Approach	0RU30JZ	Supplement Cervical Vertebral Disc with Synthetic Substitute, Open Approach
0RU047Z	Supplement Occipital-cervical Joint with Autologous Tissue Substitute, Percutaneous Endoscopic Approach	0RU13JZ	Supplement Cervical Vertebral Joint with Synthetic Substitute, Percutaneous Approach	0RU30KZ	Supplement Cervical Vertebral Disc with Nonautologous Tissue Substitute, Open Approach

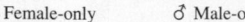

♀ Female-only   ♂ Male-only   ▲ Limited Coverage   ● Non-OR   ▥ HAC-associated procedure   ▲ Non-covered procedures   ✚ Combination

U337Z	Supplement Cervical Vertebral Disc with Autologous Tissue Substitute, Percutaneous Approach
U33JZ	Supplement Cervical Vertebral Disc with Synthetic Substitute, Percutaneous Approach
U33KZ	Supplement Cervical Vertebral Disc with Nonautologous Tissue Substitute, Percutaneous Approach
U347Z	Supplement Cervical Vertebral Disc with Autologous Tissue Substitute, Percutaneous Endoscopic Approach
U34JZ	Supplement Cervical Vertebral Disc with Synthetic Substitute, Percutaneous Endoscopic Approach
U34KZ	Supplement Cervical Vertebral Disc with Nonautologous Tissue Substitute, Percutaneous Endoscopic Approach
U407Z	Supplement Cervicothoracic Vertebral Joint with Autologous Tissue Substitute, Open Approach
U40JZ	Supplement Cervicothoracic Vertebral Joint with Synthetic Substitute, Open Approach
U40KZ	Supplement Cervicothoracic Vertebral Joint with Nonautologous Tissue Substitute, Open Approach
U437Z	Supplement Cervicothoracic Vertebral Joint with Autologous Tissue Substitute, Percutaneous Approach
U43JZ	Supplement Cervicothoracic Vertebral Joint with Synthetic Substitute, Percutaneous Approach
U43KZ	Supplement Cervicothoracic Vertebral Joint with Nonautologous Tissue Substitute, Percutaneous Approach
U447Z	Supplement Cervicothoracic Vertebral Joint with Autologous Tissue Substitute, Percutaneous Endoscopic Approach
U44JZ	Supplement Cervicothoracic Vertebral Joint with Synthetic Substitute, Percutaneous Endoscopic Approach
U44KZ	Supplement Cervicothoracic Vertebral Joint with Nonautologous Tissue Substitute, Percutaneous Endoscopic Approach
U507Z	Supplement Cervicothoracic Vertebral Disc with Autologous Tissue Substitute, Open Approach
U50JZ	Supplement Cervicothoracic Vertebral Disc with Synthetic Substitute, Open Approach
U50KZ	Supplement Cervicothoracic Vertebral Disc with Nonautologous Tissue Substitute, Open Approach
U537Z	Supplement Cervicothoracic Vertebral Disc with Autologous Tissue Substitute, Percutaneous Approach
U53JZ	Supplement Cervicothoracic Vertebral Disc with Synthetic Substitute, Percutaneous Approach
U53KZ	Supplement Cervicothoracic Vertebral Disc with Nonautologous Tissue Substitute, Percutaneous Approach
U547Z	Supplement Cervicothoracic Vertebral Disc with Autologous Tissue Substitute, Percutaneous Endoscopic Approach
U54JZ	Supplement Cervicothoracic Vertebral Disc with Synthetic Substitute, Percutaneous Endoscopic Approach
U54KZ	Supplement Cervicothoracic Vertebral Disc with Nonautologous Tissue Substitute, Percutaneous Endoscopic Approach
RU607Z	Supplement Thoracic Vertebral Joint with Autologous Tissue Substitute, Open Approach
RU60JZ	Supplement Thoracic Vertebral Joint with Synthetic Substitute, Open Approach
0RU60KZ	Supplement Thoracic Vertebral Joint with Nonautologous Tissue Substitute, Open Approach
0RU637Z	Supplement Thoracic Vertebral Joint with Autologous Tissue Substitute, Percutaneous Approach
0RU63JZ	Supplement Thoracic Vertebral Joint with Synthetic Substitute, Percutaneous Approach
0RU63KZ	Supplement Thoracic Vertebral Joint with Nonautologous Tissue Substitute, Percutaneous Approach
0RU647Z	Supplement Thoracic Vertebral Joint with Autologous Tissue Substitute, Percutaneous Endoscopic Approach
0RU64JZ	Supplement Thoracic Vertebral Joint with Synthetic Substitute, Percutaneous Endoscopic Approach
0RU64KZ	Supplement Thoracic Vertebral Joint with Nonautologous Tissue Substitute, Percutaneous Endoscopic Approach
0RU907Z	Supplement Thoracic Vertebral Disc with Autologous Tissue Substitute, Open Approach
0RU90JZ	Supplement Thoracic Vertebral Disc with Synthetic Substitute, Open Approach
0RU90KZ	Supplement Thoracic Vertebral Disc with Nonautologous Tissue Substitute, Open Approach
0RU937Z	Supplement Thoracic Vertebral Disc with Autologous Tissue Substitute, Percutaneous Approach
0RU93JZ	Supplement Thoracic Vertebral Disc with Synthetic Substitute, Percutaneous Approach
0RU93KZ	Supplement Thoracic Vertebral Disc with Nonautologous Tissue Substitute, Percutaneous Approach
0RU947Z	Supplement Thoracic Vertebral Disc with Autologous Tissue Substitute, Percutaneous Endoscopic Approach
0RU94JZ	Supplement Thoracic Vertebral Disc with Synthetic Substitute, Percutaneous Endoscopic Approach
0RU94KZ	Supplement Thoracic Vertebral Disc with Nonautologous Tissue Substitute, Percutaneous Endoscopic Approach
0RUA07Z	Supplement Thoracolumbar Vertebral Joint with Autologous Tissue Substitute, Open Approach
0RUA0JZ	Supplement Thoracolumbar Vertebral Joint with Synthetic Substitute, Open Approach
0RUA0KZ	Supplement Thoracolumbar Vertebral Joint with Nonautologous Tissue Substitute, Open Approach
0RUA37Z	Supplement Thoracolumbar Vertebral Joint with Autologous Tissue Substitute, Percutaneous Approach
0RUA3JZ	Supplement Thoracolumbar Vertebral Joint with Synthetic Substitute, Percutaneous Approach
0RUA3KZ	Supplement Thoracolumbar Vertebral Joint with Nonautologous Tissue Substitute, Percutaneous Approach
0RUA47Z	Supplement Thoracolumbar Vertebral Joint with Autologous Tissue Substitute, Percutaneous Endoscopic Approach
0RUA4JZ	Supplement Thoracolumbar Vertebral Joint with Synthetic Substitute, Percutaneous Endoscopic Approach
0RUA4KZ	Supplement Thoracolumbar Vertebral Joint with Nonautologous Tissue Substitute, Percutaneous Endoscopic Approach
0RUB07Z	Supplement Thoracolumbar Vertebral Disc with Autologous Tissue Substitute, Open Approach
0RUB0JZ	Supplement Thoracolumbar Vertebral Disc with Synthetic Substitute, Open Approach
0RUB0KZ	Supplement Thoracolumbar Vertebral Disc with Nonautologous Tissue Substitute, Open Approach
0RUB37Z	Supplement Thoracolumbar Vertebral Disc with Autologous Tissue Substitute, Percutaneous Approach
0RUB3JZ	Supplement Thoracolumbar Vertebral Disc with Synthetic Substitute, Percutaneous Approach
0RUB3KZ	Supplement Thoracolumbar Vertebral Disc with Nonautologous Tissue Substitute, Percutaneous Approach
0RUB47Z	Supplement Thoracolumbar Vertebral Disc with Autologous Tissue Substitute, Percutaneous Endoscopic Approach
0RUB4JZ	Supplement Thoracolumbar Vertebral Disc with Synthetic Substitute, Percutaneous Endoscopic Approach
0RUB4KZ	Supplement Thoracolumbar Vertebral Disc with Nonautologous Tissue Substitute, Percutaneous Endoscopic Approach
0RUC07Z	Supplement Right Temporomandibular Joint with Autologous Tissue Substitute, Open Approach
0RUC0JZ	Supplement Right Temporomandibular Joint with Synthetic Substitute, Open Approach
0RUC0KZ	Supplement Right Temporomandibular Joint with Nonautologous Tissue Substitute, Open Approach
0RUC37Z	Supplement Right Temporomandibular Joint with Autologous Tissue Substitute, Percutaneous Approach
0RUC3JZ	Supplement Right Temporomandibular Joint with Synthetic Substitute, Percutaneous Approach
0RUC3KZ	Supplement Right Temporomandibular Joint with Nonautologous Tissue Substitute, Percutaneous Approach
0RUC47Z	Supplement Right Temporomandibular Joint with Autologous Tissue Substitute, Percutaneous Endoscopic Approach
0RUC4JZ	Supplement Right Temporomandibular Joint with Synthetic Substitute, Percutaneous Endoscopic Approach
0RUC4KZ	Supplement Right Temporomandibular Joint with Nonautologous Tissue Substitute, Percutaneous Endoscopic Approach
0RUD07Z	Supplement Left Temporomandibular Joint with Autologous Tissue Substitute, Open Approach
0RUD0JZ	Supplement Left Temporomandibular Joint with Synthetic Substitute, Open Approach
0RUD0KZ	Supplement Left Temporomandibular Joint with Nonautologous Tissue Substitute, Open Approach
0RUD37Z	Supplement Left Temporomandibular Joint with Autologous Tissue Substitute, Percutaneous Approach
0RUD3JZ	Supplement Left Temporomandibular Joint with Synthetic Substitute, Percutaneous Approach
0RUD3KZ	Supplement Left Temporomandibular Joint with Nonautologous Tissue Substitute, Percutaneous Approach
0RUD47Z	Supplement Left Temporomandibular Joint with Autologous Tissue Substitute, Percutaneous Endoscopic Approach
0RUD4JZ	Supplement Left Temporomandibular Joint with Synthetic Substitute, Percutaneous Endoscopic Approach

949

0RUD4KZ Supplement Left Temporomandibular Joint with Nonautologous Tissue Substitute, Percutaneous Endoscopic Approach

0RUE07Z Supplement Right Sternoclavicular Joint with Autologous Tissue Substitute, Open Approach

　　When reported with secondary diagnosis code T84.60XA, T84.610A, T84.611A, T84.612A, T84.613A, T84.614A, T84.615A, T84.619A, T84.63XA, T84.69XA, T84.7XXA

0RUE0JZ Supplement Right Sternoclavicular Joint with Synthetic Substitute, Open Approach

　　When reported with secondary diagnosis code T84.60XA, T84.610A, T84.611A, T84.612A, T84.613A, T84.614A, T84.615A, T84.619A, T84.63XA, T84.69XA, T84.7XXA

0RUE0KZ Supplement Right Sternoclavicular Joint with Nonautologous Tissue Substitute, Open Approach

　　When reported with secondary diagnosis code T84.60XA, T84.610A, T84.611A, T84.612A, T84.613A, T84.614A, T84.615A, T84.619A, T84.63XA, T84.69XA, T84.7XXA

0RUE37Z Supplement Right Sternoclavicular Joint with Autologous Tissue Substitute, Percutaneous Approach

　　When reported with secondary diagnosis code T84.60XA, T84.610A, T84.611A, T84.612A, T84.613A, T84.614A, T84.615A, T84.619A, T84.63XA, T84.69XA, T84.7XXA

0RUE3JZ Supplement Right Sternoclavicular Joint with Synthetic Substitute, Percutaneous Approach

　　When reported with secondary diagnosis code T84.60XA, T84.610A, T84.611A, T84.612A, T84.613A, T84.614A, T84.615A, T84.619A, T84.63XA, T84.69XA, T84.7XXA

0RUE3KZ Supplement Right Sternoclavicular Joint with Nonautologous Tissue Substitute, Percutaneous Approach

　　When reported with secondary diagnosis code T84.60XA, T84.610A, T84.611A, T84.612A, T84.613A, T84.614A, T84.615A, T84.619A, T84.63XA, T84.69XA, T84.7XXA

0RUE47Z Supplement Right Sternoclavicular Joint with Autologous Tissue Substitute, Percutaneous Endoscopic Approach

　　When reported with secondary diagnosis code T84.60XA, T84.610A, T84.611A, T84.612A, T84.613A, T84.614A, T84.615A, T84.619A, T84.63XA, T84.69XA, T84.7XXA

0RUE4JZ Supplement Right Sternoclavicular Joint with Synthetic Substitute, Percutaneous Endoscopic Approach

　　When reported with secondary diagnosis code T84.60XA, T84.610A, T84.611A, T84.612A, T84.613A, T84.614A, T84.615A, T84.619A, T84.63XA, T84.69XA, T84.7XXA

0RUE4KZ Supplement Right Sternoclavicular Joint with Nonautologous Tissue Substitute, Percutaneous Endoscopic Approach

　　When reported with secondary diagnosis code T84.60XA, T84.610A, T84.611A, T84.612A, T84.613A, T84.614A, T84.615A, T84.619A, T84.63XA, T84.69XA, T84.7XXA

0RUF07Z Supplement Left Sternoclavicular Joint with Autologous Tissue Substitute, Open Approach

　　When reported with secondary diagnosis code T84.60XA, T84.610A, T84.611A, T84.612A, T84.613A, T84.614A, T84.615A, T84.619A, T84.63XA, T84.69XA, T84.7XXA

0RUF0JZ Supplement Left Sternoclavicular Joint with Synthetic Substitute, Open Approach

　　When reported with secondary diagnosis code T84.60XA, T84.610A, T84.611A, T84.612A, T84.613A, T84.614A, T84.615A, T84.619A, T84.63XA, T84.69XA, T84.7XXA

0RUF0KZ Supplement Left Sternoclavicular Joint with Nonautologous Tissue Substitute, Open Approach

　　When reported with secondary diagnosis code T84.60XA, T84.610A, T84.611A, T84.612A, T84.613A, T84.614A, T84.615A, T84.619A, T84.63XA, T84.69XA, T84.7XXA

0RUF37Z Supplement Left Sternoclavicular Joint with Autologous Tissue Substitute, Percutaneous Approach

　　When reported with secondary diagnosis code T84.60XA, T84.610A, T84.611A, T84.612A, T84.613A, T84.614A, T84.615A, T84.619A, T84.63XA, T84.69XA, T84.7XXA

0RUF3JZ Supplement Left Sternoclavicular Joint with Synthetic Substitute, Percutaneous Approach

　　When reported with secondary diagnosis code T84.60XA, T84.610A, T84.611A, T84.612A, T84.613A, T84.614A, T84.615A, T84.619A, T84.63XA, T84.69XA, T84.7XXA

0RUF3KZ Supplement Left Sternoclavicular Joint with Nonautologous Tissue Substitute, Percutaneous Approach

　　When reported with secondary diagnosis code T84.60XA, T84.610A, T84.611A, T84.612A, T84.613A, T84.614A, T84.615A, T84.619A, T84.63XA, T84.69XA, T84.7XXA

0RUF47Z Supplement Left Sternoclavicular Joint with Autologous Tissue Substitute, Percutaneous Endoscopic Approach

　　When reported with secondary diagnosis code T84.60XA, T84.610A, T84.611A, T84.612A, T84.613A, T84.614A, T84.615A, T84.619A, T84.63XA, T84.69XA, T84.7XXA

0RUF4JZ Supplement Left Sternoclavicular Joint with Synthetic Substitute, Percutaneous Endoscopic Approach

　　When reported with secondary diagnosis code T84.60XA, T84.610A, T84.611A, T84.612A, T84.613A, T84.614A, T84.615A, T84.619A, T84.63XA, T84.69XA, T84.7XXA

0RUF4KZ Supplement Left Sternoclavicular Joint with Nonautologous Tissue Substitute, Percutaneous Endoscopic Approach

　　When reported with secondary diagnosis code T84.60XA, T84.610A, T84.611A, T84.612A, T84.613A, T84.614A, T84.615A, T84.619A, T84.63XA, T84.69XA, T84.7XXA

0RUG07Z Supplement Right Acromioclavicular Joint with Autologous Tissue Substitute, Open Approach

　　When reported with secondary diagnosis code T84.60XA, T84.610A, T84.611A,

T84.612A, T84.613A, T84.614A, T84.615A, T84.619A, T84.63XA, T84.69XA, T84.7XXA

0RUG0JZ Supplement Right Acromioclavicular Joint with Synthetic Substitute, Open Approach

　　When reported with secondary diagnosis code T84.60XA, T84.610A, T84.611A, T84.612A, T84.613A, T84.614A, T84.615A, T84.619A, T84.63XA, T84.69XA, T84.7XXA

0RUG0KZ Supplement Right Acromioclavicular Joint with Nonautologous Tissue Substitute, Open Approach

　　When reported with secondary diagnosis code T84.60XA, T84.610A, T84.611A, T84.612A, T84.613A, T84.614A, T84.615A, T84.619A, T84.63XA, T84.69XA, T84.7XXA

0RUG37Z Supplement Right Acromioclavicular Joint with Autologous Tissue Substitute Percutaneous Approach

　　When reported with secondary diagnosis code T84.60XA, T84.610A, T84.611A, T84.612A, T84.613A, T84.614A, T84.615A, T84.619A, T84.63XA, T84.69XA, T84.7XXA

0RUG3JZ Supplement Right Acromioclavicular Joint with Synthetic Substitute, Percutaneous Approach

　　When reported with secondary diagnosis code T84.60XA, T84.610A, T84.611A, T84.612A, T84.613A, T84.614A, T84.615A, T84.619A, T84.63XA, T84.69XA, T84.7XXA

0RUG3KZ Supplement Right Acromioclavicular Joint with Nonautologous Tissue Substitute, Percutaneous Approach

　　When reported with secondary diagnosis code T84.60XA, T84.610A, T84.611A, T84.612A, T84.613A, T84.614A, T84.615A, T84.619A, T84.63XA, T84.69XA, T84.7XXA

0RUG47Z Supplement Right Acromioclavicular Joint with Autologous Tissue Substitute, Percutaneous Endoscopic Approach

　　When reported with secondary diagnosis code T84.60XA, T84.610A, T84.611A, T84.612A, T84.613A, T84.614A, T84.615A, T84.619A, T84.63XA, T84.69XA, T84.7XXA

0RUG4JZ Supplement Right Acromioclavicular Joint with Synthetic Substitute, Percutaneous Endoscopic Approach

　　When reported with secondary diagnosis code T84.60XA, T84.610A, T84.611A, T84.612A, T84.613A, T84.614A, T84.615A, T84.619A, T84.63XA, T84.69XA, T84.7XXA

0RUG4KZ Supplement Right Acromioclavicular Joint with Nonautologous Tissue Substitute, Percutaneous Endoscopic Approach

　　When reported with secondary diagnosis code T84.60XA, T84.610A, T84.611A, T84.612A, T84.613A, T84.614A, T84.615A, T84.619A, T84.63XA, T84.69XA, T84.7XXA

0RUH07Z Supplement Left Acromioclavicular Joint with Autologous Tissue Substitute, Open Approach

　　When reported with secondary diagnosis code T84.60XA, T84.610A, T84.611A, T84.612A, T84.613A, T84.614A, T84.615A, T84.619A, T84.63XA, T84.69XA, T84.7XXA

0RUH0JZ Supplement Left Acromioclavicular Joint with Synthetic Substitute, Open Approach
- [HAC] When reported with secondary diagnosis code T84.60XA, T84.610A, T84.611A, T84.612A, T84.613A, T84.614A, T84.615A, T84.619A, T84.63XA, T84.69XA, T84.7XXA

0RUH0KZ Supplement Left Acromioclavicular Joint with Nonautologous Tissue Substitute, Open Approach
- [HAC] When reported with secondary diagnosis code T84.60XA, T84.610A, T84.611A, T84.612A, T84.613A, T84.614A, T84.615A, T84.619A, T84.63XA, T84.69XA, T84.7XXA

0RUH37Z Supplement Left Acromioclavicular Joint with Autologous Tissue Substitute, Percutaneous Approach
- [HAC] When reported with secondary diagnosis code T84.60XA, T84.610A, T84.611A, T84.612A, T84.613A, T84.614A, T84.615A, T84.619A, T84.63XA, T84.69XA, T84.7XXA

0RUH3JZ Supplement Left Acromioclavicular Joint with Synthetic Substitute, Percutaneous Approach
- [HAC] When reported with secondary diagnosis code T84.60XA, T84.610A, T84.611A, T84.612A, T84.613A, T84.614A, T84.615A, T84.619A, T84.63XA, T84.69XA, T84.7XXA

0RUH3KZ Supplement Left Acromioclavicular Joint with Nonautologous Tissue Substitute, Percutaneous Approach
- [HAC] When reported with secondary diagnosis code T84.60XA, T84.610A, T84.611A, T84.612A, T84.613A, T84.614A, T84.615A, T84.619A, T84.63XA, T84.69XA, T84.7XXA

0RUH47Z Supplement Left Acromioclavicular Joint with Autologous Tissue Substitute, Percutaneous Endoscopic Approach
- [HAC] When reported with secondary diagnosis code T84.60XA, T84.610A, T84.611A, T84.612A, T84.613A, T84.614A, T84.615A, T84.619A, T84.63XA, T84.69XA, T84.7XXA

0RUH4JZ Supplement Left Acromioclavicular Joint with Synthetic Substitute, Percutaneous Endoscopic Approach
- [HAC] When reported with secondary diagnosis code T84.60XA, T84.610A, T84.611A, T84.612A, T84.613A, T84.614A, T84.615A, T84.619A, T84.63XA, T84.69XA, T84.7XXA

0RUH4KZ Supplement Left Acromioclavicular Joint with Nonautologous Tissue Substitute, Percutaneous Endoscopic Approach
- [HAC] When reported with secondary diagnosis code T84.60XA, T84.610A, T84.611A, T84.612A, T84.613A, T84.614A, T84.615A, T84.619A, T84.63XA, T84.69XA, T84.7XXA

0RUJ07Z Supplement Right Shoulder Joint with Autologous Tissue Substitute, Open Approach
- [HAC] When reported with secondary diagnosis code T84.60XA, T84.610A, T84.611A, T84.612A, T84.613A, T84.614A, T84.615A, T84.619A, T84.63XA, T84.69XA, T84.7XXA

0RUJ0JZ Supplement Right Shoulder Joint with Synthetic Substitute, Open Approach
- [HAC] When reported with secondary diagnosis code T84.60XA, T84.610A, T84.611A, T84.612A, T84.613A, T84.614A, T84.615A, T84.619A, T84.63XA, T84.69XA, T84.7XXA

0RUJ0KZ Supplement Right Shoulder Joint with Nonautologous Tissue Substitute, Open Approach
- [HAC] When reported with secondary diagnosis code T84.60XA, T84.610A, T84.611A, T84.612A, T84.613A, T84.614A, T84.615A, T84.619A, T84.63XA, T84.69XA, T84.7XXA

0RUJ37Z Supplement Right Shoulder Joint with Autologous Tissue Substitute, Percutaneous Approach
- [HAC] When reported with secondary diagnosis code T84.60XA, T84.610A, T84.611A, T84.612A, T84.613A, T84.614A, T84.615A, T84.619A, T84.63XA, T84.69XA, T84.7XXA

0RUJ3JZ Supplement Right Shoulder Joint with Synthetic Substitute, Percutaneous Approach
- [HAC] When reported with secondary diagnosis code T84.60XA, T84.610A, T84.611A, T84.612A, T84.613A, T84.614A, T84.615A, T84.619A, T84.63XA, T84.69XA, T84.7XXA

0RUJ3KZ Supplement Right Shoulder Joint with Nonautologous Tissue Substitute, Percutaneous Approach
- [HAC] When reported with secondary diagnosis code T84.60XA, T84.610A, T84.611A, T84.612A, T84.613A, T84.614A, T84.615A, T84.619A, T84.63XA, T84.69XA, T84.7XXA

0RUJ47Z Supplement Right Shoulder Joint with Autologous Tissue Substitute, Percutaneous Endoscopic Approach
- [HAC] When reported with secondary diagnosis code T84.60XA, T84.610A, T84.611A, T84.612A, T84.613A, T84.614A, T84.615A, T84.619A, T84.63XA, T84.69XA, T84.7XXA

0RUJ4JZ Supplement Right Shoulder Joint with Synthetic Substitute, Percutaneous Endoscopic Approach
- [HAC] When reported with secondary diagnosis code T84.60XA, T84.610A, T84.611A, T84.612A, T84.613A, T84.614A, T84.615A, T84.619A, T84.63XA, T84.69XA, T84.7XXA

0RUJ4KZ Supplement Right Shoulder Joint with Nonautologous Tissue Substitute, Percutaneous Endoscopic Approach
- [HAC] When reported with secondary diagnosis code T84.60XA, T84.610A, T84.611A, T84.612A, T84.613A, T84.614A, T84.615A, T84.619A, T84.63XA, T84.69XA, T84.7XXA

0RUK07Z Supplement Left Shoulder Joint with Autologous Tissue Substitute, Open Approach
- [HAC] When reported with secondary diagnosis code T84.60XA, T84.610A, T84.611A, T84.612A, T84.613A, T84.614A, T84.615A, T84.619A, T84.63XA, T84.69XA, T84.7XXA

0RUK0JZ Supplement Left Shoulder Joint with Synthetic Substitute, Open Approach
- [HAC] When reported with secondary diagnosis code T84.60XA, T84.610A, T84.611A, T84.612A, T84.613A, T84.614A, T84.615A, T84.619A, T84.63XA, T84.69XA, T84.7XXA

0RUK0KZ Supplement Left Shoulder Joint with Nonautologous Tissue Substitute, Open Approach
- [HAC] When reported with secondary diagnosis code T84.60XA, T84.610A, T84.611A, T84.612A, T84.613A, T84.614A, T84.615A, T84.619A, T84.63XA, T84.69XA, T84.7XXA

0RUK37Z Supplement Left Shoulder Joint with Autologous Tissue Substitute, Percutaneous Approach
- [HAC] When reported with secondary diagnosis code T84.60XA, T84.610A, T84.611A, T84.612A, T84.613A, T84.614A, T84.615A, T84.619A, T84.63XA, T84.69XA, T84.7XXA

0RUK3JZ Supplement Left Shoulder Joint with Synthetic Substitute, Percutaneous Approach
- [HAC] When reported with secondary diagnosis code T84.60XA, T84.610A, T84.611A, T84.612A, T84.613A, T84.614A, T84.615A, T84.619A, T84.63XA, T84.69XA, T84.7XXA

0RUK3KZ Supplement Left Shoulder Joint with Nonautologous Tissue Substitute, Percutaneous Approach
- [HAC] When reported with secondary diagnosis code T84.60XA, T84.610A, T84.611A, T84.612A, T84.613A, T84.614A, T84.615A, T84.619A, T84.63XA, T84.69XA, T84.7XXA

0RUK47Z Supplement Left Shoulder Joint with Autologous Tissue Substitute, Percutaneous Endoscopic Approach
- [HAC] When reported with secondary diagnosis code T84.60XA, T84.610A, T84.611A, T84.612A, T84.613A, T84.614A, T84.615A, T84.619A, T84.63XA, T84.69XA, T84.7XXA

0RUK4JZ Supplement Left Shoulder Joint with Synthetic Substitute, Percutaneous Endoscopic Approach
- [HAC] When reported with secondary diagnosis code T84.60XA, T84.610A, T84.611A, T84.612A, T84.613A, T84.614A, T84.615A, T84.619A, T84.63XA, T84.69XA, T84.7XXA

0RUK4KZ Supplement Left Shoulder Joint with Nonautologous Tissue Substitute, Percutaneous Endoscopic Approach
- [HAC] When reported with secondary diagnosis code T84.60XA, T84.610A, T84.611A, T84.612A, T84.613A, T84.614A, T84.615A, T84.619A, T84.63XA, T84.69XA, T84.7XXA

0RUL07Z Supplement Right Elbow Joint with Autologous Tissue Substitute, Open Approach
- [HAC] When reported with secondary diagnosis code T84.60XA, T84.610A, T84.611A, T84.612A, T84.613A, T84.614A, T84.615A, T84.619A, T84.63XA, T84.69XA, T84.7XXA

0RUL0JZ Supplement Right Elbow Joint with Synthetic Substitute, Open Approach
- [HAC] When reported with secondary diagnosis code T84.60XA, T84.610A, T84.611A, T84.612A, T84.613A, T84.614A, T84.615A, T84.619A, T84.63XA, T84.69XA, T84.7XXA

0RUL0KZ Supplement Right Elbow Joint with Nonautologous Tissue Substitute, Open Approach
- [HAC] When reported with secondary diagnosis code T84.60XA, T84.610A, T84.611A, T84.612A, T84.613A, T84.614A, T84.615A, T84.619A, T84.63XA, T84.69XA, T84.7XXA

♀ Female-only   ♂ Male-only   ▲ Limited Coverage   ● Non-OR   [HAC] HAC-associated procedure   ▲ Non-covered procedures   ✚ Combination

0RUL37Z Supplement Right Elbow Joint with Autologous Tissue Substitute, Percutaneous Approach
- ⬛ When reported with secondary diagnosis code T84.60XA, T84.610A, T84.611A, T84.612A, T84.613A, T84.614A, T84.615A, T84.619A, T84.63XA, T84.69XA, T84.7XXA

0RUL3JZ Supplement Right Elbow Joint with Synthetic Substitute, Percutaneous Approach
- ⬛ When reported with secondary diagnosis code T84.60XA, T84.610A, T84.611A, T84.612A, T84.613A, T84.614A, T84.615A, T84.619A, T84.63XA, T84.69XA, T84.7XXA

0RUL3KZ Supplement Right Elbow Joint with Nonautologous Tissue Substitute, Percutaneous Approach
- ⬛ When reported with secondary diagnosis code T84.60XA, T84.610A, T84.611A, T84.612A, T84.613A, T84.614A, T84.615A, T84.619A, T84.63XA, T84.69XA, T84.7XXA

0RUL47Z Supplement Right Elbow Joint with Autologous Tissue Substitute, Percutaneous Endoscopic Approach
- ⬛ When reported with secondary diagnosis code T84.60XA, T84.610A, T84.611A, T84.612A, T84.613A, T84.614A, T84.615A, T84.619A, T84.63XA, T84.69XA, T84.7XXA

0RUL4JZ Supplement Right Elbow Joint with Synthetic Substitute, Percutaneous Endoscopic Approach
- ⬛ When reported with secondary diagnosis code T84.60XA, T84.610A, T84.611A, T84.612A, T84.613A, T84.614A, T84.615A, T84.619A, T84.63XA, T84.69XA, T84.7XXA

0RUL4KZ Supplement Right Elbow Joint with Nonautologous Tissue Substitute, Percutaneous Endoscopic Approach
- ⬛ When reported with secondary diagnosis code T84.60XA, T84.610A, T84.611A, T84.612A, T84.613A, T84.614A, T84.615A, T84.619A, T84.63XA, T84.69XA, T84.7XXA

0RUM07Z Supplement Left Elbow Joint with Autologous Tissue Substitute, Open Approach
- ⬛ When reported with secondary diagnosis code T84.60XA, T84.610A, T84.611A, T84.612A, T84.613A, T84.614A, T84.615A, T84.619A, T84.63XA, T84.69XA, T84.7XXA

0RUM0JZ Supplement Left Elbow Joint with Synthetic Substitute, Open Approach
- ⬛ When reported with secondary diagnosis code T84.60XA, T84.610A, T84.611A, T84.612A, T84.613A, T84.614A, T84.615A, T84.619A, T84.63XA, T84.69XA, T84.7XXA

0RUM0KZ Supplement Left Elbow Joint with Nonautologous Tissue Substitute, Open Approach
- ⬛ When reported with secondary diagnosis code T84.60XA, T84.610A, T84.611A, T84.612A, T84.613A, T84.614A, T84.615A, T84.619A, T84.63XA, T84.69XA, T84.7XXA

0RUM37Z Supplement Left Elbow Joint with Autologous Tissue Substitute, Percutaneous Approach
- ⬛ When reported with secondary diagnosis code T84.60XA, T84.610A, T84.611A, T84.612A, T84.613A, T84.614A, T84.615A, T84.619A, T84.63XA, T84.69XA, T84.7XXA

0RUM3JZ Supplement Left Elbow Joint with Synthetic Substitute, Percutaneous Approach
- ⬛ When reported with secondary diagnosis code T84.60XA, T84.610A, T84.611A, T84.612A, T84.613A, T84.614A, T84.615A, T84.619A, T84.63XA, T84.69XA, T84.7XXA

0RUM3KZ Supplement Left Elbow Joint with Nonautologous Tissue Substitute, Percutaneous Approach
- ⬛ When reported with secondary diagnosis code T84.60XA, T84.610A, T84.611A, T84.612A, T84.613A, T84.614A, T84.615A, T84.619A, T84.63XA, T84.69XA, T84.7XXA

0RUM47Z Supplement Left Elbow Joint with Autologous Tissue Substitute, Percutaneous Endoscopic Approach
- ⬛ When reported with secondary diagnosis code T84.60XA, T84.610A, T84.611A, T84.612A, T84.613A, T84.614A, T84.615A, T84.619A, T84.63XA, T84.69XA, T84.7XXA

0RUM4JZ Supplement Left Elbow Joint with Synthetic Substitute, Percutaneous Endoscopic Approach
- ⬛ When reported with secondary diagnosis code T84.60XA, T84.610A, T84.611A, T84.612A, T84.613A, T84.614A, T84.615A, T84.619A, T84.63XA, T84.69XA, T84.7XXA

0RUM4KZ Supplement Left Elbow Joint with Nonautologous Tissue Substitute, Percutaneous Endoscopic Approach
- ⬛ When reported with secondary diagnosis code T84.60XA, T84.610A, T84.611A, T84.612A, T84.613A, T84.614A, T84.615A, T84.619A, T84.63XA, T84.69XA, T84.7XXA

0RUN07Z Supplement Right Wrist Joint with Autologous Tissue Substitute, Open Approach

0RUN0JZ Supplement Right Wrist Joint with Synthetic Substitute, Open Approach

0RUN0KZ Supplement Right Wrist Joint with Nonautologous Tissue Substitute, Open Approach

0RUN37Z Supplement Right Wrist Joint with Autologous Tissue Substitute, Percutaneous Approach

0RUN3JZ Supplement Right Wrist Joint with Synthetic Substitute, Percutaneous Approach

0RUN3KZ Supplement Right Wrist Joint with Nonautologous Tissue Substitute, Percutaneous Approach

0RUN47Z Supplement Right Wrist Joint with Autologous Tissue Substitute, Percutaneous Endoscopic Approach

0RUN4JZ Supplement Right Wrist Joint with Synthetic Substitute, Percutaneous Endoscopic Approach

0RUN4KZ Supplement Right Wrist Joint with Nonautologous Tissue Substitute, Percutaneous Endoscopic Approach

0RUP07Z Supplement Left Wrist Joint with Autologous Tissue Substitute, Open Approach

0RUP0JZ Supplement Left Wrist Joint with Synthetic Substitute, Open Approach

0RUP0KZ Supplement Left Wrist Joint with Nonautologous Tissue Substitute, Open Approach

0RUP37Z Supplement Left Wrist Joint with Autologous Tissue Substitute, Percutaneous Approach

0RUP3JZ Supplement Left Wrist Joint with Synthetic Substitute, Percutaneous Approach

0RUP3KZ Supplement Left Wrist Joint with Nonautologous Tissue Substitute, Percutaneous Approach

0RUP47Z Supplement Left Wrist Joint with Autologous Tissue Substitute, Percutaneous Endoscopic Approach

0RUP4JZ Supplement Left Wrist Joint with Synthetic Substitute, Percutaneous Endoscopic Approach

0RUP4KZ Supplement Left Wrist Joint with Nonautologous Tissue Substitute, Percutaneous Endoscopic Approach

0RUQ07Z Supplement Right Carpal Joint with Autologous Tissue Substitute, Open Approach

0RUQ0JZ Supplement Right Carpal Joint with Synthetic Substitute, Open Approach

0RUQ0KZ Supplement Right Carpal Joint with Nonautologous Tissue Substitute, Open Approach

0RUQ37Z Supplement Right Carpal Joint with Autologous Tissue Substitute, Percutaneous Approach

0RUQ3JZ Supplement Right Carpal Joint with Synthetic Substitute, Percutaneous Approach

0RUQ3KZ Supplement Right Carpal Joint with Nonautologous Tissue Substitute, Percutaneous Approach

0RUQ47Z Supplement Right Carpal Joint with Autologous Tissue Substitute, Percutaneous Endoscopic Approach

0RUQ4JZ Supplement Right Carpal Joint with Synthetic Substitute, Percutaneous Endoscopic Approach

0RUQ4KZ Supplement Right Carpal Joint with Nonautologous Tissue Substitute, Percutaneous Endoscopic Approach

0RUR07Z Supplement Left Carpal Joint with Autologous Tissue Substitute, Open Approach

0RUR0JZ Supplement Left Carpal Joint with Synthetic Substitute, Open Approach

0RUR0KZ Supplement Left Carpal Joint with Nonautologous Tissue Substitute, Open Approach

0RUR37Z Supplement Left Carpal Joint with Autologous Tissue Substitute, Percutaneous Approach

0RUR3JZ Supplement Left Carpal Joint with Synthetic Substitute, Percutaneous Approach

0RUR3KZ Supplement Left Carpal Joint with Nonautologous Tissue Substitute, Percutaneous Approach

0RUR47Z Supplement Left Carpal Joint with Autologous Tissue Substitute, Percutaneous Endoscopic Approach

0RUR4JZ Supplement Left Carpal Joint with Synthetic Substitute, Percutaneous Endoscopic Approach

0RUR4KZ Supplement Left Carpal Joint with Nonautologous Tissue Substitute, Percutaneous Endoscopic Approach

0RUS07Z Supplement Right Metacarpocarpal Joint with Autologous Tissue Substitute, Open Approach

♀ Female-only   ♂ Male-only   ▲ Limited Coverage   ● Non-OR   ⬛ HAC-associated procedure   ▲ Non-covered procedures   ➕ Combination

US0JZ   Supplement Right Metacarpocarpal Joint with Synthetic Substitute, Open Approach

US0KZ   Supplement Right Metacarpocarpal Joint with Nonautologous Tissue Substitute, Open Approach

US37Z   Supplement Right Metacarpocarpal Joint with Autologous Tissue Substitute, Percutaneous Approach

US3JZ   Supplement Right Metacarpocarpal Joint with Synthetic Substitute, Percutaneous Approach

US3KZ   Supplement Right Metacarpocarpal Joint with Nonautologous Tissue Substitute, Percutaneous Approach

US47Z   Supplement Right Metacarpocarpal Joint with Autologous Tissue Substitute, Percutaneous Endoscopic Approach

RUS4JZ   Supplement Right Metacarpocarpal Joint with Synthetic Substitute, Percutaneous Endoscopic Approach

RUS4KZ   Supplement Right Metacarpocarpal Joint with Nonautologous Tissue Substitute, Percutaneous Endoscopic Approach

RUT07Z   Supplement Left Metacarpocarpal Joint with Autologous Tissue Substitute, Open Approach

RUT0JZ   Supplement Left Metacarpocarpal Joint with Synthetic Substitute, Open Approach

RUT0KZ   Supplement Left Metacarpocarpal Joint with Nonautologous Tissue Substitute, Open Approach

RUT37Z   Supplement Left Metacarpocarpal Joint with Autologous Tissue Substitute, Percutaneous Approach

RUT3JZ   Supplement Left Metacarpocarpal Joint with Synthetic Substitute, Percutaneous Approach

RUT3KZ   Supplement Left Metacarpocarpal Joint with Nonautologous Tissue Substitute, Percutaneous Approach

RUT47Z   Supplement Left Metacarpocarpal Joint with Autologous Tissue Substitute, Percutaneous Endoscopic Approach

RUT4JZ   Supplement Left Metacarpocarpal Joint with Synthetic Substitute, Percutaneous Endoscopic Approach

RUT4KZ   Supplement Left Metacarpocarpal Joint with Nonautologous Tissue Substitute, Percutaneous Endoscopic Approach

RUU07Z   Supplement Right Metacarpophalangeal Joint with Autologous Tissue Substitute, Open Approach

0RUU0JZ   Supplement Right Metacarpophalangeal Joint with Synthetic Substitute, Open Approach

0RUU0KZ   Supplement Right Metacarpophalangeal Joint with Nonautologous Tissue Substitute, Open Approach

0RUU37Z   Supplement Right Metacarpophalangeal Joint with Autologous Tissue Substitute, Percutaneous Approach

0RUU3JZ   Supplement Right Metacarpophalangeal Joint with Synthetic Substitute, Percutaneous Approach

0RUU3KZ   Supplement Right Metacarpophalangeal Joint with Nonautologous Tissue Substitute, Percutaneous Approach

0RUU47Z   Supplement Right Metacarpophalangeal Joint with Autologous Tissue Substitute, Percutaneous Endoscopic Approach

0RUU4JZ   Supplement Right Metacarpophalangeal Joint with Synthetic Substitute, Percutaneous Endoscopic Approach

0RUU4KZ   Supplement Right Metacarpophalangeal Joint with Nonautologous Tissue Substitute, Percutaneous Endoscopic Approach

0RUV07Z   Supplement Left Metacarpophalangeal Joint with Autologous Tissue Substitute, Open Approach

0RUV0JZ   Supplement Left Metacarpophalangeal Joint with Synthetic Substitute, Open Approach

0RUV0KZ   Supplement Left Metacarpophalangeal Joint with Nonautologous Tissue Substitute, Open Approach

0RUV37Z   Supplement Left Metacarpophalangeal Joint with Autologous Tissue Substitute, Percutaneous Approach

0RUV3JZ   Supplement Left Metacarpophalangeal Joint with Synthetic Substitute, Percutaneous Approach

0RUV3KZ   Supplement Left Metacarpophalangeal Joint with Nonautologous Tissue Substitute, Percutaneous Approach

0RUV47Z   Supplement Left Metacarpophalangeal Joint with Autologous Tissue Substitute, Percutaneous Endoscopic Approach

0RUV4JZ   Supplement Left Metacarpophalangeal Joint with Synthetic Substitute, Percutaneous Endoscopic Approach

0RUV4KZ   Supplement Left Metacarpophalangeal Joint with Nonautologous Tissue Substitute, Percutaneous Endoscopic Approach

0RUW07Z   Supplement Right Finger Phalangeal Joint with Autologous Tissue Substitute, Open Approach

0RUW0JZ   Supplement Right Finger Phalangeal Joint with Synthetic Substitute, Open Approach

0RUW0KZ   Supplement Right Finger Phalangeal Joint with Nonautologous Tissue Substitute, Open Approach

0RUW37Z   Supplement Right Finger Phalangeal Joint with Autologous Tissue Substitute, Percutaneous Approach

0RUW3JZ   Supplement Right Finger Phalangeal Joint with Synthetic Substitute, Percutaneous Approach

0RUW3KZ   Supplement Right Finger Phalangeal Joint with Nonautologous Tissue Substitute, Percutaneous Approach

0RUW47Z   Supplement Right Finger Phalangeal Joint with Autologous Tissue Substitute, Percutaneous Endoscopic Approach

0RUW4JZ   Supplement Right Finger Phalangeal Joint with Synthetic Substitute, Percutaneous Endoscopic Approach

0RUW4KZ   Supplement Right Finger Phalangeal Joint with Nonautologous Tissue Substitute, Percutaneous Endoscopic Approach

0RUX07Z   Supplement Left Finger Phalangeal Joint with Autologous Tissue Substitute, Open Approach

0RUX0JZ   Supplement Left Finger Phalangeal Joint with Synthetic Substitute, Open Approach

0RUX0KZ   Supplement Left Finger Phalangeal Joint with Nonautologous Tissue Substitute, Open Approach

0RUX37Z   Supplement Left Finger Phalangeal Joint with Autologous Tissue Substitute, Percutaneous Approach

0RUX3JZ   Supplement Left Finger Phalangeal Joint with Synthetic Substitute, Percutaneous Approach

0RUX3KZ   Supplement Left Finger Phalangeal Joint with Nonautologous Tissue Substitute, Percutaneous Approach

0RUX47Z   Supplement Left Finger Phalangeal Joint with Autologous Tissue Substitute, Percutaneous Endoscopic Approach

0RUX4JZ   Supplement Left Finger Phalangeal Joint with Synthetic Substitute, Percutaneous Endoscopic Approach

0RUX4KZ   Supplement Left Finger Phalangeal Joint with Nonautologous Tissue Substitute, Percutaneous Endoscopic Approach

RW – Upper Joints, Revision

Review Coding Guideline B6.1c

RW000Z   Revision of Drainage Device in Occipital-cervical Joint, Open Approach

RW003Z   Revision of Infusion Device in Occipital-cervical Joint, Open Approach

RW004Z   Revision of Internal Fixation Device in Occipital-cervical Joint, Open Approach

RW007Z   Revision of Autologous Tissue Substitute in Occipital-cervical Joint, Open Approach

RW008Z   Revision of Spacer in Occipital-cervical Joint, Open Approach

RW00AZ   Revision of Interbody Fusion Device in Occipital-cervical Joint, Open Approach

RW00JZ   Revision of Synthetic Substitute in Occipital-cervical Joint, Open Approach

RW00KZ   Revision of Nonautologous Tissue Substitute in Occipital-cervical Joint, Open Approach

0RW030Z   Revision of Drainage Device in Occipital-cervical Joint, Percutaneous Approach

0RW033Z   Revision of Infusion Device in Occipital-cervical Joint, Percutaneous Approach

0RW034Z   Revision of Internal Fixation Device in Occipital-cervical Joint, Percutaneous Approach

0RW037Z   Revision of Autologous Tissue Substitute in Occipital-cervical Joint, Percutaneous Approach

0RW038Z   Revision of Spacer in Occipital-cervical Joint, Percutaneous Approach

0RW03AZ   Revision of Interbody Fusion Device in Occipital-cervical Joint, Percutaneous Approach

0RW03JZ   Revision of Synthetic Substitute in Occipital-cervical Joint, Percutaneous Approach

0RW03KZ   Revision of Nonautologous Tissue Substitute in Occipital-cervical Joint, Percutaneous Approach

0RW040Z   Revision of Drainage Device in Occipital-cervical Joint, Percutaneous Endoscopic Approach

0RW043Z   Revision of Infusion Device in Occipital-cervical Joint, Percutaneous Endoscopic Approach

0RW044Z   Revision of Internal Fixation Device in Occipital-cervical Joint, Percutaneous Endoscopic Approach

0RW047Z   Revision of Autologous Tissue Substitute in Occipital-cervical Joint, Percutaneous Endoscopic Approach

0RW048Z   Revision of Spacer in Occipital-cervical Joint, Percutaneous Endoscopic Approach

0RW04AZ	Revision of Interbody Fusion Device in Occipital-cervical Joint, Percutaneous Endoscopic Approach
0RW04JZ	Revision of Synthetic Substitute in Occipital-cervical Joint, Percutaneous Endoscopic Approach
0RW04KZ	Revision of Nonautologous Tissue Substitute in Occipital-cervical Joint, Percutaneous Endoscopic Approach
0RW0X0Z	Revision of Drainage Device in Occipital-cervical Joint, External Approach
0RW0X3Z	Revision of Infusion Device in Occipital-cervical Joint, External Approach
0RW0X4Z	Revision of Internal Fixation Device in Occipital-cervical Joint, External Approach
0RW0X7Z	Revision of Autologous Tissue Substitute in Occipital-cervical Joint, External Approach
0RW0X8Z	Revision of Spacer in Occipital-cervical Joint, External Approach
0RW0XAZ	Revision of Interbody Fusion Device in Occipital-cervical Joint, External Approach
0RW0XJZ	Revision of Synthetic Substitute in Occipital-cervical Joint, External Approach
0RW0XKZ	Revision of Nonautologous Tissue Substitute in Occipital-cervical Joint, External Approach
0RW100Z	Revision of Drainage Device in Cervical Vertebral Joint, Open Approach
0RW103Z	Revision of Infusion Device in Cervical Vertebral Joint, Open Approach
0RW104Z	Revision of Internal Fixation Device in Cervical Vertebral Joint, Open Approach
0RW107Z	Revision of Autologous Tissue Substitute in Cervical Vertebral Joint, Open Approach
0RW108Z	Revision of Spacer in Cervical Vertebral Joint, Open Approach
0RW10AZ	Revision of Interbody Fusion Device in Cervical Vertebral Joint, Open Approach
0RW10JZ	Revision of Synthetic Substitute in Cervical Vertebral Joint, Open Approach
0RW10KZ	Revision of Nonautologous Tissue Substitute in Cervical Vertebral Joint, Open Approach
0RW130Z	Revision of Drainage Device in Cervical Vertebral Joint, Percutaneous Approach
0RW133Z	Revision of Infusion Device in Cervical Vertebral Joint, Percutaneous Approach
0RW134Z	Revision of Internal Fixation Device in Cervical Vertebral Joint, Percutaneous Approach
0RW137Z	Revision of Autologous Tissue Substitute in Cervical Vertebral Joint, Percutaneous Approach
0RW138Z	Revision of Spacer in Cervical Vertebral Joint, Percutaneous Approach
0RW13AZ	Revision of Interbody Fusion Device in Cervical Vertebral Joint, Percutaneous Approach
0RW13JZ	Revision of Synthetic Substitute in Cervical Vertebral Joint, Percutaneous Approach
0RW13KZ	Revision of Nonautologous Tissue Substitute in Cervical Vertebral Joint, Percutaneous Approach
0RW140Z	Revision of Drainage Device in Cervical Vertebral Joint, Percutaneous Endoscopic Approach
0RW143Z	Revision of Infusion Device in Cervical Vertebral Joint, Percutaneous Endoscopic Approach
0RW144Z	Revision of Internal Fixation Device in Cervical Vertebral Joint, Percutaneous Endoscopic Approach
0RW147Z	Revision of Autologous Tissue Substitute in Cervical Vertebral Joint, Percutaneous Endoscopic Approach
0RW148Z	Revision of Spacer in Cervical Vertebral Joint, Percutaneous Endoscopic Approach
0RW14AZ	Revision of Interbody Fusion Device in Cervical Vertebral Joint, Percutaneous Endoscopic Approach
0RW14JZ	Revision of Synthetic Substitute in Cervical Vertebral Joint, Percutaneous Endoscopic Approach
0RW14KZ	Revision of Nonautologous Tissue Substitute in Cervical Vertebral Joint, Percutaneous Endoscopic Approach
0RW1X0Z	Revision of Drainage Device in Cervical Vertebral Joint, External Approach
0RW1X3Z	Revision of Infusion Device in Cervical Vertebral Joint, External Approach
0RW1X4Z	Revision of Internal Fixation Device in Cervical Vertebral Joint, External Approach
0RW1X7Z	Revision of Autologous Tissue Substitute in Cervical Vertebral Joint, External Approach
0RW1X8Z	Revision of Spacer in Cervical Vertebral Joint, External Approach
0RW1XAZ	Revision of Interbody Fusion Device in Cervical Vertebral Joint, External Approach
0RW1XJZ	Revision of Synthetic Substitute in Cervical Vertebral Joint, External Approach
0RW1XKZ	Revision of Nonautologous Tissue Substitute in Cervical Vertebral Joint, External Approach
0RW300Z	Revision of Drainage Device in Cervical Vertebral Disc, Open Approach
0RW303Z	Revision of Infusion Device in Cervical Vertebral Disc, Open Approach
0RW307Z	Revision of Autologous Tissue Substitute in Cervical Vertebral Disc, Open Approach
0RW30JZ	Revision of Synthetic Substitute in Cervical Vertebral Disc, Open Approach
0RW30KZ	Revision of Nonautologous Tissue Substitute in Cervical Vertebral Disc, Open Approach
0RW330Z	Revision of Drainage Device in Cervical Vertebral Disc, Percutaneous Approach
0RW333Z	Revision of Infusion Device in Cervical Vertebral Disc, Percutaneous Approach
0RW337Z	Revision of Autologous Tissue Substitute in Cervical Vertebral Disc, Percutaneous Approach
0RW33JZ	Revision of Synthetic Substitute in Cervical Vertebral Disc, Percutaneous Approach
0RW33KZ	Revision of Nonautologous Tissue Substitute in Cervical Vertebral Disc, Percutaneous Approach
0RW340Z	Revision of Drainage Device in Cervical Vertebral Disc, Percutaneous Endoscopic Approach
0RW343Z	Revision of Infusion Device in Cervical Vertebral Disc, Percutaneous Endoscopic Approach
0RW347Z	Revision of Autologous Tissue Substitute in Cervical Vertebral Disc, Percutaneous Endoscopic Approach
0RW34JZ	Revision of Synthetic Substitute in Cervical Vertebral Disc, Percutaneous Endoscopic Approach
0RW34KZ	Revision of Nonautologous Tissue Substitute in Cervical Vertebral Disc, Percutaneous Endoscopic Approach
0RW3X0Z	Revision of Drainage Device in Cervical Vertebral Disc, External Approach
0RW3X3Z	Revision of Infusion Device in Cervical Vertebral Disc, External Approach
0RW3X7Z	Revision of Autologous Tissue Substitute in Cervical Vertebral Disc, External Approach
0RW3XJZ	Revision of Synthetic Substitute in Cervical Vertebral Disc, External Approach
0RW3XKZ	Revision of Nonautologous Tissue Substitute in Cervical Vertebral Disc, External Approach
0RW400Z	Revision of Drainage Device in Cervicothoracic Vertebral Joint, Open Approach
0RW403Z	Revision of Infusion Device in Cervicothoracic Vertebral Joint, Open Approach
0RW404Z	Revision of Internal Fixation Device in Cervicothoracic Vertebral Joint, Open Approach
0RW407Z	Revision of Autologous Tissue Substitute in Cervicothoracic Vertebral Joint, Open Approach
0RW408Z	Revision of Spacer in Cervicothoracic Vertebral Joint, Open Approach
0RW40AZ	Revision of Interbody Fusion Device in Cervicothoracic Vertebral Joint, Open Approach
0RW40JZ	Revision of Synthetic Substitute in Cervicothoracic Vertebral Joint, Open Approach
0RW40KZ	Revision of Nonautologous Tissue Substitute in Cervicothoracic Vertebral Joint, Open Approach
0RW430Z	Revision of Drainage Device in Cervicothoracic Vertebral Joint, Percutaneous Approach
0RW433Z	Revision of Infusion Device in Cervicothoracic Vertebral Joint, Percutaneous Approach
0RW434Z	Revision of Internal Fixation Device in Cervicothoracic Vertebral Joint, Percutaneous Approach
0RW437Z	Revision of Autologous Tissue Substitute in Cervicothoracic Vertebral Joint, Percutaneous Approach
0RW438Z	Revision of Spacer in Cervicothoracic Vertebral Joint, Percutaneous Approach
0RW43AZ	Revision of Interbody Fusion Device in Cervicothoracic Vertebral Joint, Percutaneous Approach
0RW43JZ	Revision of Synthetic Substitute in Cervicothoracic Vertebral Joint, Percutaneous Approach
0RW43KZ	Revision of Nonautologous Tissue Substitute in Cervicothoracic Vertebral Joint, Percutaneous Approach
0RW440Z	Revision of Drainage Device in Cervicothoracic Vertebral Joint, Percutaneous Endoscopic Approach
0RW443Z	Revision of Infusion Device in Cervicothoracic Vertebral Joint, Percutaneous Endoscopic Approach
0RW444Z	Revision of Internal Fixation Device in Cervicothoracic Vertebral Joint, Percutaneous Endoscopic Approach
0RW447Z	Revision of Autologous Tissue Substitute in Cervicothoracic Vertebral Joint, Percutaneous Endoscopic Approach
0RW448Z	Revision of Spacer in Cervicothoracic Vertebral Joint, Percutaneous Endoscopic Approach
0RW44AZ	Revision of Interbody Fusion Device in Cervicothoracic Vertebral Joint, Percutaneous Endoscopic Approach

♀ Female-only   ♂ Male-only   ▲ Limited Coverage   ● Non-OR   ▬ HAC-associated procedure   ▲ Non-covered procedures   ✚ Combination

0RW44JZ Revision of Synthetic Substitute in Cervicothoracic Vertebral Joint, Percutaneous Endoscopic Approach

0RW44KZ Revision of Nonautologous Tissue Substitute in Cervicothoracic Vertebral Joint, Percutaneous Endoscopic Approach

0RW4X0Z Revision of Drainage Device in Cervicothoracic Vertebral Joint, External Approach

0RW4X3Z Revision of Infusion Device in Cervicothoracic Vertebral Joint, External Approach

0RW4X4Z Revision of Internal Fixation Device in Cervicothoracic Vertebral Joint, External Approach

0RW4X7Z Revision of Autologous Tissue Substitute in Cervicothoracic Vertebral Joint, External Approach

0RW4X8Z Revision of Spacer in Cervicothoracic Vertebral Joint, External Approach

0RW4XAZ Revision of Interbody Fusion Device in Cervicothoracic Vertebral Joint, External Approach

0RW4XJZ Revision of Synthetic Substitute in Cervicothoracic Vertebral Joint, External Approach

0RW4XKZ Revision of Nonautologous Tissue Substitute in Cervicothoracic Vertebral Joint, External Approach

0RW500Z Revision of Drainage Device in Cervicothoracic Vertebral Disc, Open Approach

0RW503Z Revision of Infusion Device in Cervicothoracic Vertebral Disc, Open Approach

0RW507Z Revision of Autologous Tissue Substitute in Cervicothoracic Vertebral Disc, Open Approach

0RW50JZ Revision of Synthetic Substitute in Cervicothoracic Vertebral Disc, Open Approach

0RW50KZ Revision of Nonautologous Tissue Substitute in Cervicothoracic Vertebral Disc, Open Approach

0RW530Z Revision of Drainage Device in Cervicothoracic Vertebral Disc, Percutaneous Approach

0RW533Z Revision of Infusion Device in Cervicothoracic Vertebral Disc, Percutaneous Approach

0RW537Z Revision of Autologous Tissue Substitute in Cervicothoracic Vertebral Disc, Percutaneous Approach

0RW53JZ Revision of Synthetic Substitute in Cervicothoracic Vertebral Disc, Percutaneous Approach

0RW53KZ Revision of Nonautologous Tissue Substitute in Cervicothoracic Vertebral Disc, Percutaneous Approach

0RW540Z Revision of Drainage Device in Cervicothoracic Vertebral Disc, Percutaneous Endoscopic Approach

0RW543Z Revision of Infusion Device in Cervicothoracic Vertebral Disc, Percutaneous Endoscopic Approach

0RW547Z Revision of Autologous Tissue Substitute in Cervicothoracic Vertebral Disc, Percutaneous Endoscopic Approach

0RW54JZ Revision of Synthetic Substitute in Cervicothoracic Vertebral Disc, Percutaneous Endoscopic Approach

0RW54KZ Revision of Nonautologous Tissue Substitute in Cervicothoracic Vertebral Disc, Percutaneous Endoscopic Approach

0RW5X0Z Revision of Drainage Device in Cervicothoracic Vertebral Disc, External Approach

0RW5X3Z Revision of Infusion Device in Cervicothoracic Vertebral Disc, External Approach

0RW5X7Z Revision of Autologous Tissue Substitute in Cervicothoracic Vertebral Disc, External Approach

0RW5XJZ Revision of Synthetic Substitute in Cervicothoracic Vertebral Disc, External Approach

0RW5XKZ Revision of Nonautologous Tissue Substitute in Cervicothoracic Vertebral Disc, External Approach

0RW600Z Revision of Drainage Device in Thoracic Vertebral Joint, Open Approach

0RW603Z Revision of Infusion Device in Thoracic Vertebral Joint, Open Approach

0RW604Z Revision of Internal Fixation Device in Thoracic Vertebral Joint, Open Approach

0RW607Z Revision of Autologous Tissue Substitute in Thoracic Vertebral Joint, Open Approach

0RW608Z Revision of Spacer in Thoracic Vertebral Joint, Open Approach

0RW60AZ Revision of Interbody Fusion Device in Thoracic Vertebral Joint, Open Approach

0RW60JZ Revision of Synthetic Substitute in Thoracic Vertebral Joint, Open Approach

0RW60KZ Revision of Nonautologous Tissue Substitute in Thoracic Vertebral Joint, Open Approach

0RW630Z Revision of Drainage Device in Thoracic Vertebral Joint, Percutaneous Approach

0RW633Z Revision of Infusion Device in Thoracic Vertebral Joint, Percutaneous Approach

0RW634Z Revision of Internal Fixation Device in Thoracic Vertebral Joint, Percutaneous Approach

0RW637Z Revision of Autologous Tissue Substitute in Thoracic Vertebral Joint, Percutaneous Approach

0RW638Z Revision of Spacer in Thoracic Vertebral Joint, Percutaneous Approach

0RW63AZ Revision of Interbody Fusion Device in Thoracic Vertebral Joint, Percutaneous Approach

0RW63JZ Revision of Synthetic Substitute in Thoracic Vertebral Joint, Percutaneous Approach

0RW63KZ Revision of Nonautologous Tissue Substitute in Thoracic Vertebral Joint, Percutaneous Approach

0RW640Z Revision of Drainage Device in Thoracic Vertebral Joint, Percutaneous Endoscopic Approach

0RW643Z Revision of Infusion Device in Thoracic Vertebral Joint, Percutaneous Endoscopic Approach

0RW644Z Revision of Internal Fixation Device in Thoracic Vertebral Joint, Percutaneous Endoscopic Approach

0RW647Z Revision of Autologous Tissue Substitute in Thoracic Vertebral Joint, Percutaneous Endoscopic Approach

0RW648Z Revision of Spacer in Thoracic Vertebral Joint, Percutaneous Endoscopic Approach

0RW64AZ Revision of Interbody Fusion Device in Thoracic Vertebral Joint, Percutaneous Endoscopic Approach

0RW64JZ Revision of Synthetic Substitute in Thoracic Vertebral Joint, Percutaneous Endoscopic Approach

0RW64KZ Revision of Nonautologous Tissue Substitute in Thoracic Vertebral Joint, Percutaneous Endoscopic Approach

0RW6X0Z Revision of Drainage Device in Thoracic Vertebral Joint, External Approach

0RW6X3Z Revision of Infusion Device in Thoracic Vertebral Joint, External Approach

0RW6X4Z Revision of Internal Fixation Device in Thoracic Vertebral Joint, External Approach

0RW6X7Z Revision of Autologous Tissue Substitute in Thoracic Vertebral Joint, External Approach

0RW6X8Z Revision of Spacer in Thoracic Vertebral Joint, External Approach

0RW6XAZ Revision of Interbody Fusion Device in Thoracic Vertebral Joint, External Approach

0RW6XJZ Revision of Synthetic Substitute in Thoracic Vertebral Joint, External Approach

0RW6XKZ Revision of Nonautologous Tissue Substitute in Thoracic Vertebral Joint, External Approach

0RW900Z Revision of Drainage Device in Thoracic Vertebral Disc, Open Approach

0RW903Z Revision of Infusion Device in Thoracic Vertebral Disc, Open Approach

0RW907Z Revision of Autologous Tissue Substitute in Thoracic Vertebral Disc, Open Approach

0RW90JZ Revision of Synthetic Substitute in Thoracic Vertebral Disc, Open Approach

0RW90KZ Revision of Nonautologous Tissue Substitute in Thoracic Vertebral Disc, Open Approach

0RW930Z Revision of Drainage Device in Thoracic Vertebral Disc, Percutaneous Approach

0RW933Z Revision of Infusion Device in Thoracic Vertebral Disc, Percutaneous Approach

0RW937Z Revision of Autologous Tissue Substitute in Thoracic Vertebral Disc, Percutaneous Approach

0RW93JZ Revision of Synthetic Substitute in Thoracic Vertebral Disc, Percutaneous Approach

0RW93KZ Revision of Nonautologous Tissue Substitute in Thoracic Vertebral Disc, Percutaneous Approach

0RW940Z Revision of Drainage Device in Thoracic Vertebral Disc, Percutaneous Endoscopic Approach

0RW943Z Revision of Infusion Device in Thoracic Vertebral Disc, Percutaneous Endoscopic Approach

0RW947Z Revision of Autologous Tissue Substitute in Thoracic Vertebral Disc, Percutaneous Endoscopic Approach

0RW94JZ Revision of Synthetic Substitute in Thoracic Vertebral Disc, Percutaneous Endoscopic Approach

0RW94KZ Revision of Nonautologous Tissue Substitute in Thoracic Vertebral Disc, Percutaneous Endoscopic Approach

0RW9X0Z Revision of Drainage Device in Thoracic Vertebral Disc, External Approach

0RW9X3Z Revision of Infusion Device in Thoracic Vertebral Disc, External Approach

0RW9X7Z Revision of Autologous Tissue Substitute in Thoracic Vertebral Disc, External Approach

0RW9XJZ Revision of Synthetic Substitute in Thoracic Vertebral Disc, External Approach

0RW9XKZ Revision of Nonautologous Tissue Substitute in Thoracic Vertebral Disc, External Approach

* Female-only   ♂ Male-only   ▲ Limited Coverage   ● Non-OR   ▣ HAC-associated procedure   ▲ Non-covered procedures   ✛ Combination

0RWA00Z	Revision of Drainage Device in Thoracolumbar Vertebral Joint, Open Approach
0RWA03Z	Revision of Infusion Device in Thoracolumbar Vertebral Joint, Open Approach
0RWA04Z	Revision of Internal Fixation Device in Thoracolumbar Vertebral Joint, Open Approach
0RWA07Z	Revision of Autologous Tissue Substitute in Thoracolumbar Vertebral Joint, Open Approach
0RWA08Z	Revision of Spacer in Thoracolumbar Vertebral Joint, Open Approach
0RWA0AZ	Revision of Interbody Fusion Device in Thoracolumbar Vertebral Joint, Open Approach
0RWA0JZ	Revision of Synthetic Substitute in Thoracolumbar Vertebral Joint, Open Approach
0RWA0KZ	Revision of Nonautologous Tissue Substitute in Thoracolumbar Vertebral Joint, Open Approach
0RWA30Z	Revision of Drainage Device in Thoracolumbar Vertebral Joint, Percutaneous Approach
0RWA33Z	Revision of Infusion Device in Thoracolumbar Vertebral Joint, Percutaneous Approach
0RWA34Z	Revision of Internal Fixation Device in Thoracolumbar Vertebral Joint, Percutaneous Approach
0RWA37Z	Revision of Autologous Tissue Substitute in Thoracolumbar Vertebral Joint, Percutaneous Approach
0RWA38Z	Revision of Spacer in Thoracolumbar Vertebral Joint, Percutaneous Approach
0RWA3AZ	Revision of Interbody Fusion Device in Thoracolumbar Vertebral Joint, Percutaneous Approach
0RWA3JZ	Revision of Synthetic Substitute in Thoracolumbar Vertebral Joint, Percutaneous Approach
0RWA3KZ	Revision of Nonautologous Tissue Substitute in Thoracolumbar Vertebral Joint, Percutaneous Approach
0RWA40Z	Revision of Drainage Device in Thoracolumbar Vertebral Joint, Percutaneous Endoscopic Approach
0RWA43Z	Revision of Infusion Device in Thoracolumbar Vertebral Joint, Percutaneous Endoscopic Approach
0RWA44Z	Revision of Internal Fixation Device in Thoracolumbar Vertebral Joint, Percutaneous Endoscopic Approach
0RWA47Z	Revision of Autologous Tissue Substitute in Thoracolumbar Vertebral Joint, Percutaneous Endoscopic Approach
0RWA48Z	Revision of Spacer in Thoracolumbar Vertebral Joint, Percutaneous Endoscopic Approach
0RWA4AZ	Revision of Interbody Fusion Device in Thoracolumbar Vertebral Joint, Percutaneous Endoscopic Approach
0RWA4JZ	Revision of Synthetic Substitute in Thoracolumbar Vertebral Joint, Percutaneous Endoscopic Approach
0RWA4KZ	Revision of Nonautologous Tissue Substitute in Thoracolumbar Vertebral Joint, Percutaneous Endoscopic Approach
0RWAX0Z	Revision of Drainage Device in Thoracolumbar Vertebral Joint, External Approach
0RWAX3Z	Revision of Infusion Device in Thoracolumbar Vertebral Joint, External Approach
0RWAX4Z	Revision of Internal Fixation Device in Thoracolumbar Vertebral Joint, External Approach
0RWAX7Z	Revision of Autologous Tissue Substitute in Thoracolumbar Vertebral Joint, External Approach
0RWAX8Z	Revision of Spacer in Thoracolumbar Vertebral Joint, External Approach
0RWAXAZ	Revision of Interbody Fusion Device in Thoracolumbar Vertebral Joint, External Approach
0RWAXJZ	Revision of Synthetic Substitute in Thoracolumbar Vertebral Joint, External Approach
0RWAXKZ	Revision of Nonautologous Tissue Substitute in Thoracolumbar Vertebral Joint, External Approach
0RWB00Z	Revision of Drainage Device in Thoracolumbar Vertebral Disc, Open Approach
0RWB03Z	Revision of Infusion Device in Thoracolumbar Vertebral Disc, Open Approach
0RWB07Z	Revision of Autologous Tissue Substitute in Thoracolumbar Vertebral Disc, Open Approach
0RWB0JZ	Revision of Synthetic Substitute in Thoracolumbar Vertebral Disc, Open Approach
0RWB0KZ	Revision of Nonautologous Tissue Substitute in Thoracolumbar Vertebral Disc, Open Approach
0RWB30Z	Revision of Drainage Device in Thoracolumbar Vertebral Disc, Percutaneous Approach
0RWB33Z	Revision of Infusion Device in Thoracolumbar Vertebral Disc, Percutaneous Approach
0RWB37Z	Revision of Autologous Tissue Substitute in Thoracolumbar Vertebral Disc, Percutaneous Approach
0RWB3JZ	Revision of Synthetic Substitute in Thoracolumbar Vertebral Disc, Percutaneous Approach
0RWB3KZ	Revision of Nonautologous Tissue Substitute in Thoracolumbar Vertebral Disc, Percutaneous Approach
0RWB40Z	Revision of Drainage Device in Thoracolumbar Vertebral Disc, Percutaneous Endoscopic Approach
0RWB43Z	Revision of Infusion Device in Thoracolumbar Vertebral Disc, Percutaneous Endoscopic Approach
0RWB47Z	Revision of Autologous Tissue Substitute in Thoracolumbar Vertebral Disc, Percutaneous Endoscopic Approach
0RWB4JZ	Revision of Synthetic Substitute in Thoracolumbar Vertebral Disc, Percutaneous Endoscopic Approach
0RWB4KZ	Revision of Nonautologous Tissue Substitute in Thoracolumbar Vertebral Disc, Percutaneous Endoscopic Approach
0RWBX0Z	Revision of Drainage Device in Thoracolumbar Vertebral Disc, External Approach
0RWBX3Z	Revision of Infusion Device in Thoracolumbar Vertebral Disc, External Approach
0RWBX7Z	Revision of Autologous Tissue Substitute in Thoracolumbar Vertebral Disc, External Approach
0RWBXJZ	Revision of Synthetic Substitute in Thoracolumbar Vertebral Disc, External Approach
0RWBXKZ	Revision of Nonautologous Tissue Substitute in Thoracolumbar Vertebral Disc, External Approach
0RWC00Z	Revision of Drainage Device in Right Temporomandibular Joint, Open Approach
0RWC03Z	Revision of Infusion Device in Right Temporomandibular Joint, Open Approach
0RWC04Z	Revision of Internal Fixation Device in Right Temporomandibular Joint, Open Approach
0RWC07Z	Revision of Autologous Tissue Substitute in Right Temporomandibular Joint, Open Approach
0RWC08Z	Revision of Spacer in Right Temporomandibular Joint, Open Approach
0RWC0JZ	Revision of Synthetic Substitute in Right Temporomandibular Joint, Open Approach
0RWC0KZ	Revision of Nonautologous Tissue Substitute in Right Temporomandibular Joint, Open Approach
0RWC30Z	Revision of Drainage Device in Right Temporomandibular Joint, Percutaneous Approach
0RWC33Z	Revision of Infusion Device in Right Temporomandibular Joint, Percutaneous Approach
0RWC34Z	Revision of Internal Fixation Device in Right Temporomandibular Joint, Percutaneous Approach
0RWC37Z	Revision of Autologous Tissue Substitute in Right Temporomandibular Joint, Percutaneous Approach
0RWC38Z	Revision of Spacer in Right Temporomandibular Joint, Percutaneous Approach
0RWC3JZ	Revision of Synthetic Substitute in Right Temporomandibular Joint, Percutaneous Approach
0RWC3KZ	Revision of Nonautologous Tissue Substitute in Right Temporomandibular Joint, Percutaneous Approach
0RWC40Z	Revision of Drainage Device in Right Temporomandibular Joint, Percutaneous Endoscopic Approach
0RWC43Z	Revision of Infusion Device in Right Temporomandibular Joint, Percutaneous Endoscopic Approach
0RWC44Z	Revision of Internal Fixation Device in Right Temporomandibular Joint, Percutaneous Endoscopic Approach
0RWC47Z	Revision of Autologous Tissue Substitute in Right Temporomandibular Joint, Percutaneous Endoscopic Approach
0RWC48Z	Revision of Spacer in Right Temporomandibular Joint, Percutaneous Endoscopic Approach
0RWC4JZ	Revision of Synthetic Substitute in Right Temporomandibular Joint, Percutaneous Endoscopic Approach
0RWC4KZ	Revision of Nonautologous Tissue Substitute in Right Temporomandibular Joint, Percutaneous Endoscopic Approach
0RWCX0Z	Revision of Drainage Device in Right Temporomandibular Joint, External Approach
0RWCX3Z	Revision of Infusion Device in Right Temporomandibular Joint, External Approach
0RWCX4Z	Revision of Internal Fixation Device in Right Temporomandibular Joint, External Approach

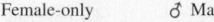

♀ Female-only   ♂ Male-only   ▲ Limited Coverage   ● Non-OR   ▦ HAC-associated procedure   ▲ Non-covered procedures   ✚ Combinatio

WCX7Z Revision of Autologous Tissue Substitute in Right Temporomandibular Joint, External Approach

WCX8Z Revision of Spacer in Right Temporomandibular Joint, External Approach

WCXJZ Revision of Synthetic Substitute in Right Temporomandibular Joint, External Approach

WCXKZ Revision of Nonautologous Tissue Substitute in Right Temporomandibular Joint, External Approach

WD00Z Revision of Drainage Device in Left Temporomandibular Joint, Open Approach

WD03Z Revision of Infusion Device in Left Temporomandibular Joint, Open Approach

WD04Z Revision of Internal Fixation Device in Left Temporomandibular Joint, Open Approach

WD07Z Revision of Autologous Tissue Substitute in Left Temporomandibular Joint, Open Approach

WD08Z Revision of Spacer in Left Temporomandibular Joint, Open Approach

WD0JZ Revision of Synthetic Substitute in Left Temporomandibular Joint, Open Approach

WD0KZ Revision of Nonautologous Tissue Substitute in Left Temporomandibular Joint, Open Approach

WD30Z Revision of Drainage Device in Left Temporomandibular Joint, Percutaneous Approach

WD33Z Revision of Infusion Device in Left Temporomandibular Joint, Percutaneous Approach

WD34Z Revision of Internal Fixation Device in Left Temporomandibular Joint, Percutaneous Approach

WD37Z Revision of Autologous Tissue Substitute in Left Temporomandibular Joint, Percutaneous Approach

WD38Z Revision of Spacer in Left Temporomandibular Joint, Percutaneous Approach

WD3JZ Revision of Synthetic Substitute in Left Temporomandibular Joint, Percutaneous Approach

WD3KZ Revision of Nonautologous Tissue Substitute in Left Temporomandibular Joint, Percutaneous Approach

WD40Z Revision of Drainage Device in Left Temporomandibular Joint, Percutaneous Endoscopic Approach

WD43Z Revision of Infusion Device in Left Temporomandibular Joint, Percutaneous Endoscopic Approach

WD44Z Revision of Internal Fixation Device in Left Temporomandibular Joint, Percutaneous Endoscopic Approach

WD47Z Revision of Autologous Tissue Substitute in Left Temporomandibular Joint, Percutaneous Endoscopic Approach

WD48Z Revision of Spacer in Left Temporomandibular Joint, Percutaneous Endoscopic Approach

WD4JZ Revision of Synthetic Substitute in Left Temporomandibular Joint, Percutaneous Endoscopic Approach

WD4KZ Revision of Nonautologous Tissue Substitute in Left Temporomandibular Joint, Percutaneous Endoscopic Approach

RWDX0Z Revision of Drainage Device in Left Temporomandibular Joint, External Approach

0RWDX3Z Revision of Infusion Device in Left Temporomandibular Joint, External Approach

0RWDX4Z Revision of Internal Fixation Device in Left Temporomandibular Joint, External Approach

0RWDX7Z Revision of Autologous Tissue Substitute in Left Temporomandibular Joint, External Approach

0RWDX8Z Revision of Spacer in Left Temporomandibular Joint, External Approach

0RWDXJZ Revision of Synthetic Substitute in Left Temporomandibular Joint, External Approach

0RWDXKZ Revision of Nonautologous Tissue Substitute in Left Temporomandibular Joint, External Approach

0RWE00Z Revision of Drainage Device in Right Sternoclavicular Joint, Open Approach

0RWE03Z Revision of Infusion Device in Right Sternoclavicular Joint, Open Approach

0RWE04Z Revision of Internal Fixation Device in Right Sternoclavicular Joint, Open Approach

0RWE07Z Revision of Autologous Tissue Substitute in Right Sternoclavicular Joint, Open Approach

0RWE08Z Revision of Spacer in Right Sternoclavicular Joint, Open Approach

0RWE0JZ Revision of Synthetic Substitute in Right Sternoclavicular Joint, Open Approach

0RWE0KZ Revision of Nonautologous Tissue Substitute in Right Sternoclavicular Joint, Open Approach

0RWE30Z Revision of Drainage Device in Right Sternoclavicular Joint, Percutaneous Approach

0RWE33Z Revision of Infusion Device in Right Sternoclavicular Joint, Percutaneous Approach

0RWE34Z Revision of Internal Fixation Device in Right Sternoclavicular Joint, Percutaneous Approach

0RWE37Z Revision of Autologous Tissue Substitute in Right Sternoclavicular Joint, Percutaneous Approach

0RWE38Z Revision of Spacer in Right Sternoclavicular Joint, Percutaneous Approach

0RWE3JZ Revision of Synthetic Substitute in Right Sternoclavicular Joint, Percutaneous Approach

0RWE3KZ Revision of Nonautologous Tissue Substitute in Right Sternoclavicular Joint, Percutaneous Approach

0RWE40Z Revision of Drainage Device in Right Sternoclavicular Joint, Percutaneous Endoscopic Approach

0RWE43Z Revision of Infusion Device in Right Sternoclavicular Joint, Percutaneous Endoscopic Approach

0RWE44Z Revision of Internal Fixation Device in Right Sternoclavicular Joint, Percutaneous Endoscopic Approach

0RWE47Z Revision of Autologous Tissue Substitute in Right Sternoclavicular Joint, Percutaneous Endoscopic Approach

0RWE48Z Revision of Spacer in Right Sternoclavicular Joint, Percutaneous Endoscopic Approach

0RWE4JZ Revision of Synthetic Substitute in Right Sternoclavicular Joint, Percutaneous Endoscopic Approach

0RWE4KZ Revision of Nonautologous Tissue Substitute in Right Sternoclavicular Joint, Percutaneous Endoscopic Approach

0RWEX0Z Revision of Drainage Device in Right Sternoclavicular Joint, External Approach

0RWEX3Z Revision of Infusion Device in Right Sternoclavicular Joint, External Approach

0RWEX4Z Revision of Internal Fixation Device in Right Sternoclavicular Joint, External Approach

0RWEX7Z Revision of Autologous Tissue Substitute in Right Sternoclavicular Joint, External Approach

0RWEX8Z Revision of Spacer in Right Sternoclavicular Joint, External Approach

0RWEXJZ Revision of Synthetic Substitute in Right Sternoclavicular Joint, External Approach

0RWEXKZ Revision of Nonautologous Tissue Substitute in Right Sternoclavicular Joint, External Approach

0RWF00Z Revision of Drainage Device in Left Sternoclavicular Joint, Open Approach

0RWF03Z Revision of Infusion Device in Left Sternoclavicular Joint, Open Approach

0RWF04Z Revision of Internal Fixation Device in Left Sternoclavicular Joint, Open Approach

0RWF07Z Revision of Autologous Tissue Substitute in Left Sternoclavicular Joint, Open Approach

0RWF08Z Revision of Spacer in Left Sternoclavicular Joint, Open Approach

0RWF0JZ Revision of Synthetic Substitute in Left Sternoclavicular Joint, Open Approach

0RWF0KZ Revision of Nonautologous Tissue Substitute in Left Sternoclavicular Joint, Open Approach

0RWF30Z Revision of Drainage Device in Left Sternoclavicular Joint, Percutaneous Approach

0RWF33Z Revision of Infusion Device in Left Sternoclavicular Joint, Percutaneous Approach

0RWF34Z Revision of Internal Fixation Device in Left Sternoclavicular Joint, Percutaneous Approach

0RWF37Z Revision of Autologous Tissue Substitute in Left Sternoclavicular Joint, Percutaneous Approach

0RWF38Z Revision of Spacer in Left Sternoclavicular Joint, Percutaneous Approach

0RWF3JZ Revision of Synthetic Substitute in Left Sternoclavicular Joint, Percutaneous Approach

0RWF3KZ Revision of Nonautologous Tissue Substitute in Left Sternoclavicular Joint, Percutaneous Approach

0RWF40Z Revision of Drainage Device in Left Sternoclavicular Joint, Percutaneous Endoscopic Approach

0RWF43Z Revision of Infusion Device in Left Sternoclavicular Joint, Percutaneous Endoscopic Approach

0RWF44Z Revision of Internal Fixation Device in Left Sternoclavicular Joint, Percutaneous Endoscopic Approach

0RWF47Z Revision of Autologous Tissue Substitute in Left Sternoclavicular Joint, Percutaneous Endoscopic Approach

0RWF48Z Revision of Spacer in Left Sternoclavicular Joint, Percutaneous Endoscopic Approach

0RWF4JZ Revision of Synthetic Substitute in Left Sternoclavicular Joint, Percutaneous Endoscopic Approach

0RWF4KZ Revision of Nonautologous Tissue Substitute in Left Sternoclavicular Joint, Percutaneous Endoscopic Approach

0RWFX0Z Revision of Drainage Device in Left Sternoclavicular Joint, External Approach

0RWFX3Z Revision of Infusion Device in Left Sternoclavicular Joint, External Approach

0RWFX4Z Revision of Internal Fixation Device in Left Sternoclavicular Joint, External Approach

0RWFX7Z Revision of Autologous Tissue Substitute in Left Sternoclavicular Joint, External Approach

0RWFX8Z Revision of Spacer in Left Sternoclavicular Joint, External Approach

0RWFXJZ Revision of Synthetic Substitute in Left Sternoclavicular Joint, External Approach

0RWFXKZ Revision of Nonautologous Tissue Substitute in Left Sternoclavicular Joint, External Approach

0RWG00Z Revision of Drainage Device in Right Acromioclavicular Joint, Open Approach

0RWG03Z Revision of Infusion Device in Right Acromioclavicular Joint, Open Approach

0RWG04Z Revision of Internal Fixation Device in Right Acromioclavicular Joint, Open Approach

0RWG07Z Revision of Autologous Tissue Substitute in Right Acromioclavicular Joint, Open Approach

0RWG08Z Revision of Spacer in Right Acromioclavicular Joint, Open Approach

0RWG0JZ Revision of Synthetic Substitute in Right Acromioclavicular Joint, Open Approach

0RWG0KZ Revision of Nonautologous Tissue Substitute in Right Acromioclavicular Joint, Open Approach

0RWG30Z Revision of Drainage Device in Right Acromioclavicular Joint, Percutaneous Approach

0RWG33Z Revision of Infusion Device in Right Acromioclavicular Joint, Percutaneous Approach

0RWG34Z Revision of Internal Fixation Device in Right Acromioclavicular Joint, Percutaneous Approach

0RWG37Z Revision of Autologous Tissue Substitute in Right Acromioclavicular Joint, Percutaneous Approach

0RWG38Z Revision of Spacer in Right Acromioclavicular Joint, Percutaneous Approach

0RWG3JZ Revision of Synthetic Substitute in Right Acromioclavicular Joint, Percutaneous Approach

0RWG3KZ Revision of Nonautologous Tissue Substitute in Right Acromioclavicular Joint, Percutaneous Approach

0RWG40Z Revision of Drainage Device in Right Acromioclavicular Joint, Percutaneous Endoscopic Approach

0RWG43Z Revision of Infusion Device in Right Acromioclavicular Joint, Percutaneous Endoscopic Approach

0RWG44Z Revision of Internal Fixation Device in Right Acromioclavicular Joint, Percutaneous Endoscopic Approach

0RWG47Z Revision of Autologous Tissue Substitute in Right Acromioclavicular Joint, Percutaneous Endoscopic Approach

0RWG48Z Revision of Spacer in Right Acromioclavicular Joint, Percutaneous Endoscopic Approach

0RWG4JZ Revision of Synthetic Substitute in Right Acromioclavicular Joint, Percutaneous Endoscopic Approach

0RWG4KZ Revision of Nonautologous Tissue Substitute in Right Acromioclavicular Joint, Percutaneous Endoscopic Approach

0RWGX0Z Revision of Drainage Device in Right Acromioclavicular Joint, External Approach

0RWGX3Z Revision of Infusion Device in Right Acromioclavicular Joint, External Approach

0RWGX4Z Revision of Internal Fixation Device in Right Acromioclavicular Joint, External Approach

0RWGX7Z Revision of Autologous Tissue Substitute in Right Acromioclavicular Joint, External Approach

0RWGX8Z Revision of Spacer in Right Acromioclavicular Joint, External Approach

0RWGXJZ Revision of Synthetic Substitute in Right Acromioclavicular Joint, External Approach

0RWGXKZ Revision of Nonautologous Tissue Substitute in Right Acromioclavicular Joint, External Approach

0RWH00Z Revision of Drainage Device in Left Acromioclavicular Joint, Open Approach

0RWH03Z Revision of Infusion Device in Left Acromioclavicular Joint, Open Approach

0RWH04Z Revision of Internal Fixation Device in Left Acromioclavicular Joint, Open Approach

0RWH07Z Revision of Autologous Tissue Substitute in Left Acromioclavicular Joint, Open Approach

0RWH08Z Revision of Spacer in Left Acromioclavicular Joint, Open Approach

0RWH0JZ Revision of Synthetic Substitute in Left Acromioclavicular Joint, Open Approach

0RWH0KZ Revision of Nonautologous Tissue Substitute in Left Acromioclavicular Joint, Open Approach

0RWH30Z Revision of Drainage Device in Left Acromioclavicular Joint, Percutaneous Approach

0RWH33Z Revision of Infusion Device in Left Acromioclavicular Joint, Percutaneous Approach

0RWH34Z Revision of Internal Fixation Device in Left Acromioclavicular Joint, Percutaneous Approach

0RWH37Z Revision of Autologous Tissue Substitute in Left Acromioclavicular Joint, Percutaneous Approach

0RWH38Z Revision of Spacer in Left Acromioclavicular Joint, Percutaneous Approach

0RWH3JZ Revision of Synthetic Substitute in Left Acromioclavicular Joint, Percutaneous Approach

0RWH3KZ Revision of Nonautologous Tissue Substitute in Left Acromioclavicular Joint, Percutaneous Approach

0RWH40Z Revision of Drainage Device in Left Acromioclavicular Joint, Percutaneous Endoscopic Approach

0RWH43Z Revision of Infusion Device in Left Acromioclavicular Joint, Percutaneous Endoscopic Approach

0RWH44Z Revision of Internal Fixation Device in Left Acromioclavicular Joint, Percutaneous Endoscopic Approach

0RWH47Z Revision of Autologous Tissue Substitute in Left Acromioclavicular Joint, Percutaneous Endoscopic Approach

0RWH48Z Revision of Spacer in Left Acromioclavicular Joint, Percutaneous Endoscopic Approach

0RWH4JZ Revision of Synthetic Substitute in Left Acromioclavicular Joint, Percutaneous Endoscopic Approach

0RWH4KZ Revision of Nonautologous Tissue Substitute in Left Acromioclavicular Joint, Percutaneous Endoscopic Approach

0RWHX0Z Revision of Drainage Device in Left Acromioclavicular Joint, External Approach

0RWHX3Z Revision of Infusion Device in Left Acromioclavicular Joint, External Approach

0RWHX4Z Revision of Internal Fixation Device in Left Acromioclavicular Joint, External Approach

0RWHX7Z Revision of Autologous Tissue Substitute in Left Acromioclavicular Joint, External Approach

0RWHX8Z Revision of Spacer in Left Acromioclavicular Joint, External Approach

0RWHXJZ Revision of Synthetic Substitute in Left Acromioclavicular Joint, External Approach

0RWHXKZ Revision of Nonautologous Tissue Substitute in Left Acromioclavicular Joint, External Approach

0RWJ00Z Revision of Drainage Device in Right Shoulder Joint, Open Approach

0RWJ03Z Revision of Infusion Device in Right Shoulder Joint, Open Approach

0RWJ04Z Revision of Internal Fixation Device in Right Shoulder Joint, Open Approach

0RWJ07Z Revision of Autologous Tissue Substitute in Right Shoulder Joint, Open Approach

0RWJ08Z Revision of Spacer in Right Shoulder Joint, Open Approach

0RWJ0JZ Revision of Synthetic Substitute in Right Shoulder Joint, Open Approach

0RWJ0KZ Revision of Nonautologous Tissue Substitute in Right Shoulder Joint, Open Approach

0RWJ30Z Revision of Drainage Device in Right Shoulder Joint, Percutaneous Approach

0RWJ33Z Revision of Infusion Device in Right Shoulder Joint, Percutaneous Approach

0RWJ34Z Revision of Internal Fixation Device in Right Shoulder Joint, Percutaneous Approach

0RWJ37Z Revision of Autologous Tissue Substitute in Right Shoulder Joint, Percutaneous Approach

0RWJ38Z Revision of Spacer in Right Shoulder Joint, Percutaneous Approach

0RWJ3JZ Revision of Synthetic Substitute in Right Shoulder Joint, Percutaneous Approach

0RWJ3KZ Revision of Nonautologous Tissue Substitute in Right Shoulder Joint, Percutaneous Approach

0RWJ40Z Revision of Drainage Device in Right Shoulder Joint, Percutaneous Endoscopic Approach

0RWJ43Z Revision of Infusion Device in Right Shoulder Joint, Percutaneous Endoscopic Approach

0RWJ44Z Revision of Internal Fixation Device in Right Shoulder Joint, Percutaneous Endoscopic Approach

0RWJ47Z Revision of Autologous Tissue Substitute in Right Shoulder Joint, Percutaneous Endoscopic Approach

0RWJ48Z Revision of Spacer in Right Shoulder Joint, Percutaneous Endoscopic Approach

0RWJ4JZ Revision of Synthetic Substitute in Right Shoulder Joint, Percutaneous Endoscopic Approach

♀ Female-only   ♂ Male-only   ▲ Limited Coverage   ● Non-OR   ▬ HAC-associated procedure   ▲ Non-covered procedures   + Combination

VJ4KZ Revision of Nonautologous Tissue Substitute in Right Shoulder Joint, Percutaneous Endoscopic Approach

VJX0Z Revision of Drainage Device in Right Shoulder Joint, External Approach

VJX3Z Revision of Infusion Device in Right Shoulder Joint, External Approach

VJX4Z Revision of Internal Fixation Device in Right Shoulder Joint, External Approach

VJX7Z Revision of Autologous Tissue Substitute in Right Shoulder Joint, External Approach

VJX8Z Revision of Spacer in Right Shoulder Joint, External Approach

VJXJZ Revision of Synthetic Substitute in Right Shoulder Joint, External Approach

VJXKZ Revision of Nonautologous Tissue Substitute in Right Shoulder Joint, External Approach

VK00Z Revision of Drainage Device in Left Shoulder Joint, Open Approach

VK03Z Revision of Infusion Device in Left Shoulder Joint, Open Approach

VK04Z Revision of Internal Fixation Device in Left Shoulder Joint, Open Approach

VK07Z Revision of Autologous Tissue Substitute in Left Shoulder Joint, Open Approach

VK08Z Revision of Spacer in Left Shoulder Joint, Open Approach

VK0JZ Revision of Synthetic Substitute in Left Shoulder Joint, Open Approach

VK0KZ Revision of Nonautologous Tissue Substitute in Left Shoulder Joint, Open Approach

VK30Z Revision of Drainage Device in Left Shoulder Joint, Percutaneous Approach

VK33Z Revision of Infusion Device in Left Shoulder Joint, Percutaneous Approach

VK34Z Revision of Internal Fixation Device in Left Shoulder Joint, Percutaneous Approach

VK37Z Revision of Autologous Tissue Substitute in Left Shoulder Joint, Percutaneous Approach

VK38Z Revision of Spacer in Left Shoulder Joint, Percutaneous Approach

VK3JZ Revision of Synthetic Substitute in Left Shoulder Joint, Percutaneous Approach

VK3KZ Revision of Nonautologous Tissue Substitute in Left Shoulder Joint, Percutaneous Approach

VK40Z Revision of Drainage Device in Left Shoulder Joint, Percutaneous Endoscopic Approach

VK43Z Revision of Infusion Device in Left Shoulder Joint, Percutaneous Endoscopic Approach

VK44Z Revision of Internal Fixation Device in Left Shoulder Joint, Percutaneous Endoscopic Approach

VK47Z Revision of Autologous Tissue Substitute in Left Shoulder Joint, Percutaneous Endoscopic Approach

VK48Z Revision of Spacer in Left Shoulder Joint, Percutaneous Endoscopic Approach

VK4JZ Revision of Synthetic Substitute in Left Shoulder Joint, Percutaneous Endoscopic Approach

VK4KZ Revision of Nonautologous Tissue Substitute in Left Shoulder Joint, Percutaneous Endoscopic Approach

VKX0Z Revision of Drainage Device in Left Shoulder Joint, External Approach

VKX3Z Revision of Infusion Device in Left Shoulder Joint, External Approach

0RWKX4Z Revision of Internal Fixation Device in Left Shoulder Joint, External Approach

0RWKX7Z Revision of Autologous Tissue Substitute in Left Shoulder Joint, External Approach

0RWKX8Z Revision of Spacer in Left Shoulder Joint, External Approach

0RWKXJZ Revision of Synthetic Substitute in Left Shoulder Joint, External Approach

0RWKXKZ Revision of Nonautologous Tissue Substitute in Left Shoulder Joint, External Approach

0RWL00Z Revision of Drainage Device in Right Elbow Joint, Open Approach

0RWL03Z Revision of Infusion Device in Right Elbow Joint, Open Approach

0RWL04Z Revision of Internal Fixation Device in Right Elbow Joint, Open Approach

0RWL05Z Revision of External Fixation Device in Right Elbow Joint, Open Approach

0RWL07Z Revision of Autologous Tissue Substitute in Right Elbow Joint, Open Approach

0RWL08Z Revision of Spacer in Right Elbow Joint, Open Approach

0RWL0JZ Revision of Synthetic Substitute in Right Elbow Joint, Open Approach

0RWL0KZ Revision of Nonautologous Tissue Substitute in Right Elbow Joint, Open Approach

0RWL30Z Revision of Drainage Device in Right Elbow Joint, Percutaneous Approach

0RWL33Z Revision of Infusion Device in Right Elbow Joint, Percutaneous Approach

0RWL34Z Revision of Internal Fixation Device in Right Elbow Joint, Percutaneous Approach

0RWL35Z Revision of External Fixation Device in Right Elbow Joint, Percutaneous Approach

0RWL37Z Revision of Autologous Tissue Substitute in Right Elbow Joint, Percutaneous Approach

0RWL38Z Revision of Spacer in Right Elbow Joint, Percutaneous Approach

0RWL3JZ Revision of Synthetic Substitute in Right Elbow Joint, Percutaneous Approach

0RWL3KZ Revision of Nonautologous Tissue Substitute in Right Elbow Joint, Percutaneous Approach

0RWL40Z Revision of Drainage Device in Right Elbow Joint, Percutaneous Endoscopic Approach

0RWL43Z Revision of Infusion Device in Right Elbow Joint, Percutaneous Endoscopic Approach

0RWL44Z Revision of Internal Fixation Device in Right Elbow Joint, Percutaneous Endoscopic Approach

0RWL45Z Revision of External Fixation Device in Right Elbow Joint, Percutaneous Endoscopic Approach

0RWL47Z Revision of Autologous Tissue Substitute in Right Elbow Joint, Percutaneous Endoscopic Approach

0RWL48Z Revision of Spacer in Right Elbow Joint, Percutaneous Endoscopic Approach

0RWL4JZ Revision of Synthetic Substitute in Right Elbow Joint, Percutaneous Endoscopic Approach

0RWL4KZ Revision of Nonautologous Tissue Substitute in Right Elbow Joint, Percutaneous Endoscopic Approach

0RWLX0Z Revision of Drainage Device in Right Elbow Joint, External Approach

0RWLX3Z Revision of Infusion Device in Right Elbow Joint, External Approach

0RWLX4Z Revision of Internal Fixation Device in Right Elbow Joint, External Approach

0RWLX5Z Revision of External Fixation Device in Right Elbow Joint, External Approach

0RWLX7Z Revision of Autologous Tissue Substitute in Right Elbow Joint, External Approach

0RWLX8Z Revision of Spacer in Right Elbow Joint, External Approach

0RWLXJZ Revision of Synthetic Substitute in Right Elbow Joint, External Approach

0RWLXKZ Revision of Nonautologous Tissue Substitute in Right Elbow Joint, External Approach

0RWM00Z Revision of Drainage Device in Left Elbow Joint, Open Approach

0RWM03Z Revision of Infusion Device in Left Elbow Joint, Open Approach

0RWM04Z Revision of Internal Fixation Device in Left Elbow Joint, Open Approach

0RWM05Z Revision of External Fixation Device in Left Elbow Joint, Open Approach

0RWM07Z Revision of Autologous Tissue Substitute in Left Elbow Joint, Open Approach

0RWM08Z Revision of Spacer in Left Elbow Joint, Open Approach

0RWM0JZ Revision of Synthetic Substitute in Left Elbow Joint, Open Approach

0RWM0KZ Revision of Nonautologous Tissue Substitute in Left Elbow Joint, Open Approach

0RWM30Z Revision of Drainage Device in Left Elbow Joint, Percutaneous Approach

0RWM33Z Revision of Infusion Device in Left Elbow Joint, Percutaneous Approach

0RWM34Z Revision of Internal Fixation Device in Left Elbow Joint, Percutaneous Approach

0RWM35Z Revision of External Fixation Device in Left Elbow Joint, Percutaneous Approach

0RWM37Z Revision of Autologous Tissue Substitute in Left Elbow Joint, Percutaneous Approach

0RWM38Z Revision of Spacer in Left Elbow Joint, Percutaneous Approach

0RWM3JZ Revision of Synthetic Substitute in Left Elbow Joint, Percutaneous Approach

0RWM3KZ Revision of Nonautologous Tissue Substitute in Left Elbow Joint, Percutaneous Approach

0RWM40Z Revision of Drainage Device in Left Elbow Joint, Percutaneous Endoscopic Approach

0RWM43Z Revision of Infusion Device in Left Elbow Joint, Percutaneous Endoscopic Approach

0RWM44Z Revision of Internal Fixation Device in Left Elbow Joint, Percutaneous Endoscopic Approach

0RWM45Z Revision of External Fixation Device in Left Elbow Joint, Percutaneous Endoscopic Approach

0RWM47Z Revision of Autologous Tissue Substitute in Left Elbow Joint, Percutaneous Endoscopic Approach

0RWM48Z Revision of Spacer in Left Elbow Joint, Percutaneous Endoscopic Approach

0RWM4JZ Revision of Synthetic Substitute in Left Elbow Joint, Percutaneous Endoscopic Approach

0RWM4KZ Revision of Nonautologous Tissue Substitute in Left Elbow Joint, Percutaneous Endoscopic Approach

0RWMX0Z Revision of Drainage Device in Left Elbow Joint, External Approach

Female-only　　♂ Male-only　　▲ Limited Coverage　　● Non-OR　　■ HAC-associated procedure　　▲ Non-covered procedures　　＋ Combination

0RWMX3Z Revision of Infusion Device in Left Elbow Joint, External Approach

0RWMX4Z Revision of Internal Fixation Device in Left Elbow Joint, External Approach

0RWMX5Z Revision of External Fixation Device in Left Elbow Joint, External Approach

0RWMX7Z Revision of Autologous Tissue Substitute in Left Elbow Joint, External Approach

0RWMX8Z Revision of Spacer in Left Elbow Joint, External Approach

0RWMXJZ Revision of Synthetic Substitute in Left Elbow Joint, External Approach

0RWMXKZ Revision of Nonautologous Tissue Substitute in Left Elbow Joint, External Approach

0RWN00Z Revision of Drainage Device in Right Wrist Joint, Open Approach

0RWN03Z Revision of Infusion Device in Right Wrist Joint, Open Approach

0RWN04Z Revision of Internal Fixation Device in Right Wrist Joint, Open Approach

0RWN05Z Revision of External Fixation Device in Right Wrist Joint, Open Approach

0RWN07Z Revision of Autologous Tissue Substitute in Right Wrist Joint, Open Approach

0RWN08Z Revision of Spacer in Right Wrist Joint, Open Approach

0RWN0JZ Revision of Synthetic Substitute in Right Wrist Joint, Open Approach

0RWN0KZ Revision of Nonautologous Tissue Substitute in Right Wrist Joint, Open Approach

0RWN30Z Revision of Drainage Device in Right Wrist Joint, Percutaneous Approach

0RWN33Z Revision of Infusion Device in Right Wrist Joint, Percutaneous Approach

0RWN34Z Revision of Internal Fixation Device in Right Wrist Joint, Percutaneous Approach

0RWN35Z Revision of External Fixation Device in Right Wrist Joint, Percutaneous Approach

0RWN37Z Revision of Autologous Tissue Substitute in Right Wrist Joint, Percutaneous Approach

0RWN38Z Revision of Spacer in Right Wrist Joint, Percutaneous Approach

0RWN3JZ Revision of Synthetic Substitute in Right Wrist Joint, Percutaneous Approach

0RWN3KZ Revision of Nonautologous Tissue Substitute in Right Wrist Joint, Percutaneous Approach

0RWN40Z Revision of Drainage Device in Right Wrist Joint, Percutaneous Endoscopic Approach

0RWN43Z Revision of Infusion Device in Right Wrist Joint, Percutaneous Endoscopic Approach

0RWN44Z Revision of Internal Fixation Device in Right Wrist Joint, Percutaneous Endoscopic Approach

0RWN45Z Revision of External Fixation Device in Right Wrist Joint, Percutaneous Endoscopic Approach

0RWN47Z Revision of Autologous Tissue Substitute in Right Wrist Joint, Percutaneous Endoscopic Approach

0RWN48Z Revision of Spacer in Right Wrist Joint, Percutaneous Endoscopic Approach

0RWN4JZ Revision of Synthetic Substitute in Right Wrist Joint, Percutaneous Endoscopic Approach

0RWN4KZ Revision of Nonautologous Tissue Substitute in Right Wrist Joint, Percutaneous Endoscopic Approach

0RWNX0Z Revision of Drainage Device in Right Wrist Joint, External Approach

0RWNX3Z Revision of Infusion Device in Right Wrist Joint, External Approach

0RWNX4Z Revision of Internal Fixation Device in Right Wrist Joint, External Approach

0RWNX5Z Revision of External Fixation Device in Right Wrist Joint, External Approach

0RWNX7Z Revision of Autologous Tissue Substitute in Right Wrist Joint, External Approach

0RWNX8Z Revision of Spacer in Right Wrist Joint, External Approach

0RWNXJZ Revision of Synthetic Substitute in Right Wrist Joint, External Approach

0RWNXKZ Revision of Nonautologous Tissue Substitute in Right Wrist Joint, External Approach

0RWP00Z Revision of Drainage Device in Left Wrist Joint, Open Approach

0RWP03Z Revision of Infusion Device in Left Wrist Joint, Open Approach

0RWP04Z Revision of Internal Fixation Device in Left Wrist Joint, Open Approach

0RWP05Z Revision of External Fixation Device in Left Wrist Joint, Open Approach

0RWP07Z Revision of Autologous Tissue Substitute in Left Wrist Joint, Open Approach

0RWP08Z Revision of Spacer in Left Wrist Joint, Open Approach

0RWP0JZ Revision of Synthetic Substitute in Left Wrist Joint, Open Approach

0RWP0KZ Revision of Nonautologous Tissue Substitute in Left Wrist Joint, Open Approach

0RWP30Z Revision of Drainage Device in Left Wrist Joint, Percutaneous Approach

0RWP33Z Revision of Infusion Device in Left Wrist Joint, Percutaneous Approach

0RWP34Z Revision of Internal Fixation Device in Left Wrist Joint, Percutaneous Approach

0RWP35Z Revision of External Fixation Device in Left Wrist Joint, Percutaneous Approach

0RWP37Z Revision of Autologous Tissue Substitute in Left Wrist Joint, Percutaneous Approach

0RWP38Z Revision of Spacer in Left Wrist Joint, Percutaneous Approach

0RWP3JZ Revision of Synthetic Substitute in Left Wrist Joint, Percutaneous Approach

0RWP3KZ Revision of Nonautologous Tissue Substitute in Left Wrist Joint, Percutaneous Approach

0RWP40Z Revision of Drainage Device in Left Wrist Joint, Percutaneous Endoscopic Approach

0RWP43Z Revision of Infusion Device in Left Wrist Joint, Percutaneous Endoscopic Approach

0RWP44Z Revision of Internal Fixation Device in Left Wrist Joint, Percutaneous Endoscopic Approach

0RWP45Z Revision of External Fixation Device in Left Wrist Joint, Percutaneous Endoscopic Approach

0RWP47Z Revision of Autologous Tissue Substitute in Left Wrist Joint, Percutaneous Endoscopic Approach

0RWP48Z Revision of Spacer in Left Wrist Joint, Percutaneous Endoscopic Approach

0RWP4JZ Revision of Synthetic Substitute in Left Wrist Joint, Percutaneous Endoscopic Approach

0RWP4KZ Revision of Nonautologous Tissue Substitute in Left Wrist Joint, Percutaneous Endoscopic Approach

0RWPX0Z Revision of Drainage Device in Left Wrist Joint, External Approach

0RWPX3Z Revision of Infusion Device in Left Wrist Joint, External Approach

0RWPX4Z Revision of Internal Fixation Device Left Wrist Joint, External Approach

0RWPX5Z Revision of External Fixation Device Left Wrist Joint, External Approach

0RWPX7Z Revision of Autologous Tissue Substitute in Left Wrist Joint, External Approach

0RWPX8Z Revision of Spacer in Left Wrist Joint, External Approach

0RWPXJZ Revision of Synthetic Substitute in Left Wrist Joint, External Approach

0RWPXKZ Revision of Nonautologous Tissue Substitute in Left Wrist Joint, External Approach

0RWQ00Z Revision of Drainage Device in Right Carpal Joint, Open Approach

0RWQ03Z Revision of Infusion Device in Right Carpal Joint, Open Approach

0RWQ04Z Revision of Internal Fixation Device in Right Carpal Joint, Open Approach

0RWQ05Z Revision of External Fixation Device Right Carpal Joint, Open Approach

0RWQ07Z Revision of Autologous Tissue Substitute in Right Carpal Joint, Open Approach

0RWQ08Z Revision of Spacer in Right Carpal Joint, Open Approach

0RWQ0JZ Revision of Synthetic Substitute in Right Carpal Joint, Open Approach

0RWQ0KZ Revision of Nonautologous Tissue Substitute in Right Carpal Joint, Open Approach

0RWQ30Z Revision of Drainage Device in Right Carpal Joint, Percutaneous Approach

0RWQ33Z Revision of Infusion Device in Right Carpal Joint, Percutaneous Approach

0RWQ34Z Revision of Internal Fixation Device in Right Carpal Joint, Percutaneous Approach

0RWQ35Z Revision of External Fixation Device in Right Carpal Joint, Percutaneous Approach

0RWQ37Z Revision of Autologous Tissue Substitute in Right Carpal Joint, Percutaneous Approach

0RWQ38Z Revision of Spacer in Right Carpal Joint Percutaneous Approach

0RWQ3JZ Revision of Synthetic Substitute in Right Carpal Joint, Percutaneous Approach

0RWQ3KZ Revision of Nonautologous Tissue Substitute in Right Carpal Joint, Percutaneous Approach

0RWQ40Z Revision of Drainage Device in Right Carpal Joint, Percutaneous Endoscopic Approach

0RWQ43Z Revision of Infusion Device in Right Carpal Joint, Percutaneous Endoscopic Approach

0RWQ44Z Revision of Internal Fixation Device in Right Carpal Joint, Percutaneous Endoscopic Approach

0RWQ45Z Revision of External Fixation Device in Right Carpal Joint, Percutaneous Endoscopic Approach

0RWQ47Z Revision of Autologous Tissue Substitute in Right Carpal Joint, Percutaneous Endoscopic Approach

0RWQ48Z Revision of Spacer in Right Carpal Joint, Percutaneous Endoscopic Approach

0RWQ4JZ Revision of Synthetic Substitute in Right Carpal Joint, Percutaneous Endoscopic Approach

0RWQ4KZ Revision of Nonautologous Tissue Substitute in Right Carpal Joint, Percutaneous Endoscopic Approach

0RWQX0Z Revision of Drainage Device in Right Carpal Joint, External Approach

0RWQX3Z Revision of Infusion Device in Right Carpal Joint, External Approach

0RWQX4Z Revision of Internal Fixation Device in Right Carpal Joint, External Approach

0RWQX5Z Revision of External Fixation Device in Right Carpal Joint, External Approach

0RWQX7Z Revision of Autologous Tissue Substitute in Right Carpal Joint, External Approach

0RWQX8Z Revision of Spacer in Right Carpal Joint, External Approach

0RWQXJZ Revision of Synthetic Substitute in Right Carpal Joint, External Approach

0RWQXKZ Revision of Nonautologous Tissue Substitute in Right Carpal Joint, External Approach

0RWR00Z Revision of Drainage Device in Left Carpal Joint, Open Approach

0RWR03Z Revision of Infusion Device in Left Carpal Joint, Open Approach

0RWR04Z Revision of Internal Fixation Device in Left Carpal Joint, Open Approach

0RWR05Z Revision of External Fixation Device in Left Carpal Joint, Open Approach

0RWR07Z Revision of Autologous Tissue Substitute in Left Carpal Joint, Open Approach

0RWR08Z Revision of Spacer in Left Carpal Joint, Open Approach

0RWR0JZ Revision of Synthetic Substitute in Left Carpal Joint, Open Approach

0RWR0KZ Revision of Nonautologous Tissue Substitute in Left Carpal Joint, Open Approach

0RWR30Z Revision of Drainage Device in Left Carpal Joint, Percutaneous Approach

0RWR33Z Revision of Infusion Device in Left Carpal Joint, Percutaneous Approach

0RWR34Z Revision of Internal Fixation Device in Left Carpal Joint, Percutaneous Approach

0RWR35Z Revision of External Fixation Device in Left Carpal Joint, Percutaneous Approach

0RWR37Z Revision of Autologous Tissue Substitute in Left Carpal Joint, Percutaneous Approach

0RWR38Z Revision of Spacer in Left Carpal Joint, Percutaneous Approach

0RWR3JZ Revision of Synthetic Substitute in Left Carpal Joint, Percutaneous Approach

0RWR3KZ Revision of Nonautologous Tissue Substitute in Left Carpal Joint, Percutaneous Approach

0RWR40Z Revision of Drainage Device in Left Carpal Joint, Percutaneous Endoscopic Approach

0RWR43Z Revision of Infusion Device in Left Carpal Joint, Percutaneous Endoscopic Approach

0RWR44Z Revision of Internal Fixation Device in Left Carpal Joint, Percutaneous Endoscopic Approach

0RWR45Z Revision of External Fixation Device in Left Carpal Joint, Percutaneous Endoscopic Approach

0RWR47Z Revision of Autologous Tissue Substitute in Left Carpal Joint, Percutaneous Endoscopic Approach

0RWR48Z Revision of Spacer in Left Carpal Joint, Percutaneous Endoscopic Approach

0RWR4JZ Revision of Synthetic Substitute in Left Carpal Joint, Percutaneous Endoscopic Approach

0RWR4KZ Revision of Nonautologous Tissue Substitute in Left Carpal Joint, Percutaneous Endoscopic Approach

0RWRX0Z Revision of Drainage Device in Left Carpal Joint, External Approach

0RWRX3Z Revision of Infusion Device in Left Carpal Joint, External Approach

0RWRX4Z Revision of Internal Fixation Device in Left Carpal Joint, External Approach

0RWRX5Z Revision of External Fixation Device in Left Carpal Joint, External Approach

0RWRX7Z Revision of Autologous Tissue Substitute in Left Carpal Joint, External Approach

0RWRX8Z Revision of Spacer in Left Carpal Joint, External Approach

0RWRXJZ Revision of Synthetic Substitute in Left Carpal Joint, External Approach

0RWRXKZ Revision of Nonautologous Tissue Substitute in Left Carpal Joint, External Approach

0RWS00Z Revision of Drainage Device in Right Metacarpocarpal Joint, Open Approach

0RWS03Z Revision of Infusion Device in Right Metacarpocarpal Joint, Open Approach

0RWS04Z Revision of Internal Fixation Device in Right Metacarpocarpal Joint, Open Approach

0RWS05Z Revision of External Fixation Device in Right Metacarpocarpal Joint, Open Approach

0RWS07Z Revision of Autologous Tissue Substitute in Right Metacarpocarpal Joint, Open Approach

0RWS08Z Revision of Spacer in Right Metacarpocarpal Joint, Open Approach

0RWS0JZ Revision of Synthetic Substitute in Right Metacarpocarpal Joint, Open Approach

0RWS0KZ Revision of Nonautologous Tissue Substitute in Right Metacarpocarpal Joint, Open Approach

0RWS30Z Revision of Drainage Device in Right Metacarpocarpal Joint, Percutaneous Approach

0RWS33Z Revision of Infusion Device in Right Metacarpocarpal Joint, Percutaneous Approach

0RWS34Z Revision of Internal Fixation Device in Right Metacarpocarpal Joint, Percutaneous Approach

0RWS35Z Revision of External Fixation Device in Right Metacarpocarpal Joint, Percutaneous Approach

0RWS37Z Revision of Autologous Tissue Substitute in Right Metacarpocarpal Joint, Percutaneous Approach

0RWS38Z Revision of Spacer in Right Metacarpocarpal Joint, Percutaneous Approach

0RWS3JZ Revision of Synthetic Substitute in Right Metacarpocarpal Joint, Percutaneous Approach

0RWS3KZ Revision of Nonautologous Tissue Substitute in Right Metacarpocarpal Joint, Percutaneous Approach

0RWS40Z Revision of Drainage Device in Right Metacarpocarpal Joint, Percutaneous Endoscopic Approach

0RWS43Z Revision of Infusion Device in Right Metacarpocarpal Joint, Percutaneous Endoscopic Approach

0RWS44Z Revision of Internal Fixation Device in Right Metacarpocarpal Joint, Percutaneous Endoscopic Approach

0RWS45Z Revision of External Fixation Device in Right Metacarpocarpal Joint, Percutaneous Endoscopic Approach

0RWS47Z Revision of Autologous Tissue Substitute in Right Metacarpocarpal Joint, Percutaneous Endoscopic Approach

0RWS48Z Revision of Spacer in Right Metacarpocarpal Joint, Percutaneous Endoscopic Approach

0RWS4JZ Revision of Synthetic Substitute in Right Metacarpocarpal Joint, Percutaneous Endoscopic Approach

0RWS4KZ Revision of Nonautologous Tissue Substitute in Right Metacarpocarpal Joint, Percutaneous Endoscopic Approach

0RWSX0Z Revision of Drainage Device in Right Metacarpocarpal Joint, External Approach

0RWSX3Z Revision of Infusion Device in Right Metacarpocarpal Joint, External Approach

0RWSX4Z Revision of Internal Fixation Device in Right Metacarpocarpal Joint, External Approach

0RWSX5Z Revision of External Fixation Device in Right Metacarpocarpal Joint, External Approach

0RWSX7Z Revision of Autologous Tissue Substitute in Right Metacarpocarpal Joint, External Approach

0RWSX8Z Revision of Spacer in Right Metacarpocarpal Joint, External Approach

0RWSXJZ Revision of Synthetic Substitute in Right Metacarpocarpal Joint, External Approach

0RWSXKZ Revision of Nonautologous Tissue Substitute in Right Metacarpocarpal Joint, External Approach

0RWT00Z Revision of Drainage Device in Left Metacarpocarpal Joint, Open Approach

0RWT03Z Revision of Infusion Device in Left Metacarpocarpal Joint, Open Approach

0RWT04Z Revision of Internal Fixation Device in Left Metacarpocarpal Joint, Open Approach

0RWT05Z Revision of External Fixation Device in Left Metacarpocarpal Joint, Open Approach

0RWT07Z Revision of Autologous Tissue Substitute in Left Metacarpocarpal Joint, Open Approach

0RWT08Z Revision of Spacer in Left Metacarpocarpal Joint, Open Approach

0RWT0JZ Revision of Synthetic Substitute in Left Metacarpocarpal Joint, Open Approach

0RWT0KZ Revision of Nonautologous Tissue Substitute in Left Metacarpocarpal Joint, Open Approach

0RWT30Z Revision of Drainage Device in Left Metacarpocarpal Joint, Percutaneous Approach

0RWT33Z Revision of Infusion Device in Left Metacarpocarpal Joint, Percutaneous Approach

0RWT34Z Revision of Internal Fixation Device in Left Metacarpocarpal Joint, Percutaneous Approach

0RWT35Z Revision of External Fixation Device in Left Metacarpocarpal Joint, Percutaneous Approach

0RWT37Z Revision of Autologous Tissue Substitute in Left Metacarpocarpal Joint, Percutaneous Approach

0RWT38Z Revision of Spacer in Left Metacarpocarpal Joint, Percutaneous Approach

0RWT3JZ Revision of Synthetic Substitute in Left Metacarpocarpal Joint, Percutaneous Approach

0RWT3KZ Revision of Nonautologous Tissue Substitute in Left Metacarpocarpal Joint, Percutaneous Approach

0RWT40Z Revision of Drainage Device in Left Metacarpocarpal Joint, Percutaneous Endoscopic Approach

0RWT43Z Revision of Infusion Device in Left Metacarpocarpal Joint, Percutaneous Endoscopic Approach

0RWT44Z Revision of Internal Fixation Device in Left Metacarpocarpal Joint, Percutaneous Endoscopic Approach

0RWT45Z Revision of External Fixation Device in Left Metacarpocarpal Joint, Percutaneous Endoscopic Approach

0RWT47Z Revision of Autologous Tissue Substitute in Left Metacarpocarpal Joint, Percutaneous Endoscopic Approach

0RWT48Z Revision of Spacer in Left Metacarpocarpal Joint, Percutaneous Endoscopic Approach

0RWT4JZ Revision of Synthetic Substitute in Left Metacarpocarpal Joint, Percutaneous Endoscopic Approach

0RWT4KZ Revision of Nonautologous Tissue Substitute in Left Metacarpocarpal Joint, Percutaneous Endoscopic Approach

0RWTX0Z Revision of Drainage Device in Left Metacarpocarpal Joint, External Approach

0RWTX3Z Revision of Infusion Device in Left Metacarpocarpal Joint, External Approach

0RWTX4Z Revision of Internal Fixation Device in Left Metacarpocarpal Joint, External Approach

0RWTX5Z Revision of External Fixation Device in Left Metacarpocarpal Joint, External Approach

0RWTX7Z Revision of Autologous Tissue Substitute in Left Metacarpocarpal Joint, External Approach

0RWTX8Z Revision of Spacer in Left Metacarpocarpal Joint, External Approach

0RWTXJZ Revision of Synthetic Substitute in Left Metacarpocarpal Joint, External Approach

0RWTXKZ Revision of Nonautologous Tissue Substitute in Left Metacarpocarpal Joint, External Approach

0RWU00Z Revision of Drainage Device in Right Metacarpophalangeal Joint, Open Approach

0RWU03Z Revision of Infusion Device in Right Metacarpophalangeal Joint, Open Approach

0RWU04Z Revision of Internal Fixation Device in Right Metacarpophalangeal Joint, Open Approach

0RWU05Z Revision of External Fixation Device in Right Metacarpophalangeal Joint, Open Approach

0RWU07Z Revision of Autologous Tissue Substitute in Right Metacarpophalangeal Joint, Open Approach

0RWU08Z Revision of Spacer in Right Metacarpophalangeal Joint, Open Approach

0RWU0JZ Revision of Synthetic Substitute in Right Metacarpophalangeal Joint, Open Approach

0RWU0KZ Revision of Nonautologous Tissue Substitute in Right Metacarpophalangeal Joint, Open Approach

0RWU30Z Revision of Drainage Device in Right Metacarpophalangeal Joint, Percutaneous Approach

0RWU33Z Revision of Infusion Device in Right Metacarpophalangeal Joint, Percutaneous Approach

0RWU34Z Revision of Internal Fixation Device in Right Metacarpophalangeal Joint, Percutaneous Approach

0RWU35Z Revision of External Fixation Device in Right Metacarpophalangeal Joint, Percutaneous Approach

0RWU37Z Revision of Autologous Tissue Substitute in Right Metacarpophalangeal Joint, Percutaneous Approach

0RWU38Z Revision of Spacer in Right Metacarpophalangeal Joint, Percutaneous Approach

0RWU3JZ Revision of Synthetic Substitute in Right Metacarpophalangeal Joint, Percutaneous Approach

0RWU3KZ Revision of Nonautologous Tissue Substitute in Right Metacarpophalangeal Joint, Percutaneous Approach

0RWU40Z Revision of Drainage Device in Right Metacarpophalangeal Joint, Percutaneous Endoscopic Approach

0RWU43Z Revision of Infusion Device in Right Metacarpophalangeal Joint, Percutaneous Endoscopic Approach

0RWU44Z Revision of Internal Fixation Device in Right Metacarpophalangeal Joint, Percutaneous Endoscopic Approach

0RWU45Z Revision of External Fixation Device in Right Metacarpophalangeal Joint, Percutaneous Endoscopic Approach

0RWU47Z Revision of Autologous Tissue Substitute in Right Metacarpophalangeal Joint, Percutaneous Endoscopic Approach

0RWU48Z Revision of Spacer in Right Metacarpophalangeal Joint, Percutaneous Endoscopic Approach

0RWU4JZ Revision of Synthetic Substitute in Right Metacarpophalangeal Joint, Percutaneous Endoscopic Approach

0RWU4KZ Revision of Nonautologous Tissue Substitute in Right Metacarpophalangeal Joint, Percutaneous Endoscopic Approach

0RWUX0Z Revision of Drainage Device in Right Metacarpophalangeal Joint, External Approach

0RWUX3Z Revision of Infusion Device in Right Metacarpophalangeal Joint, External Approach

0RWUX4Z Revision of Internal Fixation Device in Right Metacarpophalangeal Joint, External Approach

0RWUX5Z Revision of External Fixation Device in Right Metacarpophalangeal Joint, External Approach

0RWUX7Z Revision of Autologous Tissue Substitute in Right Metacarpophalangeal Joint, External Approach

0RWUX8Z Revision of Spacer in Right Metacarpophalangeal Joint, External Approach

0RWUXJZ Revision of Synthetic Substitute in Right Metacarpophalangeal Joint, External Approach

0RWUXKZ Revision of Nonautologous Tissue Substitute in Right Metacarpophalangeal Joint, External Approach

0RWV00Z Revision of Drainage Device in Left Metacarpophalangeal Joint, Open Approach

0RWV03Z Revision of Infusion Device in Left Metacarpophalangeal Joint, Open Approach

0RWV04Z Revision of Internal Fixation Device in Left Metacarpophalangeal Joint, Open Approach

0RWV05Z Revision of External Fixation Device in Left Metacarpophalangeal Joint, Open Approach

0RWV07Z Revision of Autologous Tissue Substitute in Left Metacarpophalangeal Joint, Open Approach

0RWV08Z Revision of Spacer in Left Metacarpophalangeal Joint, Open Approach

0RWV0JZ Revision of Synthetic Substitute in Left Metacarpophalangeal Joint, Open Approach

0RWV0KZ Revision of Nonautologous Tissue Substitute in Left Metacarpophalangeal Joint, Open Approach

0RWV30Z Revision of Drainage Device in Left Metacarpophalangeal Joint, Percutaneous Approach

0RWV33Z Revision of Infusion Device in Left Metacarpophalangeal Joint, Percutaneous Approach

0RWV34Z Revision of Internal Fixation Device in Left Metacarpophalangeal Joint, Percutaneous Approach

0RWV35Z Revision of External Fixation Device in Left Metacarpophalangeal Joint, Percutaneous Approach

0RWV37Z Revision of Autologous Tissue Substitute in Left Metacarpophalangeal Joint, Percutaneous Approach

0RWV38Z Revision of Spacer in Left Metacarpophalangeal Joint, Percutaneous Approach

0RWV3JZ Revision of Synthetic Substitute in Left Metacarpophalangeal Joint, Percutaneous Approach

0RWV3KZ Revision of Nonautologous Tissue Substitute in Left Metacarpophalangeal Joint, Percutaneous Approach

0RWV40Z Revision of Drainage Device in Left Metacarpophalangeal Joint, Percutaneous Endoscopic Approach

0RWV43Z Revision of Infusion Device in Left Metacarpophalangeal Joint, Percutaneous Endoscopic Approach

0RWV44Z Revision of Internal Fixation Device in Left Metacarpophalangeal Joint, Percutaneous Endoscopic Approach

0RWV45Z Revision of External Fixation Device in Left Metacarpophalangeal Joint, Percutaneous Endoscopic Approach

0RWV47Z Revision of Autologous Tissue Substitute in Left Metacarpophalangeal Joint, Percutaneous Endoscopic Approach

0RWV48Z Revision of Spacer in Left Metacarpophalangeal Joint, Percutaneous Endoscopic Approach

0RWV4JZ Revision of Synthetic Substitute in Left Metacarpophalangeal Joint, Percutaneous Endoscopic Approach

0RWV4KZ Revision of Nonautologous Tissue Substitute in Left Metacarpophalangeal Joint, Percutaneous Endoscopic Approach

0RWVX0Z Revision of Drainage Device in Left Metacarpophalangeal Joint, External Approach

WVX3Z	Revision of Infusion Device in Left Metacarpophalangeal Joint, External Approach
WVX4Z	Revision of Internal Fixation Device in Left Metacarpophalangeal Joint, External Approach
WVX5Z	Revision of External Fixation Device in Left Metacarpophalangeal Joint, External Approach
WVX7Z	Revision of Autologous Tissue Substitute in Left Metacarpophalangeal Joint, External Approach
WVX8Z	Revision of Spacer in Left Metacarpophalangeal Joint, External Approach
WVXJZ	Revision of Synthetic Substitute in Left Metacarpophalangeal Joint, External Approach
RWVXKZ	Revision of Nonautologous Tissue Substitute in Left Metacarpophalangeal Joint, External Approach
RWW00Z	Revision of Drainage Device in Right Finger Phalangeal Joint, Open Approach
RWW03Z	Revision of Infusion Device in Right Finger Phalangeal Joint, Open Approach
RWW04Z	Revision of Internal Fixation Device in Right Finger Phalangeal Joint, Open Approach
RWW05Z	Revision of External Fixation Device in Right Finger Phalangeal Joint, Open Approach
RWW07Z	Revision of Autologous Tissue Substitute in Right Finger Phalangeal Joint, Open Approach
RWW08Z	Revision of Spacer in Right Finger Phalangeal Joint, Open Approach
RWW0JZ	Revision of Synthetic Substitute in Right Finger Phalangeal Joint, Open Approach
RWW0KZ	Revision of Nonautologous Tissue Substitute in Right Finger Phalangeal Joint, Open Approach
RWW30Z	Revision of Drainage Device in Right Finger Phalangeal Joint, Percutaneous Approach
RWW33Z	Revision of Infusion Device in Right Finger Phalangeal Joint, Percutaneous Approach
RWW34Z	Revision of Internal Fixation Device in Right Finger Phalangeal Joint, Percutaneous Approach
RWW35Z	Revision of External Fixation Device in Right Finger Phalangeal Joint, Percutaneous Approach
RWW37Z	Revision of Autologous Tissue Substitute in Right Finger Phalangeal Joint, Percutaneous Approach
RWW38Z	Revision of Spacer in Right Finger Phalangeal Joint, Percutaneous Approach
RWW3JZ	Revision of Synthetic Substitute in Right Finger Phalangeal Joint, Percutaneous Approach
RWW3KZ	Revision of Nonautologous Tissue Substitute in Right Finger Phalangeal Joint, Percutaneous Approach
RWW40Z	Revision of Drainage Device in Right Finger Phalangeal Joint, Percutaneous Endoscopic Approach
0RWW43Z	Revision of Infusion Device in Right Finger Phalangeal Joint, Percutaneous Endoscopic Approach
0RWW44Z	Revision of Internal Fixation Device in Right Finger Phalangeal Joint, Percutaneous Endoscopic Approach
0RWW45Z	Revision of External Fixation Device in Right Finger Phalangeal Joint, Percutaneous Endoscopic Approach
0RWW47Z	Revision of Autologous Tissue Substitute in Right Finger Phalangeal Joint, Percutaneous Endoscopic Approach
0RWW48Z	Revision of Spacer in Right Finger Phalangeal Joint, Percutaneous Endoscopic Approach
0RWW4JZ	Revision of Synthetic Substitute in Right Finger Phalangeal Joint, Percutaneous Endoscopic Approach
0RWW4KZ	Revision of Nonautologous Tissue Substitute in Right Finger Phalangeal Joint, Percutaneous Endoscopic Approach
0RWWX0Z	Revision of Drainage Device in Right Finger Phalangeal Joint, External Approach
0RWWX3Z	Revision of Infusion Device in Right Finger Phalangeal Joint, External Approach
0RWWX4Z	Revision of Internal Fixation Device in Right Finger Phalangeal Joint, External Approach
0RWWX5Z	Revision of External Fixation Device in Right Finger Phalangeal Joint, External Approach
0RWWX7Z	Revision of Autologous Tissue Substitute in Right Finger Phalangeal Joint, External Approach
0RWWX8Z	Revision of Spacer in Right Finger Phalangeal Joint, External Approach
0RWWXJZ	Revision of Synthetic Substitute in Right Finger Phalangeal Joint, External Approach
0RWWXKZ	Revision of Nonautologous Tissue Substitute in Right Finger Phalangeal Joint, External Approach
0RWX00Z	Revision of Drainage Device in Left Finger Phalangeal Joint, Open Approach
0RWX03Z	Revision of Infusion Device in Left Finger Phalangeal Joint, Open Approach
0RWX04Z	Revision of Internal Fixation Device in Left Finger Phalangeal Joint, Open Approach
0RWX05Z	Revision of External Fixation Device in Left Finger Phalangeal Joint, Open Approach
0RWX07Z	Revision of Autologous Tissue Substitute in Left Finger Phalangeal Joint, Open Approach
0RWX08Z	Revision of Spacer in Left Finger Phalangeal Joint, Open Approach
0RWX0JZ	Revision of Synthetic Substitute in Left Finger Phalangeal Joint, Open Approach
0RWX0KZ	Revision of Nonautologous Tissue Substitute in Left Finger Phalangeal Joint, Open Approach
0RWX30Z	Revision of Drainage Device in Left Finger Phalangeal Joint, Percutaneous Approach
0RWX33Z	Revision of Infusion Device in Left Finger Phalangeal Joint, Percutaneous Approach
0RWX34Z	Revision of Internal Fixation Device in Left Finger Phalangeal Joint, Percutaneous Approach
0RWX35Z	Revision of External Fixation Device in Left Finger Phalangeal Joint, Percutaneous Approach
0RWX37Z	Revision of Autologous Tissue Substitute in Left Finger Phalangeal Joint, Percutaneous Approach
0RWX38Z	Revision of Spacer in Left Finger Phalangeal Joint, Percutaneous Approach
0RWX3JZ	Revision of Synthetic Substitute in Left Finger Phalangeal Joint, Percutaneous Approach
0RWX3KZ	Revision of Nonautologous Tissue Substitute in Left Finger Phalangeal Joint, Percutaneous Approach
0RWX40Z	Revision of Drainage Device in Left Finger Phalangeal Joint, Percutaneous Endoscopic Approach
0RWX43Z	Revision of Infusion Device in Left Finger Phalangeal Joint, Percutaneous Endoscopic Approach
0RWX44Z	Revision of Internal Fixation Device in Left Finger Phalangeal Joint, Percutaneous Endoscopic Approach
0RWX45Z	Revision of External Fixation Device in Left Finger Phalangeal Joint, Percutaneous Endoscopic Approach
0RWX47Z	Revision of Autologous Tissue Substitute in Left Finger Phalangeal Joint, Percutaneous Endoscopic Approach
0RWX48Z	Revision of Spacer in Left Finger Phalangeal Joint, Percutaneous Endoscopic Approach
0RWX4JZ	Revision of Synthetic Substitute in Left Finger Phalangeal Joint, Percutaneous Endoscopic Approach
0RWX4KZ	Revision of Nonautologous Tissue Substitute in Left Finger Phalangeal Joint, Percutaneous Endoscopic Approach
0RWXX0Z	Revision of Drainage Device in Left Finger Phalangeal Joint, External Approach
0RWXX3Z	Revision of Infusion Device in Left Finger Phalangeal Joint, External Approach
0RWXX4Z	Revision of Internal Fixation Device in Left Finger Phalangeal Joint, External Approach
0RWXX5Z	Revision of External Fixation Device in Left Finger Phalangeal Joint, External Approach
0RWXX7Z	Revision of Autologous Tissue Substitute in Left Finger Phalangeal Joint, External Approach
0RWXX8Z	Revision of Spacer in Left Finger Phalangeal Joint, External Approach
0RWXXJZ	Revision of Synthetic Substitute in Left Finger Phalangeal Joint, External Approach
0RWXXKZ	Revision of Nonautologous Tissue Substitute in Left Finger Phalangeal Joint, External Approach

Intervertebral Joint

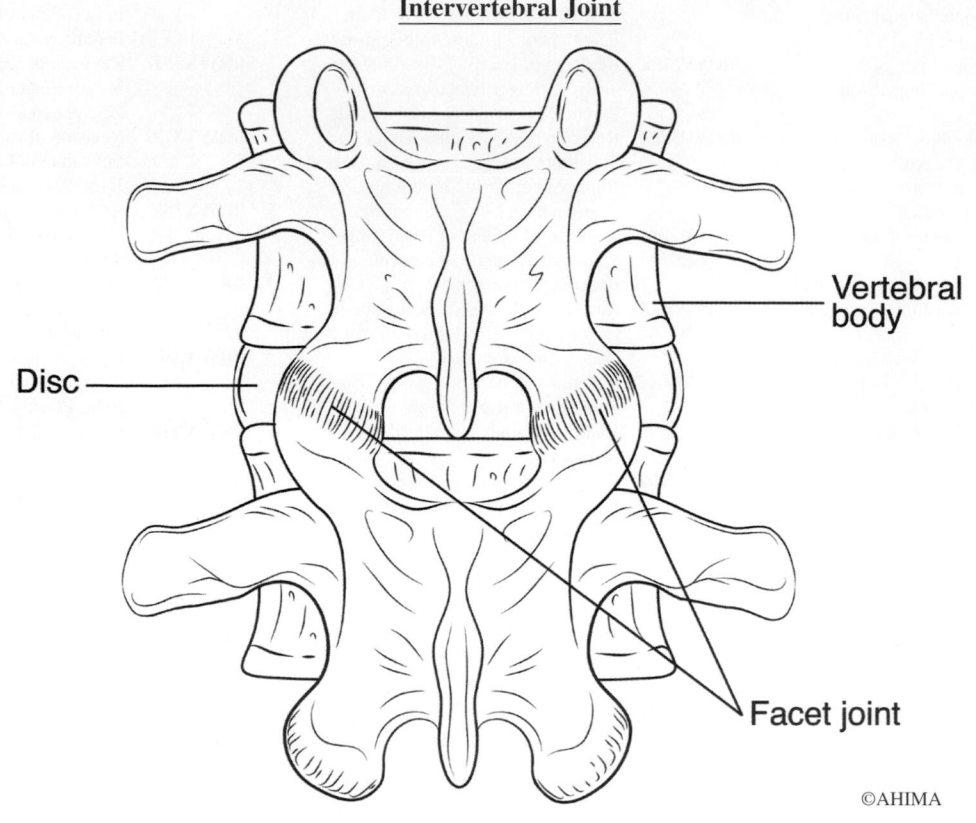

Vertebral body

Disc

Facet joint

©AHIMA

Hip

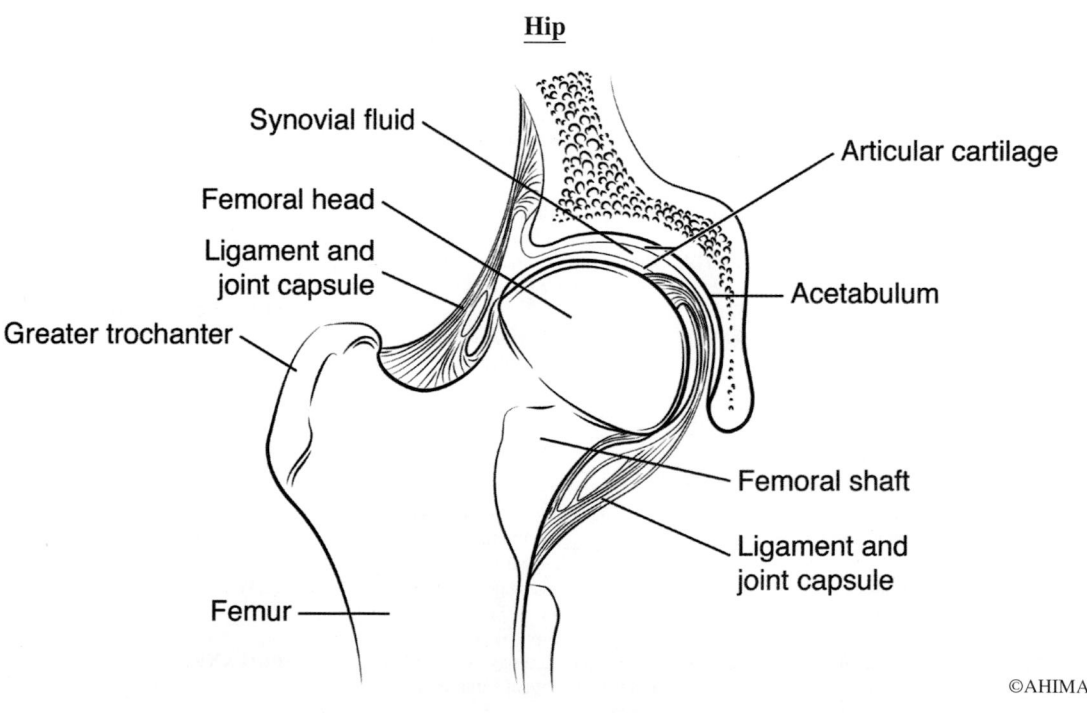

Synovial fluid

Femoral head

Ligament and joint capsule

Greater trochanter

Femur

Articular cartilage

Acetabulum

Femoral shaft

Ligament and joint capsule

©AHIMA

Knee Joint

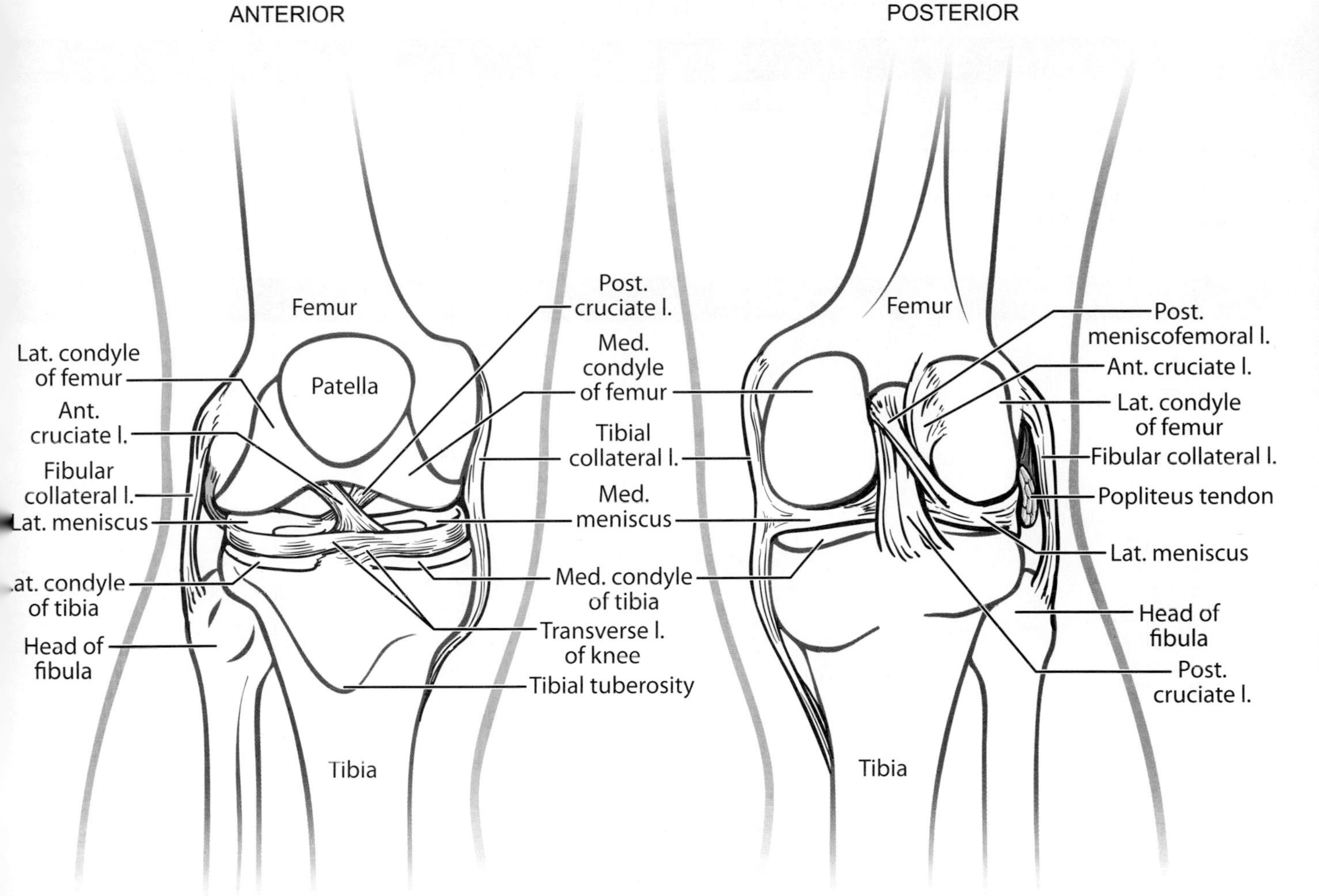

ANTERIOR

Femur

Patella

Lat. condyle of femur

Ant. cruciate l.

Fibular collateral l.

Lat. meniscus

Lat. condyle of tibia

Head of fibula

Tibia

Post. cruciate l.

Med. condyle of femur

Tibial collateral l.

Med. meniscus

Med. condyle of tibia

Transverse l. of knee

Tibial tuberosity

POSTERIOR

Femur

Post. meniscofemoral l.

Ant. cruciate l.

Lat. condyle of femur

Fibular collateral l.

Popliteus tendon

Lat. meniscus

Head of fibula

Post. cruciate l.

Tibia

©AHIMA

Ankle

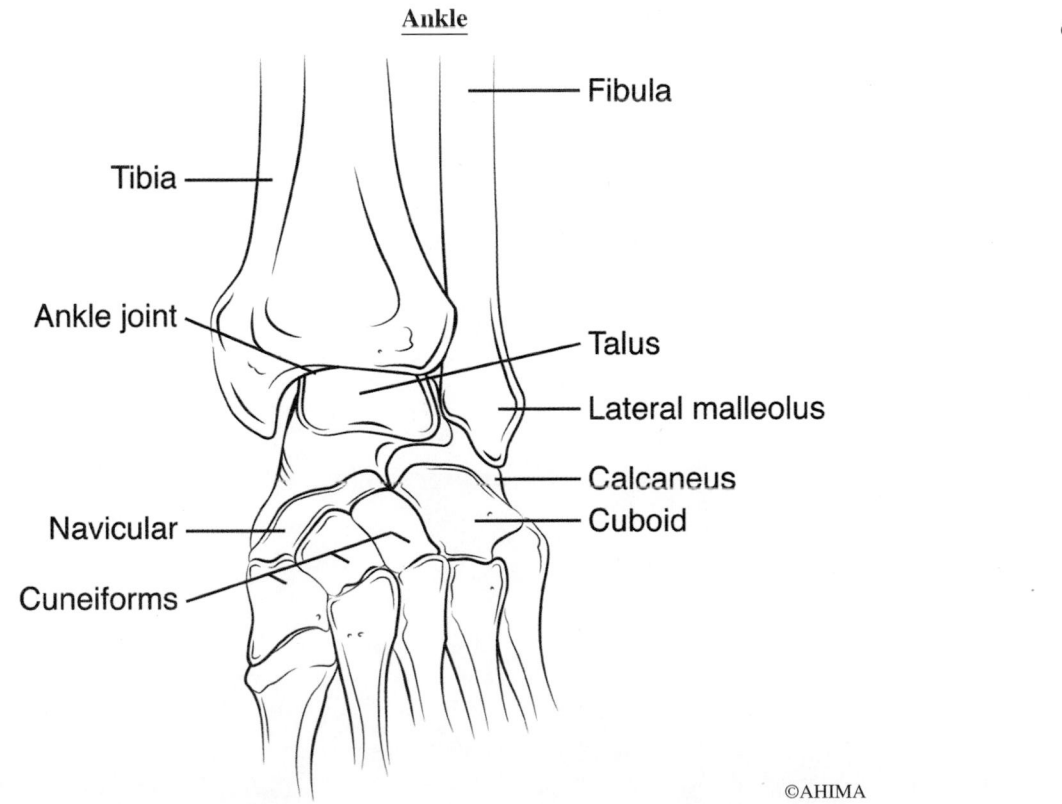

Fibula

Tibia

Ankle joint

Talus

Lateral malleolus

Calcaneus

Cuboid

Navicular

Cuneiforms

©AHIMA

Section	0	Medical and Surgical
Body System	S	Lower Joints
Operation	2	Change: Taking out or off a device from a body part and putting back an identical or similar device in or on the same body part without cutting or puncturing the skin or a mucous membrane

Body Part (4ᵗʰ)	Approach (5ᵗʰ)	Device (6ᵗʰ)	Qualifier (7ᵗʰ)
Y Lower Joint	X External	0 Drainage Device Y Other Device	Z No Qualifier

Section	0	Medical and Surgical
Body System	S	Lower Joints
Operation	5	Destruction: Physical eradication of all or a portion of a body part by the direct use of energy, force, or a destructive agent

Body Part (4ᵗʰ)	Approach (5ᵗʰ)	Device (6ᵗʰ)	Qualifier (7ᵗʰ)
0 Lumbar Vertebral Joint 2 Lumbar Vertebral Disc 3 Lumbosacral Joint 4 Lumbosacral Disc 5 Sacrococcygeal Joint 6 Coccygeal Joint 7 Sacroiliac Joint, Right 8 Sacroiliac Joint, Left 9 Hip Joint, Right B Hip Joint, Left C Knee Joint, Right D Knee Joint, Left F Ankle Joint, Right G Ankle Joint, Left H Tarsal Joint, Right J Tarsal Joint, Left K Metatarsal-Tarsal Joint, Right L Metatarsal-Tarsal Joint, Left M Metatarsal-Phalangeal Joint, Right N Metatarsal-Phalangeal Joint, Left P Toe Phalangeal Joint, Right Q Toe Phalangeal Joint, Left	0 Open 3 Percutaneous 4 Percutaneous Endoscopic	Z No Device	Z No Qualifier

Section	0	Medical and Surgical
Body System	S	Lower Joints
Operation	9	**Drainage:** Taking or letting out fluids and/or gases from a body part

Body Part (4th)	Approach (5th)	Device (6th)	Qualifier (7th)
0 Lumbar Vertebral Joint 1 Lumbar Vertebral Disc 2 Lumbosacral Joint 4 Lumbosacral Disc 5 Sacrococcygeal Joint 6 Coccygeal Joint 7 Sacroiliac Joint, Right 8 Sacroiliac Joint, Left 9 Hip Joint, Right B Hip Joint, Left C Knee Joint, Right D Knee Joint, Left F Ankle Joint, Right G Ankle Joint, Left H Tarsal Joint, Right J Tarsal Joint, Left K Metatarsal-Tarsal Joint, Right L Metatarsal-Tarsal Joint, Left L Metatarsal-Tarsal Joint, Left M Metatarsal-Phalangeal Joint, Right N Metatarsal-Phalangeal Joint, Left P Toe Phalangeal Joint, Right Q Toe Phalangeal Joint, Left	0 Open 3 Percutaneous 4 Percutaneous Endoscopic	0 Drainage Device	Z No Qualifier
0 Lumbar Vertebral Joint 2 Lumbar Vertebral Disc 3 Lumbosacral Joint 4 Lumbosacral Disc 5 Sacrococcygeal Joint 6 Coccygeal Joint 7 Sacroiliac Joint, Right 8 Sacroiliac Joint, Left 9 Hip Joint, Right B Hip Joint, Left C Knee Joint, Right D Knee Joint, Left F Ankle Joint, Right G Ankle Joint, Left H Tarsal Joint, Right J Tarsal Joint, Left K Metatarsal-Tarsal Joint, Right L Metatarsal-Tarsal Joint, Left M Metatarsal-Phalangeal Joint, Right N Metatarsal-Phalangeal Joint, Left P Toe Phalangeal Joint, Right Q Toe Phalangeal Joint, Left	0 Open 3 Percutaneous 4 Percutaneous Endoscopic	Z No Device	X Diagnostic Z No Qualifier

Section	0	Medical and Surgical
Body System	S	Lower Joints
Operation	B	Excision: Cutting out or off, without replacement, a portion of a body part

Body Part (4th)	Approach (5th)	Device (6th)	Qualifier (7th)
0 Lumbar Vertebral Joint	0 Open	Z No Device	X Diagnostic
2 Lumbar Vertebral Disc	3 Percutaneous		Z No Qualifier
3 Lumbosacral Joint	4 Percutaneous Endoscopic		
4 Lumbosacral Disc			
5 Sacrococcygeal Joint			
6 Coccygeal Joint			
7 Sacroiliac Joint, Right			
8 Sacroiliac Joint, Left			
9 Hip Joint, Right			
B Hip Joint, Left			
C Knee Joint, Right			
D Knee Joint, Left			
F Ankle Joint, Right			
G Ankle Joint, Left			
H Tarsal Joint, Right			
J Tarsal Joint, Left			
K Metatarsal-Tarsal Joint, Right			
L Metatarsal-Tarsal Joint, Left			
M Metatarsal-Phalangeal Joint, Right			
N Metatarsal-Phalangeal Joint, Left			
P Toe Phalangeal Joint, Right			
Q Toe Phalangeal Joint, Left			

Section	0	Medical and Surgical
Body System	S	Lower Joints
Operation	C	Extirpation: Taking or cutting out solid matter from a body part

Body Part (4th)	Approach (5th)	Device (6th)	Qualifier (7th)
0 Lumbar Vertebral Joint	0 Open	Z No Device	Z No Qualifier
2 Lumbar Vertebral Disc	3 Percutaneous		
3 Lumbosacral Joint	4 Percutaneous Endoscopic		
4 Lumbosacral Disc			
5 Sacrococcygeal Joint			
6 Coccygeal Joint			
7 Sacroiliac Joint, Right			
8 Sacroiliac Joint, Left			
9 Hip Joint, Right			
B Hip Joint, Left			
C Knee Joint, Right			
D Knee Joint, Left			
F Ankle Joint, Right			
G Ankle Joint, Left			
H Tarsal Joint, Right			
J Tarsal Joint, Left			
K Metatarsal-Tarsal Joint, Right			
L Metatarsal-Tarsal Joint, Left			
M Metatarsal-Phalangeal Joint, Right			
N Metatarsal-Phalangeal Joint, Left			
P Toe Phalangeal Joint, Right			
Q Toe Phalangeal Joint, Left			

Section 0 **Medical and Surgical**
Body System S **Lower Joints**
Operation G **Fusion:** Joining together portions of an articular body part rendering the articular body part immobile

Body Part (4th)	Approach (5th)	Device (6th)	Qualifier (7th)
Lumbar Vertebral Joint Lumbar Vertebral Joints, 2 or more Lumbosacral Joint	0 Open 3 Percutaneous 4 Percutaneous Endoscopic	7 Autologous Tissue Substitute A Interbody Fusion Device J Synthetic Substitute K Nonautologous Tissue Substitute Z No Device	0 Anterior Approach, Anterior Column 1 Posterior Approach, Posterior Column J Posterior Approach, Anterior Column
Sacrococcygeal Joint Coccygeal Joint Sacroiliac Joint, Right Sacroiliac Joint, Left	0 Open 3 Percutaneous 4 Percutaneous Endoscopic	4 Internal Fixation Device 7 Autologous Tissue Substitute J Synthetic Substitute K Nonautologous Tissue Substitute Z No Device	Z No Qualifier
Hip Joint, Right Hip Joint, Left Knee Joint, Right Knee Joint, Left Ankle Joint, Right Ankle Joint, Left Tarsal Joint, Right Tarsal Joint, Left Metatarsal-Tarsal Joint, Right Metatarsal-Tarsal Joint, Left Metatarsal-Phalangeal Joint, Right Metatarsal-Phalangeal Joint, Left Toe Phalangeal Joint, Right Toe Phalangeal Joint, Left	0 Open 3 Percutaneous 4 Percutaneous Endoscopic	4 Internal Fixation Device 5 External Fixation Device 7 Autologous Tissue Substitute J Synthetic Substitute K Nonautologous Tissue Substitute Z No Device	Z No Qualifier

Section 0 **Medical and Surgical**
Body System S **Lower Joints**
Operation H **Insertion:** Putting in a nonbiological appliance that monitors, assists, performs, or prevents a physiological function but does not physically take the place of a body part

Body Part (4th)	Approach (5th)	Device (6th)	Qualifier (7th)
0 Lumbar Vertebral Joint 3 Lumbosacral Joint	0 Open 3 Percutaneous 4 Percutaneous Endoscopic	3 Infusion Device 4 Internal Fixation Device 8 Spacer B Spinal Stabilization Device, Interspinous Process C Spinal Stabilization Device, Pedicle-Based D Spinal Stabilization Device, Facet Replacement	Z No Qualifier
2 Lumbar Vertebral Disc 4 Lumbosacral Disc	0 Open 3 Percutaneous 4 Percutaneous Endoscopic	3 Infusion Device 8 Spacer	Z No Qualifier
5 Sacrococcygeal Joint 6 Coccygeal Joint 7 Sacroiliac Joint, Right 8 Sacroiliac Joint, Left	0 Open 3 Percutaneous 4 Percutaneous Endoscopic	3 Infusion Device 4 Internal Fixation Device 8 Spacer	Z No Qualifier

Continued →

Section	0	Medical and Surgical
Body System	S	Lower Joints
Operation	H	**Insertion:** Putting in a nonbiological appliance that monitors, assists, performs, or prevents a physiological function but doe not physically take the place of a body part

Body Part (4th)	Approach (5th)	Device (6th)	Qualifier (7th)
9 Hip Joint, Right B Hip Joint, Left C Knee Joint, Right D Knee Joint, Left F Ankle Joint, Right G Ankle Joint, Left H Tarsal Joint, Right J Tarsal Joint, Left K Metatarsal-Tarsal Joint, Right L Metatarsal-Tarsal Joint, Left M Metatarsal-Phalangeal Joint, Right N Metatarsal-Phalangeal Joint, Left P Toe Phalangeal Joint, Right Q Toe Phalangeal Joint, Left	0 Open 3 Percutaneous 4 Percutaneous Endoscopic	3 Infusion Device 4 Internal Fixation Device 5 External Fixation Device 8 Spacer	Z No Qualifier

Section	0	Medical and Surgical
Body System	S	Lower Joints
Operation	J	**Inspection:** Visually and/or manually exploring a body part

Body Part (4th)	Approach (5th)	Device (6th)	Qualifier (7th)
0 Lumbar Vertebral Joint 2 Lumbar Vertebral Disc 3 Lumbosacral Joint 4 Lumbosacral Disc 5 Sacrococcygeal Joint 6 Coccygeal Joint 7 Sacroiliac Joint, Right 8 Sacroiliac Joint, Left 9 Hip Joint, Right B Hip Joint, Left C Knee Joint, Right D Knee Joint, Left F Ankle Joint, Right G Ankle Joint, Left H Tarsal Joint, Right J Tarsal Joint, Left K Metatarsal-Tarsal Joint, Right L Metatarsal-Tarsal Joint, Left M Metatarsal-Phalangeal Joint, Right N Metatarsal-Phalangeal Joint, Left P Toe Phalangeal Joint, Right Q Toe Phalangeal Joint, Left	0 Open 3 Percutaneous 4 Percutaneous Endoscopic X External	Z No Device	Z No Qualifier

:tion	0	Medical and Surgical
dy System	S	Lower Joints
eration	N	**Release:** Freeing a body part from an abnormal physical constraint by cutting or by the use of force

Body Part (4th)	Approach (5th)	Device (6th)	Qualifier (7th)
Lumbar Vertebral Joint Lumbar Vertebral Disc Lumbosacral Joint Lumbosacral Disc Sacrococcygeal Joint Coccygeal Joint Sacroiliac Joint, Right Sacroiliac Joint, Left Hip Joint, Right Hip Joint, Left C Knee Joint, Right D Knee Joint, Left F Ankle Joint, Right G Ankle Joint, Left H Tarsal Joint, Right J Tarsal Joint, Left K Metatarsal-Tarsal Joint, Right L Metatarsal-Tarsal Joint, Left M Metatarsal-Phalangeal Joint, Right N Metatarsal-Phalangeal Joint, Left P Toe Phalangeal Joint, Right Q Toe Phalangeal Joint, Left	0 Open 3 Percutaneous 4 Percutaneous Endoscopic X External	Z No Device	Z No Qualifier

:tion	0	Medical and Surgical
dy System	S	Lower Joints
eration	P	**Removal:** Taking out or off a device from a body part

Body Part (4th)	Approach (5th)	Device (6th)	Qualifier (7th)
0 Lumbar Vertebral Joint 3 Lumbosacral Joint	0 Open 3 Percutaneous 4 Percutaneous Endoscopic	0 Drainage Device 3 Infusion Device 4 Internal Fixation Device 7 Autologous Tissue Substitute 8 Spacer A Interbody Fusion Device J Synthetic Substitute K Nonautologous Tissue Substitute	Z No Qualifier
0 Lumbar Vertebral Joint 3 Lumbosacral Joint	X External	0 Drainage Device 3 Infusion Device 4 Internal Fixation Device	Z No Qualifier
2 Lumbar Vertebral Disc 4 Lumbosacral Disc	0 Open 3 Percutaneous 4 Percutaneous Endoscopic	0 Drainage Device 3 Infusion Device 7 Autologous Tissue Substitute J Synthetic Substitute K Nonautologous Tissue Substitute	Z No Qualifier
2 Lumbar Vertebral Disc 4 Lumbosacral Disc	X External	0 Drainage Device 3 Infusion Device	Z No Qualifier
5 Sacrococcygeal Joint 6 Coccygeal Joint 7 Sacroiliac Joint, Right 8 Sacroiliac Joint, Left	0 Open 3 Percutaneous 4 Percutaneous Endoscopic	0 Drainage Device 3 Infusion Device 4 Internal Fixation Device 7 Autologous Tissue Substitute 8 Spacer J Synthetic Substitute K Nonautologous Tissue Substitute	Z No Qualifier

Continued →

Section	0	**Medical and Surgical**
Body System	S	**Lower Joints**
Operation	P	**Removal:** Taking out or off a device from a body part

Body Part (4ᵗʰ)	Approach (5ᵗʰ)	Device (6ᵗʰ)	Qualifier (7ᵗʰ)
5 Sacrococcygeal Joint 6 Coccygeal Joint 7 Sacroiliac Joint, Right 8 Sacroiliac Joint, Left	X External	0 Drainage Device 3 Infusion Device 4 Internal Fixation Device	Z No Qualifier
9 Hip Joint, Right B Hip Joint, Left	0 Open	0 Drainage Device 3 Infusion Device 4 Internal Fixation Device 5 External Fixation Device 7 Autologous Tissue Substitute 8 Spacer 9 Liner B Resurfacing Device J Synthetic Substitute K Nonautologous Tissue Substitute	Z No Qualifier
9 Hip Joint, Right B Hip Joint, Left	3 Percutaneous 4 Percutaneous Endoscopic	0 Drainage Device 3 Infusion Device 4 Internal Fixation Device 5 External Fixation Device 7 Autologous Tissue Substitute 8 Spacer J Synthetic Substitute K Nonautologous Tissue Substitute	Z No Qualifier
9 Hip Joint, Right B Hip Joint, Left	X External	0 Drainage Device 3 Infusion Device 4 Internal Fixation Device 5 External Fixation Device	Z No Qualifier
C Knee Joint, Right D Knee Joint, Left	0 Open	0 Drainage Device 3 Infusion Device 4 Internal Fixation Device 5 External Fixation Device 7 Autologous Tissue Substitute 8 Spacer 9 Liner J Synthetic Substitute K Nonautologous Tissue Substitute	Z No Qualifier
C Knee Joint, Right D Knee Joint, Left	3 Percutaneous 4 Percutaneous Endoscopic	0 Drainage Device 3 Infusion Device 4 Internal Fixation Device 5 External Fixation Device 7 Autologous Tissue Substitute 8 Spacer J Synthetic Substitute K Nonautologous Tissue Substitute	Z No Qualifier
C Knee Joint, Right D Knee Joint, Left	X External	0 Drainage Device 3 Infusion Device 4 Internal Fixation Device 5 External Fixation Device	Z No Qualifier
F Ankle Joint, Right G Ankle Joint, Left H Tarsal Joint, Right J Tarsal Joint, Left K Metatarsal-Tarsal Joint, Right L Metatarsal-Tarsal Joint, Left M Metatarsal-Phalangeal Joint, Right N Metatarsal-Phalangeal Joint, Left P Toe Phalangeal Joint, Right Q Toe Phalangeal Joint, Left	0 Open 3 Percutaneous 4 Percutaneous Endoscopic	0 Drainage Device 3 Infusion Device 4 Internal Fixation Device 5 External Fixation Device 7 Autologous Tissue Substitute 8 Spacer J Synthetic Substitute K Nonautologous Tissue Substitute	Z No Qualifier

Continued →

Section	0	Medical and Surgical
Body System	S	Lower Joints
Operation	P	**Removal:** Taking out or off a device from a body part

Body Part (4th)	Approach (5th)	Device (6th)	Qualifier (7th)
F Ankle Joint, Right G Ankle Joint, Left H Tarsal Joint, Right J Tarsal Joint, Left K Metatarsal-Tarsal Joint, Right L Metatarsal-Tarsal Joint, Left M Metatarsal-Phalangeal Joint, Right N Metatarsal-Phalangeal Joint, Left P Toe Phalangeal Joint, Right Q Toe Phalangeal Joint, Left	X External	0 Drainage Device 3 Infusion Device 4 Internal Fixation Device 5 External Fixation Device	Z No Qualifier

Section	0	Medical and Surgical
Body System	S	Lower Joints
Operation	Q	**Repair:** Restoring, to the extent possible, a body part to its normal anatomic structure and function

Body Part (4th)	Approach (5th)	Device (6th)	Qualifier (7th)
0 Lumbar Vertebral Joint 2 Lumbar Vertebral Disc 3 Lumbosacral Joint 4 Lumbosacral Disc 5 Sacrococcygeal Joint 6 Coccygeal Joint 7 Sacroiliac Joint, Right 8 Sacroiliac Joint, Left 9 Hip Joint, Right B Hip Joint, Left C Knee Joint, Right D Knee Joint, Left F Ankle Joint, Right G Ankle Joint, Left H Tarsal Joint, Right J Tarsal Joint, Left K Metatarsal-Tarsal Joint, Right L Metatarsal-Tarsal Joint, Left M Metatarsal-Phalangeal Joint, Right N Metatarsal-Phalangeal Joint, Left P Toe Phalangeal Joint, Right Q Toe Phalangeal Joint, Left	0 Open 3 Percutaneous 4 Percutaneous Endoscopic X External	Z No Device	Z No Qualifier

Section	0	Medical and Surgical
Body System	S	Lower Joints
Operation	R	**Replacement:** Putting in or on biological or synthetic material that physically takes the place and/or function of all or a portion of a body part

Body Part (4th)	Approach (5th)	Device (6th)	Qualifier (7th)
0 Lumbar Vertebral Joint 2 Lumbar Vertebral Disc 3 Lumbosacral Joint 4 Lumbosacral Disc 5 Sacrococcygeal Joint 6 Coccygeal Joint 7 Sacroiliac Joint, Right 8 Sacroiliac Joint, Left H Tarsal Joint, Right J Tarsal Joint, Left K Metatarsal-Tarsal Joint, Right L Metatarsal-Tarsal Joint, Left M Metatarsal-Phalangeal Joint, Right N Metatarsal-Phalangeal Joint, Left P Toe Phalangeal Joint, Right Q Toe Phalangeal Joint, Left	0 Open	7 Autologous Tissue Substitute J Synthetic Substitute K Nonautologous Tissue Substitute	Z No Qualifier

Continued →

Section   **0**   **Medical and Surgical**
Body System   **S**   **Lower Joints**
Operation   **R**   **Replacement:** Putting in or on biological or synthetic material that physically takes the place and/or function of all or a portion of a body part

Body Part (4th)	Approach (5th)	Device (6th)	Qualifier (7th)
9 Hip Joint, Right B Hip Joint, Left	0 Open	1 Synthetic Substitute, Metal 2 Synthetic Substitute, Metal on Polyethylene 3 Synthetic Substitute, Ceramic 4 Synthetic Substitute, Ceramic on Polyethylene J Synthetic Substitute	9 Cemented A Uncemented Z No Qualifier
9 Hip Joint, Right B Hip Joint, Left	0 Open	7 Autologous Tissue Substitute K Nonautologous Tissue Substitute	Z No Qualifier
A Hip Joint, Acetabular Surface, Right E Hip Joint, Acetabular Surface, Left	0 Open	0 Synthetic Substitute, Polyethylene 1 Synthetic Substitute, Metal 3 Synthetic Substitute, Ceramic J Synthetic Substitute	9 Cemented A Uncemented Z No Qualifier
A Hip Joint, Acetabular Surface, Right E Hip Joint, Acetabular Surface, Left	0 Open	7 Autologous Tissue Substitute K Nonautologous Tissue Substitute	Z No Qualifier
C Knee Joint, Right D Knee Joint, Left F Ankle Joint, Right G Ankle Joint, Left T Knee Joint, Femoral Surface, Right U Knee Joint, Femoral Surface, Left V Knee Joint, Tibial Surface, Right W Knee Joint, Tibial Surface, Left	0 Open	7 Autologous Tissue Substitute K Nonautologous Tissue Substitute	Z No Qualifier
C Knee Joint, Right D Knee Joint, Left F Ankle Joint, Right G Ankle Joint, Left T Knee Joint, Femoral Surface, Right U Knee Joint, Femoral Surface, Left V Knee Joint, Tibial Surface, Right W Knee Joint, Tibial Surface, Left	0 Open	J Synthetic Substitute	9 Cemented A Uncemented Z No Qualifier
R Hip Joint, Femoral Surface, Right S Hip Joint, Femoral Surface, Left	0 Open	1 Synthetic Substitute, Metal 3 Synthetic Substitute, Ceramic J Synthetic Substitute	9 Cemented A Uncemented Z No Qualifier
R Hip Joint, Femoral Surface, Right S Hip Joint, Femoral Surface, Left	0 Open	7 Autologous Tissue Substitute K Nonautologous Tissue Substitute	Z No Qualifier

Section   **0**   **Medical and Surgical**
Body System   **S**   **Lower Joints**
Operation   **S**   **Reposition:** Moving to its normal location, or other suitable location, all or a portion of a body part

Body Part (4th)	Approach (5th)	Device (6th)	Qualifier (7th)
0 Lumbar Vertebral Joint 3 Lumbosacral Joint 5 Sacrococcygeal Joint 6 Coccygeal Joint 7 Sacroiliac Joint, Right 8 Sacroiliac Joint, Left	0 Open 3 Percutaneous 4 Percutaneous Endoscopic X External	4 Internal Fixation Device Z No Device	Z No Qualifier

Continued →

Section | 0 | Medical and Surgical
Body System | S | Lower Joints
Operation | S | **Reposition:** Moving to its normal location, or other suitable location, all or a portion of a body part

Body Part (4th)	Approach (5th)	Device (6th)	Qualifier (7th)
9 Hip Joint, Right	0 Open	4 Internal Fixation Device	Z No Qualifier
B Hip Joint, Left	3 Percutaneous	5 External Fixation Device	
C Knee Joint, Right	4 Percutaneous Endoscopic	Z No Device	
D Knee Joint, Left	X External		
F Ankle Joint, Right			
G Ankle Joint, Left			
H Tarsal Joint, Right			
J Tarsal Joint, Left			
K Metatarsal-Tarsal Joint, Right			
L Metatarsal-Tarsal Joint, Left			
M Metatarsal-Phalangeal Joint, Right			
N Metatarsal-Phalangeal Joint, Left			
P Toe Phalangeal Joint, Right			
Q Toe Phalangeal Joint, Left			

Section | 0 | Medical and Surgical
Body System | S | Lower Joints
Operation | T | **Resection:** Cutting out or off, without replacement, all of a body part

Body Part (4th)	Approach (5th)	Device (6th)	Qualifier (7th)
2 Lumbar Vertebral Disc	0 Open	Z No Device	Z No Qualifier
4 Lumbosacral Disc			
5 Sacrococcygeal Joint			
6 Coccygeal Joint			
7 Sacroiliac Joint, Right			
8 Sacroiliac Joint, Left			
9 Hip Joint, Right			
B Hip Joint, Left			
C Knee Joint, Right			
D Knee Joint, Left			
F Ankle Joint, Right			
G Ankle Joint, Left			
H Tarsal Joint, Right			
J Tarsal Joint, Left			
K Metatarsal-Tarsal Joint, Right			
L Metatarsal-Tarsal Joint, Left			
M Metatarsal-Phalangeal Joint, Right			
N Metatarsal-Phalangeal Joint, Left			
P Toe Phalangeal Joint, Right			
Q Toe Phalangeal Joint, Left			

Section   **0**   **Medical and Surgical**
Body System   **S**   **Lower Joints**
Operation   **U**   **Supplement:** Putting in or on biological or synthetic material that physically reinforces and/or augments the function of a portion of a body part

Body Part (4th)	Approach (5th)	Device (6th)	Qualifier (7th)
0 Lumbar Vertebral Joint 2 Lumbar Vertebral Disc 3 Lumbosacral Joint 4 Lumbosacral Disc 5 Sacrococcygeal Joint 6 Coccygeal Joint 7 Sacroiliac Joint, Right 8 Sacroiliac Joint, Left F Ankle Joint, Right G Ankle Joint, Left H Tarsal Joint, Right J Tarsal Joint, Left K Metatarsal-Tarsal Joint, Right L Metatarsal-Tarsal Joint, Left M Metatarsal-Phalangeal Joint, Right N Metatarsal-Phalangeal Joint, Left P Toe Phalangeal Joint, Right Q Toe Phalangeal Joint, Left	0 Open 3 Percutaneous 4 Percutaneous Endoscopic	7 Autologous Tissue Substitute J Synthetic Substitute K Nonautologous Tissue Substitute	Z No Qualifier
9 Hip Joint, Right B Hip Joint, Left	0 Open	7 Autologous Tissue Substitute 9 Liner B Resurfacing Device J Synthetic Substitute K Nonautologous Tissue Substitute	Z No Qualifier
9 Hip Joint, Right B Hip Joint, Left	3 Percutaneous 4 Percutaneous Endoscopic	7 Autologous Tissue Substitute J Synthetic Substitute K Nonautologous Tissue Substitute	Z No Qualifier
A Hip Joint, Acetabular Surface, Right E Hip Joint, Acetabular Surface, Left R Hip Joint, Femoral Surface, Right S Hip Joint, Femoral Surface, Left	0 Open	9 Liner B Resurfacing Device	Z No Qualifier
C Knee Joint, Right D Knee Joint, Left	0 Open	7 Autologous Tissue Substitute J Synthetic Substitute K Nonautologous Tissue Substitute	Z No Qualifier
C Knee Joint, Right D Knee Joint, Left	0 Open	9 Liner	C Patellar Surface Z No Qualifier
C Knee Joint, Right D Knee Joint, Left	3 Percutaneous 4 Percutaneous Endoscopic	7 Autologous Tissue Substitute J Synthetic Substitute K Nonautologous Tissue Substitute	Z No Qualifier
T Knee Joint, Femoral Surface, Right U Knee Joint, Femoral Surface, Left V Knee Joint, Tibial Surface, Right W Knee Joint, Tibial Surface, Left	0 Open	9 Liner	Z No Qualifier

		Section	0	Medical and Surgical
		Body System	S	Lower Joints
		Operation	W	Revision: Correcting, to the extent possible, a portion of a malfunctioning device or the position of a displaced device

Body Part (4th)	Approach (5th)	Device (6th)	Qualifier (7th)
0 Lumbar Vertebral Joint 3 Lumbosacral Joint	0 Open 3 Percutaneous 4 Percutaneous Endoscopic X External	0 Drainage Device 3 Infusion Device 4 Internal Fixation Device 7 Autologous Tissue Substitute 8 Spacer A Interbody Fusion Device J Synthetic Substitute K Nonautologous Tissue Substitute	Z No Qualifier
2 Lumbar Vertebral Disc 4 Lumbosacral Disc	0 Open 3 Percutaneous 4 Percutaneous Endoscopic X External	0 Drainage Device 3 Infusion Device 7 Autologous Tissue Substitute J Synthetic Substitute K Nonautologous Tissue Substitute	Z No Qualifier
5 Sacrococcygeal Joint 6 Coccygeal Joint 7 Sacroiliac Joint, Right 8 Sacroiliac Joint, Left	0 Open 3 Percutaneous 4 Percutaneous Endoscopic X External	0 Drainage Device 3 Infusion Device 4 Internal Fixation Device 7 Autologous Tissue Substitute 8 Spacer J Synthetic Substitute K Nonautologous Tissue Substitute	Z No Qualifier
9 Hip Joint, Right B Hip Joint, Left	0 Open	0 Drainage Device 3 Infusion Device 4 Internal Fixation Device 5 External Fixation Device 7 Autologous Tissue Substitute 8 Spacer 9 Liner B Resurfacing Device J Synthetic Substitute K Nonautologous Tissue Substitute	Z No Qualifier
9 Hip Joint, Right B Hip Joint, Left	3 Percutaneous 4 Percutaneous Endoscopic X External	0 Drainage Device 3 Infusion Device 4 Internal Fixation Device 5 External Fixation Device 7 Autologous Tissue Substitute 8 Spacer J Synthetic Substitute K Nonautologous Tissue Substitute	Z No Qualifier
C Knee Joint, Right D Knee Joint, Left	0 Open	0 Drainage Device 3 Infusion Device 4 Internal Fixation Device 5 External Fixation Device 7 Autologous Tissue Substitute 8 Spacer 9 Liner J Synthetic Substitute K Nonautologous Tissue Substitute	Z No Qualifier
C Knee Joint, Right D Knee Joint, Left	3 Percutaneous 4 Percutaneous Endoscopic X External	0 Drainage Device 3 Infusion Device 4 Internal Fixation Device 5 External Fixation Device 7 Autologous Tissue Substitute 8 Spacer J Synthetic Substitute K Nonautologous Tissue Substitute	Z No Qualifier

Continued →

Section	0	Medical and Surgical
Body System	S	Lower Joints
Operation	W	**Revision:** Correcting, to the extent possible, a portion of a malfunctioning device or the position of a displaced device

Body Part (4th)	Approach (5th)	Device (6th)	Qualifier (7th)
F Ankle Joint, Right G Ankle Joint, Left H Tarsal Joint, Right J Tarsal Joint, Left K Metatarsal-Tarsal Joint, Right L Metatarsal-Tarsal Joint, Left M Metatarsal-Phalangeal Joint, Right N Metatarsal-Phalangeal Joint, Left P Toe Phalangeal Joint, Right Q Toe Phalangeal Joint, Left	0 Open 3 Percutaneous 4 Percutaneous Endoscopic X External	0 Drainage Device 3 Infusion Device 4 Internal Fixation Device 5 External Fixation Device 7 Autologous Tissue Substitute 8 Spacer J Synthetic Substitute K Nonautologous Tissue Substitute	Z No Qualifier

Lower Joints Code Listing 0S2–0SW

Review Coding Guideline B4.5

0S2 – Lower Joints, Change

Review Coding Guideline B6.1c

0S2YX0Z Change Drainage Device in Lower Joint, External Approach

0S2YXYZ Change Other Device in Lower Joint, External Approach

0S5 – Lower Joints, Destruction

0S500ZZ Destruction of Lumbar Vertebral Joint, Open Approach
0S503ZZ Destruction of Lumbar Vertebral Joint, Percutaneous Approach
0S504ZZ Destruction of Lumbar Vertebral Joint, Percutaneous Endoscopic Approach
0S520ZZ Destruction of Lumbar Vertebral Disc, Open Approach
0S523ZZ Destruction of Lumbar Vertebral Disc, Percutaneous Approach
0S524ZZ Destruction of Lumbar Vertebral Disc, Percutaneous Endoscopic Approach
0S530ZZ Destruction of Lumbosacral Joint, Open Approach
0S533ZZ Destruction of Lumbosacral Joint, Percutaneous Approach
0S534ZZ Destruction of Lumbosacral Joint, Percutaneous Endoscopic Approach
0S540ZZ Destruction of Lumbosacral Disc, Open Approach
0S543ZZ Destruction of Lumbosacral Disc, Percutaneous Approach
0S544ZZ Destruction of Lumbosacral Disc, Percutaneous Endoscopic Approach
0S550ZZ Destruction of Sacrococcygeal Joint, Open Approach
0S553ZZ Destruction of Sacrococcygeal Joint, Percutaneous Approach
0S554ZZ Destruction of Sacrococcygeal Joint, Percutaneous Endoscopic Approach
0S560ZZ Destruction of Coccygeal Joint, Open Approach
0S563ZZ Destruction of Coccygeal Joint, Percutaneous Approach
0S564ZZ Destruction of Coccygeal Joint, Percutaneous Endoscopic Approach
0S570ZZ Destruction of Right Sacroiliac Joint, Open Approach
0S573ZZ Destruction of Right Sacroiliac Joint, Percutaneous Approach
0S574ZZ Destruction of Right Sacroiliac Joint, Percutaneous Endoscopic Approach

0S580ZZ Destruction of Left Sacroiliac Joint, Open Approach
0S583ZZ Destruction of Left Sacroiliac Joint, Percutaneous Approach
0S584ZZ Destruction of Left Sacroiliac Joint, Percutaneous Endoscopic Approach
0S590ZZ Destruction of Right Hip Joint, Open Approach
0S593ZZ Destruction of Right Hip Joint, Percutaneous Approach
0S594ZZ Destruction of Right Hip Joint, Percutaneous Endoscopic Approach
0S5B0ZZ Destruction of Left Hip Joint, Open Approach
0S5B3ZZ Destruction of Left Hip Joint, Percutaneous Approach
0S5B4ZZ Destruction of Left Hip Joint, Percutaneous Endoscopic Approach
0S5C0ZZ Destruction of Right Knee Joint, Open Approach
0S5C3ZZ Destruction of Right Knee Joint, Percutaneous Approach
0S5C4ZZ Destruction of Right Knee Joint, Percutaneous Endoscopic Approach
0S5D0ZZ Destruction of Left Knee Joint, Open Approach
0S5D3ZZ Destruction of Left Knee Joint, Percutaneous Approach
0S5D4ZZ Destruction of Left Knee Joint, Percutaneous Endoscopic Approach
0S5F0ZZ Destruction of Right Ankle Joint, Open Approach
0S5F3ZZ Destruction of Right Ankle Joint, Percutaneous Approach
0S5F4ZZ Destruction of Right Ankle Joint, Percutaneous Endoscopic Approach
0S5G0ZZ Destruction of Left Ankle Joint, Open Approach
0S5G3ZZ Destruction of Left Ankle Joint, Percutaneous Approach
0S5G4ZZ Destruction of Left Ankle Joint, Percutaneous Endoscopic Approach

0S5H0ZZ Destruction of Right Tarsal Joint, Open Approach
0S5H3ZZ Destruction of Right Tarsal Joint, Percutaneous Approach
0S5H4ZZ Destruction of Right Tarsal Joint, Percutaneous Endoscopic Approach
0S5J0ZZ Destruction of Left Tarsal Joint, Open Approach
0S5J3ZZ Destruction of Left Tarsal Joint, Percutaneous Approach
0S5J4ZZ Destruction of Left Tarsal Joint, Percutaneous Endoscopic Approach
0S5K0ZZ Destruction of Right Metatarsal-Tarsal Joint, Open Approach
0S5K3ZZ Destruction of Right Metatarsal-Tarsal Joint, Percutaneous Approach
0S5K4ZZ Destruction of Right Metatarsal-Tarsal Joint, Percutaneous Endoscopic Approach
0S5L0ZZ Destruction of Left Metatarsal-Tarsal Joint, Open Approach
0S5L3ZZ Destruction of Left Metatarsal-Tarsal Joint, Percutaneous Approach
0S5L4ZZ Destruction of Left Metatarsal-Tarsal Joint, Percutaneous Endoscopic Approach
0S5M0ZZ Destruction of Right Metatarsal-Phalangeal Joint, Open Approach
0S5M3ZZ Destruction of Right Metatarsal-Phalangeal Joint, Percutaneous Approach
0S5M4ZZ Destruction of Right Metatarsal-Phalangeal Joint, Percutaneous Endoscopic Approach
0S5N0ZZ Destruction of Left Metatarsal-Phalangeal Joint, Open Approach
0S5N3ZZ Destruction of Left Metatarsal-Phalangeal Joint, Percutaneous Approach
0S5N4ZZ Destruction of Left Metatarsal-Phalangeal Joint, Percutaneous Endoscopic Approach

5P0ZZ	Destruction of Right Toe Phalangeal Joint, Open Approach	**0S5P4ZZ**	Destruction of Right Toe Phalangeal Joint, Percutaneous Endoscopic Approach	**0S5Q3ZZ**	Destruction of Left Toe Phalangeal Joint, Percutaneous Approach
5P3ZZ	Destruction of Right Toe Phalangeal Joint, Percutaneous Approach	**0S5Q0ZZ**	Destruction of Left Toe Phalangeal Joint, Open Approach	**0S5Q4ZZ**	Destruction of Left Toe Phalangeal Joint, Percutaneous Endoscopic Approach

S9 – Lower Joints, Drainage

eview Coding Guidelines B3.4a and B3.4b

eview Coding Guideline B6.2

S9000Z	Drainage of Lumbar Vertebral Joint with Drainage Device, Open Approach	**0S9430Z**	Drainage of Lumbosacral Disc with Drainage Device, Percutaneous Approach	**0S9740Z**	Drainage of Right Sacroiliac Joint with Drainage Device, Percutaneous Endoscopic Approach
S900ZX	Drainage of Lumbar Vertebral Joint, Open Approach, Diagnostic	**0S943ZX**	Drainage of Lumbosacral Disc, Percutaneous Approach, Diagnostic	**0S974ZX**	Drainage of Right Sacroiliac Joint, Percutaneous Endoscopic Approach, Diagnostic
S900ZZ	Drainage of Lumbar Vertebral Joint, Open Approach	**0S943ZZ**	Drainage of Lumbosacral Disc, Percutaneous Approach	**0S974ZZ**	Drainage of Right Sacroiliac Joint, Percutaneous Endoscopic Approach
S9030Z	Drainage of Lumbar Vertebral Joint with Drainage Device, Percutaneous Approach	**0S9440Z**	Drainage of Lumbosacral Disc with Drainage Device, Percutaneous Endoscopic Approach	**0S9800Z**	Drainage of Left Sacroiliac Joint with Drainage Device, Open Approach
S903ZX	Drainage of Lumbar Vertebral Joint, Percutaneous Approach, Diagnostic	**0S944ZX**	Drainage of Lumbosacral Disc, Percutaneous Endoscopic Approach, Diagnostic	**0S980ZX**	Drainage of Left Sacroiliac Joint, Open Approach, Diagnostic
S903ZZ	Drainage of Lumbar Vertebral Joint, Percutaneous Approach	**0S944ZZ**	Drainage of Lumbosacral Disc, Percutaneous Endoscopic Approach	**0S980ZZ**	Drainage of Left Sacroiliac Joint, Open Approach
S9040Z	Drainage of Lumbar Vertebral Joint with Drainage Device, Percutaneous Endoscopic Approach	**0S9500Z**	Drainage of Sacrococcygeal Joint with Drainage Device, Open Approach	**0S9830Z**	Drainage of Left Sacroiliac Joint with Drainage Device, Percutaneous Approach
S904ZX	Drainage of Lumbar Vertebral Joint, Percutaneous Endoscopic Approach, Diagnostic	**0S9500ZX**	Drainage of Sacrococcygeal Joint, Open Approach, Diagnostic	**0S983ZX**	Drainage of Left Sacroiliac Joint, Percutaneous Approach, Diagnostic
S904ZZ	Drainage of Lumbar Vertebral Joint, Percutaneous Endoscopic Approach	**0S9500ZZ**	Drainage of Sacrococcygeal Joint, Open Approach	**0S983ZZ**	Drainage of Left Sacroiliac Joint, Percutaneous Approach
S9200Z	Drainage of Lumbar Vertebral Disc with Drainage Device, Open Approach	**0S9530Z**	Drainage of Sacrococcygeal Joint with Drainage Device, Percutaneous Approach	**0S9840Z**	Drainage of Left Sacroiliac Joint with Drainage Device, Percutaneous Endoscopic Approach
S920ZX	Drainage of Lumbar Vertebral Disc, Open Approach, Diagnostic	**0S953ZX**	Drainage of Sacrococcygeal Joint, Percutaneous Approach, Diagnostic	**0S984ZX**	Drainage of Left Sacroiliac Joint, Percutaneous Endoscopic Approach, Diagnostic
S920ZZ	Drainage of Lumbar Vertebral Disc, Open Approach	**0S953ZZ**	Drainage of Sacrococcygeal Joint, Percutaneous Approach	**0S984ZZ**	Drainage of Left Sacroiliac Joint, Percutaneous Endoscopic Approach
S9230Z	Drainage of Lumbar Vertebral Disc with Drainage Device, Percutaneous Approach	**0S9540Z**	Drainage of Sacrococcygeal Joint with Drainage Device, Percutaneous Endoscopic Approach	**0S9900Z**	Drainage of Right Hip Joint with Drainage Device, Open Approach
S923ZX	Drainage of Lumbar Vertebral Disc, Percutaneous Approach, Diagnostic	**0S954ZX**	Drainage of Sacrococcygeal Joint, Percutaneous Endoscopic Approach, Diagnostic	**0S990ZX**	Drainage of Right Hip Joint, Open Approach, Diagnostic
S923ZZ	Drainage of Lumbar Vertebral Disc, Percutaneous Approach	**0S954ZZ**	Drainage of Sacrococcygeal Joint, Percutaneous Endoscopic Approach	**0S990ZZ**	Drainage of Right Hip Joint, Open Approach
S9240Z	Drainage of Lumbar Vertebral Disc with Drainage Device, Percutaneous Endoscopic Approach	**0S9600Z**	Drainage of Coccygeal Joint with Drainage Device, Open Approach	**0S9930Z**	Drainage of Right Hip Joint with Drainage Device, Percutaneous Approach
S924ZX	Drainage of Lumbar Vertebral Disc, Percutaneous Endoscopic Approach, Diagnostic	**0S960ZX**	Drainage of Coccygeal Joint, Open Approach, Diagnostic	**0S993ZX**	Drainage of Right Hip Joint, Percutaneous Approach, Diagnostic
S924ZZ	Drainage of Lumbar Vertebral Disc, Percutaneous Endoscopic Approach	**0S960ZZ**	Drainage of Coccygeal Joint, Open Approach	**0S993ZZ**	Drainage of Right Hip Joint, Percutaneous Approach
S9300Z	Drainage of Lumbosacral Joint with Drainage Device, Open Approach	**0S9630Z**	Drainage of Coccygeal Joint with Drainage Device, Percutaneous Approach	**0S9940Z**	Drainage of Right Hip Joint with Drainage Device, Percutaneous Endoscopic Approach
S930ZX	Drainage of Lumbosacral Joint, Open Approach, Diagnostic	**0S963ZX**	Drainage of Coccygeal Joint, Percutaneous Approach, Diagnostic		
0S930ZZ	Drainage of Lumbosacral Joint, Open Approach	**0S963ZZ**	Drainage of Coccygeal Joint, Percutaneous Approach	**0S994ZX**	Drainage of Right Hip Joint, Percutaneous Endoscopic Approach, Diagnostic
0S9330Z	Drainage of Lumbosacral Joint with Drainage Device, Percutaneous Approach	**0S9640Z**	Drainage of Coccygeal Joint with Drainage Device, Percutaneous Endoscopic Approach	**0S994ZZ**	Drainage of Right Hip Joint, Percutaneous Endoscopic Approach
0S933ZX	Drainage of Lumbosacral Joint, Percutaneous Approach, Diagnostic	**0S964ZX**	Drainage of Coccygeal Joint, Percutaneous Endoscopic Approach, Diagnostic	**0S9B00Z**	Drainage of Left Hip Joint with Drainage Device, Open Approach
0S933ZZ	Drainage of Lumbosacral Joint, Percutaneous Approach	**0S964ZZ**	Drainage of Coccygeal Joint, Percutaneous Endoscopic Approach	**0S9B0ZX**	Drainage of Left Hip Joint, Open Approach, Diagnostic
0S9340Z	Drainage of Lumbosacral Joint with Drainage Device, Percutaneous Endoscopic Approach	**0S9700Z**	Drainage of Right Sacroiliac Joint with Drainage Device, Open Approach	**0S9B0ZZ**	Drainage of Left Hip Joint, Open Approach
0S934ZX	Drainage of Lumbosacral Joint, Percutaneous Endoscopic Approach, Diagnostic	**0S970ZX**	Drainage of Right Sacroiliac Joint, Open Approach, Diagnostic	**0S9B30Z**	Drainage of Left Hip Joint with Drainage Device, Percutaneous Approach
0S934ZZ	Drainage of Lumbosacral Joint, Percutaneous Endoscopic Approach	**0S970ZZ**	Drainage of Right Sacroiliac Joint, Open Approach	**0S9B3ZX**	Drainage of Left Hip Joint, Percutaneous Approach, Diagnostic
0S9400Z	Drainage of Lumbosacral Disc with Drainage Device, Open Approach	**0S9730Z**	Drainage of Right Sacroiliac Joint with Drainage Device, Percutaneous Approach	**0S9B3ZZ**	Drainage of Left Hip Joint, Percutaneous Approach
0S940ZX	Drainage of Lumbosacral Disc, Open Approach, Diagnostic	**0S973ZX**	Drainage of Right Sacroiliac Joint, Percutaneous Approach, Diagnostic	**0S9B40Z**	Drainage of Left Hip Joint with Drainage Device, Percutaneous Endoscopic Approach
0S940ZZ	Drainage of Lumbosacral Disc, Open Approach	**0S973ZZ**	Drainage of Right Sacroiliac Joint, Percutaneous Approach	**0S9B4ZX**	Drainage of Left Hip Joint, Percutaneous Endoscopic Approach, Diagnostic
				0S9B4ZZ	Drainage of Left Hip Joint, Percutaneous Endoscopic Approach

♀ Female-only	♂ Male-only	▲ Limited Coverage	● Non-OR	▰ HAC-associated procedure	▲ Non-covered procedures	✚ Combination

0S9C00Z	Drainage of Right Knee Joint with Drainage Device, Open Approach
0S9C0ZX	Drainage of Right Knee Joint, Open Approach, Diagnostic
0S9C0ZZ	Drainage of Right Knee Joint, Open Approach
0S9C30Z	Drainage of Right Knee Joint with Drainage Device, Percutaneous Approach
0S9C3ZX	Drainage of Right Knee Joint, Percutaneous Approach, Diagnostic
0S9C3ZZ	Drainage of Right Knee Joint, Percutaneous Approach
0S9C40Z	Drainage of Right Knee Joint with Drainage Device, Percutaneous Endoscopic Approach
0S9C4ZX	Drainage of Right Knee Joint, Percutaneous Endoscopic Approach, Diagnostic
0S9C4ZZ	Drainage of Right Knee Joint, Percutaneous Endoscopic Approach
0S9D00Z	Drainage of Left Knee Joint with Drainage Device, Open Approach
0S9D0ZX	Drainage of Left Knee Joint, Open Approach, Diagnostic
0S9D0ZZ	Drainage of Left Knee Joint, Open Approach
0S9D30Z	Drainage of Left Knee Joint with Drainage Device, Percutaneous Approach
0S9D3ZX	Drainage of Left Knee Joint, Percutaneous Approach, Diagnostic
0S9D3ZZ	Drainage of Left Knee Joint, Percutaneous Approach
0S9D40Z	Drainage of Left Knee Joint with Drainage Device, Percutaneous Endoscopic Approach
0S9D4ZX	Drainage of Left Knee Joint, Percutaneous Endoscopic Approach, Diagnostic
0S9D4ZZ	Drainage of Left Knee Joint, Percutaneous Endoscopic Approach
0S9F00Z	Drainage of Right Ankle Joint with Drainage Device, Open Approach
0S9F0ZX	Drainage of Right Ankle Joint, Open Approach, Diagnostic
0S9F0ZZ	Drainage of Right Ankle Joint, Open Approach
0S9F30Z	Drainage of Right Ankle Joint with Drainage Device, Percutaneous Approach
0S9F3ZX	Drainage of Right Ankle Joint, Percutaneous Approach, Diagnostic
0S9F3ZZ	Drainage of Right Ankle Joint, Percutaneous Approach
0S9F40Z	Drainage of Right Ankle Joint with Drainage Device, Percutaneous Endoscopic Approach
0S9F4ZX	Drainage of Right Ankle Joint, Percutaneous Endoscopic Approach, Diagnostic
0S9F4ZZ	Drainage of Right Ankle Joint, Percutaneous Endoscopic Approach
0S9G00Z	Drainage of Left Ankle Joint with Drainage Device, Open Approach
0S9G0ZX	Drainage of Left Ankle Joint, Open Approach, Diagnostic
0S9G0ZZ	Drainage of Left Ankle Joint, Open Approach
0S9G30Z	Drainage of Left Ankle Joint with Drainage Device, Percutaneous Approach
0S9G3ZX	Drainage of Left Ankle Joint, Percutaneous Approach, Diagnostic
0S9G3ZZ	Drainage of Left Ankle Joint, Percutaneous Approach
0S9G40Z	Drainage of Left Ankle Joint with Drainage Device, Percutaneous Endoscopic Approach
0S9G4ZX	Drainage of Left Ankle Joint, Percutaneous Endoscopic Approach, Diagnostic

0S9G4ZZ	Drainage of Left Ankle Joint, Percutaneous Endoscopic Approach
0S9H00Z	Drainage of Right Tarsal Joint with Drainage Device, Open Approach
0S9H0ZX	Drainage of Right Tarsal Joint, Open Approach, Diagnostic
0S9H0ZZ	Drainage of Right Tarsal Joint, Open Approach
0S9H30Z	Drainage of Right Tarsal Joint with Drainage Device, Percutaneous Approach
0S9H3ZX	Drainage of Right Tarsal Joint, Percutaneous Approach, Diagnostic
0S9H3ZZ	Drainage of Right Tarsal Joint, Percutaneous Approach
0S9H40Z	Drainage of Right Tarsal Joint with Drainage Device, Percutaneous Endoscopic Approach
0S9H4ZX	Drainage of Right Tarsal Joint, Percutaneous Endoscopic Approach, Diagnostic
0S9H4ZZ	Drainage of Right Tarsal Joint, Percutaneous Endoscopic Approach
0S9J00Z	Drainage of Left Tarsal Joint with Drainage Device, Open Approach
0S9J0ZX	Drainage of Left Tarsal Joint, Open Approach, Diagnostic
0S9J0ZZ	Drainage of Left Tarsal Joint, Open Approach
0S9J30Z	Drainage of Left Tarsal Joint with Drainage Device, Percutaneous Approach
0S9J3ZX	Drainage of Left Tarsal Joint, Percutaneous Approach, Diagnostic
0S9J3ZZ	Drainage of Left Tarsal Joint, Percutaneous Approach
0S9J40Z	Drainage of Left Tarsal Joint with Drainage Device, Percutaneous Endoscopic Approach
0S9J4ZX	Drainage of Left Tarsal Joint, Percutaneous Endoscopic Approach, Diagnostic
0S9J4ZZ	Drainage of Left Tarsal Joint, Percutaneous Endoscopic Approach
0S9K00Z	Drainage of Right Metatarsal-Tarsal Joint with Drainage Device, Open Approach
0S9K0ZX	Drainage of Right Metatarsal-Tarsal Joint, Open Approach, Diagnostic
0S9K0ZZ	Drainage of Right Metatarsal-Tarsal Joint, Open Approach
0S9K30Z	Drainage of Right Metatarsal-Tarsal Joint with Drainage Device, Percutaneous Approach
0S9K3ZX	Drainage of Right Metatarsal-Tarsal Joint, Percutaneous Approach, Diagnostic
0S9K3ZZ	Drainage of Right Metatarsal-Tarsal Joint, Percutaneous Approach
0S9K40Z	Drainage of Right Metatarsal-Tarsal Joint with Drainage Device, Percutaneous Endoscopic Approach
0S9K4ZX	Drainage of Right Metatarsal-Tarsal Joint, Percutaneous Endoscopic Approach, Diagnostic
0S9K4ZZ	Drainage of Right Metatarsal-Tarsal Joint, Percutaneous Endoscopic Approach
0S9L00Z	Drainage of Left Metatarsal-Tarsal Joint with Drainage Device, Open Approach
0.0S9L0ZZ	Drainage of Left Metatarsal-Tarsal Joint, Open Approach
0S9L30Z	Drainage of Left Metatarsal-Tarsal Joint with Drainage Device, Percutaneous Approach
0S9L3ZX	Drainage of Left Metatarsal-Tarsal Joint, Percutaneous Approach, Diagnostic
0S9L3ZZ	Drainage of Left Metatarsal-Tarsal Joint, Percutaneous Approach
0S9L40Z	Drainage of Left Metatarsal-Tarsal Joint with Drainage Device, Percutaneous Endoscopic Approach

0S9L4ZX	Drainage of Left Metatarsal-Tarsal Joint Percutaneous Endoscopic Approach, Diagnostic
0S9L4ZZ	Drainage of Left Metatarsal-Tarsal Joint Percutaneous Endoscopic Approach
0S9M00Z	Drainage of Right Metatarsal-Phalangeal Joint with Drainage Device, Open Approach
0S9M0ZX	Drainage of Right Metatarsal-Phalangeal Joint, Open Approach, Diagnostic
0S9M0ZZ	Drainage of Right Metatarsal-Phalangeal Joint, Open Approach
0S9M30Z	Drainage of Right Metatarsal-Phalangeal Joint with Drainage Device, Percutaneous Approach
0S9M3ZX	Drainage of Right Metatarsal-Phalangeal Joint, Percutaneous Approach, Diagnostic
0S9M3ZZ	Drainage of Right Metatarsal-Phalangeal Joint, Percutaneous Approach
0S9M40Z	Drainage of Right Metatarsal-Phalangeal Joint with Drainage Device, Percutaneous Endoscopic Approach
0S9M4ZX	Drainage of Right Metatarsal-Phalangeal Joint, Percutaneous Endoscopic Approach, Diagnostic
0S9M4ZZ	Drainage of Right Metatarsal-Phalangeal Joint, Percutaneous Endoscopic Approach
0S9N00Z	Drainage of Left Metatarsal-Phalangeal Joint with Drainage Device, Open Approach
0S9N0ZX	Drainage of Left Metatarsal-Phalangeal Joint, Open Approach, Diagnostic
0S9N0ZZ	Drainage of Left Metatarsal-Phalangeal Joint, Open Approach
0S9N30Z	Drainage of Left Metatarsal-Phalangeal Joint with Drainage Device, Percutaneous Approach
0S9N3ZX	Drainage of Left Metatarsal-Phalangeal Joint, Percutaneous Approach, Diagnostic
0S9N3ZZ	Drainage of Left Metatarsal-Phalangeal Joint, Percutaneous Approach
0S9N40Z	Drainage of Left Metatarsal-Phalangeal Joint with Drainage Device, Percutaneous Endoscopic Approach
0S9N4ZX	Drainage of Left Metatarsal-Phalangeal Joint, Percutaneous Endoscopic Approach, Diagnostic
0S9N4ZZ	Drainage of Left Metatarsal-Phalangeal Joint, Percutaneous Endoscopic Approach
0S9P00Z	Drainage of Right Toe Phalangeal Joint with Drainage Device, Open Approach
0S9P0ZX	Drainage of Right Toe Phalangeal Joint, Open Approach, Diagnostic
0S9P0ZZ	Drainage of Right Toe Phalangeal Joint, Open Approach
0S9P30Z	Drainage of Right Toe Phalangeal Joint with Drainage Device, Percutaneous Approach
0S9P3ZX	Drainage of Right Toe Phalangeal Joint, Percutaneous Approach, Diagnostic
0S9P3ZZ	Drainage of Right Toe Phalangeal Joint, Percutaneous Approach
0S9P40Z	Drainage of Right Toe Phalangeal Joint with Drainage Device, Percutaneous Endoscopic Approach
0S9P4ZX	Drainage of Right Toe Phalangeal Joint, Percutaneous Endoscopic Approach, Diagnostic
0S9P4ZZ	Drainage of Right Toe Phalangeal Joint, Percutaneous Endoscopic Approach
0S9Q00Z	Drainage of Left Toe Phalangeal Joint with Drainage Device, Open Approach
0S9Q0ZX	Drainage of Left Toe Phalangeal Joint, Open Approach, Diagnostic
0S9Q0ZZ	Drainage of Left Toe Phalangeal Joint, Open Approach

♀ Female-only   ♂ Male-only   ▲ Limited Coverage   ● Non-OR   ▦ HAC-associated procedure   ▲ Non-covered procedures   ✚ Combination

9Q30Z	Drainage of Left Toe Phalangeal Joint with Drainage Device, Percutaneous Approach
9Q3ZX	Drainage of Left Toe Phalangeal Joint, Percutaneous Approach, Diagnostic

0S9Q3ZZ	Drainage of Left Toe Phalangeal Joint, Percutaneous Approach
0S9Q40Z	Drainage of Left Toe Phalangeal Joint with Drainage Device, Percutaneous Endoscopic Approach

0S9Q4ZX	Drainage of Left Toe Phalangeal Joint, Percutaneous Endoscopic Approach, Diagnostic
0S9Q4ZZ	Drainage of Left Toe Phalangeal Joint, Percutaneous Endoscopic Approach

SB – Lower Joints, Excision

eview Coding Guidelines B3.4a and B3.4b

eview Coding Guideline B3.5

eview Coding Guideline B3.8

SB00ZX	Excision of Lumbar Vertebral Joint, Open Approach, Diagnostic
SB00ZZ	Excision of Lumbar Vertebral Joint, Open Approach
SB03ZX	Excision of Lumbar Vertebral Joint, Percutaneous Approach, Diagnostic
SB03ZZ	Excision of Lumbar Vertebral Joint, Percutaneous Approach
SB04ZX	Excision of Lumbar Vertebral Joint, Percutaneous Endoscopic Approach, Diagnostic
SB04ZZ	Excision of Lumbar Vertebral Joint, Percutaneous Endoscopic Approach
SB20ZX	Excision of Lumbar Vertebral Disc, Open Approach, Diagnostic
SB20ZZ	Excision of Lumbar Vertebral Disc, Open Approach
	AHA CC: 2Q, 2014, 6-7
SB23ZX	Excision of Lumbar Vertebral Disc, Percutaneous Approach, Diagnostic
SB23ZZ	Excision of Lumbar Vertebral Disc, Percutaneous Approach
SB24ZX	Excision of Lumbar Vertebral Disc, Percutaneous Endoscopic Approach, Diagnostic
SB24ZZ	Excision of Lumbar Vertebral Disc, Percutaneous Endoscopic Approach
SB30ZX	Excision of Lumbosacral Joint, Open Approach, Diagnostic
SB30ZZ	Excision of Lumbosacral Joint, Open Approach
SB33ZX	Excision of Lumbosacral Joint, Percutaneous Approach, Diagnostic
0SB33ZZ	Excision of Lumbosacral Joint, Percutaneous Approach
0SB34ZX	Excision of Lumbosacral Joint, Percutaneous Endoscopic Approach, Diagnostic
0SB34ZZ	Excision of Lumbosacral Joint, Percutaneous Endoscopic Approach
0SB40ZX	Excision of Lumbosacral Disc, Open Approach, Diagnostic
0SB40ZZ	Excision of Lumbosacral Disc, Open Approach
0SB43ZX	Excision of Lumbosacral Disc, Percutaneous Approach, Diagnostic
0SB43ZZ	Excision of Lumbosacral Disc, Percutaneous Approach
0SB44ZX	Excision of Lumbosacral Disc, Percutaneous Endoscopic Approach, Diagnostic
0SB44ZZ	Excision of Lumbosacral Disc, Percutaneous Endoscopic Approach
0SB50ZX	Excision of Sacrococcygeal Joint, Open Approach, Diagnostic
0SB50ZZ	Excision of Sacrococcygeal Joint, Open Approach
0SB53ZX	Excision of Sacrococcygeal Joint, Percutaneous Approach, Diagnostic
0SB53ZZ	Excision of Sacrococcygeal Joint, Percutaneous Approach
0SB54ZX	Excision of Sacrococcygeal Joint, Percutaneous Endoscopic Approach, Diagnostic

0SB54ZZ	Excision of Sacrococcygeal Joint, Percutaneous Endoscopic Approach
0SB60ZX	Excision of Coccygeal Joint, Open Approach, Diagnostic
0SB60ZZ	Excision of Coccygeal Joint, Open Approach
0SB63ZX	Excision of Coccygeal Joint, Percutaneous Approach, Diagnostic
0SB63ZZ	Excision of Coccygeal Joint, Percutaneous Approach
0SB64ZX	Excision of Coccygeal Joint, Percutaneous Endoscopic Approach, Diagnostic
0SB64ZZ	Excision of Coccygeal Joint, Percutaneous Endoscopic Approach
0SB70ZX	Excision of Right Sacroiliac Joint, Open Approach, Diagnostic
0SB70ZZ	Excision of Right Sacroiliac Joint, Open Approach
0SB73ZX	Excision of Right Sacroiliac Joint, Percutaneous Approach, Diagnostic
0SB73ZZ	Excision of Right Sacroiliac Joint, Percutaneous Approach
0SB74ZX	Excision of Right Sacroiliac Joint, Percutaneous Endoscopic Approach, Diagnostic
0SB74ZZ	Excision of Right Sacroiliac Joint, Percutaneous Endoscopic Approach
0SB80ZX	Excision of Left Sacroiliac Joint, Open Approach, Diagnostic
0SB80ZZ	Excision of Left Sacroiliac Joint, Open Approach
0SB83ZX	Excision of Left Sacroiliac Joint, Percutaneous Approach, Diagnostic
0SB83ZZ	Excision of Left Sacroiliac Joint, Percutaneous Approach
0SB84ZX	Excision of Left Sacroiliac Joint, Percutaneous Endoscopic Approach, Diagnostic
0SB84ZZ	Excision of Left Sacroiliac Joint, Percutaneous Endoscopic Approach
0SB90ZX	Excision of Right Hip Joint, Open Approach, Diagnostic
0SB90ZZ	Excision of Right Hip Joint, Open Approach
0SB93ZX	Excision of Right Hip Joint, Percutaneous Approach, Diagnostic
0SB93ZZ	Excision of Right Hip Joint, Percutaneous Approach
0SB94ZX	Excision of Right Hip Joint, Percutaneous Endoscopic Approach, Diagnostic
0SB94ZZ	Excision of Right Hip Joint, Percutaneous Endoscopic Approach
0SBB0ZX	Excision of Left Hip Joint, Open Approach, Diagnostic
0SBB0ZZ	Excision of Left Hip Joint, Open Approach
0SBB3ZX	Excision of Left Hip Joint, Percutaneous Approach, Diagnostic
0SBB3ZZ	Excision of Left Hip Joint, Percutaneous Approach
0SBB4ZX	Excision of Left Hip Joint, Percutaneous Endoscopic Approach, Diagnostic
0SBB4ZZ	Excision of Left Hip Joint, Percutaneous Endoscopic Approach
0SBC0ZX	Excision of Right Knee Joint, Open Approach, Diagnostic

0SBC0ZZ	Excision of Right Knee Joint, Open Approach
0SBC3ZX	Excision of Right Knee Joint, Percutaneous Approach, Diagnostic
0SBC3ZZ	Excision of Right Knee Joint, Percutaneous Approach
0SBC4ZX	Excision of Right Knee Joint, Percutaneous Endoscopic Approach, Diagnostic
0SBC4ZZ	Excision of Right Knee Joint, Percutaneous Endoscopic Approach
0SBD0ZX	Excision of Left Knee Joint, Open Approach, Diagnostic
0SBD0ZZ	Excision of Left Knee Joint, Open Approach
0SBD3ZX	Excision of Left Knee Joint, Percutaneous Approach, Diagnostic
0SBD3ZZ	Excision of Left Knee Joint, Percutaneous Approach
0SBD4ZX	Excision of Left Knee Joint, Percutaneous Endoscopic Approach, Diagnostic
0SBD4ZZ	Excision of Left Knee Joint, Percutaneous Endoscopic Approach
	AHA CC: 1Q, 2015, 34
0SBF0ZX	Excision of Right Ankle Joint, Open Approach, Diagnostic
0SBF0ZZ	Excision of Right Ankle Joint, Open Approach
0SBF3ZX	Excision of Right Ankle Joint, Percutaneous Approach, Diagnostic
0SBF3ZZ	Excision of Right Ankle Joint, Percutaneous Approach
0SBF4ZX	Excision of Right Ankle Joint, Percutaneous Endoscopic Approach, Diagnostic
0SBF4ZZ	Excision of Right Ankle Joint, Percutaneous Endoscopic Approach
0SBG0ZX	Excision of Left Ankle Joint, Open Approach, Diagnostic
0SBG0ZZ	Excision of Left Ankle Joint, Open Approach
0SBG3ZX	Excision of Left Ankle Joint, Percutaneous Approach, Diagnostic
0SBG3ZZ	Excision of Left Ankle Joint, Percutaneous Approach
0SBG4ZX	Excision of Left Ankle Joint, Percutaneous Endoscopic Approach, Diagnostic
0SBG4ZZ	Excision of Left Ankle Joint, Percutaneous Endoscopic Approach
0SBH0ZX	Excision of Right Tarsal Joint, Open Approach, Diagnostic
0SBH0ZZ	Excision of Right Tarsal Joint, Open Approach
0SBH3ZX	Excision of Right Tarsal Joint, Percutaneous Approach, Diagnostic
0SBH3ZZ	Excision of Right Tarsal Joint, Percutaneous Approach
0SBH4ZX	Excision of Right Tarsal Joint, Percutaneous Endoscopic Approach, Diagnostic
0SBH4ZZ	Excision of Right Tarsal Joint, Percutaneous Endoscopic Approach
0SBJ0ZX	Excision of Left Tarsal Joint, Open Approach, Diagnostic

♀ Female-only   ♂ Male-only   ▲ Limited Coverage   ● Non-OR   ▨ HAC-associated procedure   ▲ Non-covered procedures   + Combination

0SBJ0ZZ Excision of Left Tarsal Joint, Open Approach

0SBJ3ZX Excision of Left Tarsal Joint, Percutaneous Approach, Diagnostic

0SBJ3ZZ Excision of Left Tarsal Joint, Percutaneous Approach

0SBJ4ZX Excision of Left Tarsal Joint, Percutaneous Endoscopic Approach, Diagnostic

0SBJ4ZZ Excision of Left Tarsal Joint, Percutaneous Endoscopic Approach

0SBK0ZX Excision of Right Metatarsal-Tarsal Joint, Open Approach, Diagnostic

0SBK0ZZ Excision of Right Metatarsal-Tarsal Joint, Open Approach

0SBK3ZX Excision of Right Metatarsal-Tarsal Joint, Percutaneous Approach, Diagnostic

0SBK3ZZ Excision of Right Metatarsal-Tarsal Joint, Percutaneous Approach

0SBK4ZX Excision of Right Metatarsal-Tarsal Joint, Percutaneous Endoscopic Approach, Diagnostic

0SBK4ZZ Excision of Right Metatarsal-Tarsal Joint, Percutaneous Endoscopic Approach

0SBL0ZX Excision of Left Metatarsal-Tarsal Joint, Open Approach, Diagnostic

0SBL0ZZ Excision of Left Metatarsal-Tarsal Joint, Open Approach

0SBL3ZX Excision of Left Metatarsal-Tarsal Joint, Percutaneous Approach, Diagnostic

0SBL3ZZ Excision of Left Metatarsal-Tarsal Joint, Percutaneous Approach

0SBL4ZX Excision of Left Metatarsal-Tarsal Joint, Percutaneous Endoscopic Approach, Diagnostic

0SBL4ZZ Excision of Left Metatarsal-Tarsal Joint, Percutaneous Endoscopic Approach

0SBM0ZX Excision of Right Metatarsal-Phalangeal Joint, Open Approach, Diagnostic

0SBM0ZZ Excision of Right Metatarsal-Phalangeal Joint, Open Approach

0SBM3ZX Excision of Right Metatarsal-Phalangeal Joint, Percutaneous Approach, Diagnostic

0SBM3ZZ Excision of Right Metatarsal-Phalangeal Joint, Percutaneous Approach

0SBM4ZX Excision of Right Metatarsal-Phalangeal Joint, Percutaneous Endoscopic Approach, Diagnostic

0SBM4ZZ Excision of Right Metatarsal-Phalangeal Joint, Percutaneous Endoscopic Approach

0SBN0ZX Excision of Left Metatarsal-Phalangeal Joint, Open Approach, Diagnostic

0SBN0ZZ Excision of Left Metatarsal-Phalangeal Joint, Open Approach

0SBN3ZX Excision of Left Metatarsal-Phalangeal Joint, Percutaneous Approach, Diagnostic

0SBN3ZZ Excision of Left Metatarsal-Phalangeal Joint, Percutaneous Approach

0SBN4ZX Excision of Left Metatarsal-Phalangeal Joint, Percutaneous Endoscopic Approach, Diagnostic

0SBN4ZZ Excision of Left Metatarsal-Phalangeal Joint, Percutaneous Endoscopic Approach

0SBP0ZX Excision of Right Toe Phalangeal Joint, Open Approach, Diagnostic

0SBP0ZZ Excision of Right Toe Phalangeal Joint, Open Approach

0SBP3ZX Excision of Right Toe Phalangeal Joint, Percutaneous Approach, Diagnostic

0SBP3ZZ Excision of Right Toe Phalangeal Joint, Percutaneous Approach

0SBP4ZX Excision of Right Toe Phalangeal Joint, Percutaneous Endoscopic Approach, Diagnostic

0SBP4ZZ Excision of Right Toe Phalangeal Joint, Percutaneous Endoscopic Approach

0SBQ0ZX Excision of Left Toe Phalangeal Joint, Open Approach, Diagnostic

0SBQ0ZZ Excision of Left Toe Phalangeal Joint, Open Approach

0SBQ3ZX Excision of Left Toe Phalangeal Joint, Percutaneous Approach, Diagnostic

0SBQ3ZZ Excision of Left Toe Phalangeal Joint, Percutaneous Approach

0SBQ4ZX Excision of Left Toe Phalangeal Joint, Percutaneous Endoscopic Approach, Diagnostic

0SBQ4ZZ Excision of Left Toe Phalangeal Joint, Percutaneous Endoscopic Approach

0SC – Lower Joints, Extirpation

0SC00ZZ Extirpation of Matter from Lumbar Vertebral Joint, Open Approach

0SC03ZZ Extirpation of Matter from Lumbar Vertebral Joint, Percutaneous Approach

0SC04ZZ Extirpation of Matter from Lumbar Vertebral Joint, Percutaneous Endoscopic Approach

0SC20ZZ Extirpation of Matter from Lumbar Vertebral Disc, Open Approach

0SC23ZZ Extirpation of Matter from Lumbar Vertebral Disc, Percutaneous Approach

0SC24ZZ Extirpation of Matter from Lumbar Vertebral Disc, Percutaneous Endoscopic Approach

0SC30ZZ Extirpation of Matter from Lumbosacral Joint, Open Approach

0SC33ZZ Extirpation of Matter from Lumbosacral Joint, Percutaneous Approach

0SC34ZZ Extirpation of Matter from Lumbosacral Joint, Percutaneous Endoscopic Approach

0SC40ZZ Extirpation of Matter from Lumbosacral Disc, Open Approach

0SC43ZZ Extirpation of Matter from Lumbosacral Disc, Percutaneous Approach

0SC44ZZ Extirpation of Matter from Lumbosacral Disc, Percutaneous Endoscopic Approach

0SC50ZZ Extirpation of Matter from Sacrococcygeal Joint, Open Approach

0SC53ZZ Extirpation of Matter from Sacrococcygeal Joint, Percutaneous Approach

0SC54ZZ Extirpation of Matter from Sacrococcygeal Joint, Percutaneous Endoscopic Approach

0SC60ZZ Extirpation of Matter from Coccygeal Joint, Open Approach

0SC63ZZ Extirpation of Matter from Coccygeal Joint, Percutaneous Approach

0SC64ZZ Extirpation of Matter from Coccygeal Joint, Percutaneous Endoscopic Approach

0SC70ZZ Extirpation of Matter from Right Sacroiliac Joint, Open Approach

0SC73ZZ Extirpation of Matter from Right Sacroiliac Joint, Percutaneous Approach

0SC74ZZ Extirpation of Matter from Right Sacroiliac Joint, Percutaneous Endoscopic Approach

0SC80ZZ Extirpation of Matter from Left Sacroiliac Joint, Open Approach

0SC83ZZ Extirpation of Matter from Left Sacroiliac Joint, Percutaneous Approach

0SC84ZZ Extirpation of Matter from Left Sacroiliac Joint, Percutaneous Endoscopic Approach

0SC90ZZ Extirpation of Matter from Right Hip Joint, Open Approach

0SC93ZZ Extirpation of Matter from Right Hip Joint, Percutaneous Approach

0SC94ZZ Extirpation of Matter from Right Hip Joint, Percutaneous Endoscopic Approach

0SCB0ZZ Extirpation of Matter from Left Hip Joint, Open Approach

0SCB3ZZ Extirpation of Matter from Left Hip Joint, Percutaneous Approach

0SCB4ZZ Extirpation of Matter from Left Hip Joint, Percutaneous Endoscopic Approach

0SCC0ZZ Extirpation of Matter from Right Knee Joint, Open Approach

0SCC3ZZ Extirpation of Matter from Right Knee Joint, Percutaneous Approach

0SCC4ZZ Extirpation of Matter from Right Knee Joint, Percutaneous Endoscopic Approach

0SCD0ZZ Extirpation of Matter from Left Knee Joint, Open Approach

0SCD3ZZ Extirpation of Matter from Left Knee Joint, Percutaneous Approach

0SCD4ZZ Extirpation of Matter from Left Knee Joint, Percutaneous Endoscopic Approach

0SCF0ZZ Extirpation of Matter from Right Ankle Joint, Open Approach

0SCF3ZZ Extirpation of Matter from Right Ankle Joint, Percutaneous Approach

0SCF4ZZ Extirpation of Matter from Right Ankle Joint, Percutaneous Endoscopic Approach

0SCG0ZZ Extirpation of Matter from Left Ankle Joint, Open Approach

0SCG3ZZ Extirpation of Matter from Left Ankle Joint, Percutaneous Approach

0SCG4ZZ Extirpation of Matter from Left Ankle Joint, Percutaneous Endoscopic Approach

0SCH0ZZ Extirpation of Matter from Right Tarsal Joint, Open Approach

0SCH3ZZ Extirpation of Matter from Right Tarsal Joint, Percutaneous Approach

0SCH4ZZ Extirpation of Matter from Right Tarsal Joint, Percutaneous Endoscopic Approach

0SCJ0ZZ Extirpation of Matter from Left Tarsal Joint, Open Approach

0SCJ3ZZ Extirpation of Matter from Left Tarsal Joint, Percutaneous Approach

0SCJ4ZZ Extirpation of Matter from Left Tarsal Joint, Percutaneous Endoscopic Approach

0SCK0ZZ Extirpation of Matter from Right Metatarsal-Tarsal Joint, Open Approach

0SCK3ZZ Extirpation of Matter from Right Metatarsal-Tarsal Joint, Percutaneous Approach

0SCK4ZZ Extirpation of Matter from Right Metatarsal-Tarsal Joint, Percutaneous Endoscopic Approach

0SCL0ZZ Extirpation of Matter from Left Metatarsal-Tarsal Joint, Open Approach

0SCL3ZZ Extirpation of Matter from Left Metatarsal-Tarsal Joint, Percutaneous Approach

0SCL4ZZ Extirpation of Matter from Left Metatarsal-Tarsal Joint, Percutaneous Endoscopic Approach

0SCM0ZZ Extirpation of Matter from Right Metatarsal-Phalangeal Joint, Open Approach

0SCM3ZZ Extirpation of Matter from Right Metatarsal-Phalangeal Joint, Percutaneous Approach

0SCM4ZZ Extirpation of Matter from Right Metatarsal-Phalangeal Joint, Percutaneous Endoscopic Approach

0SCN0ZZ Extirpation of Matter from Left Metatarsal-Phalangeal Joint, Open Approach

♀ Female-only   ♂ Male-only   ▲ Limited Coverage   ● Non-OR   ▦ HAC-associated procedure   ▲ Non-covered procedures   ✚ Combination

CN3ZZ   Extirpation of Matter from Left Metatarsal-Phalangeal Joint, Percutaneous Approach

CN4ZZ   Extirpation of Matter from Left Metatarsal-Phalangeal Joint, Percutaneous Endoscopic Approach

CP0ZZ   Extirpation of Matter from Right Toe Phalangeal Joint, Open Approach

0SCP3ZZ   Extirpation of Matter from Right Toe Phalangeal Joint, Percutaneous Approach

0SCP4ZZ   Extirpation of Matter from Right Toe Phalangeal Joint, Percutaneous Endoscopic Approach

0SCQ0ZZ   Extirpation of Matter from Left Toe Phalangeal Joint, Open Approach

0SCQ3ZZ   Extirpation of Matter from Left Toe Phalangeal Joint, Percutaneous Approach

0SCQ4ZZ   Extirpation of Matter from Left Toe Phalangeal Joint, Percutaneous Endoscopic Approach

SG – Lower Joints, Fusion

or Fusion procedures involving the vertebral joints

eview Coding Guidelines B3.10a, B3.10b and B3.10c

SG0070   Fusion of Lumbar Vertebral Joint with Autologous Tissue Substitute, Anterior Approach, Anterior Column, Open Approach
- When reported with secondary diagnosis code T84.60XA, T84.610A, T84.611A, T84.612A, T84.613A, T84.614A, T84.615A, T84.619A, T84.63XA, T84.69XA, T84.7XXA

SG0071   Fusion of Lumbar Vertebral Joint with Autologous Tissue Substitute, Posterior Approach, Posterior Column, Open Approach
AHA CC: 1Q, 2013, 21-23; 3Q, 2013, 25-26
- When reported with secondary diagnosis code T84.60XA, T84.610A, T84.611A, T84.612A, T84.613A, T84.614A, T84.615A, T84.619A, T84.63XA, T84.69XA, T84.7XXA

SG007J   Fusion of Lumbar Vertebral Joint with Autologous Tissue Substitute, Posterior Approach, Anterior Column, Open Approach
- When reported with secondary diagnosis code T84.60XA, T84.610A, T84.611A, T84.612A, T84.613A, T84.614A, T84.615A, T84.619A, T84.63XA, T84.69XA, T84.7XXA

SG00A0   Fusion of Lumbar Vertebral Joint with Interbody Fusion Device, Anterior Approach, Anterior Column, Open Approach
- When reported with secondary diagnosis code T84.60XA, T84.610A, T84.611A, T84.612A, T84.613A, T84.614A, T84.615A, T84.619A, T84.63XA, T84.69XA, T84.7XXA

SG00A1   Fusion of Lumbar Vertebral Joint with Interbody Fusion Device, Posterior Approach, Posterior Column, Open Approach
- When reported with secondary diagnosis code T84.60XA, T84.610A, T84.611A, T84.612A, T84.613A, T84.614A, T84.615A, T84.619A, T84.63XA, T84.69XA, T84.7XXA

SG00AJ   Fusion of Lumbar Vertebral Joint with Interbody Fusion Device, Posterior Approach, Anterior Column, Open Approach
AHA CC: 3Q, 2013, 25-26
- When reported with secondary diagnosis code T84.60XA, T84.610A, T84.611A, T84.612A, T84.613A, T84.614A, T84.615A, T84.619A, T84.63XA, T84.69XA, T84.7XXA

0SG00J0   Fusion of Lumbar Vertebral Joint with Synthetic Substitute, Anterior Approach, Anterior Column, Open Approach
- When reported with secondary diagnosis code T84.60XA, T84.610A, T84.611A, T84.612A, T84.613A, T84.614A, T84.615A, T84.619A, T84.63XA, T84.69XA, T84.7XXA

0SG00J1   Fusion of Lumbar Vertebral Joint with Synthetic Substitute, Posterior Approach, Posterior Column, Open Approach
- When reported with secondary diagnosis code T84.60XA, T84.610A, T84.611A, T84.612A, T84.613A, T84.614A, T84.615A, T84.619A, T84.63XA, T84.69XA, T84.7XXA

0SG00JJ   Fusion of Lumbar Vertebral Joint with Synthetic Substitute, Posterior Approach, Anterior Column, Open Approach
- When reported with secondary diagnosis code T84.60XA, T84.610A, T84.611A, T84.612A, T84.613A, T84.614A, T84.615A, T84.619A, T84.63XA, T84.69XA, T84.7XXA

0SG00K0   Fusion of Lumbar Vertebral Joint with Nonautologous Tissue Substitute, Anterior Approach, Anterior Column, Open Approach
- When reported with secondary diagnosis code T84.60XA, T84.610A, T84.611A, T84.612A, T84.613A, T84.614A, T84.615A, T84.619A, T84.63XA, T84.69XA, T84.7XXA

0SG00K1   Fusion of Lumbar Vertebral Joint with Nonautologous Tissue Substitute, Posterior Approach, Posterior Column, Open Approach
- When reported with secondary diagnosis code T84.60XA, T84.610A, T84.611A, T84.612A, T84.613A, T84.614A, T84.615A, T84.619A, T84.63XA, T84.69XA, T84.7XXA

0SG00KJ   Fusion of Lumbar Vertebral Joint with Nonautologous Tissue Substitute, Posterior Approach, Anterior Column, Open Approach
- When reported with secondary diagnosis code T84.60XA, T84.610A, T84.611A, T84.612A, T84.613A, T84.614A, T84.615A, T84.619A, T84.63XA, T84.69XA, T84.7XXA

0SG00Z0   Fusion of Lumbar Vertebral Joint, Anterior Approach, Anterior Column, Open Approach
- When reported with secondary diagnosis code T84.60XA, T84.610A, T84.611A, T84.612A, T84.613A, T84.614A, T84.615A, T84.619A, T84.63XA, T84.69XA, T84.7XXA

0SG00Z1   Fusion of Lumbar Vertebral Joint, Posterior Approach, Posterior Column, Open Approach
- When reported with secondary diagnosis code T84.60XA, T84.610A, T84.611A, T84.612A, T84.613A, T84.614A, T84.615A, T84.619A, T84.63XA, T84.69XA, T84.7XXA

0SG00ZJ   Fusion of Lumbar Vertebral Joint, Posterior Approach, Anterior Column, Open Approach
- When reported with secondary diagnosis code T84.60XA, T84.610A, T84.611A, T84.612A, T84.613A, T84.614A, T84.615A, T84.619A, T84.63XA, T84.69XA, T84.7XXA

0SG0370   Fusion of Lumbar Vertebral Joint with Autologous Tissue Substitute, Anterior Approach, Anterior Column, Percutaneous Approach
- When reported with secondary diagnosis code T84.60XA, T84.610A, T84.611A, T84.612A, T84.613A, T84.614A, T84.615A, T84.619A, T84.63XA, T84.69XA, T84.7XXA

0SG0371   Fusion of Lumbar Vertebral Joint with Autologous Tissue Substitute, Posterior Approach, Posterior Column, Percutaneous Approach
- When reported with secondary diagnosis code T84.60XA, T84.610A, T84.611A, T84.612A, T84.613A, T84.614A, T84.615A, T84.619A, T84.63XA, T84.69XA, T84.7XXA

0SG037J   Fusion of Lumbar Vertebral Joint with Autologous Tissue Substitute, Posterior Approach, Anterior Column, Percutaneous Approach
- When reported with secondary diagnosis code T84.60XA, T84.610A, T84.611A, T84.612A, T84.613A, T84.614A, T84.615A, T84.619A, T84.63XA, T84.69XA, T84.7XXA

0SG03A0   Fusion of Lumbar Vertebral Joint with Interbody Fusion Device, Anterior Approach, Anterior Column, Percutaneous Approach
- When reported with secondary diagnosis code T84.60XA, T84.610A, T84.611A, T84.612A, T84.613A, T84.614A, T84.615A, T84.619A, T84.63XA, T84.69XA, T84.7XXA

0SG03A1   Fusion of Lumbar Vertebral Joint with Interbody Fusion Device, Posterior Approach, Posterior Column, Percutaneous Approach
- When reported with secondary diagnosis code T84.60XA, T84.610A, T84.611A, T84.612A, T84.613A, T84.614A, T84.615A, T84.619A, T84.63XA, T84.69XA, T84.7XXA

0SG03AJ   Fusion of Lumbar Vertebral Joint with Interbody Fusion Device, Posterior Approach, Anterior Column, Percutaneous Approach
- When reported with secondary diagnosis code T84.60XA, T84.610A, T84.611A, T84.612A, T84.613A, T84.614A, T84.615A, T84.619A, T84.63XA, T84.69XA, T84.7XXA

♀ Female-only   ♂ Male-only   ▲ Limited Coverage   ● Non-OR   ▣ HAC-associated procedure   ▲ Non-covered procedures   ✚ Combination

0SG03J0 Fusion of Lumbar Vertebral Joint with Synthetic Substitute, Anterior Approach, Anterior Column, Percutaneous Approach
When reported with secondary diagnosis code T84.60XA, T84.610A, T84.611A, T84.612A, T84.613A, T84.614A, T84.615A, T84.619A, T84.63XA, T84.69XA, T84.7XXA

0SG03J1 Fusion of Lumbar Vertebral Joint with Synthetic Substitute, Posterior Approach, Posterior Column, Percutaneous Approach
When reported with secondary diagnosis code T84.60XA, T84.610A, T84.611A, T84.612A, T84.613A, T84.614A, T84.615A, T84.619A, T84.63XA, T84.69XA, T84.7XXA

0SG03JJ Fusion of Lumbar Vertebral Joint with Synthetic Substitute, Posterior Approach, Anterior Column, Percutaneous Approach
When reported with secondary diagnosis code T84.60XA, T84.610A, T84.611A, T84.612A, T84.613A, T84.614A, T84.615A, T84.619A, T84.63XA, T84.69XA, T84.7XXA

0SG03K0 Fusion of Lumbar Vertebral Joint with Nonautologous Tissue Substitute, Anterior Approach, Anterior Column, Percutaneous Approach
When reported with secondary diagnosis code T84.60XA, T84.610A, T84.611A, T84.612A, T84.613A, T84.614A, T84.615A, T84.619A, T84.63XA, T84.69XA, T84.7XXA

0SG03K1 Fusion of Lumbar Vertebral Joint with Nonautologous Tissue Substitute, Posterior Approach, Posterior Column, Percutaneous Approach
When reported with secondary diagnosis code T84.60XA, T84.610A, T84.611A, T84.612A, T84.613A, T84.614A, T84.615A, T84.619A, T84.63XA, T84.69XA, T84.7XXA

0SG03KJ Fusion of Lumbar Vertebral Joint with Nonautologous Tissue Substitute, Posterior Approach, Anterior Column, Percutaneous Approach
When reported with secondary diagnosis code T84.60XA, T84.610A, T84.611A, T84.612A, T84.613A, T84.614A, T84.615A, T84.619A, T84.63XA, T84.69XA, T84.7XXA

0SG03Z0 Fusion of Lumbar Vertebral Joint, Anterior Approach, Anterior Column, Percutaneous Approach
When reported with secondary diagnosis code T84.60XA, T84.610A, T84.611A, T84.612A, T84.613A, T84.614A, T84.615A, T84.619A, T84.63XA, T84.69XA, T84.7XXA

0SG03Z1 Fusion of Lumbar Vertebral Joint, Posterior Approach, Posterior Column, Percutaneous Approach
When reported with secondary diagnosis code T84.60XA, T84.610A, T84.611A, T84.612A, T84.613A, T84.614A, T84.615A, T84.619A, T84.63XA, T84.69XA, T84.7XXA

0SG03ZJ Fusion of Lumbar Vertebral Joint, Posterior Approach, Anterior Column, Percutaneous Approach
When reported with secondary diagnosis code T84.60XA, T84.610A, T84.611A, T84.612A, T84.613A, T84.614A, T84.615A, T84.619A, T84.63XA, T84.69XA, T84.7XXA

0SG0470 Fusion of Lumbar Vertebral Joint with Autologous Tissue Substitute, Anterior Approach, Anterior Column, Percutaneous Endoscopic Approach
When reported with secondary diagnosis code T84.60XA, T84.610A, T84.611A, T84.612A, T84.613A, T84.614A, T84.615A, T84.619A, T84.63XA, T84.69XA, T84.7XXA

0SG0471 Fusion of Lumbar Vertebral Joint with Autologous Tissue Substitute, Posterior Approach, Posterior Column, Percutaneous Endoscopic Approach
When reported with secondary diagnosis code T84.60XA, T84.610A, T84.611A, T84.612A, T84.613A, T84.614A, T84.615A, T84.619A, T84.63XA, T84.69XA, T84.7XXA

0SG047J Fusion of Lumbar Vertebral Joint with Autologous Tissue Substitute, Posterior Approach, Anterior Column, Percutaneous Endoscopic Approach
When reported with secondary diagnosis code T84.60XA, T84.610A, T84.611A, T84.612A, T84.613A, T84.614A, T84.615A, T84.619A, T84.63XA, T84.69XA, T84.7XXA

0SG04A0 Fusion of Lumbar Vertebral Joint with Interbody Fusion Device, Anterior Approach, Anterior Column, Percutaneous Endoscopic Approach
When reported with secondary diagnosis code T84.60XA, T84.610A, T84.611A, T84.612A, T84.613A, T84.614A, T84.615A, T84.619A, T84.63XA, T84.69XA, T84.7XXA

0SG04A1 Fusion of Lumbar Vertebral Joint with Interbody Fusion Device, Posterior Approach, Posterior Column, Percutaneous Endoscopic Approach
When reported with secondary diagnosis code T84.60XA, T84.610A, T84.611A, T84.612A, T84.613A, T84.614A, T84.615A, T84.619A, T84.63XA, T84.69XA, T84.7XXA

0SG04AJ Fusion of Lumbar Vertebral Joint with Interbody Fusion Device, Posterior Approach, Anterior Column, Percutaneous Endoscopic Approach
When reported with secondary diagnosis code T84.60XA, T84.610A, T84.611A, T84.612A, T84.613A, T84.614A, T84.615A, T84.619A, T84.63XA, T84.69XA, T84.7XXA

0SG04J0 Fusion of Lumbar Vertebral Joint with Synthetic Substitute, Anterior Approach, Anterior Column, Percutaneous Endoscopic Approach
When reported with secondary diagnosis code T84.60XA, T84.610A, T84.611A, T84.612A, T84.613A, T84.614A, T84.615A, T84.619A, T84.63XA, T84.69XA, T84.7XXA

0SG04J1 Fusion of Lumbar Vertebral Joint with Synthetic Substitute, Posterior Approach, Posterior Column, Percutaneous Endoscopic Approach
When reported with secondary diagnosis code T84.60XA, T84.610A, T84.611A, T84.612A, T84.613A, T84.614A, T84.615A, T84.619A, T84.63XA, T84.69XA, T84.7XXA

0SG04JJ Fusion of Lumbar Vertebral Joint with Synthetic Substitute, Posterior Approach, Anterior Column, Percutaneous Endoscopic Approach

When reported with secondary diagnosis code T84.60XA, T84.610A, T84.611A, T84.612A, T84.613A, T84.614A, T84.615A, T84.619A, T84.63XA, T84.69XA, T84.7XXA

0SG04K0 Fusion of Lumbar Vertebral Joint with Nonautologous Tissue Substitute, Anterior Approach, Anterior Column, Percutaneous Endoscopic Approach
When reported with secondary diagnosis code T84.60XA, T84.610A, T84.611A, T84.612A, T84.613A, T84.614A, T84.615A, T84.619A, T84.63XA, T84.69XA, T84.7XXA

0SG04K1 Fusion of Lumbar Vertebral Joint with Nonautologous Tissue Substitute, Posterior Approach, Posterior Column, Percutaneous Endoscopic Approach
When reported with secondary diagnosis code T84.60XA, T84.610A, T84.611A, T84.612A, T84.613A, T84.614A, T84.615A, T84.619A, T84.63XA, T84.69XA, T84.7XXA

0SG04KJ Fusion of Lumbar Vertebral Joint with Nonautologous Tissue Substitute, Posterior Approach, Anterior Column, Percutaneous Endoscopic Approach
When reported with secondary diagnosis code T84.60XA, T84.610A, T84.611A, T84.612A, T84.613A, T84.614A, T84.615A, T84.619A, T84.63XA, T84.69XA, T84.7XXA

0SG04Z0 Fusion of Lumbar Vertebral Joint, Anterior Approach, Anterior Column, Percutaneous Endoscopic Approach
When reported with secondary diagnosis code T84.60XA, T84.610A, T84.611A, T84.612A, T84.613A, T84.614A, T84.615A, T84.619A, T84.63XA, T84.69XA, T84.7XXA

0SG04Z1 Fusion of Lumbar Vertebral Joint, Posterior Approach, Posterior Column, Percutaneous Endoscopic Approach
When reported with secondary diagnosis code T84.60XA, T84.610A, T84.611A, T84.612A, T84.613A, T84.614A, T84.615A, T84.619A, T84.63XA, T84.69XA, T84.7XXA

0SG04ZJ Fusion of Lumbar Vertebral Joint, Posterior Approach, Anterior Column, Percutaneous Endoscopic Approach
When reported with secondary diagnosis code T84.60XA, T84.610A, T84.611A, T84.612A, T84.613A, T84.614A, T84.615A, T84.619A, T84.63XA, T84.69XA, T84.7XXA

0SG1070 Fusion of 2 or more Lumbar Vertebral Joints with Autologous Tissue Substitute, Anterior Approach, Anterior Column, Open Approach
When reported with secondary diagnosis code T84.60XA, T84.610A, T84.611A, T84.612A, T84.613A, T84.614A, T84.615A, T84.619A, T84.63XA, T84.69XA, T84.7XXA

0SG1071 Fusion of 2 or more Lumbar Vertebral Joints with Autologous Tissue Substitute, Posterior Approach, Posterior Column, Open Approach
When reported with secondary diagnosis code T84.60XA, T84.610A, T84.611A, T84.612A, T84.613A, T84.614A, T84.615A, T84.619A, T84.63XA, T84.69XA, T84.7XXA

0SG107J Fusion of 2 or more Lumbar Vertebral Joints with Autologous Tissue Substitute, Posterior Approach, Anterior Column, Open Approach
AHA CC: 3Q, 2014, 36

Note Continued

♀ Female-only   ♂ Male-only   ▲ Limited Coverage   ● Non-OR   ■ HAC-associated procedure   ▲ Non-covered procedures   ✚ Combination

SG107J Continued Note

When reported with secondary diagnosis code T84.60XA, T84.610A, T84.611A, T84.612A, T84.613A, T84.614A, T84.615A, T84.619A, T84.63XA, T84.69XA, T84.7XXA

SG10A0 Fusion of 2 or more Lumbar Vertebral Joints with Interbody Fusion Device, Anterior Approach, Anterior Column, Open Approach

When reported with secondary diagnosis code T84.60XA, T84.610A, T84.611A, T84.612A, T84.613A, T84.614A, T84.615A, T84.619A, T84.63XA, T84.69XA, T84.7XXA

SG10A1 Fusion of 2 or more Lumbar Vertebral Joints with Interbody Fusion Device, Posterior Approach, Posterior Column, Open Approach

When reported with secondary diagnosis code T84.60XA, T84.610A, T84.611A, T84.612A, T84.613A, T84.614A, T84.615A, T84.619A, T84.63XA, T84.69XA, T84.7XXA

SG10AJ Fusion of 2 or more Lumbar Vertebral Joints with Interbody Fusion Device, Posterior Approach, Anterior Column, Open Approach

When reported with secondary diagnosis code T84.60XA, T84.610A, T84.611A, T84.612A, T84.613A, T84.614A, T84.615A, T84.619A, T84.63XA, T84.69XA, T84.7XXA

SG10J0 Fusion of 2 or more Lumbar Vertebral Joints with Synthetic Substitute, Anterior Approach, Anterior Column, Open Approach

When reported with secondary diagnosis code T84.60XA, T84.610A, T84.611A, T84.612A, T84.613A, T84.614A, T84.615A, T84.619A, T84.63XA, T84.69XA, T84.7XXA

SG10J1 Fusion of 2 or more Lumbar Vertebral Joints with Synthetic Substitute, Posterior Approach, Posterior Column, Open Approach

When reported with secondary diagnosis code T84.60XA, T84.610A, T84.611A, T84.612A, T84.613A, T84.614A, T84.615A, T84.619A, T84.63XA, T84.69XA, T84.7XXA

SG10JJ Fusion of 2 or more Lumbar Vertebral Joints with Synthetic Substitute, Posterior Approach, Anterior Column, Open Approach

When reported with secondary diagnosis code T84.60XA, T84.610A, T84.611A, T84.612A, T84.613A, T84.614A, T84.615A, T84.619A, T84.63XA, T84.69XA, T84.7XXA

0SG10K0 Fusion of 2 or more Lumbar Vertebral Joints with Nonautologous Tissue Substitute, Anterior Approach, Anterior Column, Open Approach

When reported with secondary diagnosis code T84.60XA, T84.610A, T84.611A, T84.612A, T84.613A, T84.614A, T84.615A, T84.619A, T84.63XA, T84.69XA, T84.7XXA

0SG10K1 Fusion of 2 or more Lumbar Vertebral Joints with Nonautologous Tissue Substitute, Posterior Approach, Posterior Column, Open Approach

When reported with secondary diagnosis code T84.60XA, T84.610A, T84.611A, T84.612A, T84.613A, T84.614A, T84.615A, T84.619A, T84.63XA, T84.69XA, T84.7XXA

0SG10KJ Fusion of 2 or more Lumbar Vertebral Joints with Nonautologous Tissue Substitute, Posterior Approach, Anterior Column, Open Approach

When reported with secondary diagnosis code T84.60XA, T84.610A, T84.611A, T84.612A, T84.613A, T84.614A, T84.615A, T84.619A, T84.63XA, T84.69XA, T84.7XXA

0SG10Z0 Fusion of 2 or more Lumbar Vertebral Joints, Anterior Approach, Anterior Column, Open Approach

When reported with secondary diagnosis code T84.60XA, T84.610A, T84.611A, T84.612A, T84.613A, T84.614A, T84.615A, T84.619A, T84.63XA, T84.69XA, T84.7XXA

0SG10Z1 Fusion of 2 or more Lumbar Vertebral Joints, Posterior Approach, Posterior Column, Open Approach

When reported with secondary diagnosis code T84.60XA, T84.610A, T84.611A, T84.612A, T84.613A, T84.614A, T84.615A, T84.619A, T84.63XA, T84.69XA, T84.7XXA

0SG10ZJ Fusion of 2 or more Lumbar Vertebral Joints, Posterior Approach, Anterior Column, Open Approach

When reported with secondary diagnosis code T84.60XA, T84.610A, T84.611A, T84.612A, T84.613A, T84.614A, T84.615A, T84.619A, T84.63XA, T84.69XA, T84.7XXA

0SG1370 Fusion of 2 or more Lumbar Vertebral Joints with Autologous Tissue Substitute, Anterior Approach, Anterior Column, Percutaneous Approach

When reported with secondary diagnosis code T84.60XA, T84.610A, T84.611A, T84.612A, T84.613A, T84.614A, T84.615A, T84.619A, T84.63XA, T84.69XA, T84.7XXA

0SG1371 Fusion of 2 or more Lumbar Vertebral Joints with Autologous Tissue Substitute, Posterior Approach, Posterior Column, Percutaneous Approach

When reported with secondary diagnosis code T84.60XA, T84.610A, T84.611A, T84.612A, T84.613A, T84.614A, T84.615A, T84.619A, T84.63XA, T84.69XA, T84.7XXA

0SG137J Fusion of 2 or more Lumbar Vertebral Joints with Autologous Tissue Substitute, Posterior Approach, Anterior Column, Percutaneous Approach

When reported with secondary diagnosis code T84.60XA, T84.610A, T84.611A, T84.612A, T84.613A, T84.614A, T84.615A, T84.619A, T84.63XA, T84.69XA, T84.7XXA

0SG13A0 Fusion of 2 or more Lumbar Vertebral Joints with Interbody Fusion Device, Anterior Approach, Anterior Column, Percutaneous Approach

When reported with secondary diagnosis code T84.60XA, T84.610A, T84.611A, T84.612A, T84.613A, T84.614A, T84.615A, T84.619A, T84.63XA, T84.69XA, T84.7XXA

0SG13A1 Fusion of 2 or more Lumbar Vertebral Joints with Interbody Fusion Device, Posterior Approach, Posterior Column, Percutaneous Approach

When reported with secondary diagnosis code T84.60XA, T84.610A, T84.611A, T84.612A, T84.613A, T84.614A, T84.615A, T84.619A, T84.63XA, T84.69XA, T84.7XXA

0SG13AJ Fusion of 2 or more Lumbar Vertebral Joints with Interbody Fusion Device, Posterior Approach, Anterior Column, Percutaneous Approach

When reported with secondary diagnosis code T84.60XA, T84.610A, T84.611A, T84.612A, T84.613A, T84.614A, T84.615A, T84.619A, T84.63XA, T84.69XA, T84.7XXA

0SG13J0 Fusion of 2 or more Lumbar Vertebral Joints with Synthetic Substitute, Anterior Approach, Anterior Column, Percutaneous Approach

When reported with secondary diagnosis code T84.60XA, T84.610A, T84.611A, T84.612A, T84.613A, T84.614A, T84.615A, T84.619A, T84.63XA, T84.69XA, T84.7XXA

0SG13J1 Fusion of 2 or more Lumbar Vertebral Joints with Synthetic Substitute, Posterior Approach, Posterior Column, Percutaneous Approach

When reported with secondary diagnosis code T84.60XA, T84.610A, T84.611A, T84.612A, T84.613A, T84.614A, T84.615A, T84.619A, T84.63XA, T84.69XA, T84.7XXA

0SG13JJ Fusion of 2 or more Lumbar Vertebral Joints with Synthetic Substitute, Posterior Approach, Anterior Column, Percutaneous Approach

When reported with secondary diagnosis code T84.60XA, T84.610A, T84.611A, T84.612A, T84.613A, T84.614A, T84.615A, T84.619A, T84.63XA, T84.69XA, T84.7XXA

0SG13K0 Fusion of 2 or more Lumbar Vertebral Joints with Nonautologous Tissue Substitute, Anterior Approach, Anterior Column, Percutaneous Approach

When reported with secondary diagnosis code T84.60XA, T84.610A, T84.611A, T84.612A, T84.613A, T84.614A, T84.615A, T84.619A, T84.63XA, T84.69XA, T84.7XXA

0SG13K1 Fusion of 2 or more Lumbar Vertebral Joints with Nonautologous Tissue Substitute, Posterior Approach, Posterior Column, Percutaneous Approach

When reported with secondary diagnosis code T84.60XA, T84.610A, T84.611A, T84.612A, T84.613A, T84.614A, T84.615A, T84.619A, T84.63XA, T84.69XA, T84.7XXA

0SG13KJ Fusion of 2 or more Lumbar Vertebral Joints with Nonautologous Tissue Substitute, Posterior Approach, Anterior Column, Percutaneous Approach

When reported with secondary diagnosis code T84.60XA, T84.610A, T84.611A, T84.612A, T84.613A, T84.614A, T84.615A, T84.619A, T84.63XA, T84.69XA, T84.7XXA

0SG13Z0 Fusion of 2 or more Lumbar Vertebral Joints, Anterior Approach, Anterior Column, Percutaneous Approach

When reported with secondary diagnosis code T84.60XA, T84.610A, T84.611A, T84.612A, T84.613A, T84.614A, T84.615A, T84.619A, T84.63XA, T84.69XA, T84.7XXA

0SG13Z1 Fusion of 2 or more Lumbar Vertebral Joints, Posterior Approach, Posterior Column, Percutaneous Approach

Note Continued

♀ Female-only   ♂ Male-only   ▲ Limited Coverage   ● Non-OR   ▦ HAC-associated procedure   ▲ Non-covered procedures   ✚ Combination

0SG13Z1 Continued Note

⬛ When reported with secondary diagnosis code T84.60XA, T84.610A, T84.611A, T84.612A, T84.613A, T84.614A, T84.615A, T84.619A, T84.63XA, T84.69XA, T84.7XXA

0SG13ZJ Fusion of 2 or more Lumbar Vertebral Joints, Posterior Approach, Anterior Column, Percutaneous Approach

⬛ When reported with secondary diagnosis code T84.60XA, T84.610A, T84.611A, T84.612A, T84.613A, T84.614A, T84.615A, T84.619A, T84.63XA, T84.69XA, T84.7XXA

0SG1470 Fusion of 2 or more Lumbar Vertebral Joints with Autologous Tissue Substitute, Anterior Approach, Anterior Column, Percutaneous Endoscopic Approach

⬛ When reported with secondary diagnosis code T84.60XA, T84.610A, T84.611A, T84.612A, T84.613A, T84.614A, T84.615A, T84.619A, T84.63XA, T84.69XA, T84.7XXA

0SG1471 Fusion of 2 or more Lumbar Vertebral Joints with Autologous Tissue Substitute, Posterior Approach, Posterior Column, Percutaneous Endoscopic Approach

⬛ When reported with secondary diagnosis code T84.60XA, T84.610A, T84.611A, T84.612A, T84.613A, T84.614A, T84.615A, T84.619A, T84.63XA, T84.69XA, T84.7XXA

0SG147J Fusion of 2 or more Lumbar Vertebral Joints with Autologous Tissue Substitute, Posterior Approach, Anterior Column, Percutaneous Endoscopic Approach

⬛ When reported with secondary diagnosis code T84.60XA, T84.610A, T84.611A, T84.612A, T84.613A, T84.614A, T84.615A, T84.619A, T84.63XA, T84.69XA, T84.7XXA

0SG14A0 Fusion of 2 or more Lumbar Vertebral Joints with Interbody Fusion Device, Anterior Approach, Anterior Column, Percutaneous Endoscopic Approach

⬛ When reported with secondary diagnosis code T84.60XA, T84.610A, T84.611A, T84.612A, T84.613A, T84.614A, T84.615A, T84.619A, T84.63XA, T84.69XA, T84.7XXA

0SG14A1 Fusion of 2 or more Lumbar Vertebral Joints with Interbody Fusion Device, Posterior Approach, Posterior Column, Percutaneous Endoscopic Approach

⬛ When reported with secondary diagnosis code T84.60XA, T84.610A, T84.611A, T84.612A, T84.613A, T84.614A, T84.615A, T84.619A, T84.63XA, T84.69XA, T84.7XXA

0SG14AJ Fusion of 2 or more Lumbar Vertebral Joints with Interbody Fusion Device, Posterior Approach, Anterior Column, Percutaneous Endoscopic Approach

⬛ When reported with secondary diagnosis code T84.60XA, T84.610A, T84.611A, T84.612A, T84.613A, T84.614A, T84.615A, T84.619A, T84.63XA, T84.69XA, T84.7XXA

0SG14J0 Fusion of 2 or more Lumbar Vertebral Joints with Synthetic Substitute, Anterior Approach, Anterior Column, Percutaneous Endoscopic Approach

⬛ When reported with secondary diagnosis code T84.60XA, T84.610A, T84.611A, T84.612A, T84.613A, T84.614A, T84.615A, T84.619A, T84.63XA, T84.69XA, T84.7XXA

0SG14J1 Fusion of 2 or more Lumbar Vertebral Joints with Synthetic Substitute,

Posterior Approach, Posterior Column, Percutaneous Endoscopic Approach

⬛ When reported with secondary diagnosis code T84.60XA, T84.610A, T84.611A, T84.612A, T84.613A, T84.614A, T84.615A, T84.619A, T84.63XA, T84.69XA, T84.7XXA

0SG14JJ Fusion of 2 or more Lumbar Vertebral Joints with Synthetic Substitute, Posterior Approach, Anterior Column, Percutaneous Endoscopic Approach

⬛ When reported with secondary diagnosis code T84.60XA, T84.610A, T84.611A, T84.612A, T84.613A, T84.614A, T84.615A, T84.619A, T84.63XA, T84.69XA, T84.7XXA

0SG14K0 Fusion of 2 or more Lumbar Vertebral Joints with Nonautologous Tissue Substitute, Anterior Approach, Anterior Column, Percutaneous Endoscopic Approach

⬛ When reported with secondary diagnosis code T84.60XA, T84.610A, T84.611A, T84.612A, T84.613A, T84.614A, T84.615A, T84.619A, T84.63XA, T84.69XA, T84.7XXA

0SG14K1 Fusion of 2 or more Lumbar Vertebral Joints with Nonautologous Tissue Substitute, Posterior Approach, Posterior Column, Percutaneous Endoscopic Approach

⬛ When reported with secondary diagnosis code T84.60XA, T84.610A, T84.611A, T84.612A, T84.613A, T84.614A, T84.615A, T84.619A, T84.63XA, T84.69XA, T84.7XXA

0SG14KJ Fusion of 2 or more Lumbar Vertebral Joints with Nonautologous Tissue Substitute, Posterior Approach, Anterior Column, Percutaneous Endoscopic Approach

⬛ When reported with secondary diagnosis code T84.60XA, T84.610A, T84.611A, T84.612A, T84.613A, T84.614A, T84.615A, T84.619A, T84.63XA, T84.69XA, T84.7XXA

0SG14Z0 Fusion of 2 or more Lumbar Vertebral Joints, Anterior Approach, Anterior Column, Percutaneous Endoscopic Approach

⬛ When reported with secondary diagnosis code T84.60XA, T84.610A, T84.611A, T84.612A, T84.613A, T84.614A, T84.615A, T84.619A, T84.63XA, T84.69XA, T84.7XXA

0SG14Z1 Fusion of 2 or more Lumbar Vertebral Joints, Posterior Approach, Posterior Column, Percutaneous Endoscopic Approach

⬛ When reported with secondary diagnosis code T84.60XA, T84.610A, T84.611A, T84.612A, T84.613A, T84.614A, T84.615A, T84.619A, T84.63XA, T84.69XA, T84.7XXA

0SG14ZJ Fusion of 2 or more Lumbar Vertebral Joints, Posterior Approach, Anterior Column, Percutaneous Endoscopic Approach

⬛ When reported with secondary diagnosis code T84.60XA, T84.610A, T84.611A, T84.612A, T84.613A, T84.614A, T84.615A, T84.619A, T84.63XA, T84.69XA, T84.7XXA

0SG3070 Fusion of Lumbosacral Joint with Autologous Tissue Substitute, Anterior Approach, Anterior Column, Open Approach

⬛ When reported with secondary diagnosis code T84.60XA, T84.610A, T84.611A, T84.612A, T84.613A, T84.614A, T84.615A, T84.619A, T84.63XA, T84.69XA, T84.7XXA

0SG3071 Fusion of Lumbosacral Joint with Autologous Tissue Substitute, Posterior Approach, Posterior Column, Open Approach

⬛ When reported with secondary diagnosis code T84.60XA, T84.610A, T84.611A, T84.612A, T84.613A, T84.614A, T84.615A, T84.619A, T84.63XA, T84.69XA, T84.7XXA

0SG307J Fusion of Lumbosacral Joint with Autologous Tissue Substitute, Posterior Approach, Anterior Column, Open Approach

⬛ When reported with secondary diagnosis code T84.60XA, T84.610A, T84.611A, T84.612A, T84.613A, T84.614A, T84.615A, T84.619A, T84.63XA, T84.69XA, T84.7XXA

0SG30A0 Fusion of Lumbosacral Joint with Interbody Fusion Device, Anterior Approach, Anterior Column, Open Approach

⬛ When reported with secondary diagnosis code T84.60XA, T84.610A, T84.611A, T84.612A, T84.613A, T84.614A, T84.615A, T84.619A, T84.63XA, T84.69XA, T84.7XXA

0SG30A1 Fusion of Lumbosacral Joint with Interbody Fusion Device, Posterior Approach, Posterior Column, Open Approach

⬛ When reported with secondary diagnosis code T84.60XA, T84.610A, T84.611A, T84.612A, T84.613A, T84.614A, T84.615A, T84.619A, T84.63XA, T84.69XA, T84.7XXA

0SG30AJ Fusion of Lumbosacral Joint with Interbody Fusion Device, Posterior Approach, Anterior Column, Open Approach

⬛ When reported with secondary diagnosis code T84.60XA, T84.610A, T84.611A, T84.612A, T84.613A, T84.614A, T84.615A, T84.619A, T84.63XA, T84.69XA, T84.7XXA

0SG30J0 Fusion of Lumbosacral Joint with Synthetic Substitute, Anterior Approach, Anterior Column, Open Approach

⬛ When reported with secondary diagnosis code T84.60XA, T84.610A, T84.611A, T84.612A, T84.613A, T84.614A, T84.615A, T84.619A, T84.63XA, T84.69XA, T84.7XXA

0SG30J1 Fusion of Lumbosacral Joint with Synthetic Substitute, Posterior Approach, Posterior Column, Open Approach

⬛ When reported with secondary diagnosis code T84.60XA, T84.610A, T84.611A, T84.612A, T84.613A, T84.614A, T84.615A, T84.619A, T84.63XA, T84.69XA, T84.7XXA

0SG30JJ Fusion of Lumbosacral Joint with Synthetic Substitute, Posterior Approach, Anterior Column, Open Approach

⬛ When reported with secondary diagnosis code T84.60XA, T84.610A, T84.611A, T84.612A, T84.613A, T84.614A, T84.615A, T84.619A, T84.63XA, T84.69XA, T84.7XXA

0SG30K0 Fusion of Lumbosacral Joint with Nonautologous Tissue Substitute, Anterior Approach, Anterior Column, Open Approach

Note Continued

♀ Female-only   ♂ Male-only   ▲ Limited Coverage   ● Non-OR   ⬛ HAC-associated procedure   ▲ Non-covered procedures   ✚ Combination

0SG30K0 Continued Note

When reported with secondary diagnosis code T84.60XA, T84.610A, T84.611A, T84.612A, T84.613A, T84.614A, T84.615A, T84.619A, T84.63XA, T84.69XA, T84.7XXA

0SG30K1 Fusion of Lumbosacral Joint with Nonautologous Tissue Substitute, Posterior Approach, Posterior Column, Open Approach

When reported with secondary diagnosis code T84.60XA, T84.610A, T84.611A, T84.612A, T84.613A, T84.614A, T84.615A, T84.619A, T84.63XA, T84.69XA, T84.7XXA

0SG30KJ Fusion of Lumbosacral Joint with Nonautologous Tissue Substitute, Posterior Approach, Anterior Column, Open Approach

When reported with secondary diagnosis code T84.60XA, T84.610A, T84.611A, T84.612A, T84.613A, T84.614A, T84.615A, T84.619A, T84.63XA, T84.69XA, T84.7XXA

0SG30Z0 Fusion of Lumbosacral Joint, Anterior Approach, Anterior Column, Open Approach

When reported with secondary diagnosis code T84.60XA, T84.610A, T84.611A, T84.612A, T84.613A, T84.614A, T84.615A, T84.619A, T84.63XA, T84.69XA, T84.7XXA

0SG30Z1 Fusion of Lumbosacral Joint, Posterior Approach, Posterior Column, Open Approach

When reported with secondary diagnosis code T84.60XA, T84.610A, T84.611A, T84.612A, T84.613A, T84.614A, T84.615A, T84.619A, T84.63XA, T84.69XA, T84.7XXA

0SG30ZJ Fusion of Lumbosacral Joint, Posterior Approach, Anterior Column, Open Approach

When reported with secondary diagnosis code T84.60XA, T84.610A, T84.611A, T84.612A, T84.613A, T84.614A, T84.615A, T84.619A, T84.63XA, T84.69XA, T84.7XXA

0SG3370 Fusion of Lumbosacral Joint with Autologous Tissue Substitute, Anterior Approach, Anterior Column, Percutaneous Approach

When reported with secondary diagnosis code T84.60XA, T84.610A, T84.611A, T84.612A, T84.613A, T84.614A, T84.615A, T84.619A, T84.63XA, T84.69XA, T84.7XXA

0SG3371 Fusion of Lumbosacral Joint with Autologous Tissue Substitute, Posterior Approach, Posterior Column, Percutaneous Approach

When reported with secondary diagnosis code T84.60XA, T84.610A, T84.611A, T84.612A, T84.613A, T84.614A, T84.615A, T84.619A, T84.63XA, T84.69XA, T84.7XXA

0SG337J Fusion of Lumbosacral Joint with Autologous Tissue Substitute, Posterior Approach, Anterior Column, Percutaneous Approach

When reported with secondary diagnosis code T84.60XA, T84.610A, T84.611A, T84.612A, T84.613A, T84.614A, T84.615A, T84.619A, T84.63XA, T84.69XA, T84.7XXA

0SG33A0 Fusion of Lumbosacral Joint with Interbody Fusion Device, Anterior Approach, Anterior Column, Percutaneous Approach

When reported with secondary diagnosis code T84.60XA, T84.610A, T84.611A, T84.612A, T84.613A, T84.614A, T84.615A, T84.619A, T84.63XA, T84.69XA, T84.7XXA

0SG33A1 Fusion of Lumbosacral Joint with Interbody Fusion Device, Posterior Approach, Posterior Column, Percutaneous Approach

When reported with secondary diagnosis code T84.60XA, T84.610A, T84.611A, T84.612A, T84.613A, T84.614A, T84.615A, T84.619A, T84.63XA, T84.69XA, T84.7XXA

0SG33AJ Fusion of Lumbosacral Joint with Interbody Fusion Device, Posterior Approach, Anterior Column, Percutaneous Approach

When reported with secondary diagnosis code T84.60XA, T84.610A, T84.611A, T84.612A, T84.613A, T84.614A, T84.615A, T84.619A, T84.63XA, T84.69XA, T84.7XXA

0SG33J0 Fusion of Lumbosacral Joint with Synthetic Substitute, Anterior Approach, Anterior Column, Percutaneous Approach

When reported with secondary diagnosis code T84.60XA, T84.610A, T84.611A, T84.612A, T84.613A, T84.614A, T84.615A, T84.619A, T84.63XA, T84.69XA, T84.7XXA

0SG33J1 Fusion of Lumbosacral Joint with Synthetic Substitute, Posterior Approach, Posterior Column, Percutaneous Approach

When reported with secondary diagnosis code T84.60XA, T84.610A, T84.611A, T84.612A, T84.613A, T84.614A, T84.615A, T84.619A, T84.63XA, T84.69XA, T84.7XXA

0SG33JJ Fusion of Lumbosacral Joint with Synthetic Substitute, Posterior Approach, Anterior Column, Percutaneous Approach

When reported with secondary diagnosis code T84.60XA, T84.610A, T84.611A, T84.612A, T84.613A, T84.614A, T84.615A, T84.619A, T84.63XA, T84.69XA, T84.7XXA

0SG33K0 Fusion of Lumbosacral Joint with Nonautologous Tissue Substitute, Anterior Approach, Anterior Column, Percutaneous Approach

When reported with secondary diagnosis code T84.60XA, T84.610A, T84.611A, T84.612A, T84.613A, T84.614A, T84.615A, T84.619A, T84.63XA, T84.69XA, T84.7XXA

0SG33K1 Fusion of Lumbosacral Joint with Nonautologous Tissue Substitute, Posterior Approach, Posterior Column, Percutaneous Approach

When reported with secondary diagnosis code T84.60XA, T84.610A, T84.611A, T84.612A, T84.613A, T84.614A, T84.615A, T84.619A, T84.63XA, T84.69XA, T84.7XXA

0SG33KJ Fusion of Lumbosacral Joint with Nonautologous Tissue Substitute, Posterior Approach, Anterior Column, Percutaneous Approach

When reported with secondary diagnosis code T84.60XA, T84.610A, T84.611A, T84.612A, T84.613A, T84.614A, T84.615A, T84.619A, T84.63XA, T84.69XA, T84.7XXA

0SG33Z0 Fusion of Lumbosacral Joint, Anterior Approach, Anterior Column, Percutaneous Approach

When reported with secondary diagnosis code T84.60XA, T84.610A, T84.611A,

0SG33Z1 Fusion of Lumbosacral Joint, Posterior Approach, Posterior Column, Percutaneous Approach

When reported with secondary diagnosis code T84.60XA, T84.610A, T84.611A, T84.612A, T84.613A, T84.614A, T84.615A, T84.619A, T84.63XA, T84.69XA, T84.7XXA

0SG33ZJ Fusion of Lumbosacral Joint, Posterior Approach, Anterior Column, Percutaneous Approach

When reported with secondary diagnosis code T84.60XA, T84.610A, T84.611A, T84.612A, T84.613A, T84.614A, T84.615A, T84.619A, T84.63XA, T84.69XA, T84.7XXA

0SG3470 Fusion of Lumbosacral Joint with Autologous Tissue Substitute, Anterior Approach, Anterior Column, Percutaneous Endoscopic Approach

When reported with secondary diagnosis code T84.60XA, T84.610A, T84.611A, T84.612A, T84.613A, T84.614A, T84.615A, T84.619A, T84.63XA, T84.69XA, T84.7XXA

0SG3471 Fusion of Lumbosacral Joint with Autologous Tissue Substitute, Posterior Approach, Posterior Column, Percutaneous Endoscopic Approach

When reported with secondary diagnosis code T84.60XA, T84.610A, T84.611A, T84.612A, T84.613A, T84.614A, T84.615A, T84.619A, T84.63XA, T84.69XA, T84.7XXA

0SG347J Fusion of Lumbosacral Joint with Autologous Tissue Substitute, Posterior Approach, Anterior Column, Percutaneous Endoscopic Approach

When reported with secondary diagnosis code T84.60XA, T84.610A, T84.611A, T84.612A, T84.613A, T84.614A, T84.615A, T84.619A, T84.63XA, T84.69XA, T84.7XXA

0SG34A0 Fusion of Lumbosacral Joint with Interbody Fusion Device, Anterior Approach, Anterior Column, Percutaneous Endoscopic Approach

When reported with secondary diagnosis code T84.60XA, T84.610A, T84.611A, T84.612A, T84.613A, T84.614A, T84.615A, T84.619A, T84.63XA, T84.69XA, T84.7XXA

0SG34A1 Fusion of Lumbosacral Joint with Interbody Fusion Device, Posterior Approach, Posterior Column, Percutaneous Endoscopic Approach

When reported with secondary diagnosis code T84.60XA, T84.610A, T84.611A, T84.612A, T84.613A, T84.614A, T84.615A, T84.619A, T84.63XA, T84.69XA, T84.7XXA

0SG34AJ Fusion of Lumbosacral Joint with Interbody Fusion Device, Posterior Approach, Anterior Column, Percutaneous Endoscopic Approach

When reported with secondary diagnosis code T84.60XA, T84.610A, T84.611A, T84.612A, T84.613A, T84.614A, T84.615A, T84.619A, T84.63XA, T84.69XA, T84.7XXA

0SG34J0 Fusion of Lumbosacral Joint with Synthetic Substitute, Anterior Approach, Anterior Column, Percutaneous Endoscopic Approach

Note Continued
987

0SG34J0 Continued Note

    When reported with secondary diagnosis code T84.60XA, T84.610A, T84.611A, T84.612A, T84.613A, T84.614A, T84.615A, T84.619A, T84.63XA, T84.69XA, T84.7XXA

0SG34J1 Fusion of Lumbosacral Joint with Synthetic Substitute, Posterior Approach, Posterior Column, Percutaneous Endoscopic Approach

    When reported with secondary diagnosis code T84.60XA, T84.610A, T84.611A, T84.612A, T84.613A, T84.614A, T84.615A, T84.619A, T84.63XA, T84.69XA, T84.7XXA

0SG34JJ Fusion of Lumbosacral Joint with Synthetic Substitute, Posterior Approach, Anterior Column, Percutaneous Endoscopic Approach

    When reported with secondary diagnosis code T84.60XA, T84.610A, T84.611A, T84.612A, T84.613A, T84.614A, T84.615A, T84.619A, T84.63XA, T84.69XA, T84.7XXA

0SG34K0 Fusion of Lumbosacral Joint with Nonautologous Tissue Substitute, Anterior Approach, Anterior Column, Percutaneous Endoscopic Approach

    When reported with secondary diagnosis code T84.60XA, T84.610A, T84.611A, T84.612A, T84.613A, T84.614A, T84.615A, T84.619A, T84.63XA, T84.69XA, T84.7XXA

0SG34K1 Fusion of Lumbosacral Joint with Nonautologous Tissue Substitute, Posterior Approach, Posterior Column, Percutaneous Endoscopic Approach

    When reported with secondary diagnosis code T84.60XA, T84.610A, T84.611A, T84.612A, T84.613A, T84.614A, T84.615A, T84.619A, T84.63XA, T84.69XA, T84.7XXA

0SG34KJ Fusion of Lumbosacral Joint with Nonautologous Tissue Substitute, Posterior Approach, Anterior Column, Percutaneous Endoscopic Approach

    When reported with secondary diagnosis code T84.60XA, T84.610A, T84.611A, T84.612A, T84.613A, T84.614A, T84.615A, T84.619A, T84.63XA, T84.69XA, T84.7XXA

0SG34Z0 Fusion of Lumbosacral Joint, Anterior Approach, Anterior Column, Percutaneous Endoscopic Approach

    When reported with secondary diagnosis code T84.60XA, T84.610A, T84.611A, T84.612A, T84.613A, T84.614A, T84.615A, T84.619A, T84.63XA, T84.69XA, T84.7XXA

0SG34Z1 Fusion of Lumbosacral Joint, Posterior Approach, Posterior Column, Percutaneous Endoscopic Approach

    When reported with secondary diagnosis code T84.60XA, T84.610A, T84.611A, T84.612A, T84.613A, T84.614A, T84.615A, T84.619A, T84.63XA, T84.69XA, T84.7XXA

0SG34ZJ Fusion of Lumbosacral Joint, Posterior Approach, Anterior Column, Percutaneous Endoscopic Approach

    When reported with secondary diagnosis code T84.60XA, T84.610A, T84.611A, T84.612A, T84.613A, T84.614A, T84.615A, T84.619A, T84.63XA, T84.69XA, T84.7XXA

0SG504Z Fusion of Sacrococcygeal Joint with Internal Fixation Device, Open Approach

0SG507Z Fusion of Sacrococcygeal Joint with Autologous Tissue Substitute, Open Approach

0SG50JZ Fusion of Sacrococcygeal Joint with Synthetic Substitute, Open Approach

0SG50KZ Fusion of Sacrococcygeal Joint with Nonautologous Tissue Substitute, Open Approach

0SG50ZZ Fusion of Sacrococcygeal Joint, Open Approach

0SG534Z Fusion of Sacrococcygeal Joint with Internal Fixation Device, Percutaneous Approach

0SG537Z Fusion of Sacrococcygeal Joint with Autologous Tissue Substitute, Percutaneous Approach

0SG53JZ Fusion of Sacrococcygeal Joint with Synthetic Substitute, Percutaneous Approach

0SG53KZ Fusion of Sacrococcygeal Joint with Nonautologous Tissue Substitute, Percutaneous Approach

0SG53ZZ Fusion of Sacrococcygeal Joint, Percutaneous Approach

0SG544Z Fusion of Sacrococcygeal Joint with Internal Fixation Device, Percutaneous Endoscopic Approach

0SG547Z Fusion of Sacrococcygeal Joint with Autologous Tissue Substitute, Percutaneous Endoscopic Approach

0SG54JZ Fusion of Sacrococcygeal Joint with Synthetic Substitute, Percutaneous Endoscopic Approach

0SG54KZ Fusion of Sacrococcygeal Joint with Nonautologous Tissue Substitute, Percutaneous Endoscopic Approach

0SG54ZZ Fusion of Sacrococcygeal Joint, Percutaneous Endoscopic Approach

0SG604Z Fusion of Coccygeal Joint with Internal Fixation Device, Open Approach

0SG607Z Fusion of Coccygeal Joint with Autologous Tissue Substitute, Open Approach

0SG60JZ Fusion of Coccygeal Joint with Synthetic Substitute, Open Approach

0SG60KZ Fusion of Coccygeal Joint with Nonautologous Tissue Substitute, Open Approach

0SG60ZZ Fusion of Coccygeal Joint, Open Approach

0SG634Z Fusion of Coccygeal Joint with Internal Fixation Device, Percutaneous Approach

0SG637Z Fusion of Coccygeal Joint with Autologous Tissue Substitute, Percutaneous Approach

0SG63JZ Fusion of Coccygeal Joint with Synthetic Substitute, Percutaneous Approach

0SG63KZ Fusion of Coccygeal Joint with Nonautologous Tissue Substitute, Percutaneous Approach

0SG63ZZ Fusion of Coccygeal Joint, Percutaneous Approach

0SG644Z Fusion of Coccygeal Joint with Internal Fixation Device, Percutaneous Endoscopic Approach

0SG647Z Fusion of Coccygeal Joint with Autologous Tissue Substitute, Percutaneous Endoscopic Approach

0SG64JZ Fusion of Coccygeal Joint with Synthetic Substitute, Percutaneous Endoscopic Approach

0SG64KZ Fusion of Coccygeal Joint with Nonautologous Tissue Substitute, Percutaneous Endoscopic Approach

0SG64ZZ Fusion of Coccygeal Joint, Percutaneous Endoscopic Approach

0SG704Z Fusion of Right Sacroiliac Joint with Internal Fixation Device, Open Approach

    When reported with secondary diagnosis code T84.60XA, T84.610A, T84.611A, T84.612A, T84.613A, T84.614A, T84.615A, T84.619A, T84.63XA, T84.69XA, T84.7XXA

0SG707Z Fusion of Right Sacroiliac Joint with Autologous Tissue Substitute, Open Approach

    When reported with secondary diagnosis code T84.60XA, T84.610A, T84.611A, T84.612A, T84.613A, T84.614A, T84.615A, T84.619A, T84.63XA, T84.69XA, T84.7XXA

0SG70JZ Fusion of Right Sacroiliac Joint with Synthetic Substitute, Open Approach

    When reported with secondary diagnosis code T84.60XA, T84.610A, T84.611A, T84.612A, T84.613A, T84.614A, T84.615A, T84.619A, T84.63XA, T84.69XA, T84.7XXA

0SG70KZ Fusion of Right Sacroiliac Joint with Nonautologous Tissue Substitute, Open Approach

    When reported with secondary diagnosis code T84.60XA, T84.610A, T84.611A, T84.612A, T84.613A, T84.614A, T84.615A, T84.619A, T84.63XA, T84.69XA, T84.7XXA

0SG70ZZ Fusion of Right Sacroiliac Joint, Open Approach

    When reported with secondary diagnosis code T84.60XA, T84.610A, T84.611A, T84.612A, T84.613A, T84.614A, T84.615A, T84.619A, T84.63XA, T84.69XA, T84.7XXA

0SG734Z Fusion of Right Sacroiliac Joint with Internal Fixation Device, Percutaneous Approach

    When reported with secondary diagnosis code T84.60XA, T84.610A, T84.611A, T84.612A, T84.613A, T84.614A, T84.615A, T84.619A, T84.63XA, T84.69XA, T84.7XXA

0SG737Z Fusion of Right Sacroiliac Joint with Autologous Tissue Substitute, Percutaneous Approach

    When reported with secondary diagnosis code T84.60XA, T84.610A, T84.611A, T84.612A, T84.613A, T84.614A, T84.615A, T84.619A, T84.63XA, T84.69XA, T84.7XXA

0SG73JZ Fusion of Right Sacroiliac Joint with Synthetic Substitute, Percutaneous Approach

    When reported with secondary diagnosis code T84.60XA, T84.610A, T84.611A, T84.612A, T84.613A, T84.614A, T84.615A, T84.619A, T84.63XA, T84.69XA, T84.7XXA

0SG73KZ Fusion of Right Sacroiliac Joint with Nonautologous Tissue Substitute, Percutaneous Approach

    When reported with secondary diagnosis code T84.60XA, T84.610A, T84.611A, T84.612A, T84.613A, T84.614A, T84.615A, T84.619A, T84.63XA, T84.69XA, T84.7XXA

0SG73ZZ Fusion of Right Sacroiliac Joint, Percutaneous Approach

    When reported with secondary diagnosis code T84.60XA, T84.610A, T84.611A, T84.612A, T84.613A, T84.614A, T84.615A, T84.619A, T84.63XA, T84.69XA, T84.7XXA

0SG744Z Fusion of Right Sacroiliac Joint with Internal Fixation Device, Percutaneous Endoscopic Approach

Note Continued

♀ Female-only   ♂ Male-only   ▲ Limited Coverage   ● Non-OR   ▨ HAC-associated procedure   ▲ Non-covered procedures   ✚ Combination

G744Z Continued Note

⬛ When reported with secondary diagnosis code T84.60XA, T84.610A, T84.611A, T84.612A, T84.613A, T84.614A, T84.615A, T84.619A, T84.63XA, T84.69XA, T84.7XXA

G747Z Fusion of Right Sacroiliac Joint with Autologous Tissue Substitute, Percutaneous Endoscopic Approach

⬛ When reported with secondary diagnosis code T84.60XA, T84.610A, T84.611A, T84.612A, T84.613A, T84.614A, T84.615A, T84.619A, T84.63XA, T84.69XA, T84.7XXA

G74JZ Fusion of Right Sacroiliac Joint with Synthetic Substitute, Percutaneous Endoscopic Approach

⬛ When reported with secondary diagnosis code T84.60XA, T84.610A, T84.611A, T84.612A, T84.613A, T84.614A, T84.615A, T84.619A, T84.63XA, T84.69XA, T84.7XXA

G74KZ Fusion of Right Sacroiliac Joint with Nonautologous Tissue Substitute, Percutaneous Endoscopic Approach

⬛ When reported with secondary diagnosis code T84.60XA, T84.610A, T84.611A, T84.612A, T84.613A, T84.614A, T84.615A, T84.619A, T84.63XA, T84.69XA, T84.7XXA

G74ZZ Fusion of Right Sacroiliac Joint, Percutaneous Endoscopic Approach

⬛ When reported with secondary diagnosis code T84.60XA, T84.610A, T84.611A, T84.612A, T84.613A, T84.614A, T84.615A, T84.619A, T84.63XA, T84.69XA, T84.7XXA

SG804Z Fusion of Left Sacroiliac Joint with Internal Fixation Device, Open Approach

⬛ When reported with secondary diagnosis code T84.60XA, T84.610A, T84.611A, T84.612A, T84.613A, T84.614A, T84.615A, T84.619A, T84.63XA, T84.69XA, T84.7XXA

SG807Z Fusion of Left Sacroiliac Joint with Autologous Tissue Substitute, Open Approach

⬛ When reported with secondary diagnosis code T84.60XA, T84.610A, T84.611A, T84.612A, T84.613A, T84.614A, T84.615A, T84.619A, T84.63XA, T84.69XA, T84.7XXA

SG80JZ Fusion of Left Sacroiliac Joint with Synthetic Substitute, Open Approach

⬛ When reported with secondary diagnosis code T84.60XA, T84.610A, T84.611A, T84.612A, T84.613A, T84.614A, T84.615A, T84.619A, T84.63XA, T84.69XA, T84.7XXA

SG80KZ Fusion of Left Sacroiliac Joint with Nonautologous Tissue Substitute, Open Approach

⬛ When reported with secondary diagnosis code T84.60XA, T84.610A, T84.611A, T84.612A, T84.613A, T84.614A, T84.615A, T84.619A, T84.63XA, T84.69XA, T84.7XXA

SG80ZZ Fusion of Left Sacroiliac Joint, Open Approach

⬛ When reported with secondary diagnosis code T84.60XA, T84.610A, T84.611A, T84.612A, T84.613A, T84.614A, T84.615A, T84.619A, T84.63XA, T84.69XA, T84.7XXA

SG834Z Fusion of Left Sacroiliac Joint with Internal Fixation Device, Percutaneous Approach

⬛ When reported with secondary diagnosis code T84.60XA, T84.610A, T84.611A, T84.612A, T84.613A, T84.614A, T84.615A, T84.619A, T84.63XA, T84.69XA, T84.7XXA

0SG837Z Fusion of Left Sacroiliac Joint with Autologous Tissue Substitute, Percutaneous Approach

⬛ When reported with secondary diagnosis code T84.60XA, T84.610A, T84.611A, T84.612A, T84.613A, T84.614A, T84.615A, T84.619A, T84.63XA, T84.69XA, T84.7XXA

0SG83JZ Fusion of Left Sacroiliac Joint with Synthetic Substitute, Percutaneous Approach

⬛ When reported with secondary diagnosis code T84.60XA, T84.610A, T84.611A, T84.612A, T84.613A, T84.614A, T84.615A, T84.619A, T84.63XA, T84.69XA, T84.7XXA

0SG83KZ Fusion of Left Sacroiliac Joint with Nonautologous Tissue Substitute, Percutaneous Approach

⬛ When reported with secondary diagnosis code T84.60XA, T84.610A, T84.611A, T84.612A, T84.613A, T84.614A, T84.615A, T84.619A, T84.63XA, T84.69XA, T84.7XXA

0SG83ZZ Fusion of Left Sacroiliac Joint, Percutaneous Approach

⬛ When reported with secondary diagnosis code T84.60XA, T84.610A, T84.611A, T84.612A, T84.613A, T84.614A, T84.615A, T84.619A, T84.63XA, T84.69XA, T84.7XXA

0SG844Z Fusion of Left Sacroiliac Joint with Internal Fixation Device, Percutaneous Endoscopic Approach

⬛ When reported with secondary diagnosis code T84.60XA, T84.610A, T84.611A, T84.612A, T84.613A, T84.614A, T84.615A, T84.619A, T84.63XA, T84.69XA, T84.7XXA

0SG847Z Fusion of Left Sacroiliac Joint with Autologous Tissue Substitute, Percutaneous Endoscopic Approach

⬛ When reported with secondary diagnosis code T84.60XA, T84.610A, T84.611A, T84.612A, T84.613A, T84.614A, T84.615A, T84.619A, T84.63XA, T84.69XA, T84.7XXA

0SG84JZ Fusion of Left Sacroiliac Joint with Synthetic Substitute, Percutaneous Endoscopic Approach

⬛ When reported with secondary diagnosis code T84.60XA, T84.610A, T84.611A, T84.612A, T84.613A, T84.614A, T84.615A, T84.619A, T84.63XA, T84.69XA, T84.7XXA

0SG84KZ Fusion of Left Sacroiliac Joint with Nonautologous Tissue Substitute, Percutaneous Endoscopic Approach

⬛ When reported with secondary diagnosis code T84.60XA, T84.610A, T84.611A, T84.612A, T84.613A, T84.614A, T84.615A, T84.619A, T84.63XA, T84.69XA, T84.7XXA

0SG84ZZ Fusion of Left Sacroiliac Joint, Percutaneous Endoscopic Approach

⬛ When reported with secondary diagnosis code T84.60XA, T84.610A, T84.611A, T84.612A, T84.613A, T84.614A, T84.615A, T84.619A, T84.63XA, T84.69XA, T84.7XXA

0SG904Z Fusion of Right Hip Joint with Internal Fixation Device, Open Approach

0SG905Z Fusion of Right Hip Joint with External Fixation Device, Open Approach

0SG907Z Fusion of Right Hip Joint with Autologous Tissue Substitute, Open Approach

0SG90JZ Fusion of Right Hip Joint with Synthetic Substitute, Open Approach

0SG90KZ Fusion of Right Hip Joint with Nonautologous Tissue Substitute, Open Approach

0SG90ZZ Fusion of Right Hip Joint, Open Approach

0SG934Z Fusion of Right Hip Joint with Internal Fixation Device, Percutaneous Approach

0SG935Z Fusion of Right Hip Joint with External Fixation Device, Percutaneous Approach

0SG937Z Fusion of Right Hip Joint with Autologous Tissue Substitute, Percutaneous Approach

0SG93JZ Fusion of Right Hip Joint with Synthetic Substitute, Percutaneous Approach

0SG93KZ Fusion of Right Hip Joint with Nonautologous Tissue Substitute, Percutaneous Approach

0SG93ZZ Fusion of Right Hip Joint, Percutaneous Approach

0SG944Z Fusion of Right Hip Joint with Internal Fixation Device, Percutaneous Endoscopic Approach

0SG945Z Fusion of Right Hip Joint with External Fixation Device, Percutaneous Endoscopic Approach

0SG947Z Fusion of Right Hip Joint with Autologous Tissue Substitute, Percutaneous Endoscopic Approach

0SG94JZ Fusion of Right Hip Joint with Synthetic Substitute, Percutaneous Endoscopic Approach

0SG94KZ Fusion of Right Hip Joint with Nonautologous Tissue Substitute, Percutaneous Endoscopic Approach

0SG94ZZ Fusion of Right Hip Joint, Percutaneous Endoscopic Approach

0SGB04Z Fusion of Left Hip Joint with Internal Fixation Device, Open Approach

0SGB05Z Fusion of Left Hip Joint with External Fixation Device, Open Approach

0SGB07Z Fusion of Left Hip Joint with Autologous Tissue Substitute, Open Approach

0SGB0JZ Fusion of Left Hip Joint with Synthetic Substitute, Open Approach

0SGB0KZ Fusion of Left Hip Joint with Nonautologous Tissue Substitute, Open Approach

0SGB0ZZ Fusion of Left Hip Joint, Open Approach

0SGB34Z Fusion of Left Hip Joint with Internal Fixation Device, Percutaneous Approach

0SGB35Z Fusion of Left Hip Joint with External Fixation Device, Percutaneous Approach

0SGB37Z Fusion of Left Hip Joint with Autologous Tissue Substitute, Percutaneous Approach

0SGB3JZ Fusion of Left Hip Joint with Synthetic Substitute, Percutaneous Approach

0SGB3KZ Fusion of Left Hip Joint with Nonautologous Tissue Substitute, Percutaneous Approach

0SGB3ZZ Fusion of Left Hip Joint, Percutaneous Approach

0SGB44Z Fusion of Left Hip Joint with Internal Fixation Device, Percutaneous Endoscopic Approach

0SGB45Z Fusion of Left Hip Joint with External Fixation Device, Percutaneous Endoscopic Approach

0SGB47Z Fusion of Left Hip Joint with Autologous Tissue Substitute, Percutaneous Endoscopic Approach

♀ Female-only   ♂ Male-only   ▲ Limited Coverage   ● Non-OR   ⬛ HAC-associated procedure   ▲ Non-covered procedures   ✚ Combination

0SGB4JZ Fusion of Left Hip Joint with Synthetic Substitute, Percutaneous Endoscopic Approach

0SGB4KZ Fusion of Left Hip Joint with Nonautologous Tissue Substitute, Percutaneous Endoscopic Approach

0SGB4ZZ Fusion of Left Hip Joint, Percutaneous Endoscopic Approach

0SGC04Z Fusion of Right Knee Joint with Internal Fixation Device, Open Approach

0SGC05Z Fusion of Right Knee Joint with External Fixation Device, Open Approach

0SGC07Z Fusion of Right Knee Joint with Autologous Tissue Substitute, Open Approach

0SGC0JZ Fusion of Right Knee Joint with Synthetic Substitute, Open Approach

0SGC0KZ Fusion of Right Knee Joint with Nonautologous Tissue Substitute, Open Approach

0SGC0ZZ Fusion of Right Knee Joint, Open Approach

0SGC34Z Fusion of Right Knee Joint with Internal Fixation Device, Percutaneous Approach

0SGC35Z Fusion of Right Knee Joint with External Fixation Device, Percutaneous Approach

0SGC37Z Fusion of Right Knee Joint with Autologous Tissue Substitute, Percutaneous Approach

0SGC3JZ Fusion of Right Knee Joint with Synthetic Substitute, Percutaneous Approach

0SGC3KZ Fusion of Right Knee Joint with Nonautologous Tissue Substitute, Percutaneous Approach

0SGC3ZZ Fusion of Right Knee Joint, Percutaneous Approach

0SGC44Z Fusion of Right Knee Joint with Internal Fixation Device, Percutaneous Endoscopic Approach

0SGC45Z Fusion of Right Knee Joint with External Fixation Device, Percutaneous Endoscopic Approach

0SGC47Z Fusion of Right Knee Joint with Autologous Tissue Substitute, Percutaneous Endoscopic Approach

0SGC4JZ Fusion of Right Knee Joint with Synthetic Substitute, Percutaneous Endoscopic Approach

0SGC4KZ Fusion of Right Knee Joint with Nonautologous Tissue Substitute, Percutaneous Endoscopic Approach

0SGC4ZZ Fusion of Right Knee Joint, Percutaneous Endoscopic Approach

0SGD04Z Fusion of Left Knee Joint with Internal Fixation Device, Open Approach

0SGD05Z Fusion of Left Knee Joint with External Fixation Device, Open Approach

0SGD07Z Fusion of Left Knee Joint with Autologous Tissue Substitute, Open Approach

0SGD0JZ Fusion of Left Knee Joint with Synthetic Substitute, Open Approach

0SGD0KZ Fusion of Left Knee Joint with Nonautologous Tissue Substitute, Open Approach

0SGD0ZZ Fusion of Left Knee Joint, Open Approach

0SGD34Z Fusion of Left Knee Joint with Internal Fixation Device, Percutaneous Approach

0SGD35Z Fusion of Left Knee Joint with External Fixation Device, Percutaneous Approach

0SGD37Z Fusion of Left Knee Joint with Autologous Tissue Substitute, Percutaneous Approach

0SGD3JZ Fusion of Left Knee Joint with Synthetic Substitute, Percutaneous Approach

0SGD3KZ Fusion of Left Knee Joint with Nonautologous Tissue Substitute, Percutaneous Approach

0SGD3ZZ Fusion of Left Knee Joint, Percutaneous Approach

0SGD44Z Fusion of Left Knee Joint with Internal Fixation Device, Percutaneous Endoscopic Approach

0SGD45Z Fusion of Left Knee Joint with External Fixation Device, Percutaneous Endoscopic Approach

0SGD47Z Fusion of Left Knee Joint with Autologous Tissue Substitute, Percutaneous Endoscopic Approach

0SGD4JZ Fusion of Left Knee Joint with Synthetic Substitute, Percutaneous Endoscopic Approach

0SGD4KZ Fusion of Left Knee Joint with Nonautologous Tissue Substitute, Percutaneous Endoscopic Approach

0SGD4ZZ Fusion of Left Knee Joint, Percutaneous Endoscopic Approach

0SGF04Z Fusion of Right Ankle Joint with Internal Fixation Device, Open Approach

0SGF05Z Fusion of Right Ankle Joint with External Fixation Device, Open Approach

0SGF07Z Fusion of Right Ankle Joint with Autologous Tissue Substitute, Open Approach

0SGF0JZ Fusion of Right Ankle Joint with Synthetic Substitute, Open Approach

0SGF0KZ Fusion of Right Ankle Joint with Nonautologous Tissue Substitute, Open Approach

0SGF0ZZ Fusion of Right Ankle Joint, Open Approach

0SGF34Z Fusion of Right Ankle Joint with Internal Fixation Device, Percutaneous Approach

0SGF35Z Fusion of Right Ankle Joint with External Fixation Device, Percutaneous Approach

0SGF37Z Fusion of Right Ankle Joint with Autologous Tissue Substitute, Percutaneous Approach

0SGF3JZ Fusion of Right Ankle Joint with Synthetic Substitute, Percutaneous Approach

0SGF3KZ Fusion of Right Ankle Joint with Nonautologous Tissue Substitute, Percutaneous Approach

0SGF3ZZ Fusion of Right Ankle Joint, Percutaneous Approach

0SGF44Z Fusion of Right Ankle Joint with Internal Fixation Device, Percutaneous Endoscopic Approach

0SGF45Z Fusion of Right Ankle Joint with External Fixation Device, Percutaneous Endoscopic Approach

0SGF47Z Fusion of Right Ankle Joint with Autologous Tissue Substitute, Percutaneous Endoscopic Approach

0SGF4JZ Fusion of Right Ankle Joint with Synthetic Substitute, Percutaneous Endoscopic Approach

0SGF4KZ Fusion of Right Ankle Joint with Nonautologous Tissue Substitute, Percutaneous Endoscopic Approach

0SGF4ZZ Fusion of Right Ankle Joint, Percutaneous Endoscopic Approach

0SGG04Z Fusion of Left Ankle Joint with Internal Fixation Device, Open Approach

AHA CC: 2Q, 2013, 39-40

0SGG05Z Fusion of Left Ankle Joint with External Fixation Device, Open Approach

0SGG07Z Fusion of Left Ankle Joint with Autologous Tissue Substitute, Open Approach

AHA CC: 2Q, 2013, 39-40

0SGG0JZ Fusion of Left Ankle Joint with Synthetic Substitute, Open Approach

0SGG0KZ Fusion of Left Ankle Joint with Nonautologous Tissue Substitute, Open Approach

0SGG0ZZ Fusion of Left Ankle Joint, Open Approach

0SGG34Z Fusion of Left Ankle Joint with Internal Fixation Device, Percutaneous Approach

0SGG35Z Fusion of Left Ankle Joint with External Fixation Device, Percutaneous Approach

0SGG37Z Fusion of Left Ankle Joint with Autologous Tissue Substitute, Percutaneous Approach

0SGG3JZ Fusion of Left Ankle Joint with Synthetic Substitute, Percutaneous Approach

0SGG3KZ Fusion of Left Ankle Joint with Nonautologous Tissue Substitute, Percutaneous Approach

0SGG3ZZ Fusion of Left Ankle Joint, Percutaneous Approach

0SGG44Z Fusion of Left Ankle Joint with Internal Fixation Device, Percutaneous Endoscopic Approach

0SGG45Z Fusion of Left Ankle Joint with External Fixation Device, Percutaneous Endoscopic Approach

0SGG47Z Fusion of Left Ankle Joint with Autologous Tissue Substitute, Percutaneous Endoscopic Approach

0SGG4JZ Fusion of Left Ankle Joint with Synthetic Substitute, Percutaneous Endoscopic Approach

0SGG4KZ Fusion of Left Ankle Joint with Nonautologous Tissue Substitute, Percutaneous Endoscopic Approach

0SGG4ZZ Fusion of Left Ankle Joint, Percutaneous Endoscopic Approach

0SGH04Z Fusion of Right Tarsal Joint with Internal Fixation Device, Open Approach

0SGH05Z Fusion of Right Tarsal Joint with External Fixation Device, Open Approach

0SGH07Z Fusion of Right Tarsal Joint with Autologous Tissue Substitute, Open Approach

0SGH0JZ Fusion of Right Tarsal Joint with Synthetic Substitute, Open Approach

0SGH0KZ Fusion of Right Tarsal Joint with Nonautologous Tissue Substitute, Open Approach

0SGH0ZZ Fusion of Right Tarsal Joint, Open Approach

0SGH34Z Fusion of Right Tarsal Joint with Internal Fixation Device, Percutaneous Approach

0SGH35Z Fusion of Right Tarsal Joint with External Fixation Device, Percutaneous Approach

0SGH37Z Fusion of Right Tarsal Joint with Autologous Tissue Substitute, Percutaneous Approach

0SGH3JZ Fusion of Right Tarsal Joint with Synthetic Substitute, Percutaneous Approach

0SGH3KZ Fusion of Right Tarsal Joint with Nonautologous Tissue Substitute, Percutaneous Approach

0SGH3ZZ Fusion of Right Tarsal Joint, Percutaneous Approach

0SGH44Z Fusion of Right Tarsal Joint with Internal Fixation Device, Percutaneous Endoscopic Approach

0SGH45Z Fusion of Right Tarsal Joint with External Fixation Device, Percutaneous Endoscopic Approach

0SGH47Z Fusion of Right Tarsal Joint with Autologous Tissue Substitute, Percutaneous Endoscopic Approach

0SGH4JZ Fusion of Right Tarsal Joint with Synthetic Substitute, Percutaneous Endoscopic Approach

0SGH4KZ Fusion of Right Tarsal Joint with Nonautologous Tissue Substitute, Percutaneous Endoscopic Approach

0SGH4ZZ Fusion of Right Tarsal Joint, Percutaneous Endoscopic Approach

♀ Female-only   ♂ Male-only   ▲ Limited Coverage   ● Non-OR   ■ HAC-associated procedure   ▲ Non-covered procedures   ✚ Combination

0GJ04Z   Fusion of Left Tarsal Joint with Internal Fixation Device, Open Approach

0GJ05Z   Fusion of Left Tarsal Joint with External Fixation Device, Open Approach

0GJ07Z   Fusion of Left Tarsal Joint with Autologous Tissue Substitute, Open Approach

0GJ0JZ   Fusion of Left Tarsal Joint with Synthetic Substitute, Open Approach

0GJ0KZ   Fusion of Left Tarsal Joint with Nonautologous Tissue Substitute, Open Approach

0GJ0ZZ   Fusion of Left Tarsal Joint, Open Approach

0GJ34Z   Fusion of Left Tarsal Joint with Internal Fixation Device, Percutaneous Approach

0GJ35Z   Fusion of Left Tarsal Joint with External Fixation Device, Percutaneous Approach

0GJ37Z   Fusion of Left Tarsal Joint with Autologous Tissue Substitute, Percutaneous Approach

0GJ3JZ   Fusion of Left Tarsal Joint with Synthetic Substitute, Percutaneous Approach

0GJ3KZ   Fusion of Left Tarsal Joint with Nonautologous Tissue Substitute, Percutaneous Approach

0GJ3ZZ   Fusion of Left Tarsal Joint, Percutaneous Approach

0GJ44Z   Fusion of Left Tarsal Joint with Internal Fixation Device, Percutaneous Endoscopic Approach

0GJ45Z   Fusion of Left Tarsal Joint with External Fixation Device, Percutaneous Endoscopic Approach

0GJ47Z   Fusion of Left Tarsal Joint with Autologous Tissue Substitute, Percutaneous Endoscopic Approach

0GJ4JZ   Fusion of Left Tarsal Joint with Synthetic Substitute, Percutaneous Endoscopic Approach

0GJ4KZ   Fusion of Left Tarsal Joint with Nonautologous Tissue Substitute, Percutaneous Endoscopic Approach

0GJ4ZZ   Fusion of Left Tarsal Joint, Percutaneous Endoscopic Approach

SGK04Z   Fusion of Right Metatarsal-Tarsal Joint with Internal Fixation Device, Open Approach

SGK05Z   Fusion of Right Metatarsal-Tarsal Joint with External Fixation Device, Open Approach

SGK07Z   Fusion of Right Metatarsal-Tarsal Joint with Autologous Tissue Substitute, Open Approach

SGK0JZ   Fusion of Right Metatarsal-Tarsal Joint with Synthetic Substitute, Open Approach

SGK0KZ   Fusion of Right Metatarsal-Tarsal Joint with Nonautologous Tissue Substitute, Open Approach

SGK0ZZ   Fusion of Right Metatarsal-Tarsal Joint, Open Approach

SGK34Z   Fusion of Right Metatarsal-Tarsal Joint with Internal Fixation Device, Percutaneous Approach

SGK35Z   Fusion of Right Metatarsal-Tarsal Joint with External Fixation Device, Percutaneous Approach

SGK37Z   Fusion of Right Metatarsal-Tarsal Joint with Autologous Tissue Substitute, Percutaneous Approach

SGK3JZ   Fusion of Right Metatarsal-Tarsal Joint with Synthetic Substitute, Percutaneous Approach

SGK3KZ   Fusion of Right Metatarsal-Tarsal Joint with Nonautologous Tissue Substitute, Percutaneous Approach

SGK3ZZ   Fusion of Right Metatarsal-Tarsal Joint, Percutaneous Approach

0SGK44Z   Fusion of Right Metatarsal-Tarsal Joint with Internal Fixation Device, Percutaneous Endoscopic Approach

0SGK45Z   Fusion of Right Metatarsal-Tarsal Joint with External Fixation Device, Percutaneous Endoscopic Approach

0SGK47Z   Fusion of Right Metatarsal-Tarsal Joint with Autologous Tissue Substitute, Percutaneous Endoscopic Approach

0SGK4JZ   Fusion of Right Metatarsal-Tarsal Joint with Synthetic Substitute, Percutaneous Endoscopic Approach

0SGK4KZ   Fusion of Right Metatarsal-Tarsal Joint with Nonautologous Tissue Substitute, Percutaneous Endoscopic Approach

0SGK4ZZ   Fusion of Right Metatarsal-Tarsal Joint, Percutaneous Endoscopic Approach

0SGL04Z   Fusion of Left Metatarsal-Tarsal Joint with Internal Fixation Device, Open Approach

0SGL05Z   Fusion of Left Metatarsal-Tarsal Joint with External Fixation Device, Open Approach

0SGL07Z   Fusion of Left Metatarsal-Tarsal Joint with Autologous Tissue Substitute, Open Approach

0SGL0JZ   Fusion of Left Metatarsal-Tarsal Joint with Synthetic Substitute, Open Approach

0SGL0KZ   Fusion of Left Metatarsal-Tarsal Joint with Nonautologous Tissue Substitute, Open Approach

0SGL0ZZ   Fusion of Left Metatarsal-Tarsal Joint, Open Approach

0SGL34Z   Fusion of Left Metatarsal-Tarsal Joint with Internal Fixation Device, Percutaneous Approach

0SGL35Z   Fusion of Left Metatarsal-Tarsal Joint with External Fixation Device, Percutaneous Approach

0SGL37Z   Fusion of Left Metatarsal-Tarsal Joint with Autologous Tissue Substitute, Percutaneous Approach

0SGL3JZ   Fusion of Left Metatarsal-Tarsal Joint with Synthetic Substitute, Percutaneous Approach

0SGL3KZ   Fusion of Left Metatarsal-Tarsal Joint with Nonautologous Tissue Substitute, Percutaneous Approach

0SGL3ZZ   Fusion of Left Metatarsal-Tarsal Joint, Percutaneous Approach

0SGL44Z   Fusion of Left Metatarsal-Tarsal Joint with Internal Fixation Device, Percutaneous Endoscopic Approach

0SGL45Z   Fusion of Left Metatarsal-Tarsal Joint with External Fixation Device, Percutaneous Endoscopic Approach

0SGL47Z   Fusion of Left Metatarsal-Tarsal Joint with Autologous Tissue Substitute, Percutaneous Endoscopic Approach

0SGL4JZ   Fusion of Left Metatarsal-Tarsal Joint with Synthetic Substitute, Percutaneous Endoscopic Approach

0SGL4KZ   Fusion of Left Metatarsal-Tarsal Joint with Nonautologous Tissue Substitute, Percutaneous Endoscopic Approach

0SGL4ZZ   Fusion of Left Metatarsal-Tarsal Joint, Percutaneous Endoscopic Approach

0SGM04Z   Fusion of Right Metatarsal-Phalangeal Joint with Internal Fixation Device, Open Approach

0SGM05Z   Fusion of Right Metatarsal-Phalangeal Joint with External Fixation Device, Open Approach

0SGM07Z   Fusion of Right Metatarsal-Phalangeal Joint with Autologous Tissue Substitute, Open Approach

0SGM0JZ   Fusion of Right Metatarsal-Phalangeal Joint with Synthetic Substitute, Open Approach

0SGM0KZ   Fusion of Right Metatarsal-Phalangeal Joint with Nonautologous Tissue Substitute, Open Approach

0SGM0ZZ   Fusion of Right Metatarsal-Phalangeal Joint, Open Approach

0SGM34Z   Fusion of Right Metatarsal-Phalangeal Joint with Internal Fixation Device, Percutaneous Approach

0SGM35Z   Fusion of Right Metatarsal-Phalangeal Joint with External Fixation Device, Percutaneous Approach

0SGM37Z   Fusion of Right Metatarsal-Phalangeal Joint with Autologous Tissue Substitute, Percutaneous Approach

0SGM3JZ   Fusion of Right Metatarsal-Phalangeal Joint with Synthetic Substitute, Percutaneous Approach

0SGM3KZ   Fusion of Right Metatarsal-Phalangeal Joint with Nonautologous Tissue Substitute, Percutaneous Approach

0SGM3ZZ   Fusion of Right Metatarsal-Phalangeal Joint, Percutaneous Approach

0SGM44Z   Fusion of Right Metatarsal-Phalangeal Joint with Internal Fixation Device, Percutaneous Endoscopic Approach

0SGM45Z   Fusion of Right Metatarsal-Phalangeal Joint with External Fixation Device, Percutaneous Endoscopic Approach

0SGM47Z   Fusion of Right Metatarsal-Phalangeal Joint with Autologous Tissue Substitute, Percutaneous Endoscopic Approach

0SGM4JZ   Fusion of Right Metatarsal-Phalangeal Joint with Synthetic Substitute, Percutaneous Endoscopic Approach

0SGM4KZ   Fusion of Right Metatarsal-Phalangeal Joint with Nonautologous Tissue Substitute, Percutaneous Endoscopic Approach

0SGM4ZZ   Fusion of Right Metatarsal-Phalangeal Joint, Percutaneous Endoscopic Approach

0SGN04Z   Fusion of Left Metatarsal-Phalangeal Joint with Internal Fixation Device, Open Approach

0SGN05Z   Fusion of Left Metatarsal-Phalangeal Joint with External Fixation Device, Open Approach

0SGN07Z   Fusion of Left Metatarsal-Phalangeal Joint with Autologous Tissue Substitute, Open Approach

0SGN0JZ   Fusion of Left Metatarsal-Phalangeal Joint with Synthetic Substitute, Open Approach

0SGN0KZ   Fusion of Left Metatarsal-Phalangeal Joint with Nonautologous Tissue Substitute, Open Approach

0SGN0ZZ   Fusion of Left Metatarsal-Phalangeal Joint, Open Approach

0SGN34Z   Fusion of Left Metatarsal-Phalangeal Joint with Internal Fixation Device, Percutaneous Approach

0SGN35Z   Fusion of Left Metatarsal-Phalangeal Joint with External Fixation Device, Percutaneous Approach

0SGN37Z   Fusion of Left Metatarsal-Phalangeal Joint with Autologous Tissue Substitute, Percutaneous Approach

0SGN3JZ   Fusion of Left Metatarsal-Phalangeal Joint with Synthetic Substitute, Percutaneous Approach

0SGN3KZ   Fusion of Left Metatarsal-Phalangeal Joint with Nonautologous Tissue Substitute, Percutaneous Approach

0SGN3ZZ   Fusion of Left Metatarsal-Phalangeal Joint, Percutaneous Approach

0SGN44Z   Fusion of Left Metatarsal-Phalangeal Joint with Internal Fixation Device, Percutaneous Endoscopic Approach

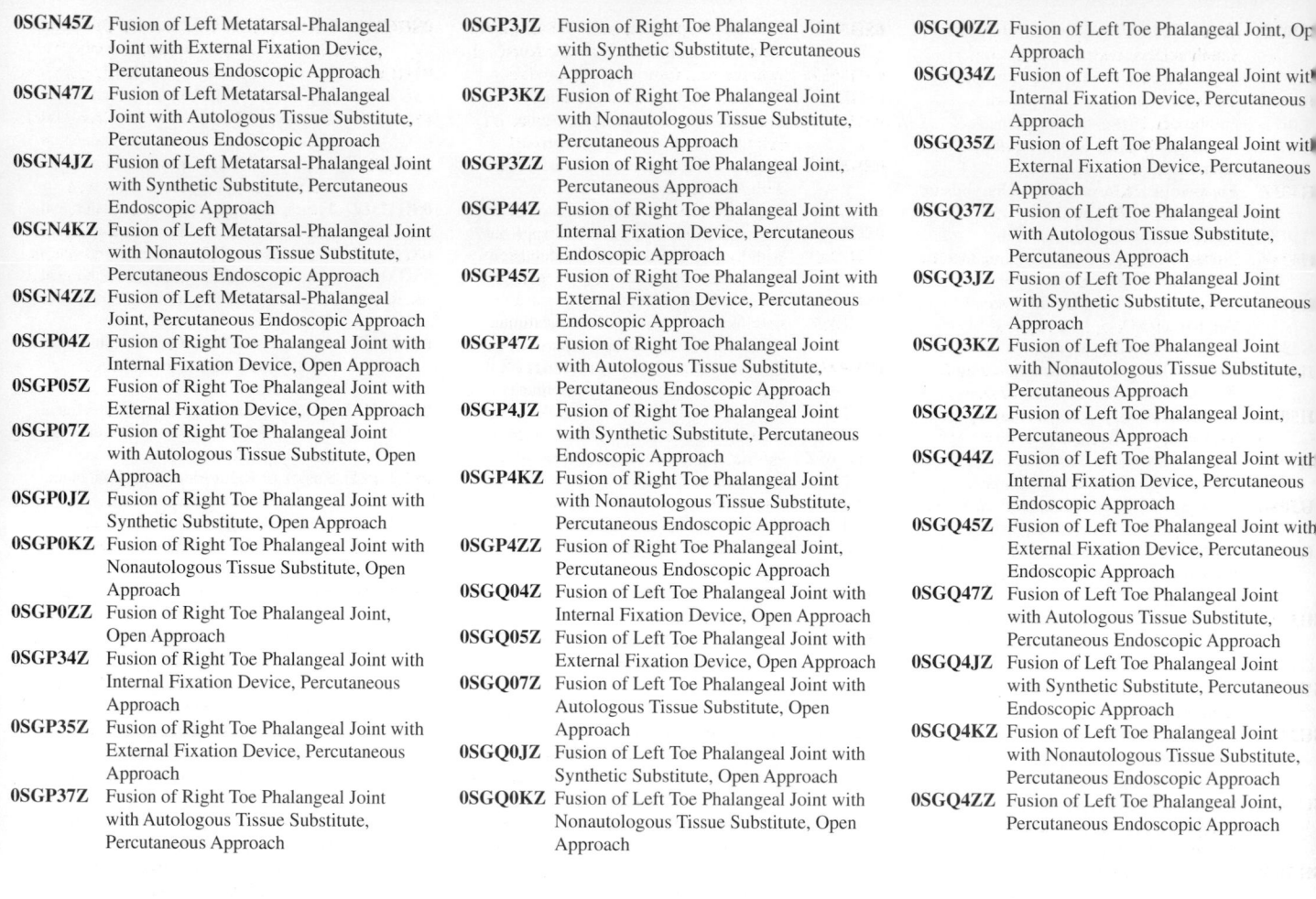

0SGN45Z Fusion of Left Metatarsal-Phalangeal Joint with External Fixation Device, Percutaneous Endoscopic Approach

0SGN47Z Fusion of Left Metatarsal-Phalangeal Joint with Autologous Tissue Substitute, Percutaneous Endoscopic Approach

0SGN4JZ Fusion of Left Metatarsal-Phalangeal Joint with Synthetic Substitute, Percutaneous Endoscopic Approach

0SGN4KZ Fusion of Left Metatarsal-Phalangeal Joint with Nonautologous Tissue Substitute, Percutaneous Endoscopic Approach

0SGN4ZZ Fusion of Left Metatarsal-Phalangeal Joint, Percutaneous Endoscopic Approach

0SGP04Z Fusion of Right Toe Phalangeal Joint with Internal Fixation Device, Open Approach

0SGP05Z Fusion of Right Toe Phalangeal Joint with External Fixation Device, Open Approach

0SGP07Z Fusion of Right Toe Phalangeal Joint with Autologous Tissue Substitute, Open Approach

0SGP0JZ Fusion of Right Toe Phalangeal Joint with Synthetic Substitute, Open Approach

0SGP0KZ Fusion of Right Toe Phalangeal Joint with Nonautologous Tissue Substitute, Open Approach

0SGP0ZZ Fusion of Right Toe Phalangeal Joint, Open Approach

0SGP34Z Fusion of Right Toe Phalangeal Joint with Internal Fixation Device, Percutaneous Approach

0SGP35Z Fusion of Right Toe Phalangeal Joint with External Fixation Device, Percutaneous Approach

0SGP37Z Fusion of Right Toe Phalangeal Joint with Autologous Tissue Substitute, Percutaneous Approach

0SGP3JZ Fusion of Right Toe Phalangeal Joint with Synthetic Substitute, Percutaneous Approach

0SGP3KZ Fusion of Right Toe Phalangeal Joint with Nonautologous Tissue Substitute, Percutaneous Approach

0SGP3ZZ Fusion of Right Toe Phalangeal Joint, Percutaneous Approach

0SGP44Z Fusion of Right Toe Phalangeal Joint with Internal Fixation Device, Percutaneous Endoscopic Approach

0SGP45Z Fusion of Right Toe Phalangeal Joint with External Fixation Device, Percutaneous Endoscopic Approach

0SGP47Z Fusion of Right Toe Phalangeal Joint with Autologous Tissue Substitute, Percutaneous Endoscopic Approach

0SGP4JZ Fusion of Right Toe Phalangeal Joint with Synthetic Substitute, Percutaneous Endoscopic Approach

0SGP4KZ Fusion of Right Toe Phalangeal Joint with Nonautologous Tissue Substitute, Percutaneous Endoscopic Approach

0SGP4ZZ Fusion of Right Toe Phalangeal Joint, Percutaneous Endoscopic Approach

0SGQ04Z Fusion of Left Toe Phalangeal Joint with Internal Fixation Device, Open Approach

0SGQ05Z Fusion of Left Toe Phalangeal Joint with External Fixation Device, Open Approach

0SGQ07Z Fusion of Left Toe Phalangeal Joint with Autologous Tissue Substitute, Open Approach

0SGQ0JZ Fusion of Left Toe Phalangeal Joint with Synthetic Substitute, Open Approach

0SGQ0KZ Fusion of Left Toe Phalangeal Joint with Nonautologous Tissue Substitute, Open Approach

0SGQ0ZZ Fusion of Left Toe Phalangeal Joint, Open Approach

0SGQ34Z Fusion of Left Toe Phalangeal Joint with Internal Fixation Device, Percutaneous Approach

0SGQ35Z Fusion of Left Toe Phalangeal Joint with External Fixation Device, Percutaneous Approach

0SGQ37Z Fusion of Left Toe Phalangeal Joint with Autologous Tissue Substitute, Percutaneous Approach

0SGQ3JZ Fusion of Left Toe Phalangeal Joint with Synthetic Substitute, Percutaneous Approach

0SGQ3KZ Fusion of Left Toe Phalangeal Joint with Nonautologous Tissue Substitute, Percutaneous Approach

0SGQ3ZZ Fusion of Left Toe Phalangeal Joint, Percutaneous Approach

0SGQ44Z Fusion of Left Toe Phalangeal Joint with Internal Fixation Device, Percutaneous Endoscopic Approach

0SGQ45Z Fusion of Left Toe Phalangeal Joint with External Fixation Device, Percutaneous Endoscopic Approach

0SGQ47Z Fusion of Left Toe Phalangeal Joint with Autologous Tissue Substitute, Percutaneous Endoscopic Approach

0SGQ4JZ Fusion of Left Toe Phalangeal Joint with Synthetic Substitute, Percutaneous Endoscopic Approach

0SGQ4KZ Fusion of Left Toe Phalangeal Joint with Nonautologous Tissue Substitute, Percutaneous Endoscopic Approach

0SGQ4ZZ Fusion of Left Toe Phalangeal Joint, Percutaneous Endoscopic Approach

0SH – Lower Joints, Insertion

0SH003Z Insertion of Infusion Device into Lumbar Vertebral Joint, Open Approach

0SH004Z Insertion of Internal Fixation Device into Lumbar Vertebral Joint, Open Approach

0SH008Z Insertion of Spacer into Lumbar Vertebral Joint, Open Approach

0SH00BZ Insertion of Interspinous Process Spinal Stabilization Device into Lumbar Vertebral Joint, Open Approach

0SH00CZ Insertion of Pedicle-Based Spinal Stabilization Device into Lumbar Vertebral Joint, Open Approach

0SH00DZ Insertion of Facet Replacement Spinal Stabilization Device into Lumbar Vertebral Joint, Open Approach

0SH033Z Insertion of Infusion Device into Lumbar Vertebral Joint, Percutaneous Approach

0SH034Z Insertion of Internal Fixation Device into Lumbar Vertebral Joint, Percutaneous Approach

0SH038Z Insertion of Spacer into Lumbar Vertebral Joint, Percutaneous Approach

0SH03BZ Insertion of Interspinous Process Spinal Stabilization Device into Lumbar Vertebral Joint, Percutaneous Approach

0SH03CZ Insertion of Pedicle-Based Spinal Stabilization Device into Lumbar Vertebral Joint, Percutaneous Approach

0SH03DZ Insertion of Facet Replacement Spinal Stabilization Device into Lumbar Vertebral Joint, Percutaneous Approach

0SH043Z Insertion of Infusion Device into Lumbar Vertebral Joint, Percutaneous Endoscopic Approach

0SH044Z Insertion of Internal Fixation Device into Lumbar Vertebral Joint, Percutaneous Endoscopic Approach

0SH048Z Insertion of Spacer into Lumbar Vertebral Joint, Percutaneous Endoscopic Approach

0SH04BZ Insertion of Interspinous Process Spinal Stabilization Device into Lumbar Vertebral Joint, Percutaneous Endoscopic Approach

0SH04CZ Insertion of Pedicle-Based Spinal Stabilization Device into Lumbar Vertebral Joint, Percutaneous Endoscopic Approach

0SH04DZ Insertion of Facet Replacement Spinal Stabilization Device into Lumbar Vertebral Joint, Percutaneous Endoscopic Approach

0SH203Z Insertion of Infusion Device into Lumbar Vertebral Disc, Open Approach

0SH208Z Insertion of Spacer into Lumbar Vertebral Disc, Open Approach

0SH233Z Insertion of Infusion Device into Lumbar Vertebral Disc, Percutaneous Approach

0SH238Z Insertion of Spacer into Lumbar Vertebral Disc, Percutaneous Approach

0SH243Z Insertion of Infusion Device into Lumbar Vertebral Disc, Percutaneous Endoscopic Approach

0SH248Z Insertion of Spacer into Lumbar Vertebral Disc, Percutaneous Endoscopic Approach

0SH303Z Insertion of Infusion Device into Lumbosacral Joint, Open Approach

0SH304Z Insertion of Internal Fixation Device into Lumbosacral Joint, Open Approach

0SH308Z Insertion of Spacer into Lumbosacral Joint, Open Approach

0SH30BZ Insertion of Interspinous Process Spinal Stabilization Device into Lumbosacral Joint, Open Approach

0SH30CZ Insertion of Pedicle-Based Spinal Stabilization Device into Lumbosacral Joint, Open Approach

0SH30DZ Insertion of Facet Replacement Spinal Stabilization Device into Lumbosacral Joint, Open Approach

0SH333Z Insertion of Infusion Device into Lumbosacral Joint, Percutaneous Approach

0SH334Z Insertion of Internal Fixation Device into Lumbosacral Joint, Percutaneous Approach

0SH338Z Insertion of Spacer into Lumbosacral Joint, Percutaneous Approach

0SH33BZ Insertion of Interspinous Process Spinal Stabilization Device into Lumbosacral Joint, Percutaneous Approach

0SH33CZ Insertion of Pedicle-Based Spinal Stabilization Device into Lumbosacral Joint, Percutaneous Approach

0SH33DZ Insertion of Facet Replacement Spinal Stabilization Device into Lumbosacral Joint, Percutaneous Approach

0SH343Z Insertion of Infusion Device into Lumbosacral Joint, Percutaneous Endoscopic Approach

0SH344Z Insertion of Internal Fixation Device into Lumbosacral Joint, Percutaneous Endoscopic Approach

0SH348Z Insertion of Spacer into Lumbosacral Joint, Percutaneous Endoscopic Approach

0SH34BZ Insertion of Interspinous Process Spinal Stabilization Device into Lumbosacral Joint, Percutaneous Endoscopic Approach

0SH34CZ Insertion of Pedicle-Based Spinal Stabilization Device into Lumbosacral Joint, Percutaneous Endoscopic Approach

♀ Female-only   ♂ Male-only   ▲ Limited Coverage   ● Non-OR   HAC HAC-associated procedure   ▲ Non-covered procedures   ✚ Combination

0H34DZ   Insertion of Facet Replacement Spinal Stabilization Device into Lumbosacral Joint, Percutaneous Endoscopic Approach

0H403Z   Insertion of Infusion Device into Lumbosacral Disc, Open Approach

0H408Z   Insertion of Spacer into Lumbosacral Disc, Open Approach

0H433Z   Insertion of Infusion Device into Lumbosacral Disc, Percutaneous Approach

0H438Z   Insertion of Spacer into Lumbosacral Disc, Percutaneous Approach

0H443Z   Insertion of Infusion Device into Lumbosacral Disc, Percutaneous Endoscopic Approach

0H448Z   Insertion of Spacer into Lumbosacral Disc, Percutaneous Endoscopic Approach

0H503Z   Insertion of Infusion Device into Sacrococcygeal Joint, Open Approach

0H504Z   Insertion of Internal Fixation Device into Sacrococcygeal Joint, Open Approach

0H508Z   Insertion of Spacer into Sacrococcygeal Joint, Open Approach

0H533Z   Insertion of Infusion Device into Sacrococcygeal Joint, Percutaneous Approach

0H534Z   Insertion of Internal Fixation Device into Sacrococcygeal Joint, Percutaneous Approach

0H538Z   Insertion of Spacer into Sacrococcygeal Joint, Percutaneous Approach

0H543Z   Insertion of Infusion Device into Sacrococcygeal Joint, Percutaneous Endoscopic Approach

0H544Z   Insertion of Internal Fixation Device into Sacrococcygeal Joint, Percutaneous Endoscopic Approach

0H548Z   Insertion of Spacer into Sacrococcygeal Joint, Percutaneous Endoscopic Approach

0H603Z   Insertion of Infusion Device into Coccygeal Joint, Open Approach

0H604Z   Insertion of Internal Fixation Device into Coccygeal Joint, Open Approach

0H608Z   Insertion of Spacer into Coccygeal Joint, Open Approach

0H633Z   Insertion of Infusion Device into Coccygeal Joint, Percutaneous Approach

0H634Z   Insertion of Internal Fixation Device into Coccygeal Joint, Percutaneous Approach

0H638Z   Insertion of Spacer into Coccygeal Joint, Percutaneous Approach

0H643Z   Insertion of Infusion Device into Coccygeal Joint, Percutaneous Endoscopic Approach

0H644Z   Insertion of Internal Fixation Device into Coccygeal Joint, Percutaneous Endoscopic Approach

0H648Z   Insertion of Spacer into Coccygeal Joint, Percutaneous Endoscopic Approach

0H703Z   Insertion of Infusion Device into Right Sacroiliac Joint, Open Approach

0H704Z   Insertion of Internal Fixation Device into Right Sacroiliac Joint, Open Approach

0H708Z   Insertion of Spacer into Right Sacroiliac Joint, Open Approach

0H733Z   Insertion of Infusion Device into Right Sacroiliac Joint, Percutaneous Approach

0H734Z   Insertion of Internal Fixation Device into Right Sacroiliac Joint, Percutaneous Approach

0H738Z   Insertion of Spacer into Right Sacroiliac Joint, Percutaneous Approach

0H743Z   Insertion of Infusion Device into Right Sacroiliac Joint, Percutaneous Endoscopic Approach

0H744Z   Insertion of Internal Fixation Device into Right Sacroiliac Joint, Percutaneous Endoscopic Approach

0SH748Z   Insertion of Spacer into Right Sacroiliac Joint, Percutaneous Endoscopic Approach

0SH803Z   Insertion of Infusion Device into Left Sacroiliac Joint, Open Approach

0SH804Z   Insertion of Internal Fixation Device into Left Sacroiliac Joint, Open Approach

0SH808Z   Insertion of Spacer into Left Sacroiliac Joint, Open Approach

0SH833Z   Insertion of Infusion Device into Left Sacroiliac Joint, Percutaneous Approach

0SH834Z   Insertion of Internal Fixation Device into Left Sacroiliac Joint, Percutaneous Approach

0SH838Z   Insertion of Spacer into Left Sacroiliac Joint, Percutaneous Approach

0SH843Z   Insertion of Infusion Device into Left Sacroiliac Joint, Percutaneous Endoscopic Approach

0SH844Z   Insertion of Internal Fixation Device into Left Sacroiliac Joint, Percutaneous Endoscopic Approach

0SH848Z   Insertion of Spacer into Left Sacroiliac Joint, Percutaneous Endoscopic Approach

0SH903Z   Insertion of Infusion Device into Right Hip Joint, Open Approach

0SH904Z   Insertion of Internal Fixation Device into Right Hip Joint, Open Approach

0SH905Z   Insertion of External Fixation Device into Right Hip Joint, Open Approach

0SH908Z   Insertion of Spacer into Right Hip Joint, Open Approach

0SH933Z   Insertion of Infusion Device into Right Hip Joint, Percutaneous Approach

0SH934Z   Insertion of Internal Fixation Device into Right Hip Joint, Percutaneous Approach

0SH935Z   Insertion of External Fixation Device into Right Hip Joint, Percutaneous Approach

0SH938Z   Insertion of Spacer into Right Hip Joint, Percutaneous Approach

0SH943Z   Insertion of Infusion Device into Right Hip Joint, Percutaneous Endoscopic Approach

0SH944Z   Insertion of Internal Fixation Device into Right Hip Joint, Percutaneous Endoscopic Approach

0SH945Z   Insertion of External Fixation Device into Right Hip Joint, Percutaneous Endoscopic Approach

0SH948Z   Insertion of Spacer into Right Hip Joint, Percutaneous Endoscopic Approach

0SHB03Z   Insertion of Infusion Device into Left Hip Joint, Open Approach

0SHB04Z   Insertion of Internal Fixation Device into Left Hip Joint, Open Approach

0SHB05Z   Insertion of External Fixation Device into Left Hip Joint, Open Approach

0SHB08Z   Insertion of Spacer into Left Hip Joint, Open Approach

0SHB33Z   Insertion of Infusion Device into Left Hip Joint, Percutaneous Approach

0SHB34Z   Insertion of Internal Fixation Device into Left Hip Joint, Percutaneous Approach

0SHB35Z   Insertion of External Fixation Device into Left Hip Joint, Percutaneous Approach

0SHB38Z   Insertion of Spacer into Left Hip Joint, Percutaneous Approach

0SHB43Z   Insertion of Infusion Device into Left Hip Joint, Percutaneous Endoscopic Approach

0SHB44Z   Insertion of Internal Fixation Device into Left Hip Joint, Percutaneous Endoscopic Approach

0SHB45Z   Insertion of External Fixation Device into Left Hip Joint, Percutaneous Endoscopic Approach

0SHB48Z   Insertion of Spacer into Left Hip Joint, Percutaneous Endoscopic Approach

0SHC03Z   Insertion of Infusion Device into Right Knee Joint, Open Approach

0SHC04Z   Insertion of Internal Fixation Device into Right Knee Joint, Open Approach

0SHC05Z   Insertion of External Fixation Device into Right Knee Joint, Open Approach

0SHC08Z   Insertion of Spacer into Right Knee Joint, Open Approach

0SHC33Z   Insertion of Infusion Device into Right Knee Joint, Percutaneous Approach

0SHC34Z   Insertion of Internal Fixation Device into Right Knee Joint, Percutaneous Approach

0SHC35Z   Insertion of External Fixation Device into Right Knee Joint, Percutaneous Approach

0SHC38Z   Insertion of Spacer into Right Knee Joint, Percutaneous Approach

0SHC43Z   Insertion of Infusion Device into Right Knee Joint, Percutaneous Endoscopic Approach

0SHC44Z   Insertion of Internal Fixation Device into Right Knee Joint, Percutaneous Endoscopic Approach

0SHC45Z   Insertion of External Fixation Device into Right Knee Joint, Percutaneous Endoscopic Approach

0SHC48Z   Insertion of Spacer into Right Knee Joint, Percutaneous Endoscopic Approach

0SHD03Z   Insertion of Infusion Device into Left Knee Joint, Open Approach

0SHD04Z   Insertion of Internal Fixation Device into Left Knee Joint, Open Approach

0SHD05Z   Insertion of External Fixation Device into Left Knee Joint, Open Approach

0SHD08Z   Insertion of Spacer into Left Knee Joint, Open Approach

0SHD33Z   Insertion of Infusion Device into Left Knee Joint, Percutaneous Approach

0SHD34Z   Insertion of Internal Fixation Device into Left Knee Joint, Percutaneous Approach

0SHD35Z   Insertion of External Fixation Device into Left Knee Joint, Percutaneous Approach

0SHD38Z   Insertion of Spacer into Left Knee Joint, Percutaneous Approach

0SHD43Z   Insertion of Infusion Device into Left Knee Joint, Percutaneous Endoscopic Approach

0SHD44Z   Insertion of Internal Fixation Device into Left Knee Joint, Percutaneous Endoscopic Approach

0SHD45Z   Insertion of External Fixation Device into Left Knee Joint, Percutaneous Endoscopic Approach

0SHD48Z   Insertion of Spacer into Left Knee Joint, Percutaneous Endoscopic Approach

0SHF03Z   Insertion of Infusion Device into Right Ankle Joint, Open Approach

0SHF04Z   Insertion of Internal Fixation Device into Right Ankle Joint, Open Approach

0SHF05Z   Insertion of External Fixation Device into Right Ankle Joint, Open Approach

0SHF08Z   Insertion of Spacer into Right Ankle Joint, Open Approach

0SHF33Z   Insertion of Infusion Device into Right Ankle Joint, Percutaneous Approach

0SHF34Z   Insertion of Internal Fixation Device into Right Ankle Joint, Percutaneous Approach

0SHF35Z   Insertion of External Fixation Device into Right Ankle Joint, Percutaneous Approach

0SHF38Z   Insertion of Spacer into Right Ankle Joint, Percutaneous Approach

0SHF43Z   Insertion of Infusion Device into Right Ankle Joint, Percutaneous Endoscopic Approach

0SHF44Z   Insertion of Internal Fixation Device into Right Ankle Joint, Percutaneous Endoscopic Approach

0SHF45Z   Insertion of External Fixation Device into Right Ankle Joint, Percutaneous Endoscopic Approach

0SHF48Z   Insertion of Spacer into Right Ankle Joint, Percutaneous Endoscopic Approach

♀ Female-only   ♂ Male-only   ▲ Limited Coverage   ● Non-OR   ■ HAC-associated procedure   ▲ Non-covered procedures   ✚ Combination

0SHG03Z Insertion of Infusion Device into Left Ankle Joint, Open Approach

0SHG04Z Insertion of Internal Fixation Device into Left Ankle Joint, Open Approach

0SHG05Z Insertion of External Fixation Device into Left Ankle Joint, Open Approach

0SHG08Z Insertion of Spacer into Left Ankle Joint, Open Approach

0SHG33Z Insertion of Infusion Device into Left Ankle Joint, Percutaneous Approach

0SHG34Z Insertion of Internal Fixation Device into Left Ankle Joint, Percutaneous Approach

0SHG35Z Insertion of External Fixation Device into Left Ankle Joint, Percutaneous Approach

0SHG38Z Insertion of Spacer into Left Ankle Joint, Percutaneous Approach

0SHG43Z Insertion of Infusion Device into Left Ankle Joint, Percutaneous Endoscopic Approach

0SHG44Z Insertion of Internal Fixation Device into Left Ankle Joint, Percutaneous Endoscopic Approach

0SHG45Z Insertion of External Fixation Device into Left Ankle Joint, Percutaneous Endoscopic Approach

0SHG48Z Insertion of Spacer into Left Ankle Joint, Percutaneous Endoscopic Approach

0SHH03Z Insertion of Infusion Device into Right Tarsal Joint, Open Approach

0SHH04Z Insertion of Internal Fixation Device into Right Tarsal Joint, Open Approach

0SHH05Z Insertion of External Fixation Device into Right Tarsal Joint, Open Approach

0SHH08Z Insertion of Spacer into Right Tarsal Joint, Open Approach

0SHH33Z Insertion of Infusion Device into Right Tarsal Joint, Percutaneous Approach

0SHH34Z Insertion of Internal Fixation Device into Right Tarsal Joint, Percutaneous Approach

0SHH35Z Insertion of External Fixation Device into Right Tarsal Joint, Percutaneous Approach

0SHH38Z Insertion of Spacer into Right Tarsal Joint, Percutaneous Approach

0SHH43Z Insertion of Infusion Device into Right Tarsal Joint, Percutaneous Endoscopic Approach

0SHH44Z Insertion of Internal Fixation Device into Right Tarsal Joint, Percutaneous Endoscopic Approach

0SHH45Z Insertion of External Fixation Device into Right Tarsal Joint, Percutaneous Endoscopic Approach

0SHH48Z Insertion of Spacer into Right Tarsal Joint, Percutaneous Endoscopic Approach

0SHJ03Z Insertion of Infusion Device into Left Tarsal Joint, Open Approach

0SHJ04Z Insertion of Internal Fixation Device into Left Tarsal Joint, Open Approach

0SHJ05Z Insertion of External Fixation Device into Left Tarsal Joint, Open Approach

0SHJ08Z Insertion of Spacer into Left Tarsal Joint, Open Approach

0SHJ33Z Insertion of Infusion Device into Left Tarsal Joint, Percutaneous Approach

0SHJ34Z Insertion of Internal Fixation Device into Left Tarsal Joint, Percutaneous Approach

0SHJ35Z Insertion of External Fixation Device into Left Tarsal Joint, Percutaneous Approach

0SHJ38Z Insertion of Spacer into Left Tarsal Joint, Percutaneous Approach

0SHJ43Z Insertion of Infusion Device into Left Tarsal Joint, Percutaneous Endoscopic Approach

0SHJ44Z Insertion of Internal Fixation Device into Left Tarsal Joint, Percutaneous Endoscopic Approach

0SHJ45Z Insertion of External Fixation Device into Left Tarsal Joint, Percutaneous Endoscopic Approach

0SHJ48Z Insertion of Spacer into Left Tarsal Joint, Percutaneous Endoscopic Approach

0SHK03Z Insertion of Infusion Device into Right Metatarsal-Tarsal Joint, Open Approach

0SHK04Z Insertion of Internal Fixation Device into Right Metatarsal-Tarsal Joint, Open Approach

0SHK05Z Insertion of External Fixation Device into Right Metatarsal-Tarsal Joint, Open Approach

0SHK08Z Insertion of Spacer into Right Metatarsal-Tarsal Joint, Open Approach

0SHK33Z Insertion of Infusion Device into Right Metatarsal-Tarsal Joint, Percutaneous Approach

0SHK34Z Insertion of Internal Fixation Device into Right Metatarsal-Tarsal Joint, Percutaneous Approach

0SHK35Z Insertion of External Fixation Device into Right Metatarsal-Tarsal Joint, Percutaneous Approach

0SHK38Z Insertion of Spacer into Right Metatarsal-Tarsal Joint, Percutaneous Approach

0SHK43Z Insertion of Infusion Device into Right Metatarsal-Tarsal Joint, Percutaneous Endoscopic Approach

0SHK44Z Insertion of Internal Fixation Device into Right Metatarsal-Tarsal Joint, Percutaneous Endoscopic Approach

0SHK45Z Insertion of External Fixation Device into Right Metatarsal-Tarsal Joint, Percutaneous Endoscopic Approach

0SHK48Z Insertion of Spacer into Right Metatarsal-Tarsal Joint, Percutaneous Endoscopic Approach

0SHL03Z Insertion of Infusion Device into Left Metatarsal-Tarsal Joint, Open Approach

0SHL04Z Insertion of Internal Fixation Device into Left Metatarsal-Tarsal Joint, Open Approach

0SHL05Z Insertion of External Fixation Device into Left Metatarsal-Tarsal Joint, Open Approach

0SHL08Z Insertion of Spacer into Left Metatarsal-Tarsal Joint, Open Approach

0SHL33Z Insertion of Infusion Device into Left Metatarsal-Tarsal Joint, Percutaneous Approach

0SHL34Z Insertion of Internal Fixation Device into Left Metatarsal-Tarsal Joint, Percutaneous Approach

0SHL35Z Insertion of External Fixation Device into Left Metatarsal-Tarsal Joint, Percutaneous Approach

0SHL38Z Insertion of Spacer into Left Metatarsal-Tarsal Joint, Percutaneous Approach

0SHL43Z Insertion of Infusion Device into Left Metatarsal-Tarsal Joint, Percutaneous Endoscopic Approach

0SHL44Z Insertion of Internal Fixation Device into Left Metatarsal-Tarsal Joint, Percutaneous Endoscopic Approach

0SHL45Z Insertion of External Fixation Device into Left Metatarsal-Tarsal Joint, Percutaneous Endoscopic Approach

0SHL48Z Insertion of Spacer into Left Metatarsal-Tarsal Joint, Percutaneous Endoscopic Approach

0SHM03Z Insertion of Infusion Device into Right Metatarsal-Phalangeal Joint, Open Approach

0SHM04Z Insertion of Internal Fixation Device into Right Metatarsal-Phalangeal Joint, Open Approach

0SHM05Z Insertion of External Fixation Device into Right Metatarsal-Phalangeal Joint, Open Approach

0SHM08Z Insertion of Spacer into Right Metatarsal-Phalangeal Joint, Open Approach

0SHM33Z Insertion of Infusion Device into Right Metatarsal-Phalangeal Joint, Percutaneous Approach

0SHM34Z Insertion of Internal Fixation Device into Right Metatarsal-Phalangeal Joint, Percutaneous Approach

0SHM35Z Insertion of External Fixation Device into Right Metatarsal-Phalangeal Joint, Percutaneous Approach

0SHM38Z Insertion of Spacer into Right Metatarsal-Phalangeal Joint, Percutaneous Approach

0SHM43Z Insertion of Infusion Device into Right Metatarsal-Phalangeal Joint, Percutaneous Endoscopic Approach

0SHM44Z Insertion of Internal Fixation Device into Right Metatarsal-Phalangeal Joint, Percutaneous Endoscopic Approach

0SHM45Z Insertion of External Fixation Device into Right Metatarsal-Phalangeal Joint, Percutaneous Endoscopic Approach

0SHM48Z Insertion of Spacer into Right Metatarsal-Phalangeal Joint, Percutaneous Endoscopic Approach

0SHN03Z Insertion of Infusion Device into Left Metatarsal-Phalangeal Joint, Open Approach

0SHN04Z Insertion of Internal Fixation Device into Left Metatarsal-Phalangeal Joint, Open Approach

0SHN05Z Insertion of External Fixation Device into Left Metatarsal-Phalangeal Joint, Open Approach

0SHN08Z Insertion of Spacer into Left Metatarsal-Phalangeal Joint, Open Approach

0SHN33Z Insertion of Infusion Device into Left Metatarsal-Phalangeal Joint, Percutaneous Approach

0SHN34Z Insertion of Internal Fixation Device into Left Metatarsal-Phalangeal Joint, Percutaneous Approach

0SHN35Z Insertion of External Fixation Device into Left Metatarsal-Phalangeal Joint, Percutaneous Approach

0SHN38Z Insertion of Spacer into Left Metatarsal-Phalangeal Joint, Percutaneous Approach

0SHN43Z Insertion of Infusion Device into Left Metatarsal-Phalangeal Joint, Percutaneous Endoscopic Approach

0SHN44Z Insertion of Internal Fixation Device into Left Metatarsal-Phalangeal Joint, Percutaneous Endoscopic Approach

0SHN45Z Insertion of External Fixation Device into Left Metatarsal-Phalangeal Joint, Percutaneous Endoscopic Approach

0SHN48Z Insertion of Spacer into Left Metatarsal-Phalangeal Joint, Percutaneous Endoscopic Approach

0SHP03Z Insertion of Infusion Device into Right Toe Phalangeal Joint, Open Approach

0SHP04Z Insertion of Internal Fixation Device into Right Toe Phalangeal Joint, Open Approach

0SHP05Z Insertion of External Fixation Device into Right Toe Phalangeal Joint, Open Approach

0SHP08Z Insertion of Spacer into Right Toe Phalangeal Joint, Open Approach

0SHP33Z Insertion of Infusion Device into Right Toe Phalangeal Joint, Percutaneous Approach

0SHP34Z Insertion of Internal Fixation Device into Right Toe Phalangeal Joint, Percutaneous Approach

♀ Female-only   ♂ Male-only   ▲ Limited Coverage   ● Non-OR   🅷🅰🅲 HAC-associated procedure   ▲ Non-covered procedures   ✚ Combination

0SHP35Z Insertion of External Fixation Device into Right Toe Phalangeal Joint, Percutaneous Approach

0SHP38Z Insertion of Spacer into Right Toe Phalangeal Joint, Percutaneous Approach

0SHP43Z Insertion of Infusion Device into Right Toe Phalangeal Joint, Percutaneous Endoscopic Approach

0SHP44Z Insertion of Internal Fixation Device into Right Toe Phalangeal Joint, Percutaneous Endoscopic Approach

0SHP45Z Insertion of External Fixation Device into Right Toe Phalangeal Joint, Percutaneous Endoscopic Approach

0SHP48Z Insertion of Spacer into Right Toe Phalangeal Joint, Percutaneous Endoscopic Approach

0SHQ03Z Insertion of Infusion Device into Left Toe Phalangeal Joint, Open Approach

0SHQ04Z Insertion of Internal Fixation Device into Left Toe Phalangeal Joint, Open Approach

0SHQ05Z Insertion of External Fixation Device into Left Toe Phalangeal Joint, Open Approach

0SHQ08Z Insertion of Spacer into Left Toe Phalangeal Joint, Open Approach

0SHQ33Z Insertion of Infusion Device into Left Toe Phalangeal Joint, Percutaneous Approach

0SHQ34Z Insertion of Internal Fixation Device into Left Toe Phalangeal Joint, Percutaneous Approach

0SHQ35Z Insertion of External Fixation Device into Left Toe Phalangeal Joint, Percutaneous Approach

0SHQ38Z Insertion of Spacer into Left Toe Phalangeal Joint, Percutaneous Approach

0SHQ43Z Insertion of Infusion Device into Left Toe Phalangeal Joint, Percutaneous Endoscopic Approach

0SHQ44Z Insertion of Internal Fixation Device into Left Toe Phalangeal Joint, Percutaneous Endoscopic Approach

0SHQ45Z Insertion of External Fixation Device into Left Toe Phalangeal Joint, Percutaneous Endoscopic Approach

0SHQ48Z Insertion of Spacer into Left Toe Phalangeal Joint, Percutaneous Endoscopic Approach

J – Lower Joints, Inspection

view Coding Guideline B3.5

view Coding Guidelines B3.11a, B3.11b and B3.11c

0SJ00ZZ Inspection of Lumbar Vertebral Joint, Open Approach

0SJ03ZZ Inspection of Lumbar Vertebral Joint, Percutaneous Approach

0SJ04ZZ Inspection of Lumbar Vertebral Joint, Percutaneous Endoscopic Approach

0SJ0XZZ Inspection of Lumbar Vertebral Joint, External Approach

0SJ20ZZ Inspection of Lumbar Vertebral Disc, Open Approach

0SJ23ZZ Inspection of Lumbar Vertebral Disc, Percutaneous Approach

0SJ24ZZ Inspection of Lumbar Vertebral Disc, Percutaneous Endoscopic Approach

0SJ2XZZ Inspection of Lumbar Vertebral Disc, External Approach

0SJ30ZZ Inspection of Lumbosacral Joint, Open Approach

0SJ33ZZ Inspection of Lumbosacral Joint, Percutaneous Approach

0SJ34ZZ Inspection of Lumbosacral Joint, Percutaneous Endoscopic Approach

0SJ3XZZ Inspection of Lumbosacral Joint, External Approach

0SJ40ZZ Inspection of Lumbosacral Disc, Open Approach

0SJ43ZZ Inspection of Lumbosacral Disc, Percutaneous Approach

0SJ44ZZ Inspection of Lumbosacral Disc, Percutaneous Endoscopic Approach

0SJ4XZZ Inspection of Lumbosacral Disc, External Approach

0SJ50ZZ Inspection of Sacrococcygeal Joint, Open Approach

0SJ53ZZ Inspection of Sacrococcygeal Joint, Percutaneous Approach

0SJ54ZZ Inspection of Sacrococcygeal Joint, Percutaneous Endoscopic Approach

0SJ5XZZ Inspection of Sacrococcygeal Joint, External Approach

0SJ60ZZ Inspection of Coccygeal Joint, Open Approach

0SJ63ZZ Inspection of Coccygeal Joint, Percutaneous Approach

0SJ64ZZ Inspection of Coccygeal Joint, Percutaneous Endoscopic Approach

0SJ6XZZ Inspection of Coccygeal Joint, External Approach

0SJ70ZZ Inspection of Right Sacroiliac Joint, Open Approach

0SJ73ZZ Inspection of Right Sacroiliac Joint, Percutaneous Approach

0SJ74ZZ Inspection of Right Sacroiliac Joint, Percutaneous Endoscopic Approach

0SJ7XZZ Inspection of Right Sacroiliac Joint, External Approach

0SJ80ZZ Inspection of Left Sacroiliac Joint, Open Approach

0SJ83ZZ Inspection of Left Sacroiliac Joint, Percutaneous Approach

0SJ84ZZ Inspection of Left Sacroiliac Joint, Percutaneous Endoscopic Approach

0SJ8XZZ Inspection of Left Sacroiliac Joint, External Approach

0SJ90ZZ Inspection of Right Hip Joint, Open Approach

0SJ93ZZ Inspection of Right Hip Joint, Percutaneous Approach

0SJ94ZZ Inspection of Right Hip Joint, Percutaneous Endoscopic Approach

0SJ9XZZ Inspection of Right Hip Joint, External Approach

0SJB0ZZ Inspection of Left Hip Joint, Open Approach

0SJB3ZZ Inspection of Left Hip Joint, Percutaneous Approach

0SJB4ZZ Inspection of Left Hip Joint, Percutaneous Endoscopic Approach

0SJBXZZ Inspection of Left Hip Joint, External Approach

0SJC0ZZ Inspection of Right Knee Joint, Open Approach

0SJC3ZZ Inspection of Right Knee Joint, Percutaneous Approach

0SJC4ZZ Inspection of Right Knee Joint, Percutaneous Endoscopic Approach

0SJCXZZ Inspection of Right Knee Joint, External Approach

0SJD0ZZ Inspection of Left Knee Joint, Open Approach

0SJD3ZZ Inspection of Left Knee Joint, Percutaneous Approach

0SJD4ZZ Inspection of Left Knee Joint, Percutaneous Endoscopic Approach

0SJDXZZ Inspection of Left Knee Joint, External Approach

0SJF0ZZ Inspection of Right Ankle Joint, Open Approach

0SJF3ZZ Inspection of Right Ankle Joint, Percutaneous Approach

0SJF4ZZ Inspection of Right Ankle Joint, Percutaneous Endoscopic Approach

0SJFXZZ Inspection of Right Ankle Joint, External Approach

0SJG0ZZ Inspection of Left Ankle Joint, Open Approach

0SJG3ZZ Inspection of Left Ankle Joint, Percutaneous Approach

0SJG4ZZ Inspection of Left Ankle Joint, Percutaneous Endoscopic Approach

0SJGXZZ Inspection of Left Ankle Joint, External Approach

0SJH0ZZ Inspection of Right Tarsal Joint, Open Approach

0SJH3ZZ Inspection of Right Tarsal Joint, Percutaneous Approach

0SJH4ZZ Inspection of Right Tarsal Joint, Percutaneous Endoscopic Approach

0SJHXZZ Inspection of Right Tarsal Joint, External Approach

0SJJ0ZZ Inspection of Left Tarsal Joint, Open Approach

0SJJ3ZZ Inspection of Left Tarsal Joint, Percutaneous Approach

0SJJ4ZZ Inspection of Left Tarsal Joint, Percutaneous Endoscopic Approach

0SJJXZZ Inspection of Left Tarsal Joint, External Approach

0SJK0ZZ Inspection of Right Metatarsal-Tarsal Joint, Open Approach

0SJK3ZZ Inspection of Right Metatarsal-Tarsal Joint, Percutaneous Approach

0SJK4ZZ Inspection of Right Metatarsal-Tarsal Joint, Percutaneous Endoscopic Approach

0SJKXZZ Inspection of Right Metatarsal-Tarsal Joint, External Approach

0SJL0ZZ Inspection of Left Metatarsal-Tarsal Joint, Open Approach

0SJL3ZZ Inspection of Left Metatarsal-Tarsal Joint, Percutaneous Approach

0SJL4ZZ Inspection of Left Metatarsal-Tarsal Joint, Percutaneous Endoscopic Approach

0SJLXZZ Inspection of Left Metatarsal-Tarsal Joint, External Approach

0SJM0ZZ Inspection of Right Metatarsal-Phalangeal Joint, Open Approach

0SJM3ZZ Inspection of Right Metatarsal-Phalangeal Joint, Percutaneous Approach

0SJM4ZZ Inspection of Right Metatarsal-Phalangeal Joint, Percutaneous Endoscopic Approach

0SJMXZZ Inspection of Right Metatarsal-Phalangeal Joint, External Approach

0SJN0ZZ Inspection of Left Metatarsal-Phalangeal Joint, Open Approach

0SJN3ZZ Inspection of Left Metatarsal-Phalangeal Joint, Percutaneous Approach

0SJN4ZZ Inspection of Left Metatarsal-Phalangeal Joint, Percutaneous Endoscopic Approach

0SJNXZZ Inspection of Left Metatarsal-Phalangeal Joint, External Approach

♀ Female-only   ♂ Male-only   ▲ Limited Coverage   ● Non-OR   ▦ HAC-associated procedure   ▲ Non-covered procedures   ✚ Combination

0SJP0ZZ Inspection of Right Toe Phalangeal Joint, Open Approach	**0SJPXZZ** Inspection of Right Toe Phalangeal Joint, External Approach	**0SJQ4ZZ** Inspection of Left Toe Phalangeal Joint, Percutaneous Endoscopic Approach
0SJP3ZZ Inspection of Right Toe Phalangeal Joint, Percutaneous Approach	**0SJQ0ZZ** Inspection of Left Toe Phalangeal Joint, Open Approach	**0SJQXZZ** Inspection of Left Toe Phalangeal Joint, External Approach
0SJP4ZZ Inspection of Right Toe Phalangeal Joint, Percutaneous Endoscopic Approach	**0SJQ3ZZ** Inspection of Left Toe Phalangeal Joint, Percutaneous Approach	

0SN – Lower Joints, Release

Review Coding Guideline B3.13

0SN00ZZ Release Lumbar Vertebral Joint, Open Approach	**0SN80ZZ** Release Left Sacroiliac Joint, Open Approach	**0SNJ0ZZ** Release Left Tarsal Joint, Open Approach
0SN03ZZ Release Lumbar Vertebral Joint, Percutaneous Approach	**0SN83ZZ** Release Left Sacroiliac Joint, Percutaneous Approach	**0SNJ3ZZ** Release Left Tarsal Joint, Percutaneous Approach
0SN04ZZ Release Lumbar Vertebral Joint, Percutaneous Endoscopic Approach	**0SN84ZZ** Release Left Sacroiliac Joint, Percutaneous Endoscopic Approach	**0SNJ4ZZ** Release Left Tarsal Joint, Percutaneous Endoscopic Approach
0SN0XZZ Release Lumbar Vertebral Joint, External Approach	**0SN8XZZ** Release Left Sacroiliac Joint, External Approach	**0SNJXZZ** Release Left Tarsal Joint, External Approach
0SN20ZZ Release Lumbar Vertebral Disc, Open Approach	**0SN90ZZ** Release Right Hip Joint, Open Approach	**0SNK0ZZ** Release Right Metatarsal-Tarsal Joint, Open Approach
0SN23ZZ Release Lumbar Vertebral Disc, Percutaneous Approach	**0SN93ZZ** Release Right Hip Joint, Percutaneous Approach	**0SNK3ZZ** Release Right Metatarsal-Tarsal Joint, Percutaneous Approach
0SN24ZZ Release Lumbar Vertebral Disc, Percutaneous Endoscopic Approach	**0SN94ZZ** Release Right Hip Joint, Percutaneous Endoscopic Approach	**0SNK4ZZ** Release Right Metatarsal-Tarsal Joint, Percutaneous Endoscopic Approach
0SN2XZZ Release Lumbar Vertebral Disc, External Approach	**0SN9XZZ** Release Right Hip Joint, External Approach	**0SNKXZZ** Release Right Metatarsal-Tarsal Joint, External Approach
0SN30ZZ Release Lumbosacral Joint, Open Approach	**0SNB0ZZ** Release Left Hip Joint, Open Approach	**0SNL0ZZ** Release Left Metatarsal-Tarsal Joint, Open Approach
0SN33ZZ Release Lumbosacral Joint, Percutaneous Approach	**0SNB3ZZ** Release Left Hip Joint, Percutaneous Approach	**0SNL3ZZ** Release Left Metatarsal-Tarsal Joint, Percutaneous Approach
0SN34ZZ Release Lumbosacral Joint, Percutaneous Endoscopic Approach	**0SNB4ZZ** Release Left Hip Joint, Percutaneous Endoscopic Approach	**0SNL4ZZ** Release Left Metatarsal-Tarsal Joint, Percutaneous Endoscopic Approach
0SN3XZZ Release Lumbosacral Joint, External Approach	**0SNBXZZ** Release Left Hip Joint, External Approach	**0SNLXZZ** Release Left Metatarsal-Tarsal Joint, External Approach
0SN40ZZ Release Lumbosacral Disc, Open Approach	**0SNC0ZZ** Release Right Knee Joint, Open Approach	**0SNM0ZZ** Release Right Metatarsal-Phalangeal Joint, Open Approach
0SN43ZZ Release Lumbosacral Disc, Percutaneous Approach	**0SNC3ZZ** Release Right Knee Joint, Percutaneous Approach	**0SNM3ZZ** Release Right Metatarsal-Phalangeal Joint, Percutaneous Approach
0SN44ZZ Release Lumbosacral Disc, Percutaneous Endoscopic Approach	**0SNC4ZZ** Release Right Knee Joint, Percutaneous Endoscopic Approach	**0SNM4ZZ** Release Right Metatarsal-Phalangeal Joint, Percutaneous Endoscopic Approach
0SN4XZZ Release Lumbosacral Disc, External Approach	**0SNCXZZ** Release Right Knee Joint, External Approach	**0SNMXZZ** Release Right Metatarsal-Phalangeal Joint, External Approach
0SN50ZZ Release Sacrococcygeal Joint, Open Approach	**0SND0ZZ** Release Left Knee Joint, Open Approach	**0SNN0ZZ** Release Left Metatarsal-Phalangeal Joint, Open Approach
0SN53ZZ Release Sacrococcygeal Joint, Percutaneous Approach	**0SND3ZZ** Release Left Knee Joint, Percutaneous Approach	**0SNN3ZZ** Release Left Metatarsal-Phalangeal Joint, Percutaneous Approach
0SN54ZZ Release Sacrococcygeal Joint, Percutaneous Endoscopic Approach	**0SND4ZZ** Release Left Knee Joint, Percutaneous Endoscopic Approach	**0SNN4ZZ** Release Left Metatarsal-Phalangeal Joint, Percutaneous Endoscopic Approach
0SN5XZZ Release Sacrococcygeal Joint, External Approach	**0SNDXZZ** Release Left Knee Joint, External Approach	**0SNNXZZ** Release Left Metatarsal-Phalangeal Joint, External Approach
0SN60ZZ Release Coccygeal Joint, Open Approach	**0SNF0ZZ** Release Right Ankle Joint, Open Approach	**0SNP0ZZ** Release Right Toe Phalangeal Joint, Open Approach
0SN63ZZ Release Coccygeal Joint, Percutaneous Approach	**0SNF3ZZ** Release Right Ankle Joint, Percutaneous Approach	**0SNP3ZZ** Release Right Toe Phalangeal Joint, Percutaneous Approach
0SN64ZZ Release Coccygeal Joint, Percutaneous Endoscopic Approach	**0SNF4ZZ** Release Right Ankle Joint, Percutaneous Endoscopic Approach	**0SNP4ZZ** Release Right Toe Phalangeal Joint, Percutaneous Endoscopic Approach
0SN6XZZ Release Coccygeal Joint, External Approach	**0SNFXZZ** Release Right Ankle Joint, External Approach	**0SNPXZZ** Release Right Toe Phalangeal Joint, External Approach
0SN70ZZ Release Right Sacroiliac Joint, Open Approach	**0SNG0ZZ** Release Left Ankle Joint, Open Approach	**0SNQ0ZZ** Release Left Toe Phalangeal Joint, Open Approach
0SN73ZZ Release Right Sacroiliac Joint, Percutaneous Approach	**0SNG3ZZ** Release Left Ankle Joint, Percutaneous Approach	**0SNQ3ZZ** Release Left Toe Phalangeal Joint, Percutaneous Approach
0SN74ZZ Release Right Sacroiliac Joint, Percutaneous Endoscopic Approach	**0SNG4ZZ** Release Left Ankle Joint, Percutaneous Endoscopic Approach	**0SNQ4ZZ** Release Left Toe Phalangeal Joint, Percutaneous Endoscopic Approach
0SN7XZZ Release Right Sacroiliac Joint, External Approach	**0SNGXZZ** Release Left Ankle Joint, External Approach	**0SNQXZZ** Release Left Toe Phalangeal Joint, External Approach
	0SNH0ZZ Release Right Tarsal Joint, Open Approach	
	0SNH3ZZ Release Right Tarsal Joint, Percutaneous Approach	
	0SNH4ZZ Release Right Tarsal Joint, Percutaneous Endoscopic Approach	
	0SNHXZZ Release Right Tarsal Joint, External Approach	

0SP – Lower Joints, Removal

Review Coding Guideline B6.1c

0SP000Z Removal of Drainage Device from Lumbar Vertebral Joint, Open Approach	**0SP007Z** Removal of Autologous Tissue Substitute from Lumbar Vertebral Joint, Open Approach	**0SP00JZ** Removal of Synthetic Substitute from Lumbar Vertebral Joint, Open Approach
0SP003Z Removal of Infusion Device from Lumbar Vertebral Joint, Open Approach	**0SP008Z** Removal of Spacer from Lumbar Vertebral Joint, Open Approach	**0SP00KZ** Removal of Nonautologous Tissue Substitute from Lumbar Vertebral Joint, Open Approach
0SP004Z Removal of Internal Fixation Device from Lumbar Vertebral Joint, Open Approach	**0SP00AZ** Removal of Interbody Fusion Device from Lumbar Vertebral Joint, Open Approach	**0SP030Z** Removal of Drainage Device from Lumbar Vertebral Joint, Percutaneous Approach

♀ Female-only   ♂ Male-only   ▲ Limited Coverage   ● Non-OR   ▰ HAC-associated procedure   ▲ Non-covered procedures   ✚ Combination

0SP033Z Removal of Infusion Device from Lumbar Vertebral Joint, Percutaneous Approach
0SP034Z Removal of Internal Fixation Device from Lumbar Vertebral Joint, Percutaneous Approach
0SP037Z Removal of Autologous Tissue Substitute from Lumbar Vertebral Joint, Percutaneous Approach
0SP038Z Removal of Spacer from Lumbar Vertebral Joint, Percutaneous Approach
0SP03AZ Removal of Interbody Fusion Device from Lumbar Vertebral Joint, Percutaneous Approach
0SP03JZ Removal of Synthetic Substitute from Lumbar Vertebral Joint, Percutaneous Approach
0SP03KZ Removal of Nonautologous Tissue Substitute from Lumbar Vertebral Joint, Percutaneous Approach
0SP040Z Removal of Drainage Device from Lumbar Vertebral Joint, Percutaneous Endoscopic Approach
0SP043Z Removal of Infusion Device from Lumbar Vertebral Joint, Percutaneous Endoscopic Approach
0SP044Z Removal of Internal Fixation Device from Lumbar Vertebral Joint, Percutaneous Endoscopic Approach
0SP047Z Removal of Autologous Tissue Substitute from Lumbar Vertebral Joint, Percutaneous Endoscopic Approach
0SP048Z Removal of Spacer from Lumbar Vertebral Joint, Percutaneous Endoscopic Approach
0SP04AZ Removal of Interbody Fusion Device from Lumbar Vertebral Joint, Percutaneous Endoscopic Approach
0SP04JZ Removal of Synthetic Substitute from Lumbar Vertebral Joint, Percutaneous Endoscopic Approach
0SP04KZ Removal of Nonautologous Tissue Substitute from Lumbar Vertebral Joint, Percutaneous Endoscopic Approach
0SP0X0Z Removal of Drainage Device from Lumbar Vertebral Joint, External Approach
0SP0X3Z Removal of Infusion Device from Lumbar Vertebral Joint, External Approach
0SP0X4Z Removal of Internal Fixation Device from Lumbar Vertebral Joint, External Approach
0SP200Z Removal of Drainage Device from Lumbar Vertebral Disc, Open Approach
0SP203Z Removal of Infusion Device from Lumbar Vertebral Disc, Open Approach
0SP207Z Removal of Autologous Tissue Substitute from Lumbar Vertebral Disc, Open Approach
0SP20JZ Removal of Synthetic Substitute from Lumbar Vertebral Disc, Open Approach
0SP20KZ Removal of Nonautologous Tissue Substitute from Lumbar Vertebral Disc, Open Approach
0SP230Z Removal of Drainage Device from Lumbar Vertebral Disc, Percutaneous Approach
0SP233Z Removal of Infusion Device from Lumbar Vertebral Disc, Percutaneous Approach
0SP237Z Removal of Autologous Tissue Substitute from Lumbar Vertebral Disc, Percutaneous Approach
0SP23JZ Removal of Synthetic Substitute from Lumbar Vertebral Disc, Percutaneous Approach
0SP23KZ Removal of Nonautologous Tissue Substitute from Lumbar Vertebral Disc, Percutaneous Approach
0SP240Z Removal of Drainage Device from Lumbar Vertebral Disc, Percutaneous Endoscopic Approach
0SP243Z Removal of Infusion Device from Lumbar Vertebral Disc, Percutaneous Endoscopic Approach

0SP247Z Removal of Autologous Tissue Substitute from Lumbar Vertebral Disc, Percutaneous Endoscopic Approach
0SP24JZ Removal of Synthetic Substitute from Lumbar Vertebral Disc, Percutaneous Endoscopic Approach
0SP24KZ Removal of Nonautologous Tissue Substitute from Lumbar Vertebral Disc, Percutaneous Endoscopic Approach
0SP2X0Z Removal of Drainage Device from Lumbar Vertebral Disc, External Approach
0SP2X3Z Removal of Infusion Device from Lumbar Vertebral Disc, External Approach
0SP300Z Removal of Drainage Device from Lumbosacral Joint, Open Approach
0SP303Z Removal of Infusion Device from Lumbosacral Joint, Open Approach
0SP304Z Removal of Internal Fixation Device from Lumbosacral Joint, Open Approach
0SP307Z Removal of Autologous Tissue Substitute from Lumbosacral Joint, Open Approach
0SP308Z Removal of Spacer from Lumbosacral Joint, Open Approach
0SP30AZ Removal of Interbody Fusion Device from Lumbosacral Joint, Open Approach
0SP30JZ Removal of Synthetic Substitute from Lumbosacral Joint, Open Approach
0SP30KZ Removal of Nonautologous Tissue Substitute from Lumbosacral Joint, Open Approach
0SP330Z Removal of Drainage Device from Lumbosacral Joint, Percutaneous Approach
0SP333Z Removal of Infusion Device from Lumbosacral Joint, Percutaneous Approach
0SP334Z Removal of Internal Fixation Device from Lumbosacral Joint, Percutaneous Approach
0SP337Z Removal of Autologous Tissue Substitute from Lumbosacral Joint, Percutaneous Approach
0SP338Z Removal of Spacer from Lumbosacral Joint, Percutaneous Approach
0SP33AZ Removal of Interbody Fusion Device from Lumbosacral Joint, Percutaneous Approach
0SP33JZ Removal of Synthetic Substitute from Lumbosacral Joint, Percutaneous Approach
0SP33KZ Removal of Nonautologous Tissue Substitute from Lumbosacral Joint, Percutaneous Approach
0SP340Z Removal of Drainage Device from Lumbosacral Joint, Percutaneous Endoscopic Approach
0SP343Z Removal of Infusion Device from Lumbosacral Joint, Percutaneous Endoscopic Approach
0SP344Z Removal of Internal Fixation Device from Lumbosacral Joint, Percutaneous Endoscopic Approach
0SP347Z Removal of Autologous Tissue Substitute from Lumbosacral Joint, Percutaneous Endoscopic Approach
0SP348Z Removal of Spacer from Lumbosacral Joint, Percutaneous Endoscopic Approach
0SP34AZ Removal of Interbody Fusion Device from Lumbosacral Joint, Percutaneous Endoscopic Approach
0SP34JZ Removal of Synthetic Substitute from Lumbosacral Joint, Percutaneous Endoscopic Approach
0SP34KZ Removal of Nonautologous Tissue Substitute from Lumbosacral Joint, Percutaneous Endoscopic Approach
0SP3X0Z Removal of Drainage Device from Lumbosacral Joint, External Approach

0SP3X3Z Removal of Infusion Device from Lumbosacral Joint, External Approach
0SP3X4Z Removal of Internal Fixation Device from Lumbosacral Joint, External Approach
0SP400Z Removal of Drainage Device from Lumbosacral Disc, Open Approach
0SP403Z Removal of Infusion Device from Lumbosacral Disc, Open Approach
0SP407Z Removal of Autologous Tissue Substitute from Lumbosacral Disc, Open Approach
0SP40JZ Removal of Synthetic Substitute from Lumbosacral Disc, Open Approach
0SP40KZ Removal of Nonautologous Tissue Substitute from Lumbosacral Disc, Open Approach
0SP430Z Removal of Drainage Device from Lumbosacral Disc, Percutaneous Approach
0SP433Z Removal of Infusion Device from Lumbosacral Disc, Percutaneous Approach
0SP437Z Removal of Autologous Tissue Substitute from Lumbosacral Disc, Percutaneous Approach
0SP43JZ Removal of Synthetic Substitute from Lumbosacral Disc, Percutaneous Approach
0SP43KZ Removal of Nonautologous Tissue Substitute from Lumbosacral Disc, Percutaneous Approach
0SP440Z Removal of Drainage Device from Lumbosacral Disc, Percutaneous Endoscopic Approach
0SP443Z Removal of Infusion Device from Lumbosacral Disc, Percutaneous Endoscopic Approach
0SP447Z Removal of Autologous Tissue Substitute from Lumbosacral Disc, Percutaneous Endoscopic Approach
0SP44JZ Removal of Synthetic Substitute from Lumbosacral Disc, Percutaneous Endoscopic Approach
0SP44KZ Removal of Nonautologous Tissue Substitute from Lumbosacral Disc, Percutaneous Endoscopic Approach
0SP4X0Z Removal of Drainage Device from Lumbosacral Disc, External Approach
0SP4X3Z Removal of Infusion Device from Lumbosacral Disc, External Approach
0SP500Z Removal of Drainage Device from Sacrococcygeal Joint, Open Approach
0SP503Z Removal of Infusion Device from Sacrococcygeal Joint, Open Approach
0SP504Z Removal of Internal Fixation Device from Sacrococcygeal Joint, Open Approach
0SP507Z Removal of Autologous Tissue Substitute from Sacrococcygeal Joint, Open Approach
0SP508Z Removal of Spacer from Sacrococcygeal Joint, Open Approach
0SP50JZ Removal of Synthetic Substitute from Sacrococcygeal Joint, Open Approach
0SP50KZ Removal of Nonautologous Tissue Substitute from Sacrococcygeal Joint, Open Approach
0SP530Z Removal of Drainage Device from Sacrococcygeal Joint, Percutaneous Approach
0SP533Z Removal of Infusion Device from Sacrococcygeal Joint, Percutaneous Approach
0SP534Z Removal of Internal Fixation Device from Sacrococcygeal Joint, Percutaneous Approach
0SP537Z Removal of Autologous Tissue Substitute from Sacrococcygeal Joint, Percutaneous Approach

Female-only   ♂ Male-only   ▲ Limited Coverage   ● Non-OR   ▨ HAC-associated procedure   ▲ Non-covered procedures   ✚ Combination

0SP538Z Removal of Spacer from Sacrococcygeal Joint, Percutaneous Approach

0SP53JZ Removal of Synthetic Substitute from Sacrococcygeal Joint, Percutaneous Approach

0SP53KZ Removal of Nonautologous Tissue Substitute from Sacrococcygeal Joint, Percutaneous Approach

0SP540Z Removal of Drainage Device from Sacrococcygeal Joint, Percutaneous Endoscopic Approach

0SP543Z Removal of Infusion Device from Sacrococcygeal Joint, Percutaneous Endoscopic Approach

0SP544Z Removal of Internal Fixation Device from Sacrococcygeal Joint, Percutaneous Endoscopic Approach

0SP547Z Removal of Autologous Tissue Substitute from Sacrococcygeal Joint, Percutaneous Endoscopic Approach

0SP548Z Removal of Spacer from Sacrococcygeal Joint, Percutaneous Endoscopic Approach

0SP54JZ Removal of Synthetic Substitute from Sacrococcygeal Joint, Percutaneous Endoscopic Approach

0SP54KZ Removal of Nonautologous Tissue Substitute from Sacrococcygeal Joint, Percutaneous Endoscopic Approach

0SP5X0Z Removal of Drainage Device from Sacrococcygeal Joint, External Approach

0SP5X3Z Removal of Infusion Device from Sacrococcygeal Joint, External Approach

0SP5X4Z Removal of Internal Fixation Device from Sacrococcygeal Joint, External Approach

0SP600Z Removal of Drainage Device from Coccygeal Joint, Open Approach

0SP603Z Removal of Infusion Device from Coccygeal Joint, Open Approach

0SP604Z Removal of Internal Fixation Device from Coccygeal Joint, Open Approach

0SP607Z Removal of Autologous Tissue Substitute from Coccygeal Joint, Open Approach

0SP608Z Removal of Spacer from Coccygeal Joint, Open Approach

0SP60JZ Removal of Synthetic Substitute from Coccygeal Joint, Open Approach

0SP60KZ Removal of Nonautologous Tissue Substitute from Coccygeal Joint, Open Approach

0SP630Z Removal of Drainage Device from Coccygeal Joint, Percutaneous Approach

0SP633Z Removal of Infusion Device from Coccygeal Joint, Percutaneous Approach

0SP634Z Removal of Internal Fixation Device from Coccygeal Joint, Percutaneous Approach

0SP637Z Removal of Autologous Tissue Substitute from Coccygeal Joint, Percutaneous Approach

0SP638Z Removal of Spacer from Coccygeal Joint, Percutaneous Approach

0SP63JZ Removal of Synthetic Substitute from Coccygeal Joint, Percutaneous Approach

0SP63KZ Removal of Nonautologous Tissue Substitute from Coccygeal Joint, Percutaneous Approach

0SP640Z Removal of Drainage Device from Coccygeal Joint, Percutaneous Endoscopic Approach

0SP643Z Removal of Infusion Device from Coccygeal Joint, Percutaneous Endoscopic Approach

0SP644Z Removal of Internal Fixation Device from Coccygeal Joint, Percutaneous Endoscopic Approach

0SP647Z Removal of Autologous Tissue Substitute from Coccygeal Joint, Percutaneous Endoscopic Approach

0SP648Z Removal of Spacer from Coccygeal Joint, Percutaneous Endoscopic Approach

0SP64JZ Removal of Synthetic Substitute from Coccygeal Joint, Percutaneous Endoscopic Approach

0SP64KZ Removal of Nonautologous Tissue Substitute from Coccygeal Joint, Percutaneous Endoscopic Approach

0SP6X0Z Removal of Drainage Device from Coccygeal Joint, External Approach

0SP6X3Z Removal of Infusion Device from Coccygeal Joint, External Approach

0SP6X4Z Removal of Internal Fixation Device from Coccygeal Joint, External Approach

0SP700Z Removal of Drainage Device from Right Sacroiliac Joint, Open Approach

0SP703Z Removal of Infusion Device from Right Sacroiliac Joint, Open Approach

0SP704Z Removal of Internal Fixation Device from Right Sacroiliac Joint, Open Approach

0SP707Z Removal of Autologous Tissue Substitute from Right Sacroiliac Joint, Open Approach

0SP708Z Removal of Spacer from Right Sacroiliac Joint, Open Approach

0SP70JZ Removal of Synthetic Substitute from Right Sacroiliac Joint, Open Approach

0SP70KZ Removal of Nonautologous Tissue Substitute from Right Sacroiliac Joint, Open Approach

0SP730Z Removal of Drainage Device from Right Sacroiliac Joint, Percutaneous Approach

0SP733Z Removal of Infusion Device from Right Sacroiliac Joint, Percutaneous Approach

0SP734Z Removal of Internal Fixation Device from Right Sacroiliac Joint, Percutaneous Approach

0SP737Z Removal of Autologous Tissue Substitute from Right Sacroiliac Joint, Percutaneous Approach

0SP738Z Removal of Spacer from Right Sacroiliac Joint, Percutaneous Approach

0SP73JZ Removal of Synthetic Substitute from Right Sacroiliac Joint, Percutaneous Approach

0SP73KZ Removal of Nonautologous Tissue Substitute from Right Sacroiliac Joint, Percutaneous Approach

0SP740Z Removal of Drainage Device from Right Sacroiliac Joint, Percutaneous Endoscopic Approach

0SP743Z Removal of Infusion Device from Right Sacroiliac Joint, Percutaneous Endoscopic Approach

0SP744Z Removal of Internal Fixation Device from Right Sacroiliac Joint, Percutaneous Endoscopic Approach

0SP747Z Removal of Autologous Tissue Substitute from Right Sacroiliac Joint, Percutaneous Endoscopic Approach

0SP748Z Removal of Spacer from Right Sacroiliac Joint, Percutaneous Endoscopic Approach

0SP74JZ Removal of Synthetic Substitute from Right Sacroiliac Joint, Percutaneous Endoscopic Approach

0SP74KZ Removal of Nonautologous Tissue Substitute from Right Sacroiliac Joint, Percutaneous Endoscopic Approach

0SP7X0Z Removal of Drainage Device from Right Sacroiliac Joint, External Approach

0SP7X3Z Removal of Infusion Device from Right Sacroiliac Joint, External Approach

0SP7X4Z Removal of Internal Fixation Device from Right Sacroiliac Joint, External Approach

0SP800Z Removal of Drainage Device from Left Sacroiliac Joint, Open Approach

0SP803Z Removal of Infusion Device from Left Sacroiliac Joint, Open Approach

0SP804Z Removal of Internal Fixation Device from Left Sacroiliac Joint, Open Approach

0SP807Z Removal of Autologous Tissue Substitute from Left Sacroiliac Joint, Open Approach

0SP808Z Removal of Spacer from Left Sacroiliac Joint, Open Approach

0SP80JZ Removal of Synthetic Substitute from Left Sacroiliac Joint, Open Approach

0SP80KZ Removal of Nonautologous Tissue Substitute from Left Sacroiliac Joint, Open Approach

0SP830Z Removal of Drainage Device from Left Sacroiliac Joint, Percutaneous Approach

0SP833Z Removal of Infusion Device from Left Sacroiliac Joint, Percutaneous Approach

0SP834Z Removal of Internal Fixation Device from Left Sacroiliac Joint, Percutaneous Approach

0SP837Z Removal of Autologous Tissue Substitute from Left Sacroiliac Joint, Percutaneous Approach

0SP838Z Removal of Spacer from Left Sacroiliac Joint, Percutaneous Approach

0SP83JZ Removal of Synthetic Substitute from Left Sacroiliac Joint, Percutaneous Approach

0SP83KZ Removal of Nonautologous Tissue Substitute from Left Sacroiliac Joint, Percutaneous Approach

0SP840Z Removal of Drainage Device from Left Sacroiliac Joint, Percutaneous Endoscopic Approach

0SP843Z Removal of Infusion Device from Left Sacroiliac Joint, Percutaneous Endoscopic Approach

0SP844Z Removal of Internal Fixation Device from Left Sacroiliac Joint, Percutaneous Endoscopic Approach

0SP847Z Removal of Autologous Tissue Substitute from Left Sacroiliac Joint, Percutaneous Endoscopic Approach

0SP848Z Removal of Spacer from Left Sacroiliac Joint, Percutaneous Endoscopic Approach

0SP84JZ Removal of Synthetic Substitute from Left Sacroiliac Joint, Percutaneous Endoscopic Approach

0SP84KZ Removal of Nonautologous Tissue Substitute from Left Sacroiliac Joint, Percutaneous Endoscopic Approach

0SP8X0Z Removal of Drainage Device from Left Sacroiliac Joint, External Approach

0SP8X3Z Removal of Infusion Device from Left Sacroiliac Joint, External Approach

0SP8X4Z Removal of Internal Fixation Device from Left Sacroiliac Joint, External Approach

0SP900Z Removal of Drainage Device from Right Hip Joint, Open Approach

0SP903Z Removal of Infusion Device from Right Hip Joint, Open Approach

0SP904Z Removal of Internal Fixation Device from Right Hip Joint, Open Approach

0SP905Z Removal of External Fixation Device from Right Hip Joint, Open Approach

0SP907Z Removal of Autologous Tissue Substitute from Right Hip Joint, Open Approach

0SP908Z Removal of Spacer from Right Hip Joint, Open Approach

0SP909Z Removal of Liner from Right Hip Joint, Open Approach

➕ *If replacement, see table 0SU to construct a code for Supplement with liner.*

0SP90BZ Removal of Resurfacing Device from Right Hip Joint, Open Approach

0SP90JZ Removal of Synthetic Substitute from Right Hip Joint, Open Approach

➕ *If replacement see table 0SR to construct code for the Replacement of the device.*

0SP90KZ Removal of Nonautologous Tissue Substitute from Right Hip Joint, Open Approach

♀ Female-only　　♂ Male-only　　▲ Limited Coverage　　● Non-OR　　▨ HAC-associated procedure　　▲ Non-covered procedures　　➕ Combinati

?930Z	Removal of Drainage Device from Right Hip Joint, Percutaneous Approach
?933Z	Removal of Infusion Device from Right Hip Joint, Percutaneous Approach
?934Z	Removal of Internal Fixation Device from Right Hip Joint, Percutaneous Approach
?935Z	Removal of External Fixation Device from Right Hip Joint, Percutaneous Approach
?937Z	Removal of Autologous Tissue Substitute from Right Hip Joint, Percutaneous Approach
?938Z	Removal of Spacer from Right Hip Joint, Percutaneous Approach
?93JZ	Removal of Synthetic Substitute from Right Hip Joint, Percutaneous Approach
?93KZ	Removal of Nonautologous Tissue Substitute from Right Hip Joint, Percutaneous Approach
?940Z	Removal of Drainage Device from Right Hip Joint, Percutaneous Endoscopic Approach
?943Z	Removal of Infusion Device from Right Hip Joint, Percutaneous Endoscopic Approach
?944Z	Removal of Internal Fixation Device from Right Hip Joint, Percutaneous Endoscopic Approach
P945Z	Removal of External Fixation Device from Right Hip Joint, Percutaneous Endoscopic Approach
P947Z	Removal of Autologous Tissue Substitute from Right Hip Joint, Percutaneous Endoscopic Approach
P948Z	Removal of Spacer from Right Hip Joint, Percutaneous Endoscopic Approach
P94JZ	Removal of Synthetic Substitute from Right Hip Joint, Percutaneous Endoscopic Approach
?P94KZ	Removal of Nonautologous Tissue Substitute from Right Hip Joint, Percutaneous Endoscopic Approach
?P9X0Z	Removal of Drainage Device from Right Hip Joint, External Approach
?P9X3Z	Removal of Infusion Device from Right Hip Joint, External Approach
?P9X4Z	Removal of Internal Fixation Device from Right Hip Joint, External Approach
P9X5Z	Removal of External Fixation Device from Right Hip Joint, External Approach
SPB00Z	Removal of Drainage Device from Left Hip Joint, Open Approach
SPB03Z	Removal of Infusion Device from Left Hip Joint, Open Approach
SPB04Z	Removal of Internal Fixation Device from Left Hip Joint, Open Approach
SPB05Z	Removal of External Fixation Device from Left Hip Joint, Open Approach
SPB07Z	Removal of Autologous Tissue Substitute from Left Hip Joint, Open Approach
SPB08Z	Removal of Spacer from Left Hip Joint, Open Approach
SPB09Z	Removal of Liner from Left Hip Joint, Open Approach
✚	*If replacement, see table 0SU to construct a code for Supplement with liner.*
SPB0BZ	Removal of Resurfacing Device from Left Hip Joint, Open Approach
SPB0JZ	Removal of Synthetic Substitute from Left Hip Joint, Open Approach
✚	*If replacement see table 0SR to construct a code for the Replacement of the device.*
SPB0KZ	Removal of Nonautologous Tissue Substitute from Left Hip Joint, Open Approach
SPB30Z	Removal of Drainage Device from Left Hip Joint, Percutaneous Approach
SPB33Z	Removal of Infusion Device from Left Hip Joint, Percutaneous Approach

0SPB34Z	Removal of Internal Fixation Device from Left Hip Joint, Percutaneous Approach
0SPB35Z	Removal of External Fixation Device from Left Hip Joint, Percutaneous Approach
0SPB37Z	Removal of Autologous Tissue Substitute from Left Hip Joint, Percutaneous Approach
0SPB38Z	Removal of Spacer from Left Hip Joint, Percutaneous Approach
0SPB3JZ	Removal of Synthetic Substitute from Left Hip Joint, Percutaneous Approach
0SPB3KZ	Removal of Nonautologous Tissue Substitute from Left Hip Joint, Percutaneous Approach
0SPB40Z	Removal of Drainage Device from Left Hip Joint, Percutaneous Endoscopic Approach
0SPB43Z	Removal of Infusion Device from Left Hip Joint, Percutaneous Endoscopic Approach
0SPB44Z	Removal of Internal Fixation Device from Left Hip Joint, Percutaneous Endoscopic Approach
0SPB45Z	Removal of External Fixation Device from Left Hip Joint, Percutaneous Endoscopic Approach
0SPB47Z	Removal of Autologous Tissue Substitute from Left Hip Joint, Percutaneous Endoscopic Approach
0SPB48Z	Removal of Spacer from Left Hip Joint, Percutaneous Endoscopic Approach
0SPB4JZ	Removal of Synthetic Substitute from Left Hip Joint, Percutaneous Endoscopic Approach
0SPB4KZ	Removal of Nonautologous Tissue Substitute from Left Hip Joint, Percutaneous Endoscopic Approach
0SPBX0Z	Removal of Drainage Device from Left Hip Joint, External Approach
0SPBX3Z	Removal of Infusion Device from Left Hip Joint, External Approach
0SPBX4Z	Removal of Internal Fixation Device from Left Hip Joint, External Approach
0SPBX5Z	Removal of External Fixation Device from Left Hip Joint, External Approach
0SPC00Z	Removal of Drainage Device from Right Knee Joint, Open Approach
0SPC03Z	Removal of Infusion Device from Right Knee Joint, Open Approach
0SPC04Z	Removal of Internal Fixation Device from Right Knee Joint, Open Approach
0SPC05Z	Removal of External Fixation Device from Right Knee Joint, Open Approach
0SPC07Z	Removal of Autologous Tissue Substitute from Right Knee Joint, Open Approach
0SPC08Z	Removal of Spacer from Right Knee Joint, Open Approach
0SPC09Z	Removal of Liner from Right Knee Joint, Open Approach
✚	*If replacement, see table 0SU to construct a code for Supplement with liner.*
0SPC0JZ	Removal of Synthetic Substitute from Right Knee Joint, Open Approach
✚	*If replacement see table 0SR to construct a code for the Replacement of the device.*
0SPC0KZ	Removal of Nonautologous Tissue Substitute from Right Knee Joint, Open Approach
0SPC30Z	Removal of Drainage Device from Right Knee Joint, Percutaneous Approach
0SPC33Z	Removal of Infusion Device from Right Knee Joint, Percutaneous Approach
0SPC34Z	Removal of Internal Fixation Device from Right Knee Joint, Percutaneous Approach
0SPC35Z	Removal of External Fixation Device from Right Knee Joint, Percutaneous Approach
0SPC37Z	Removal of Autologous Tissue Substitute from Right Knee Joint, Percutaneous Approach

0SPC38Z	Removal of Spacer from Right Knee Joint, Percutaneous Approach
0SPC3JZ	Removal of Synthetic Substitute from Right Knee Joint, Percutaneous Approach
0SPC3KZ	Removal of Nonautologous Tissue Substitute from Right Knee Joint, Percutaneous Approach
0SPC40Z	Removal of Drainage Device from Right Knee Joint, Percutaneous Endoscopic Approach
0SPC43Z	Removal of Infusion Device from Right Knee Joint, Percutaneous Endoscopic Approach
0SPC44Z	Removal of Internal Fixation Device from Right Knee Joint, Percutaneous Endoscopic Approach
0SPC45Z	Removal of External Fixation Device from Right Knee Joint, Percutaneous Endoscopic Approach
0SPC47Z	Removal of Autologous Tissue Substitute from Right Knee Joint, Percutaneous Endoscopic Approach
0SPC48Z	Removal of Spacer from Right Knee Joint, Percutaneous Endoscopic Approach
0SPC4JZ	Removal of Synthetic Substitute from Right Knee Joint, Percutaneous Endoscopic Approach
✚	*If replacement see table 0SR to construct a code for the Replacement of the device.*
0SPC4KZ	Removal of Nonautologous Tissue Substitute from Right Knee Joint, Percutaneous Endoscopic Approach
0SPCX0Z	Removal of Drainage Device from Right Knee Joint, External Approach
0SPCX3Z	Removal of Infusion Device from Right Knee Joint, External Approach
0SPCX4Z	Removal of Internal Fixation Device from Right Knee Joint, External Approach
0SPCX5Z	Removal of External Fixation Device from Right Knee Joint, External Approach
0SPD00Z	Removal of Drainage Device from Left Knee Joint, Open Approach
0SPD03Z	Removal of Infusion Device from Left Knee Joint, Open Approach
0SPD04Z	Removal of Internal Fixation Device from Left Knee Joint, Open Approach
0SPD05Z	Removal of External Fixation Device from Left Knee Joint, Open Approach
0SPD07Z	Removal of Autologous Tissue Substitute from Left Knee Joint, Open Approach
0SPD08Z	Removal of Spacer from Left Knee Joint, Open Approach
0SPD09Z	Removal of Liner from Left Knee Joint, Open Approach
✚	*If replacement, see table 0SU to construct a code for Supplement with liner.*
0SPD0JZ	Removal of Synthetic Substitute from Left Knee Joint, Open Approach
✚	*If replacement see table 0SR to construct a code for the Replacement of the device.*
0SPD0KZ	Removal of Nonautologous Tissue Substitute from Left Knee Joint, Open Approach
0SPD30Z	Removal of Drainage Device from Left Knee Joint, Percutaneous Approach
0SPD33Z	Removal of Infusion Device from Left Knee Joint, Percutaneous Approach
0SPD34Z	Removal of Internal Fixation Device from Left Knee Joint, Percutaneous Approach
0SPD35Z	Removal of External Fixation Device from Left Knee Joint, Percutaneous Approach
0SPD37Z	Removal of Autologous Tissue Substitute from Left Knee Joint, Percutaneous Approach
0SPD38Z	Removal of Spacer from Left Knee Joint, Percutaneous Approach
0SPD3JZ	Removal of Synthetic Substitute from Left Knee Joint, Percutaneous Approach

999

Female-only	♂ Male-only	▲ Limited Coverage	● Non-OR	▦ HAC-associated procedure	▲ Non-covered procedures	✚ Combination

0SPD3KZ Removal of Nonautologous Tissue Substitute from Left Knee Joint, Percutaneous Approach

0SPD40Z Removal of Drainage Device from Left Knee Joint, Percutaneous Endoscopic Approach

0SPD43Z Removal of Infusion Device from Left Knee Joint, Percutaneous Endoscopic Approach

0SPD44Z Removal of Internal Fixation Device from Left Knee Joint, Percutaneous Endoscopic Approach

0SPD45Z Removal of External Fixation Device from Left Knee Joint, Percutaneous Endoscopic Approach

0SPD47Z Removal of Autologous Tissue Substitute from Left Knee Joint, Percutaneous Endoscopic Approach

0SPD48Z Removal of Spacer from Left Knee Joint, Percutaneous Endoscopic Approach

0SPD4JZ Removal of Synthetic Substitute from Left Knee Joint, Percutaneous Endoscopic Approach

⊞ *If replacement see table 0SR to construct a code for the Replacement of the device.*

0SPD4KZ Removal of Nonautologous Tissue Substitute from Left Knee Joint, Percutaneous Endoscopic Approach

0SPDX0Z Removal of Drainage Device from Left Knee Joint, External Approach

0SPDX3Z Removal of Infusion Device from Left Knee Joint, External Approach

0SPDX4Z Removal of Internal Fixation Device from Left Knee Joint, External Approach

0SPDX5Z Removal of External Fixation Device from Left Knee Joint, External Approach

0SPF00Z Removal of Drainage Device from Right Ankle Joint, Open Approach

0SPF03Z Removal of Infusion Device from Right Ankle Joint, Open Approach

0SPF04Z Removal of Internal Fixation Device from Right Ankle Joint, Open Approach

0SPF05Z Removal of External Fixation Device from Right Ankle Joint, Open Approach

0SPF07Z Removal of Autologous Tissue Substitute from Right Ankle Joint, Open Approach

0SPF08Z Removal of Spacer from Right Ankle Joint, Open Approach

0SPF0JZ Removal of Synthetic Substitute from Right Ankle Joint, Open Approach

0SPF0KZ Removal of Nonautologous Tissue Substitute from Right Ankle Joint, Open Approach

0SPF30Z Removal of Drainage Device from Right Ankle Joint, Percutaneous Approach

0SPF33Z Removal of Infusion Device from Right Ankle Joint, Percutaneous Approach

0SPF34Z Removal of Internal Fixation Device from Right Ankle Joint, Percutaneous Approach

0SPF35Z Removal of External Fixation Device from Right Ankle Joint, Percutaneous Approach

0SPF37Z Removal of Autologous Tissue Substitute from Right Ankle Joint, Percutaneous Approach

0SPF38Z Removal of Spacer from Right Ankle Joint, Percutaneous Approach

0SPF3JZ Removal of Synthetic Substitute from Right Ankle Joint, Percutaneous Approach

0SPF3KZ Removal of Nonautologous Tissue Substitute from Right Ankle Joint, Percutaneous Approach

0SPF40Z Removal of Drainage Device from Right Ankle Joint, Percutaneous Endoscopic Approach

0SPF43Z Removal of Infusion Device from Right Ankle Joint, Percutaneous Endoscopic Approach

0SPF44Z Removal of Internal Fixation Device from Right Ankle Joint, Percutaneous Endoscopic Approach

0SPF45Z Removal of External Fixation Device from Right Ankle Joint, Percutaneous Endoscopic Approach

0SPF47Z Removal of Autologous Tissue Substitute from Right Ankle Joint, Percutaneous Endoscopic Approach

0SPF48Z Removal of Spacer from Right Ankle Joint, Percutaneous Endoscopic Approach

0SPF4JZ Removal of Synthetic Substitute from Right Ankle Joint, Percutaneous Endoscopic Approach

0SPF4KZ Removal of Nonautologous Tissue Substitute from Right Ankle Joint, Percutaneous Endoscopic Approach

0SPFX0Z Removal of Drainage Device from Right Ankle Joint, External Approach

0SPFX3Z Removal of Infusion Device from Right Ankle Joint, External Approach

0SPFX4Z Removal of Internal Fixation Device from Right Ankle Joint, External Approach

0SPFX5Z Removal of External Fixation Device from Right Ankle Joint, External Approach

0SPG00Z Removal of Drainage Device from Left Ankle Joint, Open Approach

0SPG03Z Removal of Infusion Device from Left Ankle Joint, Open Approach

0SPG04Z Removal of Internal Fixation Device from Left Ankle Joint, Open Approach

AHA CC: 2Q, 2013, 39-40

0SPG05Z Removal of External Fixation Device from Left Ankle Joint, Open Approach

0SPG07Z Removal of Autologous Tissue Substitute from Left Ankle Joint, Open Approach

0SPG08Z Removal of Spacer from Left Ankle Joint, Open Approach

0SPG0JZ Removal of Synthetic Substitute from Left Ankle Joint, Open Approach

0SPG0KZ Removal of Nonautologous Tissue Substitute from Left Ankle Joint, Open Approach

0SPG30Z Removal of Drainage Device from Left Ankle Joint, Percutaneous Approach

0SPG33Z Removal of Infusion Device from Left Ankle Joint, Percutaneous Approach

0SPG34Z Removal of Internal Fixation Device from Left Ankle Joint, Percutaneous Approach

0SPG35Z Removal of External Fixation Device from Left Ankle Joint, Percutaneous Approach

0SPG37Z Removal of Autologous Tissue Substitute from Left Ankle Joint, Percutaneous Approach

0SPG38Z Removal of Spacer from Left Ankle Joint, Percutaneous Approach

0SPG3JZ Removal of Synthetic Substitute from Left Ankle Joint, Percutaneous Approach

0SPG3KZ Removal of Nonautologous Tissue Substitute from Left Ankle Joint, Percutaneous Approach

0SPG40Z Removal of Drainage Device from Left Ankle Joint, Percutaneous Endoscopic Approach

0SPG43Z Removal of Infusion Device from Left Ankle Joint, Percutaneous Endoscopic Approach

0SPG44Z Removal of Internal Fixation Device from Left Ankle Joint, Percutaneous Endoscopic Approach

0SPG45Z Removal of External Fixation Device from Left Ankle Joint, Percutaneous Endoscopic Approach

0SPG47Z Removal of Autologous Tissue Substitute from Left Ankle Joint, Percutaneous Endoscopic Approach

0SPG48Z Removal of Spacer from Left Ankle Joint, Percutaneous Endoscopic Approach

0SPG4JZ Removal of Synthetic Substitute from Left Ankle Joint, Percutaneous Endoscopic Approach

0SPG4KZ Removal of Nonautologous Tissue Substitute from Left Ankle Joint, Percutaneous Endoscopic Approach

0SPGX0Z Removal of Drainage Device from Left Ankle Joint, External Approach

0SPGX3Z Removal of Infusion Device from Left Ankle Joint, External Approach

0SPGX4Z Removal of Internal Fixation Device from Left Ankle Joint, External Approach

0SPGX5Z Removal of External Fixation Device from Left Ankle Joint, External Approach

0SPH00Z Removal of Drainage Device from Right Tarsal Joint, Open Approach

0SPH03Z Removal of Infusion Device from Right Tarsal Joint, Open Approach

0SPH04Z Removal of Internal Fixation Device from Right Tarsal Joint, Open Approach

0SPH05Z Removal of External Fixation Device from Right Tarsal Joint, Open Approach

0SPH07Z Removal of Autologous Tissue Substitute from Right Tarsal Joint, Open Approach

0SPH08Z Removal of Spacer from Right Tarsal Joint, Open Approach

0SPH0JZ Removal of Synthetic Substitute from Right Tarsal Joint, Open Approach

0SPH0KZ Removal of Nonautologous Tissue Substitute from Right Tarsal Joint, Open Approach

0SPH30Z Removal of Drainage Device from Right Tarsal Joint, Percutaneous Approach

0SPH33Z Removal of Infusion Device from Right Tarsal Joint, Percutaneous Approach

0SPH34Z Removal of Internal Fixation Device from Right Tarsal Joint, Percutaneous Approach

0SPH35Z Removal of External Fixation Device from Right Tarsal Joint, Percutaneous Approach

0SPH37Z Removal of Autologous Tissue Substitute from Right Tarsal Joint, Percutaneous Approach

0SPH38Z Removal of Spacer from Right Tarsal Joint, Percutaneous Approach

0SPH3JZ Removal of Synthetic Substitute from Right Tarsal Joint, Percutaneous Approach

0SPH3KZ Removal of Nonautologous Tissue Substitute from Right Tarsal Joint, Percutaneous Approach

0SPH40Z Removal of Drainage Device from Right Tarsal Joint, Percutaneous Endoscopic Approach

0SPH43Z Removal of Infusion Device from Right Tarsal Joint, Percutaneous Endoscopic Approach

0SPH44Z Removal of Internal Fixation Device from Right Tarsal Joint, Percutaneous Endoscopic Approach

0SPH45Z Removal of External Fixation Device from Right Tarsal Joint, Percutaneous Endoscopic Approach

0SPH47Z Removal of Autologous Tissue Substitute from Right Tarsal Joint, Percutaneous Endoscopic Approach

0SPH48Z Removal of Spacer from Right Tarsal Joint, Percutaneous Endoscopic Approach

0SPH4JZ Removal of Synthetic Substitute from Right Tarsal Joint, Percutaneous Endoscopic Approach

0SPH4KZ Removal of Nonautologous Tissue Substitute from Right Tarsal Joint, Percutaneous Endoscopic Approach

0SPHX0Z Removal of Drainage Device from Right Tarsal Joint, External Approach

0SPHX3Z Removal of Infusion Device from Right Tarsal Joint, External Approach

♀ Female-only   ♂ Male-only   ▲ Limited Coverage   ● Non-OR   ▬ HAC-associated procedure   ▲ Non-covered procedures   ⊞ Combination

0SPHX4Z	Removal of Internal Fixation Device from Right Tarsal Joint, External Approach
0SPHX5Z	Removal of External Fixation Device from Right Tarsal Joint, External Approach
0SPJ00Z	Removal of Drainage Device from Left Tarsal Joint, Open Approach
0SPJ03Z	Removal of Infusion Device from Left Tarsal Joint, Open Approach
0SPJ04Z	Removal of Internal Fixation Device from Left Tarsal Joint, Open Approach
0SPJ05Z	Removal of External Fixation Device from Left Tarsal Joint, Open Approach
0SPJ07Z	Removal of Autologous Tissue Substitute from Left Tarsal Joint, Open Approach
0SPJ08Z	Removal of Spacer from Left Tarsal Joint, Open Approach
0SPJ0JZ	Removal of Synthetic Substitute from Left Tarsal Joint, Open Approach
0SPJ0KZ	Removal of Nonautologous Tissue Substitute from Left Tarsal Joint, Open Approach
0SPJ30Z	Removal of Drainage Device from Left Tarsal Joint, Percutaneous Approach
0SPJ33Z	Removal of Infusion Device from Left Tarsal Joint, Percutaneous Approach
0SPJ34Z	Removal of Internal Fixation Device from Left Tarsal Joint, Percutaneous Approach
0SPJ35Z	Removal of External Fixation Device from Left Tarsal Joint, Percutaneous Approach
0SPJ37Z	Removal of Autologous Tissue Substitute from Left Tarsal Joint, Percutaneous Approach
0SPJ38Z	Removal of Spacer from Left Tarsal Joint, Percutaneous Approach
0SPJ3JZ	Removal of Synthetic Substitute from Left Tarsal Joint, Percutaneous Approach
0SPJ3KZ	Removal of Nonautologous Tissue Substitute from Left Tarsal Joint, Percutaneous Approach
0SPJ40Z	Removal of Drainage Device from Left Tarsal Joint, Percutaneous Endoscopic Approach
0SPJ43Z	Removal of Infusion Device from Left Tarsal Joint, Percutaneous Endoscopic Approach
0SPJ44Z	Removal of Internal Fixation Device from Left Tarsal Joint, Percutaneous Endoscopic Approach
0SPJ45Z	Removal of External Fixation Device from Left Tarsal Joint, Percutaneous Endoscopic Approach
0SPJ47Z	Removal of Autologous Tissue Substitute from Left Tarsal Joint, Percutaneous Endoscopic Approach
0SPJ48Z	Removal of Spacer from Left Tarsal Joint, Percutaneous Endoscopic Approach
0SPJ4JZ	Removal of Synthetic Substitute from Left Tarsal Joint, Percutaneous Endoscopic Approach
0SPJ4KZ	Removal of Nonautologous Tissue Substitute from Left Tarsal Joint, Percutaneous Endoscopic Approach
0SPJX0Z	Removal of Drainage Device from Left Tarsal Joint, External Approach
0SPJX3Z	Removal of Infusion Device from Left Tarsal Joint, External Approach
0SPJX4Z	Removal of Internal Fixation Device from Left Tarsal Joint, External Approach
0SPJX5Z	Removal of External Fixation Device from Left Tarsal Joint, External Approach
0SPK00Z	Removal of Drainage Device from Right Metatarsal-Tarsal Joint, Open Approach
0SPK03Z	Removal of Infusion Device from Right Metatarsal-Tarsal Joint, Open Approach
0SPK04Z	Removal of Internal Fixation Device from Right Metatarsal-Tarsal Joint, Open Approach
0SPK05Z	Removal of External Fixation Device from Right Metatarsal-Tarsal Joint, Open Approach
0SPK07Z	Removal of Autologous Tissue Substitute from Right Metatarsal-Tarsal Joint, Open Approach
0SPK08Z	Removal of Spacer from Right Metatarsal-Tarsal Joint, Open Approach
0SPK0JZ	Removal of Synthetic Substitute from Right Metatarsal-Tarsal Joint, Open Approach
0SPK0KZ	Removal of Nonautologous Tissue Substitute from Right Metatarsal-Tarsal Joint, Open Approach
0SPK30Z	Removal of Drainage Device from Right Metatarsal-Tarsal Joint, Percutaneous Approach
0SPK33Z	Removal of Infusion Device from Right Metatarsal-Tarsal Joint, Percutaneous Approach
0SPK34Z	Removal of Internal Fixation Device from Right Metatarsal-Tarsal Joint, Percutaneous Approach
0SPK35Z	Removal of External Fixation Device from Right Metatarsal-Tarsal Joint, Percutaneous Approach
0SPK37Z	Removal of Autologous Tissue Substitute from Right Metatarsal-Tarsal Joint, Percutaneous Approach
0SPK38Z	Removal of Spacer from Right Metatarsal-Tarsal Joint, Percutaneous Approach
0SPK3JZ	Removal of Synthetic Substitute from Right Metatarsal-Tarsal Joint, Percutaneous Approach
0SPK3KZ	Removal of Nonautologous Tissue Substitute from Right Metatarsal-Tarsal Joint, Percutaneous Approach
0SPK40Z	Removal of Drainage Device from Right Metatarsal-Tarsal Joint, Percutaneous Endoscopic Approach
0SPK43Z	Removal of Infusion Device from Right Metatarsal-Tarsal Joint, Percutaneous Endoscopic Approach
0SPK44Z	Removal of Internal Fixation Device from Right Metatarsal-Tarsal Joint, Percutaneous Endoscopic Approach
0SPK45Z	Removal of External Fixation Device from Right Metatarsal-Tarsal Joint, Percutaneous Endoscopic Approach
0SPK47Z	Removal of Autologous Tissue Substitute from Right Metatarsal-Tarsal Joint, Percutaneous Endoscopic Approach
0SPK48Z	Removal of Spacer from Right Metatarsal-Tarsal Joint, Percutaneous Endoscopic Approach
0SPK4JZ	Removal of Synthetic Substitute from Right Metatarsal-Tarsal Joint, Percutaneous Endoscopic Approach
0SPK4KZ	Removal of Nonautologous Tissue Substitute from Right Metatarsal-Tarsal Joint, Percutaneous Endoscopic Approach
0SPKX0Z	Removal of Drainage Device from Right Metatarsal-Tarsal Joint, External Approach
0SPKX3Z	Removal of Infusion Device from Right Metatarsal-Tarsal Joint, External Approach
0SPKX4Z	Removal of Internal Fixation Device from Right Metatarsal-Tarsal Joint, External Approach
0SPKX5Z	Removal of External Fixation Device from Right Metatarsal-Tarsal Joint, External Approach
0SPL00Z	Removal of Drainage Device from Left Metatarsal-Tarsal Joint, Open Approach
0SPL03Z	Removal of Infusion Device from Left Metatarsal-Tarsal Joint, Open Approach
0SPL04Z	Removal of Internal Fixation Device from Left Metatarsal-Tarsal Joint, Open Approach
0SPL05Z	Removal of External Fixation Device from Left Metatarsal-Tarsal Joint, Open Approach
0SPL07Z	Removal of Autologous Tissue Substitute from Left Metatarsal-Tarsal Joint, Open Approach
0SPL08Z	Removal of Spacer from Left Metatarsal-Tarsal Joint, Open Approach
0SPL0JZ	Removal of Synthetic Substitute from Left Metatarsal-Tarsal Joint, Open Approach
0SPL0KZ	Removal of Nonautologous Tissue Substitute from Left Metatarsal-Tarsal Joint, Open Approach
0SPL30Z	Removal of Drainage Device from Left Metatarsal-Tarsal Joint, Percutaneous Approach
0SPL33Z	Removal of Infusion Device from Left Metatarsal-Tarsal Joint, Percutaneous Approach
0SPL34Z	Removal of Internal Fixation Device from Left Metatarsal-Tarsal Joint, Percutaneous Approach
0SPL35Z	Removal of External Fixation Device from Left Metatarsal-Tarsal Joint, Percutaneous Approach
0SPL37Z	Removal of Autologous Tissue Substitute from Left Metatarsal-Tarsal Joint, Percutaneous Approach
0SPL38Z	Removal of Spacer from Left Metatarsal-Tarsal Joint, Percutaneous Approach
0SPL3JZ	Removal of Synthetic Substitute from Left Metatarsal-Tarsal Joint, Percutaneous Approach
0SPL3KZ	Removal of Nonautologous Tissue Substitute from Left Metatarsal-Tarsal Joint, Percutaneous Approach
0SPL40Z	Removal of Drainage Device from Left Metatarsal-Tarsal Joint, Percutaneous Endoscopic Approach
0SPL43Z	Removal of Infusion Device from Left Metatarsal-Tarsal Joint, Percutaneous Endoscopic Approach
0SPL44Z	Removal of Internal Fixation Device from Left Metatarsal-Tarsal Joint, Percutaneous Endoscopic Approach
0SPL45Z	Removal of External Fixation Device from Left Metatarsal-Tarsal Joint, Percutaneous Endoscopic Approach
0SPL47Z	Removal of Autologous Tissue Substitute from Left Metatarsal-Tarsal Joint, Percutaneous Endoscopic Approach
0SPL48Z	Removal of Spacer from Left Metatarsal-Tarsal Joint, Percutaneous Endoscopic Approach
0SPL4JZ	Removal of Synthetic Substitute from Left Metatarsal-Tarsal Joint, Percutaneous Endoscopic Approach
0SPL4KZ	Removal of Nonautologous Tissue Substitute from Left Metatarsal-Tarsal Joint, Percutaneous Endoscopic Approach
0SPLX0Z	Removal of Drainage Device from Left Metatarsal-Tarsal Joint, External Approach
0SPLX3Z	Removal of Infusion Device from Left Metatarsal-Tarsal Joint, External Approach
0SPLX4Z	Removal of Internal Fixation Device from Left Metatarsal-Tarsal Joint, External Approach
0SPLX5Z	Removal of External Fixation Device from Left Metatarsal-Tarsal Joint, External Approach
0SPM00Z	Removal of Drainage Device from Right Metatarsal-Phalangeal Joint, Open Approach
0SPM03Z	Removal of Infusion Device from Right Metatarsal-Phalangeal Joint, Open Approach
0SPM04Z	Removal of Internal Fixation Device from Right Metatarsal-Phalangeal Joint, Open Approach

1001

0SPM05Z Removal of External Fixation Device from Right Metatarsal-Phalangeal Joint, Open Approach

0SPM07Z Removal of Autologous Tissue Substitute from Right Metatarsal-Phalangeal Joint, Open Approach

0SPM08Z Removal of Spacer from Right Metatarsal-Phalangeal Joint, Open Approach

0SPM0JZ Removal of Synthetic Substitute from Right Metatarsal-Phalangeal Joint, Open Approach

0SPM0KZ Removal of Nonautologous Tissue Substitute from Right Metatarsal-Phalangeal Joint, Open Approach

0SPM30Z Removal of Drainage Device from Right Metatarsal-Phalangeal Joint, Percutaneous Approach

0SPM33Z Removal of Infusion Device from Right Metatarsal-Phalangeal Joint, Percutaneous Approach

0SPM34Z Removal of Internal Fixation Device from Right Metatarsal-Phalangeal Joint, Percutaneous Approach

0SPM35Z Removal of External Fixation Device from Right Metatarsal-Phalangeal Joint, Percutaneous Approach

0SPM37Z Removal of Autologous Tissue Substitute from Right Metatarsal-Phalangeal Joint, Percutaneous Approach

0SPM38Z Removal of Spacer from Right Metatarsal-Phalangeal Joint, Percutaneous Approach

0SPM3JZ Removal of Synthetic Substitute from Right Metatarsal-Phalangeal Joint, Percutaneous Approach

0SPM3KZ Removal of Nonautologous Tissue Substitute from Right Metatarsal-Phalangeal Joint, Percutaneous Approach

0SPM40Z Removal of Drainage Device from Right Metatarsal-Phalangeal Joint, Percutaneous Endoscopic Approach

0SPM43Z Removal of Infusion Device from Right Metatarsal-Phalangeal Joint, Percutaneous Endoscopic Approach

0SPM44Z Removal of Internal Fixation Device from Right Metatarsal-Phalangeal Joint, Percutaneous Endoscopic Approach

0SPM45Z Removal of External Fixation Device from Right Metatarsal-Phalangeal Joint, Percutaneous Endoscopic Approach

0SPM47Z Removal of Autologous Tissue Substitute from Right Metatarsal-Phalangeal Joint, Percutaneous Endoscopic Approach

0SPM48Z Removal of Spacer from Right Metatarsal-Phalangeal Joint, Percutaneous Endoscopic Approach

0SPM4JZ Removal of Synthetic Substitute from Right Metatarsal-Phalangeal Joint, Percutaneous Endoscopic Approach

0SPM4KZ Removal of Nonautologous Tissue Substitute from Right Metatarsal-Phalangeal Joint, Percutaneous Endoscopic Approach

0SPMX0Z Removal of Drainage Device from Right Metatarsal-Phalangeal Joint, External Approach

0SPMX3Z Removal of Infusion Device from Right Metatarsal-Phalangeal Joint, External Approach

0SPMX4Z Removal of Internal Fixation Device from Right Metatarsal-Phalangeal Joint, External Approach

0SPMX5Z Removal of External Fixation Device from Right Metatarsal-Phalangeal Joint, External Approach

0SPN00Z Removal of Drainage Device from Left Metatarsal-Phalangeal Joint, Open Approach

0SPN03Z Removal of Infusion Device from Left Metatarsal-Phalangeal Joint, Open Approach

0SPN04Z Removal of Internal Fixation Device from Left Metatarsal-Phalangeal Joint, Open Approach

0SPN05Z Removal of External Fixation Device from Left Metatarsal-Phalangeal Joint, Open Approach

0SPN07Z Removal of Autologous Tissue Substitute from Left Metatarsal-Phalangeal Joint, Open Approach

0SPN08Z Removal of Spacer from Left Metatarsal-Phalangeal Joint, Open Approach

0SPN0JZ Removal of Synthetic Substitute from Left Metatarsal-Phalangeal Joint, Open Approach

0SPN0KZ Removal of Nonautologous Tissue Substitute from Left Metatarsal-Phalangeal Joint, Open Approach

0SPN30Z Removal of Drainage Device from Left Metatarsal-Phalangeal Joint, Percutaneous Approach

0SPN33Z Removal of Infusion Device from Left Metatarsal-Phalangeal Joint, Percutaneous Approach

0SPN34Z Removal of Internal Fixation Device from Left Metatarsal-Phalangeal Joint, Percutaneous Approach

0SPN35Z Removal of External Fixation Device from Left Metatarsal-Phalangeal Joint, Percutaneous Approach

0SPN37Z Removal of Autologous Tissue Substitute from Left Metatarsal-Phalangeal Joint, Percutaneous Approach

0SPN38Z Removal of Spacer from Left Metatarsal-Phalangeal Joint, Percutaneous Approach

0SPN3JZ Removal of Synthetic Substitute from Left Metatarsal-Phalangeal Joint, Percutaneous Approach

0SPN3KZ Removal of Nonautologous Tissue Substitute from Left Metatarsal-Phalangeal Joint, Percutaneous Approach

0SPN40Z Removal of Drainage Device from Left Metatarsal-Phalangeal Joint, Percutaneous Endoscopic Approach

0SPN43Z Removal of Infusion Device from Left Metatarsal-Phalangeal Joint, Percutaneous Endoscopic Approach

0SPN44Z Removal of Internal Fixation Device from Left Metatarsal-Phalangeal Joint, Percutaneous Endoscopic Approach

0SPN45Z Removal of External Fixation Device from Left Metatarsal-Phalangeal Joint, Percutaneous Endoscopic Approach

0SPN47Z Removal of Autologous Tissue Substitute from Left Metatarsal-Phalangeal Joint, Percutaneous Endoscopic Approach

0SPN48Z Removal of Spacer from Left Metatarsal-Phalangeal Joint, Percutaneous Endoscopic Approach

0SPN4JZ Removal of Synthetic Substitute from Left Metatarsal-Phalangeal Joint, Percutaneous Endoscopic Approach

0SPN4KZ Removal of Nonautologous Tissue Substitute from Left Metatarsal-Phalangeal Joint, Percutaneous Endoscopic Approach

0SPNX0Z Removal of Drainage Device from Left Metatarsal-Phalangeal Joint, External Approach

0SPNX3Z Removal of Infusion Device from Left Metatarsal-Phalangeal Joint, External Approach

0SPNX4Z Removal of Internal Fixation Device from Left Metatarsal-Phalangeal Joint, External Approach

0SPNX5Z Removal of External Fixation Device from Left Metatarsal-Phalangeal Joint, External Approach

0SPP00Z Removal of Drainage Device from Right Toe Phalangeal Joint, Open Approach

0SPP03Z Removal of Infusion Device from Right Toe Phalangeal Joint, Open Approach

0SPP04Z Removal of Internal Fixation Device from Right Toe Phalangeal Joint, Open Approach

0SPP05Z Removal of External Fixation Device from Right Toe Phalangeal Joint, Open Approach

0SPP07Z Removal of Autologous Tissue Substitute from Right Toe Phalangeal Joint, Open Approach

0SPP08Z Removal of Spacer from Right Toe Phalangeal Joint, Open Approach

0SPP0JZ Removal of Synthetic Substitute from Right Toe Phalangeal Joint, Open Approach

0SPP0KZ Removal of Nonautologous Tissue Substitute from Right Toe Phalangeal Joint, Open Approach

0SPP30Z Removal of Drainage Device from Right Toe Phalangeal Joint, Percutaneous Approach

0SPP33Z Removal of Infusion Device from Right Toe Phalangeal Joint, Percutaneous Approach

0SPP34Z Removal of Internal Fixation Device from Right Toe Phalangeal Joint, Percutaneous Approach

0SPP35Z Removal of External Fixation Device from Right Toe Phalangeal Joint, Percutaneous Approach

0SPP37Z Removal of Autologous Tissue Substitute from Right Toe Phalangeal Joint, Percutaneous Approach

0SPP38Z Removal of Spacer from Right Toe Phalangeal Joint, Percutaneous Approach

0SPP3JZ Removal of Synthetic Substitute from Right Toe Phalangeal Joint, Percutaneous Approach

0SPP3KZ Removal of Nonautologous Tissue Substitute from Right Toe Phalangeal Joint, Percutaneous Approach

0SPP40Z Removal of Drainage Device from Right Toe Phalangeal Joint, Percutaneous Endoscopic Approach

0SPP43Z Removal of Infusion Device from Right Toe Phalangeal Joint, Percutaneous Endoscopic Approach

0SPP44Z Removal of Internal Fixation Device from Right Toe Phalangeal Joint, Percutaneous Endoscopic Approach

0SPP45Z Removal of External Fixation Device from Right Toe Phalangeal Joint, Percutaneous Endoscopic Approach

0SPP47Z Removal of Autologous Tissue Substitute from Right Toe Phalangeal Joint, Percutaneous Endoscopic Approach

0SPP48Z Removal of Spacer from Right Toe Phalangeal Joint, Percutaneous Endoscopic Approach

0SPP4JZ Removal of Synthetic Substitute from Right Toe Phalangeal Joint, Percutaneous Endoscopic Approach

0SPP4KZ Removal of Nonautologous Tissue Substitute from Right Toe Phalangeal Joint, Percutaneous Endoscopic Approach

0SPPX0Z Removal of Drainage Device from Right Toe Phalangeal Joint, External Approach

0SPPX3Z Removal of Infusion Device from Right Toe Phalangeal Joint, External Approach

0SPPX4Z Removal of Internal Fixation Device from Right Toe Phalangeal Joint, External Approach

♀ Female-only   ♂ Male-only   ▲ Limited Coverage   ● Non-OR   ▬ HAC-associated procedure   ▲ Non-covered procedures   ✛ Combinatio

PX5Z	Removal of External Fixation Device from Right Toe Phalangeal Joint, External Approach
PQ00Z	Removal of Drainage Device from Left Toe Phalangeal Joint, Open Approach
PQ03Z	Removal of Infusion Device from Left Toe Phalangeal Joint, Open Approach
PQ04Z	Removal of Internal Fixation Device from Left Toe Phalangeal Joint, Open Approach
PQ05Z	Removal of External Fixation Device from Left Toe Phalangeal Joint, Open Approach
PQ07Z	Removal of Autologous Tissue Substitute from Left Toe Phalangeal Joint, Open Approach
PQ08Z	Removal of Spacer from Left Toe Phalangeal Joint, Open Approach
PQ0JZ	Removal of Synthetic Substitute from Left Toe Phalangeal Joint, Open Approach
PQ0KZ	Removal of Nonautologous Tissue Substitute from Left Toe Phalangeal Joint, Open Approach
PQ30Z	Removal of Drainage Device from Left Toe Phalangeal Joint, Percutaneous Approach
PQ33Z	Removal of Infusion Device from Left Toe Phalangeal Joint, Percutaneous Approach

0SPQ34Z	Removal of Internal Fixation Device from Left Toe Phalangeal Joint, Percutaneous Approach
0SPQ35Z	Removal of External Fixation Device from Left Toe Phalangeal Joint, Percutaneous Approach
0SPQ37Z	Removal of Autologous Tissue Substitute from Left Toe Phalangeal Joint, Percutaneous Approach
0SPQ38Z	Removal of Spacer from Left Toe Phalangeal Joint, Percutaneous Approach
0SPQ3JZ	Removal of Synthetic Substitute from Left Toe Phalangeal Joint, Percutaneous Approach
0SPQ3KZ	Removal of Nonautologous Tissue Substitute from Left Toe Phalangeal Joint, Percutaneous Approach
0SPQ40Z	Removal of Drainage Device from Left Toe Phalangeal Joint, Percutaneous Endoscopic Approach
0SPQ43Z	Removal of Infusion Device from Left Toe Phalangeal Joint, Percutaneous Endoscopic Approach
0SPQ44Z	Removal of Internal Fixation Device from Left Toe Phalangeal Joint, Percutaneous Endoscopic Approach

0SPQ45Z	Removal of External Fixation Device from Left Toe Phalangeal Joint, Percutaneous Endoscopic Approach
0SPQ47Z	Removal of Autologous Tissue Substitute from Left Toe Phalangeal Joint, Percutaneous Endoscopic Approach
0SPQ48Z	Removal of Spacer from Left Toe Phalangeal Joint, Percutaneous Endoscopic Approach
0SPQ4JZ	Removal of Synthetic Substitute from Left Toe Phalangeal Joint, Percutaneous Endoscopic Approach
0SPQ4KZ	Removal of Nonautologous Tissue Substitute from Left Toe Phalangeal Joint, Percutaneous Endoscopic Approach
0SPQX0Z	Removal of Drainage Device from Left Toe Phalangeal Joint, External Approach
0SPQX3Z	Removal of Infusion Device from Left Toe Phalangeal Joint, External Approach
0SPQX4Z	Removal of Internal Fixation Device from Left Toe Phalangeal Joint, External Approach
0SPQX5Z	Removal of External Fixation Device from Left Toe Phalangeal Joint, External Approach

SQ – Lower Joints, Repair

Review Coding Guideline B3.5

Q00ZZ	Repair Lumbar Vertebral Joint, Open Approach
Q03ZZ	Repair Lumbar Vertebral Joint, Percutaneous Approach
Q04ZZ	Repair Lumbar Vertebral Joint, Percutaneous Endoscopic Approach
Q0XZZ	Repair Lumbar Vertebral Joint, External Approach
Q20ZZ	Repair Lumbar Vertebral Disc, Open Approach
Q23ZZ	Repair Lumbar Vertebral Disc, Percutaneous Approach
Q24ZZ	Repair Lumbar Vertebral Disc, Percutaneous Endoscopic Approach
Q2XZZ	Repair Lumbar Vertebral Disc, External Approach
Q30ZZ	Repair Lumbosacral Joint, Open Approach
Q33ZZ	Repair Lumbosacral Joint, Percutaneous Approach
Q34ZZ	Repair Lumbosacral Joint, Percutaneous Endoscopic Approach
Q3XZZ	Repair Lumbosacral Joint, External Approach
Q40ZZ	Repair Lumbosacral Disc, Open Approach
Q43ZZ	Repair Lumbosacral Disc, Percutaneous Approach
Q44ZZ	Repair Lumbosacral Disc, Percutaneous Endoscopic Approach
Q4XZZ	Repair Lumbosacral Disc, External Approach
Q50ZZ	Repair Sacrococcygeal Joint, Open Approach
Q53ZZ	Repair Sacrococcygeal Joint, Percutaneous Approach
Q54ZZ	Repair Sacrococcygeal Joint, Percutaneous Endoscopic Approach
Q5XZZ	Repair Sacrococcygeal Joint, External Approach
SQ60ZZ	Repair Coccygeal Joint, Open Approach
SQ63ZZ	Repair Coccygeal Joint, Percutaneous Approach
SQ64ZZ	Repair Coccygeal Joint, Percutaneous Endoscopic Approach
SQ6XZZ	Repair Coccygeal Joint, External Approach

0SQ70ZZ	Repair Right Sacroiliac Joint, Open Approach
0SQ73ZZ	Repair Right Sacroiliac Joint, Percutaneous Approach
0SQ74ZZ	Repair Right Sacroiliac Joint, Percutaneous Endoscopic Approach
0SQ7XZZ	Repair Right Sacroiliac Joint, External Approach
0SQ80ZZ	Repair Left Sacroiliac Joint, Open Approach
0SQ83ZZ	Repair Left Sacroiliac Joint, Percutaneous Approach
0SQ84ZZ	Repair Left Sacroiliac Joint, Percutaneous Endoscopic Approach
0SQ8XZZ	Repair Left Sacroiliac Joint, External Approach
0SQ90ZZ	Repair Right Hip Joint, Open Approach
0SQ93ZZ	Repair Right Hip Joint, Percutaneous Approach
0SQ94ZZ	Repair Right Hip Joint, Percutaneous Endoscopic Approach
0SQ9XZZ	Repair Right Hip Joint, External Approach
0SQB0ZZ	Repair Left Hip Joint, Open Approach
0SQB3ZZ	Repair Left Hip Joint, Percutaneous Approach
0SQB4ZZ	Repair Left Hip Joint, Percutaneous Endoscopic Approach

AHA CC: 4Q, 2014, 25-26

0SQBXZZ	Repair Left Hip Joint, External Approach
0SQC0ZZ	Repair Right Knee Joint, Open Approach
0SQC3ZZ	Repair Right Knee Joint, Percutaneous Approach
0SQC4ZZ	Repair Right Knee Joint, Percutaneous Endoscopic Approach
0SQCXZZ	Repair Right Knee Joint, External Approach
0SQD0ZZ	Repair Left Knee Joint, Open Approach
0SQD3ZZ	Repair Left Knee Joint, Percutaneous Approach
0SQD4ZZ	Repair Left Knee Joint, Percutaneous Endoscopic Approach
0SQDXZZ	Repair Left Knee Joint, External Approach
0SQF0ZZ	Repair Right Ankle Joint, Open Approach
0SQF3ZZ	Repair Right Ankle Joint, Percutaneous Approach
0SQF4ZZ	Repair Right Ankle Joint, Percutaneous Endoscopic Approach

0SQFXZZ	Repair Right Ankle Joint, External Approach
0SQG0ZZ	Repair Left Ankle Joint, Open Approach
0SQG3ZZ	Repair Left Ankle Joint, Percutaneous Approach
0SQG4ZZ	Repair Left Ankle Joint, Percutaneous Endoscopic Approach
0SQGXZZ	Repair Left Ankle Joint, External Approach
0SQH0ZZ	Repair Right Tarsal Joint, Open Approach
0SQH3ZZ	Repair Right Tarsal Joint, Percutaneous Approach
0SQH4ZZ	Repair Right Tarsal Joint, Percutaneous Endoscopic Approach
0SQHXZZ	Repair Right Tarsal Joint, External Approach
0SQJ0ZZ	Repair Left Tarsal Joint, Open Approach
0SQJ3ZZ	Repair Left Tarsal Joint, Percutaneous Approach
0SQJ4ZZ	Repair Left Tarsal Joint, Percutaneous Endoscopic Approach
0SQJXZZ	Repair Left Tarsal Joint, External Approach
0SQK0ZZ	Repair Right Metatarsal-Tarsal Joint, Open Approach
0SQK3ZZ	Repair Right Metatarsal-Tarsal Joint, Percutaneous Approach
0SQK4ZZ	Repair Right Metatarsal-Tarsal Joint, Percutaneous Endoscopic Approach
0SQKXZZ	Repair Right Metatarsal-Tarsal Joint, External Approach
0SQL0ZZ	Repair Left Metatarsal-Tarsal Joint, Open Approach
0SQL3ZZ	Repair Left Metatarsal-Tarsal Joint, Percutaneous Approach
0SQL4ZZ	Repair Left Metatarsal-Tarsal Joint, Percutaneous Endoscopic Approach
0SQLXZZ	Repair Left Metatarsal-Tarsal Joint, External Approach
0SQM0ZZ	Repair Right Metatarsal-Phalangeal Joint, Open Approach
0SQM3ZZ	Repair Right Metatarsal-Phalangeal Joint, Percutaneous Approach
0SQM4ZZ	Repair Right Metatarsal-Phalangeal Joint, Percutaneous Endoscopic Approach
0SQMXZZ	Repair Right Metatarsal-Phalangeal Joint, External Approach

| ♀ Female-only | ♂ Male-only | ▲ Limited Coverage | ● Non-OR | ■ HAC-associated procedure | ▲ Non-covered procedures | ✚ Combination |

0SQN0ZZ Repair Left Metatarsal-Phalangeal Joint, Open Approach

0SQN3ZZ Repair Left Metatarsal-Phalangeal Joint, Percutaneous Approach

0SQN4ZZ Repair Left Metatarsal-Phalangeal Joint, Percutaneous Endoscopic Approach

0SQNXZZ Repair Left Metatarsal-Phalangeal Joint, External Approach

0SQP0ZZ Repair Right Toe Phalangeal Joint, Open Approach

0SQP3ZZ Repair Right Toe Phalangeal Joint, Percutaneous Approach

0SQP4ZZ Repair Right Toe Phalangeal Joint, Percutaneous Endoscopic Approach

0SQPXZZ Repair Right Toe Phalangeal Joint, External Approach

0SQQ0ZZ Repair Left Toe Phalangeal Joint, Open Approach

0SQQ3ZZ Repair Left Toe Phalangeal Joint, Percutaneous Approach

0SQQ4ZZ Repair Left Toe Phalangeal Joint, Percutaneous Endoscopic Approach

0SQQXZZ Repair Left Toe Phalangeal Joint, Exter Approach

0SR – Lower Joints, Replacement

0SR007Z Replacement of Lumbar Vertebral Joint with Autologous Tissue Substitute, Open Approach

0SR00JZ Replacement of Lumbar Vertebral Joint with Synthetic Substitute, Open Approach

0SR00KZ Replacement of Lumbar Vertebral Joint with Nonautologous Tissue Substitute, Open Approach

0SR207Z Replacement of Lumbar Vertebral Disc with Autologous Tissue Substitute, Open Approach

0SR20JZ Replacement of Lumbar Vertebral Disc with Synthetic Substitute, Open Approach
  ▲ *When the patients age is greater than 60 years old*

0SR20KZ Replacement of Lumbar Vertebral Disc with Nonautologous Tissue Substitute, Open Approach

0SR307Z Replacement of Lumbosacral Joint with Autologous Tissue Substitute, Open Approach

0SR30JZ Replacement of Lumbosacral Joint with Synthetic Substitute, Open Approach

0SR30KZ Replacement of Lumbosacral Joint with Nonautologous Tissue Substitute, Open Approach

0SR407Z Replacement of Lumbosacral Disc with Autologous Tissue Substitute, Open Approach

0SR40JZ Replacement of Lumbosacral Disc with Synthetic Substitute, Open Approach
  ▲ *When the patients age is greater than 60 years old*

0SR40KZ Replacement of Lumbosacral Disc with Nonautologous Tissue Substitute, Open Approach

0SR507Z Replacement of Sacrococcygeal Joint with Autologous Tissue Substitute, Open Approach

0SR50JZ Replacement of Sacrococcygeal Joint with Synthetic Substitute, Open Approach

0SR50KZ Replacement of Sacrococcygeal Joint with Nonautologous Tissue Substitute, Open Approach

0SR607Z Replacement of Coccygeal Joint with Autologous Tissue Substitute, Open Approach

0SR60JZ Replacement of Coccygeal Joint with Synthetic Substitute, Open Approach

0SR60KZ Replacement of Coccygeal Joint with Nonautologous Tissue Substitute, Open Approach

0SR707Z Replacement of Right Sacroiliac Joint with Autologous Tissue Substitute, Open Approach

0SR70JZ Replacement of Right Sacroiliac Joint with Synthetic Substitute, Open Approach

0SR70KZ Replacement of Right Sacroiliac Joint with Nonautologous Tissue Substitute, Open Approach

0SR807Z Replacement of Left Sacroiliac Joint with Autologous Tissue Substitute, Open Approach

0SR80JZ Replacement of Left Sacroiliac Joint with Synthetic Substitute, Open Approach

0SR80KZ Replacement of Left Sacroiliac Joint with Nonautologous Tissue Substitute, Open Approach

0SR9019 Replacement of Right Hip Joint with Metal Synthetic Substitute, Cemented, Open Approach

0SR901A Replacement of Right Hip Joint with Metal Synthetic Substitute, Uncemented, Open Approach

0SR901Z Replacement of Right Hip Joint with Metal Synthetic Substitute, Open Approach

0SR9029 Replacement of Right Hip Joint with Metal on Polyethylene Synthetic Substitute, Cemented, Open Approach

0SR902A Replacement of Right Hip Joint with Metal on Polyethylene Synthetic Substitute, Uncemented, Open Approach

0SR902Z Replacement of Right Hip Joint with Metal on Polyethylene Synthetic Substitute, Open Approach

0SR9039 Replacement of Right Hip Joint with Ceramic Synthetic Substitute, Cemented, Open Approach

0SR903A Replacement of Right Hip Joint with Ceramic Synthetic Substitute, Uncemented, Open Approach

0SR903Z Replacement of Right Hip Joint with Ceramic Synthetic Substitute, Open Approach

0SR9049 Replacement of Right Hip Joint with Ceramic on Polyethylene Synthetic Substitute, Cemented, Open Approach

0SR904A Replacement of Right Hip Joint with Ceramic on Polyethylene Synthetic Substitute, Uncemented, Open Approach

0SR904Z Replacement of Right Hip Joint with Ceramic on Polyethylene Synthetic Substitute, Open Approach

0SR907Z Replacement of Right Hip Joint with Autologous Tissue Substitute, Open Approach

0SR90J9 Replacement of Right Hip Joint with Synthetic Substitute, Cemented, Open Approach

0SR90JA Replacement of Right Hip Joint with Synthetic Substitute, Uncemented, Open Approach

0SR90JZ Replacement of Right Hip Joint with Synthetic Substitute, Open Approach

0SR90KZ Replacement of Right Hip Joint with Nonautologous Tissue Substitute, Open Approach

0SRA009 Replacement of Right Hip Joint, Acetabular Surface with Polyethylene Synthetic Substitute, Cemented, Open Approach

0SRA00A Replacement of Right Hip Joint, Acetabular Surface with Polyethylene Synthetic Substitute, Uncemented, Open Approach

0SRA00Z Replacement of Right Hip Joint, Acetabular Surface with Polyethylene Synthetic Substitute, Open Approach

0SRA019 Replacement of Right Hip Joint, Acetabular Surface with Metal Syntheti Substitute, Cemented, Open Approach

0SRA01A Replacement of Right Hip Joint, Acetabular Surface with Metal Syntheti Substitute, Uncemented, Open Approac

0SRA01Z Replacement of Right Hip Joint, Acetabular Surface with Metal Syntheti Substitute, Open Approach

0SRA039 Replacement of Right Hip Joint, Acetabular Surface with Ceramic Synthetic Substitute, Cemented, Open Approach

0SRA03A Replacement of Right Hip Joint, Acetabular Surface with Ceramic Synthe Substitute, Uncemented, Open Approach

0SRA03Z Replacement of Right Hip Joint, Acetabular Surface with Ceramic Synthetic Substitute, Open Approach

0SRA07Z Replacement of Right Hip Joint, Acetabular Surface with Autologous Tissue Substitute, Open Approach

0SRA0J9 Replacement of Right Hip Joint, Acetabular Surface with Synthetic Substitute, Cemented, Open Approach

0SRA0JA Replacement of Right Hip Joint, Acetabular Surface with Synthetic Substitute, Uncemented, Open Approac

0SRA0JZ Replacement of Right Hip Joint, Acetabular Surface with Synthetic Substitute, Open Approach

0SRA0KZ Replacement of Right Hip Joint, Acetabular Surface with Nonautologous Tissue Substitute, Open Approach

0SRB019 Replacement of Left Hip Joint with Met Synthetic Substitute, Cemented, Open Approach

0SRB01A Replacement of Left Hip Joint with Met Synthetic Substitute, Uncemented, Open Approach

0SRB01Z Replacement of Left Hip Joint with Met Synthetic Substitute, Open Approach

0SRB029 Replacement of Left Hip Joint with Met on Polyethylene Synthetic Substitute, Cemented, Open Approach

0SRB02A Replacement of Left Hip Joint with Met on Polyethylene Synthetic Substitute, Uncemented, Open Approach

0SRB02Z Replacement of Left Hip Joint with Met on Polyethylene Synthetic Substitute, Open Approach

0SRB039 Replacement of Left Hip Joint with Ceramic Synthetic Substitute, Cemented, Open Approach

0SRB03A Replacement of Left Hip Joint with Ceramic Synthetic Substitute, Uncemented, Open Approach

0SRB03Z Replacement of Left Hip Joint with Ceramic Synthetic Substitute, Open Approach

0SRB049 Replacement of Left Hip Joint with Ceramic on Polyethylene Synthetic Substitute, Cemented, Open Approach

0SRB04A Replacement of Left Hip Joint with Ceramic on Polyethylene Synthetic Substitute, Uncemented, Open Approach

♀ Female-only ♂ Male-only ▲ Limited Coverage ● Non-OR ▨ HAC-associated procedure ▲ Non-covered procedures ✛ Combinatio

RB04Z	Replacement of Left Hip Joint with Ceramic on Polyethylene Synthetic Substitute, Open Approach
RB07Z	Replacement of Left Hip Joint with Autologous Tissue Substitute, Open Approach
RB0J9	Replacement of Left Hip Joint with Synthetic Substitute, Cemented, Open Approach
RB0JA	Replacement of Left Hip Joint with Synthetic Substitute, Uncemented, Open Approach
RB0JZ	Replacement of Left Hip Joint with Synthetic Substitute, Open Approach
RB0KZ	Replacement of Left Hip Joint with Nonautologous Tissue Substitute, Open Approach
RC07Z	Replacement of Right Knee Joint with Autologous Tissue Substitute, Open Approach
RC0J9	Replacement of Right Knee Joint with Synthetic Substitute, Cemented, Open Approach
RC0JA	Replacement of Right Knee Joint with Synthetic Substitute, Uncemented, Open Approach
RC0JZ	Replacement of Right Knee Joint with Synthetic Substitute, Open Approach
RC0KZ	Replacement of Right Knee Joint with Nonautologous Tissue Substitute, Open Approach
RD07Z	Replacement of Left Knee Joint with Autologous Tissue Substitute, Open Approach
RD0J9	Replacement of Left Knee Joint with Synthetic Substitute, Cemented, Open Approach
RD0JA	Replacement of Left Knee Joint with Synthetic Substitute, Uncemented, Open Approach
RD0JZ	Replacement of Left Knee Joint with Synthetic Substitute, Open Approach
RD0KZ	Replacement of Left Knee Joint with Nonautologous Tissue Substitute, Open Approach
RE009	Replacement of Left Hip Joint, Acetabular Surface with Polyethylene Synthetic Substitute, Cemented, Open Approach
RE00A	Replacement of Left Hip Joint, Acetabular Surface with Polyethylene Synthetic Substitute, Uncemented, Open Approach
RE00Z	Replacement of Left Hip Joint, Acetabular Surface with Polyethylene Synthetic Substitute, Open Approach
RE019	Replacement of Left Hip Joint, Acetabular Surface with Metal Synthetic Substitute, Cemented, Open Approach
RE01A	Replacement of Left Hip Joint, Acetabular Surface with Metal Synthetic Substitute, Uncemented, Open Approach
RE01Z	Replacement of Left Hip Joint, Acetabular Surface with Metal Synthetic Substitute, Open Approach
RE039	Replacement of Left Hip Joint, Acetabular Surface with Ceramic Synthetic Substitute, Cemented, Open Approach
RE03A	Replacement of Left Hip Joint, Acetabular Surface with Ceramic Synthetic Substitute, Uncemented, Open Approach
RE03Z	Replacement of Left Hip Joint, Acetabular Surface with Ceramic Synthetic Substitute, Open Approach
RE07Z	Replacement of Left Hip Joint, Acetabular Surface with Autologous Tissue Substitute, Open Approach
RE0J9	Replacement of Left Hip Joint, Acetabular Surface with Synthetic Substitute, Cemented, Open Approach

0SRE0JA	Replacement of Left Hip Joint, Acetabular Surface with Synthetic Substitute, Uncemented, Open Approach
0SRE0JZ	Replacement of Left Hip Joint, Acetabular Surface with Synthetic Substitute, Open Approach
0SRE0KZ	Replacement of Left Hip Joint, Acetabular Surface with Nonautologous Tissue Substitute, Open Approach
0SRF07Z	Replacement of Right Ankle Joint with Autologous Tissue Substitute, Open Approach
0SRF0J9	Replacement of Right Ankle Joint with Synthetic Substitute, Cemented, Open Approach
0SRF0JA	Replacement of Right Ankle Joint with Synthetic Substitute, Uncemented, Open Approach
0SRF0JZ	Replacement of Right Ankle Joint with Synthetic Substitute, Open Approach
0SRF0KZ	Replacement of Right Ankle Joint with Nonautologous Tissue Substitute, Open Approach
0SRG07Z	Replacement of Left Ankle Joint with Autologous Tissue Substitute, Open Approach
0SRG0J9	Replacement of Left Ankle Joint with Synthetic Substitute, Cemented, Open Approach
0SRG0JA	Replacement of Left Ankle Joint with Synthetic Substitute, Uncemented, Open Approach
0SRG0JZ	Replacement of Left Ankle Joint with Synthetic Substitute, Open Approach
0SRG0KZ	Replacement of Left Ankle Joint with Nonautologous Tissue Substitute, Open Approach
0SRH07Z	Replacement of Right Tarsal Joint with Autologous Tissue Substitute, Open Approach
0SRH0JZ	Replacement of Right Tarsal Joint with Synthetic Substitute, Open Approach
0SRH0KZ	Replacement of Right Tarsal Joint with Nonautologous Tissue Substitute, Open Approach
0SRJ07Z	Replacement of Left Tarsal Joint with Autologous Tissue Substitute, Open Approach
0SRJ0JZ	Replacement of Left Tarsal Joint with Synthetic Substitute, Open Approach
0SRJ0KZ	Replacement of Left Tarsal Joint with Nonautologous Tissue Substitute, Open Approach
0SRK07Z	Replacement of Right Metatarsal-Tarsal Joint with Autologous Tissue Substitute, Open Approach
0SRK0JZ	Replacement of Right Metatarsal-Tarsal Joint with Synthetic Substitute, Open Approach
0SRK0KZ	Replacement of Right Metatarsal-Tarsal Joint with Nonautologous Tissue Substitute, Open Approach
0SRL07Z	Replacement of Left Metatarsal-Tarsal Joint with Autologous Tissue Substitute, Open Approach
0SRL0JZ	Replacement of Left Metatarsal-Tarsal Joint with Synthetic Substitute, Open Approach
0SRL0KZ	Replacement of Left Metatarsal-Tarsal Joint with Nonautologous Tissue Substitute, Open Approach
0SRM07Z	Replacement of Right Metatarsal-Phalangeal Joint with Autologous Tissue Substitute, Open Approach
0SRM0JZ	Replacement of Right Metatarsal-Phalangeal Joint with Synthetic Substitute, Open Approach

0SRM0KZ	Replacement of Right Metatarsal-Phalangeal Joint with Nonautologous Tissue Substitute, Open Approach
0SRN07Z	Replacement of Left Metatarsal-Phalangeal Joint with Autologous Tissue Substitute, Open Approach
0SRN0JZ	Replacement of Left Metatarsal-Phalangeal Joint with Synthetic Substitute, Open Approach
0SRN0KZ	Replacement of Left Metatarsal-Phalangeal Joint with Nonautologous Tissue Substitute, Open Approach
0SRP07Z	Replacement of Right Toe Phalangeal Joint with Autologous Tissue Substitute, Open Approach
0SRP0JZ	Replacement of Right Toe Phalangeal Joint with Synthetic Substitute, Open Approach
0SRP0KZ	Replacement of Right Toe Phalangeal Joint with Nonautologous Tissue Substitute, Open Approach
0SRQ07Z	Replacement of Left Toe Phalangeal Joint with Autologous Tissue Substitute, Open Approach
0SRQ0JZ	Replacement of Left Toe Phalangeal Joint with Synthetic Substitute, Open Approach
0SRQ0KZ	Replacement of Left Toe Phalangeal Joint with Nonautologous Tissue Substitute, Open Approach
0SRR019	Replacement of Right Hip Joint, Femoral Surface with Metal Synthetic Substitute, Cemented, Open Approach
0SRR01A	Replacement of Right Hip Joint, Femoral Surface with Metal Synthetic Substitute, Uncemented, Open Approach
0SRR01Z	Replacement of Right Hip Joint, Femoral Surface with Metal Synthetic Substitute, Open Approach
0SRR039	Replacement of Right Hip Joint, Femoral Surface with Ceramic Synthetic Substitute, Cemented, Open Approach
0SRR03A	Replacement of Right Hip Joint, Femoral Surface with Ceramic Synthetic Substitute, Uncemented, Open Approach
0SRR03Z	Replacement of Right Hip Joint, Femoral Surface with Ceramic Synthetic Substitute, Open Approach
0SRR07Z	Replacement of Right Hip Joint, Femoral Surface with Autologous Tissue Substitute, Open Approach
0SRR0J9	Replacement of Right Hip Joint, Femoral Surface with Synthetic Substitute, Cemented, Open Approach
0SRR0JA	Replacement of Right Hip Joint, Femoral Surface with Synthetic Substitute, Uncemented, Open Approach
0SRR0JZ	Replacement of Right Hip Joint, Femoral Surface with Synthetic Substitute, Open Approach
0SRR0KZ	Replacement of Right Hip Joint, Femoral Surface with Nonautologous Tissue Substitute, Open Approach
0SRS019	Replacement of Left Hip Joint, Femoral Surface with Metal Synthetic Substitute, Cemented, Open Approach
0SRS01A	Replacement of Left Hip Joint, Femoral Surface with Metal Synthetic Substitute, Uncemented, Open Approach
0SRS01Z	Replacement of Left Hip Joint, Femoral Surface with Metal Synthetic Substitute, Open Approach
0SRS039	Replacement of Left Hip Joint, Femoral Surface with Ceramic Synthetic Substitute, Cemented, Open Approach
0SRS03A	Replacement of Left Hip Joint, Femoral Surface with Ceramic Synthetic Substitute, Uncemented, Open Approach

1005

Female-only	♂ Male-only	▲ Limited Coverage	● Non-OR	▨ HAC-associated procedure	▲ Non-covered procedures	＋ Combination

0SRS03Z	Replacement of Left Hip Joint, Femoral Surface with Ceramic Synthetic Substitute, Open Approach	**0SRT0JZ**	Replacement of Right Knee Joint, Femoral Surface with Synthetic Substitute, Open Approach	**0SRV0JA**	Replacement of Right Knee Joint, Tibial Surface with Synthetic Substitute, Uncemented, Open Approach
0SRS07Z	Replacement of Left Hip Joint, Femoral Surface with Autologous Tissue Substitute, Open Approach	**0SRT0KZ**	Replacement of Right Knee Joint, Femoral Surface with Nonautologous Tissue Substitute, Open Approach	**0SRV0JZ**	Replacement of Right Knee Joint, Tibial Surface with Synthetic Substitute, Open Approach
0SRS0J9	Replacement of Left Hip Joint, Femoral Surface with Synthetic Substitute, Cemented, Open Approach	**0SRU07Z**	Replacement of Left Knee Joint, Femoral Surface with Autologous Tissue Substitute, Open Approach	**0SRV0KZ**	Replacement of Right Knee Joint, Tibial Surface with Nonautologous Tissue Substitute, Open Approach
0SRS0JA	Replacement of Left Hip Joint, Femoral Surface with Synthetic Substitute, Uncemented, Open Approach	**0SRU0J9**	Replacement of Left Knee Joint, Femoral Surface with Synthetic Substitute, Cemented, Open Approach	**0SRW07Z**	Replacement of Left Knee Joint, Tibial Surface with Autologous Tissue Substitute, Open Approach
0SRS0JZ	Replacement of Left Hip Joint, Femoral Surface with Synthetic Substitute, Open Approach	**0SRU0JA**	Replacement of Left Knee Joint, Femoral Surface with Synthetic Substitute, Uncemented, Open Approach	**0SRW0J9**	Replacement of Left Knee Joint, Tibial Surface with Synthetic Substitute, Cemented, Open Approach
0SRS0KZ	Replacement of Left Hip Joint, Femoral Surface with Nonautologous Tissue Substitute, Open Approach	**0SRU0JZ**	Replacement of Left Knee Joint, Femoral Surface with Synthetic Substitute, Open Approach	**0SRW0JA**	Replacement of Left Knee Joint, Tibial Surface with Synthetic Substitute, Uncemented, Open Approach
0SRT07Z	Replacement of Right Knee Joint, Femoral Surface with Autologous Tissue Substitute, Open Approach	**0SRU0KZ**	Replacement of Left Knee Joint, Femoral Surface with Nonautologous Tissue Substitute, Open Approach	**0SRW0JZ**	Replacement of Left Knee Joint, Tibial Surface with Synthetic Substitute, Open Approach
0SRT0J9	Replacement of Right Knee Joint, Femoral Surface with Synthetic Substitute, Cemented, Open Approach	**0SRV07Z**	Replacement of Right Knee Joint, Tibial Surface with Autologous Tissue Substitute, Open Approach	**0SRW0KZ**	Replacement of Left Knee Joint, Tibial Surface with Nonautologous Tissue Substitute, Open Approach
0SRT0JA	Replacement of Right Knee Joint, Femoral Surface with Synthetic Substitute, Uncemented, Open Approach	**0SRV0J9**	Replacement of Right Knee Joint, Tibial Surface with Synthetic Substitute, Cemented, Open Approach		

0SS – Lower Joints, Reposition

0SS004Z	Reposition Lumbar Vertebral Joint with Internal Fixation Device, Open Approach	**0SS544Z**	Reposition Sacrococcygeal Joint with Internal Fixation Device, Percutaneous Endoscopic Approach	**0SS80ZZ**	Reposition Left Sacroiliac Joint, Open Approach
0SS00ZZ	Reposition Lumbar Vertebral Joint, Open Approach	**0SS54ZZ**	Reposition Sacrococcygeal Joint, Percutaneous Endoscopic Approach	**0SS834Z**	Reposition Left Sacroiliac Joint with Internal Fixation Device, Percutaneous Approach
0SS034Z	Reposition Lumbar Vertebral Joint with Internal Fixation Device, Percutaneous Approach	**0SS5X4Z**	Reposition Sacrococcygeal Joint with Internal Fixation Device, External Approach	**0SS83ZZ**	Reposition Left Sacroiliac Joint, Percutaneous Approach
0SS03ZZ	Reposition Lumbar Vertebral Joint, Percutaneous Approach	**0SS5XZZ**	Reposition Sacrococcygeal Joint, External Approach	**0SS844Z**	Reposition Left Sacroiliac Joint with Internal Fixation Device, Percutaneous Endoscopic Approach
0SS044Z	Reposition Lumbar Vertebral Joint with Internal Fixation Device, Percutaneous Endoscopic Approach	**0SS604Z**	Reposition Coccygeal Joint with Internal Fixation Device, Open Approach	**0SS84ZZ**	Reposition Left Sacroiliac Joint, Percutaneous Endoscopic Approach
0SS04ZZ	Reposition Lumbar Vertebral Joint, Percutaneous Endoscopic Approach	**0SS60ZZ**	Reposition Coccygeal Joint, Open Approach	**0SS8X4Z**	Reposition Left Sacroiliac Joint with Internal Fixation Device, External Approach
0SS0X4Z	Reposition Lumbar Vertebral Joint with Internal Fixation Device, External Approach	**0SS634Z**	Reposition Coccygeal Joint with Internal Fixation Device, Percutaneous Approach	**0SS8XZZ**	Reposition Left Sacroiliac Joint, External Approach
0SS0XZZ	Reposition Lumbar Vertebral Joint, External Approach	**0SS63ZZ**	Reposition Coccygeal Joint, Percutaneous Approach	**0SS904Z**	Reposition Right Hip Joint with Internal Fixation Device, Open Approach
0SS304Z	Reposition Lumbosacral Joint with Internal Fixation Device, Open Approach	**0SS644Z**	Reposition Coccygeal Joint with Internal Fixation Device, Percutaneous Endoscopic Approach	**0SS905Z**	Reposition Right Hip Joint with External Fixation Device, Open Approach
0SS30ZZ	Reposition Lumbosacral Joint, Open Approach	**0SS64ZZ**	Reposition Coccygeal Joint, Percutaneous Endoscopic Approach	**0SS90ZZ**	Reposition Right Hip Joint, Open Approach
0SS334Z	Reposition Lumbosacral Joint with Internal Fixation Device, Percutaneous Approach	**0SS6X4Z**	Reposition Coccygeal Joint with Internal Fixation Device, External Approach	**0SS934Z**	Reposition Right Hip Joint with Internal Fixation Device, Percutaneous Approach
0SS33ZZ	Reposition Lumbosacral Joint, Percutaneous Approach	**0SS6XZZ**	Reposition Coccygeal Joint, External Approach	**0SS935Z**	Reposition Right Hip Joint with External Fixation Device, Percutaneous Approach
0SS344Z	Reposition Lumbosacral Joint with Internal Fixation Device, Percutaneous Endoscopic Approach	**0SS704Z**	Reposition Right Sacroiliac Joint with Internal Fixation Device, Open Approach	**0SS93ZZ**	Reposition Right Hip Joint, Percutaneous Approach
0SS34ZZ	Reposition Lumbosacral Joint, Percutaneous Endoscopic Approach	**0SS70ZZ**	Reposition Right Sacroiliac Joint, Open Approach	**0SS944Z**	Reposition Right Hip Joint with Internal Fixation Device, Percutaneous Endoscopic Approach
0SS3X4Z	Reposition Lumbosacral Joint with Internal Fixation Device, External Approach	**0SS734Z**	Reposition Right Sacroiliac Joint with Internal Fixation Device, Percutaneous Approach	**0SS945Z**	Reposition Right Hip Joint with External Fixation Device, Percutaneous Endoscopic Approach
0SS3XZZ	Reposition Lumbosacral Joint, External Approach	**0SS73ZZ**	Reposition Right Sacroiliac Joint, Percutaneous Approach	**0SS94ZZ**	Reposition Right Hip Joint, Percutaneous Endoscopic Approach
0SS504Z	Reposition Sacrococcygeal Joint with Internal Fixation Device, Open Approach	**0SS744Z**	Reposition Right Sacroiliac Joint with Internal Fixation Device, Percutaneous Endoscopic Approach	**0SS9X4Z**	Reposition Right Hip Joint with Internal Fixation Device, External Approach
0SS50ZZ	Reposition Sacrococcygeal Joint, Open Approach	**0SS74ZZ**	Reposition Right Sacroiliac Joint, Percutaneous Endoscopic Approach	**0SS9X5Z**	Reposition Right Hip Joint with External Fixation Device, External Approach
0SS534Z	Reposition Sacrococcygeal Joint with Internal Fixation Device, Percutaneous Approach	**0SS7X4Z**	Reposition Right Sacroiliac Joint with Internal Fixation Device, External Approach	**0SS9XZZ**	Reposition Right Hip Joint, External Approach
0SS53ZZ	Reposition Sacrococcygeal Joint, Percutaneous Approach	**0SS7XZZ**	Reposition Right Sacroiliac Joint, External Approach	**0SSB04Z**	Reposition Left Hip Joint with Internal Fixation Device, Open Approach
		0SS804Z	Reposition Left Sacroiliac Joint with Internal Fixation Device, Open Approach	**0SSB05Z**	Reposition Left Hip Joint with External Fixation Device, Open Approach
				0SSB0ZZ	Reposition Left Hip Joint, Open Approach

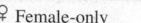

♀ Female-only   ♂ Male-only   ▲ Limited Coverage   ● Non-OR   ▦ HAC-associated procedure   ▲ Non-covered procedures   ✚ Combination

B34Z Reposition Left Hip Joint with Internal Fixation Device, Percutaneous Approach

B35Z Reposition Left Hip Joint with External Fixation Device, Percutaneous Approach

B3ZZ Reposition Left Hip Joint, Percutaneous Approach

B44Z Reposition Left Hip Joint with Internal Fixation Device, Percutaneous Endoscopic Approach

B45Z Reposition Left Hip Joint with External Fixation Device, Percutaneous Endoscopic Approach

B4ZZ Reposition Left Hip Joint, Percutaneous Endoscopic Approach

BX4Z Reposition Left Hip Joint with Internal Fixation Device, External Approach

BX5Z Reposition Left Hip Joint with External Fixation Device, External Approach

BXZZ Reposition Left Hip Joint, External Approach

C04Z Reposition Right Knee Joint with Internal Fixation Device, Open Approach

C05Z Reposition Right Knee Joint with External Fixation Device, Open Approach

C0ZZ Reposition Right Knee Joint, Open Approach

C34Z Reposition Right Knee Joint with Internal Fixation Device, Percutaneous Approach

C35Z Reposition Right Knee Joint with External Fixation Device, Percutaneous Approach

C3ZZ Reposition Right Knee Joint, Percutaneous Approach

C44Z Reposition Right Knee Joint with Internal Fixation Device, Percutaneous Endoscopic Approach

C45Z Reposition Right Knee Joint with External Fixation Device, Percutaneous Endoscopic Approach

C4ZZ Reposition Right Knee Joint, Percutaneous Endoscopic Approach

CX4Z Reposition Right Knee Joint with Internal Fixation Device, External Approach

CX5Z Reposition Right Knee Joint with External Fixation Device, External Approach

CXZZ Reposition Right Knee Joint, External Approach

D04Z Reposition Left Knee Joint with Internal Fixation Device, Open Approach

SD05Z Reposition Left Knee Joint with External Fixation Device, Open Approach

SD0ZZ Reposition Left Knee Joint, Open Approach

SD34Z Reposition Left Knee Joint with Internal Fixation Device, Percutaneous Approach

SD35Z Reposition Left Knee Joint with External Fixation Device, Percutaneous Approach

SD3ZZ Reposition Left Knee Joint, Percutaneous Approach

SD44Z Reposition Left Knee Joint with Internal Fixation Device, Percutaneous Endoscopic Approach

SD45Z Reposition Left Knee Joint with External Fixation Device, Percutaneous Endoscopic Approach

SD4ZZ Reposition Left Knee Joint, Percutaneous Endoscopic Approach

SDX4Z Reposition Left Knee Joint with Internal Fixation Device, External Approach

SDX5Z Reposition Left Knee Joint with External Fixation Device, External Approach

SDXZZ Reposition Left Knee Joint, External Approach

SSF04Z Reposition Right Ankle Joint with Internal Fixation Device, Open Approach

SSF05Z Reposition Right Ankle Joint with External Fixation Device, Open Approach

SSF0ZZ Reposition Right Ankle Joint, Open Approach

0SSF34Z Reposition Right Ankle Joint with Internal Fixation Device, Percutaneous Approach

0SSF35Z Reposition Right Ankle Joint with External Fixation Device, Percutaneous Approach

0SSF3ZZ Reposition Right Ankle Joint, Percutaneous Approach

0SSF44Z Reposition Right Ankle Joint with Internal Fixation Device, Percutaneous Endoscopic Approach

0SSF45Z Reposition Right Ankle Joint with External Fixation Device, Percutaneous Endoscopic Approach

0SSF4ZZ Reposition Right Ankle Joint, Percutaneous Endoscopic Approach

0SSFX4Z Reposition Right Ankle Joint with Internal Fixation Device, External Approach

0SSFX5Z Reposition Right Ankle Joint with External Fixation Device, External Approach

0SSFXZZ Reposition Right Ankle Joint, External Approach

0SSG04Z Reposition Left Ankle Joint with Internal Fixation Device, Open Approach

0SSG05Z Reposition Left Ankle Joint with External Fixation Device, Open Approach

0SSG0ZZ Reposition Left Ankle Joint, Open Approach

0SSG34Z Reposition Left Ankle Joint with Internal Fixation Device, Percutaneous Approach

0SSG35Z Reposition Left Ankle Joint with External Fixation Device, Percutaneous Approach

0SSG3ZZ Reposition Left Ankle Joint, Percutaneous Approach

0SSG44Z Reposition Left Ankle Joint with Internal Fixation Device, Percutaneous Endoscopic Approach

0SSG45Z Reposition Left Ankle Joint with External Fixation Device, Percutaneous Endoscopic Approach

0SSG4ZZ Reposition Left Ankle Joint, Percutaneous Endoscopic Approach

0SSGX4Z Reposition Left Ankle Joint with Internal Fixation Device, External Approach

0SSGX5Z Reposition Left Ankle Joint with External Fixation Device, External Approach

0SSGXZZ Reposition Left Ankle Joint, External Approach

0SSH04Z Reposition Right Tarsal Joint with Internal Fixation Device, Open Approach

0SSH05Z Reposition Right Tarsal Joint with External Fixation Device, Open Approach

0SSH0ZZ Reposition Right Tarsal Joint, Open Approach

0SSH34Z Reposition Right Tarsal Joint with Internal Fixation Device, Percutaneous Approach

0SSH35Z Reposition Right Tarsal Joint with External Fixation Device, Percutaneous Approach

0SSH3ZZ Reposition Right Tarsal Joint, Percutaneous Approach

0SSH44Z Reposition Right Tarsal Joint with Internal Fixation Device, Percutaneous Endoscopic Approach

0SSH45Z Reposition Right Tarsal Joint with External Fixation Device, Percutaneous Endoscopic Approach

0SSH4ZZ Reposition Right Tarsal Joint, Percutaneous Endoscopic Approach

0SSHX4Z Reposition Right Tarsal Joint with Internal Fixation Device, External Approach

0SSHX5Z Reposition Right Tarsal Joint with External Fixation Device, External Approach

0SSHXZZ Reposition Right Tarsal Joint, External Approach

0SSJ04Z Reposition Left Tarsal Joint with Internal Fixation Device, Open Approach

0SSJ05Z Reposition Left Tarsal Joint with External Fixation Device, Open Approach

0SSJ0ZZ Reposition Left Tarsal Joint, Open Approach

0SSJ34Z Reposition Left Tarsal Joint with Internal Fixation Device, Percutaneous Approach

0SSJ35Z Reposition Left Tarsal Joint with External Fixation Device, Percutaneous Approach

0SSJ3ZZ Reposition Left Tarsal Joint, Percutaneous Approach

0SSJ44Z Reposition Left Tarsal Joint with Internal Fixation Device, Percutaneous Endoscopic Approach

0SSJ45Z Reposition Left Tarsal Joint with External Fixation Device, Percutaneous Endoscopic Approach

0SSJ4ZZ Reposition Left Tarsal Joint, Percutaneous Endoscopic Approach

0SSJX4Z Reposition Left Tarsal Joint with Internal Fixation Device, External Approach

0SSJX5Z Reposition Left Tarsal Joint with External Fixation Device, External Approach

0SSJXZZ Reposition Left Tarsal Joint, External Approach

0SSK04Z Reposition Right Metatarsal-Tarsal Joint with Internal Fixation Device, Open Approach

0SSK05Z Reposition Right Metatarsal-Tarsal Joint with External Fixation Device, Open Approach

0SSK0ZZ Reposition Right Metatarsal-Tarsal Joint, Open Approach

0SSK34Z Reposition Right Metatarsal-Tarsal Joint with Internal Fixation Device, Percutaneous Approach

0SSK35Z Reposition Right Metatarsal-Tarsal Joint with External Fixation Device, Percutaneous Approach

0SSK3ZZ Reposition Right Metatarsal-Tarsal Joint, Percutaneous Approach

0SSK44Z Reposition Right Metatarsal-Tarsal Joint with Internal Fixation Device, Percutaneous Endoscopic Approach

0SSK45Z Reposition Right Metatarsal-Tarsal Joint with External Fixation Device, Percutaneous Endoscopic Approach

0SSK4ZZ Reposition Right Metatarsal-Tarsal Joint, Percutaneous Endoscopic Approach

0SSKX4Z Reposition Right Metatarsal-Tarsal Joint with Internal Fixation Device, External Approach

0SSKX5Z Reposition Right Metatarsal-Tarsal Joint with External Fixation Device, External Approach

0SSKXZZ Reposition Right Metatarsal-Tarsal Joint, External Approach

0SSL04Z Reposition Left Metatarsal-Tarsal Joint with Internal Fixation Device, Open Approach

0SSL05Z Reposition Left Metatarsal-Tarsal Joint with External Fixation Device, Open Approach

0SSL0ZZ Reposition Left Metatarsal-Tarsal Joint, Open Approach

0SSL34Z Reposition Left Metatarsal-Tarsal Joint with Internal Fixation Device, Percutaneous Approach

0SSL35Z Reposition Left Metatarsal-Tarsal Joint with External Fixation Device, Percutaneous Approach

0SSL3ZZ Reposition Left Metatarsal-Tarsal Joint, Percutaneous Approach

1007

Female-only   ♂ Male-only   ▲ Limited Coverage   ● Non-OR   ▓ HAC-associated procedure   ▲ Non-covered procedures   ✚ Combination

0SSL44Z Reposition Left Metatarsal-Tarsal Joint with Internal Fixation Device, Percutaneous Endoscopic Approach

0SSL45Z Reposition Left Metatarsal-Tarsal Joint with External Fixation Device, Percutaneous Endoscopic Approach

0SSL4ZZ Reposition Left Metatarsal-Tarsal Joint, Percutaneous Endoscopic Approach

0SSLX4Z Reposition Left Metatarsal-Tarsal Joint with Internal Fixation Device, External Approach

0SSLX5Z Reposition Left Metatarsal-Tarsal Joint with External Fixation Device, External Approach

0SSLXZZ Reposition Left Metatarsal-Tarsal Joint, External Approach

0SSM04Z Reposition Right Metatarsal-Phalangeal Joint with Internal Fixation Device, Open Approach

0SSM05Z Reposition Right Metatarsal-Phalangeal Joint with External Fixation Device, Open Approach

0SSM0ZZ Reposition Right Metatarsal-Phalangeal Joint, Open Approach

0SSM34Z Reposition Right Metatarsal-Phalangeal Joint with Internal Fixation Device, Percutaneous Approach

0SSM35Z Reposition Right Metatarsal-Phalangeal Joint with External Fixation Device, Percutaneous Approach

0SSM3ZZ Reposition Right Metatarsal-Phalangeal Joint, Percutaneous Approach

0SSM44Z Reposition Right Metatarsal-Phalangeal Joint with Internal Fixation Device, Percutaneous Endoscopic Approach

0SSM45Z Reposition Right Metatarsal-Phalangeal Joint with External Fixation Device, Percutaneous Endoscopic Approach

0SSM4ZZ Reposition Right Metatarsal-Phalangeal Joint, Percutaneous Endoscopic Approach

0SSMX4Z Reposition Right Metatarsal-Phalangeal Joint with Internal Fixation Device, External Approach

0SSMX5Z Reposition Right Metatarsal-Phalangeal Joint with External Fixation Device, External Approach

0SSMXZZ Reposition Right Metatarsal-Phalangeal Joint, External Approach

0SSN04Z Reposition Left Metatarsal-Phalangeal Joint with Internal Fixation Device, Open Approach

0SSN05Z Reposition Left Metatarsal-Phalangeal Joint with External Fixation Device, Open Approach

0SSN0ZZ Reposition Left Metatarsal-Phalangeal Joint, Open Approach

0SSN34Z Reposition Left Metatarsal-Phalangeal Joint with Internal Fixation Device, Percutaneous Approach

0SSN35Z Reposition Left Metatarsal-Phalangeal Joint with External Fixation Device, Percutaneous Approach

0SSN3ZZ Reposition Left Metatarsal-Phalangeal Joint, Percutaneous Approach

0SSN44Z Reposition Left Metatarsal-Phalangeal Joint with Internal Fixation Device, Percutaneous Endoscopic Approach

0SSN45Z Reposition Left Metatarsal-Phalangeal Joint with External Fixation Device, Percutaneous Endoscopic Approach

0SSN4ZZ Reposition Left Metatarsal-Phalangeal Joint, Percutaneous Endoscopic Approach

0SSNX4Z Reposition Left Metatarsal-Phalangeal Joint with Internal Fixation Device, External Approach

0SSNX5Z Reposition Left Metatarsal-Phalangeal Joint with External Fixation Device, External Approach

0SSNXZZ Reposition Left Metatarsal-Phalangeal Joint, External Approach

0SSP04Z Reposition Right Toe Phalangeal Joint with Internal Fixation Device, Open Approach

0SSP05Z Reposition Right Toe Phalangeal Joint with External Fixation Device, Open Approach

0SSP0ZZ Reposition Right Toe Phalangeal Joint, Open Approach

0SSP34Z Reposition Right Toe Phalangeal Joint with Internal Fixation Device, Percutaneous Approach

0SSP35Z Reposition Right Toe Phalangeal Joint with External Fixation Device, Percutaneous Approach

0SSP3ZZ Reposition Right Toe Phalangeal Joint, Percutaneous Approach

0SSP44Z Reposition Right Toe Phalangeal Joint with Internal Fixation Device, Percutaneous Endoscopic Approach

0SSP45Z Reposition Right Toe Phalangeal Joint with External Fixation Device, Percutaneous Endoscopic Approach

0SSP4ZZ Reposition Right Toe Phalangeal Joint, Percutaneous Endoscopic Approach

0SSPX4Z Reposition Right Toe Phalangeal Joint with Internal Fixation Device, External Approach

0SSPX5Z Reposition Right Toe Phalangeal Joint with External Fixation Device, External Approach

0SSPXZZ Reposition Right Toe Phalangeal Joint, External Approach

0SSQ04Z Reposition Left Toe Phalangeal Joint with Internal Fixation Device, Open Approach

0SSQ05Z Reposition Left Toe Phalangeal Joint with External Fixation Device, Open Approach

0SSQ0ZZ Reposition Left Toe Phalangeal Joint, Open Approach

0SSQ34Z Reposition Left Toe Phalangeal Joint with Internal Fixation Device, Percutaneous Approach

0SSQ35Z Reposition Left Toe Phalangeal Joint with External Fixation Device, Percutaneous Approach

0SSQ3ZZ Reposition Left Toe Phalangeal Joint, Percutaneous Approach

0SSQ44Z Reposition Left Toe Phalangeal Joint with Internal Fixation Device, Percutaneous Endoscopic Approach

0SSQ45Z Reposition Left Toe Phalangeal Joint with External Fixation Device, Percutaneous Endoscopic Approach

0SSQ4ZZ Reposition Left Toe Phalangeal Joint, Percutaneous Endoscopic Approach

0SSQX4Z Reposition Left Toe Phalangeal Joint with Internal Fixation Device, External Approach

0SSQX5Z Reposition Left Toe Phalangeal Joint with External Fixation Device, External Approach

0SSQXZZ Reposition Left Toe Phalangeal Joint, External Approach

0ST – Lower Joints, Resection

Review Coding Guideline B3.8

0ST20ZZ Resection of Lumbar Vertebral Disc, Open Approach

0ST40ZZ Resection of Lumbosacral Disc, Open Approach

0ST50ZZ Resection of Sacrococcygeal Joint, Open Approach

0ST60ZZ Resection of Coccygeal Joint, Open Approach

0ST70ZZ Resection of Right Sacroiliac Joint, Open Approach

0ST80ZZ Resection of Left Sacroiliac Joint, Open Approach

0ST90ZZ Resection of Right Hip Joint, Open Approach

0STB0ZZ Resection of Left Hip Joint, Open Approach

0STC0ZZ Resection of Right Knee Joint, Open Approach

0STD0ZZ Resection of Left Knee Joint, Open Approach
   AHA CC: 4Q, 2014, 30-31

0STF0ZZ Resection of Right Ankle Joint, Open Approach

0STG0ZZ Resection of Left Ankle Joint, Open Approach

0STH0ZZ Resection of Right Tarsal Joint, Open Approach

0STJ0ZZ Resection of Left Tarsal Joint, Open Approach

0STK0ZZ Resection of Right Metatarsal-Tarsal Joint, Open Approach

0STL0ZZ Resection of Left Metatarsal-Tarsal Joint, Open Approach

0STM0ZZ Resection of Right Metatarsal-Phalangeal Joint, Open Approach

0STN0ZZ Resection of Left Metatarsal-Phalangeal Joint, Open Approach

0STP0ZZ Resection of Right Toe Phalangeal Joint, Open Approach

0STQ0ZZ Resection of Left Toe Phalangeal Joint, Open Approach

0SU – Lower Joints, Supplement

0SU007Z Supplement Lumbar Vertebral Joint with Autologous Tissue Substitute, Open Approach

0SU00JZ Supplement Lumbar Vertebral Joint with Synthetic Substitute, Open Approach

0SU00KZ Supplement Lumbar Vertebral Joint with Nonautologous Tissue Substitute, Open Approach

0SU037Z Supplement Lumbar Vertebral Joint with Autologous Tissue Substitute, Percutaneous Approach

0SU03JZ Supplement Lumbar Vertebral Joint with Synthetic Substitute, Percutaneous Approach

0SU03KZ Supplement Lumbar Vertebral Joint with Nonautologous Tissue Substitute, Percutaneous Approach

0SU047Z Supplement Lumbar Vertebral Joint with Autologous Tissue Substitute, Percutaneous Endoscopic Approach

0SU04JZ Supplement Lumbar Vertebral Joint with Synthetic Substitute, Percutaneous Endoscopic Approach

0SU04KZ Supplement Lumbar Vertebral Joint with Nonautologous Tissue Substitute, Percutaneous Endoscopic Approach

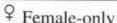

207Z	Supplement Lumbar Vertebral Disc with Autologous Tissue Substitute, Open Approach
J20JZ	Supplement Lumbar Vertebral Disc with Synthetic Substitute, Open Approach
J20KZ	Supplement Lumbar Vertebral Disc with Nonautologous Tissue Substitute, Open Approach
J237Z	Supplement Lumbar Vertebral Disc with Autologous Tissue Substitute, Percutaneous Approach
J23JZ	Supplement Lumbar Vertebral Disc with Synthetic Substitute, Percutaneous Approach
J23KZ	Supplement Lumbar Vertebral Disc with Nonautologous Tissue Substitute, Percutaneous Approach
J247Z	Supplement Lumbar Vertebral Disc with Autologous Tissue Substitute, Percutaneous Endoscopic Approach
J24JZ	Supplement Lumbar Vertebral Disc with Synthetic Substitute, Percutaneous Endoscopic Approach
J24KZ	Supplement Lumbar Vertebral Disc with Nonautologous Tissue Substitute, Percutaneous Endoscopic Approach
U307Z	Supplement Lumbosacral Joint with Autologous Tissue Substitute, Open Approach
U30JZ	Supplement Lumbosacral Joint with Synthetic Substitute, Open Approach
U30KZ	Supplement Lumbosacral Joint with Nonautologous Tissue Substitute, Open Approach
U337Z	Supplement Lumbosacral Joint with Autologous Tissue Substitute, Percutaneous Approach
U33JZ	Supplement Lumbosacral Joint with Synthetic Substitute, Percutaneous Approach
U33KZ	Supplement Lumbosacral Joint with Nonautologous Tissue Substitute, Percutaneous Approach
U347Z	Supplement Lumbosacral Joint with Autologous Tissue Substitute, Percutaneous Endoscopic Approach
U34JZ	Supplement Lumbosacral Joint with Synthetic Substitute, Percutaneous Endoscopic Approach
U34KZ	Supplement Lumbosacral Joint with Nonautologous Tissue Substitute, Percutaneous Endoscopic Approach
U407Z	Supplement Lumbosacral Disc with Autologous Tissue Substitute, Open Approach
U40JZ	Supplement Lumbosacral Disc with Synthetic Substitute, Open Approach
U40KZ	Supplement Lumbosacral Disc with Nonautologous Tissue Substitute, Open Approach
U437Z	Supplement Lumbosacral Disc with Autologous Tissue Substitute, Percutaneous Approach
U43JZ	Supplement Lumbosacral Disc with Synthetic Substitute, Percutaneous Approach
U43KZ	Supplement Lumbosacral Disc with Nonautologous Tissue Substitute, Percutaneous Approach
U447Z	Supplement Lumbosacral Disc with Autologous Tissue Substitute, Percutaneous Endoscopic Approach
U44JZ	Supplement Lumbosacral Disc with Synthetic Substitute, Percutaneous Endoscopic Approach
U44KZ	Supplement Lumbosacral Disc with Nonautologous Tissue Substitute, Percutaneous Endoscopic Approach
0SU507Z	Supplement Sacrococcygeal Joint with Autologous Tissue Substitute, Open Approach
0SU50JZ	Supplement Sacrococcygeal Joint with Synthetic Substitute, Open Approach
0SU50KZ	Supplement Sacrococcygeal Joint with Nonautologous Tissue Substitute, Open Approach
0SU537Z	Supplement Sacrococcygeal Joint with Autologous Tissue Substitute, Percutaneous Approach
0SU53JZ	Supplement Sacrococcygeal Joint with Synthetic Substitute, Percutaneous Approach
0SU53KZ	Supplement Sacrococcygeal Joint with Nonautologous Tissue Substitute, Percutaneous Approach
0SU547Z	Supplement Sacrococcygeal Joint with Autologous Tissue Substitute, Percutaneous Endoscopic Approach
0SU54JZ	Supplement Sacrococcygeal Joint with Synthetic Substitute, Percutaneous Endoscopic Approach
0SU54KZ	Supplement Sacrococcygeal Joint with Nonautologous Tissue Substitute, Percutaneous Endoscopic Approach
0SU607Z	Supplement Coccygeal Joint with Autologous Tissue Substitute, Open Approach
0SU60JZ	Supplement Coccygeal Joint with Synthetic Substitute, Open Approach
0SU60KZ	Supplement Coccygeal Joint with Nonautologous Tissue Substitute, Open Approach
0SU637Z	Supplement Coccygeal Joint with Autologous Tissue Substitute, Percutaneous Approach
0SU63JZ	Supplement Coccygeal Joint with Synthetic Substitute, Percutaneous Approach
0SU63KZ	Supplement Coccygeal Joint with Nonautologous Tissue Substitute, Percutaneous Approach
0SU647Z	Supplement Coccygeal Joint with Autologous Tissue Substitute, Percutaneous Endoscopic Approach
0SU64JZ	Supplement Coccygeal Joint with Synthetic Substitute, Percutaneous Endoscopic Approach
0SU64KZ	Supplement Coccygeal Joint with Nonautologous Tissue Substitute, Percutaneous Endoscopic Approach
0SU707Z	Supplement Right Sacroiliac Joint with Autologous Tissue Substitute, Open Approach
0SU70JZ	Supplement Right Sacroiliac Joint with Synthetic Substitute, Open Approach
0SU70KZ	Supplement Right Sacroiliac Joint with Nonautologous Tissue Substitute, Open Approach
0SU737Z	Supplement Right Sacroiliac Joint with Autologous Tissue Substitute, Percutaneous Approach
0SU73JZ	Supplement Right Sacroiliac Joint with Synthetic Substitute, Percutaneous Approach
0SU73KZ	Supplement Right Sacroiliac Joint with Nonautologous Tissue Substitute, Percutaneous Approach
0SU747Z	Supplement Right Sacroiliac Joint with Autologous Tissue Substitute, Percutaneous Endoscopic Approach
0SU74JZ	Supplement Right Sacroiliac Joint with Synthetic Substitute, Percutaneous Endoscopic Approach
0SU74KZ	Supplement Right Sacroiliac Joint with Nonautologous Tissue Substitute, Percutaneous Endoscopic Approach
0SU807Z	Supplement Left Sacroiliac Joint with Autologous Tissue Substitute, Open Approach
0SU80JZ	Supplement Left Sacroiliac Joint with Synthetic Substitute, Open Approach
0SU80KZ	Supplement Left Sacroiliac Joint with Nonautologous Tissue Substitute, Open Approach
0SU837Z	Supplement Left Sacroiliac Joint with Autologous Tissue Substitute, Percutaneous Approach
0SU83JZ	Supplement Left Sacroiliac Joint with Synthetic Substitute, Percutaneous Approach
0SU83KZ	Supplement Left Sacroiliac Joint with Nonautologous Tissue Substitute, Percutaneous Approach
0SU847Z	Supplement Left Sacroiliac Joint with Autologous Tissue Substitute, Percutaneous Endoscopic Approach
0SU84JZ	Supplement Left Sacroiliac Joint with Synthetic Substitute, Percutaneous Endoscopic Approach
0SU84KZ	Supplement Left Sacroiliac Joint with Nonautologous Tissue Substitute, Percutaneous Endoscopic Approach
0SU907Z	Supplement Right Hip Joint with Autologous Tissue Substitute, Open Approach
0SU909Z	Supplement Right Hip Joint with Liner, Open Approach
0SU90BZ	Supplement Right Hip Joint with Resurfacing Device, Open Approach
HAC	When reported with secondary diagnosis code I26.02, I26.09, I26.92, I26.99, I82.401-I82.4Z9
0SU90JZ	Supplement Right Hip Joint with Synthetic Substitute, Open Approach
0SU90KZ	Supplement Right Hip Joint with Nonautologous Tissue Substitute, Open Approach
0SU937Z	Supplement Right Hip Joint with Autologous Tissue Substitute, Percutaneous Approach
0SU93JZ	Supplement Right Hip Joint with Synthetic Substitute, Percutaneous Approach
0SU93KZ	Supplement Right Hip Joint with Nonautologous Tissue Substitute, Percutaneous Approach
0SU947Z	Supplement Right Hip Joint with Autologous Tissue Substitute, Percutaneous Endoscopic Approach
0SU94JZ	Supplement Right Hip Joint with Synthetic Substitute, Percutaneous Endoscopic Approach
0SU94KZ	Supplement Right Hip Joint with Nonautologous Tissue Substitute, Percutaneous Endoscopic Approach
0SUA09Z	Supplement Right Hip Joint, Acetabular Surface with Liner, Open Approach
0SUA0BZ	Supplement Right Hip Joint, Acetabular Surface with Resurfacing Device, Open Approach
HAC	When reported with secondary diagnosis code I26.02, I26.09, I26.92, I26.99, I82.401-I82.4Z9
0SUB07Z	Supplement Left Hip Joint with Autologous Tissue Substitute, Open Approach
0SUB09Z	Supplement Left Hip Joint with Liner, Open Approach
0SUB0BZ	Supplement Left Hip Joint with Resurfacing Device, Open Approach
HAC	When reported with secondary diagnosis code I26.02, I26.09, I26.92, I26.99, I82.401-I82.4Z9
0SUB0JZ	Supplement Left Hip Joint with Synthetic Substitute, Open Approach

1009

Female-only   ♂ Male-only   ▲ Limited Coverage   ● Non-OR   ᴴᴬᶜ HAC-associated procedure   ▲ Non-covered procedures   ✚ Combination

0SUB0KZ	Supplement Left Hip Joint with Nonautologous Tissue Substitute, Open Approach
0SUB37Z	Supplement Left Hip Joint with Autologous Tissue Substitute, Percutaneous Approach
0SUB3JZ	Supplement Left Hip Joint with Synthetic Substitute, Percutaneous Approach
0SUB3KZ	Supplement Left Hip Joint with Nonautologous Tissue Substitute, Percutaneous Approach
0SUB47Z	Supplement Left Hip Joint with Autologous Tissue Substitute, Percutaneous Endoscopic Approach
0SUB4JZ	Supplement Left Hip Joint with Synthetic Substitute, Percutaneous Endoscopic Approach
0SUB4KZ	Supplement Left Hip Joint with Nonautologous Tissue Substitute, Percutaneous Endoscopic Approach
0SUC07Z	Supplement Right Knee Joint with Autologous Tissue Substitute, Open Approach
0SUC09C	Supplement Right Knee Joint with Liner, Patellar Surface, Open Approach
0SUC09Z	Supplement Right Knee Joint with Liner, Open Approach
0SUC0JZ	Supplement Right Knee Joint with Synthetic Substitute, Open Approach
0SUC0KZ	Supplement Right Knee Joint with Nonautologous Tissue Substitute, Open Approach
0SUC37Z	Supplement Right Knee Joint with Autologous Tissue Substitute, Percutaneous Approach
0SUC3JZ	Supplement Right Knee Joint with Synthetic Substitute, Percutaneous Approach
0SUC3KZ	Supplement Right Knee Joint with Nonautologous Tissue Substitute, Percutaneous Approach
0SUC47Z	Supplement Right Knee Joint with Autologous Tissue Substitute, Percutaneous Endoscopic Approach
0SUC4JZ	Supplement Right Knee Joint with Synthetic Substitute, Percutaneous Endoscopic Approach
0SUC4KZ	Supplement Right Knee Joint with Nonautologous Tissue Substitute, Percutaneous Endoscopic Approach
0SUD07Z	Supplement Left Knee Joint with Autologous Tissue Substitute, Open Approach
0SUD09C	Supplement Left Knee Joint with Liner, Patellar Surface, Open Approach
0SUD09Z	Supplement Left Knee Joint with Liner, Open Approach
0SUD0JZ	Supplement Left Knee Joint with Synthetic Substitute, Open Approach
0SUD0KZ	Supplement Left Knee Joint with Nonautologous Tissue Substitute, Open Approach
0SUD37Z	Supplement Left Knee Joint with Autologous Tissue Substitute, Percutaneous Approach
0SUD3JZ	Supplement Left Knee Joint with Synthetic Substitute, Percutaneous Approach
0SUD3KZ	Supplement Left Knee Joint with Nonautologous Tissue Substitute, Percutaneous Approach
0SUD47Z	Supplement Left Knee Joint with Autologous Tissue Substitute, Percutaneous Endoscopic Approach
0SUD4JZ	Supplement Left Knee Joint with Synthetic Substitute, Percutaneous Endoscopic Approach

0SUD4KZ	Supplement Left Knee Joint with Nonautologous Tissue Substitute, Percutaneous Endoscopic Approach
0SUE09Z	Supplement Left Hip Joint, Acetabular Surface with Liner, Open Approach
0SUE0BZ	Supplement Left Hip Joint, Acetabular Surface with Resurfacing Device, Open Approach
HAC	When reported with secondary diagnosis code I26.02, I26.09, I26.92, I26.99, I82.401-I82.4Z9
0SUF07Z	Supplement Right Ankle Joint with Autologous Tissue Substitute, Open Approach
0SUF0JZ	Supplement Right Ankle Joint with Synthetic Substitute, Open Approach
0SUF0KZ	Supplement Right Ankle Joint with Nonautologous Tissue Substitute, Open Approach
0SUF37Z	Supplement Right Ankle Joint with Autologous Tissue Substitute, Percutaneous Approach
0SUF3JZ	Supplement Right Ankle Joint with Synthetic Substitute, Percutaneous Approach
0SUF3KZ	Supplement Right Ankle Joint with Nonautologous Tissue Substitute, Percutaneous Approach
0SUF47Z	Supplement Right Ankle Joint with Autologous Tissue Substitute, Percutaneous Endoscopic Approach
0SUF4JZ	Supplement Right Ankle Joint with Synthetic Substitute, Percutaneous Endoscopic Approach
0SUF4KZ	Supplement Right Ankle Joint with Nonautologous Tissue Substitute, Percutaneous Endoscopic Approach
0SUG07Z	Supplement Left Ankle Joint with Autologous Tissue Substitute, Open Approach
0SUG0JZ	Supplement Left Ankle Joint with Synthetic Substitute, Open Approach
0SUG0KZ	Supplement Left Ankle Joint with Nonautologous Tissue Substitute, Open Approach
0SUG37Z	Supplement Left Ankle Joint with Autologous Tissue Substitute, Percutaneous Approach
0SUG3JZ	Supplement Left Ankle Joint with Synthetic Substitute, Percutaneous Approach
0SUG3KZ	Supplement Left Ankle Joint with Nonautologous Tissue Substitute, Percutaneous Approach
0SUG47Z	Supplement Left Ankle Joint with Autologous Tissue Substitute, Percutaneous Endoscopic Approach
0SUG4JZ	Supplement Left Ankle Joint with Synthetic Substitute, Percutaneous Endoscopic Approach
0SUG4KZ	Supplement Left Ankle Joint with Nonautologous Tissue Substitute, Percutaneous Endoscopic Approach
0SUH07Z	Supplement Right Tarsal Joint with Autologous Tissue Substitute, Open Approach
0SUH0JZ	Supplement Right Tarsal Joint with Synthetic Substitute, Open Approach
0SUH0KZ	Supplement Right Tarsal Joint with Nonautologous Tissue Substitute, Open Approach
0SUH37Z	Supplement Right Tarsal Joint with Autologous Tissue Substitute, Percutaneous Approach
0SUH3JZ	Supplement Right Tarsal Joint with Synthetic Substitute, Percutaneous Approach

0SUH3KZ	Supplement Right Tarsal Joint with Nonautologous Tissue Substitute, Percutaneous Approach
0SUH47Z	Supplement Right Tarsal Joint with Autologous Tissue Substitute, Percutaneous Endoscopic Approach
0SUH4JZ	Supplement Right Tarsal Joint with Synthetic Substitute, Percutaneous Endoscopic Approach
0SUH4KZ	Supplement Right Tarsal Joint with Nonautologous Tissue Substitute, Percutaneous Endoscopic Approach
0SUJ07Z	Supplement Left Tarsal Joint with Autologous Tissue Substitute, Open Approach
0SUJ0JZ	Supplement Left Tarsal Joint with Synthetic Substitute, Open Approach
0SUJ0KZ	Supplement Left Tarsal Joint with Nonautologous Tissue Substitute, Open Approach
0SUJ37Z	Supplement Left Tarsal Joint with Autologous Tissue Substitute, Percutaneous Approach
0SUJ3JZ	Supplement Left Tarsal Joint with Synthetic Substitute, Percutaneous Approach
0SUJ3KZ	Supplement Left Tarsal Joint with Nonautologous Tissue Substitute, Percutaneous Approach
0SUJ47Z	Supplement Left Tarsal Joint with Autologous Tissue Substitute, Percutaneous Endoscopic Approach
0SUJ4JZ	Supplement Left Tarsal Joint with Synthetic Substitute, Percutaneous Endoscopic Approach
0SUJ4KZ	Supplement Left Tarsal Joint with Nonautologous Tissue Substitute, Percutaneous Endoscopic Approach
0SUK07Z	Supplement Right Metatarsal-Tarsal Joint with Autologous Tissue Substitute, Open Approach
0SUK0JZ	Supplement Right Metatarsal-Tarsal Joint with Synthetic Substitute, Open Approach
0SUK0KZ	Supplement Right Metatarsal-Tarsal Joint with Nonautologous Tissue Substitute, Open Approach
0SUK37Z	Supplement Right Metatarsal-Tarsal Joint with Autologous Tissue Substitute, Percutaneous Approach
0SUK3JZ	Supplement Right Metatarsal-Tarsal Joint with Synthetic Substitute, Percutaneous Approach
0SUK3KZ	Supplement Right Metatarsal-Tarsal Joint with Nonautologous Tissue Substitute, Percutaneous Approach
0SUK47Z	Supplement Right Metatarsal-Tarsal Joint with Autologous Tissue Substitute, Percutaneous Endoscopic Approach
0SUK4JZ	Supplement Right Metatarsal-Tarsal Joint with Synthetic Substitute, Percutaneous Endoscopic Approach
0SUK4KZ	Supplement Right Metatarsal-Tarsal Joint with Nonautologous Tissue Substitute, Percutaneous Endoscopic Approach
0SUL07Z	Supplement Left Metatarsal-Tarsal Joint with Autologous Tissue Substitute, Open Approach
0SUL0JZ	Supplement Left Metatarsal-Tarsal Joint with Synthetic Substitute, Open Approach
0SUL0KZ	Supplement Left Metatarsal-Tarsal Joint with Nonautologous Tissue Substitute, Open Approach
0SUL37Z	Supplement Left Metatarsal-Tarsal Joint with Autologous Tissue Substitute, Percutaneous Approach
0SUL3JZ	Supplement Left Metatarsal-Tarsal Joint with Synthetic Substitute, Percutaneous Approach

♀ Female-only   ♂ Male-only   ▲ Limited Coverage   ● Non-OR   HAC HAC-associated procedure   ▲ Non-covered procedures   ➕ Combination

L3KZ Supplement Left Metatarsal-Tarsal Joint with Nonautologous Tissue Substitute, Percutaneous Approach

L47Z Supplement Left Metatarsal-Tarsal Joint with Autologous Tissue Substitute, Percutaneous Endoscopic Approach

L4JZ Supplement Left Metatarsal-Tarsal Joint with Synthetic Substitute, Percutaneous Endoscopic Approach

L4KZ Supplement Left Metatarsal-Tarsal Joint with Nonautologous Tissue Substitute, Percutaneous Endoscopic Approach

M07Z Supplement Right Metatarsal-Phalangeal Joint with Autologous Tissue Substitute, Open Approach

M0JZ Supplement Right Metatarsal-Phalangeal Joint with Synthetic Substitute, Open Approach

M0KZ Supplement Right Metatarsal-Phalangeal Joint with Nonautologous Tissue Substitute, Open Approach

JM37Z Supplement Right Metatarsal-Phalangeal Joint with Autologous Tissue Substitute, Percutaneous Approach

JM3JZ Supplement Right Metatarsal-Phalangeal Joint with Synthetic Substitute, Percutaneous Approach

JM3KZ Supplement Right Metatarsal-Phalangeal Joint with Nonautologous Tissue Substitute, Percutaneous Approach

JM47Z Supplement Right Metatarsal-Phalangeal Joint with Autologous Tissue Substitute, Percutaneous Endoscopic Approach

JM4JZ Supplement Right Metatarsal-Phalangeal Joint with Synthetic Substitute, Percutaneous Endoscopic Approach

JM4KZ Supplement Right Metatarsal-Phalangeal Joint with Nonautologous Tissue Substitute, Percutaneous Endoscopic Approach

JN07Z Supplement Left Metatarsal-Phalangeal Joint with Autologous Tissue Substitute, Open Approach

JN0JZ Supplement Left Metatarsal-Phalangeal Joint with Synthetic Substitute, Open Approach

JN0KZ Supplement Left Metatarsal-Phalangeal Joint with Nonautologous Tissue Substitute, Open Approach

0SUN37Z Supplement Left Metatarsal-Phalangeal Joint with Autologous Tissue Substitute, Percutaneous Approach

0SUN3JZ Supplement Left Metatarsal-Phalangeal Joint with Synthetic Substitute, Percutaneous Approach

0SUN3KZ Supplement Left Metatarsal-Phalangeal Joint with Nonautologous Tissue Substitute, Percutaneous Approach

0SUN47Z Supplement Left Metatarsal-Phalangeal Joint with Autologous Tissue Substitute, Percutaneous Endoscopic Approach

0SUN4JZ Supplement Left Metatarsal-Phalangeal Joint with Synthetic Substitute, Percutaneous Endoscopic Approach

0SUN4KZ Supplement Left Metatarsal-Phalangeal Joint with Nonautologous Tissue Substitute, Percutaneous Endoscopic Approach

0SUP07Z Supplement Right Toe Phalangeal Joint with Autologous Tissue Substitute, Open Approach

0SUP0JZ Supplement Right Toe Phalangeal Joint with Synthetic Substitute, Open Approach

0SUP0KZ Supplement Right Toe Phalangeal Joint with Nonautologous Tissue Substitute, Open Approach

0SUP37Z Supplement Right Toe Phalangeal Joint with Autologous Tissue Substitute, Percutaneous Approach

0SUP3JZ Supplement Right Toe Phalangeal Joint with Synthetic Substitute, Percutaneous Approach

0SUP3KZ Supplement Right Toe Phalangeal Joint with Nonautologous Tissue Substitute, Percutaneous Approach

0SUP47Z Supplement Right Toe Phalangeal Joint with Autologous Tissue Substitute, Percutaneous Endoscopic Approach

0SUP4JZ Supplement Right Toe Phalangeal Joint with Synthetic Substitute, Percutaneous Endoscopic Approach

0SUP4KZ Supplement Right Toe Phalangeal Joint with Nonautologous Tissue Substitute, Percutaneous Endoscopic Approach

0SUQ07Z Supplement Left Toe Phalangeal Joint with Autologous Tissue Substitute, Open Approach

0SUQ0JZ Supplement Left Toe Phalangeal Joint with Synthetic Substitute, Open Approach

0SUQ0KZ Supplement Left Toe Phalangeal Joint with Nonautologous Tissue Substitute, Open Approach

0SUQ37Z Supplement Left Toe Phalangeal Joint with Autologous Tissue Substitute, Percutaneous Approach

0SUQ3JZ Supplement Left Toe Phalangeal Joint with Synthetic Substitute, Percutaneous Approach

0SUQ3KZ Supplement Left Toe Phalangeal Joint with Nonautologous Tissue Substitute, Percutaneous Approach

0SUQ47Z Supplement Left Toe Phalangeal Joint with Autologous Tissue Substitute, Percutaneous Endoscopic Approach

0SUQ4JZ Supplement Left Toe Phalangeal Joint with Synthetic Substitute, Percutaneous Endoscopic Approach

0SUQ4KZ Supplement Left Toe Phalangeal Joint with Nonautologous Tissue Substitute, Percutaneous Endoscopic Approach

0SUR09Z Supplement Right Hip Joint, Femoral Surface with Liner, Open Approach

0SUR0BZ Supplement Right Hip Joint, Femoral Surface with Resurfacing Device, Open Approach

■ When reported with secondary diagnosis code I26.02, I26.09, I26.92, I26.99, I82.401-I82.4Z9

0SUS09Z Supplement Left Hip Joint, Femoral Surface with Liner, Open Approach

0SUS0BZ Supplement Left Hip Joint, Femoral Surface with Resurfacing Device, Open Approach

■ When reported with secondary diagnosis code I26.02, I26.09, I26.92, I26.99, I82.401-I82.4Z9

0SUT09Z Supplement Right Knee Joint, Femoral Surface with Liner, Open Approach

0SUU09Z Supplement Left Knee Joint, Femoral Surface with Liner, Open Approach

0SUV09Z Supplement Right Knee Joint, Tibial Surface with Liner, Open Approach

0SUW09Z Supplement Left Knee Joint, Tibial Surface with Liner, Open Approach

SW – Lower Joints, Revision

review Coding Guideline B6.1c

W000Z Revision of Drainage Device in Lumbar Vertebral Joint, Open Approach

W003Z Revision of Infusion Device in Lumbar Vertebral Joint, Open Approach

W004Z Revision of Internal Fixation Device in Lumbar Vertebral Joint, Open Approach

W007Z Revision of Autologous Tissue Substitute in Lumbar Vertebral Joint, Open Approach

W008Z Revision of Spacer in Lumbar Vertebral Joint, Open Approach

W00AZ Revision of Interbody Fusion Device in Lumbar Vertebral Joint, Open Approach

W00JZ Revision of Synthetic Substitute in Lumbar Vertebral Joint, Open Approach

W00KZ Revision of Nonautologous Tissue Substitute in Lumbar Vertebral Joint, Open Approach

W030Z Revision of Drainage Device in Lumbar Vertebral Joint, Percutaneous Approach

W033Z Revision of Infusion Device in Lumbar Vertebral Joint, Percutaneous Approach

W034Z Revision of Internal Fixation Device in Lumbar Vertebral Joint, Percutaneous Approach

0SW037Z Revision of Autologous Tissue Substitute in Lumbar Vertebral Joint, Percutaneous Approach

0SW038Z Revision of Spacer in Lumbar Vertebral Joint, Percutaneous Approach

0SW03AZ Revision of Interbody Fusion Device in Lumbar Vertebral Joint, Percutaneous Approach

0SW03JZ Revision of Synthetic Substitute in Lumbar Vertebral Joint, Percutaneous Approach

0SW03KZ Revision of Nonautologous Tissue Substitute in Lumbar Vertebral Joint, Percutaneous Approach

0SW040Z Revision of Drainage Device in Lumbar Vertebral Joint, Percutaneous Endoscopic Approach

0SW043Z Revision of Infusion Device in Lumbar Vertebral Joint, Percutaneous Endoscopic Approach

0SW044Z Revision of Internal Fixation Device in Lumbar Vertebral Joint, Percutaneous Endoscopic Approach

0SW047Z Revision of Autologous Tissue Substitute in Lumbar Vertebral Joint, Percutaneous Endoscopic Approach

0SW048Z Revision of Spacer in Lumbar Vertebral Joint, Percutaneous Endoscopic Approach

0SW04AZ Revision of Interbody Fusion Device in Lumbar Vertebral Joint, Percutaneous Endoscopic Approach

0SW04JZ Revision of Synthetic Substitute in Lumbar Vertebral Joint, Percutaneous Endoscopic Approach

0SW04KZ Revision of Nonautologous Tissue Substitute in Lumbar Vertebral Joint, Percutaneous Endoscopic Approach

0SW0X0Z Revision of Drainage Device in Lumbar Vertebral Joint, External Approach

0SW0X3Z Revision of Infusion Device in Lumbar Vertebral Joint, External Approach

0SW0X4Z Revision of Internal Fixation Device in Lumbar Vertebral Joint, External Approach

0SW0X7Z Revision of Autologous Tissue Substitute in Lumbar Vertebral Joint, External Approach

Female-only ♂ Male-only ▲ Limited Coverage ● Non-OR ▦ HAC-associated procedure ▲ Non-covered procedures ✛ Combination

0SW0X8Z Revision of Spacer in Lumbar Vertebral Joint, External Approach

0SW0XAZ Revision of Interbody Fusion Device in Lumbar Vertebral Joint, External Approach

0SW0XJZ Revision of Synthetic Substitute in Lumbar Vertebral Joint, External Approach

0SW0XKZ Revision of Nonautologous Tissue Substitute in Lumbar Vertebral Joint, External Approach

0SW200Z Revision of Drainage Device in Lumbar Vertebral Disc, Open Approach

0SW203Z Revision of Infusion Device in Lumbar Vertebral Disc, Open Approach

0SW207Z Revision of Autologous Tissue Substitute in Lumbar Vertebral Disc, Open Approach

0SW20JZ Revision of Synthetic Substitute in Lumbar Vertebral Disc, Open Approach

0SW20KZ Revision of Nonautologous Tissue Substitute in Lumbar Vertebral Disc, Open Approach

0SW230Z Revision of Drainage Device in Lumbar Vertebral Disc, Percutaneous Approach

0SW233Z Revision of Infusion Device in Lumbar Vertebral Disc, Percutaneous Approach

0SW237Z Revision of Autologous Tissue Substitute in Lumbar Vertebral Disc, Percutaneous Approach

0SW23JZ Revision of Synthetic Substitute in Lumbar Vertebral Disc, Percutaneous Approach

0SW23KZ Revision of Nonautologous Tissue Substitute in Lumbar Vertebral Disc, Percutaneous Approach

0SW240Z Revision of Drainage Device in Lumbar Vertebral Disc, Percutaneous Endoscopic Approach

0SW243Z Revision of Infusion Device in Lumbar Vertebral Disc, Percutaneous Endoscopic Approach

0SW247Z Revision of Autologous Tissue Substitute in Lumbar Vertebral Disc, Percutaneous Endoscopic Approach

0SW24JZ Revision of Synthetic Substitute in Lumbar Vertebral Disc, Percutaneous Endoscopic Approach

0SW24KZ Revision of Nonautologous Tissue Substitute in Lumbar Vertebral Disc, Percutaneous Endoscopic Approach

0SW2X0Z Revision of Drainage Device in Lumbar Vertebral Disc, External Approach

0SW2X3Z Revision of Infusion Device in Lumbar Vertebral Disc, External Approach

0SW2X7Z Revision of Autologous Tissue Substitute in Lumbar Vertebral Disc, External Approach

0SW2XJZ Revision of Synthetic Substitute in Lumbar Vertebral Disc, External Approach

0SW2XKZ Revision of Nonautologous Tissue Substitute in Lumbar Vertebral Disc, External Approach

0SW300Z Revision of Drainage Device in Lumbosacral Joint, Open Approach

0SW303Z Revision of Infusion Device in Lumbosacral Joint, Open Approach

0SW304Z Revision of Internal Fixation Device in Lumbosacral Joint, Open Approach

0SW307Z Revision of Autologous Tissue Substitute in Lumbosacral Joint, Open Approach

0SW308Z Revision of Spacer in Lumbosacral Joint, Open Approach

0SW30AZ Revision of Interbody Fusion Device in Lumbosacral Joint, Open Approach

0SW30JZ Revision of Synthetic Substitute in Lumbosacral Joint, Open Approach

0SW30KZ Revision of Nonautologous Tissue Substitute in Lumbosacral Joint, Open Approach

0SW330Z Revision of Drainage Device in Lumbosacral Joint, Percutaneous Approach

0SW333Z Revision of Infusion Device in Lumbosacral Joint, Percutaneous Approach

0SW334Z Revision of Internal Fixation Device in Lumbosacral Joint, Percutaneous Approach

0SW337Z Revision of Autologous Tissue Substitute in Lumbosacral Joint, Percutaneous Approach

0SW338Z Revision of Spacer in Lumbosacral Joint, Percutaneous Approach

0SW33AZ Revision of Interbody Fusion Device in Lumbosacral Joint, Percutaneous Approach

0SW33JZ Revision of Synthetic Substitute in Lumbosacral Joint, Percutaneous Approach

0SW33KZ Revision of Nonautologous Tissue Substitute in Lumbosacral Joint, Percutaneous Approach

0SW340Z Revision of Drainage Device in Lumbosacral Joint, Percutaneous Endoscopic Approach

0SW343Z Revision of Infusion Device in Lumbosacral Joint, Percutaneous Endoscopic Approach

0SW344Z Revision of Internal Fixation Device in Lumbosacral Joint, Percutaneous Endoscopic Approach

0SW347Z Revision of Autologous Tissue Substitute in Lumbosacral Joint, Percutaneous Endoscopic Approach

0SW348Z Revision of Spacer in Lumbosacral Joint, Percutaneous Endoscopic Approach

0SW34AZ Revision of Interbody Fusion Device in Lumbosacral Joint, Percutaneous Endoscopic Approach

0SW34JZ Revision of Synthetic Substitute in Lumbosacral Joint, Percutaneous Endoscopic Approach

0SW34KZ Revision of Nonautologous Tissue Substitute in Lumbosacral Joint, Percutaneous Endoscopic Approach

0SW3X0Z Revision of Drainage Device in Lumbosacral Joint, External Approach

0SW3X3Z Revision of Infusion Device in Lumbosacral Joint, External Approach

0SW3X4Z Revision of Internal Fixation Device in Lumbosacral Joint, External Approach

0SW3X7Z Revision of Autologous Tissue Substitute in Lumbosacral Joint, External Approach

0SW3X8Z Revision of Spacer in Lumbosacral Joint, External Approach

0SW3XAZ Revision of Interbody Fusion Device in Lumbosacral Joint, External Approach

0SW3XJZ Revision of Synthetic Substitute in Lumbosacral Joint, External Approach

0SW3XKZ Revision of Nonautologous Tissue Substitute in Lumbosacral Joint, External Approach

0SW400Z Revision of Drainage Device in Lumbosacral Disc, Open Approach

0SW403Z Revision of Infusion Device in Lumbosacral Disc, Open Approach

0SW407Z Revision of Autologous Tissue Substitute in Lumbosacral Disc, Open Approach

0SW40JZ Revision of Synthetic Substitute in Lumbosacral Disc, Open Approach

0SW40KZ Revision of Nonautologous Tissue Substitute in Lumbosacral Disc, Open Approach

0SW430Z Revision of Drainage Device in Lumbosacral Disc, Percutaneous Approach

0SW433Z Revision of Infusion Device in Lumbosacral Disc, Percutaneous Approach

0SW437Z Revision of Autologous Tissue Substitute in Lumbosacral Disc, Percutaneous Approach

0SW43JZ Revision of Synthetic Substitute in Lumbosacral Disc, Percutaneous Approach

0SW43KZ Revision of Nonautologous Tissue Substitute in Lumbosacral Disc, Percutaneous Approach

0SW440Z Revision of Drainage Device in Lumbosacral Disc, Percutaneous Endoscopic Approach

0SW443Z Revision of Infusion Device in Lumbosacral Disc, Percutaneous Endoscopic Approach

0SW447Z Revision of Autologous Tissue Substitute in Lumbosacral Disc, Percutaneous Endoscopic Approach

0SW44JZ Revision of Synthetic Substitute in Lumbosacral Disc, Percutaneous Endoscopic Approach

0SW44KZ Revision of Nonautologous Tissue Substitute in Lumbosacral Disc, Percutaneous Endoscopic Approach

0SW4X0Z Revision of Drainage Device in Lumbosacral Disc, External Approach

0SW4X3Z Revision of Infusion Device in Lumbosacral Disc, External Approach

0SW4X7Z Revision of Autologous Tissue Substitute in Lumbosacral Disc, External Approach

0SW4XJZ Revision of Synthetic Substitute in Lumbosacral Disc, External Approach

0SW4XKZ Revision of Nonautologous Tissue Substitute in Lumbosacral Disc, External Approach

0SW500Z Revision of Drainage Device in Sacrococcygeal Joint, Open Approach

0SW503Z Revision of Infusion Device in Sacrococcygeal Joint, Open Approach

0SW504Z Revision of Internal Fixation Device in Sacrococcygeal Joint, Open Approach

0SW507Z Revision of Autologous Tissue Substitute in Sacrococcygeal Joint, Open Approach

0SW508Z Revision of Spacer in Sacrococcygeal Joint, Open Approach

0SW50JZ Revision of Synthetic Substitute in Sacrococcygeal Joint, Open Approach

0SW50KZ Revision of Nonautologous Tissue Substitute in Sacrococcygeal Joint, Open Approach

0SW530Z Revision of Drainage Device in Sacrococcygeal Joint, Percutaneous Approach

0SW533Z Revision of Infusion Device in Sacrococcygeal Joint, Percutaneous Approach

0SW534Z Revision of Internal Fixation Device in Sacrococcygeal Joint, Percutaneous Approach

0SW537Z Revision of Autologous Tissue Substitute in Sacrococcygeal Joint, Percutaneous Approach

0SW538Z Revision of Spacer in Sacrococcygeal Joint, Percutaneous Approach

0SW53JZ Revision of Synthetic Substitute in Sacrococcygeal Joint, Percutaneous Approach

0SW53KZ Revision of Nonautologous Tissue Substitute in Sacrococcygeal Joint, Percutaneous Approach

540Z	Revision of Drainage Device in Sacrococcygeal Joint, Percutaneous Endoscopic Approach
543Z	Revision of Infusion Device in Sacrococcygeal Joint, Percutaneous Endoscopic Approach
544Z	Revision of Internal Fixation Device in Sacrococcygeal Joint, Percutaneous Endoscopic Approach
547Z	Revision of Autologous Tissue Substitute in Sacrococcygeal Joint, Percutaneous Endoscopic Approach
548Z	Revision of Spacer in Sacrococcygeal Joint, Percutaneous Endoscopic Approach
54JZ	Revision of Synthetic Substitute in Sacrococcygeal Joint, Percutaneous Endoscopic Approach
54KZ	Revision of Nonautologous Tissue Substitute in Sacrococcygeal Joint, Percutaneous Endoscopic Approach
5X0Z	Revision of Drainage Device in Sacrococcygeal Joint, External Approach
5X3Z	Revision of Infusion Device in Sacrococcygeal Joint, External Approach
5X4Z	Revision of Internal Fixation Device in Sacrococcygeal Joint, External Approach
5X7Z	Revision of Autologous Tissue Substitute in Sacrococcygeal Joint, External Approach
5X8Z	Revision of Spacer in Sacrococcygeal Joint, External Approach
5XJZ	Revision of Synthetic Substitute in Sacrococcygeal Joint, External Approach
5XKZ	Revision of Nonautologous Tissue Substitute in Sacrococcygeal Joint, External Approach
W600Z	Revision of Drainage Device in Coccygeal Joint, Open Approach
W603Z	Revision of Infusion Device in Coccygeal Joint, Open Approach
W604Z	Revision of Internal Fixation Device in Coccygeal Joint, Open Approach
W607Z	Revision of Autologous Tissue Substitute in Coccygeal Joint, Open Approach
W608Z	Revision of Spacer in Coccygeal Joint, Open Approach
W60JZ	Revision of Synthetic Substitute in Coccygeal Joint, Open Approach
W60KZ	Revision of Nonautologous Tissue Substitute in Coccygeal Joint, Open Approach
W630Z	Revision of Drainage Device in Coccygeal Joint, Percutaneous Approach
W633Z	Revision of Infusion Device in Coccygeal Joint, Percutaneous Approach
W634Z	Revision of Internal Fixation Device in Coccygeal Joint, Percutaneous Approach
W637Z	Revision of Autologous Tissue Substitute in Coccygeal Joint, Percutaneous Approach
W638Z	Revision of Spacer in Coccygeal Joint, Percutaneous Approach
W63JZ	Revision of Synthetic Substitute in Coccygeal Joint, Percutaneous Approach
W63KZ	Revision of Nonautologous Tissue Substitute in Coccygeal Joint, Percutaneous Approach
W640Z	Revision of Drainage Device in Coccygeal Joint, Percutaneous Endoscopic Approach
W643Z	Revision of Infusion Device in Coccygeal Joint, Percutaneous Endoscopic Approach
W644Z	Revision of Internal Fixation Device in Coccygeal Joint, Percutaneous Endoscopic Approach
W647Z	Revision of Autologous Tissue Substitute in Coccygeal Joint, Percutaneous Endoscopic Approach

0SW648Z	Revision of Spacer in Coccygeal Joint, Percutaneous Endoscopic Approach
0SW64JZ	Revision of Synthetic Substitute in Coccygeal Joint, Percutaneous Endoscopic Approach
0SW64KZ	Revision of Nonautologous Tissue Substitute in Coccygeal Joint, Percutaneous Endoscopic Approach
0SW6X0Z	Revision of Drainage Device in Coccygeal Joint, External Approach
0SW6X3Z	Revision of Infusion Device in Coccygeal Joint, External Approach
0SW6X4Z	Revision of Internal Fixation Device in Coccygeal Joint, External Approach
0SW6X7Z	Revision of Autologous Tissue Substitute in Coccygeal Joint, External Approach
0SW6X8Z	Revision of Spacer in Coccygeal Joint, External Approach
0SW6XJZ	Revision of Synthetic Substitute in Coccygeal Joint, External Approach
0SW6XKZ	Revision of Nonautologous Tissue Substitute in Coccygeal Joint, External Approach
0SW700Z	Revision of Drainage Device in Right Sacroiliac Joint, Open Approach
0SW703Z	Revision of Infusion Device in Right Sacroiliac Joint, Open Approach
0SW704Z	Revision of Internal Fixation Device in Right Sacroiliac Joint, Open Approach
0SW707Z	Revision of Autologous Tissue Substitute in Right Sacroiliac Joint, Open Approach
0SW708Z	Revision of Spacer in Right Sacroiliac Joint, Open Approach
0SW70JZ	Revision of Synthetic Substitute in Right Sacroiliac Joint, Open Approach
0SW70KZ	Revision of Nonautologous Tissue Substitute in Right Sacroiliac Joint, Open Approach
0SW730Z	Revision of Drainage Device in Right Sacroiliac Joint, Percutaneous Approach
0SW733Z	Revision of Infusion Device in Right Sacroiliac Joint, Percutaneous Approach
0SW734Z	Revision of Internal Fixation Device in Right Sacroiliac Joint, Percutaneous Approach
0SW737Z	Revision of Autologous Tissue Substitute in Right Sacroiliac Joint, Percutaneous Approach
0SW738Z	Revision of Spacer in Right Sacroiliac Joint, Percutaneous Approach
0SW73JZ	Revision of Synthetic Substitute in Right Sacroiliac Joint, Percutaneous Approach
0SW73KZ	Revision of Nonautologous Tissue Substitute in Right Sacroiliac Joint, Percutaneous Approach
0SW740Z	Revision of Drainage Device in Right Sacroiliac Joint, Percutaneous Endoscopic Approach
0SW743Z	Revision of Infusion Device in Right Sacroiliac Joint, Percutaneous Endoscopic Approach
0SW744Z	Revision of Internal Fixation Device in Right Sacroiliac Joint, Percutaneous Endoscopic Approach
0SW747Z	Revision of Autologous Tissue Substitute in Right Sacroiliac Joint, Percutaneous Endoscopic Approach
0SW748Z	Revision of Spacer in Right Sacroiliac Joint, Percutaneous Endoscopic Approach
0SW74JZ	Revision of Synthetic Substitute in Right Sacroiliac Joint, Percutaneous Endoscopic Approach
0SW74KZ	Revision of Nonautologous Tissue Substitute in Right Sacroiliac Joint, Percutaneous Endoscopic Approach
0SW7X0Z	Revision of Drainage Device in Right Sacroiliac Joint, External Approach

0SW7X3Z	Revision of Infusion Device in Right Sacroiliac Joint, External Approach
0SW7X4Z	Revision of Internal Fixation Device in Right Sacroiliac Joint, External Approach
0SW7X7Z	Revision of Autologous Tissue Substitute in Right Sacroiliac Joint, External Approach
0SW7X8Z	Revision of Spacer in Right Sacroiliac Joint, External Approach
0SW7XJZ	Revision of Synthetic Substitute in Right Sacroiliac Joint, External Approach
0SW7XKZ	Revision of Nonautologous Tissue Substitute in Right Sacroiliac Joint, External Approach
0SW800Z	Revision of Drainage Device in Left Sacroiliac Joint, Open Approach
0SW803Z	Revision of Infusion Device in Left Sacroiliac Joint, Open Approach
0SW804Z	Revision of Internal Fixation Device in Left Sacroiliac Joint, Open Approach
0SW807Z	Revision of Autologous Tissue Substitute in Left Sacroiliac Joint, Open Approach
0SW808Z	Revision of Spacer in Left Sacroiliac Joint, Open Approach
0SW80JZ	Revision of Synthetic Substitute in Left Sacroiliac Joint, Open Approach
0SW80KZ	Revision of Nonautologous Tissue Substitute in Left Sacroiliac Joint, Open Approach
0SW830Z	Revision of Drainage Device in Left Sacroiliac Joint, Percutaneous Approach
0SW833Z	Revision of Infusion Device in Left Sacroiliac Joint, Percutaneous Approach
0SW834Z	Revision of Internal Fixation Device in Left Sacroiliac Joint, Percutaneous Approach
0SW837Z	Revision of Autologous Tissue Substitute in Left Sacroiliac Joint, Percutaneous Approach
0SW838Z	Revision of Spacer in Left Sacroiliac Joint, Percutaneous Approach
0SW83JZ	Revision of Synthetic Substitute in Left Sacroiliac Joint, Percutaneous Approach
0SW83KZ	Revision of Nonautologous Tissue Substitute in Left Sacroiliac Joint, Percutaneous Approach
0SW840Z	Revision of Drainage Device in Left Sacroiliac Joint, Percutaneous Endoscopic Approach
0SW843Z	Revision of Infusion Device in Left Sacroiliac Joint, Percutaneous Endoscopic Approach
0SW844Z	Revision of Internal Fixation Device in Left Sacroiliac Joint, Percutaneous Endoscopic Approach
0SW847Z	Revision of Autologous Tissue Substitute in Left Sacroiliac Joint, Percutaneous Endoscopic Approach
0SW848Z	Revision of Spacer in Left Sacroiliac Joint, Percutaneous Endoscopic Approach
0SW84JZ	Revision of Synthetic Substitute in Left Sacroiliac Joint, Percutaneous Endoscopic Approach
0SW84KZ	Revision of Nonautologous Tissue Substitute in Left Sacroiliac Joint, Percutaneous Endoscopic Approach
0SW8X0Z	Revision of Drainage Device in Left Sacroiliac Joint, External Approach
0SW8X3Z	Revision of Infusion Device in Left Sacroiliac Joint, External Approach
0SW8X4Z	Revision of Internal Fixation Device in Left Sacroiliac Joint, External Approach
0SW8X7Z	Revision of Autologous Tissue Substitute in Left Sacroiliac Joint, External Approach
0SW8X8Z	Revision of Spacer in Left Sacroiliac Joint, External Approach

Female-only   ♂ Male-only   ▲ Limited Coverage   ● Non-OR   ■ HAC-associated procedure   ▲ Non-covered procedures   ✚ Combination

0SW8XJZ	Revision of Synthetic Substitute in Left Sacroiliac Joint, External Approach
0SW8XKZ	Revision of Nonautologous Tissue Substitute in Left Sacroiliac Joint, External Approach
0SW900Z	Revision of Drainage Device in Right Hip Joint, Open Approach
0SW903Z	Revision of Infusion Device in Right Hip Joint, Open Approach
0SW904Z	Revision of Internal Fixation Device in Right Hip Joint, Open Approach
0SW905Z	Revision of External Fixation Device in Right Hip Joint, Open Approach
0SW907Z	Revision of Autologous Tissue Substitute in Right Hip Joint, Open Approach
0SW908Z	Revision of Spacer in Right Hip Joint, Open Approach
0SW909Z	Revision of Liner in Right Hip Joint, Open Approach
0SW90BZ	Revision of Resurfacing Device in Right Hip Joint, Open Approach
0SW90JZ	Revision of Synthetic Substitute in Right Hip Joint, Open Approach
0SW90KZ	Revision of Nonautologous Tissue Substitute in Right Hip Joint, Open Approach
0SW930Z	Revision of Drainage Device in Right Hip Joint, Percutaneous Approach
0SW933Z	Revision of Infusion Device in Right Hip Joint, Percutaneous Approach
0SW934Z	Revision of Internal Fixation Device in Right Hip Joint, Percutaneous Approach
0SW935Z	Revision of External Fixation Device in Right Hip Joint, Percutaneous Approach
0SW937Z	Revision of Autologous Tissue Substitute in Right Hip Joint, Percutaneous Approach
0SW938Z	Revision of Spacer in Right Hip Joint, Percutaneous Approach
0SW93JZ	Revision of Synthetic Substitute in Right Hip Joint, Percutaneous Approach
0SW93KZ	Revision of Nonautologous Tissue Substitute in Right Hip Joint, Percutaneous Approach
0SW940Z	Revision of Drainage Device in Right Hip Joint, Percutaneous Endoscopic Approach
0SW943Z	Revision of Infusion Device in Right Hip Joint, Percutaneous Endoscopic Approach
0SW944Z	Revision of Internal Fixation Device in Right Hip Joint, Percutaneous Endoscopic Approach
0SW945Z	Revision of External Fixation Device in Right Hip Joint, Percutaneous Endoscopic Approach
0SW947Z	Revision of Autologous Tissue Substitute in Right Hip Joint, Percutaneous Endoscopic Approach
0SW948Z	Revision of Spacer in Right Hip Joint, Percutaneous Endoscopic Approach
0SW94JZ	Revision of Synthetic Substitute in Right Hip Joint, Percutaneous Endoscopic Approach
0SW94KZ	Revision of Nonautologous Tissue Substitute in Right Hip Joint, Percutaneous Endoscopic Approach
0SW9X0Z	Revision of Drainage Device in Right Hip Joint, External Approach
0SW9X3Z	Revision of Infusion Device in Right Hip Joint, External Approach
0SW9X4Z	Revision of Internal Fixation Device in Right Hip Joint, External Approach
0SW9X5Z	Revision of External Fixation Device in Right Hip Joint, External Approach
0SW9X7Z	Revision of Autologous Tissue Substitute in Right Hip Joint, External Approach
0SW9X8Z	Revision of Spacer in Right Hip Joint, External Approach
0SW9XJZ	Revision of Synthetic Substitute in Right Hip Joint, External Approach
0SW9XKZ	Revision of Nonautologous Tissue Substitute in Right Hip Joint, External Approach
0SWB00Z	Revision of Drainage Device in Left Hip Joint, Open Approach
0SWB03Z	Revision of Infusion Device in Left Hip Joint, Open Approach
0SWB04Z	Revision of Internal Fixation Device in Left Hip Joint, Open Approach
0SWB05Z	Revision of External Fixation Device in Left Hip Joint, Open Approach
0SWB07Z	Revision of Autologous Tissue Substitute in Left Hip Joint, Open Approach
0SWB08Z	Revision of Spacer in Left Hip Joint, Open Approach
0SWB09Z	Revision of Liner in Left Hip Joint, Open Approach
0SWB0BZ	Revision of Resurfacing Device in Left Hip Joint, Open Approach
0SWB0JZ	Revision of Synthetic Substitute in Left Hip Joint, Open Approach
0SWB0KZ	Revision of Nonautologous Tissue Substitute in Left Hip Joint, Open Approach
0SWB30Z	Revision of Drainage Device in Left Hip Joint, Percutaneous Approach
0SWB33Z	Revision of Infusion Device in Left Hip Joint, Percutaneous Approach
0SWB34Z	Revision of Internal Fixation Device in Left Hip Joint, Percutaneous Approach
0SWB35Z	Revision of External Fixation Device in Left Hip Joint, Percutaneous Approach
0SWB37Z	Revision of Autologous Tissue Substitute in Left Hip Joint, Percutaneous Approach
0SWB38Z	Revision of Spacer in Left Hip Joint, Percutaneous Approach
0SWB3JZ	Revision of Synthetic Substitute in Left Hip Joint, Percutaneous Approach
0SWB3KZ	Revision of Nonautologous Tissue Substitute in Left Hip Joint, Percutaneous Approach
0SWB40Z	Revision of Drainage Device in Left Hip Joint, Percutaneous Endoscopic Approach
0SWB43Z	Revision of Infusion Device in Left Hip Joint, Percutaneous Endoscopic Approach
0SWB44Z	Revision of Internal Fixation Device in Left Hip Joint, Percutaneous Endoscopic Approach
0SWB45Z	Revision of External Fixation Device in Left Hip Joint, Percutaneous Endoscopic Approach
0SWB47Z	Revision of Autologous Tissue Substitute in Left Hip Joint, Percutaneous Endoscopic Approach
0SWB48Z	Revision of Spacer in Left Hip Joint, Percutaneous Endoscopic Approach
0SWB4JZ	Revision of Synthetic Substitute in Left Hip Joint, Percutaneous Endoscopic Approach
0SWB4KZ	Revision of Nonautologous Tissue Substitute in Left Hip Joint, Percutaneous Endoscopic Approach
0SWBX0Z	Revision of Drainage Device in Left Hip Joint, External Approach
0SWBX3Z	Revision of Infusion Device in Left Hip Joint, External Approach
0SWBX4Z	Revision of Internal Fixation Device in Left Hip Joint, External Approach
0SWBX5Z	Revision of External Fixation Device in Left Hip Joint, External Approach
0SWBX7Z	Revision of Autologous Tissue Substitute in Left Hip Joint, External Approach
0SWBX8Z	Revision of Spacer in Left Hip Joint, External Approach
0SWBXJZ	Revision of Synthetic Substitute in Left Hip Joint, External Approach
0SWBXKZ	Revision of Nonautologous Tissue Substitute in Left Hip Joint, External Approach
0SWC00Z	Revision of Drainage Device in Right Knee Joint, Open Approach
0SWC03Z	Revision of Infusion Device in Right Knee Joint, Open Approach
0SWC04Z	Revision of Internal Fixation Device in Right Knee Joint, Open Approach
0SWC05Z	Revision of External Fixation Device in Right Knee Joint, Open Approach
0SWC07Z	Revision of Autologous Tissue Substitute in Right Knee Joint, Open Approach
0SWC08Z	Revision of Spacer in Right Knee Joint, Open Approach
0SWC09Z	Revision of Liner in Right Knee Joint, Open Approach
0SWC0JZ	Revision of Synthetic Substitute in Right Knee Joint, Open Approach
0SWC0KZ	Revision of Nonautologous Tissue Substitute in Right Knee Joint, Open Approach
0SWC30Z	Revision of Drainage Device in Right Knee Joint, Percutaneous Approach
0SWC33Z	Revision of Infusion Device in Right Knee Joint, Percutaneous Approach
0SWC34Z	Revision of Internal Fixation Device in Right Knee Joint, Percutaneous Approach
0SWC35Z	Revision of External Fixation Device in Right Knee Joint, Percutaneous Approach
0SWC37Z	Revision of Autologous Tissue Substitute in Right Knee Joint, Percutaneous Approach
0SWC38Z	Revision of Spacer in Right Knee Joint, Percutaneous Approach
0SWC3JZ	Revision of Synthetic Substitute in Right Knee Joint, Percutaneous Approach
0SWC3KZ	Revision of Nonautologous Tissue Substitute in Right Knee Joint, Percutaneous Approach
0SWC40Z	Revision of Drainage Device in Right Knee Joint, Percutaneous Endoscopic Approach
0SWC43Z	Revision of Infusion Device in Right Knee Joint, Percutaneous Endoscopic Approach
0SWC44Z	Revision of Internal Fixation Device in Right Knee Joint, Percutaneous Endoscopic Approach
0SWC45Z	Revision of External Fixation Device in Right Knee Joint, Percutaneous Endoscopic Approach
0SWC47Z	Revision of Autologous Tissue Substitute in Right Knee Joint, Percutaneous Endoscopic Approach
0SWC48Z	Revision of Spacer in Right Knee Joint, Percutaneous Endoscopic Approach
0SWC4JZ	Revision of Synthetic Substitute in Right Knee Joint, Percutaneous Endoscopic Approach
0SWC4KZ	Revision of Nonautologous Tissue Substitute in Right Knee Joint, Percutaneous Endoscopic Approach
0SWCX0Z	Revision of Drainage Device in Right Knee Joint, External Approach
0SWCX3Z	Revision of Infusion Device in Right Knee Joint, External Approach
0SWCX4Z	Revision of Internal Fixation Device in Right Knee Joint, External Approach
0SWCX5Z	Revision of External Fixation Device in Right Knee Joint, External Approach
0SWCX7Z	Revision of Autologous Tissue Substitute in Right Knee Joint, External Approach
0SWCX8Z	Revision of Spacer in Right Knee Joint, External Approach
0SWCXJZ	Revision of Synthetic Substitute in Right Knee Joint, External Approach

0SWCXKZ Revision of Nonautologous Tissue Substitute in Right Knee Joint, External Approach

0SWD00Z Revision of Drainage Device in Left Knee Joint, Open Approach

0SWD03Z Revision of Infusion Device in Left Knee Joint, Open Approach

0SWD04Z Revision of Internal Fixation Device in Left Knee Joint, Open Approach

0SWD05Z Revision of External Fixation Device in Left Knee Joint, Open Approach

0SWD07Z Revision of Autologous Tissue Substitute in Left Knee Joint, Open Approach

0SWD08Z Revision of Spacer in Left Knee Joint, Open Approach

0SWD09Z Revision of Liner in Left Knee Joint, Open Approach

0SWD0JZ Revision of Synthetic Substitute in Left Knee Joint, Open Approach

0SWD0KZ Revision of Nonautologous Tissue Substitute in Left Knee Joint, Open Approach

0SWD30Z Revision of Drainage Device in Left Knee Joint, Percutaneous Approach

0SWD33Z Revision of Infusion Device in Left Knee Joint, Percutaneous Approach

0SWD34Z Revision of Internal Fixation Device in Left Knee Joint, Percutaneous Approach

0SWD35Z Revision of External Fixation Device in Left Knee Joint, Percutaneous Approach

0SWD37Z Revision of Autologous Tissue Substitute in Left Knee Joint, Percutaneous Approach

0SWD38Z Revision of Spacer in Left Knee Joint, Percutaneous Approach

0SWD3JZ Revision of Synthetic Substitute in Left Knee Joint, Percutaneous Approach

0SWD3KZ Revision of Nonautologous Tissue Substitute in Left Knee Joint, Percutaneous Approach

0SWD40Z Revision of Drainage Device in Left Knee Joint, Percutaneous Endoscopic Approach

0SWD43Z Revision of Infusion Device in Left Knee Joint, Percutaneous Endoscopic Approach

0SWD44Z Revision of Internal Fixation Device in Left Knee Joint, Percutaneous Endoscopic Approach

0SWD45Z Revision of External Fixation Device in Left Knee Joint, Percutaneous Endoscopic Approach

0SWD47Z Revision of Autologous Tissue Substitute in Left Knee Joint, Percutaneous Endoscopic Approach

0SWD48Z Revision of Spacer in Left Knee Joint, Percutaneous Endoscopic Approach

0SWD4JZ Revision of Synthetic Substitute in Left Knee Joint, Percutaneous Endoscopic Approach

0SWD4KZ Revision of Nonautologous Tissue Substitute in Left Knee Joint, Percutaneous Endoscopic Approach

0SWDX0Z Revision of Drainage Device in Left Knee Joint, External Approach

0SWDX3Z Revision of Infusion Device in Left Knee Joint, External Approach

0SWDX4Z Revision of Internal Fixation Device in Left Knee Joint, External Approach

0SWDX5Z Revision of External Fixation Device in Left Knee Joint, External Approach

0SWDX7Z Revision of Autologous Tissue Substitute in Left Knee Joint, External Approach

0SWDX8Z Revision of Spacer in Left Knee Joint, External Approach

0SWDXJZ Revision of Synthetic Substitute in Left Knee Joint, External Approach

0SWDXKZ Revision of Nonautologous Tissue Substitute in Left Knee Joint, External Approach

0SWF00Z Revision of Drainage Device in Right Ankle Joint, Open Approach

0SWF03Z Revision of Infusion Device in Right Ankle Joint, Open Approach

0SWF04Z Revision of Internal Fixation Device in Right Ankle Joint, Open Approach

0SWF05Z Revision of External Fixation Device in Right Ankle Joint, Open Approach

0SWF07Z Revision of Autologous Tissue Substitute in Right Ankle Joint, Open Approach

0SWF08Z Revision of Spacer in Right Ankle Joint, Open Approach

0SWF0JZ Revision of Synthetic Substitute in Right Ankle Joint, Open Approach

0SWF0KZ Revision of Nonautologous Tissue Substitute in Right Ankle Joint, Open Approach

0SWF30Z Revision of Drainage Device in Right Ankle Joint, Percutaneous Approach

0SWF33Z Revision of Infusion Device in Right Ankle Joint, Percutaneous Approach

0SWF34Z Revision of Internal Fixation Device in Right Ankle Joint, Percutaneous Approach

0SWF35Z Revision of External Fixation Device in Right Ankle Joint, Percutaneous Approach

0SWF37Z Revision of Autologous Tissue Substitute in Right Ankle Joint, Percutaneous Approach

0SWF38Z Revision of Spacer in Right Ankle Joint, Percutaneous Approach

0SWF3JZ Revision of Synthetic Substitute in Right Ankle Joint, Percutaneous Approach

0SWF3KZ Revision of Nonautologous Tissue Substitute in Right Ankle Joint, Percutaneous Approach

0SWF40Z Revision of Drainage Device in Right Ankle Joint, Percutaneous Endoscopic Approach

0SWF43Z Revision of Infusion Device in Right Ankle Joint, Percutaneous Endoscopic Approach

0SWF44Z Revision of Internal Fixation Device in Right Ankle Joint, Percutaneous Endoscopic Approach

0SWF45Z Revision of External Fixation Device in Right Ankle Joint, Percutaneous Endoscopic Approach

0SWF47Z Revision of Autologous Tissue Substitute in Right Ankle Joint, Percutaneous Endoscopic Approach

0SWF48Z Revision of Spacer in Right Ankle Joint, Percutaneous Endoscopic Approach

0SWF4JZ Revision of Synthetic Substitute in Right Ankle Joint, Percutaneous Endoscopic Approach

0SWF4KZ Revision of Nonautologous Tissue Substitute in Right Ankle Joint, Percutaneous Endoscopic Approach

0SWFX0Z Revision of Drainage Device in Right Ankle Joint, External Approach

0SWFX3Z Revision of Infusion Device in Right Ankle Joint, External Approach

0SWFX4Z Revision of Internal Fixation Device in Right Ankle Joint, External Approach

0SWFX5Z Revision of External Fixation Device in Right Ankle Joint, External Approach

0SWFX7Z Revision of Autologous Tissue Substitute in Right Ankle Joint, External Approach

0SWFX8Z Revision of Spacer in Right Ankle Joint, External Approach

0SWFXJZ Revision of Synthetic Substitute in Right Ankle Joint, External Approach

0SWFXKZ Revision of Nonautologous Tissue Substitute in Right Ankle Joint, External Approach

0SWG00Z Revision of Drainage Device in Left Ankle Joint, Open Approach

0SWG03Z Revision of Infusion Device in Left Ankle Joint, Open Approach

0SWG04Z Revision of Internal Fixation Device in Left Ankle Joint, Open Approach

0SWG05Z Revision of External Fixation Device in Left Ankle Joint, Open Approach

0SWG07Z Revision of Autologous Tissue Substitute in Left Ankle Joint, Open Approach

0SWG08Z Revision of Spacer in Left Ankle Joint, Open Approach

0SWG0JZ Revision of Synthetic Substitute in Left Ankle Joint, Open Approach

0SWG0KZ Revision of Nonautologous Tissue Substitute in Left Ankle Joint, Open Approach

0SWG30Z Revision of Drainage Device in Left Ankle Joint, Percutaneous Approach

0SWG33Z Revision of Infusion Device in Left Ankle Joint, Percutaneous Approach

0SWG34Z Revision of Internal Fixation Device in Left Ankle Joint, Percutaneous Approach

0SWG35Z Revision of External Fixation Device in Left Ankle Joint, Percutaneous Approach

0SWG37Z Revision of Autologous Tissue Substitute in Left Ankle Joint, Percutaneous Approach

0SWG38Z Revision of Spacer in Left Ankle Joint, Percutaneous Approach

0SWG3JZ Revision of Synthetic Substitute in Left Ankle Joint, Percutaneous Approach

0SWG3KZ Revision of Nonautologous Tissue Substitute in Left Ankle Joint, Percutaneous Approach

0SWG40Z Revision of Drainage Device in Left Ankle Joint, Percutaneous Endoscopic Approach

0SWG43Z Revision of Infusion Device in Left Ankle Joint, Percutaneous Endoscopic Approach

0SWG44Z Revision of Internal Fixation Device in Left Ankle Joint, Percutaneous Endoscopic Approach

0SWG45Z Revision of External Fixation Device in Left Ankle Joint, Percutaneous Endoscopic Approach

0SWG47Z Revision of Autologous Tissue Substitute in Left Ankle Joint, Percutaneous Endoscopic Approach

0SWG48Z Revision of Spacer in Left Ankle Joint, Percutaneous Endoscopic Approach

0SWG4JZ Revision of Synthetic Substitute in Left Ankle Joint, Percutaneous Endoscopic Approach

0SWG4KZ Revision of Nonautologous Tissue Substitute in Left Ankle Joint, Percutaneous Endoscopic Approach

0SWGX0Z Revision of Drainage Device in Left Ankle Joint, External Approach

0SWGX3Z Revision of Infusion Device in Left Ankle Joint, External Approach

0SWGX4Z Revision of Internal Fixation Device in Left Ankle Joint, External Approach

0SWGX5Z Revision of External Fixation Device in Left Ankle Joint, External Approach

0SWGX7Z Revision of Autologous Tissue Substitute in Left Ankle Joint, External Approach

0SWGX8Z Revision of Spacer in Left Ankle Joint, External Approach

0SWGXJZ Revision of Synthetic Substitute in Left Ankle Joint, External Approach

0SWGXKZ Revision of Nonautologous Tissue Substitute in Left Ankle Joint, External Approach

0SWH00Z Revision of Drainage Device in Right Tarsal Joint, Open Approach

0SWH03Z Revision of Infusion Device in Right Tarsal Joint, Open Approach

Female-only   ♂ Male-only   ▲ Limited Coverage   ● Non-OR   ▨ HAC-associated procedure   ▲ Non-covered procedures   ✚ Combination

0SWH04Z Revision of Internal Fixation Device in Right Tarsal Joint, Open Approach

0SWH05Z Revision of External Fixation Device in Right Tarsal Joint, Open Approach

0SWH07Z Revision of Autologous Tissue Substitute in Right Tarsal Joint, Open Approach

0SWH08Z Revision of Spacer in Right Tarsal Joint, Open Approach

0SWH0JZ Revision of Synthetic Substitute in Right Tarsal Joint, Open Approach

0SWH0KZ Revision of Nonautologous Tissue Substitute in Right Tarsal Joint, Open Approach

0SWH30Z Revision of Drainage Device in Right Tarsal Joint, Percutaneous Approach

0SWH33Z Revision of Infusion Device in Right Tarsal Joint, Percutaneous Approach

0SWH34Z Revision of Internal Fixation Device in Right Tarsal Joint, Percutaneous Approach

0SWH35Z Revision of External Fixation Device in Right Tarsal Joint, Percutaneous Approach

0SWH37Z Revision of Autologous Tissue Substitute in Right Tarsal Joint, Percutaneous Approach

0SWH38Z Revision of Spacer in Right Tarsal Joint, Percutaneous Approach

0SWH3JZ Revision of Synthetic Substitute in Right Tarsal Joint, Percutaneous Approach

0SWH3KZ Revision of Nonautologous Tissue Substitute in Right Tarsal Joint, Percutaneous Approach

0SWH40Z Revision of Drainage Device in Right Tarsal Joint, Percutaneous Endoscopic Approach

0SWH43Z Revision of Infusion Device in Right Tarsal Joint, Percutaneous Endoscopic Approach

0SWH44Z Revision of Internal Fixation Device in Right Tarsal Joint, Percutaneous Endoscopic Approach

0SWH45Z Revision of External Fixation Device in Right Tarsal Joint, Percutaneous Endoscopic Approach

0SWH47Z Revision of Autologous Tissue Substitute in Right Tarsal Joint, Percutaneous Endoscopic Approach

0SWH48Z Revision of Spacer in Right Tarsal Joint, Percutaneous Endoscopic Approach

0SWH4JZ Revision of Synthetic Substitute in Right Tarsal Joint, Percutaneous Endoscopic Approach

0SWH4KZ Revision of Nonautologous Tissue Substitute in Right Tarsal Joint, Percutaneous Endoscopic Approach

0SWHX0Z Revision of Drainage Device in Right Tarsal Joint, External Approach

0SWHX3Z Revision of Infusion Device in Right Tarsal Joint, External Approach

0SWHX4Z Revision of Internal Fixation Device in Right Tarsal Joint, External Approach

0SWHX5Z Revision of External Fixation Device in Right Tarsal Joint, External Approach

0SWHX7Z Revision of Autologous Tissue Substitute in Right Tarsal Joint, External Approach

0SWHX8Z Revision of Spacer in Right Tarsal Joint, External Approach

0SWHXJZ Revision of Synthetic Substitute in Right Tarsal Joint, External Approach

0SWHXKZ Revision of Nonautologous Tissue Substitute in Right Tarsal Joint, External Approach

0SWJ00Z Revision of Drainage Device in Left Tarsal Joint, Open Approach

0SWJ03Z Revision of Infusion Device in Left Tarsal Joint, Open Approach

0SWJ04Z Revision of Internal Fixation Device in Left Tarsal Joint, Open Approach

0SWJ05Z Revision of External Fixation Device in Left Tarsal Joint, Open Approach

0SWJ07Z Revision of Autologous Tissue Substitute in Left Tarsal Joint, Open Approach

0SWJ08Z Revision of Spacer in Left Tarsal Joint, Open Approach

0SWJ0JZ Revision of Synthetic Substitute in Left Tarsal Joint, Open Approach

0SWJ0KZ Revision of Nonautologous Tissue Substitute in Left Tarsal Joint, Open Approach

0SWJ30Z Revision of Drainage Device in Left Tarsal Joint, Percutaneous Approach

0SWJ33Z Revision of Infusion Device in Left Tarsal Joint, Percutaneous Approach

0SWJ34Z Revision of Internal Fixation Device in Left Tarsal Joint, Percutaneous Approach

0SWJ35Z Revision of External Fixation Device in Left Tarsal Joint, Percutaneous Approach

0SWJ37Z Revision of Autologous Tissue Substitute in Left Tarsal Joint, Percutaneous Approach

0SWJ38Z Revision of Spacer in Left Tarsal Joint, Percutaneous Approach

0SWJ3JZ Revision of Synthetic Substitute in Left Tarsal Joint, Percutaneous Approach

0SWJ3KZ Revision of Nonautologous Tissue Substitute in Left Tarsal Joint, Percutaneous Approach

0SWJ40Z Revision of Drainage Device in Left Tarsal Joint, Percutaneous Endoscopic Approach

0SWJ43Z Revision of Infusion Device in Left Tarsal Joint, Percutaneous Endoscopic Approach

0SWJ44Z Revision of Internal Fixation Device in Left Tarsal Joint, Percutaneous Endoscopic Approach

0SWJ45Z Revision of External Fixation Device in Left Tarsal Joint, Percutaneous Endoscopic Approach

0SWJ47Z Revision of Autologous Tissue Substitute in Left Tarsal Joint, Percutaneous Endoscopic Approach

0SWJ48Z Revision of Spacer in Left Tarsal Joint, Percutaneous Endoscopic Approach

0SWJ4JZ Revision of Synthetic Substitute in Left Tarsal Joint, Percutaneous Endoscopic Approach

0SWJ4KZ Revision of Nonautologous Tissue Substitute in Left Tarsal Joint, Percutaneous Endoscopic Approach

0SWJX0Z Revision of Drainage Device in Left Tarsal Joint, External Approach

0SWJX3Z Revision of Infusion Device in Left Tarsal Joint, External Approach

0SWJX4Z Revision of Internal Fixation Device in Left Tarsal Joint, External Approach

0SWJX5Z Revision of External Fixation Device in Left Tarsal Joint, External Approach

0SWJX7Z Revision of Autologous Tissue Substitute in Left Tarsal Joint, External Approach

0SWJX8Z Revision of Spacer in Left Tarsal Joint, External Approach

0SWJXJZ Revision of Synthetic Substitute in Left Tarsal Joint, External Approach

0SWJXKZ Revision of Nonautologous Tissue Substitute in Left Tarsal Joint, External Approach

0SWK00Z Revision of Drainage Device in Right Metatarsal-Tarsal Joint, Open Approach

0SWK03Z Revision of Infusion Device in Right Metatarsal-Tarsal Joint, Open Approach

0SWK04Z Revision of Internal Fixation Device in Right Metatarsal-Tarsal Joint, Open Approach

0SWK05Z Revision of External Fixation Device in Right Metatarsal-Tarsal Joint, Open Approach

0SWK07Z Revision of Autologous Tissue Substitute in Right Metatarsal-Tarsal Joint, Open Approach

0SWK08Z Revision of Spacer in Right Metatarsal-Tarsal Joint, Open Approach

0SWK0JZ Revision of Synthetic Substitute in Right Metatarsal-Tarsal Joint, Open Approach

0SWK0KZ Revision of Nonautologous Tissue Substitute in Right Metatarsal-Tarsal Joint, Open Approach

0SWK30Z Revision of Drainage Device in Right Metatarsal-Tarsal Joint, Percutaneous Approach

0SWK33Z Revision of Infusion Device in Right Metatarsal-Tarsal Joint, Percutaneous Approach

0SWK34Z Revision of Internal Fixation Device in Right Metatarsal-Tarsal Joint, Percutaneous Approach

0SWK35Z Revision of External Fixation Device in Right Metatarsal-Tarsal Joint, Percutaneous Approach

0SWK37Z Revision of Autologous Tissue Substitute in Right Metatarsal-Tarsal Joint, Percutaneous Approach

0SWK38Z Revision of Spacer in Right Metatarsal-Tarsal Joint, Percutaneous Approach

0SWK3JZ Revision of Synthetic Substitute in Right Metatarsal-Tarsal Joint, Percutaneous Approach

0SWK3KZ Revision of Nonautologous Tissue Substitute in Right Metatarsal-Tarsal Joint, Percutaneous Approach

0SWK40Z Revision of Drainage Device in Right Metatarsal-Tarsal Joint, Percutaneous Endoscopic Approach

0SWK43Z Revision of Infusion Device in Right Metatarsal-Tarsal Joint, Percutaneous Endoscopic Approach

0SWK44Z Revision of Internal Fixation Device in Right Metatarsal-Tarsal Joint, Percutaneous Endoscopic Approach

0SWK45Z Revision of External Fixation Device in Right Metatarsal-Tarsal Joint, Percutaneous Endoscopic Approach

0SWK47Z Revision of Autologous Tissue Substitute in Right Metatarsal-Tarsal Joint, Percutaneous Endoscopic Approach

0SWK48Z Revision of Spacer in Right Metatarsal-Tarsal Joint, Percutaneous Endoscopic Approach

0SWK4JZ Revision of Synthetic Substitute in Right Metatarsal-Tarsal Joint, Percutaneous Endoscopic Approach

0SWK4KZ Revision of Nonautologous Tissue Substitute in Right Metatarsal-Tarsal Joint, Percutaneous Endoscopic Approach

0SWKX0Z Revision of Drainage Device in Right Metatarsal-Tarsal Joint, External Approach

0SWKX3Z Revision of Infusion Device in Right Metatarsal-Tarsal Joint, External Approach

0SWKX4Z Revision of Internal Fixation Device in Right Metatarsal-Tarsal Joint, External Approach

0SWKX5Z Revision of External Fixation Device in Right Metatarsal-Tarsal Joint, External Approach

♀ Female-only   ♂ Male-only   ▲ Limited Coverage   ● Non-OR   ▨ HAC-associated procedure   ▲ Non-covered procedures   ✚ Combination

0WKX7Z Revision of Autologous Tissue Substitute in Right Metatarsal-Tarsal Joint, External Approach

0WKX8Z Revision of Spacer in Right Metatarsal-Tarsal Joint, External Approach

0WKXJZ Revision of Synthetic Substitute in Right Metatarsal-Tarsal Joint, External Approach

0WKXKZ Revision of Nonautologous Tissue Substitute in Right Metatarsal-Tarsal Joint, External Approach

0WL00Z Revision of Drainage Device in Left Metatarsal-Tarsal Joint, Open Approach

0WL03Z Revision of Infusion Device in Left Metatarsal-Tarsal Joint, Open Approach

0WL04Z Revision of Internal Fixation Device in Left Metatarsal-Tarsal Joint, Open Approach

0WL05Z Revision of External Fixation Device in Left Metatarsal-Tarsal Joint, Open Approach

0WL07Z Revision of Autologous Tissue Substitute in Left Metatarsal-Tarsal Joint, Open Approach

0WL08Z Revision of Spacer in Left Metatarsal-Tarsal Joint, Open Approach

0WL0JZ Revision of Synthetic Substitute in Left Metatarsal-Tarsal Joint, Open Approach

0WL0KZ Revision of Nonautologous Tissue Substitute in Left Metatarsal-Tarsal Joint, Open Approach

0WL30Z Revision of Drainage Device in Left Metatarsal-Tarsal Joint, Percutaneous Approach

0WL33Z Revision of Infusion Device in Left Metatarsal-Tarsal Joint, Percutaneous Approach

0WL34Z Revision of Internal Fixation Device in Left Metatarsal-Tarsal Joint, Percutaneous Approach

0WL35Z Revision of External Fixation Device in Left Metatarsal-Tarsal Joint, Percutaneous Approach

0WL37Z Revision of Autologous Tissue Substitute in Left Metatarsal-Tarsal Joint, Percutaneous Approach

0WL38Z Revision of Spacer in Left Metatarsal-Tarsal Joint, Percutaneous Approach

0WL3JZ Revision of Synthetic Substitute in Left Metatarsal-Tarsal Joint, Percutaneous Approach

0WL3KZ Revision of Nonautologous Tissue Substitute in Left Metatarsal-Tarsal Joint, Percutaneous Approach

0WL40Z Revision of Drainage Device in Left Metatarsal-Tarsal Joint, Percutaneous Endoscopic Approach

0WL43Z Revision of Infusion Device in Left Metatarsal-Tarsal Joint, Percutaneous Endoscopic Approach

0WL44Z Revision of Internal Fixation Device in Left Metatarsal-Tarsal Joint, Percutaneous Endoscopic Approach

0WL45Z Revision of External Fixation Device in Left Metatarsal-Tarsal Joint, Percutaneous Endoscopic Approach

0WL47Z Revision of Autologous Tissue Substitute in Left Metatarsal-Tarsal Joint, Percutaneous Endoscopic Approach

0WL48Z Revision of Spacer in Left Metatarsal-Tarsal Joint, Percutaneous Endoscopic Approach

0WL4JZ Revision of Synthetic Substitute in Left Metatarsal-Tarsal Joint, Percutaneous Endoscopic Approach

0WL4KZ Revision of Nonautologous Tissue Substitute in Left Metatarsal-Tarsal Joint, Percutaneous Endoscopic Approach

0SWLX0Z Revision of Drainage Device in Left Metatarsal-Tarsal Joint, External Approach

0SWLX3Z Revision of Infusion Device in Left Metatarsal-Tarsal Joint, External Approach

0SWLX4Z Revision of Internal Fixation Device in Left Metatarsal-Tarsal Joint, External Approach

0SWLX5Z Revision of External Fixation Device in Left Metatarsal-Tarsal Joint, External Approach

0SWLX7Z Revision of Autologous Tissue Substitute in Left Metatarsal-Tarsal Joint, External Approach

0SWLX8Z Revision of Spacer in Left Metatarsal-Tarsal Joint, External Approach

0SWLXJZ Revision of Synthetic Substitute in Left Metatarsal-Tarsal Joint, External Approach

0SWLXKZ Revision of Nonautologous Tissue Substitute in Left Metatarsal-Tarsal Joint, External Approach

0SWM00Z Revision of Drainage Device in Right Metatarsal-Phalangeal Joint, Open Approach

0SWM03Z Revision of Infusion Device in Right Metatarsal-Phalangeal Joint, Open Approach

0SWM04Z Revision of Internal Fixation Device in Right Metatarsal-Phalangeal Joint, Open Approach

0SWM05Z Revision of External Fixation Device in Right Metatarsal-Phalangeal Joint, Open Approach

0SWM07Z Revision of Autologous Tissue Substitute in Right Metatarsal-Phalangeal Joint, Open Approach

0SWM08Z Revision of Spacer in Right Metatarsal-Phalangeal Joint, Open Approach

0SWM0JZ Revision of Synthetic Substitute in Right Metatarsal-Phalangeal Joint, Open Approach

0SWM0KZ Revision of Nonautologous Tissue Substitute in Right Metatarsal-Phalangeal Joint, Open Approach

0SWM30Z Revision of Drainage Device in Right Metatarsal-Phalangeal Joint, Percutaneous Approach

0SWM33Z Revision of Infusion Device in Right Metatarsal-Phalangeal Joint, Percutaneous Approach

0SWM34Z Revision of Internal Fixation Device in Right Metatarsal-Phalangeal Joint, Percutaneous Approach

0SWM35Z Revision of External Fixation Device in Right Metatarsal-Phalangeal Joint, Percutaneous Approach

0SWM37Z Revision of Autologous Tissue Substitute in Right Metatarsal-Phalangeal Joint, Percutaneous Approach

0SWM38Z Revision of Spacer in Right Metatarsal-Phalangeal Joint, Percutaneous Approach

0SWM3JZ Revision of Synthetic Substitute in Right Metatarsal-Phalangeal Joint, Percutaneous Approach

0SWM3KZ Revision of Nonautologous Tissue Substitute in Right Metatarsal-Phalangeal Joint, Percutaneous Approach

0SWM40Z Revision of Drainage Device in Right Metatarsal-Phalangeal Joint, Percutaneous Endoscopic Approach

0SWM43Z Revision of Infusion Device in Right Metatarsal-Phalangeal Joint, Percutaneous Endoscopic Approach

0SWM44Z Revision of Internal Fixation Device in Right Metatarsal-Phalangeal Joint, Percutaneous Endoscopic Approach

0SWM45Z Revision of External Fixation Device in Right Metatarsal-Phalangeal Joint, Percutaneous Endoscopic Approach

0SWM47Z Revision of Autologous Tissue Substitute in Right Metatarsal-Phalangeal Joint, Percutaneous Endoscopic Approach

0SWM48Z Revision of Spacer in Right Metatarsal-Phalangeal Joint, Percutaneous Endoscopic Approach

0SWM4JZ Revision of Synthetic Substitute in Right Metatarsal-Phalangeal Joint, Percutaneous Endoscopic Approach

0SWM4KZ Revision of Nonautologous Tissue Substitute in Right Metatarsal-Phalangeal Joint, Percutaneous Endoscopic Approach

0SWMX0Z Revision of Drainage Device in Right Metatarsal-Phalangeal Joint, External Approach

0SWMX3Z Revision of Infusion Device in Right Metatarsal-Phalangeal Joint, External Approach

0SWMX4Z Revision of Internal Fixation Device in Right Metatarsal-Phalangeal Joint, External Approach

0SWMX5Z Revision of External Fixation Device in Right Metatarsal-Phalangeal Joint, External Approach

0SWMX7Z Revision of Autologous Tissue Substitute in Right Metatarsal-Phalangeal Joint, External Approach

0SWMX8Z Revision of Spacer in Right Metatarsal-Phalangeal Joint, External Approach

0SWMXJZ Revision of Synthetic Substitute in Right Metatarsal-Phalangeal Joint, External Approach

0SWMXKZ Revision of Nonautologous Tissue Substitute in Right Metatarsal-Phalangeal Joint, External Approach

0SWN00Z Revision of Drainage Device in Left Metatarsal-Phalangeal Joint, Open Approach

0SWN03Z Revision of Infusion Device in Left Metatarsal-Phalangeal Joint, Open Approach

0SWN04Z Revision of Internal Fixation Device in Left Metatarsal-Phalangeal Joint, Open Approach

0SWN05Z Revision of External Fixation Device in Left Metatarsal-Phalangeal Joint, Open Approach

0SWN07Z Revision of Autologous Tissue Substitute in Left Metatarsal-Phalangeal Joint, Open Approach

0SWN08Z Revision of Spacer in Left Metatarsal-Phalangeal Joint, Open Approach

0SWN0JZ Revision of Synthetic Substitute in Left Metatarsal-Phalangeal Joint, Open Approach

0SWN0KZ Revision of Nonautologous Tissue Substitute in Left Metatarsal-Phalangeal Joint, Open Approach

0SWN30Z Revision of Drainage Device in Left Metatarsal-Phalangeal Joint, Percutaneous Approach

0SWN33Z Revision of Infusion Device in Left Metatarsal-Phalangeal Joint, Percutaneous Approach

0SWN34Z Revision of Internal Fixation Device in Left Metatarsal-Phalangeal Joint, Percutaneous Approach

0SWN35Z Revision of External Fixation Device in Left Metatarsal-Phalangeal Joint, Percutaneous Approach

0SWN37Z Revision of Autologous Tissue Substitute in Left Metatarsal-Phalangeal Joint, Percutaneous Approach

Female-only   ♂ Male-only   ▲ Limited Coverage   ● Non-OR   ▨ HAC-associated procedure   ▲ Non-covered procedures   ✚ Combination

0SWN38Z Revision of Spacer in Left Metatarsal-Phalangeal Joint, Percutaneous Approach

0SWN3JZ Revision of Synthetic Substitute in Left Metatarsal-Phalangeal Joint, Percutaneous Approach

0SWN3KZ Revision of Nonautologous Tissue Substitute in Left Metatarsal-Phalangeal Joint, Percutaneous Approach

0SWN40Z Revision of Drainage Device in Left Metatarsal-Phalangeal Joint, Percutaneous Endoscopic Approach

0SWN43Z Revision of Infusion Device in Left Metatarsal-Phalangeal Joint, Percutaneous Endoscopic Approach

0SWN44Z Revision of Internal Fixation Device in Left Metatarsal-Phalangeal Joint, Percutaneous Endoscopic Approach

0SWN45Z Revision of External Fixation Device in Left Metatarsal-Phalangeal Joint, Percutaneous Endoscopic Approach

0SWN47Z Revision of Autologous Tissue Substitute in Left Metatarsal-Phalangeal Joint, Percutaneous Endoscopic Approach

0SWN48Z Revision of Spacer in Left Metatarsal-Phalangeal Joint, Percutaneous Endoscopic Approach

0SWN4JZ Revision of Synthetic Substitute in Left Metatarsal-Phalangeal Joint, Percutaneous Endoscopic Approach

0SWN4KZ Revision of Nonautologous Tissue Substitute in Left Metatarsal-Phalangeal Joint, Percutaneous Endoscopic Approach

0SWNX0Z Revision of Drainage Device in Left Metatarsal-Phalangeal Joint, External Approach

0SWNX3Z Revision of Infusion Device in Left Metatarsal-Phalangeal Joint, External Approach

0SWNX4Z Revision of Internal Fixation Device in Left Metatarsal-Phalangeal Joint, External Approach

0SWNX5Z Revision of External Fixation Device in Left Metatarsal-Phalangeal Joint, External Approach

0SWNX7Z Revision of Autologous Tissue Substitute in Left Metatarsal-Phalangeal Joint, External Approach

0SWNX8Z Revision of Spacer in Left Metatarsal-Phalangeal Joint, External Approach

0SWNXJZ Revision of Synthetic Substitute in Left Metatarsal-Phalangeal Joint, External Approach

0SWNXKZ Revision of Nonautologous Tissue Substitute in Left Metatarsal-Phalangeal Joint, External Approach

0SWP00Z Revision of Drainage Device in Right Toe Phalangeal Joint, Open Approach

0SWP03Z Revision of Infusion Device in Right Toe Phalangeal Joint, Open Approach

0SWP04Z Revision of Internal Fixation Device in Right Toe Phalangeal Joint, Open Approach

0SWP05Z Revision of External Fixation Device in Right Toe Phalangeal Joint, Open Approach

0SWP07Z Revision of Autologous Tissue Substitute in Right Toe Phalangeal Joint, Open Approach

0SWP08Z Revision of Spacer in Right Toe Phalangeal Joint, Open Approach

0SWP0JZ Revision of Synthetic Substitute in Right Toe Phalangeal Joint, Open Approach

0SWP0KZ Revision of Nonautologous Tissue Substitute in Right Toe Phalangeal Joint, Open Approach

0SWP30Z Revision of Drainage Device in Right Toe Phalangeal Joint, Percutaneous Approach

0SWP33Z Revision of Infusion Device in Right Toe Phalangeal Joint, Percutaneous Approach

0SWP34Z Revision of Internal Fixation Device in Right Toe Phalangeal Joint, Percutaneous Approach

0SWP35Z Revision of External Fixation Device in Right Toe Phalangeal Joint, Percutaneous Approach

0SWP37Z Revision of Autologous Tissue Substitute in Right Toe Phalangeal Joint, Percutaneous Approach

0SWP38Z Revision of Spacer in Right Toe Phalangeal Joint, Percutaneous Approach

0SWP3JZ Revision of Synthetic Substitute in Right Toe Phalangeal Joint, Percutaneous Approach

0SWP3KZ Revision of Nonautologous Tissue Substitute in Right Toe Phalangeal Joint, Percutaneous Approach

0SWP40Z Revision of Drainage Device in Right Toe Phalangeal Joint, Percutaneous Endoscopic Approach

0SWP43Z Revision of Infusion Device in Right Toe Phalangeal Joint, Percutaneous Endoscopic Approach

0SWP44Z Revision of Internal Fixation Device in Right Toe Phalangeal Joint, Percutaneous Endoscopic Approach

0SWP45Z Revision of External Fixation Device in Right Toe Phalangeal Joint, Percutaneous Endoscopic Approach

0SWP47Z Revision of Autologous Tissue Substitute in Right Toe Phalangeal Joint, Percutaneous Endoscopic Approach

0SWP48Z Revision of Spacer in Right Toe Phalangeal Joint, Percutaneous Endoscopic Approach

0SWP4JZ Revision of Synthetic Substitute in Right Toe Phalangeal Joint, Percutaneous Endoscopic Approach

0SWP4KZ Revision of Nonautologous Tissue Substitute in Right Toe Phalangeal Joint, Percutaneous Endoscopic Approach

0SWPX0Z Revision of Drainage Device in Right Toe Phalangeal Joint, External Approach

0SWPX3Z Revision of Infusion Device in Right Toe Phalangeal Joint, External Approach

0SWPX4Z Revision of Internal Fixation Device in Right Toe Phalangeal Joint, External Approach

0SWPX5Z Revision of External Fixation Device in Right Toe Phalangeal Joint, External Approach

0SWPX7Z Revision of Autologous Tissue Substitute in Right Toe Phalangeal Joint, External Approach

0SWPX8Z Revision of Spacer in Right Toe Phalangeal Joint, External Approach

0SWPXJZ Revision of Synthetic Substitute in Right Toe Phalangeal Joint, External Approach

0SWPXKZ Revision of Nonautologous Tissue Substitute in Right Toe Phalangeal Joint, External Approach

0SWQ00Z Revision of Drainage Device in Left Toe Phalangeal Joint, Open Approach

0SWQ03Z Revision of Infusion Device in Left Toe Phalangeal Joint, Open Approach

0SWQ04Z Revision of Internal Fixation Device in Left Toe Phalangeal Joint, Open Approach

0SWQ05Z Revision of External Fixation Device in Left Toe Phalangeal Joint, Open Approach

0SWQ07Z Revision of Autologous Tissue Substitute in Left Toe Phalangeal Joint, Open Approach

0SWQ08Z Revision of Spacer in Left Toe Phalangeal Joint, Open Approach

0SWQ0JZ Revision of Synthetic Substitute in Left Toe Phalangeal Joint, Open Approach

0SWQ0KZ Revision of Nonautologous Tissue Substitute in Left Toe Phalangeal Joint, Open Approach

0SWQ30Z Revision of Drainage Device in Left Toe Phalangeal Joint, Percutaneous Approach

0SWQ33Z Revision of Infusion Device in Left Toe Phalangeal Joint, Percutaneous Approach

0SWQ34Z Revision of Internal Fixation Device in Left Toe Phalangeal Joint, Percutaneous Approach

0SWQ35Z Revision of External Fixation Device in Left Toe Phalangeal Joint, Percutaneous Approach

0SWQ37Z Revision of Autologous Tissue Substitute in Left Toe Phalangeal Joint, Percutaneous Approach

0SWQ38Z Revision of Spacer in Left Toe Phalangeal Joint, Percutaneous Approach

0SWQ3JZ Revision of Synthetic Substitute in Left Toe Phalangeal Joint, Percutaneous Approach

0SWQ3KZ Revision of Nonautologous Tissue Substitute in Left Toe Phalangeal Joint, Percutaneous Approach

0SWQ40Z Revision of Drainage Device in Left Toe Phalangeal Joint, Percutaneous Endoscopic Approach

0SWQ43Z Revision of Infusion Device in Left Toe Phalangeal Joint, Percutaneous Endoscopic Approach

0SWQ44Z Revision of Internal Fixation Device in Left Toe Phalangeal Joint, Percutaneous Endoscopic Approach

0SWQ45Z Revision of External Fixation Device in Left Toe Phalangeal Joint, Percutaneous Endoscopic Approach

0SWQ47Z Revision of Autologous Tissue Substitute in Left Toe Phalangeal Joint, Percutaneous Endoscopic Approach

0SWQ48Z Revision of Spacer in Left Toe Phalangeal Joint, Percutaneous Endoscopic Approach

0SWQ4JZ Revision of Synthetic Substitute in Left Toe Phalangeal Joint, Percutaneous Endoscopic Approach

0SWQ4KZ Revision of Nonautologous Tissue Substitute in Left Toe Phalangeal Joint, Percutaneous Endoscopic Approach

0SWQX0Z Revision of Drainage Device in Left Toe Phalangeal Joint, External Approach

0SWQX3Z Revision of Infusion Device in Left Toe Phalangeal Joint, External Approach

0SWQX4Z Revision of Internal Fixation Device in Left Toe Phalangeal Joint, External Approach

0SWQX5Z Revision of External Fixation Device in Left Toe Phalangeal Joint, External Approach

0SWQX7Z Revision of Autologous Tissue Substitute in Left Toe Phalangeal Joint, External Approach

0SWQX8Z Revision of Spacer in Left Toe Phalangeal Joint, External Approach

0SWQXJZ Revision of Synthetic Substitute in Left Toe Phalangeal Joint, External Approach

0SWQXKZ Revision of Nonautologous Tissue Substitute in Left Toe Phalangeal Joint, External Approach

Urinary System

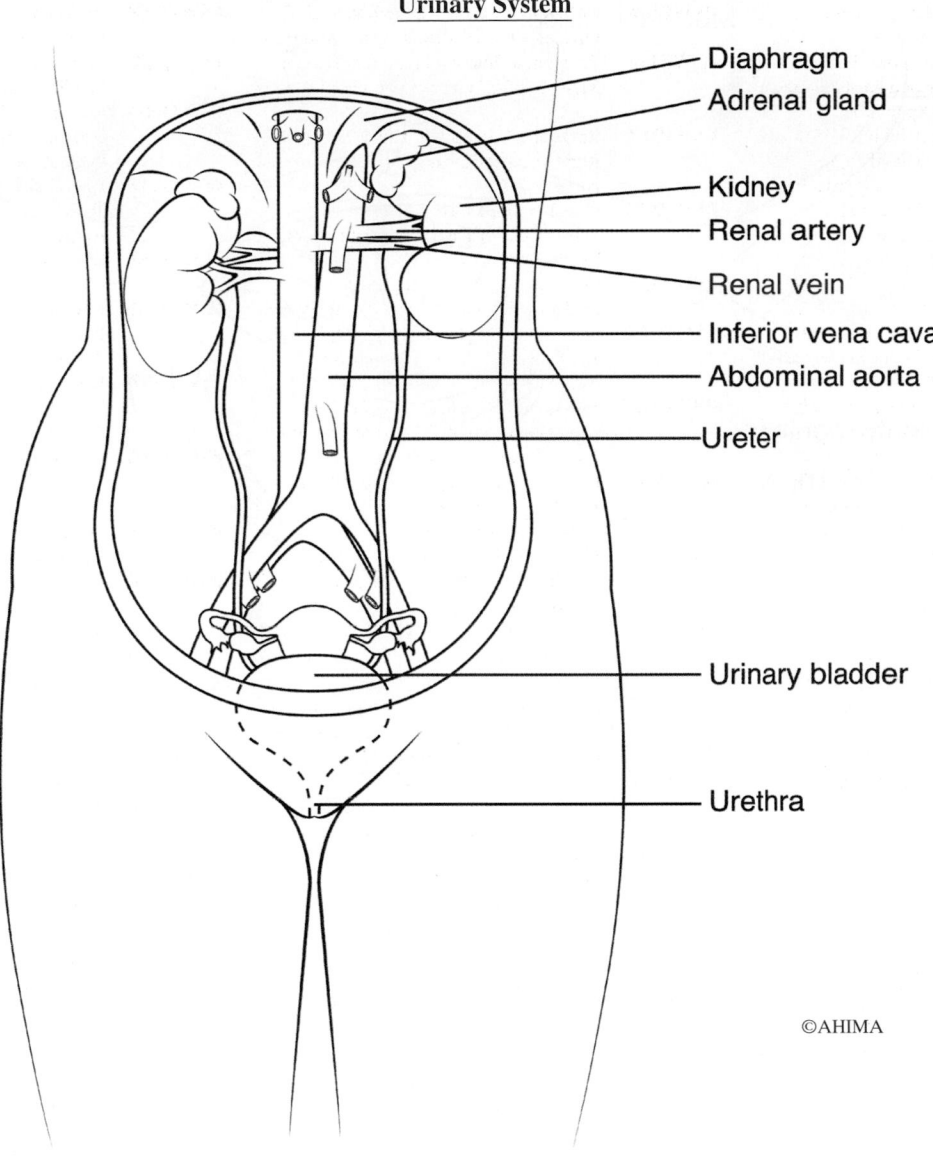

- Diaphragm
- Adrenal gland
- Kidney
- Renal artery
- Renal vein
- Inferior vena cava
- Abdominal aorta
- Ureter
- Urinary bladder
- Urethra

©AHIMA

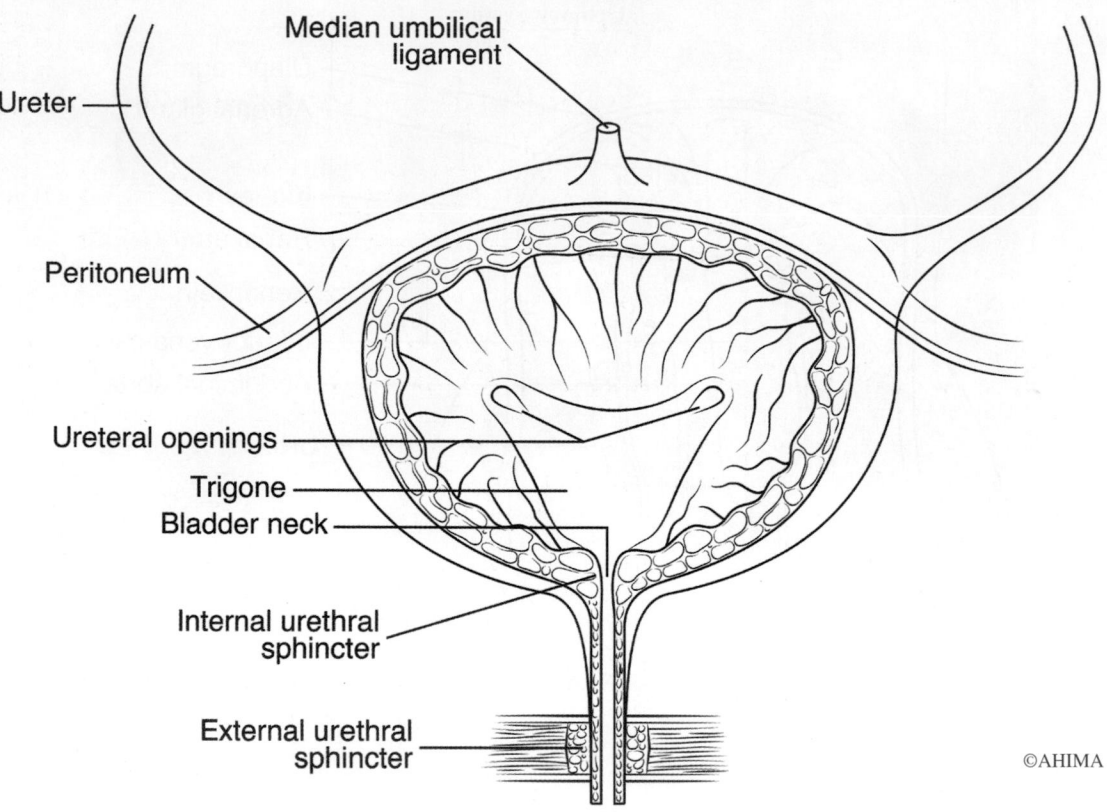

Median umbilical ligament

Ureter

Peritoneum

Ureteral openings

Trigone

Bladder neck

Internal urethral sphincter

External urethral sphincter

©AHIMA

Kidney

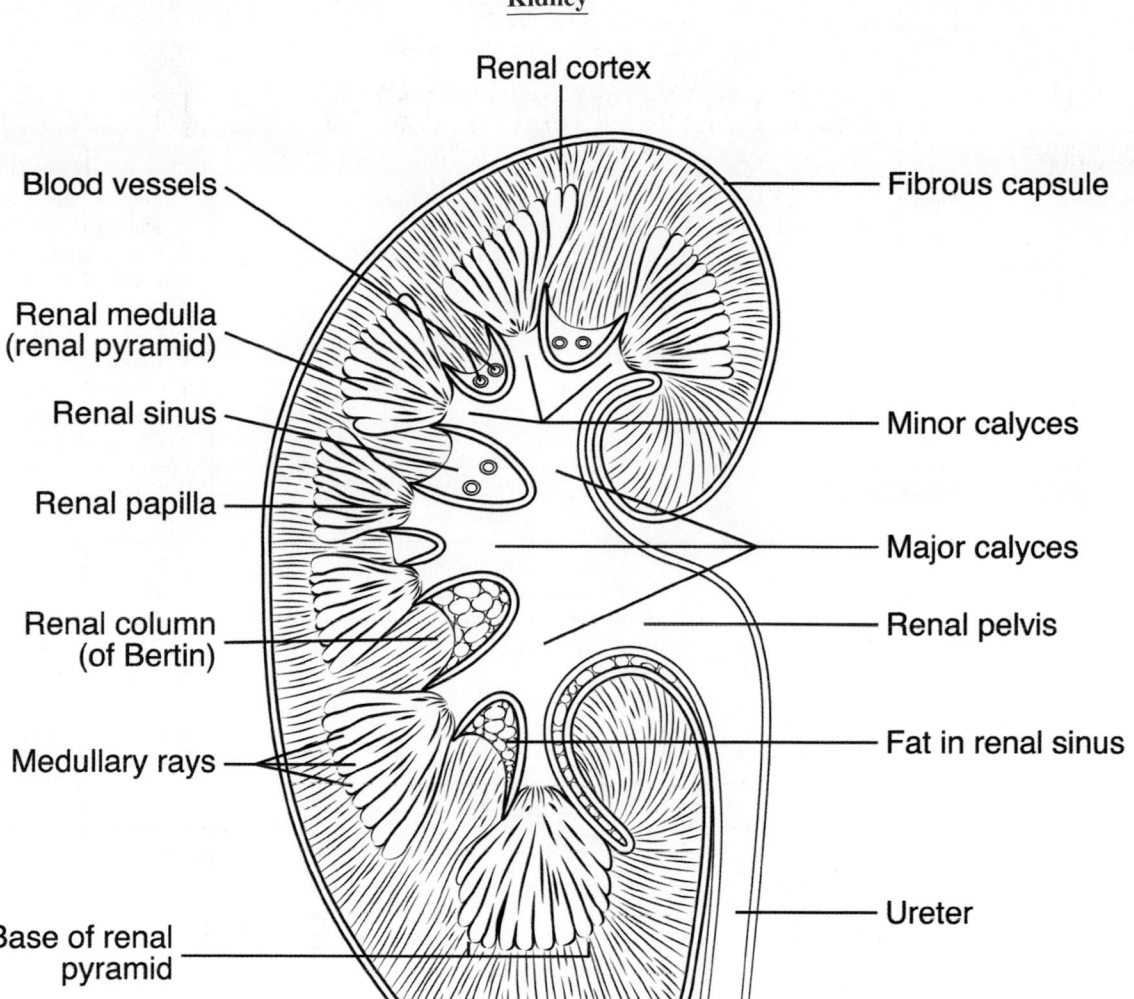

Renal cortex

Blood vessels

Renal medulla
(renal pyramid)

Renal sinus

Renal papilla

Renal column
(of Bertin)

Medullary rays

Base of renal
pyramid

Fibrous capsule

Minor calyces

Major calyces

Renal pelvis

Fat in renal sinus

Ureter

©AHIMA

Urinary System Tables 0T1–0TY

Section 0 **Medical and Surgical**
Body System T **Urinary System**
Operation 1 **Bypass:** Altering the route of passage of the contents of a tubular body part

Body Part (4ᵗʰ)	Approach (5ᵗʰ)	Device (6ᵗʰ)	Qualifier (7ᵗʰ)
3 Kidney Pelvis, Right 4 Kidney Pelvis, Left	0 Open 4 Percutaneous Endoscopic	7 Autologous Tissue Substitute J Synthetic Substitute K Nonautologous Tissue Substitute Z No Device	3 Kidney Pelvis, Right 4 Kidney Pelvis, Left 6 Ureter, Right 7 Ureter, Left 8 Colon 9 Colocutaneous A Ileum B Bladder C Ileocutaneous D Cutaneous
3 Kidney Pelvis, Right 4 Kidney Pelvis, Left	3 Percutaneous	J Synthetic Substitute	D Cutaneous
6 Ureter, Right 7 Ureter, Left 8 Ureters, Bilateral	0 Open 4 Percutaneous Endoscopic	7 Autologous Tissue Substitute J Synthetic Substitute K Nonautologous Tissue Substitute Z No Device	6 Ureter, Right 7 Ureter, Left 8 Colon 9 Colocutaneous A Ileum B Bladder C Ileocutaneous D Cutaneous
6 Ureter, Right 7 Ureter, Left 8 Ureters, Bilateral	3 Percutaneous	J Synthetic Substitute	D Cutaneous
B Bladder	0 Open 4 Percutaneous Endoscopic	7 Autologous Tissue Substitute J Synthetic Substitute K Nonautologous Tissue Substitute Z No Device	9 Colocutaneous C Ileocutaneous D Cutaneous
B Bladder	3 Percutaneous	J Synthetic Substitute	D Cutaneous

Section 0 **Medical and Surgical**
Body System T **Urinary System**
Operation 2 **Change:** Taking out or off a device from a body part and putting back an identical or similar device in or on the same body part without cutting or puncturing the skin or a mucous membrane

Body Part (4ᵗʰ)	Approach (5ᵗʰ)	Device (6ᵗʰ)	Qualifier (7ᵗʰ)
5 Kidney 9 Ureter B Bladder D Urethra	X External	0 Drainage Device Y Other Device	Z No Qualifier

Section 0 **Medical and Surgical**
Body System T **Urinary System**
Operation 5 **Destruction:** Physical eradication of all or a portion of a body part by the direct use of energy, force, or a destructive agent

Body Part (4ᵗʰ)	Approach (5ᵗʰ)	Device (6ᵗʰ)	Qualifier (7ᵗʰ)
0 Kidney, Right 1 Kidney, Left 3 Kidney Pelvis, Right 4 Kidney Pelvis, Left 6 Ureter, Right 7 Ureter, Left B Bladder C Bladder Neck	0 Open 3 Percutaneous 4 Percutaneous Endoscopic 7 Via Natural or Artificial Opening 8 Via Natural or Artificial Opening Endoscopic	Z No Device	Z No Qualifier

Continued →

Section	0	Medical and Surgical
Body System	T	Urinary System
Operation	5	**Destruction:** Physical eradication of all or a portion of a body part by the direct use of energy, force, or a destructive agent

Body Part (4ᵗʰ)	Approach (5ᵗʰ)	Device (6ᵗʰ)	Qualifier (7ᵗʰ)
D Urethra	0 Open 3 Percutaneous 4 Percutaneous Endoscopic 7 Via Natural or Artificial Opening 8 Via Natural or Artificial Opening Endoscopic X External	Z No Device	Z No Qualifier

Section	0	Medical and Surgical
Body System	T	Urinary System
Operation	7	**Dilation:** Expanding an orifice or the lumen of a tubular body part

Body Part (4ᵗʰ)	Approach (5ᵗʰ)	Device (6ᵗʰ)	Qualifier (7ᵗʰ)
3 Kidney Pelvis, Right 4 Kidney Pelvis, Left 6 Ureter, Right 7 Ureter, Left 8 Ureters, Bilateral B Bladder C Bladder Neck D Urethra	0 Open 3 Percutaneous 4 Percutaneous Endoscopic 7 Via Natural or Artificial Opening 8 Via Natural or Artificial Opening Endoscopic	D Intraluminal Device Z No Device	Z No Qualifier

Section	0	Medical and Surgical
Body System	T	Urinary System
Operation	8	**Division:** Cutting into a body part, without draining fluids and/or gases from the body part, in order to separate or transect a body part

Body Part (4ᵗʰ)	Approach (5ᵗʰ)	Device (6ᵗʰ)	Qualifier (7ᵗʰ)
2 Kidneys, Bilateral C Bladder Neck	0 Open 3 Percutaneous 4 Percutaneous Endoscopic	Z No Device	Z No Qualifier

Section	0	Medical and Surgical
Body System	T	Urinary System
Operation	9	**Drainage:** Taking or letting out fluids and/or gases from a body part

Body Part (4ᵗʰ)	Approach (5ᵗʰ)	Device (6ᵗʰ)	Qualifier (7ᵗʰ)
0 Kidney, Right 1 Kidney, Left 3 Kidney Pelvis, Right 4 Kidney Pelvis, Left 6 Ureter, Right 7 Ureter, Left 8 Ureters, Bilateral B Bladder C Bladder Neck	0 Open 3 Percutaneous 4 Percutaneous Endoscopic 7 Via Natural or Artificial Opening 8 Via Natural or Artificial Opening Endoscopic	0 Drainage Device	Z No Qualifier
0 Kidney, Right 1 Kidney, Left 3 Kidney Pelvis, Right 4 Kidney Pelvis, Left 6 Ureter, Right 7 Ureter, Left 8 Ureters, Bilateral B Bladder C Bladder Neck	0 Open 3 Percutaneous 4 Percutaneous Endoscopic 7 Via Natural or Artificial Opening 8 Via Natural or Artificial Opening Endoscopic	Z No Device	X Diagnostic Z No Qualifier

Continued ➤

Section	0	Medical and Surgical
Body System	T	Urinary System
Operation	9	Drainage: Taking or letting out fluids and/or gases from a body part

Body Part (4th)	Approach (5th)	Device (6th)	Qualifier (7th)
D Urethra	0 Open 3 Percutaneous 4 Percutaneous Endoscopic 7 Via Natural or Artificial Opening 8 Via Natural or Artificial Opening Endoscopic X External	0 Drainage Device	Z No Qualifier
D Urethra	0 Open 3 Percutaneous 4 Percutaneous Endoscopic 7 Via Natural or Artificial Opening 8 Via Natural or Artificial Opening Endoscopic X External	Z No Device	X Diagnostic Z No Qualifier

Section	0	Medical and Surgical
Body System	T	Urinary System
Operation	B	Excision: Cutting out or off, without replacement, a portion of a body part

Body Part (4th)	Approach (5th)	Device (6th)	Qualifier (7th)
0 Kidney, Right 1 Kidney, Left 3 Kidney Pelvis, Right 4 Kidney Pelvis, Left 6 Ureter, Right 7 Ureter, Left B Bladder C Bladder Neck	0 Open 3 Percutaneous 4 Percutaneous Endoscopic 7 Via Natural or Artificial Opening 8 Via Natural or Artificial Opening Endoscopic	Z No Device	X Diagnostic Z No Qualifier
D Urethra	0 Open 3 Percutaneous 4 Percutaneous Endoscopic 7 Via Natural or Artificial Opening 8 Via Natural or Artificial Opening Endoscopic X External	Z No Device	X Diagnostic Z No Qualifier

Section	0	Medical and Surgical
Body System	T	Urinary System
Operation	C	Extirpation: Taking or cutting out solid matter from a body part

Body Part (4th)	Approach (5th)	Device (6th)	Qualifier (7th)
0 Kidney, Right 1 Kidney, Left 3 Kidney Pelvis, Right 4 Kidney Pelvis, Left 6 Ureter, Right 7 Ureter, Left B Bladder C Bladder Neck	0 Open 3 Percutaneous 4 Percutaneous Endoscopic 7 Via Natural or Artificial Opening 8 Via Natural or Artificial Opening Endoscopic	Z No Device	Z No Qualifier
D Urethra	0 Open 3 Percutaneous 4 Percutaneous Endoscopic 7 Via Natural or Artificial Opening 8 Via Natural or Artificial Opening Endoscopic X External	Z No Device	Z No Qualifier

Section	0	Medical and Surgical
Body System	T	Urinary System
Operation	D	**Extraction:** Pulling or stripping out or off all or a portion of a body part by the use of force

Body Part (4th)	Approach (5th)	Device (6th)	Qualifier (7th)
0 Kidney, Right 1 Kidney, Left	0 Open 3 Percutaneous 4 Percutaneous Endoscopic	Z No Device	Z No Qualifier

Section	0	Medical and Surgical
Body System	T	Urinary System
Operation	F	**Fragmentation:** Breaking solid matter in a body part into pieces

Body Part (4th)	Approach (5th)	Device (6th)	Qualifier (7th)
3 Kidney Pelvis, Right 4 Kidney Pelvis, Left 6 Ureter, Right 7 Ureter, Left B Bladder C Bladder Neck D Urethra	0 Open 3 Percutaneous 4 Percutaneous Endoscopic 7 Via Natural or Artificial Opening 8 Via Natural or Artificial Opening Endoscopic X External	Z No Device	Z No Qualifier

Section	0	Medical and Surgical
Body System	T	Urinary System
Operation	H	**Insertion:** Putting in a nonbiological appliance that monitors, assists, performs, or prevents a physiological function but does not physically take the place of a body part

Body Part (4th)	Approach (5th)	Device (6th)	Qualifier (7th)
5 Kidney	0 Open 3 Percutaneous 4 Percutaneous Endoscopic 7 Via Natural or Artificial Opening 8 Via Natural or Artificial Opening Endoscopic	2 Monitoring Device 3 Infusion Device	Z No Qualifier
9 Ureter	0 Open 3 Percutaneous 4 Percutaneous Endoscopic 7 Via Natural or Artificial Opening 8 Via Natural or Artificial Opening Endoscopic	2 Monitoring Device 3 Infusion Device M Stimulator Lead	Z No Qualifier
B Bladder	0 Open 3 Percutaneous 4 Percutaneous Endoscopic 7 Via Natural or Artificial Opening 8 Via Natural or Artificial Opening Endoscopic	2 Monitoring Device 3 Infusion Device L Artificial Sphincter M Stimulator Lead	Z No Qualifier
C Bladder Neck	0 Open 3 Percutaneous 4 Percutaneous Endoscopic 7 Via Natural or Artificial Opening 8 Via Natural or Artificial Opening Endoscopic	L Artificial Sphincter	Z No Qualifier
D Urethra	0 Open 3 Percutaneous 4 Percutaneous Endoscopic 7 Via Natural or Artificial Opening 8 Via Natural or Artificial Opening Endoscopic X External	2 Monitoring Device 3 Infusion Device L Artificial Sphincter	Z No Qualifier

Section	0	Medical and Surgical
Body System	T	Urinary System
Operation	J	Inspection: Visually and/or manually exploring a body part

Body Part (4ᵗʰ)	Approach (5ᵗʰ)	Device (6ᵗʰ)	Qualifier (7ᵗʰ)
5 Kidney 9 Ureter B Bladder D Urethra	0 Open 3 Percutaneous 4 Percutaneous Endoscopic 7 Via Natural or Artificial Opening 8 Via Natural or Artificial Opening Endoscopic X External	Z No Device	Z No Qualifier

Section	0	Medical and Surgical
Body System	T	Urinary System
Operation	L	Occlusion: Completely closing an orifice or the lumen of a tubular body part

Body Part (4ᵗʰ)	Approach (5ᵗʰ)	Device (6ᵗʰ)	Qualifier (7ᵗʰ)
3 Kidney Pelvis, Right 4 Kidney Pelvis, Left 6 Ureter, Right 7 Ureter, Left B Bladder C Bladder Neck	0 Open 3 Percutaneous 4 Percutaneous Endoscopic	C Extraluminal Device D Intraluminal Device Z No Device	Z No Qualifier
3 Kidney Pelvis, Right 4 Kidney Pelvis, Left 6 Ureter, Right 7 Ureter, Left B Bladder C Bladder Neck	7 Via Natural or Artificial Opening 8 Via Natural or Artificial Opening Endoscopic	D Intraluminal Device Z No Device	Z No Qualifier
D Urethra	0 Open 3 Percutaneous 4 Percutaneous Endoscopic X External	C Extraluminal Device D Intraluminal Device Z No Device	Z No Qualifier
D Urethra	7 Via Natural or Artificial Opening 8 Via Natural or Artificial Opening Endoscopic	D Intraluminal Device Z No Device	Z No Qualifier

Section	0	Medical and Surgical
Body System	T	Urinary System
Operation	M	Reattachment: Putting back in or on all or a portion of a separated body part to its normal location or other suitable location

Body Part (4ᵗʰ)	Approach (5ᵗʰ)	Device (6ᵗʰ)	Qualifier (7ᵗʰ)
0 Kidney, Right 1 Kidney, Left 2 Kidneys, Bilateral 3 Kidney Pelvis, Right 4 Kidney Pelvis, Left 6 Ureter, Right 7 Ureter, Left 8 Ureters, Bilateral B Bladder C Bladder Neck D Urethra	0 Open 4 Percutaneous Endoscopic	Z No Device	Z No Qualifier

Section 0 Medical and Surgical
Body System T Urinary System
Operation N Release: Freeing a body part from an abnormal physical constraint by cutting or by the use of force

Body Part (4th)	Approach (5th)	Device (6th)	Qualifier (7th)
0 Kidney, Right 1 Kidney, Left 3 Kidney Pelvis, Right 4 Kidney Pelvis, Left 6 Ureter, Right 7 Ureter, Left B Bladder C Bladder Neck	0 Open 3 Percutaneous 4 Percutaneous Endoscopic 7 Via Natural or Artificial Opening 8 Via Natural or Artificial Opening Endoscopic	Z No Device	Z No Qualifier
D Urethra	0 Open 3 Percutaneous 4 Percutaneous Endoscopic 7 Via Natural or Artificial Opening 8 Via Natural or Artificial Opening Endoscopic X External	Z No Device	Z No Qualifier

Section 0 Medical and Surgical
Body System T Urinary System
Operation P Removal: Taking out or off a device from a body part

Body Part (4th)	Approach (5th)	Device (6th)	Qualifier (7th)
5 Kidney	0 Open 3 Percutaneous 4 Percutaneous Endoscopic 7 Via Natural or Artificial Opening 8 Via Natural or Artificial Opening Endoscopic	0 Drainage Device 2 Monitoring Device 3 Infusion Device 7 Autologous Tissue Substitute C Extraluminal Device D Intraluminal Device J Synthetic Substitute K Nonautologous Tissue Substitute	Z No Qualifier
5 Kidney	X External	0 Drainage Device 2 Monitoring Device 3 Infusion Device D Intraluminal Device	Z No Qualifier
9 Ureter	0 Open 3 Percutaneous 4 Percutaneous Endoscopic 7 Via Natural or Artificial Opening 8 Via Natural or Artificial Opening Endoscopic	0 Drainage Device 2 Monitoring Device 3 Infusion Device 7 Autologous Tissue Substitute C Extraluminal Device D Intraluminal Device J Synthetic Substitute K Nonautologous Tissue Substitute M Stimulator Lead	Z No Qualifier
9 Ureter	X External	0 Drainage Device 2 Monitoring Device 3 Infusion Device D Intraluminal Device M Stimulator Lead	Z No Qualifier
B Bladder	0 Open 3 Percutaneous 4 Percutaneous Endoscopic 7 Via Natural or Artificial Opening 8 Via Natural or Artificial Opening Endoscopic	0 Drainage Device 2 Monitoring Device 3 Infusion Device 7 Autologous Tissue Substitute C Extraluminal Device D Intraluminal Device J Synthetic Substitute K Nonautologous Tissue Substitute L Artificial Sphincter M Stimulator Lead	Z No Qualifier

Continued →

Section	0	Medical and Surgical
Body System	T	Urinary System
Operation	P	**Removal:** Taking out or off a device from a body part

Body Part (4th)	Approach (5th)	Device (6th)	Qualifier (7th)
B Bladder	**X** External	**0** Drainage Device **2** Monitoring Device **3** Infusion Device **D** Intraluminal Device **L** Artificial Sphincter **M** Stimulator Lead	**Z** No Qualifier
D Urethra	**0** Open **3** Percutaneous **4** Percutaneous Endoscopic **7** Via Natural or Artificial Opening **8** Via Natural or Artificial Opening Endoscopic	**0** Drainage Device **2** Monitoring Device **3** Infusion Device **7** Autologous Tissue Substitute **C** Extraluminal Device **D** Intraluminal Device **J** Synthetic Substitute **K** Nonautologous Tissue Substitute **L** Artificial Sphincter	**Z** No Qualifier
D Urethra	**X** External	**0** Drainage Device **2** Monitoring Device **3** Infusion Device **D** Intraluminal Device **L** Artificial Sphincter	**Z** No Qualifier

Section	0	Medical and Surgical
Body System	T	Urinary System
Operation	Q	**Repair:** Restoring, to the extent possible, a body part to its normal anatomic structure and function

Body Part (4th)	Approach (5th)	Device (6th)	Qualifier (7th)
0 Kidney, Right **1** Kidney, Left **3** Kidney Pelvis, Right **4** Kidney Pelvis, Left **6** Ureter, Right **7** Ureter, Left **B** Bladder **C** Bladder Neck	**0** Open **3** Percutaneous **4** Percutaneous Endoscopic **7** Via Natural or Artificial Opening **8** Via Natural or Artificial Opening Endoscopic	**Z** No Device	**Z** No Qualifier
D Urethra	**0** Open **3** Percutaneous **4** Percutaneous Endoscopic **7** Via Natural or Artificial Opening **8** Via Natural or Artificial Opening Endoscopic **X** External	**Z** No Device	**Z** No Qualifier

Section	0	Medical and Surgical
Body System	T	Urinary System
Operation	R	**Replacement:** Putting in or on biological or synthetic material that physically takes the place and/or function of all or a portion of a body part

Body Part (4th)	Approach (5th)	Device (6th)	Qualifier (7th)
3 Kidney Pelvis, Right **4** Kidney Pelvis, Left **6** Ureter, Right **7** Ureter, Left **B** Bladder **C** Bladder Neck	**0** Open **4** Percutaneous Endoscopic **7** Via Natural or Artificial Opening **8** Via Natural or Artificial Opening Endoscopic	**7** Autologous Tissue Substitute **J** Synthetic Substitute **K** Nonautologous Tissue Substitute	**Z** No Qualifier
D Urethra	**0** Open **4** Percutaneous Endoscopic **7** Via Natural or Artificial Opening **8** Via Natural or Artificial Opening Endoscopic **X** External	**7** Autologous Tissue Substitute **J** Synthetic Substitute **K** Nonautologous Tissue Substitute	**Z** No Qualifier

Section	0	Medical and Surgical
Body System	T	Urinary System
Operation	S	Reposition: Moving to its normal location, or other suitable location, all or a portion of a body part

Body Part (4th)	Approach (5th)	Device (6th)	Qualifier (7th)
0 Kidney, Right 1 Kidney, Left 2 Kidneys, Bilateral 3 Kidney Pelvis, Right 4 Kidney Pelvis, Left 6 Ureter, Right 7 Ureter, Left 8 Ureters, Bilateral B Bladder C Bladder Neck D Urethra	0 Open 4 Percutaneous Endoscopic	Z No Device	Z No Qualifier

Section	0	Medical and Surgical
Body System	T	Urinary System
Operation	T	Resection: Cutting out or off, without replacement, all of a body part

Body Part (4th)	Approach (5th)	Device (6th)	Qualifier (7th)
0 Kidney, Right 1 Kidney, Left 2 Kidneys, Bilateral	0 Open 4 Percutaneous Endoscopic	Z No Device	Z No Qualifier
3 Kidney Pelvis, Right 4 Kidney Pelvis, Left 6 Ureter, Right 7 Ureter, Left B Bladder C Bladder Neck D Urethra	0 Open 4 Percutaneous Endoscopic 7 Via Natural or Artificial Opening 8 Via Natural or Artificial Opening Endoscopic	Z No Device	Z No Qualifier

Section	0	Medical and Surgical
Body System	T	Urinary System
Operation	U	Supplement: Putting in or on biological or synthetic material that physically reinforces and/or augments the function of a portion of a body part

Body Part (4th)	Approach (5th)	Device (6th)	Qualifier (7th)
3 Kidney Pelvis, Right 4 Kidney Pelvis, Left 6 Ureter, Right 7 Ureter, Left B Bladder C Bladder Neck	0 Open 4 Percutaneous Endoscopic 7 Via Natural or Artificial Opening 8 Via Natural or Artificial Opening Endoscopic	7 Autologous Tissue Substitute J Synthetic Substitute K Nonautologous Tissue Substitute	Z No Qualifier
D Urethra	0 Open 4 Percutaneous Endoscopic 7 Via Natural or Artificial Opening 8 Via Natural or Artificial Opening Endoscopic X External	7 Autologous Tissue Substitute J Synthetic Substitute K Nonautologous Tissue Substitute	Z No Qualifier

Section	0	Medical and Surgical
Body System	T	Urinary System
Operation	V	Restriction: Partially closing an orifice or the lumen of a tubular body part

Body Part (4th)	Approach (5th)	Device (6th)	Qualifier (7th)
3 Kidney Pelvis, Right 4 Kidney Pelvis, Left 6 Ureter, Right 7 Ureter, Left B Bladder C Bladder Neck	0 Open 3 Percutaneous 4 Percutaneous Endoscopic	C Extraluminal Device D Intraluminal Device Z No Device	Z No Qualifier

Continued →

Section	0	Medical and Surgical
Body System	T	Urinary System
Operation	V	Restriction: Partially closing an orifice or the lumen of a tubular body part

Body Part (4th)	Approach (5th)	Device (6th)	Qualifier (7th)
3 Kidney Pelvis, Right 4 Kidney Pelvis, Left 6 Ureter, Right 7 Ureter, Left B Bladder C Bladder Neck	7 Via Natural or Artificial Opening 8 Via Natural or Artificial Opening Endoscopic	D Intraluminal Device Z No Device	Z No Qualifier
D Urethra	0 Open 3 Percutaneous 4 Percutaneous Endoscopic	C Extraluminal Device D Intraluminal Device Z No Device	Z No Qualifier
D Urethra	7 Via Natural or Artificial Opening 8 Via Natural or Artificial Opening Endoscopic	D Intraluminal Device Z No Device	Z No Qualifier
D Urethra	X External	Z No Device	Z No Qualifier

Section	0	Medical and Surgical
Body System	T	Urinary System
Operation	W	Revision: Correcting, to the extent possible, a portion of a malfunctioning device or the position of a displaced device

Body Part (4th)	Approach (5th)	Device (6th)	Qualifier (7th)
5 Kidney	0 Open 3 Percutaneous 4 Percutaneous Endoscopic 7 Via Natural or Artificial Opening 8 Via Natural or Artificial Opening Endoscopic X External	0 Drainage Device 2 Monitoring Device 3 Infusion Device 7 Autologous Tissue Substitute C Extraluminal Device D Intraluminal Device J Synthetic Substitute K Nonautologous Tissue Substitute	Z No Qualifier
9 Ureter	0 Open 3 Percutaneous 4 Percutaneous Endoscopic 7 Via Natural or Artificial Opening 8 Via Natural or Artificial Opening Endoscopic X External	0 Drainage Device 2 Monitoring Device 3 Infusion Device 7 Autologous Tissue Substitute C Extraluminal Device D Intraluminal Device J Synthetic Substitute K Nonautologous Tissue Substitute M Stimulator Lead	Z No Qualifier
B Bladder	0 Open 3 Percutaneous 4 Percutaneous Endoscopic 7 Via Natural or Artificial Opening 8 Via Natural or Artificial Opening Endoscopic X External	0 Drainage Device 2 Monitoring Device 3 Infusion Device 7 Autologous Tissue Substitute C Extraluminal Device D Intraluminal Device J Synthetic Substitute K Nonautologous Tissue Substitute L Artificial Sphincter M Stimulator Lead	Z No Qualifier
D Urethra	0 Open 3 Percutaneous 4 Percutaneous Endoscopic 7 Via Natural or Artificial Opening 8 Via Natural or Artificial Opening Endoscopic X External	0 Drainage Device 2 Monitoring Device 3 Infusion Device 7 Autologous Tissue Substitute C Extraluminal Device D Intraluminal Device J Synthetic Substitute K Nonautologous Tissue Substitute L Artificial Sphincter	Z No Qualifier

Section	0	Medical and Surgical
Body System	T	Urinary System
Operation	Y	**Transplantation:** Putting in or on all or a portion of a living body part taken from another individual or animal to physically take the place and/or function of all or a portion of a similar body part

Body Part (4th)	Approach (5th)	Device (6th)	Qualifier (7th)
0 Kidney, Right 1 Kidney, Left	0 Open	Z No Device	0 Allogeneic 1 Syngeneic 2 Zooplastic

Urinary System Code Listing 0T1–0TY

0T1 – Urinary System, Bypass

Review Coding Guideline B3.6a

0T13073 Bypass Right Kidney Pelvis to Right Kidney Pelvis with Autologous Tissue Substitute, Open Approach

0T13074 Bypass Right Kidney Pelvis to Left Kidney Pelvis with Autologous Tissue Substitute, Open Approach

0T13076 Bypass Right Kidney Pelvis to Right Ureter with Autologous Tissue Substitute, Open Approach

0T13077 Bypass Right Kidney Pelvis to Left Ureter with Autologous Tissue Substitute, Open Approach

0T13078 Bypass Right Kidney Pelvis to Colon with Autologous Tissue Substitute, Open Approach

0T13079 Bypass Right Kidney Pelvis to Colocutaneous with Autologous Tissue Substitute, Open Approach

0T1307A Bypass Right Kidney Pelvis to Ileum with Autologous Tissue Substitute, Open Approach

0T1307B Bypass Right Kidney Pelvis to Bladder with Autologous Tissue Substitute, Open Approach

0T1307C Bypass Right Kidney Pelvis to Ileocutaneous with Autologous Tissue Substitute, Open Approach

0T1307D Bypass Right Kidney Pelvis to Cutaneous with Autologous Tissue Substitute, Open Approach

0T130J3 Bypass Right Kidney Pelvis to Right Kidney Pelvis with Synthetic Substitute, Open Approach

0T130J4 Bypass Right Kidney Pelvis to Left Kidney Pelvis with Synthetic Substitute, Open Approach

0T130J6 Bypass Right Kidney Pelvis to Right Ureter with Synthetic Substitute, Open Approach

0T130J7 Bypass Right Kidney Pelvis to Left Ureter with Synthetic Substitute, Open Approach

0T130J8 Bypass Right Kidney Pelvis to Colon with Synthetic Substitute, Open Approach

0T130J9 Bypass Right Kidney Pelvis to Colocutaneous with Synthetic Substitute, Open Approach

0T130JA Bypass Right Kidney Pelvis to Ileum with Synthetic Substitute, Open Approach

0T130JB Bypass Right Kidney Pelvis to Bladder with Synthetic Substitute, Open Approach

0T130JC Bypass Right Kidney Pelvis to Ileocutaneous with Synthetic Substitute, Open Approach

0T130JD Bypass Right Kidney Pelvis to Cutaneous with Synthetic Substitute, Open Approach

0T130K3 Bypass Right Kidney Pelvis to Right Kidney Pelvis with Nonautologous Tissue Substitute, Open Approach

0T130K4 Bypass Right Kidney Pelvis to Left Kidney Pelvis with Nonautologous Tissue Substitute, Open Approach

0T130K6 Bypass Right Kidney Pelvis to Right Ureter with Nonautologous Tissue Substitute, Open Approach

0T130K7 Bypass Right Kidney Pelvis to Left Ureter with Nonautologous Tissue Substitute, Open Approach

0T130K8 Bypass Right Kidney Pelvis to Colon with Nonautologous Tissue Substitute, Open Approach

0T130K9 Bypass Right Kidney Pelvis to Colocutaneous with Nonautologous Tissue Substitute, Open Approach

0T130KA Bypass Right Kidney Pelvis to Ileum with Nonautologous Tissue Substitute, Open Approach

0T130KB Bypass Right Kidney Pelvis to Bladder with Nonautologous Tissue Substitute, Open Approach

0T130KC Bypass Right Kidney Pelvis to Ileocutaneous with Nonautologous Tissue Substitute, Open Approach

0T130KD Bypass Right Kidney Pelvis to Cutaneous with Nonautologous Tissue Substitute, Open Approach

0T130Z3 Bypass Right Kidney Pelvis to Right Kidney Pelvis, Open Approach

0T130Z4 Bypass Right Kidney Pelvis to Left Kidney Pelvis, Open Approach

0T130Z6 Bypass Right Kidney Pelvis to Right Ureter, Open Approach

0T130Z7 Bypass Right Kidney Pelvis to Left Ureter, Open Approach

0T130Z8 Bypass Right Kidney Pelvis to Colon, Open Approach

0T130Z9 Bypass Right Kidney Pelvis to Colocutaneous, Open Approach

0T130ZA Bypass Right Kidney Pelvis to Ileum, Open Approach

0T130ZB Bypass Right Kidney Pelvis to Bladder, Open Approach

0T130ZC Bypass Right Kidney Pelvis to Ileocutaneous, Open Approach

0T130ZD Bypass Right Kidney Pelvis to Cutaneous, Open Approach

0T133JD Bypass Right Kidney Pelvis to Cutaneous with Synthetic Substitute, Percutaneous Approach

0T13473 Bypass Right Kidney Pelvis to Right Kidney Pelvis with Autologous Tissue Substitute, Percutaneous Endoscopic Approach

0T13474 Bypass Right Kidney Pelvis to Left Kidney Pelvis with Autologous Tissue Substitute, Percutaneous Endoscopic Approach

0T13476 Bypass Right Kidney Pelvis to Right Ureter with Autologous Tissue Substitute, Percutaneous Endoscopic Approach

0T13477 Bypass Right Kidney Pelvis to Left Ureter with Autologous Tissue Substitute, Percutaneous Endoscopic Approach

0T13478 Bypass Right Kidney Pelvis to Colon with Autologous Tissue Substitute, Percutaneous Endoscopic Approach

0T13479 Bypass Right Kidney Pelvis to Colocutaneous with Autologous Tissue Substitute, Percutaneous Endoscopic Approach

0T1347A Bypass Right Kidney Pelvis to Ileum with Autologous Tissue Substitute, Percutaneous Endoscopic Approach

0T1347B Bypass Right Kidney Pelvis to Bladder with Autologous Tissue Substitute, Percutaneous Endoscopic Approach

0T1347C Bypass Right Kidney Pelvis to Ileocutaneous with Autologous Tissue Substitute, Percutaneous Endoscopic Approach

0T1347D Bypass Right Kidney Pelvis to Cutaneous with Autologous Tissue Substitute, Percutaneous Endoscopic Approach

0T134J3 Bypass Right Kidney Pelvis to Right Kidney Pelvis with Synthetic Substitute, Percutaneous Endoscopic Approach

0T134J4 Bypass Right Kidney Pelvis to Left Kidney Pelvis with Synthetic Substitute, Percutaneous Endoscopic Approach

0T134J6 Bypass Right Kidney Pelvis to Right Ureter with Synthetic Substitute, Percutaneous Endoscopic Approach

0T134J7 Bypass Right Kidney Pelvis to Left Ureter with Synthetic Substitute, Percutaneous Endoscopic Approach

0T134J8 Bypass Right Kidney Pelvis to Colon with Synthetic Substitute, Percutaneous Endoscopic Approach

0T134J9 Bypass Right Kidney Pelvis to Colocutaneous with Synthetic Substitute, Percutaneous Endoscopic Approach

0T134JA Bypass Right Kidney Pelvis to Ileum with Synthetic Substitute, Percutaneous Endoscopic Approach

0T134JB Bypass Right Kidney Pelvis to Bladder with Synthetic Substitute, Percutaneous Endoscopic Approach

0T134JC Bypass Right Kidney Pelvis to Ileocutaneous with Synthetic Substitute, Percutaneous Endoscopic Approach

0T134JD Bypass Right Kidney Pelvis to Cutaneous with Synthetic Substitute, Percutaneous Endoscopic Approach

0T134K3 Bypass Right Kidney Pelvis to Right Kidney Pelvis with Nonautologous Tissue Substitute, Percutaneous Endoscopic Approach

♀ Female-only	♂ Male-only	▲ Limited Coverage	● Non-OR	▬ HAC-associated procedure	▲ Non-covered procedures	➕ Combination

0T134K4 Bypass Right Kidney Pelvis to Left Kidney Pelvis with Nonautologous Tissue Substitute, Percutaneous Endoscopic Approach

0T134K6 Bypass Right Kidney Pelvis to Right Ureter with Nonautologous Tissue Substitute, Percutaneous Endoscopic Approach

0T134K7 Bypass Right Kidney Pelvis to Left Ureter with Nonautologous Tissue Substitute, Percutaneous Endoscopic Approach

0T134K8 Bypass Right Kidney Pelvis to Colon with Nonautologous Tissue Substitute, Percutaneous Endoscopic Approach

0T134K9 Bypass Right Kidney Pelvis to Colocutaneous with Nonautologous Tissue Substitute, Percutaneous Endoscopic Approach

0T134KA Bypass Right Kidney Pelvis to Ileum with Nonautologous Tissue Substitute, Percutaneous Endoscopic Approach

0T134KB Bypass Right Kidney Pelvis to Bladder with Nonautologous Tissue Substitute, Percutaneous Endoscopic Approach

0T134KC Bypass Right Kidney Pelvis to Ileocutaneous with Nonautologous Tissue Substitute, Percutaneous Endoscopic Approach

0T134KD Bypass Right Kidney Pelvis to Cutaneous with Nonautologous Tissue Substitute, Percutaneous Endoscopic Approach

0T134Z3 Bypass Right Kidney Pelvis to Right Kidney Pelvis, Percutaneous Endoscopic Approach

0T134Z4 Bypass Right Kidney Pelvis to Left Kidney Pelvis, Percutaneous Endoscopic Approach

0T134Z6 Bypass Right Kidney Pelvis to Right Ureter, Percutaneous Endoscopic Approach

0T134Z7 Bypass Right Kidney Pelvis to Left Ureter, Percutaneous Endoscopic Approach

0T134Z8 Bypass Right Kidney Pelvis to Colon, Percutaneous Endoscopic Approach

0T134Z9 Bypass Right Kidney Pelvis to Colocutaneous, Percutaneous Endoscopic Approach

0T134ZA Bypass Right Kidney Pelvis to Ileum, Percutaneous Endoscopic Approach

0T134ZB Bypass Right Kidney Pelvis to Bladder, Percutaneous Endoscopic Approach

0T134ZC Bypass Right Kidney Pelvis to Ileocutaneous, Percutaneous Endoscopic Approach

0T134ZD Bypass Right Kidney Pelvis to Cutaneous, Percutaneous Endoscopic Approach

0T14073 Bypass Left Kidney Pelvis to Right Kidney Pelvis with Autologous Tissue Substitute, Open Approach

0T14074 Bypass Left Kidney Pelvis to Left Kidney Pelvis with Autologous Tissue Substitute, Open Approach

0T14076 Bypass Left Kidney Pelvis to Right Ureter with Autologous Tissue Substitute, Open Approach

0T14077 Bypass Left Kidney Pelvis to Left Ureter with Autologous Tissue Substitute, Open Approach

0T14078 Bypass Left Kidney Pelvis to Colon with Autologous Tissue Substitute, Open Approach

0T14079 Bypass Left Kidney Pelvis to Colocutaneous with Autologous Tissue Substitute, Open Approach

0T1407A Bypass Left Kidney Pelvis to Ileum with Autologous Tissue Substitute, Open Approach

0T1407B Bypass Left Kidney Pelvis to Bladder with Autologous Tissue Substitute, Open Approach

0T1407C Bypass Left Kidney Pelvis to Ileocutaneous with Autologous Tissue Substitute, Open Approach

0T1407D Bypass Left Kidney Pelvis to Cutaneous with Autologous Tissue Substitute, Open Approach

0T140J3 Bypass Left Kidney Pelvis to Right Kidney Pelvis with Synthetic Substitute, Open Approach

0T140J4 Bypass Left Kidney Pelvis to Left Kidney Pelvis with Synthetic Substitute, Open Approach

0T140J6 Bypass Left Kidney Pelvis to Right Ureter with Synthetic Substitute, Open Approach

0T140J7 Bypass Left Kidney Pelvis to Left Ureter with Synthetic Substitute, Open Approach

0T140J8 Bypass Left Kidney Pelvis to Colon with Synthetic Substitute, Open Approach

0T140J9 Bypass Left Kidney Pelvis to Colocutaneous with Synthetic Substitute, Open Approach

0T140JA Bypass Left Kidney Pelvis to Ileum with Synthetic Substitute, Open Approach

0T140JB Bypass Left Kidney Pelvis to Bladder with Synthetic Substitute, Open Approach

0T140JC Bypass Left Kidney Pelvis to Ileocutaneous with Synthetic Substitute, Open Approach

0T140JD Bypass Left Kidney Pelvis to Cutaneous with Synthetic Substitute, Open Approach

0T140K3 Bypass Left Kidney Pelvis to Right Kidney Pelvis with Nonautologous Tissue Substitute, Open Approach

0T140K4 Bypass Left Kidney Pelvis to Left Kidney Pelvis with Nonautologous Tissue Substitute, Open Approach

0T140K6 Bypass Left Kidney Pelvis to Right Ureter with Nonautologous Tissue Substitute, Open Approach

0T140K7 Bypass Left Kidney Pelvis to Left Ureter with Nonautologous Tissue Substitute, Open Approach

0T140K8 Bypass Left Kidney Pelvis to Colon with Nonautologous Tissue Substitute, Open Approach

0T140K9 Bypass Left Kidney Pelvis to Colocutaneous with Nonautologous Tissue Substitute, Open Approach

0T140KA Bypass Left Kidney Pelvis to Ileum with Nonautologous Tissue Substitute, Open Approach

0T140KB Bypass Left Kidney Pelvis to Bladder with Nonautologous Tissue Substitute, Open Approach

0T140KC Bypass Left Kidney Pelvis to Ileocutaneous with Nonautologous Tissue Substitute, Open Approach

0T140KD Bypass Left Kidney Pelvis to Cutaneous with Nonautologous Tissue Substitute, Open Approach

0T140Z3 Bypass Left Kidney Pelvis to Right Kidney Pelvis, Open Approach

0T140Z4 Bypass Left Kidney Pelvis to Left Kidney Pelvis, Open Approach

0T140Z6 Bypass Left Kidney Pelvis to Right Ureter, Open Approach

0T140Z7 Bypass Left Kidney Pelvis to Left Ureter, Open Approach

0T140Z8 Bypass Left Kidney Pelvis to Colon, Open Approach

0T140Z9 Bypass Left Kidney Pelvis to Colocutaneous, Open Approach

0T140ZA Bypass Left Kidney Pelvis to Ileum, Open Approach

0T140ZB Bypass Left Kidney Pelvis to Bladder, Open Approach

0T140ZC Bypass Left Kidney Pelvis to Ileocutaneous, Open Approach

0T140ZD Bypass Left Kidney Pelvis to Cutaneous, Open Approach

0T143JD Bypass Left Kidney Pelvis to Cutaneous with Synthetic Substitute, Percutaneous Approach

0T14473 Bypass Left Kidney Pelvis to Right Kidney Pelvis with Autologous Tissue Substitute, Percutaneous Endoscopic Approach

0T14474 Bypass Left Kidney Pelvis to Left Kidney Pelvis with Autologous Tissue Substitute, Percutaneous Endoscopic Approach

0T14476 Bypass Left Kidney Pelvis to Right Ureter with Autologous Tissue Substitute, Percutaneous Endoscopic Approach

0T14477 Bypass Left Kidney Pelvis to Left Ureter with Autologous Tissue Substitute, Percutaneous Endoscopic Approach

0T14478 Bypass Left Kidney Pelvis to Colon with Autologous Tissue Substitute, Percutaneous Endoscopic Approach

0T14479 Bypass Left Kidney Pelvis to Colocutaneous with Autologous Tissue Substitute, Percutaneous Endoscopic Approach

0T1447A Bypass Left Kidney Pelvis to Ileum with Autologous Tissue Substitute, Percutaneous Endoscopic Approach

0T1447B Bypass Left Kidney Pelvis to Bladder with Autologous Tissue Substitute, Percutaneous Endoscopic Approach

0T1447C Bypass Left Kidney Pelvis to Ileocutaneous with Autologous Tissue Substitute, Percutaneous Endoscopic Approach

0T1447D Bypass Left Kidney Pelvis to Cutaneous with Autologous Tissue Substitute, Percutaneous Endoscopic Approach

0T144J3 Bypass Left Kidney Pelvis to Right Kidney Pelvis with Synthetic Substitute, Percutaneous Endoscopic Approach

0T144J4 Bypass Left Kidney Pelvis to Left Kidney Pelvis with Synthetic Substitute, Percutaneous Endoscopic Approach

0T144J6 Bypass Left Kidney Pelvis to Right Ureter with Synthetic Substitute, Percutaneous Endoscopic Approach

0T144J7 Bypass Left Kidney Pelvis to Left Ureter with Synthetic Substitute, Percutaneous Endoscopic Approach

0T144J8 Bypass Left Kidney Pelvis to Colon with Synthetic Substitute, Percutaneous Endoscopic Approach

0T144J9 Bypass Left Kidney Pelvis to Colocutaneous with Synthetic Substitute, Percutaneous Endoscopic Approach

0T144JA Bypass Left Kidney Pelvis to Ileum with Synthetic Substitute, Percutaneous Endoscopic Approach

0T144JB Bypass Left Kidney Pelvis to Bladder with Synthetic Substitute, Percutaneous Endoscopic Approach

0T144JC Bypass Left Kidney Pelvis to Ileocutaneous with Synthetic Substitute, Percutaneous Endoscopic Approach

0T144JD Bypass Left Kidney Pelvis to Cutaneous with Synthetic Substitute, Percutaneous Endoscopic Approach

0T144K3 Bypass Left Kidney Pelvis to Right Kidney Pelvis with Nonautologous Tissue Substitute, Percutaneous Endoscopic Approach

144K4	Bypass Left Kidney Pelvis to Left Kidney Pelvis with Nonautologous Tissue Substitute, Percutaneous Endoscopic Approach	0T160J6	Bypass Right Ureter to Right Ureter with Synthetic Substitute, Open Approach
144K6	Bypass Left Kidney Pelvis to Right Ureter with Nonautologous Tissue Substitute, Percutaneous Endoscopic Approach	0T160J7	Bypass Right Ureter to Left Ureter with Synthetic Substitute, Open Approach

0T1647C Bypass Right Ureter to Ileocutaneous with Autologous Tissue Substitute, Percutaneous Endoscopic Approach

0T1647D Bypass Right Ureter to Cutaneous with Autologous Tissue Substitute, Percutaneous Endoscopic Approach

144K4 Bypass Left Kidney Pelvis to Left Kidney Pelvis with Nonautologous Tissue Substitute, Percutaneous Endoscopic Approach

144K6 Bypass Left Kidney Pelvis to Right Ureter with Nonautologous Tissue Substitute, Percutaneous Endoscopic Approach

144K7 Bypass Left Kidney Pelvis to Left Ureter with Nonautologous Tissue Substitute, Percutaneous Endoscopic Approach

144K8 Bypass Left Kidney Pelvis to Colon with Nonautologous Tissue Substitute, Percutaneous Endoscopic Approach

144K9 Bypass Left Kidney Pelvis to Colocutaneous with Nonautologous Tissue Substitute, Percutaneous Endoscopic Approach

144KA Bypass Left Kidney Pelvis to Ileum with Nonautologous Tissue Substitute, Percutaneous Endoscopic Approach

144KB Bypass Left Kidney Pelvis to Bladder with Nonautologous Tissue Substitute, Percutaneous Endoscopic Approach

144KC Bypass Left Kidney Pelvis to Ileocutaneous with Nonautologous Tissue Substitute, Percutaneous Endoscopic Approach

144KD Bypass Left Kidney Pelvis to Cutaneous with Nonautologous Tissue Substitute, Percutaneous Endoscopic Approach

144Z3 Bypass Left Kidney Pelvis to Right Kidney Pelvis, Percutaneous Endoscopic Approach

144Z4 Bypass Left Kidney Pelvis to Left Kidney Pelvis, Percutaneous Endoscopic Approach

144Z6 Bypass Left Kidney Pelvis to Right Ureter, Percutaneous Endoscopic Approach

144Z7 Bypass Left Kidney Pelvis to Left Ureter, Percutaneous Endoscopic Approach

144Z8 Bypass Left Kidney Pelvis to Colon, Percutaneous Endoscopic Approach

144Z9 Bypass Left Kidney Pelvis to Colocutaneous, Percutaneous Endoscopic Approach

144ZA Bypass Left Kidney Pelvis to Ileum, Percutaneous Endoscopic Approach

144ZB Bypass Left Kidney Pelvis to Bladder, Percutaneous Endoscopic Approach

144ZC Bypass Left Kidney Pelvis to Ileocutaneous, Percutaneous Endoscopic Approach

144ZD Bypass Left Kidney Pelvis to Cutaneous, Percutaneous Endoscopic Approach

T16076 Bypass Right Ureter to Right Ureter with Autologous Tissue Substitute, Open Approach

T16077 Bypass Right Ureter to Left Ureter with Autologous Tissue Substitute, Open Approach

T16078 Bypass Right Ureter to Colon with Autologous Tissue Substitute, Open Approach

T16079 Bypass Right Ureter to Colocutaneous with Autologous Tissue Substitute, Open Approach

T1607A Bypass Right Ureter to Ileum with Autologous Tissue Substitute, Open Approach

T1607B Bypass Right Ureter to Bladder with Autologous Tissue Substitute, Open Approach

T1607C Bypass Right Ureter to Ileocutaneous with Autologous Tissue Substitute, Open Approach

T1607D Bypass Right Ureter to Cutaneous with Autologous Tissue Substitute, Open Approach

0T160J6 Bypass Right Ureter to Right Ureter with Synthetic Substitute, Open Approach

0T160J7 Bypass Right Ureter to Left Ureter with Synthetic Substitute, Open Approach

0T160J8 Bypass Right Ureter to Colon with Synthetic Substitute, Open Approach

0T160J9 Bypass Right Ureter to Colocutaneous with Synthetic Substitute, Open Approach

0T160JA Bypass Right Ureter to Ileum with Synthetic Substitute, Open Approach

0T160JB Bypass Right Ureter to Bladder with Synthetic Substitute, Open Approach

0T160JC Bypass Right Ureter to Ileocutaneous with Synthetic Substitute, Open Approach

0T160JD Bypass Right Ureter to Cutaneous with Synthetic Substitute, Open Approach

0T160K6 Bypass Right Ureter to Right Ureter with Nonautologous Tissue Substitute, Open Approach

0T160K7 Bypass Right Ureter to Left Ureter with Nonautologous Tissue Substitute, Open Approach

0T160K8 Bypass Right Ureter to Colon with Nonautologous Tissue Substitute, Open Approach

0T160K9 Bypass Right Ureter to Colocutaneous with Nonautologous Tissue Substitute, Open Approach

0T160KA Bypass Right Ureter to Ileum with Nonautologous Tissue Substitute, Open Approach

0T160KB Bypass Right Ureter to Bladder with Nonautologous Tissue Substitute, Open Approach

0T160KC Bypass Right Ureter to Ileocutaneous with Nonautologous Tissue Substitute, Open Approach

0T160KD Bypass Right Ureter to Cutaneous with Nonautologous Tissue Substitute, Open Approach

0T160Z6 Bypass Right Ureter to Right Ureter, Open Approach

0T160Z7 Bypass Right Ureter to Left Ureter, Open Approach

0T160Z8 Bypass Right Ureter to Colon, Open Approach

0T160Z9 Bypass Right Ureter to Colocutaneous, Open Approach

0T160ZA Bypass Right Ureter to Ileum, Open Approach

0T160ZB Bypass Right Ureter to Bladder, Open Approach

0T160ZC Bypass Right Ureter to Ileocutaneous, Open Approach

0T160ZD Bypass Right Ureter to Cutaneous, Open Approach

0T163JD Bypass Right Ureter to Cutaneous with Synthetic Substitute, Percutaneous Approach

0T16476 Bypass Right Ureter to Right Ureter with Autologous Tissue Substitute, Percutaneous Endoscopic Approach

0T16477 Bypass Right Ureter to Left Ureter with Autologous Tissue Substitute, Percutaneous Endoscopic Approach

0T16478 Bypass Right Ureter to Colon with Autologous Tissue Substitute, Percutaneous Endoscopic Approach

0T16479 Bypass Right Ureter to Colocutaneous with Autologous Tissue Substitute, Percutaneous Endoscopic Approach

0T1647A Bypass Right Ureter to Ileum with Autologous Tissue Substitute, Percutaneous Endoscopic Approach

0T1647B Bypass Right Ureter to Bladder with Autologous Tissue Substitute, Percutaneous Endoscopic Approach

0T1647C Bypass Right Ureter to Ileocutaneous with Autologous Tissue Substitute, Percutaneous Endoscopic Approach

0T1647D Bypass Right Ureter to Cutaneous with Autologous Tissue Substitute, Percutaneous Endoscopic Approach

0T164J6 Bypass Right Ureter to Right Ureter with Synthetic Substitute, Percutaneous Endoscopic Approach

0T164J7 Bypass Right Ureter to Left Ureter with Synthetic Substitute, Percutaneous Endoscopic Approach

0T164J8 Bypass Right Ureter to Colon with Synthetic Substitute, Percutaneous Endoscopic Approach

0T164J9 Bypass Right Ureter to Colocutaneous with Synthetic Substitute, Percutaneous Endoscopic Approach

0T164JA Bypass Right Ureter to Ileum with Synthetic Substitute, Percutaneous Endoscopic Approach

0T164JB Bypass Right Ureter to Bladder with Synthetic Substitute, Percutaneous Endoscopic Approach

0T164JC Bypass Right Ureter to Ileocutaneous with Synthetic Substitute, Percutaneous Endoscopic Approach

0T164JD Bypass Right Ureter to Cutaneous with Synthetic Substitute, Percutaneous Endoscopic Approach

0T164K6 Bypass Right Ureter to Right Ureter with Nonautologous Tissue Substitute, Percutaneous Endoscopic Approach

0T164K7 Bypass Right Ureter to Left Ureter with Nonautologous Tissue Substitute, Percutaneous Endoscopic Approach

0T164K8 Bypass Right Ureter to Colon with Nonautologous Tissue Substitute, Percutaneous Endoscopic Approach

0T164K9 Bypass Right Ureter to Colocutaneous with Nonautologous Tissue Substitute, Percutaneous Endoscopic Approach

0T164KA Bypass Right Ureter to Ileum with Nonautologous Tissue Substitute, Percutaneous Endoscopic Approach

0T164KB Bypass Right Ureter to Bladder with Nonautologous Tissue Substitute, Percutaneous Endoscopic Approach

0T164KC Bypass Right Ureter to Ileocutaneous with Nonautologous Tissue Substitute, Percutaneous Endoscopic Approach

0T164KD Bypass Right Ureter to Cutaneous with Nonautologous Tissue Substitute, Percutaneous Endoscopic Approach

0T164Z6 Bypass Right Ureter to Right Ureter, Percutaneous Endoscopic Approach

0T164Z7 Bypass Right Ureter to Left Ureter, Percutaneous Endoscopic Approach

0T164Z8 Bypass Right Ureter to Colon, Percutaneous Endoscopic Approach

0T164Z9 Bypass Right Ureter to Colocutaneous, Percutaneous Endoscopic Approach

0T164ZA Bypass Right Ureter to Ileum, Percutaneous Endoscopic Approach

0T164ZB Bypass Right Ureter to Bladder, Percutaneous Endoscopic Approach

0T164ZC Bypass Right Ureter to Ileocutaneous, Percutaneous Endoscopic Approach

0T164ZD Bypass Right Ureter to Cutaneous, Percutaneous Endoscopic Approach

0T17076 Bypass Left Ureter to Right Ureter with Autologous Tissue Substitute, Open Approach

0T17077 Bypass Left Ureter to Left Ureter with Autologous Tissue Substitute, Open Approach

---

Female-only   ♂ Male-only   ▲ Limited Coverage   ● Non-OR   ▦ HAC-associated procedure   ▲ Non-covered procedures   ✚ Combination

0T17078 Bypass Left Ureter to Colon with Autologous Tissue Substitute, Open Approach

0T17079 Bypass Left Ureter to Colocutaneous with Autologous Tissue Substitute, Open Approach

0T1707A Bypass Left Ureter to Ileum with Autologous Tissue Substitute, Open Approach

0T1707B Bypass Left Ureter to Bladder with Autologous Tissue Substitute, Open Approach

0T1707C Bypass Left Ureter to Ileocutaneous with Autologous Tissue Substitute, Open Approach

0T1707D Bypass Left Ureter to Cutaneous with Autologous Tissue Substitute, Open Approach

0T170J6 Bypass Left Ureter to Right Ureter with Synthetic Substitute, Open Approach

0T170J7 Bypass Left Ureter to Left Ureter with Synthetic Substitute, Open Approach

0T170J8 Bypass Left Ureter to Colon with Synthetic Substitute, Open Approach

0T170J9 Bypass Left Ureter to Colocutaneous with Synthetic Substitute, Open Approach

0T170JA Bypass Left Ureter to Ileum with Synthetic Substitute, Open Approach

0T170JB Bypass Left Ureter to Bladder with Synthetic Substitute, Open Approach

0T170JC Bypass Left Ureter to Ileocutaneous with Synthetic Substitute, Open Approach

0T170JD Bypass Left Ureter to Cutaneous with Synthetic Substitute, Open Approach

0T170K6 Bypass Left Ureter to Right Ureter with Nonautologous Tissue Substitute, Open Approach

0T170K7 Bypass Left Ureter to Left Ureter with Nonautologous Tissue Substitute, Open Approach

0T170K8 Bypass Left Ureter to Colon with Nonautologous Tissue Substitute, Open Approach

0T170K9 Bypass Left Ureter to Colocutaneous with Nonautologous Tissue Substitute, Open Approach

0T170KA Bypass Left Ureter to Ileum with Nonautologous Tissue Substitute, Open Approach

0T170KB Bypass Left Ureter to Bladder with Nonautologous Tissue Substitute, Open Approach

0T170KC Bypass Left Ureter to Ileocutaneous with Nonautologous Tissue Substitute, Open Approach

0T170KD Bypass Left Ureter to Cutaneous with Nonautologous Tissue Substitute, Open Approach

0T170Z6 Bypass Left Ureter to Right Ureter, Open Approach

0T170Z7 Bypass Left Ureter to Left Ureter, Open Approach

0T170Z8 Bypass Left Ureter to Colon, Open Approach

0T170Z9 Bypass Left Ureter to Colocutaneous, Open Approach

0T170ZA Bypass Left Ureter to Ileum, Open Approach

0T170ZB Bypass Left Ureter to Bladder, Open Approach

0T170ZC Bypass Left Ureter to Ileocutaneous, Open Approach

0T170ZD Bypass Left Ureter to Cutaneous, Open Approach

0T173JD Bypass Left Ureter to Cutaneous with Synthetic Substitute, Percutaneous Approach

0T17476 Bypass Left Ureter to Right Ureter with Autologous Tissue Substitute, Percutaneous Endoscopic Approach

0T17477 Bypass Left Ureter to Left Ureter with Autologous Tissue Substitute, Percutaneous Endoscopic Approach

0T17478 Bypass Left Ureter to Colon with Autologous Tissue Substitute, Percutaneous Endoscopic Approach

0T17479 Bypass Left Ureter to Colocutaneous with Autologous Tissue Substitute, Percutaneous Endoscopic Approach

0T1747A Bypass Left Ureter to Ileum with Autologous Tissue Substitute, Percutaneous Endoscopic Approach

0T1747B Bypass Left Ureter to Bladder with Autologous Tissue Substitute, Percutaneous Endoscopic Approach

0T1747C Bypass Left Ureter to Ileocutaneous with Autologous Tissue Substitute, Percutaneous Endoscopic Approach

0T1747D Bypass Left Ureter to Cutaneous with Autologous Tissue Substitute, Percutaneous Endoscopic Approach

0T174J6 Bypass Left Ureter to Right Ureter with Synthetic Substitute, Percutaneous Endoscopic Approach

0T174J7 Bypass Left Ureter to Left Ureter with Synthetic Substitute, Percutaneous Endoscopic Approach

0T174J8 Bypass Left Ureter to Colon with Synthetic Substitute, Percutaneous Endoscopic Approach

0T174J9 Bypass Left Ureter to Colocutaneous with Synthetic Substitute, Percutaneous Endoscopic Approach

0T174JA Bypass Left Ureter to Ileum with Synthetic Substitute, Percutaneous Endoscopic Approach

0T174JB Bypass Left Ureter to Bladder with Synthetic Substitute, Percutaneous Endoscopic Approach

0T174JC Bypass Left Ureter to Ileocutaneous with Synthetic Substitute, Percutaneous Endoscopic Approach

0T174JD Bypass Left Ureter to Cutaneous with Synthetic Substitute, Percutaneous Endoscopic Approach

0T174K6 Bypass Left Ureter to Right Ureter with Nonautologous Tissue Substitute, Percutaneous Endoscopic Approach

0T174K7 Bypass Left Ureter to Left Ureter with Nonautologous Tissue Substitute, Percutaneous Endoscopic Approach

0T174K8 Bypass Left Ureter to Colon with Nonautologous Tissue Substitute, Percutaneous Endoscopic Approach

0T174K9 Bypass Left Ureter to Colocutaneous with Nonautologous Tissue Substitute, Percutaneous Endoscopic Approach

0T174KA Bypass Left Ureter to Ileum with Nonautologous Tissue Substitute, Percutaneous Endoscopic Approach

0T174KB Bypass Left Ureter to Bladder with Nonautologous Tissue Substitute, Percutaneous Endoscopic Approach

0T174KC Bypass Left Ureter to Ileocutaneous with Nonautologous Tissue Substitute, Percutaneous Endoscopic Approach

0T174KD Bypass Left Ureter to Cutaneous with Nonautologous Tissue Substitute, Percutaneous Endoscopic Approach

0T174Z6 Bypass Left Ureter to Right Ureter, Percutaneous Endoscopic Approach

0T174Z7 Bypass Left Ureter to Left Ureter, Percutaneous Endoscopic Approach

0T174Z8 Bypass Left Ureter to Colon, Percutaneous Endoscopic Approach

0T174Z9 Bypass Left Ureter to Colocutaneous, Percutaneous Endoscopic Approach

0T174ZA Bypass Left Ureter to Ileum, Percutaneous Endoscopic Approach

0T174ZB Bypass Left Ureter to Bladder, Percutaneous Endoscopic Approach

0T174ZC Bypass Left Ureter to Ileocutaneous, Percutaneous Endoscopic Approach

0T174ZD Bypass Left Ureter to Cutaneous, Percutaneous Endoscopic Approach

0T18076 Bypass Bilateral Ureters to Right Ureter with Autologous Tissue Substitute, Open Approach

0T18077 Bypass Bilateral Ureters to Left Ureter with Autologous Tissue Substitute, Open Approach

0T18078 Bypass Bilateral Ureters to Colon with Autologous Tissue Substitute, Open Approach

0T18079 Bypass Bilateral Ureters to Colocutaneous with Autologous Tissue Substitute, Open Approach

0T1807A Bypass Bilateral Ureters to Ileum with Autologous Tissue Substitute, Open Approach

0T1807B Bypass Bilateral Ureters to Bladder with Autologous Tissue Substitute, Open Approach

0T1807C Bypass Bilateral Ureters to Ileocutaneous with Autologous Tissue Substitute, Open Approach

0T1807D Bypass Bilateral Ureters to Cutaneous with Autologous Tissue Substitute, Open Approach

0T180J6 Bypass Bilateral Ureters to Right Ureter with Synthetic Substitute, Open Approach

0T180J7 Bypass Bilateral Ureters to Left Ureter with Synthetic Substitute, Open Approach

0T180J8 Bypass Bilateral Ureters to Colon with Synthetic Substitute, Open Approach

0T180J9 Bypass Bilateral Ureters to Colocutaneous with Synthetic Substitute, Open Approach

0T180JA Bypass Bilateral Ureters to Ileum with Synthetic Substitute, Open Approach

0T180JB Bypass Bilateral Ureters to Bladder with Synthetic Substitute, Open Approach

0T180JC Bypass Bilateral Ureters to Ileocutaneous with Synthetic Substitute, Open Approach

0T180JD Bypass Bilateral Ureters to Cutaneous with Synthetic Substitute, Open Approach

0T180K6 Bypass Bilateral Ureters to Right Ureter with Nonautologous Tissue Substitute, Open Approach

0T180K7 Bypass Bilateral Ureters to Left Ureter with Nonautologous Tissue Substitute, Open Approach

0T180K8 Bypass Bilateral Ureters to Colon with Nonautologous Tissue Substitute, Open Approach

0T180K9 Bypass Bilateral Ureters to Colocutaneous with Nonautologous Tissue Substitute, Open Approach

0T180KA Bypass Bilateral Ureters to Ileum with Nonautologous Tissue Substitute, Open Approach

0T180KB Bypass Bilateral Ureters to Bladder with Nonautologous Tissue Substitute, Open Approach

0T180KC Bypass Bilateral Ureters to Ileocutaneous with Nonautologous Tissue Substitute, Open Approach

0T180KD Bypass Bilateral Ureters to Cutaneous with Nonautologous Tissue Substitute, Open Approach

0T180Z6 Bypass Bilateral Ureters to Right Ureter, Open Approach

0T180Z7 Bypass Bilateral Ureters to Left Ureter, Open Approach

0T180Z8	Bypass Bilateral Ureters to Colon, Open Approach
0T180Z9	Bypass Bilateral Ureters to Colocutaneous, Open Approach
0T180ZA	Bypass Bilateral Ureters to Ileum, Open Approach
0T180ZB	Bypass Bilateral Ureters to Bladder, Open Approach
0T180ZC	Bypass Bilateral Ureters to Ileocutaneous, Open Approach
0T180ZD	Bypass Bilateral Ureters to Cutaneous, Open Approach
0T183JD	Bypass Bilateral Ureters to Cutaneous with Synthetic Substitute, Percutaneous Approach
0T18476	Bypass Bilateral Ureters to Right Ureter with Autologous Tissue Substitute, Percutaneous Endoscopic Approach
0T18477	Bypass Bilateral Ureters to Left Ureter with Autologous Tissue Substitute, Percutaneous Endoscopic Approach
0T18478	Bypass Bilateral Ureters to Colon with Autologous Tissue Substitute, Percutaneous Endoscopic Approach
0T18479	Bypass Bilateral Ureters to Colocutaneous with Autologous Tissue Substitute, Percutaneous Endoscopic Approach
0T1847A	Bypass Bilateral Ureters to Ileum with Autologous Tissue Substitute, Percutaneous Endoscopic Approach
0T1847B	Bypass Bilateral Ureters to Bladder with Autologous Tissue Substitute, Percutaneous Endoscopic Approach
0T1847C	Bypass Bilateral Ureters to Ileocutaneous with Autologous Tissue Substitute, Percutaneous Endoscopic Approach
0T1847D	Bypass Bilateral Ureters to Cutaneous with Autologous Tissue Substitute, Percutaneous Endoscopic Approach
0T184J6	Bypass Bilateral Ureters to Right Ureter with Synthetic Substitute, Percutaneous Endoscopic Approach
0T184J7	Bypass Bilateral Ureters to Left Ureter with Synthetic Substitute, Percutaneous Endoscopic Approach
0T184J8	Bypass Bilateral Ureters to Colon with Synthetic Substitute, Percutaneous Endoscopic Approach
0T184J9	Bypass Bilateral Ureters to Colocutaneous with Synthetic Substitute, Percutaneous Endoscopic Approach
0T184JA	Bypass Bilateral Ureters to Ileum with Synthetic Substitute, Percutaneous Endoscopic Approach
0T184JB	Bypass Bilateral Ureters to Bladder with Synthetic Substitute, Percutaneous Endoscopic Approach
0T184JC	Bypass Bilateral Ureters to Ileocutaneous with Synthetic Substitute, Percutaneous Endoscopic Approach
0T184JD	Bypass Bilateral Ureters to Cutaneous with Synthetic Substitute, Percutaneous Endoscopic Approach
0T184K6	Bypass Bilateral Ureters to Right Ureter with Nonautologous Tissue Substitute, Percutaneous Endoscopic Approach
0T184K7	Bypass Bilateral Ureters to Left Ureter with Nonautologous Tissue Substitute, Percutaneous Endoscopic Approach
0T184K8	Bypass Bilateral Ureters to Colon with Nonautologous Tissue Substitute, Percutaneous Endoscopic Approach
0T184K9	Bypass Bilateral Ureters to Colocutaneous with Nonautologous Tissue Substitute, Percutaneous Endoscopic Approach
0T184KA	Bypass Bilateral Ureters to Ileum with Nonautologous Tissue Substitute, Percutaneous Endoscopic Approach
0T184KB	Bypass Bilateral Ureters to Bladder with Nonautologous Tissue Substitute, Percutaneous Endoscopic Approach
0T184KC	Bypass Bilateral Ureters to Ileocutaneous with Nonautologous Tissue Substitute, Percutaneous Endoscopic Approach
0T184KD	Bypass Bilateral Ureters to Cutaneous with Nonautologous Tissue Substitute, Percutaneous Endoscopic Approach
0T184Z6	Bypass Bilateral Ureters to Right Ureter, Percutaneous Endoscopic Approach
0T184Z7	Bypass Bilateral Ureters to Left Ureter, Percutaneous Endoscopic Approach
0T184Z8	Bypass Bilateral Ureters to Colon, Percutaneous Endoscopic Approach
0T184Z9	Bypass Bilateral Ureters to Colocutaneous, Percutaneous Endoscopic Approach
0T184ZA	Bypass Bilateral Ureters to Ileum, Percutaneous Endoscopic Approach
0T184ZB	Bypass Bilateral Ureters to Bladder, Percutaneous Endoscopic Approach
0T184ZC	Bypass Bilateral Ureters to Ileocutaneous, Percutaneous Endoscopic Approach
0T184ZD	Bypass Bilateral Ureters to Cutaneous, Percutaneous Endoscopic Approach
0T1B079	Bypass Bladder to Colocutaneous with Autologous Tissue Substitute, Open Approach
0T1B07C	Bypass Bladder to Ileocutaneous with Autologous Tissue Substitute, Open Approach
0T1B07D	Bypass Bladder to Cutaneous with Autologous Tissue Substitute, Open Approach
0T1B0J9	Bypass Bladder to Colocutaneous with Synthetic Substitute, Open Approach
0T1B0JC	Bypass Bladder to Ileocutaneous with Synthetic Substitute, Open Approach
0T1B0JD	Bypass Bladder to Cutaneous with Synthetic Substitute, Open Approach
0T1B0K9	Bypass Bladder to Colocutaneous with Nonautologous Tissue Substitute, Open Approach
0T1B0KC	Bypass Bladder to Ileocutaneous with Nonautologous Tissue Substitute, Open Approach
0T1B0KD	Bypass Bladder to Cutaneous with Nonautologous Tissue Substitute, Open Approach
0T1B0Z9	Bypass Bladder to Colocutaneous, Open Approach
0T1B0ZC	Bypass Bladder to Ileocutaneous, Open Approach
0T1B0ZD	Bypass Bladder to Cutaneous, Open Approach
0T1B3JD	Bypass Bladder to Cutaneous with Synthetic Substitute, Percutaneous Approach
0T1B479	Bypass Bladder to Colocutaneous with Autologous Tissue Substitute, Percutaneous Endoscopic Approach
0T1B47C	Bypass Bladder to Ileocutaneous with Autologous Tissue Substitute, Percutaneous Endoscopic Approach
0T1B47D	Bypass Bladder to Cutaneous with Autologous Tissue Substitute, Percutaneous Endoscopic Approach
0T1B4J9	Bypass Bladder to Colocutaneous with Synthetic Substitute, Percutaneous Endoscopic Approach
0T1B4JC	Bypass Bladder to Ileocutaneous with Synthetic Substitute, Percutaneous Endoscopic Approach
0T1B4JD	Bypass Bladder to Cutaneous with Synthetic Substitute, Percutaneous Endoscopic Approach
0T1B4K9	Bypass Bladder to Colocutaneous with Nonautologous Tissue Substitute, Percutaneous Endoscopic Approach
0T1B4KC	Bypass Bladder to Ileocutaneous with Nonautologous Tissue Substitute, Percutaneous Endoscopic Approach
0T1B4KD	Bypass Bladder to Cutaneous with Nonautologous Tissue Substitute, Percutaneous Endoscopic Approach
0T1B4Z9	Bypass Bladder to Colocutaneous, Percutaneous Endoscopic Approach
0T1B4ZC	Bypass Bladder to Ileocutaneous, Percutaneous Endoscopic Approach
0T1B4ZD	Bypass Bladder to Cutaneous, Percutaneous Endoscopic Approach

0T2 – Urinary System, Change

Review Coding Guideline B6.1c

0T25X0Z	Change Drainage Device in Kidney, External Approach
0T25XYZ	Change Other Device in Kidney, External Approach
0T29X0Z	Change Drainage Device in Ureter, External Approach
0T29XYZ	Change Other Device in Ureter, External Approach
0T2BX0Z	Change Drainage Device in Bladder, External Approach
0T2BXYZ	Change Other Device in Bladder, External Approach
0T2DX0Z	Change Drainage Device in Urethra, External Approach
0T2DXYZ	Change Other Device in Urethra, External Approach

0T5 – Urinary System, Destruction

0T500ZZ	Destruction of Right Kidney, Open Approach
0T503ZZ	Destruction of Right Kidney, Percutaneous Approach
0T504ZZ	Destruction of Right Kidney, Percutaneous Endoscopic Approach
0T507ZZ	Destruction of Right Kidney, Via Natural or Artificial Opening
0T508ZZ	Destruction of Right Kidney, Via Natural or Artificial Opening Endoscopic
0T510ZZ	Destruction of Left Kidney, Open Approach
0T513ZZ	Destruction of Left Kidney, Percutaneous Approach
0T514ZZ	Destruction of Left Kidney, Percutaneous Endoscopic Approach
0T517ZZ	Destruction of Left Kidney, Via Natural or Artificial Opening

♀ Female-only ♂ Male-only ▲ Limited Coverage ● Non-OR HAC HAC-associated procedure ▲ Non-covered procedures ⊞ Combination

0T518ZZ	Destruction of Left Kidney, Via Natural or Artificial Opening Endoscopic	0T563ZZ	Destruction of Right Ureter, Percutaneous Approach	0T5B8ZZ	Destruction of Bladder, Via Natural or Artificial Opening Endoscopic

0T518ZZ Destruction of Left Kidney, Via Natural or Artificial Opening Endoscopic
0T530ZZ Destruction of Right Kidney Pelvis, Open Approach
0T533ZZ Destruction of Right Kidney Pelvis, Percutaneous Approach
0T534ZZ Destruction of Right Kidney Pelvis, Percutaneous Endoscopic Approach
0T537ZZ Destruction of Right Kidney Pelvis, Via Natural or Artificial Opening
0T538ZZ Destruction of Right Kidney Pelvis, Via Natural or Artificial Opening Endoscopic
0T540ZZ Destruction of Left Kidney Pelvis, Open Approach
0T543ZZ Destruction of Left Kidney Pelvis, Percutaneous Approach
0T544ZZ Destruction of Left Kidney Pelvis, Percutaneous Endoscopic Approach
0T547ZZ Destruction of Left Kidney Pelvis, Via Natural or Artificial Opening
0T548ZZ Destruction of Left Kidney Pelvis, Via Natural or Artificial Opening Endoscopic
0T560ZZ Destruction of Right Ureter, Open Approach

0T563ZZ Destruction of Right Ureter, Percutaneous Approach
0T564ZZ Destruction of Right Ureter, Percutaneous Endoscopic Approach
0T567ZZ Destruction of Right Ureter, Via Natural or Artificial Opening
0T568ZZ Destruction of Right Ureter, Via Natural or Artificial Opening Endoscopic
0T570ZZ Destruction of Left Ureter, Open Approach
0T573ZZ Destruction of Left Ureter, Percutaneous Approach
0T574ZZ Destruction of Left Ureter, Percutaneous Endoscopic Approach
0T577ZZ Destruction of Left Ureter, Via Natural or Artificial Opening
0T578ZZ Destruction of Left Ureter, Via Natural or Artificial Opening Endoscopic
0T5B0ZZ Destruction of Bladder, Open Approach
0T5B3ZZ Destruction of Bladder, Percutaneous Approach
0T5B4ZZ Destruction of Bladder, Percutaneous Endoscopic Approach
0T5B7ZZ Destruction of Bladder, Via Natural or Artificial Opening

0T5B8ZZ Destruction of Bladder, Via Natural or Artificial Opening Endoscopic
0T5C0ZZ Destruction of Bladder Neck, Open Approach
0T5C3ZZ Destruction of Bladder Neck, Percutaneous Approach
0T5C4ZZ Destruction of Bladder Neck, Percutaneous Endoscopic Approach
0T5C7ZZ Destruction of Bladder Neck, Via Natural or Artificial Opening
0T5C8ZZ Destruction of Bladder Neck, Via Natural or Artificial Opening Endoscopic
0T5D0ZZ Destruction of Urethra, Open Approach
0T5D3ZZ Destruction of Urethra, Percutaneous Approach
0T5D4ZZ Destruction of Urethra, Percutaneous Endoscopic Approach
0T5D7ZZ Destruction of Urethra, Via Natural or Artificial Opening
0T5D8ZZ Destruction of Urethra, Via Natural or Artificial Opening Endoscopic
0T5DXZZ Destruction of Urethra, External Approach

0T7 – Urinary System, Dilation

0T730DZ Dilation of Right Kidney Pelvis with Intraluminal Device, Open Approach
0T730ZZ Dilation of Right Kidney Pelvis, Open Approach
0T733DZ Dilation of Right Kidney Pelvis with Intraluminal Device, Percutaneous Approach
0T733ZZ Dilation of Right Kidney Pelvis, Percutaneous Approach
0T734DZ Dilation of Right Kidney Pelvis with Intraluminal Device, Percutaneous Endoscopic Approach
0T734ZZ Dilation of Right Kidney Pelvis, Percutaneous Endoscopic Approach
0T737DZ Dilation of Right Kidney Pelvis with Intraluminal Device, Via Natural or Artificial Opening
0T737ZZ Dilation of Right Kidney Pelvis, Via Natural or Artificial Opening
0T738DZ Dilation of Right Kidney Pelvis with Intraluminal Device, Via Natural or Artificial Opening Endoscopic
0T738ZZ Dilation of Right Kidney Pelvis, Via Natural or Artificial Opening Endoscopic
0T740DZ Dilation of Left Kidney Pelvis with Intraluminal Device, Open Approach
0T740ZZ Dilation of Left Kidney Pelvis, Open Approach
0T743DZ Dilation of Left Kidney Pelvis with Intraluminal Device, Percutaneous Approach
0T743ZZ Dilation of Left Kidney Pelvis, Percutaneous Approach
0T744DZ Dilation of Left Kidney Pelvis with Intraluminal Device, Percutaneous Endoscopic Approach
0T744ZZ Dilation of Left Kidney Pelvis, Percutaneous Endoscopic Approach
0T747DZ Dilation of Left Kidney Pelvis with Intraluminal Device, Via Natural or Artificial Opening
0T747ZZ Dilation of Left Kidney Pelvis, Via Natural or Artificial Opening
0T748DZ Dilation of Left Kidney Pelvis with Intraluminal Device, Via Natural or Artificial Opening Endoscopic
0T748ZZ Dilation of Left Kidney Pelvis, Via Natural or Artificial Opening Endoscopic
0T760DZ Dilation of Right Ureter with Intraluminal Device, Open Approach
0T760ZZ Dilation of Right Ureter, Open Approach

0T763DZ Dilation of Right Ureter with Intraluminal Device, Percutaneous Approach
0T763ZZ Dilation of Right Ureter, Percutaneous Approach
0T764DZ Dilation of Right Ureter with Intraluminal Device, Percutaneous Endoscopic Approach
0T764ZZ Dilation of Right Ureter, Percutaneous Endoscopic Approach
0T767DZ Dilation of Right Ureter with Intraluminal Device, Via Natural or Artificial Opening
0T767ZZ Dilation of Right Ureter, Via Natural or Artificial Opening
0T768DZ Dilation of Right Ureter with Intraluminal Device, Via Natural or Artificial Opening Endoscopic
0T768ZZ Dilation of Right Ureter, Via Natural or Artificial Opening Endoscopic
0T770DZ Dilation of Left Ureter with Intraluminal Device, Open Approach
0T770ZZ Dilation of Left Ureter, Open Approach
0T773DZ Dilation of Left Ureter with Intraluminal Device, Percutaneous Approach
0T773ZZ Dilation of Left Ureter, Percutaneous Approach
0T774DZ Dilation of Left Ureter with Intraluminal Device, Percutaneous Endoscopic Approach
0T774ZZ Dilation of Left Ureter, Percutaneous Endoscopic Approach
0T777DZ Dilation of Left Ureter with Intraluminal Device, Via Natural or Artificial Opening
0T777ZZ Dilation of Left Ureter, Via Natural or Artificial Opening
0T778DZ Dilation of Left Ureter with Intraluminal Device, Via Natural or Artificial Opening Endoscopic
0T778ZZ Dilation of Left Ureter, Via Natural or Artificial Opening Endoscopic
0T780DZ Dilation of Bilateral Ureters with Intraluminal Device, Open Approach
0T780ZZ Dilation of Bilateral Ureters, Open Approach
0T783DZ Dilation of Bilateral Ureters with Intraluminal Device, Percutaneous Approach
0T783ZZ Dilation of Bilateral Ureters, Percutaneous Approach
0T784DZ Dilation of Bilateral Ureters with Intraluminal Device, Percutaneous Endoscopic Approach

0T784ZZ Dilation of Bilateral Ureters, Percutaneous Endoscopic Approach
0T787DZ Dilation of Bilateral Ureters with Intraluminal Device, Via Natural or Artificial Opening
0T787ZZ Dilation of Bilateral Ureters, Via Natural or Artificial Opening
0T788DZ Dilation of Bilateral Ureters with Intraluminal Device, Via Natural or Artificial Opening Endoscopic
0T788ZZ Dilation of Bilateral Ureters, Via Natural or Artificial Opening Endoscopic
0T7B0DZ Dilation of Bladder with Intraluminal Device, Open Approach
0T7B0ZZ Dilation of Bladder, Open Approach
0T7B3DZ Dilation of Bladder with Intraluminal Device, Percutaneous Approach
0T7B3ZZ Dilation of Bladder, Percutaneous Approach
0T7B4DZ Dilation of Bladder with Intraluminal Device, Percutaneous Endoscopic Approach
0T7B4ZZ Dilation of Bladder, Percutaneous Endoscopic Approach
0T7B7DZ Dilation of Bladder with Intraluminal Device, Via Natural or Artificial Opening
0T7B7ZZ Dilation of Bladder, Via Natural or Artificial Opening
0T7B8DZ Dilation of Bladder with Intraluminal Device, Via Natural or Artificial Opening Endoscopic
0T7B8ZZ Dilation of Bladder, Via Natural or Artificial Opening Endoscopic
0T7C0DZ Dilation of Bladder Neck with Intraluminal Device, Open Approach
0T7C0ZZ Dilation of Bladder Neck, Open Approach
0T7C3DZ Dilation of Bladder Neck with Intraluminal Device, Percutaneous Approach
0T7C3ZZ Dilation of Bladder Neck, Percutaneous Approach
0T7C4DZ Dilation of Bladder Neck with Intraluminal Device, Percutaneous Endoscopic Approach
0T7C4ZZ Dilation of Bladder Neck, Percutaneous Endoscopic Approach
0T7C7DZ Dilation of Bladder Neck with Intraluminal Device, Via Natural or Artificial Opening
0T7C7ZZ Dilation of Bladder Neck, Via Natural or Artificial Opening

♀ Female-only   ♂ Male-only   ▲ Limited Coverage   ● Non-OR   ▦ HAC-associated procedure   ▲ Non-covered procedures   ✚ Combination

7C8DZ Dilation of Bladder Neck with Intraluminal Device, Via Natural or Artificial Opening Endoscopic	**0T7D3ZZ** Dilation of Urethra, Percutaneous Approach	**0T7D7ZZ** Dilation of Urethra, Via Natural or Artificial Opening
7C8ZZ Dilation of Bladder Neck, Via Natural or Artificial Opening Endoscopic	**0T7D4DZ** Dilation of Urethra with Intraluminal Device, Percutaneous Endoscopic Approach	**0T7D8DZ** Dilation of Urethra with Intraluminal Device, Via Natural or Artificial Opening Endoscopic
7D0DZ Dilation of Urethra with Intraluminal Device, Open Approach	**0T7D4ZZ** Dilation of Urethra, Percutaneous Endoscopic Approach	*AHA CC: 4Q, 2013, 123*
7D0ZZ Dilation of Urethra, Open Approach	**0T7D7DZ** Dilation of Urethra with Intraluminal Device, Via Natural or Artificial Opening	**0T7D8ZZ** Dilation of Urethra, Via Natural or Artificial Opening Endoscopic
7D3DZ Dilation of Urethra with Intraluminal Device, Percutaneous Approach		

T8 – Urinary System, Division

eview Coding Guideline B3.14

820ZZ Division of Bilateral Kidneys, Open Approach	**0T824ZZ** Division of Bilateral Kidneys, Percutaneous Endoscopic Approach	**0T8C3ZZ** Division of Bladder Neck, Percutaneous Approach
823ZZ Division of Bilateral Kidneys, Percutaneous Approach	**0T8C0ZZ** Division of Bladder Neck, Open Approach	**0T8C4ZZ** Division of Bladder Neck, Percutaneous Endoscopic Approach

T9 – Urinary System, Drainage

eview Coding Guidelines B3.4a and B3.4b

eview Coding Guideline B6.2

9000Z Drainage of Right Kidney with Drainage Device, Open Approach	**0T917ZX** Drainage of Left Kidney, Via Natural or Artificial Opening, Diagnostic	**0T9430Z** Drainage of Left Kidney Pelvis with Drainage Device, Percutaneous Approach
900ZX Drainage of Right Kidney, Open Approach, Diagnostic	**0T917ZZ** Drainage of Left Kidney, Via Natural or Artificial Opening	**0T943ZX** Drainage of Left Kidney Pelvis, Percutaneous Approach, Diagnostic
900ZZ Drainage of Right Kidney, Open Approach	**0T9180Z** Drainage of Left Kidney with Drainage Device, Via Natural or Artificial Opening Endoscopic	**0T943ZZ** Drainage of Left Kidney Pelvis, Percutaneous Approach
9030Z Drainage of Right Kidney with Drainage Device, Percutaneous Approach	**0T918ZX** Drainage of Left Kidney, Via Natural or Artificial Opening Endoscopic, Diagnostic	**0T9440Z** Drainage of Left Kidney Pelvis with Drainage Device, Percutaneous Endoscopic Approach
903ZX Drainage of Right Kidney, Percutaneous Approach, Diagnostic	**0T918ZZ** Drainage of Left Kidney, Via Natural or Artificial Opening Endoscopic	**0T944ZX** Drainage of Left Kidney Pelvis, Percutaneous Endoscopic Approach, Diagnostic
903ZZ Drainage of Right Kidney, Percutaneous Approach	**0T9300Z** Drainage of Right Kidney Pelvis with Drainage Device, Open Approach	**0T944ZZ** Drainage of Left Kidney Pelvis, Percutaneous Endoscopic Approach
9040Z Drainage of Right Kidney with Drainage Device, Percutaneous Endoscopic Approach	**0T930ZX** Drainage of Right Kidney Pelvis, Open Approach, Diagnostic	**0T9470Z** Drainage of Left Kidney Pelvis with Drainage Device, Via Natural or Artificial Opening
904ZX Drainage of Right Kidney, Percutaneous Endoscopic Approach, Diagnostic	**0T930ZZ** Drainage of Right Kidney Pelvis, Open Approach	**0T947ZX** Drainage of Left Kidney Pelvis, Via Natural or Artificial Opening, Diagnostic
904ZZ Drainage of Right Kidney, Percutaneous Endoscopic Approach	**0T9330Z** Drainage of Right Kidney Pelvis with Drainage Device, Percutaneous Approach	**0T947ZZ** Drainage of Left Kidney Pelvis, Via Natural or Artificial Opening
9070Z Drainage of Right Kidney with Drainage Device, Via Natural or Artificial Opening	**0T933ZX** Drainage of Right Kidney Pelvis, Percutaneous Approach, Diagnostic	**0T9480Z** Drainage of Left Kidney Pelvis with Drainage Device, Via Natural or Artificial Opening Endoscopic
907ZX Drainage of Right Kidney, Via Natural or Artificial Opening, Diagnostic	**0T933ZZ** Drainage of Right Kidney Pelvis, Percutaneous Approach	**0T948ZX** Drainage of Left Kidney Pelvis, Via Natural or Artificial Opening Endoscopic, Diagnostic
907ZZ Drainage of Right Kidney, Via Natural or Artificial Opening	**0T9340Z** Drainage of Right Kidney Pelvis with Drainage Device, Percutaneous Endoscopic Approach	**0T948ZZ** Drainage of Left Kidney Pelvis, Via Natural or Artificial Opening Endoscopic
9080Z Drainage of Right Kidney with Drainage Device, Via Natural or Artificial Opening Endoscopic	**0T934ZX** Drainage of Right Kidney Pelvis, Percutaneous Endoscopic Approach, Diagnostic	**0T9600Z** Drainage of Right Ureter with Drainage Device, Open Approach
908ZX Drainage of Right Kidney, Via Natural or Artificial Opening Endoscopic, Diagnostic	**0T934ZZ** Drainage of Right Kidney Pelvis, Percutaneous Endoscopic Approach	**0T960ZX** Drainage of Right Ureter, Open Approach, Diagnostic
908ZZ Drainage of Right Kidney, Via Natural or Artificial Opening Endoscopic	**0T9370Z** Drainage of Right Kidney Pelvis with Drainage Device, Via Natural or Artificial Opening	**0T960ZZ** Drainage of Right Ureter, Open Approach
9100Z Drainage of Left Kidney with Drainage Device, Open Approach	**0T937ZX** Drainage of Right Kidney Pelvis, Via Natural or Artificial Opening, Diagnostic	**0T9630Z** Drainage of Right Ureter with Drainage Device, Percutaneous Approach
910ZX Drainage of Left Kidney, Open Approach, Diagnostic	**0T937ZZ** Drainage of Right Kidney Pelvis, Via Natural or Artificial Opening	**0T963ZX** Drainage of Right Ureter, Percutaneous Approach, Diagnostic
910ZZ Drainage of Left Kidney, Open Approach	**0T9380Z** Drainage of Right Kidney Pelvis with Drainage Device, Via Natural or Artificial Opening Endoscopic	**0T963ZZ** Drainage of Right Ureter, Percutaneous Approach
9130Z Drainage of Left Kidney with Drainage Device, Percutaneous Approach	**0T938ZX** Drainage of Right Kidney Pelvis, Via Natural or Artificial Opening Endoscopic, Diagnostic	**0T9640Z** Drainage of Right Ureter with Drainage Device, Percutaneous Endoscopic Approach
913ZX Drainage of Left Kidney, Percutaneous Approach, Diagnostic	**0T938ZZ** Drainage of Right Kidney Pelvis, Via Natural or Artificial Opening Endoscopic	**0T964ZX** Drainage of Right Ureter, Percutaneous Endoscopic Approach, Diagnostic
913ZZ Drainage of Left Kidney, Percutaneous Approach	**0T9400Z** Drainage of Left Kidney Pelvis with Drainage Device, Open Approach	**0T964ZZ** Drainage of Right Ureter, Percutaneous Endoscopic Approach
9140Z Drainage of Left Kidney with Drainage Device, Percutaneous Endoscopic Approach	**0T940ZX** Drainage of Left Kidney Pelvis, Open Approach, Diagnostic	**0T9670Z** Drainage of Right Ureter with Drainage Device, Via Natural or Artificial Opening
914ZX Drainage of Left Kidney, Percutaneous Endoscopic Approach, Diagnostic	**0T940ZZ** Drainage of Left Kidney Pelvis, Open Approach	**0T967ZX** Drainage of Right Ureter, Via Natural or Artificial Opening, Diagnostic
914ZZ Drainage of Left Kidney, Percutaneous Endoscopic Approach		
9170Z Drainage of Left Kidney with Drainage Device, Via Natural or Artificial Opening		

0T967ZZ	Drainage of Right Ureter, Via Natural or Artificial Opening
0T9680Z	Drainage of Right Ureter with Drainage Device, Via Natural or Artificial Opening Endoscopic
0T968ZX	Drainage of Right Ureter, Via Natural or Artificial Opening Endoscopic, Diagnostic
0T968ZZ	Drainage of Right Ureter, Via Natural or Artificial Opening Endoscopic
0T9700Z	Drainage of Left Ureter with Drainage Device, Open Approach
0T970ZX	Drainage of Left Ureter, Open Approach, Diagnostic
0T970ZZ	Drainage of Left Ureter, Open Approach
0T9730Z	Drainage of Left Ureter with Drainage Device, Percutaneous Approach
0T973ZX	Drainage of Left Ureter, Percutaneous Approach, Diagnostic
0T973ZZ	Drainage of Left Ureter, Percutaneous Approach
0T9740Z	Drainage of Left Ureter with Drainage Device, Percutaneous Endoscopic Approach
0T974ZX	Drainage of Left Ureter, Percutaneous Endoscopic Approach, Diagnostic
0T974ZZ	Drainage of Left Ureter, Percutaneous Endoscopic Approach
0T9770Z	Drainage of Left Ureter with Drainage Device, Via Natural or Artificial Opening
0T977ZX	Drainage of Left Ureter, Via Natural or Artificial Opening, Diagnostic
0T977ZZ	Drainage of Left Ureter, Via Natural or Artificial Opening
0T9780Z	Drainage of Left Ureter with Drainage Device, Via Natural or Artificial Opening Endoscopic
0T978ZX	Drainage of Left Ureter, Via Natural or Artificial Opening Endoscopic, Diagnostic
0T978ZZ	Drainage of Left Ureter, Via Natural or Artificial Opening Endoscopic
0T9800Z	Drainage of Bilateral Ureters with Drainage Device, Open Approach
0T980ZX	Drainage of Bilateral Ureters, Open Approach, Diagnostic
0T980ZZ	Drainage of Bilateral Ureters, Open Approach
0T9830Z	Drainage of Bilateral Ureters with Drainage Device, Percutaneous Approach
0T983ZX	Drainage of Bilateral Ureters, Percutaneous Approach, Diagnostic
0T983ZZ	Drainage of Bilateral Ureters, Percutaneous Approach
0T9840Z	Drainage of Bilateral Ureters with Drainage Device, Percutaneous Endoscopic Approach
0T984ZX	Drainage of Bilateral Ureters, Percutaneous Endoscopic Approach, Diagnostic

0T984ZZ	Drainage of Bilateral Ureters, Percutaneous Endoscopic Approach
0T9870Z	Drainage of Bilateral Ureters with Drainage Device, Via Natural or Artificial Opening
0T987ZX	Drainage of Bilateral Ureters, Via Natural or Artificial Opening, Diagnostic
0T987ZZ	Drainage of Bilateral Ureters, Via Natural or Artificial Opening
0T9880Z	Drainage of Bilateral Ureters with Drainage Device, Via Natural or Artificial Opening Endoscopic
0T988ZX	Drainage of Bilateral Ureters, Via Natural or Artificial Opening Endoscopic, Diagnostic
0T988ZZ	Drainage of Bilateral Ureters, Via Natural or Artificial Opening Endoscopic
0T9B00Z	Drainage of Bladder with Drainage Device, Open Approach
0T9B0ZX	Drainage of Bladder, Open Approach, Diagnostic
0T9B0ZZ	Drainage of Bladder, Open Approach
0T9B30Z	Drainage of Bladder with Drainage Device, Percutaneous Approach
0T9B3ZX	Drainage of Bladder, Percutaneous Approach, Diagnostic
0T9B3ZZ	Drainage of Bladder, Percutaneous Approach
0T9B40Z	Drainage of Bladder with Drainage Device, Percutaneous Endoscopic Approach
0T9B4ZX	Drainage of Bladder, Percutaneous Endoscopic Approach, Diagnostic
0T9B4ZZ	Drainage of Bladder, Percutaneous Endoscopic Approach
0T9B70Z	Drainage of Bladder with Drainage Device, Via Natural or Artificial Opening
0T9B7ZX	Drainage of Bladder, Via Natural or Artificial Opening, Diagnostic
0T9B7ZZ	Drainage of Bladder, Via Natural or Artificial Opening
0T9B80Z	Drainage of Bladder with Drainage Device, Via Natural or Artificial Opening Endoscopic
0T9B8ZX	Drainage of Bladder, Via Natural or Artificial Opening Endoscopic, Diagnostic
0T9B8ZZ	Drainage of Bladder, Via Natural or Artificial Opening Endoscopic
0T9C00Z	Drainage of Bladder Neck with Drainage Device, Open Approach
0T9C0ZX	Drainage of Bladder Neck, Open Approach, Diagnostic
0T9C0ZZ	Drainage of Bladder Neck, Open Approach
0T9C30Z	Drainage of Bladder Neck with Drainage Device, Percutaneous Approach
0T9C3ZX	Drainage of Bladder Neck, Percutaneous Approach, Diagnostic

0T9C3ZZ	Drainage of Bladder Neck, Percutaneou Approach
0T9C40Z	Drainage of Bladder Neck with Drainag Device, Percutaneous Endoscopic Approach
0T9C4ZX	Drainage of Bladder Neck, Percutaneou Endoscopic Approach, Diagnostic
0T9C4ZZ	Drainage of Bladder Neck, Percutaneou Endoscopic Approach
0T9C70Z	Drainage of Bladder Neck with Drainag Device, Via Natural or Artificial Openin
0T9C7ZX	Drainage of Bladder Neck, Via Natural Artificial Opening, Diagnostic
0T9C7ZZ	Drainage of Bladder Neck, Via Natural Artificial Opening
0T9C80Z	Drainage of Bladder Neck with Drainag Device, Via Natural or Artificial Openin Endoscopic
0T9C8ZX	Drainage of Bladder Neck, Via Natural Artificial Opening Endoscopic, Diagnos
0T9C8ZZ	Drainage of Bladder Neck, Via Natural Artificial Opening Endoscopic
0T9D00Z	Drainage of Urethra with Drainage Device, Open Approach
0T9D0ZX	Drainage of Urethra, Open Approach, Diagnostic
0T9D0ZZ	Drainage of Urethra, Open Approach
0T9D30Z	Drainage of Urethra with Drainage Device, Percutaneous Approach
0T9D3ZX	Drainage of Urethra, Percutaneous Approach, Diagnostic
0T9D3ZZ	Drainage of Urethra, Percutaneous Approach
0T9D40Z	Drainage of Urethra with Drainage Device, Percutaneous Endoscopic Approach
0T9D4ZX	Drainage of Urethra, Percutaneous Endoscopic Approach, Diagnostic
0T9D4ZZ	Drainage of Urethra, Percutaneous Endoscopic Approach
0T9D70Z	Drainage of Urethra with Drainage Device, Via Natural or Artificial Opening
0T9D7ZX	Drainage of Urethra, Via Natural or Artificial Opening, Diagnostic
0T9D7ZZ	Drainage of Urethra, Via Natural or Artificial Opening
0T9D80Z	Drainage of Urethra with Drainage Device, Via Natural or Artificial Opening Endoscopic
0T9D8ZX	Drainage of Urethra, Via Natural or Artificial Opening Endoscopic, Diagnosti
0T9D8ZZ	Drainage of Urethra, Via Natural or Artificial Opening Endoscopic
0T9DX0Z	Drainage of Urethra with Drainage Device, External Approach
0T9DXZX	Drainage of Urethra, External Approach, Diagnostic
0T9DXZZ	Drainage of Urethra, External Approach

0TB – Urinary System, Excision

Review Coding Guidelines B3.4a and B3.4b

Review Coding Guideline B3.8

0TB00ZX	Excision of Right Kidney, Open Approach, Diagnostic
0TB00ZZ	Excision of Right Kidney, Open Approach
0TB03ZX	Excision of Right Kidney, Percutaneous Approach, Diagnostic
0TB03ZZ	Excision of Right Kidney, Percutaneous Approach
0TB04ZX	Excision of Right Kidney, Percutaneous Endoscopic Approach, Diagnostic
0TB04ZZ	Excision of Right Kidney, Percutaneous Endoscopic Approach
0TB07ZX	Excision of Right Kidney, Via Natural or Artificial Opening, Diagnostic

0TB07ZZ	Excision of Right Kidney, Via Natural or Artificial Opening
0TB08ZX	Excision of Right Kidney, Via Natural or Artificial Opening Endoscopic, Diagnostic
0TB08ZZ	Excision of Right Kidney, Via Natural or Artificial Opening Endoscopic
0TB10ZX	Excision of Left Kidney, Open Approach, Diagnostic
0TB10ZZ	Excision of Left Kidney, Open Approach
0TB13ZX	Excision of Left Kidney, Percutaneous Approach, Diagnostic
0TB13ZZ	Excision of Left Kidney, Percutaneous Approach

0TB14ZX	Excision of Left Kidney, Percutaneous Endoscopic Approach, Diagnostic
0TB14ZZ	Excision of Left Kidney, Percutaneous Endoscopic Approach
0TB17ZX	Excision of Left Kidney, Via Natural or Artificial Opening, Diagnostic
0TB17ZZ	Excision of Left Kidney, Via Natural or Artificial Opening
0TB18ZX	Excision of Left Kidney, Via Natural or Artificial Opening Endoscopic, Diagnostic
0TB18ZZ	Excision of Left Kidney, Via Natural or Artificial Opening Endoscopic

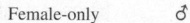

TB30ZX	Excision of Right Kidney Pelvis, Open Approach, Diagnostic
TB30ZZ	Excision of Right Kidney Pelvis, Open Approach
TB33ZX	Excision of Right Kidney Pelvis, Percutaneous Approach, Diagnostic
TB33ZZ	Excision of Right Kidney Pelvis, Percutaneous Approach
TB34ZX	Excision of Right Kidney Pelvis, Percutaneous Endoscopic Approach, Diagnostic
TB34ZZ	Excision of Right Kidney Pelvis, Percutaneous Endoscopic Approach
TB37ZX	Excision of Right Kidney Pelvis, Via Natural or Artificial Opening, Diagnostic
TB37ZZ	Excision of Right Kidney Pelvis, Via Natural or Artificial Opening
TB38ZX	Excision of Right Kidney Pelvis, Via Natural or Artificial Opening Endoscopic, Diagnostic
TB38ZZ	Excision of Right Kidney Pelvis, Via Natural or Artificial Opening Endoscopic
TB40ZX	Excision of Left Kidney Pelvis, Open Approach, Diagnostic
TB40ZZ	Excision of Left Kidney Pelvis, Open Approach
TB43ZX	Excision of Left Kidney Pelvis, Percutaneous Approach, Diagnostic
TB43ZZ	Excision of Left Kidney Pelvis, Percutaneous Approach
TB44ZX	Excision of Left Kidney Pelvis, Percutaneous Endoscopic Approach, Diagnostic
TB44ZZ	Excision of Left Kidney Pelvis, Percutaneous Endoscopic Approach
TB47ZX	Excision of Left Kidney Pelvis, Via Natural or Artificial Opening, Diagnostic
TB47ZZ	Excision of Left Kidney Pelvis, Via Natural or Artificial Opening
TB48ZX	Excision of Left Kidney Pelvis, Via Natural or Artificial Opening Endoscopic, Diagnostic
TB48ZZ	Excision of Left Kidney Pelvis, Via Natural or Artificial Opening Endoscopic
0TB60ZX	Excision of Right Ureter, Open Approach, Diagnostic
0TB60ZZ	Excision of Right Ureter, Open Approach
0TB63ZX	Excision of Right Ureter, Percutaneous Approach, Diagnostic

0TB63ZZ	Excision of Right Ureter, Percutaneous Approach
0TB64ZX	Excision of Right Ureter, Percutaneous Endoscopic Approach, Diagnostic
0TB64ZZ	Excision of Right Ureter, Percutaneous Endoscopic Approach
0TB67ZX	Excision of Right Ureter, Via Natural or Artificial Opening, Diagnostic
0TB67ZZ	Excision of Right Ureter, Via Natural or Artificial Opening
0TB68ZX	Excision of Right Ureter, Via Natural or Artificial Opening Endoscopic, Diagnostic
0TB68ZZ	Excision of Right Ureter, Via Natural or Artificial Opening Endoscopic
0TB70ZX	Excision of Left Ureter, Open Approach, Diagnostic
0TB70ZZ	Excision of Left Ureter, Open Approach
0TB73ZX	Excision of Left Ureter, Percutaneous Approach, Diagnostic
0TB73ZZ	Excision of Left Ureter, Percutaneous Approach
0TB74ZX	Excision of Left Ureter, Percutaneous Endoscopic Approach, Diagnostic
0TB74ZZ	Excision of Left Ureter, Percutaneous Endoscopic Approach
0TB77ZX	Excision of Left Ureter, Via Natural or Artificial Opening, Diagnostic
0TB77ZZ	Excision of Left Ureter, Via Natural or Artificial Opening
0TB78ZX	Excision of Left Ureter, Via Natural or Artificial Opening Endoscopic, Diagnostic
0TB78ZZ	Excision of Left Ureter, Via Natural or Artificial Opening Endoscopic
0TBB0ZX	Excision of Bladder, Open Approach, Diagnostic
0TBB0ZZ	Excision of Bladder, Open Approach
0TBB3ZX	Excision of Bladder, Percutaneous Approach, Diagnostic
0TBB3ZZ	Excision of Bladder, Percutaneous Approach
0TBB4ZX	Excision of Bladder, Percutaneous Endoscopic Approach, Diagnostic
0TBB4ZZ	Excision of Bladder, Percutaneous Endoscopic Approach
0TBB7ZX	Excision of Bladder, Via Natural or Artificial Opening, Diagnostic
0TBB7ZZ	Excision of Bladder, Via Natural or Artificial Opening

0TBB8ZX	Excision of Bladder, Via Natural or Artificial Opening Endoscopic, Diagnostic
0TBB8ZZ	Excision of Bladder, Via Natural or Artificial Opening Endoscopic
	AHA CC: 2Q, 2014, 8
0TBC0ZX	Excision of Bladder Neck, Open Approach, Diagnostic
0TBC0ZZ	Excision of Bladder Neck, Open Approach
0TBC3ZX	Excision of Bladder Neck, Percutaneous Approach, Diagnostic
0TBC3ZZ	Excision of Bladder Neck, Percutaneous Approach
0TBC4ZX	Excision of Bladder Neck, Percutaneous Endoscopic Approach, Diagnostic
0TBC4ZZ	Excision of Bladder Neck, Percutaneous Endoscopic Approach
0TBC7ZX	Excision of Bladder Neck, Via Natural or Artificial Opening, Diagnostic
0TBC7ZZ	Excision of Bladder Neck, Via Natural or Artificial Opening
0TBC8ZX	Excision of Bladder Neck, Via Natural or Artificial Opening Endoscopic, Diagnostic
0TBC8ZZ	Excision of Bladder Neck, Via Natural or Artificial Opening Endoscopic
0TBD0ZX	Excision of Urethra, Open Approach, Diagnostic
0TBD0ZZ	Excision of Urethra, Open Approach
0TBD3ZX	Excision of Urethra, Percutaneous Approach, Diagnostic
0TBD3ZZ	Excision of Urethra, Percutaneous Approach
0TBD4ZX	Excision of Urethra, Percutaneous Endoscopic Approach, Diagnostic
0TBD4ZZ	Excision of Urethra, Percutaneous Endoscopic Approach
0TBD7ZX	Excision of Urethra, Via Natural or Artificial Opening, Diagnostic
0TBD7ZZ	Excision of Urethra, Via Natural or Artificial Opening
0TBD8ZX	Excision of Urethra, Via Natural or Artificial Opening Endoscopic, Diagnostic
0TBD8ZZ	Excision of Urethra, Via Natural or Artificial Opening Endoscopic
0TBDXZX	Excision of Urethra, External Approach, Diagnostic
0TBDXZZ	Excision of Urethra, External Approach

0TC – Urinary System, Extirpation

0TC00ZZ	Extirpation of Matter from Right Kidney, Open Approach
0TC03ZZ	Extirpation of Matter from Right Kidney, Percutaneous Approach
0TC04ZZ	Extirpation of Matter from Right Kidney, Percutaneous Endoscopic Approach
0TC07ZZ	Extirpation of Matter from Right Kidney, Via Natural or Artificial Opening
0TC08ZZ	Extirpation of Matter from Right Kidney, Via Natural or Artificial Opening Endoscopic
0TC10ZZ	Extirpation of Matter from Left Kidney, Open Approach
0TC13ZZ	Extirpation of Matter from Left Kidney, Percutaneous Approach
0TC14ZZ	Extirpation of Matter from Left Kidney, Percutaneous Endoscopic Approach
0TC17ZZ	Extirpation of Matter from Left Kidney, Via Natural or Artificial Opening
0TC18ZZ	Extirpation of Matter from Left Kidney, Via Natural or Artificial Opening Endoscopic
0TC30ZZ	Extirpation of Matter from Right Kidney Pelvis, Open Approach

0TC33ZZ	Extirpation of Matter from Right Kidney Pelvis, Percutaneous Approach
0TC34ZZ	Extirpation of Matter from Right Kidney Pelvis, Percutaneous Endoscopic Approach
0TC37ZZ	Extirpation of Matter from Right Kidney Pelvis, Via Natural or Artificial Opening
0TC38ZZ	Extirpation of Matter from Right Kidney Pelvis, Via Natural or Artificial Opening Endoscopic
0TC40ZZ	Extirpation of Matter from Left Kidney Pelvis, Open Approach
0TC43ZZ	Extirpation of Matter from Left Kidney Pelvis, Percutaneous Approach
0TC44ZZ	Extirpation of Matter from Left Kidney Pelvis, Percutaneous Endoscopic Approach
0TC47ZZ	Extirpation of Matter from Left Kidney Pelvis, Via Natural or Artificial Opening
0TC48ZZ	Extirpation of Matter from Left Kidney Pelvis, Via Natural or Artificial Opening Endoscopic
0TC60ZZ	Extirpation of Matter from Right Ureter, Open Approach

0TC63ZZ	Extirpation of Matter from Right Ureter, Percutaneous Approach
0TC64ZZ	Extirpation of Matter from Right Ureter, Percutaneous Endoscopic Approach
0TC67ZZ	Extirpation of Matter from Right Ureter, Via Natural or Artificial Opening
0TC68ZZ	Extirpation of Matter from Right Ureter, Via Natural or Artificial Opening Endoscopic
	AHA CC: 4Q, 2013, 122-123
0TC70ZZ	Extirpation of Matter from Left Ureter, Open Approach
0TC73ZZ	Extirpation of Matter from Left Ureter, Percutaneous Approach
0TC74ZZ	Extirpation of Matter from Left Ureter, Percutaneous Endoscopic Approach
0TC77ZZ	Extirpation of Matter from Left Ureter, Via Natural or Artificial Opening
0TC78ZZ	Extirpation of Matter from Left Ureter, Via Natural or Artificial Opening Endoscopic
0TCB0ZZ	Extirpation of Matter from Bladder, Open Approach

♀ Female-only	♂ Male-only	▲ Limited Coverage	● Non-OR	▨ HAC-associated procedure	▲ Non-covered procedures	✚ Combination

0TCB3ZZ Extirpation of Matter from Bladder, Percutaneous Approach

0TCB4ZZ Extirpation of Matter from Bladder, Percutaneous Endoscopic Approach

0TCB7ZZ Extirpation of Matter from Bladder, Via Natural or Artificial Opening

0TCB8ZZ Extirpation of Matter from Bladder, Via Natural or Artificial Opening Endoscopic

0TCC0ZZ Extirpation of Matter from Bladder Neck, Open Approach

0TCC3ZZ Extirpation of Matter from Bladder Neck, Percutaneous Approach

0TCC4ZZ Extirpation of Matter from Bladder Neck, Percutaneous Endoscopic Approach

0TCC7ZZ Extirpation of Matter from Bladder Neck, Via Natural or Artificial Opening

0TCC8ZZ Extirpation of Matter from Bladder Neck, Via Natural or Artificial Opening Endoscopic

0TCD0ZZ Extirpation of Matter from Urethra, Open Approach

0TCD3ZZ Extirpation of Matter from Urethra, Percutaneous Approach

0TCD4ZZ Extirpation of Matter from Urethra, Percutaneous Endoscopic Approach

0TCD7ZZ Extirpation of Matter from Urethra, Via Natural or Artificial Opening

0TCD8ZZ Extirpation of Matter from Urethra, Via Natural or Artificial Opening Endoscopic

0TCDXZZ Extirpation of Matter from Urethra, External Approach

0TD – Urinary System, Extraction

0TD00ZZ Extraction of Right Kidney, Open Approach

0TD03ZZ Extraction of Right Kidney, Percutaneous Approach

0TD04ZZ Extraction of Right Kidney, Percutaneous Endoscopic Approach

0TD10ZZ Extraction of Left Kidney, Open Approach

0TD13ZZ Extraction of Left Kidney, Percutaneous Approach

0TD14ZZ Extraction of Left Kidney, Percutaneous Endoscopic Approach

0TF – Urinary System, Fragmentation

0TF30ZZ Fragmentation in Right Kidney Pelvis, Open Approach

0TF33ZZ Fragmentation in Right Kidney Pelvis, Percutaneous Approach

0TF34ZZ Fragmentation in Right Kidney Pelvis, Percutaneous Endoscopic Approach

0TF37ZZ Fragmentation in Right Kidney Pelvis, Via Natural or Artificial Opening

0TF38ZZ Fragmentation in Right Kidney Pelvis, Via Natural or Artificial Opening Endoscopic

● **0TF3XZZ** Fragmentation in Right Kidney Pelvis, External Approach
AHA CC: 4Q, 2013, 122

0TF40ZZ Fragmentation in Left Kidney Pelvis, Open Approach

0TF43ZZ Fragmentation in Left Kidney Pelvis, Percutaneous Approach

0TF44ZZ Fragmentation in Left Kidney Pelvis, Percutaneous Endoscopic Approach

0TF47ZZ Fragmentation in Left Kidney Pelvis, Via Natural or Artificial Opening

0TF48ZZ Fragmentation in Left Kidney Pelvis, Via Natural or Artificial Opening Endoscopic

● **0TF4XZZ** Fragmentation in Left Kidney Pelvis, External Approach

0TF60ZZ Fragmentation in Right Ureter, Open Approach

0TF63ZZ Fragmentation in Right Ureter, Percutaneous Approach

0TF64ZZ Fragmentation in Right Ureter, Percutaneous Endoscopic Approach

0TF67ZZ Fragmentation in Right Ureter, Via Natural or Artificial Opening

0TF68ZZ Fragmentation in Right Ureter, Via Natural or Artificial Opening Endoscopic

● **0TF6XZZ** Fragmentation in Right Ureter, External Approach

0TF70ZZ Fragmentation in Left Ureter, Open Approach

0TF73ZZ Fragmentation in Left Ureter, Percutaneous Approach

0TF74ZZ Fragmentation in Left Ureter, Percutaneous Endoscopic Approach

0TF77ZZ Fragmentation in Left Ureter, Via Natural or Artificial Opening

0TF78ZZ Fragmentation in Left Ureter, Via Natural or Artificial Opening Endoscopic

● **0TF7XZZ** Fragmentation in Left Ureter, External Approach

0TFB0ZZ Fragmentation in Bladder, Open Approach

0TFB3ZZ Fragmentation in Bladder, Percutaneous Approach

0TFB4ZZ Fragmentation in Bladder, Percutaneous Endoscopic Approach

0TFB7ZZ Fragmentation in Bladder, Via Natural or Artificial Opening

0TFB8ZZ Fragmentation in Bladder, Via Natural or Artificial Opening Endoscopic

● **0TFBXZZ** Fragmentation in Bladder, External Approach

0TFC0ZZ Fragmentation in Bladder Neck, Open Approach

0TFC3ZZ Fragmentation in Bladder Neck, Percutaneous Approach

0TFC4ZZ Fragmentation in Bladder Neck, Percutaneous Endoscopic Approach

0TFC7ZZ Fragmentation in Bladder Neck, Via Natural or Artificial Opening

0TFC8ZZ Fragmentation in Bladder Neck, Via Natural or Artificial Opening Endoscopic

● **0TFCXZZ** Fragmentation in Bladder Neck, External Approach

0TFD0ZZ Fragmentation in Urethra, Open Approach

0TFD3ZZ Fragmentation in Urethra, Percutaneous Approach

0TFD4ZZ Fragmentation in Urethra, Percutaneous Endoscopic Approach

0TFD7ZZ Fragmentation in Urethra, Via Natural or Artificial Opening

▲ **0TFD8ZZ** Fragmentation in Urethra, Via Natural or Artificial Opening Endoscopic

0TFDXZZ Fragmentation in Urethra, External Approach

0TH – Urinary System, Insertion

0TH502Z Insertion of Monitoring Device into Kidney, Open Approach

0TH503Z Insertion of Infusion Device into Kidney, Open Approach

0TH532Z Insertion of Monitoring Device into Kidney, Percutaneous Approach

0TH533Z Insertion of Infusion Device into Kidney, Percutaneous Approach

0TH542Z Insertion of Monitoring Device into Kidney, Percutaneous Endoscopic Approach

0TH543Z Insertion of Infusion Device into Kidney, Percutaneous Endoscopic Approach

0TH572Z Insertion of Monitoring Device into Kidney, Via Natural or Artificial Opening

0TH573Z Insertion of Infusion Device into Kidney, Via Natural or Artificial Opening

0TH582Z Insertion of Monitoring Device into Kidney, Via Natural or Artificial Opening Endoscopic

0TH583Z Insertion of Infusion Device into Kidney, Via Natural or Artificial Opening Endoscopic

0TH902Z Insertion of Monitoring Device into Ureter, Open Approach

0TH903Z Insertion of Infusion Device into Ureter, Open Approach

0TH90MZ Insertion of Stimulator Lead into Ureter, Open Approach

0TH932Z Insertion of Monitoring Device into Ureter, Percutaneous Approach

0TH933Z Insertion of Infusion Device into Ureter, Percutaneous Approach

0TH93MZ Insertion of Stimulator Lead into Ureter, Percutaneous Approach

0TH942Z Insertion of Monitoring Device into Ureter, Percutaneous Endoscopic Approach

0TH943Z Insertion of Infusion Device into Ureter, Percutaneous Endoscopic Approach

0TH94MZ Insertion of Stimulator Lead into Ureter, Percutaneous Endoscopic Approach

0TH972Z Insertion of Monitoring Device into Ureter, Via Natural or Artificial Opening

0TH973Z Insertion of Infusion Device into Ureter, Via Natural or Artificial Opening

0TH97MZ Insertion of Stimulator Lead into Ureter, Via Natural or Artificial Opening

0TH982Z Insertion of Monitoring Device into Ureter, Via Natural or Artificial Opening Endoscopic

0TH983Z Insertion of Infusion Device into Ureter, Via Natural or Artificial Opening Endoscopic

0TH98MZ Insertion of Stimulator Lead into Ureter, Via Natural or Artificial Opening Endoscopic

0THB02Z Insertion of Monitoring Device into Bladder, Open Approach

0THB03Z Insertion of Infusion Device into Bladder, Open Approach

0THB0LZ Insertion of Artificial Sphincter into Bladder, Open Approach

▲ **0THB0MZ** Insertion of Stimulator Lead into Bladder, Open Approach

0THB32Z Insertion of Monitoring Device into Bladder, Percutaneous Approach

0THB33Z Insertion of Infusion Device into Bladder, Percutaneous Approach

0THB3LZ	Insertion of Artificial Sphincter into Bladder, Percutaneous Approach	0THB8LZ	Insertion of Artificial Sphincter into Bladder, Via Natural or Artificial Opening Endoscopic	0THD42Z	Insertion of Monitoring Device into Urethra, Percutaneous Endoscopic Approach

0THB3MZ Insertion of Stimulator Lead into Bladder, Percutaneous Approach

0THB42Z Insertion of Monitoring Device into Bladder, Percutaneous Endoscopic Approach

0THB43Z Insertion of Infusion Device into Bladder, Percutaneous Endoscopic Approach

0THB4LZ Insertion of Artificial Sphincter into Bladder, Percutaneous Endoscopic Approach

0THB4MZ Insertion of Stimulator Lead into Bladder, Percutaneous Endoscopic Approach

0THB72Z Insertion of Monitoring Device into Bladder, Via Natural or Artificial Opening

0THB73Z Insertion of Infusion Device into Bladder, Via Natural or Artificial Opening

0THB7LZ Insertion of Artificial Sphincter into Bladder, Via Natural or Artificial Opening

0THB7MZ Insertion of Stimulator Lead into Bladder, Via Natural or Artificial Opening

0THB82Z Insertion of Monitoring Device into Bladder, Via Natural or Artificial Opening Endoscopic

0THB83Z Insertion of Infusion Device into Bladder, Via Natural or Artificial Opening Endoscopic

0THB8LZ Insertion of Artificial Sphincter into Bladder, Via Natural or Artificial Opening Endoscopic

▲ 0THB8MZ Insertion of Stimulator Lead into Bladder, Via Natural or Artificial Opening Endoscopic

0THC0LZ Insertion of Artificial Sphincter into Bladder Neck, Open Approach

0THC3LZ Insertion of Artificial Sphincter into Bladder Neck, Percutaneous Approach

0THC4LZ Insertion of Artificial Sphincter into Bladder Neck, Percutaneous Endoscopic Approach

0THC7LZ Insertion of Artificial Sphincter into Bladder Neck, Via Natural or Artificial Opening

0THC8LZ Insertion of Artificial Sphincter into Bladder Neck, Via Natural or Artificial Opening Endoscopic

0THD02Z Insertion of Monitoring Device into Urethra, Open Approach

0THD03Z Insertion of Infusion Device into Urethra, Open Approach

0THD0LZ Insertion of Artificial Sphincter into Urethra, Open Approach

0THD32Z Insertion of Monitoring Device into Urethra, Percutaneous Approach

0THD33Z Insertion of Infusion Device into Urethra, Percutaneous Approach

0THD3LZ Insertion of Artificial Sphincter into Urethra, Percutaneous Approach

0THD42Z Insertion of Monitoring Device into Urethra, Percutaneous Endoscopic Approach

0THD43Z Insertion of Infusion Device into Urethra, Percutaneous Endoscopic Approach

0THD4LZ Insertion of Artificial Sphincter into Urethra, Percutaneous Endoscopic Approach

0THD72Z Insertion of Monitoring Device into Urethra, Via Natural or Artificial Opening

0THD73Z Insertion of Infusion Device into Urethra, Via Natural or Artificial Opening

0THD7LZ Insertion of Artificial Sphincter into Urethra, Via Natural or Artificial Opening

0THD82Z Insertion of Monitoring Device into Urethra, Via Natural or Artificial Opening Endoscopic

0THD83Z Insertion of Infusion Device into Urethra, Via Natural or Artificial Opening Endoscopic

0THD8LZ Insertion of Artificial Sphincter into Urethra, Via Natural or Artificial Opening Endoscopic

0THDX2Z Insertion of Monitoring Device into Urethra, External Approach

0THDX3Z Insertion of Infusion Device into Urethra, External Approach

0THDXLZ Insertion of Artificial Sphincter into Urethra, External Approach

0TJ – Urinary System, Inspection

Review Coding Guidelines B3.11a, B3.11b and B3.11c

0TJ50ZZ Inspection of Kidney, Open Approach

0TJ53ZZ Inspection of Kidney, Percutaneous Approach

0TJ54ZZ Inspection of Kidney, Percutaneous Endoscopic Approach

0TJ57ZZ Inspection of Kidney, Via Natural or Artificial Opening

0TJ58ZZ Inspection of Kidney, Via Natural or Artificial Opening Endoscopic

0TJ5XZZ Inspection of Kidney, External Approach

0TJ90ZZ Inspection of Ureter, Open Approach

0TJ93ZZ Inspection of Ureter, Percutaneous Approach

0TJ94ZZ Inspection of Ureter, Percutaneous Endoscopic Approach

0TJ97ZZ Inspection of Ureter, Via Natural or Artificial Opening

0TJ98ZZ Inspection of Ureter, Via Natural or Artificial Opening Endoscopic

0TJ9XZZ Inspection of Ureter, External Approach

0TJB0ZZ Inspection of Bladder, Open Approach

0TJB3ZZ Inspection of Bladder, Percutaneous Approach

0TJB4ZZ Inspection of Bladder, Percutaneous Endoscopic Approach

0TJB7ZZ Inspection of Bladder, Via Natural or Artificial Opening

0TJB8ZZ Inspection of Bladder, Via Natural or Artificial Opening Endoscopic

0TJBXZZ Inspection of Bladder, External Approach

0TJD0ZZ Inspection of Urethra, Open Approach

0TJD3ZZ Inspection of Urethra, Percutaneous Approach

0TJD4ZZ Inspection of Urethra, Percutaneous Endoscopic Approach

0TJD7ZZ Inspection of Urethra, Via Natural or Artificial Opening

0TJD8ZZ Inspection of Urethra, Via Natural or Artificial Opening Endoscopic

0TJDXZZ Inspection of Urethra, External Approach

0TL – Urinary System, Occlusion

0TL30CZ Occlusion of Right Kidney Pelvis with Extraluminal Device, Open Approach

0TL30DZ Occlusion of Right Kidney Pelvis with Intraluminal Device, Open Approach

0TL30ZZ Occlusion of Right Kidney Pelvis, Open Approach

0TL33CZ Occlusion of Right Kidney Pelvis with Extraluminal Device, Percutaneous Approach

0TL33DZ Occlusion of Right Kidney Pelvis with Intraluminal Device, Percutaneous Approach

0TL33ZZ Occlusion of Right Kidney Pelvis, Percutaneous Approach

0TL34CZ Occlusion of Right Kidney Pelvis with Extraluminal Device, Percutaneous Endoscopic Approach

0TL34DZ Occlusion of Right Kidney Pelvis with Intraluminal Device, Percutaneous Endoscopic Approach

0TL34ZZ Occlusion of Right Kidney Pelvis, Percutaneous Endoscopic Approach

0TL37DZ Occlusion of Right Kidney Pelvis with Intraluminal Device, Via Natural or Artificial Opening

0TL37ZZ Occlusion of Right Kidney Pelvis, Via Natural or Artificial Opening

0TL38DZ Occlusion of Right Kidney Pelvis with Intraluminal Device, Via Natural or Artificial Opening Endoscopic

0TL38ZZ Occlusion of Right Kidney Pelvis, Via Natural or Artificial Opening Endoscopic

0TL40CZ Occlusion of Left Kidney Pelvis with Extraluminal Device, Open Approach

0TL40DZ Occlusion of Left Kidney Pelvis with Intraluminal Device, Open Approach

0TL40ZZ Occlusion of Left Kidney Pelvis, Open Approach

0TL43CZ Occlusion of Left Kidney Pelvis with Extraluminal Device, Percutaneous Approach

0TL43DZ Occlusion of Left Kidney Pelvis with Intraluminal Device, Percutaneous Approach

0TL43ZZ Occlusion of Left Kidney Pelvis, Percutaneous Approach

0TL44CZ Occlusion of Left Kidney Pelvis with Extraluminal Device, Percutaneous Endoscopic Approach

0TL44DZ Occlusion of Left Kidney Pelvis with Intraluminal Device, Percutaneous Endoscopic Approach

0TL44ZZ Occlusion of Left Kidney Pelvis, Percutaneous Endoscopic Approach

0TL47DZ Occlusion of Left Kidney Pelvis with Intraluminal Device, Via Natural or Artificial Opening

0TL47ZZ Occlusion of Left Kidney Pelvis, Via Natural or Artificial Opening

0TL48DZ Occlusion of Left Kidney Pelvis with Intraluminal Device, Via Natural or Artificial Opening Endoscopic

0TL48ZZ Occlusion of Left Kidney Pelvis, Via Natural or Artificial Opening Endoscopic

0TL60CZ Occlusion of Right Ureter with Extraluminal Device, Open Approach

♀ Female-only   ♂ Male-only   ▲ Limited Coverage   ● Non-OR   ▨ HAC-associated procedure   ▲ Non-covered procedures   ✛ Combination

Code	Description	Code	Description	Code	Description
0TL60DZ	Occlusion of Right Ureter with Intraluminal Device, Open Approach	0TL77DZ	Occlusion of Left Ureter with Intraluminal Device, Via Natural or Artificial Opening	0TLC4CZ	Occlusion of Bladder Neck with Extraluminal Device, Percutaneous Endoscopic Approach
0TL60ZZ	Occlusion of Right Ureter, Open Approach	0TL77ZZ	Occlusion of Left Ureter, Via Natural or Artificial Opening	0TLC4DZ	Occlusion of Bladder Neck with Intraluminal Device, Percutaneous Endoscopic Approach
0TL63CZ	Occlusion of Right Ureter with Extraluminal Device, Percutaneous Approach	0TL78DZ	Occlusion of Left Ureter with Intraluminal Device, Via Natural or Artificial Opening Endoscopic	0TLC4ZZ	Occlusion of Bladder Neck, Percutaneous Endoscopic Approach
0TL63DZ	Occlusion of Right Ureter with Intraluminal Device, Percutaneous Approach	0TL78ZZ	Occlusion of Left Ureter, Via Natural or Artificial Opening Endoscopic	0TLC7DZ	Occlusion of Bladder Neck with Intraluminal Device, Via Natural or Artificial Opening
0TL63ZZ	Occlusion of Right Ureter, Percutaneous Approach	0TLB0CZ	Occlusion of Bladder with Extraluminal Device, Open Approach	0TLC7ZZ	Occlusion of Bladder Neck, Via Natural or Artificial Opening
0TL64CZ	Occlusion of Right Ureter with Extraluminal Device, Percutaneous Endoscopic Approach	0TLB0DZ	Occlusion of Bladder with Intraluminal Device, Open Approach	0TLC8DZ	Occlusion of Bladder Neck with Intraluminal Device, Via Natural or Artificial Opening Endoscopic
0TL64DZ	Occlusion of Right Ureter with Intraluminal Device, Percutaneous Endoscopic Approach	0TLB0ZZ	Occlusion of Bladder, Open Approach	0TLC8ZZ	Occlusion of Bladder Neck, Via Natural or Artificial Opening Endoscopic
0TL64ZZ	Occlusion of Right Ureter, Percutaneous Endoscopic Approach	0TLB3CZ	Occlusion of Bladder with Extraluminal Device, Percutaneous Approach	0TLD0CZ	Occlusion of Urethra with Extraluminal Device, Open Approach
0TL67DZ	Occlusion of Right Ureter with Intraluminal Device, Via Natural or Artificial Opening	0TLB3DZ	Occlusion of Bladder with Intraluminal Device, Percutaneous Approach	0TLD0DZ	Occlusion of Urethra with Intraluminal Device, Open Approach
0TL67ZZ	Occlusion of Right Ureter, Via Natural or Artificial Opening	0TLB3ZZ	Occlusion of Bladder, Percutaneous Approach	0TLD0ZZ	Occlusion of Urethra, Open Approach
0TL68DZ	Occlusion of Right Ureter with Intraluminal Device, Via Natural or Artificial Opening Endoscopic	0TLB4CZ	Occlusion of Bladder with Extraluminal Device, Percutaneous Endoscopic Approach	0TLD3CZ	Occlusion of Urethra with Extraluminal Device, Percutaneous Approach
0TL68ZZ	Occlusion of Right Ureter, Via Natural or Artificial Opening Endoscopic	0TLB4DZ	Occlusion of Bladder with Intraluminal Device, Percutaneous Endoscopic Approach	0TLD3DZ	Occlusion of Urethra with Intraluminal Device, Percutaneous Approach
0TL70CZ	Occlusion of Left Ureter with Extraluminal Device, Open Approach	0TLB4ZZ	Occlusion of Bladder, Percutaneous Endoscopic Approach	0TLD3ZZ	Occlusion of Urethra, Percutaneous Approach
0TL70DZ	Occlusion of Left Ureter with Intraluminal Device, Open Approach	0TLB7DZ	Occlusion of Bladder with Intraluminal Device, Via Natural or Artificial Opening	0TLD4CZ	Occlusion of Urethra with Extraluminal Device, Percutaneous Endoscopic Approach
0TL70ZZ	Occlusion of Left Ureter, Open Approach	0TLB7ZZ	Occlusion of Bladder, Via Natural or Artificial Opening	0TLD4DZ	Occlusion of Urethra with Intraluminal Device, Percutaneous Endoscopic Approach
0TL73CZ	Occlusion of Left Ureter with Extraluminal Device, Percutaneous Approach	0TLB8DZ	Occlusion of Bladder with Intraluminal Device, Via Natural or Artificial Opening Endoscopic	0TLD4ZZ	Occlusion of Urethra, Percutaneous Endoscopic Approach
0TL73DZ	Occlusion of Left Ureter with Intraluminal Device, Percutaneous Approach	0TLB8ZZ	Occlusion of Bladder, Via Natural or Artificial Opening Endoscopic	0TLD7DZ	Occlusion of Urethra with Intraluminal Device, Via Natural or Artificial Opening
0TL73ZZ	Occlusion of Left Ureter, Percutaneous Approach	0TLC0CZ	Occlusion of Bladder Neck with Extraluminal Device, Open Approach	0TLD7ZZ	Occlusion of Urethra, Via Natural or Artificial Opening
0TL74CZ	Occlusion of Left Ureter with Extraluminal Device, Percutaneous Endoscopic Approach	0TLC0DZ	Occlusion of Bladder Neck with Intraluminal Device, Open Approach	0TLD8DZ	Occlusion of Urethra with Intraluminal Device, Via Natural or Artificial Opening Endoscopic
0TL74DZ	Occlusion of Left Ureter with Intraluminal Device, Percutaneous Endoscopic Approach	0TLC0ZZ	Occlusion of Bladder Neck, Open Approach	0TLD8ZZ	Occlusion of Urethra, Via Natural or Artificial Opening Endoscopic
0TL74ZZ	Occlusion of Left Ureter, Percutaneous Endoscopic Approach	0TLC3CZ	Occlusion of Bladder Neck with Extraluminal Device, Percutaneous Approach	0TLDXCZ	Occlusion of Urethra with Extraluminal Device, External Approach
		0TLC3DZ	Occlusion of Bladder Neck with Intraluminal Device, Percutaneous Approach	0TLDXDZ	Occlusion of Urethra with Intraluminal Device, External Approach
		0TLC3ZZ	Occlusion of Bladder Neck, Percutaneous Approach	0TLDXZZ	Occlusion of Urethra, External Approach

0TM – Urinary System, Reattachment

Code	Description	Code	Description	Code	Description
0TM00ZZ	Reattachment of Right Kidney, Open Approach	0TM34ZZ	Reattachment of Right Kidney Pelvis, Percutaneous Endoscopic Approach	0TM80ZZ	Reattachment of Bilateral Ureters, Open Approach
0TM04ZZ	Reattachment of Right Kidney, Percutaneous Endoscopic Approach	0TM40ZZ	Reattachment of Left Kidney Pelvis, Open Approach	0TM84ZZ	Reattachment of Bilateral Ureters, Percutaneous Endoscopic Approach
0TM10ZZ	Reattachment of Left Kidney, Open Approach	0TM44ZZ	Reattachment of Left Kidney Pelvis, Percutaneous Endoscopic Approach	0TMB0ZZ	Reattachment of Bladder, Open Approach
0TM14ZZ	Reattachment of Left Kidney, Percutaneous Endoscopic Approach	0TM60ZZ	Reattachment of Right Ureter, Open Approach	0TMB4ZZ	Reattachment of Bladder, Percutaneous Endoscopic Approach
0TM20ZZ	Reattachment of Bilateral Kidneys, Open Approach	0TM64ZZ	Reattachment of Right Ureter, Percutaneous Endoscopic Approach	0TMC0ZZ	Reattachment of Bladder Neck, Open Approach
0TM24ZZ	Reattachment of Bilateral Kidneys, Percutaneous Endoscopic Approach	0TM70ZZ	Reattachment of Left Ureter, Open Approach	0TMC4ZZ	Reattachment of Bladder Neck, Percutaneous Endoscopic Approach
0TM30ZZ	Reattachment of Right Kidney Pelvis, Open Approach	0TM74ZZ	Reattachment of Left Ureter, Percutaneous Endoscopic Approach	0TMD0ZZ	Reattachment of Urethra, Open Approach
				0TMD4ZZ	Reattachment of Urethra, Percutaneous Endoscopic Approach

0TN – Urinary System, Release

Review Coding Guideline B3.13

Review Coding Guideline B3.14

Code	Description	Code	Description	Code	Description
0TN00ZZ	Release Right Kidney, Open Approach	0TN03ZZ	Release Right Kidney, Percutaneous Approach	0TN04ZZ	Release Right Kidney, Percutaneous Endoscopic Approach

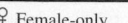 Female-only   ♂ Male-only   ▲ Limited Coverage   ● Non-OR   ▦ HAC-associated procedure   ▲ Non-covered procedures   ✚ Combination

0TN07ZZ	Release Right Kidney, Via Natural or Artificial Opening	0TN43ZZ	Release Left Kidney Pelvis, Percutaneous Approach	0TNB0ZZ	Release Bladder, Open Approach
0TN08ZZ	Release Right Kidney, Via Natural or Artificial Opening Endoscopic	0TN44ZZ	Release Left Kidney Pelvis, Percutaneous Endoscopic Approach	0TNB3ZZ	Release Bladder, Percutaneous Approach
0TN10ZZ	Release Left Kidney, Open Approach			0TNB4ZZ	Release Bladder, Percutaneous Endoscopic Approach
0TN13ZZ	Release Left Kidney, Percutaneous Approach	0TN47ZZ	Release Left Kidney Pelvis, Via Natural or Artificial Opening	0TNB7ZZ	Release Bladder, Via Natural or Artificial Opening
0TN14ZZ	Release Left Kidney, Percutaneous Endoscopic Approach	0TN48ZZ	Release Left Kidney Pelvis, Via Natural or Artificial Opening Endoscopic	0TNB8ZZ	Release Bladder, Via Natural or Artificial Opening Endoscopic
0TN17ZZ	Release Left Kidney, Via Natural or Artificial Opening	0TN60ZZ	Release Right Ureter, Open Approach	0TNC0ZZ	Release Bladder Neck, Open Approach
0TN18ZZ	Release Left Kidney, Via Natural or Artificial Opening Endoscopic	0TN63ZZ	Release Right Ureter, Percutaneous Approach	0TNC3ZZ	Release Bladder Neck, Percutaneous Approach
0TN30ZZ	Release Right Kidney Pelvis, Open Approach	0TN64ZZ	Release Right Ureter, Percutaneous Endoscopic Approach	0TNC4ZZ	Release Bladder Neck, Percutaneous Endoscopic Approach
0TN33ZZ	Release Right Kidney Pelvis, Percutaneous Approach	0TN67ZZ	Release Right Ureter, Via Natural or Artificial Opening	0TNC7ZZ	Release Bladder Neck, Via Natural or Artificial Opening
0TN34ZZ	Release Right Kidney Pelvis, Percutaneous Endoscopic Approach	0TN68ZZ	Release Right Ureter, Via Natural or Artificial Opening Endoscopic	0TNC8ZZ	Release Bladder Neck, Via Natural or Artificial Opening Endoscopic
0TN37ZZ	Release Right Kidney Pelvis, Via Natural or Artificial Opening	0TN70ZZ	Release Left Ureter, Open Approach	0TND0ZZ	Release Urethra, Open Approach
0TN38ZZ	Release Right Kidney Pelvis, Via Natural or Artificial Opening Endoscopic	0TN73ZZ	Release Left Ureter, Percutaneous Approach	0TND3ZZ	Release Urethra, Percutaneous Approach
0TN40ZZ	Release Left Kidney Pelvis, Open Approach	0TN74ZZ	Release Left Ureter, Percutaneous Endoscopic Approach	0TND4ZZ	Release Urethra, Percutaneous Endoscopic Approach
		0TN77ZZ	Release Left Ureter, Via Natural or Artificial Opening	0TND7ZZ	Release Urethra, Via Natural or Artificial Opening
		0TN78ZZ	Release Left Ureter, Via Natural or Artificial Opening Endoscopic	0TND8ZZ	Release Urethra, Via Natural or Artificial Opening Endoscopic
				0TNDXZZ	Release Urethra, External Approach

0TP – Urinary System, Removal

Review Coding Guideline B6.1c

0TP500Z	Removal of Drainage Device from Kidney, Open Approach	0TP54DZ	Removal of Intraluminal Device from Kidney, Percutaneous Endoscopic Approach	0TP58JZ	Removal of Synthetic Substitute from Kidney, Via Natural or Artificial Opening Endoscopic
0TP502Z	Removal of Monitoring Device from Kidney, Open Approach	0TP54JZ	Removal of Synthetic Substitute from Kidney, Percutaneous Endoscopic Approach	0TP58KZ	Removal of Nonautologous Tissue Substitute from Kidney, Via Natural or Artificial Opening Endoscopic
0TP503Z	Removal of Infusion Device from Kidney, Open Approach	0TP54KZ	Removal of Nonautologous Tissue Substitute from Kidney, Percutaneous Endoscopic Approach	0TP5X0Z	Removal of Drainage Device from Kidney, External Approach
0TP507Z	Removal of Autologous Tissue Substitute from Kidney, Open Approach	0TP570Z	Removal of Drainage Device from Kidney, Via Natural or Artificial Opening	0TP5X2Z	Removal of Monitoring Device from Kidney, External Approach
0TP50CZ	Removal of Extraluminal Device from Kidney, Open Approach	0TP572Z	Removal of Monitoring Device from Kidney, Via Natural or Artificial Opening	0TP5X3Z	Removal of Infusion Device from Kidney, External Approach
0TP50DZ	Removal of Intraluminal Device from Kidney, Open Approach	0TP573Z	Removal of Infusion Device from Kidney, Via Natural or Artificial Opening	0TP5XDZ	Removal of Intraluminal Device from Kidney, External Approach
0TP50JZ	Removal of Synthetic Substitute from Kidney, Open Approach	0TP577Z	Removal of Autologous Tissue Substitute from Kidney, Via Natural or Artificial Opening	0TP900Z	Removal of Drainage Device from Ureter, Open Approach
0TP50KZ	Removal of Nonautologous Tissue Substitute from Kidney, Open Approach	0TP57CZ	Removal of Extraluminal Device from Kidney, Via Natural or Artificial Opening	0TP902Z	Removal of Monitoring Device from Ureter, Open Approach
0TP530Z	Removal of Drainage Device from Kidney, Percutaneous Approach	0TP57DZ	Removal of Intraluminal Device from Kidney, Via Natural or Artificial Opening	0TP903Z	Removal of Infusion Device from Ureter, Open Approach
0TP532Z	Removal of Monitoring Device from Kidney, Percutaneous Approach	0TP57JZ	Removal of Synthetic Substitute from Kidney, Via Natural or Artificial Opening	0TP907Z	Removal of Autologous Tissue Substitute from Ureter, Open Approach
0TP533Z	Removal of Infusion Device from Kidney, Percutaneous Approach	0TP57KZ	Removal of Nonautologous Tissue Substitute from Kidney, Via Natural or Artificial Opening	0TP90CZ	Removal of Extraluminal Device from Ureter, Open Approach
0TP537Z	Removal of Autologous Tissue Substitute from Kidney, Percutaneous Approach	0TP580Z	Removal of Drainage Device from Kidney, Via Natural or Artificial Opening Endoscopic	0TP90DZ	Removal of Intraluminal Device from Ureter, Open Approach
0TP53CZ	Removal of Extraluminal Device from Kidney, Percutaneous Approach	0TP582Z	Removal of Monitoring Device from Kidney, Via Natural or Artificial Opening Endoscopic	0TP90JZ	Removal of Synthetic Substitute from Ureter, Open Approach
0TP53DZ	Removal of Intraluminal Device from Kidney, Percutaneous Approach	0TP583Z	Removal of Infusion Device from Kidney, Via Natural or Artificial Opening Endoscopic	0TP90KZ	Removal of Nonautologous Tissue Substitute from Ureter, Open Approach
0TP53JZ	Removal of Synthetic Substitute from Kidney, Percutaneous Approach	0TP587Z	Removal of Autologous Tissue Substitute from Kidney, Via Natural or Artificial Opening Endoscopic	0TP90MZ	Removal of Stimulator Lead from Ureter, Open Approach
0TP53KZ	Removal of Nonautologous Tissue Substitute from Kidney, Percutaneous Approach	0TP58CZ	Removal of Extraluminal Device from Kidney, Via Natural or Artificial Opening Endoscopic	0TP930Z	Removal of Drainage Device from Ureter, Percutaneous Approach
0TP540Z	Removal of Drainage Device from Kidney, Percutaneous Endoscopic Approach	0TP58DZ	Removal of Intraluminal Device from Kidney, Via Natural or Artificial Opening Endoscopic	0TP932Z	Removal of Monitoring Device from Ureter, Percutaneous Approach
0TP542Z	Removal of Monitoring Device from Kidney, Percutaneous Endoscopic Approach			0TP933Z	Removal of Infusion Device from Ureter, Percutaneous Approach
0TP543Z	Removal of Infusion Device from Kidney, Percutaneous Endoscopic Approach			0TP937Z	Removal of Autologous Tissue Substitute from Ureter, Percutaneous Approach
0TP547Z	Removal of Autologous Tissue Substitute from Kidney, Percutaneous Endoscopic Approach			0TP93CZ	Removal of Extraluminal Device from Ureter, Percutaneous Approach
0TP54CZ	Removal of Extraluminal Device from Kidney, Percutaneous Endoscopic Approach			0TP93DZ	Removal of Intraluminal Device from Ureter, Percutaneous Approach
				0TP93JZ	Removal of Synthetic Substitute from Ureter, Percutaneous Approach

♀ Female-only ♂ Male-only ▲ Limited Coverage ● Non-OR ▨ HAC-associated procedure ▲ Non-covered procedures ✚ Combination

0TP93KZ	Removal of Nonautologous Tissue Substitute from Ureter, Percutaneous Approach	**0TP9X0Z**	Removal of Drainage Device from Ureter, External Approach	**0TPB4LZ**	Removal of Artificial Sphincter from Bladder, Percutaneous Endoscopic Approach
0TP93MZ	Removal of Stimulator Lead from Ureter, Percutaneous Approach	**0TP9X2Z**	Removal of Monitoring Device from Ureter, External Approach	▲ **0TPB4MZ**	Removal of Stimulator Lead from Bladder, Percutaneous Endoscopic Approach
0TP940Z	Removal of Drainage Device from Ureter, Percutaneous Endoscopic Approach	**0TP9X3Z**	Removal of Infusion Device from Ureter, External Approach	**0TPB70Z**	Removal of Drainage Device from Bladder, Via Natural or Artificial Opening
0TP942Z	Removal of Monitoring Device from Ureter, Percutaneous Endoscopic Approach	**0TP9XDZ**	Removal of Intraluminal Device from Ureter, External Approach	**0TPB72Z**	Removal of Monitoring Device from Bladder, Via Natural or Artificial Opening
0TP943Z	Removal of Infusion Device from Ureter, Percutaneous Endoscopic Approach	**0TP9XMZ**	Removal of Stimulator Lead from Ureter, External Approach	**0TPB73Z**	Removal of Infusion Device from Bladder, Via Natural or Artificial Opening
0TP947Z	Removal of Autologous Tissue Substitute from Ureter, Percutaneous Endoscopic Approach	**0TPB00Z**	Removal of Drainage Device from Bladder, Open Approach	**0TPB77Z**	Removal of Autologous Tissue Substitute from Bladder, Via Natural or Artificial Opening
0TP94CZ	Removal of Extraluminal Device from Ureter, Percutaneous Endoscopic Approach	**0TPB02Z**	Removal of Monitoring Device from Bladder, Open Approach	**0TPB7CZ**	Removal of Extraluminal Device from Bladder, Via Natural or Artificial Opening
0TP94DZ	Removal of Intraluminal Device from Ureter, Percutaneous Endoscopic Approach	**0TPB03Z**	Removal of Infusion Device from Bladder, Open Approach	**0TPB7DZ**	Removal of Intraluminal Device from Bladder, Via Natural or Artificial Opening
0TP94JZ	Removal of Synthetic Substitute from Ureter, Percutaneous Endoscopic Approach	**0TPB07Z**	Removal of Autologous Tissue Substitute from Bladder, Open Approach	**0TPB7JZ**	Removal of Synthetic Substitute from Bladder, Via Natural or Artificial Opening
0TP94KZ	Removal of Nonautologous Tissue Substitute from Ureter, Percutaneous Endoscopic Approach	**0TPB0CZ**	Removal of Extraluminal Device from Bladder, Open Approach	**0TPB7KZ**	Removal of Nonautologous Tissue Substitute from Bladder, Via Natural or Artificial Opening
0TP94MZ	Removal of Stimulator Lead from Ureter, Percutaneous Endoscopic Approach	**0TPB0DZ**	Removal of Intraluminal Device from Bladder, Open Approach	**0TPB7LZ**	Removal of Artificial Sphincter from Bladder, Via Natural or Artificial Opening
0TP970Z	Removal of Drainage Device from Ureter, Via Natural or Artificial Opening	**0TPB0JZ**	Removal of Synthetic Substitute from Bladder, Open Approach	▲ **0TPB7MZ**	Removal of Stimulator Lead from Bladder, Via Natural or Artificial Opening
0TP972Z	Removal of Monitoring Device from Ureter, Via Natural or Artificial Opening	**0TPB0KZ**	Removal of Nonautologous Tissue Substitute from Bladder, Open Approach	**0TPB80Z**	Removal of Drainage Device from Bladder, Via Natural or Artificial Opening Endoscopic
0TP973Z	Removal of Infusion Device from Ureter, Via Natural or Artificial Opening	**0TPB0LZ**	Removal of Artificial Sphincter from Bladder, Open Approach	**0TPB82Z**	Removal of Monitoring Device from Bladder, Via Natural or Artificial Opening Endoscopic
0TP977Z	Removal of Autologous Tissue Substitute from Ureter, Via Natural or Artificial Opening	▲ **0TPB0MZ**	Removal of Stimulator Lead from Bladder, Open Approach	**0TPB83Z**	Removal of Infusion Device from Bladder, Via Natural or Artificial Opening Endoscopic
0TP97CZ	Removal of Extraluminal Device from Ureter, Via Natural or Artificial Opening	**0TPB30Z**	Removal of Drainage Device from Bladder, Percutaneous Approach	**0TPB87Z**	Removal of Autologous Tissue Substitute from Bladder, Via Natural or Artificial Opening Endoscopic
0TP97DZ	Removal of Intraluminal Device from Ureter, Via Natural or Artificial Opening	**0TPB32Z**	Removal of Monitoring Device from Bladder, Percutaneous Approach	**0TPB8CZ**	Removal of Extraluminal Device from Bladder, Via Natural or Artificial Opening Endoscopic
0TP97JZ	Removal of Synthetic Substitute from Ureter, Via Natural or Artificial Opening	**0TPB33Z**	Removal of Infusion Device from Bladder, Percutaneous Approach	**0TPB8DZ**	Removal of Intraluminal Device from Bladder, Via Natural or Artificial Opening Endoscopic
0TP97KZ	Removal of Nonautologous Tissue Substitute from Ureter, Via Natural or Artificial Opening	**0TPB37Z**	Removal of Autologous Tissue Substitute from Bladder, Percutaneous Approach	**0TPB8JZ**	Removal of Synthetic Substitute from Bladder, Via Natural or Artificial Opening Endoscopic
0TP97MZ	Removal of Stimulator Lead from Ureter, Via Natural or Artificial Opening	**0TPB3CZ**	Removal of Extraluminal Device from Bladder, Percutaneous Approach	**0TPB8KZ**	Removal of Nonautologous Tissue Substitute from Bladder, Via Natural or Artificial Opening Endoscopic
0TP980Z	Removal of Drainage Device from Ureter, Via Natural or Artificial Opening Endoscopic	**0TPB3DZ**	Removal of Intraluminal Device from Bladder, Percutaneous Approach	**0TPB8LZ**	Removal of Artificial Sphincter from Bladder, Via Natural or Artificial Opening Endoscopic
0TP982Z	Removal of Monitoring Device from Ureter, Via Natural or Artificial Opening Endoscopic	**0TPB3JZ**	Removal of Synthetic Substitute from Bladder, Percutaneous Approach	▲ **0TPB8MZ**	Removal of Stimulator Lead from Bladder, Via Natural or Artificial Opening Endoscopic
0TP983Z	Removal of Infusion Device from Ureter, Via Natural or Artificial Opening Endoscopic	**0TPB3KZ**	Removal of Nonautologous Tissue Substitute from Bladder, Percutaneous Approach	**0TPBX0Z**	Removal of Drainage Device from Bladder, External Approach
0TP987Z	Removal of Autologous Tissue Substitute from Ureter, Via Natural or Artificial Opening Endoscopic	**0TPB3LZ**	Removal of Artificial Sphincter from Bladder, Percutaneous Approach	**0TPBX2Z**	Removal of Monitoring Device from Bladder, External Approach
0TP98CZ	Removal of Extraluminal Device from Ureter, Via Natural or Artificial Opening Endoscopic	▲ **0TPB3MZ**	Removal of Stimulator Lead from Bladder, Percutaneous Approach	**0TPBX3Z**	Removal of Infusion Device from Bladder, External Approach
0TP98DZ	Removal of Intraluminal Device from Ureter, Via Natural or Artificial Opening Endoscopic	**0TPB40Z**	Removal of Drainage Device from Bladder, Percutaneous Endoscopic Approach	**0TPBXDZ**	Removal of Intraluminal Device from Bladder, External Approach
0TP98JZ	Removal of Synthetic Substitute from Ureter, Via Natural or Artificial Opening Endoscopic	**0TPB42Z**	Removal of Monitoring Device from Bladder, Percutaneous Endoscopic Approach	**0TPBXLZ**	Removal of Artificial Sphincter from Bladder, External Approach
0TP98KZ	Removal of Nonautologous Tissue Substitute from Ureter, Via Natural or Artificial Opening Endoscopic	**0TPB43Z**	Removal of Infusion Device from Bladder, Percutaneous Endoscopic Approach	**0TPBXMZ**	Removal of Stimulator Lead from Bladder, External Approach
0TP98MZ	Removal of Stimulator Lead from Ureter, Via Natural or Artificial Opening Endoscopic	**0TPB47Z**	Removal of Autologous Tissue Substitute from Bladder, Percutaneous Endoscopic Approach		
		0TPB4CZ	Removal of Extraluminal Device from Bladder, Percutaneous Endoscopic Approach		
		0TPB4DZ	Removal of Intraluminal Device from Bladder, Percutaneous Endoscopic Approach		
		0TPB4JZ	Removal of Synthetic Substitute from Bladder, Percutaneous Endoscopic Approach		
		0TPB4KZ	Removal of Nonautologous Tissue Substitute from Bladder, Percutaneous Endoscopic Approach		

♀ Female-only　　　♂ Male-only　　　▲ Limited Coverage　　　● Non-OR　　　■ HAC-associated procedure　　　▲ Non-covered procedures　　　✚ Combination

0TPD00Z Removal of Drainage Device from Urethra, Open Approach

0TPD02Z Removal of Monitoring Device from Urethra, Open Approach

0TPD03Z Removal of Infusion Device from Urethra, Open Approach

0TPD07Z Removal of Autologous Tissue Substitute from Urethra, Open Approach

0TPD0CZ Removal of Extraluminal Device from Urethra, Open Approach

0TPD0DZ Removal of Intraluminal Device from Urethra, Open Approach

0TPD0JZ Removal of Synthetic Substitute from Urethra, Open Approach

0TPD0KZ Removal of Nonautologous Tissue Substitute from Urethra, Open Approach

0TPD0LZ Removal of Artificial Sphincter from Urethra, Open Approach

0TPD30Z Removal of Drainage Device from Urethra, Percutaneous Approach

0TPD32Z Removal of Monitoring Device from Urethra, Percutaneous Approach

0TPD33Z Removal of Infusion Device from Urethra, Percutaneous Approach

0TPD37Z Removal of Autologous Tissue Substitute from Urethra, Percutaneous Approach

0TPD3CZ Removal of Extraluminal Device from Urethra, Percutaneous Approach

0TPD3DZ Removal of Intraluminal Device from Urethra, Percutaneous Approach

0TPD3JZ Removal of Synthetic Substitute from Urethra, Percutaneous Approach

0TPD3KZ Removal of Nonautologous Tissue Substitute from Urethra, Percutaneous Approach

0TPD3LZ Removal of Artificial Sphincter from Urethra, Percutaneous Approach

0TPD40Z Removal of Drainage Device from Urethra, Percutaneous Endoscopic Approach

0TPD42Z Removal of Monitoring Device from Urethra, Percutaneous Endoscopic Approach

0TPD43Z Removal of Infusion Device from Urethra, Percutaneous Endoscopic Approach

0TPD47Z Removal of Autologous Tissue Substitute from Urethra, Percutaneous Endoscopic Approach

0TPD4CZ Removal of Extraluminal Device from Urethra, Percutaneous Endoscopic Approach

0TPD4DZ Removal of Intraluminal Device from Urethra, Percutaneous Endoscopic Approach

0TPD4JZ Removal of Synthetic Substitute from Urethra, Percutaneous Endoscopic Approach

0TPD4KZ Removal of Nonautologous Tissue Substitute from Urethra, Percutaneous Endoscopic Approach

0TPD4LZ Removal of Artificial Sphincter from Urethra, Percutaneous Endoscopic Approach

0TPD70Z Removal of Drainage Device from Urethra, Via Natural or Artificial Opening

0TPD72Z Removal of Monitoring Device from Urethra, Via Natural or Artificial Opening

0TPD73Z Removal of Infusion Device from Urethra, Via Natural or Artificial Opening

0TPD77Z Removal of Autologous Tissue Substitute from Urethra, Via Natural or Artificial Opening

0TPD7CZ Removal of Extraluminal Device from Urethra, Via Natural or Artificial Opening

0TPD7DZ Removal of Intraluminal Device from Urethra, Via Natural or Artificial Opening

0TPD7JZ Removal of Synthetic Substitute from Urethra, Via Natural or Artificial Opening

0TPD7KZ Removal of Nonautologous Tissue Substitute from Urethra, Via Natural or Artificial Opening

0TPD7LZ Removal of Artificial Sphincter from Urethra, Via Natural or Artificial Opening

0TPD80Z Removal of Drainage Device from Urethra, Via Natural or Artificial Opening Endoscopic

0TPD82Z Removal of Monitoring Device from Urethra, Via Natural or Artificial Opening Endoscopic

0TPD83Z Removal of Infusion Device from Urethra, Via Natural or Artificial Opening Endoscopic

0TPD87Z Removal of Autologous Tissue Substitute from Urethra, Via Natural or Artificial Opening Endoscopic

0TPD8CZ Removal of Extraluminal Device from Urethra, Via Natural or Artificial Opening Endoscopic

0TPD8DZ Removal of Intraluminal Device from Urethra, Via Natural or Artificial Opening Endoscopic

0TPD8JZ Removal of Synthetic Substitute from Urethra, Via Natural or Artificial Opening Endoscopic

0TPD8KZ Removal of Nonautologous Tissue Substitute from Urethra, Via Natural or Artificial Opening Endoscopic

0TPD8LZ Removal of Artificial Sphincter from Urethra, Via Natural or Artificial Opening Endoscopic

0TPDX0Z Removal of Drainage Device from Urethra, External Approach

0TPDX2Z Removal of Monitoring Device from Urethra, External Approach

0TPDX3Z Removal of Infusion Device from Urethra, External Approach

0TPDXDZ Removal of Intraluminal Device from Urethra, External Approach

0TPDXLZ Removal of Artificial Sphincter from Urethra, External Approach

0TQ – Urinary System, Repair

0TQ00ZZ Repair Right Kidney, Open Approach
0TQ03ZZ Repair Right Kidney, Percutaneous Approach
0TQ04ZZ Repair Right Kidney, Percutaneous Endoscopic Approach
0TQ07ZZ Repair Right Kidney, Via Natural or Artificial Opening
0TQ08ZZ Repair Right Kidney, Via Natural or Artificial Opening Endoscopic
0TQ10ZZ Repair Left Kidney, Open Approach
0TQ13ZZ Repair Left Kidney, Percutaneous Approach
0TQ14ZZ Repair Left Kidney, Percutaneous Endoscopic Approach
0TQ17ZZ Repair Left Kidney, Via Natural or Artificial Opening
0TQ18ZZ Repair Left Kidney, Via Natural or Artificial Opening Endoscopic
0TQ30ZZ Repair Right Kidney Pelvis, Open Approach
0TQ33ZZ Repair Right Kidney Pelvis, Percutaneous Approach
0TQ34ZZ Repair Right Kidney Pelvis, Percutaneous Endoscopic Approach
0TQ37ZZ Repair Right Kidney Pelvis, Via Natural or Artificial Opening
0TQ38ZZ Repair Right Kidney Pelvis, Via Natural or Artificial Opening Endoscopic
0TQ40ZZ Repair Left Kidney Pelvis, Open Approach
0TQ43ZZ Repair Left Kidney Pelvis, Percutaneous Approach
0TQ44ZZ Repair Left Kidney Pelvis, Percutaneous Endoscopic Approach

0TQ47ZZ Repair Left Kidney Pelvis, Via Natural or Artificial Opening
0TQ48ZZ Repair Left Kidney Pelvis, Via Natural or Artificial Opening Endoscopic
0TQ60ZZ Repair Right Ureter, Open Approach
0TQ63ZZ Repair Right Ureter, Percutaneous Approach
0TQ64ZZ Repair Right Ureter, Percutaneous Endoscopic Approach
0TQ67ZZ Repair Right Ureter, Via Natural or Artificial Opening
0TQ68ZZ Repair Right Ureter, Via Natural or Artificial Opening Endoscopic
0TQ70ZZ Repair Left Ureter, Open Approach
0TQ73ZZ Repair Left Ureter, Percutaneous Approach
0TQ74ZZ Repair Left Ureter, Percutaneous Endoscopic Approach
0TQ77ZZ Repair Left Ureter, Via Natural or Artificial Opening
0TQ78ZZ Repair Left Ureter, Via Natural or Artificial Opening Endoscopic
0TQB0ZZ Repair Bladder, Open Approach
➕ Urostomy takedown when performed with code 0WQFXZ2, Repair of abdominal wall, stoma, external approach or 0WQFXZZ, Repair of abdominal wall, external approach.
0TQB3ZZ Repair Bladder, Percutaneous Approach
➕ Urostomy takedown when performed with code 0WQFXZ2, Repair of abdominal wall, stoma, external approach or 0WQFXZZ, Repair of abdominal wall, external approach.

0TQB4ZZ Repair Bladder, Percutaneous Endoscopic Approach
➕ Urostomy takedown when performed with code 0WQFXZ2, Repair of abdominal wall, stoma, external approach or 0WQFXZZ, Repair of abdominal wall, external approach.
0TQB7ZZ Repair Bladder, Via Natural or Artificial Opening
0TQB8ZZ Repair Bladder, Via Natural or Artificial Opening Endoscopic
0TQC0ZZ Repair Bladder Neck, Open Approach
0TQC3ZZ Repair Bladder Neck, Percutaneous Approach
0TQC4ZZ Repair Bladder Neck, Percutaneous Endoscopic Approach
0TQC7ZZ Repair Bladder Neck, Via Natural or Artificial Opening
0TQC8ZZ Repair Bladder Neck, Via Natural or Artificial Opening Endoscopic
0TQD0ZZ Repair Urethra, Open Approach
0TQD3ZZ Repair Urethra, Percutaneous Approach
0TQD4ZZ Repair Urethra, Percutaneous Endoscopic Approach
0TQD7ZZ Repair Urethra, Via Natural or Artificial Opening
0TQD8ZZ Repair Urethra, Via Natural or Artificial Opening Endoscopic
0TQDXZZ Repair Urethra, External Approach

♀ Female-only ♂ Male-only ▲ Limited Coverage ● Non-OR ▥ HAC-associated procedure ▲ Non-covered procedures ➕ Combination

0TR – Urinary System, Replacement

0TR307Z Replacement of Right Kidney Pelvis with Autologous Tissue Substitute, Open Approach

0TR30JZ Replacement of Right Kidney Pelvis with Synthetic Substitute, Open Approach

0TR30KZ Replacement of Right Kidney Pelvis with Nonautologous Tissue Substitute, Open Approach

0TR347Z Replacement of Right Kidney Pelvis with Autologous Tissue Substitute, Percutaneous Endoscopic Approach

0TR34JZ Replacement of Right Kidney Pelvis with Synthetic Substitute, Percutaneous Endoscopic Approach

0TR34KZ Replacement of Right Kidney Pelvis with Nonautologous Tissue Substitute, Percutaneous Endoscopic Approach

0TR377Z Replacement of Right Kidney Pelvis with Autologous Tissue Substitute, Via Natural or Artificial Opening

0TR37JZ Replacement of Right Kidney Pelvis with Synthetic Substitute, Via Natural or Artificial Opening

0TR37KZ Replacement of Right Kidney Pelvis with Nonautologous Tissue Substitute, Via Natural or Artificial Opening

0TR387Z Replacement of Right Kidney Pelvis with Autologous Tissue Substitute, Via Natural or Artificial Opening Endoscopic

0TR38JZ Replacement of Right Kidney Pelvis with Synthetic Substitute, Via Natural or Artificial Opening Endoscopic

0TR38KZ Replacement of Right Kidney Pelvis with Nonautologous Tissue Substitute, Via Natural or Artificial Opening Endoscopic

0TR407Z Replacement of Left Kidney Pelvis with Autologous Tissue Substitute, Open Approach

0TR40JZ Replacement of Left Kidney Pelvis with Synthetic Substitute, Open Approach

0TR40KZ Replacement of Left Kidney Pelvis with Nonautologous Tissue Substitute, Open Approach

0TR447Z Replacement of Left Kidney Pelvis with Autologous Tissue Substitute, Percutaneous Endoscopic Approach

0TR44JZ Replacement of Left Kidney Pelvis with Synthetic Substitute, Percutaneous Endoscopic Approach

0TR44KZ Replacement of Left Kidney Pelvis with Nonautologous Tissue Substitute, Percutaneous Endoscopic Approach

0TR477Z Replacement of Left Kidney Pelvis with Autologous Tissue Substitute, Via Natural or Artificial Opening

0TR47JZ Replacement of Left Kidney Pelvis with Synthetic Substitute, Via Natural or Artificial Opening

0TR47KZ Replacement of Left Kidney Pelvis with Nonautologous Tissue Substitute, Via Natural or Artificial Opening

0TR487Z Replacement of Left Kidney Pelvis with Autologous Tissue Substitute, Via Natural or Artificial Opening Endoscopic

0TR48JZ Replacement of Left Kidney Pelvis with Synthetic Substitute, Via Natural or Artificial Opening Endoscopic

0TR48KZ Replacement of Left Kidney Pelvis with Nonautologous Tissue Substitute, Via Natural or Artificial Opening Endoscopic

0TR607Z Replacement of Right Ureter with Autologous Tissue Substitute, Open Approach

0TR60JZ Replacement of Right Ureter with Synthetic Substitute, Open Approach

0TR60KZ Replacement of Right Ureter with Nonautologous Tissue Substitute, Open Approach

0TR647Z Replacement of Right Ureter with Autologous Tissue Substitute, Percutaneous Endoscopic Approach

0TR64JZ Replacement of Right Ureter with Synthetic Substitute, Percutaneous Endoscopic Approach

0TR64KZ Replacement of Right Ureter with Nonautologous Tissue Substitute, Percutaneous Endoscopic Approach

0TR677Z Replacement of Right Ureter with Autologous Tissue Substitute, Via Natural or Artificial Opening

0TR67JZ Replacement of Right Ureter with Synthetic Substitute, Via Natural or Artificial Opening

0TR67KZ Replacement of Right Ureter with Nonautologous Tissue Substitute, Via Natural or Artificial Opening

0TR687Z Replacement of Right Ureter with Autologous Tissue Substitute, Via Natural or Artificial Opening Endoscopic

0TR68JZ Replacement of Right Ureter with Synthetic Substitute, Via Natural or Artificial Opening Endoscopic

0TR68KZ Replacement of Right Ureter with Nonautologous Tissue Substitute, Via Natural or Artificial Opening Endoscopic

0TR707Z Replacement of Left Ureter with Autologous Tissue Substitute, Open Approach

0TR70JZ Replacement of Left Ureter with Synthetic Substitute, Open Approach

0TR70KZ Replacement of Left Ureter with Nonautologous Tissue Substitute, Open Approach

0TR747Z Replacement of Left Ureter with Autologous Tissue Substitute, Percutaneous Endoscopic Approach

0TR74JZ Replacement of Left Ureter with Synthetic Substitute, Percutaneous Endoscopic Approach

0TR74KZ Replacement of Left Ureter with Nonautologous Tissue Substitute, Percutaneous Endoscopic Approach

0TR777Z Replacement of Left Ureter with Autologous Tissue Substitute, Via Natural or Artificial Opening

0TR77JZ Replacement of Left Ureter with Synthetic Substitute, Via Natural or Artificial Opening

0TR77KZ Replacement of Left Ureter with Nonautologous Tissue Substitute, Via Natural or Artificial Opening

0TR787Z Replacement of Left Ureter with Autologous Tissue Substitute, Via Natural or Artificial Opening Endoscopic

0TR78JZ Replacement of Left Ureter with Synthetic Substitute, Via Natural or Artificial Opening Endoscopic

0TR78KZ Replacement of Left Ureter with Nonautologous Tissue Substitute, Via Natural or Artificial Opening Endoscopic

0TRB07Z Replacement of Bladder with Autologous Tissue Substitute, Open Approach

0TRB0JZ Replacement of Bladder with Synthetic Substitute, Open Approach

0TRB0KZ Replacement of Bladder with Nonautologous Tissue Substitute, Open Approach

0TRB47Z Replacement of Bladder with Autologous Tissue Substitute, Percutaneous Endoscopic Approach

0TRB4JZ Replacement of Bladder with Synthetic Substitute, Percutaneous Endoscopic Approach

0TRB4KZ Replacement of Bladder with Nonautologous Tissue Substitute, Percutaneous Endoscopic Approach

0TRB77Z Replacement of Bladder with Autologous Tissue Substitute, Via Natural or Artificial Opening

0TRB7JZ Replacement of Bladder with Synthetic Substitute, Via Natural or Artificial Opening

0TRB7KZ Replacement of Bladder with Nonautologous Tissue Substitute, Via Natural or Artificial Opening

0TRB87Z Replacement of Bladder with Autologous Tissue Substitute, Via Natural or Artificial Opening Endoscopic

0TRB8JZ Replacement of Bladder with Synthetic Substitute, Via Natural or Artificial Opening Endoscopic

0TRB8KZ Replacement of Bladder with Nonautologous Tissue Substitute, Via Natural or Artificial Opening Endoscopic

0TRC07Z Replacement of Bladder Neck with Autologous Tissue Substitute, Open Approach

0TRC0JZ Replacement of Bladder Neck with Synthetic Substitute, Open Approach

0TRC0KZ Replacement of Bladder Neck with Nonautologous Tissue Substitute, Open Approach

0TRC47Z Replacement of Bladder Neck with Autologous Tissue Substitute, Percutaneous Endoscopic Approach

0TRC4JZ Replacement of Bladder Neck with Synthetic Substitute, Percutaneous Endoscopic Approach

0TRC4KZ Replacement of Bladder Neck with Nonautologous Tissue Substitute, Percutaneous Endoscopic Approach

0TRC77Z Replacement of Bladder Neck with Autologous Tissue Substitute, Via Natural or Artificial Opening

0TRC7JZ Replacement of Bladder Neck with Synthetic Substitute, Via Natural or Artificial Opening

0TRC7KZ Replacement of Bladder Neck with Nonautologous Tissue Substitute, Via Natural or Artificial Opening

0TRC87Z Replacement of Bladder Neck with Autologous Tissue Substitute, Via Natural or Artificial Opening Endoscopic

0TRC8JZ Replacement of Bladder Neck with Synthetic Substitute, Via Natural or Artificial Opening Endoscopic

0TRC8KZ Replacement of Bladder Neck with Nonautologous Tissue Substitute, Via Natural or Artificial Opening Endoscopic

0TRD07Z Replacement of Urethra with Autologous Tissue Substitute, Open Approach

0TRD0JZ Replacement of Urethra with Synthetic Substitute, Open Approach

0TRD0KZ Replacement of Urethra with Nonautologous Tissue Substitute, Open Approach

0TRD47Z Replacement of Urethra with Autologous Tissue Substitute, Percutaneous Endoscopic Approach

0TRD4JZ Replacement of Urethra with Synthetic Substitute, Percutaneous Endoscopic Approach

RD4KZ Replacement of Urethra with Nonautologous Tissue Substitute, Percutaneous Endoscopic Approach

0TRD7KZ Replacement of Urethra with Nonautologous Tissue Substitute, Via Natural or Artificial Opening

0TRD8KZ Replacement of Urethra with Nonautologous Tissue Substitute, Via Natural or Artificial Opening Endoscopic

RD77Z Replacement of Urethra with Autologous Tissue Substitute, Via Natural or Artificial Opening

0TRD87Z Replacement of Urethra with Autologous Tissue Substitute, Via Natural or Artificial Opening Endoscopic

0TRDX7Z Replacement of Urethra with Autologous Tissue Substitute, External Approach

RD7JZ Replacement of Urethra with Synthetic Substitute, Via Natural or Artificial Opening

0TRD8JZ Replacement of Urethra with Synthetic Substitute, Via Natural or Artificial Opening Endoscopic

0TRDXJZ Replacement of Urethra with Synthetic Substitute, External Approach

0TRDXKZ Replacement of Urethra with Nonautologous Tissue Substitute, External Approach

'S – Urinary System, Reposition

S00ZZ Reposition Right Kidney, Open Approach
S04ZZ Reposition Right Kidney, Percutaneous Endoscopic Approach
S10ZZ Reposition Left Kidney, Open Approach
S14ZZ Reposition Left Kidney, Percutaneous Endoscopic Approach
S20ZZ Reposition Bilateral Kidneys, Open Approach
S24ZZ Reposition Bilateral Kidneys, Percutaneous Endoscopic Approach
S30ZZ Reposition Right Kidney Pelvis, Open Approach

0TS34ZZ Reposition Right Kidney Pelvis, Percutaneous Endoscopic Approach
0TS40ZZ Reposition Left Kidney Pelvis, Open Approach
0TS44ZZ Reposition Left Kidney Pelvis, Percutaneous Endoscopic Approach
0TS60ZZ Reposition Right Ureter, Open Approach
0TS64ZZ Reposition Right Ureter, Percutaneous Endoscopic Approach
0TS70ZZ Reposition Left Ureter, Open Approach
0TS74ZZ Reposition Left Ureter, Percutaneous Endoscopic Approach

0TS80ZZ Reposition Bilateral Ureters, Open Approach
0TS84ZZ Reposition Bilateral Ureters, Percutaneous Endoscopic Approach
0TSB0ZZ Reposition Bladder, Open Approach
0TSB4ZZ Reposition Bladder, Percutaneous Endoscopic Approach
0TSC0ZZ Reposition Bladder Neck, Open Approach
0TSC4ZZ Reposition Bladder Neck, Percutaneous Endoscopic Approach
0TSD0ZZ Reposition Urethra, Open Approach
0TSD4ZZ Reposition Urethra, Percutaneous Endoscopic Approach

TT – Urinary System, Resection

eview Coding Guideline B3.8

T00ZZ Resection of Right Kidney, Open Approach
T04ZZ Resection of Right Kidney, Percutaneous Endoscopic Approach
T10ZZ Resection of Left Kidney, Open Approach
AHA CC: 3Q, 2014, 16
T14ZZ Resection of Left Kidney, Percutaneous Endoscopic Approach
T20ZZ Resection of Bilateral Kidneys, Open Approach
T24ZZ Resection of Bilateral Kidneys, Percutaneous Endoscopic Approach
T30ZZ Resection of Right Kidney Pelvis, Open Approach
TT34ZZ Resection of Right Kidney Pelvis, Percutaneous Endoscopic Approach
TT37ZZ Resection of Right Kidney Pelvis, Via Natural or Artificial Opening
TT38ZZ Resection of Right Kidney Pelvis, Via Natural or Artificial Opening Endoscopic
TT40ZZ Resection of Left Kidney Pelvis, Open Approach
TT44ZZ Resection of Left Kidney Pelvis, Percutaneous Endoscopic Approach

0TT47ZZ Resection of Left Kidney Pelvis, Via Natural or Artificial Opening
0TT48ZZ Resection of Left Kidney Pelvis, Via Natural or Artificial Opening Endoscopic
0TT60ZZ Resection of Right Ureter, Open Approach
0TT64ZZ Resection of Right Ureter, Percutaneous Endoscopic Approach
0TT67ZZ Resection of Right Ureter, Via Natural or Artificial Opening
0TT68ZZ Resection of Right Ureter, Via Natural or Artificial Opening Endoscopic
0TT70ZZ Resection of Left Ureter, Open Approach
AHA CC: 3Q, 2014, 16
0TT74ZZ Resection of Left Ureter, Percutaneous Endoscopic Approach
0TT77ZZ Resection of Left Ureter, Via Natural or Artificial Opening
0TT78ZZ Resection of Left Ureter, Via Natural or Artificial Opening Endoscopic
0TTB0ZZ Resection of Bladder, Open Approach
➕ Pelvic evisceration when reported with Resection of urethra, bilateral ovaries, bilateral fallopian tubes, uterus, cervix

and vagina. *See tables 0TT and 0UT to construct the Resection codes.*
0TTB4ZZ Resection of Bladder, Percutaneous Endoscopic Approach
0TTB7ZZ Resection of Bladder, Via Natural or Artificial Opening
0TTB8ZZ Resection of Bladder, Via Natural or Artificial Opening Endoscopic
0TTC0ZZ Resection of Bladder Neck, Open Approach
0TTC4ZZ Resection of Bladder Neck, Percutaneous Endoscopic Approach
0TTC7ZZ Resection of Bladder Neck, Via Natural or Artificial Opening
0TTC8ZZ Resection of Bladder Neck, Via Natural or Artificial Opening Endoscopic
● **0TTD0ZZ** Resection of Urethra, Open Approach
0TTD4ZZ Resection of Urethra, Percutaneous Endoscopic Approach
0TTD7ZZ Resection of Urethra, Via Natural or Artificial Opening
0TTD8ZZ Resection of Urethra, Via Natural or Artificial Opening Endoscopic

TU – Urinary System, Supplement

TU307Z Supplement Right Kidney Pelvis with Autologous Tissue Substitute, Open Approach
TU30JZ Supplement Right Kidney Pelvis with Synthetic Substitute, Open Approach
TU30KZ Supplement Right Kidney Pelvis with Nonautologous Tissue Substitute, Open Approach
TU347Z Supplement Right Kidney Pelvis with Autologous Tissue Substitute, Percutaneous Endoscopic Approach
TU34JZ Supplement Right Kidney Pelvis with Synthetic Substitute, Percutaneous Endoscopic Approach
TU34KZ Supplement Right Kidney Pelvis with Nonautologous Tissue Substitute, Percutaneous Endoscopic Approach

0TU377Z Supplement Right Kidney Pelvis with Autologous Tissue Substitute, Via Natural or Artificial Opening
0TU37JZ Supplement Right Kidney Pelvis with Synthetic Substitute, Via Natural or Artificial Opening
0TU37KZ Supplement Right Kidney Pelvis with Nonautologous Tissue Substitute, Via Natural or Artificial Opening
0TU387Z Supplement Right Kidney Pelvis with Autologous Tissue Substitute, Via Natural or Artificial Opening Endoscopic
0TU38JZ Supplement Right Kidney Pelvis with Synthetic Substitute, Via Natural or Artificial Opening Endoscopic
0TU38KZ Supplement Right Kidney Pelvis with Nonautologous Tissue Substitute, Via Natural or Artificial Opening Endoscopic

0TU407Z Supplement Left Kidney Pelvis with Autologous Tissue Substitute, Open Approach
0TU40JZ Supplement Left Kidney Pelvis with Synthetic Substitute, Open Approach
0TU40KZ Supplement Left Kidney Pelvis with Nonautologous Tissue Substitute, Open Approach
0TU447Z Supplement Left Kidney Pelvis with Autologous Tissue Substitute, Percutaneous Endoscopic Approach
0TU44JZ Supplement Left Kidney Pelvis with Synthetic Substitute, Percutaneous Endoscopic Approach
0TU44KZ Supplement Left Kidney Pelvis with Nonautologous Tissue Substitute, Percutaneous Endoscopic Approach

♀ Female-only   ♂ Male-only   ▲ Limited Coverage   ● Non-OR   ▦ HAC-associated procedure   ▲ Non-covered procedures   ➕ Combination

0TU477Z Supplement Left Kidney Pelvis with Autologous Tissue Substitute, Via Natural or Artificial Opening

0TU47JZ Supplement Left Kidney Pelvis with Synthetic Substitute, Via Natural or Artificial Opening

0TU47KZ Supplement Left Kidney Pelvis with Nonautologous Tissue Substitute, Via Natural or Artificial Opening

0TU487Z Supplement Left Kidney Pelvis with Autologous Tissue Substitute, Via Natural or Artificial Opening Endoscopic

0TU48JZ Supplement Left Kidney Pelvis with Synthetic Substitute, Via Natural or Artificial Opening Endoscopic

0TU48KZ Supplement Left Kidney Pelvis with Nonautologous Tissue Substitute, Via Natural or Artificial Opening Endoscopic

0TU607Z Supplement Right Ureter with Autologous Tissue Substitute, Open Approach

0TU60JZ Supplement Right Ureter with Synthetic Substitute, Open Approach

0TU60KZ Supplement Right Ureter with Nonautologous Tissue Substitute, Open Approach

0TU647Z Supplement Right Ureter with Autologous Tissue Substitute, Percutaneous Endoscopic Approach

0TU64JZ Supplement Right Ureter with Synthetic Substitute, Percutaneous Endoscopic Approach

0TU64KZ Supplement Right Ureter with Nonautologous Tissue Substitute, Percutaneous Endoscopic Approach

0TU677Z Supplement Right Ureter with Autologous Tissue Substitute, Via Natural or Artificial Opening

0TU67JZ Supplement Right Ureter with Synthetic Substitute, Via Natural or Artificial Opening

0TU67KZ Supplement Right Ureter with Nonautologous Tissue Substitute, Via Natural or Artificial Opening

0TU687Z Supplement Right Ureter with Autologous Tissue Substitute, Via Natural or Artificial Opening Endoscopic

0TU68JZ Supplement Right Ureter with Synthetic Substitute, Via Natural or Artificial Opening Endoscopic

0TU68KZ Supplement Right Ureter with Nonautologous Tissue Substitute, Via Natural or Artificial Opening Endoscopic

0TU707Z Supplement Left Ureter with Autologous Tissue Substitute, Open Approach

0TU70JZ Supplement Left Ureter with Synthetic Substitute, Open Approach

0TU70KZ Supplement Left Ureter with Nonautologous Tissue Substitute, Open Approach

0TU747Z Supplement Left Ureter with Autologous Tissue Substitute, Percutaneous Endoscopic Approach

0TU74JZ Supplement Left Ureter with Synthetic Substitute, Percutaneous Endoscopic Approach

0TU74KZ Supplement Left Ureter with Nonautologous Tissue Substitute, Percutaneous Endoscopic Approach

0TU777Z Supplement Left Ureter with Autologous Tissue Substitute, Via Natural or Artificial Opening

0TU77JZ Supplement Left Ureter with Synthetic Substitute, Via Natural or Artificial Opening

0TU77KZ Supplement Left Ureter with Nonautologous Tissue Substitute, Via Natural or Artificial Opening

0TU787Z Supplement Left Ureter with Autologous Tissue Substitute, Via Natural or Artificial Opening Endoscopic

0TU78JZ Supplement Left Ureter with Synthetic Substitute, Via Natural or Artificial Opening Endoscopic

0TU78KZ Supplement Left Ureter with Nonautologous Tissue Substitute, Via Natural or Artificial Opening Endoscopic

0TUB07Z Supplement Bladder with Autologous Tissue Substitute, Open Approach

0TUB0JZ Supplement Bladder with Synthetic Substitute, Open Approach

0TUB0KZ Supplement Bladder with Nonautologous Tissue Substitute, Open Approach

0TUB47Z Supplement Bladder with Autologous Tissue Substitute, Percutaneous Endoscopic Approach

0TUB4JZ Supplement Bladder with Synthetic Substitute, Percutaneous Endoscopic Approach

0TUB4KZ Supplement Bladder with Nonautologous Tissue Substitute, Percutaneous Endoscopic Approach

0TUB77Z Supplement Bladder with Autologous Tissue Substitute, Via Natural or Artificial Opening

0TUB7JZ Supplement Bladder with Synthetic Substitute, Via Natural or Artificial Opening

0TUB7KZ Supplement Bladder with Nonautologous Tissue Substitute, Via Natural or Artificial Opening

0TUB87Z Supplement Bladder with Autologous Tissue Substitute, Via Natural or Artificial Opening Endoscopic

0TUB8JZ Supplement Bladder with Synthetic Substitute, Via Natural or Artificial Opening Endoscopic

0TUB8KZ Supplement Bladder with Nonautologous Tissue Substitute, Via Natural or Artificial Opening Endoscopic

0TUC07Z Supplement Bladder Neck with Autologous Tissue Substitute, Open Approach

0TUC0JZ Supplement Bladder Neck with Synthetic Substitute, Open Approach

0TUC0KZ Supplement Bladder Neck with Nonautologous Tissue Substitute, Open Approach

0TUC47Z Supplement Bladder Neck with Autologous Tissue Substitute, Percutaneous Endoscopic Approach

0TUC4JZ Supplement Bladder Neck with Synthetic Substitute, Percutaneous Endoscopic Approach

0TUC4KZ Supplement Bladder Neck with Nonautologous Tissue Substitute, Percutaneous Endoscopic Approach

0TUC77Z Supplement Bladder Neck with Autologous Tissue Substitute, Via Natural or Artificial Opening

0TUC7JZ Supplement Bladder Neck with Synthetic Substitute, Via Natural or Artificial Opening

0TUC7KZ Supplement Bladder Neck with Nonautologous Tissue Substitute, Via Natural or Artificial Opening

0TUC87Z Supplement Bladder Neck with Autologous Tissue Substitute, Via Natural or Artificial Opening Endoscopic

0TUC8JZ Supplement Bladder Neck with Synthetic Substitute, Via Natural or Artificial Opening Endoscopic

0TUC8KZ Supplement Bladder Neck with Nonautologous Tissue Substitute, Via Natural or Artificial Opening Endoscopic

0TUD07Z Supplement Urethra with Autologous Tissue Substitute, Open Approach

0TUD0JZ Supplement Urethra with Synthetic Substitute, Open Approach

0TUD0KZ Supplement Urethra with Nonautologous Tissue Substitute, Open Approach

0TUD47Z Supplement Urethra with Autologous Tissue Substitute, Percutaneous Endoscopic Approach

0TUD4JZ Supplement Urethra with Synthetic Substitute, Percutaneous Endoscopic Approach

0TUD4KZ Supplement Urethra with Nonautologous Tissue Substitute, Percutaneous Endoscopic Approach

0TUD77Z Supplement Urethra with Autologous Tissue Substitute, Via Natural or Artificial Opening

0TUD7JZ Supplement Urethra with Synthetic Substitute, Via Natural or Artificial Opening

0TUD7KZ Supplement Urethra with Nonautologous Tissue Substitute, Via Natural or Artificial Opening

0TUD87Z Supplement Urethra with Autologous Tissue Substitute, Via Natural or Artificial Opening Endoscopic

0TUD8JZ Supplement Urethra with Synthetic Substitute, Via Natural or Artificial Opening Endoscopic

0TUD8KZ Supplement Urethra with Nonautologous Tissue Substitute, Via Natural or Artificial Opening Endoscopic

0TUDX7Z Supplement Urethra with Autologous Tissue Substitute, External Approach

0TUDXJZ Supplement Urethra with Synthetic Substitute, External Approach

0TUDXKZ Supplement Urethra with Nonautologous Tissue Substitute, External Approach

0TV – Urinary System, Restriction

0TV30CZ Restriction of Right Kidney Pelvis with Extraluminal Device, Open Approach

0TV30DZ Restriction of Right Kidney Pelvis with Intraluminal Device, Open Approach

0TV30ZZ Restriction of Right Kidney Pelvis, Open Approach

0TV33CZ Restriction of Right Kidney Pelvis with Extraluminal Device, Percutaneous Approach

0TV33DZ Restriction of Right Kidney Pelvis with Intraluminal Device, Percutaneous Approach

0TV33ZZ Restriction of Right Kidney Pelvis, Percutaneous Approach

0TV34CZ Restriction of Right Kidney Pelvis with Extraluminal Device, Percutaneous Endoscopic Approach

0TV34DZ Restriction of Right Kidney Pelvis with Intraluminal Device, Percutaneous Endoscopic Approach

0TV34ZZ Restriction of Right Kidney Pelvis, Percutaneous Endoscopic Approach

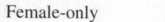

♀ Female-only   ♂ Male-only   ▲ Limited Coverage   ● Non-OR   ▰ HAC-associated procedure   ▲ Non-covered procedures   ✛ Combination

0TV37DZ Restriction of Right Kidney Pelvis with Intraluminal Device, Via Natural or Artificial Opening

0TV37ZZ Restriction of Right Kidney Pelvis, Via Natural or Artificial Opening

0TV38DZ Restriction of Right Kidney Pelvis with Intraluminal Device, Via Natural or Artificial Opening Endoscopic

0TV38ZZ Restriction of Right Kidney Pelvis, Via Natural or Artificial Opening Endoscopic

0TV40CZ Restriction of Left Kidney Pelvis with Extraluminal Device, Open Approach

0TV40DZ Restriction of Left Kidney Pelvis with Intraluminal Device, Open Approach

0TV40ZZ Restriction of Left Kidney Pelvis, Open Approach

0TV43CZ Restriction of Left Kidney Pelvis with Extraluminal Device, Percutaneous Approach

0TV43DZ Restriction of Left Kidney Pelvis with Intraluminal Device, Percutaneous Approach

0TV43ZZ Restriction of Left Kidney Pelvis, Percutaneous Approach

0TV44CZ Restriction of Left Kidney Pelvis with Extraluminal Device, Percutaneous Endoscopic Approach

0TV44DZ Restriction of Left Kidney Pelvis with Intraluminal Device, Percutaneous Endoscopic Approach

0TV44ZZ Restriction of Left Kidney Pelvis, Percutaneous Endoscopic Approach

0TV47DZ Restriction of Left Kidney Pelvis with Intraluminal Device, Via Natural or Artificial Opening

0TV47ZZ Restriction of Left Kidney Pelvis, Via Natural or Artificial Opening

0TV48DZ Restriction of Left Kidney Pelvis with Intraluminal Device, Via Natural or Artificial Opening Endoscopic

0TV48ZZ Restriction of Left Kidney Pelvis, Via Natural or Artificial Opening Endoscopic

0TV60CZ Restriction of Right Ureter with Extraluminal Device, Open Approach

0TV60DZ Restriction of Right Ureter with Intraluminal Device, Open Approach

0TV60ZZ Restriction of Right Ureter, Open Approach

0TV63CZ Restriction of Right Ureter with Extraluminal Device, Percutaneous Approach

0TV63DZ Restriction of Right Ureter with Intraluminal Device, Percutaneous Approach

0TV63ZZ Restriction of Right Ureter, Percutaneous Approach

0TV64CZ Restriction of Right Ureter with Extraluminal Device, Percutaneous Endoscopic Approach

0TV64DZ Restriction of Right Ureter with Intraluminal Device, Percutaneous Endoscopic Approach

0TV64ZZ Restriction of Right Ureter, Percutaneous Endoscopic Approach

0TV67DZ Restriction of Right Ureter with Intraluminal Device, Via Natural or Artificial Opening

0TV67ZZ Restriction of Right Ureter, Via Natural or Artificial Opening

0TV68DZ Restriction of Right Ureter with Intraluminal Device, Via Natural or Artificial Opening Endoscopic

0TV68ZZ Restriction of Right Ureter, Via Natural or Artificial Opening Endoscopic

0TV70CZ Restriction of Left Ureter with Extraluminal Device, Open Approach

0TV70DZ Restriction of Left Ureter with Intraluminal Device, Open Approach

0TV70ZZ Restriction of Left Ureter, Open Approach

0TV73CZ Restriction of Left Ureter with Extraluminal Device, Percutaneous Approach

0TV73DZ Restriction of Left Ureter with Intraluminal Device, Percutaneous Approach

0TV73ZZ Restriction of Left Ureter, Percutaneous Approach

0TV74CZ Restriction of Left Ureter with Extraluminal Device, Percutaneous Endoscopic Approach

0TV74DZ Restriction of Left Ureter with Intraluminal Device, Percutaneous Endoscopic Approach

0TV74ZZ Restriction of Left Ureter, Percutaneous Endoscopic Approach

0TV77DZ Restriction of Left Ureter with Intraluminal Device, Via Natural or Artificial Opening

0TV77ZZ Restriction of Left Ureter, Via Natural or Artificial Opening

0TV78DZ Restriction of Left Ureter with Intraluminal Device, Via Natural or Artificial Opening Endoscopic

0TV78ZZ Restriction of Left Ureter, Via Natural or Artificial Opening Endoscopic

0TVB0CZ Restriction of Bladder with Extraluminal Device, Open Approach

0TVB0DZ Restriction of Bladder with Intraluminal Device, Open Approach

0TVB0ZZ Restriction of Bladder, Open Approach

0TVB3CZ Restriction of Bladder with Extraluminal Device, Percutaneous Approach

0TVB3DZ Restriction of Bladder with Intraluminal Device, Percutaneous Approach

0TVB3ZZ Restriction of Bladder, Percutaneous Approach

0TVB4CZ Restriction of Bladder with Extraluminal Device, Percutaneous Endoscopic Approach

0TVB4DZ Restriction of Bladder with Intraluminal Device, Percutaneous Endoscopic Approach

0TVB4ZZ Restriction of Bladder, Percutaneous Endoscopic Approach

0TVB7DZ Restriction of Bladder with Intraluminal Device, Via Natural or Artificial Opening

0TVB7ZZ Restriction of Bladder, Via Natural or Artificial Opening

0TVB8DZ Restriction of Bladder with Intraluminal Device, Via Natural or Artificial Opening Endoscopic

0TVB8ZZ Restriction of Bladder, Via Natural or Artificial Opening Endoscopic

0TVC0CZ Restriction of Bladder Neck with Extraluminal Device, Open Approach

0TVC0DZ Restriction of Bladder Neck with Intraluminal Device, Open Approach

0TVC0ZZ Restriction of Bladder Neck, Open Approach

0TVC3CZ Restriction of Bladder Neck with Extraluminal Device, Percutaneous Approach

0TVC3DZ Restriction of Bladder Neck with Intraluminal Device, Percutaneous Approach

0TVC3ZZ Restriction of Bladder Neck, Percutaneous Approach

0TVC4CZ Restriction of Bladder Neck with Extraluminal Device, Percutaneous Endoscopic Approach

0TVC4DZ Restriction of Bladder Neck with Intraluminal Device, Percutaneous Endoscopic Approach

0TVC4ZZ Restriction of Bladder Neck, Percutaneous Endoscopic Approach

0TVC7DZ Restriction of Bladder Neck with Intraluminal Device, Via Natural or Artificial Opening

0TVC7ZZ Restriction of Bladder Neck, Via Natural or Artificial Opening

0TVC8DZ Restriction of Bladder Neck with Intraluminal Device, Via Natural or Artificial Opening Endoscopic

0TVC8ZZ Restriction of Bladder Neck, Via Natural or Artificial Opening Endoscopic

0TVD0CZ Restriction of Urethra with Extraluminal Device, Open Approach

0TVD0DZ Restriction of Urethra with Intraluminal Device, Open Approach

0TVD0ZZ Restriction of Urethra, Open Approach

0TVD3CZ Restriction of Urethra with Extraluminal Device, Percutaneous Approach

0TVD3DZ Restriction of Urethra with Intraluminal Device, Percutaneous Approach

0TVD3ZZ Restriction of Urethra, Percutaneous Approach

0TVD4CZ Restriction of Urethra with Extraluminal Device, Percutaneous Endoscopic Approach

0TVD4DZ Restriction of Urethra with Intraluminal Device, Percutaneous Endoscopic Approach

0TVD4ZZ Restriction of Urethra, Percutaneous Endoscopic Approach

0TVD7DZ Restriction of Urethra with Intraluminal Device, Via Natural or Artificial Opening

0TVD7ZZ Restriction of Urethra, Via Natural or Artificial Opening

0TVD8DZ Restriction of Urethra with Intraluminal Device, Via Natural or Artificial Opening Endoscopic

0TVD8ZZ Restriction of Urethra, Via Natural or Artificial Opening Endoscopic

0TVDXZZ Restriction of Urethra, External Approach

0TW – Urinary System, Revision

Review Coding Guideline B6.1c

0TW500Z Revision of Drainage Device in Kidney, Open Approach

0TW502Z Revision of Monitoring Device in Kidney, Open Approach

0TW503Z Revision of Infusion Device in Kidney, Open Approach

0TW507Z Revision of Autologous Tissue Substitute in Kidney, Open Approach

0TW50CZ Revision of Extraluminal Device in Kidney, Open Approach

0TW50DZ Revision of Intraluminal Device in Kidney, Open Approach

0TW50JZ Revision of Synthetic Substitute in Kidney, Open Approach

0TW50KZ Revision of Nonautologous Tissue Substitute in Kidney, Open Approach

0TW530Z Revision of Drainage Device in Kidney, Percutaneous Approach

♀ Female-only　　♂ Male-only　　▲ Limited Coverage　　● Non-OR　　HAC HAC-associated procedure　　▲ Non-covered procedures　　✚ Combination

0TW532Z	Revision of Monitoring Device in Kidney, Percutaneous Approach
0TW533Z	Revision of Infusion Device in Kidney, Percutaneous Approach
0TW537Z	Revision of Autologous Tissue Substitute in Kidney, Percutaneous Approach
0TW53CZ	Revision of Extraluminal Device in Kidney, Percutaneous Approach
0TW53DZ	Revision of Intraluminal Device in Kidney, Percutaneous Approach
0TW53JZ	Revision of Synthetic Substitute in Kidney, Percutaneous Approach
0TW53KZ	Revision of Nonautologous Tissue Substitute in Kidney, Percutaneous Approach
0TW540Z	Revision of Drainage Device in Kidney, Percutaneous Endoscopic Approach
0TW542Z	Revision of Monitoring Device in Kidney, Percutaneous Endoscopic Approach
0TW543Z	Revision of Infusion Device in Kidney, Percutaneous Endoscopic Approach
0TW547Z	Revision of Autologous Tissue Substitute in Kidney, Percutaneous Endoscopic Approach
0TW54CZ	Revision of Extraluminal Device in Kidney, Percutaneous Endoscopic Approach
0TW54DZ	Revision of Intraluminal Device in Kidney, Percutaneous Endoscopic Approach
0TW54JZ	Revision of Synthetic Substitute in Kidney, Percutaneous Endoscopic Approach
0TW54KZ	Revision of Nonautologous Tissue Substitute in Kidney, Percutaneous Endoscopic Approach
0TW570Z	Revision of Drainage Device in Kidney, Via Natural or Artificial Opening
0TW570Z	Revision of Monitoring Device in Kidney, Via Natural or Artificial Opening
0TW573Z	Revision of Infusion Device in Kidney, Via Natural or Artificial Opening
0TW577Z	Revision of Autologous Tissue Substitute in Kidney, Via Natural or Artificial Opening
0TW57CZ	Revision of Extraluminal Device in Kidney, Via Natural or Artificial Opening
0TW57DZ	Revision of Intraluminal Device in Kidney, Via Natural or Artificial Opening
0TW57JZ	Revision of Synthetic Substitute in Kidney, Via Natural or Artificial Opening
0TW57KZ	Revision of Nonautologous Tissue Substitute in Kidney, Via Natural or Artificial Opening
0TW580Z	Revision of Drainage Device in Kidney, Via Natural or Artificial Opening Endoscopic
0TW582Z	Revision of Monitoring Device in Kidney, Via Natural or Artificial Opening Endoscopic
0TW583Z	Revision of Infusion Device in Kidney, Via Natural or Artificial Opening Endoscopic
0TW587Z	Revision of Autologous Tissue Substitute in Kidney, Via Natural or Artificial Opening Endoscopic
0TW58CZ	Revision of Extraluminal Device in Kidney, Via Natural or Artificial Opening Endoscopic
0TW58DZ	Revision of Intraluminal Device in Kidney, Via Natural or Artificial Opening Endoscopic
0TW58JZ	Revision of Synthetic Substitute in Kidney, Via Natural or Artificial Opening Endoscopic
0TW58KZ	Revision of Nonautologous Tissue Substitute in Kidney, Via Natural or Artificial Opening Endoscopic

0TW5X0Z	Revision of Drainage Device in Kidney, External Approach
0TW5X2Z	Revision of Monitoring Device in Kidney, External Approach
0TW5X3Z	Revision of Infusion Device in Kidney, External Approach
0TW5X7Z	Revision of Autologous Tissue Substitute in Kidney, External Approach
0TW5XCZ	Revision of Extraluminal Device in Kidney, External Approach
0TW5XDZ	Revision of Intraluminal Device in Kidney, External Approach
0TW5XJZ	Revision of Synthetic Substitute in Kidney, External Approach
0TW5XKZ	Revision of Nonautologous Tissue Substitute in Kidney, External Approach
0TW900Z	Revision of Drainage Device in Ureter, Open Approach
0TW902Z	Revision of Monitoring Device in Ureter, Open Approach
0TW903Z	Revision of Infusion Device in Ureter, Open Approach
0TW907Z	Revision of Autologous Tissue Substitute in Ureter, Open Approach
0TW90CZ	Revision of Extraluminal Device in Ureter, Open Approach
0TW90DZ	Revision of Intraluminal Device in Ureter, Open Approach
0TW90JZ	Revision of Synthetic Substitute in Ureter, Open Approach
0TW90KZ	Revision of Nonautologous Tissue Substitute in Ureter, Open Approach
0TW90MZ	Revision of Stimulator Lead in Ureter, Open Approach
0TW930Z	Revision of Drainage Device in Ureter, Percutaneous Approach
0TW932Z	Revision of Monitoring Device in Ureter, Percutaneous Approach
0TW933Z	Revision of Infusion Device in Ureter, Percutaneous Approach
0TW937Z	Revision of Autologous Tissue Substitute in Ureter, Percutaneous Approach
0TW93CZ	Revision of Extraluminal Device in Ureter, Percutaneous Approach
0TW93DZ	Revision of Intraluminal Device in Ureter, Percutaneous Approach
0TW93JZ	Revision of Synthetic Substitute in Ureter, Percutaneous Approach
0TW93KZ	Revision of Nonautologous Tissue Substitute in Ureter, Percutaneous Approach
0TW93MZ	Revision of Stimulator Lead in Ureter, Percutaneous Approach
0TW940Z	Revision of Drainage Device in Ureter, Percutaneous Endoscopic Approach
0TW942Z	Revision of Monitoring Device in Ureter, Percutaneous Endoscopic Approach
0TW943Z	Revision of Infusion Device in Ureter, Percutaneous Endoscopic Approach
0TW947Z	Revision of Autologous Tissue Substitute in Ureter, Percutaneous Endoscopic Approach
0TW94CZ	Revision of Extraluminal Device in Ureter, Percutaneous Endoscopic Approach
0TW94DZ	Revision of Intraluminal Device in Ureter, Percutaneous Endoscopic Approach
0TW94JZ	Revision of Synthetic Substitute in Ureter, Percutaneous Endoscopic Approach
0TW94KZ	Revision of Nonautologous Tissue Substitute in Ureter, Percutaneous Endoscopic Approach
0TW94MZ	Revision of Stimulator Lead in Ureter, Percutaneous Endoscopic Approach
0TW970Z	Revision of Drainage Device in Ureter, Via Natural or Artificial Opening

0TW972Z	Revision of Monitoring Device in Ureter Via Natural or Artificial Opening
0TW973Z	Revision of Infusion Device in Ureter, Via Natural or Artificial Opening
0TW977Z	Revision of Autologous Tissue Substitut in Ureter, Via Natural or Artificial Opening
0TW97CZ	Revision of Extraluminal Device in Ureter, Via Natural or Artificial Opening
0TW97DZ	Revision of Intraluminal Device in Ureter, Via Natural or Artificial Opening
0TW97JZ	Revision of Synthetic Substitute in Ureter, Via Natural or Artificial Opening
0TW97KZ	Revision of Nonautologous Tissue Substitute in Ureter, Via Natural or Artificial Opening
0TW97MZ	Revision of Stimulator Lead in Ureter, Via Natural or Artificial Opening
0TW980Z	Revision of Drainage Device in Ureter, Via Natural or Artificial Opening Endoscopic
0TW982Z	Revision of Monitoring Device in Ureter, Via Natural or Artificial Opening Endoscopic
0TW983Z	Revision of Infusion Device in Ureter, Via Natural or Artificial Opening Endoscopic
0TW987Z	Revision of Autologous Tissue Substitute in Ureter, Via Natural or Artificial Opening Endoscopic
0TW98CZ	Revision of Extraluminal Device in Ureter, Via Natural or Artificial Opening Endoscopic
0TW98DZ	Revision of Intraluminal Device in Ureter, Via Natural or Artificial Opening Endoscopic
0TW98JZ	Revision of Synthetic Substitute in Ureter, Via Natural or Artificial Opening Endoscopic
0TW98KZ	Revision of Nonautologous Tissue Substitute in Ureter, Via Natural or Artificial Opening Endoscopic
0TW98MZ	Revision of Stimulator Lead in Ureter, Via Natural or Artificial Opening Endoscopic
0TW9X0Z	Revision of Drainage Device in Ureter, External Approach
0TW9X2Z	Revision of Monitoring Device in Ureter, External Approach
0TW9X3Z	Revision of Infusion Device in Ureter, External Approach
0TW9X7Z	Revision of Autologous Tissue Substitute in Ureter, External Approach
0TW9XCZ	Revision of Extraluminal Device in Ureter, External Approach
0TW9XDZ	Revision of Intraluminal Device in Ureter, External Approach
0TW9XJZ	Revision of Synthetic Substitute in Ureter, External Approach
0TW9XKZ	Revision of Nonautologous Tissue Substitute in Ureter, External Approach
0TW9XMZ	Revision of Stimulator Lead in Ureter, External Approach
0TWB00Z	Revision of Drainage Device in Bladder, Open Approach
0TWB02Z	Revision of Monitoring Device in Bladder, Open Approach
0TWB03Z	Revision of Infusion Device in Bladder, Open Approach
0TWB07Z	Revision of Autologous Tissue Substitute in Bladder, Open Approach
0TWB0CZ	Revision of Extraluminal Device in Bladder, Open Approach
0TWB0DZ	Revision of Intraluminal Device in Bladder, Open Approach
0TWB0JZ	Revision of Synthetic Substitute in Bladder, Open Approach

WB0KZ	Revision of Nonautologous Tissue Substitute in Bladder, Open Approach
WB0LZ	Revision of Artificial Sphincter in Bladder, Open Approach
WB0MZ	Revision of Stimulator Lead in Bladder, Open Approach
WB30Z	Revision of Drainage Device in Bladder, Percutaneous Approach
WB32Z	Revision of Monitoring Device in Bladder, Percutaneous Approach
WB33Z	Revision of Infusion Device in Bladder, Percutaneous Approach
WB37Z	Revision of Autologous Tissue Substitute in Bladder, Percutaneous Approach
WB3CZ	Revision of Extraluminal Device in Bladder, Percutaneous Approach
WB3DZ	Revision of Intraluminal Device in Bladder, Percutaneous Approach
WB3JZ	Revision of Synthetic Substitute in Bladder, Percutaneous Approach
TWB3KZ	Revision of Nonautologous Tissue Substitute in Bladder, Percutaneous Approach
TWB3LZ	Revision of Artificial Sphincter in Bladder, Percutaneous Approach
TWB3MZ	Revision of Stimulator Lead in Bladder, Percutaneous Approach
TWB40Z	Revision of Drainage Device in Bladder, Percutaneous Endoscopic Approach
TWB42Z	Revision of Monitoring Device in Bladder, Percutaneous Endoscopic Approach
TWB43Z	Revision of Infusion Device in Bladder, Percutaneous Endoscopic Approach
TWB47Z	Revision of Autologous Tissue Substitute in Bladder, Percutaneous Endoscopic Approach
TWB4CZ	Revision of Extraluminal Device in Bladder, Percutaneous Endoscopic Approach
TWB4DZ	Revision of Intraluminal Device in Bladder, Percutaneous Endoscopic Approach
TWB4JZ	Revision of Synthetic Substitute in Bladder, Percutaneous Endoscopic Approach
TWB4KZ	Revision of Nonautologous Tissue Substitute in Bladder, Percutaneous Endoscopic Approach
TWB4LZ	Revision of Artificial Sphincter in Bladder, Percutaneous Endoscopic Approach
TWB4MZ	Revision of Stimulator Lead in Bladder, Percutaneous Endoscopic Approach
TWB70Z	Revision of Drainage Device in Bladder, Via Natural or Artificial Opening
TWB72Z	Revision of Monitoring Device in Bladder, Via Natural or Artificial Opening
TWB73Z	Revision of Infusion Device in Bladder, Via Natural or Artificial Opening
TWB77Z	Revision of Autologous Tissue Substitute in Bladder, Via Natural or Artificial Opening
0TWB7CZ	Revision of Extraluminal Device in Bladder, Via Natural or Artificial Opening
0TWB7DZ	Revision of Intraluminal Device in Bladder, Via Natural or Artificial Opening
0TWB7JZ	Revision of Synthetic Substitute in Bladder, Via Natural or Artificial Opening
0TWB7KZ	Revision of Nonautologous Tissue Substitute in Bladder, Via Natural or Artificial Opening

0TWB7LZ	Revision of Artificial Sphincter in Bladder, Via Natural or Artificial Opening
0TWB7MZ	Revision of Stimulator Lead in Bladder, Via Natural or Artificial Opening
0TWB80Z	Revision of Drainage Device in Bladder, Via Natural or Artificial Opening Endoscopic
0TWB82Z	Revision of Monitoring Device in Bladder, Via Natural or Artificial Opening Endoscopic
0TWB83Z	Revision of Infusion Device in Bladder, Via Natural or Artificial Opening Endoscopic
0TWB87Z	Revision of Autologous Tissue Substitute in Bladder, Via Natural or Artificial Opening Endoscopic
0TWB8CZ	Revision of Extraluminal Device in Bladder, Via Natural or Artificial Opening Endoscopic
0TWB8DZ	Revision of Intraluminal Device in Bladder, Via Natural or Artificial Opening Endoscopic
0TWB8JZ	Revision of Synthetic Substitute in Bladder, Via Natural or Artificial Opening Endoscopic
0TWB8KZ	Revision of Nonautologous Tissue Substitute in Bladder, Via Natural or Artificial Opening Endoscopic
0TWB8LZ	Revision of Artificial Sphincter in Bladder, Via Natural or Artificial Opening Endoscopic
0TWB8MZ	Revision of Stimulator Lead in Bladder, Via Natural or Artificial Opening Endoscopic
0TWBX0Z	Revision of Drainage Device in Bladder, External Approach
0TWBX2Z	Revision of Monitoring Device in Bladder, External Approach
0TWBX3Z	Revision of Infusion Device in Bladder, External Approach
0TWBX7Z	Revision of Autologous Tissue Substitute in Bladder, External Approach
0TWBXCZ	Revision of Extraluminal Device in Bladder, External Approach
0TWBXDZ	Revision of Intraluminal Device in Bladder, External Approach
0TWBXJZ	Revision of Synthetic Substitute in Bladder, External Approach
0TWBXKZ	Revision of Nonautologous Tissue Substitute in Bladder, External Approach
0TWBXLZ	Revision of Artificial Sphincter in Bladder, External Approach
0TWBXMZ	Revision of Stimulator Lead in Bladder, External Approach
0TWD00Z	Revision of Drainage Device in Urethra, Open Approach
0TWD02Z	Revision of Monitoring Device in Urethra, Open Approach
0TWD03Z	Revision of Infusion Device in Urethra, Open Approach
0TWD07Z	Revision of Autologous Tissue Substitute in Urethra, Open Approach
0TWD0CZ	Revision of Extraluminal Device in Urethra, Open Approach
0TWD0DZ	Revision of Intraluminal Device in Urethra, Open Approach
0TWD0JZ	Revision of Synthetic Substitute in Urethra, Open Approach
0TWD0KZ	Revision of Nonautologous Tissue Substitute in Urethra, Open Approach
0TWD0LZ	Revision of Artificial Sphincter in Urethra, Open Approach
0TWD30Z	Revision of Drainage Device in Urethra, Percutaneous Approach
0TWD32Z	Revision of Monitoring Device in Urethra, Percutaneous Approach

0TWD33Z	Revision of Infusion Device in Urethra, Percutaneous Approach
0TWD37Z	Revision of Autologous Tissue Substitute in Urethra, Percutaneous Approach
0TWD3CZ	Revision of Extraluminal Device in Urethra, Percutaneous Approach
0TWD3DZ	Revision of Intraluminal Device in Urethra, Percutaneous Approach
0TWD3JZ	Revision of Synthetic Substitute in Urethra, Percutaneous Approach
0TWD3KZ	Revision of Nonautologous Tissue Substitute in Urethra, Percutaneous Approach
0TWD3LZ	Revision of Artificial Sphincter in Urethra, Percutaneous Approach
0TWD40Z	Revision of Drainage Device in Urethra, Percutaneous Endoscopic Approach
0TWD42Z	Revision of Monitoring Device in Urethra, Percutaneous Endoscopic Approach
0TWD43Z	Revision of Infusion Device in Urethra, Percutaneous Endoscopic Approach
0TWD47Z	Revision of Autologous Tissue Substitute in Urethra, Percutaneous Endoscopic Approach
0TWD4CZ	Revision of Extraluminal Device in Urethra, Percutaneous Endoscopic Approach
0TWD4DZ	Revision of Intraluminal Device in Urethra, Percutaneous Endoscopic Approach
0TWD4JZ	Revision of Synthetic Substitute in Urethra, Percutaneous Endoscopic Approach
0TWD4KZ	Revision of Nonautologous Tissue Substitute in Urethra, Percutaneous Endoscopic Approach
0TWD4LZ	Revision of Artificial Sphincter in Urethra, Percutaneous Endoscopic Approach
0TWD70Z	Revision of Drainage Device in Urethra, Via Natural or Artificial Opening
0TWD72Z	Revision of Monitoring Device in Urethra, Via Natural or Artificial Opening
0TWD73Z	Revision of Infusion Device in Urethra, Via Natural or Artificial Opening
0TWD77Z	Revision of Autologous Tissue Substitute in Urethra, Via Natural or Artificial Opening
0TWD7CZ	Revision of Extraluminal Device in Urethra, Via Natural or Artificial Opening
0TWD7DZ	Revision of Intraluminal Device in Urethra, Via Natural or Artificial Opening
0TWD7JZ	Revision of Synthetic Substitute in Urethra, Via Natural or Artificial Opening
0TWD7KZ	Revision of Nonautologous Tissue Substitute in Urethra, Via Natural or Artificial Opening
0TWD7LZ	Revision of Artificial Sphincter in Urethra, Via Natural or Artificial Opening
0TWD80Z	Revision of Drainage Device in Urethra, Via Natural or Artificial Opening Endoscopic
0TWD82Z	Revision of Monitoring Device in Urethra, Via Natural or Artificial Opening Endoscopic
0TWD83Z	Revision of Infusion Device in Urethra, Via Natural or Artificial Opening Endoscopic
0TWD87Z	Revision of Autologous Tissue Substitute in Urethra, Via Natural or Artificial Opening Endoscopic

♀ Female-only   ♂ Male-only   ▲ Limited Coverage   ● Non-OR   ■ HAC-associated procedure   ▲ Non-covered procedures   ✚ Combination

0TWD8CZ	Revision of Extraluminal Device in Urethra, Via Natural or Artificial Opening Endoscopic
0TWD8DZ	Revision of Intraluminal Device in Urethra, Via Natural or Artificial Opening Endoscopic
0TWD8JZ	Revision of Synthetic Substitute in Urethra, Via Natural or Artificial Opening Endoscopic
0TWD8KZ	Revision of Nonautologous Tissue Substitute in Urethra, Via Natural or Artificial Opening Endoscopic

0TWD8LZ	Revision of Artificial Sphincter in Urethra, Via Natural or Artificial Opening Endoscopic
0TWDX0Z	Revision of Drainage Device in Urethra, External Approach
0TWDX2Z	Revision of Monitoring Device in Urethra, External Approach
0TWDX3Z	Revision of Infusion Device in Urethra, External Approach
0TWDX7Z	Revision of Autologous Tissue Substitute in Urethra, External Approach

0TWDXCZ	Revision of Extraluminal Device in Urethra, External Approach
0TWDXDZ	Revision of Intraluminal Device in Urethra, External Approach
0TWDXJZ	Revision of Synthetic Substitute in Urethra, External Approach
0TWDXKZ	Revision of Nonautologous Tissue Substitute in Urethra, External Approach
0TWDXLZ	Revision of Artificial Sphincter in Urethra, External Approach

0TY – Urinary System, Transplantation

Review Coding Guideline B3.16

0TY00Z0 Transplantation of Right Kidney, Allogeneic, Open Approach
➕ Kidney/Pancreas transplant when reported with Transplant of the Pancreas. *See table 0FY to construct the Transplantation code.*

0TY00Z1 Transplantation of Right Kidney, Syngeneic, Open Approach
➕ Kidney/Pancreas transplant when reported with Transplant of the Pancreas. *See table 0FY to construct the Transplantation code.*

0TY00Z2 Transplantation of Right Kidney, Zooplastic, Open Approach
➕ Kidney/Pancreas transplant when reported with Transplant of the Pancreas. *See table 0FY to construct the Transplantation code.*

0TY10Z0 Transplantation of Left Kidney, Allogeneic, Open Approach
➕ Kidney/Pancreas transplant when reported with Transplant of the Pancreas. *See table 0FY to construct the Transplantation code.*

0TY10Z1 Transplantation of Left Kidney, Syngeneic, Open Approach
➕ Kidney/Pancreas transplant when reported with Transplant of the Pancreas. *See table 0FY to construct the Transplantation code.*

0TY10Z2 Transplantation of Left Kidney, Zooplastic, Open Approach
➕ Kidney/Pancreas transplant when reported with Transplant of the Pancreas. *See table 0FY to construct the Transplantation code.*

♀ Female-only   ♂ Male-only   ▲ Limited Coverage   ● Non-OR   ▨ HAC-associated procedure   ▲ Non-covered procedures   ➕ Combination

Female Reproductive System

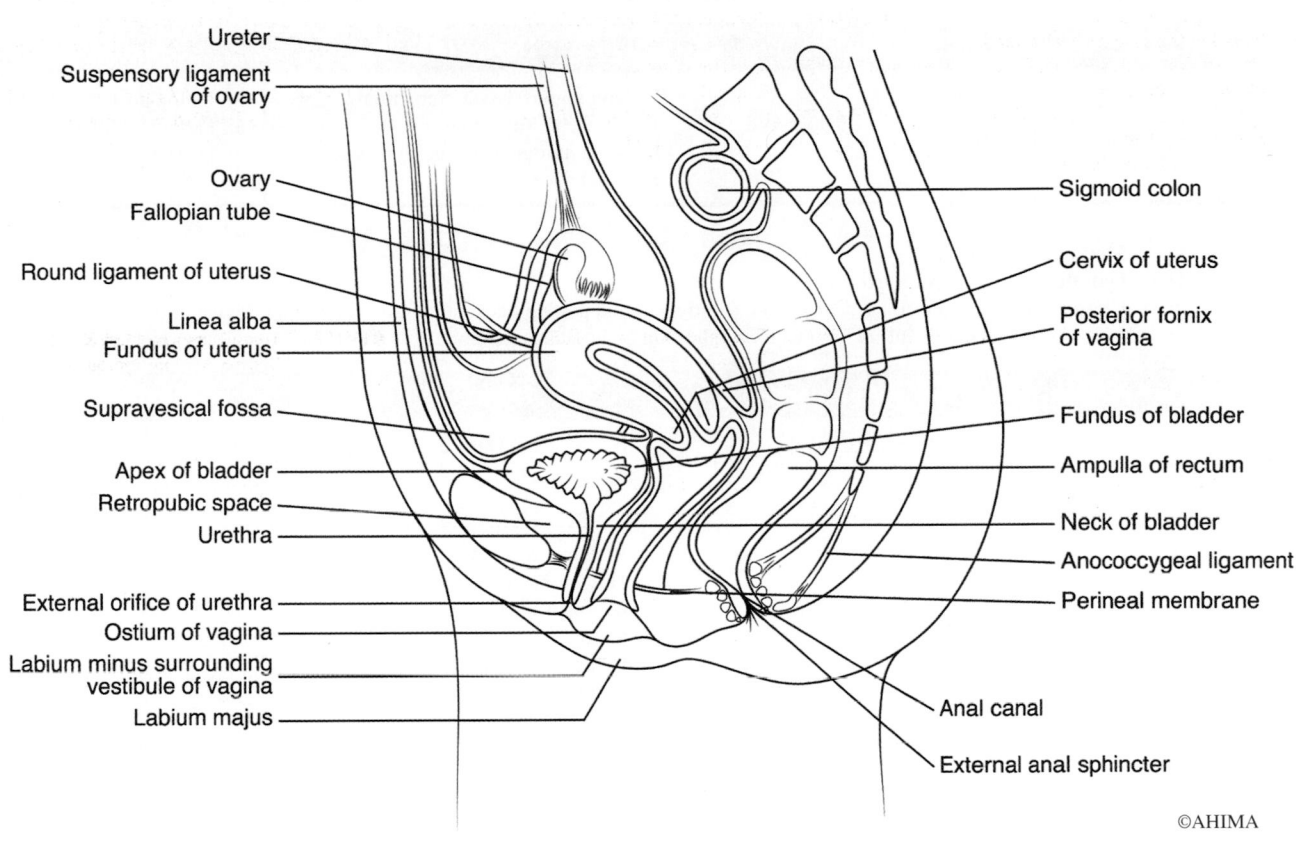

Ureter
Suspensory ligament of ovary
Ovary
Fallopian tube
Round ligament of uterus
Linea alba
Fundus of uterus
Supravesical fossa
Apex of bladder
Retropubic space
Urethra
External orifice of urethra
Ostium of vagina
Labium minus surrounding vestibule of vagina
Labium majus

Sigmoid colon
Cervix of uterus
Posterior fornix of vagina
Fundus of bladder
Ampulla of rectum
Neck of bladder
Anococcygeal ligament
Perineal membrane
Anal canal
External anal sphincter

©AHIMA

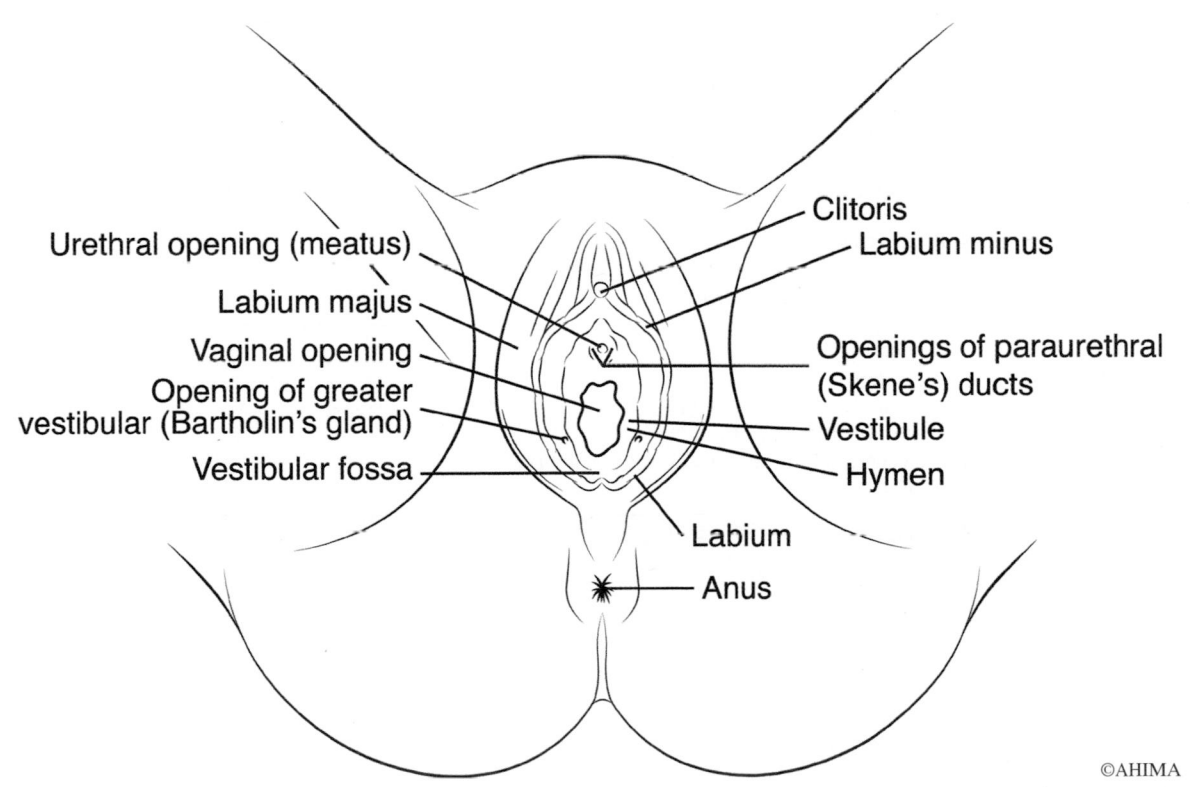

Urethral opening (meatus)
Labium majus
Vaginal opening
Opening of greater vestibular (Bartholin's gland)
Vestibular fossa

Clitoris
Labium minus
Openings of paraurethral (Skene's) ducts
Vestibule
Hymen
Labium
Anus

©AHIMA

Female Reproductive System Tables 0U1–0UY

Section	0	Medical and Surgical
Body System	U	Female Reproductive System
Operation	1	**Bypass:** Altering the route of passage of the contents of a tubular body part

Body Part (4th)	Approach (5th)	Device (6th)	Qualifier (7th)
5 Fallopian Tube, Right 6 Fallopian Tube, Left	0 Open 4 Percutaneous Endoscopic	7 Autologous Tissue Substitute J Synthetic Substitute K Nonautologous Tissue Substitute Z No Device	5 Fallopian Tube, Right 6 Fallopian Tube, Left 9 Uterus

Section	0	Medical and Surgical
Body System	U	Female Reproductive System
Operation	2	**Change:** Taking out or off a device from a body part and putting back an identical or similar device in or on the same body part without cutting or puncturing the skin or a mucous membrane

Body Part (4th)	Approach (5th)	Device (6th)	Qualifier (7th)
3 Ovary 8 Fallopian Tube M Vulva	X External	0 Drainage Device Y Other Device	Z No Qualifier
D Uterus and Cervix	X External	0 Drainage Device H Contraceptive Device Y Other Device	Z No Qualifier
H Vagina and Cul-de-sac	X External	0 Drainage Device G Intraluminal Device, Pessary Y Other Device	Z No Qualifier

Section	0	Medical and Surgical
Body System	U	Female Reproductive System
Operation	5	**Destruction:** Physical eradication of all or a portion of a body part by the direct use of energy, force, or a destructive agent

Body Part (4th)	Approach (5th)	Device (6th)	Qualifier (7th)
0 Ovary, Right 1 Ovary, Left 2 Ovaries, Bilateral 4 Uterine Supporting Structure	0 Open 3 Percutaneous 4 Percutaneous Endoscopic	Z No Device	Z No Qualifier
5 Fallopian Tube, Right 6 Fallopian Tube, Left 7 Fallopian Tubes, Bilateral 9 Uterus B Endometrium C Cervix F Cul-de-sac	0 Open 3 Percutaneous 4 Percutaneous Endoscopic 7 Via Natural or Artificial Opening 8 Via Natural or Artificial Opening Endoscopic	Z No Device	Z No Qualifier
G Vagina K Hymen	0 Open 3 Percutaneous 4 Percutaneous Endoscopic 7 Via Natural or Artificial Opening 8 Via Natural or Artificial Opening Endoscopic X External	Z No Device	Z No Qualifier
J Clitoris L Vestibular Gland M Vulva	0 Open X External	Z No Device	Z No Qualifier

Section	0	Medical and Surgical
Body System	U	Female Reproductive System
Operation	7	Dilation: Expanding an orifice or the lumen of a tubular body part

Body Part (4th)	Approach (5th)	Device (6th)	Qualifier (7th)
Fallopian Tube, Right Fallopian Tube, Left Fallopian Tubes, Bilateral Uterus Cervix Vagina	0 Open 3 Percutaneous 4 Percutaneous Endoscopic 7 Via Natural or Artificial Opening 8 Via Natural or Artificial Opening Endoscopic	D Intraluminal Device Z No Device	Z No Qualifier
Hymen	0 Open 3 Percutaneous 4 Percutaneous Endoscopic 7 Via Natural or Artificial Opening 8 Via Natural or Artificial Opening Endoscopic X External	D Intraluminal Device Z No Device	Z No Qualifier

Section	0	Medical and Surgical
Body System	U	Female Reproductive System
Operation	8	Division: Cutting into a body part, without draining fluids and/or gases from the body part, in order to separate or transect a body part

Body Part (4th)	Approach (5th)	Device (6th)	Qualifier (7th)
Ovary, Right Ovary, Left Ovaries, Bilateral Uterine Supporting Structure	0 Open 3 Percutaneous 4 Percutaneous Endoscopic	Z No Device	Z No Qualifier
Hymen	7 Via Natural or Artificial Opening 8 Via Natural or Artificial Opening Endoscopic X External	Z No Device	Z No Qualifier

Section	0	Medical and Surgical
Body System	U	Female Reproductive System
Operation	9	Drainage: Taking or letting out fluids and/or gases from a body part

Body Part (4th)	Approach (5th)	Device (6th)	Qualifier (7th)
0 Ovary, Right 1 Ovary, Left 2 Ovaries, Bilateral	0 Open 3 Percutaneous 4 Percutaneous Endoscopic	0 Drainage Device	Z No Qualifier
0 Ovary, Right 1 Ovary, Left 2 Ovaries, Bilateral	0 Open 3 Percutaneous 4 Percutaneous Endoscopic	Z No Device	X Diagnostic Z No Qualifier
0 Ovary, Right 1 Ovary, Left 2 Ovaries, Bilateral	X External	Z No Device	Z No Qualifier
4 Uterine Supporting Structure	0 Open 3 Percutaneous 4 Percutaneous Endoscopic	0 Drainage Device	Z No Qualifier
4 Uterine Supporting Structure	0 Open 3 Percutaneous 4 Percutaneous Endoscopic	Z No Device	X Diagnostic Z No Qualifier
5 Fallopian Tube, Right 6 Fallopian Tube, Left 7 Fallopian Tubes, Bilateral 9 Uterus C Cervix F Cul-de-sac	0 Open 3 Percutaneous 4 Percutaneous Endoscopic 7 Via Natural or Artificial Opening 8 Via Natural or Artificial Opening Endoscopic	0 Drainage Device	Z No Qualifier

Continued →

Section 0 **Medical and Surgical**
Body System U **Female Reproductive System**
Operation 9 **Drainage:** Taking or letting out fluids and/or gases from a body part

Body Part (4th)	Approach (5th)	Device (6th)	Qualifier (7th)
5 Fallopian Tube, Right 6 Fallopian Tube, Left 7 Fallopian Tubes, Bilateral 9 Uterus C Cervix F Cul-de-sac	0 Open 3 Percutaneous 4 Percutaneous Endoscopic 7 Via Natural or Artificial Opening 8 Via Natural or Artificial Opening Endoscopic	Z No Device	X Diagnostic Z No Qualifier
G Vagina K Hymen	0 Open 3 Percutaneous 4 Percutaneous Endoscopic 7 Via Natural or Artificial Opening 8 Via Natural or Artificial Opening Endoscopic X External	0 Drainage Device	Z No Qualifier
G Vagina K Hymen	0 Open 3 Percutaneous 4 Percutaneous Endoscopic 7 Via Natural or Artificial Opening 8 Via Natural or Artificial Opening Endoscopic X External	Z No Device	X Diagnostic Z No Qualifier
J Clitoris L Vestibular Gland M Vulva	0 Open X External	0 Drainage Device	Z No Qualifier
J Clitoris L Vestibular Gland M Vulva	0 Open X External	Z No Device	X Diagnostic Z No Qualifier

Section 0 **Medical and Surgical**
Body System U **Female Reproductive System**
Operation B **Excision:** Cutting out or off, without replacement, a portion of a body part

Body Part (4th)	Approach (5th)	Device (6th)	Qualifier (7th)
0 Ovary, Right 1 Ovary, Left 2 Ovaries, Bilateral 4 Uterine Supporting Structure 5 Fallopian Tube, Right 6 Fallopian Tube, Left 7 Fallopian Tubes, Bilateral 9 Uterus C Cervix F Cul-de-sac	0 Open 3 Percutaneous 4 Percutaneous Endoscopic 7 Via Natural or Artificial Opening 8 Via Natural or Artificial Opening Endoscopic	Z No Device	X Diagnostic Z No Qualifier
G Vagina K Hymen	0 Open 3 Percutaneous 4 Percutaneous Endoscopic 7 Via Natural or Artificial Opening 8 Via Natural or Artificial Opening Endoscopic X External	Z No Device	X Diagnostic Z No Qualifier
J Clitoris L Vestibular Gland M Vulva	0 Open X External	Z No Device	X Diagnostic Z No Qualifier

Section 0 Medical and Surgical
Body System U Female Reproductive System
Operation C Extirpation: Taking or cutting out solid matter from a body part

Body Part (4th)	Approach (5th)	Device (6th)	Qualifier (7th)
0 Ovary, Right 1 Ovary, Left 2 Ovaries, Bilateral 4 Uterine Supporting Structure	0 Open 3 Percutaneous 4 Percutaneous Endoscopic	Z No Device	Z No Qualifier
5 Fallopian Tube, Right 6 Fallopian Tube, Left 7 Fallopian Tubes, Bilateral 9 Uterus B Endometrium C Cervix F Cul-de-sac	0 Open 3 Percutaneous 4 Percutaneous Endoscopic 7 Via Natural or Artificial Opening 8 Via Natural or Artificial Opening Endoscopic	Z No Device	Z No Qualifier
G Vagina K Hymen	0 Open 3 Percutaneous 4 Percutaneous Endoscopic 7 Via Natural or Artificial Opening 8 Via Natural or Artificial Opening Endoscopic X External	Z No Device	Z No Qualifier
J Clitoris L Vestibular Gland M Vulva	0 Open X External	Z No Device	Z No Qualifier

Section 0 Medical and Surgical
Body System U Female Reproductive System
Operation D Extraction: Pulling or stripping out or off all or a portion of a body part by the use of force

Body Part (4th)	Approach (5th)	Device (6th)	Qualifier (7th)
B Endometrium	7 Via Natural or Artificial Opening 8 Via Natural or Artificial Opening Endoscopic	Z No Device	X Diagnostic Z No Qualifier
N Ova	0 Open 3 Percutaneous 4 Percutaneous Endoscopic	Z No Device	Z No Qualifier

Section 0 Medical and Surgical
Body System U Female Reproductive System
Operation F Fragmentation: Breaking solid matter in a body part into pieces

Body Part (4th)	Approach (5th)	Device (6th)	Qualifier (7th)
5 Fallopian Tube, Right 6 Fallopian Tube, Left 7 Fallopian Tubes, Bilateral 9 Uterus	0 Open 3 Percutaneous 4 Percutaneous Endoscopic 7 Via Natural or Artificial Opening 8 Via Natural or Artificial Opening Endoscopic X External	Z No Device	Z No Qualifier

Section   0   **Medical and Surgical**
Body System   U   **Female Reproductive System**
Operation   H   **Insertion:** Putting in a nonbiological appliance that monitors, assists, performs, or prevents a physiological function but does not physically take the place of a body part

Body Part (4th)	Approach (5th)	Device (6th)	Qualifier (7th)
3 Ovary	0 Open 3 Percutaneous 4 Percutaneous Endoscopic	3 Infusion Device	Z No Qualifier
8 Fallopian Tube D Uterus and Cervix H Vagina and Cul-de-sac	0 Open 3 Percutaneous 4 Percutaneous Endoscopic 7 Via Natural or Artificial Opening 8 Via Natural or Artificial Opening Endoscopic	3 Infusion Device	Z No Qualifier
9 Uterus	7 Via Natural or Artificial Opening 8 Via Natural or Artificial Opening Endoscopic	H Contraceptive Device	Z No Qualifier
C Cervix	0 Open 3 Percutaneous 4 Percutaneous Endoscopic	1 Radioactive Element	Z No Qualifier
C Cervix	7 Via Natural or Artificial Opening 8 Via Natural or Artificial Opening Endoscopic	1 Radioactive Element H Contraceptive Device	Z No Qualifier
F Cul-de-sac	7 Via Natural or Artificial Opening 8 Via Natural or Artificial Opening Endoscopic	G Intraluminal Device, Pessary	Z No Qualifier
G Vagina	0 Open 3 Percutaneous 4 Percutaneous Endoscopic X External	1 Radioactive Element	Z No Qualifier
G Vagina	7 Via Natural or Artificial Opening 8 Via Natural or Artificial Opening Endoscopic	1 Radioactive Element G Intraluminal Device, Pessary	Z No Qualifier

Section   0   **Medical and Surgical**
Body System   U   **Female Reproductive System**
Operation   J   **Inspection:** Visually and/or manually exploring a body part

Body Part (4th)	Approach (5th)	Device (6th)	Qualifier (7th)
3 Ovary	0 Open 3 Percutaneous 4 Percutaneous Endoscopic X External	Z No Device	Z No Qualifier
8 Fallopian Tube D Uterus and Cervix H Vagina and Cul-de-sac	0 Open 3 Percutaneous 4 Percutaneous Endoscopic 7 Via Natural or Artificial Opening 8 Via Natural or Artificial Opening Endoscopic X External	Z No Device	Z No Qualifier
M Vulva	0 Open X External	Z No Device	Z No Qualifier

Section   0   **Medical and Surgical**
Body System   U   **Female Reproductive System**
Operation   L   **Occlusion:** Completely closing an orifice or the lumen of a tubular body part

Body Part (4th)	Approach (5th)	Device (6th)	Qualifier (7th)
5 Fallopian Tube, Right 6 Fallopian Tube, Left 7 Fallopian Tubes, Bilateral	0 Open 3 Percutaneous 4 Percutaneous Endoscopic	C Extraluminal Device D Intraluminal Device Z No Device	Z No Qualifier

Continued →

Section | 0 | Medical and Surgical
Body System | U | Female Reproductive System
Operation | L | Occlusion: Completely closing an orifice or the lumen of a tubular body part

Body Part (4th)	Approach (5th)	Device (6th)	Qualifier (7th)
Fallopian Tube, Right Fallopian Tube, Left Fallopian Tubes, Bilateral	7 Via Natural or Artificial Opening 8 Via Natural or Artificial Opening Endoscopic	D Intraluminal Device Z No Device	Z No Qualifier
Cul-de-sac Vagina	7 Via Natural or Artificial Opening 8 Via Natural or Artificial Opening Endoscopic	D Intraluminal Device Z No Device	Z No Qualifier

Section | 0 | Medical and Surgical
Body System | U | Female Reproductive System
Operation | M | Reattachment: Putting back in or on all or a portion of a separated body part to its normal location or other suitable location

Body Part (4th)	Approach (5th)	Device (6th)	Qualifier (7th)
0 Ovary, Right 1 Ovary, Left 2 Ovaries, Bilateral 4 Uterine Supporting Structure 5 Fallopian Tube, Right 6 Fallopian Tube, Left 7 Fallopian Tubes, Bilateral 9 Uterus C Cervix F Cul-de-sac G Vagina	0 Open 4 Percutaneous Endoscopic	Z No Device	Z No Qualifier
Clitoris M Vulva	X External	Z No Device	Z No Qualifier
K Hymen	0 Open 4 Percutaneous Endoscopic X External	Z No Device	Z No Qualifier

Section | 0 | Medical and Surgical
Body System | U | Female Reproductive System
Operation | N | Release: Freeing a body part from an abnormal physical constraint by cutting or by the use of force

Body Part (4th)	Approach (5th)	Device (6th)	Qualifier (7th)
0 Ovary, Right 1 Ovary, Left 2 Ovaries, Bilateral 4 Uterine Supporting Structure	0 Open 3 Percutaneous 4 Percutaneous Endoscopic	Z No Device	Z No Qualifier
5 Fallopian Tube, Right 6 Fallopian Tube, Left 7 Fallopian Tubes, Bilateral 9 Uterus C Cervix F Cul-de-sac	0 Open 3 Percutaneous 4 Percutaneous Endoscopic 7 Via Natural or Artificial Opening 8 Via Natural or Artificial Opening Endoscopic	Z No Device	Z No Qualifier
G Vagina K Hymen	0 Open 3 Percutaneous 4 Percutaneous Endoscopic 7 Via Natural or Artificial Opening 8 Via Natural or Artificial Opening Endoscopic X External	Z No Device	Z No Qualifier
J Clitoris L Vestibular Gland M Vulva	0 Open X External	Z No Device	Z No Qualifier

Section	0	Medical and Surgical
Body System	U	Female Reproductive System
Operation	P	**Removal:** Taking out or off a device from a body part

Body Part (4th)	Approach (5th)	Device (6th)	Qualifier (7th)
3 Ovary	0 Open 3 Percutaneous 4 Percutaneous Endoscopic X External	0 Drainage Device 3 Infusion Device	Z No Qualifier
8 Fallopian Tube	0 Open 3 Percutaneous 4 Percutaneous Endoscopic 7 Via Natural or Artificial Opening 8 Via Natural or Artificial Opening Endoscopic	0 Drainage Device 3 Infusion Device 7 Autologous Tissue Substitute C Extraluminal Device D Intraluminal Device J Synthetic Substitute K Nonautologous Tissue Substitute	Z No Qualifier
8 Fallopian Tube	X External	0 Drainage Device 3 Infusion Device D Intraluminal Device	Z No Qualifier
D Uterus and Cervix	0 Open 3 Percutaneous 4 Percutaneous Endoscopic 7 Via Natural or Artificial Opening 8 Via Natural or Artificial Opening Endoscopic	0 Drainage Device 1 Radioactive Element 3 Infusion Device 7 Autologous Tissue Substitute C Extraluminal Device D Intraluminal Device H Contraceptive Device J Synthetic Substitute K Nonautologous Tissue Substitute	Z No Qualifier
D Uterus and Cervix	X External	0 Drainage Device 3 Infusion Device D Intraluminal Device H Contraceptive Device	Z No Qualifier
H Vagina and Cul-de-sac	0 Open 3 Percutaneous 4 Percutaneous Endoscopic 7 Via Natural or Artificial Opening 8 Via Natural or Artificial Opening Endoscopic	0 Drainage Device 1 Radioactive Element 3 Infusion Device 7 Autologous Tissue Substitute D Intraluminal Device J Synthetic Substitute K Nonautologous Tissue Substitute	Z No Qualifier
H Vagina and Cul-de-sac	X External	0 Drainage Device 1 Radioactive Element 3 Infusion Device D Intraluminal Device	Z No Qualifier
M Vulva	0 Open	0 Drainage Device 7 Autologous Tissue Substitute J Synthetic Substitute K Nonautologous Tissue Substitute	Z No Qualifier
M Vulva	X External	0 Drainage Device	Z No Qualifier

Section	0	Medical and Surgical
Body System	U	Female Reproductive System
Operation	Q	**Repair:** Restoring, to the extent possible, a body part to its normal anatomic structure and function

Body Part (4th)	Approach (5th)	Device (6th)	Qualifier (7th)
0 Ovary, Right 1 Ovary, Left 2 Ovaries, Bilateral 4 Uterine Supporting Structure	0 Open 3 Percutaneous 4 Percutaneous Endoscopic	Z No Device	Z No Qualifier

Continued →

	Section	0	Medical and Surgical
	Body System	U	Female Reproductive System
	Operation	Q	Repair: Restoring, to the extent possible, a body part to its normal anatomic structure and function

Body Part (4th)	Approach (5th)	Device (6th)	Qualifier (7th)
Fallopian Tube, Right Fallopian Tube, Left Fallopian Tubes, Bilateral Uterus C Cervix Cul-de-sac	0 Open 3 Percutaneous 4 Percutaneous Endoscopic 7 Via Natural or Artificial Opening 8 Via Natural or Artificial Opening Endoscopic	Z No Device	Z No Qualifier
G Vagina K Hymen	0 Open 3 Percutaneous 4 Percutaneous Endoscopic 7 Via Natural or Artificial Opening 8 Via Natural or Artificial Opening Endoscopic X External	Z No Device	Z No Qualifier
Clitoris Vestibular Gland M Vulva	0 Open X External	Z No Device	Z No Qualifier

	Section	0	Medical and Surgical
	Body System	U	Female Reproductive System
	Operation	S	Reposition: Moving to its normal location, or other suitable location, all or a portion of a body part

Body Part (4th)	Approach (5th)	Device (6th)	Qualifier (7th)
0 Ovary, Right 1 Ovary, Left 2 Ovaries, Bilateral 4 Uterine Supporting Structure 5 Fallopian Tube, Right 6 Fallopian Tube, Left 7 Fallopian Tubes, Bilateral C Cervix F Cul-de-sac	0 Open 4 Percutaneous Endoscopic	Z No Device	Z No Qualifier
9 Uterus G Vagina	0 Open 4 Percutaneous Endoscopic X External	Z No Device	Z No Qualifier

	Section	0	Medical and Surgical
	Body System	U	Female Reproductive System
	Operation	T	Resection: Cutting out or off, without replacement, all of a body part

Body Part (4th)	Approach (5th)	Device (6th)	Qualifier (7th)
0 Ovary, Right 1 Ovary, Left 2 Ovaries, Bilateral 5 Fallopian Tube, Right 6 Fallopian Tube, Left 7 Fallopian Tubes, Bilateral 9 Uterus	0 Open 4 Percutaneous Endoscopic 7 Via Natural or Artificial Opening 8 Via Natural or Artificial Opening Endoscopic F Via Natural or Artificial Opening With Percutaneous Endoscopic Assistance	Z No Device	Z No Qualifier
4 Uterine Supporting Structure C Cervix F Cul-de-sac G Vagina	0 Open 4 Percutaneous Endoscopic 7 Via Natural or Artificial Opening 8 Via Natural or Artificial Opening Endoscopic	Z No Device	Z No Qualifier
J Clitoris L Vestibular Gland M Vulva	0 Open X External	Z No Device	Z No Qualifier

Continued →

Section	0	Medical and Surgical
Body System	U	Female Reproductive System
Operation	T	Resection: Cutting out or off, without replacement, all of a body part

Body Part (4th)	Approach (5th)	Device (6th)	Qualifier (7th)
K Hymen	0 Open 4 Percutaneous Endoscopic 7 Via Natural or Artificial Opening 8 Via Natural or Artificial Opening Endoscopic X External	Z No Device	Z No Qualifier

Section	0	Medical and Surgical
Body System	U	Female Reproductive System
Operation	U	Supplement: Putting in or on biological or synthetic material that physically reinforces and/or augments the function of a portion of a body part

Body Part (4th)	Approach (5th)	Device (6th)	Qualifier (7th)
4 Uterine Supporting Structure	0 Open 4 Percutaneous Endoscopic	7 Autologous Tissue Substitute J Synthetic Substitute K Nonautologous Tissue Substitute	Z No Qualifier
5 Fallopian Tube, Right 6 Fallopian Tube, Left 7 Fallopian Tubes, Bilateral F Cul-de-sac	0 Open 4 Percutaneous Endoscopic 7 Via Natural or Artificial Opening 8 Via Natural or Artificial Opening Endoscopic	7 Autologous Tissue Substitute J Synthetic Substitute K Nonautologous Tissue Substitute	Z No Qualifier
G Vagina K Hymen	0 Open 4 Percutaneous Endoscopic 7 Via Natural or Artificial Opening 8 Via Natural or Artificial Opening Endoscopic X External	7 Autologous Tissue Substitute J Synthetic Substitute K Nonautologous Tissue Substitute	Z No Qualifier
J Clitoris M Vulva	0 Open X External	7 Autologous Tissue Substitute J Synthetic Substitute K Nonautologous Tissue Substitute	Z No Qualifier

Section	0	Medical and Surgical
Body System	U	Female Reproductive System
Operation	V	Restriction: Partially closing an orifice or the lumen of a tubular body part

Body Part (4th)	Approach (5th)	Device (6th)	Qualifier (7th)
C Cervix	0 Open 3 Percutaneous 4 Percutaneous Endoscopic	C Extraluminal Device D Intraluminal Device Z No Device	Z No Qualifier
C Cervix	7 Via Natural or Artificial Opening 8 Via Natural or Artificial Opening Endoscopic	D Intraluminal Device Z No Device	Z No Qualifier

Section	0	Medical and Surgical
Body System	U	Female Reproductive System
Operation	W	Revision: Correcting, to the extent possible, a portion of a malfunctioning device or the position of a displaced device

Body Part (4th)	Approach (5th)	Device (6th)	Qualifier (7th)
3 Ovary	0 Open 3 Percutaneous 4 Percutaneous Endoscopic X External	0 Drainage Device 3 Infusion Device	Z No Qualifier

Continued →

Section	0	Medical and Surgical
Body System	U	Female Reproductive System
Operation	W	Revision: Correcting, to the extent possible, a portion of a malfunctioning device or the position of a displaced device

Body Part (4th)	Approach (5th)	Device (6th)	Qualifier (7th)
8 Fallopian Tube	0 Open 3 Percutaneous 4 Percutaneous Endoscopic 7 Via Natural or Artificial Opening 8 Via Natural or Artificial Opening Endoscopic X External	0 Drainage Device 3 Infusion Device 7 Autologous Tissue Substitute C Extraluminal Device D Intraluminal Device J Synthetic Substitute K Nonautologous Tissue Substitute	Z No Qualifier
D Uterus and Cervix	0 Open 3 Percutaneous 4 Percutaneous Endoscopic 7 Via Natural or Artificial Opening 8 Via Natural or Artificial Opening Endoscopic	0 Drainage Device 1 Radioactive Element 3 Infusion Device 7 Autologous Tissue Substitute C Extraluminal Device D Intraluminal Device H Contraceptive Device J Synthetic Substitute K Nonautologous Tissue Substitute	Z No Qualifier
D Uterus and Cervix	X External	0 Drainage Device 3 Infusion Device 7 Autologous Tissue Substitute C Extraluminal Device D Intraluminal Device H Contraceptive Device J Synthetic Substitute K Nonautologous Tissue Substitute	Z No Qualifier
H Vagina and Cul-de-sac	0 Open 3 Percutaneous 4 Percutaneous Endoscopic 7 Via Natural or Artificial Opening 8 Via Natural or Artificial Opening Endoscopic	0 Drainage Device 1 Radioactive Element 3 Infusion Device 7 Autologous Tissue Substitute D Intraluminal Device J Synthetic Substitute K Nonautologous Tissue Substitute	Z No Qualifier
H Vagina and Cul-de-sac	X External	0 Drainage Device 3 Infusion Device 7 Autologous Tissue Substitute D Intraluminal Device J Synthetic Substitute K Nonautologous Tissue Substitute	Z No Qualifier
M Vulva	0 Open X External	0 Drainage Device 7 Autologous Tissue Substitute J Synthetic Substitute K Nonautologous Tissue Substitute	Z No Qualifier

Section	0	Medical and Surgical
Body System	U	Female Reproductive System
Operation	Y	Transplantation: Putting in or on all or a portion of a living body part taken from another individual or animal to physically take the place and/or function of all or a portion of a similar body part

Body Part (4th)	Approach (5th)	Device (6th)	Qualifier (7th)
0 Ovary, Right 1 Ovary, Left	0 Open	Z No Device	0 Allogeneic 1 Syngeneic 2 Zooplastic

Female Reproductive System Code Listing 0U1–0UY

0U1 – Female Reproductive System, Bypass

Review Coding Guideline B3.6a

♀ **0U15075** Bypass Right Fallopian Tube to Right Fallopian Tube with Autologous Tissue Substitute, Open Approach

♀ **0U15076** Bypass Right Fallopian Tube to Left Fallopian Tube with Autologous Tissue Substitute, Open Approach

♀ **0U15079** Bypass Right Fallopian Tube to Uterus with Autologous Tissue Substitute, Open Approach

♀ **0U150J5** Bypass Right Fallopian Tube to Right Fallopian Tube with Synthetic Substitute, Open Approach

♀ **0U150J6** Bypass Right Fallopian Tube to Left Fallopian Tube with Synthetic Substitute, Open Approach

♀ **0U150J9** Bypass Right Fallopian Tube to Uterus with Synthetic Substitute, Open Approach

♀ **0U150K5** Bypass Right Fallopian Tube to Right Fallopian Tube with Nonautologous Tissue Substitute, Open Approach

♀ **0U150K6** Bypass Right Fallopian Tube to Left Fallopian Tube with Nonautologous Tissue Substitute, Open Approach

♀ **0U150K9** Bypass Right Fallopian Tube to Uterus with Nonautologous Tissue Substitute, Open Approach

♀ **0U150Z5** Bypass Right Fallopian Tube to Right Fallopian Tube, Open Approach

♀ **0U150Z6** Bypass Right Fallopian Tube to Left Fallopian Tube, Open Approach

♀ **0U150Z9** Bypass Right Fallopian Tube to Uterus, Open Approach

♀ **0U15475** Bypass Right Fallopian Tube to Right Fallopian Tube with Autologous Tissue Substitute, Percutaneous Endoscopic Approach

♀ **0U15476** Bypass Right Fallopian Tube to Left Fallopian Tube with Autologous Tissue Substitute, Percutaneous Endoscopic Approach

♀ **0U15479** Bypass Right Fallopian Tube to Uterus with Autologous Tissue Substitute, Percutaneous Endoscopic Approach

♀ **0U154J5** Bypass Right Fallopian Tube to Right Fallopian Tube with Synthetic Substitute, Percutaneous Endoscopic Approach

♀ **0U154J6** Bypass Right Fallopian Tube to Left Fallopian Tube with Synthetic Substitute, Percutaneous Endoscopic Approach

♀ **0U154J9** Bypass Right Fallopian Tube to Uterus with Synthetic Substitute, Percutaneous Endoscopic Approach

♀ **0U154K5** Bypass Right Fallopian Tube to Right Fallopian Tube with Nonautologous Tissue Substitute, Percutaneous Endoscopic Approach

♀ **0U154K6** Bypass Right Fallopian Tube to Left Fallopian Tube with Nonautologous Tissue Substitute, Percutaneous Endoscopic Approach

♀ **0U154K9** Bypass Right Fallopian Tube to Uterus with Nonautologous Tissue Substitute, Percutaneous Endoscopic Approach

♀ **0U154Z5** Bypass Right Fallopian Tube to Right Fallopian Tube, Percutaneous Endoscopic Approach

♀ **0U154Z6** Bypass Right Fallopian Tube to Left Fallopian Tube, Percutaneous Endoscopic Approach

♀ **0U154Z9** Bypass Right Fallopian Tube to Uterus, Percutaneous Endoscopic Approach

♀ **0U16075** Bypass Left Fallopian Tube to Right Fallopian Tube with Autologous Tissue Substitute, Open Approach

♀ **0U16076** Bypass Left Fallopian Tube to Left Fallopian Tube with Autologous Tissue Substitute, Open Approach

♀ **0U16079** Bypass Left Fallopian Tube to Uterus with Autologous Tissue Substitute, Open Approach

♀ **0U160J5** Bypass Left Fallopian Tube to Right Fallopian Tube with Synthetic Substitute, Open Approach

♀ **0U160J6** Bypass Left Fallopian Tube to Left Fallopian Tube with Synthetic Substitute, Open Approach

♀ **0U160J9** Bypass Left Fallopian Tube to Uterus with Synthetic Substitute, Open Approach

♀ **0U160K5** Bypass Left Fallopian Tube to Right Fallopian Tube with Nonautologous Tissue Substitute, Open Approach

♀ **0U160K6** Bypass Left Fallopian Tube to Left Fallopian Tube with Nonautologous Tissue Substitute, Open Approach

♀ **0U160K9** Bypass Left Fallopian Tube to Uterus with Nonautologous Tissue Substitute, Open Approach

♀ **0U160Z5** Bypass Left Fallopian Tube to Right Fallopian Tube, Open Approach

♀ **0U160Z6** Bypass Left Fallopian Tube to Left Fallopian Tube, Open Approach

♀ **0U160Z9** Bypass Left Fallopian Tube to Uterus, Open Approach

♀ **0U16475** Bypass Left Fallopian Tube to Right Fallopian Tube with Autologous Tissue Substitute, Percutaneous Endoscopic Approach

♀ **0U16476** Bypass Left Fallopian Tube to Left Fallopian Tube with Autologous Tissue Substitute, Percutaneous Endoscopic Approach

♀ **0U16479** Bypass Left Fallopian Tube to Uterus with Autologous Tissue Substitute, Percutaneous Endoscopic Approach

♀ **0U164J5** Bypass Left Fallopian Tube to Right Fallopian Tube with Synthetic Substitute, Percutaneous Endoscopic Approach

♀ **0U164J6** Bypass Left Fallopian Tube to Left Fallopian Tube with Synthetic Substitute, Percutaneous Endoscopic Approach

♀ **0U164J9** Bypass Left Fallopian Tube to Uterus with Synthetic Substitute, Percutaneous Endoscopic Approach

♀ **0U164K5** Bypass Left Fallopian Tube to Right Fallopian Tube with Nonautologous Tissue Substitute, Percutaneous Endoscopic Approach

♀ **0U164K6** Bypass Left Fallopian Tube to Left Fallopian Tube with Nonautologous Tissue Substitute, Percutaneous Endoscopic Approach

♀ **0U164K9** Bypass Left Fallopian Tube to Uterus with Nonautologous Tissue Substitute, Percutaneous Endoscopic Approach

♀ **0U164Z5** Bypass Left Fallopian Tube to Right Fallopian Tube, Percutaneous Endoscopic Approach

♀ **0U164Z6** Bypass Left Fallopian Tube to Left Fallopian Tube, Percutaneous Endoscopic Approach

♀ **0U164Z9** Bypass Left Fallopian Tube to Uterus, Percutaneous Endoscopic Approach

0U2 – Female Reproductive System, Change

Review Coding Guideline B6.1c

♀ **0U23X0Z** Change Drainage Device in Ovary, External Approach

♀ **0U23XYZ** Change Other Device in Ovary, External Approach

♀ **0U28X0Z** Change Drainage Device in Fallopian Tube, External Approach

♀ **0U28XYZ** Change Other Device in Fallopian Tube, External Approach

♀ **0U2DX0Z** Change Drainage Device in Uterus and Cervix, External Approach

♀ **0U2DXHZ** Change Contraceptive Device in Uterus and Cervix, External Approach

♀ **0U2DXYZ** Change Other Device in Uterus and Cervix, External Approach

♀ **0U2HX0Z** Change Drainage Device in Vagina and Cul-de-sac, External Approach

♀ **0U2HXGZ** Change Pessary in Vagina and Cul-de-sac, External Approach

♀ **0U2HXYZ** Change Other Device in Vagina and Cul-de-sac, External Approach

♀ **0U2MX0Z** Change Drainage Device in Vulva, External Approach

♀ **0U2MXYZ** Change Other Device in Vulva, External Approach

0U5 – Female Reproductive System, Destruction

♀ **0U500ZZ** Destruction of Right Ovary, Open Approach

♀ **0U503ZZ** Destruction of Right Ovary, Percutaneous Approach

♀ **0U504ZZ** Destruction of Right Ovary, Percutaneous Endoscopic Approach

♀ **0U510ZZ** Destruction of Left Ovary, Open Approach

♀ **0U513ZZ** Destruction of Left Ovary, Percutaneous Approach

♀ **0U514ZZ** Destruction of Left Ovary, Percutaneous Endoscopic Approach

♀ **0U520ZZ** Destruction of Bilateral Ovaries, Open Approach

♀ **0U523ZZ** Destruction of Bilateral Ovaries, Percutaneous Approach

♀ **0U524ZZ** Destruction of Bilateral Ovaries, Percutaneous Endoscopic Approach

♀ **0U540ZZ** Destruction of Uterine Supporting Structure, Open Approach

♀ **0U543ZZ** Destruction of Uterine Supporting Structure, Percutaneous Approach

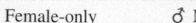

544ZZ Destruction of Uterine Supporting Structure, Percutaneous Endoscopic Approach	♀ 0U590ZZ Destruction of Uterus, Open Approach	♀ 0U5F7ZZ Destruction of Cul-de-sac, Via Natural or Artificial Opening
550ZZ Destruction of Right Fallopian Tube, Open Approach	♀ 0U593ZZ Destruction of Uterus, Percutaneous Approach	♀ 0U5F8ZZ Destruction of Cul-de-sac, Via Natural or Artificial Opening Endoscopic
553ZZ Destruction of Right Fallopian Tube, Percutaneous Approach	♀ 0U594ZZ Destruction of Uterus, Percutaneous Endoscopic Approach	♀ 0U5G0ZZ Destruction of Vagina, Open Approach
554ZZ Destruction of Right Fallopian Tube, Percutaneous Endoscopic Approach	♀ 0U597ZZ Destruction of Uterus, Via Natural or Artificial Opening	♀ 0U5G3ZZ Destruction of Vagina, Percutaneous Approach
557ZZ Destruction of Right Fallopian Tube, Via Natural or Artificial Opening	♀ 0U598ZZ Destruction of Uterus, Via Natural or Artificial Opening Endoscopic	♀ 0U5G4ZZ Destruction of Vagina, Percutaneous Endoscopic Approach
558ZZ Destruction of Right Fallopian Tube, Via Natural or Artificial Opening Endoscopic	♀ 0U5B0ZZ Destruction of Endometrium, Open Approach	♀ 0U5G7ZZ Destruction of Vagina, Via Natural or Artificial Opening
560ZZ Destruction of Left Fallopian Tube, Open Approach	♀ 0U5B3ZZ Destruction of Endometrium, Percutaneous Approach	♀ 0U5G8ZZ Destruction of Vagina, Via Natural or Artificial Opening Endoscopic
563ZZ Destruction of Left Fallopian Tube, Percutaneous Approach	♀ 0U5B4ZZ Destruction of Endometrium, Percutaneous Endoscopic Approach	♀ 0U5GXZZ Destruction of Vagina, External Approach
564ZZ Destruction of Left Fallopian Tube, Percutaneous Endoscopic Approach	♀ 0U5B7ZZ Destruction of Endometrium, Via Natural or Artificial Opening	♀ 0U5J0ZZ Destruction of Clitoris, Open Approach
567ZZ Destruction of Left Fallopian Tube, Via Natural or Artificial Opening	♀ 0U5B8ZZ Destruction of Endometrium, Via Natural or Artificial Opening Endoscopic	♀ 0U5JXZZ Destruction of Clitoris, External Approach
568ZZ Destruction of Left Fallopian Tube, Via Natural or Artificial Opening Endoscopic	♀ 0U5C0ZZ Destruction of Cervix, Open Approach	♀ 0U5K0ZZ Destruction of Hymen, Open Approach
570ZZ Destruction of Bilateral Fallopian Tubes, Open Approach	♀ 0U5C3ZZ Destruction of Cervix, Percutaneous Approach	♀ 0U5K3ZZ Destruction of Hymen, Percutaneous Approach
573ZZ Destruction of Bilateral Fallopian Tubes, Percutaneous Approach	♀ 0U5C4ZZ Destruction of Cervix, Percutaneous Endoscopic Approach	♀ 0U5K4ZZ Destruction of Hymen, Percutaneous Endoscopic Approach
574ZZ Destruction of Bilateral Fallopian Tubes, Percutaneous Endoscopic Approach	♀ 0U5C7ZZ Destruction of Cervix, Via Natural or Artificial Opening	♀ 0U5K7ZZ Destruction of Hymen, Via Natural or Artificial Opening
577ZZ Destruction of Bilateral Fallopian Tubes, Via Natural or Artificial Opening	♀ 0U5C8ZZ Destruction of Cervix, Via Natural or Artificial Opening Endoscopic	♀ 0U5K8ZZ ▲ Destruction of Hymen, Via Natural or Artificial Opening Endoscopic
578ZZ Destruction of Bilateral Fallopian Tubes, Via Natural or Artificial Opening Endoscopic	♀ 0U5F0ZZ Destruction of Cul-de-sac, Open Approach	♀ 0U5KXZZ Destruction of Hymen, External Approach
	♀ 0U5F3ZZ Destruction of Cul-de-sac, Percutaneous Approach	♀ 0U5L0ZZ Destruction of Vestibular Gland, Open Approach
	♀ 0U5F4ZZ Destruction of Cul-de-sac, Percutaneous Endoscopic Approach	♀ 0U5LXZZ Destruction of Vestibular Gland, External Approach
		♀ 0U5M0ZZ Destruction of Vulva, Open Approach
		♀ 0U5MXZZ Destruction of Vulva, External Approach

J7 – Female Reproductive System, Dilation

750DZ Dilation of Right Fallopian Tube with Intraluminal Device, Open Approach	♀ 0U767DZ Dilation of Left Fallopian Tube with Intraluminal Device, Via Natural or Artificial Opening	♀ 0U794DZ Dilation of Uterus with Intraluminal Device, Percutaneous Endoscopic Approach
750ZZ Dilation of Right Fallopian Tube, Open Approach	♀ 0U767ZZ Dilation of Left Fallopian Tube, Via Natural or Artificial Opening	♀ 0U794ZZ Dilation of Uterus, Percutaneous Endoscopic Approach
753DZ Dilation of Right Fallopian Tube with Intraluminal Device, Percutaneous Approach	♀ 0U768DZ Dilation of Left Fallopian Tube with Intraluminal Device, Via Natural or Artificial Opening Endoscopic	♀ 0U797DZ Dilation of Uterus with Intraluminal Device, Via Natural or Artificial Opening
753ZZ Dilation of Right Fallopian Tube, Percutaneous Approach	♀ 0U768ZZ Dilation of Left Fallopian Tube, Via Natural or Artificial Opening Endoscopic	♀ 0U797ZZ Dilation of Uterus, Via Natural or Artificial Opening
754DZ Dilation of Right Fallopian Tube with Intraluminal Device, Percutaneous Endoscopic Approach	♀ 0U770DZ Dilation of Bilateral Fallopian Tubes with Intraluminal Device, Open Approach	♀ 0U798DZ Dilation of Uterus with Intraluminal Device, Via Natural or Artificial Opening Endoscopic
754ZZ Dilation of Right Fallopian Tube, Percutaneous Endoscopic Approach	♀ 0U770ZZ Dilation of Bilateral Fallopian Tubes, Open Approach	♀ 0U798ZZ Dilation of Uterus, Via Natural or Artificial Opening Endoscopic
757DZ Dilation of Right Fallopian Tube with Intraluminal Device, Via Natural or Artificial Opening	♀ 0U773DZ Dilation of Bilateral Fallopian Tubes with Intraluminal Device, Percutaneous Approach	♀ 0U7C0DZ Dilation of Cervix with Intraluminal Device, Open Approach
757ZZ Dilation of Right Fallopian Tube, Via Natural or Artificial Opening	♀ 0U773ZZ Dilation of Bilateral Fallopian Tubes, Percutaneous Approach	♀ 0U7C0ZZ Dilation of Cervix, Open Approach
758DZ Dilation of Right Fallopian Tube with Intraluminal Device, Via Natural or Artificial Opening Endoscopic	♀ 0U774DZ Dilation of Bilateral Fallopian Tubes with Intraluminal Device, Percutaneous Endoscopic Approach	♀ 0U7C3DZ Dilation of Cervix with Intraluminal Device, Percutaneous Approach
758ZZ Dilation of Right Fallopian Tube, Via Natural or Artificial Opening Endoscopic	♀ 0U774ZZ Dilation of Bilateral Fallopian Tubes, Percutaneous Endoscopic Approach	♀ 0U7C3ZZ Dilation of Cervix, Percutaneous Approach
760DZ Dilation of Left Fallopian Tube with Intraluminal Device, Open Approach	♀ 0U777DZ Dilation of Bilateral Fallopian Tubes with Intraluminal Device, Via Natural or Artificial Opening	♀ 0U7C4DZ Dilation of Cervix with Intraluminal Device, Percutaneous Endoscopic Approach
760ZZ Dilation of Left Fallopian Tube, Open Approach	♀ 0U777ZZ Dilation of Bilateral Fallopian Tubes, Via Natural or Artificial Opening	♀ 0U7C4ZZ Dilation of Cervix, Percutaneous Endoscopic Approach
763DZ Dilation of Left Fallopian Tube with Intraluminal Device, Percutaneous Approach	♀ 0U778DZ Dilation of Bilateral Fallopian Tubes with Intraluminal Device, Via Natural or Artificial Opening Endoscopic	♀ 0U7C7DZ Dilation of Cervix with Intraluminal Device, Via Natural or Artificial Opening
763ZZ Dilation of Left Fallopian Tube, Percutaneous Approach	♀ 0U778ZZ Dilation of Bilateral Fallopian Tubes, Via Natural or Artificial Opening Endoscopic	♀ 0U7C7ZZ Dilation of Cervix, Via Natural or Artificial Opening
764DZ Dilation of Left Fallopian Tube with Intraluminal Device, Percutaneous Endoscopic Approach	♀ 0U790DZ Dilation of Uterus with Intraluminal Device, Open Approach	♀ 0U7C8DZ Dilation of Cervix with Intraluminal Device, Via Natural or Artificial Opening Endoscopic
764ZZ Dilation of Left Fallopian Tube, Percutaneous Endoscopic Approach	♀ 0U790ZZ Dilation of Uterus, Open Approach	♀ 0U7C8ZZ Dilation of Cervix, Via Natural or Artificial Opening Endoscopic
	♀ 0U793DZ Dilation of Uterus with Intraluminal Device, Percutaneous Approach	♀ 0U7G0DZ Dilation of Vagina with Intraluminal Device, Open Approach
	♀ 0U793ZZ Dilation of Uterus, Percutaneous Approach	♀ 0U7G0ZZ Dilation of Vagina, Open Approach
		♀ 0U7G3DZ Dilation of Vagina with Intraluminal Device, Percutaneous Approach

Female-only   ♂ Male-only   ▲ Limited Coverage   ● Non-OR   ▦ HAC-associated procedure   ▲ Non-covered procedures   ✚ Combination

♀ **0U7G3ZZ** Dilation of Vagina, Percutaneous Approach
♀ **0U7G4DZ** Dilation of Vagina with Intraluminal Device, Percutaneous Endoscopic Approach
♀ **0U7G4ZZ** Dilation of Vagina, Percutaneous Endoscopic Approach
♀ **0U7G7DZ** Dilation of Vagina with Intraluminal Device, Via Natural or Artificial Opening
♀ **0U7G7ZZ** Dilation of Vagina, Via Natural or Artificial Opening
♀ **0U7G8DZ** Dilation of Vagina with Intraluminal Device, Via Natural or Artificial Opening Endoscopic

♀ **0U7G8ZZ** Dilation of Vagina, Via Natural or Artificial Opening Endoscopic
♀ **0U7K0DZ** Dilation of Hymen with Intraluminal Device, Open Approach
♀ **0U7K0ZZ** Dilation of Hymen, Open Approach
♀ **0U7K3DZ** Dilation of Hymen with Intraluminal Device, Percutaneous Approach
♀ **0U7K3ZZ** Dilation of Hymen, Percutaneous Approach
♀ **0U7K4DZ** Dilation of Hymen with Intraluminal Device, Percutaneous Endoscopic Approach
♀ **0U7K4ZZ** Dilation of Hymen, Percutaneous Endoscopic Approach

♀ **0U7K7DZ** Dilation of Hymen with Intraluminal Device, Via Natural or Artificial Openi
♀ **0U7K7ZZ** Dilation of Hymen, Via Natural or Artificial Opening
♀ **0U7K8DZ** Dilation of Hymen with Intraluminal Device, Via Natural or Artificial Openi Endoscopic
♀ **0U7K8ZZ** Dilation of Hymen, Via Natural or Artificial Opening Endoscopic
♀ **0U7KXDZ** Dilation of Hymen with Intraluminal Device, External Approach
♀ **0U7KXZZ** Dilation of Hymen, External Approach

0U8 – Female Reproductive System, Division

Review Coding Guideline B3.14

♀ **0U800ZZ** Division of Right Ovary, Open Approach
♀ **0U803ZZ** Division of Right Ovary, Percutaneous Approach
♀ **0U804ZZ** Division of Right Ovary, Percutaneous Endoscopic Approach
♀ **0U810ZZ** Division of Left Ovary, Open Approach
♀ **0U813ZZ** Division of Left Ovary, Percutaneous Approach
♀ **0U814ZZ** Division of Left Ovary, Percutaneous Endoscopic Approach

♀ **0U820ZZ** Division of Bilateral Ovaries, Open Approach
♀ **0U823ZZ** Division of Bilateral Ovaries, Percutaneous Approach
♀ **0U824ZZ** Division of Bilateral Ovaries, Percutaneous Endoscopic Approach
♀ **0U840ZZ** Division of Uterine Supporting Structure, Open Approach
♀ **0U843ZZ** Division of Uterine Supporting Structure, Percutaneous Approach

♀ **0U844ZZ** Division of Uterine Supporting Structu Percutaneous Endoscopic Approach
♀ **0U8K7ZZ** Division of Hymen, Via Natural or Artificial Opening
♀ **0U8K8ZZ** Division of Hymen, Via Natural or Artificial Opening Endoscopic
♀ **0U8KXZZ** Division of Hymen, External Approach

0U9 – Female Reproductive System, Drainage

Review Coding Guidelines B3.4a and B3.4b

Review Coding Guideline B6.2

♀ **0U9000Z** Drainage of Right Ovary with Drainage Device, Open Approach
♀ **0U900ZX** Drainage of Right Ovary, Open Approach, Diagnostic
♀ **0U900ZZ** Drainage of Right Ovary, Open Approach
♀ **0U9030Z** Drainage of Right Ovary with Drainage Device, Percutaneous Approach
♀ **0U903ZX** Drainage of Right Ovary, Percutaneous Approach, Diagnostic
♀ **0U903ZZ** Drainage of Right Ovary, Percutaneous Approach
♀ **0U9040Z** Drainage of Right Ovary with Drainage Device, Percutaneous Endoscopic Approach
♀ **0U904ZX** Drainage of Right Ovary, Percutaneous Endoscopic Approach, Diagnostic
♀ **0U904ZZ** Drainage of Right Ovary, Percutaneous Endoscopic Approach
♀ **0U90XZZ** Drainage of Right Ovary, External Approach
♀ **0U9100Z** Drainage of Left Ovary with Drainage Device, Open Approach
♀ **0U910ZX** Drainage of Left Ovary, Open Approach, Diagnostic
♀ **0U910ZZ** Drainage of Left Ovary, Open Approach
♀ **0U9130Z** Drainage of Left Ovary with Drainage Device, Percutaneous Approach
♀ **0U913ZX** Drainage of Left Ovary, Percutaneous Approach, Diagnostic
♀ **0U913ZZ** Drainage of Left Ovary, Percutaneous Approach
♀ **0U9140Z** Drainage of Left Ovary with Drainage Device, Percutaneous Endoscopic Approach
♀ **0U914ZX** Drainage of Left Ovary, Percutaneous Endoscopic Approach, Diagnostic
♀ **0U914ZZ** Drainage of Left Ovary, Percutaneous Endoscopic Approach
♀ **0U91XZZ** Drainage of Left Ovary, External Approach
♀ **0U9200Z** Drainage of Bilateral Ovaries with Drainage Device, Open Approach

♀ **0U920ZX** Drainage of Bilateral Ovaries, Open Approach, Diagnostic
♀ **0U920ZZ** Drainage of Bilateral Ovaries, Open Approach
♀ **0U9230Z** Drainage of Bilateral Ovaries with Drainage Device, Percutaneous Approach
♀ **0U923ZX** Drainage of Bilateral Ovaries, Percutaneous Approach, Diagnostic
♀ **0U923ZZ** Drainage of Bilateral Ovaries, Percutaneous Approach
♀ **0U9240Z** Drainage of Bilateral Ovaries with Drainage Device, Percutaneous Endoscopic Approach
♀ **0U924ZX** Drainage of Bilateral Ovaries, Percutaneous Endoscopic Approach, Diagnostic
♀ **0U924ZZ** Drainage of Bilateral Ovaries, Percutaneous Endoscopic Approach
♀ **0U92XZZ** Drainage of Bilateral Ovaries, External Approach
♀ **0U9400Z** Drainage of Uterine Supporting Structure with Drainage Device, Open Approach
♀ **0U940ZX** Drainage of Uterine Supporting Structure, Open Approach, Diagnostic
♀ **0U940ZZ** Drainage of Uterine Supporting Structure, Open Approach
♀ **0U9430Z** Drainage of Uterine Supporting Structure with Drainage Device, Percutaneous Approach
♀ **0U943ZX** Drainage of Uterine Supporting Structure, Percutaneous Approach, Diagnostic
♀ **0U943ZZ** Drainage of Uterine Supporting Structure, Percutaneous Approach
♀ **0U9440Z** Drainage of Uterine Supporting Structure with Drainage Device, Percutaneous Endoscopic Approach
♀ **0U944ZX** Drainage of Uterine Supporting Structure, Percutaneous Endoscopic Approach, Diagnostic
♀ **0U944ZZ** Drainage of Uterine Supporting Structure, Percutaneous Endoscopic Approach

♀ **0U9500Z** Drainage of Right Fallopian Tube with Drainage Device, Open Approach
♀ **0U950ZX** Drainage of Right Fallopian Tube, Open Approach, Diagnostic
♀ **0U950ZZ** Drainage of Right Fallopian Tube, Oper Approach
♀ **0U9530Z** Drainage of Right Fallopian Tube with Drainage Device, Percutaneous Approac
♀ **0U953ZX** Drainage of Right Fallopian Tube, Percutaneous Approach, Diagnostic
♀ **0U953ZZ** Drainage of Right Fallopian Tube, Percutaneous Approach
♀ **0U9540Z** Drainage of Right Fallopian Tube with Drainage Device, Percutaneous Endoscopic Approach
♀ **0U954ZX** Drainage of Right Fallopian Tube, Percutaneous Endoscopic Approach, Diagnostic
♀ **0U954ZZ** Drainage of Right Fallopian Tube, Percutaneous Endoscopic Approach
♀ **0U9570Z** Drainage of Right Fallopian Tube with Drainage Device, Via Natural or Artificia Opening
♀ **0U957ZX** Drainage of Right Fallopian Tube, Via Natural or Artificial Opening, Diagnostic
♀ **0U957ZZ** Drainage of Right Fallopian Tube, Via Natural or Artificial Opening
♀ **0U9580Z** Drainage of Right Fallopian Tube with Drainage Device, Via Natural or Artificia Opening Endoscopic
♀ **0U958ZX** Drainage of Right Fallopian Tube, Via Natural or Artificial Opening Endoscopic Diagnostic
♀ **0U958ZZ** Drainage of Right Fallopian Tube, Via Natural or Artificial Opening Endoscopic
♀ **0U9600Z** Drainage of Left Fallopian Tube with Drainage Device, Open Approach
♀ **0U960ZX** Drainage of Left Fallopian Tube, Open Approach, Diagnostic
♀ **0U960ZZ** Drainage of Left Fallopian Tube, Open Approach

1066

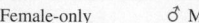

U9630Z Drainage of Left Fallopian Tube with Drainage Device, Percutaneous Approach

U963ZX Drainage of Left Fallopian Tube, Percutaneous Approach, Diagnostic

U963ZZ Drainage of Left Fallopian Tube, Percutaneous Approach

U9640Z Drainage of Left Fallopian Tube with Drainage Device, Percutaneous Endoscopic Approach

U964ZX Drainage of Left Fallopian Tube, Percutaneous Endoscopic Approach, Diagnostic

U964ZZ Drainage of Left Fallopian Tube, Percutaneous Endoscopic Approach

U9670Z Drainage of Left Fallopian Tube with Drainage Device, Via Natural or Artificial Opening

U967ZX Drainage of Left Fallopian Tube, Via Natural or Artificial Opening, Diagnostic

U967ZZ Drainage of Left Fallopian Tube, Via Natural or Artificial Opening

U9680Z Drainage of Left Fallopian Tube with Drainage Device, Via Natural or Artificial Opening Endoscopic

U968ZX Drainage of Left Fallopian Tube, Via Natural or Artificial Opening Endoscopic, Diagnostic

U968ZZ Drainage of Left Fallopian Tube, Via Natural or Artificial Opening Endoscopic

U9700Z Drainage of Bilateral Fallopian Tubes with Drainage Device, Open Approach

U970ZX Drainage of Bilateral Fallopian Tubes, Open Approach, Diagnostic

U970ZZ Drainage of Bilateral Fallopian Tubes, Open Approach

U9730Z Drainage of Bilateral Fallopian Tubes with Drainage Device, Percutaneous Approach

U973ZX Drainage of Bilateral Fallopian Tubes, Percutaneous Approach, Diagnostic

U973ZZ Drainage of Bilateral Fallopian Tubes, Percutaneous Approach

U9740Z Drainage of Bilateral Fallopian Tubes with Drainage Device, Percutaneous Endoscopic Approach

U974ZX Drainage of Bilateral Fallopian Tubes, Percutaneous Endoscopic Approach, Diagnostic

U974ZZ Drainage of Bilateral Fallopian Tubes, Percutaneous Endoscopic Approach

U9770Z Drainage of Bilateral Fallopian Tubes with Drainage Device, Via Natural or Artificial Opening

U977ZX Drainage of Bilateral Fallopian Tubes, Via Natural or Artificial Opening, Diagnostic

U977ZZ Drainage of Bilateral Fallopian Tubes, Via Natural or Artificial Opening

U9780Z Drainage of Bilateral Fallopian Tubes with Drainage Device, Via Natural or Artificial Opening Endoscopic

U978ZX Drainage of Bilateral Fallopian Tubes, Via Natural or Artificial Opening Endoscopic, Diagnostic

U978ZZ Drainage of Bilateral Fallopian Tubes, Via Natural or Artificial Opening Endoscopic

0U9900Z Drainage of Uterus with Drainage Device, Open Approach

0U990ZX Drainage of Uterus, Open Approach, Diagnostic

0U990ZZ Drainage of Uterus, Open Approach

0U9930Z Drainage of Uterus with Drainage Device, Percutaneous Approach

0U993ZX Drainage of Uterus, Percutaneous Approach, Diagnostic

0U993ZZ Drainage of Uterus, Percutaneous Approach

0U9940Z Drainage of Uterus with Drainage Device, Percutaneous Endoscopic Approach

♀ 0U994ZX Drainage of Uterus, Percutaneous Endoscopic Approach, Diagnostic

♀ 0U994ZZ Drainage of Uterus, Percutaneous Endoscopic Approach

♀ 0U9970Z Drainage of Uterus with Drainage Device, Via Natural or Artificial Opening

♀ 0U997ZX Drainage of Uterus, Via Natural or Artificial Opening, Diagnostic

♀ 0U997ZZ Drainage of Uterus, Via Natural or Artificial Opening

♀ 0U9980Z Drainage of Uterus with Drainage Device, Via Natural or Artificial Opening Endoscopic

♀ 0U998ZX Drainage of Uterus, Via Natural or Artificial Opening Endoscopic, Diagnostic

♀ 0U998ZZ Drainage of Uterus, Via Natural or Artificial Opening Endoscopic

♀ 0U9C00Z Drainage of Cervix with Drainage Device, Open Approach

♀ 0U9C0ZX Drainage of Cervix, Open Approach, Diagnostic

♀ 0U9C0ZZ Drainage of Cervix, Open Approach

♀ 0U9C30Z Drainage of Cervix with Drainage Device, Percutaneous Approach

♀ 0U9C3ZX Drainage of Cervix, Percutaneous Approach, Diagnostic

♀ 0U9C3ZZ Drainage of Cervix, Percutaneous Approach

♀ 0U9C40Z Drainage of Cervix with Drainage Device, Percutaneous Endoscopic Approach

♀ 0U9C4ZX Drainage of Cervix, Percutaneous Endoscopic Approach, Diagnostic

♀ 0U9C4ZZ Drainage of Cervix, Percutaneous Endoscopic Approach

♀ 0U9C70Z Drainage of Cervix with Drainage Device, Via Natural or Artificial Opening

♀ 0U9C7ZX Drainage of Cervix, Via Natural or Artificial Opening, Diagnostic

♀ 0U9C7ZZ Drainage of Cervix, Via Natural or Artificial Opening

♀ 0U9C80Z Drainage of Cervix with Drainage Device, Via Natural or Artificial Opening Endoscopic

♀ 0U9C8ZX Drainage of Cervix, Via Natural or Artificial Opening Endoscopic, Diagnostic

♀ 0U9C8ZZ Drainage of Cervix, Via Natural or Artificial Opening Endoscopic

♀ 0U9F00Z Drainage of Cul-de-sac with Drainage Device, Open Approach

♀ 0U9F0ZX Drainage of Cul-de-sac, Open Approach, Diagnostic

♀ 0U9F0ZZ Drainage of Cul-de-sac, Open Approach

♀ 0U9F30Z Drainage of Cul-de-sac with Drainage Device, Percutaneous Approach

♀ 0U9F3ZX Drainage of Cul-de-sac, Percutaneous Approach, Diagnostic

♀ 0U9F3ZZ Drainage of Cul-de-sac, Percutaneous Approach

♀ 0U9F40Z Drainage of Cul-de-sac with Drainage Device, Percutaneous Endoscopic Approach

♀ 0U9F4ZX Drainage of Cul-de-sac, Percutaneous Endoscopic Approach, Diagnostic

♀ 0U9F4ZZ Drainage of Cul-de-sac, Percutaneous Endoscopic Approach

♀ 0U9F70Z Drainage of Cul-de-sac with Drainage Device, Via Natural or Artificial Opening

♀ 0U9F7ZX Drainage of Cul-de-sac, Via Natural or Artificial Opening, Diagnostic

♀ 0U9F7ZZ Drainage of Cul-de-sac, Via Natural or Artificial Opening

♀ 0U9F80Z Drainage of Cul-de-sac with Drainage Device, Via Natural or Artificial Opening Endoscopic

♀ 0U9F8ZX Drainage of Cul-de-sac, Via Natural or Artificial Opening Endoscopic, Diagnostic

♀ 0U9F8ZZ Drainage of Cul-de-sac, Via Natural or Artificial Opening Endoscopic

♀ 0U9G00Z Drainage of Vagina with Drainage Device, Open Approach

♀ 0U9G0ZX Drainage of Vagina, Open Approach, Diagnostic

♀ 0U9G0ZZ Drainage of Vagina, Open Approach

♀ 0U9G30Z Drainage of Vagina with Drainage Device, Percutaneous Approach

♀ 0U9G3ZX Drainage of Vagina, Percutaneous Approach, Diagnostic

♀ 0U9G3ZZ Drainage of Vagina, Percutaneous Approach

♀ 0U9G40Z Drainage of Vagina with Drainage Device, Percutaneous Endoscopic Approach

♀ 0U9G4ZX Drainage of Vagina, Percutaneous Endoscopic Approach, Diagnostic

♀ 0U9G4ZZ Drainage of Vagina, Percutaneous Endoscopic Approach

♀ 0U9G70Z Drainage of Vagina with Drainage Device, Via Natural or Artificial Opening

♀ 0U9G7ZX Drainage of Vagina, Via Natural or Artificial Opening, Diagnostic

♀ 0U9G7ZZ Drainage of Vagina, Via Natural or Artificial Opening

♀ 0U9G80Z Drainage of Vagina with Drainage Device, Via Natural or Artificial Opening Endoscopic

♀ 0U9G8ZX Drainage of Vagina, Via Natural or Artificial Opening Endoscopic, Diagnostic

♀ 0U9G8ZZ Drainage of Vagina, Via Natural or Artificial Opening Endoscopic

♀ 0U9GX0Z Drainage of Vagina with Drainage Device, External Approach

♀ 0U9GXZX Drainage of Vagina, External Approach, Diagnostic

♀ 0U9GXZZ Drainage of Vagina, External Approach

♀ 0U9J00Z Drainage of Clitoris with Drainage Device, Open Approach

♀ 0U9J0ZX Drainage of Clitoris, Open Approach, Diagnostic

♀ 0U9J0ZZ Drainage of Clitoris, Open Approach

♀ 0U9JX0Z Drainage of Clitoris with Drainage Device, External Approach

♀ 0U9JXZX Drainage of Clitoris, External Approach, Diagnostic

♀ 0U9JXZZ Drainage of Clitoris, External Approach

♀ 0U9K00Z Drainage of Hymen with Drainage Device, Open Approach

♀ 0U9K0ZX Drainage of Hymen, Open Approach, Diagnostic

♀ 0U9K0ZZ Drainage of Hymen, Open Approach

♀ 0U9K30Z Drainage of Hymen with Drainage Device, Percutaneous Approach

♀ 0U9K3ZX Drainage of Hymen, Percutaneous Approach, Diagnostic

♀ 0U9K3ZZ Drainage of Hymen, Percutaneous Approach

♀ 0U9K40Z Drainage of Hymen with Drainage Device, Percutaneous Endoscopic Approach

♀ 0U9K4ZX Drainage of Hymen, Percutaneous Endoscopic Approach, Diagnostic

♀ 0U9K4ZZ Drainage of Hymen, Percutaneous Endoscopic Approach

♀ 0U9K70Z Drainage of Hymen with Drainage Device, Via Natural or Artificial Opening

♀ 0U9K7ZX Drainage of Hymen, Via Natural or Artificial Opening, Diagnostic

♀ 0U9K7ZZ Drainage of Hymen, Via Natural or Artificial Opening

♀ 0U9K80Z Drainage of Hymen with Drainage Device, Via Natural or Artificial Opening Endoscopic

♀ 0U9K8ZX Drainage of Hymen, Via Natural or Artificial Opening Endoscopic, Diagnostic

♀ 0U9K8ZZ Drainage of Hymen, Via Natural or Artificial Opening Endoscopic

♀ Female-only   ♂ Male-only   ▲ Limited Coverage   ● Non-OR   ▨ HAC-associated procedure   ▲ Non-covered procedures   ⊞ Combination

♀ **0U9KX0Z** Drainage of Hymen with Drainage Device, External Approach

♀ **0U9KXZX** Drainage of Hymen, External Approach, Diagnostic

♀ **0U9KXZZ** Drainage of Hymen, External Approach

♀ **0U9L00Z** Drainage of Vestibular Gland with Drainage Device, Open Approach

♀ **0U9L0ZX** Drainage of Vestibular Gland, Open Approach, Diagnostic

♀ **0U9L0ZZ** Drainage of Vestibular Gland, Open Approach

♀ **0U9LX0Z** Drainage of Vestibular Gland with Drainage Device, External Approach

♀ **0U9LXZX** Drainage of Vestibular Gland, External Approach, Diagnostic

♀ **0U9LXZZ** Drainage of Vestibular Gland, External Approach

♀ **0U9M00Z** Drainage of Vulva with Drainage Device, Open Approach

♀ **0U9M0ZX** Drainage of Vulva, Open Approach, Diagnostic

♀ **0U9M0ZZ** Drainage of Vulva, Open Approach

♀ **0U9MX0Z** Drainage of Vulva with Drainage Device, External Approach

♀ **0U9MXZX** Drainage of Vulva, External Approach, Diagnostic

♀ **0U9MXZZ** Drainage of Vulva, External Approach

0UB – Female Reproductive System, Excision

Review Coding Guidelines B3.4a and B3.4b

Review Coding Guideline B3.8

♀ **0UB00ZX** Excision of Right Ovary, Open Approach, Diagnostic

♀ **0UB00ZZ** Excision of Right Ovary, Open Approach

♀ **0UB03ZX** Excision of Right Ovary, Percutaneous Approach, Diagnostic

♀ **0UB03ZZ** Excision of Right Ovary, Percutaneous Approach

♀ **0UB04ZX** Excision of Right Ovary, Percutaneous Endoscopic Approach, Diagnostic

♀ **0UB04ZZ** Excision of Right Ovary, Percutaneous Endoscopic Approach

♀ **0UB07ZX** Excision of Right Ovary, Via Natural or Artificial Opening, Diagnostic

♀ **0UB07ZZ** Excision of Right Ovary, Via Natural or Artificial Opening

♀ **0UB08ZX** Excision of Right Ovary, Via Natural or Artificial Opening Endoscopic, Diagnostic

♀ **0UB08ZZ** Excision of Right Ovary, Via Natural or Artificial Opening Endoscopic

♀ **0UB10ZX** Excision of Left Ovary, Open Approach, Diagnostic

♀ **0UB10ZZ** Excision of Left Ovary, Open Approach

♀ **0UB13ZX** Excision of Left Ovary, Percutaneous Approach, Diagnostic

♀ **0UB13ZZ** Excision of Left Ovary, Percutaneous Approach

♀ **0UB14ZX** Excision of Left Ovary, Percutaneous Endoscopic Approach, Diagnostic

♀ **0UB14ZZ** Excision of Left Ovary, Percutaneous Endoscopic Approach

♀ **0UB17ZX** Excision of Left Ovary, Via Natural or Artificial Opening, Diagnostic

♀ **0UB17ZZ** Excision of Left Ovary, Via Natural or Artificial Opening

♀ **0UB18ZX** Excision of Left Ovary, Via Natural or Artificial Opening Endoscopic, Diagnostic

♀ **0UB18ZZ** Excision of Left Ovary, Via Natural or Artificial Opening Endoscopic

♀ **0UB20ZX** Excision of Bilateral Ovaries, Open Approach, Diagnostic

♀ **0UB20ZZ** Excision of Bilateral Ovaries, Open Approach

♀ **0UB23ZX** Excision of Bilateral Ovaries, Percutaneous Approach, Diagnostic

♀ **0UB23ZZ** Excision of Bilateral Ovaries, Percutaneous Approach

♀ **0UB24ZX** Excision of Bilateral Ovaries, Percutaneous Endoscopic Approach, Diagnostic

♀ **0UB24ZZ** Excision of Bilateral Ovaries, Percutaneous Endoscopic Approach

♀ **0UB27ZX** Excision of Bilateral Ovaries, Via Natural or Artificial Opening, Diagnostic

♀ **0UB27ZZ** Excision of Bilateral Ovaries, Via Natural or Artificial Opening

♀ **0UB28ZX** Excision of Bilateral Ovaries, Via Natural or Artificial Opening Endoscopic, Diagnostic

♀ **0UB28ZZ** Excision of Bilateral Ovaries, Via Natural or Artificial Opening Endoscopic

♀ **0UB40ZX** Excision of Uterine Supporting Structure, Open Approach, Diagnostic

♀ **0UB40ZZ** Excision of Uterine Supporting Structure, Open Approach

♀ **0UB43ZX** Excision of Uterine Supporting Structure, Percutaneous Approach, Diagnostic

♀ **0UB43ZZ** Excision of Uterine Supporting Structure, Percutaneous Approach

♀ **0UB44ZX** Excision of Uterine Supporting Structure, Percutaneous Endoscopic Approach, Diagnostic

♀ **0UB44ZZ** Excision of Uterine Supporting Structure, Percutaneous Endoscopic Approach

♀ **0UB47ZX** Excision of Uterine Supporting Structure, Via Natural or Artificial Opening, Diagnostic

♀ **0UB47ZZ** Excision of Uterine Supporting Structure, Via Natural or Artificial Opening

♀ **0UB48ZX** Excision of Uterine Supporting Structure, Via Natural or Artificial Opening Endoscopic, Diagnostic

♀ **0UB48ZZ** Excision of Uterine Supporting Structure, Via Natural or Artificial Opening Endoscopic

♀ **0UB50ZX** Excision of Right Fallopian Tube, Open Approach, Diagnostic

♀ **0UB50ZZ** Excision of Right Fallopian Tube, Open Approach

♀ **0UB53ZX** Excision of Right Fallopian Tube, Percutaneous Approach, Diagnostic

♀ **0UB53ZZ** Excision of Right Fallopian Tube, Percutaneous Approach

♀ **0UB54ZX** Excision of Right Fallopian Tube, Percutaneous Endoscopic Approach, Diagnostic

♀ **0UB54ZZ** Excision of Right Fallopian Tube, Percutaneous Endoscopic Approach

♀ **0UB57ZX** Excision of Right Fallopian Tube, Via Natural or Artificial Opening, Diagnostic

♀ **0UB57ZZ** Excision of Right Fallopian Tube, Via Natural or Artificial Opening

♀ **0UB58ZX** Excision of Right Fallopian Tube, Via Natural or Artificial Opening Endoscopic, Diagnostic

♀ **0UB58ZZ** Excision of Right Fallopian Tube, Via Natural or Artificial Opening Endoscopic

♀ **0UB60ZX** Excision of Left Fallopian Tube, Open Approach, Diagnostic

♀ **0UB60ZZ** Excision of Left Fallopian Tube, Open Approach

♀ **0UB63ZX** Excision of Left Fallopian Tube, Percutaneous Approach, Diagnostic

♀ **0UB63ZZ** Excision of Left Fallopian Tube, Percutaneous Approach

♀ **0UB64ZX** Excision of Left Fallopian Tube, Percutaneous Endoscopic Approach, Diagnostic

♀ **0UB64ZZ** Excision of Left Fallopian Tube, Percutaneous Endoscopic Approach

♀ **0UB67ZX** Excision of Left Fallopian Tube, Via Natural or Artificial Opening, Diagnostic

♀ **0UB67ZZ** Excision of Left Fallopian Tube, Via Natural or Artificial Opening

♀ **0UB68ZX** Excision of Left Fallopian Tube, Via Natural or Artificial Opening Endoscopic Diagnostic

♀ **0UB68ZZ** Excision of Left Fallopian Tube, Via Natural or Artificial Opening Endoscopic

♀ **0UB70ZX** Excision of Bilateral Fallopian Tubes, Open Approach, Diagnostic

♀ **0UB70ZZ** Excision of Bilateral Fallopian Tubes, Open Approach

♀ **0UB73ZX** Excision of Bilateral Fallopian Tubes, Percutaneous Approach, Diagnost

♀ **0UB73ZZ** Excision of Bilateral Fallopian Tubes, Percutaneous Approach

♀ **0UB74ZX** Excision of Bilateral Fallopian Tubes, Percutaneous Endoscopic Approach, Diagnostic

♀ **0UB74ZZ** Excision of Bilateral Fallopian Tubes, Percutaneous Endoscopic Approach

♀ **0UB77ZX** Excision of Bilateral Fallopian Tubes, Via Natural or Artificial Opening, Diagnostic

♀ **0UB77ZZ** Excision of Bilateral Fallopian Tubes, Via Natural or Artificial Opening

♀ **0UB78ZX** Excision of Bilateral Fallopian Tubes, Via Natural or Artificial Opening Endoscopic Diagnostic

♀ **0UB78ZZ** Excision of Bilateral Fallopian Tubes, Via Natural or Artificial Opening Endoscopic

♀ **0UB90ZX** Excision of Uterus, Open Approach, Diagnostic

♀ **0UB90ZZ** Excision of Uterus, Open Approach
AHA CC: 4Q, 2014, 16

♀ **0UB93ZX** Excision of Uterus, Percutaneous Approach, Diagnostic

♀ **0UB93ZZ** Excision of Uterus, Percutaneous Approach

♀ **0UB94ZX** Excision of Uterus, Percutaneous Endoscopic Approach, Diagnostic

♀ **0UB94ZZ** Excision of Uterus, Percutaneous Endoscopic Approach

♀ **0UB97ZX** Excision of Uterus, Via Natural or Artificial Opening, Diagnostic

♀ **0UB97ZZ** Excision of Uterus, Via Natural or Artificial Opening

♀ **0UB98ZX** Excision of Uterus, Via Natural or Artificial Opening Endoscopic, Diagnostic

♀ **0UB98ZZ** Excision of Uterus, Via Natural or Artificial Opening Endoscopic

♀ **0UBC0ZX** Excision of Cervix, Open Approach, Diagnostic

♀ **0UBC0ZZ** Excision of Cervix, Open Approach

♀ **0UBC3ZX** Excision of Cervix, Percutaneous Approach, Diagnostic

♀ **0UBC3ZZ** Excision of Cervix, Percutaneous Approach

♀ **0UBC4ZX** Excision of Cervix, Percutaneous Endoscopic Approach, Diagnostic

♀ Female-only　　♂ Male-only　　▲ Limited Coverage　　● Non-OR　　▦ HAC-associated procedure　　▲ Non-covered procedures　　✚ Combination

BC4ZZ	Excision of Cervix, Percutaneous Endoscopic Approach	♀ 0UBG0ZZ Excision of Vagina, Open Approach	♀ 0UBK3ZZ Excision of Hymen, Percutaneous Approach

BC4ZZ Excision of Cervix, Percutaneous Endoscopic Approach

BC7ZX Excision of Cervix, Via Natural or Artificial Opening, Diagnostic

BC7ZZ Excision of Cervix, Via Natural or Artificial Opening

BC8ZX Excision of Cervix, Via Natural or Artificial Opening Endoscopic, Diagnostic

BC8ZZ Excision of Cervix, Via Natural or Artificial Opening Endoscopic

BF0ZX Excision of Cul-de-sac, Open Approach, Diagnostic

BF0ZZ Excision of Cul-de-sac, Open Approach

BF3ZX Excision of Cul-de-sac, Percutaneous Approach, Diagnostic

BF3ZZ Excision of Cul-de-sac, Percutaneous Approach

BF4ZX Excision of Cul-de-sac, Percutaneous Endoscopic Approach, Diagnostic

BF4ZZ Excision of Cul-de-sac, Percutaneous Endoscopic Approach

BF7ZX Excision of Cul-de-sac, Via Natural or Artificial Opening, Diagnostic

BF7ZZ Excision of Cul-de-sac, Via Natural or Artificial Opening

BF8ZX Excision of Cul-de-sac, Via Natural or Artificial Opening Endoscopic, Diagnostic

BF8ZZ Excision of Cul-de-sac, Via Natural or Artificial Opening Endoscopic

BG0ZX Excision of Vagina, Open Approach, Diagnostic

♀ 0UBG0ZZ Excision of Vagina, Open Approach

♀ 0UBG3ZX Excision of Vagina, Percutaneous Approach, Diagnostic

♀ 0UBG3ZZ Excision of Vagina, Percutaneous Approach

♀ 0UBG4ZX Excision of Vagina, Percutaneous Endoscopic Approach, Diagnostic

♀ 0UBG4ZZ Excision of Vagina, Percutaneous Endoscopic Approach

♀ 0UBG7ZX Excision of Vagina, Via Natural or Artificial Opening, Diagnostic

♀ 0UBG7ZZ Excision of Vagina, Via Natural or Artificial Opening

♀ 0UBG8ZX Excision of Vagina, Via Natural or Artificial Opening Endoscopic, Diagnostic

♀ 0UBG8ZZ Excision of Vagina, Via Natural or Artificial Opening Endoscopic

♀ 0UBGXZX Excision of Vagina, External Approach, Diagnostic

♀ 0UBGXZZ Excision of Vagina, External Approach

♀ 0UBJ0ZX Excision of Clitoris, Open Approach, Diagnostic

♀ 0UBJ0ZZ Excision of Clitoris, Open Approach

♀ 0UBJXZX Excision of Clitoris, External Approach, Diagnostic

♀ 0UBJXZZ Excision of Clitoris, External Approach

♀ 0UBK0ZX Excision of Hymen, Open Approach, Diagnostic

♀ 0UBK0ZZ Excision of Hymen, Open Approach

♀ 0UBK3ZX Excision of Hymen, Percutaneous Approach, Diagnostic

♀ 0UBK3ZZ Excision of Hymen, Percutaneous Approach

♀ 0UBK4ZX Excision of Hymen, Percutaneous Endoscopic Approach, Diagnostic

♀ 0UBK4ZZ Excision of Hymen, Percutaneous Endoscopic Approach

♀ 0UBK7ZX Excision of Hymen, Via Natural or Artificial Opening, Diagnostic

♀ 0UBK7ZZ Excision of Hymen, Via Natural or Artificial Opening

♀ 0UBK8ZX Excision of Hymen, Via Natural or Artificial Opening Endoscopic, Diagnostic

♀ 0UBK8ZZ Excision of Hymen, Via Natural or Artificial Opening Endoscopic

♀ 0UBKXZX Excision of Hymen, External Approach, Diagnostic

♀ 0UBKXZZ Excision of Hymen, External Approach

♀ 0UBL0ZX Excision of Vestibular Gland, Open Approach, Diagnostic

♀ 0UBL0ZZ Excision of Vestibular Gland, Open Approach

♀ 0UBLXZX Excision of Vestibular Gland, External Approach, Diagnostic

♀ 0UBLXZZ Excision of Vestibular Gland, External Approach

♀ 0UBM0ZX Excision of Vulva, Open Approach, Diagnostic

♀ 0UBM0ZZ Excision of Vulva, Open Approach

♀ 0UBMXZX Excision of Vulva, External Approach, Diagnostic

♀ 0UBMXZZ Excision of Vulva, External Approach
AHA CC: 3Q, 2014, 12

0UC – Female Reproductive System, Extirpation

UC00ZZ Extirpation of Matter from Right Ovary, Open Approach

UC03ZZ Extirpation of Matter from Right Ovary, Percutaneous Approach

UC04ZZ Extirpation of Matter from Right Ovary, Percutaneous Endoscopic Approach

UC10ZZ Extirpation of Matter from Left Ovary, Open Approach

UC13ZZ Extirpation of Matter from Left Ovary, Percutaneous Approach

UC14ZZ Extirpation of Matter from Left Ovary, Percutaneous Endoscopic Approach

UC20ZZ Extirpation of Matter from Bilateral Ovaries, Open Approach

UC23ZZ Extirpation of Matter from Bilateral Ovaries, Percutaneous Approach

UC24ZZ Extirpation of Matter from Bilateral Ovaries, Percutaneous Endoscopic Approach

UC40ZZ Extirpation of Matter from Uterine Supporting Structure, Open Approach

UC43ZZ Extirpation of Matter from Uterine Supporting Structure, Percutaneous Approach

UC44ZZ Extirpation of Matter from Uterine Supporting Structure, Percutaneous Endoscopic Approach

UC50ZZ Extirpation of Matter from Right Fallopian Tube, Open Approach

UC53ZZ Extirpation of Matter from Right Fallopian Tube, Percutaneous Approach

UC54ZZ Extirpation of Matter from Right Fallopian Tube, Percutaneous Endoscopic Approach

UC57ZZ Extirpation of Matter from Right Fallopian Tube, Via Natural or Artificial Opening

UC58ZZ Extirpation of Matter from Right Fallopian Tube, Via Natural or Artificial Opening Endoscopic

UC60ZZ Extirpation of Matter from Left Fallopian Tube, Open Approach

♀ 0UC63ZZ Extirpation of Matter from Left Fallopian Tube, Percutaneous Approach

♀ 0UC64ZZ Extirpation of Matter from Left Fallopian Tube, Percutaneous Endoscopic Approach

♀ 0UC67ZZ Extirpation of Matter from Left Fallopian Tube, Via Natural or Artificial Opening

♀ 0UC68ZZ Extirpation of Matter from Left Fallopian Tube, Via Natural or Artificial Opening Endoscopic

♀ 0UC70ZZ Extirpation of Matter from Bilateral Fallopian Tubes, Open Approach

♀ 0UC73ZZ Extirpation of Matter from Bilateral Fallopian Tubes, Percutaneous Approach

♀ 0UC74ZZ Extirpation of Matter from Bilateral Fallopian Tubes, Percutaneous Endoscopic Approach

♀ 0UC77ZZ Extirpation of Matter from Bilateral Fallopian Tubes, Via Natural or Artificial Opening

♀ 0UC78ZZ Extirpation of Matter from Bilateral Fallopian Tubes, Via Natural or Artificial Opening Endoscopic

♀ 0UC90ZZ Extirpation of Matter from Uterus, Open Approach

♀ 0UC93ZZ Extirpation of Matter from Uterus, Percutaneous Approach

♀ 0UC94ZZ Extirpation of Matter from Uterus, Percutaneous Endoscopic Approach

♀ 0UC97ZZ Extirpation of Matter from Uterus, Via Natural or Artificial Opening
AHA CC: 2Q, 2013, 38

♀ 0UC98ZZ Extirpation of Matter from Uterus, Via Natural or Artificial Opening Endoscopic

♀ 0UCB0ZZ Extirpation of Matter from Endometrium, Open Approach

♀ 0UCB3ZZ Extirpation of Matter from Endometrium, Percutaneous Approach

♀ 0UCB4ZZ Extirpation of Matter from Endometrium, Percutaneous Endoscopic Approach

♀ 0UCB7ZZ Extirpation of Matter from Endometrium, Via Natural or Artificial Opening

♀ 0UCB8ZZ Extirpation of Matter from Endometrium, Via Natural or Artificial Opening Endoscopic

♀ 0UCC0ZZ Extirpation of Matter from Cervix, Open Approach

♀ 0UCC3ZZ Extirpation of Matter from Cervix, Percutaneous Approach

♀ 0UCC4ZZ Extirpation of Matter from Cervix, Percutaneous Endoscopic Approach

♀ 0UCC7ZZ Extirpation of Matter from Cervix, Via Natural or Artificial Opening

♀ 0UCC8ZZ Extirpation of Matter from Cervix, Via Natural or Artificial Opening Endoscopic

♀ 0UCF0ZZ Extirpation of Matter from Cul-de-sac, Open Approach

♀ 0UCF3ZZ Extirpation of Matter from Cul-de-sac, Percutaneous Approach

♀ 0UCF4ZZ Extirpation of Matter from Cul-de-sac, Percutaneous Endoscopic Approach

♀ 0UCF7ZZ Extirpation of Matter from Cul-de-sac, Via Natural or Artificial Opening

♀ 0UCF8ZZ Extirpation of Matter from Cul-de-sac, Via Natural or Artificial Opening Endoscopic

♀ 0UCG0ZZ Extirpation of Matter from Vagina, Open Approach

♀ 0UCG3ZZ Extirpation of Matter from Vagina, Percutaneous Approach

♀ 0UCG4ZZ Extirpation of Matter from Vagina, Percutaneous Endoscopic Approach

♀ 0UCG7ZZ Extirpation of Matter from Vagina, Via Natural or Artificial Opening

♀ 0UCG8ZZ Extirpation of Matter from Vagina, Via Natural or Artificial Opening Endoscopic

♀ 0UCGXZZ Extirpation of Matter from Vagina, External Approach

♀ 0UCJ0ZZ Extirpation of Matter from Clitoris, Open Approach

♀ Female-only ♂ Male-only ▲ Limited Coverage ● Non-OR ▨ HAC-associated procedure ▲ Non-covered procedures ✚ Combination

♀ **0UCJXZZ** Extirpation of Matter from Clitoris, External Approach

♀ **0UCK0ZZ** Extirpation of Matter from Hymen, Open Approach

♀ **0UCK3ZZ** Extirpation of Matter from Hymen, Percutaneous Approach

♀ **0UCK4ZZ** Extirpation of Matter from Hymen, Percutaneous Endoscopic Approach

♀ **0UCK7ZZ** Extirpation of Matter from Hymen, Via Natural or Artificial Opening

♀ **0UCK8ZZ** Extirpation of Matter from Hymen, Via Natural or Artificial Opening Endoscopic

♀ **0UCKXZZ** Extirpation of Matter from Hymen, External Approach

♀ **0UCL0ZZ** Extirpation of Matter from Vestibular Gland, Open Approach

♀ **0UCLXZZ** Extirpation of Matter from Vestibular Gland, External Approach

♀ **0UCM0ZZ** Extirpation of Matter from Vulva, Open Approach

♀ **0UCMXZZ** Extirpation of Matter from Vulva, External Approach

0UD – Female Reproductive System, Extraction

Review Coding Guidelines B3.4a and B3.4b

Review Coding Guideline C2

♀ **0UDB7ZX** Extraction of Endometrium, Via Natural or Artificial Opening, Diagnostic

♀ **0UDB7ZZ** Extraction of Endometrium, Via Natural or Artificial Opening

♀ **0UDB8ZX** Extraction of Endometrium, Via Natural or Artificial Opening Endoscopic, Diagnostic

♀ **0UDB8ZZ** Extraction of Endometrium, Via Natural or Artificial Opening Endoscopic

♀ **0UDN0ZZ** Extraction of Ova, Open

♀ **0UDN3ZZ** Extraction of Ova, Percutaneous

♀ **0UDN4ZZ** Extraction of Ova, Percutaneous Endoscopic

0UF – Female Reproductive System, Fragmentation

♀ **0UF50ZZ** Fragmentation in Right Fallopian Tube, Open Approach

♀ **0UF53ZZ** Fragmentation in Right Fallopian Tube, Percutaneous Approach

♀ **0UF54ZZ** Fragmentation in Right Fallopian Tube, Percutaneous Endoscopic Approach

♀ **0UF57ZZ** Fragmentation in Right Fallopian Tube, Via Natural or Artificial Opening

♀ **0UF58ZZ** Fragmentation in Right Fallopian Tube, Via Natural or Artificial Opening Endoscopic

♀ ▲ **0UF5XZZ** Fragmentation in Right Fallopian Tube, External Approach

♀ **0UF60ZZ** Fragmentation in Left Fallopian Tube, Open Approach

♀ **0UF63ZZ** Fragmentation in Left Fallopian Tube, Percutaneous Approach

♀ **0UF64ZZ** Fragmentation in Left Fallopian Tube, Percutaneous Endoscopic Approach

♀ **0UF67ZZ** Fragmentation in Left Fallopian Tube, Via Natural or Artificial Opening

♀ **0UF68ZZ** Fragmentation in Left Fallopian Tube, Via Natural or Artificial Opening Endoscopic

♀ ▲ **0UF6XZZ** Fragmentation in Left Fallopian Tube, External Approach

♀ **0UF70ZZ** Fragmentation in Bilateral Fallopian Tubes, Open Approach

♀ **0UF73ZZ** Fragmentation in Bilateral Fallopian Tubes, Percutaneous Approach

♀ **0UF74ZZ** Fragmentation in Bilateral Fallopian Tubes, Percutaneous Endoscopic Approach

♀ **0UF77ZZ** Fragmentation in Bilateral Fallopian Tubes, Via Natural or Artificial Opening

♀ **0UF78ZZ** Fragmentation in Bilateral Fallopian Tubes, Via Natural or Artificial Opening Endoscopic

♀ ▲ **0UF7XZZ** Fragmentation in Bilateral Fallopian Tubes, External Approach

♀ **0UF90ZZ** Fragmentation in Uterus, Open Approach

♀ **0UF93ZZ** Fragmentation in Uterus, Percutaneous Approach

♀ **0UF94ZZ** Fragmentation in Uterus, Percutaneous Endoscopic Approach

♀ **0UF97ZZ** Fragmentation in Uterus, Via Natural or Artificial Opening

♀ **0UF98ZZ** Fragmentation in Uterus, Via Natural or Artificial Opening Endoscopic

♀ ▲ **0UF9XZZ** Fragmentation in Uterus, External Approach

0UH – Female Reproductive System, Insertion

♀ **0UH303Z** Insertion of Infusion Device into Ovary, Open Approach

♀ **0UH333Z** Insertion of Infusion Device into Ovary, Percutaneous Approach

♀ **0UH343Z** Insertion of Infusion Device into Ovary, Percutaneous Endoscopic Approach

♀ **0UH803Z** Insertion of Infusion Device into Fallopian Tube, Open Approach

♀ **0UH833Z** Insertion of Infusion Device into Fallopian Tube, Percutaneous Approach

♀ **0UH843Z** Insertion of Infusion Device into Fallopian Tube, Percutaneous Endoscopic Approach

♀ **0UH873Z** Insertion of Infusion Device into Fallopian Tube, Via Natural or Artificial Opening

♀ **0UH883Z** Insertion of Infusion Device into Fallopian Tube, Via Natural or Artificial Opening Endoscopic

♀ **0UH97HZ** Insertion of Contraceptive Device into Uterus, Via Natural or Artificial Opening

AHA CC: 2Q, 2013, 34

♀ **0UH98HZ** Insertion of Contraceptive Device into Uterus, Via Natural or Artificial Opening Endoscopic

♀ **0UHC01Z** Insertion of Radioactive Element into Cervix, Open Approach

♀ **0UHC31Z** Insertion of Radioactive Element into Cervix, Percutaneous Approach

♀ **0UHC41Z** Insertion of Radioactive Element into Cervix, Percutaneous Endoscopic Approach

♀ **0UHC71Z** Insertion of Radioactive Element into Cervix, Via Natural or Artificial Opening

♀ **0UHC7HZ** Insertion of Contraceptive Device into Cervix, Via Natural or Artificial Opening

♀ **0UHC81Z** Insertion of Radioactive Element into Cervix, Via Natural or Artificial Opening Endoscopic

♀ **0UHC8HZ** Insertion of Contraceptive Device into Cervix, Via Natural or Artificial Opening Endoscopic

♀ **0UHD03Z** Insertion of Infusion Device into Uterus and Cervix, Open Approach

♀ **0UHD33Z** Insertion of Infusion Device into Uterus and Cervix, Percutaneous Approach

♀ **0UHD43Z** Insertion of Infusion Device into Uterus and Cervix, Percutaneous Endoscopic Approach

♀ **0UHD73Z** Insertion of Infusion Device into Uterus and Cervix, Via Natural or Artificial Opening

♀ **0UHD83Z** Insertion of Infusion Device into Uterus and Cervix, Via Natural or Artificial Opening Endoscopic

♀ **0UHF7GZ** Insertion of Pessary into Cul-de-sac, Via Natural or Artificial Opening

♀ **0UHF8GZ** Insertion of Pessary into Cul-de-sac, Via Natural or Artificial Opening Endoscopic

♀ **0UHG01Z** Insertion of Radioactive Element into Vagina, Open Approach

♀ **0UHG31Z** Insertion of Radioactive Element into Vagina, Percutaneous Approach

♀ **0UHG41Z** Insertion of Radioactive Element into Vagina, Percutaneous Endoscopic Approach

♀ **0UHG71Z** Insertion of Radioactive Element into Vagina, Via Natural or Artificial Opening

♀ **0UHG7GZ** Insertion of Pessary into Vagina, Via Natural or Artificial Opening

♀ **0UHG81Z** Insertion of Radioactive Element into Vagina, Via Natural or Artificial Opening Endoscopic

♀ **0UHG8GZ** Insertion of Pessary into Vagina, Via Natural or Artificial Opening Endoscopic

♀ **0UHGX1Z** Insertion of Radioactive Element into Vagina, External Approach

♀ **0UHH03Z** Insertion of Infusion Device into Vagina and Cul-de-sac, Open Approach

♀ **0UHH33Z** Insertion of Infusion Device into Vagina and Cul-de-sac, Percutaneous Approach

♀ **0UHH43Z** Insertion of Infusion Device into Vagina and Cul-de-sac, Percutaneous Endoscopic Approach

♀ **0UHH73Z** Insertion of Infusion Device into Vagina and Cul-de-sac, Via Natural or Artificial Opening

♀ **0UHH83Z** Insertion of Infusion Device into Vagina and Cul-de-sac, Via Natural or Artificial Opening Endoscopic

0UJ – Female Reproductive System, Inspection

Review Coding Guidelines B3.11a, B3.11b and B3.11c

♀ **0UJ30ZZ** Inspection of Ovary, Open Approach

♀ **0UJ33ZZ** Inspection of Ovary, Percutaneous Approach

♀ **0UJ34ZZ** Inspection of Ovary, Percutaneous Endoscopic Approach

♀ Female-only   ♂ Male-only   ▲ Limited Coverage   ● Non-OR   ▬ HAC-associated procedure   ▲ Non-covered procedures   ✚ Combination

0J3XZZ Inspection of Ovary, External Approach

J80ZZ Inspection of Fallopian Tube, Open Approach

J83ZZ Inspection of Fallopian Tube, Percutaneous Approach

J84ZZ Inspection of Fallopian Tube, Percutaneous Endoscopic Approach

J87ZZ Inspection of Fallopian Tube, Via Natural or Artificial Opening

J88ZZ Inspection of Fallopian Tube, Via Natural or Artificial Opening Endoscopic

J8XZZ Inspection of Fallopian Tube, External Approach

♀ 0UJD0ZZ Inspection of Uterus and Cervix, Open Approach

♀ 0UJD3ZZ Inspection of Uterus and Cervix, Percutaneous Approach

♀ 0UJD4ZZ Inspection of Uterus and Cervix, Percutaneous Endoscopic Approach
AHA CC: 1Q, 2015, 33-34

♀ 0UJD7ZZ Inspection of Uterus and Cervix, Via Natural or Artificial Opening

♀ 0UJD8ZZ Inspection of Uterus and Cervix, Via Natural or Artificial Opening Endoscopic

♀ 0UJDXZZ Inspection of Uterus and Cervix, External Approach

♀ 0UJH0ZZ Inspection of Vagina and Cul-de-sac, Open Approach

♀ 0UJH3ZZ Inspection of Vagina and Cul-de-sac, Percutaneous Approach

♀ 0UJH4ZZ Inspection of Vagina and Cul-de-sac, Percutaneous Endoscopic Approach

♀ 0UJH7ZZ Inspection of Vagina and Cul-de-sac, Via Natural or Artificial Opening

♀ 0UJH8ZZ Inspection of Vagina and Cul-de-sac, Via Natural or Artificial Opening Endoscopic

♀ 0UJHXZZ Inspection of Vagina and Cul-de-sac, External Approach

♀ 0UJM0ZZ Inspection of Vulva, Open Approach

♀ 0UJMXZZ Inspection of Vulva, External Approach

UL – Female Reproductive System, Occlusion

0UL50CZ Occlusion of Right Fallopian Tube with Extraluminal Device, Open Approach

0UL50DZ Occlusion of Right Fallopian Tube with Intraluminal Device, Open Approach

0UL50ZZ Occlusion of Right Fallopian Tube, Open Approach

0UL53CZ Occlusion of Right Fallopian Tube with Extraluminal Device, Percutaneous Approach

0UL53DZ Occlusion of Right Fallopian Tube with Intraluminal Device, Percutaneous Approach

0UL53ZZ Occlusion of Right Fallopian Tube, Percutaneous Approach

0UL54CZ Occlusion of Right Fallopian Tube with Extraluminal Device, Percutaneous Endoscopic Approach

0UL54DZ Occlusion of Right Fallopian Tube with Intraluminal Device, Percutaneous Endoscopic Approach

0UL54ZZ Occlusion of Right Fallopian Tube, Percutaneous Endoscopic Approach

0UL57DZ Occlusion of Right Fallopian Tube with Intraluminal Device, Via Natural or Artificial Opening

0UL57ZZ Occlusion of Right Fallopian Tube, Via Natural or Artificial Opening

0UL58DZ Occlusion of Right Fallopian Tube with Intraluminal Device, Via Natural or Artificial Opening Endoscopic

0UL58ZZ Occlusion of Right Fallopian Tube, Via Natural or Artificial Opening Endoscopic

0UL60CZ Occlusion of Left Fallopian Tube with Extraluminal Device, Open Approach

0UL60DZ Occlusion of Left Fallopian Tube with Intraluminal Device, Open Approach

0UL60ZZ Occlusion of Left Fallopian Tube, Open Approach

♀ 0UL63CZ Occlusion of Left Fallopian Tube with Extraluminal Device, Percutaneous Approach

♀ 0UL63DZ Occlusion of Left Fallopian Tube with Intraluminal Device, Percutaneous Approach

♀ 0UL63ZZ Occlusion of Left Fallopian Tube, Percutaneous Approach

♀ 0UL64CZ Occlusion of Left Fallopian Tube with Extraluminal Device, Percutaneous Endoscopic Approach

♀ 0UL64DZ Occlusion of Left Fallopian Tube with Intraluminal Device, Percutaneous Endoscopic Approach

♀ 0UL64ZZ Occlusion of Left Fallopian Tube, Percutaneous Endoscopic Approach

♀ 0UL67DZ Occlusion of Left Fallopian Tube with Intraluminal Device, Via Natural or Artificial Opening

♀ 0UL67ZZ Occlusion of Left Fallopian Tube, Via Natural or Artificial Opening

♀ 0UL68DZ Occlusion of Left Fallopian Tube with Intraluminal Device, Via Natural or Artificial Opening Endoscopic

♀ 0UL68ZZ Occlusion of Left Fallopian Tube, Via Natural or Artificial Opening Endoscopic

♀ ▲ 0UL70CZ Occlusion of Bilateral Fallopian Tubes with Extraluminal Device, Open Approach

♀ ▲ 0UL70DZ Occlusion of Bilateral Fallopian Tubes with Intraluminal Device, Open Approach

♀ ▲ 0UL70ZZ Occlusion of Bilateral Fallopian Tubes, Open Approach

♀ ▲ 0UL73CZ Occlusion of Bilateral Fallopian Tubes with Extraluminal Device, Percutaneous Approach

♀ ▲ 0UL73DZ Occlusion of Bilateral Fallopian Tubes with Intraluminal Device, Percutaneous Approach

♀ ▲ 0UL73ZZ Occlusion of Bilateral Fallopian Tubes, Percutaneous Approach

♀ ▲ 0UL74CZ Occlusion of Bilateral Fallopian Tubes with Extraluminal Device, Percutaneous Endoscopic Approach

♀ ▲ 0UL74DZ Occlusion of Bilateral Fallopian Tubes with Intraluminal Device, Percutaneous Endoscopic Approach

♀ ▲ 0UL74ZZ Occlusion of Bilateral Fallopian Tubes, Percutaneous Endoscopic Approach

♀ ▲ 0UL77DZ Occlusion of Bilateral Fallopian Tubes with Intraluminal Device, Via Natural or Artificial Opening

♀ ▲ 0UL77ZZ Occlusion of Bilateral Fallopian Tubes, Via Natural or Artificial Opening

♀ ▲ 0UL78DZ Occlusion of Bilateral Fallopian Tubes with Intraluminal Device, Via Natural or Artificial Opening Endoscopic

♀ ▲ 0UL78ZZ Occlusion of Bilateral Fallopian Tubes, Via Natural or Artificial Opening Endoscopic

♀ 0ULF7DZ Occlusion of Cul-de-sac with Intraluminal Device, Via Natural or Artificial Opening

♀ 0ULF7ZZ Occlusion of Cul-de-sac, Via Natural or Artificial Opening

♀ 0ULF8DZ Occlusion of Cul-de-sac with Intraluminal Device, Via Natural or Artificial Opening Endoscopic

♀ 0ULF8ZZ Occlusion of Cul-de-sac, Via Natural or Artificial Opening Endoscopic

♀ 0ULG7DZ Occlusion of Vagina with Intraluminal Device, Via Natural or Artificial Opening

♀ 0ULG7ZZ Occlusion of Vagina, Via Natural or Artificial Opening

♀ 0ULG8DZ Occlusion of Vagina with Intraluminal Device, Via Natural or Artificial Opening Endoscopic

♀ 0ULG8ZZ Occlusion of Vagina, Via Natural or Artificial Opening Endoscopic

UM – Female Reproductive System, Reattachment

0UM00ZZ Reattachment of Right Ovary, Open Approach

0UM04ZZ Reattachment of Right Ovary, Percutaneous Endoscopic Approach

0UM10ZZ Reattachment of Left Ovary, Open Approach

0UM14ZZ Reattachment of Left Ovary, Percutaneous Endoscopic Approach

0UM20ZZ Reattachment of Bilateral Ovaries, Open Approach

0UM24ZZ Reattachment of Bilateral Ovaries, Percutaneous Endoscopic Approach

0UM40ZZ Reattachment of Uterine Supporting Structure, Open Approach

0UM44ZZ Reattachment of Uterine Supporting Structure, Percutaneous Endoscopic Approach

♀ 0UM50ZZ Reattachment of Right Fallopian Tube, Open Approach

♀ 0UM54ZZ Reattachment of Right Fallopian Tube, Percutaneous Endoscopic Approach

♀ 0UM60ZZ Reattachment of Left Fallopian Tube, Open Approach

♀ 0UM64ZZ Reattachment of Left Fallopian Tube, Percutaneous Endoscopic Approach

♀ 0UM70ZZ Reattachment of Bilateral Fallopian Tubes, Open Approach

♀ 0UM74ZZ Reattachment of Bilateral Fallopian Tubes, Percutaneous Endoscopic Approach

♀ 0UM90ZZ Reattachment of Uterus, Open Approach

♀ 0UM94ZZ Reattachment of Uterus, Percutaneous Endoscopic Approach

♀ 0UMC0ZZ Reattachment of Cervix, Open Approach

♀ 0UMC4ZZ Reattachment of Cervix, Percutaneous Endoscopic Approach

♀ 0UMF0ZZ Reattachment of Cul-de-sac, Open Approach

♀ 0UMF4ZZ Reattachment of Cul-de-sac, Percutaneous Endoscopic Approach

♀ 0UMG0ZZ Reattachment of Vagina, Open Approach

♀ 0UMG4ZZ Reattachment of Vagina, Percutaneous Endoscopic Approach

♀ 0UMJXZZ Reattachment of Clitoris, External Approach

♀ 0UMK0ZZ Reattachment of Hymen, Open Approach

♀ 0UMK4ZZ Reattachment of Hymen, Percutaneous Endoscopic Approach

♀ 0UMKXZZ Reattachment of Hymen, External Approach

♀ 0UMMXZZ Reattachment of Vulva, External Approach

♀ Female-only   ♂ Male-only   ▲ Limited Coverage   ● Non-OR   ▨ HAC-associated procedure   ▲ Non-covered procedures   ✚ Combination

0UN – Female Reproductive System, Release

Review Coding Guideline B3.13

Review Coding Guideline B3.14

♀ 0UN00ZZ Release Right Ovary, Open Approach
♀ 0UN03ZZ Release Right Ovary, Percutaneous Approach
♀ 0UN04ZZ Release Right Ovary, Percutaneous Endoscopic Approach
♀ 0UN10ZZ Release Left Ovary, Open Approach
♀ 0UN13ZZ Release Left Ovary, Percutaneous Approach
♀ 0UN14ZZ Release Left Ovary, Percutaneous Endoscopic Approach
♀ 0UN20ZZ Release Bilateral Ovaries, Open Approach
♀ 0UN23ZZ Release Bilateral Ovaries, Percutaneous Approach
♀ 0UN24ZZ Release Bilateral Ovaries, Percutaneous Endoscopic Approach
♀ 0UN40ZZ Release Uterine Supporting Structure, Open Approach
♀ 0UN43ZZ Release Uterine Supporting Structure, Percutaneous Approach
♀ 0UN44ZZ Release Uterine Supporting Structure, Percutaneous Endoscopic Approach
♀ 0UN50ZZ Release Right Fallopian Tube, Open Approach
♀ 0UN53ZZ Release Right Fallopian Tube, Percutaneous Approach
♀ 0UN54ZZ Release Right Fallopian Tube, Percutaneous Endoscopic Approach
♀ 0UN57ZZ Release Right Fallopian Tube, Via Natural or Artificial Opening
♀ 0UN58ZZ Release Right Fallopian Tube, Via Natural or Artificial Opening Endoscopic
♀ 0UN60ZZ Release Left Fallopian Tube, Open Approach
♀ 0UN63ZZ Release Left Fallopian Tube, Percutaneous Approach

♀ 0UN64ZZ Release Left Fallopian Tube, Percutaneous Endoscopic Approach
♀ 0UN67ZZ Release Left Fallopian Tube, Via Natural or Artificial Opening
♀ 0UN68ZZ Release Left Fallopian Tube, Via Natural or Artificial Opening Endoscopic
♀ 0UN70ZZ Release Bilateral Fallopian Tubes, Open Approach
♀ 0UN73ZZ Release Bilateral Fallopian Tubes, Percutaneous Approach
♀ 0UN74ZZ Release Bilateral Fallopian Tubes, Percutaneous Endoscopic Approach
♀ 0UN77ZZ Release Bilateral Fallopian Tubes, Via Natural or Artificial Opening
♀ 0UN78ZZ Release Bilateral Fallopian Tubes, Via Natural or Artificial Opening Endoscopic
♀ 0UN90ZZ Release Uterus, Open Approach
♀ 0UN93ZZ Release Uterus, Percutaneous Approach
♀ 0UN94ZZ Release Uterus, Percutaneous Endoscopic Approach
♀ 0UN97ZZ Release Uterus, Via Natural or Artificial Opening
♀ 0UN98ZZ Release Uterus, Via Natural or Artificial Opening Endoscopic
♀ 0UNC0ZZ Release Cervix, Open Approach
♀ 0UNC3ZZ Release Cervix, Percutaneous Approach
♀ 0UNC4ZZ Release Cervix, Percutaneous Endoscopic Approach
♀ 0UNC7ZZ Release Cervix, Via Natural or Artificial Opening
♀ 0UNC8ZZ Release Cervix, Via Natural or Artificial Opening Endoscopic
♀ 0UNF0ZZ Release Cul-de-sac, Open Approach
♀ 0UNF3ZZ Release Cul-de-sac, Percutaneous Approach

♀ 0UNF4ZZ Release Cul-de-sac, Percutaneous Endoscopic Approach
♀ 0UNF7ZZ Release Cul-de-sac, Via Natural or Artificial Opening
♀ 0UNF8ZZ Release Cul-de-sac, Via Natural or Artificial Opening Endoscopic
♀ 0UNG0ZZ Release Vagina, Open Approach
♀ 0UNG3ZZ Release Vagina, Percutaneous Approa
♀ 0UNG4ZZ Release Vagina, Percutaneous Endoscopic Approach
♀ 0UNG7ZZ Release Vagina, Via Natural or Artifici Opening
♀ 0UNG8ZZ Release Vagina, Via Natural or Artifici Opening Endoscopic
♀ 0UNGXZZ Release Vagina, External Approach
♀ 0UNJ0ZZ Release Clitoris, Open Approach
♀ 0UNJXZZ Release Clitoris, External Approach
♀ 0UNK0ZZ Release Hymen, Open Approach
♀ 0UNK3ZZ Release Hymen, Percutaneous Approa
♀ 0UNK4ZZ Release Hymen, Percutaneous Endoscopic Approach
♀ 0UNK7ZZ Release Hymen, Via Natural or Artific Opening
♀ 0UNK8ZZ Release Hymen, Via Natural or Artifici Opening Endoscopic
♀ 0UNKXZZ Release Hymen, External Approach
♀ 0UNL0ZZ Release Vestibular Gland, Open Approach
♀ 0UNLXZZ Release Vestibular Gland, External Approach
♀ 0UNM0ZZ Release Vulva, Open Approach
♀ 0UNMXZZ Release Vulva, External Approach

0UP – Female Reproductive System, Removal

Review Coding Guideline B6.1c

♀ 0UP300Z Removal of Drainage Device from Ovary, Open Approach
♀ 0UP303Z Removal of Infusion Device from Ovary, Open Approach
♀ 0UP330Z Removal of Drainage Device from Ovary, Percutaneous Approach
♀ 0UP333Z Removal of Infusion Device from Ovary, Percutaneous Approach
♀ 0UP340Z Removal of Drainage Device from Ovary, Percutaneous Endoscopic Approach
♀ 0UP343Z Removal of Infusion Device from Ovary, Percutaneous Endoscopic Approach
♀ 0UP3X0Z Removal of Drainage Device from Ovary, External Approach
♀ 0UP3X3Z Removal of Infusion Device from Ovary, External Approach
♀ 0UP800Z Removal of Drainage Device from Fallopian Tube, Open Approach
♀ 0UP803Z Removal of Infusion Device from Fallopian Tube, Open Approach
♀ 0UP807Z Removal of Autologous Tissue Substitute from Fallopian Tube, Open Approach
♀ 0UP80CZ Removal of Extraluminal Device from Fallopian Tube, Open Approach
♀ 0UP80DZ Removal of Intraluminal Device from Fallopian Tube, Open Approach
♀ 0UP80JZ Removal of Synthetic Substitute from Fallopian Tube, Open Approach
♀ 0UP80KZ Removal of Nonautologous Tissue Substitute from Fallopian Tube, Open Approach

♀ 0UP830Z Removal of Drainage Device from Fallopian Tube, Percutaneous Approach
♀ 0UP833Z Removal of Infusion Device from Fallopian Tube, Percutaneous Approach
♀ 0UP837Z Removal of Autologous Tissue Substitute from Fallopian Tube, Percutaneous Approach
♀ 0UP83CZ Removal of Extraluminal Device from Fallopian Tube, Percutaneous Approach
♀ 0UP83DZ Removal of Intraluminal Device from Fallopian Tube, Percutaneous Approach
♀ 0UP83JZ Removal of Synthetic Substitute from Fallopian Tube, Percutaneous Approach
♀ 0UP83KZ Removal of Nonautologous Tissue Substitute from Fallopian Tube, Percutaneous Approach
♀ 0UP840Z Removal of Drainage Device from Fallopian Tube, Percutaneous Endoscopic Approach
♀ 0UP843Z Removal of Infusion Device from Fallopian Tube, Percutaneous Endoscopic Approach
♀ 0UP847Z Removal of Autologous Tissue Substitute from Fallopian Tube, Percutaneous Endoscopic Approach
♀ 0UP84CZ Removal of Extraluminal Device from Fallopian Tube, Percutaneous Endoscopic Approach
♀ 0UP84DZ Removal of Intraluminal Device from Fallopian Tube, Percutaneous Endoscopic Approach

♀ 0UP84JZ Removal of Synthetic Substitute from Fallopian Tube, Percutaneous Endoscopic Approach
♀ 0UP84KZ Removal of Nonautologous Tissue Substitute from Fallopian Tube, Percutaneous Endoscopic Approach
♀ 0UP870Z Removal of Drainage Device from Fallopian Tube, Via Natural or Artificial Opening
♀ 0UP873Z Removal of Infusion Device from Fallopian Tube, Via Natural or Artificial Opening
♀ 0UP877Z Removal of Autologous Tissue Substitute from Fallopian Tube, Via Natural or Artificial Opening
♀ 0UP87CZ Removal of Extraluminal Device from Fallopian Tube, Via Natural or Artificial Opening
♀ 0UP87DZ Removal of Intraluminal Device from Fallopian Tube, Via Natural or Artificial Opening
♀ 0UP87JZ Removal of Synthetic Substitute from Fallopian Tube, Via Natural or Artificial Opening
♀ 0UP87KZ Removal of Nonautologous Tissue Substitute from Fallopian Tube, Via Natural or Artificial Opening
♀ 0UP880Z Removal of Drainage Device from Fallopian Tube, Via Natural or Artificial Opening Endoscopic

♀ Female-only   ♂ Male-only   ▲ Limited Coverage   ● Non-OR   HAC-associated procedure   ▲ Non-covered procedures   + Combination

P883Z Removal of Infusion Device from Fallopian Tube, Via Natural or Artificial Opening Endoscopic

P887Z Removal of Autologous Tissue Substitute from Fallopian Tube, Via Natural or Artificial Opening Endoscopic

P88CZ Removal of Extraluminal Device from Fallopian Tube, Via Natural or Artificial Opening Endoscopic

P88DZ Removal of Intraluminal Device from Fallopian Tube, Via Natural or Artificial Opening Endoscopic

P88JZ Removal of Synthetic Substitute from Fallopian Tube, Via Natural or Artificial Opening Endoscopic

P88KZ Removal of Nonautologous Tissue Substitute from Fallopian Tube, Via Natural or Artificial Opening Endoscopic

P8X0Z Removal of Drainage Device from Fallopian Tube, External Approach

P8X3Z Removal of Infusion Device from Fallopian Tube, External Approach

P8XDZ Removal of Intraluminal Device from Fallopian Tube, External Approach

JPD00Z Removal of Drainage Device from Uterus and Cervix, Open Approach

JPD01Z Removal of Radioactive Element from Uterus and Cervix, Open Approach

JPD03Z Removal of Infusion Device from Uterus and Cervix, Open Approach

JPD07Z Removal of Autologous Tissue Substitute from Uterus and Cervix, Open Approach

JPD0CZ Removal of Extraluminal Device from Uterus and Cervix, Open Approach

JPD0DZ Removal of Intraluminal Device from Uterus and Cervix, Open Approach

JPD0HZ Removal of Contraceptive Device from Uterus and Cervix, Open Approach

JPD0JZ Removal of Synthetic Substitute from Uterus and Cervix, Open Approach

JPD0KZ Removal of Nonautologous Tissue Substitute from Uterus and Cervix, Open Approach

JPD30Z Removal of Drainage Device from Uterus and Cervix, Percutaneous Approach

JPD31Z Removal of Radioactive Element from Uterus and Cervix, Percutaneous Approach

JPD33Z Removal of Infusion Device from Uterus and Cervix, Percutaneous Approach

JPD37Z Removal of Autologous Tissue Substitute from Uterus and Cervix, Percutaneous Approach

UPD3CZ Removal of Extraluminal Device from Uterus and Cervix, Percutaneous Approach

UPD3DZ Removal of Intraluminal Device from Uterus and Cervix, Percutaneous Approach

UPD3HZ Removal of Contraceptive Device from Uterus and Cervix, Percutaneous Approach

UPD3JZ Removal of Synthetic Substitute from Uterus and Cervix, Percutaneous Approach

UPD3KZ Removal of Nonautologous Tissue Substitute from Uterus and Cervix, Percutaneous Approach

UPD40Z Removal of Drainage Device from Uterus and Cervix, Percutaneous Endoscopic Approach

UPD41Z Removal of Radioactive Element from Uterus and Cervix, Percutaneous Endoscopic Approach

UPD43Z Removal of Infusion Device from Uterus and Cervix, Percutaneous Endoscopic Approach

♀ 0UPD47Z Removal of Autologous Tissue Substitute from Uterus and Cervix, Percutaneous Endoscopic Approach

♀ 0UPD4CZ Removal of Extraluminal Device from Uterus and Cervix, Percutaneous Endoscopic Approach

♀ 0UPD4DZ Removal of Intraluminal Device from Uterus and Cervix, Percutaneous Endoscopic Approach

♀ 0UPD4HZ Removal of Contraceptive Device from Uterus and Cervix, Percutaneous Endoscopic Approach

♀ 0UPD4JZ Removal of Synthetic Substitute from Uterus and Cervix, Percutaneous Endoscopic Approach

♀ 0UPD4KZ Removal of Nonautologous Tissue Substitute from Uterus and Cervix, Percutaneous Endoscopic Approach

♀ 0UPD70Z Removal of Drainage Device from Uterus and Cervix, Via Natural or Artificial Opening

♀ 0UPD71Z Removal of Radioactive Element from Uterus and Cervix, Via Natural or Artificial Opening

♀ 0UPD73Z Removal of Infusion Device from Uterus and Cervix, Via Natural or Artificial Opening

♀ 0UPD77Z Removal of Autologous Tissue Substitute from Uterus and Cervix, Via Natural or Artificial Opening

♀ 0UPD7CZ Removal of Extraluminal Device from Uterus and Cervix, Via Natural or Artificial Opening

♀ 0UPD7DZ Removal of Intraluminal Device from Uterus and Cervix, Via Natural or Artificial Opening

♀ 0UPD7HZ Removal of Contraceptive Device from Uterus and Cervix, Via Natural or Artificial Opening

♀ 0UPD7JZ Removal of Synthetic Substitute from Uterus and Cervix, Via Natural or Artificial Opening

♀ 0UPD7KZ Removal of Nonautologous Tissue Substitute from Uterus and Cervix, Via Natural or Artificial Opening

♀ 0UPD80Z Removal of Drainage Device from Uterus and Cervix, Via Natural or Artificial Opening Endoscopic

♀ 0UPD81Z Removal of Radioactive Element from Uterus and Cervix, Via Natural or Artificial Opening Endoscopic

♀ 0UPD83Z Removal of Infusion Device from Uterus and Cervix, Via Natural or Artificial Opening Endoscopic

♀ 0UPD87Z Removal of Autologous Tissue Substitute from Uterus and Cervix, Via Natural or Artificial Opening Endoscopic

♀ 0UPD8CZ Removal of Extraluminal Device from Uterus and Cervix, Via Natural or Artificial Opening Endoscopic

♀ 0UPD8DZ Removal of Intraluminal Device from Uterus and Cervix, Via Natural or Artificial Opening Endoscopic

♀ 0UPD8HZ Removal of Contraceptive Device from Uterus and Cervix, Via Natural or Artificial Opening Endoscopic

♀ 0UPD8JZ Removal of Synthetic Substitute from Uterus and Cervix, Via Natural or Artificial Opening Endoscopic

♀ 0UPD8KZ Removal of Nonautologous Tissue Substitute from Uterus and Cervix, Via Natural or Artificial Opening Endoscopic

♀ 0UPDX0Z Removal of Drainage Device from Uterus and Cervix, External Approach

♀ 0UPDX3Z Removal of Infusion Device from Uterus and Cervix, External Approach

♀ 0UPDXDZ Removal of Intraluminal Device from Uterus and Cervix, External Approach

♀ 0UPDXHZ Removal of Contraceptive Device from Uterus and Cervix, External Approach

♀ 0UPH00Z Removal of Drainage Device from Vagina and Cul-de-sac, Open Approach

♀ 0UPH01Z Removal of Radioactive Element from Vagina and Cul-de-sac, Open Approach

♀ 0UPH03Z Removal of Infusion Device from Vagina and Cul-de-sac, Open Approach

♀ 0UPH07Z Removal of Autologous Tissue Substitute from Vagina and Cul-de-sac, Open Approach

♀ 0UPH0DZ Removal of Intraluminal Device from Vagina and Cul-de-sac, Open Approach

♀ 0UPH0JZ Removal of Synthetic Substitute from Vagina and Cul-de-sac, Open Approach

♀ 0UPH0KZ Removal of Nonautologous Tissue Substitute from Vagina and Cul-de-sac, Open Approach

♀ 0UPH30Z Removal of Drainage Device from Vagina and Cul-de-sac, Percutaneous Approach

♀ 0UPH31Z Removal of Radioactive Element from Vagina and Cul-de-sac, Percutaneous Approach

♀ 0UPH33Z Removal of Infusion Device from Vagina and Cul-de-sac, Percutaneous Approach

♀ 0UPH37Z Removal of Autologous Tissue Substitute from Vagina and Cul-de-sac, Percutaneous Approach

♀ 0UPH3DZ Removal of Intraluminal Device from Vagina and Cul-de-sac, Percutaneous Approach

♀ 0UPH3JZ Removal of Synthetic Substitute from Vagina and Cul-de-sac, Percutaneous Approach

♀ 0UPH3KZ Removal of Nonautologous Tissue Substitute from Vagina and Cul-de-sac, Percutaneous Approach

♀ 0UPH40Z Removal of Drainage Device from Vagina and Cul-de-sac, Percutaneous Endoscopic Approach

♀ 0UPH41Z Removal of Radioactive Element from Vagina and Cul-de-sac, Percutaneous Endoscopic Approach

♀ 0UPH43Z Removal of Infusion Device from Vagina and Cul-de-sac, Percutaneous Endoscopic Approach

♀ 0UPH47Z Removal of Autologous Tissue Substitute from Vagina and Cul-de-sac, Percutaneous Endoscopic Approach

♀ 0UPH4DZ Removal of Intraluminal Device from Vagina and Cul-de-sac, Percutaneous Endoscopic Approach

♀ 0UPH4JZ Removal of Synthetic Substitute from Vagina and Cul-de-sac, Percutaneous Endoscopic Approach

♀ 0UPH4KZ Removal of Nonautologous Tissue Substitute from Vagina and Cul-de-sac, Percutaneous Endoscopic Approach

♀ 0UPH70Z Removal of Drainage Device from Vagina and Cul-de-sac, Via Natural or Artificial Opening

♀ 0UPH71Z Removal of Radioactive Element from Vagina and Cul-de-sac, Via Natural or Artificial Opening

♀ 0UPH73Z Removal of Infusion Device from Vagina and Cul-de-sac, Via Natural or Artificial Opening

♀ 0UPH77Z Removal of Autologous Tissue Substitute from Vagina and Cul-de-sac, Via Natural or Artificial Opening

♀ 0UPH7DZ Removal of Intraluminal Device from Vagina and Cul-de-sac, Via Natural or Artificial Opening

♀ Female-only   ♂ Male-only   ▲ Limited Coverage   ● Non-OR   ▨ HAC-associated procedure   ▲ Non-covered procedures   ✚ Combination

♀ 0UPH7JZ Removal of Synthetic Substitute from Vagina and Cul-de-sac, Via Natural or Artificial Opening
♀ 0UPH7KZ Removal of Nonautologous Tissue Substitute from Vagina and Cul-de-sac, Via Natural or Artificial Opening
♀ 0UPH80Z Removal of Drainage Device from Vagina and Cul-de-sac, Via Natural or Artificial Opening Endoscopic
♀ 0UPH81Z Removal of Radioactive Element from Vagina and Cul-de-sac, Via Natural or Artificial Opening Endoscopic
♀ 0UPH83Z Removal of Infusion Device from Vagina and Cul-de-sac, Via Natural or Artificial Opening Endoscopic

♀ 0UPH87Z Removal of Autologous Tissue Substitute from Vagina and Cul-de-sac, Via Natural or Artificial Opening Endoscopic
♀ 0UPH8DZ Removal of Intraluminal Device from Vagina and Cul-de-sac, Via Natural or Artificial Opening Endoscopic
♀ 0UPH8JZ Removal of Synthetic Substitute from Vagina and Cul-de-sac, Via Natural or Artificial Opening Endoscopic
♀ 0UPH8KZ Removal of Nonautologous Tissue Substitute from Vagina and Cul-de-sac, Via Natural or Artificial Opening Endoscopic
♀ 0UPHX0Z Removal of Drainage Device from Vagina and Cul-de-sac, External Approach

♀ 0UPHX1Z Removal of Radioactive Element from Vagina and Cul-de-sac, External Approach
♀ 0UPHX3Z Removal of Infusion Device from Vagina and Cul-de-sac, External Approach
♀ 0UPHXDZ Removal of Intraluminal Device from Vagina and Cul-de-sac, External Approach
♀ 0UPM00Z Removal of Drainage Device from Vulva, Open Approach
♀ 0UPM07Z Removal of Autologous Tissue Substitute from Vulva, Open Approach
♀ 0UPM0JZ Removal of Synthetic Substitute from Vulva, Open Approach
♀ 0UPM0KZ Removal of Nonautologous Tissue Substitute from Vulva, Open Approach
♀ 0UPMX0Z Removal of Drainage Device from Vulva, External Approach

0UQ – Female Reproductive System, Repair

♀ 0UQ00ZZ Repair Right Ovary, Open Approach
♀ 0UQ03ZZ Repair Right Ovary, Percutaneous Approach
♀ 0UQ04ZZ Repair Right Ovary, Percutaneous Endoscopic Approach
♀ 0UQ10ZZ Repair Left Ovary, Open Approach
♀ 0UQ13ZZ Repair Left Ovary, Percutaneous Approach
♀ 0UQ14ZZ Repair Left Ovary, Percutaneous Endoscopic Approach
♀ 0UQ20ZZ Repair Bilateral Ovaries, Open Approach
♀ 0UQ23ZZ Repair Bilateral Ovaries, Percutaneous Approach
♀ 0UQ24ZZ Repair Bilateral Ovaries, Percutaneous Endoscopic Approach
♀ 0UQ40ZZ Repair Uterine Supporting Structure, Open Approach
♀ 0UQ43ZZ Repair Uterine Supporting Structure, Percutaneous Approach
♀ 0UQ44ZZ Repair Uterine Supporting Structure, Percutaneous Endoscopic Approach
♀ 0UQ50ZZ Repair Right Fallopian Tube, Open Approach
♀ 0UQ53ZZ Repair Right Fallopian Tube, Percutaneous Approach
♀ 0UQ54ZZ Repair Right Fallopian Tube, Percutaneous Endoscopic Approach
♀ 0UQ57ZZ Repair Right Fallopian Tube, Via Natural or Artificial Opening
♀ 0UQ58ZZ Repair Right Fallopian Tube, Via Natural or Artificial Opening Endoscopic
♀ 0UQ60ZZ Repair Left Fallopian Tube, Open Approach
♀ 0UQ63ZZ Repair Left Fallopian Tube, Percutaneous Approach

♀ 0UQ64ZZ Repair Left Fallopian Tube, Percutaneous Endoscopic Approach
♀ 0UQ67ZZ Repair Left Fallopian Tube, Via Natural or Artificial Opening
♀ 0UQ68ZZ Repair Left Fallopian Tube, Via Natural or Artificial Opening Endoscopic
♀ 0UQ70ZZ Repair Bilateral Fallopian Tubes, Open Approach
♀ 0UQ73ZZ Repair Bilateral Fallopian Tubes, Percutaneous Approach
♀ 0UQ74ZZ Repair Bilateral Fallopian Tubes, Percutaneous Endoscopic Approach
♀ 0UQ77ZZ Repair Bilateral Fallopian Tubes, Via Natural or Artificial Opening
♀ 0UQ78ZZ Repair Bilateral Fallopian Tubes, Via Natural or Artificial Opening Endoscopic
♀ 0UQ90ZZ Repair Uterus, Open Approach
♀ 0UQ93ZZ Repair Uterus, Percutaneous Approach
♀ 0UQ94ZZ Repair Uterus, Percutaneous Endoscopic Approach
♀ 0UQ97ZZ Repair Uterus, Via Natural or Artificial Opening
♀ 0UQ98ZZ Repair Uterus, Via Natural or Artificial Opening Endoscopic
♀ 0UQC0ZZ Repair Cervix, Open Approach
♀ 0UQC3ZZ Repair Cervix, Percutaneous Approach
♀ 0UQC4ZZ Repair Cervix, Percutaneous Endoscopic Approach
♀ 0UQC7ZZ Repair Cervix, Via Natural or Artificial Opening
♀ 0UQC8ZZ Repair Cervix, Via Natural or Artificial Opening Endoscopic
♀ 0UQF0ZZ Repair Cul-de-sac, Open Approach
♀ 0UQF3ZZ Repair Cul-de-sac, Percutaneous Approach

♀ 0UQF4ZZ Repair Cul-de-sac, Percutaneous Endoscopic Approach
♀ 0UQF7ZZ Repair Cul-de-sac, Via Natural or Artificial Opening
♀ 0UQF8ZZ Repair Cul-de-sac, Via Natural or Artificial Opening Endoscopic
♀ 0UQG0ZZ Repair Vagina, Open Approach
♀ 0UQG3ZZ Repair Vagina, Percutaneous Approach
♀ 0UQG4ZZ Repair Vagina, Percutaneous Endoscopic Approach
●♀ 0UQG7ZZ Repair Vagina, Via Natural or Artificial Opening
●♀ 0UQG8ZZ Repair Vagina, Via Natural or Artificial Opening Endoscopic
●♀ 0UQGXZZ Repair Vagina, External Approach
♀ 0UQJ0ZZ Repair Clitoris, Open Approach
♀ 0UQJXZZ Repair Clitoris, External Approach
AHA CC: 4Q, 2013, 120-121
♀ 0UQK0ZZ Repair Hymen, Open Approach
♀ 0UQK3ZZ Repair Hymen, Percutaneous Approach
♀ 0UQK4ZZ Repair Hymen, Percutaneous Endoscopic Approach
♀ 0UQK7ZZ Repair Hymen, Via Natural or Artificial Opening
♀ 0UQK8ZZ Repair Hymen, Via Natural or Artificial Opening Endoscopic
♀ 0UQKXZZ Repair Hymen, External Approach
♀ 0UQL0ZZ Repair Vestibular Gland, Open Approach
♀ 0UQLXZZ Repair Vestibular Gland, External Approach
●♀ 0UQM0ZZ Repair Vulva, Open Approach
●♀ 0UQMXZZ Repair Vulva, External Approach
AHA CC: 4Q, 2014, 18-19

0US – Female Reproductive System, Reposition

♀ 0US00ZZ Reposition Right Ovary, Open Approach
♀ 0US04ZZ Reposition Right Ovary, Percutaneous Endoscopic Approach
♀ 0US10ZZ Reposition Left Ovary, Open Approach
♀ 0US14ZZ Reposition Left Ovary, Percutaneous Endoscopic Approach
♀ 0US20ZZ Reposition Bilateral Ovaries, Open Approach
♀ 0US24ZZ Reposition Bilateral Ovaries, Percutaneous Endoscopic Approach
♀ 0US40ZZ Reposition Uterine Supporting Structure, Open Approach
♀ 0US44ZZ Reposition Uterine Supporting Structure, Percutaneous Endoscopic Approach

♀ 0US50ZZ Reposition Right Fallopian Tube, Open Approach
♀ 0US54ZZ Reposition Right Fallopian Tube, Percutaneous Endoscopic Approach
♀ 0US60ZZ Reposition Left Fallopian Tube, Open Approach
♀ 0US64ZZ Reposition Left Fallopian Tube, Percutaneous Endoscopic Approach
♀ 0US70ZZ Reposition Bilateral Fallopian Tubes, Open Approach
♀ 0US74ZZ Reposition Bilateral Fallopian Tubes, Percutaneous Endoscopic Approach
♀ 0US90ZZ Reposition Uterus, Open Approach

♀ 0US94ZZ Reposition Uterus, Percutaneous Endoscopic Approach
♀ 0US9XZZ Reposition Uterus, External Approach
♀ 0USC0ZZ Reposition Cervix, Open Approach
♀ 0USC4ZZ Reposition Cervix, Percutaneous Endoscopic Approach
♀ 0USF0ZZ Reposition Cul-de-sac, Open Approach
♀ 0USF4ZZ Reposition Cul-de-sac, Percutaneous Endoscopic Approach
♀ 0USG0ZZ Reposition Vagina, Open Approach
♀ 0USG4ZZ Reposition Vagina, Percutaneous Endoscopic Approach
♀ 0USGXZZ Reposition Vagina, External Approach

0UT – Female Reproductive System, Resection

Review Coding Guideline B3.8

♀ 0UT00ZZ Resection of Right Ovary, Open Approach
AHA CC: 1Q, 2013, 24

♀ 0UT04ZZ Resection of Right Ovary, Percutaneous Endoscopic Approach

♀ 0UT07ZZ Resection of Right Ovary, Via Natural or Artificial Opening

♀ Female-only   ♂ Male-only   ▲ Limited Coverage   ● Non-OR   ▦ HAC-associated procedure   ▲ Non-covered procedures   ✚ Combination

♀ **T08ZZ** Resection of Right Ovary, Via Natural or Artificial Opening Endoscopic

T0FZZ Resection of Right Ovary, Via Natural or Artificial Opening With Percutaneous Endoscopic Assistance

T10ZZ Resection of Left Ovary, Open Approach

T14ZZ Resection of Left Ovary, Percutaneous Endoscopic Approach

T17ZZ Resection of Left Ovary, Via Natural or Artificial Opening

T18ZZ Resection of Left Ovary, Via Natural or Artificial Opening Endoscopic

T1FZZ Resection of Left Ovary, Via Natural or Artificial Opening With Percutaneous Endoscopic Assistance

T20ZZ Resection of Bilateral Ovaries, Open Approach
AHA CC: 1Q, 2015, 33-34

T24ZZ Resection of Bilateral Ovaries, Percutaneous Endoscopic Approach

T27ZZ Resection of Bilateral Ovaries, Via Natural or Artificial Opening

T28ZZ Resection of Bilateral Ovaries, Via Natural or Artificial Opening Endoscopic

T2FZZ Resection of Bilateral Ovaries, Via Natural or Artificial Opening With Percutaneous Endoscopic Assistance

T40ZZ Resection of Uterine Supporting Structure, Open Approach
+ Radical hysterectomy when reported with resection of the uterus and cervix. *See table 0UT to construct the Resection codes.*

T44ZZ Resection of Uterine Supporting Structure, Percutaneous Endoscopic Approach
+ Radical hysterectomy when reported with resection of the uterus and cervix. *See table 0UT to construct the Resection codes.*

T47ZZ Resection of Uterine Supporting Structure, Via Natural or Artificial Opening
+ Radical hysterectomy when reported with resection of the uterus and cervix. *See table 0UT to construct the Resection codes.*

♀ **0UT48ZZ** Resection of Uterine Supporting Structure, Via Natural or Artificial Opening Endoscopic
+ Radical hysterectomy when reported with resection of the uterus and cervix. *See table 0UT to construct the Resection codes.*

♀ **0UT50ZZ** Resection of Right Fallopian Tube, Open Approach

♀ **0UT54ZZ** Resection of Right Fallopian Tube, Percutaneous Endoscopic Approach

♀ **0UT57ZZ** Resection of Right Fallopian Tube, Via Natural or Artificial Opening

♀ **0UT58ZZ** Resection of Right Fallopian Tube, Via Natural or Artificial Opening Endoscopic

♀ **0UT5FZZ** Resection of Right Fallopian Tube, Via Natural or Artificial Opening With Percutaneous Endoscopic Assistance

♀ **0UT60ZZ** Resection of Left Fallopian Tube, Open Approach

♀ **0UT64ZZ** Resection of Left Fallopian Tube, Percutaneous Endoscopic Approach

♀ **0UT67ZZ** Resection of Left Fallopian Tube, Via Natural or Artificial Opening

♀ **0UT68ZZ** Resection of Left Fallopian Tube, Via Natural or Artificial Opening Endoscopic

♀ **0UT6FZZ** Resection of Left Fallopian Tube, Via Natural or Artificial Opening With Percutaneous Endoscopic Assistance

♀ **0UT70ZZ** Resection of Bilateral Fallopian Tubes, Open Approach
AHA CC: 1Q, 2015, 33-34

♀ **0UT74ZZ** Resection of Bilateral Fallopian Tubes, Percutaneous Endoscopic Approach

♀ **0UT77ZZ** Resection of Bilateral Fallopian Tubes, Via Natural or Artificial Opening

♀ **0UT78ZZ** Resection of Bilateral Fallopian Tubes, Via Natural or Artificial Opening Endoscopic

♀ **0UT7FZZ** Resection of Bilateral Fallopian Tubes, Via Natural or Artificial Opening With Percutaneous Endoscopic Assistance

♀ **0UT90ZZ** Resection of Uterus, Open Approach
AHA CC: 3Q, 2013, 28; 1Q, 2015, 33-34

♀ **0UT94ZZ** Resection of Uterus, Percutaneous Endoscopic Approach

♀ **0UT97ZZ** Resection of Uterus, Via Natural or Artificial Opening

♀ **0UT98ZZ** Resection of Uterus, Via Natural or Artificial Opening Endoscopic

♀ **0UT9FZZ** Resection of Uterus, Via Natural or Artificial Opening With Percutaneous Endoscopic Assistance

♀ **0UTC0ZZ** Resection of Cervix, Open Approach
AHA CC: 3Q, 2013, 28; 1Q, 2015, 33-34

♀ **0UTC4ZZ** Resection of Cervix, Percutaneous Endoscopic Approach

♀ **0UTC7ZZ** Resection of Cervix, Via Natural or Artificial Opening

♀ **0UTC8ZZ** Resection of Cervix, Via Natural or Artificial Opening Endoscopic

♀ **0UTF0ZZ** Resection of Cul-de-sac, Open Approach

♀ **0UTF4ZZ** Resection of Cul-de-sac, Percutaneous Endoscopic Approach

♀ **0UTF7ZZ** Resection of Cul-de-sac, Via Natural or Artificial Opening

♀ **0UTF8ZZ** Resection of Cul-de-sac, Via Natural or Artificial Opening Endoscopic

♀ **0UTG0ZZ** Resection of Vagina, Open Approach

♀ **0UTG4ZZ** Resection of Vagina, Percutaneous Endoscopic Approach

♀ **0UTG7ZZ** Resection of Vagina, Via Natural or Artificial Opening

♀ **0UTG8ZZ** Resection of Vagina, Via Natural or Artificial Opening Endoscopic

♀ **0UTJ0ZZ** Resection of Clitoris, Open Approach

♀ **0UTJXZZ** Resection of Clitoris, External Approach

♀ **0UTK0ZZ** Resection of Hymen, Open Approach

♀ **0UTK4ZZ** Resection of Hymen, Percutaneous Endoscopic Approach

♀ **0UTK7ZZ** Resection of Hymen, Via Natural or Artificial Opening

♀ **0UTK8ZZ** Resection of Hymen, Via Natural or Artificial Opening Endoscopic

♀ **0UTKXZZ** Resection of Hymen, External Approach

♀ **0UTL0ZZ** Resection of Vestibular Gland, Open Approach

♀ **0UTLXZZ** Resection of Vestibular Gland, External Approach

♀ **0UTM0ZZ** Resection of Vulva, Open Approach

♀ **0UTMXZZ** Resection of Vulva, External Approach

0U – Female Reproductive System, Supplement

UU407Z Supplement Uterine Supporting Structure with Autologous Tissue Substitute, Open Approach

UU40JZ Supplement Uterine Supporting Structure with Synthetic Substitute, Open Approach

UU40KZ Supplement Uterine Supporting Structure with Nonautologous Tissue Substitute, Open Approach

UU447Z Supplement Uterine Supporting Structure with Autologous Tissue Substitute, Percutaneous Endoscopic Approach

UU44JZ Supplement Uterine Supporting Structure with Synthetic Substitute, Percutaneous Endoscopic Approach

UU44KZ Supplement Uterine Supporting Structure with Nonautologous Tissue Substitute, Percutaneous Endoscopic Approach

UU507Z Supplement Right Fallopian Tube with Autologous Tissue Substitute, Open Approach

UU50JZ Supplement Right Fallopian Tube with Synthetic Substitute, Open Approach

UU50KZ Supplement Right Fallopian Tube with Nonautologous Tissue Substitute, Open Approach

UU547Z Supplement Right Fallopian Tube with Autologous Tissue Substitute, Percutaneous Endoscopic Approach

♀ **0UU54JZ** Supplement Right Fallopian Tube with Synthetic Substitute, Percutaneous Endoscopic Approach

♀ **0UU54KZ** Supplement Right Fallopian Tube with Nonautologous Tissue Substitute, Percutaneous Endoscopic Approach

♀ **0UU577Z** Supplement Right Fallopian Tube with Autologous Tissue Substitute, Via Natural or Artificial Opening

♀ **0UU57JZ** Supplement Right Fallopian Tube with Synthetic Substitute, Via Natural or Artificial Opening

♀ **0UU57KZ** Supplement Right Fallopian Tube with Nonautologous Tissue Substitute, Via Natural or Artificial Opening

♀ **0UU587Z** Supplement Right Fallopian Tube with Autologous Tissue Substitute, Via Natural or Artificial Opening Endoscopic

♀ **0UU58JZ** Supplement Right Fallopian Tube with Synthetic Substitute, Via Natural or Artificial Opening Endoscopic

♀ **0UU58KZ** Supplement Right Fallopian Tube with Nonautologous Tissue Substitute, Via Natural or Artificial Opening Endoscopic

♀ **0UU607Z** Supplement Left Fallopian Tube with Autologous Tissue Substitute, Open Approach

♀ **0UU60JZ** Supplement Left Fallopian Tube with Synthetic Substitute, Open Approach

♀ **0UU60KZ** Supplement Left Fallopian Tube with Nonautologous Tissue Substitute, Open Approach

♀ **0UU647Z** Supplement Left Fallopian Tube with Autologous Tissue Substitute, Percutaneous Endoscopic Approach

♀ **0UU64JZ** Supplement Left Fallopian Tube with Synthetic Substitute, Percutaneous Endoscopic Approach

♀ **0UU64KZ** Supplement Left Fallopian Tube with Nonautologous Tissue Substitute, Percutaneous Endoscopic Approach

♀ **0UU677Z** Supplement Left Fallopian Tube with Autologous Tissue Substitute, Via Natural or Artificial Opening

♀ **0UU67JZ** Supplement Left Fallopian Tube with Synthetic Substitute, Via Natural or Artificial Opening

♀ **0UU67KZ** Supplement Left Fallopian Tube with Nonautologous Tissue Substitute, Via Natural or Artificial Opening

♀ **0UU687Z** Supplement Left Fallopian Tube with Autologous Tissue Substitute, Via Natural or Artificial Opening Endoscopic

♀ **0UU68JZ** Supplement Left Fallopian Tube with Synthetic Substitute, Via Natural or Artificial Opening Endoscopic

♀ **0UU68KZ** Supplement Left Fallopian Tube with Nonautologous Tissue Substitute, Via Natural or Artificial Opening Endoscopic

♀ Female-only ♂ Male-only ▲ Limited Coverage ● Non-OR ▨ HAC-associated procedure ▲ Non-covered procedures + Combination

♀ **0UU707Z** Supplement Bilateral Fallopian Tubes with Autologous Tissue Substitute, Open Approach

♀ **0UU70JZ** Supplement Bilateral Fallopian Tubes with Synthetic Substitute, Open Approach

♀ **0UU70KZ** Supplement Bilateral Fallopian Tubes with Nonautologous Tissue Substitute, Open Approach

♀ **0UU747Z** Supplement Bilateral Fallopian Tubes with Autologous Tissue Substitute, Percutaneous Endoscopic Approach

♀ **0UU74JZ** Supplement Bilateral Fallopian Tubes with Synthetic Substitute, Percutaneous Endoscopic Approach

♀ **0UU74KZ** Supplement Bilateral Fallopian Tubes with Nonautologous Tissue Substitute, Percutaneous Endoscopic Approach

♀ **0UU777Z** Supplement Bilateral Fallopian Tubes with Autologous Tissue Substitute, Via Natural or Artificial Opening

♀ **0UU77JZ** Supplement Bilateral Fallopian Tubes with Synthetic Substitute, Via Natural or Artificial Opening

♀ **0UU77KZ** Supplement Bilateral Fallopian Tubes with Nonautologous Tissue Substitute, Via Natural or Artificial Opening

♀ **0UU787Z** Supplement Bilateral Fallopian Tubes with Autologous Tissue Substitute, Via Natural or Artificial Opening Endoscopic

♀ **0UU78JZ** Supplement Bilateral Fallopian Tubes with Synthetic Substitute, Via Natural or Artificial Opening Endoscopic

♀ **0UU78KZ** Supplement Bilateral Fallopian Tubes with Nonautologous Tissue Substitute, Via Natural or Artificial Opening Endoscopic

♀ **0UUF07Z** Supplement Cul-de-sac with Autologous Tissue Substitute, Open Approach

♀ **0UUF0JZ** Supplement Cul-de-sac with Synthetic Substitute, Open Approach

♀ **0UUF0KZ** Supplement Cul-de-sac with Nonautologous Tissue Substitute, Open Approach

♀ **0UUF47Z** Supplement Cul-de-sac with Autologous Tissue Substitute, Percutaneous Endoscopic Approach

♀ **0UUF4JZ** Supplement Cul-de-sac with Synthetic Substitute, Percutaneous Endoscopic Approach

♀ **0UUF4KZ** Supplement Cul-de-sac with Nonautologous Tissue Substitute, Percutaneous Endoscopic Approach

♀ **0UUF77Z** Supplement Cul-de-sac with Autologous Tissue Substitute, Via Natural or Artificial Opening

♀ **0UUF7JZ** Supplement Cul-de-sac with Synthetic Substitute, Via Natural or Artificial Opening

♀ **0UUF7KZ** Supplement Cul-de-sac with Nonautologous Tissue Substitute, Via Natural or Artificial Opening

♀ **0UUF87Z** Supplement Cul-de-sac with Autologous Tissue Substitute, Via Natural or Artificial Opening Endoscopic

♀ **0UUF8JZ** Supplement Cul-de-sac with Synthetic Substitute, Via Natural or Artificial Opening Endoscopic

♀ **0UUF8KZ** Supplement Cul-de-sac with Nonautologous Tissue Substitute, Via Natural or Artificial Opening Endoscopic

♀ **0UUG07Z** Supplement Vagina with Autologous Tissue Substitute, Open Approach

♀ **0UUG0JZ** Supplement Vagina with Synthetic Substitute, Open Approach

♀ **0UUG0KZ** Supplement Vagina with Nonautologous Tissue Substitute, Open Approach

♀ **0UUG47Z** Supplement Vagina with Autologous Tissue Substitute, Percutaneous Endoscopic Approach

♀ **0UUG4JZ** Supplement Vagina with Synthetic Substitute, Percutaneous Endoscopic Approach

♀ **0UUG4KZ** Supplement Vagina with Nonautologous Tissue Substitute, Percutaneous Endoscopic Approach

♀ **0UUG77Z** Supplement Vagina with Autologous Tissue Substitute, Via Natural or Artificial Opening

♀ **0UUG7JZ** Supplement Vagina with Synthetic Substitute, Via Natural or Artificial Opening

♀ **0UUG7KZ** Supplement Vagina with Nonautologous Tissue Substitute, Via Natural or Artificial Opening

♀ **0UUG87Z** Supplement Vagina with Autologous Tissue Substitute, Via Natural or Artificial Opening Endoscopic

♀ **0UUG8JZ** Supplement Vagina with Synthetic Substitute, Via Natural or Artificial Opening Endoscopic

♀ **0UUG8KZ** Supplement Vagina with Nonautologous Tissue Substitute, Via Natural or Artificial Opening Endoscopic

♀ **0UUGX7Z** Supplement Vagina with Autologous Tissue Substitute, External Approach

♀ **0UUGXJZ** Supplement Vagina with Synthetic Substitute, External Approach

♀ **0UUGXKZ** Supplement Vagina with Nonautologous Tissue Substitute, External Approach

♀ **0UUJ07Z** Supplement Clitoris with Autologous Tissue Substitute, Open Approach

♀ **0UUJ0JZ** Supplement Clitoris with Synthetic Substitute, Open Approach

♀ **0UUJ0KZ** Supplement Clitoris with Nonautologous Tissue Substitute, Open Approach

♀ **0UUJX7Z** Supplement Clitoris with Autologous Tissue Substitute, External Approach

♀ **0UUJXJZ** Supplement Clitoris with Synthetic Substitute, External Approach

♀ **0UUJXKZ** Supplement Clitoris with Nonautologous Tissue Substitute, External Approach

♀ **0UUK07Z** Supplement Hymen with Autologous Tissue Substitute, Open Approach

♀ **0UUK0JZ** Supplement Hymen with Synthetic Substitute, Open Approach

♀ **0UUK0KZ** Supplement Hymen with Nonautologous Tissue Substitute, Open Approach

♀ **0UUK47Z** Supplement Hymen with Autologous Tissue Substitute, Percutaneous Endoscopic Approach

♀ **0UUK4JZ** Supplement Hymen with Synthetic Substitute, Percutaneous Endoscopic Approach

♀ **0UUK4KZ** Supplement Hymen with Nonautologous Tissue Substitute, Percutaneous Endoscopic Approach

♀ **0UUK77Z** Supplement Hymen with Autologous Tissue Substitute, Via Natural or Artificial Opening

♀ **0UUK7JZ** Supplement Hymen with Synthetic Substitute, Via Natural or Artificial Opening

♀ **0UUK7KZ** Supplement Hymen with Nonautologous Tissue Substitute, Via Natural or Artificial Opening

♀ **0UUK87Z** Supplement Hymen with Autologous Tissue Substitute, Via Natural or Artificial Opening Endoscopic

♀ **0UUK8JZ** Supplement Hymen with Synthetic Substitute, Via Natural or Artificial Opening Endoscopic

♀ **0UUK8KZ** Supplement Hymen with Nonautologous Tissue Substitute, Via Natural or Artificial Opening Endoscopic

♀ **0UUKX7Z** Supplement Hymen with Autologous Tissue Substitute, External Approach

♀ **0UUKXJZ** Supplement Hymen with Synthetic Substitute, External Approach

♀ **0UUKXKZ** Supplement Hymen with Nonautologous Tissue Substitute, External Approach

♀ **0UUM07Z** Supplement Vulva with Autologous Tissue Substitute, Open Approach

♀ **0UUM0JZ** Supplement Vulva with Synthetic Substitute, Open Approach

♀ **0UUM0KZ** Supplement Vulva with Nonautologous Tissue Substitute, Open Approach

♀ **0UUMX7Z** Supplement Vulva with Autologous Tissue Substitute, External Approach

♀ **0UUMXJZ** Supplement Vulva with Synthetic Substitute, External Approach

♀ **0UUMXKZ** Supplement Vulva with Nonautologous Tissue Substitute, External Approach

0UV – Female Reproductive System, Restriction

♀ **0UVC0CZ** Restriction of Cervix with Extraluminal Device, Open Approach

♀ **0UVC0DZ** Restriction of Cervix with Intraluminal Device, Open Approach

♀ **0UVC0ZZ** Restriction of Cervix, Open Approach

♀ **0UVC3CZ** Restriction of Cervix with Extraluminal Device, Percutaneous Approach

♀ **0UVC3DZ** Restriction of Cervix with Intraluminal Device, Percutaneous Approach

♀ **0UVC3ZZ** Restriction of Cervix, Percutaneous Approach

♀ **0UVC4CZ** Restriction of Cervix with Extraluminal Device, Percutaneous Endoscopic Approach

♀ **0UVC4DZ** Restriction of Cervix with Intraluminal Device, Percutaneous Endoscopic Approach

♀ **0UVC4ZZ** Restriction of Cervix, Percutaneous Endoscopic Approach

♀ **0UVC7DZ** Restriction of Cervix with Intraluminal Device, Via Natural or Artificial Opening

♀ **0UVC7ZZ** Restriction of Cervix, Via Natural or Artificial Opening

♀ **0UVC8DZ** Restriction of Cervix with Intraluminal Device, Via Natural or Artificial Opening Endoscopic

♀ **0UVC8ZZ** Restriction of Cervix, Via Natural or Artificial Opening Endoscopic

0UW – Female Reproductive System, Revision

Review Coding Guideline B6.1c

♀ **0UW300Z** Revision of Drainage Device in Ovary, Open Approach

♀ **0UW303Z** Revision of Infusion Device in Ovary, Open Approach

♀ **0UW330Z** Revision of Drainage Device in Ovary, Percutaneous Approach

W333Z	Revision of Infusion Device in Ovary, Percutaneous Approach
W340Z	Revision of Drainage Device in Ovary, Percutaneous Endoscopic Approach
W343Z	Revision of Infusion Device in Ovary, Percutaneous Endoscopic Approach
W3X0Z	Revision of Drainage Device in Ovary, External Approach
W3X3Z	Revision of Infusion Device in Ovary, External Approach
W800Z	Revision of Drainage Device in Fallopian Tube, Open Approach
W803Z	Revision of Infusion Device in Fallopian Tube, Open Approach
W807Z	Revision of Autologous Tissue Substitute in Fallopian Tube, Open Approach
W80CZ	Revision of Extraluminal Device in Fallopian Tube, Open Approach
W80DZ	Revision of Intraluminal Device in Fallopian Tube, Open Approach
W80JZ	Revision of Synthetic Substitute in Fallopian Tube, Open Approach
W80KZ	Revision of Nonautologous Tissue Substitute in Fallopian Tube, Open Approach
W830Z	Revision of Drainage Device in Fallopian Tube, Percutaneous Approach
JW833Z	Revision of Infusion Device in Fallopian Tube, Percutaneous Approach
JW837Z	Revision of Autologous Tissue Substitute in Fallopian Tube, Percutaneous Approach
JW83CZ	Revision of Extraluminal Device in Fallopian Tube, Percutaneous Approach
JW83DZ	Revision of Intraluminal Device in Fallopian Tube, Percutaneous Approach
JW83JZ	Revision of Synthetic Substitute in Fallopian Tube, Percutaneous Approach
JW83KZ	Revision of Nonautologous Tissue Substitute in Fallopian Tube, Percutaneous Approach
JW840Z	Revision of Drainage Device in Fallopian Tube, Percutaneous Endoscopic Approach
JW843Z	Revision of Infusion Device in Fallopian Tube, Percutaneous Endoscopic Approach
JW847Z	Revision of Autologous Tissue Substitute in Fallopian Tube, Percutaneous Endoscopic Approach
JW84CZ	Revision of Extraluminal Device in Fallopian Tube, Percutaneous Endoscopic Approach
UW84DZ	Revision of Intraluminal Device in Fallopian Tube, Percutaneous Endoscopic Approach
UW84JZ	Revision of Synthetic Substitute in Fallopian Tube, Percutaneous Endoscopic Approach
UW84KZ	Revision of Nonautologous Tissue Substitute in Fallopian Tube, Percutaneous Endoscopic Approach
UW870Z	Revision of Drainage Device in Fallopian Tube, Via Natural or Artificial Opening
UW873Z	Revision of Infusion Device in Fallopian Tube, Via Natural or Artificial Opening
UW877Z	Revision of Autologous Tissue Substitute in Fallopian Tube, Via Natural or Artificial Opening
UW87CZ	Revision of Extraluminal Device in Fallopian Tube, Via Natural or Artificial Opening
UW87DZ	Revision of Intraluminal Device in Fallopian Tube, Via Natural or Artificial Opening
UW87JZ	Revision of Synthetic Substitute in Fallopian Tube, Via Natural or Artificial Opening
UW87KZ	Revision of Nonautologous Tissue Substitute in Fallopian Tube, Via Natural or Artificial Opening

♀	0UW880Z	Revision of Drainage Device in Fallopian Tube, Via Natural or Artificial Opening Endoscopic
♀	0UW883Z	Revision of Infusion Device in Fallopian Tube, Via Natural or Artificial Opening Endoscopic
♀	0UW887Z	Revision of Autologous Tissue Substitute in Fallopian Tube, Via Natural or Artificial Opening Endoscopic
♀	0UW88CZ	Revision of Extraluminal Device in Fallopian Tube, Via Natural or Artificial Opening Endoscopic
♀	0UW88DZ	Revision of Intraluminal Device in Fallopian Tube, Via Natural or Artificial Opening Endoscopic
♀	0UW88JZ	Revision of Synthetic Substitute in Fallopian Tube, Via Natural or Artificial Opening Endoscopic
♀	0UW88KZ	Revision of Nonautologous Tissue Substitute in Fallopian Tube, Via Natural or Artificial Opening Endoscopic
♀	0UW8X0Z	Revision of Drainage Device in Fallopian Tube, External Approach
♀	0UW8X3Z	Revision of Infusion Device in Fallopian Tube, External Approach
♀	0UW8X7Z	Revision of Autologous Tissue Substitute in Fallopian Tube, External Approach
♀	0UW8XCZ	Revision of Extraluminal Device in Fallopian Tube, External Approach
♀	0UW8XDZ	Revision of Intraluminal Device in Fallopian Tube, External Approach
♀	0UW8XJZ	Revision of Synthetic Substitute in Fallopian Tube, External Approach
♀	0UW8XKZ	Revision of Nonautologous Tissue Substitute in Fallopian Tube, External Approach
♀	0UWD00Z	Revision of Drainage Device in Uterus and Cervix, Open Approach
♀	0UWD01Z	Revision of Radioactive Element in Uterus and Cervix, Open Approach
♀	0UWD03Z	Revision of Infusion Device in Uterus and Cervix, Open Approach
♀	0UWD07Z	Revision of Autologous Tissue Substitute in Uterus and Cervix, Open Approach
♀	0UWD0CZ	Revision of Extraluminal Device in Uterus and Cervix, Open Approach
♀	0UWD0DZ	Revision of Intraluminal Device in Uterus and Cervix, Open Approach
♀	0UWD0HZ	Revision of Contraceptive Device in Uterus and Cervix, Open Approach
♀	0UWD0JZ	Revision of Synthetic Substitute in Uterus and Cervix, Open Approach
♀	0UWD0KZ	Revision of Nonautologous Tissue Substitute in Uterus and Cervix, Open Approach
♀	0UWD30Z	Revision of Drainage Device in Uterus and Cervix, Percutaneous Approach
♀	0UWD31Z	Revision of Radioactive Element in Uterus and Cervix, Percutaneous Approach
♀	0UWD33Z	Revision of Infusion Device in Uterus and Cervix, Percutaneous Approach
♀	0UWD37Z	Revision of Autologous Tissue Substitute in Uterus and Cervix, Percutaneous Approach
♀	0UWD3CZ	Revision of Extraluminal Device in Uterus and Cervix, Percutaneous Approach
♀	0UWD3DZ	Revision of Intraluminal Device in Uterus and Cervix, Percutaneous Approach
♀	0UWD3HZ	Revision of Contraceptive Device in Uterus and Cervix, Percutaneous Approach
♀	0UWD3JZ	Revision of Synthetic Substitute in Uterus and Cervix, Percutaneous Approach

♀	0UWD3KZ	Revision of Nonautologous Tissue Substitute in Uterus and Cervix, Percutaneous Approach
♀	0UWD40Z	Revision of Drainage Device in Uterus and Cervix, Percutaneous Endoscopic Approach
♀	0UWD41Z	Revision of Radioactive Element in Uterus and Cervix, Percutaneous Endoscopic Approach
♀	0UWD43Z	Revision of Infusion Device in Uterus and Cervix, Percutaneous Endoscopic Approach
♀	0UWD47Z	Revision of Autologous Tissue Substitute in Uterus and Cervix, Percutaneous Endoscopic Approach
♀	0UWD4CZ	Revision of Extraluminal Device in Uterus and Cervix, Percutaneous Endoscopic Approach
♀	0UWD4DZ	Revision of Intraluminal Device in Uterus and Cervix, Percutaneous Endoscopic Approach
♀	0UWD4HZ	Revision of Contraceptive Device in Uterus and Cervix, Percutaneous Endoscopic Approach
♀	0UWD4JZ	Revision of Synthetic Substitute in Uterus and Cervix, Percutaneous Endoscopic Approach
♀	0UWD4KZ	Revision of Nonautologous Tissue Substitute in Uterus and Cervix, Percutaneous Endoscopic Approach
♀	0UWD70Z	Revision of Drainage Device in Uterus and Cervix, Via Natural or Artificial Opening
♀	0UWD71Z	Revision of Radioactive Element in Uterus and Cervix, Via Natural or Artificial Opening
♀	0UWD73Z	Revision of Infusion Device in Uterus and Cervix, Via Natural or Artificial Opening
♀	0UWD77Z	Revision of Autologous Tissue Substitute in Uterus and Cervix, Via Natural or Artificial Opening
♀	0UWD7CZ	Revision of Extraluminal Device in Uterus and Cervix, Via Natural or Artificial Opening
♀	0UWD7DZ	Revision of Intraluminal Device in Uterus and Cervix, Via Natural or Artificial Opening
♀	0UWD7HZ	Revision of Contraceptive Device in Uterus and Cervix, Via Natural or Artificial Opening
♀	0UWD7JZ	Revision of Synthetic Substitute in Uterus and Cervix, Via Natural or Artificial Opening
♀	0UWD7KZ	Revision of Nonautologous Tissue Substitute in Uterus and Cervix, Via Natural or Artificial Opening
♀	0UWD80Z	Revision of Drainage Device in Uterus and Cervix, Via Natural or Artificial Opening Endoscopic
♀	0UWD81Z	Revision of Radioactive Element in Uterus and Cervix, Via Natural or Artificial Opening Endoscopic
♀	0UWD83Z	Revision of Infusion Device in Uterus and Cervix, Via Natural or Artificial Opening Endoscopic
♀	0UWD87Z	Revision of Autologous Tissue Substitute in Uterus and Cervix, Via Natural or Artificial Opening Endoscopic
♀	0UWD8CZ	Revision of Extraluminal Device in Uterus and Cervix, Via Natural or Artificial Opening Endoscopic
♀	0UWD8DZ	Revision of Intraluminal Device in Uterus and Cervix, Via Natural or Artificial Opening Endoscopic
♀	0UWD8HZ	Revision of Contraceptive Device in Uterus and Cervix, Via Natural or Artificial Opening Endoscopic

♀ Female-only   ♂ Male-only   ▲ Limited Coverage   ● Non-OR   ▬ HAC-associated procedure   ▲ Non-covered procedures   ✛ Combination

♀ **0UWD8JZ** Revision of Synthetic Substitute in Uterus and Cervix, Via Natural or Artificial Opening Endoscopic

♀ **0UWD8KZ** Revision of Nonautologous Tissue Substitute in Uterus and Cervix, Via Natural or Artificial Opening Endoscopic

♀ **0UWDX0Z** Revision of Drainage Device in Uterus and Cervix, External Approach

♀ **0UWDX3Z** Revision of Infusion Device in Uterus and Cervix, External Approach

♀ **0UWDX7Z** Revision of Autologous Tissue Substitute in Uterus and Cervix, External Approach

♀ **0UWDXCZ** Revision of Extraluminal Device in Uterus and Cervix, External Approach

♀ **0UWDXDZ** Revision of Intraluminal Device in Uterus and Cervix, External Approach

♀ **0UWDXHZ** Revision of Contraceptive Device in Uterus and Cervix, External Approach

♀ **0UWDXJZ** Revision of Synthetic Substitute in Uterus and Cervix, External Approach

♀ **0UWDXKZ** Revision of Nonautologous Tissue Substitute in Uterus and Cervix, External Approach

♀ **0UWH00Z** Revision of Drainage Device in Vagina and Cul-de-sac, Open Approach

♀ **0UWH01Z** Revision of Radioactive Element in Vagina and Cul-de-sac, Open Approach

♀ **0UWH03Z** Revision of Infusion Device in Vagina and Cul-de-sac, Open Approach

♀ **0UWH07Z** Revision of Autologous Tissue Substitute in Vagina and Cul-de-sac, Open Approach

♀ **0UWH0DZ** Revision of Intraluminal Device in Vagina and Cul-de-sac, Open Approach

♀ **0UWH0JZ** Revision of Synthetic Substitute in Vagina and Cul-de-sac, Open Approach

♀ **0UWH0KZ** Revision of Nonautologous Tissue Substitute in Vagina and Cul-de-sac, Open Approach

♀ **0UWH30Z** Revision of Drainage Device in Vagina and Cul-de-sac, Percutaneous Approach

♀ **0UWH31Z** Revision of Radioactive Element in Vagina and Cul-de-sac, Percutaneous Approach

♀ **0UWH33Z** Revision of Infusion Device in Vagina and Cul-de-sac, Percutaneous Approach

♀ **0UWH37Z** Revision of Autologous Tissue Substitute in Vagina and Cul-de-sac, Percutaneous Approach

♀ **0UWH3DZ** Revision of Intraluminal Device in Vagina and Cul-de-sac, Percutaneous Approach

♀ **0UWH3JZ** Revision of Synthetic Substitute in Vagina and Cul-de-sac, Percutaneous Approach

♀ **0UWH3KZ** Revision of Nonautologous Tissue Substitute in Vagina and Cul-de-sac, Percutaneous Approach

♀ **0UWH40Z** Revision of Drainage Device in Vagina and Cul-de-sac, Percutaneous Endoscopic Approach

♀ **0UWH41Z** Revision of Radioactive Element in Vagina and Cul-de-sac, Percutaneous Endoscopic Approach

♀ **0UWH43Z** Revision of Infusion Device in Vagina and Cul-de-sac, Percutaneous Endoscopic Approach

♀ **0UWH47Z** Revision of Autologous Tissue Substitute in Vagina and Cul-de-sac, Percutaneous Endoscopic Approach

♀ **0UWH4DZ** Revision of Intraluminal Device in Vagina and Cul-de-sac, Percutaneous Endoscopic Approach

♀ **0UWH4JZ** Revision of Synthetic Substitute in Vagina and Cul-de-sac, Percutaneous Endoscopic Approach

♀ **0UWH4KZ** Revision of Nonautologous Tissue Substitute in Vagina and Cul-de-sac, Percutaneous Endoscopic Approach

♀ **0UWH70Z** Revision of Drainage Device in Vagina and Cul-de-sac, Via Natural or Artificial Opening

♀ **0UWH71Z** Revision of Radioactive Element in Vagina and Cul-de-sac, Via Natural or Artificial Opening

♀ **0UWH73Z** Revision of Infusion Device in Vagina and Cul-de-sac, Via Natural or Artificial Opening

♀ **0UWH77Z** Revision of Autologous Tissue Substitute in Vagina and Cul-de-sac, Via Natural or Artificial Opening

♀ **0UWH7DZ** Revision of Intraluminal Device in Vagina and Cul-de-sac, Via Natural or Artificial Opening

♀ **0UWH7JZ** Revision of Synthetic Substitute in Vagina and Cul-de-sac, Via Natural or Artificial Opening

♀ **0UWH7KZ** Revision of Nonautologous Tissue Substitute in Vagina and Cul-de-sac, Via Natural or Artificial Opening

♀ **0UWH80Z** Revision of Drainage Device in Vagina and Cul-de-sac, Via Natural or Artificial Opening Endoscopic

♀ **0UWH81Z** Revision of Radioactive Element in Vagina and Cul-de-sac, Via Natural or Artificial Opening Endoscopic

♀ **0UWH83Z** Revision of Infusion Device in Vagina and Cul-de-sac, Via Natural or Artificial Opening Endoscopic

♀ **0UWH87Z** Revision of Autologous Tissue Substitute in Vagina and Cul-de-sac, Natural or Artificial Opening Endoscopic

♀ **0UWH8DZ** Revision of Intraluminal Device in Vagina and Cul-de-sac, Via Natural or Artificial Opening Endoscopic

♀ **0UWH8JZ** Revision of Synthetic Substitute in Vagina and Cul-de-sac, Via Natural or Artificial Opening Endoscopic

♀ **0UWH8KZ** Revision of Nonautologous Tissue Substitute in Vagina and Cul-de-sac, Natural or Artificial Opening Endoscopic

♀ **0UWHX0Z** Revision of Drainage Device in Vagina and Cul-de-sac, External Approach

♀ **0UWHX3Z** Revision of Infusion Device in Vagina and Cul-de-sac, External Approach

♀ **0UWHX7Z** Revision of Autologous Tissue Substitute in Vagina and Cul-de-sac, External Approach

♀ **0UWHXDZ** Revision of Intraluminal Device in Vagina and Cul-de-sac, External Approach

♀ **0UWHXJZ** Revision of Synthetic Substitute in Vagina and Cul-de-sac, External Approach

♀ **0UWHXKZ** Revision of Nonautologous Tissue Substitute in Vagina and Cul-de-sac, External Approach

♀ **0UWM00Z** Revision of Drainage Device in Vulva, Open Approach

♀ **0UWM07Z** Revision of Autologous Tissue Substitute in Vulva, Open Approach

♀ **0UWM0JZ** Revision of Synthetic Substitute in Vulva, Open Approach

♀ **0UWM0KZ** Revision of Nonautologous Tissue Substitute in Vulva, Open Approach

♀ **0UWMX0Z** Revision of Drainage Device in Vulva, External Approach

♀ **0UWMX7Z** Revision of Autologous Tissue Substitute in Vulva, External Approach

♀ **0UWMXJZ** Revision of Synthetic Substitute in Vulva, External Approach

♀ **0UWMXKZ** Revision of Nonautologous Tissue Substitute in Vulva, External Approach

0UY – Female Reproductive System, Transplantation

Review Coding Guideline B3.16

♀ **0UY00Z0** Transplantation of Right Ovary, Allogeneic, Open Approach

♀ **0UY00Z1** Transplantation of Right Ovary, Syngeneic, Open Approach

♀ **0UY00Z2** Transplantation of Right Ovary, Zooplastic, Open Approach

♀ **0UY10Z0** Transplantation of Left Ovary, Allogeneic, Open Approach

♀ **0UY10Z1** Transplantation of Left Ovary, Syngeneic, Open Approach

♀ **0UY10Z2** Transplantation of Left Ovary, Zooplastic, Open Approach

♀ Female-only   ♂ Male-only   ▲ Limited Coverage   ● Non-OR   ▰ HAC-associated procedure   ▲ Non-covered procedures   ✚ Combinati

Male Reproductive System

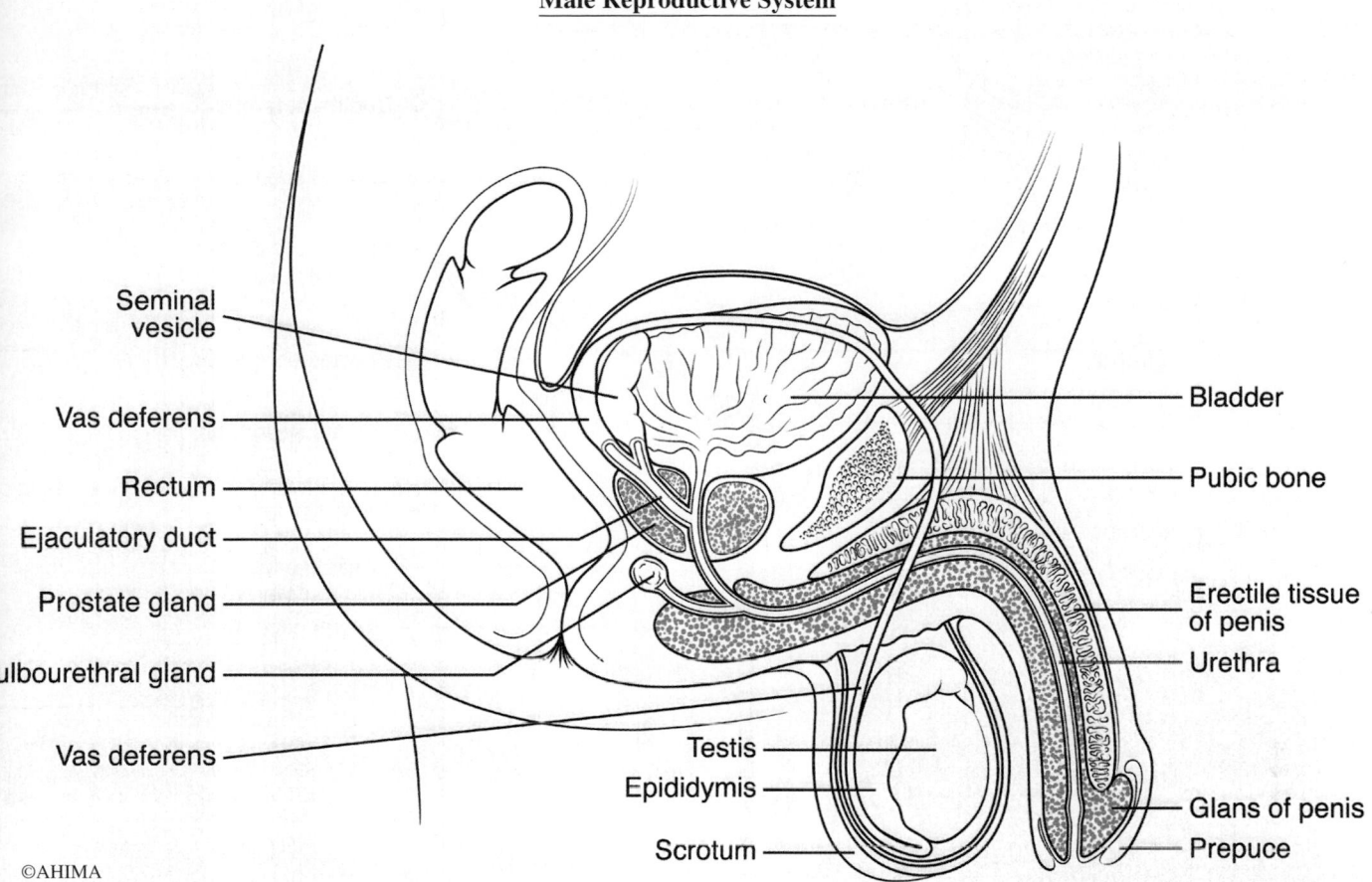

Seminal vesicle

Vas deferens

Rectum

Ejaculatory duct

Prostate gland

Bulbourethral gland

Vas deferens

Testis

Epididymis

Scrotum

Bladder

Pubic bone

Erectile tissue of penis

Urethra

Glans of penis

Prepuce

©AHIMA

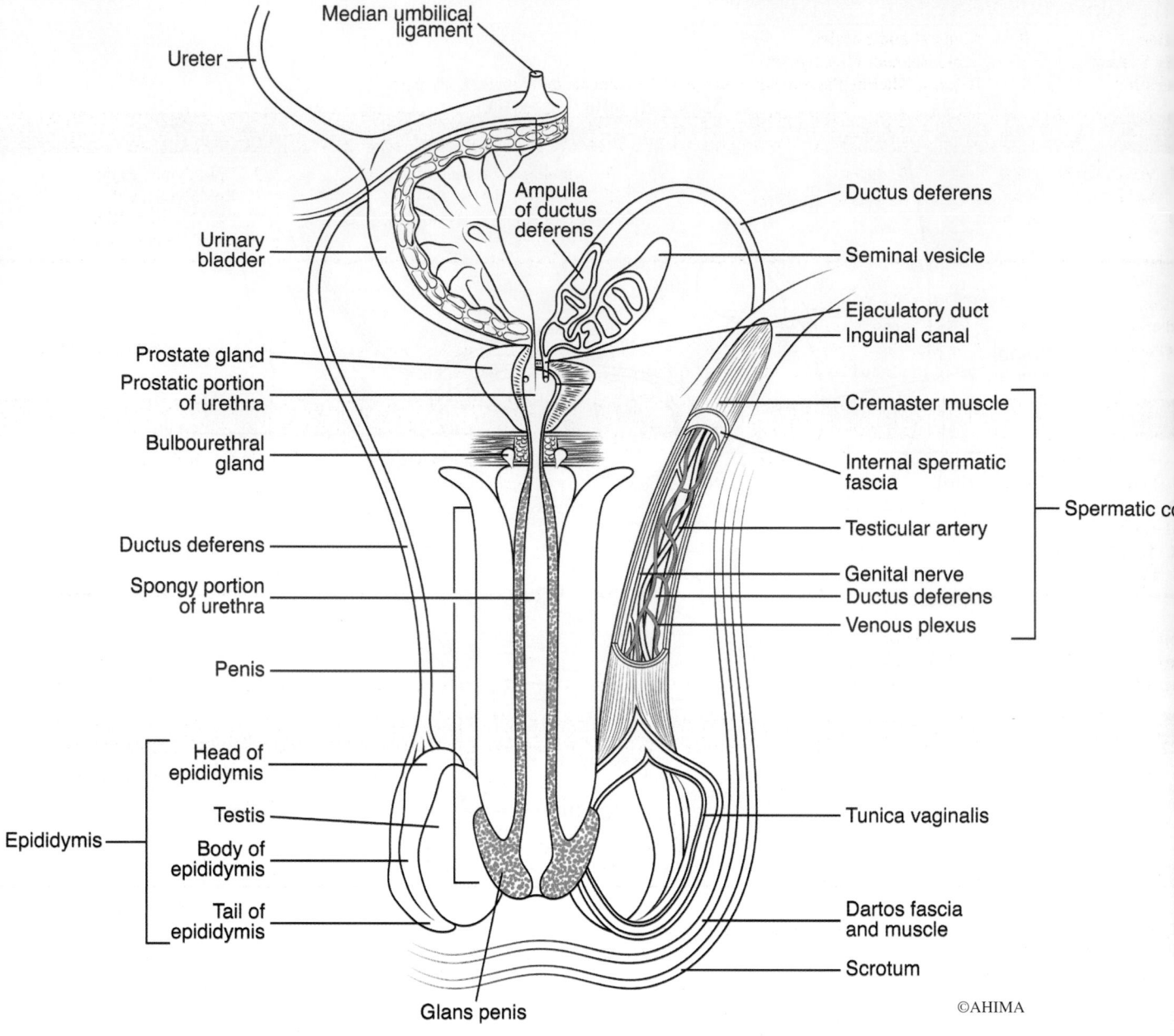

Median umbilical ligament

Ureter

Urinary bladder

Prostate gland

Prostatic portion of urethra

Bulbourethral gland

Ductus deferens

Spongy portion of urethra

Penis

Head of epididymis

Epididymis

Testis

Body of epididymis

Tail of epididymis

Glans penis

Ampulla of ductus deferens

Ductus deferens

Seminal vesicle

Ejaculatory duct

Inguinal canal

Cremaster muscle

Internal spermatic fascia

Spermatic c̲

Testicular artery

Genital nerve

Ductus deferens

Venous plexus

Tunica vaginalis

Dartos fascia and muscle

Scrotum

©AHIMA

tion	0	Medical and Surgical
ly System	V	Male Reproductive System
eration	1	**Bypass:** Altering the route of passage of the contents of a tubular body part

Body Part (4ᵗʰ)	Approach (5ᵗʰ)	Device (6ᵗʰ)	Qualifier (7ᵗʰ)
Vas Deferens, Right Vas Deferens, Left Vas Deferens, Bilateral	0 Open 4 Percutaneous Endoscopic	7 Autologous Tissue Substitute J Synthetic Substitute K Nonautologous Tissue Substitute Z No Device	J Epididymis, Right K Epididymis, Left N Vas Deferens, Right P Vas Deferens, Left

tion	0	Medical and Surgical
dy System	V	Male Reproductive System
eration	2	**Change:** Taking out or off a device from a body part and putting back an identical or similar device in or on the same body part without cutting or puncturing the skin or a mucous membrane

Body Part (4ᵗʰ)	Approach (5ᵗʰ)	Device (6ᵗʰ)	Qualifier (7ᵗʰ)
Prostate and Seminal Vesicles Scrotum and Tunica Vaginalis Testis Epididymis and Spermatic Cord Vas Deferens Penis	X External	0 Drainage Device Y Other Device	Z No Qualifier

ction	0	Medical and Surgical
dy System	V	Male Reproductive System
eration	5	**Destruction:** Physical eradication of all or a portion of a body part by the direct use of energy, force, or a destructive agent

Body Part (4ᵗʰ)	Approach (5ᵗʰ)	Device (6ᵗʰ)	Qualifier (7ᵗʰ)
Prostate	0 Open 3 Percutaneous 4 Percutaneous Endoscopic 7 Via Natural or Artificial Opening 8 Via Natural or Artificial Opening Endoscopic	Z No Device	Z No Qualifier
Seminal Vesicle, Right Seminal Vesicle, Left Seminal Vesicles, Bilateral Tunica Vaginalis, Right Tunica Vaginalis, Left Testis, Right Testis, Left Testes, Bilateral Spermatic Cord, Right Spermatic Cord, Left Spermatic Cords, Bilateral Epididymis, Right Epididymis, Left Epididymis, Bilateral Vas Deferens, Right Vas Deferens, Left Vas Deferens, Bilateral	0 Open 3 Percutaneous 4 Percutaneous Endoscopic	Z No Device	Z No Qualifier
Scrotum Penis Prepuce	0 Open 3 Percutaneous 4 Percutaneous Endoscopic X External	Z No Device	Z No Qualifier

Section	0	Medical and Surgical
Body System	V	Male Reproductive System
Operation	7	Dilation: Expanding an orifice or the lumen of a tubular body part

Body Part (4th)	Approach (5th)	Device (6th)	Qualifier (7th)
N Vas Deferens, Right P Vas Deferens, Left Q Vas Deferens, Bilateral	0 Open 3 Percutaneous 4 Percutaneous Endoscopic	D Intraluminal Device Z No Device	Z No Qualifier

Section	0	Medical and Surgical
Body System	V	Male Reproductive System
Operation	9	Drainage: Taking or letting out fluids and/or gases from a body part

Body Part (4th)	Approach (5th)	Device (6th)	Qualifier (7th)
0 Prostate	0 Open 3 Percutaneous 4 Percutaneous Endoscopic 7 Via Natural or Artificial Opening 8 Via Natural or Artificial Opening Endoscopic	0 Drainage Device	Z No Qualifier
0 Prostate	0 Open 3 Percutaneous 4 Percutaneous Endoscopic 7 Via Natural or Artificial Opening 8 Via Natural or Artificial Opening Endoscopic	Z No Device	X Diagnostic Z No Qualifier
1 Seminal Vesicle, Right 2 Seminal Vesicle, Left 3 Seminal Vesicles, Bilateral 6 Tunica Vaginalis, Right 7 Tunica Vaginalis, Left 9 Testis, Right B Testis, Left C Testes, Bilateral F Spermatic Cord, Right G Spermatic Cord, Left H Spermatic Cords, Bilateral J Epididymis, Right K Epididymis, Left L Epididymis, Bilateral N Vas Deferens, Right P Vas Deferens, Left Q Vas Deferens, Bilateral	0 Open 3 Percutaneous 4 Percutaneous Endoscopic	0 Drainage Device	Z No Qualifier
1 Seminal Vesicle, Right 2 Seminal Vesicle, Left 3 Seminal Vesicles, Bilateral 6 Tunica Vaginalis, Right 7 Tunica Vaginalis, Left 9 Testis, Right B Testis, Left C Testes, Bilateral F Spermatic Cord, Right G Spermatic Cord, Left H Spermatic Cords, Bilateral J Epididymis, Right K Epididymis, Left L Epididymis, Bilateral N Vas Deferens, Right P Vas Deferens, Left Q Vas Deferens, Bilateral	0 Open 3 Percutaneous 4 Percutaneous Endoscopic	Z No Device	X Diagnostic Z No Qualifier
5 Scrotum S Penis T Prepuce	0 Open 3 Percutaneous 4 Percutaneous Endoscopic X External	0 Drainage Device	Z No Qualifier

Continued →

~~tion~~	0	Medical and Surgical	
~~y System~~	V	Male Reproductive System	
~~eration~~	9	Drainage: Taking or letting out fluids and/or gases from a body part	

Body Part (4th)	Approach (5th)	Device (6th)	Qualifier (7th)
Scrotum Penis Prepuce	0 Open 3 Percutaneous 4 Percutaneous Endoscopic X External	Z No Device	X Diagnostic Z No Qualifier

~~tion~~	0	Medical and Surgical	
~~dy System~~	V	Male Reproductive System	
~~eration~~	B	Excision: Cutting out or off, without replacement, a portion of a body part	

Body Part (4th)	Approach (5th)	Device (6th)	Qualifier (7th)
Prostate	0 Open 3 Percutaneous 4 Percutaneous Endoscopic 7 Via Natural or Artificial Opening 8 Via Natural or Artificial Opening Endoscopic	Z No Device	X Diagnostic Z No Qualifier
Seminal Vesicle, Right Seminal Vesicle, Left Seminal Vesicles, Bilateral Tunica Vaginalis, Right Tunica Vaginalis, Left Testis, Right Testis, Left Testes, Bilateral Spermatic Cord, Right Spermatic Cord, Left Spermatic Cords, Bilateral Epididymis, Right Epididymis, Left Epididymis, Bilateral Vas Deferens, Right Vas Deferens, Left Vas Deferens, Bilateral	0 Open 3 Percutaneous 4 Percutaneous Endoscopic	Z No Device	X Diagnostic Z No Qualifier
Scrotum Penis Prepuce	0 Open 3 Percutaneous 4 Percutaneous Endoscopic X External	Z No Device	X Diagnostic Z No Qualifier

~~ction~~	0	Medical and Surgical	
~~dy System~~	V	Male Reproductive System	
~~eration~~	C	Extirpation: Taking or cutting out solid matter from a body part	

Body Part (4th)	Approach (5th)	Device (6th)	Qualifier (7th)
Prostate	0 Open 3 Percutaneous 4 Percutaneous Endoscopic 7 Via Natural or Artificial Opening 8 Via Natural or Artificial Opening Endoscopic	Z No Device	Z No Qualifier

Continued →

Section	0	Medical and Surgical
Body System	V	Male Reproductive System
Operation	C	**Extirpation:** Taking or cutting out solid matter from a body part

Body Part (4th)	Approach (5th)	Device (6th)	Qualifier (7th)
1 Seminal Vesicle, Right 2 Seminal Vesicle, Left 3 Seminal Vesicles, Bilateral 6 Tunica Vaginalis, Right 7 Tunica Vaginalis, Left 9 Testis, Right B Testis, Left C Testes, Bilateral F Spermatic Cord, Right G Spermatic Cord, Left H Spermatic Cords, Bilateral J Epididymis, Right K Epididymis, Left L Epididymis, Bilateral N Vas Deferens, Right P Vas Deferens, Left Q Vas Deferens, Bilateral	0 Open 3 Percutaneous 4 Percutaneous Endoscopic	Z No Device	Z No Qualifier
5 Scrotum S Penis T Prepuce	0 Open 3 Percutaneous 4 Percutaneous Endoscopic X External	Z No Device	Z No Qualifier

Section	0	Medical and Surgical
Body System	V	Male Reproductive System
Operation	H	**Insertion:** Putting in a nonbiological appliance that monitors, assists, performs, or prevents a physiological function but does not physically take the place of a body part

Body Part (4th)	Approach (5th)	Device (6th)	Qualifier (7th)
0 Prostate	0 Open 3 Percutaneous 4 Percutaneous Endoscopic 7 Via Natural or Artificial Opening 8 Via Natural or Artificial Opening Endoscopic	1 Radioactive Element	Z No Qualifier
4 Prostate and Seminal Vesicles 8 Scrotum and Tunica Vaginalis D Testis M Epididymis and Spermatic Cord R Vas Deferens	0 Open 3 Percutaneous 4 Percutaneous Endoscopic 7 Via Natural or Artificial Opening 8 Via Natural or Artificial Opening Endoscopic	3 Infusion Device	Z No Qualifier
S Penis	0 Open 3 Percutaneous 4 Percutaneous Endoscopic X External	3 Infusion Device	Z No Qualifier

Section	0	Medical and Surgical
Body System	V	Male Reproductive System
Operation	J	**Inspection:** Visually and/or manually exploring a body part

Body Part (4th)	Approach (5th)	Device (6th)	Qualifier (7th)
4 Prostate and Seminal Vesicles 8 Scrotum and Tunica Vaginalis D Testis M Epididymis and Spermatic Cord R Vas Deferens S Penis	0 Open 3 Percutaneous 4 Percutaneous Endoscopic X External	Z No Device	Z No Qualifier

Section	0	Medical and Surgical
Body System	V	Male Reproductive System
Operation	L	**Occlusion:** Completely closing an orifice or the lumen of a tubular body part

Body Part (4th)	Approach (5th)	Device (6th)	Qualifier (7th)
Spermatic Cord, Right Spermatic Cord, Left Spermatic Cords, Bilateral Vas Deferens, Right Vas Deferens, Left Vas Deferens, Bilateral	0 Open 3 Percutaneous 4 Percutaneous Endoscopic	C Extraluminal Device D Intraluminal Device Z No Device	Z No Qualifier

Section	0	Medical and Surgical
Body System	V	Male Reproductive System
Operation	M	**Reattachment:** Putting back in or on all or a portion of a separated body part to its normal location or other suitable location

Body Part (4th)	Approach (5th)	Device (6th)	Qualifier (7th)
Scrotum Penis	X External	Z No Device	Z No Qualifier
Tunica Vaginalis, Right Tunica Vaginalis, Left Testis, Right Testis, Left Testes, Bilateral Spermatic Cord, Right Spermatic Cord, Left Spermatic Cords, Bilateral	0 Open 4 Percutaneous Endoscopic	Z No Device	Z No Qualifier

Section	0	Medical and Surgical
Body System	V	Male Reproductive System
Operation	N	**Release:** Freeing a body part from an abnormal physical constraint by cutting or by the use of force

Body Part (4th)	Approach (5th)	Device (6th)	Qualifier (7th)
0 Prostate	0 Open 3 Percutaneous 4 Percutaneous Endoscopic 7 Via Natural or Artificial Opening 8 Via Natural or Artificial Opening Endoscopic	Z No Device	Z No Qualifier
1 Seminal Vesicle, Right 2 Seminal Vesicle, Left 3 Seminal Vesicles, Bilateral 6 Tunica Vaginalis, Right 7 Tunica Vaginalis, Left 9 Testis, Right B Testis, Left C Testes, Bilateral F Spermatic Cord, Right G Spermatic Cord, Left H Spermatic Cords, Bilateral J Epididymis, Right K Epididymis, Left L Epididymis, Bilateral N Vas Deferens, Right P Vas Deferens, Left Q Vas Deferens, Bilateral	0 Open 3 Percutaneous 4 Percutaneous Endoscopic	Z No Device	Z No Qualifier
5 Scrotum S Penis T Prepuce	0 Open 3 Percutaneous 4 Percutaneous Endoscopic X External	Z No Device	Z No Qualifier

Body Part (4th)	Approach (5th)	Device (6th)	Qualifier (7th)
4 Prostate and Seminal Vesicles	0 Open 3 Percutaneous 4 Percutaneous Endoscopic 7 Via Natural or Artificial Opening 8 Via Natural or Artificial Opening Endoscopic	0 Drainage Device 1 Radioactive Element 3 Infusion Device 7 Autologous Tissue Substitute J Synthetic Substitute K Nonautologous Tissue Substitute	Z No Qualifier
4 Prostate and Seminal Vesicles	X External	0 Drainage Device 1 Radioactive Element 3 Infusion Device	Z No Qualifier
8 Scrotum and Tunica Vaginalis D Testis S Penis	0 Open 3 Percutaneous 4 Percutaneous Endoscopic 7 Via Natural or Artificial Opening 8 Via Natural or Artificial Opening Endoscopic	0 Drainage Device 3 Infusion Device 7 Autologous Tissue Substitute J Synthetic Substitute K Nonautologous Tissue Substitute	Z No Qualifier
8 Scrotum and Tunica Vaginalis D Testis S Penis	X External	0 Drainage Device 3 Infusion Device	Z No Qualifier
M Epididymis and Spermatic Cord	0 Open 3 Percutaneous 4 Percutaneous Endoscopic 7 Via Natural or Artificial Opening 8 Via Natural or Artificial Opening Endoscopic	0 Drainage Device 3 Infusion Device 7 Autologous Tissue Substitute C Extraluminal Device J Synthetic Substitute K Nonautologous Tissue Substitute	Z No Qualifier
M Epididymis and Spermatic Cord	X External	0 Drainage Device 3 Infusion Device	Z No Qualifier
R Vas Deferens	0 Open 3 Percutaneous 4 Percutaneous Endoscopic 7 Via Natural or Artificial Opening 8 Via Natural or Artificial Opening Endoscopic	0 Drainage Device 3 Infusion Device 7 Autologous Tissue Substitute C Extraluminal Device D Intraluminal Device J Synthetic Substitute K Nonautologous Tissue Substitute	Z No Qualifier
R Vas Deferens	X External	0 Drainage Device 3 Infusion Device D Intraluminal Device	Z No Qualifier

Body Part (4th)	Approach (5th)	Device (6th)	Qualifier (7th)
0 Prostate	0 Open 3 Percutaneous 4 Percutaneous Endoscopic 7 Via Natural or Artificial Opening 8 Via Natural or Artificial Opening Endoscopic	Z No Device	Z No Qualifier

Continued →

Section	0	Medical and Surgical
Body System	V	Male Reproductive System
Operation	Q	Repair: Restoring, to the extent possible, a body part to its normal anatomic structure and function

Body Part (4th)	Approach (5th)	Device (6th)	Qualifier (7th)
Seminal Vesicle, Right Seminal Vesicle, Left Seminal Vesicles, Bilateral Tunica Vaginalis, Right Tunica Vaginalis, Left Testis, Right Testis, Left Testes, Bilateral Spermatic Cord, Right Spermatic Cord, Left Spermatic Cords, Bilateral Epididymis, Right Epididymis, Left Epididymis, Bilateral Vas Deferens, Right Vas Deferens, Left Vas Deferens, Bilateral	0 Open 3 Percutaneous 4 Percutaneous Endoscopic	Z No Device	Z No Qualifier
Scrotum Penis Prepuce	0 Open 3 Percutaneous 4 Percutaneous Endoscopic X External	Z No Device	Z No Qualifier

Section	0	Medical and Surgical
Body System	V	Male Reproductive System
Operation	R	Replacement: Putting in or on biological or synthetic material that physically takes the place and/or function of all or a portion of a body part

Body Part (4th)	Approach (5th)	Device (6th)	Qualifier (7th)
9 Testis, Right B Testis, Left C Testes, Bilateral	0 Open	J Synthetic Substitute	Z No Qualifier

Section	0	Medical and Surgical
Body System	V	Male Reproductive System
Operation	S	Reposition: Moving to its normal location, or other suitable location, all or a portion of a body part

Body Part (4th)	Approach (5th)	Device (6th)	Qualifier (7th)
9 Testis, Right B Testis, Left C Testes, Bilateral F Spermatic Cord, Right G Spermatic Cord, Left H Spermatic Cords, Bilateral	0 Open 3 Percutaneous 4 Percutaneous Endoscopic	Z No Device	Z No Qualifier

Section	0	Medical and Surgical
Body System	V	Male Reproductive System
Operation	T	Resection: Cutting out or off, without replacement, all of a body part

Body Part (4th)	Approach (5th)	Device (6th)	Qualifier (7th)
0 Prostate	0 Open 4 Percutaneous Endoscopic 7 Via Natural or Artificial Opening 8 Via Natural or Artificial Opening Endoscopic	Z No Device	Z No Qualifier

Continued →

Section	0	Medical and Surgical
Body System	V	Male Reproductive System
Operation	T	**Resection:** Cutting out or off, without replacement, all of a body part

Body Part (4th)	Approach (5th)	Device (6th)	Qualifier (7th)
1 Seminal Vesicle, Right 2 Seminal Vesicle, Left 3 Seminal Vesicles, Bilateral 6 Tunica Vaginalis, Right 7 Tunica Vaginalis, Left 9 Testis, Right B Testis, Left C Testes, Bilateral F Spermatic Cord, Right G Spermatic Cord, Left H Spermatic Cords, Bilateral J Epididymis, Right K Epididymis, Left L Epididymis, Bilateral N Vas Deferens, Right P Vas Deferens, Left Q Vas Deferens, Bilateral	0 Open 4 Percutaneous Endoscopic	Z No Device	Z No Qualifier
5 Scrotum S Penis T Prepuce	0 Open 4 Percutaneous Endoscopic X External	Z No Device	Z No Qualifier

Section	0	Medical and Surgical
Body System	V	Male Reproductive System
Operation	U	**Supplement:** Putting in or on biological or synthetic material that physically reinforces and/or augments the function of a portion of a body part

Body Part (4th)	Approach (5th)	Device (6th)	Qualifier (7th)
1 Seminal Vesicle, Right 2 Seminal Vesicle, Left 3 Seminal Vesicles, Bilateral 6 Tunica Vaginalis, Right 7 Tunica Vaginalis, Left F Spermatic Cord, Right G Spermatic Cord, Left H Spermatic Cords, Bilateral J Epididymis, Right K Epididymis, Left L Epididymis, Bilateral N Vas Deferens, Right P Vas Deferens, Left Q Vas Deferens, Bilateral	0 Open 4 Percutaneous Endoscopic	7 Autologous Tissue Substitute J Synthetic Substitute K Nonautologous Tissue Substitute	Z No Qualifier
5 Scrotum S Penis T Prepuce	0 Open 4 Percutaneous Endoscopic X External	7 Autologous Tissue Substitute J Synthetic Substitute K Nonautologous Tissue Substitute	Z No Qualifier
9 Testis, Right B Testis, Left C Testes, Bilateral	0 Open	7 Autologous Tissue Substitute J Synthetic Substitute K Nonautologous Tissue Substitute	Z No Qualifier

tion	0	**Medical and Surgical**
dy System	V	**Male Reproductive System**
eration	W	**Revision:** Correcting, to the extent possible, a portion of a malfunctioning device or the position of a displaced device

Body Part (4ᵗʰ)	Approach (5ᵗʰ)	Device (6ᵗʰ)	Qualifier (7ᵗʰ)
Prostate and Seminal Vesicles Scrotum and Tunica Vaginalis) Testis . Penis	0 Open 3 Percutaneous 4 Percutaneous Endoscopic 7 Via Natural or Artificial Opening 8 Via Natural or Artificial Opening Endoscopic X External	0 Drainage Device 3 Infusion Device 7 Autologous Tissue Substitute J Synthetic Substitute K Nonautologous Tissue Substitute	Z No Qualifier
M Epididymis and Spermatic Cord	0 Open 3 Percutaneous 4 Percutaneous Endoscopic 7 Via Natural or Artificial Opening 8 Via Natural or Artificial Opening Endoscopic X External	0 Drainage Device 3 Infusion Device 7 Autologous Tissue Substitute C Extraluminal Device J Synthetic Substitute K Nonautologous Tissue Substitute	Z No Qualifier
R Vas Deferens	0 Open 3 Percutaneous 4 Percutaneous Endoscopic 7 Via Natural or Artificial Opening 8 Via Natural or Artificial Opening Endoscopic X External	0 Drainage Device 3 Infusion Device 7 Autologous Tissue Substitute C Extraluminal Device D Intraluminal Device J Synthetic Substitute K Nonautologous Tissue Substitute	Z No Qualifier

Iale Reproductive System Code Listing 0V1–0VW

V1 – Male Reproductive System, Bypass

eview Coding Guideline B3.6a

V1N07J Bypass Right Vas Deferens to Right Epididymis with Autologous Tissue Substitute, Open Approach

V1N07K Bypass Right Vas Deferens to Left Epididymis with Autologous Tissue Substitute, Open Approach

V1N07N Bypass Right Vas Deferens to Right Vas Deferens with Autologous Tissue Substitute, Open Approach

V1N07P Bypass Right Vas Deferens to Left Vas Deferens with Autologous Tissue Substitute, Open Approach

V1N0JJ Bypass Right Vas Deferens to Right Epididymis with Synthetic Substitute, Open Approach

0V1N0JK Bypass Right Vas Deferens to Left Epididymis with Synthetic Substitute, Open Approach

0V1N0JN Bypass Right Vas Deferens to Right Vas Deferens with Synthetic Substitute, Open Approach

0V1N0JP Bypass Right Vas Deferens to Left Vas Deferens with Synthetic Substitute, Open Approach

0V1N0KJ Bypass Right Vas Deferens to Right Epididymis with Nonautologous Tissue Substitute, Open Approach

0V1N0KK Bypass Right Vas Deferens to Left Epididymis with Nonautologous Tissue Substitute, Open Approach

0V1N0KN Bypass Right Vas Deferens to Right Vas Deferens with Nonautologous Tissue Substitute, Open Approach

0V1N0KP Bypass Right Vas Deferens to Left Vas Deferens with Nonautologous Tissue Substitute, Open Approach

0V1N0ZJ Bypass Right Vas Deferens to Right Epididymis, Open Approach

♂ 0V1N0ZK Bypass Right Vas Deferens to Left Epididymis, Open Approach

♂ 0V1N0ZN Bypass Right Vas Deferens to Right Vas Deferens, Open Approach

♂ 0V1N0ZP Bypass Right Vas Deferens to Left Vas Deferens, Open Approach

♂ 0V1N47J Bypass Right Vas Deferens to Right Epididymis with Autologous Tissue Substitute, Percutaneous Endoscopic Approach

♂ 0V1N47K Bypass Right Vas Deferens to Left Epididymis with Autologous Tissue Substitute, Percutaneous Endoscopic Approach

♂ 0V1N47N Bypass Right Vas Deferens to Right Vas Deferens with Autologous Tissue Substitute, Percutaneous Endoscopic Approach

♂ 0V1N47P Bypass Right Vas Deferens to Left Vas Deferens with Autologous Tissue Substitute, Percutaneous Endoscopic Approach

♂ 0V1N4JJ Bypass Right Vas Deferens to Right Epididymis with Synthetic Substitute, Percutaneous Endoscopic Approach

♂ 0V1N4JK Bypass Right Vas Deferens to Left Epididymis with Synthetic Substitute, Percutaneous Endoscopic Approach

♂ 0V1N4JN Bypass Right Vas Deferens to Right Vas Deferens with Synthetic Substitute, Percutaneous Endoscopic Approach

♂ 0V1N4JP Bypass Right Vas Deferens to Left Vas Deferens with Synthetic Substitute, Percutaneous Endoscopic Approach

♂ 0V1N4KJ Bypass Right Vas Deferens to Right Epididymis with Nonautologous Tissue Substitute, Percutaneous Endoscopic Approach

♂ 0V1N4KK Bypass Right Vas Deferens to Left Epididymis with Nonautologous Tissue Substitute, Percutaneous Endoscopic Approach

♂ 0V1N4KN Bypass Right Vas Deferens to Right Vas Deferens with Nonautologous Tissue Substitute, Percutaneous Endoscopic Approach

♂ 0V1N4KP Bypass Right Vas Deferens to Left Vas Deferens with Nonautologous Tissue Substitute, Percutaneous Endoscopic Approach

♂ 0V1N4ZJ Bypass Right Vas Deferens to Right Epididymis, Percutaneous Endoscopic Approach

♂ 0V1N4ZK Bypass Right Vas Deferens to Left Epididymis, Percutaneous Endoscopic Approach

♂ 0V1N4ZN Bypass Right Vas Deferens to Right Vas Deferens, Percutaneous Endoscopic Approach

♂ 0V1N4ZP Bypass Right Vas Deferens to Left Vas Deferens, Percutaneous Endoscopic Approach

♂ 0V1P07J Bypass Left Vas Deferens to Right Epididymis with Autologous Tissue Substitute, Open Approach

♂ 0V1P07K Bypass Left Vas Deferens to Left Epididymis with Autologous Tissue Substitute, Open Approach

♂ 0V1P07N Bypass Left Vas Deferens to Right Vas Deferens with Autologous Tissue Substitute, Open Approach

♂ 0V1P07P Bypass Left Vas Deferens to Left Vas Deferens with Autologous Tissue Substitute, Open Approach

♀ Female-only   ♂ Male-only   ▲ Limited Coverage   ● Non-OR   ▬ HAC-associated procedure   ▲ Non-covered procedures   ✚ Combination

♂ **0V1P0JJ** Bypass Left Vas Deferens to Right Epididymis with Synthetic Substitute, Open Approach

♂ **0V1P0JK** Bypass Left Vas Deferens to Left Epididymis with Synthetic Substitute, Open Approach

♂ **0V1P0JN** Bypass Left Vas Deferens to Right Vas Deferens with Synthetic Substitute, Open Approach

♂ **0V1P0JP** Bypass Left Vas Deferens to Left Vas Deferens with Synthetic Substitute, Open Approach

♂ **0V1P0KJ** Bypass Left Vas Deferens to Right Epididymis with Nonautologous Tissue Substitute, Open Approach

♂ **0V1P0KK** Bypass Left Vas Deferens to Left Epididymis with Nonautologous Tissue Substitute, Open Approach

♂ **0V1P0KN** Bypass Left Vas Deferens to Right Vas Deferens with Nonautologous Tissue Substitute, Open Approach

♂ **0V1P0KP** Bypass Left Vas Deferens to Left Vas Deferens with Nonautologous Tissue Substitute, Open Approach

♂ **0V1P0ZJ** Bypass Left Vas Deferens to Right Epididymis, Open Approach

♂ **0V1P0ZK** Bypass Left Vas Deferens to Left Epididymis, Open Approach

♂ **0V1P0ZN** Bypass Left Vas Deferens to Right Vas Deferens, Open Approach

♂ **0V1P0ZP** Bypass Left Vas Deferens to Left Vas Deferens, Open Approach

♂ **0V1P47J** Bypass Left Vas Deferens to Right Epididymis with Autologous Tissue Substitute, Percutaneous Endoscopic Approach

♂ **0V1P47K** Bypass Left Vas Deferens to Left Epididymis with Autologous Tissue Substitute, Percutaneous Endoscopic Approach

♂ **0V1P47N** Bypass Left Vas Deferens to Right Vas Deferens with Autologous Tissue Substitute, Percutaneous Endoscopic Approach

♂ **0V1P47P** Bypass Left Vas Deferens to Left Vas Deferens with Autologous Tissue Substitute, Percutaneous Endoscopic Approach

♂ **0V1P4JJ** Bypass Left Vas Deferens to Right Epididymis with Synthetic Substitute, Percutaneous Endoscopic Approach

♂ **0V1P4JK** Bypass Left Vas Deferens to Left Epididymis with Synthetic Substitute, Percutaneous Endoscopic Approach

♂ **0V1P4JN** Bypass Left Vas Deferens to Right Vas Deferens with Synthetic Substitute, Percutaneous Endoscopic Approach

♂ **0V1P4JP** Bypass Left Vas Deferens to Left Vas Deferens with Synthetic Substitute, Percutaneous Endoscopic Approach

♂ **0V1P4KJ** Bypass Left Vas Deferens to Right Epididymis with Nonautologous Tissue Substitute, Percutaneous Endoscopic Approach

♂ **0V1P4KK** Bypass Left Vas Deferens to Left Epididymis with Nonautologous Tissue Substitute, Percutaneous Endoscopic Approach

♂ **0V1P4KN** Bypass Left Vas Deferens to Right Vas Deferens with Nonautologous Tissue Substitute, Percutaneous Endoscopic Approach

♂ **0V1P4KP** Bypass Left Vas Deferens to Left Vas Deferens with Nonautologous Tissue Substitute, Percutaneous Endoscopic Approach

♂ **0V1P4ZJ** Bypass Left Vas Deferens to Right Epididymis, Percutaneous Endoscopic Approach

♂ **0V1P4ZK** Bypass Left Vas Deferens to Left Epididymis, Percutaneous Endoscopic Approach

♂ **0V1P4ZN** Bypass Left Vas Deferens to Right Vas Deferens, Percutaneous Endoscopic Approach

♂ **0V1P4ZP** Bypass Left Vas Deferens to Left Vas Deferens, Percutaneous Endoscopic Approach

♂ **0V1Q07J** Bypass Bilateral Vas Deferens to Right Epididymis with Autologous Tissue Substitute, Open Approach

♂ **0V1Q07K** Bypass Bilateral Vas Deferens to Left Epididymis with Autologous Tissue Substitute, Open Approach

♂ **0V1Q07N** Bypass Bilateral Vas Deferens to Right Vas Deferens with Autologous Tissue Substitute, Open Approach

♂ **0V1Q07P** Bypass Bilateral Vas Deferens to Left Vas Deferens with Autologous Tissue Substitute, Open Approach

♂ **0V1Q0JJ** Bypass Bilateral Vas Deferens to Right Epididymis with Synthetic Substitute, Open Approach

♂ **0V1Q0JK** Bypass Bilateral Vas Deferens to Left Epididymis with Synthetic Substitute, Open Approach

♂ **0V1Q0JN** Bypass Bilateral Vas Deferens to Right Vas Deferens with Synthetic Substitute, Open Approach

♂ **0V1Q0JP** Bypass Bilateral Vas Deferens to Left Vas Deferens with Synthetic Substitute, Open Approach

♂ **0V1Q0KJ** Bypass Bilateral Vas Deferens to Right Epididymis with Nonautologous Tissue Substitute, Open Approach

♂ **0V1Q0KK** Bypass Bilateral Vas Deferens to Left Epididymis with Nonautologous Tissue Substitute, Open Approach

♂ **0V1Q0KN** Bypass Bilateral Vas Deferens to Right Vas Deferens with Nonautologous Tissue Substitute, Open Approach

♂ **0V1Q0KP** Bypass Bilateral Vas Deferens to Left Vas Deferens with Nonautologous Tissue Substitute, Open Approach

♂ **0V1Q0ZJ** Bypass Bilateral Vas Deferens to Right Epididymis, Open Approach

♂ **0V1Q0ZK** Bypass Bilateral Vas Deferens to Left Epididymis, Open Approach

♂ **0V1Q0ZN** Bypass Bilateral Vas Deferens to Right Vas Deferens, Open Approach

♂ **0V1Q0ZP** Bypass Bilateral Vas Deferens to Left Vas Deferens, Open Approach

♂ **0V1Q47J** Bypass Bilateral Vas Deferens to Right Epididymis with Autologous Tissue Substitute, Percutaneous Endoscopic Approach

♂ **0V1Q47K** Bypass Bilateral Vas Deferens to Left Epididymis with Autologous Tissue Substitute, Percutaneous Endoscopic Approach

♂ **0V1Q47N** Bypass Bilateral Vas Deferens to Right Vas Deferens with Autologous Tissue Substitute, Percutaneous Endoscopic Approach

♂ **0V1Q47P** Bypass Bilateral Vas Deferens to Left Vas Deferens with Autologous Tissue Substitute, Percutaneous Endoscopic Approach

♂ **0V1Q4JJ** Bypass Bilateral Vas Deferens to Right Epididymis with Synthetic Substitute, Percutaneous Endoscopic Approach

♂ **0V1Q4JK** Bypass Bilateral Vas Deferens to Left Epididymis with Synthetic Substitute, Percutaneous Endoscopic Approach

♂ **0V1Q4JN** Bypass Bilateral Vas Deferens to Right Vas Deferens with Synthetic Substitute, Percutaneous Endoscopic Approach

♂ **0V1Q4JP** Bypass Bilateral Vas Deferens to Left Vas Deferens with Synthetic Substitute, Percutaneous Endoscopic Approach

♂ **0V1Q4KJ** Bypass Bilateral Vas Deferens to Right Epididymis with Nonautologous Tissue Substitute, Percutaneous Endoscopic Approach

♂ **0V1Q4KK** Bypass Bilateral Vas Deferens to Left Epididymis with Nonautologous Tissue Substitute, Percutaneous Endoscopic Approach

♂ **0V1Q4KN** Bypass Bilateral Vas Deferens to Right Vas Deferens with Nonautologous Tissue Substitute, Percutaneous Endoscopic Approach

♂ **0V1Q4KP** Bypass Bilateral Vas Deferens to Left Vas Deferens with Nonautologous Tissue Substitute, Percutaneous Endoscopic Approach

♂ **0V1Q4ZJ** Bypass Bilateral Vas Deferens to Right Epididymis, Percutaneous Endoscopic Approach

♂ **0V1Q4ZK** Bypass Bilateral Vas Deferens to Left Epididymis, Percutaneous Endoscopic Approach

♂ **0V1Q4ZN** Bypass Bilateral Vas Deferens to Right Vas Deferens, Percutaneous Endoscopic Approach

♂ **0V1Q4ZP** Bypass Bilateral Vas Deferens to Left Vas Deferens, Percutaneous Endoscopic Approach

0V2 – Male Reproductive System, Change

Review Coding Guideline B6.1c

♂ **0V24X0Z** Change Drainage Device in Prostate and Seminal Vesicles, External Approach

♂ **0V24XYZ** Change Other Device in Prostate and Seminal Vesicles, External Approach

♂ **0V28X0Z** Change Drainage Device in Scrotum and Tunica Vaginalis, External Approach

♂ **0V28XYZ** Change Other Device in Scrotum and Tunica Vaginalis, External Approach

♂ **0V2DX0Z** Change Drainage Device in Testis, External Approach

♂ **0V2DXYZ** Change Other Device in Testis, External Approach

♂ **0V2MX0Z** Change Drainage Device in Epididymis and Spermatic Cord, External Approach

♂ **0V2MXYZ** Change Other Device in Epididymis and Spermatic Cord, External Approach

♂ **0V2RX0Z** Change Drainage Device in Vas Deferens, External Approach

♂ **0V2RXYZ** Change Other Device in Vas Deferens, External Approach

♂ **0V2SX0Z** Change Drainage Device in Penis, External Approach

♂ **0V2SXYZ** Change Other Device in Penis, External Approach

5 – Male Reproductive System, Destruction

♂ 0V500ZZ Destruction of Prostate, Open Approach
♂ 0V503ZZ Destruction of Prostate, Percutaneous Approach
♂ 0V504ZZ Destruction of Prostate, Percutaneous Endoscopic Approach
♂ 0V507ZZ Destruction of Prostate, Via Natural or Artificial Opening
♂ 0V508ZZ Destruction of Prostate, Via Natural or Artificial Opening Endoscopic
♂ 0V510ZZ Destruction of Right Seminal Vesicle, Open Approach
♂ 0V513ZZ Destruction of Right Seminal Vesicle, Percutaneous Approach
♂ 0V514ZZ Destruction of Right Seminal Vesicle, Percutaneous Endoscopic Approach
♂ 0V520ZZ Destruction of Left Seminal Vesicle, Open Approach
♂ 0V523ZZ Destruction of Left Seminal Vesicle, Percutaneous Approach
♂ 0V524ZZ Destruction of Left Seminal Vesicle, Percutaneous Endoscopic Approach
♂ 0V530ZZ Destruction of Bilateral Seminal Vesicles, Open Approach
♂ 0V533ZZ Destruction of Bilateral Seminal Vesicles, Percutaneous Approach
♂ 0V534ZZ Destruction of Bilateral Seminal Vesicles, Percutaneous Endoscopic Approach
♂ 0V550ZZ Destruction of Scrotum, Open Approach
♂ 0V553ZZ Destruction of Scrotum, Percutaneous Approach
♂ 0V554ZZ Destruction of Scrotum, Percutaneous Endoscopic Approach
♂ 0V55XZZ Destruction of Scrotum, External Approach
♂ 0V560ZZ Destruction of Right Tunica Vaginalis, Open Approach
♂ 0V563ZZ Destruction of Right Tunica Vaginalis, Percutaneous Approach
♂ 0V564ZZ Destruction of Right Tunica Vaginalis, Percutaneous Endoscopic Approach
♂ 0V570ZZ Destruction of Left Tunica Vaginalis, Open Approach
♂ 0V573ZZ Destruction of Left Tunica Vaginalis, Percutaneous Approach

♂ 0V574ZZ Destruction of Left Tunica Vaginalis, Percutaneous Endoscopic Approach
♂ 0V590ZZ Destruction of Right Testis, Open Approach
♂ 0V593ZZ Destruction of Right Testis, Percutaneous Approach
♂ 0V594ZZ Destruction of Right Testis, Percutaneous Endoscopic Approach
♂ 0V5B0ZZ Destruction of Left Testis, Open Approach
♂ 0V5B3ZZ Destruction of Left Testis, Percutaneous Approach
♂ 0V5B4ZZ Destruction of Left Testis, Percutaneous Endoscopic Approach
♂ 0V5C0ZZ Destruction of Bilateral Testes, Open Approach
♂ 0V5C3ZZ Destruction of Bilateral Testes, Percutaneous Approach
♂ 0V5C4ZZ Destruction of Bilateral Testes, Percutaneous Endoscopic Approach
♂ 0V5F0ZZ Destruction of Right Spermatic Cord, Open Approach
♂ 0V5F3ZZ Destruction of Right Spermatic Cord, Percutaneous Approach
♂ 0V5F4ZZ Destruction of Right Spermatic Cord, Percutaneous Endoscopic Approach
♂ 0V5G0ZZ Destruction of Left Spermatic Cord, Open Approach
♂ 0V5G3ZZ Destruction of Left Spermatic Cord, Percutaneous Approach
♂ 0V5G4ZZ Destruction of Left Spermatic Cord, Percutaneous Endoscopic Approach
♂ 0V5H0ZZ Destruction of Bilateral Spermatic Cords, Open Approach
♂ 0V5H3ZZ Destruction of Bilateral Spermatic Cords, Percutaneous Approach
♂ 0V5H4ZZ Destruction of Bilateral Spermatic Cords, Percutaneous Endoscopic Approach
♂ 0V5J0ZZ Destruction of Right Epididymis, Open Approach
♂ 0V5J3ZZ Destruction of Right Epididymis, Percutaneous Approach
♂ 0V5J4ZZ Destruction of Right Epididymis, Percutaneous Endoscopic Approach

♂ 0V5K0ZZ Destruction of Left Epididymis, Open Approach
♂ 0V5K3ZZ Destruction of Left Epididymis, Percutaneous Approach
♂ 0V5K4ZZ Destruction of Left Epididymis, Percutaneous Endoscopic Approach
♂ 0V5L0ZZ Destruction of Bilateral Epididymis, Open Approach
♂ 0V5L3ZZ Destruction of Bilateral Epididymis, Percutaneous Approach
♂ 0V5L4ZZ Destruction of Bilateral Epididymis, Percutaneous Endoscopic Approach
♂▲ 0V5N0ZZ Destruction of Right Vas Deferens, Open Approach
♂▲ 0V5N3ZZ Destruction of Right Vas Deferens, Percutaneous Approach
♂▲ 0V5N4ZZ Destruction of Right Vas Deferens, Percutaneous Endoscopic Approach
♂▲ 0V5P0ZZ Destruction of Left Vas Deferens, Open Approach
♂▲ 0V5P3ZZ Destruction of Left Vas Deferens, Percutaneous Approach
♂▲ 0V5P4ZZ Destruction of Left Vas Deferens, Percutaneous Endoscopic Approach
♂ 0V5Q0ZZ Destruction of Bilateral Vas Deferens, Open Approach
♂ 0V5Q3ZZ Destruction of Bilateral Vas Deferens, Percutaneous Approach
♂ 0V5Q4ZZ Destruction of Bilateral Vas Deferens, Percutaneous Endoscopic Approach
♂ 0V5S0ZZ Destruction of Penis, Open Approach
♂ 0V5S3ZZ Destruction of Penis, Percutaneous Approach
♂ 0V5S4ZZ Destruction of Penis, Percutaneous Endoscopic Approach
♂ 0V5SXZZ Destruction of Penis, External Approach
♂ 0V5T0ZZ Destruction of Prepuce, Open Approach
♂ 0V5T3ZZ Destruction of Prepuce, Percutaneous Approach
♂ 0V5T4ZZ Destruction of Prepuce, Percutaneous Endoscopic Approach
♂ 0V5TXZZ Destruction of Prepuce, External Approach

V7 – Male Reproductive System, Dilation

♂ 0V7N0DZ Dilation of Right Vas Deferens with Intraluminal Device, Open Approach
♂ 0V7N0ZZ Dilation of Right Vas Deferens, Open Approach
♂ 0V7N3DZ Dilation of Right Vas Deferens with Intraluminal Device, Percutaneous Approach
♂ 0V7N3ZZ Dilation of Right Vas Deferens, Percutaneous Approach
♂ 0V7N4DZ Dilation of Right Vas Deferens with Intraluminal Device, Percutaneous Endoscopic Approach
♂ 0V7N4ZZ Dilation of Right Vas Deferens, Percutaneous Endoscopic Approach

♂ 0V7P0DZ Dilation of Left Vas Deferens with Intraluminal Device, Open Approach
♂ 0V7P0ZZ Dilation of Left Vas Deferens, Open Approach
♂ 0V7P3DZ Dilation of Left Vas Deferens with Intraluminal Device, Percutaneous Approach
♂ 0V7P3ZZ Dilation of Left Vas Deferens, Percutaneous Approach
♂ 0V7P4DZ Dilation of Left Vas Deferens with Intraluminal Device, Percutaneous Endoscopic Approach
♂ 0V7P4ZZ Dilation of Left Vas Deferens, Percutaneous Endoscopic Approach

♂ 0V7Q0DZ Dilation of Bilateral Vas Deferens with Intraluminal Device, Open Approach
♂ 0V7Q0ZZ Dilation of Bilateral Vas Deferens, Open Approach
♂ 0V7Q3DZ Dilation of Bilateral Vas Deferens with Intraluminal Device, Percutaneous Approach
♂ 0V7Q3ZZ Dilation of Bilateral Vas Deferens, Percutaneous Approach
♂ 0V7Q4DZ Dilation of Bilateral Vas Deferens with Intraluminal Device, Percutaneous Endoscopic Approach
♂ 0V7Q4ZZ Dilation of Bilateral Vas Deferens, Percutaneous Endoscopic Approach

0V9 – Male Reproductive System, Drainage

Review Coding Guidelines B3.4a and B3.4b

Review Coding Guideline B6.2

♂ 0V9000Z Drainage of Prostate with Drainage Device, Open Approach
♂ 0V900ZX Drainage of Prostate, Open Approach, Diagnostic
♂ 0V900ZZ Drainage of Prostate, Open Approach
♂ 0V9030Z Drainage of Prostate with Drainage Device, Percutaneous Approach
♂ 0V903ZX Drainage of Prostate, Percutaneous Approach, Diagnostic

♂ 0V903ZZ Drainage of Prostate, Percutaneous Approach
♂ 0V9040Z Drainage of Prostate with Drainage Device, Percutaneous Endoscopic Approach
♂ 0V904ZX Drainage of Prostate, Percutaneous Endoscopic Approach, Diagnostic
♂ 0V904ZZ Drainage of Prostate, Percutaneous Endoscopic Approach

♂ 0V9070Z Drainage of Prostate with Drainage Device, Via Natural or Artificial Opening
♂ 0V907ZX Drainage of Prostate, Via Natural or Artificial Opening, Diagnostic
♂ 0V907ZZ Drainage of Prostate, Via Natural or Artificial Opening
♂ 0V9080Z Drainage of Prostate with Drainage Device, Via Natural or Artificial Opening Endoscopic

♀ Female-only   ♂ Male-only   ▲ Limited Coverage   ● Non-OR   ▬ HAC-associated procedure   ▲ Non-covered procedures   ✛ Combination

♂ **0V908ZX** Drainage of Prostate, Via Natural or Artificial Opening Endoscopic, Diagnostic

♂ **0V908ZZ** Drainage of Prostate, Via Natural or Artificial Opening Endoscopic

♂ **0V9100Z** Drainage of Right Seminal Vesicle with Drainage Device, Open Approach

♂ **0V910ZX** Drainage of Right Seminal Vesicle, Open Approach, Diagnostic

♂ **0V910ZZ** Drainage of Right Seminal Vesicle, Open Approach

♂ **0V9130Z** Drainage of Right Seminal Vesicle with Drainage Device, Percutaneous Approach

♂ **0V913ZX** Drainage of Right Seminal Vesicle, Percutaneous Approach, Diagnostic

♂ **0V913ZZ** Drainage of Right Seminal Vesicle, Percutaneous Approach

♂ **0V9140Z** Drainage of Right Seminal Vesicle with Drainage Device, Percutaneous Endoscopic Approach

♂ **0V914ZX** Drainage of Right Seminal Vesicle, Percutaneous Endoscopic Approach, Diagnostic

♂ **0V914ZZ** Drainage of Right Seminal Vesicle, Percutaneous Endoscopic Approach

♂ **0V9200Z** Drainage of Left Seminal Vesicle with Drainage Device, Open Approach

♂ **0V920ZX** Drainage of Left Seminal Vesicle, Open Approach, Diagnostic

♂ **0V920ZZ** Drainage of Left Seminal Vesicle, Open Approach

♂ **0V9230Z** Drainage of Left Seminal Vesicle with Drainage Device, Percutaneous Approach

♂ **0V923ZX** Drainage of Left Seminal Vesicle, Percutaneous Approach, Diagnostic

♂ **0V923ZZ** Drainage of Left Seminal Vesicle, Percutaneous Approach

♂ **0V9240Z** Drainage of Left Seminal Vesicle with Drainage Device, Percutaneous Endoscopic Approach

♂ **0V924ZX** Drainage of Left Seminal Vesicle, Percutaneous Endoscopic Approach, Diagnostic

♂ **0V924ZZ** Drainage of Left Seminal Vesicle, Percutaneous Endoscopic Approach

♂ **0V9300Z** Drainage of Bilateral Seminal Vesicles with Drainage Device, Open Approach

♂ **0V930ZX** Drainage of Bilateral Seminal Vesicles, Open Approach, Diagnostic

♂ **0V930ZZ** Drainage of Bilateral Seminal Vesicles, Open Approach

♂ **0V9330Z** Drainage of Bilateral Seminal Vesicles with Drainage Device, Percutaneous Approach

♂ **0V933ZX** Drainage of Bilateral Seminal Vesicles, Percutaneous Approach, Diagnostic

♂ **0V933ZZ** Drainage of Bilateral Seminal Vesicles, Percutaneous Approach

♂ **0V9340Z** Drainage of Bilateral Seminal Vesicles with Drainage Device, Percutaneous Endoscopic Approach

♂ **0V934ZX** Drainage of Bilateral Seminal Vesicles, Percutaneous Endoscopic Approach, Diagnostic

♂ **0V934ZZ** Drainage of Bilateral Seminal Vesicles, Percutaneous Endoscopic Approach

♂ **0V9500Z** Drainage of Scrotum with Drainage Device, Open Approach

♂ **0V950ZX** Drainage of Scrotum, Open Approach, Diagnostic

♂ **0V950ZZ** Drainage of Scrotum, Open Approach

♂ **0V9530Z** Drainage of Scrotum with Drainage Device, Percutaneous Approach

♂ **0V953ZX** Drainage of Scrotum, Percutaneous Approach, Diagnostic

♂ **0V953ZZ** Drainage of Scrotum, Percutaneous Approach

♂ **0V9540Z** Drainage of Scrotum with Drainage Device, Percutaneous Endoscopic Approach

♂ **0V954ZX** Drainage of Scrotum, Percutaneous Endoscopic Approach, Diagnostic

♂ **0V954ZZ** Drainage of Scrotum, Percutaneous Endoscopic Approach

♂ **0V95X0Z** Drainage of Scrotum with Drainage Device, External Approach

♂ **0V95XZX** Drainage of Scrotum, External Approach, Diagnostic

♂ **0V95XZZ** Drainage of Scrotum, External Approach

♂ **0V9600Z** Drainage of Right Tunica Vaginalis with Drainage Device, Open Approach

♂ **0V960ZX** Drainage of Right Tunica Vaginalis, Open Approach, Diagnostic

♂ **0V960ZZ** Drainage of Right Tunica Vaginalis, Open Approach

♂ **0V9630Z** Drainage of Right Tunica Vaginalis with Drainage Device, Percutaneous Approach

♂ **0V963ZX** Drainage of Right Tunica Vaginalis, Percutaneous Approach, Diagnostic

♂ **0V963ZZ** Drainage of Right Tunica Vaginalis, Percutaneous Approach

♂ **0V9640Z** Drainage of Right Tunica Vaginalis with Drainage Device, Percutaneous Endoscopic Approach

♂ **0V964ZX** Drainage of Right Tunica Vaginalis, Percutaneous Endoscopic Approach, Diagnostic

♂ **0V964ZZ** Drainage of Right Tunica Vaginalis, Percutaneous Endoscopic Approach

♂ **0V9700Z** Drainage of Left Tunica Vaginalis with Drainage Device, Open Approach

♂ **0V970ZX** Drainage of Left Tunica Vaginalis, Open Approach, Diagnostic

♂ **0V970ZZ** Drainage of Left Tunica Vaginalis, Open Approach

♂ **0V9730Z** Drainage of Left Tunica Vaginalis with Drainage Device, Percutaneous Approach

♂ **0V973ZX** Drainage of Left Tunica Vaginalis, Percutaneous Approach, Diagnostic

♂ **0V973ZZ** Drainage of Left Tunica Vaginalis, Percutaneous Approach

♂ **0V9740Z** Drainage of Left Tunica Vaginalis with Drainage Device, Percutaneous Endoscopic Approach

♂ **0V974ZX** Drainage of Left Tunica Vaginalis, Percutaneous Endoscopic Approach, Diagnostic

♂ **0V974ZZ** Drainage of Left Tunica Vaginalis, Percutaneous Endoscopic Approach

♂ **0V9900Z** Drainage of Right Testis with Drainage Device, Open Approach

♂ **0V990ZX** Drainage of Right Testis, Open Approach, Diagnostic

♂ **0V990ZZ** Drainage of Right Testis, Open Approach

♂ **0V9930Z** Drainage of Right Testis with Drainage Device, Percutaneous Approach

♂ **0V993ZX** Drainage of Right Testis, Percutaneous Approach, Diagnostic

♂ **0V993ZZ** Drainage of Right Testis, Percutaneous Approach

♂ **0V9940Z** Drainage of Right Testis with Drainage Device, Percutaneous Endoscopic Approach

♂ **0V994ZX** Drainage of Right Testis, Percutaneous Endoscopic Approach, Diagnostic

♂ **0V994ZZ** Drainage of Right Testis, Percutaneous Endoscopic Approach

♂ **0V9B00Z** Drainage of Left Testis with Drainage Device, Open Approach

♂ **0V9B0ZX** Drainage of Left Testis, Open Approach, Diagnostic

♂ **0V9B0ZZ** Drainage of Left Testis, Open Approach

♂ **0V9B30Z** Drainage of Left Testis with Drainage Device, Percutaneous Approach

♂ **0V9B3ZX** Drainage of Left Testis, Percutaneous Approach, Diagnostic

♂ **0V9B3ZZ** Drainage of Left Testis, Percutaneous Approach

♂ **0V9B40Z** Drainage of Left Testis with Drainage Device, Percutaneous Endoscopic Approach

♂ **0V9B4ZX** Drainage of Left Testis, Percutaneous Endoscopic Approach, Diagnostic

♂ **0V9B4ZZ** Drainage of Left Testis, Percutaneous Endoscopic Approach

♂ **0V9C00Z** Drainage of Bilateral Testes with Drainage Device, Open Approach

♂ **0V9C0ZX** Drainage of Bilateral Testes, Open Approach, Diagnostic

♂ **0V9C0ZZ** Drainage of Bilateral Testes, Open Approach

♂ **0V9C30Z** Drainage of Bilateral Testes with Drainage Device, Percutaneous Approach

♂ **0V9C3ZX** Drainage of Bilateral Testes, Percutaneous Approach, Diagnostic

♂ **0V9C3ZZ** Drainage of Bilateral Testes, Percutaneous Approach

♂ **0V9C40Z** Drainage of Bilateral Testes with Drainage Device, Percutaneous Endoscopic Approach

♂ **0V9C4ZX** Drainage of Bilateral Testes, Percutaneous Endoscopic Approach, Diagnostic

♂ **0V9C4ZZ** Drainage of Bilateral Testes, Percutaneous Endoscopic Approach

♂ **0V9F00Z** Drainage of Right Spermatic Cord with Drainage Device, Open Approach

♂ **0V9F0ZX** Drainage of Right Spermatic Cord, Open Approach, Diagnostic

♂ **0V9F0ZZ** Drainage of Right Spermatic Cord, Open Approach

♂ **0V9F30Z** Drainage of Right Spermatic Cord with Drainage Device, Percutaneous Approach

♂ **0V9F3ZX** Drainage of Right Spermatic Cord, Percutaneous Approach, Diagnostic

♂ **0V9F3ZZ** Drainage of Right Spermatic Cord, Percutaneous Approach

♂ **0V9F40Z** Drainage of Right Spermatic Cord with Drainage Device, Percutaneous Endoscopic Approach

♂ **0V9F4ZX** Drainage of Right Spermatic Cord, Percutaneous Endoscopic Approach, Diagnostic

♂ **0V9F4ZZ** Drainage of Right Spermatic Cord, Percutaneous Endoscopic Approach

♂ **0V9G00Z** Drainage of Left Spermatic Cord with Drainage Device, Open Approach

♂ **0V9G0ZX** Drainage of Left Spermatic Cord, Open Approach, Diagnostic

♂ **0V9G0ZZ** Drainage of Left Spermatic Cord, Open Approach

♂ **0V9G30Z** Drainage of Left Spermatic Cord with Drainage Device, Percutaneous Approach

♂ **0V9G3ZX** Drainage of Left Spermatic Cord, Percutaneous Approach, Diagnostic

♂ **0V9G3ZZ** Drainage of Left Spermatic Cord, Percutaneous Approach

♂ **0V9G40Z** Drainage of Left Spermatic Cord with Drainage Device, Percutaneous Endoscopic Approach

♂ **0V9G4ZX** Drainage of Left Spermatic Cord, Percutaneous Endoscopic Approach, Diagnostic

♂ **0V9G4ZZ** Drainage of Left Spermatic Cord, Percutaneous Endoscopic Approach

♂ **0V9H00Z** Drainage of Bilateral Spermatic Cords with Drainage Device, Open Approach

♂ **0V9H0ZX** Drainage of Bilateral Spermatic Cords, Open Approach, Diagnostic

♂ **0V9H0ZZ** Drainage of Bilateral Spermatic Cords, Open Approach

♀ Female-only   ♂ Male-only   ▲ Limited Coverage   ● Non-OR   ▰ HAC-associated procedure   ▲ Non-covered procedures   ✚ Combination

0V9H30Z Drainage of Bilateral Spermatic Cords with Drainage Device, Percutaneous Approach

♂ 0V9L0ZZ Drainage of Bilateral Epididymis, Open Approach

♂ 0V9Q0ZZ Drainage of Bilateral Vas Deferens, Open Approach

0V9H3ZX Drainage of Bilateral Spermatic Cords, Percutaneous Approach, Diagnostic

♂ 0V9L30Z Drainage of Bilateral Epididymis with Drainage Device, Percutaneous Approach

♂ 0V9Q30Z Drainage of Bilateral Vas Deferens with Drainage Device, Percutaneous Approach

0V9H3ZZ Drainage of Bilateral Spermatic Cords, Percutaneous Approach

♂ 0V9L3ZX Drainage of Bilateral Epididymis, Percutaneous Approach, Diagnostic

♂ 0V9Q3ZX Drainage of Bilateral Vas Deferens, Percutaneous Approach, Diagnostic

0V9H40Z Drainage of Bilateral Spermatic Cords with Drainage Device, Percutaneous Endoscopic Approach

♂ 0V9L3ZZ Drainage of Bilateral Epididymis, Percutaneous Approach

♂ 0V9Q3ZZ Drainage of Bilateral Vas Deferens, Percutaneous Approach

0V9H4ZX Drainage of Bilateral Spermatic Cords, Percutaneous Endoscopic Approach, Diagnostic

♂ 0V9L40Z Drainage of Bilateral Epididymis with Drainage Device, Percutaneous Endoscopic Approach

♂ 0V9Q40Z Drainage of Bilateral Vas Deferens with Drainage Device, Percutaneous Endoscopic Approach

0V9H4ZZ Drainage of Bilateral Spermatic Cords, Percutaneous Endoscopic Approach

♂ 0V9L4ZX Drainage of Bilateral Epididymis, Percutaneous Endoscopic Approach, Diagnostic

♂ 0V9Q4ZX Drainage of Bilateral Vas Deferens, Percutaneous Endoscopic Approach, Diagnostic

0V9J00Z Drainage of Right Epididymis with Drainage Device, Open Approach

♂ 0V9L4ZZ Drainage of Bilateral Epididymis, Percutaneous Endoscopic Approach

♂ 0V9Q4ZZ Drainage of Bilateral Vas Deferens, Percutaneous Endoscopic Approach

0V9J0ZX Drainage of Right Epididymis, Open Approach, Diagnostic

♂ 0V9N00Z Drainage of Right Vas Deferens with Drainage Device, Open Approach

♂ 0V9S00Z Drainage of Penis with Drainage Device, Open Approach

0V9J0ZZ Drainage of Right Epididymis, Open Approach

♂ 0V9N0ZX Drainage of Right Vas Deferens, Open Approach, Diagnostic

♂ 0V9S0ZX Drainage of Penis, Open Approach, Diagnostic

0V9J30Z Drainage of Right Epididymis with Drainage Device, Percutaneous Approach

♂ 0V9N0ZZ Drainage of Right Vas Deferens, Open Approach

♂ 0V9S0ZZ Drainage of Penis, Open Approach

0V9J3ZX Drainage of Right Epididymis, Percutaneous Approach, Diagnostic

♂ 0V9N30Z Drainage of Right Vas Deferens with Drainage Device, Percutaneous Approach

♂ 0V9S30Z Drainage of Penis with Drainage Device, Percutaneous Approach

0V9J3ZZ Drainage of Right Epididymis, Percutaneous Approach

♂ 0V9N3ZX Drainage of Right Vas Deferens, Percutaneous Approach, Diagnostic

♂ 0V9S3ZX Drainage of Penis, Percutaneous Approach, Diagnostic

0V9J40Z Drainage of Right Epididymis with Drainage Device, Percutaneous Endoscopic Approach

♂ 0V9N3ZZ Drainage of Right Vas Deferens, Percutaneous Approach

♂ 0V9S3ZZ Drainage of Penis, Percutaneous Approach

0V9J4ZX Drainage of Right Epididymis, Percutaneous Endoscopic Approach, Diagnostic

♂ 0V9N40Z Drainage of Right Vas Deferens with Drainage Device, Percutaneous Endoscopic Approach

♂ 0V9S40Z Drainage of Penis with Drainage Device, Percutaneous Endoscopic Approach

0V9J4ZZ Drainage of Right Epididymis, Percutaneous Endoscopic Approach

♂ 0V9N4ZX Drainage of Right Vas Deferens, Percutaneous Endoscopic Approach, Diagnostic

♂ 0V9S4ZX Drainage of Penis, Percutaneous Endoscopic Approach, Diagnostic

0V9K00Z Drainage of Left Epididymis with Drainage Device, Open Approach

♂ 0V9N4ZZ Drainage of Right Vas Deferens, Percutaneous Endoscopic Approach

♂ 0V9S4ZZ Drainage of Penis, Percutaneous Endoscopic Approach

0V9K0ZX Drainage of Left Epididymis, Open Approach, Diagnostic

♂ 0V9P00Z Drainage of Left Vas Deferens with Drainage Device, Open Approach

♂ 0V9SX0Z Drainage of Penis with Drainage Device, External Approach

0V9K0ZZ Drainage of Left Epididymis, Open Approach

♂ 0V9P0ZX Drainage of Left Vas Deferens, Open Approach, Diagnostic

♂ 0V9SXZX Drainage of Penis, External Approach, Diagnostic

0V9K30Z Drainage of Left Epididymis with Drainage Device, Percutaneous Approach

♂ 0V9P0ZZ Drainage of Left Vas Deferens, Open Approach

♂ 0V9SXZZ Drainage of Penis, External Approach

0V9K3ZX Drainage of Left Epididymis, Percutaneous Approach, Diagnostic

♂ 0V9P30Z Drainage of Left Vas Deferens with Drainage Device, Percutaneous Approach

♂ 0V9T00Z Drainage of Prepuce with Drainage Device, Open Approach

0V9K3ZZ Drainage of Left Epididymis, Percutaneous Approach

♂ 0V9P3ZX Drainage of Left Vas Deferens, Percutaneous Approach, Diagnostic

♂ 0V9T0ZX Drainage of Prepuce, Open Approach, Diagnostic

0V9K40Z Drainage of Left Epididymis with Drainage Device, Percutaneous Endoscopic Approach

♂ 0V9P3ZZ Drainage of Left Vas Deferens, Percutaneous Approach

♂ 0V9T0ZZ Drainage of Prepuce, Open Approach

0V9K4ZX Drainage of Left Epididymis, Percutaneous Endoscopic Approach, Diagnostic

♂ 0V9P40Z Drainage of Left Vas Deferens with Drainage Device, Percutaneous Endoscopic Approach

♂ 0V9T30Z Drainage of Prepuce with Drainage Device, Percutaneous Approach

0V9K4ZZ Drainage of Left Epididymis, Percutaneous Endoscopic Approach

♂ 0V9P4ZX Drainage of Left Vas Deferens, Percutaneous Endoscopic Approach, Diagnostic

♂ 0V9T3ZX Drainage of Prepuce, Percutaneous Approach, Diagnostic

0V9L00Z Drainage of Bilateral Epididymis with Drainage Device, Open Approach

♂ 0V9P4ZZ Drainage of Left Vas Deferens, Percutaneous Endoscopic Approach

♂ 0V9T3ZZ Drainage of Prepuce, Percutaneous Approach

0V9L0ZX Drainage of Bilateral Epididymis, Open Approach, Diagnostic

♂ 0V9Q00Z Drainage of Bilateral Vas Deferens with Drainage Device, Open Approach

♂ 0V9T40Z Drainage of Prepuce with Drainage Device, Percutaneous Endoscopic Approach

♂ 0V9Q0ZX Drainage of Bilateral Vas Deferens, Open Approach, Diagnostic

♂ 0V9T4ZX Drainage of Prepuce, Percutaneous Endoscopic Approach, Diagnostic

♂ 0V9T4ZZ Drainage of Prepuce, Percutaneous Endoscopic Approach

♂ 0V9TX0Z Drainage of Prepuce with Drainage Device, External Approach

♂ 0V9TXZX Drainage of Prepuce, External Approach, Diagnostic

♂ 0V9TXZZ Drainage of Prepuce, External Approach

0VB – Male Reproductive System, Excision

Review Coding Guidelines B3.4a and B3.4b

Review Coding Guideline B3.8

0VB00ZX Excision of Prostate, Open Approach, Diagnostic

♂ 0VB07ZX Excision of Prostate, Via Natural or Artificial Opening, Diagnostic

♂ 0VB10ZZ Excision of Right Seminal Vesicle, Open Approach

0VB00ZZ Excision of Prostate, Open Approach

♂ 0VB07ZZ Excision of Prostate, Via Natural or Artificial Opening

♂ 0VB13ZX Excision of Right Seminal Vesicle, Percutaneous Approach, Diagnostic

0VB03ZX Excision of Prostate, Percutaneous Approach, Diagnostic

♂ 0VB08ZX Excision of Prostate, Via Natural or Artificial Opening Endoscopic, Diagnostic

♂ 0VB13ZZ Excision of Right Seminal Vesicle, Percutaneous Approach

0VB03ZZ Excision of Prostate, Percutaneous Approach

♂ 0VB08ZZ Excision of Prostate, Via Natural or Artificial Opening Endoscopic

♂ 0VB14ZX Excision of Right Seminal Vesicle, Percutaneous Endoscopic Approach, Diagnostic

0VB04ZX Excision of Prostate, Percutaneous Endoscopic Approach, Diagnostic

♂ 0VB10ZX Excision of Right Seminal Vesicle, Open Approach, Diagnostic

♂ 0VB14ZZ Excision of Right Seminal Vesicle, Percutaneous Endoscopic Approach

0VB04ZZ Excision of Prostate, Percutaneous Endoscopic Approach

♀ Female-only   ♂ Male-only   ▲ Limited Coverage   ● Non-OR   ■ HAC-associated procedure   ▲ Non-covered procedures   ➕ Combination

♂ 0VB20ZX Excision of Left Seminal Vesicle, Open Approach, Diagnostic

♂ 0VB20ZZ Excision of Left Seminal Vesicle, Open Approach

♂ 0VB23ZX Excision of Left Seminal Vesicle, Percutaneous Approach, Diagnostic

♂ 0VB23ZZ Excision of Left Seminal Vesicle, Percutaneous Approach

♂ 0VB24ZX Excision of Left Seminal Vesicle, Percutaneous Endoscopic Approach, Diagnostic

♂ 0VB24ZZ Excision of Left Seminal Vesicle, Percutaneous Endoscopic Approach

♂ 0VB30ZX Excision of Bilateral Seminal Vesicles, Open Approach, Diagnostic

♂ 0VB30ZZ Excision of Bilateral Seminal Vesicles, Open Approach

♂ 0VB33ZX Excision of Bilateral Seminal Vesicles, Percutaneous Approach, Diagnostic

♂ 0VB33ZZ Excision of Bilateral Seminal Vesicles, Percutaneous Approach

♂ 0VB34ZX Excision of Bilateral Seminal Vesicles, Percutaneous Endoscopic Approach, Diagnostic

♂ 0VB34ZZ Excision of Bilateral Seminal Vesicles, Percutaneous Endoscopic Approach

♂ 0VB50ZX Excision of Scrotum, Open Approach, Diagnostic

♂ 0VB50ZZ Excision of Scrotum, Open Approach

♂ 0VB53ZX Excision of Scrotum, Percutaneous Approach, Diagnostic

♂ 0VB53ZZ Excision of Scrotum, Percutaneous Approach

♂ 0VB54ZX Excision of Scrotum, Percutaneous Endoscopic Approach, Diagnostic

♂ 0VB54ZZ Excision of Scrotum, Percutaneous Endoscopic Approach

♂ 0VB5XZX Excision of Scrotum, External Approach, Diagnostic

♂ 0VB5XZZ Excision of Scrotum, External Approach

♂ 0VB60ZX Excision of Right Tunica Vaginalis, Open Approach, Diagnostic

♂ 0VB60ZZ Excision of Right Tunica Vaginalis, Open Approach

♂ 0VB63ZX Excision of Right Tunica Vaginalis, Percutaneous Approach, Diagnostic

♂ 0VB63ZZ Excision of Right Tunica Vaginalis, Percutaneous Approach

♂ 0VB64ZX Excision of Right Tunica Vaginalis, Percutaneous Endoscopic Approach, Diagnostic

♂ 0VB64ZZ Excision of Right Tunica Vaginalis, Percutaneous Endoscopic Approach

♂ 0VB70ZX Excision of Left Tunica Vaginalis, Open Approach, Diagnostic

♂ 0VB70ZZ Excision of Left Tunica Vaginalis, Open Approach

♂ 0VB73ZX Excision of Left Tunica Vaginalis, Percutaneous Approach, Diagnostic

♂ 0VB73ZZ Excision of Left Tunica Vaginalis, Percutaneous Approach

♂ 0VB74ZX Excision of Left Tunica Vaginalis, Percutaneous Endoscopic Approach, Diagnostic

♂ 0VB74ZZ Excision of Left Tunica Vaginalis, Percutaneous Endoscopic Approach

♂ 0VB90ZX Excision of Right Testis, Open Approach, Diagnostic

♂ 0VB90ZZ Excision of Right Testis, Open Approach

♂ 0VB93ZX Excision of Right Testis, Percutaneous Approach, Diagnostic

♂ 0VB93ZZ Excision of Right Testis, Percutaneous Approach

♂ 0VB94ZX Excision of Right Testis, Percutaneous Endoscopic Approach, Diagnostic

♂ 0VB94ZZ Excision of Right Testis, Percutaneous Endoscopic Approach

♂ 0VBB0ZX Excision of Left Testis, Open Approach, Diagnostic

♂ 0VBB0ZZ Excision of Left Testis, Open Approach

♂ 0VBB3ZX Excision of Left Testis, Percutaneous Approach, Diagnostic

♂ 0VBB3ZZ Excision of Left Testis, Percutaneous Approach

♂ 0VBB4ZX Excision of Left Testis, Percutaneous Endoscopic Approach, Diagnostic

♂ 0VBB4ZZ Excision of Left Testis, Percutaneous Endoscopic Approach

♂ 0VBC0ZX Excision of Bilateral Testes, Open Approach, Diagnostic

♂ 0VBC0ZZ Excision of Bilateral Testes, Open Approach

♂ 0VBC3ZX Excision of Bilateral Testes, Percutaneous Approach, Diagnostic

♂ 0VBC3ZZ Excision of Bilateral Testes, Percutaneous Approach

♂ 0VBC4ZX Excision of Bilateral Testes, Percutaneous Endoscopic Approach, Diagnostic

♂ 0VBC4ZZ Excision of Bilateral Testes, Percutaneous Endoscopic Approach

♂ 0VBF0ZX Excision of Right Spermatic Cord, Open Approach, Diagnostic

♂ 0VBF0ZZ Excision of Right Spermatic Cord, Open Approach

♂ 0VBF3ZX Excision of Right Spermatic Cord, Percutaneous Approach, Diagnostic

♂ 0VBF3ZZ Excision of Right Spermatic Cord, Percutaneous Approach

♂ 0VBF4ZX Excision of Right Spermatic Cord, Percutaneous Endoscopic Approach, Diagnostic

♂ 0VBF4ZZ Excision of Right Spermatic Cord, Percutaneous Endoscopic Approach

♂ 0VBG0ZX Excision of Left Spermatic Cord, Open Approach, Diagnostic

♂ 0VBG0ZZ Excision of Left Spermatic Cord, Open Approach

♂ 0VBG3ZX Excision of Left Spermatic Cord, Percutaneous Approach, Diagnostic

♂ 0VBG3ZZ Excision of Left Spermatic Cord, Percutaneous Approach

♂ 0VBG4ZX Excision of Left Spermatic Cord, Percutaneous Endoscopic Approach, Diagnostic

♂ 0VBG4ZZ Excision of Left Spermatic Cord, Percutaneous Endoscopic Approach

♂ 0VBH0ZX Excision of Bilateral Spermatic Cords, Open Approach, vDiagnostic

♂ 0VBH0ZZ Excision of Bilateral Spermatic Cords, Open Approach

♂ 0VBH3ZX Excision of Bilateral Spermatic Cords, Percutaneous Approach, Diagnostic

♂ 0VBH3ZZ Excision of Bilateral Spermatic Cords, Percutaneous Approach

♂ 0VBH4ZX Excision of Bilateral Spermatic Cords, Percutaneous Endoscopic Approach, Diagnostic

♂ 0VBH4ZZ Excision of Bilateral Spermatic Cords, Percutaneous Endoscopic Approach

♂ 0VBJ0ZX Excision of Right Epididymis, Open Approach, Diagnostic

♂ 0VBJ0ZZ Excision of Right Epididymis, Open Approach

♂ 0VBJ3ZX Excision of Right Epididymis, Percutaneous Approach, Diagnostic

♂ 0VBJ3ZZ Excision of Right Epididymis, Percutaneous Approach

♂ 0VBJ4ZX Excision of Right Epididymis, Percutaneous Endoscopic Approach, Diagnostic

♂ 0VBJ4ZZ Excision of Right Epididymis, Percutaneous Endoscopic Approach

♂ 0VBK0ZX Excision of Left Epididymis, Open Approach, Diagnostic

♂ 0VBK0ZZ Excision of Left Epididymis, Open Approach

♂ 0VBK3ZX Excision of Left Epididymis, Percutaneous Approach, Diagnostic

♂ 0VBK3ZZ Excision of Left Epididymis, Percutaneous Approach

♂ 0VBK4ZX Excision of Left Epididymis, Percutaneous Endoscopic Approach, Diagnostic

♂ 0VBK4ZZ Excision of Left Epididymis, Percutaneous Endoscopic Approach

♂ 0VBL0ZX Excision of Bilateral Epididymis, Open Approach, Diagnostic

♂ 0VBL0ZZ Excision of Bilateral Epididymis, Open Approach

♂ 0VBL3ZX Excision of Bilateral Epididymis, Percutaneous Approach, Diagnostic

♂ 0VBL3ZZ Excision of Bilateral Epididymis, Percutaneous Approach

♂ 0VBL4ZX Excision of Bilateral Epididymis, Percutaneous Endoscopic Approach, Diagnostic

♂ 0VBL4ZZ Excision of Bilateral Epididymis, Percutaneous Endoscopic Approach

♂ 0VBN0ZX Excision of Right Vas Deferens, Open Approach, Diagnostic

♂ 0VBN0ZZ Excision of Right Vas Deferens, Open Approach
▲

♂ 0VBN3ZX Excision of Right Vas Deferens, Percutaneous Approach, Diagnostic

♂ 0VBN3ZZ Excision of Right Vas Deferens, Percutaneous Approach
▲

♂ 0VBN4ZX Excision of Right Vas Deferens, Percutaneous Endoscopic Approach, Diagnostic

♂ 0VBN4ZZ Excision of Right Vas Deferens, Percutaneous Endoscopic Approach
▲

♂ 0VBP0ZX Excision of Left Vas Deferens, Open Approach, Diagnostic

♂ 0VBP0ZZ Excision of Left Vas Deferens, Open Approach

♂ 0VBP3ZX Excision of Left Vas Deferens, Percutaneous Approach, Diagnostic

♂ 0VBP3ZZ Excision of Left Vas Deferens, Percutaneous Approach
▲

♂ 0VBP4ZX Excision of Left Vas Deferens, Percutaneous Endoscopic Approach, Diagnostic

♂ 0VBP4ZZ Excision of Left Vas Deferens, Percutaneous Endoscopic Approach
▲

♂ 0VBQ0ZX Excision of Bilateral Vas Deferens, Open Approach, Diagnostic

♂ 0VBQ0ZZ Excision of Bilateral Vas Deferens, Open Approach
▲

♂ 0VBQ3ZX Excision of Bilateral Vas Deferens, Percutaneous Approach, Diagnostic

♂ 0VBQ3ZZ Excision of Bilateral Vas Deferens, Percutaneous Approach
▲

♂ 0VBQ4ZX Excision of Bilateral Vas Deferens, Percutaneous Endoscopic Approach, Diagnostic

♂ 0VBQ4ZZ Excision of Bilateral Vas Deferens, Percutaneous Endoscopic Approach
▲

AHA CC: 4Q, 2014, 33-34

♂ 0VBS0ZX Excision of Penis, Open Approach, Diagnostic

♂ 0VBS0ZZ Excision of Penis, Open Approach

♂ 0VBS3ZX Excision of Penis, Percutaneous Approach, Diagnostic

♂ 0VBS3ZZ Excision of Penis, Percutaneous Approach

♂ 0VBS4ZX Excision of Penis, Percutaneous Endoscopic Approach, Diagnostic

♂ 0VBS4ZZ Excision of Penis, Percutaneous Endoscopic Approach

♂ 0VBSXZX Excision of Penis, External Approach, Diagnostic

♂ 0VBSXZZ Excision of Penis, External Approach

♂ 0VBT0ZX Excision of Prepuce, Open Approach, Diagnostic

BT0ZZ Excision of Prepuce, Open Approach
BT3ZX Excision of Prepuce, Percutaneous
Approach, Diagnostic
BT3ZZ Excision of Prepuce, Percutaneous
Approach

♂ 0VBT4ZX Excision of Prepuce, Percutaneous
Endoscopic Approach, Diagnostic
♂ 0VBT4ZZ Excision of Prepuce, Percutaneous
Endoscopic Approach

♂ 0VBTXZX Excision of Prepuce, External Approach,
Diagnostic
♂ 0VBTXZZ Excision of Prepuce, External Approach

C – Male Reproductive System, Extirpation

VC00ZZ Extirpation of Matter from Prostate, Open
Approach
VC03ZZ Extirpation of Matter from Prostate,
Percutaneous Approach
VC04ZZ Extirpation of Matter from Prostate,
Percutaneous Endoscopic Approach
VC07ZZ Extirpation of Matter from Prostate, Via
Natural or Artificial Opening
VC08ZZ Extirpation of Matter from Prostate, Via
Natural or Artificial Opening Endoscopic
VC10ZZ Extirpation of Matter from Right Seminal
Vesicle, Open Approach
VC13ZZ Extirpation of Matter from Right Seminal
Vesicle, Percutaneous Approach
VC14ZZ Extirpation of Matter from Right Seminal
Vesicle, Percutaneous Endoscopic
Approach
VC20ZZ Extirpation of Matter from Left Seminal
Vesicle, Open Approach
VC23ZZ Extirpation of Matter from Left Seminal
Vesicle, Percutaneous Approach
VC24ZZ Extirpation of Matter from Left Seminal
Vesicle, Percutaneous Endoscopic
Approach
VC30ZZ Extirpation of Matter from Bilateral
Seminal Vesicles, Open Approach
VC33ZZ Extirpation of Matter from Bilateral
Seminal Vesicles, Percutaneous Approach
VC34ZZ Extirpation of Matter from Bilateral
Seminal Vesicles, Percutaneous
Endoscopic Approach
VC50ZZ Extirpation of Matter from Scrotum,
Open Approach
VC53ZZ Extirpation of Matter from Scrotum,
Percutaneous Approach
VC54ZZ Extirpation of Matter from Scrotum,
Percutaneous Endoscopic Approach
VC5XZZ Extirpation of Matter from Scrotum,
External Approach
VC60ZZ Extirpation of Matter from Right Tunica
Vaginalis, Open Approach
VC63ZZ Extirpation of Matter from Right Tunica
Vaginalis, Percutaneous Approach
VC64ZZ Extirpation of Matter from Right Tunica
Vaginalis, Percutaneous Endoscopic
Approach
VC70ZZ Extirpation of Matter from Left Tunica
Vaginalis, Open Approach
VC73ZZ Extirpation of Matter from Left Tunica
Vaginalis, Percutaneous Approach

♂ 0VC74ZZ Extirpation of Matter from Left Tunica
Vaginalis, Percutaneous Endoscopic
Approach
♂ 0VC90ZZ Extirpation of Matter from Right Testis,
Open Approach
♂ 0VC93ZZ Extirpation of Matter from Right Testis,
Percutaneous Approach
♂ 0VC94ZZ Extirpation of Matter from Right Testis,
Percutaneous Endoscopic Approach
♂ 0VCB0ZZ Extirpation of Matter from Left Testis,
Open Approach
♂ 0VCB3ZZ Extirpation of Matter from Left Testis,
Percutaneous Approach
♂ 0VCB4ZZ Extirpation of Matter from Left Testis,
Percutaneous Endoscopic Approach
♂ 0VCC0ZZ Extirpation of Matter from Bilateral
Testes, Open Approach
♂ 0VCC3ZZ Extirpation of Matter from Bilateral
Testes, Percutaneous Approach
♂ 0VCC4ZZ Extirpation of Matter from Bilateral Testes,
Percutaneous Endoscopic Approach
♂ 0VCF0ZZ Extirpation of Matter from Right
Spermatic Cord, Open Approach
♂ 0VCF3ZZ Extirpation of Matter from Right
Spermatic Cord, Percutaneous Approach
♂ 0VCF4ZZ Extirpation of Matter from Right
Spermatic Cord, Percutaneous
Endoscopic Approach
♂ 0VCG0ZZ Extirpation of Matter from Left Spermatic
Cord, Open Approach
♂ 0VCG3ZZ Extirpation of Matter from Left Spermatic
Cord, Percutaneous Approach
♂ 0VCG4ZZ Extirpation of Matter from Left Spermatic
Cord, Percutaneous Endoscopic Approach
♂ 0VCH0ZZ Extirpation of Matter from Bilateral
Spermatic Cords, Open Approach
♂ 0VCH3ZZ Extirpation of Matter from Bilateral
Spermatic Cords, Percutaneous Approach
♂ 0VCH4ZZ Extirpation of Matter from Bilateral
Spermatic Cords, Percutaneous
Endoscopic Approach
♂ 0VCJ0ZZ Extirpation of Matter from Right
Epididymis, Open Approach
♂ 0VCJ3ZZ Extirpation of Matter from Right
Epididymis, Percutaneous Approach
♂ 0VCJ4ZZ Extirpation of Matter from Right
Epididymis, Percutaneous Endoscopic
Approach
♂ 0VCK0ZZ Extirpation of Matter from Left
Epididymis, Open Approach

♂ 0VCK3ZZ Extirpation of Matter from Left
Epididymis, Percutaneous Approach
♂ 0VCK4ZZ Extirpation of Matter from Left
Epididymis, Percutaneous Endoscopic
Approach
♂ 0VCL0ZZ Extirpation of Matter from Bilateral
Epididymis, Open Approach
♂ 0VCL3ZZ Extirpation of Matter from Bilateral
Epididymis, Percutaneous Approach
♂ 0VCL4ZZ Extirpation of Matter from Bilateral
Epididymis, Percutaneous Endoscopic
Approach
♂ 0VCN0ZZ Extirpation of Matter from Right Vas
Deferens, Open Approach
♂ 0VCN3ZZ Extirpation of Matter from Right Vas
Deferens, Percutaneous Approach
♂ 0VCN4ZZ Extirpation of Matter from Right Vas
Deferens, Percutaneous Endoscopic
Approach
♂ 0VCP0ZZ Extirpation of Matter from Left Vas
Deferens, Open Approach
♂ 0VCP3ZZ Extirpation of Matter from Left Vas
Deferens, Percutaneous Approach
♂ 0VCP4ZZ Extirpation of Matter from Left Vas
Deferens, Percutaneous Endoscopic
Approach
♂ 0VCQ0ZZ Extirpation of Matter from Bilateral Vas
Deferens, Open Approach
♂ 0VCQ3ZZ Extirpation of Matter from Bilateral Vas
Deferens, Percutaneous Approach
♂ 0VCQ4ZZ Extirpation of Matter from Bilateral
Vas Deferens, Percutaneous Endoscopic
Approach
♂ 0VCS0ZZ Extirpation of Matter from Penis, Open
Approach
♂ 0VCS3ZZ Extirpation of Matter from Penis,
Percutaneous Approach
♂ 0VCS4ZZ Extirpation of Matter from Penis,
Percutaneous Endoscopic Approach
♂ 0VCSXZZ Extirpation of Matter from Penis, External
Approach
♂ 0VCT0ZZ Extirpation of Matter from Prepuce, Open
Approach
♂ 0VCT3ZZ Extirpation of Matter from Prepuce,
Percutaneous Approach
♂ 0VCT4ZZ Extirpation of Matter from Prepuce,
Percutaneous Endoscopic Approach
♂ 0VCTXZZ Extirpation of Matter from Prepuce,
External Approach

VH – Male Reproductive System, Insertion

0VH001Z Insertion of Radioactive Element into
Prostate, Open Approach
0VH031Z Insertion of Radioactive Element into
Prostate, Percutaneous Approach
0VH041Z Insertion of Radioactive Element into
Prostate, Percutaneous Endoscopic
Approach
0VH071Z Insertion of Radioactive Element into
Prostate, Via Natural or Artificial Opening
0VH081Z Insertion of Radioactive Element into
Prostate, Via Natural or Artificial Opening
Endoscopic
0VH403Z Insertion of Infusion Device into Prostate
and Seminal Vesicles, Open Approach
0VH433Z Insertion of Infusion Device into Prostate
and Seminal Vesicles, Percutaneous
Approach

♂ 0VH443Z Insertion of Infusion Device into Prostate
and Seminal Vesicles, Percutaneous
Endoscopic Approach
♂ 0VH473Z Insertion of Infusion Device into Prostate
and Seminal Vesicles, Via Natural or
Artificial Opening
♂ 0VH483Z Insertion of Infusion Device into Prostate
and Seminal Vesicles, Via Natural or
Artificial Opening Endoscopic
♂ 0VH803Z Insertion of Infusion Device into Scrotum
and Tunica Vaginalis, Open Approach
♂ 0VH833Z Insertion of Infusion Device into Scrotum
and Tunica Vaginalis, Percutaneous
Approach
♂ 0VH843Z Insertion of Infusion Device into Scrotum
and Tunica Vaginalis, Percutaneous
Endoscopic Approach

♂ 0VH873Z Insertion of Infusion Device into Scrotum
and Tunica Vaginalis, Via Natural or
Artificial Opening
♂ 0VH883Z Insertion of Infusion Device into Scrotum
and Tunica Vaginalis, Via Natural or
Artificial Opening Endoscopic
♂ 0VHD03Z Insertion of Infusion Device into Testis,
Open Approach
♂ 0VHD33Z Insertion of Infusion Device into Testis,
Percutaneous Approach
♂ 0VHD43Z Insertion of Infusion Device into Testis,
Percutaneous Endoscopic Approach
♂ 0VHD73Z Insertion of Infusion Device into Testis,
Via Natural or Artificial Opening
♂ 0VHD83Z Insertion of Infusion Device into Testis,
Via Natural or Artificial Opening
Endoscopic

1095

♀ Female-only   ♂ Male-only   ▲ Limited Coverage   ● Non-OR   ▨ HAC-associated procedure   ▲ Non-covered procedures   ✚ Combination

♂ **0VHM03Z** Insertion of Infusion Device into Epididymis and Spermatic Cord, Open Approach

♂ **0VHM33Z** Insertion of Infusion Device into Epididymis and Spermatic Cord, Percutaneous Approach

♂ **0VHM43Z** Insertion of Infusion Device into Epididymis and Spermatic Cord, Percutaneous Endoscopic Approach

♂ **0VHM73Z** Insertion of Infusion Device into Epididymis and Spermatic Cord, Via Natural or Artificial Opening

♂ **0VHM83Z** Insertion of Infusion Device into Epididymis and Spermatic Cord, Via Natural or Artificial Opening Endoscopic

♂ **0VHR03Z** Insertion of Infusion Device into Vas Deferens, Open Approach

♂ **0VHR33Z** Insertion of Infusion Device into Vas Deferens, Percutaneous Approach

♂ **0VHR43Z** Insertion of Infusion Device into Vas Deferens, Percutaneous Endoscopic Approach

♂ **0VHR73Z** Insertion of Infusion Device into Vas Deferens, Via Natural or Artificial Opening

♂ **0VHR83Z** Insertion of Infusion Device into Vas Deferens, Via Natural or Artificial Opening Endoscopic

♂ **0VHS03Z** Insertion of Infusion Device into Penis Open Approach

♂ **0VHS33Z** Insertion of Infusion Device into Penis, Percutaneous Approach

♂ **0VHS43Z** Insertion of Infusion Device into Penis, Percutaneous Endoscopic Approach

♂ **0VHSX3Z** Insertion of Infusion Device into Penis, External Approach

0VJ – Male Reproductive System, Inspection

Review Coding Guidelines B3.11a, B3.11b and B3.11c

♂ **0VJ40ZZ** Inspection of Prostate and Seminal Vesicles, Open Approach

♂ **0VJ43ZZ** Inspection of Prostate and Seminal Vesicles, Percutaneous Approach

♂ **0VJ44ZZ** Inspection of Prostate and Seminal Vesicles, Percutaneous Endoscopic Approach

♂ **0VJ4XZZ** Inspection of Prostate and Seminal Vesicles, External Approach

♂ **0VJ80ZZ** Inspection of Scrotum and Tunica Vaginalis, Open Approach

♂ **0VJ83ZZ** Inspection of Scrotum and Tunica Vaginalis, Percutaneous Approach

♂ **0VJ84ZZ** Inspection of Scrotum and Tunica Vaginalis, Percutaneous Endoscopic Approach

♂ **0VJ8XZZ** Inspection of Scrotum and Tunica Vaginalis, External Approach

♂ **0VJD0ZZ** Inspection of Testis, Open Approach

♂ **0VJD3ZZ** Inspection of Testis, Percutaneous Approach

♂ **0VJD4ZZ** Inspection of Testis, Percutaneous Endoscopic Approach

♂ **0VJDXZZ** Inspection of Testis, External Approach

♂ **0VJM0ZZ** Inspection of Epididymis and Spermatic Cord, Open Approach

♂ **0VJM3ZZ** Inspection of Epididymis and Spermatic Cord, Percutaneous Approach

♂ **0VJM4ZZ** Inspection of Epididymis and Spermatic Cord, Percutaneous Endoscopic Approach

♂ **0VJMXZZ** Inspection of Epididymis and Spermatic Cord, External Approach

♂ **0VJR0ZZ** Inspection of Vas Deferens, Open Approach

♂ **0VJR3ZZ** Inspection of Vas Deferens, Percutaneous Approach

♂ **0VJR4ZZ** Inspection of Vas Deferens, Percutaneous Endoscopic Approach

♂ **0VJRXZZ** Inspection of Vas Deferens, External Approach

♂ **0VJS0ZZ** Inspection of Penis, Open Approach

♂ **0VJS3ZZ** Inspection of Penis, Percutaneous Approach

♂ **0VJS4ZZ** Inspection of Penis, Percutaneous Endoscopic Approach

♂ **0VJSXZZ** Inspection of Penis, External Approach

0VL – Male Reproductive System, Occlusion

♂ **0VLF0CZ** Occlusion of Right Spermatic Cord with Extraluminal Device, Open Approach

♂ **0VLF0DZ** Occlusion of Right Spermatic Cord with Intraluminal Device, Open Approach

♂ **0VLF0ZZ** Occlusion of Right Spermatic Cord, Open Approach

♂ **0VLF3CZ** Occlusion of Right Spermatic Cord with Extraluminal Device, Percutaneous Approach

♂ **0VLF3DZ** Occlusion of Right Spermatic Cord with Intraluminal Device, Percutaneous Approach

♂ **0VLF3ZZ** Occlusion of Right Spermatic Cord, Percutaneous Approach

♂ **0VLF4CZ** Occlusion of Right Spermatic Cord with Extraluminal Device, Percutaneous Endoscopic Approach

♂ **0VLF4DZ** Occlusion of Right Spermatic Cord with Intraluminal Device, Percutaneous Endoscopic Approach

♂ **0VLF4ZZ** Occlusion of Right Spermatic Cord, Percutaneous Endoscopic Approach

♂ **0VLG0CZ** Occlusion of Left Spermatic Cord with Extraluminal Device, Open Approach

♂ **0VLG0DZ** Occlusion of Left Spermatic Cord with Intraluminal Device, Open Approach

♂ **0VLG0ZZ** Occlusion of Left Spermatic Cord, Open Approach

♂ **0VLG3CZ** Occlusion of Left Spermatic Cord with Extraluminal Device, Percutaneous Approach

♂ **0VLG3DZ** Occlusion of Left Spermatic Cord with Intraluminal Device, Percutaneous Approach

♂ **0VLG3ZZ** Occlusion of Left Spermatic Cord, Percutaneous Approach

♂ **0VLG4CZ** Occlusion of Left Spermatic Cord with Extraluminal Device, Percutaneous Endoscopic Approach

♂ **0VLG4DZ** Occlusion of Left Spermatic Cord with Intraluminal Device, Percutaneous Endoscopic Approach

♂ **0VLG4ZZ** Occlusion of Left Spermatic Cord, Percutaneous Endoscopic Approach

♂ **0VLH0CZ** Occlusion of Bilateral Spermatic Cords with Extraluminal Device, Open Approach

♂ **0VLH0DZ** Occlusion of Bilateral Spermatic Cords with Intraluminal Device, Open Approach

♂ **0VLH0ZZ** Occlusion of Bilateral Spermatic Cords, Open Approach

♂ **0VLH3CZ** Occlusion of Bilateral Spermatic Cords with Extraluminal Device, Percutaneous Approach

♂ **0VLH3DZ** Occlusion of Bilateral Spermatic Cords with Intraluminal Device, Percutaneous Approach

♂ **0VLH3ZZ** Occlusion of Bilateral Spermatic Cords, Percutaneous Approach

♂ **0VLH4CZ** Occlusion of Bilateral Spermatic Cords with Extraluminal Device, Percutaneous Endoscopic Approach

♂ **0VLH4DZ** Occlusion of Bilateral Spermatic Cords with Intraluminal Device, Percutaneous Endoscopic Approach

♂ **0VLH4ZZ** Occlusion of Bilateral Spermatic Cords, Percutaneous Endoscopic Approach

♂ **0VLN0CZ** Occlusion of Right Vas Deferens with Extraluminal Device, Open Approach

♂ **0VLN0DZ** Occlusion of Right Vas Deferens with Intraluminal Device, Open Approach

♂ **0VLN0ZZ** Occlusion of Right Vas Deferens, Open Approach

♂ **0VLN3CZ** Occlusion of Right Vas Deferens with Extraluminal Device, Percutaneous Approach

♂ **0VLN3DZ** Occlusion of Right Vas Deferens with Intraluminal Device, Percutaneous Approach

♂ **0VLN3ZZ** Occlusion of Right Vas Deferens, Percutaneous Approach

♂ **0VLN4CZ** Occlusion of Right Vas Deferens with Extraluminal Device, Percutaneous Endoscopic Approach

♂ **0VLN4DZ** Occlusion of Right Vas Deferens with Intraluminal Device, Percutaneous Endoscopic Approach

♂ **0VLN4ZZ** Occlusion of Right Vas Deferens, Percutaneous Endoscopic Approach

♂ **0VLP0CZ** Occlusion of Left Vas Deferens with Extraluminal Device, Open Approach

♂ **0VLP0DZ** Occlusion of Left Vas Deferens with Intraluminal Device, Open Approach

♂ **0VLP0ZZ** Occlusion of Left Vas Deferens, Open Approach

♂ **0VLP3CZ** Occlusion of Left Vas Deferens with Extraluminal Device, Percutaneous Approach

♂ **0VLP3DZ** Occlusion of Left Vas Deferens with Intraluminal Device, Percutaneous Approach

♂ **0VLP3ZZ** Occlusion of Left Vas Deferens, Percutaneous Approach

♂ **0VLP4CZ** Occlusion of Left Vas Deferens with Extraluminal Device, Percutaneous Endoscopic Approach

♂ **0VLP4DZ** Occlusion of Left Vas Deferens with Intraluminal Device, Percutaneous Endoscopic Approach

♂ **0VLP4ZZ** Occlusion of Left Vas Deferens, Percutaneous Endoscopic Approach

♂ **0VLQ0CZ** Occlusion of Bilateral Vas Deferens with Extraluminal Device, Open Approach

♂ **0VLQ0DZ** Occlusion of Bilateral Vas Deferens with Intraluminal Device, Open Approach

♂ **0VLQ0ZZ** Occlusion of Bilateral Vas Deferens, Open Approach

♂ **0VLQ3CZ** Occlusion of Bilateral Vas Deferens with Extraluminal Device, Percutaneous Approach

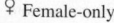

LQ3DZ Occlusion of Bilateral Vas Deferens with Intraluminal Device, Percutaneous Approach

♂ 0VLQ4CZ Occlusion of Bilateral Vas Deferens with Extraluminal Device, Percutaneous Endoscopic Approach ▲

♂ 0VLQ4DZ Occlusion of Bilateral Vas Deferens with Intraluminal Device, Percutaneous Endoscopic Approach

LQ3ZZ Occlusion of Bilateral Vas Deferens, Percutaneous Approach

♂ 0VLQ4ZZ Occlusion of Bilateral Vas Deferens, Percutaneous Endoscopic Approach ▲

M – Male Reproductive System, Reattachment

M5XZZ Reattachment of Scrotum, External Approach

♂ 0VM94ZZ Reattachment of Right Testis, Percutaneous Endoscopic Approach

♂ 0VMF4ZZ Reattachment of Right Spermatic Cord, Percutaneous Endoscopic Approach

M60ZZ Reattachment of Right Tunica Vaginalis, Open Approach

♂ 0VMB0ZZ Reattachment of Left Testis, Open Approach

♂ 0VMG0ZZ Reattachment of Left Spermatic Cord, Open Approach

M64ZZ Reattachment of Right Tunica Vaginalis, Percutaneous Endoscopic Approach

♂ 0VMB4ZZ Reattachment of Left Testis, Percutaneous Endoscopic Approach

♂ 0VMG4ZZ Reattachment of Left Spermatic Cord, Percutaneous Endoscopic Approach

M70ZZ Reattachment of Left Tunica Vaginalis, Open Approach

♂ 0VMC0ZZ Reattachment of Bilateral Testes, Open Approach

♂ 0VMH0ZZ Reattachment of Bilateral Spermatic Cords, Open Approach

M74ZZ Reattachment of Left Tunica Vaginalis, Percutaneous Endoscopic Approach

♂ 0VMC4ZZ Reattachment of Bilateral Testes, Percutaneous Endoscopic Approach

♂ 0VMH4ZZ Reattachment of Bilateral Spermatic Cords, Percutaneous Endoscopic Approach

M90ZZ Reattachment of Right Testis, Open Approach

♂ 0VMF0ZZ Reattachment of Right Spermatic Cord, Open Approach

♂ 0VMSXZZ Reattachment of Penis, External Approach

N – Male Reproductive System, Release

Review Coding Guideline B3.13

VN00ZZ Release Prostate, Open Approach

♂ 0VN74ZZ Release Left Tunica Vaginalis, Percutaneous Endoscopic Approach

♂ 0VNK3ZZ Release Left Epididymis, Percutaneous Approach

VN03ZZ Release Prostate, Percutaneous Approach

♂ 0VN90ZZ Release Right Testis, Open Approach

♂ 0VNK4ZZ Release Left Epididymis, Percutaneous Endoscopic Approach

VN04ZZ Release Prostate, Percutaneous Endoscopic Approach

♂ 0VN93ZZ Release Right Testis, Percutaneous Approach

♂ 0VNL0ZZ Release Bilateral Epididymis, Open Approach

VN07ZZ Release Prostate, Via Natural or Artificial Opening

♂ 0VN94ZZ Release Right Testis, Percutaneous Endoscopic Approach

♂ 0VNL3ZZ Release Bilateral Epididymis, Percutaneous Approach

VN08ZZ Release Prostate, Via Natural or Artificial Opening Endoscopic

♂ 0VNB0ZZ Release Left Testis, Open Approach

♂ 0VNL4ZZ Release Bilateral Epididymis, Percutaneous Endoscopic Approach

VN10ZZ Release Right Seminal Vesicle, Open Approach

♂ 0VNB3ZZ Release Left Testis, Percutaneous Approach

♂ 0VNN0ZZ Release Right Vas Deferens, Open Approach

VN13ZZ Release Right Seminal Vesicle, Percutaneous Approach

♂ 0VNB4ZZ Release Left Testis, Percutaneous Endoscopic Approach

♂ 0VNN3ZZ Release Right Vas Deferens, Percutaneous Approach

VN14ZZ Release Right Seminal Vesicle, Percutaneous Endoscopic Approach

♂ 0VNC0ZZ Release Bilateral Testes, Open Approach

♂ 0VNN4ZZ Release Right Vas Deferens, Percutaneous Endoscopic Approach

VN20ZZ Release Left Seminal Vesicle, Open Approach

♂ 0VNC3ZZ Release Bilateral Testes, Percutaneous Approach

♂ 0VNP0ZZ Release Left Vas Deferens, Open Approach

VN23ZZ Release Left Seminal Vesicle, Percutaneous Approach

♂ 0VNC4ZZ Release Bilateral Testes, Percutaneous Endoscopic Approach

♂ 0VNP3ZZ Release Left Vas Deferens, Percutaneous Approach

VN24ZZ Release Left Seminal Vesicle, Percutaneous Endoscopic Approach

♂ 0VNF0ZZ Release Right Spermatic Cord, Open Approach

♂ 0VNP4ZZ Release Left Vas Deferens, Percutaneous Endoscopic Approach

VN30ZZ Release Bilateral Seminal Vesicles, Open Approach

♂ 0VNF3ZZ Release Right Spermatic Cord, Percutaneous Approach

♂ 0VNQ0ZZ Release Bilateral Vas Deferens, Open Approach

VN33ZZ Release Bilateral Seminal Vesicles, Percutaneous Approach

♂ 0VNF4ZZ Release Right Spermatic Cord, Percutaneous Endoscopic Approach

♂ 0VNQ3ZZ Release Bilateral Vas Deferens, Percutaneous Approach

VN34ZZ Release Bilateral Seminal Vesicles, Percutaneous Endoscopic Approach

♂ 0VNG0ZZ Release Left Spermatic Cord, Open Approach

♂ 0VNQ4ZZ Release Bilateral Vas Deferens, Percutaneous Endoscopic Approach

VN50ZZ Release Scrotum, Open Approach

♂ 0VNG3ZZ Release Left Spermatic Cord, Percutaneous Approach

♂ 0VNS0ZZ Release Penis, Open Approach

VN53ZZ Release Scrotum, Percutaneous Approach

♂ 0VNG4ZZ Release Left Spermatic Cord, Percutaneous Endoscopic Approach

♂ 0VNS3ZZ Release Penis, Percutaneous Approach

VN54ZZ Release Scrotum, Percutaneous Endoscopic Approach

♂ 0VNH0ZZ Release Bilateral Spermatic Cords, Open Approach

♂ 0VNS4ZZ Release Penis, Percutaneous Endoscopic Approach

VN5XZZ Release Scrotum, External Approach

♂ 0VNH3ZZ Release Bilateral Spermatic Cords, Percutaneous Approach

♂ 0VNSXZZ Release Penis, External Approach

VN60ZZ Release Right Tunica Vaginalis, Open Approach

♂ 0VNH4ZZ Release Bilateral Spermatic Cords, Percutaneous Endoscopic Approach

♂ 0VNT0ZZ Release Prepuce, Open Approach

VN63ZZ Release Right Tunica Vaginalis, Percutaneous Approach

♂ 0VNJ0ZZ Release Right Epididymis, Open Approach

♂ 0VNT3ZZ Release Prepuce, Percutaneous Approach

VN64ZZ Release Right Tunica Vaginalis, Percutaneous Endoscopic Approach

♂ 0VNJ3ZZ Release Right Epididymis, Percutaneous Approach

♂ 0VNT4ZZ Release Prepuce, Percutaneous Endoscopic Approach

VN70ZZ Release Left Tunica Vaginalis, Open Approach

♂ 0VNJ4ZZ Release Right Epididymis, Percutaneous Endoscopic Approach

♂ 0VNTXZZ Release Prepuce, External Approach

VN73ZZ Release Left Tunica Vaginalis, Percutaneous Approach

♂ 0VNK0ZZ Release Left Epididymis, Open Approach

VP – Male Reproductive System, Removal

Review Coding Guideline B6.1c

0VP400Z Removal of Drainage Device from Prostate and Seminal Vesicles, Open Approach

♂ 0VP403Z Removal of Infusion Device from Prostate and Seminal Vesicles, Open Approach

♂ 0VP40JZ Removal of Synthetic Substitute from Prostate and Seminal Vesicles, Open Approach

0VP401Z Removal of Radioactive Element from Prostate and Seminal Vesicles, Open Approach

♂ 0VP407Z Removal of Autologous Tissue Substitute from Prostate and Seminal Vesicles, Open Approach

Female-only ♂ Male-only ▲ Limited Coverage ● Non-OR ▥ HAC-associated procedure ▲ Non-covered procedures ✚ Combination

♂ **0VP40KZ** Removal of Nonautologous Tissue Substitute from Prostate and Seminal Vesicles, Open Approach

♂ **0VP430Z** Removal of Drainage Device from Prostate and Seminal Vesicles, Percutaneous Approach

♂ **0VP431Z** Removal of Radioactive Element from Prostate and Seminal Vesicles, Percutaneous Approach

♂ **0VP433Z** Removal of Infusion Device from Prostate and Seminal Vesicles, Percutaneous Approach

♂ **0VP437Z** Removal of Autologous Tissue Substitute from Prostate and Seminal Vesicles, Percutaneous Approach

♂ **0VP43JZ** Removal of Synthetic Substitute from Prostate and Seminal Vesicles, Percutaneous Approach

♂ **0VP43KZ** Removal of Nonautologous Tissue Substitute from Prostate and Seminal Vesicles, Percutaneous Approach

♂ **0VP440Z** Removal of Drainage Device from Prostate and Seminal Vesicles, Percutaneous Endoscopic Approach

♂ **0VP441Z** Removal of Radioactive Element from Prostate and Seminal Vesicles, Percutaneous Endoscopic Approach

♂ **0VP443Z** Removal of Infusion Device from Prostate and Seminal Vesicles, Percutaneous Endoscopic Approach

♂ **0VP447Z** Removal of Autologous Tissue Substitute from Prostate and Seminal Vesicles, Percutaneous Endoscopic Approach

♂ **0VP44JZ** Removal of Synthetic Substitute from Prostate and Seminal Vesicles, Percutaneous Endoscopic Approach

♂ **0VP44KZ** Removal of Nonautologous Tissue Substitute from Prostate and Seminal Vesicles, Percutaneous Endoscopic Approach

♂ **0VP470Z** Removal of Drainage Device from Prostate and Seminal Vesicles, Via Natural or Artificial Opening

♂ **0VP471Z** Removal of Radioactive Element from Prostate and Seminal Vesicles, Via Natural or Artificial Opening

♂ **0VP473Z** Removal of Infusion Device from Prostate and Seminal Vesicles, Via Natural or Artificial Opening

♂ **0VP477Z** Removal of Autologous Tissue Substitute from Prostate and Seminal Vesicles, Via Natural or Artificial Opening

♂ **0VP47JZ** Removal of Synthetic Substitute from Prostate and Seminal Vesicles, Via Natural or Artificial Opening

♂ **0VP47KZ** Removal of Nonautologous Tissue Substitute from Prostate and Seminal Vesicles, Via Natural or Artificial Opening

♂ **0VP480Z** Removal of Drainage Device from Prostate and Seminal Vesicles, Via Natural or Artificial Opening Endoscopic

♂ **0VP481Z** Removal of Radioactive Element from Prostate and Seminal Vesicles, Via Natural or Artificial Opening Endoscopic

♂ **0VP483Z** Removal of Infusion Device from Prostate and Seminal Vesicles, Via Natural or Artificial Opening Endoscopic

♂ **0VP487Z** Removal of Autologous Tissue Substitute from Prostate and Seminal Vesicles, Via Natural or Artificial Opening Endoscopic

♂ **0VP48JZ** Removal of Synthetic Substitute from Prostate and Seminal Vesicles, Via Natural or Artificial Opening Endoscopic

♂ **0VP48KZ** Removal of Nonautologous Tissue Substitute from Prostate and Seminal Vesicles, Via Natural or Artificial Opening Endoscopic

♂ **0VP4X0Z** Removal of Drainage Device from Prostate and Seminal Vesicles, External Approach

♂ **0VP4X1Z** Removal of Radioactive Element from Prostate and Seminal Vesicles, External Approach

♂ **0VP4X3Z** Removal of Infusion Device from Prostate and Seminal Vesicles, External Approach

♂ **0VP800Z** Removal of Drainage Device from Scrotum and Tunica Vaginalis, Open Approach

♂ **0VP803Z** Removal of Infusion Device from Scrotum and Tunica Vaginalis, Open Approach

♂ **0VP807Z** Removal of Autologous Tissue Substitute from Scrotum and Tunica Vaginalis, Open Approach

♂ **0VP80JZ** Removal of Synthetic Substitute from Scrotum and Tunica Vaginalis, Open Approach

♂ **0VP80KZ** Removal of Nonautologous Tissue Substitute from Scrotum and Tunica Vaginalis, Open Approach

♂ **0VP830Z** Removal of Drainage Device from Scrotum and Tunica Vaginalis, Percutaneous Approach

♂ **0VP833Z** Removal of Infusion Device from Scrotum and Tunica Vaginalis, Percutaneous Approach

♂ **0VP837Z** Removal of Autologous Tissue Substitute from Scrotum and Tunica Vaginalis, Percutaneous Approach

♂ **0VP83JZ** Removal of Synthetic Substitute from Scrotum and Tunica Vaginalis, Percutaneous Approach

♂ **0VP83KZ** Removal of Nonautologous Tissue Substitute from Scrotum and Tunica Vaginalis, Percutaneous Approach

♂ **0VP840Z** Removal of Drainage Device from Scrotum and Tunica Vaginalis, Percutaneous Endoscopic Approach

♂ **0VP843Z** Removal of Infusion Device from Scrotum and Tunica Vaginalis, Percutaneous Endoscopic Approach

♂ **0VP847Z** Removal of Autologous Tissue Substitute from Scrotum and Tunica Vaginalis, Percutaneous Endoscopic Approach

♂ **0VP84JZ** Removal of Synthetic Substitute from Scrotum and Tunica Vaginalis, Percutaneous Endoscopic Approach

♂ **0VP84KZ** Removal of Nonautologous Tissue Substitute from Scrotum and Tunica Vaginalis, Percutaneous Endoscopic Approach

♂ **0VP870Z** Removal of Drainage Device from Scrotum and Tunica Vaginalis, Via Natural or Artificial Opening

♂ **0VP873Z** Removal of Infusion Device from Scrotum and Tunica Vaginalis, Via Natural or Artificial Opening

♂ **0VP877Z** Removal of Autologous Tissue Substitute from Scrotum and Tunica Vaginalis, Via Natural or Artificial Opening

♂ **0VP87JZ** Removal of Synthetic Substitute from Scrotum and Tunica Vaginalis, Via Natural or Artificial Opening

♂ **0VP87KZ** Removal of Nonautologous Tissue Substitute from Scrotum and Tunica Vaginalis, Via Natural or Artificial Opening

♂ **0VP880Z** Removal of Drainage Device from Scrotum and Tunica Vaginalis, Via Natural or Artificial Opening Endoscopic

♂ **0VP883Z** Removal of Infusion Device from Scrotum and Tunica Vaginalis, Via Natural or Artificial Opening Endoscopic

♂ **0VP887Z** Removal of Autologous Tissue Substitute from Scrotum and Tunica Vaginalis, Via Natural or Artificial Opening Endoscopic

♂ **0VP88JZ** Removal of Synthetic Substitute from Scrotum and Tunica Vaginalis, Via Natural or Artificial Opening Endoscopic

♂ **0VP88KZ** Removal of Nonautologous Tissue Substitute from Scrotum and Tunica Vaginalis, Via Natural or Artificial Opening Endoscopic

♂ **0VP8X0Z** Removal of Drainage Device from Scrotum and Tunica Vaginalis, External Approach

♂ **0VP8X3Z** Removal of Infusion Device from Scrotum and Tunica Vaginalis, External Approach

♂ **0VPD00Z** Removal of Drainage Device from Testis, Open Approach

♂ **0VPD03Z** Removal of Infusion Device from Testis, Open Approach

♂ **0VPD07Z** Removal of Autologous Tissue Substitute from Testis, Open Approach

♂ **0VPD0JZ** Removal of Synthetic Substitute from Testis, Open Approach

♂ **0VPD0KZ** Removal of Nonautologous Tissue Substitute from Testis, Open Approach

♂ **0VPD30Z** Removal of Drainage Device from Testis, Percutaneous Approach

♂ **0VPD33Z** Removal of Infusion Device from Testis, Percutaneous Approach

♂ **0VPD37Z** Removal of Autologous Tissue Substitute from Testis, Percutaneous Approach

♂ **0VPD3JZ** Removal of Synthetic Substitute from Testis, Percutaneous Approach

♂ **0VPD3KZ** Removal of Nonautologous Tissue Substitute from Testis, Percutaneous Approach

♂ **0VPD40Z** Removal of Drainage Device from Testis, Percutaneous Endoscopic Approach

♂ **0VPD43Z** Removal of Infusion Device from Testis, Percutaneous Endoscopic Approach

♂ **0VPD47Z** Removal of Autologous Tissue Substitute from Testis, Percutaneous Endoscopic Approach

♂ **0VPD4JZ** Removal of Synthetic Substitute from Testis, Percutaneous Endoscopic Approach

♂ **0VPD4KZ** Removal of Nonautologous Tissue Substitute from Testis, Percutaneous Endoscopic Approach

♂ **0VPD70Z** Removal of Drainage Device from Testis, Via Natural or Artificial Opening

♂ **0VPD73Z** Removal of Infusion Device from Testis, Via Natural or Artificial Opening

♂ **0VPD77Z** Removal of Autologous Tissue Substitute from Testis, Via Natural or Artificial Opening

♂ **0VPD7JZ** Removal of Synthetic Substitute from Testis, Via Natural or Artificial Opening

♂ **0VPD7KZ** Removal of Nonautologous Tissue Substitute from Testis, Via Natural or Artificial Opening

♂ **0VPD80Z** Removal of Drainage Device from Testis, Via Natural or Artificial Opening Endoscopic

♂ **0VPD83Z** Removal of Infusion Device from Testis, Via Natural or Artificial Opening Endoscopic

♂ **0VPD87Z** Removal of Autologous Tissue Substitute from Testis, Via Natural or Artificial Opening Endoscopic

♂ **0VPD8JZ** Removal of Synthetic Substitute from Testis, Via Natural or Artificial Opening Endoscopic

♂ **0VPD8KZ** Removal of Nonautologous Tissue Substitute from Testis, Via Natural or Artificial Opening Endoscopic

♂ **0VPDX0Z** Removal of Drainage Device from Testis, External Approach

♂ **0VPDX3Z** Removal of Infusion Device from Testis, External Approach

♀ Female-only　　♂ Male-only　　▲ Limited Coverage　　● Non-OR　　▨ HAC-associated procedure　　▲ Non-covered procedures　　➕ Combination

PM00Z Removal of Drainage Device from Epididymis and Spermatic Cord, Open Approach

PM03Z Removal of Infusion Device from Epididymis and Spermatic Cord, Open Approach

PM07Z Removal of Autologous Tissue Substitute from Epididymis and Spermatic Cord, Open Approach

PM0CZ Removal of Extraluminal Device from Epididymis and Spermatic Cord, Open Approach

VPM0JZ Removal of Synthetic Substitute from Epididymis and Spermatic Cord, Open Approach

VPM0KZ Removal of Nonautologous Tissue Substitute from Epididymis and Spermatic Cord, Open Approach

VPM30Z Removal of Drainage Device from Epididymis and Spermatic Cord, Percutaneous Approach

VPM33Z Removal of Infusion Device from Epididymis and Spermatic Cord, Percutaneous Approach

VPM37Z Removal of Autologous Tissue Substitute from Epididymis and Spermatic Cord, Percutaneous Approach

VPM3CZ Removal of Extraluminal Device from Epididymis and Spermatic Cord, Percutaneous Approach

VPM3JZ Removal of Synthetic Substitute from Epididymis and Spermatic Cord, Percutaneous Approach

VPM3KZ Removal of Nonautologous Tissue Substitute from Epididymis and Spermatic Cord, Percutaneous Approach

VPM40Z Removal of Drainage Device from Epididymis and Spermatic Cord, Percutaneous Endoscopic Approach

VPM43Z Removal of Infusion Device from Epididymis and Spermatic Cord, Percutaneous Endoscopic Approach

VPM47Z Removal of Autologous Tissue Substitute from Epididymis and Spermatic Cord, Percutaneous Endoscopic Approach

VPM4CZ Removal of Extraluminal Device from Epididymis and Spermatic Cord, Percutaneous Endoscopic Approach

VPM4JZ Removal of Synthetic Substitute from Epididymis and Spermatic Cord, Percutaneous Endoscopic Approach

VPM4KZ Removal of Nonautologous Tissue Substitute from Epididymis and Spermatic Cord, Percutaneous Endoscopic Approach

0VPM70Z Removal of Drainage Device from Epididymis and Spermatic Cord, Via Natural or Artificial Opening

0VPM73Z Removal of Infusion Device from Epididymis and Spermatic Cord, Via Natural or Artificial Opening

0VPM77Z Removal of Autologous Tissue Substitute from Epididymis and Spermatic Cord, Via Natural or Artificial Opening

0VPM7CZ Removal of Extraluminal Device from Epididymis and Spermatic Cord, Via Natural or Artificial Opening

0VPM7JZ Removal of Synthetic Substitute from Epididymis and Spermatic Cord, Via Natural or Artificial Opening

0VPM7KZ Removal of Nonautologous Tissue Substitute from Epididymis and Spermatic Cord, Via Natural or Artificial Opening

0VPM80Z Removal of Drainage Device from Epididymis and Spermatic Cord, Via Natural or Artificial Opening Endoscopic

♂ 0VPM83Z Removal of Infusion Device from Epididymis and Spermatic Cord, Via Natural or Artificial Opening Endoscopic

♂ 0VPM87Z Removal of Autologous Tissue Substitute from Epididymis and Spermatic Cord, Via Natural or Artificial Opening Endoscopic

♂ 0VPM8CZ Removal of Extraluminal Device from Epididymis and Spermatic Cord, Via Natural or Artificial Opening Endoscopic

♂ 0VPM8JZ Removal of Synthetic Substitute from Epididymis and Spermatic Cord, Via Natural or Artificial Opening Endoscopic

♂ 0VPM8KZ Removal of Nonautologous Tissue Substitute from Epididymis and Spermatic Cord, Via Natural or Artificial Opening Endoscopic

♂ 0VPMX0Z Removal of Drainage Device from Epididymis and Spermatic Cord, External Approach

♂ 0VPMX3Z Removal of Infusion Device from Epididymis and Spermatic Cord, External Approach

♂ 0VPR00Z Removal of Drainage Device from Vas Deferens, Open Approach

♂ 0VPR03Z Removal of Infusion Device from Vas Deferens, Open Approach

♂ 0VPR07Z Removal of Autologous Tissue Substitute from Vas Deferens, Open Approach

♂ 0VPR0CZ Removal of Extraluminal Device from Vas Deferens, Open Approach

♂ 0VPR0DZ Removal of Intraluminal Device from Vas Deferens, Open Approach

♂ 0VPR0JZ Removal of Synthetic Substitute from Vas Deferens, Open Approach

♂ 0VPR0KZ Removal of Nonautologous Tissue Substitute from Vas Deferens, Open Approach

♂ 0VPR30Z Removal of Drainage Device from Vas Deferens, Percutaneous Approach

♂ 0VPR33Z Removal of Infusion Device from Vas Deferens, Percutaneous Approach

♂ 0VPR37Z Removal of Autologous Tissue Substitute from Vas Deferens, Percutaneous Approach

♂ 0VPR3CZ Removal of Extraluminal Device from Vas Deferens, Percutaneous Approach

♂ 0VPR3DZ Removal of Intraluminal Device from Vas Deferens, Percutaneous Approach

♂ 0VPR3JZ Removal of Synthetic Substitute from Vas Deferens, Percutaneous Approach

♂ 0VPR3KZ Removal of Nonautologous Tissue Substitute from Vas Deferens, Percutaneous Approach

♂ 0VPR40Z Removal of Drainage Device from Vas Deferens, Percutaneous Endoscopic Approach

♂ 0VPR43Z Removal of Infusion Device from Vas Deferens, Percutaneous Endoscopic Approach

♂ 0VPR47Z Removal of Autologous Tissue Substitute from Vas Deferens, Percutaneous Endoscopic Approach

♂ 0VPR4CZ Removal of Extraluminal Device from Vas Deferens, Percutaneous Endoscopic Approach

♂ 0VPR4DZ Removal of Intraluminal Device from Vas Deferens, Percutaneous Endoscopic Approach

♂ 0VPR4JZ Removal of Synthetic Substitute from Vas Deferens, Percutaneous Endoscopic Approach

♂ 0VPR4KZ Removal of Nonautologous Tissue Substitute from Vas Deferens, Percutaneous Endoscopic Approach

♂ 0VPR70Z Removal of Drainage Device from Vas Deferens, Via Natural or Artificial Opening

♂ 0VPR73Z Removal of Infusion Device from Vas Deferens, Via Natural or Artificial Opening

♂ 0VPR77Z Removal of Autologous Tissue Substitute from Vas Deferens, Via Natural or Artificial Opening

♂ 0VPR7CZ Removal of Extraluminal Device from Vas Deferens, Via Natural or Artificial Opening

♂ 0VPR7DZ Removal of Intraluminal Device from Vas Deferens, Via Natural or Artificial Opening

♂ 0VPR7JZ Removal of Synthetic Substitute from Vas Deferens, Via Natural or Artificial Opening

♂ 0VPR7KZ Removal of Nonautologous Tissue Substitute from Vas Deferens, Via Natural or Artificial Opening

♂ 0VPR80Z Removal of Drainage Device from Vas Deferens, Via Natural or Artificial Opening Endoscopic

♂ 0VPR83Z Removal of Infusion Device from Vas Deferens, Via Natural or Artificial Opening Endoscopic

♂ 0VPR87Z Removal of Autologous Tissue Substitute from Vas Deferens, Via Natural or Artificial Opening Endoscopic

♂ 0VPR8CZ Removal of Extraluminal Device from Vas Deferens, Via Natural or Artificial Opening Endoscopic

♂ 0VPR8DZ Removal of Intraluminal Device from Vas Deferens, Via Natural or Artificial Opening Endoscopic

♂ 0VPR8JZ Removal of Synthetic Substitute from Vas Deferens, Via Natural or Artificial Opening Endoscopic

♂ 0VPR8KZ Removal of Nonautologous Tissue Substitute from Vas Deferens, Via Natural or Artificial Opening Endoscopic

♂ 0VPRX0Z Removal of Drainage Device from Vas Deferens, External Approach

♂ 0VPRX3Z Removal of Infusion Device from Vas Deferens, External Approach

♂ 0VPRXDZ Removal of Intraluminal Device from Vas Deferens, External Approach

♂ 0VPS00Z Removal of Drainage Device from Penis, Open Approach

♂ 0VPS03Z Removal of Infusion Device from Penis, Open Approach

♂ 0VPS07Z Removal of Autologous Tissue Substitute from Penis, Open Approach

♂ 0VPS0JZ Removal of Synthetic Substitute from Penis, Open Approach

♂ 0VPS0KZ Removal of Nonautologous Tissue Substitute from Penis, Open Approach

♂ 0VPS30Z Removal of Drainage Device from Penis, Percutaneous Approach

♂ 0VPS33Z Removal of Infusion Device from Penis, Percutaneous Approach

♂ 0VPS37Z Removal of Autologous Tissue Substitute from Penis, Percutaneous Approach

♂ 0VPS3JZ Removal of Synthetic Substitute from Penis, Percutaneous Approach

♂ 0VPS3KZ Removal of Nonautologous Tissue Substitute from Penis, Percutaneous Approach

♂ 0VPS40Z Removal of Drainage Device from Penis, Percutaneous Endoscopic Approach

♂ 0VPS43Z Removal of Infusion Device from Penis, Percutaneous Endoscopic Approach

♀ Female-only   ♂ Male-only   ▲ Limited Coverage   ● Non-OR   ▨ HAC-associated procedure   ▲ Non-covered procedures   ➕ Combination

♂ 0VPS47Z Removal of Autologous Tissue Substitute from Penis, Percutaneous Endoscopic Approach

♂ 0VPS4JZ Removal of Synthetic Substitute from Penis, Percutaneous Endoscopic Approach

♂ 0VPS4KZ Removal of Nonautologous Tissue Substitute from Penis, Percutaneous Endoscopic Approach

♂ 0VPS70Z Removal of Drainage Device from Penis, Via Natural or Artificial Opening

♂ 0VPS73Z Removal of Infusion Device from Penis, Via Natural or Artificial Opening

♂ 0VPS77Z Removal of Autologous Tissue Substitute from Penis, Via Natural or Artificial Opening

♂ 0VPS7JZ Removal of Synthetic Substitute from Penis, Via Natural or Artificial Opening

♂ 0VPS7KZ Removal of Nonautologous Tissue Substitute from Penis, Via Natural or Artificial Opening

♂ 0VPS80Z Removal of Drainage Device from Penis, Via Natural or Artificial Opening Endoscopic

♂ 0VPS83Z Removal of Infusion Device from Penis, Via Natural or Artificial Opening Endoscopic

♂ 0VPS87Z Removal of Autologous Tissue Substitute from Penis, Via Natural or Artificial Opening Endoscopic

♂ 0VPS8JZ Removal of Synthetic Substitute from Penis, Via Natural or Artificial Opening Endoscopic

♂ 0VPS8KZ Removal of Nonautologous Tissue Substitute from Penis, Via Natural or Artificial Opening Endoscopic

♂ 0VPSX0Z Removal of Drainage Device from Penis, External Approach

♂ 0VPSX3Z Removal of Infusion Device from Penis, External Approach

0VQ – Male Reproductive System, Repair

♂ 0VQ00ZZ Repair Prostate, Open Approach
♂ 0VQ03ZZ Repair Prostate, Percutaneous Approach
♂ 0VQ04ZZ Repair Prostate, Percutaneous Endoscopic Approach
♂ 0VQ07ZZ Repair Prostate, Via Natural or Artificial Opening
♂ 0VQ08ZZ Repair Prostate, Via Natural or Artificial Opening Endoscopic
♂ 0VQ10ZZ Repair Right Seminal Vesicle, Open Approach
♂ 0VQ13ZZ Repair Right Seminal Vesicle, Percutaneous Approach
♂ 0VQ14ZZ Repair Right Seminal Vesicle, Percutaneous Endoscopic Approach
♂ 0VQ20ZZ Repair Left Seminal Vesicle, Open Approach
♂ 0VQ23ZZ Repair Left Seminal Vesicle, Percutaneous Approach
♂ 0VQ24ZZ Repair Left Seminal Vesicle, Percutaneous Endoscopic Approach
♂ 0VQ30ZZ Repair Bilateral Seminal Vesicles, Open Approach
♂ 0VQ33ZZ Repair Bilateral Seminal Vesicles, Percutaneous Approach
♂ 0VQ34ZZ Repair Bilateral Seminal Vesicles, Percutaneous Endoscopic Approach
♂ 0VQ50ZZ Repair Scrotum, Open Approach
♂ 0VQ53ZZ Repair Scrotum, Percutaneous Approach
♂ 0VQ54ZZ Repair Scrotum, Percutaneous Endoscopic Approach
♂ 0VQ5XZZ Repair Scrotum, External Approach
♂ 0VQ60ZZ Repair Right Tunica Vaginalis, Open Approach
♂ 0VQ63ZZ Repair Right Tunica Vaginalis, Percutaneous Approach
♂ 0VQ64ZZ Repair Right Tunica Vaginalis, Percutaneous Endoscopic Approach
♂ 0VQ70ZZ Repair Left Tunica Vaginalis, Open Approach

♂ 0VQ73ZZ Repair Left Tunica Vaginalis, Percutaneous Approach
♂ 0VQ74ZZ Repair Left Tunica Vaginalis, Percutaneous Endoscopic Approach
♂ 0VQ90ZZ Repair Right Testis, Open Approach
♂ 0VQ93ZZ Repair Right Testis, Percutaneous Approach
♂ 0VQ94ZZ Repair Right Testis, Percutaneous Endoscopic Approach
♂ 0VQB0ZZ Repair Left Testis, Open Approach
♂ 0VQB3ZZ Repair Left Testis, Percutaneous Approach
♂ 0VQB4ZZ Repair Left Testis, Percutaneous Endoscopic Approach
♂ 0VQC0ZZ Repair Bilateral Testes, Open Approach
♂ 0VQC3ZZ Repair Bilateral Testes, Percutaneous Approach
♂ 0VQC4ZZ Repair Bilateral Testes, Percutaneous Endoscopic Approach
♂ 0VQF0ZZ Repair Right Spermatic Cord, Open Approach
♂ 0VQF3ZZ Repair Right Spermatic Cord, Percutaneous Approach
♂ 0VQF4ZZ Repair Right Spermatic Cord, Percutaneous Endoscopic Approach
♂ 0VQG0ZZ Repair Left Spermatic Cord, Open Approach
♂ 0VQG3ZZ Repair Left Spermatic Cord, Percutaneous Approach
♂ 0VQG4ZZ Repair Left Spermatic Cord, Percutaneous Endoscopic Approach
♂ 0VQH0ZZ Repair Bilateral Spermatic Cords, Open Approach
♂ 0VQH3ZZ Repair Bilateral Spermatic Cords, Percutaneous Approach
♂ 0VQH4ZZ Repair Bilateral Spermatic Cords, Percutaneous Endoscopic Approach
♂ 0VQJ0ZZ Repair Right Epididymis, Open Approach
♂ 0VQJ3ZZ Repair Right Epididymis, Percutaneous Approach

♂ 0VQJ4ZZ Repair Right Epididymis, Percutaneous Endoscopic Approach
♂ 0VQK0ZZ Repair Left Epididymis, Open Approach
♂ 0VQK3ZZ Repair Left Epididymis, Percutaneous Approach
♂ 0VQK4ZZ Repair Left Epididymis, Percutaneous Endoscopic Approach
♂ 0VQL0ZZ Repair Bilateral Epididymis, Open Approach
♂ 0VQL3ZZ Repair Bilateral Epididymis, Percutaneous Approach
♂ 0VQL4ZZ Repair Bilateral Epididymis, Percutaneous Endoscopic Approach
♂ 0VQN0ZZ Repair Right Vas Deferens, Open Approach
♂ 0VQN3ZZ Repair Right Vas Deferens, Percutaneous Approach
♂ 0VQN4ZZ Repair Right Vas Deferens, Percutaneous Endoscopic Approach
♂ 0VQP0ZZ Repair Left Vas Deferens, Open Approach
♂ 0VQP3ZZ Repair Left Vas Deferens, Percutaneous Approach
♂ 0VQP4ZZ Repair Left Vas Deferens, Percutaneous Endoscopic Approach
♂ 0VQQ0ZZ Repair Bilateral Vas Deferens, Open Approach
♂ 0VQQ3ZZ Repair Bilateral Vas Deferens, Percutaneous Approach
♂ 0VQQ4ZZ Repair Bilateral Vas Deferens, Percutaneous Endoscopic Approach
♂ 0VQS0ZZ Repair Penis, Open Approach
♂ 0VQS3ZZ Repair Penis, Percutaneous Approach
♂ 0VQS4ZZ Repair Penis, Percutaneous Endoscopic Approach
♂ 0VQSXZZ Repair Penis, External Approach
♂ 0VQT0ZZ Repair Prepuce, Open Approach
♂ 0VQT3ZZ Repair Prepuce, Percutaneous Approach
♂ 0VQT4ZZ Repair Prepuce, Percutaneous Endoscopic Approach
♂ 0VQTXZZ Repair Prepuce, External Approach

0VR – Male Reproductive System, Replacement

♂ 0VR90JZ Replacement of Right Testis with Synthetic Substitute, Open Approach

♂ 0VRB0JZ Replacement of Left Testis with Synthetic Substitute, Open Approach

♂ 0VRC0JZ Replacement of Bilateral Testes with Synthetic Substitute, Open Approach

0VS – Male Reproductive System, Reposition

♂ 0VS90ZZ Reposition Right Testis, Open Approach
♂ 0VS93ZZ Reposition Right Testis, Percutaneous Approach
♂ 0VS94ZZ Reposition Right Testis, Percutaneous Endoscopic Approach
♂ 0VSB0ZZ Reposition Left Testis, Open Approach
♂ 0VSB3ZZ Reposition Left Testis, Percutaneous Approach
♂ 0VSB4ZZ Reposition Left Testis, Percutaneous Endoscopic Approach
♂ 0VSC0ZZ Reposition Bilateral Testes, Open Approach

♂ 0VSC3ZZ Reposition Bilateral Testes, Percutaneous Approach
♂ 0VSC4ZZ Reposition Bilateral Testes, Percutaneous Endoscopic Approach
♂ 0VSF0ZZ Reposition Right Spermatic Cord, Open Approach
♂ 0VSF3ZZ Reposition Right Spermatic Cord, Percutaneous Approach
♂ 0VSF4ZZ Reposition Right Spermatic Cord, Percutaneous Endoscopic Approach
♂ 0VSG0ZZ Reposition Left Spermatic Cord, Open Approach

♂ 0VSG3ZZ Reposition Left Spermatic Cord, Percutaneous Approach
♂ 0VSG4ZZ Reposition Left Spermatic Cord, Percutaneous Endoscopic Approach
♂ 0VSH0ZZ Reposition Bilateral Spermatic Cords, Open Approach
♂ 0VSH3ZZ Reposition Bilateral Spermatic Cords, Percutaneous Approach
♂ 0VSH4ZZ Reposition Bilateral Spermatic Cords, Percutaneous Endoscopic Approach

♀ Female-only   ♂ Male-only   ▲ Limited Coverage   ● Non-OR   ▦ HAC-associated procedure   ▲ Non-covered procedures   ✚ Combination

0VT – Male Reproductive System, Resection

Review Coding Guideline B3.8

0VT00ZZ	Resection of Prostate, Open Approach	♂ **0VT50ZZ**	Resection of Scrotum, Open Approach	♂ **0VTJ0ZZ**	Resection of Right Epididymis, Open Approach
⊞	Radical prostatectomy when reported with Resection of bilateral seminal vesicles. *See table 0VT to construct the Resection code.*	♂ **0VT54ZZ**	Resection of Scrotum, Percutaneous Endoscopic Approach	♂ **0VTJ4ZZ**	Resection of Right Epididymis, Percutaneous Endoscopic Approach
0VT04ZZ	Resection of Prostate, Percutaneous Endoscopic Approach	♂ **0VT5XZZ**	Resection of Scrotum, External Approach	♂ **0VTK0ZZ**	Resection of Left Epididymis, Open Approach
		♂ **0VT60ZZ**	Resection of Right Tunica Vaginalis, Open Approach	♂ **0VTK4ZZ**	Resection of Left Epididymis, Percutaneous Endoscopic Approach
⊞	Radical prostatectomy when reported with Resection of bilateral seminal vesicles. *See table 0VT to construct the Resection code.*	♂ **0VT64ZZ**	Resection of Right Tunica Vaginalis, Percutaneous Endoscopic Approach	♂ **0VTL0ZZ**	Resection of Bilateral Epididymis, Open Approach
	AHA CC: 4Q, 2014, 33-34	♂ **0VT70ZZ**	Resection of Left Tunica Vaginalis, Open Approach	♂ **0VTL4ZZ**	Resection of Bilateral Epididymis, Percutaneous Endoscopic Approach
0VT07ZZ	Resection of Prostate, Via Natural or Artificial Opening	♂ **0VT74ZZ**	Resection of Left Tunica Vaginalis, Percutaneous Endoscopic Approach	♂ **0VTN0ZZ** ▲	Resection of Right Vas Deferens, Open Approach
⊞	Radical prostatectomy when reported with Resection of bilateral seminal vesicles. *See table 0VT to construct the Resection code.*	♂ **0VT90ZZ**	Resection of Right Testis, Open Approach	♂ **0VTN4ZZ** ▲	Resection of Right Vas Deferens, Percutaneous Endoscopic Approach
		♂ **0VT94ZZ**	Resection of Right Testis, Percutaneous Endoscopic Approach	♂ **0VTP0ZZ** ▲	Resection of Left Vas Deferens, Open Approach
0VT08ZZ	Resection of Prostate, Via Natural or Artificial Opening Endoscopic	♂ **0VTB0ZZ**	Resection of Left Testis, Open Approach	♂ **0VTP4ZZ** ▲	Resection of Left Vas Deferens, Percutaneous Endoscopic Approach
⊞	Radical prostatectomy when reported with Resection of bilateral seminal vesicles. *See table 0VT to construct the Resection code.*	♂ **0VTB4ZZ**	Resection of Left Testis, Percutaneous Endoscopic Approach	♂ **0VTQ0ZZ** ▲	Resection of Bilateral Vas Deferens, Open Approach
		♂ **0VTC0ZZ**	Resection of Bilateral Testes, Open Approach	♂ **0VTQ4ZZ** ▲	Resection of Bilateral Vas Deferens, Percutaneous Endoscopic Approach
0VT10ZZ	Resection of Right Seminal Vesicle, Open Approach	♂ **0VTC4ZZ**	Resection of Bilateral Testes, Percutaneous Endoscopic Approach	♂ **0VTS0ZZ**	Resection of Penis, Open Approach
0VT14ZZ	Resection of Right Seminal Vesicle, Percutaneous Endoscopic Approach	♂ **0VTF0ZZ**	Resection of Right Spermatic Cord, Open Approach	♂ **0VTS4ZZ**	Resection of Penis, Percutaneous Endoscopic Approach
0VT20ZZ	Resection of Left Seminal Vesicle, Open Approach	♂ **0VTF4ZZ**	Resection of Right Spermatic Cord, Percutaneous Endoscopic Approach	♂ **0VTSXZZ**	Resection of Penis, External Approach
0VT24ZZ	Resection of Left Seminal Vesicle, Percutaneous Endoscopic Approach	♂ **0VTG0ZZ**	Resection of Left Spermatic Cord, Open Approach	♂ **0VTT0ZZ**	Resection of Prepuce, Open Approach
0VT30ZZ	Resection of Bilateral Seminal Vesicles, Open Approach	♂ **0VTG4ZZ**	Resection of Left Spermatic Cord, Percutaneous Endoscopic Approach	♂ **0VTT4ZZ**	Resection of Prepuce, Percutaneous Endoscopic Approach
0VT34ZZ	Resection of Bilateral Seminal Vesicles, Percutaneous Endoscopic Approach	♂ **0VTH0ZZ**	Resection of Bilateral Spermatic Cords, Open Approach	♂ **0VTTXZZ**	Resection of Prepuce, External Approach
	AHA CC: 4Q, 2014, 33-34	♂ **0VTH4ZZ**	Resection of Bilateral Spermatic Cords, Percutaneous Endoscopic Approach		

0VU – Male Reproductive System, Supplement

0VU107Z	Supplement Right Seminal Vesicle with Autologous Tissue Substitute, Open Approach	♂ **0VU30JZ**	Supplement Bilateral Seminal Vesicles with Synthetic Substitute, Open Approach	♂ **0VU60JZ**	Supplement Right Tunica Vaginalis with Synthetic Substitute, Open Approach
0VU10JZ	Supplement Right Seminal Vesicle with Synthetic Substitute, Open Approach	♂ **0VU30KZ**	Supplement Bilateral Seminal Vesicles with Nonautologous Tissue Substitute, Open Approach	♂ **0VU60KZ**	Supplement Right Tunica Vaginalis with Nonautologous Tissue Substitute, Open Approach
0VU10KZ	Supplement Right Seminal Vesicle with Nonautologous Tissue Substitute, Open Approach	♂ **0VU347Z**	Supplement Bilateral Seminal Vesicles with Autologous Tissue Substitute, Percutaneous Endoscopic Approach	♂ **0VU647Z**	Supplement Right Tunica Vaginalis with Autologous Tissue Substitute, Percutaneous Endoscopic Approach
0VU147Z	Supplement Right Seminal Vesicle with Autologous Tissue Substitute, Percutaneous Endoscopic Approach	♂ **0VU34JZ**	Supplement Bilateral Seminal Vesicles with Synthetic Substitute, Percutaneous Endoscopic Approach	♂ **0VU64JZ**	Supplement Right Tunica Vaginalis with Synthetic Substitute, Percutaneous Endoscopic Approach
0VU14JZ	Supplement Right Seminal Vesicle with Synthetic Substitute, Percutaneous Endoscopic Approach	♂ **0VU34KZ**	Supplement Bilateral Seminal Vesicles with Nonautologous Tissue Substitute, Percutaneous Endoscopic Approach	♂ **0VU64KZ**	Supplement Right Tunica Vaginalis with Nonautologous Tissue Substitute, Percutaneous Endoscopic Approach
0VU14KZ	Supplement Right Seminal Vesicle with Nonautologous Tissue Substitute, Percutaneous Endoscopic Approach	♂ **0VU507Z**	Supplement Scrotum with Autologous Tissue Substitute, Open Approach	♂ **0VU707Z**	Supplement Left Tunica Vaginalis with Autologous Tissue Substitute, Open Approach
0VU207Z	Supplement Left Seminal Vesicle with Autologous Tissue Substitute, Open Approach	♂ **0VU50JZ**	Supplement Scrotum with Synthetic Substitute, Open Approach	♂ **0VU70JZ**	Supplement Left Tunica Vaginalis with Synthetic Substitute, Open Approach
0VU20JZ	Supplement Left Seminal Vesicle with Synthetic Substitute, Open Approach	♂ **0VU50KZ**	Supplement Scrotum with Nonautologous Tissue Substitute, Open Approach	♂ **0VU70KZ**	Supplement Left Tunica Vaginalis with Nonautologous Tissue Substitute, Open Approach
0VU20KZ	Supplement Left Seminal Vesicle with Nonautologous Tissue Substitute, Open Approach	♂ **0VU547Z**	Supplement Scrotum with Autologous Tissue Substitute, Percutaneous Endoscopic Approach	♂ **0VU747Z**	Supplement Left Tunica Vaginalis with Autologous Tissue Substitute, Percutaneous Endoscopic Approach
0VU247Z	Supplement Left Seminal Vesicle with Autologous Tissue Substitute, Percutaneous Endoscopic Approach	♂ **0VU54JZ**	Supplement Scrotum with Synthetic Substitute, Percutaneous Endoscopic Approach	♂ **0VU74JZ**	Supplement Left Tunica Vaginalis with Synthetic Substitute, Percutaneous Endoscopic Approach
0VU24JZ	Supplement Left Seminal Vesicle with Synthetic Substitute, Percutaneous Endoscopic Approach	♂ **0VU54KZ**	Supplement Scrotum with Nonautologous Tissue Substitute, Percutaneous Endoscopic Approach	♂ **0VU74KZ**	Supplement Left Tunica Vaginalis with Nonautologous Tissue Substitute, Percutaneous Endoscopic Approach
0VU24KZ	Supplement Left Seminal Vesicle with Nonautologous Tissue Substitute, Percutaneous Endoscopic Approach	♂ **0VU5X7Z**	Supplement Scrotum with Autologous Tissue Substitute, External Approach	♂ **0VU907Z**	Supplement Right Testis with Autologous Tissue Substitute, Open Approach
0VU307Z	Supplement Bilateral Seminal Vesicles with Autologous Tissue Substitute, Open Approach	♂ **0VU5XJZ**	Supplement Scrotum with Synthetic Substitute, External Approach	♂ **0VU90JZ**	Supplement Right Testis with Synthetic Substitute, Open Approach
		♂ **0VU5XKZ**	Supplement Scrotum with Nonautologous Tissue Substitute, External Approach		
		♂ **0VU607Z**	Supplement Right Tunica Vaginalis with Autologous Tissue Substitute, Open Approach		

1101

♀ Female-only   ♂ Male-only   ▲ Limited Coverage   ● Non-OR   ▥ HAC-associated procedure   ▲ Non-covered procedures   ⊞ Combination

♂ 0VU90KZ Supplement Right Testis with Nonautologous Tissue Substitute, Open Approach

♂ 0VUB07Z Supplement Left Testis with Autologous Tissue Substitute, Open Approach

♂ 0VUB0JZ Supplement Left Testis with Synthetic Substitute, Open Approach

♂ 0VUB0KZ Supplement Left Testis with Nonautologous Tissue Substitute, Open Approach

♂ 0VUC07Z Supplement Bilateral Testes with Autologous Tissue Substitute, Open Approach

♂ 0VUC0JZ Supplement Bilateral Testes with Synthetic Substitute, Open Approach

♂ 0VUC0KZ Supplement Bilateral Testes with Nonautologous Tissue Substitute, Open Approach

♂ 0VUF07Z Supplement Right Spermatic Cord with Autologous Tissue Substitute, Open Approach

♂ 0VUF0JZ Supplement Right Spermatic Cord with Synthetic Substitute, Open Approach

♂ 0VUF0KZ Supplement Right Spermatic Cord with Nonautologous Tissue Substitute, Open Approach

♂ 0VUF47Z Supplement Right Spermatic Cord with Autologous Tissue Substitute, Percutaneous Endoscopic Approach

♂ 0VUF4JZ Supplement Right Spermatic Cord with Synthetic Substitute, Percutaneous Endoscopic Approach

♂ 0VUF4KZ Supplement Right Spermatic Cord with Nonautologous Tissue Substitute, Percutaneous Endoscopic Approach

♂ 0VUG07Z Supplement Left Spermatic Cord with Autologous Tissue Substitute, Open Approach

♂ 0VUG0JZ Supplement Left Spermatic Cord with Synthetic Substitute, Open Approach

♂ 0VUG0KZ Supplement Left Spermatic Cord with Nonautologous Tissue Substitute, Open Approach

♂ 0VUG47Z Supplement Left Spermatic Cord with Autologous Tissue Substitute, Percutaneous Endoscopic Approach

♂ 0VUG4JZ Supplement Left Spermatic Cord with Synthetic Substitute, Percutaneous Endoscopic Approach

♂ 0VUG4KZ Supplement Left Spermatic Cord with Nonautologous Tissue Substitute, Percutaneous Endoscopic Approach

♂ 0VUH07Z Supplement Bilateral Spermatic Cords with Autologous Tissue Substitute, Open Approach

♂ 0VUH0JZ Supplement Bilateral Spermatic Cords with Synthetic Substitute, Open Approach

♂ 0VUH0KZ Supplement Bilateral Spermatic Cords with Nonautologous Tissue Substitute, Open Approach

♂ 0VUH47Z Supplement Bilateral Spermatic Cords with Autologous Tissue Substitute, Percutaneous Endoscopic Approach

♂ 0VUH4JZ Supplement Bilateral Spermatic Cords with Synthetic Substitute, Percutaneous Endoscopic Approach

♂ 0VUH4KZ Supplement Bilateral Spermatic Cords with Nonautologous Tissue Substitute, Percutaneous Endoscopic Approach

♂ 0VUJ07Z Supplement Right Epididymis with Autologous Tissue Substitute, Open Approach

♂ 0VUJ0JZ Supplement Right Epididymis with Synthetic Substitute, Open Approach

♂ 0VUJ0KZ Supplement Right Epididymis with Nonautologous Tissue Substitute, Open Approach

♂ 0VUJ47Z Supplement Right Epididymis with Autologous Tissue Substitute, Percutaneous Endoscopic Approach

♂ 0VUJ4JZ Supplement Right Epididymis with Synthetic Substitute, Percutaneous Endoscopic Approach

♂ 0VUJ4KZ Supplement Right Epididymis with Nonautologous Tissue Substitute, Percutaneous Endoscopic Approach

♂ 0VUK07Z Supplement Left Epididymis with Autologous Tissue Substitute, Open Approach

♂ 0VUK0JZ Supplement Left Epididymis with Synthetic Substitute, Open Approach

♂ 0VUK0KZ Supplement Left Epididymis with Nonautologous Tissue Substitute, Open Approach

♂ 0VUK47Z Supplement Left Epididymis with Autologous Tissue Substitute, Percutaneous Endoscopic Approach

♂ 0VUK4JZ Supplement Left Epididymis with Synthetic Substitute, Percutaneous Endoscopic Approach

♂ 0VUK4KZ Supplement Left Epididymis with Nonautologous Tissue Substitute, Percutaneous Endoscopic Approach

♂ 0VUL07Z Supplement Bilateral Epididymis with Autologous Tissue Substitute, Open Approach

♂ 0VUL0JZ Supplement Bilateral Epididymis with Synthetic Substitute, Open Approach

♂ 0VUL0KZ Supplement Bilateral Epididymis with Nonautologous Tissue Substitute, Open Approach

♂ 0VUL47Z Supplement Bilateral Epididymis with Autologous Tissue Substitute, Percutaneous Endoscopic Approach

♂ 0VUL4JZ Supplement Bilateral Epididymis with Synthetic Substitute, Percutaneous Endoscopic Approach

♂ 0VUL4KZ Supplement Bilateral Epididymis with Nonautologous Tissue Substitute, Percutaneous Endoscopic Approach

♂ 0VUN07Z Supplement Right Vas Deferens with Autologous Tissue Substitute, Open Approach

♂ 0VUN0JZ Supplement Right Vas Deferens with Synthetic Substitute, Open Approach

♂ 0VUN0KZ Supplement Right Vas Deferens with Nonautologous Tissue Substitute, Open Approach

♂ 0VUN47Z Supplement Right Vas Deferens with Autologous Tissue Substitute, Percutaneous Endoscopic Approach

♂ 0VUN4JZ Supplement Right Vas Deferens with Synthetic Substitute, Percutaneous Endoscopic Approach

♂ 0VUN4KZ Supplement Right Vas Deferens with Nonautologous Tissue Substitute, Percutaneous Endoscopic Approach

♂ 0VUP07Z Supplement Left Vas Deferens with Autologous Tissue Substitute, Open Approach

♂ 0VUP0JZ Supplement Left Vas Deferens with Synthetic Substitute, Open Approach

♂ 0VUP0KZ Supplement Left Vas Deferens with Nonautologous Tissue Substitute, Open Approach

♂ 0VUP47Z Supplement Left Vas Deferens with Autologous Tissue Substitute, Percutaneous Endoscopic Approach

♂ 0VUP4JZ Supplement Left Vas Deferens with Synthetic Substitute, Percutaneous Endoscopic Approach

♂ 0VUP4KZ Supplement Left Vas Deferens with Nonautologous Tissue Substitute, Percutaneous Endoscopic Approach

♂ 0VUQ07Z Supplement Bilateral Vas Deferens with Autologous Tissue Substitute, Open Approach

♂ 0VUQ0JZ Supplement Bilateral Vas Deferens with Synthetic Substitute, Open Approach

♂ 0VUQ0KZ Supplement Bilateral Vas Deferens with Nonautologous Tissue Substitute, Open Approach

♂ 0VUQ47Z Supplement Bilateral Vas Deferens with Autologous Tissue Substitute, Percutaneous Endoscopic Approach

♂ 0VUQ4JZ Supplement Bilateral Vas Deferens with Synthetic Substitute, Percutaneous Endoscopic Approach

♂ 0VUQ4KZ Supplement Bilateral Vas Deferens with Nonautologous Tissue Substitute, Percutaneous Endoscopic Approach

♂ 0VUS07Z Supplement Penis with Autologous Tissue Substitute, Open Approach

♂ 0VUS0JZ Supplement Penis with Synthetic Substitute, Open Approach

♂ 0VUS0KZ Supplement Penis with Nonautologous Tissue Substitute, Open Approach

♂ 0VUS47Z Supplement Penis with Autologous Tissue Substitute, Percutaneous Endoscopic Approach

♂ 0VUS4JZ Supplement Penis with Synthetic Substitute, Percutaneous Endoscopic Approach

♂ 0VUS4KZ Supplement Penis with Nonautologous Tissue Substitute, Percutaneous Endoscopic Approach

♂ 0VUSX7Z Supplement Penis with Autologous Tissue Substitute, External Approach

♂ 0VUSXJZ Supplement Penis with Synthetic Substitute, External Approach

♂ 0VUSXKZ Supplement Penis with Nonautologous Tissue Substitute, External Approach

♂ 0VUT07Z Supplement Prepuce with Autologous Tissue Substitute, Open Approach

♂ 0VUT0JZ Supplement Prepuce with Synthetic Substitute, Open Approach

♂ 0VUT0KZ Supplement Prepuce with Nonautologous Tissue Substitute, Open Approach

♂ 0VUT47Z Supplement Prepuce with Autologous Tissue Substitute, Percutaneous Endoscopic Approach

♂ 0VUT4JZ Supplement Prepuce with Synthetic Substitute, Percutaneous Endoscopic Approach

♂ 0VUT4KZ Supplement Prepuce with Nonautologous Tissue Substitute, Percutaneous Endoscopic Approach

♂ 0VUTX7Z Supplement Prepuce with Autologous Tissue Substitute, External Approach

♂ 0VUTXJZ Supplement Prepuce with Synthetic Substitute, External Approach

♂ 0VUTXKZ Supplement Prepuce with Nonautologous Tissue Substitute, External Approach

♀ Female-only   ♂ Male-only   ▲ Limited Coverage   ● Non-OR   ᴴᴬᶜ HAC-associated procedure   ▲ Non-covered procedures   ✛ Combination

0VW400Z Revision of Drainage Device in Prostate and Seminal Vesicles, Open Approach

0VW403Z Revision of Infusion Device in Prostate and Seminal Vesicles, Open Approach

0VW407Z Revision of Autologous Tissue Substitute in Prostate and Seminal Vesicles, Open Approach

0VW40JZ Revision of Synthetic Substitute in Prostate and Seminal Vesicles, Open Approach

0VW40KZ Revision of Nonautologous Tissue Substitute in Prostate and Seminal Vesicles, Open Approach

0VW430Z Revision of Drainage Device in Prostate and Seminal Vesicles, Percutaneous Approach

0VW433Z Revision of Infusion Device in Prostate and Seminal Vesicles, Percutaneous Approach

0VW437Z Revision of Autologous Tissue Substitute in Prostate and Seminal Vesicles, Percutaneous Approach

0VW43JZ Revision of Synthetic Substitute in Prostate and Seminal Vesicles, Percutaneous Approach

0VW43KZ Revision of Nonautologous Tissue Substitute in Prostate and Seminal Vesicles, Percutaneous Approach

0VW440Z Revision of Drainage Device in Prostate and Seminal Vesicles, Percutaneous Endoscopic Approach

0VW443Z Revision of Infusion Device in Prostate and Seminal Vesicles, Percutaneous Endoscopic Approach

0VW447Z Revision of Autologous Tissue Substitute in Prostate and Seminal Vesicles, Percutaneous Endoscopic Approach

0VW44JZ Revision of Synthetic Substitute in Prostate and Seminal Vesicles, Percutaneous Endoscopic Approach

0VW44KZ Revision of Nonautologous Tissue Substitute in Prostate and Seminal Vesicles, Percutaneous Endoscopic Approach

0VW470Z Revision of Drainage Device in Prostate and Seminal Vesicles, Via Natural or Artificial Opening

0VW473Z Revision of Infusion Device in Prostate and Seminal Vesicles, Via Natural or Artificial Opening

0VW477Z Revision of Autologous Tissue Substitute in Prostate and Seminal Vesicles, Via Natural or Artificial Opening

0VW47JZ Revision of Synthetic Substitute in Prostate and Seminal Vesicles, Via Natural or Artificial Opening

0VW47KZ Revision of Nonautologous Tissue Substitute in Prostate and Seminal Vesicles, Via Natural or Artificial Opening

0VW480Z Revision of Drainage Device in Prostate and Seminal Vesicles, Via Natural or Artificial Opening Endoscopic

0VW483Z Revision of Infusion Device in Prostate and Seminal Vesicles, Via Natural or Artificial Opening Endoscopic

0VW487Z Revision of Autologous Tissue Substitute in Prostate and Seminal Vesicles, Via Natural or Artificial Opening Endoscopic

0VW48JZ Revision of Synthetic Substitute in Prostate and Seminal Vesicles, Via Natural or Artificial Opening Endoscopic

♂ 0VW48KZ Revision of Nonautologous Tissue Substitute in Prostate and Seminal Vesicles, Via Natural or Artificial Opening Endoscopic

♂ 0VW4X0Z Revision of Drainage Device in Prostate and Seminal Vesicles, External Approach

♂ 0VW4X3Z Revision of Infusion Device in Prostate and Seminal Vesicles, External Approach

♂ 0VW4X7Z Revision of Autologous Tissue Substitute in Prostate and Seminal Vesicles, External Approach

♂ 0VW4XJZ Revision of Synthetic Substitute in Prostate and Seminal Vesicles, External Approach

♂ 0VW4XKZ Revision of Nonautologous Tissue Substitute in Prostate and Seminal Vesicles, External Approach

♂ 0VW800Z Revision of Drainage Device in Scrotum and Tunica Vaginalis, Open Approach

♂ 0VW803Z Revision of Infusion Device in Scrotum and Tunica Vaginalis, Open Approach

♂ 0VW807Z Revision of Autologous Tissue Substitute in Scrotum and Tunica Vaginalis, Open Approach

♂ 0VW80JZ Revision of Synthetic Substitute in Scrotum and Tunica Vaginalis, Open Approach

♂ 0VW80KZ Revision of Nonautologous Tissue Substitute in Scrotum and Tunica Vaginalis, Open Approach

♂ 0VW830Z Revision of Drainage Device in Scrotum and Tunica Vaginalis, Percutaneous Approach

♂ 0VW833Z Revision of Infusion Device in Scrotum and Tunica Vaginalis, Percutaneous Approach

♂ 0VW837Z Revision of Autologous Tissue Substitute in Scrotum and Tunica Vaginalis, Percutaneous Approach

♂ 0VW83JZ Revision of Synthetic Substitute in Scrotum and Tunica Vaginalis, Percutaneous Approach

♂ 0VW83KZ Revision of Nonautologous Tissue Substitute in Scrotum and Tunica Vaginalis, Percutaneous Approach

♂ 0VW840Z Revision of Drainage Device in Scrotum and Tunica Vaginalis, Percutaneous Endoscopic Approach

♂ 0VW843Z Revision of Infusion Device in Scrotum and Tunica Vaginalis, Percutaneous Endoscopic Approach

♂ 0VW847Z Revision of Autologous Tissue Substitute in Scrotum and Tunica Vaginalis, Percutaneous Endoscopic Approach

♂ 0VW84JZ Revision of Synthetic Substitute in Scrotum and Tunica Vaginalis, Percutaneous Endoscopic Approach

♂ 0VW84KZ Revision of Nonautologous Tissue Substitute in Scrotum and Tunica Vaginalis, Percutaneous Endoscopic Approach

♂ 0VW870Z Revision of Drainage Device in Scrotum and Tunica Vaginalis, Via Natural or Artificial Opening

♂ 0VW873Z Revision of Infusion Device in Scrotum and Tunica Vaginalis, Via Natural or Artificial Opening

♂ 0VW877Z Revision of Autologous Tissue Substitute in Scrotum and Tunica Vaginalis, Via Natural or Artificial Opening

♂ 0VW87JZ Revision of Synthetic Substitute in Scrotum and Tunica Vaginalis, Via Natural or Artificial Opening

♂ 0VW87KZ Revision of Nonautologous Tissue Substitute in Scrotum and Tunica Vaginalis, Via Natural or Artificial Opening

♂ 0VW880Z Revision of Drainage Device in Scrotum and Tunica Vaginalis, Via Natural or Artificial Opening Endoscopic

♂ 0VW883Z Revision of Infusion Device in Scrotum and Tunica Vaginalis, Via Natural or Artificial Opening Endoscopic

♂ 0VW887Z Revision of Autologous Tissue Substitute in Scrotum and Tunica Vaginalis, Via Natural or Artificial Opening Endoscopic

♂ 0VW88JZ Revision of Synthetic Substitute in Scrotum and Tunica Vaginalis, Via Natural or Artificial Opening Endoscopic

♂ 0VW88KZ Revision of Nonautologous Tissue Substitute in Scrotum and Tunica Vaginalis, Via Natural or Artificial Opening Endoscopic

♂ 0VW8X0Z Revision of Drainage Device in Scrotum and Tunica Vaginalis, External Approach

♂ 0VW8X3Z Revision of Infusion Device in Scrotum and Tunica Vaginalis, External Approach

♂ 0VW8X7Z Revision of Autologous Tissue Substitute in Scrotum and Tunica Vaginalis, External Approach

♂ 0VW8XJZ Revision of Synthetic Substitute in Scrotum and Tunica Vaginalis, External Approach

♂ 0VW8XKZ Revision of Nonautologous Tissue Substitute in Scrotum and Tunica Vaginalis, External Approach

♂ 0VWD00Z Revision of Drainage Device in Testis, Open Approach

♂ 0VWD03Z Revision of Infusion Device in Testis, Open Approach

♂ 0VWD07Z Revision of Autologous Tissue Substitute in Testis, Open Approach

♂ 0VWD0JZ Revision of Synthetic Substitute in Testis, Open Approach

♂ 0VWD0KZ Revision of Nonautologous Tissue Substitute in Testis, Open Approach

♂ 0VWD30Z Revision of Drainage Device in Testis, Percutaneous Approach

♂ 0VWD33Z Revision of Infusion Device in Testis, Percutaneous Approach

♂ 0VWD37Z Revision of Autologous Tissue Substitute in Testis, Percutaneous Approach

♂ 0VWD3JZ Revision of Synthetic Substitute in Testis, Percutaneous Approach

♂ 0VWD3KZ Revision of Nonautologous Tissue Substitute in Testis, Percutaneous Approach

♂ 0VWD40Z Revision of Drainage Device in Testis, Percutaneous Endoscopic Approach

♂ 0VWD43Z Revision of Infusion Device in Testis, Percutaneous Endoscopic Approach

♂ 0VWD47Z Revision of Autologous Tissue Substitute in Testis, Percutaneous Endoscopic Approach

♂ 0VWD4JZ Revision of Synthetic Substitute in Testis, Percutaneous Endoscopic Approach

♂ 0VWD4KZ Revision of Nonautologous Tissue Substitute in Testis, Percutaneous Endoscopic Approach

♂ 0VWD70Z Revision of Drainage Device in Testis, Via Natural or Artificial Opening

♂ 0VWD73Z Revision of Infusion Device in Testis, Via Natural or Artificial Opening

♂ 0VWD77Z Revision of Autologous Tissue Substitute in Testis, Via Natural or Artificial Opening

♀ Female-only   ♂ Male-only   ▲ Limited Coverage   ● Non-OR   ▥ HAC-associated procedure   ▲ Non-covered procedures   ✛ Combination

♂ **0VWD7JZ** Revision of Synthetic Substitute in Testis, Via Natural or Artificial Opening

♂ **0VWD7KZ** Revision of Nonautologous Tissue Substitute in Testis, Via Natural or Artificial Opening

♂ **0VWD80Z** Revision of Drainage Device in Testis, Via Natural or Artificial Opening Endoscopic

♂ **0VWD83Z** Revision of Infusion Device in Testis, Via Natural or Artificial Opening Endoscopic

♂ **0VWD87Z** Revision of Autologous Tissue Substitute in Testis, Via Natural or Artificial Opening Endoscopic

♂ **0VWD8JZ** Revision of Synthetic Substitute in Testis, Via Natural or Artificial Opening Endoscopic

♂ **0VWD8KZ** Revision of Nonautologous Tissue Substitute in Testis, Via Natural or Artificial Opening Endoscopic

♂ **0VWDX0Z** Revision of Drainage Device in Testis, External Approach

♂ **0VWDX3Z** Revision of Infusion Device in Testis, External Approach

♂ **0VWDX7Z** Revision of Autologous Tissue Substitute in Testis, External Approach

♂ **0VWDXJZ** Revision of Synthetic Substitute in Testis, External Approach

♂ **0VWDXKZ** Revision of Nonautologous Tissue Substitute in Testis, External Approach

♂ **0VWM00Z** Revision of Drainage Device in Epididymis and Spermatic Cord, Open Approach

♂ **0VWM03Z** Revision of Infusion Device in Epididymis and Spermatic Cord, Open Approach

♂ **0VWM07Z** Revision of Autologous Tissue Substitute in Epididymis and Spermatic Cord, Open Approach

♂ **0VWM0CZ** Revision of Extraluminal Device in Epididymis and Spermatic Cord, Open Approach

♂ **0VWM0JZ** Revision of Synthetic Substitute in Epididymis and Spermatic Cord, Open Approach

♂ **0VWM0KZ** Revision of Nonautologous Tissue Substitute in Epididymis and Spermatic Cord, Open Approach

♂ **0VWM30Z** Revision of Drainage Device in Epididymis and Spermatic Cord, Percutaneous Approach

♂ **0VWM33Z** Revision of Infusion Device in Epididymis and Spermatic Cord, Percutaneous Approach

♂ **0VWM37Z** Revision of Autologous Tissue Substitute in Epididymis and Spermatic Cord, Percutaneous Approach

♂ **0VWM3CZ** Revision of Extraluminal Device in Epididymis and Spermatic Cord, Percutaneous Approach

♂ **0VWM3JZ** Revision of Synthetic Substitute in Epididymis and Spermatic Cord, Percutaneous Approach

♂ **0VWM3KZ** Revision of Nonautologous Tissue Substitute in Epididymis and Spermatic Cord, Percutaneous Approach

♂ **0VWM40Z** Revision of Drainage Device in Epididymis and Spermatic Cord, Percutaneous Endoscopic Approach

♂ **0VWM43Z** Revision of Infusion Device in Epididymis and Spermatic Cord, Percutaneous Endoscopic Approach

♂ **0VWM47Z** Revision of Autologous Tissue Substitute in Epididymis and Spermatic Cord, Percutaneous Endoscopic Approach

♂ **0VWM4CZ** Revision of Extraluminal Device in Epididymis and Spermatic Cord, Percutaneous Endoscopic Approach

♂ **0VWM4JZ** Revision of Synthetic Substitute in Epididymis and Spermatic Cord, Percutaneous Endoscopic Approach

♂ **0VWM4KZ** Revision of Nonautologous Tissue Substitute in Epididymis and Spermatic Cord, Percutaneous Endoscopic Approach

♂ **0VWM70Z** Revision of Drainage Device in Epididymis and Spermatic Cord, Via Natural or Artificial Opening

♂ **0VWM73Z** Revision of Infusion Device in Epididymis and Spermatic Cord, Via Natural or Artificial Opening

♂ **0VWM77Z** Revision of Autologous Tissue Substitute in Epididymis and Spermatic Cord, Via Natural or Artificial Opening

♂ **0VWM7CZ** Revision of Extraluminal Device in Epididymis and Spermatic Cord, Via Natural or Artificial Opening

♂ **0VWM7JZ** Revision of Synthetic Substitute in Epididymis and Spermatic Cord, Via Natural or Artificial Opening

♂ **0VWM7KZ** Revision of Nonautologous Tissue Substitute in Epididymis and Spermatic Cord, Via Natural or Artificial Opening

♂ **0VWM80Z** Revision of Drainage Device in Epididymis and Spermatic Cord, Via Natural or Artificial Opening Endoscopic

♂ **0VWM83Z** Revision of Infusion Device in Epididymis and Spermatic Cord, Via Natural or Artificial Opening Endoscopic

♂ **0VWM87Z** Revision of Autologous Tissue Substitute in Epididymis and Spermatic Cord, Via Natural or Artificial Opening Endoscopic

♂ **0VWM8CZ** Revision of Extraluminal Device in Epididymis and Spermatic Cord, Via Natural or Artificial Opening Endoscopic

♂ **0VWM8JZ** Revision of Synthetic Substitute in Epididymis and Spermatic Cord, Via Natural or Artificial Opening Endoscopic

♂ **0VWM8KZ** Revision of Nonautologous Tissue Substitute in Epididymis and Spermatic Cord, Via Natural or Artificial Opening Endoscopic

♂ **0VWMX0Z** Revision of Drainage Device in Epididymis and Spermatic Cord, External Approach

♂ **0VWMX3Z** Revision of Infusion Device in Epididymis and Spermatic Cord, External Approach

♂ **0VWMX7Z** Revision of Autologous Tissue Substitute in Epididymis and Spermatic Cord, External Approach

♂ **0VWMXCZ** Revision of Extraluminal Device in Epididymis and Spermatic Cord, External Approach

♂ **0VWMXJZ** Revision of Synthetic Substitute in Epididymis and Spermatic Cord, External Approach

♂ **0VWMXKZ** Revision of Nonautologous Tissue Substitute in Epididymis and Spermatic Cord, External Approach

♂ **0VWR00Z** Revision of Drainage Device in Vas Deferens, Open Approach

♂ **0VWR03Z** Revision of Infusion Device in Vas Deferens, Open Approach

♂ **0VWR07Z** Revision of Autologous Tissue Substitute in Vas Deferens, Open Approach

♂ **0VWR0CZ** Revision of Extraluminal Device in Vas Deferens, Open Approach

♂ **0VWR0DZ** Revision of Intraluminal Device in Vas Deferens, Open Approach

♂ **0VWR0JZ** Revision of Synthetic Substitute in Vas Deferens, Open Approach

♂ **0VWR0KZ** Revision of Nonautologous Tissue Substitute in Vas Deferens, Open Approach

♂ **0VWR30Z** Revision of Drainage Device in Vas Deferens, Percutaneous Approach

♂ **0VWR33Z** Revision of Infusion Device in Vas Deferens, Percutaneous Approach

♂ **0VWR37Z** Revision of Autologous Tissue Substitute in Vas Deferens, Percutaneo[us] Approach

♂ **0VWR3CZ** Revision of Extraluminal Device in Va[s] Deferens, Percutaneous Approach

♂ **0VWR3DZ** Revision of Intraluminal Device in Vas Deferens, Percutaneous Approach

♂ **0VWR3JZ** Revision of Synthetic Substitute in Vas Deferens, Percutaneous Approach

♂ **0VWR3KZ** Revision of Nonautologous Tissue Substitute in Vas Deferens, Percutaneo[us] Approach

♂ **0VWR40Z** Revision of Drainage Device in Vas Deferens, Percutaneous Endoscopic Approach

♂ **0VWR43Z** Revision of Infusion Device in Vas Deferens, Percutaneous Endoscopic Approach

♂ **0VWR47Z** Revision of Autologous Tissue Substitute in Vas Deferens, Percutaneo[us] Endoscopic Approach

♂ **0VWR4CZ** Revision of Extraluminal Device in Vas Deferens, Percutaneous Endoscopic Approach

♂ **0VWR4DZ** Revision of Intraluminal Device in Vas Deferens, Percutaneous Endoscopic Approach

♂ **0VWR4JZ** Revision of Synthetic Substitute in Vas Deferens, Percutaneous Endoscopic Approach

♂ **0VWR4KZ** Revision of Nonautologous Tissue Substitute in Vas Deferens, Percutaneo[us] Endoscopic Approach

♂ **0VWR70Z** Revision of Drainage Device in Vas Deferens, Via Natural or Artificial Opening

♂ **0VWR73Z** Revision of Infusion Device in Vas Deferens, Via Natural or Artificial Opening

♂ **0VWR77Z** Revision of Autologous Tissue Substitute in Vas Deferens, Via Natural or Artificial Opening

♂ **0VWR7CZ** Revision of Extraluminal Device in Vas Deferens, Via Natural or Artificial Opening

♂ **0VWR7DZ** Revision of Intraluminal Device in Vas Deferens, Via Natural or Artificial Opening

♂ **0VWR7JZ** Revision of Synthetic Substitute in Vas Deferens, Via Natural or Artificial Opening

♂ **0VWR7KZ** Revision of Nonautologous Tissue Substitute in Vas Deferens, Via Natural or Artificial Opening

♂ **0VWR80Z** Revision of Drainage Device in Vas Deferens, Via Natural or Artificial Opening Endoscopic

♂ **0VWR83Z** Revision of Infusion Device in Vas Deferens, Via Natural or Artificial Opening Endoscopic

♂ **0VWR87Z** Revision of Autologous Tissue Substitute in Vas Deferens, Via Natural or Artificial Opening Endoscopic

♂ **0VWR8CZ** Revision of Extraluminal Device in Vas Deferens, Via Natural or Artificial Opening Endoscopic

♂ **0VWR8DZ** Revision of Intraluminal Device in Vas Deferens, Via Natural or Artificial Opening Endoscopic

♀ Female-only   ♂ Male-only   ▲ Limited Coverage   ● Non-OR   ▦ HAC-associated procedure   ▲ Non-covered procedures   ➕ Combination

VWR8JZ	Revision of Synthetic Substitute in Vas Deferens, Via Natural or Artificial Opening Endoscopic	♂ **0VWS0KZ**	Revision of Nonautologous Tissue Substitute in Penis, Open Approach	♂ **0VWS77Z**	Revision of Autologous Tissue Substitute in Penis, Via Natural or Artificial Opening
VWR8KZ	Revision of Nonautologous Tissue Substitute in Vas Deferens, Via Natural or Artificial Opening Endoscopic	♂ **0VWS30Z**	Revision of Drainage Device in Penis, Percutaneous Approach	♂ **0VWS7JZ**	Revision of Synthetic Substitute in Penis, Via Natural or Artificial Opening
VWRX0Z	Revision of Drainage Device in Vas Deferens, External Approach	♂ **0VWS33Z**	Revision of Infusion Device in Penis, Percutaneous Approach	♂ **0VWS7KZ**	Revision of Nonautologous Tissue Substitute in Penis, Via Natural or Artificial Opening
VWRX3Z	Revision of Infusion Device in Vas Deferens, External Approach	♂ **0VWS37Z**	Revision of Autologous Tissue Substitute in Penis, Percutaneous Approach	♂ **0VWS80Z**	Revision of Drainage Device in Penis, Via Natural or Artificial Opening Endoscopic
VWRX7Z	Revision of Autologous Tissue Substitute in Vas Deferens, External Approach	♂ **0VWS3JZ**	Revision of Synthetic Substitute in Penis, Percutaneous Approach	♂ **0VWS83Z**	Revision of Infusion Device in Penis, Via Natural or Artificial Opening Endoscopic
0VWRXCZ	Revision of Extraluminal Device in Vas Deferens, External Approach	♂ **0VWS3KZ**	Revision of Nonautologous Tissue Substitute in Penis, Percutaneous Approach	♂ **0VWS87Z**	Revision of Autologous Tissue Substitute in Penis, Via Natural or Artificial Opening Endoscopic
0VWRXDZ	Revision of Intraluminal Device in Vas Deferens, External Approach	♂ **0VWS40Z**	Revision of Drainage Device in Penis, Percutaneous Endoscopic Approach	♂ **0VWS8JZ**	Revision of Synthetic Substitute in Penis, Via Natural or Artificial Opening Endoscopic
0VWRXJZ	Revision of Synthetic Substitute in Vas Deferens, External Approach	♂ **0VWS43Z**	Revision of Infusion Device in Penis, Percutaneous Endoscopic Approach	♂ **0VWS8KZ**	Revision of Nonautologous Tissue Substitute in Penis, Via Natural or Artificial Opening Endoscopic
0VWRXKZ	Revision of Nonautologous Tissue Substitute in Vas Deferens, External Approach	♂ **0VWS47Z**	Revision of Autologous Tissue Substitute in Penis, Percutaneous Endoscopic Approach	♂ **0VWSX0Z**	Revision of Drainage Device in Penis, External Approach
0VWS00Z	Revision of Drainage Device in Penis, Open Approach	♂ **0VWS4JZ**	Revision of Synthetic Substitute in Penis, Percutaneous Endoscopic Approach	♂ **0VWSX3Z**	Revision of Infusion Device in Penis, External Approach
0VWS03Z	Revision of Infusion Device in Penis, Open Approach	♂ **0VWS4KZ**	Revision of Nonautologous Tissue Substitute in Penis, Percutaneous Endoscopic Approach	♂ **0VWSX7Z**	Revision of Autologous Tissue Substitute in Penis, External Approach
0VWS07Z	Revision of Autologous Tissue Substitute in Penis, Open Approach	♂ **0VWS70Z**	Revision of Drainage Device in Penis, Via Natural or Artificial Opening	♂ **0VWSXJZ**	Revision of Synthetic Substitute in Penis, External Approach
0VWS0JZ	Revision of Synthetic Substitute in Penis, Open Approach	♂ **0VWS73Z**	Revision of Infusion Device in Penis, Via Natural or Artificial Opening	♂ **0VWSXKZ**	Revision of Nonautologous Tissue Substitute in Penis, External Approach

---

♀ Female-only ♂ Male-only ▲ Limited Coverage ● Non-OR ▆ HAC-associated procedure ▲ Non-covered procedures ✚ Combination

Body Cavities

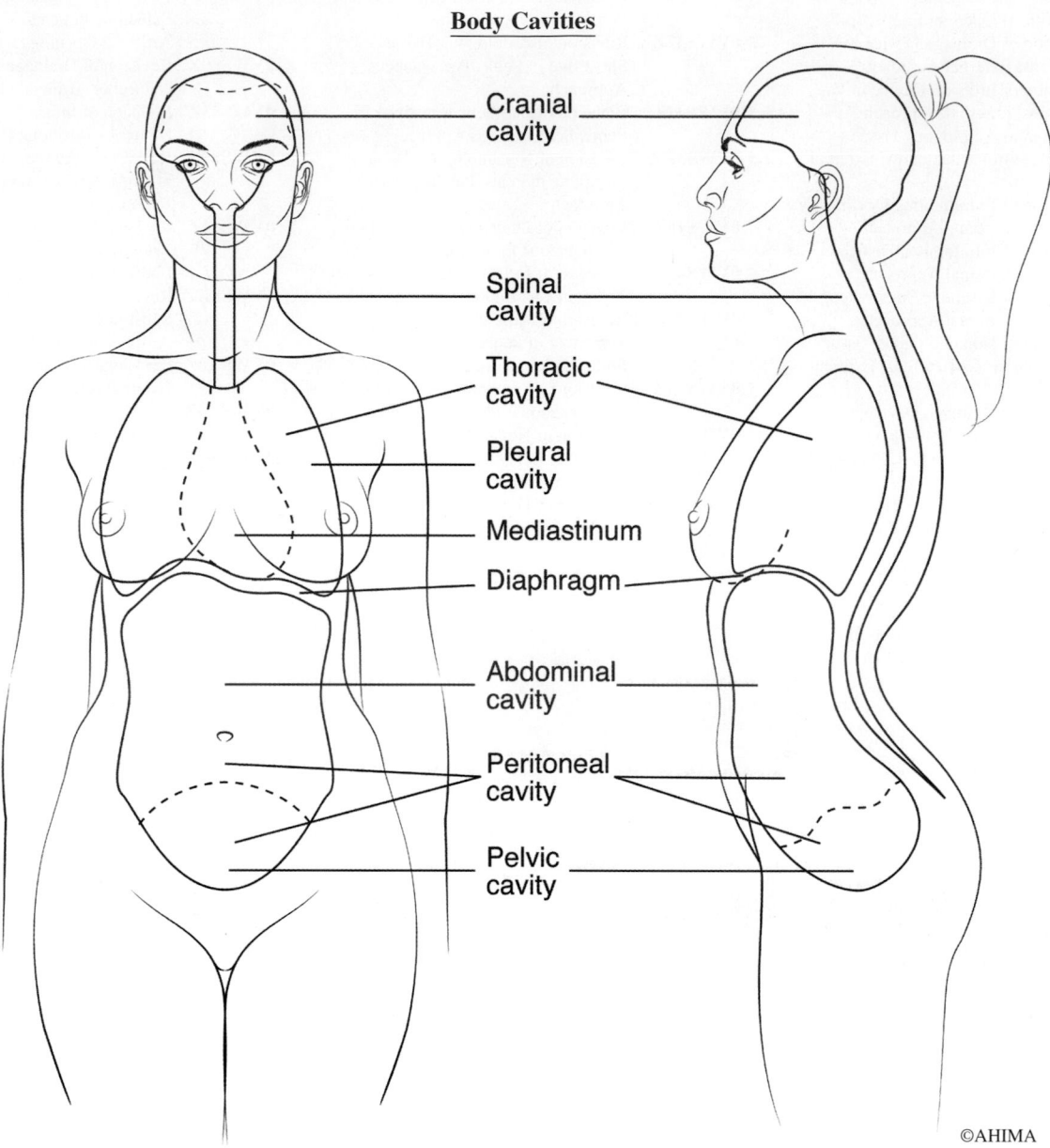

Cranial cavity

Spinal cavity

Thoracic cavity

Pleural cavity

Mediastinum

Diaphragm

Abdominal cavity

Peritoneal cavity

Pelvic cavity

©AHIMA

Body Areas

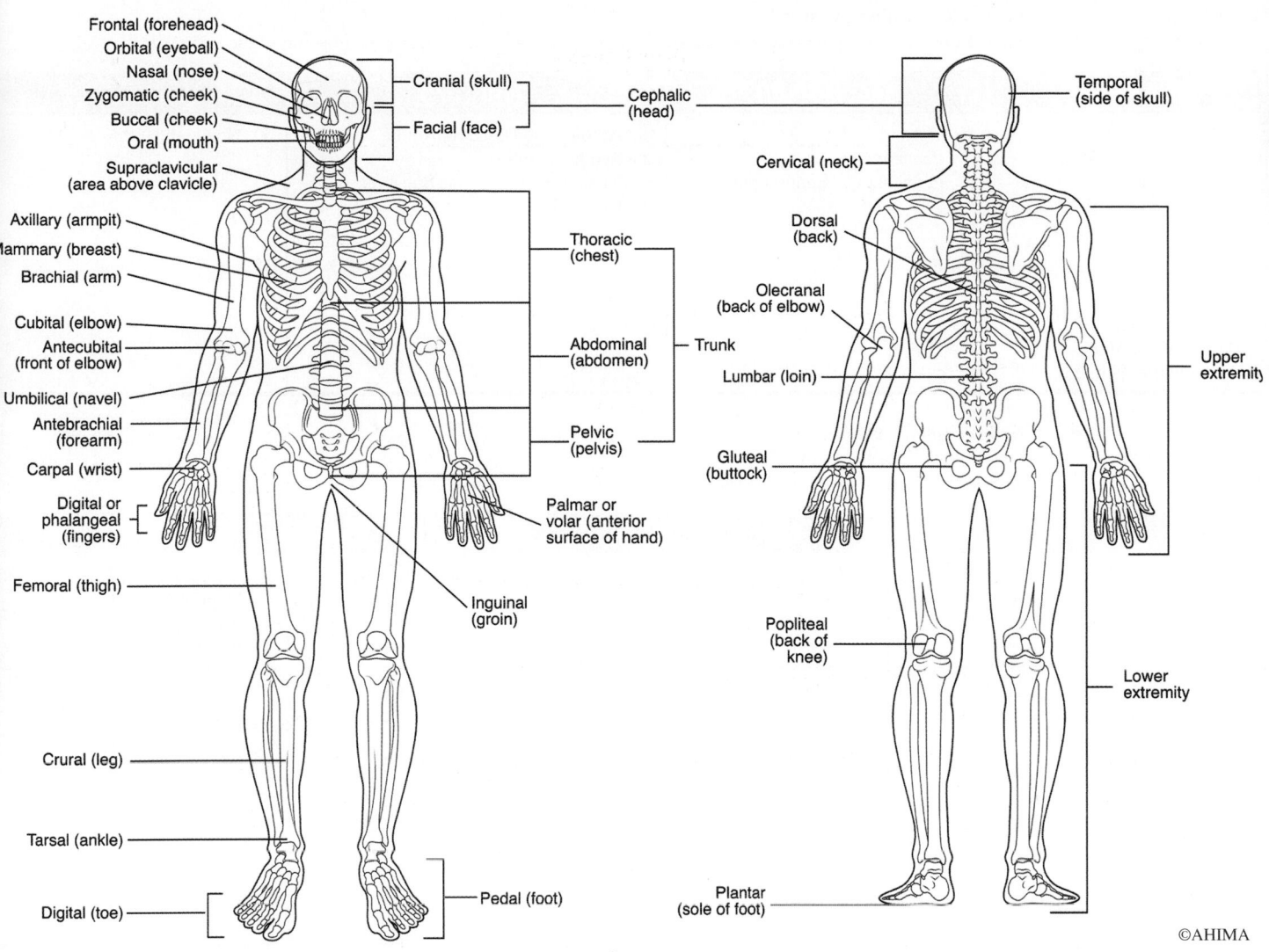

Frontal (forehead)
Orbital (eyeball)
Nasal (nose)
Zygomatic (cheek)
Buccal (cheek)
Oral (mouth)
Supraclavicular (area above clavicle)

Axillary (armpit)
Mammary (breast)
Brachial (arm)

Cubital (elbow)
Antecubital (front of elbow)

Umbilical (navel)
Antebrachial (forearm)

Carpal (wrist)

Digital or phalangeal (fingers)

Femoral (thigh)

Crural (leg)

Tarsal (ankle)

Digital (toe)

Cranial (skull)
Facial (face)

Cephalic (head)

Thoracic (chest)

Abdominal (abdomen)

Trunk

Pelvic (pelvis)

Palmar or volar (anterior surface of hand)

Inguinal (groin)

Pedal (foot)

Temporal (side of skull)

Cervical (neck)

Dorsal (back)

Olecranal (back of elbow)

Lumbar (loin)

Gluteal (buttock)

Popliteal (back of knee)

Plantar (sole of foot)

Upper extremity

Lower extremity

©AHIMA

Anatomical Regions, General Tables 0W0–0WW

Section	0	Medical and Surgical
Body System	W	Anatomical Regions, General
Operation	0	**Alteration:** Modifying the anatomic structure of a body part without affecting the function of the body part

Body Part (4th)	Approach (5th)	Device (6th)	Qualifier (7th)
0 Head	0 Open	7 Autologous Tissue Substitute	Z No Qualifier
2 Face	3 Percutaneous	J Synthetic Substitute	
4 Upper Jaw	4 Percutaneous Endoscopic	K Nonautologous Tissue Substitute	
5 Lower Jaw		Z No Device	
6 Neck			
8 Chest Wall			
F Abdominal Wall			
K Upper Back			
L Lower Back			
M Perineum, Male			
N Perineum, Female			

Section	0	Medical and Surgical
Body System	W	Anatomical Regions, General
Operation	1	**Bypass:** Altering the route of passage of the contents of a tubular body part

Body Part (4th)	Approach (5th)	Device (6th)	Qualifier (7th)
1 Cranial Cavity	0 Open	J Synthetic Substitute	9 Pleural Cavity, Right B Pleural Cavity, Left G Peritoneal Cavity J Pelvic Cavity
9 Pleural Cavity, Right B Pleural Cavity, Left G Peritoneal Cavity J Pelvic Cavity	0 Open 4 Percutaneous Endoscopic	J Synthetic Substitute	4 Cutaneous 9 Pleural Cavity, Right B Pleural Cavity, Left G Peritoneal Cavity J Pelvic Cavity Y Lower Vein
9 Pleural Cavity, Right B Pleural Cavity, Left G Peritoneal Cavity J Pelvic Cavity	3 Percutaneous	J Synthetic Substitute	4 Cutaneous

Section	0	Medical and Surgical
Body System	W	Anatomical Regions, General
Operation	2	**Change:** Taking out or off a device from a body part and putting back an identical or similar device in or on the same body part without cutting or puncturing the skin or a mucous membrane

Body Part (4th)	Approach (5th)	Device (6th)	Qualifier (7th)
0 Head	X External	0 Drainage Device	Z No Qualifier
1 Cranial Cavity		Y Other Device	
2 Face			
4 Upper Jaw			
5 Lower Jaw			
6 Neck			
8 Chest Wall			
9 Pleural Cavity, Right			
B Pleural Cavity, Left			
C Mediastinum			
D Pericardial Cavity			
F Abdominal Wall			
G Peritoneal Cavity			
H Retroperitoneum			
J Pelvic Cavity			
K Upper Back			
L Lower Back			
M Perineum, Male			
N Perineum, Female			

Section	0	Medical and Surgical
Body System	W	Anatomical Regions, General
Operation	3	Control: Stopping, or attempting to stop, postprocedural bleeding

Body Part (4th)	Approach (5th)	Device (6th)	Qualifier (7th)
0 Head 1 Cranial Cavity 2 Face 4 Upper Jaw 5 Lower Jaw 6 Neck 8 Chest Wall 9 Pleural Cavity, Right B Pleural Cavity, Left C Mediastinum D Pericardial Cavity F Abdominal Wall G Peritoneal Cavity H Retroperitoneum J Pelvic Cavity K Upper Back L Lower Back M Perineum, Male N Perineum, Female	0 Open 3 Percutaneous 4 Percutaneous Endoscopic	Z No Device	Z No Qualifier
3 Oral Cavity and Throat	0 Open 3 Percutaneous 4 Percutaneous Endoscopic 7 Via Natural or Artificial Opening 8 Via Natural or Artificial Opening Endoscopic X External	Z No Device	Z No Qualifier
P Gastrointestinal Tract Q Respiratory Tract R Genitourinary Tract	0 Open 3 Percutaneous 4 Percutaneous Endoscopic 7 Via Natural or Artificial Opening 8 Via Natural or Artificial Opening Endoscopic	Z No Device	Z No Qualifier

Section	0	Medical and Surgical
Body System	W	Anatomical Regions, General
Operation	4	Creation: Making a new genital structure that does not take over the function of a body part

Body Part (4th)	Approach (5th)	Device (6th)	Qualifier (7th)
M Perineum, Male	0 Open	7 Autologous Tissue Substitute J Synthetic Substitute K Nonautologous Tissue Substitute Z No Device	0 Vagina
N Perineum, Female	0 Open	7 Autologous Tissue Substitute J Synthetic Substitute K Nonautologous Tissue Substitute Z No Device	1 Penis

Section	0	Medical and Surgical
Body System	W	Anatomical Regions, General
Operation	8	Division: Cutting into a body part, without draining fluids and/or gases from the body part, in order to separate or transect a body part

Body Part (4th)	Approach (5th)	Device (6th)	Qualifier (7th)
N Perineum, Female	X External	Z No Device	Z No Qualifier

Section   0   **Medical and Surgical**
Body System   W   **Anatomical Regions, General**
Operation   9   **Drainage:** Taking or letting out fluids and/or gases from a body part

Body Part (4th)	Approach (5th)	Device (6th)	Qualifier (7th)
0 Head 1 Cranial Cavity 2 Face 3 Oral Cavity and Throat 4 Upper Jaw 5 Lower Jaw 6 Neck 8 Chest Wall 9 Pleural Cavity, Right B Pleural Cavity, Left C Mediastinum D Pericardial Cavity F Abdominal Wall G Peritoneal Cavity H Retroperitoneum J Pelvic Cavity K Upper Back L Lower Back M Perineum, Male N Perineum, Female	0 Open 3 Percutaneous 4 Percutaneous Endoscopic	0 Drainage Device	Z No Qualifier
0 Head 1 Cranial Cavity 2 Face 3 Oral Cavity and Throat 4 Upper Jaw 5 Lower Jaw 6 Neck 8 Chest Wall 9 Pleural Cavity, Right B Pleural Cavity, Left C Mediastinum D Pericardial Cavity F Abdominal Wall G Peritoneal Cavity H Retroperitoneum J Pelvic Cavity K Upper Back L Lower Back M Perineum, Male N Perineum, Female	0 Open 3 Percutaneous 4 Percutaneous Endoscopic	Z No Device	X Diagnostic Z No Qualifier

Section   0   **Medical and Surgical**
Body System   W   **Anatomical Regions, General**
Operation   B   **Excision:** Cutting out or off, without replacement, a portion of a body part

Body Part (4th)	Approach (5th)	Device (6th)	Qualifier (7th)
0 Head 2 Face 4 Upper Jaw 5 Lower Jaw 8 Chest Wall K Upper Back L Lower Back M Perineum, Male N Perineum, Female	0 Open 3 Percutaneous 4 Percutaneous Endoscopic X External	Z No Device	X Diagnostic Z No Qualifier
6 Neck F Abdominal Wall	0 Open 3 Percutaneous 4 Percutaneous Endoscopic	Z No Device	X Diagnostic Z No Qualifier

Continued →

Section	0	Medical and Surgical
Body System	W	Anatomical Regions, General
Operation	B	Excision: Cutting out or off, without replacement, a portion of a body part

Body Part (4th)	Approach (5th)	Device (6th)	Qualifier (7th)
6 Neck F Abdominal Wall	X External	Z No Device	2 Stoma X Diagnostic Z No Qualifier
C Mediastinum H Retroperitoneum	0 Open 3 Percutaneous 4 Percutaneous Endoscopic	Z No Device	X Diagnostic Z No Qualifier

Section	0	Medical and Surgical
Body System	W	Anatomical Regions, General
Operation	C	Extirpation: Taking or cutting out solid matter from a body part

Body Part (4th)	Approach (5th)	Device (6th)	Qualifier (7th)
1 Cranial Cavity 3 Oral Cavity and Throat 9 Pleural Cavity, Right B Pleural Cavity, Left C Mediastinum D Pericardial Cavity G Peritoneal Cavity J Pelvic Cavity	0 Open 3 Percutaneous 4 Percutaneous Endoscopic X External	Z No Device	Z No Qualifier
P Gastrointestinal Tract Q Respiratory Tract R Genitourinary Tract	0 Open 3 Percutaneous 4 Percutaneous Endoscopic 7 Via Natural or Artificial Opening 8 Via Natural or Artificial Opening Endoscopic X External	Z No Device	Z No Qualifier

Section	0	Medical and Surgical
Body System	W	Anatomical Regions, General
Operation	F	Fragmentation: Breaking solid matter in a body part into pieces

Body Part (4th)	Approach (5th)	Device (6th)	Qualifier (7th)
1 Cranial Cavity 3 Oral Cavity and Throat 9 Pleural Cavity, Right B Pleural Cavity, Left C Mediastinum D Pericardial Cavity G Peritoneal Cavity J Pelvic Cavity	0 Open 3 Percutaneous 4 Percutaneous Endoscopic X External	Z No Device	Z No Qualifier
P Gastrointestinal Tract Q Respiratory Tract R Genitourinary Tract	0 Open 3 Percutaneous 4 Percutaneous Endoscopic 7 Via Natural or Artificial Opening 8 Via Natural or Artificial Opening Endoscopic X External	Z No Device	Z No Qualifier

Section   **0**   **Medical and Surgical**
Body System   **W**   **Anatomical Regions, General**
Operation   **H**   **Insertion:** Putting in a nonbiological appliance that monitors, assists, performs, or prevents a physiological function but does not physically take the place of a body part

Body Part (4th)	Approach (5th)	Device (6th)	Qualifier (7th)
0 Head 1 Cranial Cavity 2 Face 3 Oral Cavity and Throat 4 Upper Jaw 5 Lower Jaw 6 Neck 8 Chest Wall 9 Pleural Cavity, Right B Pleural Cavity, Left C Mediastinum D Pericardial Cavity F Abdominal Wall G Peritoneal Cavity H Retroperitoneum J Pelvic Cavity K Upper Back L Lower Back M Perineum, Male N Perineum, Female	0 Open 3 Percutaneous 4 Percutaneous Endoscopic	1 Radioactive Element 3 Infusion Device Y Other Device	Z No Qualifier
P Gastrointestinal Tract Q Respiratory Tract R Genitourinary Tract	0 Open 3 Percutaneous 4 Percutaneous Endoscopic 7 Via Natural or Artificial Opening 8 Via Natural or Artificial Opening Endoscopic	1 Radioactive Element 3 Infusion Device Y Other Device	Z No Qualifier

Section   **0**   **Medical and Surgical**
Body System   **W**   **Anatomical Regions, General**
Operation   **J**   **Inspection:** Visually and/or manually exploring a body part

Body Part (4th)	Approach (5th)	Device (6th)	Qualifier (7th)
0 Head 2 Face 3 Oral Cavity and Throat 4 Upper Jaw 5 Lower Jaw 6 Neck 8 Chest Wall F Abdominal Wall K Upper Back L Lower Back M Perineum, Male N Perineum, Female	0 Open 3 Percutaneous 4 Percutaneous Endoscopic X External	Z No Device	Z No Qualifier
1 Cranial Cavity 9 Pleural Cavity, Right B Pleural Cavity, Left C Mediastinum D Pericardial Cavity G Peritoneal Cavity H Retroperitoneum J Pelvic Cavity	0 Open 3 Percutaneous 4 Percutaneous Endoscopic	Z No Device	Z No Qualifier
P Gastrointestinal Tract Q Respiratory Tract R Genitourinary Tract	0 Open 3 Percutaneous 4 Percutaneous Endoscopic 7 Via Natural or Artificial Opening 8 Via Natural or Artificial Opening Endoscopic	Z No Device	Z No Qualifier

Section 0 Medical and Surgical
Body System W Anatomical Regions, General
Operation M Reattachment: Putting back in or on all or a portion of a separated body part to its normal location or other suitable location

Body Part (4th)	Approach (5th)	Device (6th)	Qualifier (7th)
2 Face 4 Upper Jaw 5 Lower Jaw 6 Neck 8 Chest Wall F Abdominal Wall K Upper Back L Lower Back M Perineum, Male N Perineum, Female	0 Open	Z No Device	Z No Qualifier

Section 0 Medical and Surgical
Body System W Anatomical Regions, General
Operation P Removal: Taking out or off a device from a body part

Body Part (4th)	Approach (5th)	Device (6th)	Qualifier (7th)
0 Head 2 Face 4 Upper Jaw 5 Lower Jaw 6 Neck 8 Chest Wall C Mediastinum F Abdominal Wall K Upper Back L Lower Back M Perineum, Male N Perineum, Female	0 Open 3 Percutaneous 4 Percutaneous Endoscopic X External	0 Drainage Device 1 Radioactive Element 3 Infusion Device 7 Autologous Tissue Substitute J Synthetic Substitute K Nonautologous Tissue Substitute Y Other Device	Z No Qualifier
1 Cranial Cavity 9 Pleural Cavity, Right B Pleural Cavity, Left G Peritoneal Cavity J Pelvic Cavity	0 Open 3 Percutaneous 4 Percutaneous Endoscopic	0 Drainage Device 1 Radioactive Element 3 Infusion Device J Synthetic Substitute Y Other Device	Z No Qualifier
1 Cranial Cavity 9 Pleural Cavity, Right B Pleural Cavity, Left G Peritoneal Cavity J Pelvic Cavity	X External	0 Drainage Device 1 Radioactive Element 3 Infusion Device	Z No Qualifier
D Pericardial Cavity H Retroperitoneum	0 Open 3 Percutaneous 4 Percutaneous Endoscopic	0 Drainage Device 1 Radioactive Element 3 Infusion Device Y Other Device	Z No Qualifier
D Pericardial Cavity H Retroperitoneum	X External	0 Drainage Device 1 Radioactive Element 3 Infusion Device	Z No Qualifier
P Gastrointestinal Tract Q Respiratory Tract R Genitourinary Tract	0 Open 3 Percutaneous 4 Percutaneous Endoscopic 7 Via Natural or Artificial Opening 8 Via Natural or Artificial Opening Endoscopic X External	1 Radioactive Element 3 Infusion Device Y Other Device	Z No Qualifier

Section   **0**   **Medical and Surgical**
Body System   **W**   **Anatomical Regions, General**
Operation   **Q**   **Repair:** Restoring, to the extent possible, a body part to its normal anatomic structure and function

Body Part (4th)	Approach (5th)	Device (6th)	Qualifier (7th)
0 Head 2 Face 4 Upper Jaw 5 Lower Jaw 8 Chest Wall K Upper Back L Lower Back M Perineum, Male N Perineum, Female	0 Open 3 Percutaneous 4 Percutaneous Endoscopic X External	Z No Device	Z No Qualifier
6 Neck F Abdominal Wall	0 Open 3 Percutaneous 4 Percutaneous Endoscopic	Z No Device	Z No Qualifier
6 Neck F Abdominal Wall	X External	Z No Device	2 Stoma Z No Qualifier
C Mediastinum	0 Open 3 Percutaneous 4 Percutaneous Endoscopic	Z No Device	Z No Qualifier

Section   **0**   **Medical and Surgical**
Body System   **W**   **Anatomical Regions, General**
Operation   **U**   **Supplement:** Putting in or on biological or synthetic material that physically reinforces and/or augments the function of a portion of a body part

Body Part (4th)	Approach (5th)	Device (6th)	Qualifier (7th)
0 Head 2 Face 4 Upper Jaw 5 Lower Jaw 6 Neck 8 Chest Wall C Mediastinum F Abdominal Wall K Upper Back L Lower Back M Perineum, Male N Perineum, Female	0 Open 4 Percutaneous Endoscopic	7 Autologous Tissue Substitute J Synthetic Substitute K Nonautologous Tissue Substitute	Z No Qualifier

Section   **0**   **Medical and Surgical**
Body System   **W**   **Anatomical Regions, General**
Operation   **W**   **Revision:** Correcting, to the extent possible, a portion of a malfunctioning device or the position of a displaced device

Body Part (4th)	Approach (5th)	Device (6th)	Qualifier (7th)
0 Head 2 Face 4 Upper Jaw 5 Lower Jaw 6 Neck 8 Chest Wall C Mediastinum F Abdominal Wall K Upper Back L Lower Back M Perineum, Male N Perineum, Female	0 Open 3 Percutaneous 4 Percutaneous Endoscopic X External	0 Drainage Device 1 Radioactive Element 3 Infusion Device 7 Autologous Tissue Substitute J Synthetic Substitute K Nonautologous Tissue Substitute Y Other Device	Z No Qualifier

Continued →

				Section	0	Medical and Surgical	

Section   0   **Medical and Surgical**
Body System   W   **Anatomical Regions, General**
Operation   W   **Revision:** Correcting, to the extent possible, a portion of a malfunctioning device or the position of a displaced device

Body Part (4th)	Approach (5th)	Device (6th)	Qualifier (7th)
1 Cranial Cavity 9 Pleural Cavity, Right B Pleural Cavity, Left G Peritoneal Cavity J Pelvic Cavity	0 Open 3 Percutaneous 4 Percutaneous Endoscopic X External	0 Drainage Device 1 Radioactive Element 3 Infusion Device J Synthetic Substitute Y Other Device	Z No Qualifier
D Pericardial Cavity H Retroperitoneum	0 Open 3 Percutaneous 4 Percutaneous Endoscopic X External	0 Drainage Device 1 Radioactive Element 3 Infusion Device Y Other Device	Z No Qualifier
P Gastrointestinal Tract Q Respiratory Tract R Genitourinary Tract	0 Open 3 Percutaneous 4 Percutaneous Endoscopic 7 Via Natural or Artificial Opening 8 Via Natural or Artificial Opening Endoscopic X External	1 Radioactive Element 3 Infusion Device Y Other Device	Z No Qualifier

Anatomical Regions, General Code Listing 0W0–0WW

0W0 – Anatomical Regions, General, Alteration

0W0007Z   Alteration of Head with Autologous Tissue Substitute, Open Approach
0W000JZ   Alteration of Head with Synthetic Substitute, Open Approach
0W000KZ   Alteration of Head with Nonautologous Tissue Substitute, Open Approach
0W000ZZ   Alteration of Head, Open Approach
0W0037Z   Alteration of Head with Autologous Tissue Substitute, Percutaneous Approach
0W003JZ   Alteration of Head with Synthetic Substitute, Percutaneous Approach
0W003KZ   Alteration of Head with Nonautologous Tissue Substitute, Percutaneous Approach
0W003ZZ   Alteration of Head, Percutaneous Approach
0W0047Z   Alteration of Head with Autologous Tissue Substitute, Percutaneous Endoscopic Approach
0W004JZ   Alteration of Head with Synthetic Substitute, Percutaneous Endoscopic Approach
0W004KZ   Alteration of Head with Nonautologous Tissue Substitute, Percutaneous Endoscopic Approach
0W004ZZ   Alteration of Head, Percutaneous Endoscopic Approach
0W0207Z   Alteration of Face with Autologous Tissue Substitute, Open Approach
0W020JZ   Alteration of Face with Synthetic Substitute, Open Approach
0W020KZ   Alteration of Face with Nonautologous Tissue Substitute, Open Approach
0W020ZZ   Alteration of Face, Open Approach
    AHA CC: 1Q, 2015, 31
0W0237Z   Alteration of Face with Autologous Tissue Substitute, Percutaneous Approach
0W023JZ   Alteration of Face with Synthetic Substitute, Percutaneous Approach
0W023KZ   Alteration of Face with Nonautologous Tissue Substitute, Percutaneous Approach
0W023ZZ   Alteration of Face, Percutaneous Approach
0W0247Z   Alteration of Face with Autologous Tissue Substitute, Percutaneous Endoscopic Approach

0W024JZ   Alteration of Face with Synthetic Substitute, Percutaneous Endoscopic Approach
0W024KZ   Alteration of Face with Nonautologous Tissue Substitute, Percutaneous Endoscopic Approach
0W024ZZ   Alteration of Face, Percutaneous Endoscopic Approach
0W0407Z   Alteration of Upper Jaw with Autologous Tissue Substitute, Open Approach
0W040JZ   Alteration of Upper Jaw with Synthetic Substitute, Open Approach
0W040KZ   Alteration of Upper Jaw with Nonautologous Tissue Substitute, Open Approach
0W040ZZ   Alteration of Upper Jaw, Open Approach
0W0437Z   Alteration of Upper Jaw with Autologous Tissue Substitute, Percutaneous Approach
0W043JZ   Alteration of Upper Jaw with Synthetic Substitute, Percutaneous Approach
0W043KZ   Alteration of Upper Jaw with Nonautologous Tissue Substitute, Percutaneous Approach
0W043ZZ   Alteration of Upper Jaw, Percutaneous Approach
0W0447Z   Alteration of Upper Jaw with Autologous Tissue Substitute, Percutaneous Endoscopic Approach
0W044JZ   Alteration of Upper Jaw with Synthetic Substitute, Percutaneous Endoscopic Approach
0W044KZ   Alteration of Upper Jaw with Nonautologous Tissue Substitute, Percutaneous Endoscopic Approach
0W044ZZ   Alteration of Upper Jaw, Percutaneous Endoscopic Approach
0W0507Z   Alteration of Lower Jaw with Autologous Tissue Substitute, Open Approach
0W050JZ   Alteration of Lower Jaw with Synthetic Substitute, Open Approach
0W050KZ   Alteration of Lower Jaw with Nonautologous Tissue Substitute, Open Approach
0W050ZZ   Alteration of Lower Jaw, Open Approach

0W0537Z   Alteration of Lower Jaw with Autologous Tissue Substitute, Percutaneous Approach
0W053JZ   Alteration of Lower Jaw with Synthetic Substitute, Percutaneous Approach
0W053KZ   Alteration of Lower Jaw with Nonautologous Tissue Substitute, Percutaneous Approach
0W053ZZ   Alteration of Lower Jaw, Percutaneous Approach
0W0547Z   Alteration of Lower Jaw with Autologous Tissue Substitute, Percutaneous Endoscopic Approach
0W054JZ   Alteration of Lower Jaw with Synthetic Substitute, Percutaneous Endoscopic Approach
0W054KZ   Alteration of Lower Jaw with Nonautologous Tissue Substitute, Percutaneous Endoscopic Approach
0W054ZZ   Alteration of Lower Jaw, Percutaneous Endoscopic Approach
0W0607Z   Alteration of Neck with Autologous Tissue Substitute, Open Approach
0W060JZ   Alteration of Neck with Synthetic Substitute, Open Approach
0W060KZ   Alteration of Neck with Nonautologous Tissue Substitute, Open Approach
0W060ZZ   Alteration of Neck, Open Approach
0W0637Z   Alteration of Neck with Autologous Tissue Substitute, Percutaneous Approach
0W063JZ   Alteration of Neck with Synthetic Substitute, Percutaneous Approach
0W063KZ   Alteration of Neck with Nonautologous Tissue Substitute, Percutaneous Approach
0W063ZZ   Alteration of Neck, Percutaneous Approach
0W0647Z   Alteration of Neck with Autologous Tissue Substitute, Percutaneous Endoscopic Approach
0W064JZ   Alteration of Neck with Synthetic Substitute, Percutaneous Endoscopic Approach
0W064KZ   Alteration of Neck with Nonautologous Tissue Substitute, Percutaneous Endoscopic Approach

♀ Female-only   ♂ Male-only   ▲ Limited Coverage   ● Non-OR   ▦ HAC-associated procedure   ▲ Non-covered procedures   ✚ Combination

0W064ZZ Alteration of Neck, Percutaneous Endoscopic Approach

0W0807Z Alteration of Chest Wall with Autologous Tissue Substitute, Open Approach

0W080JZ Alteration of Chest Wall with Synthetic Substitute, Open Approach

0W080KZ Alteration of Chest Wall with Nonautologous Tissue Substitute, Open Approach

0W080ZZ Alteration of Chest Wall, Open Approach

0W0837Z Alteration of Chest Wall with Autologous Tissue Substitute, Percutaneous Approach

0W083JZ Alteration of Chest Wall with Synthetic Substitute, Percutaneous Approach

0W083KZ Alteration of Chest Wall with Nonautologous Tissue Substitute, Percutaneous Approach

0W083ZZ Alteration of Chest Wall, Percutaneous Approach

0W0847Z Alteration of Chest Wall with Autologous Tissue Substitute, Percutaneous Endoscopic Approach

0W084JZ Alteration of Chest Wall with Synthetic Substitute, Percutaneous Endoscopic Approach

0W084KZ Alteration of Chest Wall with Nonautologous Tissue Substitute, Percutaneous Endoscopic Approach

0W084ZZ Alteration of Chest Wall, Percutaneous Endoscopic Approach

0W0F07Z Alteration of Abdominal Wall with Autologous Tissue Substitute, Open Approach

0W0F0JZ Alteration of Abdominal Wall with Synthetic Substitute, Open Approach

0W0F0KZ Alteration of Abdominal Wall with Nonautologous Tissue Substitute, Open Approach

0W0F0ZZ Alteration of Abdominal Wall, Open Approach

0W0F37Z Alteration of Abdominal Wall with Autologous Tissue Substitute, Percutaneous Approach

0W0F3JZ Alteration of Abdominal Wall with Synthetic Substitute, Percutaneous Approach

0W0F3KZ Alteration of Abdominal Wall with Nonautologous Tissue Substitute, Percutaneous Approach

0W0F3ZZ Alteration of Abdominal Wall, Percutaneous Approach

0W0F47Z Alteration of Abdominal Wall with Autologous Tissue Substitute, Percutaneous Endoscopic Approach

0W0F4JZ Alteration of Abdominal Wall with Synthetic Substitute, Percutaneous Endoscopic Approach

0W0F4KZ Alteration of Abdominal Wall with Nonautologous Tissue Substitute, Percutaneous Endoscopic Approach

0W0F4ZZ Alteration of Abdominal Wall, Percutaneous Endoscopic Approach

0W0K07Z Alteration of Upper Back with Autologous Tissue Substitute, Open Approach

0W0K0JZ Alteration of Upper Back with Synthetic Substitute, Open Approach

0W0K0KZ Alteration of Upper Back with Nonautologous Tissue Substitute, Open Approach

0W0K0ZZ Alteration of Upper Back, Open Approach

0W0K37Z Alteration of Upper Back with Autologous Tissue Substitute, Percutaneous Approach

0W0K3JZ Alteration of Upper Back with Synthetic Substitute, Percutaneous Approach

0W0K3KZ Alteration of Upper Back with Nonautologous Tissue Substitute, Percutaneous Approach

0W0K3ZZ Alteration of Upper Back, Percutaneous Approach

0W0K47Z Alteration of Upper Back with Autologous Tissue Substitute, Percutaneous Endoscopic Approach

0W0K4JZ Alteration of Upper Back with Synthetic Substitute, Percutaneous Endoscopic Approach

0W0K4KZ Alteration of Upper Back with Nonautologous Tissue Substitute, Percutaneous Endoscopic Approach

0W0K4ZZ Alteration of Upper Back, Percutaneous Endoscopic Approach

0W0L07Z Alteration of Lower Back with Autologous Tissue Substitute, Open Approach

0W0L0JZ Alteration of Lower Back with Synthetic Substitute, Open Approach

0W0L0KZ Alteration of Lower Back with Nonautologous Tissue Substitute, Open Approach

0W0L0ZZ Alteration of Lower Back, Open Approach

0W0L37Z Alteration of Lower Back with Autologous Tissue Substitute, Percutaneous Approach

0W0L3JZ Alteration of Lower Back with Synthetic Substitute, Percutaneous Approach

0W0L3KZ Alteration of Lower Back with Nonautologous Tissue Substitute, Percutaneous Approach

0W0L3ZZ Alteration of Lower Back, Percutaneous Approach

0W0L47Z Alteration of Lower Back with Autologous Tissue Substitute, Percutaneous Endoscopic Approach

0W0L4JZ Alteration of Lower Back with Synthetic Substitute, Percutaneous Endoscopic Approach

0W0L4KZ Alteration of Lower Back with Nonautologous Tissue Substitute, Percutaneous Endoscopic Approach

0W0L4ZZ Alteration of Lower Back, Percutaneous Endoscopic Approach

♂ **0W0M07Z** Alteration of Male Perineum with Autologous Tissue Substitute, Open Approach

♂ **0W0M0JZ** Alteration of Male Perineum with Synthetic Substitute, Open Approach

♂ **0W0M0KZ** Alteration of Male Perineum with Nonautologous Tissue Substitute, Open Approach

♂ **0W0M0ZZ** Alteration of Male Perineum, Open Approach

♂ **0W0M37Z** Alteration of Male Perineum with Autologous Tissue Substitute, Percutaneous Approach

♂ **0W0M3JZ** Alteration of Male Perineum with Synthetic Substitute, Percutaneous Approach

♂ **0W0M3KZ** Alteration of Male Perineum with Nonautologous Tissue Substitute, Percutaneous Approach

♂ **0W0M3ZZ** Alteration of Male Perineum, Percutaneous Approach

♂ **0W0M47Z** Alteration of Male Perineum with Autologous Tissue Substitute, Percutaneous Endoscopic Approach

♂ **0W0M4JZ** Alteration of Male Perineum with Synthetic Substitute, Percutaneous Endoscopic Approach

♂ **0W0M4KZ** Alteration of Male Perineum with Nonautologous Tissue Substitute, Percutaneous Endoscopic Approach

♂ **0W0M4ZZ** Alteration of Male Perineum, Percutaneous Endoscopic Approach

♀ **0W0N07Z** Alteration of Female Perineum with Autologous Tissue Substitute, Open Approach

♀ **0W0N0JZ** Alteration of Female Perineum with Synthetic Substitute, Open Approach

♀ **0W0N0KZ** Alteration of Female Perineum with Nonautologous Tissue Substitute, Open Approach

♀ **0W0N0ZZ** Alteration of Female Perineum, Open Approach

♀ **0W0N37Z** Alteration of Female Perineum with Autologous Tissue Substitute, Percutaneous Approach

♀ **0W0N3JZ** Alteration of Female Perineum with Synthetic Substitute, Percutaneous Approach

♀ **0W0N3KZ** Alteration of Female Perineum with Nonautologous Tissue Substitute, Percutaneous Approach

♀ **0W0N3ZZ** Alteration of Female Perineum, Percutaneous Approach

♀ **0W0N47Z** Alteration of Female Perineum with Autologous Tissue Substitute, Percutaneous Endoscopic Approach

♀ **0W0N4JZ** Alteration of Female Perineum with Synthetic Substitute, Percutaneous Endoscopic Approach

♀ **0W0N4KZ** Alteration of Female Perineum with Nonautologous Tissue Substitute, Percutaneous Endoscopic Approach

♀ **0W0N4ZZ** Alteration of Female Perineum, Percutaneous Endoscopic Approach

0W1 – Anatomical Regions, General, Bypass

Review Coding Guideline B3.6a

0W110J9 Bypass Cranial Cavity to Right Pleural Cavity with Synthetic Substitute, Open Approach

0W110JB Bypass Cranial Cavity to Left Pleural Cavity with Synthetic Substitute, Open Approach

0W110JG Bypass Cranial Cavity to Peritoneal Cavity with Synthetic Substitute, Open Approach

0W110JJ Bypass Cranial Cavity to Pelvic Cavity with Synthetic Substitute, Open Approach

0W190J4 Bypass Right Pleural Cavity to Cutaneous with Synthetic Substitute, Open Approach

0W190J9 Bypass Right Pleural Cavity to Right Pleural Cavity with Synthetic Substitute, Open Approach

0W190JB Bypass Right Pleural Cavity to Left Pleural Cavity with Synthetic Substitute, Open Approach

0W190JG Bypass Right Pleural Cavity to Peritoneal Cavity with Synthetic Substitute, Open Approach

0W190JJ Bypass Right Pleural Cavity to Pelvic Cavity with Synthetic Substitute, Open Approach

0W190JY Bypass Right Pleural Cavity to Lower Vein with Synthetic Substitute, Open Approach

0W193J4 Bypass Right Pleural Cavity to Cutaneous with Synthetic Substitute, Percutaneous Approach

0W194J4 Bypass Right Pleural Cavity to Cutaneous with Synthetic Substitute, Percutaneous Endoscopic Approach

194J9	Bypass Right Pleural Cavity to Right Pleural Cavity with Synthetic Substitute, Percutaneous Endoscopic Approach
194JB	Bypass Right Pleural Cavity to Left Pleural Cavity with Synthetic Substitute, Percutaneous Endoscopic Approach
194JG	Bypass Right Pleural Cavity to Peritoneal Cavity with Synthetic Substitute, Percutaneous Endoscopic Approach
194JJ	Bypass Right Pleural Cavity to Pelvic Cavity with Synthetic Substitute, Percutaneous Endoscopic Approach
194JY	Bypass Right Pleural Cavity to Lower Vein with Synthetic Substitute, Percutaneous Endoscopic Approach
1B0J4	Bypass Left Pleural Cavity to Cutaneous with Synthetic Substitute, Open Approach
1B0J9	Bypass Left Pleural Cavity to Right Pleural Cavity with Synthetic Substitute, Open Approach
1B0JB	Bypass Left Pleural Cavity to Left Pleural Cavity with Synthetic Substitute, Open Approach
1B0JG	Bypass Left Pleural Cavity to Peritoneal Cavity with Synthetic Substitute, Open Approach
1B0JJ	Bypass Left Pleural Cavity to Pelvic Cavity with Synthetic Substitute, Open Approach
1B0JY	Bypass Left Pleural Cavity to Lower Vein with Synthetic Substitute, Open Approach
1B3J4	Bypass Left Pleural Cavity to Cutaneous with Synthetic Substitute, Percutaneous Approach
1B4J4	Bypass Left Pleural Cavity to Cutaneous with Synthetic Substitute, Percutaneous Endoscopic Approach
1B4J9	Bypass Left Pleural Cavity to Right Pleural Cavity with Synthetic Substitute, Percutaneous Endoscopic Approach
1B4JB	Bypass Left Pleural Cavity to Left Pleural Cavity with Synthetic Substitute, Percutaneous Endoscopic Approach

0W1B4JG	Bypass Left Pleural Cavity to Peritoneal Cavity with Synthetic Substitute, Percutaneous Endoscopic Approach
0W1B4JJ	Bypass Left Pleural Cavity to Pelvic Cavity with Synthetic Substitute, Percutaneous Endoscopic Approach
0W1B4JY	Bypass Left Pleural Cavity to Lower Vein with Synthetic Substitute, Percutaneous Endoscopic Approach
0W1G0J4	Bypass Peritoneal Cavity to Cutaneous with Synthetic Substitute, Open Approach
0W1G0J9	Bypass Peritoneal Cavity to Right Pleural Cavity with Synthetic Substitute, Open Approach
0W1G0JB	Bypass Peritoneal Cavity to Left Pleural Cavity with Synthetic Substitute, Open Approach
0W1G0JG	Bypass Peritoneal Cavity to Peritoneal Cavity with Synthetic Substitute, Open Approach
0W1G0JJ	Bypass Peritoneal Cavity to Pelvic Cavity with Synthetic Substitute, Open Approach
0W1G0JY	Bypass Peritoneal Cavity to Lower Vein with Synthetic Substitute, Open Approach
0W1G3J4	Bypass Peritoneal Cavity to Cutaneous with Synthetic Substitute, Percutaneous Approach *AHA CC: 4Q, 2013, 126 127*
0W1G4J4	Bypass Peritoneal Cavity to Cutaneous with Synthetic Substitute, Percutaneous Endoscopic Approach *AHA CC: 4Q, 2013, 127*
0W1G4J9	Bypass Peritoneal Cavity to Right Pleural Cavity with Synthetic Substitute, Percutaneous Endoscopic Approach
0W1G4JB	Bypass Peritoneal Cavity to Left Pleural Cavity with Synthetic Substitute, Percutaneous Endoscopic Approach
0W1G4JG	Bypass Peritoneal Cavity to Peritoneal Cavity with Synthetic Substitute, Percutaneous Endoscopic Approach
0W1G4JJ	Bypass Peritoneal Cavity to Pelvic Cavity with Synthetic Substitute, Percutaneous Endoscopic Approach

0W1G4JY	Bypass Peritoneal Cavity to Lower Vein with Synthetic Substitute, Percutaneous Endoscopic Approach
♀ 0W1J0J4	Bypass Pelvic Cavity to Cutaneous with Synthetic Substitute, Open Approach
♀ 0W1J0J9	Bypass Pelvic Cavity to Right Pleural Cavity with Synthetic Substitute, Open Approach
♀ 0W1J0JB	Bypass Pelvic Cavity to Left Pleural Cavity with Synthetic Substitute, Open Approach
♀ 0W1J0JG	Bypass Pelvic Cavity to Peritoneal Cavity with Synthetic Substitute, Open Approach
♀ 0W1J0JJ	Bypass Pelvic Cavity to Pelvic Cavity with Synthetic Substitute, Open Approach
♀ 0W1J0JY	Bypass Pelvic Cavity to Lower Vein with Synthetic Substitute, Open Approach
♀ 0W1J3J4	Bypass Pelvic Cavity to Cutaneous with Synthetic Substitute, Percutaneous Approach
♀ 0W1J4J4	Bypass Pelvic Cavity to Cutaneous with Synthetic Substitute, Percutaneous Endoscopic Approach
♀ 0W1J4J9	Bypass Pelvic Cavity to Right Pleural Cavity with Synthetic Substitute, Percutaneous Endoscopic Approach
♀ 0W1J4JB	Bypass Pelvic Cavity to Left Pleural Cavity with Synthetic Substitute, Percutaneous Endoscopic Approach
♀ 0W1J4JG	Bypass Pelvic Cavity to Peritoneal Cavity with Synthetic Substitute, Percutaneous Endoscopic Approach
♀ 0W1J4JJ	Bypass Pelvic Cavity to Pelvic Cavity with Synthetic Substitute, Percutaneous Endoscopic Approach
♀ 0W1J4JY	Bypass Pelvic Cavity to Lower Vein with Synthetic Substitute, Percutaneous Endoscopic Approach

This is a female-only service, however, it is not included in the female-only edit logic for MCE V30

W2 – Anatomical Regions, General, Change

Review Coding Guideline B6.1c

W20X0Z	Change Drainage Device in Head, External Approach
W20XYZ	Change Other Device in Head, External Approach
W21X0Z	Change Drainage Device in Cranial Cavity, External Approach
W21XYZ	Change Other Device in Cranial Cavity, External Approach
W22X0Z	Change Drainage Device in Face, External Approach
W22XYZ	Change Other Device in Face, External Approach
W24X0Z	Change Drainage Device in Upper Jaw, External Approach
W24XYZ	Change Other Device in Upper Jaw, External Approach
W25X0Z	Change Drainage Device in Lower Jaw, External Approach
W25XYZ	Change Other Device in Lower Jaw, External Approach
W26X0Z	Change Drainage Device in Neck, External Approach
W26XYZ	Change Other Device in Neck, External Approach
W28X0Z	Change Drainage Device in Chest Wall, External Approach

0W28XYZ	Change Other Device in Chest Wall, External Approach
0W29X0Z	Change Drainage Device in Right Pleural Cavity, External Approach
0W29XYZ	Change Other Device in Right Pleural Cavity, External Approach
0W2BX0Z	Change Drainage Device in Left Pleural Cavity, External Approach
0W2BXYZ	Change Other Device in Left Pleural Cavity, External Approach
0W2CX0Z	Change Drainage Device in Mediastinum, External Approach
0W2CXYZ	Change Other Device in Mediastinum, External Approach
0W2DX0Z	Change Drainage Device in Pericardial Cavity, External Approach
0W2DXYZ	Change Other Device in Pericardial Cavity, External Approach
0W2FX0Z	Change Drainage Device in Abdominal Wall, External Approach
0W2FXYZ	Change Other Device in Abdominal Wall, External Approach
0W2GX0Z	Change Drainage Device in Peritoneal Cavity, External Approach
0W2GXYZ	Change Other Device in Peritoneal Cavity, External Approach

0W2HX0Z	Change Drainage Device in Retroperitoneum, External Approach
0W2HXYZ	Change Other Device in Retroperitoneum, External Approach
0W2JX0Z	Change Drainage Device in Pelvic Cavity, External Approach
0W2JXYZ	Change Other Device in Pelvic Cavity, External Approach
0W2KX0Z	Change Drainage Device in Upper Back, External Approach
0W2KXYZ	Change Other Device in Upper Back, External Approach
0W2LX0Z	Change Drainage Device in Lower Back, External Approach
0W2LXYZ	Change Other Device in Lower Back, External Approach
0W2MX0Z	Change Drainage Device in Male Perineum, External Approach
0W2MXYZ	Change Other Device in Male Perineum, External Approach
0W2NX0Z	Change Drainage Device in Female Perineum, External Approach
0W2NXYZ	Change Other Device in Female Perineum, External Approach

♀ Female-only   ♂ Male-only   ▲ Limited Coverage   ● Non-OR   ▦ HAC-associated procedure   ▲ Non-covered procedures   ✚ Combination

0W3 – Anatomical Regions, General, Control

Review Coding Guideline B3.7

0W300ZZ Control Bleeding in Head, Open Approach	**0W384ZZ** Control Bleeding in Chest Wall, Percutaneous Endoscopic Approach	**0W3K4ZZ** Control Bleeding in Upper Back, Percutaneous Endoscopic Approach
0W303ZZ Control Bleeding in Head, Percutaneous Approach	**0W390ZZ** Control Bleeding in Right Pleural Cavity, Open Approach	**0W3L0ZZ** Control Bleeding in Lower Back, Open Approach
0W304ZZ Control Bleeding in Head, Percutaneous Endoscopic Approach	**0W393ZZ** Control Bleeding in Right Pleural Cavity, Percutaneous Approach	**0W3L3ZZ** Control Bleeding in Lower Back, Percutaneous Approach
0W310ZZ Control Bleeding in Cranial Cavity, Open Approach	**0W394ZZ** Control Bleeding in Right Pleural Cavity, Percutaneous Endoscopic Approach	**0W3L4ZZ** Control Bleeding in Lower Back, Percutaneous Endoscopic Approach
0W313ZZ Control Bleeding in Cranial Cavity, Percutaneous Approach	**0W3B0ZZ** Control Bleeding in Left Pleural Cavity, Open Approach	**0W3M0ZZ** Control Bleeding in Male Perineum, Open Approach
0W314ZZ Control Bleeding in Cranial Cavity, Percutaneous Endoscopic Approach	**0W3B3ZZ** Control Bleeding in Left Pleural Cavity, Percutaneous Approach	**0W3M3ZZ** Control Bleeding in Male Perineum, Percutaneous Approach
0W320ZZ Control Bleeding in Face, Open Approach	**0W3B4ZZ** Control Bleeding in Left Pleural Cavity, Percutaneous Endoscopic Approach	**0W3M4ZZ** Control Bleeding in Male Perineum, Percutaneous Endoscopic Approach
0W323ZZ Control Bleeding in Face, Percutaneous Approach	**0W3C0ZZ** Control Bleeding in Mediastinum, Open Approach	**0W3N0ZZ** Control Bleeding in Female Perineum, Open Approach
0W324ZZ Control Bleeding in Face, Percutaneous Endoscopic Approach	**0W3C3ZZ** Control Bleeding in Mediastinum, Percutaneous Approach	**0W3N3ZZ** Control Bleeding in Female Perineum, Percutaneous Approach
0W330ZZ Control Bleeding in Oral Cavity and Throat, Open Approach	**0W3C4ZZ** Control Bleeding in Mediastinum, Percutaneous Endoscopic Approach	**0W3N4ZZ** Control Bleeding in Female Perineum, Percutaneous Endoscopic Approach
0W333ZZ Control Bleeding in Oral Cavity and Throat, Percutaneous Approach	**0W3D0ZZ** Control Bleeding in Pericardial Cavity, Open Approach	**0W3P0ZZ** Control Bleeding in Gastrointestinal Tract, Open Approach
0W334ZZ Control Bleeding in Oral Cavity and Throat, Percutaneous Endoscopic Approach	**0W3D3ZZ** Control Bleeding in Pericardial Cavity, Percutaneous Approach	**0W3P3ZZ** Control Bleeding in Gastrointestinal Tract, Percutaneous Approach
0W337ZZ Control Bleeding in Oral Cavity and Throat, Via Natural or Artificial Opening	**0W3D4ZZ** Control Bleeding in Pericardial Cavity, Percutaneous Endoscopic Approach	**0W3P4ZZ** Control Bleeding in Gastrointestinal Tract, Percutaneous Endoscopic Approach
0W338ZZ Control Bleeding in Oral Cavity and Throat, Via Natural or Artificial Opening Endoscopic	**0W3F0ZZ** Control Bleeding in Abdominal Wall, Open Approach	**0W3P7ZZ** Control Bleeding in Gastrointestinal Tract, Via Natural or Artificial Opening
0W33XZZ Control Bleeding in Oral Cavity and Throat, External Approach	**0W3F3ZZ** Control Bleeding in Abdominal Wall, Percutaneous Approach	**0W3P8ZZ** Control Bleeding in Gastrointestinal Tract, Via Natural or Artificial Opening Endoscopic
0W340ZZ Control Bleeding in Upper Jaw, Open Approach	**0W3F4ZZ** Control Bleeding in Abdominal Wall, Percutaneous Endoscopic Approach	**0W3Q0ZZ** Control Bleeding in Respiratory Tract, Open Approach
0W343ZZ Control Bleeding in Upper Jaw, Percutaneous Approach	**0W3G0ZZ** Control Bleeding in Peritoneal Cavity, Open Approach	**0W3Q3ZZ** Control Bleeding in Respiratory Tract, Percutaneous Approach
0W344ZZ Control Bleeding in Upper Jaw, Percutaneous Endoscopic Approach	**0W3G3ZZ** Control Bleeding in Peritoneal Cavity, Percutaneous Approach	**0W3Q4ZZ** Control Bleeding in Respiratory Tract, Percutaneous Endoscopic Approach
0W350ZZ Control Bleeding in Lower Jaw, Open Approach	**0W3G4ZZ** Control Bleeding in Peritoneal Cavity, Percutaneous Endoscopic Approach	**0W3Q7ZZ** Control Bleeding in Respiratory Tract, Via Natural or Artificial Opening
0W353ZZ Control Bleeding in Lower Jaw, Percutaneous Approach	**0W3H0ZZ** Control Bleeding in Retroperitoneum, Open Approach	**0W3Q8ZZ** Control Bleeding in Respiratory Tract, Via Natural or Artificial Opening Endoscopic
0W354ZZ Control Bleeding in Lower Jaw, Percutaneous Endoscopic Approach	**0W3H3ZZ** Control Bleeding in Retroperitoneum, Percutaneous Approach	**0W3R0ZZ** Control Bleeding in Genitourinary Tract, Open Approach
0W360ZZ Control Bleeding in Neck, Open Approach	**0W3H4ZZ** Control Bleeding in Retroperitoneum, Percutaneous Endoscopic Approach	**0W3R3ZZ** Control Bleeding in Genitourinary Tract, Percutaneous Approach
0W363ZZ Control Bleeding in Neck, Percutaneous Approach	**0W3J0ZZ** Control Bleeding in Pelvic Cavity, Open Approach	**0W3R4ZZ** Control Bleeding in Genitourinary Tract, Percutaneous Endoscopic Approach
0W364ZZ Control Bleeding in Neck, Percutaneous Endoscopic Approach	**0W3J3ZZ** Control Bleeding in Pelvic Cavity, Percutaneous Approach	**0W3R7ZZ** Control Bleeding in Genitourinary Tract, Via Natural or Artificial Opening
0W380ZZ Control Bleeding in Chest Wall, Open Approach	**0W3J4ZZ** Control Bleeding in Pelvic Cavity, Percutaneous Endoscopic Approach	*AHA CC: 4Q, 2014, 44*
0W383ZZ Control Bleeding in Chest Wall, Percutaneous Approach	**0W3K0ZZ** Control Bleeding in Upper Back, Open Approach	**0W3R8ZZ** Control Bleeding in Genitourinary Tract, Via Natural or Artificial Opening Endoscopic
	0W3K3ZZ Control Bleeding in Upper Back, Percutaneous Approach	

0W4 – Anatomical Regions, General, Creation

♂ ▲ **0W4M070** Creation of Vagina in Male Perineum with Autologous Tissue Substitute, Open Approach

♂ ▲ **0W4M0J0** Creation of Vagina in Male Perineum with Synthetic Substitute, Open Approach

♂ ▲ **0W4M0K0** Creation of Vagina in Male Perineum with Nonautologous Tissue Substitute, Open Approach

♂ ▲ **0W4M0Z0** Creation of Vagina in Male Perineum, Open Approach

♀ ▲ **0W4N071** Creation of Penis in Female Perineum with Autologous Tissue Substitute, Open Approach

♀ ▲ **0W4N0J1** Creation of Penis in Female Perineum with Synthetic Substitute, Open Approach

♀ ▲ **0W4N0K1** Creation of Penis in Female Perineum with Nonautologous Tissue Substitute, Open Approach

♀ ▲ **0W4N0Z1** Creation of Penis in Female Perineum, Open Approach

0W8 – Anatomical Regions, General, Division

♀ **0W8NXZZ** Division of Female Perineum, External Approach

eview Coding Guidelines B3.4a and B3.4b

eview Coding Guideline B6.2

W9000Z Drainage of Head with Drainage Device, Open Approach

V900ZX Drainage of Head, Open Approach, Diagnostic

V900ZZ Drainage of Head, Open Approach

V9030Z Drainage of Head with Drainage Device, Percutaneous Approach

V903ZX Drainage of Head, Percutaneous Approach, Diagnostic

V903ZZ Drainage of Head, Percutaneous Approach

V9040Z Drainage of Head with Drainage Device, Percutaneous Endoscopic Approach

V904ZX Drainage of Head, Percutaneous Endoscopic Approach, Diagnostic

V904ZZ Drainage of Head, Percutaneous Endoscopic Approach

V9100Z Drainage of Cranial Cavity with Drainage Device, Open Approach

W910ZX Drainage of Cranial Cavity, Open Approach, Diagnostic

W910ZZ Drainage of Cranial Cavity, Open Approach

W9130Z Drainage of Cranial Cavity with Drainage Device, Percutaneous Approach

W913ZX Drainage of Cranial Cavity, Percutaneous Approach, Diagnostic

W913ZZ Drainage of Cranial Cavity, Percutaneous Approach

W9140Z Drainage of Cranial Cavity with Drainage Device, Percutaneous Endoscopic Approach

W914ZX Drainage of Cranial Cavity, Percutaneous Endoscopic Approach, Diagnostic

W914ZZ Drainage of Cranial Cavity, Percutaneous Endoscopic Approach

W9200Z Drainage of Face with Drainage Device, Open Approach

W920ZX Drainage of Face, Open Approach, Diagnostic

W920ZZ Drainage of Face, Open Approach

W9230Z Drainage of Face with Drainage Device, Percutaneous Approach

W923ZX Drainage of Face, Percutaneous Approach, Diagnostic

W923ZZ Drainage of Face, Percutaneous Approach

W9240Z Drainage of Face with Drainage Device, Percutaneous Endoscopic Approach

W924ZX Drainage of Face, Percutaneous Endoscopic Approach, Diagnostic

W924ZZ Drainage of Face, Percutaneous Endoscopic Approach

W9300Z Drainage of Oral Cavity and Throat with Drainage Device, Open Approach

W930ZX Drainage of Oral Cavity and Throat, Open Approach, Diagnostic

W930ZZ Drainage of Oral Cavity and Throat, Open Approach

W9330Z Drainage of Oral Cavity and Throat with Drainage Device, Percutaneous Approach

W933ZX Drainage of Oral Cavity and Throat, Percutaneous Approach, Diagnostic

W933ZZ Drainage of Oral Cavity and Throat, Percutaneous Approach

W9340Z Drainage of Oral Cavity and Throat with Drainage Device, Percutaneous Endoscopic Approach

W934ZX Drainage of Oral Cavity and Throat, Percutaneous Endoscopic Approach, Diagnostic

0W934ZZ Drainage of Oral Cavity and Throat, Percutaneous Endoscopic Approach

0W9400Z Drainage of Upper Jaw with Drainage Device, Open Approach

0W940ZX Drainage of Upper Jaw, Open Approach, Diagnostic

0W940ZZ Drainage of Upper Jaw, Open Approach

0W9430Z Drainage of Upper Jaw with Drainage Device, Percutaneous Approach

0W943ZX Drainage of Upper Jaw, Percutaneous Approach, Diagnostic

0W943ZZ Drainage of Upper Jaw, Percutaneous Approach

0W9440Z Drainage of Upper Jaw with Drainage Device, Percutaneous Endoscopic Approach

0W944ZX Drainage of Upper Jaw, Percutaneous Endoscopic Approach, Diagnostic

0W944ZZ Drainage of Upper Jaw, Percutaneous Endoscopic Approach

0W9500Z Drainage of Lower Jaw with Drainage Device, Open Approach

0W950ZX Drainage of Lower Jaw, Open Approach, Diagnostic

0W950ZZ Drainage of Lower Jaw, Open Approach

0W9530Z Drainage of Lower Jaw with Drainage Device, Percutaneous Approach

0W953ZX Drainage of Lower Jaw, Percutaneous Approach, Diagnostic

0W953ZZ Drainage of Lower Jaw, Percutaneous Approach

0W9540Z Drainage of Lower Jaw with Drainage Device, Percutaneous Endoscopic Approach

0W954ZX Drainage of Lower Jaw, Percutaneous Endoscopic Approach, Diagnostic

0W954ZZ Drainage of Lower Jaw, Percutaneous Endoscopic Approach

0W9600Z Drainage of Neck with Drainage Device, Open Approach

0W960ZX Drainage of Neck, Open Approach, Diagnostic

0W960ZZ Drainage of Neck, Open Approach

0W9630Z Drainage of Neck with Drainage Device, Percutaneous Approach

0W963ZX Drainage of Neck, Percutaneous Approach, Diagnostic

0W963ZZ Drainage of Neck, Percutaneous Approach

0W9640Z Drainage of Neck with Drainage Device, Percutaneous Endoscopic Approach

0W964ZX Drainage of Neck, Percutaneous Endoscopic Approach, Diagnostic

0W964ZZ Drainage of Neck, Percutaneous Endoscopic Approach

0W9800Z Drainage of Chest Wall with Drainage Device, Open Approach

0W980ZX Drainage of Chest Wall, Open Approach, Diagnostic

0W980ZZ Drainage of Chest Wall, Open Approach

0W9830Z Drainage of Chest Wall with Drainage Device, Percutaneous Approach

0W983ZX Drainage of Chest Wall, Percutaneous Approach, Diagnostic

0W983ZZ Drainage of Chest Wall, Percutaneous Approach

0W9840Z Drainage of Chest Wall with Drainage Device, Percutaneous Endoscopic Approach

0W984ZX Drainage of Chest Wall, Percutaneous Endoscopic Approach, Diagnostic

0W984ZZ Drainage of Chest Wall, Percutaneous Endoscopic Approach

0W9900Z Drainage of Right Pleural Cavity with Drainage Device, Open Approach

0W990ZX Drainage of Right Pleural Cavity, Open Approach, Diagnostic

0W990ZZ Drainage of Right Pleural Cavity, Open Approach

0W9930Z Drainage of Right Pleural Cavity with Drainage Device, Percutaneous Approach

0W993ZX Drainage of Right Pleural Cavity, Percutaneous Approach, Diagnostic

0W993ZZ Drainage of Right Pleural Cavity, Percutaneous Approach

0W9940Z Drainage of Right Pleural Cavity with Drainage Device, Percutaneous Endoscopic Approach

0W994ZX Drainage of Right Pleural Cavity, Percutaneous Endoscopic Approach, Diagnostic

0W994ZZ Drainage of Right Pleural Cavity, Percutaneous Endoscopic Approach

0W9B00Z Drainage of Left Pleural Cavity with Drainage Device, Open Approach

0W9B0ZX Drainage of Left Pleural Cavity, Open Approach, Diagnostic

0W9B0ZZ Drainage of Left Pleural Cavity, Open Approach

0W9B30Z Drainage of Left Pleural Cavity with Drainage Device, Percutaneous Approach

0W9B3ZX Drainage of Left Pleural Cavity, Percutaneous Approach, Diagnostic

0W9B3ZZ Drainage of Left Pleural Cavity, Percutaneous Approach

0W9B40Z Drainage of Left Pleural Cavity with Drainage Device, Percutaneous Endoscopic Approach

0W9B4ZX Drainage of Left Pleural Cavity, Percutaneous Endoscopic Approach, Diagnostic

0W9B4ZZ Drainage of Left Pleural Cavity, Percutaneous Endoscopic Approach

0W9C00Z Drainage of Mediastinum with Drainage Device, Open Approach

0W9C0ZX Drainage of Mediastinum, Open Approach, Diagnostic

0W9C0ZZ Drainage of Mediastinum, Open Approach

0W9C30Z Drainage of Mediastinum with Drainage Device, Percutaneous Approach

0W9C3ZX Drainage of Mediastinum, Percutaneous Approach, Diagnostic

0W9C3ZZ Drainage of Mediastinum, Percutaneous Approach

0W9C40Z Drainage of Mediastinum with Drainage Device, Percutaneous Endoscopic Approach

0W9C4ZX Drainage of Mediastinum, Percutaneous Endoscopic Approach, Diagnostic

0W9C4ZZ Drainage of Mediastinum, Percutaneous Endoscopic Approach

0W9D00Z Drainage of Pericardial Cavity with Drainage Device, Open Approach

0W9D0ZX Drainage of Pericardial Cavity, Open Approach, Diagnostic

0W9D0ZZ Drainage of Pericardial Cavity, Open Approach

0W9D30Z Drainage of Pericardial Cavity with Drainage Device, Percutaneous Approach

0W9D3ZX Drainage of Pericardial Cavity, Percutaneous Approach, Diagnostic

0W9D3ZZ Drainage of Pericardial Cavity, Percutaneous Approach

0W9D40Z Drainage of Pericardial Cavity with Drainage Device, Percutaneous Endoscopic Approach

♀ Female-only   ♂ Male-only   ▲ Limited Coverage   ● Non-OR   ▬ HAC-associated procedure   ▲ Non-covered procedures   ➕ Combination

0W9D4ZX	Drainage of Pericardial Cavity, Percutaneous Endoscopic Approach, Diagnostic	
0W9D4ZZ	Drainage of Pericardial Cavity, Percutaneous Endoscopic Approach	
0W9F00Z	Drainage of Abdominal Wall with Drainage Device, Open Approach	
0W9F0ZX	Drainage of Abdominal Wall, Open Approach, Diagnostic	
0W9F0ZZ	Drainage of Abdominal Wall, Open Approach	
0W9F30Z	Drainage of Abdominal Wall with Drainage Device, Percutaneous Approach	
0W9F3ZX	Drainage of Abdominal Wall, Percutaneous Approach, Diagnostic	
0W9F3ZZ	Drainage of Abdominal Wall, Percutaneous Approach	
0W9F40Z	Drainage of Abdominal Wall with Drainage Device, Percutaneous Endoscopic Approach	
0W9F4ZX	Drainage of Abdominal Wall, Percutaneous Endoscopic Approach, Diagnostic	
0W9F4ZZ	Drainage of Abdominal Wall, Percutaneous Endoscopic Approach	
0W9G00Z	Drainage of Peritoneal Cavity with Drainage Device, Open Approach	
0W9G0ZX	Drainage of Peritoneal Cavity, Open Approach, Diagnostic	
0W9G0ZZ	Drainage of Peritoneal Cavity, Open Approach	
0W9G30Z	Drainage of Peritoneal Cavity with Drainage Device, Percutaneous Approach	
0W9G3ZX	Drainage of Peritoneal Cavity, Percutaneous Approach, Diagnostic	
0W9G3ZZ	Drainage of Peritoneal Cavity, Percutaneous Approach	
0W9G40Z	Drainage of Peritoneal Cavity with Drainage Device, Percutaneous Endoscopic Approach	
0W9G4ZX	Drainage of Peritoneal Cavity, Percutaneous Endoscopic Approach, Diagnostic	
0W9G4ZZ	Drainage of Peritoneal Cavity, Percutaneous Endoscopic Approach	
0W9H00Z	Drainage of Retroperitoneum with Drainage Device, Open Approach	
0W9H0ZX	Drainage of Retroperitoneum, Open Approach, Diagnostic	
0W9H0ZZ	Drainage of Retroperitoneum, Open Approach	
0W9H30Z	Drainage of Retroperitoneum with Drainage Device, Percutaneous Approach	
0W9H3ZX	Drainage of Retroperitoneum, Percutaneous Approach, Diagnostic	

0W9H3ZZ	Drainage of Retroperitoneum, Percutaneous Approach	
0W9H40Z	Drainage of Retroperitoneum with Drainage Device, Percutaneous Endoscopic Approach	
0W9H4ZX	Drainage of Retroperitoneum, Percutaneous Endoscopic Approach, Diagnostic	
0W9H4ZZ	Drainage of Retroperitoneum, Percutaneous Endoscopic Approach	
0W9J00Z	Drainage of Pelvic Cavity with Drainage Device, Open Approach	
0W9J0ZX	Drainage of Pelvic Cavity, Open Approach, Diagnostic	
0W9J0ZZ	Drainage of Pelvic Cavity, Open Approach	
0W9J30Z	Drainage of Pelvic Cavity with Drainage Device, Percutaneous Approach	
0W9J3ZX	Drainage of Pelvic Cavity, Percutaneous Approach, Diagnostic	
0W9J3ZZ	Drainage of Pelvic Cavity, Percutaneous Approach	
0W9J40Z	Drainage of Pelvic Cavity with Drainage Device, Percutaneous Endoscopic Approach	
0W9J4ZX	Drainage of Pelvic Cavity, Percutaneous Endoscopic Approach, Diagnostic	
0W9J4ZZ	Drainage of Pelvic Cavity, Percutaneous Endoscopic Approach	
0W9K00Z	Drainage of Upper Back with Drainage Device, Open Approach	
0W9K0ZX	Drainage of Upper Back, Open Approach, Diagnostic	
0W9K0ZZ	Drainage of Upper Back, Open Approach	
0W9K30Z	Drainage of Upper Back with Drainage Device, Percutaneous Approach	
0W9K3ZX	Drainage of Upper Back, Percutaneous Approach, Diagnostic	
0W9K3ZZ	Drainage of Upper Back, Percutaneous Approach	
0W9K40Z	Drainage of Upper Back with Drainage Device, Percutaneous Endoscopic Approach	
0W9K4ZX	Drainage of Upper Back, Percutaneous Endoscopic Approach, Diagnostic	
0W9K4ZZ	Drainage of Upper Back, Percutaneous Endoscopic Approach	
0W9L00Z	Drainage of Lower Back with Drainage Device, Open Approach	
0W9L0ZX	Drainage of Lower Back, Open Approach, Diagnostic	
0W9L0ZZ	Drainage of Lower Back, Open Approach	
0W9L30Z	Drainage of Lower Back with Drainage Device, Percutaneous Approach	

0W9L3ZX	Drainage of Lower Back, Percutaneous Approach, Diagnostic	
0W9L3ZZ	Drainage of Lower Back, Percutaneous Approach	
0W9L40Z	Drainage of Lower Back with Drainage Device, Percutaneous Endoscopic Approach	
0W9L4ZX	Drainage of Lower Back, Percutaneous Endoscopic Approach, Diagnostic	
0W9L4ZZ	Drainage of Lower Back, Percutaneous Endoscopic Approach	
♂ **0W9M00Z**	Drainage of Male Perineum with Drainage Device, Open Approach	
♂ **0W9M0ZX**	Drainage of Male Perineum, Open Approach, Diagnostic	
♂ **0W9M0ZZ**	Drainage of Male Perineum, Open Approach	
♂ **0W9M30Z**	Drainage of Male Perineum with Drainage Device, Percutaneous Approach	
♂ **0W9M3ZX**	Drainage of Male Perineum, Percutaneous Approach, Diagnostic	
♂ **0W9M3ZZ**	Drainage of Male Perineum, Percutaneous Approach	
♂ **0W9M40Z**	Drainage of Male Perineum with Drainage Device, Percutaneous Endoscopic Approach	
♂ **0W9M4ZX**	Drainage of Male Perineum, Percutaneous Endoscopic Approach, Diagnostic	
♂ **0W9M4ZZ**	Drainage of Male Perineum, Percutaneous Endoscopic Approach	
♀ **0W9N00Z**	Drainage of Female Perineum with Drainage Device, Open Approach	
♀ **0W9N0ZX**	Drainage of Female Perineum, Open Approach, Diagnostic	
♀ **0W9N0ZZ**	Drainage of Female Perineum, Open Approach	
♀ **0W9N30Z**	Drainage of Female Perineum with Drainage Device, Percutaneous Approach	
♀ **0W9N3ZX**	Drainage of Female Perineum, Percutaneous Approach, Diagnostic	
♀ **0W9N3ZZ**	Drainage of Female Perineum, Percutaneous Approach	
♀ **0W9N40Z**	Drainage of Female Perineum with Drainage Device, Percutaneous Endoscopic Approach	
♀ **0W9N4ZX**	Drainage of Female Perineum, Percutaneous Endoscopic Approach, Diagnostic	
	This is a female-only service, however, it is not included in the female-only edit logic for MCE V30	
♀ **0W9N4ZZ**	Drainage of Female Perineum, Percutaneous Endoscopic Approach	

0WB – Anatomical Regions, General, Excision

Review Coding Guidelines B3.4a and B3.4b

0WB00ZX	Excision of Head, Open Approach, Diagnostic	
0WB00ZZ	Excision of Head, Open Approach	
0WB03ZX	Excision of Head, Percutaneous Approach, Diagnostic	
0WB03ZZ	Excision of Head, Percutaneous Approach	
0WB04ZX	Excision of Head, Percutaneous Endoscopic Approach, Diagnostic	
0WB04ZZ	Excision of Head, Percutaneous Endoscopic Approach	
0WB0XZX	Excision of Head, External Approach, Diagnostic	
0WB0XZZ	Excision of Head, External Approach	
0WB20ZX	Excision of Face, Open Approach, Diagnostic	
0WB20ZZ	Excision of Face, Open Approach	

0WB23ZX	Excision of Face, Percutaneous Approach, Diagnostic	
0WB23ZZ	Excision of Face, Percutaneous Approach	
0WB24ZX	Excision of Face, Percutaneous Endoscopic Approach, Diagnostic	
0WB24ZZ	Excision of Face, Percutaneous Endoscopic Approach	
0WB2XZX	Excision of Face, External Approach, Diagnostic	
0WB2XZZ	Excision of Face, External Approach	
0WB40ZX	Excision of Upper Jaw, Open Approach, Diagnostic	
0WB40ZZ	Excision of Upper Jaw, Open Approach	
0WB43ZX	Excision of Upper Jaw, Percutaneous Approach, Diagnostic	
0WB43ZZ	Excision of Upper Jaw, Percutaneous Approach	

0WB44ZX	Excision of Upper Jaw, Percutaneous Endoscopic Approach, Diagnostic	
0WB44ZZ	Excision of Upper Jaw, Percutaneous Endoscopic Approach	
0WB4XZX	Excision of Upper Jaw, External Approach, Diagnostic	
0WB4XZZ	Excision of Upper Jaw, External Approach	
0WB50ZX	Excision of Lower Jaw, Open Approach, Diagnostic	
0WB50ZZ	Excision of Lower Jaw, Open Approach	
0WB53ZX	Excision of Lower Jaw, Percutaneous Approach, Diagnostic	
0WB53ZZ	Excision of Lower Jaw, Percutaneous Approach	
0WB54ZX	Excision of Lower Jaw, Percutaneous Endoscopic Approach, Diagnostic	

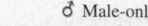

♀ Female-only   ♂ Male-only   ▲ Limited Coverage   ● Non-OR   ▩ HAC-associated procedure   ▲ Non-covered procedures   ✛ Combination

0WB54ZZ Excision of Lower Jaw, Percutaneous Endoscopic Approach
0WB5XZX Excision of Lower Jaw, External Approach, Diagnostic
0WB5XZZ Excision of Lower Jaw, External Approach
0WB60ZX Excision of Neck, Open Approach, Diagnostic
0WB60ZZ Excision of Neck, Open Approach
0WB63ZX Excision of Neck, Percutaneous Approach, Diagnostic
0WB63ZZ Excision of Neck, Percutaneous Approach
0WB64ZX Excision of Neck, Percutaneous Endoscopic Approach, Diagnostic
0WB64ZZ Excision of Neck, Percutaneous Endoscopic Approach
0WB6XZ2 Excision of Neck, Stoma, External Approach
0WB6XZX Excision of Neck, External Approach, Diagnostic
0WB6XZZ Excision of Neck, External Approach
0WB80ZX Excision of Chest Wall, Open Approach, Diagnostic
0WB80ZZ Excision of Chest Wall, Open Approach
0WB83ZX Excision of Chest Wall, Percutaneous Approach, Diagnostic
0WB83ZZ Excision of Chest Wall, Percutaneous Approach
0WB84ZX Excision of Chest Wall, Percutaneous Endoscopic Approach, Diagnostic
0WB84ZZ Excision of Chest Wall, Percutaneous Endoscopic Approach
0WB8XZX Excision of Chest Wall, External Approach, Diagnostic
0WB8XZZ Excision of Chest Wall, External Approach
0WBC0ZX Excision of Mediastinum, Open Approach, Diagnostic
0WBC0ZZ Excision of Mediastinum, Open Approach
0WBC3ZX Excision of Mediastinum, Percutaneous Approach, Diagnostic
0WBC3ZZ Excision of Mediastinum, Percutaneous Approach
0WBC4ZX Excision of Mediastinum, Percutaneous Endoscopic Approach, Diagnostic
0WBC4ZZ Excision of Mediastinum, Percutaneous Endoscopic Approach
0WBF0ZX Excision of Abdominal Wall, Open Approach, Diagnostic

0WBF0ZZ Excision of Abdominal Wall, Open Approach
0WBF3ZX Excision of Abdominal Wall, Percutaneous Approach, Diagnostic
0WBF3ZZ Excision of Abdominal Wall, Percutaneous Approach
0WBF4ZX Excision of Abdominal Wall, Percutaneous Endoscopic Approach, Diagnostic
0WBF4ZZ Excision of Abdominal Wall, Percutaneous Endoscopic Approach
0WBFXZ2 Excision of Abdominal Wall, Stoma, External Approach
0WBFXZX Excision of Abdominal Wall, External Approach, Diagnostic
0WBFXZZ Excision of Abdominal Wall, External Approach
0WBH0ZX Excision of Retroperitoneum, Open Approach, Diagnostic
0WBH0ZZ Excision of Retroperitoneum, Open Approach
0WBH3ZX Excision of Retroperitoneum, Percutaneous Approach, Diagnostic
0WBH3ZZ Excision of Retroperitoneum, Percutaneous Approach
0WBH4ZX Excision of Retroperitoneum, Percutaneous Endoscopic Approach, Diagnostic
0WBH4ZZ Excision of Retroperitoneum, Percutaneous Endoscopic Approach
0WBK0ZX Excision of Upper Back, Open Approach, Diagnostic
0WBK0ZZ Excision of Upper Back, Open Approach
0WBK3ZX Excision of Upper Back, Percutaneous Approach, Diagnostic
0WBK3ZZ Excision of Upper Back, Percutaneous Approach
0WBK4ZX Excision of Upper Back, Percutaneous Endoscopic Approach, Diagnostic
0WBK4ZZ Excision of Upper Back, Percutaneous Endoscopic Approach
0WBKXZX Excision of Upper Back, External Approach, Diagnostic
0WBKXZZ Excision of Upper Back, External Approach
0WBL0ZX Excision of Lower Back, Open Approach, Diagnostic
0WBL0ZZ Excision of Lower Back, Open Approach

0WBL3ZX Excision of Lower Back, Percutaneous Approach, Diagnostic
0WBL3ZZ Excision of Lower Back, Percutaneous Approach
0WBL4ZX Excision of Lower Back, Percutaneous Endoscopic Approach, Diagnostic
0WBL4ZZ Excision of Lower Back, Percutaneous Endoscopic Approach
0WBLXZX Excision of Lower Back, External Approach, Diagnostic
0WBLXZZ Excision of Lower Back, External Approach
♂ 0WBM0ZX Excision of Male Perineum, Open Approach, Diagnostic
♂ 0WBM0ZZ Excision of Male Perineum, Open Approach
♂ 0WBM3ZX Excision of Male Perineum, Percutaneous Approach, Diagnostic
♂ 0WBM3ZZ Excision of Male Perineum, Percutaneous Approach
♂ 0WBM4ZX Excision of Male Perineum, Percutaneous Endoscopic Approach, Diagnostic
♂ 0WBM4ZZ Excision of Male Perineum, Percutaneous Endoscopic Approach
♂ 0WBMXZX Excision of Male Perineum, External Approach, Diagnostic
♂ 0WBMXZZ Excision of Male Perineum, External Approach
♀ 0WBN0ZX Excision of Female Perineum, Open Approach, Diagnostic
♀ 0WBN0ZZ Excision of Female Perineum, Open Approach
♀ 0WBN3ZX Excision of Female Perineum, Percutaneous Approach, Diagnostic
♀ 0WBN3ZZ Excision of Female Perineum, Percutaneous Approach
♀ 0WBN4ZX Excision of Female Perineum, Percutaneous Endoscopic Approach, Diagnostic
♀ 0WBN4ZZ Excision of Female Perineum, Percutaneous Endoscopic Approach
♀ 0WBNXZX Excision of Female Perineum, External Approach, Diagnostic
♀ 0WBNXZZ Excision of Female Perineum, External Approach

AHA CC: 4Q, 2013, 119 120

WC – Anatomical Regions, General, Extirpation

0WC10ZZ Extirpation of Matter from Cranial Cavity, Open Approach
0WC13ZZ Extirpation of Matter from Cranial Cavity, Percutaneous Approach
0WC14ZZ Extirpation of Matter from Cranial Cavity, Percutaneous Endoscopic Approach
0WC1XZZ Extirpation of Matter from Cranial Cavity, External Approach
0WC30ZZ Extirpation of Matter from Oral Cavity and Throat, Open Approach
0WC33ZZ Extirpation of Matter from Oral Cavity and Throat, Percutaneous Approach
0WC34ZZ Extirpation of Matter from Oral Cavity and Throat, Percutaneous Endoscopic Approach
0WC3XZZ Extirpation of Matter from Oral Cavity and Throat, External Approach
0WC90ZZ Extirpation of Matter from Right Pleural Cavity, Open Approach
0WC93ZZ Extirpation of Matter from Right Pleural Cavity, Percutaneous Approach
0WC94ZZ Extirpation of Matter from Right Pleural Cavity, Percutaneous Endoscopic Approach
0WC9XZZ Extirpation of Matter from Right Pleural Cavity, External Approach

0WCB0ZZ Extirpation of Matter from Left Pleural Cavity, Open Approach
0WCB3ZZ Extirpation of Matter from Left Pleural Cavity, Percutaneous Approach
0WCB4ZZ Extirpation of Matter from Left Pleural Cavity, Percutaneous Endoscopic Approach
0WCBXZZ Extirpation of Matter from Left Pleural Cavity, External Approach
0WCC0ZZ Extirpation of Matter from Mediastinum, Open Approach
0WCC3ZZ Extirpation of Matter from Mediastinum, Percutaneous Approach
0WCC4ZZ Extirpation of Matter from Mediastinum, Percutaneous Endoscopic Approach
0WCCXZZ Extirpation of Matter from Mediastinum, External Approach
0WCD0ZZ Extirpation of Matter from Pericardial Cavity, Open Approach
0WCD3ZZ Extirpation of Matter from Pericardial Cavity, Percutaneous Approach
0WCD4ZZ Extirpation of Matter from Pericardial Cavity, Percutaneous Endoscopic Approach
0WCDXZZ Extirpation of Matter from Pericardial Cavity, External Approach

0WCG0ZZ Extirpation of Matter from Peritoneal Cavity, Open Approach
0WCG3ZZ Extirpation of Matter from Peritoneal Cavity, Percutaneous Approach
0WCG4ZZ Extirpation of Matter from Peritoneal Cavity, Percutaneous Endoscopic Approach
0WCGXZZ Extirpation of Matter from Peritoneal Cavity, External Approach
0WCJ0ZZ Extirpation of Matter from Pelvic Cavity, Open Approach
0WCJ3ZZ Extirpation of Matter from Pelvic Cavity, Percutaneous Approach
0WCJ4ZZ Extirpation of Matter from Pelvic Cavity, Percutaneous Endoscopic Approach
0WCJXZZ Extirpation of Matter from Pelvic Cavity, External Approach
0WCP0ZZ Extirpation of Matter from Gastrointestinal Tract, Open Approach
0WCP3ZZ Extirpation of Matter from Gastrointestinal Tract, Percutaneous Approach
0WCP4ZZ Extirpation of Matter from Gastrointestinal Tract, Percutaneous Endoscopic Approach
0WCP7ZZ Extirpation of Matter from Gastrointestinal Tract, Via Natural or Artificial Opening

♀ Female-only ♂ Male-only ▲ Limited Coverage ● Non-OR ▨ HAC-associated procedure ▲ Non-covered procedures ✚ Combination

0WCP8ZZ	Extirpation of Matter from Gastrointestinal Tract, Via Natural or Artificial Opening Endoscopic	
0WCPXZZ	Extirpation of Matter from Gastrointestinal Tract, External Approach	
0WCQ0ZZ	Extirpation of Matter from Respiratory Tract, Open Approach	
0WCQ3ZZ	Extirpation of Matter from Respiratory Tract, Percutaneous Approach	
0WCQ4ZZ	Extirpation of Matter from Respiratory Tract, Percutaneous Endoscopic Approach	

0WCQ7ZZ — Extirpation of Matter from Respiratory Tract, Via Natural or Artificial Opening

0WCQ8ZZ — Extirpation of Matter from Respiratory Tract, Via Natural or Artificial Opening Endoscopic

0WCQXZZ — Extirpation of Matter from Respiratory Tract, External Approach

0WCR0ZZ — Extirpation of Matter from Genitourinary Tract, Open Approach

0WCR3ZZ — Extirpation of Matter from Genitourinary Tract, Percutaneous Approach

0WCR4ZZ — Extirpation of Matter from Genitourinary Tract, Percutaneous Endoscopic Approach

0WCR7ZZ — Extirpation of Matter from Genitourinary Tract, Via Natural or Artificial Opening

0WCR8ZZ — Extirpation of Matter from Genitourinary Tract, Via Natural or Artificial Opening Endoscopic

0WCRXZZ — Extirpation of Matter from Genitourinary Tract, External Approach

0WF – Anatomical Regions, General, Fragmentation

0WF10ZZ — Fragmentation in Cranial Cavity, Open Approach

0WF13ZZ — Fragmentation in Cranial Cavity, Percutaneous Approach

0WF14ZZ — Fragmentation in Cranial Cavity, Percutaneous Endoscopic Approach

▲ 0WF1XZZ — Fragmentation in Cranial Cavity, External Approach

0WF30ZZ — Fragmentation in Oral Cavity and Throat, Open Approach

0WF33ZZ — Fragmentation in Oral Cavity and Throat, Percutaneous Approach

0WF34ZZ — Fragmentation in Oral Cavity and Throat, Percutaneous Endoscopic Approach

▲ 0WF3XZZ — Fragmentation in Oral Cavity and Throat, External Approach

0WF90ZZ — Fragmentation in Right Pleural Cavity, Open Approach

0WF93ZZ — Fragmentation in Right Pleural Cavity, Percutaneous Approach

0WF94ZZ — Fragmentation in Right Pleural Cavity, Percutaneous Endoscopic Approach

▲ 0WF9XZZ — Fragmentation in Right Pleural Cavity, External Approach

0WFB0ZZ — Fragmentation in Left Pleural Cavity, Open Approach

0WFB3ZZ — Fragmentation in Left Pleural Cavity, Percutaneous Approach

0WFB4ZZ — Fragmentation in Left Pleural Cavity, Percutaneous Endoscopic Approach

▲ 0WFBXZZ — Fragmentation in Left Pleural Cavity, External Approach

0WFC0ZZ — Fragmentation in Mediastinum, Open Approach

0WFC3ZZ — Fragmentation in Mediastinum, Percutaneous Approach

0WFC4ZZ — Fragmentation in Mediastinum, Percutaneous Endoscopic Approach

▲ 0WFCXZZ — Fragmentation in Mediastinum, External Approach

0WFD0ZZ — Fragmentation in Pericardial Cavity, Open Approach

0WFD3ZZ — Fragmentation in Pericardial Cavity, Percutaneous Approach

0WFD4ZZ — Fragmentation in Pericardial Cavity, Percutaneous Endoscopic Approach

0WFDXZZ — Fragmentation in Pericardial Cavity, External Approach

0WFG0ZZ — Fragmentation in Peritoneal Cavity, Open Approach

0WFG3ZZ — Fragmentation in Peritoneal Cavity, Percutaneous Approach

0WFG4ZZ — Fragmentation in Peritoneal Cavity, Percutaneous Endoscopic Approach

▲ 0WFGXZZ — Fragmentation in Peritoneal Cavity, External Approach

0WFJ0ZZ — Fragmentation in Pelvic Cavity, Open Approach

0WFJ3ZZ — Fragmentation in Pelvic Cavity, Percutaneous Approach

0WFJ4ZZ — Fragmentation in Pelvic Cavity, Percutaneous Endoscopic Approach

▲ 0WFJXZZ — Fragmentation in Pelvic Cavity, External Approach

0WFP0ZZ — Fragmentation in Gastrointestinal Tract, Open Approach

0WFP3ZZ — Fragmentation in Gastrointestinal Tract, Percutaneous Approach

0WFP4ZZ — Fragmentation in Gastrointestinal Tract Percutaneous Endoscopic Approach

0WFP7ZZ — Fragmentation in Gastrointestinal Tract Via Natural or Artificial Opening

0WFP8ZZ — Fragmentation in Gastrointestinal Tract, Via Natural or Artificial Opening Endoscopic

▲ 0WFPXZZ — Fragmentation in Gastrointestinal Tract External Approach

0WFQ0ZZ — Fragmentation in Respiratory Tract, Open Approach

0WFQ3ZZ — Fragmentation in Respiratory Tract, Percutaneous Approach

0WFQ4ZZ — Fragmentation in Respiratory Tract, Percutaneous Endoscopic Approach

0WFQ7ZZ — Fragmentation in Respiratory Tract, Via Natural or Artificial Opening

0WFQ8ZZ — Fragmentation in Respiratory Tract, Via Natural or Artificial Opening Endoscopic

▲ 0WFQXZZ — Fragmentation in Respiratory Tract, External Approach

0WFR0ZZ — Fragmentation in Genitourinary Tract, Open Approach

0WFR3ZZ — Fragmentation in Genitourinary Tract, Percutaneous Approach

0WFR4ZZ — Fragmentation in Genitourinary Tract, Percutaneous Endoscopic Approach

0WFR7ZZ — Fragmentation in Genitourinary Tract, Via Natural or Artificial Opening

0WFR8ZZ — Fragmentation in Genitourinary Tract, Via Natural or Artificial Opening Endoscopic

● 0WFRXZZ — Fragmentation in Genitourinary Tract, External Approach

0WH – Anatomical Regions, General, Insertion

0WH001Z — Insertion of Radioactive Element into Head, Open Approach

● 0WH003Z — Insertion of Infusion Device into Head, Open Approach

● 0WH00YZ — Insertion of Other Device into Head, Open Approach

0WH031Z — Insertion of Radioactive Element into Head, Percutaneous Approach

● 0WH033Z — Insertion of Infusion Device into Head, Percutaneous Approach

● 0WH03YZ — Insertion of Other Device into Head, Percutaneous Approach

0WH041Z — Insertion of Radioactive Element into Head, Percutaneous Endoscopic Approach

● 0WH043Z — Insertion of Infusion Device into Head, Percutaneous Endoscopic Approach

● 0WH04YZ — Insertion of Other Device into Head, Percutaneous Endoscopic Approach

0WH101Z — Insertion of Radioactive Element into Cranial Cavity, Open Approach

0WH103Z — Insertion of Infusion Device into Cranial Cavity, Open Approach

0WH10YZ — Insertion of Other Device into Cranial Cavity, Open Approach

0WH131Z — Insertion of Radioactive Element into Cranial Cavity, Percutaneous Approach

0WH133Z — Insertion of Infusion Device into Cranial Cavity, Percutaneous Approach

0WH13YZ — Insertion of Other Device into Cranial Cavity, Percutaneous Approach

0WH141Z — Insertion of Radioactive Element into Cranial Cavity, Percutaneous Endoscopic Approach

0WH143Z — Insertion of Infusion Device into Cranial Cavity, Percutaneous Endoscopic Approach

0WH14YZ — Insertion of Other Device into Cranial Cavity, Percutaneous Endoscopic Approach

0WH201Z — Insertion of Radioactive Element into Face, Open Approach

● 0WH203Z — Insertion of Infusion Device into Face, Open Approach

● 0WH20YZ — Insertion of Other Device into Face, Open Approach

0WH231Z — Insertion of Radioactive Element into Face, Percutaneous Approach

● 0WH233Z — Insertion of Infusion Device into Face, Percutaneous Approach

● 0WH23YZ — Insertion of Other Device into Face, Percutaneous Approach

0WH241Z — Insertion of Radioactive Element into Face, Percutaneous Endoscopic Approach

● 0WH243Z — Insertion of Infusion Device into Face, Percutaneous Endoscopic Approach

● 0WH24YZ — Insertion of Other Device into Face, Percutaneous Endoscopic Approach

0WH301Z — Insertion of Radioactive Element into Oral Cavity and Throat, Open Approach

0WH303Z — Insertion of Infusion Device into Oral Cavity and Throat, Open Approach

0WH30YZ — Insertion of Other Device into Oral Cavity and Throat, Open Approach

0WH331Z — Insertion of Radioactive Element into Oral Cavity and Throat, Percutaneous Approach

0WH333Z — Insertion of Infusion Device into Oral Cavity and Throat, Percutaneous Approach

0WH33YZ — Insertion of Other Device into Oral Cavity and Throat, Percutaneous Approach

'H341Z	Insertion of Radioactive Element into Oral Cavity and Throat, Percutaneous Endoscopic Approach
'H343Z	Insertion of Infusion Device into Oral Cavity and Throat, Percutaneous Endoscopic Approach
'H34YZ	Insertion of Other Device into Oral Cavity and Throat, Percutaneous Endoscopic Approach
'H401Z	Insertion of Radioactive Element into Upper Jaw, Open Approach
WH403Z	Insertion of Infusion Device into Upper Jaw, Open Approach
WH40YZ	Insertion of Other Device into Upper Jaw, Open Approach
H431Z	Insertion of Radioactive Element into Upper Jaw, Percutaneous Approach
WH433Z	Insertion of Infusion Device into Upper Jaw, Percutaneous Approach
WH43YZ	Insertion of Other Device into Upper Jaw, Percutaneous Approach
H441Z	Insertion of Radioactive Element into Upper Jaw, Percutaneous Endoscopic Approach
WH443Z	Insertion of Infusion Device into Upper Jaw, Percutaneous Endoscopic Approach
WH44YZ	Insertion of Other Device into Upper Jaw, Percutaneous Endoscopic Approach
H501Z	Insertion of Radioactive Element into Lower Jaw, Open Approach
WH503Z	Insertion of Infusion Device into Lower Jaw, Open Approach
WH50YZ	Insertion of Other Device into Lower Jaw, Open Approach
H531Z	Insertion of Radioactive Element into Lower Jaw, Percutaneous Approach
WH533Z	Insertion of Infusion Device into Lower Jaw, Percutaneous Approach
WH53YZ	Insertion of Other Device into Lower Jaw, Percutaneous Approach
H541Z	Insertion of Radioactive Element into Lower Jaw, Percutaneous Endoscopic Approach
WH543Z	Insertion of Infusion Device into Lower Jaw, Percutaneous Endoscopic Approach
WH54YZ	Insertion of Other Device into Lower Jaw, Percutaneous Endoscopic Approach
H601Z	Insertion of Radioactive Element into Neck, Open Approach
WH603Z	Insertion of Infusion Device into Neck, Open Approach
WH60YZ	Insertion of Other Device into Neck, Open Approach
H631Z	Insertion of Radioactive Element into Neck, Percutaneous Approach
0WH633Z	Insertion of Infusion Device into Neck, Percutaneous Approach
0WH63YZ	Insertion of Other Device into Neck, Percutaneous Approach
WH641Z	Insertion of Radioactive Element into Neck, Percutaneous Endoscopic Approach
0WH643Z	Insertion of Infusion Device into Neck, Percutaneous Endoscopic Approach
0WH64YZ	Insertion of Other Device into Neck, Percutaneous Endoscopic Approach
WH801Z	Insertion of Radioactive Element into Chest Wall, Open Approach
WH803Z	Insertion of Infusion Device into Chest Wall, Open Approach
WH80YZ	Insertion of Other Device into Chest Wall, Open Approach
WH831Z	Insertion of Radioactive Element into Chest Wall, Percutaneous Approach
WH833Z	Insertion of Infusion Device into Chest Wall, Percutaneous Approach
WH83YZ	Insertion of Other Device into Chest Wall, Percutaneous Approach
0WH841Z	Insertion of Radioactive Element into Chest Wall, Percutaneous Endoscopic Approach
0WH843Z	Insertion of Infusion Device into Chest Wall, Percutaneous Endoscopic Approach
0WH84YZ	Insertion of Other Device into Chest Wall, Percutaneous Endoscopic Approach
0WH901Z	Insertion of Radioactive Element into Right Pleural Cavity, Open Approach
0WH903Z	Insertion of Infusion Device into Right Pleural Cavity, Open Approach
0WH90YZ	Insertion of Other Device into Right Pleural Cavity, Open Approach
0WH931Z	Insertion of Radioactive Element into Right Pleural Cavity, Percutaneous Approach
0WH933Z	Insertion of Infusion Device into Right Pleural Cavity, Percutaneous Approach
0WH93YZ	Insertion of Other Device into Right Pleural Cavity, Percutaneous Approach
0WH941Z	Insertion of Radioactive Element into Right Pleural Cavity, Percutaneous Endoscopic Approach
0WH943Z	Insertion of Infusion Device into Right Pleural Cavity, Percutaneous Endoscopic Approach
0WH94YZ	Insertion of Other Device into Right Pleural Cavity, Percutaneous Endoscopic Approach
0WHB01Z	Insertion of Radioactive Element into Left Pleural Cavity, Open Approach
0WHB03Z	Insertion of Infusion Device into Left Pleural Cavity, Open Approach
0WHB0YZ	Insertion of Other Device into Left Pleural Cavity, Open Approach
0WHB31Z	Insertion of Radioactive Element into Left Pleural Cavity, Percutaneous Approach
0WHB33Z	Insertion of Infusion Device into Left Pleural Cavity, Percutaneous Approach
0WHB3YZ	Insertion of Other Device into Left Pleural Cavity, Percutaneous Approach
0WHB41Z	Insertion of Radioactive Element into Left Pleural Cavity, Percutaneous Endoscopic Approach
0WHB43Z	Insertion of Infusion Device into Left Pleural Cavity, Percutaneous Endoscopic Approach
0WHB4YZ	Insertion of Other Device into Left Pleural Cavity, Percutaneous Endoscopic Approach
0WHC01Z	Insertion of Radioactive Element into Mediastinum, Open Approach
0WHC03Z	Insertion of Infusion Device into Mediastinum, Open Approach
0WHC0YZ	Insertion of Other Device into Mediastinum, Open Approach
0WHC31Z	Insertion of Radioactive Element into Mediastinum, Percutaneous Approach
0WHC33Z	Insertion of Infusion Device into Mediastinum, Percutaneous Approach
0WHC3YZ	Insertion of Other Device into Mediastinum, Percutaneous Approach
0WHC41Z	Insertion of Radioactive Element into Mediastinum, Percutaneous Endoscopic Approach
0WHC43Z	Insertion of Infusion Device into Mediastinum, Percutaneous Endoscopic Approach
0WHC4YZ	Insertion of Other Device into Mediastinum, Percutaneous Endoscopic Approach
0WHD01Z	Insertion of Radioactive Element into Pericardial Cavity, Open Approach
0WHD03Z	Insertion of Infusion Device into Pericardial Cavity, Open Approach
0WHD0YZ	Insertion of Other Device into Pericardial Cavity, Open Approach
0WHD31Z	Insertion of Radioactive Element into Pericardial Cavity, Percutaneous Approach
0WHD33Z	Insertion of Infusion Device into Pericardial Cavity, Percutaneous Approach
0WHD3YZ	Insertion of Other Device into Pericardial Cavity, Percutaneous Approach
0WHD41Z	Insertion of Radioactive Element into Pericardial Cavity, Percutaneous Endoscopic Approach
0WHD43Z	Insertion of Infusion Device into Pericardial Cavity, Percutaneous Endoscopic Approach
0WHD4YZ	Insertion of Other Device into Pericardial Cavity, Percutaneous Endoscopic Approach
0WHF01Z	Insertion of Radioactive Element into Abdominal Wall, Open Approach
0WHF03Z	Insertion of Infusion Device into Abdominal Wall, Open Approach
0WHF0YZ	Insertion of Other Device into Abdominal Wall, Open Approach
0WHF31Z	Insertion of Radioactive Element into Abdominal Wall, Percutaneous Approach
0WHF33Z	Insertion of Infusion Device into Abdominal Wall, Percutaneous Approach
0WHF3YZ	Insertion of Other Device into Abdominal Wall, Percutaneous Approach
0WHF41Z	Insertion of Radioactive Element into Abdominal Wall, Percutaneous Endoscopic Approach
0WHF43Z	Insertion of Infusion Device into Abdominal Wall, Percutaneous Endoscopic Approach
0WHF4YZ	Insertion of Other Device into Abdominal Wall, Percutaneous Endoscopic Approach
0WHG01Z	Insertion of Radioactive Element into Peritoneal Cavity, Open Approach
0WHG03Z	Insertion of Infusion Device into Peritoneal Cavity, Open Approach
0WHG0YZ	Insertion of Other Device into Peritoneal Cavity, Open Approach
0WHG31Z	Insertion of Radioactive Element into Peritoneal Cavity, Percutaneous Approach
0WHG33Z	Insertion of Infusion Device into Peritoneal Cavity, Percutaneous Approach
0WHG3YZ	Insertion of Other Device into Peritoneal Cavity, Percutaneous Approach
0WHG41Z	Insertion of Radioactive Element into Peritoneal Cavity, Percutaneous Endoscopic Approach
0WHG43Z	Insertion of Infusion Device into Peritoneal Cavity, Percutaneous Endoscopic Approach
0WHG4YZ	Insertion of Other Device into Peritoneal Cavity, Percutaneous Endoscopic Approach
0WHH01Z	Insertion of Radioactive Element into Retroperitoneum, Open Approach
0WHH03Z	Insertion of Infusion Device into Retroperitoneum, Open Approach
0WHH0YZ	Insertion of Other Device into Retroperitoneum, Open Approach
0WHH31Z	Insertion of Radioactive Element into Retroperitoneum, Percutaneous Approach
0WHH33Z	Insertion of Infusion Device into Retroperitoneum, Percutaneous Approach
0WHH3YZ	Insertion of Other Device into Retroperitoneum, Percutaneous Approach
0WHH41Z	Insertion of Radioactive Element into Retroperitoneum, Percutaneous Endoscopic Approach
0WHH43Z	Insertion of Infusion Device into Retroperitoneum, Percutaneous Endoscopic Approach
0WHH4YZ	Insertion of Other Device into Retroperitoneum, Percutaneous Endoscopic Approach

Female-only　　♂ Male-only　　▲ Limited Coverage　　● Non-OR　　▨ HAC-associated procedure　　▲ Non-covered procedures　　▦ Combination

0WHJ01Z Insertion of Radioactive Element into Pelvic Cavity, Open Approach

0WHJ03Z Insertion of Infusion Device into Pelvic Cavity, Open Approach

0WHJ0YZ Insertion of Other Device into Pelvic Cavity, Open Approach

0WHJ31Z Insertion of Radioactive Element into Pelvic Cavity, Percutaneous Approach

0WHJ33Z Insertion of Infusion Device into Pelvic Cavity, Percutaneous Approach

0WHJ3YZ Insertion of Other Device into Pelvic Cavity, Percutaneous Approach

0WHJ41Z Insertion of Radioactive Element into Pelvic Cavity, Percutaneous Endoscopic Approach

0WHJ43Z Insertion of Infusion Device into Pelvic Cavity, Percutaneous Endoscopic Approach

0WHJ4YZ Insertion of Other Device into Pelvic Cavity, Percutaneous Endoscopic Approach

0WHK01Z Insertion of Radioactive Element into Upper Back, Open Approach

● **0WHK03Z** Insertion of Infusion Device into Upper Back, Open Approach

● **0WHK0YZ** Insertion of Other Device into Upper Back, Open Approach

0WHK31Z Insertion of Radioactive Element into Upper Back, Percutaneous Approach

● **0WHK33Z** Insertion of Infusion Device into Upper Back, Percutaneous Approach

● **0WHK3YZ** Insertion of Other Device into Upper Back, Percutaneous Approach

0WHK41Z Insertion of Radioactive Element into Upper Back, Percutaneous Endoscopic Approach

● **0WHK43Z** Insertion of Infusion Device into Upper Back, Percutaneous Endoscopic Approach

● **0WHK4YZ** Insertion of Other Device into Upper Back, Percutaneous Endoscopic Approach

0WHL01Z Insertion of Radioactive Element into Lower Back, Open Approach

● **0WHL03Z** Insertion of Infusion Device into Lower Back, Open Approach

● **0WHL0YZ** Insertion of Other Device into Lower Back, Open Approach

0WHL31Z Insertion of Radioactive Element into Lower Back, Percutaneous Approach

● **0WHL33Z** Insertion of Infusion Device into Lower Back, Percutaneous Approach

● **0WHL3YZ** Insertion of Other Device into Lower Back, Percutaneous Approach

0WHL41Z Insertion of Radioactive Element into Lower Back, Percutaneous Endoscopic Approach

● **0WHL43Z** Insertion of Infusion Device into Lower Back, Percutaneous Endoscopic Approach

● **0WHL4YZ** Insertion of Other Device into Lower Back, Percutaneous Endoscopic Approach

♂ **0WHM01Z** Insertion of Radioactive Element into Male Perineum, Open Approach
This is a male-only service, however, it is not included in the male-only edit logic for MCE V30

♂● **0WHM03Z** Insertion of Infusion Device into Male Perineum, Open Approach
This is a male-only service, however, it is not included in the male-only edit logic for MCE V30

♂● **0WHM0YZ** Insertion of Other Device into Male Perineum, Open Approach
This is a male-only service, however, it is not included in the male-only edit logic for MCE V30

♂ **0WHM31Z** Insertion of Radioactive Element into Male Perineum, Percutaneous Approach

♂● **0WHM33Z** Insertion of Infusion Device into Male Perineum, Percutaneous Approach
This is a male-only service, however, it is not included in the male-only edit logic for MCE V30

♂● **0WHM3YZ** Insertion of Other Device into Male Perineum, Percutaneous Approach
This is a male-only service, however, it is not included in the male-only edit logic for MCE V30

♂ **0WHM41Z** Insertion of Radioactive Element into Male Perineum, Percutaneous Endoscopic Approach
This is a male-only service, however, it is not included in the male-only edit logic for MCE V30

♂● **0WHM43Z** Insertion of Infusion Device into Male Perineum, Percutaneous Endoscopic Approach
This is a male-only service, however, it is not included in the male-only edit logic for MCE V30

♂● **0WHM4YZ** Insertion of Other Device into Male Perineum, Percutaneous Endoscopic Approach
This is a male-only service, however, it is not included in the male-only edit logic for MCE V30

♀ **0WHN01Z** Insertion of Radioactive Element into Female Perineum, Open Approach
This is a female-only service, however, it is not included in the female-only edit logic for MCE V30

♀ **0WHN03Z** Insertion of Infusion Device into Female Perineum, Open Approach

♀ **0WHN0YZ** Insertion of Other Device into Female Perineum, Open Approach

♀ **0WHN31Z** Insertion of Radioactive Element into Female Perineum, Percutaneous Approach
This is a female-only service, however, it is not included in the female-only edit logic for MCE V30

♀ **0WHN33Z** Insertion of Infusion Device into Female Perineum, Percutaneous Approach

♀ **0WHN3YZ** Insertion of Other Device into Female Perineum, Percutaneous Approach

♀ **0WHN41Z** Insertion of Radioactive Element into Female Perineum, Percutaneous Endoscopic Approach
This is a female-only service, however, it is not included in the female-only edit logic for MCE V30

♀ **0WHN43Z** Insertion of Infusion Device into Female Perineum, Percutaneous Endoscopic Approach

♀ **0WHN4YZ** Insertion of Other Device into Female Perineum, Percutaneous Endoscopic Approach

0WHP01Z Insertion of Radioactive Element into Gastrointestinal Tract, Open Approach

0WHP03Z Insertion of Infusion Device into Gastrointestinal Tract, Open Approach

0WHP0YZ Insertion of Other Device into Gastrointestinal Tract, Open Approach

0WHP31Z Insertion of Radioactive Element into Gastrointestinal Tract, Percutaneous Approach

0WHP33Z Insertion of Infusion Device into Gastrointestinal Tract, Percutaneous Approach

0WHP3YZ Insertion of Other Device into Gastrointestinal Tract, Percutaneous Approach

0WHP41Z Insertion of Radioactive Element into Gastrointestinal Tract, Percutaneous Endoscopic Approach

0WHP43Z Insertion of Infusion Device into Gastrointestinal Tract, Percutaneous Endoscopic Approach

0WHP4YZ Insertion of Other Device into Gastrointestinal Tract, Percutaneous Endoscopic Approach

0WHP71Z Insertion of Radioactive Element into Gastrointestinal Tract, Via Natural or Artificial Opening

0WHP73Z Insertion of Infusion Device into Gastrointestinal Tract, Via Natural or Artificial Opening

0WHP7YZ Insertion of Other Device into Gastrointestinal Tract, Via Natural or Artificial Opening

0WHP81Z Insertion of Radioactive Element into Gastrointestinal Tract, Via Natural or Artificial Opening Endoscopic

0WHP83Z Insertion of Infusion Device into Gastrointestinal Tract, Via Natural or Artificial Opening Endoscopic

0WHP8YZ Insertion of Other Device into Gastrointestinal Tract, Via Natural or Artificial Opening Endoscopic

0WHQ01Z Insertion of Radioactive Element into Respiratory Tract, Open Approach

0WHQ03Z Insertion of Infusion Device into Respiratory Tract, Open Approach

0WHQ0YZ Insertion of Other Device into Respiratory Tract, Open Approach

0WHQ31Z Insertion of Radioactive Element into Respiratory Tract, Percutaneous Approach

0WHQ33Z Insertion of Infusion Device into Respiratory Tract, Percutaneous Approach

0WHQ3YZ Insertion of Other Device into Respiratory Tract, Percutaneous Approach

0WHQ41Z Insertion of Radioactive Element into Respiratory Tract, Percutaneous Endoscopic Approach

0WHQ43Z Insertion of Infusion Device into Respiratory Tract, Percutaneous Endoscopic Approach

0WHQ4YZ Insertion of Other Device into Respiratory Tract, Percutaneous Endoscopic Approach

0WHQ71Z Insertion of Radioactive Element into Respiratory Tract, Via Natural or Artificial Opening

0WHQ73Z Insertion of Infusion Device into Respiratory Tract, Via Natural or Artificial Opening

0WHQ7YZ Insertion of Other Device into Respiratory Tract, Via Natural or Artificial Opening

0WHQ81Z Insertion of Radioactive Element into Respiratory Tract, Via Natural or Artificial Opening Endoscopic

0WHQ83Z Insertion of Infusion Device into Respiratory Tract, Via Natural or Artificial Opening Endoscopic

0WHQ8YZ Insertion of Other Device into Respiratory Tract, Via Natural or Artificial Opening Endoscopic

0WHR01Z Insertion of Radioactive Element into Genitourinary Tract, Open Approach

0WHR03Z Insertion of Infusion Device into Genitourinary Tract, Open Approach

0WHR0YZ Insertion of Other Device into Genitourinary Tract, Open Approach

0WHR31Z Insertion of Radioactive Element into Genitourinary Tract, Percutaneous Approach

0WHR33Z Insertion of Infusion Device into Genitourinary Tract, Percutaneous Approach

♀ Female-only   ♂ Male-only   ▲ Limited Coverage   ● Non-OR   ▨ HAC-associated procedure   ▲ Non-covered procedures   + Combination

0WHR3YZ Insertion of Other Device into Genitourinary Tract, Percutaneous Approach

0WHR41Z Insertion of Radioactive Element into Genitourinary Tract, Percutaneous Endoscopic Approach

0WHR43Z Insertion of Infusion Device into Genitourinary Tract, Percutaneous Endoscopic Approach

0WHR4YZ Insertion of Other Device into Genitourinary Tract, Percutaneous Endoscopic Approach

0WHR71Z Insertion of Radioactive Element into Genitourinary Tract, Via Natural or Artificial Opening

0WHR73Z Insertion of Infusion Device into Genitourinary Tract, Via Natural or Artificial Opening

0WHR7YZ Insertion of Other Device into Genitourinary Tract, Via Natural or Artificial Opening

0WHR81Z Insertion of Radioactive Element into Genitourinary Tract, Via Natural or Artificial Opening Endoscopic

0WHR83Z Insertion of Infusion Device into Genitourinary Tract, Via Natural or Artificial Opening Endoscopic

0WHR8YZ Insertion of Other Device into Genitourinary Tract, Via Natural or Artificial Opening Endoscopic

0WJ – Anatomical Regions, General, Inspection

Review Coding Guidelines B3.11a, B3.11b and B3.11c

0WJ00ZZ Inspection of Head, Open Approach

0WJ03ZZ Inspection of Head, Percutaneous Approach

0WJ04ZZ Inspection of Head, Percutaneous Endoscopic Approach

0WJ0XZZ Inspection of Head, External Approach

0WJ10ZZ Inspection of Cranial Cavity, Open Approach

0WJ13ZZ Inspection of Cranial Cavity, Percutaneous Approach

0WJ14ZZ Inspection of Cranial Cavity, Percutaneous Endoscopic Approach

0WJ20ZZ Inspection of Face, Open Approach

0WJ23ZZ Inspection of Face, Percutaneous Approach

0WJ24ZZ Inspection of Face, Percutaneous Endoscopic Approach

0WJ2XZZ Inspection of Face, External Approach

0WJ30ZZ Inspection of Oral Cavity and Throat, Open Approach

0WJ33ZZ Inspection of Oral Cavity and Throat, Percutaneous Approach

0WJ34ZZ Inspection of Oral Cavity and Throat, Percutaneous Endoscopic Approach

0WJ3XZZ Inspection of Oral Cavity and Throat, External Approach

0WJ40ZZ Inspection of Upper Jaw, Open Approach

0WJ43ZZ Inspection of Upper Jaw, Percutaneous Approach

0WJ44ZZ Inspection of Upper Jaw, Percutaneous Endoscopic Approach

0WJ4XZZ Inspection of Upper Jaw, External Approach

0WJ50ZZ Inspection of Lower Jaw, Open Approach

0WJ53ZZ Inspection of Lower Jaw, Percutaneous Approach

0WJ54ZZ Inspection of Lower Jaw, Percutaneous Endoscopic Approach

0WJ5XZZ Inspection of Lower Jaw, External Approach

0WJ60ZZ Inspection of Neck, Open Approach

0WJ63ZZ Inspection of Neck, Percutaneous Approach

0WJ64ZZ Inspection of Neck, Percutaneous Endoscopic Approach

0WJ6XZZ Inspection of Neck, External Approach

0WJ80ZZ Inspection of Chest Wall, Open Approach

0WJ83ZZ Inspection of Chest Wall, Percutaneous Approach

0WJ84ZZ Inspection of Chest Wall, Percutaneous Endoscopic Approach

0WJ8XZZ Inspection of Chest Wall, External Approach

0WJ90ZZ Inspection of Right Pleural Cavity, Open Approach

0WJ93ZZ Inspection of Right Pleural Cavity, Percutaneous Approach

0WJ94ZZ Inspection of Right Pleural Cavity, Percutaneous Endoscopic Approach

0WJB0ZZ Inspection of Left Pleural Cavity, Open Approach

0WJB3ZZ Inspection of Left Pleural Cavity, Percutaneous Approach

0WJB4ZZ Inspection of Left Pleural Cavity, Percutaneous Endoscopic Approach

0WJC0ZZ Inspection of Mediastinum, Open Approach

0WJC3ZZ Inspection of Mediastinum, Percutaneous Approach

0WJC4ZZ Inspection of Mediastinum, Percutaneous Endoscopic Approach

0WJD0ZZ Inspection of Pericardial Cavity, Open Approach

0WJD3ZZ Inspection of Pericardial Cavity, Percutaneous Approach

0WJD4ZZ Inspection of Pericardial Cavity, Percutaneous Endoscopic Approach

0WJF0ZZ Inspection of Abdominal Wall, Open Approach

0WJF3ZZ Inspection of Abdominal Wall, Percutaneous Approach

0WJF4ZZ Inspection of Abdominal Wall, Percutaneous Endoscopic Approach

0WJFXZZ Inspection of Abdominal Wall, External Approach

0WJG0ZZ Inspection of Peritoneal Cavity, Open Approach

0WJG3ZZ Inspection of Peritoneal Cavity, Percutaneous Approach

0WJG4ZZ Inspection of Peritoneal Cavity, Percutaneous Endoscopic Approach

AHA CC: 2Q, 2013, 36-37

0WJH0ZZ Inspection of Retroperitoneum, Open Approach

0WJH3ZZ Inspection of Retroperitoneum, Percutaneous Approach

0WJH4ZZ Inspection of Retroperitoneum, Percutaneous Endoscopic Approach

0WJJ0ZZ Inspection of Pelvic Cavity, Open Approach

0WJJ3ZZ Inspection of Pelvic Cavity, Percutaneous Approach

0WJJ4ZZ Inspection of Pelvic Cavity, Percutaneous Endoscopic Approach

● **0WJK0ZZ** Inspection of Upper Back, Open Approach

0WJK3ZZ Inspection of Upper Back, Percutaneous Approach

0WJK4ZZ Inspection of Upper Back, Percutaneous Endoscopic Approach

0WJKXZZ Inspection of Upper Back, External Approach

● **0WJL0ZZ** Inspection of Lower Back, Open Approach

0WJL3ZZ Inspection of Lower Back, Percutaneous Approach

0WJL4ZZ Inspection of Lower Back, Percutaneous Endoscopic Approach

0WJLXZZ Inspection of Lower Back, External Approach

♂ **0WJM0ZZ** Inspection of Male Perineum, Open Approach

♂ **0WJM3ZZ** Inspection of Male Perineum, Percutaneous Approach

♂ **0WJM4ZZ** Inspection of Male Perineum, Percutaneous Endoscopic Approach

♂ **0WJMXZZ** Inspection of Male Perineum, External Approach

♀ **0WJN0ZZ** Inspection of Female Perineum, Open Approach

♀ **0WJN3ZZ** Inspection of Female Perineum, Percutaneous Approach

♀ **0WJN4ZZ** Inspection of Female Perineum, Percutaneous Endoscopic Approach

♀ **0WJNXZZ** Inspection of Female Perineum, External Approach

0WJP0ZZ Inspection of Gastrointestinal Tract, Open Approach

0WJP3ZZ Inspection of Gastrointestinal Tract, Percutaneous Approach

0WJP4ZZ Inspection of Gastrointestinal Tract, Percutaneous Endoscopic Approach

0WJP7ZZ Inspection of Gastrointestinal Tract, Via Natural or Artificial Opening Approach

0WJP8ZZ Inspection of Gastrointestinal Tract, Via Natural or Artificial Opening Endoscopic Approach

0WJQ0ZZ Inspection of Respiratory Tract, Open Approach

0WJQ3ZZ Inspection of Respiratory Tract, Percutaneous Approach

0WJQ4ZZ Inspection of Respiratory Tract, Percutaneous Endoscopic Approach

0WJQ7ZZ Inspection of Respiratory Tract, Via Natural or Artificial Opening Approach

0WJQ8ZZ Inspection of Respiratory Tract, Via Natural or Artificial Opening Endoscopic Approach

0WJR0ZZ Inspection of Genitourinary Tract, Open Approach

0WJR3ZZ Inspection of Genitourinary Tract, Percutaneous Approach

0WJR4ZZ Inspection of Genitourinary Tract, Percutaneous Endoscopic Approach

0WJR7ZZ Inspection of Genitourinary Tract, Via Natural or Artificial Opening Approach

0WJR8ZZ Inspection of Genitourinary Tract, Via Natural or Artificial Opening Endoscopic Approach

● Female-only　♂ Male-only　▲ Limited Coverage　● Non-OR　▬ HAC-associated procedure　▲ Non-covered procedures　✚ Combination

0WM – Anatomical Regions, General, Reattachment

0WM20ZZ	Reattachment of Face, Open Approach	
0WM40ZZ	Reattachment of Upper Jaw, Open Approach	
0WM50ZZ	Reattachment of Lower Jaw, Open Approach	
0WM60ZZ	Reattachment of Neck, Open Approach	

0WM80ZZ	Reattachment of Chest Wall, Open Approach
0WMF0ZZ	Reattachment of Abdominal Wall, Open Approach
0WMK0ZZ	Reattachment of Upper Back, Open Approach

0WML0ZZ	Reattachment of Lower Back, Open Approach
♂ 0WMM0ZZ	Reattachment of Male Perineum, Open Approach
♀ 0WMN0ZZ	Reattachment of Female Perineum, Open Approach

0WP – Anatomical Regions, General, Removal

Review Coding Guideline B6.1c

0WP000Z	Removal of Drainage Device from Head, Open Approach
0WP001Z	Removal of Radioactive Element from Head, Open Approach
0WP003Z	Removal of Infusion Device from Head, Open Approach
0WP007Z	Removal of Autologous Tissue Substitute from Head, Open Approach
0WP00JZ	Removal of Synthetic Substitute from Head, Open Approach
0WP00KZ	Removal of Nonautologous Tissue Substitute from Head, Open Approach
0WP00YZ	Removal of Other Device from Head, Open Approach
0WP030Z	Removal of Drainage Device from Head, Percutaneous Approach
0WP031Z	Removal of Radioactive Element from Head, Percutaneous Approach
0WP033Z	Removal of Infusion Device from Head, Percutaneous Approach
0WP037Z	Removal of Autologous Tissue Substitute from Head, Percutaneous Approach
0WP03JZ	Removal of Synthetic Substitute from Head, Percutaneous Approach
0WP03KZ	Removal of Nonautologous Tissue Substitute from Head, Percutaneous Approach
0WP03YZ	Removal of Other Device from Head, Percutaneous Approach
0WP040Z	Removal of Drainage Device from Head, Percutaneous Endoscopic Approach
0WP041Z	Removal of Radioactive Element from Head, Percutaneous Endoscopic Approach
0WP043Z	Removal of Infusion Device from Head, Percutaneous Endoscopic Approach
0WP047Z	Removal of Autologous Tissue Substitute from Head, Percutaneous Endoscopic Approach
0WP04JZ	Removal of Synthetic Substitute from Head, Percutaneous Endoscopic Approach
0WP04KZ	Removal of Nonautologous Tissue Substitute from Head, Percutaneous Endoscopic Approach
0WP04YZ	Removal of Other Device from Head, Percutaneous Endoscopic Approach
0WP0X0Z	Removal of Drainage Device from Head, External Approach
0WP0X1Z	Removal of Radioactive Element from Head, External Approach
0WP0X3Z	Removal of Infusion Device from Head, External Approach
0WP0X7Z	Removal of Autologous Tissue Substitute from Head, External Approach
0WP0XJZ	Removal of Synthetic Substitute from Head, External Approach
0WP0XKZ	Removal of Nonautologous Tissue Substitute from Head, External Approach
0WP0XYZ	Removal of Other Device from Head, External Approach
0WP100Z	Removal of Drainage Device from Cranial Cavity, Open Approach
0WP101Z	Removal of Radioactive Element from Cranial Cavity, Open Approach

0WP103Z	Removal of Infusion Device from Cranial Cavity, Open Approach
0WP10JZ	Removal of Synthetic Substitute from Cranial Cavity, Open Approach
0WP10YZ	Removal of Other Device from Cranial Cavity, Open Approach
0WP130Z	Removal of Drainage Device from Cranial Cavity, Percutaneous Approach
0WP131Z	Removal of Radioactive Element from Cranial Cavity, Percutaneous Approach
0WP133Z	Removal of Infusion Device from Cranial Cavity, Percutaneous Approach
0WP13JZ	Removal of Synthetic Substitute from Cranial Cavity, Percutaneous Approach
0WP13YZ	Removal of Other Device from Cranial Cavity, Percutaneous Approach
0WP140Z	Removal of Drainage Device from Cranial Cavity, Percutaneous Endoscopic Approach
0WP141Z	Removal of Radioactive Element from Cranial Cavity, Percutaneous Endoscopic Approach
0WP143Z	Removal of Infusion Device from Cranial Cavity, Percutaneous Endoscopic Approach
0WP14JZ	Removal of Synthetic Substitute from Cranial Cavity, Percutaneous Endoscopic Approach
0WP14YZ	Removal of Other Device from Cranial Cavity, Percutaneous Endoscopic Approach
0WP1X0Z	Removal of Drainage Device from Cranial Cavity, External Approach
0WP1X1Z	Removal of Radioactive Element from Cranial Cavity, External Approach
0WP1X3Z	Removal of Infusion Device from Cranial Cavity, External Approach
0WP200Z	Removal of Drainage Device from Face, Open Approach
0WP201Z	Removal of Radioactive Element from Face, Open Approach
0WP203Z	Removal of Infusion Device from Face, Open Approach
0WP207Z	Removal of Autologous Tissue Substitute from Face, Open Approach
0WP20JZ	Removal of Synthetic Substitute from Face, Open Approach
0WP20KZ	Removal of Nonautologous Tissue Substitute from Face, Open Approach
0WP20YZ	Removal of Other Device from Face, Open Approach
0WP230Z	Removal of Drainage Device from Face, Percutaneous Approach
0WP231Z	Removal of Radioactive Element from Face, Percutaneous Approach
0WP233Z	Removal of Infusion Device from Face, Percutaneous Approach
0WP237Z	Removal of Autologous Tissue Substitute from Face, Percutaneous Approach
0WP23JZ	Removal of Synthetic Substitute from Face, Percutaneous Approach
0WP23KZ	Removal of Nonautologous Tissue Substitute from Face, Percutaneous Approach

0WP23YZ	Removal of Other Device from Face, Percutaneous Approach
0WP240Z	Removal of Drainage Device from Face, Percutaneous Endoscopic Approach
0WP241Z	Removal of Radioactive Element from Face, Percutaneous Endoscopic Approach
0WP243Z	Removal of Infusion Device from Face, Percutaneous Endoscopic Approach
0WP247Z	Removal of Autologous Tissue Substitute from Face, Percutaneous Endoscopic Approach
0WP24JZ	Removal of Synthetic Substitute from Face, Percutaneous Endoscopic Approach
0WP24KZ	Removal of Nonautologous Tissue Substitute from Face, Percutaneous Endoscopic Approach
0WP24YZ	Removal of Other Device from Face, Percutaneous Endoscopic Approach
0WP2X0Z	Removal of Drainage Device from Face, External Approach
0WP2X1Z	Removal of Radioactive Element from Face, External Approach
0WP2X3Z	Removal of Infusion Device from Face, External Approach
0WP2X7Z	Removal of Autologous Tissue Substitute from Face, External Approach
0WP2XJZ	Removal of Synthetic Substitute from Face, External Approach
0WP2XKZ	Removal of Nonautologous Tissue Substitute from Face, External Approach
0WP2XYZ	Removal of Other Device from Face, External Approach
0WP400Z	Removal of Drainage Device from Upper Jaw, Open Approach
0WP401Z	Removal of Radioactive Element from Upper Jaw, Open Approach
0WP403Z	Removal of Infusion Device from Upper Jaw, Open Approach
0WP407Z	Removal of Autologous Tissue Substitute from Upper Jaw, Open Approach
0WP40JZ	Removal of Synthetic Substitute from Upper Jaw, Open Approach
0WP40KZ	Removal of Nonautologous Tissue Substitute from Upper Jaw, Open Approach
0WP40YZ	Removal of Other Device from Upper Jaw, Open Approach
0WP430Z	Removal of Drainage Device from Upper Jaw, Percutaneous Approach
0WP431Z	Removal of Radioactive Element from Upper Jaw, Percutaneous Approach
0WP433Z	Removal of Infusion Device from Upper Jaw, Percutaneous Approach
0WP437Z	Removal of Autologous Tissue Substitute from Upper Jaw, Percutaneous Approach
0WP43JZ	Removal of Synthetic Substitute from Upper Jaw, Percutaneous Approach
0WP43KZ	Removal of Nonautologous Tissue Substitute from Upper Jaw, Percutaneous Approach
0WP43YZ	Removal of Other Device from Upper Jaw, Percutaneous Approach
0WP440Z	Removal of Drainage Device from Upper Jaw, Percutaneous Endoscopic Approach

♀ Female-only	♂ Male-only	▲ Limited Coverage	● Non-OR	▩ HAC-associated procedure	▲ Non-covered procedures	✚ Combination

0WP441Z Removal of Radioactive Element from Upper Jaw, Percutaneous Endoscopic Approach

0WP443Z Removal of Infusion Device from Upper Jaw, Percutaneous Endoscopic Approach

0WP447Z Removal of Autologous Tissue Substitute from Upper Jaw, Percutaneous Endoscopic Approach

0WP44JZ Removal of Synthetic Substitute from Upper Jaw, Percutaneous Endoscopic Approach

0WP44KZ Removal of Nonautologous Tissue Substitute from Upper Jaw, Percutaneous Endoscopic Approach

0WP44YZ Removal of Other Device from Upper Jaw, Percutaneous Endoscopic Approach

0WP4X0Z Removal of Drainage Device from Upper Jaw, External Approach

0WP4X1Z Removal of Radioactive Element from Upper Jaw, External Approach

0WP4X3Z Removal of Infusion Device from Upper Jaw, External Approach

0WP4X7Z Removal of Autologous Tissue Substitute from Upper Jaw, External Approach

0WP4XJZ Removal of Synthetic Substitute from Upper Jaw, External Approach

0WP4XKZ Removal of Nonautologous Tissue Substitute from Upper Jaw, External Approach

0WP4XYZ Removal of Other Device from Upper Jaw, External Approach

0WP500Z Removal of Drainage Device from Lower Jaw, Open Approach

0WP501Z Removal of Radioactive Element from Lower Jaw, Open Approach

0WP503Z Removal of Infusion Device from Lower Jaw, Open Approach

0WP507Z Removal of Autologous Tissue Substitute from Lower Jaw, Open Approach

0WP50JZ Removal of Synthetic Substitute from Lower Jaw, Open Approach

0WP50KZ Removal of Nonautologous Tissue Substitute from Lower Jaw, Open Approach

0WP50YZ Removal of Other Device from Lower Jaw, Open Approach

0WP530Z Removal of Drainage Device from Lower Jaw, Percutaneous Approach

0WP531Z Removal of Radioactive Element from Lower Jaw, Percutaneous Approach

0WP533Z Removal of Infusion Device from Lower Jaw, Percutaneous Approach

0WP537Z Removal of Autologous Tissue Substitute from Lower Jaw, Percutaneous Approach

0WP53JZ Removal of Synthetic Substitute from Lower Jaw, Percutaneous Approach

0WP53KZ Removal of Nonautologous Tissue Substitute from Lower Jaw, Percutaneous Approach

0WP53YZ Removal of Other Device from Lower Jaw, Percutaneous Approach

0WP540Z Removal of Drainage Device from Lower Jaw, Percutaneous Endoscopic Approach

0WP541Z Removal of Radioactive Element from Lower Jaw, Percutaneous Endoscopic Approach

0WP543Z Removal of Infusion Device from Lower Jaw, Percutaneous Endoscopic Approach

0WP547Z Removal of Autologous Tissue Substitute from Lower Jaw, Percutaneous Endoscopic Approach

0WP54JZ Removal of Synthetic Substitute from Lower Jaw, Percutaneous Endoscopic Approach

0WP54KZ Removal of Nonautologous Tissue Substitute from Lower Jaw, Percutaneous Endoscopic Approach

0WP54YZ Removal of Other Device from Lower Jaw, Percutaneous Endoscopic Approach

0WP5X0Z Removal of Drainage Device from Lower Jaw, External Approach

0WP5X1Z Removal of Radioactive Element from Lower Jaw, External Approach

0WP5X3Z Removal of Infusion Device from Lower Jaw, External Approach

0WP5X7Z Removal of Autologous Tissue Substitute from Lower Jaw, External Approach

0WP5XJZ Removal of Synthetic Substitute from Lower Jaw, External Approach

0WP5XKZ Removal of Nonautologous Tissue Substitute from Lower Jaw, External Approach

0WP5XYZ Removal of Other Device from Lower Jaw, External Approach

0WP600Z Removal of Drainage Device from Neck, Open Approach

0WP601Z Removal of Radioactive Element from Neck, Open Approach

0WP603Z Removal of Infusion Device from Neck, Open Approach

0WP607Z Removal of Autologous Tissue Substitute from Neck, Open Approach

0WP60JZ Removal of Synthetic Substitute from Neck, Open Approach

0WP60KZ Removal of Nonautologous Tissue Substitute from Neck, Open Approach

0WP60YZ Removal of Other Device from Neck, Open Approach

0WP630Z Removal of Drainage Device from Neck, Percutaneous Approach

0WP631Z Removal of Radioactive Element from Neck, Percutaneous Approach

0WP633Z Removal of Infusion Device from Neck, Percutaneous Approach

0WP637Z Removal of Autologous Tissue Substitute from Neck, Percutaneous Approach

0WP63JZ Removal of Synthetic Substitute from Neck, Percutaneous Approach

0WP63KZ Removal of Nonautologous Tissue Substitute from Neck, Percutaneous Approach

0WP63YZ Removal of Other Device from Neck, Percutaneous Approach

0WP640Z Removal of Drainage Device from Neck, Percutaneous Endoscopic Approach

0WP641Z Removal of Radioactive Element from Neck, Percutaneous Endoscopic Approach

0WP643Z Removal of Infusion Device from Neck, Percutaneous Endoscopic Approach

0WP647Z Removal of Autologous Tissue Substitute from Neck, Percutaneous Endoscopic Approach

0WP64JZ Removal of Synthetic Substitute from Neck, Percutaneous Endoscopic Approach

0WP64KZ Removal of Nonautologous Tissue Substitute from Neck, Percutaneous Endoscopic Approach

0WP64YZ Removal of Other Device from Neck, Percutaneous Endoscopic Approach

0WP6X0Z Removal of Drainage Device from Neck, External Approach

0WP6X1Z Removal of Radioactive Element from Neck, External Approach

0WP6X3Z Removal of Infusion Device from Neck, External Approach

0WP6X7Z Removal of Autologous Tissue Substitute from Neck, External Approach

0WP6XJZ Removal of Synthetic Substitute from Neck, External Approach

0WP6XKZ Removal of Nonautologous Tissue Substitute from Neck, External Approach

0WP6XYZ Removal of Other Device from Neck, External Approach

0WP800Z Removal of Drainage Device from Chest Wall, Open Approach

0WP801Z Removal of Radioactive Element from Chest Wall, Open Approach

0WP803Z Removal of Infusion Device from Chest Wall, Open Approach

0WP807Z Removal of Autologous Tissue Substitute from Chest Wall, Open Approach

0WP80JZ Removal of Synthetic Substitute from Chest Wall, Open Approach

0WP80KZ Removal of Nonautologous Tissue Substitute from Chest Wall, Open Approach

0WP80YZ Removal of Other Device from Chest Wall, Open Approach

0WP830Z Removal of Drainage Device from Chest Wall, Percutaneous Approach

0WP831Z Removal of Radioactive Element from Chest Wall, Percutaneous Approach

0WP833Z Removal of Infusion Device from Chest Wall, Percutaneous Approach

0WP837Z Removal of Autologous Tissue Substitute from Chest Wall, Percutaneous Approach

0WP83JZ Removal of Synthetic Substitute from Chest Wall, Percutaneous Approach

0WP83KZ Removal of Nonautologous Tissue Substitute from Chest Wall, Percutaneous Approach

0WP83YZ Removal of Other Device from Chest Wall, Percutaneous Approach

0WP840Z Removal of Drainage Device from Chest Wall, Percutaneous Endoscopic Approach

0WP841Z Removal of Radioactive Element from Chest Wall, Percutaneous Endoscopic Approach

0WP843Z Removal of Infusion Device from Chest Wall, Percutaneous Endoscopic Approach

0WP847Z Removal of Autologous Tissue Substitute from Chest Wall, Percutaneous Endoscopic Approach

0WP84JZ Removal of Synthetic Substitute from Chest Wall, Percutaneous Endoscopic Approach

0WP84KZ Removal of Nonautologous Tissue Substitute from Chest Wall, Percutaneous Endoscopic Approach

0WP84YZ Removal of Other Device from Chest Wall, Percutaneous Endoscopic Approach

0WP8X0Z Removal of Drainage Device from Chest Wall, External Approach

0WP8X1Z Removal of Radioactive Element from Chest Wall, External Approach

0WP8X3Z Removal of Infusion Device from Chest Wall, External Approach

0WP8X7Z Removal of Autologous Tissue Substitute from Chest Wall, External Approach

0WP8XJZ Removal of Synthetic Substitute from Chest Wall, External Approach

0WP8XKZ Removal of Nonautologous Tissue Substitute from Chest Wall, External Approach

0WP8XYZ Removal of Other Device from Chest Wall, External Approach

0WP900Z Removal of Drainage Device from Right Pleural Cavity, Open Approach

0WP901Z Removal of Radioactive Element from Right Pleural Cavity, Open Approach

0WP903Z Removal of Infusion Device from Right Pleural Cavity, Open Approach

0WP90JZ Removal of Synthetic Substitute from Right Pleural Cavity, Open Approach

0WP90YZ Removal of Other Device from Right Pleural Cavity, Open Approach

0WP930Z Removal of Drainage Device from Right Pleural Cavity, Percutaneous Approach

♀ Female-only   ♂ Male-only   ▲ Limited Coverage   ● Non-OR   ▆ HAC-associated procedure   ▲ Non-covered procedures   ✚ Combination

0WP931Z	Removal of Radioactive Element from Right Pleural Cavity, Percutaneous Approach
0WP933Z	Removal of Infusion Device from Right Pleural Cavity, Percutaneous Approach
0WP93JZ	Removal of Synthetic Substitute from Right Pleural Cavity, Percutaneous Approach
0WP93YZ	Removal of Other Device from Right Pleural Cavity, Percutaneous Approach
0WP940Z	Removal of Drainage Device from Right Pleural Cavity, Percutaneous Endoscopic Approach
0WP941Z	Removal of Radioactive Element from Right Pleural Cavity, Percutaneous Endoscopic Approach
0WP943Z	Removal of Infusion Device from Right Pleural Cavity, Percutaneous Endoscopic Approach
0WP94JZ	Removal of Synthetic Substitute from Right Pleural Cavity, Percutaneous Endoscopic Approach
0WP94YZ	Removal of Other Device from Right Pleural Cavity, Percutaneous Endoscopic Approach
0WP9X0Z	Removal of Drainage Device from Right Pleural Cavity, External Approach
0WP9X1Z	Removal of Radioactive Element from Right Pleural Cavity, External Approach
0WP9X3Z	Removal of Infusion Device from Right Pleural Cavity, External Approach
0WPB00Z	Removal of Drainage Device from Left Pleural Cavity, Open Approach
0WPB01Z	Removal of Radioactive Element from Left Pleural Cavity, Open Approach
0WPB03Z	Removal of Infusion Device from Left Pleural Cavity, Open Approach
0WPB0JZ	Removal of Synthetic Substitute from Left Pleural Cavity, Open Approach
0WPB0YZ	Removal of Other Device from Left Pleural Cavity, Open Approach
0WPB30Z	Removal of Drainage Device from Left Pleural Cavity, Percutaneous Approach
0WPB31Z	Removal of Radioactive Element from Left Pleural Cavity, Percutaneous Approach
0WPB33Z	Removal of Infusion Device from Left Pleural Cavity, Percutaneous Approach
0WPB3JZ	Removal of Synthetic Substitute from Left Pleural Cavity, Percutaneous Approach
0WPB3YZ	Removal of Other Device from Left Pleural Cavity, Percutaneous Approach
0WPB40Z	Removal of Drainage Device from Left Pleural Cavity, Percutaneous Endoscopic Approach
0WPB41Z	Removal of Radioactive Element from Left Pleural Cavity, Percutaneous Endoscopic Approach
0WPB43Z	Removal of Infusion Device from Left Pleural Cavity, Percutaneous Endoscopic Approach
0WPB4JZ	Removal of Synthetic Substitute from Left Pleural Cavity, Percutaneous Endoscopic Approach
0WPB4YZ	Removal of Other Device from Left Pleural Cavity, Percutaneous Endoscopic Approach
0WPBX0Z	Removal of Drainage Device from Left Pleural Cavity, External Approach
0WPBX1Z	Removal of Radioactive Element from Left Pleural Cavity, External Approach
0WPBX3Z	Removal of Infusion Device from Left Pleural Cavity, External Approach
0WPC00Z	Removal of Drainage Device from Mediastinum, Open Approach
0WPC01Z	Removal of Radioactive Element from Mediastinum, Open Approach

0WPC03Z	Removal of Infusion Device from Mediastinum, Open Approach
0WPC07Z	Removal of Autologous Tissue Substitute from Mediastinum, Open Approach
0WPC0JZ	Removal of Synthetic Substitute from Mediastinum, Open Approach
0WPC0KZ	Removal of Nonautologous Tissue Substitute from Mediastinum, Open Approach
0WPC0YZ	Removal of Other Device from Mediastinum, Open Approach
0WPC30Z	Removal of Drainage Device from Mediastinum, Percutaneous Approach
0WPC31Z	Removal of Radioactive Element from Mediastinum, Percutaneous Approach
0WPC33Z	Removal of Infusion Device from Mediastinum, Percutaneous Approach
0WPC37Z	Removal of Autologous Tissue Substitute from Mediastinum, Percutaneous Approach
0WPC3JZ	Removal of Synthetic Substitute from Mediastinum, Percutaneous Approach
0WPC3KZ	Removal of Nonautologous Tissue Substitute from Mediastinum, Percutaneous Approach
0WPC3YZ	Removal of Other Device from Mediastinum, Percutaneous Approach
0WPC40Z	Removal of Drainage Device from Mediastinum, Percutaneous Endoscopic Approach
0WPC41Z	Removal of Radioactive Element from Mediastinum, Percutaneous Endoscopic Approach
0WPC43Z	Removal of Infusion Device from Mediastinum, Percutaneous Endoscopic Approach
0WPC47Z	Removal of Autologous Tissue Substitute from Mediastinum, Percutaneous Endoscopic Approach
0WPC4JZ	Removal of Synthetic Substitute from Mediastinum, Percutaneous Endoscopic Approach
0WPC4KZ	Removal of Nonautologous Tissue Substitute from Mediastinum, Percutaneous Endoscopic Approach
0WPC4YZ	Removal of Other Device from Mediastinum, Percutaneous Endoscopic Approach
0WPCX0Z	Removal of Drainage Device from Mediastinum, External Approach
0WPCX1Z	Removal of Radioactive Element from Mediastinum, External Approach
0WPCX3Z	Removal of Infusion Device from Mediastinum, External Approach
0WPCX7Z	Removal of Autologous Tissue Substitute from Mediastinum, External Approach
0WPCXJZ	Removal of Synthetic Substitute from Mediastinum, External Approach
0WPCXKZ	Removal of Nonautologous Tissue Substitute from Mediastinum, External Approach
0WPCXYZ	Removal of Other Device from Mediastinum, External Approach
0WPD00Z	Removal of Drainage Device from Pericardial Cavity, Open Approach
0WPD01Z	Removal of Radioactive Element from Pericardial Cavity, Open Approach
0WPD03Z	Removal of Infusion Device from Pericardial Cavity, Open Approach
0WPD0YZ	Removal of Other Device from Pericardial Cavity, Open Approach
0WPD30Z	Removal of Drainage Device from Pericardial Cavity, Percutaneous Approach
0WPD31Z	Removal of Radioactive Element from Pericardial Cavity, Percutaneous Approach

0WPD33Z	Removal of Infusion Device from Pericardial Cavity, Percutaneous Approach
0WPD3YZ	Removal of Other Device from Pericardial Cavity, Percutaneous Approach
0WPD40Z	Removal of Drainage Device from Pericardial Cavity, Percutaneous Endoscopic Approach
0WPD41Z	Removal of Radioactive Element from Pericardial Cavity, Percutaneous Endoscopic Approach
0WPD43Z	Removal of Infusion Device from Pericardial Cavity, Percutaneous Endoscopic Approach
0WPD4YZ	Removal of Other Device from Pericardial Cavity, Percutaneous Endoscopic Approach
0WPDX0Z	Removal of Drainage Device from Pericardial Cavity, External Approach
0WPDX1Z	Removal of Radioactive Element from Pericardial Cavity, External Approach
0WPDX3Z	Removal of Infusion Device from Pericardial Cavity, External Approach
0WPF00Z	Removal of Drainage Device from Abdominal Wall, Open Approach
0WPF01Z	Removal of Radioactive Element from Abdominal Wall, Open Approach
0WPF03Z	Removal of Infusion Device from Abdominal Wall, Open Approach
0WPF07Z	Removal of Autologous Tissue Substitute from Abdominal Wall, Open Approach
0WPF0JZ	Removal of Synthetic Substitute from Abdominal Wall, Open Approach
0WPF0KZ	Removal of Nonautologous Tissue Substitute from Abdominal Wall, Open Approach
0WPF0YZ	Removal of Other Device from Abdominal Wall, Open Approach
0WPF30Z	Removal of Drainage Device from Abdominal Wall, Percutaneous Approach
0WPF31Z	Removal of Radioactive Element from Abdominal Wall, Percutaneous Approach
0WPF33Z	Removal of Infusion Device from Abdominal Wall, Percutaneous Approach
0WPF37Z	Removal of Autologous Tissue Substitute from Abdominal Wall, Percutaneous Approach
0WPF3JZ	Removal of Synthetic Substitute from Abdominal Wall, Percutaneous Approach
0WPF3KZ	Removal of Nonautologous Tissue Substitute from Abdominal Wall, Percutaneous Approach
0WPF3YZ	Removal of Other Device from Abdominal Wall, Percutaneous Approach
0WPF40Z	Removal of Drainage Device from Abdominal Wall, Percutaneous Endoscopic Approach
0WPF41Z	Removal of Radioactive Element from Abdominal Wall, Percutaneous Endoscopic Approach
0WPF43Z	Removal of Infusion Device from Abdominal Wall, Percutaneous Endoscopic Approach
0WPF47Z	Removal of Autologous Tissue Substitute from Abdominal Wall, Percutaneous Endoscopic Approach
0WPF4JZ	Removal of Synthetic Substitute from Abdominal Wall, Percutaneous Endoscopic Approach
0WPF4KZ	Removal of Nonautologous Tissue Substitute from Abdominal Wall, Percutaneous Endoscopic Approach
0WPF4YZ	Removal of Other Device from Abdominal Wall, Percutaneous Endoscopic Approach
0WPFX0Z	Removal of Drainage Device from Abdominal Wall, External Approach

0WPFX1Z	Removal of Radioactive Element from Abdominal Wall, External Approach
0WPFX3Z	Removal of Infusion Device from Abdominal Wall, External Approach
0WPFX7Z	Removal of Autologous Tissue Substitute from Abdominal Wall, External Approach
0WPFXJZ	Removal of Synthetic Substitute from Abdominal Wall, External Approach
0WPFXKZ	Removal of Nonautologous Tissue Substitute from Abdominal Wall, External Approach
0WPFXYZ	Removal of Other Device from Abdominal Wall, External Approach
0WPG00Z	Removal of Drainage Device from Peritoneal Cavity, Open Approach
0WPG01Z	Removal of Radioactive Element from Peritoneal Cavity, Open Approach
0WPG03Z	Removal of Infusion Device from Peritoneal Cavity, Open Approach
0WPG0JZ	Removal of Synthetic Substitute from Peritoneal Cavity, Open Approach
0WPG0YZ	Removal of Other Device from Peritoneal Cavity, Open Approach
0WPG30Z	Removal of Drainage Device from Peritoneal Cavity, Percutaneous Approach
0WPG31Z	Removal of Radioactive Element from Peritoneal Cavity, Percutaneous Approach
0WPG33Z	Removal of Infusion Device from Peritoneal Cavity, Percutaneous Approach
0WPG3JZ	Removal of Synthetic Substitute from Peritoneal Cavity, Percutaneous Approach
0WPG3YZ	Removal of Other Device from Peritoneal Cavity, Percutaneous Approach
0WPG40Z	Removal of Drainage Device from Peritoneal Cavity, Percutaneous Endoscopic Approach
0WPG41Z	Removal of Radioactive Element from Peritoneal Cavity, Percutaneous Endoscopic Approach
0WPG43Z	Removal of Infusion Device from Peritoneal Cavity, Percutaneous Endoscopic Approach
0WPG4JZ	Removal of Synthetic Substitute from Peritoneal Cavity, Percutaneous Endoscopic Approach
0WPG4YZ	Removal of Other Device from Peritoneal Cavity, Percutaneous Endoscopic Approach
0WPGX0Z	Removal of Drainage Device from Peritoneal Cavity, External Approach
0WPGX1Z	Removal of Radioactive Element from Peritoneal Cavity, External Approach
0WPGX3Z	Removal of Infusion Device from Peritoneal Cavity, External Approach
0WPH00Z	Removal of Drainage Device from Retroperitoneum, Open Approach
0WPH01Z	Removal of Radioactive Element from Retroperitoneum, Open Approach
0WPH03Z	Removal of Infusion Device from Retroperitoneum, Open Approach
0WPH0YZ	Removal of Other Device from Retroperitoneum, Open Approach
0WPH30Z	Removal of Drainage Device from Retroperitoneum, Percutaneous Approach
0WPH31Z	Removal of Radioactive Element from Retroperitoneum, Percutaneous Approach
0WPH33Z	Removal of Infusion Device from Retroperitoneum, Percutaneous Approach
0WPH3YZ	Removal of Other Device from Retroperitoneum, Percutaneous Approach
0WPH40Z	Removal of Drainage Device from Retroperitoneum, Percutaneous Endoscopic Approach

0WPH41Z	Removal of Radioactive Element from Retroperitoneum, Percutaneous Endoscopic Approach
0WPH43Z	Removal of Infusion Device from Retroperitoneum, Percutaneous Endoscopic Approach
0WPH4YZ	Removal of Other Device from Retroperitoneum, Percutaneous Endoscopic Approach
0WPHX0Z	Removal of Drainage Device from Retroperitoneum, External Approach
0WPHX1Z	Removal of Radioactive Element from Retroperitoneum, External Approach
0WPHX3Z	Removal of Infusion Device from Retroperitoneum, External Approach
0WPJ00Z	Removal of Drainage Device from Pelvic Cavity, Open Approach
0WPJ01Z	Removal of Radioactive Element from Pelvic Cavity, Open Approach
0WPJ03Z	Removal of Infusion Device from Pelvic Cavity, Open Approach
0WPJ0JZ	Removal of Synthetic Substitute from Pelvic Cavity, Open Approach
0WPJ0YZ	Removal of Other Device from Pelvic Cavity, Open Approach
0WPJ30Z	Removal of Drainage Device from Pelvic Cavity, Percutaneous Approach
0WPJ31Z	Removal of Radioactive Element from Pelvic Cavity, Percutaneous Approach
0WPJ33Z	Removal of Infusion Device from Pelvic Cavity, Percutaneous Approach
0WPJ3JZ	Removal of Synthetic Substitute from Pelvic Cavity, Percutaneous Approach
0WPJ3YZ	Removal of Other Device from Pelvic Cavity, Percutaneous Approach
0WPJ40Z	Removal of Drainage Device from Pelvic Cavity, Percutaneous Endoscopic Approach
0WPJ41Z	Removal of Radioactive Element from Pelvic Cavity, Percutaneous Endoscopic Approach
0WPJ43Z	Removal of Infusion Device from Pelvic Cavity, Percutaneous Endoscopic Approach
0WPJ4JZ	Removal of Synthetic Substitute from Pelvic Cavity, Percutaneous Endoscopic Approach
0WPJ4YZ	Removal of Other Device from Pelvic Cavity, Percutaneous Endoscopic Approach
0WPJX0Z	Removal of Drainage Device from Pelvic Cavity, External Approach
0WPJX1Z	Removal of Radioactive Element from Pelvic Cavity, External Approach
0WPJX3Z	Removal of Infusion Device from Pelvic Cavity, External Approach
0WPK00Z	Removal of Drainage Device from Upper Back, Open Approach
0WPK01Z	Removal of Radioactive Element from Upper Back, Open Approach
0WPK03Z	Removal of Infusion Device from Upper Back, Open Approach
0WPK07Z	Removal of Autologous Tissue Substitute from Upper Back, Open Approach
0WPK0JZ	Removal of Synthetic Substitute from Upper Back, Open Approach
0WPK0KZ	Removal of Nonautologous Tissue Substitute from Upper Back, Open Approach
0WPK0YZ	Removal of Other Device from Upper Back, Open Approach
0WPK30Z	Removal of Drainage Device from Upper Back, Percutaneous Approach
0WPK31Z	Removal of Radioactive Element from Upper Back, Percutaneous Approach
0WPK33Z	Removal of Infusion Device from Upper Back, Percutaneous Approach

0WPK37Z	Removal of Autologous Tissue Substitute from Upper Back, Percutaneous Approach
0WPK3JZ	Removal of Synthetic Substitute from Upper Back, Percutaneous Approach
0WPK3KZ	Removal of Nonautologous Tissue Substitute from Upper Back, Percutaneous Approach
0WPK3YZ	Removal of Other Device from Upper Back, Percutaneous Approach
0WPK40Z	Removal of Drainage Device from Upper Back, Percutaneous Endoscopic Approach
0WPK41Z	Removal of Radioactive Element from Upper Back, Percutaneous Endoscopic Approach
0WPK43Z	Removal of Infusion Device from Upper Back, Percutaneous Endoscopic Approach
0WPK47Z	Removal of Autologous Tissue Substitute from Upper Back, Percutaneous Endoscopic Approach
0WPK4JZ	Removal of Synthetic Substitute from Upper Back, Percutaneous Endoscopic Approach
0WPK4KZ	Removal of Nonautologous Tissue Substitute from Upper Back, Percutaneous Endoscopic Approach
0WPK4YZ	Removal of Other Device from Upper Back, Percutaneous Endoscopic Approach
0WPKX0Z	Removal of Drainage Device from Upper Back, External Approach
0WPKX1Z	Removal of Radioactive Element from Upper Back, External Approach
0WPKX3Z	Removal of Infusion Device from Upper Back, External Approach
0WPKX7Z	Removal of Autologous Tissue Substitute from Upper Back, External Approach
0WPKXJZ	Removal of Synthetic Substitute from Upper Back, External Approach
0WPKXKZ	Removal of Nonautologous Tissue Substitute from Upper Back, External Approach
0WPKXYZ	Removal of Other Device from Upper Back, External Approach
0WPL00Z	Removal of Drainage Device from Lower Back, Open Approach
0WPL01Z	Removal of Radioactive Element from Lower Back, Open Approach
0WPL03Z	Removal of Infusion Device from Lower Back, Open Approach
0WPL07Z	Removal of Autologous Tissue Substitute from Lower Back, Open Approach
0WPL0JZ	Removal of Synthetic Substitute from Lower Back, Open Approach
0WPL0KZ	Removal of Nonautologous Tissue Substitute from Lower Back, Open Approach
0WPL0YZ	Removal of Other Device from Lower Back, Open Approach
0WPL30Z	Removal of Drainage Device from Lower Back, Percutaneous Approach
0WPL31Z	Removal of Radioactive Element from Lower Back, Percutaneous Approach
0WPL33Z	Removal of Infusion Device from Lower Back, Percutaneous Approach
0WPL37Z	Removal of Autologous Tissue Substitute from Lower Back, Percutaneous Approach
0WPL3JZ	Removal of Synthetic Substitute from Lower Back, Percutaneous Approach
0WPL3KZ	Removal of Nonautologous Tissue Substitute from Lower Back, Percutaneous Approach
0WPL3YZ	Removal of Other Device from Lower Back, Percutaneous Approach

♀ Female-only ♂ Male-only ▲ Limited Coverage ● Non-OR ▦ HAC-associated procedure ▲ Non-covered procedures ✚ Combination

0WPL40Z	Removal of Drainage Device from Lower Back, Percutaneous Endoscopic Approach
0WPL41Z	Removal of Radioactive Element from Lower Back, Percutaneous Endoscopic Approach
0WPL43Z	Removal of Infusion Device from Lower Back, Percutaneous Endoscopic Approach
0WPL47Z	Removal of Autologous Tissue Substitute from Lower Back, Percutaneous Endoscopic Approach
0WPL4JZ	Removal of Synthetic Substitute from Lower Back, Percutaneous Endoscopic Approach
0WPL4KZ	Removal of Nonautologous Tissue Substitute from Lower Back, Percutaneous Endoscopic Approach
0WPL4YZ	Removal of Other Device from Lower Back, Percutaneous Endoscopic Approach
0WPLX0Z	Removal of Drainage Device from Lower Back, External Approach
0WPLX1Z	Removal of Radioactive Element from Lower Back, External Approach
0WPLX3Z	Removal of Infusion Device from Lower Back, External Approach
0WPLX7Z	Removal of Autologous Tissue Substitute from Lower Back, External Approach
0WPLXJZ	Removal of Synthetic Substitute from Lower Back, External Approach
0WPLXKZ	Removal of Nonautologous Tissue Substitute from Lower Back, External Approach
0WPLXYZ	Removal of Other Device from Lower Back, External Approach
♂ 0WPM00Z	Removal of Drainage Device from Male Perineum, Open Approach
♂ 0WPM01Z	Removal of Radioactive Element from Male Perineum, Open Approach
♂ 0WPM03Z	Removal of Infusion Device from Male Perineum, Open Approach
♂ 0WPM07Z	Removal of Autologous Tissue Substitute from Male Perineum, Open Approach
♂ 0WPM0JZ	Removal of Synthetic Substitute from Male Perineum, Open Approach
♂ 0WPM0KZ	Removal of Nonautologous Tissue Substitute from Male Perineum, Open Approach
♂ 0WPM0YZ	Removal of Other Device from Male Perineum, Open Approach
♂ 0WPM30Z	Removal of Drainage Device from Male Perineum, Percutaneous Approach
♂ 0WPM31Z	Removal of Radioactive Element from Male Perineum, Percutaneous Approach
♂ 0WPM33Z	Removal of Infusion Device from Male Perineum, Percutaneous Approach
♂ 0WPM37Z	Removal of Autologous Tissue Substitute from Male Perineum, Percutaneous Approach
♂ 0WPM3JZ	Removal of Synthetic Substitute from Male Perineum, Percutaneous Approach
♂ 0WPM3KZ	Removal of Nonautologous Tissue Substitute from Male Perineum, Percutaneous Approach
♂ 0WPM3YZ	Removal of Other Device from Male Perineum, Percutaneous Approach
♂ 0WPM40Z	Removal of Drainage Device from Male Perineum, Percutaneous Endoscopic Approach
♂ 0WPM41Z	Removal of Radioactive Element from Male Perineum, Percutaneous Endoscopic Approach
♂ 0WPM43Z	Removal of Infusion Device from Male Perineum, Percutaneous Endoscopic Approach

♂ 0WPM47Z	Removal of Autologous Tissue Substitute from Male Perineum, Percutaneous Endoscopic Approach
♂ 0WPM4JZ	Removal of Synthetic Substitute from Male Perineum, Percutaneous Endoscopic Approach
♂ 0WPM4KZ	Removal of Nonautologous Tissue Substitute from Male Perineum, Percutaneous Endoscopic Approach
♂ 0WPM4YZ	Removal of Other Device from Male Perineum, Percutaneous Endoscopic Approach
♂ 0WPMX0Z	Removal of Drainage Device from Male Perineum, External Approach
♂ 0WPMX1Z	Removal of Radioactive Element from Male Perineum, External Approach
♂ 0WPMX3Z	Removal of Infusion Device from Male Perineum, External Approach
♂ 0WPMX7Z	Removal of Autologous Tissue Substitute from Male Perineum, External Approach
♂ 0WPMXJZ	Removal of Synthetic Substitute from Male Perineum, External Approach
♂ 0WPMXKZ	Removal of Nonautologous Tissue Substitute from Male Perineum, External Approach
♂ 0WPMXYZ	Removal of Other Device from Male Perineum, External Approach
♀ 0WPN00Z	Removal of Drainage Device from Female Perineum, Open Approach
♀ 0WPN01Z	Removal of Radioactive Element from Female Perineum, Open Approach
♀ 0WPN03Z	Removal of Infusion Device from Female Perineum, Open Approach
♀ 0WPN07Z	Removal of Autologous Tissue Substitute from Female Perineum, Open Approach
♀ 0WPN0JZ	Removal of Synthetic Substitute from Female Perineum, Open Approach
♀ 0WPN0KZ	Removal of Nonautologous Tissue Substitute from Female Perineum, Open Approach
♀ 0WPN0YZ	Removal of Other Device from Female Perineum, Open Approach
♀ 0WPN30Z	Removal of Drainage Device from Female Perineum, Percutaneous Approach
♀ 0WPN31Z	Removal of Radioactive Element from Female Perineum, Percutaneous Approach
♀ 0WPN33Z	Removal of Infusion Device from Female Perineum, Percutaneous Approach
♀ 0WPN37Z	Removal of Autologous Tissue Substitute from Female Perineum, Percutaneous Approach
♀ 0WPN3JZ	Removal of Synthetic Substitute from Female Perineum, Percutaneous Approach
♀ 0WPN3KZ	Removal of Nonautologous Tissue Substitute from Female Perineum, Percutaneous Approach
♀ 0WPN3YZ	Removal of Other Device from Female Perineum, Percutaneous Approach
♀ 0WPN40Z	Removal of Drainage Device from Female Perineum, Percutaneous Endoscopic Approach
♀ 0WPN41Z	Removal of Radioactive Element from Female Perineum, Percutaneous Endoscopic Approach
♀ 0WPN43Z	Removal of Infusion Device from Female Perineum, Percutaneous Endoscopic Approach
♀ 0WPN47Z	Removal of Autologous Tissue Substitute from Female Perineum, Percutaneous Endoscopic Approach
♀ 0WPN4JZ	Removal of Synthetic Substitute from Female Perineum, Percutaneous Endoscopic Approach

♀ 0WPN4KZ	Removal of Nonautologous Tissue Substitute from Female Perineum, Percutaneous Endoscopic Approach
♀ 0WPN4YZ	Removal of Other Device from Female Perineum, Percutaneous Endoscopic Approach
♀ 0WPNX0Z	Removal of Drainage Device from Female Perineum, External Approach
♀ 0WPNX1Z	Removal of Radioactive Element from Female Perineum, External Approach
♀ 0WPNX3Z	Removal of Infusion Device from Fem Perineum, External Approach
♀ 0WPNX7Z	Removal of Autologous Tissue Substitu from Female Perineum, External Approach
♀ 0WPNXJZ	Removal of Synthetic Substitute from Female Perineum, External Approach
♀ 0WPNXKZ	Removal of Nonautologous Tissue Substitute from Female Perineum, External Approach
♀ 0WPNXYZ	Removal of Other Device from Female Perineum, External Approach
0WPP01Z	Removal of Radioactive Element from Gastrointestinal Tract, Open Approach
0WPP03Z	Removal of Infusion Device from Gastrointestinal Tract, Open Approach
0WPP0YZ	Removal of Other Device from Gastrointestinal Tract, Open Approach
0WPP31Z	Removal of Radioactive Element from Gastrointestinal Tract, Percutaneous Approach
0WPP33Z	Removal of Infusion Device from Gastrointestinal Tract, Percutaneous Approach
0WPP3YZ	Removal of Other Device from Gastrointestinal Tract, Percutaneous Approach
0WPP41Z	Removal of Radioactive Element from Gastrointestinal Tract, Percutaneous Endoscopic Approach
0WPP43Z	Removal of Infusion Device from Gastrointestinal Tract, Percutaneous Endoscopic Approach
0WPP4YZ	Removal of Other Device from Gastrointestinal Tract, Percutaneous Endoscopic Approach
0WPP71Z	Removal of Radioactive Element from Gastrointestinal Tract, Via Natural or Artificial Opening
0WPP73Z	Removal of Infusion Device from Gastrointestinal Tract, Via Natural or Artificial Opening
0WPP7YZ	Removal of Other Device from Gastrointestinal Tract, Via Natural or Artificial Opening
0WPP81Z	Removal of Radioactive Element from Gastrointestinal Tract, Via Natural or Artificial Opening Endoscopic
0WPP83Z	Removal of Infusion Device from Gastrointestinal Tract, Via Natural or Artificial Opening Endoscopic
0WPP8YZ	Removal of Other Device from Gastrointestinal Tract, Via Natural or Artificial Opening Endoscopic
0WPPX1Z	Removal of Radioactive Element from Gastrointestinal Tract, External Approach
0WPPX3Z	Removal of Infusion Device from Gastrointestinal Tract, External Approach
0WPPXYZ	Removal of Other Device from Gastrointestinal Tract, External Approach
0WPQ01Z	Removal of Radioactive Element from Respiratory Tract, Open Approach
0WPQ03Z	Removal of Infusion Device from Respiratory Tract, Open Approach
0WPQ0YZ	Removal of Other Device from Respiratory Tract, Open Approach

♀ Female-only   ♂ Male-only   ▲ Limited Coverage   ● Non-OR   ▬ HAC-associated procedure   ▲ Non-covered procedures   ✚ Combination

Code	Description	Code	Description	Code	Description
PQ31Z	Removal of Radioactive Element from Respiratory Tract, Percutaneous Approach	0WPQ83Z	Removal of Infusion Device from Respiratory Tract, Via Natural or Artificial Opening Endoscopic	0WPR43Z	Removal of Infusion Device from Genitourinary Tract, Percutaneous Endoscopic Approach
PQ33Z	Removal of Infusion Device from Respiratory Tract, Percutaneous Approach	0WPQ8YZ	Removal of Other Device from Respiratory Tract, Via Natural or Artificial Opening Endoscopic	0WPR4YZ	Removal of Other Device from Genitourinary Tract, Percutaneous Endoscopic Approach
PQ3YZ	Removal of Other Device from Respiratory Tract, Percutaneous Approach	0WPQX1Z	Removal of Radioactive Element from Respiratory Tract, External Approach	0WPR71Z	Removal of Radioactive Element from Genitourinary Tract, Via Natural or Artificial Opening
PQ41Z	Removal of Radioactive Element from Respiratory Tract, Percutaneous Endoscopic Approach	0WPQX3Z	Removal of Infusion Device from Respiratory Tract, External Approach	0WPR73Z	Removal of Infusion Device from Genitourinary Tract, Via Natural or Artificial Opening
PQ43Z	Removal of Infusion Device from Respiratory Tract, Percutaneous Endoscopic Approach	0WPQXYZ	Removal of Other Device from Respiratory Tract, External Approach	0WPR7YZ	Removal of Other Device from Genitourinary Tract, Via Natural or Artificial Opening
PQ4YZ	Removal of Other Device from Respiratory Tract, Percutaneous Endoscopic Approach	0WPR01Z	Removal of Radioactive Element from Genitourinary Tract, Open Approach	0WPR81Z	Removal of Radioactive Element from Genitourinary Tract, Via Natural or Artificial Opening Endoscopic
PQ71Z	Removal of Radioactive Element from Respiratory Tract, Via Natural or Artificial Opening	0WPR03Z	Removal of Infusion Device from Genitourinary Tract, Open Approach	0WPR83Z	Removal of Infusion Device from Genitourinary Tract, Via Natural or Artificial Opening Endoscopic
PQ73Z	Removal of Infusion Device from Respiratory Tract, Via Natural or Artificial Opening	0WPR0YZ	Removal of Other Device from Genitourinary Tract, Open Approach	0WPR8YZ	Removal of Other Device from Genitourinary Tract, Via Natural or Artificial Opening Endoscopic
PQ7YZ	Removal of Other Device from Respiratory Tract, Via Natural or Artificial Opening	0WPR31Z	Removal of Radioactive Element from Genitourinary Tract, Percutaneous Approach	0WPRX1Z	Removal of Radioactive Element from Genitourinary Tract, External Approach
PQ81Z	Removal of Radioactive Element from Respiratory Tract, Via Natural or Artificial Opening Endoscopic	0WPR33Z	Removal of Infusion Device from Genitourinary Tract, Percutaneous Approach	0WPRX3Z	Removal of Infusion Device from Genitourinary Tract, External Approach
		0WPR3YZ	Removal of Other Device from Genitourinary Tract, Percutaneous Approach	0WPRXYZ	Removal of Other Device from Genitourinary Tract, External Approach
		0WPR41Z	Removal of Radioactive Element from Genitourinary Tract, Percutaneous Endoscopic Approach		

WQ – Anatomical Regions, General, Repair

Code	Description	Code	Description	Code	Description
WQ00ZZ	Repair Head, Open Approach	0WQ83ZZ	Repair Chest Wall, Percutaneous Approach	0WQL4ZZ	Repair Lower Back, Percutaneous Endoscopic Approach
WQ03ZZ	Repair Head, Percutaneous Approach	0WQ84ZZ	Repair Chest Wall, Percutaneous Endoscopic Approach	0WQLXZZ	Repair Lower Back, External Approach
WQ04ZZ	Repair Head, Percutaneous Endoscopic Approach	0WQ8XZZ	Repair Chest Wall, External Approach	♂ 0WQM0ZZ	Repair Male Perineum, Open Approach *This is a male-only service, however, it is not included in the male-only edit logic for MCE V30*
WQ0XZZ	Repair Head, External Approach	0WQC0ZZ	Repair Mediastinum, Open Approach		
WQ20ZZ	Repair Face, Open Approach	0WQC3ZZ	Repair Mediastinum, Percutaneous Approach	♂ 0WQM3ZZ	Repair Male Perineum, Percutaneous Approach *This is a male-only service, however, it is not included in the male-only edit logic for MCE V30*
WQ23ZZ	Repair Face, Percutaneous Approach	0WQC4ZZ	Repair Mediastinum, Percutaneous Endoscopic Approach		
WQ24ZZ	Repair Face, Percutaneous Endoscopic Approach	0WQF0ZZ	Repair Abdominal Wall, Open Approach *AHA CC: 4Q, 2014, 38-39; 3Q, 2014, 28-29*	♂ 0WQM4ZZ	Repair Male Perineum, Percutaneous Endoscopic Approach *This is a male-only service, however, it is not included in the male-only edit logic for MCE V30*
WQ2XZZ	Repair Face, External Approach				
WQ40ZZ	Repair Upper Jaw, Open Approach	0WQF3ZZ	Repair Abdominal Wall, Percutaneous Approach		
WQ43ZZ	Repair Upper Jaw, Percutaneous Approach	0WQF4ZZ	Repair Abdominal Wall, Percutaneous Endoscopic Approach	♂ 0WQMXZZ	Repair Male Perineum, External Approach *This is a male-only service, however, it is not included in the male-only edit logic for MCE V30*
WQ44ZZ	Repair Upper Jaw, Percutaneous Endoscopic Approach	0WQFXZ2	Repair Abdominal Wall, Stoma, External Approach		
WQ4XZZ	Repair Upper Jaw, External Approach	0WQFXZZ	Repair Abdominal Wall, External Approach	♀ 0WQN0ZZ	Repair Female Perineum, Open Approach
WQ50ZZ	Repair Lower Jaw, Open Approach	0WQK0ZZ	Repair Upper Back, Open Approach	♀ 0WQN3ZZ	Repair Female Perineum, Percutaneous Approach
WQ53ZZ	Repair Lower Jaw, Percutaneous Approach	0WQK3ZZ	Repair Upper Back, Percutaneous Approach		
WQ54ZZ	Repair Lower Jaw, Percutaneous Endoscopic Approach	0WQK4ZZ	Repair Upper Back, Percutaneous Endoscopic Approach	♀ 0WQN4ZZ	Repair Female Perineum, Percutaneous Endoscopic Approach
WQ5XZZ	Repair Lower Jaw, External Approach	0WQKXZZ	Repair Upper Back, External Approach	♀ 0WQNXZZ	Repair Female Perineum, External Approach
WQ60ZZ	Repair Neck, Open Approach	0WQL0ZZ	Repair Lower Back, Open Approach		
WQ63ZZ	Repair Neck, Percutaneous Approach	0WQL3ZZ	Repair Lower Back, Percutaneous Approach		
WQ64ZZ	Repair Neck, Percutaneous Endoscopic Approach				
WQ6XZ2	Repair Neck, Stoma, External Approach				
WQ6XZZ	Repair Neck, External Approach				
WQ80ZZ	Repair Chest Wall, Open Approach				

WU – Anatomical Regions, General, Supplement

WU007Z	Supplement Head with Autologous Tissue Substitute, Open Approach	0WU04KZ	Supplement Head with Nonautologous Tissue Substitute, Percutaneous Endoscopic Approach	0WU24JZ	Supplement Face with Synthetic Substitute, Percutaneous Endoscopic Approach
WU00JZ	Supplement Head with Synthetic Substitute, Open Approach	0WU207Z	Supplement Face with Autologous Tissue Substitute, Open Approach	0WU24KZ	Supplement Face with Nonautologous Tissue Substitute, Percutaneous Endoscopic Approach
WU00KZ	Supplement Head with Nonautologous Tissue Substitute, Open Approach	0WU20JZ	Supplement Face with Synthetic Substitute, Open Approach	0WU407Z	Supplement Upper Jaw with Autologous Tissue Substitute, Open Approach
WU047Z	Supplement Head with Autologous Tissue Substitute, Percutaneous Endoscopic Approach	0WU20KZ	Supplement Face with Nonautologous Tissue Substitute, Open Approach	0WU40JZ	Supplement Upper Jaw with Synthetic Substitute, Open Approach
WU04JZ	Supplement Head with Synthetic Substitute, Percutaneous Endoscopic Approach	0WU247Z	Supplement Face with Autologous Tissue Substitute, Percutaneous Endoscopic Approach	0WU40KZ	Supplement Upper Jaw with Nonautologous Tissue Substitute, Open Approach

♀ Female-only	♂ Male-only	▲ Limited Coverage	● Non-OR	▧ HAC-associated procedure	▲ Non-covered procedures	✚ Combination

0WU447Z	Supplement Upper Jaw with Autologous Tissue Substitute, Percutaneous Endoscopic Approach
0WU44JZ	Supplement Upper Jaw with Synthetic Substitute, Percutaneous Endoscopic Approach
0WU44KZ	Supplement Upper Jaw with Nonautologous Tissue Substitute, Percutaneous Endoscopic Approach
0WU507Z	Supplement Lower Jaw with Autologous Tissue Substitute, Open Approach
0WU50JZ	Supplement Lower Jaw with Synthetic Substitute, Open Approach
0WU50KZ	Supplement Lower Jaw with Nonautologous Tissue Substitute, Open Approach
0WU547Z	Supplement Lower Jaw with Autologous Tissue Substitute, Percutaneous Endoscopic Approach
0WU54JZ	Supplement Lower Jaw with Synthetic Substitute, Percutaneous Endoscopic Approach
0WU54KZ	Supplement Lower Jaw with Nonautologous Tissue Substitute, Percutaneous Endoscopic Approach
0WU607Z	Supplement Neck with Autologous Tissue Substitute, Open Approach
0WU60JZ	Supplement Neck with Synthetic Substitute, Open Approach
0WU60KZ	Supplement Neck with Nonautologous Tissue Substitute, Open Approach
0WU647Z	Supplement Neck with Autologous Tissue Substitute, Percutaneous Endoscopic Approach
0WU64JZ	Supplement Neck with Synthetic Substitute, Percutaneous Endoscopic Approach
0WU64KZ	Supplement Neck with Nonautologous Tissue Substitute, Percutaneous Endoscopic Approach
0WU807Z	Supplement Chest Wall with Autologous Tissue Substitute, Open Approach
0WU80JZ	Supplement Chest Wall with Synthetic Substitute, Open Approach

AHA CC: 4Q, 2012, 101-102

0WU80KZ	Supplement Chest Wall with Nonautologous Tissue Substitute, Open Approach
0WU847Z	Supplement Chest Wall with Autologous Tissue Substitute, Percutaneous Endoscopic Approach
0WU84JZ	Supplement Chest Wall with Synthetic Substitute, Percutaneous Endoscopic Approach

0WU84KZ	Supplement Chest Wall with Nonautologous Tissue Substitute, Percutaneous Endoscopic Approach
0WUC07Z	Supplement Mediastinum with Autologous Tissue Substitute, Open Approach
0WUC0JZ	Supplement Mediastinum with Synthetic Substitute, Open Approach
0WUC0KZ	Supplement Mediastinum with Nonautologous Tissue Substitute, Open Approach
0WUC47Z	Supplement Mediastinum with Autologous Tissue Substitute, Percutaneous Endoscopic Approach
0WUC4JZ	Supplement Mediastinum with Synthetic Substitute, Percutaneous Endoscopic Approach
0WUC4KZ	Supplement Mediastinum with Nonautologous Tissue Substitute, Percutaneous Endoscopic Approach
0WUF07Z	Supplement Abdominal Wall with Autologous Tissue Substitute, Open Approach
0WUF0JZ	Supplement Abdominal Wall with Synthetic Substitute, Open Approach

AHA CC: 4Q, 2014, 39-40

0WUF0KZ	Supplement Abdominal Wall with Nonautologous Tissue Substitute, Open Approach
0WUF47Z	Supplement Abdominal Wall with Autologous Tissue Substitute, Percutaneous Endoscopic Approach
0WUF4JZ	Supplement Abdominal Wall with Synthetic Substitute, Percutaneous Endoscopic Approach
0WUF4KZ	Supplement Abdominal Wall with Nonautologous Tissue Substitute, Percutaneous Endoscopic Approach
0WUK07Z	Supplement Upper Back with Autologous Tissue Substitute, Open Approach
0WUK0JZ	Supplement Upper Back with Synthetic Substitute, Open Approach
0WUK0KZ	Supplement Upper Back with Nonautologous Tissue Substitute, Open Approach
0WUK47Z	Supplement Upper Back with Autologous Tissue Substitute, Percutaneous Endoscopic Approach
0WUK4JZ	Supplement Upper Back with Synthetic Substitute, Percutaneous Endoscopic Approach
0WUK4KZ	Supplement Upper Back with Nonautologous Tissue Substitute, Percutaneous Endoscopic Approach

0WUL07Z	Supplement Lower Back with Autologous Tissue Substitute, Open Approach
0WUL0JZ	Supplement Lower Back with Synthetic Substitute, Open Approach
0WUL0KZ	Supplement Lower Back with Nonautologous Tissue Substitute, Open Approach
0WUL47Z	Supplement Lower Back with Autologous Tissue Substitute, Percutaneous Endoscopic Approach
0WUL4JZ	Supplement Lower Back with Synthetic Substitute, Percutaneous Endoscopic Approach
0WUL4KZ	Supplement Lower Back with Nonautologous Tissue Substitute, Percutaneous Endoscopic Approach
♂ 0WUM07Z	Supplement Male Perineum with Autologous Tissue Substitute, Open Approach
♂ 0WUM0JZ	Supplement Male Perineum with Synthetic Substitute, Open Approach
♂ 0WUM0KZ	Supplement Male Perineum with Nonautologous Tissue Substitute, Open Approach
♂ 0WUM47Z	Supplement Male Perineum with Autologous Tissue Substitute, Percutaneous Endoscopic Approach
♂ 0WUM4JZ	Supplement Male Perineum with Synthetic Substitute, Percutaneous Endoscopic Approach
♂ 0WUM4KZ	Supplement Male Perineum with Nonautologous Tissue Substitute, Percutaneous Endoscopic Approach
♀ 0WUN07Z	Supplement Female Perineum with Autologous Tissue Substitute, Open Approach
♀ 0WUN0JZ	Supplement Female Perineum with Synthetic Substitute, Open Approach
♀ 0WUN0KZ	Supplement Female Perineum with Nonautologous Tissue Substitute, Open Approach
♀ 0WUN47Z	Supplement Female Perineum with Autologous Tissue Substitute, Percutaneous Endoscopic Approach
♀ 0WUN4JZ	Supplement Female Perineum with Synthetic Substitute, Percutaneous Endoscopic Approach
♀ 0WUN4KZ	Supplement Female Perineum with Nonautologous Tissue Substitute, Percutaneous Endoscopic Approach

0WW – Anatomical Regions, General, Revision

Review Coding Guideline B6.1c

● 0WW000Z	Revision of Drainage Device in Head, Open Approach
● 0WW001Z	Revision of Radioactive Element in Head, Open Approach
● 0WW003Z	Revision of Infusion Device in Head, Open Approach
● 0WW007Z	Revision of Autologous Tissue Substitute in Head, Open Approach
● 0WW00JZ	Revision of Synthetic Substitute in Head, Open Approach
● 0WW00KZ	Revision of Nonautologous Tissue Substitute in Head, Open Approach
● 0WW00YZ	Revision of Other Device in Head, Open Approach
● 0WW030Z	Revision of Drainage Device in Head, Percutaneous Approach
● 0WW031Z	Revision of Radioactive Element in Head, Percutaneous Approach

● 0WW033Z	Revision of Infusion Device in Head, Percutaneous Approach
● 0WW037Z	Revision of Autologous Tissue Substitute in Head, Percutaneous Approach
● 0WW03JZ	Revision of Synthetic Substitute in Head, Percutaneous Approach
● 0WW03KZ	Revision of Nonautologous Tissue Substitute in Head, Percutaneous Approach
● 0WW03YZ	Revision of Other Device in Head, Percutaneous Approach
● 0WW040Z	Revision of Drainage Device in Head, Percutaneous Endoscopic Approach
● 0WW041Z	Revision of Radioactive Element in Head, Percutaneous Endoscopic Approach
● 0WW043Z	Revision of Infusion Device in Head, Percutaneous Endoscopic Approach

● 0WW047Z	Revision of Autologous Tissue Substitute in Head, Percutaneous Endoscopic Approach
● 0WW04JZ	Revision of Synthetic Substitute in Head, Percutaneous Endoscopic Approach
● 0WW04KZ	Revision of Nonautologous Tissue Substitute in Head, Percutaneous Endoscopic Approach
● 0WW04YZ	Revision of Other Device in Head, Percutaneous Endoscopic Approach
0WW0X0Z	Revision of Drainage Device in Head, External Approach
0WW0X1Z	Revision of Radioactive Element in Head, External Approach
0WW0X3Z	Revision of Infusion Device in Head, External Approach
0WW0X7Z	Revision of Autologous Tissue Substitute in Head, External Approach

0WW0XJZ Revision of Synthetic Substitute in Head, External Approach

0WW0XKZ Revision of Nonautologous Tissue Substitute in Head, External Approach

0WW0XYZ Revision of Other Device in Head, External Approach

0WW100Z Revision of Drainage Device in Cranial Cavity, Open Approach

0WW101Z Revision of Radioactive Element in Cranial Cavity, Open Approach

0WW103Z Revision of Infusion Device in Cranial Cavity, Open Approach

0WW10JZ Revision of Synthetic Substitute in Cranial Cavity, Open Approach

0WW10YZ Revision of Other Device in Cranial Cavity, Open Approach

0WW130Z Revision of Drainage Device in Cranial Cavity, Percutaneous Approach

0WW131Z Revision of Radioactive Element in Cranial Cavity, Percutaneous Approach

0WW133Z Revision of Infusion Device in Cranial Cavity, Percutaneous Approach

0WW13JZ Revision of Synthetic Substitute in Cranial Cavity, Percutaneous Approach

0WW13YZ Revision of Other Device in Cranial Cavity, Percutaneous Approach

0WW140Z Revision of Drainage Device in Cranial Cavity, Percutaneous Endoscopic Approach

0WW141Z Revision of Radioactive Element in Cranial Cavity, Percutaneous Endoscopic Approach

0WW143Z Revision of Infusion Device in Cranial Cavity, Percutaneous Endoscopic Approach

0WW14JZ Revision of Synthetic Substitute in Cranial Cavity, Percutaneous Endoscopic Approach

0WW14YZ Revision of Other Device in Cranial Cavity, Percutaneous Endoscopic Approach

0WW1X0Z Revision of Drainage Device in Cranial Cavity, External Approach

0WW1X1Z Revision of Radioactive Element in Cranial Cavity, External Approach

0WW1X3Z Revision of Infusion Device in Cranial Cavity, External Approach

0WW1XJZ Revision of Synthetic Substitute in Cranial Cavity, External Approach

0WW1XYZ Revision of Other Device in Cranial Cavity, External Approach

0WW200Z Revision of Drainage Device in Face, Open Approach

0WW201Z Revision of Radioactive Element in Face, Open Approach

0WW203Z Revision of Infusion Device in Face, Open Approach

0WW207Z Revision of Autologous Tissue Substitute in Face, Open Approach

0WW20JZ Revision of Synthetic Substitute in Face, Open Approach

0WW20KZ Revision of Nonautologous Tissue Substitute in Face, Open Approach

0WW20YZ Revision of Other Device in Face, Open Approach

0WW230Z Revision of Drainage Device in Face, Percutaneous Approach

0WW231Z Revision of Radioactive Element in Face, Percutaneous Approach

0WW233Z Revision of Infusion Device in Face, Percutaneous Approach

0WW237Z Revision of Autologous Tissue Substitute in Face, Percutaneous Approach

0WW23JZ Revision of Synthetic Substitute in Face, Percutaneous Approach

0WW23KZ Revision of Nonautologous Tissue Substitute in Face, Percutaneous Approach

● 0WW23YZ Revision of Other Device in Face, Percutaneous Approach

● 0WW240Z Revision of Drainage Device in Face, Percutaneous Endoscopic Approach

● 0WW241Z Revision of Radioactive Element in Face, Percutaneous Endoscopic Approach

● 0WW243Z Revision of Infusion Device in Face, Percutaneous Endoscopic Approach

● 0WW247Z Revision of Autologous Tissue Substitute in Face, Percutaneous Endoscopic Approach

● 0WW24JZ Revision of Synthetic Substitute in Face, Percutaneous Endoscopic Approach

● 0WW24KZ Revision of Nonautologous Tissue Substitute in Face, Percutaneous Endoscopic Approach

● 0WW24YZ Revision of Other Device in Face, Percutaneous Endoscopic Approach

0WW2X0Z Revision of Drainage Device in Face, External Approach

0WW2X1Z Revision of Radioactive Element in Face, External Approach

0WW2X3Z Revision of Infusion Device in Face, External Approach

0WW2X7Z Revision of Autologous Tissue Substitute in Face, External Approach

0WW2XJZ Revision of Synthetic Substitute in Face, External Approach

0WW2XKZ Revision of Nonautologous Tissue Substitute in Face, External Approach

0WW2XYZ Revision of Other Device in Face, External Approach

● 0WW400Z Revision of Drainage Device in Upper Jaw, Open Approach

● 0WW401Z Revision of Radioactive Element in Upper Jaw, Open Approach

● 0WW403Z Revision of Infusion Device in Upper Jaw, Open Approach

● 0WW407Z Revision of Autologous Tissue Substitute in Upper Jaw, Open Approach

● 0WW40JZ Revision of Synthetic Substitute in Upper Jaw, Open Approach

● 0WW40KZ Revision of Nonautologous Tissue Substitute in Upper Jaw, Open Approach

● 0WW40YZ Revision of Other Device in Upper Jaw, Open Approach

● 0WW430Z Revision of Drainage Device in Upper Jaw, Percutaneous Approach

● 0WW431Z Revision of Radioactive Element in Upper Jaw, Percutaneous Approach

● 0WW433Z Revision of Infusion Device in Upper Jaw, Percutaneous Approach

● 0WW437Z Revision of Autologous Tissue Substitute in Upper Jaw, Percutaneous Approach

● 0WW43JZ Revision of Synthetic Substitute in Upper Jaw, Percutaneous Approach

● 0WW43KZ Revision of Nonautologous Tissue Substitute in Upper Jaw, Percutaneous Approach

● 0WW43YZ Revision of Other Device in Upper Jaw, Percutaneous Approach

● 0WW440Z Revision of Drainage Device in Upper Jaw, Percutaneous Endoscopic Approach

● 0WW441Z Revision of Radioactive Element in Upper Jaw, Percutaneous Endoscopic Approach

● 0WW443Z Revision of Infusion Device in Upper Jaw, Percutaneous Endoscopic Approach

● 0WW447Z Revision of Autologous Tissue Substitute in Upper Jaw, Percutaneous Endoscopic Approach

● 0WW44JZ Revision of Synthetic Substitute in Upper Jaw, Percutaneous Endoscopic Approach

● 0WW44KZ Revision of Nonautologous Tissue Substitute in Upper Jaw, Percutaneous Endoscopic Approach

● 0WW44YZ Revision of Other Device in Upper Jaw, Percutaneous Endoscopic Approach

0WW4X0Z Revision of Drainage Device in Upper Jaw, External Approach

0WW4X1Z Revision of Radioactive Element in Upper Jaw, External Approach

0WW4X3Z Revision of Infusion Device in Upper Jaw, External Approach

0WW4X7Z Revision of Autologous Tissue Substitute in Upper Jaw, External Approach

0WW4XJZ Revision of Synthetic Substitute in Upper Jaw, External Approach

0WW4XKZ Revision of Nonautologous Tissue Substitute in Upper Jaw, External Approach

0WW4XYZ Revision of Other Device in Upper Jaw, External Approach

● 0WW500Z Revision of Drainage Device in Lower Jaw, Open Approach

● 0WW501Z Revision of Radioactive Element in Lower Jaw, Open Approach

● 0WW503Z Revision of Infusion Device in Lower Jaw, Open Approach

● 0WW507Z Revision of Autologous Tissue Substitute in Lower Jaw, Open Approach

● 0WW50JZ Revision of Synthetic Substitute in Lower Jaw, Open Approach

● 0WW50KZ Revision of Nonautologous Tissue Substitute in Lower Jaw, Open Approach

● 0WW50YZ Revision of Other Device in Lower Jaw, Open Approach

● 0WW530Z Revision of Drainage Device in Lower Jaw, Percutaneous Approach

● 0WW531Z Revision of Radioactive Element in Lower Jaw, Percutaneous Approach

● 0WW533Z Revision of Infusion Device in Lower Jaw, Percutaneous Approach

● 0WW537Z Revision of Autologous Tissue Substitute in Lower Jaw, Percutaneous Approach

● 0WW53JZ Revision of Synthetic Substitute in Lower Jaw, Percutaneous Approach

● 0WW53KZ Revision of Nonautologous Tissue Substitute in Lower Jaw, Percutaneous Approach

● 0WW53YZ Revision of Other Device in Lower Jaw, Percutaneous Approach

● 0WW540Z Revision of Drainage Device in Lower Jaw, Percutaneous Endoscopic Approach

● 0WW541Z Revision of Radioactive Element in Lower Jaw, Percutaneous Endoscopic Approach

● 0WW543Z Revision of Infusion Device in Lower Jaw, Percutaneous Endoscopic Approach

● 0WW547Z Revision of Autologous Tissue Substitute in Lower Jaw, Percutaneous Endoscopic Approach

● 0WW54JZ Revision of Synthetic Substitute in Lower Jaw, Percutaneous Endoscopic Approach

● 0WW54KZ Revision of Nonautologous Tissue Substitute in Lower Jaw, Percutaneous Endoscopic Approach

● 0WW54YZ Revision of Other Device in Lower Jaw, Percutaneous Endoscopic Approach

0WW5X0Z Revision of Drainage Device in Lower Jaw, External Approach

0WW5X1Z Revision of Radioactive Element in Lower Jaw, External Approach

0WW5X3Z Revision of Infusion Device in Lower Jaw, External Approach

0WW5X7Z Revision of Autologous Tissue Substitute in Lower Jaw, External Approach

0WW5XJZ Revision of Synthetic Substitute in Lower Jaw, External Approach

♀ Female-only ♂ Male-only ▲ Limited Coverage ● Non-OR ▥ HAC-associated procedure ▲ Non-covered procedures ✚ Combination

0WW5XKZ Revision of Nonautologous Tissue Substitute in Lower Jaw, External Approach

0WW5XYZ Revision of Other Device in Lower Jaw, External Approach

● **0WW600Z** Revision of Drainage Device in Neck, Open Approach

● **0WW601Z** Revision of Radioactive Element in Neck, Open Approach

● **0WW603Z** Revision of Infusion Device in Neck, Open Approach

● **0WW607Z** Revision of Autologous Tissue Substitute in Neck, Open Approach

● **0WW60JZ** Revision of Synthetic Substitute in Neck, Open Approach

● **0WW60KZ** Revision of Nonautologous Tissue Substitute in Neck, Open Approach

● **0WW60YZ** Revision of Other Device in Neck, Open Approach

● **0WW630Z** Revision of Drainage Device in Neck, Percutaneous Approach

● **0WW631Z** Revision of Radioactive Element in Neck, Percutaneous Approach

● **0WW633Z** Revision of Infusion Device in Neck, Percutaneous Approach

● **0WW637Z** Revision of Autologous Tissue Substitute in Neck, Percutaneous Approach

● **0WW63JZ** Revision of Synthetic Substitute in Neck, Percutaneous Approach

● **0WW63KZ** Revision of Nonautologous Tissue Substitute in Neck, Percutaneous Approach

● **0WW63YZ** Revision of Other Device in Neck, Percutaneous Approach

● **0WW640Z** Revision of Drainage Device in Neck, Percutaneous Endoscopic Approach

● **0WW641Z** Revision of Radioactive Element in Neck, Percutaneous Endoscopic Approach

● **0WW643Z** Revision of Infusion Device in Neck, Percutaneous Endoscopic Approach

● **0WW647Z** Revision of Autologous Tissue Substitute in Neck, Percutaneous Endoscopic Approach

● **0WW64JZ** Revision of Synthetic Substitute in Neck, Percutaneous Endoscopic Approach

● **0WW64KZ** Revision of Nonautologous Tissue Substitute in Neck, Percutaneous Endoscopic Approach

● **0WW64YZ** Revision of Other Device in Neck, Percutaneous Endoscopic Approach

0WW6X0Z Revision of Drainage Device in Neck, External Approach

0WW6X1Z Revision of Radioactive Element in Neck, External Approach

0WW6X3Z Revision of Infusion Device in Neck, External Approach

0WW6X7Z Revision of Autologous Tissue Substitute in Neck, External Approach

0WW6XJZ Revision of Synthetic Substitute in Neck, External Approach

0WW6XKZ Revision of Nonautologous Tissue Substitute in Neck, External Approach

0WW6XYZ Revision of Other Device in Neck, External Approach

0WW800Z Revision of Drainage Device in Chest Wall, Open Approach

0WW801Z Revision of Radioactive Element in Chest Wall, Open Approach

0WW803Z Revision of Infusion Device in Chest Wall, Open Approach

0WW807Z Revision of Autologous Tissue Substitute in Chest Wall, Open Approach

0WW80JZ Revision of Synthetic Substitute in Chest Wall, Open Approach

0WW80KZ Revision of Nonautologous Tissue Substitute in Chest Wall, Open Approach

0WW80YZ Revision of Other Device in Chest Wall, Open Approach

0WW830Z Revision of Drainage Device in Chest Wall, Percutaneous Approach

0WW831Z Revision of Radioactive Element in Chest Wall, Percutaneous Approach

0WW833Z Revision of Infusion Device in Chest Wall, Percutaneous Approach

0WW837Z Revision of Autologous Tissue Substitute in Chest Wall, Percutaneous Approach

0WW83JZ Revision of Synthetic Substitute in Chest Wall, Percutaneous Approach

0WW83KZ Revision of Nonautologous Tissue Substitute in Chest Wall, Percutaneous Approach

0WW83YZ Revision of Other Device in Chest Wall, Percutaneous Approach

0WW840Z Revision of Drainage Device in Chest Wall, Percutaneous Endoscopic Approach

0WW841Z Revision of Radioactive Element in Chest Wall, Percutaneous Endoscopic Approach

0WW843Z Revision of Infusion Device in Chest Wall, Percutaneous Endoscopic Approach

0WW847Z Revision of Autologous Tissue Substitute in Chest Wall, Percutaneous Endoscopic Approach

0WW84JZ Revision of Synthetic Substitute in Chest Wall, Percutaneous Endoscopic Approach

0WW84KZ Revision of Nonautologous Tissue Substitute in Chest Wall, Percutaneous Endoscopic Approach

0WW84YZ Revision of Other Device in Chest Wall, Percutaneous Endoscopic Approach

0WW8X0Z Revision of Drainage Device in Chest Wall, External Approach

0WW8X1Z Revision of Radioactive Element in Chest Wall, External Approach

0WW8X3Z Revision of Infusion Device in Chest Wall, External Approach

0WW8X7Z Revision of Autologous Tissue Substitute in Chest Wall, External Approach

0WW8XJZ Revision of Synthetic Substitute in Chest Wall, External Approach

0WW8XKZ Revision of Nonautologous Tissue Substitute in Chest Wall, External Approach

0WW8XYZ Revision of Other Device in Chest Wall, External Approach

0WW900Z Revision of Drainage Device in Right Pleural Cavity, Open Approach

0WW901Z Revision of Radioactive Element in Right Pleural Cavity, Open Approach

0WW903Z Revision of Infusion Device in Right Pleural Cavity, Open Approach

0WW90JZ Revision of Synthetic Substitute in Right Pleural Cavity, Open Approach

0WW90YZ Revision of Other Device in Right Pleural Cavity, Open Approach

0WW930Z Revision of Drainage Device in Right Pleural Cavity, Percutaneous Approach

0WW931Z Revision of Radioactive Element in Right Pleural Cavity, Percutaneous Approach

0WW933Z Revision of Infusion Device in Right Pleural Cavity, Percutaneous Approach

0WW93JZ Revision of Synthetic Substitute in Right Pleural Cavity, Percutaneous Approach

0WW93YZ Revision of Other Device in Right Pleural Cavity, Percutaneous Approach

0WW940Z Revision of Drainage Device in Right Pleural Cavity, Percutaneous Endoscopic Approach

0WW941Z Revision of Radioactive Element in Right Pleural Cavity, Percutaneous Endoscopic Approach

0WW943Z Revision of Infusion Device in Right Pleural Cavity, Percutaneous Endoscopic Approach

0WW94JZ Revision of Synthetic Substitute in Right Pleural Cavity, Percutaneous Endoscopic Approach

0WW94YZ Revision of Other Device in Right Pleural Cavity, Percutaneous Endoscopic Approach

0WW9X0Z Revision of Drainage Device in Right Pleural Cavity, External Approach

0WW9X1Z Revision of Radioactive Element in Right Pleural Cavity, External Approach

0WW9X3Z Revision of Infusion Device in Right Pleural Cavity, External Approach

0WW9XJZ Revision of Synthetic Substitute in Right Pleural Cavity, External Approach

0WW9XYZ Revision of Other Device in Right Pleural Cavity, External Approach

0WWB00Z Revision of Drainage Device in Left Pleural Cavity, Open Approach

0WWB01Z Revision of Radioactive Element in Left Pleural Cavity, Open Approach

0WWB03Z Revision of Infusion Device in Left Pleural Cavity, Open Approach

0WWB0JZ Revision of Synthetic Substitute in Left Pleural Cavity, Open Approach

0WWB0YZ Revision of Other Device in Left Pleural Cavity, Open Approach

0WWB30Z Revision of Drainage Device in Left Pleural Cavity, Percutaneous Approach

0WWB31Z Revision of Radioactive Element in Left Pleural Cavity, Percutaneous Approach

0WWB33Z Revision of Infusion Device in Left Pleural Cavity, Percutaneous Approach

0WWB3JZ Revision of Synthetic Substitute in Left Pleural Cavity, Percutaneous Approach

0WWB3YZ Revision of Other Device in Left Pleural Cavity, Percutaneous Approach

0WWB40Z Revision of Drainage Device in Left Pleural Cavity, Percutaneous Endoscopic Approach

0WWB41Z Revision of Radioactive Element in Left Pleural Cavity, Percutaneous Endoscopic Approach

0WWB43Z Revision of Infusion Device in Left Pleural Cavity, Percutaneous Endoscopic Approach

0WWB4JZ Revision of Synthetic Substitute in Left Pleural Cavity, Percutaneous Endoscopic Approach

0WWB4YZ Revision of Other Device in Left Pleural Cavity, Percutaneous Endoscopic Approach

0WWBX0Z Revision of Drainage Device in Left Pleural Cavity, External Approach

0WWBX1Z Revision of Radioactive Element in Left Pleural Cavity, External Approach

0WWBX3Z Revision of Infusion Device in Left Pleural Cavity, External Approach

0WWBXJZ Revision of Synthetic Substitute in Left Pleural Cavity, External Approach

0WWBXYZ Revision of Other Device in Left Pleural Cavity, External Approach

0WWC00Z Revision of Drainage Device in Mediastinum, Open Approach

0WWC01Z Revision of Radioactive Element in Mediastinum, Open Approach

0WWC03Z Revision of Infusion Device in Mediastinum, Open Approach

0WWC07Z Revision of Autologous Tissue Substitute in Mediastinum, Open Approach

0WWC0JZ Revision of Synthetic Substitute in Mediastinum, Open Approach

♀ Female-only   ♂ Male-only   ▲ Limited Coverage   ● Non-OR   ▥ HAC-associated procedure   ▲ Non-covered procedures   ✛ Combination

0WWC0KZ	Revision of Nonautologous Tissue Substitute in Mediastinum, Open Approach	
0WWC0YZ	Revision of Other Device in Mediastinum, Open Approach	
0WWC30Z	Revision of Drainage Device in Mediastinum, Percutaneous Approach	
0WWC31Z	Revision of Radioactive Element in Mediastinum, Percutaneous Approach	
0WWC33Z	Revision of Infusion Device in Mediastinum, Percutaneous Approach	
0WWC37Z	Revision of Autologous Tissue Substitute in Mediastinum, Percutaneous Approach	
0WWC3JZ	Revision of Synthetic Substitute in Mediastinum, Percutaneous Approach	
0WWC3KZ	Revision of Nonautologous Tissue Substitute in Mediastinum, Percutaneous Approach	
0WWC3YZ	Revision of Other Device in Mediastinum, Percutaneous Approach	
0WWC40Z	Revision of Drainage Device in Mediastinum, Percutaneous Endoscopic Approach	
0WWC41Z	Revision of Radioactive Element in Mediastinum, Percutaneous Endoscopic Approach	
0WWC43Z	Revision of Infusion Device in Mediastinum, Percutaneous Endoscopic Approach	
0WWC47Z	Revision of Autologous Tissue Substitute in Mediastinum, Percutaneous Endoscopic Approach	
0WWC4JZ	Revision of Synthetic Substitute in Mediastinum, Percutaneous Endoscopic Approach	
0WWC4KZ	Revision of Nonautologous Tissue Substitute in Mediastinum, Percutaneous Endoscopic Approach	
0WWC4YZ	Revision of Other Device in Mediastinum, Percutaneous Endoscopic Approach	
0WWCX0Z	Revision of Drainage Device in Mediastinum, External Approach	
0WWCX1Z	Revision of Radioactive Element in Mediastinum, External Approach	
0WWCX3Z	Revision of Infusion Device in Mediastinum, External Approach	
0WWCX7Z	Revision of Autologous Tissue Substitute in Mediastinum, External Approach	
0WWCXJZ	Revision of Synthetic Substitute in Mediastinum, External Approach	
0WWCXKZ	Revision of Nonautologous Tissue Substitute in Mediastinum, External Approach	
0WWCXYZ	Revision of Other Device in Mediastinum, External Approach	
0WWD00Z	Revision of Drainage Device in Pericardial Cavity, Open Approach	
0WWD01Z	Revision of Radioactive Element in Pericardial Cavity, Open Approach	
0WWD03Z	Revision of Infusion Device in Pericardial Cavity, Open Approach	
0WWD0YZ	Revision of Other Device in Pericardial Cavity, Open Approach	
0WWD30Z	Revision of Drainage Device in Pericardial Cavity, Percutaneous Approach	
0WWD31Z	Revision of Radioactive Element in Pericardial Cavity, Percutaneous Approach	
0WWD33Z	Revision of Infusion Device in Pericardial Cavity, Percutaneous Approach	
0WWD3YZ	Revision of Other Device in Pericardial Cavity, Percutaneous Approach	
0WWD40Z	Revision of Drainage Device in Pericardial Cavity, Percutaneous Endoscopic Approach	

0WWD41Z	Revision of Radioactive Element in Pericardial Cavity, Percutaneous Endoscopic Approach
0WWD43Z	Revision of Infusion Device in Pericardial Cavity, Percutaneous Endoscopic Approach
0WWD4YZ	Revision of Other Device in Pericardial Cavity, Percutaneous Endoscopic Approach
0WWDX0Z	Revision of Drainage Device in Pericardial Cavity, External Approach
0WWDX1Z	Revision of Radioactive Element in Pericardial Cavity, External Approach
0WWDX3Z	Revision of Infusion Device in Pericardial Cavity, External Approach
0WWDXYZ	Revision of Other Device in Pericardial Cavity, External Approach
0WWF00Z	Revision of Drainage Device in Abdominal Wall, Open Approach
0WWF01Z	Revision of Radioactive Element in Abdominal Wall, Open Approach
0WWF03Z	Revision of Infusion Device in Abdominal Wall, Open Approach
0WWF07Z	Revision of Autologous Tissue Substitute in Abdominal Wall, Open Approach
0WWF0JZ	Revision of Synthetic Substitute in Abdominal Wall, Open Approach
0WWF0KZ	Revision of Nonautologous Tissue Substitute in Abdominal Wall, Open Approach
0WWF0YZ	Revision of Other Device in Abdominal Wall, Open Approach
0WWF30Z	Revision of Drainage Device in Abdominal Wall, Percutaneous Approach
0WWF31Z	Revision of Radioactive Element in Abdominal Wall, Percutaneous Approach
0WWF33Z	Revision of Infusion Device in Abdominal Wall, Percutaneous Approach
0WWF37Z	Revision of Autologous Tissue Substitute in Abdominal Wall, Percutaneous Approach
0WWF3JZ	Revision of Synthetic Substitute in Abdominal Wall, Percutaneous Approach
0WWF3KZ	Revision of Nonautologous Tissue Substitute in Abdominal Wall, Percutaneous Approach
0WWF3YZ	Revision of Other Device in Abdominal Wall, Percutaneous Approach
0WWF40Z	Revision of Drainage Device in Abdominal Wall, Percutaneous Endoscopic Approach
0WWF41Z	Revision of Radioactive Element in Abdominal Wall, Percutaneous Endoscopic Approach
0WWF43Z	Revision of Infusion Device in Abdominal Wall, Percutaneous Endoscopic Approach
0WWF47Z	Revision of Autologous Tissue Substitute in Abdominal Wall, Percutaneous Endoscopic Approach
0WWF4JZ	Revision of Synthetic Substitute in Abdominal Wall, Percutaneous Endoscopic Approach
0WWF4KZ	Revision of Nonautologous Tissue Substitute in Abdominal Wall, Percutaneous Endoscopic Approach
0WWF4YZ	Revision of Other Device in Abdominal Wall, Percutaneous Endoscopic Approach
0WWFX0Z	Revision of Drainage Device in Abdominal Wall, External Approach
0WWFX1Z	Revision of Radioactive Element in Abdominal Wall, External Approach
0WWFX3Z	Revision of Infusion Device in Abdominal Wall, External Approach
0WWFX7Z	Revision of Autologous Tissue Substitute in Abdominal Wall, External Approach
0WWFXJZ	Revision of Synthetic Substitute in Abdominal Wall, External Approach

0WWFXKZ	Revision of Nonautologous Tissue Substitute in Abdominal Wall, External Approach
0WWFXYZ	Revision of Other Device in Abdominal Wall, External Approach
0WWG00Z	Revision of Drainage Device in Peritoneal Cavity, Open Approach
0WWG01Z	Revision of Radioactive Element in Peritoneal Cavity, Open Approach
0WWG03Z	Revision of Infusion Device in Peritoneal Cavity, Open Approach
0WWG0JZ	Revision of Synthetic Substitute in Peritoneal Cavity, Open Approach
0WWG0YZ	Revision of Other Device in Peritoneal Cavity, Open Approach
0WWG30Z	Revision of Drainage Device in Peritoneal Cavity, Percutaneous Approach
0WWG31Z	Revision of Radioactive Element in Peritoneal Cavity, Percutaneous Approach
0WWG33Z	Revision of Infusion Device in Peritoneal Cavity, Percutaneous Approach
0WWG3JZ	Revision of Synthetic Substitute in Peritoneal Cavity, Percutaneous Approach
0WWG3YZ	Revision of Other Device in Peritoneal Cavity, Percutaneous Approach
0WWG40Z	Revision of Drainage Device in Peritoneal Cavity, Percutaneous Endoscopic Approach
0WWG41Z	Revision of Radioactive Element in Peritoneal Cavity, Percutaneous Endoscopic Approach
0WWG43Z	Revision of Infusion Device in Peritoneal Cavity, Percutaneous Endoscopic Approach
0WWG4JZ	Revision of Synthetic Substitute in Peritoneal Cavity, Percutaneous Endoscopic Approach
0WWG4YZ	Revision of Other Device in Peritoneal Cavity, Percutaneous Endoscopic Approach
0WWGX0Z	Revision of Drainage Device in Peritoneal Cavity, External Approach
0WWGX1Z	Revision of Radioactive Element in Peritoneal Cavity, External Approach
0WWGX3Z	Revision of Infusion Device in Peritoneal Cavity, External Approach
0WWGXJZ	Revision of Synthetic Substitute in Peritoneal Cavity, External Approach
0WWGXYZ	Revision of Other Device in Peritoneal Cavity, External Approach
0WWH00Z	Revision of Drainage Device in Retroperitoneum, Open Approach
0WWH01Z	Revision of Radioactive Element in Retroperitoneum, Open Approach
0WWH03Z	Revision of Infusion Device in Retroperitoneum, Open Approach
0WWH0YZ	Revision of Other Device in Retroperitoneum, Open Approach
0WWH30Z	Revision of Drainage Device in Retroperitoneum, Percutaneous Approach
0WWH31Z	Revision of Radioactive Element in Retroperitoneum, Percutaneous Approach
0WWH33Z	Revision of Infusion Device in Retroperitoneum, Percutaneous Approach
0WWH3YZ	Revision of Other Device in Retroperitoneum, Percutaneous Approach
0WWH40Z	Revision of Drainage Device in Retroperitoneum, Percutaneous Endoscopic Approach
0WWH41Z	Revision of Radioactive Element in Retroperitoneum, Percutaneous Endoscopic Approach
0WWH43Z	Revision of Infusion Device in Retroperitoneum, Percutaneous Endoscopic Approach

Medical and Surgical, Anatomical Regions, General Code Listings

1135

♀ Female-only	♂ Male-only	▲ Limited Coverage	● Non-OR	HAC-associated procedure	▲ Non-covered procedures	✚ Combination

0WWH4YZ Revision of Other Device in Retroperitoneum, Percutaneous Endoscopic Approach

0WWHX0Z Revision of Drainage Device in Retroperitoneum, External Approach

0WWHX1Z Revision of Radioactive Element in Retroperitoneum, External Approach

0WWHX3Z Revision of Infusion Device in Retroperitoneum, External Approach

0WWHXYZ Revision of Other Device in Retroperitoneum, External Approach

0WWJ00Z Revision of Drainage Device in Pelvic Cavity, Open Approach

0WWJ01Z Revision of Radioactive Element in Pelvic Cavity, Open Approach

0WWJ03Z Revision of Infusion Device in Pelvic Cavity, Open Approach

0WWJ0JZ Revision of Synthetic Substitute in Pelvic Cavity, Open Approach

0WWJ0YZ Revision of Other Device in Pelvic Cavity, Open Approach

0WWJ30Z Revision of Drainage Device in Pelvic Cavity, Percutaneous Approach

0WWJ31Z Revision of Radioactive Element in Pelvic Cavity, Percutaneous Approach

0WWJ33Z Revision of Infusion Device in Pelvic Cavity, Percutaneous Approach

0WWJ3JZ Revision of Synthetic Substitute in Pelvic Cavity, Percutaneous Approach

0WWJ3YZ Revision of Other Device in Pelvic Cavity, Percutaneous Approach

0WWJ40Z Revision of Drainage Device in Pelvic Cavity, Percutaneous Endoscopic Approach

0WWJ41Z Revision of Radioactive Element in Pelvic Cavity, Percutaneous Endoscopic Approach

0WWJ43Z Revision of Infusion Device in Pelvic Cavity, Percutaneous Endoscopic Approach

0WWJ4JZ Revision of Synthetic Substitute in Pelvic Cavity, Percutaneous Endoscopic Approach

0WWJ4YZ Revision of Other Device in Pelvic Cavity, Percutaneous Endoscopic Approach

0WWJX0Z Revision of Drainage Device in Pelvic Cavity, External Approach

0WWJX1Z Revision of Radioactive Element in Pelvic Cavity, External Approach

0WWJX3Z Revision of Infusion Device in Pelvic Cavity, External Approach

0WWJXJZ Revision of Synthetic Substitute in Pelvic Cavity, External Approach

0WWJXYZ Revision of Other Device in Pelvic Cavity, External Approach

● **0WWK00Z** Revision of Drainage Device in Upper Back, Open Approach

● **0WWK01Z** Revision of Radioactive Element in Upper Back, Open Approach

● **0WWK03Z** Revision of Infusion Device in Upper Back, Open Approach

● **0WWK07Z** Revision of Autologous Tissue Substitute in Upper Back, Open Approach

● **0WWK0JZ** Revision of Synthetic Substitute in Upper Back, Open Approach

● **0WWK0KZ** Revision of Nonautologous Tissue Substitute in Upper Back, Open Approach

● **0WWK0YZ** Revision of Other Device in Upper Back, Open Approach

● **0WWK30Z** Revision of Drainage Device in Upper Back, Percutaneous Approach

● **0WWK31Z** Revision of Radioactive Element in Upper Back, Percutaneous Approach

● **0WWK33Z** Revision of Infusion Device in Upper Back, Percutaneous Approach

● **0WWK37Z** Revision of Autologous Tissue Substitute in Upper Back, Percutaneous Approach

● **0WWK3JZ** Revision of Synthetic Substitute in Upper Back, Percutaneous Approach

● **0WWK3KZ** Revision of Nonautologous Tissue Substitute in Upper Back, Percutaneous Approach

● **0WWK3YZ** Revision of Other Device in Upper Back, Percutaneous Approach

● **0WWK40Z** Revision of Drainage Device in Upper Back, Percutaneous Endoscopic Approach

● **0WWK41Z** Revision of Radioactive Element in Upper Back, Percutaneous Endoscopic Approach

● **0WWK43Z** Revision of Infusion Device in Upper Back, Percutaneous Endoscopic Approach

● **0WWK47Z** Revision of Autologous Tissue Substitute in Upper Back, Percutaneous Endoscopic Approach

● **0WWK4JZ** Revision of Synthetic Substitute in Upper Back, Percutaneous Endoscopic Approach

● **0WWK4KZ** Revision of Nonautologous Tissue Substitute in Upper Back, Percutaneous Endoscopic Approach

● **0WWK4YZ** Revision of Other Device in Upper Back, Percutaneous Endoscopic Approach

0WWKX0Z Revision of Drainage Device in Upper Back, External Approach

0WWKX1Z Revision of Radioactive Element in Upper Back, External Approach

0WWKX3Z Revision of Infusion Device in Upper Back, External Approach

0WWKX7Z Revision of Autologous Tissue Substitute in Upper Back, External Approach

0WWKXJZ Revision of Synthetic Substitute in Upper Back, External Approach

0WWKXKZ Revision of Nonautologous Tissue Substitute in Upper Back, External Approach

0WWKXYZ Revision of Other Device in Upper Back, External Approach

● **0WWL00Z** Revision of Drainage Device in Lower Back, Open Approach

● **0WWL01Z** Revision of Radioactive Element in Lower Back, Open Approach

● **0WWL03Z** Revision of Infusion Device in Lower Back, Open Approach

● **0WWL07Z** Revision of Autologous Tissue Substitute in Lower Back, Open Approach

● **0WWL0JZ** Revision of Synthetic Substitute in Lower Back, Open Approach

● **0WWL0KZ** Revision of Nonautologous Tissue Substitute in Lower Back, Open Approach

● **0WWL0YZ** Revision of Other Device in Lower Back, Open Approach

● **0WWL30Z** Revision of Drainage Device in Lower Back, Percutaneous Approach

● **0WWL31Z** Revision of Radioactive Element in Lower Back, Percutaneous Approach

● **0WWL33Z** Revision of Infusion Device in Lower Back, Percutaneous Approach

● **0WWL37Z** Revision of Autologous Tissue Substitute in Lower Back, Percutaneous Approach

● **0WWL3JZ** Revision of Synthetic Substitute in Lower Back, Percutaneous Approach

● **0WWL3KZ** Revision of Nonautologous Tissue Substitute in Lower Back, Percutaneous Approach

● **0WWL3YZ** Revision of Other Device in Lower Back, Percutaneous Approach

● **0WWL40Z** Revision of Drainage Device in Lower Back, Percutaneous Endoscopic Approach

● **0WWL41Z** Revision of Radioactive Element in Lower Back, Percutaneous Endoscopic Approach

● **0WWL43Z** Revision of Infusion Device in Lower Back, Percutaneous Endoscopic Approach

● **0WWL47Z** Revision of Autologous Tissue Substitute in Lower Back, Percutaneous Endoscopic Approach

● **0WWL4JZ** Revision of Synthetic Substitute in Lower Back, Percutaneous Endoscopic Approach

● **0WWL4KZ** Revision of Nonautologous Tissue Substitute in Lower Back, Percutaneous Endoscopic Approach

● **0WWL4YZ** Revision of Other Device in Lower Back, Percutaneous Endoscopic Approach

0WWLX0Z Revision of Drainage Device in Lower Back, External Approach

0WWLX1Z Revision of Radioactive Element in Lower Back, External Approach

0WWLX3Z Revision of Infusion Device in Lower Back, External Approach

0WWLX7Z Revision of Autologous Tissue Substitute in Lower Back, External Approach

0WWLXJZ Revision of Synthetic Substitute in Lower Back, External Approach

0WWLXKZ Revision of Nonautologous Tissue Substitute in Lower Back, External Approach

0WWLXYZ Revision of Other Device in Lower Back, External Approach

♂ **0WWM00Z** Revision of Drainage Device in Male Perineum, Open Approach

♂ **0WWM01Z** Revision of Radioactive Element in Male Perineum, Open Approach

♂ **0WWM03Z** Revision of Infusion Device in Male Perineum, Open Approach

♂ **0WWM07Z** Revision of Autologous Tissue Substitute in Male Perineum, Open Approach

♂ **0WWM0JZ** Revision of Synthetic Substitute in Male Perineum, Open Approach

♂ **0WWM0KZ** Revision of Nonautologous Tissue Substitute in Male Perineum, Open Approach

♂ **0WWM0YZ** Revision of Other Device in Male Perineum, Open Approach

♂ **0WWM30Z** Revision of Drainage Device in Male Perineum, Percutaneous Approach

♂ **0WWM31Z** Revision of Radioactive Element in Male Perineum, Percutaneous Approach

♂ **0WWM33Z** Revision of Infusion Device in Male Perineum, Percutaneous Approach

♂ **0WWM37Z** Revision of Autologous Tissue Substitute in Male Perineum, Percutaneous Approach

♂ **0WWM3JZ** Revision of Synthetic Substitute in Male Perineum, Percutaneous Approach

♂ **0WWM3KZ** Revision of Nonautologous Tissue Substitute in Male Perineum, Percutaneous Approach

♂ **0WWM3YZ** Revision of Other Device in Male Perineum, Percutaneous Approach

♂ **0WWM40Z** Revision of Drainage Device in Male Perineum, Percutaneous Endoscopic Approach

♂ **0WWM41Z** Revision of Radioactive Element in Male Perineum, Percutaneous Endoscopic Approach

♂ **0WWM43Z** Revision of Infusion Device in Male Perineum, Percutaneous Endoscopic Approach

♂ **0WWM47Z** Revision of Autologous Tissue Substitute in Male Perineum, Percutaneous Endoscopic Approach

♂ **0WWM4JZ** Revision of Synthetic Substitute in Male Perineum, Percutaneous Endoscopic Approach

♀ Female-only   ♂ Male-only   ▲ Limited Coverage   ● Non-OR   ▨ HAC-associated procedure   ▲ Non-covered procedures   ✚ Combination

WWM4KZ	Revision of Nonautologous Tissue Substitute in Male Perineum, Percutaneous Endoscopic Approach
WWM4YZ	Revision of Other Device in Male Perineum, Percutaneous Endoscopic Approach
WWMX0Z	Revision of Drainage Device in Male Perineum, External Approach
WWMX1Z	Revision of Radioactive Element in Male Perineum, External Approach
WWMX3Z	Revision of Infusion Device in Male Perineum, External Approach
WWMX7Z	Revision of Autologous Tissue Substitute in Male Perineum, External Approach
WWMXJZ	Revision of Synthetic Substitute in Male Perineum, External Approach
WWMXKZ	Revision of Nonautologous Tissue Substitute in Male Perineum, External Approach *This is a male-only service, however, it is not included in the male-only edit logic for MCE V30*
WWMXYZ	Revision of Other Device in Male Perineum, External Approach *This is a male-only service, however, it is not included in the male-only edit logic for MCE V30*
WWN00Z	Revision of Drainage Device in Female Perineum, Open Approach
WWN01Z	Revision of Radioactive Element in Female Perineum, Open Approach
WWN03Z	Revision of Infusion Device in Female Perineum, Open Approach
WWN07Z	Revision of Autologous Tissue Substitute in Female Perineum, Open Approach
WWN0JZ	Revision of Synthetic Substitute in Female Perineum, Open Approach
WWN0KZ	Revision of Nonautologous Tissue Substitute in Female Perineum, Open Approach
WWN0YZ	Revision of Other Device in Female Perineum, Open Approach
WWN30Z	Revision of Drainage Device in Female Perineum, Percutaneous Approach
WWN31Z	Revision of Radioactive Element in Female Perineum, Percutaneous Approach
WWN33Z	Revision of Infusion Device in Female Perineum, Percutaneous Approach
WWN37Z	Revision of Autologous Tissue Substitute in Female Perineum, Percutaneous Approach
WWN3JZ	Revision of Synthetic Substitute in Female Perineum, Percutaneous Approach
WWN3KZ	Revision of Nonautologous Tissue Substitute in Female Perineum, Percutaneous Approach
WWN3YZ	Revision of Other Device in Female Perineum, Percutaneous Approach
WWN40Z	Revision of Drainage Device in Female Perineum, Percutaneous Endoscopic Approach
WWN41Z	Revision of Radioactive Element in Female Perineum, Percutaneous Endoscopic Approach
WWN43Z	Revision of Infusion Device in Female Perineum, Percutaneous Endoscopic Approach
WWN47Z	Revision of Autologous Tissue Substitute in Female Perineum, Percutaneous Endoscopic Approach
WWN4JZ	Revision of Synthetic Substitute in Female Perineum, Percutaneous Endoscopic Approach

♀ 0WWN4KZ	Revision of Nonautologous Tissue Substitute in Female Perineum, Percutaneous Endoscopic Approach
♀ 0WWN4YZ	Revision of Other Device in Female Perineum, Percutaneous Endoscopic Approach
♀ 0WWNX0Z	Revision of Drainage Device in Female Perineum, External Approach
♀ 0WWNX1Z	Revision of Radioactive Element in Female Perineum, External Approach
♀ 0WWNX3Z	Revision of Infusion Device in Female Perineum, External Approach
♀ 0WWNX7Z	Revision of Autologous Tissue Substitute in Female Perineum, External Approach
♀ 0WWNXJZ	Revision of Synthetic Substitute in Female Perineum, External Approach
♀ 0WWNXKZ	Revision of Nonautologous Tissue Substitute in Female Perineum, External Approach
♀ 0WWNXYZ	Revision of Other Device in Female Perineum, External Approach
0WWP01Z	Revision of Radioactive Element in Gastrointestinal Tract, Open Approach
0WWP03Z	Revision of Infusion Device in Gastrointestinal Tract, Open Approach
0WWP0YZ	Revision of Other Device in Gastrointestinal Tract, Open Approach
0WWP31Z	Revision of Radioactive Element in Gastrointestinal Tract, Percutaneous Approach
0WWP33Z	Revision of Infusion Device in Gastrointestinal Tract, Percutaneous Approach
0WWP3YZ	Revision of Other Device in Gastrointestinal Tract, Percutaneous Approach
0WWP41Z	Revision of Radioactive Element in Gastrointestinal Tract, Percutaneous Endoscopic Approach
0WWP43Z	Revision of Infusion Device in Gastrointestinal Tract, Percutaneous Endoscopic Approach
0WWP4YZ	Revision of Other Device in Gastrointestinal Tract, Percutaneous Endoscopic Approach
0WWP71Z	Revision of Radioactive Element in Gastrointestinal Tract, Via Natural or Artificial Opening
0WWP73Z	Revision of Infusion Device in Gastrointestinal Tract, Via Natural or Artificial Opening
0WWP7YZ	Revision of Other Device in Gastrointestinal Tract, Via Natural or Artificial Opening
0WWP81Z	Revision of Radioactive Element in Gastrointestinal Tract, Via Natural or Artificial Opening Endoscopic
0WWP83Z	Revision of Infusion Device in Gastrointestinal Tract, Via Natural or Artificial Opening Endoscopic
0WWP8YZ	Revision of Other Device in Gastrointestinal Tract, Via Natural or Artificial Opening Endoscopic
0WWPX1Z	Revision of Radioactive Element in Gastrointestinal Tract, External Approach
0WWPX3Z	Revision of Infusion Device in Gastrointestinal Tract, External Approach
0WWPXYZ	Revision of Other Device in Gastrointestinal Tract, External Approach
0WWQ01Z	Revision of Radioactive Element in Respiratory Tract, Open Approach
0WWQ03Z	Revision of Infusion Device in Respiratory Tract, Open Approach

0WWQ0YZ	Revision of Other Device in Respiratory Tract, Open Approach
0WWQ31Z	Revision of Radioactive Element in Respiratory Tract, Percutaneous Approach
0WWQ33Z	Revision of Infusion Device in Respiratory Tract, Percutaneous Approach
0WWQ3YZ	Revision of Other Device in Respiratory Tract, Percutaneous Approach
0WWQ41Z	Revision of Radioactive Element in Respiratory Tract, Percutaneous Endoscopic Approach
0WWQ43Z	Revision of Infusion Device in Respiratory Tract, Percutaneous Endoscopic Approach
0WWQ4YZ	Revision of Other Device in Respiratory Tract, Percutaneous Endoscopic Approach
0WWQ71Z	Revision of Radioactive Element in Respiratory Tract, Via Natural or Artificial Opening
0WWQ73Z	Revision of Infusion Device in Respiratory Tract, Via Natural or Artificial Opening
0WWQ7YZ	Revision of Other Device in Respiratory Tract, Via Natural or Artificial Opening
0WWQ81Z	Revision of Radioactive Element in Respiratory Tract, Via Natural or Artificial Opening Endoscopic
0WWQ83Z	Revision of Infusion Device in Respiratory Tract, Via Natural or Artificial Opening Endoscopic
0WWQ8YZ	Revision of Other Device in Respiratory Tract, Via Natural or Artificial Opening Endoscopic
0WWQX1Z	Revision of Radioactive Element in Respiratory Tract, External Approach
0WWQX3Z	Revision of Infusion Device in Respiratory Tract, External Approach
0WWQXYZ	Revision of Other Device in Respiratory Tract, External Approach
0WWR01Z	Revision of Radioactive Element in Genitourinary Tract, Open Approach
0WWR03Z	Revision of Infusion Device in Genitourinary Tract, Open Approach
0WWR0YZ	Revision of Other Device in Genitourinary Tract, Open Approach
0WWR31Z	Revision of Radioactive Element in Genitourinary Tract, Percutaneous Approach
0WWR33Z	Revision of Infusion Device in Genitourinary Tract, Percutaneous Approach
0WWR3YZ	Revision of Other Device in Genitourinary Tract, Percutaneous Approach
0WWR41Z	Revision of Radioactive Element in Genitourinary Tract, Percutaneous Endoscopic Approach
0WWR43Z	Revision of Infusion Device in Genitourinary Tract, Percutaneous Endoscopic Approach
0WWR4YZ	Revision of Other Device in Genitourinary Tract, Percutaneous Endoscopic Approach
0WWR71Z	Revision of Radioactive Element in Genitourinary Tract, Via Natural or Artificial Opening
0WWR73Z	Revision of Infusion Device in Genitourinary Tract, Via Natural or Artificial Opening
0WWR7YZ	Revision of Other Device in Genitourinary Tract, Via Natural or Artificial Opening

0WWR81Z Revision of Radioactive Element in Genitourinary Tract, Via Natural or Artificial Opening Endoscopic

0WWR83Z Revision of Infusion Device in Genitourinary Tract, Via Natural or Artificial Opening Endoscopic

0WWR8YZ Revision of Other Device in Genitourinary Tract, Via Natural or Artificial Opening Endoscopic

0WWRX1Z Revision of Radioactive Element in Genitourinary Tract, External Approach

0WWRX3Z Revision of Infusion Device in Genitourinary Tract, External Approa

0WWRXYZ Revision of Other Device in Genitourinary Tract, External Approa

♀ Female-only   ♂ Male-only   ▲ Limited Coverage   ● Non-OR   ▨ HAC-associated procedure   ▲ Non-covered procedures   ✚ Combinatio

Anatomical Regions, Upper Extremities Tables 0X0–0XX

Section	0	Medical and Surgical
Body System	X	Anatomical Regions, Upper Extremities
Operation	0	**Alteration:** Modifying the anatomic structure of a body part without affecting the function of the body part

Body Part (4th)	Approach (5th)	Device (6th)	Qualifier (7th)
2 Shoulder Region, Right 3 Shoulder Region, Left 4 Axilla, Right 5 Axilla, Left 6 Upper Extremity, Right 7 Upper Extremity, Left 8 Upper Arm, Right 9 Upper Arm, Left B Elbow Region, Right C Elbow Region, Left D Lower Arm, Right F Lower Arm, Left G Wrist Region, Right H Wrist Region, Left	0 Open 3 Percutaneous 4 Percutaneous Endoscopic	7 Autologous Tissue Substitute J Synthetic Substitute K Nonautologous Tissue Substitute Z No Device	Z No Qualifier

Section	0	Medical and Surgical
Body System	X	Anatomical Regions, Upper Extremities
Operation	2	**Change:** Taking out or off a device from a body part and putting back an identical or similar device in or on the same body part without cutting or puncturing the skin or a mucous membrane

Body Part (4th)	Approach (5th)	Device (6th)	Qualifier (7th)
6 Upper Extremity, Right 7 Upper Extremity, Left	X External	0 Drainage Device Y Other Device	Z No Qualifier

Section	0	Medical and Surgical
Body System	X	Anatomical Regions, Upper Extremities
Operation	3	**Control:** Stopping, or attempting to stop, postprocedural bleeding

Body Part (4th)	Approach (5th)	Device (6th)	Qualifier (7th)
2 Shoulder Region, Right 3 Shoulder Region, Left 4 Axilla, Right 5 Axilla, Left 6 Upper Extremity, Right 7 Upper Extremity, Left 8 Upper Arm, Right 9 Upper Arm, Left B Elbow Region, Right C Elbow Region, Left D Lower Arm, Right F Lower Arm, Left G Wrist Region, Right H Wrist Region, Left J Hand, Right K Hand, Left	0 Open 3 Percutaneous 4 Percutaneous Endoscopic	Z No Device	Z No Qualifier

Section	0	Medical and Surgical
Body System	X	Anatomical Regions, Upper Extremities
Operation	6	Detachment: Cutting off all or a portion of the upper or lower extremities

Body Part (4th)	Approach (5th)	Device (6th)	Qualifier (7th)
0 Forequarter, Right 1 Forequarter, Left 2 Shoulder Region, Right 3 Shoulder Region, Left B Elbow Region, Right C Elbow Region, Left	0 Open	Z No Device	Z No Qualifier
8 Upper Arm, Right 9 Upper Arm, Left D Lower Arm, Right F Lower Arm, Left	0 Open	Z No Device	1 High 2 Mid 3 Low
J Hand, Right K Hand, Left	0 Open	Z No Device	0 Complete 4 Complete 1st Ray 5 Complete 2nd Ray 6 Complete 3rd Ray 7 Complete 4th Ray 8 Complete 5th Ray 9 Partial 1st Ray B Partial 2nd Ray C Partial 3rd Ray D Partial 4th Ray F Partial 5th Ray
L Thumb, Right M Thumb, Left N Index Finger, Right P Index Finger, Left Q Middle Finger, Right R Middle Finger, Left S Ring Finger, Right T Ring Finger, Left V Little Finger, Right W Little Finger, Left	0 Open	Z No Device	0 Complete 1 High 2 Mid 3 Low

Section	0	Medical and Surgical
Body System	X	Anatomical Regions, Upper Extremities
Operation	9	Drainage: Taking or letting out fluids and/or gases from a body part

Body Part (4th)	Approach (5th)	Device (6th)	Qualifier (7th)
2 Shoulder Region, Right 3 Shoulder Region, Left 4 Axilla, Right 5 Axilla, Left 6 Upper Extremity, Right 7 Upper Extremity, Left 8 Upper Arm, Right 9 Upper Arm, Left B Elbow Region, Right C Elbow Region, Left D Lower Arm, Right F Lower Arm, Left G Wrist Region, Right H Wrist Region, Left J Hand, Right K Hand, Left	0 Open 3 Percutaneous 4 Percutaneous Endoscopic	0 Drainage Device	Z No Qualifier

Continued →

Section 0 **Medical and Surgical**
Body System X **Anatomical Regions, Upper Extremities**
Operation 9 **Drainage:** Taking or letting out fluids and/or gases from a body part

Body Part (4ᵗʰ)	Approach (5ᵗʰ)	Device (6ᵗʰ)	Qualifier (7ᵗʰ)
2 Shoulder Region, Right	0 Open	Z No Device	X Diagnostic
3 Shoulder Region, Left	3 Percutaneous		Z No Qualifier
4 Axilla, Right	4 Percutaneous Endoscopic		
5 Axilla, Left			
6 Upper Extremity, Right			
7 Upper Extremity, Left			
8 Upper Arm, Right			
9 Upper Arm, Left			
B Elbow Region, Right			
C Elbow Region, Left			
D Lower Arm, Right			
F Lower Arm, Left			
G Wrist Region, Right			
H Wrist Region, Left			
J Hand, Right			
K Hand, Left			

Section 0 **Medical and Surgical**
Body System X **Anatomical Regions, Upper Extremities**
Operation B **Excision:** Cutting out or off, without replacement, a portion of a body part

Body Part (4ᵗʰ)	Approach (5ᵗʰ)	Device (6ᵗʰ)	Qualifier (7ᵗʰ)
2 Shoulder Region, Right	0 Open	Z No Device	X Diagnostic
3 Shoulder Region, Left	3 Percutaneous		Z No Qualifier
4 Axilla, Right	4 Percutaneous Endoscopic		
5 Axilla, Left			
6 Upper Extremity, Right			
7 Upper Extremity, Left			
8 Upper Arm, Right			
9 Upper Arm, Left			
B Elbow Region, Right			
C Elbow Region, Left			
D Lower Arm, Right			
F Lower Arm, Left			
G Wrist Region, Right			
H Wrist Region, Left			
J Hand, Right			
K Hand, Left			

Section 0 **Medical and Surgical**
Body System X **Anatomical Regions, Upper Extremities**
Operation H **Insertion:** Putting in a nonbiological appliance that monitors, assists, performs, or prevents a physiological function but does not physically take the place of a body part

Body Part (4ᵗʰ)	Approach (5ᵗʰ)	Device (6ᵗʰ)	Qualifier (7ᵗʰ)
2 Shoulder Region, Right	0 Open	1 Radioactive Element	Z No Qualifier
3 Shoulder Region, Left	3 Percutaneous	3 Infusion Device	
4 Axilla, Right	4 Percutaneous Endoscopic	Y Other Device	
5 Axilla, Left			
6 Upper Extremity, Right			
7 Upper Extremity, Left			
8 Upper Arm, Right			
9 Upper Arm, Left			
B Elbow Region, Right			
C Elbow Region, Left			
D Lower Arm, Right			
F Lower Arm, Left			
G Wrist Region, Right			
H Wrist Region, Left			
J Hand, Right			
K Hand, Left			

Section	0	Medical and Surgical
Body System	X	Anatomical Regions, Upper Extremities
Operation	J	Inspection: Visually and/or manually exploring a body part

Body Part (4th)	Approach (5th)	Device (6th)	Qualifier (7th)
2 Shoulder Region, Right 3 Shoulder Region, Left 4 Axilla, Right 5 Axilla, Left 6 Upper Extremity, Right 7 Upper Extremity, Left 8 Upper Arm, Right 9 Upper Arm, Left B Elbow Region, Right C Elbow Region, Left D Lower Arm, Right F Lower Arm, Left G Wrist Region, Right H Wrist Region, Left J Hand, Right K Hand, Left	0 Open 3 Percutaneous 4 Percutaneous Endoscopic X External	Z No Device	Z No Qualifier

Section	0	Medical and Surgical
Body System	X	Anatomical Regions, Upper Extremities
Operation	M	Reattachment: Putting back in or on all or a portion of a separated body part to its normal location or other suitable location

Body Part (4th)	Approach (5th)	Device (6th)	Qualifier (7th)
0 Forequarter, Right 1 Forequarter, Left 2 Shoulder Region, Right 3 Shoulder Region, Left 4 Axilla, Right 5 Axilla, Left 6 Upper Extremity, Right 7 Upper Extremity, Left 8 Upper Arm, Right 9 Upper Arm, Left B Elbow Region, Right C Elbow Region, Left D Lower Arm, Right F Lower Arm, Left G Wrist Region, Right H Wrist Region, Left J Hand, Right K Hand, Left L Thumb, Right M Thumb, Left N Index Finger, Right P Index Finger, Left Q Middle Finger, Right R Middle Finger, Left S Ring Finger, Right T Ring Finger, Left V Little Finger, Right W Little Finger, Left	0 Open	Z No Device	Z No Qualifier

Section	**0**	**Medical and Surgical**	
Body System	**X**	**Anatomical Regions, Upper Extremities**	
Operation	**P**	**Removal:** Taking out or off a device from a body part	

Body Part (4th)	Approach (5th)	Device (6th)	Qualifier (7th)
Upper Extremity, Right Upper Extremity, Left	0 Open 3 Percutaneous 4 Percutaneous Endoscopic X External	0 Drainage Device 1 Radioactive Element 3 Infusion Device 7 Autologous Tissue Substitute J Synthetic Substitute K Nonautologous Tissue Substitute Y Other Device	Z No Qualifier

Section	**0**	**Medical and Surgical**	
Body System	**X**	**Anatomical Regions, Upper Extremities**	
Operation	**Q**	**Repair:** Restoring, to the extent possible, a body part to its normal anatomic structure and function	

Body Part (4th)	Approach (5th)	Device (6th)	Qualifier (7th)
2 Shoulder Region, Right 3 Shoulder Region, Left 4 Axilla, Right 5 Axilla, Left 6 Upper Extremity, Right 7 Upper Extremity, Left 8 Upper Arm, Right 9 Upper Arm, Left B Elbow Region, Right C Elbow Region, Left D Lower Arm, Right F Lower Arm, Left G Wrist Region, Right H Wrist Region, Left J Hand, Right K Hand, Left L Thumb, Right M Thumb, Left N Index Finger, Right P Index Finger, Left Q Middle Finger, Right R Middle Finger, Left S Ring Finger, Right T Ring Finger, Left V Little Finger, Right W Little Finger, Left	0 Open 3 Percutaneous 4 Percutaneous Endoscopic X External	Z No Device	Z No Qualifier

Section	**0**	**Medical and Surgical**	
Body System	**X**	**Anatomical Regions, Upper Extremities**	
Operation	**R**	**Replacement:** Putting in or on biological or synthetic material that physically takes the place and/or function of all or a portion of a body part	

Body Part (4th)	Approach (5th)	Device (6th)	Qualifier (7th)
L Thumb, Right M Thumb, Left	0 Open 4 Percutaneous Endoscopic	7 Autologous Tissue Substitute	N Toe, Right P Toe, Left

Section	0	Medical and Surgical
Body System	X	Anatomical Regions, Upper Extremities
Operation	U	Supplement: Putting in or on biological or synthetic material that physically reinforces and/or augments the function of a portion of a body part

Body Part (4th)	Approach (5th)	Device (6th)	Qualifier (7th)
2 Shoulder Region, Right 3 Shoulder Region, Left 4 Axilla, Right 5 Axilla, Left 6 Upper Extremity, Right 7 Upper Extremity, Left 8 Upper Arm, Right 9 Upper Arm, Left B Elbow Region, Right C Elbow Region, Left D Lower Arm, Right F Lower Arm, Left G Wrist Region, Right H Wrist Region, Left J Hand, Right K Hand, Left L Thumb, Right M Thumb, Left N Index Finger, Right P Index Finger, Left Q Middle Finger, Right R Middle Finger, Left S Ring Finger, Right T Ring Finger, Left V Little Finger, Right W Little Finger, Left	0 Open 4 Percutaneous Endoscopic	7 Autologous Tissue Substitute J Synthetic Substitute K Nonautologous Tissue Substitute	Z No Qualifier

Section	0	Medical and Surgical
Body System	X	Anatomical Regions, Upper Extremities
Operation	W	Revision: Correcting, to the extent possible, a portion of a malfunctioning device or the position of a displaced device

Body Part (4th)	Approach (5th)	Device (6th)	Qualifier (7th)
6 Upper Extremity, Right 7 Upper Extremity, Left	0 Open 3 Percutaneous 4 Percutaneous Endoscopic X External	0 Drainage Device 3 Infusion Device 7 Autologous Tissue Substitute J Synthetic Substitute K Nonautologous Tissue Substitute Y Other Device	Z No Qualifier

Section	0	Medical and Surgical
Body System	X	Anatomical Regions, Upper Extremities
Operation	X	Transfer: Moving, without taking out, all or a portion of a body part to another location to take over the function of all or a portion of a body part

Body Part (4th)	Approach (5th)	Device (6th)	Qualifier (7th)
N Index Finger, Right	0 Open	Z No Device	L Thumb, Right
P Index Finger, Left	0 Open	Z No Device	M Thumb, Left

0X0207Z Alteration of Right Shoulder Region with Autologous Tissue Substitute, Open Approach

0X020JZ Alteration of Right Shoulder Region with Synthetic Substitute, Open Approach

0X020KZ Alteration of Right Shoulder Region with Nonautologous Tissue Substitute, Open Approach

0X020ZZ Alteration of Right Shoulder Region, Open Approach

0X0237Z Alteration of Right Shoulder Region with Autologous Tissue Substitute, Percutaneous Approach

0X023JZ Alteration of Right Shoulder Region with Synthetic Substitute, Percutaneous Approach

0X023KZ Alteration of Right Shoulder Region with Nonautologous Tissue Substitute, Percutaneous Approach

0X023ZZ Alteration of Right Shoulder Region, Percutaneous Approach

0X0247Z Alteration of Right Shoulder Region with Autologous Tissue Substitute, Percutaneous Endoscopic Approach

0X024JZ Alteration of Right Shoulder Region with Synthetic Substitute, Percutaneous Endoscopic Approach

0X024KZ Alteration of Right Shoulder Region with Nonautologous Tissue Substitute, Percutaneous Endoscopic Approach

0X024ZZ Alteration of Right Shoulder Region, Percutaneous Endoscopic Approach

0X0307Z Alteration of Left Shoulder Region with Autologous Tissue Substitute, Open Approach

0X030JZ Alteration of Left Shoulder Region with Synthetic Substitute, Open Approach

0X030KZ Alteration of Left Shoulder Region with Nonautologous Tissue Substitute, Open Approach

0X030ZZ Alteration of Left Shoulder Region, Open Approach

0X0337Z Alteration of Left Shoulder Region with Autologous Tissue Substitute, Percutaneous Approach

0X033JZ Alteration of Left Shoulder Region with Synthetic Substitute, Percutaneous Approach

0X033KZ Alteration of Left Shoulder Region with Nonautologous Tissue Substitute, Percutaneous Approach

0X033ZZ Alteration of Left Shoulder Region, Percutaneous Approach

0X0347Z Alteration of Left Shoulder Region with Autologous Tissue Substitute, Percutaneous Endoscopic Approach

0X034JZ Alteration of Left Shoulder Region with Synthetic Substitute, Percutaneous Endoscopic Approach

0X034KZ Alteration of Left Shoulder Region with Nonautologous Tissue Substitute, Percutaneous Endoscopic Approach

0X034ZZ Alteration of Left Shoulder Region, Percutaneous Endoscopic Approach

0X0407Z Alteration of Right Axilla with Autologous Tissue Substitute, Open Approach

0X040JZ Alteration of Right Axilla with Synthetic Substitute, Open Approach

0X040KZ Alteration of Right Axilla with Nonautologous Tissue Substitute, Open Approach

0X040ZZ Alteration of Right Axilla, Open Approach

0X0437Z Alteration of Right Axilla with Autologous Tissue Substitute, Percutaneous Approach

0X043JZ Alteration of Right Axilla with Synthetic Substitute, Percutaneous Approach

0X043KZ Alteration of Right Axilla with Nonautologous Tissue Substitute, Percutaneous Approach

0X043ZZ Alteration of Right Axilla, Percutaneous Approach

0X0447Z Alteration of Right Axilla with Autologous Tissue Substitute, Percutaneous Endoscopic Approach

0X044JZ Alteration of Right Axilla with Synthetic Substitute, Percutaneous Endoscopic Approach

0X044KZ Alteration of Right Axilla with Nonautologous Tissue Substitute, Percutaneous Endoscopic Approach

0X044ZZ Alteration of Right Axilla, Percutaneous Endoscopic Approach

0X0507Z Alteration of Left Axilla with Autologous Tissue Substitute, Open Approach

0X050JZ Alteration of Left Axilla with Synthetic Substitute, Open Approach

0X050KZ Alteration of Left Axilla with Nonautologous Tissue Substitute, Open Approach

0X050ZZ Alteration of Left Axilla, Open Approach

0X0537Z Alteration of Left Axilla with Autologous Tissue Substitute, Percutaneous Approach

0X053JZ Alteration of Left Axilla with Synthetic Substitute, Percutaneous Approach

0X053KZ Alteration of Left Axilla with Nonautologous Tissue Substitute, Percutaneous Approach

0X053ZZ Alteration of Left Axilla, Percutaneous Approach

0X0547Z Alteration of Left Axilla with Autologous Tissue Substitute, Percutaneous Endoscopic Approach

0X054JZ Alteration of Left Axilla with Synthetic Substitute, Percutaneous Endoscopic Approach

0X054KZ Alteration of Left Axilla with Nonautologous Tissue Substitute, Percutaneous Endoscopic Approach

0X054ZZ Alteration of Left Axilla, Percutaneous Endoscopic Approach

0X0607Z Alteration of Right Upper Extremity with Autologous Tissue Substitute, Open Approach

0X060JZ Alteration of Right Upper Extremity with Synthetic Substitute, Open Approach

0X060KZ Alteration of Right Upper Extremity with Nonautologous Tissue Substitute, Open Approach

0X060ZZ Alteration of Right Upper Extremity, Open Approach

0X0637Z Alteration of Right Upper Extremity with Autologous Tissue Substitute, Percutaneous Approach

0X063JZ Alteration of Right Upper Extremity with Synthetic Substitute, Percutaneous Approach

0X063KZ Alteration of Right Upper Extremity with Nonautologous Tissue Substitute, Percutaneous Approach

0X063ZZ Alteration of Right Upper Extremity, Percutaneous Approach

0X0647Z Alteration of Right Upper Extremity with Autologous Tissue Substitute, Percutaneous Endoscopic Approach

0X064JZ Alteration of Right Upper Extremity with Synthetic Substitute, Percutaneous Endoscopic Approach

0X064KZ Alteration of Right Upper Extremity with Nonautologous Tissue Substitute, Percutaneous Endoscopic Approach

0X064ZZ Alteration of Right Upper Extremity, Percutaneous Endoscopic Approach

0X0707Z Alteration of Left Upper Extremity with Autologous Tissue Substitute, Open Approach

0X070JZ Alteration of Left Upper Extremity with Synthetic Substitute, Open Approach

0X070KZ Alteration of Left Upper Extremity with Nonautologous Tissue Substitute, Open Approach

0X070ZZ Alteration of Left Upper Extremity, Open Approach

0X0737Z Alteration of Left Upper Extremity with Autologous Tissue Substitute, Percutaneous Approach

0X073JZ Alteration of Left Upper Extremity with Synthetic Substitute, Percutaneous Approach

0X073KZ Alteration of Left Upper Extremity with Nonautologous Tissue Substitute, Percutaneous Approach

0X073ZZ Alteration of Left Upper Extremity, Percutaneous Approach

0X0747Z Alteration of Left Upper Extremity with Autologous Tissue Substitute, Percutaneous Endoscopic Approach

0X074JZ Alteration of Left Upper Extremity with Synthetic Substitute, Percutaneous Endoscopic Approach

0X074KZ Alteration of Left Upper Extremity with Nonautologous Tissue Substitute, Percutaneous Endoscopic Approach

0X074ZZ Alteration of Left Upper Extremity, Percutaneous Endoscopic Approach

0X0807Z Alteration of Right Upper Arm with Autologous Tissue Substitute, Open Approach

0X080JZ Alteration of Right Upper Arm with Synthetic Substitute, Open Approach

0X080KZ Alteration of Right Upper Arm with Nonautologous Tissue Substitute, Open Approach

0X080ZZ Alteration of Right Upper Arm, Open Approach

0X0837Z Alteration of Right Upper Arm with Autologous Tissue Substitute, Percutaneous Approach

0X083JZ Alteration of Right Upper Arm with Synthetic Substitute, Percutaneous Approach

0X083KZ Alteration of Right Upper Arm with Nonautologous Tissue Substitute, Percutaneous Approach

0X083ZZ Alteration of Right Upper Arm, Percutaneous Approach

0X0847Z Alteration of Right Upper Arm with Autologous Tissue Substitute, Percutaneous Endoscopic Approach

0X084JZ Alteration of Right Upper Arm with Synthetic Substitute, Percutaneous Endoscopic Approach

0X084KZ Alteration of Right Upper Arm with Nonautologous Tissue Substitute, Percutaneous Endoscopic Approach

0X084ZZ Alteration of Right Upper Arm, Percutaneous Endoscopic Approach

0X0907Z Alteration of Left Upper Arm with Autologous Tissue Substitute, Open Approach

0X090JZ Alteration of Left Upper Arm with Synthetic Substitute, Open Approach

0X090KZ Alteration of Left Upper Arm with Nonautologous Tissue Substitute, Open Approach

0X090ZZ Alteration of Left Upper Arm, Open Approach

0X0937Z Alteration of Left Upper Arm with Autologous Tissue Substitute, Percutaneous Approach

0X093JZ Alteration of Left Upper Arm with Synthetic Substitute, Percutaneous Approach

0X093KZ Alteration of Left Upper Arm with Nonautologous Tissue Substitute, Percutaneous Approach

0X093ZZ Alteration of Left Upper Arm, Percutaneous Approach

0X0947Z Alteration of Left Upper Arm with Autologous Tissue Substitute, Percutaneous Endoscopic Approach

0X094JZ Alteration of Left Upper Arm with Synthetic Substitute, Percutaneous Endoscopic Approach

0X094KZ Alteration of Left Upper Arm with Nonautologous Tissue Substitute, Percutaneous Endoscopic Approach

0X094ZZ Alteration of Left Upper Arm, Percutaneous Endoscopic Approach

0X0B07Z Alteration of Right Elbow Region with Autologous Tissue Substitute, Open Approach

0X0B0JZ Alteration of Right Elbow Region with Synthetic Substitute, Open Approach

0X0B0KZ Alteration of Right Elbow Region with Nonautologous Tissue Substitute, Open Approach

0X0B0ZZ Alteration of Right Elbow Region, Open Approach

0X0B37Z Alteration of Right Elbow Region with Autologous Tissue Substitute, Percutaneous Approach

0X0B3JZ Alteration of Right Elbow Region with Synthetic Substitute, Percutaneous Approach

0X0B3KZ Alteration of Right Elbow Region with Nonautologous Tissue Substitute, Percutaneous Approach

0X0B3ZZ Alteration of Right Elbow Region, Percutaneous Approach

0X0B47Z Alteration of Right Elbow Region with Autologous Tissue Substitute, Percutaneous Endoscopic Approach

0X0B4JZ Alteration of Right Elbow Region with Synthetic Substitute, Percutaneous Endoscopic Approach

0X0B4KZ Alteration of Right Elbow Region with Nonautologous Tissue Substitute, Percutaneous Endoscopic Approach

0X0B4ZZ Alteration of Right Elbow Region, Percutaneous Endoscopic Approach

0X0C07Z Alteration of Left Elbow Region with Autologous Tissue Substitute, Open Approach

0X0C0JZ Alteration of Left Elbow Region with Synthetic Substitute, Open Approach

0X0C0KZ Alteration of Left Elbow Region with Nonautologous Tissue Substitute, Open Approach

0X0C0ZZ Alteration of Left Elbow Region, Open Approach

0X0C37Z Alteration of Left Elbow Region with Autologous Tissue Substitute, Percutaneous Approach

0X0C3JZ Alteration of Left Elbow Region with Synthetic Substitute, Percutaneous Approach

0X0C3KZ Alteration of Left Elbow Region with Nonautologous Tissue Substitute, Percutaneous Approach

0X0C3ZZ Alteration of Left Elbow Region, Percutaneous Approach

0X0C47Z Alteration of Left Elbow Region with Autologous Tissue Substitute, Percutaneous Endoscopic Approach

0X0C4JZ Alteration of Left Elbow Region with Synthetic Substitute, Percutaneous Endoscopic Approach

0X0C4KZ Alteration of Left Elbow Region with Nonautologous Tissue Substitute, Percutaneous Endoscopic Approach

0X0C4ZZ Alteration of Left Elbow Region, Percutaneous Endoscopic Approach

0X0D07Z Alteration of Right Lower Arm with Autologous Tissue Substitute, Open Approach

0X0D0JZ Alteration of Right Lower Arm with Synthetic Substitute, Open Approach

0X0D0KZ Alteration of Right Lower Arm with Nonautologous Tissue Substitute, Open Approach

0X0D0ZZ Alteration of Right Lower Arm, Open Approach

0X0D37Z Alteration of Right Lower Arm with Autologous Tissue Substitute, Percutaneous Approach

0X0D3JZ Alteration of Right Lower Arm with Synthetic Substitute, Percutaneous Approach

0X0D3KZ Alteration of Right Lower Arm with Nonautologous Tissue Substitute, Percutaneous Approach

0X0D3ZZ Alteration of Right Lower Arm, Percutaneous Approach

0X0D47Z Alteration of Right Lower Arm with Autologous Tissue Substitute, Percutaneous Endoscopic Approach

0X0D4JZ Alteration of Right Lower Arm with Synthetic Substitute, Percutaneous Endoscopic Approach

0X0D4KZ Alteration of Right Lower Arm with Nonautologous Tissue Substitute, Percutaneous Endoscopic Approach

0X0D4ZZ Alteration of Right Lower Arm, Percutaneous Endoscopic Approach

0X0F07Z Alteration of Left Lower Arm with Autologous Tissue Substitute, Open Approach

0X0F0JZ Alteration of Left Lower Arm with Synthetic Substitute, Open Approach

0X0F0KZ Alteration of Left Lower Arm with Nonautologous Tissue Substitute, Open Approach

0X0F0ZZ Alteration of Left Lower Arm, Open Approach

0X0F37Z Alteration of Left Lower Arm with Autologous Tissue Substitute, Percutaneous Approach

0X0F3JZ Alteration of Left Lower Arm with Synthetic Substitute, Percutaneous Approach

0X0F3KZ Alteration of Left Lower Arm with Nonautologous Tissue Substitute, Percutaneous Approach

0X0F3ZZ Alteration of Left Lower Arm, Percutaneous Approach

0X0F47Z Alteration of Left Lower Arm with Autologous Tissue Substitute, Percutaneous Endoscopic Approach

0X0F4JZ Alteration of Left Lower Arm with Synthetic Substitute, Percutaneous Endoscopic Approach

0X0F4KZ Alteration of Left Lower Arm with Nonautologous Tissue Substitute, Percutaneous Endoscopic Approach

0X0F4ZZ Alteration of Left Lower Arm, Percutaneous Endoscopic Approach

0X0G07Z Alteration of Right Wrist Region with Autologous Tissue Substitute, Open Approach

0X0G0JZ Alteration of Right Wrist Region with Synthetic Substitute, Open Approach

0X0G0KZ Alteration of Right Wrist Region with Nonautologous Tissue Substitute, Open Approach

0X0G0ZZ Alteration of Right Wrist Region, Open Approach

0X0G37Z Alteration of Right Wrist Region with Autologous Tissue Substitute, Percutaneous Approach

0X0G3JZ Alteration of Right Wrist Region with Synthetic Substitute, Percutaneous Approach

0X0G3KZ Alteration of Right Wrist Region with Nonautologous Tissue Substitute, Percutaneous Approach

0X0G3ZZ Alteration of Right Wrist Region, Percutaneous Approach

0X0G47Z Alteration of Right Wrist Region with Autologous Tissue Substitute, Percutaneous Endoscopic Approach

0X0G4JZ Alteration of Right Wrist Region with Synthetic Substitute, Percutaneous Endoscopic Approach

0X0G4KZ Alteration of Right Wrist Region with Nonautologous Tissue Substitute, Percutaneous Endoscopic Approach

0X0G4ZZ Alteration of Right Wrist Region, Percutaneous Endoscopic Approach

0X0H07Z Alteration of Left Wrist Region with Autologous Tissue Substitute, Open Approach

0X0H0JZ Alteration of Left Wrist Region with Synthetic Substitute, Open Approach

0X0H0KZ Alteration of Left Wrist Region with Nonautologous Tissue Substitute, Open Approach

0X0H0ZZ Alteration of Left Wrist Region, Open Approach

0X0H37Z Alteration of Left Wrist Region with Autologous Tissue Substitute, Percutaneous Approach

0X0H3JZ Alteration of Left Wrist Region with Synthetic Substitute, Percutaneous Approach

0X0H3KZ Alteration of Left Wrist Region with Nonautologous Tissue Substitute, Percutaneous Approach

0X0H3ZZ Alteration of Left Wrist Region, Percutaneous Approach

0X0H47Z Alteration of Left Wrist Region with Autologous Tissue Substitute, Percutaneous Endoscopic Approach

0X0H4JZ Alteration of Left Wrist Region with Synthetic Substitute, Percutaneous Endoscopic Approach

0X0H4KZ Alteration of Left Wrist Region with Nonautologous Tissue Substitute, Percutaneous Endoscopic Approach

0X0H4ZZ Alteration of Left Wrist Region, Percutaneous Endoscopic Approach

2 – Anatomical Regions, Upper Extremities, Change

view Coding Guideline B6.1c

26X0Z Change Drainage Device in Right Upper Extremity, External Approach
0X27X0Z Change Drainage Device in Left Upper Extremity, External Approach
26XYZ Change Other Device in Right Upper Extremity, External Approach
0X27XYZ Change Other Device in Left Upper Extremity, External Approach

3 – Anatomical Regions, Upper Extremities, Control

view Coding Guideline B3.7

320ZZ Control Bleeding in Right Shoulder Region, Open Approach
323ZZ Control Bleeding in Right Shoulder Region, Percutaneous Approach
324ZZ Control Bleeding in Right Shoulder Region, Percutaneous Endoscopic Approach
330ZZ Control Bleeding in Left Shoulder Region, Open Approach
333ZZ Control Bleeding in Left Shoulder Region, Percutaneous Approach
334ZZ Control Bleeding in Left Shoulder Region, Percutaneous Endoscopic Approach
340ZZ Control Bleeding in Right Axilla, Open Approach
343ZZ Control Bleeding in Right Axilla, Percutaneous Approach
344ZZ Control Bleeding in Right Axilla, Percutaneous Endoscopic Approach
350ZZ Control Bleeding in Left Axilla, Open Approach
353ZZ Control Bleeding in Left Axilla, Percutaneous Approach
354ZZ Control Bleeding in Left Axilla, Percutaneous Endoscopic Approach
360ZZ Control Bleeding in Right Upper Extremity, Open Approach
363ZZ Control Bleeding in Right Upper Extremity, Percutaneous Approach
364ZZ Control Bleeding in Right Upper Extremity, Percutaneous Endoscopic Approach
370ZZ Control Bleeding in Left Upper Extremity, Open Approach

AHA CC: 1Q, 2015, 35

0X373ZZ Control Bleeding in Left Upper Extremity, Percutaneous Approach
0X374ZZ Control Bleeding in Left Upper Extremity, Percutaneous Endoscopic Approach
0X380ZZ Control Bleeding in Right Upper Arm, Open Approach
0X383ZZ Control Bleeding in Right Upper Arm, Percutaneous Approach
0X384ZZ Control Bleeding in Right Upper Arm, Percutaneous Endoscopic Approach
0X390ZZ Control Bleeding in Left Upper Arm, Open Approach
0X393ZZ Control Bleeding in Left Upper Arm, Percutaneous Approach
0X394ZZ Control Bleeding in Left Upper Arm, Percutaneous Endoscopic Approach
0X3B0ZZ Control Bleeding in Right Elbow Region, Open Approach
0X3B3ZZ Control Bleeding in Right Elbow Region, Percutaneous Approach
0X3B4ZZ Control Bleeding in Right Elbow Region, Percutaneous Endoscopic Approach
0X3C0ZZ Control Bleeding in Left Elbow Region, Open Approach
0X3C3ZZ Control Bleeding in Left Elbow Region, Percutaneous Approach
0X3C4ZZ Control Bleeding in Left Elbow Region, Percutaneous Endoscopic Approach
0X3D0ZZ Control Bleeding in Right Lower Arm, Open Approach
0X3D3ZZ Control Bleeding in Right Lower Arm, Percutaneous Approach

0X3D4ZZ Control Bleeding in Right Lower Arm, Percutaneous Endoscopic Approach
0X3F0ZZ Control Bleeding in Left Lower Arm, Open Approach
0X3F3ZZ Control Bleeding in Left Lower Arm, Percutaneous Approach
0X3F4ZZ Control Bleeding in Left Lower Arm, Percutaneous Endoscopic Approach
0X3G0ZZ Control Bleeding in Right Wrist Region, Open Approach
0X3G3ZZ Control Bleeding in Right Wrist Region, Percutaneous Approach
0X3G4ZZ Control Bleeding in Right Wrist Region, Percutaneous Endoscopic Approach
0X3H0ZZ Control Bleeding in Left Wrist Region, Open Approach
0X3H3ZZ Control Bleeding in Left Wrist Region, Percutaneous Approach
0X3H4ZZ Control Bleeding in Left Wrist Region, Percutaneous Endoscopic Approach
0X3J0ZZ Control Bleeding in Right Hand, Open Approach
0X3J3ZZ Control Bleeding in Right Hand, Percutaneous Approach
0X3J4ZZ Control Bleeding in Right Hand, Percutaneous Endoscopic Approach
0X3K0ZZ Control Bleeding in Left Hand, Open Approach
0X3K3ZZ Control Bleeding in Left Hand, Percutaneous Approach
0X3K4ZZ Control Bleeding in Left Hand, Percutaneous Endoscopic Approach

X6 – Anatomical Regions, Upper Extremities, Detachment

X600ZZ Detachment at Right Forequarter, Open Approach
X610ZZ Detachment at Left Forequarter, Open Approach
X620ZZ Detachment at Right Shoulder Region, Open Approach
X630ZZ Detachment at Left Shoulder Region, Open Approach
X680Z1 Detachment at Right Upper Arm, High, Open Approach
X680Z2 Detachment at Right Upper Arm, Mid, Open Approach
X680Z3 Detachment at Right Upper Arm, Low, Open Approach
X690Z1 Detachment at Left Upper Arm, High, Open Approach
X690Z2 Detachment at Left Upper Arm, Mid, Open Approach
X690Z3 Detachment at Left Upper Arm, Low, Open Approach
X6B0ZZ Detachment at Right Elbow Region, Open Approach
X6C0ZZ Detachment at Left Elbow Region, Open Approach
X6D0Z1 Detachment at Right Lower Arm, High, Open Approach

0X6D0Z2 Detachment at Right Lower Arm, Mid, Open Approach
0X6D0Z3 Detachment at Right Lower Arm, Low, Open Approach
0X6F0Z1 Detachment at Left Lower Arm, High, Open Approach
0X6F0Z2 Detachment at Left Lower Arm, Mid, Open Approach
0X6F0Z3 Detachment at Left Lower Arm, Low, Open Approach
0X6J0Z0 Detachment at Right Hand, Complete, Open Approach
0X6J0Z4 Detachment at Right Hand, Complete 1st Ray, Open Approach
0X6J0Z5 Detachment at Right Hand, Complete 2nd Ray, Open Approach
0X6J0Z6 Detachment at Right Hand, Complete 3rd Ray, Open Approach
0X6J0Z7 Detachment at Right Hand, Complete 4th Ray, Open Approach
0X6J0Z8 Detachment at Right Hand, Complete 5th Ray, Open Approach
0X6J0Z9 Detachment at Right Hand, Partial 1st Ray, Open Approach
0X6J0ZB Detachment at Right Hand, Partial 2nd Ray, Open Approach

0X6J0ZC Detachment at Right Hand, Partial 3rd Ray, Open Approach
0X6J0ZD Detachment at Right Hand, Partial 4th Ray, Open Approach
0X6J0ZF Detachment at Right Hand, Partial 5th Ray, Open Approach
0X6K0Z0 Detachment at Left Hand, Complete, Open Approach
0X6K0Z4 Detachment at Left Hand, Complete 1st Ray, Open Approach
0X6K0Z5 Detachment at Left Hand, Complete 2nd Ray, Open Approach
0X6K0Z6 Detachment at Left Hand, Complete 3rd Ray, Open Approach
0X6K0Z7 Detachment at Left Hand, Complete 4th Ray, Open Approach
0X6K0Z8 Detachment at Left Hand, Complete 5th Ray, Open Approach
0X6K0Z9 Detachment at Left Hand, Partial 1st Ray, Open Approach
0X6K0ZB Detachment at Left Hand, Partial 2nd Ray, Open Approach
0X6K0ZC Detachment at Left Hand, Partial 3rd Ray, Open Approach
0X6K0ZD Detachment at Left Hand, Partial 4th Ray, Open Approach

Female-only   ♂ Male-only   ▲ Limited Coverage   ● Non-OR   ▩ HAC-associated procedure   ▲ Non-covered procedures   ✚ Combination

0X6K0ZF	Detachment at Left Hand, Partial 5th Ray, Open Approach
0X6L0Z0	Detachment at Right Thumb, Complete, Open Approach
0X6L0Z1	Detachment at Right Thumb, High, Open Approach
0X6L0Z2	Detachment at Right Thumb, Mid, Open Approach
0X6L0Z3	Detachment at Right Thumb, Low, Open Approach
0X6M0Z0	Detachment at Left Thumb, Complete, Open Approach
0X6M0Z1	Detachment at Left Thumb, High, Open Approach
0X6M0Z2	Detachment at Left Thumb, Mid, Open Approach
0X6M0Z3	Detachment at Left Thumb, Low, Open Approach
0X6N0Z0	Detachment at Right Index Finger, Complete, Open Approach
0X6N0Z1	Detachment at Right Index Finger, High, Open Approach
0X6N0Z2	Detachment at Right Index Finger, Mid, Open Approach
0X6N0Z3	Detachment at Right Index Finger, Low, Open Approach
0X6P0Z0	Detachment at Left Index Finger, Complete, Open Approach
0X6P0Z1	Detachment at Left Index Finger, High, Open Approach
0X6P0Z2	Detachment at Left Index Finger, Mid, Open Approach
0X6P0Z3	Detachment at Left Index Finger, Low, Open Approach
0X6Q0Z0	Detachment at Right Middle Finger, Complete, Open Approach
0X6Q0Z1	Detachment at Right Middle Finger, High, Open Approach
0X6Q0Z2	Detachment at Right Middle Finger, Mid, Open Approach
0X6Q0Z3	Detachment at Right Middle Finger, Low, Open Approach
0X6R0Z0	Detachment at Left Middle Finger, Complete, Open Approach
0X6R0Z1	Detachment at Left Middle Finger, High, Open Approach
0X6R0Z2	Detachment at Left Middle Finger, Mid, Open Approach
0X6R0Z3	Detachment at Left Middle Finger, Low, Open Approach
0X6S0Z0	Detachment at Right Ring Finger, Complete, Open Approach
0X6S0Z1	Detachment at Right Ring Finger, High, Open Approach
0X6S0Z2	Detachment at Right Ring Finger, Mid, Open Approach
0X6S0Z3	Detachment at Right Ring Finger, Low, Open Approach
0X6T0Z0	Detachment at Left Ring Finger, Complete, Open Approach
0X6T0Z1	Detachment at Left Ring Finger, High, Open Approach
0X6T0Z2	Detachment at Left Ring Finger, Mid, Open Approach
0X6T0Z3	Detachment at Left Ring Finger, Low, Open Approach
0X6V0Z0	Detachment at Right Little Finger, Complete, Open Approach
0X6V0Z1	Detachment at Right Little Finger, High, Open Approach
0X6V0Z2	Detachment at Right Little Finger, Mid, Open Approach
0X6V0Z3	Detachment at Right Little Finger, Low, Open Approach
0X6W0Z0	Detachment at Left Little Finger, Complete, Open Approach
0X6W0Z1	Detachment at Left Little Finger, High, Open Approach
0X6W0Z2	Detachment at Left Little Finger, Mid, Open Approach
0X6W0Z3	Detachment at Left Little Finger, Low, Open Approach

0X9 – Anatomical Regions, Upper Extremities, Drainage

Review Coding Guidelines B3.4a and B3.4b

Review Coding Guideline B6.2

0X9200Z	Drainage of Right Shoulder Region with Drainage Device, Open Approach
0X920ZX	Drainage of Right Shoulder Region, Open Approach, Diagnostic
0X920ZZ	Drainage of Right Shoulder Region, Open Approach
0X9230Z	Drainage of Right Shoulder Region with Drainage Device, Percutaneous Approach
0X923ZX	Drainage of Right Shoulder Region, Percutaneous Approach, Diagnostic
0X923ZZ	Drainage of Right Shoulder Region, Percutaneous Approach
0X9240Z	Drainage of Right Shoulder Region with Drainage Device, Percutaneous Endoscopic Approach
0X924ZX	Drainage of Right Shoulder Region, Percutaneous Endoscopic Approach, Diagnostic
0X924ZZ	Drainage of Right Shoulder Region, Percutaneous Endoscopic Approach
0X9300Z	Drainage of Left Shoulder Region with Drainage Device, Open Approach
0X930ZX	Drainage of Left Shoulder Region, Open Approach, Diagnostic
0X930ZZ	Drainage of Left Shoulder Region, Open Approach
0X9330Z	Drainage of Left Shoulder Region with Drainage Device, Percutaneous Approach
0X933ZX	Drainage of Left Shoulder Region, Percutaneous Approach, Diagnostic
0X933ZZ	Drainage of Left Shoulder Region, Percutaneous Approach
0X9340Z	Drainage of Left Shoulder Region with Drainage Device, Percutaneous Endoscopic Approach
0X934ZX	Drainage of Left Shoulder Region, Percutaneous Endoscopic Approach, Diagnostic
0X934ZZ	Drainage of Left Shoulder Region, Percutaneous Endoscopic Approach
0X9400Z	Drainage of Right Axilla with Drainage Device, Open Approach
0X940ZX	Drainage of Right Axilla, Open Approach, Diagnostic
0X940ZZ	Drainage of Right Axilla, Open Approach
0X9430Z	Drainage of Right Axilla with Drainage Device, Percutaneous Approach
0X943ZX	Drainage of Right Axilla, Percutaneous Approach, Diagnostic
0X943ZZ	Drainage of Right Axilla, Percutaneous Approach
0X9440Z	Drainage of Right Axilla with Drainage Device, Percutaneous Endoscopic Approach
0X944ZX	Drainage of Right Axilla, Percutaneous Endoscopic Approach, Diagnostic
0X944ZZ	Drainage of Right Axilla, Percutaneous Endoscopic Approach
0X9500Z	Drainage of Left Axilla with Drainage Device, Open Approach
0X950ZX	Drainage of Left Axilla, Open Approach, Diagnostic
0X950ZZ	Drainage of Left Axilla, Open Approach
0X9530Z	Drainage of Left Axilla with Drainage Device, Percutaneous Approach
0X953ZX	Drainage of Left Axilla, Percutaneous Approach, Diagnostic
0X953ZZ	Drainage of Left Axilla, Percutaneous Approach
0X9540Z	Drainage of Left Axilla with Drainage Device, Percutaneous Endoscopic Approach
0X954ZX	Drainage of Left Axilla, Percutaneous Endoscopic Approach, Diagnostic
0X954ZZ	Drainage of Left Axilla, Percutaneous Endoscopic Approach
0X9600Z	Drainage of Right Upper Extremity with Drainage Device, Open Approach
0X960ZX	Drainage of Right Upper Extremity, Open Approach, Diagnostic
0X960ZZ	Drainage of Right Upper Extremity, Open Approach
0X9630Z	Drainage of Right Upper Extremity with Drainage Device, Percutaneous Approach
0X963ZX	Drainage of Right Upper Extremity, Percutaneous Approach, Diagnostic
0X963ZZ	Drainage of Right Upper Extremity, Percutaneous Approach
0X9640Z	Drainage of Right Upper Extremity with Drainage Device, Percutaneous Endoscopic Approach
0X964ZX	Drainage of Right Upper Extremity, Percutaneous Endoscopic Approach, Diagnostic
0X964ZZ	Drainage of Right Upper Extremity, Percutaneous Endoscopic Approach
0X9700Z	Drainage of Left Upper Extremity with Drainage Device, Open Approach
0X970ZX	Drainage of Left Upper Extremity, Open Approach, Diagnostic
0X970ZZ	Drainage of Left Upper Extremity, Open Approach
0X9730Z	Drainage of Left Upper Extremity with Drainage Device, Percutaneous Approach
0X973ZX	Drainage of Left Upper Extremity, Percutaneous Approach, Diagnostic
0X973ZZ	Drainage of Left Upper Extremity, Percutaneous Approach
0X9740Z	Drainage of Left Upper Extremity with Drainage Device, Percutaneous Endoscopic Approach
0X974ZX	Drainage of Left Upper Extremity, Percutaneous Endoscopic Approach, Diagnostic
0X974ZZ	Drainage of Left Upper Extremity, Percutaneous Endoscopic Approach
0X9800Z	Drainage of Right Upper Arm with Drainage Device, Open Approach
0X980ZX	Drainage of Right Upper Arm, Open Approach, Diagnostic
0X980ZZ	Drainage of Right Upper Arm, Open Approach
0X9830Z	Drainage of Right Upper Arm with Drainage Device, Percutaneous Approach
0X983ZX	Drainage of Right Upper Arm, Percutaneous Approach, Diagnostic

♀ Female-only   ♂ Male-only   ▲ Limited Coverage   ● Non-OR   ▨ HAC-associated procedure   ▲ Non-covered procedures   ✚ Combinati

983ZZ Drainage of Right Upper Arm, Percutaneous Approach

9840Z Drainage of Right Upper Arm with Drainage Device, Percutaneous Endoscopic Approach

984ZX Drainage of Right Upper Arm, Percutaneous Endoscopic Approach, Diagnostic

984ZZ Drainage of Right Upper Arm, Percutaneous Endoscopic Approach

9900Z Drainage of Left Upper Arm with Drainage Device, Open Approach

990ZX Drainage of Left Upper Arm, Open Approach, Diagnostic

990ZZ Drainage of Left Upper Arm, Open Approach

9930Z Drainage of Left Upper Arm with Drainage Device, Percutaneous Approach

993ZX Drainage of Left Upper Arm, Percutaneous Approach, Diagnostic

993ZZ Drainage of Left Upper Arm, Percutaneous Approach

9940Z Drainage of Left Upper Arm with Drainage Device, Percutaneous Endoscopic Approach

994ZX Drainage of Left Upper Arm, Percutaneous Endoscopic Approach, Diagnostic

994ZZ Drainage of Left Upper Arm, Percutaneous Endoscopic Approach

9B00Z Drainage of Right Elbow Region with Drainage Device, Open Approach

9B0ZX Drainage of Right Elbow Region, Open Approach, Diagnostic

9B0ZZ Drainage of Right Elbow Region, Open Approach

9B30Z Drainage of Right Elbow Region with Drainage Device, Percutaneous Approach

9B3ZX Drainage of Right Elbow Region, Percutaneous Approach, Diagnostic

9B3ZZ Drainage of Right Elbow Region, Percutaneous Approach

9B40Z Drainage of Right Elbow Region with Drainage Device, Percutaneous Endoscopic Approach

9B4ZX Drainage of Right Elbow Region, Percutaneous Endoscopic Approach, Diagnostic

9B4ZZ Drainage of Right Elbow Region, Percutaneous Endoscopic Approach

9C00Z Drainage of Left Elbow Region with Drainage Device, Open Approach

9C0ZX Drainage of Left Elbow Region, Open Approach, Diagnostic

9C0ZZ Drainage of Left Elbow Region, Open Approach

9C30Z Drainage of Left Elbow Region with Drainage Device, Percutaneous Approach

9C3ZX Drainage of Left Elbow Region, Percutaneous Approach, Diagnostic

9C3ZZ Drainage of Left Elbow Region, Percutaneous Approach

0X9C40Z Drainage of Left Elbow Region with Drainage Device, Percutaneous Endoscopic Approach

0X9C4ZX Drainage of Left Elbow Region, Percutaneous Endoscopic Approach, Diagnostic

0X9C4ZZ Drainage of Left Elbow Region, Percutaneous Endoscopic Approach

0X9D00Z Drainage of Right Lower Arm with Drainage Device, Open Approach

0X9D0ZX Drainage of Right Lower Arm, Open Approach, Diagnostic

0X9D0ZZ Drainage of Right Lower Arm, Open Approach

0X9D30Z Drainage of Right Lower Arm with Drainage Device, Percutaneous Approach

0X9D3ZX Drainage of Right Lower Arm, Percutaneous Approach, Diagnostic

0X9D3ZZ Drainage of Right Lower Arm, Percutaneous Approach

0X9D40Z Drainage of Right Lower Arm with Drainage Device, Percutaneous Endoscopic Approach

0X9D4ZX Drainage of Right Lower Arm, Percutaneous Endoscopic Approach, Diagnostic

0X9D4ZZ Drainage of Right Lower Arm, Percutaneous Endoscopic Approach

0X9F00Z Drainage of Left Lower Arm with Drainage Device, Open Approach

0X9F0ZX Drainage of Left Lower Arm, Open Approach, Diagnostic

0X9F0ZZ Drainage of Left Lower Arm, Open Approach

0X9F30Z Drainage of Left Lower Arm with Drainage Device, Percutaneous Approach

0X9F3ZX Drainage of Left Lower Arm, Percutaneous Approach, Diagnostic

0X9F3ZZ Drainage of Left Lower Arm, Percutaneous Approach

0X9F40Z Drainage of Left Lower Arm with Drainage Device, Percutaneous Endoscopic Approach

0X9F4ZX Drainage of Left Lower Arm, Percutaneous Endoscopic Approach, Diagnostic

0X9F4ZZ Drainage of Left Lower Arm, Percutaneous Endoscopic Approach

0X9G00Z Drainage of Right Wrist Region with Drainage Device, Open Approach

0X9G0ZX Drainage of Right Wrist Region, Open Approach, Diagnostic

0X9G0ZZ Drainage of Right Wrist Region, Open Approach

0X9G30Z Drainage of Right Wrist Region with Drainage Device, Percutaneous Approach

0X9G3ZX Drainage of Right Wrist Region, Percutaneous Approach, Diagnostic

0X9G3ZZ Drainage of Right Wrist Region, Percutaneous Approach

0X9G40Z Drainage of Right Wrist Region with Drainage Device, Percutaneous Endoscopic Approach

0X9G4ZX Drainage of Right Wrist Region, Percutaneous Endoscopic Approach, Diagnostic

0X9G4ZZ Drainage of Right Wrist Region, Percutaneous Endoscopic Approach

0X9H00Z Drainage of Left Wrist Region with Drainage Device, Open Approach

0X9H0ZX Drainage of Left Wrist Region, Open Approach, Diagnostic

0X9H0ZZ Drainage of Left Wrist Region, Open Approach

0X9H30Z Drainage of Left Wrist Region with Drainage Device, Percutaneous Approach

0X9H3ZX Drainage of Left Wrist Region, Percutaneous Approach, Diagnostic

0X9H3ZZ Drainage of Left Wrist Region, Percutaneous Approach

0X9H40Z Drainage of Left Wrist Region with Drainage Device, Percutaneous Endoscopic Approach

0X9H4ZX Drainage of Left Wrist Region, Percutaneous Endoscopic Approach, Diagnostic

0X9H4ZZ Drainage of Left Wrist Region, Percutaneous Endoscopic Approach

0X9J00Z Drainage of Right Hand with Drainage Device, Open Approach

0X9J0ZX Drainage of Right Hand, Open Approach, Diagnostic

0X9J0ZZ Drainage of Right Hand, Open Approach

0X9J30Z Drainage of Right Hand with Drainage Device, Percutaneous Approach

0X9J3ZX Drainage of Right Hand, Percutaneous Approach, Diagnostic

0X9J3ZZ Drainage of Right Hand, Percutaneous Approach

0X9J40Z Drainage of Right Hand with Drainage Device, Percutaneous Endoscopic Approach

0X9J4ZX Drainage of Right Hand, Percutaneous Endoscopic Approach, Diagnostic

0X9J4ZZ Drainage of Right Hand, Percutaneous Endoscopic Approach

0X9K00Z Drainage of Left Hand with Drainage Device, Open Approach

0X9K0ZX Drainage of Left Hand, Open Approach, Diagnostic

0X9K0ZZ Drainage of Left Hand, Open Approach

0X9K30Z Drainage of Left Hand with Drainage Device, Percutaneous Approach

0X9K3ZX Drainage of Left Hand, Percutaneous Approach, Diagnostic

0X9K3ZZ Drainage of Left Hand, Percutaneous Approach

0X9K40Z Drainage of Left Hand with Drainage Device, Percutaneous Endoscopic Approach

0X9K4ZX Drainage of Left Hand, Percutaneous Endoscopic Approach, Diagnostic

0X9K4ZZ Drainage of Left Hand, Percutaneous Endoscopic Approach

XB – Anatomical Regions, Upper Extremities, Excision

Review Coding Guidelines B3.4a and B3.4b

0XB20ZX Excision of Right Shoulder Region, Open Approach, Diagnostic

0XB20ZZ Excision of Right Shoulder Region, Open Approach

0XB23ZX Excision of Right Shoulder Region, Percutaneous Approach, Diagnostic

0XB23ZZ Excision of Right Shoulder Region, Percutaneous Approach

0XB24ZX Excision of Right Shoulder Region, Percutaneous Endoscopic Approach, Diagnostic

0XB24ZZ Excision of Right Shoulder Region, Percutaneous Endoscopic Approach

0XB30ZX Excision of Left Shoulder Region, Open Approach, Diagnostic

0XB30ZZ Excision of Left Shoulder Region, Open Approach

0XB33ZX Excision of Left Shoulder Region, Percutaneous Approach, Diagnostic

0XB33ZZ Excision of Left Shoulder Region, Percutaneous Approach

0XB34ZX Excision of Left Shoulder Region, Percutaneous Endoscopic Approach, Diagnostic

0XB34ZZ Excision of Left Shoulder Region, Percutaneous Endoscopic Approach

♀ Female-only   ♂ Male-only   ▲ Limited Coverage   ● Non-OR   ▓ HAC-associated procedure   ▲ Non-covered procedures   ✚ Combination

0XB40ZX Excision of Right Axilla, Open Approach, Diagnostic

0XB40ZZ Excision of Right Axilla, Open Approach

0XB43ZX Excision of Right Axilla, Percutaneous Approach, Diagnostic

0XB43ZZ Excision of Right Axilla, Percutaneous Approach

0XB44ZX Excision of Right Axilla, Percutaneous Endoscopic Approach, Diagnostic

0XB44ZZ Excision of Right Axilla, Percutaneous Endoscopic Approach

0XB50ZX Excision of Left Axilla, Open Approach, Diagnostic

0XB50ZZ Excision of Left Axilla, Open Approach

0XB53ZX Excision of Left Axilla, Percutaneous Approach, Diagnostic

0XB53ZZ Excision of Left Axilla, Percutaneous Approach

0XB54ZX Excision of Left Axilla, Percutaneous Endoscopic Approach, Diagnostic

0XB54ZZ Excision of Left Axilla, Percutaneous Endoscopic Approach

0XB60ZX Excision of Right Upper Extremity, Open Approach, Diagnostic

0XB60ZZ Excision of Right Upper Extremity, Open Approach

0XB63ZX Excision of Right Upper Extremity, Percutaneous Approach, Diagnostic

0XB63ZZ Excision of Right Upper Extremity, Percutaneous Approach

0XB64ZX Excision of Right Upper Extremity, Percutaneous Endoscopic Approach, Diagnostic

0XB64ZZ Excision of Right Upper Extremity, Percutaneous Endoscopic Approach

0XB70ZX Excision of Left Upper Extremity, Open Approach, Diagnostic

0XB70ZZ Excision of Left Upper Extremity, Open Approach

0XB73ZX Excision of Left Upper Extremity, Percutaneous Approach, Diagnostic

0XB73ZZ Excision of Left Upper Extremity, Percutaneous Approach

0XB74ZX Excision of Left Upper Extremity, Percutaneous Endoscopic Approach, Diagnostic

0XB74ZZ Excision of Left Upper Extremity, Percutaneous Endoscopic Approach

0XB80ZX Excision of Right Upper Arm, Open Approach, Diagnostic

0XB80ZZ Excision of Right Upper Arm, Open Approach

0XB83ZX Excision of Right Upper Arm, Percutaneous Approach, Diagnostic

0XB83ZZ Excision of Right Upper Arm, Percutaneous Approach

0XB84ZX Excision of Right Upper Arm, Percutaneous Endoscopic Approach, Diagnostic

0XB84ZZ Excision of Right Upper Arm, Percutaneous Endoscopic Approach

0XB90ZX Excision of Left Upper Arm, Open Approach, Diagnostic

0XB90ZZ Excision of Left Upper Arm, Open Approach

0XB93ZX Excision of Left Upper Arm, Percutaneous Approach, Diagnostic

0XB93ZZ Excision of Left Upper Arm, Percutaneous Approach

0XB94ZX Excision of Left Upper Arm, Percutaneous Endoscopic Approach, Diagnostic

0XB94ZZ Excision of Left Upper Arm, Percutaneous Endoscopic Approach

0XBB0ZX Excision of Right Elbow Region, Open Approach, Diagnostic

0XBB0ZZ Excision of Right Elbow Region, Open Approach

0XBB3ZX Excision of Right Elbow Region, Percutaneous Approach, Diagnostic

0XBB3ZZ Excision of Right Elbow Region, Percutaneous Approach

0XBB4ZX Excision of Right Elbow Region, Percutaneous Endoscopic Approach, Diagnostic

0XBB4ZZ Excision of Right Elbow Region, Percutaneous Endoscopic Approach

0XBC0ZX Excision of Left Elbow Region, Open Approach, Diagnostic

0XBC0ZZ Excision of Left Elbow Region, Open Approach

0XBC3ZX Excision of Left Elbow Region, Percutaneous Approach, Diagnostic

0XBC3ZZ Excision of Left Elbow Region, Percutaneous Approach

0XBC4ZX Excision of Left Elbow Region, Percutaneous Endoscopic Approach, Diagnostic

0XBC4ZZ Excision of Left Elbow Region, Percutaneous Endoscopic Approach

0XBD0ZX Excision of Right Lower Arm, Open Approach, Diagnostic

0XBD0ZZ Excision of Right Lower Arm, Open Approach

0XBD3ZX Excision of Right Lower Arm, Percutaneous Approach, Diagnostic

0XBD3ZZ Excision of Right Lower Arm, Percutaneous Approach

0XBD4ZX Excision of Right Lower Arm, Percutaneous Endoscopic Approach, Diagnostic

0XBD4ZZ Excision of Right Lower Arm, Percutaneous Endoscopic Approach

0XBF0ZX Excision of Left Lower Arm, Open Approach, Diagnostic

0XBF0ZZ Excision of Left Lower Arm, Open Approach

0XBF3ZX Excision of Left Lower Arm, Percutane Approach, Diagnostic

0XBF3ZZ Excision of Left Lower Arm, Percutane Approach

0XBF4ZX Excision of Left Lower Arm, Percutane Endoscopic Approach, Diagnostic

0XBF4ZZ Excision of Left Lower Arm, Percutane Endoscopic Approach

0XBG0ZX Excision of Right Wrist Region, Open Approach, Diagnostic

0XBG0ZZ Excision of Right Wrist Region, Open Approach

0XBG3ZX Excision of Right Wrist Region, Percutaneous Approach, Diagnostic

0XBG3ZZ Excision of Right Wrist Region, Percutaneous Approach

0XBG4ZX Excision of Right Wrist Region, Percutaneous Endoscopic Approach, Diagnostic

0XBG4ZZ Excision of Right Wrist Region, Percutaneous Endoscopic Approach

0XBH0ZX Excision of Left Wrist Region, Open Approach, Diagnostic

0XBH0ZZ Excision of Left Wrist Region, Open Approach

0XBH3ZX Excision of Left Wrist Region, Percutaneous Approach, Diagnostic

0XBH3ZZ Excision of Left Wrist Region, Percutaneous Approach

0XBH4ZX Excision of Left Wrist Region, Percutaneous Endoscopic Approach, Diagnostic

0XBH4ZZ Excision of Left Wrist Region, Percutaneous Endoscopic Approach

0XBJ0ZX Excision of Right Hand, Open Approach Diagnostic

0XBJ0ZZ Excision of Right Hand, Open Approach

0XBJ3ZX Excision of Right Hand, Percutaneous Approach, Diagnostic

0XBJ3ZZ Excision of Right Hand, Percutaneous Approach

0XBJ4ZX Excision of Right Hand, Percutaneous Endoscopic Approach, Diagnostic

0XBJ4ZZ Excision of Right Hand, Percutaneous Endoscopic Approach

0XBK0ZX Excision of Left Hand, Open Approach, Diagnostic

0XBK0ZZ Excision of Left Hand, Open Approach

0XBK3ZX Excision of Left Hand, Percutaneous Approach, Diagnostic

0XBK3ZZ Excision of Left Hand, Percutaneous Approach

0XBK4ZX Excision of Left Hand, Percutaneous Endoscopic Approach, Diagnostic

0XBK4ZZ Excision of Left Hand, Percutaneous Endoscopic Approach

0XH – Anatomical Regions, Upper Extremities, Insertion

0XH201Z Insertion of Radioactive Element into Right Shoulder Region, Open Approach

● 0XH203Z Insertion of Infusion Device into Right Shoulder Region, Open Approach

● 0XH20YZ Insertion of Other Device into Right Shoulder Region, Open Approach

0XH231Z Insertion of Radioactive Element into Right Shoulder Region, Percutaneous Approach

● 0XH233Z Insertion of Infusion Device into Right Shoulder Region, Percutaneous Approach

● 0XH23YZ Insertion of Other Device into Right Shoulder Region, Percutaneous Approach

0XH241Z Insertion of Radioactive Element into Right Shoulder Region, Percutaneous Endoscopic Approach

● 0XH243Z Insertion of Infusion Device into Right Shoulder Region, Percutaneous Endoscopic Approach

● 0XH24YZ Insertion of Other Device into Right Shoulder Region, Percutaneous Endoscopic Approach

0XH301Z Insertion of Radioactive Element into Left Shoulder Region, Open Approach

● 0XH303Z Insertion of Infusion Device into Left Shoulder Region, Open Approach

● 0XH30YZ Insertion of Other Device into Left Shoulder Region, Open Approach

0XH331Z Insertion of Radioactive Element into Left Shoulder Region, Percutaneous Approach

● 0XH333Z Insertion of Infusion Device into Left Shoulder Region, Percutaneous Approach

● 0XH33YZ Insertion of Other Device into Left Shoulder Region, Percutaneous Approach

0XH341Z Insertion of Radioactive Element into Left Shoulder Region, Percutaneous Endoscopic Approach

● 0XH343Z Insertion of Infusion Device into Left Shoulder Region, Percutaneous Endoscopic Approach

● 0XH34YZ Insertion of Other Device into Left Shoulder Region, Percutaneous Endoscopic Approach

0XH401Z Insertion of Radioactive Element into Right Axilla, Open Approach

● 0XH403Z Insertion of Infusion Device into Right Axilla, Open Approach

XH40YZ Insertion of Other Device into Right Axilla, Open Approach

H431Z Insertion of Radioactive Element into Right Axilla, Percutaneous Approach

XH433Z Insertion of Infusion Device into Right Axilla, Percutaneous Approach

XH43YZ Insertion of Other Device into Right Axilla, Percutaneous Approach

H441Z Insertion of Radioactive Element into Right Axilla, Percutaneous Endoscopic Approach

XH443Z Insertion of Infusion Device into Right Axilla, Percutaneous Endoscopic Approach

XH44YZ Insertion of Other Device into Right Axilla, Percutaneous Endoscopic Approach

H501Z Insertion of Radioactive Element into Left Axilla, Open Approach

XH503Z Insertion of Infusion Device into Left Axilla, Open Approach

XH50YZ Insertion of Other Device into Left Axilla, Open Approach

H531Z Insertion of Radioactive Element into Left Axilla, Percutaneous Approach

XH533Z Insertion of Infusion Device into Left Axilla, Percutaneous Approach

XH53YZ Insertion of Other Device into Left Axilla, Percutaneous Approach

H541Z Insertion of Radioactive Element into Left Axilla, Percutaneous Endoscopic Approach

XH543Z Insertion of Infusion Device into Left Axilla, Percutaneous Endoscopic Approach

XH54YZ Insertion of Other Device into Left Axilla, Percutaneous Endoscopic Approach

XH601Z Insertion of Radioactive Element into Right Upper Extremity, Open Approach

XH603Z Insertion of Infusion Device into Right Upper Extremity, Open Approach

XH60YZ Insertion of Other Device into Right Upper Extremity, Open Approach

XH631Z Insertion of Radioactive Element into Right Upper Extremity, Percutaneous Approach

XH633Z Insertion of Infusion Device into Right Upper Extremity, Percutaneous Approach

XH63YZ Insertion of Other Device into Right Upper Extremity, Percutaneous Approach

XH641Z Insertion of Radioactive Element into Right Upper Extremity, Percutaneous Endoscopic Approach

XH643Z Insertion of Infusion Device into Right Upper Extremity, Percutaneous Endoscopic Approach

XH64YZ Insertion of Other Device into Right Upper Extremity, Percutaneous Endoscopic Approach

XH701Z Insertion of Radioactive Element into Left Upper Extremity, Open Approach

XH703Z Insertion of Infusion Device into Left Upper Extremity, Open Approach

XH70YZ Insertion of Other Device into Left Upper Extremity, Open Approach

XH731Z Insertion of Radioactive Element into Left Upper Extremity, Percutaneous Approach

XH733Z Insertion of Infusion Device into Left Upper Extremity, Percutaneous Approach

XH73YZ Insertion of Other Device into Left Upper Extremity, Percutaneous Approach

XH741Z Insertion of Radioactive Element into Left Upper Extremity, Percutaneous Endoscopic Approach

XH743Z Insertion of Infusion Device into Left Upper Extremity, Percutaneous Endoscopic Approach

XH74YZ Insertion of Other Device into Left Upper Extremity, Percutaneous Endoscopic Approach

0XH801Z Insertion of Radioactive Element into Right Upper Arm, Open Approach

● 0XH803Z Insertion of Infusion Device into Right Upper Arm, Open Approach

● 0XH80YZ Insertion of Other Device into Right Upper Arm, Open Approach

0XH831Z Insertion of Radioactive Element into Right Upper Arm, Percutaneous Approach

● 0XH833Z Insertion of Infusion Device into Right Upper Arm, Percutaneous Approach

● 0XH83YZ Insertion of Other Device into Right Upper Arm, Percutaneous Approach

0XH841Z Insertion of Radioactive Element into Right Upper Arm, Percutaneous Endoscopic Approach

● 0XH843Z Insertion of Infusion Device into Right Upper Arm, Percutaneous Endoscopic Approach

● 0XH84YZ Insertion of Other Device into Right Upper Arm, Percutaneous Endoscopic Approach

0XH901Z Insertion of Radioactive Element into Left Upper Arm, Open Approach

● 0XH903Z Insertion of Infusion Device into Left Upper Arm, Open Approach

● 0XH90YZ Insertion of Other Device into Left Upper Arm, Open Approach

0XH931Z Insertion of Radioactive Element into Left Upper Arm, Percutaneous Approach

● 0XH933Z Insertion of Infusion Device into Left Upper Arm, Percutaneous Approach

● 0XH93YZ Insertion of Other Device into Left Upper Arm, Percutaneous Approach

0XH941Z Insertion of Radioactive Element into Left Upper Arm, Percutaneous Endoscopic Approach

● 0XH943Z Insertion of Infusion Device into Left Upper Arm, Percutaneous Endoscopic Approach

● 0XH94YZ Insertion of Other Device into Left Upper Arm, Percutaneous Endoscopic Approach

0XHB01Z Insertion of Radioactive Element into Right Elbow Region, Open Approach

● 0XHB03Z Insertion of Infusion Device into Right Elbow Region, Open Approach

● 0XHB0YZ Insertion of Other Device into Right Elbow Region, Open Approach

0XHB31Z Insertion of Radioactive Element into Right Elbow Region, Percutaneous Approach

● 0XHB33Z Insertion of Infusion Device into Right Elbow Region, Percutaneous Approach

● 0XHB3YZ Insertion of Other Device into Right Elbow Region, Percutaneous Approach

0XHB41Z Insertion of Radioactive Element into Right Elbow Region, Percutaneous Endoscopic Approach

● 0XHB43Z Insertion of Infusion Device into Right Elbow Region, Percutaneous Endoscopic Approach

● 0XHB4YZ Insertion of Other Device into Right Elbow Region, Percutaneous Endoscopic Approach

0XHC01Z Insertion of Radioactive Element into Left Elbow Region, Open Approach

● 0XHC03Z Insertion of Infusion Device into Left Elbow Region, Open Approach

● 0XHC0YZ Insertion of Other Device into Left Elbow Region, Open Approach

0XHC31Z Insertion of Radioactive Element into Left Elbow Region, Percutaneous Approach

● 0XHC33Z Insertion of Infusion Device into Left Elbow Region, Percutaneous Approach

● 0XHC3YZ Insertion of Other Device into Left Elbow Region, Percutaneous Approach

0XHC41Z Insertion of Radioactive Element into Left Elbow Region, Percutaneous Endoscopic Approach

● 0XHC43Z Insertion of Infusion Device into Left Elbow Region, Percutaneous Endoscopic Approach

● 0XHC4YZ Insertion of Other Device into Left Elbow Region, Percutaneous Endoscopic Approach

0XHD01Z Insertion of Radioactive Element into Right Lower Arm, Open Approach

● 0XHD03Z Insertion of Infusion Device into Right Lower Arm, Open Approach

● 0XHD0YZ Insertion of Other Device into Right Lower Arm, Open Approach

0XHD31Z Insertion of Radioactive Element into Right Lower Arm, Percutaneous Approach

● 0XHD33Z Insertion of Infusion Device into Right Lower Arm, Percutaneous Approach

● 0XHD3YZ Insertion of Other Device into Right Lower Arm, Percutaneous Approach

0XHD41Z Insertion of Radioactive Element into Right Lower Arm, Percutaneous Endoscopic Approach

● 0XHD43Z Insertion of Infusion Device into Right Lower Arm, Percutaneous Endoscopic Approach

● 0XHD4YZ Insertion of Other Device into Right Lower Arm, Percutaneous Endoscopic Approach

0XHF01Z Insertion of Radioactive Element into Left Lower Arm, Open Approach

● 0XHF03Z Insertion of Infusion Device into Left Lower Arm, Open Approach

● 0XHF0YZ Insertion of Other Device into Left Lower Arm, Open Approach

0XHF31Z Insertion of Radioactive Element into Left Lower Arm, Percutaneous Approach

● 0XHF33Z Insertion of Infusion Device into Left Lower Arm, Percutaneous Approach

● 0XHF3YZ Insertion of Other Device into Left Lower Arm, Percutaneous Approach

0XHF41Z Insertion of Radioactive Element into Left Lower Arm, Percutaneous Endoscopic Approach

● 0XHF43Z Insertion of Infusion Device into Left Lower Arm, Percutaneous Endoscopic Approach

● 0XHF4YZ Insertion of Other Device into Left Lower Arm, Percutaneous Endoscopic Approach

0XHG01Z Insertion of Radioactive Element into Right Wrist Region, Open Approach

● 0XHG03Z Insertion of Infusion Device into Right Wrist Region, Open Approach

● 0XHG0YZ Insertion of Other Device into Right Wrist Region, Open Approach

0XHG31Z Insertion of Radioactive Element into Right Wrist Region, Percutaneous Approach

● 0XHG33Z Insertion of Infusion Device into Right Wrist Region, Percutaneous Approach

● 0XHG3YZ Insertion of Other Device into Right Wrist Region, Percutaneous Approach

0XHG41Z Insertion of Radioactive Element into Right Wrist Region, Percutaneous Endoscopic Approach

● 0XHG43Z Insertion of Infusion Device into Right Wrist Region, Percutaneous Endoscopic Approach

● 0XHG4YZ Insertion of Other Device into Right Wrist Region, Percutaneous Endoscopic Approach

0XHH01Z Insertion of Radioactive Element into Left Wrist Region, Open Approach

● 0XHH03Z Insertion of Infusion Device into Left Wrist Region, Open Approach

● 0XHH0YZ Insertion of Other Device into Left Wrist Region, Open Approach

0XHH31Z Insertion of Radioactive Element into Left Wrist Region, Percutaneous Approach

Female-only   ♂ Male-only   ▲ Limited Coverage   ● Non-OR   ▨ HAC-associated procedure   ▲ Non-covered procedures   ✚ Combination

● **0XHH33Z** Insertion of Infusion Device into Left Wrist Region, Percutaneous Approach

● **0XHH3YZ** Insertion of Other Device into Left Wrist Region, Percutaneous Approach

0XHH41Z Insertion of Radioactive Element into Left Wrist Region, Percutaneous Endoscopic Approach

● **0XHH43Z** Insertion of Infusion Device into Left Wrist Region, Percutaneous Endoscopic Approach

● **0XHH4YZ** Insertion of Other Device into Left Wrist Region, Percutaneous Endoscopic Approach

0XHJ01Z Insertion of Radioactive Element into Right Hand, Open Approach

● **0XHJ03Z** Insertion of Infusion Device into Right Hand, Open Approach

● **0XHJ0YZ** Insertion of Other Device into Right Hand, Open Approach

0XHJ31Z Insertion of Radioactive Element into Right Hand, Percutaneous Approach

● **0XHJ33Z** Insertion of Infusion Device into Right Hand, Percutaneous Approach

● **0XHJ3YZ** Insertion of Other Device into Right Hand, Percutaneous Approach

0XHJ41Z Insertion of Radioactive Element into Right Hand, Percutaneous Endoscopic Approach

● **0XHJ43Z** Insertion of Infusion Device into Right Hand, Percutaneous Endoscopic Approach

● **0XHJ4YZ** Insertion of Other Device into Right Hand, Percutaneous Endoscopic Approach

0XHK01Z Insertion of Radioactive Element into Left Hand, Open Approach

● **0XHK03Z** Insertion of Infusion Device into Left Hand, Open Approach

● **0XHK0YZ** Insertion of Other Device into Left Hand, Open Approach

0XHK31Z Insertion of Radioactive Element into Left Hand, Percutaneous Approach

● **0XHK33Z** Insertion of Infusion Device into Left Hand, Percutaneous Approach

● **0XHK3YZ** Insertion of Other Device into Left Hand, Percutaneous Approach

● **0XHK41Z** Insertion of Radioactive Element into Left Hand, Percutaneous Endoscopic Approach

● **0XHK43Z** Insertion of Infusion Device into Left Hand, Percutaneous Endoscopic Approach

● **0XHK4YZ** Insertion of Other Device into Left Hand, Percutaneous Endoscopic Approach

0XJ – Anatomical Regions, Upper Extremities, Inspection

Review Coding Guidelines B3.11a, B3.11b and B3.11c

● **0XJ20ZZ** Inspection of Right Shoulder Region, Open Approach

0XJ23ZZ Inspection of Right Shoulder Region, Percutaneous Approach

0XJ24ZZ Inspection of Right Shoulder Region, Percutaneous Endoscopic Approach

0XJ2XZZ Inspection of Right Shoulder Region, External Approach

● **0XJ30ZZ** Inspection of Left Shoulder Region, Open Approach

0XJ33ZZ Inspection of Left Shoulder Region, Percutaneous Approach

0XJ34ZZ Inspection of Left Shoulder Region, Percutaneous Endoscopic Approach

0XJ3XZZ Inspection of Left Shoulder Region, External Approach

● **0XJ40ZZ** Inspection of Right Axilla, Open Approach

0XJ43ZZ Inspection of Right Axilla, Percutaneous Approach

0XJ44ZZ Inspection of Right Axilla, Percutaneous Endoscopic Approach

0XJ4XZZ Inspection of Right Axilla, External Approach

● **0XJ50ZZ** Inspection of Left Axilla, Open Approach

0XJ53ZZ Inspection of Left Axilla, Percutaneous Approach

0XJ54ZZ Inspection of Left Axilla, Percutaneous Endoscopic Approach

0XJ5XZZ Inspection of Left Axilla, External Approach

● **0XJ60ZZ** Inspection of Right Upper Extremity, Open Approach

0XJ63ZZ Inspection of Right Upper Extremity, Percutaneous Approach

0XJ64ZZ Inspection of Right Upper Extremity, Percutaneous Endoscopic Approach

0XJ6XZZ Inspection of Right Upper Extremity, External Approach

● **0XJ70ZZ** Inspection of Left Upper Extremity, Open Approach

0XJ73ZZ Inspection of Left Upper Extremity, Percutaneous Approach

0XJ74ZZ Inspection of Left Upper Extremity, Percutaneous Endoscopic Approach

0XJ7XZZ Inspection of Left Upper Extremity, External Approach

● **0XJ80ZZ** Inspection of Right Upper Arm, Open Approach

0XJ83ZZ Inspection of Right Upper Arm, Percutaneous Approach

0XJ84ZZ Inspection of Right Upper Arm, Percutaneous Endoscopic Approach

0XJ8XZZ Inspection of Right Upper Arm, External Approach

● **0XJ90ZZ** Inspection of Left Upper Arm, Open Approach

0XJ93ZZ Inspection of Left Upper Arm, Percutaneous Approach

0XJ94ZZ Inspection of Left Upper Arm, Percutaneous Endoscopic Approach

0XJ9XZZ Inspection of Left Upper Arm, External Approach

● **0XJB0ZZ** Inspection of Right Elbow Region, Open Approach

0XJB3ZZ Inspection of Right Elbow Region, Percutaneous Approach

0XJB4ZZ Inspection of Right Elbow Region, Percutaneous Endoscopic Approach

0XJBXZZ Inspection of Right Elbow Region, External Approach

● **0XJC0ZZ** Inspection of Left Elbow Region, Open Approach

0XJC3ZZ Inspection of Left Elbow Region, Percutaneous Approach

0XJC4ZZ Inspection of Left Elbow Region, Percutaneous Endoscopic Approach

0XJCXZZ Inspection of Left Elbow Region, External Approach

● **0XJD0ZZ** Inspection of Right Lower Arm, Open Approach

0XJD3ZZ Inspection of Right Lower Arm, Percutaneous Approach

0XJD4ZZ Inspection of Right Lower Arm, Percutaneous Endoscopic Approach

0XJDXZZ Inspection of Right Lower Arm, External Approach

● **0XJF0ZZ** Inspection of Left Lower Arm, Open Approach

0XJF3ZZ Inspection of Left Lower Arm, Percutaneous Approach

0XJF4ZZ Inspection of Left Lower Arm, Percutaneous Endoscopic Approach

0XJFXZZ Inspection of Left Lower Arm, External Approach

● **0XJG0ZZ** Inspection of Right Wrist Region, Open Approach

0XJG3ZZ Inspection of Right Wrist Region, Percutaneous Approach

0XJG4ZZ Inspection of Right Wrist Region, Percutaneous Endoscopic Approach

0XJGXZZ Inspection of Right Wrist Region, External Approach

● **0XJH0ZZ** Inspection of Left Wrist Region, Open Approach

0XJH3ZZ Inspection of Left Wrist Region, Percutaneous Approach

0XJH4ZZ Inspection of Left Wrist Region, Percutaneous Endoscopic Approach

0XJHXZZ Inspection of Left Wrist Region, External Approach

● **0XJJ0ZZ** Inspection of Right Hand, Open Approach

0XJJ3ZZ Inspection of Right Hand, Percutaneous Approach

0XJJ4ZZ Inspection of Right Hand, Percutaneous Endoscopic Approach

0XJJXZZ Inspection of Right Hand, External Approach

● **0XJK0ZZ** Inspection of Left Hand, Open Approach

0XJK3ZZ Inspection of Left Hand, Percutaneous Approach

0XJK4ZZ Inspection of Left Hand, Percutaneous Endoscopic Approach

0XJKXZZ Inspection of Left Hand, External Approach

0XM – Anatomical Regions, Upper Extremities, Reattachment

0XM00ZZ Reattachment of Right Forequarter, Open Approach

0XM10ZZ Reattachment of Left Forequarter, Open Approach

0XM20ZZ Reattachment of Right Shoulder Region, Open Approach

0XM30ZZ Reattachment of Left Shoulder Region, Open Approach

0XM40ZZ Reattachment of Right Axilla, Open Approach

0XM50ZZ Reattachment of Left Axilla, Open Approach

0XM60ZZ Reattachment of Right Upper Extremity, Open Approach

0XM70ZZ Reattachment of Left Upper Extremity, Open Approach

0XM80ZZ Reattachment of Right Upper Arm, Open Approach

0XM90ZZ Reattachment of Left Upper Arm, Open Approach

0XMB0ZZ Reattachment of Right Elbow Region, Open Approach

0XMC0ZZ Reattachment of Left Elbow Region, Open Approach

0XMD0ZZ Reattachment of Right Lower Arm, Open Approach

0XMF0ZZ Reattachment of Left Lower Arm, Open Approach

0XMG0ZZ Reattachment of Right Wrist Region, Open Approach

MH0ZZ	Reattachment of Left Wrist Region, Open Approach	0XMN0ZZ	Reattachment of Right Index Finger, Open Approach	0XMS0ZZ	Reattachment of Right Ring Finger, Open Approach
MJ0ZZ	Reattachment of Right Hand, Open Approach	0XMP0ZZ	Reattachment of Left Index Finger, Open Approach	0XMT0ZZ	Reattachment of Left Ring Finger, Open Approach
MK0ZZ	Reattachment of Left Hand, Open Approach	0XMQ0ZZ	Reattachment of Right Middle Finger, Open Approach	0XMV0ZZ	Reattachment of Right Little Finger, Open Approach
ML0ZZ	Reattachment of Right Thumb, Open Approach	0XMR0ZZ	Reattachment of Left Middle Finger, Open Approach	0XMW0ZZ	Reattachment of Left Little Finger, Open Approach
MM0ZZ	Reattachment of Left Thumb, Open Approach				

XP – Anatomical Regions, Upper Extremities, Removal

view Coding Guideline B6.1c

P600Z	Removal of Drainage Device from Right Upper Extremity, Open Approach	0XP64JZ	Removal of Synthetic Substitute from Right Upper Extremity, Percutaneous Endoscopic Approach	0XP737Z	Removal of Autologous Tissue Substitute from Left Upper Extremity, Percutaneous Approach
P601Z	Removal of Radioactive Element from Right Upper Extremity, Open Approach	0XP64KZ	Removal of Nonautologous Tissue Substitute from Right Upper Extremity, Percutaneous Endoscopic Approach	0XP73JZ	Removal of Synthetic Substitute from Left Upper Extremity, Percutaneous Approach
P603Z	Removal of Infusion Device from Right Upper Extremity, Open Approach	0XP64YZ	Removal of Other Device from Right Upper Extremity, Percutaneous Endoscopic Approach	0XP73KZ	Removal of Nonautologous Tissue Substitute from Left Upper Extremity, Percutaneous Approach
P607Z	Removal of Autologous Tissue Substitute from Right Upper Extremity, Open Approach	0XP6X0Z	Removal of Drainage Device from Right Upper Extremity, External Approach	0XP73YZ	Removal of Other Device from Left Upper Extremity, Percutaneous Approach
P60JZ	Removal of Synthetic Substitute from Right Upper Extremity, Open Approach	0XP6X1Z	Removal of Radioactive Element from Right Upper Extremity, External Approach	0XP740Z	Removal of Drainage Device from Left Upper Extremity, Percutaneous Endoscopic Approach
P60KZ	Removal of Nonautologous Tissue Substitute from Right Upper Extremity, Open Approach	0XP6X3Z	Removal of Infusion Device from Right Upper Extremity, External Approach	0XP741Z	Removal of Radioactive Element from Left Upper Extremity, Percutaneous Endoscopic Approach
P60YZ	Removal of Other Device from Right Upper Extremity, Open Approach	0XP6X7Z	Removal of Autologous Tissue Substitute from Right Upper Extremity, External Approach	0XP743Z	Removal of Infusion Device from Left Upper Extremity, Percutaneous Endoscopic Approach
P630Z	Removal of Drainage Device from Right Upper Extremity, Percutaneous Approach	0XP6XJZ	Removal of Synthetic Substitute from Right Upper Extremity, External Approach	0XP747Z	Removal of Autologous Tissue Substitute from Left Upper Extremity, Percutaneous Endoscopic Approach
P631Z	Removal of Radioactive Element from Right Upper Extremity, Percutaneous Approach	0XP6XKZ	Removal of Nonautologous Tissue Substitute from Right Upper Extremity, External Approach	0XP74JZ	Removal of Synthetic Substitute from Left Upper Extremity, Percutaneous Endoscopic Approach
P633Z	Removal of Infusion Device from Right Upper Extremity, Percutaneous Approach	0XP6XYZ	Removal of Other Device from Right Upper Extremity, External Approach	0XP74KZ	Removal of Nonautologous Tissue Substitute from Left Upper Extremity, Percutaneous Endoscopic Approach
P637Z	Removal of Autologous Tissue Substitute from Right Upper Extremity, Percutaneous Approach	0XP700Z	Removal of Drainage Device from Left Upper Extremity, Open Approach	0XP74YZ	Removal of Other Device from Left Upper Extremity, Percutaneous Endoscopic Approach
P63JZ	Removal of Synthetic Substitute from Right Upper Extremity, Percutaneous Approach	0XP701Z	Removal of Radioactive Element from Left Upper Extremity, Open Approach	0XP7X0Z	Removal of Drainage Device from Left Upper Extremity, External Approach
P63KZ	Removal of Nonautologous Tissue Substitute from Right Upper Extremity, Percutaneous Approach	0XP703Z	Removal of Infusion Device from Left Upper Extremity, Open Approach	0XP7X1Z	Removal of Radioactive Element from Left Upper Extremity, External Approach
P63YZ	Removal of Other Device from Right Upper Extremity, Percutaneous Approach	0XP707Z	Removal of Autologous Tissue Substitute from Left Upper Extremity, Open Approach	0XP7X3Z	Removal of Infusion Device from Left Upper Extremity, External Approach
P640Z	Removal of Drainage Device from Right Upper Extremity, Percutaneous Endoscopic Approach	0XP70JZ	Removal of Synthetic Substitute from Left Upper Extremity, Open Approach	0XP7X7Z	Removal of Autologous Tissue Substitute from Left Upper Extremity, External Approach
P641Z	Removal of Radioactive Element from Right Upper Extremity, Percutaneous Endoscopic Approach	0XP70KZ	Removal of Nonautologous Tissue Substitute from Left Upper Extremity, Open Approach	0XP7XJZ	Removal of Synthetic Substitute from Left Upper Extremity, External Approach
P643Z	Removal of Infusion Device from Right Upper Extremity, Percutaneous Endoscopic Approach	0XP70YZ	Removal of Other Device from Left Upper Extremity, Open Approach	0XP7XKZ	Removal of Nonautologous Tissue Substitute from Left Upper Extremity, External Approach
P647Z	Removal of Autologous Tissue Substitute from Right Upper Extremity, Percutaneous Endoscopic Approach	0XP730Z	Removal of Drainage Device from Left Upper Extremity, Percutaneous Approach	0XP7XYZ	Removal of Other Device from Left Upper Extremity, External Approach
		0XP731Z	Removal of Radioactive Element from Left Upper Extremity, Percutaneous Approach		
		0XP733Z	Removal of Infusion Device from Left Upper Extremity, Percutaneous Approach		

XQ – Anatomical Regions, Upper Extremities, Repair

XQ20ZZ	Repair Right Shoulder Region, Open Approach	0XQ33ZZ	Repair Left Shoulder Region, Percutaneous Approach	0XQ4XZZ	Repair Right Axilla, External Approach
XQ23ZZ	Repair Right Shoulder Region, Percutaneous Approach	0XQ34ZZ	Repair Left Shoulder Region, Percutaneous Endoscopic Approach	0XQ50ZZ	Repair Left Axilla, Open Approach
XQ24ZZ	Repair Right Shoulder Region, Percutaneous Endoscopic Approach	0XQ3XZZ	Repair Left Shoulder Region, External Approach	0XQ53ZZ	Repair Left Axilla, Percutaneous Approach
XQ2XZZ	Repair Right Shoulder Region, External Approach	0XQ40ZZ	Repair Right Axilla, Open Approach	0XQ54ZZ	Repair Left Axilla, Percutaneous Endoscopic Approach
XQ30ZZ	Repair Left Shoulder Region, Open Approach	0XQ43ZZ	Repair Right Axilla, Percutaneous Approach	0XQ5XZZ	Repair Left Axilla, External Approach
		0XQ44ZZ	Repair Right Axilla, Percutaneous Endoscopic Approach	0XQ60ZZ	Repair Right Upper Extremity, Open Approach
				0XQ63ZZ	Repair Right Upper Extremity, Percutaneous Approach

Female-only   ♂ Male-only   ▲ Limited Coverage   ● Non-OR   ▥ HAC-associated procedure   ▲ Non-covered procedures   ✚ Combination

0XQ64ZZ	Repair Right Upper Extremity, Percutaneous Endoscopic Approach
0XQ6XZZ	Repair Right Upper Extremity, External Approach
0XQ70ZZ	Repair Left Upper Extremity, Open Approach
0XQ73ZZ	Repair Left Upper Extremity, Percutaneous Approach
0XQ74ZZ	Repair Left Upper Extremity, Percutaneous Endoscopic Approach
0XQ7XZZ	Repair Left Upper Extremity, External Approach
0XQ80ZZ	Repair Right Upper Arm, Open Approach
0XQ83ZZ	Repair Right Upper Arm, Percutaneous Approach
0XQ84ZZ	Repair Right Upper Arm, Percutaneous Endoscopic Approach
0XQ8XZZ	Repair Right Upper Arm, External Approach
0XQ90ZZ	Repair Left Upper Arm, Open Approach
0XQ93ZZ	Repair Left Upper Arm, Percutaneous Approach
0XQ94ZZ	Repair Left Upper Arm, Percutaneous Endoscopic Approach
0XQ9XZZ	Repair Left Upper Arm, External Approach
0XQB0ZZ	Repair Right Elbow Region, Open Approach
0XQB3ZZ	Repair Right Elbow Region, Percutaneous Approach
0XQB4ZZ	Repair Right Elbow Region, Percutaneous Endoscopic Approach
0XQBXZZ	Repair Right Elbow Region, External Approach
0XQC0ZZ	Repair Left Elbow Region, Open Approach
0XQC3ZZ	Repair Left Elbow Region, Percutaneous Approach
0XQC4ZZ	Repair Left Elbow Region, Percutaneous Endoscopic Approach
0XQCXZZ	Repair Left Elbow Region, External Approach
0XQD0ZZ	Repair Right Lower Arm, Open Approach
0XQD3ZZ	Repair Right Lower Arm, Percutaneous Approach
0XQD4ZZ	Repair Right Lower Arm, Percutaneous Endoscopic Approach
0XQDXZZ	Repair Right Lower Arm, External Approach
0XQF0ZZ	Repair Left Lower Arm, Open Approach
0XQF3ZZ	Repair Left Lower Arm, Percutaneous Approach
0XQF4ZZ	Repair Left Lower Arm, Percutaneous Endoscopic Approach
0XQFXZZ	Repair Left Lower Arm, External Approach
0XQG0ZZ	Repair Right Wrist Region, Open Approach
0XQG3ZZ	Repair Right Wrist Region, Percutaneous Approach
0XQG4ZZ	Repair Right Wrist Region, Percutaneous Endoscopic Approach
0XQGXZZ	Repair Right Wrist Region, External Approach
0XQH0ZZ	Repair Left Wrist Region, Open Approach
0XQH3ZZ	Repair Left Wrist Region, Percutaneous Approach
0XQH4ZZ	Repair Left Wrist Region, Percutaneous Endoscopic Approach
0XQHXZZ	Repair Left Wrist Region, External Approach
0XQJ0ZZ	Repair Right Hand, Open Approach
0XQJ3ZZ	Repair Right Hand, Percutaneous Approach
0XQJ4ZZ	Repair Right Hand, Percutaneous Endoscopic Approach
0XQJXZZ	Repair Right Hand, External Approach
0XQK0ZZ	Repair Left Hand, Open Approach
0XQK3ZZ	Repair Left Hand, Percutaneous Approach
0XQK4ZZ	Repair Left Hand, Percutaneous Endoscopic Approach
0XQKXZZ	Repair Left Hand, External Approach
0XQL0ZZ	Repair Right Thumb, Open Approach
0XQL3ZZ	Repair Right Thumb, Percutaneous Approach
0XQL4ZZ	Repair Right Thumb, Percutaneous Endoscopic Approach
0XQLXZZ	Repair Right Thumb, External Approach
0XQM0ZZ	Repair Left Thumb, Open Approach
0XQM3ZZ	Repair Left Thumb, Percutaneous Approach
0XQM4ZZ	Repair Left Thumb, Percutaneous Endoscopic Approach
0XQMXZZ	Repair Left Thumb, External Approach
0XQN0ZZ	Repair Right Index Finger, Open Approach
0XQN3ZZ	Repair Right Index Finger, Percutaneous Approach
0XQN4ZZ	Repair Right Index Finger, Percutaneous Endoscopic Approach
0XQNXZZ	Repair Right Index Finger, External Approach
0XQP0ZZ	Repair Left Index Finger, Open Approach
0XQP3ZZ	Repair Left Index Finger, Percutaneous Approach
0XQP4ZZ	Repair Left Index Finger, Percutaneous Endoscopic Approach
0XQPXZZ	Repair Left Index Finger, External Approach
0XQQ0ZZ	Repair Right Middle Finger, Open Approach
0XQQ3ZZ	Repair Right Middle Finger, Percutaneous Approach
0XQQ4ZZ	Repair Right Middle Finger, Percutaneous Endoscopic Approach
0XQQXZZ	Repair Right Middle Finger, External Approach
0XQR0ZZ	Repair Left Middle Finger, Open Approach
0XQR3ZZ	Repair Left Middle Finger, Percutaneous Approach
0XQR4ZZ	Repair Left Middle Finger, Percutaneous Endoscopic Approach
0XQRXZZ	Repair Left Middle Finger, External Approach
0XQS0ZZ	Repair Right Ring Finger, Open Approach
0XQS3ZZ	Repair Right Ring Finger, Percutaneous Approach
0XQS4ZZ	Repair Right Ring Finger, Percutaneous Endoscopic Approach
0XQSXZZ	Repair Right Ring Finger, External Approach
0XQT0ZZ	Repair Left Ring Finger, Open Approach
0XQT3ZZ	Repair Left Ring Finger, Percutaneous Approach
0XQT4ZZ	Repair Left Ring Finger, Percutaneous Endoscopic Approach
0XQTXZZ	Repair Left Ring Finger, External Approach
0XQV0ZZ	Repair Right Little Finger, Open Approach
0XQV3ZZ	Repair Right Little Finger, Percutaneous Approach
0XQV4ZZ	Repair Right Little Finger, Percutaneous Endoscopic Approach
0XQVXZZ	Repair Right Little Finger, External Approach
0XQW0ZZ	Repair Left Little Finger, Open Approach
0XQW3ZZ	Repair Left Little Finger, Percutaneous Approach
0XQW4ZZ	Repair Left Little Finger, Percutaneous Endoscopic Approach
0XQWXZZ	Repair Left Little Finger, External Approach

0XR – Anatomical Regions, Upper Extremities, Replacement

0XRL07N	Replacement of Right Thumb with Right Toe, Autologous Tissue Substitute, Open Approach
0XRL07P	Replacement of Right Thumb with Left Toe, Autologous Tissue Substitute, Open Approach
0XRL47N	Replacement of Right Thumb with Right Toe, Autologous Tissue Substitute, Percutaneous Endoscopic Approach
0XRL47P	Replacement of Right Thumb with Left Toe, Autologous Tissue Substitute, Percutaneous Endoscopic Approach
0XRM07N	Replacement of Left Thumb with Right Toe, Autologous Tissue Substitute, Open Approach
0XRM07P	Replacement of Left Thumb with Left Toe, Autologous Tissue Substitute, Open Approach
0XRM47N	Replacement of Left Thumb with Right Toe, Autologous Tissue Substitute, Percutaneous Endoscopic Approach
0XRM47P	Replacement of Left Thumb with Left Toe, Autologous Tissue Substitute, Percutaneous Endoscopic Approach

0XU – Anatomical Regions, Upper Extremities, Supplement

0XU207Z	Supplement Right Shoulder Region with Autologous Tissue Substitute, Open Approach
0XU20JZ	Supplement Right Shoulder Region with Synthetic Substitute, Open Approach
0XU20KZ	Supplement Right Shoulder Region with Nonautologous Tissue Substitute, Open Approach
0XU247Z	Supplement Right Shoulder Region with Autologous Tissue Substitute, Percutaneous Endoscopic Approach
0XU24JZ	Supplement Right Shoulder Region with Synthetic Substitute, Percutaneous Endoscopic Approach
0XU24KZ	Supplement Right Shoulder Region with Nonautologous Tissue Substitute, Percutaneous Endoscopic Approach
0XU307Z	Supplement Left Shoulder Region with Autologous Tissue Substitute, Open Approach
0XU30JZ	Supplement Left Shoulder Region with Synthetic Substitute, Open Approach
0XU30KZ	Supplement Left Shoulder Region with Nonautologous Tissue Substitute, Open Approach

0XU347Z Supplement Left Shoulder Region with Autologous Tissue Substitute, Percutaneous Endoscopic Approach

0XU34JZ Supplement Left Shoulder Region with Synthetic Substitute, Percutaneous Endoscopic Approach

0XU34KZ Supplement Left Shoulder Region with Nonautologous Tissue Substitute, Percutaneous Endoscopic Approach

0XU407Z Supplement Right Axilla with Autologous Tissue Substitute, Open Approach

0XU40JZ Supplement Right Axilla with Synthetic Substitute, Open Approach

0XU40KZ Supplement Right Axilla with Nonautologous Tissue Substitute, Open Approach

0XU447Z Supplement Right Axilla with Autologous Tissue Substitute, Percutaneous Endoscopic Approach

0XU44JZ Supplement Right Axilla with Synthetic Substitute, Percutaneous Endoscopic Approach

0XU44KZ Supplement Right Axilla with Nonautologous Tissue Substitute, Percutaneous Endoscopic Approach

0XU507Z Supplement Left Axilla with Autologous Tissue Substitute, Open Approach

0XU50JZ Supplement Left Axilla with Synthetic Substitute, Open Approach

0XU50KZ Supplement Left Axilla with Nonautologous Tissue Substitute, Open Approach

0XU547Z Supplement Left Axilla with Autologous Tissue Substitute, Percutaneous Endoscopic Approach

0XU54JZ Supplement Left Axilla with Synthetic Substitute, Percutaneous Endoscopic Approach

0XU54KZ Supplement Left Axilla with Nonautologous Tissue Substitute, Percutaneous Endoscopic Approach

0XU607Z Supplement Right Upper Extremity with Autologous Tissue Substitute, Open Approach

0XU60JZ Supplement Right Upper Extremity with Synthetic Substitute, Open Approach

0XU60KZ Supplement Right Upper Extremity with Nonautologous Tissue Substitute, Open Approach

0XU647Z Supplement Right Upper Extremity with Autologous Tissue Substitute, Percutaneous Endoscopic Approach

0XU64JZ Supplement Right Upper Extremity with Synthetic Substitute, Percutaneous Endoscopic Approach

0XU64KZ Supplement Right Upper Extremity with Nonautologous Tissue Substitute, Percutaneous Endoscopic Approach

0XU707Z Supplement Left Upper Extremity with Autologous Tissue Substitute, Open Approach

0XU70JZ Supplement Left Upper Extremity with Synthetic Substitute, Open Approach

0XU70KZ Supplement Left Upper Extremity with Nonautologous Tissue Substitute, Open Approach

0XU747Z Supplement Left Upper Extremity with Autologous Tissue Substitute, Percutaneous Endoscopic Approach

0XU74JZ Supplement Left Upper Extremity with Synthetic Substitute, Percutaneous Endoscopic Approach

0XU74KZ Supplement Left Upper Extremity with Nonautologous Tissue Substitute, Percutaneous Endoscopic Approach

0XU807Z Supplement Right Upper Arm with Autologous Tissue Substitute, Open Approach

0XU80JZ Supplement Right Upper Arm with Synthetic Substitute, Open Approach

0XU80KZ Supplement Right Upper Arm with Nonautologous Tissue Substitute, Open Approach

0XU847Z Supplement Right Upper Arm with Autologous Tissue Substitute, Percutaneous Endoscopic Approach

0XU84JZ Supplement Right Upper Arm with Synthetic Substitute, Percutaneous Endoscopic Approach

0XU84KZ Supplement Right Upper Arm with Nonautologous Tissue Substitute, Percutaneous Endoscopic Approach

0XU907Z Supplement Left Upper Arm with Autologous Tissue Substitute, Open Approach

0XU90JZ Supplement Left Upper Arm with Synthetic Substitute, Open Approach

0XU90KZ Supplement Left Upper Arm with Nonautologous Tissue Substitute, Open Approach

0XU947Z Supplement Left Upper Arm with Autologous Tissue Substitute, Percutaneous Endoscopic Approach

0XU94JZ Supplement Left Upper Arm with Synthetic Substitute, Percutaneous Endoscopic Approach

0XU94KZ Supplement Left Upper Arm with Nonautologous Tissue Substitute, Percutaneous Endoscopic Approach

0XUB07Z Supplement Right Elbow Region with Autologous Tissue Substitute, Open Approach

0XUB0JZ Supplement Right Elbow Region with Synthetic Substitute, Open Approach

0XUB0KZ Supplement Right Elbow Region with Nonautologous Tissue Substitute, Open Approach

0XUB47Z Supplement Right Elbow Region with Autologous Tissue Substitute, Percutaneous Endoscopic Approach

0XUB4JZ Supplement Right Elbow Region with Synthetic Substitute, Percutaneous Endoscopic Approach

0XUB4KZ Supplement Right Elbow Region with Nonautologous Tissue Substitute, Percutaneous Endoscopic Approach

0XUC07Z Supplement Left Elbow Region with Autologous Tissue Substitute, Open Approach

0XUC0JZ Supplement Left Elbow Region with Synthetic Substitute, Open Approach

0XUC0KZ Supplement Left Elbow Region with Nonautologous Tissue Substitute, Open Approach

0XUC47Z Supplement Left Elbow Region with Autologous Tissue Substitute, Percutaneous Endoscopic Approach

0XUC4JZ Supplement Left Elbow Region with Synthetic Substitute, Percutaneous Endoscopic Approach

0XUC4KZ Supplement Left Elbow Region with Nonautologous Tissue Substitute, Percutaneous Endoscopic Approach

0XUD07Z Supplement Right Lower Arm with Autologous Tissue Substitute, Open Approach

0XUD0JZ Supplement Right Lower Arm with Synthetic Substitute, Open Approach

0XUD0KZ Supplement Right Lower Arm with Nonautologous Tissue Substitute, Open Approach

0XUD47Z Supplement Right Lower Arm with Autologous Tissue Substitute, Percutaneous Endoscopic Approach

0XUD4JZ Supplement Right Lower Arm with Synthetic Substitute, Percutaneous Endoscopic Approach

0XUD4KZ Supplement Right Lower Arm with Nonautologous Tissue Substitute, Percutaneous Endoscopic Approach

0XUF07Z Supplement Left Lower Arm with Autologous Tissue Substitute, Open Approach

0XUF0JZ Supplement Left Lower Arm with Synthetic Substitute, Open Approach

0XUF0KZ Supplement Left Lower Arm with Nonautologous Tissue Substitute, Open Approach

0XUF47Z Supplement Left Lower Arm with Autologous Tissue Substitute, Percutaneous Endoscopic Approach

0XUF4JZ Supplement Left Lower Arm with Synthetic Substitute, Percutaneous Endoscopic Approach

0XUF4KZ Supplement Left Lower Arm with Nonautologous Tissue Substitute, Percutaneous Endoscopic Approach

0XUG07Z Supplement Right Wrist Region with Autologous Tissue Substitute, Open Approach

0XUG0JZ Supplement Right Wrist Region with Synthetic Substitute, Open Approach

0XUG0KZ Supplement Right Wrist Region with Nonautologous Tissue Substitute, Open Approach

0XUG47Z Supplement Right Wrist Region with Autologous Tissue Substitute, Percutaneous Endoscopic Approach

0XUG4JZ Supplement Right Wrist Region with Synthetic Substitute, Percutaneous Endoscopic Approach

0XUG4KZ Supplement Right Wrist Region with Nonautologous Tissue Substitute, Percutaneous Endoscopic Approach

0XUH07Z Supplement Left Wrist Region with Autologous Tissue Substitute, Open Approach

0XUH0JZ Supplement Left Wrist Region with Synthetic Substitute, Open Approach

0XUH0KZ Supplement Left Wrist Region with Nonautologous Tissue Substitute, Open Approach

0XUH47Z Supplement Left Wrist Region with Autologous Tissue Substitute, Percutaneous Endoscopic Approach

0XUH4JZ Supplement Left Wrist Region with Synthetic Substitute, Percutaneous Endoscopic Approach

0XUH4KZ Supplement Left Wrist Region with Nonautologous Tissue Substitute, Percutaneous Endoscopic Approach

0XUJ07Z Supplement Right Hand with Autologous Tissue Substitute, Open Approach

0XUJ0JZ Supplement Right Hand with Synthetic Substitute, Open Approach

0XUJ0KZ Supplement Right Hand with Nonautologous Tissue Substitute, Open Approach

0XUJ47Z Supplement Right Hand with Autologous Tissue Substitute, Percutaneous Endoscopic Approach

0XUJ4JZ Supplement Right Hand with Synthetic Substitute, Percutaneous Endoscopic Approach

0XUJ4KZ Supplement Right Hand with Nonautologous Tissue Substitute, Percutaneous Endoscopic Approach

0XUK07Z Supplement Left Hand with Autologous Tissue Substitute, Open Approach

0XUK0JZ Supplement Left Hand with Synthetic Substitute, Open Approach

0XUK0KZ	Supplement Left Hand with Nonautologous Tissue Substitute, Open Approach
0XUK47Z	Supplement Left Hand with Autologous Tissue Substitute, Percutaneous Endoscopic Approach
0XUK4JZ	Supplement Left Hand with Synthetic Substitute, Percutaneous Endoscopic Approach
0XUK4KZ	Supplement Left Hand with Nonautologous Tissue Substitute, Percutaneous Endoscopic Approach
0XUL07Z	Supplement Right Thumb with Autologous Tissue Substitute, Open Approach
0XUL0JZ	Supplement Right Thumb with Synthetic Substitute, Open Approach
0XUL0KZ	Supplement Right Thumb with Nonautologous Tissue Substitute, Open Approach
0XUL47Z	Supplement Right Thumb with Autologous Tissue Substitute, Percutaneous Endoscopic Approach
0XUL4JZ	Supplement Right Thumb with Synthetic Substitute, Percutaneous Endoscopic Approach
0XUL4KZ	Supplement Right Thumb with Nonautologous Tissue Substitute, Percutaneous Endoscopic Approach
0XUM07Z	Supplement Left Thumb with Autologous Tissue Substitute, Open Approach
0XUM0JZ	Supplement Left Thumb with Synthetic Substitute, Open Approach
0XUM0KZ	Supplement Left Thumb with Nonautologous Tissue Substitute, Open Approach
0XUM47Z	Supplement Left Thumb with Autologous Tissue Substitute, Percutaneous Endoscopic Approach
0XUM4JZ	Supplement Left Thumb with Synthetic Substitute, Percutaneous Endoscopic Approach
0XUM4KZ	Supplement Left Thumb with Nonautologous Tissue Substitute, Percutaneous Endoscopic Approach
0XUN07Z	Supplement Right Index Finger with Autologous Tissue Substitute, Open Approach
0XUN0JZ	Supplement Right Index Finger with Synthetic Substitute, Open Approach
0XUN0KZ	Supplement Right Index Finger with Nonautologous Tissue Substitute, Open Approach
0XUN47Z	Supplement Right Index Finger with Autologous Tissue Substitute, Percutaneous Endoscopic Approach
0XUN4JZ	Supplement Right Index Finger with Synthetic Substitute, Percutaneous Endoscopic Approach
0XUN4KZ	Supplement Right Index Finger with Nonautologous Tissue Substitute, Percutaneous Endoscopic Approach

0XUP07Z	Supplement Left Index Finger with Autologous Tissue Substitute, Open Approach
0XUP0JZ	Supplement Left Index Finger with Synthetic Substitute, Open Approach
0XUP0KZ	Supplement Left Index Finger with Nonautologous Tissue Substitute, Open Approach
0XUP47Z	Supplement Left Index Finger with Autologous Tissue Substitute, Percutaneous Endoscopic Approach
0XUP4JZ	Supplement Left Index Finger with Synthetic Substitute, Percutaneous Endoscopic Approach
0XUP4KZ	Supplement Left Index Finger with Nonautologous Tissue Substitute, Percutaneous Endoscopic Approach
0XUQ07Z	Supplement Right Middle Finger with Autologous Tissue Substitute, Open Approach
0XUQ0JZ	Supplement Right Middle Finger with Synthetic Substitute, Open Approach
0XUQ0KZ	Supplement Right Middle Finger with Nonautologous Tissue Substitute, Open Approach
0XUQ47Z	Supplement Right Middle Finger with Autologous Tissue Substitute, Percutaneous Endoscopic Approach
0XUQ4JZ	Supplement Right Middle Finger with Synthetic Substitute, Percutaneous Endoscopic Approach
0XUQ4KZ	Supplement Right Middle Finger with Nonautologous Tissue Substitute, Percutaneous Endoscopic Approach
0XUR07Z	Supplement Left Middle Finger with Autologous Tissue Substitute, Open Approach
0XUR0JZ	Supplement Left Middle Finger with Synthetic Substitute, Open Approach
0XUR0KZ	Supplement Left Middle Finger with Nonautologous Tissue Substitute, Open Approach
0XUR47Z	Supplement Left Middle Finger with Autologous Tissue Substitute, Percutaneous Endoscopic Approach
0XUR4JZ	Supplement Left Middle Finger with Synthetic Substitute, Percutaneous Endoscopic Approach
0XUR4KZ	Supplement Left Middle Finger with Nonautologous Tissue Substitute, Percutaneous Endoscopic Approach
0XUS07Z	Supplement Right Ring Finger with Autologous Tissue Substitute, Open Approach
0XUS0JZ	Supplement Right Ring Finger with Synthetic Substitute, Open Approach
0XUS0KZ	Supplement Right Ring Finger with Nonautologous Tissue Substitute, Open Approach
0XUS47Z	Supplement Right Ring Finger with Autologous Tissue Substitute, Percutaneous Endoscopic Approach

0XUS4JZ	Supplement Right Ring Finger with Synthetic Substitute, Percutaneous Endoscopic Approach
0XUS4KZ	Supplement Right Ring Finger with Nonautologous Tissue Substitute, Percutaneous Endoscopic Approach
0XUT07Z	Supplement Left Ring Finger with Autologous Tissue Substitute, Open Approach
0XUT0JZ	Supplement Left Ring Finger with Synthetic Substitute, Open Approach
0XUT0KZ	Supplement Left Ring Finger with Nonautologous Tissue Substitute, Open Approach
0XUT47Z	Supplement Left Ring Finger with Autologous Tissue Substitute, Percutaneous Endoscopic Approach
0XUT4JZ	Supplement Left Ring Finger with Synthetic Substitute, Percutaneous Endoscopic Approach
0XUT4KZ	Supplement Left Ring Finger with Nonautologous Tissue Substitute, Percutaneous Endoscopic Approach
0XUV07Z	Supplement Right Little Finger with Autologous Tissue Substitute, Open Approach
0XUV0JZ	Supplement Right Little Finger with Synthetic Substitute, Open Approach
0XUV0KZ	Supplement Right Little Finger with Nonautologous Tissue Substitute, Open Approach
0XUV47Z	Supplement Right Little Finger with Autologous Tissue Substitute, Percutaneous Endoscopic Approach
0XUV4JZ	Supplement Right Little Finger with Synthetic Substitute, Percutaneous Endoscopic Approach
0XUV4KZ	Supplement Right Little Finger with Nonautologous Tissue Substitute, Percutaneous Endoscopic Approach
0XUW07Z	Supplement Left Little Finger with Autologous Tissue Substitute, Open Approach
0XUW0JZ	Supplement Left Little Finger with Synthetic Substitute, Open Approach
0XUW0KZ	Supplement Left Little Finger with Nonautologous Tissue Substitute, Open Approach
0XUW47Z	Supplement Left Little Finger with Autologous Tissue Substitute, Percutaneous Endoscopic Approach
0XUW4JZ	Supplement Left Little Finger with Synthetic Substitute, Percutaneous Endoscopic Approach
0XUW4KZ	Supplement Left Little Finger with Nonautologous Tissue Substitute, Percutaneous Endoscopic Approach

0XW – Anatomical Regions, Upper Extremities, Revision

Review Coding Guideline B6.1c

● 0XW600Z	Revision of Drainage Device in Right Upper Extremity, Open Approach
● 0XW603Z	Revision of Infusion Device in Right Upper Extremity, Open Approach
● 0XW607Z	Revision of Autologous Tissue Substitute in Right Upper Extremity, Open Approach
● 0XW60JZ	Revision of Synthetic Substitute in Right Upper Extremity, Open Approach

● 0XW60KZ	Revision of Nonautologous Tissue Substitute in Right Upper Extremity, Open Approach
● 0XW60YZ	Revision of Other Device in Right Upper Extremity, Open Approach
● 0XW630Z	Revision of Drainage Device in Right Upper Extremity, Percutaneous Approach
● 0XW633Z	Revision of Infusion Device in Right Upper Extremity, Percutaneous Approach

● 0XW637Z	Revision of Autologous Tissue Substitute in Right Upper Extremity, Percutaneous Approach
● 0XW63JZ	Revision of Synthetic Substitute in Right Upper Extremity, Percutaneous Approach
● 0XW63KZ	Revision of Nonautologous Tissue Substitute in Right Upper Extremity, Percutaneous Approach
● 0XW63YZ	Revision of Other Device in Right Upper Extremity, Percutaneous Approach

♀ Female-only	♂ Male-only	▲ Limited Coverage	● Non-OR	▨ HAC-associated procedure	▲ Non-covered procedures	+ Combinatio

0XW640Z	Revision of Drainage Device in Right Upper Extremity, Percutaneous Endoscopic Approach	0XW6XYZ	Revision of Other Device in Right Upper Extremity, External Approach	● 0XW743Z	Revision of Infusion Device in Left Upper Extremity, Percutaneous Endoscopic Approach
0XW643Z	Revision of Infusion Device in Right Upper Extremity, Percutaneous Endoscopic Approach	● 0XW700Z	Revision of Drainage Device in Left Upper Extremity, Open Approach	● 0XW747Z	Revision of Autologous Tissue Substitute in Left Upper Extremity, Percutaneous Endoscopic Approach
0XW647Z	Revision of Autologous Tissue Substitute in Right Upper Extremity, Percutaneous Endoscopic Approach	● 0XW703Z	Revision of Infusion Device in Left Upper Extremity, Open Approach	● 0XW74JZ	Revision of Synthetic Substitute in Left Upper Extremity, Percutaneous Endoscopic Approach
0XW64JZ	Revision of Synthetic Substitute in Right Upper Extremity, Percutaneous Endoscopic Approach	● 0XW707Z	Revision of Autologous Tissue Substitute in Left Upper Extremity, Open Approach	● 0XW74KZ	Revision of Nonautologous Tissue Substitute in Left Upper Extremity, Percutaneous Endoscopic Approach
● 0XW64KZ	Revision of Nonautologous Tissue Substitute in Right Upper Extremity, Percutaneous Endoscopic Approach	● 0XW70JZ	Revision of Synthetic Substitute in Left Upper Extremity, Open Approach	● 0XW74YZ	Revision of Other Device in Left Upper Extremity, Percutaneous Endoscopic Approach
● 0XW64YZ	Revision of Other Device in Right Upper Extremity, Percutaneous Endoscopic Approach	● 0XW70KZ	Revision of Nonautologous Tissue Substitute in Left Upper Extremity, Open Approach	0XW7X0Z	Revision of Drainage Device in Left Upper Extremity, External Approach
0XW6X0Z	Revision of Drainage Device in Right Upper Extremity, External Approach	● 0XW70YZ	Revision of Other Device in Left Upper Extremity, Open Approach	0XW7X3Z	Revision of Infusion Device in Left Upper Extremity, External Approach
0XW6X3Z	Revision of Infusion Device in Right Upper Extremity, External Approach	● 0XW730Z	Revision of Drainage Device in Left Upper Extremity, Percutaneous Approach	0XW7X7Z	Revision of Autologous Tissue Substitute in Left Upper Extremity, External Approach
0XW6X7Z	Revision of Autologous Tissue Substitute in Right Upper Extremity, External Approach	● 0XW733Z	Revision of Infusion Device in Left Upper Extremity, Percutaneous Approach		
		● 0XW737Z	Revision of Autologous Tissue Substitute in Left Upper Extremity, Percutaneous Approach	0XW7XJZ	Revision of Synthetic Substitute in Left Upper Extremity, External Approach
0XW6XJZ	Revision of Synthetic Substitute in Right Upper Extremity, External Approach	● 0XW73JZ	Revision of Synthetic Substitute in Left Upper Extremity, Percutaneous Approach	0XW7XKZ	Revision of Nonautologous Tissue Substitute in Left Upper Extremity, External Approach
0XW6XKZ	Revision of Nonautologous Tissue Substitute in Right Upper Extremity, External Approach	● 0XW73KZ	Revision of Nonautologous Tissue Substitute in Left Upper Extremity, Percutaneous Approach	0XW7XYZ	Revision of Other Device in Left Upper Extremity, External Approach
		● 0XW73YZ	Revision of Other Device in Left Upper Extremity, Percutaneous Approach		
		● 0XW740Z	Revision of Drainage Device in Left Upper Extremity, Percutaneous Endoscopic Approach		

XX – Anatomical Regions, Upper Extremities, Transfer

| 0XXN0ZL | Transfer Right Index Finger to Right Thumb, Open Approach | 0XXP0ZM | Transfer Left Index Finger to Left Thumb, Open Approach |

♀ Female-only   ♂ Male-only   ▲ Limited Coverage   ● Non-OR   ▨ HAC-associated procedure   ▲ Non-covered procedures   ✛ Combination

Anatomical Regions, Lower Extremities 0Y0–0YW

Section	0	Medical and Surgical
Body System	Y	Anatomical Regions, Lower Extremities
Operation	0	**Alteration:** Modifying the anatomic structure of a body part without affecting the function of the body part

Body Part (4th)	Approach (5th)	Device (6th)	Qualifier (7th)
0 Buttock, Right 1 Buttock, Left 9 Lower Extremity, Right B Lower Extremity, Left C Upper Leg, Right D Upper Leg, Left F Knee Region, Right G Knee Region, Left H Lower Leg, Right J Lower Leg, Left K Ankle Region, Right L Ankle Region, Left	0 Open 3 Percutaneous 4 Percutaneous Endoscopic	7 Autologous Tissue Substitute J Synthetic Substitute K Nonautologous Tissue Substitute Z No Device	Z No Qualifier

Section	0	Medical and Surgical
Body System	Y	Anatomical Regions, Lower Extremities
Operation	2	**Change:** Taking out or off a device from a body part and putting back an identical or similar device in or on the same body part without cutting or puncturing the skin or a mucous membrane

Body Part (4th)	Approach (5th)	Device (6th)	Qualifier (7th)
9 Lower Extremity, Right B Lower Extremity, Left	X External	0 Drainage Device Y Other Device	Z No Qualifier

Section	0	Medical and Surgical
Body System	Y	Anatomical Regions, Lower Extremities
Operation	3	**Control:** Stopping, or attempting to stop, postprocedural bleeding

Body Part (4th)	Approach (5th)	Device (6th)	Qualifier (7th)
0 Buttock, Right 1 Buttock, Left 5 Inguinal Region, Right 6 Inguinal Region, Left 7 Femoral Region, Right 8 Femoral Region, Left 9 Lower Extremity, Right B Lower Extremity, Left C Upper Leg, Right D Upper Leg, Left F Knee Region, Right G Knee Region, Left H Lower Leg, Right J Lower Leg, Left K Ankle Region, Right L Ankle Region, Left M Foot, Right N Foot, Left	0 Open 3 Percutaneous 4 Percutaneous Endoscopic	Z No Device	Z No Qualifier

Section	0	Medical and Surgical
Body System	Y	Anatomical Regions, Lower Extremities
Operation	6	Detachment: Cutting off all or a portion of the upper or lower extremities

Body Part (4th)	Approach (5th)	Device (6th)	Qualifier (7th)
2 Hindquarter, Right 3 Hindquarter, Left 4 Hindquarter, Bilateral 7 Femoral Region, Right 8 Femoral Region, Left F Knee Region, Right G Knee Region, Left	0 Open	Z No Device	Z No Qualifier
C Upper Leg, Right D Upper Leg, Left H Lower Leg, Right J Lower Leg, Left	0 Open	Z No Device	1 High 2 Mid 3 Low
M Foot, Right N Foot, Left	0 Open	Z No Device	0 Complete 4 Complete 1st Ray 5 Complete 2nd Ray 6 Complete 3rd Ray 7 Complete 4th Ray 8 Complete 5th Ray 9 Partial 1st Ray B Partial 2nd Ray C Partial 3rd Ray D Partial 4th Ray F Partial 5th Ray
P 1st Toe, Right Q 1st Toe, Left R 2nd Toe, Right S 2nd Toe, Left T 3rd Toe, Right U 3rd Toe, Left V 4th Toe, Right W 4th Toe, Left X 5th Toe, Right Y 5th Toe, Left	0 Open	Z No Device	0 Complete 1 High 2 Mid 3 Low

Section	0	Medical and Surgical
Body System	Y	Anatomical Regions, Lower Extremities
Operation	9	Drainage: Taking or letting out fluids and/or gases from a body part

Body Part (4th)	Approach (5th)	Device (6th)	Qualifier (7th)
0 Buttock, Right 1 Buttock, Left 5 Inguinal Region, Right 6 Inguinal Region, Left 7 Femoral Region, Right 8 Femoral Region, Left 9 Lower Extremity, Right B Lower Extremity, Left C Upper Leg, Right D Upper Leg, Left F Knee Region, Right G Knee Region, Left H Lower Leg, Right J Lower Leg, Left K Ankle Region, Right L Ankle Region, Left M Foot, Right N Foot, Left	0 Open 3 Percutaneous 4 Percutaneous Endoscopic	0 Drainage Device	Z No Qualifier

Continued →

Section	0	Medical and Surgical
Body System	Y	Anatomical Regions, Lower Extremities
Operation	9	Drainage: Taking or letting out fluids and/or gases from a body part

Body Part (4th)	Approach (5th)	Device (6th)	Qualifier (7th)
0 Buttock, Right 1 Buttock, Left 5 Inguinal Region, Right 6 Inguinal Region, Left 7 Femoral Region, Right 8 Femoral Region, Left 9 Lower Extremity, Right B Lower Extremity, Left C Upper Leg, Right D Upper Leg, Left F Knee Region, Right G Knee Region, Left H Lower Leg, Right J Lower Leg, Left K Ankle Region, Right L Ankle Region, Left M Foot, Right N Foot, Left	0 Open 3 Percutaneous 4 Percutaneous Endoscopic	Z No Device	X Diagnostic Z No Qualifier

Section	0	Medical and Surgical
Body System	Y	Anatomical Regions, Lower Extremities
Operation	B	Excision: Cutting out or off, without replacement, a portion of a body part

Body Part (4th)	Approach (5th)	Device (6th)	Qualifier (7th)
0 Buttock, Right 1 Buttock, Left 5 Inguinal Region, Right 6 Inguinal Region, Left 7 Femoral Region, Right 8 Femoral Region, Left 9 Lower Extremity, Right B Lower Extremity, Left C Upper Leg, Right D Upper Leg, Left F Knee Region, Right G Knee Region, Left H Lower Leg, Right J Lower Leg, Left K Ankle Region, Right L Ankle Region, Left M Foot, Right N Foot, Left	0 Open 3 Percutaneous 4 Percutaneous Endoscopic	Z No Device	X Diagnostic Z No Qualifier

Section 0 Medical and Surgical
Body System Y Anatomical Regions, Lower Extremities
Operation H Insertion: Putting in a nonbiological appliance that monitors, assists, performs, or prevents a physiological function but does not physically take the place of a body part

Body Part (4th)	Approach (5th)	Device (6th)	Qualifier (7th)
0 Buttock, Right	0 Open	1 Radioactive Element	Z No Qualifier
1 Buttock, Left	3 Percutaneous	3 Infusion Device	
5 Inguinal Region, Right	4 Percutaneous Endoscopic	Y Other Device	
6 Inguinal Region, Left			
7 Femoral Region, Right			
8 Femoral Region, Left			
9 Lower Extremity, Right			
B Lower Extremity, Left			
C Upper Leg, Right			
D Upper Leg, Left			
F Knee Region, Right			
G Knee Region, Left			
H Lower Leg, Right			
J Lower Leg, Left			
K Ankle Region, Right			
L Ankle Region, Left			
M Foot, Right			
N Foot, Left			

Section 0 Medical and Surgical
Body System Y Anatomical Regions, Lower Extremities
Operation J Inspection: Visually and/or manually exploring a body part

Body Part (4th)	Approach (5th)	Device (6th)	Qualifier (7th)
0 Buttock, Right	0 Open	Z No Device	Z No Qualifier
1 Buttock, Left	3 Percutaneous		
5 Inguinal Region, Right	4 Percutaneous Endoscopic		
6 Inguinal Region, Left	X External		
7 Femoral Region, Right			
8 Femoral Region, Left			
9 Lower Extremity, Right			
A Inguinal Region, Bilateral			
B Lower Extremity, Left			
C Upper Leg, Right			
D Upper Leg, Left			
E Femoral Region, Bilateral			
F Knee Region, Right			
G Knee Region, Left			
H Lower Leg, Right			
J Lower Leg, Left			
K Ankle Region, Right			
L Ankle Region, Left			
M Foot, Right			
N Foot, Left			

Section	0	Medical and Surgical
Body System	Y	Anatomical Regions, Lower Extremities
Operation	M	Reattachment: Putting back in or on all or a portion of a separated body part to its normal location or other suitable location

Body Part (4th)	Approach (5th)	Device (6th)	Qualifier (7th)
0 Buttock, Right	0 Open	Z No Device	Z No Qualifier
1 Buttock, Left			
2 Hindquarter, Right			
3 Hindquarter, Left			
4 Hindquarter, Bilateral			
5 Inguinal Region, Right			
6 Inguinal Region, Left			
7 Femoral Region, Right			
8 Femoral Region, Left			
9 Lower Extremity, Right			
B Lower Extremity, Left			
C Upper Leg, Right			
D Upper Leg, Left			
F Knee Region, Right			
G Knee Region, Left			
H Lower Leg, Right			
J Lower Leg, Left			
K Ankle Region, Right			
L Ankle Region, Left			
M Foot, Right			
N Foot, Left			
P 1st Toe, Right			
Q 1st Toe, Left			
R 2nd Toe, Right			
S 2nd Toe, Left			
T 3rd Toe, Right			
U 3rd Toe, Left			
V 4th Toe, Right			
W 4th Toe, Left			
X 5th Toe, Right			
Y 5th Toe, Left			

Section	0	Medical and Surgical
Body System	Y	Anatomical Regions, Lower Extremities
Operation	P	Removal: Taking out or off a device from a body part

Body Part (4th)	Approach (5th)	Device (6th)	Qualifier (7th)
9 Lower Extremity, Right	0 Open	0 Drainage Device	Z No Qualifier
B Lower Extremity, Left	3 Percutaneous	1 Radioactive Element	
	4 Percutaneous Endoscopic	3 Infusion Device	
	X External	7 Autologous Tissue Substitute	
		J Synthetic Substitute	
		K Nonautologous Tissue Substitute	
		Y Other Device	

ction	**0**	**Medical and Surgical**	
dy System	**Y**	**Anatomical Regions, Lower Extremities**	
eration	**Q**	**Repair:** Restoring, to the extent possible, a body part to its normal anatomic structure and function	

Body Part (4ᵗʰ)	Approach (5ᵗʰ)	Device (6ᵗʰ)	Qualifier (7ᵗʰ)
0 Buttock, Right	0 Open	Z No Device	Z No Qualifier
4 Buttock, Left	3 Percutaneous		
5 Inguinal Region, Right	4 Percutaneous Endoscopic		
6 Inguinal Region, Left	X External		
7 Femoral Region, Right			
8 Femoral Region, Left			
9 Lower Extremity, Right			
A Inguinal Region, Bilateral			
B Lower Extremity, Left			
C Upper Leg, Right			
D Upper Leg, Left			
E Femoral Region, Bilateral			
F Knee Region, Right			
G Knee Region, Left			
H Lower Leg, Right			
J Lower Leg, Left			
K Ankle Region, Right			
L Ankle Region, Left			
M Foot, Right			
N Foot, Left			
P 1st Toe, Right			
Q 1st Toe, Left			
R 2nd Toe, Right			
S 2nd Toe, Left			
T 3rd Toe, Right			
U 3rd Toe, Left			
V 4th Toe, Right			
W 4th Toe, Left			
X 5th Toe, Right			
Y 5th Toe, Left			

Section	0	Medical and Surgical
Body System	Y	Anatomical Regions, Lower Extremities
Operation	U	Supplement: Putting in or on biological or synthetic material that physically reinforces and/or augments the function of a portion of a body part

Body Part (4th)	Approach (5th)	Device (6th)	Qualifier (7th)
0 Buttock, Right 1 Buttock, Left 5 Inguinal Region, Right 6 Inguinal Region, Left 7 Femoral Region, Right 8 Femoral Region, Left 9 Lower Extremity, Right A Inguinal Region, Bilateral B Lower Extremity, Left C Upper Leg, Right D Upper Leg, Left E Femoral Region, Bilateral F Knee Region, Right G Knee Region, Left H Lower Leg, Right J Lower Leg, Left K Ankle Region, Right L Ankle Region, Left M Foot, Right N Foot, Left P 1st Toe, Right Q 1st Toe, Left R 2nd Toe, Right S 2nd Toe, Left T 3rd Toe, Right U 3rd Toe, Left V 4th Toe, Right W 4th Toe, Left X 5th Toe, Right Y 5th Toe, Left	0 Open 4 Percutaneous Endoscopic	7 Autologous Tissue Substitute J Synthetic Substitute K Nonautologous Tissue Substitute	Z No Qualifier

Section	0	Medical and Surgical
Body System	Y	Anatomical Regions, Lower Extremities
Operation	W	Revision: Correcting, to the extent possible, a portion of a malfunctioning device or the position of a displaced device

Body Part (4th)	Approach (5th)	Device (6th)	Qualifier (7th)
9 Lower Extremity, Right B Lower Extremity, Left	0 Open 3 Percutaneous 4 Percutaneous Endoscopic X External	0 Drainage Device 3 Infusion Device 7 Autologous Tissue Substitute J Synthetic Substitute K Nonautologous Tissue Substitute Y Other Device	Z No Qualifier

Anatomical Regions, Lower Extremities Code Listing 0Y0–0YW

0Y0 – Anatomical Regions, Lower Extremities, Alteration

0Y0007Z Alteration of Right Buttock with Autologous Tissue Substitute, Open Approach
0Y000JZ Alteration of Right Buttock with Synthetic Substitute, Open Approach
0Y000KZ Alteration of Right Buttock with Nonautologous Tissue Substitute, Open Approach
0Y000ZZ Alteration of Right Buttock, Open Approach
0Y0037Z Alteration of Right Buttock with Autologous Tissue Substitute, Percutaneous Approach
0Y003JZ Alteration of Right Buttock with Synthetic Substitute, Percutaneous Approach
0Y003KZ Alteration of Right Buttock with Nonautologous Tissue Substitute, Percutaneous Approach

0Y003ZZ Alteration of Right Buttock, Percutaneous Approach
0Y0047Z Alteration of Right Buttock with Autologous Tissue Substitute, Percutaneous Endoscopic Approach
0Y004JZ Alteration of Right Buttock with Synthetic Substitute, Percutaneous Endoscopic Approach
0Y004KZ Alteration of Right Buttock with Nonautologous Tissue Substitute, Percutaneous Endoscopic Approach
0Y004ZZ Alteration of Right Buttock, Percutaneous Endoscopic Approach
0Y0107Z Alteration of Left Buttock with Autologous Tissue Substitute, Open Approach

0Y010JZ Alteration of Left Buttock with Synthetic Substitute, Open Approach
0Y010KZ Alteration of Left Buttock with Nonautologous Tissue Substitute, Open Approach
0Y010ZZ Alteration of Left Buttock, Open Approach
0Y0137Z Alteration of Left Buttock with Autologous Tissue Substitute, Percutaneous Approach
0Y013JZ Alteration of Left Buttock with Synthetic Substitute, Percutaneous Approach
0Y013KZ Alteration of Left Buttock with Nonautologous Tissue Substitute, Percutaneous Approach

0Y013ZZ	Alteration of Left Buttock, Percutaneous Approach
0Y0147Z	Alteration of Left Buttock with Autologous Tissue Substitute, Percutaneous Endoscopic Approach
0Y014JZ	Alteration of Left Buttock with Synthetic Substitute, Percutaneous Endoscopic Approach
0Y014KZ	Alteration of Left Buttock with Nonautologous Tissue Substitute, Percutaneous Endoscopic Approach
0Y014ZZ	Alteration of Left Buttock, Percutaneous Endoscopic Approach
0Y0907Z	Alteration of Right Lower Extremity with Autologous Tissue Substitute, Open Approach
0Y090JZ	Alteration of Right Lower Extremity with Synthetic Substitute, Open Approach
0Y090KZ	Alteration of Right Lower Extremity with Nonautologous Tissue Substitute, Open Approach
0Y090ZZ	Alteration of Right Lower Extremity, Open Approach
0Y0937Z	Alteration of Right Lower Extremity with Autologous Tissue Substitute, Percutaneous Approach
0Y093JZ	Alteration of Right Lower Extremity with Synthetic Substitute, Percutaneous Approach
0Y093KZ	Alteration of Right Lower Extremity with Nonautologous Tissue Substitute, Percutaneous Approach
0Y093ZZ	Alteration of Right Lower Extremity, Percutaneous Approach
0Y0947Z	Alteration of Right Lower Extremity with Autologous Tissue Substitute, Percutaneous Endoscopic Approach
0Y094JZ	Alteration of Right Lower Extremity with Synthetic Substitute, Percutaneous Endoscopic Approach
0Y094KZ	Alteration of Right Lower Extremity with Nonautologous Tissue Substitute, Percutaneous Endoscopic Approach
0Y094ZZ	Alteration of Right Lower Extremity, Percutaneous Endoscopic Approach
0Y0B07Z	Alteration of Left Lower Extremity with Autologous Tissue Substitute, Open Approach
0Y0B0JZ	Alteration of Left Lower Extremity with Synthetic Substitute, Open Approach
0Y0B0KZ	Alteration of Left Lower Extremity with Nonautologous Tissue Substitute, Open Approach
0Y0B0ZZ	Alteration of Left Lower Extremity, Open Approach
0Y0B37Z	Alteration of Left Lower Extremity with Autologous Tissue Substitute, Percutaneous Approach
0Y0B3JZ	Alteration of Left Lower Extremity with Synthetic Substitute, Percutaneous Approach
0Y0B3KZ	Alteration of Left Lower Extremity with Nonautologous Tissue Substitute, Percutaneous Approach
0Y0B3ZZ	Alteration of Left Lower Extremity, Percutaneous Approach
0Y0B47Z	Alteration of Left Lower Extremity with Autologous Tissue Substitute, Percutaneous Endoscopic Approach
0Y0B4JZ	Alteration of Left Lower Extremity with Synthetic Substitute, Percutaneous Endoscopic Approach
0Y0B4KZ	Alteration of Left Lower Extremity with Nonautologous Tissue Substitute, Percutaneous Endoscopic Approach
0Y0B4ZZ	Alteration of Left Lower Extremity, Percutaneous Endoscopic Approach
0Y0C07Z	Alteration of Right Upper Leg with Autologous Tissue Substitute, Open Approach
0Y0C0JZ	Alteration of Right Upper Leg with Synthetic Substitute, Open Approach
0Y0C0KZ	Alteration of Right Upper Leg with Nonautologous Tissue Substitute, Open Approach
0Y0C0ZZ	Alteration of Right Upper Leg, Open Approach
0Y0C37Z	Alteration of Right Upper Leg with Autologous Tissue Substitute, Percutaneous Approach
0Y0C3JZ	Alteration of Right Upper Leg with Synthetic Substitute, Percutaneous Approach
0Y0C3KZ	Alteration of Right Upper Leg with Nonautologous Tissue Substitute, Percutaneous Approach
0Y0C3ZZ	Alteration of Right Upper Leg, Percutaneous Approach
0Y0C47Z	Alteration of Right Upper Leg with Autologous Tissue Substitute, Percutaneous Endoscopic Approach
0Y0C4JZ	Alteration of Right Upper Leg with Synthetic Substitute, Percutaneous Endoscopic Approach
0Y0C4KZ	Alteration of Right Upper Leg with Nonautologous Tissue Substitute, Percutaneous Endoscopic Approach
0Y0C4ZZ	Alteration of Right Upper Leg, Percutaneous Endoscopic Approach
0Y0D07Z	Alteration of Left Upper Leg with Autologous Tissue Substitute, Open Approach
0Y0D0JZ	Alteration of Left Upper Leg with Synthetic Substitute, Open Approach
0Y0D0KZ	Alteration of Left Upper Leg with Nonautologous Tissue Substitute, Open Approach
0Y0D0ZZ	Alteration of Left Upper Leg, Open Approach
0Y0D37Z	Alteration of Left Upper Leg with Autologous Tissue Substitute, Percutaneous Approach
0Y0D3JZ	Alteration of Left Upper Leg with Synthetic Substitute, Percutaneous Approach
0Y0D3KZ	Alteration of Left Upper Leg with Nonautologous Tissue Substitute, Percutaneous Approach
0Y0D3ZZ	Alteration of Left Upper Leg, Percutaneous Approach
0Y0D47Z	Alteration of Left Upper Leg with Autologous Tissue Substitute, Percutaneous Endoscopic Approach
0Y0D4JZ	Alteration of Left Upper Leg with Synthetic Substitute, Percutaneous Endoscopic Approach
0Y0D4KZ	Alteration of Left Upper Leg with Nonautologous Tissue Substitute, Percutaneous Endoscopic Approach
0Y0D4ZZ	Alteration of Left Upper Leg, Percutaneous Endoscopic Approach
0Y0F07Z	Alteration of Right Knee Region with Autologous Tissue Substitute, Open Approach
0Y0F0JZ	Alteration of Right Knee Region with Synthetic Substitute, Open Approach
0Y0F0KZ	Alteration of Right Knee Region with Nonautologous Tissue Substitute, Open Approach
0Y0F0ZZ	Alteration of Right Knee Region, Open Approach
0Y0F37Z	Alteration of Right Knee Region with Autologous Tissue Substitute, Percutaneous Approach
0Y0F3JZ	Alteration of Right Knee Region with Synthetic Substitute, Percutaneous Approach
0Y0F3KZ	Alteration of Right Knee Region with Nonautologous Tissue Substitute, Percutaneous Approach
0Y0F3ZZ	Alteration of Right Knee Region, Percutaneous Approach
0Y0F47Z	Alteration of Right Knee Region with Autologous Tissue Substitute, Percutaneous Endoscopic Approach
0Y0F4JZ	Alteration of Right Knee Region with Synthetic Substitute, Percutaneous Endoscopic Approach
0Y0F4KZ	Alteration of Right Knee Region with Nonautologous Tissue Substitute, Percutaneous Endoscopic Approach
0Y0F4ZZ	Alteration of Right Knee Region, Percutaneous Endoscopic Approach
0Y0G07Z	Alteration of Left Knee Region with Autologous Tissue Substitute, Open Approach
0Y0G0JZ	Alteration of Left Knee Region with Synthetic Substitute, Open Approach
0Y0G0KZ	Alteration of Left Knee Region with Nonautologous Tissue Substitute, Open Approach
0Y0G0ZZ	Alteration of Left Knee Region, Open Approach
0Y0G37Z	Alteration of Left Knee Region with Autologous Tissue Substitute, Percutaneous Approach
0Y0G3JZ	Alteration of Left Knee Region with Synthetic Substitute, Percutaneous Approach
0Y0G3KZ	Alteration of Left Knee Region with Nonautologous Tissue Substitute, Percutaneous Approach
0Y0G3ZZ	Alteration of Left Knee Region, Percutaneous Approach
0Y0G47Z	Alteration of Left Knee Region with Autologous Tissue Substitute, Percutaneous Endoscopic Approach
0Y0G4JZ	Alteration of Left Knee Region with Synthetic Substitute, Percutaneous Endoscopic Approach
0Y0G4KZ	Alteration of Left Knee Region with Nonautologous Tissue Substitute, Percutaneous Endoscopic Approach
0Y0G4ZZ	Alteration of Left Knee Region, Percutaneous Endoscopic Approach
0Y0H07Z	Alteration of Right Lower Leg with Autologous Tissue Substitute, Open Approach
0Y0H0JZ	Alteration of Right Lower Leg with Synthetic Substitute, Open Approach
0Y0H0KZ	Alteration of Right Lower Leg with Nonautologous Tissue Substitute, Open Approach
0Y0H0ZZ	Alteration of Right Lower Leg, Open Approach
0Y0H37Z	Alteration of Right Lower Leg with Autologous Tissue Substitute, Percutaneous Approach
0Y0H3JZ	Alteration of Right Lower Leg with Synthetic Substitute, Percutaneous Approach
0Y0H3KZ	Alteration of Right Lower Leg with Nonautologous Tissue Substitute, Percutaneous Approach
0Y0H3ZZ	Alteration of Right Lower Leg, Percutaneous Approach
0Y0H47Z	Alteration of Right Lower Leg with Autologous Tissue Substitute, Percutaneous Endoscopic Approach
0Y0H4JZ	Alteration of Right Lower Leg with Synthetic Substitute, Percutaneous Endoscopic Approach

Female-only ♂ Male-only ▲ Limited Coverage ● Non-OR ▦ HAC-associated procedure ▲ Non-covered procedures ✚ Combination

0Y0H4KZ	Alteration of Right Lower Leg with Nonautologous Tissue Substitute, Percutaneous Endoscopic Approach
0Y0H4ZZ	Alteration of Right Lower Leg, Percutaneous Endoscopic Approach
0Y0J07Z	Alteration of Left Lower Leg with Autologous Tissue Substitute, Open Approach
0Y0J0JZ	Alteration of Left Lower Leg with Synthetic Substitute, Open Approach
0Y0J0KZ	Alteration of Left Lower Leg with Nonautologous Tissue Substitute, Open Approach
0Y0J0ZZ	Alteration of Left Lower Leg, Open Approach
0Y0J37Z	Alteration of Left Lower Leg with Autologous Tissue Substitute, Percutaneous Approach
0Y0J3JZ	Alteration of Left Lower Leg with Synthetic Substitute, Percutaneous Approach
0Y0J3KZ	Alteration of Left Lower Leg with Nonautologous Tissue Substitute, Percutaneous Approach
0Y0J3ZZ	Alteration of Left Lower Leg, Percutaneous Approach
0Y0J47Z	Alteration of Left Lower Leg with Autologous Tissue Substitute, Percutaneous Endoscopic Approach
0Y0J4JZ	Alteration of Left Lower Leg with Synthetic Substitute, Percutaneous Endoscopic Approach
0Y0J4KZ	Alteration of Left Lower Leg with Nonautologous Tissue Substitute, Percutaneous Endoscopic Approach
0Y0J4ZZ	Alteration of Left Lower Leg, Percutaneous Endoscopic Approach
0Y0K07Z	Alteration of Right Ankle Region with Autologous Tissue Substitute, Open Approach
0Y0K0JZ	Alteration of Right Ankle Region with Synthetic Substitute, Open Approach
0Y0K0KZ	Alteration of Right Ankle Region with Nonautologous Tissue Substitute, Open Approach
0Y0K0ZZ	Alteration of Right Ankle Region, Open Approach
0Y0K37Z	Alteration of Right Ankle Region with Autologous Tissue Substitute, Percutaneous Approach
0Y0K3JZ	Alteration of Right Ankle Region with Synthetic Substitute, Percutaneous Approach
0Y0K3KZ	Alteration of Right Ankle Region with Nonautologous Tissue Substitute, Percutaneous Approach
0Y0K3ZZ	Alteration of Right Ankle Region, Percutaneous Approach
0Y0K47Z	Alteration of Right Ankle Region with Autologous Tissue Substitute, Percutaneous Endoscopic Approach
0Y0K4JZ	Alteration of Right Ankle Region with Synthetic Substitute, Percutaneous Endoscopic Approach
0Y0K4KZ	Alteration of Right Ankle Region with Nonautologous Tissue Substitute, Percutaneous Endoscopic Approach
0Y0K4ZZ	Alteration of Right Ankle Region, Percutaneous Endoscopic Approach
0Y0L07Z	Alteration of Left Ankle Region with Autologous Tissue Substitute, Open Approach
0Y0L0JZ	Alteration of Left Ankle Region with Synthetic Substitute, Open Approach
0Y0L0KZ	Alteration of Left Ankle Region with Nonautologous Tissue Substitute, Open Approach
0Y0L0ZZ	Alteration of Left Ankle Region, Open Approach
0Y0L37Z	Alteration of Left Ankle Region with Autologous Tissue Substitute, Percutaneous Approach
0Y0L3JZ	Alteration of Left Ankle Region with Synthetic Substitute, Percutaneous Approach
0Y0L3KZ	Alteration of Left Ankle Region with Nonautologous Tissue Substitute, Percutaneous Approach
0Y0L3ZZ	Alteration of Left Ankle Region, Percutaneous Approach
0Y0L47Z	Alteration of Left Ankle Region with Autologous Tissue Substitute, Percutaneous Endoscopic Approach
0Y0L4JZ	Alteration of Left Ankle Region with Synthetic Substitute, Percutaneous Endoscopic Approach
0Y0L4KZ	Alteration of Left Ankle Region with Nonautologous Tissue Substitute, Percutaneous Endoscopic Approach
0Y0L4ZZ	Alteration of Left Ankle Region, Percutaneous Endoscopic Approach

0Y2 – Anatomical Regions, Lower Extremities, Change

Review Coding Guideline B6.1c

0Y29X0Z	Change Drainage Device in Right Lower Extremity, External Approach
0Y29XYZ	Change Other Device in Right Lower Extremity, External Approach
0Y2BX0Z	Change Drainage Device in Left Lower Extremity, External Approach
0Y2BXYZ	Change Other Device in Left Lower Extremity, External Approach

0Y3 – Anatomical Regions, Lower Extremities, Control

Review Coding Guideline B3.7

0Y300ZZ	Control Bleeding in Right Buttock, Open Approach
0Y303ZZ	Control Bleeding in Right Buttock, Percutaneous Approach
0Y304ZZ	Control Bleeding in Right Buttock, Percutaneous Endoscopic Approach
0Y310ZZ	Control Bleeding in Left Buttock, Open Approach
0Y313ZZ	Control Bleeding in Left Buttock, Percutaneous Approach
0Y314ZZ	Control Bleeding in Left Buttock, Percutaneous Endoscopic Approach
0Y350ZZ	Control Bleeding in Right Inguinal Region, Open Approach
0Y353ZZ	Control Bleeding in Right Inguinal Region, Percutaneous Approach
0Y354ZZ	Control Bleeding in Right Inguinal Region, Percutaneous Endoscopic Approach
0Y360ZZ	Control Bleeding in Left Inguinal Region, Open Approach
0Y363ZZ	Control Bleeding in Left Inguinal Region, Percutaneous Approach
0Y364ZZ	Control Bleeding in Left Inguinal Region, Percutaneous Endoscopic Approach
0Y370ZZ	Control Bleeding in Right Femoral Region, Open Approach
0Y373ZZ	Control Bleeding in Right Femoral Region, Percutaneous Approach
0Y374ZZ	Control Bleeding in Right Femoral Region, Percutaneous Endoscopic Approach
0Y380ZZ	Control Bleeding in Left Femoral Region, Open Approach
0Y383ZZ	Control Bleeding in Left Femoral Region, Percutaneous Approach
0Y384ZZ	Control Bleeding in Left Femoral Region, Percutaneous Endoscopic Approach
0Y390ZZ	Control Bleeding in Right Lower Extremity, Open Approach
0Y393ZZ	Control Bleeding in Right Lower Extremity, Percutaneous Approach
0Y394ZZ	Control Bleeding in Right Lower Extremity, Percutaneous Endoscopic Approach
0Y3B0ZZ	Control Bleeding in Left Lower Extremity, Open Approach
0Y3B3ZZ	Control Bleeding in Left Lower Extremity, Percutaneous Approach
0Y3B4ZZ	Control Bleeding in Left Lower Extremity, Percutaneous Endoscopic Approach
0Y3C0ZZ	Control Bleeding in Right Upper Leg, Open Approach
0Y3C3ZZ	Control Bleeding in Right Upper Leg, Percutaneous Approach
0Y3C4ZZ	Control Bleeding in Right Upper Leg, Percutaneous Endoscopic Approach
0Y3D0ZZ	Control Bleeding in Left Upper Leg, Open Approach
0Y3D3ZZ	Control Bleeding in Left Upper Leg, Percutaneous Approach
0Y3D4ZZ	Control Bleeding in Left Upper Leg, Percutaneous Endoscopic Approach
0Y3F0ZZ	Control Bleeding in Right Knee Region, Open Approach
0Y3F3ZZ	Control Bleeding in Right Knee Region, Percutaneous Approach
0Y3F4ZZ	Control Bleeding in Right Knee Region, Percutaneous Endoscopic Approach
0Y3G0ZZ	Control Bleeding in Left Knee Region, Open Approach
0Y3G3ZZ	Control Bleeding in Left Knee Region, Percutaneous Approach
0Y3G4ZZ	Control Bleeding in Left Knee Region, Percutaneous Endoscopic Approach
0Y3H0ZZ	Control Bleeding in Right Lower Leg, Open Approach
0Y3H3ZZ	Control Bleeding in Right Lower Leg, Percutaneous Approach
0Y3H4ZZ	Control Bleeding in Right Lower Leg, Percutaneous Endoscopic Approach
0Y3J0ZZ	Control Bleeding in Left Lower Leg, Open Approach
0Y3J3ZZ	Control Bleeding in Left Lower Leg, Percutaneous Approach

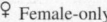

♀ Female-only   ♂ Male-only   ▲ Limited Coverage   ● Non-OR   ▦ HAC-associated procedure   ▲ Non-covered procedures   ✛ Combination

Y3J4ZZ	Control Bleeding in Left Lower Leg, Percutaneous Endoscopic Approach	0Y3L3ZZ	Control Bleeding in Left Ankle Region, Percutaneous Approach	0Y3N0ZZ	Control Bleeding in Left Foot, Open Approach
Y3K0ZZ	Control Bleeding in Right Ankle Region, Open Approach	0Y3L4ZZ	Control Bleeding in Left Ankle Region, Percutaneous Endoscopic Approach	0Y3N3ZZ	Control Bleeding in Left Foot, Percutaneous Approach
Y3K3ZZ	Control Bleeding in Right Ankle Region, Percutaneous Approach	0Y3M0ZZ	Control Bleeding in Right Foot, Open Approach	0Y3N4ZZ	Control Bleeding in Left Foot, Percutaneous Endoscopic Approach
Y3K4ZZ	Control Bleeding in Right Ankle Region, Percutaneous Endoscopic Approach	0Y3M3ZZ	Control Bleeding in Right Foot, Percutaneous Approach		
Y3L0ZZ	Control Bleeding in Left Ankle Region, Open Approach	0Y3M4ZZ	Control Bleeding in Right Foot, Percutaneous Endoscopic Approach		

Y6 – Anatomical Regions, Lower Extremities, Detachment

Y620ZZ	Detachment at Right Hindquarter, Open Approach	0Y6M0ZC	Detachment at Right Foot, Partial 3rd Ray, Open Approach	0Y6S0Z1	Detachment at Left 2nd Toe, High, Open Approach
Y630ZZ	Detachment at Left Hindquarter, Open Approach	0Y6M0ZD	Detachment at Right Foot, Partial 4th Ray, Open Approach	0Y6S0Z2	Detachment at Left 2nd Toe, Mid, Open Approach
Y640ZZ	Detachment at Bilateral Hindquarter, Open Approach	0Y6M0ZF	Detachment at Right Foot, Partial 5th Ray, Open Approach	0Y6S0Z3	Detachment at Left 2nd Toe, Low, Open Approach
Y670ZZ	Detachment at Right Femoral Region, Open Approach	0Y6N0Z0	Detachment at Left Foot, Complete, Open Approach	0Y6T0Z0	Detachment at Right 3rd Toe, Complete, Open Approach
Y680ZZ	Detachment at Left Femoral Region, Open Approach		*AHA CC: 1Q, 2015, 28*	0Y6T0Z1	Detachment at Right 3rd Toe, High, Open Approach
Y6C0Z1	Detachment at Right Upper Leg, High, Open Approach	0Y6N0Z4	Detachment at Left Foot, Complete 1st Ray, Open Approach	0Y6T0Z2	Detachment at Right 3rd Toe, Mid, Open Approach
Y6C0Z2	Detachment at Right Upper Leg, Mid, Open Approach	0Y6N0Z5	Detachment at Left Foot, Complete 2nd Ray, Open Approach	0Y6T0Z3	Detachment at Right 3rd Toe, Low, Open Approach
Y6C0Z3	Detachment at Right Upper Leg, Low, Open Approach	0Y6N0Z6	Detachment at Left Foot, Complete 3rd Ray, Open Approach	0Y6U0Z0	Detachment at Left 3rd Toe, Complete, Open Approach
Y6D0Z1	Detachment at Left Upper Leg, High, Open Approach	0Y6N0Z7	Detachment at Left Foot, Complete 4th Ray, Open Approach	0Y6U0Z1	Detachment at Left 3rd Toe, High, Open Approach
Y6D0Z2	Detachment at Left Upper Leg, Mid, Open Approach	0Y6N0Z8	Detachment at Left Foot, Complete 5th Ray, Open Approach	0Y6U0Z2	Detachment at Left 3rd Toe, Mid, Open Approach
Y6D0Z3	Detachment at Left Upper Leg, Low, Open Approach	0Y6N0Z9	Detachment at Left Foot, Partial 1st Ray, Open Approach	0Y6U0Z3	Detachment at Left 3rd Toe, Low, Open Approach
Y6F0ZZ	Detachment at Right Knee Region, Open Approach	0Y6N0ZB	Detachment at Left Foot, Partial 2nd Ray, Open Approach	0Y6V0Z0	Detachment at Right 4th Toe, Complete, Open Approach
Y6G0ZZ	Detachment at Left Knee Region, Open Approach	0Y6N0ZC	Detachment at Left Foot, Partial 3rd Ray, Open Approach	0Y6V0Z1	Detachment at Right 4th Toe, High, Open Approach
0Y6H0Z1	Detachment at Right Lower Leg, High, Open Approach	0Y6N0ZD	Detachment at Left Foot, Partial 4th Ray, Open Approach	0Y6V0Z2	Detachment at Right 4th Toe, Mid, Open Approach
0Y6H0Z2	Detachment at Right Lower Leg, Mid, Open Approach	0Y6N0ZF	Detachment at Left Foot, Partial 5th Ray, Open Approach	0Y6V0Z3	Detachment at Right 4th Toe, Low, Open Approach
0Y6H0Z3	Detachment at Right Lower Leg, Low, Open Approach	0Y6P0Z0	Detachment at Right 1st Toe, Complete, Open Approach	0Y6W0Z0	Detachment at Left 4th Toe, Complete, Open Approach
0Y6J0Z1	Detachment at Left Lower Leg, High, Open Approach	0Y6P0Z1	Detachment at Right 1st Toe, High, Open Approach	0Y6W0Z1	Detachment at Left 4th Toe, High, Open Approach
0Y6J0Z2	Detachment at Left Lower Leg, Mid, Open Approach	0Y6P0Z2	Detachment at Right 1st Toe, Mid, Open Approach	0Y6W0Z2	Detachment at Left 4th Toe, Mid, Open Approach
0Y6J0Z3	Detachment at Left Lower Leg, Low, Open Approach	0Y6P0Z3	Detachment at Right 1st Toe, Low, Open Approach	0Y6W0Z3	Detachment at Left 4th Toe, Low, Open Approach
0Y6M0Z0	Detachment at Right Foot, Complete, Open Approach	0Y6Q0Z0	Detachment at Left 1st Toe, Complete, Open Approach	0Y6X0Z0	Detachment at Right 5th Toe, Complete, Open Approach
0Y6M0Z4	Detachment at Right Foot, Complete 1st Ray, Open Approach	0Y6Q0Z1	Detachment at Left 1st Toe, High, Open Approach	0Y6X0Z1	Detachment at Right 5th Toe, High, Open Approach
0Y6M0Z5	Detachment at Right Foot, Complete 2nd Ray, Open Approach	0Y6Q0Z2	Detachment at Left 1st Toe, Mid, Open Approach	0Y6X0Z2	Detachment at Right 5th Toe, Mid, Open Approach
0Y6M0Z6	Detachment at Right Foot, Complete 3rd Ray, Open Approach	0Y6Q0Z3	Detachment at Left 1st Toe, Low, Open Approach	0Y6X0Z3	Detachment at Right 5th Toe, Low, Open Approach
0Y6M0Z7	Detachment at Right Foot, Complete 4th Ray, Open Approach	0Y6R0Z0	Detachment at Right 2nd Toe, Complete, Open Approach	0Y6Y0Z0	Detachment at Left 5th Toe, Complete, Open Approach
0Y6M0Z8	Detachment at Right Foot, Complete 5th Ray, Open Approach	0Y6R0Z1	Detachment at Right 2nd Toe, High, Open Approach	0Y6Y0Z1	Detachment at Left 5th Toe, High, Open Approach
0Y6M0Z9	Detachment at Right Foot, Partial 1st Ray, Open Approach	0Y6R0Z2	Detachment at Right 2nd Toe, Mid, Open Approach	0Y6Y0Z2	Detachment at Left 5th Toe, Mid, Open Approach
0Y6M0ZB	Detachment at Right Foot, Partial 2nd Ray, Open Approach	0Y6R0Z3	Detachment at Right 2nd Toe, Low, Open Approach	0Y6Y0Z3	Detachment at Left 5th Toe, Low, Open Approach
		0Y6S0Z0	Detachment at Left 2nd Toe, Complete, Open Approach		

0Y9 – Anatomical Regions, Lower Extremities, Drainage

Review Coding Guidelines B3.4a and B3.4b

Review Coding Guideline B6.2

0Y9000Z	Drainage of Right Buttock with Drainage Device, Open Approach	0Y900ZX	Drainage of Right Buttock, Open Approach, Diagnostic	0Y900ZZ	Drainage of Right Buttock, Open Approach

♀ Female-only	♂ Male-only	▲ Limited Coverage	● Non-OR	▪ HAC-associated procedure	▲ Non-covered procedures	Combination

0Y9030Z Drainage of Right Buttock with Drainage Device, Percutaneous Approach

0Y903ZX Drainage of Right Buttock, Percutaneous Approach, Diagnostic

0Y903ZZ Drainage of Right Buttock, Percutaneous Approach

0Y9040Z Drainage of Right Buttock with Drainage Device, Percutaneous Endoscopic Approach

0Y904ZX Drainage of Right Buttock, Percutaneous Endoscopic Approach, Diagnostic

0Y904ZZ Drainage of Right Buttock, Percutaneous Endoscopic Approach

0Y9100Z Drainage of Left Buttock with Drainage Device, Open Approach

0Y910ZX Drainage of Left Buttock, Open Approach, Diagnostic

0Y910ZZ Drainage of Left Buttock, Open Approach

0Y9130Z Drainage of Left Buttock with Drainage Device, Percutaneous Approach

0Y913ZX Drainage of Left Buttock, Percutaneous Approach, Diagnostic

0Y913ZZ Drainage of Left Buttock, Percutaneous Approach

0Y9140Z Drainage of Left Buttock with Drainage Device, Percutaneous Endoscopic Approach

0Y914ZX Drainage of Left Buttock, Percutaneous Endoscopic Approach, Diagnostic

0Y914ZZ Drainage of Left Buttock, Percutaneous Endoscopic Approach

0Y9500Z Drainage of Right Inguinal Region with Drainage Device, Open Approach

0Y950ZX Drainage of Right Inguinal Region, Open Approach, Diagnostic

0Y950ZZ Drainage of Right Inguinal Region, Open Approach

AHA CC: 1Q, 2015, 23

0Y9530Z Drainage of Right Inguinal Region with Drainage Device, Percutaneous Approach

0Y953ZX Drainage of Right Inguinal Region, Percutaneous Approach, Diagnostic

0Y953ZZ Drainage of Right Inguinal Region, Percutaneous Approach

0Y9540Z Drainage of Right Inguinal Region with Drainage Device, Percutaneous Endoscopic Approach

0Y954ZX Drainage of Right Inguinal Region, Percutaneous Endoscopic Approach, Diagnostic

0Y954ZZ Drainage of Right Inguinal Region, Percutaneous Endoscopic Approach

0Y9600Z Drainage of Left Inguinal Region with Drainage Device, Open Approach

0Y960ZX Drainage of Left Inguinal Region, Open Approach, Diagnostic

0Y960ZZ Drainage of Left Inguinal Region, Open Approach

0Y9630Z Drainage of Left Inguinal Region with Drainage Device, Percutaneous Approach

0Y963ZX Drainage of Left Inguinal Region, Percutaneous Approach, Diagnostic

0Y963ZZ Drainage of Left Inguinal Region, Percutaneous Approach

0Y9640Z Drainage of Left Inguinal Region with Drainage Device, Percutaneous Endoscopic Approach

0Y964ZX Drainage of Left Inguinal Region, Percutaneous Endoscopic Approach, Diagnostic

0Y964ZZ Drainage of Left Inguinal Region, Percutaneous Endoscopic Approach

0Y9700Z Drainage of Right Femoral Region with Drainage Device, Open Approach

0Y970ZX Drainage of Right Femoral Region, Open Approach, Diagnostic

0Y970ZZ Drainage of Right Femoral Region, Open Approach

0Y9730Z Drainage of Right Femoral Region with Drainage Device, Percutaneous Approach

0Y973ZX Drainage of Right Femoral Region, Percutaneous Approach, Diagnostic

0Y973ZZ Drainage of Right Femoral Region, Percutaneous Approach

0Y9740Z Drainage of Right Femoral Region with Drainage Device, Percutaneous Endoscopic Approach

0Y974ZX Drainage of Right Femoral Region, Percutaneous Endoscopic Approach, Diagnostic

0Y974ZZ Drainage of Right Femoral Region, Percutaneous Endoscopic Approach

0Y9800Z Drainage of Left Femoral Region with Drainage Device, Open Approach

0Y980ZX Drainage of Left Femoral Region, Open Approach, Diagnostic

0Y980ZZ Drainage of Left Femoral Region, Open Approach

AHA CC: 1Q, 2015, 22

0Y9830Z Drainage of Left Femoral Region with Drainage Device, Percutaneous Approach

0Y983ZX Drainage of Left Femoral Region, Percutaneous Approach, Diagnostic

0Y983ZZ Drainage of Left Femoral Region, Percutaneous Approach

0Y9840Z Drainage of Left Femoral Region with Drainage Device, Percutaneous Endoscopic Approach

0Y984ZX Drainage of Left Femoral Region, Percutaneous Endoscopic Approach, Diagnostic

0Y984ZZ Drainage of Left Femoral Region, Percutaneous Endoscopic Approach

0Y9900Z Drainage of Right Lower Extremity with Drainage Device, Open Approach

0Y990ZX Drainage of Right Lower Extremity, Open Approach, Diagnostic

0Y990ZZ Drainage of Right Lower Extremity, Open Approach

0Y9930Z Drainage of Right Lower Extremity with Drainage Device, Percutaneous Approach

0Y993ZX Drainage of Right Lower Extremity, Percutaneous Approach, Diagnostic

0Y993ZZ Drainage of Right Lower Extremity, Percutaneous Approach

0Y9940Z Drainage of Right Lower Extremity with Drainage Device, Percutaneous Endoscopic Approach

0Y994ZX Drainage of Right Lower Extremity, Percutaneous Endoscopic Approach, Diagnostic

0Y994ZZ Drainage of Right Lower Extremity, Percutaneous Endoscopic Approach

0Y9B00Z Drainage of Left Lower Extremity with Drainage Device, Open Approach

0Y9B0ZX Drainage of Left Lower Extremity, Open Approach, Diagnostic

0Y9B0ZZ Drainage of Left Lower Extremity, Open Approach

0Y9B30Z Drainage of Left Lower Extremity with Drainage Device, Percutaneous Approach

0Y9B3ZX Drainage of Left Lower Extremity, Percutaneous Approach, Diagnostic

0Y9B3ZZ Drainage of Left Lower Extremity, Percutaneous Approach

0Y9B40Z Drainage of Left Lower Extremity with Drainage Device, Percutaneous Endoscopic Approach

0Y9B4ZX Drainage of Left Lower Extremity, Percutaneous Endoscopic Approach, Diagnostic

0Y9B4ZZ Drainage of Left Lower Extremity, Percutaneous Endoscopic Approach

0Y9C00Z Drainage of Right Upper Leg with Drainage Device, Open Approach

0Y9C0ZX Drainage of Right Upper Leg, Open Approach, Diagnostic

0Y9C0ZZ Drainage of Right Upper Leg, Open Approach

0Y9C30Z Drainage of Right Upper Leg with Drainage Device, Percutaneous Approach

0Y9C3ZX Drainage of Right Upper Leg, Percutaneous Approach, Diagnostic

0Y9C3ZZ Drainage of Right Upper Leg, Percutaneous Approach

0Y9C40Z Drainage of Right Upper Leg with Drainage Device, Percutaneous Endoscopic Approach

0Y9C4ZX Drainage of Right Upper Leg, Percutaneous Endoscopic Approach, Diagnostic

0Y9C4ZZ Drainage of Right Upper Leg, Percutaneous Endoscopic Approach

0Y9D00Z Drainage of Left Upper Leg with Drainage Device, Open Approach

0Y9D0ZX Drainage of Left Upper Leg, Open Approach, Diagnostic

0Y9D0ZZ Drainage of Left Upper Leg, Open Approach

0Y9D30Z Drainage of Left Upper Leg with Drainage Device, Percutaneous Approach

0Y9D3ZX Drainage of Left Upper Leg, Percutaneous Approach, Diagnostic

0Y9D3ZZ Drainage of Left Upper Leg, Percutaneous Approach

0Y9D40Z Drainage of Left Upper Leg with Drainage Device, Percutaneous Endoscopic Approach

0Y9D4ZX Drainage of Left Upper Leg, Percutaneous Endoscopic Approach, Diagnostic

0Y9D4ZZ Drainage of Left Upper Leg, Percutaneous Endoscopic Approach

0Y9F00Z Drainage of Right Knee Region with Drainage Device, Open Approach

0Y9F0ZX Drainage of Right Knee Region, Open Approach, Diagnostic

0Y9F0ZZ Drainage of Right Knee Region, Open Approach

0Y9F30Z Drainage of Right Knee Region with Drainage Device, Percutaneous Approach

0Y9F3ZX Drainage of Right Knee Region, Percutaneous Approach, Diagnostic

0Y9F3ZZ Drainage of Right Knee Region, Percutaneous Approach

0Y9F40Z Drainage of Right Knee Region with Drainage Device, Percutaneous Endoscopic Approach

0Y9F4ZX Drainage of Right Knee Region, Percutaneous Endoscopic Approach, Diagnostic

0Y9F4ZZ Drainage of Right Knee Region, Percutaneous Endoscopic Approach

0Y9G00Z Drainage of Left Knee Region with Drainage Device, Open Approach

0Y9G0ZX Drainage of Left Knee Region, Open Approach, Diagnostic

0Y9G0ZZ Drainage of Left Knee Region, Open Approach

0Y9G30Z Drainage of Left Knee Region with Drainage Device, Percutaneous Approach

0Y9G3ZX Drainage of Left Knee Region, Percutaneous Approach, Diagnostic

0Y9G3ZZ Drainage of Left Knee Region, Percutaneous Approach

0Y9G40Z Drainage of Left Knee Region with Drainage Device, Percutaneous Endoscopic Approach

0Y9G4ZX Drainage of Left Knee Region, Percutaneous Endoscopic Approach, Diagnostic

0Y9G4ZZ Drainage of Left Knee Region, Percutaneous Endoscopic Approach

Y9H00Z Drainage of Right Lower Leg with Drainage Device, Open Approach	**0Y9K00Z** Drainage of Right Ankle Region with Drainage Device, Open Approach	**0Y9L4ZZ** Drainage of Left Ankle Region, Percutaneous Endoscopic Approach
Y9H0ZX Drainage of Right Lower Leg, Open Approach, Diagnostic	**0Y9K0ZX** Drainage of Right Ankle Region, Open Approach, Diagnostic	**0Y9M00Z** Drainage of Right Foot with Drainage Device, Open Approach
Y9H0ZZ Drainage of Right Lower Leg, Open Approach	**0Y9K0ZZ** Drainage of Right Ankle Region, Open Approach	**0Y9M0ZX** Drainage of Right Foot, Open Approach, Diagnostic
Y9H30Z Drainage of Right Lower Leg with Drainage Device, Percutaneous Approach	**0Y9K30Z** Drainage of Right Ankle Region with Drainage Device, Percutaneous Approach	**0Y9M0ZZ** Drainage of Right Foot, Open Approach
Y9H3ZX Drainage of Right Lower Leg, Percutaneous Approach, Diagnostic	**0Y9K3ZX** Drainage of Right Ankle Region, Percutaneous Approach, Diagnostic	**0Y9M30Z** Drainage of Right Foot with Drainage Device, Percutaneous Approach
Y9H3ZZ Drainage of Right Lower Leg, Percutaneous Approach	**0Y9K3ZZ** Drainage of Right Ankle Region, Percutaneous Approach	**0Y9M3ZX** Drainage of Right Foot, Percutaneous Approach, Diagnostic
Y9H40Z Drainage of Right Lower Leg with Drainage Device, Percutaneous Endoscopic Approach	**0Y9K40Z** Drainage of Right Ankle Region with Drainage Device, Percutaneous Endoscopic Approach	**0Y9M3ZZ** Drainage of Right Foot, Percutaneous Approach
Y9H4ZX Drainage of Right Lower Leg, Percutaneous Endoscopic Approach, Diagnostic	**0Y9K4ZX** Drainage of Right Ankle Region, Percutaneous Endoscopic Approach, Diagnostic	**0Y9M40Z** Drainage of Right Foot with Drainage Device, Percutaneous Endoscopic Approach
Y9H4ZZ Drainage of Right Lower Leg, Percutaneous Endoscopic Approach	**0Y9K4ZZ** Drainage of Right Ankle Region, Percutaneous Endoscopic Approach	**0Y9M4ZX** Drainage of Right Foot, Percutaneous Endoscopic Approach, Diagnostic
Y9J00Z Drainage of Left Lower Leg with Drainage Device, Open Approach	**0Y9L00Z** Drainage of Left Ankle Region with Drainage Device, Open Approach	**0Y9M4ZZ** Drainage of Right Foot, Percutaneous Endoscopic Approach
Y9J0ZX Drainage of Left Lower Leg, Open Approach, Diagnostic	**0Y9L0ZX** Drainage of Left Ankle Region, Open Approach, Diagnostic	**0Y9N00Z** Drainage of Left Foot with Drainage Device, Open Approach
Y9J0ZZ Drainage of Left Lower Leg, Open Approach	**0Y9L0ZZ** Drainage of Left Ankle Region, Open Approach	**0Y9N0ZX** Drainage of Left Foot, Open Approach, Diagnostic
Y9J30Z Drainage of Left Lower Leg with Drainage Device, Percutaneous Approach	**0Y9L30Z** Drainage of Left Ankle Region with Drainage Device, Percutaneous Approach	**0Y9N0ZZ** Drainage of Left Foot, Open Approach
Y9J3ZX Drainage of Left Lower Leg, Percutaneous Approach, Diagnostic	**0Y9L3ZX** Drainage of Left Ankle Region, Percutaneous Approach, Diagnostic	**0Y9N30Z** Drainage of Left Foot with Drainage Device, Percutaneous Approach
Y9J3ZZ Drainage of Left Lower Leg, Percutaneous Approach	**0Y9L3ZZ** Drainage of Left Ankle Region, Percutaneous Approach	**0Y9N3ZX** Drainage of Left Foot, Percutaneous Approach, Diagnostic
Y9J40Z Drainage of Left Lower Leg with Drainage Device, Percutaneous Endoscopic Approach	**0Y9L40Z** Drainage of Left Ankle Region with Drainage Device, Percutaneous Endoscopic Approach	**0Y9N3ZZ** Drainage of Left Foot, Percutaneous Approach
Y9J4ZX Drainage of Left Lower Leg, Percutaneous Endoscopic Approach, Diagnostic	**0Y9L4ZX** Drainage of Left Ankle Region, Percutaneous Endoscopic Approach, Diagnostic	**0Y9N40Z** Drainage of Left Foot with Drainage Device, Percutaneous Endoscopic Approach
Y9J4ZZ Drainage of Left Lower Leg, Percutaneous Endoscopic Approach		**0Y9N4ZX** Drainage of Left Foot, Percutaneous Endoscopic Approach, Diagnostic
		0Y9N4ZZ Drainage of Left Foot, Percutaneous Endoscopic Approach

0YB – Anatomical Regions, Lower Extremities, Excision

Review Coding Guidelines B3.4a and B3.4b

YB00ZX Excision of Right Buttock, Open Approach, Diagnostic	**0YB54ZX** Excision of Right Inguinal Region, Percutaneous Endoscopic Approach, Diagnostic	**0YB80ZZ** Excision of Left Femoral Region, Open Approach
YB00ZZ Excision of Right Buttock, Open Approach	**0YB54ZZ** Excision of Right Inguinal Region, Percutaneous Endoscopic Approach	**0YB83ZX** Excision of Left Femoral Region, Percutaneous Approach, Diagnostic
YB03ZX Excision of Right Buttock, Percutaneous Approach, Diagnostic	**0YB60ZX** Excision of Left Inguinal Region, Open Approach, Diagnostic	**0YB83ZZ** Excision of Left Femoral Region, Percutaneous Approach
YB03ZZ Excision of Right Buttock, Percutaneous Approach	**0YB60ZZ** Excision of Left Inguinal Region, Open Approach	**0YB84ZX** Excision of Left Femoral Region, Percutaneous Endoscopic Approach, Diagnostic
YB04ZX Excision of Right Buttock, Percutaneous Endoscopic Approach, Diagnostic	**0YB63ZX** Excision of Left Inguinal Region, Percutaneous Approach, Diagnostic	**0YB84ZZ** Excision of Left Femoral Region, Percutaneous Endoscopic Approach
YB04ZZ Excision of Right Buttock, Percutaneous Endoscopic Approach	**0YB63ZZ** Excision of Left Inguinal Region, Percutaneous Approach	**0YB90ZX** Excision of Right Lower Extremity, Open Approach, Diagnostic
YB10ZX Excision of Left Buttock, Open Approach, Diagnostic	**0YB64ZX** Excision of Left Inguinal Region, Percutaneous Endoscopic Approach, Diagnostic	**0YB90ZZ** Excision of Right Lower Extremity, Open Approach
YB10ZZ Excision of Left Buttock, Open Approach	**0YB64ZZ** Excision of Left Inguinal Region, Percutaneous Endoscopic Approach	**0YB93ZX** Excision of Right Lower Extremity, Percutaneous Approach, Diagnostic
YB13ZX Excision of Left Buttock, Percutaneous Approach, Diagnostic	**0YB70ZX** Excision of Right Femoral Region, Open Approach, Diagnostic	**0YB93ZZ** Excision of Right Lower Extremity, Percutaneous Approach
YB13ZZ Excision of Left Buttock, Percutaneous Approach	**0YB70ZZ** Excision of Right Femoral Region, Open Approach	**0YB94ZX** Excision of Right Lower Extremity, Percutaneous Endoscopic Approach, Diagnostic
YB14ZX Excision of Left Buttock, Percutaneous Endoscopic Approach, Diagnostic	**0YB73ZX** Excision of Right Femoral Region, Percutaneous Approach, Diagnostic	**0YB94ZZ** Excision of Right Lower Extremity, Percutaneous Endoscopic Approach
YB14ZZ Excision of Left Buttock, Percutaneous Endoscopic Approach	**0YB73ZZ** Excision of Right Femoral Region, Percutaneous Approach	**0YBB0ZX** Excision of Left Lower Extremity, Open Approach, Diagnostic
YB50ZX Excision of Right Inguinal Region, Open Approach, Diagnostic	**0YB74ZX** Excision of Right Femoral Region, Percutaneous Endoscopic Approach, Diagnostic	**0YBB0ZZ** Excision of Left Lower Extremity, Open Approach
YB50ZZ Excision of Right Inguinal Region, Open Approach	**0YB74ZZ** Excision of Right Femoral Region, Percutaneous Endoscopic Approach	**0YBB3ZX** Excision of Left Lower Extremity, Percutaneous Approach, Diagnostic
YB53ZX Excision of Right Inguinal Region, Percutaneous Approach, Diagnostic	**0YB80ZX** Excision of Left Femoral Region, Open Approach, Diagnostic	**0YBB3ZZ** Excision of Left Lower Extremity, Percutaneous Approach
YB53ZZ Excision of Right Inguinal Region, Percutaneous Approach		

♀ Female-only   ♂ Male-only   ▲ Limited Coverage   ● Non-OR   ▨ HAC-associated procedure   ▲ Non-covered procedures   ➕ Combination

0YBB4ZX Excision of Left Lower Extremity, Percutaneous Endoscopic Approach, Diagnostic

0YBB4ZZ Excision of Left Lower Extremity, Percutaneous Endoscopic Approach

0YBC0ZX Excision of Right Upper Leg, Open Approach, Diagnostic

0YBC0ZZ Excision of Right Upper Leg, Open Approach

0YBC3ZX Excision of Right Upper Leg, Percutaneous Approach, Diagnostic

0YBC3ZZ Excision of Right Upper Leg, Percutaneous Approach

0YBC4ZX Excision of Right Upper Leg, Percutaneous Endoscopic Approach, Diagnostic

0YBC4ZZ Excision of Right Upper Leg, Percutaneous Endoscopic Approach

0YBD0ZX Excision of Left Upper Leg, Open Approach, Diagnostic

0YBD0ZZ Excision of Left Upper Leg, Open Approach

0YBD3ZX Excision of Left Upper Leg, Percutaneous Approach, Diagnostic

0YBD3ZZ Excision of Left Upper Leg, Percutaneous Approach

0YBD4ZX Excision of Left Upper Leg, Percutaneous Endoscopic Approach, Diagnostic

0YBD4ZZ Excision of Left Upper Leg, Percutaneous Endoscopic Approach

0YBF0ZX Excision of Right Knee Region, Open Approach, Diagnostic

0YBF0ZZ Excision of Right Knee Region, Open Approach

0YBF3ZX Excision of Right Knee Region, Percutaneous Approach, Diagnostic

0YBF3ZZ Excision of Right Knee Region, Percutaneous Approach

0YBF4ZX Excision of Right Knee Region, Percutaneous Endoscopic Approach, Diagnostic

0YBF4ZZ Excision of Right Knee Region, Percutaneous Endoscopic Approach

0YBG0ZX Excision of Left Knee Region, Open Approach, Diagnostic

0YBG0ZZ Excision of Left Knee Region, Open Approach

0YBG3ZX Excision of Left Knee Region, Percutaneous Approach, Diagnostic

0YBG3ZZ Excision of Left Knee Region, Percutaneous Approach

0YBG4ZX Excision of Left Knee Region, Percutaneous Endoscopic Approach, Diagnostic

0YBG4ZZ Excision of Left Knee Region, Percutaneous Endoscopic Approach

0YBH0ZX Excision of Right Lower Leg, Open Approach, Diagnostic

0YBH0ZZ Excision of Right Lower Leg, Open Approach

0YBH3ZX Excision of Right Lower Leg, Percutaneous Approach, Diagnostic

0YBH3ZZ Excision of Right Lower Leg, Percutaneous Approach

0YBH4ZX Excision of Right Lower Leg, Percutaneous Endoscopic Approach, Diagnostic

0YBH4ZZ Excision of Right Lower Leg, Percutaneous Endoscopic Approach

0YBJ0ZX Excision of Left Lower Leg, Open Approach, Diagnostic

0YBJ0ZZ Excision of Left Lower Leg, Open Approach

0YBJ3ZX Excision of Left Lower Leg, Percutaneous Approach, Diagnostic

0YBJ3ZZ Excision of Left Lower Leg, Percutaneous Approach

0YBJ4ZX Excision of Left Lower Leg, Percutaneous Endoscopic Approach, Diagnostic

0YBJ4ZZ Excision of Left Lower Leg, Percutaneous Endoscopic Approach

0YBK0ZX Excision of Right Ankle Region, Open Approach, Diagnostic

0YBK0ZZ Excision of Right Ankle Region, Open Approach

0YBK3ZX Excision of Right Ankle Region, Percutaneous Approach, Diagnostic

0YBK3ZZ Excision of Right Ankle Region, Percutaneous Approach

0YBK4ZX Excision of Right Ankle Region, Percutaneous Endoscopic Approach, Diagnostic

0YBK4ZZ Excision of Right Ankle Region, Percutaneous Endoscopic Approach

0YBL0ZX Excision of Left Ankle Region, Open Approach, Diagnostic

0YBL0ZZ Excision of Left Ankle Region, Open Approach

0YBL3ZX Excision of Left Ankle Region, Percutaneous Approach, Diagnostic

0YBL3ZZ Excision of Left Ankle Region, Percutaneous Approach

0YBL4ZX Excision of Left Ankle Region, Percutaneous Endoscopic Approach, Diagnostic

0YBL4ZZ Excision of Left Ankle Region, Percutaneous Endoscopic Approach

0YBM0ZX Excision of Right Foot, Open Approach, Diagnostic

0YBM0ZZ Excision of Right Foot, Open Approach

0YBM3ZX Excision of Right Foot, Percutaneous Approach, Diagnostic

0YBM3ZZ Excision of Right Foot, Percutaneous Approach

0YBM4ZX Excision of Right Foot, Percutaneous Endoscopic Approach, Diagnostic

0YBM4ZZ Excision of Right Foot, Percutaneous Endoscopic Approach

0YBN0ZX Excision of Left Foot, Open Approach, Diagnostic

0YBN0ZZ Excision of Left Foot, Open Approach

0YBN3ZX Excision of Left Foot, Percutaneous Approach, Diagnostic

0YBN3ZZ Excision of Left Foot, Percutaneous Approach

0YBN4ZX Excision of Left Foot, Percutaneous Endoscopic Approach, Diagnostic

0YBN4ZZ Excision of Left Foot, Percutaneous Endoscopic Approach

0YH – Anatomical Regions, Lower Extremities, Insertion

0YH001Z Insertion of Radioactive Element into Right Buttock, Open Approach

● **0YH003Z** Insertion of Infusion Device into Right Buttock, Open Approach

● **0YH00YZ** Insertion of Other Device into Right Buttock, Open Approach

0YH031Z Insertion of Radioactive Element into Right Buttock, Percutaneous Approach

● **0YH033Z** Insertion of Infusion Device into Right Buttock, Percutaneous Approach

● **0YH03YZ** Insertion of Other Device into Right Buttock, Percutaneous Approach

0YH041Z Insertion of Radioactive Element into Right Buttock, Percutaneous Endoscopic Approach

● **0YH043Z** Insertion of Infusion Device into Right Buttock, Percutaneous Endoscopic Approach

● **0YH04YZ** Insertion of Other Device into Right Buttock, Percutaneous Endoscopic Approach

0YH101Z Insertion of Radioactive Element into Left Buttock, Open Approach

● **0YH103Z** Insertion of Infusion Device into Left Buttock, Open Approach

● **0YH10YZ** Insertion of Other Device into Left Buttock, Open Approach

0YH131Z Insertion of Radioactive Element into Left Buttock, Percutaneous Approach

● **0YH133Z** Insertion of Infusion Device into Left Buttock, Percutaneous Approach

● **0YH13YZ** Insertion of Other Device into Left Buttock, Percutaneous Approach

0YH141Z Insertion of Radioactive Element into Left Buttock, Percutaneous Endoscopic Approach

● **0YH143Z** Insertion of Infusion Device into Left Buttock, Percutaneous Endoscopic Approach

● **0YH14YZ** Insertion of Other Device into Left Buttock, Percutaneous Endoscopic Approach

0YH501Z Insertion of Radioactive Element into Right Inguinal Region, Open Approach

● **0YH503Z** Insertion of Infusion Device into Right Inguinal Region, Open Approach

● **0YH50YZ** Insertion of Other Device into Right Inguinal Region, Open Approach

0YH531Z Insertion of Radioactive Element into Right Inguinal Region, Percutaneous Approach

● **0YH533Z** Insertion of Infusion Device into Right Inguinal Region, Percutaneous Approach

● **0YH53YZ** Insertion of Other Device into Right Inguinal Region, Percutaneous Approach

0YH541Z Insertion of Radioactive Element into Right Inguinal Region, Percutaneous Endoscopic Approach

● **0YH543Z** Insertion of Infusion Device into Right Inguinal Region, Percutaneous Endoscopic Approach

● **0YH54YZ** Insertion of Other Device into Right Inguinal Region, Percutaneous Endoscopic Approach

0YH601Z Insertion of Radioactive Element into Left Inguinal Region, Open Approach

● **0YH603Z** Insertion of Infusion Device into Left Inguinal Region, Open Approach

● **0YH60YZ** Insertion of Other Device into Left Inguinal Region, Open Approach

0YH631Z Insertion of Radioactive Element into Left Inguinal Region, Percutaneous Approach

● **0YH633Z** Insertion of Infusion Device into Left Inguinal Region, Percutaneous Approach

● **0YH63YZ** Insertion of Other Device into Left Inguinal Region, Percutaneous Approach

0YH641Z Insertion of Radioactive Element into Left Inguinal Region, Percutaneous Endoscopic Approach

● **0YH643Z** Insertion of Infusion Device into Left Inguinal Region, Percutaneous Endoscopic Approach

● **0YH64YZ** Insertion of Other Device into Left Inguinal Region, Percutaneous Endoscopic Approach

0YH701Z Insertion of Radioactive Element into Right Femoral Region, Open Approach

● **0YH703Z** Insertion of Infusion Device into Right Femoral Region, Open Approach

● **0YH70YZ** Insertion of Other Device into Right Femoral Region, Open Approach

♀ Female-only   ♂ Male-only   ▲ Limited Coverage   ● Non-OR   ▨ HAC-associated procedure   ▲ Non-covered procedures   ✚ Combination

0YH731Z Insertion of Radioactive Element into Right Femoral Region, Percutaneous Approach

● **0YH733Z** Insertion of Infusion Device into Right Femoral Region, Percutaneous Approach

● **0YH73YZ** Insertion of Other Device into Right Femoral Region, Percutaneous Approach

● **0YH741Z** Insertion of Radioactive Element into Right Femoral Region, Percutaneous Endoscopic Approach

● **0YH743Z** Insertion of Infusion Device into Right Femoral Region, Percutaneous Endoscopic Approach

● **0YH74YZ** Insertion of Other Device into Right Femoral Region, Percutaneous Endoscopic Approach

0YH801Z Insertion of Radioactive Element into Left Femoral Region, Open Approach

● **0YH803Z** Insertion of Infusion Device into Left Femoral Region, Open Approach

● **0YH80YZ** Insertion of Other Device into Left Femoral Region, Open Approach

0YH831Z Insertion of Radioactive Element into Left Femoral Region, Percutaneous Approach

● **0YH833Z** Insertion of Infusion Device into Left Femoral Region, Percutaneous Approach

● **0YH83YZ** Insertion of Other Device into Left Femoral Region, Percutaneous Approach

0YH841Z Insertion of Radioactive Element into Left Femoral Region, Percutaneous Endoscopic Approach

● **0YH843Z** Insertion of Infusion Device into Left Femoral Region, Percutaneous Endoscopic Approach

● **0YH84YZ** Insertion of Other Device into Left Femoral Region, Percutaneous Endoscopic Approach

0YH901Z Insertion of Radioactive Element into Right Lower Extremity, Open Approach

● **0YH903Z** Insertion of Infusion Device into Right Lower Extremity, Open Approach

● **0YH90YZ** Insertion of Other Device into Right Lower Extremity, Open Approach

0YH931Z Insertion of Radioactive Element into Right Lower Extremity, Percutaneous Approach

● **0YH933Z** Insertion of Infusion Device into Right Lower Extremity, Percutaneous Approach

● **0YH93YZ** Insertion of Other Device into Right Lower Extremity, Percutaneous Approach

0YH941Z Insertion of Radioactive Element into Right Lower Extremity, Percutaneous Endoscopic Approach

● **0YH943Z** Insertion of Infusion Device into Right Lower Extremity, Percutaneous Endoscopic Approach

● **0YH94YZ** Insertion of Other Device into Right Lower Extremity, Percutaneous Endoscopic Approach

0YHB01Z Insertion of Radioactive Element into Left Lower Extremity, Open Approach

● **0YHB03Z** Insertion of Infusion Device into Left Lower Extremity, Open Approach

● **0YHB0YZ** Insertion of Other Device into Left Lower Extremity, Open Approach

0YHB31Z Insertion of Radioactive Element into Left Lower Extremity, Percutaneous Approach

● **0YHB33Z** Insertion of Infusion Device into Left Lower Extremity, Percutaneous Approach

● **0YHB3YZ** Insertion of Other Device into Left Lower Extremity, Percutaneous Approach

0YHB41Z Insertion of Radioactive Element into Left Lower Extremity, Percutaneous Endoscopic Approach

● **0YHB43Z** Insertion of Infusion Device into Left Lower Extremity, Percutaneous Endoscopic Approach

● **0YHB4YZ** Insertion of Other Device into Left Lower Extremity, Percutaneous Endoscopic Approach

0YHC01Z Insertion of Radioactive Element into Right Upper Leg, Open Approach

● **0YHC03Z** Insertion of Infusion Device into Right Upper Leg, Open Approach

● **0YHC0YZ** Insertion of Other Device into Right Upper Leg, Open Approach

0YHC31Z Insertion of Radioactive Element into Right Upper Leg, Percutaneous Approach

● **0YHC33Z** Insertion of Infusion Device into Right Upper Leg, Percutaneous Approach

● **0YHC3YZ** Insertion of Other Device into Right Upper Leg, Percutaneous Approach

0YHC41Z Insertion of Radioactive Element into Right Upper Leg, Percutaneous Endoscopic Approach

● **0YHC43Z** Insertion of Infusion Device into Right Upper Leg, Percutaneous Endoscopic Approach

● **0YHC4YZ** Insertion of Other Device into Right Upper Leg, Percutaneous Endoscopic Approach

0YHD01Z Insertion of Radioactive Element into Left Upper Leg, Open Approach

● **0YHD03Z** Insertion of Infusion Device into Left Upper Leg, Open Approach

● **0YHD0YZ** Insertion of Other Device into Left Upper Leg, Open Approach

0YHD31Z Insertion of Radioactive Element into Left Upper Leg, Percutaneous Approach

● **0YHD33Z** Insertion of Infusion Device into Left Upper Leg, Percutaneous Approach

● **0YHD3YZ** Insertion of Other Device into Left Upper Leg, Percutaneous Approach

0YHD41Z Insertion of Radioactive Element into Left Upper Leg, Percutaneous Endoscopic Approach

● **0YHD43Z** Insertion of Infusion Device into Left Upper Leg, Percutaneous Endoscopic Approach

● **0YHD4YZ** Insertion of Other Device into Left Upper Leg, Percutaneous Endoscopic Approach

0YHF01Z Insertion of Radioactive Element into Right Knee Region, Open Approach

● **0YHF03Z** Insertion of Infusion Device into Right Knee Region, Open Approach

● **0YHF0YZ** Insertion of Other Device into Right Knee Region, Open Approach

0YHF31Z Insertion of Radioactive Element into Right Knee Region, Percutaneous Approach

● **0YHF33Z** Insertion of Infusion Device into Right Knee Region, Percutaneous Approach

● **0YHF3YZ** Insertion of Other Device into Right Knee Region, Percutaneous Approach

0YHF41Z Insertion of Radioactive Element into Right Knee Region, Percutaneous Endoscopic Approach

● **0YHF43Z** Insertion of Infusion Device into Right Knee Region, Percutaneous Endoscopic Approach

● **0YHF4YZ** Insertion of Other Device into Right Knee Region, Percutaneous Endoscopic Approach

0YHG01Z Insertion of Radioactive Element into Left Knee Region, Open Approach

● **0YHG03Z** Insertion of Infusion Device into Left Knee Region, Open Approach

● **0YHG0YZ** Insertion of Other Device into Left Knee Region, Open Approach

0YHG31Z Insertion of Radioactive Element into Left Knee Region, Percutaneous Approach

● **0YHG33Z** Insertion of Infusion Device into Left Knee Region, Percutaneous Approach

● **0YHG3YZ** Insertion of Other Device into Left Knee Region, Percutaneous Approach

0YHG41Z Insertion of Radioactive Element into Left Knee Region, Percutaneous Endoscopic Approach

● **0YHG43Z** Insertion of Infusion Device into Left Knee Region, Percutaneous Endoscopic Approach

● **0YHG4YZ** Insertion of Other Device into Left Knee Region, Percutaneous Endoscopic Approach

0YHH01Z Insertion of Radioactive Element into Right Lower Leg, Open Approach

● **0YHH03Z** Insertion of Infusion Device into Right Lower Leg, Open Approach

● **0YHH0YZ** Insertion of Other Device into Right Lower Leg, Open Approach

0YHH31Z Insertion of Radioactive Element into Right Lower Leg, Percutaneous Approach

● **0YHH33Z** Insertion of Infusion Device into Right Lower Leg, Percutaneous Approach

● **0YHH3YZ** Insertion of Other Device into Right Lower Leg, Percutaneous Approach

0YHH41Z Insertion of Radioactive Element into Right Lower Leg, Percutaneous Endoscopic Approach

● **0YHH43Z** Insertion of Infusion Device into Right Lower Leg, Percutaneous Endoscopic Approach

● **0YHH4YZ** Insertion of Other Device into Right Lower Leg, Percutaneous Endoscopic Approach

0YHJ01Z Insertion of Radioactive Element into Left Lower Leg, Open Approach

● **0YHJ03Z** Insertion of Infusion Device into Left Lower Leg, Open Approach

● **0YHJ0YZ** Insertion of Other Device into Left Lower Leg, Open Approach

0YHJ31Z Insertion of Radioactive Element into Left Lower Leg, Percutaneous Approach

● **0YHJ33Z** Insertion of Infusion Device into Left Lower Leg, Percutaneous Approach

● **0YHJ3YZ** Insertion of Other Device into Left Lower Leg, Percutaneous Approach

0YHJ41Z Insertion of Radioactive Element into Left Lower Leg, Percutaneous Endoscopic Approach

● **0YHJ43Z** Insertion of Infusion Device into Left Lower Leg, Percutaneous Endoscopic Approach

● **0YHJ4YZ** Insertion of Other Device into Left Lower Leg, Percutaneous Endoscopic Approach

0YHK01Z Insertion of Radioactive Element into Right Ankle Region, Open Approach

● **0YHK03Z** Insertion of Infusion Device into Right Ankle Region, Open Approach

● **0YHK0YZ** Insertion of Other Device into Right Ankle Region, Open Approach

0YHK31Z Insertion of Radioactive Element into Right Ankle Region, Percutaneous Approach

● **0YHK33Z** Insertion of Infusion Device into Right Ankle Region, Percutaneous Approach

● **0YHK3YZ** Insertion of Other Device into Right Ankle Region, Percutaneous Approach

0YHK41Z Insertion of Radioactive Element into Right Ankle Region, Percutaneous Endoscopic Approach

● **0YHK43Z** Insertion of Infusion Device into Right Ankle Region, Percutaneous Endoscopic Approach

● **0YHK4YZ** Insertion of Other Device into Right Ankle Region, Percutaneous Endoscopic Approach

♀ Female-only   ♂ Male-only   ▲ Limited Coverage   ● Non-OR   ▰ HAC-associated procedure   ▲ Non-covered procedures   ✚ Combination

● 0YHL01Z Insertion of Radioactive Element into Left Ankle Region, Open Approach

● 0YHL03Z Insertion of Infusion Device into Left Ankle Region, Open Approach

● 0YHL0YZ Insertion of Other Device into Left Ankle Region, Open Approach

0YHL31Z Insertion of Radioactive Element into Left Ankle Region, Percutaneous Approach

● 0YHL33Z Insertion of Infusion Device into Left Ankle Region, Percutaneous Approach

● 0YHL3YZ Insertion of Other Device into Left Ankle Region, Percutaneous Approach

0YHL41Z Insertion of Radioactive Element into Left Ankle Region, Percutaneous Endoscopic Approach

● 0YHL43Z Insertion of Infusion Device into Left Ankle Region, Percutaneous Endoscopic Approach

● 0YHL4YZ Insertion of Other Device into Left Ankle Region, Percutaneous Endoscopic Approach

0YHM01Z Insertion of Radioactive Element into Right Foot, Open Approach

● 0YHM03Z Insertion of Infusion Device into Right Foot, Open Approach

● 0YHM0YZ Insertion of Other Device into Right Foot, Open Approach

0YHM31Z Insertion of Radioactive Element into Right Foot, Percutaneous Approach

● 0YHM33Z Insertion of Infusion Device into Right Foot, Percutaneous Approach

● 0YHM3YZ Insertion of Other Device into Right Foot, Percutaneous Approach

0YHM41Z Insertion of Radioactive Element into Right Foot, Percutaneous Endoscopic Approach

● 0YHM43Z Insertion of Infusion Device into Right Foot, Percutaneous Endoscopic Approach

● 0YHM4YZ Insertion of Other Device into Right Foot, Percutaneous Endoscopic Approach

0YHN01Z Insertion of Radioactive Element into Left Foot, Open Approach

● 0YHN03Z Insertion of Infusion Device into Left Foot, Open Approach

● 0YHN0YZ Insertion of Other Device into Left Foot, Open Approach

0YHN31Z Insertion of Radioactive Element into Left Foot, Percutaneous Approach

● 0YHN33Z Insertion of Infusion Device into Left Foot, Percutaneous Approach

● 0YHN3YZ Insertion of Other Device into Left Foot, Percutaneous Approach

0YHN41Z Insertion of Radioactive Element into Left Foot, Percutaneous Endoscopic Approach

● 0YHN43Z Insertion of Infusion Device into Left Foot, Percutaneous Endoscopic Approach

● 0YHN4YZ Insertion of Other Device into Left Foot, Percutaneous Endoscopic Approach

0YJ – Anatomical Regions, Lower Extremities, Inspection

Review Coding Guidelines B3.11a, B3.11b and B3.11c

● 0YJ00ZZ Inspection of Right Buttock, Open Approach

0YJ03ZZ Inspection of Right Buttock, Percutaneous Approach

0YJ04ZZ Inspection of Right Buttock, Percutaneous Endoscopic Approach

0YJ0XZZ Inspection of Right Buttock, External Approach

● 0YJ10ZZ Inspection of Left Buttock, Open Approach

0YJ13ZZ Inspection of Left Buttock, Percutaneous Approach

0YJ14ZZ Inspection of Left Buttock, Percutaneous Endoscopic Approach

0YJ1XZZ Inspection of Left Buttock, External Approach

0YJ50ZZ Inspection of Right Inguinal Region, Open Approach

0YJ53ZZ Inspection of Right Inguinal Region, Percutaneous Approach

0YJ54ZZ Inspection of Right Inguinal Region, Percutaneous Endoscopic Approach

0YJ5XZZ Inspection of Right Inguinal Region, External Approach

0YJ60ZZ Inspection of Left Inguinal Region, Open Approach

0YJ63ZZ Inspection of Left Inguinal Region, Percutaneous Approach

0YJ64ZZ Inspection of Left Inguinal Region, Percutaneous Endoscopic Approach

0YJ6XZZ Inspection of Left Inguinal Region, External Approach

0YJ70ZZ Inspection of Right Femoral Region, Open Approach

0YJ73ZZ Inspection of Right Femoral Region, Percutaneous Approach

0YJ74ZZ Inspection of Right Femoral Region, Percutaneous Endoscopic Approach

0YJ7XZZ Inspection of Right Femoral Region, External Approach

● 0YJ80ZZ Inspection of Left Femoral Region, Open Approach

0YJ83ZZ Inspection of Left Femoral Region, Percutaneous Approach

0YJ84ZZ Inspection of Left Femoral Region, Percutaneous Endoscopic Approach

0YJ8XZZ Inspection of Left Femoral Region, External Approach

● 0YJ90ZZ Inspection of Right Lower Extremity, Open Approach

0YJ93ZZ Inspection of Right Lower Extremity, Percutaneous Approach

0YJ94ZZ Inspection of Right Lower Extremity, Percutaneous Endoscopic Approach

0YJ9XZZ Inspection of Right Lower Extremity, External Approach

0YJA0ZZ Inspection of Bilateral Inguinal Region, Open Approach

0YJA3ZZ Inspection of Bilateral Inguinal Region, Percutaneous Approach

0YJA4ZZ Inspection of Bilateral Inguinal Region, Percutaneous Endoscopic Approach

0YJAXZZ Inspection of Bilateral Inguinal Region, External Approach

● 0YJB0ZZ Inspection of Left Lower Extremity, Open Approach

0YJB3ZZ Inspection of Left Lower Extremity, Percutaneous Approach

0YJB4ZZ Inspection of Left Lower Extremity, Percutaneous Endoscopic Approach

0YJBXZZ Inspection of Left Lower Extremity, External Approach

● 0YJC0ZZ Inspection of Right Upper Leg, Open Approach

0YJC3ZZ Inspection of Right Upper Leg, Percutaneous Approach

0YJC4ZZ Inspection of Right Upper Leg, Percutaneous Endoscopic Approach

0YJCXZZ Inspection of Right Upper Leg, External Approach

● 0YJD0ZZ Inspection of Left Upper Leg, Open Approach

0YJD3ZZ Inspection of Left Upper Leg, Percutaneous Approach

0YJD4ZZ Inspection of Left Upper Leg, Percutaneous Endoscopic Approach

0YJDXZZ Inspection of Left Upper Leg, External Approach

● 0YJE0ZZ Inspection of Bilateral Femoral Region, Open Approach

0YJE3ZZ Inspection of Bilateral Femoral Region, Percutaneous Approach

0YJE4ZZ Inspection of Bilateral Femoral Region, Percutaneous Endoscopic Approach

0YJEXZZ Inspection of Bilateral Femoral Region, External Approach

● 0YJF0ZZ Inspection of Right Knee Region, Open Approach

0YJF3ZZ Inspection of Right Knee Region, Percutaneous Approach

0YJF4ZZ Inspection of Right Knee Region, Percutaneous Endoscopic Approach

0YJFXZZ Inspection of Right Knee Region, External Approach

● 0YJG0ZZ Inspection of Left Knee Region, Open Approach

0YJG3ZZ Inspection of Left Knee Region, Percutaneous Approach

0YJG4ZZ Inspection of Left Knee Region, Percutaneous Endoscopic Approach

0YJGXZZ Inspection of Left Knee Region, External Approach

● 0YJH0ZZ Inspection of Right Lower Leg, Open Approach

0YJH3ZZ Inspection of Right Lower Leg, Percutaneous Approach

0YJH4ZZ Inspection of Right Lower Leg, Percutaneous Endoscopic Approach

0YJHXZZ Inspection of Right Lower Leg, External Approach

● 0YJJ0ZZ Inspection of Left Lower Leg, Open Approach

0YJJ3ZZ Inspection of Left Lower Leg, Percutaneous Approach

0YJJ4ZZ Inspection of Left Lower Leg, Percutaneous Endoscopic Approach

0YJJXZZ Inspection of Left Lower Leg, External Approach

● 0YJK0ZZ Inspection of Right Ankle Region, Open Approach

0YJK3ZZ Inspection of Right Ankle Region, Percutaneous Approach

0YJK4ZZ Inspection of Right Ankle Region, Percutaneous Endoscopic Approach

0YJKXZZ Inspection of Right Ankle Region, External Approach

● 0YJL0ZZ Inspection of Left Ankle Region, Open Approach

0YJL3ZZ Inspection of Left Ankle Region, Percutaneous Approach

0YJL4ZZ Inspection of Left Ankle Region, Percutaneous Endoscopic Approach

0YJLXZZ Inspection of Left Ankle Region, External Approach

● 0YJM0ZZ Inspection of Right Foot, Open Approach

0YJM3ZZ Inspection of Right Foot, Percutaneous Approach

0YJM4ZZ Inspection of Right Foot, Percutaneous Endoscopic Approach

0YJMXZZ Inspection of Right Foot, External Approach

♀ Female-only ♂ Male-only ▲ Limited Coverage ● Non-OR ■ HAC-associated procedure ▲ Non-covered procedures ✚ Combination

0YJN0ZZ Inspection of Left Foot, Open Approach	0YJN4ZZ Inspection of Left Foot, Percutaneous Endoscopic Approach	0YJNXZZ Inspection of Left Foot, External Approach
0YJN3ZZ Inspection of Left Foot, Percutaneous Approach		

0YM – Anatomical Regions, Lower Extremities, Reattachment

0YM00ZZ Reattachment of Right Buttock, Open Approach	0YMC0ZZ Reattachment of Right Upper Leg, Open Approach	0YMQ0ZZ Reattachment of Left 1st Toe, Open Approach
0YM10ZZ Reattachment of Left Buttock, Open Approach	0YMD0ZZ Reattachment of Left Upper Leg, Open Approach	0YMR0ZZ Reattachment of Right 2nd Toe, Open Approach
0YM20ZZ Reattachment of Right Hindquarter, Open Approach	0YMF0ZZ Reattachment of Right Knee Region, Open Approach	0YMS0ZZ Reattachment of Left 2nd Toe, Open Approach
0YM30ZZ Reattachment of Left Hindquarter, Open Approach	0YMG0ZZ Reattachment of Left Knee Region, Open Approach	0YMT0ZZ Reattachment of Right 3rd Toe, Open Approach
0YM40ZZ Reattachment of Bilateral Hindquarter, Open Approach	0YMH0ZZ Reattachment of Right Lower Leg, Open Approach	0YMU0ZZ Reattachment of Left 3rd Toe, Open Approach
0YM50ZZ Reattachment of Right Inguinal Region, Open Approach	0YMJ0ZZ Reattachment of Left Lower Leg, Open Approach	0YMV0ZZ Reattachment of Right 4th Toe, Open Approach
0YM60ZZ Reattachment of Left Inguinal Region, Open Approach	0YMK0ZZ Reattachment of Right Ankle Region, Open Approach	0YMW0ZZ Reattachment of Left 4th Toe, Open Approach
0YM70ZZ Reattachment of Right Femoral Region, Open Approach	0YML0ZZ Reattachment of Left Ankle Region, Open Approach	0YMX0ZZ Reattachment of Right 5th Toe, Open Approach
0YM80ZZ Reattachment of Left Femoral Region, Open Approach	0YMM0ZZ Reattachment of Right Foot, Open Approach	0YMY0ZZ Reattachment of Left 5th Toe, Open Approach
0YM90ZZ Reattachment of Right Lower Extremity, Open Approach	0YMN0ZZ Reattachment of Left Foot, Open Approach	
0YMB0ZZ Reattachment of Left Lower Extremity, Open Approach	0YMP0ZZ Reattachment of Right 1st Toe, Open Approach	

0YP – Anatomical Regions, Lower Extremities, Removal

Review Coding Guideline B6.1c

0YP900Z Removal of Drainage Device from Right Lower Extremity, Open Approach	0YP947Z Removal of Autologous Tissue Substitute from Right Lower Extremity, Percutaneous Endoscopic Approach	0YPB0YZ Removal of Other Device from Left Lower Extremity, Open Approach
0YP901Z Removal of Radioactive Element from Right Lower Extremity, Open Approach	0YP94JZ Removal of Synthetic Substitute from Right Lower Extremity, Percutaneous Endoscopic Approach	0YPB30Z Removal of Drainage Device from Left Lower Extremity, Percutaneous Approach
0YP903Z Removal of Infusion Device from Right Lower Extremity, Open Approach	0YP94KZ Removal of Nonautologous Tissue Substitute from Right Lower Extremity, Percutaneous Endoscopic Approach	0YPB31Z Removal of Radioactive Element from Left Lower Extremity, Percutaneous Approach
0YP907Z Removal of Autologous Tissue Substitute from Right Lower Extremity, Open Approach	0YP94YZ Removal of Other Device from Right Lower Extremity, Percutaneous Endoscopic Approach	0YPB33Z Removal of Infusion Device from Left Lower Extremity, Percutaneous Approach
0YP90JZ Removal of Synthetic Substitute from Right Lower Extremity, Open Approach	0YP9X0Z Removal of Drainage Device from Right Lower Extremity, External Approach	0YPB37Z Removal of Autologous Tissue Substitute from Left Lower Extremity, Percutaneous Approach
0YP90KZ Removal of Nonautologous Tissue Substitute from Right Lower Extremity, Open Approach	0YP9X1Z Removal of Radioactive Element from Right Lower Extremity, External Approach	0YPB3JZ Removal of Synthetic Substitute from Left Lower Extremity, Percutaneous Approach
0YP90YZ Removal of Other Device from Right Lower Extremity, Open Approach	0YP9X3Z Removal of Infusion Device from Right Lower Extremity, External Approach	0YPB3KZ Removal of Nonautologous Tissue Substitute from Left Lower Extremity, Percutaneous Approach
0YP930Z Removal of Drainage Device from Right Lower Extremity, Percutaneous Approach	0YP9X7Z Removal of Autologous Tissue Substitute from Right Lower Extremity, External Approach	0YPB3YZ Removal of Other Device from Left Lower Extremity, Percutaneous Approach
0YP931Z Removal of Radioactive Element from Right Lower Extremity, Percutaneous Approach	0YP9XJZ Removal of Synthetic Substitute from Right Lower Extremity, External Approach	0YPB40Z Removal of Drainage Device from Left Lower Extremity, Percutaneous Endoscopic Approach
0YP933Z Removal of Infusion Device from Right Lower Extremity, Percutaneous Approach	0YP9XKZ Removal of Nonautologous Tissue Substitute from Right Lower Extremity, External Approach	0YPB41Z Removal of Radioactive Element from Left Lower Extremity, Percutaneous Endoscopic Approach
0YP937Z Removal of Autologous Tissue Substitute from Right Lower Extremity, Percutaneous Approach	0YP9XYZ Removal of Other Device from Right Lower Extremity, External Approach	0YPB43Z Removal of Infusion Device from Left Lower Extremity, Percutaneous Endoscopic Approach
0YP93JZ Removal of Synthetic Substitute from Right Lower Extremity, Percutaneous Approach	0YPB00Z Removal of Drainage Device from Left Lower Extremity, Open Approach	0YPB47Z Removal of Autologous Tissue Substitute from Left Lower Extremity, Percutaneous Endoscopic Approach
0YP93KZ Removal of Nonautologous Tissue Substitute from Right Lower Extremity, Percutaneous Approach	0YPB01Z Removal of Radioactive Element from Left Lower Extremity, Open Approach	0YPB4JZ Removal of Synthetic Substitute from Left Lower Extremity, Percutaneous Endoscopic Approach
0YP93YZ Removal of Other Device from Right Lower Extremity, Percutaneous Approach	0YPB03Z Removal of Infusion Device from Left Lower Extremity, Open Approach	0YPB4KZ Removal of Nonautologous Tissue Substitute from Left Lower Extremity, Percutaneous Endoscopic Approach
0YP940Z Removal of Drainage Device from Right Lower Extremity, Percutaneous Endoscopic Approach	0YPB07Z Removal of Autologous Tissue Substitute from Left Lower Extremity, Open Approach	0YPB4YZ Removal of Other Device from Left Lower Extremity, Percutaneous Endoscopic Approach
0YP941Z Removal of Radioactive Element from Right Lower Extremity, Percutaneous Endoscopic Approach	0YPB0JZ Removal of Synthetic Substitute from Left Lower Extremity, Open Approach	0YPBX0Z Removal of Drainage Device from Left Lower Extremity, External Approach
0YP943Z Removal of Infusion Device from Right Lower Extremity, Percutaneous Endoscopic Approach	0YPB0KZ Removal of Nonautologous Tissue Substitute from Left Lower Extremity, Open Approach	0YPBX1Z Removal of Radioactive Element from Left Lower Extremity, External Approach

♀ Female-only	♂ Male-only	▲ Limited Coverage	● Non-OR	▧ HAC-associated procedure	▲ Non-covered procedures	✚ Combination

0YPBX3Z	Removal of Infusion Device from Left Lower Extremity, External Approach
0YPBX7Z	Removal of Autologous Tissue Substitute from Left Lower Extremity, External Approach
0YPBXJZ	Removal of Synthetic Substitute from Left Lower Extremity, External Approach
0YPBXKZ	Removal of Nonautologous Tissue Substitute from Left Lower Extremity, External Approach
0YPBXYZ	Removal of Other Device from Left Lower Extremity, External Approach

0YQ – Anatomical Regions, Lower Extremities, Repair

0YQ00ZZ	Repair Right Buttock, Open Approach
0YQ03ZZ	Repair Right Buttock, Percutaneous Approach
0YQ04ZZ	Repair Right Buttock, Percutaneous Endoscopic Approach
0YQ0XZZ	Repair Right Buttock, External Approach
0YQ10ZZ	Repair Left Buttock, Open Approach
0YQ13ZZ	Repair Left Buttock, Percutaneous Approach
0YQ14ZZ	Repair Left Buttock, Percutaneous Endoscopic Approach
0YQ1XZZ	Repair Left Buttock, External Approach
0YQ50ZZ	Repair Right Inguinal Region, Open Approach
0YQ53ZZ	Repair Right Inguinal Region, Percutaneous Approach
0YQ54ZZ	Repair Right Inguinal Region, Percutaneous Endoscopic Approach
0YQ5XZZ	Repair Right Inguinal Region, External Approach
0YQ60ZZ	Repair Left Inguinal Region, Open Approach
0YQ63ZZ	Repair Left Inguinal Region, Percutaneous Approach
0YQ64ZZ	Repair Left Inguinal Region, Percutaneous Endoscopic Approach
0YQ6XZZ	Repair Left Inguinal Region, External Approach
0YQ70ZZ	Repair Right Femoral Region, Open Approach
0YQ73ZZ	Repair Right Femoral Region, Percutaneous Approach
0YQ74ZZ	Repair Right Femoral Region, Percutaneous Endoscopic Approach
0YQ7XZZ	Repair Right Femoral Region, External Approach
0YQ80ZZ	Repair Left Femoral Region, Open Approach
0YQ83ZZ	Repair Left Femoral Region, Percutaneous Approach
0YQ84ZZ	Repair Left Femoral Region, Percutaneous Endoscopic Approach
0YQ8XZZ	Repair Left Femoral Region, External Approach
0YQ90ZZ	Repair Right Lower Extremity, Open Approach
0YQ93ZZ	Repair Right Lower Extremity, Percutaneous Approach
0YQ94ZZ	Repair Right Lower Extremity, Percutaneous Endoscopic Approach
0YQ9XZZ	Repair Right Lower Extremity, External Approach
0YQA0ZZ	Repair Bilateral Inguinal Region, Open Approach
0YQA3ZZ	Repair Bilateral Inguinal Region, Percutaneous Approach
0YQA4ZZ	Repair Bilateral Inguinal Region, Percutaneous Endoscopic Approach
0YQAXZZ	Repair Bilateral Inguinal Region, External Approach
0YQB0ZZ	Repair Left Lower Extremity, Open Approach
0YQB3ZZ	Repair Left Lower Extremity, Percutaneous Approach
0YQB4ZZ	Repair Left Lower Extremity, Percutaneous Endoscopic Approach
0YQBXZZ	Repair Left Lower Extremity, External Approach
0YQC0ZZ	Repair Right Upper Leg, Open Approach
0YQC3ZZ	Repair Right Upper Leg, Percutaneous Approach
0YQC4ZZ	Repair Right Upper Leg, Percutaneous Endoscopic Approach
0YQCXZZ	Repair Right Upper Leg, External Approach
0YQD0ZZ	Repair Left Upper Leg, Open Approach
0YQD3ZZ	Repair Left Upper Leg, Percutaneous Approach
0YQD4ZZ	Repair Left Upper Leg, Percutaneous Endoscopic Approach
0YQDXZZ	Repair Left Upper Leg, External Approach
0YQE0ZZ	Repair Bilateral Femoral Region, Open Approach
0YQE3ZZ	Repair Bilateral Femoral Region, Percutaneous Approach
0YQE4ZZ	Repair Bilateral Femoral Region, Percutaneous Endoscopic Approach
0YQEXZZ	Repair Bilateral Femoral Region, External Approach
0YQF0ZZ	Repair Right Knee Region, Open Approach
0YQF3ZZ	Repair Right Knee Region, Percutaneous Approach
0YQF4ZZ	Repair Right Knee Region, Percutaneous Endoscopic Approach
0YQFXZZ	Repair Right Knee Region, External Approach
0YQG0ZZ	Repair Left Knee Region, Open Approach
0YQG3ZZ	Repair Left Knee Region, Percutaneous Approach
0YQG4ZZ	Repair Left Knee Region, Percutaneous Endoscopic Approach
0YQGXZZ	Repair Left Knee Region, External Approach
0YQH0ZZ	Repair Right Lower Leg, Open Approach
0YQH3ZZ	Repair Right Lower Leg, Percutaneous Approach
0YQH4ZZ	Repair Right Lower Leg, Percutaneous Endoscopic Approach
0YQHXZZ	Repair Right Lower Leg, External Approach
0YQJ0ZZ	Repair Left Lower Leg, Open Approach
0YQJ3ZZ	Repair Left Lower Leg, Percutaneous Approach
0YQJ4ZZ	Repair Left Lower Leg, Percutaneous Endoscopic Approach
0YQJXZZ	Repair Left Lower Leg, External Approach
0YQK0ZZ	Repair Right Ankle Region, Open Approach
0YQK3ZZ	Repair Right Ankle Region, Percutaneous Approach
0YQK4ZZ	Repair Right Ankle Region, Percutaneous Endoscopic Approach
0YQKXZZ	Repair Right Ankle Region, External Approach
0YQL0ZZ	Repair Left Ankle Region, Open Approach
0YQL3ZZ	Repair Left Ankle Region, Percutaneous Approach
0YQL4ZZ	Repair Left Ankle Region, Percutaneous Endoscopic Approach
0YQLXZZ	Repair Left Ankle Region, External Approach
0YQM0ZZ	Repair Right Foot, Open Approach
0YQM3ZZ	Repair Right Foot, Percutaneous Approach
0YQM4ZZ	Repair Right Foot, Percutaneous Endoscopic Approach
0YQMXZZ	Repair Right Foot, External Approach
0YQN0ZZ	Repair Left Foot, Open Approach
0YQN3ZZ	Repair Left Foot, Percutaneous Approach
0YQN4ZZ	Repair Left Foot, Percutaneous Endoscopic Approach
0YQNXZZ	Repair Left Foot, External Approach
0YQP0ZZ	Repair Right 1st Toe, Open Approach
0YQP3ZZ	Repair Right 1st Toe, Percutaneous Approach
0YQP4ZZ	Repair Right 1st Toe, Percutaneous Endoscopic Approach
0YQPXZZ	Repair Right 1st Toe, External Approach
0YQQ0ZZ	Repair Left 1st Toe, Open Approach
0YQQ3ZZ	Repair Left 1st Toe, Percutaneous Approach
0YQQ4ZZ	Repair Left 1st Toe, Percutaneous Endoscopic Approach
0YQQXZZ	Repair Left 1st Toe, External Approach
0YQR0ZZ	Repair Right 2nd Toe, Open Approach
0YQR3ZZ	Repair Right 2nd Toe, Percutaneous Approach
0YQR4ZZ	Repair Right 2nd Toe, Percutaneous Endoscopic Approach
0YQRXZZ	Repair Right 2nd Toe, External Approach
0YQS0ZZ	Repair Left 2nd Toe, Open Approach
0YQS3ZZ	Repair Left 2nd Toe, Percutaneous Approach
0YQS4ZZ	Repair Left 2nd Toe, Percutaneous Endoscopic Approach
0YQSXZZ	Repair Left 2nd Toe, External Approach
0YQT0ZZ	Repair Right 3rd Toe, Open Approach
0YQT3ZZ	Repair Right 3rd Toe, Percutaneous Approach
0YQT4ZZ	Repair Right 3rd Toe, Percutaneous Endoscopic Approach
0YQTXZZ	Repair Right 3rd Toe, External Approach
0YQU0ZZ	Repair Left 3rd Toe, Open Approach
0YQU3ZZ	Repair Left 3rd Toe, Percutaneous Approach
0YQU4ZZ	Repair Left 3rd Toe, Percutaneous Endoscopic Approach
0YQUXZZ	Repair Left 3rd Toe, External Approach
0YQV0ZZ	Repair Right 4th Toe, Open Approach
0YQV3ZZ	Repair Right 4th Toe, Percutaneous Approach
0YQV4ZZ	Repair Right 4th Toe, Percutaneous Endoscopic Approach
0YQVXZZ	Repair Right 4th Toe, External Approach
0YQW0ZZ	Repair Left 4th Toe, Open Approach
0YQW3ZZ	Repair Left 4th Toe, Percutaneous Approach
0YQW4ZZ	Repair Left 4th Toe, Percutaneous Endoscopic Approach
0YQWXZZ	Repair Left 4th Toe, External Approach
0YQX0ZZ	Repair Right 5th Toe, Open Approach
0YQX3ZZ	Repair Right 5th Toe, Percutaneous Approach
0YQX4ZZ	Repair Right 5th Toe, Percutaneous Endoscopic Approach
0YQXXZZ	Repair Right 5th Toe, External Approach
0YQY0ZZ	Repair Left 5th Toe, Open Approach
0YQY3ZZ	Repair Left 5th Toe, Percutaneous Approach
0YQY4ZZ	Repair Left 5th Toe, Percutaneous Endoscopic Approach
0YQYXZZ	Repair Left 5th Toe, External Approach

0YU007Z Supplement Right Buttock with Autologous Tissue Substitute, Open Approach

0YU00JZ Supplement Right Buttock with Synthetic Substitute, Open Approach

0YU00KZ Supplement Right Buttock with Nonautologous Tissue Substitute, Open Approach

0YU047Z Supplement Right Buttock with Autologous Tissue Substitute, Percutaneous Endoscopic Approach

0YU04JZ Supplement Right Buttock with Synthetic Substitute, Percutaneous Endoscopic Approach

0YU04KZ Supplement Right Buttock with Nonautologous Tissue Substitute, Percutaneous Endoscopic Approach

0YU107Z Supplement Left Buttock with Autologous Tissue Substitute, Open Approach

0YU10JZ Supplement Left Buttock with Synthetic Substitute, Open Approach

0YU10KZ Supplement Left Buttock with Nonautologous Tissue Substitute, Open Approach

0YU147Z Supplement Left Buttock with Autologous Tissue Substitute, Percutaneous Endoscopic Approach

0YU14JZ Supplement Left Buttock with Synthetic Substitute, Percutaneous Endoscopic Approach

0YU14KZ Supplement Left Buttock with Nonautologous Tissue Substitute, Percutaneous Endoscopic Approach

0YU507Z Supplement Right Inguinal Region with Autologous Tissue Substitute, Open Approach

0YU50JZ Supplement Right Inguinal Region with Synthetic Substitute, Open Approach

0YU50KZ Supplement Right Inguinal Region with Nonautologous Tissue Substitute, Open Approach

0YU547Z Supplement Right Inguinal Region with Autologous Tissue Substitute, Percutaneous Endoscopic Approach

0YU54JZ Supplement Right Inguinal Region with Synthetic Substitute, Percutaneous Endoscopic Approach

0YU54KZ Supplement Right Inguinal Region with Nonautologous Tissue Substitute, Percutaneous Endoscopic Approach

0YU607Z Supplement Left Inguinal Region with Autologous Tissue Substitute, Open Approach

0YU60JZ Supplement Left Inguinal Region with Synthetic Substitute, Open Approach

0YU60KZ Supplement Left Inguinal Region with Nonautologous Tissue Substitute, Open Approach

0YU647Z Supplement Left Inguinal Region with Autologous Tissue Substitute, Percutaneous Endoscopic Approach

0YU64JZ Supplement Left Inguinal Region with Synthetic Substitute, Percutaneous Endoscopic Approach

0YU64KZ Supplement Left Inguinal Region with Nonautologous Tissue Substitute, Percutaneous Endoscopic Approach

0YU707Z Supplement Right Femoral Region with Autologous Tissue Substitute, Open Approach

0YU70JZ Supplement Right Femoral Region with Synthetic Substitute, Open Approach

0YU70KZ Supplement Right Femoral Region with Nonautologous Tissue Substitute, Open Approach

0YU747Z Supplement Right Femoral Region with Autologous Tissue Substitute, Percutaneous Endoscopic Approach

0YU74JZ Supplement Right Femoral Region with Synthetic Substitute, Percutaneous Endoscopic Approach

0YU74KZ Supplement Right Femoral Region with Nonautologous Tissue Substitute, Percutaneous Endoscopic Approach

0YU807Z Supplement Left Femoral Region with Autologous Tissue Substitute, Open Approach

0YU80JZ Supplement Left Femoral Region with Synthetic Substitute, Open Approach

0YU80KZ Supplement Left Femoral Region with Nonautologous Tissue Substitute, Open Approach

0YU847Z Supplement Left Femoral Region with Autologous Tissue Substitute, Percutaneous Endoscopic Approach

0YU84JZ Supplement Left Femoral Region with Synthetic Substitute, Percutaneous Endoscopic Approach

0YU84KZ Supplement Left Femoral Region with Nonautologous Tissue Substitute, Percutaneous Endoscopic Approach

0YU907Z Supplement Right Lower Extremity with Autologous Tissue Substitute, Open Approach

0YU90JZ Supplement Right Lower Extremity with Synthetic Substitute, Open Approach

0YU90KZ Supplement Right Lower Extremity with Nonautologous Tissue Substitute, Open Approach

0YU947Z Supplement Right Lower Extremity with Autologous Tissue Substitute, Percutaneous Endoscopic Approach

0YU94JZ Supplement Right Lower Extremity with Synthetic Substitute, Percutaneous Endoscopic Approach

0YU94KZ Supplement Right Lower Extremity with Nonautologous Tissue Substitute, Percutaneous Endoscopic Approach

0YUA07Z Supplement Bilateral Inguinal Region with Autologous Tissue Substitute, Open Approach

0YUA0JZ Supplement Bilateral Inguinal Region with Synthetic Substitute, Open Approach

0YUA0KZ Supplement Bilateral Inguinal Region with Nonautologous Tissue Substitute, Open Approach

0YUA47Z Supplement Bilateral Inguinal Region with Autologous Tissue Substitute, Percutaneous Endoscopic Approach

0YUA4JZ Supplement Bilateral Inguinal Region with Synthetic Substitute, Percutaneous Endoscopic Approach

0YUA4KZ Supplement Bilateral Inguinal Region with Nonautologous Tissue Substitute, Percutaneous Endoscopic Approach

0YUB07Z Supplement Left Lower Extremity with Autologous Tissue Substitute, Open Approach

0YUB0JZ Supplement Left Lower Extremity with Synthetic Substitute, Open Approach

0YUB0KZ Supplement Left Lower Extremity with Nonautologous Tissue Substitute, Open Approach

0YUB47Z Supplement Left Lower Extremity with Autologous Tissue Substitute, Percutaneous Endoscopic Approach

0YUB4JZ Supplement Left Lower Extremity with Synthetic Substitute, Percutaneous Endoscopic Approach

0YUB4KZ Supplement Left Lower Extremity with Nonautologous Tissue Substitute, Percutaneous Endoscopic Approach

0YUC07Z Supplement Right Upper Leg with Autologous Tissue Substitute, Open Approach

0YUC0JZ Supplement Right Upper Leg with Synthetic Substitute, Open Approach

0YUC0KZ Supplement Right Upper Leg with Nonautologous Tissue Substitute, Open Approach

0YUC47Z Supplement Right Upper Leg with Autologous Tissue Substitute, Percutaneous Endoscopic Approach

0YUC4JZ Supplement Right Upper Leg with Synthetic Substitute, Percutaneous Endoscopic Approach

0YUC4KZ Supplement Right Upper Leg with Nonautologous Tissue Substitute, Percutaneous Endoscopic Approach

0YUD07Z Supplement Left Upper Leg with Autologous Tissue Substitute, Open Approach

0YUD0JZ Supplement Left Upper Leg with Synthetic Substitute, Open Approach

0YUD0KZ Supplement Left Upper Leg with Nonautologous Tissue Substitute, Open Approach

0YUD47Z Supplement Left Upper Leg with Autologous Tissue Substitute, Percutaneous Endoscopic Approach

0YUD4JZ Supplement Left Upper Leg with Synthetic Substitute, Percutaneous Endoscopic Approach

0YUD4KZ Supplement Left Upper Leg with Nonautologous Tissue Substitute, Percutaneous Endoscopic Approach

0YUE07Z Supplement Bilateral Femoral Region with Autologous Tissue Substitute, Open Approach

0YUE0JZ Supplement Bilateral Femoral Region with Synthetic Substitute, Open Approach

0YUE0KZ Supplement Bilateral Femoral Region with Nonautologous Tissue Substitute, Open Approach

0YUE47Z Supplement Bilateral Femoral Region with Autologous Tissue Substitute, Percutaneous Endoscopic Approach

0YUE4JZ Supplement Bilateral Femoral Region with Synthetic Substitute, Percutaneous Endoscopic Approach

0YUE4KZ Supplement Bilateral Femoral Region with Nonautologous Tissue Substitute, Percutaneous Endoscopic Approach

0YUF07Z Supplement Right Knee Region with Autologous Tissue Substitute, Open Approach

0YUF0JZ Supplement Right Knee Region with Synthetic Substitute, Open Approach

0YUF0KZ Supplement Right Knee Region with Nonautologous Tissue Substitute, Open Approach

0YUF47Z Supplement Right Knee Region with Autologous Tissue Substitute, Percutaneous Endoscopic Approach

0YUF4JZ Supplement Right Knee Region with Synthetic Substitute, Percutaneous Endoscopic Approach

0YUF4KZ Supplement Right Knee Region with Nonautologous Tissue Substitute, Percutaneous Endoscopic Approach

0YUG07Z Supplement Left Knee Region with Autologous Tissue Substitute, Open Approach

0YUG0JZ Supplement Left Knee Region with Synthetic Substitute, Open Approach

♀ Female-only   ♂ Male-only   ▲ Limited Coverage   ● Non-OR   ▥ HAC-associated procedure   ▲ Non-covered procedures   ✚ Combination

0YUG0KZ	Supplement Left Knee Region with Nonautologous Tissue Substitute, Open Approach
0YUG47Z	Supplement Left Knee Region with Autologous Tissue Substitute, Percutaneous Endoscopic Approach
0YUG4JZ	Supplement Left Knee Region with Synthetic Substitute, Percutaneous Endoscopic Approach
0YUG4KZ	Supplement Left Knee Region with Nonautologous Tissue Substitute, Percutaneous Endoscopic Approach
0YUH07Z	Supplement Right Lower Leg with Autologous Tissue Substitute, Open Approach
0YUH0JZ	Supplement Right Lower Leg with Synthetic Substitute, Open Approach
0YUH0KZ	Supplement Right Lower Leg with Nonautologous Tissue Substitute, Open Approach
0YUH47Z	Supplement Right Lower Leg with Autologous Tissue Substitute, Percutaneous Endoscopic Approach
0YUH4JZ	Supplement Right Lower Leg with Synthetic Substitute, Percutaneous Endoscopic Approach
0YUH4KZ	Supplement Right Lower Leg with Nonautologous Tissue Substitute, Percutaneous Endoscopic Approach
0YUJ07Z	Supplement Left Lower Leg with Autologous Tissue Substitute, Open Approach
0YUJ0JZ	Supplement Left Lower Leg with Synthetic Substitute, Open Approach
0YUJ0KZ	Supplement Left Lower Leg with Nonautologous Tissue Substitute, Open Approach
0YUJ47Z	Supplement Left Lower Leg with Autologous Tissue Substitute, Percutaneous Endoscopic Approach
0YUJ4JZ	Supplement Left Lower Leg with Synthetic Substitute, Percutaneous Endoscopic Approach
0YUJ4KZ	Supplement Left Lower Leg with Nonautologous Tissue Substitute, Percutaneous Endoscopic Approach
0YUK07Z	Supplement Right Ankle Region with Autologous Tissue Substitute, Open Approach
0YUK0JZ	Supplement Right Ankle Region with Synthetic Substitute, Open Approach
0YUK0KZ	Supplement Right Ankle Region with Nonautologous Tissue Substitute, Open Approach
0YUK47Z	Supplement Right Ankle Region with Autologous Tissue Substitute, Percutaneous Endoscopic Approach
0YUK4JZ	Supplement Right Ankle Region with Synthetic Substitute, Percutaneous Endoscopic Approach
0YUK4KZ	Supplement Right Ankle Region with Nonautologous Tissue Substitute, Percutaneous Endoscopic Approach
0YUL07Z	Supplement Left Ankle Region with Autologous Tissue Substitute, Open Approach
0YUL0JZ	Supplement Left Ankle Region with Synthetic Substitute, Open Approach
0YUL0KZ	Supplement Left Ankle Region with Nonautologous Tissue Substitute, Open Approach
0YUL47Z	Supplement Left Ankle Region with Autologous Tissue Substitute, Percutaneous Endoscopic Approach
0YUL4JZ	Supplement Left Ankle Region with Synthetic Substitute, Percutaneous Endoscopic Approach
0YUL4KZ	Supplement Left Ankle Region with Nonautologous Tissue Substitute, Percutaneous Endoscopic Approach
0YUM07Z	Supplement Right Foot with Autologous Tissue Substitute, Open Approach
0YUM0JZ	Supplement Right Foot with Synthetic Substitute, Open Approach
0YUM0KZ	Supplement Right Foot with Nonautologous Tissue Substitute, Open Approach
0YUM47Z	Supplement Right Foot with Autologous Tissue Substitute, Percutaneous Endoscopic Approach
0YUM4JZ	Supplement Right Foot with Synthetic Substitute, Percutaneous Endoscopic Approach
0YUM4KZ	Supplement Right Foot with Nonautologous Tissue Substitute, Percutaneous Endoscopic Approach
0YUN07Z	Supplement Left Foot with Autologous Tissue Substitute, Open Approach
0YUN0JZ	Supplement Left Foot with Synthetic Substitute, Open Approach
0YUN0KZ	Supplement Left Foot with Nonautologous Tissue Substitute, Open Approach
0YUN47Z	Supplement Left Foot with Autologous Tissue Substitute, Percutaneous Endoscopic Approach
0YUN4JZ	Supplement Left Foot with Synthetic Substitute, Percutaneous Endoscopic Approach
0YUN4KZ	Supplement Left Foot with Nonautologous Tissue Substitute, Percutaneous Endoscopic Approach
0YUP07Z	Supplement Right 1st Toe with Autologous Tissue Substitute, Open Approach
0YUP0JZ	Supplement Right 1st Toe with Synthetic Substitute, Open Approach
0YUP0KZ	Supplement Right 1st Toe with Nonautologous Tissue Substitute, Open Approach
0YUP47Z	Supplement Right 1st Toe with Autologous Tissue Substitute, Percutaneous Endoscopic Approach
0YUP4JZ	Supplement Right 1st Toe with Synthetic Substitute, Percutaneous Endoscopic Approach
0YUP4KZ	Supplement Right 1st Toe with Nonautologous Tissue Substitute, Percutaneous Endoscopic Approach
0YUQ07Z	Supplement Left 1st Toe with Autologous Tissue Substitute, Open Approach
0YUQ0JZ	Supplement Left 1st Toe with Synthetic Substitute, Open Approach
0YUQ0KZ	Supplement Left 1st Toe with Nonautologous Tissue Substitute, Open Approach
0YUQ47Z	Supplement Left 1st Toe with Autologous Tissue Substitute, Percutaneous Endoscopic Approach
0YUQ4JZ	Supplement Left 1st Toe with Synthetic Substitute, Percutaneous Endoscopic Approach
0YUQ4KZ	Supplement Left 1st Toe with Nonautologous Tissue Substitute, Percutaneous Endoscopic Approach
0YUR07Z	Supplement Right 2nd Toe with Autologous Tissue Substitute, Open Approach
0YUR0JZ	Supplement Right 2nd Toe with Synthetic Substitute, Open Approach
0YUR0KZ	Supplement Right 2nd Toe with Nonautologous Tissue Substitute, Open Approach
0YUR47Z	Supplement Right 2nd Toe with Autologous Tissue Substitute, Percutaneous Endoscopic Approach
0YUR4JZ	Supplement Right 2nd Toe with Synthetic Substitute, Percutaneous Endoscopic Approach
0YUR4KZ	Supplement Right 2nd Toe with Nonautologous Tissue Substitute, Percutaneous Endoscopic Approach
0YUS07Z	Supplement Left 2nd Toe with Autologous Tissue Substitute, Open Approach
0YUS0JZ	Supplement Left 2nd Toe with Synthetic Substitute, Open Approach
0YUS0KZ	Supplement Left 2nd Toe with Nonautologous Tissue Substitute, Open Approach
0YUS47Z	Supplement Left 2nd Toe with Autologous Tissue Substitute, Percutaneous Endoscopic Approach
0YUS4JZ	Supplement Left 2nd Toe with Synthetic Substitute, Percutaneous Endoscopic Approach
0YUS4KZ	Supplement Left 2nd Toe with Nonautologous Tissue Substitute, Percutaneous Endoscopic Approach
0YUT07Z	Supplement Right 3rd Toe with Autologous Tissue Substitute, Open Approach
0YUT0JZ	Supplement Right 3rd Toe with Synthetic Substitute, Open Approach
0YUT0KZ	Supplement Right 3rd Toe with Nonautologous Tissue Substitute, Open Approach
0YUT47Z	Supplement Right 3rd Toe with Autologous Tissue Substitute, Percutaneous Endoscopic Approach
0YUT4JZ	Supplement Right 3rd Toe with Synthetic Substitute, Percutaneous Endoscopic Approach
0YUT4KZ	Supplement Right 3rd Toe with Nonautologous Tissue Substitute, Percutaneous Endoscopic Approach
0YUU07Z	Supplement Left 3rd Toe with Autologous Tissue Substitute, Open Approach
0YUU0JZ	Supplement Left 3rd Toe with Synthetic Substitute, Open Approach
0YUU0KZ	Supplement Left 3rd Toe with Nonautologous Tissue Substitute, Open Approach
0YUU47Z	Supplement Left 3rd Toe with Autologous Tissue Substitute, Percutaneous Endoscopic Approach
0YUU4JZ	Supplement Left 3rd Toe with Synthetic Substitute, Percutaneous Endoscopic Approach
0YUU4KZ	Supplement Left 3rd Toe with Nonautologous Tissue Substitute, Percutaneous Endoscopic Approach
0YUV07Z	Supplement Right 4th Toe with Autologous Tissue Substitute, Open Approach
0YUV0JZ	Supplement Right 4th Toe with Synthetic Substitute, Open Approach
0YUV0KZ	Supplement Right 4th Toe with Nonautologous Tissue Substitute, Open Approach
0YUV47Z	Supplement Right 4th Toe with Autologous Tissue Substitute, Percutaneous Endoscopic Approach
0YUV4JZ	Supplement Right 4th Toe with Synthetic Substitute, Percutaneous Endoscopic Approach
0YUV4KZ	Supplement Right 4th Toe with Nonautologous Tissue Substitute, Percutaneous Endoscopic Approach

♀ Female-only   ♂ Male-only   ▲ Limited Coverage   ● Non-OR   ▆ HAC-associated procedure   ▲ Non-covered procedures   ✚ Combination

0YUW07Z	Supplement Left 4th Toe with Autologous Tissue Substitute, Open Approach	0YUX07Z	Supplement Right 5th Toe with Autologous Tissue Substitute, Open Approach	0YUY07Z	Supplement Left 5th Toe with Autologous Tissue Substitute, Open Approach
0YUW0JZ	Supplement Left 4th Toe with Synthetic Substitute, Open Approach	0YUX0JZ	Supplement Right 5th Toe with Synthetic Substitute, Open Approach	0YUY0JZ	Supplement Left 5th Toe with Synthetic Substitute, Open Approach
0YUW0KZ	Supplement Left 4th Toe with Nonautologous Tissue Substitute, Open Approach	0YUX0KZ	Supplement Right 5th Toe with Nonautologous Tissue Substitute, Open Approach	0YUY0KZ	Supplement Left 5th Toe with Nonautologous Tissue Substitute, Open Approach
0YUW47Z	Supplement Left 4th Toe with Autologous Tissue Substitute, Percutaneous Endoscopic Approach	0YUX47Z	Supplement Right 5th Toe with Autologous Tissue Substitute, Percutaneous Endoscopic Approach	0YUY47Z	Supplement Left 5th Toe with Autologous Tissue Substitute, Percutaneous Endoscopic Approach
0YUW4JZ	Supplement Left 4th Toe with Synthetic Substitute, Percutaneous Endoscopic Approach	0YUX4JZ	Supplement Right 5th Toe with Synthetic Substitute, Percutaneous Endoscopic Approach	0YUY4JZ	Supplement Left 5th Toe with Synthetic Substitute, Percutaneous Endoscopic Approach
0YUW4KZ	Supplement Left 4th Toe with Nonautologous Tissue Substitute, Percutaneous Endoscopic Approach	0YUX4KZ	Supplement Right 5th Toe with Nonautologous Tissue Substitute, Percutaneous Endoscopic Approach	0YUY4KZ	Supplement Left 5th Toe with Nonautologous Tissue Substitute, Percutaneous Endoscopic Approach

0YW – Anatomical Regions, Lower Extremities, Revision

Review Coding Guideline B6.1c

- **0YW900Z** Revision of Drainage Device in Right Lower Extremity, Open Approach
- **0YW903Z** Revision of Infusion Device in Right Lower Extremity, Open Approach
- **0YW907Z** Revision of Autologous Tissue Substitute in Right Lower Extremity, Open Approach
- **0YW90JZ** Revision of Synthetic Substitute in Right Lower Extremity, Open Approach
- **0YW90KZ** Revision of Nonautologous Tissue Substitute in Right Lower Extremity, Open Approach
- **0YW90YZ** Revision of Other Device in Right Lower Extremity, Open Approach
- **0YW930Z** Revision of Drainage Device in Right Lower Extremity, Percutaneous Approach
- **0YW933Z** Revision of Infusion Device in Right Lower Extremity, Percutaneous Approach
- **0YW937Z** Revision of Autologous Tissue Substitute in Right Lower Extremity, Percutaneous Approach
- **0YW93JZ** Revision of Synthetic Substitute in Right Lower Extremity, Percutaneous Approach
- **0YW93KZ** Revision of Nonautologous Tissue Substitute in Right Lower Extremity, Percutaneous Approach
- **0YW93YZ** Revision of Other Device in Right Lower Extremity, Percutaneous Approach
- **0YW940Z** Revision of Drainage Device in Right Lower Extremity, Percutaneous Endoscopic Approach
- **0YW943Z** Revision of Infusion Device in Right Lower Extremity, Percutaneous Endoscopic Approach
- **0YW947Z** Revision of Autologous Tissue Substitute in Right Lower Extremity, Percutaneous Endoscopic Approach
- **0YW94JZ** Revision of Synthetic Substitute in Right Lower Extremity, Percutaneous Endoscopic Approach
- **0YW94KZ** Revision of Nonautologous Tissue Substitute in Right Lower Extremity, Percutaneous Endoscopic Approach

- **0YW94YZ** Revision of Other Device in Right Lower Extremity, Percutaneous Endoscopic Approach
- **0YW9X0Z** Revision of Drainage Device in Right Lower Extremity, External Approach
- **0YW9X3Z** Revision of Infusion Device in Right Lower Extremity, External Approach
- **0YW9X7Z** Revision of Autologous Tissue Substitute in Right Lower Extremity, External Approach
- **0YW9XJZ** Revision of Synthetic Substitute in Right Lower Extremity, External Approach
- **0YW9XKZ** Revision of Nonautologous Tissue Substitute in Right Lower Extremity, External Approach
- **0YW9XYZ** Revision of Other Device in Right Lower Extremity, External Approach
- ● **0YWB00Z** Revision of Drainage Device in Left Lower Extremity, Open Approach
- ● **0YWB03Z** Revision of Infusion Device in Left Lower Extremity, Open Approach
- ● **0YWB07Z** Revision of Autologous Tissue Substitute in Left Lower Extremity, Open Approach
- ● **0YWB0JZ** Revision of Synthetic Substitute in Left Lower Extremity, Open Approach
- ● **0YWB0KZ** Revision of Nonautologous Tissue Substitute in Left Lower Extremity, Open Approach
- ● **0YWB0YZ** Revision of Other Device in Left Lower Extremity, Open Approach
- ● **0YWB30Z** Revision of Drainage Device in Left Lower Extremity, Percutaneous Approach
- ● **0YWB33Z** Revision of Infusion Device in Left Lower Extremity, Percutaneous Approach
- ● **0YWB37Z** Revision of Autologous Tissue Substitute in Left Lower Extremity, Percutaneous Approach
- ● **0YWB3JZ** Revision of Synthetic Substitute in Left Lower Extremity, Percutaneous Approach
- ● **0YWB3KZ** Revision of Nonautologous Tissue Substitute in Left Lower Extremity, Percutaneous Approach

- ● **0YWB3YZ** Revision of Other Device in Left Lower Extremity, Percutaneous Approach
- ● **0YWB40Z** Revision of Drainage Device in Left Lower Extremity, Percutaneous Endoscopic Approach
- ● **0YWB43Z** Revision of Infusion Device in Left Lower Extremity, Percutaneous Endoscopic Approach
- ● **0YWB47Z** Revision of Autologous Tissue Substitute in Left Lower Extremity, Percutaneous Endoscopic Approach
- ● **0YWB4JZ** Revision of Synthetic Substitute in Left Lower Extremity, Percutaneous Endoscopic Approach
- ● **0YWB4KZ** Revision of Nonautologous Tissue Substitute in Left Lower Extremity, Percutaneous Endoscopic Approach
- ● **0YWB4YZ** Revision of Other Device in Left Lower Extremity, Percutaneous Endoscopic Approach
- **0YWBX0Z** Revision of Drainage Device in Left Lower Extremity, External Approach
- **0YWBX3Z** Revision of Infusion Device in Left Lower Extremity, External Approach
- **0YWBX7Z** Revision of Autologous Tissue Substitute in Left Lower Extremity, External Approach
- **0YWBXJZ** Revision of Synthetic Substitute in Left Lower Extremity, External Approach
- **0YWBXKZ** Revision of Nonautologous Tissue Substitute in Left Lower Extremity, External Approach
- **0YWBXYZ** Revision of Other Device in Left Lower Extremity, External Approach

♀ Female-only	♂ Male-only	▲ Limited Coverage	● Non-OR	HAC HAC-associated procedure	▲ Non-covered procedures	✚ Combination

Within each section of ICD-10-PCS the characters have different meanings. The seven character meanings for the Obstetrics section are illustrated here through the procedure example of *Manually-assisted delivery.*

Section	Body System	Root Operation	Body Part	Approach	Device	Qualifier
Obstetrics	Pregnancy	Delivery	Products of Conception	External	None	None
1	0	E	0	X	Z	Z

Section (Character 1)

All Obstetric procedure codes have a first character value of 1.

Body System (Character 2)

The alphanumeric character for the body system is placed in the second position. The body system applicable to the Obstetrics section is Pregnancy and has a character value of 0.

Root Operations (Character 3)

The alphanumeric character value for root operations is placed in the third position. Listed below are the root operations applicable to the Obstetrics section with their associated meaning.

Character Value	Root Operation	Root Operation Definition
2	Change	Taking out or off a device from a body part and putting back an identical or similar device in or on the same body part without cutting or puncturing the skin or a mucous membrane
9	Drainage	Taking or letting out fluids and/or gases from a body part
A	Abortion	Artificially terminating a pregnancy
D	Extraction	Pulling or stripping out or off all or a portion of a body part by the use of force
E	Delivery	Assisting the passage of the products of conception from the genital canal
H	Insertion	Putting in a nonbiological appliance that monitors, assists, performs, or prevents a physiological function but does not physically take the place of a body part
J	Inspection	Visually and/or manually exploring a body part
P	Removal	Taking out or off a device from a body part, region or orifice
Q	Repair	Restoring, to the extent possible, a body part to its normal anatomic structure and function
S	Reposition	Moving to its normal location, or other suitable location, all or a portion of a body part
T	Resection	Cutting out or off, without replacement, all of a body part
Y	Transplantation	Putting in or on all or a portion of a living body part taken from another individual or animal to physically take the place and/or function of all or a portion of a similar body part

Body Part (Character 4)

For each body system the applicable body part character values will be available for procedure code construction. An example of a body part is Products of Conception.

Approach (Character 5)

The approach is the technique used to reach the procedure site. The following are the approach character values for the Obstetrics section with the associated definitions.

Character Value	Approach	Approach Definition
0	Open	Cutting through the skin or mucous membrane and any other body layers necessary to expose the site of the procedure
3	Percutaneous	Entry, by puncture or minor incision, of instrumentation through the skin or mucous membrane and any other body layers necessary to reach the site of the procedure

Continued →

Character Value	Approach	Approach Definition
4	Percutaneous Endoscopic	Entry, by puncture or minor incision, of instrumentation through the skin or mucous membrane and any other body layers necessary to reach and visualize the site of the procedure
7	Via Natural or Artificial Opening	Entry of instrumentation through a natural or artificial external opening to reach the site of the procedure
8	Via Natural or Artificial Opening Endoscopic	Entry of instrumentation through a natural or artificial external opening to reach and visualize the site of the procedure
X	External	Procedures performed directly on the skin or mucous membrane and procedures performed indirectly by the application of external force through the skin or mucous membrane

Device (Character 6)

Depending on the procedure performed there may or may not be a device used. There are two types of devices included in the Obstetrics section: monitoring electrode and other device. When a device is not utilized during the procedure, the placeholder Z is the character value that should be reported.

Qualifier (Character 7)

The qualifier represents an additional attribute for the procedure when applicable. For example, drainage procedures in this section include several qualifiers including fetal cerebrospinal fluid that is reported with the character value of A. If there is no qualifier for a procedure, the placeholder Z is the character valve that should be reported.

Obstetric Section Guidelines (section 1)

C. Obstetrics Section

Products of Conception

C1. Procedures performed on the products of conception are coded to the Obstetrics section. Procedures performed on the pregnant female other than the products of conception are coded to the appropriate root operation in the Medical and Surgical section.

Example: Amniocentesis is coded to the products of conception body part in the Obstetrics section. Repair of obstetric urethral laceration is coded to the urethra body part in the Medical and Surgical section.

Procedures following delivery or abortion

C2. Procedures performed following a delivery or abortion for curettage of the endometrium or evacuation of retained products of conception are all coded in the Obstetrics section, to the root operation Extraction and the body part Products of Conception, Retained. Diagnostic or therapeutic dilation and curettage performed during times other than the postpartum or post-abortion period are all coded in the Medical and Surgical section, to the root operation Extraction and the body part Endometrium.

Obstetrics Section Tables and Code Listings

Obstetrics Tables 102–10Y

Section	1	Obstetrics
Body System	0	Pregnancy
Operation	2	**Change:** Taking out or off a device from a body part and putting back an identical or similar device in or on the same body part without cutting or puncturing the skin or a mucous membrane

Body Part (4th)	Approach (5th)	Device (6th)	Qualifier (7th)
0 Products of Conception	7 Via Natural or Artificial Opening	3 Monitoring Electrode Y Other Device	Z No Qualifier

Section   1   **Obstetrics**
Body System   0   **Pregnancy**
Operation   9   **Drainage:** Taking or letting out fluids and/or gases from a body part

Body Part (4th)	Approach (5th)	Device (6th)	Qualifier (7th)
0 Products of Conception	0 Open 3 Percutaneous 4 Percutaneous Endoscopic 7 Via Natural or Artificial Opening 8 Via Natural or Artificial Opening Endoscopic	Z No Device	9 Fetal Blood A Fetal Cerebrospinal Fluid B Fetal Fluid, Other C Amniotic Fluid, Therapeutic D Fluid, Other U Amniotic Fluid, Diagnostic

Section   1   **Obstetrics**
Body System   0   **Pregnancy**
Operation   A   **Abortion:** Artificially terminating a pregnancy

Body Part (4th)	Approach (5th)	Device (6th)	Qualifier (7th)
0 Products of Conception	0 Open 3 Percutaneous 4 Percutaneous Endoscopic 8 Via Natural or Artificial Opening Endoscopic	Z No Device	Z No Qualifier
0 Products of Conception	7 Via Natural or Artificial Opening	Z No Device	6 Vacuum W Laminaria X Abortifacient Z No Qualifier

Section   1   **Obstetrics**
Body System   0   **Pregnancy**
Operation   D   **Extraction:** Pulling or stripping out or off all or a portion of a body part by the use of force

Body Part (4th)	Approach (5th)	Device (6th)	Qualifier (7th)
0 Products of Conception	0 Open	Z No Device	0 Classical 1 Low Cervical 2 Extraperitoneal
0 Products of Conception	7 Via Natural or Artificial Opening	Z No Device	3 Low Forceps 4 Mid Forceps 5 High Forceps 6 Vacuum 7 Internal Version 8 Other
1 Products of Conception, Retained 2 Products of Conception, Ectopic	7 Via Natural or Artificial Opening 8 Via Natural or Artificial Opening Endoscopic	Z No Device	Z No Qualifier

Section   1   **Obstetrics**
Body System   0   **Pregnancy**
Operation   E   **Delivery:** Assisting the passage of the products of conception from the genital canal

Body Part (4th)	Approach (5th)	Device (6th)	Qualifier (7th)
0 Products of Conception	X External	Z No Device	Z No Qualifier

Section	1	Obstetrics
Body System	0	Pregnancy
Operation	H	**Insertion:** Putting in a nonbiological appliance that monitors, assists, performs, or prevents a physiological function but does not physically take the place of a body part

Body Part (4th)	Approach (5th)	Device (6th)	Qualifier (7th)
0 Products of Conception	0 Open 7 Via Natural or Artificial Opening	3 Monitoring Electrode Y Other Device	Z No Qualifier

Section	1	Obstetrics
Body System	0	Pregnancy
Operation	J	**Inspection:** Visually and/or manually exploring a body part

Body Part (4th)	Approach (5th)	Device (6th)	Qualifier (7th)
0 Products of Conception 1 Products of Conception, Retained 2 Products of Conception, Ectopic	0 Open 3 Percutaneous 4 Percutaneous Endoscopic 7 Via Natural or Artificial Opening 8 Via Natural or Artificial Opening Endoscopic X External	Z No Device	Z No Qualifier

Section	1	Obstetrics
Body System	0	Pregnancy
Operation	P	**Removal:** Taking out or off a device from a body part, region or orifice

Body Part (4th)	Approach (5th)	Device (6th)	Qualifier (7th)
0 Products of Conception	0 Open 7 Via Natural or Artificial Opening	3 Monitoring Electrode Y Other Device	Z No Qualifier

Section	1	Obstetrics
Body System	0	Pregnancy
Operation	Q	**Repair:** Restoring, to the extent possible, a body part to its normal anatomic structure and function

Body Part (4th)	Approach (5th)	Device (6th)	Qualifier (7th)
0 Products of Conception	0 Open 3 Percutaneous 4 Percutaneous Endoscopic 7 Via Natural or Artificial Opening 8 Via Natural or Artificial Opening Endoscopic	Y Other Device Z No Device	E Nervous System F Cardiovascular System G Lymphatics and Hemic H Eye J Ear, Nose and Sinus K Respiratory System L Mouth and Throat M Gastrointestinal System N Hepatobiliary and Pancreas P Endocrine System Q Skin R Musculoskeletal System S Urinary System T Female Reproductive System V Male Reproductive System Y Other Body System

Section   1   **Obstetrics**
Body System   0   **Pregnancy**
Operation   S   **Reposition:** Moving to its normal location, or other suitable location, all or a portion of a body part

Body Part (4th)	Approach (5th)	Device (6th)	Qualifier (7th)
0 Products of Conception	7 Via Natural or Artificial Opening X External	Z No Device	Z No Qualifier
2 Products of Conception, Ectopic	0 Open 3 Percutaneous 4 Percutaneous Endoscopic 7 Via Natural or Artificial Opening 8 Via Natural or Artificial Opening Endoscopic	Z No Device	Z No Qualifier

Section   1   **Obstetrics**
Body System   0   **Pregnancy**
Operation   T   **Resection:** Cutting out or off, without replacement, all of a body part

Body Part (4th)	Approach (5th)	Device (6th)	Qualifier (7th)
2 Products of Conception, Ectopic	0 Open 3 Percutaneous 4 Percutaneous Endoscopic 7 Via Natural or Artificial Opening 8 Via Natural or Artificial Opening Endoscopic	Z No Device	Z No Qualifier

Section   1   **Obstetrics**
Body System   0   **Pregnancy**
Operation   Y   **Transplantation:** Putting in or on all or a portion of a living body part taken from another individual or animal to physically take the place and/or function of all or a portion of a similar body part

Body Part (4th)	Approach (5th)	Device (6th)	Qualifier (7th)
0 Products of Conception	3 Percutaneous 4 Percutaneous Endoscopic 7 Via Natural or Artificial Opening	Z No Device	E Nervous System F Cardiovascular System G Lymphatics and Hemic H Eye J Ear, Nose and Sinus K Respiratory System L Mouth and Throat M Gastrointestinal System N Hepatobiliary and Pancreas P Endocrine System Q Skin R Musculoskeletal System S Urinary System T Female Reproductive System V Male Reproductive System Y Other Body System

102 – Obstetrics, Pregnancy, Change

Review Coding Guideline C1

102073Z Change Monitoring Electrode in Products of Conception, Via Natural or Artificial Opening

♀ 10207YZ Change Other Device in Products of Conception, Via Natural or Artificial Opening

109 – Obstetrics, Pregnancy, Drainage

10900Z9 Drainage of Fetal Blood from Products of Conception, Open Approach

10900ZA Drainage of Fetal Cerebrospinal Fluid from Products of Conception, Open Approach

10900ZB Drainage of Other Fetal Fluid from Products of Conception, Open Approach

10900ZC Drainage of Amniotic Fluid, Therapeutic from Products of Conception, Open Approach

10900ZD Drainage of Other Fluid from Products of Conception, Open Approach

10900ZU Drainage of Amniotic Fluid, Diagnostic from Products of Conception, Open Approach

10903Z9 Drainage of Fetal Blood from Products of Conception, Percutaneous Approach

10903ZA Drainage of Fetal Cerebrospinal Fluid from Products of Conception, Percutaneous Approach

10903ZB Drainage of Other Fetal Fluid from Products of Conception, Percutaneous Approach

10903ZC Drainage of Amniotic Fluid, Therapeutic from Products of Conception, Percutaneous Approach

10903ZD Drainage of Other Fluid from Products of Conception, Percutaneous Approach

10903ZU Drainage of Amniotic Fluid, Diagnostic from Products of Conception, Percutaneous Approach

♀ 10904Z9 Drainage of Fetal Blood from Products of Conception, Percutaneous Endoscopic Approach

♀ 10904ZA Drainage of Fetal Cerebrospinal Fluid from Products of Conception, Percutaneous Endoscopic Approach

♀ 10904ZB Drainage of Other Fetal Fluid from Products of Conception, Percutaneous Endoscopic Approach

♀ 10904ZC Drainage of Amniotic Fluid, Therapeutic from Products of Conception, Percutaneous Endoscopic Approach
AHA CC: 3Q, 2014, 12-13

♀ 10904ZD Drainage of Other Fluid from Products of Conception, Percutaneous Endoscopic Approach

♀ 10904ZU Drainage of Amniotic Fluid, Diagnostic from Products of Conception, Percutaneous Endoscopic Approach

♀ 10907Z9 Drainage of Fetal Blood from Products of Conception, Via Natural or Artificial Opening

♀ 10907ZA Drainage of Fetal Cerebrospinal Fluid from Products of Conception, Via Natural or Artificial Opening

♀ 10907ZB Drainage of Other Fetal Fluid from Products of Conception, Via Natural or Artificial Opening

♀ 10907ZC Drainage of Amniotic Fluid, Therapeutic from Products of Conception, Via Natural or Artificial Opening
AHA CC: 2Q, 2014, 9-10

♀ 10907ZD Drainage of Other Fluid from Products of Conception, Via Natural or Artificial Opening

♀ 10907ZU Drainage of Amniotic Fluid, Diagnostic from Products of Conception, Via Natural or Artificial Opening

♀ 10908Z9 Drainage of Fetal Blood from Products of Conception, Via Natural or Artificial Opening Endoscopic

♀ 10908ZA Drainage of Fetal Cerebrospinal Fluid from Products of Conception, Via Natural or Artificial Opening Endoscopic

♀ 10908ZB Drainage of Other Fetal Fluid from Products of Conception, Via Natural or Artificial Opening Endoscopic

♀ 10908ZC Drainage of Amniotic Fluid, Therapeutic from Products of Conception, Via Natural or Artificial Opening Endoscopic

♀ 10908ZD Drainage of Other Fluid from Products of Conception, Via Natural or Artificial Opening Endoscopic

♀ 10908ZU Drainage of Amniotic Fluid, Diagnostic from Products of Conception, Via Natural or Artificial Opening Endoscopic

10A – Obstetrics, Pregnancy, Abortion

10A00ZZ Abortion of Products of Conception, Open Approach

10A03ZZ Abortion of Products of Conception, Percutaneous Approach

10A04ZZ Abortion of Products of Conception, Percutaneous Endoscopic Approach

♀● 10A07Z6 Abortion of Products of Conception, Vacuum, Via Natural or Artificial Opening

♀ 10A07ZW Abortion of Products of Conception, Laminaria, Via Natural or Artificial Opening

♀ 10A07ZX Abortion of Products of Conception, Abortifacient, Via Natural or Artificial Opening

♀ 10A07ZZ Abortion of Products of Conception, Via Natural or Artificial Opening

♀ 10A08ZZ Abortion of Products of Conception, Via Natural or Artificial Opening Endoscopic

10D – Obstetrics, Pregnancy, Extraction

Review Coding Guideline C2

10D00Z0 Extraction of Products of Conception, Classical, Open Approach

10D00Z1 Extraction of Products of Conception, Low Cervical, Open Approach

10D00Z2 Extraction of Products of Conception, Extraperitoneal, Open Approach

10D07Z3 Extraction of Products of Conception, Low Forceps, Via Natural or Artificial Opening

●10D07Z4 Extraction of Products of Conception, Mid Forceps, Via Natural or Artificial Opening

♀● 10D07Z5 Extraction of Products of Conception, High Forceps, Via Natural or Artificial Opening

♀● 10D07Z6 Extraction of Products of Conception, Vacuum, Via Natural or Artificial Opening
AHA CC: 4Q, 2014, 43

♀● 10D07Z7 Extraction of Products of Conception, Internal Version, Via Natural or Artificial Opening

♀ 10D07Z8 Extraction of Products of Conception, Other, Via Natural or Artificial Opening

♀ 10D17ZZ Extraction of Products of Conception, Retained, Via Natural or Artificial Opening

♀ 10D18ZZ Extraction of Products of Conception, Retained, Via Natural or Artificial Opening Endoscopic

♀ 10D27ZZ Extraction of Products of Conception, Ectopic, Via Natural or Artificial Opening

♀ 10D28ZZ Extraction of Products of Conception, Ectopic, Via Natural or Artificial Opening Endoscopic

10E – Obstetrics, Pregnancy, Delivery

●10E0XZZ Delivery of Products of Conception, External Approach
AHA CC: 2Q, 2014, 9-10; 4Q, 2014, 17-18

♀ Female-only   ♂ Male-only   ▲ Limited Coverage   ● Non-OR   ▬ HAC-associated procedure   ▲ Non-covered procedures   ✛ Combination

10H – Obstetrics, Pregnancy, Insertion

♀ **10H003Z** Insertion of Monitoring Electrode into Products of Conception, Open Approach

♀ **10H00YZ** Insertion of Other Device into Products of Conception, Open Approach

♀ **10H073Z** Insertion of Monitoring Electrode into Products of Conception, Via Natural or Artificial Opening

♀ **10H07YZ** Insertion of Other Device into Products of Conception, Via Natural or Artificial Opening
AHA CC: 2Q, 2013, 36

10J – Obstetrics, Pregnancy, Inspection

♀ **10J00ZZ** Inspection of Products of Conception, Open Approach

♀ **10J03ZZ** Inspection of Products of Conception, Percutaneous Approach

♀ **10J04ZZ** Inspection of Products of Conception, Percutaneous Endoscopic Approach

♀ **10J07ZZ** Inspection of Products of Conception, Via Natural or Artificial Opening

♀ **10J08ZZ** Inspection of Products of Conception, Via Natural or Artificial Opening Endoscopic

♀ **10J0XZZ** Inspection of Products of Conception, External Approach

♀ **10J10ZZ** Inspection of Products of Conception, Retained, Open Approach

♀ **10J13ZZ** Inspection of Products of Conception, Retained, Percutaneous Approach

♀ **10J14ZZ** Inspection of Products of Conception, Retained, Percutaneous Endoscopic Approach

♀ **10J17ZZ** Inspection of Products of Conception, Retained, Via Natural or Artificial Opening

♀ **10J18ZZ** Inspection of Products of Conception, Retained, Via Natural or Artificial Opening Endoscopic

♀ **10J1XZZ** Inspection of Products of Conception, Retained, External Approach

♀ **10J20ZZ** Inspection of Products of Conception, Ectopic, Open Approach

♀ **10J23ZZ** Inspection of Products of Conception, Ectopic, Percutaneous Approach

♀ **10J24ZZ** Inspection of Products of Conception, Ectopic, Percutaneous Endoscopic Approach

♀ **10J27ZZ** Inspection of Products of Conception, Ectopic, Via Natural or Artificial Openin

♀ **10J28ZZ** Inspection of Products of Conception, Ectopic, Via Natural or Artificial Opening Endoscopic

♀ **10J2XZZ** Inspection of Products of Conception, Ectopic, External Approach

10P – Obstetrics, Pregnancy, Removal

♀ **10P003Z** Removal of Monitoring Electrode from Products of Conception, Open Approach

♀ **10P00YZ** Removal of Other Device from Products of Conception, Open Approach

♀ **10P073Z** Removal of Monitoring Electrode from Products of Conception, Via Natural or Artificial Opening

♀ **10P07YZ** Removal of Other Device from Products of Conception, Via Natural or Artificial Opening

10Q – Obstetrics, Pregnancy, Repair

♀ **10Q00YE** Repair Nervous System in Products of Conception with Other Device, Open Approach

♀ **10Q00YF** Repair Cardiovascular System in Products of Conception with Other Device, Open Approach

♀ **10Q00YG** Repair Lymphatics and Hemic in Products of Conception with Other Device, Open Approach

♀ **10Q00YH** Repair Eye in Products of Conception with Other Device, Open Approach

♀ **10Q00YJ** Repair Ear, Nose and Sinus in Products of Conception with Other Device, Open Approach

♀ **10Q00YK** Repair Respiratory System in Products of Conception with Other Device, Open Approach

♀ **10Q00YL** Repair Mouth and Throat in Products of Conception with Other Device, Open Approach

♀ **10Q00YM** Repair Gastrointestinal System in Products of Conception with Other Device, Open Approach

♀ **10Q00YN** Repair Hepatobiliary and Pancreas in Products of Conception with Other Device, Open Approach

♀ **10Q00YP** Repair Endocrine System in Products of Conception with Other Device, Open Approach

♀ **10Q00YQ** Repair Skin in Products of Conception with Other Device, Open Approach

♀ **10Q00YR** Repair Musculoskeletal System in Products of Conception with Other Device, Open Approach

♀ **10Q00YS** Repair Urinary System in Products of Conception with Other Device, Open Approach

♀ **10Q00YT** Repair Female Reproductive System in Products of Conception with Other Device, Open Approach

♀ **10Q00YV** Repair Male Reproductive System in Products of Conception with Other Device, Open Approach

♀ **10Q00YY** Repair Other Body System in Products of Conception with Other Device, Open Approach

♀ **10Q00ZE** Repair Nervous System in Products of Conception, Open Approach

♀ **10Q00ZF** Repair Cardiovascular System in Products of Conception, Open Approach

♀ **10Q00ZG** Repair Lymphatics and Hemic in Products of Conception, Open Approach

♀ **10Q00ZH** Repair Eye in Products of Conception, Open Approach

♀ **10Q00ZJ** Repair Ear, Nose and Sinus in Products of Conception, Open Approach

♀ **10Q00ZK** Repair Respiratory System in Products of Conception, Open Approach

♀ **10Q00ZL** Repair Mouth and Throat in Products of Conception, Open Approach

♀ **10Q00ZM** Repair Gastrointestinal System in Products of Conception, Open Approach

♀ **10Q00ZN** Repair Hepatobiliary and Pancreas in Products of Conception, Open Approach

♀ **10Q00ZP** Repair Endocrine System in Products of Conception, Open Approach

♀ **10Q00ZQ** Repair Skin in Products of Conception, Open Approach

♀ **10Q00ZR** Repair Musculoskeletal System in Products of Conception, Open Approach

♀ **10Q00ZS** Repair Urinary System in Products of Conception, Open Approach

♀ **10Q00ZT** Repair Female Reproductive System in Products of Conception, Open Approach

♀ **10Q00ZV** Repair Male Reproductive System in Products of Conception, Open Approach

♀ **10Q00ZY** Repair Other Body System in Products of Conception, Open Approach

♀ **10Q03YE** Repair Nervous System in Products of Conception with Other Device, Percutaneous Approach

♀ **10Q03YF** Repair Cardiovascular System in Products of Conception with Other Device, Percutaneous Approach

♀ **10Q03YG** Repair Lymphatics and Hemic in Products of Conception with Other Device, Percutaneous Approach

♀ **10Q03YH** Repair Eye in Products of Conception with Other Device, Percutaneous Approach

♀ **10Q03YJ** Repair Ear, Nose and Sinus in Products of Conception with Other Device, Percutaneous Approach

♀ **10Q03YK** Repair Respiratory System in Products of Conception with Other Device, Percutaneous Approach

♀ **10Q03YL** Repair Mouth and Throat in Products of Conception with Other Device, Percutaneous Approach

♀ **10Q03YM** Repair Gastrointestinal System in Products of Conception with Other Device, Percutaneous Approach

♀ **10Q03YN** Repair Hepatobiliary and Pancreas in Products of Conception with Other Device, Percutaneous Approach

♀ **10Q03YP** Repair Endocrine System in Products of Conception with Other Device, Percutaneous Approach

♀ **10Q03YQ** Repair Skin in Products of Conception with Other Device, Percutaneous Approach

♀ **10Q03YR** Repair Musculoskeletal System in Products of Conception with Other Device, Percutaneous Approach

♀ **10Q03YS** Repair Urinary System in Products of Conception with Other Device, Percutaneous Approach

♀ **10Q03YT** Repair Female Reproductive System in Products of Conception with Other Device, Percutaneous Approach

♀ **10Q03YV** Repair Male Reproductive System in Products of Conception with Other Device, Percutaneous Approach

♀ **10Q03YY** Repair Other Body System in Products of Conception with Other Device, Percutaneous Approach

♀ **10Q03ZE** Repair Nervous System in Products of Conception, Percutaneous Approach

♀ **10Q03ZF** Repair Cardiovascular System in Products of Conception, Percutaneous Approach

♀ Female-only   ♂ Male-only   ▲ Limited Coverage   ● Non-OR   ▬ HAC-associated procedure   ▲ Non-covered procedures   ✚ Combination

0Q03ZG Repair Lymphatics and Hemic in Products of Conception, Percutaneous Approach

0Q03ZH Repair Eye in Products of Conception, Percutaneous Approach

0Q03ZJ Repair Ear, Nose and Sinus in Products of Conception, Percutaneous Approach

0Q03ZK Repair Respiratory System in Products of Conception, Percutaneous Approach

0Q03ZL Repair Mouth and Throat in Products of Conception, Percutaneous Approach

0Q03ZM Repair Gastrointestinal System in Products of Conception, Percutaneous Approach

0Q03ZN Repair Hepatobiliary and Pancreas in Products of Conception, Percutaneous Approach

0Q03ZP Repair Endocrine System in Products of Conception, Percutaneous Approach

10Q03ZQ Repair Skin in Products of Conception, Percutaneous Approach

10Q03ZR Repair Musculoskeletal System in Products of Conception, Percutaneous Approach

10Q03ZS Repair Urinary System in Products of Conception, Percutaneous Approach

10Q03ZT Repair Female Reproductive System in Products of Conception, Percutaneous Approach

10Q03ZV Repair Male Reproductive System in Products of Conception, Percutaneous Approach

10Q03ZY Repair Other Body System in Products of Conception, Percutaneous Approach

10Q04YE Repair Nervous System in Products of Conception with Other Device, Percutaneous Endoscopic Approach

10Q04YF Repair Cardiovascular System in Products of Conception with Other Device, Percutaneous Endoscopic Approach

10Q04YG Repair Lymphatics and Hemic in Products of Conception with Other Device, Percutaneous Endoscopic Approach

10Q04YH Repair Eye in Products of Conception with Other Device, Percutaneous Endoscopic Approach

10Q04YJ Repair Ear, Nose and Sinus in Products of Conception with Other Device, Percutaneous Endoscopic Approach

10Q04YK Repair Respiratory System in Products of Conception with Other Device, Percutaneous Endoscopic Approach

10Q04YL Repair Mouth and Throat in Products of Conception with Other Device, Percutaneous Endoscopic Approach

10Q04YM Repair Gastrointestinal System in Products of Conception with Other Device, Percutaneous Endoscopic Approach

10Q04YN Repair Hepatobiliary and Pancreas in Products of Conception with Other Device, Percutaneous Endoscopic Approach

10Q04YP Repair Endocrine System in Products of Conception with Other Device, Percutaneous Endoscopic Approach

10Q04YQ Repair Skin in Products of Conception with Other Device, Percutaneous Endoscopic Approach

10Q04YR Repair Musculoskeletal System in Products of Conception with Other Device, Percutaneous Endoscopic Approach

10Q04YS Repair Urinary System in Products of Conception with Other Device, Percutaneous Endoscopic Approach

♀10Q04YT Repair Female Reproductive System in Products of Conception with Other Device, Percutaneous Endoscopic Approach

♀ 10Q04YV Repair Male Reproductive System in Products of Conception with Other Device, Percutaneous Endoscopic Approach

♀ 10Q04YY Repair Other Body System in Products of Conception with Other Device, Percutaneous Endoscopic Approach

♀ 10Q04ZE Repair Nervous System in Products of Conception, Percutaneous Endoscopic Approach

♀ 10Q04ZF Repair Cardiovascular System in Products of Conception, Percutaneous Endoscopic Approach

♀ 10Q04ZG Repair Lymphatics and Hemic in Products of Conception, Percutaneous Endoscopic Approach

♀ 10Q04ZH Repair Eye in Products of Conception, Percutaneous Endoscopic Approach

♀ 10Q04ZJ Repair Ear, Nose and Sinus in Products of Conception, Percutaneous Endoscopic Approach

♀ 10Q04ZK Repair Respiratory System in Products of Conception, Percutaneous Endoscopic Approach

♀ 10Q04ZL Repair Mouth and Throat in Products of Conception, Percutaneous Endoscopic Approach

♀ 10Q04ZM Repair Gastrointestinal System in Products of Conception, Percutaneous Endoscopic Approach

♀ 10Q04ZN Repair Hepatobiliary and Pancreas in Products of Conception, Percutaneous Endoscopic Approach

♀ 10Q04ZP Repair Endocrine System in Products of Conception, Percutaneous Endoscopic Approach

♀ 10Q04ZQ Repair Skin in Products of Conception, Percutaneous Endoscopic Approach

♀ 10Q04ZR Repair Musculoskeletal System in Products of Conception, Percutaneous Endoscopic Approach

♀ 10Q04ZS Repair Urinary System in Products of Conception, Percutaneous Endoscopic Approach

♀ 10Q04ZT Repair Female Reproductive System in Products of Conception, Percutaneous Endoscopic Approach

♀ 10Q04ZV Repair Male Reproductive System in Products of Conception, Percutaneous Endoscopic Approach

♀ 10Q04ZY Repair Other Body System in Products of Conception, Percutaneous Endoscopic Approach

AHA CC: 3Q, 2014, 12-13

♀ 10Q07YE Repair Nervous System in Products of Conception with Other Device, Via Natural or Artificial Opening

♀ 10Q07YF Repair Cardiovascular System in Products of Conception with Other Device, Via Natural or Artificial Opening

♀ 10Q07YG Repair Lymphatics and Hemic in Products of Conception with Other Device, Via Natural or Artificial Opening

♀ 10Q07YH Repair Eye in Products of Conception with Other Device, Via Natural or Artificial Opening

♀ 10Q07YJ Repair Ear, Nose and Sinus in Products of Conception with Other Device, Via Natural or Artificial Opening

♀ 10Q07YK Repair Respiratory System in Products of Conception with Other Device, Via Natural or Artificial Opening

♀ 10Q07YL Repair Mouth and Throat in Products of Conception with Other Device, Via Natural or Artificial Opening

♀ 10Q07YM Repair Gastrointestinal System in Products of Conception with Other Device, Via Natural or Artificial Opening

♀ 10Q07YN Repair Hepatobiliary and Pancreas in Products of Conception with Other Device, Via Natural or Artificial Opening

♀ 10Q07YP Repair Endocrine System in Products of Conception with Other Device, Via Natural or Artificial Opening

♀ 10Q07YQ Repair Skin in Products of Conception with Other Device, Via Natural or Artificial Opening

♀ 10Q07YR Repair Musculoskeletal System in Products of Conception with Other Device, Via Natural or Artificial Opening

♀ 10Q07YS Repair Urinary System in Products of Conception with Other Device, Via Natural or Artificial Opening

♀ 10Q07YT Repair Female Reproductive System in Products of Conception with Other Device, Via Natural or Artificial Opening

♀ 10Q07YV Repair Male Reproductive System in Products of Conception with Other Device, Via Natural or Artificial Opening

♀ 10Q07YY Repair Other Body System in Products of Conception with Other Device, Via Natural or Artificial Opening

♀ 10Q07ZE Repair Nervous System in Products of Conception, Via Natural or Artificial Opening

♀ 10Q07ZF Repair Cardiovascular System in Products of Conception, Via Natural or Artificial Opening

♀ 10Q07ZG Repair Lymphatics and Hemic in Products of Conception, Via Natural or Artificial Opening

♀ 10Q07ZH Repair Eye in Products of Conception, Via Natural or Artificial Opening

♀ 10Q07ZJ Repair Ear, Nose and Sinus in Products of Conception, Via Natural or Artificial Opening

♀ 10Q07ZK Repair Respiratory System in Products of Conception, Via Natural or Artificial Opening

♀ 10Q07ZL Repair Mouth and Throat in Products of Conception, Via Natural or Artificial Opening

♀ 10Q07ZM Repair Gastrointestinal System in Products of Conception, Via Natural or Artificial Opening

♀ 10Q07ZN Repair Hepatobiliary and Pancreas in Products of Conception, Via Natural or Artificial Opening

♀ 10Q07ZP Repair Endocrine System in Products of Conception, Via Natural or Artificial Opening

♀ 10Q07ZQ Repair Skin in Products of Conception, Via Natural or Artificial Opening

♀ 10Q07ZR Repair Musculoskeletal System in Products of Conception, Via Natural or Artificial Opening

♀ 10Q07ZS Repair Urinary System in Products of Conception, Via Natural or Artificial Opening

♀ 10Q07ZT Repair Female Reproductive System in Products of Conception, Via Natural or Artificial Opening

♀ 10Q07ZV Repair Male Reproductive System in Products of Conception, Via Natural or Artificial Opening

♀ 10Q07ZY Repair Other Body System in Products of Conception, Via Natural or Artificial Opening

♀ 10Q08YE Repair Nervous System in Products of Conception with Other Device, Via Natural or Artificial Opening Endoscopic

♀ 10Q08YF Repair Cardiovascular System in Products of Conception with Other Device, Via Natural or Artificial Opening Endoscopic

1185

♀ **10Q08YG** Repair Lymphatics and Hemic in Products of Conception with Other Device, Via Natural or Artificial Opening Endoscopic

♀ **10Q08YH** Repair Eye in Products of Conception with Other Device, Via Natural or Artificial Opening Endoscopic

♀ **10Q08YJ** Repair Ear, Nose and Sinus in Products of Conception with Other Device, Via Natural or Artificial Opening Endoscopic

♀ **10Q08YK** Repair Respiratory System in Products of Conception with Other Device, Via Natural or Artificial Opening Endoscopic

♀ **10Q08YL** Repair Mouth and Throat in Products of Conception with Other Device, Via Natural or Artificial Opening Endoscopic

♀ **10Q08YM** Repair Gastrointestinal System in Products of Conception with Other Device, Via Natural or Artificial Opening Endoscopic

♀ **10Q08YN** Repair Hepatobiliary and Pancreas in Products of Conception with Other Device, Via Natural or Artificial Opening Endoscopic

♀ **10Q08YP** Repair Endocrine System in Products of Conception with Other Device, Via Natural or Artificial Opening Endoscopic

♀ **10Q08YQ** Repair Skin in Products of Conception with Other Device, Via Natural or Artificial Opening Endoscopic

♀ **10Q08YR** Repair Musculoskeletal System in Products of Conception with Other Device, Via Natural or Artificial Opening Endoscopic

♀ **10Q08YS** Repair Urinary System in Products of Conception with Other Device, Via Natural or Artificial Opening Endoscopic

♀ **10Q08YT** Repair Female Reproductive System in Products of Conception with Other Device, Via Natural or Artificial Opening Endoscopic

♀ **10Q08YV** Repair Male Reproductive System in Products of Conception with Other Device, Via Natural or Artificial Opening Endoscopic

♀ **10Q08YY** Repair Other Body System in Products of Conception with Other Device, Via Natural or Artificial Opening Endoscopic

♀ **10Q08ZE** Repair Nervous System in Products of Conception, Via Natural or Artificial Opening Endoscopic

♀ **10Q08ZF** Repair Cardiovascular System in Products of Conception, Via Natural or Artificial Opening Endoscopic

♀ **10Q08ZG** Repair Lymphatics and Hemic in Products of Conception, Via Natural or Artificial Opening Endoscopic

♀ **10Q08ZH** Repair Eye in Products of Conception, Via Natural or Artificial Opening Endoscopic

♀ **10Q08ZJ** Repair Ear, Nose and Sinus in Products of Conception, Via Natural or Artificial Opening Endoscopic

♀ **10Q08ZK** Repair Respiratory System in Products of Conception, Via Natural or Artificial Opening Endoscopic

♀ **10Q08ZL** Repair Mouth and Throat in Products of Conception, Via Natural or Artificial Opening Endoscopic

♀ **10Q08ZM** Repair Gastrointestinal System in Products of Conception, Via Natural or Artificial Opening Endoscopic

♀ **10Q08ZN** Repair Hepatobiliary and Pancreas in Products of Conception, Via Natural or Artificial Opening Endoscopic

♀ **10Q08ZP** Repair Endocrine System in Products of Conception, Via Natural or Artificial Opening Endoscopic

♀ **10Q08ZQ** Repair Skin in Products of Conception, Via Natural or Artificial Opening Endoscopic

♀ **10Q08ZR** Repair Musculoskeletal System in Products of Conception, Via Natural or Artificial Opening Endoscopic

♀ **10Q08ZS** Repair Urinary System in Products of Conception, Via Natural or Artificial Opening Endoscopic

♀ **10Q08ZT** Repair Female Reproductive System in Products of Conception, Via Natural or Artificial Opening Endoscopic

♀ **10Q08ZV** Repair Male Reproductive System in Products of Conception, Via Natural or Artificial Opening Endoscopic

♀ **10Q08ZY** Repair Other Body System in Products of Conception, Via Natural or Artificial Opening Endoscopic

10S – Obstetrics, Pregnancy, Reposition

♀● **10S07ZZ** Reposition Products of Conception, Via Natural or Artificial Opening

♀ **10S0XZZ** Reposition Products of Conception, External Approach

♀ **10S20ZZ** Reposition Products of Conception, Ectopic, Open Approach

♀ **10S23ZZ** Reposition Products of Conception, Ectopic, Percutaneous Approach

♀ **10S24ZZ** Reposition Products of Conception, Ectopic, Percutaneous Endoscopic Approach

♀ **10S27ZZ** Reposition Products of Conception, Ectopic, Via Natural or Artificial Opening

♀ **10S28ZZ** Reposition Products of Conception, Ectopic, Via Natural or Artificial Opening Endoscopic

10T – Obstetrics, Pregnancy, Resection

♀ **10T20ZZ** Resection of Products of Conception, Ectopic, Open Approach

♀ **10T23ZZ** Resection of Products of Conception, Ectopic, Percutaneous Approach

♀ **10T24ZZ** Resection of Products of Conception, Ectopic, Percutaneous Endoscopic Approach

♀ **10T27ZZ** Resection of Products of Conception, Ectopic, Via Natural or Artificial Opening

♀ **10T28ZZ** Resection of Products of Conception, Ectopic, Via Natural or Artificial Opening Endoscopic

10Y – Obstetrics, Pregnancy, Transplantation

♀ **10Y03ZE** Transplantation of Nervous System into Products of Conception, Percutaneous Approach

♀ **10Y03ZF** Transplantation of Cardiovascular System into Products of Conception, Percutaneous Approach

♀ **10Y03ZG** Transplantation of Lymphatics and Hemic into Products of Conception, Percutaneous Approach

♀ **10Y03ZH** Transplantation of Eye into Products of Conception, Percutaneous Approach

♀ **10Y03ZJ** Transplantation of Ear, Nose and Sinus into Products of Conception, Percutaneous Approach

♀ **10Y03ZK** Transplantation of Respiratory System into Products of Conception, Percutaneous Approach

♀ **10Y03ZL** Transplantation of Mouth and Throat into Products of Conception, Percutaneous Approach

♀ **10Y03ZM** Transplantation of Gastrointestinal System into Products of Conception, Percutaneous Approach

♀ **10Y03ZN** Transplantation of Hepatobiliary and Pancreas into Products of Conception, Percutaneous Approach

♀ **10Y03ZP** Transplantation of Endocrine System into Products of Conception, Percutaneous Approach

♀ **10Y03ZQ** Transplantation of Skin into Products of Conception, Percutaneous Approach

♀ **10Y03ZR** Transplantation of Musculoskeletal System into Products of Conception, Percutaneous Approach

♀ **10Y03ZS** Transplantation of Urinary System into Products of Conception, Percutaneous Approach

♀ **10Y03ZT** Transplantation of Female Reproductive System into Products of Conception, Percutaneous Approach

♀ **10Y03ZV** Transplantation of Male Reproductive System into Products of Conception, Percutaneous Approach

♀ **10Y03ZY** Transplantation of Other Body System into Products of Conception, Percutaneous Approach

♀ **10Y04ZE** Transplantation of Nervous System into Products of Conception, Percutaneous Endoscopic Approach

♀ **10Y04ZF** Transplantation of Cardiovascular System into Products of Conception, Percutaneous Endoscopic Approach

♀ **10Y04ZG** Transplantation of Lymphatics and Hemic into Products of Conception, Percutaneous Endoscopic Approach

♀ **10Y04ZH** Transplantation of Eye into Products of Conception, Percutaneous Endoscopic Approach

♀ **10Y04ZJ** Transplantation of Ear, Nose and Sinus into Products of Conception, Percutaneous Endoscopic Approach

♀ **10Y04ZK** Transplantation of Respiratory System into Products of Conception, Percutaneous Endoscopic Approach

♀ **10Y04ZL** Transplantation of Mouth and Throat into Products of Conception, Percutaneous Endoscopic Approach

♀ **10Y04ZM** Transplantation of Gastrointestinal System into Products of Conception, Percutaneous Endoscopic Approach

♀ **10Y04ZN** Transplantation of Hepatobiliary and Pancreas into Products of Conception, Percutaneous Endoscopic Approach

♀ **10Y04ZP** Transplantation of Endocrine System into Products of Conception, Percutaneous Endoscopic Approach

♀ Female-only　　♂ Male-only　　▲ Limited Coverage　　● Non-OR　　▨ HAC-associated procedure　　▲ Non-covered procedures　　✚ Combination

Y04ZQ Transplantation of Skin into Products of Conception, Percutaneous Endoscopic Approach

Y04ZR Transplantation of Musculoskeletal System into Products of Conception, Percutaneous Endoscopic Approach

Y04ZS Transplantation of Urinary System into Products of Conception, Percutaneous Endoscopic Approach

Y04ZT Transplantation of Female Reproductive System into Products of Conception, Percutaneous Endoscopic Approach

Y04ZV Transplantation of Male Reproductive System into Products of Conception, Percutaneous Endoscopic Approach

Y04ZY Transplantation of Other Body System into Products of Conception, Percutaneous Endoscopic Approach

Y07ZE Transplantation of Nervous System into Products of Conception, Via Natural or Artificial Opening

♀ **10Y07ZF** Transplantation of Cardiovascular System into Products of Conception, Via Natural or Artificial Opening

♀ **10Y07ZG** Transplantation of Lymphatics and Hemic into Products of Conception, Via Natural or Artificial Opening

♀ **10Y07ZH** Transplantation of Eye into Products of Conception, Via Natural or Artificial Opening

♀ **10Y07ZJ** Transplantation of Ear, Nose and Sinus into Products of Conception, Via Natural or Artificial Opening

♀ **10Y07ZK** Transplantation of Respiratory System into Products of Conception, Via Natural or Artificial Opening

♀ **10Y07ZL** Transplantation of Mouth and Throat into Products of Conception, Via Natural or Artificial Opening

♀ **10Y07ZM** Transplantation of Gastrointestinal System into Products of Conception, Via Natural or Artificial Opening

♀ **10Y07ZN** Transplantation of Hepatobiliary and Pancreas into Products of Conception, Via Natural or Artificial Opening

♀ **10Y07ZP** Transplantation of Endocrine System into Products of Conception, Via Natural or Artificial Opening

♀ **10Y07ZQ** Transplantation of Skin into Products of Conception, Via Natural or Artificial Opening

♀ **10Y07ZR** Transplantation of Musculoskeletal System into Products of Conception, Via Natural or Artificial Opening

♀ **10Y07ZS** Transplantation of Urinary System into Products of Conception, Via Natural or Artificial Opening

♀ **10Y07ZT** Transplantation of Female Reproductive System into Products of Conception, Via Natural or Artificial Opening

♀ **10Y07ZV** Transplantation of Male Reproductive System into Products of Conception, Via Natural or Artificial Opening

♀ **10Y07ZY** Transplantation of Other Body System into Products of Conception, Via Natural or Artificial Opening

Within each section of ICD-10-PCS the characters have different meanings. The seven character meanings for the Placement section illustrated below through the procedure example of *Placement of pressure dressing on abdominal wall*.

Section	Body System	Root Operation	Body Region	Approach	Device	Qualifier
Placement	Anatomical Regions	Compression	Abdominal Wall	External	Pressure Dressing	None
2	W	1	3	X	6	Z

Section (Character 1)

All Placement procedure codes have a first character value of 2.

Body System (Character 2)

The alphanumeric character for the body system is placed in the second position. There are two character values applicable for the Placement section. The character value of W is reported for anatomical regions. The character value Y is reported for anatomical orifices.

Root Operations (Character 3)

The alphanumeric character value for root operations is placed in the third position. The following are the root operations applicable to the Placement section with their associated meaning.

Character Value	Root Operation	Root Operation Definition
0	Change	Taking out or off a device from a body part and putting back an identical or similar device in or on the same body part without cutting or puncturing the skin or a mucous membrane
1	Compression	Putting pressure on a body region
2	Dressing	Putting material on a body region for protection
3	Immobilization	Limiting or preventing motion of a body region
4	Packing	Putting material in a body region or orifice
5	Removal	Taking out or off a device from a body part
6	Traction	Exerting a pulling force on a body region in a distal direction

Body Region (Character 4)

For each body system the applicable body part character values will be available for procedure code construction. An example of a body region is Chest Wall.

Approach (Character 5)

The only approach technique utilized for the Placement section is External approach and is reported with the character value of X.

Character Value	Approach	Approach Definition
X	External	Procedures performed directly on the skin or mucous membrane and procedures performed indirectly by the application of external force through the skin or mucous membrane

Device (Character 6)

Depending on the procedure performed there may or may not be a device used. There are several types of devices included in the Placement section. Here is a sample list of the devices included in this section:

- Cast
- Packing material
- Pressure dressing
- Traction apparatus

en a device is not utilized during the procedure, the placeholder Z is the character value that should be reported.

ualifier (Character 7)

e qualifier represents an additional attribute for the procedure when applicable. Currently, there are no qualifiers in the Placement section; refore, the placeholder character value of Z should be reported.

ction Notes

fore reporting Change and Removal procedures in this section users should *Review coding guideline B6.1c.*

HA Coding Clinic

/60X0Z Traction of Head using Traction Apparatus - AHA CC: 2Q, 2013, 39

lacement Section Tables

acement Tables 2W0–2Y5

ction	2	**Placement**
dy System	W	**Anatomical Regions**
peration	0	**Change:** Taking out or off a device from a body part and putting back an identical or similar device in or on the same body part without cutting or puncturing the skin or a mucous membrane

Body Region (4ᵗʰ)	Approach (5ᵗʰ)	Device (6ᵗʰ)	Qualifier (7ᵗʰ)
0 Head	X External	0 Traction Apparatus	Z No Qualifier
2 Neck		1 Splint	
3 Abdominal Wall		2 Cast	
4 Chest Wall		3 Brace	
5 Back		4 Bandage	
6 Inguinal Region, Right		5 Packing Material	
7 Inguinal Region, Left		6 Pressure Dressing	
8 Upper Extremity, Right		7 Intermittent Pressure	
9 Upper Extremity, Left		Device	
A Upper Arm, Right		Y Other Device	
B Upper Arm, Left			
C Lower Arm, Right			
D Lower Arm, Left			
E Hand, Right			
F Hand, Left			
G Thumb, Right			
H Thumb, Left			
J Finger, Right			
K Finger, Left			
L Lower Extremity, Right			
M Lower Extremity, Left			
N Upper Leg, Right			
P Upper Leg, Left			
Q Lower Leg, Right			
R Lower Leg, Left			
S Foot, Right			
T Foot, Left			
U Toe, Right			
V Toe, Left			
1 Face	X External	0 Traction Apparatus	Z No Qualifier
		1 Splint	
		2 Cast	
		3 Brace	
		4 Bandage	
		5 Packing Material	
		6 Pressure Dressing	
		7 Intermittent Pressure Device	
		9 Wire	
		Y Other Device	

Section	2	Placement
Body System	W	Anatomical Regions
Operation	1	Compression: Putting pressure on a body region

Body Region (4th)	Approach (5th)	Device (6th)	Qualifier (7th)
0 Head	X External	6 Pressure Dressing	Z No Qualifier
1 Face		7 Intermittent Pressure Device	
2 Neck			
3 Abdominal Wall			
4 Chest Wall			
5 Back			
6 Inguinal Region, Right			
7 Inguinal Region, Left			
8 Upper Extremity, Right			
9 Upper Extremity, Left			
A Upper Arm, Right			
B Upper Arm, Left			
C Lower Arm, Right			
D Lower Arm, Left			
E Hand, Right			
F Hand, Left			
G Thumb, Right			
H Thumb, Left			
J Finger, Right			
K Finger, Left			
L Lower Extremity, Right			
M Lower Extremity, Left			
N Upper Leg, Right			
P Upper Leg, Left			
Q Lower Leg, Right			
R Lower Leg, Left			
S Foot, Right			
T Foot, Left			
U Toe, Right			
V Toe, Left			

Section	2	Placement
Body System	W	Anatomical Regions
Operation	2	**Dressing:** Putting material on a body region for protection

Body Region (4ᵗʰ)	Approach (5ᵗʰ)	Device (6ᵗʰ)	Qualifier (7ᵗʰ)
0 Head	X External	4 Bandage	Z No Qualifier
1 Face			
2 Neck			
3 Abdominal Wall			
4 Chest Wall			
5 Back			
6 Inguinal Region, Right			
7 Inguinal Region, Left			
8 Upper Extremity, Right			
9 Upper Extremity, Left			
A Upper Arm, Right			
B Upper Arm, Left			
C Lower Arm, Right			
D Lower Arm, Left			
E Hand, Right			
F Hand, Left			
G Thumb, Right			
H Thumb, Left			
J Finger, Right			
K Finger, Left			
L Lower Extremity, Right			
M Lower Extremity, Left			
N Upper Leg, Right			
P Upper Leg, Left			
Q Lower Leg, Right			
R Lower Leg, Left			
S Foot, Right			
T Foot, Left			
U Toe, Right			
V Toe, Left			

Section   2   Placement
Body System   W   Anatomical Regions
Operation   3   **Immobilization:** Limiting or preventing motion of a body region

Body Region (4th)	Approach (5th)	Device (6th)	Qualifier (7th)
0 Head 2 Neck 3 Abdominal Wall 4 Chest Wall 5 Back 6 Inguinal Region, Right 7 Inguinal Region, Left 8 Upper Extremity, Right 9 Upper Extremity, Left A Upper Arm, Right B Upper Arm, Left C Lower Arm, Right D Lower Arm, Left E Hand, Right F Hand, Left G Thumb, Right H Thumb, Left J Finger, Right K Finger, Left L Lower Extremity, Right M Lower Extremity, Left N Upper Leg, Right P Upper Leg, Left Q Lower Leg, Right R Lower Leg, Left S Foot, Right T Foot, Left U Toe, Right V Toe, Left	X External	1 Splint 2 Cast 3 Brace Y Other Device	Z No Qualifier
1 Face	X External	1 Splint 2 Cast 3 Brace 9 Wire Y Other Device	Z No Qualifier

Section	2	Placement
Body System	W	Anatomical Regions
Operation	4	Packing: Putting material in a body region or orifice

Body Region (4th)	Approach (5th)	Device (6th)	Qualifier (7th)
0 Head	X External	5 Packing Material	Z No Qualifier
1 Face			
2 Neck			
3 Abdominal Wall			
4 Chest Wall			
5 Back			
6 Inguinal Region, Right			
7 Inguinal Region, Left			
8 Upper Extremity, Right			
9 Upper Extremity, Left			
A Upper Arm, Right			
B Upper Arm, Left			
C Lower Arm, Right			
D Lower Arm, Left			
E Hand, Right			
F Hand, Left			
G Thumb, Right			
H Thumb, Left			
J Finger, Right			
K Finger, Left			
L Lower Extremity, Right			
M Lower Extremity, Left			
N Upper Leg, Right			
P Upper Leg, Left			
Q Lower Leg, Right			
R Lower Leg, Left			
S Foot, Right			
T Foot, Left			
U Toe, Right			
V Toe, Left			

Section	2	Placement
Body System	W	Anatomical Regions
Operation	5	Removal: Taking out or off a device from a body part

Body Region (4ᵗʰ)	Approach (5ᵗʰ)	Device (6ᵗʰ)	Qualifier (7ᵗʰ)
0 Head 2 Neck 3 Abdominal Wall 4 Chest Wall 5 Back 6 Inguinal Region, Right 7 Inguinal Region, Left 8 Upper Extremity, Right 9 Upper Extremity, Left A Upper Arm, Right B Upper Arm, Left C Lower Arm, Right D Lower Arm, Left E Hand, Right F Hand, Left G Thumb, Right H Thumb, Left J Finger, Right K Finger, Left L Lower Extremity, Right M Lower Extremity, Left N Upper Leg, Right P Upper Leg, Left Q Lower Leg, Right R Lower Leg, Left S Foot, Right T Foot, Left U Toe, Right V Toe, Left	X External	0 Traction Apparatus 1 Splint 2 Cast 3 Brace 4 Bandage 5 Packing Material 6 Pressure Dressing 7 Intermittent Pressure Device Y Other Device	Z No Qualifier
1 Face	X External	0 Traction Apparatus 1 Splint 2 Cast 3 Brace 4 Bandage 5 Packing Material 6 Pressure Dressing 7 Intermittent Pressure Device 9 Wire Y Other Device	Z No Qualifier

Section	2	Placement
Body System	W	Anatomical Regions
Operation	6	Traction: Exerting a pulling force on a body region in a distal direction

Body Region (4th)	Approach (5th)	Device (6th)	Qualifier (7th)
0 Head	X External	0 Traction Apparatus	Z No Qualifier
1 Face		Z No Device	
2 Neck			
3 Abdominal Wall			
4 Chest Wall			
5 Back			
6 Inguinal Region, Right			
7 Inguinal Region, Left			
8 Upper Extremity, Right			
9 Upper Extremity, Left			
A Upper Arm, Right			
B Upper Arm, Left			
C Lower Arm, Right			
D Lower Arm, Left			
E Hand, Right			
F Hand, Left			
G Thumb, Right			
H Thumb, Left			
J Finger, Right			
K Finger, Left			
L Lower Extremity, Right			
M Lower Extremity, Left			
N Upper Leg, Right			
P Upper Leg, Left			
Q Lower Leg, Right			
R Lower Leg, Left			
S Foot, Right			
T Foot, Left			
U Toe, Right			
V Toe, Left			

Section	2	Placement
Body System	Y	Anatomical Orifices
Operation	0	Change: Taking out or off a device from a body part and putting back an identical or similar device in or on the same body part without cutting or puncturing the skin or a mucous membrane

Body Region (4th)	Approach (5th)	Device (6th)	Qualifier (7th)
0 Mouth and Pharynx	X External	5 Packing Material	Z No Qualifier
1 Nasal			
2 Ear			
3 Anorectal			
4 Female Genital Tract			
5 Urethra			

Section	2	Placement
Body System	Y	Anatomical Orifices
Operation	4	Packing: Putting material in a body region or orifice

Body Region (4th)	Approach (5th)	Device (6th)	Qualifier (7th)
0 Mouth and Pharynx	X External	5 Packing Material	Z No Qualifier
1 Nasal			
2 Ear			
3 Anorectal			
4 Female Genital Tract			
5 Urethra			

Section   2   Placement
Body System   Y   Anatomical Orifices
Operation   5   Removal: Taking out or off a device from a body part

Body Region (4th)	Approach (5th)	Device (6th)	Qualifier (7th)
0 Mouth and Pharynx 1 Nasal 2 Ear 3 Anorectal 4 Female Genital Tract 5 Urethra	X External	5 Packing Material	Z No Qualifier

0 Mouth and Pharynx	X External	5 Packing Material	Z No Qualifier

Within each section of ICD-10-PCS, the characters have different meanings. The seven character meanings for the Administration section are illustrated here through the procedure example of *Nerve block injection to median nerve*.

Section	Body System	Root Operation	Body System/ Region	Approach	Substance	Qualifier
Administration	Physiological System and Anatomical Region	Introduction	Peripheral Nerves and Plexi	Percutaneous	Regional Anesthetic	None
3	E	0	T	3	C	Z

Section (Character 1)

All Administration procedure codes have a first character value of 3.

Body System (Character 2)

The alphanumeric character for the body system is placed in the second position. There are three character values applicable for the Administration section.

Character Value	Character Value Description
0	Circulatory
C	Indwelling Device
E	Physiological System and Anatomical Region

Root Operations (Character 3)

The alphanumeric character value for root operations is placed in the third position. Listed here are the root operations applicable to the Administration section with their associated meaning.

Character Value	Root Operation	Root Operation Definition
0	Introduction	Putting in or on a therapeutic, diagnostic, nutritional, physiological, or prophylactic substance except blood or blood products
1	Irrigation	Putting in or on a cleansing substance
2	Transfusion	Putting in blood or blood products

Body System/Region (Character 4)

For each body system the applicable body part character values will be available for procedure code construction. An example of a body region is upper GI.

Approach (Character 5)

The approach is the technique used to reach the procedure site. Listed here are the approach character values for the Administration with the associated definitions.

Character Value	Approach	Approach Definition
0	Open	Cutting through the skin or mucous membrane and any other body layers necessary to expose the site of the procedure
3	Percutaneous	Entry, by puncture or minor incision, of instrumentation through the skin or mucous membrane and any other body layers necessary to reach the site of the procedure
7	Via Natural or Artificial Opening	Entry of instrumentation through a natural or artificial external opening to reach the site of the procedure
8	Via Natural or Artificial Opening Endoscopic	Entry of instrumentation through a natural or artificial external opening to reach and visualize the site of the procedure
X	External	Procedures performed directly on the skin or mucous membrane and procedures performed indirectly by the application of external force through the skin or mucous membrane

Substance (Character 6)

In the Administration section a substance is always utilized. The substance is reported in the sixth character position by the type of substance utilized. The following is a sample list of the substances included in this section:

- Anti-inflammatory
- Antineoplastic
- Bone marrow
- Platelet inhibitor
- Whole blood

Qualifier (Character 7)

The qualifier represents an additional attribute for the procedure when applicable. There are several qualifiers included in the Administration section. For example, transfusion procedures in this section include qualifiers including Autologous and Nonautologous that are reported with the character values of 0 and 1, respectively. If there is no qualifier for a procedure, the placeholder Z is the character value that should be reported.

If a coder is unsure of which option to select for the substance qualifier utilized during the procedure, Appendix F can be used to guide the selection. It is important to note that not all substance qualifier categories are provided by CMS in Appendix F. However, for example, the coding scenario indicates that Clolar was introduced percutaneously via the peripheral vein. The coder references Table 3E0 (Introduction in Physiological Systems and Anatomical Regions) under the peripheral vein, percutaneous approach, anti-neoplastic. Clolar is not a substance qualifier choice. However, the coder can then locate the substance qualifier categories in Appendix F. The category Clofarabine includes Clolar. Therefore, the coder should select P - Clofarabine for the 7th character.

Important Definitions for the Administration Section

Administration Root Operation	Qualifier	Definition
Transfusion (302)	0 - Autologous	Derived or transferred from the same individual's body*
	1 - Nonautologous	Derived or transferred from another individual's body

*Taken from The Free Dictionary by Farlex at www.thefreedictionary.com

Section Notes

Before reporting Transfusion procedures for embryonic stem cells (6th character A), bone marrow (6th character G), cord blood stem cells (6th character X) or hematopoietic stem cells (6th character Y) users should *Review coding guideline B3.16.*

Before reporting Administration codes for all Biliary and Pancreatic Tract (4th character value of J) procedures with a 6th character value of U (Pancreatic Islet Cells), users should *Review coding guideline B3.16.*

Before reporting Irrigation procedures in this section, users should *Review coding guideline B6.1c.*

Medicare Non-Covered Administration Codes

Non-Covered with pdx or sdx C91.00, C92.00, C92.10, C92.11, C92.40, C92.50, C92.60, C92.A0, C93.00, C94.00 or C95.00

30230AZ	30233AZ	30240AZ	30243AZ	30250G0	30253Y0	30263G0
30230G0	30233G0	30240G0	30243G0	30250Y0	30260G0	30263Y0
30230Y0	30233Y0	30240Y0	30243Y0	30253G0	30260Y0	

Non-Covered with pdx or sdx C90.00 or C90.01

30230G1	30233Y1	30243G1	30250Y1	30260G1	30263G1	
30230Y1	30240G1	30243Y1	30253G1	30260Y1	30263Y1	
30233G1	30240Y1	30250G1	30253Y1	30263G1		

AHA Coding Clinic

3E013GC Introduction of Other Therapeutic Substance into Subcutaneous Tissue, Percutaneous Approach - AHA CC 2Q, 2014, 10

3E0234Z Introduction of Serum, Toxoid and Vaccine into Muscle, Percutaneous Approach - AHA CC: 4Q, 2014, 16

3E03317 Introduction of Other Thrombolytic into Peripheral Vein, Percutaneous Approach - AHA CC 4Q, 2013, 124

3E033VJ Introduction of Other Hormone into Peripheral Vein, Percutaneous Approach - AHA CC: 4Q, 2014, 17-18

3E05305 Introduction of Other Antineoplastic into Peripheral Artery, Percutaneous Approach - AHA CC: 1Q, 2015, 38

3E06317 Introduction of Other Thrombolytic into Central Artery, Percutaneous Approach - AHA CC: 4Q, 2014, 19-20 2015, 38

3E0G8TZ Introduction of Destructive Agent into Upper GI, Via Natural or Artificial Opening Endoscopic - AHA CC 1Q, 2013, 27

3E0M3GC Introduction of Other Therapeutic Substance into Peritoneal Cavity, Percutaneous Approach - AJA CC: 4Q, 2014, 38

3E0P7GC Introduction of Other Therapeutic Substance into Female Reproductive, Via Natural or Artificial Opening - AHA CC 2Q, 2014, 8-9

3E0Q305 Introduction of Other Antineoplastic into Cranial Cavity and Brain, Percutaneous Approach - AHA CC: 4Q, 2014, 34-35

3E0R305 Introduction of Other Antineoplastic into Spinal Canal, Percutaneous Approach - AHA CC: 1Q, 2015, 31

Administration Tables 302–3E1

Section	3	**Administration**
Body System	0	**Circulatory**
Operation	2	**Transfusion:** Putting in blood or blood products

Body System / Region (4th)		Approach (5th)		Substance (6th)		Qualifier (7th)	
3	Peripheral Vein	0	Open	A	Stem Cells, Embryonic	Z	No Qualifier
4	Central Vein	3	Percutaneous				
3	Peripheral Vein	0	Open	G	Bone Marrow	0	Autologous
4	Central Vein	3	Percutaneous	H	Whole Blood	1	Nonautologous
				J	Serum Albumin		
				K	Frozen Plasma		
				L	Fresh Plasma		
				M	Plasma Cryoprecipitate		
				N	Red Blood Cells		
				P	Frozen Red Cells		
				Q	White Cells		
				R	Platelets		
				S	Globulin		
				T	Fibrinogen		
				V	Antihemophilic Factors		
				W	Factor IX		
				X	Stem Cells, Cord Blood		
				Y	Stem Cells, Hematopoietic		
5	Peripheral Artery	0	Open	G	Bone Marrow	0	Autologous
6	Central Artery	3	Percutaneous	H	Whole Blood	1	Nonautologous
				J	Serum Albumin		
				K	Frozen Plasma		
				L	Fresh Plasma		
				M	Plasma Cryoprecipitate		
				N	Red Blood Cells		
				P	Frozen Red Cells		
				Q	White Cells		
				R	Platelets		
				S	Globulin		
				T	Fibrinogen		
				V	Antihemophilic Factors		
				W	Factor IX		
				X	Stem Cells, Cord Blood		
				Y	Stem Cells, Hematopoietic		
7	Products of Conception, Circulatory	3	Percutaneous	H	Whole Blood	1	Nonautologous
		7	Via Natural or Artificial Opening	J	Serum Albumin		
				K	Frozen Plasma		
				L	Fresh Plasma		
				M	Plasma Cryoprecipitate		
				N	Red Blood Cells		
				P	Frozen Red Cells		
				Q	White Cells		
				R	Platelets		
				S	Globulin		
				T	Fibrinogen		
				V	Antihemophilic Factors		
				W	Factor IX		
8	Vein	0	Open	B	4-Factor Prothrombin Complex Concentrate	1	Nonautologous
		3	Percutaneous				

Section	3	Administration
Body System	C	Indwelling Device
Operation	1	Irrigation: Putting in or on a cleansing substance

Body System / Region (4th)	Approach (5th)	Substance (6th)	Qualifier (7th)
Z None	X External	8 Irrigating Substance	Z No Qualifier

Section	3	Administration
Body System	E	Physiological Systems and Anatomical Regions
Operation	0	Introduction: Putting in or on a therapeutic, diagnostic, nutritional, physiological, or prophylactic substance except blood or blood products

Body System / Region (4th)	Approach (5th)	Substance (6th)	Qualifier (7th)
0 Skin and Mucous Membranes	X External	0 Antineoplastic	5 Other Antineoplastic M Monoclonal Antibody
0 Skin and Mucous Membranes	X External	2 Anti-infective	8 Oxazolidinones 9 Other Anti-infective
0 Skin and Mucous Membranes	X External	3 Anti-inflammatory 4 Serum, Toxoid and Vaccine B Local Anesthetic K Other Diagnostic Substance M Pigment N Analgesics, Hypnotics, Sedatives T Destructive Agent	Z No Qualifier
0 Skin and Mucous Membranes	X External	G Other Therapeutic Substance	C Other Substance
1 Subcutaneous Tissue	0 Open	2 Anti-infective	A Anti-Infective Envelope
1 Subcutaneous Tissue	3 Percutaneous	0 Antineoplastic	5 Other Antineoplastic M Monoclonal Antibody
1 Subcutaneous Tissue	3 Percutaneous	2 Anti-infective	8 Oxazolidinones 9 Other Anti-infective A Anti-Infective Envelope
1 Subcutaneous Tissue	3 Percutaneous	3 Anti-inflammatory 4 Serum, Toxoid and Vaccine 6 Nutritional Substance 7 Electrolytic and Water Balance Substance B Local Anesthetic H Radioactive Substance K Other Diagnostic Substance N Analgesics, Hypnotics, Sedatives T Destructive Agent	Z No Qualifier
1 Subcutaneous Tissue	3 Percutaneous	G Other Therapeutic Substance	C Other Substance
1 Subcutaneous Tissue	3 Percutaneous	V Hormone	G Insulin J Other Hormone
2 Muscle	3 Percutaneous	0 Antineoplastic	5 Other Antineoplastic M Monoclonal Antibody
2 Muscle	3 Percutaneous	2 Anti-infective	8 Oxazolidinones 9 Other Anti-infective

Continued →

Section 3 Administration

Body System E Physiological Systems and Anatomical Regions

Operation 0 Introduction: Putting in or on a therapeutic, diagnostic, nutritional, physiological, or prophylactic substance except blood or blood products

Body System / Region (4th)	Approach (5th)	Substance (6th)	Qualifier (7th)
2 Muscle	3 Percutaneous	3 Anti-inflammatory 4 Serum, Toxoid and Vaccine 6 Nutritional Substance 7 Electrolytic and Water Balance Substance B Local Anesthetic H Radioactive Substance K Other Diagnostic Substance N Analgesics, Hypnotics, Sedatives T Destructive Agent	Z No Qualifier
2 Muscle	3 Percutaneous	G Other Therapeutic Substance	C Other Substance
3 Peripheral Vein	0 Open	0 Antineoplastic	2 High-dose Interleukin-2 3 Low-dose Interleukin-2 5 Other Antineoplastic M Monoclonal Antibody P Clofarabine
3 Peripheral Vein	0 Open	1 Thrombolytic	6 Recombinant Human-activated Protein C 7 Other Thrombolytic
3 Peripheral Vein	0 Open	2 Anti-infective	8 Oxazolidinones 9 Other Anti-infective
3 Peripheral Vein	0 Open	3 Anti-inflammatory 4 Serum, Toxoid and Vaccine 6 Nutritional Substance 7 Electrolytic and Water Balance Substance F Intracirculatory Anesthetic H Radioactive Substance K Other Diagnostic Substance N Analgesics, Hypnotics, Sedatives P Platelet Inhibitor R Antiarrhythmic T Destructive Agent X Vasopressor	Z No Qualifier
3 Peripheral Vein	0 Open	G Other Therapeutic Substance	C Other Substance N Blood Brain Barrier Disruption
3 Peripheral Vein	0 Open	U Pancreatic Islet Cells	0 Autologous 1 Nonautologous
3 Peripheral Vein	0 Open	V Hormone	G Insulin H Human B-type Natriuretic Peptide J Other Hormone
3 Peripheral Vein	0 Open	W Immunotherapeutic	K Immunostimulator L Immunosuppressive
3 Peripheral Vein	3 Percutaneous	0 Antineoplastic	2 High-dose Interleukin-2 3 Low-dose Interleukin-2 5 Other Antineoplastic M Monoclonal Antibody P Clofarabine
3 Peripheral Vein	3 Percutaneous	1 Thrombolytic	6 Recombinant Human-activated Protein C 7 Other Thrombolytic

Continued →

Section 3 Administration
Body System E Physiological Systems and Anatomical Regions
Operation 0 Introduction: Putting in or on a therapeutic, diagnostic, nutritional, physiological, or prophylactic substance except blood or blood products

Body System / Region (4ᵗʰ)	Approach (5ᵗʰ)	Substance (6ᵗʰ)	Qualifier (7ᵗʰ)
3 Peripheral Vein	3 Percutaneous	2 Anti-infective	8 Oxazolidinones 9 Other Anti-infective
3 Peripheral Vein	3 Percutaneous	3 Anti-inflammatory 4 Serum, Toxoid and Vaccine 6 Nutritional Substance 7 Electrolytic and Water Balance Substance F Intracirculatory Anesthetic H Radioactive Substance K Other Diagnostic Substance N Analgesics, Hypnotics, Sedatives P Platelet Inhibitor R Antiarrhythmic T Destructive Agent X Vasopressor	Z No Qualifier
3 Peripheral Vein	3 Percutaneous	G Other Therapeutic Substance	C Other Substance N Blood Brain Barrier Disruption Q Glucarpidase
3 Peripheral Vein	3 Percutaneous	U Pancreatic Islet Cells	0 Autologous 1 Nonautologous
3 Peripheral Vein	3 Percutaneous	V Hormone	G Insulin H Human B-type Natriuretic Peptide J Other Hormone
3 Peripheral Vein	3 Percutaneous	W Immunotherapeutic	K Immunostimulator L Immunosuppressive
4 Central Vein	0 Open	0 Antineoplastic	2 High-dose Interleukin-2 3 Low-dose Interleukin-2 5 Other Antineoplastic M Monoclonal Antibody P Clofarabine
4 Central Vein	0 Open	1 Thrombolytic	6 Recombinant Human-activated Protein C 7 Other Thrombolytic
4 Central Vein	0 Open	2 Anti-infective	8 Oxazolidinones 9 Other Anti-infective
4 Central Vein	0 Open	3 Anti-inflammatory 4 Serum, Toxoid and Vaccine 6 Nutritional Substance 7 Electrolytic and Water Balance Substance F Intracirculatory Anesthetic H Radioactive Substance K Other Diagnostic Substance N Analgesics, Hypnotics, Sedatives P Platelet Inhibitor R Antiarrhythmic T Destructive Agent X Vasopressor	Z No Qualifier
4 Central Vein	0 Open	G Other Therapeutic Substance	C Other Substance N Blood Brain Barrier Disruption

Continued →

Section 3 Administration
Body System E Physiological Systems and Anatomical Regions
Operation 0 Introduction: Putting in or on a therapeutic, diagnostic, nutritional, physiological, or prophylactic substance except blood or blood products

3E0 Continued

3E0

Body System / Region (4th)	Approach (5th)	Substance (6th)	Qualifier (7th)
4 Central Vein	0 Open	V Hormone	G Insulin H Human B-type Natriuretic Peptide J Other Hormone
4 Central Vein	0 Open	W Immunotherapeutic	K Immunostimulator L Immunosuppressive
4 Central Vein	3 Percutaneous	0 Antineoplastic	2 High-dose Interleukin-2 3 Low-dose Interleukin-2 5 Other Antineoplastic M Monoclonal Antibody P Clofarabine
4 Central Vein	3 Percutaneous	1 Thrombolytic	6 Recombinant Human-activated Protein C 7 Other Thrombolytic
4 Central Vein	3 Percutaneous	2 Anti-infective	8 Oxazolidinones 9 Other Anti-infective
4 Central Vein	3 Percutaneous	3 Anti-inflammatory 4 Serum, Toxoid and Vaccine 6 Nutritional Substance 7 Electrolytic and Water Balance Substance F Intracirculatory Anesthetic H Radioactive Substance K Other Diagnostic Substance N Analgesics, Hypnotics, Sedatives P Platelet Inhibitor R Antiarrhythmic T Destructive Agent X Vasopressor	Z No Qualifier
4 Central Vein	3 Percutaneous	G Other Therapeutic Substance	C Other Substance N Blood Brain Barrier Disruption Q Glucarpidase
4 Central Vein	3 Percutaneous	V Hormone	G Insulin H Human B-type Natriuretic Peptide J Other Hormone
4 Central Vein	3 Percutaneous	W Immunotherapeutic	K Immunostimulator L Immunosuppressive
5 Peripheral Artery 6 Central Artery	0 Open 3 Percutaneous	0 Antineoplastic	2 High-dose Interleukin-2 3 Low-dose Interleukin-2 5 Other Antineoplastic M Monoclonal Antibody P Clofarabine
5 Peripheral Artery 6 Central Artery	0 Open 3 Percutaneous	1 Thrombolytic	6 Recombinant Human-activated Protein C 7 Other Thrombolytic
5 Peripheral Artery 6 Central Artery	0 Open 3 Percutaneous	2 Anti-infective	8 Oxazolidinones 9 Other Anti-infective

Continued →

Section   **3**   **Administration**
Body System   **E**   **Physiological Systems and Anatomical Regions**
Operation   **0**   **Introduction:** Putting in or on a therapeutic, diagnostic, nutritional, physiological, or prophylactic substance except blood or blood products

Body System / Region (4th)	Approach (5th)	Substance (6th)	Qualifier (7th)
5 Peripheral Artery 6 Central Artery	0 Open 3 Percutaneous	3 Anti-inflammatory 4 Serum, Toxoid and Vaccine 6 Nutritional Substance 7 Electrolytic and Water Balance Substance F Intracirculatory Anesthetic H Radioactive Substance K Other Diagnostic Substance N Analgesics, Hypnotics, Sedatives P Platelet Inhibitor R Antiarrhythmic T Destructive Agent X Vasopressor	Z No Qualifier
5 Peripheral Artery 6 Central Artery	0 Open 3 Percutaneous	G Other Therapeutic Substance	C Other Substance N Blood Brain Barrier Disruption
5 Peripheral Artery 6 Central Artery	0 Open 3 Percutaneous	V Hormone	G Insulin H Human B-type Natriuretic Peptide J Other Hormone
5 Peripheral Artery 6 Central Artery	0 Open 3 Percutaneous	W Immunotherapeutic	K Immunostimulator L Immunosuppressive
7 Coronary Artery 8 Heart	0 Open 3 Percutaneous	1 Thrombolytic	6 Recombinant Human-activated Protein C 7 Other Thrombolytic
7 Coronary Artery 8 Heart	0 Open 3 Percutaneous	G Other Therapeutic Substance	C Other Substance
7 Coronary Artery 8 Heart	0 Open 3 Percutaneous	K Other Diagnostic Substance P Platelet Inhibitor	Z No Qualifier
9 Nose	3 Percutaneous 7 Via Natural or Artificial Opening X External	0 Antineoplastic	5 Other Antineoplastic M Monoclonal Antibody
9 Nose	3 Percutaneous 7 Via Natural or Artificial Opening X External	2 Anti-infective	8 Oxazolidinones 9 Other Anti-infective
9 Nose	3 Percutaneous 7 Via Natural or Artificial Opening X External	3 Anti-inflammatory 4 Serum, Toxoid and Vaccine B Local Anesthetic H Radioactive Substance K Other Diagnostic Substance N Analgesics, Hypnotics, Sedatives T Destructive Agent	Z No Qualifier
9 Nose	3 Percutaneous 7 Via Natural or Artificial Opening X External	G Other Therapeutic Substance	C Other Substance
A Bone Marrow	3 Percutaneous	0 Antineoplastic	5 Other Antineoplastic M Monoclonal Antibody
A Bone Marrow	3 Percutaneous	G Other Therapeutic Substance	C Other Substance

Continued →

Section 3 **Administration**
Body System E **Physiological Systems and Anatomical Regions**
Operation 0 **Introduction:** Putting in or on a therapeutic, diagnostic, nutritional, physiological, or prophylactic substance except blood or blood products

Body System / Region (4th)	Approach (5th)	Substance (6th)	Qualifier (7th)
B Ear	3 Percutaneous 7 Via Natural or Artificial Opening X External	0 Antineoplastic	4 Liquid Brachytherapy Radioisotope 5 Other Antineoplastic M Monoclonal Antibody
B Ear	3 Percutaneous 7 Via Natural or Artificial Opening X External	2 Anti-infective	8 Oxazolidinones 9 Other Anti-infective
B Ear	3 Percutaneous 7 Via Natural or Artificial Opening X External	3 Anti-inflammatory B Local Anesthetic H Radioactive Substance K Other Diagnostic Substance N Analgesics, Hypnotics, Sedatives T Destructive Agent	Z No Qualifier
B Ear	3 Percutaneous 7 Via Natural or Artificial Opening X External	G Other Therapeutic Substance	C Other Substance
C Eye	3 Percutaneous 7 Via Natural or Artificial Opening X External	0 Antineoplastic	4 Liquid Brachytherapy Radioisotope 5 Other Antineoplastic M Monoclonal Antibody
C Eye	3 Percutaneous 7 Via Natural or Artificial Opening X External	2 Anti-infective	8 Oxazolidinones 9 Other Anti-infective
C Eye	3 Percutaneous 7 Via Natural or Artificial Opening X External	3 Anti-inflammatory B Local Anesthetic H Radioactive Substance K Other Diagnostic Substance M Pigment N Analgesics, Hypnotics, Sedatives T Destructive Agent	Z No Qualifier
C Eye	3 Percutaneous 7 Via Natural or Artificial Opening X External	G Other Therapeutic Substance	C Other Substance
C Eye	3 Percutaneous 7 Via Natural or Artificial Opening X External	S Gas	F Other Gas
D Mouth and Pharynx	3 Percutaneous 7 Via Natural or Artificial Opening X External	0 Antineoplastic	4 Liquid Brachytherapy Radioisotope 5 Other Antineoplastic M Monoclonal Antibody
D Mouth and Pharynx	3 Percutaneous 7 Via Natural or Artificial Opening X External	2 Anti-infective	8 Oxazolidinones 9 Other Anti-infective

Continued →

Section 3 Administration
Body System E Physiological Systems and Anatomical Regions
Operation 0 Introduction: Putting in or on a therapeutic, diagnostic, nutritional, physiological, or prophylactic substance except blood or blood products

Body System / Region (4th)	Approach (5th)	Substance (6th)	Qualifier (7th)
D Mouth and Pharynx	**3** Percutaneous **7** Via Natural or Artificial Opening **X** External	**3** Anti-inflammatory **4** Serum, Toxoid and Vaccine **6** Nutritional Substance **7** Electrolytic and Water Balance Substance **B** Local Anesthetic **H** Radioactive Substance **K** Other Diagnostic Substance **N** Analgesics, Hypnotics, Sedatives **R** Antiarrhythmic **T** Destructive Agent	**Z** No Qualifier
D Mouth and Pharynx	**3** Percutaneous **7** Via Natural or Artificial Opening **X** External	**G** Other Therapeutic Substance	**C** Other Substance
E Products of Conception **G** Upper GI **H** Lower GI **K** Genitourinary Tract **N** Male Reproductive	**3** Percutaneous **7** Via Natural or Artificial Opening **8** Via Natural or Artificial Opening Endoscopic	**0** Antineoplastic	**4** Liquid Brachytherapy Radioisotope **5** Other Antineoplastic **M** Monoclonal Antibody
E Products of Conception **G** Upper GI **H** Lower GI **K** Genitourinary Tract **N** Male Reproductive	**3** Percutaneous **7** Via Natural or Artificial Opening **8** Via Natural or Artificial Opening Endoscopic	**2** Anti-infective	**8** Oxazolidinones **9** Other Anti-infective
E Products of Conception **G** Upper GI **H** Lower GI **K** Genitourinary Tract **N** Male Reproductive	**3** Percutaneous **7** Via Natural or Artificial Opening **8** Via Natural or Artificial Opening Endoscopic	**3** Anti-inflammatory **6** Nutritional Substance **7** Electrolytic and Water Balance Substance **B** Local Anesthetic **H** Radioactive Substance **K** Other Diagnostic Substance **N** Analgesics, Hypnotics, Sedatives **T** Destructive Agent	**Z** No Qualifier
E Products of Conception **G** Upper GI **H** Lower GI **K** Genitourinary Tract **N** Male Reproductive	**3** Percutaneous **7** Via Natural or Artificial Opening **8** Via Natural or Artificial Opening Endoscopic	**G** Other Therapeutic Substance	**C** Other Substance
E Products of Conception **G** Upper GI **H** Lower GI **K** Genitourinary Tract **N** Male Reproductive	**3** Percutaneous **7** Via Natural or Artificial Opening **8** Via Natural or Artificial Opening Endoscopic	**S** Gas	**F** Other Gas
F Respiratory Tract	**3** Percutaneous	**0** Antineoplastic	**4** Liquid Brachytherapy Radioisotope **5** Other Antineoplastic **M** Monoclonal Antibody
F Respiratory Tract	**3** Percutaneous	**2** Anti-infective	**8** Oxazolidinones **9** Other Anti-infective

Continued →

Section 3 Administration
Body System E Physiological Systems and Anatomical Regions
Operation 0 Introduction: Putting in or on a therapeutic, diagnostic, nutritional, physiological, or prophylactic substance except blood or blood products

3E0 Continued

3E0

Body System / Region (4th)	Approach (5th)	Substance (6th)	Qualifier (7th)
F Respiratory Tract	3 Percutaneous	3 Anti-inflammatory 6 Nutritional Substance 7 Electrolytic and Water Balance Substance B Local Anesthetic H Radioactive Substance K Other Diagnostic Substance N Analgesics, Hypnotics, Sedatives T Destructive Agent	Z No Qualifier
F Respiratory Tract	3 Percutaneous	G Other Therapeutic Substance	C Other Substance
F Respiratory Tract	3 Percutaneous	S Gas	D Nitric Oxide F Other Gas
F Respiratory Tract	7 Via Natural or Artificial Opening 8 Via Natural or Artificial Opening Endoscopic	0 Antineoplastic	4 Liquid Brachytherapy Radioisotope 5 Other Antineoplastic M Monoclonal Antibody
F Respiratory Tract	7 Via Natural or Artificial Opening 8 Via Natural or Artificial Opening Endoscopic	2 Anti-infective	8 Oxazolidinones 9 Other Anti-infective
F Respiratory Tract	7 Via Natural or Artificial Opening 8 Via Natural or Artificial Opening Endoscopic	3 Anti-inflammatory 6 Nutritional Substance 7 Electrolytic and Water Balance Substance B Local Anesthetic D Inhalation Anesthetic H Radioactive Substance K Other Diagnostic Substance N Analgesics, Hypnotics, Sedatives T Destructive Agent	Z No Qualifier
F Respiratory Tract	7 Via Natural or Artificial Opening 8 Via Natural or Artificial Opening Endoscopic	G Other Therapeutic Substance	C Other Substance
F Respiratory Tract	7 Via Natural or Artificial Opening 8 Via Natural or Artificial Opening Endoscopic	S Gas	D Nitric Oxide F Other Gas
J Biliary and Pancreatic Tract	3 Percutaneous 7 Via Natural or Artificial Opening 8 Via Natural or Artificial Opening Endoscopic	0 Antineoplastic	4 Liquid Brachytherapy Radioisotope 5 Other Antineoplastic M Monoclonal Antibody
J Biliary and Pancreatic Tract	3 Percutaneous 7 Via Natural or Artificial Opening 8 Via Natural or Artificial Opening Endoscopic	2 Anti-infective	8 Oxazolidinones 9 Other Anti-infective

Continued →

3E0

Section 3 **Administration**
Body System E **Physiological Systems and Anatomical Regions**
Operation 0 **Introduction:** Putting in or on a therapeutic, diagnostic, nutritional, physiological, or prophylactic substance except blood or blood products

3E0 Continu

Body System / Region (4th)	Approach (5th)	Substance (6th)	Qualifier (7th)
J Biliary and Pancreatic Tract	**3** Percutaneous **7** Via Natural or Artificial Opening **8** Via Natural or Artificial Opening Endoscopic	**3** Anti-inflammatory **6** Nutritional Substance **7** Electrolytic and Water Balance Substance **B** Local Anesthetic **H** Radioactive Substance **K** Other Diagnostic Substance **N** Analgesics, Hypnotics, Sedatives **T** Destructive Agent	**Z** No Qualifier
J Biliary and Pancreatic Tract	**3** Percutaneous **7** Via Natural or Artificial Opening **8** Via Natural or Artificial Opening Endoscopic	**G** Other Therapeutic Substance	**C** Other Substance
J Biliary and Pancreatic Tract	**3** Percutaneous **7** Via Natural or Artificial Opening **8** Via Natural or Artificial Opening Endoscopic	**S** Gas	**F** Other Gas
J Biliary and Pancreatic Tract	**3** Percutaneous **7** Via Natural or Artificial Opening **8** Via Natural or Artificial Opening Endoscopic	**U** Pancreatic Islet Cells	**0** Autologous **1** Nonautologous
L Pleural Cavity **M** Peritoneal Cavity	**0** Open	**5** Adhesion Barrier	**Z** No Qualifier
L Pleural Cavity **M** Peritoneal Cavity	**3** Percutaneous	**0** Antineoplastic	**4** Liquid Brachytherapy Radioisotope **5** Other Antineoplastic **M** Monoclonal Antibody
L Pleural Cavity **M** Peritoneal Cavity	**3** Percutaneous	**2** Anti-infective	**8** Oxazolidinones **9** Other Anti-infective
L Pleural Cavity **M** Peritoneal Cavity	**3** Percutaneous	**3** Anti-inflammatory **6** Nutritional Substance **7** Electrolytic and Water Balance Substance **B** Local Anesthetic **H** Radioactive Substance **K** Other Diagnostic Substance **N** Analgesics, Hypnotics, Sedatives **T** Destructive Agent	**Z** No Qualifier
L Pleural Cavity **M** Peritoneal Cavity	**3** Percutaneous	**G** Other Therapeutic Substance	**C** Other Substance
L Pleural Cavity **M** Peritoneal Cavity	**3** Percutaneous	**S** Gas	**F** Other Gas
L Pleural Cavity **M** Peritoneal Cavity	**7** Via Natural or Artificial Opening	**0** Antineoplastic	**4** Liquid Brachytherapy Radioisotope **5** Other Antineoplastic **M** Monoclonal Antibody

Continued →

Section 3 Administration
Body System E Physiological Systems and Anatomical Regions
Operation 0 Introduction: Putting in or on a therapeutic, diagnostic, nutritional, physiological,
or prophylactic substance except blood or blood products

3E0 Continued

3E0

Body System / Region (4th)	Approach (5th)	Substance (6th)	Qualifier (7th)
L Pleural Cavity M Peritoneal Cavity	7 Via Natural or Artificial Opening	S Gas	F Other Gas
P Female Reproductive	0 Open	5 Adhesion Barrier	Z No Qualifier
P Female Reproductive	3 Percutaneous 7 Via Natural or Artificial Opening	0 Antineoplastic	4 Liquid Brachytherapy Radioisotope 5 Other Antineoplastic M Monoclonal Antibody
P Female Reproductive	3 Percutaneous 7 Via Natural or Artificial Opening	2 Anti-infective	8 Oxazolidinones 9 Other Anti-infective
P Female Reproductive	3 Percutaneous 7 Via Natural or Artificial Opening	3 Anti-inflammatory 6 Nutritional Substance 7 Electrolytic and Water Balance Substance B Local Anesthetic H Radioactive Substance K Other Diagnostic Substance L Sperm N Analgesics, Hypnotics, Sedatives T Destructive Agent	Z No Qualifier
P Female Reproductive	3 Percutaneous 7 Via Natural or Artificial Opening	G Other Therapeutic Substance	C Other Substance
P Female Reproductive	3 Percutaneous 7 Via Natural or Artificial Opening	Q Fertilized Ovum	0 Autologous 1 Nonautologous
P Female Reproductive	3 Percutaneous 7 Via Natural or Artificial Opening	S Gas	F Other Gas
P Female Reproductive	8 Via Natural or Artificial Opening Endoscopic	0 Antineoplastic	4 Liquid Brachytherapy Radioisotope 5 Other Antineoplastic M Monoclonal Antibody
P Female Reproductive	8 Via Natural or Artificial Opening Endoscopic	2 Anti-infective	8 Oxazolidinones 9 Other Anti-infective
P Female Reproductive	8 Via Natural or Artificial Opening Endoscopic	3 Anti-inflammatory 6 Nutritional Substance 7 Electrolytic and Water Balance Substance B Local Anesthetic H Radioactive Substance K Other Diagnostic Substance N Analgesics, Hypnotics, Sedatives T Destructive Agent	Z No Qualifier
P Female Reproductive	8 Via Natural or Artificial Opening Endoscopic	G Other Therapeutic Substance	C Other Substance
P Female Reproductive	8 Via Natural or Artificial Opening Endoscopic	S Gas	F Other Gas
Q Cranial Cavity and Brain	0 Open	A Stem Cells, Embryonic	Z No Qualifier

Continued →

3E0

Section 3 Administration
Body System E Physiological Systems and Anatomical Regions
Operation 0 Introduction: Putting in or on a therapeutic, diagnostic, nutritional, physiological,
or prophylactic substance except blood or blood products

3E0 Continu

Body System / Region (4th)	Approach (5th)	Substance (6th)	Qualifier (7th)
Q Cranial Cavity and Brain	0 Open	E Stem Cells, Somatic	0 Autologous 1 Nonautologous
Q Cranial Cavity and Brain	3 Percutaneous	0 Antineoplastic	4 Liquid Brachytherapy Radioisotope 5 Other Antineoplastic M Monoclonal Antibody
Q Cranial Cavity and Brain	3 Percutaneous	2 Anti-infective	8 Oxazolidinones 9 Other Anti-infective
Q Cranial Cavity and Brain	3 Percutaneous	3 Anti-inflammatory 6 Nutritional Substance 7 Electrolytic and Water Balance Substance A Stem Cells, Embryonic B Local Anesthetic H Radioactive Substance K Other Diagnostic Substance N Analgesics, Hypnotics, Sedatives T Destructive Agent	Z No Qualifier
Q Cranial Cavity and Brain	3 Percutaneous	E Stem Cells, Somatic	0 Autologous 1 Nonautologous
Q Cranial Cavity and Brain	3 Percutaneous	G Other Therapeutic Substance	C Other Substance
Q Cranial Cavity and Brain	3 Percutaneous	S Gas	F Other Gas
Q Cranial Cavity and Brain	7 Via Natural or Artificial Opening	0 Antineoplastic	4 Liquid Brachytherapy Radioisotope 5 Other Antineoplastic M Monoclonal Antibody
Q Cranial Cavity and Brain	7 Via Natural or Artificial Opening	S Gas	F Other Gas
R Spinal Canal	0 Open	A Stem Cells, Embryonic	Z No Qualifier
R Spinal Canal	0 Open	E Stem Cells, Somatic	0 Autologous 1 Nonautologous
R Spinal Canal	3 Percutaneous	0 Antineoplastic	2 High-dose Interleukin-2 3 Low-dose Interleukin-2 4 Liquid Brachytherapy Radioisotope 5 Other Antineoplastic M Monoclonal Antibody
R Spinal Canal	3 Percutaneous	2 Anti-infective	8 Oxazolidinones 9 Other Anti-infective
R Spinal Canal	3 Percutaneous	3 Anti-inflammatory 6 Nutritional Substance 7 Electrolytic and Water Balance Substance A Stem Cells, Embryonic B Local Anesthetic C Regional Anesthetic H Radioactive Substance K Other Diagnostic Substance N Analgesics, Hypnotics, Sedatives T Destructive Agent	Z No Qualifier

Continued -

Section 3 Administration
Body System E Physiological Systems and Anatomical Regions
Operation 0 Introduction: Putting in or on a therapeutic, diagnostic, nutritional, physiological, or prophylactic substance except blood or blood products

3E0 Continued

3E0

Body System / Region (4ᵗʰ)	Approach (5ᵗʰ)	Substance (6ᵗʰ)	Qualifier (7ᵗʰ)
R Spinal Canal	3 Percutaneous	E Stem Cells, Somatic	0 Autologous 1 Nonautologous
R Spinal Canal	3 Percutaneous	G Other Therapeutic Substance	C Other Substance
R Spinal Canal	3 Percutaneous	S Gas	F Other Gas
R Spinal Canal	7 Via Natural or Artificial Opening	S Gas	F Other Gas
S Epidural Space	3 Percutaneous	0 Antineoplastic	2 High-dose Interleukin-2 3 Low-dose Interleukin-2 4 Liquid Brachytherapy Radioisotope 5 Other Antineoplastic M Monoclonal Antibody
S Epidural Space	3 Percutaneous	2 Anti-infective	8 Oxazolidinones 9 Other Anti-infective
S Epidural Space	3 Percutaneous	3 Anti-inflammatory 6 Nutritional Substance 7 Electrolytic and Water Balance Substance B Local Anesthetic C Regional Anesthetic H Radioactive Substance K Other Diagnostic Substance N Analgesics, Hypnotics, Sedatives T Destructive Agent	Z No Qualifier
S Epidural Space	3 Percutaneous	G Other Therapeutic Substance	C Other Substance
S Epidural Space	3 Percutaneous	S Gas	F Other Gas
S Epidural Space	7 Via Natural or Artificial Opening	S Gas	F Other Gas
T Peripheral Nerves and Plexi X Cranial Nerves	3 Percutaneous	3 Anti-inflammatory B Local Anesthetic C Regional Anesthetic T Destructive Agent	Z No Qualifier
T Peripheral Nerves and Plexi X Cranial Nerves	3 Percutaneous	G Other Therapeutic Substance	C Other Substance
U Joints	0 Open	2 Anti-infective	8 Oxazolidinones 9 Other Anti-infective
U Joints	0 Open	G Other Therapeutic Substance	B Recombinant Bone Morphogenetic Protein
U Joints	3 Percutaneous	0 Antineoplastic	4 Liquid Brachytherapy Radioisotope 5 Other Antineoplastic M Monoclonal Antibody
U Joints	3 Percutaneous	2 Anti-infective	8 Oxazolidinones 9 Other Anti-infective

Continued →

Body System / Region (4th)	Approach (5th)	Substance (6th)	Qualifier (7th)
U Joints	3 Percutaneous	3 Anti-inflammatory 6 Nutritional Substance 7 Electrolytic and Water Balance Substance B Local Anesthetic H Radioactive Substance K Other Diagnostic Substance N Analgesics, Hypnotics, Sedatives T Destructive Agent	Z No Qualifier
U Joints	3 Percutaneous	G Other Therapeutic Substance	B Recombinant Bone Morphogenetic Protein C Other Substance
U Joints	3 Percutaneous	S Gas	F Other Gas
V Bones	0 Open	G Other Therapeutic Substance	B Recombinant Bone Morphogenetic Protein
V Bones	3 Percutaneous	0 Antineoplastic	5 Other Antineoplastic M Monoclonal Antibody
V Bones	3 Percutaneous	2 Anti-infective	8 Oxazolidinones 9 Other Anti-infective
V Bones	3 Percutaneous	3 Anti-inflammatory 6 Nutritional Substance 7 Electrolytic and Water Balance Substance B Local Anesthetic H Radioactive Substance K Other Diagnostic Substance N Analgesics, Hypnotics, Sedatives T Destructive Agent	Z No Qualifier
V Bones	3 Percutaneous	G Other Therapeutic Substance	B Recombinant Bone Morphogenetic Protein C Other Substance
W Lymphatics	3 Percutaneous	0 Antineoplastic	5 Other Antineoplastic M Monoclonal Antibody
W Lymphatics	3 Percutaneous	2 Anti-infective	8 Oxazolidinones 9 Other Anti-infective
W Lymphatics	3 Percutaneous	3 Anti-inflammatory 6 Nutritional Substance 7 Electrolytic and Water Balance Substance B Local Anesthetic H Radioactive Substance K Other Diagnostic Substance N Analgesics, Hypnotics, Sedatives T Destructive Agent	Z No Qualifier
W Lymphatics	3 Percutaneous	G Other Therapeutic Substance	C Other Substance
Y Pericardial Cavity	3 Percutaneous	0 Antineoplastic	4 Liquid Brachytherapy Radioisotope 5 Other Antineoplastic M Monoclonal Antibody
Y Pericardial Cavity	3 Percutaneous	2 Anti-infective	8 Oxazolidinones 9 Other Anti-infective

Continued →

Section 3 **Administration**
Body System E **Physiological Systems and Anatomical Regions**
Operation 0 **Introduction:** Putting in or on a therapeutic, diagnostic, nutritional, physiological, or prophylactic substance except blood or blood products

Body System / Region (4th)	Approach (5th)	Substance (6th)	Qualifier (7th)
Y Pericardial Cavity	3 Percutaneous	3 Anti-inflammatory 6 Nutritional Substance 7 Electrolytic and Water Balance Substance B Local Anesthetic H Radioactive Substance K Other Diagnostic Substance N Analgesics, Hypnotics, Sedatives T Destructive Agent	Z No Qualifier
Y Pericardial Cavity	3 Percutaneous	G Other Therapeutic Substance	C Other Substance
Y Pericardial Cavity	3 Percutaneous	S Gas	F Other Gas
Y Pericardial Cavity	7 Via Natural or Artificial Opening	0 Antineoplastic	4 Liquid Brachytherapy Radioisotope 5 Other Antineoplastic M Monoclonal Antibody
Y Pericardial Cavity	7 Via Natural or Artificial Opening	S Gas	F Other Gas

Section 3 **Administration**
Body System E **Physiological Systems and Anatomical Regions**
Operation 1 **Irrigation:** Putting in or on a cleansing substance

Body System / Region (4th)	Approach (5th)	Substance (6th)	Qualifier (7th)
0 Skin and Mucous Membranes C Eye	3 Percutaneous X External	8 Irrigating Substance	X Diagnostic Z No Qualifier
9 Nose B Ear F Respiratory Tract G Upper GI H Lower GI J Biliary and Pancreatic Tract K Genitourinary Tract N Male Reproductive P Female Reproductive	3 Percutaneous 7 Via Natural or Artificial Opening 8 Via Natural or Artificial Opening Endoscopic	8 Irrigating Substance	X Diagnostic Z No Qualifier
L Pleural Cavity Q Cranial Cavity and Brain R Spinal Canal S Epidural Space U Joints Y Pericardial Cavity	3 Percutaneous	8 Irrigating Substance	X Diagnostic Z No Qualifier
M Peritoneal Cavity	3 Percutaneous	8 Irrigating Substance	X Diagnostic Z No Qualifier
M Peritoneal Cavity	3 Percutaneous	9 Dialysate	Z No Qualifier

Within each section of ICD-10-PCS the characters have different meanings. The seven character meanings for the Measurement and Monitoring section are illustrated here through the procedure example of *External electrocardiogram (EKG), single reading*.

Section	Body System	Root Operation	Body System	Approach	Function / Device	Qualifier
Measurement and Monitoring	Physiological Systems	Measurement	Cardiac	External	Electrical Activity	None
4	A	0	2	X	4	Z

Section (Character 1)

All Measurement and Monitoring procedure codes have a first character value of 4.

Body System (Character 2)

The alphanumeric character for the body system is placed in the second position. There are two character values applicable for the Measurement and Monitoring section. The character value of A is reported for physiological systems. The character value B is reported for physiological devices.

Root Operations (Character 3)

The alphanumeric character value for root operations is placed in the third position. Listed here are the root operations applicable to the Measurement and Monitoring section with their associated meaning.

Character Value	Root Operation	Root Operation Definition
0	Measurement	Determining the level of a physiological or physical function at a point in time
1	Monitoring	Determining the level of a physiological or physical function repetitively over a period of time

Body System/Region (Character 4)

For each body system the applicable body part character values will be available for procedure code construction. An example of a body region for this section is Respiratory.

Approach (Character 5)

The approach is the technique used to reach the procedure site. The following are the approach character values for the Measurement and Monitoring section with the associated definitions.

Character Value	Approach	Approach Definition
0	Open	Cutting through the skin or mucous membrane and any other body layers necessary to expose the site of the procedure
3	Percutaneous	Entry, by puncture or minor incision, of instrumentation through the skin or mucous membrane and any other body layers necessary to reach the site of the procedure
4	Percutaneous Endoscopic	Entry, by puncture or minor incision, of instrumentation through the skin or mucous membrane and any other body layers necessary to reach and visualize the site of the procedure
7	Via Natural or Artificial Opening	Entry of instrumentation through a natural or artificial external opening to reach the site of the procedure
8	Via Natural or Artificial Opening Endoscopic	Entry of instrumentation through a natural or artificial external opening to reach and visualize the site of the procedure
X	External	Procedures performed directly on the skin or mucous membrane and procedures performed indirectly by the application of external force through the skin or mucous membrane

unction/Device (Character 6)

the Measurement and Monitoring section a function or device is always utilized. The function or device is reported in the sixth character osition by the type of function monitored or measured or by the device utilized. The following is a sample list of the functions and devices cluded in this section:

- Conductivity
- Flow
- Metabolism
- Pressure
- Sound

ualifier (Character 7)

he qualifier represents an additional attribute for the procedure when applicable. There are several qualifiers included in the Measurement nd Monitoring section. For example, measurement procedures in this section include several qualifiers including stress that is reported with ne character value of 4. If there is no qualifier for a procedure, the placeholder Z is the character valve that should be reported.

HA Coding Clinic

A1134G Monitoring of Peripheral Nervous Electrical Activity, Intraoperative, Percutaneous Approach - AHA CC: 4Q, 2015, 28-29
A11X4G Monitoring of Peripheral Nervous Electrical Activity, Intraoperative, External Approach - AHA CC: 1Q, 2015, 26

Measurement and Monitoring Section Tables

Measurement and Monitoring Tables 4A0–4B0

ection	4	**Measurement and Monitoring**
ody System	A	**Physiological Systems**
peration	0	**Measurement:** Determining the level of a physiological or physical function at a point in time

Body System (4th)	Approach (5th)	Function / Device (6th)	Qualifier (7th)
0 Central Nervous	0 Open	2 Conductivity 4 Electrical Activity B Pressure	Z No Qualifier
0 Central Nervous	3 Percutaneous	4 Electrical Activity	Z No Qualifier
0 Central Nervous	3 Percutaneous	B Pressure K Temperature R Saturation	D Intracranial
0 Central Nervous	7 Via Natural or Artificial Opening	B Pressure K Temperature R Saturation	D Intracranial
0 Central Nervous	X External	2 Conductivity 4 Electrical Activity	Z No Qualifier
1 Peripheral Nervous	0 Open 3 Percutaneous X External	2 Conductivity	9 Sensory B Motor
1 Peripheral Nervous	0 Open 3 Percutaneous X External	4 Electrical Activity	Z No Qualifier
2 Cardiac	0 Open 3 Percutaneous	4 Electrical Activity 9 Output C Rate F Rhythm H Sound P Action Currents	Z No Qualifier
2 Cardiac	0 Open 3 Percutaneous	N Sampling and Pressure	6 Right Heart 7 Left Heart 8 Bilateral

Continued →

Section   **4**   **Measurement and Monitoring**
Body System   **A**   **Physiological Systems**
Operation   **0**   **Measurement:** Determining the level of a physiological or physical function at a point in time

Body System (4th)	Approach (5th)	Function / Device (6th)	Qualifier (7th)
2 Cardiac	X External	4 Electrical Activity	A Guidance Z No Qualifier
2 Cardiac	X External	9 Output C Rate F Rhythm H Sound P Action Currents	Z No Qualifier
2 Cardiac	X External	M Total Activity	4 Stress
3 Arterial	0 Open 3 Percutaneous	5 Flow J Pulse	1 Peripheral 3 Pulmonary C Coronary
3 Arterial	0 Open 3 Percutaneous	B Pressure	1 Peripheral 3 Pulmonary C Coronary F Other Thoracic
3 Arterial	0 Open 3 Percutaneous	H Sound R Saturation	1 Peripheral
3 Arterial	X External	5 Flow B Pressure H Sound J Pulse R Saturation	1 Peripheral
4 Venous	0 Open 3 Percutaneous	5 Flow B Pressure J Pulse	0 Central 1 Peripheral 2 Portal 3 Pulmonary
4 Venous	0 Open 3 Percutaneous	R Saturation	1 Peripheral
4 Venous	X External	5 Flow B Pressure J Pulse R Saturation	1 Peripheral
5 Circulatory	X External	L Volume	Z No Qualifier
6 Lymphatic	0 Open 3 Percutaneous	5 Flow B Pressure	Z No Qualifier
7 Visual	X External	0 Acuity 7 Mobility B Pressure	Z No Qualifier
8 Olfactory	X External	0 Acuity	Z No Qualifier
9 Respiratory	7 Via Natural or Artificial Opening 8 Via Natural or Artificial Opening Endoscopic X External	1 Capacity 5 Flow C Rate D Resistance L Volume M Total Activity	Z No Qualifier
B Gastrointestinal	7 Via Natural or Artificial Opening 8 Via Natural or Artificial Opening Endoscopic	8 Motility B Pressure G Secretion	Z No Qualifier

Continued →

Section 4 **Measurement and Monitoring**
Body System A **Physiological Systems**
Operation 0 **Measurement: Determining the level of a physiological or physical function at a point in time**

Body System (4th)	Approach (5th)	Function / Device (6th)	Qualifier (7th)
C Biliary	**3** Percutaneous **4** Percutaneous Endoscopic **7** Via Natural or Artificial Opening **8** Via Natural or Artificial Opening Endoscopic	**5** Flow **B** Pressure	**Z** No Qualifier
D Urinary	**7** Via Natural or Artificial Opening	**3** Contractility **5** Flow **B** Pressure **D** Resistance **L** Volume	**Z** No Qualifier
F Musculoskeletal	**3** Percutaneous **X** External	**3** Contractility	**Z** No Qualifier
H Products of Conception, Cardiac	**7** Via Natural or Artificial Opening **8** Via Natural or Artificial Opening Endoscopic **X** External	**4** Electrical Activity **C** Rate **F** Rhythm **H** Sound	**Z** No Qualifier
J Products of Conception, Nervous	**7** Via Natural or Artificial Opening **8** Via Natural or Artificial Opening Endoscopic **X** External	**2** Conductivity **4** Electrical Activity **B** Pressure	**Z** No Qualifier
Z None	**7** Via Natural or Artificial Opening	**6** Metabolism **K** Temperature	**Z** No Qualifier
Z None	**X** External	**6** Metabolism **K** Temperature **Q** Sleep	**Z** No Qualifier

Section 4 **Measurement and Monitoring**
Body System A **Physiological Systems**
Operation 1 **Monitoring: Determining the level of a physiological or physical function repetitively over a period of time**

Body System (4th)	Approach (5th)	Function / Device (6th)	Qualifier (7th)
0 Central Nervous	**0** Open	**2** Conductivity **B** Pressure	**Z** No Qualifier
0 Central Nervous	**0** Open	**4** Electrical Activity	**G** Intraoperative **Z** No Qualifier
0 Central Nervous	**3** Percutaneous	**4** Electrical Activity	**G** Intraoperative **Z** No Qualifier
0 Central Nervous	**3** Percutaneous	**B** Pressure **K** Temperature **R** Saturation	**D** Intracranial
0 Central Nervous	**7** Via Natural or Artificial Opening	**B** Pressure **K** Temperature **R** Saturation	**D** Intracranial
0 Central Nervous	**X** External	**2** Conductivity	**Z** No Qualifier
0 Central Nervous	**X** External	**4** Electrical Activity	**G** Intraoperative **Z** No Qualifier
1 Peripheral Nervous	**0** Open **3** Percutaneous **X** External	**2** Conductivity	**9** Sensory **B** Motor

Continued →

Section **4** **Measurement and Monitoring**
Body System **A** **Physiological Systems**
Operation **1** **Monitoring:** Determining the level of a physiological or physical function repetitively over a period of time

Body System (4th)	Approach (5th)	Function / Device (6th)	Qualifier (7th)
1 Peripheral Nervous	0 Open 3 Percutaneous X External	4 Electrical Activity	G Intraoperative Z No Qualifier
2 Cardiac	0 Open 3 Percutaneous	4 Electrical Activity 9 Output C Rate F Rhythm H Sound	Z No Qualifier
2 Cardiac	X External	4 Electrical Activity	5 Ambulatory Z No Qualifier
2 Cardiac	X External	9 Output C Rate F Rhythm H Sound	Z No Qualifier
2 Cardiac	X External	M Total Activity	4 Stress
3 Arterial	0 Open 3 Percutaneous	5 Flow B Pressure J Pulse	1 Peripheral 3 Pulmonary C Coronary
3 Arterial	0 Open 3 Percutaneous	H Sound R Saturation	1 Peripheral
3 Arterial	X External	5 Flow B Pressure H Sound J Pulse R Saturation	1 Peripheral
4 Venous	0 Open 3 Percutaneous	5 Flow B Pressure J Pulse	0 Central 1 Peripheral 2 Portal 3 Pulmonary
4 Venous	0 Open 3 Percutaneous	R Saturation	0 Central 2 Portal 3 Pulmonary
4 Venous	X External	5 Flow B Pressure J Pulse	1 Peripheral
6 Lymphatic	0 Open 3 Percutaneous	5 Flow B Pressure	Z No Qualifier
9 Respiratory	7 Via Natural or Artificial Opening X External	1 Capacity 5 Flow C Rate D Resistance L Volume	Z No Qualifier
B Gastrointestinal	7 Via Natural or Artificial Opening 8 Via Natural or Artificial Opening Endoscopic	8 Motility B Pressure G Secretion	Z No Qualifier

Continued →

Section 4 Measurement and Monitoring
Body System A Physiological Systems
Operation 1 Monitoring: Determining the level of a physiological or physical function repetitively over a period of time

4A1 Continued

4A1–4B0

Body System (4th)	Approach (5th)	Function / Device (6th)	Qualifier (7th)
D Urinary	7 Via Natural or Artificial Opening	3 Contractility 5 Flow B Pressure D Resistance L Volume	Z No Qualifier
H Products of Conception, Cardiac	7 Via Natural or Artificial Opening 8 Via Natural or Artificial Opening Endoscopic X External	4 Electrical Activity C Rate F Rhythm H Sound	Z No Qualifier
J Products of Conception, Nervous	7 Via Natural or Artificial Opening 8 Via Natural or Artificial Opening Endoscopic X External	2 Conductivity 4 Electrical Activity B Pressure	Z No Qualifier
Z None	7 Via Natural or Artificial Opening	K Temperature	Z No Qualifier
Z None	X External	K Temperature Q Sleep	Z No Qualifier

Section 4 Measurement and Monitoring
Body System B Physiological Devices
Operation 0 Measurement: Determining the level of a physiological or physical function at a point in time

Body System (4th)	Approach (5th)	Function / Device (6th)	Qualifier (7th)
0 Central Nervous 1 Peripheral Nervous F Musculoskeletal	X External	V Stimulator	Z No Qualifier
2 Cardiac	X External	S Pacemaker T Defibrillator	Z No Qualifier
9 Respiratory	X External	S Pacemaker	Z No Qualifier

Within each section of ICD-10-PCS the characters have different meanings. The seven character meanings for the Extracorporeal Assistance and Performance section are illustrated here through the procedure example of *Hyperbaric oxygenation of wound*.

Section	Body System	Root Operation	Body System	Duration	Function	Qualifier
Extracorporeal Assistance and Performance	Physiological Systems	Assistance	Circulatory	Intermittent	Oxygenation	Hyperbaric
5	A	0	5	1	2	1

Section (Character 1)

All Extracorporeal Assistance and Performance procedure codes have a first character value of 5.

Body System (Character 2)

The alphanumeric character for the body system is placed in the second position. There is one character value applicable for the Extracorporeal Assistance and Performance section. The character value of A is reported for physiological systems.

Root Operations (Character 3)

The alphanumeric character value for root operations is placed in the third position. Listed here are the root operations applicable to the Extracorporeal Assistance and Performance section with their associated meaning.

Character Value	Root Operation	Root Operation Definition
0	Assistance	Taking over a portion of a physiological function by extracorporeal means
1	Performance	Completely taking over a physiological function by extracorporeal means
2	Restoration	Returning, or attempting to return, a physiological function to its original state by extracorporeal means

Body System (Character 4)

For each body system, the applicable body part character values will be available for procedure code construction. An example of a body region for this section is respiratory.

Duration (Character 5)

The duration represents the length of time or frequency for which the assistance or performance is utilized. Some examples of duration are Intermittent, Continuous, or Less than 24 consecutive hours.

Function (Character 6)

In the Extracorporeal Assistance and Performance section a function is always reported. The function is reported in the sixth character position. The following is a sample list of the functions utilized in this section:

- Output
- Oxygenation
- Pacing
- Ventilation

Qualifier (Character 7)

The qualifier represents an additional attribute for the procedure when applicable. There are several qualifiers included in the Extracorporeal Assistance and Performance section. For example, assistance procedures in this section include several qualifiers including Balloon Pump, which is reported with the character value of 0. If there is no qualifier for a procedure, the placeholder Z is the character valve that should be reported.

HA Coding Clinic

A02210 Assistance with Cardiac Output using Balloon Pump, Continuous - AHA CC: 3Q, 2013, 18-19
A0221D Assistance with Cardiac Output using Impeller Pump, Continuous - AHA CC: 3Q, 2014, 19
A09357 Assistance with Respiratory Ventilation, <24 Hrs, CPAP - AHA CC: 4Q, 2014, 9-10
A09457 Assistance with Respiratory Ventilation, 24-96 Hrs, CPAP - AHA CC: 4Q, 2014, 9-10
A09557 Assistance with Respiratory Ventilation, >96 Hrs, CPAP - AHA CC: 4Q, 2014, 9-10
A1221Z Performance of Cardiac Output, Continuous - AHA CC: 3Q, 2013, 18-19; 1Q, 2014, 10-11; 3Q, 2014, 16-17, 20-21
A1223Z Performance of Cardiac Pacing, Continuous - AHA CC: 3Q, 2013, 18-19
A1935Z Respiratory Ventilation, Less than 24 Consecutive Hours - AHA CC: 4Q, 2014, 3-15
A1945Z Respiratory Ventilation, 24-96 Consecutive Hours - AHA CC: 4Q, 2014, 3-15
A1955Z Respiratory Ventilation, Greater than 96 Consecutive Hours - AHA CC: 4Q, 2014, 3-15

Extracorporeal Assistance and Performance Section Tables

Extracorporeal Assistance and Performance Tables 5A0–5A2

Section	5	Extracorporeal Assistance and Performance
Body System	A	Physiological Systems
Operation	0	Assistance: Taking over a portion of a physiological function by extracorporeal means

Body System (4th)	Duration (5th)	Function (6th)	Qualifier (7th)
2 Cardiac	1 Intermittent 2 Continuous	1 Output	0 Balloon Pump 5 Pulsatile Compression 6 Other Pump D Impeller Pump
5 Circulatory	1 Intermittent 2 Continuous	2 Oxygenation	1 Hyperbaric C Supersaturated
9 Respiratory	3 Less than 24 Consecutive Hours 4 24-96 Consecutive Hours 5 Greater than 96 Consecutive Hours	5 Ventilation	7 Continuous Positive Airway Pressure 8 Intermittent Positive Airway Pressure 9 Continuous Negative Airway Pressure B Intermittent Negative Airway Pressure Z No Qualifier

Section	5	Extracorporeal Assistance and Performance
Body System	A	Physiological Systems
Operation	1	Performance: Completely taking over a physiological function by extracorporeal means

Body System (4th)	Duration (5th)	Function (6th)	Qualifier (7th)
2 Cardiac	0 Single	1 Output	2 Manual
2 Cardiac	1 Intermittent	3 Pacing	Z No Qualifier
2 Cardiac	2 Continuous	1 Output 3 Pacing	Z No Qualifier
5 Circulatory	2 Continuous	2 Oxygenation	3 Membrane
9 Respiratory	0 Single	5 Ventilation	4 Nonmechanical
9 Respiratory	3 Less than 24 Consecutive Hours 4 24-96 Consecutive Hours 5 Greater than 96 Consecutive Hours	5 Ventilation	Z No Qualifier
C Biliary D Urinary	0 Single 6 Multiple	0 Filtration	Z No Qualifier

Section	5	Extracorporeal Assistance and Performance
Body System	A	Physiological Systems
Operation	2	Restoration: Returning, or attempting to return, a physiological function to its original state by extracorporeal means.

Body System (4th)	Duration (5th)	Function (6th)	Qualifier (7th)
2 Cardiac	0 Single	4 Rhythm	Z No Qualifier

Within each section of ICD-10-PCS the characters have different meanings. The seven character meanings for the Extracorporeal Therapies section are illustrated here through the procedure example of *Ultraviolet light phototherapy, series treatment*.

Section	Body System	Root Operation	Body System	Duration	Qualifier	Qualifier
Extracorporeal Therapies	Physiological Systems	UV Light Therapy	Skin	Multiple	None	None
6	A	8	0	1	Z	Z

Section (Character 1)

All Extracorporeal Therapies procedure codes have a first character value of 6.

Body System (Character 2)

The alphanumeric character for the body system is placed in the second position. There is one character value applicable for the Extracorporeal Therapies section. The character value of A is reported for physiological systems.

Root Operations (Character 3)

The alphanumeric character value for root operations is placed in the third position. Listed below are the root operations applicable to the Extracorporeal Therapies section with their associated meaning.

Character Value	Root Operation	Root Operation Definition
0	Atmospheric Control	Extracorporeal control of atmospheric pressure and composition
1	Decompression	Extracorporeal elimination of undissolved gas from body fluids
2	Electromagnetic Therapy	Extracorporeal treatment by electromagnetic rays
3	Hyperthermia	Extracorporeal raising of body temperature
4	Hypothermia	Extracorporeal lowering of body temperature
5	Pheresis	Extracorporeal separation of blood products
6	Phototherapy	Extracorporeal treatment by light rays
7	Ultrasound Therapy	Extracorporeal treatment by ultrasound
8	Ultraviolet Light Therapy	Extracorporeal treatment by ultraviolet light
9	Shock Wave Therapy	Extracorporeal treatment by shock waves

Body System (Character 4)

For each body system the applicable body part character values will be available for procedure code construction. An example of a body region for this section is Skin.

Duration (Character 5)

The duration represents the number of therapy sessions performed. Single is reported with character value 0; Multiple is reported with character value 1.

Qualifier (Character 6)

Character 6 is the first of two qualifier characters for the Extracorporeal Therapies section. The qualifier represents an additional attribute for the procedure when applicable. There are currently no qualifier values for the sixth character position, so the character value of Z is always reported.

Qualifier (Character 7)

Character 7 is the second of two qualifier characters for the Extracorporeal Therapies section. The qualifier represents an additional attribute for the procedure when applicable. There are some qualifiers included in the Extracorporeal Therapies section. For example, pheresis procedures in this section include several qualifiers including Plasma that is reported with the character value of 3. If there is no qualifier for a procedure, the placeholder Z is the character valve that should be reported.

AHA Coding Clinic

6A750Z7 Ultrasound Therapy of Other Vessels, Single - AHA CC: 4Q, 2014, 19-20

Extracorporeal Therapies Tables

Extracorporeal Therapies Tables 6A0–6A9

Section	6	Extracorporeal Therapies
Body System	A	Physiological Systems
Operation	0	Atmospheric Control: Extracorporeal control of atmospheric pressure and composition

Body System (4th)	Duration (5th)	Qualifier (6th)	Qualifier (7th)
Z None	0 Single 1 Multiple	Z No Qualifier	Z No Qualifier

Section	6	Extracorporeal Therapies
Body System	A	Physiological Systems
Operation	1	Decompression: Extracorporeal elimination of undissolved gas from body fluids

Body System (4th)	Duration (5th)	Qualifier (6th)	Qualifier (7th)
5 Circulatory	0 Single 1 Multiple	Z No Qualifier	Z No Qualifier

Section	6	Extracorporeal Therapies
Body System	A	Physiological Systems
Operation	2	Electromagnetic Therapy: Extracorporeal treatment by electromagnetic rays

Body System (4th)	Duration (5th)	Qualifier (6th)	Qualifier (7th)
1 Urinary 2 Central Nervous	0 Single 1 Multiple	Z No Qualifier	Z No Qualifier

Section	6	Extracorporeal Therapies
Body System	A	Physiological Systems
Operation	3	Hyperthermia: Extracorporeal raising of body temperature

Body System (4th)	Duration (5th)	Qualifier (6th)	Qualifier (7th)
Z None	0 Single 1 Multiple	Z No Qualifier	Z No Qualifier

Section	6	Extracorporeal Therapies
Body System	A	Physiological Systems
Operation	4	Hypothermia: Extracorporeal lowering of body temperature

Body System (4th)	Duration (5th)	Qualifier (6th)	Qualifier (7th)
Z None	0 Single 1 Multiple	Z No Qualifier	Z No Qualifier

Section	6	Extracorporeal Therapies
Body System	A	Physiological Systems
Operation	5	Pheresis: Extracorporeal separation of blood products

Body System (4th)	Duration (5th)	Qualifier (6th)	Qualifier (7th)
5 Circulatory	0 Single 1 Multiple	Z No Qualifier	0 Erythrocytes 1 Leukocytes 2 Platelets 3 Plasma T Stem Cells, Cord Blood V Stem Cells, Hematopoietic

Section	6	Extracorporeal Therapies
Body System	A	Physiological Systems
Operation	6	Phototherapy: Extracorporeal treatment by light rays

Body System (4th)	Duration (5th)	Qualifier (6th)	Qualifier (7th)
0 Skin 5 Circulatory	0 Single 1 Multiple	Z No Qualifier	Z No Qualifier

Section	6	Extracorporeal Therapies
Body System	A	Physiological Systems
Operation	7	Ultrasound Therapy: Extracorporeal treatment by ultrasound

Body System (4th)	Duration (5th)	Qualifier (6th)	Qualifier (7th)
5 Circulatory	0 Single 1 Multiple	Z No Qualifier	4 Head and Neck Vessels 5 Heart 6 Peripheral Vessels 7 Other Vessels Z No Qualifier

Section	6	Extracorporeal Therapies
Body System	A	Physiological Systems
Operation	8	Ultraviolet Light Therapy: Extracorporeal treatment by ultraviolet light

Body System (4th)	Duration (5th)	Qualifier (6th)	Qualifier (7th)
0 Skin	0 Single 1 Multiple	Z No Qualifier	Z No Qualifier

Section	6	Extracorporeal Therapies
Body System	A	Physiological Systems
Operation	9	Shock Wave Therapy: Extracorporeal treatment by shock waves

Body System (4th)	Duration (5th)	Qualifier (6th)	Qualifier (7th)
3 Musculoskeletal	0 Single 1 Multiple	Z No Qualifier	Z No Qualifier

Within each section of ICD-10-PCS, the characters have different meanings. The seven character meanings for the Osteopathic section are illustrated below through the procedure example of Indirect osteopathic treatment of sacrum.

Section	Body System	Root Operation	Body Region	Approach	Method	Qualifier
Osteopathic	Anatomical Regions	Treatment	Sacrum	External	Indirect	None
7	W	0	4	X	4	Z

Section (Character 1)

All Osteopathic procedure codes have a first character value of 7.

Body System (Character 2)

The alphanumeric character for the body system is placed in the second position. There is one character value applicable for the Osteopathic section. The character value of W is reported for anatomical regions.

Root Operations (Character 3)

The alphanumeric character value for root operations is placed in the third position. Listed here is the root operation applicable to the Osteopathic section with its associated meaning.

Character Value	Root Operation	Root Operation Definition
0	Treatment	Manual treatment to eliminate or alleviate somatic dysfunction and related disorders

Body Region (Character 4)

For each body region the applicable body part character values will be available for procedure code construction. An example of a body region for this section is Head.

Approach (Character 5)

The approach is the technique used to reach the procedure site. The following are the approach character values for the Osteopathic section with the associated definitions.

Character Value	Approach	Approach Definition
X	External	Procedures performed directly on the skin or mucous membrane and procedures performed indirectly by the application of external force through the skin or mucous membrane

Method (Character 6)

The method identifies the treatment method used to complete the osteopathic procedure. The available methods are:

- Articulatory-Raising
- Fascial Release
- General Mobilization
- High Velocity-Low Amplitude
- Indirect
- Low Velocity-High Amplitude
- Lymphatic Pump
- Muscle Energy-Isometric
- Muscle Energy-Isotonic
- Other

Qualifier (Character 7)

The qualifier represents an additional attribute for the procedure when applicable. Currently, there are no qualifiers in the Osteopath section; therefore, the placeholder character value of Z should be reported.

Osteopathic Section Table

Osteopathic Table 7W0

Section 7 **Osteopathic**
Body System W **Anatomical Regions**
Operation 0 **Treatment:** Manual treatment to eliminate or alleviate somatic dysfunction and related disorders

Body Region (4th)	Approach (5th)	Method (6th)	Qualifier (7th)
0 Head	X External	0 Articulatory-Raising	Z None
1 Cervical		1 Fascial Release	
2 Thoracic		2 General Mobilization	
3 Lumbar		3 High Velocity-Low Amplitude	
4 Sacrum		4 Indirect	
5 Pelvis		5 Low Velocity-High Amplitude	
6 Lower Extremities		6 Lymphatic Pump	
7 Upper Extremities		7 Muscle Energy-Isometric	
8 Rib Cage		8 Muscle Energy-Isotonic	
9 Abdomen		9 Other Method	

Within each section of ICD-10-PCS the characters have different meanings. The seven character meanings for the Other Procedures section are illustrated here through the procedure example of Yoga therapy.

Section	Body System	Root Operation	Body Region	Approach	Method	Qualifier
Other Procedures	Physiological Systems and Anatomical Regions	Other Procedures	None	External	Other Method	Yoga Therapy
8	E	0	Z	X	Y	4

Section (Character 1)

All Other Procedures codes have a first character value of 8.

Body System (Character 2)

The alphanumeric character for the body system is placed in the second position. There are two character values applicable for the Other Procedures section. The character value of C is reported for indwelling device. Th character value of E is reported for physiological system and anatomical regions.

Root Operations (Character 3)

The alphanumeric character value for root operations is placed in the third position. Listed here is the root operation applicable to the Other Procedures section with its associated meaning.

Character Value	Root Operation	Root Operation Definition
0	Other Procedures	Methodologies which attempt to remediate or cure a disorder or disease

Body Region (Character 4)

For each body region the applicable body part character values will be available for procedure code construction. An example of a body region for this section is Lower Extremity.

Approach (Character 5)

The approach is the technique used to reach the procedure site. The following are the approach character values for the Other Procedures section with the associated definitions.

Character Value	Approach	Approach Definition
0	Open	Cutting through the skin or mucous membrane and any other body layers necessary to expose the site of the procedure
3	Percutaneous	Entry, by puncture or minor incision, of instrumentation through the skin or mucous membrane and any other body layers necessary to reach the site of the procedure
4	Percutaneous Endoscopic	Entry, by puncture or minor incision, of instrumentation through the skin or mucous membrane and any other body layers necessary to reach and visualize the site of the procedure
7	Via Natural or Artificial Opening	Entry of instrumentation through a natural or artificial external opening to reach the site of the procedure
8	Via Natural or Artificial Opening Endoscopic	Entry of instrumentation through a natural or artificial external opening to reach and visualize the site of the procedure
X	External	Procedures performed directly on the skin or mucous membrane and procedures performed indirectly by the application of external force through the skin or mucous membrane

Method (Character 6)

The method identifies the treatment method used to complete the other procedure. The available methods are:

- Acupuncture
- Collection
- Computer Assisted Procedure
- Near Infrared Spectroscopy
- Robotic Assisted procedure
- Therapeutic Massage
- Other

Qualifier (Character 7)

The qualifier represents an additional attribute for the procedure when applicable. In the preceding example of Yoga therapy, the qualifier of 4 was used to report that the other procedure was Yoga therapy. If there is no qualifier for a procedure, the placeholder Z is the character valve that should be reported.

AHA Coding Clinic

8E0W4CZ Robotic Assisted Procedure of Trunk Region, Percutaneous Endoscopic Approach - AHA CC: 4Q, 2014, 33-34; 1Q, 2015, 33-34

Other Procedures Section Tables

Other Procedures Tables 8C0–8E0

Section	8	Other Procedures
Body System	C	Indwelling Device
Operation	0	Other Procedures: Methodologies which attempt to remediate or cure a disorder or disease

Body Region (4th)	Approach (5th)	Method (6th)	Qualifier (7th)
1 Nervous System	X External	6 Collection	J Cerebrospinal Fluid L Other Fluid
2 Circulatory System	X External	6 Collection	K Blood L Other Fluid

Section	8	Other Procedures
Body System	E	Physiological Systems and Anatomical Regions
Operation	0	Other Procedures: Methodologies which attempt to remediate or cure a disorder or disease

Body Region (4th)	Approach (5th)	Method (6th)	Qualifier (7th)
1 Nervous System U Female Reproductive System	X External	Y Other Method	7 Examination
2 Circulatory System	3 Percutaneous	D Near Infrared Spectroscopy	Z No Qualifier
9 Head and Neck Region W Trunk Region	0 Open 3 Percutaneous 4 Percutaneous Endoscopic 7 Via Natural or Artificial Opening 8 Via Natural or Artificial Opening Endoscopic	C Robotic Assisted Procedure	Z No Qualifier
9 Head and Neck Region W Trunk Region	X External	B Computer Assisted Procedure	F With Fluoroscopy G With Computerized Tomography H With Magnetic Resonance Imaging Z No Qualifier
9 Head and Neck Region W Trunk Region	X External	C Robotic Assisted Procedure	Z No Qualifier

Continued →

Section 8 Other Procedures *8E0 Continued*
Body System E Physiological Systems and Anatomical Regions
Operation 0 Other Procedures: Methodologies which attempt to remediate or cure a disorder or disease

8E0

Body Region (4th)	Approach (5th)	Method (6th)	Qualifier (7th)
9 Head and Neck Region W Trunk Region	X External	Y Other Method	8 Suture Removal
H Integumentary System and Breast	3 Percutaneous	0 Acupuncture	0 Anesthesia Z No Qualifier
H Integumentary System and Breast	X External	6 Collection	2 Breast Milk
H Integumentary System and Breast	X External	Y Other Method	9 Piercing
K Musculoskeletal System	X External	1 Therapeutic Massage	Z No Qualifier
K Musculoskeletal System	X External	Y Other Method	7 Examination
V Male Reproductive System	X External	1 Therapeutic Massage	C Prostate D Rectum
V Male Reproductive System	X External	6 Collection	3 Sperm
X Upper Extremity Y Lower Extremity	0 Open 3 Percutaneous 4 Percutaneous Endoscopic	C Robotic Assisted Procedure	Z No Qualifier
X Upper Extremity Y Lower Extremity	X External	B Computer Assisted Procedure	F With Fluoroscopy G With Computerized Tomography H With Magnetic Resonance Imaging Z No Qualifier
X Upper Extremity Y Lower Extremity	X External	C Robotic Assisted Procedure	Z No Qualifier
X Upper Extremity Y Lower Extremity	X External	Y Other Method	8 Suture Removal
Z None	X External	Y Other Method	1 In Vitro Fertilization 4 Yoga Therapy 5 Meditation 6 Isolation

Within each section of ICD-10-PCS the characters have different meanings. The seven character meanings for the Chiropractic section are illustrated here through the procedure example of Chiropractic treatment of cervical spine, short lever specific contact.

Section	Body System	Root Operation	Body Region	Approach	Method	Qualifier
Chiropractic	Anatomical Regions	Manipulation	Cervical	External	Short Lever Specific Contact	None
9	W	B	1	X	H	Z

Section (Character 1)

All Chiropractic procedure codes have a first character value of 9.

Body System (Character 2)

The alphanumeric character for the body system is placed in the second position. There is one character value applicable for the Chiropractic section. The character value of W is reported for anatomical regions.

Root Operations (Character 3)

The alphanumeric character value for root operations is placed in the third position. The following is the root operation applicable to the Chiropractic section with its associated meaning.

Character Value	Root Operation	Root Operation Definition
B	Manipulation	Manual procedure that involves a directed thrust to move a joint past the physiological range of motion, without exceeding the anatomical limit

Body Region (Character 4)

For each body region the applicable body part character values will be available for procedure code construction. An example of a body region for this section is Rib Cage.

Approach (Character 5)

The approach is the technique used to reach the procedure site. The following are the approach character values for the Chiropractic section with the associated definitions.

Character Value	Approach	Approach Definition
X	External	Procedures performed directly on the skin or mucous membrane and procedures performed indirectly by the application of external force through the skin or mucous membrane

Method (Character 6)

The method identifies the treatment method used to complete the chiropractic procedure. The available methods are:

- Non-Manual
- Indirect Visceral
- Extra-Articular
- Direct-Visual
- Long Lever Specific Contact
- Short Lever Specific Contact
- Long and Short Lever Specific Contact
- Mechanically Assisted
- Other

Qualifier (Character 7)

The qualifier represents an additional attribute for the procedure when applicable. Currently, there are no qualifiers in the Chiropractic section; therefore, the placeholder character value of Z should be reported.

Chiropractic Section Table

Chiropractic Table 9WB

Section	9	Chiropractic
Body System	W	Anatomical Regions
Operation	B	Manipulation: Manual procedure that involves a directed thrust to move a joint past the physiological range of motion, without exceeding the anatomical limit

Body Region (4th)	Approach (5th)	Method (6th)	Qualifier (7th)
0 Head	X External	B Non-Manual	Z None
1 Cervical		C Indirect Visceral	
2 Thoracic		D Extra-Articular	
3 Lumbar		F Direct Visceral	
4 Sacrum		G Long Lever Specific Contact	
5 Pelvis		H Short Lever Specific Contact	
6 Lower Extremities		J Long and Short Lever Specific Contact	
7 Upper Extremities		K Mechanically Assisted	
8 Rib Cage		L Other Method	
9 Abdomen			

Within each section of ICD-10-PCS the characters have different meanings. The seven character meanings for the Imaging section ar illustrated here through the procedure example of X-ray right clavicle, limited study.

Section	Body System	Root Type	Body Part	Contrast	Qualifier	Qualifier
Imaging	Non-Axial Upper Bones	Plain Radiography	Clavicle, right	None	None	None
B	P	0	4	Z	Z	Z

Section (Character 1)

All Imaging procedure codes have a first character value of B.

Body System (Character 2)

The alphanumeric character for the body system is placed in the second position. The following are the body systems applicable to th Imaging section.

Character Value	Character Value Description
0	Central Nervous System
2	Heart
3	Upper Arteries
4	Lower Arteries
5	Veins
7	Lymphatic System
8	Eye
9	Ear, Nose, Mouth and Throat
B	Respiratory System
D	Gastrointestinal System
F	Hepatobiliary System and Pancreas
G	Endocrine System
H	Skin, Subcutaneous Tissue and Breast
L	Connective Tissue
N	Skull and Facial Bones
P	Non-Axial Upper Bones
Q	Non-Axial Lower Bones
R	Axial Skeleton, Except Skull and Facial Bones
T	Urinary System
U	Female Reproductive System
V	Male Reproductive System
W	Anatomical Regions
Y	Fetus and Obstetrical

Root Types (Character 3)

The alphanumeric character value for root types is placed in the third position. Listed here are the root types applicable to the Imaging section with their associated meaning.

Character Value	Root Type	Root Type Definition
0	Plain Radiography	Planar display of an image developed from the capture of external ionizing radiation on photographic or photoconductive plate
1	Fluoroscopy	Single plane or bi-plane real time display of an image developed from the capture of external ionizing radiation on a fluorescent screen. The image may also be stored by either digital or analog means

Continued →

Character Value	Root Type	Root Type Definition
2	Computerized Tomography (CT Scan)	Computer reformatted digital display of multiplanar images developed from the capture of multiple exposures of external ionizing radiation
3	Magnetic Resonance Imaging (MRI)	Computer reformatted digital display of multiplanar images developed from the capture of radiofrequency signals emitted by nuclei in a body site excited within a magnetic field
4	Ultrasonography	Real time display of images of anatomy or flow information developed from the capture of reflected and attenuated high frequency sound waves

Body Part (Character 4)

For each body part the applicable body part character values will be available for procedure code construction. An example of a body part for this section is Spinal Cord.

Contrast (Character 5)

When contrast is utilized during an imaging procedure, the corresponding contrast character value should be reported in the fifth character position. The following are the contrast character values for the Imaging section:

- High Osmolar
- Low Osmolar
- Other Contrast

If contrast is not utilized, the placeholder character value of Z should be reported.

Qualifier (Character 6)

This qualifier character specifies when an image taken without contrast is followed by one with contrast. The character value of 0 is reported for Unenhanced and Enhanced.

Qualifier (Character 7)

The qualifier represents an additional attribute for the procedure when applicable. For example, ultrasonography procedures in this section include the qualifier Densitometry that is reported with the character value of 1 for some body parts. If there is no qualifier for a procedure, the placeholder Z is the character value that should be reported.

Imaging Section Tables

Imaging Tables B00–BY4

Section	B	Imaging
Body System	0	Central Nervous System
Type	0	Plain Radiography: Planar display of an image developed from the capture of external ionizing radiation on photographic or photoconductive plate

Body Part (4th)	Contrast (5th)	Qualifier (6th)	Qualifier (7th)
B Spinal Cord	0 High Osmolar 1 Low Osmolar Y Other Contrast Z None	Z None	Z None

Section	B	Imaging
Body System	0	Central Nervous System
Type	1	Fluoroscopy: Single plane or bi-plane real time display of an image developed from the capture of external ionizing radiation on a fluorescent screen. The image may also be stored by either digital or analog means

Body Part (4th)	Contrast (5th)	Qualifier (6th)	Qualifier (7th)
B Spinal Cord	0 High Osmolar 1 Low Osmolar Y Other Contrast Z None	Z None	Z None

Section	B	Imaging
Body System	0	Central Nervous System
Type	2	Computerized Tomography (CT Scan): Computer reformatted digital display of multiplanar images developed from the capture of multiple exposures of external ionizing radiation

Body Part (4th)	Contrast (5th)	Qualifier (6th)	Qualifier (7th)
0 Brain 7 Cisterna 8 Cerebral Ventricle(s) 9 Sella Turcica/Pituitary Gland B Spinal Cord	0 High Osmolar 1 Low Osmolar Y Other Contrast	0 Unenhanced and Enhanced Z None	Z None
0 Brain 7 Cisterna 8 Cerebral Ventricle(s) 9 Sella Turcica/Pituitary Gland B Spinal Cord	Z None	Z None	Z None

Section	B	Imaging
Body System	0	Central Nervous System
Type	3	Magnetic Resonance Imaging (MRI): Computer reformatted digital display of multiplanar images developed from the capture of radiofrequency signals emitted by nuclei in a body site excited within a magnetic field

Body Part (4th)	Contrast (5th)	Qualifier (6th)	Qualifier (7th)
0 Brain 9 Sella Turcica/Pituitary Gland B Spinal Cord C Acoustic Nerves	Y Other Contrast	0 Unenhanced and Enhanced Z None	Z None
0 Brain 9 Sella Turcica/Pituitary Gland B Spinal Cord C Acoustic Nerves	Z None	Z None	Z None

Section	B	Imaging
Body System	0	Central Nervous System
Type	4	Ultrasonography: Real time display of images of anatomy or flow information developed from the capture of reflected and attenuated high frequency sound waves

Body Part (4th)	Contrast (5th)	Qualifier (6th)	Qualifier (7th)
0 Brain B Spinal Cord	Z None	Z None	Z None

Section	B	Imaging
Body System	2	Heart
Type	0	Plain Radiography: Planar display of an image developed from the capture of external ionizing radiation on photographic or photoconductive plate

Body Part (4th)	Contrast (5th)	Qualifier (6th)	Qualifier (7th)
0 Coronary Artery, Single 1 Coronary Arteries, Multiple 2 Coronary Artery Bypass Graft, Single 3 Coronary Artery Bypass Grafts, Multiple 4 Heart, Right 5 Heart, Left 6 Heart, Right and Left 7 Internal Mammary Bypass Graft, Right 8 Internal Mammary Bypass Graft, Left F Bypass Graft, Other	0 High Osmolar 1 Low Osmolar Y Other Contrast	Z None	Z None

Section   **B**   **Imaging**
Body System   **2**   **Heart**
Type   **1**   **Fluoroscopy:** Single plane or bi-plane real time display of an image developed from the capture of external ionizing radiation on a fluorescent screen. The image may also be stored by either digital or analog means

Body Part (4th)	Contrast (5th)	Qualifier (6th)	Qualifier (7th)
0 Coronary Artery, Single 1 Coronary Arteries, Multiple 2 Coronary Artery Bypass Graft, Single 3 Coronary Artery Bypass Grafts, Multiple	0 High Osmolar 1 Low Osmolar Y Other Contrast	1 Laser	0 Intraoperative
0 Coronary Artery, Single 1 Coronary Arteries, Multiple 2 Coronary Artery Bypass Graft, Single 3 Coronary Artery Bypass Grafts, Multiple	0 High Osmolar 1 Low Osmolar Y Other Contrast	Z None	Z None
4 Heart, Right 5 Heart, Left 6 Heart, Right and Left 7 Internal Mammary Bypass Graft, Right 8 Internal Mammary Bypass Graft, Left F Bypass Graft, Other	0 High Osmolar 1 Low Osmolar Y Other Contrast	Z None	Z None

Section   **B**   **Imaging**
Body System   **2**   **Heart**
Type   **2**   **Computerized Tomography (CT Scan):** Computer reformatted digital display of multiplanar images developed from the capture of multiple exposures of external ionizing radiation

Body Part (4th)	Contrast (5th)	Qualifier (6th)	Qualifier (7th)
1 Coronary Arteries, Multiple 3 Coronary Artery Bypass Grafts, Multiple 6 Heart, Right and Left	0 High Osmolar 1 Low Osmolar Y Other Contrast	0 Unenhanced and Enhanced Z None	Z None
1 Coronary Arteries, Multiple 3 Coronary Artery Bypass Grafts, Multiple 6 Heart, Right and Left	Z None	2 Intravascular Optical Coherence Z None	Z None

Section   **B**   **Imaging**
Body System   **2**   **Heart**
Type   **3**   **Magnetic Resonance Imaging (MRI):** Computer reformatted digital display of multiplanar images developed from the capture of radiofrequency signals emitted by nuclei in a body site excited within a magnetic field

Body Part (4th)	Contrast (5th)	Qualifier (6th)	Qualifier (7th)
1 Coronary Arteries, Multiple 3 Coronary Artery Bypass Grafts, Multiple 6 Heart, Right and Left	Y Other Contrast	0 Unenhanced and Enhanced Z None	Z None
1 Coronary Arteries, Multiple 3 Coronary Artery Bypass Grafts, Multiple 6 Heart, Right and Left	Z None	Z None	Z None

Section	B	Imaging
Body System	2	Heart
Type	4	**Ultrasonography:** Real time display of images of anatomy or flow information developed from the capture of reflected and attenuated high frequency sound waves

Body Part (4th)	Contrast (5th)	Qualifier (6th)	Qualifier (7th)
0 Coronary Artery, Single 1 Coronary Arteries, Multiple 4 Heart, Right 5 Heart, Left 6 Heart, Right and Left B Heart with Aorta C Pericardium D Pediatric Heart	Y Other Contrast	Z None	Z None
0 Coronary Artery, Single 1 Coronary Arteries, Multiple 4 Heart, Right 5 Heart, Left 6 Heart, Right and Left B Heart with Aorta C Pericardium D Pediatric Heart	Z None	Z None	3 Intravascular 4 Transesophageal Z None

Section	B	Imaging
Body System	3	Upper Arteries
Type	0	**Plain Radiography:** Planar display of an image developed from the capture of external ionizing radiation on photographic or photoconductive plate

Body Part (4th)	Contrast (5th)	Qualifier (6th)	Qualifier (7th)
0 Thoracic Aorta 1 Brachiocephalic-Subclavian Artery, Right 2 Subclavian Artery, Left 3 Common Carotid Artery, Right 4 Common Carotid Artery, Left 5 Common Carotid Arteries, Bilateral 6 Internal Carotid Artery, Right 7 Internal Carotid Artery, Left 8 Internal Carotid Arteries, Bilateral 9 External Carotid Artery, Right B External Carotid Artery, Left C External Carotid Arteries, Bilateral D Vertebral Artery, Right F Vertebral Artery, Left G Vertebral Arteries, Bilateral H Upper Extremity Arteries, Right J Upper Extremity Arteries, Left K Upper Extremity Arteries, Bilateral L Intercostal and Bronchial Arteries M Spinal Arteries N Upper Arteries, Other P Thoraco-Abdominal Aorta Q Cervico-Cerebral Arch R Intracranial Arteries S Pulmonary Artery, Right T Pulmonary Artery, Left	0 High Osmolar 1 Low Osmolar Y Other Contrast Z None	Z None	Z None

Section	B	Imaging
Body System	3	Upper Arteries
Type	1	**Fluoroscopy:** Single plane or bi-plane real time display of an image developed from the capture of external ionizing radiation on a fluorescent screen. The image may also be stored by either digital or analog means

Body Part (4th)	Contrast (5th)	Qualifier (6th)	Qualifier (7th)
0 Thoracic Aorta	0 High Osmolar	1 Laser	0 Intraoperative
1 Brachiocephalic-Subclavian Artery, Right	1 Low Osmolar		
2 Subclavian Artery, Left	Y Other Contrast		
3 Common Carotid Artery, Right			
4 Common Carotid Artery, Left			
5 Common Carotid Arteries, Bilateral			
6 Internal Carotid Artery, Right			
7 Internal Carotid Artery, Left			
8 Internal Carotid Arteries, Bilateral			
9 External Carotid Artery, Right			
B External Carotid Artery, Left			
C External Carotid Arteries, Bilateral			
D Vertebral Artery, Right			
F Vertebral Artery, Left			
G Vertebral Arteries, Bilateral			
H Upper Extremity Arteries, Right			
J Upper Extremity Arteries, Left			
K Upper Extremity Arteries, Bilateral			
L Intercostal and Bronchial Arteries			
M Spinal Arteries			
N Upper Arteries, Other			
P Thoraco-Abdominal Aorta			
Q Cervico-Cerebral Arch			
R Intracranial Arteries			
S Pulmonary Artery, Right			
T Pulmonary Artery, Left			
0 Thoracic Aorta	0 High Osmolar	Z None	Z None
1 Brachiocephalic-Subclavian Artery, Right	1 Low Osmolar		
2 Subclavian Artery, Left	Y Other Contrast		
3 Common Carotid Artery, Right			
4 Common Carotid Artery, Left			
5 Common Carotid Arteries, Bilateral			
6 Internal Carotid Artery, Right			
7 Internal Carotid Artery, Left			
8 Internal Carotid Arteries, Bilateral			
9 External Carotid Artery, Right			
B External Carotid Artery, Left			
C External Carotid Arteries, Bilateral			
D Vertebral Artery, Right			
F Vertebral Artery, Left			
G Vertebral Arteries, Bilateral			
H Upper Extremity Arteries, Right			
J Upper Extremity Arteries, Left			
K Upper Extremity Arteries, Bilateral			
L Intercostal and Bronchial Arteries			
M Spinal Arteries			
N Upper Arteries, Other			
P Thoraco-Abdominal Aorta			
Q Cervico-Cerebral Arch			
R Intracranial Arteries			
S Pulmonary Artery, Right			
T Pulmonary Artery, Left			

Continued →

Section	B	Imaging
Body System	3	Upper Arteries
Type	1	**Fluoroscopy:** Single plane or bi-plane real time display of an image developed from the capture of external ionizing radiation on a fluorescent screen. The image may also be stored by either digital or analog means

Body Part (4th)	Contrast (5th)	Qualifier (6th)	Qualifier (7th)
0 Thoracic Aorta 1 Brachiocephalic-Subclavian Artery, Right 2 Subclavian Artery, Left 3 Common Carotid Artery, Right 4 Common Carotid Artery, Left 5 Common Carotid Arteries, Bilateral 6 Internal Carotid Artery, Right 7 Internal Carotid Artery, Left 8 Internal Carotid Arteries, Bilateral 9 External Carotid Artery, Right B External Carotid Artery, Left C External Carotid Arteries, Bilateral D Vertebral Artery, Right F Vertebral Artery, Left G Vertebral Arteries, Bilateral H Upper Extremity Arteries, Right J Upper Extremity Arteries, Left K Upper Extremity Arteries, Bilateral L Intercostal and Bronchial Arteries M Spinal Arteries N Upper Arteries, Other P Thoraco-Abdominal Aorta Q Cervico-Cerebral Arch R Intracranial Arteries S Pulmonary Artery, Right T Pulmonary Artery, Left	Z None	Z None	Z None

Section	B	Imaging
Body System	3	Upper Arteries
Type	2	**Computerized Tomography (CT Scan):** Computer reformatted digital display of multiplanar images developed from the capture of multiple exposures of external ionizing radiation

Body Part (4th)	Contrast (5th)	Qualifier (6th)	Qualifier (7th)
0 Thoracic Aorta 5 Common Carotid Arteries, Bilateral 8 Internal Carotid Arteries, Bilateral G Vertebral Arteries, Bilateral R Intracranial Arteries S Pulmonary Artery, Right T Pulmonary Artery, Left	0 High Osmolar 1 Low Osmolar Y Other Contrast	Z None	Z None
0 Thoracic Aorta 5 Common Carotid Arteries, Bilateral 8 Internal Carotid Arteries, Bilateral G Vertebral Arteries, Bilateral R Intracranial Arteries S Pulmonary Artery, Right T Pulmonary Artery, Left	Z None	2 Intravascular Optical Coherence Z None	Z None

Section   **B**   **Imaging**
Body System   **3**   **Upper Arteries**
Type   **3**   **Magnetic Resonance Imaging (MRI):** Computer reformatted digital display of multiplanar images developed from the capture of radiofrequency signals emitted by nuclei in a body site excited within a magnetic field

Body Part (4ᵗʰ)	Contrast (5ᵗʰ)	Qualifier (6ᵗʰ)	Qualifier (7ᵗʰ)
0 Thoracic Aorta **5** Common Carotid Arteries, Bilateral **8** Internal Carotid Arteries, Bilateral **G** Vertebral Arteries, Bilateral **H** Upper Extremity Arteries, Right **J** Upper Extremity Arteries, Left **K** Upper Extremity Arteries, Bilateral **M** Spinal Arteries **Q** Cervico-Cerebral Arch **R** Intracranial Arteries	**Y** Other Contrast	**0** Unenhanced and Enhanced **Z** None	**Z** None
0 Thoracic Aorta **5** Common Carotid Arteries, Bilateral **8** Internal Carotid Arteries, Bilateral **G** Vertebral Arteries, Bilateral **H** Upper Extremity Arteries, Right **J** Upper Extremity Arteries, Left **K** Upper Extremity Arteries, Bilateral **M** Spinal Arteries **Q** Cervico-Cerebral Arch **R** Intracranial Arteries	**Z** None	**Z** None	**Z** None

Section   **B**   **Imaging**
Body System   **3**   **Upper Arteries**
Type   **4**   **Ultrasonography:** Real time display of images of anatomy or flow information developed from the capture of reflected and attenuated high frequency sound waves

Body Part (4ᵗʰ)	Contrast (5ᵗʰ)	Qualifier (6ᵗʰ)	Qualifier (7ᵗʰ)
0 Thoracic Aorta **1** Brachiocephalic-Subclavian Artery, Right **2** Subclavian Artery, Left **3** Common Carotid Artery, Right **4** Common Carotid Artery, Left **5** Common Carotid Arteries, Bilateral **6** Internal Carotid Artery, Right **7** Internal Carotid Artery, Left **8** Internal Carotid Arteries, Bilateral **H** Upper Extremity Arteries, Right **J** Upper Extremity Arteries, Left **K** Upper Extremity Arteries, Bilateral **R** Intracranial Arteries **S** Pulmonary Artery, Right **T** Pulmonary Artery, Left **V** Ophthalmic Arteries	**Z** None	**Z** None	**3** Intravascular **Z** None

Section | B | Imaging
Body System | 4 | Lower Arteries
Type | 0 | **Plain Radiography:** Planar display of an image developed from the capture of external ionizing radiation on photographic or photoconductive plate

Body Part (4th)	Contrast (5th)	Qualifier (6th)	Qualifier (7th)
0 Abdominal Aorta 2 Hepatic Artery 3 Splenic Arteries 4 Superior Mesenteric Artery 5 Inferior Mesenteric Artery 6 Renal Artery, Right 7 Renal Artery, Left 8 Renal Arteries, Bilateral 9 Lumbar Arteries B Intra-Abdominal Arteries, Other C Pelvic Arteries D Aorta and Bilateral Lower Extremity Arteries F Lower Extremity Arteries, Right G Lower Extremity Arteries, Left J Lower Arteries, Other M Renal Artery Transplant	0 High Osmolar 1 Low Osmolar Y Other Contrast	Z None	Z None

Section | B | Imaging
Body System | 4 | Lower Arteries
Type | 1 | **Fluoroscopy:** Single plane or bi-plane real time display of an image developed from the capture of external ionizing radiation on a fluorescent screen. The image may also be stored by either digital or analog means

Body Part (4th)	Contrast (5th)	Qualifier (6th)	Qualifier (7th)
0 Abdominal Aorta 2 Hepatic Artery 3 Splenic Arteries 4 Superior Mesenteric Artery 5 Inferior Mesenteric Artery 6 Renal Artery, Right 7 Renal Artery, Left 8 Renal Arteries, Bilateral 9 Lumbar Arteries B Intra-Abdominal Arteries, Other C Pelvic Arteries D Aorta and Bilateral Lower Extremity Arteries F Lower Extremity Arteries, Right G Lower Extremity Arteries, Left J Lower Arteries, Other	0 High Osmolar 1 Low Osmolar Y Other Contrast	1 Laser	0 Intraoperative
0 Abdominal Aorta 2 Hepatic Artery 3 Splenic Arteries 4 Superior Mesenteric Artery 5 Inferior Mesenteric Artery 6 Renal Artery, Right 7 Renal Artery, Left 8 Renal Arteries, Bilateral 9 Lumbar Arteries B Intra-Abdominal Arteries, Other C Pelvic Arteries D Aorta and Bilateral Lower Extremity Arteries F Lower Extremity Arteries, Right G Lower Extremity Arteries, Left J Lower Arteries, Other	0 High Osmolar 1 Low Osmolar Y Other Contrast	Z None	Z None

Continued →

Section	B	Imaging
Body System	4	Lower Arteries
Type	1	**Fluoroscopy:** Single plane or bi-plane real time display of an image developed from the capture of external ionizing radiation on a fluorescent screen. The image may also be stored by either digital or analog means

Body Part (4th)	Contrast (5th)	Qualifier (6th)	Qualifier (7th)
0 Abdominal Aorta 2 Hepatic Artery 3 Splenic Arteries 4 Superior Mesenteric Artery 5 Inferior Mesenteric Artery 6 Renal Artery, Right 7 Renal Artery, Left 8 Renal Arteries, Bilateral 9 Lumbar Arteries B Intra-Abdominal Arteries, Other C Pelvic Arteries D Aorta and Bilateral Lower Extremity Arteries F Lower Extremity Arteries, Right G Lower Extremity Arteries, Left J Lower Arteries, Other	Z None	Z None	Z None

Section	B	Imaging
Body System	4	Lower Arteries
Type	2	**Computerized Tomography (CT Scan):** Computer reformatted digital display of multiplanar images developed from the capture of multiple exposures of external ionizing radiation

Body Part (4th)	Contrast (5th)	Qualifier (6th)	Qualifier (7th)
0 Abdominal Aorta 1 Celiac Artery 4 Superior Mesenteric Artery 8 Renal Arteries, Bilateral C Pelvic Arteries F Lower Extremity Arteries, Right G Lower Extremity Arteries, Left H Lower Extremity Arteries, Bilateral M Renal Artery Transplant	0 High Osmolar 1 Low Osmolar Y Other Contrast	Z None	Z None
0 Abdominal Aorta 1 Celiac Artery 4 Superior Mesenteric Artery 8 Renal Arteries, Bilateral C Pelvic Arteries F Lower Extremity Arteries, Right G Lower Extremity Arteries, Left H Lower Extremity Arteries, Bilateral M Renal Artery Transplant	Z None	2 Intravascular Optical Coherence Z None	Z None

Section	B	Imaging
Body System	4	Lower Arteries
Type	3	**Magnetic Resonance Imaging (MRI):** Computer reformatted digital display of multiplanar images developed from the capture of radiofrequency signals emitted by nuclei in a body site excited within a magnetic field

Body Part (4th)	Contrast (5th)	Qualifier (6th)	Qualifier (7th)
0 Abdominal Aorta 1 Celiac Artery 4 Superior Mesenteric Artery 8 Renal Arteries, Bilateral C Pelvic Arteries F Lower Extremity Arteries, Right G Lower Extremity Arteries, Left H Lower Extremity Arteries, Bilateral	Y Other Contrast	0 Unenhanced and Enhanced Z None	Z None

Continued →

Section   B   **Imaging**
Body System   4   **Lower Arteries**
Type   3   **Magnetic Resonance Imaging (MRI):** Computer reformatted digital display of multiplanar images developed from the capture of radiofrequency signals emitted by nuclei in a body site excited within a magnetic field

Body Part (4th)	Contrast (5th)	Qualifier (6th)	Qualifier (7th)
0 Abdominal Aorta **1** Celiac Artery **4** Superior Mesenteric Artery **8** Renal Arteries, Bilateral **C** Pelvic Arteries **F** Lower Extremity Arteries, Right **G** Lower Extremity Arteries, Left **H** Lower Extremity Arteries, Bilateral	**Z** None	**Z** None	**Z** None

Section   B   **Imaging**
Body System   4   **Lower Arteries**
Type   4   **Ultrasonography:** Real time display of images of anatomy or flow information developed from the capture of reflected and attenuated high frequency sound waves

Body Part (4th)	Contrast (5th)	Qualifier (6th)	Qualifier (7th)
0 Abdominal Aorta **4** Superior Mesenteric Artery **5** Inferior Mesenteric Artery **6** Renal Artery, Right **7** Renal Artery, Left **8** Renal Arteries, Bilateral **B** Intra-Abdominal Arteries, Other **F** Lower Extremity Arteries, Right **G** Lower Extremity Arteries, Left **H** Lower Extremity Arteries, Bilateral **K** Celiac and Mesenteric Arteries **L** Femoral Artery **N** Penile Arteries	**Z** None	**Z** None	**3** Intravascular **Z** None

Section	B	Imaging
Body System	5	Veins
Type	0	**Plain Radiography:** Planar display of an image developed from the capture of external ionizing radiation on photographic or photoconductive plate

Body Part (4th)	Contrast (5th)	Qualifier (6th)	Qualifier (7th)
0 Epidural Veins	0 High Osmolar	Z None	Z None
1 Cerebral and Cerebellar Veins	1 Low Osmolar		
2 Intracranial Sinuses	Y Other Contrast		
3 Jugular Veins, Right			
4 Jugular Veins, Left			
5 Jugular Veins, Bilateral			
6 Subclavian Vein, Right			
7 Subclavian Vein, Left			
8 Superior Vena Cava			
9 Inferior Vena Cava			
B Lower Extremity Veins, Right			
C Lower Extremity Veins, Left			
D Lower Extremity Veins, Bilateral			
F Pelvic (Iliac) Veins, Right			
G Pelvic (Iliac) Veins, Left			
H Pelvic (Iliac) Veins, Bilateral			
J Renal Vein, Right			
K Renal Vein, Left			
L Renal Veins, Bilateral			
M Upper Extremity Veins, Right			
N Upper Extremity Veins, Left			
P Upper Extremity Veins, Bilateral			
Q Pulmonary Vein, Right			
R Pulmonary Vein, Left			
S Pulmonary Veins, Bilateral			
T Portal and Splanchnic Veins			
V Veins, Other			
W Dialysis Shunt/Fistula			

Section	B	Imaging
Body System	5	Veins
Type	1	**Fluoroscopy:** Single plane or bi-plane real time display of an image developed from the capture of external ionizing radiation on a fluorescent screen. The image may also be stored by either digital or analog means

Body Part (4th)	Contrast (5th)	Qualifier (6th)	Qualifier (7th)
0 Epidural Veins	0 High Osmolar	Z None	A Guidance
1 Cerebral and Cerebellar Veins	1 Low Osmolar		Z None
2 Intracranial Sinuses	Y Other Contrast		
3 Jugular Veins, Right	Z None		
4 Jugular Veins, Left			
5 Jugular Veins, Bilateral			
6 Subclavian Vein, Right			
7 Subclavian Vein, Left			
8 Superior Vena Cava			
9 Inferior Vena Cava			
B Lower Extremity Veins, Right			
C Lower Extremity Veins, Left			
D Lower Extremity Veins, Bilateral			
F Pelvic (Iliac) Veins, Right			
G Pelvic (Iliac) Veins, Left			
H Pelvic (Iliac) Veins, Bilateral			
J Renal Vein, Right			
K Renal Vein, Left			
L Renal Veins, Bilateral			
M Upper Extremity Veins, Right			
N Upper Extremity Veins, Left			
P Upper Extremity Veins, Bilateral			
Q Pulmonary Vein, Right			
R Pulmonary Vein, Left			
S Pulmonary Veins, Bilateral			
T Portal and Splanchnic Veins			
V Veins, Other			
W Dialysis Shunt/Fistula			

Section   **B**   **Imaging**
Body System   **5**   **Veins**
Type   **2**   **Computerized Tomography (CT Scan):** Computer reformatted digital display of multiplanar images developed from the capture of multiple exposures of external ionizing radiation

Body Part (4th)	Contrast (5th)	Qualifier (6th)	Qualifier (7th)
2 Intracranial Sinuses 8 Superior Vena Cava 9 Inferior Vena Cava F Pelvic (Iliac) Veins, Right G Pelvic (Iliac) Veins, Left H Pelvic (Iliac) Veins, Bilateral J Renal Vein, Right K Renal Vein, Left L Renal Veins, Bilateral Q Pulmonary Vein, Right R Pulmonary Vein, Left S Pulmonary Veins, Bilateral T Portal and Splanchnic Veins	0 High Osmolar 1 Low Osmolar Y Other Contrast	0 Unenhanced and Enhanced Z None	Z None
2 Intracranial Sinuses 8 Superior Vena Cava 9 Inferior Vena Cava F Pelvic (Iliac) Veins, Right G Pelvic (Iliac) Veins, Left H Pelvic (Iliac) Veins, Bilateral J Renal Vein, Right	Z None	2 Intravascular Optical Coherence Z None	Z None
K Renal Vein, Left L Renal Veins, Bilateral Q Pulmonary Vein, Right R Pulmonary Vein, Left S Pulmonary Veins, Bilateral T Portal and Splanchnic Veins			

Section   **B**   **Imaging**
Body System   **5**   **Veins**
Type   **3**   **Magnetic Resonance Imaging (MRI):** Computer reformatted digital display of multiplanar images developed from the capture of radiofrequency signals emitted by nuclei in a body site excited within a magnetic field

Body Part (4th)	Contrast (5th)	Qualifier (6th)	Qualifier (7th)
1 Cerebral and Cerebellar Veins 2 Intracranial Sinuses 5 Jugular Veins, Bilateral 8 Superior Vena Cava 9 Inferior Vena Cava B Lower Extremity Veins, Right C Lower Extremity Veins, Left D Lower Extremity Veins, Bilateral H Pelvic (Iliac) Veins, Bilateral L Renal Veins, Bilateral M Upper Extremity Veins, Right N Upper Extremity Veins, Left P Upper Extremity Veins, Bilateral S Pulmonary Veins, Bilateral T Portal and Splanchnic Veins V Veins, Other	Y Other Contrast	0 Unenhanced and Enhanced Z None	Z None

Continued →

Section   B   Imaging
Body System   5   Veins
Type   3   **Magnetic Resonance Imaging (MRI):** Computer reformatted digital display of multiplanar images developed from the capture of radiofrequency signals emitted by nuclei in a body site excited within a magnetic field

Body Part (4th)	Contrast (5th)	Qualifier (6th)	Qualifier (7th)
1 Cerebral and Cerebellar Veins	Z None	Z None	Z None
2 Intracranial Sinuses			
5 Jugular Veins, Bilateral			
8 Superior Vena Cava			
9 Inferior Vena Cava			
B Lower Extremity Veins, Right			
C Lower Extremity Veins, Left			
D Lower Extremity Veins, Bilateral			
H Pelvic (Iliac) Veins, Bilateral			
L Renal Veins, Bilateral			
M Upper Extremity Veins, Right			
N Upper Extremity Veins, Left			
P Upper Extremity Veins, Bilateral			
S Pulmonary Veins, Bilateral			
T Portal and Splanchnic Veins			
V Veins, Other			

Section   B   Imaging
Body System   5   Veins
Type   4   **Ultrasonography:** Real time display of images of anatomy or flow information developed from the capture of reflected and attenuated high frequency sound waves

Body Part (4th)	Contrast (5th)	Qualifier (6th)	Qualifier (7th)
3 Jugular Veins, Right	Z None	Z None	3 Intravascular
4 Jugular Veins, Left			A Guidance
6 Subclavian Vein, Right			Z None
7 Subclavian Vein, Left			
8 Superior Vena Cava			
9 Inferior Vena Cava			
B Lower Extremity Veins, Right			
C Lower Extremity Veins, Left			
D Lower Extremity Veins, Bilateral			
J Renal Vein, Right			
K Renal Vein, Left			
L Renal Veins, Bilateral			
M Upper Extremity Veins, Right			
N Upper Extremity Veins, Left			
P Upper Extremity Veins, Bilateral			
T Portal and Splanchnic Veins			

Section   B   Imaging
Body System   7   Lymphatic System
Type   0   **Plain Radiography:** Planar display of an image developed from the capture of external ionizing radiation on photographic or photoconductive plate

Body Part (4th)	Contrast (5th)	Qualifier (6th)	Qualifier (7th)
0 Abdominal/Retroperitoneal Lymphatics, Unilateral	0 High Osmolar	Z None	Z None
1 Abdominal/Retroperitoneal Lymphatics, Bilateral	1 Low Osmolar		
4 Lymphatics, Head and Neck	Y Other Contrast		
5 Upper Extremity Lymphatics, Right			
6 Upper Extremity Lymphatics, Left			
7 Upper Extremity Lymphatics, Bilateral			
8 Lower Extremity Lymphatics, Right			
9 Lower Extremity Lymphatics, Left			
B Lower Extremity Lymphatics, Bilateral			
C Lymphatics, Pelvic			

Section	B	Imaging
Body System	8	Eye
Type	0	**Plain Radiography:** Planar display of an image developed from the capture of external ionizing radiation on photographic or photoconductive plate

Body Part (4th)	Contrast (5th)	Qualifier (6th)	Qualifier (7th)
0 Lacrimal Duct, Right 1 Lacrimal Duct, Left 2 Lacrimal Ducts, Bilateral	0 High Osmolar 1 Low Osmolar Y Other Contrast	Z None	Z None
3 Optic Foramina, Right 4 Optic Foramina, Left 5 Eye, Right 6 Eye, Left 7 Eyes, Bilateral	Z None	Z None	Z None

Section	B	Imaging
Body System	8	Eye
Type	2	**Computerized Tomography (CT Scan):** Computer reformatted digital display of multiplanar images developed from the capture of multiple exposures of external ionizing radiation

Body Part (4th)	Contrast (5th)	Qualifier (6th)	Qualifier (7th)
5 Eye, Right 6 Eye, Left 7 Eyes, Bilateral	0 High Osmolar 1 Low Osmolar Y Other Contrast	0 Unenhanced and Enhanced Z None	Z None
5 Eye, Right 6 Eye, Left 7 Eyes, Bilateral	Z None	Z None	Z None

Section	B	Imaging
Body System	8	Eye
Type	3	**Magnetic Resonance Imaging (MRI):** Computer reformatted digital display of multiplanar images developed from the capture of radiofrequency signals emitted by nuclei in a body site excited within a magnetic field

Body Part (4th)	Contrast (5th)	Qualifier (6th)	Qualifier (7th)
5 Eye, Right 6 Eye, Left 7 Eyes, Bilateral	Y Other Contrast	0 Unenhanced and Enhanced Z None	Z None
5 Eye, Right 6 Eye, Left 7 Eyes, Bilateral	Z None	Z None	Z None

Section	B	Imaging
Body System	8	Eye
Type	4	**Ultrasonography:** Real time display of images of anatomy or flow information developed from the capture of reflected and attenuated high frequency sound waves

Body Part (4th)	Contrast (5th)	Qualifier (6th)	Qualifier (7th)
5 Eye, Right 6 Eye, Left 7 Eyes, Bilateral	Z None	Z None	Z None

Section	B	Imaging
Body System	9	Ear, Nose, Mouth and Throat
Type	0	**Plain Radiography:** Planar display of an image developed from the capture of external ionizing radiation on photographic or photoconductive plate

Body Part (4th)	Contrast (5th)	Qualifier (6th)	Qualifier (7th)
2 Paranasal Sinuses F Nasopharynx/Oropharynx H Mastoids	Z None	Z None	Z None
4 Parotid Gland, Right 5 Parotid Gland, Left 6 Parotid Glands, Bilateral 7 Submandibular Gland, Right 8 Submandibular Gland, Left 9 Submandibular Glands, Bilateral B Salivary Gland, Right C Salivary Gland, Left D Salivary Glands, Bilateral	0 High Osmolar 1 Low Osmolar Y Other Contrast	Z None	Z None

Section	B	Imaging
Body System	9	Ear, Nose, Mouth and Throat
Type	1	**Fluoroscopy:** Single plane or bi-plane real time display of an image developed from the capture of external ionizing radiation on a fluorescent screen. The image may also be stored by either digital or analog means

Body Part (4th)	Contrast (5th)	Qualifier (6th)	Qualifier (7th)
G Pharynx and Epiglottis J Larynx	Y Other Contrast Z None	Z None	Z None

Section	B	Imaging
Body System	9	Ear, Nose, Mouth and Throat
Type	2	**Computerized Tomography (CT Scan):** Computer reformatted digital display of multiplanar images developed from the capture of multiple exposures of external ionizing radiation

Body Part (4th)	Contrast (5th)	Qualifier (6th)	Qualifier (7th)
0 Ear 2 Paranasal Sinuses 6 Parotid Glands, Bilateral 9 Submandibular Glands, Bilateral D Salivary Glands, Bilateral F Nasopharynx/Oropharynx J Larynx	0 High Osmolar 1 Low Osmolar Y Other Contrast	0 Unenhanced and Enhanced Z None	Z None
0 Ear 2 Paranasal Sinuses 6 Parotid Glands, Bilateral 9 Submandibular Glands, Bilateral D Salivary Glands, Bilateral F Nasopharynx/Oropharynx J Larynx	Z None	Z None	Z None

Section	B	Imaging
Body System	9	Ear, Nose, Mouth and Throat
Type	3	**Magnetic Resonance Imaging (MRI):** Computer reformatted digital display of multiplanar images developed from the capture of radiofrequency signals emitted by nuclei in a body site excited within a magnetic field

Body Part (4th)	Contrast (5th)	Qualifier (6th)	Qualifier (7th)
0 Ear 2 Paranasal Sinuses 6 Parotid Glands, Bilateral 9 Submandibular Glands, Bilateral D Salivary Glands, Bilateral F Nasopharynx/Oropharynx J Larynx	Y Other Contrast	0 Unenhanced and Enhanced Z None	Z None

Continued →

Section   B   **Imaging**
Body System   9   **Ear, Nose, Mouth and Throat**
Type   3   **Magnetic Resonance Imaging (MRI):** Computer reformatted digital display of multiplanar images developed from the capture of radiofrequency signals emitted by nuclei in a body site excited within a magnetic field

Body Part (4th)	Contrast (5th)	Qualifier (6th)	Qualifier (7th)
0 Ear **2** Paranasal Sinuses **6** Parotid Glands, Bilateral **9** Submandibular Glands, Bilateral **D** Salivary Glands, Bilateral **F** Nasopharynx/Oropharynx **J** Larynx	**Z** None	**Z** None	**Z** None

Section   B   **Imaging**
Body System   B   **Respiratory System**
Type   0   **Plain Radiography:** Planar display of an image developed from the capture of external ionizing radiation on photographic or photoconductive plate

Body Part (4th)	Contrast (5th)	Qualifier (6th)	Qualifier (7th)
7 Tracheobronchial Tree, Right **8** Tracheobronchial Tree, Left **9** Tracheobronchial Trees, Bilateral	**Y** Other Contrast	**Z** None	**Z** None
D Upper Airways	**Z** None	**Z** None	**Z** None

Section   B   **Imaging**
Body System   B   **Respiratory System**
Type   1   **Fluoroscopy:** Single plane or bi-plane real time display of an image developed from the capture of external ionizing radiation on a fluorescent screen. The image may also be stored by either digital or analog means

Body Part (4th)	Contrast (5th)	Qualifier (6th)	Qualifier (7th)
2 Lung, Right **3** Lung, Left **4** Lungs, Bilateral **6** Diaphragm **C** Mediastinum **D** Upper Airways	**Z** None	**Z** None	**Z** None
7 Tracheobronchial Tree, Right **8** Tracheobronchial Tree, Left **9** Tracheobronchial Trees, Bilateral	**Y** Other Contrast	**Z** None	**Z** None

Section   B   **Imaging**
Body System   B   **Respiratory System**
Type   2   **Computerized Tomography (CT Scan):** Computer reformatted digital display of multiplanar images developed from the capture of multiple exposures of external ionizing radiation

Body Part (4th)	Contrast (5th)	Qualifier (6th)	Qualifier (7th)
4 Lungs, Bilateral **7** Tracheobronchial Tree, Right **8** Tracheobronchial Tree, Left **9** Tracheobronchial Trees, Bilateral **F** Trachea/Airways	**0** High Osmolar **1** Low Osmolar **Y** Other Contrast	**0** Unenhanced and Enhanced **Z** None	**Z** None
4 Lungs, Bilateral **7** Tracheobronchial Tree, Right **8** Tracheobronchial Tree, Left **9** Tracheobronchial Trees, Bilateral **F** Trachea/Airways	**Z** None	**Z** None	**Z** None

Section	B	Imaging
Body System	B	Respiratory System
Type	3	Magnetic Resonance Imaging (MRI): Computer reformatted digital display of multiplanar images developed from the capture of radiofrequency signals emitted by nuclei in a body site excited within a magnetic field

Body Part (4th)	Contrast (5th)	Qualifier (6th)	Qualifier (7th)
G Lung Apices	Y Other Contrast	0 Unenhanced and Enhanced Z None	Z None
G Lung Apices	Z None	Z None	Z None

Section	B	Imaging
Body System	B	Respiratory System
Type	4	Ultrasonography: Real time display of images of anatomy or flow information developed from the capture of reflected and attenuated high frequency sound waves

Body Part (4th)	Contrast (5th)	Qualifier (6th)	Qualifier (7th)
B Pleura C Mediastinum	Z None	Z None	Z None

Section	B	Imaging
Body System	D	Gastrointestinal System
Type	1	Fluoroscopy: Single plane or bi-plane real time display of an image developed from the capture of external ionizing radiation on a fluorescent screen. The image may also be stored by either digital or analog means

Body Part (4th)	Contrast (5th)	Qualifier (6th)	Qualifier (7th)
1 Esophagus 2 Stomach 3 Small Bowel 4 Colon 5 Upper GI 6 Upper GI and Small Bowel 9 Duodenum B Mouth/Oropharynx	Y Other Contrast Z None	Z None	Z None

Section	B	Imaging
Body System	D	Gastrointestinal System
Type	2	Computerized Tomography (CT Scan): Computer reformatted digital display of multiplanar images developed from the capture of multiple exposures of external ionizing radiation

Body Part (4th)	Contrast (5th)	Qualifier (6th)	Qualifier (7th)
4 Colon	0 High Osmolar 1 Low Osmolar Y Other Contrast	0 Unenhanced and Enhanced Z None	Z None
4 Colon	Z None	Z None	Z None

Section	B	Imaging
Body System	D	Gastrointestinal System
Type	4	Ultrasonography: Real time display of images of anatomy or flow information developed from the capture of reflected and attenuated high frequency sound waves

Body Part (4th)	Contrast (5th)	Qualifier (6th)	Qualifier (7th)
1 Esophagus 2 Stomach 7 Gastrointestinal Tract 8 Appendix 9 Duodenum C Rectum	Z None	Z None	Z None

Section   **B**   **Imaging**
Body System   **F**   **Hepatobiliary System and Pancreas**
Type   **0**   **Plain Radiography:** Planar display of an image developed from the capture of external ionizing radiation on photographic or photoconductive plate

Body Part (4th)	Contrast (5th)	Qualifier (6th)	Qualifier (7th)
0 Bile Ducts 3 Gallbladder and Bile Ducts C Hepatobiliary System, All	0 High Osmolar 1 Low Osmolar Y Other Contrast	Z None	Z None

Section   **B**   **Imaging**
Body System   **F**   **Hepatobiliary System and Pancreas**
Type   **1**   **Fluoroscopy:** Single plane or bi-plane real time display of an image developed from the capture of external ionizing radiation on a fluorescent screen. The image may also be stored by either digital or analog means

Body Part (4th)	Contrast (5th)	Qualifier (6th)	Qualifier (7th)
0 Bile Ducts 1 Biliary and Pancreatic Ducts 2 Gallbladder 3 Gallbladder and Bile Ducts 4 Gallbladder, Bile Ducts and Pancreatic Ducts 8 Pancreatic Ducts	0 High Osmolar 1 Low Osmolar Y Other Contrast	Z None	Z None

Section   **B**   **Imaging**
Body System   **F**   **Hepatobiliary System and Pancreas**
Type   **2**   **Computerized Tomography (CT Scan):** Computer reformatted digital display of multiplanar images developed from the capture of multiple exposures of external ionizing radiation

Body Part (4th)	Contrast (5th)	Qualifier (6th)	Qualifier (7th)
5 Liver 6 Liver and Spleen 7 Pancreas C Hepatobiliary System, All	0 High Osmolar 1 Low Osmolar Y Other Contrast	0 Unenhanced and Enhanced Z None	Z None
5 Liver 6 Liver and Spleen 7 Pancreas C Hepatobiliary System, All	Z None	Z None	Z None

Section   **B**   **Imaging**
Body System   **F**   **Hepatobiliary System and Pancreas**
Type   **3**   **Magnetic Resonance Imaging (MRI):** Computer reformatted digital display of multiplanar images developed from the capture of radiofrequency signals emitted by nuclei in a body site excited within a magnetic field

Body Part (4th)	Contrast (5th)	Qualifier (6th)	Qualifier (7th)
5 Liver 6 Liver and Spleen 7 Pancreas	Y Other Contrast	0 Unenhanced and Enhanced Z None	Z None
5 Liver 6 Liver and Spleen 7 Pancreas	Z None	Z None	Z None

Section	B	Imaging
Body System	F	Hepatobiliary System and Pancreas
Type	4	Ultrasonography: Real time display of images of anatomy or flow information developed from the capture of reflected and attenuated high frequency sound waves

Body Part (4th)	Contrast (5th)	Qualifier (6th)	Qualifier (7th)
0 Bile Ducts 2 Gallbladder 3 Gallbladder and Bile Ducts 5 Liver 6 Liver and Spleen 7 Pancreas C Hepatobiliary System, All	Z None	Z None	Z None

Section	B	Imaging
Body System	G	Endocrine System
Type	2	Computerized Tomography (CT Scan): Computer reformatted digital display of multiplanar images developed from the capture of multiple exposures of external ionizing radiation

Body Part (4th)	Contrast (5th)	Qualifier (6th)	Qualifier (7th)
2 Adrenal Glands, Bilateral 3 Parathyroid Glands 4 Thyroid Gland	0 High Osmolar 1 Low Osmolar Y Other Contrast	0 Unenhanced and Enhanced Z None	Z None
2 Adrenal Glands, Bilateral 3 Parathyroid Glands 4 Thyroid Gland	Z None	Z None	Z None

Section	B	Imaging
Body System	G	Endocrine System
Type	3	Magnetic Resonance Imaging (MRI): Computer reformatted digital display of multiplanar images developed from the capture of radiofrequency signals emitted by nuclei in a body site excited within a magnetic field

Body Part (4th)	Contrast (5th)	Qualifier (6th)	Qualifier (7th)
2 Adrenal Glands, Bilateral 3 Parathyroid Glands 4 Thyroid Gland	Y Other Contrast	0 Unenhanced and Enhanced Z None	Z None
2 Adrenal Glands, Bilateral 3 Parathyroid Glands 4 Thyroid Gland	Z None	Z None	Z None

Section	B	Imaging
Body System	G	Endocrine System
Type	4	Ultrasonography: Real time display of images of anatomy or flow information developed from the capture of reflected and attenuated high frequency sound waves

Body Part (4th)	Contrast (5th)	Qualifier (6th)	Qualifier (7th)
0 Adrenal Gland, Right 1 Adrenal Gland, Left 2 Adrenal Glands, Bilateral 3 Parathyroid Glands 4 Thyroid Gland	Z None	Z None	Z None

Section	B	Imaging
Body System	H	Skin, Subcutaneous Tissue and Breast
Type	0	**Plain Radiography:** Planar display of an image developed from the capture of external ionizing radiation on photographic or photoconductive plate

Body Part (4th)	Contrast (5th)	Qualifier (6th)	Qualifier (7th)
0 Breast, Right 1 Breast, Left 2 Breasts, Bilateral	Z None	Z None	Z None
3 Single Mammary Duct, Right 4 Single Mammary Duct, Left 5 Multiple Mammary Ducts, Right 6 Multiple Mammary Ducts, Left	0 High Osmolar 1 Low Osmolar Y Other Contrast Z None	Z None	Z None

Section	B	Imaging
Body System	H	Skin, Subcutaneous Tissue and Breast
Type	3	**Magnetic Resonance Imaging (MRI):** Computer reformatted digital display of multiplanar images developed from the capture of radiofrequency signals emitted by nuclei in a body site excited within a magnetic field

Body Part (4th)	Contrast (5th)	Qualifier (6th)	Qualifier (7th)
0 Breast, Right 1 Breast, Left 2 Breasts, Bilateral D Subcutaneous Tissue, Head/Neck F Subcutaneous Tissue, Upper Extremity G Subcutaneous Tissue, Thorax H Subcutaneous Tissue, Abdomen and Pelvis J Subcutaneous Tissue, Lower Extremity	Y Other Contrast	0 Unenhanced and Enhanced Z None	Z None
0 Breast, Right 1 Breast, Left 2 Breasts, Bilateral D Subcutaneous Tissue, Head/Neck F Subcutaneous Tissue, Upper Extremity G Subcutaneous Tissue, Thorax H Subcutaneous Tissue, Abdomen and Pelvis J Subcutaneous Tissue, Lower Extremity	Z None	Z None	Z None

Section	B	Imaging
Body System	H	Skin, Subcutaneous Tissue and Breast
Type	4	**Ultrasonography:** Real time display of images of anatomy or flow information developed from the capture of reflected and attenuated high frequency sound waves

Body Part (4th)	Contrast (5th)	Qualifier (6th)	Qualifier (7th)
0 Breast, Right 1 Breast, Left 2 Breasts, Bilateral 7 Extremity, Upper 8 Extremity, Lower 9 Abdominal Wall B Chest Wall C Head and Neck	Z None	Z None	Z None

Section | B | Imaging
Body System | L | Connective Tissue
Type | 3 | **Magnetic Resonance Imaging (MRI):** Computer reformatted digital display of multiplanar images developed from the capture of radiofrequency signals emitted by nuclei in a body site excited within a magnetic field

Body Part (4th)	Contrast (5th)	Qualifier (6th)	Qualifier (7th)
0 Connective Tissue, Upper Extremity 1 Connective Tissue, Lower Extremity 2 Tendons, Upper Extremity 3 Tendons, Lower Extremity	Y Other Contrast	0 Unenhanced and Enhanced Z None	Z None
0 Connective Tissue, Upper Extremity 1 Connective Tissue, Lower Extremity 2 Tendons, Upper Extremity 3 Tendons, Lower Extremity	Z None	Z None	Z None

Section | B | Imaging
Body System | L | Connective Tissue
Type | 4 | **Ultrasonography:** Real time display of images of anatomy or flow information developed from the capture of reflected and attenuated high frequency sound waves

Body Part (4th)	Contrast (5th)	Qualifier (6th)	Qualifier (7th)
0 Connective Tissue, Upper Extremity 1 Connective Tissue, Lower Extremity 2 Tendons, Upper Extremity 3 Tendons, Lower Extremity	Z None	Z None	Z None

Section | B | Imaging
Body System | N | Skull and Facial Bones
Type | 0 | **Plain Radiography:** Planar display of an image developed from the capture of external ionizing radiation on photographic or photoconductive plate

Body Part (4th)	Contrast (5th)	Qualifier (6th)	Qualifier (7th)
0 Skull 1 Orbit, Right 2 Orbit, Left 3 Orbits, Bilateral 4 Nasal Bones 5 Facial Bones 6 Mandible B Zygomatic Arch, Right C Zygomatic Arch, Left D Zygomatic Arches, Bilateral G Tooth, Single H Teeth, Multiple J Teeth, All	Z None	Z None	Z None
7 Temporomandibular Joint, Right 8 Temporomandibular Joint, Left 9 Temporomandibular Joints, Bilateral	0 High Osmolar 1 Low Osmolar Y Other Contrast Z None	Z None	Z None

Section | B | Imaging
Body System | N | Skull and Facial Bones
Type | 1 | **Fluoroscopy:** Single plane or bi-plane real time display of an image developed from the capture of external ionizing radiation on a fluorescent screen. The image may also be stored by either digital or analog means

Body Part (4th)	Contrast (5th)	Qualifier (6th)	Qualifier (7th)
7 Temporomandibular Joint, Right 8 Temporomandibular Joint, Left 9 Temporomandibular Joints, Bilateral	0 High Osmolar 1 Low Osmolar Y Other Contrast Z None	Z None	Z None

Section	B	Imaging
Body System	N	Skull and Facial Bones
Type	2	**Computerized Tomography (CT Scan):** Computer reformatted digital display of multiplanar images developed from the capture of multiple exposures of external ionizing radiation

Body Part (4th)	Contrast (5th)	Qualifier (6th)	Qualifier (7th)
0 Skull 3 Orbits, Bilateral 5 Facial Bones 6 Mandible 9 Temporomandibular Joints, Bilateral F Temporal Bones	0 High Osmolar 1 Low Osmolar Y Other Contrast Z None	Z None	Z None

Section	B	Imaging
Body System	N	Skull and Facial Bones
Type	3	**Magnetic Resonance Imaging (MRI):** Computer reformatted digital display of multiplanar images developed from the capture of radiofrequency signals emitted by nuclei in a body site excited within a magnetic field

Body Part (4th)	Contrast (5th)	Qualifier (6th)	Qualifier (7th)
9 Temporomandibular Joints, Bilateral	Y Other Contrast Z None	Z None	Z None

Section	B	Imaging
Body System	P	Non-Axial Upper Bones
Type	0	**Plain Radiography:** Planar display of an image developed from the capture of external ionizing radiation on photographic or photoconductive plate

Body Part (4th)	Contrast (5th)	Qualifier (6th)	Qualifier (7th)
0 Sternoclavicular Joint, Right 1 Sternoclavicular Joint, Left 2 Sternoclavicular Joints, Bilateral 3 Acromioclavicular Joints, Bilateral 4 Clavicle, Right 5 Clavicle, Left 6 Scapula, Right 7 Scapula, Left A Humerus, Right B Humerus, Left E Upper Arm, Right F Upper Arm, Left J Forearm, Right K Forearm, Left N Hand, Right P Hand, Left R Finger(s), Right S Finger(s), Left X Ribs, Right Y Ribs, Left	Z None	Z None	Z None
8 Shoulder, Right 9 Shoulder, Left C Hand/Finger Joint, Right D Hand/Finger Joint, Left G Elbow, Right H Elbow, Left L Wrist, Right M Wrist, Left	0 High Osmolar 1 Low Osmolar Y Other Contrast Z None	Z None	Z None

Section   **B**   **Imaging**

Body System   **P**   **Non-Axial Upper Bones**

Type   **1**   **Fluoroscopy:** Single plane or bi-plane real time display of an image developed from the capture of external ionizing radiation on a fluorescent screen. The image may also be stored by either digital or analog means

Body Part (4th)	Contrast (5th)	Qualifier (6th)	Qualifier (7th)
0 Sternoclavicular Joint, Right **1** Sternoclavicular Joint, Left **2** Sternoclavicular Joints, Bilateral **3** Acromioclavicular Joints, Bilateral **4** Clavicle, Right **5** Clavicle, Left **6** Scapula, Right **7** Scapula, Left **A** Humerus, Right **B** Humerus, Left **E** Upper Arm, Right **F** Upper Arm, Left **J** Forearm, Right **K** Forearm, Left **N** Hand, Right **P** Hand, Left **R** Finger(s), Right **S** Finger(s), Left **X** Ribs, Right **Y** Ribs, Left	**Z** None	**Z** None	**Z** None
8 Shoulder, Right **9** Shoulder, Left **L** Wrist, Right **M** Wrist, Left	**0** High Osmolar **1** Low Osmolar **Y** Other Contrast **Z** None	**Z** None	**Z** None
C Hand/Finger Joint, Right **D** Hand/Finger Joint, Left **G** Elbow, Right **H** Elbow, Left	**0** High Osmolar **1** Low Osmolar **Y** Other Contrast	**Z** None	**Z** None

Section   **B**   **Imaging**

Body System   **P**   **Non-Axial Upper Bones**

Type   **2**   **Computerized Tomography (CT Scan):** Computer reformatted digital display of multiplanar images developed from the capture of multiple exposures of external ionizing radiation

Body Part (4th)	Contrast (5th)	Qualifier (6th)	Qualifier (7th)
0 Sternoclavicular Joint, Right **1** Sternoclavicular Joint, Left **W** Thorax	**0** High Osmolar **1** Low Osmolar **Y** Other Contrast	**Z** None	**Z** None

Continued →

Section   **B**   **Imaging**
Body System   **P**   **Non-Axial Upper Bones**
Type   **2**   **Computerized Tomography (CT Scan):** Computer reformatted digital display of multiplanar images developed from the capture of multiple exposures of external ionizing radiation

Body Part (4th)	Contrast (5th)	Qualifier (6th)	Qualifier (7th)
2 Sternoclavicular Joints, Bilateral	0 High Osmolar	Z None	Z None
3 Acromioclavicular Joints, Bilateral	1 Low Osmolar		
4 Clavicle, Right	Y Other Contrast		
5 Clavicle, Left	Z None		
6 Scapula, Right			
7 Scapula, Left			
8 Shoulder, Right			
9 Shoulder, Left			
A Humerus, Right			
B Humerus, Left			
E Upper Arm, Right			
F Upper Arm, Left			
G Elbow, Right			
H Elbow, Left			
J Forearm, Right			
K Forearm, Left			
L Wrist, Right			
M Wrist, Left			
N Hand, Right			
P Hand, Left			
Q Hands and Wrists, Bilateral			
R Finger(s), Right			
S Finger(s), Left			
T Upper Extremity, Right			
U Upper Extremity, Left			
V Upper Extremities, Bilateral			
X Ribs, Right			
Y Ribs, Left			
C Hand/Finger Joint, Right	Z None	Z None	Z None
D Hand/Finger Joint, Left			

Section   **B**   **Imaging**
Body System   **P**   **Non-Axial Upper Bones**
Type   **3**   **Magnetic Resonance Imaging (MRI):** Computer reformatted digital display of multiplanar images developed from the capture of radiofrequency signals emitted by nuclei in a body site excited within a magnetic field

Body Part (4th)	Contrast (5th)	Qualifier (6th)	Qualifier (7th)
8 Shoulder, Right	Y Other Contrast	0 Unenhanced and Enhanced	Z None
9 Shoulder, Left		Z None	
C Hand/Finger Joint, Right			
D Hand/Finger Joint, Left			
E Upper Arm, Right			
F Upper Arm, Left			
G Elbow, Right			
H Elbow, Left			
J Forearm, Right			
K Forearm, Left			
L Wrist, Right			
M Wrist, Left			

Continued →

Section   B   Imaging
Body System   P   Non-Axial Upper Bones
Type   3   **Magnetic Resonance Imaging (MRI):** Computer reformatted digital display of multiplanar images developed from the capture of radiofrequency signals emitted by nuclei in a body site excited within a magnetic field

Body Part (4th)	Contrast (5th)	Qualifier (6th)	Qualifier (7th)
8 Shoulder, Right 9 Shoulder, Left C Hand/Finger Joint, Right D Hand/Finger Joint, Left E Upper Arm, Right F Upper Arm, Left G Elbow, Right H Elbow, Left J Forearm, Right K Forearm, Left L Wrist, Right M Wrist, Left	Z None	Z None	Z None

Section   B   Imaging
Body System   P   Non-Axial Upper Bones
Type   4   **Ultrasonography:** Real time display of images of anatomy or flow information developed from the capture of reflected and attenuated high frequency sound waves

Body Part (4th)	Contrast (5th)	Qualifier (6th)	Qualifier (7th)
8 Shoulder, Right 9 Shoulder, Left G Elbow, Right H Elbow, Left L Wrist, Right M Wrist, Left N Hand, Right P Hand, Left	Z None	Z None	1 Densitometry Z None

Section   B   Imaging
Body System   Q   Non-Axial Lower Bones
Type   0   **Plain Radiography:** Planar display of an image developed from the capture of external ionizing radiation on photographic or photoconductive plate

Body Part (4th)	Contrast (5th)	Qualifier (6th)	Qualifier (7th)
0 Hip, Right 1 Hip, Left	0 High Osmolar 1 Low Osmolar Y Other Contrast	Z None	Z None
0 Hip, Right 1 Hip, Left	Z None	Z None	1 Densitometry Z None
3 Femur, Right 4 Femur, Left	Z None	Z None	1 Densitometry Z None
7 Knee, Right 8 Knee, Left G Ankle, Right H Ankle, Left	0 High Osmolar 1 Low Osmolar Y Other Contrast Z None	Z None	Z None
D Lower Leg, Right F Lower Leg, Left J Calcaneus, Right K Calcaneus, Left L Foot, Right M Foot, Left P Toe(s), Right Q Toe(s), Left V Patella, Right W Patella, Left	Z None	Z None	Z None

Continued →

Section	B	Imaging
Body System	Q	Non-Axial Lower Bones
Type	0	**Plain Radiography:** Planar display of an image developed from the capture of external ionizing radiation on photographic or photoconductive plate

Body Part (4th)	Contrast (5th)	Qualifier (6th)	Qualifier (7th)
X Foot/Toe Joint, Right Y Foot/Toe Joint, Left	0 High Osmolar 1 Low Osmolar Y Other Contrast	Z None	Z None

Section	B	Imaging
Body System	Q	Non-Axial Lower Bones
Type	1	**Fluoroscopy:** Single plane or bi-plane real time display of an image developed from the capture of external ionizing radiation on a fluorescent screen. The image may also be stored by either digital or analog means

Body Part (4th)	Contrast (5th)	Qualifier (6th)	Qualifier (7th)
0 Hip, Right 1 Hip, Left 7 Knee, Right 8 Knee, Left G Ankle, Right H Ankle, Left X Foot/Toe Joint, Right Y Foot/Toe Joint, Left	0 High Osmolar 1 Low Osmolar Y Other Contrast Z None	Z None	Z None
3 Femur, Right 4 Femur, Left D Lower Leg, Right F Lower Leg, Left J Calcaneus, Right K Calcaneus, Left L Foot, Right M Foot, Left P Toe(s), Right Q Toe(s), Left V Patella, Right W Patella, Left	Z None	Z None	Z None

Section	B	Imaging
Body System	Q	Non-Axial Lower Bones
Type	2	**Computerized Tomography (CT Scan):** Computer reformatted digital display of multiplanar images developed from the capture of multiple exposures of external ionizing radiation

Body Part (4th)	Contrast (5th)	Qualifier (6th)	Qualifier (7th)
0 Hip, Right 1 Hip, Left 3 Femur, Right 4 Femur, Left 7 Knee, Right 8 Knee, Left D Lower Leg, Right F Lower Leg, Left G Ankle, Right H Ankle, Left J Calcaneus, Right K Calcaneus, Left L Foot, Right M Foot, Left P Toe(s), Right Q Toe(s), Left R Lower Extremity, Right S Lower Extremity, Left V Patella, Right W Patella, Left X Foot/Toe Joint, Right Y Foot/Toe Joint, Left	0 High Osmolar 1 Low Osmolar Y Other Contrast Z None	Z None	Z None

Continued →

Section	B	Imaging
Body System	Q	Non-Axial Lower Bones
Type	2	Computerized Tomography (CT Scan): Computer reformatted digital display of multiplanar images developed from the capture of multiple exposures of external ionizing radiation

Body Part (4ᵗʰ)	Contrast (5ᵗʰ)	Qualifier (6ᵗʰ)	Qualifier (7ᵗʰ)
B Tibia/Fibula, Right C Tibia/Fibula, Left	0 High Osmolar 1 Low Osmolar Y Other Contrast	Z None	Z None

Section	B	Imaging
Body System	Q	Non-Axial Lower Bones
Type	3	Magnetic Resonance Imaging (MRI): Computer reformatted digital display of multiplanar images developed from the capture of radiofrequency signals emitted by nuclei in a body site excited within a magnetic field

Body Part (4ᵗʰ)	Contrast (5ᵗʰ)	Qualifier (6ᵗʰ)	Qualifier (7ᵗʰ)
0 Hip, Right 1 Hip, Left 3 Femur, Right 4 Femur, Left 7 Knee, Right 8 Knee, Left D Lower Leg, Right F Lower Leg, Left G Ankle, Right H Ankle, Left J Calcaneus, Right K Calcaneus, Left L Foot, Right M Foot, Left P Toe(s), Right Q Toe(s), Left V Patella, Right W Patella, Left	Y Other Contrast	0 Unenhanced and Enhanced Z None	Z None
0 Hip, Right 1 Hip, Left 3 Femur, Right 4 Femur, Left 7 Knee, Right 8 Knee, Left D Lower Leg, Right F Lower Leg, Left G Ankle, Right H Ankle, Left J Calcaneus, Right K Calcaneus, Left L Foot, Right M Foot, Left P Toe(s), Right Q Toe(s), Left V Patella, Right W Patella, Left	Z None	Z None	Z None

Section	B	Imaging
Body System	Q	Non-Axial Lower Bones
Type	4	**Ultrasonography:** Real time display of images of anatomy or flow information developed from the capture of reflected and attenuated high frequency sound waves

Body Part (4ᵗʰ)	Contrast (5ᵗʰ)	Qualifier (6ᵗʰ)	Qualifier (7ᵗʰ)
0 Hip, Right 1 Hip, Left 2 Hips, Bilateral 7 Knee, Right 8 Knee, Left 9 Knees, Bilateral	Z None	Z None	Z None

Section	B	Imaging
Body System	R	Axial Skeleton, Except Skull and Facial Bones
Type	0	**Plain Radiography:** Planar display of an image developed from the capture of external ionizing radiation on photographic or photoconductive plate

Body Part (4ᵗʰ)	Contrast (5ᵗʰ)	Qualifier (6ᵗʰ)	Qualifier (7ᵗʰ)
0 Cervical Spine 7 Thoracic Spine 9 Lumbar Spine G Whole Spine	Z None	Z None	1 Densitometry Z None
1 Cervical Disc(s) 2 Thoracic Disc(s) 3 Lumbar Disc(s) 4 Cervical Facet Joint(s) 5 Thoracic Facet Joint(s) 6 Lumbar Facet Joint(s) D Sacroiliac Joints	0 High Osmolar 1 Low Osmolar Y Other Contrast Z None	Z None	Z None
8 Thoracolumbar Joint B Lumbosacral Joint C Pelvis F Sacrum and Coccyx H Sternum	Z None	Z None	Z None

Section	B	Imaging
Body System	R	Axial Skeleton, Except Skull and Facial Bones
Type	1	**Fluoroscopy:** Single plane or bi-plane real time display of an image developed from the capture of external ionizing radiation on a fluorescent screen. The image may also be stored by either digital or analog means

Body Part (4ᵗʰ)	Contrast (5ᵗʰ)	Qualifier (6ᵗʰ)	Qualifier (7ᵗʰ)
0 Cervical Spine 1 Cervical Disc(s) 2 Thoracic Disc(s) 3 Lumbar Disc(s) 4 Cervical Facet Joint(s) 5 Thoracic Facet Joint(s) 6 Lumbar Facet Joint(s) 7 Thoracic Spine 8 Thoracolumbar Joint 9 Lumbar Spine B Lumbosacral Joint C Pelvis D Sacroiliac Joints F Sacrum and Coccyx G Whole Spine H Sternum	0 High Osmolar 1 Low Osmolar Y Other Contrast Z None	Z None	Z None

	Section	B	Imaging
	Body System	R	Axial Skeleton, Except Skull and Facial Bones
	Type	2	Computerized Tomography (CT Scan): Computer reformatted digital display of multiplanar images developed from the capture of multiple exposures of external ionizing radiation

Body Part (4th)	Contrast (5th)	Qualifier (6th)	Qualifier (7th)
0 Cervical Spine 7 Thoracic Spine 9 Lumbar Spine C Pelvis D Sacroiliac Joints F Sacrum and Coccyx	0 High Osmolar 1 Low Osmolar Y Other Contrast Z None	Z None	Z None

	Section	B	Imaging
	Body System	R	Axial Skeleton, Except Skull and Facial Bones
	Type	3	Magnetic Resonance Imaging (MRI): Computer reformatted digital display of multiplanar images developed from the capture of radiofrequency signals emitted by nuclei in a body site excited within a magnetic field

Body Part (4th)	Contrast (5th)	Qualifier (6th)	Qualifier (7th)
0 Cervical Spine 1 Cervical Disc(s) 2 Thoracic Disc(s) 3 Lumbar Disc(s) 7 Thoracic Spine 9 Lumbar Spine C Pelvis F Sacrum and Coccyx	Y Other Contrast	0 Unenhanced and Enhanced Z None	Z None
0 Cervical Spine 1 Cervical Disc(s) 2 Thoracic Disc(s) 3 Lumbar Disc(s) 7 Thoracic Spine 9 Lumbar Spine C Pelvis F Sacrum and Coccyx	Z None	Z None	Z None

	Section	B	Imaging
	Body System	R	Axial Skeleton, Except Skull and Facial Bones
	Type	4	Ultrasonography: Real time display of images of anatomy or flow information developed from the capture of reflected and attenuated high frequency sound waves

Body Part (4th)	Contrast (5th)	Qualifier (6th)	Qualifier (7th)
0 Cervical Spine 7 Thoracic Spine 9 Lumbar Spine F Sacrum and Coccyx	Z None	Z None	Z None

	Section	B	Imaging
	Body System	T	Urinary System
	Type	0	Plain Radiography: Planar display of an image developed from the capture of external ionizing radiation on photographic or photoconductive plate

Body Part (4th)	Contrast (5th)	Qualifier (6th)	Qualifier (7th)
0 Bladder 1 Kidney, Right 2 Kidney, Left 3 Kidneys, Bilateral 4 Kidneys, Ureters and Bladder 5 Urethra 6 Ureter, Right 7 Ureter, Left 8 Ureters, Bilateral B Bladder and Urethra C Ileal Diversion Loop	0 High Osmolar 1 Low Osmolar Y Other Contrast Z None	Z None	Z None

1261

Section   **B**   **Imaging**
Body System   **T**   **Urinary System**
Type   **1**   **Fluoroscopy:** Single plane or bi-plane real time display of an image developed from the capture of external ionizing radiation on a fluorescent screen. The image may also be stored by either digital or analog means

Body Part (4th)	Contrast (5th)	Qualifier (6th)	Qualifier (7th)
0 Bladder 1 Kidney, Right 2 Kidney, Left 3 Kidneys, Bilateral 4 Kidneys, Ureters and Bladder 5 Urethra 6 Ureter, Right 7 Ureter, Left B Bladder and Urethra C Ileal Diversion Loop D Kidney, Ureter and Bladder, Right F Kidney, Ureter and Bladder, Left G Ileal Loop, Ureters and Kidneys	0 High Osmolar 1 Low Osmolar Y Other Contrast Z None	Z None	Z None

Section   **B**   **Imaging**
Body System   **T**   **Urinary System**
Type   **2**   **Computerized Tomography (CT Scan):** Computer reformatted digital display of multiplanar images developed from the capture of multiple exposures of external ionizing radiation

Body Part (4th)	Contrast (5th)	Qualifier (6th)	Qualifier (7th)
0 Bladder 1 Kidney, Right 2 Kidney, Left 3 Kidneys, Bilateral 9 Kidney Transplant	0 High Osmolar 1 Low Osmolar Y Other Contrast	0 Unenhanced and Enhanced Z None	Z None
0 Bladder 1 Kidney, Right 2 Kidney, Left 3 Kidneys, Bilateral 9 Kidney Transplant	Z None	Z None	Z None

Section   **B**   **Imaging**
Body System   **T**   **Urinary System**
Type   **3**   **Magnetic Resonance Imaging (MRI):** Computer reformatted digital display of multiplanar images developed from the capture of radiofrequency signals emitted by nuclei in a body site excited within a magnetic field

Body Part (4th)	Contrast (5th)	Qualifier (6th)	Qualifier (7th)
0 Bladder 1 Kidney, Right 2 Kidney, Left 3 Kidneys, Bilateral 9 Kidney Transplant	Y Other Contrast	0 Unenhanced and Enhanced Z None	Z None
0 Bladder 1 Kidney, Right 2 Kidney, Left 3 Kidneys, Bilateral 9 Kidney Transplant	Z None	Z None	Z None

Section   B   **Imaging**
Body System   T   **Urinary System**
Type   4   **Ultrasonography:** Real time display of images of anatomy or flow information developed from the capture of reflected and attenuated high frequency sound waves

Body Part (4ᵗʰ)	Contrast (5ᵗʰ)	Qualifier (6ᵗʰ)	Qualifier (7ᵗʰ)
0 Bladder	Z None	Z None	Z None
1 Kidney, Right			
2 Kidney, Left			
3 Kidneys, Bilateral			
5 Urethra			
6 Ureter, Right			
7 Ureter, Left			
8 Ureters, Bilateral			
9 Kidney Transplant			
J Kidneys and Bladder			

Section   B   **Imaging**
Body System   U   **Female Reproductive System**
Type   0   **Plain Radiography:** Planar display of an image developed from the capture of external ionizing radiation on photographic or photoconductive plate

Body Part (4ᵗʰ)	Contrast (5ᵗʰ)	Qualifier (6ᵗʰ)	Qualifier (7ᵗʰ)
0 Fallopian Tube, Right	0 High Osmolar	Z None	Z None
1 Fallopian Tube, Left	1 Low Osmolar		
2 Fallopian Tubes, Bilateral	Y Other Contrast		
6 Uterus			
8 Uterus and Fallopian Tubes			
9 Vagina			

Section   B   **Imaging**
Body System   U   **Female Reproductive System**
Type   1   **Fluoroscopy:** Single plane or bi-plane real time display of an image developed from the capture of external ionizing radiation on a fluorescent screen. The image may also be stored by either digital or analog means

Body Part (4ᵗʰ)	Contrast (5ᵗʰ)	Qualifier (6ᵗʰ)	Qualifier (7ᵗʰ)
0 Fallopian Tube, Right	0 High Osmolar	Z None	Z None
1 Fallopian Tube, Left	1 Low Osmolar		
2 Fallopian Tubes, Bilateral	Y Other Contrast		
6 Uterus	Z None		
8 Uterus and Fallopian Tubes			
9 Vagina			

Section   B   **Imaging**
Body System   U   **Female Reproductive System**
Type   3   **Magnetic Resonance Imaging (MRI):** Computer reformatted digital display of multiplanar images developed from the capture of radiofrequency signals emitted by nuclei in a body site excited within a magnetic field

Body Part (4ᵗʰ)	Contrast (5ᵗʰ)	Qualifier (6ᵗʰ)	Qualifier (7ᵗʰ)
3 Ovary, Right	Y Other Contrast	0 Unenhanced and Enhanced	Z None
4 Ovary, Left		Z None	
5 Ovaries, Bilateral			
6 Uterus			
9 Vagina			
B Pregnant Uterus			
C Uterus and Ovaries			
3 Ovary, Right	Z None	Z None	Z None
4 Ovary, Left			
5 Ovaries, Bilateral			
6 Uterus			
9 Vagina			
B Pregnant Uterus			
C Uterus and Ovaries			

Section **B** **Imaging**
Body System **U** **Female Reproductive System**
Type **4** **Ultrasonography:** Real time display of images of anatomy or flow information developed from the capture of reflected and attenuated high frequency sound waves

Body Part (4th)	Contrast (5th)	Qualifier (6th)	Qualifier (7th)
0 Fallopian Tube, Right 1 Fallopian Tube, Left 2 Fallopian Tubes, Bilateral 3 Ovary, Right 4 Ovary, Left 5 Ovaries, Bilateral 6 Uterus C Uterus and Ovaries	Y Other Contrast Z None	Z None	Z None

Section **B** **Imaging**
Body System **V** **Male Reproductive System**
Type **0** **Plain Radiography:** Planar display of an image developed from the capture of external ionizing radiation on photographic or photoconductive plate

Body Part (4th)	Contrast (5th)	Qualifier (6th)	Qualifier (7th)
0 Corpora Cavernosa 1 Epididymis, Right 2 Epididymis, Left 3 Prostate 5 Testicle, Right 6 Testicle, Left 8 Vasa Vasorum	0 High Osmolar 1 Low Osmolar Y Other Contrast	Z None	Z None

Section **B** **Imaging**
Body System **V** **Male Reproductive System**
Type **1** **Fluoroscopy:** Single plane or bi-plane real time display of an image developed from the capture of external ionizing radiation on a fluorescent screen. The image may also be stored by either digital or analog means

Body Part (4th)	Contrast (5th)	Qualifier (6th)	Qualifier (7th)
0 Corpora Cavernosa 8 Vasa Vasorum	0 High Osmolar 1 Low Osmolar Y Other Contrast Z None	Z None	Z None

Section **B** **Imaging**
Body System **V** **Male Reproductive System**
Type **2** **Computerized Tomography (CT Scan):** Computer reformatted digital display of multiplanar images developed from the capture of multiple exposures of external ionizing radiation

Body Part (4th)	Contrast (5th)	Qualifier (6th)	Qualifier (7th)
3 Prostate	0 High Osmolar 1 Low Osmolar Y Other Contrast	0 Unenhanced and Enhanced Z None	Z None
3 Prostate	Z None	Z None	Z None

Section   **B**   **Imaging**
Body System **V**   **Male Reproductive System**
Type   **3**   **Magnetic Resonance Imaging (MRI):** Computer reformatted digital display of multiplanar images developed from the capture of radiofrequency signals emitted by nuclei in a body site excited within a magnetic field

Body Part (4th)	Contrast (5th)	Qualifier (6th)	Qualifier (7th)
0 Corpora Cavernosa 3 Prostate 4 Scrotum 5 Testicle, Right 6 Testicle, Left 7 Testicles, Bilateral	Y Other Contrast	0 Unenhanced and Enhanced Z None	Z None
0 Corpora Cavernosa 3 Prostate 4 Scrotum 5 Testicle, Right 6 Testicle, Left 7 Testicles, Bilateral	Z None	Z None	Z None

Section   **B**   **Imaging**
Body System **V**   **Male Reproductive System**
Type   **4**   **Ultrasonography:** Real time display of images of anatomy or flow information developed from the capture of reflected and attenuated high frequency sound waves

Body Part (4th)	Contrast (5th)	Qualifier (6th)	Qualifier (7th)
4 Scrotum 9 Prostate and Seminal Vesicles B Penis	Z None	Z None	Z None

Section   **B**   **Imaging**
Body System **W**   **Anatomical Regions**
Type   **0**   **Plain Radiography:** Planar display of an image developed from the capture of external ionizing radiation on photographic or photoconductive plate

Body Part (4th)	Contrast (5th)	Qualifier (6th)	Qualifier (7th)
0 Abdomen 1 Abdomen and Pelvis 3 Chest B Long Bones, All C Lower Extremity J Upper Extremity K Whole Body L Whole Skeleton M Whole Body, Infant	Z None	Z None	Z None

Section   **B**   **Imaging**
Body System **W**   **Anatomical Regions**
Type   **1**   **Fluoroscopy:** Single plane or bi-plane real time display of an image developed from the capture of external ionizing radiation on a fluorescent screen. The image may also be stored by either digital or analog means

Body Part (4th)	Contrast (5th)	Qualifier (6th)	Qualifier (7th)
1 Abdomen and Pelvis 9 Head and Neck C Lower Extremity J Upper Extremity	0 High Osmolar 1 Low Osmolar Y Other Contrast Z None	Z None	Z None

Section   **B**   **Imaging**
Body System   **W**   **Anatomical Regions**
Type   **2**   **Computerized Tomography (CT Scan):** Computer reformatted digital display of multiplanar images developed from the capture of multiple exposures of external ionizing radiation

Body Part (4th)	Contrast (5th)	Qualifier (6th)	Qualifier (7th)
0 Abdomen **1** Abdomen and Pelvis **4** Chest and Abdomen **5** Chest, Abdomen and Pelvis **8** Head **9** Head and Neck **F** Neck **G** Pelvic Region	**0** High Osmolar **1** Low Osmolar **Y** Other Contrast	**0** Unenhanced and Enhanced **Z** None	**Z** None
0 Abdomen **1** Abdomen and Pelvis **4** Chest and Abdomen **5** Chest, Abdomen and Pelvis **8** Head **9** Head and Neck **F** Neck **G** Pelvic Region	**Z** None	**Z** None	**Z** None

Section   **B**   **Imaging**
Body System   **W**   **Anatomical Regions**
Type   **3**   **Magnetic Resonance Imaging (MRI):** Computer reformatted digital display of multiplanar images developed from the capture of radiofrequency signals emitted by nuclei in a body site excited within a magnetic field

Body Part (4th)	Contrast (5th)	Qualifier (6th)	Qualifier (7th)
0 Abdomen **8** Head **F** Neck **G** Pelvic Region **H** Retroperitoneum **P** Brachial Plexus	**Y** Other Contrast	**0** Unenhanced and Enhanced **Z** None	**Z** None
0 Abdomen **8** Head **F** Neck **G** Pelvic Region **H** Retroperitoneum **P** Brachial Plexus	**Z** None	**Z** None	**Z** None
3 Chest	**Y** Other Contrast	**0** Unenhanced and Enhanced **Z** None	**Z** None

Section   **B**   **Imaging**
Body System   **W**   **Anatomical Regions**
Type   **4**   **Ultrasonography:** Real time display of images of anatomy or flow information developed from the capture of reflected and attenuated high frequency sound waves

Body Part (4th)	Contrast (5th)	Qualifier (6th)	Qualifier (7th)
0 Abdomen **1** Abdomen and Pelvis **F** Neck **G** Pelvic Region	**Z** None	**Z** None	**Z** None

Section   **B**   **Imaging**
Body System   **Y**   **Fetus and Obstetrical**
Type   **3**   **Magnetic Resonance Imaging (MRI):** Computer reformatted digital display of multiplanar images developed from the capture of radiofrequency signals emitted by nuclei in a body site excited within a magnetic field

Body Part (4th)	Contrast (5th)	Qualifier (6th)	Qualifier (7th)
0 Fetal Head 1 Fetal Heart 2 Fetal Thorax 3 Fetal Abdomen 4 Fetal Spine 5 Fetal Extremities 6 Whole Fetus	Y Other Contrast	0 Unenhanced and Enhanced Z None	Z None
0 Fetal Head 1 Fetal Heart 2 Fetal Thorax 3 Fetal Abdomen 4 Fetal Spine 5 Fetal Extremities 6 Whole Fetus	Z None	Z None	Z None

Section   **B**   **Imaging**
Body System   **Y**   **Fetus and Obstetrical**
Type   **4**   **Ultrasonography:** Real time display of images of anatomy or flow information developed from the capture of reflected and attenuated high frequency sound waves

Body Part (4th)	Contrast (5th)	Qualifier (6th)	Qualifier (7th)
7 Fetal Umbilical Cord 8 Placenta 9 First Trimester, Single Fetus B First Trimester, Multiple Gestation C Second Trimester, Single Fetus D Second Trimester, Multiple Gestation F Third Trimester, Single Fetus G Third Trimester, Multiple Gestation	Z None	Z None	Z None

Within each section of ICD-10-PCS the characters have different meanings. The seven character meanings for the Nuclear Medicine section are illustrated here through the procedure example of *Technetium tomo scan of liver*.

Section	Body System	Root Type	Body Part	Radionuclide	Qualifier	Qualifier
Nuclear Medicine	Hepatobiliary and Pancreas	Tomographic (Tomo)	Liver	Technetium 99m	None	None
C	F	2	5	1	Z	Z

Section (Character 1)

All Nuclear Medicine procedure codes have a first character value of C.

Body System (Character 2)

The alphanumeric character for the body system is placed in the second position. The following are the body systems applicable to the Nuclear Medicine section.

Character Value	Character Value Description
0	Central Nervous System
2	Heart
5	Veins
7	Lymphatic System
8	Eye
9	Ear, Nose, Mouth and Throat
B	Respiratory System
D	Gastrointestinal System
F	Hepatobiliary System and Pancreas
G	Endocrine System
H	Skin, Subcutaneous Tissue and Breast
P	Musculoskeletral
T	Urinary System
V	Male Reproductive System
W	Anatomical Regions

Root Types (Character 3)

The alphanumeric character value for root types is placed in the third position. The following are the root types applicable to the Nuclear Medicine section with their associated meaning.

Character Value	Root Type	Root Type Definition
1	Planar Nuclear Medicine Imaging	Introduction of radioactive materials into the body for single plane display of images developed from the capture of radioactive emissions
2	Tomographic (Tomo) Nuclear Medicine Imaging	Introduction of radioactive materials into the body for three dimensional display of images developed from the capture of radioactive emissions
3	Positron Emission Tomographic (PET) Imaging	Introduction of radioactive materials into the body for three dimensional display of images developed from the simultaneous capture, 180 degrees apart, of radioactive emissions
4	Nonimaging Nuclear Medicine Uptake	Introduction of radioactive materials into the body for measurements of organ function, from the detection of radioactive emissions
5	Nonimaging Nuclear Medicine Probe	Introduction of radioactive materials into the body for the study of distribution and fate of certain substances by the detection of radioactive emissions; or, alternatively, measurement of absorption of radioactive emissions from an external source

Continued →

Character Value	Root Type	Root Type Definition
6	Nonimaging Nuclear Medicine Assay	Introduction of radioactive materials into the body for the study of body fluids and blood elements, by the detection of radioactive emissions
7	Systemic Nuclear Medicine Therapy	Introduction of unsealed radioactive materials into the body for treatment

Body Part (Character 4)

For each body part the applicable body part character values will be available for procedure code construction. An example of a body part is Cerebrospinal Fluid.

Radionuclide (Character 5)

When radionuclide is utilized during a nuclear medicine procedure, the corresponding radionuclide character value should be reported in the fifth character position. The following are examples of the radionuclide character values available for the Nuclear Medicine section.

- Krypton (Kr-81m)
- Technetium 99m (Tc-99m)
- Xenon 127 (Xe-127)
- Xenon 133 (Xe-133)
- Other Radionuclide

If radionuclide is not utilized, the placeholder character value of Z should be reported.

Qualifier (Character 6)

The qualifier represents an additional attribute for the procedure when applicable. Currently, there are no qualifiers in the Nuclear Medicine section; therefore, the placeholder character value of Z should be reported.

Qualifier (Character 7)

The qualifier represents an additional attribute for the procedure when applicable. Currently, there are no qualifiers in the Nuclear Medicine section; therefore, the placeholder character value of Z should be reported.

Nuclear Medicine Section Tables

Nuclear Medicine Tables C01–CW7

Section   C   **Nuclear Medicine**
Body System   0   **Central Nervous System**
Type   1   **Planar Nuclear Medicine Imaging:** Introduction of radioactive materials into the body for single plane display of images developed from the capture of radioactive emissions

Body Part (4th)	Radionuclide (5th)	Qualifier (6th)	Qualifier (7th)
0 Brain	1 Technetium 99m (Tc-99m) Y Other Radionuclide	Z None	Z None
5 Cerebrospinal Fluid	D Indium 111 (In-111) Y Other Radionuclide	Z None	Z None
Y Central Nervous System	Y Other Radionuclide	Z None	Z None

Section	C	Nuclear Medicine
Body System	0	Central Nervous System
Type	2	Tomographic (Tomo) Nuclear Medicine Imaging: Introduction of radioactive materials into the body for three dimensional display of images developed from the capture of radioactive emissions

Body Part (4th)	Radionuclide (5th)	Qualifier (6th)	Qualifier (7th)
0 Brain	1 Technetium 99m (Tc-99m) F Iodine 123 (I-123) S Thallium 201 (Tl-201) Y Other Radionuclide	Z None	Z None
5 Cerebrospinal Fluid	D Indium 111 (In-111) Y Other Radionuclide	Z None	Z None
Y Central Nervous System	Y Other Radionuclide	Z None	Z None

Section	C	Nuclear Medicine
Body System	0	Central Nervous System
Type	3	Positron Emission Tomographic (PET) Imaging: Introduction of radioactive materials into the body for three dimensional display of images developed from the simultaneous capture, 180 degrees apart, of radioactive emissions

Body Part (4th)	Radionuclide (5th)	Qualifier (6th)	Qualifier (7th)
0 Brain	B Carbon 11 (C-11) K Fluorine 18 (F-18) M Oxygen 15 (O-15) Y Other Radionuclide	Z None	Z None
Y Central Nervous System	Y Other Radionuclide	Z None	Z None

Section	C	Nuclear Medicine
Body System	0	Central Nervous System
Type	5	Nonimaging Nuclear Medicine Probe: Introduction of radioactive materials into the body for the study of distribution and fate of certain substances by the detection of radioactive emissions; or, alternatively, measurement of absorption of radioactive emissions from an external source

Body Part (4th)	Radionuclide (5th)	Qualifier (6th)	Qualifier (7th)
0 Brain	V Xenon 133 (Xe-133) Y Other Radionuclide	Z None	Z None
Y Central Nervous System	Y Other Radionuclide	Z None	Z None

Section	C	Nuclear Medicine
Body System	2	Heart
Type	1	Planar Nuclear Medicine Imaging: Introduction of radioactive materials into the body for single plane display of images developed from the capture of radioactive emissions

Body Part (4th)	Radionuclide (5th)	Qualifier (6th)	Qualifier (7th)
6 Heart, Right and Left	1 Technetium 99m (Tc-99m) Y Other Radionuclide	Z None	Z None
G Myocardium	1 Technetium 99m (Tc-99m) D Indium 111 (In-111) S Thallium 201 (Tl-201) Y Other Radionuclide Z None	Z None	Z None
Y Heart	Y Other Radionuclide	Z None	Z None

Section	C	Nuclear Medicine
Body System	2	Heart
Type	2	Tomographic (Tomo) Nuclear Medicine Imaging: Introduction of radioactive materials into the body for three dimensional display of images developed from the capture of radioactive emissions

Body Part (4th)	Radionuclide (5th)	Qualifier (6th)	Qualifier (7th)
6 Heart, Right and Left	1 Technetium 99m (Tc-99m) Y Other Radionuclide	Z None	Z None
G Myocardium	1 Technetium 99m (Tc-99m) D Indium 111 (In-111) K Fluorine 18 (F-18) S Thallium 201 (Tl-201) Y Other Radionuclide Z None	Z None	Z None
Y Heart	Y Other Radionuclide	Z None	Z None

Section	C	Nuclear Medicine
Body System	2	Heart
Type	3	Positron Emission Tomographic (PET) Imaging: Introduction of radioactive materials into the body for three dimensional display of images developed from the simultaneous capture, 180 degrees apart, of radioactive emissions

Body Part (4th)	Radionuclide (5th)	Qualifier (6th)	Qualifier (7th)
G Myocardium	K Fluorine 18 (F-18) M Oxygen 15 (O-15) Q Rubidium 82 (Rb-82) R Nitrogen 13 (N-13) Y Other Radionuclide	Z None	Z None
Y Heart	Y Other Radionuclide	Z None	Z None

Section	C	Nuclear Medicine
Body System	2	Heart
Type	5	Nonimaging Nuclear Medicine Probe: Introduction of radioactive materials into the body for the study of distribution and fate of certain substances by the detection of radioactive emissions; or, alternatively, measurement of absorption of radioactive emissions from an external source

Body Part (4th)	Radionuclide (5th)	Qualifier (6th)	Qualifier (7th)
6 Heart, Right and Left	1 Technetium 99m (Tc-99m) Y Other Radionuclide	Z None	Z None
Y Heart	Y Other Radionuclide	Z None	Z None

Section	C	Nuclear Medicine
Body System	5	Veins
Type	1	Planar Nuclear Medicine Imaging: Introduction of radioactive materials into the body for single plane display of images developed from the capture of radioactive emissions

Body Part (4th)	Radionuclide (5th)	Qualifier (6th)	Qualifier (7th)
B Lower Extremity Veins, Right C Lower Extremity Veins, Left D Lower Extremity Veins, Bilateral N Upper Extremity Veins, Right P Upper Extremity Veins, Left Q Upper Extremity Veins, Bilateral R Central Veins	1 Technetium 99m (Tc-99m) Y Other Radionuclide	Z None	Z None
Y Veins	Y Other Radionuclide	Z None	Z None

Section	C	Nuclear Medicine
Body System	7	Lymphatic and Hematologic System
Type	1	**Planar Nuclear Medicine Imaging:** Introduction of radioactive materials into the body for single plane display of images developed from the capture of radioactive emissions

Body Part (4th)	Radionuclide (5th)	Qualifier (6th)	Qualifier (7th)
0 Bone Marrow	1 Technetium 99m (Tc-99m) D Indium 111 (In-111) Y Other Radionuclide	Z None	Z None
2 Spleen 5 Lymphatics, Head and Neck D Lymphatics, Pelvic J Lymphatics, Head K Lymphatics, Neck L Lymphatics, Upper Chest M Lymphatics, Trunk N Lymphatics, Upper Extremity P Lymphatics, Lower Extremity	1 Technetium 99m (Tc-99m) Y Other Radionuclide	Z None	Z None
3 Blood	D Indium 111 (In-111) Y Other Radionuclide	Z None	Z None
Y Lymphatic and Hematologic System	Y Other Radionuclide	Z None	Z None

Section	C	Nuclear Medicine
Body System	7	Lymphatic and Hematologic System
Type	2	**Tomographic (Tomo) Nuclear Medicine Imaging:** Introduction of radioactive materials into the body for three dimensional display of images developed from the capture of radioactive emissions

Body Part (4th)	Radionuclide (5th)	Qualifier (6th)	Qualifier (7th)
2 Spleen	1 Technetium 99m (Tc-99m) Y Other Radionuclide	Z None	Z None
Y Lymphatic and Hematologic System	Y Other Radionuclide	Z None	Z None

Section	C	Nuclear Medicine
Body System	7	Lymphatic and Hematologic System
Type	5	**Nonimaging Nuclear Medicine Probe:** Introduction of radioactive materials into the body for the study of distribution and fate of certain substances by the detection of radioactive emissions; or, alternatively, measurement of absorption of radioactive emissions from an external source

Body Part (4th)	Radionuclide (5th)	Qualifier (6th)	Qualifier (7th)
5 Lymphatics, Head and Neck D Lymphatics, Pelvic J Lymphatics, Head K Lymphatics, Neck L Lymphatics, Upper Chest M Lymphatics, Trunk N Lymphatics, Upper Extremity P Lymphatics, Lower Extremity	1 Technetium 99m (Tc-99m) Y Other Radionuclide	Z None	Z None
Y Lymphatic and Hematologic System	Y Other Radionuclide	Z None	Z None

Section	C	Nuclear Medicine
Body System	7	Lymphatic and Hematologic System
Type	6	Nonimaging Nuclear Medicine Assay: Introduction of radioactive materials into the body for the study of body fluids and blood elements, by the detection of radioactive emissions

Body Part (4th)	Radionuclide (5th)	Qualifier (6th)	Qualifier (7th)
3 Blood	1 Technetium 99m (Tc-99m) 7 Cobalt 58 (Co-58) C Cobalt 57 (Co-57) D Indium 111 (In-111) H Iodine 125 (I-125) W Chromium (Cr-51) Y Other Radionuclide	Z None	Z None
Y Lymphatic and Hematologic System	Y Other Radionuclide	Z None	Z None

Section	C	Nuclear Medicine
Body System	8	Eye
Type	1	Planar Nuclear Medicine Imaging: Introduction of radioactive materials into the body for single plane display of images developed from the capture of radioactive emissions

Body Part (4th)	Radionuclide (5th)	Qualifier (6th)	Qualifier (7th)
9 Lacrimal Ducts, Bilateral	1 Technetium 99m (Tc-99m) Y Other Radionuclide	Z None	Z None
Y Eye	Y Other Radionuclide	Z None	Z None

Section	C	Nuclear Medicine
Body System	9	Ear, Nose, Mouth and Throat
Type	1	Planar Nuclear Medicine Imaging: Introduction of radioactive materials into the body for single plane display of images developed from the capture of radioactive emissions

Body Part (4th)	Radionuclide (5th)	Qualifier (6th)	Qualifier (7th)
B Salivary Glands, Bilateral	1 Technetium 99m (Tc-99m) Y Other Radionuclide	Z None	Z None
Y Ear, Nose, Mouth and Throat	Y Other Radionuclide	Z None	Z None

Section	C	Nuclear Medicine
Body System	B	Respiratory System
Type	1	Planar Nuclear Medicine Imaging: Introduction of radioactive materials into the body for single plane display of images developed from the capture of radioactive emissions

Body Part (4th)	Radionuclide (5th)	Qualifier (6th)	Qualifier (7th)
2 Lungs and Bronchi	1 Technetium 99m (Tc-99m) 9 Krypton (Kr-81m) T Xenon 127 (Xe-127) V Xenon 133 (Xe-133) Y Other Radionuclide	Z None	Z None
Y Respiratory System	Y Other Radionuclide	Z None	Z None

Section	C	Nuclear Medicine
Body System	B	Respiratory System
Type	2	**Tomographic (Tomo) Nuclear Medicine Imaging:** Introduction of radioactive materials into the body for three dimensional display of images developed from the capture of radioactive emissions

Body Part (4ᵗʰ)	Radionuclide (5ᵗʰ)	Qualifier (6ᵗʰ)	Qualifier (7ᵗʰ)
2 Lungs and Bronchi	1 Technetium 99m (Tc-99m) 9 Krypton (Kr-81m) Y Other Radionuclide	Z None	Z None
Y Respiratory System	Y Other Radionuclide	Z None	Z None

Section	C	Nuclear Medicine
Body System	B	Respiratory System
Type	3	**Positron Emission Tomographic (PET) Imaging:** Introduction of radioactive materials into the body for three dimensional display of images developed from the simultaneous capture, 180 degrees apart, of radioactive emissions

Body Part (4ᵗʰ)	Radionuclide (5ᵗʰ)	Qualifier (6ᵗʰ)	Qualifier (7ᵗʰ)
2 Lungs and Bronchi	K Fluorine 18 (F-18) Y Other Radionuclide	Z None	Z None
Y Respiratory System	Y Other Radionuclide	Z None	Z None

Section	C	Nuclear Medicine
Body System	D	Gastrointestinal System
Type	1	**Planar Nuclear Medicine Imaging:** Introduction of radioactive materials into the body for single plane display of images developed from the capture of radioactive emissions

Body Part (4ᵗʰ)	Radionuclide (5ᵗʰ)	Qualifier (6ᵗʰ)	Qualifier (7ᵗʰ)
5 Upper Gastrointestinal Tract 7 Gastrointestinal Tract	1 Technetium 99m (Tc-99m) D Indium 111 (In-111) Y Other Radionuclide	Z None	Z None
Y Digestive System	Y Other Radionuclide	Z None	Z None

Section	C	Nuclear Medicine
Body System	D	Gastrointestinal System
Type	2	**Tomographic (Tomo) Nuclear Medicine Imaging:** Introduction of radioactive materials into the body for three dimensional display of images developed from the capture of radioactive emissions

Body Part (4ᵗʰ)	Radionuclide (5ᵗʰ)	Qualifier (6ᵗʰ)	Qualifier (7ᵗʰ)
7 Gastrointestinal Tract	1 Technetium 99m (Tc-99m) D Indium 111 (In-111) Y Other Radionuclide	Z None	Z None
Y Digestive System	Y Other Radionuclide	Z None	Z None

Section	C	Nuclear Medicine
Body System	F	Hepatobiliary System and Pancreas
Type	1	**Planar Nuclear Medicine Imaging:** Introduction of radioactive materials into the body for single plane display of images developed from the capture of radioactive emissions

Body Part (4ᵗʰ)	Radionuclide (5ᵗʰ)	Qualifier (6ᵗʰ)	Qualifier (7ᵗʰ)
4 Gallbladder 5 Liver 6 Liver and Spleen C Hepatobiliary System, All	1 Technetium 99m (Tc-99m) Y Other Radionuclide	Z None	Z None
Y Hepatobiliary System and Pancreas	Y Other Radionuclide	Z None	Z None

Section	C	Nuclear Medicine
Body System	F	Hepatobiliary System and Pancreas
Type	2	Tomographic (Tomo) Nuclear Medicine Imaging: Introduction of radioactive materials into the body for three dimensional display of images developed from the capture of radioactive emissions

Body Part (4th)	Radionuclide (5th)	Qualifier (6th)	Qualifier (7th)
4 Gallbladder 5 Liver 6 Liver and Spleen	1 Technetium 99m (Tc-99m) Y Other Radionuclide	Z None	Z None
Y Hepatobiliary System and Pancreas	Y Other Radionuclide	Z None	Z None

Section	C	Nuclear Medicine
Body System	G	Endocrine System
Type	1	Planar Nuclear Medicine Imaging: Introduction of radioactive materials into the body for single plane display of images developed from the capture of radioactive emissions

Body Part (4th)	Radionuclide (5th)	Qualifier (6th)	Qualifier (7th)
1 Parathyroid Glands	1 Technetium 99m (Tc-99m) S Thallium 201 (Tl-201) Y Other Radionuclide	Z None	Z None
2 Thyroid Gland	1 Technetium 99m (Tc-99m) F Iodine 123 (I-123) G Iodine 131 (I-131) Y Other Radionuclide	Z None	Z None
4 Adrenal Glands, Bilateral	G Iodine 131 (I-131) Y Other Radionuclide	Z None	Z None
Y Endocrine System	Y Other Radionuclide	Z None	Z None

Section	C	Nuclear Medicine
Body System	G	Endocrine System
Type	2	Tomographic (Tomo) Nuclear Medicine Imaging: Introduction of radioactive materials into the body for three dimensional display of images developed from the capture of radioactive emissions

Body Part (4th)	Radionuclide (5th)	Qualifier (6th)	Qualifier (7th)
1 Parathyroid Glands	1 Technctium 99m (Tc-99m) S Thallium 201 (Tl-201) Y Other Radionuclide	Z None	Z None
Y Endocrine System	Y Other Radionuclide	Z None	Z None

Section	C	Nuclear Medicine
Body System	G	Endocrine System
Type	4	Nonimaging Nuclear Medicine Uptake: Introduction of radioactive materials into the body for measurements of organ function, from the detection of radioactive emissions

Body Part (4th)	Radionuclide (5th)	Qualifier (6th)	Qualifier (7th)
2 Thyroid Gland	1 Technetium 99m (Tc-99m) F Iodine 123 (I-123) G Iodine 131 (I-131) Y Other Radionuclide	Z None	Z None
Y Endocrine System	Y Other Radionuclide	Z None	Z None

Section   **C**   **Nuclear Medicine**
Body System   **H**   **Skin, Subcutaneous Tissue and Breast**
Type   **1**   **Planar Nuclear Medicine Imaging:** Introduction of radioactive materials into the body for single plane display of images developed from the capture of radioactive emissions

Body Part (4th)	Radionuclide (5th)	Qualifier (6th)	Qualifier (7th)
0 Breast, Right 1 Breast, Left 2 Breasts, Bilateral	1 Technetium 99m (Tc-99m) S Thallium 201 (Tl-201) Y Other Radionuclide	Z None	Z None
Y Skin, Subcutaneous Tissue and Breast	Y Other Radionuclide	Z None	Z None

Section   **C**   **Nuclear Medicine**
Body System   **H**   **Skin, Subcutaneous Tissue and Breast**
Type   **2**   **Tomographic (Tomo) Nuclear Medicine Imaging:** Introduction of radioactive materials into the body for three dimensional display of images developed from the capture of radioactive emissions

Body Part (4th)	Radionuclide (5th)	Qualifier (6th)	Qualifier (7th)
0 Breast, Right 1 Breast, Left 2 Breasts, Bilateral	1 Technetium 99m (Tc-99m) S Thallium 201 (Tl-201) Y Other Radionuclide	Z None	Z None
Y Skin, Subcutaneous Tissue and Breast	Y Other Radionuclide	Z None	Z None

Section   **C**   **Nuclear Medicine**
Body System   **P**   **Musculoskeletal System**
Type   **1**   **Planar Nuclear Medicine Imaging:** Introduction of radioactive materials into the body for single plane display of images developed from the capture of radioactive emissions

Body Part (4th)	Radionuclide (5th)	Qualifier (6th)	Qualifier (7th)
1 Skull 4 Thorax 5 Spine 6 Pelvis 7 Spine and Pelvis 8 Upper Extremity, Right 9 Upper Extremity, Left B Upper Extremities, Bilateral C Lower Extremity, Right D Lower Extremity, Left F Lower Extremities, Bilateral Z Musculoskeletal System, All	1 Technetium 99m (Tc-99m) Y Other Radionuclide	Z None	Z None
Y Musculoskeletal System, Other	Y Other Radionuclide	Z None	Z None

Section   C   **Nuclear Medicine**
Body System   P   **Musculoskeletal System**
Type   2   **Tomographic (Tomo) Nuclear Medicine Imaging:** Introduction of radioactive materials into the body for three dimensional display of images developed from the capture of radioactive emissions

Body Part (4th)	Radionuclide (5th)	Qualifier (6th)	Qualifier (7th)
1 Skull 2 Cervical Spine 3 Skull and Cervical Spine 4 Thorax 6 Pelvis 7 Spine and Pelvis 8 Upper Extremity, Right 9 Upper Extremity, Left B Upper Extremities, Bilateral C Lower Extremity, Right D Lower Extremity, Left F Lower Extremities, Bilateral G Thoracic Spine H Lumbar Spine J Thoracolumbar Spine	1 Technetium 99m (Tc-99m) Y Other Radionuclide	Z None	Z None
Y Musculoskeletal System, Other	Y Other Radionuclide	Z None	Z None

Section   C   **Nuclear Medicine**
Body System   P   **Musculoskeletal System**
Type   5   **Nonimaging Nuclear Medicine Probe:** Introduction of radioactive materials into the body for the study of distribution and fate of certain substances by the detection of radioactive emissions; or, alternatively, measurement of absorption of radioactive emissions from an external source

Body Part (4th)	Radionuclide (5th)	Qualifier (6th)	Qualifier (7th)
5 Spine N Upper Extremities P Lower Extremities	Z None	Z None	Z None
Y Musculoskeletal System, Other	Y Other Radionuclide	Z None	Z None

Section   C   **Nuclear Medicine**
Body System   T   **Urinary System**
Type   1   **Planar Nuclear Medicine Imaging:** Introduction of radioactive materials into the body for single plane display of images developed from the capture of radioactive emissions

Body Part (4th)	Radionuclide (5th)	Qualifier (6th)	Qualifier (7th)
3 Kidneys, Ureters and Bladder	1 Technetium 99m (Tc-99m) F Iodine 123 (I-123) G Iodine 131 (I-131) Y Other Radionuclide	Z None	Z None
H Bladder and Ureters	1 Technetium 99m (Tc-99m) Y Other Radionuclide	Z None	Z None
Y Urinary System	Y Other Radionuclide	Z None	Z None

Section   C   **Nuclear Medicine**
Body System   T   **Urinary System**
Type   2   **Tomographic (Tomo) Nuclear Medicine Imaging:** Introduction of radioactive materials into the body for three dimensional display of images developed from the capture of radioactive emissions

Body Part (4th)	Radionuclide (5th)	Qualifier (6th)	Qualifier (7th)
3 Kidneys, Ureters and Bladder	1 Technetium 99m (Tc-99m) Y Other Radionuclide	Z None	Z None
Y Urinary System	Y Other Radionuclide	Z None	Z None

Section   **C**   **Nuclear Medicine**
Body System   **T**   **Urinary System**
Type   **6**   **Nonimaging Nuclear Medicine Assay:** Introduction of radioactive materials into the body for the study of body fluids and blood elements, by the detection of radioactive emissions

Body Part (4th)	Radionuclide (5th)	Qualifier (6th)	Qualifier (7th)
3 Kidneys, Ureters and Bladder	**1** Technetium 99m (Tc-99m) **F** Iodine 123 (I-123) **G** Iodine 131 (I-131) **H** Iodine 125 (I-125) **Y** Other Radionuclide	**Z** None	**Z** None
Y Urinary System	**Y** Other Radionuclide	**Z** None	**Z** None

Section   **C**   **Nuclear Medicine**
Body System   **V**   **Male Reproductive System**
Type   **1**   **Planar Nuclear Medicine Imaging:** Introduction of radioactive materials into the body for single plane display of images developed from the capture of radioactive emissions

Body Part (4th)	Radionuclide (5th)	Qualifier (6th)	Qualifier (7th)
9 Testicles, Bilateral	**1** Technetium 99m (Tc-99m) **Y** Other Radionuclide	**Z** None	**Z** None
Y Male Reproductive System	**Y** Other Radionuclide	**Z** None	**Z** None

Section   **C**   **Nuclear Medicine**
Body System   **W**   **Anatomical Regions**
Type   **1**   **Planar Nuclear Medicine Imaging:** Introduction of radioactive materials into the body for single plane display of images developed from the capture of radioactive emissions

Body Part (4th)	Radionuclide (5th)	Qualifier (6th)	Qualifier (7th)
0 Abdomen **1** Abdomen and Pelvis **4** Chest and Abdomen **6** Chest and Neck **B** Head and Neck **D** Lower Extremity **J** Pelvic Region **M** Upper Extremity **N** Whole Body	**1** Technetium 99m (Tc-99m) **D** Indium 111 (In-111) **F** Iodine 123 (I-123) **G** Iodine 131 (I-131) **L** Gallium 67 (Ga-67) **S** Thallium 201 (Tl-201) **Y** Other Radionuclide	**Z** None	**Z** None
3 Chest	**1** Technetium 99m (Tc-99m) **D** Indium 111 (In-111) **F** Iodine 123 (I-123) **G** Iodine 131 (I-131) **K** Fluorine 18 (F-18) **L** Gallium 67 (Ga-67) **S** Thallium 201 (Tl-201) **Y** Other Radionuclide	**Z** None	**Z** None
Y Anatomical Regions, Multiple	**Y** Other Radionuclide	**Z** None	**Z** None
Z Anatomical Region, Other	**Z** None	**Z** None	**Z** None

Section	C	Nuclear Medicine
Body System	W	Anatomical Regions
Type	2	**Tomographic (Tomo) Nuclear Medicine Imaging:** Introduction of radioactive materials into the body for three dimensional display of images developed from the capture of radioactive emissions

Body Part (4th)	Radionuclide (5th)	Qualifier (6th)	Qualifier (7th)
0 Abdomen 1 Abdomen and Pelvis 3 Chest 4 Chest and Abdomen 6 Chest and Neck B Head and Neck D Lower Extremity J Pelvic Region M Upper Extremity	1 Technetium 99m (Tc-99m) D Indium 111 (In-111) F Iodine 123 (I-123) G Iodine 131 (I-131) K Fluorine 18 (F-18) L Gallium 67 (Ga-67) S Thallium 201 (Tl-201) Y Other Radionuclide	Z None	Z None
Y Anatomical Regions, Multiple	Y Other Radionuclide	Z None	Z None

Section	C	Nuclear Medicine
Body System	W	Anatomical Regions
Type	3	**Positron Emission Tomographic (PET) Imaging:** Introduction of radioactive materials into the body for three dimensional display of images developed from the simultaneous capture, 180 degrees apart, of radioactive emissions

Body Part (4th)	Radionuclide (5th)	Qualifier (6th)	Qualifier (7th)
N Whole Body	Y Other Radionuclide	Z None	Z None

Section	C	Nuclear Medicine
Body System	W	Anatomical Regions
Type	5	**Nonimaging Nuclear Medicine Probe:** Introduction of radioactive materials into the body for the study of distribution and fate of certain substances by the detection of radioactive emissions; or, alternatively, measurement of absorption of radioactive emissions from an external source

Body Part (4th)	Radionuclide (5th)	Qualifier (6th)	Qualifier (7th)
0 Abdomen 1 Abdomen and Pelvis 3 Chest 4 Chest and Abdomen 6 Chest and Neck B Head and Neck D Lower Extremity J Pelvic Region M Upper Extremity	1 Technetium 99m (Tc-99m) D Indium 111 (In-111) Y Other Radionuclide	Z None	Z None

Section	C	Nuclear Medicine
Body System	W	Anatomical Regions
Type	7	**Systemic Nuclear Medicine Therapy:** Introduction of unsealed radioactive materials into the body for treatment

Body Part (4th)	Radionuclide (5th)	Qualifier (6th)	Qualifier (7th)
0 Abdomen 3 Chest	N Phosphorus 32 (P-32) Y Other Radionuclide	Z None	Z None
G Thyroid	G Iodine 131 (I-131) Y Other Radionuclide	Z None	Z None
N Whole Body	8 Samarium 153 (Sm-153) G Iodine 131 (I-131) N Phosphorus 32 (P-32) P Strontium 89 (Sr-89) Y Other Radionuclide	Z None	Z None
Y Anatomical Regions, Multiple	Y Other Radionuclide	Z None	Z None

Within each section of ICD-10-PCS the characters have different meanings. The seven character meanings for the Radiation Therapy section are illustrated here through the procedure example of *HDR brachytherapy of prostate using Palladium 103*.

Section	Body System	Modality	Treatment Site	Modality Qualifier	Isotope	Qualifier
Radiation Therapy	Male Reproductive System	Brachytherapy	Prostate	High Dose Rate (HDR)	Palladium 103	None
D	V	1	0	9	B	Z

Section (Character 1)

All Radiation Therapy procedure codes have a first character value of D.

Body System (Character 2)

The alphanumeric character for the body system is placed in the second position. The following are the body systems applicable to the Radiation Therapy section.

Character Value	Character Value Description
0	Central and Peripheral Nervous System
7	Lymphatic and hematologic System
8	Eye
9	Ear, Nose, Mouth and Throat
B	Respiratory System
D	Gastrointestinal System
F	Hepatobiliary System and Pancreas
G	Endocrine System
H	Skin
M	Breast
P	Musculoskeletral
T	Urinary System
U	Female Reproductive System
V	Male Reproductive System
W	Anatomical Regions

Modality (Character 3)

The alphanumeric character value for root types is placed in the third position. The following are the root types applicable to the Radiation Therapy section with their associated meaning.

Character Value	Modality	Modality Definition
0	Beam Radiation	The external use of high-energy radiation such as x-rays, photons, electrons, or protons
1	Brachytherapy	The use of radioactive sources placed directly into a tumor bearing area to generate local regions of high intensity radiation
2	Stereotactic Radiosurgery	The use of external radiation sources either from a linear accelerator or a special Cobalt-60 irradiator to deliver many beams of radiation directly to an internal structure in a single fraction
Y	Other Radiation	Other types of radiation therapy such as hyperthermia, contact radiation and plaque radiation. *See Modality qualifier, character 5, for specified types of other radiation.*

Source: CSI Navigator for Radiation Oncology, 2010

Treatment Site (Character 4)

For each treatment site the applicable body part character values will be available for procedure code construction. An example of a treatment site for this section is Brain Stem.

Modality Qualifier (Character 5)

The modality qualifier further specifies the treatment modality. The following are examples of the modality qualifier values available for the Radiation Therapy section:

- Photons >10 MeV
- Neutrons
- Electrons
- High Dose Rate
- Hyperthermia

Isotope (Character 6)

When an isotope is utilized during a radiation oncology procedure, the corresponding isotope character value should be reported in the sixth character position. The following are examples of the isotope character values available for the Radiation Therapy section:

- Iridium 192 (Ir-192)
- Iodine 125 (I-125)
- Californium 252 (Cf-252)

Qualifier (Character 7)

The qualifier represents an additional attribute for the procedure when applicable. For example, beam radiation procedures in this section include the qualifier Intraoperative that is reported with the character value of 0 for some body parts. If there is no qualifier for a procedure, the placeholder Z is the character valve that should be reported.

Radiation Therapy Section Tables

Radiation Therapy Tables D00–DWY

Section	D	Radiation Therapy
Body System	0	Central and Peripheral Nervous System
Modality	0	Beam Radiation

Treatment Site (4th)	Modality Qualifier (5th)	Isotope (6th)	Qualifier (7th)
0 Brain 1 Brain Stem 6 Spinal Cord 7 Peripheral Nerve	0 Photons <1 MeV 1 Photons 1 - 10 MeV 2 Photons >10 MeV 4 Heavy Particles (Protons,Ions) 5 Neutrons 6 Neutron Capture	Z None	Z None
0 Brain 1 Brain Stem 6 Spinal Cord 7 Peripheral Nerve	3 Electrons	Z None	0 Intraoperative Z None

Section	D	Radiation Therapy
Body System	0	Central and Peripheral Nervous System
Modality	1	Brachytherapy

Treatment Site (4th)	Modality Qualifier (5th)	Isotope (6th)	Qualifier (7th)
0 Brain 1 Brain Stem 6 Spinal Cord 7 Peripheral Nerve	9 High Dose Rate (HDR) B Low Dose Rate (LDR)	7 Cesium 137 (Cs-137) 8 Iridium 192 (Ir-192) 9 Iodine 125 (I-125) B Palladium 103 (Pd-103) C Californium 252 (Cf-252) Y Other Isotope	Z None

Section	D	Radiation Therapy
Body System	0	Central and Peripheral Nervous System
Modality	2	Stereotactic Radiosurgery

Treatment Site (4th)	Modality Qualifier (5th)	Isotope (6th)	Qualifier (7th)
0 Brain 1 Brain Stem 6 Spinal Cord 7 Peripheral Nerve	D Stereotactic Other Photon Radiosurgery H Stereotactic Particulate Radiosurgery J Stereotactic Gamma Beam Radiosurgery	Z None	Z None

Section	D	Radiation Therapy
Body System	0	Central and Peripheral Nervous System
Modality	Y	Other Radiation

Treatment Site (4th)	Modality Qualifier (5th)	Isotope (6th)	Qualifier (7th)
0 Brain 1 Brain Stem 6 Spinal Cord 7 Peripheral Nerve	7 Contact Radiation 8 Hyperthermia F Plaque Radiation K Laser Interstitial Thermal Therapy	Z None	Z None

Section	D	Radiation Therapy
Body System	7	Lymphatic and Hematologic System
Modality	0	Beam Radiation

Treatment Site (4th)	Modality Qualifier (5th)	Isotope (6th)	Qualifier (7th)
0 Bone Marrow 1 Thymus 2 Spleen 3 Lymphatics, Neck 4 Lymphatics, Axillary 5 Lymphatics, Thorax 6 Lymphatics, Abdomen 7 Lymphatics, Pelvis 8 Lymphatics, Inguinal	0 Photons <1 MeV 1 Photons 1 - 10 MeV 2 Photons >10 MeV 4 Heavy Particles (Protons,Ions) 5 Neutrons 6 Neutron Capture	Z None	Z None
0 Bone Marrow 1 Thymus 2 Spleen 3 Lymphatics, Neck 4 Lymphatics, Axillary 5 Lymphatics, Thorax 6 Lymphatics, Abdomen 7 Lymphatics, Pelvis 8 Lymphatics, Inguinal	3 Electrons	Z None	0 Intraoperative Z None

Section	D	Radiation Therapy
Body System	7	Lymphatic and Hematologic System
Modality	1	Brachytherapy

Treatment Site (4th)	Modality Qualifier (5th)	Isotope (6th)	Qualifier (7th)
0 Bone Marrow 1 Thymus 2 Spleen 3 Lymphatics, Neck 4 Lymphatics, Axillary 5 Lymphatics, Thorax 6 Lymphatics, Abdomen 7 Lymphatics, Pelvis 8 Lymphatics, Inguinal	9 High Dose Rate (HDR) B Low Dose Rate (LDR)	7 Cesium 137 (Cs-137) 8 Iridium 192 (Ir-192) 9 Iodine 125 (I-125) B Palladium 103 (Pd-103) C Californium 252 (Cf-252) Y Other Isotope	Z None

Section | D | Radiation Therapy
Body System | 7 | Lymphatic and Hematologic System
Modality | 2 | Stereotactic Radiosurgery

Treatment Site (4th)	Modality Qualifier (5th)	Isotope (6th)	Qualifier (7th)
0 Bone Marrow 1 Thymus 2 Spleen 3 Lymphatics, Neck 4 Lymphatics, Axillary 5 Lymphatics, Thorax 6 Lymphatics, Abdomen 7 Lymphatics, Pelvis 8 Lymphatics, Inguinal	D Stereotactic Other Photon Radiosurgery H Stereotactic Particulate Radiosurgery J Stereotactic Gamma Beam Radiosurgery	Z None	Z None

Section | D | Radiation Therapy
Body System | 7 | Lymphatic and Hematologic System
Modality | Y | Other Radiation

Treatment Site (4th)	Modality Qualifier (5th)	Isotope (6th)	Qualifier (7th)
0 Bone Marrow 1 Thymus 2 Spleen 3 Lymphatics, Neck 4 Lymphatics, Axillary 5 Lymphatics, Thorax 6 Lymphatics, Abdomen 7 Lymphatics, Pelvis 8 Lymphatics, Inguinal	8 Hyperthermia F Plaque Radiation	Z None	Z None

Section | D | Radiation Therapy
Body System | 8 | Eye
Modality | 0 | Beam Radiation

Treatment Site (4th)	Modality Qualifier (5th)	Isotope (6th)	Qualifier (7th)
0 Eye	0 Photons <1 MeV 1 Photons 1 - 10 MeV 2 Photons >10 MeV 4 Heavy Particles (Protons,Ions) 5 Neutrons 6 Neutron Capture	Z None	Z None
0 Eye	3 Electrons	Z None	0 Intraoperative Z None

Section | D | Radiation Therapy
Body System | 8 | Eye
Modality | 1 | Brachytherapy

Treatment Site (4th)	Modality Qualifier (5th)	Isotope (6th)	Qualifier (7th)
0 Eye	9 High Dose Rate (HDR) B Low Dose Rate (LDR)	7 Cesium 137 (Cs-137) 8 Iridium 192 (Ir-192) 9 Iodine 125 (I-125) B Palladium 103 (Pd-103) C Californium 252 (Cf-252) Y Other Isotope	Z None

Section	D	Radiation Therapy
Body System	8	Eye
Modality	2	Stereotactic Radiosurgery

Treatment Site (4th)	Modality Qualifier (5th)	Isotope (6th)	Qualifier (7th)
0 Eye	D Stereotactic Other Photon Radiosurgery H Stereotactic Particulate Radiosurgery J Stereotactic Gamma Beam Radiosurgery	Z None	Z None

Section	D	Radiation Therapy
Body System	8	Eye
Modality	Y	Other Radiation

Treatment Site (4th)	Modality Qualifier (5th)	Isotope (6th)	Qualifier (7th)
0 Eye	7 Contact Radiation 8 Hyperthermia F Plaque Radiation	Z None	Z None

Section	D	Radiation Therapy
Body System	9	Ear, Nose, Mouth and Throat
Modality	0	Beam Radiation

Treatment Site (4th)	Modality Qualifier (5th)	Isotope (6th)	Qualifier (7th)
0 Ear 1 Nose 3 Hypopharynx 4 Mouth 5 Tongue 6 Salivary Glands 7 Sinuses 8 Hard Palate 9 Soft Palate B Larynx D Nasopharynx F Oropharynx	0 Photons <1 MeV 1 Photons 1 - 10 MeV 2 Photons >10 MeV 4 Heavy Particles (Protons,Ions) 5 Neutrons 6 Neutron Capture	Z None	Z None
0 Ear 1 Nose 3 Hypopharynx 4 Mouth 5 Tongue 6 Salivary Glands 7 Sinuses 8 Hard Palate 9 Soft Palate B Larynx D Nasopharynx F Oropharynx	3 Electrons	Z None	0 Intraoperative Z None

Section **D** Radiation Therapy
Body System **9** Ear, Nose, Mouth and Throat
Modality **1** Brachytherapy

Treatment Site (4th)	Modality Qualifier (5th)	Isotope (6th)	Qualifier (7th)
0 Ear	**9** High Dose Rate (HDR)	**7** Cesium 137 (Cs-137)	**Z** None
1 Nose	**B** Low Dose Rate (LDR)	**8** Iridium 192 (Ir-192)	
3 Hypopharynx		**9** Iodine 125 (I-125)	
4 Mouth		**B** Palladium 103 (Pd-103)	
5 Tongue		**C** Californium 252 (Cf-252)	
6 Salivary Glands		**Y** Other Isotope	
7 Sinuses			
8 Hard Palate			
9 Soft Palate			
B Larynx			
D Nasopharynx			
F Oropharynx			

Section **D** Radiation Therapy
Body System **9** Ear, Nose, Mouth and Throat
Modality **2** Stereotactic Radiosurgery

Treatment Site (4th)	Modality Qualifier (5th)	Isotope (6th)	Qualifier (7th)
0 Ear	**D** Stereotactic Other Photon Radiosurgery	**Z** None	**Z** None
1 Nose	**H** Stereotactic Particulate Radiosurgery		
4 Mouth	**J** Stereotactic Gamma Beam Radiosurgery		
5 Tongue			
6 Salivary Glands			
7 Sinuses			
8 Hard Palate			
9 Soft Palate			
B Larynx			
C Pharynx			
D Nasopharynx			

Section **D** Radiation Therapy
Body System **9** Ear, Nose, Mouth and Throat
Modality **Y** Other Radiation

Treatment Site (4th)	Modality Qualifier (5th)	Isotope (6th)	Qualifier (7th)
0 Ear	**7** Contact Radiation	**Z** None	**Z** None
1 Nose	**8** Hyperthermia		
5 Tongue	**F** Plaque Radiation		
6 Salivary Glands			
7 Sinuses			
8 Hard Palate			
9 Soft Palate			
3 Hypopharynx	**7** Contact Radiation	**Z** None	**Z** None
F Oropharynx	**8** Hyperthermia		
4 Mouth	**7** Contact Radiation	**Z** None	**Z** None
B Larynx	**8** Hyperthermia		
D Nasopharynx	**C** Intraoperative Radiation Therapy (IORT)		
	F Plaque Radiation		
C Pharynx	**C** Intraoperative Radiation Therapy (IORT)	**Z** None	**Z** None
	F Plaque Radiation		

Section	D	Radiation Therapy
Body System	B	Respiratory System
Modality	0	Beam Radiation

Treatment Site (4th)	Modality Qualifier (5th)	Isotope (6th)	Qualifier (7th)
0 Trachea 1 Bronchus 2 Lung 5 Pleura 6 Mediastinum 7 Chest Wall 8 Diaphragm	0 Photons <1 MeV 1 Photons 1 - 10 MeV 2 Photons >10 MeV 4 Heavy Particles (Protons,Ions) 5 Neutrons 6 Neutron Capture	Z None	Z None
0 Trachea 1 Bronchus 2 Lung 5 Pleura 6 Mediastinum 7 Chest Wall 8 Diaphragm	3 Electrons	Z None	0 Intraoperative Z None

Section	D	Radiation Therapy
Body System	B	Respiratory System
Modality	1	Brachytherapy

Treatment Site (4th)	Modality Qualifier (5th)	Isotope (6th)	Qualifier (7th)
0 Trachea 1 Bronchus 2 Lung 5 Pleura 6 Mediastinum 7 Chest Wall 8 Diaphragm	9 High Dose Rate (HDR) B Low Dose Rate (LDR)	7 Cesium 137 (Cs-137) 8 Iridium 192 (Ir-192) 9 Iodine 125 (I-125) B Palladium 103 (Pd-103) C Californium 252 (Cf-252) Y Other Isotope	Z None

Section	D	Radiation Therapy
Body System	B	Respiratory System
Modality	2	Stereotactic Radiosurgery

Treatment Site (4th)	Modality Qualifier (5th)	Isotope (6th)	Qualifier (7th)
0 Trachea 1 Bronchus 2 Lung 5 Pleura 6 Mediastinum 7 Chest Wall 8 Diaphragm	D Stereotactic Other Photon Radiosurgery H Stereotactic Particulate Radiosurgery J Stereotactic Gamma Beam Radiosurgery	Z None	Z None

Section	D	Radiation Therapy
Body System	B	Respiratory System
Modality	Y	Other Radiation

Treatment Site (4th)	Modality Qualifier (5th)	Isotope (6th)	Qualifier (7th)
0 Trachea 1 Bronchus 2 Lung 5 Pleura 6 Mediastinum 7 Chest Wall 8 Diaphragm	7 Contact Radiation 8 Hyperthermia F Plaque Radiation K Laser Interstitial Thermal Therapy	Z None	Z None

Section   D   Radiation Therapy
Body System   D   Gastrointestinal System
Modality   0   Beam Radiation

Treatment Site (4th)	Modality Qualifier (5th)	Isotope (6th)	Qualifier (7th)
0 Esophagus 1 Stomach 2 Duodenum 3 Jejunum 4 Ileum 5 Colon 7 Rectum	0 Photons <1 MeV 1 Photons 1 - 10 MeV 2 Photons >10 MeV 4 Heavy Particles (Protons,Ions) 5 Neutrons 6 Neutron Capture	Z None	Z None
0 Esophagus 1 Stomach 2 Duodenum 3 Jejunum 4 Ileum 5 Colon 7 Rectum	3 Electrons	Z None	0 Intraoperative Z None

Section   D   Radiation Therapy
Body System   D   Gastrointestinal System
Modality   1   Brachytherapy

Treatment Site (4th)	Modality Qualifier (5th)	Isotope (6th)	Qualifier (7th)
0 Esophagus 1 Stomach 2 Duodenum 3 Jejunum 4 Ileum 5 Colon 7 Rectum	9 High Dose Rate (HDR) B Low Dose Rate (LDR)	7 Cesium 137 (Cs-137) 8 Iridium 192 (Ir-192) 9 Iodine 125 (I-125) B Palladium 103 (Pd-103) C Californium 252 (Cf-252) Y Other Isotope	Z None

Section   D   Radiation Therapy
Body System   D   Gastrointestinal System
Modality   2   Stereotactic Radiosurgery

Treatment Site (4th)	Modality Qualifier (5th)	Isotope (6th)	Qualifier (7th)
0 Esophagus 1 Stomach 2 Duodenum 3 Jejunum 4 Ileum 5 Colon 7 Rectum	D Stereotactic Other Photon Radiosurgery H Stereotactic Particulate Radiosurgery J Stereotactic Gamma Beam Radiosurgery	Z None	Z None

Section   D   Radiation Therapy
Body System   D   Gastrointestinal System
Modality   Y   Other Radiation

Treatment Site (4th)	Modality Qualifier (5th)	Isotope (6th)	Qualifier (7th)
0 Esophagus	7 Contact Radiation 8 Hyperthermia F Plaque Radiation K Laser Interstitial Thermal Therapy	Z None	Z None
1 Stomach 2 Duodenum 3 Jejunum 4 Ileum 5 Colon 7 Rectum	7 Contact Radiation 8 Hyperthermia C Intraoperative Radiation Therapy (IORT) F Plaque Radiation K Laser Interstitial Thermal Therapy	Z None	Z None

Continued →

Section	D	Radiation Therapy
Body System	D	Gastrointestinal System
Modality	Y	Other Radiation

Treatment Site (4th)	Modality Qualifier (5th)	Isotope (6th)	Qualifier (7th)
8 Anus	C Intraoperative Radiation Therapy (IORT) F Plaque Radiation K Laser Interstitial Thermal Therapy	Z None	Z None

Section	D	Radiation Therapy
Body System	F	Hepatobiliary System and Pancreas
Modality	0	Beam Radiation

Treatment Site (4th)	Modality Qualifier (5th)	Isotope (6th)	Qualifier (7th)
0 Liver 1 Gallbladder 2 Bile Ducts 3 Pancreas	0 Photons <1 MeV 1 Photons 1 - 10 MeV 2 Photons >10 MeV 4 Heavy Particles (Protons,Ions) 5 Neutrons 6 Neutron Capture	Z None	Z None
0 Liver 1 Gallbladder 2 Bile Ducts 3 Pancreas	3 Electrons	Z None	0 Intraoperative Z None

Section	D	Radiation Therapy
Body System	F	Hepatobiliary System and Pancreas
Modality	1	Brachytherapy

Treatment Site (4th)	Modality Qualifier (5th)	Isotope (6th)	Qualifier (7th)
0 Liver 1 Gallbladder 2 Bile Ducts 3 Pancreas	9 High Dose Rate (HDR) B Low Dose Rate (LDR)	7 Cesium 137 (Cs-137) 8 Iridium 192 (Ir-192) 9 Iodine 125 (I-125) B Palladium 103 (Pd-103) C Californium 252 (Cf-252) Y Other Isotope	Z None

Section	D	Radiation Therapy
Body System	F	Hepatobiliary System and Pancreas
Modality	2	Stereotactic Radiosurgery

Treatment Site (4th)	Modality Qualifier (5th)	Isotope (6th)	Qualifier (7th)
0 Liver 1 Gallbladder 2 Bile Ducts 3 Pancreas	D Stereotactic Other Photon Radiosurgery H Stereotactic Particulate Radiosurgery J Stereotactic Gamma Beam Radiosurgery	Z None	Z None

Section	D	Radiation Therapy
Body System	F	Hepatobiliary System and Pancreas
Modality	Y	Other Radiation

Treatment Site (4th)	Modality Qualifier (5th)	Isotope (6th)	Qualifier (7th)
0 Liver 1 Gallbladder 2 Bile Ducts 3 Pancreas	7 Contact Radiation 8 Hyperthermia C Intraoperative Radiation Therapy (IORT) F Plaque Radiation K Laser Interstitial Thermal Therapy	Z None	Z None

Section	D	Radiation Therapy
Body System	G	Endocrine System
Modality	0	Beam Radiation

Treatment Site (4th)	Modality Qualifier (5th)	Isotope (6th)	Qualifier (7th)
0 Pituitary Gland 1 Pineal Body 2 Adrenal Glands 4 Parathyroid Glands 5 Thyroid	0 Photons <1 MeV 1 Photons 1 - 10 MeV 2 Photons >10 MeV 5 Neutrons 6 Neutron Capture	Z None	Z None
0 Pituitary Gland 1 Pineal Body 2 Adrenal Glands 4 Parathyroid Glands 5 Thyroid	3 Electrons	Z None	0 Intraoperative Z None

Section	D	Radiation Therapy
Body System	G	Endocrine System
Modality	1	Brachytherapy

Treatment Site (4th)	Modality Qualifier (5th)	Isotope (6th)	Qualifier (7th)
0 Pituitary Gland 1 Pineal Body 2 Adrenal Glands 4 Parathyroid Glands 5 Thyroid	9 High Dose Rate (HDR) B Low Dose Rate (LDR)	7 Cesium 137 (Cs-137) 8 Iridium 192 (Ir-192) 9 Iodine 125 (I-125) B Palladium 103 (Pd-103) C Californium 252 (Cf-252) Y Other Isotope	Z None

Section	D	Radiation Therapy
Body System	G	Endocrine System
Modality	2	Stereotactic Radiosurgery

Treatment Site (4th)	Modality Qualifier (5th)	Isotope (6th)	Qualifier (7th)
0 Pituitary Gland 1 Pineal Body 2 Adrenal Glands 4 Parathyroid Glands 5 Thyroid	D Stereotactic Other Photon Radiosurgery H Stereotactic Particulate Radiosurgery J Stereotactic Gamma Beam Radiosurgery	Z None	Z None

Section	D	Radiation Therapy
Body System	G	Endocrine System
Modality	Y	Other Radiation

Treatment Site (4th)	Modality Qualifier (5th)	Isotope (6th)	Qualifier (7th)
0 Pituitary Gland 1 Pineal Body 2 Adrenal Glands 4 Parathyroid Glands 5 Thyroid	7 Contact Radiation 8 Hyperthermia F Plaque Radiation K Laser Interstitial Thermal Therapy	Z None	Z None

Section	D	Radiation Therapy
Body System	H	Skin
Modality	0	Beam Radiation

Treatment Site (4th)	Modality Qualifier (5th)	Isotope (6th)	Qualifier (7th)
2 Skin, Face 3 Skin, Neck 4 Skin, Arm 6 Skin, Chest 7 Skin, Back 8 Skin, Abdomen 9 Skin, Buttock B Skin, Leg	0 Photons <1 MeV 1 Photons 1 - 10 MeV 2 Photons >10 MeV 4 Heavy Particles (Protons,Ions) 5 Neutrons 6 Neutron Capture	Z None	Z None
2 Skin, Face 3 Skin, Neck 4 Skin, Arm 6 Skin, Chest 7 Skin, Back 8 Skin, Abdomen 9 Skin, Buttock B Skin, Leg	3 Electrons	Z None	0 Intraoperative Z None

Section	D	Radiation Therapy
Body System	H	Skin
Modality	Y	Other Radiation

Treatment Site (4th)	Modality Qualifier (5th)	Isotope (6th)	Qualifier (7th)
2 Skin, Face 3 Skin, Neck 4 Skin, Arm 6 Skin, Chest 7 Skin, Back 8 Skin, Abdomen 9 Skin, Buttock B Skin, Leg	7 Contact Radiation 8 Hyperthermia F Plaque Radiation	Z None	Z None
5 Skin, Hand C Skin, Foot	F Plaque Radiation	Z None	Z None

Section	D	Radiation Therapy
Body System	M	Breast
Modality	0	Beam Radiation

Treatment Site (4th)	Modality Qualifier (5th)	Isotope (6th)	Qualifier (7th)
0 Breast, Left 1 Breast, Right	0 Photons <1 MeV 1 Photons 1 - 10 MeV 2 Photons >10 MeV 4 Heavy Particles (Protons,Ions) 5 Neutrons 6 Neutron Capture	Z None	Z None
0 Breast, Left 1 Breast, Right	3 Electrons	Z None	0 Intraoperative Z None

Section	D	Radiation Therapy
Body System	M	Breast
Modality	1	Brachytherapy

Treatment Site (4th)	Modality Qualifier (5th)	Isotope (6th)	Qualifier (7th)
0 Breast, Left 1 Breast, Right	9 High Dose Rate (HDR) B Low Dose Rate (LDR)	7 Cesium 137 (Cs-137) 8 Iridium 192 (Ir-192) 9 Iodine 125 (I-125) B Palladium 103 (Pd-103) C Californium 252 (Cf-252) Y Other Isotope	Z None

Section	D	Radiation Therapy
Body System	M	Breast
Modality	2	Stereotactic Radiosurgery

Treatment Site (4th)	Modality Qualifier (5th)	Isotope (6th)	Qualifier (7th)
0 Breast, Left 1 Breast, Right	D Stereotactic Other Photon Radiosurgery H Stereotactic Particulate Radiosurgery J Stereotactic Gamma Beam Radiosurgery	Z None	Z None

Section	D	Radiation Therapy
Body System	M	Breast
Modality	Y	Other Radiation

Treatment Site (4th)	Modality Qualifier (5th)	Isotope (6th)	Qualifier (7th)
0 Breast, Left 1 Breast, Right	7 Contact Radiation 8 Hyperthermia F Plaque Radiation K Laser Interstitial Thermal Therapy	Z None	Z None

Section	D	Radiation Therapy
Body System	P	Musculoskeletal System
Modality	0	Beam Radiation

Treatment Site (4th)	Modality Qualifier (5th)	Isotope (6th)	Qualifier (7th)
0 Skull 2 Maxilla 3 Mandible 4 Sternum 5 Rib(s) 6 Humerus 7 Radius/Ulna 8 Pelvic Bones 9 Femur B Tibia/Fibula C Other Bone	0 Photons <1 MeV 1 Photons 1 - 10 MeV 2 Photons >10 MeV 4 Heavy Particles (Protons,Ions) 5 Neutrons 6 Neutron Capture	Z None	Z None
0 Skull 2 Maxilla 3 Mandible 4 Sternum 5 Rib(s) 6 Humerus 7 Radius/Ulna 8 Pelvic Bones 9 Femur B Tibia/Fibula C Other Bone	3 Electrons	Z None	0 Intraoperative Z None

Section	D	Radiation Therapy
Body System	P	Musculoskeletal System
Modality	Y	Other Radiation

Treatment Site (4th)	Modality Qualifier (5th)	Isotope (6th)	Qualifier (7th)
0 Skull 2 Maxilla 3 Mandible 4 Sternum 5 Rib(s) 6 Humerus 7 Radius/Ulna 8 Pelvic Bones 9 Femur B Tibia/Fibula C Other Bone	7 Contact Radiation 8 Hyperthermia F Plaque Radiation	Z None	Z None

Section	D	Radiation Therapy
Body System	T	Urinary System
Modality	0	Beam Radiation

Treatment Site (4th)	Modality Qualifier (5th)	Isotope (6th)	Qualifier (7th)
0 Kidney 1 Ureter 2 Bladder 3 Urethra	0 Photons <1 MeV 1 Photons 1 - 10 MeV 2 Photons >10 MeV 4 Heavy Particles (Protons,Ions) 5 Neutrons 6 Neutron Capture	Z None	Z None
0 Kidney 1 Ureter 2 Bladder 3 Urethra	3 Electrons	Z None	0 Intraoperative Z None

Section	D	Radiation Therapy
Body System	T	Urinary System
Modality	1	Brachytherapy

Treatment Site (4th)	Modality Qualifier (5th)	Isotope (6th)	Qualifier (7th)
0 Kidney 1 Ureter 2 Bladder 3 Urethra	9 High Dose Rate (HDR) B Low Dose Rate (LDR)	7 Cesium 137 (Cs-137) 8 Iridium 192 (Ir-192) 9 Iodine 125 (I-125) B Palladium 103 (Pd-103) C Californium 252 (Cf-252) Y Other Isotope	Z None

Section	D	Radiation Therapy
Body System	T	Urinary System
Modality	2	Stereotactic Radiosurgery

Treatment Site (4th)	Modality Qualifier (5th)	Isotope (6th)	Qualifier (7th)
0 Kidney 1 Ureter 2 Bladder 3 Urethra	D Stereotactic Other Photon Radiosurgery H Stereotactic Particulate Radiosurgery J Stereotactic Gamma Beam Radiosurgery	Z None	Z None

Section	D	Radiation Therapy
Body System	T	Urinary System
Modality	Y	Other Radiation

Treatment Site (4th)	Modality Qualifier (5th)	Isotope (6th)	Qualifier (7th)
0 Kidney 1 Ureter 2 Bladder 3 Urethra	7 Contact Radiation 8 Hyperthermia C Intraoperative Radiation Therapy (IORT) F Plaque Radiation	Z None	Z None

Section	D	Radiation Therapy
Body System	U	Female Reproductive System
Modality	0	Beam Radiation

Treatment Site (4th)	Modality Qualifier (5th)	Isotope (6th)	Qualifier (7th)
0 Ovary 1 Cervix 2 Uterus	0 Photons <1 MeV 1 Photons 1 - 10 MeV 2 Photons >10 MeV 4 Heavy Particles (Protons,Ions) 5 Neutrons 6 Neutron Capture	Z None	Z None

Continued →

Section   D   Radiation Therapy
Body System   U   Female Reproductive System
Modality   0   Beam Radiation

DU0 Continued

DU0–DV0

Radiation Therapy Section Tables

Treatment Site (4ᵗʰ)	Modality Qualifier (5ᵗʰ)	Isotope (6ᵗʰ)	Qualifier (7ᵗʰ)
0 Ovary 1 Cervix 2 Uterus	3 Electrons	Z None	0 Intraoperative Z None

Section   D   Radiation Therapy
Body System   U   Female Reproductive System
Modality   1   Brachytherapy

Treatment Site (4ᵗʰ)	Modality Qualifier (5ᵗʰ)	Isotope (6ᵗʰ)	Qualifier (7ᵗʰ)
0 Ovary 1 Cervix 2 Uterus	9 High Dose Rate (HDR) B Low Dose Rate (LDR)	7 Cesium 137 (Cs-137) 8 Iridium 192 (Ir-192) 9 Iodine 125 (I-125) B Palladium 103 (Pd-103) C Californium 252 (Cf-252) Y Other Isotope	Z None

Section   D   Radiation Therapy
Body System   U   Female Reproductive System
Modality   2   Stereotactic Radiosurgery

Treatment Site (4ᵗʰ)	Modality Qualifier (5ᵗʰ)	Isotope (6ᵗʰ)	Qualifier (7ᵗʰ)
0 Ovary 1 Cervix 2 Uterus	D Stereotactic Other Photon Radiosurgery H Stereotactic Particulate Radiosurgery J Stereotactic Gamma Beam Radiosurgery	Z None	Z None

Section   D   Radiation Therapy
Body System   U   Female Reproductive System
Modality   Y   Other Radiation

Treatment Site (4ᵗʰ)	Modality Qualifier (5ᵗʰ)	Isotope (6ᵗʰ)	Qualifier (7ᵗʰ)
0 Ovary 1 Cervix 2 Uterus	7 Contact Radiation 8 Hyperthermia C Intraoperative Radiation Therapy (IORT) F Plaque Radiation	Z None	Z None

Section   D   Radiation Therapy
Body System   V   Male Reproductive System
Modality   0   Beam Radiation

Treatment Site (4ᵗʰ)	Modality Qualifier (5ᵗʰ)	Isotope (6ᵗʰ)	Qualifier (7ᵗʰ)
0 Prostate 1 Testis	0 Photons <1 MeV 1 Photons 1 - 10 MeV 2 Photons >10 MeV 4 Heavy Particles (Protons,Ions) 5 Neutrons 6 Neutron Capture	Z None	Z None
0 Prostate 1 Testis	3 Electrons	Z None	0 Intraoperative Z None

Section	D	Radiation Therapy
Body System	V	Male Reproductive System
Modality	1	Brachytherapy

Treatment Site (4th)	Modality Qualifier (5th)	Isotope (6th)	Qualifier (7th)
0 Prostate 1 Testis	9 High Dose Rate (HDR) B Low Dose Rate (LDR)	7 Cesium 137 (Cs-137) 8 Iridium 192 (Ir-192) 9 Iodine 125 (I-125) B Palladium 103 (Pd-103) C Californium 252 (Cf-252) Y Other Isotope	Z None

Section	D	Radiation Therapy
Body System	V	Male Reproductive System
Modality	2	Stereotactic Radiosurgery

Treatment Site (4th)	Modality Qualifier (5th)	Isotope (6th)	Qualifier (7th)
0 Prostate 1 Testis	D Stereotactic Other Photon Radiosurgery H Stereotactic Particulate Radiosurgery J Stereotactic Gamma Beam Radiosurgery	Z None	Z None

Section	D	Radiation Therapy
Body System	V	Male Reproductive System
Modality	Y	Other Radiation

Treatment Site (4th)	Modality Qualifier (5th)	Isotope (6th)	Qualifier (7th)
0 Prostate	7 Contact Radiation 8 Hyperthermia C Intraoperative Radiation Therapy (IORT) F Plaque Radiation K Laser Interstitial Thermal Therapy	Z None	Z None
1 Testis	7 Contact Radiation 8 Hyperthermia F Plaque Radiation	Z None	Z None

Section	D	Radiation Therapy
Body System	W	Anatomical Regions
Modality	0	Beam Radiation

Treatment Site (4th)	Modality Qualifier (5th)	Isotope (6th)	Qualifier (7th)
1 Head and Neck 2 Chest 3 Abdomen 4 Hemibody 5 Whole Body 6 Pelvic Region	0 Photons <1 MeV 1 Photons 1 - 10 MeV 2 Photons >10 MeV 4 Heavy Particles (Protons,Ions) 5 Neutrons 6 Neutron Capture	Z None	Z None
1 Head and Neck 2 Chest 3 Abdomen 4 Hemibody 5 Whole Body 6 Pelvic Region	3 Electrons	Z None	0 Intraoperative Z None

Section   **D**   **Radiation Therapy**
Body System   **W**   **Anatomical Regions**
Modality   **1**   **Brachytherapy**

Treatment Site (4ᵗʰ)	Modality Qualifier (5ᵗʰ)	Isotope (6ᵗʰ)	Qualifier (7ᵗʰ)
1 Head and Neck **2** Chest **3** Abdomen **6** Pelvic Region	**9** High Dose Rate (HDR) **B** Low Dose Rate (LDR)	**7** Cesium 137 (Cs-137) **8** Iridium 192 (Ir-192) **9** Iodine 125 (I-125) **B** Palladium 103 (Pd-103) **C** Californium 252 (Cf-252) **Y** Other Isotope	**Z** None

Section   **D**   **Radiation Therapy**
Body System   **W**   **Anatomical Regions**
Modality   **2**   **Stereotactic Radiosurgery**

Treatment Site (4ᵗʰ)	Modality Qualifier (5ᵗʰ)	Isotope (6ᵗʰ)	Qualifier (7ᵗʰ)
1 Head and Neck **2** Chest **3** Abdomen **6** Pelvic Region	**D** Stereotactic Other Photon Radiosurgery **H** Stereotactic Particulate Radiosurgery **J** Stereotactic Gamma Beam Radiosurgery	**Z** None	**Z** None

Section   **D**   **Radiation Therapy**
Body System   **W**   **Anatomical Regions**
Modality   **Y**   **Other Radiation**

Treatment Site (4ᵗʰ)	Modality Qualifier (5ᵗʰ)	Isotope (6ᵗʰ)	Qualifier (7ᵗʰ)
1 Head and Neck **2** Chest **3** Abdomen **4** Hemibody **6** Pelvic Region	**7** Contact Radiation **8** Hyperthermia **F** Plaque Radiation	**Z** None	**Z** None
5 Whole Body	**7** Contact Radiation **8** Hyperthermia **F** Plaque Radiation	**Z** None	**Z** None
5 Whole Body	**G** Isotope Administration	**D** Iodine 131 (I-131) **F** Phosphorus 32 (P-32) **G** Strontium 89 (Sr-89) **H** Strontium 90 (Sr-90) **Y** Other Isotope	**Z** None

Physical Rehabilitation and Diagnostic Audiology Section (F00–F15)

Within each section of ICD-10-PCS the characters have different meanings. The seven character meanings for the Physical Rehabilitation and Diagnostic Audiology section are illustrated below through the procedure example of *Individual fitting of moveable brace, right knee.*

Section	Section Qualifier	Root Type	Body System/Region	Type Qualifier	Equipment	Qualifier
Physical Rehabilitation and Diagnostic Audiology	Rehabilitation	Device Fitting	None	Dynamic Orthosis	Orthosis	None
F	0	D	Z	6	E	Z

Section (Character 1)

All Physical Rehabilitation and Diagnostic Audiology procedure codes have a first character value of F.

Section Qualifier (Character 2)

The alphanumeric character in the second character position identifies if the procedure is a physical rehabilitation procedure or a diagnostic audiology procedure. Physical rehabilitation is reported with character value 0, and diagnostic audiology is reported with character value 1.

Root Type (Character 3)

The alphanumeric character value for root types is placed in the third position. The following are the root types applicable to the Physical Rehabilitation and Diagnostic Audiology section with their associated meaning.

Character Value	Root Type	Root Type Definition
0	Speech Assessment	Measurement of speech and related functions
1	Motor and/or Nerve Function Assessment	Measurement of motor, nerve, and related functions
2	Activities of Daily Living Assessment	Measurement of functional level for activities of daily living
3	Hearing Assessment	Measurement of hearing and related functions
4	Hearing Aid Assessment	Measurement of the appropriateness and/or effectiveness of a hearing device
5	Vestibular Assessment	Measurement of the vestibular system and related functions
6	Speech Treatment	Application of techniques to improve, augment, or compensate for speech and related functional impairment
7	Motor Treatment	Exercise or activities to increase or facilitate motor function
8	Activities of Daily Living Treatment	Exercise or activities to facilitate functional competence for activities of daily living
9	Hearing Treatment	Application of techniques to improve, augment, or compensate for hearing and related functional impairment
B	Cochlear Implant Treatment	Application of techniques to improve the communication abilities of individuals with cochlear implant
C	Vestibular Treatment	Application of techniques to improve, augment, or compensate for vestibular and related functional impairment
D	Device Fitting	Fitting of a device designed to facilitate or support achievement of a higher level of function
F	Caregiver Training	Training in activities to support patient's optimal level of function

Body System/Region (Character 4)

For each body system/region the applicable body part character values will be available for procedure code construction. An example of a body region for this section is Musculoskeletal System—Lower Back/Lower Extremity.

Type Qualifier (Character 5)

Type qualifier further specifies the root type procedure. For example, the type qualifier of Gait Training/Functional Ambulation is used with Motor Treatment (character value 7) when applicable.

Equipment (Character 6)

If equipment is utilized during the procedure character six is used to report the type. Some examples of equipment are

- Aerobic Endurance and Conditioning
- Electrotherapeutic
- Mechanical
- Orthosis
- Prosthesis

If equipment is not utilized, the placeholder character value of Z should be reported.

Qualifier (Character 7)

The qualifier represents an additional attribute for the procedure when applicable. Currently, there are no qualifiers in the Physical Rehabilitation and Diagnostic Audiology section; therefore, the placeholder character value of Z should be reported.

Physical Rehabilitation and Diagnostic Audiology Section Tables

Physical Rehabilitation and Diagnostic Audiology Tables F00–F15

Section	F	Physical Rehabilitation and Diagnostic Audiology
Section Qualifier	0	Rehabilitation
Type	0	Speech Assessment: Measurement of speech and related functions

Body System / Region (4th)	Type Qualifier (5th)	Equipment (6th)	Qualifier (7th)
3 Neurological System - Whole Body	G Communicative/Cognitive Integration Skills	K Audiovisual M Augmentative / Alternative Communication P Computer Y Other Equipment Z None	Z None
Z None	0 Filtered Speech 3 Staggered Spondaic Word Q Performance Intensity Phonetically Balanced Speech Discrimination R Brief Tone Stimuli S Distorted Speech T Dichotic Stimuli V Temporal Ordering of Stimuli W Masking Patterns	1 Audiometer 2 Sound Field / Booth K Audiovisual Z None	Z None
Z None	1 Speech Threshold 2 Speech/Word Recognition	1 Audiometer 2 Sound Field / Booth 9 Cochlear Implant K Audiovisual Z None	Z None
Z None	4 Sensorineural Acuity Level	1 Audiometer 2 Sound Field / Booth Z None	Z None
Z None	5 Synthetic Sentence Identification	1 Audiometer 2 Sound Field / Booth 9 Cochlear Implant K Audiovisual	Z None
Z None	6 Speech and/or Language Screening 7 Nonspoken Language 8 Receptive/Expressive Language C Aphasia G Communicative/Cognitive Integration Skills L Augmentative/Alternative Communication System	K Audiovisual M Augmentative / Alternative Communication P Computer Y Other Equipment Z None	Z None

Continued →

Section   F   **Physical Rehabilitation and Diagnostic Audiology**
Section Qualifier   0   **Rehabilitation**
Type   0   **Speech Assessment:** Measurement of speech and related functions

Body System / Region (4th)	Type Qualifier (5th)	Equipment (6th)	Qualifier (7th)
Z None	9 Articulation/Phonology	K Audiovisual P Computer Q Speech Analysis Y Other Equipment Z None	Z None
Z None	B Motor Speech	K Audiovisual N Biosensory Feedback P Computer Q Speech Analysis T Aerodynamic Function Y Other Equipment Z None	Z None
Z None	D Fluency	K Audiovisual N Biosensory Feedback P Computer Q Speech Analysis S Voice Analysis T Aerodynamic Function Y Other Equipment Z None	Z None
Z None	F Voice	K Audiovisual N Biosensory Feedback P Computer S Voice Analysis T Aerodynamic Function Y Other Equipment Z None	Z None
Z None	H Bedside Swallowing and Oral Function P Oral Peripheral Mechanism	Y Other Equipment Z None	Z None
Z None	J Instrumental Swallowing and Oral Function	T Aerodynamic Function W Swallowing Y Other Equipment	Z None
Z None	K Orofacial Myofunctional	K Audiovisual P Computer Y Other Equipment Z None	Z None
Z None	M Voice Prosthetic	K Audiovisual P Computer S Voice Analysis V Speech Prosthesis Y Other Equipment Z None	Z None
Z None	N Non-invasive Instrumental Status	N Biosensory Feedback P Computer Q Speech Analysis S Voice Analysis T Aerodynamic Function Y Other Equipment	Z None
Z None	X Other Specified Central Auditory Processing	Z None	Z None

Section   F   Physical Rehabilitation and Diagnostic Audiology
Section Qualifier   0   Rehabilitation
Type   1   Motor and/or Nerve Function Assessment: Measurement of motor, nerve, and related functions

Body System / Region (4th)	Type Qualifier (5th)	Equipment (6th)	Qualifier (7th)
0 Neurological System - Head and Neck **1** Neurological System - Upper Back / Upper Extremity **2** Neurological System - Lower Back / Lower Extremity **3** Neurological System - Whole Body	**0** Muscle Performance	**E** Orthosis **F** Assistive, Adaptive, Supportive or Protective **U** Prosthesis **Y** Other Equipment **Z** None	**Z** None
0 Neurological System - Head and Neck **1** Neurological System - Upper Back / Upper Extremity **2** Neurological System - Lower Back / Lower Extremity **3** Neurological System - Whole Body	**1** Integumentary Integrity **3** Coordination/Dexterity **4** Motor Function **G** Reflex Integrity	**Z** None	**Z** None
0 Neurological System - Head and Neck **1** Neurological System - Upper Back / Upper Extremity **2** Neurological System - Lower Back / Lower Extremity **3** Neurological System - Whole Body	**5** Range of Motion and Joint Integrity **6** Sensory Awareness/ Processing/Integrity	**Y** Other Equipment **Z** None	**Z** None
D Integumentary System - Head and Neck **F** Integumentary System - Upper Back / Upper Extremity **G** Integumentary System - Lower Back / Lower Extremity **H** Integumentary System - Whole Body **J** Musculoskeletal System - Head and Neck **K** Musculoskeletal System - Upper Back / Upper Extremity **L** Musculoskeletal System - Lower Back / Lower Extremity **M** Musculoskeletal System - Whole Body	**0** Muscle Performance	**E** Orthosis **F** Assistive, Adaptive, Supportive or Protective **U** Prosthesis **Y** Other Equipment **Z** None	**Z** None
D Integumentary System - Head and Neck **F** Integumentary System - Upper Back / Upper Extremity **G** Integumentary System - Lower Back / Lower Extremity **H** Integumentary System - Whole Body **J** Musculoskeletal System - Head and Neck **K** Musculoskeletal System - Upper Back / Upper Extremity **L** Musculoskeletal System - Lower Back / Lower Extremity **M** Musculoskeletal System - Whole Body	**1** Integumentary Integrity	**Z** None	**Z** None
D Integumentary System - Head and Neck **F** Integumentary System - Upper Back / Upper Extremity **G** Integumentary System - Lower Back / Lower Extremity **H** Integumentary System - Whole Body **J** Musculoskeletal System - Head and Neck **K** Musculoskeletal System - Upper Back / Upper Extremity **L** Musculoskeletal System - Lower Back / Lower Extremity **M** Musculoskeletal System - Whole Body	**5** Range of Motion and Joint Integrity **6** Sensory Awareness/ Processing/Integrity	**Y** Other Equipment **Z** None	**Z** None

Continued →

Section	F	Physical Rehabilitation and Diagnostic Audiology
Section Qualifier	0	Rehabilitation
Type	1	**Motor and/or Nerve Function Assessment:** Measurement of motor, nerve, and related functions

Body System / Region (4th)	Type Qualifier (5th)	Equipment (6th)	Qualifier (7th)
N Genitourinary System	0 Muscle Performance	E Orthosis F Assistive, Adaptive, Supportive or Protective U Prosthesis Y Other Equipment Z None	Z None
Z None	2 Visual Motor Integration	K Audiovisual M Augmentative / Alternative Communication N Biosensory Feedback P Computer Q Speech Analysis S Voice Analysis Y Other Equipment Z None	Z None
Z None	7 Facial Nerve Function	7 Electrophysiologic	Z None
Z None	9 Somatosensory Evoked Potentials	J Somatosensory	Z None
Z None	B Bed Mobility C Transfer F Wheelchair Mobility	E Orthosis F Assistive, Adaptive, Supportive or Protective U Prosthesis Z None	Z None
Z None	D Gait and/or Balance	E Orthosis F Assistive, Adaptive, Supportive or Protective U Prosthesis Y Other Equipment Z None	Z None

Section	F	Physical Rehabilitation and Diagnostic Audiology
Section Qualifier	0	Rehabilitation
Type	2	**Activities of Daily Living Assessment:** Measurement of functional level for activities of daily living

Body System / Region (4th)	Type Qualifier (5th)	Equipment (6th)	Qualifier (7th)
0 Neurological System - Head and Neck	9 Cranial Nerve Integrity D Neuromotor Development	Y Other Equipment Z None	Z None
1 Neurological System - Upper Back / Upper Extremity 2 Neurological System - Lower Back / Lower Extremity 3 Neurological System - Whole Body	D Neuromotor Development	Y Other Equipment Z None	Z None
4 Circulatory System - Head and Neck 5 Circulatory System - Upper Back / Upper Extremity 6 Circulatory System - Lower Back / Lower Extremity 8 Respiratory System - Head and Neck 9 Respiratory System - Upper Back / Upper Extremity B Respiratory System - Lower Back / Lower Extremity	G Ventilation, Respiration and Circulation	C Mechanical G Aerobic Endurance and Conditioning Y Other Equipment Z None	Z None

Continued →

Section F Physical Rehabilitation and Diagnostic Audiology
Section Qualifier 0 Rehabilitation
Type 2 **Activities of Daily Living Assessment:** Measurement of functional level for activities of daily living

Body System / Region (4th)	Type Qualifier (5th)	Equipment (6th)	Qualifier (7th)
7 Circulatory System - Whole Body C Respiratory System - Whole Body	7 Aerobic Capacity and Endurance	E Orthosis G Aerobic Endurance and Conditioning U Prosthesis Y Other Equipment Z None	Z None
7 Circulatory System - Whole Body C Respiratory System - Whole Body	G Ventilation, Respiration and Circulation	C Mechanical G Aerobic Endurance and Conditioning Y Other Equipment Z None	Z None
Z None	0 Bathing/Showering 1 Dressing 3 Grooming/Personal Hygiene 4 Home Management	E Orthosis F Assistive, Adaptive, Supportive or Protective U Prosthesis Z None	Z None
Z None	2 Feeding/Eating 8 Anthropometric Characteristics F Pain	Y Other Equipment Z None	Z None
Z None	5 Perceptual Processing	K Audiovisual M Augmentative / Alternative Communication N Biosensory Feedback P Computer Q Speech Analysis S Voice Analysis Y Other Equipment Z None	Z None
Z None	6 Psychosocial Skills	Z None	Z None
Z None	B Environmental, Home and Work Barriers C Ergonomics and Body Mechanics	E Orthosis F Assistive, Adaptive, Supportive or Protective U Prosthesis Y Other Equipment Z None	Z None
Z None	H Vocational Activities and Functional Community or Work Reintegration Skills	E Orthosis F Assistive, Adaptive, Supportive or Protective G Aerobic Endurance and Conditioning U Prosthesis Y Other Equipment Z None	Z None

Section F Physical Rehabilitation and Diagnostic Audiology
Section Qualifier 0 Rehabilitation
Type 6 **Speech Treatment:** Application of techniques to improve, augment, or compensate for speech and related functional impairment

Body System / Region (4th)	Type Qualifier (5th)	Equipment (6th)	Qualifier (7th)
3 Neurological System - Whole Body	6 Communicative/Cognitive Integration Skills	K Audiovisual M Augmentative / Alternative Communication P Computer Y Other Equipment Z None	Z None

Continued →

Section	F	Physical Rehabilitation and Diagnostic Audiology
Section Qualifier	0	Rehabilitation
Type	6	**Speech Treatment:** Application of techniques to improve, augment, or compensate for speech and related functional impairment

Body System / Region (4th)	Type Qualifier (5th)	Equipment (6th)	Qualifier (7th)
Z None	**0** Nonspoken Language **3** Aphasia **6** Communicative/Cognitive Integration Skills	**K** Audiovisual **M** Augmentative / Alternative Communication **P** Computer **Y** Other Equipment **Z** None	**Z** None
Z None	**1** Speech-Language Pathology and Related Disorders Counseling **2** Speech-Language Pathology and Related Disorders Prevention	**K** Audiovisual **Z** None	**Z** None
Z None	**4** Articulation/Phonology	**K** Audiovisual **P** Computer **Q** Speech Analysis **T** Aerodynamic Function **Y** Other Equipment **Z** None	**Z** None
Z None	**5** Aural Rehabilitation	**K** Audiovisual **L** Assistive Listening **M** Augmentative / Alternative Communication **N** Biosensory Feedback **P** Computer **Q** Speech Analysis **S** Voice Analysis **Y** Other Equipment **Z** None	**Z** None
Z None	**7** Fluency	**4** Electroacoustic Immitance / Acoustic Reflex **K** Audiovisual **N** Biosensory Feedback **Q** Speech Analysis **S** Voice Analysis **T** Aerodynamic Function **Y** Other Equipment **Z** None	**Z** None
Z None	**8** Motor Speech	**K** Audiovisual **N** Biosensory Feedback **P** Computer **Q** Speech Analysis **S** Voice Analysis **T** Aerodynamic Function **Y** Other Equipment **Z** None	**Z** None
Z None	**9** Orofacial Myofunctional	**K** Audiovisual **P** Computer **Y** Other Equipment **Z** None	**Z** None
Z None	**B** Receptive/Expressive Language	**K** Audiovisual **L** Assistive Listening **M** Augmentative / Alternative Communication **P** Computer **Y** Other Equipment **Z** None	**Z** None

Continued →

Section	F	Physical Rehabilitation and Diagnostic Audiology		*F06 Continued*
Section Qualifier	0	Rehabilitation		
Type	6	Speech Treatment: Application of techniques to improve, augment, or compensate for speech and related functional impairment		

Body System / Region (4th)	Type Qualifier (5th)	Equipment (6th)	Qualifier (7th)
Z None	C Voice	K Audiovisual N Biosensory Feedback P Computer S Voice Analysis T Aerodynamic Function V Speech Prosthesis Y Other Equipment Z None	Z None
Z None	D Swallowing Dysfunction	M Augmentative / Alternative Communication T Aerodynamic Function V Speech Prosthesis Y Other Equipment Z None	Z None

Section	F	Physical Rehabilitation and Diagnostic Audiology		
Section Qualifier	0	Rehabilitation		
Type	7	Motor Treatment: Exercise or activities to increase or facilitate motor function		

Body System / Region (4th)	Type Qualifier (5th)	Equipment (6th)	Qualifier (7th)
0 Neurological System - Head and Neck 1 Neurological System - Upper Back / Upper Extremity 2 Neurological System - Lower Back / Lower Extremity 3 Neurological System - Whole Body D Integumentary System - Head and Neck F Integumentary System - Upper Back / Upper Extremity G Integumentary System - Lower Back / Lower Extremity H Integumentary System - Whole Body J Musculoskeletal System - Head and Neck K Musculoskeletal System - Upper Back / Upper Extremity L Musculoskeletal System - Lower Back / Lower Extremity M Musculoskeletal System - Whole Body	0 Range of Motion and Joint Mobility 1 Muscle Performance 2 Coordination/Dexterity 3 Motor Function	E Orthosis F Assistive, Adaptive, Supportive or Protective U Prosthesis Y Other Equipment Z None	Z None
0 Neurological System - Head and Neck 1 Neurological System - Upper Back / Upper Extremity 2 Neurological System - Lower Back / Lower Extremity 3 Neurological System - Whole Body D Integumentary System - Head and Neck F Integumentary System - Upper Back / Upper Extremity G Integumentary System - Lower Back / Lower Extremity H Integumentary System - Whole Body J Musculoskeletal System - Head and Neck K Musculoskeletal System - Upper Back / Upper Extremity L Musculoskeletal System - Lower Back / Lower Extremity M Musculoskeletal System - Whole Body	6 Therapeutic Exercise	B Physical Agents C Mechanical D Electrotherapeutic E Orthosis F Assistive, Adaptive, Supportive or Protective G Aerobic Endurance and Conditioning H Mechanical or Electromechanical U Prosthesis Y Other Equipment Z None	Z None
0 Neurological System - Head and Neck 1 Neurological System - Upper Back / Upper Extremity 2 Neurological System - Lower Back / Lower Extremity 3 Neurological System - Whole Body D Integumentary System - Head and Neck F Integumentary System - Upper Back / Upper Extremity G Integumentary System - Lower Back / Lower Extremity H Integumentary System - Whole Body J Musculoskeletal System - Head and Neck K Musculoskeletal System - Upper Back / Upper Extremity L Musculoskeletal System - Lower Back / Lower Extremity M Musculoskeletal System - Whole Body	7 Manual Therapy Techniques	Z None	Z None

Continued →

Section | F | Physical Rehabilitation and Diagnostic Audiology
Section Qualifier | 0 | Rehabilitation
Type | 7 | **Motor Treatment:** Exercise or activities to increase or facilitate motor function

Body System / Region (4th)	Type Qualifier (5th)	Equipment (6th)	Qualifier (7th)
4 Circulatory System - Head and Neck 5 Circulatory System - Upper Back / Upper Extremity 6 Circulatory System - Lower Back / Lower Extremity 7 Circulatory System - Whole Body 8 Respiratory System - Head and Neck 9 Respiratory System - Upper Back / Upper Extremity B Respiratory System - Lower Back / Lower Extremity C Respiratory System - Whole Body	6 Therapeutic Exercise	B Physical Agents C Mechanical D Electrotherapeutic E Orthosis F Assistive, Adaptive, Supportive or Protective G Aerobic Endurance and Conditioning H Mechanical or Electromechanical U Prosthesis Y Other Equipment Z None	Z None
N Genitourinary System	1 Muscle Performance	E Orthosis F Assistive, Adaptive, Supportive or Protective U Prosthesis Y Other Equipment Z None	Z None
N Genitourinary System	6 Therapeutic Exercise	B Physical Agents C Mechanical D Electrotherapeutic E Orthosis F Assistive, Adaptive, Supportive or Protective G Aerobic Endurance and Conditioning H Mechanical or Electromechanical U Prosthesis Y Other Equipment Z None	Z None
Z None	4 Wheelchair Mobility	D Electrotherapeutic E Orthosis F Assistive, Adaptive, Supportive or Protective U Prosthesis Y Other Equipment Z None	Z None
Z None	5 Bed Mobility	C Mechanical E Orthosis F Assistive, Adaptive, Supportive or Protective U Prosthesis Y Other Equipment Z None	Z None
Z None	8 Transfer Training	C Mechanical D Electrotherapeutic E Orthosis F Assistive, Adaptive, Supportive or Protective U Prosthesis Y Other Equipment Z None	Z None

Continued →

Body System / Region (4th)	Type Qualifier (5th)	Equipment (6th)	Qualifier (7th)
Z None	9 Gait Training/Functional Ambulation	C Mechanical D Electrotherapeutic E Orthosis F Assistive, Adaptive, Supportive or Protective G Aerobic Endurance and Conditioning U Prosthesis Y Other Equipment Z None	Z None

Section   F   Physical Rehabilitation and Diagnostic Audiology

Section Qualifier   0   Rehabilitation

Type   8   Activities of Daily Living Treatment: Exercise or activities to facilitate functional competence for activities of daily living

Body System / Region (4th)	Type Qualifier (5th)	Equipment (6th)	Qualifier (7th)
D Integumentary System - Head and Neck F Integumentary System - Upper Back / Upper Extremity G Integumentary System - Lower Back / Lower Extremity H Integumentary System - Whole Body J Musculoskeletal System - Head and Neck K Musculoskeletal System - Upper Back / Upper Extremity L Musculoskeletal System - Lower Back / Lower Extremity M Musculoskeletal System - Whole Body	5 Wound Management	B Physical Agents C Mechanical D Electrotherapeutic E Orthosis F Assistive, Adaptive, Supportive or Protective U Prosthesis Y Other Equipment Z None	Z None
Z None	0 Bathing/Showering Techniques 1 Dressing Techniques 2 Grooming/Personal Hygiene	E Orthosis F Assistive, Adaptive, Supportive or Protective U Prosthesis Y Other Equipment Z None	Z None
Z None	3 Feeding/Eating	C Mechanical D Electrotherapeutic E Orthosis F Assistive, Adaptive, Supportive or Protective U Prosthesis Y Other Equipment Z None	Z None
Z None	4 Home Management	D Electrotherapeutic E Orthosis F Assistive, Adaptive, Supportive or Protective U Prosthesis Y Other Equipment Z None	Z None
Z None	6 Psychosocial Skills	Z None	Z None

Continued →

Physical Rehabilitation and Diagnostic Audiology Section Tables

Section	F	Physical Rehabilitation and Diagnostic Audiology
Section Qualifier	0	Rehabilitation
Type	8	**Activities of Daily Living Treatment:** Exercise or activities to facilitate functional competence for activities of daily living

Body System / Region (4th)	Type Qualifier (5th)	Equipment (6th)	Qualifier (7th)
Z None	7 Vocational Activities and Functional Community or Work Reintegration Skills	B Physical Agents C Mechanical D Electrotherapeutic E Orthosis F Assistive, Adaptive, Supportive or Protective G Aerobic Endurance and Conditioning U Prosthesis Y Other Equipment Z None	Z None

Section	F	Physical Rehabilitation and Diagnostic Audiology
Section Qualifier	0	Rehabilitation
Type	9	**Hearing Treatment:** Application of techniques to improve, augment, or compensate for hearing and related functional impairment

Body System / Region (4th)	Type Qualifier (5th)	Equipment (6th)	Qualifier (7th)
Z None	0 Hearing and Related Disorders Counseling 1 Hearing and Related Disorders Prevention	K Audiovisual Z None	Z None
Z None	2 Auditory Processing	K Audiovisual L Assistive Listening P Computer Y Other Equipment Z None	Z None
Z None	3 Cerumen Management	X Cerumen Management Z None	Z None

Section	F	Physical Rehabilitation and Diagnostic Audiology
Section Qualifier	0	Rehabilitation
Type	B	**Cochlear Implant Treatment:** Application of techniques to improve the communication abilities of individuals with cochlear implant

Body System / Region (4th)	Type Qualifier (5th)	Equipment (6th)	Qualifier (7th)
Z None	0 Cochlear Implant Rehabilitation	1 Audiometer 2 Sound Field / Booth 9 Cochlear Implant K Audiovisual P Computer Y Other Equipment	Z None

Section	F	Physical Rehabilitation and Diagnostic Audiology
Section Qualifier	0	Rehabilitation
Type	C	**Vestibular Treatment:** Application of techniques to improve, augment, or compensate for vestibular and related functional impairment

Body System / Region (4th)	Type Qualifier (5th)	Equipment (6th)	Qualifier (7th)
3 Neurological System - Whole Body H Integumentary System - Whole Body M Musculoskeletal System - Whole Body	3 Postural Control	E Orthosis F Assistive, Adaptive, Supportive or Protective U Prosthesis Y Other Equipment Z None	Z None

Continued →

Section **F** **Physical Rehabilitation and Diagnostic Audiology**
Section Qualifier **0** **Rehabilitation**
Type **C** **Vestibular Treatment:** Application of techniques to improve, augment, or compensate for vestibular and related functional impairment

Body System / Region (4th)	Type Qualifier (5th)	Equipment (6th)	Qualifier (7th)
Z None	**0** Vestibular	**8** Vestibular / Balance **Z** None	**Z** None
Z None	**1** Perceptual Processing **2** Visual Motor Integration	**K** Audiovisual **L** Assistive Listening **N** Biosensory Feedback **P** Computer **Q** Speech Analysis **S** Voice Analysis **T** Aerodynamic Function **Y** Other Equipment **Z** None	**Z** None

Section **F** **Physical Rehabilitation and Diagnostic Audiology**
Section Qualifier **0** **Rehabilitation**
Type **D** **Device Fitting:** Fitting of a device designed to facilitate or support achievement of a higher level of function

Body System / Region (4th)	Type Qualifier (5th)	Equipment (6th)	Qualifier (7th)
Z None	**0** Tinnitus Masker	**5** Hearing Aid Selection / Fitting / Test **Z** None	**Z** None
Z None	**1** Monaural Hearing Aid **2** Binaural Hearing Aid **5** Assistive Listening Device	**1** Audiometer **2** Sound Field / Booth **5** Hearing Aid Selection / Fitting / Test **K** Audiovisual **L** Assistive Listening **Z** None	**Z** None
Z None	**3** Augmentative/Alternative Communication System	**M** Augmentative / Alternative Communication	**Z** None
Z None	**4** Voice Prosthetic	**S** Voice Analysis **V** Speech Prosthesis	**Z** None
Z None	**6** Dynamic Orthosis **7** Static Orthosis **8** Prosthesis **9** Assistive, Adaptive, Supportive or Protective Devices	**E** Orthosis **F** Assistive, Adaptive, Supportive or Protective **U** Prosthesis **Z** None	**Z** None

Section	F	Physical Rehabilitation and Diagnostic Audiology
Section Qualifier	0	Rehabilitation
Type	F	Caregiver Training: Training in activities to support patient's optimal level of function

Body System / Region (4th)	Type Qualifier (5th)	Equipment (6th)	Qualifier (7th)
Z None	0 Bathing/Showering Technique 1 Dressing 2 Feeding and Eating 3 Grooming/Personal Hygiene 4 Bed Mobility 5 Transfer 6 Wheelchair Mobility 7 Therapeutic Exercise 8 Airway Clearance Techniques 9 Wound Management B Vocational Activities and Functional Community or Work Reintegration Skills C Gait Training/Functional Ambulation D Application, Proper Use and Care of Devices F Application, Proper Use and Care of Orthoses G Application, Proper Use and Care of Prosthesis H Home Management	E Orthosis F Assistive, Adaptive, Supportive or Protective U Prosthesis Z None	Z None
Z None	J Communication Skills	K Audiovisual L Assistive Listening M Augmentative / Alternative Communication P Computer Z None	Z None

Section	F	Physical Rehabilitation and Diagnostic Audiology
Section Qualifier	1	Diagnostic Audiology
Type	3	Hearing Assessment: Measurement of hearing and related functions

Body System / Region (4th)	Type Qualifier (5th)	Equipment (6th)	Qualifier (7th)
Z None	0 Hearing Screening	0 Occupational Hearing 1 Audiometer 2 Sound Field / Booth 3 Tympanometer 8 Vestibular / Balance 9 Cochlear Implant Z None	Z None
Z None	1 Pure Tone Audiometry, Air 2 Pure Tone Audiometry, Air and Bone	0 Occupational Hearing 1 Audiometer 2 Sound Field / Booth Z None	Z None
Z None	3 Bekesy Audiometry 6 Visual Reinforcement Audiometry 9 Short Increment Sensitivity Index B Stenger C Pure Tone Stenger	1 Audiometer 2 Sound Field / Booth Z None	Z None
Z None	4 Conditioned Play Audiometry 5 Select Picture Audiometry	1 Audiometer 2 Sound Field / Booth K Audiovisual Z None	Z None
Z None	7 Alternate Binaural or Monaural Loudness Balance	1 Audiometer K Audiovisual Z None	Z None

Continued →

Section | F | Physical Rehabilitation and Diagnostic Audiology | *F13 Continued*
Section Qualifier | 1 | Diagnostic Audiology
Type | 3 | **Hearing Assessment:** Measurement of hearing and related functions

Body System / Region (4th)	Type Qualifier (5th)	Equipment (6th)	Qualifier (7th)
Z None	8 Tone Decay D Tympanometry F Eustachian Tube Function G Acoustic Reflex Patterns H Acoustic Reflex Threshold J Acoustic Reflex Decay	3 Tympanometer 4 Electroacoustic Immitance / Acoustic Reflex Z None	Z None
Z None	K Electrocochleography L Auditory Evoked Potentials	7 Electrophysiologic Z None	Z None
Z None	M Evoked Otoacoustic Emissions, Screening N Evoked Otoacoustic Emissions, Diagnostic	6 Otoacoustic Emission (OAE) Z None	Z None
Z None	P Aural Rehabilitation Status	1 Audiometer 2 Sound Field / Booth 4 Electroacoustic Immitance / Acoustic Reflex 9 Cochlear Implant K Audiovisual L Assistive Listening P Computer Z None	Z None
Z None	Q Auditory Processing	K Audiovisual P Computer Y Other Equipment Z None	Z None

Section | F | Physical Rehabilitation and Diagnostic Audiology
Section Qualifier | 1 | Diagnostic Audiology
Type | 4 | **Hearing Aid Assessment:** Measurement of the appropriateness and/or effectiveness of a hearing device

Body System / Region (4th)	Type Qualifier (5th)	Equipment (6th)	Qualifier (7th)
Z None	0 Cochlear Implant	1 Audiometer 2 Sound Field / Booth 3 Tympanometer 4 Electroacoustic Immitance / Acoustic Reflex 5 Hearing Aid Selection / Fitting / Test 7 Electrophysiologic 9 Cochlear Implant K Audiovisual L Assistive Listening P Computer Y Other Equipment Z None	Z None
Z None	1 Ear Canal Probe Microphone 6 Binaural Electroacoustic Hearing Aid Check 8 Monaural Electroacoustic Hearing Aid Check	5 Hearing Aid Selection / Fitting / Test Z None	Z None

Continued →

Section   **F**   **Physical Rehabilitation and Diagnostic Audiology**
Section Qualifier   **1**   **Diagnostic Audiology**
Type   **4**   **Hearing Aid Assessment:** Measurement of the appropriateness and/or effectiveness of a hearing device

Body System / Region (4th)	Type Qualifier (5th)	Equipment (6th)	Qualifier (7th)
Z None	2 Monaural Hearing Aid 3 Binaural Hearing Aid	1 Audiometer 2 Sound Field / Booth 3 Tympanometer 4 Electroacoustic Immitance / Acoustic Reflex 5 Hearing Aid Selection / Fitting / Test K Audiovisual L Assistive Listening P Computer Z None	Z None
Z None	4 Assistive Listening System/ Device Selection	1 Audiometer 2 Sound Field / Booth 3 Tympanometer 4 Electroacoustic Immitance / Acoustic Reflex K Audiovisual L Assistive Listening Z None	Z None
Z None	5 Sensory Aids	1 Audiometer 2 Sound Field / Booth 3 Tympanometer 4 Electroacoustic Immitance / Acoustic Reflex 5 Hearing Aid Selection / Fitting / Test K Audiovisual L Assistive Listening Z None	Z None
Z None	7 Ear Protector Attentuation	0 Occupational Hearing Z None	Z None

Section   **F**   **Physical Rehabilitation and Diagnostic Audiology**
Section Qualifier   **1**   **Diagnostic Audiology**
Type   **5**   **Vestibular Assessment:** Measurement of the vestibular system and related functions

Body System / Region (4th)	Type Qualifier (5th)	Equipment (6th)	Qualifier (7th)
Z None	0 Bithermal, Binaural Caloric Irrigation 1 Bithermal, Monaural Caloric Irrigation 2 Unithermal Binaural Screen 3 Oscillating Tracking 4 Sinusoidal Vertical Axis Rotational 5 Dix-Hallpike Dynamic 6 Computerized Dynamic Posturography	8 Vestibular / Balance Z None	Z None
Z None	7 Tinnitus Masker	5 Hearing Aid Selection / Fitting / Test Z None	Z None

Within each section of ICD-10-PCS the characters have different meanings. The seven character meanings for the Mental Health section are illustrated here through the procedure example of *Crisis intervention*.

Section	Body System	Root Type	Qualifier	Qualifier	Qualifier	Qualifier
Mental Health	None	Crisis Intervention	None	None	None	None
G	Z	2	Z	Z	Z	Z

Section (Character 1)

All Mental Health procedure codes have a first character value of G.

Body System (Character 2)

The body system is not specified for mental health; therefore, the placeholder character value of Z is reported in the second character position.

Root Type (Character 3)

The alphanumeric character value for root types is placed in the third position. Listed below are the root types applicable to the Mental Health section with their associated meaning.

Character Value	Root Type	Root Type Definition
1	Psychological Tests	The administration and interpretation of standardized psychological tests and measurement instruments for the assessment of psychological function
2	Crisis Intervention	Treatment of a traumatized, acutely disturbed or distressed individual for the purpose of short-term stabilization
3	Medication Management	Monitoring and adjusting the use of medications for the treatment of a mental health disorder
5	Individual Psychotherapy	Treatment of an individual with a mental health disorder by behavioral, cognitive, psychoanalytic, psychodynamic or psychophysiological means to improve functioning or well-being
6	Counseling	The application of psychological methods to treat an individual with normal developmental issues and psychological problems in order to increase function, improve well-being, alleviate distress, maladjustment or resolve crises
7	Family Psychotherapy	Treatment that includes one or more family members of an individual with a mental health disorder by behavioral, cognitive, psychoanalytic, psychodynamic or psychophysiological means to improve functioning or well-being
B	Electroconvulsive Therapy	The application of controlled electrical voltages to treat a mental health disorder
C	Biofeedback	Provision of information from the monitoring and regulating of physiological processes in conjunction with cognitive-behavioral techniques to improve patient functioning or well-being
F	Hypnosis	Induction of a state of heightened suggestibility by auditory, visual and tactile techniques to elicit an emotional or behavioral response
G	Narcosynthesis	Administration of intravenous barbiturates in order to release suppressed or repressed thoughts
H	Group Psychotherapy	Treatment of two or more individuals with a mental health disorder by behavioral, cognitive, psychoanalytic, psychodynamic or psychophysiological means to improve functioning or well-being
J	Light Therapy	Application of specialized light treatments to improve functioning or well-being

Qualifier (Character 4)

This qualifier further specifies the root type procedure. For example, the qualifier of Development further specifies the type of Psychological Tests.

Qualifier (Character 5)

The qualifier represents an additional attribute for the procedure when applicable. Currently, there are no qualifiers in the Mental Health section; therefore, the placeholder character value of Z should be reported.

Qualifier (Character 6)

The qualifier represents an additional attribute for the procedure when applicable. Currently, there are no qualifiers in the Mental Health section; therefore, the placeholder character value of Z should be reported.

Qualifier (Character 7)

The qualifier represents an additional attribute for the procedure when applicable. Currently, there are no qualifiers in the Mental Health section; therefore, the placeholder character value of Z should be reported.

Mental Health Tables

Mental Health Tables GZ1–GZJ

Section   **G**   **Mental Health**
Body System   **Z**   **None**
Type   **1**   **Psychological Tests:** The administration and interpretation of standardized psychological tests and measurement instruments for the assessment of psychological function

Qualifier (4ᵗʰ)	Qualifier (5ᵗʰ)	Qualifier (6ᵗʰ)	Qualifier (7ᵗʰ)
0 Developmental 1 Personality and Behavioral 2 Intellectual and Psychoeducational 3 Neuropsychological 4 Neurobehavioral and Cognitive Status	Z None	Z None	Z None

Section   **G**   **Mental Health**
Body System   **Z**   **None**
Type   **2**   **Crisis Intervention:** Treatment of a traumatized, acutely disturbed or distressed individual for the purpose of short-term stabilization

Qualifier (4ᵗʰ)	Qualifier (5ᵗʰ)	Qualifier (6ᵗʰ)	Qualifier (7ᵗʰ)
Z None	Z None	Z None	Z None

Section   **G**   **Mental Health**
Body System   **Z**   **None**
Type   **3**   **Medication Management:** Monitoring and adjusting the use of medications for the treatment of a mental health disorder

Qualifier (4ᵗʰ)	Qualifier (5ᵗʰ)	Qualifier (6ᵗʰ)	Qualifier (7ᵗʰ)
Z None	Z None	Z None	Z None

Section   **G**   **Mental Health**
Body System   **Z**   **None**
Type   **5**   **Individual Psychotherapy:** Treatment of an individual with a mental health disorder by behavioral, cognitive, psychoanalytic, psychodynamic or psychophysiological means to improve functioning or well-being

Qualifier (4ᵗʰ)	Qualifier (5ᵗʰ)	Qualifier (6ᵗʰ)	Qualifier (7ᵗʰ)
0 Interactive 1 Behavioral 2 Cognitive 3 Interpersonal 4 Psychoanalysis 5 Psychodynamic 6 Supportive 8 Cognitive-Behavioral 9 Psychophysiological	Z None	Z None	Z None

Section G **Mental Health**
Body System Z **None**
Type 6 **Counseling:** The application of psychological methods to treat an individual with normal developmental issues and psychological problems in order to increase function, improve well-being, alleviate distress, maladjustment or resolve crises

Qualifier (4th)	Qualifier (5th)	Qualifier (6th)	Qualifier (7th)
0 Educational 1 Vocational 3 Other Counseling	Z None	Z None	Z None

Section G **Mental Health**
Body System Z **None**
Type 7 **Family Psychotherapy:** Treatment that includes one or more family members of an individual with a mental health disorder by behavioral, cognitive, psychoanalytic, psychodynamic or psychophysiological means to improve functioning or well-being

Qualifier (4th)	Qualifier (5th)	Qualifier (6th)	Qualifier (7th)
2 Other Family Psychotherapy	Z None	Z None	Z None

Section G **Mental Health**
Body System Z **None**
Type B **Electroconvulsive Therapy:** The application of controlled electrical voltages to treat a mental health disorder

Qualifier (4th)	Qualifier (5th)	Qualifier (6th)	Qualifier (7th)
0 Unilateral-Single Seizure 1 Unilateral-Multiple Seizure 2 Bilateral-Single Seizure 3 Bilateral-Multiple Seizure 4 Other Electroconvulsive Therapy	Z None	Z None	Z None

Section G **Mental Health**
Body System Z **None**
Type C **Biofeedback:** Provision of information from the monitoring and regulating of physiological processes in conjunction with cognitive-behavioral techniques to improve patient functioning or well-being

Qualifier (4th)	Qualifier (5th)	Qualifier (6th)	Qualifier (7th)
9 Other Biofeedback	Z None	Z None	Z None

Section G **Mental Health**
Body System Z **None**
Type F **Hypnosis:** Induction of a state of heightened suggestibility by auditory, visual and tactile techniques to elicit an emotional or behavioral response

Qualifier (4th)	Qualifier (5th)	Qualifier (6th)	Qualifier (7th)
Z None	Z None	Z None	Z None

Section G **Mental Health**
Body System Z **None**
Type G **Narcosynthesis:** Administration of intravenous barbiturates in order to release suppressed or repressed thoughts

Qualifier (4th)	Qualifier (5th)	Qualifier (6th)	Qualifier (7th)
Z None	Z None	Z None	Z None

Section   G   **Mental Health**
Body System   Z   **None**
Type   H   **Group Psychotherapy:** Treatment of two or more individuals with a mental health disorder by behavioral, cognitive, psychoanalytic, psychodynamic or psychophysiological means to improve functioning or well-being

Qualifier (4th)	Qualifier (5th)	Qualifier (6th)	Qualifier (7th)
Z None	**Z** None	**Z** None	**Z** None

Section   G   **Mental Health**
Body System   Z   **None**
Type   J   **Light Therapy:** Application of specialized light treatments to improve functioning or well-being

Qualifier (4th)	Qualifier (5th)	Qualifier (6th)	Qualifier (7th)
Z None	**Z** None	**Z** None	**Z** None

Within each section of ICD-10-PCS the characters have different meanings. The seven character meanings for the Substance Abuse section are illustrated below through the procedure example of *Substance abuse family counseling*.

Section	Body System	Root Type	Qualifier	Qualifier	Qualifier	Qualifier
Substance Abuse	None	Family Counseling	Other Family Counseling	None	None	None
H	Z	6	3	Z	Z	Z

Section (Character 1)

All Substance Abuse procedure codes have a first character value of H.

Body System (Character 2)

The body system is not specified for substance abuse; therefore, the placeholder character value of Z is reported in the second character position.

Root Type (Character 3)

The alphanumeric character value for root types is placed in the third position. The following are the root types applicable to the Substance Abuse section with their associated meaning.

Character Value	Root Type	Root Type Definition
2	Detoxification Services	Detoxification from alcohol and/or drugs
3	Individual Counseling	The application of psychological methods to treat an individual with addictive behavior
4	Group Counseling	The application of psychological methods to treat two or more individuals with addictive behavior
5	Individual Psychotherapy	Treatment of an individual with addictive behavior by behavioral, cognitive, psychoanalytic, psychodynamic or psychophysiological means
6	Family Counseling	The application of psychological methods that includes one or more family members to treat an individual with addictive behavior
8	Medication Management	Monitoring and adjusting the use of replacement medications for the treatment of addiction
9	Pharmacotherapy	The use of replacement medications for the treatment of addiction

Qualifier (Character 4)

This qualifier further specifies the root type procedure. For example, the qualifier of Cognitive further specifies the type of Individual counseling.

Qualifier (Character 5)

The qualifier represents an additional attribute for the procedure when applicable. Currently, there are no qualifiers in the Substance Abuse section; therefore, the placeholder character value of Z should be reported.

Qualifier (Character 6)

The qualifier represents an additional attribute for the procedure when applicable. Currently, there are no qualifiers in the Substance Abuse section; therefore, the placeholder character value of Z should be reported.

Qualifier (Character 7)

The qualifier represents an additional attribute for the procedure when applicable. Currently, there are no qualifiers in the Substance Abuse section; therefore, the placeholder character value of Z should be reported.

Substance Abuse Treatment Section Tables

Substance Abuse Treatment Tables HZ2–HZ9

Section	H	Substance Abuse Treatment
Body System	Z	None
Type	2	**Detoxification Services:** Detoxification from alcohol and/or drugs

Qualifier (4th)	Qualifier (5th)	Qualifier (6th)	Qualifier (7th)
Z None	**Z** None	**Z** None	**Z** None

Section	H	Substance Abuse Treatment
Body System	Z	None
Type	3	**Individual Counseling:** The application of psychological methods to treat an individual with addictive behavior

Qualifier (4th)	Qualifier (5th)	Qualifier (6th)	Qualifier (7th)
0 Cognitive **1** Behavioral **2** Cognitive-Behavioral **3** 12-Step **4** Interpersonal **5** Vocational **6** Psychoeducation **7** Motivational Enhancement **8** Confrontational **9** Continuing Care **B** Spiritual **C** Pre/Post-Test Infectious Disease	**Z** None	**Z** None	**Z** None

Section	H	Substance Abuse Treatment
Body System	Z	None
Type	4	**Group Counseling:** The application of psychological methods to treat two or more individuals with addictive behavior

Qualifier (4th)	Qualifier (5th)	Qualifier (6th)	Qualifier (7th)
0 Cognitive **1** Behavioral **2** Cognitive-Behavioral **3** 12-Step **4** Interpersonal **5** Vocational **6** Psychoeducation **7** Motivational Enhancement **8** Confrontational **9** Continuing Care **B** Spiritual **C** Pre/Post-Test Infectious Disease	**Z** None	**Z** None	**Z** None

Section   **H**   **Substance Abuse Treatment**
Body System   **Z**   **None**
Type   **5**   **Individual Psychotherapy:** Treatment of an individual with addictive behavior by behavioral, cognitive, psychoanalytic, psychodynamic or psychophysiological means

Qualifier (4ᵗʰ)	Qualifier (5ᵗʰ)	Qualifier (6ᵗʰ)	Qualifier (7ᵗʰ)
0 Cognitive 1 Behavioral 2 Cognitive-Behavioral 3 12-Step 4 Interpersonal 5 Interactive 6 Psychoeducation 7 Motivational Enhancement 8 Confrontational 9 Supportive B Psychoanalysis C Psychodynamic D Psychophysiological	Z None	Z None	Z None

Section   **H**   **Substance Abuse Treatment**
Body System   **Z**   **None**
Type   **6**   **Family Counseling:** The application of psychological methods that includes one or more family members to treat an individual with addictive behavior

Qualifier (4ᵗʰ)	Qualifier (5ᵗʰ)	Qualifier (6ᵗʰ)	Qualifier (7ᵗʰ)
3 Other Family Counseling	Z None	Z None	Z None

Section   **H**   **Substance Abuse Treatment**
Body System   **Z**   **None**
Type   **8**   **Medication Management:** Monitoring and adjusting the use of replacement medications for the treatment of addiction

Qualifier (4ᵗʰ)	Qualifier (5ᵗʰ)	Qualifier (6ᵗʰ)	Qualifier (7ᵗʰ)
0 Nicotine Replacement 1 Methadone Maintenance 2 Levo-alpha-acetyl-methadol (LAAM) 3 Antabuse 4 Naltrexone 5 Naloxone 6 Clonidine 7 Bupropion 8 Psychiatric Medication 9 Other Replacement Medication	Z None	Z None	Z None

Section   **H**   **Substance Abuse Treatment**
Body System   **Z**   **None**
Type   **9**   **Pharmacotherapy:** The use of replacement medications for the treatment of addiction

Qualifier (4ᵗʰ)	Qualifier (5ᵗʰ)	Qualifier (6ᵗʰ)	Qualifier (7ᵗʰ)
0 Nicotine Replacement 1 Methadone Maintenance 2 Levo-alpha-acetyl-methadol (LAAM) 3 Antabuse 4 Naltrexone 5 Naloxone 6 Clonidine 7 Bupropion 8 Psychiatric Medication 9 Other Replacement Medication	Z None	Z None	Z None

New Technology (X2C–XW0)

Within each section of ICD-10-PCS the characters have different meanings. The seven character meanings for the New Technology section are illustrated below through the procedure example of *Introduction of ceftazidime-avibactam anti-infective into peripheral vein, percutaneous approach.*

Section	Body System	Root Operation	Body Part	Approach	Device / Substance / Technology	Qualifier
New Technology	Anatomical Regions	Introduction	Peripheral Vein	Percutaneous	Ceftazidime-Avibactam Anti-infective	New Technology Group 1
X	W	0	3	3	2	1

Section (Character 1)

All New Technology procedure codes have a first character value of X.

Body System (Character 2)

For each body system the applicable body part character values will be available for procedure code construction.

Root Operations (Character 3)

The alphanumeric character value for root operations is placed in the third position. Listed below are the root operations applicable to the New Technology section with their associated meaning.

Character Value	Root Operation	Root Operation Definition
C	Extirpation	Taking or cutting out solid matter from a body part
0	Introduction	Putting in or on a therapeutic, diagnostic, nutritional, physiological, or prophylactic substance except blood or blood products
2	Monitoring	Determining the level of a physiological or physical function repetitively

Body Part (Character 4)

For each body system the applicable body part character values will be available for procedure code construction.

Approach (Character 5)

The approach is the technique used to reach the procedure site. Listed below are the approach character values for the New Technology section with the associated definitions.

Character Value	Approach	Approach Definition
0	Open	Cutting through the skin or mucous membrane and any other body layers necessary to expose the site of the procedure
3	Percutaneous	Entry, by puncture or minor incision, of instrumentation through the skin or mucous membrane and any other body layers necessary to reach the site of the procedure
4	Percutaneous Endoscopic	Entry, by puncture or minor incision, of instrumentation through the skin or mucous membrane and any other body layers necessary to reach and visualize the site of the procedure
X	External	Procedures performed directly on the skin or mucous membrane and procedures performed indirectly by the application of external force through the skin or mucous membrane

Device/Substance/Technology (Character 6)

The New Technology section created a place within ICD-10-PCS to include procedure codes for new services that utilize a specific new device, substance, or technology. Procedures in this section may be part of the Inpatient Prospective Payment System (IPPS) new technology add-on payment mechanism. Depending on the procedure performed there is either a device, substance, or new technology utilized.

Qualifier (Character 7)

The qualifier represents the category year in which the new device, substance, or technology was added to the coding system. In federal fiscal year 2016 (October 1, 2015) the first group of device, substance, and technology was added and therefore are labeled as New Technology Group 1.

New Technology Section Guidelines (section X)

D. New Technology Section

General Guidelines

D1. Section X codes are standalone codes. They are not supplemental codes. Section X codes fully represent the specific procedure described in the code title, and do not require any additional codes from other sections of ICD-10-PCS. When section X contains a code title which describes a specific new technology procedure, only that X code is reported for the procedure. There is no need to report a broader, non-specific code in another section of ICD-10-PCS.

Example: XW04321 Introduction of Ceftazidime-Avibactam Anti-infective into Central Vein, Percutaneous Approach, New Technology Group 1 can be coded to indicate that Ceftazidime-Avibactam Anti-infective was administered via a central vein. A separate code from table 3E0 in the Administration section of ICD-10-PCS is not coded in addition to this code.

New Technology Section Tables

New Technology Tables X2C–XW0

Section	X	New Technology
Body System	2	Cardiovascular System
Operation	C	**Extirpation:** Taking or cutting out solid matter from a body part

Body Part	Approach	Device / Substance / Technology	Qualifier
0 Coronary Artery, One Site **1** Coronary Artery, Two Sites **2** Coronary Artery, Three Sites **3** Coronary Artery, Four or More Sites	**3** Percutaneous	**6** Orbital Atherectomy Technology	**1** New Technology Group 1

Section	X	New Technology
Body System	R	Joints
Operation	2	**Monitoring:** Determining the level of a physiological or physical function repetitively over a period of time

Body Part	Approach	Device / Substance / Technology	Qualifier
G Knee Joint, Right **H** Knee Joint, Left	**0** Open	**2** Intraoperative Knee Replacement Sensor	**1** New Technology Group 1

Section	X	New Technology
Body System	W	Anatomical Regions
Operation	0	**Introduction:** Putting in or on a therapeutic, diagnostic, nutritional, physiological, or prophylactic substance except blood or blood products

Body Part	Approach	Device / Substance / Technology	Qualifier
3 Peripheral Vein **4** Central Vein	**3** Percutaneous	**2** Ceftazidime-Avibactam Anti-infective **3** Idarucizumab, Dabigatran Reversal Agent **4** Isavuconazole Anti-infective **5** Blinatumomab Antineoplastic Immunotherapy	**1** New Technology Group 1

Appendix A: Root Operations Definitions

Section 0 - Medical and Surgical — Character 3 - Root Operation

Alteration (0)	**Definition:** Modifying the anatomic structure of a body part without affecting the function of the body part **Explanation:** Principal purpose is to improve appearance **Includes/Examples:** Face lift, breast augmentation
Bypass (1)	**Definition:** Altering the route of passage of the contents of a tubular body part **Explanation:** Rerouting contents of a body part to a downstream area of the normal route, to a similar route and body part, or to an abnormal route and dissimilar body part. Includes one or more anastomoses, with or without the use of a device **Includes/Examples:** Coronary artery bypass, colostomy formation
Change (2)	**Definition:** Taking out or off a device from a body part and putting back an identical or similar device in or on the same body part without cutting or puncturing the skin or a mucous membrane **Explanation:** All CHANGE procedures are coded using the approach EXTERNAL **Includes/Examples:** Urinary catheter change, gastrostomy tube change
Control (3)	**Definition:** Stopping, or attempting to stop, postprocedural bleeding **Explanation:** The site of the bleeding is coded as an anatomical region and not to a specific body part **Includes/Examples:** Control of post-prostatectomy hemorrhage, control of post-tonsillectomy hemorrhage
Creation (4)	**Definition:** Making a new genital structure that does not take over the function of a body part **Explanation:** Used only for sex change operations **Includes/Examples:** Creation of vagina in a male, creation of penis in a female
Destruction (5)	**Definition:** Physical eradication of all or a portion of a body part by the direct use of energy, force, or a destructive agent **Explanation:** None of the body part is physically taken out **Includes/Examples:** Fulguration of rectal polyp, cautery of skin lesion
Detachment (6)	**Definition:** Cutting off all or a portion of the upper or lower extremities **Explanation:** The body part value is the site of the detachment, with a qualifier if applicable to further specify the level where the extremity was detached **Includes/Examples:** Below knee amputation, disarticulation of shoulder
Dilation (7)	**Definition:** Expanding an orifice or the lumen of a tubular body part **Explanation:** The orifice can be a natural orifice or an artificially created orifice. Accomplished by stretching a tubular body part using intraluminal pressure or by cutting part of the orifice or wall of the tubular body part **Includes/Examples:** Percutaneous transluminal angioplasty, pyloromyotomy
Division (8)	**Definition:** Cutting into a body part, without draining fluids and/or gases from the body part, in order to separate or transect a body part **Explanation:** All or a portion of the body part is separated into two or more portions **Includes/Examples:** Spinal cordotomy, osteotomy
Drainage (9)	**Definition:** Taking or letting out fluids and/or gases from a body part **Explanation:** The qualifier DIAGNOSTIC is used to identify drainage procedures that are biopsies **Includes/Examples:** Thoracentesis, incision and drainage
Excision (B)	**Definition:** Cutting out or off, without replacement, a portion of a body part **Explanation:** The qualifier DIAGNOSTIC is used to identify excision procedures that are biopsies **Includes/Examples:** Partial nephrectomy, liver biopsy
Extirpation (C)	**Definition:** Taking or cutting out solid matter from a body part **Explanation:** The solid matter may be an abnormal byproduct of a biological function or a foreign body; it may be imbedded in a body part or in the lumen of a tubular body part. The solid matter may or may not have been previously broken into pieces **Includes/Examples:** Thrombectomy, choledocholithotomy
Extraction (D)	**Definition:** Pulling or stripping out or off all or a portion of a body part by the use of force **Explanation:** The qualifier DIAGNOSTIC is used to identify extraction procedures that are biopsies **Includes/Examples:** Dilation and curettage, vein stripping
Fragmentation (F)	**Definition:** Breaking solid matter in a body part into pieces **Explanation:** Physical force (e.g., manual, ultrasonic) applied directly or indirectly is used to break the solid matter into pieces. The solid matter may be an abnormal byproduct of a biological function or a foreign body. The pieces of solid matter are not taken out **Includes/Examples:** Extracorporeal shockwave lithotripsy, transurethral lithotripsy
Fusion (G)	**Definition:** Joining together portions of an articular body part rendering the articular body part immobile **Explanation:** The body part is joined together by fixation device, bone graft, or other means **Includes/Examples:** Spinal fusion, ankle arthrodesis
Insertion (H)	**Definition:** Putting in a nonbiological appliance that monitors, assists, performs, or prevents a physiological function but does not physically take the place of a body part **Includes/Examples:** Insertion of radioactive implant, insertion of central venous catheter

Continued →

Inspection (J)	**Definition:** Visually and/or manually exploring a body part **Explanation:** Visual exploration may be performed with or without optical instrumentation. Manual exploration may be performed directly or through intervening body layers **Includes/Examples:** Diagnostic arthroscopy, exploratory laparotomy
Map (K)	**Definition:** Locating the route of passage of electrical impulses and/or locating functional areas in a body part **Explanation:** Applicable only to the cardiac conduction mechanism and the central nervous system **Includes/Examples:** Cardiac mapping, cortical mapping
Occlusion (L)	**Definition:** Completely closing an orifice or the lumen of a tubular body part **Explanation:** The orifice can be a natural orifice or an artificially created orifice **Includes/Examples:** Fallopian tube ligation, ligation of inferior vena cava
Reattachment (M)	**Definition:** Putting back in or on all or a portion of a separated body part to its normal location or other suitable location **Explanation:** Vascular circulation and nervous pathways may or may not be reestablished **Includes/Examples:** Reattachment of hand, reattachment of avulsed kidney
Release (N)	**Definition:** Freeing a body part from an abnormal physical constraint by cutting or by the use of force **Explanation:** Some of the restraining tissue may be taken out but none of the body part is taken out **Includes/Examples:** Adhesiolysis, carpal tunnel release
Removal (P)	**Definition:** Taking out or off a device from a body part **Explanation:** If a device is taken out and a similar device put in without cutting or puncturing the skin or mucous membrane, the procedure is coded to the root operation CHANGE. Otherwise, the procedure for taking out a device is coded to the root operation REMOVAL **Includes/Examples:** Drainage tube removal, cardiac pacemaker removal
Repair (Q)	**Definition:** Restoring, to the extent possible, a body part to its normal anatomic structure and function **Explanation:** Used only when the method to accomplish the repair is not one of the other root operations **Includes/Examples:** Colostomy takedown, suture of laceration
Replacement (R)	**Definition:** Putting in or on biological or synthetic material that physically takes the place and/or function of all or a portion of a body part **Explanation:** The body part may have been taken out or replaced, or may be taken out, physically eradicated, or rendered nonfunctional during the Replacement procedure. A Removal procedure is coded for taking out the device used in a previous replacement procedure **Includes/Examples:** Total hip replacement, bone graft, free skin graft
Reposition (S)	**Definition:** Moving to its normal location, or other suitable location, all or a portion of a body part **Explanation:** The body part is moved to a new location from an abnormal location, or from a normal location where it is not functioning correctly. The body part may or may not be cut out or off to be moved to the new location **Includes/Examples:** Reposition of undescended testicle, fracture reduction
Resection (T)	**Definition:** Cutting out or off, without replacement, all of a body part **Includes/Examples:** Total nephrectomy, total lobectomy of lung
Restriction (V)	**Definition:** Partially closing an orifice or the lumen of a tubular body part **Explanation:** The orifice can be a natural orifice or an artificially created orifice **Includes/Examples:** Esophagogastric fundoplication, cervical cerclage
Revision (W)	**Definition:** Correcting, to the extent possible, a portion of a malfunctioning device or the position of a displaced device **Explanation:** Revision can include correcting a malfunctioning or displaced device by taking out or putting in components of the device such as a screw or pin **Includes/Examples:** Adjustment of position of pacemaker lead, recementing of hip prosthesis
Supplement (U)	**Definition:** Putting in or on biological or synthetic material that physically reinforces and/or augments the function of a portion of a body part **Explanation:** The biological material is non-living, or is living and from the same individual. The body part may have been previously replaced, and the Supplement procedure is performed to physically reinforce and/or augment the function of the replaced body part **Includes/Examples:** Herniorrhaphy using mesh, free nerve graft, mitral valve ring annuloplasty, put a new acetabular liner in a previous hip replacement
Transfer (X)	**Definition:** Moving, without taking out, all or a portion of a body part to another location to take over the function of all or a portion of a body part **Explanation:** The body part transferred remains connected to its vascular and nervous supply **Includes/Examples:** Tendon transfer, skin pedicle flap transfer
Transplantation (Y)	**Definition:** Putting in or on all or a portion of a living body part taken from another individual or animal to physically take the place and/or function of all or a portion of a similar body part **Explanation:** The native body part may or may not be taken out, and the transplanted body part may take over all or a portion of its function **Includes/Examples:** Kidney transplant, heart transplant

Section 1 - Obstetrics — Character 3 - Root Operations Unique to Obstetrics

Abortion (A)	**Definition:** Artificially terminating a pregnancy **Explanation:** Subdivided according to whether an additional device such as a laminaria or abortifacient is used, or whether the abortion was performed by mechanical means **Includes/Example:** Transvaginal abortion using vacuum aspiration technique

Continued →

Section 1 - Obstetrics — Character 3 - Root Operations Unique to Obstetrics

Delivery (E)	**Definition:** Assisting the passage of the products of conception from the genital canal **Explanation:** Applies only to manually-assisted, vaginal delivery **Includes/Example:** Manually-assisted delivery

Section 2 - Placement — Character 3 - Root Operation

Change (0)	**Definition:** Taking out or off a device from a body part and putting back an identical or similar device in or on the same body part without cutting or puncturing the skin or a mucous membrane **Includes/Example:** Change of vaginal packing
Compression (1)	**Definition:** Putting pressure on a body region **Includes/Example:** Placement of pressure dressing on abdominal wall
Dressing (2)	**Definition:** Putting material on a body region for protection **Includes/Example:** Application of sterile dressing to head wound
Immobilization (3)	**Definition:** Limiting or preventing motion of a body region **Includes/Example:** Placement of splint on left finger
Packing (4)	**Definition:** Putting material in a body region or orifice **Includes/Example:** Placement of nasal packing
Removal (5)	**Definition:** Taking out or off a device from a body part **Includes/Example:** Removal of cast from right lower leg
Traction (6)	**Definition:** Exerting a pulling force on a body region in a distal direction **Includes/Example:** Lumbar traction using motorized split-traction table

Section 3 - Administration — Character 3 - Root Operation

Introduction (0)	**Definition:** Putting in or on a therapeutic, diagnostic, nutritional, physiological, or prophylactic substance except blood or blood products **Includes/Example:** Nerve block injection to median nerve
Irrigation (1)	**Definition:** Putting in or on a cleansing substance **Includes/Example:** Flushing of eye
Transfusion (2)	**Definition:** Putting in blood or blood products **Includes/Example:** Transfusion of cell saver red cells into central venous line

Section 4 - Measurement and Monitoring — Character 3 - Root Operation

Measurement (0)	**Definition:** Determining the level of a physiological or physical function at a point in time **Includes/Example:** External electrocardiogram (EKG), single reading
Monitoring (1)	**Definition:** Determining the level of a physiological or physical function repetitively over a period of time **Includes/Example:** Urinary pressure monitoring

Section 5 - Extracorporeal Assistance and Performance — Character 3 - Root Operation

Assistance (0)	**Definition:** Taking over a portion of a physiological function by extracorporeal means **Includes/Example:** Hyperbaric oxygenation of wound
Performance (1)	**Definition:** Completely taking over a physiological function by extracorporeal means **Includes/Example:** Cardiopulmonary bypass in conjunction with CABG
Restoration (2)	**Definition:** Returning, or attempting to return, a physiological function to its original state by extracorporeal means. **Includes/Example:** Attempted cardiac defibrillation, unsuccessful

Section 6 - Extracorporeal Therapies — Character 3 - Root Operation

Atmospheric Control (0)	**Definition:** Extracorporeal control of atmospheric pressure and composition **Includes/Example:** Atmospheric control, single treatment
Decompression (1)	**Definition:** Extracorporeal elimination of undissolved gas from body fluids **Includes/Example:** Hyperbaric decompression treatment, single
Electromagnetic Therapy (2)	**Definition:** Extracorporeal treatment by electromagnetic rays **Includes/Example:** Electromagnetic therapy, central nervous, multiple treatments
Hyperthermia (3)	**Definition:** Extracorporeal raising of body temperature **Includes/Example:** Hyperthermia, single treatment

Continued →

Section 6 - Extracorporeal Therapies — Character 3 - Root Operation

Hypothermia (4)	**Definition:** Extracorporeal lowering of body temperature **Includes/Example:** Whole body hypothermia treatment for temperature imbalances, series treatment
Pheresis (5)	**Definition:** Extracorporeal separation of blood products **Includes/Example:** Therapeutic leukopheresis, single treatment
Phototherapy (6)	**Definition:** Extracorporeal treatment by light rays **Includes/Example:** Phototherapy of circulatory system, series treatment
Shock Wave Therapy (7)	**Definition:** Extracorporeal treatment by shock waves **Includes/Example:** Shock wave therapy, musculoskeletal, single treatment
Ultrasound Therapy (8)	**Definition:** Extracorporeal treatment by ultrasound **Includes/Example:** Ultrasound therapy of the heart, single treatment
Ultraviolet Light Therapy (9)	**Definition:** Extracorporeal treatment by ultraviolet light **Includes/Example:** Ultraviolet light phototherapy, series treatment

Section 7 - Osteopathic — Character 3 - Root Operation

Treatment (0)	**Definition:** Manual treatment to eliminate or alleviate somatic dysfunction and related disorders **Includes/Example:** Fascial release of abdomen, osteopathic treatment

Section 8 - Other Procedures — Character 3 - Root Operation

Other Procedures (0)	**Definition:** Methodologies which attempt to remediate or cure a disorder or disease **Includes/Example:** Acupuncture

Section 9 - Chiropractic — Character 3 - Root Operation

Manipulation (B)	**Definition:** Manual procedure that involves a directed thrust to move a joint past the physiological range of motion, without exceeding the anatomical limit **Includes/Example:** Chiropractic treatment of cervical spine, short lever specific contact

Section X - New Technology — Character 3 - Root Operation

Extirpation	**Definition:** Taking or cutting out solid matter from a body part **Explanation:** The solid matter may be an abnormal by product of a biological function or a foreign body; it may be imbedded in a body part or in the lumen of a tubular body part. The solid matter may or may not have been previously broken into pieces **Includes/Example:** Thrombectomy, choledocholithotomy
Introduction	**Definition:** Putting in or on a therapeutic, diagnostic, nutritional, physiological, or prophylactic substance except blood or blood products
Monitoring	**Definition:** Determining the level of a physiological or physical function repetitively over a period of time

Appendix B: Type and Qualifier Definitions

Section B - Imaging — Character 3 - Root Type

Computerized Tomography (CT Scan)	**Definition:** Computer reformatted digital display of multiplanar images developed from the capture of multiple exposures of external ionizing radiation
Fluoroscopy	**Definition:** Single plane or bi-plane real time display of an image developed from the capture of external ionizing radiation on a fluorescent screen. The image may also be stored by either digital or analog means
Magnetic Resonance Imaging (MRI)	**Definition:** Computer reformatted digital display of multiplanar images developed from the capture of radiofrequency signals emitted by nuclei in a body site excited within a magnetic field
Plain Radiography	**Definition:** Planar display of an image developed from the capture of external ionizing radiation on photographic or photoconductive plate
Ultrasonography	**Definition:** Real time display of images of anatomy or flow information developed from the capture of reflected and attenuated high frequency sound waves

Section C - Nuclear Medicine — Character 3 - Root Type

Nonimaging Nuclear Medicine Assay	**Definition:** Introduction of radioactive materials into the body for the study of body fluids and blood elements, by the detection of radioactive emissions

Continued →

Section C - Nuclear Medicine — Character 3 - Root Type

Nonimaging Nuclear Medicine Probe	**Definition:** Introduction of radioactive materials into the body for the study of distribution and fate of certain substances by the detection of radioactive emissions; or, alternatively, measurement of absorption of radioactive emissions from an external source
Nonimaging Nuclear Medicine Uptake	**Definition:** Introduction of radioactive materials into the body for measurements of organ function, from the detection of radioactive emissions
Planar Nuclear Medicine Imaging	**Definition:** Introduction of radioactive materials into the body for single plane display of images developed from the capture of radioactive emissions
Positron Emission Tomographic (PET) Imaging	**Definition:** Introduction of radioactive materials into the body for three dimensional display of images developed from the simultaneous capture, 180 degrees apart, of radioactive emissions
Systemic Nuclear Medicine Therapy	**Definition:** Introduction of unsealed radioactive materials into the body for treatment
Tomographic (Tomo) Nuclear Medicine Imaging	**Definition:** Introduction of radioactive materials into the body for three dimensional display of images developed from the capture of radioactive emissions

Section F - Physical Rehabilitation and Diagnostic Audiology — Character 3 - Root Type

Activities of Daily Living Assessment	**Definition:** Measurement of functional level for activities of daily living
Activities of Daily Living Treatment	**Definition:** Exercise or activities to facilitate functional competence for activities of daily living
Caregiver Training	**Definition:** Training in activities to support patient's optimal level of function
Cochlear Implant Treatment	**Definition:** Application of techniques to improve the communication abilities of individuals with cochlear implant
Device Fitting	**Definition:** Fitting of a device designed to facilitate or support achievement of a higher level of function
Hearing Aid Assessment	**Definition:** Measurement of the appropriateness and/or effectiveness of a hearing device
Hearing Assessment	**Definition:** Measurement of hearing and related functions
Hearing Treatment	**Definition:** Application of techniques to improve, augment, or compensate for hearing and related functional impairment
Motor and/or Nerve Function Assessment	**Definition:** Measurement of motor, nerve, and related functions
Motor Treatment	**Definition:** Exercise or activities to increase or facilitate motor function
Speech Assessment	**Definition:** Measurement of speech and related functions
Speech Treatment	**Definition:** Application of techniques to improve, augment, or compensate for speech and related functional impairment
Vestibular Assessment	**Definition:** Measurement of the vestibular system and related functions
Vestibular Treatment	**Definition:** Application of techniques to improve, augment, or compensate for vestibular and related functional impairment

Section F - Physical Rehabilitation and Diagnostic Audiology — Character 5 - Type Qualifier

Acoustic Reflex Decay	**Definition:** Measures reduction in size/strength of acoustic reflex over time **Includes/Examples:** Includes site of lesion test
Acoustic Reflex Patterns	**Definition:** Defines site of lesion based upon presence/absence of acoustic reflexes with ipsilateral vs. contralateral stimulation
Acoustic Reflex Threshold	**Definition:** Determines minimal intensity that acoustic reflex occurs with ipsilateral and/or contralateral stimulation
Aerobic Capacity and Endurance	**Definition:** Measures autonomic responses to positional changes; perceived exertion, dyspnea or angina during activity; performance during exercise protocols; standard vital signs; and blood gas analysis or oxygen consumption
Alternate Binaural or Monaural Loudness Balance	**Definition:** Determines auditory stimulus parameter that yields the same objective sensation **Includes/Examples:** Sound intensities that yield same loudness perception
Anthropometric Characteristics	**Definition:** Measures edema, body fat composition, height, weight, length and girth
Aphasia (Assessment)	**Definition:** Measures expressive and receptive speech and language function including reading and writing
Aphasia (Treatment)	**Definition:** Applying techniques to improve, augment, or compensate for receptive/ expressive language impairments
Articulation/Phonology (Assessment)	**Definition:** Measures speech production
Articulation/Phonology (Treatment)	**Definition:** Applying techniques to correct, improve, or compensate for speech productive impairment
Assistive Listening Device	**Definition:** Assists in use of effective and appropriate assistive listening device/system
Assistive Listening System/Device Selection	**Definition:** Measures the effectiveness and appropriateness of assistive listening systems/devices
Assistive, Adaptive, Supportive or Protective Devices	**Explanation:** Devices to facilitate or support achievement of a higher level of function in wheelchair mobility; bed mobility; transfer or ambulation ability; bath and showering ability; dressing; grooming; personal hygiene; play or leisure

Continued →

Auditory Evoked Potentials	**Definition:** Measures electric responses produced by the VIIIth cranial nerve and brainstem following auditory stimulation
Auditory Processing (Assessment)	**Definition:** Evaluates ability to receive and process auditory information and comprehension of spoken language
Auditory Processing (Treatment)	**Definition:** Applying techniques to improve the receiving and processing of auditory information and comprehension of spoken language
Augmentative/Alternative Communication System (Assessment)	**Definition:** Determines the appropriateness of aids, techniques, symbols, and/or strategies to augment or replace speech and enhance communication **Includes/Examples:** Includes the use of telephones, writing equipment, emergency equipment, and TDD
Augmentative/Alternative Communication System (Treatment)	**Includes/Examples:** Includes augmentative communication devices and aids
Aural Rehabilitation	**Definition:** Applying techniques to improve the communication abilities associated with hearing loss
Aural Rehabilitation Status	**Definition:** Measures impact of a hearing loss including evaluation of receptive and expressive communication skills
Bathing/Showering	**Includes/Examples:** Includes obtaining and using supplies; soaping, rinsing, and drying body parts; maintaining bathing position; and transferring to and from bathing positions
Bathing/Showering Techniques	**Definition:** Activities to facilitate obtaining and using supplies, soaping, rinsing and drying body parts, maintaining bathing position, and transferring to and from bathing positions
Bed Mobility (Assessment)	**Definition:** Transitional movement within bed
Bed Mobility (Treatment)	**Definition:** Exercise or activities to facilitate transitional movements within bed
Bedside Swallowing and Oral Function	**Includes/Examples:** Bedside swallowing includes assessment of sucking, masticating, coughing, and swallowing. Oral function includes assessment of musculature for controlled movements, structures and functions to determine coordination and phonation
Bekesy Audiometry	**Definition:** Uses an instrument that provides a choice of discrete or continuously varying pure tones; choice of pulsed or continuous signal
Binaural Electroacoustic Hearing Aid Check	**Definition:** Determines mechanical and electroacoustic function of bilateral hearing aids using hearing aid test box
Binaural Hearing Aid (Assessment)	**Definition:** Measures the candidacy, effectiveness, and appropriateness of a hearing aids **Explanation:** Measures bilateral fit
Binaural Hearing Aid (Treatment)	**Explanation:** Assists in achieving maximum understanding and performance
Bithermal, Binaural Caloric Irrigation	**Definition:** Measures the rhythmic eye movements stimulated by changing the temperature of the vestibular system
Bithermal, Monaural Caloric Irrigation	**Definition:** Measures the rhythmic eye movements stimulated by changing the temperature of the vestibular system in one ear
Brief Tone Stimuli	**Definition:** Measures specific central auditory process
Cerumen Management	**Definition:** Includes examination of external auditory canal and tympanic membrane and removal of cerumen from external ear canal
Cochlear Implant	**Definition:** Measures candidacy for cochlear implant
Cochlear Implant Rehabilitation	**Definition:** Applying techniques to improve the communication abilities of individuals with cochlear implant; includes programming the device, providing patients/families with information
Communicative/Cognitive Integration Skills (Assessment)	**Definition:** Measures ability to use higher cortical functions **Includes/Examples:** Includes orientation, recognition, attention span, initiation and termination of activity, memory, sequencing, categorizing, concept formation, spatial operations, judgment, problem solving, generalization and pragmatic communication
Communicative/Cognitive Integration Skills (Treatment)	**Definition:** Activities to facilitate the use of higher cortical functions **Includes/Examples:** Includes level of arousal, orientation, recognition, attention span, initiation and termination of activity, memory sequencing, judgment and problem solving, learning and generalization, and pragmatic communication
Computerized Dynamic Posturography	**Definition:** Measures the status of the peripheral and central vestibular system and the sensory/motor component of balance; evaluates the efficacy of vestibular rehabilitation
Conditioned Play Audiometry	**Definition:** Behavioral measures using nonspeech and speech stimuli to obtain frequency-specific and ear-specific information on auditory status from the patient **Explanation:** Obtains speech reception threshold by having patient point to pictures of spondaic words
Coordination/Dexterity (Assessment)	**Definition:** Measures large and small muscle groups for controlled goal-directed movements **Explanation:** Dexterity includes object manipulation

Continued →

Coordination/Dexterity (Treatment)	**Definition:** Exercise or activities to facilitate gross coordination and fine coordination
Cranial Nerve Integrity	**Definition:** Measures cranial nerve sensory and motor functions, including tastes, smell and facial expression
Dichotic Stimuli	**Definition:** Measures specific central auditory process
Distorted Speech	**Definition:** Measures specific central auditory process
Dix-Hallpike Dynamic	**Definition:** Measures nystagmus following Dix-Hallpike maneuver
Dressing	**Includes/Examples:** Includes selecting clothing and accessories, obtaining clothing from storage, dressing and, fastening and adjusting clothing and shoes, and applying and removing personal devices, prosthesis or orthosis
Dressing Techniques	**Definition:** Activities to facilitate selecting clothing and accessories, dressing and undressing, adjusting clothing and shoes, applying and removing devices, prostheses or orthoses
Dynamic Orthosis	**Includes/Examples:** Includes customized and prefabricated splints, inhibitory casts, spinal and other braces, and protective devices; allows motion through transfer of movement from other body parts or by use of outside forces
Ear Canal Probe Microphone	**Definition:** Real ear measures
Ear Protector Attentuation	**Definition:** Measures ear protector fit and effectiveness
Electrocochleography	**Definition:** Measures the VIIIth cranial nerve action potential
Environmental, Home and Work Barriers	**Definition:** Measures current and potential barriers to optimal function, including safety hazards, access problems and home or office design
Ergonomics and Body Mechanics	**Definition:** Ergonomic measurement of job tasks, work hardening or work conditioning needs; functional capacity; and body mechanics
Eustachian Tube Function	**Definition:** Measures eustachian tube function and patency of eustachian tube
Evoked Otoacoustic Emissions, Diagnostic	**Definition:** Measures auditory evoked potentials in a diagnostic format
Evoked Otoacoustic Emissions, Screening	**Definition:** Measures auditory evoked potentials in a screening format
Facial Nerve Function	**Definition:** Measures electrical activity of the VIIth cranial nerve (facial nerve)
Feeding/Eating (Assessment)	**Includes/Examples:** Includes setting up food, selecting and using utensils and tableware, bringing food or drink to mouth, cleaning face, hands, and clothing, and management of alternative methods of nourishment
Feeding/Eating (Treatment)	**Definition:** Exercise or activities to facilitate setting up food, selecting and using utensils and tableware, bringing food or drink to mouth, cleaning face, hands, and clothing, and management of alternative methods of nourishment
Filtered Speech	**Definition:** Uses high or low pass filtered speech stimuli to assess central auditory processing disorders, site of lesion testing
Fluency (Assessment)	**Definition:** Measures speech fluency or stuttering
Fluency (Treatment)	**Definition:** Applying techniques to improve and augment fluent speech
Gait and/or Balance	**Definition:** Measures biomechanical, arthrokinematic and other spatial and temporal characteristics of gait and balance
Gait Training/Functional Ambulation	**Definition:** Exercise or activities to facilitate ambulation on a variety of surfaces and in a variety of environments
Grooming/Personal Hygiene (Assessment)	**Includes/Examples:** Includes ability to obtain and use supplies in a sequential fashion, general grooming, oral hygiene, toilet hygiene, personal care devices, including care for artificial airways
Grooming/Personal Hygiene (Treatment)	**Definition:** Activities to facilitate obtaining and using supplies in a sequential fashion: general grooming, oral hygiene, toilet hygiene, cleaning body, and personal care devices, including artificial airways
Hearing and Related Disorders Counseling	**Definition:** Provides patients/families/caregivers with information, support, referrals to facilitate recovery from a communication disorder **Includes/Examples:** Includes strategies for psychosocial adjustment to hearing loss for clients and families/caregivers
Hearing and Related Disorders Prevention	**Definition:** Provides patients/families/caregivers with information and support to prevent communication disorders
Hearing Screening	**Definition:** Pass/refer measures designed to identify need for further audiologic assessment
Home Management (Assessment)	**Definition:** Obtaining and maintaining personal and household possessions and environment **Includes/Examples:** Includes clothing care, cleaning, meal preparation and cleanup, shopping, money management, household maintenance, safety procedures, and childcare/parenting

Continued →

Home Management (Treatment)	**Definition:** Activities to facilitate obtaining and maintaining personal household possessions and environment **Includes/Examples:** Includes clothing care, cleaning, meal preparation and clean-up, shopping, money management, household maintenance, safety procedures, childcare/parenting
Instrumental Swallowing and Oral Function	**Definition:** Measures swallowing function using instrumental diagnostic procedures **Explanation:** Methods include videofluoroscopy, ultrasound, manometry, endoscopy
Integumentary Integrity	**Includes/Examples:** Includes burns, skin conditions, ecchymosis, bleeding, blisters, scar tissue, wounds and other traumas, tissue mobility, turgor and texture
Manual Therapy Techniques	**Definition:** Techniques in which the therapist uses his/her hands to administer skilled movements **Includes/Examples:** Includes connective tissue massage, joint mobilization and manipulation, manual lymph drainage, manual traction, soft tissue mobilization and manipulation
Masking Patterns	**Definition:** Measures central auditory processing status
Monaural Electroacoustic Hearing Aid Check	**Definition:** Determines mechanical and electroacoustic function of one hearing aid using hearing aid test box
Monaural Hearing Aid (Assessment)	**Definition:** Measures the candidacy, effectiveness, and appropriateness of a hearing aid **Explanation:** Measures unilateral fit
Monaural Hearing Aid (Treatment)	**Explanation:** Assists in achieving maximum understanding and performance
Motor Function (Assessment)	**Definition:** Measures the body's functional and versatile movement patterns **Includes/Examples:** Includes motor assessment scales, analysis of head, trunk and limb movement, and assessment of motor learning
Motor Function (Treatment)	**Definition:** Exercise or activities to facilitate crossing midline, laterality, bilateral integration, praxis, neuromuscular relaxation, inhibition, facilitation, motor function and motor learning
Motor Speech (Assessment)	**Definition:** Measures neurological motor aspects of speech production
Motor Speech (Treatment)	**Definition:** Applying techniques to improve and augment the impaired neurological motor aspects of speech production
Muscle Performance (Assessment)	**Definition:** Measures muscle strength, power and endurance using manual testing, dynamometry or computer-assisted electromechanical muscle test; functional muscle strength, power and endurance; muscle pain, tone, or soreness; or pelvic-floor musculature **Explanation:** Muscle endurance refers to the ability to contract a muscle repeatedly over time
Muscle Performance (Treatment)	**Definition:** Exercise or activities to increase the capacity of a muscle to do work in terms of strength, power, and/or endurance **Explanation:** Muscle strength is the force exerted to overcome resistance in one maximal effort. Muscle power is work produced per unit of time, or the product of strength and speed. Muscle endurance is the ability to contract a muscle repeatedly over time
Neuromotor Development	**Definition:** Measures motor development, righting and equilibrium reactions, and reflex and equilibrium reactions
Neurophysiologic Intraoperative	**Definition:** Monitors neural status during surgery
Non-invasive Instrumental Status	**Definition:** Instrumental measures of oral, nasal, vocal, and velopharyngeal functions as they pertain to speech production
Nonspoken Language (Assessment)	**Definition:** Measures nonspoken language (print, sign, symbols) for communication
Nonspoken Language (Treatment)	**Definition:** Applying techniques that improve, augment, or compensate spoken communication
Oral Peripheral Mechanism	**Definition:** Structural measures of face, jaw, lips, tongue, teeth, hard and soft palate, pharynx as related to speech production
Orofacial Myofunctional (Assessment)	**Definition:** Measures orofacial myofunctional patterns for speech and related functions
Orofacial Myofunctional (Treatment)	**Definition:** Applying techniques to improve, alter, or augment impaired orofacial myofunctional patterns and related speech production errors
Oscillating Tracking	**Definition:** Measures ability to visually track
Pain	**Definition:** Measures muscle soreness, pain and soreness with joint movement, and pain perception **Includes/Examples:** Includes questionnaires, graphs, symptom magnification scales or visual analog scales
Perceptual Processing (Assessment)	**Definition:** Measures stereognosis, kinesthesia, body schema, right-left discrimination, form constancy, position in space, visual closure, figure-ground, depth perception, spatial relations and topographical orientation

Continued →

Perceptual Processing (Treatment)	**Definition:** Exercise and activities to facilitate perceptual processing **Explanation:** Includes stereognosis, kinesthesia, body schema, right-left discrimination, form constancy, position in space, visual closure, figure-ground, depth perception, spatial relations, and topographical orientation **Includes/Examples:** Includes stereognosis, kinesthesia, body schema, right-left discrimination, form constancy, position in space, visual closure, figure-ground, depth perception, spatial relations, and topographical orientation
Performance Intensity Phonetically Balanced Speech Discrimination	**Definition:** Measures word recognition over varying intensity levels
Postural Control	**Definition:** Exercise or activities to increase postural alignment and control
Prosthesis	**Explanation:** Artificial substitutes for missing body parts that augment performance or function
Psychosocial Skills (Assessment)	**Definition:** The ability to interact in society and to process emotions **Includes/Examples:** Includes psychological (values, interests, self-concept); social (role performance, social conduct, interpersonal skills, self expression); self-management (coping skills, time management, self-control)
Psychosocial Skills (Treatment)	**Definition:** The ability to interact in society and to process emotions **Includes/Examples:** Includes psychological (values, interests, self-concept); social (role performance, social conduct, interpersonal skills, self expression); self-management (coping skills, time management, self-control)
Pure Tone Audiometry, Air	**Definition:** Air-conduction pure tone threshold measures with appropriate masking
Pure Tone Audiometry, Air and Bone	**Definition:** Air-conduction and bone-conduction pure tone threshold measures with appropriate masking
Pure Tone Stenger	**Definition:** Measures unilateral nonorganic hearing loss based on simultaneous presentation of pure tones of differing volume
Range of Motion and Joint Integrity	**Definition:** Measures quantity, quality, grade, and classification of joint movement and/or mobility **Explanation:** Range of Motion is the space, distance or angle through which movement occurs at a joint or series of joints. Joint integrity is the conformance of joints to expected anatomic, biomechanical and kinematic norms
Range of Motion and Joint Mobility	**Definition:** Exercise or activities to increase muscle length and joint mobility
Receptive/Expressive Language (Assessment)	**Definition:** Measures receptive and expressive language
Receptive/Expressive Language (Treatment)	**Definition:** Applying techniques tot improve and augment receptive/expressive language
Reflex Integrity	**Definition:** Measures the presence, absence, or exaggeration of developmentally appropriate, pathologic or normal reflexes
Select Picture Audiometry	**Definition:** Establishes hearing threshold levels for speech using pictures
Sensorineural Acuity Level	**Definition:** Measures sensorineural acuity masking presented via bone conduction
Sensory Aids	**Definition:** Determines the appropriateness of a sensory prosthetic device, other than a hearing aid or assistive listening system/device
Sensory Awareness/Processing/Integrity	**Includes/Examples:** Includes light touch, pressure, temperature, pain, sharp/dull, proprioception, vestibular, visual, auditory, gustatory, and olfactory
Short Increment Sensitivity Index	**Definition:** Measures the ear's ability to detect small intensity changes; site of lesion test requiring a behavioral response
Sinusoidal Vertical Axis Rotational	**Definition:** Measures nystagmus following rotation
Somatosensory Evoked Potentials	**Definition:** Measures neural activity from sites throughout the body
Speech and/or Language Screening	**Definition:** Identifies need for further speech and/or language evaluation
Speech Threshold	**Definition:** Measures minimal intensity needed to repeat spondaic words
Speech-Language Pathology and Related Disorders Counseling	**Definition:** Provides patients/families with information, support, referrals to facilitate recovery from a communication disorder
Speech-Language Pathology and Related Disorders Prevention	**Definition:** Applying techniques to avoid or minimize onset and/or development of a communication disorder
Speech/Word Recognition	**Definition:** Measures ability to repeat/identify single syllable words; scores given as a percentage; includes word recognition/speech discrimination
Staggered Spondaic Word	**Definition:** Measures central auditory processing site of lesion based upon dichotic presentation of spondaic words
Static Orthosis	**Includes/Examples:** Includes customized and prefabricated splints, inhibitory casts, spinal and other braces, and protective devices; has no moving parts, maintains joint(s) in desired position

Continued →

Appendix B

Stenger	**Definition:** Measures unilateral nonorganic hearing loss based on simultaneous presentation of signals of differing volume
Swallowing Dysfunction	**Definition:** Activities to improve swallowing function in coordination with respiratory function **Includes/Examples:** Includes function and coordination of sucking, mastication, coughing, swallowing
Synthetic Sentence Identification	**Definition:** Measures central auditory dysfunction using identification of third order approximations of sentences and competing messages
Temporal Ordering of Stimuli	**Definition:** Measures specific central auditory process
Therapeutic Exercise	**Definition:** Exercise or activities to facilitate sensory awareness, sensory processing, sensory integration, balance training, conditioning, reconditioning **Includes/Examples:** Includes developmental activities, breathing exercises, aerobic endurance activities, aquatic exercises, stretching and ventilatory muscle training
Tinnitus Masker (Assessment)	**Definition:** Determines candidacy for tinnitus masker
Tinnitus Masker (Treatment)	**Explanation:** Used to verify physical fit, acoustic appropriateness, and benefit; assists in achieving maximum benefit
Tone Decay	**Definition:** Measures decrease in hearing sensitivity to a tone; site of lesion test requiring a behavioral response
Transfer	**Definition:** Transitional movement from one surface to another
Transfer Training	**Definition:** Exercise or activities to facilitate movement from one surface to another
Tympanometry	**Definition:** Measures the integrity of the middle ear; measures ease at which sound flows through the tympanic membrane while air pressure against the membrane is varied
Unithermal Binaural Screen	**Definition:** Measures the rhythmic eye movements stimulated by changing the temperature of the vestibular system in both ears using warm water, screening format
Ventilation, Respiration and Circulation	**Definition:** Measures ventilatory muscle strength, power and endurance, pulmonary function and ventilatory mechanics **Includes/Examples:** Includes ability to clear airway, activities that aggravate or relieve edema, pain, dyspnea or other symptoms, chest wall mobility, cardiopulmonary response to performance of ADL and IAD, cough and sputum, standard vital signs
Vestibular	**Definition:** Applying techniques to compensate for balance disorders; includes habituation, exercise therapy, and balance retraining
Visual Motor Integration (Assessment)	**Definition:** Coordinating the interaction of information from the eyes with body movement during activity
Visual Motor Integration (Treatment)	**Definition:** Exercise or activities to facilitate coordinating the interaction of information from eyes with body movement during activity
Visual Reinforcement Audiometry	**Definition:** Behavioral measures using nonspeech and speech stimuli to obtain frequency/ear-specific information on auditory status **Includes/Examples:** Includes a conditioned response of looking toward a visual reinforcer (e.g., lights, animated toy) every time auditory stimuli are heard
Vocational Activities and Functional Community or Work Reintegration Skills (Assessment)	**Definition:** Measures environmental, home, work (job/school/play) barriers that keep patients from functioning optimally in their environment **Includes/Examples:** Includes assessment of vocational skill and interests, environment of work (job/school/play), injury potential and injury prevention or reduction, ergonomic stressors, transportation skills, and ability to access and use community resources
Vocational Activities and Functional Community or Work Reintegration Skills (Treatment)	**Definition:** Activities to facilitate vocational exploration, body mechanics training, job acquisition, and environmental or work (job/school/play) task adaptation **Includes/Examples:** Includes injury prevention and reduction, ergonomic stressor reduction, job coaching and simulation, work hardening and conditioning, driving training, transportation skills, and use of community resources
Voice (Assessment)	**Definition:** Measures vocal structure, function and production
Voice (Treatment)	**Definition:** Applying techniques to improve voice and vocal function
Voice Prosthetic (Assessment)	**Definition:** Determines the appropriateness of voice prosthetic/adaptive device to enhance or facilitate communication
Voice Prosthetic (Treatment)	**Includes/Examples:** Includes electrolarynx, and other assistive, adaptive, supportive devices
Wheelchair Mobility (Assessment)	**Definition:** Measures fit and functional abilities within wheelchair in a variety of environments
Wheelchair Mobility (Treatment)	**Definition:** Management, maintenance and controlled operation of a wheelchair, scooter or other device, in and on a variety of surfaces and environments
Wound Management	**Includes/Examples:** Includes non-selective and selective debridement (enzymes, autolysis, sharp debridement), dressings (wound coverings, hydrogel, vacuum-assisted closure), topical agents, etc.

Biofeedback	**Definition:** Provision of information from the monitoring and regulating of physiological processes in conjunction with cognitive-behavioral techniques to improve patient functioning or well-being **Includes/Examples:** Includes EEG, blood pressure, skin temperature or peripheral blood flow, ECG, electrooculogram, EMG, respirometry or capnometry, GSR/EDR, perineometry to monitor/regulate bowel/bladder activity, electrogastrogram to monitor/regulate gastric motility
Counseling	**Definition:** The application of psychological methods to treat an individual with normal developmental issues and psychological problems in order to increase function, improve well-being, alleviate distress, maladjustment or resolve crises
Crisis Intervention	**Definition:** Treatment of a traumatized, acutely disturbed or distressed individual for the purpose of short-term stabilization **Includes/Examples:** Includes defusing, debriefing, counseling, psychotherapy and/or coordination of care with other providers or agencies
Electroconvulsive Therapy	**Definition:** The application of controlled electrical voltages to treat a mental health disorder **Includes/Examples:** Includes appropriate sedation and other preparation of the individual
Family Psychotherapy	**Definition:** Treatment that includes one or more family members of an individual with a mental health disorder by behavioral, cognitive, psychoanalytic, psychodynamic or psychophysiological means to improve functioning or well-being **Explanation:** Remediation of emotional or behavioral problems presented by one or more family members in cases where psychotherapy with more than one family member is indicated
Group Psychotherapy	**Definition:** Treatment of two or more individuals with a mental health disorder by behavioral, cognitive, psychoanalytic, psychodynamic or psychophysiological means to improve functioning or well-being
Hypnosis	**Definition:** Induction of a state of heightened suggestibility by auditory, visual and tactile techniques to elicit an emotional or behavioral response
Individual Psychotherapy	**Definition:** Treatment of an individual with a mental health disorder by behavioral, cognitive, psychoanalytic, psychodynamic or psychophysiological means to improve functioning or well-being
Light Therapy	**Definition:** Application of specialized light treatments to improve functioning or well-being
Medication Management	**Definition:** Monitoring and adjusting the use of medications for the treatment of a mental health disorder
Narcosynthesis	**Definition:** Administration of intravenous barbiturates in order to release suppressed or repressed thoughts
Psychological Tests	**Definition:** The administration and interpretation of standardized psychological tests and measurement instruments for the assessment of psychological function

Section G - Mental Health — Character 4 - Type Qualifier

Behavioral	**Definition:** Primarily to modify behavior **Includes/Examples:** Includes modeling and role playing, positive reinforcement of target behaviors, response cost, and training of self-management skills
Cognitive	**Definition:** Primarily to correct cognitive distortions and errors
Cognitive-Behavioral	**Definition:** Combining cognitive and behavioral treatment strategies to improve functioning **Explanation:** Maladaptive responses are examined to determine how cognitions relate to behavior patterns in response to an event. Uses learning principles and information-processing models
Developmental	**Definition:** Age-normed developmental status of cognitive, social and adaptive behavior skills
Intellectual and Psychoeducational	**Definition:** Intellectual abilities, academic achievement and learning capabilities (including behaviors and emotional factors affecting learning
Interactive	**Definition:** Uses primarily physical aids and other forms of non-oral interaction with a patient who is physically, psychologically or developmentally unable to use ordinary language for communication **Includes/Examples:** Includes. the use of toys in symbolic play
Interpersonal	**Definition:** Helps an individual make changes in interpersonal behaviors to reduce psychological dysfunction **Includes/Examples:** Includes exploratory techniques, encouragement of affective expression, clarification of patient statements, analysis of communication patterns, use of therapy relationship and behavior change techniques
Neurobehavioral and Cognitive Status	**Definition:** Includes neurobehavioral status exam, interview(s), and observation for the clinical assessment of thinking, reasoning and judgment, acquired knowledge, attention, memory, visual spatial abilities, language functions, and planning
Neuropsychological	**Definition:** Thinking, reasoning and judgment, acquired knowledge, attention, memory, visual spatial abilities, language functions, planning
Personality and Behavioral	**Definition:** Mood, emotion, behavior, social functioning, psychopathological conditions, personality traits and characteristics

Continued →

Section G - Mental Health — Character 4 - Type Qualifier

Psychoanalysis	**Definition:** Methods of obtaining a detailed account of past and present mental and emotional experiences to determine the source and eliminate or diminish the undesirable effects of unconscious conflicts **Explanation:** Accomplished by making the individual aware of their existence, origin, and inappropriate expression in emotions and behavior
Psychodynamic	**Definition:** Exploration of past and present emotional experiences to understand motives and drives using insight-oriented techniques to reduce the undesirable effects of internal conflicts on emotions and behavior **Explanation:** Techniques include empathetic listening, clarifying self-defeating behavior patterns, and exploring adaptive alternatives
Psychophysiological	**Definition:** Monitoring and alteration of physiological processes to help the individual associate physiological reactions combined with cognitive and behavioral strategies to gain improved control of these processes to help the individual cope more effectively
Supportive	**Definition:** Formation of therapeutic relationship primarily for providing emotional support to prevent further deterioration in functioning during periods of particular stress **Explanation:** Often used in conjunction with other therapeutic approaches
Vocational	**Definition:** Exploration of vocational interests, aptitudes and required adaptive behavior skills to develop and carry out a plan for achieving a successful vocational placement **Includes/Examples:** Includes enhancing work related adjustment and/or pursuing viable options in training education or preparation

Section H - Substance Abuse Treatment — Character 3 - Root Type

Detoxification Services	**Definition:** Detoxification from alcohol and/or drugs **Explanation:** Not a treatment modality, but helps the patient stabilize physically and psychologically until the body becomes free of drugs and the effects of alcohol
Family Counseling	**Definition:** The application of psychological methods that includes one or more family members to treat an individual with addictive behavior **Explanation:** Provides support and education for family members of addicted individuals. Family member participation is seen as a critical area of substance abuse treatment
Group Counseling	**Definition:** The application of psychological methods to treat two or more individuals with addictive behavior **Explanation:** Provides structured group counseling sessions and healing power through the connection with others
Individual Counseling	**Definition:** The application of psychological methods to treat an individual with addictive behavior **Explanation:** Comprised of several different techniques, which apply various strategies to address drug addiction
Individual Psychotherapy	**Definition:** Treatment of an individual with addictive behavior by behavioral, cognitive, psychoanalytic, psychodynamic or psychophysiological means
Medication Management	**Definition:** Monitoring and adjusting the use of replacement medications for the treatment of addiction
Pharmacotherapy	**Definition:** The use of replacement medications for the treatment of addiction

Appendix C: Approach Definitions

Section 0 - Medical and Surgical — Character 5 - Approach

External (X)	**Definition:** Procedures performed directly on the skin or mucous membrane and procedures performed indirectly by the application of external force through the skin or mucous membrane
Open (0)	**Definition:** Cutting through the skin or mucous membrane and any other body layers necessary to expose the site of the procedure
Percutaneous (3)	**Definition:** Entry, by puncture or minor incision, of instrumentation through the skin or mucous membrane and any other body layers necessary to reach the site of the procedure
Percutaneous Endoscopic (4)	**Definition:** Entry, by puncture or minor incision, of instrumentation through the skin or mucous membrane and any other body layers necessary to reach and visualize the site of the procedure
Via Natural or Artificial Opening (7)	**Definition:** Entry of instrumentation through a natural or artificial external opening to reach the site of the procedure
Via Natural or Artificial Opening Endoscopic (8)	**Definition:** Entry of instrumentation through a natural or artificial external opening to reach and visualize the site of the procedure
Via Natural or Artificial Opening With Percutaneous Endoscopic Assistance (F)	**Definition:** Entry of instrumentation through a natural or artificial external opening and entry, by puncture or minor incision, of instrumentation through the skin or mucous membrane and any other body layers necessary to aid in the performance of the procedure

Section 1 - Obstetrics — Character 5 - Approach

External (X)	**Definition:** Procedures performed directly on the skin or mucous membrane and procedures performed indirectly by the application of external force through the skin or mucous membrane
Open (0)	**Definition:** Cutting through the skin or mucous membrane and any other body layers necessary to expose the site of the procedure
Percutaneous (3)	**Definition:** Entry, by puncture or minor incision, of instrumentation through the skin or mucous membrane and any other body layers necessary to reach the site of the procedure
Percutaneous Endoscopic (4)	**Definition:** Entry, by puncture or minor incision, of instrumentation through the skin or mucous membrane and any other body layers necessary to reach and visualize the site of the procedure
Via Natural or Artificial Opening (7)	**Definition:** Entry of instrumentation through a natural or artificial external opening to reach the site of the procedure
Via Natural or Artificial Opening Endoscopic (8)	**Definition:** Entry of instrumentation through a natural or artificial external opening to reach and visualize the site of the procedure

Section 2 - Placement — Character 5 - Approach

External (X)	**Definition:** Procedures performed directly on the skin or mucous membrane and procedures performed indirectly by the application of external force through the skin or mucous membrane

Section 3 - Administration — Character 5 - Approach

External (X)	**Definition:** Procedures performed directly on the skin or mucous membrane and procedures performed indirectly by the application of external force through the skin or mucous membrane
Open (0)	**Definition:** Cutting through the skin or mucous membrane and any other body layers necessary to expose the site of the procedure
Percutaneous (3)	**Definition:** Entry, by puncture or minor incision, of instrumentation through the skin or mucous membrane and any other body layers necessary to reach the site of the procedure
Via Natural or Artificial Opening (7)	**Definition:** Entry of instrumentation through a natural or artificial external opening to reach the site of the procedure
Via Natural or Artificial Opening Endoscopic (8)	**Definition:** Entry of instrumentation through a natural or artificial external opening to reach and visualize the site of the procedure

Section 4 - Measurement and Monitoring — Character 5 - Approach

External (X)	**Definition:** Procedures performed directly on the skin or mucous membrane and procedures performed indirectly by the application of external force through the skin or mucous membrane
Open (0)	**Definition:** Cutting through the skin or mucous membrane and any other body layers necessary to expose the site of the procedure
Percutaneous (3)	**Definition:** Entry, by puncture or minor incision, of instrumentation through the skin or mucous membrane and any other body layers necessary to reach the site of the procedure
Percutaneous Endoscopic (4)	**Definition:** Entry, by puncture or minor incision, of instrumentation through the skin or mucous membrane and any other body layers necessary to reach and visualize the site of the procedure
Via Natural or Artificial Opening (7)	**Definition:** Entry of instrumentation through a natural or artificial external opening to reach the site of the procedure
Via Natural or Artificial Opening Endoscopic (8)	**Definition:** Entry of instrumentation through a natural or artificial external opening to reach and visualize the site of the procedure

Section 7 - Osteopathic — Character 5 - Approach

External (X)	**Definition:** Procedures performed directly on the skin or mucous membrane and procedures performed indirectly by the application of external force through the skin or mucous membrane

Section 8 - Other Procedures — Character 5 - Approach

External (X)	**Definition:** Procedures performed directly on the skin or mucous membrane and procedures performed indirectly by the application of external force through the skin or mucous membrane
Open (0)	**Definition:** Cutting through the skin or mucous membrane and any other body layers necessary to expose the site of the procedure
Percutaneous (3)	**Definition:** Entry, by puncture or minor incision, of instrumentation through the skin or mucous membrane and any other body layers necessary to reach the site of the procedure
Percutaneous Endoscopic (4)	**Definition:** Entry, by puncture or minor incision, of instrumentation through the skin or mucous membrane and any other body layers necessary to reach and visualize the site of the procedure
Via Natural or Artificial Opening (7)	**Definition:** Entry of instrumentation through a natural or artificial external opening to reach the site of the procedure
Via Natural or Artificial Opening Endoscopic (8)	**Definition:** Entry of instrumentation through a natural or artificial external opening to reach and visualize the site of the procedure

Continued →

Section 9 - Chiropractic — Character 5 - Approach

External (X)	**Definition:** Procedures performed directly on the skin or mucous membrane and procedures performed indirectly by the application of external force through the skin or mucous membrane

Section X - New Technology — Character 5 - Approach

External	**Definition:** Procedures performed directly on the skin or mucous membrane and procedures performed indirectly by the application of external force through the skin or mucous membrane
Open	**Definition:** Cutting through the skin or mucous membrane and any other body layers necessary to expose the site of the procedure
Percutaneous	**Definition:** Entry, by puncture or minor incision, of instrumentation through the skin or mucous membrane and any other body layers necessary to reach the site of the procedure
Percutaneous Endoscopic	**Definition:** Entry, by puncture or minor incision, of instrumentation through the skin or mucous membrane and any other body layers necessary to reach and visualize the site of the procedure

Appendix D: Medical and Surgical Body Parts

Appendices D–F are structured to assist coders with confirming character selections within the Tables. For example, if the coder is considering the body part of Abdomen Muscle, appendix D can be referenced to identify all of the muscles that are included in the body part Abdomen Muscle (see row 2 in the table below). After reviewing the information, the coder can determine if the body part under consideration is correct or if another body part should be reviewed. The same process can be followed for devices which are included in appendix E and substances which are included in appendix F.

Section 0 - Medical and Surgical — Character 4 - Body Part

1st Toe, Left **1st** Toe, Right	**Includes:** Hallux
Abdomen Muscle, Left **Abdomen** Muscle, Right	**Includes:** External oblique muscle Internal oblique muscle Pyramidalis muscle Rectus abdominis muscle Transversus abdominis muscle
Abdominal Aorta	**Includes:** Inferior phrenic artery Lumbar artery Median sacral artery Middle suprarenal artery Ovarian artery Testicular artery
Abdominal Sympathetic Nerve	**Includes:** **Abdominal** aortic plexus Auerbach's (myenteric) plexus Celiac (solar) plexus Celiac ganglion Gastric plexus Hepatic plexus Inferior hypogastric plexus Inferior mesenteric ganglion Inferior mesenteric plexus Meissner's (submucous) plexus Myenteric (Auerbach's) plexus Pancreatic plexus Pelvic splanchnic nerve Renal plexus Solar (celiac) plexus Splenic plexus Submucous (Meissner's) plexus Superior hypogastric plexus Superior mesenteric ganglion Superior mesenteric plexus Suprarenal plexus

Section 0 - Medical and Surgical — Character 4 - Body Part

Abducens Nerve	**Includes:** Sixth cranial nerve
Accessory Nerve	**Includes:** Eleventh cranial nerve
Acoustic Nerve	**Includes:** Cochlear nerve Eighth cranial nerve Scarpa's (vestibular) ganglion Spiral ganglion Vestibular (Scarpa's) ganglion Vestibular nerve Vestibulocochlear nerve
Adenoids	**Includes:** Pharyngeal tonsil
Adrenal Gland **Adrenal** Gland, Left **Adrenal** Gland, Right **Adrenal** Glands, Bilateral	**Includes:** Suprarenal gland
Ampulla of Vater	**Includes:** Duodenal ampulla Hepatopancreatic ampulla
Anal Sphincter	**Includes:** External anal sphincter Internal anal sphincter
Ankle Bursa and Ligament, Left **Ankle** Bursa and Ligament, Right	**Includes:** Calcaneofibular ligament Deltoid ligament Ligament of the lateral malleolus Talofibular ligament
Ankle Joint, Left **Ankle** Joint, Right	**Includes:** Inferior tibiofibular joint Talocrural joint

Continued →

Anterior Chamber, Left **Anterior** Chamber, Right	**Includes:** Aqueous humour
Anterior Tibial Artery, Left **Anterior** Tibial Artery, Right	**Includes:** Anterior lateral malleolar artery Anterior medial malleolar artery Anterior tibial recurrent artery Dorsalis pedis artery Posterior tibial recurrent artery
Anus	**Includes:** Anal orifice
Aortic Valve	**Includes:** Aortic annulus
Appendix	**Includes:** Vermiform appendix
Ascending Colon	**Includes:** Hepatic flexure
Atrial Septum	**Includes:** Interatrial septum
Atrium, Left	**Includes:** Atrium pulmonale Left auricular appendix
Atrium, Right	**Includes:** Atrium dextrum cordis Right auricular appendix Sinus venosus
Auditory Ossicle, Left **Auditory** Ossicle, Right	**Includes:** Incus Malleus Ossicular chain Stapes
Axillary Artery, Left **Axillary** Artery, Right	**Includes:** Anterior circumflex humeral artery Lateral thoracic artery Posterior circumflex humeral artery Subscapular artery Superior thoracic artery Thoracoacromial artery
Azygos Vein	**Includes:** Right ascending lumbar vein Right subcostal vein
Basal Ganglia	**Includes:** Basal nuclei Claustrum Corpus striatum Globus pallidus Substantia nigra Subthalamic nucleus
Basilic Vein, Left **Basilic** Vein, Right	**Includes:** Median antebrachial vein Median cubital vein
Bladder	**Includes:** Trigone of bladder
Brachial Artery, Left **Brachial** Artery, Right	**Includes:** Inferior ulnar collateral artery Profunda brachii Superior ulnar collateral artery

Brachial Plexus	**Includes:** Axillary nerve Dorsal scapular nerve First intercostal nerve Long thoracic nerve Musculocutaneous nerve Subclavius nerve Suprascapular nerve
Brachial Vein, Left **Brachial** Vein, Right	**Includes:** Radial vein Ulnar vein
Brain	**Includes:** Cerebrum Corpus callosum Encephalon
Breast, Bilateral **Breast,** Left **Breast,** Right	**Includes:** Mammary duct Mammary gland
Buccal Mucosa	**Includes:** Buccal gland Molar gland Palatine gland
Carotid Bodies, Bilateral **Carotid** Body, Left **Carotid** Body, Right	**Includes:** Carotid glomus
Carpal Joint, Left **Carpal** Joint, Right	**Includes:** Intercarpal joint Midcarpal joint
Carpal, Left **Carpal,** Right	**Includes:** Capitate bone Hamate bone Lunate bone Pisiform bone Scaphoid bone Trapezium bone Trapezoid bone Triquetral bone
Celiac Artery	**Includes:** Celiac trunk
Cephalic Vein, Left **Cephalic** Vein, Right	**Includes:** Accessory cephalic vein
Cerebellum	**Includes:** Culmen
Cerebral Hemisphere	**Includes:** Frontal lobe Occipital lobe Parietal lobe Temporal lobe
Cerebral Meninges	**Includes:** Arachnoid mater, intracranial Leptomeninges, intracranial Pia mater, intracranial

Continued →

Cerebral Ventricle	**Includes:** Aqueduct of Sylvius Cerebral aqueduct (Sylvius) Choroid plexus Ependyma Foramen of Monro (intraventricular) Fourth ventricle Interventricular foramen (Monro) Left lateral ventricle Right lateral ventricle Third ventricle
Cervical Nerve	**Includes:** Greater occipital nerve Spinal nerve, cervical Suboccipital nerve Third occipital nerve
Cervical Plexus	**Includes:** Ansa cervicalis Cutaneous (transverse) cervical nerve Great auricular nerve Lesser occipital nerve Supraclavicular nerve Transverse (cutaneous) cervical nerve
Cervical Vertebra	**Includes:** Spinous process Vertebral arch Vertebral foramen Vertebral lamina Vertebral pedicle
Cervical Vertebral Joint	**Includes:** Atlantoaxial joint Cervical facet joint
Cervical Vertebral Joints, 2 or more	**Includes:** Cervical facet joint
Cervicothoracic Vertebral Joint	**Includes:** Cervicothoracic facet joint
Cisterna Chyli	**Includes:** Intestinal lymphatic trunk Lumbar lymphatic trunk
Coccygeal Glomus	**Includes:** Coccygeal body
Colic Vein	**Includes:** Ileocolic vein Left colic vein Middle colic vein Right colic vein
Conduction Mechanism	**Includes:** Atrioventricular node Bundle of His Bundle of Kent Sinoatrial node
Conjunctiva, Left **Conjunctiva,** Right	**Includes:** Plica semilunaris

Dura Mater	**Includes:** Diaphragma sellae Dura mater, intracranial Falx cerebri Tentorium cerebelli
Elbow Bursa and Ligament, Left **Elbow** Bursa and Ligament, Right	**Includes:** Annular ligament Olecranon bursa Radial collateral ligament Ulnar collateral ligament
Elbow Joint, Left **Elbow** Joint, Right	**Includes:** Distal humerus, involving joint Humeroradial joint Humeroulnar joint Proximal radioulnar joint
Epidural Space	**Includes:** Epidural space, intracranial Extradural space, intracranial
Epiglottis	**Includes:** Glossoepiglottic fold
Esophagogastric Junction	**Includes:** Cardia Cardioesophageal junction Gastroesophageal (GE) junction
Esophagus, Lower	**Includes:** Abdominal esophagus
Esophagus, Middle	**Includes:** Thoracic esophagus
Esophagus, Upper	**Includes:** Cervical esophagus
Ethmoid Bone, Left **Ethmoid** Bone, Right	**Includes:** Cribriform plate
Ethmoid Sinus, Left **Ethmoid** Sinus, Right	**Includes:** Ethmoidal air cell
Eustachian Tube, Left **Eustachian** Tube, Right	**Includes:** Auditory tube Pharyngotympanic tube
External Auditory Canal, Left **External** Auditory Canal, Right	**Includes:** External auditory meatus
External Carotid Artery, Left **External** Carotid Artery, Right	**Includes:** Ascending pharyngeal artery Internal maxillary artery Lingual artery Maxillary artery Occipital artery Posterior auricular artery Superior thyroid artery

Continued →

External Ear, Bilateral **External** Ear, Left **External** Ear, Right	**Includes:** Antihelix Antitragus Auricle Earlobe Helix Pinna Tragus
External Iliac Artery, Left **External** Iliac Artery, Right	**Includes:** Deep circumflex iliac artery Inferior epigastric artery
External Jugular Vein, Left **External** Jugular Vein, Right	**Includes:** Posterior auricular vein
Extraocular Muscle, Left **Extraocular** Muscle, Right	**Includes:** Inferior oblique muscle Inferior rectus muscle Lateral rectus muscle Medial rectus muscle Superior oblique muscle Superior rectus muscle
Eye, Left **Eye**, Right	**Includes:** Ciliary body Posterior chamber
Face Artery	**Includes:** Angular artery Ascending palatine artery External maxillary artery Facial artery Inferior labial artery Submental artery Superior labial artery
Face Vein, Left **Face** Vein, Right	**Includes:** Angular vein Anterior facial vein Common facial vein Deep facial vein Frontal vein Posterior facial (retromandibular) vein Supraorbital vein
Facial Muscle	**Includes:** Buccinator muscle Corrugator supercilii muscle Depressor anguli oris muscle Depressor labii inferioris muscle Depressor septi nasi muscle Depressor supercilii muscle Levator anguli oris muscle Levator labii superioris alaeque nasi Levator labii superioris alaeque nasi Levator labii superioris alaeque nasi Levator labii superioris muscle Mentalis muscle Nasalis muscle Occipitofrontalis muscle Orbicularis oris muscle Procerus muscle Risorius muscle Zygomaticus muscle

Facial Nerve	**Includes:** Chorda tympani Geniculate ganglion Greater superficial petrosal nerve Nerve to the stapedius Parotid plexus Posterior auricular nerve Seventh cranial nerve Submandibular ganglion
Fallopian Tube, Left **Fallopian** Tube, Right	**Includes:** Oviduct Salpinx Uterine tube
Femoral Artery, Left **Femoral** Artery, Right	**Includes:** Circumflex iliac artery Deep femoral artery Descending genicular artery External pudendal artery Superficial epigastric artery
Femoral Nerve	**Includes:** Anterior crural nerve Saphenous nerve
Femoral Shaft, Left **Femoral** Shaft, Right	**Includes:** Body of femur
Femoral Vein, Left **Femoral** Vein, Right	**Includes:** Deep femoral (profunda femoris) vein Popliteal vein Profunda femoris (deep femoral) vein
Fibula, Left **Fibula**, Right	**Includes:** Body of fibula Head of fibula Lateral malleolus
Finger Nail	**Includes:** Nail bed Nail plate
Finger Phalangeal Joint, Left **Finger** Phalangeal Joint, Right	**Includes:** Interphalangeal (IP) joint
Foot Artery, Left **Foot** Artery, Right	**Includes:** Arcuate artery Dorsal metatarsal artery Lateral plantar artery Lateral tarsal artery Medial plantar artery
Foot Bursa and Ligament, Left **Foot** Bursa and Ligament, Right	**Includes:** Calcaneocuboid ligament Cuneonavicular ligament Intercuneiform ligament Interphalangeal ligament Metatarsal ligament Metatarsophalangeal ligament Subtalar ligament Talocalcaneal ligament Talocalcaneonavicular ligament Tarsometatarsal ligament

Continued →

Foot Muscle, Left **Foot** Muscle, Right	**Includes:** Abductor hallucis muscle Adductor hallucis muscle Extensor digitorum brevis muscle Extensor hallucis brevis muscle Flexor digitorum brevis muscle Flexor hallucis brevis muscle Quadratus plantae muscle
Foot Vein, Left **Foot** Vein, Right	**Includes:** Common digital vein Dorsal metatarsal vein Dorsal venous arch Plantar digital vein Plantar metatarsal vein Plantar venous arch
Frontal Bone, Left **Frontal** Bone, Right	**Includes:** Zygomatic process of frontal bone
Gastric Artery	**Includes:** Left gastric artery Right gastric artery
Glenoid Cavity, Left **Glenoid** Cavity, Right	**Includes:** Glenoid fossa (of scapula)
Glomus Jugulare	**Includes:** Jugular body
Glossopharyngeal Nerve	**Includes:** Carotid sinus nerve Ninth cranial nerve Tympanic nerve
Greater Omentum	**Includes:** Gastrocolic ligament Gastrocolic omentum Gastrophrenic ligament Gastrosplenic ligament
Greater Saphenous Vein, Left **Greater** Saphenous Vein, Right	**Includes:** External pudendal vein Great saphenous vein Superficial circumflex iliac vein Superficial epigastric vein
Hand Artery, Left **Hand** Artery, Right	**Includes:** Deep palmar arch Princeps pollicis artery Radialis indicis Superficial palmar arch
Hand Bursa and Ligament, Left **Hand** Bursa and Ligament, Right	**Includes:** Carpometacarpal ligament Intercarpal ligament Interphalangeal ligament Lunotriquetral ligament Metacarpal ligament Metacarpophalangeal ligament Pisohamate ligament Pisometacarpal ligament Scapholunate ligament Scaphotrapezium ligament
Hand Muscle, Left **Hand** Muscle, Right	**Includes:** Hypothenar muscle Palmar interosseous muscle Thenar muscle

Hand Vein, Left **Hand** Vein, Right	**Includes:** Dorsal metacarpal vein Palmar (volar) digital vein Palmar (volar) metacarpal vein Superficial palmar venous arch Volar (palmar) digital vein Volar (palmar) metacarpal vein
Head and Neck Bursa and Ligament	**Includes:** Alar ligament of axis Cervical interspinous ligament Cervical intertransverse ligament Cervical ligamentum flavum Interspinous ligament Lateral temporomandibular ligament Sphenomandibular ligament Stylomandibular ligament Transverse ligament of atlas
Head and Neck Sympathetic Nerve	**Includes:** Cavernous plexus Cervical ganglion Ciliary ganglion Internal carotid plexus Otic ganglion Pterygopalatine (sphenopalatine) ganglion Sphenopalatine (pterygopalatine) ganglion Stellate ganglion Submandibular ganglion Submaxillary ganglion
Head Muscle	**Includes:** Auricularis muscle Masseter muscle Pterygoid muscle Splenius capitis muscle Temporalis muscle Temporoparietalis muscle
Heart, Left	**Includes:** Left coronary sulcus Obtuse margin
Heart, Right	**Includes:** Right coronary sulcus
Hemiazygos Vein	**Includes:** Left ascending lumbar vein Left subcostal vein
Hepatic Artery	**Includes:** Common hepatic artery Gastroduodenal artery Hepatic artery proper
Hip Bursa and Ligament, Left **Hip** Bursa and Ligament, Right	**Includes:** Iliofemoral ligament Ischiofemoral ligament Pubofemoral ligament Transverse acetabular ligament Trochanteric bursa
Hip Joint, Left **Hip** Joint, Right	**Includes:** Acetabulofemoral joint

Continued →

Hip Muscle, Left **Hip** Muscle, Right	**Includes:** Gemellus muscle Gluteus maximus muscle Gluteus medius muscle Gluteus minimus muscle Iliacus muscle Obturator muscle Piriformis muscle Psoas muscle Quadratus femoris muscle Tensor fasciae latae muscle
Humeral Head, Left **Humeral** Head, Right	**Includes:** Greater tuberosity Lesser tuberosity Neck of humerus (anatomical)(surgical)
Humeral Shaft, Left **Humeral** Shaft, Right	**Includes:** Distal humerus Humerus, distal Lateral epicondyle of humerus Medial epicondyle of humerus
Hypogastric Vein, Left **Hypogastric** Vein, Right	**Includes:** Gluteal vein Internal iliac vein Internal pudendal vein Lateral sacral vein Middle hemorrhoidal vein Obturator vein Uterine vein Vaginal vein Vesical vein
Hypoglossal Nerve	**Includes:** Twelfth cranial nerve
Hypothalamus	**Includes:** Mammillary body
Inferior Mesenteric Artery	**Includes:** Sigmoid artery Superior rectal artery
Inferior Mesenteric Vein	**Includes:** Sigmoid vein Superior rectal vein
Inferior Vena Cava	**Includes:** Postcava Right inferior phrenic vein Right ovarian vein Right second lumbar vein Right suprarenal vein Right testicular vein
Inguinal Region, Bilateral **Inguinal** Region, Left **Inguinal** Region, Right	**Includes:** Inguinal canal Inguinal triangle
Inner Ear, Left **Inner** Ear, Right	**Includes:** Bony labyrinth Bony vestibule Cochlea Round window Semicircular canal
Innominate Artery	**Includes:** Brachiocephalic artery Brachiocephalic trunk

**Section 0 - Medical and Surgical —
Character 4 - Body Part**

Innominate Vein, Left **Innominate** Vein, Right	**Includes:** Brachiocephalic vein Inferior thyroid vein
Internal Carotid Artery, Left **Internal** Carotid Artery, Right	**Includes:** Caroticotympanic artery Carotid sinus Ophthalmic artery
Internal Iliac Artery, Left **Internal** Iliac Artery, Right	**Includes:** Deferential artery Hypogastric artery Iliolumbar artery Inferior gluteal artery Inferior vesical artery Internal pudendal artery Lateral sacral artery Middle rectal artery Obturator artery Superior gluteal artery Umbilical artery Uterine artery Vaginal artery
Internal Mammary Artery, Left **Internal** Mammary Artery, Right	**Includes:** Anterior intercostal artery Internal thoracic artery Musculophrenic artery Pericardiophrenic artery Superior epigastric artery
Intracranial Artery	**Includes:** Anterior cerebral artery Anterior choroidal artery Anterior communicating artery Basilar artery Circle of Willis Middle cerebral artery Posterior cerebral artery Posterior communicating artery Posterior inferior cerebellar artery (PICA)
Intracranial Vein	**Includes:** Anterior cerebral vein Basal (internal) cerebral vein Dural venous sinus Great cerebral vein Inferior cerebellar vein Inferior cerebral vein Internal (basal) cerebral vein Middle cerebral vein Ophthalmic vein Superior cerebellar vein Superior cerebral vein
Jejunum	**Includes:** Duodenojejunal flexure
Kidney	**Includes:** Renal calyx Renal capsule Renal cortex Renal segment
Kidney Pelvis, Left **Kidney** Pelvis, Right	**Includes:** Ureteropelvic junction (UPJ)

Continued →

Kidney, Left **Kidney,** Right **Kidneys,** Bilateral	**Includes:** Renal calyx Renal capsule Renal cortex Renal segment
Knee Bursa and Ligament, Left **Knee** Bursa and Ligament, Right	**Includes:** Anterior cruciate ligament (ACL) Lateral collateral ligament (LCL) Ligament of head of fibula Medial collateral ligament (MCL) Patellar ligament Popliteal ligament Posterior cruciate ligament (PCL) Prepatellar bursa
Knee Joint, Femoral Surface, Left **Knee** Joint, Femoral Surface, Right	**Includes:** Femoropatellar joint Patellofemoral joint
Knee Joint, Left **Knee** Joint, Right	**Includes:** Femoropatellar joint Femorotibial joint Lateral meniscus Medial meniscus Patellofemoral joint Tibiofemoral joint
Knee Joint, Tibial Surface, Left **Knee** Joint, Tibial Surface, Right	**Includes:** Femorotibial joint Tibiofemoral joint
Knee Tendon, Left **Knee** Tendon, Right	**Includes:** Patellar tendon
Lacrimal Duct, Left **Lacrimal** Duct, Right	**Includes:** Lacrimal canaliculus Lacrimal punctum Lacrimal sac Nasolacrimal duct
Larynx	**Includes:** Aryepiglottic fold Arytenoid cartilage Corniculate cartilage Cuneiform cartilage False vocal cord Glottis Rima glottidis Thyroid cartilage Ventricular fold
Lens, Left **Lens,** Right	**Includes:** Zonule of Zinn
Lesser Omentum	**Includes:** Gastrohepatic omentum Hepatogastric ligament
Lesser Saphenous Vein, Left **Lesser** Saphenous Vein, Right	**Includes:** Small saphenous vein
Liver	**Includes:** Quadrate lobe

Lower Arm and Wrist Muscle, Left **Lower** Arm and Wrist Muscle, Right	**Includes:** Anatomical snuffbox Brachioradialis muscle Extensor carpi radialis muscle Extensor carpi ulnaris muscle Flexor carpi radialis muscle Flexor carpi ulnaris muscle Flexor pollicis longus muscle Palmaris longus muscle Pronator quadratus muscle Pronator teres muscle
Lower Eyelid, Left **Lower** Eyelid, Right	**Includes:** Inferior tarsal plate Medial canthus
Lower Femur, Left **Lower** Femur, Right	**Includes:** Lateral condyle of femur Lateral epicondyle of femur Medial condyle of femur Medial epicondyle of femur
Lower Leg Muscle, Left **Lower** Leg Muscle, Right	**Includes:** Extensor digitorum longus muscle Extensor hallucis longus muscle Fibularis brevis muscle Fibularis longus muscle Flexor digitorum longus muscle Flexor hallucis longus muscle Gastrocnemius muscle Peroneus brevis muscle Peroneus longus muscle Popliteus muscle Soleus muscle Tibialis anterior muscle Tibialis posterior muscle
Lower Leg Tendon, Left **Lower** Leg Tendon, Right	**Includes:** Achilles tendon
Lower Lip	**Includes:** Frenulum labii inferioris Labial gland Vermilion border
Lumbar Nerve	**Includes:** Lumbosacral trunk Spinal nerve, lumbar Superior clunic (cluneal) nerve
Lumbar Plexus	**Includes:** Accessory obturator nerve Genitofemoral nerve Iliohypogastric nerve Ilioinguinal nerve Lateral femoral cutaneous nerve Obturator nerve Superior gluteal nerve
Lumbar Spinal Cord	**Includes:** Cauda equina Conus medullaris
Lumbar Sympathetic Nerve	**Includes:** Lumbar ganglion Lumbar splanchnic nerve

Continued →

Lumbar Vertebra	**Includes:** Spinous process Vertebral arch Vertebral foramen Vertebral lamina Vertebral pedicle
Lumbar Vertebral Joint	**Includes:** Lumbar facet joint
Lumbosacral Joint	**Includes:** Lumbosacral facet joint
Lymphatic, Aortic	**Includes:** Celiac lymph node Gastric lymph node Hepatic lymph node Lumbar lymph node Pancreaticosplenic lymph node Paraaortic lymph node Retroperitoneal lymph node
Lymphatic, Head	**Includes:** Buccinator lymph node Infraauricular lymph node Infraparotid lymph node Parotid lymph node Preauricular lymph node Submandibular lymph node Submaxillary lymph node Submental lymph node Subparotid lymph node Suprahyoid lymph node
Lymphatic, Left Axillary	**Includes:** Anterior (pectoral) lymph node Apical (subclavicular) lymph node Brachial (lateral) lymph node Central axillary lymph node Lateral (brachial) lymph node Pectoral (anterior) lymph node Posterior (subscapular) lymph node Subclavicular (apical) lymph node Subscapular (posterior) lymph node
Lymphatic, Left Lower Extremity	**Includes:** Femoral lymph node Popliteal lymph node
Lymphatic, Left Neck	**Includes:** Cervical lymph node Jugular lymph node Mastoid (postauricular) lymph node Occipital lymph node Postauricular (mastoid) lymph node Retropharyngeal lymph node Supraclavicular (Virchow's) lymph node Virchow's (supraclavicular) lymph node
Lymphatic, Left Upper Extremity	**Includes:** Cubital lymph node Deltopectoral (infraclavicular) lymph node Epitrochlear lymph node Infraclavicular (deltopectoral) lymph node Supratrochlear lymph node

Lymphatic, Mesenteric	**Includes:** Inferior mesenteric lymph node Pararectal lymph node Superior mesenteric lymph node
Lymphatic, Pelvis	**Includes:** Common iliac (subaortic) lymph node Gluteal lymph node Iliac lymph node Inferior epigastric lymph node Obturator lymph node Sacral lymph node Subaortic (common iliac) lymph node Suprainguinal lymph node
Lymphatic, Right Axillary	**Includes:** Anterior (pectoral) lymph node Apical (subclavicular) lymph node Brachial (lateral) lymph node Central axillary lymph node Lateral (brachial) lymph node Pectoral (anterior) lymph node Posterior (subscapular) lymph node Subclavicular (apical) lymph node Subscapular (posterior) lymph node
Lymphatic, Right Lower Extremity	**Includes:** Femoral lymph node Popliteal lymph node
Lymphatic, Right Neck	**Includes:** Cervical lymph node Jugular lymph node Mastoid (postauricular) lymph node Occipital lymph node Postauricular (mastoid) lymph node Retropharyngeal lymph node Right jugular trunk Right lymphatic duct Right subclavian trunk Supraclavicular (Virchow's) lymph node Virchow's (supraclavicular) lymph node
Lymphatic, Right Upper Extremity	**Includes:** Cubital lymph node Deltopectoral (infraclavicular) lymph node Epitrochlear lymph node Infraclavicular (deltopectoral) lymph node Supratrochlear lymph node
Lymphatic, Thorax	**Includes:** Intercostal lymph node Mediastinal lymph node Parasternal lymph node Paratracheal lymph node Tracheobronchial lymph node
Mandible, Left **Mandible,** Right	**Includes:** Alveolar process of mandible Condyloid process Mandibular notch Mental foramen
Mastoid Sinus, Left **Mastoid** Sinus, Right	**Includes:** Mastoid air cells

Continued →

Maxilla, Left **Maxilla,** Right	**Includes:** Alveolar process of maxilla
Maxillary Sinus, Left **Maxillary** Sinus, Right	**Includes:** Antrum of Highmore
Median Nerve	**Includes:** Anterior interosseous nerve Palmar cutaneous nerve
Medulla Oblongata	**Includes:** Myelencephalon
Mesentery	**Includes:** Mesoappendix Mesocolon
Metacarpocarpal Joint, Left **Metacarpocarpal** Joint, Right	**Includes:** Carpometacarpal (CMC) joint
Metatarsal-Phalangeal Joint, Left **Metatarsal-Phalangeal** Joint, Right	**Includes:** Metatarsophalangeal (MTP) joint
Metatarsal-Tarsal Joint, Left **Metatarsal-Tarsal** Joint, Right	**Includes:** Tarsometatarsal joint
Middle Ear, Left **Middle** Ear, Right	**Includes:** Oval window Tympanic cavity
Minor Salivary Gland	**Includes:** Anterior lingual gland
Mitral Valve	**Includes:** Bicuspid valve Left atrioventricular valve Mitral annulus
Nasal Bone	**Includes:** Vomer of nasal septum
Nasal Septum	**Includes:** Quadrangular cartilage Septal cartilage Vomer bone
Nasal Turbinate	**Includes:** Inferior turbinate Middle turbinate Nasal concha Superior turbinate
Nasopharynx	**Includes:** Choana Fossa of Rosenmuller Pharyngeal recess Rhinopharynx

Neck Muscle, Left **Neck** Muscle, Right	**Includes:** Anterior vertebral muscle Arytenoid muscle Cricothyroid muscle Infrahyoid muscle Levator scapulae muscle Platysma muscle Scalene muscle Splenius cervicis muscle Sternocleidomastoid muscle Suprahyoid muscle Thyroarytenoid muscle
Nipple, Left **Nipple,** Right	**Includes:** Areola
Nose	**Includes:** Columella External naris Greater alar cartilage Internal naris Lateral nasal cartilage Lesser alar cartilage Nasal cavity Nostril
Occipital Bone, Left **Occipital** Bone, Right	**Includes:** Foramen magnum
Oculomotor Nerve	**Includes:** Third cranial nerve
Olfactory Nerve	**Includes:** First cranial nerve Olfactory bulb
Optic Nerve	**Includes:** Optic chiasma Second cranial nerve
Orbit, Left **Orbit,** Right	**Includes:** Bony orbit Orbital portion of ethmoid bone Orbital portion of frontal bone Orbital portion of lacrimal bone Orbital portion of maxilla Orbital portion of palatine bone Orbital portion of sphenoid bone Orbital portion of zygomatic bone
Pancreatic Duct	**Includes:** Duct of Wirsung
Pancreatic Duct, Accessory	**Includes:** Duct of Santorini
Parotid Duct, Left **Parotid** Duct, Right	**Includes:** Stensen's duct
Pelvic Bone, Left **Pelvic** Bone, Right	**Includes:** Iliac crest Ilium Ischium Pubis
Pelvic Cavity	**Includes:** Retropubic space
Penis	**Includes:** Corpus cavernosum Corpus spongiosum

Continued →

Perineum Muscle	**Includes:** Bulbospongiosus muscle Cremaster muscle Deep transverse perineal muscle Ischiocavernosus muscle Superficial transverse perineal muscle
Peritoneum	**Includes:** Epiploic foramen
Peroneal Artery, Left **Peroneal** Artery, Right	**Includes:** Fibular artery
Peroneal Nerve	**Includes:** Common fibular nerve Common peroneal nerve External popliteal nerve Lateral sural cutaneous nerve
Pharynx	**Includes:** Hypopharynx Laryngopharynx Oropharynx Piriform recess (sinus)
Phrenic Nerve	**Includes:** Accessory phrenic nerve
Pituitary Gland	**Includes:** Adenohypophysis Hypophysis Neurohypophysis
Pons	**Includes:** Apneustic center Basis pontis Locus ceruleus Pneumotaxic center Pontine tegmentum Superior olivary nucleus
Popliteal Artery, Left **Popliteal** Artery, Right	**Includes:** Inferior genicular artery Middle genicular artery Superior genicular artery Sural artery
Portal Vein	**Includes:** Hepatic portal vein
Prepuce	**Includes:** Foreskin Glans penis
Pudendal Nerve	**Includes:** Posterior labial nerve Posterior scrotal nerve
Pulmonary Artery, Left	**Includes:** Arterial canal (duct) Botallo's duct Pulmoaortic canal
Pulmonary Valve	**Includes:** Pulmonary annulus Pulmonic valve
Pulmonary Vein, Left	**Includes:** Left inferior pulmonary vein Left superior pulmonary vein

Pulmonary Vein, Right	**Includes:** Right inferior pulmonary vein Right superior pulmonary vein
Radial Artery, Left **Radial** Artery, Right	**Includes:** Radial recurrent artery
Radial Nerve	**Includes:** Dorsal digital nerve Musculospiral nerve Palmar cutaneous nerve Posterior interosseous nerve
Radius, Left **Radius,** Right	**Includes:** Ulnar notch
Rectum	**Includes:** Anorectal junction
Renal Artery, Left **Renal** Artery, Right	**Includes:** Inferior suprarenal artery Renal segmental artery
Renal Vein, Left	**Includes:** Left inferior phrenic vein Left ovarian vein Left second lumbar vein Left suprarenal vein Left testicular vein
Retina, Left **Retina,** Right	**Includes:** Fovea Macula Optic disc
Retroperitoneum	**Includes:** Retroperitoneal space
Sacral Nerve	**Includes:** Spinal nerve, sacral
Sacral Plexus	**Includes:** Inferior gluteal nerve Posterior femoral cutaneous nerve Pudendal nerve
Sacral Sympathetic Nerve	**Includes:** Ganglion impar (ganglion of Walther) Pelvic splanchnic nerve Sacral ganglion Sacral splanchnic nerve
Sacrococcygeal Joint	**Includes:** Sacrococcygeal symphysis
Scapula, Left **Scapula,** Right	**Includes:** Acromion (process) Coracoid process
Sciatic Nerve	**Includes:** Ischiatic nerve

Continued →

Shoulder Bursa and Ligament, Left **Shoulder** Bursa and Ligament, Right	**Includes:** Acromioclavicular ligament Coracoacromial ligament Coracoclavicular ligament Coracohumeral ligament Costoclavicular ligament Glenohumeral ligament Interclavicular ligament Sternoclavicular ligament Subacromial bursa Transverse humeral ligament Transverse scapular ligament
Shoulder Joint, Left **Shoulder** Joint, Right	**Includes:** Glenohumeral joint Glenoid ligament (labrum)
Shoulder Muscle, Left **Shoulder** Muscle, Right	**Includes:** Deltoid muscle Infraspinatus muscle Subscapularis muscle Supraspinatus muscle Teres major muscle Teres minor muscle
Sigmoid Colon	**Includes:** Rectosigmoid junction Sigmoid flexure
Skin	**Includes:** Dermis Epidermis Sebaceous gland Sweat gland
Sphenoid Bone, Left **Sphenoid** Bone, Right	**Includes:** Greater wing Lesser wing Optic foramen Pterygoid process Sella turcica
Spinal Canal	**Includes:** Epidural space, spinal Extradural space, spinal Subarachnoid space, spinal Subdural space, spinal Vertebral canal
Spinal Meninges	**Includes:** Arachnoid mater, spinal Denticulate (dentate) ligament Dura mater, spinal Leptomeninges, spinal Pia mater, spinal
Spleen	**Includes:** Accessory spleen
Splenic Artery	**Includes:** Left gastroepiploic artery Pancreatic artery Short gastric artery
Splenic Vein	**Includes:** Left gastroepiploic vein Pancreatic vein
Sternum	**Includes:** Manubrium Suprasternal notch Xiphoid process

Stomach, Pylorus	**Includes:** Pyloric antrum Pyloric canal Pyloric sphincter
Subarachnoid Space	**Includes:** Subarachnoid space, intracranial
Subclavian Artery, Left **Subclavian** Artery, Right	**Includes:** Costocervical trunk Dorsal scapular artery Internal thoracic artery
Subcutaneous Tissue and Fascia, Anterior Neck	**Includes:** Deep cervical fascia Pretracheal fascia
Subcutaneous Tissue and Fascia, Chest	**Includes:** Pectoral fascia
Subcutaneous Tissue and Fascia, Face	**Includes:** Masseteric fascia Orbital fascia
Subcutaneous Tissue and Fascia, Left Foot	**Includes:** Plantar fascia (aponeurosis)
Subcutaneous Tissue and Fascia, Left Hand	**Includes:** Palmar fascia (aponeurosis)
Subcutaneous Tissue and Fascia, Left Lower Arm	**Includes:** Antebrachial fascia Bicipital aponeurosis
Subcutaneous Tissue and Fascia, Left Upper Arm	**Includes:** Axillary fascia Deltoid fascia Infraspinatus fascia Subscapular aponeurosis Supraspinatus fascia
Subcutaneous Tissue and Fascia, Left Upper Leg	**Includes:** Crural fascia Fascia lata Iliac fascia Iliotibial tract (band)
Subcutaneous Tissue and Fascia, Posterior Neck	**Includes:** Prevertebral fascia
Subcutaneous Tissue and Fascia, Right Foot	**Includes:** Plantar fascia (aponeurosis)
Subcutaneous Tissue and Fascia, Right Hand	**Includes:** Palmar fascia (aponeurosis)
Subcutaneous Tissue and Fascia, Right Lower Arm	**Includes:** Antebrachial fascia Bicipital aponeurosis
Subcutaneous Tissue and Fascia, Right Upper Arm	**Includes:** Axillary fascia Deltoid fascia Infraspinatus fascia Subscapular aponeurosis Supraspinatus fascia
Subcutaneous Tissue and Fascia, Right Upper Leg	**Includes:** Crural fascia Fascia lata Iliac fascia Iliotibial tract (band)
Subcutaneous Tissue and Fascia, Scalp	**Includes:** Galea aponeurotica

Continued →

Subcutaneous Tissue and Fascia, Trunk	**Includes:** External oblique aponeurosis Transversalis fascia
Subdural Space	**Includes:** Subdural space, intracranial
Submaxillary Gland, Left **Submaxillary** Gland, Right	**Includes:** Submandibular gland
Superior Mesenteric Artery	**Includes:** Ileal artery Ileocolic artery Inferior pancreaticoduodenal artery Jejunal artery
Superior Mesenteric Vein	**Includes:** Right gastroepiploic vein
Superior Vena Cava	**Includes:** Precava
Tarsal Joint, Left **Tarsal** Joint, Right	**Includes:** Calcaneocuboid joint Cuboideonavicular joint Cuneonavicular joint Intercuneiform joint Subtalar (talocalcaneal) joint Talocalcaneal (subtalar) joint Talocalcaneonavicular joint
Tarsal, Left **Tarsal,** Right	**Includes:** Calcaneus Cuboid bone Intermediate cuneiform bone Lateral cuneiform bone Medial cuneiform bone Navicular bone Talus bone
Temporal Artery, Left **Temporal** Artery, Right	**Includes:** Middle temporal artery Superficial temporal artery Transverse facial artery
Temporal Bone, Left **Temporal** Bone, Right	**Includes:** Mastoid process Petrous part of temporal bone Tympanic part of temoporal bone Zygomatic process of temporal bone
Thalamus	**Includes:** Epithalamus Geniculate nucleus Metathalamus Pulvinar
Thoracic Aorta	**Includes:** Aortic arch Aortic intercostal artery Ascending aorta Bronchial artery Esophageal artery Subcostal artery
Thoracic Duct	**Includes:** Left jugular trunk Left subclavian trunk

Thoracic Nerve	**Includes:** Intercostal nerve Intercostobrachial nerve Spinal nerve, thoracic Subcostal nerve
Thoracic Sympathetic Nerve	**Includes:** Cardiac plexus Esophageal plexus Greater splanchnic nerve Inferior cardiac nerve Least splanchnic nerve Lesser splanchnic nerve Middle cardiac nerve Pulmonary plexus Superior cardiac nerve Thoracic aortic plexus Thoracic ganglion
Thoracic Vertebra	**Includes:** **Spinous** process **Vertebral** arch **Vertebral** foramen **Vertebral** lamina **Vertebral** pedicle
Thoracic Vertebral Joint	**Includes:** **Costotransverse** joint **Costovertebral** joint **Thoracic** facet joint
Thoracolumbar Vertebral Joint	**Includes:** **Thoracolumbar** facet joint
Thorax Bursa and Ligament, Left **Thorax** Bursa and Ligament, Right	**Includes:** **Costotransverse** ligament **Costoxiphoid** ligament **Sternocostal** ligament
Thorax Muscle, Left **Thorax** Muscle, Right	**Includes:** **Intercostal** muscle **Levatores** costarum muscle **Pectoralis** major muscle **Pectoralis** minor muscle **Serratus** anterior muscle **Subclavius** muscle **Subcostal** muscle **Transverse** thoracis muscle
Thymus	**Includes:** **Thymus** gland
Thyroid Artery, Left **Thyroid** Artery, Right	**Includes:** **Cricothyroid** artery **Hyoid** artery **Sternocleidomastoid** artery **Superior** laryngeal artery **Superior** thyroid artery **Thyrocervical** trunk
Tibia, Left **Tibia,** Right	**Includes:** **Lateral** condyle of tibia **Medial** condyle of tibia **Medial** malleolus
Tibial Nerve	**Includes:** **Lateral** plantar nerve **Medial** plantar nerve **Medial** popliteal nerve **Medial** sural cutaneous nerve

Continued →

	Includes:
Toe Nail	Nail bed Nail plate
Toe Phalangeal Joint, Left **Toe** Phalangeal Joint, Right	Includes: Interphalangeal (IP) joint
Tongue	Includes: Frenulum linguae Lingual tonsil
Tongue, Palate, Pharynx Muscle	Includes: Chondroglossus muscle Genioglossus muscle Hyoglossus muscle Inferior longitudinal muscle Levator veli palatini muscle Palatoglossal muscle Palatopharyngeal muscle Pharyngeal constrictor muscle Salpingopharyngeus muscle Styloglossus muscle Stylopharyngeus muscle Superior longitudinal muscle Tensor veli palatini muscle
Tonsils	Includes: Palatine tonsil
Trachea	Includes: Cricoid cartilage
Transverse Colon	Includes: Splenic flexure
Tricuspid Valve	Includes: Right atrioventricular valve Tricuspid annulus
Trigeminal Nerve	Includes: Fifth cranial nerve Gasserian ganglion Mandibular nerve Maxillary nerve Ophthalmic nerve Trifacial nerve
Trochlear Nerve	Includes: Fourth cranial nerve
Trunk Bursa and Ligament, Left **Trunk** Bursa and Ligament, Right	Includes: Iliolumbar ligament Interspinous ligament Intertransverse ligament Ligamentum flavum Pubic ligament Sacrococcygeal ligament Sacroiliac ligament Sacrospinous ligament Sacrotuberous ligament Supraspinous ligament
Trunk Muscle, Left **Trunk** Muscle, Right	Includes: Coccygeus muscle Erector spinae muscle Interspinalis muscle Intertransversarius muscle Latissimus dorsi muscle Levator ani muscle Quadratus lumborum muscle Rhomboid major muscle Rhomboid minor muscle Serratus posterior muscle Transversospinalis muscle Trapezius muscle

	Includes:
Tympanic Membrane, Left **Tympanic** Membrane, Right	Includes: Pars flaccida
Ulna, Left **Ulna,** Right	Includes: Olecranon process Radial notch
Ulnar Artery, Left **Ulnar** Artery, Right	Includes: Anterior ulnar recurrent artery Common interosseous artery Posterior ulnar recurrent artery
Ulnar Nerve	Includes: Cubital nerve
Upper Arm Muscle, Left **Upper** Arm Muscle, Right	Includes: Biceps brachii muscle Brachialis muscle Coracobrachialis muscle Triceps brachii muscle
Upper Eyelid, Left **Upper** Eyelid, Right	Includes: Lateral canthus Levator palpebrae superioris muscle Orbicularis oculi muscle Superior tarsal plate
Upper Femur, Left **Upper** Femur, Right	Includes: Femoral head Greater trochanter Lesser trochanter Neck of femur
Upper Leg Muscle, Left **Upper** Leg Muscle, Right	Includes: Adductor brevis muscle Adductor longus muscle Adductor magnus muscle Biceps femoris muscle Gracilis muscle Pectineus muscle Quadriceps (femoris) Rectus femoris muscle Sartorius muscle Semimembranosus muscle Semitendinosus muscle Vastus intermedius muscle Vastus lateralis muscle Vastus medialis muscle
Upper Lip	Includes: Frenulum labii superioris Labial gland Vermilion border
Ureter **Ureter,** Left **Ureter,** Right **Ureters,** Bilateral	Includes: Ureteral orifice Ureterovesical orifice
Urethra	Includes: Bulbourethral (Cowper's) gland Cowper's (bulbourethral) gland External urethral sphincter Internal urethral sphincter Membranous urethra Penile urethra Prostatic urethra

Continued →

Section 0 - Medical and Surgical — Character 4 - Body Part	
Uterine Supporting Structure	**Includes:** Broad ligament Infundibulopelvic ligament Ovarian ligament Round ligament of uterus
Uterus	**Includes:** Fundus uteri Myometrium Perimetrium Uterine cornu
Uvula	**Includes:** Palatine uvula
Vagus Nerve	**Includes:** Anterior vagal trunk Pharyngeal plexus Pneumogastric nerve Posterior vagal trunk Pulmonary plexus Recurrent laryngeal nerve Superior laryngeal nerve Tenth cranial nerve
Vas Deferens **Vas** Deferens, Bilateral **Vas** Deferens, Left **Vas** Deferens, Right	**Includes:** Ductus deferens Ejaculatory duct
Ventricle, Right	**Includes:** Conus arteriosus
Ventricular Septum	**Includes:** Interventricular septum

Section 0 - Medical and Surgical — Character 4 - Body Part	
Vertebral Artery, Left **Vertebral** Artery, Right	**Includes:** Anterior spinal artery Posterior spinal artery
Vertebral Vein, Left **Vertebral** Vein, Right	**Includes:** Deep cervical vein Suboccipital venous plexus
Vestibular Gland	**Includes:** Bartholin's (greater vestibular) gland Greater vestibular (Bartholin's) gland Paraurethral (Skene's) gland Skene's (paraurethral) gland
Vitreous, Left **Vitreous,** Right	**Includes:** Vitreous body
Vocal Cord, Left **Vocal** Cord, Right	**Includes:** Vocal fold
Vulva	**Includes:** Labia majora Labia minora
Wrist Bursa and Ligament, Left **Wrist** Bursa and Ligament, Right	**Includes:** Palmar ulnocarpal ligament Radial collateral carpal ligament Radiocarpal ligament Radioulnar ligament Ulnar collateral carpal ligament
Wrist Joint, Left **Wrist** Joint, Right	**Includes:** Distal radioulnar joint Radiocarpal joint

Appendix E: Medical and Surgical Device Table (Device Key) and Device Aggregation Table

Section 0 - Medical and Surgical — Character 6 - Device	
Artificial Sphincter in Gastrointestinal System	**Includes:** Artificial anal sphincter (AAS) Artificial bowel sphincter (neosphincter)
Artificial Sphincter in Urinary System	**Includes:** AMS 800® Urinary Control System Artificial urinary sphincter (AUS)
Autologous Arterial Tissue in Heart and Great Vessels	**Includes:** Autologous artery graft
Autologous Arterial Tissue in Lower Arteries	**Includes:** Autologous artery graft
Autologous Arterial Tissue in Lower Veins	**Includes:** Autologous artery graft
Autologous Arterial Tissue in Upper Arteries	**Includes:** Autologous artery graft
Autologous Arterial Tissue in Upper Veins	**Includes:** Autologous artery graft

Section 0 - Medical and Surgical — Character 6 - Device	
Autologous Tissue Substitute	**Includes:** Autograft Cultured epidermal cell autograft Epicel® cultured epidermal autograft
Autologous Venous Tissue in Heart and Great Vessels	**Includes:** Autologous vein graft
Autologous Venous Tissue in Lower Arteries	**Includes:** Autologous vein graft
Autologous Venous Tissue in Lower Veins	**Includes:** Autologous vein graft
Autologous Venous Tissue in Upper Arteries	**Includes:** Autologous vein graft
Autologous Venous Tissue in Upper Veins	**Includes:** Autologous vein graft

Continued →

Bone Growth Stimulator in Head and Facial Bones	**Includes:** Electrical bone growth stimulator (EBGS) Ultrasonic osteogenic stimulator Ultrasound bone healing system
Bone Growth Stimulator in Lower Bones	**Includes:** Electrical bone growth stimulator (EBGS) Ultrasonic osteogenic stimulator Ultrasound bone healing system
Bone Growth Stimulator in Upper Bones	**Includes:** Electrical bone growth stimulator (EBGS) Ultrasonic osteogenic stimulator Ultrasound bone healing system
Cardiac Lead in Heart and Great Vessels	**Includes:** Cardiac contractility modulation lead
Cardiac Lead, Defibrillator for Insertion in Heart and Great Vessels	**Includes:** ACUITY™ Steerable Lead Attain Ability® lead Attain StarFix® (OTW) lead Cardiac resynchronization therapy (CRT) lead Corox (OTW) Bipolar Lead Durata® Defibrillation Lead ENDOTAK RELIANCE® (G) Defibrillation Lead
Cardiac Lead, Pacemaker for Insertion in Heart and Great Vessels	**Includes:** ACUITY™ Steerable Lead Attain Ability® lead Attain StarFix® (OTW) lead Cardiac resynchronization therapy (CRT) lead Corox (OTW) Bipolar Lead
Cardiac Resynchronization Defibrillator Pulse Generator for Insertion in Subcutaneous Tissue and Fascia	**Includes:** COGNIS® CRT-D Concerto II CRT-D Consulta CRT-D CONTAK RENEWAL® 3 RF (HE) CRT-D LIVIAN™ CRT-D Maximo II DR CRT-D Ovatio™ CRT-D Protecta XT CRT-D Viva (XT)(S)
Cardiac Resynchronization Pacemaker Pulse Generator for Insertion in Subcutaneous Tissue and Fascia	**Includes:** Consulta CRT-P Stratos LV Synchra CRT-P
Contraceptive Device in Female Reproductive System	**Includes:** Intrauterine device (IUD)
Contraceptive Device in Subcutaneous Tissue and Fascia	**Includes:** Subdermal progesterone implant
Contractility Modulation Device for Insertion in Subcutaneous Tissue and Fascia	**Includes:** Optimizer™ III implantable pulse generator
Defibrillator Generator for Insertion in Subcutaneous Tissue and Fascia	**Includes:** Evera (XT)(S)(DR/VR) Implantable cardioverter-defibrillator (ICD) Maximo II DR (VR) Protecta XT DR (XT VR) Secura (DR) (VR) Virtuoso (II) (DR) (VR)
Diaphragmatic Pacemaker Lead in Respiratory System	**Includes:** Phrenic nerve stimulator lead
Drainage Device	**Includes:** Cystostomy tube Foley catheter Percutaneous nephrostomy catheter Thoracostomy tube
External Fixation Device in Head and Facial Bones	**Includes:** External fixator
External Fixation Device in Lower Bones	**Includes:** External fixator
External Fixation Device in Lower Joints	**Includes:** External fixator
External Fixation Device in Upper Bones	**Includes:** External fixator
External Fixation Device in Upper Joints	**Includes:** External fixator
External Fixation Device, Hybrid for Insertion in Upper Bones	**Includes:** Delta frame external fixator Sheffield hybrid external fixator
External Fixation Device, Hybrid for Insertion in Lower Bones	**Includes:** Delta frame external fixator Sheffield hybrid external fixator
External Fixation Device, Hybrid for Reposition in Upper Bones	**Includes:** Delta frame external fixator Sheffield hybrid external fixator
External Fixation Device, Hybrid for Reposition in Lower Bones	**Includes:** Delta frame external fixator Sheffield hybrid external fixator
External Fixation Device, Limb Lengthening for Insertion in Upper Bones	**Includes:** Ilizarov-Vecklich device
External Fixation Device, Limb Lengthening for Insertion in Lower Bones	**Includes:** Ilizarov-Vecklich device
External Fixation Device, Monoplanar for Insertion in Upper Bones	**Includes:** Uniplanar external fixator
External Fixation Device, Monoplanar for Insertion in Lower Bones	**Includes:** Uniplanar external fixator
External Fixation Device, Monoplanar for Reposition in Upper Bones	**Includes:** Uniplanar external fixator
External Fixation Device, Monoplanar for Reposition in Lower Bones	**Includes:** Uniplanar external fixator

Continued →

Appendix E

External Fixation Device, Ring for Insertion in Upper Bones	**Includes:** Ilizarov external fixator Sheffield ring external fixator
External Fixation Device, Ring for Insertion in Lower Bones	**Includes:** Ilizarov external fixator Sheffield ring external fixator
External Fixation Device, Ring for Reposition in Upper Bones	**Includes:** Ilizarov external fixator Sheffield ring external fixator
External Fixation Device, Ring for Reposition in Lower Bones	**Includes:** Ilizarov external fixator Sheffield ring external fixator
External Heart Assist System in Heart and Great Vessels	**Includes:** Biventricular external heart assist system BVS 5000 Ventricular Assist Device Centrimag(R) Blood Pump TandemHeart® System Thoratec Paracorporeal Ventricular Assist Device
Extraluminal Device	**Includes:** LAP-BAND® adjustable gastric banding system REALIZE® Adjustable Gastric Band TigerPaw® system for closure of left atrial appendage
Feeding Device in Gastrointestinal System	**Includes:** Percutaneous endoscopic gastrojejunostomy (PEG/J) tube Percutaneous endoscopic gastrostomy (PEG) tube
Hearing Device in Ear, Nose, Sinus	**Includes:** Esteem® implantable hearing system
Hearing Device in Head and Facial Bones	**Includes:** Bone anchored hearing device
Hearing Device, Bone Conduction for Insertion in Ear, Nose, Sinus	**Includes:** Bone anchored hearing device
Hearing Device, Multiple Channel Cochlear Prosthesis for Insertion in Ear, Nose, Sinus	**Includes:** Cochlear implant (CI), multiple channel (electrode)
Hearing Device, Single Channel Cochlear Prosthesis for Insertion in Ear, Nose, Sinus	**Includes:** Cochlear implant (CI), single channel (electrode)
Implantable Heart Assist System in Heart and Great Vessels	**Includes:** Berlin Heart Ventricular Assist Device DeBakey Left Ventricular Assist Device DuraHeart Left Ventricular Assist System HeartMate II® Left Ventricular Assist Device (LVAD) HeartMate XVE® Left Ventricular Assist Device (LVAD) MicroMed HeartAssist Novacor Left Ventricular Assist Device Thoratec IVAD (Implantable Ventricular Assist Device)

Infusion Device	**Includes:** Ascenda Intrathecal Catheter InDura, intrathecal catheter (1P) (spinal) Non-tunneled central venous catheter Peripherally inserted central catheter (PICC) Tunneled spinal (intrathecal) catheter
Infusion Device, Pump in Subcutaneous Tissue and Fascia	**Includes:** Implantable drug infusion pump (anti-spasmodic)(chemotherapy)(pain) Injection reservoir, pump Pump reservoir Subcutaneous injection reservoir, pump SynchroMed pump
Interbody Fusion Device in Lower Joints	**Includes:** Axial Lumbar Interbody Fusion System AxiaLIF® System CoRoent® XL Direct Lateral Interbody Fusion (DLIF) device EXtreme Lateral Interbody Fusion (XLIF) device Interbody fusion (spine) cage XLIF® System
Interbody Fusion Device in Upper Joints	**Includes:** BAK/C® Interbody Cervical Fusion System Interbody fusion (spine) cage
Internal Fixation Device in Head and Facial Bones	**Includes:** Bone screw (interlocking)(lag)(pedicle) (recessed) Kirschner wire (K-wire) Neutralization plate
Internal Fixation Device in Lower Bones	**Includes:** Bone screw (interlocking)(lag)(pedicle) (recessed) Clamp and rod internal fixation system (CRIF) Kirschner wire (K-wire) Neutralization plate
Internal Fixation Device in Lower Joints	**Includes:** Fusion screw (compression)(lag)(locking) Joint fixation plate Kirschner wire (K-wire)
Internal Fixation Device in Upper Bones	**Includes:** Bone screw (interlocking)(lag)(pedicle) (recessed) Clamp and rod internal fixation system (CRIF) Kirschner wire (K-wire) Neutralization plate
Internal Fixation Device in Upper Joints	**Includes:** Fusion screw (compression)(lag)(locking) Joint fixation plate Kirschner wire (K-wire)
Internal Fixation Device, Intramedullary in Lower Bones	**Includes:** Intramedullary (IM) rod (nail) Intramedullary skeletal kinetic distractor (ISKD) Kuntscher nail

Continued →

Internal Fixation Device, Intramedullary in Upper Bones	**Includes:** Intramedullary (IM) rod (nail) Intramedullary skeletal kinetic distractor (ISKD) Kuntscher nail
Internal Fixation Device, Rigid Plate for Insertion in Upper Bones	**Includes:** Titanium Sternal Fixation System (TSFS)
Internal Fixation Device, Rigid Plate for Reposition in Upper Bones	**Includes:** Titanium Sternal Fixation System (TSFS)
Intraluminal Device	**Includes:** Absolute Pro Vascular (OTW) Self-Expanding Stent System Acculink (RX) Carotid Stent System AneuRx® AAA Advantage® Assurant (Cobalt) stent Carotid WALLSTENT® Monorail® Endoprosthesis CoAxia NeuroFlo catheter Colonic Z-Stent® Complete (SE) stent Driver stent (RX) (OTW) E-Luminexx™ (Biliary)(Vascular) Stent Embolization coil(s) Endurant® Endovascular Stent Graft Express® (LD) Premounted Stent System Express® Biliary SD Monorail® Premounted Stent System Express® SD Renal Monorail® Premounted Stent System FLAIR® Endovascular Stent Graft Formula™ Balloon-Expandable Renal Stent System Herculink (RX) Elite Renal Stent System LifeStent® (Flexstar)(XL) Vascular Stent System Micro-Driver stent (RX) (OTW) MULTI-LINK (VISION)(MINI-VISION) (ULTRA) Coronary Stent System Omnilink Elite Vascular Balloon Expandable Stent System Pipeline™ Embolization device (PED) Protégé® RX Carotid Stent System Stent, intraluminal (cardiovascular) (gastrointestinal)(hepatobiliary)(urinary) Talent® Converter Talent® Occluder Talent® Stent Graft (abdominal)(thoracic) Therapeutic occlusion coil(s) Ultraflex™ Precision Colonic Stent System Valiant Thoracic Stent Graft WALLSTENT® Endoprosthesis Xact Carotid Stent System Zenith Flex® AAA Endovascular Graft Zenith® Renu™ AAA Ancillary Graft Zenith TX2® TAA Endovascular Graft
Intraluminal Device, Airway in Ear, Nose, Sinus	**Includes:** Nasopharyngeal airway (NPA)
Intraluminal Device, Airway in Gastrointestinal System	**Includes:** Esophageal obturator airway (EOA)

Intraluminal Device, Airway in Mouth and Throat	**Includes:** Guedel airway Oropharyngeal airway (OPA)
Intraluminal Device, Bioactive in Upper Arteries	**Includes:** Bioactive embolization coil(s) Micrus CERECYTE microcoil
Intraluminal Device, Drug-eluting in Heart and Great Vessels	**Includes:** CYPHER® Stent Endeavor® (III)(IV) (Sprint) Zotarolimus-eluting Coronary Stent System Everolimus-eluting coronary stent Paclitaxel-eluting coronary stent Sirolimus-eluting coronary stent TAXUS® Liberté® Paclitaxel-eluting Coronary Stent System XIENCE Everolimus Eluting Coronary Stent System Zotarolimus-eluting coronary stent
Intraluminal Device, Drug-eluting in Lower Arteries	**Includes:** Paclitaxel-eluting peripheral stent Zilver® PTX® (paclitaxel) Drug-Eluting Peripheral Stent
Intraluminal Device, Drug-eluting in Upper Arteries	**Includes:** Paclitaxel-eluting peripheral stent Zilver® PTX® (paclitaxel) Drug-Eluting Peripheral Stent
Intraluminal Device, Endobronchial Valve in Respiratory System	**Includes:** Spiration IBV™ Valve System
Intraluminal Device, Pessary in Female Reproductive System	**Includes:** Pessary ring Vaginal pessary
Intraluminal Device, Endotracheal Airway in Respiratory System	**Includes:** Endotracheal tube (cuffed)(double-lumen)
Liner in Lower Joints	**Includes:** Acetabular cup Hip (joint) liner Joint liner (insert) Knee (implant) insert Tibial insert
Monitoring Device	**Includes:** Blood glucose monitoring system Cardiac event recorder Continuous Glucose Monitoring (CGM) device Implantable glucose monitoring device Loop recorder, implantable Reveal (DX)(XT)
Monitoring Device, Hemodynamic for Insertion in Subcutaneous Tissue and Fascia	**Includes:** Implantable hemodynamic monitor (IIIM) Implantable hemodynamic monitoring system (IHMS)
Monitoring Device, Pressure Sensor for Insertion in Heart and Great Vessels	**Includes:** CardioMEMS® pressure sensor EndoSure® sensor

Continued →

Appendix E

1349

Neurostimulator Lead in Central Nervous System	**Includes:** Cortical strip neurostimulator lead DBS lead Deep brain neurostimulator lead RNS System lead Spinal cord neurostimulator lead
Neurostimulator Lead in Peripheral Nervous System	**Includes:** InterStim® Therapy lead
Neurostimulator Generator in Head and Facial Bones	**Includes:** RNS system neurostimulator generator
Nonautologous Tissue Substitute	**Includes:** Acellular Hydrated Dermis Bone bank bone graft Tissue bank graft
Pacemaker, Dual Chamber for Insertion in Subcutaneous Tissue and Fascia	**Includes:** Advisa (MRI) EnRhythm Kappa Revo MRI™ SureScan® pacemaker Two lead pacemaker Versa
Pacemaker, Single Chamber for Insertion in Subcutaneous Tissue and Fascia	**Includes:** Single lead pacemaker (atrium)(ventricle)
Pacemaker, Single Chamber Rate Responsive for Insertion in Subcutaneous Tissue and Fascia	**Includes:** Single lead rate responsive pacemaker (atrium)(ventricle)
Radioactive Element	**Includes:** Brachytherapy seeds
Resurfacing Device in Lower Joints	**Includes:** CONSERVE® PLUS Total Resurfacing Hip System Cormet Hip Resurfacing System
Spacer in Lower Joints	**Includes:** Joint spacer (antibiotic)
Spacer in Upper Joints	**Includes:** Joint spacer (antibiotic)
Spinal Stabilization Device, Facet Replacement for Insertion in Upper Joints	**Includes:** Facet replacement spinal stabilization device
Spinal Stabilization Device, Facet Replacement for Insertion in Lower Joints	**Includes:** Facet replacement spinal stabilization device
Spinal Stabilization Device, Interspinous Process for Insertion in Upper Joints	**Includes:** Interspinous process spinal stabilization device X-STOP® Spacer
Spinal Stabilization Device, Interspinous Process for Insertion in Lower Joints	**Includes:** Interspinous process spinal stabilization device X-STOP® Spacer
Spinal Stabilization Device, Pedicle-Based for Insertion in Upper Joints	**Includes:** Dynesys® Dynamic Stabilization System Pedicle-based dynamic stabilization device
Spinal Stabilization Device, Pedicle-Based for Insertion in Lower Joints	**Includes:** Dynesys® Dynamic Stabilization System Pedicle-based dynamic stabilization device

Stimulator Generator in Subcutaneous Tissue and Fascia	**Includes:** Baroreflex Activation Therapy(R) (BAT(R)) Diaphragmatic pacemaker generator Mark IV Breathing Pacemaker System Phrenic nerve stimulator generator Rheos(R) System device
Stimulator Generator, Multiple Array for Insertion in Subcutaneous Tissue and Fascia	**Includes:** Activa PC neurostimulator Enterra gastric neurostimulator Neurostimulator generator, multiple channel PrimeAdvanced neurostimulator (SureScan)(MRI Safe)
Stimulator Generator, Multiple Array Rechargeable for Insertion in Subcutaneous Tissue and Fascia	**Includes:** Activa RC neurostimulator Neurostimulator generator, multiple channel rechargeable RestoreAdvanced neurostimulator (SureScan)(MRI Safe) RestoreSensor neurostimulator (SureScan) (MRI Safe) RestoreUltra neurostimulator (SureScan) (MRI Safe)
Stimulator Generator, Single Array for Insertion in Subcutaneous Tissue and Fascia	**Includes:** Activa SC neurostimulator InterStim® Therapy neurostimulator Itrel (3)(4) neurostimulator Neurostimulator generator, single channel
Stimulator Generator, Single Array Rechargeable for Insertion in Subcutaneous Tissue and Fascia	**Includes:** Neurostimulator generator, single channel rechargeable
Stimulator Lead in Gastrointestinal System	**Includes:** Gastric electrical stimulation (GES) lead Gastric pacemaker lead
Stimulator Lead in Muscles	**Includes:** Electrical muscle stimulation (EMS) lead Electronic muscle stimulator lead Neuromuscular electrical stimulation (NEMS) lead
Stimulator Lead in Upper Arteries	**Includes:** Baroreflex Activation Therapy® (BAT®) Carotid (artery) sinus (baroreceptor) lead Rheos® System lead
Stimulator Lead in Urinary System	**Includes:** Sacral nerve modulation (SNM) lead Sacral neuromodulation lead Urinary incontinence stimulator lead

Continued →

Appendix E

Synthetic Substitute	**Includes:** **AbioCor®** Total Replacement Heart **AMPLATZER®** Muscular VSD Occluder **Annuloplasty** ring **Bard®** Composix® (E/X)(LP) mesh **Bard®** Composix® Kugel® patch **Bard®** Dulex™ mesh **Bard®** Ventralex™ hernia patch **BRYAN®** Cervical Disc System **Ex-PRESS™** mini glaucoma shunt **Flexible** Composite Mesh **GORE®** DUALMESH® **Holter** valve ventricular shunt **MitraClip** valve repair system **Nitinol** framed polymer mesh **Open** Pivot Aortic Valve Graft (AVG) **Open** Pivot (mechanical) valve **Partially** absorbable mesh **PHYSIOMESH™** Flexible Composite Mesh **Polymethylmethacrylate** (PMMA) **Polypropylene** mesh **PRESTIGE®** Cervical Disc **PROCEED™** Ventral Patch **Prodisc-C** **Prodisc-L** **PROLENE** Polypropylene Hernia System (PHS) **Rebound** HRD® (Hernia Repair Device) **SynCardia** Total Artificial Heart **Total** artificial (replacement) heart **ULTRAPRO** Hernia System (UHS) **ULTRAPRO** Partially Absorbable Lightweight Mesh **ULTRAPRO** Plug **Ventrio™** Hernia Patch **Zimmer®** NexGen® LPS Mobile Bearing Knee **Zimmer®** NexGen® LPS-Flex Mobile Knee
Synthetic Substitute, Ceramic for Replacement in Lower Joints	**Includes:** **Novation®** Ceramic AHS® (Articulation Hip System)
Synthetic Substitute, Ceramic on Polyethylene for Replacement in Lower Joints	**Includes:** **Oxidized** zirconium ceramic hip bearing surface
Synthetic Substitute, Intraocular Telescope for Replacement in Eye	**Includes:** **Implantable** Miniature Telescope™ (IMT)
Synthetic Substitute, Metal for Replacement in Lower Joints	**Includes:** **Cobalt/chromium** head and socket

Synthetic Substitute, Metal on Polyethylene for Replacement in Lower Joints	**Includes:** Cobalt/chromium head and polyethylene socket
Synthetic Substitute, Polyethylene for Replacement in Lower Joints	**Includes:** Polyethylene socket
Synthetic Substitute, Reverse Ball and Socket for Replacement in Upper Joints	**Includes:** Delta III Reverse shoulder prosthesis Reverse® Shoulder Prosthesis
Tissue Expander in Skin and Breast	**Includes:** Tissue expander (inflatable)(injectable)
Tissue Expander in Subcutaneous Tissue and Fascia	**Includes:** Tissue expander (inflatable)(injectable)
Tracheostomy Device in Respiratory System	**Includes:** Tracheostomy tube
Vascular Access Device in Subcutaneous Tissue and Fascia	**Includes:** Tunneled central venous catheter Vectra® Vascular Access Graft
Vascular Access Device, Reservoir in Subcutaneous Tissue and Fascia	**Includes:** Implanted (venous)(access) port Injection reservoir, port Subcutaneous injection reservoir, port
Zooplastic Tissue in Heart and Great Vessels	**Includes:** 3f (Aortic) Bioprosthesis valve Bovine pericardial valve Bovine pericardium graft Contegra Pulmonary Valved Conduit CoreValve transcatheter aortic valve Epic™ Stented Tissue Valve (aortic) Freestyle (Stentless) Aortic Root Bioprosthesis Hancock Bioprosthesis (aortic) (mitral) valve Hancock Bioprosthetic Valved Conduit Melody® transcatheter pulmonary valve Mitroflow® Aortic Pericardial Heart Valve Mosaic Bioprosthesis (aortic) (mitral) valve Porcine (bioprosthetic) valve SAPIEN transcatheter aortic valve SJM Biocor® Stented Valve System Stented tissue valve Trifecta™ Valve (aortic) Xenograft

Device Aggregation Table

Specific Device	for Operation	in Body System	General Device
Autologous Arterial Tissue	All applicable	Heart and Great Vessels Lower Arteries Lower Veins Upper Arteries Upper Veins	**7** Autologous Tissue Substitute
Autologous Venous Tissue	All applicable	Heart and Great Vessels Lower Arteries Lower Veins Upper Arteries Upper Veins	**7** Autologous Tissue Substitute
Cardiac Lead, Defibrillator	Insertion	Heart and Great Vessels	**M** Cardiac Lead
Cardiac Lead, Pacemaker	Insertion	Heart and Great Vessels	**M** Cardiac Lead
Cardiac Resynchronization Defibrillator Pulse Generator	Insertion	Subcutaneous Tissue and Fascia	**P** Cardiac Rhythm Related Device
Cardiac Resynchronization Pacemaker Pulse Generator	Insertion	Subcutaneous Tissue and Fascia	**P** Cardiac Rhythm Related Device
Contractility Modulation Device	Insertion	Subcutaneous Tissue and Fascia	**P** Cardiac Rhythm Related Device
Defibrillator Generator	Insertion	Subcutaneous Tissue and Fascia	**P** Cardiac Rhythm Related Device
Epiretinal Visual Prosthesis	All applicable	Eye	**J** Synthetic Substitute
External Fixation Device, Hybrid	Insertion	Lower Bones Upper Bones	**5** External Fixation Device
External Fixation Device, Hybrid	Reposition	Lower Bones Upper Bones	**5** External Fixation Device
External Fixation Device, Limb Lengthening	Insertion	Lower Bones Upper Bones	**5** External Fixation Device
External Fixation Device, Monoplanar	Insertion	Lower Bones Upper Bones	**5** External Fixation Device
External Fixation Device, Monoplanar	Reposition	Lower Bones Upper Bones	**5** External Fixation Device
External Fixation Device, Ring	Insertion	Lower Bones Upper Bones	**5** External Fixation Device
External Fixation Device, Ring	Reposition	Lower Bones Upper Bones	**5** External Fixation Device
Hearing Device, Bone Conduction	Insertion	Ear, Nose, Sinus	**S** Hearing Device
Hearing Device, Multiple Channel Cochlear Prosthesis	Insertion	Ear, Nose, Sinus	**S** Hearing Device
Hearing Device, Single Channel Cochlear Prosthesis	Insertion	Ear, Nose, Sinus	**S** Hearing Device
Internal Fixation Device, Intramedullary	All applicable	Lower Bones Upper Bones	**4** Internal Fixation Device
Internal Fixation Device, Rigid Plate	Insertion	Upper Bones	**4** Internal Fixation Device
Internal Fixation Device, Rigid Plate	Reposition	Upper Bones	**4** Internal Fixation Device
Intraluminal Device, Pessary	All applicable	Female Reproductive System	**D** Intraluminal Device

Specific Device	for Operation	in Body System	General Device	
Intraluminal Device, Airway	All applicable	Ear, Nose, Sinus Gastrointestinal System Mouth and Throat	D	Intraluminal Device
Intraluminal Device, Bioactive	All applicable	Upper Arteries	D	Intraluminal Device
Intraluminal Device, Drug-eluting	All applicable	Heart and Great Vessels Lower Arteries Upper Arteries	D	Intraluminal Device
Intraluminal Device, Endobronchial Valve	All applicable	Respiratory System	D	Intraluminal Device
Intraluminal Device, Endotracheal Airway	All applicable	Respiratory System	D	Intraluminal Device
Intraluminal Device, Radioactive	All applicable	Heart and Great Vessels	D	Intraluminal Device
Monitoring Device, Hemodynamic	Insertion	Subcutaneous Tissue and Fascia	2	Monitoring Device
Monitoring Device, Pressure Sensor	Insertion	Heart and Great Vessels	2	Monitoring Device
Pacemaker, Dual Chamber	Insertion	Subcutaneous Tissue and Fascia	P	Cardiac Rhythm Related Device
Pacemaker, Single Chamber	Insertion	Subcutaneous Tissue and Fascia	P	Cardiac Rhythm Related Device
Pacemaker, Single Chamber Rate Responsive	Insertion	Subcutaneous Tissue and Fascia	P	Cardiac Rhythm Related Device
Spinal Stabilization Device, Facet Replacement	Insertion	Lower Joints Upper Joints	4	Internal Fixation Device
Spinal Stabilization Device, Interspinous Process	Insertion	Lower Joints Upper Joints	4	Internal Fixation Device
Spinal Stabilization Device, Pedicle-Based	Insertion	Lower Joints Upper Joints	4	Internal Fixation Device
Stimulator Generator, Multiple Array	Insertion	Subcutaneous Tissue and Fascia	M	Stimulator Generator
Stimulator Generator, Multiple Array Rechargeable	Insertion	Subcutaneous Tissue and Fascia	M	Stimulator Generator
Stimulator Generator, Single Array	Insertion	Subcutaneous Tissue and Fascia	M	Stimulator Generator
Stimulator Generator, Single Array Rechargeable	Insertion	Subcutaneous Tissue and Fascia	M	Stimulator Generator
Synthetic Substitute, Ceramic	Replacement	Lower Joints	J	Synthetic Substitute
Synthetic Substitute, Ceramic on Polyethylene	Replacement	Lower Joints	J	Synthetic Substitute
Synthetic Substitute, Intraocular Telescope	Replacement	Eye	J	Synthetic Substitute
Synthetic Substitute, Metal	Replacement	Lower Joints	J	Synthetic Substitute
Synthetic Substitute, Metal on Polyethylene	Replacement	Lower Joints	J	Synthetic Substitute
Synthetic Substitute, Polyethylene	Replacement	Lower Joints	J	Synthetic Substitute
Synthetic Substitute, Reverse Ball and Socket	Replacement	Upper Joints	J	Synthetic Substitute

Section 3 – Administration Character 6 – Substance

4-Factor Prothrombin Complex Concentrate	**Includes:** Kcentra
Adhesion Barrier	**Includes:** Seprafilm
Anti-Infective Envelope	**Includes:** AIGISRx Antibacterial Envelope Antimicrobial envelope
Clofarabine	**Includes:** Clolar
Glucarpidase	**Includes:** Voraxaze
Human B-type Natriuretic Peptide	**Includes:** Nesiritide
Other Thrombolytic	**Includes:** Tissue Plasinogen Activator (tPA)(r-tPA)
Oxazolidinones	**Includes:** Zyvox
Recombinant Bone Morphogenetic Protein	**Includes:** Bone morphogenetic protein 2 (BMP 2) rhBMP-2